S0-AFO-115

Principles *and* Practice *of* RADIATION ONCOLOGY

Carlos A. Perez, M.D.
Director, Radiation Oncology Center
Mallinckrodt Institute of Radiology
Washington University Medical Center
St. Louis, Missouri

Luther W. Brady, M.D.
Professor and Chairman
Department of Radiation Oncology and Nuclear Medicine
Hahnemann University
Philadelphia, Pennsylvania

With 94 Additional Contributors

Assistants to the Editors
Alice Becker
Carl G. Karsch
Connie Povilat

Principles *and* Practice *of* RADIATION ONCOLOGY

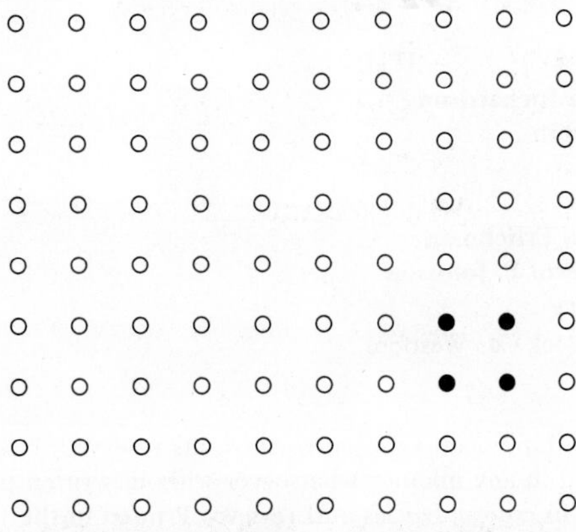

Second Edition

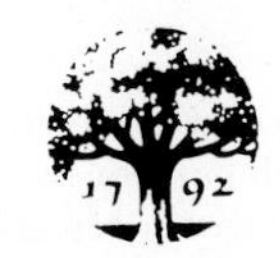

J. B. Lippincott Company
Philadelphia
New York London Hagerstown

Developmental Editor: **Julia Richardson**
Project Editor: **Dina K. Rubin**
Indexer: **Julia Figures**
Designer: **Doug Smock**
Production Manager: **Caren Erlichman**
Production Coordinator: **Kevin P. Johnson**
Compositor: **Circle Graphics**
Printer/Binder: The Courier Book Co./Westford

2nd Edition
 Printed in the United States of America. For information write J. B. Lippincott Company, East Washington Square, Philadelphia, Pennsylvania 19105.

6 5 4 3 2

Library of Congress Cataloging-in-Publication Data

Principles and practice of radiation oncology / [editors] Carlos A.
Perez, Luther W. Brady ; with 94 additional contributors ;
assistants to the editors, Alice Becker, Carl G. Karsch, Connie
Povilat. — 2nd ed.
p. cm.
Includes bibliographical references and index.
ISBN 0-397-51162-0
1. Cancer—Radiotherapy. I. Perez, Carlos A., 1934–
II. Brady, Luther W., 1925– .
[DNLM: 1. Neoplasms—radiotherapy. QZ 269 P957]
RC271.R3P73 1992
616.99'40642—dc20
DNLM/DLC
for Library of Congress 91-25387
CIP

The authors and publisher have exerted every effort to ensure that drug selection and dosage set forth in this text are in accord with current recommendations and practice at the time of publication. However, in view of ongoing research, changes in government regulations, and the constant flow of information relating to drug therapy and drug reactions, the reader is urged to check the package insert for each drug for any change in indications and dosage and for added warnings and precautions. This is particularly important when the recommended agent is a new or infrequently employed drug.

To our patients, who taught us with their courage and suffering
To our teachers and forebears, who inspired us with their knowledge and insight
To our trainees, who will advance the field further
To our families, who unselfishly endured our endeavors

CONTRIBUTORS

Beatriz E. Amendola, M.D.
South Miami Hospital, Miami, Florida

K. Kian Ang, M.D., Ph.D.
Professor of Radiotherapy, Department of Clinical Radiotherapy, University of Texas, M.D. Anderson Cancer Center, Houston, Texas

John Antoniades, M.D.
Professor, Hahnemann University; Chief, Department of Radiation Oncology, Lankenau Hospital, Philadelphia, Pennsylvania

James J. Augsburger, M.D.
Associate Clinical Professor of Ophthalmology, Jefferson Medical College, Thomas Jefferson University; Attending Surgeon, Oncology Unit, Retina Service, Wills Eye Hospital, Philadelphia, Pennsylvania

Hassan Aziz, M.D.
Clinical Associate Professor, State University of New York, Health Science Center at Brooklyn, Long Island College Hospital, Brooklyn, New York

Robert J. Bertoli, M.D.
Assistant Professor, Radiation Oncology, Hahnemann University; Associate Radiation Oncologist to the Hospital, Pennsylvania Hospital, Philadelphia, Pennsylvania

Steven A. Binnick, M.D.
Associate Professor of Medicine, Division of Dermatology, Hahnemann University, Philadelphia, Pennsylvania

Luther W. Brady, M.D.
Hylda Cohn/American Cancer Society Professor of Clinical Oncology; Chairman, Department of Radiation Oncology and Nuclear Medicine, Hahnemann University, Philadelphia, Pennsylvania

John D. Busowski, M.S., M.D.
Chairman, Obstetrics and Gynecology, The Byerly Hospital, Hartsville, South Carolina

Felipe A. Calvo, M.D.
Director, Department of Radiation Oncology, Clinica Universitaria, University of Navarra School of Medicine, Pamplona, Spain

Nicholas J. Cassisi, D.D.S., M.D.
Professor and Chairman, Department of Otolaryngology, University of Florida College of Medicine, Shands Hospital, Gainesville, Florida

Louis S. Constine, M.D.
Associate Professor, University of Rochester, Strong Memorial Hospital, Rochester, New York

Jay S. Cooper, M.D., F.A.C.R.
Professor of Radiology; Director of Radiation Oncology, New York University Medical Center, New York, New York

Bernard J. Cummings, M.B., Ch.B., F.R.C.P.C.
Professor, Department of Radiology, University of Toronto; Radiation Oncologist, The Princess Margaret Hospital, Toronto, Ontario, Canada

Giulio J. D'Angio, M.D.
Professor of Radiology; Professor of Radiation Oncology; Professor of Pediatric Oncology, University of Pennsylvania School of Medicine; Vice Chairman and Clinical Director, Hospital of the University of Pennsylvania, Philadelphia, Pennsylvania

Lawrence W. Davis, M.D.
Professor and Chairman, Albert Einstein College of Medicine, Montefiore Medical Center, Bronx, New York

John L. Day, Ph.D. (Deceased)
Department of Radiation Oncology and Nuclear Medicine, Hahnemann University, Philadelphia, Pennsylvania

Luis Delclos, M.D.
Professor of Radiotherapy, Margaret and Ben Love Professorship in Honor of Dr. Charles LeMaistre, M.D. Anderson Cancer Center, University of Texas, Houston, Texas

V. Rao Devineni, M.D.
Assistant Professor of Radiology, Radiation Oncology Center, Mallinckrodt Institute of Radiology, Washington University Medical Center; Associate Radiation Oncologist, Barnes Hospital and DePaul Health Center, St. Louis, Missouri

Sarah S. Donaldson, M.D., F.A.C.R.
Professor of Radiation Oncology, Stanford University School of Medicine, Stanford University Hospital, Stanford, California

Robert E. Drzymala, Ph.D.
Assistant Professor, Mallinckrodt Institute of Radiology, Washington University School of Medicine, St. Louis, Missouri

Bahman Emami, M.D., F.A.C.R.
Professor of Radiology, Washington University School of Medicine, St. Louis, Missouri

Luis Felippe Fajardo L-G, M.D.
Professor of Pathology, Stanford University School of Medicine; Chief of Laboratory Service, Veterans Affairs Medical Center, Palo Alto, California

Scot Fisher, D.O.
Assistant Professor, Department of Radiation Oncology and Nuclear Medicine, Hahnemann University Hospital; Director, Radiation Oncology, The Graduate Hospital, Philadelphia, Pennsylvania

Peter J. Fitzpatrick, M.B., B.S., F.R.C.P.(C), F.R.C.R.
Professor and Chairman of Radiation Oncology, Dalhousie University; Physician-in-Chief, Cancer Treatment Research Foundation of Nova Scotia, Halifax, Nova Scotia

Karen K. Fu, M.D., F.A.C.R.
Professor, Department of Radiation Oncology, University of California, San Francisco, San Francisco, California

Delia M. Garcia, M.D.
Radiation Oncology Center, Mallinckrodt Institute of Radiology, Washington University Medical Center, St. Louis, Missouri

Glenn P. Glasgow, Ph.D.
Professor, Division of Medical Physics, Loyola/Hines Department of Radiotherapy, Stritch School of Medicine, Loyola University of Chicago, Maywood, Illinois

John R. Glassburn, M.D., F.A.C.R.
Adjunct Professor of Radiation Oncology, University of Pennsylvania; Professor of Radiation Oncology, Hahnemann University Hospital, Chief of the Section of Radiation Oncology, Pennsylvania Hospital, Philadelphia, Pennsylvania

Eli Glatstein, M.D.
Chief, Radiation Oncology Branch, Professor of Radiology, Uniform Services, University of Health Sciences, National Cancer Institute, Bethesda, Maryland

Larry D. Greenfield, M.D., F.A.M.W.A., F.A.C.N.P.
Clinical Associate Professor of Radiological Sciences, UCLA Medical Center, Los Angeles, California; Chairman, Department of Medical Imaging, Rancho Los Amigos Medical Center, Downey, California

Thomas W. Griffin, M.D.
Professor and Chairman, Department of Radiation Oncology, University of Washington School of Medicine; Director, University Cancer Center, University of Washington Medical Center, Seattle, Washington

Perry W. Grigsby, M.D., M.B.A.
Associate Professor of Radiology, Radiation Oncology Center, Mallinckrodt Institute of Radiology, Washington University Medical Center; Clinical Chief, MIR, Radiation Oncology Center, Barnes Hospital, St. Louis, Missouri

Leonard L. Gunderson, M.D., M.S.
Chairman in Oncology, Mayo Medical School; Chairman of Radiation Oncology, Mayo Clinic, Rochester, Minnesota

Richard T. Hoppe, M.D., F.A.C.R.
Professor, Department of Radiation Oncology, Stanford University School of Medicine, Stanford, California

Carolyn J. Horowitz, M.D., Ph.D.
Medical Director, The Radiation Oncology Center at Marlton, Marlton, New Jersey

A. Robert Kagan, M.D., F.A.C.R.
Clinical Professor, Radiation Oncology, University of California, Los Angeles; Chief, Radiation Oncology, Southern California Permanente Medical Group, Los Angeles, California

Ulf L. Karlsson, M.D., Ph.D.
Associate Professor and Director, Department of Radiation Oncology, University of New Mexico Cancer Center, Albuquerque, New Mexico

James W. Keller, M.D.
Assistant Professor, University of Rochester, Strong Memorial Hospital, Rochester, New York

Morton M. Kligerman, M.D., F.A.C.R.
Henry K. Pancoast Professor Emeritus of Research Oncology, University of Pennsylvania Medical School, Philadelphia, Pennsylvania

Larry E. Kun, M.D.
Chairman, Department of Radiation Oncology, St. Jude Children's Research Hospital; Professor, Departments of Radiology and Pediatrics, University of Tennessee College of Medicine, Memphis, Tennessee

Robert R. Kuske, M.D.
Chairman, Department of Radiation Oncology, Ochsner Clinic, New Orleans, Louisiana

Peter P. Lai, Ph.D., M.D.
Associate Professor of Radiology, Mallinckrodt Institute of Radiology, Washington University School of Medicine; Associate Radiation Oncologist, Barnes Hospital, St. Louis, Missouri

David A. Larson, M.D., Ph.D.
Associate Professor and Vice Chairman, Department of Radiation Oncology, University of California, San Francisco, San Francisco, California

Theodore S. Lawrence, M.D., Ph.D.
Assistant Professor, University of Michigan Medical Center, Ann Arbor, Michigan

Steven A. Leibel, M.D.
Attending Radiation Oncologist, Department of Radiation Oncology, Memorial Sloan-Kettering Cancer Center, New York, New York

Seymour H. Levitt, M.D.
Professor and Head, Department of Therapeutic Radiology–Radiation Oncology, University of Minnesota Hospital and Clinic, Minneapolis, Minnesota

Allen S. Lichter, M.D.
Professor of Radiation Therapy; Chair, Department of Radiation Therapy, University of Michigan Medical Center, Ann Arbor, Michigan

David A. Lightfoot, M.A.
Professor, Hahnemann University, Philadelphia, Pennsylvania

Hsiu-san Lin, M.D., Ph.D.
Professor of Radiology, Mallinckrodt Institute of Radiology, Washington University School of Medicine, St. Louis, Missouri

Robert Lindberg, M.D.
Professor and Chairman, Department of Radiation Oncology, Brown Cancer Center, University of Louisville, Louisville, Kentucky

Kenneth H. Luk, M.D.
Clinical Professor; Chairman, Division of Radiation Oncology, Department of Radiology, University of California, Irvine, Duarte, California

Anthony Mancuso, M.D.
Professor of Radiology, Department of Radiology, University of Florida, Shands Teaching Hospital and Clinic, Gainesville, Florida

Victor A. Marcial-Vega, M.D.
Clinical Assistant Professor, Department of Radiation Oncology, University of Miami Medical Center; Radiation Oncologist, Baptist Hospital of Miami, Cancer Treatment Center, Miami, Florida

Arnold M. Markoe, M.D., Sc.D.
Associate Professor, University of Miami Medical Center; Clinic Director, Jackson Memorial Hospital, Miami, Florida

James E. Marks, M.D.
Professor and Chairman, Department of Radiotherapy, Loyola University of Chicago, Stritch School of Medicine, Loyola University Medical Center, Maywood, Illinois

James A. Martenson, Jr., M.D.
Assistant Professor of Oncology, Mayo Graduate School of Medicine; Consultant, Mayo Clinic, Rochester, Minnesota

Sandra McDonald, M.D.
Assistant Professor, University of Rochester, Strong Memorial Hospital, Rochester, New York

William M. Mendenhall, M.D.
Associate Professor, Department of Radiation Oncology, University of Florida College of Medicine, Shands Teaching Hospital, Gainesville, Florida

Bizhan Micaily, M.D.
Associate Professor of Radiation Oncology, Department of Radiation Oncology, Hahnemann University, Philadelphia, Pennsylvania

Rodney R. Million, M.D.
Professor and Chairman, Department of Radiation Oncology, University of Florida College of Medicine, University of Florida Cancer Center, Gainesville, Florida

David Monyak, M.D.
Assistant Professor, University of Minnesota; Assistant Professor, University of Minnesota Hospital and Clinic, Minneapolis, Minnesota

Robert J. Myerson, Ph.D., M.D.
Assistant Professor, Mallinckrodt Institute of Radiology, Washington University School of Medicine, St. Louis, Missouri

Diana F. Nelson, M.D.
Associate Professor, University of Rochester, Highland Hospital, Rochester, New York

Stanley E. Order, M.D., Sc.D., F.A.C.R.
Professor of Radiation Oncology, The Johns Hopkins School of Medicine, Director, Radiation Oncology, The Johns Hopkins Hospital, Baltimore, Maryland

Thomas F. Pajak, Ph.D.
Director, Statistical Unit, American College of Radiology, Philadelphia, Pennsylvania

William J. Pao, M.D.
Division of Radiation Oncology, St. Luke's Hospital, Milwaukee, Wisconsin

James T. Parsons, M.D.
The Rodney R. Million, M.D., Professor of Radiation Oncology, Associate Professor, Department of Radiation Oncology, University of Florida College of Medicine; Therapeutic Radiologist, Shands Teaching Hospital, Gainesville, Florida

Carlos A. Perez, M.D.
Director, Radiation Oncology Center, Mallinckrodt Institute of Radiology, Washington University Medical Center, St. Louis, Missouri

Lester J. Peters, M.D.
Professor of Radiotherapy; Head, Division of Radiotherapy, John G. and Marie Stella Kenedy Chair, University of Texas, M.D. Anderson Cancer Center, Houston, Texas

Miljenko V. Pilepich, M.D.
Head, Department of Radiation Oncology, Catherine McAuley Health Systems, Ann Arbor, Michigan

James A. Purdy, Ph.D.
Professor and Associate Director, Radiation Oncology Center, Washington University School of Medicine, Mallinckrodt Institute of Radiology, St. Louis, Missouri

Joseph L. Roti Roti, Ph.D.
Professor of Radiology, Chief, Section of Cancer Biology, Mallinckrodt Institute of Radiology, Washington University School of Medicine, St. Louis, Missouri

Marvin Rotman, M.D.
Professor, Regional Chairman, State University of New York, Health Science Center at Brooklyn, Brooklyn, New York

Philip Rubin, M.D., F.A.C.R.
Professor, Department of Radiation Oncology, University of Rochester; Chairman, Division of Radiation Oncology, Rochester, New York

William Serber, M.D., F.A.C.R.
Professor of Clinical Radiation Oncology, Hahnemann University, Department of Radiation Oncology and Nuclear Medicine, Hahnemann University Hospital, Philadelphia, Pennsylvania

Glenn E. Sheline, M.D., Ph.D. (Deceased)
Professor and Vice-Chairman, Department of Radiation Oncology, University of California, San Francisco, California

Jerry A. Shields, M.D.
Professor of Ophthalmology, Thomas Jefferson University; Director, Ocular Oncology Service, Wills Eye Hospital, Philadelphia, Pennsylvania

Joseph R. Simpson, M.D., Ph.D.
Associate Professor of Radiology, Washington University School of Medicine; Clinical Chief, Radiation Oncology Center, Missouri Baptist Medical Center; Associate Radiation Oncologist, Barnes Hospital, Jewish Hospital, Children's Hospital, St. Louis, Missouri

Larry D. Simpson, Ph.D.
Professor and Chief, Radiation Physics Division, Department of Radiation Oncology and Nuclear Medicine, Hahnemann University, Philadelphia, Pennsylvania

Stephen R. Smalley, M.D.
Associate Professor, University of Kansas Medical Center, Kansas City, Kansas

Merrill J. Solan, M.D.
Assistant Professor, Department of Radiation Oncology and Nuclear Medicine, Hahnemann University, Philadelphia, Pennsylvania; Mercy Catholic Medical Center, Darby, Pennsylvania

J. Gershon Spector, M.D.
Professor of Otolaryngology, Washington University School of Medicine, St. Louis, Missouri

Scott P. Stringer, M.D.
Assistant Professor for Surgery and Otolaryngology; Medical Director of ENT Physician's Clinic, University of Florida, Gainesville, Florida

Samuel Strober, M.D.
Professor of Medicine, Division of Immunology, Stanford University Hospital, Stanford, California

Norah duV. Tapley, M.D. (Deceased)
M.D. Anderson Cancer Center, University of Texas System Cancer Center, Houston, Texas

Joel E. Tepper, M.D.
Professor and Chair, Department of Radiation Oncology, University of North Carolina School of Medicine; Chair, Department of Radiation Oncology, University of North Carolina Hospital, Chapel Hill, North Carolina

Howard D. Thames, Ph.D.
Professor of Biomathematics, Department of Biomathematics, Helen Buchanan and Stanley Joseph Seegar Research Professor, University of Texas, M.D. Anderson Cancer Center, Houston, Texas

Gillian M. Thomas, M.D.
Associate Professor, Departments of Radiology and Obstetrics and Gynecology, University of Toronto, Toronto-Bayview Regional Cancer Centre, University of Toronto, Canada

Patrick R. M. Thomas, M.B., B.S.
Professor and Chairman, Department of Radiation Oncology, Temple University School of Medicine, Philadelphia, Pennsylvania

Richard J. Torpie, M.D.
Clinical Associate Professor, Hahnemann University, Philadelphia, Pennsylvania; Chief, Division of Radiation Oncology, St. Luke's Hospital, Bethlehem, Pennsylvania

Eric C. Vonderheid, M.D.
Professor of Medicine, Division of Dermatology, Hahnemann University, Philadelphia, Pennsylvania

Kent Wallner, M.D., B.A.
Assistant Professor, Attending Radiation Oncologist, Department of Radiation Oncology, Memorial Sloan-Kettering Cancer Center, New York, New York

C. C. Wang, M.D.
Professor of Radiation Therapy, Harvard Medical School; Head, Division of Clinical Services, Department of Radiation Oncology, Massachusetts General Hospital, Boston, Massachusetts

Todd H. Wasserman, M.D.
Professor of Radiation Oncology, Radiation Oncology Center, Mallinckrodt Institute of Radiology, Washington University Medical Center; Chairman, Department of Radiation Oncology, Jewish Hospital of St. Louis, St. Louis, Missouri

Christopher G. Willett, M.D.
Assistant Professor in Radiation Oncology, Harvard Medical School; Assistant Radiation Oncologist, Department of Radiation Oncology, Massachusetts General Hospital, Boston, Massachusetts

Stephen D. Williams, M.D.
Professor of Medicine, Indiana University; Chief, Hematology Oncology, Indianapolis Veterans Administration Medical Center, Indianapolis, Indiana

Jeffrey F. Williamson, Ph.D.
Associate Professor, Chief, Brachytherapy Physics Service, Washington University School of Medicine; Barnes Hospital, Mallinckrodt Institute of Radiology, St. Louis, Missouri

H. Rodney Withers, M.D., D.Sc.
Professor of Radiation Oncology, Head, Division of Experimental Radiation Oncology, UCLA Medical Center, Los Angeles, California

PREFACE

Approximately 60% of all cancer patients in the United States receive radiation therapy each year as definitive therapy for palliation, or as an adjunct to surgery or chemotherapy. In 1991, according to American Cancer Society estimates, one million new cases of invasive cancer, 50,000 new cases of carcinoma *in situ* of the uterine cervix, 15,000 new cases of carcinoma *in situ* of the female breast, and 600,000 new cases of nonmelanomatous skin cancer were diagnosed in the United States. Approximately 70% of patients with invasive cancer present with disease apparently limited to the local region; 30% have metastases at the time of the initial presentation. Of those who present with locoregional disease, 56% will be cured and 44% will develop recurrent cancer. Therefore, a substantial portion of the resources in cancer care is devoted to control of the locoregional tumor, including the optimal use of radiation therapy.

Management of the patient with cancer has evolved into a complex, closely integrated application of fundamental concepts and sophisticated technology to evaluate and stage the tumor and, using various modalities, to obtain the best therapeutic results, emphasizing the quality of life of the patient. *Principles and Practice of Radiation Oncology* is designed to contribute to a better understanding of the natural history of cancer, the physical methods of radiation application, the effects of irradiation on normal tissues, and the most judicious ways in which radiation therapy can be employed in the treatment of any particular patient, either as a single modality or as part of a multimodality treatment program.

Chapters on basic radiation biology, radiation therapy physics and treatment planning, multimodal integrated programs for patient management, and such technical applications of irradiation as electron beam therapy, brachytherapy, and high linear energy transfer radiations have been updated to incorporate newer concepts.

New chapters have been added, reflecting recent technologic advances in total body and hemibody irradiation, concomitant chemotherapy and irradiation, and acquired immunodeficiency syndrome-related Kaposi's sarcoma. A new section on stereotactic irradiation was added to the brain tumor chapter, and the remote control afterloading material has been expanded substantially. To allow for more in-depth coverage of the subjects, several chapters have been divided to include new chapters on treatment of stage T1–T2 breast cancer, locally advanced breast tumors, spinal canal lesions, and pediatric brain tumors. The second edition also contains two excellent chapters on normal tissue effects of irradiation.

The chapters discussing disease by anatomic site cover pertinent information on each tumor. The format includes sections on epidemiology, pathology, diagnostic workup, treatment techniques, applications of surgery and chemotherapy, end results of treatment, and pertinent clinical trials. The second edition has been revised extensively to include many reports on new techniques and results.

We recognize that there is a great deal of individuality in the techniques of irradiation, and we have attempted to include descriptions of various technical approaches, leaving to the individual reader the critical task of selecting the most appropriate one for the particular patient under consideration. The comprehensive and rigorous assessment of each tumor site set forth in this text provides the foundation for proper application of radiation therapy techniques and multimodal programs in the treatment of patients with cancer.

We sincerely hope that *Principles and Practice of Radiation Oncology* will continue to advance clinical and research activities in cancer management. It is our expectation that this updated and expanded edition will help foster new knowledge that will improve delivery of radiation therapy and ultimately will result in a reduction in the time lost from other activities, in cost to the health care system, and in the human suffering occasioned by cancer.

ACKNOWLEDGMENTS

We are deeply indebted and most appreciative of the efforts of all of the contributors whose expertise, lucid presentation, and promptness eased the task of preparing this volume. Particularly, an expression of thanks and dedication is due to their families who endured our efforts in the preparation of the book; to the faculty and residents in our departments who were very supportive and supplied continued intellectual stimulation, valuable suggestions, and materials toward the completion of the book; to the editorial and secretarial staff—Alice Becker, Connie Davis, Josephine Garcia, Jane Meyer, and Connie Povilat—who took on the herculean task of preparing the manuscript; and to our mentors, who set the standards by which we practice and pursue our professional endeavors.

Without the uncompromising devotion of each of them to the project, it would not have been completed. To every one of them, we owe our everlasting gratitude.

Carlos A. Perez, M.D.
Luther W. Brady, M.D.

CONTENTS

Principles *and* Practice *of* RADIATION ONCOLOGY

1

○ ○ ○ • • •

Overview

Carlos A. Perez
Luther W. Brady

HISTORICAL PERSPECTIVE

Roentgen described x-rays in 1895,[303] and the Curies reported their discovery of radium in 1898.[57] Almost immediately, the biologic effects of ionizing radiations were recognized. The first patient cured by radiation therapy was reported on in 1899, after which clinical radiation therapy had a long and challenging growth period in the early 1920s. Technologic advances accumulated more rapidly than did basic biologic knowledge. By 1913 Coolidge had developed an x-ray tube with a peak energy of 140 kV, and by 1922, 200 kV x-rays were available for deep therapy.

Clinical radiation therapy as a medical discipline began at the International Congress of Oncology in Paris in 1922 when Coutard and Hautant presented evidence that advanced laryngeal cancer could be cured without disastrous, treatment-induced sequelae.[51] By 1934 Coutard had developed a protracted, fractionated scheme that remains the basis for current radiation therapy,[52] and in 1936 Paterson[261] published results in the treatment of cancer with x-rays. The treatment of malignant tumors in many anatomic locations with brachytherapy, starting with ^{226}Ra needles and tubes, has increased steadily since 1910. With time, ionizing radiation became more precise, high-energy protons and electrons were available, and treatment planning and delivery became more accurate and reproducible.

There has been exponential growth in the knowledge of radiation physics, radiation biology, clinical treatment planning, and the use of computers in radiation therapy. In the last two decades considerable advances have been made in the treatment of cancer, with cure now being a realistic therapeutic objective in over 50% of newly diagnosed patients.[65,318] This improvement in therapy can be attributed to progress in several major areas:

1. Greater dissemination of information to physicians and the public and innovative screening and diagnostic tools that increase awareness and early cancer detection
2. Multiple therapeutic approaches for a variety of tumors
3. Advanced surgical techniques and irradiation equipment and more effective cytotoxic drugs
4. Greater interaction among cancer surgeons, radiation oncologists, medical oncologists, and pathologists stressing the combined modality approach in treatment
5. Closer interaction among physicians and basic scientists, allowing the transfer of clinically relevent biomedical discoveries to the bedside
6. Broad use of appropriate clinical trial methodology to evaluate innovative or alternative treatment programs.

RADIATION ONCOLOGY IN CANCER MANAGEMENT

Radiation oncology is a clinical and scientific endeavor devoted to management of patients with cancer (and other diseases) by ionizing radiation, alone or combined with other modalities, investigation of the biologic and physical basis of radiation therapy, and training of professionals in the field. *Radiation therapy* is a clinical specialty dealing with the use of ionizing radiations in the treatment of patients with malignant neoplasias (and occasionally benign conditions). The aim of radiation therapy is to deliver a precisely measured dose of radiation to a defined tumor volume with as minimal damage as possible to surrounding healthy tissue, resulting in eradication of the tumor, a high quality of life, and prolongation of survival at reasonable cost.

In addition to curative efforts, irradiation plays a major role in cancer management in the effective palliation or prevention of symptoms of the disease: Pain can be alleviated, luminal patency restored, skeletal integrity preserved, and organ function reestablished with minimal morbidity in a variety of clinical circumstances.[48]

Buschke[31] defined a *radiotherapist* as a physician who limited his or her practice to radiation therapy; he emphasized the active role of the radiation oncologist:

> While the patient is under our care we take full and exclusive responsibility, exactly as does the surgeon who takes care of a patient with cancer. This means that we examine the patient personally, review the microscopic material, perform examinations and take a biopsy if necessary. On the basis of this thorough clinical investigation we consider the plan of treatment and suggest it to the referring physician and to the patient. We reserve for ourselves the right to an independent opinion regarding diagnosis and advisable therapy and if necessary, the right of disagreement with the referring physician. . . . During the course of treatment, we ourselves direct any additional medication that may be necessary . . . and are ready to be called in an emergency at any time.

Buschke went on to indicate that in order to integrate the various disciplines and provide better care to patients it was extremely important for the radiation therapist to cooperate closely with specialists in other fields in management of the patient.

These concepts were reinforced and amplified by Bush[32] in his dissertation, "The Compleat Oncologist" and del Regato[62] in his 1975 ASTR presidential address.

Today radiation oncology is recognized as a separate specialty by the American Board of Radiology, the American College of Radiology, and the American Board of Medical Specialties.

THE PROCESS OF RADIATION THERAPY

As illustrated in Figure 1-1, the clinical use of irradiation is a complex process that involves many professionals and a variety of interrelated functions. The aim of therapy should be defined at the onset of the formulation of therapeutic strategy as

Curative, in which it is projected that the patient has a probability of surviving after adequate therapy, even if that chance is low (as in T4 tumors of the head and neck or in carcinoma of the lung)

Palliative, in which there is no hope of the patient surviving for extended periods. Nevertheless symptoms that produce discomfort or an impending condition that may impair the comfort or self-sufficiency of the patient require treatment.

In curative therapy a certain probability of significant side effects, even though undesirable, may be acceptable. However, the same is not generally true in palliative treatment, in which no major iatrogenic conditions should be seen. Nevertheless, it is necessary to remember that in the palliation of primary tumors, relatively high doses of radiation are required to control the tumor for the survival period of the patient (sometimes 75% to 80% of curative dose).

In a curative setting it is extremely important for the radiation oncologist to deliver the highest possible dose to the tumor volume to ensure maximum tumor control while at the same time keeping to the lowest possible level any severe sequelae of radiation treatment in the surrounding normal tissues. The concept is illustrated when using one treatment regimen—for instance, parallel opposed portals—in which the normal tissues receive a significantly higher radiation dose than with an optimized multiple field plan.

The prescription of radiation is based on the following principles:

1. Evaluation of the full extent of the tumor (staging) by whatever means available, including radiographic, radioisotope, and other studies
2. Knowledge of the pathologic characteristics of the disease,

KEY STAFF FUNCTION IN RADIATION THERAPY

	KEY STAFF	SUPPORTIVE ROLE
1. CLINICAL EVALUATION	Rad. Oncologist	
2. THERAPEUTIC DECISION	Rad. Oncologist	
3. TARGET VOLUME LOCALIZATION		
Tumor Volume	Rad. Oncologist	Sim. Tech./Dosimetrist
Sensitive Critical Organs	Rad. Oncologist	Sim. Tech./Dosimetrist
Patient Contour	Dosimetrist	Sim. Tech./Dosimetrist
4. TREATMENT PLANNING		
Beam Data-Computerization	Physicist	
Computation of Beams	Physicist	Dosimetrist
Shielding Blocks, Treatment Aids, etc.	Dosimetrist/ Mold Room Tech.	Rad. Oncologist/ Physicist
Analysis of Alternate Plans	Rad. Oncologist/ Physicist	Dosimetrist
Selection of Treatment Plan	Rad. Oncologist/ Physicist	
Dose Calculation	Dosimetrist	Physicist
5. SIMULATION/VERIFICATION OF TREATMENT PLAN	Rad. Oncologist/ Sim. Tech.	Dosimetrist/ Physicist
6. TREATMENT		
First Day Set-Up	Rad. Oncologist/ Physicist/ Therapy Tech.s	Dosimetrist/ Physicist
Localization Films	Rad. Oncologist/ Therapy Tech.s	
Dosimetry Checks/ Initial Chart Review	Physicist/ Rad. Oncologist	Dosimetrist/ Chief Tech.
Repositioning/Retreatment	Therapy Tech.s	Dosimetrist/ Chief Tech.
7. PERIODIC EVALUATION (During Treatment)		
Tumor Response/Tolerance	Rad. Oncologist	Nurses/RTTs
8. FOLLOW-UP EVALUATION	Rad. Oncologist	Nurses

FIGURE 1–1. Functions involved in radiation therapy. (Inter-Society Council for Radiation Oncology: Radiation Oncology in Integrated Cancer Management. Philadelphia, American College of Radiology, November 1986)

including potential areas of spread, that may influence choice of therapy, (*i.e.*, rationale for elective irradiation of the lymphatics in the neck or the pelvis)
3. Definition of goals of therapy (cure *versus* palliation)
4. Selection of appropriate treatment modalities, which may be irradiation alone or combined with surgery, chemotherapy, or both. The choice has a significant impact on the volume treated and the doses of radiation delivered.
5. Determination of the optimal dose of radiation and the volume to be treated, which is made according to the anatomic location, histologic type, stage, and other characteristics of the tumor, and the normal structures present in the region. The radiation oncologist should never hesitate to modify established policies in order to tailor the treatment plan to the needs of the patient.
6. Periodic evaluation of the patient's general condition, tumor response, and status of the normal tissues treated

The radiation oncologist must work closely with the physics, treatment planning, and dosimetry staffs to ensure the greatest possible accuracy and practicality in the design of treatment plans and computation of dose distributions. The ultimate responsibility for treatment decisions and the technical execution of the therapy, as well as its consequences, always rest with the radiation oncologist.[265] No computer calculations or physics procedures can correct the errors of clinical judgment, misunderstanding of physical concepts, or unsatisfactory planning and execution of radiation therapy. The skills of the clinician can never be completely replaced by technologic developments in physics, computers, or other technical aspects of radiation therapy; however, more accurate techniques ensure that the best possible treatment is being executed and that the possibility of subjective interpretations or inaccuracies is reduced to a minimum.

PRESCRIPTION OF IRRADIATION AND TREATMENT PLANNING

It should be stressed that different doses of radiation are required for given probabilities of tumor control, depending on the type and initial number of clonogenic cells present. Therefore, varying radiation doses may be delivered to certain portions of the tumor (periphery, central portion); doses may vary also in cases in which all gross tumor has been surgically removed.[105]

From a cell burden standpoint, a clinical tumor can be considered to encompass the following compartments: macroscopic (visible or palpable), microextensions into adjacent tissues, and subclinical disease, presumed to be present but not detectable even under the microscope. The treatment portals must adequately cover all three compartments in addition to a margin to compensate for geometric inaccuracies during radiation exposure (Fig. 1-2).

Sensitive structures within the irradiated volume should be clearly identified, and the maximum doses to be delivered to them must be specified. Simulation is necessary in most instances to accurately identify the tumor volume and the sensitive structures and to document the configuration of the portals and target volume to be irradiated.[76]

Treatment aids, such as shielding blocks, molds, masks, immobilization devices, and compensators, are extremely important in treatment planning and delivery of optimal dose distribution. The radiation oncologist should be familiar with the physical characteristics of these devices and use them (discriminately, for economic reasons) to achieve optimal therapeutic results. Simpler treatment delivery techniques that yield an acceptable radiation dose distribution should be preferred over more complex ones, in which a greater margin of error on a day-to-day treatment basis may be present. Repositioning and immobilization are critical, because the only effective irradiation is that which strikes the clonogenic tumor cells. Therefore in fractionated irradiation, accurate setup should enable the patient to maintain the desired position during every daily treatment. Repositioning and immobilization devices, such as the Alfa cradle, plaster casts, thermoplast molds, bite blocks, and arm boards, are invaluable in assisting technologists in patient positioning. Accuracy is periodically assessed with portal (localization) films.[380]

Rabinowitz and colleagues[296] reported on the analysis of simulator and portal films of 71 patients, 25 of whom were analyzed retrospectively, 39 prospectively, and seven with daily portal films. Some discrepancies were noted between the simulator and the localization (treatment) portal films. The researchers offered three explanations for the discrepancies: the portal films may allow the physician more mature judgment of what is desirable in the patient's treatment; the discrepancies

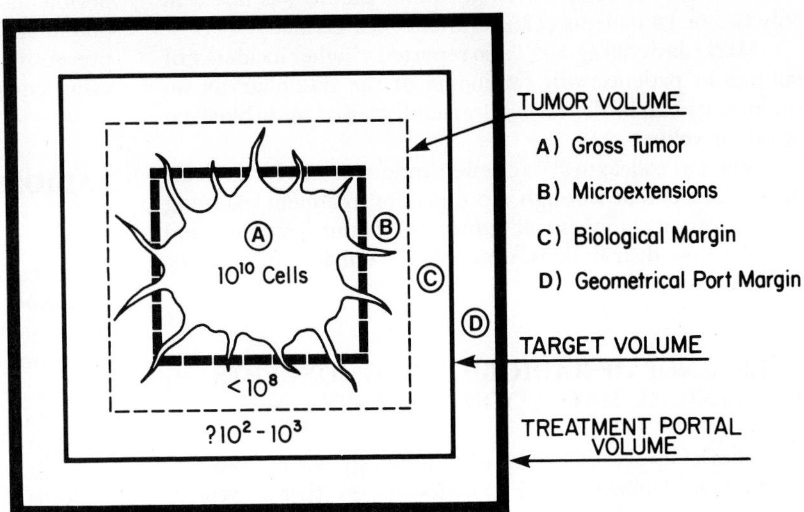

FIGURE 1–2. Schematic representation of tumor volume and target volume. The treatment volume includes the tumor volume, potential areas of local and regional microscopic disease around the tumor, and a margin of surrounding normal tissue. (Perez CA, Purdy JA: Rationale for treatment planning in radiation therapy. In Levitt SH [ed]: Technological Basis of Radiation Therapy: Practical Clinical Applications, 2nd ed. Philadelphia, Lea & Febiger)

are true measures of systematic positioning errors, and the discrepancies are a result of errors in data analysis. Fortunately, with an average value of 3 mm standard deviation of the variations, the mean worst case discrepancy averaged 3.5 mm in the head and neck region, 9.2 mm in the thorax, 5.1 mm in the abdomen, 8.4 mm in the pelvis, and 6.9 mm in the extremities. Other authors have documented similar localization errors on the basis of portal film review analysis.[33,170,212,213,296]

Hendrickson[146] reported a 3.5% incidence of error in multiple parameters (setting of field size, timer, gantry and collimator angles, and patient positioning) with one technologist working. The error rate declined to 2.8% when two technologists worked together. Marks and co-workers[212,213] demonstrated, by systematic use of verification films, a high incidence of localization errors on patients irradiated for head and neck cancer or malignant lymphomas. These errors were corrected with improved immobilization of the patients. For instance, the use of a bite block in patients with head and neck tumors reduced localization incidence of errors from 16% to 1%.[212]

Hulshof and associates[157] analyzed the incidence and magnitude of localization errors detected by verification films during mantle field irradiation for Hodgkin's disease in 126 treatment setups. The first verification film at the beginning of treatment showed localization errors of over 1 cm in 13% of the cases leading to a critical margin between the shielding block and the tumor-bearing area in 9% of treatment setups. After the first correction, an adequate treatment setup was obtained in 60% of the cases and after two corrections in 84%, thus demonstrating the usefulness of verification films in improving the localization of portals and monitoring of subsequent corrections.

Byhardt and associates[33] and Rabinowitz and co-workers[296] observed relatively few errors resulting from block misplacement. Obviously, if adequate margins have been built into the design of the portals, these positioning errors may not critically affect outcome. However, some studies have pointed out that setup errors may correlate with decreased tumor control. Kinzie and co-workers,[170] in the Patterns of Care Study review of patients with Hodgkin's disease treated with radiation therapy alone, found that 33% of patients whose treatment portals were inadequate subsequently developed in-field or marginal recurrences, in comparison with only 7% of those treated with adequate portals. Similar observations were reported by Marks and associates.[213] Doss,[73] in a study of patients with upper airway carcinoma, showed that in 21 of 28 patients (75%) with treatments in which 30% or more portals exhibited a blocking error, a recurrence developed, whereas tumor failure was noted in only two of 12 patients (17%) without such errors.

Marks and colleagues[211] also reported a higher incidence of failures in patients with carcinoma of the nasopharynx on whom shielding of the ear inadvertently caused some blocking of tumor volume.

Suit and colleagues[349] reviewed various recent technologic developments that through more precise treatment planning and delivery techniques will reduce the volume irradiated and improve dose distributions, which should enhance therapeutic outcome.

RELEVANCE OF RADIOBIOLOGIC CONCEPTS IN CLINICAL RADIATION THERAPY

The clinical application of radiation therapy has evolved primarily from empiricism. Nevertheless, in the past 30 years a major effort has been applied to the potential use of radiobiologic concepts in designing safer and more effective therapeutic strategies. Kaplan[167] pointed out that in the first three decades of this century radiobiologists worked closely with radiotherapists in attempting to describe and understand the biologic phenomena induced by ionizing radiations. Although direct extrapolation from *in vitro* and *in vivo* experimental data may not have resulted in spectacular advances in clinical radiation therapy, it should be stressed that these biologic concepts have greatly enhanced our understanding of the principles surrounding the clinical use of ionizing radiation. Experiments on radiation damage to DNA (both single and double-strand scissions) and its repair have facilitated understanding of repair of sublethal and potentially lethal damage[86,395] and provided the rationale for manipulation of dose-time relationship and the trials of chemical modifiers or protectors in radiation therapy of human tumors.[109]

One of the most significant contributions of radiation biology has been the theory of cell kill as a function of increasing doses of a cytocidal agent, as well as the demonstration of repair of sublethal or potentially lethal damage after irradiation.[88,293,395] This concept has led to a better understanding of dose-response curves for tumor control probability and effect on normal tissues and application of dose-time concepts to fractionation. The demonstration of hypoxic cells in tumors and their different sensitivity to irradiation[289] has been another important contribution leading to the concept of reoxygenation[166] and the potential use of hyperbaric oxygen or hypoxic radiation sensitizers in clinical radiation therapy.[69,393]

The study of cell proliferation kinetics, the biologic basis of cell kill by irradiation or chemotherapeutic agents, and the effectiveness of each modality in specific cellular compartments has strengthened understanding of combination therapy.[347,368,369] The same can be said for the use of various combinations of irradiation and surgery to decrease locoregional recurrences or to exploit the specific ability of each modality to eradicate tumor cells in different compartments, such as in the excision of gross tumor and irradiation of the tumor bed and regional microextensions.[288]

Similarly, interest in high linear energy transfer radiations and hyperthermia has been rekindled recently, largely because of promising experimental results in the laboratory.[108]

Fletcher[104] reviewed the application of various radiobiologic concepts to clinical radiation therapy and strongly recommended that the teaching of radiobiology and cell kinetics should be expanded considerably in the training of the radiation oncologist to enhance our clinical skills. Furthermore, experimental models in the laboratory should indicate avenues for potential advancement and may warn of pitfalls to avoid, thus preventing disastrous therapeutic results in the design of innovative clinical trials.

RADIOSENSITIVITY AND RADIOCURABILITY

In 1906, Bergonie and Tribondeau[17] formulated a law, relating radiosensitivity to reproductive capacity of the cells, based on their experiments on rat testis in which they were able to destroy the germinal cells, whereas the interstitial tissue and Sertoli syncytium remained unimpaired:

> X-rays are more effective on cells which have a greater reproductive activity; the effectiveness is greater on those cells which have a longer dividing future ahead, on those cells the morphology and the function of which are least fixed. From this law, it is easy to understand that roentgen

radiation destroys tumors without destroying healthy tissues.

According to Fletcher,[103] this law, which linked radiosensitivity of the tumor to that of the mother organ, did much harm to clinical radiation therapy, leading to the concept that undifferentiated tumors with mitotic activity were radiosensitive and that differentiated tumors were radioresistant.

In 1914, Schwarz[324] postulated that it was inefficient to give the total radiation dose in one treatment because some cells were in different states of radiosensitivity and because there was a better chance that multiple exposures could hit the cells in a radiosensitive phase, which at that time was thought to be mitosis. He also initiated the concept of therapeutic ratio, on the assumption that fractionation increased the tolerance of normal tissues and not that of the tumor, because the malignant cells had a greater reproductive capacity and therefore were more likely to be in a radiosensitive phase.

Radiocurability refers to the eradication of tumor at the primary or regional site and reflects a direct effect of the irradiation, which may not parallel the patient's ultimate outcome. *Radiosensitivity* expresses the response (degree and speed of regression) of the tumor to irradiation.

The response of human tumors to irradiation is a key question for radiation oncologists that has been addressed by many leading radiobiologists. At least four explanations have been considered to explain the different radiosensitivities of tumors:

Hypoxia. To explain the spectrum of clinical radioresponsiveness on the basis of hypoxia, one must believe that the less responsive tumors have a high hypoxic fraction or have failed to reoxygenate during fractionated treatment or both.[346] Although it is not possible to prove that hypoxia is unimportant in conventional radiation therapy, some doubts about its importance have been expressed with the limited success of neutron therapy or hypoxic cell radiosensitizers.[70,77]

Proportion of clonogenic cells. Proliferating cells are highly radiosensitive.

Inherent radiosensitivity of tumor cells. Fertil and Malaise[95] and Deacon and colleagues[59] established a positive correlation between the steepness of the initial slope of the oxic cell survival curve for human tumor cells and their response to radiation. The magnitude of differences among cell lines at low doses is sufficient to explain the range of curability observed clinically.[346] Steel and Peacock[346] analyzed human tumor radiosensitivity in light of existing concepts of cell kill based on the linear quadratic equation.

Repair of radiation damage. Repair of sublethal damage (split-course) is found in almost all tumor cell lines.[87] Potentially lethal damage (PLD) has been found to vary considerably from one cell line to another and has been reputed by Weichselbaum and Little[396] to correlate with clinical radiocurability, with the less curable tumors showing the greatest degree of PLD recovery.

No significant correlation exists between the responsiveness of a tumor to irradiation and radiocurability; thus, a tumor may be radiosensitive and yet incurable, or *vice versa,* relatively radioresistant and still curable by irradiation alone or in combination with other modalities.

Some authors have reported a correlation between the response of a tumor 6 weeks after the completion of radiation treatment with ultimate probability of local tumor control.[350] Of course, for this analysis to be valid it is necessary to compare patients with the same initial stage because, in general, the more advanced lesions have a greater probability of tumor persistence at the completion of radiation therapy and local recurrence may be more frequent. Barkley and Fletcher[12] reported an 82% probability of tumor control in 88 patients with tumors of the oropharynx that had regressed completely at the end of therapy, in contrast to 41% in 237 patients with persistent tumor at completion of therapy. Sobel and colleagues[340] concluded that local tumor control probability in head and neck tumors could be predicted with the greatest accuracy and consistency between 1 and 3 months after completion of radiation treatment. They noted that the prediction was 80% accurate in favorable tumors (T1, T2) but decreased to 50% to 60% in more advanced primary lesions. They also emphasized that complete tumor clearance is a more accurate predictor of tumor control in the oral cavity and oropharynx, where the sites are accessible to visual and palpable evaluation, than in the hypopharynx.

We observed a good correlation between the probability of local tumor control and the complete or partial regression of tumor at completion of irradiation in over 800 patients with varying stages of carcinoma of the uterine cervix[160,271] but no correlation of these parameters in patients with localized carcinoma of the prostate treated with irradiation.[273]

Tumor Radiosensitivity and Predictive Assays

Since the inception of the use of ionizing radiation, many authors have categorized the response of tumors according to their sensitivity to irradiation, starting with Wetterer[400] in 1913, who characterized tumor radiation sensitivity based on histologic types. Paterson[263] divided all tumors into three groups: radiosensitive, intermediate, and radioresistant. The first category included embryonic tumors and reticuloses; the second, squamous cell and adenocarcinomas; and the third group, soft tissue and bone sarcomas and melanomas. Table 1-1 categorizes different tumors according to their response to radiation therapy.

Attempts have been made to predict the response of tumors to radiation depending on several parameters, such as the assay proposed by Glucksmann,[124] consisting of differential cell counts of mitotic, resting, and degenerating cells from biopsies of the growing edge of the tumor before and after initiation of irradiation. It is generally accepted that many, if not all, tumors contain mixed cell populations of stem cells with differing sensitivity to antineoplastic agents and that therapy can be selected for resistant cell populations or, in the case of certain cytotoxic agents, induce cellular resistance.[35] Peters and colleagues[280] have recently described an innovative predictive assay to assess tumor response *in vitro.* They reviewed the subject of inherent radiosensitivity in tumor and normal tissues as a predictor of human tumor response and the difficulties in predicting the probability of tumor control by irradiation in a given patient.[279] They believe that it is not unreasonable to expect that cellular radiosensitivity and other radiobiologically based predictive assays will refine the discrimination of existing prognostic factors and offer better means to select therapeutic strategies on a more rational basis.

Probability of Tumor Control

It is axiomatic in radiation therapy that higher doses of irradiation produce better tumor control, and numerous dose-response curves in a variety of tumors have been published. The

TABLE 1–1
Curative Doses of Radiation for Different Tumor Types

2000–3000 cGy
- Seminoma
- Dysgerminoma
- Acute lymphocytic leukemia

3000–4000 cGy
- Seminoma (bulky)
- Wilms' tumor
- Neuroblastoma

4000–4500 cGy
- Hodgkin's disease
- Lymphosarcoma
- Histiocytic cell sarcoma
- Skin cancer (basal cell)

5000–6000 cGy
- Lymph nodes, metastatic (N_0, N_1)
- Squamous cell carcinoma, cervix cancer, and head and neck cancer
- Embryonal cancer
- Breast cancer, ovarian cancer
- Medulloblastoma
- Retinoblastoma
- Ewing's tumor
- Breast cancer (excised)

6000–6500 cGy
- Larynx (<1 cm)
- Breast cancer (T_1)

7000–7500 cGy
- Oral cavity (<2 cm, 2–4 cm)
- Oro-naso-laryngo-pharyngeal cancers
- Breast cancer (T_2)
- Bladder cancers
- Cervix cancer
- Uterine fundal cancer
- Ovarian cancer
- Lymph nodes, metastatic (1–3 cm)
- Lung cancer (<3 cm)

8000 cGy OR ABOVE
- Head and neck cancer (>4 cm)
- Breast cancer (>5 cm)
- Glioblastomas (gliomas)
- Osteogenic sarcomas (bone sarcomas)
- Melanomas
- Soft tissue sarcomas (>5 cm)
- Thyroid cancer
- Lymph nodes, metastatic (>6 cm)

(Modified from Rubin P: Clinical Oncology: A Multidisciplinary Approach, 6th ed, p 64. New York, American Cancer Society, 1983)

first dose-response data were reported for skin cancer by Miescher[227] in 1934; 10 years later Strandqvist[348] published a dose-response curve for skin cancer. As Fletcher[103] points out, dose-response curves can be elicited only when a group of homogeneous tumors is given a range of radiation doses, indicating that tumor control is a probabilistic event. For every increment of radiation dose a certain fraction of cells will be killed. Therefore the total number of surviving cells will be proportional to the initial number present and the fraction killed with each dose.[103] Thus it is apparent that various levels of irradiation yield a different probability of tumor control, depending on the extent of the lesion (number of clonogenic cells present). For subclinical disease in squamous cell carcinoma of the upper respiratory tract or for adenocarcinoma of the breast, doses of 4500 cGy to 5000 cGy result in control of the disease in over 90% of patients.[104,223] Subclinical disease has been referred to as deposits of tumor cells that are too small to be detected clinically and even microscopically but, if left untreated, may evolve to clinically apparent tumor.[257] It must be emphasized that microscopic evidence of tumor, such as at the surgical margin, should not be regarded as subclinical disease. Cell aggregates greater than $10^6/cm^3$ or higher are required for the

TABLE 1-2
Tumor Control Probability Correlated with Radiation Dose and Volume of Cancer

DOSE	SQUAMOUS CELL CARCINOMA OF THE UPPER RESPIRATORY AND DIGESTIVE TRACTS	ADENOCARCINOMA OF THE BREAST
5000 cGy*	>90% subclinical[102]	>90% Subclinical[101]
	60% T1 lesions of nasopharynx[230]	
	≈50% 1–3 cm neck nodes[245]	
6000 cGy*	≈90% T1 lesions of pharynx and larynx†	
	≈50% T3 and T4 lesions of tonsillar fossa[94,266]	
	≈90% 1–3 cm neck nodes[322]	90% Clinically positive axillary nodes 2.5–3 cm‡[101]
	≈70% 3–5 cm neck nodes[385]	
7000 cGy*	≈90% T2 lesions of tonsillar fossa and supraglottic larynx[329,331]	
	≈80% T3 and T4 lesions of tonsillar fossa[331]	
		65% 2–3 cm primary[36]
7000–8000 cGy (8–9 wk)	→	30% >5 cm primary[36]
8000–9000 cGy (8–10 wk)	→	56% >5 cm primary[36]
8000–10,000 cGy (10–12 wk)	→	75% 5–15 cm primary[418]

* *1000 cGy in five fractions each week*
† *Universal experience*
‡ *The control rate is corrected for the percentage of nodes that would be positive histologically had a dissection of the axilla been done.*
(Fletcher GH, Shukovsky LJ: J Radiol Electrol 56:383, 1975)

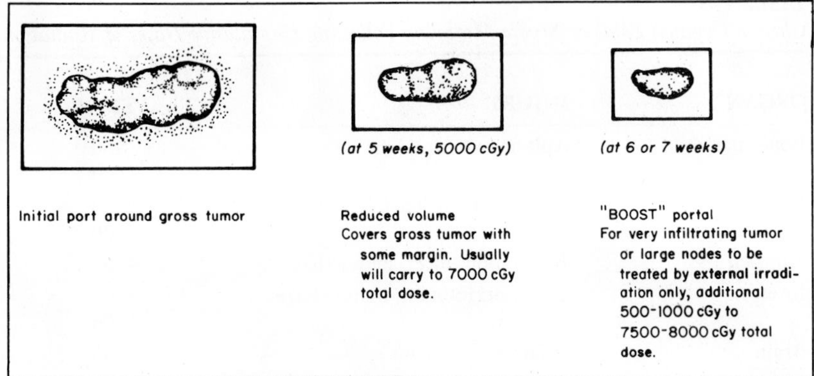

(at 5 weeks, 5000 cGy)
(at 6 or 7 weeks)
Initial port around gross tumor
Reduced volume
Covers gross tumor with some margin. Usually will carry to 7000 cGy total dose.
"BOOST" portal
For very infiltrating tumor or large nodes to be treated by external irradiation only, additional 500-1000 cGy to 7500-8000 cGy total dose.

FIGURE 1–3. Shrinking field technique. (Modified from Fletcher GH: Textbook of Radiotherapy, 3rd ed, p 228. Philadelphia, Lea & Febiger, 1983)

pathologist to detect them. Therefore these volumes must receive higher doses of radiation, in the range of 6000 cGy to 6500 cGy in 6 to 7 weeks for epithelial tumors.

For clinically palpable tumors, doses of 6000 cGy (for T1) to 7500 cGy to 8000 cGy (for T4 tumors) are required (200 cGy/day, five fractions weekly). This dose range and probability of tumor control have been documented for squamous cell and adenocarcinoma[103, 106, 225, 329] (Table 1-2).

Even with preoperative irradiation, the dose effect on probability of tumor control can be documented. At Memorial Hospital, New York, with doses of 2000 cGy (400 cGy/day for 1 week) to the neck combined with radical neck dissection, the failure rate was 22%, whereas it was only 7% when 5000 cGy was given in 5 weeks postoperatively.[383] At Washington University in carcinoma of the rectosigmoid, the failure rate with 2000 cGy given in 1 week was 20% compared with less than 5% with 4500 cGy tolerance dose (TD), both administered preoperatively.[391]

Baclesse[9, 10] initiated the concept of the different doses of radiation for various portions of the tumor. The dose administered through small portals to residual disease is called a *boost* but not in a biologic sense because it is given to obtain the same probability of control as for subclinical aggregates.[103]

One consequence of the concepts just discussed is the use of portals that are progressively reduced in size ("shrinking field" technique) to administer progressively higher doses of radiation to the central portion of the tumor where more clonogenic cells (presumably hypoxic) are present, in comparison with lesser doses that would be required to eradicate the disease in the periphery where a lower number of and better oxygenated tumor cells are assumed to be present (Fig. 1-3).

Normal Tissue Effects

A variety of changes in normal tissues are induced by ionizing radiations, depending on the total dose, fractionation schedule (daily dose and time), and volume treated; these factors are closely interrelated (Fig. 1-4). Structural alterations without anatomic or functional impairment may be noted, whereas in other instances substantial injuries with tissue destruction, severe dysfunction, or even death may take place. Normal tissues have a substantial capacity to recover from sublethal or potentially lethal damage induced by radiation (at tolerable dose levels). Cells may go through several divisions before somatic death takes place, although they may be biologically nonclonogenic immediately after the radiation exposure. Injury to the normal tissues may be caused by the radiation effect on the microvasculature or the support tissues[368] (stromal or parenchymal cells). Table 1-3 illustrates the tolerance of a variety of normal tissues to cumulative doses of radiation delivered with standard fractionation (about 200 cGy TD/day, five fractions weekly). In recent years several authors have reported higher tolerance doses for a variety of organs,[210, 217, 235, 268, 285, 286] which stresses the importance of updating this information in the light of more precise treatment planning and delivery of radiation and more accurate evaluation and recording of sequelae.

Rubin[320] has indicated the usefulness of assigning a certain percentage of risk complication, depending on the dose of the radiation. The minimal tolerance dose is defined as $TD_{5/5}$, which represents the dose of radiation that could cause no more than a 5% severe complication rate within 5 years after treatment. An acceptable complication rate for severe injury could be 5% to 10% in most clinical situations. Moderate-degree sequelae are noted in varying proportions (10% to 25% of patients), depending on the doses of radiation given and the organs at risk.

Chronologically, the effects of irradiation have been subdivided as *acute* (first 6 months), *subacute* (second 6 months), or *late* (depending on the time they are observed; Fig. 1-5). The gross manifestations depend on the kinetic properties of the cells (slow or rapid renewal) and the dose of radiation given.[319]

For a specified dose of radiation the normal tissue tolerance has been reported to decrease with larger volumes. This was demonstrated for skin by Paterson[262] in a graph plotting doses delivered with orthovoltage x-rays that would produce moist desquamation (Fig. 1-6). The same phenomenon was later reported with supervoltage radiation for other organs[344] and for brachytherapy. However, in a recent review of 268 patients with head and neck tumors treated with various total doses and fractions Maciejewski and associates[203] observed no difference in acute or late effects in patients treated with small (50 cm^2 to 80 cm^2) or large fields (100 cm^2 to 140 cm^2).

Coutard[51] observed varying degrees of mucositis and moist desquamation with varying doses and fractionations in patients treated for head and neck tumors. He noticed that regrowth of the mucosa and skin would come not only from the periphery of the irradiated field, but from cells surviving in the center of the

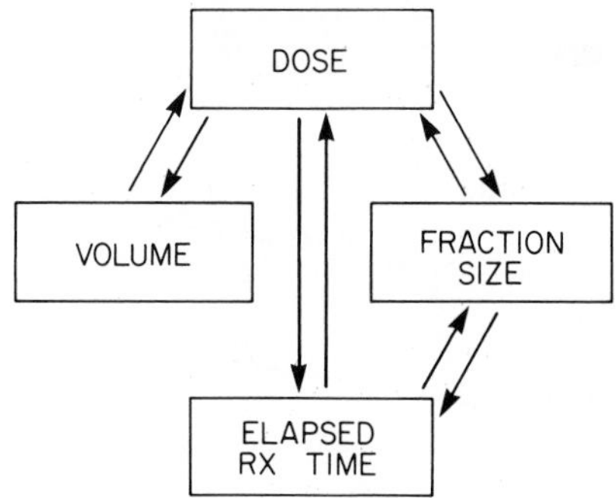

FIGURE 1–4. Basic dosimetric parameters determining normal tissue effects in radiation therapy.

TABLE 1–3
Class 1 Organs: Fatal or Severe Morbidity Following Cumulative Doses of Radiation Delivered With Standard Fractionation

ORGAN	INJURY	$TD_{5/5}$*	$TD_{50/5}$†	WHOLE OR PARTIAL ORGAN (FIELD SIZE OR LENGTH)
Bone marrow	Aplasia, pancytopenia	250	450	Whole
		3000	4000	Segmental
Liver	Acute and chronic hepatitis	2500	4000	Whole
		1500	2000	Whole (strip)
Stomach	Perforation, ulcer, hemorrhage	4500	5500	100 cm
Intestine	Ulcer, perforation, hemorrhage	4500	5500	400 cm
		5000	6500	100 cm
Brain	Infarction, necrosis	5000	6000	Whole
Spinal cord	Infarction, necrosis	4500	5500	10 cm
Heart	Pericarditis, pancarditis	4500	5500	60%
		7000	8000	25%
Lung	Acute and chronic pneumonitis	3000	3500	100 cm
		1500	2500	Whole
Kidney	Acute and chronic nephrosclerosis	1500	2000	Whole (strip)
		2000	2500	Whole
Fetus	Death	200	400	Whole

* *$TD_{5/5}$: minimal tolerance dose—the dose to which a given population of patients is exposed under a standard set of treatment conditions resulting in no more than a 5% severe complication rate within 5 years of treatment*
† *$TD_{50/5}$: the maximal tolerance dose—the dose to which a given population of patients is exposed under a standard set of treatment conditions resulting in a 50% severe complication rate within 5 years after treatment*
(Rubin P, Cooper R, Phillips TL [eds]: Radiation Biology and Radiation Pathology Syllabus. Set RT 1:Radiation Oncology. Chicago, American College of Radiology, 1975)

field. On the basis of these observations, Baclesse[9] designed a fractionation schedule for carcinoma of the breast with lower daily doses, which extended for 10 to 12 weeks, in an effort to avoid the acute mucositis and moist desquamation so that higher doses of radiation could be given. Even though acute reactions were decreased, a large number of the patients developed severe late tissue damage.[343] As Fletcher[103] noted, with the advent of megavoltage radiation, with its skin-sparing effect, radiation oncologists are not as familiar with the skin reactions previously noted, unless glancing fields are used. With the increasing use of electron beams, particularly at higher energies, skin reactions are frequently seen in clinical practice today.

No correlation has been established between the incidence and severity of acute reactions and the same parameters for late effects. Withers[408] compiled data depicting isoeffect lines for acute or late effects in several organs. The slopes for late reactions were steeper than for acute effects, and a lack of correlation was found between the doses required for acute or late effects. This may be due to the difference in the slopes of cell survival curves for acute or late effects[107] (Fig. 1-7).

Combining radiation therapy with surgery or cytotoxic agents frequently decreases the tolerance of normal tissues to a given dose of radiation (Fig. 1-8), which may necessitate adjustments in the treatment planning.

Therapeutic Ratio (Gain)

It is apparent that there is (or should be) an optimal dose that produces the maximal probability of tumor control with a minimal (reasonably acceptable) incidence of complications (preferably called *sequelae of therapy*).

The farther the two curves diverge, the more favorable is the therapeutic ratio (Fig. 1-9). The therapeutic ratio or therapeutic gain factor (TGF) of a given regimen could be expressed as follows:

$$\text{TGF} = \frac{\%\ \text{tumor control A versus B therapy}}{\%\ \text{major complications A versus B therapy}}$$

The higher the TGF, the more efficient the particular

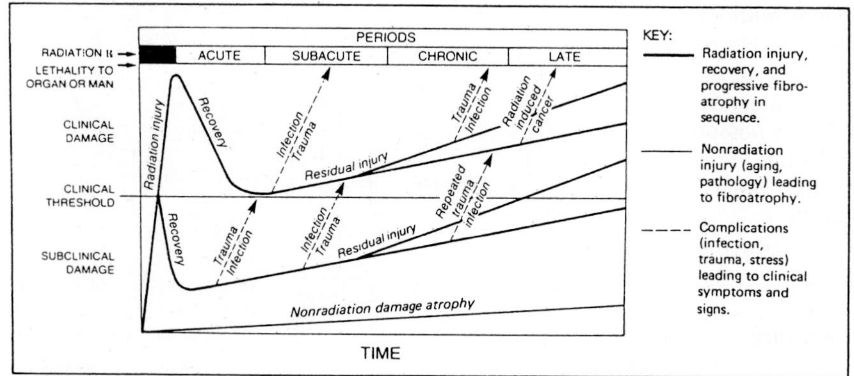

FIGURE 1–5. Sequence of clinical events after radiation therapy. (Rubin P, Casarett GW: Clinical Radiation Pathology, vols 1 and 2. Philadelphia, WB Saunders, 1968)

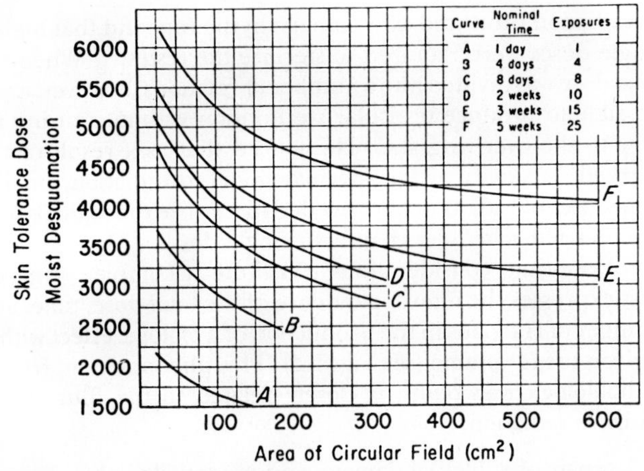

FIGURE 1–6. Graph showing relationship between dose and size of area irradiated (healthy skin in an average site) to produce moist desquamation for various overall treatment times (daily irradiation at about 50 R/minute for each exposure with radiation of half-value layer 1.5 mm Cu). (Paterson R: The Treatment of Malignant Disease by Radium and X-rays, p 39. Baltimore, Williams & Wilkins, 1949)

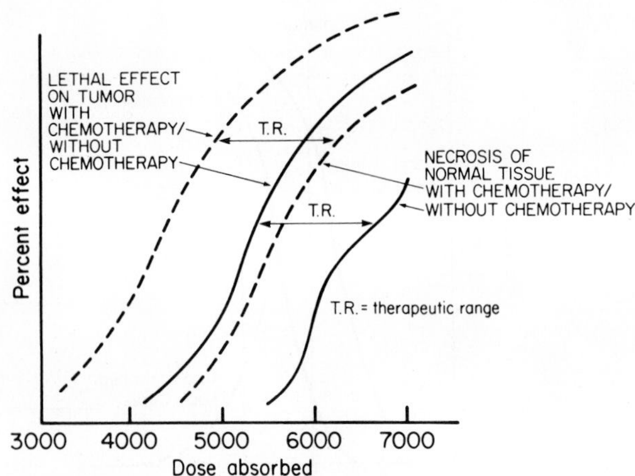

FIGURE 1–8. Theoretic curves for tumor control and complications as a function of radiation dose both with and without chemotherapy. TR: therapeutic ratio, or the difference between tumor control and complication frequency. (Perez CA, Thomas PRM: Radiation therapy: basic concepts and clinical implications. In Sutow WW, Fernbach DJ, Vietti TJ [eds]: Clinical Pediatric Oncology, 3rd ed, pp 167–209. St. Louis, CV Mosby, 1984)

therapy is. Such a quantitative expression could be used to compare different therapeutic strategies. Mendelsohn[221] has expressed this concept in terms of "uncomplicated tumor ablation" (Fig. 1-10). The selection of a dose must weigh the probability of major complications for any potential enhancement of tumor control. Models for decision making, using Bayes' theorem, incorporate values assigned to positive or negative outcomes[222]: positive outcome—uncomplicated cure; negative outcome—complicated cure, uncomplicated recurrence, complicated recurrence.

Moore and Mendelsohn[236] addressed the definition of optimal treatment levels in radiation therapy by an analysis of the receiver-operating characteristics (ROC). The concept of isoutility based on risk preference was developed further by Prewitt.[291] Metz and co-workers[226] applied the ROC optimization analysis to the probability of tumor control and complications in carcinoma of the nasopharynx.

Andrews[7,8] emphasized that in radiation therapy, even though it is recognized that a correlation exists between total dose delivered to the tumor and probability of control, efforts to reduce the risk of failure cannot be made at the cost of increasing the risk of injury (beyond reasonable levels). This principle

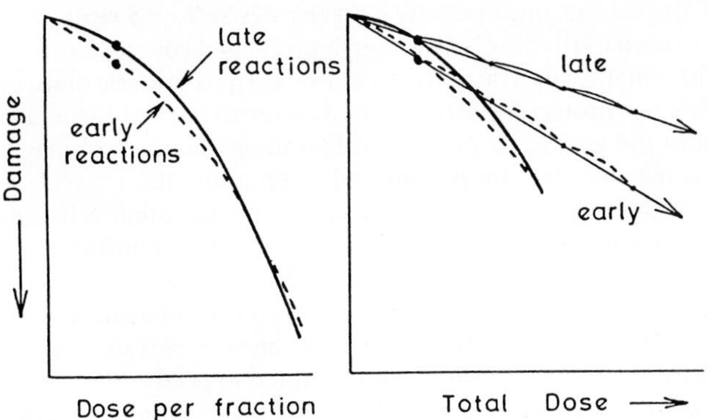

FIGURE 1–7. Difference in cell survival curves for acute and late radiation effects with single or multifractionated doses of irradiation. (Fowler JF: Fractionation and therapeutic gain. In Steel GG, Adams GE, Peckham MT [eds]: Biological Basis of Radiotherapy, pp 181–194. Amsterdam, Elsevier Science, 1983)

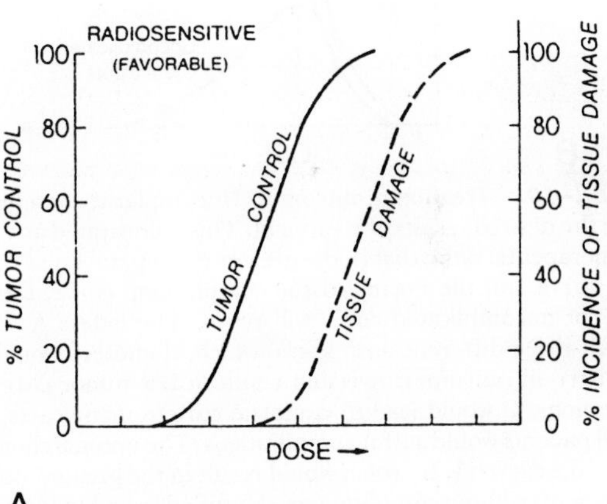

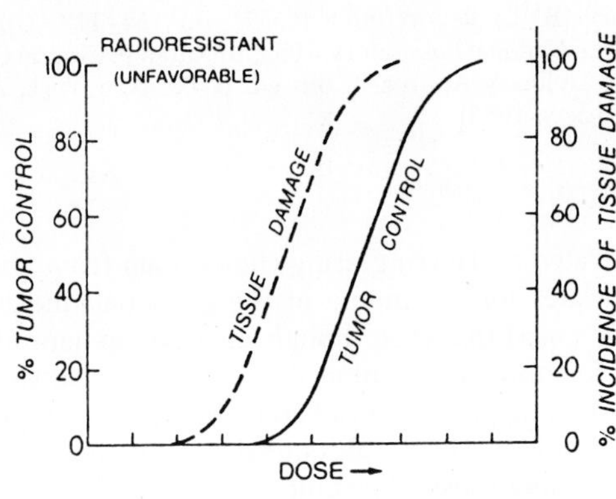

FIGURE 1–9. Different therapeutic ratios exist in different clinical circumstances depending on the radiosensitivity (dose-response curves) for the tumor versus critical normal tissue in the treatment field. (**A**) Favorable. (**B**) Unfavorable. (Rubin P: Clinical Oncology: A Multidisciplinary Approach, 6th ed. p. 63. New York, American Cancer Society, 1983)

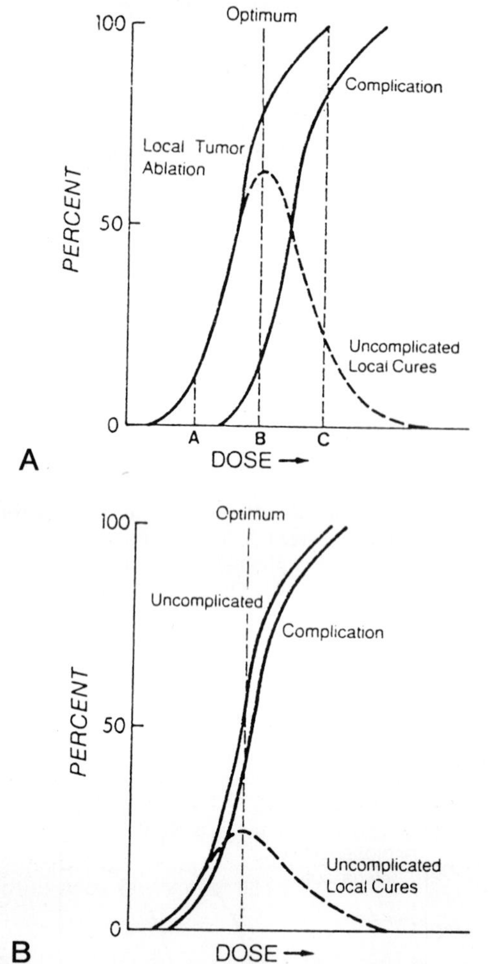

FIGURE 1–10. Treatment outcomes. Uncomplicated curves (*dashed line*) are the desired results of treatment. This is illustrated as a function of the therapeutic ratio; that is, the greater the separation of the tumor control curve and the normal tissue complication curve, the greater number of uncomplicated cures will result. The letters A, B, and C represent three different dose levels, which, if chosen, would lead to three different outcomes: A would result in few tumor cures but no complications; C would lead to complete cure in many cases, but virtually all patients would suffer complications. The optimal choice in this group of dose levels is B, which would result in the greatest number of cured patients without complications. (Modified from Mendelsohn ML: The biology of dose-limiting tissues. In Time and Dose Relationships in Radiation Biology as Applied to Radiotherapy, Brookhaven National Laboratory [BNL] Report 5023 [C-57], pp 154–173. Upton, NY, Brookhaven National Laboratory, 1969; In Rubin P: Clinical Oncology: A Multidisciplinary Approach, 6th ed. p. 69. New York, American Cancer Society, 1983)

was illustrated by Herring using clinical data from Shukovsky and associates for carcinoma of the glossopalatine sulcus.[330] Andrews[8] noted that even though the development of a ROC formula for optimal radiation therapy is a logical step in the decision-making process in radiation therapy, this optimization formula should not be the absolute determinant, because clinical considerations are important.

DOSE-TIME FACTORS

In an attempt to increase the therapeutic ratio, various fractionation schedules have been used in radiation therapy delivery. At the turn of the century, Regaud noted that a single dose of radiation produced skin damage in the ram and that higher single doses were required to sterilize the testes.[298] When the total dose was divided into a number of fractions, however, it was possible to produce testicular sterilization without causing injury to the overlying skin. He noticed that as a result of the marked sensitivity of the spermatogonia to radiation, smaller total doses of radiation were needed to sterilize the animals with fractionated schedules than with single doses.

Dose-time considerations constitute a complex function that expresses the interdependence of the total dose, time, and number of fractions in the production of a biologic effect within a given tissue volume (see Fig. 1-4). This phenomenon, from a radiobiologic viewpoint, is closely related to the four R's of ionizing radiation:

- repair of sublethal damage and potentially lethal damage
- repopulation of cells between fractions
- redistribution of cells throughout the cell cycle (partially due to radiation-induced synchrony)
- reoxygenation observed after one or more exposures to radiation

Moss and associates[237] noted the following advantages of dose fractionation:

Reduction in the number of hypoxic cells is brought about through cell kill and reoxygenation. Cater and Silver[37] demonstrated increased oxygenation in the tumor after irradiation, whereas changes in normal tissue oxygen were found to be slight or nonexistent.

Reduction in the absolute number of tumor cells is achieved by the initial fractions with the initial killing of the better-oxygenated cells. If the amount of available oxygen remains constant and there are fewer cancer cells, the amount of oxygen per remaining cell increases.

Blood vessels compressed by a growing cancer are decompressed as the cancer shrinks, permitting better oxygenation. The distance that oxygen must diffuse through tissue is reduced with each fraction.

Fractionation exploits the difference in recovery rate between normal tissues and tumors. Radiation-induced redistribution of cells within the cell cycle tends to sensitize rapidly proliferating cells.

The acute effects of single doses of radiation can be decreased with fractionation. The patient's symptomatic tolerance improves with fractionated irradiation.

In general, fractionation of irradiation spares acute reactions because of compensatory proliferation in the epithelium of the skin or mucosa, which accelerates at 2 or 3 weeks after initiation of therapy.[63] However, a prolonged course of therapy with small daily fractions decreases early acute reactions but does not protect for serious late damage to normal tissue, may allow the growth of rapidly proliferating tumors, and may be inconvenient for the patient and uneconomical.

The choice of optimal dose/time/fractionation schedules for various tumors should be individualized according to cell kinetic characteristics and clinical observations.[54,370] Recently Fowler[111] published theoretic considerations based on a series of assumptions of the values used in the linear quadratic equation with a time factor in which he attempted to predict the optimal dose fractionation schedules for tumors with various cell doubling times. He concluded that optimal overall times depend primarily on the doubling time of the tumor cells and the intrinsic radiosensitivity, α (assumed to be proportional to α/β). Short overall times are required for tumors with a high α/β ratio or fast proliferation. For median potential proliferation, dou-

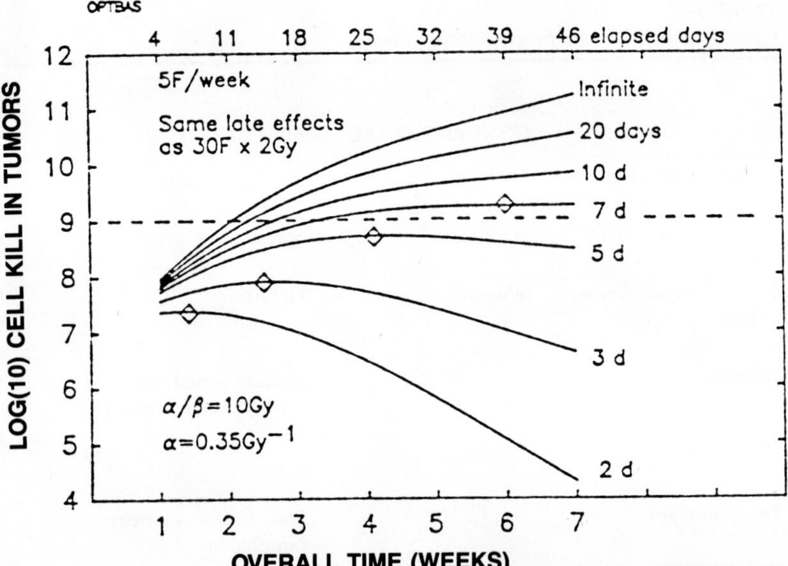

FIGURE 1–11. Log cell kill in tumors as a function of overall time, for schedules using five fractions per week to a total dose that gives the same late effects as 30 fractions of 2 Gy (assuming α/β = 3 Gy for late effects). Each curve is for the stated proliferation doubling time (average over the overall time). The diamond-shaped symbols show the maximum cell kill for that doubling time at the optimum overall time for that number of fractions per week. If there is no diamond, the optimum overall time is more than 7 weeks. The dashed line is drawn arbitrarily at 9 logs of cell kill. (Fowler JF: Radiother Oncol 18:165–181, 1990)

bling times of 5 days and intermediate radiosensitivity overall times of 2.5 to 4 weeks would be optimal. More slowly proliferating tumors should be treated with longer overall times (Fig. 1-11). With regard to fractionation Fowler believes that five fractions per week are preferable to three fractions, because less log cell kill occurs with the latter schedule (about one log for all, except 1 or 2 weeks overall time). He stressed that clinical trials should be carried out to logically select appropriate dose-time schedules. Flow cytometry and other *in vitro* techniques to assess tumor radiosensitivity in biopsy specimens may be helpful in this endeavor.

Altered Fractionation

Without solid biologic basis and because of empiricism and convenience, the "standard fractionation" for radiation therapy has evolved into five fractions weekly. Other fractionation schedules have been proposed, which deliver several fractions daily or which use a split-course regimen. The various types of schedules are shown in Figure 1-12, and the characteristics for hyperfractionation, accelerated fractionation, or split-course schedules as well as potential advantages or disadvantages are summarized in Table 1-4. Peschel and Fischer[278] reviewed the rationale for multiple daily fractionation schedules. They emphasized that any alteration in fractionation schedule is potentially harmful and must be approached with great caution. They listed the following radiobiologic principles that are pertinent when one is selecting treatment schedules to maximize the eradication of tumor cells, while taking into account the tolerance of normal cells:

Prolongation of overall treatment time favors a rapidly proliferating over a slowly proliferating cell population and provides for reoxygenation of originally hypoxic cells.

Increase in the number of treatment fractions favors a cell population that repairs sublethal damage and provides opportunity for redistribution of cells throughout the cell cycle between treatments.

Close spacing (hours) of the radiation treatments could significantly favor a subpopulation of cells that repairs sublethal damage more rapidly.

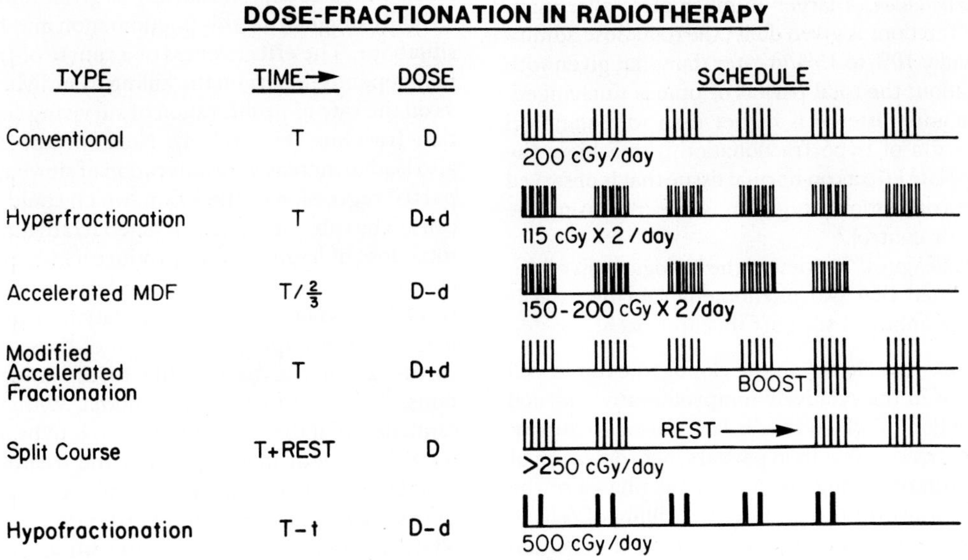

DOSE-FRACTIONATION IN RADIOTHERAPY

TYPE	TIME →	DOSE	SCHEDULE
Conventional	T	D	200 cGy/day
Hyperfractionation	T	D+d	115 cGy X 2 / day
Accelerated MDF	T/$\frac{2}{3}$	D−d	150-200 cGy X 2 /day
Modified Accelerated Fractionation	T	D+d	BOOST
Split Course	T+REST	D	REST → >250 cGy/day
Hypofractionation	T−t	D−d	500 cGy/day

FIGURE 1–12. Various types of fractionation used in radiation therapy.

TABLE 1–4
Comparison of Various Fractionation Schedules

	CONVENTIONAL	SPLIT-COURSE	(ACCELERATED) MULTIPLE DAILY FRACTIONS	HYPERFRACTIONATION
Indication in tumors of growth rate	Average	Average or slow	Rapid	Slow (with large cell loss factors)
Normal tissue effects, acute	Standard	Standard or greater	Greater	Standard or greater
Normal tissue effects, late	Standard	Greater	Standard (if complete repair of SLD occurs) or greater	Lower
Advantages		Shorter actual treatment time (fewer fractions)	Destroys more tumor cells; prevents tumor cell repopulation; less overall treatment time	(?) Lower OER with small doses (4); spares late damage; allows reoxygenation; allows stem cell repopulation
Disadvantages		May permit tumor repopulation		More fractions

SLD: sublethal damage; OER: oxygen enhancement ratio

Thus, theoretically, multiple daily fractionation (MDF) could be more effective in rapidly growing tumors with a high growth fraction, whereas less-than-daily fractionation (one, two, or three doses/week) and higher doses may be more efficacious for slow-growing tumors (large D_o cell populations) or for tumor cells with a large D_q (melanoma).

Normal tissues behave as actively proliferating cells for expression of acute reactions but as slowly proliferating cells in the manifestation of late injury.[408]

Several biologic studies have suggested that a minimum of 4 and preferably 6 or even 8 hours should be allowed between fractions when multiple daily fractionation is used to allow maximum repair of normal tissues.[110,405]

With *accelerated fractionation,* several fractions of radiation are given daily over a shorter total period. Some reduction in the total dose administered must be introduced. These schedules appear to be preferable for use with hypoxic cell sensitizers or other chemical modifiers of radiation response that require the presence of a high concentration of the compound in the tumor at the time of the radiation exposure.

With *hyperfractionation,* a larger number of smaller-than-conventional dose fractions is given daily; the total dose administered daily is usually 10% to 15% greater than that given with standard fractionation; the total period of time is unchanged, and the total dose administered is higher than with standard fractionation. The aim of hyperfractionation is to achieve the same percentage of late effects on normal tissue that is observed with a comparable conventional regimen, while increasing the probability of tumor control.[405]

Withers and colleagues[405] reviewed the biologic basis of this regimen and indicated that two phenomena (not necessarily independent of one another) support this approach:

Greater division cycle asynchrony in the clonogenic tumor cell population than in the relatively nonproliferative normal cells, the depletion of which causes late normal tissue injury. Each dose fraction results in partial synchronization of the surviving tumor clonogens in resistant phases of the division cycle because of the preferential killing of cells in sensitive phases at the time of irradiation. Redistribution toward asynchrony results in a net loss of resistant-phase survivors into sensitive phases of the cycle, with a potential for a greater number of tumor cells likely to be killed by the next fraction of radiation.

An inherent difference in the radiosensitivity of actively proliferating cells (existing in some normal tissues and in the growth fraction of most tumors) and slowly proliferating cells (those found in the tissues that manifest late injury). Slowly proliferating cells become relatively more resistant as the dose per fraction is decreased.[364] This increasing relative resistance of the slowly proliferating target cells with decreasing dose of radiation leads to preferential sparing of late tissue effects, as illustrated by a steeper slope of isoeffect curves for late effects (see Fig. 1-7).

Accelerated Repopulation

Withers and associates[406] have described experimental observations documenting accelerated repopulation of tumor cells after fractionated radiation therapy is given and discontinued and strongly suggest that this phenomenon may take place in clinical situations. The effectiveness of a course of fractionated irradiation depends in part on the killing by individual fractions as well as on the rate of proliferation of surviving cells between irradiation fractions (Fig. 1-13*A*). Neoadjuvant chemotherapy may also lead to increased proliferation of surviving tumor cells after partial regression of the lesion, which could result in decreased cell kill by subsequent fractionated irradiation (Fig. 1-13*B*). The total dose of irradiation to produce a 50% probability of tumor control must be increased when fractionation is prolonged beyond 4 weeks because of repopulation of surviving cells, which may result in improved nutrition of those cells following early shrinkage of the tumor due to the initial irradiation fractions.[139,148] In a hypothetical model, Withers and associates[406] estimated that the dose of radiation is to be increased by 60 cGy for every day of interruption of the treatment.

Taylor and associates[360] found a close correlation between the estimated increment in isoeffect dose per day and the overall treatment time in 473 patients with squamous cell carcinoma of the head and neck treated with radiation. Taking into consid-

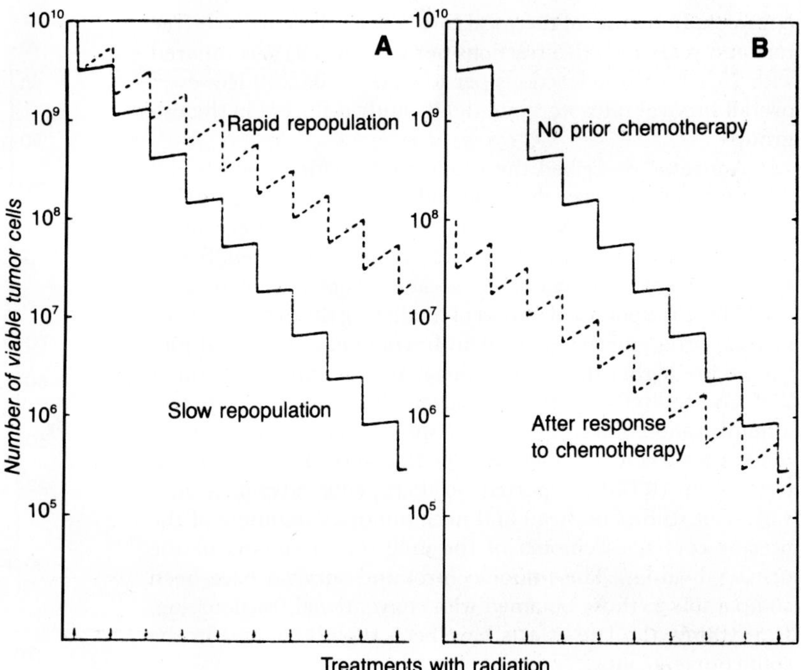

FIGURE 1–13. (**A**) Schematic diagram indicating that cell survival during a course of fractionated irradiation depends not only on the proportion of cells killed with each dose (equal for the two curves shown) but also on the rate of proliferation of surviving cells between dose fractions, which differs for the two curves. (**B**) Hypothetical diagram to illustrate the number of surviving cells in a tumor during treatment with irradiation alone (*solid line*) or during radiation treatment delivered to a tumor that has responded to chemotherapy (*i.e.*, cell number reduced to 1% at start of radiation treatment), but where proliferation has been stimulated (*broken line*). Note that cell survival is similar after fractionated irradiation, despite the initial response to drugs. (Tannock IF: Radiother Oncol 16:83–101, 1989)

eration that this study was a retrospective analysis, some variations among the various anatomic sites were noted, and the increment in isoeffect dose per day was estimated to be larger than 100 cGy (consistent with Withers' estimate of 60 cGy). In contrast, Lai and associates[181] in a large number of patients treated with definitive irradiation for carcinoma of the prostate noted no significant impact of short interruptions (less than 1 week) or overall length of treatment on local tumor control, suggesting that accelerated repopulation may not occur in slowly proliferating tumors.

Clinical Observations on Dose Time and Tumor Control

Different fractionation schedules have been shown to affect therapeutic outcome with low linear energy transfer (LET) radiations (photons and electrons). Fowler and co-workers,[112] in experiments using a mammary murine adenocarcinoma, demonstrated that with different fractionated schedules of radiation an optimal time of approximately 10 days was needed to obtain tumor control in about 50% of the animals with the various schedules. With a shorter time, only the multiple daily fraction schedule (nine fractions) was effective. If a longer period was allowed (18 days), the probability of tumor control decreased even with multiple fraction schedules (15 fractions) because of tumor proliferation. Fowler and colleagues,[109,112] on the other hand, showed no significant impact of fractionation on tumor control or survival rate in mice irradiated with neutrons.

Eichhorn[84] reported on patients with unresectable bronchogenic carcinomas treated with either 250 cGy five times per week or 600 cGy every fifth day to a dose of 5500 cGy delivered with x-rays. Tumor destruction was determined by microscopic examination of autopsy specimens. The lowest destruction of tumor cells was observed in the patients treated with 400 cGy, 600 cGy, or 1000 cGy fractions. Eichhorn concluded that "in spontaneous human tumors, the size of the proliferating compartment has a greater influence on radiosensitivity than hypoxia."[84] Nonproliferating cells are transferred into the proliferating compartment, which respond to daily doses below 300 cGy. Higher doses are less efficient because the nonproliferating compartment is more resistant to irradiation.

Byhardt and associates[34] reported on 96 patients with squamous carcinoma of the oral cavity and oropharynx treated with five fractions per week to total doses ranging from 6000 cGy in 30 fractions over 46 days to 7200 cGy in 36 fractions over 51 days, or with three fractions per week with total doses ranging from 5400 cGy in 18 fractions over 42 days to 7200 cGy in 24 fractions over 61 to 77 days. The nominal standard dose (NSD) for the two groups was relatively similar. The local tumor control by T-stage was significantly lower in patients treated with three fractions per week (three of 26) than in those receiving five fractions (28 of 43). Effects on normal tissues were not evaluated.

Equivalency of two different time-dose regimens of radiation has been reported by Weissberg and co-workers[398] in a prospective randomized trial involving 64 patients with advanced carcinoma of the head and neck. Patients were treated with five fractions of 200 cGy per day to 6000 cGy to 7000 cGy in 6 to 7 weeks, or with 400 cGy daily to a total dose of 4400 cGy in 2 to 3 weeks. Acute skin and mucosal reactions occurred earlier in patients receiving 400 cGy daily. However, the reactions were of the same intensity as in those patients receiving five fractions per week. Tumor control, palliation rate, and normal tissue reactions were similar in both groups.

Kok[175] used three *versus* five fractions of radiation per week in the treatment of Stage I carcinoma of the larynx; all patients received the same minimum tumor dose of 6300 cGy. The 3-year local tumor control rate was 89% in 18 patients receiving five fractions per week and 62% in 42 patients treated with three fractions per week.

Wiernik and The British Institute of Radiology[402] reported on a randomized trial of three *versus* five fractions of radiation per week in 732 patients with carcinoma of the laryngopharynx, each receiving different total doses of radiation with approximately the same TDF values. The radiation doses ranged from 5000 cGy to 5300 cGy for the three fractions per week and from 5400 cGy to 6100 cGy for the patients receiving five fractions per week. In tumors of the vocal cord, the local recurrence-free rate at 8 years with five fractions per week was 91% compared with 75% for three fractions per week ($P = 0.026$). However, overall survival rates were not significantly different in the two groups.

Andrews[6] described the results in 43 patients with squamous cell carcinoma of the head and neck treated with 8000 to 10,000 cGy with 2 MV x-rays, three fractions per week in an overall time of 14 weeks. Only nine patients were cured, five of whom had early tumors of the vocal cords or nasopharynx.

There is a potential impact of modifying the overall time by *split-course* regimen when the daily fractions of radiation administered are higher than conventional, that is, administration of 250 cGy to 300 cGy TD for ten fractions, 2 or 3 weeks of rest, and administration of a second course similar to the first one for a total of 5000 cGy or 6000 cGy. The Radiation Therapy Oncology Group (RTOG) reported no therapeutic advantage in a variety of studies on head and neck tumors, carcinoma of the uterine cervix, carcinoma of the lung, or carcinoma of the urinary bladder. The tumor control and survival have been comparable to those obtained with conventional fractionation. If anything, the late effects have been slightly greater in the split-course groups.[208]

On the other hand, reports have been published by the University of Florida on patients with carcinoma of the head and neck, uterine cervix, and prostate who were treated to definitive doses of radiation therapy with conventional fractionation but with a rest period halfway through the course of therapy.[258,259] Some of the groups of patients in the split-course regimen showed lower tumor control and survival.[258] This is probably a result of the repopulation of clonogenic surviving cells in the tumor during the rest period.

Jampolis and colleagues[161] and Wang[392] have reported the results of studies using hyperfractionation at their respective institutions, but no randomized comparison with "standard fractionation" was made. Horiot and colleagues[155] reviewed the results of several cooperative clinical trials with altered fractionation schedules and noted that hyperfractionation yielded better 2- and 3-year locoregional tumor control than conventional fractionation in T2–T3 oropharyngeal carcinoma.

The RTOG has conducted several clinical trials with either hyperfractionated or accelerated fractionation schedules in a variety of tumors and normal tissues.[209] It is necessary to wait for some time for the late effects on normal tissues to manifest themselves before drawing definite conclusions on the safety of these altered fractionation schedules.

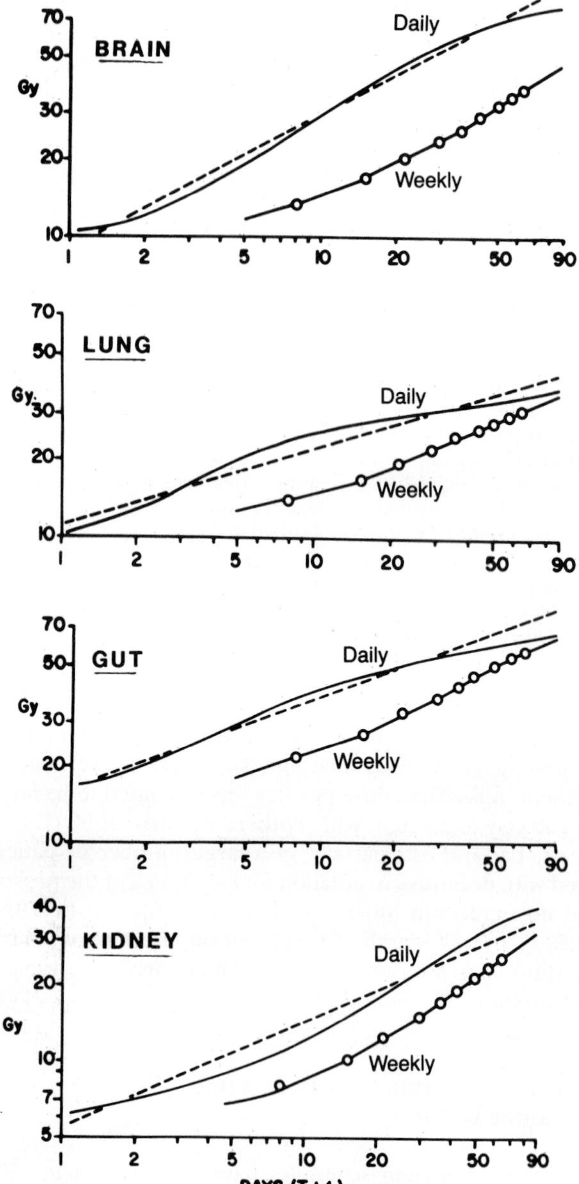

FIGURE 1–14. Isoeffect functions for 5% risk of injury to irradiated organs. Lines shown are related to "daily" (five times a week) and once-weekly treatment. (Cohen L, Creditor M: Int J Radiat Oncol Biol Phys 9:233–241, 1983)

Clinical Observations on Dose Time and Normal Tissue Effects

Several studies have been implemented in a variety of human tissues in an effort to determine the dose-time relationship.[43] Figure 1-14 illustrates the various tolerance limits for several organs.[45] Cohen and Creditor[45] explained the reasons to support their hypothesis that computed, tissue-specific isoeffect tables based on cell kinetics parameters are better predictors of radiation effects on normal tissues than the standard time-dose equations.

Examples of the effects of different fractionations and normal tissue effects have been reported for several different organs. The difference in incidence of necrosis of the skin observed with both a small and a larger number of fractions was illustrated by Traenkle and Malay.[367]

Turesson and Notter[372] treated two parasternal fields in each patient with carcinoma of the breast. One portal received daily radiation fractions of 254 cGy (16 fractions) and the other 729 cGy (four fractions). They matched the acute doses using the cumulative radiation effect (CRE) formula. Figure 1-15 discloses no significant difference in the acute reactions with either schedule. However, with time the late effects of the larger fractions (telangiectasis and fibrosis) become evident.

In 1965 Andrews[6] reported on 20 patients with squamous cell carcinoma of the upper respiratory and digestive tracts treated with a single dose of 2000 cGy to 2700 cGy, with most patients receiving 2500 cGy. Only four of the patients had no evidence of disease at 1 year, and complications were severe in a large proportion (*e.g.,* seven patients had mucositis; eight, ulceration; four, laryngeal edema; two, cartilage necrosis). Four patients required tracheostomy. At Washington University, 47 patients with advanced carcinoma of the breast were treated

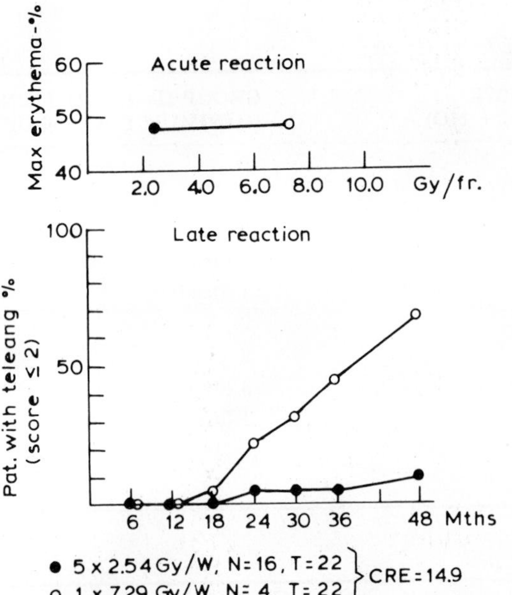

FIGURE 1–15. The upper panel shows the maximal skin erythema (mean of the upper, middle, and lower parasternal regions), and the lower panel shows the number of patients with telangiectasia (score ≤ 2) with daily (*solid circles*) and once-a-week (*open circles*) fractions. (Turesson I, Notter G: Int J Radiat Oncol Biol Phys 10:593–598, 1984)

with 2500 cGy given on 2 consecutive days.[83] Severe fibrosis, frozen shoulder, lymphedema, and radiation pneumonitis were noted in most patients, particularly the long-term survivors.

Dische and co-workers[71] used 500 cGy to 600 cGy TD per fraction twice weekly for total radiation doses of 3400 cGy to 3600 cGy in 18 days for advanced carcinoma of the lung. Of 70 patients who survived for a minimum of 6 months, eight (11%) developed radiation myelopathy. Similar experience was reported by the RTOG with a comparable dose schedule; of 12 patients surviving longer than 1 year, five (41%) developed myelopathy.[332]

Montague[233] treated a large number of patients with preoperative ^{60}Co radiation before radical mastectomy with either three or five fractions of radiation per week. The regional lymphatics received 4500 cGy TD and the breast 3500 cGy to 4000 cGy TD in 4 weeks. Table 1-5 shows a significantly higher incidence of complications in patients treated with three weekly fractions. Also, a smaller group of patients were treated with radiation alone to doses of approximately 6000 cGy TD to the breast and 5000 cGy to the regional lymph nodes (with a boost when necessary).

Singh[334] described more serious late complications after five weekly radiation doses of 580 cGy in patients with Stage III carcinoma of the uterine cervix, using equal NSD in rets (TDF = 66), when compared with patients receiving 200 cGy daily, five times per week (Table 1-6).

Meoz and associates[224] reported on 30 patients with advanced pelvic malignancy who were treated with three once-weekly radiation doses of 1000 cGy, preceded by 4 g/m^2 dose of misonidazole. Five major complications resulted (three bowel obstructions, one bowel perforation, and one vesicovaginal fistula), which is considered excessive for palliative situations.

In contrast, Spanos and associates[342] reported on a phase II study of daily multifraction split-course irradiation in 142 patients (50% had recurrent or metastatic disease in the pelvis only and the other 50% had associated extrapelvic metastases) receiving 370 cGy per fraction given twice daily for two consecutive days, repeated at 3- to 6-week intervals for a total of three courses, aiming to a total tumor dose of 4440 cGy. The dose was based on linear quadratic equation considerations of acute late effects, assuming and α/β ratio of 10 for acute and 4 for late effects. Twenty-seven patients survived for more than 1 year; only two cases of grade 3 toxicity (lower GI) were recorded.

Lower-fraction protracted irradiation does not necessarily protect normal tissues, and the effects are dependent on the total dose delivered. Spanos and colleagues[343] reported on 158 patients with Stage III and Stage IV breast cancer treated with doses ranging from 6000 cGy in 8 weeks to over 10,000 cGy in 13 weeks (Baclesse technique). All patients developed some fibrosis. The incidence of necrosis with doses of 8000 cGy or less was about 5%, whereas with doses above this level necrosis occurred in 14% of the patients.

The effect of dose fractionation on normal tissue has recently been emphasized by experimental and clinical observations on late effects in animals and patients treated with single-dose intraoperative radiation therapy. Powers and associates[287] indicated that intraoperative radiation doses of 1000 cGy to 1500 cGy have an effect five times or greater than the same amount of radiation given in 200 cGy fractions. Osteosarcoma occurred in 21% (eight of 38) of dogs that received doses greater than 2500 cGy intraoperatively. However, only one of

TABLE 1–5
Incidence of Complications of Wound Healing in Patients with Primary Radical Mastectomy

		PREOPERATIVE IRRADIATION	
COMPLICATIONS	NO PREOPERATIVE IRRADIATION—644 PATIENTS (%)	^{60}CO 5×/WK—274 PATIENTS 1954–SEPT. 1962 (%)	^{60}CO 3×/WK—59 PATIENTS* OCT. 1962–JULY 1964 (%)
Delayed wound healing	3.5	6.0	15.0
Moderate slough	8.0	3.0	13.5
Severe slough with graft	2.0	1.5	7.0
Rib necrosis	0.2	1.0	3.0
Infection	0.5	2.0	17.0
Total (% patients)	14.0	13.0	56.0

* *Seven additional patients, 3×/wk: two radical mastectomies canceled, five simple mastectomies.*
(Montague ED: Radiology 90:962–966, 1968)

TABLE 1–6
Late Reactions or Complications Following Radiation Therapy of Carcinoma of Uterine Cervix

COMPLICATIONS	GROUP I—5 FRACTIONS/WK (MINIMUM FOLLOW-UP 2+ MO)	GROUP II—1 FRACTION/WK (MINIMUM FOLLOW-UP 12 MO)
No complications	11	0
Proctitis lasting over 6 mo	8	8
Severe proctitis requiring colostomy	0	6 (1 dead*)
Perforation of small bowel	0	1 (dead*)
Vesicovaginal fistula	0	1 (dead*)
Rectovaginal fistula	0	2
Edema of vulva, mons, etc.	0	2
Residual disease	3 (dead)	3 (dead)
Death from metastasis	1 (lung)	1 (liver)
Death from local recurrence	1	0
Total	24	24

* *Died after surgery.*
(Singh K: Br J Radiol 51:357–362, 1978)

four dogs that received 2500 cGy intraoperative radiation combined with 5000 cGy external beam radiation developed a tumor, and no tumors occurred at doses below this level. LeCouteur and associates[185] reported severe peripheral neuropathy in dogs receiving doses of intraoperative radiation in the range of 2000 cGy, whereas dogs treated with less than 1500 cGy had no evidence of neuropathy. Likewise, Shaw and colleagues[326] noted peripheral neuropathy in 32% of 50 patients who received intraoperative irradiation as a component of therapy in primary or recurrent pelvic cancer; the development of neurotoxicity was more common with radiation doses of 1500 cGy to 2500 cGy than with doses of 1000 cGy to 1250 cGy.

The impact of altered fractionation schedules on late normal tissue effects is also under close scrutiny. Olmi and coworkers[246] reported on 161 patients with advanced head and neck cancer treated with accelerated fractionation (4800 cGy to 5200 cGy delivered in three daily fractions of 200 cGy of radiation with a 4-hour interval between each session for 11 to 12 days). The local tumor control rate, stage by stage, was similar to that observed by the authors in historical controls treated with conventional fractionation. Acute mucosal reactions were more pronounced with conventional fractionation 2 weeks after initiation of treatment and complete recovery after 6 to 10 weeks. The actuarial 5-year risk of severe late damage with accelerated cancer (squamous cell and basal cell carcinoma); most tumors were treated within 14 and 29 days and only one within 45 days. An isoeffect line was drawn, with a slope of 0.22. He fitted the recovery factors of MacComb and Quimby and Reisner using an extrapolated value of 0.35 day as the time for a single dose. He fractionation was 24%; 16% of the patients (eight of 53) had osteonecrosis. Most late complications developed within 2 years, with the incidence being higher than in historical, conventionally treated patients.

Isoeffect Graphs

To express an equal biologic effect produced by various fractionation schedules, isoeffect lines have been generated. Fletcher,[103] in his textbook, noted that Kronig and Friedrich[179] published the first report on the observation that a specific physical dose of radiation is less biologically effective if given in multiple fractions, which embodies the original concept of recovery *between* fractions. Later MacComb and Quimby[202] and Reisner[299] established the rate of recovery in experimentally produced skin reactions in patients.

In 1944, Strandqvist[348] published a monograph describing the results of radiation treatment of 280 patients with skin also produced a graph for various degrees of radiation reaction on the skin, ranging from erythema to necrosis (Fig. 1-16). It should be emphasized that in these curves the vertical coordinate represents the total dose given and the abscissa the total

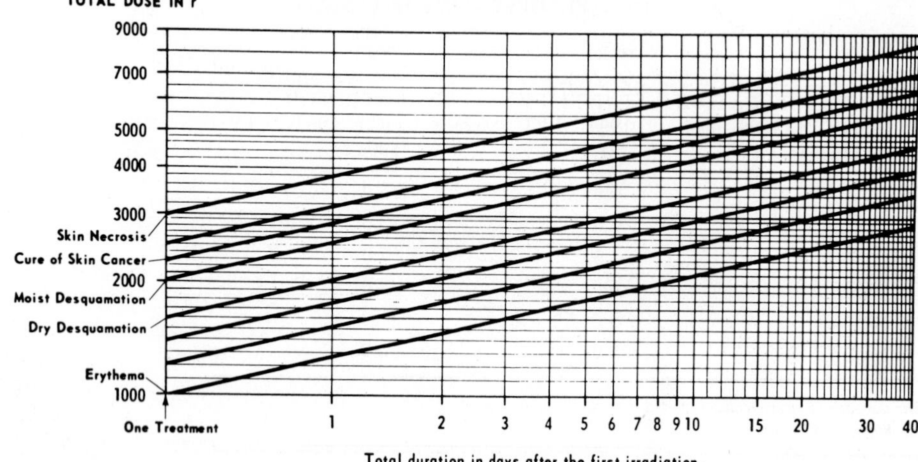

FIGURE 1–16. Strandqvist's curves on log paper. The slope of the curves (0.22) is the same for the tumoricidal dose for squamous cell carcinoma for various degrees of skin reactions. (Strandqvist M: Acta Radiol [Stockh] [Suppl] 55:1–300, 1944)

duration in days after the first irradiation. However, some authors have plotted similar graphs representing the number of fractions in the horizontal coordinate. It is critical to identify these two parameters, because one could deliver 6000 cGy in 6 weeks in 30 fractions given five times weekly or the same dose delivered in 18 fractions given three times weekly. The effects on normal tissue certainly would be different.

Von Essen,[384] using the Strandqvist data as well as his own, pointed out the importance of the volume irradiated when isoeffect parameters are studied. A graphic, three-dimensional display of these data has been published. The reader is referred to Von Essen's publication for the mathematical explanation of the model.[384]

Dutreix and co-workers[80] published observations on the influence of fraction size in fractionated irradiation for patients with cancer of the lung, in which one of the supraclavicular areas of one patient received a single exposure and the other area two exposures separated by 6 hours. They noticed that two fractions of 100 cGy produced the same skin reaction as one fraction of 200 cGy. As the fraction size increased, however, it took a higher dose in the two-fraction schedule to produce the same reaction as with the single-fraction schedule. At M.D. Anderson Hospital, with mucositis of the faucial arch used as an end point, it was observed that 1000 cGy per week given in five fractions of 200 cGy is equivalent to 1100 cGy given in ten fractions, twice a day, separated by 3 hours.[103]

Analysis of other data by Cohen and co-workers[42] has demonstrated that the radiation reaction slopes for various normal tissues differ, as do slopes of tumor curability and normal tissue late effects. In general, the slope for tumor curability is less steep than that for normal tissue reactions.[42] Fletcher and colleagues,[106] Ghossein and colleagues,[121] Spanos and co-workers,[344] and Shukovsky[329] reported isoeffect lines for various squamous cell carcinomas of the head and neck, for different stages, with slopes varying from 0.33 to 0.38. Table 1-7 illustrates the influence of the isoeffect exponent on the total dose of various treatment schedules (4 to 8 weeks) with five fractions weekly.[103] The radiation doses are equivalent to 6000 cGy delivered in 6 weeks with one daily fraction five times per week. Fletcher emphasized that equivalent single doses cannot be used legitimately to facilitate an analysis when various doses, number of fractions, and times are used.

Furthermore, as stated earlier, tolerance of normal tissues is strongly related to the volume irradiated. A total tumor dose of 6200 cGy in 25 fractions over 33 days is equivalent to 1900 ret nominal standard dose, which, according to Ellis's formula,[89] is equal to 7000 cGy in 35 fractions over 47 days. Whereas 6000 cGy could be given safely in 5 weeks for a small glottic tumor with a 5-cm × 5-cm portal, the same dose delivered in the same period for a supraglottic carcinoma, with a larger portal covering the entire larynx, would result in prohibitive acute and late sequelae.[106]

TABLE 1–7
Equivalent Doses for Daily Fractionated Courses of From 4 to 8 Weeks Using Different Isoeffect Exponents*

ISOEFFCT EXPONENT	DURATION OF TREATMENT (5 FRACTIONS/WK)				
	4 WK	5 WK	6 WK	7 WK	8 WK
0.25	5400	5725	6000	6250	6450
0.30	5275	5650	6000	6300	6550
0.35	5150	5600	6000	6350	6650
0.40	5050	5550	6000	6400	6725

** Calculated to nearest 25 cGy by the formula: Equivalent dose in x days = Antilog [Log 6000 − isoeffect component (Log 40 − Log x)]; 40 = overall time in days for 30 daily fractions (Fletcher GH [ed]: Textbook of Radiotherapy, 3rd ed. Philadelphia, Lea & Febiger, 1980)*

Nominal Standard Dose

Although of historical interest today, radiation oncologists should be familiar with some of the details relative to the nominal standard dose (NSD), which for 20 years was frequently found in the literature to express equivalency of clinical doses of radiation. In 1969 Ellis[91] suggested that if one number could be used to represent the dose of radiation that reached normal tissue tolerance, this would be advantageous in comparing different techniques. This figure represented the normal connective tissue tolerance because this was, in his thinking, the limiting factor in most tumor therapy. Because of the difficulty in using radiobiologic data for clinical purposes, Ellis used human data based on skin tolerance and curability for squamous cell carcinoma. From a paper by Cohen,[44] he pointed out that the regression coefficient for squamous cell carcinoma was different from that of normal skin (0.24).

The NSD is expressed as a constant of proportionality, the dimensions including dose, time, and number of fractions administered

$$D = (NSD)\ T^{0.11} \times N^{0.24}$$

where

D = total dose of irradiation
NSD = nominal standard dose (rets)
T = total time in days in which the total dose of radiation is administered
N = number of radiation fractions

The unit for NSD expression is the ret. It should never be assumed that the NSD value represents a "single equivalent dose" because the isoeffect time calculated by Ellis used data from four to 30 fractions. Another flaw of the NSD calculation is that it does not allow for the effect of variations in volume treated or for interruptions of therapy (split-course therapy). Orton[250] estimated that NSD calculations were misused about 50% of the time by unaware clinicians comparing different radiation therapy regimens.

The NSD formula has been the subject of much evaluation and controversy. Berry and associates[18, 19] irradiated domestic swine with 250 kVp x-rays in courses of 1, 6, and 30 fractions to various TDs to ascertain the validity of this formula. They found that the NSD was a poor predictor of early skin response. Late skin tolerance was not closely correlated with the level of early response, but skin necrosis was well predicted by the NSD formula. They also evaluated subcutaneous fibrosis after the same doses and fractionation of irradiation and noted that the NSD formula did not predict correctly the doses required to produce a given effect. The slope of the isoeffect curve between six and 30 fractions was 0.46 compared with the 0.33 coefficient in the NSD formula. Furthermore, the degree of late fibrosis did not correlate with the severity of the early skin reaction.

Hopewell and co-workers[152] used an experiment on the pig with the same number of fractions used by Berry to assess the application of the NSD formula to kidney tolerance. They also found that the renal tolerance was 30% to 45% lower for the six-fraction treatment than in the other two fractionation groups.

They concluded that the widely differing partial tolerance doses observed suggested that the NSD system could not be applied to predict variation in radiation dose and fractionation when damage to the kidney is studied.

Later Withers and colleagues[407] found that the NSD formula did not predict isoeffect in pig skin irradiation with ^{60}Co using two or five fractions per week. Moreover, early reactions did not predict the magnitude of late damage when dose fractionation was altered from conventional daily schedules.

Dutreix and colleagues[80] analyzed skin reactions in the same patient treated in two fields with different dose schedules in 44 patients who received x-ray doses ranging from 1100 cGy to 1500 cGy. Other patients were treated with single or split doses ranging from 1200 cGy to 1350 cGy. They concluded that under typical regimens of radiation therapy, when the number of fractions and overall time are simultaneously increased, the dose increase is mainly associated with cellular recovery if the number of fractions is small, and to cellular repopulation when the dose per fraction becomes small and the number of fractions is larger (>15). Dutreix and colleagues compared their data with the NSD formula, stating that in the NSD formula the role of the number of fractions (N) is overestimated and that the role of overall time (T) is underestimated for a large number of small fractions.

Cohen,[43,44] using a mathematical model and data derived from skin reactions and doses yielding cures in epidermoid carcinoma, concluded that a formula describing the cellular response to irradiation of tissues and tumor required at least three exponential components: irreversible, single-hit damage; multitarget inactivation with early repair; and cellular repopulation factor to conform to empirically observed dose-time relationships.

Time-Dose Factor

In 1973 Orton and Ellis[254] published a simplification of the NSD concept more applicable to clinical radiation therapy, stating that when a treatment did not result in normal connective tissue tolerance, treatment effectiveness should be described in terms of partial tolerance. For further details the reader is referred to the original publication.[254]

Although there is no definite basis for application of the time-dose factor (TDF) concept to clinical radiation therapy, equivalency of various dose schedules is constantly sought. For split-course regimens the TDF values can be used by adding the TDF value for each of the partial tolerance factors corresponding to each component of the treatment and by correcting for the decay of the first part of the treatment TDF.

Time-Dose Factor in Brachytherapy

In 1974 Orton[249] defined TDF values for continuous irradiation, which could be used with temporary or permanent brachytherapy implants, using various isotopes. The reader is referred to the original publication for the derivation of the equations. A standard radium therapy regimen used for comparison with other equivalent techniques was 6000 cGy in 168 hours. According to Ellis,[89] this was equivalent to 1800 rets of fractionated external irradiation.

Data to accommodate the isoeffect curve for various dose rates (cGy/hour) was derived from previous clinical observations reported by Paterson, Green, and Mitchell[249] (Fig. 1-17). Tables with TDF values for constant dose rates for temporary and some permanent implants were generated. Orton and Webber[251] described the use of the TDF concept for calculation of equivalent doses using permanent ^{125}I implants combined with external irradiation. They pointed out that the physical doses could not be added and that a biologic effectiveness representation of the dose was needed because of the low dose rate of the ^{125}I implants.

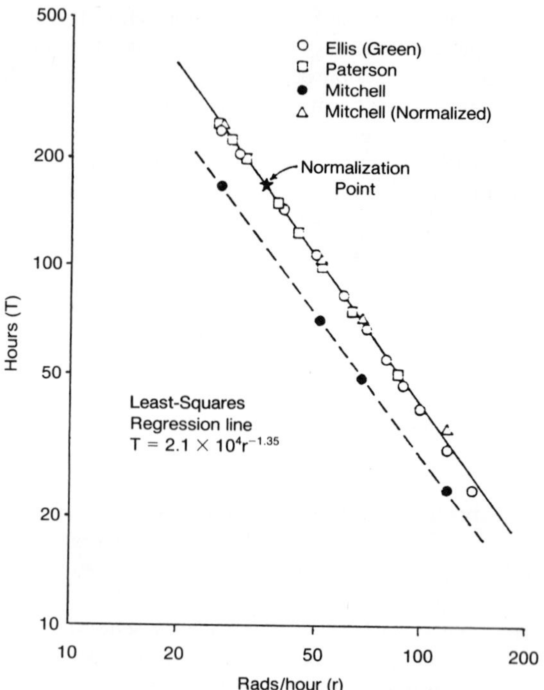

FIGURE 1–17. Treatment times at different dose rates that result in biologic effects equivalent to those produced in 168 hours at 35.7 cGy/hour. These data are used for calculation of TDF factors for brachytherapy. (Orton CG: Br J Radiol 47:603–607, 1974)

In 1985 Ellis[92] wrote an article in which he reviewed the rationale and analyzed the usefulness of the NSD-TDF concept in radiation therapy. He pointed out that in addition to photons, this formula can be used for other radiations with different relative biologic efficiency (RBE), such as neutrons or π-mesons. He concluded that the NSD-TDF concept has broad application in radiation therapy but that clinical testing and observation of effects based on meticulous dosimetry, planning, and delivery must be the ultimate criteria by which the usefulness of the concept is judged.

Cumulative Radiation Effect

Kirk and co-workers[171] formulated the concept of cumulative radiation effect (CRE) to assess the biologic effect of various fractionated regimens on the basis of the accumulated subtolerance radiation damage. This is a generalized form of the NSD concept described by Ellis. They stated that the NSD formula could be written as follows:

$$D = R_f \times N^{0.24} \times T^{0.11}$$

where R_f is a positive constant of proportionality, which assumes different values representing the isoeffect curves of a variety of radiation effects. The value of R_f increases with the severity of the effect. The dose is expressed in reu (radiation effect unit). For more details on the mathematical derivation of the formula, refer to the original publication.

Turesson and Notter[371] suggested the use of the CRE correction factors for predicting late normal tissue damage. Hopewell and Gunn[152] criticized the interpretation of the data and concluded that it could not be used to obtain a correction factor for calculations involving establishment of safe tolerance doses for late effects in patients. Their conclusions were based on the viewpoint that only injury due to vascular damage qualified as "late effects." Peters and Withers,[281] however, indicate that many clinical late effects are the result of depletion of slowly proliferating parenchymal cells rather than vascular injury. Although they reject the criticisms of Hopewell and Gunn, they also point out that no single set of correction factors can be universally applied to an exact relationship of dose, time, and late effect and that good clinical observation and judgment are necessary in dealing with this issue.

Linear Quadratic Equation

Besides the isoeffect concepts previously shown, more recently formulations based on dose survival models have been proposed to evaluate the biologic equivalence of various doses and fractionation schedules. These assumptions are based on a linear quadratic (α/β ratio) survival curve represented by the equation:

$$\text{Log}_e\ S = \alpha D + \beta D^2$$

in which α represents the linear, nonreparable component of log cell kill, and β represents cell kill after some repair process has been eliminated with increasing dose. Thus β represents a reparable (more than a few hours) component of cell damage (Fig. 1-18). The dose at which the two components of cell kill are equal constitutes the α/β ratio.

In a study of 17 human tumor cell lines, Steel and Peacock[346] observed that the average surviving fraction at 200 cGy from the α component is 0.44 and from the β component 0.88. The β effect at that dose level appears to be similar in radiosensitive and radioresistant tumors; thus among radiosensitive tumors in which the survival from the α component is below 0.3, the β effect makes a very small contribution to overall radiosensitivity in the lower dose region. The overall effect of many small fractions is to amplify the dominance of the α component. The β effect is unimportant because repair will be almost complete. The most radiocurable tumors have higher β values than the less curable tumors.

The shape of the dose survival curve with photons differs for acutely and slowly responding normal tissues, although this phenomenon is not observed with neutrons (Fig. 1-19). The severity of the late effects changes more rapidly with a variation in the size of dose per fraction when a total dose is selected to yield equivalent acute effects. With a decreasing size of dose per fraction, the total dose required to achieve a certain isoeffect increases more for late-responding tissues than for acutely responding tissues. Thus, in hyperfractionated regimens, the toleration dose would be increased more for late effects than for acute effects. Conversely, if large doses per fraction are used, the total dose required to achieve isoeffects in late-responding tissues would be reduced more for late effects than for acute effects. In general, acutely reacting tissues have a high α/β ratio (between 8 Gy and 15 Gy), whereas those tissues involved in late effects have a low α/β ratio (1 Gy to 5 Gy). Some of these values obtained in animal experiments are summarized in Table 1-8.

The values for α and β can be obtained from graphs in which the reciprocal of the total dose (Gy-1) and the dose per fraction (Gy) are plotted (Fig. 1-20). A straight line is obtained. The intercept of this line with the zero dose per fraction axis is

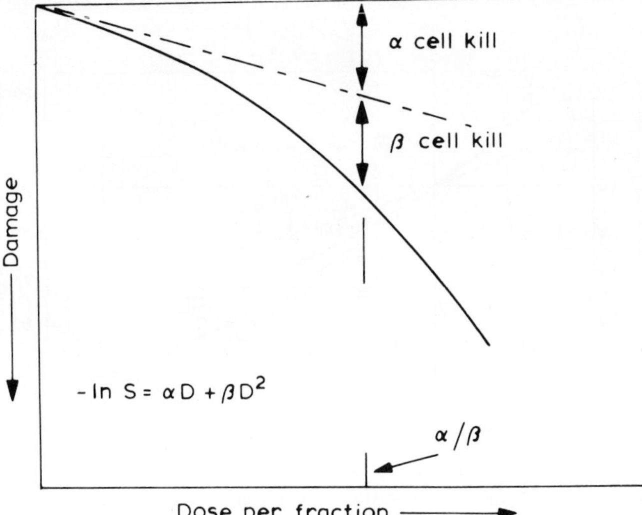

FIGURE 1–18. At a dose equal to the α/β ratio, the log cell kill due to the α-process (nonreparable) is equal to that due to the β-process (reparable injury); α/β is thus a measure of how soon the survival curve begins to bend over significantly. (Fowler JR: Fractionation and therapeutic gain. In Steel GG, Adams GE, Peckham MJ [eds]: Biological Basis of Radiotherapy, pp 181–194. Amsterdam, Elsevier Science, 1983)

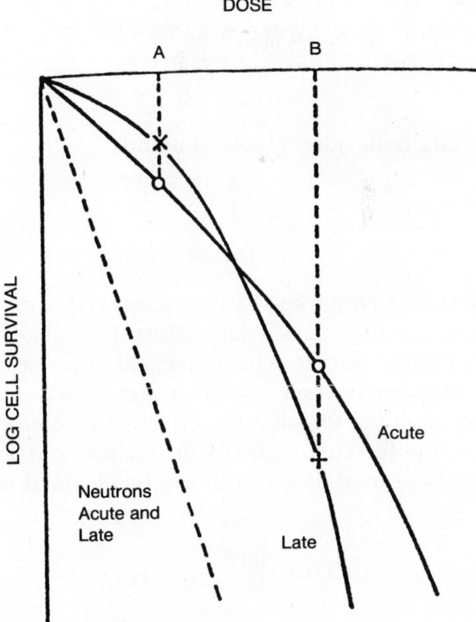

FIGURE 1–19. Hypothetical survival curves for the target cells for acute and late effects in normal tissues exposed to x-rays or neutrons. The α/β ratio in the equation for surviving fractions ($SF = e^{-\alpha D + \beta D^2}$) is higher for late effects than for acute effects in x-irradiated tissues, resulting in a greater rate of change in effect in late-responding tissues with change in dose. At dose *A*, survival of target cells is higher in late-effects than in acute-effects tissues, whereas at dose *B*, the reverse is true. Therefore increasing the dose per fraction from A to B results in a relatively greater increase in late rather than acute injury. In the case of neutrons, the α/β ratio is low, with no detectable influence on the quadratic function (βD^2) over the first two decades of reduction in cell survival, implying that accumulation of sublethal injury plays a negligible role in cell killing by doses of neutrons of clinical interest. At these doses, the RBE is higher for late effects than it is for acute effects. (Fowler JR: Fractionation and therapeutic gain. In Steel GG, Adams GE, Peckham MJ [eds]: The Biological Basis of Radiotherapy, pp 181--194. Amsterdam, Elsevier Science, 1983)

TABLE 1–8
Ratio of Linear (α) to Quadratic (β) Terms from Multifraction Experiments and Clinical Data

TISSUE	α/β RATIO (Gy) EXPERIMENTAL	CLINICAL*
Early reactions		
Skin/subcutaneous tissues	9–12	5–10
Jejunum	6–10	2.2–8
Colon	10–11	—
Testis	12–13	—
Callus	9–10	—
Late reactions		
Spinal cord	1.0–4.9	3.3
Kidney	1.5–2.4	—
Lung	2.4–6.3	4.2–4.7
Bladder	3.1–7.0	3.4–4.5

* *Based on data from Turesson and Notter[372], Dische and associates[71], Sause and associates[321]*
(Modified from Fowler JF: Fractionation and therapeutic gain. In Steel GG, Adams GE, Peckham MJ [eds]: The Biological Basis of Radiotherapy, pp 181–194. Amsterdam, Elsevier Science, 1983)

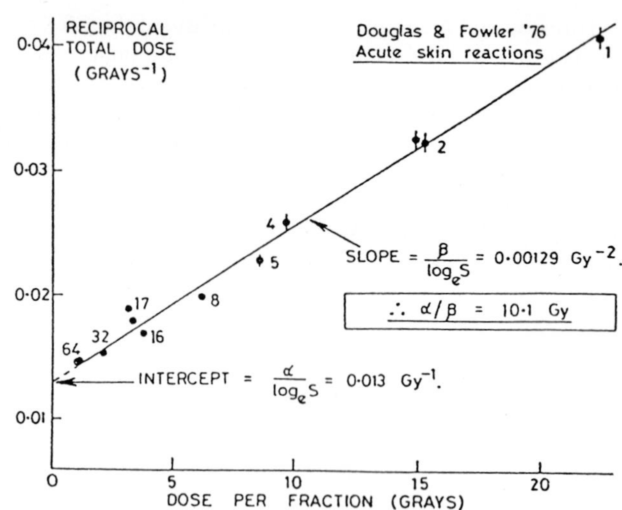

FIGURE 1–20. Values of α and β. If the reciprocal of total dose (for several multifraction schedules) is plotted against dose per fraction, a straight line will be obtained. The intercept of this line with the zero dose-per-fraction axis is proportional to α (α/ln S). The slope is proportional to β (β/ln S). The α/β ratio is readily determined. For absolute values of α and β, clonogenic assay is necessary for the endpoint. (Fowler JR: Fractionation and therapeutic gain. In Steel GG, Adams GE, Peckham MJ [eds.]: The Biological Basis of Radiotherapy, pp 181–194. Amsterdam, Elsevier Science, 1983)

proportional to α (α/ln S), which is the natural logarithm of survival. The slope is proportional to β (β/ln S).[75,363]

The algebraic functions to derive the straight line from the reciprocal total dose per fraction plot are shown below:

Multiple fractions of d, each xn:

$$-\ln S = n(\alpha d + \beta d^2)$$
$$= \alpha nd + \beta nd^2$$
$$= nd(\alpha + \beta d)$$

Dividing both sides by total dose nd:

$$\frac{-\ln S}{nd} = \underset{\text{Intercept}}{\alpha} + \underset{\text{Slope}}{\beta d}$$

Withers and co-workers[409] have proposed a method for using these survival curve parameters for calculating the change in TD necessary to achieve an equal response in a tissue when the dose per fraction is varied, using the α/β ratios. This calculation accounts for only the effect of repair of cellular injury. The isoeffect curves vary for different tissues (Fig. 1-21). An extrapolated total dose (ETD) can be obtained using this formula:

$$ETD = \frac{-\ln S}{\alpha}$$

$$ETD = nd[1 + d/(\alpha/\beta)]$$

If one wishes to compare two treatment regimens, the following formula can be used:

$$\frac{Dr}{Dx} = \frac{\alpha/\beta + dx}{\alpha/\beta + dr}$$

in which

Dr = known total dose (reference dose)
Dx = new total dose (with different fractionation schedule)
dr = known fractionation (reference)
dx = new fractionation schedule

Example of use of this formula: Suppose that 5000 cGy (50 Gy) in 25 fractions is delivered to yield a given biologic effect. If one assumes that the subcutaneous tissue is the limiting parameter (late reaction), it is desirable to know what the total dose to be administered will be using 4 Gy fractions. Assume α/β = 5 Gy.

Using the latter formula,

$$Dx = Dr\frac{\alpha/\beta + dr}{\alpha/\beta + dx}$$

Thus

$$Dx = 50\text{ Gy}\left(\frac{5+2}{5+4}\right) = 39\text{ Gy}$$

Yaes[416] proposed a modification of the linear quadratic isoeffect model in which the effect of proliferation is taken into account for multiple daily fractionation schedules. The pro-

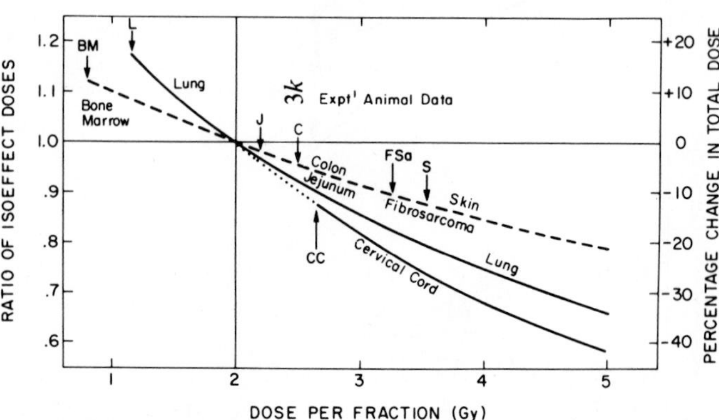

FIGURE 1–21. Isoeffect curves derived from data from experimental animal systems. The lowest dose per fraction used in experiments with the various tissues is marked by an *arrow.* Given the accuracy needed in determining isoeffective doses in human tissues, it is clear that more appropriate experimental animal data are needed. The isoeffect curves indicate, however, that changes in total dose with changes in fraction size vary with the tissue considered critical and are greater for slowly responding tissues. (Withers HR, Thames HD, Peters LJ: Radiother Oncol 1:187–191, 1983)

posed isoeffect relationship involves the fraction size and the total dose of irradiation and predicts higher isoeffect doses for small dose fractions.

Linear quadratic models may be used to calculate the α/β ratio in some clinical situations.[58] For instance, Bentzen and associates,[15] studying 163 patients receiving postmastectomy irradiation (3660 cGy in 12 fractions, two fractions per week, or 4092 cGy in 22 fractions, five fractions per week), analyzed the occurrence of impaired shoulder movement resulting from fibrosis. The α/β ratio was estimated at 3.5 Gy. A dose-response relationship was clearly demonstrated in addition to the effect of the fractionation schedule.

DOSE RATE

The dose rate with which irradiation is delivered may significantly influence the biologic response to a given dose, particularly in the case of sparsely ionizing radiations, such as x-rays and τ-rays.[140] Three main biologic processes are involved in the dose rate effect (Fig. 1-22):

Repair of sublethal damage, which occurs when radiation is delivered at a low dose rate and treatment time is extended to a point at which it is comparable to the repair half-time. As the dose rate is reduced, more repair of sublethal damage occurs because the radiation injury is spread out over a longer period. The cell survival curves become progressively less steep, and at the same time the extrapolation number approaches unity.

Cell proliferation, which occurs during the course of protracted radiation exposure if the dose rate is low enough or the cell cycle time is short enough

Redistribution and accumulation of cells throughout the proliferative cycle, which occurs with a low dose rate in which proliferation is decreased because cells are arrested and accumulate in G_2. This is a relatively radiosensitive phase of the cycle. As a result, cell kill may be greater for a lower dose rate.

With the advent of moderate and high dose rate remote control afterloading devices, an increased emphasis has been placed on the biologic effects of irradiation dose rate. Many *in vitro* and *in vivo* experimental observations indicate variations in cell kill and repair of sublethal or potentially lethal damage with varying dose rates of ionizing radiations. The so-called dose rate effect is most dramatic between 1 cGy/minute and 100 cGy/minute.[141] Recently Dutreix[79] reviewed the role of the dose rate on biologic effects as assessed by the ability of the cell to repair radiation damage (α/β ratio) and the repair kinetics (repair time constant). The biologic effect achieved by a given radiation dose decreases as the dose rate diminishes, chiefly as a result of the increase in cell repair that occurs during continuous prolonged irradiation. This occurs because cell proliferation is virtually negligible in the range of treatment times used in curie therapy.[79]

In some experiments a bending of the cell survival curve at very low dose rates has been noted, instead of the expected exponential, possibly because of cell redistribution[417] or a decline in the repair capacity of the cell with large doses.[378] Dutreix[79] states that the variation of the isoeffect dose occurs mainly in the range of medium dose rates (100 to 1000 cGy/hour) and it vanishes at a very high dose rate because the cell repair is negligible during the short treatment time. At a very low dose rate, because the cell kill is caused only by direct lethal events that are considered independent of the dose rate, cell repair is also negligible. The induction of sublethal injury is relatively slow compared with the rate of repair, and cell kill by accumulation of sublethal injury remains minimal. Dutreix[79] quantifies the dose-rate effect based on a method proposed by Liversage,[198] equating it with continuous irradiation. For an analysis of detailed mathematical formula derivations and clinical applications, refer to the original publication.[79]

The dose-rate effect in clinical brachytherapy was described initially by Green[90, 249] and by Paterson.[263] The historical isoeffect curve showed a significant increase in dose when time was increased from 2 to 7 days. However, the validity of Paterson's curve was questioned by Pierquin and associates,[283] who used the same dose of 7000 cGy with treatment times ranging from 3 to 8 days for the treatment of head and neck tumors with ^{192}Ir implants and did not observe any difference in the control rate or incidence of necrosis. Figure 1-23 shows computed isoeffect curves with reference to 6000 cGy in 7 days. The agreement with Paterson's curve is acceptable when the α/β value equals 3 Gy and T_r (repair half-time) equals 1.5 hours, but the curve is shallower when α/β equals 10 Gy and T_r equals 1 hour. Paterson's curve should be expected to correspond to late reactions and to overestimate the variation for early reactions and control of squamous cell carcinoma.

Hall and Brenner[142] recently published an excellent review of radiobiologic effects and clinical relevance of dose rate. Included were several important concepts:

1. At ultra-high doses and instantaneous dose rates (1000 cGy pulsed in nanoseconds), the rapid deposition of radiant energy consumes oxygen very quickly for diffusion to maintain an adequate level of oxygenation, and dose-response curves are characteristic of hypoxia. Interest in clinical application of this approach has waned.
2. Based on laboratory data, it may be possible to design schedules with a pulse width of several minutes and a pulse interval of about 1 hour to achieve cell kill equivalent to that obtained with continuous 3000 cGy in 60 hours (50 cGy/hour).
3. Using the linear quadratic equation, it is possible to estimate the equivalency of high and low dose-rate exposures, with a variety of fractionation schedules (remembering that lower number of fractions may result in enhanced late effects).

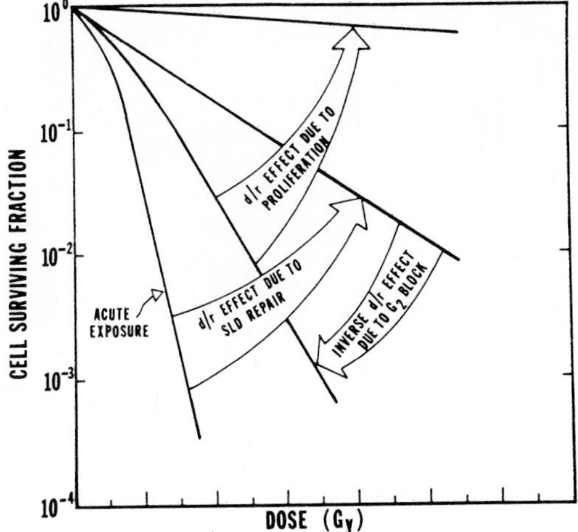

FIGURE 1–22. Factors that govern the dose-rate effect. Sublethal damage (SLD) repair, cellular proliferation, and redistribution and accumulation that lead to an inverse dose-rate effect. (Hall EJ: Radiobiology for the Radiologist, 3rd ed. Philadelphia, JB Lippincott, 1988)

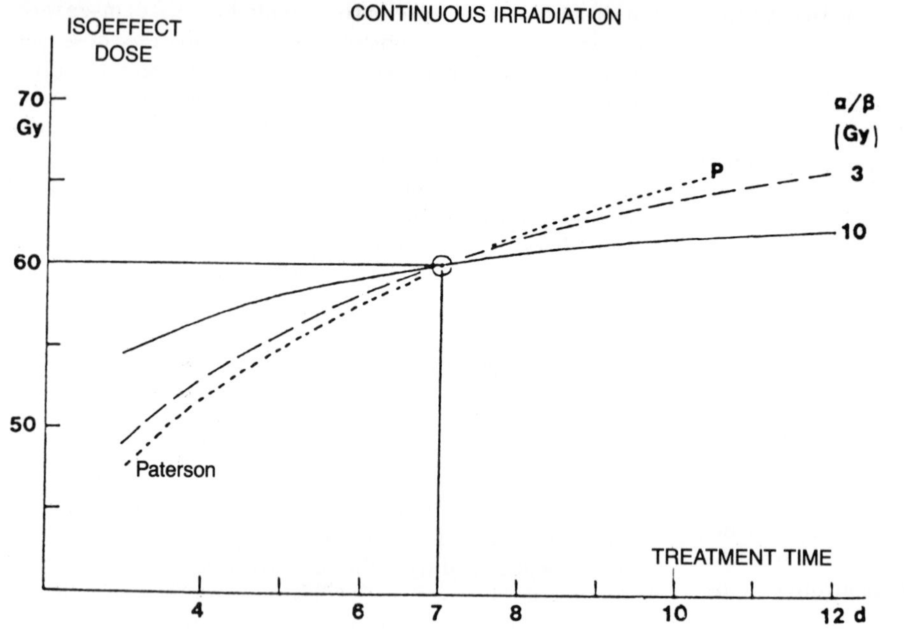

FIGURE 1–23. Low-dose rate irradiation. Isoeffect dose equivalent to 60 Gy in 7 days. Two sets of parameters have been considered for the computation, which would presumably correspond to skin and mucosa early reactions and to the effect on the epithelioma (α/β = 10 Gy, T_r = 1 hour) and to late reactions (α/β = 3 Gy, T_r = 1.5 hour). (Dutreix J: Radiother Oncol 15:25–37, 1989)

Special consideration should be given to the effect of high dose-rate brachytherapy on normal tissues. Thus the tumor dose must be adjusted (12% to 25% decrease) compared with that delivered with conventional low dose rates.[253]

There has been special interest in continuous low dose-rate irradiation with external cobalt units.[282,404] Pierquin[282] used a modified ^{60}Co unit with a small industrial source (activity 45 Ci). Radiation was delivered at 100 cGy to 139 cGy per hour to administer daily tumor doses of 800 cGy to 1000 cGy in 7 to 8 hours. A minimum of five treatments was given per week, although occasionally weekends and holidays caused schedule modifications. Patients were given short rest periods every 1 or 2 hours. Tumor doses of approximately 6300 cGy were delivered in eight to 11 fractions, with the volume reduced to 8 cm × 10 cm after 4500 cGy. Nineteen patients with advanced tumors of the mouth and pharynx were treated in the primary lesion and the upper cervical lymph nodes with two parallel opposed portals. In seven patients split-course irradiation was administered. In 15 of the 19 patients no evidence of tumor was found 3 months after treatment. Only three patients developed recurrences. Of the 19 patients, two developed moist and six developed dry desquamation; the others had erythema only. No significant late effects on the skin or subcutaneous tissue were noted; 16 of the 19 patients developed severe mucositis. Seven patients developed necrosis, six in large areas of the oral cavity and pharynx, in several instances at the tumor site.

IMPORTANCE OF TREATMENT PLANNING IN RADIATION THERAPY

Herring[149] discussed the theoretic consequences of fitting dose-response curves for tumor control and normal tissue injury. He emphasized that the predicted consequences are based on the precision with which the dose and the volume irradiated are defined. For instance, an imprecise treatment system could lead to a high incidence of necrosis with, paradoxically, a low probability of tumor control[252] (Fig. 1-24). Reducing radiation doses in an effort to avoid complications further reduces the probability of achieving tumor control if such action is based on the wrong assumption that the tumor control/complication ratio is related only to radiation dose levels. Cunningham[56] recently pointed out that the goal recommended by ICRU[158] of a ± 5% accuracy for dose delivery computations is difficult to achieve. However, every effort should be made to develop accurate dose calculation algorithms, including methods to correct for inho-

3-Dimensional Treatment Planning

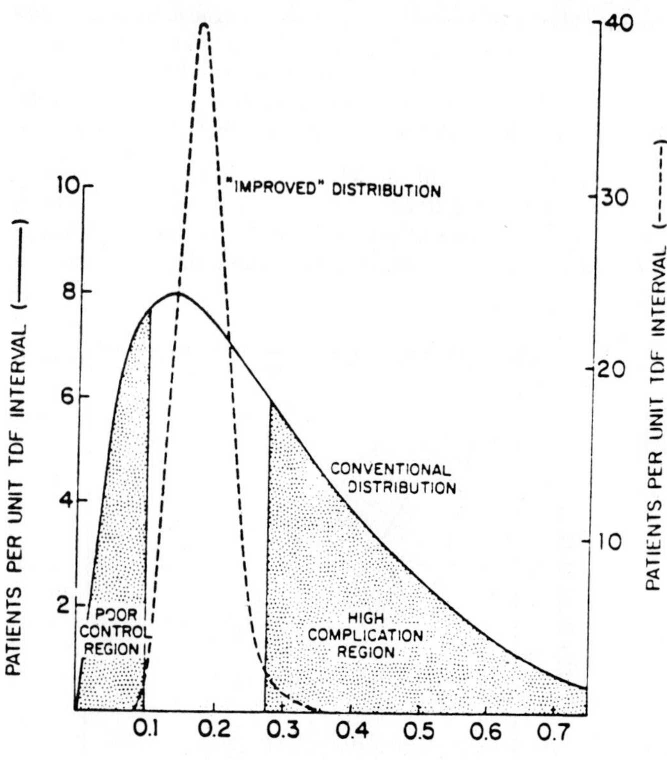

FIGURE 1–24. Frequency distribution of patients treated to different probabilities of complication. (Orton CG: Other considerations in 3-dimensional treatment planning. In Bagne F [ed]: Computerized Treatment Planning Systems, pp 136–141. HHS Publications FDA 84-8223, 1984)

mogeneities in tissue density and the shape of the patient's body, and to develop practical treatment planning capabilities to obtain the highest possible dose optimization in the irradiated volume (tumor and normal tissues).

Suit and co-workers[349] pointed out the benefits of reducing the treatment volume in an effort to deliver higher doses of irradiation, which may improve the quality of tumor control without excessively irradiating surrounding normal tissues, thereby decreasing treatment-related morbidity.

Various steps can be taken to decrease toxicity in normal tissues, including precise treatment planning and irradiation techniques, selective decreased volume receiving higher doses dictated by estimated cell burden, and maneuvers to exclude sensitive organs from the irradiated volume. For instance, Gallagher and associates[119] described a technique of abdominal wall compression in the prone position combined with bladder distention to treat patients with pelvic tumors to displace the small bowel from the pelvic fields. The severity of acute gastrointestinal effects correlated positively with the small bowel volume receiving doses greater than 4500 cGy.

Furthermore, with the emphasis on organ preservation (which is being applied to patients with tumors in the head and neck, breast, and rectosigmoid areas as well as soft tissue sarcomas), treatment planning is critical to achieve these goals with maximum tumor control probability and satisfactory cosmetic results.

Conditions for Optimization of External Beam Irradiation

Kitebatake and associates[172] outlined definite requirements for optimal dose distribution with external irradiation in both tumor and normal tissues. The following is a slightly modified list of factors published by these authors:

Small entrance and exit dose (except with superficial tumors). Ideally, when the maximum dose is not required at the skin or subcutaneous tissues, the higher dose should be at the target volume, with lower dose to the skin and subcutaneous tissues at the entrance and exit sites.

Small side-scattering dose. High-energy photon beams produce minimal amounts of side-scattered irradiation.

Small differential tissue absorption. With 250 kV x-rays, absorption of irradiation is significantly greater in bone than in soft tissues.[162] This phenomenon disappears with high-energy x-rays because of the decreasing importance of the photoelectric effect and the increasing Compton effect between 1 MV and 10 MV. At energies of 20 MeV, however, an increase of 5% in the dose in the soft tissues near a bone (high Z) interface may occur.

Optimal tumor (target) dose. The aim of good treatment planning is to exploit the maximum therapeutic ratio of beam arrangement. The target volume should receive a homogeneous dose while delivering as little dose as possible to the surrounding normal tissue.

Small integral dose. The ideal situation is represented by an optimal dose to the target volume with a minimum dose contribution to the rest of the patient.

Optimal dose distribution may be achieved by a combination of multiple stationary beams or by moving-beam therapy, such as in arc or full rotational techniques. In addition, the optimal dose distribution in many tumors requires more than one-beam energy or multiple-beam arrangements. A combination of external beams and intracavitary or interstitial therapy may also be required, depending on the location of the tumor and the beam type and energies used.

New Approaches to Treatment Planning

Advances in medical imaging, primarily computed tomography (CT), have made the necessary data available to accurately model the patient, both spatially and in terms of density, for treatment planning. This development, along with advances in computer and graphic display technologies, has stimulated the development of treatment planning systems that address a much broader range of problems than just dose calculation.[126,294] Such systems, called three-dimensional (3D), aim to provide the following capabilities: relevant diagnostic information in evaluating the patient's disease; delineation of normal tissues; definition of tumor and target volume; simulation of therapy with generation of digital reconstructed radiographs; design of treatment aids (compensators, blocks); calculation of 3D dose distributions and dose optimization; critical evaluation of treatment plan.

The potential benefits from such 3D systems could be great, even when limited to specific disease sites and treatment situations only; research efforts in this area are growing. Currently, several groups in the United States are investigating the use of advanced computer and display technologies for simulation of therapy purposes.[127,295] In these prototype systems, contiguous CT slices are used to define anatomic structures and target volumes. External radiation beams of any possible orientation are allowed. A significant feature of these systems is the so-called beam's eye-view (BEV) in which patient contours are viewed as if the observer's eye is placed at the source of radiation looking out along the axis of the radiation beam[127,219] (Fig. 1-25*A*).

The reader should understand that although BEV is a necessary mode of viewing for 3D treatment planning systems, it alone is not sufficient for optimum planning, especially when multibeam arrangements or noncoplanar beam techniques are used. Instead, the ability to view the beam setup from any arbitrary position, including BEV, is needed (FIG. 1-25*B*). The high visibility of image presentation has spurred development of computer graphics in the new generation 3D treatment planning systems.[220,294] Although these systems allow the simulation of the geometric setup, the evaluation of the plan is still made on the merits of the dose distributions.

In an attempt to attain the goal of 3% accuracy, a new generation of dose calculation methods has been proposed. These are the Δ-Volume method,[412,413] differential pencil beam method,[232] dose spread array method,[204] and the Fourier convolution method.[27] They all employ theoretically calculated absorbed dose arrays as input data. In particular, the latter three methods rely on similar Monte Carlo-generated data, which include electron transport information. These methods are undergoing critical evaluations and have not been implemented into commercial treatment planning systems as yet.

Current efforts in the display of 3D dose data include multilevel 2D displays showing isodose lines superimposed on CT images; the display of dose as a spectrum of colors superimposed on anatomic information represented by modulation of intensity; a "movie" or film-loop display in which sequential transverse CT sections are viewed in rapid sequence resulting in a simulated film-loop mode, and display of dose levels in terms of 3D surfaces.[126] In addition, dose-volume histograms (DVHs)

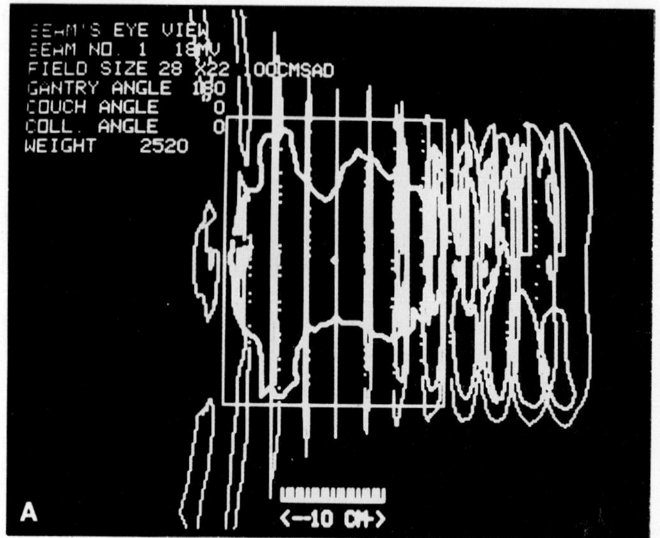

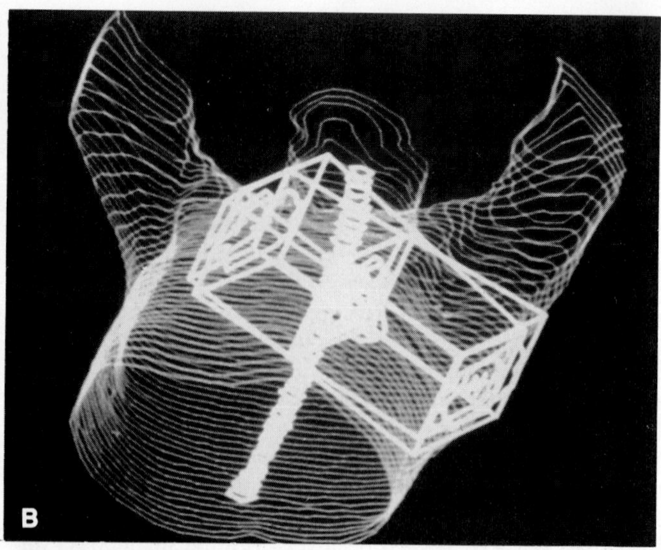

FIGURE 1–25. (**A**) A significant feature of 3D treatment planning systems is the "beam's eye-view" (BEV) display in which patient contours are viewed as if the observer's eye were placed at the source of radiation looking out along the axis of the radiation beam. (**B**) A real-time interactive physician's eye-view (PEV) showing the patient and all the radiation beams is ideal for demonstrating proper handling of multibeam arrangements, field abutments, and gaps. (Perez CA, Purdy JA: Rationale for treatment planning in radiation therapy. In Levitt SH [ed]: Technological Basis of Radiation Therapy: Practical Clinical Applications, 2nd ed. Philadelphia, Lea & FebIger, in press)

are proving to be extremely useful as a means of dose display. DVHs are particularly useful in assessing several treatment plan dose distributions.[39] They provide a complete summary of the entire 3D dose matrix showing the amount of target volume or critical structure receiving more than a specified dose level (Fig. 1-26). Dose-volume histograms do not provide spatial information; thus they cannot replace the other methods of dose display, but can complement them only.

Treatment verification is another area in which 3D treatment planning systems are likely to play an important role. The increased sophistication in treatment planning requires parallel development in precise patient repositioning and immobilization techniques so that an optimal dose can be delivered to selected target volumes.[349] Portal films used for geometric/topographic verification are generally of poor quality, making accurate identification of internal landmarks difficult. Recently, several real-time, on-line verification systems have been described, which allow for the monitoring of the position of the area to be treated during the radiation exposure.[411] An example of a portal obtained with a fiberoptic system developed at Washington University is shown in Figure 1-27. This method allows for an improved precision in delivery of multiple fractions of external irradiation.[133,411] In 3D treatment planning systems, reconstruction of sequential CT slice data can be used to generate a simulation film, which in turn can be used to aid in localization and comparison with the treatment portal film for verifying treatment geometry.[40,127] It should be noted that geometric verification primarily ensures reproducibility. Noninvasive techniques to actually verify dosimetrically the implementation of an optimized treatment plan are scarce.

Improved accuracy in treatment planning and delivery may give credence to a long-heralded goal of optimizing the

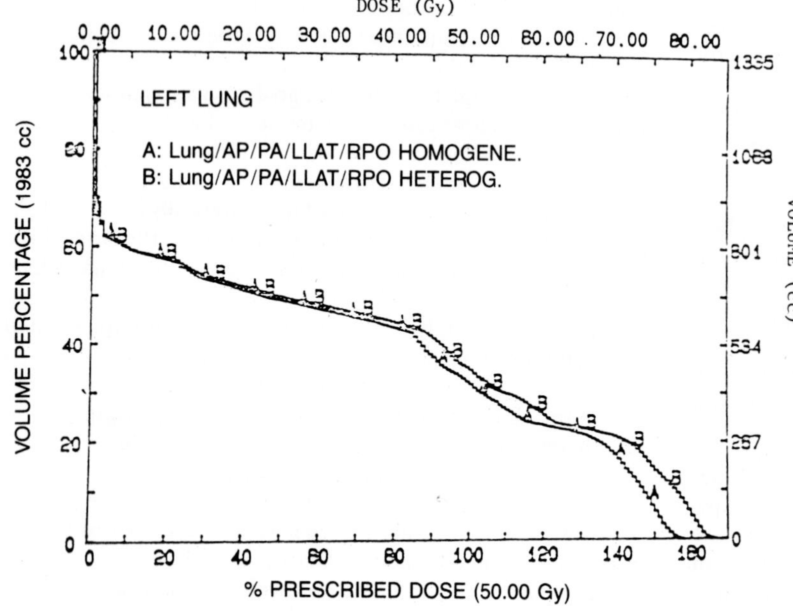

FIGURE 1–26. The dose-volume histogram (DVH) provides a complete summary of the entire 3D dose matrix showing the amount of target volume or critical structure receiving more or less than a specified dose level. Shown here is a DVH for the right lung of a patient with lung cancer. The dose distribution was calculated with (plan A) and without (plan B) correction for heterogeneities. (Perez CA, Purdy JA: Rationale for treatment planning in radiation therapy. In Levitt SH [ed]: Technological Basis of Radiation Therapy: Practical Clinical Applications, 2nd ed. Philadelphia, Lea & Febiger, in press)

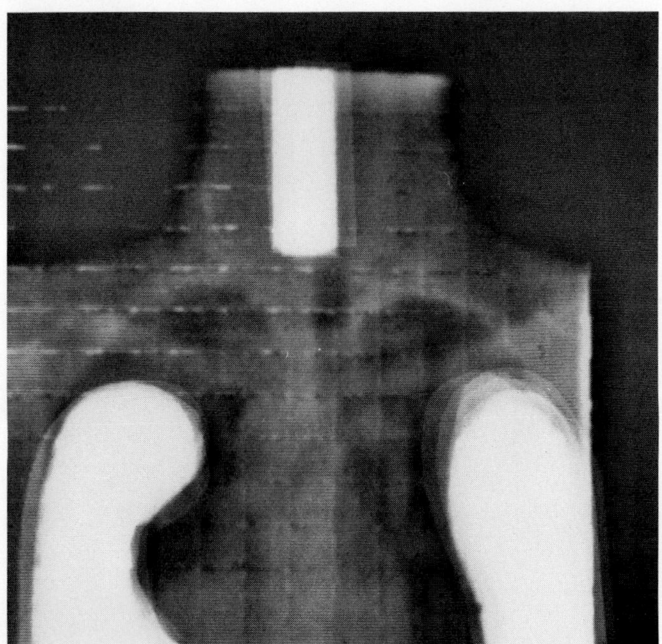

FIGURE 1–27. Real-time verification images of a mantle portal using an innovative fiberoptic system. Superimposition of several exposures is illustrated.

dose of radiation given to a patient through conformational dynamic therapy (Fig. 1-28). Recently, multileaf collimators have been produced commercially, and computer interplay between the simulator and the radiation therapy machines is feasible. The highly complex treatment plan generated by computational techniques can be transferred to the patient on a CT simulator, and this information subsequently is fed to the treatment machine through a computer interface, which conforms to the shape of the collimator as the therapy is delivered. As Lichter and co-workers[188] indicated, although dynamic conformational therapy will be commercially available within the next 10 years, potential problems need to be addressed to make it a practical therapeutic modality.

IMPACT OF LOCAL TUMOR CONTROL ON SURVIVAL

Suit and colleagues[352] have reported that experimentally, in animal tumor models, the incidence of distant metastases is usually higher in those animals with local failure than in those with local tumor control. We observed a similar phenomenon in patients with carcinoma of the lung,[267] prostate,[273] and uterine cervix.[271]

Because of the emphasis on the control of systemic disease, mostly by medical oncologists,[66] assessment of the importance of locoregional tumor control in patients with malignant tumors has been relatively underemphasized. Table 1-9, compiled from data reported by the American Cancer Society,[2] illustrates the fact that in a large proportion of patients with cancer seen in the United States, locoregional recurrence is just as prevalent (68% of the patients dying with disease) as distant metastases. Noteworthy, a large proportion of patients (50%) have *both* locoregional recurrence and distant metastases.

Suit and co-workers[352] pointed out that in the United States, elimination of locoregional failures in patients without distant metastases at the time of diagnosis would result in a significant increase in survivors *per annum,* including 2700 uterine cervix patients, including those with the following malignancies: uterine cervix, 2700; oral cavity and oropharynx, 2000; ovarian, 4000; and colorectal, 17,000.

Suit and co-workers[352] also noted that long-term disease-free survival after salvage treatment of patients with local fail-

TABLE 1–9
Estimated Incidence, Mortality, and Sites of Failure of the Most Common Types of Cancer in the United States in 1990

			DISTRIBUTION OF FAILURES (DEATHS)			
ORGAN	**NEW CASES/YR**	**DEATHS/YR**	L-R ONLY	COMB. L-R + DM	DM ONLY	TOTAL DEATHS L-R TUMOR
Lung	157,000	142,000	49,700	49,700	42,600	99,400
Colon and rectum	155,000	60,900	6090	14,225	39,585	21,315
Breast	150,900	44,300	6645	26,580	11,075	33,225
Prostate	106,000	30,000	4500	19,500	6000	24,000
Uterus*	46,500	10,000	2000	5000	3000	7000
Oral, pharynx, larynx	42,800	12,100	6050	3630	2420	9680
Bladder	49,000	9700	2910	2425	4365	5335
Lymphomas	54,800	28,700	5740	5740	17,220	11,480
Pancreas, biliary	42,700	36,900	7380	22,140	7380	29,520
Esophagus, stomach	33,800	23,200	6960	11,600	4640	18,560
Leukemia	27,800	18,100	7240	7240	3620	14,480
Ovary	20,500	12,400	11,160	620	620	11,780
Brain, CNS	15,600	11,100	10,711	278	111	10,989
Total	902,400	439,400	127,086	169,678	142,636	296,764 (68%)

* *Cervix, invasive and endometrium*
L-R: local-regional tumor
DM: distant metastases
(Data from American Cancer Society, Cancer Facts and Figures, 1990)

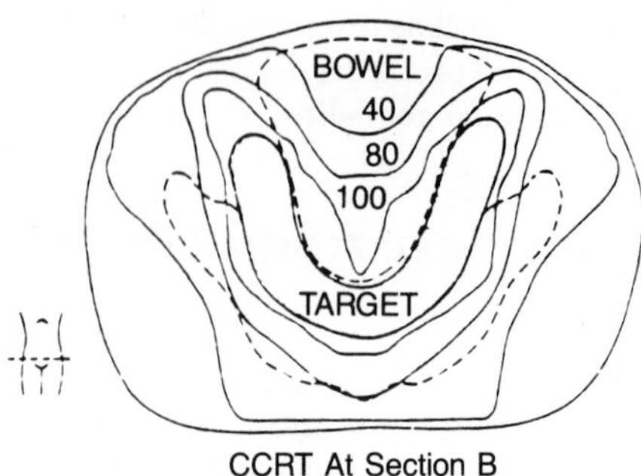

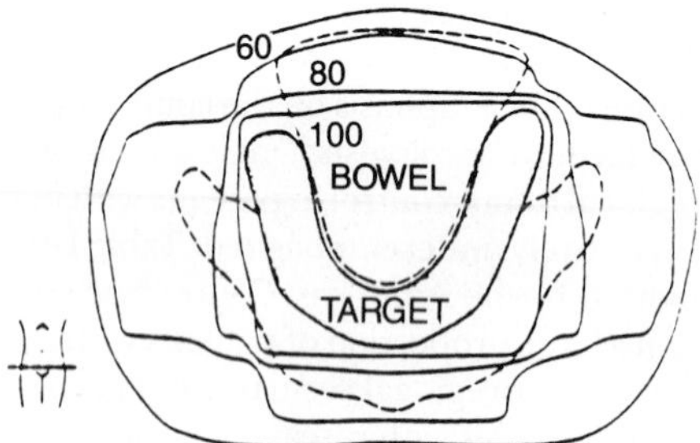

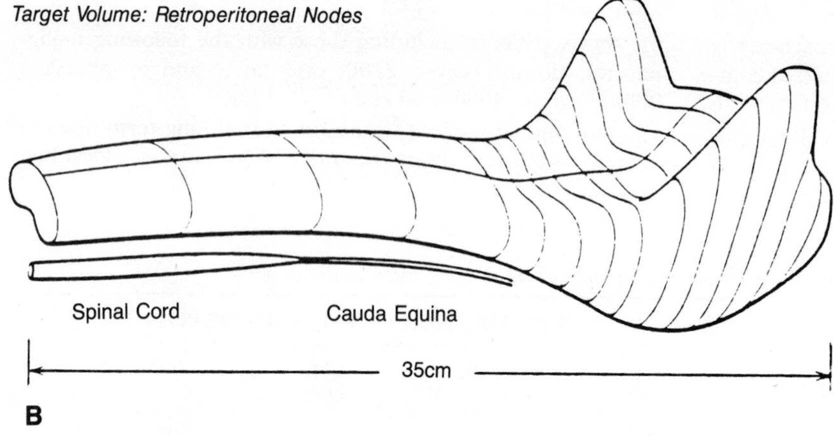

FIGURE 1–28. (**A**) Dose distribution (top) in a transverse cut through the pelvis using conformational therapy techniques. Dose distribution (bottom) from a conventional treatment technique. (**B**) Schematic representation of a target volume consisting of the retroperitoneal and pelvic nodes. Proximity to the spinal cord is indicated. (Bjarngard BE, Chin LM, Kijewski PK: Dynamic treatment planning. In Bagne F [ed]: Computerized Treatment Planning Systems, pp 110–123. HHS publication FDA 84–8223, 1984)

ure only should be viewed as proof that improved treatment of the primary lesion results in higher survival rates, provided that the patients do not have and will not develop distant metastases. These authors presented data to indicate that in a variety of tumors, a correlation exists between the incidence of locoregional failures and the development of distant metastases (Table 1-10). Also included in the report are data that demonstrate the importance of higher doses of radiation in improving the probability of tumor control.

At Washington University, a 10% improvement in survival rate was noted in 464 patients with Stage IIB and Stage III carcinoma of the uterine cervix treated with different doses of radiation.[271] Similar observations were noted in patients treated for Stage C carcinoma of the prostate with varying doses of radiation.[273] However, Goitein and associates[125] pointed out that the impact of computed tomography treatment planning on survival is limited because a number of other factors affect the overall prognosis of the patient. Using theoretic assumptions, they calculated that the improvement in survival rate was approximately 4%. Although a conservative estimate, this represents a significant number of patients, considering that there were about 1 million new cancer patients diagnosed in the United States in 1990, and approximately 500,000 were treated with radiation therapy, with over 50% of the patients receiving treatment with a curative aim.

QUALITY ASSURANCE

A comprehensive program in quality assurance is critical in any radiation oncology center to ensure the best possible treatment for the individual patient and to establish and document all operating policies and procedures. Quality assurance procedures in radiation therapy vary, depending on whether a standard treatment or a clinical trial is carried out at single or multiple institutions. Particularly in multi-institutional studies,

TABLE 1–10
Observed and Expected Incidence of Distant Metastases in Patients with Pelvic Failure Treated by Radiation Alone for Carcinoma of Uterine Cervix

STAGE	NUMBER OF PATIENTS	OBSERVED INCIDENCE OF LOCAL FAILURE AND DISTANT METASTASES — LOCAL FAILURE (%)	EXPECTED INCIDENCE OF LOCAL CONTROL AND DISTANT METASTASES — LOCAL CONTROL
I	1801	40/141 (28.4)	3.5
IIa	1962	46/331 (14.0)	6.0
IIb	2233	106/566 (18.7)	11.4
III	1660	173/602 (28.7)	15.2
IV	171	57/112 (50.9)	25.4

(Suit HD, Westgate SJ: Int J Radiat Oncol Biol Phys 12:453–458 1986; after Perez CA, et al, 1983)

there is a need for clear instructions and standardized parameters in dosimetry procedures, treatment techniques, and treatment planning to be carried out by all participants.[270]

Many of the reports of the Patterns of Care Study demonstrate a definite correlation between the quality of the radiation therapy delivered at various types of institutions and the outcome of therapy.[143]

In general, a quality assurance program should include broad efforts in several categorical areas such as

Statistics on patient-related activities. Statistics should include total number of new patients seen and treated per year, number of retreated patients, anatomic site of tumors treated, and number of procedures performed (consultations, treatment visits, fields treated, simulations, treatment plans done, brachytherapy procedures performed, and follow-up visits).

Patient records and forms. Radiation oncology records should ideally be kept separate from the hospital records to ensure ready access to both types of records in different areas of the hospital when required. Written communications with referring physicians should be routine practice, and copies of appropriate sections of the radiation therapy record should be sent to the referring physician as well as to the hospital record room.

Every patient must have a complete *consultation note,* with a history and physical examination, description of pertinent physical findings required for staging, and laboratory and radiographic studies that may be helpful in the selection of therapy. The histologic or cytologic documentation of cancer (or compelling reason for lack of verification) should be an integral part of the record. Drawings or photographs illustrating the extent, character, location, and stage of the tumor should always be included.

The details of treatment planning, the volume treated (portals), dose prescription, calculations, simulator and periodic portal localization films, and isodose curves must be documented. The record should indicate the position of the patient, any special immobilization, shielding, or beam-modifying devices, doses of radiation given, monitoring units, time used for daily treatment, and recording of the maximum daily dose (given) and tumor doses delivered. Following is a checklist for completion of treatment chart review, suggested by the American College of Radiology[3]:

- diagnosis stated
- stage of disease recorded
- pertinent histopathology report in chart
- relevant history of the disease stated in consult note
- physical findings relevant to the disease stated
- treatment plan or prescription dated and signed by responsible physician at beginning of treatment
- planned dose and method of delivery stated
- treatment site or treatment volume specified
- fields documented by portal films
- dosimetry calculations in chart and checked by physicist
- isodose calculations in chart and checked by physicist
- treatment record checked weekly by physician
- treatment record checked weekly by physicist or dosimetrist
- evidence of weekly evaluation of patient by responsible physician
- summary or completion of therapy report prepared
- follow-up plan stated
- other comments
- name of person completing review; date

Every radiation oncology center should develop or adopt appropriate forms for patient registration, tumor staging, dose prescription and recording including brachytherapy procedures, and follow-up information. Pathology reports and laboratory data can be copied from the hospital chart or obtained from the respective departments for inclusion in the radiation oncology record. Figure 1-29 illustrates examples of dose prescription, dose computation, and daily dose recording forms used at Washington University. Forms are available for staging purposes in each of the anatomic sites, many of them designed following suggestions of the American Joint Committee.[4]

Treatment policies and treatment planning/dosimetry procedures. Each institution must develop well-defined policies of treatment for each pathologic entity to ensure uniformity of management, to ensure consistency of data for better evaluation of therapy results, and to guide the radiation oncologist in the indications for radiation therapy, depending on the anatomic location, extent (stage), histologic features of the tumor, and general condition of the patient. The description of radiation therapy must include details on the target volume, tumor doses, and fractionation schedules that should be delivered to the patient, all of which are critical elements in treatment planning.

To verify the validity of treatment administration of radiation therapy, data concerning the planned treatment techniques, technical factors, and dose prescription should

MULTIPLE DAILY FX.

DOSE SHEET # /

RADIATION ONCOLOGY CENTER
MALLINCKRODT INSTITUTE OF RADIOLOGY
WASHINGTON UNIVERSITY MEDICAL CENTER

RADIATION ONCOLOGY NO.

Name ____ (Last) (First) (M. Initial) Date ____

Diagnosis ____ Stage ____ PROTOCOL NO: ____

Rad. Oncologist ____ Resident ____ Referring M.D. ____

Aim of Rx: Curative ____ Palliative ____ Pre-Op. ____ Post-Op. ____ Chemo. ____

Instructions; (1) Fields are to be numbered consecutively for different anatomical areas (1, 2, 3, etc.). (2) Parallel opposed or isocentric fields will be designated with the number and a letter suffix (1A, 1B, etc.) (3) Field size to be specified at SSD or Isocenter (the first number represents transverse axis and second number the longitudinal axis. (4) Dose prescription must be completed before the initiation of therapy. (5) On daily dose sheet, tumor dose section, anatomical site treated and portals should be clearly labelled and all those contributions to that target added on a single row. (6) Any change of therapy plan must be entered in dose prescription section with new date.

Date	**PLAN OF THERAPY** (To be filled out by M.D.)
Staff M.D. Signature	

EXTERNAL RX PRESCRIPTION

Date	Anatomical Site Treated	Field No.	Field Description	Machine	Modality	No. of Fields Per Frac.	No. of Fx per Day	Tumor Dose per Field (cGy)	Tumor Dose per Frac	Daily TD (cGy)	Total Tumor Dose (cGy)	Fractions per Week

Dose Changed

BRACHYTHERAPY PRESCRIPTION

Type	MG-Hrs.	cGy

MAXIMUM TOLERANCE DOSE TO SECONDARY POINTS OR CRITICAL STRUCTURES:

SIMULATION SET-UP

ACQUIRED DATA	**DATE**
Comp. Filter	
Contour-Rx Plan	
CT Scan-Rx Plan	
Irreg. Measurement	
INFORMATION FILED	**DATE**
Isodoses	
Irreg. Field Calc	

Form #54A MIR-RO (5/90)

FIELD DESCRIPTIONS						
Procedure Date Sim. Tech. Init	1 Film for Block 2 Sim. for Lines 3 Block Simulator 4 Verify Port 5 Resim. Port					
Immobilization	1 Bite Block 2 Cork & Tongue Blade 3 Alpha Cradle 4 Therma. Plas. 5 Arm Stretcher					
Body	1 Supine 2 Prone 3 Oblique					
Head	1 On Table 2 On Sponge 3 Oblique 4 Facemask					
Arms	1 At Side 2 Above Head 3 On Chest					
Set-up	1 SSD 2 SAD 3 Rotation					

A

FIGURE 1–29. Forms used at Mallinckrodt Institute of Radiology. (**A**) Dose prescription. (**B**) Calculation of doses. (**C**) Daily dose record.

be reviewed by both the radiation oncologist directing the treatment and the physics/dosimetry staff. Simulation, localization films, Polaroid pictures, and so on, are required to document the appropriateness of the irradiation portals. The dosimetry review consists of initial and periodic verification of the maximum and tumor doses delivered to the tumor, draining lymphatics, and critical normal structures throughout the course of irradiation.

Equipment evaluation and calibration procedures. Each radiation oncology facility should have a formal equipment quality assurance program, developed by the chief radiation physicist in close cooperation with the radiation oncology director. Quality assurance procedures and results from periodic performance tests and calibration of all the therapy machines must be accurately documented.[48] It is strongly recommended that a log book be kept at each therapy machine console to allow the machine operator (therapy technologist) to document immediate problems related to machine performance that could affect radiation and mechanical safety. Quality assurance requirements in each of these areas are outlined in several publications.[159]

Quality Assurance Committee

The director of the radiation oncology department appoints the committee, which meets regularly to review the following: results of review and audit process; physics quality assurance program report; review of outcome studies; mortality and morbidity conference; any case of "misadministration" or error in delivery of greater than 10% of the intended dose; any chart in which an incident report is filed.

For additional details, refer to the publication by the American College of Radiology.[3]

Review Conferences and Practice Audits

A thorough clinical practice quality assurance program in a radiation oncology facility should, in addition to the previously mentioned, conduct at various predetermined times regular conferences and meetings to establish policies of treatment and procedures for the clinical operation, to set up a mechanism for regular documentation and filing of all quality assurance pro-

Date of Calculation					
Anatomical Site Treated					
Field Number					
Machine					
Modality and Energy (MeV)					
Superficial (Beam Filter)					
HVL					
Patient Diameter (cm)					
SSD (cm)					
Cone Size or Collimator Setting					
Field Size at SSD					
Eq. Sq. Field Size at SSD (cm²)					
PDD (Percent Depth Dose)					
SAD (cm) (Isocenter)					
Collimator Setting					
Field Size at Isocenter					
Eq. Sq. Field Size at Isocenter (cm²)					
Depth of Calculation (cm)					
IDD (Isocenter Depth Dose)					
IPF (Isocenter Peak Scatter Factor)					
Wedge Angle (Degree)					
Wedge Factor					
D_{fs}					
PSF (Peak-Scatter Factor)					
MU or Time/Field (Min)					
Given Max Dose (cGy)/Field					
Tumor Dose Per Field (cGy)					
Number Fields Per Fraction					
Tumor Dose Per Fraction (cGy)					
Number Fractions Per Day					
Physician Check (Initials)					
Physics Check (Initials)					

ROTATIONAL THERAPY

Machine ______ Modality ______

Field Size	Avg. Radius	Avg. TAR	Isocentric Depth
Tray Factor	D_{fs}	Dose per Field of Isocenter ______ cGy	
Arc ______ °		Start ______ ° Stop ______ °	
Monitor Units			MU/deg

DOSE CALCULATIONS - REMARKS

BRACHYTHERAPY DELIVERED

Date	Sources	MG - Hrs.

ORDERS CODE: DAILY DOSE SECTION

1. Loc. Film
2. M.D. Check Setup
3. Dosimetrist Check Setup
4. Patient to be seen in Exam Room
5. Tech. Supvr. Check Setup
6. Simulation
7. Tattoo
8. Blood Counts
9. Pt. to see Nurse
10. Pt. to see Social Service
11. Pt. to see Dietician

FIGURE 1–29. (*Continued*) **B**

cedures, to provide periodic reviews of plans of treatment and records of the patients (charts, portal films, isodose curves, and so on), and to have in-place committees that periodically review various aspects of quality assurance, including standard policies, corrective action, and deviations from quality assurance.

Conferences to be instituted are review of new patients, review of treatment techniques and portal films, weekly chart rounds of patients under treatment, and morbidity (and mortality) conference.

Staffing Requirements

Ideally, all patients with a diagnosis of cancer should get the best possible care, regardless of the location and the circumstances under which the diagnosis is made. A multidisciplinary approach to the management of the patient should be strongly advocated—at facilities with adequate staff, expertise, and resources to provide optimal care to achieve the best tumor control and lower morbidity at a reasonable cost.

The radiation oncologist should play an integral part in the evaluation and decision-making process for selection of therapy in all patients. To adequately perform all functions required in a radiation oncology facility, standards have been formulated for acquisition of equipment and staffing levels.[159] The requirements for staffing a radiation oncology facility are listed in Table 1-11. Obviously, adjustments must be made, depending on geographic location, size of the facility, and financial considerations, as long as the optimal care of the patient is not compromised.

MODIFIERS OF RADIATION RESPONSE

Several approaches have been used to enhance the therapeutic ratio in radiation therapy:

Physical modifiers of low LET radiations. Equipment improvements have led to better depth dose characteristics (high-energy photons and electrons), less side scatter, less differential absorption in bone and normal tissues, and selective energy deposition at specific depths (protons). These advances in

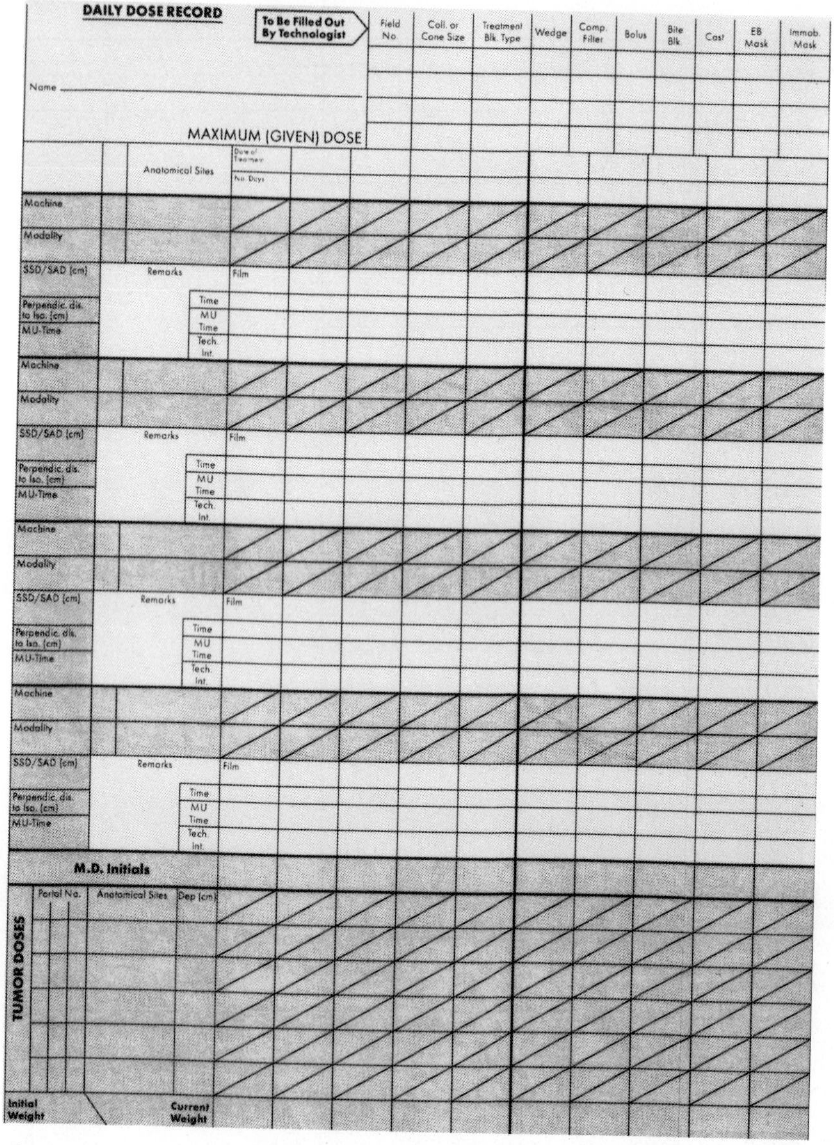

DAILY DOSE RECORD

To Be Filled Out By Technologist

Field No.	Coll. or Cone Size	Treatment Blk. Type	Wedge	Comp. Filter	Bolus	Bite Blk.	Cast	EB Mask	Immob. Mask

Name

MAXIMUM (GIVEN) DOSE

Anatomical Sites — Date of Treatment — No. Days

Machine
Modality
SSD/SAD (cm) — Remarks — Film
Perpendic. dis. to Iso. (cm) — Time
MU-Time — MU — Time — Tech. Int.

Machine
Modality
SSD/SAD (cm) — Remarks — Film
Perpendic. dis. to Iso. (cm) — Time
MU-Time — MU — Time — Tech. Int.

Machine
Modality
SSD/SAD (cm) — Remarks — Film
Perpendic. dis. to Iso. (cm) — Time
MU-Time — MU — Time — Tech. Int.

Machine
Modality
SSD/SAD (cm) — Remarks — Film
Perpendic. dis. to Iso. (cm) — Time
MU-Time — MU — Time — Tech. Int.

M.D. Initials

TUMOR DOSES — Portal No. — Anatomical Sites — Dep (cm)

Initial Weight — Current Weight

C

FIGURE 1–29. (*Continued*)

radiation delivery became possible with the advent of sophisticated high-energy linear accelerators and proton generators.

High LET radiations. Theoretically, the importance of tumor hypoxia as a factor causing unsatisfactory results is less with neutrons, π-mesons, and heavy ions than with standard doses of radiation delivered with low LET beams.[108]

Hyperbaric oxygen or tourniquet technique. These techniques involve the use of increased oxygen tension to improve the effects of radiation on the tumor[69] or the use of an orthopedic tourniquet to produce severe hypoxia in the surrounding normal tissues so that higher radiation doses can be delivered.[350] Theoretically, these approaches yield better tumor control without damaging the normal tissues, although clinical trials were not conclusive.[41,69,147,163,376]

Hypoxic sensitizers. Compounds with electron affinity from the nitroimidazole group theoretically produce free radicals in a manner similar to that of oxygen, selectively sensitizing hypoxic cells to radiation. Misonidazole (R0-07-0582) was evaluated in numerous clinical trials by the RTOG, with no evidence of clinical efficacy.[393] New compounds, such as SR-2508, have been tested in phase I studies and are under clinical evaluation.

Perfluorocarbons. These agents are administered in emulsion (they are insoluble in water) in sufficient concentrations (combined with inhalation of 95% to 100% oxygen) to enhance oxygen transport and release it in the presence of low oxygen tension.[132,341] Their potential application in the treatment of patients with cancer is under evaluation.[101,306]

Cytotoxic agents. Drugs such as dactinomycin (Actinomycin D), doxorubicin (Adriamycin), 5-fluorouracil, cyclophosphamide, cisplatin, methotrexate, bleomycin, and others have been shown to interact with radiation in several forms to maximize tumor cell kill. In some instances, increased normal tissue reactions have been observed.

Radioprotectors. Sulfhydryl-containing compounds, such as cystine and cysteamine, have been used in animals to protect normal tissues against irradiation. WR-2721,[375] a thiophosphate derivative of cysteamine, selectively has been shown to protect normal tissues, including bone marrow, salivary glands, and intestinal mucosa in animals, with little effect on tumor response to irradiation. This compound is under investigation by the RTOG in a phase I study.

Hyperthermia. Heat at temperatures above 42.5°C has been shown to kill cells by itself or to enhance the effects of radiation and numerous cytotoxic agents. Heat selectively

TABLE 1–11
Personnel Requirements for Clinical Radiation Therapy*

CATEGORY	STAFFING
Radiation Oncologist-in-Chief	One per program
Staff Radiation Oncologist	One additional for each 200–250 patients treated annually
Radiation Physicist	One per center; Additional in ratio of 1 per 400 patients treated annually
Treatment Planning Staff	One per 300 patients treated annually
Dosimetrist	
Physics Technologist	
Radiation Therapy Technologist	
Supervisor	One per center
Staff (Treatment)	2–3 per megavoltage unit up to 40 patients treated daily per unit 4–6 per megavoltage unit up to 60 patients treated daily per unit
Staff (Simulation)	1–2 per simulator
Staff (Brachytherapy)	As needed
Treatment Aide	As needed
Nurse	One per center
Additional R.N., L.V.N.	One per 300 patients treated annually
Social Worker	As needed
Dietitian	As needed
Physical Therapist	As needed
Maintenance Engineer or electronics technician	One per 2 megavoltage units

* *Additional personnel for research and education programs.*
(Inter-Society Council for Radiation Oncology: Radiation Oncology in Integrated Cancer Management. Philadelphia, American College of Radiology, 1986)

kills cells that are chronically hypoxic and nutritionally deficient and have a low pH–characteristics shared by tumor cells in comparison with the better-oxygenated and better-nourished normal cells. Furthermore, heat preferentially kills cells in the S phase of the proliferative cycle, which have been known to be resistant to radiation.[68, 362] For more complete review of these subjects, the reader is referred to the respective chapters in this text.

TUMOR BIOLOGY AND CANCER THERAPY

Malignant tumors constitute heterogeneous conglomerates of cells, not governed by homeostatic factors, with varying ranges of cellular proliferation and growth rates. It is estimated that a small tumor of 1 cm^3 (1 g) in volume has 10^9 cells. Assuming exponential growth of one clonogenic cell the tumor would have undergone 30 doubling times by the time it is clinically detected. Growth from 1 g to 1 kg requires only ten further doubling times. Tumors grow at different rates because of variations in cell proliferation kinetics related to numerous factors, including tumor vascularity and nutrition, cell loss, and host immune response.

Malignant neoplasias may invade adjacent tissues or spread to regional lymph nodes or distant sites. Metastases remain the major cause of death in patients with cancer. The mechanisms responsible for metastatic behavior are not fully understood. Tumor cell heterogeneity and capability to metastasize vary.[339] The formation of a metastatic colony is the result of a complex series of tumor-host interactions that follow primary tumor initiation and progression.[96] Following local invasion of adjacent host-tissue barriers, the tumor invades the vascular wall or lymphatic channels, after which the tumor cells in the circulation evade host defenses. A three-step hypothesis has been proposed that involves a sequence of biochemical events during tumor cell invasion of the extracellular matrix[191]: tumor cell attachment by means of cell-surface receptors that specifically bind to components of the matrix; hydrolytic enzymes locally degrading the matrix, including the attachment components; and tumor cell locomotion into the region of the matrix modified by proteolysis.

Several gene products that are augmented in metastatic cells have been identified. The laminin receptor has been shown experimentally to play a role in hematogenous metastasis.[13, 193] The role of collagenases and collagenase inhibitors in tumor cell invasion has been reviewed.[194] The unrestrained activity of collagenases may be involved in tumor cell invasion. Tumor cell motility factors also appear to be associated with metastatic cells.[192, 193] Tumor cell-surface lectins may also play a role in the metastatic process. Genes that regulate a major histocompatibility antigen on the tumor cell surface have been shown to affect the metastatic process. Other evidence indicates that tumor cells may express genes that enhance their immunogenicity with consequent suppression of metastasis.[339]

The correlation of oncogene expression with human tumor metastatic aggressiveness has recently been reviewed, and increased expression or amplification of oncogenes has been reported in a variety of tumor systems.[192] Amplification of the HER-2/neu oncogene has been correlated with metastasis in human breast cancer,[337, 377] whereas N-myc amplification has been associated with rapid progression of neuroblastomas.[325] Increased expression of ras oncogenes has been detected in various cancers, including breast and colon, and L-myc gene is amplified in small cell carcinomas of the lung.[243] Sobel[339] dis-

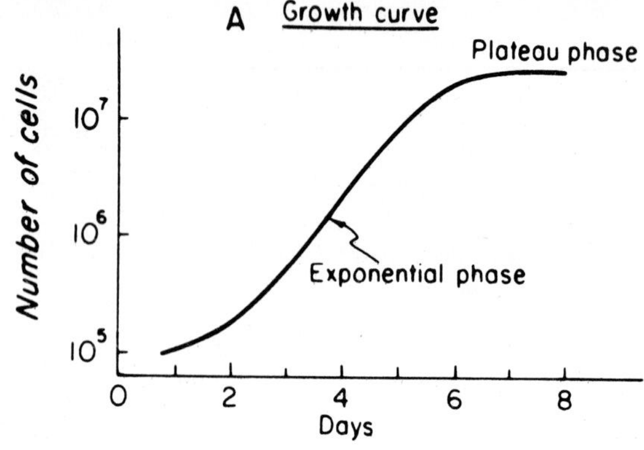

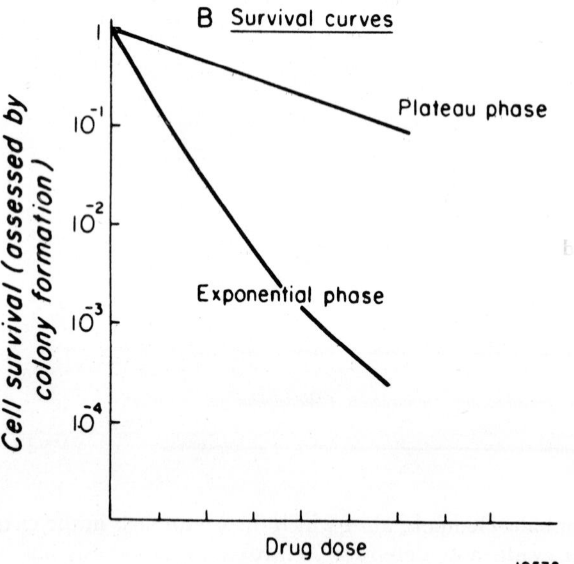

FIGURE 1–30. (**A**) Cells in tissue culture show a period of rapid proliferation and exponential growth, followed by slowing of growth and a plateau phase as nutrients are depleted and cell concentration increases. (**B**) Effect of drugs against slowly and rapidly proliferating cells can be assessed by treatment of cell cultures in the exponential and plateau phases. Cells are then replated to assess survival by colony formation. Most drugs show greater toxicity for rapidly proliferating cells in exponential growth phase, as in the example shown. (Tannock IF: Principles of cell proliferation: cell kinetics. In DeVita VT Jr, Hellman S, Rosenberg SA [eds]: Cancer: Principles and Practice of Oncology, 3rd ed, pp 3–13. Philadelphia, JB Lippincott, 1989)

cussed the possibility that genetic control of metastasis is also exerted by deactivation of specific genes, metastasis-suppressor genes, in a matter analogous to the action of tumor-suppressor genes on tumorigenicity.

Malignant tumors exhibit different sensitivity to ionizing radiations or cytotoxic agents, depending on the cellular rate of proliferation (proliferating cells are more sensitive) or even on the position of the cell in the proliferative cycle[359] (Figs. 1-30 and 1-31).

It is known that hypoxic cells are less sensitive to ionizing radiations.[137] Hypoxic cell populations in solid tumors may also be resistant to some anticancer drugs. This effect may take place because hypoxic cells tend to be slowly proliferating.[150, 354, 356] Also, the same hemodynamic factors that influence oxygen diffusion may have an impact on the ability of the cytotoxic agents to diffuse in the tumor.[38, 78, 244, 355, 399]

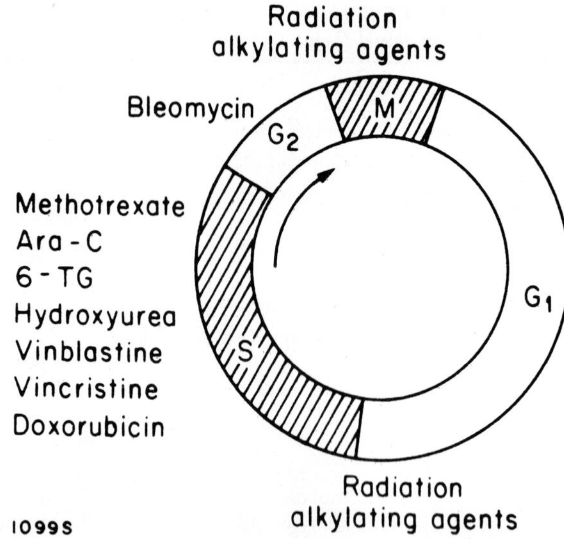

FIGURE 1–31. The position in the cell cycle at which anticancer drugs and radiation most often exert their maximum lethal toxicity. Drugs and radiation may also act to delay progression around the cycle (*e.g.*, vinblastine and vincristine induce mitotic arrest). (Tannock IF: Principles of cell proliferation: cell kinetics. In DeVita VT Jr, Hellman S, Rosenberg SA [eds]: Cancer: Principles and Practice of Oncology, 3rd ed, pp 3–13. Philadelphia, JB Lippincott, 1989)

ONCOGENES

Oncogenes were initially identified as genes capable of causing cancer. The studies were largely based on transplantable tumors in chicken, mice, and rats,[228] and oncogenes were initially described as the genetic material carried by RNA tumor viruses that resulted in rapid malignant transformation of target cells. Now it is recognized that oncogenes are normal cellular genes that may contribute to the development of the malignant cell if their expression is altered through mutation, translocation, amplification, or some other mechanism. Evidence suggests that at least two genetic changes are needed to produce a cancer cell, and oncogene studies support this concept.[228] In the 1970s it was found that RNA viruses could be classified as either rapidly transforming or slowly transforming. The rapidly transforming viruses carry genetic information capable of inducing tumors directly (oncogenes), whereas the slowly transforming viruses do not carry oncogenes and may induce tumors by inserting next to host cellular genes and in some way altering the transcription of the adjacent cellular gene. At this time over 20 viral oncogenes have been identified (Table 1-12).

A list of oncogenes not associated with RNA tumor viruses but recognized either by their activity in transformation or by their association with chromosome translocations is presented in Table 1-13.[228] When DNA probing techniques were used, it was found that sequences homologous to the oncogene region of the virus were present in the DNA of all tissues of virus-free chickens (Fig. 1-32). The normal cellular sequences have been referred to as *proto-oncogenes.*[20, 379] The oncogene carried by a virus is referred to as v-onc, whereas the proto-oncogene is referred to as c-onc. In the normal cell the expression of proto-oncogene is well controlled and appears to play a role in the growth and development of the organism. The function of some of these genes has been determined; for others, a close association between cell proliferation and gene expression has been established.[228]

TABLE 1–12
Proto-Oncogenes That Have Been Deleted in RNA Viruses

PROTO-ONCOGENE/ ONCOGENE	SPECIES OF ORIGIN	POSSIBLE SUBCELLULAR LOCATION(S) OF GENE PRODUCT	POSSIBLE FUNCTION OF GENE PRODUCT
abl	mouse	Plasma and cytoplasmic membranes	Protein-tyrosine kinase
erb-A	chicken	Cytoplasm	?
erb-B	chicken	Plasma and cytoplasmic membranes	Protein-tyrosine kinase
ets	chicken	Nucleus (fused with product of v-myb)	?
fes/fps	cat	Plasma and cytoplasmic membranes	Protein-tyrosine kinase
fgr	cat	Plasma and cytoplasmic membranes	Protein-tyrosine kinase
fms	cat	Plasma and cytoplasmic membranes	Protein-tyrosine kinase
fos	mouse	Nucleus	?
kit	mouse	?	?
mil/raf	mouse	Cytoplasm	Protein-serine/threonine kinase
mos	mouse	Cytoplasm	Protein-serine/threonine kinase
myb	chicken	Nucleus	?
myc	chicken	Nucleus	?
ras	mouse, rat	Plasma membrane	Regulator of adenylate cyclase
rel	chicken	Cytoplasm	?
ros	chicken	Plasma and cytoplasmic membranes	Protein-tyrosine kinase
sis	mouse	Cytoplasm/secreted	Analogue of PDGF-β*
ski	mouse	Nucleus	?
src	chicken	Plasma and cytoplasmic membranes	Protein-tyrosine kinase
yes	chicken	Plasma and cytoplasmic membranes	Protein-tyrosine kinase

* *β-chain of platelet-derived growth factor*
(Minden MD: Oncogenes. In Tannock IF, Hill RP (eds): The Basic Science of Oncology, pp 72–88. New York, Pergamon Press, 1987)

Stimulation of a nonmalignant cell into a proliferative state often depends on an external signal, which is received by a receptor on the cell membrane, transferred through the membrane into the cytoplasm and ultimately to the nucleus in which DNA synthesis is initiated. Proto-oncogenes have been found that function at each step of this pathway. The erb-B oncogene is homologous to the gene encoding for cell membrane receptor of epidermal growth factor (EGF). The interaction of EGF with this receptor reduces the proliferation of epidermal cells such as breast epithelium. The protein products of the proto-oncogenes, src, abl, and ras, are cytoplasmic in location. The proto-oncogene products of myc, fos, ski, and myb are nuclear in location and are believed to play an important role in the control of cell division. The expression of these genes may be responsible for the entry of the cell into DNA synthesis.

Strong evidence suggests that malignancy induction may be associated with genetic changes in the cell. Examples of this are the finding of specific chromosome abnormalities in malignant cells, association of tumor development with DNA-damaging agents such as ionizing irradiation and chemical carcinogens, and increasing incidence of cancer in hereditary diseases such as xeroderma pigmentosum and others.[228] Increased production of the normal protein products of amplified proto-oncogenes may contribute to the development of the malignant phenotype. The mechanisms that lead to amplification of genes are unknown. Gene amplification has been well characterized as a mechanism that conveys resistance of cells to drugs such as methotrexate or colchicine, and it may occur on a random basis or because the drugs interfere with DNA synthesis. The amplified gene presumably is retained because it conveys a selective advantage to the cell.[228]

Chromosome translocations occur very frequently in some types of tumors, suggesting that they may play a role in their development. Examples of translocations are the 9;22 Philadelphia chromosome in chronic myelogenous leukemia, the 15;17 in promyelocytic leukemia, and several translocations involving chromosome 8 seen in lymphatic malignancies. Common sites of translocations in malignant cells are frequently near an oncogene.[316]

Role of Proto-oncogenes in Normal and Transformed Cells

The role of proto-oncogenes in the growth and development of normal and malignant cells is not yet well known. Oncogene protein products can be grouped into several classes, depending on their location and reactivity: nuclear, cytoplasmic, and membrane protein kinases, cytoplasmic GTP (guanosine triphosphate) binding proteins, growth factors, and others. Growth factors are proteins that act at the cell surface to stimulate cell growth. No evidence suggests that *in vivo* production of a growth factor induces malignancy.

For a more detailed review of the subject, refer to other publications such as the chapter by Minden in *Basic Science of Oncology*[228] or *Oncogenes* by Burck, Liu, and Larrick.[30]

TUMOR MARKERS

Tumor markers are substances that may be detected in body fluids and are produced by or associated with a variety of tumors. These substances may be used to aid in tumor diagnosis and prognosis, to assess tumor cell burden, and to detect early

TABLE 1–13
Proto-Oncogenes That Have Not Appeared in Retroviruses

PROTO-ONCOGENE	METHOD OF IDENTIFICATION	ORIGINAL SOURCE
bcl-1	Translocation	B-cell leukemia
bcl-2	Translocation	B-cell lymphoma
Blym	Transfection	B-cell lymphoma
int-1	Insertional mutagenesis	Mammary carcinoma
int-2	Insertional mutagenesis	Mammary carcinoma
L-myc	Amplification	Lung carcinoma
mcf2	Transfection	Mammary carcinoma
mcf3	Transfection	Mammary carcinoma
met	Transfection	Chemically transformed osteosarcoma cells
Mlvi-1	Insertional mutagenesis	T-cell lymphoma
Mlvi-2	Insertional mutagenesis	T-cell lymphoma
Mlvi-3	Insertional mutagenesis	T-cell lymphoma
neu	Transfection	Neuroblastoma
N-myc	Amplification	Neuroblastoma
N-ras	Transfection	Neuroblastoma
onc-D	Transfection	Colon carcinoma
pim-1	Insertional mutagenesis	T-cell lymphoma
tcl-1	Translocation	T-cell leukemia
Tlym-1	Transfection	T-cell lymphoma
Tlym-2	Transfection	T-cell lymphoma

(Minden MD: Oncogenes. In Tannock IF, Hill RP (eds): The Basic Science of Oncology, pp 72–88. New York, Pergamon Press, 1987)

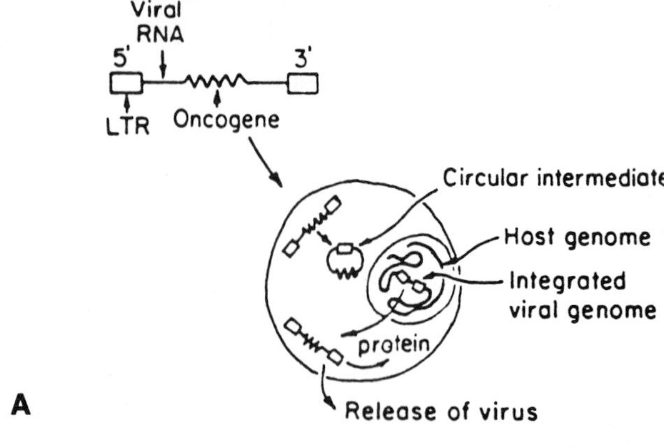

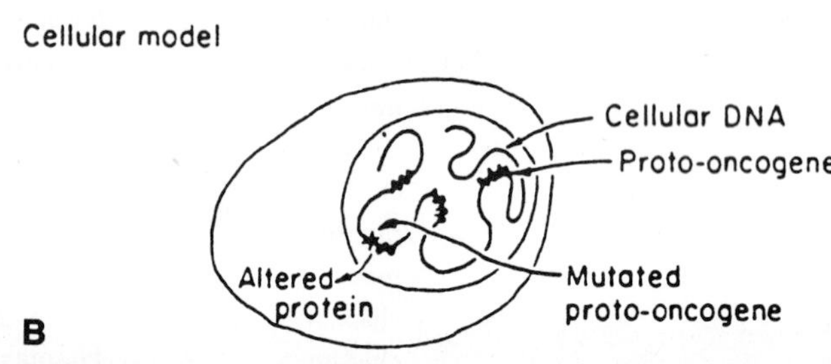

FIGURE 1–32. (**A**) In the viral oncogene model, an RNA virus carrying an oncogene enters a cell. Double-stranded DNA is made from viral RNA, using the enzyme reverse transcriptase, and may integrate into the host genome. This genetic information may be transcribed to produce an mRNA, which is packaged as a mature virus or is translated into a protein that leads to malignant transformation. (**B**) In the cellular-oncogene model, proto-oncogenes are seen as normal genes in mammalian cells. Alterations by mutation, amplification, or translocation may lead to gene products that cause malignant transformation. (Minden MD: Oncogenes. In Tannock IF, Hill RP [eds]: The Basic Science of Oncology, pp 72–88. New York, Pergamon Press, 1987)

recurrent tumors after therapy. They also may be helpful in the selection and scheduling of therapy. However, these markers are not produced uniquely by tumors, and their levels in blood differ from normal quantitatively rather than qualitatively.[207] A classification of substances used or proposed to be used as tumor markers is shown in Table 1-14. Tumor markers are present in low concentrations in the plasma and require sophisticated techniques for their detection such as radioimmunoassay, immunoradiometric assay, or enzyme-linked immunosorbent assay. All three procedures depend on the formation of antigen-antibody complexes, in which a purified preparation of a particular marker is used initially to prepare the specific antibodies (usually monoclonal); these antibodies are attached to a solid support such as Sephadex beads.

Sensitivity of a marker refers to the proportion of patients with a particular tumor who have elevated plasma levels of the marker. Specificity is indicated by the proportion of patients who do not have this particular pathologic process and who exhibit normal plasma levels of the marker. Ideally a marker has a high value of sensitivity and specificity.

Oncofetal Proteins

Oncofetal proteins are present during a variable period of normal embryonic or fetal life. They do not disappear en-

TABLE 1–14
Classification of Tumor Markers Showing Selected Examples

TUMOR MARKER	CLASSIFICATION
Oncofetal proteins	Carcinoembryonic antigen (CEA) Alpha-fetoprotein (AFP)
Hormones	Human chorionic gonadotropin (hCG) Ectopic hormones
Enzymes	Prostatic acid phosphatase Alkaline phosphatase Lactic dehydrogenase Gamma glutamyl transpeptidase (GGT)
Immunoglobulins	
Tumor-associated antigens	CA-125
Miscellaneous markers	Polyamines Nucleosides Tissue polypeptide antigen (TPA) Isoferritins Acute-phase proteins

(Malkin A: Tumor markers. In Tannock IF, Hill RP (eds): The Basic Science of Oncology, pp 192–203. New York, Pergamon Press, 1987)

tirely in the adult and may reappear with certain malignancies. Classic examples are carcinoembryonic antigen (CEA) and α-fetoprotein (AFP).

Carcinoembryonic antigen-elevated blood levels have been identified in some nonmalignant diseases such as cirrhosis and chronic obstructive pulmonary disease, and modest elevations may occur in smokers. The presence of increased levels of the protein, seen in a variety of epithelial tumors, such as colorectal, breast, lung, and pancreatic cancer, suggests that "de-repression" may be a characteristic of malignant growth or, alternatively, that stem cells or other primitive progenitor cells populate the tumor.[207] The half-life of CEA in plasma is about 6 to 8 days.

Alpha-fetoprotein is an α_1-globulin product of the fetal liver, gastrointestinal tract, and yolk sac and is normally present in fetal circulation. Marked increases in plasma AFP levels are noted in 80% of patients with hepatocellular carcinoma and about 60% of patients with nonseminomatous testicular tumors. AFP also may be elevated in the presence of nonmalignant liver disease, especially cirrhosis. AFP has a half-life in plasma of approximately 5.5 days.

Hormones

Human chorionic gonadotropin (HCG) is produced normally by the syncytiotrophoblast cells of the placenta during pregnancy. Most pregnancy tests are based on its detection in serum or urine. Elevated levels of HCG are found in the plasma of almost all women with tumors of trophoblastic origin (choriocarcinoma), in about 10% to 15% of patients with seminoma, and in 60% to 80% nonseminomatous testicular tumors. Minimal elevations of HCG are sometimes observed in patients with tumors of other organs such as breast and large bowel.

Enzymes

Prostatic acid phosphatase is an enzyme secreted by the normal prostate gland cells. Alkaline phosphatase may be produced by the liver, bone, or placenta. Lactic dehydrogenase (LDH), a tetramer comprised of combinations of two polypeptide chains designated H for heart and M for muscle, may be elevated in patients with bulky tumors such as lymphoma.

Immunoglobulin and Tumor-Associated Antigens

Immunoglobulin levels are elevated in patients with multiple myeloma and B cell lymphomas. Excessive urinary excretion of light-chain immunoglobulins is almost pathognomonic of these disorders. Protein electrophoresis of serum or urine of these patients shows a sharp peak, indicating the presence of a monoclonal protein referred to as an M protein.

Tumor-associated antigens have been described in a variety of tumors as a result of the widespread availability of techniques for production of monoclonal antibodies, including prostatic specific antigen (PSA), ovarian antigen CA-125, and others.

For further reading on this subject, the chapter by Malkin in *Basic Science of Oncology*[207] and the monograph *Tumor Marker Antigens*[151] are recommended.

MANAGEMENT OF THE PATIENT WITH CANCER

The optimal care of patients with malignant tumors is a multidisciplinary effort, which may combine two or more of the classic disciplines: surgery, radiation therapy, and chemotherapy. Many professionals, including physicians, physicists, laboratory scientists, nurses, rehabilitation staff, sociologists, and social workers, are intimately involved in the care of the patient with cancer. Pathologists, radiologists, clinical laboratory physicians, and immunologists are integral members of the team that renders the correct diagnosis. Other fields, such as biology, biochemistry, and pharmacology, have contributed greatly to the advancement of methods used to evaluate and treat patients with cancer (*e.g.*, biomarkers, cell kinetics indicators, oncogenes).

The radiation oncologist, like any other physician, must assess all conditions relative to the patient and to the tumor under consideration for treatment and must systematically review the need for diagnostic and staging procedures as well as the best therapeutic strategy. This has been well illustrated in a series of "decision trees" designed by the Patterns of Care Study Group for radiation therapy in 10 different tumors[178] (Fig. 1-33). In a subsequent analysis, Kramer[177] documented that in several instances a clear relationship existed between compliance with guidelines for diagnostic or therapeutic procedures (best current management consensus) and the outcome, as defined by survival rate, recurrence patterns, or complications of treatment.

Emphasis on screening and early diagnosis of cancer as well as improvements in therapeutic strategies have had a significant positive impact on the survival rates of patients with cancer. In the United States, the SEER results[113] have shown a small but steady improvement in survival rate for patients with a variety of tumor sites (Table 1-15). A recent article from Sweden reported a 5-year relative survival rate of 34.2% for males diagnosed from 1960 to 1964 and 47.1% for those diagnosed from 1980 to 1984. The corresponding values for women were 48.7% and 56.9%. The mean loss of expected life among cancer patients decreased from 9.6 to 7 years. Relative survival rates at various times after diagnosis are illustrated in Figure 1-34, supporting a substantial increase in survival rate of patients with cancer since 1960.[1]

As noted previously, by the time a human cancer has reached the size of 1 cm^3, approximately 10^9 cells are present. Chemotherapy that kills 90% of the tumor cells reduces cell numbers from 10^6 to 10^5, or a one-log kill. Even a 99.999% cell kill, a figure that seems enormous to clinicians, represents only a five-log reduction in cell number. Intimately connected with the cell kill concept was Skipper's realization that cell destruction by drugs followed first-order kinetics: A given dose of drug destroys a constant fraction of cells (proportional to the initial number of cells present), not a fixed number.[335] When repetitive doses of drugs are given, the tumor cell kill per treatment is the net result of the initial cell kill minus the fraction killed plus the regrowth of tumor in the interval between treatments. If sufficient time elapses, the tumor may regrow to pretreatment levels or greater, and the patient may die of the disease. Clinically this is an important concept because the cycles of chemotherapy must be timed far enough apart to allow recovery of the host from normal tissue toxicity but close enough to prevent tumor repopulation.[335]

The data of Suit and Wette[353] and Skipper[335] suggest that radiation and chemotherapy exert their effects through a re-

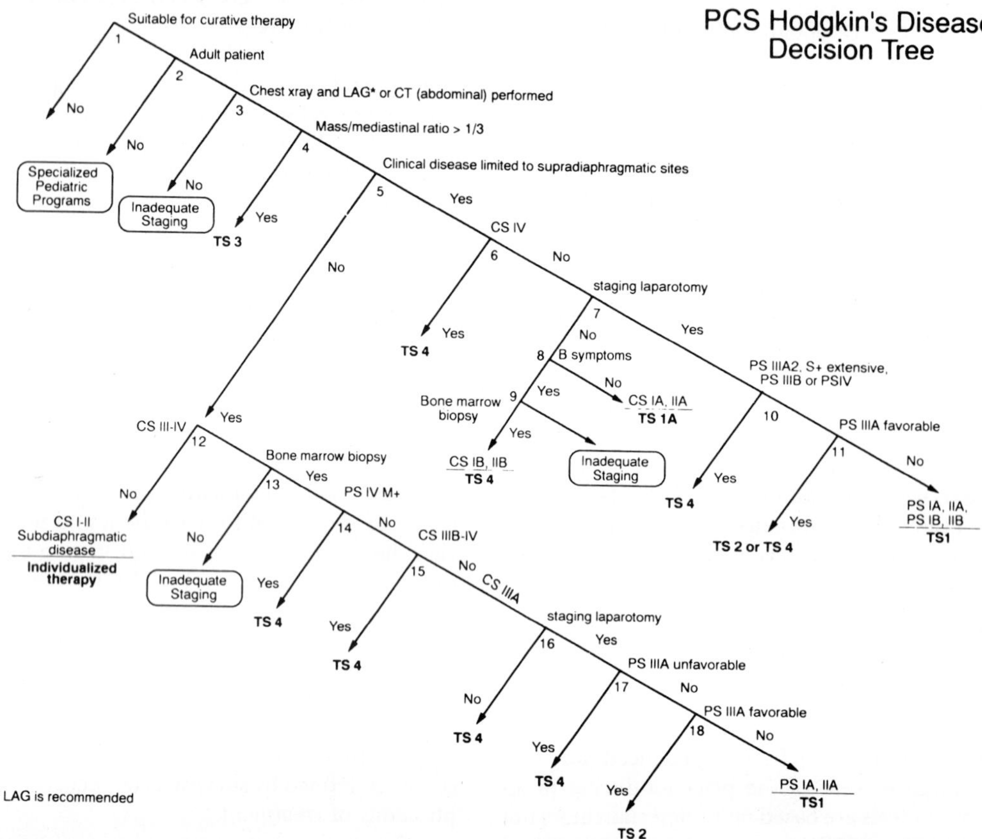

FIGURE 1–33. Example of decision tree in evaluation and treatment used by Patterns of Care Study. (Hoppe RT [ed]: Patterns of Care Process Study Newsletter [Hodgkin's Disease]. 1990–1991. Philadelphia, American College of Radiology, 1991)

duction of tumor cell burden by several logs, limited by normal tissue toxicity. Therefore proper implementation of each of these treatment modalities (concomitant or sequential) is critically important to achieving the maximum potential for cure. The aim of multiagent chemotherapy is to combine drugs that differ in biologic effect so as to attack several sites in the biosynthetic pathways or inhibit several critical cell functions, thereby producing additive or supra-additive effects without overlapping normal tissue toxicity.

Frei[114] thoroughly reviewed the rationale and evolution of chemotherapy in the management of patients with cancer. He emphasized the established or "putative" contributions of this modality to the cure of malignant tumors in the United States. Frei[114] concluded that current developments in basic tumor biology, evolving clinical innovations, and their interactions provide realistic grounds for optimism about continuing progress in the curative management of patients with cancer. Even though cancer chemotherapy has improved strikingly, primarily against hematologic, trophoblastic, testicular, and pediatric neoplasias, only marginal gains have been obtained against the most common solid tumors, including cancers of the breast, lung, and colon.

The immune response, in which regional lymphatics play a critical role,[98] is an important mechanism influencing tumor cell proliferation and dissemination.

Mathe and colleagues[214] suggested that immunotherapy is most effective when applied at a point in treatment when the tumor cell burden is 10^6 cells or less, and Wrba[414] suggests that host immunosurveillance becomes effective at a lesser tumor cell burden. The functionality of the host immune response, which may bear strongly on whether the tumor is ultimately eradicated following major cytoreductive therapies, depends on factors as diverse as the effects of tumor growth, host nutrition, and cytoreductive therapy. The effect of sequential or concomitant multimodality therapy on the capacity of the host to mount an immune response is a vitally important area for investigation.

LIMITATIONS OF CLASSIC MODALITIES OF CANCER THERAPY

Although the classic methods of cancer therapy are effective in the management of many patients, it is very important to be aware of a variety of factors that limit their effectiveness in controlling large or disseminated tumors.

Surgery

The effectiveness of surgery is limited by

- Inadequate removal of the gross tumor, leading to a local recurrence
- Inadequate resection of microextensions in tissues adjacent to gross tumor. Although radical operations may eliminate some of these microextensions, the price may be anatomic deformity and perhaps physiologic impairment
- Undetected metastasis to regional lymph nodes. Regional lymph nodes may provide an important host immunodefense against tumor cells.[98,276] At the same time, however, they may be invaded by tumor cells and, if not removed, may cause a treatment failure.

TABLE 1–15
Trends in 5-Year Relative Survival Rates for Selected Sites of Cancer Among U.S. Whites, 1960–1984

	YEAR OF DIAGNOSIS				
SITES	1960–1963* (%)	1970–1973* (%)	1974–1976† (%)	1977–1978† (%)	1979–1984† (%)
All sites	39	43	50	50	50
Oral cavity and pharynx	45	43	54	53	53
Esophagus	4	4	5	6	7
Stomach	11	13	14	15	16
Colon	43	49	50	52	54
Rectum	38	45	48	50	52
Liver	2	3	4	3	3
Pancreas	1	2	3	2	3
Larynx	53	62	66	69	66
Lung and bronchus	8	10	12	13	13
Melanoma of skin	60	68	78	80	80
Breast (females)	63	68	74	75	75
Cervix uteri	58	64	70	69	67
Corpus uteri	73	81	88	87	83
Ovary	32	36	36	37	37
Prostate	50	63	67	70	73
Testis	63	72	78	86	91
Bladder	53	61	73	75	77
Kidney	37	46	51	50	51
Brain and nervous system	18	20	22	23	23
Thyroid	83	86	92	92	92
Hodgkin's disease	40	67	71	73	74
Non-Hodgkin's lymphoma	31	41	47	48	49
Multiple myeloma	12	19	24	24	24
Leukemia	14	22	34	37	32

From National Cancer Institute: Annual Cancer Statistics Review Including Cancer Trends 1950–1985. Bethesda, MD, 1988.
** Rates based on data from the End Results Group using a series of hospital registries and one population-based registry.*
† Rates based on data from the SEER program, with follow-up of patients through 1985.

Systemic micrometastasis. Tumor cell dissemination may take place at any time, but it has been shown that more tumor cells are circulating in the peripheral blood when a tumor is manipulated. Surgical techniques minimizing the handling of tumors to prevent dissemination of tumor cells, or hypothetically the use of some substances such as warfarin or heparin or cytotoxic drugs may decrease distant metastases and improve surgical results.[216]

Radiation Therapy

As in the case of surgery, the effectiveness of irradiation is limited by

I. Tumor cell burden
   A. Inadequate depopulation of clonogens in the primary tumor, which may cause a local recurrence
   B. Regional microextensions or metastasis to the lymphatics, which may not be included in the irradiated volume
   C. Clinically unapparent distant metastasis at the time of initial therapy

II. Physical and technical factors
   A. Inaccurate tumor localization because of the radiation oncologist's inability to define the target volume adequately (geographic miss)
   B. Inadequate treatment planning, which may result in nonhomogeneous doses of radiation throughout the target volume
   C. Unreliable daily irradiation techniques, which may result in poor positioning and immobilization (inaccurate treatment)

III. Biologic factors
   A. Hypoxic cell subpopulations, which require higher doses of radiation than well-oxygenated cells for the same level of cell kill (oxygen enhancement ratio)[133]
   B. Repair of sublethal or potentially lethal damage after irradiation[88, 395]
   C. Position of the cell in the proliferative cycle. Cells in late G_1 or S phase are more resistant to irradiation than are cells in other portions of the cycle. Cells in G_0 (reversible nonclonogenic state) are also more resistant to irradiation than are rapidly proliferating cells.[362]
   D. Tumor cell repopulation during fractionated therapy or after completion of therapy. If proliferation occurs at a rate greater than that of the cells being killed by irradiation, tumor will recur. In some tumors accelerated repopulation may take place after administration of some irradiation or chemotherapy.[359]

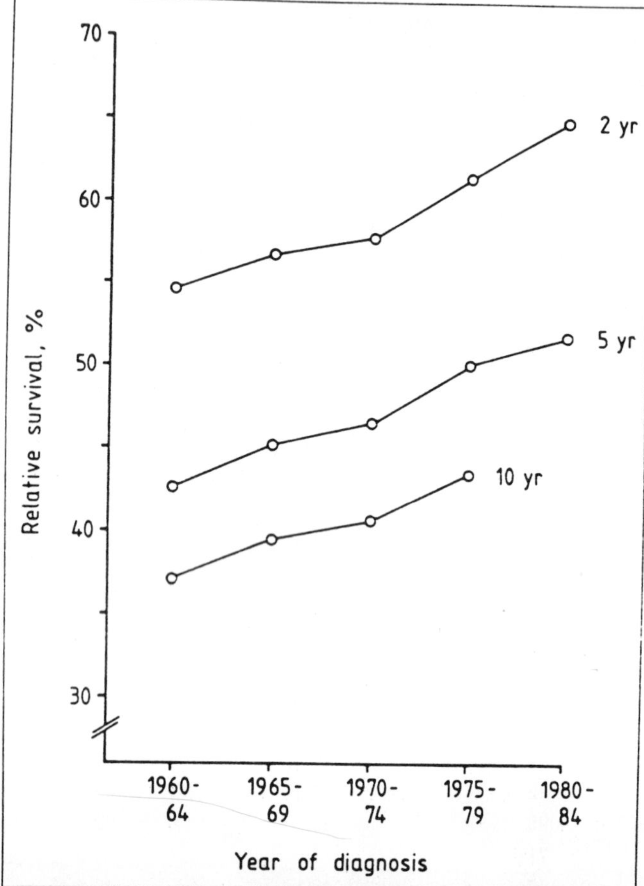

FIGURE 1–34. Relative survival rate after 2, 5, and 10 years of observation of patients diagnosed during consecutive 5-year calendar periods. (Adami H-O, Sparen P, Bergstrom R, et al: J Natl Cancer Inst 81:1640–1647, 1989)

E. Limited tolerance of the surrounding normal tissues to irradiation, thus precluding the delivery of higher doses

Chemotherapy

Some of the limitations of chemotherapy are relative to pharmacodynamic factors, such as decreased drug diffusion because of abnormal vasculature in the tumor and decreased drug incorporation and use in the cell.

Several biologic factors may significantly limit the effectiveness of cytotoxic agents:

Tumor cell burden. Chemotherapy is more effective against a smaller number of tumor cells (within a given similar type of cell).

Proportion of clonogenic cells. Cytotoxic agents are more effective in proliferating cells (growth fraction) and less efficacious in cells with low proliferative activity.

Variations of cell sensitivity to drugs throughout the proliferative cell cycle. Some drugs may be phase-specific (killing or arresting dividing cells during a specific phase of cell cycle, such as DNA synthesis), cycle-specific (killing proliferating cells more effectively than resting cells), or nonspecific (equally toxic for resting cycling cells [G_0 phase], which may be recruited into active proliferation after administration of some cytotoxic drugs and reduction of the total tumor cell burden).

Chemoresistance. Some cells that initially respond to chemotherapy may later be affected less or not at all by the same drugs or combinations, even at higher doses.[361]

Mode of administration of cytotoxic drugs (pulsed, continuous, sequential, and so on) and timing of administration of one drug in relation to the other. The timing of administration of the drugs may allow for tumor cell synchronization or for the sensitization of the tumor cells to the effects of other drugs.

Dose of chemotherapy and frequency of administration. Several studies have shown that the frequency of administration or higher doses of chemotherapy have a substantial impact on the induction and maintenance of tumor regression.[114]

The possible interactions of chemotherapy with other local modalities are summarized in Table 1-16. As stated earlier, one of the main obstacles to successful treatment of many solid tumors with cytotoxic drugs is the development of drug resistance by malignant cells. Many mechanisms are implicated in multiple drug resistance, such as alternations in drug transport, free radical detoxification, cell surface glycoprotein, and phosphoprotein accumulation and modification of membrane structure and dynamics. Increasing concentration of P-glycoprotein expression may be associated with decreased response to chemotherapy. Many other agents, including calcium channel blockers, calmodulin inhibitors, antibodies, tamoxifen, cyclosporin A, and lypophilic polycyclic compounds have been found to have multidrug resistance modulating activity *in vitro*.[238,239,361]

Combination of Therapeutic Modalities

Irradiation and Surgery

The main combinations of surgery and radiation therapy revolve around preoperative, postoperative, and intraoperative radiation therapy; use of surgery or irradiation alone to treat the primary disease and lymph node metastases; or less-than-conventional surgery followed by irradiation for regional subclinical disease. The following tumors are indications for com-

TABLE 1–16
Possible Interaction of Chemotherapy and Local Modalities

CHEMOTHERAPY EFFECT (+ OR −)	CONSEQUENCE ON LOCAL MODALITY
Downstaging (+)	Enhance operability (Surgery)
Decrease bulk (+)	Increase oxygenation (Radiation)
Decrease potential radiation repair (+)	Enhance effects if given in proximity (Radiation)
Increase lethal (+) damage (+)	Enhance effects if given together (Radiation)
Selection of resistance (−)	Decrease efficacy if cross resistant (Radiation)
Increase residual growth (−) fraction (−)	Decrease efficacy of some forms of radiation (Radiation)
Adverse host and other factors (−)	Enhances complications from local therapies (Surgery and Radiation) and/or negates favorable effects from primary tumor removal (Surgery)

(Muggia FM, Gill I: PPO Updates 4:1–12, 1990)

bined surgery and radiation therapy: tumors with low cure rates by either surgery or radiation therapy alone; tumors with great potential for local or regional recurrence; tumors with great potential for lymphatic invasion; tumors with great potential for residual disease after surgery. In addition, surgery and radiation may be indicated for the preservation of function and the enhancement of cosmesis.

The combination of surgery and radiation therapy has produced neither dramatic nor substantial improvement in the survival rate of patients with cancer. This may be due in part to the lack of analysis of reasons for locoregional failure and to the potential for disseminated metastases. Failure to demonstrate the real value of combined surgery and radiation therapy is probably also related to its indiscriminate application to all patients, including inappropriate groups such as those in whom the disease is too advanced locally and regionally and in whom there is a substantial potential for disseminated disease at the time of initial treatment.

The rationale for preoperative radiation therapy is its potential ability to eradicate subclinical disease beyond the margins of the surgical resection, to diminish tumor implantation by decreasing the number of viable cells within the operative field, to sterilize lymph node metastases outside the operative field, to decrease the potential for dissemination of clonogenic tumor cells that might produce distant metastases, and to increase the possibility of resectability. This is because tumor cells can be disseminated beyond the operative field (outside the subsequently irradiated volume) during surgery and because surgical trauma may interfere with the vascular supply of the tissues, thereby rendering hypoxic the residual tumor cells within the postoperatively irradiated volume. The main disadvantage of preoperative irradiation is that it may interfere with normal healing of the tissues affected by the radiation. Such interference, however, is minimal when the radiation doses are below 4500 cGy to 5000 cGy in 5 weeks.

The rationale for postoperative irradiation is based on the fact that it is possible to treat any residual tumor in the operative field by destroying subclinical foci of tumor cells following the surgical procedure, by eradicating adjacent subclinical foci or cancer (including lymph node metastases), and by delivering higher doses than can be achieved with preoperative irradiation—the greater dose being directed to the volume of high risk or known residual disease. For example, Vikram and Farr[382] and Fletcher[103] from M.D. Anderson Hospital reported improved survival rates in patients with head and neck tumors treated with combined therapy compared with surgery alone. Wallgren and co-workers[390] noted comparable improved survival rates in 639 patients with operable carcinoma of the breast treated with preoperative or postoperative radiation therapy, compared with 321 patients treated with radiation alone. The rate of local recurrences was 6.9% in the patients treated with combined therapy and 21.5% in those treated with surgery alone.

The potential disadvantages of postoperative irradiation are related to the delay imposed on the initiation of radiation therapy until wound healing is complete. Theoretic and experimental evidence suggest that the radiation effect may be impaired by vascular changes produced in the tumor bed by surgery. Experimental data suggest that preoperative irradiation may be more effective than postoperative irradiation.[274] However, higher doses of postoperative irradiation may be more effective than lower doses delivered preoperatively, as noted by Vikram and associates[382] in 114 patients with advanced, resectable head and neck tumors.

Furthermore, Vikram and associates[383] noted a higher locoregional recurrence rate and decreased survival rate in 41 patients with advanced head and neck tumors treated with postoperative radiation therapy that was initiated more than 6 weeks after the surgical procedure when compared with 53 patients on whom radiation therapy was started within 6 weeks of the time of the operation. Because Vikram's study was not a prospective randomized study, it is possible that more locally advanced tumors required greater surgical resections, resulting in longer healing periods.

Irradiation and Chemotherapy

Chemotherapy alone or combined with radiation may be used in several settings. *Primary chemotherapy* is used as definitive treatment, as part of the primary lesion treatment (even if later followed by other local therapy), and when the primary tumor response to the initial treatment is the key identifier of systemic effects.[238] *Adjuvant therapy* is used as an adjunct to other local modalities as part of the initial curative treatment. Frei[115] proposed the term *neoadjuvant chemotherapy* when this modality is used in the initial treatment of patients with local tumors, before surgery or radiation therapy.

The effects of combined radiation therapy and chemotherapy can be described as independent, additive, or interactive. Chemotherapy and radiation therapy can be administered sequentially or concomitantly. Wrba's data[414] suggest that sequencing of treatment at the appropriate time is significantly related to the residual tumor cell burden at the point of introduction of each new treatment program.

Administration of chemotherapy *before* radiation therapy produces some cell kill and reduction in the number of cells to be eliminated by the irradiation. The use of chemotherapy *during* radiation therapy has a strong rationale because it could interact with the local treatment (additive and even supra-additive action) and could also affect subclinical disease early in treatment. Nevertheless, it must be remembered that the combination of modalities may enhance normal tissue toxicity. Chemotherapy *after* radiation therapy, as an adjuvant, has been used primarily for control of subclinical disease. This approach, in conjunction with administration during treatment, has proven to be successful in patients with Wilms' tumor, rhabdomyosarcoma, Ewing's sarcoma, and osteogenic sarcomas, as well as in premenopausal patients with breast cancer and to some extent in those with small cell carcinoma of the lung.

In selecting combination therapy (radiation and cytotoxic drugs), it is important to assess the effectiveness of concomitant or sequential administration of two methods of therapy, the toxicity of combined modalities, and the salvage rate for patients failing initial treatment with a single modality. For instance, total nodal irradiation plus mechlorethamine, vincristine sulfate (Oncovin), procarbazine, and prednisone (MOPP) is superior to MOPP alone in the treatment of Stages IB, II, and III Hodgkin's disease in terms of length of initial disease-free survival. The difference disappears with long-term follow-up, however, because salvage therapy with irradiation and ABVD (actinomycin, bleomycin, vincristine, and doxorubicin) is superior in patients initially treated with MOPP alone.[308]

In combined treatment, when new agents with inherent toxicity are added, results may be inferior to those with the combination involving fewer agents. Toxicity may lower tumor control because the added toxicity may require lowering the doses of the effective agents, which decreases response rate, and because initial increased fatal toxicity prevents some dying patients from demonstrating tumor response that could have been observed if they had survived. Overall survival may be compromised as well.

Integrated Multimodality Cancer Management

A combined modality approach to patient management requires a broad understanding of the biologic effects of each treatment modality used. Analysis of specific prognostic factors for the individual patient improves the clinician's ability to select the most appropriate treatment. The management of a patient with a malignant tumor is conditioned by the following parameters: anatomic location of tumor, stage (extent) of the tumor, histologic type of the tumor, general condition of the patient (including immunologic response).

The following modalities have traditionally been used in the management of these patients:

Surgery, for a lesion that can be technically removed completely
Radiation therapy, for a localized lesion in which surgery may cause anatomically or physiologically undesirable sequelae and for a more extensive lesion not amenable to a surgical resection
Chemotherapy, for micrometastasis (as an adjuvant therapy) or for extensive or chemosensitive tumors (neoadjuvant, definitive) or for disseminated disease (palliative)

Combinations of two or all three modalities are frequently used to improve tumor control and patient survival. Steel and Peckham[345,347] postulated the biologic basis of cancer therapy as spatial cooperation, in which an agent is active against tumor cells spatially missed by another agent; addition of antitumor effects by two or more agents; and nonoverlapping toxicity and protection of normal tissues. Figure 1-35 illustrates the selective use of a given therapeutic modality to achieve tumor control in each compartment. Large primary tumors or metastatic lymph nodes must be removed surgically or treated with definitive

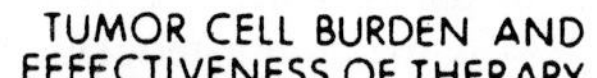

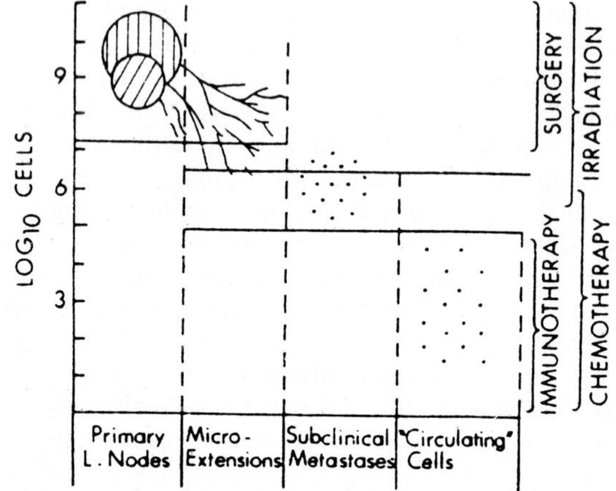

FIGURE 1–35. Diagrammatic representation of the use of different treatment modalities to eliminate a given tumor cell burden. Large primary tumors or metastatic lymph nodes must be removed surgically or by radiation therapy. Regional microextensions are effectively eliminated by irradiation, and chemotherapy is applied mainly for subclinical disease, although it also has an effect on some of the larger tumors. (Perez CA, Marks JE, Powers WE: Semin Oncol 4:387--397, 1977)

radiation therapy. Regional microextensions are eliminated effectively by irradiation without the anatomic and at times physiologic deficit produced by equivalent medical surgery. Chemotherapy is applied mainly to control disseminated subclinical disease, although it also has an effect on some of the larger tumors. A variety of patients might benefit from such an integrated, multimodal treatment program, including those with tumors of the head and neck, breast, and urinary bladder and those with bone and soft tissue sarcomas, in which the locoregional and distant metastatic components are of major significance in the disease process.

The combination of conservation surgery with radiation therapy to obtain better cosmetic results in carcinoma of the breast, the combination of limb-sparing surgical procedures with irradiation (and sometimes with chemotherapy) for the treatment of soft tissue sarcomas (and some bone tumors of the extremities), and the multimodality approach to pediatric tumors are examples of the practical application of evolving concepts.[85,97,189,234,307,381] The results obtained with these more conservative surgical approaches in combination with radiation therapy are similar in scope and outcome as those obtained with radical surgical procedures. Likewise, another example is the improved survival rates reported with adjuvant chemotherapy in premenopausal patients with carcinoma of the breast[26] or in patients with soft tissue sarcoma of the extremities. However, these encouraging results have not been documented in postmenopausal patients with breast carcinoma[187] or in patients with soft tissue sarcomas arising in other anatomic locations.[307]

Various authors[138,304,315] have reported pelvic failure rates in 10% to 15% of patients with Stage B2-C carcinoma of the rectosigmoid with surgery and irradiation in contrast to 35% to 50% with surgery alone, although no significant impact on survival rate was noted. The Gastrointestinal Tumor Study Group[120] described higher survival rates and lower incidence of pelvic failures in patients with Stage B2-C carcinoma of the rectosigmoid treated with postoperative pelvic irradiation (4000 cGy to 4500 cGy in 4 to 5 weeks) and chemotherapy (5-fluorouracil [5-FU] and methyl-CCNU) compared with a control group treated with radiation alone.

DeVita and colleagues[66] stressed the impact of combined modality therapy both in local tumor control and survival rate in a variety of tumors. Unfortunately, there remains a substantial number of tumors in which both local tumor control and survival are poor. In these neoplasms, improvement in local tumor control alone is not likely to reflect an improved survival rate because of the lack of effective therapy for micrometastases. Thus efforts must be continued to find more effective systemic treatment for these patients.

Innovative New Modalities

Many exciting biologic and technologic developments have taken place in radiation oncology in the past 30 years through clinical trials on the use of protons to enhance the physical capabilities for precise dose delivery and the use of high LET radiation, such as neutrons or heavy ions, to enhance the biologic ability to destroy tumor cells. Our capability to precisely deliver higher doses of radiation to limited volumes has been increased by means of technical advances such as computer use for treatment planning, including 3D approaches, the use of intraoperative irradiation, and stereotactic techniques for the treatment of intracranial arteriovenous malformations and tumors. These developments are reviewed in detail in other chapters in this text.

BIOLOGIC RESPONSE MODIFIERS

Biologic response modifiers (BRMs) are natural substances that enhance host defense mechanisms against tumors. The following agents have been used: active immunotherapy (nonspecific: BCG, levamisole, *C. parvum*; interferons; IL-2; and specific: tumor cell vaccines), passive immunotherapy: monoclonal antibodies; LAK; TIL (tumor infiltrating lymphocytes), and other agents: colony-stimulating factors.

BCG, levamisole, and *C. parvum* as immunotherapy substances have been ineffective, except for the use of BCG by direct instillation into the bladder for patients with superficial tumors, in whom complete responses are often seen. Recently a combination of levamisole with 5-fluorouracil (5-FU) as an adjuvant for Dukes B2 and C colon cancer was shown to improve length of survival and disease-free survival.[231]

Interferons are a family of hormone-like cellular proteins produced by virtually all eukaryotic cells in response to a wide range of stimuli. There are three types of interferons: α, β, and τ. Interferon-α was originally classified as leukocyte interferon and interferon-β as fibroblast interferon, although both are produced by most mammalian cells. In contrast, interferon-τ is made only by T lymphocytes and large granular lymphocytes.[156]

Interferons mediate their effects through the transcription of a large number of genes, which may vary according to interferon type. Interferons have their greatest effects in resting cells, but they prolong all phases of the cell cycle. Interferons also affect the expression of proto-oncogenes such as myc, ras, mos, and abl.[117]

Interferon is approved for use by the Food and Drug Administration for two indications: hairy cell leukemia (HCL) and AIDS-related Kaposi's sarcoma.[128] Chronic myelogenous leukemia (CML) is also highly responsive to interferon-α given at a higher dose than that used for HCL. Interferon-α produces objective antitumor responses, usually partial and of several months' duration, in patients with low-grade lymphoma. Interferon-α is active in superficial bladder cancers when applied intravesically, much the same as that reported for BCG. Major toxicities associated with the interferons are fever and chills, myalgia, fatigue, and weight loss.

Interleukin-2 (IL-2) is a protein produced by activated T lymphocytes in response to a signal from antigen and the cytokine interleukin-1. IL-2 was formerly known as T-cell growth factor. IL-2 interacts with cells by specific receptor binding, as the interferons do. Some of the antitumor effects are generated by the induction of lymphoid cells with the capacity to lyse fresh tumor cells (LAK cells). Clinical trials have been made possible by the cloning and production of IL-2 and the pioneering work of Rosenberg and associates.[310] Objective tumor regressions have been seen in patients with renal cell carcinoma, melanoma, colorectal cancer, non-Hodgkin's lymphoma, and low-grade lymphomas.

The toxicity of high-dose IL-2 is considerable, probably the result of lymphoid infiltration into a number of vital organs; lymphopenia and depletion of LAK precursor cells are common. IL-2 also induces a capillary leak syndrome with extravascular fluid accumulation and the secretion of the other cytokines, such as interferon-τ. The hemodynamic changes following administration of IL-2 are a drop in mean arterial pressure with associated tachycardia, followed by weight gain with interstitial edema and prerenal azotemia.

LAK cells have been described as unique killers, distinct from cytolytic T cells and NK cells. Animal models have indicated that LAK cells generated *in vitro* could be adoptively transferred, with greater antitumor effect noted when LAK and IL-2 were used together than with one either alone.[93,297,309] About 10% of patients with renal cancer and melanoma have had complete responses to IL-2 plus LAK, and responses also have been documented in colorectal cancer and non-Hodgkin's lymphoma.[311]

The treatment-associated mortality for interferons is about 2.5%. Toxicity of treatment is similar in patients receiving high dose IL-2 alone or together with LAK.

More recently, Rosenberg and colleagues[312] reported on the therapeutic efficacy of tumor-infiltrating lymphocytes (TILs). These are prepared *in vitro* by growing a single suspension of tumor together with IL-2. In contrast to LAK, TILs lysed cells through specific MHC-restricted killing and are many times more potent than LAK. Objective remission in 11 of 20 melanoma patients treated with TIL has been observed by Rosenberg's group; further studies are in progress.

Monoclonal antibodies (Mabs) are immunoglobulins that share the same variable region (idiotype). Production of monoclonal antibodies in large quantity was made possible through a hybridoma technique developed by Kohler and Milstein.[174] This technique involves harvesting spleens from immunized mice, fusing these cells with mouse plasmacytoma cells, and growing them in a medium that allows survival of fused cells only. Antitumor use of monoclonal antibody includes the possibility of conjugation to toxins, therapeutic isotopes, and chemotherapeutic drugs in addition to use of Mab alone.

Knox and colleagues[173] have pioneered Mab therapy for B-cell lymphoma. Sixteen patients treated with anti-idiotypic Mab by the Stanford group were reported on; eight had clinically significant partial or complete responses, including one complete response of 6 years' duration. Toxicity was minimal, but included transient thrombocytopenia or neutropenia, hypotension, rash, fever, and chills, often seen at the initiation of therapy.

One way of overcoming the problem of heterogeneous or weak antigen expression is the conjugation of Mab with a toxin, chemotherapeutic agent, or therapeutic radioisotope. A variety of chemotherapeutic conjugates have been studied in animal tumors. A phase I study with doxorubicin (Adriamycin) linked to Mab derived against a variety of tumors was well tolerated in 23 patients. These approaches require tumor access and are significantly hindered by a human antimouse antibody response.

Of the therapeutic radioisotopes for conjugation with Mab, ^{131}I has been used most extensively because of its availability, relatively inexpensive cost, and ease of use. However, it has low average beta energy and is relatively unstable in conjugation *in vitro* because it becomes rapidly dehalogenated. Order and colleagues[248] have pioneered the use of radiolabeled polyclonal antiferritin antibodies in Hodgkin's disease and hepatoma, achieving response rates of 40% to 50%. Press and associates[290] recently reported on the treatment of 10 refractory non-Hodgkin's lymphoma patients with ^{131}I-labeled MB-1 (anti-CD37) antibody. In four patients receiving "high-dose" (232 to 608 mCi) therapy with absorbed dose estimates to tumor sites ranging from 850 cGy to 4260 cGy, all had complete tumor regression lasting from 5 to 11 months or more. There were no significant acute toxic events, but myelosuppression led to the use of stored autologous marrow in two patients.

Another use of Mab is in the preparation of tumor vaccines, a form of active immunotherapy. This is based on the fact that anti-idiotype antibodies (antibody 2), which react with idiotype (antibody 1), bear the internal image of the antigen (with which antibody 1 reacts). Thus vaccination with antibody 2 may allow the host to make antitumor response (antibody 3 or anti-anti-idiotypes).

Hematopoietic colony-stimulating factors (CSFs) are low-molecular-weight glycoproteins that have become available for clinical use through advances in biochemistry and recombinant DNA technology.

IL-3, also known as multi-CSF and produced by T lymphocytes, may have as its major function the initiation of stem cell differentiation. IL-3 is capable of generating colonies with a variety of morphologies and is probably the least restricted of the CSFs with regard to cell lineage.

PHOTODYNAMIC THERAPY

The effect of light-activated chemicals on biologic systems has been described since 1900.[75] In 1961 Lipson and co-workers[195] reported on treatment of a patient with recurrent breast cancer with the hematoporphyrin derivative for fluorescence detection of tumor tissue that would localize exposure of the tumor to light. A comparison of photodynamic therapy (PDT) and ionizing radiation is shown in Table 1-17.

Photodynamic therapy involves the interaction of a sensitizer, light, and oxygen (Fig. 1-36). The ground state sensitizer is excited by the absorption of light and can subsequently react through a free radical mechanism or alternatively through a spin-state transition involving reactive singlet oxygen. Both pathways yield potentially cytotoxic compounds, although the singlet oxygen process is thought to be predominant in photodynamic therapy.[61] The deactivation of activated sensitizer to ground state can also occur with either liberation of heat or emission of a photon (the latter process is called *fluorescence* or *phosphorescence*, depending on the spin state of excited sensitizer). The hematoporphyrin photosensitizer is a complex mixture of porphyrins produced by the acetic acid-sulfuric acid treatment of hematoporphyrin, which in turn is manufactured commercially by the degradation of hemoglobin. Dougherty[74] later purified and characterized the most active component as dihematoporphyrin ether, although an ester bond between the hematoporphyrin units has also been proposed.[129] This material provided a higher therapeutic ratio (tumor compared with skin response) in animal testing than the previously employed hematoporphyrin.

Photofrin-2 is taken up by the reticuloendothelial system. Highest levels and longest retention are seen in the liver, spleen, kidney, and adrenals. The tumor-to-normal tissue ratio ranges from 20 to 1 in the brain, 6 to 1 in the liver, and 1 to 1 in the skin.

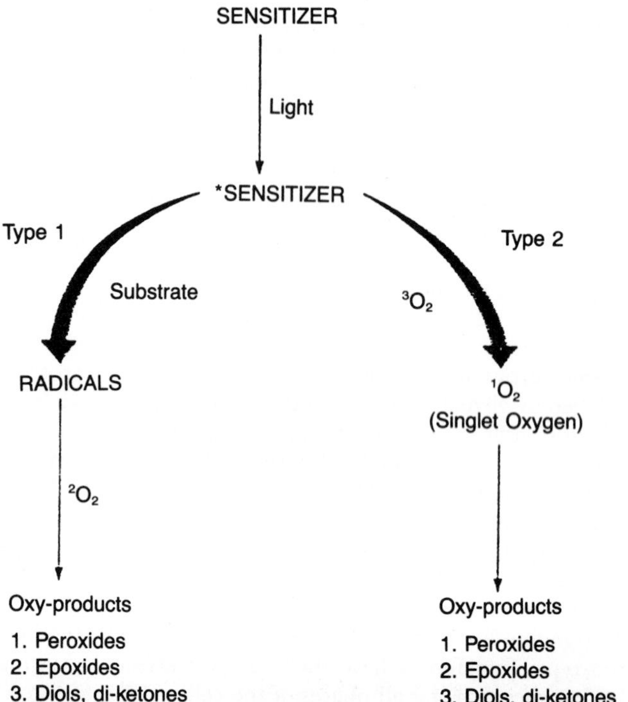

FIGURE 1–36. Light-activated photosensitizer can interact with ground state molecular oxygen by way of a type 1 (free radical) or a type 2 (singlet oxygen) oxidative pathway to yield reactive oxygen species. (Delaney TF, Glatstein EJ: Compr Ther 14:43–55, 1988)

The compound can be retained in the skin up to 8 weeks, and cutaneous photosensitivity is the only known side effect, which can be prevented by avoiding exposure to sunlight. It is advised that the drug not be used in patients with compromised hepatic function, because the liver is the primary metabolic and excretory organ for porphyrins and the site of highest accumulation of these compounds after injection.

Light-activated compounds, which selectively would localize in the tumor, are photochemically activated over a relatively narrow frequency range of light at a wavelength with appropri-

TABLE 1–17
Comparison of Photodynamic Therapy and Ionizing Irradiation

CRITERION	PDT	RT
Cellular damage	Polysystem	DNA
Tumor death	Somatic, vascular	Reproductive
Latency	Immediate	Delayed
Anoxia	Reduces effect	Reduces effect
Mutagenicity	No	Yes
Therapeutic ratio	Tumor selectively damaged	Normal tissue repair
Retreatment limits	Apparently none	Cumulative tolerance dose
Fractionation	? No benefit	Beneficial
Dose rate effects	Probably no	Yes

PDT: photodynamic therapy; RT: ionizing irradiation

ate tissue penetration. Hematoporphyrin absorbs light most strongly in the ultraviolet/visible blue region around 400 nm, with other less prominent peaks seen at or near 500 nm, 540 nm, and 580 nm. In the clinic, red light (630 nm) is most frequently used because it has deeper tissue penetration, although the excitation band is less prominent. The penetration of red light in tissue is a complex phenomenon that depends on many factors including tissue density, organ pigmentation, blood flow, surface geometry, and tissue interfaces. It is roughly estimated that the optical power density of red light falls off exponentially with the 1/e or 37% value occurring between 1 mm and 4 mm,[72] thus PDT with this light can produce tumor necrosis to a depth of 3 mm to 7 mm. PDT requires adequate light to produce effective photosensitization, the energy and wavelength being dictated by the photochemical properties of the photosensitizer, the biologic and physical characteristics of the tumor, and the mode of light delivery used. The amount of light energy delivered is generally expressed in joules and represents the product of light output or power in watts (joules/second) and the time of light exposure in seconds. Laser systems for use in clinical PDT include argon-pumped dye laser and pulsed metal vapor laser, which yield 4 to 5 watts of usable light.[72]

Tumor destruction by PDT *in vivo* has been ascribed to both direct cytotoxicity on tumor cells and indirect cytotoxicity, possibly resulting from damage to small blood vessels supplying the tumor.

Association between loss of cellular viability and inhibition of membrane transport as well as localization of HPD fluorescence in a membrane fraction suggests that membrane targets are involved in cellular inactivation by PDT.[72] Other types of cellular injury have been reported, but plasma membrane damage and mitochondrial injury appear to be the most critical for cellular destruction. DNA damage might be less pronounced than other cytotoxic effects occurring elsewhere in the cell.[130]

Preclinical trials of PDT in animal models demonstrated efficacy in several anatomic sites including eye, central nervous system, bladder, peritoneal cavity, and bronchus.[74] Patients with skin lesions such as recurrent carcinoma of the breast, basal and squamous cell carcinoma, malignant melanomas, mycosis fungoides, and Kaposi's sarcoma have been treated with this modality.[72,74,169] Treatment appears to be effective to a depth of approximately 5 mm, depending on dose delivered, concentration of sensitizer injected, and type of light delivery. Lesions thicker than 5 mm may need several external treatments or interstitial techniques. PDT has also been used with encouraging results in some patients with head and neck tumors recurrent at the primary site or in the neck, with brain gliomas, with choroidal malignant melanoma of the eye, with tumors of the tracheobronchial tree and esophagus, with carcinoma of the bladder, and with some gynecologic malignancies. Table 1-18 summarizes the results of these clinical trials.

CANCER PREVENTION

It is mandatory for the radiation oncologist to play an active role in disseminating information and counseling patients on the importance of cancer prevention and the detrimental effects of exposure to physical or chemical carcinogens.

The association of smoking with increased incidence of carcinoma of the lung and the head and neck has been reported.[373,415] About 35% of patients cured of head and neck cancer develop a second malignancy in the upper respiratory/digestive tract.[49] Long-standing sun exposure increases the incidence of skin cancer and melanoma.[176] Some reports link carcinoma of the gastrointestinal tract to dietary factors.[197,201,205,302]

Evidence is growing that multiple cellular genetic factors rather than a single initiating event are involved in the development of most human cancers.[284,397] The hypothesis that proto-oncogenes are directly involved in the induction and promotion of cancer is supported by many reports.[21,336] Oncogenes that have been associated with human malignancy include myc (Burkitt's lymphoma), ras (neuroblastoma, leukemia, sarcomas), abl (chronic myelogenous leukemia), N-myc (neuroblastoma), and Neu/eroB2 (breast cancer).[118,183]

Greenwald and associates[136] recently reviewed the potential application of chemopreventive agents that may inhibit the development of cancer by limiting exposure to initiators or promoters through stimulation of inactivation or excretion mechanisms. Exposure to carcinogenic effects may be decreased by inhibiting the activation of proto-oncogenes or by antagonizing oncogene expression. Radiation oncologists are in a unique position to actively support and recruit patients for these chemoprevention studies.

SECOND PRIMARY MALIGNANT TUMORS

Patients cured of a malignant lesion have a significant high risk of developing other cancers. Cooper and associates[49] illustrated the incidence of second malignant tumors in 928 patients with squamous cell carcinoma of the head and neck treated with radiation therapy alone. The estimated risk of developing a second tumor within 5 years from irradiation was 15%, and within 8 years the risk was 23% (Table 1-19). The development of the second malignancy decreased the probability of survival of these patients by 7% at 5 years and 14.7% at 8 years. Other authors have also shown a great propensity of patients with head and neck cancer to develop other tumors in the upper respiratory and digestive tracts[49] (Tables 1-20 and 1-21).

Patients treated with radiation for retinoblastoma, particularly the hereditary type, have an increased risk for developing second primary tumors, most commonly osteosarcoma in irradiated bones. Of 50 infants treated with radiation for retinoblastoma, seven developed osteosarcoma; one, angiosarcoma; one, rhabdomyosarcoma; one, malignant fibrosis histiocytoma; and one, an unclassified round cell tumor within the irradiated fields and three at distant sites.[338]

The induction of secondary neoplasias is directly related to the therapeutic modality used. For instance, in patients treated for Hodgkin's disease, a recent report described a relative risk of acute or nonlymphocytic leukemia of 1% in patients treated with radiation therapy alone, 9.0% in those treated with chemotherapy alone, and 7.7% when both modalities were used (Table 1-22).

For many types of neoplasms the incidence of carcinogenesis induction reaches a maximum at some intermediate dose and decreases as the dose is increased further. The dose incidence curve generally rises more steeply with high-LET radiation doses than with low-LET, especially at low dose rates (Fig. 1-37). Ron and colleagues[305] reported an increased incidence of brain/nervous system tumors (1.8 excess risk per 10,000 persons per year) in 10,834 children irradiated for tinea capitis compared with the same number of nonirradiated matched controls and 5392 siblings. Twelve malignant brain tumors were found in the irradiated patients compared with five and one suspected in nonirradiated persons. Average radiation dose received was 400 cGy in 5 consecutive days. The authors concluded that radiation doses of 100 cGy to 200 cGy significantly increased the risk of neurologic tumors.

TABLE 1–18
Photodynamic Therapy Results

STUDY	PATIENTS/ SITES	DOSE	RESPONSE (%) CR	PR/SR	COMMENTS
CUTANEOUS					
Dougherty[74]	15/50		75	25	Basal cell
Kennedy[169]	3/38		100		Basal cell; durable CR to 35 cm
Dougherty[74]	5/100		80	20	Endemic Kaposi's sarcoma
Dougherty[74]	5/10		20	75	Squamous cell
Dougherty[74]	50/100		50	30	Melanoma; CRs no pigment
Schuh[323]	14	36–288 J/cm^2	15	69	Breast; CRs durable 4–6 mo
HEAD AND NECK					
Grossweiner[137]	10	60–100 J/cm^2	80	10	Early and advanced disease
Wile[403]	21	17–91 J/cm^2	29	52	Primary site
Wile[403]	10	17–91 J/cm^2	20	30	Regional soft tissue
Hayata[145]	6	34–390 J/cm^2		100	Primary site
CENTRAL NERVOUS SYSTEM					
Laws[184]	5	810 J			No toxicity/phase I study
Kaye[168]	23	70–230 J/cm^2			No toxicity/phase I study
Muller[240]	32	8–68 J/cm^2	19	13	25% cerebral edema
EYE					
Bruce[29]	11	293–6800 J/cm^2	27	73	Follow-up less than 1 yr
Murphree[241]	9	50–400 J/cm^2	22	66	Melanoma; CR no pigment
Murphree[241]	9	50–400 J/cm^2	11	77	Retinoblastoma; all recur
BRONCHUS					
Balchum[11]	35	Variable			If tumor intraluminal, 80 % opened
Edell[82]	38/40	Variable			35% pathologic CR rate; CRs in early lesions
Hayata[145]	8	120–240 J/cm^2	75	25	Early stage
Pass[260]	10	27–250 J/cm^2			80% opening if narrowed/obstructed bronchus
ESOPHAGEAL					
McCaughan[215]	7	Variable			Improved swallowing in all patients
Thomas[365]	14	60–337 J/cm^2			14% pathologic CR; all patients improved swallowing
GASTRIC					
Hayata[144]	4	34–960 J/cm^2	100		Early stage; 75% recur 5–27 mos
Hayata[144]	12	34–960 J/cm^2			Resected post-PDT; 5/12 no tumor in specimen
BLADDER					
Benson[14]	4	Focal 150 J/cm^2	100		TIS; recur elsewhere in bladder
Tsuchiya[369]	8	Focal 120–360 J/cm^2	100		Ta–T2; recur at 6–18 mos
Hisazumi[144]	9/36	Focal 50–300 J/cm^2	50	19	Ta–T1 lesions; all CR ≤2 cm
Prout[292]	19/50	Focal 100–200 J/cm^2	24	50	Ta, T1, T1S lesions
Benson[14]	10	Whole bladder 25–45 J/cm^2	60	20	T1S or T1S + 2
GYNECOLOGIC					
Rettenmaier[300]	6/9	120–40 J/cm^2	22	44	Lesions of vagina, perineum
Corti[50]	7/7	60–240 J/cm^2	71	29	Vaginal/vault lesions
Ward[72]	5/5		40	60	CRs durable at 10, 12 mos
McCaughan[215]	5/5	Variable	100		Superficial tumor eradicated for 5–15 mos

CR: clinical complete response; PR/SR: partial or significant response; PDT: photodynamic therapy

TABLE 1–19
Rates of SMTs in Patients Who Had No Prior or Simultaneous SMTs, From Start of Radiation Therapy

			ESTIMATED % DEVELOPING SMT					
			3 YEARS		5 YEARS		8 YEARS	
	NO. EVAL	NO. SMT	%	(NO. AT RISK)	%	(NO. AT RISK)	%	(NO. AT RISK)
Overall	928	110	10	(412)	15	(288)	23	(87)
Site								
Hypopharynx	68	5	16	(11)	*	(8)	*	(2)
Oral cavity	202	24	11	(66)	22	(40)	28	(10)
Oropharynx	211	22	12	(75)	15	(41)	21	(14)
Supraglottic	110	13	8	(34)	19	(26)	*	(6)
Glottic	337	46	8	(226)	12	(173)	21	(55)
T-Stage								
T1	341	51	7	(233)	13	(173)	23	(56)
T2	317	41	14	(132)	18	(88)	21	(26)
T3	179	13	10	(39)	16	(22)	*	(5)
T4	91	5	*	(8)	*	(5)	—	—
N-Stage								
N0	660	94	10	(363)	15	(260)	24	(79)
N1	96	8	10	(28)	21	(16)	*	(6)
N2	81	2	6	(14)	*	(7)	*	(1)
N3	91	6	*	(7)	*	(5)	*	(1)
AJC Stage								
I	323	50	8	(225)	14	(168)	23	(33)
II	239	36	15	(111)	20	(74)	22	(23)
III	157	14	9	(51)	17	(32)	*	(9)
IV	209	10	7	(25)	7	(14)	*	(2)

SMT: second malignant tumor
** Estimate is unreliable because too few patients are at risk.*
(Cooper JS, Pajak TF, Rubin P, et al: Int J Radiat Oncol Biol Phys 17:449–456, 1989)

Cumberlin and associates[55] published estimates of the expected number of second malignancies induced in selected sensitive sites by scattered irradiation during radiation therapy for cancer, based on 192,761 new cancer patients treated in 1987. The model projected a 0.7% incidence for leukemia and 0.3% for solid tumors. This translates into about 1247 lifetime excess malignancies (none necessarily fatal) in the population initially irradiated. The authors stressed that the possible carcinogenesis induced by irradiation must be weighed against the risks and benefits of alternative treatments for cancer. Emphasis should be placed on the benefit of increased survival time as a result of therapy significantly outweighing the increased induction of malignant neoplasias.[47]

PSYCHOLOGIC, EMOTIONAL, AND SOMATIC SUPPORT OF RADIATION THERAPY PATIENT

Patients with cancer are often frightened, concerned with prognosis, and fearful of the procedures to be used. It is extremely important for the radiation oncologist and staff (nurse, social worker, technologist, and even receptionist) to be empathetic and to spend time with the patient discussing the nature of the tumor under treatment, the prognosis, and the procedures to be undertaken as well as side effects of therapy.

Relatives, particularly of elderly and pediatric patients, may need special psychologic or emotional support. The radiation oncologist should be available to discuss with them the particulars of the treatment, provided that this is acceptable to the patient.

Continued support of the patient during radiation therapy is mandatory, with at least one weekly evaluation by the radiation oncologist to assess the effects of treatment on the tumor and the side effects of therapy. Psychologic and emotional reinforcement, medications, dietetic counseling, oral cavity care, and skin care instructions are an integral part of the management of radiation therapy patients and should result in better therapeutic outcome.

RADIATION ONCOLOGIST AND CLINICAL TRIALS

Medical literature is replete with reports on therapeutic results ranging from case reports to retrospective studies and comparisons with historical controls to prospectively controlled randomized clinical trials.

Obviously, in situations in which small differences in outcome are anticipated, appropriately executed clinical trials are critical to develop better therapeutic strategies. Figure 1-38 illustrates the dynamics of these various studies and the role of clinical trials in improving the management of patients with cancer. In those situations in which no clear-cut management policy exists, the radiation oncologist must accept the paucity of

TABLE 1–20
Incidence and Distribution of Second Malignancies Reported in a Representative Survey of the Literature

STUDY	POPULATION STUDIED	PRIMARY TUMOR SITE	NO. CASES STUDIED	WHEN FOUND	% 2ND PRIMARIES	% IN LUNG*	% IN H & N†	% IN ESOPHAGUS‡
Black *et al*[23]	Ohio	H & N	577	M	14.7	31§	41§	12§
Boice and Fraumeni[25]	Connecticut	Larynx	4139	M	13.1	33	?	4
Cohn and Peppard[46]	Michigan	H & N	267	M	7.1	37	36§	25§
Deviri *et al*[64]	Israel	Larynx	1660	M	4.3	32	6	6
De Vries and Snow[67]	Holland	Larynx	748	A	13.9	62	?	?
Gluckman and Crissman[123]	Ohio	Larynx	2135	A	11.2	46	9	9
Gluckman and Crissman[123]	Ohio	Oral	1551	A	18.5	20	20	10
Gluckman and Crissman[123]	Ohio	Hypopharynx	324	A	14.1	27	18	20
Gluckman and Crissman[123]	Ohio	Oropharynx	880	A	10.4	12	34	8
Hordijk and De Jong[154]	Holland	Oropharynx	691	A	20.5	57	11	?
Hordijk and De Jong[154]	Holland	Oral	152	A	17.1	31	54	?
Hordijk and De Jong[154]	Holland	Hypopharynx	127	A	17.3	53	35	?
Lundgren and Olofsson[199]	Sweden	Larynx	295	M	6.8	43§	14§	10§
Maisel and Vermeersch[206]	Minnesota	H & N	449	M	9.8	39	52	2
Olsen[247]	Denmark	Larynx	3847	M	9.6	36	?	0
Parker and Enstrom[256]	California	H & N	2151	M	8.3	?	40	68
Shikhani *et al*[327]	Maryland	H & N	1864	M	5.0	?	?	?
Shons and Mc Quarrie[328]	Minnesota	H & N	405	M	12.8**	37	36	27
Vrabec[386]	Pennsylvania	H & N	1518	A	11.5	28	28	14
Wagenfeld *et al*[389]	Canada	Glottic	740	A	5.7**	52	42	6
Weichert and Schumrick[394]	Ohio	H & N	825	M	4.2	22§	61§	7§

A: All; M: metachronous; H & N: head and neck region; Oral: oral cavity
** % of all second malignancies that occurred in the lung*
† % of all second malignancies that occurred in the head and neck region
‡ % of all second malignancies that occurred in the esophagus
§ Includes patients whose disease was not metachronous
*** Includes only upper aerodigestive tract malignancies*
(Cooper JS, Pajak TF, Rubin P, et al: Int J Radiat Oncol Biol Phys 17:449–456, 1989)

data and the need to generate and participate in clinical studies. Every patient with a malignant tumor should participate in clinical investigation under the appropriate conditions and with safeguard of his or her own rights.

ETHICAL CONSIDERATIONS

The radiation oncology staff must acknowledge patients' rights and responsibilities that directly influence the quality of their care and are conducive to establishing the most desirable relationship between patients and staff.

Patients have the following rights:

The right to be treated as human beings. All patients should be treated with respect and consideration as all persons are entitled, regardless of race, sex, creed, or national origin.

The right to feel secure with their health care program. Patients must be able to obtain complete, current information concerning individual diagnosis, treatment, and prognosis in terms they can understand. If the patient is too ill, this information will be discussed with the patient's family or other appropriate persons. Patients have the right to receive information from their physicians before giving informed consent for treatment. Of course, in an emergency, treatment comes first, explanations later.

The right to privacy. Discussion of the patient's condition, as well as any consultations, examinations, or treatments is confidential and should be conducted as discreetly as possible. The medical records of patients are private and confidential. Their permission in writing is necessary, except as otherwise provided by law, before any of the information is released to such persons as lawyers, third-party payment contractors, and insurance agents or companies.

The right to service. All patients have the right to expect that their requests for services will be fulfilled, within reasonable limits.

The right to understand the cost of treatment. An explanation of all charges relating to his or her health care programs should always be readily available to the patient. It is important to provide patients with itemized statements and assist them with completing and processing insurance forms. If financial problems arise, suitable arrangements can be made for payment.

The right to be advised of education or research activities. Patients should know the identity and professional status of persons directly involved in their care and should know which physicians are primarily responsible for their care. In teaching institutions, student, intern, or resident involvement in patient care should be explained to the patient.

Patients will be advised if their participation as a subject in a research activity is desired. Of course, patients have the right to refuse to participate in such activities and retain the right to withdraw their participation at any time. The

TABLE 1–21
Second Malignant Tumors: Review of the Literature

					FREQUENCY BY SITE					
AUTHOR	**NO. TOTAL POPULATION**	**RATIO M:F**	**TIME TO SMT (YEARS)**	**NO. SMT (%)**	LUNG	H & N SMOKING/ ALCOHOL-RELATED	ESOPH-AGUS	COLO-RECTAL	PROSTATE (INCIDENTAL)	OTHER
Berg *et al*[16] (Bethesda, MD)	1651			167 (10.1)	39 (23%)	30 (17%)	11 (6%)	—	—	—
Brown[28] (Toronto)	1600	30:1	5	61 (3.8)	18 (2%)	16 (26%)	—	—	—	Skin 17 (27%)
Wagenfeld *et al*[389] (Toronto)	740			48 (6.5)	25 (52%)	16 (48%)	—	—	—	—
De Viri *et al*[64] (Israel)	1660	8:1	5.5	84 (5)	25 (29%)	5 (8.8%)	—	14 (16.2%)	—	—
Hordijk *et al*[154] (Netherlands)	691		2 (50%)	142 (20.5)	81 (57%)	16 (9.8%)	—	—	—	—
Vyas *et al*[387] (India)	Unknown	1.33:1	5	29	15 (52%)	—	—	—	—	—
Gluckman *et al*[123] (Cincinnati, OH)	2135			240 (11.2)	69 (33%)	29 (13.7%)	19 (9%)	—	—	—
Miyahara *et al*[229] (Japan)	1389		0–23	138 (9.95)	23 (15%)	43 (28.8%)	—	—	—	GI 68 (44.4%)
Boice *et al*[25] (Connecticut)	4139	7.5:1	1–4	541 (13.1)	178 (33%)	40 (7%)	—	76 (14%)	63 (12%)	—
Olsen[247] (Denmark)	3847	6.6:1	1–4	368 (9.6)	131 (36%)	16 (4%)	—	39 (11%)	31 (18%)	Stomach 30 (8%)
De Vries *et al*[67] (Netherlands)	748	20:1	4	104 (14)	64 (61.5%)	9 (8.6%)	—	—	—	—
Lundgren *et al*[199] (Sweden)	295	10:1	6.3	32 (10.8)	12 (37.5%)	10 (31.2%)	2 (6.2%)	—	—	—
Present series[218] (Rochester, NY)	235	7:1	4	50 (21)	22 (44%)	9 (18%)	—	10 (20%)	6 (12%)	—

SMT: second malignant tumor
(McDonald S, Haie C, Rubin P, et al: Int J Radiat Oncol Biol Phys 17:457–465, 1989)

TABLE 1–22
Distribution and Relative Risk of Acute or Nonlymphocytic Leukemia According to Overall Treatment Category

TREATMENT	NO. OF PATIENTS	NO. OF CONTROLS	RELATIVE RISK*	*P* VALUE
Radiation therapy only	11	158	1.0	—
Chemotherapy only	30	48	9.0 (4.1–20)	<0.001
Radiation therapy and chemotherapy	108	203	7.7 (3.9–15)	<0.001
Total	149	411†	—	—

** Values in parentheses are 95% confidence intervals.*
† Two controls were reported to have been treated with neither radiation therapy nor chemotherapy.
(Kaldor JM, Day NE, Clarke EA, et al: N Engl J Med 322:7–13, 1990)

investigational review board's approval of the protocol and signed investigational consent forms are mandatory.

The right to counseling on refusal of treatment. Patients should be advised by the physician to consider their decision carefully if they decide to decline treatments or procedures. (We routinely write a certified letter, receipt requested, to patients refusing treatment to document that they were notified of the consequences of such action.) A thorough explanation should be given so that patients understand the full extent of the consequences of their decision. It is always desirable to ask patients to sign an acknowledgment relative to discussions on this matter.

PROFESSIONAL LIABILITY AND RISK MANAGEMENT

In these days of increasing litigation and, unfortunately, growing adversarial situations between physicians and patients, it is critical for the radiation oncologist and staff to make every effort to decrease professional liability risks.

Rosenthal[313] listed the more specific geneses of medical malpractice suits as follows:

Medical accident that may not be adequately understood by the patient or explained by the treating physician

Less than successful or unexpected adverse results of treatment

Poor results from previous treatment elsewhere and ill-advised comments by other physicians or health care personnel

Rejection of plan of therapy without appropriate documentation that the physician has advised the patient of the consequences of the declining treatment. (At our Institute, we document this discussion in the chart and send the patient a certified letter advising him or her of the consequences of rejection of treatment.)

Complaint of experimentation when the patient has not been appropriately informed of the nature of the therapy to be administered

Angry patient who may find this way to vent anger or frustration about any events surrounding treatment, including lack of communication, discourteous treatment by the physician or staff, or amount of the medical bill

The best prevention against a lawsuit is based on good rapport with the patient (and relatives), effective quality assurance programs in all activities related to the management of the

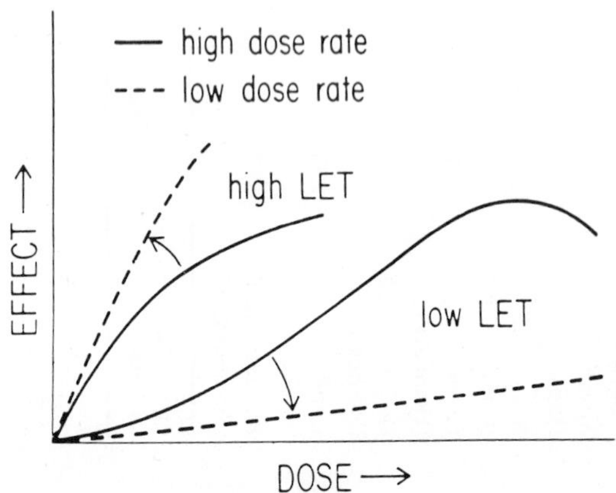

FIGURE 1–37. Schematic dose-response curves for incidence of tumors in relation to dose and dose rate of high LET and low LET radiation. LET: linear energy transfer. (Upton AC: Biological aspects of radiation carcinogenesis. In Boice JD, Fraumeni JF [eds]: Radiation Carcinogenesis: Epidemiology and Biological Significance, p 9. New York, Raven Press, 1984) see also Thomason et al[366] and Sinclair[333].

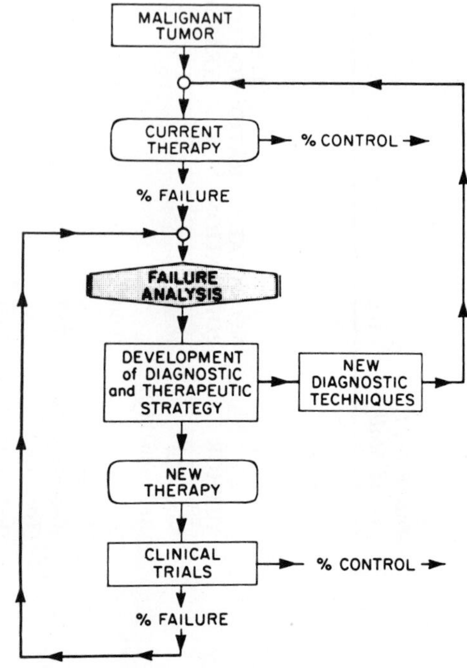

FIGURE 1–38. Relationship of failure analysis to present and future diagnostic and treatment strategies. (Cox JD: Cancer Treat Symp 2:1–3, 1983)

patient, and clear and accurate records with documentation of all procedures, discussions, and events that take place during and after the treatment of the patient.

After appropriate clinical assessment, the histologic diagnosis on the patient must be confirmed at the treating institution; this includes the review of outside pathologic slides. All procedures performed on the patient should be recorded on the chart including details of daily treatments, such as use of special treatment aids (wedges, immobilization devices) and any problems related to equipment operation. All treatment parameters and calculations should be accurately recorded and verified by a physicist or dosimetrist, in addition to the radiation oncologist. As professional liability attorneys say, "If it is not recorded on the chart, we may assume it never happened."

The physician and staff may help in their own professional liability defense, in case of a lawsuit. It is extremely important for the physician to understand and, at an appropriate time, identify early warning signs of an impending malpractice suit. The physician should promptly contact his or her attorney and insurance carrier.

The physician should prepare an incidence report in anticipation of potential litigation, describing all the details regarding the potential liability, including dates when events took place, actors and witnesses to be identified by name, affiliation, and status. It is very important that incidence reports become part of the hospital record and are not to be distributed within the institution. These reports are confidential information between the physician and the attorney/insurance carrier. The report should be prepared while the facts are still fresh so that documentation will be more likely to be optimal.

Clear and well-kept records with notes documenting every discussion and procedure that is performed on the patient should help in case of a risk-management lawsuit. A full discussion with the patient and relatives regarding planned therapy, particularly side effects of irradiation, and a well-documented informed consent form are valuable in risk management.

Informed Consent

The need to obtain informed consent for treatment is based on the patient's right to self-determination and the fiduciary relationship between the patient and the physician.[301]

The law requires that the treating physician adequately

Pelvis Only - Female with castration

PERMIT #2
MIR-RO (4/88)

RADIATION ONCOLOGY CENTER
MALLINCKRODT INSTITUTE OF RADIOLOGY
WASHINGTON UNIVERSITY MEDICAL CENTER

INFORMED CONSENT FOR TREATMENT

Date ____________

I hereby request and authorize the physicians and associated staff of the Radiation Oncology Center in charge of the care of my ____________
(Self - Wife - Husband - Child)
____________ to employ ____________
(Name of Patient)
therapy and continue treatments from time to time as they may deem necessary or advisable. Radiation therapy to the abdomen necessarily exposes many of the tissues in the treated area to the effects of the radiations. Occasionally scar tissue occurs, which produces symptoms that can be serious and may even require surgical correction. Fortunately, this is the exception rather than the rule.

I, also, grant permission to take x-ray films or perform a simulation to aid in the planning of my treatment.

Radiation therapy to the pelvis occasionally causes some transient side effects such as nausea, vomiting, diarrhea, and loss of appetite. Some organs in the pelvis are sensitive to the radiation and will be protected as much as possible. These include the small bowel, the bladder, and the rectum. Irradiation of the ovaries can produce changes in their function, with decrease in hormones and sterility. In children there is the special consideration of decreased bone growth with resulting deformity.

I understand the following specific side effects may be related to this particular treatment:

Diarrhea, bladder and rectal irritation; scar tissue in pelvis. Radiation effects and possibility of significant damage to bladder and/or rectum and/or small intestine, and/or ureters, which may require an operation which may result in a colostomy or artificial bladder. Remote possibility of abnormal opening between vagina and/or bladder and/or rectum. Castration and sterility (cessation of ovarian function). Loss of pubic hair, and skin reaction (sunburn).

I understand that no guarantee is made as to the outcome of this treatment or the course of the disease. The Staff will make every effort to obtain the best possible results.

I have been informed that written and computerized records regarding my illness, treatment, and follow-up will be kept by the Staff of the Radiation Oncology Center. Furthermore, I hereby authorize the Staff of the Radiation Oncology Center to request copies of my medical records, pathology slides, radiographs, and associated reports, or other information pertinent to my tumor, for research purposes. I also understand that computer access to and/or copies of these records is provided to authorized medical personnel at affiliated institutions where I may continue my treatments.

I have read the above, which was also fully explained to me, and give my informed consent.

Signed: ____________ Witness: ____________
(Patient or person authorized to consent for patient)

Staff Physician:

Resident Physician:

FIGURE 1–39. Informed consent form used at Mallinckrodt Institute of Radiology.

apprise every patient of the nature of the disease requiring treatment, the recommended course of therapy and details regarding it, alternative treatments available, benefits of recommended treatment, and all minor and major risks (acute and late effects) associated with the recommended therapy. It is always advisable to discuss the informed consent contents in the presence of a witness and have that person sign the informed consent form or the chart verifying that the information was discussed with the patient.

The competent adult patient or legal representative must agree to the treatment and give their approval. For minors or legally incompetent adults, informed consent must be signed by the parents, adult brothers or sisters, or a responsible close relative or legal guardian. Spouses of incompetent adults may be allowed to sign by the state. Emancipated minors may provide their own consent. It is extremely important for the radiation oncologist and the staff to spend as much time as needed to ensure that the patient and, if necessary, the relatives understand all aspects of the radiation therapy, particularly the specific description of its various potential deleterious effects. At Washington University situations are always indicated in which surgery may be required to correct a complication and specifically in which gastroscopy, colostomy, ileal bladder, or other substituting organ operation may be necessary to correct sequelae of therapy.

It must be stressed that in dealing with children or mentally incompetent adults, a thorough discussion of the plan of therapy and sequelae should be held with the parents, relatives, or legal guardian of the patient, and they must sign the informed consent.

Figure 1-39 (on preceding page) illustrates a typical informed consent form at the Mallinckrodt Institute of Radiology. Although, in case of a lawsuit, having a properly executed informed consent form in the record is helpful, more important is the incontrovertible documentation in the chart of the pertinent discussion held with the patient. Table 1-23 describes many specific sequelae in several anatomic sites that should be included in the informed consent.

TABLE 1–23
Possible Specific Sequelae of Therapy Discussed in Informed Consent

	SEQUELAE	
ANATOMIC SITE	ACUTE	LATE
Brain	Earache, headache, dizziness, hair loss, erythema	Hearing loss, damage to middle or inner ear; pituitary gland dysfunction; cataract formation; brain necrosis
Head and neck	Odynophagia, dysphagia, hoarseness, xerostomia, dysgeusia, weight loss	Subcutaneous fibrosis, skin ulceration, necrosis; thyroid dysfunction; persistent hoarseness, dysphonia, xerostomia, dysgeusia; cartilage necrosis; osteoradionecrosis of mandible; delayed wound healing, fistulae; dental decay; damage to middle ear and inner ear; apical pulmonary fibrosis Rare: myelopathy
Lung and mediastinum or esophagus	Odynophagia, dysphagia, hoarseness, cough; pneumonitis, carditis	Progressive fibrosis of lung, dyspnea, chronic cough; esophageal stricture Rare: chronic pericarditis, myelopathy
Breast or chest wall	Odynophagia, dysphagia, hoarseness, cough; pneumonitis (asymptomatic); carditis; cytopenia	Fibrosis, retraction of breast; lung fibrosis; arm edema; chronic endocarditis, myocardial infarction Rare: osteonecrosis of ribs
Abdomen or pelvis	Nausea, vomiting, abdominal pain, diarrhea; urinary frequency, dysuria, nocturia; cytopenia	Proctitis, sigmoiditis; rectal or sigmoid stricture; colonic perforation or obstruction; contracted bladder, urinary incontinence, hematuria (chronic cystitis); vesicovaginal fistula; rectovaginal fistula; leg edema; scrotal edema, sexual impotency; vaginal retraction or scarring; sterilization; sexual impotence Rare: damage to liver or kidneys
Extremities	Erythema, dry/moist desquamation	Subcutaneous fibrosis; ankylosis, edema; bone/soft tissue necrosis

QUANTIFICATION OF TREATMENT TOXICITY

For scientific and other reasons there is a critical need to accurately assess and record morbidity of treatment, because this, in addition to therapeutic efficacy, will be a crucial parameter in the evaluation of new regimens and the selection of therapy for an individual patient. Multiple schemata have been developed, although a complete consensus has not been reached as to the ideal grading scores. Tables 1-24 and 1-25 depict the toxicity grading systems for various organs developed by RTOG and EORTC (cooperative clinical trial groups).

(*Text continues on page 55*)

TABLE 1–24
Acute Radiation Morbidity Scoring Criteria (RTOG)

	SCORE				
ORGAN/TISSUE	**0**	**GRADE 1**	**GRADE 2**	**GRADE 3**	**GRADE 4**
Skin	No change over baseline	Follicular, faint or dull erythema, epilation, dry desquamation, decreased sweating	Tender or bright erythema, patchy moist desquamation, moderate edema	Confluent, moist desquamation other than skin folds, pitting edema	Ulceration, hemorrhage, necrosis
Mucous membrane	No change over baseline	Injection, may experience mild pain not requiring analgesic	Patchy mucositis that may produce an inflammatory serosanguinous discharge, may experience moderate pain requiring analgesic	Confluent fibrinous mucositis; may include severe pain requiring narcotic	Ulceration, hemorrhage, or necrosis
Eye	No change	Mild conjunctivitis with or without scleral injection, increased tearing	Moderate conjunctivitis with or without keratitis requiring steroids or antibiotics, dry eye requiring artificial tears, iritis with photophobia	Severe keratitis with corneal ulceration, objective decrease in visual acuity or in visual fields, acute glaucoma, panophthalmitis	Loss of vision (unilateral or bilateral)
Ear	No change over baseline	Mild external otitis with erythema, pruritis, secondary to dry desquamation not requiring medication. Audiogram unchanged from baseline	Moderate external otitis requiring topical medication, serous otitis medius, hypoacusis on testing only	Severe external otitis with discharge or moist desquamation, symptomatic hypoacusis, tinnitus, not drug-related	Deafness
Salivary gland	No change over baseline	Mild mouth dryness; slightly thickened saliva; may have slightly altered taste such as metallic; these changes not reflected in alteration in baseline feeding behavior, such as increased use of liquids with meals	Moderate to complete dryness; thick, sticky saliva, markedly altered taste	—	Acute salivary gland necrosis
Pharynx and esophagus	No change over baseline	Mild dysphagia or odynophagia; may require topical anesthetic or nonnarcotic analgesics; may require soft diet	Moderate dysphagia or odynophagia; may require narcotic analgesics; may require purée or liquid diet	Severe dysphagia or odynophagia with dehydration or weight loss (>15% from pretreatment baseline) requiring NG feeding tube, IV fluids, or hyperalimentation	Complete obstruction, ulceration, perforation, fistula

(*continued*)

TABLE 1–24
(Continued)

		SCORE			
ORGAN/TISSUE	**0**	**GRADE 1**	**GRADE 2**	**GRADE 3**	**GRADE 4**
Larynx	No change over baseline	Mild or intermittent hoarseness; cough not requiring antitussive; erythema of mucosa	Persistent hoarseness but able to vocalize; referred ear pain, sore throat, patchy fibrinous exudate or mild arythenoid edema not requiring narcotic; cough requiring antitussive	Whispered speech, throat pain or referred ear pain requiring narcotic; confluent fibrinous exudate, marked arytenoid edema	Marked dyspnea; stridor or hemoptysis with tracheostomy or intubation necessary
Upper GI	No change	Anorexia with ≤5% weight loss from pretreatment baseline; nausea not requiring antiemetics; abdominal discomfort not requiring parasympatholytic drugs or analgesics	Anorexia with ≤15% weight loss from pre-treatment baseline; nausea or vomiting requiring antiemetics; abdominal pain re-quiring analgesics	Anorexia with >15% weight loss from pre-treatment baseline or requiring NG tube or parenteral support; nausea or vomiting requiring NG tube or parenteral support; abdominal pain, se-vere despite medica-tion; hematemesis or melena; abdominal distention (flat plate radiograph demon-strated distended bowel loops)	Ileus, subacute or acute obstruction, perforation, GI bleeding requiring transfusion; abdominal pain requiring tube decompression or bowel diversion
Lower GI including pelvis	No change	Increased frequency or change in quality of bowel habits not requiring medication; rectal discomfort not requiring analgesics	Diarrhea requiring parasympatholytic drugs (*e.g.*, diphenox-ylate); mucous dis-charge not necessitat-ing sanitary pads; rec-tal or abdominal pain requiring analgesics	Diarrhea requiring parenteral support; severe mucous or blood discharge necessitating sanitary pads; abdominal distention (flat plate radiogrpah demonstrates distended bowel loops)	Acute or subacute obstruction, fistula or perforation, GI bleeding requiring transfusion, abdomi-nal pain or tenesmus requiring tube de-compression or bowel diversion
Lung	No change	Mild symptoms of dry cough or dyspnea on exertion	Persistent cough requiring narcotic, antitussive agents; dyspnea with minimal effort but not at rest	Severe cough unresponsive to narcotic antitussive agent or dyspnea at rest; clinical or radiologic evidence of acute pneumonitis; intermittent O_2 or steroids may be required	Severe respiratory in-sufficiency; contin-uous oxygen or assisted ventilation
Genitourinary	No change	Frequency of urination or nocturia twice pretreatment habit; dysuria, urgency not requiring medication	Frequency of urination or nocturia less frequent than every hour; dysuria, urgency, bladder spasm requiring local anesthetic (*e.g.*, phenazopyridine)	Frequency with urgency and nocturia hourly or more frequently; dysuria, pelvic pain, or bladder spasm requiring regular, frequent narcotic; gross hematuria with or without clot passage	Hematuria requiring transfusion; acute bladder obstruction not secondary to clot passage, ulceration, or necrosis
Heart	No change over baseline	Asymptomatic but objective evidence of EKG changes or peri-cardial abnormalities without evidence of other heart disease	Symptomatic with EKG changes and radiologic findings of congestive heart failure or pericardial disease; no specific treatment required	Congestive heart failure, angina pectoris, pericardial disease responding to therapy	Congestive heart failure, angina pectoris, pericardial disease, arrhythmias not responsive to nonsurgical measures

(continued)

TABLE 1–24
(Continued)

ORGAN/TISSUE	SCORE 0	GRADE 1	GRADE 2	GRADE 3	GRADE 4
CNS	No change	Fully functional status (able to work) wih minor neurologic findings; no medication needed	Neurologic findings sufficient to require home care; nursing assistance may be required; medication including steroids; antiseizure agents may be required	Neurologic findings requiring hospitalization for initial management	Serious neurologic impairment that includes paralysis, coma, or seizures >3 per wk despite medication; hospitalization required
Hematologic WBC (× 1000)	≥4.0	3.0–<4.0	2.0–<3.0	1.0–<2.0	<1.0
Platelets (× 1000)	>100	75–<100	50–<75	25–<50	<25 or spontaneous bleeding
Neutrophils (× 1000)	≥1.9	1.5–<1.9	1.0–<1.5	0.5–<1.0	<0.5 or sepsis
Hemoglobin (GM %)	>11	11–9.5	<9.5–7.5	<7.5–5.0	—
Hematocrit (%)	≥32	20–<32	20	Packed cell transfusion required	—

Guidelines
The acute morbidity criteria are used to score/grade toxicity from radiation therapy. The criteria are relevant from day 1, the commencement of therapy, through day 90. Thereafter, the EORTC/RTOG Criteria for Late Effects are to be utilized.
The evaluator must attempt to discriminate between disease and treatment-related signs and symptoms.
An accurate baseline evaluation prior to commencement of therapy is necessary.
All toxicities of Grade 3, 4, or 5 must be verified by the principal investigator.*
** Any toxicity that caused death is graded 5.*

TABLE 1–25
Late Radiation Morbidity Scoring Scheme (RTOG, EORTC)

ORGAN/TISSUE	0	GRADE 1	GRADE 2	GRADE 3	GRADE 4	GRADE 5
Skin	None	Slight atrophy, pigmentation change, some hair loss	Patchy atrophy, moderate telangiectasia, total hair loss	Marked atrophy, gross telangiectasia	Ulceration	Death directly related to radiation late effect
Subcutaneous tissue	None	Slight induration (fibrosis) and loss of subcutaneous fat	Moderate fibrosis but asymptomatic, slight field contracture; <10% linear reduction	Severe induration and loss of subcutaneous tissue; field contracture >10% linear measurement	Necrosis	
Mucous membrane	None	Slight atrophy and dryness	Moderate atrophy and telangiectasia, little mucus	Marked atrophy with complete dryness, severe telangiectasia	Ulceration	
Salivary glands	None	Slight dryness of mouth, good response on stimulation	Moderate dryness of mouth, poor response on stimulation	Complete dryness of mouth, no response on stimulation	Fibrosis	
Spinal cord	None	Mild L'hermitte's sign	Severe L'hermitte's sign	Objective neurologic findings at or below cord level treated	Mono-, para-quadriplegia	
Brain	None	Mild headache, slight lethargy	Moderate headache, great lethargy	Severe headache, severe CNS dysfunction (partial loss of power or dyskinesia)	Seizures or paralysis, coma	

(continued)

TABLE 1–25
(Continued)

ORGAN/TISSUE	0	GRADE 1	GRADE 2	GRADE 3	GRADE 4	GRADE 5
Eye	None	Asymptomatic cataract, minor corneal ulceration or keratitis	Symptomatic cataract, moderate corneal ulceration, minor retinopathy or glaucoma	Severe keratitis, severe retinopathy or detachment, severe glaucoma	Panophthalmitis, blindness	
Larynx	None	Hoarseness, slight arytenoid edema	Moderate arytenoid edema, chondritis	Severe edema, severe chondritis	Necrosis	
Lung	None	Asymptomatic or mild symptoms (dry cough), slight radiographic appearances	Moderate symptomatic fibrosis or pneumonitis (severe cough); low-grade fever, patchy radiographic appearances	Severe symptomatic fibrosis or pneumonitis, dense radiographic changes	Severe respiratory insufficiency, continuous O_2, assisted ventilation	
Heart	None	Asymptomatic or mild symptoms, transient T-wave inversion and ST changes, sinus tachycardia >110 (at rest)	Moderate angina on effort, mild pericarditis, normal heart size, persistent abnormality T wave and ST changes, low ORS	Severe angina, pericardial effusion, constrictive pericarditis, moderate heart failure, cardiac enlargement, EKG abnormalities	Tamponade, severe heart failure, severe constrictive pericarditis	
Esophagus	None	Mild fibrosis, slight difficulty in swallowing solids, no pain on swallowing	Unable to take solid food normally, swallowing semisolid food, dilatation may be indicated	Severe fibrosis, able to swallow only liquids, may have pain on swallowing; dilatation required	Necrosis, perforation, fistula	
Small/large intestine	None	Mild diarrhea, mild cramping, bowel movement 5 times daily, slight rectal discharge or bleeding	Moderate diarrhea and colic, bowel movement >5 times daily, excessive rectal mucus or intermittent bleeding	Obstruction or bleeding requiring surgery	Necrosis, perforation, fistula	
Liver	None	Mild lassitude, nausea, dyspepsia, slightly abnormal liver function	Moderate symptoms, some abnormal liver function tests, serum albumin normal	Disabling hepatitic insufficiency, liver function tests grossly abnormal, low albumin, edema or ascites	Necrosis, hepatic coma or encephalopathy	
Kidney	None	Transient albuminuria, no hypertension, mild impairment renal function, urea 25–35 mg%, creatinine 1.5–2.0 mg%, creatinine clearance >75%	Persistent moderate albuminuria (2+); mild hypertension, no related anemia, moderate impairment renal function; urea >36–60 mg%, creatinine clearance (50–74%)	Severe albuminuria, severe hypertension, persistent anemia (<100%), severe renal failure, urea >60 mg%, creatinine >4.0 mg%, creatinine clearance <50%	Malignant hypertension, uremic coma; urea >100%	
Bladder	None	Slight epithelial atrophy, mild telangiectasia (microscopic hematuria)	Moderate frequency, generalized telangiectasia, intermittent macroscopic hematuria	Severe frequency and dysuria, severe generalized telangiectasia (often with petechiae), frequent hematuria, reduction in bladder capacity (<150 cc)	Necrosis, contracted bladder (capacity <100 cc), severe hemorrhagic cystitis	

(continued)

TABLE 1–25
(Continued)

ORGAN/TISSUE	0	GRADE 1	GRADE 2	GRADE 3	GRADE 4	GRADE 5
Bone	None	Asymptomatic, no growth retardation, reduced bone density	Moderate pain or tenderness, growth retardation, irregular bone sclerosis	Severe pain or tenderness, complete arrest of bone growth, dense bone sclerosis	Necrosis, spontaneous fracture	
Joint	None	Mild joint stiffness, slight limitation of movement	Moderate stiffness, intermittent or moderate joint pain, moderate limitation of movement	Severe joint stiffness, pain with severe limitation of movement	Necrosis, complete fixation	

REFERENCES

1. Adami HO, Sparen P, Bergstrom R, et al: Increasing survival trend after cancer diagnosis in Sweden 1960–1984. J Natl Cancer Inst 81(21):1640–1674, 1989
2. American Cancer Society: Cancer Facts and Figures 1990. Atlanta, American Cancer Society, 1990
3. American College of Radiology: Draft Standards for Radiation Oncology, April 11, 1990
4. American Joint Committee on Cancer: Manual for Staging of Cancer, 3rd ed. Philadelphia, JB Lippincott, 1988
5. Amory HI, Brick IV: Irradiation damage of intestines following 1000 kV roentgen therapy: Tolerance dose. Radiology 56:49–57, 1951
6. Andrews JR: Dose-time relationships in cancer radiotherapy: A clinical radiobiology study of extremes of dose and time. Am J Roentgenol Radium Ther Nucl Med 93:56–74, 1965
7. Andrews JR: Optimization of radiotherapy: Some notes on the principles and practice of optimization of cancer treatment and implications for clinical research. Cancer Clin Trials 4:483–495, 1981
8. Andrews JR: Benefit, risk and optimization by ROC analysis in cancer radiotherapy. Int J Radiat Oncol Biol Phys 11:1557–1562, 1985
9. Baclesse F: Carcinoma of the larynx. Br J Radiol 3:1–62, 1949
10. Baclesse F: Roentgentherapy alone in the cancer of the breast. Acta Union Int Contra Cancrum 15:1023–1026, 1959
11. Balchum O, Doiron DR: Photoradiation therapy of endobronchial cancer. Clin Chest Medicine 6:255, 1985
12. Barkley HT, Fletcher GH: The significance of residual disease after external irradiation of squamous cell carcinoma of the oropharynx. Radiology 124:493–495, 1977
13. Barsky SH, Rao CN, Williams JE, et al: Laminin molecular domains which alter mestastasis in a murine model. J Clin Invest 74:843–848, 1984
14. Benson RC: Laser photodynamic therapy for bladder cancer. Mayo Clin Proc 61:859–864, 1986
15. Bentzen SM, Overgaard M, Thames HD: Fractionation sensitivity of a functional endpoint: Impaired shoulder movement after post-mastectomy radiotherapy. Int J Radiat Oncol Biol Phys 17:531–537, 1989
16. Berg JW, Schottenfeld D, Ritter F: Incidence of multiple primary cancers: III. Cancers of the respiratory and upper digestive system as multiple primary cancers. J Natl Cancer Inst 44:263–274, 1970
17. Bergonie J, Tribondeau L: Interpretation of some results of radiotherapy and an attempt at determining a logical technique of treatment. Radiat Res 11:587–588, 1959 (translation of original article in CR Acad Sci 143:983, 1906)
18. Berry RJ, Wiernik G. Patterson TJS: Skin tolerance to fractionated x-irradiation in the pig: How good a predictor is the NSD formula. Br J Radiol 47:185–190, 1974
19. Berry RJ, Wiernik G, Patterson TJS, et al: Excess late subcutaneous fibrosis after irradiation of pig skin, consequent upon application of the NSD formula. Br J Radiol 47:227–281, 1974
20. Bishop JM: Cellular oncogenes and retroviruses. Ann Rev Biochem 52:301–354, 1983
21. Bishop JM: The molecular genetics of cancer. Science 235:305–311, 1987
22. Bjarngard BE, Chin LM, Kijewski PK: Dynamic treatment planning. In Bagne F (ed): Computerized Treatment Planning Systems, pp 110–123. HHS Publication FDA 84–8223, 1984
23. Black RJ, Gluckman JL, Shumrick DA: Multiple primary tumors of the upper aerodigestive tract. Clin Otolaryngol 8:277–281, 1983
24. Boden G: Radiation myelitis of the cervical spinal cord. Br J Radiol 21:464, 1948
25. Boice JD, Fraumeni JF Jr: Second cancer following cancer of the respiratory system in Connecticut. Natl Cancer Inst Monogr 68:83–98, 1985
26. Bonadonna G, Valagussa P: Adjuvant systems therapy for resectable breast cancer. J Clin Oncol 3:259–275, 1985
27. Boyer A, Mok E: A photon dose distribution model employing convolution method. Med Phys 12:169–177, 1985
28. Brown M: Second primaries in cases of cancer of the larynx. J Laryngol Otol 92:991–996, 1978
29. Bruce BA: Evaluation of hematoporphyrin photoradiation therapy to treat choroidal melanoma. Lasers Surg Med 4:59–64, 1984
30. Burck KB, Liu ET, Larrick JW: Oncogenes: An Introduction to the Concept of Cancer Genes. New York, Springer-Verlag, 1988
31. Buschke F: What is a radiotherapist (editorial)? Radiology 79:319–321, 1962
32. Bush RS: The complete oncologist: The Buschke Lecture. Int J Radiat Oncol Biol Phys 8:1019–1027 1982
33. Byhardt RW, Cox JD, Hornburg A, et al: Weekly localization films and detection of field placement errors. Int J Radiat Oncol Biol Phys 4:881–887, 1978
34. Byhardt RW, Greenberg M, Cox JD: Local control of squamous carcinoma of oral cavity and oropharynx with 3 vs 5 treatment fractions per week. Int J Radiat Oncol Biol Phys 2:415–420, 1977
35. Calabresi P, Dexter DL. Heppner GA: Clinical and pharmacological implications of cancer cell differentiation and heterogeneity. Biochem Pharmacol 28:1933–1941, 1979
36. Calle R, Fletcher GH, Pierquin B: Le bases de la radiotherapie curative des eiptheliomas mammaires. J Radiol Electrol 54:929–938, 1973
37. Cater DB, Silver IA: Quantitative measurements of oxygen tension in normal tissues and in the tumours of patients before and after radiotherapy. Acta Radiol 53:233–256, 1960
38. Chaplin DJ, Durand RE, Olive PL: Cell selection from a murine tumour using the fluorescent probe Hoechst 33342. Br J Cancer 51:569–572, 1985

39. Chen GTY, Austin-Seymour M, Castro JR, et al: Dose volume histograms in treatment planning evaluation of carcinoma of the pancreas. In International Conference of Computers in Radiation Therapy: Proceedings of 8th International Conference. IEEE Computer Press, 1984
40. Chin LM, Siddon RL, Svensson GK, et al: Progress in 3-D treatment planning for photon beam therapy. Int J Radiat Oncol Biol Phys 11:2011–2020, 1985
41. Churchill-Davidson I: Oxygen effect on radiosensitivity. Proceedings of the Conference on Research of the Radiotherapy of Cancer. New York American Cancer Society, 1961
42. Cohen L: Clinical radiation dosage. II. Interrelation of time, area and therapeutic ratio. Br J Radiol 22:706–713, 1949
43. Cohen L: Radiation response and recovery: Radiobiological principles and their relation to clinical practice. In Schwartz EER (ed): The Biological Basis of Radiation Therapy, pp 208–348. Philadelphia, JB Lippincott, 1966
44. Cohen L: Theoretical "iso-survival" formulae for fractionated radiation therapy. Br J Radiol 41:522–528, 1968
45. Cohen L, Creditor M: Iso-effect tables for tolerance of irradiated normal human tissues. Int J Radiat Oncol Biol Phys 9:233–241, 1983
46. Cohn AM, Peppard SB: Multiple primary malignant tumors of the head and neck Am J Otolaryngol 1:411–417, 1980
47. Coltman CA Jr, Dahlberg S: Treatment-related leukemia. N Engl J Med 322:52–53, 1990
48. Committee for Radiation Oncology Studies: Criteria for Radiation Oncology in Multidisciplinary Cancer Management. Report to the Director of the National Cancer Institute, National Institutes of Health. Philadelphia, American College of Radiology, 1986
49. Cooper JS, Pajak TF, Rubin P, et al: Second malignancies in patients who have head and neck cancer: Incidence, effect on survival and implications based on the RTOG experience. Int J Radiat Oncol Biol Phys 17(3):449–456, 1989
50. Corti L, Tomio L, Maluta S, et al: Recurring gynaecologic cancer treated with photodynamic therapy. Photochem Photobiol 46:949–952, 1987
51. Coutard H: Roentgentherapy of epitheliomas of the tonsillar region, hypopharynx and larynx from 1920 to 1926. Am J Roentgenol 28:313–331, 1932
52. Coutard H: Principles of x-ray therapy of malignant diseases. Lancet 2:1–8, 1934
53. Cox JD: Failure analysis in diagnostic and treatment strategies in cancer management. Cancer Treat Symp 2:1–3, 1983
54. Cox JD: Fractionation: A paradigm for clinical research in radiation oncology. Int J Radiat Oncol Biol Phys 13:1271–1281, 1987
55. Cumberlin RL, Dritschilo A, Mossman KL: Carcinogenic effects of scattered dose associated with radiation therapy. Int J Radiat Oncol Biol Phys 17:623–629, 1989
56. Cunningham JR: Development of computer algorithms for radiation treatment planning. Int J Radiat Oncol Biol Phys 16:1367–1376, 1989
57. Curie P, Curie Mme P, Bemont G: Sur une nouvelle substance fortement radioactive contenue dans la pechblende (note presented by M Becquerel). Compt Rend Acad Sci (Paris) 127:1215–1217, 1898
58. Dale RG: The application of the linear-quadratic dose-effect equation to fractionated and protracted radiotherapy. Br J Radiol 58:515–528, 1985
59. Deacon J, Peckham MJ, Steel GG: The radioresponsiveness of human tumours and the initial slope of the cell survival curve. Radiother Oncol 2:317–323, 1984
60. Delaney TF, Glatstein JE: Photodynamic therapy of cancer. Compr Ther 14:43–55, 1988
61. DeLaney TF, Glatstein JE: Photodynamic Therapy: Theory and Practice. 31st ASTRO Scientific Meeting, Refresher Course #108, 1989
62. del Regato JA: You have come a long way . . . ! 1975 ASTR Presidential Address. Int J Radiat Oncol Biol Phys 1:383–385, 1976
63. Denekamp J: Changes in the rate of repopulation during multifraction irradiation of mouse skin. Br J Radiol 46:381–387, 1973
64. Deviri E, Bartal A, Goldsher M, et al: Occurrence of additional primary neoplasms in patients with laryngeal carcinoma in Israel (1960–1976). Ann Otol Rhinol Laryngol 91:261–265, 1982
65. DeVita VT Jr: Principles of chemotherapy. In DeVita VT Jr, Hellman S, Rosenberg SA (eds): Cancer: Principles and Practice of Oncology, 2nd ed, pp 257–285. Philadelphia, JB Lippincott, 1985
66. DeVita VT, Lippman M, Hubbard SM, et al: The effect of combined modality therapy on local control and survival. Int J Radiat Oncol Biol Phys 12:487–501, 1986
67. deVries N, Snow GB: Multiple primary tumors in laryngeal cancer. J Laryngol Otol 100:915–918, 1986
68. Dewey WC, Hopwood LE, Sapareto SA, et al: Cellular responses to combinations of hyperthermia and radiation. Radiology 123:463–474, 1977
69. Dische S: Hyperbaric oxygen: The Medical Research Council Trials and their clinical significance. Br J Radiol 51:888–894, 1979
70. Dische S: Chemical sensitizers for hypoxic cells: A decade of experience in clinical radiotherapy. Radiother Oncol 3:97–115, 1985
71. Dische S, Martin WMC, Anderson P: Radiation myelopathy in patients treated for carcinoma of the bronchus using a six fraction regime of radiotherapy. Br J Radiol 54:29–35, 1981
72. Doiron DR, Gomer CJ (eds): Porphyrin Localization and Treatment of Tumors. New York, Alan Liss, 1984
73. Doss LL: Localization error and local recurrence in upper airway carcinoma. Proceedings of the Workshop on Quality Control in the Radiotherapy Department of the Cancer and Leukemia Group B (CALGB), New York, May 31, 1979
74. Dougherty TJ: Photosensitization of malignant tumors. Semin Surg Oncol 2:24–37, 1986
75. Douglas BG, Fowler JF: The effect of multiple small doses of x-rays on skin reactions in the mouse and a basic interpretation. Radiat Res 66:401–426, 1976
76. Dritschilo A, Sherman D, Emami B, et al: The cost effectiveness of a radiation therapy simulator: A model for the determination of need. Int J Radiat Oncol Biol Phys 5:243–247, 1979
77. Duncan W: A clinical evaluation of fast neutron therapy. In Steel GG, Adams GE, Peckham MJ (eds): The Biological Basis of Radiotherapy, pp 277–286. Amsterdam, Elsevier Science BV, 1983
78. Durand RE: Chemosensitivity testing in V79 spheroids: Drug delivery and cellular microenvironment. J Natl Cancer Inst 77:247–252, 1986
79. Dutreix J: Expression of the dose rate effect in clinical curietherapy. Radiother Oncol 15:25–37, 1989
80. Dutreix J, Wambersie A, Bounik C: Cellular recovery in human skin reactions: application to dose fraction number overall time relationship in radiotherapy. Eur J Cancer 9:159–167, 1973
81. Dynes JB, Smedal MI: Radiation myeletis. Am J Roentgenol 83:78, 1960
82. Edell ES, Cortese DA: Bronchoscopic phototherapy with hematoporphyrin derivative for treatment of localized bronchogenic carcinoma: A 5-year experience. May Clin Proc 62:8–14, 1987
83. Edelman AH, Holtz S, Powers WE: Radiotherapy for inoperable carcinoma of the breast. Am J Roentgenol 9:585–599, 1965
84. Eichhorn H-J: Different fractionation schemas tested by histological examination of autopsy specimens from lung cancer patients. Br J Radiol 54:132–135, 1981
85. Eilber F: Limb salvage for skeletal and soft tissues sarcomas. Cancer 53:2579–2594, 1984
87. Elkind MM: DNA damage and cell killing: Cause and effect. Cancer 45:2123–2127, 1985
86. Elkind MM: Repair processes in the treatment and induction of cancer with radiation. Cancer 10:2165–2171, 1990
88. Elkind MM, Sutton H: Radiation response of mammalian cells grown in culture. I. Repair of x-ray damage in surviving Chinese hamster cells. Radiat Res 13:556–593, 1960
89. Ellis F: Time, fractionation, and dose rate in radiotherapy. In

Vaeth JM (ed): Frontiers of Radiation Therapy and Oncology, Vol 3, pp 131–140. Basel, S Karger, 1968
90. Ellis F: Time and Dose Relationships in Radiation Biology as Applied to Radiotherapy. Brookhaven National Laboratory, BNL50203 (C-5), p 313, 1969
91. Ellis F: Dose, time and fractionation: A clinical hypothesis. Clin Radiol 20:1–7, 1969
92. Ellis F: Is NSD-TDF useful to radiotherapy? Int J Radiat Oncol Biol Phys 11:1685–1697, 1985
93. Ettinghausen SE, Lipford EH III, Mule JJ, et al: Recombinant interleuken stimulates *in vivo* proliferation of adoptively transferred lymphokine activated killer (LAK) cells. J Immunol 135:3623–3635, 1985
94. Fayos JV, Lampe I: Radiation therapy of carcinoma of the tonsillar region. Am J Roentgenol Radium Ther Nucl Med 111:85–94, 1971
95. Fertil B, Malaise EP: Inherent cellular radiosensitivity as a basic concept for human tumor radiotherapy. Int J Radiat Oncol Biol Phys 7:621–629, 1981
96. Fidler IJ, Hart IR: Biological diversity in metastatic neoplasms: Origins and implications. Science 217:998–1003, 1982
97. Fisher B, Bauer M, Margolese R, et al: Five-year results of a randomized clinical trial comparing total mastectomy and segmental mastectomy with or without radiation in the treatment of breast cancer. N Engl J Med 320:822–828, 1989
98. Fisher B, Fisher ER: Studies concerning the regional lymph nodes in cancer: Initiation of immunity. Cancer 17:1001–1004, 1971
99. Fisher B, Ganduz N, Safter EA: Influence of the interval between primary tumor removal and chemotherapy on kinetics and growth of metastases. Cancer Res 43:1488–1492, 1983
100. Fisher JJ, Rockwell S, Martin DF: Perfluorochemicals and hyperbaric oxygen in radiation therapy. Int J Radiat Oncol Biol Phys 12:95–102, 1986
101. Fletcher GH: Local results of irradiation in the primary management of localized breast cancer. Cancer 29:545–551, 1972
102. Fletcher GH: Clinical dose-response curve of human malignant epithelial tumors. Br J Radiol 46:1–12, 1973
103. Fletcher GH (ed). Textbook of Radiotherapy, 3rd ed, Philadelphia, Lea & Febiger, 1980
104. Fletcher GH: Keynote address: The scientific basis of the present and future practice of clinical radiotherapy. Int J Radiat Oncol Biol Phys 9:1073–1082, 1983
105. Fletcher GH: Implications of the density of clonogenic infestations in radiotherapy. Int J Radiat Oncol Biol Phys 12:1675–1680, 1986
106. Fletcher GH, Shukovsky LJ: The interplay of radiocurability and tolerance in the irradiation of human cancers. J Radiol Electrol 56:383–400, 1975
107. Fowler JF: Fractionation and therapeutic gain. In Steel GE, Adams GE, Peckham MT (eds): Biological Basis of Radiotherapy, pp 181–194. Amsterdam, Elsevier Science, 1983
108. Fowler JF: Rationales for high linear energy transfer radiotherapy. In Steel GG, Adams GE, Peckham JM (eds): The Biological Basis of Radiotherapy, pp 261–268. Amsterdam, Elsevier Science, 1983
109. Fowler JF: La Ronde: Radiation sciences and medical radiology. Radiother Oncol 1:1–22, 1983
110. Fowler JF: The linear quadratic formula and progress in fractionated radiotherapy: A review. Br J Radiol 62:679–694, 1989
111. Fowler JF: How worthwhile are short schedules in radiotherapy? A series of exploratory calculations. Radiother Oncol 18:165–181, 1990
112. Fowler JF, Denekamp J, Page AL, et al: Fractionation with x-rays and neutrons in mice: Response of skin and C3H mammary tumours. Br J Radiol 45:237–249, 1972
113. Fraumeni JF Jr, Hoover RN, Devesa SS, et al: Epidemiology of cancer. In DeVita VT Jr, Hellman S, Rosenberg SA (eds): Cancer: Principles and Practice of Oncology, 3rd ed, pp 196–235. Philadelphia, JB Lippincott, 1989
114. Frei, E: Curative cancer chemotherapy. Cancer Res 45:6523–6537, 1985
115. Frei E III: What's in a name: neoadjuvant. J Natl Cancer Inst 80:1088–1089, 1989
116. Friedman M: Calculated Risks of Radiation Injury of Normal Tissue in the Treatment of Cancer of the Testis, p 390. Proc 2nd National Cancer Conference, Cincinnati, 1952
117. Friedman RM, Merigan T, Sreevalsan T (eds): Interferons as Cell Growth Inhibitors and Antitumor Factors, UCLA Symposia on Molecular and Cellular Biology, New Series Volume 50. New York, Alan Liss, 1986
118. Friend SH, Dryja TP, Weinberg RA: Oncogenes and tumor-suppressing genes. N Engl J Med 318:618–622, 1988
119. Gallagher MJ, Brereton HD, Rostock RA, et al: A prospective study of treatment techniques to minimize the volume of pelvic small bowel with reduction of acute and late effects associated with pelvic irradiation. Int J Radiat Oncol Biol Phys 12:1565–1573, 1986
120. Gastrointestinal Tumor Study Group: Prolongation of the disease-free interval in surgically treated rectal carcinoma. N Engl J Med 312:1465–1472,1985
121. Ghossein A, Bataini JP, Ennuyer A, et al: Local control and site of failure in radically irradiated supraglottic laryngeal cancer. Radiology 112:187–192, 1974
122. Gish JR, Coates EO, Du Sault L, et al: Pulmonary radiation reaction: A vital capacity and time-dose study. Radiology 73:679–683, 1959
123. Gluckman JL, Crissman JD: Survival rates in 548 patients with multiple neoplasms of the upper aerodigestive tract. Laryngoscope 93:71–74, 1983
124. Glucksmann A: Preliminary observations on the quantitative examination of human biopsy material taken from irradiated carcinomata. Br J Radiol 14:187–198, 1941
125. Goitein M: Computed tomography in planning radiation therapy. Int J Radiat Oncol Biol Phys 5:445–447, 1979
126. Goitein M, Abrams M: Multi-dimensional treatment planning. I Delineation of anatomy. Int J Radiat Oncol Biol Phys 9:777–787, 1983
127. Goitein M. Abrams M: Multi-dimensional treatment planning. II. Beam's eye-view, back projection, and projection through CT sections, Int J Radiat Oncol Biol Phys 9:789–797, 1983
128. Golomb HW, Jacobs A, Fefer A, at al: Alpha-2 interferon therapy of hairy cell leukemia: A multicenter study of 64 patients. J Clin Oncol 4:900, 1986
129. Gomer CJ: Photodynamic therapy. Photochem Photobiol 46:561–949, 1987
130. Gomer CJ, Rucker N, Banerjee A, et al: Comparison of mutagenicity and induction of sister chromatid exchange in Chinese hamster cells exposed to hematoporphyrin derivative photoradiation, ionizing radiation, or ultraviolet radiation. Cancer Res 43:2622–2627, 1983
131. Goodman RL, Moore RE, Davis ME et al: Perfluorocarbon emulsions in cancer therapy: Preliminary observations on presently available formulations. Int J Radiat Oncol Biol Phys 10:1421–1424, 1984
132. Graham ML, Cheng AY, Geer LY, et al: A method to analyze 2-dimensional daily radiotherapy portal images from an online fiber-optic imaging system. Int J Radiat Oncol Biol Phys, 20:613–619, 1991
133. Gray LH, Conger AD, Ebert M, et al: The concept of oxygen dissolved in tissues at the time of irradiation as a factor in radiotherapy. Br J Radiol 26:638–648, 1953
134. Gray MJ, Kottmeier HL: Rectal and bladder injuries following radium for carcinoma of the cervix at the Radiumhemmet. Am J Obstet Gynecol 74:1294–1303, 1957
135. Greenfield MM, Stark FM: Postirradiation neuropathy. Am J Roentgenol 60:627–622, 1948
136. Greenwald P, Nixon DW, Malone WF, et al: Concepts in cancer chemoprevention research. Cancer 65:1483–1490, 1990
137. Grossweiner LI: Membrane photosensitization by hematoporphyrin and hematoporphyrin derivative. In Doiron DR, Gomer CJ (eds): Porphyrin Localization and Treatment of Tumors, pp 391–404. New York, Alan Liss, 1984
138. Gunderson LL, Russell AH, Llewellyn HJ, et al: Treatment planning for colorectal cancer: Radiation and surgical tech-

niques and value of small-bowel films. Int J Radiat Oncol Biol Phys 11:1379–1393, 1985

139. Gunduz N, Fisher B, Saffer EA: Effect of surgical removal on the growth and kinetics of residual tumor. Cancer Res 39:3861–3865, 1979
140. Hall EJ: Radiobiology for the Radiologist, 3rd ed, pp 275–290.Philadelphia, JB Lippincott, 1988
141. Hall EJ: Dose-rate considerations. In Hilaris BS, Batata MA (eds): Brachytherapy Oncology–1983, pp 33–39. New York, Memorial Sloan-Kettering Cancer Center, 1983
142. Hall EJ, Brenner DJ: The dose-rate effect revisited: radiobiological considerations of the importance in radiotherapy. Int J Radiat Oncol Biol Phys, in press
143. Hanks GE, Kinzie JJ, White RL, et al: Patterns of care outcome studies: Results of the national practice in Hodgkin's disease. Cancer 51:569–573, 1983
144. Hayata Y, Dougherty TJ (eds): Lasers and Hematoporphyrin Derivative in Cancer. Tokyo, Igaku-Shoin, 1983
145. Hayata Y, Kato H: Applications of laser phototherapy in the diagnosis and treatment of lung cancer. Jpn Ann Thorac Surg 3:203–210, 1983
146. Hendrickson FR: Four P's of human error in treatment delivery. Int J Radiat Oncol Biol Phys 4:913–914, 1978
147. Henk JM, Smith CW: Radiotherapy and hyperbaric oxygen in head and neck cancer. Lancet 1:104–105, 1977
148. Hermens AF, Barendsen GW: The proliferative status and clonogenic capacity of tumor cells in a transplantable rhabdomyosarcoma of the rat before and after irradiation with 800 rad of x-rays. Cell Tissue Kinet 11:83–100, 1978
149. Herring DF: The consequences of dose response curves for tumor control and normal tissue injury on the precision necessary in patient management. Laryngoscope 85:1112, 1975
150. Hirst DG, Denekamp J: Tumour cell proliferation in relation to the vasculature. Cell Tissue Kinet 12:31–42, 1979
151. Holmgren J (ed): Tumor Marker Antigens. Goteborg, Sweden Studentlitteratur, 1985
152. Hopewell JW, Gunn Y: Factors for correcting the CRE formula for late effects in normal tissues: How valid are they (letter to editor)? Int J Radiat Oncol Biol Phys 7:683–684, 1981
153. Hopewell JW, Wiernik G: Tolerance of the pig kidney to fractionated x-irradiation. In Beck ERA (ed): Radiobiological Research and Radiotherapy, Proc Symp Vienna 1976, vol 1, pp 65–73. Vienna, IAEA, 1977
154. Hordijk GJ, de Jong JMA: Synchronous and metachronous tumors in patients with head and neck cancer. J Laryngol Otol 97:619–621, 1983
155. Horiot JC, van den Bogaert W, Ang KK, et al: European Organization for Research on Treatment of Cancer Trials using radiotherapy with multiple fractions per day: A 1978–1987 survey. Front Radiat Ther Oncol 22:149–161, 1988
156. Horning SJ: Biologic Repair Modifiers. Int J Radiat Oncol Biol Phys 17(Suppl 1):92–93, 1989
157. Hulshof M, Venuytsel L, van den Bogaert W, et al: Localization errors in mantle-field irradiation for Hodgkin's disease. Int J Radiat Oncol Biol Phys 17:679–683, 1989
158. ICRU: Determination of absorbed dose in a patient irradiated by beams of X or gamma rays. In Radiotherapy Procedures, ICRU Report 24. Washington, DC, International Commission of Radiation Units and Measurements, 1976
159. Inter-Society Council for Radiation Oncology: Radiation Oncology in Integrated Cancer Management. Philadelphia, American College of Radiology, November 1986
160. Jacobs AJ, Faris C, Perez CA, et al: Short-term persistence of carcinoma of the uterine cervix following radiation: An indicator of long-term prognosis. Cancer 57:944–950, 1986
161. Jampolis S, Pipard G, Horiot JC, et al: Preliminary results using twice a day fractionation in the radiotherapeutic management of advanced cancers of the head and neck. AJR 129:1091–1093, 1977
162. Johns JE, Cunningham JR: The Physics of Radiology, 3rd ed. Springfield, IL, Charles C Thomas, 1969
163. Johnson RJR: Gynecological Cancer Treated with Cobalt under Hyperbaric Conditions, pp 185–194. First Annual San Francisco Cancer Symposium, 1966
164. Jones A: Transient radiation myelopathy (with reference to Lhermitte's sign of electrical paraesthesia). Br J Radiol 37:727–744, 1964
165. Kaldor JM, Day NE, Clarke EA, et al: Leukemia following Hodgkin's disease. N Engl J Med 322:7–13, 1990
166. Kallman RF: The phenomenon of reoxygenation and its implications for fractionated radiotherapy. Radiology 105:135–142, 1972
167. Kaplan HS: Radiobiology's contribution to radiotherapy: Promise or mirage? Failla Memorial Lecture. Radiat Res 43:460–476, 1970
168. Kaye AH, Morstyn G, Brownbill HD: Adjuvant high-dose photoradiation therapy in the treatment of cerebral gliomas: A phase I–II study. J Neurosurg 67:500–505, 1987
169. Kessel D, Dougherty TJ (eds): Porphyrin Photosensitization. New York, Plenum Press, 1983
170. Kinzie JJ, Hanks GE, Maclean CJ, et al: Patterns of Care Study: Hodgkin's disease relapse rates and adequacy of portals. Cancer 52:2223–2226, 1983
171. Kirk J, Gray WM, Watson ER: Cumulative radiation effect. I. Fractionated treatment regimens. Clin Radiol 122:145–155, 1971
172. Kitabatake T, Hattori H, Okumura Y: Optimum energy in supervoltage x-ray therapy. Strahlentherapie 137:158, 1969
173. Knox SJ, Levy R, Miller RA, et al: The radiobiological effect of ^{131}I-anti-idiotype monoclonal antibody therapy (*MAB) in murine B cell lymphoma compared with continuous decaying low dose rate and acutely fractionated external beam irradiation (abstract). Int J Radiat Oncol Biol Phys 17(suppl 1):118, 1989
174. Kohler G, Milstein C: Derivation of specific antibody producing tissue culture and tumor lines by cell fusion. Eur J Immunol 6:511, 1976
175. Kok G: The influence of the size of the fraction dose on normal and tumor tissue ^{60}Co radiation treatment of carcinoma of the larynx and inoperable carcinoma of the breast. Radiol Clin Biol 40:100–115, 1971
176. Kopf AW: Prevention and early detection of skin cancer: melanoma. Cancer 62:1791, 1988
177. Kramer S: An overview of process and outcome data in the Patterns of Care Study. Int J Radiat Oncol Biol Phys 7:795–800, 1981
178. Kramer S, Herring D: The Patterns of Care Study: a nationwide evaluation of the practice of radiation therapy in cancer management. Int J Radiat Oncol Biol Phys 1:1231–1236, 1976
179. Kronig S, Friedrich W: Physikalische und biologische Grundlagen der Strahlentherapie. Sonderbtrand der Strahlentherapie, 1918
180. Kunkler PB, Farr RF, Luxton RW: The limit of renal tolerance to x-rays: An investigation into renal damage occurring following the treatment of tumours of the testis by abdominal baths. Br J Radiol 25:192–201, 1952
181. Lai PP, Shapiro SJ, Perez CA: Carcinoma of the prostate stage B and C: influence of duration of radiotherapy (abstract). Int J Radiat Oncol Biol Phys 17(Suppl 1):164, 1989
182. Lampe I: Radiation tolerance of the central nervous system. In Buschke F (ed): Progress in Radiation Therapy. New York, Grune & Stratton, 1958
183. Land H, Parada LF, Weinberg RA: Cellular oncogenes and multistep carcinogenesis. Science 222:771–778, 1983
184. Laws ER, Cortese DA, Kinsey JH, et al: Photoradiation therapy in the treatment of malignant brain tumors: A phase I (feasibility) study. Neurosurgery 9:672–678, 1981
185. LeCouteur RA, Gillette EL, Powers BE, et al: Peripheral neuropathies following experimental intraoperative radiation therapy (IORT). Int J Radiat Oncol Biol Phys 17:583–590, 1989
186. Ledingham JM, Cohen M: Hypertension following irradiation of kidneys. Lancet i:9, 1958
187. Levitt S, Potish RA: The case for adjuvant CMF chemotherapy in breast cancer: Has it been made? Cancer Clin Trials 4:363–369, 1981
188. Lichter AS, Fraass BA, McShan DL: Recent advances in radiotherapy treatment planning. Oncology 2:43–57, 1988

189. Lindberg, Martin RG, Romsdahl MM, et al: Conservative surgery and postoperative radiotherapy in 300 adults with soft-tissue sarcomas. Cancer 47:2391–2397, 1981
190. Lindgren M: On tolerance of brain tissue and sensitivity of brain tumours to irradiation. Acta Radiol (Suppl) 170:1–73, 1958
191. Liotta LA: Tumor invasion and metastases: Role of the extracellular matrix: Rhoads Memorial Award Lecture. Cancer Res 46:1–7, 1986
192. Liotta LA: Gene products which play a role in cancer invasion and metastasis. Breast Cancer Res Treat 11:113–124, 1988
193. Liotta LA, Mandler R, Murano G, et al: Tumor cell autocrine motility factor. Proc Natl Acad Sci USA 83:3302–3306, 1986
194. Liotta LA, Thorgeirsson UP, Garbisa SL: Role of collagenases in tumor cell invasion. Cancer Met Rev 1:277–288, 1982
195. Lipson RL, Baldes EJ, Olsen EM: Hematoporphyrin derivative for detection and management of cancer. Proceedings of the IX International Cancer Congress, 1966
196. Littbrand B, Edsmyr F: Hyperfractionated Radiotherapy of Carcinoma of the Urinary Bladder. Presented at Third International Meeting on Progress in Radio-Oncology, Vienna, Austria, 1985
197. Liu K, Moss D, Persky V: Dietary cholesterol, fat, and fibre, and colon-cancer mortality. Lancet 2:782, 1979
198. Liversage WE: A general formula for equating protracted and acute regimes of radiation. Br J Radiol 42:432–440, 1969
199. Lundgren J, Olofsson J: Multiple primary malignancies in patients treated for laryngeal carcinoma. J Otolaryngol 15(3):145–150, 1986
200. Luxton RW, Kunkler PB: Radiation nephritis. Acta Radiol (Ther Phys Biol) 2:169–178, 1964
201. Lyon JL, Gardner JW, West DW: Cancer incidence in Mormons and non-Mormons in Utah during 1967–75. J Natl Cancer Inst 65:1055, 1980
202. MacComb WS, Quimby EH: The rate of recovery of human skin from the effects of hard or soft roentgen rays or gamma rays. Radiology 27:196–207, 1936
203. Maciejewski B, Withers HR, Taylor JMG, Hliniak A: Dose fractionation and regeneration in radiotherapy for cancer of the oral cavity and oropharynx. II. Normal tissue responses: Acute and late effects. Int J Radiat Oncol Biol Phys 18:101–111, 1990
204. Macki TR, Scrimger JW, Battista JJ: A convolution method of calculating dose for 15 MV x-rays. Med Phys 12:188–196, 1985
205. MacLennen R, Jensen OM, Mosbech J, et al: Diet, transit time, stool weight, and colon cancer in two Scandinavian populations. Am J Clin Nutr (Suppl) 31:S239, 1978
206. Maisel RH, Vermeersch H: Panendoscopy for second primaries in head and neck cancer. Ann Otol Rhinol Laryngol 90:460–464, 1981
207. Malkin A: Tumor markers. In Tannock IF, Hill RP (eds): The Basic Science of Oncology, pp 192–203. New York, Pergamon Press, 1987
208. Marcial VA, Hanley JA, Davis LW, et al: Split-course radiation therapy of carcinoma of the base of the tongue: Results of a prospective national collaborative clinical trial of the Radiation Therapy Oncology Group. Int J Radiat Oncol Biol Phys 9:437–443, 1983
209. Marcial VA, Pajak TF, Chang C, et al: Hyperfractionated photon radiation therapy in the treatment of advanced squamous cell carcinoma of the oral cavity, pharynx, larynx, and sinuses, using radiation therapy as the only planned modality: Preliminary report by the Radiation Therapy Oncology Group (RTOG). Int J Radiat Oncol Biol Phys 13:41–47, 1987
210. Marcus RB Jr, Million RR: The incidence of myelitis after irradiation of the cervical spinal cord. Int J Radiat Oncol Biol Phys 19:3–8, 1990
211. Marks JE, Bedwinek JM, Lee F, et al: Dose-response analysis for nasopharyngeal carcinoma. Cancer 50:1042–1050, 1982
212. Marks JE, Haus AG: The effect of immobilization on localization errors in the radiotherapy of head and neck cancer. Clin Radiol 27:175–177, 1976
213. Marks JE, Haus AG, Sutton HG, et al: Localization error in the radiotherapy of Hodgkin's disease and malignant lymphoma with extended mantle fields. Cancer 34:83–90, 1974
214. Mathe G, Kamel M, Dezfulian M, et al: An experimental screening for "systemic adjuvants of immunity" applicable in cancer immunotherapy. Cancer Res 33:1987–1997, 1973
215. McCaughan JS Jr: Overview of experience with photodynamic therapy for malignancy in 192 patients. Photochem Photobiol 46:903–909, 1987
216. McCulloch P, George WD: Warfarin inhibition of metastasses: the role of anticoagulation. Br J Surg 74:879–883, 1987
217. McCunniff AJ, Laing MJ: Radiation tolerance of the cervical spinal cord. Int J Radiat Oncol Biol Phys 16:675–678, 1989
218. McDonald S, Haie C, Rubin P, et al: Second malignant tumors in patients with laryngeal carcinoma: Diagnosis, treatment, and prevention. Int J Radiat Oncol Biol Phys 17(3):457–465, 1989
219. McShan DL, Fraass BA, Lichter AS: Full integration of the beam's eye view concept into computerized treatment planning. Int J Radiat Oncol Biol Phys 18:1485–1494, 1990
220. McShan DL, Silverman A, Lanza DM, et al: A computerized three-dimensional treatment planning system utilizing interactive colour graphics. Br J Radiol 52:478–481, 1979
221. Mendelsohn ML: The biology of dose-limiting tissues. In Time and Dose Relationships in Radiation Biology as Applied to Radiotherapy, Brookhaven National Laboratory (BNL) Report 5023 (C-57), pp 154–173. Upton, NY, Brookhaven National Laboratory, 1969
222. Mendelsohn ML: Radiotherapy and tolerance. In Vaeth JM (ed): Frontiers of Radiation Therapy and Oncology, pp 512–528. Baltimore, University Park Press, 1972
223. Mendenhall WM, Million RR, Cassisi NJ: Elective neck irradiation in squamous cell carcinoma of the head and neck. Head Neck Surg 3:15–20, 1980
224. Meoz RT, Spanos WJ, Doss L, et al: Misonidazole combined with large-fraction pelvic irradiation in the treatment of patients with advanced pelvic malignancies: Preliminary report of an ongoing RTOG phase I/II study. Am J Clin Oncol 6:417–422, 1983
225. Meoz-Mendez RT, Fletcher GH, Guillamondegui OM, et al: Analysis of the results of irradiation in the treatment of squamous cell carcinomas of the pharyngeal walls. Int J Radiat Oncol Biol Phys 4:579–585, 1978
226. Metz CE, Tokars RP, Kronman HB, et al: Maximum likelihood estimation of dose-response parameters for therapeutic operating characteristic (TOC) analysis of carcinoma of the nasopharynx. Int J Radiat Oncol Biol Phys 8:1185–1192, 1983
227. Miescher G: Erfolge der karzinombehandlung an der Dermatologischen Klinik Zurich. Einzeitige Hochstdosis and Fraktionierte Behandlung. Strahlentherapie 49:65–81, 1934
228. Minden MD: Oncogenes. In Tannock IF, Hill RP (eds): The Basic Science of Oncology, pp 72–88. New York, Pergamon Press, 1987
229. Miyahara H, Yoshino K, Umatani K, et al: Multiple primary tumors in laryngeal cancer. J Laryngol Otol 99:999–1004, 1985
230. Moench HC, Phillips TL: Carcinoma of the nasopharynx: Review of 146 patients with emphasis on radiation dose and time factors. Am J Surg 124:515–518, 1972
231. Moertel CCG, Fleming TR, Macdonald JS, et al: Levamisole and fluorouracil for adjuvant therapy of resected colon carcinoma. N Engl J Med 322:352–358, 1989
232. Mohan R, Chui C, Lidofsky L: Differential pencil beam dose computation model for photons. Med Phys 13:64–73, 1986
233. Montague ED: Experience with altered fractionation in radiation therapy of breast cancer. Radiology 90:962–966, 1968
234. Montague ED: Conservation surgery and radiation therapy in the treatment of operable breast cancer. Cancer 53:700–704, 1984
235. Montana GS, Fowler WC, Varia MA, et al: Carcinoma of the cervix, stage III: Results of radiation therapy. Cancer 57:148–154, 1986
236. Moore DH, Mendelsohn ML: Optimal treatment levels in cancer therapy. Cancer 30:97–106, 1972
237. Moss WT, Brand WN, Battifora H (eds): Radiation Oncology:

Rationale, Techniques, Results, 5th ed, pp 24–25. St. Louis, CV Mosby, 1979

238. Muggia FM: Primary chemotherapy: Concepts and issues. In Wagedner DJJ, Blijham GH, Smeets JBG, Wils JA (eds): Primary Chemotherapy in Cancer Medicine, pp 377–383. New York, Alan Liss, 1985
239. Muggia FM, Gill I: Primary chemotherapy. PPO Updates 4:1–12, 1990
240. Muller PJ, Wilson BC: Photodynamic therapy of malignant primary brain tumors: Clinical effects, post-operative ICP, and light penetration of the brain. Photochem Photobiol 46:929–935, 1987
241. Murphree AL, Cote M, Gomer CJ: The evaluation of photodynamic therapy techniques in the treatment of intraocular tumors. Photochem Photobiol 46:919–923, 1987
242. National Council on Radiation Protection and Measurements: Comparative Carcinogenicity of Ionizing Radiation and Chemicals, NCRP Report No. 96. Bethesda, National Council on Radiation Protection and Measurements, 1989
243. Nau MM, Brooks BJ, Battey J, et al: L-myc, a new myc-related gene amplified and expressed in human small cell lung cancer. Nature 317:69–73, 1985
244. Nederman T, Carlsson J, Malmqvist M: Penetration of substances into tumor tissue: A methodological study on cellular spheroids. In Vitro 17:290–298, 1981
245. Northrop M, Fletcher GH, Jesse RH, et al: Evolution of neck disease in patients with primary squamous cell carcinoma of the oral tongue, floor of mouth, and palatine arch, and clinically positive neck nodes neither fixed nor bilateral. Cancer 29:23–30, 1972
246. Olmi P, Cellai E, Chiavacci A, et al: Accelerated fractionation in advanced head and neck cancer: Results and analysis of late sequelae. Radiother Oncol 17:199–207, 1990
247. Olsen JH: Second cancer following cancer of the respiratory system in Denmark, 1943–80. Natl Cancer Inst Monogr 68:309–312, 1985
248. Order S: Presidential Address: systemic radiotherapy–the new frontier. Int J Radiat Oncol Biol Phys 18:981–992, 1990
249. Orton CG: Time-dose factors (TDFs) in brachytherapy. Br J Radiol 47:603–607, 1974
250. Orton CG: Errors in applying the NSD concept. Radiology 115:233–235, 1975
251. Orton CG, Webber BM: Time-dose factor (TDF) analysis of dose rate effects in permanent implant dosimetry. Int J Radiat Oncol Biol Phys 2:55–60, 1977
252. Orton CG: Other considerations in 3-dimensional treatment planning. In Bagne F (ed): Computerized Treatment Planning Systems, pp 136–141, HHS Publications FDA 84-8223, 1984
253. Orton CG, Cohen L: A unified approach to dose-effect relationships in radiotherapy. I Modified TDF and linear quadratic equations. Int J Radiat Oncol Biol Phys 14:549–556, 1988
254. Orton CG, Ellis F: A simplification in the use of the NSD concept in practical radiotherapy. Br J Radiol 46:529–537, 1973
255. Pallis CA, Louis S, Morgan RL: Radiation myelopathy. Brain 84:460, 1961
256. Parker RG, Enstrom JE: Second primary cancers of the head and neck following treatment of initial primary head and neck cancers. Int J Radiat Oncol Biol Phys 14:561–564, 1988
257. Parsons JT: Time-dose-volume relationships in radiation therapy. In Million RR, Cassissi NJ (eds): Management of Head and Neck Cancer: A Multidisciplinary Approach, pp 137–172. Philadelphia, JB Lippincott, 1984
258. Parsons JT, Bova FJ, Million RR: A re-evaluation of split-course technique for squamous cell carcinoma of the head and neck. Int J Radiat Oncol Biol Phys 6:1645–1652, 1980
259. Parsons JT, Thar TL, Bova FJ, et al: An evaluation of split-course irradiation for pelvic malignancies. Int J Radiat Oncol Biol Phys 6:175–181, 1980
260. Pass HI, DeLaney TF, Smith PD, et al: Bronchoscopic phototherapy at comparable dose rates: Early results. Ann Thorac Surg 47:693–699, 1989
261. Paterson RP: The radical x-ray treatment of the carcinomata. Br J Radiol 9:671–679, 1936
262. Paterson R: The Treatment of Malignant Disease by Radium and X-ray: Being a Practice of Radiotherapy. Baltimore, Williams & Wilkins, 1949
263. Paterson R: Studies in optimum dosage. Br J Radiol 25:505–516, 1952
264. Paterson E, Gilbert CW, Matthews JJ: Time-intensity factors and whole body irradiation. Br J Radiol 25:427, 1952
265. Perez CA: The critical need for accurate treatment planning and quality control in radiation therapy. Int J Radiat Oncol Biol Phys 2:815–818, 1977
266. Perez CA, Ackerman LV, Mill WB, et al: Malignant tumors of the tonsil: Analysis of failures and factors affecting prognosis. Am J Roentgenol Radium Ther Nucl Med 114:43–58, 1972
267. Perez CA, Bauer M, Edelstein S, et al: Impact of tumor control on survival in carcinoma of the lung treated with irradiation. Int J Radiat Oncol Biol Phys 12:539–547, 1986
268. Perez CA, Breaux S, Bedwinek JM, et al: Radiation therapy alone in the treatment of carcinoma of the uterine cervix. II. Analysis of complications. Cancer 54:235–246, 1984
269. Perez CA, Breaux S, Madoc-Jones H, et al: Radiation therapy alone in the treatment of carcinoma of the uterine cervis. I. Analysis of tumor recurrence. Cancer 51:1393–1402, 1983
270. Perez CA, Gardner P, Glasgow GP: Radiotherapy quality assurance in clinical trials. Int J Radiat Oncol Biol Phys 10:119–125, 1984
271. Perez CA, Kuske RR, Camel HM, et al: Analysis of pelvic tumor control and impact on survival in carcinoma of the uterine cervix treated with radiation therapy alone. Int J Radiat Oncol Biol Phys 14:613–621, 1988
272. Perez CA, Marks J, Powers WE: Preoperative irradiation in head and neck cancer. Semin Oncol 4:387–397, 1977
273. Perez CA, Pilepich MV, Zivnuska F: Tumor control in definitive irradiation of localized carcinoma of the prostate. Int J Radiat Oncol Biol Phys 12:523–531, 1986
274. Perez CA, Powers WE: Studies on optimal dose of preoperative irradiation and time for surgery in the cure of a mouse lymphosarcoma. Radiology 89:116–122, 1967
275. Perez CA, Purdy JA: Rationale for treatment planning in radiation therapy. In Levitt SH (ed): Technological Basis of Radiation Therapy: Practical Clinical Applications, 2nd ed. Philadelphia, Lea & Febiger, in press
276. Perez CA, Stewart CC, Wagner B: Role of the regional lymph nodes in tumor immunity. In Proceedings of the Conference on Interaction of Radiation and Host Immune Defense Mechanism in Malignancy, pp 225–244. Upton, NY, Brookhaven National Laboratories, 1974
277. Perez CA, Thomas PRM: Radiation therapy: Basic concepts and clinical implications. In Sutow W, Fernbach DJ, Vietti TJ (eds): Clinical Pediatric Oncology, 3rd ed, pp 167–209. St. Louis, CV Mosby, 1984
278. Peschel RE, Fischer JJ: Multiple daily fractionation schedules. Int J Radiat Oncol Biol Phys 8:1811–1812, 1982
279. Peters LJ: Inherent radiosensitivity of tumor and normal tissue cells as a predictor of human tumor response. Radiother Oncol 17:177–190, 1990
280. Peters LJ, Brock WA, Chapman JD, et al: Predictive assays of tumor radiocurability. Am J Clin Oncol 11:275–287, 1988
281. Peters LJ, Withers HR: Factors for correcting the CRE-formula for late effects in normal tissues: How valid are they (letter to editor)? Int J Radiat Oncol Biol Phys 7:684–685, 1981
282. Pierquin B, Baillet F, Brown CH: Low dose irradiation in advanced tumors of head and neck. Acta Radiol 14:497–504, 1975
283. Pierquin B, Chassagne D, Baillet F, et al: Clinical observations on the time factor in interstitial radiotherapy using iridium 192. Clin Radiol 24:506–509, 1973
284. Pitot HC: Principles of cancer biology: Chemical carcinogenesis. In DeVita VT Jr, Hellman S, Rosenberg SA (eds): Cancer: Principles and Practice of Oncology, pp 79–100. Philadelphia, JB Lippincott, 1985
285. Pourquier H, Delard R, Achille E, et al: A quantified approach to the analysis and prevention of urinary complications in radiotherapeutic treatment of cancer of the cervix. Int J Radiat Oncol Biol Phys 13:1025–1033, 1987

286. Pourquier H, Dubois JB, Delard R: Cancer of the uterine cervix: Dosimetric guidelines for prevention of late rectal and rectosigmoid complications as a result of radiotherapeutic treatment. Int J Radiat Oncol Biol Phys 8:1887–1895, 1982
287. Powers BE, Gillette EL, McChesney SL, et al: Bone necrosis and tumor induction following experimental intraoperative irradiation. Int J Radiat Oncol Biol Phys 17:559–567, 1989
288. Powers WE, Tolmach LJ: Preoperative radiation therapy, biological basis and experimental investigations. Nature (Lond) 201:272–273, 1964
289. Powers WE, Tolmach LJ: Demonstration of an anoxic component in a mouse tumor-cell population by *in vivo* assay of survival following irradiation. Radiology 83:328–336, 1964
290. Press OW, Eary JF, Badger CC, et al: Treatment of refractory non-Hodgkin's lymphoma with radiolabeled MB-1 (anti-CD37) antibody. J Clin Oncol 7:1027–1038, 1989
291. Prewitt JMS: Optimization criteria and strategies for radiotherapy. I Feasibility of an alogorithmic approach. Proc San Diego Biomed 12(Suppl):175–182, 1973
292. Prout GR, Lin CW, Benson R, et al: Photodynamic therapy with hematoporphyrin derivative in the treatment of superficial transitional-cell carcinoma of the bladder. N Engl J Med 317:1251–1256, 1987
293. Puck TT, Marcus PI: Actions of x-rays on mammalian cells. J Exp Med 103:653–666, 1956
294. Purdy JA, Wong JW, Harms WB, et al: Three dimensional radiation treatment planning system. Proceedings of the 9th International Conference on the Use of Computers in Radiation Therapy, Scheveningen, The Netherlands, North Holland, Netherlands, 1987
295. Purdy JA, Wong JW, Harms WB, et al: State of the art of high energy photon treatment planning. Front Radiat Ther Oncol 21:4–24, 1987
296. Rabinowitz I, Broomberg J, Goitein M, et al: Accuracy of radiation field alignment in clinical practice. Int J Radiat Oncol Biol Phys 11:1857–1867, 1985
297. Rayner AA, Grimm EA, Lotze MT, et al: Lymphokine-activated killer (LAK) cell phenomenon: Analysis of factors relevant to the imunotherapy of human cancer. Cancer 55:1327–1333, 1985
298. Regaud C, Ferroux R: Discordance des effects de rayons X, d'une part dans le testicule, par le peau, d'autre part dans le fractionment de la dose. Compt Rend Soc Biol 97:431–434, 1927
299. Reisner A: Hauterythem und rotgenstrahlung. Ergeb Med Strahlenforsch 6:1, 1933
300. Rettenmaier MA, Berman ML, DiSaia PJ, et al: Gynecologic uses of photoradiation therapy. Adv Exp Med Biol 170:767–775, 1984
301. Reuter SR: An overview of informed consent for radiologists. AJR 148:219–227, 1987
302. Risch HA, Jain M, Choi NW, et al: Dietary factors and the incidence of cancer of the stomach. Am J Epidemiol 122:947–959, 1985
303. Roentgen WC: "On a new kind of rays (preliminary communication)." Translation of a paper read before the Physikalische-medicinischen Gesellschaft of Wurzburg on December 28, 1985. Br J Radiol 4:32, 1931
304. Romsdahl MM, Withers HR: Radiotherapy combined with curative surgery. Arch Surg 113:446–453, 1978
305. Ron E, Modan B, Boice JD, et al: Tumors of the brain and nervous system after radiotherapy in childhood. N Engl J Med 319:1033–1039, 1988
306. Rose C, Lustig R, McIntosh N, et al: A clinical trial of fluosol DA 20% in advanced squamous cell carcinoma of the head and neck. Int J Radiat Oncol Biol Phys 12:1325–1327, 1988
307. Rosenberg SA: Prospective randomized trials demonstrating the efficacy of adjuvant chemotherapy in adult patients with soft tissue sarcomas. Cancer Treat Rep 68:1067–1078, 1984
308. Rosenberg SA, Kaplan HS, Hoppe RT, et al: An overview of the rationale and results of Stanford randomized trials in the treatment of Hodgkin's disease: 1957–1980. In Jones SE, Salmon SE (eds): Adjuvant Therapy of Cancer III, pp 65–78. New York, Grune & Stratton, 1981
309. Rosenberg SA, Longo DL, Lotze MT: Principles and applications of biologic therapy. In Devita VT Jr, Hellman S, Rosenberg SA (eds): Cancer: Principles and Practice of Oncology, 3rd ed, pp 301–347. Philadelphia, JB Lippincott, 1989
310. Rosenberg SA, Lotze MT, Mule JJ: New approaches to the immunotherapy of cancer. Ann Intern Med 108;853–864, 1988
311. Rosenberg SA, Lotze MT, Muul LM, et al: A progress report on the treatment of 157 patients with advanced cancer using lymphokine-activated killer cells and interleukin-2 or high-dose interleukin-2 alone. N Engl J Med 316:889–897, 1987
312. Rosenberg SA, Packard BS, Aebersold PM, et al: Immunotherapy of patients with metastatic melanoma using tumor infiltrating lymphocytes and interleukin-2: preliminary report. N Engl J Med 319:1676–1680, 1988
313. Rosenthal RS: Malpractice: Cause and its prevention. Laryngoscope 88:1–11, 1978
314. Ross WM: The radiotherapeutic and radiological aspects of radiation fibrosis of the lungs. Thorax 11:241–248, 1956
315. Roswit B, Higgins GA Jr, Keehn RJ: Preoperative irradiation for carcinoma of the rectum and rectosigmoid colon: Report of a National Veterans Administration randomized study. Cancer 35:1597–1602, 1975
316. Rowley JD: Biological implications of consistent chromosome rearrangements in leukemia and lymphoma. Cancer Res 44:3159–3168, 1984
317. Rubin P: Clinical Oncology: A Multidisciplinary Approach, 6th ed. New York, American Cancer Society, 1983
318. Rubin P: The emergence of radiation oncology as a distinct medical specialty. Int J Radiat Oncol Biol Phys 11:1247–1270, 1985
319. Rubin P, Casarett GW: Clinical Radiation Pathology, vols 1 and 2. Philadelphia, WB Saunders, 1968
320. Rubin P, Cooper R, Phillips TL (eds): Radiation Biology and Radiation Pathology Syllabus (Set RT 1:Radiation Oncology). Chicago, American College of Radiology, 1975
321. Sause WT, Stewart JR, Plenk HP, et al: Late skin changes following twice-weekly electron beam radiation to post-mastectomy chest wall. Int J Radiat Oncol Biol Phys 7:1541–1544, 1981
322. Schneider JJ, Fletcher GH, Barkley HT Jr: Control by irradiation alone of nonfixed clinically positive lymph nodes from squamous cell carcinoma of the oral cavity, oropharynx, supraglottic larynx, and hypopharynx. Am J Roentgenol Radium Ther Med 123:42–48, 1975
323. Schuh M, Nseyo UO, Potter WR, et al: Photodynamic therapy for palliation of locally recurrent breast carcinoma. J Clin Oncol 5:1766–1799, 1987
324. Schwarz G: Heilung teifliegender Karzinome durch Rontgenbestrahlung von der Korperoberflache. Munch Med Wochenschr 61:1733, 1914
325. Seeger RC, Broudeur GM, Sather H, et al: Association of multiple copies of the N-myc oncogene in untreated human neuroblastomas. N Engl J Med 313:1111–1116, 1985
326. Shaw EG, Gunderson LL, Martin JK, et al: Peripheral nerve and unreteral tolerance to intraoperative radiation therapy: Clinical and dose-response analysis. Consensus Meeting on Phase III Trials in Intraoperative Radiation Therapy, Philadelphia, July 10–11, 1987
327. Shikhani AH, Mantanoski GM, Jones MM, et al: Multiple primary malignancies in head and neck cancer. Arch Otolaryngol Head Neck Surg 112:1172–1179, 1986
328. Shons AR, McQuarrie DG: Multiple primary epidermoid carcinomas of the upper aerodigestive tract. Arch Surg 120: 1007–1009, 1985
329. Shukovsky LJ: Dose, time, volume relationships in squamous cell carcinoma of the supraglottic larynx. Am J Roentgenol 108:27–29, 1970
330. Shukovsky LJ, Baeza MR, Fletcher GH: Results of irradiation of squamous cell carcinomas of the glossopalatine sulcus. Radiology 120:405–408, 1976
331. Shukovsky LJ, Fletcher GH: Time-dose and tumor volume relationships in the irradiation of squamous cell carcinoma of the tonsillar fossa. Radiology 107:621–626, 1973
332. Simpson JR, Perez CA, Phillips TL, et al: Large fraction radiotherapy plus misonidazole for treatment of advanced lung

cancer: Report of a phase I/II trial. Int J Radiat Oncol Biol Phys 8:303–308, 1982

333. Sinclair WK: Fifty years of neutrons in biology and medicine: The comparative effects of neutrons in biological systems. In Booz J, Ebert H (eds): Proceedings of the Eighth Symposium in Microdosimetry, p 1. Luxembourg; Eur 8395 Commission European Communities, 1983
334. Singh K: Two regimens with the same TDF but differing morbidity used in the treatment of stage III carcinoma of the cervix. Br J Radiol 51:357–362, 1978
335. Skipper HE, Schabel FM JR, Mellet LB, et al: Implications of biochemical cytokinetic, pharmacologic and toxicologic relationships in the design of optimal therapeutic schedules. Cancer Chemother Rep 54:431–450, 1950
336. Slamon DJ: Proto-oncogenes and human cancers. N Engl J Med 317:955–957, 1987
337. Slamon DJ, Clark GM, Wong SG, et al: Human breast cancer: Correlation of relapse and survival with amplification of the HER-2/neu oncogene. Science 235:177–182, 1987
338. Smith LM, Donaldson SS, Egbert PR, et al: Aggressive management of second primary tumors in survivors of hereditary retinoblastoma. Int J Radiat Oncol Biol Phys 17:499–505, 1989
339. Sobel ME: Metastasis suppressor genes. J Natl Cancer Inst 82(4):267–276, 1990
340. Sobel S, Rubin P, Keller B, Poulter C: Tumor persistence as a predictor of outcome after radiation therapy of head and neck cancers. Int J Radiat Oncol Biol Phys 1:873–880, 1976
341. Song CW, Zhang WL, Pence DM, et al: Increased radiosensitivity of tumors by perfluorochemicals and carbogen. Int J Radiat Oncol Biol Phys 11:1833–1836, 1985
342. Spanos W Jr, Guse C, Perez CA, et al: Phase II study of multiple daily fractionations in the palliation of advanced pelvic malignancies: Preliminary report of RTOG 85-02. Int J Radiat Oncol Biol Phys 17:659–661, 1989
343. Spanos WJ, Montague ED, Fletcher GH: Late complications of radiation only for advanced breast cancer. Int J Radiat Oncol Biol Phys 6:1473–1476, 1980
344. Spanos WJ Jr, Shukovsky LJ, Fletcher GH: Time, dose, and tumor volume relationships in irradiation of squamous cell carcinomas of the base of the tongue. Cancer 37:2591–2599, 1976
345. Steel GC: The combination of radiotherapy and chemotherapy. In Steel GG, Adams GE, Peckham MJ (eds): The Biological Basis of Radiotherapy, pp 239–248. Amsterdam, Elsevier Science, 1983
346. Steel GG, Peacock JH: Why are some human tumours more radiosensitive than others? Radiother Oncol 15:63–72, 1989
347. Steel GG, Peckham MJ: Exploitable mechanisms in combined radiotherapy-chemotherapy: The concept of additivity. Int J Radiat Oncol Biol Phys 5:85–91, 1979
348. Strandqvist M: Sutdien uber die kumulative wirkung der rontgenstrahlen bie frakionierung. Acta Radiol (Stockh) 55(Suppl):1–300, 1944
349. Suit HD, Becht J, Leong J, et al: Potential for improvement in radiation therapy. Int J Radiat Oncol Biol Phys 14:777–786, 1988
350. Suit H, Lindberg R: Radiation therapy administered under conditions of tourniquet-induced local tissue hypoxia. Am J Roentgenol 2:27–37, 1968
351. Suit H, Lindberg R, Fletcher GH: Prognostic significance of extent of tumor regression at completion of radiation therapy. Radiology 84:1100–1107, 1965
352. Suit HD, Westgate SJ: Impact of improved local tumor control on survival. Int J Radiat Oncol Biol Phys 12:453–458, 1986
353. Suit HD, Wette R: Theoretical considerations on the influence of dose fractionation on effectiveness of radiation therapy. Natl Cancer Inst Monogr 24:225–241, 1967
354. Tannock IF: Population kinetics of carcinoma cells, capillary endothelial cells, and fibroblasts in a transplanted mouse mammary tumor. Cancer Res 30:2470–2476, 1970
355. Tannock IF: Response of aerobic and hypoxic cell in a solid tumor to Adriamycin and cyclophosphamide, and interaction of the drugs with radiation. Cancer Res 42:4921–4926, 1982
356. Tannock IF: The relation between cell proliferation and the vascular system in a transplanted murine mammary tumour. Br J Cancer 22:258–273, 1986
357. Tannock IF: Principles of cell proliferation: Cell kinetics. In DeVita VT Jr, Hellman S, Rosenberg SA (eds): Cancer: Principles and Practice of Oncology, 3rd ed, pp 3–13. Philadelphia, JB Lippincott, 1989
358. Tannock IF: Combined modality treatment with radiotherapy and chemotherapy. Radiother Oncol 16:83–101, 1989
359. Tannock IF, Hill RP (eds): The Basic Science of Oncology. New York, Pergamon Press, 1987
360. Taylor JMG, Withers HR, Mendenhall WM: Dose-time considerations of head and neck squamous cell carcinomas treated with irradiation. Radiother Oncol 17:95–102, 1990
361. Teeter LD: Drug resistance and chemotherapy: A perspective. Cancer Bull 41:14–20, 1989
362. Terasima T, Tolmach LJ: Variations in several responses of HeLa cells to x-irradiation during the division cycle. Biophys J 3:11–33, 1963
363. Thames HD, Withers HR, Mason KA, et al: Dose-survival characteristics of mouse jejunal crypt cells. Int J Radiat Oncol Biol Phys 7:1591–1597, 1981
364. Thames HD Jr, Withers HR, Peters LJ, et al: Changes in early and late radiation responses with altered dose fractionation: Implications for dose-survival relationships. Int J Radiat Oncol Biol Phys 8:219–226, 1982
365. Thomas RJ, et al: High dose photoirradiation of esophageal cancer. Ann Surg 206:193–199, 1987
366. Thomason JF, Lombard LS, Grahn D, et al: RBE of fission neutrons for life shortening and tumorigenesis. In Broerse JJ, Gerber GB (eds): Neutron Carcinogenesis, p 75. Luxembourg, Commission of the European Communities, 1982
367. Traenkle HL, Malay D: Further observations of late radiation necrosis following therapy of skin cancer: Results of fractionation of the total dose. Arch Dermatol Syph 81:908–913, 1960
368. Travis EL: Primer of Medical Radiobiology, 2nd ed. Chicago, Year Book Medical Publishers, 1989
369. Tsuchiya A, Obara N, Makoto M, et al: Hematoporphyrin derivative and laser photoradiation in the diagnosis and treatment of bladder cancer. J Urol 130:79–82, 1982
370. Tubiana M, Richare JM, Malaise E; Kinetics of tumor growth and of cell proliferation in U.R.D.T. cancers: Therapeutic implications. Laryngoscope 85:1039–1052, 1975
371. Turesson I, Notter G: The response of pig skin to single and fractionated high dose-rate and continuous low dose-rate ^{137}Cs-irradiation. III. Re-evaluation of the CRE system and the TDF system according to the present findings. Int J Radiat Oncol Biol Phys 5:1773–1779, 1979
372. Turesson I, Notter G: The influence of fraction size in radiotherapy on the late normal tissue reaction. I. Comparison of the effects of daily and once-a-week fractionation on human skin. Int J Radiat Oncol Biol Phys 10:593–598, 1984
373. United States Department of Health and Human Services, Centers for Disease Control: Smoking-Attributable Mortality and Years of Potential Life Lost. United States. 1984 MMWR 36:693–697, 1987
374. Upton AC: Biological aspects of radiation carcinogenesis. In Boice JD, Fraumeni JF (eds): Radiation Carcinogenesis: Epidemiology and Biological Significance, p 9. New York, Raven Press, 1984
375. Utley JF, Seaver N, Newton GL, et al: Pharmacokinetics of WR-1065 in mouse tissues following treatment with WR-02721. Int J Radiat Oncol Biol Phys 10:1525, 1984
376. van den Brenk HAS: Hyperbaric oxygen in radiation therapy. Am J Roentgenol 102:8–26, 1968
377. van de Vijver M, van de Bersselaar R, Devilee P, et al: Amplification of the neu (c-erbB-2) oncogene in human mammary tumors is relatively frequent and is often accomplained by amplification of the linked c-erbA oncogene. Mol Cell Biol 7:2019–2023, 1987
378. Van Rongen E: Analysis of cell survival after multiple fractions and low dose-rate irradiation of two *in vitro* cultured rat tumor cell lines. Radiat Res 104:28–46, 1985
379. Varmus HE: The molecular genetics of cellular oncogenes. Ann Rev Genet 18:553–612, 1984

380. Verhey LV, Goitein M. McNulty P, et al: Precise positioning of patients for radiation therapy. Int J Radiat Oncol Biol Phys 8:289–294, 1982
381. Veronesi U, Banfi A, DelVecchio M, et al: Comparison of Halsted radical mastectomy with quadrantectomy, axillary dissection, and radiotherapy in early breast cancer: long-term results. Eur J Cancer Clin Oncol 22:1085–1089, 1986
382. Vikram B, Farr HW: Adjuvant radiation therapy in locally advanced head and neck cancer. Cancer 33:134–138, 1983
383. Vikram B, Strong EW, Shah JP, et al: Failure in the neck following multimodality treatment for advanced head and neck cancer. Head Neck Surg 6:724–729, 1984
384. Von Essen CF: A spatial model of time-dose-area relationships in radiation therapy. Radiology 81:881–883, 1963
385. Votava C Jr, Fletcher GH, Jesse RH Jr, et al: Management of cervical nodes, either fixed or bilateral, from squamous cell carcinoma of the oral cavity and faucial arch. Radiology 105:417–420, 1972
386. Vrabec DP: Multiple primary malignancies of the upper aerodigestive system. Ann Otol Rhinol Laryngol 88:846–854, 1979
387. Vyas JJ, Deshpande RK, Sharma S, et al: Multiple primary cancers in Indian population: Metachronous and synchronous lesions. J Surg Oncol 23(4):239–249, 1983
388. Wachowski TJ, Chenault H: Degenerative effects of large doses of roentgen rays on human brain. Radiology 45:227–246, 1945
389. Wagenfeld DJH, Harwood AH, Bryce DP, et al: Second primary respiratory tract malignancies in glottic carcinoma. Cancer 46:1883–1886, 1980
390. Wallgren A, Arner O, Bergstrom J, et al: The value of preoperative radiotherapy in operable mammary carcinoma. Int J Radiat Oncol Biol Phys 6:287–290, 1980
391. Walz BJ, Fleshman JW Jr: Adjunctive use of radiation therapy in rectal adenocarcinoma. In Kodner IJ (ed): Colon, Rectal and Anal Surgery: Current Techniques and Controversies, pp 204–217. St. Louis, CV Mosby, 1985
392. Wang CC: Improved local control for advanced oropharyngeal carcinoma following twice daily radiation therapy. Am J Clin Oncol 8:512–516, 1985
393. Wasserman TH: Hypoxic cell radiosensitizers: Present and future (editorial). Int J Radiat Oncol Biol Phys 7:849–852, 1981
394. Weichert KA, Schumrick D: Multiple malignancies in patients with primary carcinomas of the head and neck. Laryngoscope 89:988–991, 1979
395. Weichselbaum RR, Little JB: Radioresistance in some human tumor cells conferred *in vitro* by repair of potentially lethal x-ray damage. Radiology 145:511–513, 1982
396. Weichselbaum RR, Little JB: The differential response of human tumours to fractionated radiation may be due to a post-irradiation repair process. Br J Cancer 46:532–537, 1982
397. Weinstein B: The origins of human cancer: Molecular mechanisms of carcinogenesis and their implications for cancer prevention and treatment. Cancer Res 48:4135–4143, 1988
398. Weissberg JB, Son YH, Percarpio B, Fischer JJ: Randomized trial of conventional versus high fractional dose radiation therapy in the treatment of advanced head and neck cancer. Int J Radiat Oncol Biol Phys 8:179–185, 1982
399. West GW, Weichselbaum R, Little JB: Limited penetration of methotrexate into human osteosarcoma spheroids as a proposed model for solid tumor resistance to adjuvant chemotherapy. Cancer Res 40:3665–3668, 1980
400. Wetterer J: Handbuch der Rontgen Therapie. Leipzig i:176, 1913–1914
401. Whitfield AGW, Bond WH, Arnott WM: Radiation reactions in the lung. Q J Med 25:67–86, 1956
402. Wiernik G, Bleehen NM, Brindle J, et al: Sixth interim progress report on the British Institute of Radiology fractionation study of 3F/week versus 5F/week in radiotherapy of the laryngo-pharynx. Br J Radiol 51:241–250, 1978
403. Wile AG, Dahlman A, Burns RG, et al: Laser photoradiation therapy of cancer following hematoporphyrin sensitization. Lasers Surg Med 2:163–168, 1982
404. Wilson JF: Low dose rate teletherapy: review of recent clinical study. In Proceedings of 2nd International Dose-Time Conference, University of Wisconsin, Madison, September 12–14, 1984
405. Withers HR, Peters LJ, Thames HD, Fletcher GH: Hyperfractionation. Int J Radiat Oncol Biol Phys 8:1807–1809, 1982
406. Withers HR, Taylor JMF, Maciejewski B: The hazard of accelerated tumor clonogen repopulation during radiotherapy. Acta Oncol 27:131–146, 1988
407. Withers HR, Thames HD Jr, Flow BL, et al: The relationship of acute to late skin injury in 2 and 5 fractions/week x-ray therapy. Int J Radiat Oncol Biol Phys 4:595–601, 1978
408. Withers HR, Thames HD, Peters LJ: Differences in fractionation response of acutely and late responding tissues. In Karcher KH, et al (eds): Progress in Radio-Oncology II, pp 287–296. New York, Raven Press, 1982
409. Withers HR, Thames HD, Peters LJ: A new isoeffect curve for change in dose per fraction. Radiother Oncol 1:187–191, 1983
410. Wizenberger M (ed): Patterns of Care Process Study Newsletter (Hodgkin's disease). Philadelphia, American College of Radiology, 1979
411. Wong JW, Binns WR, Cheng AY, et al: On-line radiotherapy imaging with an array of fiber-optic image reducers. Int J Radiat Oncol Biol Phys 18:1477–1484, 1990
412. Wong JW, Henkelman RM: A new approach to CT-pixel-based photon dose calculations in heterogeneous media. Med Phys 10:199–208, 1983
413. Wong JW, Slessinger ED, Rosenberger FU, et al: The delta-volume method for 3-dimensional photon dose calculations. Computer Society Press, IEEE:26–30, 1984
414. Wrba E: Ubersicht uber 198 maligne pulmonale Erkankungen im Jahre 1975—Therapie und Erbenisse (Eng Abstr). Wien Medworkenscher 103(12):436–439, 1980
415. Wynder EL, Graham EA: Tobacco smoking as a possible etiologic factor in bronchogenic carcinoma: A study of 684 proved cases. JAMA 143:329–336, 1950
416. Yaes RJ: Linear-quadratic model isoeffect relations for proliferating tumor cells for treatment with multiple fractions per day. Int J Radiat Oncol Biol Phys 17(4):901–905, 1989
417. Zeeman EM, Bedford JS: Dose rate effects in mammalian cells. V. Dose fractionation effects in non-cycling C3H 10 T1/2 cells. Int J Radiat Oncol Biol Phys 10:2089–2098, 1984
418. Zimmerman KW, Montague ED, Fletcher GH: Frequency, anatomical distribution and management of local recurrences after definitive therapy for breast cancer. Cancer 19:67–74, 1966

2

○ ○ ○ • • •

Biologic Basis of Radiation Therapy

H. Rodney Withers

TISSUE RADIOBIOLOGY

Pathobiology of Radiation Injury in Normal Tissues: Target Cells

Radiation damages the DNA, and cells usually die only after their reproductive integrity is tested by one or more attempts at mitotic division.[202,203] Therefore, the rate at which injury develops is related, at least in part, to the proliferative activity of the tissue. Actively proliferating tissues (gastrointestinal mucosa, bone marrow, oropharyngeal and esophageal mucosa, skin) develop injury early, whereas tissues composed of slowly proliferating cells develop injury slowly. Examples of slowly proliferating, late-responding tissues are central and peripheral nervous system, kidney, dermis, cartilage, and bone.

Customarily, late sequelae of radiation have been ascribed to vascular injury.[117,172] However, there is no satisfactory evidence for this, and injury to tissues such as spinal cord, nerves, kidney, dermis, and bones is more logically regarded as the result of depletion of "target" cells such as oligodendrocytes in the central nervous system (CNS), Schwann cells in peripheral nerves, tubule epithelium in the kidney, endothelial cells in blood vessels, and various mesenchymal cells such as fibroblasts, osteoblasts, and chondroblasts.[260] It is not suggested that vascular injury does not occur or that it does not contribute in various ways to a reduced vitality of irradiated tissues. However, vascular injury can compound the injury without being the cause. An exception in which vascular injury is apparently the cause of injury is in the human liver (not in experimental rats or mice) in which occlusion of centrilobular veins can be a fatal result of irradiation[106,229] or of high doses of certain cytotoxic drugs (*e.g.*, methotrexate).

Functional Subunits

The "tolerance" dose for a tissue depends on its organization into functional subunits as well as the radiosensitivity of its target cells. For example, epilation occurs at doses lower than those required for desquamation of the epidermis, not because the cells in the hair differ in their radiosensitivity, follicle and basal epithelium, but because there is a smaller number of cells in the functional subunit which produces a hair than in the sheet of cells that regenerates the keratinized skin surface. Similar considerations apply to depigmentation: hair is depigmented by relatively low doses of radiation,[219] but the epidermis loses its pigmentation only after high doses. This is because each hair follicle contains a small number of melanocytes, sometimes only one, whereas melanocytes are more numerous in the epidermis and can disseminate melanin throughout a relatively large area of keratinocytes.

In the kidney, the functional subunit is the nephron.[257,268] If a tubule is completely de-epithelialized, it is lost permanently because it is not repopulated from adjacent nephrons. Therefore, the tolerance dose for the kidney is determined not by the size of the organ but by the size of its subunits (the number of tubule cells per nephron). For example, if the kidney contained 10^{11} tubule cells distributed as 10^4 cells in each of 10^7 nephrons, and any one of these 10^4 cells were capable of regenerating the tubule, then a dose that reduced survival to 10^{-4} (1 cell per 10,000) would leave one surviving cell per tubule (on average). Because of the random nature of cell survival following irradiation, some tubules would contain more than one surviving cell and others would contain none. From Poisson distribution statistics, the percentage with no survivors would be 37%. Thus, a dose that would reduce cell survival to 10^{-4} would eliminate 37% of the functional units (nephrons) of the kidney. However, if instead the organ were composed of 10^4 nephrons, each containing 10^7 cells, it would require a dose that reduced survival rate to 10^{-7} to eliminate 37% of the nephrons. In terms of a multifractionated dose regimen, during which a logarithmic decline in cell number occurs, the dose required to reduce survival to 10^{-7} is 7/4 (1.75) times greater than that required to reduce survival to 10^{-4}. This example does not suggest that kidney tolerance can be altered by changing its organization but illustrates why tolerance doses can vary so much among tissues and organs of various sizes, the target cells of which may not vary much in intrinsic radiosensitivity.

Whereas the structural organization into functional subunits for hair and kidney is easy to appreciate, it is not easy to appreciate the concept in some other tissues. For example, in mouse skin, the survival of about 10 cells per cm^2 out of a normal population of approximately 10^6 basal stem cells is required to maintain uninterrupted integrity and prevent overt desquamation.[236] Therefore, for mouse skin the functional subunit would be about 1/10 cm^2. In tissues such as lung, dermis, or spinal cord, the functional subunit is not clearly established. From knowledge of tolerance doses, it is relatively small in the lung, intermediate in the spinal cord, and large in the dermis.

Effects Other Than Cell Killing

Some sequelae of irradiation are not obviously effects of cell depletion.[12,26] For example, irradiation of the upper abdomen can cause nausea and vomiting. Erythema of the skin can develop within hours of exposure. Irradiation of the brain can cause life-threatening edema within hours, and somnolence can appear within hours and can recur, or first appear, at about 6 weeks after irradiation. Irradiation of the spinal cord can affect the meninges and lead to a positive Lhermitte's sign. Easy fatigability is common when a patient receives irradiation to a large volume, especially within the abdomen. In experimental animals, irradiation of the lungs can temporarily increase the probability of development of metastases from subsequent intravenous injection of tumor cells, but this does not appear to be a problem in clinical radiation therapy.[156] A late effect that is not explicable in terms of cell killing is the development of cancer *en cuirasse* in the skin or peritoneum in a distribution that matches precisely the radiation field size. The biology of this phenomenon may resemble that of the late-developing enhancement of metastases by preirradiation of mouse lung.[57] At a cellular level, division cycle delay is a phenomenon independent of cell killing.[20,51,63,203]

Kinetics of Radiation Responses

Acute Responses

The ultimate severity of radiation injury in a tissue depends on the extent to which its stem cell population is depleted. The total dose required to produce an injury is determined by the number of stem cells in the functional subunit and their radiosensitivity. However, the rate of development of injury and, to some extent, its severity depend on the turnover and differentiation kinetics of the tissue. For example, leukocyte and platelet numbers drop quickly after irradiation of bone marrow because they have a fast turnover rate, whereas anemia is not an obvious effect because red cells turn over slowly. This difference in radiation responses of different components of a system with a common stem cell exemplifies how rate of response is not a reliable indicator of clonogenic cell radiosensitivity.

The dependence of rate of development of injury on the kinetics of the tissue is also illustrated by the response of the testis to irradiation. Each division of a spermatogenic stem cell ultimately produces more than 1000 sperm through successive divisions of terminally differentiating spermatogonia and spermatocytes. In humans, it is more than 60 days after the division of a spermatogonial stem cell before the numerous progeny appear as sperm in the seminal vesicles. The earliest differentiating spermatogonia are extremely radiosensitive, whereas postmeiotic spermatids show little effect from irradiation. Therefore, irradiation of the testis selectively depletes early spermatogonia with little effect on more mature stages of spermatogenesis. Accordingly, sperm counts remain normal for weeks after exposure, falling steeply only at the time when the progeny of the irradiated spermatogonia would normally have reached the seminal vesicles.

In a simpler system, that is, the mucosa of the small bowel, all mitotic activity is confined to the crypts; the cells lining the villus are nonproliferative. The crypt cells divide rapidly (an average of more than once daily in humans) and hence are lost rapidly if sterilized by radiation. The villus shows no immediate effect of irradiation, with shortening becoming evident only as a result of the continuing programmed shedding of differentiated cells in the absence of renewal from the crypt.

Late Responses

Overt radiation injury develops slowly and at different rates in slowly proliferating tissues. The higher the dose—that is, the greater the radiation injury[130]—the fewer are the division cycles that the cells can successfully negotiate before their death.[202,203] Therefore, injury develops more quickly with increase in dose. Furthermore, the more rapid loss of cells may accelerate the recruitment of cells into cycle, resulting in an avalanche effect,[135] and an earlier expression of the injury. This occurs in both early- and late-responding tissues,[129,135] but is more obvious in those that respond slowly. Various intercurrent insults (chemotherapy, surgery, dental or other mechanical trauma, hyperthermia, and infection) are also capable of precipitating an early expression of radiation injury in slowly responding tissues,[83,84] presumably the result of early recruitment of stem cells into cycle.

Whereas severe early response in a rapid proliferating tissue permits adjustment of the dose schedule during a standard course of multifraction radiation therapy, tolerance doses* for late injuries, which occur after completion of therapy, must be based on the statistics of past experience. Such doses have not been precisely defined even though, in practice, there are widely accepted limits to the total doses usually considered tolerable by various organs. Some examples of these limits are given in Chapter 3.

Kinetics of Tumor Response

Most tumors, even some slow-growing ones, contain a proportion of rapidly proliferating cells and show an early response to irradiation. Although it is important to remember that some tumors respond slowly, most regress quickly. They are considered to be analogous to acutely responding normal tissues when dose fractionation effects are discussed later.

Rate of response of a tumor to irradiation depends not only on the proliferation kinetics of the malignant clonogens† but also on the programmed lifetime of terminally differentiated cells within the tumor. Thus a tumor that is growing quickly because a large proportion of its cells are highly proliferative clonogens may regress quickly (and regrow quickly if not sterilized). However, even slow-growing tumors regress quickly if

---

* *Tolerance dose is the dose that gives an acceptable probability of complications.[259] The acceptable complication rate varies with many factors, such as tissue or organ at risk (compare spinal cord with a small volume of abdominal dermis), likely outcome from treatment of disease (cure, painful recurrence, early death from metastases), patient attitude, litigiousness of the society, and so forth.*

† *Clonogen is an operational term describing a cell that (in retrospect) was capable of generating a clone. If it is malignant, it generates or regenerates a tumor; if it is normal it can regenerate a functional subunit. In tumors and many normal tissues, the clonogens are not morphologically different from some of the nonclonogenic cells.*

their slow growth results from a programmed high cell loss rate[179,259] (*e.g.*, by apoptosis,[112] shedding of differentiated cells). A practical implication of the different reasons for different rates of tumor response is that although the average local control rate may be higher for rapidly than for slowly regressing tumors of a given type,[18,122] it is not good policy to reduce the total dose just because the tumor regresses rapidly.[189]

The situation is not so clear when a tumor regresses slowly. Sometimes slow regression reflects slow proliferation and cell loss kinetics of the tumor, sometimes it indicates a mass of residual stroma, and sometimes it signals treatment failure. Some tumors, such as prostatic carcinoma, some cases of nodular sclerosing Hodgkin's disease, teratocarcinomas of testis, some soft tissue sarcomas, choroidal melanomas, pituitary adenomas, chordomas, or glomus tumors, are characteristically slow to regress even though sterilized of clonogens.

It is generally unnecessary and even misleading to obtain early postirradiation biopsies of a slowly regressing tumor. Not only do biopsies increase the risk of necrosis in heavily irradiated tissues, but they may lead to surgical "salvage" of a sterilized tumor because sterilized but still-living tumor cells are commonly histologically indistinguishable from cells with retained clonogenic capacity.

GROWTH KINETICS

Cell Loss Factor

Unless normal tissues are growing or involuting, each mitotic division results in an average of only one new cell, one daughter being lost at some future time by one of several mechanisms (*e.g.*, desquamation, apoptosis, phagocytosis). By definition, the cell loss factor in such a steady state is 1.0.[179] The *only* requirement for growth or regeneration of a cycling cell population is a decrease from 1.0 in the cell loss factor, that is, that on average, fewer than one of the two daughters of a cell division is lost. A cell loss factor less than 1.0 is therefore a characteristic of both regeneration and malignant growth. Maximum growth is achieved if the cell loss factor is reduced to zero.

A regenerating tissue usually has a shorter mean cell cycle time than when it is in steady state, but a shortened cell cycle time merely speeds up growth or regrowth and, contrary to common thinking, is not essential to it. Malignant tissues may have a mean cell cycle time shorter or longer than their normal counterparts, but even with a slower cell cycle time they grow quickly if their cell loss factor is low. The relative importance of cell cycle time and cell loss factor can be illustrated by considering that intestinal crypt cells may have an average cell cycle time of 16 to 20 hours and yet, being in steady state, an infinitely slow growth rate. If the cell loss factor were to change from 1.0 to 0, the cell number would double every 16 to 20 hours, with a single cell forming a mass as large as the whole body in about 1 month.

Tumors, especially carcinomas, usually have cell loss factors that are closer to 1.0 than to 0.[179] Their growth rate is therefore much slower than suggested by the proliferative activity detected by a mitotic count or an S-phase count (labeling index).[102] Thus, an abundance of mitotic figures in a histologic section, a high labeling index after injection of radiolabeled thymidine, or a high S-phase content in a flow microfluorometer[21,22,235] is not necessarily evidence of rapid growth. The slow-growing basal cell carcinomas of skin, in which numerous mitotic figures are commonly visible, are a classic example of this.

Tumors with a high cell production and loss rate have a high potential for early and rapid regeneration from even modest reductions in their cell loss factor after cell depletion induced by radiation or other cytotoxic insult. Therefore, even a slow-growing (but highly proliferative) tumor may regenerate rapidly. Thus, not only in rapidly growing tumors, but also in many slow-growing tumors, it is unsafe to protract treatment more than necessary.[259] Rapid repopulation in a slow-growing tumor should not seem so surprising because the same thing happens in rapidly proliferating, but, by definition, steady-state, normal tissues, such as oropharyngeal and gastrointestinal mucosa, whose normal growth rate is infinitely slow because of a cell loss factor of 1.0.

Potential Doubling Time

The proliferative activity of the total constituent cell population is a better predictor than growth rate for the potential regeneration rate of both normal tissues and tumors. The best available measure is the *potential doubling time*, or T_{pot}.[21,22,179,235] This term is usually limited to tumors but conceptually can be applied to the clonogenic cell population in normal tissues. It is the time that would be required to double the number of clonogenic cells if the cell loss factor decreased to zero. In this circumstance the doubling time would equal the cell cycle time. It is determined from knowing the average duration of the S phase (T_s) and the fraction of cells in S phase, measured by labeling index (LI):

$$T_{pot} = \lambda T_S / LI$$

where λ is a correction factor for the cell cycle distribution of the population. The term is misleading because the cell cycle time measured in an unperturbed large tumor before treatment may be longer or shorter than that relevant to a surviving subpopulation in a regressing tumor. Thus the regrowth rate of a tumor could easily exceed that predicted by the potential doubling time, just as it may never reach it. Nevertheless, characteristics such as S-phase labeling and mitotic rate are more logical predictors of the kinetics of a regenerative response than is the preirradiation growth rate alone. A relatively short lifetime of differentiating cells (that are not part of the growth fraction), a low growth fraction, a high proliferative index, or a high cell loss factor should predict for rapid regression[259] as well as for early and rapid regrowth if cells survive.

Growth Fraction

Not all cells in a tumor are proliferating. Cells apparently out of cycle have been called G_0 cells, but the techniques available for detecting proliferation do not discriminate between cells that are cycling very slowly and those that are out of cycle. The fraction of tumor cells detected to be in cycle is called the *growth fraction*,[133] and in solid tumors is usually a small proportion of the total (*e.g.*, 20%).

If the growth fraction remained constant with time, the growth rate of the whole tumor would be the same as that of the growth fraction. However, solid tumors usually grow at a progressively slower rate as they enlarge, reflecting a decrease in the growth fraction (see control curve, Fig. 2-2). The typical shape of a growth curve can be approximated by a Gompertz equation.[179] Such mathematical curve fitting describes the data but has no unique biologic rationale.

The growth fraction probably increases after cytoreductive therapy, contributing to the accelerated regrowth described later. An analogous response is found with some normal tissues (liver, dermis), which have only a small fraction of cells in cycle but in which regeneration can occur rapidly through recruitment of resting, G_0-phase cells into cycle. (Because such tissues are not growing, the small fraction of cycling cells must be in steady state and does not constitute a growth fraction.)

Regeneration (Repopulation) in Normal Tissue

The delay before onset of regeneration in irradiated tissues varies in proportion to variation in the time taken for expression of injury. Cell depletion occurs at widely different rates in different tissues for two reasons: most lethally injured cells express their injury only when they attempt division, and the natural cell loss rate is highly variable. The lag time until repopulation in a rapidly turning-over tissue such as the jejunal mucosa may be less than 24 hours. The process is slightly slower in the colon and the stomach. In renal tubules no histologic evidence of cell depletion exists for many months, and there is an unknown but long lag period before the onset of repopulation; more than 12 months is required for a single cell to reconstitute the tubule.[257] The duration of the lag time and the kinetics of repopulation are best measured by a split-dose irradiation technique in which an increase in the number of cells with time after the first dose is reflected in an increase in the dose required to produce a certain level of effect (isoeffect) in the tissue. Typical cytokinetic methods are not useful because after doses relevant to radiation therapy, most of the cells are sterilized, and the kinetics measured are those of doomed, not surviving cells.

After the lag period, repopulation proceeds quickly but at different rates in different tissues. The rate has not been well quantified in many tissues, especially in those which respond late. Some approximate doubling times in mice are 8, 12, and 22 hours for jejunum,[234] colon,[238] and skin,[232] respectively.

In humans, tissue turnover kinetics are slower than in mice and not as well quantified. They have been approximated for oropharyngeal mucosa from consideration of its responses to various dose fractionation regimens used clinically.[248,254] Mucositis begins to appear approximately 14 to 21 days after the start of a regimen of 200 cGy, five times per week.[75] However, repopulation begins before that (at about 10 to 12 days).[215] The lag period may be shortened by high initial doses, but by only 1 or 2 days. After repopulation begins, it can increase the tolerance of the mucosa to such a dose regimen by about an *average* of 100 cGy/day, approximately equivalent to a doubling of clonogenic cell number every 2 days.[248,254] If daily irradiation is suspended (*e.g.*, during a 10- to 14-day break in a split-course accelerated regimen), clonogenic cells may be able to repopulate at two or three times that rate.[8,11,215,222,224,248,249,254] These values are at best estimates quoted to provide a framework for understanding clinical radiobiology.

The critical point for understanding the role of repopulation in time-dose relationships in radiation therapy is that there is a lag period during which repopulation does not occur, followed by a phase of rapid exponential growth; in general, the lag period is shorter for chemotherapy, hyperthermia, and surgery because the cell depletion that stimulates a regenerative response usually occurs more rapidly than after irradiation.

The importance of repopulation is implicit in the history of radiation therapy: Protraction of treatment regimens to current standard overall times would have been of no benefit if regeneration were not contributing to a reduction in acute toxicity. Conversely, when attempts are made to deliver curative therapy more quickly than is now standard, acute responses become too severe unless special efforts are made to circumvent the problem (discussed later here and in Chap. 3).

Figure 2-1 shows that in some tissues, regeneration begins within 1 or 2 days of the initiation of radiation therapy, whereas in others there is no evidence for regeneration even after 2 months.

Experimental Tumor Regeneration

Hermens and Barendsen[92] showed a rapid exponential increase in clonogen number in an irradiated rat rhabdomyosarcoma after several days (Fig. 2-2). It is understandable that a clinician observing a regressing tumor would not suspect the existence of regeneration among surviving clonogens; however, Figure 2-2 reveals that the initial rapid regrowth among the 1% of surviving clonogens occurred while the tumor was still regressing. The initial effect on tumor volume of accelerated regrowth by the 1% of tumor cells surviving is not macroscopically evident.

Using a mouse mammary carcinoma, Kummermehr and Trott[115] demonstrated clones containing thousands of regenerating malignant cells easily visible in stained cross sections at a time when the tumor, consisting mainly of lethally injured, degenerating cells, was still regressing after irradiation.

Other evidence for regeneration in experimental animal tumors comes from studies showing an increase in the dose required to control the tumor with increasing overall treatment duration.[188]

Clinical Tumor Regeneration

Until recently it was not fully appreciated that accelerated regeneration by surviving tumor clonogens could occur during radiation therapy. Although hormone-sensitive tumors were an obvious exception, it was thought that tumors grew autonomously and that their growth rate was not subject to regulation by environmental conditions and homeostatic mechanisms.[233] For example, in the nominal standard dose (NSD) concept, it was postulated that the time factor did not apply to tumor responses.[67]

The only available method for quantifying clonogen growth in human tumors is the increase in dose necessary to achieve a constant rate of local tumor control as a function of extension of treatment duration (or a decrease in dose with shortening of time).

Regrowth is of concern to the planning and delivery of radiation therapy only when it occurs before the completion of treatment. Evidence for accelerated regrowth within the duration of a standard radiation therapy regimen has come mostly from analysis of results of treatment of head and neck cancer. It is likely that a repopulation response occurs in tumors in all sites, but with quantitative differences from tumor to tumor.

Accelerated repopulation by human tumor clonogens during fractionated irradiation is suggested by several observations.

RECURRENCE TIME DISTRIBUTIONS

One cell must undergo nearly 30 doublings to become detectable as a recurrence; even 10,000 surviving cells would have to undergo 15 to 17 doublings. Most recurrences for most sites are detectable within 12 months.[76,145] For a detectable recurrence to develop from 10,000 surviving cells in 6 months, or from 1 cell in 12 months, would require an *average* tumor volume doubling time of about 12 days. The median volume

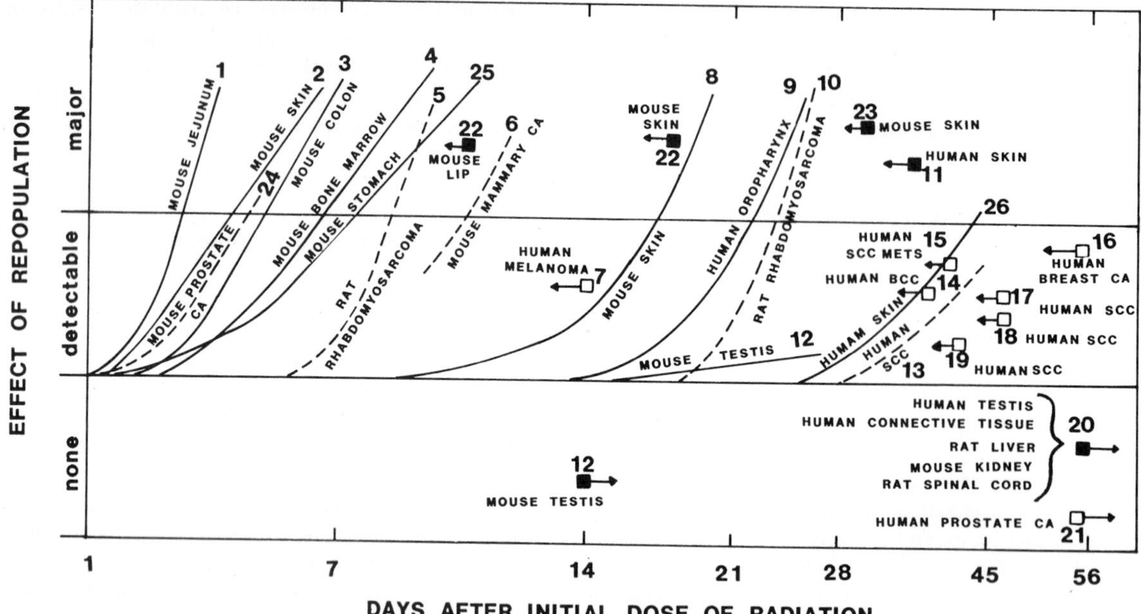

FIGURE 2–1. Representation of the approximate kinetics of regeneration of irradiated normal tissues (*solid lines, solid symbols*) and tumors (*broken lines, open symbols*). Curves are based on measurements or estimates of regeneration; symbols denote times at which an effect of regeneration has already appeared (←■) or has not yet appeared (■→). The logarithmic abscissa is for the convenience of presentation only and has no biologic rationale. In general, the human data are displaced to the right of experimental animal data reflecting a slower initiation of repopulation because human tissues proliferate more slowly than do their rodent counterparts; they were exposed to protracted dose regimens; and less sensitive endpoints were used to detect onset of repopulation in humans. (Numbers on the curve and symbols refer to the sources of data). 1: Withers,[239, 251]; 2: Withers,[237]; 3: Withers and Mason,[255]; 4:McCulloch and Till,[131]; 5: Hermens and Barendsen,[92]; 6: Suit et al,[188]; 7: Choi et al,[40]; 8: Denekamp,[49]; 9: Fletcher,[75] Horoit,[101] van der Schueren et al,[215] Wang et al,[222–224]; 10: Barendsen and Broerse,[17]; 11: Arcangeli et al,[13]; 12: Withers et al,[253], Meistrich et al,[132]; 13: Maciejewski et al,[122–126]; 14: Allen,[2]; 15: Maciejewski,[124]; 16: Barker et al,[15]; 17: Wang et al,[222–224]; 18: Parsons et al,[146]; 19: Maciejewski et al,[124]; 20: Pedrick and Hoppe,[151] Maciejewski et al,[125] Fisher and Hendry,[73] Withers and Mason,[257] van der Kogel[212, 213]; White and Hornsey,[230] 21: Withers et al,[268]; 22: Xu et al,[269] Ang et al,[11]; 23: Ang et al,[8]; 24: Kummermehr,[115]; 25: Chen and Withers,[39]; 26: Turesson and Notter.[206])

doubling time for tumors of the size presenting for radiation therapy is about 60 days.[38] Therefore, accelerated regrowth occurs as a result of treatment. A similar rapid postirradiation regrowth is seen in pulmonary metastases after subcurative doses.[217] These results do not establish that accelerated repopulation begins within the tumor before completion of therapy. They were, however, an early clue that accelerated growth of the tumor may be a problem in radiation therapy.

SPLIT-COURSE TREATMENT

When squamous cell carcinomas (SCC) of the head and neck were treated with the same total dose in continuous and split-course regimens, the local control rate in the split-course treatment was lower in every stage of disease[145, 146] and even in postoperative elective therapy.[6] This suggests that tumor growth occurred during the extended time required for the split-course regimen. However, in split-course treatment of prostate cancer there was no detectable decrease in local control, within comparable ranges of total dose,[149, 162] a result consistent with its indolent growth pattern.

PROTRACTED TREATMENT

In several retrospective analyses of the treatment of patients with head and neck cancer, protraction of treatment was associated with a decreasing rate of locoregional control.[122–126, 142, 263] This is consistent with accelerated tumor regeneration. These analyses were of two types.

SCATTERGRAM ANALYSIS. The worsening results obtained from protracting treatment are illustrated by Figure 2-3 in which individual responses (control, recurrence, persistence) for a series of patients with a relatively homogeneous stage of disease are presented as a function of total dose and overall treatment duration.[126] The curves trace the calculated values for the dose giving tumor control rates of 50% (TCD_{50}) and 90% (TCD_{90}). The data in this scattergram cover treatment durations of about 30 to 55 days and indicate that, within those time limits, each day's extension of treatment requires that the total dose be increased by about 60 cGy to achieve a constant rate of tumor control. The same pattern was seen in 11 other subsets of patients.[126] Reanalysis of scattergrams published in earlier literature showed a similar result.[126, 263]

Assuming a dose of 180 cGy to 240 cGy is required to reduce cell survival by 50% (see later in chapter), an increase of 60 cGy/day is consistent with a time of 3 to 4 days for a doubling of tumor clonogen number. Because the average doubling time of a tumor of the size presenting for treatment is about 45 to 60 days,[38, 179] the data reflect a dramatic change in growth rate at some time within 30 days of the start of radiation therapy.

TCD_{50} ANALYSIS. Figure 2-4 presents calculated TCD_{50} values for SCC of head and neck from data published in the literature.[263] Although confident estimates cannot be made from such a retrospective analysis of the literature, the TCD_{50}

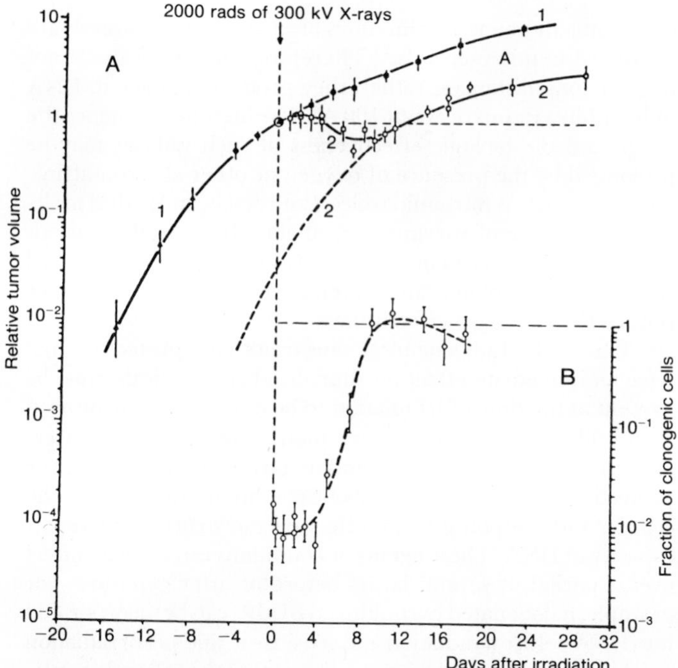

FIGURE 2–2. Growth curves for a rat rhabdomyosarcoma and for its constituent clonogenic cells after a dose that reduced survival rate to 1%. The upper curve (1) shows unperturbed growth of tumors; the middle curve (2) shows regression and regrowth of tumors irradiated on day 0 with a dose that reduced cell survival to 1%; the lower curve (B) traces the repopulation of the tumor by surviving clonogens. Exponential regrowth of the surviving clonogenic cells occurs while the gross tumor is regressing. (Hermens AF, Barendsen GW: Eur J Cancer 5:173, 1969. ©1969 Pergamon Press, Ltd)

values seem fairly independent of treatment duration up to about 28 days, after which they increase rapidly (consistent with 60 cGy/day). Our present working hypothesis is that, *on average*, squamous cell carcinomas of head and neck exhibit a lag period of about 4 weeks from the start of treatment, after which they repopulate quickly. This pattern is only an average, and it is possible that there is a broad spectrum of repopulation kinetics.

It should be reemphasized that after about 4000 cGy in 200 cGy fractions over 4 weeks, the absolute number of surviving clonogenic tumor cells is very low (*e.g.*, 1/50,000 of the initial tumor cell population). Their rapid growth would not be evident macroscopically, and inspection of the tumor, which is in the process of regressing, could mislead the oncologist into not suspecting subclinical regrowth at a rapid rate.

A lag period of up to 4 weeks and a 60 cGy/day increase in the "isocontrol" dose are not evidence that the best overall duration of radiation therapy for head and neck cancer is 4 weeks. Repopulation of the mucosa begins at about 10 to 12 days and is more rapid than in the tumor, requiring an average daily dose increment of about 100 cGy for an isoresponse.[248,263] Thus a therapeutic gain in mucosal tolerance relative to tumor control should still be achieved by extending treatment beyond 4 weeks. However, late-responding tissues do not benefit from repopulation; therefore, the response differential between them and the tumor decreases when the growth of the residual tumor accelerates. Therefore, the overall therapeutic differential should be greatest if the tolerance dose for the critical late-responding tissue is delivered in the shortest overall time consistent with an acceptable acute response.[243,248,254,263] (Dose per fraction is discussed later in chapter.)

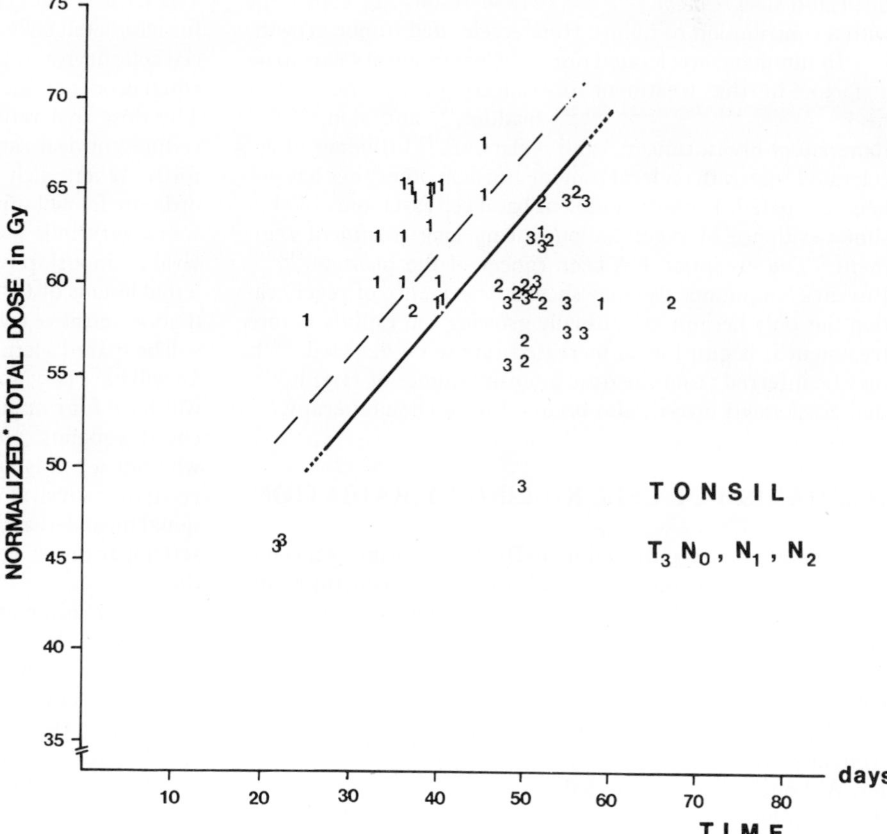

FIGURE 2–3. Scattergram with TCD_{50} and TCD_{90} (tumor control dose) curves for 3-year local control of squamous cell carcinomas of the tonsil (1: local control; 2: recurrence; 3: persistence of detectable disease). For a given total dose, local control decreased with protraction of overall treatment time. For a given overall time, local control improved with increase in dose. The total doses were normalized to be equivalent to the total dose in 2.5 Gy fractions using the linear quadratic (LQ) isoeffect curve (Fig. 2–19). An α/β value of 25 Gy was used, being the best estimate from these and other data. (Maciejewski B, Withers HR, Taylor JMH: Int J Radiat Oncol Biol Phys 16:831, 1989)

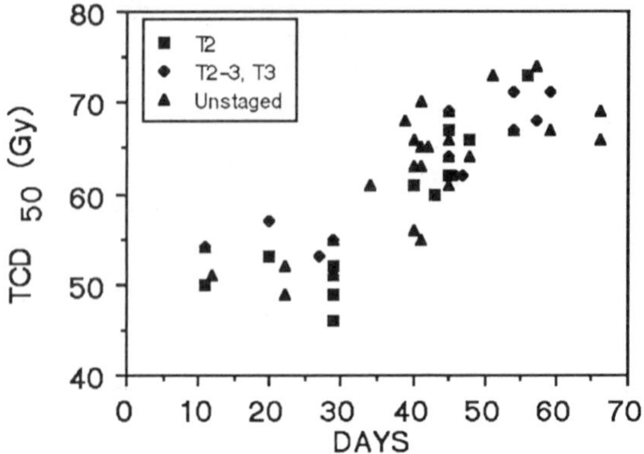

FIGURE 2–4. Estimated TCD_{50} values as a function of treatment duration from published results of radiation therapy for squamous carcinomas of head and neck excluding nasopharynx and true vocal cord. TCD_{50} values are expressed as $LQED_{2Gy}$ (linear quadratic effective dose), the equivalent dose given in 2 Gy fractions calculated using the linear-quadratic model. Total doses for an isoeffect rise steeply with protraction of treatment duration, implying accelerated repopulation by surviving tumor clonogens consistent with the 3- to 4-day average doubling time calculated from scattergrams[263] (Fig. 2-3). The relatively constant TCD_{50} value for treatments lasting up to 4 weeks is consistent with an average time of onset of accelerated growth at about 4 weeks. Growth of clonogens at the average preirradiation doubling rate of 2 months would have little detectable effect on TCD_{50} values (about 2.5 Gy increase in 8 weeks). (Modified from Withers HR, Taylor JMG, Maciejewski B: Acta Oncol 27:131, 1988)

ACCELERATED TREATMENT

In nonrandomized studies, shortening the overall duration of treatment improved the local outcome of therapy in inflammatory breast cancer,[14] melanoma metastases to brain,[40] and head and neck cancer.[113,222–224] These results are consistent with a contribution to failure from accelerated tumor growth.

In summary, accelerated tumor regeneration appears to be a factor in the treatment of cancers of the head and neck[6,7,113,122–126,145,146,222–224,263] bladder,[123] and skin,[2,95] inflammatory breast cancer,[14] and melanoma.[40] Influence of accelerated regrowth on local tumor control in other sites has not been evaluated. Even the indolent basal cell carcinoma of skin shows evidence of regeneration during long treatment regimens.[2] The exception has been cancer of the prostate.[149,162] Burkitt's lymphoma also may show little evidence of regeneration but only because it is usually growing too rapidly before treatment is begun for an increased rate to be detected.[139] It may be inferred from the dose intensity studies of Hyrniuk[104] that accelerated growth also occurs during chemotherapy.

MECHANISM OF CELL KILLING BY RADIATION

It is generally believed that injury to DNA is the primary mechanism by which radiation kills cells.[4,66] Other damage (to membranes or microtubules) may be a supplementary mechanism of cytotoxicity.[4,58] Membrane injury preceding apoptosis is thought to be important in the interphase death of mature lymphocytes.[175]

X-rays deposit their energy in a tissue through the electrons ejected from the cells' constituent molecules—mainly water. Although some of the lethal injury from x-rays is from direct ionization of the DNA molecule by a scattered electron, the predominant mechanism is indirect through lesions induced in DNA by hydroxyl radicals produced from ionization of its ambient water. The lifetimes of such hydroxyl radicals are measured in microseconds.[25] Therefore, these radicals cannot migrate long distances; rather, they produce damage in DNA only within a radius of about 100 A°. The lifetime and hence the range and the biologic effectiveness of such radicals may be prolonged by the presence of oxygen or other electron-affinic molecules such as nitroimidazoles. Conversely, sulfhydryl molecules, which are of varying natural abundance in the nucleus and can be introduced in compounds such as DMSO (dimethyl sulfoxide) or cysteine, can "scavenge" free radicals and hence reduce their biologic effectiveness.

Obviously, radiochemical sensitizers and protectors that have an immediate effect on short-lived free radicals must be present at the time of irradiation to be effective. If introduced even milliseconds later they are ineffective. These sensitizers and protectors are to be differentiated from other sensitizing or protective substances, or metabolic conditions, that modify the cellular radioresponse by an effect on the structure or repair capacity of DNA. These agents or conditions can exert an effect over a period of several hours before or after exposure. For example, halogenated pyrimidines (BUdR) can be incorporated into DNA before irradiation and sensitize it, and postirradiation conditions that suppress progression within the cell cycle (cycloheximide, nutrient-free medium) permit the cells more time to repair potentially lethal damage.

As mentioned earlier, cells lethally injured by radiation may execute one or more mitoses before death. During this period, a variety of chromosome aberrations can be found, and these have been used for quantifying radiation injury in several important experimental studies.[27,50,89,118,166,167]

RANDOM NATURE OF CELL KILLING

The earliest understanding of the dose response relationships for irradiated cells came from studies with bacteria.[4,118] Bacterial cell survival rate decreases geometrically with dose; that is, equal dose increments cause constant proportionate decreases. The dose that reduces survival rate to 50% will, if doubled, reduce survival rate to 25%, and if tripled, to 12.5%, and so forth. When such a relationship is plotted on a logarithmic ordinate for cell survival and a linear abscissa for dose (so-called semilogarithmic plot), a straight line results. Such a dose-survival relationship reflects a random process of cell killing: 100 lethal lesions distributed randomly throughout 100 equally radiation-sensitive cells will not kill them all. On average, 37 cells will be spared a lethal lesion; 37 will have one lethal lesion; about 18 will have two; about 6 will have three, and an occasional one will have four or five lethal lesions, with the total lethal lesion count equaling 100 (Fig. 2-5). Of course, it is immaterial whether a cell is killed by one or more lethal lesions, but the recurring survival rate of 37% of the survivors for each additional mean lethal dose (100 lethal events in 100 cells) ensures a semilogarithmic relationship between cell survival rate and dose.

The mathematic bent of early radiation biologists, many of whom were also physicists, caused them to describe the slope of survival curves in terms of the mean lethal dose (D_{37} or D_0), which reduces survival rate by one natural logarithm (e^{-1}), rather than D_{50} (half-dose) or D_{10} (the dose to reduce survival rate by one common logarithm, to 10%).

It is generally easier for biologists to think in terms of the halving-dose (D_{50}), analogous to half-times of randomly decaying radioisotopes, or even in terms of doses that reduce survival rate to 10% (by one common [base 10] logarithm). However, the

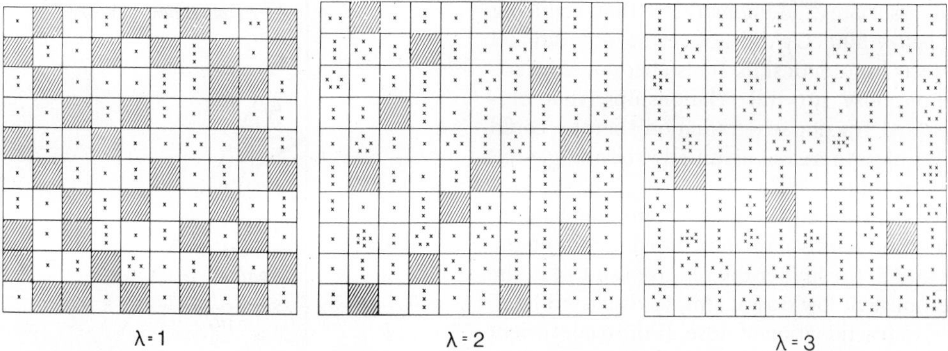

FIGURE 2–5. Random distribution in 100 equal-sized "targets" of 100, 200, or 300 "hits." The probability that any one of the 100 targets will not be struck when 100 "hits" are delivered randomly is e^{-1} or 37%. The same probability of survival applies for each equal increment in the number of hits: 200 hits would result in a probability of survival of e^{-2} or 0.37×0.37. Even after 300 hits, there is still a chance of $e^{-3} = 5\%$ that any one target will survive. This proportionate, or geometric, decrement in survival rate may be plotted as a straight line on semilogarithmic coordinates. (Withers HR, Peters LJ: Biological aspects of radiation therapy. In Fletcher GH [ed]: Textbook of Radiotherapy, 3rd ed. Philadelphia, Lea & Febiger, 1980)

nomenclature using natural logarithms is conceptually more elegant and is now firmly established. For rough approximations, a D_{50} is about 70% of D_0, and D_{10} is about 2.3 times D_0.

MAMMALIAN CELL SURVIVAL CURVE

The first survival curve for mammalian cells was published by Puck and Marcus in 1956.[165] Mammalian cells are relatively radiosensitive, with D_0 values ranging between about 75 and 200 cGy, less than one tenth of those for most bacteria. Also, unlike those for bacterial cells, mammalian cell survival curves usually have a shoulder before beginning a logarithmic decline. Such a "bending-down" shape indicates that the radiation becomes more effective per unit dose as injury accumulates within the cells. This is usually explained by assuming that cells could accumulate some radiation injury, but that this "sublethal" injury could be converted to lethal injury by additional dose. An alternative, more recent concept is that accumulated injury reduces the capacity of the cell to repair injury.[4,193]

DOSE SURVIVAL FORMULAS

Linear Quadratic (LQ) Formula

Read[167] quantified growth delay and chromosome aberrations in bean roots in terms of a linear dose coefficient (α) and a coefficient (β) for the square of the dose,

$$\text{Effect} \propto \alpha d + \beta d^2.$$

This LQ formula can be used to fit a continuously bending curve to cell survival data:

$$\text{SF (survival fraction)} = e^{-(\alpha d + \beta d^2)}$$

During the 1960s and much of the 1970s, the linear component of this dose survival relationship (αd), as it related to radiation therapy, was largely ignored. However, it dominates the response at low doses and, with radiation therapy delivered in doses per fraction of the order of 200 cGy, the linear (single-hit, or α) component assumes major significance (Fig. 2-6). The importance to radiation therapy of the initial linear region of the dose survival curve was "rediscovered" in the early 1970s

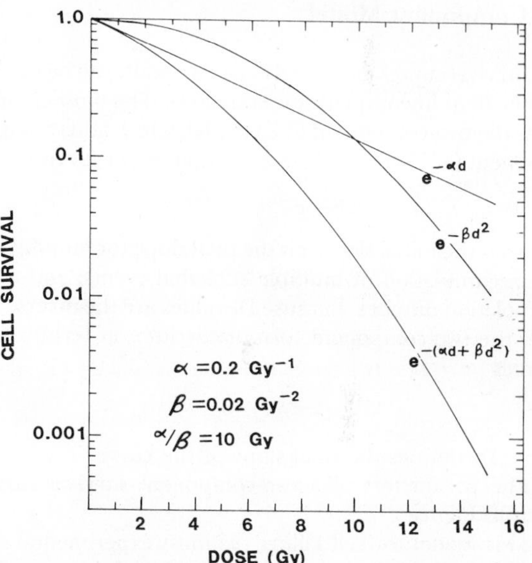

FIGURE 2–6. Model dose survival curves for mammalian cells showing that the experimentally determined curve for acute exposures (*lowest curve*) is the product of two mechanisms, single-hit injury described by an exponential curve ($e^{-\alpha d}$) and multihit, or cumulative, injury described by a continuously bending curve related by a coefficient, β, to the square of the dose. At doses of clinical relevance, cell death from the single-hit mechanism predominates. The rate at which the survival curve bends from an initial, essentially exponential region depends on the ratio (α/β) of the coefficients for single-hit and multihit killing: The lower the value, the sooner and more steeply the curve bends. The value of α/β is the dose at which single and multihit mechanisms contribute equally to cell killing: In these curves, α/β = 10 Gy, which is a value characteristic of acutely responding tissues. Target cells in late-responding normal tissues are characterized by low α/β values; hence, their survival curves are curvier. The flexure dose, D_f, is the dose at which deviation from the initial exponential part of the curve is difficult to detect and, for available biologic assay systems, is about one tenth of α/β. When doses in a multifraction regimen are less than D_f, further dose fractionation does not produce detectable "sparing" (because cell killing is essentially all the result of single-hit events, the lesions potentially contributing to multievent killing being completely repaired during the fractionation intervals). The lower the α/β value, the lower the dose at which multihit mechanisms cause cell death, the lower the value of D_f, and the lower the dose per fraction below which a sparing effect of dose fractionation is lost. The curve for single-hit killing ($e^{-\alpha d}$) can be measured experimentally using very small dose fractions or a continuous low-dose rate exposure, but the curve for multihit killing ($e^{-\beta d^2}$) can be determined only indirectly from a knowledge of the other two curves.

when Dutreix and associates[60] demonstrated that reducing doses per fraction below 300 cGy did not result in additional sparing of acute effects in human skin. It also became appreciated, from modeling dose survival relationships, that brachytherapy or standard fractionated radiation therapy could not eradicate cancer unless there was assumed to be a single-hit, nonrepairable form of injury.[30,250]

The dose range over which the linear component dominates in a linear quadratic survival relationship depends on the relative values of α and β: the higher the relative value of α, the more linear the response at low doses, and, as discussed later, the less sensitive it is to fractionation of dose. If the α coefficient is low relative to the β coefficient, the survival curve will be "curvier," bending down after a relatively small initial linear region; there will also be a marked effect of dose fractionation. In other words, a high α/β ratio implies little fractionation effect at low doses; conversely a low α/β ratio indicates that dose fractionation will have a marked sparing effect on the survival rate of a cell population (see Fig. 2-18).

Two-Component Model

Dose survival curves measured experimentally can be well fitted by other than linear quadratic equations. The most commonly used is the two-component (TC) model, which adds a single-hit component ($e^{-\alpha x}$ or $e^{-D/_1D_0}$) to a multiple-event survival model.

$$SF = e^{-\alpha x(1 - [1 - e^{\gamma x}]^{n})}$$

where α is the initial slope, τ is the final slope for multihit killing from accumulation of multiple sublethal events, and n is the extrapolation number. Because D_0 values are the inverse of the slope, the two-component formula, written in terms of dose, becomes

$$SF = [e^{-D/_1D_0}(1 - e^{-D/_nD_o n})],$$

where $_nD_o$ defines the final slope of the curve.

The parameters of a two-component survival curve are shown in Figure 2-7.

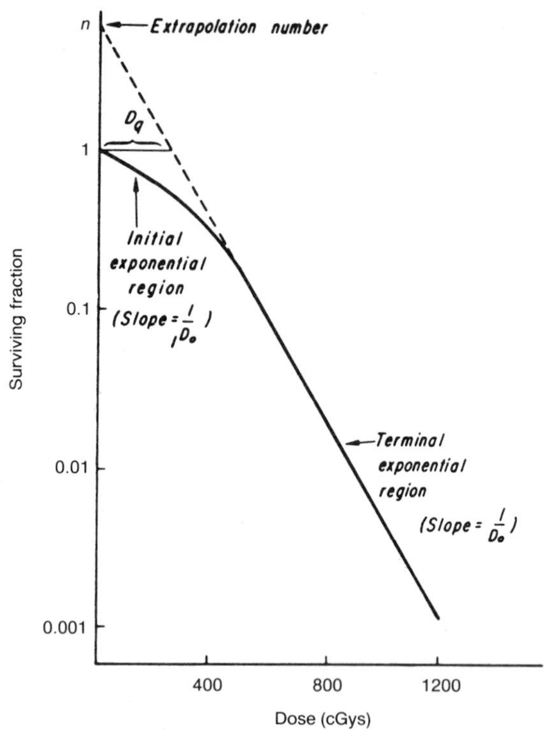

FIGURE 2–7. A two-component survival curve for mammalian cells is characterized by a "shoulder" followed by a *terminal exponential region,* the slope of which is defined by a D_o value (slope = $1/D_o$). The position of the curve on the radiation dose axis can be fixed by the intercepts of the terminal exponential region extrapolated back to the zero dose axis (*n*) or to the 100% survival level (D_q): *n* is termed the extrapolation number, and D_q the quasithreshold dose. Although *n* and *Dq* are parameters that define the width of the shoulder on the survival curve, they do not indicate its *shape,* which is of prime importance in radiation therapy. The survival curve shoulder can be considered to consist of an initial exponential region (the slope of which is defined by $_1D_o$), followed by a downward-bending segment that merges asymptotically into the final exponential region of the survival curve. (Withers HR, Peters LJ: Biological aspects of radiation therapy. In Fletcher GH [ed]: Textbook of Radiotherapy, 3rd ed. Philadelphia, Lea & Febiger, 1980)

This model for cell killing fits most experimental data at least as well as the linear quadratic model. Neither model has been proven "correct" in a biologic sense; over a limited dose range (*e.g.*, 2 Gy to 6 Gy), they can each 'fit' data indistinguishably' (Fig. 2-8). Survival curves for some mammalian cells appear to continue bending at high doses, as predicted by the linear quadratic model, whereas some curves become logarithmic (linear on a semilogarithmic plot), as predicted by the two-component model. However, the form of the survival rate response at low doses (< 300 cGy) is what matters in clinical radiation therapy; over this dose range tissue responses and cell survival rate have not been measured sufficiently accurately to know whether the LQ or the TC model is more appropriate for describing the response of tissues to the most clinically relevant doses. Unfortunately, the models give significantly different results when used to predict responses to doses below 200 cGy from responses measured at doses above 200 cGy.[109]

Comparison of Linear Quadratic and Two-Component Survival Models

Neither the LQ nor the TC model has any established biologic basis. They therefore should be viewed only as convenient methods of describing a survival curve mathematically. The LQ model predicts a survival curve that bends continuously, whereas the TC model provides a survival curve that becomes linear at high doses. Thus for the LQ model there is no value for D_0 or extrapolation number because the slope keeps increasing with increase in dose, as does the value for n. At low doses the LQ model describes a curve that bends more than a TC curve if both are to fit the same data over an intermediate dose range (200 cGy to 800 cGy). Although the difference in the survival curves may appear small on the logarithmic ordinate of a semilogarithmic survival rate plot, it can be amplified to a very large difference if a dose of 115 cGy, for example, is repeated 70 times or more, as could happen in a hyperfractionated radiation therapy regimen.

Because it is mathematically simpler, the LQ model has gained popularity.[16,55,77,111,119,170,193,199,265–268] It provides a good fit to data over the dose range 200 cGy to 800 cGy, but its great advantage and the most important reason for its popularity are that α/β ratios can be determined from multifraction experiments even though the absolute values of each coefficient remain unknown and that, conversely, the responses of tissues to dose fractionation can be predicted from just the ratio of α/β.

Repair of Sublethal Damage

In 1959, Elkind and Sutton[64] showed that the sublethal injury associated with a shoulder in the survival curve could be re-

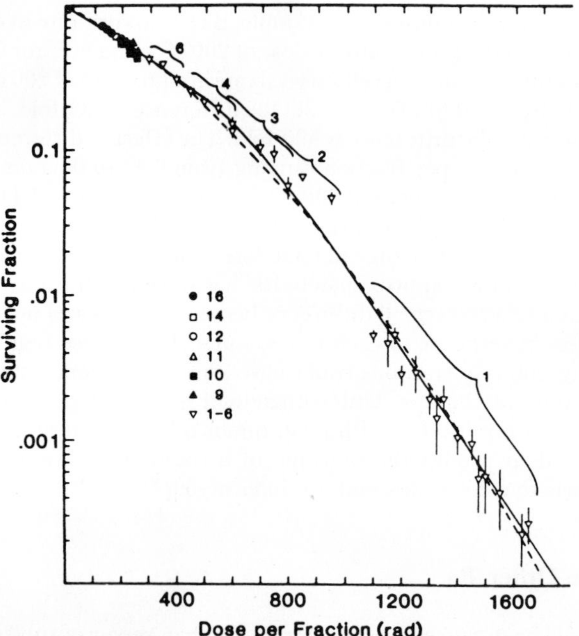

FIGURE 2–8. Effective single-dose survival curves for clonogenic cells of jejunal crypts fitted to multifraction data using linear quadratic (*broken curves*) and two-component (*solid lines*) models. (Numbered braces illustrate that the data were from experiments using that number of fractions.) Mean survival curve parameters for LQ model, $\alpha = 0.23$ Gy, $\beta = 0.018\ Gy^{-2}$, for TC model, ${}_1D_0 = 3.57$ Gy, $D_0 = 1.43$ Gy, ${}_nD_0 = 2.37$ Gy and $n = 20.4$. (Reprinted with permission from Thames HD, Withers HR, Mason KA, et al: Int J Radiat Oncol Biol Phys 71:1591, 1981 © 1981 Pergamon Pres, Ltd)

paired, given a few hours of normal metabolic activity. The repair of sublethal injury may be quantified by the increase in cell survival rate with increasing time between two fractions (survival rate ratio) or by the increase in total dose necessary to achieve a certain level of cell survival (Fig. 2-9). Thus, if two doses were separated by several hours, the survival rate of cells was that which would be predicted from summing up the independent effect of each dose, as though the survivors of the first dose had not been previously irradiated and harbored no residual (by definition, sublethal) injury. In other words, if two equal doses were given with a fractionation interval of several hours, sufficient for complete repair of sublethal injury, the net survival rate would be the product of the survival rate from each

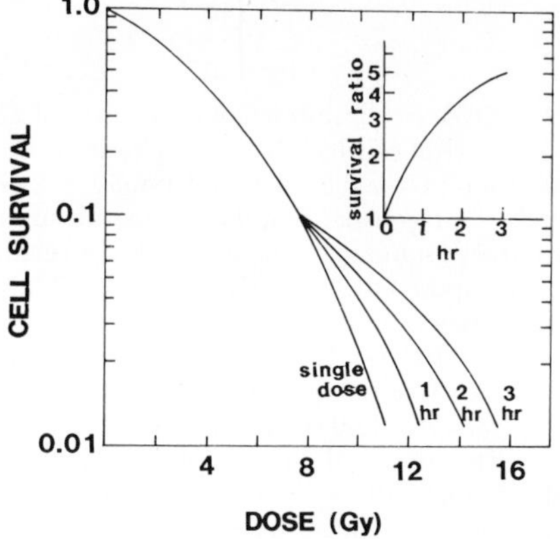

FIGURE 2–9. Recovery curves of the type first described by Elkind and Sutton.[63] The repair of sublethal injury begins immediately and can be measured in terms of survival ratio (*inset*) or the increment in dose to achieve isosurvival.

dose (Fig. 2-10). For example, if 200 cGy reduced survival rate to 50%, two doses of 200 cGy separated by a few hours would reduce survival rate to 50% of 50%, three doses to $(0.5)^3$ and n doses to $(0.5)^n$.

Initial Linear Region of Survival Curve

As mentioned earlier, mammalian cell survival curves show an initial, essentially linear region before beginning to bend down. Operationally, the downward bend results from accumulation of sublethal lesions, which interact to become lethal. In this model, the initial slope reflects single-hit lethality, and the downward bending reflects multihit or multitarget lethality. Thus, at least in an operational sense, an x-ray beam produces lethal lesions by both single-hit (α-type) and multihit (β-type) mechanisms (see Fig. 2-6). A biophysical basis for single-hit or multihit killing is not established, but it is simplest to consider it in terms of how an electron loses its energy after being ejected by a photon. The rate of deposition of energy by a charged particle is inversely proportional to its energy. Hence, along its track, the electron is initially sparsely ionizing, but as it loses its energy through collisions and scattering, it rapidly becomes increasingly more densely ionizing. The dense ionization at the end of the electron track is presumed to be sufficient to induce irreversible single-hit injury without requiring additional accumulation of ionization injury from other electron tracks.* Therefore, an x-ray beam should be regarded as a mixture of high and low linear energy transfer (LET) radiation. The survival curve measured experimentally is the net result of single-hit killing, which yields a direct exponential decline in cell survival rate, and multihit, or cumulative, injury, which yields a curve that becomes increasingly steep with increase in dose (Fig. 2-6).

At low doses, the single-hit (α-type) lethality predominates, because little opportunity exists for accumulating sufficient interactive (β-type) injury. If sufficient time (a few hours) elapses between each of a series of small dose fractions, cell killing from accumulation of sublethal injury will also be insignificant because of repeated repair during the fractionation intervals. Likewise, exposure to low dose-rate continuous irradiation results in predominantly α-type lethality because of continuous repair during the overall duration of exposure. When essentially all cell killing results from single-hit injury, the effective survival curve is linear and defined by the limiting value for D_0 characteristic of the initial part of the single-dose survival curve.

Multifraction Survival Curves

Obviously, with an equal proportionate decrease in survival rate with each equal increment in dose, even when a proportion of the killing results from β-type injury, the dose survival relationship for a series of equal dose fractions must be logarithmic; that is, the survival curve is a straight line when plotted on semilogarithmic coordinates (Fig. 2-10). Also, the curve extrapolates to 1 (or 100%) from any dose level, which is not a characteristic of a single-dose survival curve for x-rays. The slope of such a linear multifraction curve is less than that for the single-dose

** In certain conditions of postirradiation cell culture, some single-hit injury can be repaired,[209,210] but in general its repair is less efficient and effective than the repair of multihit, sublethal injury. In this chapter, single-hit injury is considered to be nonrepairable; thus the term is operational, not mechanistic.*

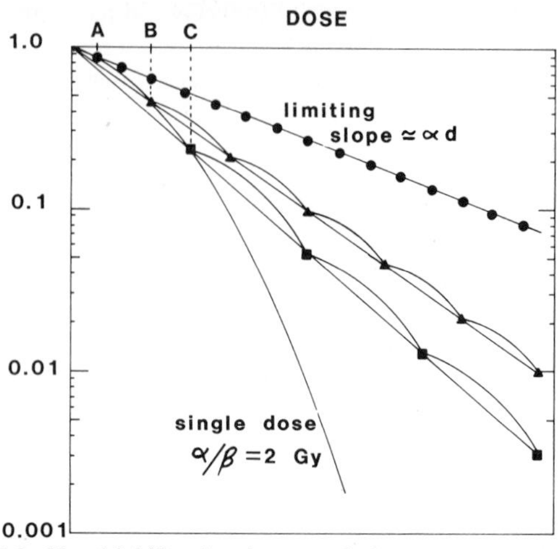

FIGURE 2–10. Multifraction-dose survival curves compared with a single-dose curve. Effective survival curves for multifraction regimens that produce an equal (proportionate) decrement in survival from each dose are linear, with shallower slopes than the single dose curve at the same dose. Slopes of the multifraction curves become less steep with decrease in fraction size until the dose per fraction is so low that multihit killing contributes negligibly and the slope is the limiting one determined by single-hit killing (and ${}_eD_o = 1/\alpha$). The dose per fraction below which the effective survival curve becomes no shallower is a function of the curviness of the single-dose survival curve and is lower with lower α/β values.

curve at equivalent total doses, and the smaller the dose per fraction, the shallower the slope of the multifraction curve.

The slope of a survival curve for a multifraction regimen that produces equal decrements in (logarithmic) survival rate can be described in terms of the "effective D_0," or $D_{0(\text{eff})}$, or ${}_{\text{eff}}D_0$ or ${}_eD_0$.[259] The values for ${}_eD_0$ are greater than the D_0 value of the single-dose curve; that is, the curve is shallower. For clinical radiation therapy, ${}_eD_0$ values for mammalian cells are relevant, whereas D_0 values are largely irrelevant. Values of ${}_eD_0$ for 2 Gy fractions are commonly in the range of 200 cGy to 500 cGy, compared with 75 cGy to 200 cGy for D_0 values. Because the survival curve is linear for multiple dose fractions (assuming each dose fraction produces an equal decrement in cell survival rate), because it originates at 1 (or 100%), and because a dose equal to the ${}_eD_0$ value reduces survival rate to e^{-1}, the surviving fraction from any total dose, D, is simply $e^{-D/{}_eD_0}$. On the basis of ${}_eD_0$ values of 250 cGy to 500 cGy, the fraction of cells surviving 200 cGy would range from 0.45 to 0.67. In mice, surviving fractions from 200 cGy are about 0.6 for jejunal crypt and spermatogenic stem cells and for colonic cells, about 0.65 to 0.7, reflecting ${}_eD_0$ values for 200 cGy fractions of about 390 cGy and 500 cGy, respectively. If one assumes that each dose fraction in a multifraction regimen produced the same decrement in cell survival rate and that regeneration did not occur (not a realistic assumption in clinical practice), a regimen of 30 fractions of 200 cGy would reduce survival rate of jejunal crypt cells to 2×10^{-7}. This can be calculated in two ways:

$$\text{SF after } 30 \times 2 \text{ Gy} = (\text{SF after } 2 \text{ Gy})^{30} = (0.6)^{30} = 2 \times 10^{-7}. \quad (1)$$

$$\text{SF after 60 Gy in 2 Gy fractions} = e^{-60/{}_eD_o} = e^{-60/3.9} = 2 \times 10^{-7}. \quad (2)$$

Small differences between different cell types in their survival rate from each dose fraction amplify into large differences after many such doses. For example, if cell survival rate in one tissue was 60% (or 0.6) after a dose of 200 cGy, and 50% (or 0.5) in another, the ratio of cell survival rate after n doses of 200 cGy would be $(0.6/0.5)^n$. For n = 30, the difference is 237-fold, and for n = 35, the difference is 590-fold. The effect of differences in survival rate per fraction ranging from 0.35 to 0.65 on the outcome of 30 fractions of 200 cGy are shown in Figure 2-11.[266] The ratio of cell survival rate after 30 × 2 Gy is shown on the ordinate, and the change in total dose to achieve the same level of survival rate (approximately 10^{-9}) is shown on the abscissa. Thus a relatively small difference between tumors and normal tissues in response to each fraction in a clinical dose regimen using 200 cGy fractions could have a major influence on the outcome of therapy. Unfortunately, it is not yet possible to measure survival rate of human tumor cells with the accuracy needed to predict the outcome of a course of therapy, but efforts to achieve this end are intensifying.[27,28,37,155,159]

The Other Rs

As will be discussed later, factors other than repair of sublethal damage and repopulation may influence survival rate from a multifraction dose regimen. The most important such phenomena occurring in surviving cells between dose fractions are *redistribution* through the division cycle[242,270] and, in hypoxic

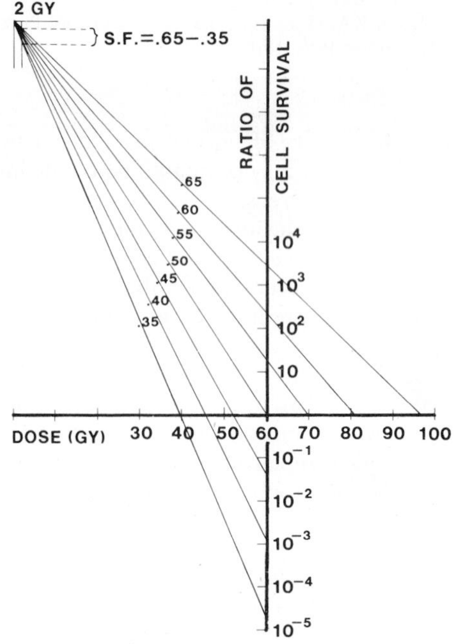

FIGURE 2–11. Effective multifraction-dose survival curves for cell populations, the survival of which from 2 Gy varies from 0.65 to 0.35. When survival from 2 Gy is 0.5, survival from 30 × 2 Gy is $(0.5)^{30}$ = approximately 10^{-9}. In constructing the figure, this survival value was taken as an arbitrary "standard" against which the relative survival of other populations exposed to 30 × 2 Gy was plotted. The abscissa at the standard survival shows the total doses in 2 Gy fractions necessary to achieve that standard survival level in different cell populations. In all cases, an equal effect per dose fraction was assumed. The ratios of cell survival after a total dose of 60 Gy illustrate the exponential amplification of survival differences with increasing dose. Thus dose fractionation can transform small differences in response at low doses (2.0 Gy) to large ultimate differences; measurements must be made accurately after a dose of 2 Gy to predict accurately the ultimate outcome of high-dose multifraction irradiation. (Reprinted with permission from Withers HR: Int J Radiat Oncol Biol Phys 12:693, 1986 © 1986 Pergamon Press, Ltd)

tumor clonogens, *reoxygenation*,[110] which complete the four Rs of dose fractionation in radiation therapy.[238,241] If the effect of such phenomena on the response to each dose were constant throughout the whole course of a multifraction regimen, the resulting survival curve would be linear but with a slope that would depend on the extent that each phenomenon affected the response to each dose fraction. More likely, the influence of the various phenomena, and particularly that of regeneration, varies with time, and, as a result, the effective rate of reduction in survival changes as treatment progresses.

Potentially Lethal Damage and Repair

If cells are held for several hours after irradiation in a nonproliferative state (by keeping them in a nutrient-free medium, in contact inhibition, or in a medium containing a drug such as cycloheximide, which inhibits protein synthesis), their survival rate is increased in relation to that observed if they are allowed to progress through the division cycle. This increase in cell survival rate from modifying the growth conditions after a single dose of x-rays (distinct from the increase in survival rate resulting from sublethal damage repair that occurs when a dose is split into two fractions) has been attributed to repair of potentially lethal damage.[24,87,120,161,209,210,225–227] The terms *sublethal damage repair* (SLDR) and *potentially lethal damage repair* (PLDR) are operational, describing repair measured in split-dose and single-dose experiments, respectively, and do not imply that the mechanisms are different or even understood. Whether the mechanisms of SLDR and PLDR are the same or different is controversial.[209,210]

Most experiments indicate that PLDR is constant at all dose levels, that is, that the ratio of doses required to produce an effect in its presence or absence is the same at all levels of injury (Fig. 2-12). However, it is difficult to measure this accurately at low doses, just as it has been difficult to measure differences in oxygen enhancement ratio at low doses.[142] For the most part, the demonstration of PLDR has been *in vitro*. Some *in vivo* transplantation assays for survival in nonproliferating normal tissues (liver[72,108] and mammary[41] cell) have shown *in situ* repair when transplantation was delayed. Some results show a greater relative increase in survival rate at low than at high doses, increasing the size of the shoulder in the survival curve, an effect that has not been observed *in vitro*, whereas others show only a shallower slope.[72] Some *in vitro* assays suggest that PLDR is less at low than at high doses.[87] Less PLDR at doses where

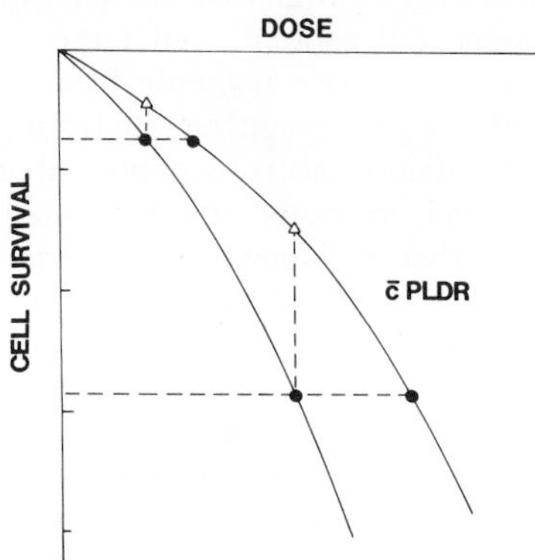

FIGURE 2–12. The typical effect of repair of potentially lethal damage (PLDR) on cell survival. The ratio of dose to produce a given level of cell survival in the presence or absence of PLDR is constant at all levels of injury (in this example, 1.4).

nonrepairable damage predominates is consistent with other observations that PLDR does not occur after high LET exposures.[24] Other studies, however, have shown that postirradiation culture conditions can reduce the slope of the initial part of the x-ray dose survival curve, that is, they can permit repair of single-hit injury.[209,210]

PLDR after x-irradiation is influenced by division cycle stage either slightly[161] or not at all.[24] This is in contrast to the large differences found for SLDR.

The significance of PLDR to radiation therapy would be in its effect on the response of nonproliferating cells: It could increase the tolerance dose for a nonproliferative cell population (*e.g.*, in the target cells for late injury), by reducing the initial slope of the survival curve.

It is frequently hypothesized that because solid tumors have a low growth fraction, their clonogenic cells repair PLD, and that this could be a cause for failure of radiation therapy.[225–227] PLDR may be a factor in the radioresistance of slowly responding tumors but is unlikely to be significant in the response of most tumors, especially after the surviving clonogenic cells accelerate their growth rate. Because it is likely that repair of PLDR could reduce the effect of x-irradiation more in late-responding normal tissues than in tumors, it would seem unwise to devise clinical schemes for reducing the effectiveness of PLDR (except in the unlikely event that such approaches could be made tumor-specific).

TUMOR CONTROL PROBABILITY

As clonogenic tumor cell survival decreases with increasing radiation dose, the probability of tumor control increases, but not linearly. Success or failure in controlling a tumor depends on killing the last surviving clonogen. Therefore, in terms of tumor control (excluding palliation), all the dose is "wasted" if even one clonogen survives; conversely, control is achieved abruptly as the last clonogen is sterilized. A plot of the probability of control *versus* dose for a single tumor is therefore one of 0% response up to a certain dose and then an immediate rise to 100% response at the death of the last clonogen. When the dose response of 100 exactly similar tumors is plotted, however, the shape of the tumor control probability (TCP) curve is different because cell killing is a random process.

Because of the randomness of cell killing, there is, after exposure of a series of identical tumors to a constant dose of radiation, a Poisson (or, strictly speaking, binomial) distribution of numbers of surviving clonogens per tumor. For example, if a certain dose reduced the cell survival to an *average* of one clonogen per tumor, there would be, on an average among the series of identical tumors, 37% with no survivors, 37% with one, 18.4% with two, 6.1% with three, and 1.5% with four or more surviving clonogens; the total number of surviving clonogens would be the same as the number of tumors irradiated (an average of one cell per tumor). Obviously, the local control rate would be 37%, not 0%.

Poisson statistics correlate probability of tumor control with cell survival rate by the formula,

$$P_{cure} = e^{-x} = e^{-(SF \cdot M)},$$

where x is the average number of surviving clonogens per tumor, which in turn is the product of SF, the fraction of cells surviving, and M, the initial cell number. If, for example, a tumor contained 10^7 clonogens initially, a reduction by a factor of 10^7 (to a cell survival rate of 10^{-7}) would be required to reduce average cell survival to one and P_{cure} to $e^{-1} = .37$ or 37%.

$$P_{cure} = e^{-(10^7 \times 10^{-7})} = e^{-1} = .37, \text{ or } 37\%.$$

If the total dose were increased by two $_eD_0$ values, cell survival would be further reduced by two natural logarithms, from 1 to $1 \times e^{-2}$, that is, to an average of 0.135 cells per tumor, and

$$P_{cure} = e^{-0.135} = .87, \text{ or } 87\%$$

It can be calculated that an increase in dose by three effective D_o values is sufficient to raise the probability of cure from 10% to 90%.

$$\text{If } P_{cure} = 10\% = .1 = e^{-x}$$
$$\text{then } x = 2.3.$$

where x is the average number of surviving clonogens per tumor. In other words, at 10% local control rate there is an average of 2.3 clonogens per tumor.

After an increase in dose by three $_eD_0$ values,

$$P_{cure} = e^{-(2.3 \times e^{-3})} = e^{-(0.115)} = .89, \text{ or } 89\%.$$

This relationship between probability of cure and dose, above a certain threshold, is described by a sigmoid curve (Fig. 2-13). It is obvious from the previous equations and calculations that the slope of the curve is a function of the $_eD_0$ values for the last few surviving tumor clonogens. It is steeper for neutrons or for single-dose x-ray treatments than for multifraction x-ray exposures, and steeper (by the OER) for euoxic than for hypoxic cells.

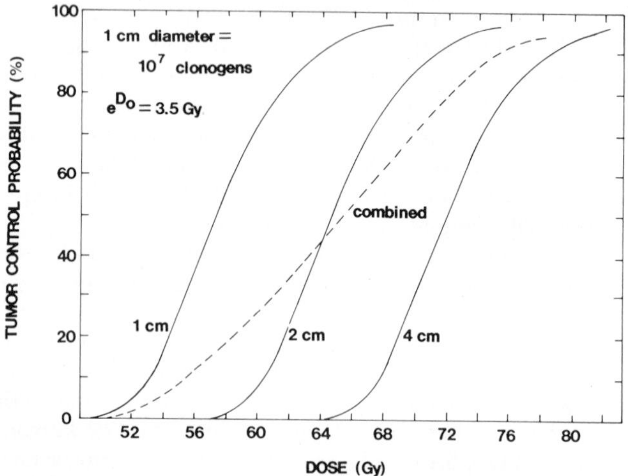

FIGURE 2–13. Theoretical tumor control probability (TCP) curves for three spherical tumors (*solid lines*) and one that would result from a study incorporating into the dose response analysis all three tumor sizes in equal proportions (*broken line*). They were calculated on the assumptions that the dose was given in 2 Gy fractions, that the $_eD_o$ value for 2 Gy per fraction was 3.5 Gy, and that a 1 cm diameter spherical tumor contained 10^7 clonogens. As tumor volume increases, so does the dose required for a certain probability of control. The cell number increases by 8 times and 64 times as the spherical tumor increases from 1 cm diameter to 2 cm and 4 cm, respectively. An exponential increase in clonogen number is related to a linear increase in dose for an isoeffect. Heterogeneity of even one factor, initial clonogen number, causes the TCP curve to be shallower (*broken line*). Retrospective clinical studies incorporate a large number of causes for heterogeneity of response.

TCP curves are sometimes plotted as logit or probit curves. Such graphs are a form of logarithmic plot in which the incidence of tumor control is plotted logarithmically on either side of the 50% value. This method is useful for mathematical analyses of data (*e.g.*, for determining TCD_{50} values) and yields straight lines instead of sigmoid curves.

The dose that yields a 50% control rate is known as the tumor control dose 50 or TCD_{50}. Any level of control can be specified, and in clinical studies a higher rate is aspired to, but for experimental studies, the TCD_{50} is useful because it is in a steep part of the curve and hence sensitive to small changes in the effectiveness of therapy. (The curve is steepest at TCD_{37}, *i.e.*, the dose at which there is an average of one surviving clonogenic cell per tumor, which would make the TCD_{37} value an even more sensitive endpoint than the TCD_{50}.)

Although TCP curves with the anticipated slope can be constructed from experimental animal data, those for human tumor control usually are shallower than predicted from estimates of tumor cell radiosensitivity.[19,74,81,90,134,157,176,177,196] This reflects heterogeneity of the clinical material and treatment prescriptions. Heterogeneity, which leads to a shallower slope because of a wider spread of tumor responses to a given (nominal) dose, is caused by different initial numbers of clonogens, differences in repair of sublethal injury and potentially lethal injury, a spectrum of redistribution and regeneration rates, variations in reoxygenation kinetics, inhomogeneities of dose distribution, differences in dose rate, geographic misses, differences in dose calculation, inconsistency of methods of dose prescription, and more.

The effect of constructing TCP curves for a series of tumors nonhomogeneous in only one characteristic is illustrated in Figure 2-13. It was assumed that otherwise similar tumors were of three sizes, varying in diameter by factors of 2. Because volume is proportional to the cube of the diameter, ($V = \pi d^3/6$), there is an eightfold difference in clonogen number for each doubling in tumor diameter. If the tumors were stratified carefully by volume, three distinct steep TCP curves would be obtained. If the analysis included tumors of all sizes and if each tumor size formed one third of the sample being analyzed in a carefully performed experiment using a range of total doses, the TCP curve obtained for the whole group would be that shown as a broken line. Although it would not be appropriate to include tumors with a 64-fold range of volumes in an analysis of clinical results, heterogeneity of such magnitude is easily possible because the range of total cell content in a certain stage of human cancer may be large and the range in clonogenic cell content even larger. Variations in clonogenic cell content derive not only from differences in tumor volume within a given stage but also from differences in extent of cell differentiation, necrosis, or normal cell infiltration (fibrovascular stroma, macrophages, or other reticuloendothelial cells). Further variation in the *effective* number of clonogens would arise from differences among tumors in the rate of repopulation of surviving cells during radiation therapy and the lag time until that acceleration begins.

Additional reasons exist for expecting relatively shallow TCP curves from analyses of clinical data. Most data were derived from retrospective studies because it is not acceptable practice to deliver a range of total doses in a prospective study merely to establish a dose response curve for that type of tumor. If radiation therapy were perfect, the doses given to a series of patients would be individualized to yield the same (high) probability of control in each patient, and the TCP curve would be flat. Even if not perfect, treatment is often individualized, which tends to flatten TCP curves from retrospective studies. Furthermore, changes in dose per fraction and overall time introduce heterogeneity into the biologically effective dose. The NSD equation has been used in efforts to normalize differences between physical and biologic isodose contours[229] and to construct TCP curves.[171, 173] However, this equation is now known to be inappropriate for these purposes.[259]

In recent analyses of tumor response, the effect of variations in tumor characteristics and in treatment parameters has been minimized.[125] Uniformity among tumors was facilitated by analyzing a body of data large enough to allow relatively homogeneous stages of disease to be studied independently. Variations in treatment parameters were minimized by analyzing subgroups of patients treated within a narrow range of overall treatment time and by correcting for size of dose per fraction using the LQ isoeffect formula. With these advantages, the analyses produced relatively steep dose response curves (see Fig. 2-3, in which 400 cGy increase TCP from 50% to 90%).

Dose response curves for the incidence of a certain effect (a specific complication) in normal tissues are also sigmoid above a certain threshold. Curves for death from bone marrow or gastrointestinal injury are well known, but any tissue effect (paralysis, fatal pneumonitis, skin desquamation) may be used as an endpoint. Such curves are used for estimating LD_{50} or ED_{50} values, the doses that cause lethality or any specified effect in 50% of cases, respectively. Because normal tissues are more homogeneous than tumors in their composition and radiation responses, complication probability curves are steeper than those for tumor control.[105, 129, 194]

The art of radiation therapy can be quantified. The probability of tumor control must be balanced against the probability of complications in a risk-benefit analysis (both represented by sigmoid curves illustrated in Fig. 1-10), with many factors relating to both the tumor and the host. This is illustrated by different points:

1. Improvements in radiation therapy require that the response curves for normal tissue and tumor responses be separated further. Increases in biologic effectiveness of therapy must be greater in the tumor than in normal tissues, or normal tissues must be preferentially spared if there is to be a therapeutic gain.
2. In the steep midrange of tumor control probability, or complication frequency, a small change in the biologic effectiveness of therapy can provide a substantial change in clinical outcome. This has a further implication: If a change in treatment produces a modest difference in effect (*e.g.*, of tumor control or of frequency of complications), that change should not be interpreted as a major change in the *biologic* effectiveness of the dose.
3. At incidences of effect less than about 10% and greater than about 85%, the changes in effect with changes in biologically effective dose are less dramatic. For example, if the TCP were already 90%, no therapeutic gain would occur and perhaps a therapeutic disadvantage would be achieved from increases in dose if there were already an associated incidence of severe complications of 5% or more.
4. In view of the closeness of dose response curves for normal tissues and most human tumors, it is inappropriate for the radiation therapist to produce no complications in practice. Clearly, devastating complications such as myelitis should be strenuously avoided, as should any unnecessary complications. Within the treatment volume, however, a certain incidence of occurrence of injury to normal tissues sufficient to be defined as a complication is a prerequisite to good curative radiation therapy.
5. If the tumor response curve is predominantly to the right of the normal tissue complications curve, tumor control without complications is unlikely and other modalities should be used, either independently or as adjuvants. For example, the TCP curves for large tumors may lie to the right of those for complications, whereas those for smaller tumors of the same type may be to the left. In this situation a therapeutic gain could result from excision of the main mass of a large tumor by surgery, or some form of chemotherapy may add to the effect of irradiation without increasing normal tissue toxicity. However, a 50% or even 90% debulking is of modest value: A 90% reduction in tumor volume represents only one decade reduction in (logarithmic) cell number, equivalent to 700 cGy to 900 cGy in 200 cGy fractions, other things being equal.

The relative shallowness of human TCP curves discussed earlier should not obscure the fact that for an individual patient, tumor eradication depends on sterilizing the last clonogen, and it is not known at what dose along the abscissa of a TCP curve the patient's chances increase from 0% to 100%. It is without biologic rationale to deny the existence of a potential benefit from maximizing the dose in a patient considered to have some finite chance of tumor control merely because retrospective studies (incorporating an inevitable heterogeneity of tumors and treatments) reveal a shallow TCP curve.[90]

OXYGEN EFFECT

Oxygen is the most potent chemical modifier of radiosensitivity.[50, 65, 85, 166] Hypoxic mammalian cells are 2.5 to 3.0 times less radiosensitive than well-oxygenated cells. Many early clinicians and radiobiologists had reported that restricting the blood flow to a tissue decreased its radiation response. They thought it was a metabolic effect, but in 1951 Read[166] showed that oxygen sensitized cells through a radiochemical mechanism that enhanced the infliction of injury.

The exact mechanisms by which oxygen sensitizes cells to radiation are not known for sure.[5, 3, 69] It is generally believed that it enhances injury by combining with an unpaired electron in the outer shell of a free radical to yield a peroxide, which is more stable and toxic than the free radical. Because the lifetime of a free radical is measured in microseconds,[25] oxygen must be present in the nucleus at the time of irradiation; adding it even 1/100 of a second after exposure produces no sensitization to radiation. The property of oxygen critical to its radiosensitizing effect is its electron affinity, and from this realization radiochemists developed oxygen-mimetic, electron-affinic radiosensitizers[1, 29, 186] such as metronidazole, misonidazole, SR2509, and other nitroimidazoles. These radiosensitizers have the potential to be more useful than oxygen in clinical radiation therapy because they are easier to administer; also because they are less rapidly metabolized, they can diffuse further from blood vessels into the hypoxic regions of the tumor.[52]

The relationship between oxygen tension and radiosensitivity, an example of which is shown in Figure 2-14,[50] varies among cell types. A radiosensitivity halfway between that of hypoxic and euoxic (aerobic) cells is achieved with oxygen concentrations ranging from about 3 mm to 10 mm Hg.[5, 47, 50, 65]

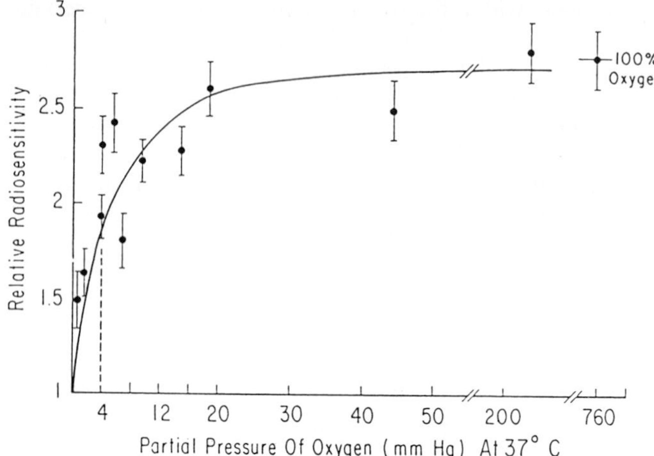

FIGURE 2–14. Curve relating cellular radiation sensitivity to partial pressure of O_2 at the time of irradiation. Data were obtained by scoring anaphase aberrations in Ehrlich ascites tumor cells,[50] but very similar curves have been obtained for cell killing of both mammalian cells[45] and bacteria.[5] About 50% of the total sensitization by O_2 is seen at a partial pressure of approximately 4 mm Hg at 37°C. (Withers HR, Peters LJ: Biological aspects of radiation therapy. In Fletcher GH [ed]: Textbook of Radiotherapy, 3rd ed. Philadelphia, Lea & Febiger, 1980)

The oxygen concentration at which half-sensitization occurs has been called the *k value.*[5] The curve relating metabolic activity to oxygen concentration is much steeper than, and to the left of that shown for radiosensitivity in Figure 2-14. Therefore, hypoxic cells with a markedly reduced radiosensitivity can be viable and metabolically normal.

Figure 2-15 shows how survival curves are modified by oxygen concentration. The ratio of doses required to produce the same effect (*e.g.*, a certain level of cell survival) in hypoxic conditions as in euoxia is called the *oxygen enhancement ratio* (OER). The OER usually varies between 2.5 and 3.0 for a wide variety of mammalian (and other) cell types exposed to x-rays or τ-rays and does not vary as cells progress through the division cycle.

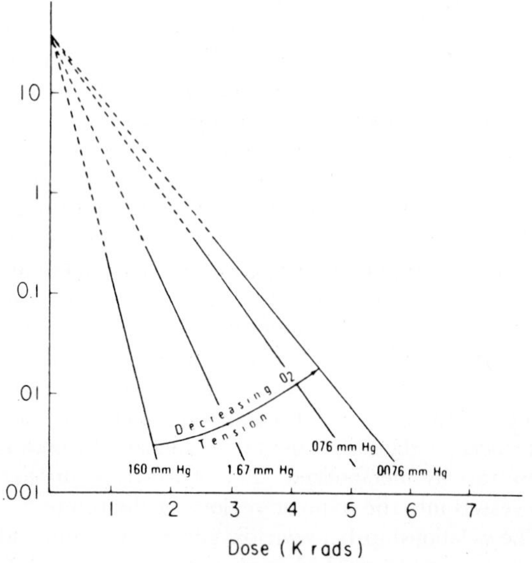

FIGURE 2–15. Survival curves for Chinese hamster cells irradiated at different O_2 tensions.[65] Decreasing $_pO_2$ reduces the slope of the final exponential region of the survival curve without changing the extrapolation number. (OER) = D_o hypoxic/D_o air. (Withers HR, Peters LJ: Biological aspects of radiation therapy. In Fletcher GH [ed]: Textbook of Radiotherapy, 3rd ed. Philadelphia, Lea & Febiger, 1980)

The OER varies with the type of radiation. For very densely ionizing radiations such as α particles or the beams of stripped nuclei produced by the Bevalac at Berkeley, the OER may be 1 or close to it. For neutrons used in clinical radiation therapy, it is approximately 1.6.

Until recently, it was generally considered that oxygen was dose-modifying; that is, OER was constant at all doses. However, evidence is mounting that at low doses[143] or low dose rates[88, 89] of x-rays or τ-rays, the OER may be slightly lower than the 2.5 to 3.0 that is characteristic at high doses. As discussed, electrons scattered by photons may be regarded operationally as a mixture of low and high LET particles. It is not unreasonable to postulate that a lower oxygen enhancement ratio at low doses or low dose rates reflects the predominance of the relatively high-LET "neutron-like" component of the scattered electrons in producing cell killing. Thus low dose rates or low fractional doses of x-rays are a form of "poor man's neutrons."[250]

Relevance of Hypoxia to Clinical Radiation Therapy

Solid tumors contain cells at oxygen tensions less than necessary for maximum radiosensitivity.[80, 95, 110, 137, 164, 188, 190, 200, 201] Oxygenation of tissues at the microscopic level is critically dependent on blood flow in capillaries, and values of arterial and venous oxygen tension are of secondary relevance if blood is stagnant or nearly stagnant, which it can be in the inefficient capillaries in tumors.[221]

Hypoxic foci in tumors may reflect not only a low ratio of total surface area of the capillary network per unit volume of tissue,[221] but also sluggish blood flow and shunting.

Tumor cell hypoxia has been demonstrated in experimental animals by a variety of methods.[137] When a tumor contains a small proportion of hypoxic cells, the dose survival curve for its constituent cells has two components: an initial, relatively rapid decline in cell survival rate from depletion of the more radiosensitive euoxic cells and then a flexure and a slower decline resulting from the radioresistance of the small proportion of hypoxic cells, which, because of their radioresistance, survive doses much higher than those tolerated by their euoxic counterparts. The influence of small proportions of hypoxic cells on responses to single and multifraction regimens will be discussed later.

Human tumors probably also contain a proportion of hypoxic cells. The pH of venous blood from tumors is usually lower than that from normal tissues, indicating that anaerobic glycolysis occurs within the tumor.[44] Histologic evidence of necrosis is seen in many tumors.[201] Average pO_2 levels measured by oxygen electrodes are lower in tumors than in normal tissues.[34, 80] Colposcopic and histologic examination of carcinoma of the cervix shows widely spaced and inefficient (sinusoidal) blood vessels.[114] More recently, metabolic breakdown products of misonidazole, characteristic of hypoxic physiology, have been found in human tumor cells.[35, 36, 208] Some observations of improved results of radiation therapy from treatment in hyperbaric oxygen[53, 91, 211] or after correction of anemia,[31, 68] and of worse results when oxygen content of the tumor is low,[80] also suggest that hypoxia may limit the radiocurability of a proportion of human cancers.[169]

Despite the probable existence of hypoxic cells within many, if not all, solid tumors of humans, hypoxia does not appear to be a constant and possibly not even a common cause of failure of radiation therapy.[261] The most likely reason for this is that the oxygenation of tumor cells varies during radiation therapy so that cells that are hypoxic one day may be euoxic at some later time during therapy. This phenomenon is called *reoxygenation,*[110] which will be discussed later.

MULTIFRACTION TISSUE RESPONSES AND ISOEFFECT RELATIONSHIPS

History

Strandqvist[185] published isoeffect curves in 1944, in which he related the probability of tumor control and of skin reactions to overall treatment time. That work preceded the demonstration by Puck and Marcus[165] in 1956 that mammalian cell survival curves had a shoulder, and by Elkind and Sutton[64] in 1959 that sublethal injury could be repaired,[64] and therefore that number of fractions, not just overall time, was important.

Fowler and Stern[78] demonstrated that varying the number of fractions (N) and overall time (T) affected the response of skin independently, and Ellis[67] developed the NSD formula to incorporate these two variables into an isoeffect curve that was hoped would be relevant to radiation therapy.

More recently, isoeffect curves have been proposed based on parameters of dose survival curves only[16, 55, 199, 267] or also including other biologic parameters, such as regeneration.[42, 43] We now understand that there can be no single universally applicable isoeffect equation or curve because tissues (and tumors) differ in their fractionation responses and repopulation kinetics.[264]

The fractionation response of tissues and tumors can be considered in terms of four Rs[241]: repair of sublethal injury, regeneration, redistribution within the division cycle, and, in tumors, reoxygenation.

Repair of Sublethal Damage: Acutely Responding versus Late-Responding Tissues

The most general biologic phenomenon among those influencing the fractionation response is the capacity for repair of sublethal injury.[64] It does, however, vary among tissues, with slowly responding tissues consistently showing a greater capacity than rapidly responding tissues.[16, 199, 265–268] A possible explanation for the systematic difference between early- and late-responding tissues is that repair in early-responding tissues is foreshortened by the progression of surviving cells within the division cycle with consequent "fixation" of injury. Regardless of the mechanism, the effect is that late-responding tissues are spared more by dose fractionation than are acutely responding tissues; that is, the dose for an isoeffect in late-responding tissues increases relatively more with dose fractionation than it does for an isoeffect in an acutely responding tissue.

The slopes of the isoeffect curves in Figure 2-16 reflect the shape of the dose survival or dose function curves for the target cells in various tissues. The steeper slopes of isoeffect curves for late responses reflect a cell-killing mechanism characterized by relatively less single-hit (α-type) injury and dominated more by accumulation of repairable (multhit or β-type) injury than in acutely responding tissues. In terms of the linear quadratic cell survival model, the target cells for late effects have a low α/β ratio, describing a survival curve that curves more than that for acutely responding tissues (Fig. 2-17). Thus, as dose per fraction is increased, there is a relatively steeper decline in survival rate of target cells in late-responding than in early-responding tissues; conversely, with decrease in dose per fraction, relatively greater sparing occurs in late-responding tissues (Fig. 2-18).

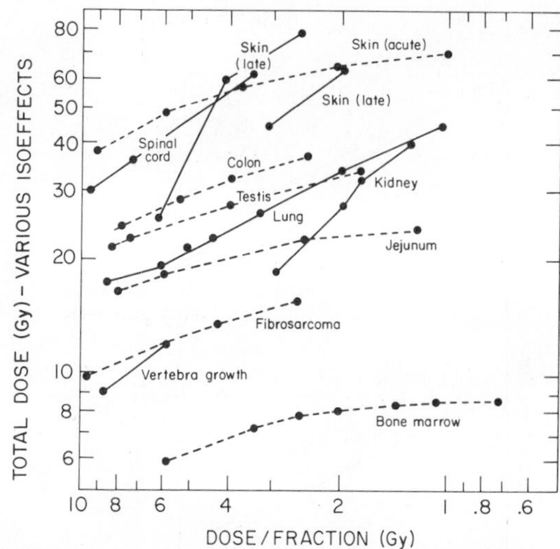

FIGURE 2–16. Isoeffect curves in which the total dose necessary for a certain effect in various tissues is plotted as a function of dose per fraction. (late effects: *solid lines*; acute effects: *broken lines*). Data were selected to exclude an influence on total dose of regeneration during multifraction experiments. The isodoses for late effects increase more rapidly with decrease in dose per fraction than is the case for acute effects. (Withers HR: Cancer 55:2086, 1985)

Also, repair of sublethal injury continues far longer in late-responding than in early-responding tissues.[9, 192, 193, 195]

The lower α/β ratios for late-responding tissues are a consistent observation in experimental systems and in clinical experience.[199, 264–266, 268] Examples of α/β values for tissues are shown in Table 2-1.

Some specific clinical implications of the differences in fractionation response between acutely and late-responding tissues are the following:

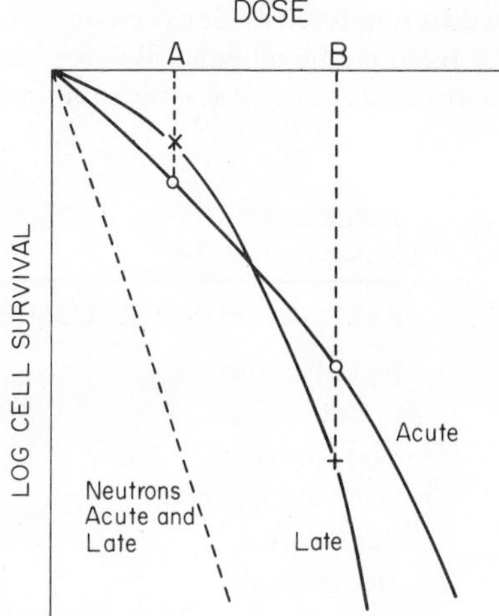

FIGURE 2–17. Hypothetical survival curves for the target cells for acute and late effects in normal tissues exposed to x-rays or neutrons. The α/β ratio is lower for late effects than for acute effects in x-irradiated tissues, resulting in a greater change in effect in late-responding tissues with a change in dose. At dose A, survival of target cells is higher in late-effects than in acute-effect tissues; at dose B, the reverse is true. Increasing the dose per fraction from A to B results in a relatively greater increase in late than acute injury. For neutrons, the α/β ratio is high with no detectable influence of the quadratic function (βd^2) over the first two decades of reduction in cell survival, implying that accumulation of sublethal injury plays a negligible role in cell killing by doses of neutrons of clinical interest. (Withers HR, Thames HD, Peters LJ: Int J Radiat Oncol Biol Phys 8:2071, 1982 © 1982 Pergamon Press, Ltd)

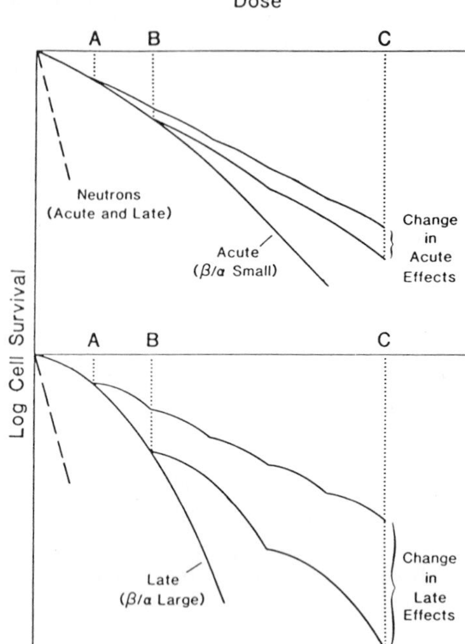

FIGURE 2–18. Hypothetical single and multifraction dose-survival curves for target cells in acutely and late-responding tissues. The single-dose curve for acute effects has a long initial exponential region, and the curve bends slowly—a response described by a high α/β ratio in the linear-quadratic (LQ) response model. The curve for late effects curves more and is described by a low α/β ratio. With changes in fraction size A to B there is relatively little change in the effective multifraction survival curve for acute effects but a large change in that for late effects. (Withers HR, Thames HD, Peters LJ: Differences in the fractionation response of acute and late responding tissues. In Karcher KH, Kogelnik HD, Reinartz G [eds]: Progress in Radio-Oncology II, pp 287–296. New York, Raven Press, 1982)

1. Large dose fractions are relatively more harmful for late-responding tissues. If the same acute reactions are achieved with two different fractionation regimens—one using large doses per fraction, the other small doses per fraction—the late responses will be more severe from the large dose per fraction regimen. This dissociation has been observed in many clinical studies.[7,127,140,141,199,206,266–268]
2. A therapeutic gain may be possible by using the smallest practical dose per fraction in treating tumors, especially the more highly proliferative ones that respond quickly. A continuing decrease in dose per fraction leads to a relatively greater increase in the "tolerance" dose for late-responding tissues than in the dose required for a specified level of tumor control; that is, the therapeutic differential between late-responding tissues and tumors increases. For example, if it were necessary to deliver two fractions of 120 cGy to achieve the same effect in a late-responding tissue as with one fraction of 200 cGy, but two fractions of only 105 cGy for an isoeffect in an acutely responding tumor, the therapeutic gain would be 1.2/1.05 = 1.14. In this example, hyperfractionation would increase the biologically effective tumor dose by 14% with no increase in the biologically effective dose to the late-responding normal tissues. If the α/β ratio for acutely responding normal tissues was the same as that for the tumor, a concomitant 14% increase would occur in biologically effective dose to the acutely responding normal tissues that would have to be tolerated. In some hyperfractionated regimens, the acute toxicity may demand an increase in the overall treatment duration to permit more regeneration by normal tissue cells. This would reduce the magnitude of the therapeutic gain from hyperfractionation.
3. To achieve the maximal potential therapeutic gain, repair of sublethal damage in late-responding tissues must be complete, implying fractionation intervals of at least 6 hours if multiple fractions are given each day.[9,158,192,193,195] For spinal cord it should be longer.
4. The relative biologic efficiency (RBE) for neutrons for late effects is high at low doses because the greater sparing effect from fractionated x-ray doses is lost. This high RBE for late effects, which has been found in clinical trials of neutron radiation therapy,[105] does not reflect an especially damaging effect of neutrons on slowly responding tissues but rather the disproportionate sparing of these tissues with fractionated doses of x-rays.[240]

TABLE 2–1
*Values for α/β (Gy)**

EARLY-RESPONDING TISSUES	α/β	LATE-RESPONDING TISSUES	α/β†
Jejunal mucosa	13	Spinal cord[86,121,174,212,213,230]	1.6–5
Colonic mucosa	7	Kidney[33,96,218,231]	0.5–5
Skin epithelium	10	Lung[71,140,144,204,216,220]	1.6–4.5
Spermatogenic cells	13	Liver[72]	1.4–3.5
Bone marrow	9	Human skin[23,140,206,207]	1.6–4.5
Melanocytes[219]	6.5	Cartilage and submucosa[127]	1.0–4.9
Mouse fibrosarcoma metastases[128]	10	Dermis[84]	2.5 ± 1.0
Human tumors[125,126,136,187,190]	6–25	Bladder[183]	5.0–10.0
		Bone[141]	1.8–2.5
Experimental tumors[232]	10–35	Mediastinum/pericardium[45,46,116]	1.0–2.5

* *Values are a synthesis from ranges of values from our own data, from references shown, and from a collection of data references elsewhere (references 77, 199, 253–256). They were mostly derived from doses per fraction <10 Gy for two reasons: clinical relevance and uncertainty about the applicability of linear quadratic model at high doses.*

† *The influence of α/β value on isoeffect dose calculations increases with decrease in the α/β ratio, but the data are least well defined for tissues characterized by low α/β values. The uncertainties of values for late effects reflect several technical difficulties in experimental assessment of fractionation responses in slowly responding tissues, and are reason for caution in using the LQ isoeffect formula, especially for doses per fraction less than 2 Gy.[11,109]*

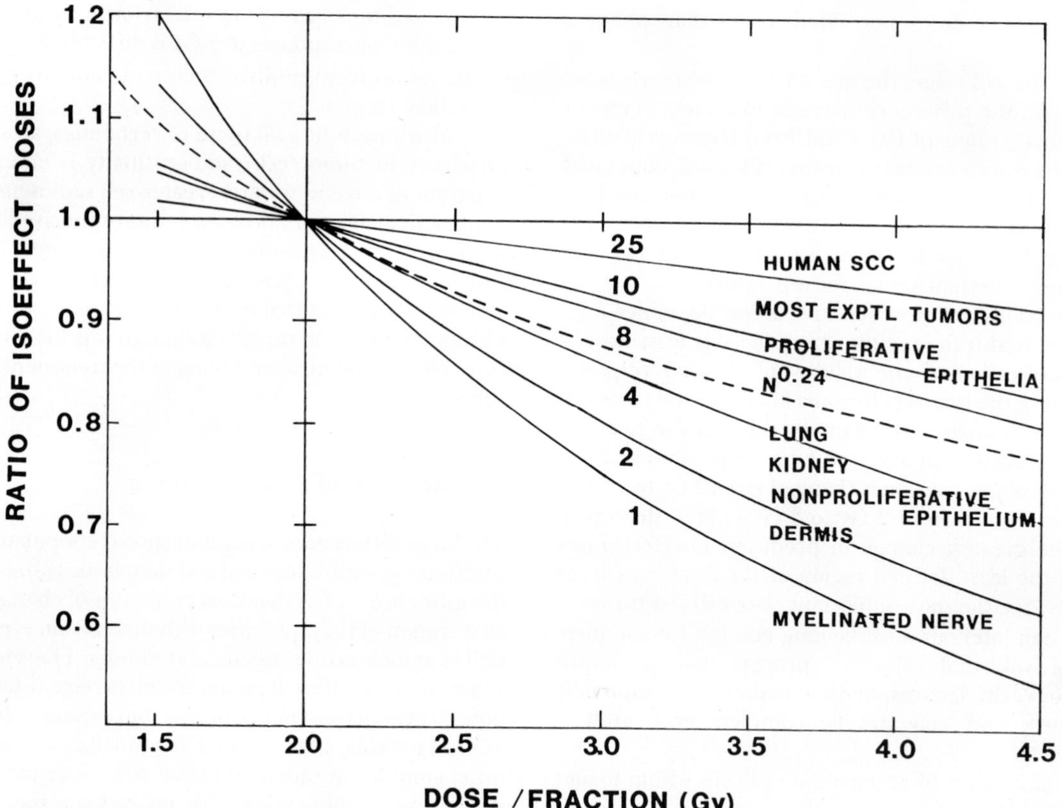

FIGURE 2–19. Isoeffect curves relating total dose to dose per fraction, total dose being expressed as a ratio of that necessary in 2 Gy fractions (*i.e.*, the $LQED_{2Gy}$). α/β ratios (in Gy) are shown on the curves. Although the α/β ratios are not yet established accurately or even precisely for most normal tissues, especially late-responding ones (see Table 2–1), the likely order of fractionation sensitivities is as shown. The broken line traces the change in dose as it would have been predicted by a factor $N^{0.24}$ in the nominal standard dose (NSD) formula. Phenomena other than repair of sublethal injury, specifically repopulation, are not accounted for by these curves. (Withers HR: Radiat Res 119:395, 1989)

Isoeffect Formula for Change in Fraction Size

It is possible (within limits) to quantify the effect of changing size of dose per fraction using a formula based on the assumption that the LQ response formula is appropriate[267]:

$$D_{new} = D_{ref} \times (\alpha/\beta + d_{ref}/\alpha/\beta + d_{new}),$$

where D_{new} is the total dose being determined for a change in size of dose per fraction to d_{new}, and D_{ref} is the total dose given previously in standard fractions of d_{ref}, and α/β is a characteristic of the dose response of the tissue in question, all doses being expressed in Gy. For example, if the new dose per fraction were to be 4 Gy and the standard fraction size was 2 Gy, the ratio of total doses to achieve the same effects in a tissue with an α/β value of 2 Gy would be .66. For a tissue with an α/β value of 10 Gy, it would be .85.

The curves in Figure 2-19 are constructed on the basis of the LQ response formula, assuming that the standard dose per fraction is 2 Gy and that the total dosage (normalized to 1) is that which would be given in 2 Gy fractions. Shown for comparison is a plot based on the NSD formula where the correction for time is ignored; that is, where $D = NSD \times N^{0.24}$. Figure 2-20 plots experimental data on the same type of isoeffect curve as shown in Figure 2-19.

The following caveats are emphasized regarding the present use of the LQ isoeffect formula and curves:

1. It has not been established that the LQ response model applies to tissue responses at all dose levels. It fits experimental data well over a limited dose range (*i.e.*, 2 Gy to 8 Gy), but its validity beyond that range has yet to be established, especially for such vital structures as spinal cord[10]

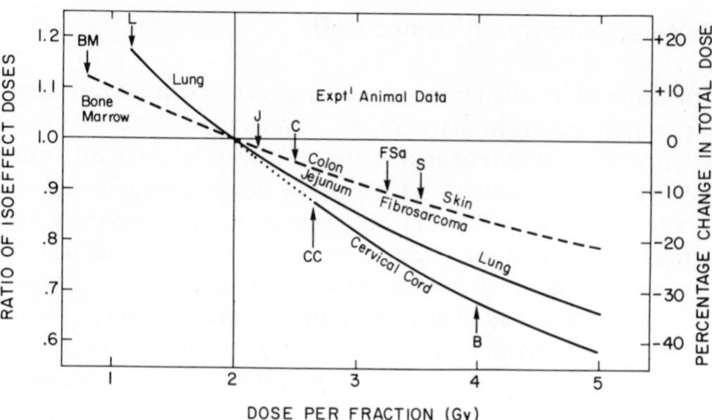

FIGURE 2–20. Isoeffect curves for experimental animal data. The lowest dose per fraction used in experiments with the various tissues is marked with an *arrow.* Variation in fractionation responses among tissues is large. Late-responding tissues require larger changes in total dose for an isoeffect when dose per fraction is changed. Responses at doses per fraction less than 2 Gy are needed before experimental animal data are useful in determining isoeffect doses for hyperfractionated regimens. (Withers HR, Thames HD, Peters LJ: Radiother Oncol 1:187, 1983)

and especially at doses per fraction less than about 2 Gy.[9,10,109]

2. The lower the α/β value, the greater the dose corrections. For example, the difference between isoeffect curves for tissues with α/β values of 10 Gy and 20 Gy is relatively small, whereas the difference between curves for α/β values of 1 Gy and 2 Gy is rather large (see Fig. 2-19). Because late-responding tissues are characterized by lower α/β values, they are at high risk for incorrect estimates of isoeffect doses using uncertain values for α/β values.
3. Dose corrections are most sensitive at low doses per fraction, which is also the region where there is least experimental verification of the validity of the LQ response model. Using the isoeffect formula above, or the curves in Figure 2-19, compare, for example, the ratios of isoeffect doses for a tissue characterized by an α/β value of 2 Gy when the dose per fraction is changed from 2 Gy to 1 Gy (a 33% increase) and from 2 Gy to 3 Gy (a 20% decrease). Hence, the greatest change in predicted isoeffect doses occurs in the least defined region of the isoeffect curves (low doses) for the most important (late effects) tissues.
4. Interfraction intervals must be long enough for complete repair of sublethal injury, a process that is significantly slower in late-responding tissues, and especially spinal cord, and may not be complete even after 6 hours.[9,158,192,193,195]
5. No account is taken of regeneration of cells within tissues during multifraction regimens.

For the previously mentioned reasons, the LQ formula or curve is of limited value. It should be used cautiously for estimating changes in total dose with change in fraction size below 2 Gy. It is useful, however, for changes between 2 Gy and 8 Gy.

Tissue responses and cell survival curves may be well defined by both the LQ and TC models over a range of doses from 2 Gy to about 8 Gy. However, at lower and higher doses the two models yield curves that diverge from one another. The clinical relevance of such a divergence is in the predicted response at low doses per fraction. If the low dose responses were better described by the TC than by the LQ model, then use of the LQ isoeffect formula would result in overdosage in hyperfractionated regimens.

Radiosensitivity of Tumor Cells

The doses of irradiation required for a certain control rate may vary widely among human tumors. Nevertheless, it is difficult to be sure to what extent malignant cells vary in their intrinsic (genetic) radiosensitivity. This is partly because epigenetic factors (*e.g.*, clonogen fraction, reoxygenation, and regrowth kinetics) probably vary greatly among tumors of the same histology and even more among tumors of different histology, obscuring the potential effects on tumor radiocurability of heterogeneity of intrinsic radiosensitivity. The uncertainty is also partly a reflection of the technical difficulties in measuring tumor cell radiosensitivity.

Recently, the intrinsic radiosensitivity of human tumor cells has received considerable experimental attention with the ultimate hope of factoring it into treatment strategy for individual patients.[27,28,37,48,70,155,159] The experimental methodology demands growth of tumor cells *in vitro* or as xenografts in immunologically tolerant (nude) mice. In most systems this involves a large cell selection factor because the "plating efficiency" (the fraction of cells that actually grows after transplantation into a culture medium or a nude mouse) is low. Furthermore, accurate quantitation of responses to 2 Gy is difficult, and measurement of $_{e}D_{o}$ values from multifraction irradiation is complicated by secondary factors.

Notwithstanding all these uncertainties, a picture of great variability in tumor cell radiosensitivity is emerging. This is apparent as a trend toward greater cell radiosensitivity among tumors that are traditionally radioresponsive,[48,70] as a wide spectrum of radiosensitivities within one tumor type,[27,28,155,159] and as variation in α/β ratios[187,190] (see Table 2-1). Most important, it is suggested that *in vitro* radiosensitivity might correlate with outcome of therapy,[159] although it is too early to apply *in vitro* cell survival measurements to the treatment of an individual patient.

Regeneration of Normal Tissue

The large differences in regeneration (repopulation) characteristics among various normal and neoplastic tissues illustrate that the influence on fractionation responses of changes in the overall duration of therapy varies with time within even one tissue as well as among various tissues and tumors. Therefore, a constant value in an isoeffect formula for a correction factor for variations in overall treatment duration (an exponent for time in days as used in NSD, CRE, or TDF formulas, *i.e.*, nominal standard dose, cumulative radiation effect, time-dose factor) is clearly a dangerous simplification with no biologic foundation.[259] For example, early regeneration of intestinal mucosa or bone marrow makes a major contribution to the net response to a treatment regimen protracted over several weeks, whereas protraction provides little or no benefit to spinal cord, kidney, or dermis.

Regeneration of Tumors

As discussed previously, the influence of overall treatment duration on local control rates in human tumors is greater than generally appreciated. Following are some clinical implications of tumor regeneration for curative radiation therapy:

Protracting treatment any longer than necessary is likely to be disadvantageous. For example, using 1.8 Gy rather than 2 Gy fractions given five times per week extends overall treatment time by about 10% and should be reserved for situations in which acute responses are likely to be dose-rate-limiting.

If a break in treatment is necessary because of acute toxicity, it should be kept as short as is tolerable.

Planned split-course therapy is inadvisable unless it is part of an accelerated treatment protocol that ultimately shortens the overall treatment duration (discussed later).

Breaks in therapy for nonmedical reasons (machine breakdown, holidays) may sometimes merit "catch-up" treatments, for example, by two treatments on 1 day in patients being treated for cure.

Obviously, rapidly growing tumors must be treated rapidly. However, it is reasonable to also accelerate to the extent possible the treatment of tumors with a high proliferative index, regardless of their growth rate because they are likely to reduce their cell loss rate and become rapidly growing during treatment as a response to the cytotoxic effect of therapy. In fact, the treatment of all tumors should be completed as quickly as possible (consistent with other considerations) because all tumors grow, and it is difficult to predict the accelerated repopulation response of individual tumors.

Redistribution

Cells vary in radiosensitivity as they traverse the division cycle.[178, 191] The survival curves in Figure 2-21 show an enormous variation in initial slopes, the difference in radiosensitivity between late S-phase and G_2-M cells being greater than that between euoxic and hypoxic cells (discussed later).

After exposure to a dose of 2 Gy, the survivors in an initially asynchronous population of cells will be partially synchronized in relatively resistant phases of the division cycle (because of the preferential killing of cells in sensitive phases). When these relatively resistant survivors resume their progression through the division cycle, they move into more sensitive phases; hence a fluctuating pattern of response results, as long as they remain synchronized.[64] It is impossible to exploit, for clinical gain, the fluctuating radiosensitivity of a synchronously progressing cell population. It is practical, however, and even unavoidable to exploit the *loss* of synchrony that results from differences in the rates at which surviving cells progress through the cell cycle.

Proliferating cells, particularly in tumors, have a wide spread in the rates at which they move from one mitosis to the next. This large variation in progression rates ensures early redistribution of partially synchronized cells toward a more asynchronous mixture. As a result, with time, a greater proportion of the surviving population will be in sensitive phases of the division cycle than was the case immediately after irradiation. Such redistribution to asynchrony produces a net "self-sensitization" within the population as a whole. Such self-sensitization does not occur in a nonproliferating cell population. Therefore, fractionation of dose would be expected to enhance the therapeutic ratio by permitting division cycle redistribution among surviving tumor cells but not among nonproliferating target cells in late-responding normal tissues.[242] The differential is greater the smaller the dose per fraction, and the differential obtained is amplified as an exponential function of the number of fractions delivered. This amplification of small differentials between cycling tumor cells

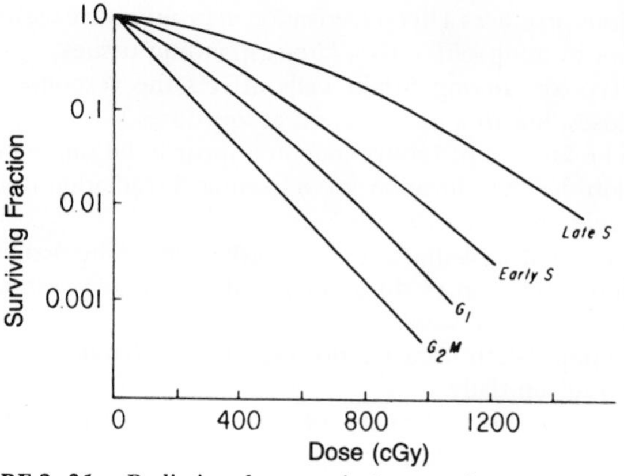

FIGURE 2–21. Radiation dose survival curves for one line of mammalian cells (V-79 Chinese hamster) synchronized in four positions in the division cycle.[178] Significant differences occur in the survival of cells at different ages, with the differences relative to absolute survival being greatest at lower doses. The survival ratio between late S and G_2M cells after 200 cGy is approximately 5. (Withers HR, Peters LJ: Biological aspects of radiation therapy. In Fletcher GH [ed]: Textbook of Radiotherapy, 3rd ed. Philadelphia, Lea & Febiger, 1980)

and the non-redistributing target cells in late-responding normal tissues was the rationale for initiating clinical trials of hyperfractionation[242] before it was appreciated that late-responding normal tissues also showed a systematically greater capacity for repair of sublethal injury.[199, 266, 268]

The effect of cell cycle redistribution on tissue and tumor responses to multifraction irradiation is difficult to demonstrate, even though variation in radiosensitivity within the division cycle has been amply demonstrated.[256] Cell cycle redistribution is probably the cause of the sensitivity of spermatogenic stem cells to split-dose irradiation[253] and can be demonstrated in jejunal crypt cells. However, in most circumstances, the effect of cell cycle distribution is subtle. It is difficult to envision that it does not influence multifraction responses in all proliferating tissues, and therefore its absence rather than its existence is difficult to demonstrate.

Reoxygenation

Commonly, about 30% of the cells in experimentally transplanted tumors in rodents are radiobiologically hypoxic, although sufficiently oxygenated to retain viability. Because these cells are radioresistant, they survive a dose of x-rays better than the 70% euoxic cells. Thus if no change occurs in the distribution of oxygenation during a course of 2 Gy fractions, the majority of cells surviving the first few fractions would be hypoxic. As a result, the fraction of cells surviving in such a hypoxic tumor cell population would not be less than 10^{-4} after 70 Gy in 2 Gy fractions. Lack of reoxygenation is not compatible with achieving high rates of tumor control with such doses.

Reoxygenation may result from several mechanisms: reduction in total tumor cell population without loss of blood vessels, resulting in a corresponding increase in vascular density; selective loss of the more radiation-sensitive euoxic cells, thus reducing the separation between the blood vessels and the more distant, previously hypoxic, cells; decreased oxygen consumption by dying cells, resulting in a shallower gradient in oxygen concentration as distance from the capillaries increases; cyclical variations in blood flow resulting from shunting; and ameboid movement of tumor cells.

The net effect of reoxygenation during fractionated irradiation is a relative sensitization of the tumor, which is in sharp contrast to the sparing effect of repair of sublethal damage. Because normal tissues are well vascularized and relatively well oxygenated to begin with, tumor reoxygenation during fractionated radiation therapy improves the therapeutic ratio relative to that achieved with single doses or a few large fractions.

The magnitude of the effect of reoxygenation on the response of a tumor to multiple dose fractions can be appreciated from Figure 2-22 and Table 2-2. To achieve the same probability of control with a series of 200 cGy fractions, the dose to a tumor that reoxygenated repeatedly to an 80-to-20 oxic-to-hypoxic cell mixture would need to be 15% higher than necessary if all tumor cells were euoxic (see Table 2-2). If the proportion of hypoxic cells were lower or if the oxygen enhancement ratio were less than 2.5, a dose increment less than 15% would be necessary. This contrasts with the nearly 250% increase (OER = 2.5) if there were no reoxygenation.

The rate at which reoxygenation occurs in human tumors is unknown. It has varied appreciably in animal experiments but in general occurs rapidly, being complete in most cases within 6 to 24 hours.[103, 200] Most studies on the kinetics of reoxygenation

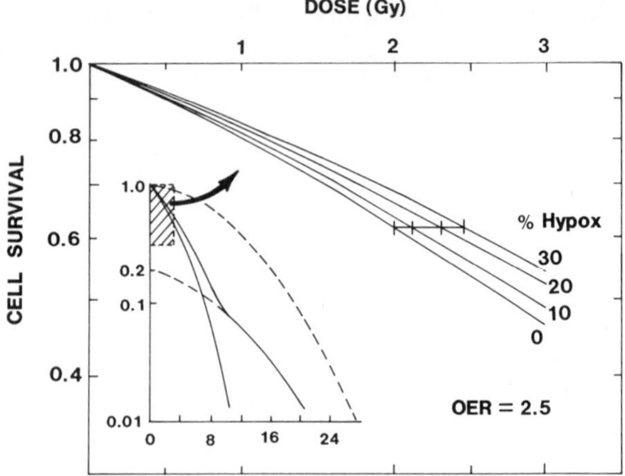

FIGURE 2–22. Survival curves to illustrate the effect of up to 30% hypoxic cells on the response to doses of clinical relevance (≤ 3 Gy). The oxygen enhancement ratio (OER) was assumed to be constant (2.5) up to 3 Gy. Dose modification factors from assuming various proportions of hypoxic cells are shown in Table 2–2. (*Inset*) Marked effect on compressed coordinates exerted by a minority (20%) of hypoxic cells after the dose is high enough to have killed most of the more sensitive, euoxic cells. For comparison, a curve for a completely hypoxic cell population is shown as a dashed line. The main figure is an enlargement of the hatched region of the inset. The numbers in Table 2–2 would be appreciably lower if the OER at low doses were less than 2.5, as suggested recently.[143]

in animal tumors have used large dose fractions. It is anticipated that reoxygenation would be more effective in a clinically relevant regimen using multiple small doses.[93]

In changing to a purely hyperfractionated regimen, the physical dose per day is increased by about 15% to 20% over that in a standard regimen, but it is given in more than one fraction. The modification of tumor radiation response by a subpopulation of hypoxic cells is least at low doses. Therefore, the kinetics of reoxygenation are not of concern in purely hyperfractionated regimens.

In accelerated treatments, the overall treatment time is shorter, and the possibility of inadequate reoxygenation arises. Nevertheless, the kinetics of reoxygenation in experimental animal systems is rapid in relation to the overall duration of even an accelerated clinical regimen. The modest shortening of overall treatment duration possible in accelerated external beam therapy seems unlikely to prejudice reoxygenation. Of more concern is the possible inability of a tumor to reoxygenate during brachytherapy of 1 to 7 days. In practice, the good results obtained with brachytherapy suggest that, even with such short treatment durations, adequate reoxygenation is achieved, an observation consistent with the few available experimental data.[94]

TABLE 2–2
*Ratios of Dose for Isosurvival Equivalent to That from 2 Gy in Oxic Conditions**

RATIO OF EUOXIC TO HYPOXIC CELLS	DOSE MODIFICATION FACTOR
100/0	1.0
90/10	1.07
80/20	1.15
70/30	1.23
60/40	1.35

**Assuming a constant OER of 2.5 at all doses.*

An area of recent interest, intraoperative radiation therapy, in which large dose fractions (1500 to 2500 cGy) are given as a single fraction, may be compromised by the existence of hypoxic tumor cells. With such large single-dose treatments, a large dose of a hypoxic cell sensitizer is a reasonable adjuvant. Similarly, the recent trend to use large dose fractions in high dose-rate brachytherapy may increase the potential for compromising the benefit of reoxygenation.

MODIFICATION OF FRACTIONATION PATTERNS

Standard radiation therapy regimens, using about 200 cGy per day 5 days per week, have developed empirically over the decades as a good overall pattern of dose fractionation. It is important to realize, however, that it may not be the best fractionation pattern and that it is certainly inappropriate in certain clinical situations.[197,243] Advances in radiation biology have made it easier to be flexible in adapting and individualizing fractionated dose regimens.

The biologic factors relevant to modifications of dose fractionation are as follows:

1. There are differences among tissues in the relative contributions to cell lethality from single-hit and multihit killing as judged by their survival rate from multiple-dose fractions (see Figs. 2-16 to 2-20). In slowly proliferative tissues the influence of repair of sublethal (multihit) injury is systematically greater than is the case with acutely responding tissues. In terms of the LQ survival curve model, the α/β ratio is lower for late-responding tissues.
2. Surviving cells in acutely responding tissues have an enormous capacity for repopulation (see Fig. 2-1).
3. Tumors show an accelerated repopulation response (see Figs. 2-2 to 2-4). Although there is probably great variability from tumor to tumor, *on the average,* the lag time before its onset is longer, and its rate thereafter slower, than the comparable parameters for acutely responding normal tissues.
4. Cell cycle redistribution to asynchrony between dose fractions produces a net sensitization in proliferative tissues but not in nonproliferative, late-responding tissues.
5. Hypoxia among tumor cells affects the response at all doses, but to a lesser extent at low doses.
6. The kinetics of reoxygenation appear to be rapid in relation to the duration of a standard radiation therapy regimen.
7. Repair of sublethal injury in slowly responding tissues continues for a longer duration than that in acutely responding tissues.
8. Repopulation occurs more rapidly if radiation therapy is not given daily.
9. The lag time to the onset of repopulation is shortened by a rapid accumulation of injury.

There are four ways in which a dose-time treatment pattern can be changed. The size of dose fractions can be increased or decreased, and the overall treatment duration can be lengthened or shortened. A modified fractionation pattern can incorporate more than one of these changes as, for example, in accelerated hyperfractionation. Two modifications, increasing the size of dose fractions and lengthening overall time, are likely to be therapeutically disadvantageous and will be discussed first.

Increasing Size of Dose per Fraction

Many clinical and experimental animal studies have shown that large dose fractions are associated with an increase in the severity of late responses in relation to acute responses[199, 266, 268] (see Figs. 2-16 and 2-20).

Radiobiologically, this dissociation between acute and late effects with increase in fraction size can be described as reflecting a lower α/β ratio for late-responding tissues than for acutely responding tissues (see Figs. 2-16 and 2-18; Table 2-1). Most tumors are actively proliferating and rapidly responding, and their fractionation response is similar to that of acutely responding normal tissues,[126, 232] although there are exceptions.[136, 187, 190] Therefore, from the viewpoint of differentials in α/β ratios, increasing the size of dose fractions (hypofractionation) would provide a therapeutic disadvantage.

For example, assume respective α/β ratios of 10 Gy and 3 Gy for the tumor and the critical late-responding normal tissue. If the standard treatment had been 6600 cGy in 200 cGy fractions, the isoeffective total dose for the late-responding tissue exposed to a 400 cGy regimen, determined using the LQ isoeffect formula, would be .71 of 6600 cGy (4700 cGy). However, to achieve a constant rate of tumor control would require that the total dose be reduced to only .86 of 6600 cGy (5660 cGy). Therefore, if the incidence and severity of late sequelae were to be maintained constant by giving only 4700 cGy, the tumor would be relatively underdosed, receiving only .71/.86 = 83% of the dose biologically equivalent to the reference dose of 6600 cGy in 200 cGy fractions. Alternatively, if the biologic effect on the tumor were to be maintained constant by giving a total of 5660 cGy, the biologic dose to the late-responding tissues would be 20% (.86/.71) too high. Obviously the therapeutic ratio will be reduced regardless of the choice made between lowering the biologic dose to the tumor or raising it for the late-responding tissue.

Increasing Overall Treatment Duration

Repopulation in acutely responding tissues would permit delivery of enormous doses if irradiation were protracted for months. In these circumstances the late–responding tissues, which are not protected by an early repopulation response, limit the tolerable dose. Because of this limit, the treatment duration should be extended only as long as it takes to deliver the tolerance dose for the critical late-responding tissue without causing intolerable acute injury.

Because many tumors show an accelerated response some time after the start of a multifraction regimen and some are already growing rapidly before treatment has begun, it is illogical to extend the overall duration of radiation therapy for longer than is necessary to limit acute normal tissue toxicity.

Hyperfractionation

Hyperfractionation may be defined as the use of smaller-than-standard doses per fraction. It can be achieved without extending the overall treatment duration by treating once a day for 6 or 7 days per week, but is usually achieved by giving two fractions per day for 5 days per week. Its major aim now is to increase the therapeutic differential between late-responding normal tissues and acutely responding tumors, exploiting differences in their α/β ratios.[199, 266, 268] Historically, however, it was introduced to exploit the "self-sensitizing" effect of cell cycle redistribution present in the tumor but absent in late-responding normal tissues.[242] A third, but minor, rationale for expecting a therapeutic gain from hyperfractionation is that the oxygen enhancement ratio is lower at low doses.[62, 89, 143] The small difference in effective oxygen enhancement ratio at doses per fraction of less than 2 Gy, especially when the proportion of hypoxic tumor cells is low, makes this a relatively minor factor (Fig. 2-22).

Hyperfractionation may not be an advantage in the treatment of slowly proliferating tumors because, like slowly proliferating normal tissues, their α/β ratio may be low. Furthermore, some tumor types may be inherently characterized by a low α/β ratio regardless of their proliferation profile, as suggested, for example, by some animal tumors[190] and by cell survival assays for some human melanomas.[28, 159]

Quantifying the dose per fraction and total doses in a hyperfractionated regimen is still uncertain. Clinical evidence suggests that if one fraction of 200 cGy/day is replaced with two fractions, the dose per fraction should be between 115 cGy and 125 cGy. For comparison, the dose per fraction necessary for an isoeffect in acutely responding tissues (and most tumors) would be between 105 cGy and 110 cGy. Assuming the isoeffect dose for late-responding tissues was increased by 20% and that for tumor by only 5%, the therapeutic differential would be increased by 1.2/1.05 = 1.14. Therefore, if two fractions of 120 cGy/day replaced one fraction of 200 cGy/day (to achieve an isoeffect in late-responding tissues), the acute responses of normal tissues, as well as of tumors, would be increased as if the dose had been increased by 14%. (Coincidentally, if the overall treatment time were unchanged, the rate of treatment would be accelerated by 14%.[247]) This should improve tumor control rates, but in some treatment situations the increase in acute toxicity may be intolerable. Thus it may be necessary in such situations to protract the overall treatment duration slightly, accepting the possibility of a lesser therapeutic gain.

When two fractions are given per day, the interfraction interval should be as long as possible. It should not be less than 6 hours if late-responding tissues are of concern.[9, 193, 195] The reason for proposing a fractionation interval as long as possible is that late-responding normal tissues continue repairing sublethal damage for a period of at least 6 hours,[9, 10, 192, 193, 195] in contrast to acutely responding tissues, which appear to terminate repair within 3 or 4 hours. In spinal cord, repair may continue for more than 12 hours.

Initial clinical results with hyperfractionation in head and neck.[107, 147, 148, 158, 228] and bladder[62] cancer have suggested a potential therapeutic gain. Nonrandomized studies have suggested that local control of head and neck cancer could be improved by about 15%. The only randomized trial to have been completed and analyzed confirms the impression of improvement suggested by nonrandomized studies[99–101]: at last report,[98] a total dose of 8050 cGy in 115 cGy fractions given twice per day provided a 20% improvement in local control over that from 7000 cGy in 200 cGy fractions, with a probable improvement in survival rate and no difference in the incidence of late sequelae.

Accelerated Treatment

Accelerated treatment may be defined as a shortening of the overall treatment duration. Its aim is to minimize the potential for tumor growth or regeneration during therapy. The difficulty is to avoid excessive toxicity in the acutely responding normal tissues. Treatment could be accelerated by using large doses per fraction, but is not advised in curative treatment for the reasons discussed earlier. Thus, in practice, accelerated regimens should use conventional doses per fraction given more frequently than in conventional treatment (six or more times per week). However, because the weekly dose rate cannot be doubled (because of acute toxicity), it is often convenient to exploit the advantages of a reduced fraction size if a patient is to be treated twice per day.

Several methods have been or are being used for delivering treatment in a shorter time period than that required for a regimen of 200 cGy per fraction, five times per week, which will be assumed to be "standard" (obviously, such a regimen is already accelerated 10% in relation to a similar treatment using 180 cGy fractions):

1. *Multiple standard fractions per day,* in which multiple fractions of approximately 200 cGy have been given in a continuous course lasting less than 2 weeks,[82, 138, 152, 168] with good local control rates but high frequency of severe complications
2. *Relative hypofractionation,* in which 5000 cGy is given in 15 fractions in 3 weeks,[61, 184] or 20 fractions in 4 weeks.[90, 91] These treatments are standard procedure in a number of centers.
3. *Concomitant boosting,* in which the boost dose to a reduced volume is given "concomitantly" with the treatment of the initial volume[113, 153, 157, 158] rather than as a sequel, as would be standard in a shrinking field treatment. The boost is given as a second dose, with an interfraction interval of at least 6 hours, on several days during the latter part of treatment.
4. *Continuous hyperfractionated accelerated radiation,* in which 5100 cGy to 5400 cGy has been given as 140 cGy or 150 cGy fractions, three times daily at 6-hour intervals for 12 consecutive days.[54, 173] Tumor control rates are encouraging, but acute toxicity is substantial. There has also been an unexpected increase in myelopathy.
5. *Split-course accelerated treatment,* in which head and neck tumors have been given about 3800 cGy in two fractions of 160 cGy per day over about 10 days and then, after a break of 12 to 14 days, an additional 2800 cGy (approximately), the total treatment lasting about 6 weeks.[222–224] The results are better than in historic controls. A similar regimen, using three fractions per day of 150 cGy to a total dose of about 3000 cGy, followed by a second course delivering about 4000 cGy given 12 to 14 days later, is at present undergoing clinical trial.[101]
6. *Brachytherapy* will be discussed separately, but is a form of accelerated therapy.

Because accelerated tumor regrowth has its greatest effect later in a standard regimen, even a 1-week shortening should be advantageous (see Figs. 2-3 and 2-4). The importance of accelerated repopulation in a treated tumor can be visualized by considering that two to three doublings of surviving clonogens should add about the same increment in tumor cell burden as a one-step increase in T-stage. (A doubling in diameter of a spherical tumor represents the equivalent of three cell doublings, whereas the doubling in diameter of a flatter superficial tumor is equivalent to between two and three doublings.)

Patients most suitable for accelerated regimens are those with rapidly growing tumors or those with a high potential for rapid regrowth.[197] Tumors with high proliferative activity or a high cell loss factor would be most likely to exhibit an early and rapid acceleration of regrowth. It may become possible to predict which tumors will repopulate early and quickly,[21, 22] but, in principle, all tumors should be treated in as short an overall time as consistent with acceptable acute morbidity. The total dose administered should not be reduced from standard levels.

Although there is potential for improved results of radiation therapy from modifying and individualizing fractionation patterns on an experimental basis, the acceleration of tumor growth, the repopulation in acutely responding tissues, and the relative repair capacities of late-responding normal tissues and tumors have important implications for everyday conventional radiation therapy.[263] For example, it is inappropriate to complete radiation therapy—at least for head and neck cancers—on a Monday after a weekend break, which represents a 3-day extension. Likewise, it is not usually advisable to begin a course of curative therapy on a Friday. In general, predictable breaks in treatment (public holidays, and so forth), if they prolong treatment significantly, should be accounted for without resorting to large fractions by delivering more than five fractions per week. Also, chemotherapy given over several weeks before the start of radiation therapy can compromise the chance for local control through the initiation of accelerated repopulation.

LOW DOSE-RATE IRRADIATION

Low dose-rate continuous irradiation has the same biologic advantages as described earlier for hyperfractionation. Additional advantages are as follows:

1. Proliferative cells may be delayed in their progression through the division cycle.[20, 51, 63, 102, 203] Such mitotic delay occurs in radiosensitive phases (*e.g.,* late G_2 and the G_1S boundary). Such a skewed redistribution could enhance self-sensitization of proliferative tissues, without such an effect in late-responding tissues.
2. The overall duration of therapy is shortened.
3. The high dose regions near the radioactive sources would have a high probability of being completely sterilized of tumor cells. When the logarithmic nature of cell killing is considered, this is not as great an advantage as it may seem initially. For example, radiation "cautery" of 50% of the tumor cells represents a gain that is equivalent to only the ${}_eD_{50}$ or about 200 cGy to 250 cGy of a standard multifraction regimen.
4. The volume of normal tissue receiving a high dose is minimized. Associated with the lower total dose beyond the treatment volume there is also a reduction in dose rate, boosting further the sparing effect, especially in the late-responding tissues.[59]

A potential biologic disadvantage (neglecting such practical considerations as feasibility) is that the relatively rapid fall-off in dose beyond the stipulated treatment volume, as well as in unintentional "cold-spots," could lead to a rapid decrease in the probability of tumor cell eradication if the tumor lay beyond the specified minimum tumor isodose. As with any radiation therapy, a geographic miss, or area of significant underdosage, negates the purpose of curative treatment.

The use of high dose-rate, high dose-per-fraction brachytherapy has advantages in terms of logistics and protection of staff, but also has biologic disadvantages: loss of therapeutic differential between slowly responding tissues and tumors because of differences in the dose survival characteristics (α/β ratios) of their target cells; reduced effect of cell cycle redistribution and division cycle (mitotic) delay, and increased potential influence on radiation response of a subpopulation of hypoxic tumor cells.

Permanent implants of radioisotopes with long half-lives (*e.g.*, ^{125}I) are also disadvantageous radiobiologically because the late-responding normal tissues accumulate enormous doses and, unlike the acutely responding normal tissues, are not spared appreciably by repopulation; and the dose rate is too low if the total dose over an extended period is to be limited. Very low dose rates facilitate "escape" of tumor clonogens through "normal" growth or accelerated regeneration, in all but the most slowly proliferative tumors.

As with high dose-rate brachytherapy, other considerations may overwhelm the radiobiologic disadvantages.

Optimal Dose Rate

As with dose per fraction in multifraction irradiation, it is impossible to specify an ideal low dose rate for brachytherapy. Considerations include competing biologic variables (repopulation, reoxygenation, and repair), logistic and other medical factors, and the vagaries of dose specification in an inhomogeneous distribution. Biologically, the considerations resemble those for hyperfractionation.

Repair of sublethal injury influences the response of mouse jejunal crypt cells with change in dose rate even at relatively high dose rates such as 10 Gy/minute (60,000 cGy/hour) to 1 Gy/minute (6000 cGy/hour). However, the sparing is most pronounced with changes among lower dose rates, especially in the range between about 1000 cGy/hour and 100 cGy/hour. At lower dose rates, the effect of repair alone is obscured by a contribution from repopulation.

In rat spinal cord, a slowly responding tissue, a major change in effectiveness occurs with change from 400 cGy/hour to 200 cGy/hour.[174] Technical factors in such experiments make investigation of lower dose rates difficult, but comparison of the 200 cGy/hour data with multifraction data[9,10,192,212,213,254] indicates potential for substantial further sparing with further decrease in dose rate. A similarly large dose rate effect is seen for lung.[56] Such a large sparing effect of reduced dose rate is to be expected in late-responding tissues for two, probably interdependent, reasons: the low α/β ratios characteristic of slowly-responding tissues imply a large capacity for repair, and the rates of repair, as expressed in half-times, are slower than in acutely responding tissues.[59,174,192] Also, there should be no significant self-sensitization by division cycle redistribution.

Thus, a differential between late-responding normal tissues and an acutely responding tumor is enhanced if the irradiation is slow enough to permit full exploitation of the large capacity for repair in the normal tissue. From experimental data currently available, it seems possible that the differential between slowly responding and rapidly responding tissues may be further amplified by even lower dose rates than a common "standard" rate of about 60 cGy/hour. Nevertheless, the standard rate may represent a reasonable compromise between the desirability of a low dose rate for optimizing repair differentials and the contrary radiobiologic, medical, and logistic reasons for favoring a short treatment time.

Low Dose-Rate Total Body Irradiation

Because bone marrow stem cells are characterized by a high α/β ratio (see Table 2-1) and other leukopoietic and leukemia cells may be similar in radiosensitivity,[93] it is reasonable to prepare patients with leukemia for bone marrow transplantation using either multiple small dose fractions or continuous low dose-rate exposure. This is supported by a great deal of clinical and experimental data.[45,160,205] However, the dose rates between about 100 cGy/hour and 700 cGy/hour chosen for various continuous low dose-rate total body irradiation regimens cover a range in which biologic effectiveness changes rapidly with change in dose rate. Thus the biologic dose rates used in various centers, though not greatly different for hematopoietic cells, and perhaps not for immunocytes, were very different for other tissues. Furthermore, experimental animal data suggest that even lower dose rates would provide a better therapeutic differential between organized and liquid tissues.[56,144,174,204,205] Because such low dose rates in a single sitting are not practical, multifraction exposures, using low doses per fraction, also commonly given at a low dose rate, have been adopted by many transplantation centers.

Equivalence in biologic dose is difficult to prescribe because the biologic effectiveness of x-rays or τ-rays is different for different tissues and changes differently with changes in fractionation pattern and dose rate. In general, low doses per fraction and low dose rates provide the best therapeutic differentials, provided that the overall treatment duration is kept short in relation to the growth rate of the leukemia cells and immunocytes.

LINEAR ENERGY TRANSFER

The rate at which a charged particle such as an electron or proton deposits its energy along its track is described as its linear energy transfer (LET). The heavier the particle, the higher its LET. Thus, electrons have a predominantly low LET, protons slightly higher, neutrons higher still, and heavy charged particles have the highest LET of clinically employed radiations.

The rate of energy transfer also increases as particles slow. Therefore, because primary and secondary particles are slowed and stopped by their interactions within the cells, a beam of radiation can be described only by an average value of LET. An average LET has relatively little meaning to the biophysics of energy deposition, but is a useful guide to the radiation therapist. Although the details of measuring and expressing LET values are controversial, suffice it to say that as the LET of a beam increases, so also does its biologic efficiency.* The oxygen enhancement ratio decreases with increasing LET.[15] Variations in division cycle-related radiosensitivity are less with high LET beams. The amount of cell killing by single-hit, nonrepairable events increases in relation to that from accumulation of sublethal injury, so that there is little sparing from dose fractionation. Compared with x-rays, linear energy transfer preferentially reduces the tolerance of late-responding tissues in relation to acutely responding tissues.[265] Also, there is little if any repair of potentially lethal injury,[24] so that tolerance of late-responding tissues may be further decreased in relation to that of acutely responding tissues.

RELATIVE BIOLOGIC EFFICIENCY

Relative biologic efficiency (RBE) of two beams is measured as a ratio of doses to produce the same effect:

RBE = dose (standard beam)/dose (test beam).

**At very high LET values, an "overkill" phenomenon results in a decreasing biologic effect per unit of measured physical dose.*

In radiation therapy, the term RBE is usually associated with a comparison of neutrons and photons, although in theory it is a much more general term with wider applicability for comparing the effectiveness of treatment approaches such as high and low dose-rate x-irradiation. It cannot be measured accurately unless the same effect is achieved by both radiations (see Fig. 2-24). Initially, the standard photon beam was 250 kVp x-rays, but now, at least from the viewpoint of radiation therapy, it is ^{60}Co (250 kVp x-rays are at least 15% more efficient than ^{60}Co in killing mammalian cells). It is not widely appreciated that even at relatively high dose rates, the photon beam effectiveness varies with dose rate and also that this is an important determinant of RBE. From these considerations it is clearly necessary that the conditions of RBE measurements be explicitly stated.

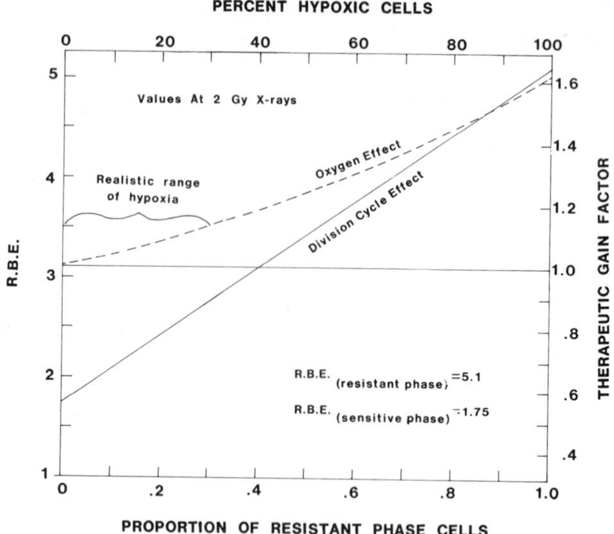

FIGURE 2–23. Comparison of therapeutic gain factor (TGF) for neutrons relative to photons as a function of different proportions of hypoxic tumor clonogens and different division cycle distributions, assuming the use of 2 Gy fractional doses of x-rays. The $RBE_{n/x}$ for dose-limiting, late-responding tissues is taken as 3.1. This was the value used for 50 $MeV_{d/Be}$ neutrons used in one clinical trial in which the doses per fraction in x-ray regimens were 1.8 Gy to 2.0 Gy. The methods used for determining the curves are published elsewhere.[240, 244, 258] Efficient division cycle redistribution could favor the use of x-rays (TGF < 1) but, if inefficient, could provide a more powerful rationale than hypoxia for expecting a therapeutic gain from substituting neutrons for x-rays. The total therapeutic gain would be compounded if both reoxygenation and redistribution were inefficient. (Withers HR: Strahlentherapie 161:739, 1985)

NEUTRONS

Neutrons deposit energy in a tissue through collisions with nuclei (mainly of hydrogen) rather than with electrons, as occurs with photon beams. Although neutrons are uncharged, the cellular injury they produce is through free radicals formed from ion pairs—the same basic mechanism as that for x-rays. The difference between neutrons and x-rays is that the column of ionization produced by the proton ejected from the nucleus by the neutron is much denser than that produced by an electron ejected by a photon. Because of the density of resulting free radicals, neutron irradiation is more likely than x-irradiation to cause irreparable injury to a double strand of DNA.

Oxygen Effect

Also associated with the density of ionization resulting from neutron irradiation is a reduced oxygen enhancement ratio. If the oxygen enhancement ratio for x-rays is 2.6 and for neutrons is 1.6, the ratio, called the *hypoxic gain factor,* would be 2.6/1.6 = 1.6. In other words, if a course of neutrons is given that produces normal tissue sequelae equivalent to those from 6600 cGy of x-rays given in 200 cGy fractions, the biologic effect of the neutrons on the completely hypoxic tumor would be equivalent to that from (1.6 × 6600 cGy) = 10,560 cGy of x-rays.

Of course, 100% of tumor cells are not hypoxic, and so the actual therapeutic gain factor is lower than the hypoxic gain factor of 1.6. The exact value of therapeutic gain factor depends on the percentage of hypoxic cells, which in a multifraction regimen is a function of the reoxygenation of the tumor, and on the dose per fraction. The lower the percentage of hypoxic cells and the lower the dose per fraction, the lower the therapeutic gain factor.[246] The relationship between percentage of hypoxic tumor cells and the therapeutic gain factor for doses per fraction equivalent to 2 Gy x-rays is shown in Figure 2-23. If a tumor was treated with a multifraction regimen of neutrons and if it reoxygenated efficiently to a constant hypoxic-euoxic cell ratio, the therapeutic gain factor value shown in Figure 2-23 would be constant. If, however, reoxygenation were inefficient, the therapeutic gain factor would rise as treatment progressed.

Division Cycle Distribution

The response of cells to neutrons is less influenced by the cells' position in the division cycle than is the case with exposure to x-rays. Therefore, the RBE is greater for cells in x-ray-resistant phases of the cell cycle than for those cells in phases that are relatively x-ray-sensitive. Depending on the relative mixtures of resistant- and sensitive-phase cells in tumors and in critical normal tissues, a therapeutic gain or loss may result from using neutrons (Fig. 2-23).[244,258] For example, if a tumor consisted entirely of cells in an x-ray-resistant phase of the cell cycle for which the RBE was 5 and if the critical normal tissue had an RBE of 3, then the neutron dose would need only to be reduced by a factor of 3 for equal toxicity. Therefore, the therapeutic gain would be 5/3 = 1.66. If, however, 100% of the tumor cells were in x-ray-sensitive phases of the cycle for which the RBE was only 1.7, the therapeutic "gain" would be 1.7/3 = 0.57; that is, there would be a therapeutic loss equivalent to reducing the x-ray dose to 57%. Thus the "kinetics gain factor" for neutrons could result in a major advantage or a disaster in neutron therapy, depending on the selection of patients for treatment.[246] A comparison of the kinetics gain factor and hypoxic gain factor is shown in Figure 2-23.

Dose Fractionation

Because of a greater contribution to cell lethality from single-hit nonrepairable events with neutrons than with x-rays, the cell survival rate is more nearly exponential over a wider dose range. It is also steeper than that for x-rays. In terms of the LQ survival curve formula, neutrons have a very high α/β value (*e.g.,* 30 to 100 Gy). Therefore, dose fractionation is of less significance in neutron radiation therapy than in x-ray therapy.

If two survival curves have the same shape, the RBE is constant at all doses. In the case of neutrons and photons, the dose survival curves have different shapes and the RBE at low doses per fraction is higher than at higher doses per fraction (Fig. 2-24).

The first trial of neutron radiation therapy was carried out before it was known that mammalian cell x-ray survival curves had a shoulder. The preclinical RBE measurements made at high doses were inappropriate for fractionated neutron therapy. Although tumor control rates were satisfactory, normal tissue sequelae were severe. The use of neutrons was discontinued until a clearer understanding of the underlying biology became available in the early 1960s.

The second generation of neutron clinical trials was initiated before it was widely appreciated that late-responding normal tissues exhibit a greater capacity for repair of x-ray injury than do acutely responding normal tissues and that neutrons show no such preferential sparing of late-responding tissues. Therefore, the early phases of the second round of neutron studies used neutron doses based on RBE values determined for acutely responding tissues. Because the RBE values for late injury were higher at the low doses per fraction employed, there was a substantial incidence of severe late sequelae.[105] In a third generation of neutron trials, RBE values are based on late-responding tissues, and because these tissues do not depend on protraction of overall time for a sparing effect of dose fractionation, overall treatment durations are shorter. Thus present-day neutron clinical trials use a smaller number of dose fractions given in a relatively short overall treatment time.

Clearly, from the viewpoint of a clinical trial of neutrons, it would be advantageous to identify poorly reoxygenating tumors and tumors with an age-density distribution skewed toward relatively x-ray-resistant phases.[246] Such a skewed age-density distribution might develop during radiation therapy in a tumor that is inefficient in cell cycle redistribution between fractions, yielding an increasing kinetics gain factor as treatment progressed. A similar effect on the hypoxic gain factor would occur in poorly reoxygenating tumors. Finally, neutrons may be better than x-rays for treating rapidly growing or rapidly regenerating tumors because treatment can be given quickly. Thus, if poorly reoxygenating, poorly redistributing, intrinsically x-ray-resistant, rapidly growing, and rapidly repopulating tumors existed and could be identified prospectively, neutrons would provide a clear improvement in their therapy. Such predictive assays would also permit more selective modification of x-ray regimens.[246]

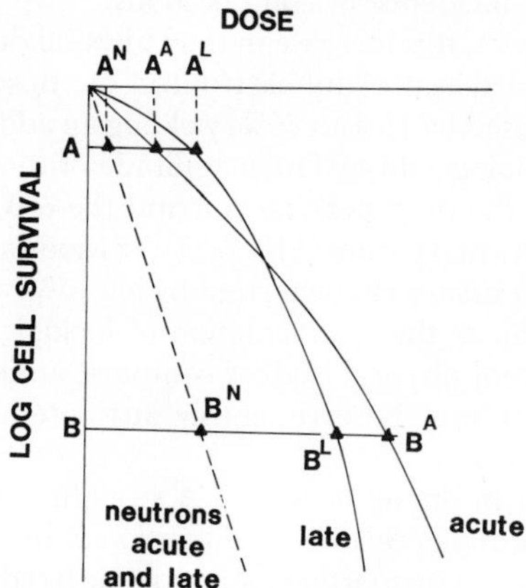

FIGURE 2–24. Model cell survival curves for acutely responding and late-responding normal tissues exposed to neutrons or x-rays. For neutrons the survival curve is the same as that for target cells in acutely responding and late-responding tissues. For x-rays the curve for late effects curves more, the α/β value being lower. $RBE_{n/x}$ values are different for different types of tissue and also change with dose. At the level of effect *A*, the $RBE_{n/x}$ values for acute and late effects are 3.3 and 5.3, respectively. At the level of effect *B*, the $RBE_{n/x}$ value for the late effects is 2.1, which is not only lower at high doses but less than the value of 2.5 for acute effects.

VOLUME EFFECT

Traditionally, radiation oncologists have reduced the total dose when treating large volumes of normal tissue. Also, the reduction from 200 cGy to 180 cGy per fraction, which is now widespread, had its origin in the volume effect because the longer treatment duration enhanced the mucosal "tolerance" to large treatment fields in the head and neck.[76] In the orthovoltage era the recommended reduction in dose with increase in treatment volume was large.[150] With the advent of skin-sparing megavoltage beams, the volume effect received less attention as an influence in selection of total dose, especially as it became more generally accepted that larger tumors required higher doses for their control.

There is no single volume effect, defined as a *decreased tolerance* when a large volume is treated. At least four types of volume effect exist.[262] Also some factors probably can be discarded as contributors to the effect. For example, there is no convincing evidence that exposure of an increased volume of an organ increases cellular radiosensitivity.[262] The radiosensitivity of skin epithelium has been shown to be constant over a 5000-fold range of treatment area.[236,262] Also no evidence exists that vascular damage plays a role.[260] Four factors likely to contribute to a volume effect are discussed here:

1. Reduced tolerance to equally severe injury with increase in volume. A patient can tolerate a small area of injury (such as ulceration) better than the same severity of injury in a large area, in which pain, exudation, and consequences of infection are more severe, healing is slower, and consequential contraction and scarring may be worse. Therefore, the effect of increasing volume in this instance is that the injury is more incapacitating to the host, even though the radiosensitivity of the "target" cells and hence the severity of the radiation response per unit area are unchanged, being independent of the area or volume treated.
2. Increased probability of a complication from the same severity of injury. If the functional subunits (FSUs) in a normal tissue are arranged in series, like links in a chain, as they are in nerve tracts, the loss of one subunit results in the overt expression of injury regardless of the state of the other subunits in the series. In this instance, the probability of injury increases with increase in the number of FSUs exposed (with treatment volume; Fig. 2-25).

   The most obvious examples of organs in which such a volume effect might occur are spinal cord, nerves, and the cylindrical sheath of peritoneum covering the small intestine. Such a volume effect has been demonstrated clinically for small bowel obstruction[163] and experimentally for myelitis.[97,214]

   The relationship between number of functional subunits irradiated (n) and probability of a complication (P) is described by the formula,

$$P = 1 - (1 - p)^n,$$

   where p is the probability of the loss of one FSU. This relationship is illustrated in Figure 2-26. Increasing the volume (number of FSUs exposed) reduces the dose neces-

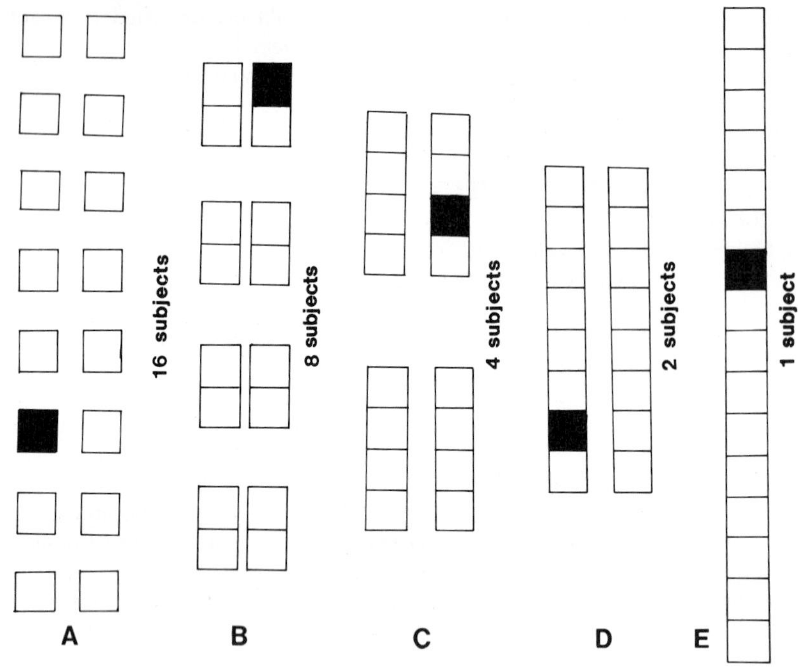

FIGURE 2–25. Diagrammatic representation of the influence on the probability of a complication from increasing the treatment volume in a tissue where functional subunits (FSUs) are arranged serially. The average survival of FSUs was 1 in 16, sterilized FSUs being denoted by the black squares. With small volumes (A), the probability of myelitis was 6% (1/16), whereas it would approach 100% if 16 FSUs in one patient were exposed (E). The actual probabilities can be calculated using the equation in the text. (Withers HR, Taylor JMG, Maciejewski B: Int J Radiat Oncol Biol Phys 1:751, 1988)

sary to produce a complication and increases the steepness of the dose-response curves. The effect becomes less marked when the number of irradiated FSUs is large. Therefore, the size of the FSU determines the range of organ volumes over which a significant volume effect will be detected. With small bowel the probability of obstruction increases even when large volumes are enlarged,[79,252] suggesting that for the peritoneal sheath the (unknown) FSU

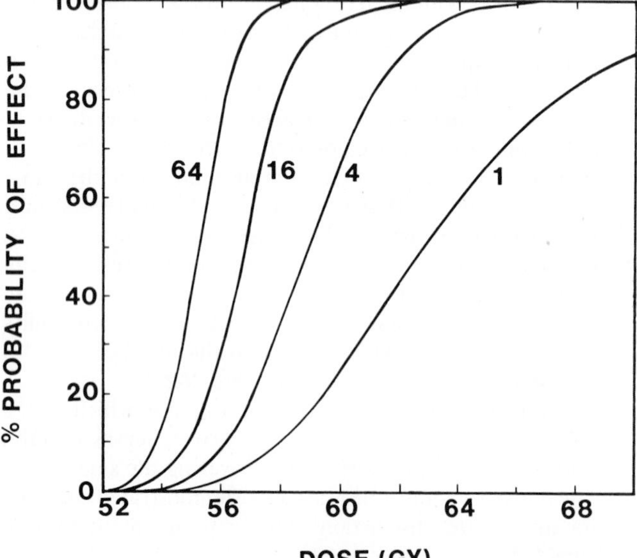

FIGURE 2–26. Curves illustrating how the probability of producing a complication increases with increase in the number of serially arranged functional subunits included in the treatment volume. The curves were positioned by assuming that 58 Gy in 2 Gy fractions sterilized 10% of functional subunits and that for a series of 2 Gy fractions the effective D_0 for the target cells was 4 Gy. The curves are shifted to the left and are steeper with increase in number of functional subunits exposed, but this effect becomes less obvious when large numbers of subunits are involved. (Modified from Withers HR, Taylor JMG, Maciejewski B: Int J Radiat Oncol Biol Phys 14:751, 1988)

that prevents adhesion formation and bowel obstruction must be large.

3. Increased heterogeneity of dose. In some situations involving treatment of large volumes, there are large gradients in dose distribution. This could occur, for example, with tangential field treatment of a large breast. Without careful planning, a tumor dose may be prescribed at the 80% level, leading to a 25% higher dose in the region of D_{max}. Also, with large fields large variations in contour may exist. These variations could result in a high dose in regions in which the patient thickness is less than was measured at the midplane as, for example, in the spinal cord at the thoracic inlet. When the threshold-sigmoid curve plotting the probability of complications against dose is steep, as is it is for normal tissues studied in experimental animals,[194] a 15% to 25% increase in total dose could produce a marked change in incidence of complications.

    However, this increase in total physical dose is further compounded by the "double trouble" of a dose per fraction also increased by 15% to 25%, yielding an additional increment in biologic dose. The magnitude of the increase depends on the dose per fraction and the α/β value of the relevant normal tissues (Fig. 2-27). Obviously, the effect is greatest in tissues characterized by low α/β values (see Table 2-1). Since the augmentation of biologic doses is not evident from physical isodose contours, an increased biologic effect may be erroneously attributed to the large volume *per se*.
4. Reduction in organ "reserve." A straightforward volume effect relates merely to the obliteration of the reserve of an organ in direct proportion to the volume irradiated, such as the lung in which the total dose required for an attempt at cure for most tumors would be sufficient to eliminate functional integrity in the treatment volume.

Acknowledgments

Jan Haas and Kathy Mason helped extensively in preparation of the manuscript.

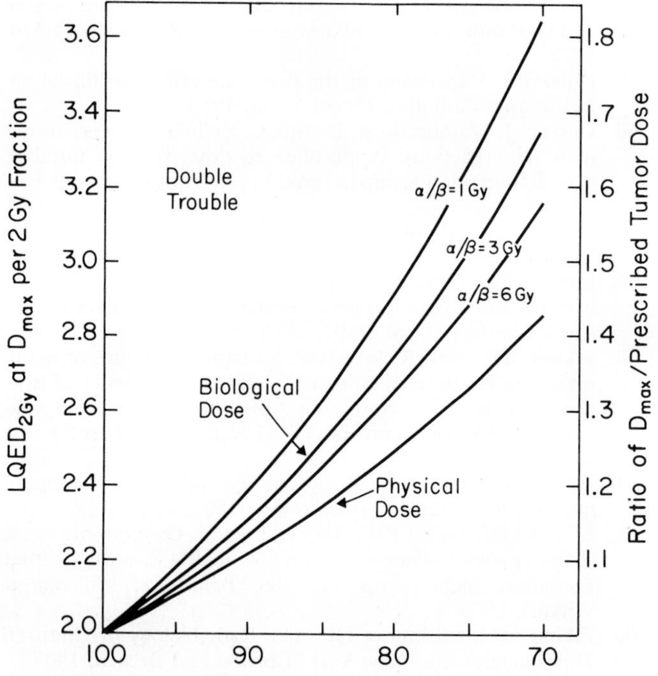

FIGURE 2–27. Influence of dose heterogeneity on physical and biologic doses as a function of the isodose line chosen for defining tumor dose and of α/β ratio of the tissue located at D_{max}. The divergence of biologic and physical doses reflects the change in biologic dose that results from change in dose per fraction that derives from the heterogeneity of dose distribution. The lower the α/β ratio, the greater the divergence between biologic and physical doses. This "double-trouble" is not reflected in physics isodose distributions and may explain not only a spurious volume effect but also may contribute to low values of tolerance doses that have appeared in the literature from time to time.

REFERENCES

1. Adams GE, Fowler JF, Wardman P: Hypoxic cell sensitizers in radiobiology and radiotherapy. Br J Cancer 37(Suppl 3):1, 1978
2. Allen EP: A trial of radiation dose prescription based on dose-cell survival formula. Australas Radiol 28:156, 1984
3. Alper T: Cell Survival After Low Doses of Radiation: Theoretical and Clinical Implications. Bristol, England, John Wiley & Sons, 1975
4. Alper T: Cellular Radiobiology. London, University Press, 1979
5. Alper T, Howard-Flanders P: The role of oxygen in modifying the radiosensitivity of *E. coli* B. Nature 178:978, 1956
6. Amdur RJ, Parsons J, Mendenhall WM, et al: Split course versus continuous course irradiation in the postoperative setting for squamous cell carcinoma of the head and neck. Int J Radiat Oncol Biol Phys 17:279, 1989
7. Andrews JR: Dose-time relationships in cancer radiotherapy: A clinical radiobiology study of extremes of dose and time. Am J Roentgenol Rad Ther Nucl Med 93:56, 1965
8. Ang KK, Landuyt W, Rijnders A, et al: Differences in repopulation kinetics in mouse skin during split-course multiple fractions per day or daily fractionated irradiation. Int J Radiat Oncol Biol Phys 10:95, 1985
9. Ang KK, van der Kogel AJ, van Dam J, et al: The kinetics of repair of sublethal damage in the rat cervical spinal cord during fractionated irradiation. Radiother Oncol 1:247, 1984
10. Ang KK, van der Kogel AJ, van der Schueren E: Lack of evidence for increased tolerance of rat spinal cord with decreasing fraction doses below 2 Gy. Int J Radiat Oncol Biol Phys 11:105, 1985
11. Ang KK, Xu FX, Vanuytsel, et al: Repopulation kinetics in irradiated mouse lip mucosa: The relative importance of treatment protraction and time distribution of irradiation. Radiat Res 101:162, 1985
12. Anno GH, Baum SJ, Withers HR, Young RW: Symptomatology of acute radiation effects in humans after exposure to doses of 0.5–30 Gy. Health Phys 56:821, 1989
13. Arcangeli G. Mauro F, Nervi C, et al: Dose survival relationship for epithelial cells of human skin after multifraction irradiation: Evaluation by a quantitative method *in vivo*. Int J Radiat Oncol Biol Phys 6:841, 1980
14. Baker JL, Montague ED, Peters LJ: Clinical experience with irradiation of inflammatory carcinoma of the breast with and without elective chemotherapy. Cancer 45:625, 1980
15. Barendsen GW: Responses of cultured cells, tumors and normal tissues to radiations in different linear energy transfer. Curr Top Radiat Res 4:295, 1968
16. Barendsen GW: Dose fractionation, dose rate and isoeffect relationships for normal tissue responses. Int J Radiat Oncol Biol Phys 8:1981, 1982
17. Barendsen GW, Broerse JJ: Experimental radiotherapy of a rat rhabdomyosarcoma with 15 MeV neutrons and 300 kV X rays. II. Effects of fractionated treatments, applied five times a week for several weeks. Eur J Cancer 6:89, 1970
18. Barkley HT, Fletcher GH: The significance of residual disease after external irradiation of squamous cell carcinoma of the oropharynx. Radiology 124:493, 1977
19. Bataini P, Brugere J, Bernier J, et al: Results of radical radiotherapeutic treatment of carcinoma of the pyriform sinus: Experience of the Institut Curie. Int J Radiat Oncol Biol Phys 8:1277, 1982
20. Bedford JS, Mitchell JB: Mitotic accumulation of HeLa cells during continuous irradiation. Radiat Res 70:173, 1977
21. Begg AC: Derivation of cell kinetic parameters from human tumours. In McNally NJ (ed): The Scientific Basis of Modern Radiotherapy, BIR Report 19, pp 115–116. London, BIR, 1989
22. Begg AC, McNally NJ, Shrieve DC, Karcher H: A method to measure the duration of DNA synthesis and the potential doubling time from a single sample. Cytometry 6:620, 1985
23. Bentzen SM, Christensen JJ, Overgaard J, et al: Some methodological problems in estimating radiobiological data from clinical data. Acta Oncol 27:105, 1988
24. Blakely EA, Chang PY, Lommel L: Cell-cycle-dependent recovery from heavy-ion damage in G_1-phase cells. Radiat Res 104(Suppl):5145, 1985
25. Boag JW: The time scale in radiobiology. In Nygaard OF, Adler HI, Sinclair WK (eds): Radiation Research, pp 9–29. Proceedings of 5th International Congress of Radiation Research. New York, Academic Press, 1975
26. Brinkman R, Lamberts HB: Radiopathology of extracellular structures. In Ebert M, Howard A (eds): Current Topics in Radiation Research, vol 2, pp 279–302. Amsterdam, Elsevier North Holland, 1966
27. Brock WA: Kinetics of micronucleus expression in synchronized irradiated Chinese hamster ovary cells. Cell Tissue Kinet 18:247, 1985
28. Brock WA: Predictive assays. In Withers HR, Peters LJ (eds): Innovations in Radiation Oncology, pp 11–24. Heidelberg, Springer-Verlag, 1988
29. Brown JM: Sensitizers in radiotherapy. In Withers HR, Peters LJ (eds): Innovations in Radiation Oncology, pp 247–264. Heidelberg, Springer-Verlag, 1988
30. Brown BW, Thompson JR, Barkley HT, et al: Theoretical considerations of dose rate factors influencing radiation strategy. Radiology 110:197, 1974
31. Bush RS, Jenkin RDT, Alh WEC, et al: Definitive evidence for hypoxic cells influencing cure in cancer therapy. Br J Cancer 37(Suppl 3):302, 1978
32. Byfield JE, Calabro-Jones P, Klisak I, et al: Pharmacologic requirements for obtaining sensitization of human tumor cells *in vitro* to combined 5-fluorouracil of ftorafur and x-rays. Int J Radiat Oncol Biol Phys 8:1923, 1982
33. Caldwell WL: Time dose factors in fatal post-irradiation nephritis. In Alper T (ed): Cell Survival After Low Doses of Radiation, pp 328–332. Bristol, John Wiley & Sons, 1975

34. Cater DB, Silver IA: Quantitative measurement of oxygen tension in normal tissues and in the tumours of patients before and after radiotherapy. Acta Radiol 53:233 1960
35. Chapman JD, Franko AJ, Koch CJ: The fraction of hypoxic clonogenic cells in tumor populations. In Fletcher GH, Nervi C, Withers HR (eds): Biological Bases and Clinical Implications of Tumor Radioresistance, p 61. New York, Masson, 1983
36. Chapman JD, Urtasun RC, Franko AJ, et al: The measurement of oxygenation status in individual tumors. In Prediction of Response in Radiation Therapy, pp 49–60. AAPM Symposium Proceeding 7, New York, American Institute of Physics, 1988
37. Chapman JD, Peters LJ, Withers HR: Prediction of Tumor Treatment Response. New York, Pergamon Press, 1989
38. Charbit A, Malaise EP, Tubiana M: Relation between the pathological nature and the growth rate of human tumors. Eur J Cancer 7:307, 1971
39. Chen KY, Withers HR: Survival characteristics of stem cells of gastric mucosa exposed to localized gamma irradiation in C_3H mice. Int J Radiat Oncol Biol Phys 21:521, 1972
40. Choi KN, Withers HR, Rotman M: Metastatic melanoma in brain: Rapid treatment or large dose fractions. Cancer 56:10, 1985
41. Clifton KH: Qualitative studies of the radiobiology of hormone-responsive normal cell populations. In Meyn R, Withers HR (eds): Radiation Biology in Cancer Research, p 501. New York, Raven Press, 1980
42. Cohen L: Theoretical "iso-survival"formulae for fractionated radiation therapy. Br J Radiol 41:522, 1968
43. Cohen L, Creditor M: Isoeffect tables for tolerance of irradiated normal human tissues. Int J Radiat Oncol Biol Phys 9:233, 1983
44. Cori CF, Cori GT: Carbohydrate metabolism of tumors: Changes in sugar, lactic acid, and CO_2-combining power of blood passing through tumor. J Biol Chem 65:397, 1925
45. Cosset JM, Baume D, Pico L, et al: Single dose versus hyperfractionationed total body irradiation before allogeneic bone marrow transplantation: A non-randomized comparative study of 54 patients at the Institut Gustave-Roussy. Radiother Oncol 15:151, 1989
46. Cosset JM, Henry-Amar M, Girinski T, et al: Late toxicity of radiotherapy in Hodgkin's disease. Acta Oncol 27:123, 1988
47. Cullen B, Lansley I: The effect of preirradiation growth conditions on the relative radiosensitivities of mammalian cells at low oxygen concentrations. Int J Radiat Biol 26:579, 1974
48. Deacon J, Peckham MJ, Steel GG: The radioresponsiveness of human tumors and the initial slope of the cell survival curve. Radiother Oncol 2:317–323, 1984
49. Denekamp J: Changes in the rate of repopulation during multifraction irradiation of mouse skin. Br J Radiol 46:381, 1973
50. Deschner EE, Gray LH: Influence of oxygen tension on x-ray-induced chromosomal damage in Ehrlich ascites tumor cells irradiated *in vitro* and *in vivo*. Radiat Res 11:115, 1959
51. Dewey WC, Robinette SM: Progression of viable and nonviable synchronized Chinese hamster cells into the S phase after X-irradiation in mitosis or the S phase. Int J Radiat Biol 16:495, 1969
52. Dische S: Review of chemical radiosensitizers: Update to 1988. In McNally NJ (ed): The Scientific Basis of Modern Radiotherapy, BIR Report 19, pp 91–96. London, BIR, 1989
53. Dische S, Anderson PJ, Sealy R, et al: Carcinoma of the cervix—anaemia, radiotherapy and hyperbaric oxygen. Br J Radiol 56:251, 1983
54. Dische S, Saunders MI: Continuous hyperfractionated accelerated radiotherapy. Br J Cancer 59:325, 1989
55. Douglas BG, Fowler JF: The effect of multiple small doses of x-rays on skin reactions in the mouse and a basic interpretation. Radiat Res 66:401, 1976
56. Down JD, Easton DF, Steel GG: Repair in the mouse lung during low dose rate irradiation. Radiother Oncol 6:29, 1986
57. Dubravsky N, Dubrawsky C, Jampolis S, et al: Long-term effects of pulmonary damage in mice on lung weight, compliance, hydroxyproline content and formation of metastases. Br J Radiol 54:1075, 1981
58. Dubravsky N, Withers HR: The effect of irradiation on free and total tubulin in L-P59 tumors in mice. Radiat Res 74:540, 1978
59. Dutreix J: Expression of the dose rate effect in clinical curietherapy. Radiother Oncol 15:25, 1989
60. Dutreix J, Wambersie A, Bounik C: Cellular recovery in human skin reactions: Application to dose, fraction number, overall time relationship in radiotherapy. Eur J Cancer 9:159, 1973
61. Easson EC, Pointon RCS: The Radiotherapy of Malignant Disease. Berlin, Springer-Verlag, 1985
62. Edsmyr F, Anderson L, Esposti PL, et al: Irradiation therapy with multiple small fractions per day in urinary bladder cancer. Radiother Oncol 4:197, 1985
63. Elkind MM, Han A, Volz KW: Radiation response of mammalian cells grown in culture. IV. Dose dependence of division delay and postirradiation growth of surviving and non-surviving Chinese hamster cells. J Natl Cancer Inst 30:705, 1963
64. Elkind MM, Sutton H: X-ray damage and recovery in mammalian cells in culture. Nature 184:1293, 1959
65. Elkind MM, Swain RW, Alescio T, et al: Oxygen, nitrogen, recovery and radiation therapy. In Shalek R, (ed): Cellular Radiation Biology, pp 442–466. Baltimore, Williams & Wilkins, 1965
66. Elkind MM, Whitmore GF: The Radiobiology of Cultured Mammalian Cells. New York, Gordon and Breach, 1967
67. Ellis F: Nominal standard dose and the ret. Br J Radiol 44:101, 1971
68. Evans JC, Per Bergsjo MD: The influence of anaemia on the results of radiotherapy in carcinoma of the cervix. Radiology 84:709, 1965
69. Ewing D, Powers EL: Oxygen-dependent sensitization of irradiated cells. In Meyn RE, Withers HR (eds): Radiation Biology in Cancer Research, pp 143–168. New York, Raven Press, 1980
70. Fertil B, Malaise EP: Intrinsic radiosensitivity of human cell lines is correlated with radioresponsiveness of human tumors. Int J Radiat Oncol Biol Phys 11:1699, 1985
71. Field SB, Hornsey S, Kutsutani Y: Effects of fractionated irradiation on mouse lung and a phenomenon of slow repair. Br J Radiol 49:700, 1976
72. Fisher DR, Hendry JH: Dose fractionation and hepatocyte clonogens. Radiat Res 113:51 1988
73. Fisher DR, Hendry JH, Scott D: Long-term repair *in vivo* of colony-forming ability and chromosomal injury in x-irradiated mouse hepatocytes. Radiat Res 113:40, 1988
74. Fletcher GH: Clinical dose-response curves of human malignant epithelial tumours. Br J Radiol 46:1, 1973
75. Fletcher GH: Textbook of Radiotherapy, p 184. Philadelphia, Lea & Febiger, 1980
76. Fletcher GH: Textbook of Radiotherapy, I, II and III. eds. Philadelphia, Lea & Febiger, 1966, 1973, 1980
77. Fowler JF: J.F. Kirk Memorial Lecture: What next in fractionated radiotherapy. Br J Cancer 49(suppl 6):285, 1984
78. Fowler JF, Stern BE: II Dose-time relationships in radiotherapy and the validity of cell survival curve models. Br J Radiol 36:163, 1963
79. Gallagher MS, Brereton HD, Rostock RA, et al: A prospective study of treatment techniques to minimize the volume of pelvic small bowel with reduction of acute and late effects associated with pelvic irradiation. Int J Radiat Oncol Biol Phys 12:1565, 1986
80. Gatenby RA, Coia LA: Oxygen distribution in squamous cell carcinoma metastases: Relationship to outcome of radiation therapy. Am J Clin Oncol 10:101, 1987
81. Ghossein NA, Bataini JP, Ennuyer A, et al: Local control and site of failure in radically irradiated supraglottic laryngeal cancer. Radiology 112:187, 1974
82. Gonzales-Gonzales B, Breur K, van der Schueren E: Preliminary results in advanced head and neck cancer in radiotherapy by multiple fractions per day. Clin Radiol 31:417, 1980
83. Gorodetsky R, McBride WH, Withers HR: Assay of radiation effects in mouse skin as expressed in wound healing. Radiat Res 116:135, 1988

84. Gorodetsky R, Mou X, Fisher DR, et al: Radiation effect in mouse skin: Dose fractionation and wound healing. Int J Radiat Oncol Biol Phys, 18:1077, 1990
85. Gray LH, Conger AD, Ebert M, et al: The concentration of oxygen dissolved in tissues at the time of irradiation as a factor in radiotherapy. Br J Radiol 26:638, 1953
86. Habermalz HJ, Valley B, Habermalz E: Radiation myelopathy of the mouse spinal cord in isoeffect correlations after fractionated radiation. Strahlenther Onkol 163:626, 1987
87. Hahn GM, Little JB: Plateau-phase cultures of mammalian cells: An *in vitro* model for human cancer. Curr Top Radiat Res Q 8:39, 1972
88. Hall EJ, Bedford JS, Oliver R: Extreme hypoxia, its effect on the survival of mammalian cells irradiated at high and low dose rates. Br J Radiol 39:302, 1966
89. Hall EJ: Radiation dose-rate: A factor of importance in radiobiology and radiotherapy. Br J Radiol 45:81, 1972
90. Harwood AR, Beale FA, Cummings JB, et al: Supraglottic laryngeal carcinoma: An analysis of dose-time-volume factors in 410 patients. Int J Radiat Oncol Biol Phys 9:311, 1983
91. Henk JM, Kunkler PB, Smith CW: Radiotherapy and hyperbaric oxygen in head and neck cancer. Lancet ii:101, 1977
92. Hermens AF, Barendsen GW: Changes of cell proliferation characteristics in a rat rhabdomyosarcoma before and after x-irradiation. Eur J Cancer 5:173, 1969
93. Hewitt HB: Fundamental aspects of the radiotherapy of cancer. In The Scientific Basis of Medicine: Annual Review, p 305. London, Athlone Pr Humanities, 1962
94. Hill RP, Bush RS: The effect of continuous or fractionated irradiation on a murine sarcoma. Br J Radiol 46:167, 1973
95. Hliniak A, Maciejewski B, Trott KR: The influence of the number of fractions, overall treatment time and field size on the local control of cancer of the skin. Br J Radiol 56:596, 1983
96. Hopewell JW, Wiernik G: Tolerance of pig kidney to fractionated x-irradiation. In Radiobiological Research and Radiotherapy, vol 1, pp 65–73, Vienna, IAEA, 1977
97. Hopewell JW, Morris AD, Dixon-Brown A: The influence of field size on the late tolerance of the rat spinal cord to single doses of X rays. Br J Radiol 60:1099, 1987
98. Horiot JC, DePauw M, von Glabbeke M: Hyperfractionation versus conventional fractionation in curative radiotherapy of oropharynx tumor: updated results of a randomized EORTC trial. Abstract 0–0290, 5th European Conference on Clinical Oncology, London, 1989
99. Horiot JC, Nabid A, Chaplain G, et al: Clinical experience with multiple daily fractionation in the radiotherapy of head and neck cancer. Cancer Bull 34:230, 1982
100. Horiot JC, Lefur R. Nguyen T, et al: Two fractions per day in the radiotherapy of oropharynx trial (Abstr). Int J Radiat Oncol Biol Phys 15(Suppl 1):178, 1988
101. Horiot JC, van den Bogaert W, Ang KK, et al: EORTC trials using radiotherapy with multiple fractions per day. Front Radiat Ther Oncol 22:148, 1988
102. Howard A, Pelc SR: Synthesis of deoxyribonucleic acid in normal and irradiated cells and its relation to chromosome breakage. Heredity 6(Suppl):261, 1952
103. Howes AE: An estimation of changes in the proportions and absolute numbers of hypoxic cells after irradiation of transplanted C_3H mammary tumours. Br J Radiol 42:441, 1969
104. Hryniuk WM: The importance of dose intensity in outcome of chemotherapy. In DeVita VT, Hellman S, Rosenberg SA (eds): Important Advances in Oncology 1988, pp 121–142. Philadelphia, JB Lippincott, 1988
105. Hussey DH, Fletcher GH: Clinical features of 16 and 50 $MeV_{d/Be}$ neutrons. Eur J Cancer 10:357, 1974
106. Ingold JA, Reed GB, Kaplan HS, et al: Radiation hepatitis. Am J Roentgenol 93:200, 1965
107. Jampolis S, Pipard G, Horiot JC, et al: Preliminary results using twice-a-day fractionation on the radiotherapeutic management of advanced cancers of the head and neck. Am J Roentgenol 129:1091, 1977
108. Jirtle RL, McLain JR, Strom SC et al: Repair of radiation damage in noncycling parenchymal hepatocytes. Br J Radiol 55:847, 1982
109. Joiner MC: The dependence of radiation response on the dose per fraction. In McNally NJ (ed): The Scientific Basis of Modern Radiotherapy, BIR Report 19, pp 20–26. London, BIR, 1989
110. Kallman RF: The phenomenon of reoxygenation and its implication for fractionated radiotherapy. Radiology 105:135, 1972
111. Kellerer AM, Rossi HH: A generalized formulation of dual radiation action. Radiat Res 75:471, 1978
112. Kerr JFR, Wyllie AH, Currie AR: Apoptosis: A basic biological phenomenon with wide-ranging implications in tissue kinetics. Br J Cancer 26:239, 1972
113. Knee R, Field RS, Peters LJ: Concomitant boost radiotherapy for advanced squamous cell carcinoma of the head and neck. Radiother Oncol 4:1, 1985
114. Kolstad P: The development of the vascular bed in tumours as seen in squamous cell carcinoma of the cervix uteri. Br J Radiol 38:216, 1965
115. Kummermehr J, Trott KR: Rate of repopulation in a slow and a fast growing mouse tumor. In Karcher KH, Kogelnik HD, Reinartz G (eds): Progress in Radio-Oncology II, p 299. New York, Raven Press, 1982
116. Lauk S, Ruth S, Trott KR: The effects of dose-fractionation on radiation-induced heart disease in rats. Radiother Oncol 8:363, 1987
117. Law MP: Radiation-induced vascular injury and its relation to late effects in normal tissues. In Lett JT, Adler H (eds): Advances in Radiation Biology, vol 9, pp 37–73. New York, Academic Press, 1981
118. Lea DE: Actions of Radiation on Living Cells, 2nd ed. Gray LH (ed): England, Cambridge University Press, 1956
119. Leith JT, DeWyngaert JK, Glicksman AS: Radiation myelopathy in the rat: An interpretation of dose effect relationships. Int J Radiat Oncol Biol Phys 7:1673, 1981
120. Little JB: Repair of potentially lethal radiation damage in mammalian cells: Enhancement by conditioned medium from stationary cultures. Int J Radiat Biol 20:87, 1971
121. Lo YC: The effect of ionizing radiation and hyperthermia on mouse spinal cord. Ph D Thesis, University of California, Los Angeles, 1989
122. Maciejewski B: Regression rate of metastatic neck lymph nodes after radiation treatment as a prognostic factor for local control. Radiother Oncol 8:301, 1987
123. Maciejewski B, Majewski S: Radiotherapy of bladder cancer. II. Dose fractionation and tumor regeneration. Acta Oncol, in press, 1990
124. Maciejewski B, Preuss-Bayer G, Trott KR: The influence of the number of fractions and overall treatment time on the local tumor control of cancer of the larynx. Int J Radiat Oncol Biol Phys 9:321, 1983
125. Maciejewski B, Taylor JMG, Withers HR: Alpha/beta value and the importance of size of dose per fraction for late complications in the supraglottic larynx. Radiother Oncol 7:323–326, 1986
126. Maciejewski B, Withers HR, Taylor JMG: Dose fractionation and regeneration in radiotherapy for cancer of the oral cavity and oropharynx. 1. Tumor dose-response and repopulation. Int J Radiat Oncol Biol Phys 16:831, 1989
127. Maciejewski B, Withers HR, Taylor JMG: Dose fractionation and regeneration in radiotherapy for cancer of the oral cavity and oropharynx. II. Acute and late effects in normal tissues. Int J Radiat Oncol Biol Phys, in press, 1990
128. Mason KA, Withers HR: RBE of neutrons generated by 50 MeV deuterons on beryllium for control of artificial pulmonary metastases of a mouse fibrosarcoma, Br J Radiol 50:652, 1977
129. Mason KA, Withers HR, Davis CA: Dose dependent latency of fatal gastrointestinal and bone marrow syndrome. Int J Radiat Biol 55:1, 1989
130. McBride WH, Withers HR: *In vitro* studies of ante-mortem proliferation kinetics. Br J Cancer 53(Suppl 7):386, 1986
131. McCulloch EA, Till JE: Proliferation of hematopoietic colony-forming cells transplanted into irradiated mice. Radiat Res 22:383, 1964
132. Meistrich ML, Hunter NR, Suzuki N, et al: Gradual regeneration of mouse testicular stem cells after ionizing radiation. Radiat Res 74:349, 1978

133. Mendelsohn ML: The growth fraction: a new concept applied to tumors. Science 132:1496, 1960
134. Meoz-Mendez RT, Fletcher GH, Guillamondegui OM, et al: Analysis of the results of irradiation in the treatment of squamous cell carcinomas of the pharyngeal walls. Int J Radiat Oncol Biol Phys 4:579, 1978
135. Michalowski A: Effects of radiation on normal tissues: Hypothetical mechanisms and limitations of *in situ* assays of clonogenicity. Radiat Environ Biophys 19:157, 1981
136. Moulder JE, Dutreix J, Rockwell S, et al: Applicability of animal tumor data to cancer therapy in humans. Int J Radiat Oncol Biol Phys 14:913, 1988
137. Moulder JE, Rockwell S: Hypoxic fractions of solid tumors: Experimental techniques, methods of analysis and a survey of existing data. Int J Radiat Oncol Biol Phys 10:695, 1984
138. Nguyen TD, Panis X, Froissart D, et al: Analysis of late complications after rapid hyperfractionated radiotherapy in advanced head and neck cancers. Int J Radiat Oncol Biol Phys 14:23, 1988
139. Norin T, Onyango J: Radiotherapy in Burkitt's lymphoma: Conventional or superfractionated regime—early results. Int J Radiat Oncol Biol Phys 2:339, 1987
140. Overgaard M: The clinical implication of non-standard fractionation. Int J Radiat Oncol Biol Phys 11:1225, 1985
141. Overgaard M: Spontaneous radiation-induced rib fractures in breast cancer patients treated with postmastectomy irradiation: A clinical radiobiological analysis of fraction size and dose response relationship in late bone damage. Acta Oncol 27:117, 1988
142. Overgaard J, Hjelm-Hansen M, Vendelbo Johansen L, Andersen AP: Comparison of conventional and split-course radiotherapy as primary treatment in carcinoma of the larynx. Acta Oncol 27:147, 1988
143. Palcic B, Skarsgard LD: Reduced oxygen enhancement ratio at low doses of ionizing radiation. Radiat Res 100:328, 1984
144. Parkins CS, Fowler JF: Repair in mouse lung of multifraction X-rays and neutrons. Br J Radiol 58:1087, 1985
145. Parsons JT: Time-dose-volume relationships in radiation therapy. In Million RR, Cassisi NJ (eds): Management of Head and Neck Cancer, pp 137–172. Philadelphia, JB Lippincott, 1984
146. Parsons JT, Bova FJ, Million RR: A reevaluation of split-course technique for squamous cell carcinoma of the head and neck. Int J Radiat Oncol Biol Phys 6:1645, 1980
147. Parsons JT, Cassisi NJ, Million RR: Results of twice-a-day irradiation of squamous cell carcinoma of the head and neck. Int J Radiat Oncol Biol Phys 10:2041, 1984
148. Parsons JT, Million RR: Radiation therapy with multiple fractions per day in the treatment of head and neck cancer. In Jacobs C (ed): Head and Neck Oncology, pp 71–91. The Hague, Martinus Nijhoff, 1987
149. Parsons JT, Thar TL, Bova FJ, et al: An evaluation of split-course irradiation for pelvic malignancies. Int J Radiat Oncol Biol Phys 6:175, 1980
150. Paterson RP: The Treatment of Malignant Disease by Radium and X Rays. London, Edward Arnold, 1948
151. Pedrick TJ, Hoppe RT: Recovery of spermatogenesis following pelvic irradiation for Hodgkin's disease. Int J Radiat Oncol Biol Phys 12:117, 1986
152. Peracchia G, Salti C: Radiotherapy with thrice-a-day fractionation in a short overall time. Int J Radiat Oncol Biol Phys 7:99, 1981
153. Peters LJ, Ang KK: Accelerated fractionation. In Withers HR, Peters LJ (eds): Innovations in Radiation Oncology, pp 231–238. Heidelberg, Springer-Verlag, 1988
154. Peters LJ, Ang KK, Thames HD: Fractionation in the treatment of head and neck cancer: A critical comparison of different strategies. Acta Radiol Oncol 27:185, 1988
155. Peters LJ, Brock WA, Chapman JD, et al: Predictive assays of tumor radiocurability. Am J Clin Oncol 11:275, 1988
156. Peters LJ, Mason KA, Withers HR: Effect of lung irradiation on metastases: Radiobiological studies and clinical correlations. In Meyn RE, Withers HR (eds): Radiation Biology in Cancer Research, pp 515–529. New York, Raven Press, 1980
157. Peters LJ, Thames HD: Dose-response relationship for supraglottic laryngeal carcinoma. Int J Radiat Oncol Biol Phys 9:421, 1983
158. Peters LJ, Ang KK, Thames HD: Altered fractionation schedules. In Perez CA, Brady LW, (eds): Principles and Practice of Radiation Oncology, pp 00–00. Philadelphia, JB Lippincott, 1991
159. Peters LJ, Tofilon PJ, Groepfert H, Brock WA: Radiosensitivity of primary tumor cultures as a determinant of human head and neck cancers. In McNally NJ (ed): The Scientific Basis of Modern Radiotherapy, BIR Report 19, pp 132–135. London, BIR, 1989
160. Peters LJ, Withers HR, Cundiff JH, et al: Radiobiological considerations in the use of total body irradiation for bone marrow transplantation. Radiology 131:243, 1979
161. Phillips RA, Tolmach LJ: Repair of potentially lethal damage in x-irradiated HeLa cells. Radiat Res 29:413, 1966
162. Pino Y, Torres JL, Lee DJ, et al: Local control and reduced complications in split course irradiation of prostatic cancer. Int J Radiat Oncol Biol Phys 7:43, 1981
163. Potish RA: Importance of predisposing factors in the development of enteric damage. Am J Clin Oncol 5:189, 1982
164. Powers WE, Tolmach LJ: A multicomponent x-ray survival curve for mouse lymphosarcoma cells irradiated *in vivo.* Nature 197:710, 1963
165. Puck TT, Marcus PI: Action of x-rays on mammalian cells. J Exp Med 103:653, 1956
166. Read J: The effect of ionizing radiation on the broad bean root. X. Br J Radiol 25:89; 154, 1952
167. Read J: Radiation Biology of Vicia Faba in Relation to the General Problem. Oxford, Blackwell Scientific Publications, 1959
168. Resouly A, Svoboda VHJ: Management of advanced head and neck squamous carcinoma by multiple daily sessions of radiotherapy. In Karcher KH (ed): Progress in Radio-Oncology II, pp 339–348. New York, Raven Press 1982
169. Rojas A: Oxygen: A clinical reality or a mirage. In McNally NJ (ed): The Scientific Basis of Modern Radiotherapy, BIR Report 19, pp 86–90. London, BIR, 1989
170. Rossi HH: A note on the effects of fractionation of high LET radiations. Radiat Res 66:170, 1976
171. Rubin P: The Franz Buschke Lecture: Late effects of chemotherapy and radiation therapy: A new hypothesis. Int J Radiat Oncol Biol Phys 10:5, 1984
172. Rubin P, Casarett GW: Clinical Radiation Pathology, vols 1 and 2. Philadelphia, WB Saunders, 1968
173. Saunders MI, Dische S: Continuous hyperfractionated accelerated radiotherapy in non-small cell carcinoma of the bronchus. In McNally NJ (ed): The Scientific Basis of Modern Radiotherapy, BIR Report 19, pp 47–52. London, BIR, 1989
174. Scalliet P, Landuyt W, van der Schueren E: Repair kinetics as a determining factor for the late tolerance of central nervous system to low dose rate irradiation. Radiother Oncol 14:345, 1989
175. Sellins KS, Cohen JJ: Gene induction by γ-irradiation leads to DNA fragmentation in lymphocytes. J Immunol 10:3199, 1987
176. Shukovsky LJ: Dose, time, volume relationships in squamous cell carcinoma of the supraglottic larynx. Am J Roentgenol 108:27, 1970
177. Shukovsky LJ, Fletcher GH: Time-dose and tumor volume relationships in the irradiation of squamous cell carcinoma of the tonsillar fossa. Radiology 107:621, 1973
178. Sinclair WK: Dependence of radiosensitivities upon cell age. In Time and Dose Relationships in Radiation Biology as Applied to Radiotherapy, p 97. Brookhaven National Lab Report 50203 (C-57), 1969
179. Steel GG: Growth Kinetics of Tumours. New York, Oxford University Press, 1977
180. Steel GG: Terminology in the description of drug-radiation interactions. Int J Radiat Oncol Biol Phys 5:1145, 1979
181. Steel GG: The combination of radiotherapy and chemotherapy. In Steel GG, Adams GE, Peckham MJ (eds): The Biological Basis of Radiotherapy, pp 239–248. Amsterdam, Elsevier, 1983
182. Stewart FA: Late normal tissue damage after combined che-

motherapy and radiotherapy. In McNally NJ (eds): The Scientific Basis of Modern Radiotherapy, BIR Report 19, p 95. London, BIR, 1989

183. Stewart FA, Randhawa VS, Michael BD: Multifraction irradiation of mouse bladders. Radiother Oncol 2:131, 1984
184. Stewart JG, Jackson AW: The steepness of the dose response curve for both tumor cure and normal tissue injury. Laryngoscope 85:1107:1975
185. Strandqvist M: Studien uber die kumulative wirking der rontgenstrahlen bei fraktionierung. Acta Radiol (Stockh) 55(Suppl):1, 1944
186. Stratford IJ, Sheldon PW, Adams GE: Hypoxic cell radiosensitizers. In Steel GG, Adams GE, Peckham MJ (eds): The Biological Basis of Radiotherapy, pp 211–223. Amsterdam, Elsevier, 1983
187. Stuschke M, Budach V, Budach W, et al: Repair capacity of human soft tissue sarcomas. In Karcher KH (ed): Progress in Radio-Oncology IV, pp 53–57. New York, Raven Press, 1988
188. Suit HD, Howes AF, Hunter N: Dependence of response of a C3H mammary carcinoma to fractionated irradiation on fractionation number and intertreatment interval. Radiat Res 72:440, 1977
189. Suit HD, Lindberg RD, Fletcher GH: Prognostic significance of extent of tumor regression at completion of radiation therapy. Radiology 84:1100, 1965
190. Suit HD, Zietman A, Miralbell R, Sedlacek R: Human tumor xenografts for study of the radiation response of human tumors. In Prediction of Radiation Response in Radiation Therapy, pp 251–262. AAPM Symposium Proceedings 7, New York, American Institute of Physics, 1989
191. Terasima T, Tolmach LJ: Variations in several responses of HeLa cells to x-irradiation during the division cycle. Biophys J 3:11, 1963
192. Thames HD, Ang KK, Stewart FA, van der Schueren E: Does incomplete repair explain the apparent failure of the basic LQ model to predict spinal cord and kidney responses to low doses per fraction? Int J Radiat Biol 54:13, 1988
193. Thames HD, Hendry JH: Fractionation in Radiotherapy. London, Taylor & Francis, 1987
194. Thames HD, Hendry JH, Moore JV, et al: The high steepness of dose-response curves for late-responding tissues. Radiother Oncol 15:49, 1989
195. Thames HD, Mason KA, Bentzen SM: Split dose recovery in mouse jejunal crypt cells. In McNally NJ (eds): The Scientific Basis of Modern Radiotherapy, BIR Report 19, pp 37–42. London, BIR, 1989
196. Thames HD, Peters LJ, Spanos W, et al: Dose response of squamous cell carcinomas of the upper respiratory and digestive tracts. Br J Cancer 41(Suppl IV):35, 1980
197. Thames HD, Peters LJ, Withers HR, et al: Accelerated fractionation vs. hyperfractionation: Rationale for several treatments per day. Int J Radiat Oncol Biol Phys 9:127, 1983
198. Thames HD, Withers, HR, Mason KA, et al: Dose-survival characteristics of mouse jejunal crypt cells. Int J Radiat Oncol Biol Phys 7:1591, 1981
199. Thames HD, Withers HR, Peters LJ, et al: Changes in early and late radiation responses with altered dose fractionation: Implications for dose-survival relationships. Int J Radiat Oncol Biol Phys 8:219, 1982
200. Thomlinson RH: Reoxygenation as a function of tumor size and histopathological type. In Time and Dose Relationships in Radiation Biology as Applied to Radiotherapy, pp 242–254. Brookhaven National Lab Report 50203 (C-57), 1970
201. Thomlinson RH, Gray LH: The histological structure of some human lung cancers and possible implications for radiotherapy. Br J Cancer 9:539, 1955
202. Thompson LH, Suit HD: Proliferation kinetics of x-irradiated mouse L cells studied with time-lapse photography. II. Int J Radiat Biol 15:347, 1969
203. Tolmach LJ: Growth patterns in irradiated HeLa cells. Ann NY Acad Sci 95:743, 1961
204. Travis EL, Parkins CS, Down JD, et al: Repair in mouse lung between multiple small doses of X rays. Radiat Res 94:326, 1983
205. Travis EL, Peters LJ, McNeill J: Effect of dose-rate on total body irradiation: Lethality and pathologic findings. Radiother Oncol 4:341, 1985
206. Turesson I, Notter G: The influence of the overall treatment time in radiotherapy on the acute reaction: Comparison of the effects of daily and twice-a-week fractionation on human skin. Int J Radiat Oncol Biol Phys 10:599, 1984
207. Turesson I, Notter G: Accelerated versus conventional fractionation. Acta Oncol 27:169, 1988
208. Urtusan RC, Chapman JD, Raleigh JA, et al: A novel technique for measuring human tissue hypoxia at the cellular level. Br J Cancer 54:453, 1986
209. Utsumi H, Elkind MM: Potentially lethal damage versus sublethal damage: Independent repair processes in actively growing Chinese hamster cells. Radiat Res 77:346, 1979
210. Utsumi H, Hill CK, Ben-Hur E, et al: "Single-hit" potentially lethal damage: Evidence of its repair in mammalian cells. Radiat Res 87:576, 1981
211. van den Brenk HAS: The oxygen effect in radiation therapy. Curr Top Radiat Res 5:197, 1969
212. van der Kogel AJ: Radiation tolerance of the rat spinal cord: Time-dose relationships. Radiology 122:505, 1977
213. van der Kogel AJ: Mechanisms of late radiation injury in the spinal cord. In Meyn R, Withers HR (eds): Radiation Biology in Cancer Research, pp 461–470. New York, Raven Press, 1980
214. van der Kogel AJ: Effect of volume and localization on rat spinal cord. In Fielden EM, Folwer JF, Hendry JH, Scott D (eds): Proceedings of the 8th International Congress of Radiation Research, p 352. London, Taylor & Francis, 1987
215. van der Schueren E, van den Bogaert W, Ang KK: Radiotherapy with multiple fractions per day. In Steel GG, Adams GE, Peckham MJ (eds): The Biological Basis of Radiotherapy, p 195. Amsterdam, Elsevier, 1983
216. van Dyk J, Mah K, Keane TJ: Radiation-induced lung damage: Dose-time fractionation considerations. Radiother Oncol 14:55, 1989
217. van Peperzeel HA: Effects of single doses of radiation on lung metastases in man and experimental animals. Eur J Cancer 8:665, 1972
218. van Rongen E, Kuijpers WC, Madhuizen HT, van der Kogel AJ: Effects of multifraction irradiation on the rat kidney. Int J Radiat Oncol Biol Phys 15:1161, 1988
219. Vegesna, V, Withers HR, Taylor JMG: The effect on depigmentation after multifraction irradiation of mouse resting hair follicle. Radiat Res 111:464, 1987
220. Vegesna V, Withers HR, Taylor JMG: Repair kinetics of mouse lung. Radiother Oncol 15:115, 1989
221. Vogel AW: Intratumoral vascular changes with increased size of a mammary adenocarcinoma: A new method and results. J Natl Cancer Inst 34:571, 1965
222. Wang CC: Accelerated fractionation. In Withers HR, Peters LJ (eds): Innovations in Radiation Oncology, pp 239–243. Heidelberg, Springer-Verlag, 1988
223. Wang CC: Accelerated hyperfractionation radiation therapy for carcinoma of the nasopharynx. Cancer 63:2461, 1989
224. Wang CC, Blitzer PH, Suit HD: Twice-a-day radiation therapy for cancer of the head and neck. Cancer 55:2100, 1985
225. Weichselbaum RR, Little JB: Repair of potentially lethal x-ray damage and possible applications to clinical radiotherapy. Int J Radiat Oncol Biol Phys 9:91, 1982
226. Weichselbaum RR: The role of DNA repair processes in the response of human tumors to fractionated radiotherapy. Int J Radiat Oncol Biol Phys 10:1127, 1984
227. Weichselbaum RR, Schmit A, Little JB: Cellular repair factors influencing radiocurability of human malignant tumours. Br J Cancer 45:10, 1982
228. Wendt CD, Peters LJ, Ang KK, et al: Hyperfractionated radiotherapy in the treatment of squamous cell carcinomas of the supraglottic larynx. Int J Radiat Oncol Biol Phys 17:1057, 1989
229. Wharton JT, Delclos L, Gallager S, et al: Radiation hepatitis induced by abdominal irradiation with cobalt 60 moving strip technique. Am J Roentgenol 117:73, 1973
230. White A, Hornsey S: Time-dependent repair of radiation

damage in the rat spinal cord after X rays and neutrons. Eur J Cancer 16:957, 1980

231. Williams MV, Denekamp J: Radiation induced renal damage in mice: Influence of fraction size. Int J Radiat Oncol Biol Phys 10:885, 1984
232. Williams MV, Denekamp J, Fowler JF: A review of α/β ratios for experimental tumors. Intl J Radiat Oncol Biol Phys 11:87, 1985
233. Willis RA: Pathology of Tumors, 4th ed. London, Butterworth, 1967
234. Wilson CS, Hall EJ: On the advisability of treating all fields each radiotherapy session. Radiology 98:419, 1971
235. Wilson GD, McNally NJ, Dische S, et al: Measurement of cell kinetics in human tumors *in vivo* using bromodeoxyuridine incorporation and flow cytometry. Br J Cancer 58:423, 1988
236. Withers HR: The dose-survival relationship for irradiation of epithelial cells of mouse skin. Br J Radiol 40:187, 1967
237. Withers HR: Recovery and repopulation *in vivo* by mouse skin epithelial cells during fractionated irradiation. Radiat Res 32:227, 1967
238. Withers HR: Capacity for repair in cells of normal and malignant tissues. In Time and Dose Relationships in Radiation Biology as Applied to Radiotherapy, pp 54–69. Brookhaven National Laboratory Report 50203 (C-57), 1970
239. Withers HR: Regeneration of intestinal mucosa after irradiation. Cancer 28:75, 1971
240. Withers HR: The biological basis for high LET radiotherapy. Radiology 108:131, 1973
241. Withers HR: The 4 R's of radiotherapy. In Lett JT, Alder H (eds): Advances in Radiation Biology, vol 5, p 241. New York, Academic Press, 1975
242. Withers HR: Cell cycle redistribution as a factor in multifraction irradiation. Radiology 114:199, 1975
243. Withers HR: Biologic basis for altered fractionation schemes. Cancer 55:2086, 1985
244. Withers HR: Neutron radiobiology and clinical consequences. Strahlentherapie 161:739, 1985
245. Withers HR: Predicting late normal tissue responses. Int J Radiat Oncol Biol Phys 12:693, 1986
246. Withers HR: Neutrons and other clinical trials: Impossible dreams? Int J Radiat Oncol Biol Phys 13:1967, 1987
247. Withers HR: Inherent acceleration of tumor dose-rate in hyperfractionated regimens. Int J Radiat Oncol Biol Phys 14:400, 1988
248. Withers HR: Contrarian concepts in the progress of radiotherapy. Radiat Res 119:395, 1989
249. Withers HR: Unpublished data
250. Withers HR, Chen KY: Poor man's neutrons? Br J Radiol 44:818, 1971
251. Withers HR, Chu AM, Reid BO, et al: Response of mouse jejunum to multifraction radiation. Int J Radiat Oncol Biol Phys 1:41, 1975
252. Withers HR, Cuasay L, Mason KA, et al: Elective radiation therapy in the curative treatment of cancer of the rectum and rectosigmoid. In Strohlein JR, Romsdahl JR (eds): Gastrointestinal Cancer, pp 351–361. New York, Raven Press, 1981
253. Withers HR, Hunter N, Barkley HT, et al: Radiation survival and regeneration of characteristics of spermatogenic stem cells of mouse testis. Radiat Res 57:88, 1974
254. Withers HR, Maciejewski B, Taylor JMG: Biology of options in dose fractionation. In McNally NJ (ed): The Scientific Basis of Modern Radiotherapy, BIR Report 19, pp 27–36. London, BIR, 1989
255. Withers HR, Mason KA: The kinetics of recovery in irradiated colonic mucosa of the mouse. Cancer 34:896, 1974
256. Withers HR, Mason KA, Reid BO, et al: Response of mouse intestine to neutrons and gamma-rays in relation to dose fractionation and division cycle. Cancer 34:39, 1974
257. Withers HR, Mason KA, Thames HD: Late radiation response of kidney assayed by tubule cell survival. Brt J Radiol 59:587, 1986
258. Withers HR, Peters LJ: Radiobiology of high LET irradiation (neutrons). In Karcher KH, Kogelnik HD, Meyer HJ (eds): Progress in Radio-Oncology, pp 1–7. Stuttgart, Georg Thieme-Verlag, 1980
259. Withers HR, Peters LJ: Biological aspects of radiation therapy. In Fletcher GH (ed): Textbook of Radiotherapy, 3rd ed, pp 103–180. Philadelphia, Lea & Febiger, 1980
260. Withers HR, Peters LJ, Kogelnik HD: The pathobiology of late effects of irradiation. In Meyn RE, Withers HR (eds): Radiation Biology in Cancer Research, pp 439–448. New York, Raven Press, 1980
261. Withers HR, Suit HD: Is oxygen important in the radiocurability of human tumors? In Friedman M (ed): The Biological and Clinical Basis of Radiosensitivity, p 548. Springfield, IL, Charles C Thomas, 1974
262. Withers HR, Taylor JMG, Maciejewski B: Treatment volume and tissue tolerance. Int J Radiat Oncol Biol Phys 14:751, 1988
263. Withers HR, Taylor JMG, Maciejewski B: The hazard of accelerated tumor clonogen repopulation during radiotherapy. Acta Oncol 27:131, 1988
264. Withers HR, Thames HD: Dose fractionation and volume effects in normal tissues and tumors. Am J Clin Oncol 11:313, 1988
265. Withers HR, Thames HD, Peters LJ: Biological bases for high RBE values for late effects of neutron irradiation. Int J Radiat Oncol Biol Phys 8:2071, 1982
266. Withers HR, Thames HD, Peters LJ: Differences in the fractionation response of acute and late responding tissues. In Karcher KH, Kogelnik HD, Reinartz G (eds): Progress in Radio-Oncology II, pp 287–296. New York, Raven Press, 1982
267. Withers HR, Thames HD, Peters LJ: A new isoeffect curve for change in dose per fraction. Radiother Oncol 1:187, 1983
268. Withers HR, Thames HD, Peters LJ, et al: Normal tissue radioresistance in clinical radiotherapy. In Fletcher GH, Nervi C, Withers HR (eds): Biological Bases and Clinical Implications of Tumor Radioresistance, p 139. New York, Masson, 1983
269. Xu F, van der Schueren E, Ang KK: Acute reactions of the lip mucosa of mice to fractionated irradiations. Radiother Oncol 1:369, 1984
270. Zeman EM, Bedford JS: Changes in early and late effects with dose-per-fraction: Alpha, beta, redistribution and repair. Int J Radiat Oncol Biol Phys 10:1039, 1984

3

Altered Fractionation Schedules

Lester J. Peters
K. Kian Ang
Howard D. Thames

The term "altered fractionation" is relative because from the earliest days of radiation therapy there has been no agreement as to what constitutes the norm. Regimens regarded as conventional differ widely in different parts of the world. For example, in the Manchester school, radical (definitive) treatments are dispensed in 16 fractions over 3 weeks, whereas in the United States, most definitive treatments are administered in 35 to 40 fractions over 7 to 8 weeks. To a large extent, the evolution of "conventional" dose fractionation schedules reflects logistic and financial considerations and the availability of equipment and staff as much as any serious effort to determine which fractionation schedule maximizes the therapeutic advantage.[84,94] Many schedules now considered unconventional have had their proponents in the past, but only recently has sufficient information been available to assess the merits of different fractionation schedules on a radiobiologic basis.

For the sake of this chapter, conventional fractionation is defined according to current practice in the United States; that is, for curative treatment for most cancers, fractional doses of 180 to 200 cGy are given once daily, Monday through Friday, to total doses determined by the tumor being treated and the tolerance of critical normal tissues within the target volume (usually in the range of 6000 to 7000 cGy).

The possible permutations by which such a conventional schedule may be altered are infinite. In this chapter, however, we shall discuss regimens using more than one dose fraction per day for all or part of the treatment course. The reason for this focus is that a sound radiobiologic rationale can be developed for either reducing the size of dose per fraction, the overall time of treatment, or both, all of which require the use of multiple fractions per day.

To categorize and discuss the radiobiologic basis of different regimens using multiple fractions per day, the following definitions are used. In *hyperfractionation* the total dose is increased, the size of dose per fraction is reduced, the number of dose fractions is increased, and overall time is relatively unchanged. *Quasi-hyperfractionation* is the same as hyperfractionation except that the total dose is not increased. This defeats the rationale of hyperfractionation. In *accelerated fractionation* overall time is reduced, and the number of dose fractions, total dose, and size of dose per fraction are either unchanged or somewhat reduced, depending on the extent of overall time reduction. *Quasi-accelerated fractionation* is the same as accelerated fractionation except that the overall time is not reduced because of a treatment interruption, which defeats the rationale of accelerated fractionation. *Accelerated hyperfractionation* incorporates features of both hyperfractionation and accelerated fractionation. Here, such regimens are classified as predominantly hyperfractionated or predominantly accelerated, according to which rationale carries the greatest weight.

BACKGROUND RADIOBIOLOGY

The basic radiobiology of fractionation is discussed at length in Chapter 2. Here only the time-dose parameters relevant to altered fractionation schedules are reviewed. In clinical practice, depending on the dose-fractionation schedule, either acute reactions or late sequelae of therapy may be dose limiting. Careful clinical observation of patients treated with conventional schedules has enabled radiation therapists to establish the expected relationship between the severity of acute and late reactions (*i.e.*, a certain probability of late normal tissue injury corresponds with a certain intensity of acute reactions). Perhaps the most important consequence of altering a fractionation schedule is that this expected relationship is no longer valid: Late effects are more sensitive to changes in size of dose per fraction, and acute reactions are more sensitive to changes in the rate of dose accumulation.

Time-Dose Parameters

The time-dose parameters that determine normal tissue tolerance are total dose, overall duration of treatment, size of dose per fraction, and frequency of dose fractions. The latter two determine the rate of dose accumulation, sometimes referred to as the "weekly dose rate." The intensity of acute reactions in epithelial and other tissues organized into stem cell, maturation, and functional compartments (such as bone marrow) reflects the balance between the rate of cell killing by irradiation and the rate of regeneration of surviving stem cells. This balance depends primarily on the rate of dose accumulation. The fraction size is also a factor in determining the severity of acute reactions (large fractions being more damaging centigray for centigray than small ones), but to a lesser extent than is the case for late reactions. After an acute reaction has peaked (*e.g.*, moist desquamation of the skin has occurred), further stem cell killing cannot produce an increase in *intensity* of the acute reaction but will manifest as an increased time to heal the reaction. If sufficient stem cells do not survive to heal an acute reaction, it may progress into a consequential late injury.[75]

Late reactions following radiation therapy occur in tissues characterized by slow cellular turnover, such as mature connective tissues and the parenchymal cells of various organs. Because cellular depletion in such tissues is not manifested until after a typical course of radiation therapy is completed, no opportunity exists for regeneration to occur during treatment, and the rate of dose accumulation and overall duration of treatment are therefore of minor significance in determining the severity of late reactions. Conversely, such reactions depend greatly on total dose, size of dose per fraction, and interfraction interval when dose fractions are closely spaced.

Repair Capacity and Repair Kinetics

Traditionally, cellular repair capacity has been estimated by measuring the width of the shoulder on the survival curve (D_q) or by measuring the difference in dose for the same biologic effect when a single dose (D_1) is split into two doses (D_2). Provided there is sufficient time between the doses for full repair (but not significant repopulation) and the size of each of the two dose fractions is sufficiently large, D_2–D_1 is equivalent to D_q. With clinically relevant dose fractionation, however, D_q is not an adequate measure of repair capacity because it reflects the *width* of the shoulder of the survival curve, whereas the *shape* of the shoulder determines the fractionation response for sizes of dose per fraction in the shoulder region. Thus, two cell types can have the same D_q and D_o, but manifest very different fractionation responses to small dose fractions because of differences in shape of survival curves in the shoulder region (Fig. 3-1). Both survival curves (A and B) in panel 1 have the same D_o and D_q; however, it is clear from panels 2 and 3 that the effect of a change in dose per fraction on the total dose of fractionated irradiation for a given level of cell kill will be higher in cells in which survival response is described by the more curvy shoulder (A) than by the straighter shoulder (B).

The linear quadratic survival curve equation has become popular because it provides a good description of the shape of the shoulder region of the survival curve with only two variables: α, which describes the linear component of cell killing and thus the initial slope of the survival curve, and β, which describes the quadratic component of cell killing that causes the bending of the survival curve at higher doses.[56] The lower the α/β ratio, the greater the curvature of the shoulder on survival curve and the greater the capacity for repair when the radiation dose is fractionated.

The relevance of cell survival parameters (*e.g.*, α and β) to the responses of organized tissues and tumors rests on the target cell hypothesis, which holds that the responses of tissues may be quantified by the survival parameters of the underlying target cells whose depletion by radiation causes observable damage. Whereas this hypothesis has been tested in only a few tissues and tumors,[94] it has been useful in practice to describe the fractionation response of many normal tissues and tumors empirically in terms of the α/β ratio of the putative target cells in those tissues.

Both the capacity to repair sublethal damage (α/β) and its rate of repair ($T^1/2$) vary among different cell lines and tissue types. Most quantitative information concerning these variables has been obtained from fractionation experiments in animals, mainly rodents. Table 3-1 lists estimates of the α/β ratio for a variety of normal tissues in animals. The general observation is that late-responding tissues have low α/β ratios and acutely responding tissues have higher α/β ratios. To realize an increase in tolerance of late-responding tissues through dose fractionation, it is essential for the time interval between the dose fractions to be long enough to allow complete repair to occur. If doses are too closely spaced, injury will accumulate between dose fractions, and successive doses will become increasingly more damaging.

It is customary for repair kinetics to be quantitated in terms of the half-time for repair, although a simple monoexponential function may not adequately describe the process.[42] Of the tissues in which repair kinetics have been studied, half-times for repair tend to be longest (1 to several hours) in the skin, kidney, and spinal cord, shortest (about half an hour) in the jejunal mucosa, and intermediate in the lung and colon.[2,4,5,31,42,48,54,79,80,94,99,102,110] The exact values vary according to experimental protocol, and considerable overlap exists in the confidence limits of repair half-time. However, it is clear that unlike repair capacity, no systematic difference in repair kinetics exists between acutely responding and late responding normal tissues. The important point is that several late responding normal tissues that one might hope to spare by hyperfractionation have long repair halftimes, and therefore an adequate interfraction interval must be ensured.

Repair kinetics is of particular importance in determining the response of the spinal cord to fractionation schedules of more than one daily fraction. In rats, experimental data have shown that complete repair (that occurring with a 24-hour interfraction interval) has not occurred even with an 8-hour interfraction interval (Ang and associates, unpublished data).[4] A recent clinical report of radiation myelopathy occurring in two patients who received 4200 cGy in 28 fractions of 150 cGy, three times per day with a 6-hour interfraction interval over 9 consecutive days, supports this observation.[28]

The data are even less clear on the dependence of repair kinetics on the size of dose per fraction. The half-time of repair appears to be independent of fraction size in the spinal cord,[4] with a slight trend toward longer half-times after larger dose fractions. Longer repair half-times after larger dose fractions have also been observed in skin, but the value of $T^1/2$ appears to be longer after smaller dose fractions in the kidney.[78] In the case of the lung, reported values of $T^1/2$ are essentially independent of fraction size except at very small doses per fraction, at which shorter half-times have been found.[42,102] No effect of fraction size on repair kinetics was observed in the jejunum.[95] Because of the variability of experimental data, it is not possible to make generalizations about repair kinetics by tissue class. For clinical applications, however, it is judicious to err on the conservative side by allowing as long a time between dose fractions as possible; a review of the clinical data[96] suggests that for practical purposes the minimum safe interval for tissues other than the spinal cord is 6 hours.

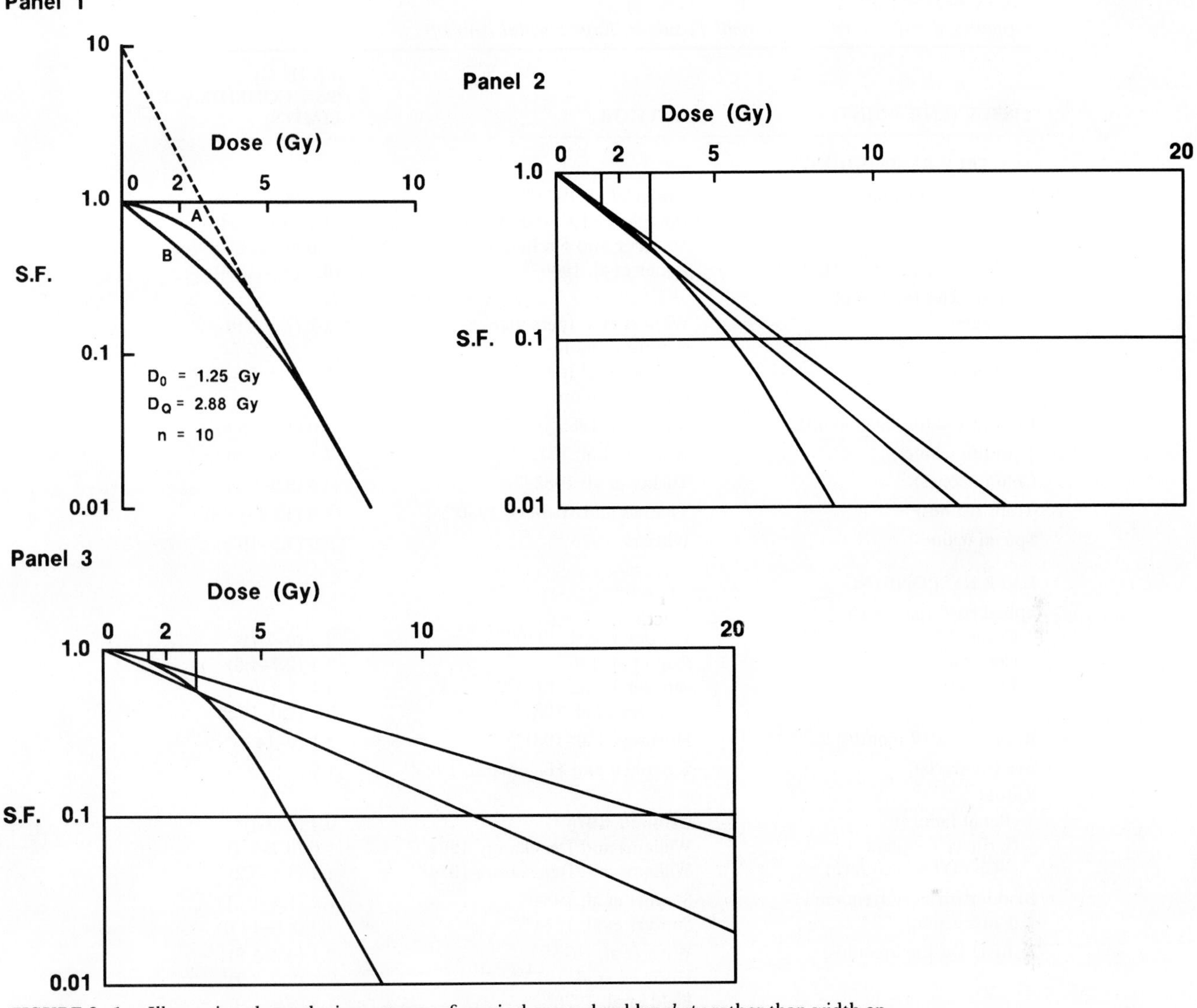

FIGURE 3–1. Illustration shows the importance of survival curve shoulder *shape* rather than width on the response to fractionated irradiation. *Panel 1.* Two survival curves with the same D_o, D_Q and n, but with different initial slopes and shoulder curvatures. In terms of the linear quadratic model of cell survival, the α/β ratio is lower for curve *A* than for curve *B*. *Panels 2* and *3*. Effect of change in fraction size on the dose required for a given isoeffect. *Panel 2* shows that when the shoulder has a steep initial slope and little curvature (high α/β), a change in dose per fraction from 3 Gy to 1.5 Gy would only slightly increase the total dose needed to produce a given survival fraction. *Panel 3* shows that when the shoulder has a shallow initial slope and marked curvature (low α/β), a much greater increase in total dose is necessary to produce a given survival fraction when the same change in dose per fraction is made. (Peters LJ, Brock WA, Travis EL: Radiation biology at clinically relevant fractions. In DeVita V, Hellman S, Rosenberg SA [eds]: Important Advances in Oncology 1990. Philadelphia, JB Lippincott, 1991)

In general, the estimated values of α/β for early and late reactions in human normal tissues are consistent with results from experimental animals. Data on repair kinetics in human normal tissues are extremely sparse, but, as indicated earlier, some human evidence suggests that interfraction recovery may be slower in humans than in rodents (Table 3-2)[93].

With regard to tumors, squamous cell carcinomas of the head and neck, cervix, skin, and non-small cell lung cancers are characterized by high α/β ratios in agreement with rodent models. However, available data from melanomas and liposarcomas suggest somewhat lower α/β ratios for these tumor types. There is also a hint that the α/β ratio for breast adenocarcinomas may be lower than those for other carcinomas listed in Table 3-2,[68] but the data are insufficient to reach any firm conclusion.

Overall Time

The importance of overall time with regard to acute normal tissue reactions has long been recognized, but it has only recently been appreciated that the curability of many cancers (particularly squamous cell carcinomas) is also highly dependent on overall treatment time. As noted previously, the intensity of acute reactions is determined primarily by the rate of dose accumulation (weekly dose rate). The importance of the

TABLE 3–1
Estimates of α/β for Various Normal Tissues in Experimental Animals

TISSUE (END POINT)	AUTHOR	α/β IN Gy (95% CONFIDENCE LIMITS)
ACUTELY RESPONDING		
Skin (desquamation)	Fowler et al, 1974[40]	9.4 (6.1–14.3)
	Douglas and Fowler, 1976[29]	11.7 (9.1–15.4)
	Moulder and Fischer, 1976[65]	21.0 (16.2–27.8)
	Joiner et al, 1986[55]	10.5 (8.5–12.5)
Hair follicles (epilation)		
Anagen	Withers et al (personal communication)	7.7 (7.4–8.0)
Telogen	Withers et al (personal communication)	5.5 (5.2–5.8)
Lip mucosa (desquamation)	Ang et al, 1985[5]	7.9 (1.8–25.8)
Jejunum (clones)	Withers et al, 1975[119]	7.1 (6.8–7.5)
Colon (clones)	Tucker et al, 1983[104]	8.4 (8.3–8.5)
Testis (clones)	Thames and Withers, 1980[98]	13.9 (13.4–14.3)
Spleen (clones)	Withers, 1975[118]	8.9 (7.5–10.9)
LATE RESPONDING		
Spinal cord (paralysis)		
Cervical	van der Kogel, 1979[108]	2.5 (0–7.7)*
Cervical	Ang et al, 1987[4]	3.4 (2.7–4.3)
Lumbar	van der Kogel, 1979[108]	4.1 (2.2–6.5)
Lumbar	Hornsey et al, 1981[53]	5.2 (2.0–10.2)
Brain (LD_{50}/10 months)	Hornsey et al, 1981[53]	2.1 (0–14.4)*
Eye (cataracts)	Schenken and Hagemann, 1975[83]	1.2 (0.6–2.1)
Kidney		
(Renal failure)	Caldwell, 1975[15]	0.4 (0–3.4)*
(Urinary frequency)	Williams and Denekamp, 1984[116]	1.6 (0.7–2.4)
(^{51}Cr-EDTA clearance)	Williams and Denekamp, 1984[116]	4.1 (3.1–5.2)
Bladder (urinary frequency)	Stewart et al, 1984[88]	7.2 (1.3–18.1)
(Contraction)	Stewart et al, 1984[88]	7.8 (2.6–17.0)
Lung (LD_{50}/pneumonitis)	Wara et al, 1973[113]	2.1 (0.2–5.2)
	Hornsey et al, 1975[52]	2.5 (2.0–3.2)
	Field et al, 1976[37]	4.3 (3.8–4.9)
	Parkins and Fowler, 1985[72]	3.0 (2.4–3.6)
	Vegesna et al, 1985[110]	3.7 (3.2–4.3)
	Travis et al, 1987[102]	3.7 (2.8–4.5)
Bowel (Stricture/perforation)	Terry and Denekamp, 1984[91]	3.0–5.0 (0–22.0)*
Dermis/subcutis—pig (contraction)	Withers et al, 1978[121]	$0.3 < \alpha/\beta < 2.4$
Total body irradiation (LD_{50}/1 yr)	Travis et al, 1985[101]	5.1 (0–15.0)*

**Lower confidence limit is negative, but is listed as 0, because a negative α/β has no biologic meaning.*
(Modified from Thames HD, Hendry JH [eds]: Fractionation in Radiotherapy. London, Taylor & Francis, 1987)

weekly dose rate is a reflection of the biologic fact that acute reactions represent a deficit in the balance between the rate of cell killing by radiation and cell regeneration from surviving stem cells. After the stem cell population is depleted to the point at which it is unable to renew the functional layers of the epithelium, the acute reaction peaks and further depopulation produces no increase in severity of the reaction. This means that the peak intensity of acute reactions is influenced more by the rate of dose accumulation than by the total dose, after a certain threshold of total dose has been reached.

Conversely, the time taken to heal, as opposed to the peak intensity of the acute reactions, is dependent on total dose, provided that the weekly dose rate exceeds the regenerative ability of the surviving stem cells. This is because healing is a function of the absolute number of stem cells surviving the course of treatment, and the higher the total dose, the fewer stem cells will survive. Although most classic late radiation sequelae (*e.g.*, spinal cord injury) show little or no dependence on overall time (provided full recovery occurs between dose fractions), overall time may be of significance for another class of late effects in which total doses were less than or similar to conventional regimens and in which a higher incidence of late reactions was observed.[74, 90, 107] To explain these results, a distinction needs to be drawn between "true" late effects and "consequential" late reactions.[75] Many of the late effects seen in these studies can be attributed to severe and prolonged epithelial denudation rather than to direct radiation injury of the mesenchymal tissues normally associated with late reactions.

TABLE 3–2
Estimates of α/β for Human Tissues and Tumors

TISSUE/TUMOR	AUTHOR	ESTIMATE OR BOUND OF α/β IN Gy (95% CONFIDENCE LIMITS WHERE APPLICABLE)
EARLY REACTIONS		
Skin		
Erythema	Turesson and Thames, 1989[106]	8.8 (6.9–11.6)
	Bentzen et al, 1988[9]	12.3 (2–23)
Desquamation (T ≤ 29 days)	Turesson and Thames, 1989[106]	11.2 (8.5–17.6)
Lung—acute	Cox, 1987[21]	>8.8
LATE REACTIONS		
Supraglottic larynx—late sequelae	Maciejewski, et al, 1986[60]	3.8 (0.8–14)
Larynx		
Cartilage necrosis	Henk and James, 1978[47]	~3.4
	Horiot et al, 1972[49]	<4.4
	Fletcher et al, 1974[38] and Stell and Morrison, 1973[87]	<4.2
Oropharynx—late sequelae	Horiot et al, 1988[51]	~4.5
Skin		
Telangiectasia	Turesson and Thames, 1989[106]	3.9 (2.7–4.8)
	Bentzen et al, 1989[12]	3.7 (0.2–4.7)
Subcutaneous fibrosis	Bentzen et al, 1989[12]	1.9 (0.8–3)
Shoulder		
Impaired movement	Bentzen et al, 1989[10]	3.5 (0.7–6.2)
Lung		
Pneumonitis	Cox, 1987[21]	<3.8
Cord		
Myelopathy	Dische et al, 1981[27]	<3.3
Brachial plexus		
Plexopathy	Powell et al, 1989[77]	<5.3
Bowel		
Stricture/perforation	Bennett, 1978[8] and Edsmyr et al, 1985[33]	2.2 < α/β < 8
TUMORS		
Vocal cord	Harrison et al, 1988[46]	>9.9
Oral cavity/oropharynx	Maciejewski et al, 1989[61]	~25
	Byhardt et al, 1977[14] and	>6.5
	Cox et al, 1980[23]	~10.3
	Handa et al, 1980[45]	>7
Lung		
Squamous cell, large cell, adenocarcinoma	Cox et al, 1980[23]	50–90
Cervix	Watson et al, 1978[114]	>13.9
Skin	Trott et al, 1984[103]	8.5 (4.5–11.3)
Melanoma	Bentzen et al, 1989[11]	0.6 (0–2.5)*
Liposarcoma	Thames and Suit, 1986[97]	0.4 (0–5.4)*

**Lower confidence limit is negative, but is listed as 0, because a negative α/β has no biologic meaning.*
(Modified from Thames HD, Bentzen SM, Turesson I, et al: Time-dose factor in radiotherapy: A review of the human data. Radiother Oncol 19:219–235, 1990)

Evidence for accelerated regeneration of surviving tumor cells after initiation of treatment comes from three principal observations: (1) time-to-recurrence data for tumors that are not sterilized by radiation therapy, (2) a comparison of split-course and continuous-course treatment regimens, and (3) an analysis of tumor-control doses as a function of time (with correction for fraction size differences).

Time-to-Recurrence

The majority of recurrences of squamous cell carcinomas of the head and neck occur within 2 years of treatment. An example of time-to-recurrence data (from patients with squamous cell carcinomas of the pyriform sinus) is provided in the report of El Badawi and associates.[35] It showed that the median time to recurrence was approximately 6 months and that 90% of all recurrences occurred within 2 years. Because the recurrences occurred from a population of tumors in which the majority were controlled, it follows that most recurrences must have arisen from one or a few surviving clonogenic cells. For one surviving clonogen to produce a clinically detectable recurrence requires about 30 volume doublings. In other words, the mean doubling time of nonsterilized tumor cells must have been only about 6 days.

Split-Course Compared With Continuous-Course Treatment

Million and Zimmerman[64] first reported inferior results with split-course treatment compared with continuous-course treatments for head and neck cancer, when daily and total doses were not adjusted to compensate for the split. Subsequently, Budhina and colleagues[13] calculated that the dose necessary to compensate for a split in treatment was approximately 50 cGy per day. A more recent report from Overgaard and coworkers[69] established that to achieve equal probability of tumor control of laryngeal cancers, a dose increment of 1100 to 1200 cGy was necessary to offset a treatment break of 3 weeks (50 to 60 cGy/day). Assuming that 200 to 300 cGy in 200 cGy fractions is necessary to reduce the surviving fractions of clonogenic cells by 50%, these data imply that four to six doublings must have occurred during the 3-week treatment split, yielding a clonogenic cell doubling time of 3.5 to 5 days.

Tumor Control Dose and Treatment Time

The most detailed analyses of the dose equivalent of regeneration occurring *during* fractionated radiation therapy are those of Withers and associates[120] and Maciejewski and colleagues.[61] These studies show that after a variable lag period, surviving tumor clonogens regenerate rapidly during fractionated radiation therapy to the extent that each additional day of treatment requires approximately 60 cGy, on average, to offset clonogenic cell regeneration. This value for the dose equivalent of regeneration during therapy is very similar to that obtained from analysis of the split-course data.

From all three types of analysis, therefore, it appears that after initiation of cytoreductive therapy, surviving clonogens in squamous cell carcinomas of the head and neck are able to regenerate with doubling times on the order of 3 to 5 days.

Currently no known method directly measures the proliferation kinetics of surviving clonogenic cells during treatment. Kummermehr and Trott[58] made an extensive study of the relationship between various pretreatment kinetic parameters and the regenerative response during treatment in a variety of experimental tumors. These experiments have shown that no single kinetic parameter can predict consistently the behavior of a tumor during treatment. The most useful, however, is the pretreatment potential doubling time (T_{pot}). T_{pot} can be determined from a measure of the labeling index and the length of S phase of the cell cycle. This type of study is now possible in humans using flow cytometric analyses of tumor cells labeled *in vivo* with bromodeoxyuridine (BrdUrd), which is tagged with a fluorescent monoclonal antibody. Preliminary data reported by Begg and associates[7] have shown that in a series of seven head and neck cancers, five had short potential doubling times (2.3 to 5.1 days), whereas two had much longer T_{pots} (13 and 25 days). Unpublished data of Terry and co-workers (1989) from a series of 28 squamous cell carcinomas of the head and neck treated at M.D. Anderson Cancer Center show a median T_{pot} of 3 to 4 days.

Isoeffect Formulas

The effect of changes of dose fractionation schedule on the total dose required to produce a certain level of biologic effect can be conveniently represented by isoeffect curves or formulas. The first clinical isoeffect curve was produced by Strandqvist, who plotted total dose against overall time of treatment for the cure of skin cancers and different degrees of skin reaction.[89] On double logarithmic coordinates, these isoeffect curves approximated a straight line, implying the existence of a power function relationship between dose and time ($D \alpha T^k$). In the early 1960s, Fowler and Stern[41] demonstrated experimentally in pigs that the time factor in radiation therapy was a composite, representing both the number of dose fractions and the overall time, and that the biologic effect was more dependent on the number of dose fractions than on the overall time *per se*. These experimental observations, along with clinical data of Cohen[18–20] that were interpreted as showing a difference of 0.11 in the time exponents for cure of squamous cell carcinoma of the skin and for acute skin reactions, led to the birth of the nominal standard dose (NSD) formula of Ellis[36]: $D \propto N^{0.24} \times T^{0.11}$ (N = number of dose fractions; T = overall time).

This formula purported to represent the effect of changing fractionation parameters on the tolerance of normal connective tissues, which were considered to impose the ultimate dose limitation for all radiation therapy. From the NSD concept, the tolerance dose formula (TDF) tables and the cumulative radiation effect (CRE) formulas were derived. In the middle and late 1970s, it was recognized that the exponents N and T used in the NSD formula were not appropriate for all tissue types: In general, isoeffect curves for late-reacting normal tissues were characterized by larger exponents of N and smaller exponents of T. These observations led to modifications of the NSD and CRE formulas on a tissue-specific basis.[105,113] Dutreix and associates[32] made the important point that isoeffect relationships depended fundamentally on size of dose per fraction and not on number of dose fractions (although the two are interrelated).

When total isoeffect doses for different normal tissue end points were plotted against dose per fraction, Withers and coworkers[118] showed that the curves for late reactions were consistently steeper than those for early reactions. This observation was given a quantitative basis by Thames and co-workers,[100] leading to the emergence of isoeffect formulas based on the linear quadratic (LQ) model of cell survival: $\ln S = N(\alpha d + \beta d^2)$. The basic isoeffect formula based on the LQ model is as follows:

$$\frac{D_1}{D_2} = \frac{\alpha/\beta + d_2}{\alpha/\beta + d_1}$$

(D = total dose for isoeffect; d = dose per fraction). This basic formula assumes complete repair between dose fractions, and no time factor is incorporated in it.

Thus, the basic formula may be used only when dose fractions are spaced widely enough apart to ensure complete repair and when the isoeffect end point is either not time-dependent (as with most late reactions) or the two schedules being compared involve the same overall time. When these conditions are not met, modifications of the formula allow the introduction of terms to compensate for incomplete repair or proliferation of target cells during treatment. These modifications, however, make the formula more difficult for the mathematically unversed.[94]

Isoeffect relationships based on the LQ model have now

been tested in a large number of experimental animal systems, and in general good agreement has been obtained for fraction sizes between 100 cGy and 1000 cGy. The exception has been with the spinal cord where, with fractional doses below 200 cGy, the LQ model overestimates tolerance, possibly because of lack of complete repair between dose fractions.[92]

Whereas the LQ-based isoeffect model is internally consistent for a wide range of tissue types and end points, clinical application of the model for derivation of new fractionation schedules is limited by the lack of precision of estimates of α/β. Even in animal systems where experimental conditions can be closely controlled, estimates of α/β showed large confidence intervals (see Table 3-1). The α/β ratios of available human data are consistent with the experimentally determined α/β ratios, but have very wide confidence bounds (see Table 3-2).

The bottom line is that no isoeffect formula is sufficiently reliable to preempt clinical judgment, and in the final analysis, each new fractionation schedule must be tested clinically to establish its safety.

RATIONALE FOR HYPERFRACTIONATION

The basic rationale of hyperfractionation is that the use of small dose fractions allows higher total doses to be administered within the tolerance of late-responding normal tissues and that this translates into a higher biologically effective dose to the tumor. For this rationale to hold, the α/β ratio for tumor cells must be greater than that for the dose-limiting normal tissue. As noted previously, acutely responding tissues as a class have higher α/β ratios than late-responding normal tissues. Because of the kinetic similarity between tumors and acutely responding normal tissues, it may be predicted that tumors also tend to have large α/β ratios. Good data exist for rodent tumors showing this to be true.[117] However, data for human tumors are sparse and imprecise.[93] As noted previously (see Table 3-2), most human tumors appear to have large α/β ratios, but there are exceptions. This is important to remember, because it would be inappropriate to use hyperfractionation in the treatment of tumors characterized by low α/β ratios.

Other rationales for hyperfractionation are radiosensitization through redistribution and lesser dependence on oxygen effect. The greater the number of dose fractions in a treatment régimen, the greater is the opportunity for tumor cells to be sensitized by redistribution in the division cycle; that is, cells in a radioresistant phase at the time of any given fraction are more likely to be caught in a sensitive phase at the time of a subsequent fraction. With small fractional doses, the influence of tumor cell hypoxia is reduced on two counts. First, the proportion of hypoxic cells needs to be higher to significantly increase the surviving fraction and, second, the oxygen enhancement ratio is lower.[71]

Because the rationale for hyperfractionation depends on tumors behaving similarly to acutely responding normal tissues, the use of this strategy inevitably will be associated with more severe acute reactions than in conventional fractionation; this is confirmed by a survey of the clinical data.[96] However, to the extent that total doses are determined by the tolerance of late-responding normal tissues, a therapeutic gain should be realized in the treatment of tumors with large α/β ratios.

Parenthetically, the same logic predicts that for tumors characterized by a large α/β ratio, a therapeutic *disadvantage* would result from the use of large dose fractions (hypofractionation). A schematic illustration of the anticipated changes in isoeffect relationships for late-responding and acutely responding normal tissues and tumors with high α/β ratios is shown in Figure 3-2.

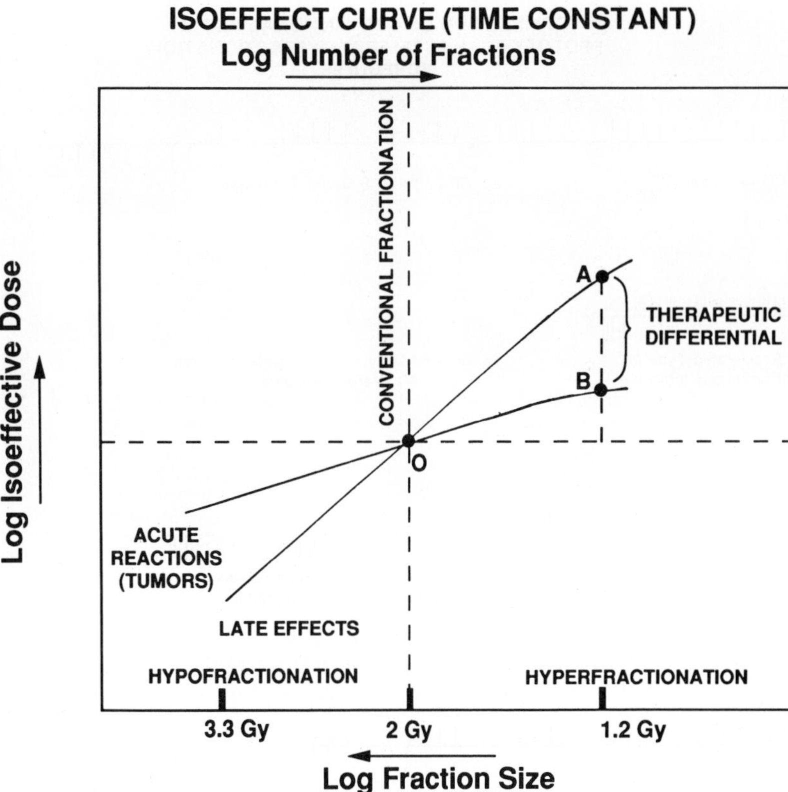

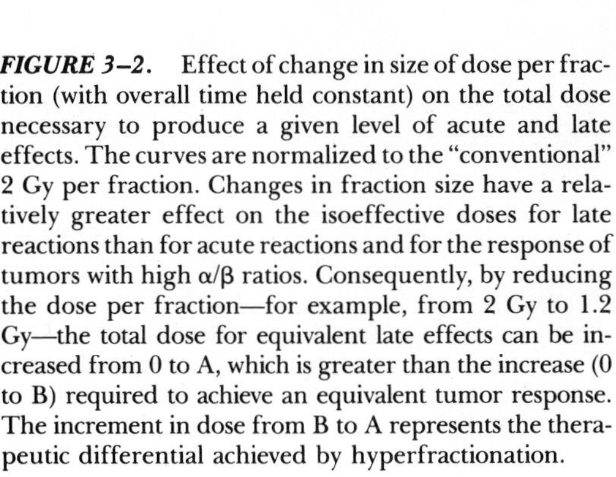

FIGURE 3–2. Effect of change in size of dose per fraction (with overall time held constant) on the total dose necessary to produce a given level of acute and late effects. The curves are normalized to the "conventional" 2 Gy per fraction. Changes in fraction size have a relatively greater effect on the isoeffective doses for late reactions than for acute reactions and for the response of tumors with high α/β ratios. Consequently, by reducing the dose per fraction—for example, from 2 Gy to 1.2 Gy—the total dose for equivalent late effects can be increased from 0 to A, which is greater than the increase (0 to B) required to achieve an equivalent tumor response. The increment in dose from B to A represents the therapeutic differential achieved by hyperfractionation.

Quasi-hyperfractionation

The strategy of hyperfractionation depends on the total dose being increased to take advantage of the improved tolerance of late-responding normal tissues to smaller fractional doses. Some authors have characterized as hyperfractionated, regimens in which small dose fractions have been delivered on a multiple-fraction-per-day basis, but in which the total dose has been limited to a level at or below that tolerated with conventional fractionation. This strategy offers no prospect of improved tumor control and is therefore termed quasi-hyperfractionation.

RATIONALE FOR ACCELERATED FRACTIONATION

The basic rationale for accelerated fractionation is that reduction in overall treatment time decreases the opportunity for tumor cell regeneration during treatment and therefore increases the probability of tumor control for a given total dose. Because overall treatment time has little influence on the probability of late normal tissue injury (provided the size of dose per fraction is not increased and the interval between dose fractions is sufficient for complete repair to take place), a therapeutic gain should be realized.

Shortening of overall treatment time without reduction in total dose should always increase the therapeutic ratio so long as acute reactions remain tolerable. However, when the overall duration of treatment is markedly reduced, it is necessary to reduce total dose to prevent excessively severe acute reactions. Under these circumstances, a therapeutic gain is realized only if the dose equivalent of regeneration of tumor cells during the time by which treatment is shortened exceeds the actual reduction in dose mandated by the maximum tolerated dose for acute reactions.

Three basic strategies for accelerated fractionation have been tested or are presently used (Fig. 3-3). Type A consists of an intensive short course of treatment in which the overall duration of treatment is markedly reduced with a corresponding substantial decrease in the total dose. Types B and C represent techniques in which the duration of treatment is more modestly reduced but the total dose is kept in the same range as for a conventional treatment. This is accomplished by using either a split-course or concomitant boost technique. These techniques are conveniently differentiated on the basis of the strategy adopted to circumvent intolerable acute reactions: for type A a reduction in dose; for type B a break in treatment; for type C a reduction in volume of mucosa exposed to accelerated treatment.

Figure 3-4 depicts an isoeffect model of the zone of therapeutic gain for each of these accelerated fractionation schedules in the treatment of head and neck cancers. The isoeffect curve for acute and consequential late reactions is based on maximum tolerated doses (MTD) for accelerated fractionation regimens reported by Saunders and colleagues[81,82] (5400 cGy in 36 fractions delivered in 12 days), Lamb and associates[59] (5940 cGy in 33 fractions delivered in 24 days), and Peters and co-workers[75] (7200 cGy in 42 fractions delivered in 40 days), and the report of Andrews[1] that there was no mucositis in a series of 43 patients treated to doses of up to 10,000 cGy in 43 to 44 fractions over 100 days. The curve for generic late (primary chronic) effects is based on abundant clinical experience that 7000 to 7200 cGy in 180 to 200 cGy fractions represents the limit of tolerance for late sequelae of head and neck irradiation. Because the time factor is negligible for primary chronic effects (provided that sufficient time is allowed between fractions for complete Elkind recovery), this isoeffect curve is drawn flat from 2 weeks onward.

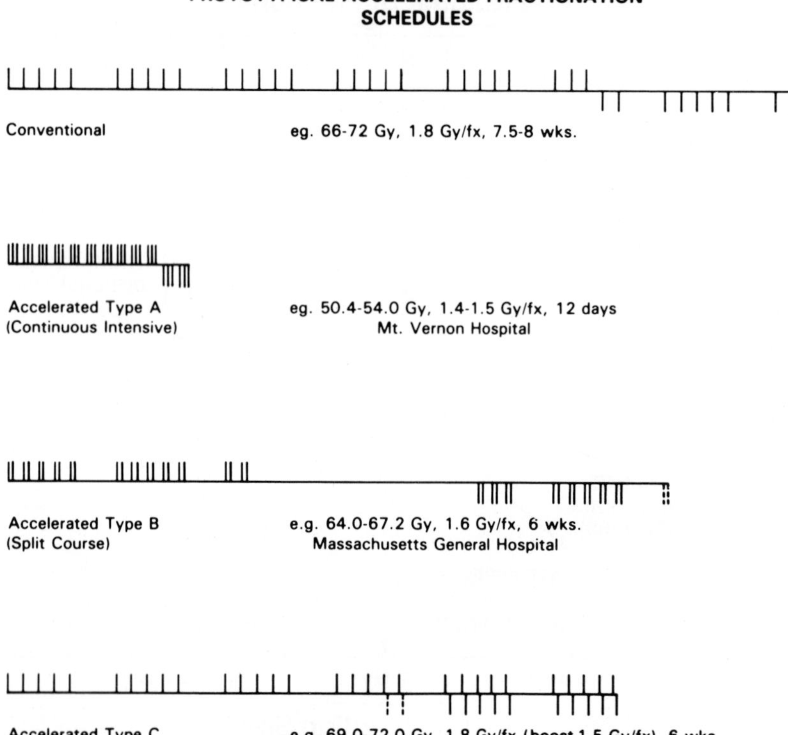

FIGURE 3–3. Conventional and accelerated fractionation schedules. For each schedule, the large field treatment is denoted by the bars above the line, and the boost field treatment by the bars below the line. The broken bars represent treatments omitted in the lower ranges of total dose. (Peters LJ, Ang KK, Thames HD: Acta Oncol 27:185, 1988)

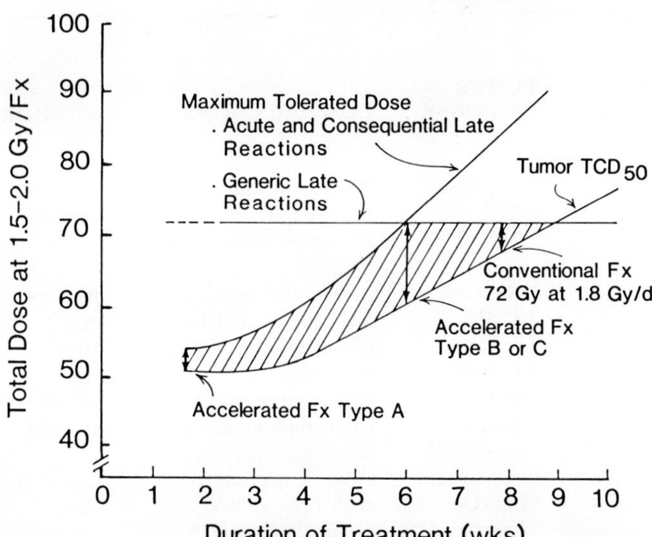

FIGURE 3–4. Zone of therapeutic gain in squamous cell carcinomas of the head and neck for different accelerated fractionation schedules. Type A is 54 Gy in 36 fractions over 12 days,[82] and Type B is 72 Gy in 42 fractions over 40 days.[75] Type C is 67.2 in 42 fractions over 42 days.[112] For explanation, see text. (Peters LJ, Brock WA, Travis EL: Radiation biology at clinically relevant fractions. In DeVita V, Hellman S, Rosenberg SA [eds]: Important Advances in Oncology 1990. Philadelphia, JB Lippincott, 1991)

The tumor TCD_{50} curve is based on the composite for all head and neck sites generated by Withers and associates[120] from a literature review. The shaded area represents the zone of therapeutic gain; the vertical separation between the isoeffect for dose-limiting normal tissue reactions and tumor control is a measure of the therapeutic gain for a given treatment. With a type A accelerated fractionation schedule, the therapeutic gain is limited by the tolerance of acutely reacting normal tissues. Conversely, with conventional fractionation it is limited by the tolerance of late-reacting normal tissues. The maximum gain is predicted with a type B or type C accelerated fractionation schedule in which the treatment time is adjusted such that both acute and late reactions are simultaneously dose-limiting, that is, when the maximum dose that can be tolerated by late-responding tissues is given in the shortest time that permits its tolerance by acutely responding tissues. This conclusion is unaffected in principle by the exact position of the tumor TCD_{50} curve. The only requirements are that the upward slope of this curve (representing regeneration of tumor clonogens) is less steep than the slope of the isoeffect curve for acute reactions and that accelerated regeneration in the tumor clonogens does not begin significantly earlier during treatment than that in the stem cells of the mucous membranes.

Quasi-accelerated Fractionation

The strategy of accelerated fractionation depends on the overall duration of treatment being reduced to take advantage of the lack of overall time dependence on the tolerance of classically late-responding normal tissues. Some authors have characterized as accelerated fractionation regimens in which *segments* of treatment have been given on an accelerated basis, but in which the overall duration of the complete course of treatment is not reduced because of the insertion of rest intervals between the accelerated segments. This strategy offers no prospects of improved tumor control through reducing tumor cell regeneration during treatment and is therefore termed quasi-accelerated fractionation.

HYPERFRACTIONATION *VERSUS* ACCELERATED FRACTIONATION

For any dose fractionation regimen, the factors determining tumor cell kill are the radiosensitivity of the tumor cells at the dose per fraction used and the regenerative response of survivors during treatment. Fowler[39] has recently published an exhaustive comparison of different fractionation schedules as a function of clonogenic cell doubling time during treatment and its time of onset. The basic conclusion of this analysis is that tumor cell kill is increased to much the same extent using both high-dose hyperfractionation and accelerated fractionation of type C. Both were significantly more effective than accelerated fractionation of type A unless the clonogen doubling time during treatment was less than approximately 2 days. The similarity of results modeled for the hyperfractionated and accelerated regimens considered is not surprising since hyperfractionated treatment at 120 cGy b.i.d. incorporates a degree of acceleration such that the overall time difference between the two strategies is minimized. Conversely, the accelerated fractionation schedules were based on fractional doses somewhat smaller than the conventional norm of 200 cGy. This reflects a convergence of rationales toward the realization that the best therapeutic strategy is likely to result from delivering the maximum dose tolerated by late-responding normal tissues in the minimum time consistent with tolerable acute reactions.

It should be remembered that for tumors with a slow clonogen regeneration rate during treatment, pure hyperfractionation to maximize the total tumor dose may be preferable, but tumor cell survival parameters also influence the choice of strategy. If the tumor α/β ratio is small, hyperfractionation is contraindicated. Under these circumstances, combined modality therapy with chemical radiosensitizers, high LET (linear energy transfer), or even hypofractionated low LET should be considered.[76]

CLINICAL STUDIES

A summary of the data from published clinical studies using altered fractionation schedules is provided in Tables 3-3 to 3-7.

Predominantly Hyperfractionation: Phases I and II

Several pilot studies and nonrandomized treatment series using predominantly hyperfractionated schedules have been reported in the following tumors sites: four, head and neck; four, brain; two, lung; and one, bladder (Table 3-3). The head and neck studies used fractional doses of 110 to 120 cGy twice daily, with interfraction intervals ranging from 3 to 8 hours. All showed an increase in mucosal reactions as predicted radiobiologically, associated with improved tumor control in relation to historic series. Parsons and colleagues[73] and Wendt and associates[115] both estimated an approximate 15 percentage point increase in tumor control probability with their hyperfractionated schedules without any overall increase in late complica-

TABLE 3–3
Clinical Studies Using Predominantly Hyperfractionation: Phase I/II

TUMOR SITE	NO. OF PATIENTS	DOSE/FX (cGy)	FX/DAY (INTER-VAL IN H)	TOTAL DOSE (cGy)	OVERALL TIME (WK)	TUMOR RESPONSE	COMPLICATIONS	AUTHOR
Head and neck (SCC)								
Various sites (advanced)	65	110–120	2 (≤3)	6000–7500	5–6.5	3-yr DFS: ~40%	Severe mucositis: 22%; late complications: 17% (3 fatal—2 after salvage surgery)	Meoz et al, 1984[63]
Various sites (T2–4)	132	120	2 (4–6)	7440–7920	6	Local control T2: 81% T3: 76% T4: 20%	Severe mucositis: 20%; NG tube: 11%; late effects: 3% moderate; 5% severe	Parsons et al, 1988[73]
Supraglottic larynx: T2, 3	38	120	2 (≥4)	7200–8060	6–7	2-yr Loco-regional control: 85%	Severe mucositis: 25%; late complications: 5% (2 cartilage necrosis)	Wendt et al, 1989[115]
Various sites (advanced)	237	120	2 (4–8)	6720–7680	5.5–6.5	Local control 6720 cGy: 25% 7200 cGy: 37% 7680 cGy: 42%	Grade 4 necrosis: 6720 cGy: 10%; 7200 cGy: 5.1%; 7680 cGy: 13.9%	Cox et al, 1990[25]
Brain								
(Glioblastoma)	30	100	3 (3–3.5)	4500–6000 + 5 × 200 cGy (boost)	4–5	MST: 40 vs 30 wk (historic control)	No evidence of brain necrosis	Douglas et al, 1982[30]
Brain stem								
(Glioma)	16	120	2 (4–8)	6480	5.5	MST: 11 mo	No evidence of radionecrosis	Packer et al, 1987[70]
(Glioma)	34	110	2 (4–6)	6600	6	MST: 11 mo	Moist skin desquamation (3 cases); otitis media/externa (9 cases). No evidence of CNS injury on biopsy/autopsy (8 cases)	Freeman et al, 1988[43]
(Glioma)	53	100	2 (4–8)	7200	7.2	MST: 17 mo	No evidence of an increase in acute or late normal tissue injury	Edwards et al, 1989[34]
Bladder (TCC)	50	120	2 (≥4)	6000–6960	5–5.5	2-yr survival: 48%	2-yr grade 3 + 4 late complications: 10%	Cox et al, 1988[24]
Lung (NSCLC)	120	120	2 (4–6)	5040–7440	4.5–6.5	CR: 13%; PR: 33%	Severe late complications 10% with doses >6000 cGy	Seydel et al, 1985[85]
Lung (NSCLC)	848	120	2 (≥4)	6000–7920	5–6.5	Doses ≥ 6960 cGy gave best results (2-yr survival: 29%) in favorable Stage III subset	Grade 3–5 pneumonitis: 6000–6480 cGy: 2.6%; 6960–7440 cGy: 5.7%; 7920 cGy: 8.1%; 2-yr actuarial risk of any grade 3+ toxicity 22% at 6960 cGy	Cox et al, 1990[22]

DFS: disease-free survival; MST: median survival time; CR: complete response; PR: partial response

tions. The risk of late complications increased, however, with total doses over 7680 cGy. The Radiation Therapy Oncology Group (RTOG) study reported by Cox and co-workers[25] shows a dose response function for tumor control as the total dose was escalated from 6720 cGy to 7680 cGy. Late normal tissue injury was comparable to that observed with conventional fractionation in previous RTOG studies.

Three of the four brain studies have focused on brain stem gliomas. Each involved two daily fractions with a minimum 4-hour interfraction interval. Fractional doses were 100 cGy (Northern California Oncology Group [NCOG]),[34] 110 cGy (Pediatric Oncology Group [POG]),[43] and 120 cGy (Children's Hospital of Pennsylvania [CHOP]).[70] All three studies were designed for dose escalation, and results have been reported with total doses of 7200 cGy (NCOG), 6600 cGy (POG), and 6480 cGy (CHOP). The NCOG study showed a significant improvement in median survival rate over historic controls, whereas the other two studies did not. None of the studies showed evidence of brain stem necrosis. A lack of necrosis in these studies may be perceived as inconsistent with the experimental data, which do not suggest a major increase in spinal cord tolerance with hyperfractionation. More likely, however, the explanation is that accepted norms for brain stem tolerance with conventional fractionation are well below the threshold for any significant incidence of this complication. Moreover, follow-up times have been short, and all patients have been receiving heavy doses of steroids. Caution should be exercised, therefore, in assuming that these regimens will be safe in long-term survivors.

In lung cancer, a large RTOG study reported by Cox and associates[22] used fractional doses of 120 cGy twice daily with a minimum 4-hour interfraction interval to total doses ranging from 6000 to 7920 cGy. The best survival rate overall was achieved with 6960 cGy total dose with an increased incidence of severe complications being observed at the highest dose level.

The bladder study was also an RTOG dose escalation protocol. Fractional doses of 120 cGy given twice daily with a minimum 4-hour interfraction interval were used to deliver 6000 to 6960 cGy to the pelvis. The 2-year actuarial incidence of grade 3 and 4 late complications was only 10%, suggesting that the tolerance of pelvic organs may be significantly increased through hyperfractionation.

Predominantly Hyperfractionation: Phase III

Three prospective randomized phase III clinical trials, two in the head and neck and one in the urinary bladder, have been reported using hyperfractionated schedules (Table 3-4). The largest of these, conducted by the European Organization for Research and Treatment of Cancer (EORTC) and reported by Horiot and others,[50,51] compared two fractions of 115 cGy with a 6- to 8-hour interfraction interval to a total dose of 8050 cGy in 7 weeks *versus* a single daily fraction of 200 cGy to a total dose of 7000 cGy in 7 weeks. The trial was limited to patients with T2–T3, N0–N1 tumors of the oropharynx to ensure homogeneity of the patient population. The overall 3-year locoregional control rate was increased from 38% to 57% by hyperfractionation ($P = 0.01$). There was no significant difference in treatment-related morbidity.

The second randomized head and neck study was reported recently by Datta and co-workers.[26] In this study, twice-daily fractions of 120 cGy with a 4- to 6-hour interfraction interval to a total dose of 7920 cGy in 6.5 weeks was compared with a single daily fraction of 200 cGy to a total dose of 6600 cGy in 6.5 weeks. Two-year locoregional control was increased from 33% to 63% by hyperfractionation ($P < 0.001$). Again, no increase in late treatment complications was observed.

Edsmyr and colleagues[33] reported a phase III randomized study in bladder cancer in which T2–T4 tumors were treated with either three daily fractions of 100 cGy with 4-hour interfraction intervals to a total dose of 8400 cGy or a single daily fraction of 200 cGy to a total dose of 6400 cGy. Both treatments were given in a split course over a total time of 8 weeks. The cystoscopic complete response rate was increased from 36% to 65% by hyperfractionation ($P < 0.001$), and 5-year survival rate was also significantly increased. In this study, however, severe late treatment complications were increased in the hyperfractionated arm, indicating that these were not isoeffect doses chosen for late normal tissue injury. From these data, the lower bound of the α/β ratio for late reactions can be set at 220 cGy. Taking a more reasonable α/β ratio of 400 cGy would yield a dose of 7700 cGy in 100 cGy fractions as being equivalent to 6400 cGy in 200 cGy fractions.

Quasi-hyperfractionation Studies

Two trials, one in the head and neck and one in the brain, have been reported using fractional doses and interfraction intervals consistent with hyperfractionation, but total doses less than those tolerated with conventional fractionation (Table 3-5). In the RTOG trial reported by Marcial and associates,[62] patients received either 120 cGy twice daily to a total dose of 6000 cGy, or 180 to 200 cGy once daily to total doses of 6600 to 7380 cGy. Despite the fact that the hyperfractionated arm was underdosed, equivalent rates of locoregional control were achieved, implying that had the hyperfractionated schedule been carried to the maximum tolerated dose, an improvement in tumor control may have been realized. Similar conclusions may be

TABLE 3–4
Clinical Studies Using Predominantly Hyperfractionation: Phase III

TUMOR SITE	NO. OF PATIENTS	DOSE/FX (cGy)	FX/DAY (INTERVAL IN H)	TOTAL DOSE (cGy)	OVERALL TIME (WK)	TUMOR RESPONSE	COMPLICATIONS	AUTHOR
Head and neck								
Oropharynx (T2–3)	158 153	115 200	2 (6–8) 1	8050 7000	7 7	5-yr Locoregional control: 57% vs 38% ($P = 0.01$)	No difference in acute mucositis grade 2–3 late effects: 32% vs 26%	Horiot et al, 1988, 1989[50,51]
Various sites (T2–3)	91 85	120 200	2 (4–6) 1	7920 6600	6.5 6.5	2-yr Locoregional control: 63% vs 33% ($P < 0.001$)	Acute mucosal and skin reactions more intense in hyperfractionation arm (requiring 3–5 days' treatment interruption in 34 pts). No difference in late complications.	Datta et al, in press[26]
Bladder (T2–T4)	83 85	100 200	3 (4) 1	8400 6400	8 (2-wk break) 8 (2-wk break)	Complete response at 6 mo: 65% vs 36% ($P < 0.001$) 5-yr survival: 34% vs 22% ($P = 0.01$)	Severe late reactions (intestinal obstructions, fistulae, bleeding): 12% vs 5%	Edsmyr et al, 1985[33]

TABLE 3–5
Clinical Studies Using Quasihyperfractionation

TUMOR SITE	NO. OF PATIENTS	DOSE/FX (cGy)	FX/DAY (INTER-VAL IN H)	TOTAL DOSE (cGy)	OVERALL TIME (WK)	TUMOR RESPONSE	COMPLICATIONS	AUTHOR
CNS								
Malignant glioma	134	48–190	1–3 (8–24)	3000–4000	1–4	No difference in median survival time	No difference in CNS complications	Simpson et al, 1976[86]
Head and Neck								
Various sites (randomized)	94 93	120 180–200	2 (3–6) 1	6000 6600–7380	5 7–8	2-yr Locoregional control: 30% vs 29%	Severe mucositis: 23% vs 13%; no difference in late effects	Marcial et al, 1987[62]
Various sites	178	90	8	6000–7200	4–6 (2- to 4-wk break)	Crude local control: 44% 2-yr overall survival: 13%	Mucosal necrosis: 14%; tracheostomy: 5%; late complications in 20/25 survivors	Nguyen et al, 1985[66]

drawn from the study of Simpson and colleagues[86] in which hyperfractionated treatment of gliomas was limited to a maximum total dose of 4000 cGy.

The third quasi-hyperfractionated study was that of Nguyen and others[66] who employed a schedule using eight fractions, each of 90 cGy with a 2-hour interfraction interval to total doses of 6000 to 7200 cGy in an overall time of 4 to 6 weeks. This study was characterized by an excessive rate of severe late complications that may be attributed to the short interfraction interval and large number of dose fractions given per day, with incomplete repair between dose fractions.

Predominantly Accelerated Fractionation Regimens

As described in the rationale for accelerated fractionation, different strategies can be employed to reduce overall time with or without a reduction in total dose (Table 3-6). The clinical data will be reviewed according to the strategy employed.

TYPE A: CONTINUOUS SHORT INTENSIVE COURSES. The pioneering study of short-course intensive accelerated fractionation was that of Norin and colleagues,[67] who showed that in the treatment of Burkitt's lymphoma three times daily treatment with fractional doses of 100 cGy to 125 cGy yielded greatly improved response rates compared with once-daily fractionation to similar total doses.

Short intensive schedules in which total doses of around 5000 cGy to 5500 cGy have been delivered in elapsed times of 2 weeks or less have been reported for three series of head and neck and one series of lung cancer patients. All three head and neck trials produced high tumor clearance rates but at the expense of severe acute reactions, usually requiring the patient to be hospitalized. In addition, significant late toxicity has been encountered. In two studies,[74,90] most of the late effects can be interpreted as consequential in nature, but in the third study[28] unexpected radiation myelopathy was also encountered at total doses well below those tolerated with conventional fractionation. Assuming no dosimetric error is uncovered, these results are

TABLE 3–6
Clinical Studies Using Predominantly Accelerated Fractionation: Phases I, II, and III

TUMOR SITE	NO. OF PATIENTS	DOSE/FX (cGy)	FX/DAY (INTER-VAL IN H)	TOTAL DOSE (cGy)	OVERALL TIME (WK)	TUMOR RESPONSE	COMPLICATIONS	AUTHOR
TYPE A: CONTINUOUS SHORT INTENSIVE SCHEDULES								
Burkitt's lymphoma	34	100–125	3 (?)	2500–3100	~2 wk	CR: ~74% (better than once-daily treatment)	None	Norin et al, 1977[67]
Head and neck								
Various sites	99	140–150	3 (6)	5040–5400	12 days	2-yr control: 51%	Severe mucositis, generally 2 wk hospitalization for nutritional support; myelopathy: 2	Dische et al, 1989[28]
Various sites	59	170–230	3 (≥3)	5000–5500	10–14 days	CR at 3 mo: 86%; 3-yr survival: 44%	Peak mucositis 5–10 days posttreatment (occasional hospitalization); severe late complications (necrosis, stenosis): 19%	Svoboda, 1984[90]

(continued)

TABLE 3–6
(Continued)

TUMOR SITE	NO. OF PATIENTS	DOSE/FX (cGy)	FX/DAY (INTER-VAL IN H)	TOTAL DOSE (cGy)	OVERALL TIME (WK)	TUMOR RESPONSE	COMPLICATIONS	AUTHOR
TYPE A: CONTINUOUS SHORT INTENSIVE SCHEDULES								
Various sites	22	200	3 (4)	4800–5400	9–11 days	CR at 8 mo: 68%	Confluent mucositis: 100%; mucosal necrosis: 55%; treatment-related deaths: 13	Perrachia and Salti, 1981[74]
Various sites	48	180	3 (≥4) 3 days/wk	5940	3.5 wk	CR at 2 mo: 56%; 2-yr DFS: 32%	Severe mucositis; patients with oral cavity lesions required hospitalization	Gray et al, 1986[44]
Breast								
Inoperable	39	140–300	3 (>3)	4000–4750	5–14 days	CR: 56%; 3-yr TC: 27%	Skin thickening and fibrosis if >4500 cGy and >160 cGy/fx. Leathering and necrosis if >4500 cGy and >300 cGy/fx.	Svoboda, 1984[90]
Inflammatory	42	127–135	2 (≥3)	5100–5400 +boost	4 wk	CR at 1–3 yr: 77%; 2-yr survival: 27%	Pneumonitis: 10%; severe fibrosis: 7%	Barker et al, 1980[6]
Lung (NSCLC)	17	180–200	2 (~3)	6600	<4 wk	CR: 40%	Acute-chronic esophagitis: 100%; severe complication: 24%	Von Rottkay, 1986[111]
Lung (NSCLC)	75	140–150	3 (6)	5040–5400	12 days	2-yr survival: 40%	Troublesome dysphagia from day 21 to 28	Dische et al, 1989[28]
Brain								
Isolated melanoma	20	300–375	2 (≥6)	3000–3750	1 wk	MST: 41 wk	Acute edema: 10%; late atrophy: 2	Choi et al, 1985[16,17]
metastases	23	190–240	2 (≥6)	3750–4800	2 wk	MST: 27 wk	Acute edema: 8%; late atrophy: 1	
TYPE B: SPLIT-COURSE ACCELERATED FRACTIONATION SCHEDULES								
Head and neck								
Various sites	321	160	2 (≥4)	6720–7200	~6.5 wk	3-yr Locoregional control: 68% (historical control: 46%)	Severe mucositis; late effects comparable to CF	Wang et al, 1985[112]
Brain								
Malignant glioma	295	200	3 (4)	6000 ±misonidazole	4 wk	MST: no difference	No difference in brain necrosis	Horiot et al, 1988[51]
(randomized)		200	1	6000	6 wk			
TYPE C: CONCOMITANT BOOST								
Head and neck								
Various sites	53	180–200 +120–150 (boost)	1–2 (3–6)	7000–7400	6 wk	2-yr Locoregional control: 65%	Severe mucositis: 35%; moderate late effects: 11% XRT only	Knee et al, 1985[57]
Oropharynx (T2–3)	79	180 +150 (boost)	1–2 (4–6)	6900–7200	6 wk (including 10–12 days boost given b.i.d.)	2-yr Locoregional control: 68%	Severe mucositis (>6 wks after treatment): 9%; NG tube: 18%; late effects: 7%; 1 carotid rupture (after salvage surg.), 2 transient bone exposures, 1 mucosal ulceration	Ang et al, 1990[3]

CR: complete response; DFS: disease-free survival; MST: median survival time

interpreted by us as evidence of the cumulative effect of incomplete repair in the spinal cord, even with 6-hour interfraction intervals when three fractions per day were given on 12 consecutive days. The study of Svoboda[90] of inoperable breast cancer with ultra-accelerated treatment was also characterized by increased late effects as a function of total dose and fraction size.

Three studies—one head and neck,[44] one inflammatory breast,[6] and one lung[111]—have used accelerated treatment regimens of approximately 4 weeks' duration. In the inflammatory breast study, local tumor control rates were significantly improved over prior experience with the protracted Baclesse technique, without any undue acute toxicity. In the lung study, however, there is indication that accelerated fractionation consisting of 180 to 200 cGy, twice daily to a total dose of 6600 cGy in 4 weeks or less, exceeds the tolerance of the esophagus: All patients developed severe acute esophagitis, and secondary severe complications occurred in 25% of patients.

The last two studies in this section involve the treatment of isolated brain metastases of malignant melanoma.[16,17] The patients received either twice-daily fractions of 300 to 375 cGy to total doses of 3000 cGy to 3750 cGy in 1 week or 190 cGy to 240 cGy per fraction to total doses of 3750 cGy to 4800 cGy in 2 weeks. The median survival time of the patients treated in 1 week was significantly improved, although whether this is a result of the time factor or the size of dose per fraction is unclear. With both regimens, the incidence of acute edema and late brain atrophy was small with the *caveat* that survival times were short.

TYPE B: SPLIT-COURSE ACCELERATED FRACTIONATION SCHEDULES. In a variety of head and neck sites, Wang and co-workers[112] have reported improved locoregional control rates compared with historic controls with accelerated split-course treatment. The regimen that Wang characterizes as b.i.d. consists of 160 cGy fractional doses given twice daily with a minimum 4-hour interfraction interval to total doses of 6720 cGy to 7200 cGy in 6.5 to 7 weeks in a split course (Fig. 3-3). In a series of 321 patients, Wang and colleagues[112] reported an overall improvement in 3-year locoregional control from 46% to 68%. Although late morbidity is poorly documented in either series, it was said to be comparable, whereas acute reactions were more severe, as expected. The EORTC conducted a randomized trial with accelerated split-course radiation for treatment of malignant gliomas.[50,51] In both arms of the trial, a tumor dose of 6000 cGy in 30 fractions was delivered in either 6 weeks with conventional fractionation or 4 weeks, using an accelerated split-course regimen. No difference in median survival time or incidence of late brain necrosis was observed.

TYPE C: CONCOMITANT BOOST. Results of the concomitant boost schedule developed at UTMDACC (see Fig. 3-3) were recently reported by Ang and co-workers[3] in a series of 79 patients, most of whom had moderately advanced oropharyngeal primary lesions. An overall 2-year locoregional control rate of 68% was realized. The study was designed to test the optimum scheduling of the concomitant boost, either at the beginning or the end, or at evenly distributed intervals throughout the basic course of treatment. The best results were obtained when the concomitant boost was given during the last 2 to 2.5 weeks of the basic treatment course; in this subset of patients the 2-year locoregional control rate was 78%. Severe acute reactions were increased compared with conventional fractionation, but no increase in late treatment complications has been observed.

Quasi-accelerated Fractionation

Two trials have been conducted in which segments of accelerated fractionation have been interrupted by treatment breaks so that no reduction in overall treatment time was achieved (Table 3-7). The first of these was a prospectively randomized trial in head and neck cancer in which a quasi-accelerated regimen consisting of 160 cGy 3 times daily in a split-course delivering 6720 cGy to 7200 cGy over 6 to 7 weeks was compared with standard fractionation.[107] Locoregional control rates and 3-year survival rates were identical in both arms of the study. However, an increased incidence of late effects occurred with the quasi-accelerated regimen, which may be attributable to the short minimum interfraction interval of 3 hours specified in this protocol.

The other study in prostate cancer employed fractional doses of 200 cGy given 3 times daily with a 4-hour interfraction interval to a total dose of 6000 cGy in 6 weeks with one or two treatment interruptions.[109] This regimen produced an unexpectly high incidence of severe late complications, again possibly attributable to incomplete repair between dose fractions.

CONCLUSIONS

Several important conclusions can be drawn from the results of clinical trials reported to date with altered fractionation schedules:

1. Pilot studies using both hyperfractionation and accelerated fractionation suggest that a therapeutic gain is possible with these strategies. However, evidence of improvement in the therapeutic ratio from prospective randomized trials is limited to hyperfractionation for head and neck cancer.
2. As predicted radiobiologically, both hyperfractionation and accelerated fractionation produce more severe acute reactions than does conventional treatment. In the case of type A accelerated fractionation regimens, acute normal tissue reactions (and their sequelae) are the major limitation to total dose.

TABLE 3–7
Clinical Studies Using Quasiaccelerated Fractionation

TUMOR SITE	NO. OF PATIENTS	DOSE/FX (cGy)	FX/DAY (INTERVAL IN H)	TOTAL DOSE (cGy)	OVERALL TIME (WK)	TUMOR RESPONSE	COMPLICATIONS	AUTHOR
Head and neck Various sites (randomized)	149	160	3 (≥3)	6720–7200	6–7 (4-wk rest)	3-yr Locoregional control: 35%; 3-yr survival: 31% (for both arms)	Severe mucositis—4 patients did not complete treatment; late effects: 20% vs 11% (ulceration, trismus, dysphagia)	Van den Bogaert et al, 1986[107]
	159	170–200	1	7000–7500	7–8			
Prostate Stage B and C	91	200	3 (4)	6000	6 (1 break of 3–4 wk or 2 breaks of 17 days)	Not stated	Severe complications (incontinence, stenosis, etc.): 19%	Vanuytsel et al, 1986[109]

3. Ultra-accelerated treatment with daily doses of 480 cGy or more have been associated with increased treatment-related deaths, sometimes associated with massive tumor hemorrhage.
4. As predicted radiobiologically, the results of accelerated regimens of type B or type C appear overall to be superior to those of type A. Prospective randomized studies comparing these strategies with best conventional fractionation are urgently needed.
5. Altered fractionation regimens may be associated with unexpected late normal tissue sequelae. The risk is related to the size of dose per fraction, the number of fractions delivered per day, and the interfraction interval. The larger the dose per fraction, the greater the number of fractions per day; the shorter the interfraction interval, the greater is the cumulative effect of incomplete repair in reducing the tolerance of late-responding normal tissues.

ACKNOWLEDGMENTS

Supported in part by Grants CA06294, CA29026, and CA16627 awarded by the National Cancer Institute, Department of Health and Human Services, USA.

REFERENCES

1. Andrews JR: Dose-time relationships in cancer radiotherapy: A clinical radiobiology study of extremes of dose and time. Am J Roentgenol 93:56–74, 1965
2. Ang KK, Landuyt W, Xu FX, et al: The effect of small radiation doses per fraction on mouse lip mucosa assessed using the concept of partial tolerance. Radiother Oncol 8:79–86, 1987
3. Ang KK, Peters LJ, Weber RS, et al: Concomitant boost radiotherapy schedules in the treatment of carcinoma of the oropharynx and nasopharynx. Int J Radiat Oncol Biol Phys 19:1339–1345, 1991
4. Ang KK, Thames HD, van der Kogel AJ, et al: Is the rate of repair of radiation-induced sublethal damage in a spinal cord dependent on the size of dose per fraction? Int J Radiat Oncol Biol Phys 13:557–562, 1987
5. Ang K, Xu FX, Landuyt W, et al: The kinetics and capacity of repair of sublethal damage in mouse lip mucosa during fractionated irradiations. Int J Radiat Oncol Biol Phys 11:1977–1985, 1985
6. Barker JL, Montague ED, Peters LJ: Clinical experience with irradiation of inflammatory carcinoma of the breast with and without elective chemotherapy. Cancer 45:625–629, 1980
7. Begg AC, Moonen L, Hofland I, et al: Human tumour cell kinetics using a monoclonal antibody against iododeoxyuridine: Intratumour sampling variations. Radiother Oncol 11:337–347, 1988
8. Bennett MR: The treatment of stage III squamous carcinoma of the cervix in air and hyperbaric oxygen. Br J Radiol 51:68, 1978
9. Bentzen SM, Juul-Christensen J, Overgaard J, et al: Some methodological problems in estimating radiobiological parameters from clinical data: Alpha/beta ratios and electron RBE for cutaneous reactions in patients treated with post-mastectomy radiotherapy. Acta Oncol 27:105–116, 1988
10. Bentzen SM, Overgaard M, Thames HD: Fractionation sensitivity of a functional endpoint: Impaired shoulder movement after post-mastectomy radiotherapy. Int J Radiat Oncol Biol Phys 17:531–537, 1989
11. Bentzen SM, Overgaard J, Thames HD, et al: Clinical radiobiology of malignant melanoma. Radiother Oncol 16:169–182, 1989
12. Bentzen SM, Thames HD, Overgaard M: Latent-time estimation for late cutaneous and subcutaneous radiation reactions in a single follow-up clinical study. Radiother Oncol 15:267–274, 1989
13. Budhina M, Skrk J, Smid L, et al: Tumor cell repopulation in the rest interval of split-course radiation treatment. Strahlentherapie 156:402, 1980
14. Byhardt RW, Greenberg M, Cox JD: Local control of squamous carcinoma of oral cavity and oropharynx with 3 vs 5 treatment fractions per week. Int J Radiat Oncol Biol Phys 2:415–420, 1977
15. Caldwell WL: Time-dose factors in fatal post-irradiation nephritis. In Alper T (ed): Cell Survival After Low Doses of Radiation, pp 328–332, Bristol, J Wright, 1975
16. Choi KN, Withers HR, Rotman M: Intracranial metastases from melanomas: clinical features and treatment by accelerated fractionation. Cancer 56:1–9, 1985
17. Choi KN, Withers HR, Rotman M: Metastatic melanoma in brain: Rapid treatment or large dose fractions. Cancer 56:10–15, 1985
18. Cohen L: Clinical radiation dosage. I. Br J Radiol 22:160–163, 1949
19. Cohen L: Clinical radiation dosage. II. Br J Radiol 22:706–713, 1949
20. Cohen L, Kerrich JE: Estimation of biological dosage factors in clinical radiotherapy. Br J Cancer 5:180–193, 1951
21. Cox JD: Presidential Address: Fractionation: a paradigm for clinical research in radiation oncology. Int J Radiat Oncol Biol Phys 13:1271–1281, 1987
22. Cox JD, Azarnia N, Byhardt RW, et al: Hyperfractionated radiation therapy (1.2 Gy b.i.d.) with 69.6 Gy total dose increases survival in favorable patients with stage III non-small cell carcinoma of the lung: report of RTOG 83–11. J Clin Oncol 8:1543–1545, 1990
23. Cox JD, Byhardt RW, Komaki R, et al: Reduced fractionation and the potential of hypoxic cell sensitizers in irradiation of malignant epithelial tumors. Int J Radiat Oncol Biol Phys 6:37–40, 1980
24. Cox JD, Guse C, Asbell S, et al: Tolerance of pelvic normal tissues to hyperfractionated radiation therapy: Results of Protocol 83-08 of the Radiation Therapy Oncology Group. Int J Radiat Oncol Biol Phys 15:1331–1336, 1988
25. Cox JD, Pajak T, Marcial VA, et al: Dose-response for local control with hyperfractionated radiation therapy in advanced carcinomas of the upper aerodigestive tracts: Preliminary report of the Radiation Therapy Oncology Group Protocol 83-13. Int J Radiat Oncol Biol Phys 18:515–521, 1990
26. Datta NR, Choudhry AD, Gupta S, et al: Twice a day versus once a day radiation therapy in head and neck cancer. Int J Radiat Oncol Biol Phys, in press
27. Dische S, Martin WMC, Anderson P: Radiation myelopathy in patients treated for carcinoma of the bronchus using a six fraction regime of radiotherapy. Br J Radiol 54:29–35, 1981
28. Dische S, Saunders MI: Continuous hyperfractionated, accelerated radiotherapy (CHART): an interim report upon late morbidity. Radiother Oncol 16:65–72, 1989
29. Douglas BG, Fowler JF: The effect of multiple small doses of x-rays on skin reactions in the mouse and a basic interpretation. Radiat Res 66:401–421, 1976
30. Douglas B, Worth A: Superfractionation in glioblastoma multiforme: results of a phase II study. Int J Radiat Oncol Biol Phys 8:1787–1794, 1982
31. Down JD, Easton DF, Steel GG: Repair in mouse lung during low dose-rate irradiation. Radiother Oncol 6:29–42, 1986
32. Dutreix J, Wambersie A, Bounik C: Cellular recovery in human skin reactions: applications to dose fraction number-overall time relationship in radiotherapy. Eur J Cancer 9:159–167, 1973
33. Edsmyr F, Andersson L, Esposti P, et al: Irradiation therapy with multiple small fractions per day in urinary bladder cancer. Radiother Oncol 4:197–203, 1985
34. Edwards MSB, Wara WM, Urtasun RC, et al: Hyperfractionated radiation therapy for brain-stem glioma: A phase I–II trial. J. Neurosurg 70:691–700, 1989
35. El Badawi SA, Goepfert H, Fletcher GH, et al: Squamous cell carcinoma of the pyriform sinus. Laryngoscope 92:357–364, 1982

36. Ellis F: Nominal standard dose and the ret. Br J Radiol 44:101–108, 1971
37. Field SB, Hornsey S, Kutsutani Y: Effects of fractionated irradiation on mouse lung and a phenomenon of slow repair. Br J Radiol 49:700–707, 1976
38. Fletcher GH, Barkley HT, Shukovsky LJ: Present status of the time factor in clinical radiotherapy. II. The nominal standard dose formula. J Radiol 55:745–751, 1974
39. Fowler JF: The linear-quadratic formula and progress in fractionated radiotherapy. Br J Radiol 62:679–694, 1989
40. Fowler JF, Denekamp J, Delapeyre C, et al: Skin reactions in mice after multifraction x-irradiation. Int J Radiat Biol 25:213, 1974
41. Fowler JF, Stern BE: Dose-time relationships in radiotherapy and the validity of cell survival curve models. Br J Radiol 36:163–173, 1963
42. Fowler JF, Whitred CA, Joiner MC: Repair kinetics in mouse lung: a fast component at 1.1 Gy per fraction. Int J Radiat Biol 56:335–353, 1989
43. Freeman CR, Krischer J, Sanford RA, et al: Hyperfractionated radiotherapy in brain stem tumors: Results of a Pediatric Oncology Group study. Int J Radiat Oncol Biol Phys 15:311–318, 1988
44. Gray AJ: Treatment of advanced head and neck cancer with accelerated fractionation. Int J Radiat Oncol Biol Phys 12:9–12, 1986
45. Handa K, Edoliya TN, Pandey RK, et al: A radiotherapeutic clinical trial of twice per week vs five times per week in oral cancer. Stralentherapie 156:626–631, 1980
46. Harrison D, Crennan E, Cruickshank D, et al: Hypofractionation reduces the therapeutic ratio in early glottic carcinoma. Int J Radiat Oncol Biol Phys 15:365–372, 1988
47. Henk JM, James KW: Comparative trials of large and small fractions in the radiotherapy of head and neck cancer. Clin Radiol 29:611–616, 1978
48. Henkleman RM, Lam GKY, Kornelsen RO, et al: Explanation of dose-rate and split-dose effects in mouse foot reaction using the same time factor. Radiat Res 84:276–289, 1980
49. Horiot JC, Fletcher GH, Ballantyne AJ, et al: Analysis of failures in early vocal cord cancer. Radiology 103:663–665, 1972
50. Horiot JC, Le Fur R, Nguygen T, et al: Hyperfractionation versus conventional fractionation in curative radiotherapy of oropharynx carcinoma: Updated results of a randomized EORTC trial. In Abstracts of the Proceedings of the 17th International Congress of Radiology, Paris, July 1–8, 1989, p. 232 (#1067)
51. Horiot J, van den Bogaert W, Ang KK, et al: European Organization for Research on Treatment of Cancer trials using radiotherapy with multiple fractions per day. A 1978–1987 survey. In Vaeth J, Meyer J (eds): Time, Dose, and Fractionation in the Radiation Therapy of Cancer. Front Radiat Ther Onco, vol 22, pp 149–161, Basel, S Karger, 1988
52. Hornsey S, Kutsutani Y, Field SB: Damage to mouse lung with fractionated neutrons and x-rays. Radiology 116:171–176, 1975
53. Hornsey S, Morris CC, Myers R, et al: Relative biological effectiveness for damage to the central nervous system by neutrons. Int J Radiat Oncol Biol Phys 7:185–189, 1981
54. Huczkowski J, Trott KR: Jejunal crypt stem cell survival after fractionated τ-irradiation performed at different dose rates. Int J Radiat Biol 51:131–137, 1987
55. Joiner MC, Denekamp J, Maughan RL: The use of "top-up" experiments to investigate the effect of very small doses per fraction in mouse skin. Int J Radiat Biol 49:565–580, 1986
56. Kellerer AM, Rossi HH: The theory of dual radiation action. Curr Topics Radiat Res 8:85–158, 1972
57. Knee R, Fields RS, Peters LJ: Concomitant boost radiotherapy for advanced squamous cell carcinoma of the head and neck. Radiother Oncol 4:1–7, 1985
58. Kummermehr J, Trott K-R: Rate of repopulation in a slow and fast growing mouse tumour. In Karcher KH, Kognelik D (eds): Progress in Radio-Oncology II, pp 299–308. New York, Raven Press, 1982
59. Lamb D, Spry N, Gray A, et al: Accelerated fractionation radiotherapy for advanced head and neck cancer. Radiother Oncol 18:107–116, 1990
60. Maciejewski B, Taylor JMG, Withers, HR: Alpha/beta value and the importance of size of dose per fraction for late complications in the supraglottic larynx. Radiother Oncol 7:323–326, 1986
61. Maciejewski B, Withers HR, Taylor JMG, et al: Dose fractionation and regeneration in radiotherapy for cancer of the oral cavity and oropharynx: Tumor dose-response and repopulation. Int J Radiat Oncol Biol Phys 16:831–843, 1989
62. Marcial V, Pajak T, Chang C, et al: Hyperfractionated photon radiation therapy in the treatment of advanced squamous cell carcinoma of the oral cavity, pharynx, larynx, and sinuses, using radiation therapy as the only planned modality: Preliminary report by the Radiation Therapy Oncology Group (RTOG). Int J Radiat Oncol Biol Phys 13:41–47, 1987
63. Meoz R, Fletcher GH, Peters LJ, et al: Twice-daily fractionation schemes for advanced head and neck cancer. Int J Radiat Oncol Biol Phys 10:831–836, 1984
64. Million RR, Zimmerman RC: Evaluation of University of Florida split-course technique for various head and neck squamous cell carcinomas. Cancer 35:1533–1536, 1975
65. Moulder JE, Fischer JJ: Radiation reaction of rat skin: The role of the number of fractions and the overall treatment time. Cancer 37:2762–2767, 1976
66. Nguyen T, Demange L, Froissart D, et al: Rapid hyperfractionated radiotherapy: Clinical results in 178 advanced squamous cell carcinomas of the head and neck. Cancer 56:16–19, 1985
67. Norin T, Onyango J: Radiotherapy in Burkitt's lymphoma: Conventional or superfractionated regime—early results. Int J Radiat Oncol Biol Phys 2:399–406, 1977
68. Notter G, Turesson I: Multiple small fractions per day versus conventional fractionation: Comparison of normal tissue reactions and effect on breast carcinoma. Radiother Oncol 1:299–308, 1984
69. Overgaard J, Hansen-Hjelm M, Johansen LV, Andersen AP; Comparison of conventional and split-course radiotherapy as primary treatment in carcinoma of the larynx. Acta Oncol 27:147–152, 1988
70. Packer R, Littman P, Sposto R, et al: Results of a pilot study of hyperfractionated radiation therapy for children with brain stem gliomas. Int J Radiat Oncol Biol Phys 13:1647–1651, 1987
71. Palcic B, Skarsgard LD: Reduced oxygen enhancement ratio at low doses of ionizing radiation. Radiat Res 100:328–339, 1984
72. Parkins CS, Fowler JF: Repair in mouse lung of multifraction x-rays and neutrons: Extension to 40 fractions. Br J Radiol 58:1097–1103, 1985
73. Parsons J, Mendenhall W, Cassisi N, et al: Hyperfractionation for head and neck cancer. Int J Radiat Oncol Biol Phys 14:649–658, 1988
74. Peracchia G, Salti C: Radiotherapy with thrice-a-day fractionation in a short overall time: Clinical experiences. Int J Radiat Oncol Biol Phys 7:99–104, 1981
75. Peters LJ, Ang KK, Thames HD: Accelerated fractionation in the radiation treatment of head and neck cancer: A critical comparison of different strategies. Acta Oncol 27:185–194, 1988
76. Peters LJ, Brock WA, Travis EL: Radiation biology at clinically relevant fractions. In DeVita V, Hellman S, Rosenberg SA (eds): Important Advances in Oncology 1990. Philadelphia, JB Lippincott, 1991
77. Powell S, Cooke J, Parsons C: Radiation induced brachial plexus injury: follow-up of two different fractionation schedules. Radiother Oncol 18:213–220, 1990
78. Rojas A, Joiner MC: The influence of dose per fraction on repair kinetics Radiother Oncol 14:329–336, 1989
79. Rojas A, Joiner M, Ninis J, et al: Rate of repair of radiation injury (kidney). Gray Laboratory Annual Report, 1986, pp 42–43
80. Rojas A, Joiner M, Ninis J, et al: Time scale of repair of radiation injury: dose dependence (skin), p 51. Gray Laboratory Annual Report, 1986

81. Saunders M, Dische S, Fowler J, et al: Radiotherapy with three fractions per day for twelve consecutive days for tumors of the thorax, head and neck. In Vaeth J, Meyer J (eds): Time, Dose and Fractionation in the Radiation Therapy of Cancer. Front Radiat Ther Oncol, vol 22, pp 99–104. Basel, S Karger, 1988
82. Saunders MI, Dische S, Fowler JF, et al: Radiotherapy employing three fractions on each of twelve consecutive days. Acta Oncol 27:163–167, 1988
83. Schenken LL, Hagemann RF: Time/dose relationships in experimental radiation cataractogenesis. Radiology 117:193–198, 1975
84. Scott O: Divergence of opinion over the linear-quadratic model. Br J Radiol 60:1042–1043, 1987
85. Seydel H, Diener-West M, Urtasun R, et al: Radiation Therapy Oncology Group (RTOG): Hyperfractionation in the radiation therapy of unresectable non-oat cell carcinoma of the lung: Preliminary report of a RTOG pilot study. Int J Radiat Oncol Biol Phys 11:1841–1847, 1985
86. Simpson WJ, Platts ME: Fractionation study in the treatment of glioblastoma multiforme. Int J Radiat Oncol Biol Phys 1:639–644, 1976
87. Stell PM, Morrison MD: Radiation necrosis of the larynx. Arch Otolaryngol 98:111–113, 1973
88. Stewart FA, Randhawa VS, Michael BD: Multifraction irradiation of mouse bladders. Radiother Oncol 2:131–140, 1984
89. Strandqvist M: Studien uber die kumulative Wirkung der Rontgenstrahlen bei Fraktionierung. Acta Radiol 55(Suppl): 1, 1944
90. Svoboda V: Accelerated fractionation: The Portsmouth experience 1972–1984. In Proceedings of Varian's Fourth European Clinac Users Meeting, Malta, May 25–26, 1984, pp. 70–75, Zug Switzerland, Varian, 1984
91. Terry NHA, Denekamp J: RBE values and repair characteristics for colo-rectal injury after caesium-137 gamma-ray and neutron irradiation. II. Fractionation up to ten doses. Br J Radiol 57:617–629, 1984
92. Thames H, Ang KK, Stewart F: Does incomplete repair explain the apparent failure of the basic LQ model to predict spinal cord and kidney response to low doses per fraction? Int J Radiat Biol 54:13–19, 1988
93. Thames HD, Bentzen SM, Turesson I, et al: Time-dose factor in radiotherapy: a review of the human data. Radiother Oncol 19:219–235, 1990
94. Thames HD, Hendry JH (eds): Fractionation in Radiotherapy. London, Taylor & Francis, 1987
95. Thames HD, Mason KA, Bentzen SM, et al: Characterization of the repair kinetics of split-dose recovery in mouse jejunal crypt cells. Br J Radiol (BIR Report) 19:37–42, 1989
96. Thames HD, Peters LJ, Ang KK: Time-dose considerations for normal-tissue tolerance. In Vaeth JM (ed): Radiation Effects on Normal Tissues: Clinical Tolerance Levels, Frontiers of Radiation Therapy and Oncology, vol 23, Basel, S Karger, 1989, pp 113–130
97. Thames HD, Suit HD: Tumor radioresponsiveness versus fractionation sensitivity. Int J Radiat Oncol Biol Phys 12:687–691, 1986
98. Thames HD, Withers HR: Test of equal effect per fraction and estimation of initial clonogen number in microcolony assays of survival after fractionated irradiation. Br J Radiol 53:1071–1077, 1980
99. Thames HD, Withers HR, Peters LJ: Tissue repair capacity and repair kinetics deduced from multi-fractionated or continuous irradiation regimens with incomplete repair. Br J Cancer 49 (suppl VI):263–269, 1984
100. Thames H, Withers HR, Peters LJ, et al: Changes in early and late radiation responses with altered dose fractionation: Implications for dose-survival relationships. Int J Radiat Oncol Biol Phys 8:219–226, 1982
101. Travis EL, Peters LJ, McNeill J, et al: Effect of dose-rate on total body irradiation: Lethality and pathologic findings. Radiother Oncol 4:341–351, 1985
102. Travis EL, Thames HD, Watkins TL, et al: The kinetics of repair in mouse lung after fractionated irradiation. Int J Radiat Biol 52:901–919, 1987
103. Trott KR, Maciejewski B, Preuss-Bayer G: Dose-response curve and split-dose recovery in human skin cancer. Radiother Oncol 2:123–130, 1984
104. Tucker SL, Withers HR, Mason KA, et al: A dose-surviving fraction curve for mouse colonic mucosa. Eur J Cancer Clin Oncol 19:433, 1983
105. Turesson I, Notter G: Skin reaction as a biological parameter for control of different dose schedules and gap correction. Acta Radiother 15:162–176, 1976
106. Turesson I, Thames HD: Repair capacity and kinetics of human skin during fractionated radiotherapy: Erythema, desquamation, and telangiectasia after 3 and 5 years' follow-up. Radiother Oncol 15:169–188, 1989
107. van de Bogaert W, van der Schueren E, Horiot J, et al: Early results of the EORTC randomized clinical trial on multiple fractions per day (MFD) and misonidazole in advanced head and neck cancer. Int J Radiat Oncol Biol Phys 12:587–591, 1986
108. van der Kogel AJ: Late effects of radiation on the spinal cord. Ph.D. Thesis, University of Amsterdam, Radiobiological Institute of the Organization for Health Research TNO, Rijswijk, The Netherlands, 1979
109. Vanuytsel L, Ang K, Vandenbussche L, et al: Radiotherapy in multiple fractions per day for prostatic carcinoma: Late complications. Int J Radiat Oncol Bio Phys 12:1589–1595, 1986
110. Vegesna V, Withers HR, Thames, HD, et al: Multifraction radiation response of mouse lung. Int J Radiat Biol 47:413–422, 1985
111. Von Rottkay P: Remission and acute toxicity during accelerated fractionated irradiation of non-small cell bronchial carcinoma. Strahlentherapie 162:300–307, 1986
112. Wang CC, Blitzer PH, Suit H: Twice-a-day radiation therapy for cancer of the head and neck. Cancer 55:2100–2104, 1985
113. Wara WM, Phillips TL, Margolis LW, Smith V: Radiation pneumonitis: a new approach to the derivation of time-dose factors. Cancer 32:547–552, 1973
114. Watson ER, Halnan KE, Dische S, et al: Hyperbaric oxygen and radiotherapy: a Medical Research Council trial in carcinoma of the cervix. Br J Radiol 51:879–887, 1978
115. Wendt CD, Peters LJ, Ang K, et al: Hyperfractionated radiotherapy in the treatment of squamous cell carcinomas of the supraglottic larynx. Int J Radiat Oncol Biol Phys, 17:1057–1062, 1989
116. Williams MV, Denekamp J: Radiation induced renal damage in mice: influence of fraction size. Int J Radiat Oncol Biol Phys 10:885–894, 1984
117. Williams MV, Denekamp J, Fowler JF: A review of α/β values for experimental tumors: Implications for clinical studies of altered fractionation. Int J Radiat Oncol Biol Phys 11:87–96, 1985
118. Withers HR: Isoeffect curves for various proliferative tissues in experimental animals. In Proceedings of Conference on Time-Dose Relationships in Clinical Radiotherapy, pp 30–38. Madison, Wisconsin, Madison Printing and Publishing, 1975
119. Withers HR, Chu AM, Reid BO, et al: Response of mouse jejunum to multifraction radiation. Int J Radiat Oncol Biol Phys 1:41–52, 1975
120. Withers HR, Taylor JMG, Maciejewski B: The hazard of accelerated tumor clonogen repopulation during radiotherapy. Acta Oncol 27:131–146, 1988
121. Withers HR, Thames HD, Flow BL, et al: The relationship of acute and late skin injury in 2 and 5 fraction/week τ-ray therapy. Int J Radiat Oncol Biol Phys 4:595–601, 1978

4

Morphology of Radiation Effects on Normal Tissues

Luis Felipe Fajardo L–G

This chapter describes the pathology of radiation injury in normal mammalian tissues, especially those of humans. The first part is a brief review of the acute lesions (those occurring hours to days after radiation exposure) observed in bone marrow, alimentary epithelia, and germinal cells of the testis. Most acute lesions have been studied in subjects exposed to whole-body, single doses in the median lethal dose (LD_{50}) range.

The second part of the chapter is a more detailed description of the delayed lesions (those usually seen months to years after exposure) that occur, mainly following exposure to x-rays or τ-rays, as used in humans for localized, fractionated clinical radiation therapy. The correlation of dose with type and severity of lesions has been made in several radiation pathology publications[3, 10, 14, 15, 21, 35, 37] and therefore will not be discussed here. It should be emphasized that there are no pathognomonic (morphologic) features of radiation injury. However, although not specific individually, combined radiation lesions are characteristic enough to be recognized.

ACUTE LESIONS

Alterations can be observed morphologically in many tissues within minutes after radiation exposure if the appropriate doses and detecting tools are used in the appropriate cells. For instance, cytoplasmic alterations of lymphocytes have been observed by electron microscopy 8 to 30 minutes after a single dose of 500 to 3000 R.[27, 36]

Hematopoietic Tissue

The bone marrow has probably been the tissue most extensively studied by radiation biologists, and it is one of the best described by pathologists working on victims of radiation accidents[1, 4, 17] or atomic warfare.[4, 7, 25]

These studies have shown that for most mammals a single, total-body exposure of 250 cGy to 800 cGy results in bone marrow failure with death of 50% of individuals (if untreated) within 60 days. The sequence of alterations is remarkably similar in most species, when the lethal dose for each species is given ($LD_{50/60}$). Such sequence, terminating in death, has been named the "acute radiation bone marrow syndrome."

From human and experimental information, the following changes occur after a single-dose (SD) total-body exposure at the $LD_{50/60}$ level (350 cGy to 1050 cGy for humans, depending on available treatment[7, 30]):

Necrosis (karyopyknosis, lysis) of the precursor cells of the three main hematopoietic lines—erythroblasts, myeloblasts, and megakaryoblasts—starts within 24 hours of exposure. As the early cells are lysed and the less sensitive, mature nucleated cells (*e.g.*, segmented granulocytes) migrate from the marrow, progressive depopulation of nucleated cells occurs, which reaches nadir by 3 to 5 days.

The normally narrow blood sinusoids suffer severe dilatation, which also becomes maximal by 2 to 3 days and results in extensive extravasation of erythrocytes into the compartment previously occupied by the nucleated cells.

Beyond 5 days the cell debris and erythrocytes are removed, and the sinusoids contract progressively. As this occurs, the adipocytes increase in number and by 8 days they occupy a large proportion of the marrow cavity.

In some individuals there is an early, abortive attempt at regeneration of nucleated cells before day 8. Beyond 8 days usually a sustained, progressive increase in cellularity occurs that is parallel with a decrease in adipocytes. By 30 days the marrow often has normal cellularity or may be hypercellular, even in individuals who will die between 30 and 60 days. Often atypical cells (especially myelocytes) are seen and, as expected, hemosiderin-laden macrophages are numerous.

The above alterations, of course, are mirrored in the blood:[1] Following an early neutrophilia and thrombocytosis, lasting for hours, a rapidly progressive neutropenia and thrombocytopenia occur, which reach nadir (<500 neutrophils/mm^3) by day 30. Lymphocytes drop rapidly and stay very low for several weeks. Red cells, as expected, decrease at a low rate; therefore by 30 days the patient may have a hemoglobin level of 8 g/dl.[1] Thus the maximum pancytopenia occurs about 3 weeks later than the maximum bone marrow depletion, and victims of total-body

Supported in part by Veterans Administration Research Funds (MRIS 2735-01).

irradiation can die of pancytopenia while having a normocellular marrow.[25]

The sequence of alterations that occurs during and after fractionated, therapeutic irradiation to a localized area of the marrow is similar to the previously mentioned sequence, but the changes occur over a much longer time span.[10,37] For instance, the nadir of cell depletion takes place at ~ 35 days instead of 3 to 5 days.[37] The delayed lesion following doses of more than 5000 cGy is unique. Instead of the fibrosis observed in most other organs, adipose tissue replaces the permanently aplastic areas[10,37] (see Fig. 4-10 and further discussion at end of chapter).

Alimentary Tract Epithelia

All segments of the alimentary tube suffer epithelial damage following total-body irradiation with single doses of 1000 cGy or above.[4,10,25,30,35,40] This damage, however, is not uniform or consistently present in each segment, except in the small intestinal (enteric) epithelium, which appears to be the most radiosensitive; it has the shortest cell cycling time of all epithelia in the adult.

Following is a sequential description of the changes that occur in the villi and crypts of the small intestine, as observed in humans and some other mammals.[4,10,25,35]

Within a few hours after exposure mitotic activity ceases in the proliferative portion of the crypts (middle third). Cell necrosis, characterized by pyknosis, karyorrhexis, and karyolysis, occurs progressively, reaching maximum by 6 to 8 hours, at which time the necrotic debris accumulates in the lumen.

The remaining cells undergo a transient attempt to divide, which results in numerous mitoses (above preirradiation level), often atypical. This proliferative burst usually occurs between 8 and 24 hours. Large, bizarre epithelial cells are often produced at this time.

Beyond 24 hours the proliferation ceases, and progressive cell loss occurs without renewal, which eventually results in denudation of the villi. To compensate this net cell loss, several mechanisms are activated[40]: shortening of the villus; contraction of the crypt; flattening of the (often large) residual cells to cover a larger area of the basal lamina; longer retention of villus cells, which become senescent while still attached to the lower part of the villus; and activation of all remaining stem cells to proliferate.

These mechanisms can compensate some of the injury; therefore in the intestine receiving 1000 cGy or less, there is progressive, rapid recovery of the enteric epithelium beyond 3 days. However, the intestine receiving 1500 cGy or more continues to lose cells, exposing more and more surface of the basal lamina over the next few days. By 7 to 10 days death occurs from electrolyte, water, and protein loss and from infection (acute intestinal radiation syndrome), provided that the bone marrow has also been irradiated.

If the individual survives, the enteric mucosa may be permanently altered, with short, blunt villi, which result in malabsorption or a protein-losing enteropathy. This enteropathy also may occur focally following fractionated therapeutic irradiation of the abdomen, especially in children.[9,38]

Gonads

Both ovaries and testes have highly radiosensitive cells: oogonia (in the embryo) and granulosa cells of the ovary, and spermatogonia and spermatocytes of the testis. Whereas the lesions of the adult ovary are best demonstrated months to years after exposure (delayed lesions), the testis shows characteristic acute *and* delayed lesions.[40] The following description refers only to the testicular parenchyma.

In humans, after a single dose of 1200 R to one testis,[8] the following sequence of lesions has occurred[8]: necrosis of germinal cells (especially spermatogonia B, spermatocytes) began at 3.5 hours and reached a peak at 5 hours. The necrotic debris of the germinal cells persisted for 10 days. Aside from this debris, syncytial masses of pyknotic nuclei have appeared in the lumina of seminiferous tubules, remaining there for months.[10] (These syncytial formations are a nonspecific response of the tubules to a variety of injurious agents.)

Spermatogonia are swollen, or karyopyknotic, when identifiable. Other changes in germ cells include fragmentation and clumping of chromosomes, absent spindles, arrested or blocked metaphases, dumbbell-shaped anaphases, and polyploid giant cells.[8]

Other studies (summarized in Fajardo[10]) have shown that these changes are not necessarily permanent following lower doses. The sterilizing single dose for humans is not known, but it is probably in the range of 500 cGy to 600 cGy. Curiously enough low dose fractionated irradiation appears to produce a faster decrease in sperm count than comparable single doses.[26]

When permanent damage occurs, all germ cells disappear. Spermatogonia and spermatocytes are destroyed *in situ,* whereas spermatids and spermatozoa migrate out. After high (several thousand cGy) doses Sertoli's cells also eventually disappear. Finally, the tubules become fibrous scars within a thickened lamina propria. The stromal Leydig's cells remain unaltered even after high doses.

Because the duration of spermatogenesis is 64 days in humans[10] and because spermatozoa are not destroyed by sterilizing doses, oligospermia does not appear for several weeks.[10] Conversely, regeneration of spermatogonia usually does not begin until 2 to 8 weeks after the injury.[35] Therefore, even when the radiation dose is not large enough to cause permanent sterility, a period of temporary oligospermia (or azoospermia) of weeks to months may intervene before recovery.[35]

DELAYED LESIONS

Unlike the conventional descriptions of radiation pathology, which are structured according to organ systems,[3,10,25,35,39,40] this chapter is organized according to the repetitive morphologic patterns observed in multiple tissues.[12] The delayed radiation-induced lesions discussed are grouped into those that occur in *epithelia* and *parenchyma* of various organs, *stroma,* and *blood vessels*[12] (Table 4-1). Because not all lesions fit into such general patterns, the exceptions are then described or mentioned separately as characteristic lesions of some organs (Table 4-2).

Epithelial and Parenchymal Lesions

Atrophy is one of the most consistent delayed effects of therapeutic irradiation. It occurs in all lining epithelia—skin, alimentary, respiratory, and urinary tracts—as well as in all glands (*e.g.,* salivary, pancreatic, mammary, cutaneous). Atrophy also affects parenchymatous tissues such as kidney, lung, and gonads.

It is clear, however, that some epithelia or parenchyma

TABLE 4–1
Patterns of Delayed Lesions In Irradiated Human Tissues

EPITHELIAL AND PARENCHYMAL

Atrophy, necrosis, ulceration, metaplasia, atypia, dysplasia, neoplasia

STROMAL

Fibrosis, atypical fibroblasts, fibrinous exudate, necrosis; lack or paucity of cellular inflammatory exudate

VASCULAR

Capillaries and sinusoids: endothelial cell damage, rupture of wall, thrombosis

Small- and medium-sized arteries: fibrinoid necrosis; medial fibrosis; myointimal proliferation, with or without lipophages; thrombosis, acute, segmental vasculitis (localized); focal scars

Large arteries: myointimal proliferation, atheromatosis, thrombosis, rupture

Small veins: intimal proliferation and fibrosis; veno-occlusive disease (liver)

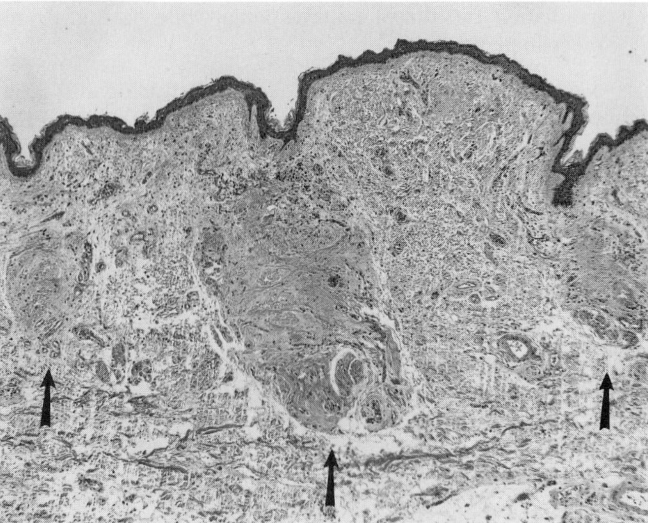

FIGURE 4–1. Atrophy and fibrosis of skin 3 months after a dose of 5000 cGy in 35 days for carcinoma of the larynx. The epidermis is thin and wrinkled but not ulcerated. There is moderate diffuse fibrosis of the dermis. The hair follicles and sebaceous glands (pilosebaceous units) are totally atrophic and replaced by bulbous masses of collagen "hanging" from the epidermis (*arrows*) (H & E, × 50)

suffer more often or more severely than others. Qualitatively such tissues may be separated into three groups.

1. Severe atrophy is seen in epidermis, sebaceous glands (perhaps the most affected in the skin), alimentary epithelium (especially intestine), urothelium, salivary glands, and germinal cells of the testis (Figs. 4-1 to 4-4).
2. Moderate atrophy occurs in the epithelia of the upper respiratory and alimentary tracts, lung, mammary glands, prostate, and kidney.
3. Atrophy is less common or less severe in sweat glands, liver, and endocrine glands. The latter are rarely affected by external electromagnetic radiation, but are seriously altered by internally administered radionuclides (thyroid) or by heavy particle beams (pituitary).

Necrosis occurs in many epithelial and a few parenchymal cells during the *acute* phase of radiation injury, but with the exception of the skin and mucosas, such early lesions are seldom seen in humans. Delayed necrosis generally results from ischemia. It causes interruption of the lining epithelia (ulcers) of variable depth and chronicity, the skin, upper alimentary and respiratory tracts, intestine, urinary tract, and genitalia (see Fig. 4-3). One of the most characteristic sites for delayed necrosis is the central nervous system (CNS), particularly the white matter of the cerebral hemispheres or of the spinal cord.[5]

Radionecrosis of the CNS is of the coagulative type: a granular, acidophilic material replaces the normal neuropil; lipophages are often present in some areas; demyelination is also present in such areas, but it is focal.

TABLE 4–2
Characteristic Organ and Tissue Lesions

Congenital malformations	Acute sialadenitis
Growth delay	Colitis cystica profunda
Bone deformity	Rapid hemopoietic and lymphopoietic depletion
Acute radiation pneumonitis	Delayed bone marrow hypoplasia or aplasia
Veno-occlusive liver disease	Cataract

Metaplasia (the replacement of one mature tissue by another) is not a common radiation effect. In a few sites, however, it occurs regularly; the replacement of the normal epithelium of the glands and ducts of the prostate by squamous epithelium is an example.

Atypia of epithelial cells is not only a striking, usually delayed alteration, but also a source of confusion and error. It may affect nucleus or cytoplasm or both. Most often there is enlargement of both nucleus and cytoplasm of individual cells. The nuclei may appear hyperchromatic but the chromatin is frequently "smudged" (not distinct). Nucleoli are often promi-

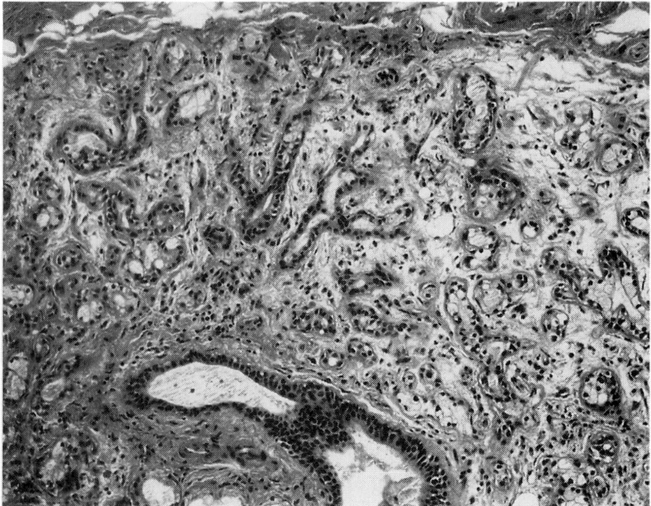

FIGURE 4–2. Atrophy is exemplified in this section of a minor salivary gland from a middle-aged male, irradiated 8 years earlier for carcinoma of the floor of the mouth. Instead of the normally crowded parenchyma containing mainly secretory acini and some ducts, the gland now is almost totally devoid of acini. The ducts are now easily seen and widely separated from each other by loose stroma containing few inflammatory cells. The ducts are dilated, particularly the main duct in the lower part of the picture (H & E, × 125).

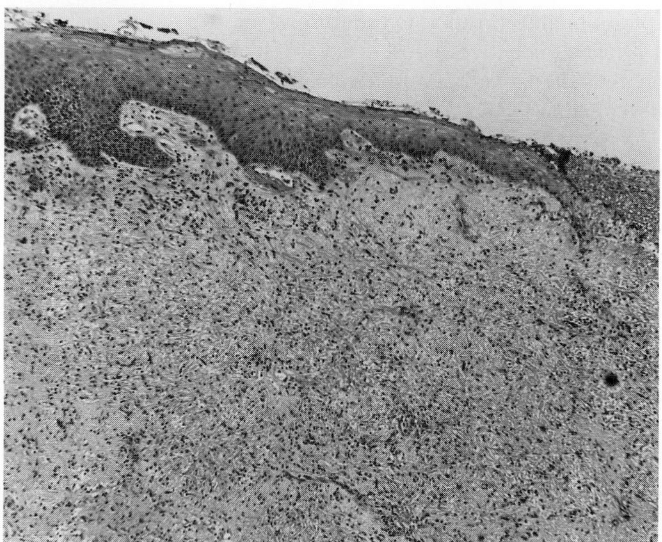

FIGURE 4–3. Fibrosis, atrophy, and ulceration are illustrated in this section of oral mucosa, irradiated (dose unknown) 6 years earlier for an adjacent neoplasm. The epithelium appears relatively normal in the left half, atrophic in the next one fourth, and ulcerated in the right one fourth; at that point it is replaced by a mass of fibrin and red cells. The normal submucosa is replaced by dense fibrous tissue; no adipose tissue is seen. Because of the ulceration more inflammatory cells are seen in the stroma than one sees ordinarily in delayed radiation injury (H & E, × 57).

nent. Generally only some of the cells of a given structure (duct, gland, epithelial surface) show atypia, and architecturally there is no suggestion of neoplasia.

Atypia has been observed in epidermis, squamous mucosas (mouth, larynx, vagina, cervix, and others), bronchi and pulmonary alveoli, stomach, minor salivary glands, endometrium, urothelium, mammary glands, and prostate. In the last three sites this atypia has caused considerable diagnostic difficulty even for experienced pathologists.

Dysplasia induced by radiation in epithelia is not uncommon in epidermis and squamous mucosas, and is rare in nonsquamous epithelia. It is a late lesion (usually several months to years after exposure) characterized by nuclear atypia, with hyperchromatism, lack of polarity (directional, organized maturation), involvement of large clones of cells, and architectural alterations. Dysplasia implies genetic damage, and abnormal ploidy can be documented. It should be differentiated from the benign atypia described earlier and should be considered premalignant, although not all cases necessarily evolve into neoplasms. In the skin and squamous mucosas, neoplasia may follow dysplasia, years after exposure.

Neoplasia resulting from radiation is well documented, yet greatly exaggerated, to the point that any tumor arising in an irradiated area is viewed by many as radiation-induced. In a recent review of radiation oncogenesis,[11] I stated the criteria necessary to accept a given neoplasm as radiation-induced. For a list of the neoplasms that, as of early 1986, had met the necessary criteria, the reader is referred to that publication.[11]

From the morphologic point of view, radiation-induced neoplasms (RIN) are no different from the corresponding neoplasms not induced by radiation. It is interesting, nevertheless, that within certain organs, radiation tends to induce only certain types of tumors, not just any type. For example, in the thyroid almost all malignant RIN are papillary carcinomas. In the lung most RIN are small cell (oat cell) carcinomas. The RIN arising in the bone marrow are usually granulocytic leukemias or, less often, multiple myeloma; there is no evidence that chronic lymphatic leukemia has ever been induced by radiation in humans.

Hypermaturation and the converse, *dedifferentiation*, of cells as the result of irradiation have been observed in carcinomas and could possibly occur in nonneoplastic epithelia, but we have not observed the latter.

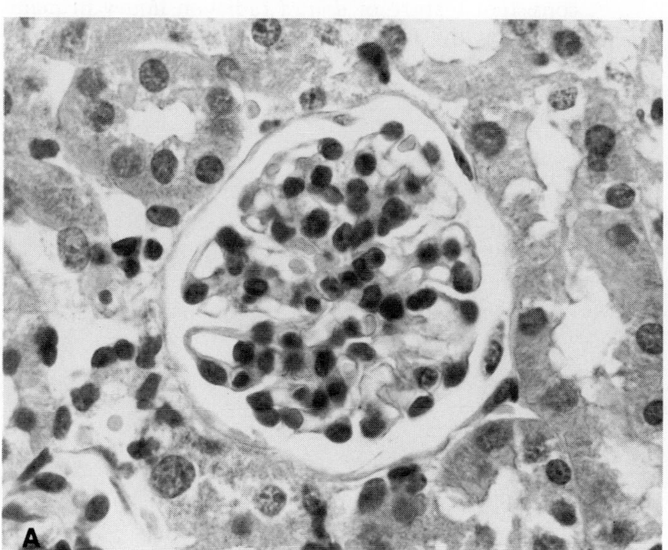

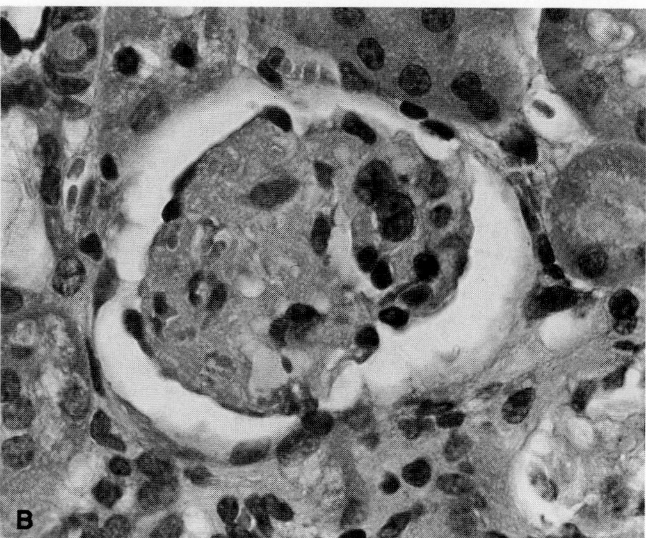

FIGURE 4–4. Radiation nephropathy. (**A**) A section of normal murine kidney, with a glomerulus in the center, surrounded by tubules (mainly proximal convoluted). Notice the regular distribution of small dense nuclei in the glomerular tuft and the multiple, well-defined capillary lumina. (**B**) Section of a kidney 9 months after 4500 cGy in 10 fractions given to the kidneys *in situ*. Notice increase in the density of the glomerular tuft, which no longer has capillary lumina. Glomerular nuclei are irregularly distributed, and some are also enlarged. Some of the tubules (upper left, lower right) are atrophic. Radiation nephropathy in humans and other mammals affects primarily glomeruli and tubules and eventually results in atrophy with fibrosis. Arteries are compromised secondarily, probably as the result of hypertension (H & E, × 650).

Stromal Lesions

Of all the lesions described here, stromal lesions are best recognized by pathologists as radiation-induced or radiation-associated. The most typical combinations of the features described below here occur in the submucosa and the deep soft tissues of the mouth, pharynx, larynx, and genitalia. Typical stromal lesions can be seen also in the skin and lower urinary tract. Some of the features occur in the lower alimentary tube. Although fibrosis is a characteristic feature of delayed radiation injury in parenchymatous organs (*e.g.*, lung, kidney), the other stromal features, such as typical fibroblasts, are rarely observed in such organs.

Fibrosis is one of the most common delayed radiation-associated manifestations (see Figs. 4-1 and 4-3). It occurs in almost all tissues and organs, and it is time- and dose-dependent, but its extent and severity vary from site to site. The typical radiation-induced fibrosis is nonhomogeneous. Some areas have very dense, acellular collagen, whereas areas next to them have only a few fibrous bands. This alteration is easiest to appreciate in adipose tissue, skeletal or cardiac muscle, or parenchymatous organs.

It is more practical to list the sites in which fibrosis does not occur, or is rare, than to list the many tissues in which it is often found. Fibrosis does not occur in the lens or in the central nervous system (gliosis, the CNS counterpart of fibrosis, does occur, but it is not a predominant feature). In the hematopoietic bone marrow, replacement by adipose tissue is the result of high doses of radiation; fibrosis does not occur unless a neoplasm or an inflammatory lesion had been present prior to the irradiation, in which case the stroma of such lesion persists in the marrow space. Radiation injury to the bone itself may lead, after high doses, to necrosis rather than fibrosis. Delayed hepatic injury shows surprisingly little fibrosis, except in areas that contained tumor before exposure. The same occurs in lymph nodes: when high doses result in lymphocyte depletion, the skeleton of the node remains, with little additional connective tissue, except in the areas that harbored tumor.

Fibrosis is much more than a mark of radiation damage; it is damaging in itself. Crippling or deforming skin retraction; esophageal, intestinal or urinary stenosis with obstruction; myocardial failure; pericardial restrictive disease; and reduction in pulmonary function are some examples of its effects.

A characteristic feature is the presence of *fibrin* in the stroma. Probably it occurs in most irradiated mesenchymal tissues, but it is only detectable by light microscopy in some soft tissues. Fibrinous exudate appears as a delicate network of acidophilic fibrils in the midst of collagen and fibroblasts. It is not seen throughout the entire area of fibrosis, but rather it occurs in widely separate foci. Special stains such as the phosphotungstic acid–hematoxylin or the Fraser–Lendrum techniques facilitate the recognition of fibrin. This finding is valuable in the differential diagnosis of delayed radiation fibrosis, but only in sites that are not ulcerated or have other causes for active inflammatory exudate. Fibrin is a component of inflammatory exudate and is expected to be present wherever there is inflammation.

Fibrinous exudate is found months to many years after exposure and in sequential biopsies of a given site, suggesting either its persistence in the stroma due to decreased fibrinolysis (because of depletion of plasminogen activator) or repeated formation of fibrin, or more likely to both mechanisms.

Atypical fibroblasts (so-called radiation fibroblasts; AF) are very characteristic of delayed radiation injury. These are large, bizarre cells, usually basophilic, with angulated and elongated cytoplasm. Triangular or even star shapes are observed, and a common configuration is reminiscent of a "swallow tail" (Fig. 4-5). The nuclei are almost invariably hyperchromatic—probably polyploid—and "smudged," but mitotic figures are almost never seen.

Atypical fibroblasts are found in delayed lesions, predominantly of the submucosa of the upper respiratory tract, the entire alimentary tract, and the lower urinary tract and genitalia. They are less common in nonulcerated skin and deep soft tissues. AF are almost never seen in deep organs such as lungs, heart, liver, or brain. Maximow,[28] who recognized them many years ago, observed that AF occurred only in sites subject to inflammation; this is still generally but not absolutely true. We have noted that AF are more common in the presence of infection.[10]

Cells almost identical with AF are seen occasionally in nonirradiated, chronically inflamed tissues, particularly at the base of chronic pressure ulcers (decubitus ulcers).

Necrosis of stromal elements is uncommon in the absence of ulceration, superimposed infection, or tumor. When it occurs, necrosis is not necessarily helpful in the diagnosis, but it may suggest severe ischemia, perhaps as the result of the vascular lesions described separately. Fat necrosis is rare. It has been described in the irradiated breast,[6] and may present as a mass clinically mimicking a recurrent tumor.[6]

Most instances of necrosis in irradiated tissues are associated with radiation-induced ulcers (see Fig. 4-3). The beds of such chronic ulcers have the usual elements: necrotic debris, granulation tissue, fibrosis, and so on. In contrast to the ulcers of other etiologies, cellular (leukocytic) exudate seems to be less prominent, and "fibrinoid" necrosis of small arteries is more common. Aside from bleeding, the inflammatory events that occur in the beds of these ulcers contribute eventually to fibrosis, deformities, stenosis, and so forth.

Vascular lesions are prominent morphologically and are very important in the pathogenesis of delayed radiation injury. Although these lesions could be considered also as stromal, the vascular changes are described separately.

A consistent feature of *delayed* radiation injury in mammalian tissues is the lack or paucity of cellular *inflammatory*

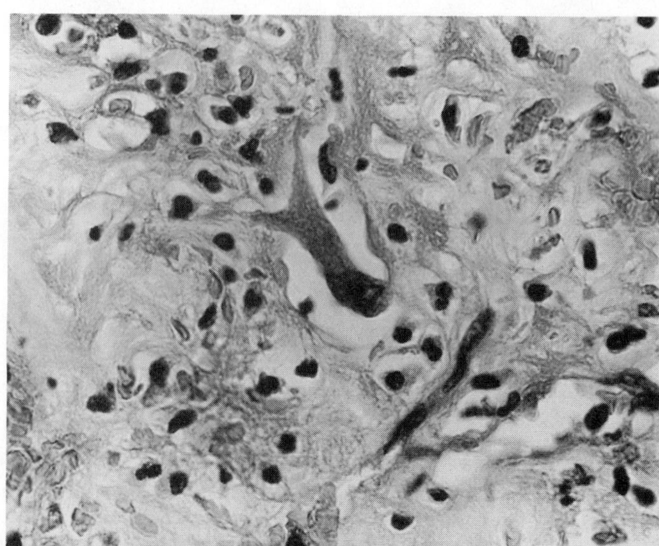

FIGURE 4–5. Atypical fibroblast in the stroma of the oral cavity many months after a dose in excess of 5000 cGy. This tripolar cell, in the center of the field, has an ill-defined ("smudged") hyperchromatic nucleus in the blunt pole (bottom right). The stroma surrounding it consists of loose collagen with moderate hemorrhage. These "radiation fibroblasts" are typical of delayed injury in tissues that suffer radiation *and* inflammation (H & E, × 600).

response. With rare exceptions (such as ulcers), the stromal reactions just described are devoid of granulocytes and contain only a few lymphocytes or macrophages. This is best seen in deep tissues such as myocardium, pericardium, and renal parenchyma (see Fig. 4-4), but to a certain degree it is present in almost all tissues, as long as there is no ulceration or superimposed infection.

The absence of cellular inflammatory response is helpful in the differential diagnosis of radiation pathology. Furthermore it supports the concept that radiation injury is not mediated through an immune mechanism.

Vascular Lesions

Alterations of the blood vessels were recognized by radiation workers as early as 1899.[20] Since then many radiation biologists have explored the functional implications of such alterations.[22,32,34] Pathologists have become familiar with the most commonly detected changes of the vasculature[13] (those in arterioles and capillaries). The vessels are described later in decreasing order of radiation sensitivity, as judged by morphologic parameters.

Blood capillaries and *sinusoids*, the narrowest and most ubiquitous elements of the vasculature, appear to be also the most radiosensitive. This is related to the sensitivity of endothelial cells, which constitute the most important part of their walls. Only some lesions of these vessels are appreciated by light microscopy. Dilatation is common and, when superficially located, can be detected clinically as telangiectasia of skin or mucous membranes; asymmetry, with irregularity of the wall; focally prominent endothelial cells; and, rarely, thrombosis (Fig. 4-6). Electron microscopy[10,13] allows detection of earlier and more subtle alterations. These are best observed in sequential experimental studies of various mammalian tissues (heart,[16] lung,[29] kidney, and others[10]) and include irregularity of cytoplasm with formation of pseudopodia or "fronds"; swelling or "blebs" of cytoplasm, often obstructing the lumen; detachment of endothelial cells from the basal lamina; cell pyknosis; rupture of plasma membrane; thrombosis; rupture of capillary wall; loss of entire capillary segments; and, in some organs, regrowth of the lost vessels.[10,16,29] These changes probably occur in many tissues, perhaps all, but have been documented in only a few.[10,13,33]

Studies of human tissues, by light or electron microscopy, do not usually reveal the most important result of the above acute damage—a reduction in the microvascular network, which ultimately results in ischemia. This has been well documented experimentally in some tissues such as myocardium, central nervous system, and skin.[2,16,23]

Small arteries (measuring up to 100 μm in external diameter) have a muscular wall, which, although thin, gives some protection from rupture. These segments may develop necrosis in the delayed phase (*e.g.*, fibrinoid necrosis of arterioles in the brain), but this is not observed often in other organs. More common are subendothelial or adventitial fibrosis, hyalinization of the media (dense, acellular, acidophilic, collagenous material), and accumulation of lipid-laden macrophages in the intima (see text that follows). Thrombosis may occur with any of these changes.

Medium arteries (100 μm to 500 μm) develop late lesions often recognized by pathologists. The most common is intimal fibrosis, characterized by deposition of collagen and fibroblasts (myofibroblasts; Fig. 4-7). Lipid-containing macrophages (foam cells) may accumulate in the intima, in variable numbers, sometimes causing narrowing or complete obstruction (Fig. 4-8). Fibrin may be present among the foam cells (Fig. 4-8), and occlusive thrombosis may occur. Spontaneous atherosclerosis often produces these foam cell plaques in large arteries, but

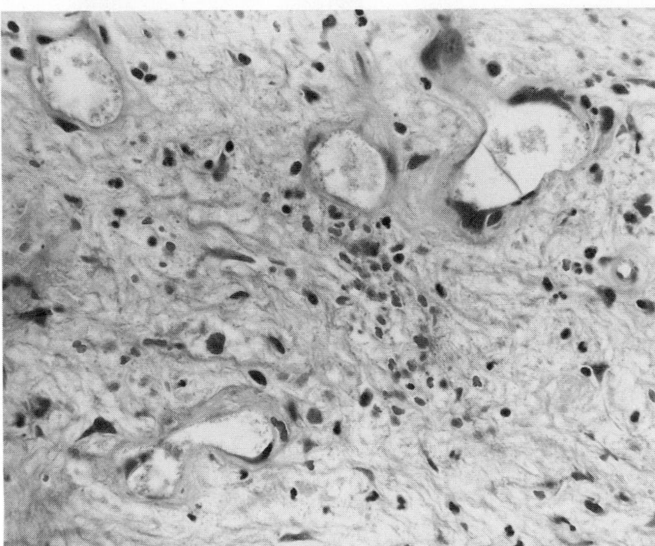

FIGURE 4–6. Telangiectasia of blood capillaries. This section of buccal mucosa, irradiated several years earlier for an adjacent squamous carcinoma, shows moderate diffuse fibrosis and mild hemorrhage. Four capillaries in this field exhibit asymmetric dilatation, and one of them (top right) shows marked enlargement of its endothelial cells, with hyperchromatic nuclei, H & E, × 300.

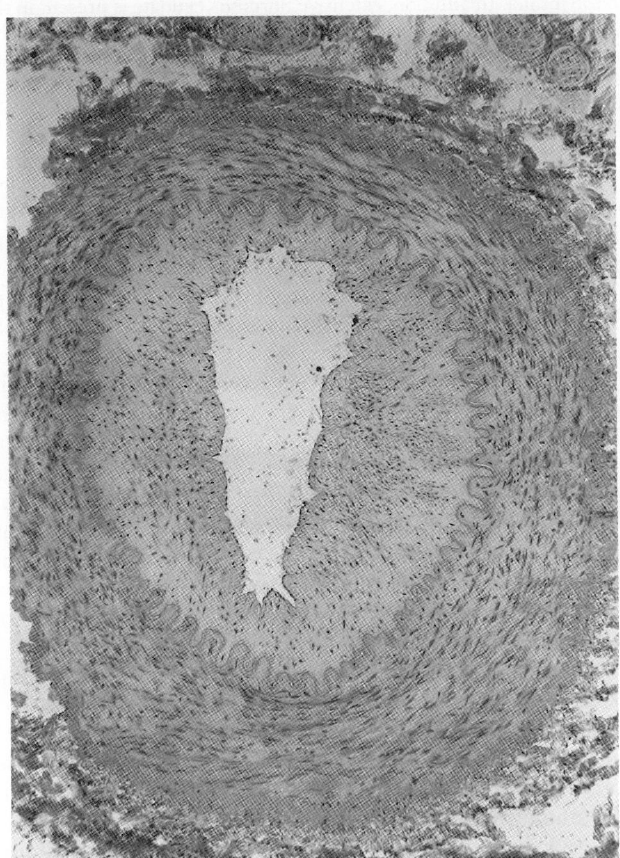

FIGURE 4–7. Gastric artery showing concentric myointimal proliferation, years after therapy (unknown dose) for adjacent neoplasm. Most of the tissue between the wavy internal elastic membrane and the reduced lumen is an abnormal growth of myocytes, fibroblasts, and collagen.

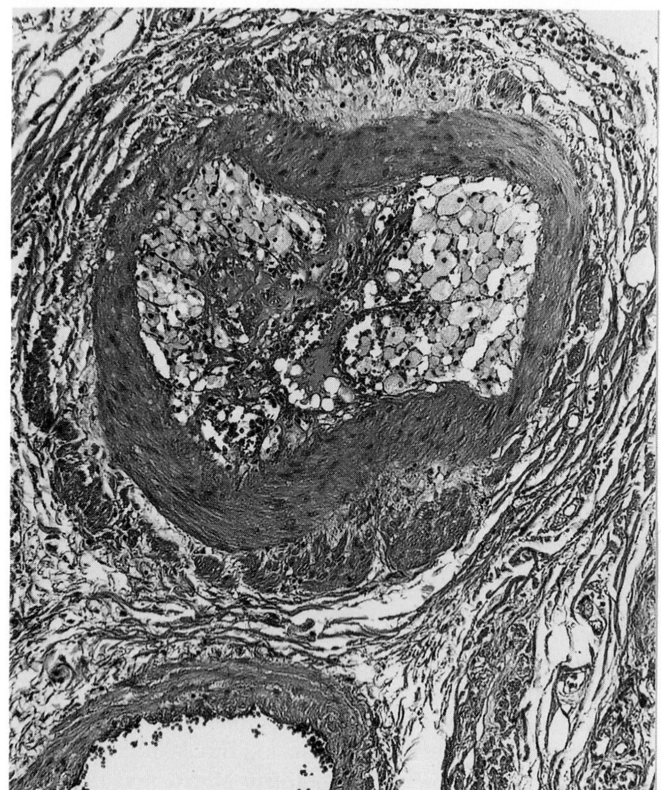

FIGURE 4–8. "Foamy" lipophages in the intima of an enteric submucosal artery, years after therapy for a pelvic neoplasm. Severe reduction of the lumen of this vessel is caused by the accumulation of lipid-containing macrophages (oval, lightly stained cells with eccentric nuclei) in the intima. In addition, extensive fibrinous exudate is present in the intima (dark-gray material to the left of the displaced lumen). This characteristic lesion is often focal; the section of vessel in the lower part of the field—presumably from the same artery—is normal (H & E, × 110).

rarely in medium and small vessels. Therefore, although not specific, foam cell plaques in medium and small arteries are highly suggestive of radiation injury. These tend to occur more often in the wall of the intestine and in the ovaries.[3,10,13]

Vasculitis may occur as a rare, delayed lesion. It is an exception to the general rule (see discussion of stromal lesions) that cellular inflammatory exudate is absent or minimal in delayed radiation pathology. We have found examples of active arteritis in the wall of the intestine, in the pelvic adipose tissue, and in the breast.[13] The infiltrate is generally lymphocytic, moderate to heavy, and localized in the media, adventitia, and, less frequently, the intima. In the latter, thrombosis may be present. We can recognize scars in these vessels (of presumed vasculitis),[13] and in the acute cases that we have been able to follow no generalized vasculitis has developed. Thus we believe that this radiation-associated vasculitis is probably self-limited and heals without therapy.[13,33]

Large arteries (> 500 μm) are less often affected than smaller vessels, perhaps because their ample lumen and thick wall, made of relatively radioresistant cells, protect them.[13,33] Nevertheless, lesions can occur and are well documented because of their dramatic effects: myointimal proliferation, with or without lipid deposits, which may be greater in irradiated sites than in the rest of the body; mural or occlusive thrombosis; and finally rupture of large arteries. Arterial rupture is often a fatal complication that tends to occur in the carotid, the femoral arteries, or the aorta.[13,15] It may not result from radiation alone, and in fact many such ruptures are clearly caused by other factors such as infections, exposure to digestive enzymes (*e.g.*, saliva), or exposure to air.[15] However, recent experimental evidence indicates that some arterial perforations may result solely from high-dose irradiation.[18]

Small veins (containing only a few layers of muscle) are affected overall less often than their arterial counterparts. Nev-

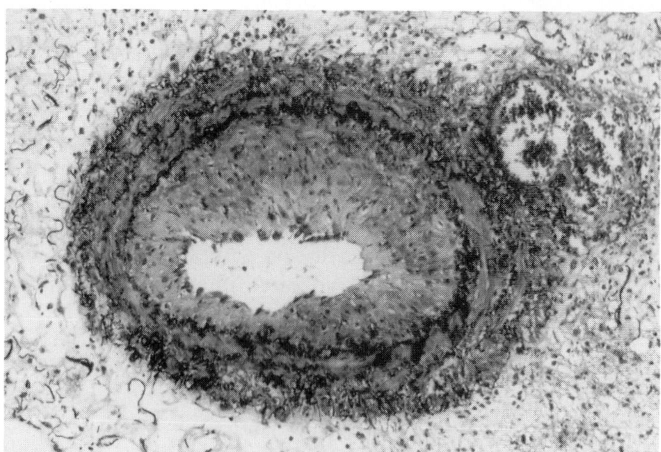

FIGURE 4–9. Mesenteric vein several years after 5000 cGy for carcinoma of the endometrium. Notice eccentric intimal proliferation that has reduced the lumen to less than half of its (vertical) diameter. Elastic lamellae (*black areas*) appear to be intact. Phlebosclerosis of this type is common in the irradiated small intestine and rare elsewhere (Verhoeff-van Gieson, × 110).

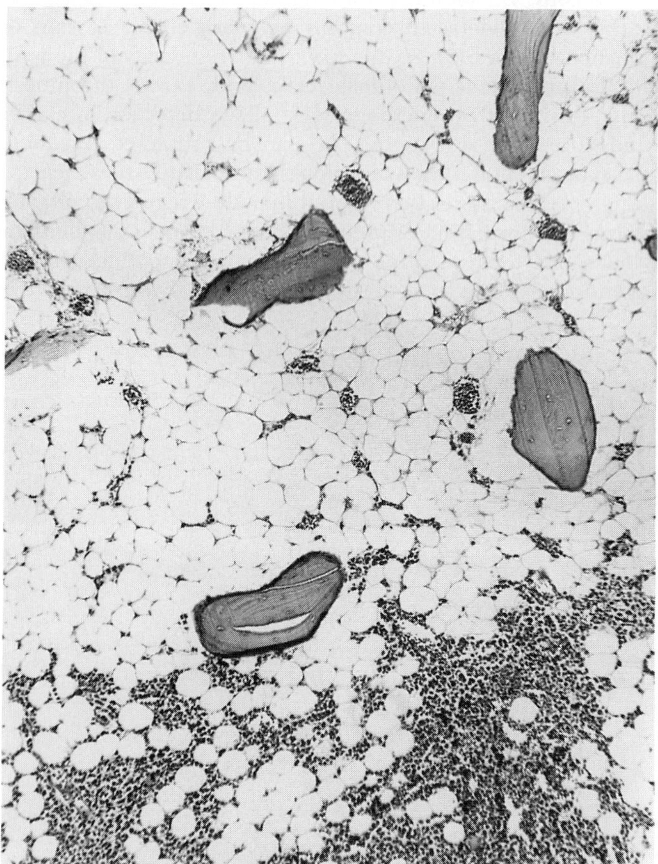

FIGURE 4–10. Delayed, permanent bone marrow aplasia. This thoracic vertebra of a 60-year-old man, after treatment 5 years earlier for pulmonary carcinoma, received a dose more than 5500 cGy to a portion of its marrow. The upper two thirds of the photograph corresponds roughly to the treated field and shows complete hemopoietic aplasia: only adipocytes and slightly dilated sinuses. The lower one third shows hemopoietic marrow with almost normal cellularity. In addition, osteoporosis (not a radiation effect) is seen (H & E, × 62).

ertheless, in the wall of the intestine intimal or medial fibrosis or even thrombosis of the veins is found as often, or more often, than similar arterial lesions[3,13] (Fig. 4-9). In the liver, radiation produces a venous rather than an arterial lesion.

Large veins (measuring 500 μm or more) seem to be the least affected of the blood vessels by radiation, whereas they are often invaded by tumors. Thus, in irradiated tissues the veins showing transmural scars are often in fact vessels that contained neoplasms before being irradiated.[10,13]

Some Characteristic Organ Lesions

It is obvious that a number of injuries do not fit into the previously described patterns. Table 4-2 lists the best-known of those lesions that are characteristic of certain organs or tissues.

Permanent *bone marrow hypoplasia or aplasia* is common. It occurs as focal, sharply circumscribed lesions, several months after total doses of fractionated radiation of more than 5000 cGy (second wave of aplasia).[37] In this case the hematopoietic cells are decreased in number or absent[37] (Fig. 4-10). Plasma cells and lymphocytes may be the only remaining cells. But these normal elements are not replaced by fibrous tissue as in other organs. They are replaced by adipocytes (Fig. 4-10). This is an exception to the rule that delayed radiation injury results in fibrosis. Furthermore, there is no fibrinous exudate, and fibroblasts (atypical or otherwise) are not seen.[10] The only areas in which collagen is found are those that existed before irradiation. The stroma of preexisting tumor nodules or inflammatory foci remains even if the neoplastic cells or the inflammatory exudate have disappeared.[10] Deposition of thorium dioxide, however, results in delayed fibrosis, but this situation is very rarely encountered today.[10]

Lymphopoietic tissues are generally quite sensitive to radiation, except for selected populations (*e.g.*, committed T-lymphocytes). As in the bone marrow, severe acute depletion of cells (lymphocytes) occurs in the spleen, lymph nodes, thymus, Peyer's patches, and so on,[10,25,27,36] following single doses, even below the LD_{50} level. Recovery from acute depletion, however, is considerably better than in the marrow, especially at the high doses. Months to years following doses of several thousand cGy (*e.g.*, those used for pelvic neoplasms), the lymph nodes show remarkable repopulation by lymphocytes (Fig. 4-11) and often appear histologically normal. As in the case of the marrow, fibrous scars in lymph nodes generally represent preirradiation lesions (tumors, granulomas, and so forth) and are not radiation-induced foci of fibrosis.

Acute radiation pneumonitis, which occurs 7 to 16 weeks after initiation of therapy, has a constellation of typical changes[10,12]: enlargement and atypia of type II pneumocytes, alveolar wall edema, variable number of alveolar macrophages, and, most prominent, hyaline membranes (mainly made of fibrin) lining alveolar ducts and alveoli (Figs. 4-12 and 4-13). These findings are the features of acute, diffuse alveolar injury or "adult respiratory distress syndrome" (ARDS), a condition that may result from many etiologies besides radiation such as shock, systemic or inhaled toxins, various drugs, and infections.[10,21] However, the morphology of acute radiation pneumonitis is characteristic enough to sometimes distinguish it from even the ARDS produced by antineoplastic compounds, which closely mimics it. As in other irradiated tissues, acute radiation pneumonitis eventually results, months later, in pulmonary fibrosis. It varies in severity from moderate septal thickening by collagen (diffuse interstitial fibrosis as in Fig. 4-14) to large, solid scars.

Veno-occlusive liver disease usually appears within 90 days of initiation of therapy. The lesion occurs in the centrilobular veins

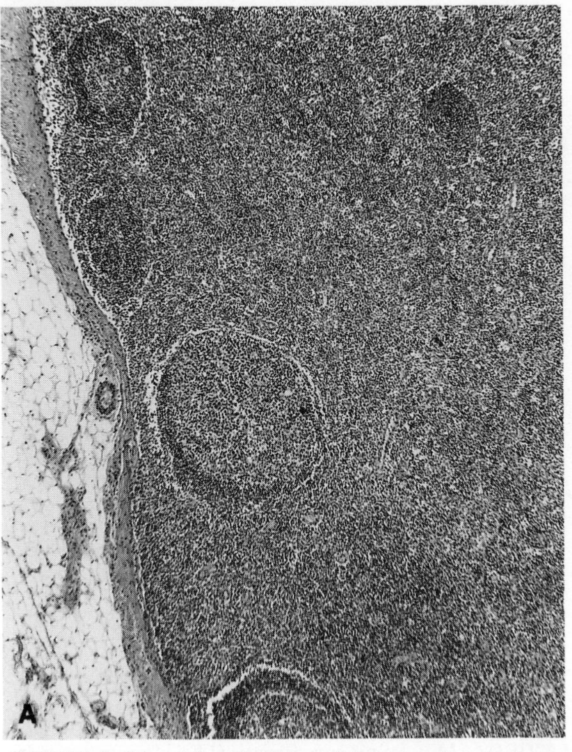

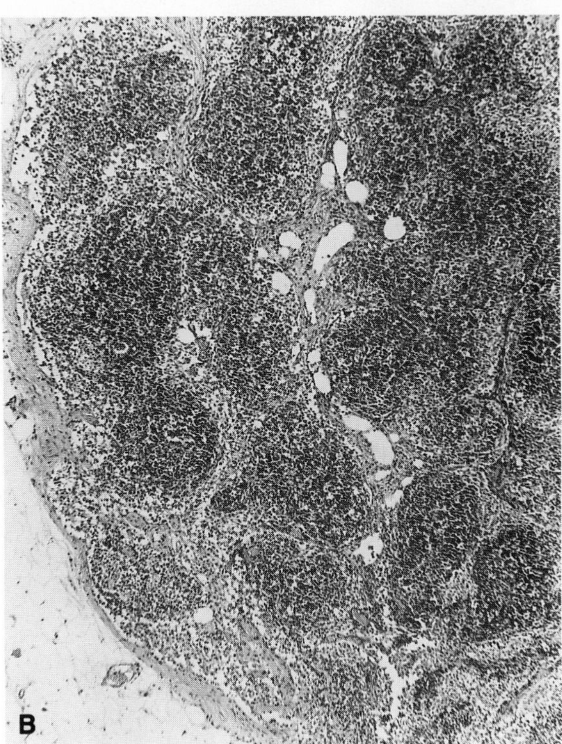

FIGURE 4–11. Delayed effects of therapeutic radiation on lymphopoietic tissue. (**A**) A normal (unirradiated) paraaortic lymph node, with cortical tissue containing prominent follicles; the mantle has many lymphocytes; the medullary sinuses are not apparent; only the subcapsular sinus is visible. (**B**) A pelvic lymph node from a field treated several years before with external radiation (? > 5000 cGy) for carcinoma of the colon. Notice moderate depletion of lymphocytes in the mantle and adjacent medulla; this depletion reveals the medullary sinuses, which appear as empty spaces in center of figure (**A** and **B,** H & E, × 50).

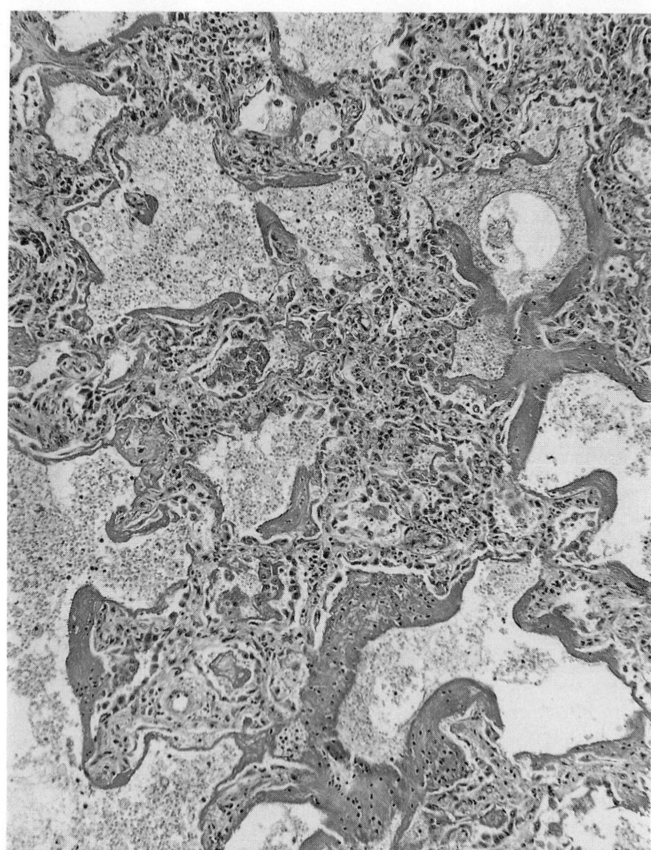

FIGURE 4–12. Acute radiation pneumonitis. Low-power micrograph of a lung from a patient who died 12 weeks after initiation of a course of 4000 cGy over 3 weeks for pulmonary carcinoma. Alveoli are either collapsed and unrecognizable (center) or inconspicuous (top). Most of the air sacs visible are alveolar ducts; these are lined by a thick layer of amorphous material—hyaline membranes (gray). The sacs also contain a granular proteinaceous "edema fluid" (H & E, × 90).

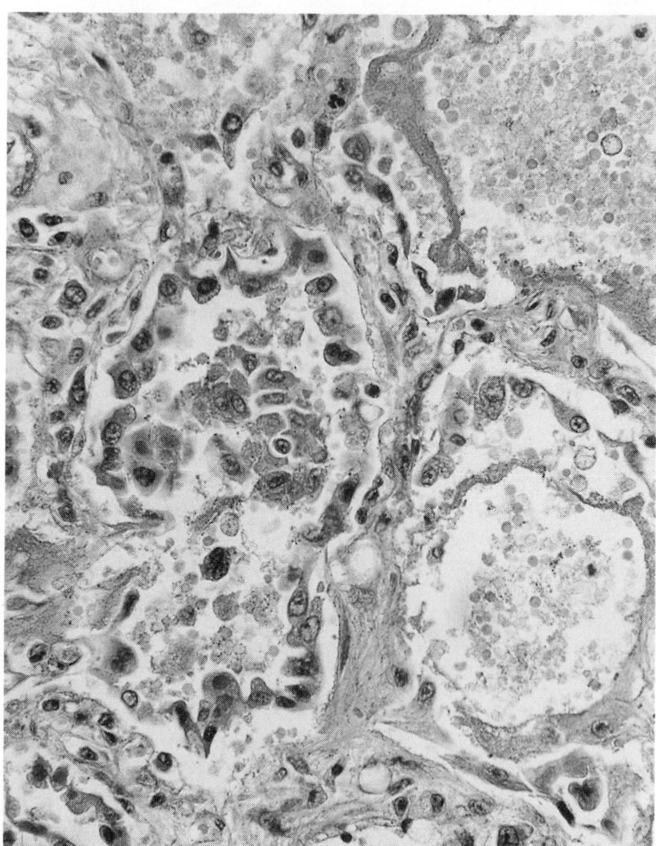

FIGURE 4–13. Detail of the lung illustrated in Figure 4–12. Two alveoli in center and right are lined by rather prominent, cuboidal, or even columnar, alveolar type II pneumocytes. This layer of pneumocytes is partially detached from the wall. In the upper right corner there is a portion of an alveolar duct lined by hyaline membrane (H & E, × 320).

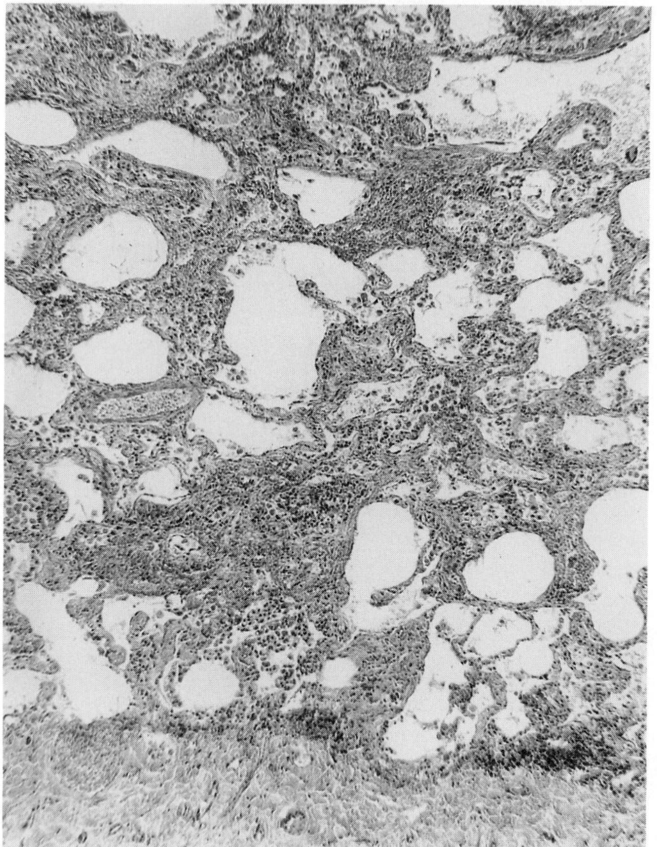

FIGURE 4–14. Pulmonary fibrosis. This lung section is from a patient who died (of unrelated disease) more than 6 years after receiving 4600 cGy to the mediastinum and adjacent lung for a lymphoma. The alveoli are moderately reduced in size and number by diffuse interstitial fibrosis, characterized in this field by increase in the thickness of the interalveolar septae. The pleura (bottom) shows diffuse fibrosis (H & E, × 63).

and the terminal portion of their afferent sinusoids, as well as in some sublobular veins.[10,14,31] Probably because of endothelial injury, delicate fibrin strands are formed in the lumen.[14] This event is followed by collagen deposition, which produces a network that obstructs the lumen and traps erythrocytes.[10,14] Acute centrilobular congestion with subsequent necrosis ensues, causing most of the clinical manifestations, if the affected area is large enough, and even leading to death.[14] However, most cases subside and heal, leaving only minimal scars.[24] It is remarkable that the liver arterioles show no evidence of damage. The veins (including some portal venules[14]) seem to bear the brunt of the injury.

Acute sialoadenitis is an uncommon clinical manifestation, appearing during the course of radiation therapy. The pathogenesis and the morphology of this lesion are poorly understood because biopsies are not obtained for obvious reasons. *Colitis cystica profunda* (CSP) associated with irradiation is also uncommon.[10,19] Unlike the more common CSP, which is usually limited to the submucosa, radiation CSP invades deep into the muscularis and may mimic a well-differentiated adenocarcinoma.[10,19]

For reasons of brevity, this review does not include pathologic descriptions of radiation-induced congenital malformations, delay in bone growth, bone deformities, or cataracts. Such descriptions can be found in various publications, including those on radiopathology.[10,35]

Acknowledgment

I appreciate the assistance of Donna L. Buckley.

REFERENCES

1. Andrews GA: Radiation accidents and their management. Radiat Res 7(Suppl):390–397, 1967
2. Archambeau J, Ines A, Fajardo LF, et al: Response of swine skin microvasculature to acute single exposures of x-rays: Quantification of endothelial changes. Radiat Res 98:37–51, 1984
3. Berthrong M, Fajardo LF: Radiation injury in surgical pathology. II. Am J Surg Pathol 5:152–178, 1981
4. Bond VP, Fliedner TM, Archambeau JO: Mammalian Radiation Lethality. New York, Academic Press, 1965
5. Burger PC, Mahaley MS, Dudka L, Vogel FS: The morphologic effects of radiation administered therapeutically for intracranial gliomas: A postmortem study of 25 cases. Cancer 44:1256–1272, 1979
6. Clarke D, Curtis JL, Martinez A, et al: Fat necrosis of the breast simulating recurrent carcinoma after primary radiotherapy in the management of early stage breast carcinoma. Cancer 52:442–445, 1983
7. Committee on the Biological Effects of Ionizing Radiation: The effects on populations of exposure to low levels of ionizing radiation: 1980, pp 265–476. Washington, DC, National Research Council-National Academy Press, 1980
8. Deschner EE, Rugh R, Grupp E: A cytological and cytochemical study of x-irradiated human testes. Milit Med 125:447–462, 1960
9. Donaldson SS: Nutritional consequences of radiotherapy. Cancer Res 37:2407–2413, 1977
10. Fajardo LF: Pathology of Radiation Injury. New York, Masson, 1982
11. Fajardo LF: Ionizing radiation and neoplasia. In Fenoglio C, Weinstein RS (eds): IAP Monograph on "New Concepts in Neoplasia as Applied to Diagnostic Pathology," pp 97–125. Baltimore, Williams & Wilkins, 1986
12. Fajardo LF: Morphologic patterns of radiation injury. Front Radiat Ther Oncol 23:75–84, 1989
13. Fajardo LF, Berthrong M: Vascular lesions following radiation. Pathol Ann 23:297–330, 1988
14. Fajardo LF, Colby TV: Pathogenesis of veno-occlusive liver disease following radiation. Arch Pathol Lab Med 104:584–588, 1980
15. Fajardo LF, Lee A: Rupture of major vessels after radiation. Cancer 36:904–913, 1975
16. Fajardo LF, Stewart JR: Pathogenesis of radiation-induced myocardial fibrosis. Lab Invest 29:244–257, 1973
17. Fanger H, Lushbaugh CC: Radiation death from cardiovascular shock following a criticality accident. Arch Pathol 83:446–460, 1967
18. Fee WE Jr, Goffinet DR, Fajardo LF, et al: Safety of ^{125}iodine and ^{192}iridium implants to the canine carotid artery: Preliminary report. Laryngoscope 95:317–320, 1985
19. Gardiner GW, McAuliffe N, Murray D: Colitis cystica profunda occurring in a radiation-induced colonic stricture. Hum Pathol 15:295–298, 1984
20. Gassmann A: Zur histologie der Roentgenulcer. Fortschr Geb Roentgenstrahlen 2:199–211, 1899
21. Gross NJ: Pulmonary effects of radiation therapy. Ann Intern Med 86:81–92, 1977
22. Hopewell JW: Radiation effects on vascular tissue. In Potten CS, Hendry JH (eds): Cytotoxic Insult to Tissue: Effects on Cell Lineages, pp 228–257. Edinburgh, Churchill-Livingstone, 1983
23. Hopewell JW, Campling D, Calvo W, et al: Vascular radiation damage: Its cellular basis and likely consequences. Br J Cancer 53 (Suppl VII):181–191, 1986
24. Lewin K, Millis RR: Human radiation hepatitis: A morphologic study with emphasis on the late change. Arch Pathol 96:21–26, 1973
25. Liebow AA, Warren S, DeCoursey E: Pathology of atomic bomb casualties. Am J Pathol 25:853–1027, 1949
26. Lushbaugh CC, Ricks RC: Some cytokinetic and histopathologic considerations of irradiated male and female gonadal tissues. Front Radiat Ther Oncol 6:228–248, 1972
27. Maisin J, Dunjic A, Maisin JR: Lymphatic system and thymus. In Berdjis CC (ed): Pathology of Irradiation, pp 496–541. Baltimore, Williams & Wilkins, 1971
28. Maximow AA: Studies on the changes produced by roentgen rays in inflamed connective tissue. J Exp Med 37:319–340, 1923
29. Phillips TL: An ultrastructural study of the development of radiation injury in the lung. Radiology 87:49–54, 1966
30. Reactor Safety Study. Appendix VI. WASH-1400 (NUREG 75/014). USNRC, 1975
31. Reed GB, Cox AJ: The human liver after radiation injury: A form of veno-occlusive disease. Am J Pathol 48:597–612, 1966
32. Reinhold HS, Business GH: Radiosensitivity of capillary endothelium. Br J Radiol 46:54–57, 1973
33. Reinhold HS, Fajardo LF, Hopewell JW: The vascular system. In Altman KI (ed): Relative Radiosensitivities of Human Organ Systems, Academic Press, London, Vol 14, pp 177–226, 1990
34. Reinhold HS, Hopewell JW: Late changes in the architecture of blood vessels in the rat brain after irradiation. Br J Radiol 53:693–696, 1980
35. Rubin P, Casarett GW: Clinical Radiation Pathology. Philadelphia, WB Saunders, 1968
36. Smith EB, White DC, Hartsock RJ, Dixon AC: Acute ultrastructural effects of 500 R on the lymph node of the mouse. Am J Pathol 50:159–175, 1967
37. Sykes MP, Chu FCH, Wilkerson WG: Local bone marrow changes secondary to therapeutic irradiation. Radiology 75:919–924, 1960
38. Vatistas S, Hornsey S: Radiation induced protein loss into the gastrointestinal tract. Br J Roengenol 39:547–550, 1966
39. Warren S: The Pathology of Ionizing Radiation. Springfield, Charles C Thomas, 1961
40. White DC: An Atlas of Radiation Histopathology. T/D-26676 Technical Information Center, Office of Public Affairs. US Energy Research and Development Administration, 1975

5

Late Effects of Cancer Treatment: Radiation and Drug Toxicity

Philip Rubin
Louis S. Constine
Diana F. Nelson

A substantial body of clinical experience and pathologic data has established the progression in time of tissue injury triggered by a course of radiation. Depending on how vital the organ is, severe morbidity or even mortality can occur. A dose response of a normal tissue needs to be evaluated in time. The "time course paradigm"[34,35] has been postulated in most normal tissues as a sequence of clinical events based on histopathologic alterations following irradiation (Fig. 5-1). Such a schema can also be applied to chemotherapy.

A major difference between chemotherapy and radiation therapy is believed to be the absence of late effects after exposure to drugs; the concern for tolerance of chemotherapy regimens is their acute and subacute toxicity.[108] The increasing documentation of late somatic changes in organs attributable to chemotherapy alone has dispelled the view that few late effects are associated with the prolonged use of drugs.[52] The basis for radiation changes is parenchymal cellular hypoplasia of stem cells and alterations in the fine vasculature and fibroconnective tissues. The late effects of chemotherapy are postulated to result predominantly from parenchymal cellular depletion of both noncycling and cycling cells also, but with sparing of the microcirculation and fibroconnective tissue stroma. A modification of the radiation time course paradigm[180] will be made to accommodate the late effects of cytotoxic drugs.

RADIOSENSITIVITY OR RESPONSIVENESS BASED ON CELL MITOTIC BEHAVIOR AND POTENTIAL

Cellular Radiosensitivity

The sequential changes that occur following irradiation in tissue are based on the mitotic behavior of the component cells and potential for either staying in cycle or differentiating.[180] The original description used to illustrate cellular radiation sensitivity was reinterpreted in current cellular kinetic terminology.[4,100] The vegetative and differentiating intermitotic cells described by Cowdry[50] are supplanted by the undifferentiated stem cell (USC) and the committed stem cell (CSC). The maturation of the cell into a fixed postmitotic cell is referred to as the functional mature cell (FMC). The cell that is difficult to define is the reverting mature cell (RMC), because it may appear to be a noncycling functional mature cell but, under appropriate stimulus, has the capacity to dedifferentiate and proliferate. The basic tenet of this concept is that the dividing or cycling cell (USC or CSC) is more vulnerable to radiation than the nondividing cell, particularly if it is a functional mature cell (FMC) or a reverting mature cell (RMC); that is, radiation cell death is expressed as a mitotically linked death and occurs only when the cell divides—with a few exceptions such as the small lymphocyte.

Cell Cycle Correlation to Radiosensitivity

The radiosensitivity of cells is based on their progression through the cell cycle. Proliferating cells are more radiosensitive than quiescent cells, particularly in early S phase and G_2M.

Organization of Tissues According to Cell Renewal

The organization of normal tissues according to cell renewal characteristics is portrayed in Figure 5-2. The parenchymal cell compartments of the various organs in the body are either rapid renewal or slow renewal systems. The epithelial tissues lining mucosal surfaces in the upper aerodigestive passages, gastrointestinal (GI) tract, urinary systems, and bone marrow are examples of rapid renewal tissues. These tissues tend to have uncom-

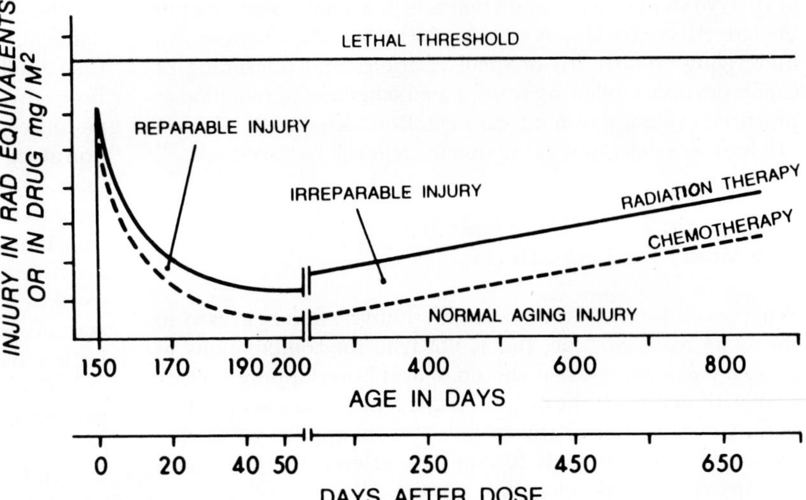

FIGURE 5–1. Late effects after exposure to radiation and chemotherapy are the residual damages that express themselves months to years in time. The slopes indicate the reparable and irreparable injury, above the aging injury, due to the persistent effects on tissues and their microcirculation. Residual damage has been a basic assumption after radiation treatment (*solid line*) and is carefully considered in designing radiation regimens. In contrast, chemotherapists assume that acute effects are completely reparable injury with no late effects, portrayed (*broken line*) as similar to the normal aging injury line. This is an illusion not consistent with currently reported findings of late effects after chemotherapy. (Rubin P: Int J Radiat Oncol Biol Phys 10:5–34, 1984)

mitted (USC) or committed stem cell (CSC) compartments that rapidly proliferate and differentiate. The functional cell is usually differentiated and is a fixed mature cell (FMC), essentially incapable of further mitotic activity.

CHEMOSENSITIVITY BASED ON CELL MITOTIC BEHAVIOR AND POTENTIAL

Drug Action as Phase- or Cycle-Specific

Cell cycle kinetics has been classically used to describe the response of cells to chemotherapeutic agents. Drug action is described either as *phase-* or *cycle-specific,* referring to cell killing either in S phase or elsewhere in the cycle.[172,231] The expression of cell lethality at time of mitosis in rapidly proliferating tissues appears clinically as an acute injury. The cells most vulnerable are those actively cycling or dividing stem cells, in contrast to those cells in G_0 or prolonged G_1, which are protected particularly from S phase-specific drugs such as hydroxyurea or methotrexate.[18,39,230]

Drug Action on Stem Cell Depletion

The dose-limiting organ is a function of drug targeting in a specific tissue. The experimental evidence of Botnik and associates[25] in a variety of tissues shows that, despite the normal appearance of regenerated cells and tissues after chemotherapy insult, some of their proliferative reserve capacity has been lost. For example, when chemotherapeutically treated bone marrow is further challenged to repopulate by serial transplantation using the Till and McCullough model,[225] the loss of stem cells is uncovered. This phenomenon of stem cell depletion has been found in other tissues, such as skin or hair follicles. The term *stem cell senescence* was introduced to describe the concept of depletion of stem cell reserve or loss of normal mitotic potential

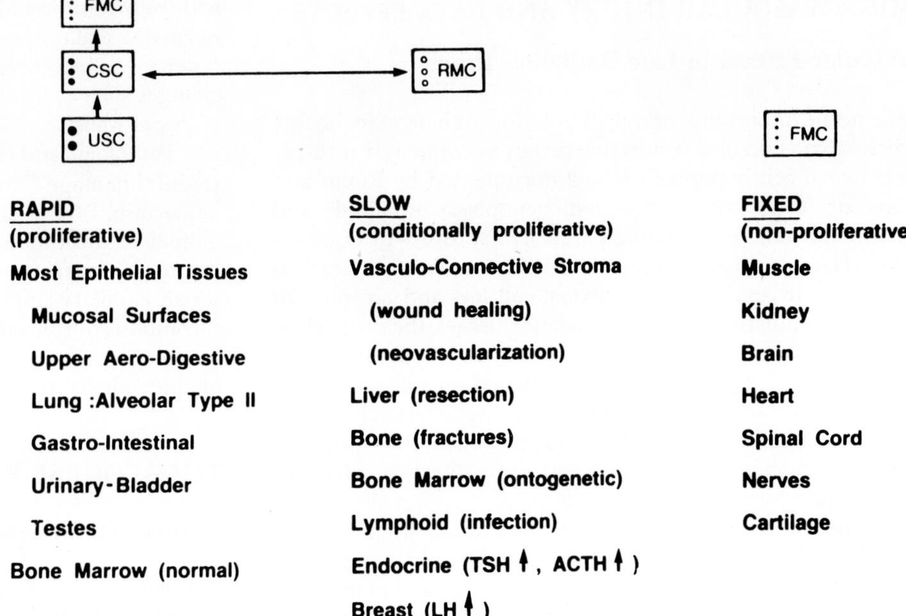

FIGURE 5–2. Normal tissues are either rapid renewal, slow renewal, or fixed renewal, that is, proliferative, conditionally proliferative (with the stimulus noted in parentheses), or nonproliferative. In the fixed renewal system, repair is possible only through connective tissue replacement. In rapid and slow renewal systems, regeneration of parenchymal cells is possible. TSH: thyroid-stimulating hormone; ACTH: adrenocorticotropic hormone; LH: lactogenic hormone. (Rubin P: Int J Radiat Oncol Biol Phys, 10:5–34, 1984)

of reserve stem cells.[188] Radiation acts in a similar fashion, but the late effects are always associated with vascular changes. An underlying endarteritis of small arterioles and thickening of capillaries occur following fractionated schedules of radiation as practiced in clinical tumor treatment. Both drugs and radiation can lead to accelerated aging due to stem cell senescence.[25,104]

Clonogenic Tumor Cell Depletion as a Model for Late Effects

Whereas all forms of radiation are additive when delivered to the same tissue volume, this is not true for combinations of agents, particularly when chosen to avoid overlapping toxicity in specific organs. If the diagrammatic representation of reduction of the number of tumor cells[152] were applied to normal tissues, theoretic models for the late effects due to chemotherapy could be developed.

The assumption is made that active drugs provide a degree of tumor cell log kill (Fig. 5-3*A*). In most multidrug regimens, the number of tumor cells is progressively reduced as the induction, consolidation, and maintenance phases of regimens are completed. If the tumor clonogenic cells are reduced to zero, cure results. If drug resistance appears, the tumor can recur. The early or late reappearances are often a function of the time at which drug resistance developed. Parallels between the phases of drug treatment and the radiation therapy regimen can be drawn. The radiation boost field and boost dose may be compared with the consolidation phase.

Stem Cell Depletion as a Basis for Normal Tissue Late Effects

When the concept of stem cell depletion is applied to normal tissues, a similar set of events can be pictured (Fig. 5-3*B*). For the cancer treatment to be successful, a differential degree tumor and normal tissue cell kill must occur. As drugs or radiation regimens deplete these stem cells, first reversible and then irreversible injury occurs. A major conceptual difference is that no known radioresistance or chemoresistance is in normal tissues as in tumors.[58]

MICROVASCULAR INJURY AND LATE EFFECTS

Vascular Effects in Late Radiation Injury

The prime importance of radiation-induced changes in the fine microcirculation and connective tissues as compared with parenchymal cell hypoplasia is well documented by Rubin and Casarett.[183] As previously stated, hypoplasia of rapidly and continually self-repopulating parenchymal tissues or organs is caused largely through direct mechanisms such as cell death at mitosis with resultant parenchymal cell loss and atrophy. In slowly repopulating or nonrepopulating tissues, the production of parenchymal hypoplasia is due both to direct cell effects and indirect effects on the fine vasculoconnective tissue stroma. In both circumstances, the slowly progressive arteriolar fibrosis and interstitial fibrosis after irradiation contribute to the delayed parenchymal hypoplasia and cause the late effects of radiation.

The essential lesion occurs in the endothelium of small vessels such as arterioles, capillaries, and venules rather than larger vessels. The resulting lesion is a consequence of inherent radiosensitivity of the relevant cells, luminal compromise due to smaller diameter of the vessels for a given tissue, or direct organ damage from parenchymal cell injury. The swelling of endothelial cells leads to a narrowing obstruction that impedes blood flow. This leads to thrombosis and regenerative attempts by the endothelial cells. The early changes are spotty in their distribution along the course of vessels, rather than uniform and continuous.[183] Hopewell[109,110] stresses the need for serial histologic sections to appreciate these lesions. Alternately, microangiography allows for fuller viewing of the fine circulation of tissues because of the loss of detail in regular microsections that are 5 μ to 10 μ. It is understandable why the observer, without proper training, may conclude that the apparent absence of such vascular lesions in a microsection is proof of their insignificance.

The progression of vascular damage and the cicatrization process interstitially leads to more and more points along the course of the affected small blood vessels that show degenerative and fibrotic change, so that more sections of small blood vessels per unit area of tissues readily reveal the changes.

Numerous investigations have substantiated one consistent change after irradiation of tissues: the appearance of irregularly spaced vascular constrictions, particularly in the walls of arterioles.[34,35,109,110,145] The possible development of such constrictions, because of slow depopulation of damaged endothelial cells and reactive hyperplasia to regenerate the loss, can lead to clones to cells at irregularly spaced intervals along the vessel wall, producing a "sausage segment" effect.[109]

In all sites studied to date, the ^{3}H-thymidine labeling index for normal endothelial cells is low—less than 1%.[109,110] This explains why the manifestation of endothelial injury, which is expressed months later, is associated with a phase of increased labeling or compensatory hyperplasia that is focal in distribution. The only other lesion that could account for these "sausage segments" is smooth muscle, which has an even lower rate of labeling—less than 0.1%.[109,110]

Focal constrictions, demonstrated in autoradiographic correlation with histologic observations represent thickening of the arteries due to endothelial hyperplasia, resulting in partial or total occlusion of the vascular lumen; this has been observed in heart, kidney, lung, brain, and dermis. Hopewell,[110] using pig dermis, has confirmed that cells in these occlusive lesions are synthesizing DNA. Three phases of this vascular injury occur in time: early, intermediate, and late. The intermediate lesions mediated through depletion of endothelial cells are associated with reduction in blood flow. Tissue atrophy reestablishes the normal vascular density. The late changes of more than 1 year observed in blood vessels are mainly characterized by arteriole changes such as hyaline, fibrinoid, and collagenous thickening of vessel walls.

Pathologic and clinical illustrations of the type of radiation vascular damage[183] are lignous fibrosis subcutaneously and telangiectasia of the skin, sclerosis of the renal arterioles and glomeruli, ulceration and infarction necrosis of fibrosis of bowel due to obliterative arteritis, ischemic necrosis of the brain, interstitial capillary injury of the myocardium, veno-occlusive thrombosis of central veins of the liver, choroidal vasculitis and hemorrhage,[12] pulmonary interstitial fibrosis, bone necrosis, bladder ulcers, telangiectasia, and contracted bladder.

TIME-COURSE PARADIGM

Clinical Pathologic Course of Events

The expression of injury in time after irradiation allows for identification of an early or acute injury, which is often repara-

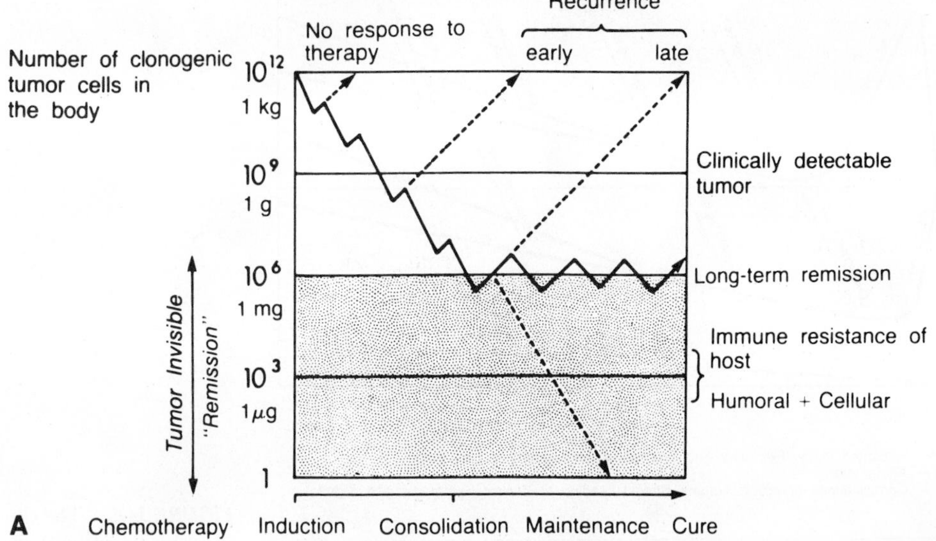

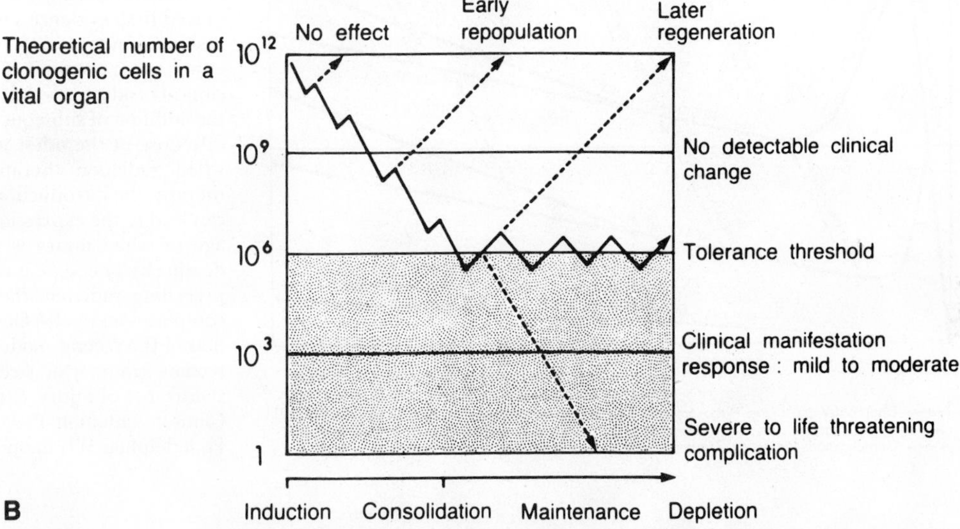

FIGURE 5–3. (**A**) Diagrammatic presentation of the reduction of the number of tumor cells by chemotherapy application. It indicates the induction, consolidation, and maintenance phases of chemotherapy required for cure. If resistance sets in, the tumor can escape and recur. A similar paradigm can be applied to irradiation curability, although as a rule, there is no maintenance phase for irradiation regimens. (**B**) If one compares the tumor clonogenic cell reduction model with the reduction of essential normal tissue stem cells, a similar model can be developed for regeneration of vital clonogenic cells versus complication, which can be mild to moderate or severe to life-threatening, depending on the depletion of the stem cells required to maintain the viability of the organ. The required number is speculative and is therefore not known or defined for various normal tissues. However, if the number of known stem cells that existed in a normal adult tissue were established, and their radiosensitivity (D_q and D_o) or chemosensitivity characteristics determined, it would be possible to calculate the doses that would deplete the organ system by irradiation or chemotherapy and lead to complications. (Rubin P: Int J Radiat Oncol Biol Phys 10:5–34, 1984)

ble, and a later component, which is irreparable (Fig. 5-1). The mechanisms of action, according to Casarett,[34,35] are presented both as a parenchymal cell loss and injury and alteration of the vasculoconnective tissue. The initial recovery on the tissue level results predominantly from parenchymal cellular repopulation. The progressive component is the arteriocapillary fibrosis that predominates in the late irreparable injury and accentuates the cellular depletion of the parenchyma. A clinical pathologic course for most normal tissues and organs has been presented by Rubin and Casarett[183] in a paradigm based on documented histopathophysiologic events in humans and *in vivo* laboratory animals. The clinical pathologic course of events is illustrated in terms of subclinical and clinical damage with a threshold that can be expressed as a radiation tolerance dose (Fig. 5-4*A*).

A similar clinical pathologic course is postulated following chemotherapy administration (Fig. 5-4*B*). Precise quantifica-

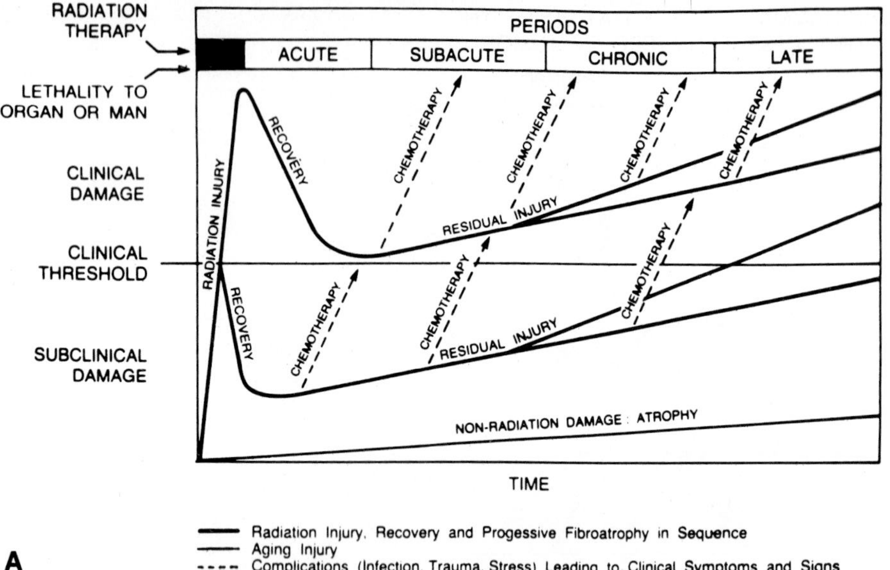

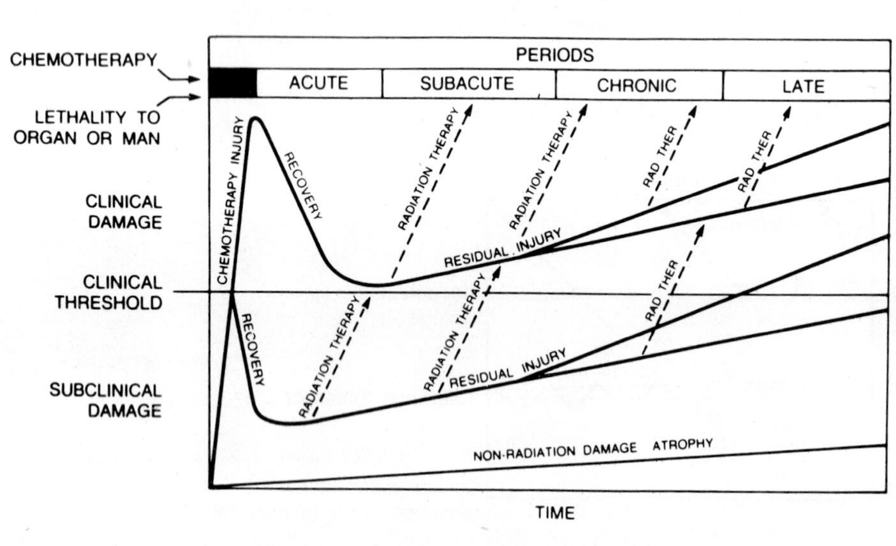

FIGURE 5–4. The clinicopathologic course of events following radiation exposure can be complicated by the addition of chemotherapy, which can augment these changes. Similarly, chemotherapy can result in a parallel set of events. Depending on which mode is employed first, evidence suggests that both leave residual injury when large enough doses of either agent are used. This can result in subclinical residuum, which may be uncovered by the addition of subsequent use of a seemingly safe dose of the other mode. (**A**) Classically, when radiation therapy precedes chemotherapy, the introduction of the second mode can lead to the expression of subclinical damage or when injury is present, can lead to death. (**B**) The same is true of chemotherapy preceding radiation therapy. In addition to complications (*broken lines*) caused by the addition of the second mode alone, associated infection, trauma, or stress can lead to overt syndromes of injury. (Rubin P, Casarett GW: Clinical Radiation Pathology, vols I and II. Philadelphia, WB Saunders, 1968)

tion of pathophysiologic injury is often difficult to define and needs solution to provide data that can be clinically useful. The search for predictive biochemical, metabolic, or physiologic parameters in terms of early events following irradiation or chemotherapy is a major direction of research and hopefully can be used to monitor the more permanent pathologic damage that will occur, or is occurring, on a subclinical level.[179]

Dose-limiting organs and tissues in radiation oncology have been segregated into three classes according to their tolerance doses.[186] The minimal tolerance dose ($TD_{5/5}$) and the maximal tissue tolerance dose ($TD_{50/5}$) refer to a severe to life-threatening complication of 5% and 50%, occurring within 5 years of therapeutic radiation treatment. The different categories of tissues stress the vital importance of the organ or tissue for survival. In the first category are those organs and tissues which, if injured irreparably, lead to death or severe morbidity; in the second category are those associated with moderate morbidity and, in exceptional circumstances, death; in the third category are those with mild transient and reparable consequences with little to no morbidity occurring.[186]

Kinetics of Cell Radiation and Chemopathology

The clinical pathologic course of events following radiation exposure can be complicated by the addition of chemotherapy, which can augment these changes. Similarly, chemotherapy followed by irradiation can result in a parallel set of events. Residual injury can result in subclinical residuum that may be uncovered by the subsequent use of a seemingly safe dose of the other modality. Thus, classically, when radiation therapy precedes chemotherapy, the introduction of the second modality can lead to the expression of subclinical damage; when frank injury is already present, increased morbidity or even death can result. The same is true of chemotherapy preceding radiation therapy. This will be further illustrated later.

Combined Effects of Drugs and Radiation

Radiation acts both on the microcirculatory systems and parenchymal cells of tissues and organs; chemotherapy acts predominantly on the cellular parenchymal component. In rapid renewal systems, the same stem cell population is affected and the increased acute toxicity of both modalities combined can usually be reduced by applying them sequentially. In slow renewal tissues, their additive effects are often due to entirely different target cell populations in the same organ system. However, the late effects may not be avoided because chemotherapy, even when delayed (in prolonged maintenance schedules), can result in additional stem cell kill and can lead to expression of subclinical radiation effects. It is necessary to be aware of the iatrogenic syndromes secondary to cancer treatment so that they are not confused with recurrent or metastatic disease.[26,52] In the pediatric setting, the many proliferating tissues are even more vulnerable than in adults in whom many normal organs are in a mature steady state with slow cell renewal kinetics.

The new hypothesis for explaining the late effects of chemotherapy and irradiation stems from the different mechanisms of action. There has been a tendency to refer to a clinical drug-radiation reaction as a "recall phenomenon" of radiation injury or an enhancement of radiation injuries. The evidence accumulating in the literature is that many chemotherapeutic agents affect either different target cell populations compared with that of irradiation or similar cell populations through entirely different pathophysiologic mechanisms. The effect on organ physiology may be additive, but it is not a simple stem cell depletion of a similar population by the two different modalities.[4] Furthermore, the regional administration of radiation results in focal injury to the vasculoconnective tissue stroma, whereas chemotherapeutic administration does not.

ORGAN TOLERANCE: DOSE-LIMITING TISSUES

Organ tolerance is determined by the radiosensitivity of the relevant stem cell subpopulations, which may not always be proliferating or dividing.[100] The functional capacity of cells is often distinct from the regenerative capacity and permits organ physiology to be preserved in the face of injury and allows for recovery or repair of the insult. Most organ systems are composed of many cell subpopulations (20 to 40 or more), each performing an important activity.[183] The most radiosensitive vital cell population determines organ tolerance and organ failure just as the degree of importance of an organ that has been irradiated determines the survival of an organism.

Heart

The functional and structural complexity of the heart is mirrored by the variety of radiation injuries that can occur. A classification system modified from Fajardo and Stewart[78] includes acute pericarditis during irradiation (rare and associated with juxtapericardial cancer); delayed pericarditis that can present abruptly or as chronic pericardial effusion; pancarditis, which includes pericardial and myocardial fibrosis with or without endocardial fibroelastosis (only after large doses); myopathy in the absence of significant pericardial disease; coronary artery disease, usually involving the left anterior descending artery; functional valvular injury; and conduction defects. Although there is occurrence of coronary artery disease, it is relatively uncommon and multifactorial. The histologic hallmark of these injuries is fibrosis in the interstitium, with normal-appearing myocytes and capillary and arterial narrowing.

Several parameters must be considered in the evaluation of radiation injuries, including relative weighting of the radiation portals and thus the amount of radiation delivered to different depths of the heart; presence of juxtapericardial tumor; volume and specific areas of the heart irradiated; total and fractional radiation dose; presence of other risk factors in each patient such as age, weight, blood pressure, family history, lipoprotein levels, and habits such as smoking; and use of specific chemotherapeutic agents.

Clinical Syndromes

Delayed acute pericarditis can be symptomatically occult or can manifest suddenly with fever, dyspnea, pleuritic chest pain, friction rub, ST and T wave changes and decreased QRS voltage.[7,218] Up to 30% of patients treated with radiation for Hodgkin's disease with a mean midplane heart dose of 4600 cGy will be affected. With equally weighted anterior and posterior fields and the use of subcarinal blocking, the incidence decreases to 2.5%.[33] A report by Stewart on 25 patients who developed cardiac damage, primarily pericarditis, shows the relevance of radiation dose and cardiac volume to the type of injury.[215] The onset of delayed acute pericarditis averages 6 months, and 92% of effusion occurs within 12 months. Although the effusion usually resolves within 1 to 10 months, it may persist for years. Up to 50% of patients develop some degree of tamponade (paradoxic pulse, Kussmaul's sign), occasionally requiring pericardiocentesis. Chronic effusive-constrictive pericarditis develops in 10% to 15% of patients and may require pericardectomy. On the other hand, constriction may present 5 to 50 years following irradiation with no antecedent acute disease.[7,32,218] Diuretics are sometimes necessary to control peripheral edema or ascites.

Pancarditis is both rare and severe and probably requires radiation doses of at least 6000 cGy.[218] Intractable congestive heart failure can result. Restrictive hemodynamics are demonstrated by catheterization.

Myocardiopathy is highly potentiated by doxorubicin, but occurs in its absence. In an autopsy study of patients who were irradiated with at least 3500 cGy—many with anterior-only portals (mean dose of 5600 cGy to anterior heart surface)—50% showed myocardial fibrosis, 75% showed fibrous thickening of the mural endocardium, and over 90% showed pericardial thickening.[29] Right ventricular end-diastolic function may also be reduced by up to 25% in asymptomatic patients.[31] Ejection fractions may be decreased in up to 33%.

Fibrous valvular endocardial thickening is found in 80% of autopsied patients treated with high radiation doses. The mitral, aortic, and tricuspid valves are most frequently affected.[29]

High degree atrioventricular conduction abnormalities are rarely seen and have been attributed to fibrosis of the atrioventricular (AV) node conducting branches.[44]

The incidence and extent of coronary artery disease (CAD) is not clear. Both autopsy and patient series have documented the occurrence of CAD after radiation doses as low as 2400 cGy and after higher doses.[29,64,134] At autopsy, patients treated with anterior weighted radiation techniques had narrowing of up to 75%, most frequently involving the proximal portion of the arteries. The media and adventitia were thickened or replaced by fibrosis tissue, either diffusely or focally. Bizarre fibroblasts, hyalinization, intimal thickening with collagen, endothelial cells, and histiocytes are seen.[29] However, a study of patients irradiated for Hodgkin's disease showed no statistically significant increase in CAD beyond that in a control population.[20] This report, however, has some methodologic weaknesses. Prospective studies are needed to address this question.

Pathophysiology

The severe cardiomyopathies encountered as a late effect of cancer treatment demonstrate the additive effects of both radiation and drugs through the action on two different populations of cells.

Radiation alters the fine vasculoconnective stroma of the myocardium.[76–78,98,135] These histopathologic and ultrastructural changes of doxorubicin alone, radiation alone, and both radiation and doxorubicin dramatically show these independent and additive organ effects[67–69,74] (Fig. 5-5).

Radiation changes in the heart are typical in humans and are experimentally reproducible and similar in rabbits and some other primates.[14,76,77,217] The hallmark is a pericardial effusion clinically and fibrosis pathologically involving a thickened collagenous pericardium and an extensive fibrinous exudate. When the myocardium is involved, diffuse interstitial fibrosis occurs, which follows the pattern of septae in the myocardium. With therapeutic doses of radiation, direct damage to myocytes in humans and animals does not occur.[217]

The coronary arteries are large enough not to be the main focus of radiation lesions, and coronary thrombosis is a relatively infrequent occurrence, found in less than 5% of patients treated. Coronary thrombosis does not differ from spontaneous arteriosclerosis in nonirradiated patients[130,216] and, therefore, is difficult to establish without a matched cohort of patients managed by other means.

In a variety of radiation schedules, serial sacrifice of rabbits yielded a predictable and identifiable sequence of lesions in the myocardial microvasculture.[76] Severe alterations in myocardial capillaries, including irregularities of the endothelial cell membranes, cytoplasmic swelling, thrombosis, and rupture of the walls, have been reported.[77] Quantitative studies showed that the ratio of capillaries to myocytes was reduced by approximately 50% over nonirradiated controls at 120 to 540 days. By pulse labeling with tritiated thymidine, a peak incorporation entirely within capillary endothelial cells was noted. Fajardo and Stewart's hypothesis is that radiation insult results in latent damage to the capillary endothelial cells. A compensatory burst of endothelial cell proliferation occurs and the cells die at mitosis. The resulting reduction in capillaries leads to ischemia and, in turn, myocardial fibrosis.[77]

Radiation Effects

Experimental studies in a rabbit model were performed by Stewart, who found that single radiation doses of 1800 cGy to

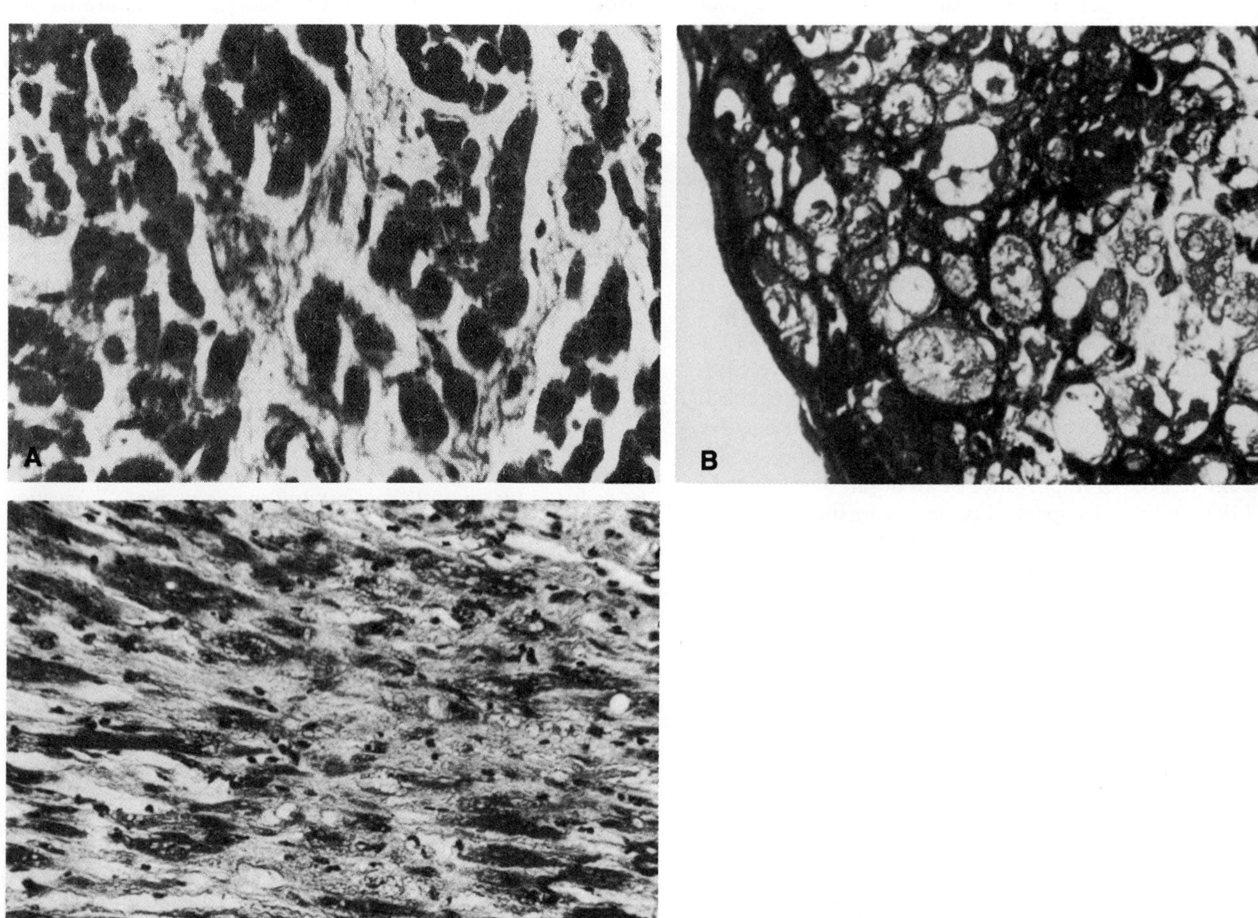

FIGURE 5–5. (**A**) Radiation therapy effects. The myocardium or cardiac myocytes are normal in appearance, with increased fibrosis in the interstitium with capillary and arterial narrowing. (**B**) Chemotherapy effects. The effect of doxorubicin (Adriamycin) is dramatic, with vacuolization selectively localized to the cardiac myocytes. The interstitium is normal in appearance, showing vascular sparing, despite dramatic cellular changes. (**C**) Combined radiation and chemotherapy effects illustrates damage to both the vascular connective tissue stroma and the cardiac myocyte. (**A** to **C**, Eltringham JR, Fajardo LF, Stewart JR: Radiology 115:471–472, 1975)

2000 cGy or fractionated doses of 5400 cGy (450 cGy × 12) caused pericarditis in all animals, whereas less than 1800 cGy (single dose) caused no damage.[77] Pathologically the following was observed: Between 6 and 48 hours following irradiation an inflammatory exudate was seen in all layers of the heart, and after 70 days progressive pericardial and myocardial fibrosis leading to tamponade and heart failure occurred in 87% of animals.[76,218] Gavin studied beagles and showed that single radiation doses of 1220 cGy resulted in pericardial effusion, whereas 1500 cGy doses caused tamponade in 50% of animals at 6 months.[88]

The relevance of radiation dose to cardiac sequelae is underscored by differences in the incidence following different radiation techniques that deliver more or less than 4000 cGy to the heart. Thus, among patients treated for Hodgkin's disease, less than 5% develop pericarditis when radiation dose of less than 4000 cGy is administered through equally weighted anterior and posterior portals, whereas a 30% incidence is seen following anteriorly weighted techniques.[32] Brosius[29] described autopsy findings in patients with Hodgkin's disease of pericardial thickening in 94%, myocardial fibrosis in 50%, fibrotic mural endocardial thickening in 75%, valvular thickening in 81%, and coronary lesions in more than 75% following a calculated dose of 5590 cGy anteriorly (3930 cGy posteriorly). The relationship of the volume of the heart irradiated and the dose administered to the occurrence of cardiac damage is suggested by early data collected by Stewart.[215]

Chemotherapy Effects

Chemotherapeutic injury, best studied and documented for doxorubicin, leads to direct cytotoxicity to cardiomyocytes.[15,16,67,237,238] No clinical manifestations are expected from low doses of 20 to 450 mg/M^2, but microscopic changes on endocardial biopsy are detectable. At 500 to 550 mg/M^2, the threshold for clinical damage is reached.[90] For elderly patients with cardiac disease or those receiving mediastinal irradiation, modified schedules to 300 to 350 mg/M^2 are advised.[237] With radiation doses in the range of 4500 cGy to 5000 cGy (standard fractionation), a threshold is reached for injury, depending on whether the whole heart volume or part of the myocardium is included.[215] A long list of other agents associated with late cardiomyopathy exists (Table 5-1).

The exact molecular lesion for doxorubicin is believed to be interference with myocardial DNA-dependent RNA synthesis at the nuclear or mitochondrial level, which could affect functional and structural proteins.[109,117] This is expressed as direct damage to myocytes that are vacuolated, and large diffuse patches of replacement fibrosis appears.

The cardiomyopathy attributed to chemotherapy usually results, however, in congestive heart failure. Many drugs[69,89] cause myocardial damage through various mechanisms, including direct toxic damage and hypersensitivity reactions (see Table 5-1). Histopathologically, the lesions of the anthracyclines differ distinctly from those of radiation. The underlying lesion is the damaged myocyte and is characterized either by loss of contractile elements (myofibrillar degeneration) or by sacrotubular vacuolization within myocytes[74]; the vasculoconnective stroma is spared. In high-risk patients, careful monitoring of left ventricular ejection fraction by radionuclide scan, particularly gaited exercise scan, cardiac catheterization, and endomyocardial biopsy should be considered.[2,67]

TABLE 5–1
Agents Causing Cardiac Toxicity

AGENTS	TOXICITY
Adriamycin, daunorubicin	Cardiomyopathy
5-fluorouracil	Myocardial infarction + ischemia
Actinomycin D	Acute hemorragic necrosis
Mithromycin	Cardiomyopathy
Cyclophosphamide (H.D.)	Diffuse myocardial necrosis + CHF
Mitomycin C	Cardiomyopathy
Imidazole carboxamide	Cardiomyopathy
VP-16-213 (+RAD)	Myocardial ischemia
MOPP (±RAD)	Myocardial ischemia + infarction
BCNU	Cardiomyopathy

(Rubin P: Int J Radiat Oncol Biol Phys 10:5–34, 1984)

Combined Modalities

The effect of combining both radiation and chemotherapy has been intensively studied by Eltringham and co-workers,[67,69] and the evidence indicates that an additive effect but no sensitization or enhancement occurs. An additive effect was found using 350 animals and three different fractionation schedules for radiation and for doxorubicin. The histopathology showed both myocardial damage and interstitial fibrosis when both modalities were used. On the basis of dose and interval of treatment used in these experiments, 250 cGy was considered equivalent to mg/M^2 of doxorubicin. The threshold dose of 450 to 500 mg/M^2 for doxorubicin parallels the 4500 cGy to 5000 cGy dose for radiation therapy. Recall of subthreshold radiation injury is time-independent, and doxorubicin administered 5 to 10 years after radiation therapy can produce cardiac decompensation.[15]

It is important to note that the threshold dose of doxorubicin that produces detectable histopathologic changes is less than that recommended clinically, that is, 200 mg/M^2. Bonadonna and Valagussa[21] recommended that the dose of doxorubicin be lowered to 300 mg/M^2 in adult women on adjuvant breast cancer trials using doxorubicin. The lesions produced by doxorubicin are different from those caused by radiation, but they are additive regarding pathophysiologic effects on cardiac function and output. In one of the few studies to assess the combined effect of doxorubicin and radiation, La Monte[132] reported on 20 adults treated with MOPP/ABVD and mantle therapy, studied at a median of 39 months following treatment. Four patients had either a decreased left ventricular ejection fraction at rest or a decreased response to exercise, and one additional patient had congestive heart failure documented by radionuclide cardiac angiography. The mean cumulative dose of doxorubicin was 176 mg/M^2 and the radiation dose was 2000 cGy.

Lung

Clinical Syndromes

The lung is one of the most sensitive organs to cancer treatment. Radiation has long been known to produce dramatic effects in lung, both relatively acute and early, as well as late.[153,158,192,226,227] The sequence of morphologic changes has been well documented and intensively studied at the microscopic and ultrastructural levels.[164,165] Radiation pneumonitis and radiation fibrosis are the two major manifestations of radiation injury. The pneumonitis phase occurs 1 to 3 months and the fibrotic phase 2 to 4 months after a course of irradiation is completed.

Two distinct, delayed lung injuries occur following irradiation in contrast to that which occurs in chemotherapy. Acute pneumonitis, seen after radiation exposure of both lungs, occurs with single doses exceeding 750 cGy with a steep dose response at up to 1000 cGy, resulting in high lethality.[187] This radiation lesion is attributable to ablation of type II alveolar cells and results in early surfactant release into the alveoli. In contrast, bleomycin affects type I cells with secondary alterations in type II alveolar cells. A different but distinct early release of surfactant occurs with bleomycin toxicity and, when combined with radiation, leads to a shift of the radiation dose-response curve to the left.[235] The true late effects of pulmonary fibrosis can be seen both with and without an acute phase. The role of vascular injury is an important aspect of interstitial fibrosis and occurs following irradiation. Septal changes are also seen after drug injury, but these may be secondary in nature, following the alveolitis they produce.

Pathophysiology

The first rather startling occurrence after lung irradiation is the immediate injury to the alveolar type II cell as detected by electron microscopy and the early release of surfactant[192] (Fig. 5-6). These two events are readily detected within minutes to hours and have no evident manifestations, clinically or radiographically.[84] If a biopsy were performed, no histopathologic changes would be seen at the microscopic level, but ultrastructural changes demonstrate that a dramatic sequence of changes is occurring. The latent period often of 1 to 3 months occurs before detectable pathologic or clinical syndromes are seen as a result of alveolar type II cell injury and eventual loss.[84] The next phase, a proliferative one for type II pneumonocytes, occurs between 1 to 3 months, and there is compensatory hypertrophy of lamellar bodies.[188] The late fibrotic phase begins at 3 to 6 months and is recognized by sclerosis of the alveolar wall and extensive endothelial damage with loss and replacement of some capillaries, and eventual replacement of alveolar spaces, and by fibrosis with loss of function.[188] With single radiation doses of 1000 cGy to 2000 cGy, a greater proportion of endothelial injury was noted[164] and less alveolar cell damage, but this was based on conventional H and E sections and light microscopy.[164] Radiation causes blistering of the capillary endothelial cells and plays an independent role in leading to both early and late pulmonary effects, and is more readily detected by electron microscopy.

Sequential ultrastructural studies[169] have identified endothelial cell changes in alveolar capillaries within 5 days of irradiation, leading to platelet thrombi and luminal obstruction. Recanalization occurs months later and is reflected in decreased pulmonary blood flow, arterial hypoxia, particularly after exercise, and altered CO diffusion. The relationship between alveolar type II cell injury and capillary damage needs to be better elucidated. Travis[226] has studied the histologic changes in mice, describing three consecutive phases (acute, intermediate, and late), and has related both the acute and the fibrotic histologic changes to a progressive increase in breathing frequency.

Numerous pulmonary function parameters are pulmonary ventilation tests, nuclear medicine techniques for aeration and blood flow, diffusion capacities and alveolar lavage for surfactant release and collagenase, and biopsy analyses for hydroxyproline content and cellular alterations. Radiographic studies include computed tomography (CT) using density and pixel numbers, and magnetic resonance imaging (MRI) promises to differentiate normal from abnormal irradiated tissues in the intact organ. Serial studies are possible and predictive parameters for sequencing modes and determination of pulmonary tolerance may be feasible in the future using surfactant release.[192]

The potential use of alveolar surfactant lavage to detect later pneumonitis is shown in experimental work on mice.[192] The steep dose-response curve for surfactant release is identical with that for lethality of the mice at 200 days (Fig. 5-7).

Radiation Effects

Single-dose radiation exposures to the lung are common as an incidental component of total-body irradiation (TBI) programs widely used in preparatory regimens for bone marrow transplant (BMT). The relatively high radiosensitivity of the lung was also noted when patients who had survived hemibody irradiation suffered fatal interstitial pneumonitis.[84] Through careful analysis, Keane and co-workers[121] determined exact dose correction factors; supervoltage and in particular telecobalt radiation therapy displayed an increased lung transmission of 15% to 20%. The dose range for lethal radiation-induced pneumonitis is firmly established at 820 cGy for a 5%, 930 cGy for a 50%, and 1100 cGy for an 80% incidence following a single high dose-rate exposure[84, 121](Fig. 5-8). This dose-response relationship is shifted to the right for protracted low dose-rate radiation as used in TBI for bone marrow transplant.[121] In mice, the single-dose survival curves are also very steep, in the range of 200 cGy for a change from an LD_{10} to an LD_{90}.[209]

Fractionated radiation dramatically improves tolerance in both experimental and clinical settings. Wara and Phillips[241] demonstrated that in a mouse model the $LD_{50/160}$ changed from 1365 cGy in a single fraction to 3820 cGy in 10 fractions for a dose modification factor of 2.79.[241] Also important is the effect of dose rate, because considerable protection is conferred by lowering the rate from 47 to 8 cGy/minute.[71] The $LD_{50/30}$ thus changes from 775 cGy to 870 cGy for a dose modification ratio of 1.12.[71] The relevance of dose rate in several animal species has been summarized by Lockhart and others.[139] The clinical data for fractionated regimens have been carefully reconstructed by Phillips and Wara, particularly for children with Wilms' tumor, many of whom received whole lung irradiation with or without Actinomycin. The dose for a 5% lethality ($TD_{5/5}$) was 2650 cGy in 20 fractions, or 770 rets, and for 50% lethality it was 3050 cGy in 20 fractions, or 992 rets. The dose modification factor for single versus fractionated doses in 3.2, demonstrating a considerable increase in tolerance for the latter.[241]

Studies in our laboratories by Siemann illustrate the effect of increasing time intervals and decreasing fraction sizes on lung injury after irradiation. Considerable protection is evident when comparison is made between single exposures and once-weekly, once-daily, or twice-daily fractionation regimens. When the end point for evaluation is not only acute pneumonitis but the late appearance of fibrosis, a similar alteration in tolerance dose-response data is again noted.[198] The appearance of the late effect without an antecedent acute effect illustrates an important principle: the need to follow animals for long intervals to truly appreciate the late effects, much as in patients. The dose to produce late-appearing interstitial septal fibrosis is lower than that for early pneumonitis, regardless of the fractionation scheme used.[187]

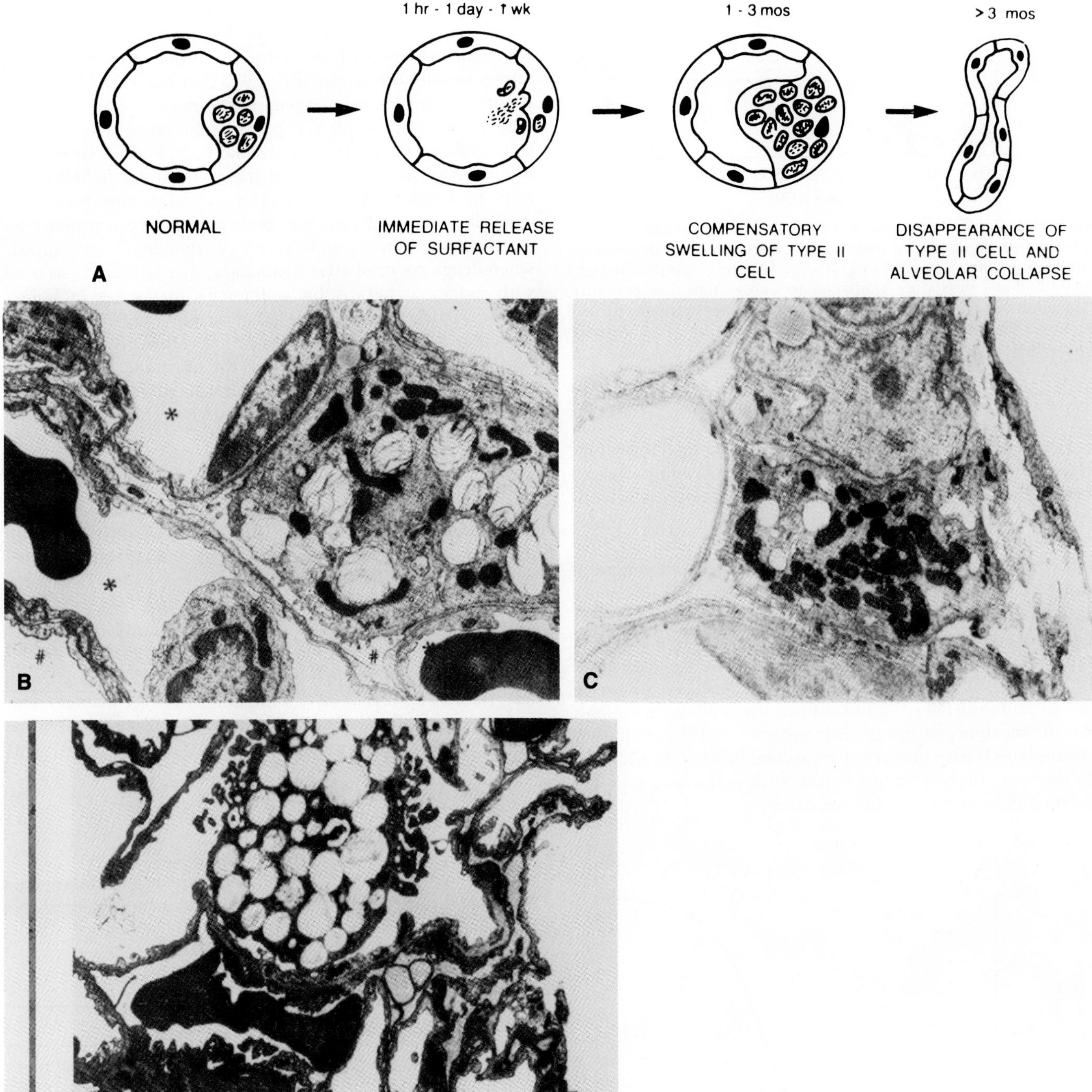

FIGURE 5–6. (**A**) Radiation pneumonitis is an alveolitis with dramatic sequential changes in the alveolar type II cells following irradiation shown diagrammatically. (**B**) The normal cell shows the large surfactant-containing globules in the cytoplasm of the type II cell, differentiating it from the flattened type I cell. (**C**) The dramatic release of the surfactant globules immediately after irradiation from 1 hour to weeks later is shown. (**D**) The compensatory accumulation of surfactant globules in the cytoplasm of the type II cell is demonstrated, occurring months later. The last step is postulated in the line diagram (**A**) and remains to be substantiated in studies: the type II cell attempts to divide and dies. Acute pneumonitis results from loss of sufficient numbers of alveolar type II cells that maintain alveolar potency. (Rubin P, Siemann DW, Shapiro D, et al: Int J Radiat Oncol Biol Phys 9:1669–1673, 1983)

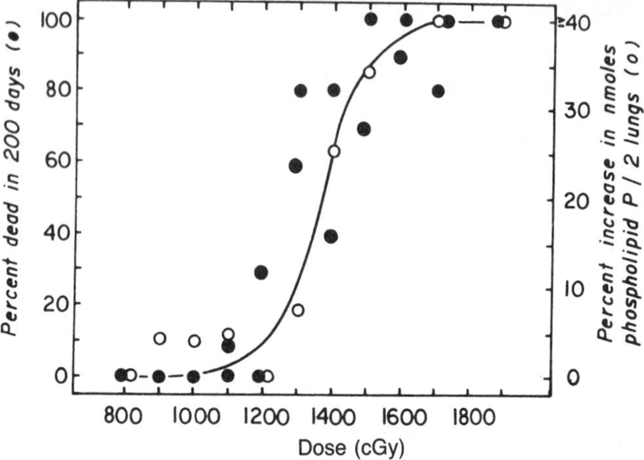

FIGURE 5–7. The dose response curve for alveolar surfactant release is steep, with no significant change until 1300 cGy when it dramatically climbs and plateaus at 1600 to 1700 cGy. This event was detected and quantified at 7 days after irradiation, following single-dose exposure, and predicted for lethality on the exact same dose response curve 4 months later. (Rubin P, Siemann DW, Shapiro D, et al: Int J Radiat Oncol Biol Phys 9:1669–1673, 1983)

Although different experiences are recorded regarding the incidence of pneumonopathy in patients with lung or breast cancer, a specific range of injurious doses has not been identified. To complicate this problem, patients with lung cancer also have pulmonary abnormalities resulting from changes produced by the cancer itself.[42] Assessment with computed tomography has more recently provided sharper end points for the recognition of fibrosis. The dose for the induction of fibrosis is 4000 cGy and increases to 5000 cGy for pneumonopathy. The impact of split-course and once-weekly irradiation schedules on the incidence of pneumonitis and fibrosis has been shown by Salazar and associates[198] and confirms the findings in animals that the incidence of fibrosis is increased in relation to that of pneumonitis if patients survive for several months. In addition, the degree of fibrosis is a function of the dose fractions as well as the total dose and total time for delivery.

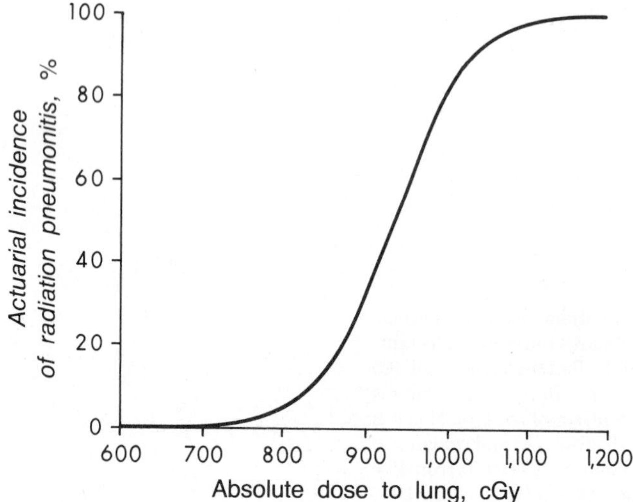

FIGURE 5–8. A best-fit curve based on a probit regression analysis of actuarial incidence of radiation pneumonitis versus absolute dose to lung for patients receiving upper hemibody irradiation. (Keane TJ, Van Dyk J, Rader WD: Int J Radiat Oncol Biol Phys 7:1365–1370, 1981)

Chemotherapy Effects

The dose-response data for both radiation and the more commonly known toxic agents are being recorded with increasing frequency in animals and humans.[121]

At least 17 chemotherapeutic agents are known to produce pulmonary damage and can probably cause a constellation of lesions[1,9,91,188,212,243] (Table 5-2). The most frequently reported agents to produce toxicity are bleomycin and BCNU.[243] Changes reported with fractional administration are alveolitis, parenchymal fibrosis, and interstitial changes. With bleomycin, the prominent lesions are seen in the nucleus of the alveolar type I cell.[9] This, in turn, triggers proliferative activity in the stem cells, which are type II alveolar cells. Further irradiation after bleomycin can heighten damage and add to lethality; this must be avoided when these cytotoxic drugs have been used clinically. The combination of both modalities can produce an intensified response, and "recall phenomenon" can appear when drugs are used after irradiation. Actinomycin D, as used with radiation therapy for pulmonary metastases in Wilms' tumor, was found to produce lethal radiation pneumonitis with radiation doses within tolerance.[137,241] More recently, it has been shown that bleomycin[243] and the nitrosoureas alone each can produce severe pneumonopathies, heighten radiation reactions, and lead to increased mortality when the two modalities are combined.

Bleomycin and BCNU toxicity is related to total accumulated dose. A steep rise in pulmonary damage with bleomycin occurs with doses between 400 and 500 units. In a multivariate analysis by Aronim and co-workers,[8] a 50% incidence of BCNU lung damage occurred at 1500 mg/M^2.[77] Their multivariate index predicts with a high degree of accuracy, those patients at risk for developing pneumonitis with increasing dose.

The presence of capillary blistering with bleomycin and endothelial cell proliferation may indicate the ability of this agent to directly damage the microvasculature.[91] However, as in any serious epithelial lesions in lung, indirect changes may occur interstitially and lead to secondary capillary alterations as part of general inflammatory response.

Kidney

Clinical Syndromes

Rubin and Casarett[183] combined autopsy and clinical data to define different periods in the progression of renal dysfunc-

TABLE 5–2
Antitumor Agents with Pulmonary Toxicity

AGENT	TOXICITY
Bleomycin (±RAD) (±O_2)	Acute/late pneumonitis/fibrosis
BCNU	Late pulmonary fibrosis
Procarbazine	Hypersensitivity
Methotrexate	Hypersensitivity
Actinomycin D (+RAD)	Acute/late pneumonitis
Cyclophosphamide	Pneumonopathy
Busulfan	Pneumonopathy
Prednisone (+RAD)	Acute/late pneumonopathy
Chlorambucil	Acute/late pneumonopathy
Mitomycin C	Acute/late pneumonopathy
VM 26	Acute/late pneumonopathy

(Rubin P: Int J Radiat Oncol Biol Phys 10:5–34, 1984)

tion following irradiation. The acute period (up to 6 months) is rarely symptomatic, and a decreased glomerular filtration rate may be present. In the subacute period (6 to 12 months) the signs and symptoms include dyspnea on exertion, headaches, ankle edema, lassitude, anemia, hypertension, albuminuria, papilledema, elevated blood urea, and urinary abnormalities (granular and hyalin casts, red blood cells). Death may occur from chronic uremia or left ventricular failure, pulmonary edema, pleural effusion, and hepatic congestion. In the chronic period (generally after 18 months) either benign or malignant hypertension is seen, depending on the severity of the renal insult. Chronic radiation nephropathy in its mildest forms may not be diagnosed until 10 to 14 years following therapy. Abnormalities may be only proteinuria and azotemia with urinary casts and mild or no hypertension. A contracted renal size (mild atrophy) is seen on intravenous pyelogram (IVP). When chronic nephropathy is severe, death may result.

The immediate acute period following fractionated therapeutic irradiation is silent clinically. The initial pathologic changes are subtle and spotty and seen mainly in the vascular bed. The essential lesion is a progressive arteriolar nephrosclerotic process. Its rate of progression is usually determined by volume, dose, and time. The manifestations of clinical radiation nephritis may be a variety of syndromes, depending on the rate and degree of the arteriolar nephrosclerotic process. Recovery from acute renal failure does not alter the underlying pathologic picture, and the prognosis remains poor.

Pathophysiology

The initial injury is clinically silent, and the major focus of change is in the arteriolar-glomerular area rather than the tubular epithelium (Fig. 5-9). The cortical tubules rather than the medullary tubules are involved, and this involvement usually follows rather than precedes vascular alterations. Microangiography dramatically indicates glomerulosclerosis as a function of increasing dose, so that complete obliteration of glomeruli occurs at single doses above 500 cGy to 2000 cGy.[145]

In the study by Glatstein and colleagues,[93] radiation-induced lesions in the kidney were detected by light microscopy and occurred as in a progressive replacement of capillary walls and lumina leading to glomerular sclerosis, which preceded tubular atrophy. Larger arteries were not affected whereas glomeruli were being lost. These observations were corroborated by 86 Rb extraction techniques,[92] which estimate total capillary blood flow within the kidneys. This blood flow was reduced significantly but was still variable 2 to 3 months after irradiation. The evidence suggests that a functional lesion is occurring in glomerular capillaries and precedes tubular depletion.[171]

Radiation Effects

The sensitivity of the kidneys to radiation-induced injury is such that these organs can limit the delivery of optimal doses to tumors in their vicinity. In humans, dose-response data following high single-dose exposure to both kidneys are scarce. Fractionated doses of 1000 cGy to 2000 cGy cause a decrease in the glomerular filtration rate, a 38% to 87% reduction in renal plasma flow, and suppression of tubular excretory capacity up to 12 months following therapy. The blood urea and maximum urinary concentrating ability, however, remain normal after these doses.[144] If the entire single kidney is treated with fractionated doses of more than 2600 cGy, a 35% decrease in creatinine clearance is seen at 5 years[244] (Table 5-3). Overall, for the kidney failure following fractionated radiation was calculated to be 2300 cGy for a $TD_{5/5}$ (5% incidence at 5 years), and 2800 cGy for a $T_{50/5}$ (50% incidence at 5 years).

Following total-body irradiation, nephrosclerotic changes occur consistent with progressive arteriolonephrosclerosis due to degeneration of arterioles or capillaries.[239] Glatstein and associates[93] performed experiments in mice showing that single radiation doses of more than 1900 cGy to both kidneys caused renal failure and death, whereas 1100 cGy allowed a 90% survival rate. Jongejan and colleagues[119] showed that in the months following single doses of up to 1500 cGy to both kidneys in rats, the glomerular filtration rates and urine osmolality progressively deteriorated, and the systolic blood pressure rose. However, recovery was observed after lower doses.

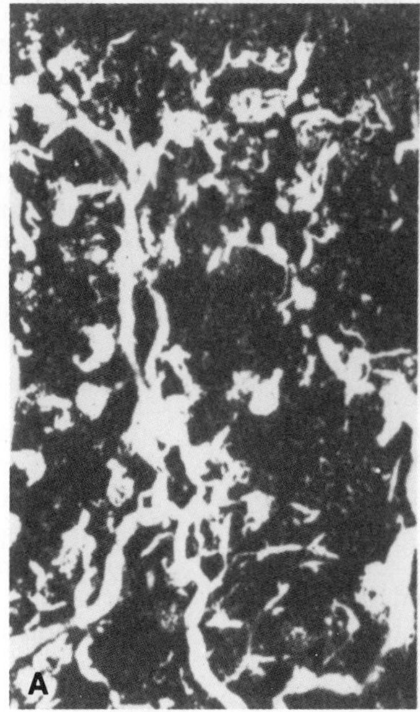

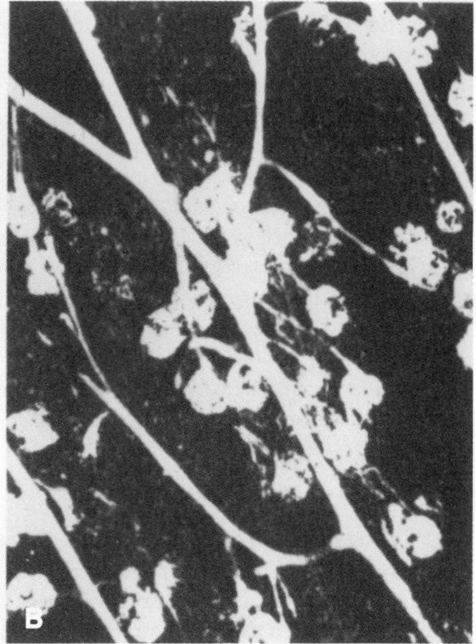

FIGURE 5–9. Radiation nephropathy. The underlying radiation pathology in the various radiation syndromes is due to the severity of the microvascular lesions, which is related to both the total dose and the volume of kidney exposed. (**A**) Following an exposure dose of 2000 cGy, a dramatic change is seen in the afferent and efferent arterioles, with scattered areas of segmental narrowing spotty in nature, and an entire disruption of the glomerular apparatus with a variety of defects and fragmentation indicting damage to their fine vasculature. (**B**) A microangiographic view of the normal renal cortex indicating normal afferent and efferent arterioles with full rounded glomerular tufts. (Maier JG, Casarett GW: University of Rochester Atomic Energy Commission Report, UR-62, 1962)

TABLE 5–3
Percentage Decrease in Mean Creatinine Clearance According to Percentage of Kidney Irradiated (>2600 cGy) and Time After Radiation Therapy

	50% KIDNEY IRRADIATED		60%–85% KIDNEY IRRADIATED		90%–100% KIDNEY IRRADIATED	
YEAR	NO. OF OBSERVATIONS	% DECREASE IN CREATININE CLEARANCE	NO. OF OBSERVATIONS	% DECREASE IN CREATININE CLEARANCE	NO. OF OBSERVATIONS	% DECREASE IN CREATININE CLEARANCE
1	8	11 (±26)	6	14 (±9)	5	26 (±33)
2	18	9 (±32)	4	12 (±18)	12	21 (±45)
3	12	21 (±28)	5	22 (±54)	5	23 (±10)
4	1	—	1	—	6	14 (±16)
5	3	3 (±44)	2	53 (±18)	6	35 (±13)
>5	6	7 (±36)	3	24 (±17)	7	29 (±18)

(Willett C, Tepper J, Orlow E, et al: Int J Radiat Oncol Biol Phys 12:1601–1604, 1986)
Numbers in parentheses indicate standard deviation.

Chemotherapy Effects

Chemotherapeutic changes are distinctly different from radiation effects and lead tonephrotoxic effects expressed as tubular damage.[61, 62, 70, 87, 156, 158, 202] Cisplatin, which is highly reactive and binds to guanine in DNA, produces acute tubular necrosis and atrophy.[52, 62, 81, 85, 96] The major concern with other chemotherapeutic agents is proximal tubular damage.[10] High dose methotrexate and streptozocin produce acute renal damage in the form of a direct effect on renotubular cells, but the evidence for late effects is not clear.[2] Avner and Inglefinger[10] noted toxicity unexpectedly encountered in 17 children treated with nitrosoureas; it consisted of extensive glomerulosclerosis, interstitial fibrosis, and tissue loss. Changes were similar to radiation changes, but "lack the vascular effect." The effect was dose-dependent and occurred in all six pediatric patients who received more than 1500 mg/M^2 and was more common in children than in adults.[102]

The potential of certain urinary enzymes to reflect nephrotoxicity suggests direct injury of drugs to tubular cells. Cisplatin given as a bolus yields a fourfold increase in urinary glucoronidase and may serve as a measure of renal damage. This is eliminated when cisplatin is given as a continuous infusion. The major clinical expression of chemotherapy injury is renal failure, reflected as a decrease in creatinine clearance rather than as hypertension and proteinuria.

The late effects following nephrotoxicity induced by drugs or cisplatin are different from radiation effects. The target cells are renal tubular cells for agents such as cisplatin, high dose methotrexate, and streptozocin in contrast to the endothelial cells of the fine microcirculation of the kidney for irradiation. Tolerance doses are well established for radiation therapy. Pediatric patients are particularly sensitive to drugs such as the nitrosoureas that cause renal growth inhibition and atrophy.[200] Irradiation produces glomerulosclerosis and thickening of the fine afferent arterioles, and such lesions tend to precede the recognition of tubular cell injury. When combined treatment is used, additive or enhanced effects can occur.

Combined Modalities

The combined effects of chemotherapy and radiation therapy have been described in Wilms' tumor patients and appear to be an enhancement of radiation changes.[62, 155] Agents used in Wilms' tumor such as dactinomycin, vincristine, cyclophosphamide, and doxorubicin lead to little injury when combined without irradiation.[45] However, when given as multiple drugs, they lead to earlier appearance of lesions with lower nontoxic radiation doses. Inhibition of renal hypertrophy as a compensatory phenomenon after nephrectomy has been noted by Donaldson and associates[61, 62] in addition to nephritis and atrophy. Changes seen at threshold doses of 2000 cGy can occur at 1000 cGy with multiagent chemotherapy. Doxorubicin can produce a chemotherapeutic nephrotoxicity in rabbits not seen in humans.[75]

Liver

Clinical Syndromes

Because the hepatic cells are relatively resistant to the direct cytocidal actions of radiation and because relatively large doses of radiation are required to cause marked acute inflammation in the liver, the acute clinical period tends to be relatively silent. However, progressive damage in the fine vasculature of the liver may eventually lead to clinically significant secondary degeneration of liver late in the acute clinical period or even after the acute period, depending on the dose and rate of progression of vascular damage.

The relative sensitivity of the liver to radiation injury precludes the eradication of infiltrating tumors from this organ by high doses to the total liver. Following such doses a series of pathologic changes occurs in the liver such as hyperemia, increase in volume, dilatation and congestion of sinusoids, atrophy of hepatocytes, and veno-occlusive lesions appearing as early as 2.5 to 6 months after irradiation.[183] The patient develops ascites, and there is an increase in hepatic size and a rise in bilirubin and alkaline phosphatase levels.

Pathophysiology

The basic lesion of radiation hepatopathy is central vein thrombosis at the lobular level; this results in retrograde congestion leading to hemorrhage and secondary alterations in surrounding hepatocytes[113, 136] (Fig. 5-10). Severe acute hepatic changes often progress to progressive fibrosis or cirrhosis and liver failure.[115] This unique veno-occlusive lesion is unlike the typical radiation-induced fine arteriolar-capillary damage seen in most other tissue injuries[179] and may represent an endothelial platelet agglutination phenomenon.[204]

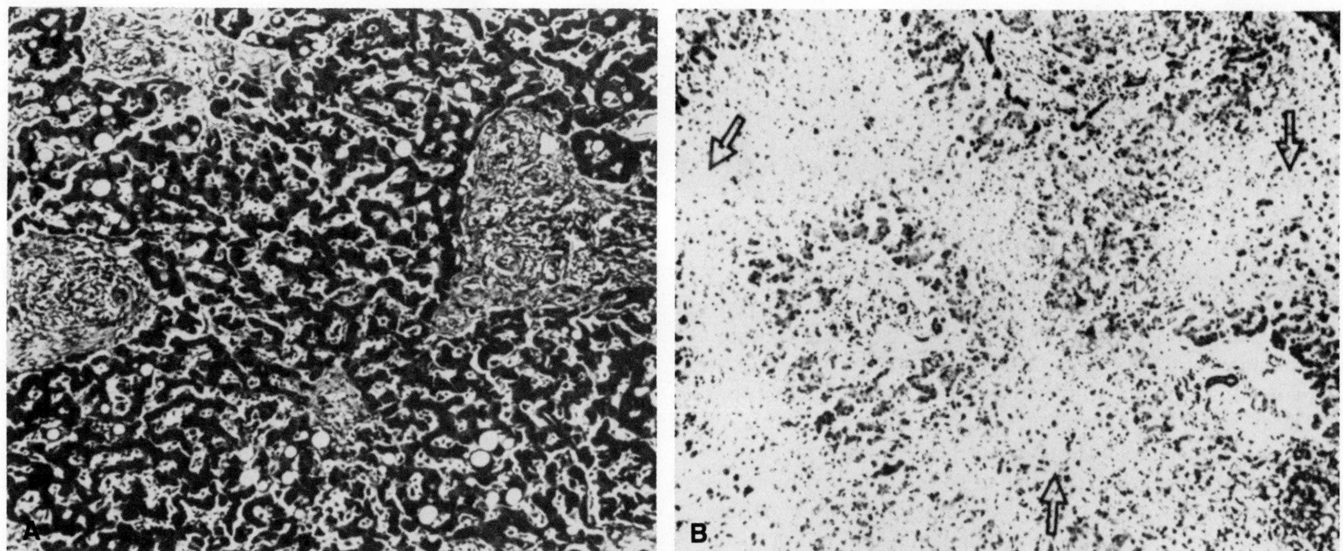

FIGURE 5–10. Radiation hepatopathy. (**A**) The difference in distribution in radiation-induced and chemotherapy-induced lesions is illustrated by chronic radiation hepatitis, showing isolated scattered islands of fibrosis surrounding the central lobular veins and secondary atrophy of surrounding hepatocytes. The rest of the lobule appears normal. (**B**) Chemotherapy (methotrexate) showing a diffuse necrosis of hepatocytes and fatty replacement with a few zones of hepatic cell viability surrounding the central portal veins. The *arrows* point to a peripheral location of the severe hepatocyte necrosis. (Minow RA, Stern MH, Casey JH, et al: Cancer 38:1524–1528, 1976)

Radiation Effects

Ingold and colleagues[115] reviewed 40 patients who received total liver irradiation in the course of therapy for ovarian carcinoma or lymphoma and found that no cases of radiation-induced liver disease occurred below a dose of 2500 cGy, whereas 21% of patients had abnormalities following a dose of 3000 cGy to 3600 cGy, and 42% following 3800 cGy to 4200 cGy (Fig. 5-11). Tefft[220] studied changes in hepatic function in children over 5 years of age. He observed that fractionated radiation doses of less than 2500 cGy caused abnormal liver function tests and radionuclide scans in approximately 50% of patients, whereas 2500 cGy to 3500 cGy doses caused abnormalities in 63%, and doses of more than 3500 cGy was highly toxic to 86% of patients. Phillips and co-workers[168] showed that in adults substantial hepatic damage occurred at fractionated radiation doses of more than 2000 to 3750 cGy, and Kim and colleagues[126] described similar changes after more than 3000 cGy. Veno-occlusive disease is an uncommon but severe complication of total-body irradiation administered in preparation for bone marrow transplant and can occur following single doses as low as 750 cGy.[246] Short, intense fractionation schedules, such as those used in ab-

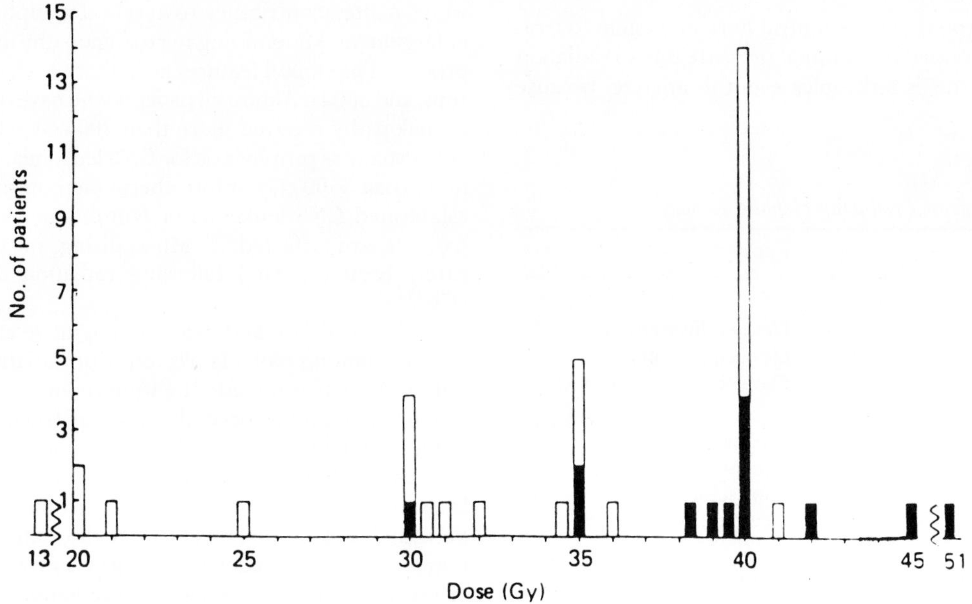

FIGURE 5–11. Dose distribution in 40 patients treated with irradiation of the entire liver at 1300 to 5100 cGy. The incidence of radiation hepatitis appears to be related to the dose of hepatic radiation given. Open columns: total number of patients; filled columns: cases of radiation hepatitis. (Modified from Ingold JA, et al: Radiation hepatitis. Am J Roentgenol 93:200–208, 1965)

dominal strip field techniques for the treatment of ovarian cancer, lower the threshold dose to 1500 cGy to 2000 cGy.[166]

Chemotherapy Effects

Chemotherapeutic injury of the liver[167] leading to hepatopathy similar to that seen in radiation injury is uncommon, although the nitrosoureas can produce severe and fatal damage that mimics radiation injury (Table 5-4). In contrast, the drug acts directly on the hepatocytes, which results in a diffuse hepatocellular necrosis and fatty replacement.[150] This occurrence was reported by Minow and co-workers[150] in 11 adults using a combination of 6 mercaptopurine and doxorubicin. Severe hepatic dysfunction is manifested by elevation in alkaline phosphatase, serum total bilirubin, and glutamic-oxaloacetic transaminase. Similar lesions have been seen with the use of antineoplastic drugs,[167] alone or in combination with irradiation, particularly busulfan, cytarabine, and 6-thioguanine; other agents are urethane,[148] arsphenamine,[129] and oral contraceptives.[3]

Combined Modalities

Another example of altered pathophysiology following liver irradiation is the inability to metabolize agents. This has been reported in Wilms' tumor patients treated on the right side of the abdomen rather than the left side.[36,220,221,222] Actinomycin D and vincristine have a longer half-life in liver-irradiated patients, due to altered metabolism, causing more dysfunction of liver and heightened marrow suppression. The pediatric patient, as noted in the young mice, is more vulnerable, leading to hepatotoxicity due to prolonged methotrexate administration.[4] Rapidly proliferating hepatoblasts induced by hepatectomy are particularly vulnerable to drugs such as dactinomycin, which block repair even more than does radiation.[81]

Central Nervous System

Clinical Syndromes

The initial response of the central nervous system to irradiation may be increased intracranial pressure due to radiation edema. However, this is a complex event to analyze, because tumor-associated cerebral edema may exist before radiation treatment is undertaken. It is not until the subacute period that the severe manifestations of infarction and gliosis appear as brain necrosis or the Brown-Séquard syndrome with transection of the cord. Children in the chronic clinical period show poor cerebration, and mental retardation may follow total-brain irradiation, as for medulloblastoma. However, preexisting hydrocephalus due to posterior fossa tumors causes cerebral atrophy and poor mentation independent of and augmenting the radiation effect. Repeated courses of radiation tend to exceed tolerance, further obliterate the vasculature, and increase the risk of brain necrosis.

Radiation necrosis (RN) occurs in 1% to 5% of patients after 5500 to 6000 cGy doses fractionated over 6 weeks. Above this rather narrow dose range the likelihood of RN substantially increases. In one of the few prospective studies, Marks and colleagues[146] reported a 5% incidence of RN in patients treated with 5400 cGy or more in 180 cGy to 200 cGy fractions (Fig. 5-12). Although the onset of symptoms can be as early as 6 months after treatment, the peak time of presentation is 1 to 2 years. Seventy-five percent of cases of radiation necrosis are apparent by 3 years. Headache and other expressions of increased intracranial pressure are frequently present in addition to focal deficits.

Radiation necrosis is visualized on CT as a mass lesion with surrounding edema.[197] Angiography may show areas of avascularity, compared with neovascularity in a recurrent tumor. Magnetic resonance imaging has recently been shown to identify a spectrum of radiation changes with great sensitivity.[48] Differentiation of radiation necrosis from recurrent tumor generally requires pathologic documentation, although metabolic positron emission tomography (PET) scans may be helpful. Radiation necrosis is often progressive and fatal. Surgical debulking is performed when possible.[245] Corticosteroids may offer transient relief. Reducing the volume of radiation is presumed to decrease the risk for RN. Although Kun's data support such a relationship in children, other reports do not.[54,131]

Leukoencephalopathy is characterized by multiple noninflammatory necrotic foci in the white matter with demyelinization and reactive astrocytosis. The demyelinization of the white matter contributes to cerebral atrophy and ventricular enlargement. Mineralizing microangiopathy may accompany the process. The clinical features are lethargy, seizures, spasticity, paresis, and ataxia. Almost all patients who have developed leukoencephalopathy received more than 200 cGy whole-brain irradiation, usually as prophylaxis for CNS leukemia. Following doses of more than 3500 cGy or intrathecal methotrexate of 150 mg for established CNS leukemia or lymphoma, as many as 50% of patients are affected.[180] Mineralizing microangiopathy has rarely been reported following radiation doses below 2000 cGy.[174]

The incidence and extent of cognitive and emotional dysfunction among patients treated with radiation are difficult to define. Variables include the underlying disease (brain tumor or leukemia) and associated pathology (such as hydrocephalus or increased intracranial pressure) and other therapies (surgery and chemotherapy). Several studies of children treated for brain tumors demonstrate an adverse neurocognitive effect of therapy (Table 5-5). The extent of the contribution of irradiation to these dysfunctions is not clear. LeBaron[133] documented effects in children treated without radiation that were almost as severe as those treated with radiation. Those patients who required radiation therapy might have more risk factors for adverse neurocognitive effects (such as a tumor with a worse prognosis and a higher risk of CNS relapse).

TABLE 5–4
Chemotherapeutic Agents Producing Hepatic Toxicity

DRUG	EFFECT
Nitrosoureas	
BCNU	Elevated liver enzymes
CCNU	Elevated liver enzymes
Streptozotocin	Elevated liver enzymes
Antimetabolites	
Methotrexate	Fibrosis, cirrhosis
6-mercaptopurine	Cholestasis, necrosis
Azathioprine	Cholestasis, necrosis
Cytosine arabinoside	Elevated liver enzymes
Antibiotics	
Mithramycin	Acute necrosis
Enzymes	
L-asparaginase	Fatty metamorphosis

(Perry MC: Semin Oncol 9:65–74, 1982)

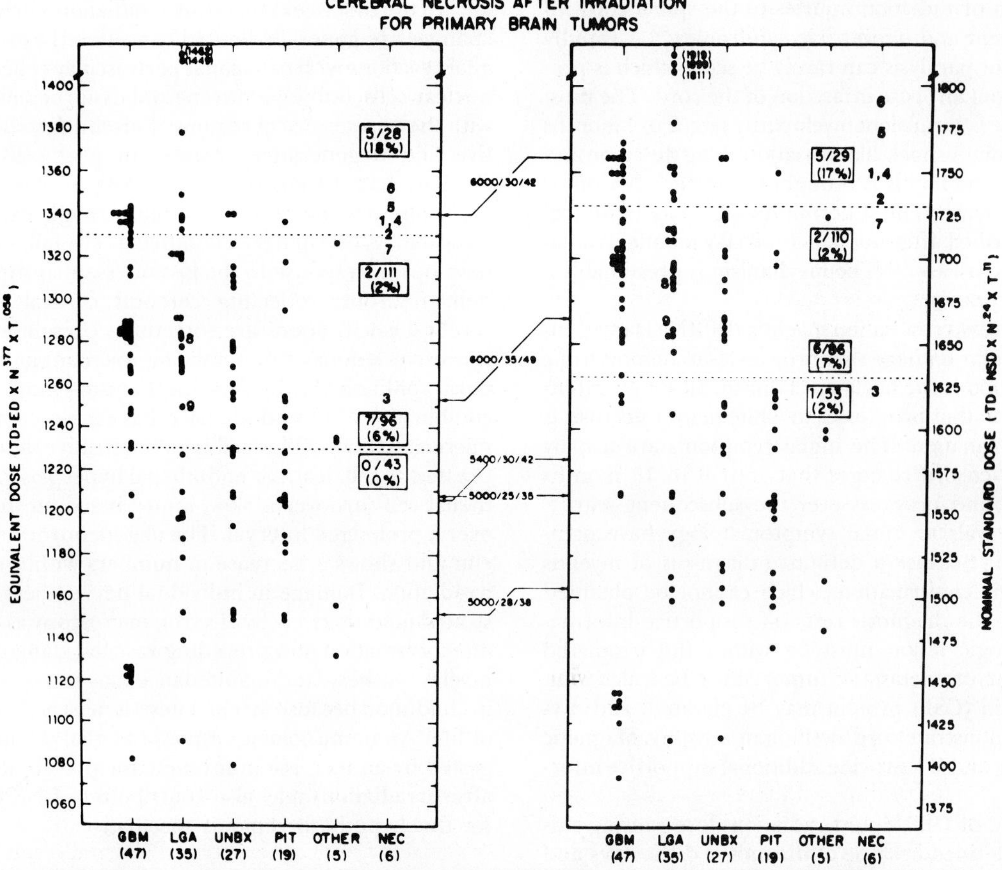

FIGURE 5–12. Scattergrams depicting nominal standard dose (NSD) and equivalent dose (ED) for all patients in each irradiated subpopulation and patients 1–9 with pathologically proven and suspected radionecrosis (NEC) of brain. The subpopulation irradiated were patients with glioblastoma multiforme (GBM), low-grade astrocytoma (LGA), unbiopsied tumors (UNBX), and pituitary tumors (PIT). The risk of radionecrosis (number with necrosis/total irradiated) is shown above and below two NSD and two ED levels, each separated by 100 ret units. (Marks JE, et al: Int J Radiat Oncol Biol Phys 7:243–252, 1981)

TABLE 5–5
Neurocognitive Effects of Radiation Therapy to the Brain

SERIES	TUMOR	NO. OF PATIENTS	RADIATION THERAPY DOSE (cGy)	OUTCOME
Hirsch et al[107]	Medullo-blastoma	28	3500 WB 5500 PF	12% had IQs > 90, 31% < 70; 93% had behavior disturbances
Danoff et al[54]	Several	38	4000–6500	17% had IQs < 70, 56% > 90; 37% had emotional difficulties
Duffner et al[63]	Posterior fossa	10	2600–4000	40% had IQs < 70, 20% > 90; 4 of 5 with IQs > 80 were learning disabled
Kun et al[131]	Several	26	4000–5800 WB 5000–5500 local	8 of 15 who underwent surgery and radiation therapy had IQs < 90; serial testing in 10 showed improvement in 2, stability in 5, and further deterioration in 3
Packer et al[160]	Medullo-blastoma	28	3500–4000 WB 5000–5500 PF	Mean IQ, 96 (range, 50–120)

WB = whole brain, PF = posterior fossa boost
(Modified from Constine LS: Tumors in children in cure with preservation of function and aesthetics. In Wilson JF [ed]: Syllabus: A Categorical Course in Radiation Therapy, pp 75–91. Oak Brook, IL, RSNA, 1988)

The spectrum of radiation injuries to the spinal cord includes both transient and irreversible syndromes.[95] A rapidly evolving permanent paralysis can rarely be seen, which is presumed to result from an acute infarction of the cord. The most common syndrome is a transient myelopathy seen 2 to 4 months following irradiation. A shock-like sensation along the spine and tingling or pain in the hands is brought on by neck flexion or stretching of the arms. This Lhermitte's sign has most frequently been described after 4000 to 4500 cGy mantle irradiation for Hodgkin's disease.[118] The mechanism is presumably a transient demyelinization.

Chronic progressive radiation myelitis (CPRM) is rare. Intramedullary vascular damage that progresses to hemorrhagic necrosis or infarction is the likely mechanism, although extensive demyelinization that progresses to white matter necrosis is an alternative explanation. The initial symptoms are usually paresthesias and sensory changes that start 9 to 15 months following therapy and progress over the subsequent year.[203] Much longer intervals to initial symptomatology have occasionally been seen. Because a definitive diagnosis of myelitis requires pathologic confirmation, which cannot be obtained except at autopsy, the diagnosis rests on supportive information. The neurologic lesion must be within the irradiated volume. Recurrent or metastatic tumor must be ruled out. Cerebrospinal fluid (CSF) protein may be elevated, and myelography can demonstrate cord swelling or atrophy. Magnetic resonance imaging and CT provide additional supportive information.

The incidence of CPRM and radiation dose causing this event are poorly defined because of diagnostic difficulties and the variety of radiation techniques (with uncertain dosimetry). Wara's review suggests that 4200 cGy in 25 fractions carries a 1% risk, 4500 cGy a 5% risk, and 6100 cGy a 50% risk.[242] Cohen's data indicate the 5% risk to be at 4900 cGy.[43]

An increased risk of myelopathy is associated with higher individual fraction sizes, shorter overall treatment time, higher total doses, and long lengths of the cord treated[95] (especially > 10 cm). Children may be more at risk for CPRM, developing it after lower radiation doses and with shorter latency periods.[203] Actinomycin D may decrease the dose threshold.[138]

Pathophysiology

In the central nervous system, the neurons and neuroganglions are considered in their mature state to be some of the most resistant cells in humans. These cells are fixed postmitotic cells and are not able to divide.[179] The vulnerable portions of the system are proliferating cells such as the oligodendrogliocytes, which produce myelin, and the fine vasculature, which, in essence, composes the interstitium along with astrocytes in the brain. Most radiation injuries reflect events occurring, not in functioning mature nerve cells, but in the vasculoconnective tissue stroma (Fig. 5-13). The radiopathologic literature is the classic "chicken and egg" argument, because the biassociation of cerebral and spinal cord necrosis and vessel thickening is evident.[179] Most of the recent literature[19,37] on cerebral atrophy following neutron therapy suggests a new mechanism of action for high linear energy transfer (LET) irradiation directly on neurons due to high lipid content of the brain and increased energy absorption. However, careful studies of late effects in the brain by Brady[26] and on the spinal cord by van der Kogel and Barendsen[234] confirm the importance of damage to the interstitium and vasculature as the major target of injury for both neutrons and photons.

In the first weeks following irradiation, early demyelinating changes are generally limited to scattered astrocytic or microglial reactions with occasional perivascular collections of mononuclear cells. Subsequently, neural tissue begins to break down with the appearance of regions of myelin destruction, proliferative and degenerative changes in glial cells, and vascular changes such as endothelial cell loss, proliferation, capillary occlusion, degeneration, and hemorrhagic exudates. When a critical mass of capillary endothelial cells fail, vasogenic edema develops in response to the loss of essential support of dependent neurons, reflecting cerebral cortical atrophy. Intracerebral calcifications are sometimes present and presumably represent lesions of mineralizing microangiopathy. The three most commonly proposed mechanisms may act alone or in combination. The endothelial cell is essential for patency of the microcirculation. This cell is radiosensitive, and damage is expressed as cell death or endothelial hyperplasia. Because endothelial cell turnover is slow, injury based on these cells occurs over a prolonged interval. The oligodendrocyte maintains myelin and shows a decrease in numbers within weeks following irradiation. Damage in individual nerve fibers can be demonstrated quantitatively by electron microscopy as early as 2 weeks after irradiation and preceding vascular damage.[232] Effects on myelin synthesis and maintenance may be especially important in childhood because myelogenesis is most active in the first year of life. An immunologic response to glial cell antigens (as suggested by an increase in myelin basic protein levels in the CSF after irradiation) may also contribute to CNS injury. Support for this hypothesis remains speculative.

Radiation Effects

A variety of data on the tolerances of the CNS to irradiation is available from animal and patient studies. Extensive fractionation studies have been performed on the tolerance of the rodent spinal cord, with a value of about 0.4 for the N exponent and essentially zero for the T exponent in the nominal standard dose (NSD) isoeffect formula.[112,224] Leith recently reviewed available data on the dose-response relationship of radiation-induced spinal cord paralysis in the rat and found that the estimated dose needed to produce paralysis in 50% of animals ranged from 1900 cGy to 2506 cGy.[135,233] Fractionated doses, however, produce paralysis over an extremely large total dose range. Ang and co-workers[6] have estimated the ED_{50} in rats to be as high as 1400 cGy in 200 cGy fractions. Thus far the applicability of such animal findings to humans in not clear.

The tolerance of the whole brain to single doses of radiation was studied by Kemper and associates[123] in the monkey. Essentially no effect was seen after radiation doses of 1000 cGy; a scatter of focal lesions was present after 1500 cGy at 26 weeks, with a confluence of lesions at 52 weeks. Extensive necrosis with ventricular enlargement and lethality occurred after 2000 cGy of radiation. The incidence of brain necrosis following single radiation doses was also studied in rabbits and was found to be strictly dependent on the volume of brain exposed. Necrosis occurred after 2100 cGy to 5000 cGy to maximal volumes.[11] Clinical data indicate that 4500 cGy to 5500 cGy to the brain and 5000 cGy to the spinal cord result in a 5% incidence of severe complications in 5 years, with 75% of cases occurring within 3 years.[208] Data for single-dose radiation are sparse, but when Hindo and co-workers[106] used single doses of 1000 cGy in patients with brain metastases, 7% of patients died within 48 hours. Following 1000 cGy total-body irradiation in preparation for bone marrow transplant, Thomas and colleagues[223] found a

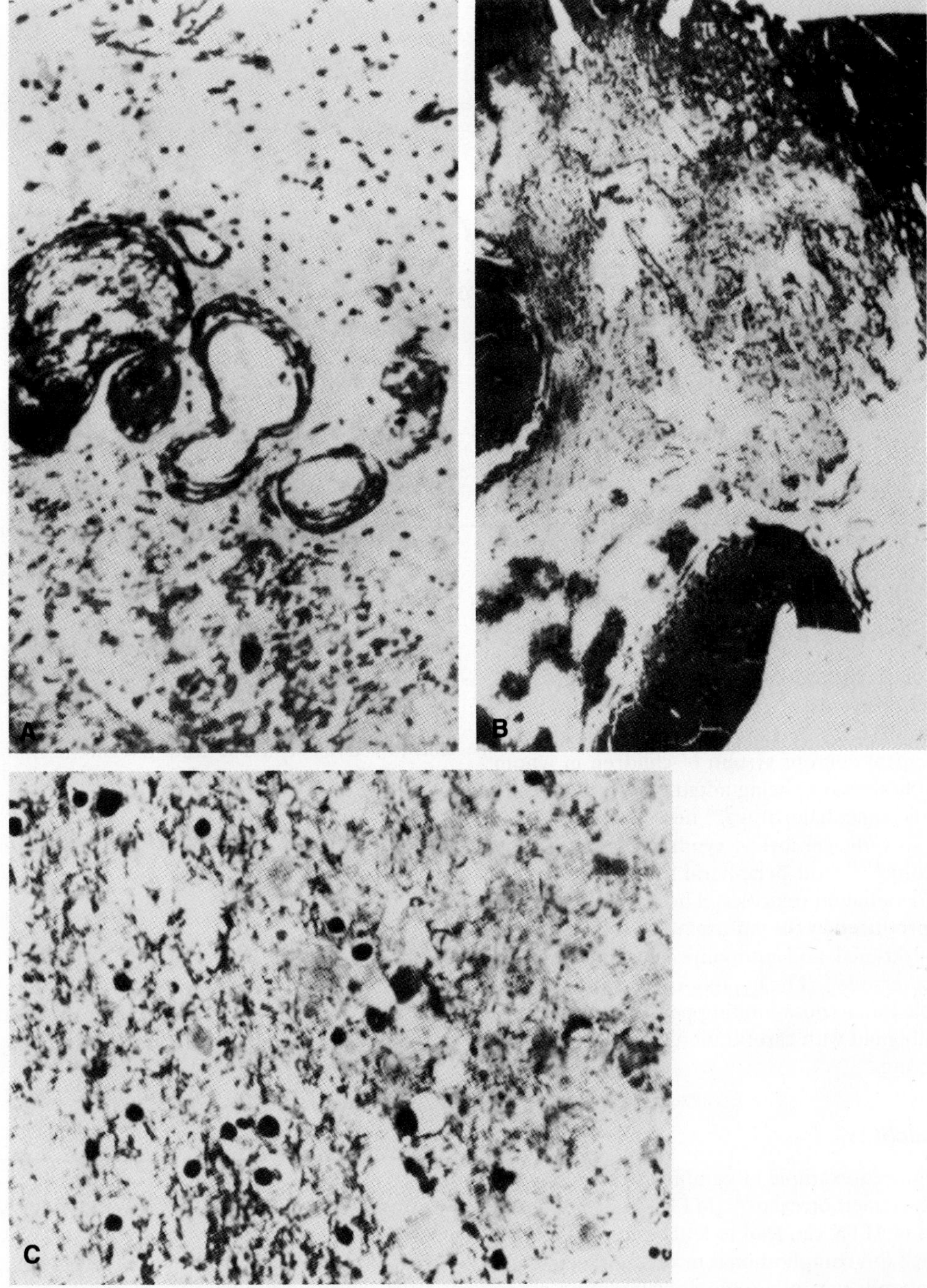

FIGURE 5–13. (**A and B**) White matter necrosis is very common with methotrexate and is diffuse, unrelated to vascularization. (**C**) In contrast, the radiation-induced lesions are oriented around vessels that are damaged, such as the dystrophic calcification of fine vessels, referred to as mineralizing microangiopathy. (**A, B** Bleyer WA, Griffin TW: White matter necrosis, mineralizing microangiography, and intellectual abilities in survivors of childhood leukemia: associations with central nervous system irradiation and methotrexate therapy. In Gilbert HA, Kagan AR [eds]: Radiation Damage to the Nervous System, pp 155–174. New York, Raven Press, 1980; **C,** Rubin P, Casarett GW: Clinical Radiation Pathology, vols I and II. Philadelphia, University Park Press, 1968)

7% incidence of leukoencephalopathy at 1 to 5 months in patients who were previously treated with 12 doses of 200 cGy for acute lymphocytic leukemia (ALL) prophylaxis.

Again, the importance of fraction size in addition to total dose and time has been stressed in determining tolerance to radiation.[12,111] Altered schedules using hypofractionation must be given more weight in formulations that determine tolerance. A number of investigators suggest that the curve representing the lowest dosage for necrosis has a slope of 0.41 and is more than indicated by the typical exponent of 0.33 in the Ellis NSD formula.[111] Sheline and co-workers,[208] in their concept of the neuroret for expressing brain tolerance, offer similar warnings about spinal cord tolerance; these also have been made by Hornsey and associates[111] (Fig. 5-14). Both groups stress the decrease of central nervous system tolerance with increase in fraction size.

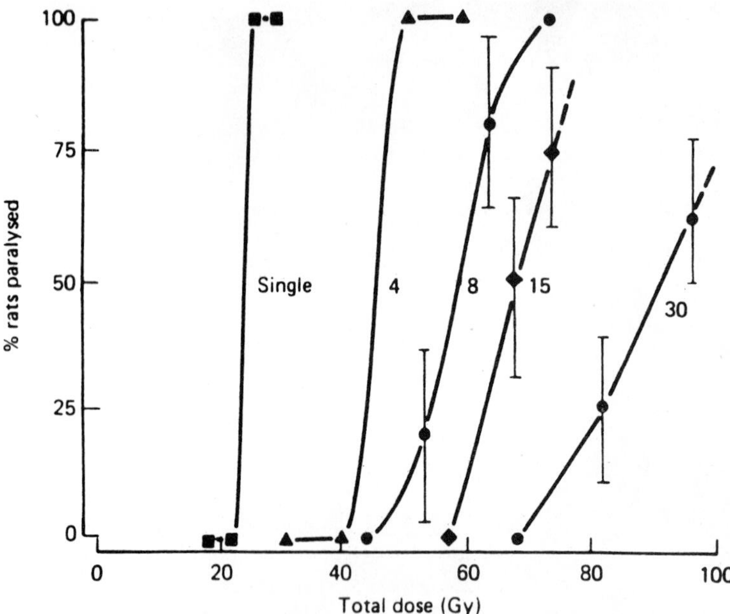

FIGURE 5–14. Probability of paralysis in rats after irradiation of a segment of the spinal cord with either a single dose or various numbers of fractions, all given in 6 weeks. (Modified from Hornsey S, White A: Br J Radiol 53:168–169, 1980)

Chemotherapy Effects

The number of acute and late syndromes related to an expanding number of agents in cancer chemotherapy is increasing[30,71,120] (Table 5-6). A factor is the increased vulnerability of the central nervous system of children in whom many of these complications are being noted.[38,174] Entities such as acute and chronic encephalopathy,[168] necrotizing leukoencephalopathy,[17,18,86] acute cerebellar syndromes,[17,18] mineralizing microgropathy,[17,18] and peripheral neuropathies[71] reflect both drug and radiation toxicities. The most well-known changes are those produced by the vincamines in their ability to produce peripheral, cranial, and autonomic neuropathies; fortunately most are reversible.[71] The hypoxic cell radiosensitizers such as misonidazole lead to dose-limiting peripheral neuropathies that are usually mild with careful monitoring, but can be severe and debilitating.[26]

Combined Modalities

The best-recognized example of combined radiation and drug effects involves methotrexate[18] (MTX; Fig. 5-15). Although large doses of MTX can lead to leukoencephalopathy, according to Bleyer,[17] this complication is most often seen when whole-brain irradiation is part of a regimen using MTX intrathecally[18] or in high doses intravenously. In contrast to radiation, most drugs supposedly do not cause late effects. This has been attributed to their inability to cross the blood-brain barriers. However, radiation alters and increases capillary permeability, facilitating the systemically administered drug, particularly MTX, to enter the brain.[99] Damage to the vascular choroid plexus can alter MTX clearance and decrease turnover, thereby leading to higher drug concentrations.[12] The ependymal connective tissue layer may be affected, allowing MTX to enter the ventricles and the central nervous system white matter. The incidence of injury is highest when all modalities are combined and is uncommonly seem when radiation or methotrexate is administered alone.

The predominance of vascular effects as the major factor in late central nervous system effects is illustrated by the distribution patterns of the brain lesions. The radiation lesions are either in close association or at a distance from the vascular lesions due to their spotty character. The distant lesions are accounted for by the terminal arborization of the fine cerebral vasculature, which leads to necrosis appearing "downstream."[179] The kinetics of vasculoconnective tissue stroma allow these cells to express radiation injury more readily than neurons because no mitotic activity occurs in the latter. Chemotherapy clearly spares the vasculature, but is cytotoxic and acts directly on the glial cells producing diffuse white matter necrosis, leading to encephalopathies not seen with radiation therapy.

Gastrointestinal Tract

Clinical Syndromes

The radiosensitivity of the gastric mucosa is reflected in the early depression of hydrochloric acid and pepsinogen secretion

TABLE 5–6
CNS: Late Effects and Chemotoxic Agents

Acute encephalopathies	Mineralizing microangiopathy
IT MTX − XRT	XRT ± IT MTX
XRT ± IT MTX	Cerebral atrophy
HDMTX ("strokelike")	IT MTS ± XRT
Asparaginases (early and late)	IT ARA-C ± XRT
HMM/PMM	Pontine myelinolysis
Ftorafur (IV)	XRT ± IT MTX
Procarbazine	Neuropathies
BCNU (intracarotid)	Vincas (VCR, VDS, VBL) also cranial
cis-DDP (intracarotid)	cis-DDP (also cranial and VIII)
Cyclophosphamide (?)	HMM/PMM
5-azacytidine	Procarbazine
PALA	5-azacytidine
Spirogermanium	VP-16-213; VM-26
Misonidazole	Misonidazole (also VIII)
High-dose ARA-C	Methyl-G
Chronic encephalopathies	
Necrotizing leukoencephalopathy	
XRT→ IT MTX	
IT or IV MTX	
IT ARA-C	

(Evans A, Bleyer A, Kaplan R, et al: Cancer Clin Trials 4[Suppl]:31–35, 1981)

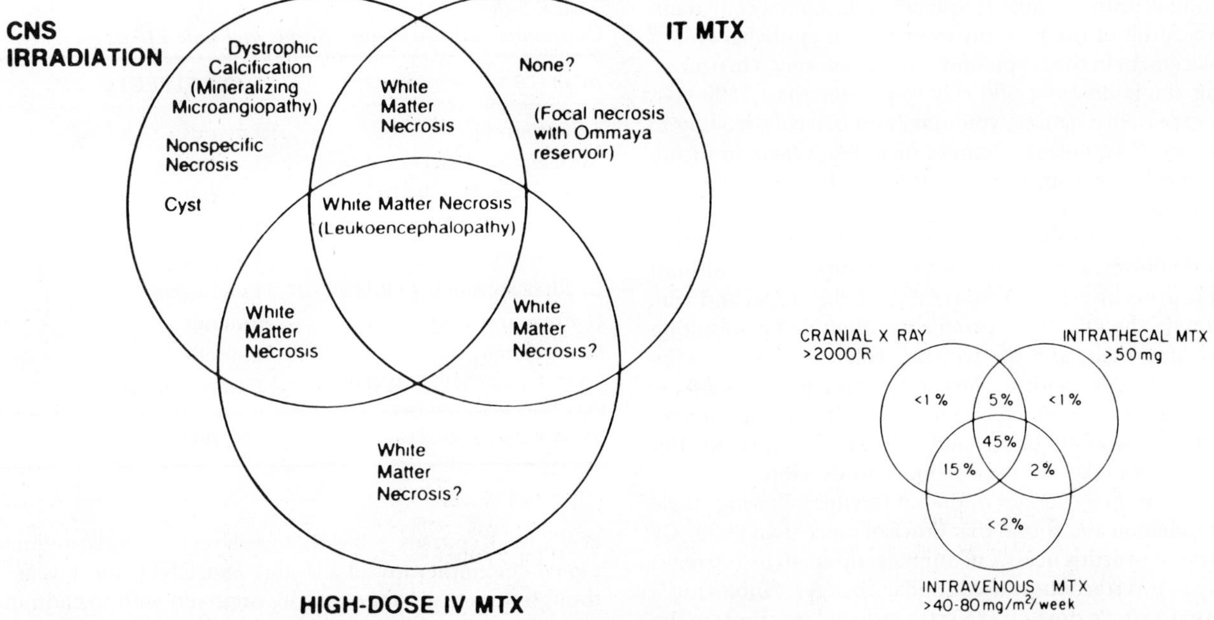

FIGURE 5–15. Encephalopathies are induced by both radiation and chemotherapy and can be both acute and chronic. (**A**) Venn diagram illustrates the pathophysiology of delayed neurotoxic sequelae months to years later, associated with CNS irradiation, intrathecal methotrexate and high-dose intravenous methotrexate, alone or in combination. (**B**) Venn diagram shows that incidence is greatest for all modes combined. In this diagram, the incidence is shown to be very low with either irradiation or chemotherapy alone, but rises considerably (to 45% of patients) when all these modes are combined. The mechanism is believed to be attributable to the alteration of the blood-brain barrier by irradiation followed by entry of methotrexate into the central nervous system, causing diffuse necrosis and damage. (Evans A, et al: Cancer Clin Trials 4[Suppl]:31–35, 1981)

after modest radiation doses of 1500 cGy to 2000 cGy. Although some recovery of cellular structure occurs, suppression continues for a longer time in many cases, yet complete recovery of function can take place within 1 year after radiation therapy. Generally at levels at or above 5000 cGy, cellular and functional recovery are never complete, and the chance of developing a radiation ulcer is high. An ulcer in this anatomic setting can lead to hemorrhage and perforation, which can be fatal. A chronically atrophic and contracted stomach may develop.

The early onset of malabsorption of fat and hypermotility after modest doses illustrates the radiosensitivity of the small intestine. Generally, recovery at lower dose levels is without stigmata although some persistence of small bowel dysfunction and mesenteric cramping can be noted. Surgical intervention and adhesions can precipitate a more serious course of events. With higher doses, the clinical threshold is crossed, resulting in diarrhea, malabsorption of fat, and leakage of albumin into the bowel. If an obliterative arteritis develops, the risk of infarction and perforation remains despite recovery. The underlying lesion is one of ulceration and segmental enteritis that can lead to stenosis of the bowel lumen, with varying degrees of obstruction during the chronic period.

The manifestations of radiation injury in the colon and rectum are less than those in the small intestine after similar doses. The initial reaction of hypermotility at modest levels of 1000 to 2000 cGy rapidly disappears. If constipation is a later complication, roughage can traumatize the bowel surface mucosa. The onset of tenesmus may be obscured by the simultaneous onset of diarrhea if a large segment of small bowel is being treated, in addition to the rectum. Higher doses can cause painless rectal bleeding that rarely is fatal 6 to 12 months after irradiation. Segmental colitis and rectal strictures are major concerns. Fortunately, severe bowel injury is not common because of improved radiation techniques and the monitoring of radium applications.

Pathophysiology

Progressive endoarteritis is the critical radiation lesion for late effects in the alimentary tract. It results in either ulceration and infarction necrosis with more rapid obliteration of vessels or an increasing slow fibrosis and stricture of bowel with gradual narrowing of the fine vasculature.[183] Unlike the acute mucosal loss and gradual return of regenerative epithelial clonogenic clusters in bowel crypts after irradiation, late ulceration is spotty and focal. The long axis of the ulcer is transverse, similar to ulcers that occur in obliterative vasculitis of other origins.[183] Fistulas and perforation are focal and transmural, representing geographic loss of a segment of mucosa and its smooth musculature. The cause of this occurrence cannot be explained by simultaneous cellular hypoplasia of two different cells: mucosa and smooth muscle. The association of obliterative endoarteritis in zones of necrosis and perforation indicate infarction necrosis of supplying vessels as the essential mechanism.[183] Surgical handling of bowel and freeing of adhesions months to years after irradiation interferes with a tenuous blood supply and can precipitate alterations in hemodynamics, which may lead to repeated operations for infarction necrosis, often resulting in death.[183] Mucosal surfaces are intact with endoarteritis as an underlying defect requiring an event such as surgical handling or trauma to result in a clinical manifestation.[124]

Radiation Effects

The gastrointestinal tract includes many organs that demonstrate a spectrum of sensitivities to radiation-induced injury.

The terminal ileum is most frequently symptomatically damaged, as a result of the high turnover rate of epithelial cells[100] (cell replacement in the crypts and villi occurs every 3 to 6 days). Following single doses of 500 cGy to greater than 1500 cGy, patients experience nausea, vomiting, and diarrhea leading to dehydration.[144] Pathologic changes include a cessation of mitosis, crypt cell pyknosis, fragmentation, and swelling and vacoulation of the cells in the enteric mucosa. After 6 to 8 hours, mucosal cells demonstrate a transient proliferation with a burst of atypical mitoses, and over the next 48 hours cell loss without renewal is progressive, with shortening of the crypts and villi. Subsequently the villi show progressive denudation resulting in a loss of protein and electrolytes. Following lower radiation doses, recovery with a chronic reaction may ensue; the submucosa is most severely affected. Collagen and bizarre fibroblasts replace fatty tissue, and vascular lesions occur. Delayed effects can take 10 years or more to develop.[100]

Trott[228] studied changes in the rat rectum following single doses of radiation and found that doses of more than 2000 cGy caused severe proctitis in 50% of animals within 40 to 200 days; 2450 cGy in two fractions caused similar changes. Hubmann[114] showed that a single dose of 2250 cGy induced strictures in the small intestine in 50% of rodents at 100 days, and 2150 cGy caused the same condition in the rectum. The incidence of rectal obstruction increased from 0 to 100%, with increasing single doses of 1500 cGy to 3000 cGy.

In humans, single radiation doses of as little as 150 cGy to 300 cGy cause acute effects with necrosis in the walls of crypts. The tolerance of the different gastrointestinal organs to fractionated radiation is shown in Table 5-7.[177]

Chemotherapy Effects

Chemotherapy alone does not apparently produce significant late gastrointestinal complications with any frequency, despite the well-documented acute toxicity caused by a long list of agents[124,151] (Table 5-8). Drugs such as 5-fluorouracil (5-FU) and semustine (MeCCNU) produce diarrhea, but late effects are seen only in combination with radiation.[56] Nausea and vomiting are caused by many of the aklyators such as nitrogen mustard and Cytoxan and by some of the antibiotics acting as intercalators such as dactinomycin and doxorubicin.[201]

Dethlefsen[56] and Schenken and colleagues[201] have studied the combinations of a variety of chemotherapeutic agents such as dactinomycin and doxorubicin with radiation as to acute changes, but this is not applicable to late events. The absence of predictive parameters for late intestinal events was demonstrated in the catastrophic complications that occurred in a carefully piloted Eastern Cooperative Oncology Group (ECOG) study using split-course radiation (6000 cGy in 10 weeks, 2000 cGy/2 week courses × 3 with 2-week rest intervals) and maintenance chemotherapy (5-FU and MeCCNU) for 1 year.[53] Although no undue acute toxicity occurred with the administration of either radiation therapy or chemotherapy, late fistulization and necrosis occurred in 29% of patients 6 months to 2 years after all therapy ceased.

TABLE 5–7
The Tolerance of Gastrointestinal Organs to Fractionated Irradiation

ORGAN (WHOLE)	$TD_{5/5}$ (cGy)	$TD_{50/5}$ (cGy)
Esophagus	6000	7500
Stomach	5000	5000
Intestine	5000	6000
Colon	5500	6500
Rectum	6000	8000

(Modified from Roswitt B, Malsky S, Reid C: Front Radiat Ther Oncol 6:160–181, 1972)

TABLE 5–8
Gastrointestinal Chemotoxic Agents and Late Effects

AGENTS	LATE EFFECTS
5-fluorouracil	Enteritis
Adriamycin (+RAD)	Esophagitis
Actinomycin D (+RAD)	Enteritis
Cisplatin (+RAD)	Enteritis
Methotrexate	Enteritis
Cyclophosphamide (+RAD)	Esophagitis
Hydroxyurea	Enteritis
Procarbazine	Enteritis
5-FU + meCCNU (+RAD)	Fistulas, perforation

(Rubin P: Int J Radiat Oncol Biol Phys 10:5–34, 1984)

Bone Marrow

Clinical Syndromes

The elements of the blood and bone marrow respond to irradiation by progressively decreasing in numbers due to the destruction of primitive radiosensitive precursor cells. The neutropenia seen in the first week results from cessation of production and rapid turnover of these cells. This is followed in 2 to 3 weeks by thrombocytopenia and in 2 to 3 months by anemia. Recovery is related to the degree of initial response and generally begins with a regeneration of the depleted stem cells. If large volumes of bone marrow have been irradiated, a hypoplastic marrow can persist and occasionally become aplastic. The latter event may also result from infiltrating the marrow and should be suspected if the depression in blood count does not occur at a predictable time or if only a limited volume of the bone marrow has been irradiated.

The bone marrow is the major dose-limiting organ, in terms of its acute toxicity, when irradiation and chemotherapy are combined. Following the sequential use of these modalities, damage may persist, despite normal-appearing peripheral blood counts after aggressive treatment by each modality separately. The effects of chemotherapy on bone marrow are readily reflected by the peripheral blood counts, with the nadir occurring 2 to 3 weeks after treatment.[104] In contrast, the effects of radiation therapy are more varied, as the compensatory mechanisms for regeneration vary both with dose and volume exposed. The repopulation and recovery of irradiated bone marrow is further confounded by the volume-dependent nature of their compensatory mechanisms and the lack of correlation between the hemogram, which is often normal, and bone marrow injury.[192]

Future refinement in assay systems for progenitor cells such as CFU-GM, BFU-a, CFM-a, and CFU-GEMM will allow study of different cell lineages.[83,147] In addition, assay systems for the connective tissue stroma (CFU-M) of bone marrow allows for a means to study the microenvironment essential for normal hematopoiesis.[40]

Radiation Effects

The bone marrow is one of the most radiosensitive organs, responding to total body doses of 150 cGy to 750 cGy with a rapid depletion of vital stem cells within 1 week of exposure.[230] Death usually occurs as a result of granulocytopenia and thrombocytopenia predisposing the patient to overwhelming infection and hemorrhage[5] (Fig. 5-16). The recent reactor safety estimates for an $LD_{50/30}$ are at variance with information from nuclear warfare estimates. Radiation doses of 300 cGy to 500 cGy result in an $LD_{50/100}$, with death rate (and shorter interval to death) more frequently resulting from 750 cGy to 1050 cGy.[176] Following bone marrow transplants, doses of 750 cGy to 1050 cGy are well tolerated, and the microvasculature of the marrow still allows for the implantation and proliferation of transferred stem cells.[125]

Fractionated radiation doses to the whole bone marrow organ are rarely used in clinical schedules except for treatment of certain leukemias, multiple myelomas, and non-Hodgkin's lymphomas, and more recently in the form of total-body irradiation for bone marrow transplant.[13,33,116,223] In chronic lymphocytic leukemia (CLL) extremely small daily doses of 5 cGy to 15 cGy were effectively used to total doses of 50 cGy to 150 cGy, with the total regimen at times administered more than once.[178] In non-Hodgkin's lymphoma the higher dose schedules were more frequently well tolerated, with 10 cGy to 15 cGy being given twice weekly to a total of 30 cGy weekly for 5 weeks to 150 cGy. Cycles of treatment were given monthly and could lead to total doses as high as 300 cGy to 450 cGy; however, severe to life-threatening hematologic toxicity sometimes occurred.[33] A process of titration of dose is essential because severe thrombocytopenia can occur, and treatment should be withheld if the platelet count falls below 100,000. Patients with multiple myeloma and CLL appear to exhibit more hematologic sensitivity to total-body irradiation than those with normal bone marrow, and death has resulted after very modest radiation doses.[13,183] Data from animal models suggest that this sensitivity is atypical. A series of experiments in rabbits documented that small daily doses of 10 cGy or 25 cGy given repeatedly to very high total doses are well tolerated, greatly exceeding the single-dose $LD_{50/30}$.[184] To explain the sensitivity seen in the above patient groups, it has been postulated that the hematopoietic cells in these diseases do not respond appropriately to an irradiation stimulus by an increase in colony-stimulating factor in the serum.[199]

The suppressive effects of radiation of bone marrow are volume-and dose-dependent and are of considerable importance clinically. Knopse and colleagues[128] reported that single doses in excess of 2000 cGy are required, whereas fractionated regimens produce aplasia only with doses greater than 3000 cGy. Rubin determined that doses of 4000 cGy are required to suppress regeneration at delayed times of 2 to 5 years (Fig. 5-17).

Following the loss of bone marrow activity in 10% to 25% of the bone marrow after radiation to this volume, the unexposed bone marrow responds by increasing its population of progenitor cells.[180] In this situation, the bone marrow may fail to regenerate the ablated portion of marrow because the compensatory process is able to meet the demands for hematopoiesis. However, when a larger volume of bone marrow is irradiated (nearly 50%) the paradoxic phenomenon of in-field regeneration is seen 2 to 5 years later, as well as extension of bone marrow into previously quiescent long bones within 1 to 2 years. This is well illustrated by the evaluation and mapping of bone marrow with nuclear scans using ^{99m}Tc-colloid undertaken in Hodgkin's disease treated with different radiation field arrangements.[189] This volume effect is best understood by reviewing the findings after subdividing clinical and experimental investigations into three arbitrary categories and examining the dose, time, and fractionation factors[154,190,192] (Table 5-9).

When less than 10% to 15% of bone marrow volume is irradiated, permanent ablation of bone marrow occurs with fractionated doses beyond 3000 cGy and single doses of 2000 cGy. The ability of the protected bone marrow to compensate by accelerating its rate of hematopoiesis is sufficient.[51]

When 25% to 50% of bone marrow is exposed to radiation, permanent ablation occurs at similar dose levels as small fields. However, all the nonirradiated marrow becomes active and remains in this state of prolonged stimulus for the ablated segment. This is best demonstrated by the failure of bone marrow to regenerate in field after mantle treatment only in Hodgkin's disease after doses of 3000 cGy to 4000 cGy.[212,229,230]

For subtotal bone marrow irradiation, in which 50% to 75% of the bone marrow is exposed, a complex series of events occurs to compensate for the large volume of bone marrow suppression (see Fig. 5-17). The length of the stimulus persists for years.

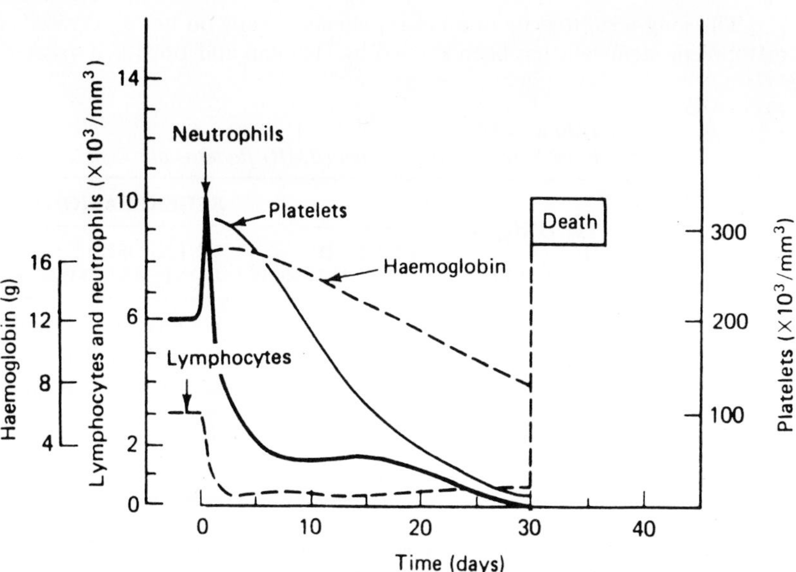

FIGURE 5–16. Expected hematologic response of a human following a single-dose, total-body exposure of 450 cGy. (Modified from Andrews GA: Radiat Res 7[Suppl]:390–397, 1967)

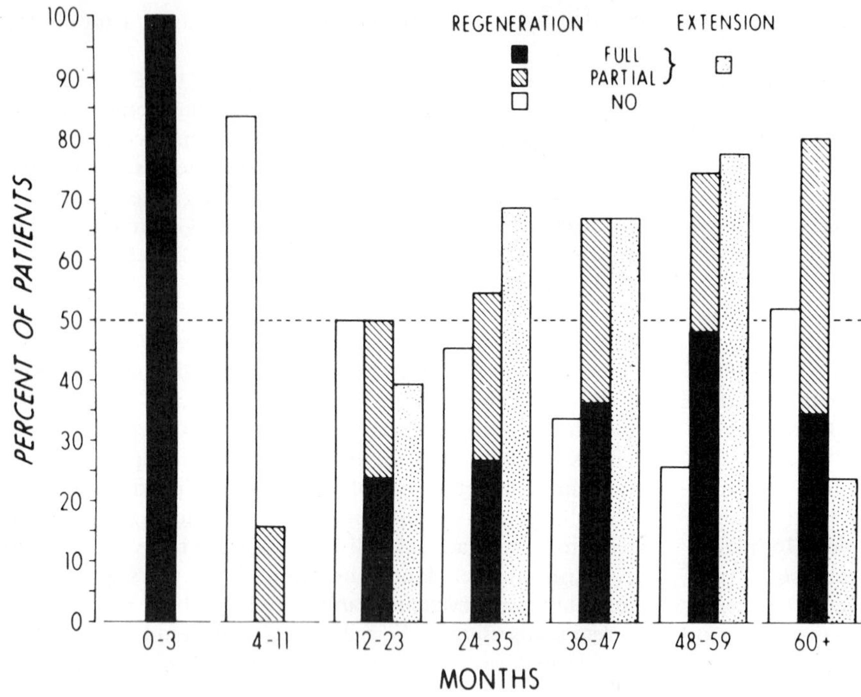

FIGURE 5–17. Radiation suppression and regeneration of bone marrow is a function of both radiation dose and volume of bone marrow irradiated. Bone marrow regeneration is determined by scanning with Tc-S colloid. The bone marrow activity was scored as similar to normal, representing full regeneration, no activity as complete suppression, and partial activity as partial regeneration (see key). Severe bone marrow suppression is seen in the first year following irradiation in patients with Hodgkin's disease receiving total nodal irradiation. In-field regeneration occurs gradually from 1 to 5 years, with the majority of patients showing some evidence of bone marrow activity at doses of 4000 cGy + 500 cGy used in these cases. Extension of bone marrow into the distal femur and proximal humerus occurs within 1 year and returns to normal or decreases only after 5 years. (Rubin P, Scarantino CW: Int J Radiat Oncol Biol Phys 4:3–23, 1978)

First, the activity increases in the protected, unexposed marrow segments. Then extension of the bone marrow compartment into the femora and humeri occurs, and, paradoxically, the irradiated bone marrow regenerates between doses of 3500 cGy to 4000 cGy.[190, 192] The $TD_{50/5}$ is 4000 cGy following large segmental marrow irradiation if more than 50% of bone marrow is exposed, or 3000 cGy if 25% of marrow is exposed. In-field bone marrow regenerates when a larger volume of bone marrow is exposed to higher doses, which suggests that the stromal vascular connective tissues are able to support bone marrow repopulation if the stimulus is large. The use of radioisotopic scans allows for *in vivo* mapping of activity. Studies from different laboratories illustrate similar findings for ^{99m}Tc-colloid,[170] ^{110}In, and ^{59}Fe. Tubiana and colleagues[230] have shown hyperactivity in the nonirradiated bone marrow 8 to 13 years after irradiation. The relationship of the response of various progenitor cells to marrow irradiation is depicted in Figure 5-18.

Chemotherapy Effects

The long-term toxicity of adjuvant chemotherapy on hematopoietic stem cells has been studied by Hellman and Botnik[104] and by Botnik and colleagues.[25] Bone marrow that appears to be normally functioning following chemotherapy is shown to have limited reserve when challenged by additional therapy. Long-term effects on the proliferation capacity of bone marrow stem cells have been identified in mice following administration of busulfan and L-phenylalanine mustard.[122] With use of serial spleen colony-counting techniques, the loss of reserve capacity of bone marrow cells was identified, particularly with busulfan rather than the other alkylating agents.

Combined Modalities

Although MOPP therapy is tolerated after total nodal irradiation (TNI), bone marrow tolerance requires modification of dose. In sequencing the two modalities, chemotherapy appears to be better tolerated preceding irradiation than following full courses of radiation.[113]

The explanation for the poor tolerance of the irradiated bone marrow organ to chemotherapy may include not only the ablation or suppression of certain segments, but also the increased sensitivity of the hyperactive unexposed marrow. With a greater proportion of bone marrow stem cells cycling in the

TABLE 5–9
Bone Marrow Regeneration (BMR) Patterns and Compensatory Mechanisms

TECHNIQUES OF IRRADIATION	REGENERATION			DOSES (cGy)	
	EXPOSED BONE MARROW	UNEXPOSED BONE MARROW	EXTENSION	DAILY	TOTAL
Small field	$\bar{0}$	Local-regional ↑ BMR	$\bar{0}$		
Large field	$\bar{0}$	Generalized ↑↑ BMR	$\bar{0}$		
Segmental field	Suppresses BMR and recovers BMR	Generalized ↑↑ BMR	↑↑		
Total body	Active	—	$\bar{0}$	5–10	>100

$\bar{0}$: Normal; ↑: increased activity; ↑↑: very increased activity
(Rubin P: Int J Radiat Oncol Biol Phys 105–34, 1984)

RADIATION KINETICS OF BMR

IRRADIATED

	CORTEX	MEDULLA		BLOOD		TIME
RADIATION	$\downarrow CFU_m$	$\downarrow\downarrow CFU_s$	$\downarrow CFU_c$	$\downarrow$ WBC	$\downarrow$ PLATELETS	3-4 WKS.
RESPONSE	$\uparrow CFU_m$	$\bar{0}\ CFU_s$	$\bar{0}\ CFU_c$	$\uparrow$ WBC	$\uparrow$ PLATELETS	1-2 MOS.
REGENERATION	$\uparrow CFU_m$	$\uparrow CFU_s$	$\uparrow CFU_c$	N WBC	N PLATELETS	1-4 YEARS

UNIRRADIATED

	CORTEX	MEDULLA		BLOOD		TIME
COMPENSATORY GENERATION	CFU_m	$\uparrow\uparrow CFU_s$	$\uparrow\uparrow CFU_c$	$\uparrow$ WBC	$\uparrow$ PLATELETS	1-2 MOS.
EXTENTION	$\uparrow CFU_m$	$\uparrow CFU_s$	$\uparrow CFU_c$	N WBC	N PLATELETS	MOS. - YEARS

FIGURE 5–18. Kinetics of bone marrow regeneration after irradiation. The bone marrow stem cell compartment is illustrated as CFU_m, which is a pleuripotential cell located in the Haversian canal system of the cortex, CFU_5 is the uncommitted pleuripotential stem cell in the bone marrow, and CFU_c is the committed cell forming granulocytes. With segmental irradiation, the major depression is the marrow CFU_s and CFU_c compartment, with some alteration in the cortical CFU_m. The nadir in the peripheral blood is manifested in 3 to 4 weeks, with a depression in white cells and platelets, followed by recovery in 1 to 2 months. Normal blood values persist for years following subtotal nodal irradiation or total nodal irradiation in Hodgkin's disease, despite prolonged marrow cell suppression. The regeneration of the irradiated bone marrow is very gradual, as indicated, with recovery occurring from 1 to 5 years. The blood count is normal, however, because compensatory regeneration occurs in the protected unirradiated bone marrow, whereas the activity is markedly increased in the CFU_s and CFU_c compartments. Eventually, extension of bone marrow into the femora and humeri occurs by ingrowth of the CFU_m into bone marrow recapitulating the ontogeny of bone marrow regeneration. It is believed that the same regenerative mechanism is operational in the irradiated cortex and marrow and accounts for the in-field recovery of bone marrow. *CFU*: colony-forming unit. (Rubin P, Scarantino CW: Int J Radiat Oncol Biol Phys 4:3–23, 1978)

unexposed segment and acting as a compensatory mechanism, these marrow cells are more chemosensitive.[191]

Full courses of chemotherapy can render the delivery of full courses of radiation difficult due to a lack of marrow reserve.[147] Thus the poorer tolerance of TNI after six cycles of MOPP in advanced Hodgkin's disease requires modification of the radiation dose to lower values. Fortunately, this sequence can be administered with clinical success using moderate doses (1500 cGy to 2000 cGy) of radiation as advocated by Prosnitz and co-workers,[175] with little further alterations in blood counts.

When both modalities need to be combined, particularly simultaneously, split courses or lower modified doses of radiation or chemotherapy are administered in short sequences. This is advocated in pediatric tumors, oat cell cancer, Hodgkin's disease, non-Hodgkin's lymphoma, and inflammatory breast cancers.[175] A short course of chemotherapy or radiation therapy is given as an induction modality, followed by full doses of the other definitive modality. In operable breast cancer, two studies using six cycles of CMF (cyclophosphamide, methotrexate, and 5-fluorouracil) and chest wall irradiation have shown some but not greater toxicity than with CMF alone. The simultaneous administration of chemotherapy and radiation therapy may in some situations be better tolerated than sequential courses that trigger compensating mechanisms. Currently, the choice of the drug combination and the use of combined radiation and drugs depend on the degree of acute toxicity, but the important determinant is the late effects on marrow reserve. Assay systems for bone marrow stem cells may be a better indication of the ultimate choice of the treatment combination. These observations are also consistent with the laboratory observation that limited doses of chemotherapy act as a bone marrow stimulus and may be a radioprotectant.[190]

Other Vital Tissues—Not Dose-Limiting

Testes

Testicular dysfunction in the form of azoospermia or hormonal alterations results from extremely low doses of radiation. It may thus occur as a consequence of the exposure to scattered radiation delivered during therapy for such highly curable conditions as Hodgkin's disease, as well as after total-body irradiation in preparatory regimens for bone marrow transplant.[211,213] This tissue sensitivity is convincingly illustrated by Heller,[103] who documented changes in sperm counts in men after various single radiation doses[32] (Fig. 5-19). The sensitivity of the sperm depends on the stage of development of this cell lineage. Lushbaugh and Casarett[140] reviewed animal data and noted that mouse spermatogonia die after single doses of less than 35 cGy, whereas 200 cGy to 1000 cGy is necessary to kill spermatocytes, and 1500 cGy to ablate the spermatid population. The sensitivity of this cell line is species-dependent, as emphasized by the observation that more than 60,000 cGy is needed to kill mature rabbit spermatids. Moreover, the time for recovery is also different in different species, with rodents recovering more quickly than humans.[213]

In humans, a differential sensitivity of sperm according to the stage of development is also seen, with single radiation doses of 15 cGy killing spermatogonia, 200 cGy killing spermatocytes, and 500 cGy to 600 cGy needed to kill mature spermatoids.[140]

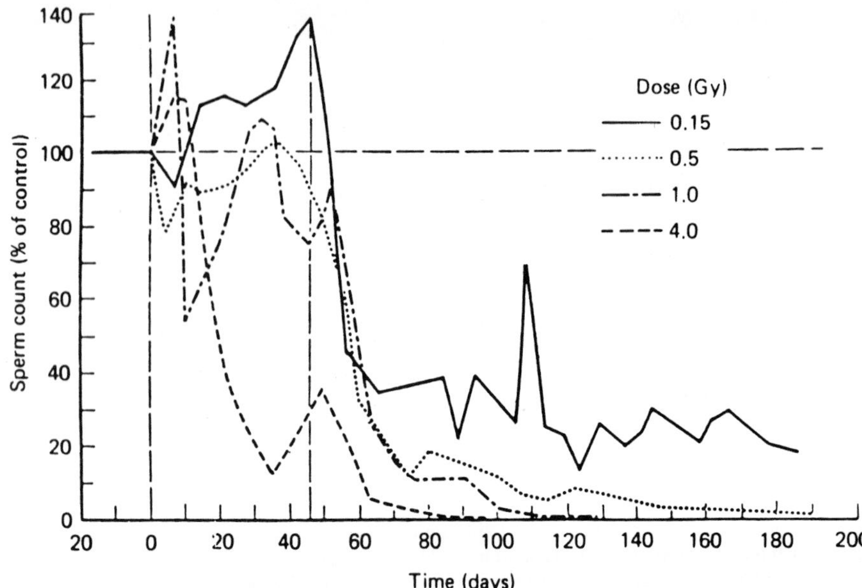

FIGURE 5–19. Sperm counts of normal men following various single high-intensity x-ray (190 kVp) exposures to testes. (Modified from Lushbaugh CG, Casarett GW: Cancer 37:1111–1120, 1976)

Oligospermia occurs after a dose as low as 50 cGy of radiation. Recovery to normal cell counts requires 9 to 18 months after doses lower than 100 cGy, 30 months after 200 cGy to 300 cGy, and 5 or more years after 400 cGy to 600 cGy. At the higher doses of radiation permanent sterility is common; at lower doses reduced sperm count is seen 60 to 80 days after exposure, which is the duration of time in which maturation would otherwise be complete.[103] Because of the kinetics of cell maturation, spermatogonia in humans and animals are more sensitive to fractionated radiation doses, with azoospermia occurring after 200 cGy to 300 cGy of scattered radiation to the testes in the course of treating Hodgkin's disease. Recovery may take 3 to 14 years.[163] In fact, doses as small as 28 cGy to 135 cGy over 45 weeks can cause temporary azoospermia; recovery from these lower doses is more rapid, taking 1 to 3 years.[163] The overall sensitivities after single doses of radiation in humans are described in Table 5-10.

Hormonal alterations after radiation therapy are also well described. Shapiro and co-workers[207] documented decreases in follicle-stimulating hormone at 6 months, with recovery over 30 months, following scattered radiation doses of 100 cGy to 2500 cGy in 25 to 30 fractions; full recovery occurred only when the total dose was less than 50 cGy. Full recovery of luteinizing hormone production occurred at doses of less than 200 cGy. Again, different observers have noted different sensitivities. Thus Shalet and colleagues[205, 206] noted that Leydig's cell function was not impaired following 270 cGy to 980 cGy (20 fractions over 4 weeks) but that failure did occur after 2400 cGy (over 16 to 22 days) of radiation.

TABLE 5–10
The Sensitivities of Sperm Production to Single Doses of Radiation

REFERENCE	$TD_{5/5}$	$TD_{50/5}$
Rubin and Casarett[183]	150–250 cGy	2000 cGy
Lushbaugh and Casarett[140]	<450 cGy	>600 cGy

(Modified from Constine LS, Rubin P: Total body irradiation: normal tissue effects. In Bleehen NM [ed]: Radiobiology in Radiotherapy, pp 95–121. New York, Springer-Verlag, 1987)

Ovaries

When girls and adult females are irradiated, the static populations of mature ovarian oocytes do not repopulate after destruction.[141] This may explain why the dose of radiation necessary to obliterate all the oocytes is larger in younger than in older women. For women over the age of 40 years, 600 cGy in fractionated doses can cause permanent menopause,[103, 137] whereas 50% of younger women become sterile after 200 cGy[103, 141](Fig. 5-20). Overall, a 5% incidence of sterility is seen at 5 years after 200 cGy to 600 cGy, and a 50% incidence following doses greater than 600 cGy to 2000 cGy, depending on patient age.[60, 140] Following 1000 cGy in a single dose, in the form of total irradiation for bone marrow transplant, prepubertal girls showed an absence of menses and development of secondary sexual characteristics; pubertal women all experienced ovarian failure, and 50% had menopausal symptoms.[211]

Animal data are again species-dependent and related to the stage of oocyte maturation. In the mouse, the least mature follicles are sensitive to less than 10 cGy of radiation, whereas more mature follicles are ablated after single doses of less than 100 cGy or fractionated doses of less than 300 cGy to 400 cGy.[140] In the dog, single doses of more than 2000 cGy are necessary, and fractionated doses (30 cGy/day) of 475 cGy.[141]

Thyroid

Thyroid dysfunction may result from direct radiation injury to this gland, as seen in patients treated for Hodgkin's disease with mantle irradiation. This is manifested by elevated serum thyrotropic hormone (TSH) with or without a concomitant decrease in thyroxine (T^4) values; these abnormalities occur more frequently as the fractionated dose to the whole gland increases from 1500 cGy to 5000 cGy.[47, 94] Different series have reported the incidence of elevated TSH to range from 4% to 88%.[47, 59, 157] Uncompensated hypothyroidism (decreased T^4 and elevated TSH) is observed to occur in 6% to 20% of patients. Data on hypothyroidism resulting from single doses of radiation are provided by Sklar and associates,[210] who found that 750 cGy administered as total-body irradiation in preparation for bone marrow transplant caused a decrease in T^4 in 9% of patients, and an elevated TSH in 35%.[210]

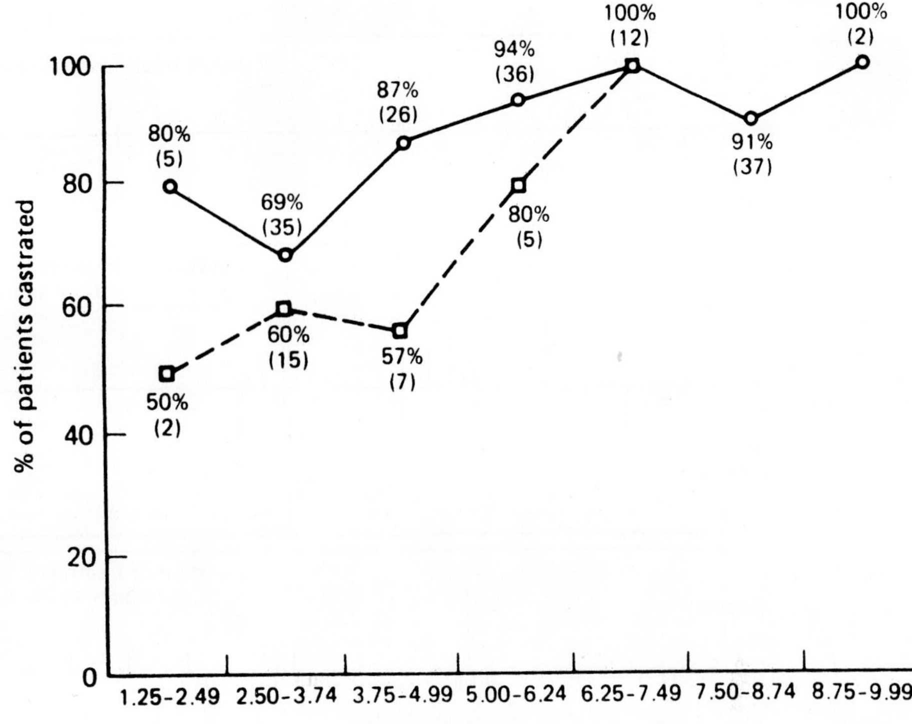

FIGURE 5–20. The efficiency of different roentgen ray doses delivered to the ovaries in producing permanent castration. *Continuous line:* all patients; *broken line:* patients less than 40 years of age. (Modified from Heller CG: Effects on the germinal epithelium of radiobiological factors in manned space flight. In Laughlin WH [ed]: NRC Publication 1487, pp 124–133. Washington, DC, National Academy of Sciences, National Research Council, 1967)

Eye

The eye is composed of several tissues that vary greatly in radiosensitivity. Acute reactions in decreasing order of severity include iridocyclitis, keratitis, conjunctivitis, and blepharitis. Delayed reactions, which generally occur after 6 months, include retinopathy, optic neuropathy, lacrimal gland atrophy or duct stenosis, glaucoma resulting from iridocyclitis, cataract, corneal vascularization and scarring, conjunctival telangiectasia, and eyelid atrophy with entropion or ectropion. These ill effects may follow the treatment of orbital rhabdomyosarcoma (Table 5-11). These several manifestations of injury translate into symptoms of pain and visual loss.

The retina is richly supplied by an end-arterial system highly vulnerable to radiation damage and with limited regenerative capacity. Retina injury begins to be expressed 1.5 to 3 years following therapy. The vessels are progressively obstructed, producing ischemia and edema. Neovascularization of the retina or optic disk may occur. If new vessels invade the vitreous as well as the retina, then traction retinal detachment or vitreous hemorrhage occurs. Telangiectasia, microaneurysms, hemorrhages, and exudates develop. Visual loss is painless unless neovascular glaucoma develops. At 180 to 200 cGy doses/fraction, the threshold for injury is 4600 cGy, although it rarely occurs below doses of 5000 cGy to 6000 cGy. As fraction size increases to 250 cGy or more, the incidence of injury increases.[240]

TABLE 5–11
Orbital Complications in Rhabdomyosarcoma

FUNCTIONAL	STRUCTURAL
Decreased/absent vision 89%	Cataracts 90%
Photophobia 35%	Orbital hypoplasia 65%
Conjunctivitis 32%	Facial asymmetry 51%
Keratitis 27%	Corneal change 27%
Dryness of globe 11%	Enophthalmos 27%
	Retinal changes 87%

(Halperin E, Kun L, Constine L, Tarbell M: Pediatric Radiation Oncology. New York, Raven Press, 1989)

When the major and accessory lacrimal glands and duct are irradiated, secondary symptoms can develop within months and can be fully developed by 1 year. When radiation injury is mild, tearing, a foreign body sensation, and photophobia secondary to corneal epithelial damage are noted. When injury is severe, corneal ulceration, opacification, and vascularization sufficient to cause visual loss occur. Injury is rare below 4500 cGy and common above 600 cGy doses of radiation.[161]

Low dose radiation damages the germinal zone of the epithelium on the equator of the lens. Abnormalities originate in the posterior pole as a small dot. As this enlarges, the center becomes clear, forming a disk just anterior to the posteror lens capsule.[73] This progresses to the anterior pole, and the cortex then becomes opaque. Merriam and Focht[149] reported an evaluation of the dose relationship in 1957 (Fig. 5-21). After single radiation doses of 200 cGy, abnormalities were detected but not clinically significant until doses of more than 400 cGy to 500 cGy. With fractionated radiation, a 60% incidence (progressive in 50%) was seen after 750 cGy to 950 cGy and 100% after 1150 cGy. Other investigators have suggested a threshold for damage of about 2000 cGy of radiation.[28] The interval to abnormality in various studies is 2 to 3 years, but ranges from 6 months to 35 years, depending on dose. Cataracts are seen after total-body irradiation for bone marrow transplantation. Deeg and colleagues[55] reported that 80% of patients were affected after a single radiation dose of 1000 cGy but only 19% after fractionated regimens to 1200 cGy to 1500 cGy.

Radiation injury to the distal nerve end produces ischemic optic neuropathy, whereas more proximal injury produces retrobulbar optic neuropathy. The peak time of onset is 1 to 1.5 years, manifested by visual field deficits or central scotoma.[127]

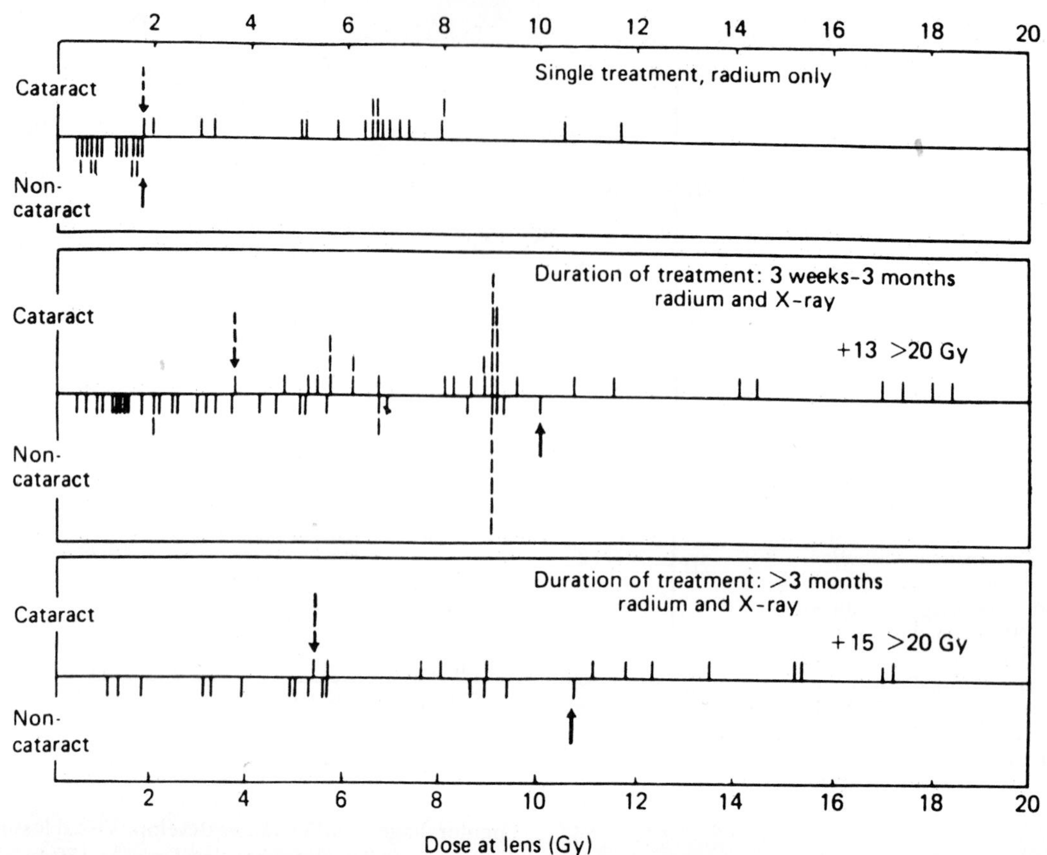

FIGURE 5–21. Doses of x- or γ-radiation to lens in 97 cases of radiation cataract and 70 cases without lens opacities. (Modified from Merriam GR, Focht EF: Am J Roentgenol 77:759–785, 1957)

Injury is rare below 5000 cGy in 180 cGy to 200 cGy fractionated doses.

The lid may epilate after fractionated radiation doses to 2000 cGy to 3000 cGy. Rounding of the lid margins is not seen after doses below 4000 cGy, and ectropion is uncommon below 5000 cGy to 6000 cGy.

TOTAL-BODY IRRADIATION

Total-body irradiation (TBI) with conditioning chemotherapy programs and bone marrow transplantation, along with the incidental exposure during space travel, has stimulated a renewed interest in the biologic effects of TBI. The lethal syndromes that follow high-intensity irradiation are related to the doses that the whole of specific sensitive organs receive.[73] Different threshold dose levels exist for irreversible injury to the stem cell populations of various organs or tissues. Once these thresholds are exceeded, the result is loss of the organ's functional integrity with an inability to repopulate or repair.[100] The degree of importance of the organ determines the survival of the patient, and the time course of the expression of injury relates to the cell kinetics and cycle time of the stem cell. The classic radiation lethality syndromes relating to bone marrow, gastrointestinal (GI) tract, and central nervous system (CNS) failure each have a tolerance dose and time course to fatality[183] (Table 5-12). When the whole body is irradiated intensively with single exposures, death occurs within minutes to months as a function of dose and the organ system affected. Damage to other organs, not directly leading to death, additionally contribute qualitatively or quantitatively to the syndrome. The prominent acute syndromes and modes of death after single-dose TBI are, in the order of occurrence and decreasing threshold dose, the CNS syndrome, the GI syndrome, and the hematopoietic syndrome.[183] Table 5-12 summarizes a variety of parameters of the acute radiation syndromes in humans.

Animal data available on these syndromes are generally consistent with observations in humans. For example, hematopoietic death occurs in 50% of humans in 30 to 60 days following single doses of 240 cGy to 750 cGy.[22] Similarly, the hematopoietic $LD_{50/30-60}$ is 600 cGy to 700 cGy in rodents, 600 cGy in rabbits, 250 cGy in pigs and goats, and 600 cGy in the macaque monkey.[22] For any particular organ-related syndrome the actual threshold dose may not be clinically relevant because the adverse effects resulting from injury to another organ system may predominate. Thus, when the dose is at the threshold for the CNS syndrome, it is far above the threshold for the GI and hematopoietic syndromes.

Clear differences exist in the timing of the development of the pathology that leads to functioned impairment from the loss of relevant cells in the determining organs. Thus, the CNS syndrome becomes apparent within a few minutes to hours after irradiation and continues to express itself during the early parts of the latent periods for the GI and hematopoietic syndromes. Similarly, when the dose permits survival of the patient through the period of the CNS syndrome but exceeds the threshold for the GI syndrome, this syndrome becomes apparent during the latent period for the hematopoietic syndrome. It should be noted that the median acute lethal dose ($LD_{50/60}$) for humans for brief, intensive total-body irradiation is not precisely known, nor is the influence of age or sex. However, this dose has been estimated to be between 300 cGy and 500 cGy,

TABLE 5–12
Some Aspects of the Acute Radiation Syndromes in Humans (After Total Body Irradiation)

	ACUTE SYNDROMES IN TOTAL BODY IRRADIATION		
ASPECTS	CENTRAL NERVOUS SYSTEM (CNS) SYNDROME	GASTRO-INTESTINAL (GI) SYNDROME	HEMOPOIETIC SYNDROME
Chief determining organ	Brain	Small intestine	Bone marrow
Syndrome threshold	2000 cGy	500 cGy	100 cGy
Syndrome latency	1–3 hours	3–5 days	2–3 weeks
Death threshold	5000 cGy	1000 cGy	200 cGy
Death time	Within 2 days	3 days to 2 weeks	3 weeks–2 months
Characteristic signs and symptoms	Lethargy, tremors, convulsions, ataxia	Malaise, anorexia, nausea, vomiting, diarrhea, GI malfunction, fever, dehydration, electrolyte loss, circulatory collapse	Malaise, fever, dyspnea on exertion, fatigue, leukopenia, thrombopenia purpura
Major underlying pathology	Vasculitis (CNS), encephalitis, meningitis, edema (CNS)	Depletion of intestinal epithelium, neutropenia (marrow damage), infection	Bone marrow atrophy, pancytopenia, infection, hemorrhage, anemia

(Modified from Rubin P, Casarett GW: Clinical Radiation Pathology, vols I and II. Philadelphia, WB Saunders, 1968)

with death primarily associated with the hematopoietic and GI syndromes.

Survival after TBI intentionally administered as preparation for bone marrow transplantation results from the infusion of viable bone marrow and intensive supportive care. Patients so treated demonstrate delayed adverse effects dependent on the tolerance of individual organs to irradiation of their entirety.

THE CHANGING ORDER OF RADIOSENSITIVITY

In this era of multimodalities, many factors affect our concepts of radiosensitivity. Rapid advances in radiation oncology, radiation biology, and radiation physics and accumulating information on the interactions of other therapeutic modalities (*e.g.*, chemotherapy, biologic response modifiers) with radiation have an impact on our understanding of normal tissue toxicities. Thus previously defined radiation tolerance doses (TD_5 and TD_{50}) remain as valuable guides, but their applicability has changed; radiation doses customarily deemed "safe" may no longer be so. When combined with another modality, such doses can lead to severe late effects in different vital organs.[159] Factors relevant to defining tolerance doses include therapy, the host, and the tumor.

Parameters of Therapy

Dose Factors

The concept of an optimal radiation dose that provides maximal curability and minimal toxicity is the basis of varying fractionation schedules[66,178,180,183] (Table 5-13). The Strandqvist lines or isoeffect plots based on varying dose-time regimens suggested that an optimal zone could be found, yielding a favorable therapeutic ratio.[214] Although these lines were drawn with parallel slopes, it became apparent to many investigators that tumors may respond differently from normal tissues, and a divergence of the isoeffect slopes occurs.[236] The importance of the volume of normal tissue[142] and dose-time factors needs to be stressed in considering tolerance of normal tissue or organ

TABLE 5–13
Tolerance Doses ($TD_{5/5}$–$TD_{50/5}$) to Whole Organ Irradiation

SINGLE DOSE (cGy)		FRACTIONATED DOSE (cGy)	
Lymphoid	200–500	Testes	100–200
Bone marrow	200–1000	Ovary	600–1000
Ovary	200–600	Eye (lens)	600–1200
Testes	200–1000	Lung	2000–3000
Eye (lens)	200–1000	Kidney	2000–3000
Lung	700–1000	Liver	3500–4000
Gastrointestinal	500–1000	Skin	3000–4000
Colorectal	1000–2000	Thyroid	3000–4000
Kidney	1000–2000	Heart	4000–5000
Bone marrow	1500–2000	Lymphoid	4000–5000
Heart	1800–2000	Bone marrow	4000–5000
Liver	1500–2000	Gastrointestinal	5000–6000
Mucosa	500–2000	VCTS*	5000–6000
VCTS*	1000–2000	Spinal cord	5000–6000
Skin	1500–2000	Peripheral nerve	6500–7700
Peripheral nerve	1500–2000	Mucosa	6500–7700
Spinal cord	1500–2000	Brain	6000–7000
Brain	1500–2500	Bone and cartilage	>7000
Bone and cartilage	>3000	Muscle	>7000
Muscle	>3000		

* *Vasculoconnective tissue systems*
(Modified from Rubin P: The law and order of radiation sensitivity, absolute vs relative. In Vaeth JM, Meyer JL [eds]: Radiation Tolerance of Normal Tissues, vol 23. Basel, Karger, 1989)

effects. Accordingly, a tabulation of the changing order of radiosensitivity is mainly based on dose, but volume is also considered. Another new modality—intraoperative radiation therapy—has led to the use of large single doses to large tissue volumes and has provided new insights into the tolerance dose.

Currently, the prescribed tolerance dose is at best a calculated estimate of the TD_5 and TD_{50}, based on recorded human and animal data.[73,100,183] The complication probability for either 5% (TD_5) and 50% (TD_{50}) assumes uniform irradiation of all or part of an organ, conventional fractionation schedules (180 to 200 cGy/fraction and five fractions/week), relatively normal organ function as a baseline, no adjuvant drugs or surgical manipulations, and age ranges that exclude children and the elderly. Because the literature is not always complete or precise,[73,183] extrapolation is inevitably involved in using either clinical or experimental animal data. The dose levels are rounded off rather than offering doses to one or two decimals, as is occasionally reported. Such accuracy can be as misleading as the general estimates of tolerance doses offered.

The following are single radiation doses to whole organs[49] (Table 5-14):

100 cGy to 1000 cGy. The cells most affected are those of lymphoid tissue, lymphocytes, bone marrow, hematopoietic stem cells, lens epithelium, ovarian oocyte, testes spermatogonia, lung type II cells and GI epithilium and villi. Most include rapidly dividing stem cells and are directly affected without injury to the microvasculature or connective tissue stroma.

1000 cGy to 2000 cGy. Most other organ systems respond to radiation, including the upper aerodigestive mucosa, kidney, heart, liver, peripheral nerves, spinal cord, and brain. Skin probably would be affected as well. These are deliberately listed as organs with effects related to both radiation damage to microcirculation and connective tissue interstitium, as well as parenchymal cells. Because of the large single doses of radiation used, it is difficult to differentiate the impact of indirect vascular injury from direct effects on parenchymal cells that are often slowly cycling.

>2000 cGy. At doses greater than 2000 cGy, a number of otherwise radioresistant structures may be affected, including bone and cartilage, muscle, endocrine organs such as the pituitary and adrenals, reproductive organs such as the uterus and prostate, and other organs such as the pancreas and biliary system.

For fractionated doses for whole and partial organ volumes[49,183,193] see Table 5-15. The greatest clinical experience is with limited field irradiation to part of an organ, and has provided insights into tissue/organ radiation sensitivity. Many dose

TABLE 5–14
Tolerance Doses (Single Dose—Whole Organ)

TARGET CELL	COMPLICATION END POINT	DOSE RANGE (cGy) TD_5–TD_{50}
RANGE: 100 TO 1000 cGy		
Lymphoid and lymphocytes	Lymphopenia	200–500
Bone marrow hematopoietic stem cells	Aplasia	200–1000
Lens epithelium	Cataract	200–800
Ovarian oocytes	Sterility	200–600
Testes spermatogonia	Sterility	200–600
Lung type II cells	Pneumonitis	700–1000
Gastrointestinal epithelial cells	Enteritis	500–1000
RANGE: 1000 TO 2000 cGy		
Range: 1000 to 2000 cGy		
Colorectal epithelial cells	Colitis	1000–2000
Upper aerodigestive mucosa	Mucositis	1500–2000
Kidney	Nephritis	1100–1900
Heart	Carditis	1800–2000
Liver	Hepatitis	1500–2000
Peripheral nerve	Neuropathy	1500–2000
Spinal cord	Myelopathy	1500–2000
Brain	Encephalopathy	1500–2000
Microcirculation	Vasculitis	1500–2000
Connective tissue stroma	Inflammation	1500–2000
RANGE: >2000 cGy		
Bone and cartilage	Osteitis/fracture	>2000
Muscle	Myositis/myopathy	>2000
Endocrines: pituitary/adrenals	Hypopituitarism	>2000
Pancreas	Addisonian	>2000
	Pancreatitis/diabetes	>2000

(Rubin P: The law and order of radiation sensitivity, absolute vs relative. In Vaeth JM, Meyer JL [eds]: Radiation Tolerance of Normal Tissues, vol 23. Basel, Karger, 1989)

TABLE 5–15
Tolerance Doses TD_5–TD_{50} (Fractionated Dose—Whole or Partial Organ)

TARGET CELL	COMPLICATION END POINT	DOSE RANGE (cGy) TD_5–TD_{50}
RANGE: 200 TO 1000 cGy		
Lymphocytes and lymphoid	Lymphopenia	200–1000
Testes spermatogonia	Sterility	100–200
Ovarian oocytes	Sterility	600–1000
Diseased bone marrow (CLL or multiple myeloma)	Severe leukopenia and thrombocytopenia	300–500
RANGE: 1000 TO 2000 cGy		
Lens	Cataract	600–1200
Bone marrow stem cell	Acute aplasia	1500–2000
RANGE: 2000 TO 3000 cGy		
Kidney: renal glomeruli	Arterionephrosclerosis	2300–2800
Lung: type II: VCTS	Pneumonitis/fibrosis	2000–3000
RANGE: 3000 TO 4000 cGy		
Liver central veins	Hepatopathy	3500–4000
Bone marrow	Hypoplasia	2500–3500
RANGE: 4000 TO 5000 cGy		
Heart/whole organ	Pericarditis and pancarditis	4300–5000
Bone marrow microenvironments, sinusitis	Permanent aplasia	4500–5000
RANGE: 5000 TO 6000 cGy		
Gastrointestinal	Infarction necrosis	5000–5500
Heart/partial organ	Cardiomyopathy	5500–6500
Spinal cord	Myelopathy	5000–6000
Brain	Encephalopathy	5400–7000
RANGE: >6000 TO 7000 cGy		
Mucosa (UAD)	Ulcer	6500–7500
Rectum	Ulcer	6500–7500
Bladder	Ulcer	6500–7500
Mature bones	Fracture	6500–7000
Pancreas	Pancreatitis	

VCTS: vasculoconnective tissue systems; UAD: upper aerodigestive tract
(Rubin P: The law and order of radiation sensitivity, absolute vs relative. In Vaeth JM, Meyer JL [eds]: Radiation Tolerance of Normal Tissues, vol 23. Basel, Karger, 1989)

ranges have been avoided in humans, and only animal data exist as guides. Unfortunately large fraction sizes and shorter time intervals are often employed in experiments and are different from conventional clinical schedules where 200 cGy daily and 1000 cGy weekly are the standard.

Volume Factors[142]

The volume of an irradiated organ or tissue may be as important as the fractionation effect in determining the total dose prescribed. Paterson[162] first quantified the impact of volume on radiation response of normal skin, showing an inverse relationship of dose and volume using similar fractionation schemata. Von Essen[236] demonstrated that an increase in the volume of tumor and normal skin leads to an adverse therapeutic ratio because the slopes for tumor curability and normal tissue tolerance were different. Fractionation of dose resulted in favorable therapeutic ratios for skin tumors less than 3 cm^2 but were virtually impossible to achieve for volumes exceeding 100 cm^2.

The concept of a "tolerance volume" (TV) needs to be defined just as tolerance dose was defined. The volume is most critical to the outcome of injury. Generally it is clinically safe to obliterate a certain volume of a vital organ with large doses, that is, exceeding the TD_{90-100}, similar to surgical resection (Table 5-16). Loss of the volume does not affect organ survival because the organ can offer compensation for such loss through regeneration or hypertrophy and remain functional for survival despite being impaired. The following definitions are used.

Tolerance volume, 5% to 25%, is reached when 5% to 25% of the organ volume irradiated can result in a life-threatening or lethal complication.

Tolerance volume, 50% to 90%, is reached when 50% to 90% of the organ volume irradiated can result in a life-threatening or lethal complication.

These tolerance volumes are generally the two levels of critical volumes for the dose-limiting or vital organs defined as class I (essential for survival). Only the GI tract and the central nervous system can have disastrous outcomes after small vol-

TABLE 5–16
Volume Effects

	% ABLATED COMPATIBLE WITH DETECTABLE EFFECT	% ABLATED INCOMPATIBLE WITH SURVIVAL	LETHAL EVENT
Bone marrow	<25	>75–100	+
Ovary	50	100	0
Testes	50	100	0
Lens	<25	>75–100	0
Lung	25–50	>75–100	+
GI	>5	?	+
Kidney	50	76	+
Heart	25	>75–100	+
Liver	25–50	>75–100	+
Mucosa	25–50	>75–100	+
Peripheral nerve	>5	?	0
Spinal cord	>5	?	+
Brain	>5	>50–100	+
Bone/cartilage	>10	?	0

(Rubin P: The law and order of radiation sensitivity, absolute vs relative. In Vaeth JM, Meyer JL [eds]: Radiation Tolerance of Normal Tissues, vol 23. Basel, Karger, 1989)

umes (TV_{5-25}) are exposed to doses exceeding tolerance (TD_{5-50}). It is important to note that necrotic bowel can be resected and on occasion necrotic foci can be successfully resected in brain. For the majority of organs often considered dose-limiting, such as bone marrow, lung, kidney, and probably heart and liver, high doses to smaller volumes are tolerated. Such organs may decompensate when more than 50% of the total volume (as applied to paired organs) is exceeded.

The dose-volume histogram is being adopted by numerous investigators to predict unfavorable outcomes as a result of volume loss in a critical structure[41] (Fig. 5-22). Thus the dose-response curves for an individual organ change is a function of volume and dose. With computerized 3D dosimetry programs, each patient's customized radiation therapy should be considered as a complete dose-response curve, rather than as one point on a dose-response curve.

Volume-modifying factors (VMF) and dose-modifying factors (DMF), can be approximated for different vital organs. Although it is beyond the scope of this chapter to present an accurate analysis of these data, the basis for such a determination is provided. These modifying factors are defined as follows:

$$\text{VMF} = \frac{TD_{5-50} \text{ for partial organ irradiation}}{TD_{5-50} \text{ for whole organ irradiation}}$$

$$\text{DMF} = \frac{TD_{5-50} \text{ for fractionated irradiation}}{TD_{5-50} \text{ for single dose irradiation}}$$

According to Lyman and colleagues,[142, 143] many authors have offered a simple model for dependence of dose on irradiated volume to cause a specified complication. This is a power-law relationship of the form:

$$TD(V) = TD(1)V^n$$

where TD = tolerance dose, V = the fraction of the volume (or the ratio of the size of irradiated tissue to some reference size), and n = a size-dependent parameter. Furthermore, Lyman presented a three-parameter model that connects the three variables of interest: complication probability (P), dose (D), and volume (V), expressed as follows:

$$P = \frac{1}{\sqrt{2\pi}} \int_{-\infty}^{t_{max}} e^{-t^2/2}\, dt$$

where $t = (D - TD_{50}(V)/(V))$ and $(V) = m^*TD_{50}(V)$. Equation 1 is used to obtain $TD_{50}(V)$, and m is the third free parameter to be determined by the data. This formula is a combination of the power law dose-volume relationship (equation 1) and an error function representation of the complication dose relationship, and gives back these equations if complication probability or volume, respectively, is held constant.

The 3D display relating dose and volume to the probability of complications is important to this clinical concept[143] (Fig. 5-23). The dose-response curve and its steepness vary as a function of volume, and organ tolerance should not be viewed or expressed simply as a function of dose; that is, a large number of dose-response curves express organ tolerance according to the volume of the irradiated organ. The probability of 5% or 50% complication rate is plotted in Figure 5-24, which graphically demonstrates that as the volume decreases, the dose required to produce a complication increases.[142]

Uniform Toxicity Scoring

To conclude on an important pragmatic note, there is a need to develop a uniform toxicity scoring for late effects.[185, 195] The introduction of multimodal management to cancer treatment has resulted in differences in reporting toxicity to treatment. The radiation oncologist in contrast to the medical oncologist is more aware of the importance of late effects after the acute phase of the reaction has been managed. However, chemotherapy produces late effects similar to those for irradiation, and these complications have been increasingly documented in the literature. Yet the focus remains on relatively acute and subacute effects. As a result, two different scoring and grading systems for toxicity have emerged. The radiation scores have

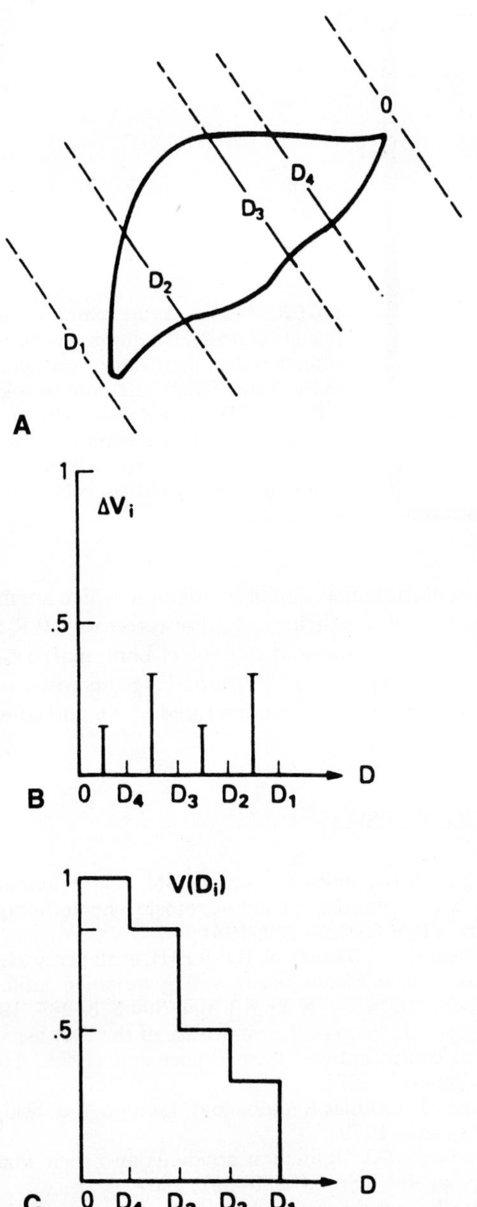

FIGURE 5–22. Creation of a dose-volume histogram. (**A**) Representation of the three-dimensional distribution of doses within a planar isodose map for the organ. Broken lines show isodose lines outside the organ under consideration. Note the convention that the index i on D_i increases with decreasing dose. (**B**) Differential dose-volume histogram derived from a complete set of such maps. (**C**) Equivalent integral, or dose-cumulative-volume, histogram. $V(D_i)$ refers to the fraction of the organ receiving dose D_i or more. (Lyman JT: Radiat Res 104[Suppl 8]: S13–S19, 1985)

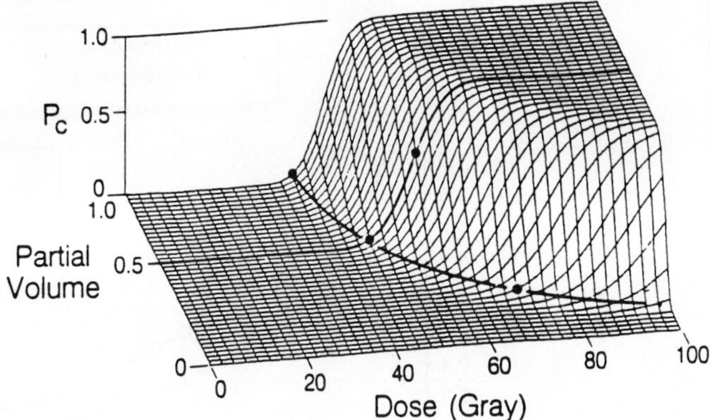

FIGURE 5–23. Each organ has a spectrum of dose response curves as a function of volume irradiated. A three-dimensional surface representation of the probability of complication for the heart as a function of the dose and the partial volume that is uniformily irradiated. (Lyman JT: Radiat Res 104 [Suppl 8]: S13–S19, 1985)

been oriented toward specific pathologic lesions, whereas chemotherapy grades usually reflect functional and physiologic changes. Toxicity reporting of multiagent chemotherapy combinations and their interaction with radiation effects has stimulated national cooperative groups to form committees to assess acute effects and develop appropriate scoring and grading systems.

A recommendation for a uniform system is the desired end product based on "consensus criteria." In September 1985, a conference on toxicity was held in Baltimore. A subcommittee, composed of representatives from several cooperative groups and the National Cancer Institute, was formed at this meeting with the aim of addressing the question of standardized toxic effects criteria. Conclusions and recommendations made by the committee are summarized here.[195]

1. There is a need for uniform toxicity scoring, both for acute and late effects but particularly with regard to late effects in vital organs.
2. The toxicity scale should consist of five grades: mild, moderate, severe, life-threatening, and fatal. The emphasis should be on grades 3, 4, and 5, with consideration for both peak grade and peak time in developing an appropriate index (Table 5-17).
3. In addition to the major modalities of radiation therapy and chemotherapy, which are known to produce such late toxicities, the effects of host co-factors, other modalities, and recurrent tumor need to be carefully considered.
4. End points need to be clearly defined in terms of somatic and genetic effects and second malignant tumors with appropriate time scales set, preferably more than 6 months following the introduction of treatment. There is a need for a working committee on late effects representing all major modalities consisting of a radiation oncologist, a medical oncologist, and a surgical oncologist, depending on the site.
5. Protocols for longitudinal studies of key dose-limiting normal tissues and organs, using appropriate standard diagnostic laboratory and imaging tests, need to be developed. These should include CT, MRI, and PET scans.
6. Actuarial risk reporting and recall of long-term survivors should be done initially in selected patients cohorts, namely, survivors beyond 2 years. Although for malignan-

TABLE 5–17
Scale/Grade

1	2	3	4	5
Mild, 10% ⇅	Moderate, 25% ⇅	Severe, 50% ⇅	Life-threatening, 75% ⇅	Fatal, 100% ⇅
Range of values: relative units				
1–3	3–5	5–8	8–10	>10
1.5 X NL	3 X NL	5 X NL	10 X NL	>10 X NL

(Rubin P, Wasserman TH: Int J Radiat Oncol Biol Phys 14[1]:529–538, 1988)

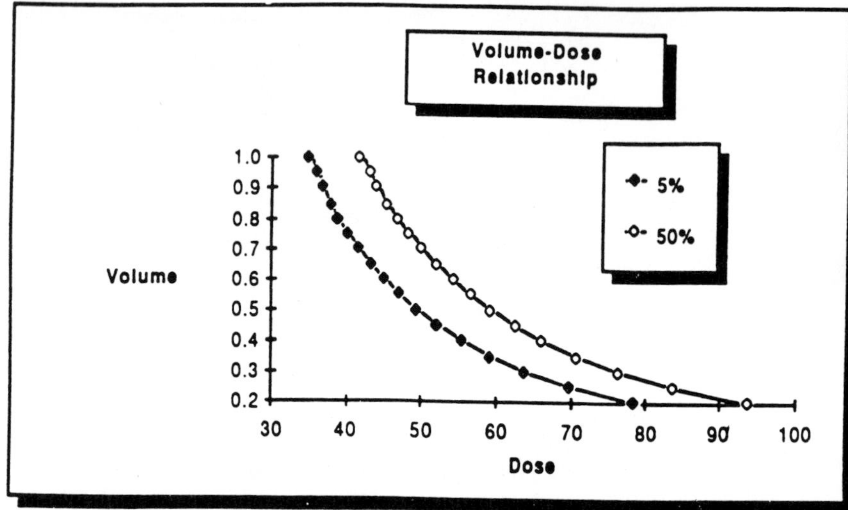

FIGURE 5–24. As the volume of an organ irradiated decreases, the dose to produce 5% or 50% complications increases. This illustrates that there is no "fixed" safe dose or tolerance dose TD_5 and TD_{50}, but it varies. (Rubin P: The law and order of radiation sensitivity, absolute as relative. In Vaeth JM, Meyer JL [eds]: Radiation Tolerance of Normal Tissues, vol 23. Basel, Karger, 1989).

cies in which a 50% survival rate has been considered most appropriate for such studies, this requirement may be too stringent; instead the assessment of adverse effects should be done in all survivors beyond 2 years. This is particularly true for highly fatal cancers for which intensive regimens of combined modalities are used.

7. Publications should routinely present therapeutic ratios and use standard toxicity and late effects scoring along with tumor response rates.[195]

Further efforts were made at Williamsburg in 1987 to develop precise criteria for categories I and II organ toxicity by defining the late-effect pathologic lesion, evaluative diagnostic tests, medical and surgical interventions, and the character of the acute and late effects according to organ site.[185] Most recently, Wittes has circulated a standardized system for acute toxicity scoring derived at a National Cancer Institute consensus meeting that was recommended by the national cooperative groups to all investigators involved in clinical trials (Wittes RE: Personal written communication, 1988). A similar standardized late effects classification needs to be more widely adopted and should be based on the available RTOG-EORTC late effects scales. Protocols need to be developed prospectively to accurately document late effects in all long-term survivors, that is, those surviving more than 2 years.[185]

Predictive Assays for Late Effects

Predictive assays are needed for late effects in vital normal tissues just as predictive assays are needed in tumors.[187] A simple biochemical test that is accurate and reproducible would be optimal. An example of this approach is the development of surfactant release as a measure or index of developing later fatal radiation pneumonitis.[192] In a number of different murine strains and different species such as the rabbit, detection of increased levels of alveolar surfactant and serum surfactant on the 7th day after irradiation correlates with later lethality at 4 months.[194] A similar assay has been developed for myelin basic protein released into the cerebrospinal fluid at 1 to 2 months after irradiation, which correlates with late myelopathy.[196] Although these are laboratory models at present, protocols are ongoing in humans. These assays are the first biochemical markers identified for later radiation effects and represent a line of study that should be extended to many other vital tissues and organs. The hypothesis is that unique proteins and other biochemical products are released into body fluids and serums during or at the conclusion of irradiation, which are measurable and useful as predictors. Radioprotectors (WR-2721 and others) have the potential to protect bone marrow, skin, mucosa, and salivary glands.[219] Dramatic results with avoidance of lung fibrosis have been demonstrated by Xu and co-workers.[247]

REFERENCES

1. Ahlgren JD, Smith FP, Kerwin DM, et al: Pulmonary disease as a complication of chlorozotocin chemotherapy. Cancer Treat Rep 65:223–229, 1981
2. Alexander J, Dainiak N, Berger HJ, et al: Serial assessment of doxorubicin cardiotoxicity with quantitative radionuclide angiocardiography. N Engl J Med 300:278–283, 1979
3. Alpert H: Veno-occlusive disease of the liver associated with oral contraceptives: Case report and review. Hum Pathol 7:709–718, 1976
4. Alpes T: Cellular Radiobiology. London, Cambridge University Press, 1979
5. Andrews GA: Radiation accidents and their management. Radiat Res 7(Suppl):390–397, 1967
6. Ang K, van der Kogel A, Van der Schueren E: Lack of evidence for increased tolerance of rat cord with decreasing fraction doses below 2 Gy. Int J Radiat Oncol Biol Phys 11:105–110, 1985
7. Applefeld M, Cole J, Pollock S, et al: The late appearance of chronic pericardial disease in patients treated by radiotherapy for Hodgkin's disease. Ann Intern Med 94:338–341, 1981
8. Aronim PA, Mahaley MS, Rudnick SA, et al: Prediction of BCNU pulmonary toxicity in patients with malignant gliomas—an assessment of risk-factors. N Engl J Med 303:183–188, 1980
9. Aso Y, Yoneda K, Kikkawa Y: Morphologic and biochemical study of pulmonary changes induced by bleomycin in mice. Lab Invest 35:558–568, 1976
10. Avner ED, Ingelfinger JR: Special considerations relating to the pediatric cancer patient. In Rieselbach RE, Garnick MB (eds): Cancer and the Kidney. Philadelphia, Lea & Febiger, 1981
11. Berg NO, Lindgren M: Relation between field size and tolerance of rabbit-s brain to roentgen irradiation (200 kV) via a slit-shaped field. Acta Radiol 1:147–168, 1963
12. Berge G, Brun A, Hakansson CH, et al: Sensitivity to irradiation of the brain stem. Irradiation myelitis in the treatment of a nasopharynx carcinoma. Cancer 33:1263–1268, 1974
13. Bergsagel DE: Total body irradiation for myelomatosis. Br Med J ii:325–327, 1971
14. Bieber CP, Jamieson S, Raney A, et al: Cardiac allograft survival in Rhesus primates treated with combined total lym-

phoid irradiation and rabbit antithymocyte globulin. Transplantation 28:347–350, 1979

15. Billingham ME: Endocardial changes. In Vaeth JM (ed): Anthracycline Treated Patients With and Without Irradiation. Frontiers of Radiation Therapy and Oncology vol 13, pp 67–81. New York, S Karger, 1979
16. Billingham ME, Bristow MR, Glatstein E, et al: Adriamycin cardiotoxicity: Endomyocardial biopsy evidence of enhancement by irradiation. Am J Surg Pathol 1(1):17–23, 1977
17. Bleyer WA: Neurologic sequelae of methotrexate ionizing radiation: A new classification. Cancer Treat Rep 65:89–98, 1981
18. Bleyer WA, Griffin TW: White matter necrosis, mineralizing microangiography, and intellectual abilities in survivors of childhood leukemia: Associations with central nervous system irradiation and methotrexate therapy In Gilbert HA, Kagan AR (eds): Radiation Damage to the Nervous System, pp 155–174. New York, Raven Press, 1980
19. Bloom HJG, Wallace ENK, Henk JM: The treatment and prognosis of medulloblastoma in children. A study of 82 verified cases. J Roentgenol 105:43–62, 1969
20. Boivin JF, et al: Coronary heart disease mortality after irradiation for Hodgkin's disease. Cancer 49:2470–2475, 1982
21. Bonadonna G, Valagussa P: Chemotherapy of breast cancer. Current views and results. Int J Radiat Oncol Biol Phys 9:279–297, 1983
22. Bond VP, Fludner TM, Archambeau JO: Mammalian radiation lethality. New York, Academic Press, 1965
23. Borch RF, Pleasants ME: Inhibition of cis-platinum nephrotoxicity by diethyldithiocarcamate rescue in a rat model. Proc Nat Acad Sci USA 76(12):6611–6614, 1979
24. Botnik LE, Hannon EC, Hellman S: Multisystem stem cell failure after apparent recovery from alkylating agents. Cancer Res 38:1942–1947, 1978
25. Botnik LE, Hannon ECM, Hellman S: Late effects of cytotoxic agents on the normal tissue of mice. In Vaeth JM (ed) Frontiers of Radiation Therapy and Oncology 13:36–47. New York, S Karger 1979
26. Brady LW (ed): Long-term normal tissue effects of cancer treatment. Can Clin Trials 4(Suppl):7;9–71, 1981
27. Bristow MR, Mason JW, Billingham ME, Daniels JR: Doxorubicin cardiomyopathy: Evaluations by phonocardiology, endomyocardial biopsy, and cardiac catheterization. Ann Intern Med 88:168–175, 1978
28. Britten M, Halman K, Meredith W: Radiation cataract—new evidence on radiation dosage to the lens. Br J Radiol 39:612–617, 1966
29. Brosius FC III, Waller BF, Roberts WC: Radiation heart disease. Analysis of 16 young (aged 15–33 years) necropsy patients who received over 3,500 rads to the heart. Am J Med 70:519–530, 1981
30. Burger PC, Kamenar E, Schold SC, et al: Encephalomyelopathy following high-dose BCNU therapy. Cancer 48:1318–1327, 1981
31. Burns RJ, Bar-Shlomo B, Druck M: Detection of radiation cardiomyopathy by gated radionuclide angiography. Am J Med 74:297–302, 1983
32. Byhardt R, Brace K, Ruckdeschel J: Dose and treatment factors in radiation related pericardial effusion associated with the mantle technique for Hodgkin's disease. Cancer 35:795, 1975
33. Carbell SC, Chaffey JT, Rosenthal DS, et al: Results of total body irradiation in the treatment of advanced non-Hodgkin's lymphoma. Cancer 43:994–1000, 1979
34. Casarett GW: Aging. In Vaeth JM (ed): Frontiers of Radiation Therapy and Oncology, vol 6, pp 479–485. New York, S Karger, 1972
35. Casarett GW: Similarities and contrasts between radiation and time pathology. In Strehler B (ed): Advances in Gerontological Research, pp 109–163. New York, Academic Press, 1964
36. Cassady JR, Carabell SC, Jaffe N: Chemotherapy irradiation related hepatic dysfunction in patients with Wilms' tumor. In Vaeth JM (ed): Frontiers of Radiation Therapy and Oncology, vol 13, pp 147–160. New York, S Karger, 1979
37. Catterall M, Bloom HCJ, Ash DV, et al: Fast neutrons compared with megavoltage X rays in the treatment or patients with supratentorial blioblastoma: A controlled pilot study. Int J Radiat Oncol Biol Phys 6:261–266, 1980
38. Ch'ien LT, Rhomes JA, Stagner S, et al: Long-term neurological implications of somnolence syndrome in children with acute lymphocytic leukemia. Ann Neurol 8:273–277, 1980
39. Chabner BA, Myers CE, Oliverio VT: Clinical pharmacology of anticancer drugs. Semin Oncol 4:217–226, 1977
40. Chaffey JT, Hellman S: Radiation fractionation as applied to murine colony forming cells in differing proliferative states. Radiology 93:1167–1172, 1969
41. Chen GTY, Austin-Seymour M, Castro JC, et al: Dose volume histograms in treatment planning evaluation of carcinoma of the pancreas. In Proceedings Eighth International Conference on Uses of Computers in Radiation Therapy, pp 264–268, 1984
42. Choi NC, Kanarek OJ, Kazemi H: Physiologic changes in pulmonary function after thoracic radiotherapy for patients with lung cancer and role of regional pulmonary function studies in predicting postradiotherapy pulmonary function before radiotherapy. Cancer Treat Symp 2:119–130, 1985
43. Cohen L, Creditor M: Isoeffect tables for tolerance of irradiated normal human tissues. Int J Radiat Oncol Biol Phys 9:233–241, 1983
44. Cohen S, Bharati S, Glass J, et al: Radiotherapy as a cause of complete atrioventricular block in Hodgkin's disease: An electrophysiological-pathological correlation. Arch Intern Med 141:676–679, 1981
45. Concannon JP, Summers RE, Cole C, Weill C: Effects on renal function. X-radiation combined with systemic actinomycin D. Am J Roentgenol 108:141–147, 1970
46. Constine LS: Tumors in children in cure with preservation of function and aesthetic. In Wilson JF (ed): Syllabus: A Categorical Course in Radiation Therapy, pp 75–91. Oak Brook, Ill, RNSA, 1988
47. Constine LS, Donaldson SS, McDougall IR, et al: Thyroid dysfunction after radiotherapy in children with Hodgkin's disease. Cancer 53:878–883, 1984
48. Constine LS, Konski A, Ekholm S, et al: Adverse effects of brain irradiation correlated with MR and CT imaging. Int J Radiat Oncol Biol Phys 15:319–330, 1988
49. Constine LS, Rubin P: Total body irradiation: normal tissue effects. In Bleehen NM (ed): Radiobiology in Radiotherapy, pp 95–121. New York, Springer-Verlag, 1987
50. Cowdry EV: Textbook of Histology, 4th ed. Philadelphia, Lea & Febiger, 1950
51. Croizat H, Friendel E, Tubiana M: Proliferative activity of stem cells in the bone marrow of mice after single and multiple irradiations (total and partial body). Int J Radiat Biol 18:347–358, 1970
52. D'Angio G (ed): Delayed Consequences of Cancer Therapy: Proven and Potential. Cancer 37:979–1236, 1976
53. Danjoux CE, Catton GE: Delayed complications in colorectal carcinoma treated by combination radiotherapy and 5-fluorouracil—Eastern Cooperative Oncology Group (ECOG) Pilot Study. Int J Radiat Oncol Biol Phys 5:311–316, 1979
54. Danoff BF, Cowchock S, Marquette C, et al: Assessment of the long-term effects of primary radiation therapy for brain tumors in children. Cancer 49:1580–1586, 1982
55. Deeg HJ, Flounoy N, Sullivan K, et al: Cataracts after total body irradiation and marrow transplant: A sparing effect of dose fractionation. Int J Radiat Oncol Biol Phys 10:957–964, 1984
56. Dethlefsen LA: Cellular recovery kinetic studies relevant to combined modality research and therapy, Int J Radiat Oncol Biol Phys 5:1175–1184, 1979
57. DeVita VT: Principles of chemotherapy. In DeVita VT, Hellman S, Rosenberg SA (eds): Cancer: Principles and Practice of Oncology, pp 132–155. Philadelphia, JB Lippincott, 1982
58. DeVita VT: The relationship between tumor mass and resistance to chemotherapy: Implications for surgical adjuvant treatment of cancer. The James Ewing Lecture delivered at the 35th annual meeting of the Society of Surgical Oncology, April 1982
59. Devney RB, Sklar CA, Nesbit ME, et al: Serial thyroid func-

tion measurements in children with Hodgkin's disease. J Pediatr 105:225–227, 1984
60. Doll R, Smith PG: The long-term effects of X-irradiation in patients treated for metropathia haemorrhagica. Br J Radiol 41:362–368, 1968
61. Donaldson SS, Moskowitz PS, Canty EL, Efron B: Radiation-induced inhibition of compensatory renal growth in the weanling mouse kidney. Radiology 128:491–495, 1978
62. Donaldson SS, Moskowitz PS, Fajardo LF: Combination radiation-adriamycin therapy: Renoprival growth, function, and structural effects in the immature mouse. Int J Radiat Oncol Biol Phys 6:851–859, 1980
63. Duffner PK, Cohen M Thomas P, Lansley S, et al: Long term effects of cranial irradiation in the central nervous system. Cancer 56:1841–1847; 1985
64. Dunsmore LD, LoPonte MA, Dunsmore RA: Radiation-induced coronary artery disease. J Am Coll Cardiol 8:239–244, 1986
65. Edwards MS, Wilson CB: Treatment of radiation necrosis. In Gilbert HA, Kagan HR (eds): Radiation Damage to the Nervous System, pp 129–144. New York, Raven Press, 1980
66. Ellis F: Is NSD-TDF useful to radiotherapy? Int J Radiat Oncol Biol Phys 11:1685–1699, 1985
67. Eltringham JR: Cardiac response to combined modality therapy. Frontiers of Radiation Therapy and Oncology 13:161–174, 1979
68. Eltringham JR, Fajardo LF, Stewart JR: Adriamycin cardiomyopathy: Enhanced cardiac damage in rabbits with combined drug and cardiac irradiation. Radiology 115:471–472, 1975
69. Eltringham JR, Fajardo LF, Stewart JR, Klauber MR: Investigation of cardiotoxicity in rabbits from adriamycin and fractionated cardiac irradiation: Preliminary results. Frontiers of Radiation Therapy and Oncology 13:21–35, 1979
70. Ercan MT, Or IS, Bekdik CF, et al: ^{99m}TC-Methyl CCNU for the static imaging of kidneys. Eur J Nucl Med 5:109–114, 1980
71. Evans A, Bleyer A, Kaplan R, et al: Central nervous system workshop. Cancer Clin Trials 4(Suppl):31–35, 1981
72. Evans RG: Radiobiologic considerations in magna-field irradiation. Int J Radiat Oncol Biol Phys 9:1907–1912, 1983
73. Fajardo LF: Pathology of Radiation Injury. New York, Masson, 1982
74. Fajardo LF, Eltingham JR, Stewart JR: Combined cardiotoxicity of adriamycin and x-radiation. Lab Invest 34(1):89–96, 1976
75. Fajardo LF, Eltingham JR, Stewart JR, Klauber, MR: Adriamycin nephrotoxicity. Lab Invest 43:242–253, 1980
76. Fajardo LF, Stewart JR: Experimental radiation-induced heart disease. 1. Light microscopic studies. Am J Pathol 59:299–316, 1970
77. Fajardo LF, Stewart JR: Pathogenesis of radiation-induced myocardial fibrosis. Lab Invest 29:244–257, 1973
78. Fajardo LF, Stewart JR, Cohn KE: Morphology of radiation-induced heart disease. Arch Pathol Lab Med 86:512–519, 1968
79. Field SB, Michalowski A: Endpoints for damage to normal tissues. Int J Radiat Oncol Biol Phys 5:1185–1196, 1979
80. Filler RM, Maddock CI, Tefft M, Vawter G, Brown B: Effects of actinomycin D and x-ray on partially hepatectomized rats. Surgical Forum 19:358–360, 1968
81. Frei E: Summary and prospective statement concerning the genitourinary workshop. Cancer Clin Trials 4:25–29, 1981
82. Friedman MA, Bozdeck MJ, Billingham ME, Rider AK: Doxorubicin cardiotoxicity: Serial endomyocardial biopsies and systolic time intervals. JAMA 15:1603–1606, 1978
83. Frindel E, Croizat H, Vassont F: Stimulating factors liberated by treated bone marrow: *In vivo* effect on CFU kinetics. Exp Hematol 4:56–61, 1976
84. Fryer CJ, Fitzpatrick PJ, Rider WD, Poon P: Radiation pneumonitis: Experience following a large single dose of irradiation. Int J Radiat Oncol Biol Phys 4:931–936, 1978
85. Fukushima S, Araio M, Cohen SM, et al: Scanning electron microscopy of cyclophosphamide induced hyperplasia of the rat urinary bladder. Lab Invest 44:89–96, 1981
86. Gangji D, Reaman GH, Cohen SR, et al: Leukoencephalopathy and elevated levels of myelin basic protein in the cerebrospinal fluid of patients with acute lymphoblastic leukemia. N Engl J Med 303:19–21, 1980
87. Garnick MB, Mayer RJ, Abelson HT: Renal failure associated with cancer chemotherapy. In Brenner BM, Lazarus JM, Myers BD (eds): Acute Renal Failure. Philadelphia, WB Saunders, 1981
88. Gavin PR, Gillette EL: Radiation response of the canine cardiovascular system. Radiat Res 90(Suppl):489–500, 1982
89. Ghione M: Cardiotoxic effects of antitumor agents. Chemother Pharmacol 1:25–34, 1978
90. Gilladoga AC, Tan CT, Phillips FC, et al: Cardiac status of 40 children receiving adriamycin over 495 mg/m^2 and animal studies. Proc Am Assoc Cancer Res 15:107, 1974
91. Ginsberg SJ, Comis RL: The pulmonary toxicity of antineoplastic agents. Semin Oncol 9:34–51, 1982
92. Glatstein E: Alterations in 86 Rubidium extraction in normal mouse tissues after irradiation. An estimate of long-term blood flow changes in kidney, lung, liver, skin and muscle. Radiat Res 53:88–101, 1973
93. Glatstein E, Fajardo LF, Brown JM: Radiation injury in the mouse kidney. 1. Sequential light microscopic studies. Int J Radiat Oncol Biol Phys 2:933–943, 1977
94. Glatstein E, McHardy-Young S, Brast N, et al: Alterations in serum thyrotropin (TSH) and thyroid function following radiotherapy in patients with malignant lymphoma. J Clin Endocrinol Metab 32:833–841, 1971
95. Goldwein JW: Radiation myelopathy: A review. Med Pediatr Oncol 15:89–95, 1987
96. Gonzalez-Vitale JC, Hayes DM, Cvitkovic E, Sternberg SS: The renal pathology in clinical trials of cisplatinum (II) diaminedichloride. Cancer 39:1362–1371, 1977
97. Goorin AM, Borow KM, Goldman A, et al: Congestive heart failure due to adriamycin cardiotoxicity: Its natural history in children. Cancer 47:2810–2816, 1981
98. Greenwood RD, Rosenthal A, Cassady R, et al: Constructive pericarditis in childhood due to mediastinal irradiation. Circulation 50:1033–1039, 1974
99. Griffin TV, Rasey JS, Bleyer WA: The effect of photon irradiation on blood-brain barrier permeability to methotrexate in mice. Cancer 40:1109–1111, 1977
100. Hall EJ: Radiobiology for the radiologist. New York, Harper & Row, 1978
101. Halperin E, Kun L, Constine L, Tarbell N: Pediatric Radiation Oncology, p 434. New York, Raven Press, 1989
102. Harmon WE, Cohen H, Schneeberger EE, Grupe WE: Chronic renal failures in children treated with methyl CCNU. N Engl J Med 300:1200–1203, 1979
103. Heller CG: Effects on the germinal epithelium of radiobiological factors in manned space flight. In Langham WH (ed): NRC Publication 1487. Washington, DC: National Academy of Sciences, National Research Council, pp 124–133, 1967
104. Hellman S, Botnik LE: Stem cell depletion: an explanation of the late effects of cytotoxins. Int J Radiat Oncol Biol Phys 2:181–184, 1977
105. Heyn R, Rozob A, Raney B: Late effects of therapy in therapy in orbital rhabdomyosarcoma. Cancer 57:1738–1743, 1986
106. Hindo WA, De Trana F, Lee M-S, et al: Large dose increment irradiation in treatment of cerebral metastases. Cancer 26:138–141, 1970
107. Hirsh J, Renier D, Czernechow P: Medulloblastoma in childhood: survival and functional results. Acta Neurochir 48:1–15, 1979
108. Holland JF, Frei E: Cancer Medicine. Philadelphia, Lea & Febiger, 1973
109. Hopewell JW: Early and late changes in the functional vascularity of the hamster cheek pouch after local irradiation. Radiat Res 63:157–164, 1975
110. Hopewell JW: Radiation Effects on Vascular Tissue. The Nonneoplastic Late Effects Session. Brussels ICR, 1981

111. Hornsey S, Morris CC, Myers R, White A: RBE for damage to the CNS by neutrons. Int J Radiat Oncol Biol Phys 1983
112. Hornsey S, White A: Isoeffect curve for radiation myelopathy. Br J Radiol 53:168–169, 1980
113. Hresnchyshyn MM: Results of the Gynecologic Oncology Group trials on ovarian cancer: Preliminary report. In Symposium on ovarian carcinoma. NCI Monograph 42:155–165, 1975
114. Hubmann FH: Effect of x-irradiation on the rectum of the rat. Br J Radiol 54:250–254, 1981
115. Ingold JA, Reed GB, Kaplan HS, Bagshaw MA: Radiation hepatitis. Am J Roentgenol 93:200–208, 1965
116. Jaffe JP, Bosch A, Raich PC: Sequential half-body radiotherapy in advanced multiple myeloma. Cancer 43:124–128, 1979
117. Jeneke RS, Dalbow DG, Bartuska BM, et al: Comparative inhibition of myocardial RNA synthesis by anthracycline antibiotics. Cancer Treat Rep, in press
118. Jones AM: Transient radiation myelopathy (with reference to L'Hermitt sign of electrical paresthesia). Br J Radiol 37:727–744, 1964
119. Jongejan H, van der Kogel A, Provoost A, et al: Radiation nephropathy in young and adult rats. Int J Radiat Oncol Biol Phys 13:225–232, 1987
120. Kaplan RS, Wiernik PH: Neurotoxicity of antineoplastic drugs. Semin Oncol 9:103–130, 1982
121. Keane TJ, Van Dyk J, Rider WD: Idiopathic interstitial pneumonia following bone marrow transplantation: The relationship with total body irradiation. Int J Radiat Oncol Biol Phys 7:1365–1370, 1981
122. Keizer MJ: Protection of hematopoetic stem cells during cytotoxic treatment, p 92. Rijswijk, Netherlands: Radiobiological Institute, 1976
123. Kemper T, O'Neill R, Caveness W: Effects of single dose supervoltage whole brain radiation in *Macaca mulatta.* J Neuropathol Exp Neurol 36:916–940, 1977
124. Ketcham A, Withers HR: Gastrointestinal workshop. Cancer Clin Trials 4:15–18, 1981
125. Kim TH, Khan FM, Galvin JM: A report of the work party: comparison of total body irradiation techniques for bone marrow transplantation. Int J Radiat Oncol Biol Phys 6:775–784, 1980
126. Kim TH, Panakon AM, Friedman M: Acute transient radiation hepatitis following whole abdominal irradiation. Clin Radiol 27:449–454, 1976
127. Kline L, Kim J, Ceballos R: Radiation optic neuropathy. Ophthalmology 92:1118–1126, 1985
128. Knopse WH, Blom J, Crosby WH: Regeneration of locally irradiated bone marrow. II. Induction or regeneration in permanently aplastic medullary cavities. Blood 31:400–405, 1968
129. Kolmer JA, Lucke B: A study of the histologic changes produced experimentally in rabbits by arsphenamine. Arch Dermatol Syphilol 3:483–514, 1921
130. Kopelson G, Herwig KJ: The etiologies of coronary artery disease in cancer patients. Int J Radiat Oncol Biol Phys 4:895–906, 1978
131. Kun LE, Mulhern RK, Crisco JJ: Quality of life in children treated for brain tumors: Intellectual, emotional and academic functions. J Neurosurg 58:1–6, 1983
132. La Monte C, Yeh S, Straus D: Long-term follow-up of cardiac function in patients with Hodgkin's disease treated with mediastinal irradiation and combination hemotherapy including doxorubicin. Cancer Treat Rep 70:439–444, 1986
133. LeBaron S, Zeltzer P, Zeltzer L, et al: Assessment of quality of survival in children with medulloblastoma and cerebellar astrocytoma. Cancer 54:135–138, 1988
134. Lederman G, Sheldon T, Chaffey J, et al: Cardiac disease after mediastinal irradiation for seminoma. Cancer 60:772–776, 1987
135. Leith JT, DeWyngaert K, Glicksman A: Radiation myelopathy in the rat: an interpretation of dose relationships. Int J Radiat Oncol Biol Phys 7:1673–1677, 1981
136. Lewin K, Millis RR: Human radiation hepatitis. A morphologic study with emphasis on the late changes. Arch Pathol 96:21–26, 1973
137. Littman P, Meadows AT, Polgar G, et al: Pulmonary function in survivors of Wilm's tumor. Cancer 37:2773–2776, 1976
138. Littman P, Rosenstock J, Bailey C: Radiation myelitis following craniospinal irradiation with concurrent actinomycin D therapy. Med Pediatr Oncol 5(1):145–151, 1978
139. Lockhart SF, Down JD, Steel GG: The effect of low dose rate and cyclophosphamide on the radiation tolerance of the mouse lung. Int J Radiat Oncol Biol Phys 12:1437–1440, 1986
140. Lushbaugh CG, Casarett GW: The effects of gonadal irradiation in clinical radiation therapy: A review. Cancer 37:1111–1120, 1976
141. Lushbaugh CG, Ricks RC: Some cytokinetic and histopathologic considerations of irradiated male and female gonadal tissues. Frontiers of Radiation Therapy and Oncology 6:228–248, 1972
142. Lyman JT: Complication probability as assessed from dose-volume histograms. Radiat Res 104(Suppl):S-13–S-19, 1985
143. Lyman JT, Wolbarst AB: Optimization of radiation therapy III: a method of assessing complication probabilities from dose-volume histograms. Int J Radiat Oncol Biol Phys 14:103–109, 1987
144. Maier JG: Effects of radiations on kidney, bladder and prostate. Frontiers of Radiation Therapy and Oncology 6:196–227, 1972
145. Maier JG, Casarett GW: Pathophysiologic aspects of radiation nephritis in dogs. University of Rochester Atomic Energy Commission Report, UR-626, 1962
146. Marks JE, Baglan RJ, Prassad SC, Blank WF: Cerebral radionecrosis: Incidence and risk in relation to dose, time, fractionation and volume. Int Radiat Oncol Biol Phys 7:243–252, 1981
147. Marsh JC: The effects of cancer chemotherapeutic agents on normal hematopoietic precursor cells: A review. Cancer Res 36:1853–1882, 1976
148. Meacham GC, Tillotson FW, Heinle RW: Liver damage after prolonged urethane therapy. Am J Clin Pathol 22:22–27, 1952
149. Merriam GR Jr, Focht EF: A clinical study of radiation cataracts and the relationship to dose. Am J Roentgenol 77:759–785, 1957
150. Minow RA, Stern MH, Casey JH, et al: Clinicopathologic correlation of liver damage in patients treated with 6-mercaptopurine and adriamycin. Cancer 38:1524–1528, 1976
151. Mitchell EP, Schien PS: Gastrointestinal toxicity of chemotherapeutic agents. Semin Oncol 9:52–64, 1982
152. Monterdini S (ed): Manual of cancer chemotherapy, 3rd ed, vol 56. UICC Technical Reprint Series. Geneva, UICC, 1981
153. Moosavi H, McDonald S, Rubin P, et al: Early radiation dose-response in lung: an ultrastructural study. Int J Radiat Oncol Biol Phys 2:921–932, 1977
154. Morandet N, Paramentier C, Flamant R: Étude par le fer 59 des effets de la radiotherapie etendue des hematosarcomes sur l'erythropoiese. Biomedicine 18:228, 1973
155. Moskowitz PS, Donaldson SS: The clinical spectrum of radiation/chemotherapy nephropathy in children treated for Wilms tumor. Am J Radiol, in press
156. Moskowitz PS, Donaldson SS, Canty EL: Chemotherapy-induced inhibition of compensatory renal growth in the immature mouse. Am J Radiol 134:491–496, 1980
157. Nelson DF, Reddy KV, O'Mara RE, et al: Thyroid abnormalities following neck irradiation for Hodgkin's disease. Cancer 42:2553–2562, 1978
158. Nichols WC, Moertel CG: Nephrotoxicity of methyl CCNU (Letter). N Engl J Med 301:1181, 1979
159. Orton CG, Cohen L: A unified approach to dose-effect relationships in radiotherapy. I: Modified TDF and linear quadratic equations. Int J Radiat Oncol Biol Phys 14:549–557, 1988
160. Parker R, Meadows A, Roche L, et al: Long term sequelae of cancer treatment on the nervous system in childhood. Med Pediatr Oncol 15:241–253, 1987

161. Parsons JJ, Fitzpatrick CR, Hood CT, et al: The effects of irradiation on the eye and optic nerve. Int J Radiat Oncol Biol Phys 9:609–622, 1983
162. Paterson R: The treatment of malignancy by radium and X-rays. Being a practice of radiotherapy. London, Edward Arnold & Co, 1947
163. Pedrick TJ, Hoppe RT: Recovery of spermatogenesis following pelvic irradiation for Hodgkin's disease. Int J Radiat Oncol Biol Phys 12:117–121, 1986
164. Penney DP, Rubin P: Specific early fine structural changes in lung following irradiation. Int J Radiat Oncol Biol Phys 2:1123–1132, 1977
165. Penney DP, Shapiro DL, Rubin P, Finkelstein J: Long-term effects of radiation on the mouse lung and potential induction of radiation pneumonitis. Int J Radiat Oncol Biol Phys, in press
166. Perez CA, Korba A, Zwnuska F, et al: ^{60}Co moving strip technique in the management of carcinoma of the ovary: Analysis of tumor control and morbidity. Int J Radiat Oncol Biol Phys 4:379–388, 1978
167. Perry MC: Hepatotoxicity of chemotherapeutic agents. Semin Oncol 9:65–74, 1982
168. Phillips R, Karnofsky D, Hamelton L, et al: Roentgen therapy of hepatic metastases. Am J Roentgenol 71:826–834, 1984
169. Phillips TL: An ultrastructural study of the development of radiation injury in the lung. Radiology 87:49–54, 1966
170. Phillips TL: Tissue toxicity of radiation-drug interactions. In Sokal GH, Maickel RP (eds): Radiation-drug interactions in the treatment of cancer. Wiley Series in Diagnostic and Therapeutic Radiology. New York, John Wiley & Sons, 1980:175–200
171. Phillips TL, Ross G: A quantitative technique for measuring renal damage after irradiation. Radiology 109:457–462, 1973
172. Pratt WB, Ruddon RW: The Anticancer Drugs. New York, Oxford University Press, 1979
173. Price RA, Birdwell DA: The central nervous system in childhood leukemia III. Mineralizing microangiopathy and dystrophic calcification. Cancer 42:717–728, 1978
174. Price RA, Jamieson PA: The central nervous system in childhood leukemia. H subacute leukoencephalopathy. Cancer 35:306–318, 1975
175. Prosnitz LR, Farber LR, Fisher JJ, et al: Long-term remissions with combined modality therapy for advanced Hodgkin's disease. Cancer 37:2826–2833, 1976
176. Reactor safety study. Appendix VI. USNRC, Washington DC1400 (NUREG 75/014), 1975
177. Roswitt B, Malsky S, Reid C: Radiation tolerance of the gastrointestinal tract. In Vaeth JM (ed): Frontiers of Radiation Therapy and Oncology 6:160–181. New York, S Karger, 1972
178. Rubin P: Radiation effect and tolerance, normal tissue. In Vaeth JM (ed): Frontiers of Radiation Therapy and Oncology, vol 6. Baltimore, University Park Press, 1972
179. Rubin P: Radiation toxicology: Quantitative radiation pathology for predicting effects. Cancer 39(Suppl):21:729–736, 1977
180. Rubin P: The Franz Buschke lecture. Late effects of chemotherapy and radiation therapy: A new hypothesis. Int J Radiat Oncol Biol Phys 10:5–34, 1984
181. Rubin P: The law and order of radiation sensitivity, absolute vs relative. In Vaeth JM, Meyer JL (eds): Radiation Tolerance of Normal Tissues, vol 23. Basel, Karger, 1989
182. Rubin P, Bennett JM, Begg C, et al: The comparison of total body irradiation versus chlorambucil and prednisone for remission induction or active chronic lymphocytic leukemia: An ECOG study. I. Total body irradiation, response and toxicity. Int J Radiat Oncol Biol Phys 7:1623–1632, 1981
183. Rubin P, Casarett GW: Clinical radiation pathology, vols. I and II. Philadelphia, WB Saunders, 1968
184. Rubin P, Constine LS, Scarantino CW: The paradoxes in patterns and mechanisms of bone marrow regeneration after irradiation. II. Total body irradiation. Radiother Oncol 2:227–233, 1984
185. Rubin P, Constine LS, Van Ess J: Late effects of toxicity scoring. NCI Monograph. 6:9–18, 1988
186. Rubin P, Cooper RA, Phillips TL (eds): Radiation biology and radiation pathology syllabus. Chicago: American College of Radiation Publications, 1978
187. Rubin P, Finkelstein JN, Siemann DW, et al: Predictive biochemical assays for late radiation effects. Int J Radiat Oncol Biol Phys 12:469–476, 1984
188. Rubin P, Keys H, Poulter CA: Changing concepts in the tolerance of radioresistance and radiosensitivity of normal tissue/organs. In Biological basis and clinical importance of tumor radioresistants. New York, Masson, 1983
189. Rubin P, Landman S, Mayer E, et al: Bone marrow regeneration and extension after extended field irradiation in Hodgkin's disease. Cancer 32:699–711, 1973
190. Rubin P, Nabila A, Elbadawi A, et al: Bone marrow regeneration from cortex following segmental fractionated irradiation. Int J Radiat Oncol Biol Phys 2:27–38, 1977
191. Rubin P, Scarantino CW: The bone marrow organ and the critical structure in radiation-drug interaction. Int J Radiat Oncol Biol Phys 4:3–23, 1978
192. Rubin P, Shapiro D, Finckelstein J, Penney D: The early release of surfactant following lung irradiation of alveolar type II cells. Int J Radiat Oncol Biol Phys 6:75–77, 1980
193. Rubin P, Siemann D: Principles of radiation oncology and cancer radiotherapy. In Rubin P (ed): Clinical Oncology. A Multidisciplinary Approach, 6th ed, pp 58–72. New York, American Cancer Society, 1983
194. Rubin P, Siemann DW, Shapiro D, et al: Surfactant release as an early measure of radiation pneumonitis. Int J Radiat Oncol Biol Phys 9:1669–1673, 1983
195. Rubin P, Wasserman TH: The late effects of toxicity scoring. Int J Radiat Oncol Biol Phys 14(1):S29–S28, 1988
196. Rubin P, Whitaker JN, Bryant RG, et al: Myelin basic protein and magnetic resonance imaging for diagnosing radiation myelopathy. Preliminary report. Int J Radiat Oncol Biol Phys 15:1371–1381, 1988
197. Safadari GH, Fuentes JM, Dubois JM, et al: Radiation necrosis of the braIn time of onset and incidence related to total dose and fractionation of radiation. Neuroradiology 27:44–47, 1985
198. Salazar OM, Van Houtte P, Rubin P: Once-a-week radiation for locally advanced lung cancer: final report. Cancer 54:719–725, 1984
199. Scarantino CE, Rubin P, Constine LS: The paradoxes in patterns and mechanisms of bone marrow regeneration after irradiation. I. Different volumes and doses. Radiother Oncol 2:215–225, 1984
200. Schacht RG, Feiner HD, Gallo GR, et al: Nephrotoxicity of nitrosoureas. Cancer 48:1328–1334, 1981
201. Schenken LL, Burdolt DR, Kovacs CJ: Adriamycin radiation induced combinations: drug induced delayed gastrointestinal radiosensitivity. Int J Radiat Oncol Biol Phys 5:1265–1270, 1979
202. Schilsky RL: Renal and metabolic toxicities of cancer chemotherapy. Semin Oncol 9:75–83, 1982
203. Schullheiss TE, Higgins EM, El-Mahdi HM: The latent period in radiation myelopathy. Int J Radiat Oncol Biol Phys 10:1109–1115, 1984
204. Schultz HP, Glatstein E, Kaplan HS: Management of presumptive or proven Hodgkin's disease of the liver. A proven radiotherapy technique. Int J Radiat Oncol Biol Phys 1:1–8, 1975
205. Shalet SM, Beardwell CG, Jacobs HG, et al: Testicular function following irradiation of the human prepubertal testis. Clin Endocrinol 9:483–490, 1978
206. Shalet SM, Horner A, Ahmed JR: Leydig cell damage after testicular irradiation for acute lymphoblastic leukemia. Med Pediatr Oncol 13:65–68, 1985
207. Shapiro E, Kinsella T, Makuch R, et al: Effect of fractionated irradiation on endocrine aspects of testicular function. J Clin Oncol 3:1232–1239, 1985
208. Sheline GE, Wara, WM, Smith V: Therapeutic irradiation and brain injury. Int J Radiat Oncol Biol Phys 6:1215–1228, 1980
209. Siemann DW, Hill RP, Penney DP: Early and late pulmonary toxicity in mice evaluated 180 and 420 days following localized lung irradiation. Radiat Res 89:396–407, 1982
210. Sklar CA, Kim TH, Ramsay NKC: Thyroid dysfunction

among long-term survivors of bone marrow transplantation. Am J Med 73:688–694, 1982

211. Sklar CA, Kim TH, Williamson IF, et al: Ovarian function after successful bone marrow transplantation in post-menarcheal females. Med Pediatr Oncol 11:361–364, 1983
212. Sorokin SP: The cell of the lungs. In Morphology of experimental respiratory carcinogenesis. Proceedings of the Biology Division, Oak Ridge National Laboratory, 1970
213. Speiser B, Rubin P, Casarett G: Aspermia following lower truncal irradiation in Hodgkin's disease. Cancer 32:692–698, 1973
214. Standqvist M: Studienuber die Kumulative Wirkung der Rontgenstrahlen bei Fraktionierung. Acta Radiol 55:1–300, 1944
215. Stewart JR, Cohen KE, Fajardo LF: Radiation-induced heart disease. A study of twenty-five patients. Radiology 89(2):302–310, 1967
216. Stewart JR, Fajardo LF: Cancer and coronary artery disease. Editorial comment. Int J Radiat Oncol Biol Phys 4:915–916, 1978
217. Stewart JR, Fajardo LF: Dose response in human and experimental radiation-induced heart disease. Radiology 99(2): 403–408, 1971
218. Stewart JR, Fajardo LF: Radiation-induced heart disease: an update. Prog Cardiovasc Dis 27:173–194, 1984
219. Takahashi I, Nagai T, Miyaishi K, et al: Clinical study of the radioprotective effects of amifostine (Ym-08310, WR-2721) on chronic radiation injury. Int J Radiat Oncol Biol Phys 12:935–939, 1986
220. Tefft M: Radiation related toxicities in National Wilms' Tumor Study Number 1. Int J Radiat Oncol Biol Phys 2:455–464, 1977
221. Tefft M, Mitus A, Das I, et al: Irradiation of the liver in children: Review of experience in the acute and chronic phases, and in the intact normal and partially resected. Am J Roentgenol 108:365–385, 1970
222. Tefft M, Traggis JD, Miller RM: Liver irradiation in children: Acute changes with transient leukopenia and thrombocytopenia. Am J Roentgenol 4:750–764, 1969
223. Thomas ED, Storb R, Buckner CD: Total body irradiation in preparation for bone marrow engraftment. Transplant Proc 8:591–593, 1976
224. Thomas ED, Storb R, Clift RA, et al: Bone marrow transplantation. N Engl J Med 292:832–843; 895–902, 1975
225. Till JE, McCullough EA: A direct measurement of the radiation sensitivity of normal mouse bone marrow cells. Radiat Res 14:213–222, 1961
226. Travis EL: The sequence of histological changes in mouse lungs after single doses of x-rays. Int J Radiat Oncol Biol Phys 6:345–347, 1980
227. Travis EL, Harley RA, Fenn JO, et al: Pathologic changes in the lung following single and multiple fraction irradiation. Int J Radiat Oncol Biol Phys 2:475–490, 1977
228. Trott K-R: Chronic damage after radiation therapy: challenge to radiation biology. Int J Radiat Oncol Biol Phys 10:907–913, 1984
229. Tubiana M, Bernard CI, Lalanne C: Modification de l'erythropoiese auprès radiotherapie pelvienne. Acta Radiol 52:321, 1959
230. Tubiana M, Friendel E, Croizat H: Effects of radiation on bone marrow. Pathol Biol (Paris) 27(6):326–334, 1979
231. Valeriote FA, Edelstein MB: The role of cell kinetics in cancer chemotherapy. Semin Oncol 4:217–226, 1977
232. van der Kogel AJ: Mechanisms of late radiation injury in the spinal cord, p 461. In Meyn RE and Withers HR (eds): Radiation Biology in Cancer Research. New York, Raven Press, 1980
233. van der Kogel AJ: Radiation tolerance of the spinal cord: time-dose relationships. Radiology 122:505–509, 1977
234. van der Kogel AJ, Barendsen GW: Late effects of spinal cord irradiation with 300 kV x-rays and 15 MeV neutrons. Br J Radiol 47:393–398, 1974
235. Van Houtte P, Rubin P, Finkelstein J, et al: The effect of bleomycin alone or in combination with radiation on surfactant release in the lung. Submitted to American Radium Society, 1982
236. Von Essen CF: Roentgen therapy of skin and lip carcinoma: factors influencing success and failure. Am J Roentgenol 83:556–570, 1960
237. Von Hoff DD, Layard MW, Basa P, et al: Risk factors for doxorubicin-induced congestive heart failure. Ann Intern Med 91:710–717, 1979
238. Von Hoff DD, Rozencweig M, Piccart M: The cardiotoxicity of anticancer agents. Semin Oncol 9:23–33, 1982
239. Wachholz BW, Casarett GW: Radiation hypertension and nephrosclerosis. Radiat Res 41:39–56, 1970
240. Wara W, Irvine A, Neger R, et al: Radiation retinopathy. Int J Radiat Oncol Biol Phys 5:81–83, 1979
241. Wara WM, Phillips TL, Margolis LW, et al: Radiation pneumonitis: a new approach to the derivation of time-dose factors. Cancer 32:547–552, 1973
242. Wara W, Phillips T, Sheline G, Schwade J: Radiation tolerance of the spinal cord. Cancer 35:1558–1562, 1975
243. Weiss BR, Muggia FM: Cytotoxic drug-induced pulmonary disease: update 1980. Am J Med 68:259–266, 1980
244. Willett C, Tepper J, Orlow E, et al: Renal complications secondary to radiation treatment of upper abdominal malignancies. Int J Radiat Oncol Biol Phys 12:1601–1604, 1986
245. Woo E, Lam K, Yu Y: Cerebral radionecrosis: Is surgery necessary? J Neuro Neurosurg Psych 50:1407–1414, 1982
246. Woods W, Dehner L, Nesbit M: Fatal veno-occlusive disease of the liver following high-dose chemotherapy, irradiation and bone marrow transplantation. Am J Med 68:285–290, 1980
247. Xu GZ, Cai WM, Qin DX, et al: Chinese herb destagnation series I: Combination of radiation and destagnation in the treatment of nasopharyngeal carcinoma (NPC)—a prospective randomized trial on 188 cases. Int J Radiat Oncol Biol Phys, in press

6

○ ○ ○ ● ● ●

Staging and Classification of Cancer: A Unified Approach

Philip Rubin
Sandra McDonald
James W. Keller

A uniform and unified classification system is necessary for the accurate staging of cancers. The TNM system introduced by Denoix more than four decades ago[8] (1943–1952) has gradually been forged to provide an international basis for categorizing cancers and to allow for comparable end results in reporting. The International Union Against Cancer (UICC) and the American Joint Committee on Cancer (AJCC) were constituted to develop a meaningful staging system using TNM categories in the early 1950s (O. Beahrs, personal communication, January, 1959). After considerable debate and dialogue, both groups published comprehensive manuals and handbooks using the same TNM language but with stages defined differently. Only in the past decade with the publication of the third edition of *Manual for Staging of Cancer* by the AJCC[2] (1988) and the fourth edition of *TNM Classification of Malignant Tumors* (1987) has true concurrence of classifications occurred on both sides of the Atlantic. Of equal importance is the fact that special staging systems widely introduced and used by international specialty oncology societies were blended into the TNM system if feasible and, if not, were adopted instead of a TNM system. Examples are the classification of malignant gynecologic tumors by FIGO and the Ann Arbor classification of Hodgkin's and non-Hodgkin's lymphomas.

Unfortunately, the cost of uniformity among the AJCC, UICC, and special interest groups has meant continued change in staging systems over the past decade (Fig. 6-1). These same TNM symbols really represent different subgroups in that the previous editions of the AJCC and UICC publications are at variance with the latest editions (fourth edition of UICC and third edition of the AJCC). Oncologists must scrupulously search out the precise TNM system and dates to ensure comparability of data when reading the literature of the 1980s.

In addition, the introduction of diagnostic imaging technology such as CT and MRI has further compounded the issue, because these technologies are not available to all oncologists, particularly in different parts of the world. Clinical staging beyond physical examination has become widely conditioned by imaging procedures and laboratory findings. Surgical pathologic staging is accepted for numerous inaccessible sites and has been introduced or added to anatomic sites previously not staged. Criteria for the staging workup at each site are available in the aforementioned manuals.

The impact of other factors beyond the anatomic extent of the cancer to ascertain the true biology of the cancer is increasingly evident in the addition of the histopathologic classification of malignancies by the WHO International Classification for Oncology.[44] For some lesions, particularly sarcomas such as glioblastoma multiforme, soft tissue sarcomas, and osteogenic sarcomas, histopathologic grade is more dominant in determining the "stage group" than the anatomic extent. With the development of precise immunoassays, new tests such as prostate-specific antigens (PSA) carry more meaning than nonspecific enzymes such as alkaline and acid phosphatase in determining prognosis. With the identification of new markers based on molecular biologic expression of cancer as in DNA histograms, oncogenes, protein adducts, trophic or growth factors, cell receptors (ER+ or ER−), a new era of prognostic factors beyond TNM is likely to develop. With flow cytometry and radiolabeling, cell kinetics, labeling index, growth fraction, and percentage of cells in different phases of the cell cycle can be readily and economically determined.

The classification staging literature of the past three decades is at variance because of changes with each edition of the AJCC and UICC manuals, and it is important that a period of

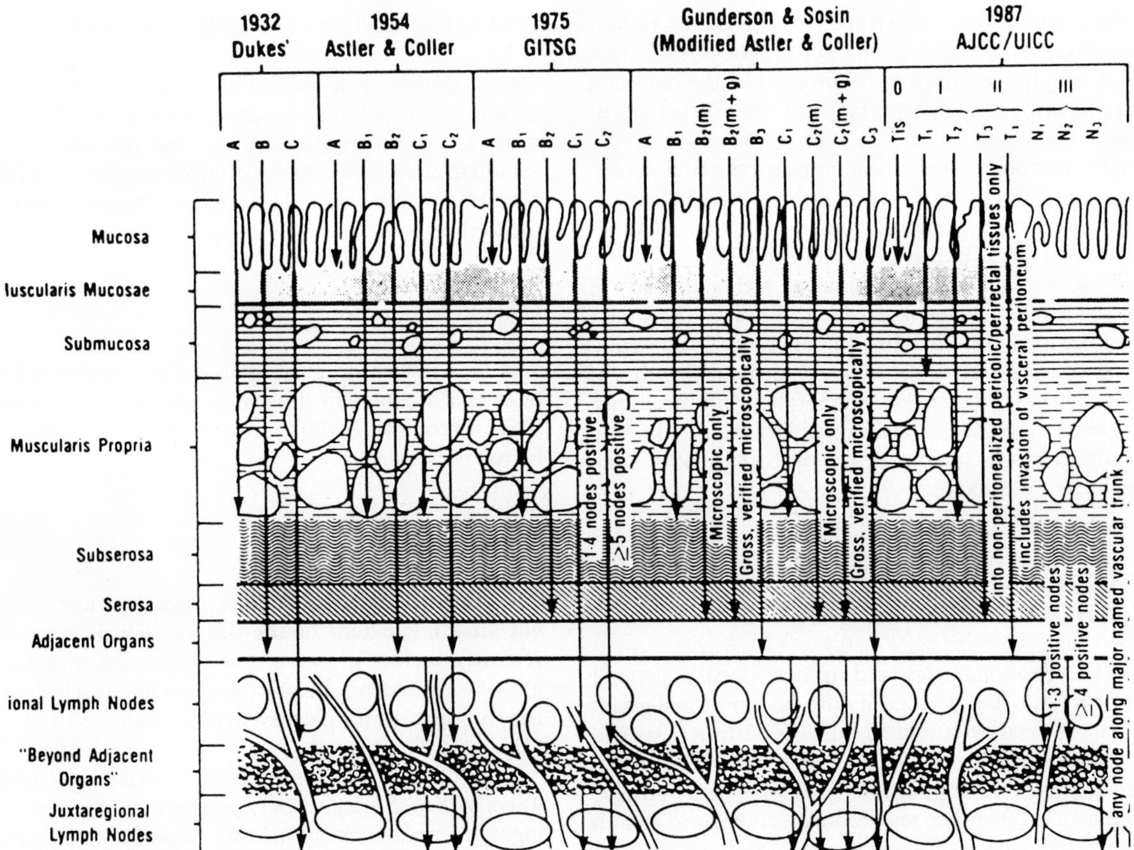

FIGURE 6–1. Schematic comparison of the various pathologic staging systems. (DeVita, VT, Hellman S, Rosenberg SA [eds]: Cancer: Principles and Practice of Oncology, 3rd ed. p. 909. Philadelphia, JB Lippincott, 1989)

stabilization is allowed before more changes are introduced. In this chapter we will provide an overview of the criteria and bases for the current classification systems and the importance of histopathology. A unified system for T, N, and M categories is offered, based on a linguistic analysis of different TNM systems at each site. Each site has a T category that advances according to size, spread patterns to subsites, and invasion of adjacent structures and surrounding viscera. N categories advance as variations based on size and number of nodes increase and ipsilateral or bilateral and contralateral spread occurs. These distinctions often differ for reasons that are not obvious, nor are investigative data based on clinical findings or results always offered to explain the basis of the change or the determining factors used.

OBJECTIVES OF A CANCER CLASSIFICATION SYSTEM

The objectives of a classification system for cancer are well stated by the UICC[42]: aiding the clinician in planning treatment, giving some indication of prognosis, assisting in the evaluation of end results, facilitating the exchange of information among treatment centers, and assisting in the continuing investigation of cancer.

The term "stages of cancer" does not imply a regular progression from Stage I to Stage IV; rather, these stages are arbitrary divisions, often related to prognosis and frequently related to treatment. Final placement into a category depends on well-defined features. However, the clinician's judgment concerning the extent of the cancer is often the most decisive factor in prognosis and selection of treatment.

Because general agreement concerning determination of the extent of disease at each anatomic site was the primary aim, the UICC chose to define the three components of the cancer and its spread, rather than work out a precise staging system. The extent of the primary tumor (T), the regional nodes (N), and the presence of metastases (M) are to be determined before treatment, should remain unchanged, and should not be altered by evidence obtained at operation. The number of T categories was set at four and the number of N categories at four; M categories were to be based on the presence or absence of metastases. No further general rules were outlined.

CURRENT CLASSIFICATION OF CANCER

It is appropriate to review the general considerations of both the UICC and the AJCC for staging cancers. The UICC statement notes that the historical practice of dividing cancer cases into groups according to stages arose because the crude survival or apparent recovery rates were higher for cases of localized disease than for cancer extending beyond the organ of origin. The designations of "early" and "late" on one hand and "localized" and "widespread" on the other were interchanged, implying some regular progression with time.

To evaluate where one modality was superior to another, two similar groups of cancer patients had to be compared. The best parameter to establish staging was thought to be the anatomic extent of disease. Therefore, the primary emphasis was placed on a precise, complete description of the primary tumor, regional lymph nodes, and distant metastases. The classification is a means of simply recording facts observed by the clinician, whereas staging implies an interpretation of these facts regarding prognosis.

The AJCC position is to establish "appropriate clinical classifications based on simplicity, practicability, and credibility." As a basis for formulating its clinical staging system, the AJCC has adopted the TNM classification system of the UICC and seeks compatibility with it so far as is consistent with standards of practice in the United States. Actually, the two systems have incompatibilities in all ten sites. In addition, many inconsistencies exist within each system regarding specific categories of involvement. If these two major committees, specifically assigned to agree and dedicated to compatibility, cannot develop congruous and uniform standards, the probability of general acceptance is even less likely.

IMPORTANCE OF HISTOPATHOLOGIC GROUPING

Histopathology is no longer ignored in most classifications of neoplasms. It is important to identify the variety of malignant processes that can occur in tissues because the pattern of spread often reflects the specific cell type, its stage of differentiation, and its anaplasticity. The language for describing histopatholoy is being standardized from two major sources: the World Health Organization's *International Classification of Diseases for Oncology*,[44] and the Armed Forces Institute of Pathology (AFIP) *Atlas of Tumor Pathology*.[29]

ANATOMIC EXTENT OF DISEASE

The adoption of the TNM system by the UICC and the AJCC has been the most important general agreement in the reporting of neoplastic disease. The proposed technique of description and classification applicable to all sites of cancer involves five steps:

A. Identification of extent of disease by use of these symbols:
  1. T, extent of primary tumor
  2. N, condition of regional nodes
  3. M, distant metastases

B. Assignment of a series of numbers to each of these three components, indicating ascending degrees of involvement, T1, T2, N1, N2, and so on

C. Indication of the presence of metastases by M+ and absence by M0. For certain sites a number of specific M categories (M1, M2, and so on) may be desirable.

D. Grouping of the TNM assignments into a smaller number of clinical stages, usually four. This system makes it possible to regroup many categories (approximately 50) into similar staging systems.

E. Addition of supplementary information based on the results of histologic examination by appending the symbol (+), for example, N+, or the addition of symbols designating a specific radiologic study, such as NL (lymphangiography).

The major criticism of this system, as it is currently used, arises from the different meanings and modifications assigned to the T and N categories by the two major committees, different cooperative groups, and various authors.

ONCOTAXONOMY: A UNIFIED APPROACH

Oncotaxonomy is a unified and uniform approach to cancer classification and staging. Paradigms or models for primary tumors (T) or lymph nodes (N) and metastases (M) are presented to assist the reader in establishing certain guiding principles. Where these principles are not followed, a comment will be offered unless it is clearly supported by clinical data.

Oncologic Anatomy

The first step in organizing an oncotaxonomy is knowing the oncologic anatomy of the tumor site, that is, the regional anatomy surrounding the organ or tissue of origin including lymphatic drainage.[37]

T Categories

The criterion for categorizing a primary tumor (T) is the apparent anatomic extent of the disease, which is based on three features: surface spread, depth of invasion, and size. Following a review of existing classifications, an attempt is made to define the clinical basis for placement of a tumor in T1, T2, T3, or T4 (Table 6-1).

Depth of invasion is the main criterion used, and it primarily consists of the degree of extension into adjacent or surrounding structures such as muscle, capsule, bone, cartilage, and other viscera. Loss of mobility or fixation of the tumor to another structure is used in most schema. Figure 6-2 illustrates the variety of tissues often involved at different primary sites. The fibrous capsule in solid organs, in contrast to the intrinsic muscle wall of hollow organs, is often the first tissue invaded by the cancer. The most difficult tasks are the clinical assignment of a structure to the "adjacent tissue" category and the distinction of adjacent tissue from "surrounding tissue." The term "adjacent tissue" often refers to an attached structure with an ill-defined boundary between it and the organ or site of origin, which performs a similar function and is of similar tissue type. In contrast, a "surrounding tissue" is most often different in tissue type and function such as another viscera.

Tumor size can be related to cell number; it can also be related to tumor age, but this is based on many assumptions. A small tumor is thought to be "early" in a clinical sense, but microscopic foci up to 1.0 cm^3 consist of 10^9 cells. Rate of growth, cell removal or loss, and host resistance are factors that affect spread patterns. Under the most controlled animal conditions, measurement of tumor volume to estimate rate of growth is fraught with error: even when time zero is known, true log growth is limited. As soon as the tumor becomes grossly palpable, changes in growth fraction and cell cycle and loss occur. On a microscopic tissue level, cancer can spread by means of three pathways—local, lymphatic, or vascular—at any point in its evolution. It can enlarge and progress from T1 to T4 with little local cell loss, or cell loss can be in the form of local cell death and tumor necrosis.

In breast, oral cavity, and cervical cancer, size differentiates T categories, but it has not been used in other locations. When size is used, a tumor 2 cm or less in diameter is assigned to T1, a tumor 2 cm to 4 or 5 cm in diameter to T2, and one greater than 4 to 5 cm in diameter to T3. Although the terms "massive" or "huge" have been applied to T4 lesions, no size is given, but a tumor 10 cm or larger in diameter would readily fall into this category.

TABLE 6–1
Specific Criteria Related to T Categories

	T1	T2	T3	T4
DEPTH OF INVASION				
Solid organs	Confined	Capsule muscle	Bone cartilage	Viscera
Hollow organs	Submucosa	Muscularis	Serosa	
Mobility	Mobile	Partial mobility	Fixed	Fixed and destructive
Neighboring structures	Not invaded	Adjacent (attached)	Surrounding (detached)	Viscera
SURFACE SPREAD				
Regions (R)	1/2 or R_1	R_1	$R_1 + R_2$	$R_1 + R_2 + R_3$
Circumference	<1/3	1/3 to 1/2	>1/2 to 2/3	>2/3
SIZE				
Diameter	<2 cm	2 to 4–5 cm	>4–5 cm	>10.0 cm

(Rubin P [ed]: Clinical Oncology: A Multidisciplinary Approach, 6th ed, p 11. New York, American Cancer Society, 1983)

There are two basic classifications for primary tumors depending on whether the organ is a solid or hollow.

Modified Classification for Solid Organs

In classification of cancer of solid organs, size of tumor is often used to categorize its extent. The importance of tumor size relates to organ size and in most situations also relates to depth of invasion.

T1: Confined to the organ of origin, usually 2 cm in its largest diameter; localized; mobile

T2: Deeply invading to adjacent structures, including muscle, ligaments, capsule; from 2 cm to 4 or 5 cm in its largest diameter; localized; mobile or partially mobile

T3: Regionally confined; usually greater than 4 cm or 5 cm but less than 10 cm; fixed. Critical criterion is fixation, most often bone and cartilage, but invasion of the extrinsic muscle walls, serosa, and skin is also included. Surrounding detached structures of different anatomy or function are in this category, but this inclusion can be debated because of the varieties of anatomic structures.

T4: A massive lesion, greater than 10 cm in diameter, destructive, not confined to the region. Invasions into major nerves, arteries, and veins are placed in this category. Destruction of bone in addition to fixation is an advanced sign.

Modified Classification for Hollow Organs

The circumferential spread of luminal compromise, as well as other features, is considered important, particularly in the gastrointestinal tract. Special organs, such as those of the upper respiratory and digestive tract, have features of both solid and hollow structures and present unique problems. The relationship of bone to the mucosal surface or to the organ of origin causes shifts in emphasis categories, as is discussed.

T1: Superficially invading, limited to mucosa or submucosa; less than one third of circumference; localized; occupying not more than one half of one region

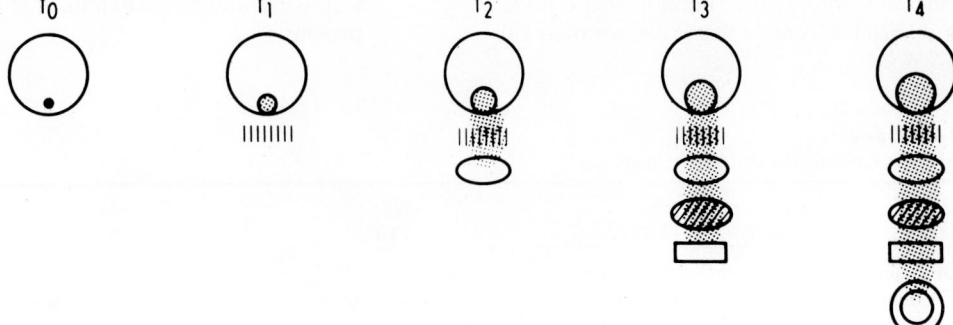

FIGURE 6–2. Classification of extent of primary tumor in solid viscera, portraying the organ (*large circle*) and the cancer (*dotted small circular areas*). The vertical lines are adjacent muscle, the clear oval an adjacent attached structure, and the lined oval a surrounding (often detached) structure. The rectangle stands for bone or cartilage and the double circle, another organ. The gravity of cancer spread or progress is identified in the sequential spread shown and is the basis of most classifications of T1, T2, T3, and T4. For a solid structure or site, T2 is deeply invading, usually 2 cm to 4 or 5 cm in its largest diameter, localized, mobile, or partially mobile; T3 is regionally confined, usually more than 4 or 5 cm but less than 10 cm, fixed; T4 is a massive lesion, more than 10 cm in diameter, destructive, not confined to the region. (Rubin P: Cancer 31:963, 1973)

T2: Deeply invading, into muscularis region; more than one third but less than one half of the luminal circumference; occupying more than one half of the region; mobile

T3: Invading all layers of the visceral wall, through serosa into surrounding structures; fixed but not necessarily to bone; covering more than one half of circumference; occupying more than one visceral region

T4: A massive, destructive lesion, causing a fistula or sinus; covering more than two thirds of circumference; resulting in complete luminal obstruction; occupying more than two visceral regions

Multiple tumors can be indicated by a numerical prefix; the tumor in the highest category is indicated by a numerical subscript.

N Categories

A unified code should be readily agreed on for grouping of nodes. The criteria are size, firmness, capsular invasion, depth of invasion, mobility or fixation, single or multiple nodes, ipsilateral, contralateral, and bilateral distribution, and distant nodes (Table 6-2).

The concept of a "regional node-bearing" area should be abandoned, as Rouviere[34] advised, because the lymph nodes in the anatomic region of a specific organ do not consistently receive all the lymph flow of that organ. Rouviere[34] introduced the terms "first echelon" and "second echelon" of lymph nodes. The *first echelon* is the first set of lymph nodes receiving the drainage of a specific organ. The *second echelon* consists of those nodes that commonly receive lymph drainage, both prograde and retrograde, from another lymph node rather than directly from the site or organ. Echelon may be interchanged (in the translator's note in Rouviere's text) with *station*, a preferred term, which refers to a regular stopping place in a stage of a progression, as in cancer spread.

The concept involves a clinical distinction. Thus in categorizing cancers of the oral cavity, oropharynx, hypopharynx, and larynx, current classification schemata of the UICC[15] and AJCC[1] refer to neck nodes as the regional nodes. An effort is made to indicate whether the drainage is unilateral or bilateral, because the assignment of contralateral nodes to N2 or N4 depends on whether such contralateral nodes drain a site directly or indirectly.

Size is one of the most important criteria in that a node must be palpable or detectable. A node that is greater than 1.0 cm and less than 3.0 cm is considered to be significant regardless of its firmness. In the UICC schema N0 refers to no evidence of palpable nodes and N1 to palpable nodes. The distinction between the "not suspected" and "suspected" nodes is noted as N1a *versus* N1b. In the AJCC schema the negative situation (nodes not suspected), which includes both N0 and N1a of the UICC schema, embodies the principle of downstaging, or giving the patient the benefit of the doubt. In the interest of reaching a common agreement, however, the AJCC has adopted the UICC designations.

Firmness is another important criterion in differentiating N0 from N1. Clearly, a hard pea-sized node (0.5 cm) may be considered significant.

Roundness refers to the measurement of nodal thickness. A discoid or flat node is usually a shotty node. The rounder the node is, the more likely it is to be firm and involved by tumor.

Number of involved lymph nodes is another variable in categorization. The presence of multiple nodes is often associated with invasion of the nodal capsule, making the nodes tend to cluster and resulting in matting and eventually loss of mobility.

Mobility is another important criterion in considering progression. The term "fixation" is often used but rarely defined in a classification schema. Loss of mobility of a lymph node results from invasion of the nodal capsule and infiltration of adjacent tissues. Invasion into muscle can be determined by loss of mobility on contraction of the muscle. Complete fixation is reserved for the N3 category and refers to fixation to bone, major blood vessels, or skin. Finally, fistulization is fixation with destruction of skin; for example, fistula and bone lysis or sclerosis refer to a proposed N4 category.

Nodal Classification

The general description is offered for all nodal sites, based on the criteria just described (Fig. 6-3).

N0: No evidence of disease in lymph nodes. This category, is a major point of conflict between the UICC and the AJCC. Palpable flat nodes usually 1.0 cm or less in diameter of little significance are N0 in the AJCC but N1a in the UICC classification. When nonpalpable nodes are examined microscopically, they should be designated as N1 when there is no evidence of microscopic foci and N+ when microscopic tumor foci are present.

TABLE 6–2
Specific Criteria Related to N Categories

	N1 FIRST	N2 FIRST	N3 FIRST	N4 SECOND
Drainage				
Unilateral	Ipsilateral	Ipsilateral	Ipsilateral	Contralateral
Bilateral	Ipsilateral	Contralateral or bilateral	Ipsilateral or contralateral	Distant
Number	Solitary	Multiple		
Size	<2–3 cm	>3 cm	>5 cm	>10 cm
Mobility	Mobile	Partial matted muscle invasion	Fixed to vessels, bone, skin	Fixed and destructive

To distinguish N0 from N1 the specific criteria include: Size—between 1 and 2 cm; Firmness—soft to hard; Roundness—0.5 to 1 cm.
(Rubin P [ed]: Clinical Oncology: A Multidisciplinary Approach, 6th ed, p 11. New York, American Cancer Society, 1983)

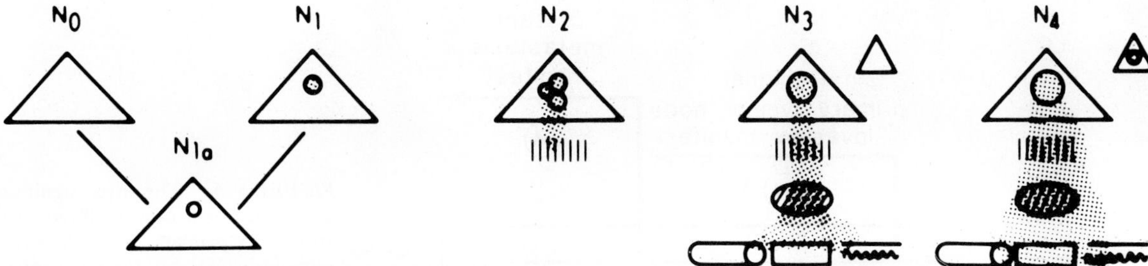

FIGURE 6–3. Classification of nodal involvement. The triangle represents a node-bearing region. The large triangle represents the first station (regional) node and the small triangle, the second station (juxtaregional) node. The small, dotted, circular areas represent the cancer. The vertical lines represent muscle; the lined oval, surrounding separate structure (s); the rectangle, bone or cartilage; the cylinder, blood vessels; and the horizontal double lines, skin. The order of progression of the cancer extends as shown with increasing involvement of surrounding structures in N1, N2, N3, and N4. (Rubin P: Cancer 31:963, 1973)

N1: Palpable and movable nodes limited to the first station. Metastases are suggested on the basis of firmness and roundness of the node and its size alone, for example, 2 cm to 3 cm in diameter. The presence of all these qualities rather than only one increases the certainty of diagnosis. The presence of multiple nodes does not change this category provided that the nodes are confined to the regional primary stations and are not matted.

N2: Firm to hard nodes, palpable and partially movable; 3 cm to 5 cm in diameter. Such nodes may show microscopic evidence of capsular invasion; clinically, they may be matted together or demonstrate partial fixation to adjacent muscle. Nodes can be contralateral or bilateral if the primary tumor drains to both sides by virtue of anatomy, but involvement is confined to the first station.

N3: Complete fixation. Invasion extends beyond the capsule, with complete fixation to bone, large blood vessels, skin (dermal lymphatic invasion), or nerves (perineural invasion).

N4: Nodes involved beyond the first station. They are in second or distant stations. If two first but distinct nodal stations are vertically arranged and both are involved, such double involvement is staged as N4. A special situation arises in two circumstances: when the primary tumor drains to midline nodes that are located on both sides of the midline (*e.g.*, testes to retroperitoneal periaortic nodes) and when the primary tumor crosses the midline and drains to both sides of the anatomy (*e.g.*, midline tongue to both sides of the neck). In such situations, two node-bearing areas are equal and, in the same horizontal plane, are both considered as primary and therefore are not N4 but N2. Extensive nodal necrosis leading to destruction of bone and skin (fistula) or massive size (10 cm) may be placed in this group.

Nx: Nodes inaccessible to clinical evaluation.

NL: Nodes evaluated by lymphangiography. L− refers to a negative study and L+ to a positive study. An equivocal finding can be referred to as L+ if equivocally positive, and L− if equivocally negative

N− or N+: Nodes evaluated by microscopic study and designated as negative or positive depending on findings

M Categories

The lack of a consistent and thorough attempt to categorize anatomic extent of metastases is conspicuous in current schema. The important feature is the presence or absence of a metastases, for example, M0 versus M1.

The designation of Mx for nonmetastatic workup should be used when the likelihood is considered low, rather than M0. Note that visceral involvement by direct extension is not considered to be a metastasis. The following classification schema is offered (Fig. 6-4):

M0: No evidence of metastases

M1: Solitary, isolated metastasis confined to one organ or anatomic site

M2: Multiple metastatic foci confined to one organ or system or one anatomic site, for example, lungs, skeleton, or liver, with minimal or no functional impairment

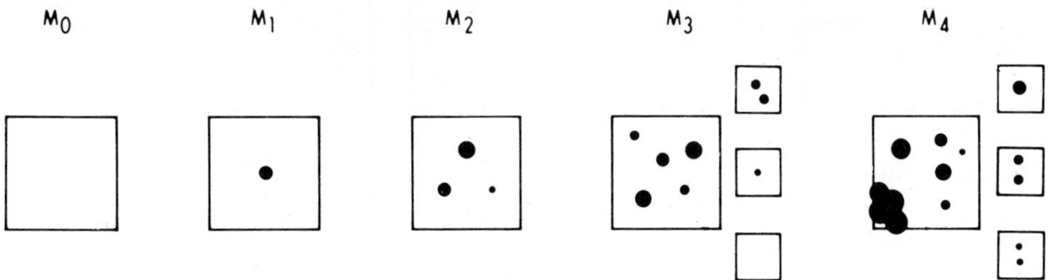

FIGURE 6–4. Classification of metastatic involvement. Each box represents a visceral organ. The number of black dots represents the number of metastatic lesions. The stages are explained in the text; the order of progression is M1a, M1b, M1c, and M1d. The number of organs and number of metastases increases. (Rubin P: Cancer 31:963, 1973)

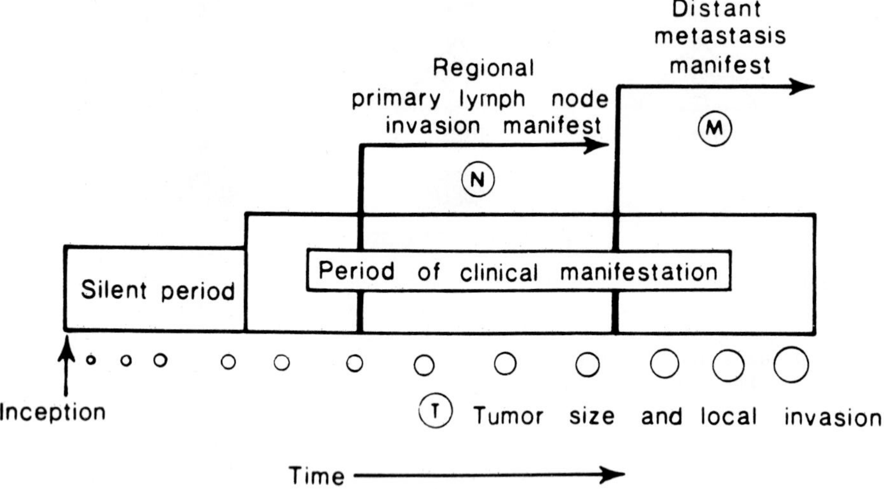

FIGURE 6–5. The three significant events in the life of a cancer—tumor growth (T), spread to primary lymph nodes (N), and metastasis (M)—are used as they appear (or do not appear) on clinical examination, before definitive therapy begins, to indicate the extension of the cancer. This shorthand method of indicating the extension of disease at a particular designated time is the stage of the cancer in its evolution. (Beahrs OH, Henson DE, Hutter RVP, Myers MH [eds]: Manual for Staging of Cancer, 3rd ed, p4. Philadelphia, Lippincott, 1988)

M3: Multiple organs involved anatomically, with no or minimal to moderate functional impairment of involved organs

M4: Multiple organs involved anatomically, with moderate to severe functional impairment of involved organs

Mx: No metastatic workup done

M: Modified to show viscera involved by appended letter: pulmonary metastases (Mp), hepatic (Mh), osseous (Mo), skin (Ms), brain (Mb), and so on

M+: Microscopic evidence of suspected metastases, confirmed by pathologic examination

UNIFIED STAGE GROUPING

A logical or orderly progression of a malignant tumor may occur in time from Stage I to Stage II to Stage III to Stage IV (Fig. 6-5), although as illustrated in Figure 6-1, cancer occasionally spreads in a predictable fashion from T1 to T4 before involved nodes appear and progress from N1 to N3; following this phase, metastases appear. In fact, node involvement or hematogenous spread can occur with T1 and T2 stages.

The problem with having five categories each for the primary tumor (T), regional nodes (N), and metastases (M) is that a patient can be placed in one of 12 different categories, which is unmanageable for the clinician. The reduction to four stage groupings has become clinical custom (Fig. 6-6).

A unified stage grouping would provide a rational basis for comparing patterns of spread based on the biology, anatomic location, organ of origin, and nodal drainage of the cancer. However, in the new editions of the UICC and AJCC manuals, the stage groupings have been frequently changed and follow no uniform set of criteria, thus require careful scrutiny before use.

CLASSIFICATION OF ILLNESS

Sporadic attempts have been made to classify the amount of illness, discomfort, or distress caused by the cancer. The devel-

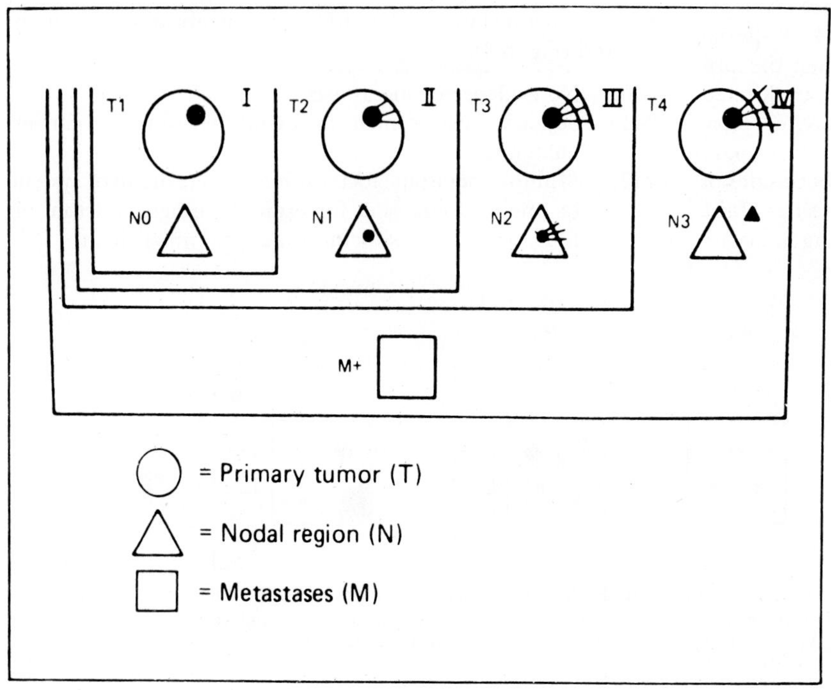

FIGURE 6–6. Stage grouping. The stage grouping is based on clustering TNM categories. (Rubin P [ed]: Clinical Oncology: A Multidisciplinary Approach, 6th ed, p 12. American Cancer Society, 1983)

opment of a clinical taxonomy has been emphasized by Feinstein[9] as a procedural step not related to anatomic or pathologic considerations. The clinical spectrum of patients consists of lanthanic types and complainants of varying degrees. Lanthanic patients are asymptomatic, that is, in a latent, occult, or subclinical phase of their disease. Complainants have symptoms that compel them to seek medical attention. The primary complaints can be divided temporarily into those of short (<1 year) or long duration (>1 year). Systemic complaints such as anorexia, weight loss, and anemia are nonspecific and can indicate metastatic disease or may represent a bodily response to a large localized mass.

A definable illness index, using capital letters as in Hodgkin's disease, could be formulated:

A: Asymptomatic or lanthanic
B: Primary complaints related to symptoms and signs produced by primary cancer and regional lymph nodes
C: Systemic complaints related to nonspecific generalized signs such as weight loss, anemia, fevers, pruritus, and night sweats
D: Paraneoplastic complaints related to metabolic disturbances such as neuropathies and dermatomyositis, resulting from hormones such as antidiuretic hormone (ADH) and corticosteroids
E: Metastatic complaints related to symptoms produced by distant metastases

CLASSIFICATION OF THE HOST

The host may have many conditional factors, in addition to the cancer, that will determine not only the treatment but also the outcome. Certain vital statistics may be used to describe the host: sex (and endocrine status with regard to menopause), age, race, religion, marital status, number of children, occupation, socioeconomic status, and familial (genetic) background.

Associated medical disease is a hidden factor determining the selection of surgical or nonsurgical methods. The patient with severe cardiac or chronic pulmonary disease, with renal or hepatic dysfunction, and with debilitating arthritis or neurologic disorder are at high risk for surgery but may require surgery therapy for cancer. Life span may be reduced in these circumstances, often independent of the outcome of cancer management.

Performance Index

It is important to determine the ability of the patient to perform daily functions. The quality of survival, rather than the quantity, needs definition, as suggested in a performance index modified by the AJCC and some of the cooperative groups (Table 6-3).

Psychologic Index

The effect of the disease on the psychology and *vice versa* has received much comment. The documentation of psychologic states and correlation with clinical course are attempted with the following rating system: appropriate response, anxiety, depression, euphoria, denial, suicidal, psychotic, other.

PROCESS OF STAGING

It is necessary to define the minimum diagnostic workup that establishes the extent of the disease. The UICC system deems acceptable all diagnostic radiologic procedures and endoscopy of any type. Operative findings are combined with pathologic specimens and are allowed in many sites such as ovary and gastrointestinal tract. The AJCC allows inclusion of all types of examinations ordinarily available to the average specialist, but surgical and pathologic findings are not to be used in assigning clinical stage, except in certain sites where specific operations are necessary for determination of the stage. There are four steps in defining the extent of tumor:

1. Clinical staging—the evaluation of the apparent extent,

TABLE 6–3
Criteria for "Performance Status" on the Karnofsky Scale

Able to carry on normal activity; no special care is needed	100	Normal; no complaints; no evidence of disease
	90	Able to carry on normal activity; minor signs or symptoms of disease
	80	Normal activity with effort; some signs or symptoms of disease
Unable to work; able to live at home and care for most personal needs; a varying amount of assistance is needed	70	Cares for self; unable to carry on normal activity or to do active work
	60	Requires occasional assistance but is able to care for most needs
	50	Requires considerable assistance and frequent medical care
Unable to care for self; requires equivalent of institutional or hospital care; disease may be progressing rapidly	40	Disabled; requires special care and assistance
	30	Severely disabled; hospitalization is indicated although death not imminent
	20	Very sick; hospitalization necessary; active supportive treatment is necessary
	10	Moribund, fatal processes progressing rapidly
	0	Dead

(Karnofsky DA, Abelmann WH, Kraver LF, et al: Cancer 1:634, 1948)

based on physical examination, routine laboratory studies, and radiographic and endoscopic procedures in different anatomic studies

2. Radiographic staging—the use of sophisticated radiography, such as selective arteriography, tomograms, air insufflation, lymphangiography, venography, and radioisotope scanning procedures
3. Surgical staging—the exploratory procedure to identify the extent of disease, such as laparotomy in Hodgkin's disease[17] or ovarian cancer
4. Pathologic staging—the use of endoscopic biopsy to determine depth of invasion as in cervical or bladder cancer; the practice of needle biopsy to establish presence or absence of nodal disease

The most recent AJCC designation for staging depends on different types of evaluative evidence used for classifying the extent of disease at different sites and at different times: *c*TNM, clinical-diagnostic staging; *s*TNM, surgical-evaluative staging; *p*TNM, postsurgical treatment-pathologic staging; *r*TNM, retreatment staging (clinical-diagnostic stage classification when restaging is necessary for additional or secondary treatment); *a*TNM, autopsy staging.

For cancers at certain accessible sites, especially those that can be treated appropriately by more than one modality, the extent of the cancer should be determined and recorded before definitive treatment is carried out. This makes it possible to compare the results of different modalities of treatment of certain lesions, such as carcinoma of the cervix,[15] oral cavity, and larynx. Postsurgical treatment-pathologic staging is used to describe the known extent of the disease following the complete examination of the therapeutically resected specimen. Amount of residual tumor, if any, following surgical resection should be recorded.

It is essential not to intermix clinical-diagnostic and surgical-pathologic staging because shifting of T and N categories purifies each stage and has an impact on reporting of end results. The results improve in all stages, but overall survival remains the same. This is illustrated in Figure 6-7 by Ulfelder in ovarian cancer staging and illustrates the importance of comparing patients by using the same criteria.

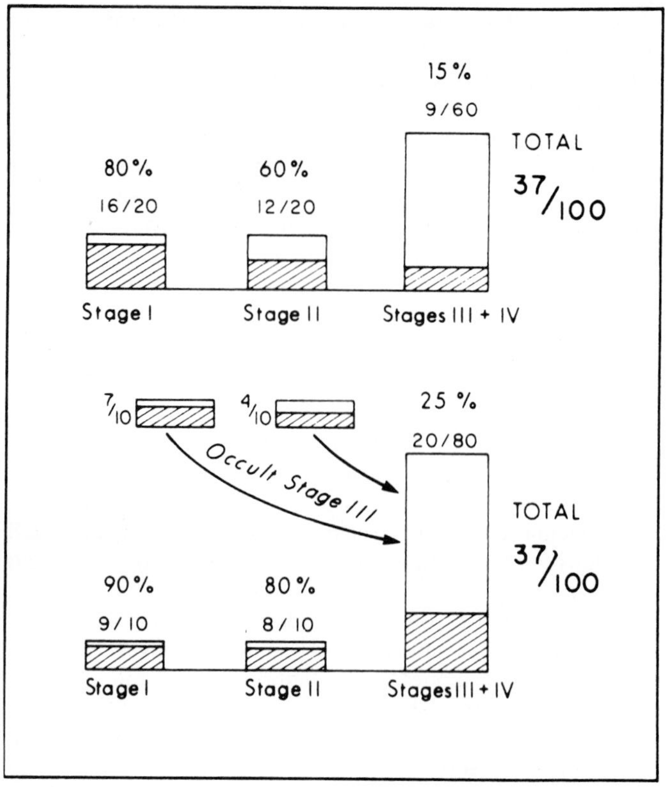

FIGURE 6–7. Hypothetical graph of 5-year survival (*shaded columns*) by stages of 100 patients with ovarian carcinoma. The upper row indicates the original staging; the lower row shows reassignment of one half of each group in Stages I and II because of the discovery of occult, biopsy-proven extension to either the diaphragmatic peritoneum or the retroperitoneal nodes. Although the overall cure rate is unchanged (37%), the rate in each column is significantly increased. (Ulfelder H: Int J Radiat Oncol Biol Phys 7:1083–1086, 1981)

Controversy and Differences in Staging Systems

It is important to recognize that considerable controversy regarding the differences in staging systems exist and that classification schemata continue to evolve. The use of the same letters (TNM) and Roman numerals (I through IV) has created a sense of uniformity in the literature. However, most systems have changed in the three decades that the UICC and AJCC have been in existence. One needs only to scan literature on the head and neck[3,4,37] to recognize the degree of divergence as well as convergence among systems in different aspects. The pragmatic adoption of the Ann Arbor system by the AJCC and UICC has led to uniformity in reporting. The histopathology is crucial to understanding non-Hodgkin's lymphomas,[5,12,19,21,28] but classifications are constantly changing. Currently histopathology is of less prognostic importance in Hodgkin's lymphoma.

Occasionally a neoplastic disease undergoes a dynamic change and a new staging system emerges,[18] as in Kaposi's sarcoma in patients with acquired immunodeficiency syndrome (AIDS). Some of the common cancer classifications respond to new imaging approaches[32,39] and require refinement and alteration, as in breast cancer,[6,41] or they change because of different diagnostic or pathologic approaches, as in colorectal cancer[7,26,33,46] or genitourinary cancers such as renal,[14] bladder,[3,31] prostate,[20,40,43] and testicular tumors.[25,27] Gynecologic cancer classification and staging systems have not changed greatly since their introduction in 1920, but they have been affected by new diagnostic operative procedures[24] such as laparotomy for staging of nodes to increase accuracy.[12,36]

Impact of New Imaging Modalities on the Staging Process

The advances and variety of new imaging modalities have made a major impact on the staging process. Computed tomography (CT) has become the standard against which other tumor imaging procedures are measured. Table 6-4 illustrates the common imaging procedures most often applied to oncologic staging. Magnetic resonance imaging (MRI) is emerging as a tumor-imaging technique that will challenge CT because it has the

---

Surgical-Pathologic Staging

Surgical-evaluative staging is used to describe the known extent of disease after a major surgical exploration, biospy, or both. It is particularly applicable to cancers at sites inaccessible to clinical evaluation, such as carcinoma of the ovary, stomach, colon, kidney, and lung. Information obtained by surgical exploration, histopathologic studies of biopsy specimens, or both may be used, along with the available clinical data, to describe the extent of disease.

TABLE 6–4
Specific Imaging Procedure: Limitations and Applications

IMAGING PROCEDURE	RELATIVE COST	RELATIVE SENSITIVITY	RELATIVE SPECIFICITY	COMMENTS
Plain film radiography	low	varied	high	Plain films have excellent sensitivity and specificity in the soft tissues (mammography) and bones. In the chest, low-contrast tumor targets are a problem.
Xerography	low	high	moderate/high	Edge enhancement and wide exposure latitude allow soft tissue application (breast, neck, appendicular soft tissues, bone, and soft tissue tumor imaging).
Contrast GI studies	moderate	high	high	Cancer screening applications can be justified for high-risk groups (esophagus, stomach, and colon).
Radionuclide liver scan	moderate	moderate	low	Displaced by CT/US as screening liver imaging modality of choice. ? still initial screen of choice.
Radionuclide bone scan	moderate	high	low	Procedure of choice in skeletal scanning. Abnormal sites must be verified by film radiography.
Radionuclide brain scan	moderate	moderate	low	CT has replaced radionuclide brain scanning except where CT access is limited.
Ultrasound abdominal scanning	moderate	high	moderate	Lack of radiation exposure, cost, and availability lend ultrasound to abdominal screening. Technique is operator dependent.
Computed tomography				
Brain	high	high	moderate	Procedure of choice for screening mass/lesion suspect using contrast enhancement only.
Lung	high	high	low	Highest sensitivity of all studies in detection of lung nodules. High false-positive rate.
Abdomen	high	high	moderate	
Angiography	high	high	moderate	Cost, invasiveness, and time limit applications.
Magnetic resonance (MR)	high	high	high(?)	Resolution similar to CT. Elimination of bone artifacts makes CNS images better than CT. In chest, tumor and hilar node imaging improved over CT. Applications elsewhere—insufficient experience.

(Bragg DG, Rubin P, Youker JE [eds]: Oncologic Imaging, p 19. New York, Pergamon Press, 1985)

advantage of three-dimensional imaging of the tumor and surrounding anatomy. The prospect of tumor and normal tissue discrimination with MRS in *in vivo* spectroscopy, particularly with surface coils, awaits the development of new and higher field strength magnets.[11] These new imaging studies are being evaluated in diagnostic clinical trials similar to therapeutic clinical trials. When a tumor is detected and a specific histopathologic diagnosis established, the development of tumor imaging strategy is needed for precise definition of the tumor (T) and lymph node (N) components. Reference to a recent comprehensive textbook on oncologic imaging is recommended to guide clinicians at specific tumor sites in the course of staging, treatment, and follow-up decisions. Each tumor site requires different imaging strategies to optimize the staging workup so that the best combination of treatment modalities is chosen.

REFERENCES

1. American Joint Committee on Cancer: Manual for Staging of Cancer, 2nd ed. Philadelphia, JB Lippincott, 1983
2. American Joint Committee on Cancer: Manual for Staging of Cancer, 3rd ed. Philadelphia, JB Lippincott, 1988
3. Baker HW: Staging of head and neck cancer. Int Adv Surg Oncol 6:1, 1983
4. Black RJ, Gluckman JL: Staging systems for cancer of the head and neck region: Comparison between AJC and UICC. Clin Otolaryngol 8:305, 1983
5. Castellino RA, Dunnick NR, Goffinet DR, et al: Predictive value of lymphography for sites of subdiaphragmatic disease encountered at staging laparotomy in newly diagnosed Hodgkin's disease and non-Hodgkin's lymphoma. J Clin Oncol 1:532, 1983
6. Cuschieri A, Irving AD, Robertson AJ, et al: Percentage of malignant involvement: A new concept in staging of breast cancer. Ann R Coll Surg Engl 65:11, 1983
7. Davis NC, Newland RC: Terminology and classification of colorectal adenocarcinoma: The Australian clinico-pathological staging system. Aust NZ J Surg 53:211, 1983
8. Denoix PF: TNM classification. Bull Inst Nat Hyg Paris 1:1–69, 1944; 5:52–82, 1944
9. Feinstein AR: Clinical Judgement. Huntington, NY, Robert E Kriega Publishing Co, 1974
10. Fryjordet A, Skatun J: Staging of urinary bladder cancer by computerized tomography compared to clinical staging and postoperative pathologic staging. J Oslo City Hosp 33:76, 1983
11. Fullerton GD Cameron IL: Nuclear magnetic resonance imaging in biological systems. Biomed Tech 3(6):458, 1985
12. Gerbie MV: Malignant tumors of the vagina: Classification and approach to treatment. Rostard Med 73:271, 1983
13. Glimelius B, Haeberg H, Sundstrom C: Morphological classification of non-Hodgkin malignant lymphoma. II. Comparison between Rappaport's classification and the Kiel classification. Scand J Haematol 30:13, 1983
14. Hata Y, Tada S, Kato Y, et al: Staging of renal cell carcinoma by computed topography. J Comput Assist Tomogr 7:828, 1983
15. International Union Against Cancer: TNM Atlas: Illustrated Guide to the Classification of Malignant Tumours. Heidelberg, Springer-Verlag, 1982
16. Jackson H Jr, Parker F Jr: Hodgkin's Disease and Allied Disorders. New York, Oxford University Press, 1947

17. Joshua DE, Dalgleish A, Kronenberg H: Is staging laparotomy necessary in patients with supradiaphragmatic Stage I and IIA Hodgkin's disease? Lancet 1:847, 1984
18. Krigel RL, Laubstein LJ, Muggia FM: Kaposi's sarcoma: a new staging classification. Cancer Treat Rep 67:531, 1983
19. Krueger GR, Medina JR, Nein HO, et al: A new working formulation of non-Hodgkin's lymphomas: A retrospective study of the new NCI classification proposal in comparison to the Rappaport and Kiel classifications. Cancer 52:833, 1983
20. Lange PH, Narayan, P: Understanding and undergrading of prostate cancer: argument for postoperative radiation as adjuvant therapy. Urology 21:113, 1983
21. Leonard RC, Cuzick J, MacLennan IC, et al: Prognostic factors in non-Hodgkin's lymphoma: The importance of symptomatic stage as adjunct to the Kiel histopathological classification. Br J Cancer 47:91, 1983
22. Lister TA, Crother D, Sutcliffe SB, et al: Report of the Committee Convened to Discuss the Evaluation and Staging of Patients with Hodgkin's Disease, Cottswald Meeting. J Clin Oncol 7:1630–1636, 1989
23. Lukes RJ, Butler BB, Hicks EB: Natural History of Hodgkin's disease as related to its pathologic picture. Cancer 19:317–344, 1966
24. Maggino T, Bonetto F, Catapano P, et al: Clinical staging versus operative staging in cervical cancer. Clin Exp Obstet Gynecol 10:201, 1983
25. Maricek, B, Brutschin P, Triller J, et al: Lymphography and computed tomography in staging nonseminomatous testicular cancer: Limited detection of early stage metastatic disease. Urol Radiol 5:243, 1983
26. Mauro MA, Lee JK, Heiken JP, et al: Radiologic staging of gastrointestinal neoplasms. Surg Clin North Am 64:67, 1984
27. McCauley RL, Javadpour N: Supraclavicular node biopsy in staging of testicular carcinoma. Cancer 51:359, 1983
28. Moir DH: War of the words: Classification of non-Hodgkin's lymphomas. Pathology 15:359, 1983
29. National Research Council Committee on Pathology: Atlas of Tumor Pathology. Washington, Armed Forces Institute of Pathology, 1950–present.
30. Nelson D.F, Deiner-West M, Horton J, et al: Combined modality approach to treatment of malignant gliomas: Reevaluation of RTOG 7401/ECOG 1374 with long-term follow-up. A joint Radiation Therapy Oncology Group (RTOG) and Eastern Cooperative Oncology Group (ECOG) study. NCI Monograph. 6:279–284;1988
31. Nelson RP: New concepts in staging and follow-up of bladder carcinoma. Urology 21:105, 1983
32. Osborne MP, Meijer WS, Yeh SD, et al: Lymphoscintigraphy in the staging of solid tumors. Surg Gynecol Obstet 156:384, 1983
33. Pheils MT: Staging of large bowel cancer. Med J Aust 1:254, 1984
34. Rouviere H: Anatomie des Lymphatiques des l'Homme. Paris, Masson, 1932
35. Rubin P: A unified classification of tumors: An oncotaxonomy with symbols. Cancer 31:963, 1973
36. Rubin P, Bragg DG: The staging and classification of cancers. In Bragg DG, Rubin P, Youker JE (eds): Oncologic Imaging, pp 1–11. New York, Pergamon Press, 1985
37. Rubin P, Keys H: The staging and classification of cancer: A unified approach. In Carter SK, Glatstein E, Livingston RB (eds): Principles of Cancer Treatment, pp 14–25. New York, McGraw-Hill, 1982
38. Sakai S, Ebihara T, Ono 1, et al: A comparison of AJC and JJC proposals on TNM classification of maxillary sinus carcinoma. Arch Otorhinolaryngol 237:139, 1983
39. Shibata HR: Lymphoscintigraphy in the staging of breast cancer. Can J Surg 26:487, 1983
40. Spirnak JP, Resnick Ml: Clinical staging of prostate cancer: New modalities. Urol Clin North Am 11:221, 1984
41. Stenkvist B, Bengtsson E, Eriksson O, et al: Histopathologic systems of breast cancer classification: Reproducibility and clinical significance. J Clin Pathol 36(Suppl):392, 1983
42. TNM Classification of Malignant Tumors, International Union Against Cancer, 4th ed. Berlin, Springer-Verlag, 1987
43. Whitmore WE Jr: Natural history and staging of prostate cancer. Urol Clin North Am 11:205, 1984
44. World Health Organization: International Classification of Diseases for Oncology. Geneva, WHO, 1976
45. World Health Organization Technical Report Series, No. 53:47–48, 1952
46. Zinkin LD: A critical review of the classification and staging of colorectal cancer. Dis Colon Rectum 26:37, 1983

7

Methodology of Clinical Trials

Thomas F. Pajak

A clinical trial is a preplanned study of the safety and efficacy of one or more potentially beneficial therapies in humans. The patients are selected according to predetermined criteria of eligibility and then observed for predefined evidence of favorable and unfavorable effects. The data are collected prospectively. A clinical trial can be conducted within a single institution or among many cooperating institutions. Although single-institution studies have the advantage of more direct supervision, there are often too few patients available in one location to conduct a definitive trial discriminating among therapies with moderate differences in improvement within a reasonable period, making multiinstitutional trials necessary.

PROSPECTIVE CLINICAL TRIALS VERSUS RETROSPECTIVE STUDIES

The evaluation of different treatment approaches can be accomplished with a prospective clinical trial. However, if a particular treatment approach has been tried in the past, a second evaluation method is to conduct a retrospective survey of those instances where it has been used.

The major strength of prospective clinical trials is that the objectives are defined in advance. The patients can be selected, treated, and evaluated in accordance with standardized procedures, and the data can be recorded in a careful manner. When the treatments are randomly assigned, the resulting data are considered to be unbiased, which permits an immediate and straightforward interpretation of the study results.

The major disadvantage in pursuing prospective trials is the length of time required to obtain an answer. For example, to evaluate the addition of breast irradiation to segmental mastectomy for women with Stage I and II breast cancer, the women would first have to be enrolled in the trial and then followed up for at least 5 years before a definitive analysis could be done. The National Surgical Adjuvant Breast and Bowel Project (NSABP) reported the results from such a similarly designed prospective trial, which took 10.0 years from the entry of the first patient to publication of the results.[14] For long-term studies, the question asked at the beginning of the trial must be carefully formulated so that the answer derived still has clinical relevance by the time it is published. The NSABP breast trial proved that segmental mastectomy followed by breast irradiation is an appropriate therapy for Stage I and Stage II breast tumors that are ≤4 cm if the margins of the resected specimens are free of tumor.

The number of questions asked in a prospective trial should be kept to a minimum. As the number of questions is increased, there is a corresponding increase in the number of patients required and the complexity of the trial, diminishing the chances of successfully completing the trial. Ideally, prospective trials should be restricted to evaluating one treatment objective.

Ancillary studies seeking to learn about disease-related processes should be appended whenever possible to treatment studies. The advantage is that patients have received a standardized protocol treatment that makes the interpretation of the results easier, enhancing acceptance of the results. For example, the Radiation Therapy Oncology Group (RTOG) conducted an ancillary clinicopathologic study of advanced inoperable head and neck tumors in conjunction with the evaluation of concomitant radiation therapy and cisplatin chemotherapy. The ancillary study found improved response and survival in patients with nonkeratinizing squamous cell carcinomas.[9]

One way to obtain an answer sooner is to conduct a retrospective survey that examines the outcomes of past patients treated in a variety of ways. These surveys may contain serious potential biases. For example, a more intensive treatment given to a patient with a poorer prognosis may artificially appear inferior. The principal problem arises from the way in which a particular treatment was selected for a patient and how it was subsequently administered. The selection of the treatment and its delivery are influenced by preexisting factors that cannot be readily documented. These undocumented factors may introduce large biases in the analysis and interpretation of the findings.

Bias can be dramatic if undocumented factors directly influence the treatment data. For example, Perez and associates[38] and Hanks and colleagues[21] reported a dose-response effect for the local control of prostatic carcinoma with radiation. The former group reported the effect for Stage C patients treated at Mallinckrodt Institute, and the latter group reported it for Stage B patients from the Patterns of Care Surveys. In both instances, the results depended on the high in-field recurrence rates for patients receiving total doses of less than 6000 cGy. For the Stage B patients, the crude in-field recurrence rate was 24% (22 of 87), and for the Stage C patients, the crude rate was 38% (5 of 13). One important consideration is the total amount of radiation therapy originally prescribed for the patients who received less than 6000 cGy. For the Patterns of Care Stage B patients, no information was provided about their originally prescribed doses or about the various institutional treatment policies. The treatment policy employed at Mallinckrodt Institute for Stage C patients called for a minimum dose of 6000 cGy to the prostate with an additional 1000 cGy, depending on the size of the prostate. For the Stage C patients, receiving a total dose of less than 6000 cGy was probably the result of general condition, poor tolerance to therapy, or disease progression during radiation treatment. Thus, the reported dose-response effect in Stage C patients may merely reflect the overall condition and tolerance of the men treated, and the claimed therapeutic effect should be questioned. If one assumes that Stage B patients from Patterns of Care Surveys were usually prescribed more than 6000 cGy, then the same question applies to their claimed dose-response effect.

In addition, the quality of the data available for the retrospective study may be inadequate, because there was originally no plan to conduct such a study when the data were collected. The most common deficiency is missing data. The RTOG experience with assessing retrospectively the quality of the surgery performed in a three-arm prospective randomized trial (RTOG 7303) for operable head and neck cancer patients illustrates the problems.[27] The data for surgical quality control review could be collected retrospectively on 155 of 223 patients having protocol surgery. Eight patients were subsequently found to have insufficient or illegible data submitted and were excluded from all analyses. All four proposed measures of surgical quality could be completely evaluated in only 115 (52%) of 223 patients.[25]

HISTORIC CONTROLS

Conducting a trial with historic controls has some very attractive aspects. Fewer patients are required to be accrued, which saves time. Because the investigators can offer a single treatment believed to be better than the standard, they are relieved of any ethical dilemma, and the patients will know that they are receiving the best treatment their doctors have to offer. The investigator also saves time because explaining a single-treatment study takes far less time than a randomized study.

Some factors diminish the reliability of historic controls.[3,40,44,45] In the interval between the treatment of the historic controls and the treatment of the patients with the new experimental approach, the diagnostic procedures, patient referral patterns, response evaluation, and supportive patient care may have changed significantly. As with retrospective studies, the data for historic controls may be inadequate, because it was not known what would be needed for evaluating a future study when the information was collected. Patients entered on the new experimental treatment are more likely to be excluded from analysis on the basis of a protocol violation found after entry. This probably would not happen in the historic control group, because the necessary data are unavailable or because the investigator did not meticulously evaluate the treatment given the controls. For these reasons, trials using historic controls are generally not accepted as definitive confirmation that a particular treatment approach is superior.

TYPES OF PROSPECTIVE TRIALS

Studies that evaluate treatments can be classified in terms of their objectives. For chemotherapy trials, three distinct "phases" (phase I, phase II, and phase III) have evolved. Radiation oncologists have adopted the terminology developed by medical oncologists with one main difference. The endpoints used in phase I and II trials of radiation therapy modalities are often broader. Late toxicity, for example, may occur many years after the completion of radiation therapy. This contrasts with the usual short-term endpoints of acute toxicity and initial tumor response typically used with chemotherapy phase I and II trials.

The sample size requirements for a radiation therapy trial with a long-term ("late") toxicity endpoint are usually two to three times larger than for a chemotherapy trial. Not all patients entered into the radiation therapy trial survive beyond the latent period for late toxicity or remain at risk long enough after the latent period. Because of the increased sample size requirements and the longer minimum follow-up period necessary, some radiation therapy phase I and phase II trials may take appreciably longer to complete than the typical chemotherapy trials.

Phase I Studies

The objective of a phase I study is to determine the maximum-tolerated dose for a single schedule and mode of administration by evaluating toxicity. Chemotherapy trials usually evaluate acute or short-term toxicity. In radiation therapy trials, the toxicity to be evaluated can be either acute or late, depending on the modality being evaluated. Trials, for example, investigating hyperthermia and radiosensitizers employ acute toxicities as the principal endpoint to determine the maximum-tolerated temperature and duration and the total dosage of a drug, respectively. Trials investigating altered radiation fractionation schemes, such as hyperfractionation (radiation twice a day), employ late toxicity as the principal endpoint to determine the maximum-tolerated total dose.

Phase II Studies

The primary goal of a phase II trial is to determine whether a particular treatment program is sufficiently effective with acceptable toxicity to warrant further testing in a large-scale phase III trial. Ideally, a phase II study would only be initiated after a phase I trial. In phase II chemotherapy trials, the usual endpoint to measure activity is the extent of tumor reduction, either partial or complete response. This endpoint can be measured relatively early. Although radiation oncologists frequently use initial tumor response as an endpoint, locoregional control of the tumor at some specified time is a more meaningful measure of antitumor activity for them. The endpoint of locoregional control requires longer patient follow-up than that of initial tumor response. Because of the late endpoints used in evaluating morbidity and antitumor effects, studies are sometimes designed to look at both endpoints simultaneously and are designated as phase I/II studies. The RTOG trials for determining the "best" total dose for altered radiation schemes in treating lung and head and neck tumors are examples of phase I/II studies.[8]

Phase III Studies

Phase III trials consist of randomized comparisons of an experimental treatment, which has already undergone phase I and II testing, with a standard treatment. Phase III trials are typically conducted using patients who have had no previous treatment for the cancer under study. Phase III trials evaluating chemotherapeutic agents typically require many more patients than phase I or II studies. The endpoints in phase III drug studies, such as response-duration and survival, take much more time than the acute toxicity and initial tumor response endpoints used in phase I and II drug studies. A larger population is not necessarily needed in radiation therapy phase III studies; a phase I/II radiation dose-searching study may require more patients than a phase III study.

PRINCIPLES AND SELECTION OF ENDPOINTS

The term *endpoints* refers to the criteria by which the efficacy or the morbidity associated with a treatment are evaluated. Explicit endpoints are required before the sample size and the duration of the study can be determined. This also ensures that the appropriate clinical observations are made in a way that does not bias the result. In a study comparing adjuvant treatment with no treatment after surgery, the patients assigned to the control arm must be evaluated as often as patients on the active treatment; otherwise, disease failures are detected sooner on the adjuvant treatment arm.

Absolute survival is usually the most objective measure of treatment because a patient is either alive or dead. It calls for no interpretation. Survival is not a good measure in situations for which there are highly effective salvage therapies that may produce dramatically prolonged disease control and survival. For example, patients with early Hodgkin's disease who have failed local field irradiation can be salvaged with combination chemotherapy so successfully now that many patients can be cured.[5] Survival may not be a good endpoint if the study population is elderly or consists of patients with early disease with the potential of long survival. This is often the case in trials for men with Stage B and Stage C prostate cancer.

Many investigators use *determinate survival* instead of absolute survival to adjust for deaths from unrelated causes. Failure for determinate survival is defined as death with active local or metastatic cancer. Deaths from any other cause with no active cancer are considered as censored observations at the point of death and not as treatment failures. Determinate survival often calls for subjective judgment on the part of the investigators and depends on the timeliness and quality of the follow-up data. Ideally, if investigators want to use determinate survival, they should also report absolute survival and summarize the causes of death so that the reader can judge the appropriateness of the data and the extent of possible biases introduced.[30] Using both endpoints in patients with carcinoma of the prostate, Laramore and associates showed that fast neutron irradiation was superior to photon radiation therapy.[30] McGowan used only determinate survival in assessing the influence of prior transurethal resection on the prognosis of men with prostate cancer treated with irradiation.[31] No information was provided in his report about the total number of patients who had died or the causes of death. The reader was, therefore, unable to assess whether deaths from intercurrent diseases may have introduced a bias into the comparison of patients with and without transurethal resection of the prostate.

There is a third type of survival often reported. It is called *disease-free survival, relapse-free survival,* or *no evidence of disease (NED) survival.* This endpoint is generally used to compare two treatment approaches after surgery, as in the NSABP trials, or two treatments that effect almost complete disappearance of the initial disease. However, there is no general agreement about what constitutes a treatment failure or how NED survival is to be estimated. One way of estimating NED survival is to consider a patient as a failure at the first reported occurrence of locally or distantly progressive disease or death from any cause. For evaluating its trials and estimating NED survival, the NSABP also considers a patient who develops a second primary tumor as a failure if the patient did not otherwise fail. Patients who do have persistent disease after treatment are problematic when NED survival is estimated. The RTOG trials in treating prostate cancers have considered patients with persistent disease as failures on day 1 for the estimation of NED survival.[42]

Other commonly used endpoints are tumor shrinkage and duration of tumor disappearance. Complete and partial response are two of the most widely used classifications of tumor shrinkage. A *complete response* occurs if all the documented pretreatment measurable disease and related symptoms have disappeared without the appearance of any new disease for at least 1 month. A *partial response* occurs if more than 50% regression of all measurable pretreatment disease is achieved for at least 1 month. These two response categories call for subjective judgment. Whether a patient achieves a partial response depends on who is doing the measurements.[35] The more closely the patients are evaluated by the investigator, the fewer are the number of complete responses and the shorter are the durations of the complete responses. It is assumed that patients with partial responses do better than those who have less than partial responses. This was not the case for head and neck patients after induction chemotherapy administered before planned surgery and radiation therapy in the RTOG 8116 study.[24] Survival of the partial responders after induction chemotherapy was similar to survival of patients not achieving partial responses. However, both groups had statistically significant worse survival than the complete responders after chemotherapy induction.

In addition to absolute or determinate survival, the endpoints most frequently used to evaluate radiation therapy schemes are locoregional tumor control and late effects. Different methods of estimating locoregional control have been used for head and neck trials. The RTOG approach is based on achieving complete response and has been consistently used since 1979. Patients not achieving a complete response are considered locoregional failures as of day 1. Patients achieving a complete response and subsequently failing are considered locoregional failures as of the date the failure was noted.[12]

The Danish Head and Neck Cancer Study Group (DAHANCA) and the European Organization for Research on Treatment of Cancer (EORTC) Radiotherapy Group have used only tumor progression to define failure.[37,48] EORTC considered patients whose tumor progressed during radiation therapy as failures at the end of irradiation. Patients whose tumor progressed after radiation therapy were classified as failures on the first reported occurrence. DAHANCA also considered a patient whose tumor progressed as a failure. Because DAHANCA started their evaluation of locoregional control from 6 months after the start of radiation, it was unclear how patients who died during the first 6 months were assessed in the estimation of locoregional control. Both the RTOG and the EORTC used the Kaplan-Meier technique to adjust for the number of patients at risk when estimating locoregional control. It is not known whether DAHANCA employed any statistical technique to adjust for the varying number of patients at risk. The EORTC method was applied to the previously reported RTOG misonidazole study.[13] Table 7-1 compares the estimates obtained by the EORTC method with the RTOG method. At 6 months, the difference between the estimates is quite striking, and by 2 years, the difference diminishes. The magnitude of differences between the two treatments using either the RTOG or the EORTC method of estimation is similar. All 147 patients who did not achieve a complete response were classified as

TABLE 7–1
Comparison of the RTOG and the EORTC Methods for Estimating Locoregional Control

		ESTIMATED RATE		
TREATMENT	METHOD	6 MO	1 YR	2 YR
RT + Misonidazole	RTOG	43%	31%	22%
	EORTC	74%	46%	31%
RT alone	RTOG	50%	37%	27%
	EORTC	76%	48%	33%

treatment failures with the RTOG method; 99 (67%) were so classified by the EORTC method. One standardized approach to estimate locoregional control must be adopted so that trials can be compared.

TARGET POPULATIONS FOR SELECTED ENDPOINTS

The patient population targeted for a study should have two characteristics. First, it should enable evaluation of the selected endpoint. If late effects are the major endpoint, the patient population targeted for the study should have a high probability of surviving long enough to observe any possible deleterious late effects. For example, the RTOG defined an optimal subset of patients with brain metastases for its investigations of various altered fractionation schedules.[10] Before a population is considered suitable for a study, there must also be ethical appraisal of the proposed treatment approach and the currently accepted approaches. Second, the population targeted for the study must be large enough so that the patient accrual can be obtained in a reasonable period.

SAMPLE SIZE AND STUDY DURATION

The feasibility of a study should be evaluated by the length of time necessary from the entry of the first patient until the time the study is ready for final analysis. This interval can be divided into two parts. The first part consists of the time needed to enter the required number of patients, and the second part is the follow-up observation to measure treatment activity.

Before the required number of patients can be calculated for a phase III study, the investigator must specify the following items:

1. Type I error (α)
2. One-tailed versus two-tailed test
3. Type II error (β)
4. Baseline expectation for the principal endpoint with the standard arm
5. Estimate of the minimum difference between the treatments

The type I error is the error of deciding that one treatment is superior to another when there is really no difference in efficacy. The rate is given as a probability of a difference occurring simply by chance alone when no treatment difference really exists. The type I error can be thought of as the false-positive rate associated with clinical trials. The type I error is often designated as the level of significance. The Greek letter alpha (α) is used to denote it. In medical research, values of less than 0.05 are considered to be evidence that chance alone cannot explain an occurrence. The smaller the value for α, the less likely it is that chance alone can explain the occurrence.

The interpretation of the type I error depends on whether the statistical test comparing the treatments is "two tailed" or "one tailed." Two-tailed tests are appropriate if the investigator wants to detect a statistically significant difference favoring one of the treatment arms, regardless of which one it happens to be. In a clinical trial comparing two distinct combination chemotherapy programs, a two-tailed approach should be used. In this situation, there are three possible results from the trial:

1. One combination is found superior, and it becomes the treatment of choice.
2. The other combination is found superior, and it becomes the treatment of choice.
3. Neither combination is found to be superior to the other, and subsequent treatment selection is based on other factors, such as toxicity or cost.

In a trial comparing an experimental treatment with a standard treatment, an investigator may consider it unnecessary and even unethical to statistically demonstrate that the experimental treatment is significantly worse than the standard treatment. The investigator is really interested in only two possible results from the clinical trial. If the experimental treatment is better than the standard treatment, then the experimental treatment becomes the treatment of choice. Alternatively, if the experimental treatment is not better, the standard treatment remains the treatment of choice.

In this situation, the investigator could use a one-tailed statistical test to establish the superiority of the experimental treatment arm. The use of the one-tailed test is somewhat controversial among statisticians. Many believe that a one-tailed test should be used only when a treatment difference in a given direction is impossible (*i.e.*, the experimental treatment is significantly less effective than the standard treatment), because the criterion for rejecting the null hypothesis of no treatment difference is more liberal for a one-tailed test than for a two-tailed test.[11] All the subsequent charts for sample sizes in this chapter are based on a two-tailed test comparing the treatments.

The type II error is the error of deciding that two or more treatments are equivalently effective, although one treatment is actually superior to the other treatment(s). This error rate is given as a probability of failing to detect a specified magnitude of difference among the treatments when the difference in outcome is actually true. The type II error can be thought of as the false-negative rate associated with clinical trials. The type II error rate is denoted by the Greek letter beta (β). The lower the beta value, the smaller is the chance of failing to detect a real difference. Generally, type II error is set at 0.20. However, if it is probable that the trial will not be duplicated, then β should be set at a lower value, such as 0.10. For example, the national phase III study testing the effectiveness of chemotherapy sandwiched between surgery and radiation therapy in patients with head and neck tumors was designed with a type II error of 0.10 because of the limited number of patients available. This study took over 5 years to accrue the necessary patients, and it is extremely unlikely that it will be repeated.[46]

Routinely, type I errors (significance levels) appear in all papers reporting treatment comparisons. Type II errors of failing to detect treatment differences are almost never reported. These are critically important when an investigator is reporting no treatment difference. Table 7-2 shows the size of type II errors for various hypothesized response rates and sample sizes. For a treatment comparison of response rates based on 25 patients on each arm, a 10% difference (between

TABLE 7–2
Type II Errors for Various Response Rates and Sample Sizes

NUMBER OF PATIENTS PER ARM	OBSERVED TWO RESPONSE RATES*			
	50% − 40% = 10%	55% − 40% = 15%	60% − 40% = 20%	65% − 40% = 25%
25	94/100†	88/100	80/100	69/100
50	88/100	75/100	56/100	36/100
100	63/100	49/100	23/100	7/100
150	37/100	30/100	8/100	1/100

* *Type II errors (missing a treatment difference) were based on binomial distribution with* $\alpha = 0.05$ *and the parameters specified in the table.*
† *A treatment difference of 10% (50% − 40%) will fail to be detected 94 out of 100 times.*

40% and 50%) will not be detected as statistically significant 94 out of 100 times (94/100). With 150 patients per treatment arm, the type II error associated with this 10% difference reduces to 37/100. If the desired type II errors associated with a 10% difference (40%–50%) are 20/100 or 10/100, respectively, the required sample sizes per treatment arm becomes 407 and 538 patients.

Consider the situation in which the investigator reports no statistical significance for a treatment difference of 25% = (65% − 40%) based on 25 patients. The associated type error II of 69/100 (Table 7-2) tells the reader that the reporting of no statistical difference in this case should be anticipated. If the reader judges the 25% difference between the two treatments to be clinically important, the interpretation should be that the difference fails to be statistically significant because of an inadequate sample size. Another clinical trial with a large enough sample to reduce the type II error should be conducted to substantiate the reported lack of a difference of 25%.

The next consideration is to estimate the baseline rate for the standard treatment arm in the population targeted for the study, either from an analysis of preceding studies or from the literature. In either case, previous results may have been based on a study population that differs somewhat from the population targeted for the new study.

The estimate of the minimum improvement in rate expected between the standard and the experimental treatment should be based on pilot data and what would be considered clinically relevant. This difference in improvement is denoted by the lower case Greek letter delta (δ). In studies of locoregional control rates, patients may die of causes other than the primary disease or may be lost to follow-up, and this must be taken into account when sample size requirements are estimated. From the analyses of previous studies or from the literature, estimates for this death rate can be obtained and the required sample size adjusted accordingly.

Table 7-3 can be used to calculate the sample size when the

TABLE 7–3
Total Number of Patients Required to Detect an Improvement in Response Rate Over the Smaller Response Rate

SMALLER RATE (P_1)	IMPROVEMENT IN RESPONSE RATES ($P_2 - P_1$)									
	0.05	0.10	0.15	0.20	0.25	0.30	0.35	0.40	0.45	0.50
0.05	1240*	412	226	148	108	84	66	54	46	38
	946†	318	176	116	86	66	54	44	36	32
0.10	1912	570	292	184	128	96	76	60	50	42
	1448	436	224	142	100	76	60	48	40	34
0.15	2500	708	348	212	146	106	82	66	52	44
	1888	538	266	164	114	84	64	52	42	36
0.20	3004	822	394	238	158	114	88	68	54	44
	2264	626	302	182	124	90	68	54	44	36
0.25	3424	918	432	254	168	120	90	70	56	46
	2578	696	330	196	130	94	72	56	44	36
0.30	3760	990	460	268	176	124	92	72	56	44
	2828	750	350	206	136	96	72	56	44	36
0.35	4012	1044	478	276	178	126	92	70	54	44
	3018	790	364	212	138	98	72	56	44	36
0.40	4180	1074	488	278	178	124	90	68	52	42
	3142	814	372	214	138	96	72	54	42	34
0.45	4264	1086	488	276	176	120	88	66	50	38
	3206	822	372	212	136	94	68	52	40	32
0.50	4264	1074	478	268	168	114	82	60	46	34
	3206	814	364	206	130	90	64	48	36	28

* *Upper figure:* $\alpha = 0.05$ *and* $\beta = 0.10$
† *Lower figure:* $\alpha = 0.05$ *and* $\beta = 0.20$

comparison is based on two proportions. It provides the number of patients required per treatment arm to satisfy the specified conditions for type I and II errors and the baseline success rate with hypothesized improvement in rate. These values were derived using the method of Casagrande and associates.[4] To illustrate use of the table, assume we wish to test the addition of chemotherapy to radiation therapy in the treatment of women with advanced cervical cancer (AJC Stages IIIA and IIIB). From a previous RTOG study of the same population, an estimated 50% survival rate at 2 years with standard radiation therapy was observed. If α is set at 0.05 and β is set at 0.20, 182 patients on each arm for a total of 364 patients will be needed if a minimum improvement of 15% is sought. The number of patients required per arm is reduced by 43% if the minimum improvement is increased to 20%. However, the number of patients is increased by 124% if the minimum improvement is decreased to 10%.

The sample size depends on the level of improvement to be detected. Thus, testing an experimental treatment with the promise of only minor improvement in the success rate is not generally feasible because of the large number of patients needed to detect the difference. On the other hand, the level of improvement should not be arbitrarily set at an unrealistically large margin to ensure that the number of patients needed for the trial is obtainable.

If a 30% minimum improvement with the addition of chemotherapy in the trial is hypothesized, only 45 patients per arm would be needed. With that number of patients, a 20% improvement would be missed 60 out of 100 times and a 15% improvement would be missed 77 out of 100 times. Thus, a better approach is to test for a moderate improvement that is clinically meaningful.

Instead of just comparing the proportion of patients alive at a specified time for two treatments, the researcher can compare their entire survival experience. To accomplish this, one has to make some assumptions about the mathematic form of the survival distribution. The logrank test is now commonly used in the analysis of cancer clinical trials. Freedman has reported tables, based on the logrank test, of the number of patients required.[18] The format of Table 7-4 is similar to that in Table 7-3, which makes it easy to use. However, this table assumes that analysis occurs at a fixed time T after the last patient has entered the study; information on patient follow-up extending beyond T is excluded. Practically, this means that if the analysis is planned 1 year after the last patient entered, all the follow-up beyond 1 year would be excluded in this analysis. Because of the exclusion of possible follow-up data, the required number of patients tends to be overestimated. Table 7-4 gives the total number of patients required per arm to detect various degrees of improvement over a baseline rate in two situations: for $\alpha = 0.05$ and $\beta = 0.20$ and for $\alpha = 0.05$ and $\beta = 0.10$. For the proposed advanced cervical study, 140 patients would be required per arm to detect at least 15% improvement in survival.

For a more precise estimate of the number of patients required and the time before the definitive analysis can be undertaken, the method described by Bernstein and Lagakos[2] or Lachin and Foulkes[28] should be used. The method specifies the usual parameters required for sample size estimates and allows specification of patient accrual rate, the length of follow-up after completion of accrual, and losses resulting from death from unrelated causes if the primary endpoint is locoregional control. These methods are more complicated, and a computer is required to implement them.

RANDOMIZATION

One reason that randomization is used in phase III studies is to minimize selection bias by the clinical investigator who enters patients on a particular study. Patients selected for randomization must be able to tolerate all the treatment programs proposed in the protocol because the investigator does not know the treatment assignment beforehand. The Eastern Cooperative Oncology Group (ECOG) conducted a single-institution pilot study to determine the maximum tolerable dose of cisplatin (DDP) as a radiosensitizer by administering it weekly during intensive radiation therapy in the treatment of locally advanced unresectable head and neck cancer. Besides establishing the dose of DDP at 20 mg/m^2, a complete response rate of 84% (27 of 32 patients) was observed.[22] With this very encouraging result, ECOG undertook a randomized trial to compare this combined program with standard radiation therapy alone. Later the trial was expanded into an intergroup effort. The preliminary analysis after completing the patient accrual for the phase III trial showed no difference in the complete response rates (34% for radiation therapy with DDP in the randomized trial versus 30% for radiation therapy alone).[23]

The phase trial III showed no response enhancement with the addition of weekly cisplatin during radiation therapy for patients able to tolerate the combined approach before randomization. The difference in the complete response rates between the phase I/II and the phase III studies may result from patient selection. The investigators in the phase I/II study may have intentionally selected patients whom they believed could tolerate the increased dose of weekly cisplatin.

Randomization tends to balance the distribution of prognostic factors, both known and unknown, among the patient groups assigned to each treatment regimen. Thus, randomization ensures that previously published results from the treatment comparisons in past studies are just as applicable today as when they were published and will still be applicable 10 years from now. Randomization lends increased credibility to the results and promotes wider acceptance among other clinical investigators.[1,29]

The simplest randomization plan calls for figuratively flipping a coin to determine the treatment assignment for each patient. Unfortunately, there is no guarantee at any intermediate point that the patients are equally balanced between the two treatments or that the assigned treatment groups have similar prognostic profiles. All that statistical theory can guarantee is that, as the total number of patients entered on the study increases, the number of patients randomized to each treatment group tends to become equal.[29] If serious imbalances occur, statistical analyses cannot completely compensate for them; furthermore, when major adjustments have to be made, the results tend to have less credibility.

To minimize the chances of imbalances that may ruin a study, a stratified randomization plan can be used. Each stratum is defined by a combination of important prognostic factors. In each stratum, the treatment assignments are evenly distributed after a specified number, which has to be a multiple of the number of different treatments and provides the size of the "block." Using the example of the proposed cervical cancer trial, there are two treatments, designated as X for radiation therapy plus chemotherapy trial and Y for radiation therapy alone. Suppose that AJC Stage (IIIB versus IVA) and pretreatment Karnofsky performance score (80 to 100 versus 50 to 70) are considered to be important prognostic factors influencing survival. Then there are a total of 4 strata (2 × 2) for which

TABLE 7–4
Total Number of Patients Required to Detect an Improvement in Survival Rate Over a Baseline Survival Rate

BASELINE	IMPROVEMENT IN SURVIVAL RATES ($P_2 - P_1$)									
P_1	0.05	0.10	0.15	0.20	0.25	0.30	0.35	0.40	0.45	0.50
0.05	664(615)*	232(209)	133(116)	92(78)	71(58)	58(46)	49(38)	43(32)	38(27)	35(24)
	497(459)†	174(156)	100(87)	69(59)	53(44)	43(34)	37(29)	32(24)	29(21)	26(18)
0.10	1289(1128)	395(335)	207(171)	135(108)	98(76)	76(57)	63(45)	53(37)	46(31)	41(26)
	963(843)	295(251)	155(128)	101(30)	73(57)	57(43)	47(34)	40(28)	35(23)	31(20)
0.15	1894(1562)	544(435)	272(211)	170(128)	120(87)	91(64)	73(49)	61(39)	52(32)	45(27)
	1415(1167)	406(325)	204(158)	127(95)	90(65)	68(48)	55(37)	46(29)	39(24)	34(20)
0.20	2445(1895)	676(507)	328(238)	200(140)	138(93)	103(67)	81(51)	66(40)	56(32)	48(26)
	1827(1416)	505(379)	245(178)	150(105)	104(70)	77(50)	61(38)	50(30)	42(24)	36(20)
0.25	2927(2122)	788(551)	375(253)	224(146)	152(95)	112(67)	87(50)	70(39)	59(31)	50(25)
	2187(1585)	589(412)	280(189)	168(109)	114(71)	84(50)	65(37)	63(29)	44(23)	38(19)
0.30	3330(2247)	879(571)	411(257)	243(145)	163(93)	118(65)	91(47)	73(36)	60(28)	51(23)
	2487(1679)	657(427)	307(192)	192(109)	122(70)	89(49)	68(36)	55(27)	45(21)	39(17)
0.35	3647(2279)	949(569)	438(251)	255(140)	169(89)	122(61)	93(44)	74(33)	60(25)	51(20)
	2724(1703)	709(425)	327(188)	191(105)	127(66)	91(45)	70(33)	55(25)	46(19)	39(15)
0.40	3876(2228)	995(547)	454(238)	262(131)	172(81)	123(55)	93(39)	73(29)	60(22)	50(17)
	2895(1665)	744(409)	339(178)	196(98)	129(61)	92(41)	70(29)	55(22)	45(17)	38(13)
0.45	4014(2107)	1019(509)	460(218)	263(118)	171(72)	121(48)	91(34)	71(24)	58(18)	48(14)
	2999(1574)	762(381)	344(163)	197(88)	128(54)	91(36)	68(25)	54(18)	44(14)	37(11)
0.50	4061(1929)	1020(459)	456(193)	258(103)	166(62)	116(40)	87(28)	67(20)	55(15)	
	3034(1441)	763(343)	341(145)	193(77)	125(46)	88(30)	65(21)	51(15)	42(11)	
0.55	4017(1707)	998(399)	441(165)	247(86)	158(51)	110(33)	81(22)	63(15)		
	3001(1275)	746(298)	330(123)	185(64)	119(38)	83(24)	61(17)	48(12)		
0.60	3881(1455)	953(333)	417(135)	231(69)	146(40)	101(25)	74(16)			
	2900(1087)	713(249)	312(101)	173(52)	110(30)	76(19)	56(12)			
0.65	3654(1187)	896(265)	382(105)	209(52)	131(29)	89(17)				
	2730(887)	663(198)	286(78)	157(39)	99(22)	68(13)				
0.70	3337(917)	796(199)	338(76)	182(36)	112(19)					
	2493(685)	596(149)	253(57)	137(27)	85(15)					
0.75	2930(659)	684(136)	284(49)	150(22)						
	2190(492)	512(102)	214(37)	114(17)						
0.80	2436(426)	551(82)	222(27)							
	1821(318)	413(62)	168(21)							
0.85	1854(231)	398(39)								
	1387(173)	300(30)								
0.90	1189(89)									
	892(66)									

* *Upper figure:* $\alpha = 0.05$, $\beta = 0.10$
† *Lower figure:* $\alpha = 0.05$, $\beta = 0.20$
(Freedman LS: Stat Med, 1; 121, 1982)

random treatment assignments must be generated. They are IIIB and KPS 80 to 100; IIIB and KPS 50 to 70; IVA and KPS 80 to 100; IVA and KPS 50 to 70. In each stratum, the researcher must decide at which point in the block there should be balance. If it is after four treatment assignments, then there are six possible sequences, XXYY, XYXY XYYX, YXXY, YXYX, and YYXX.

A random number table equating X with odd numbers and Y with even numbers can be used to generate each block in every stratum. Tables for treatment assignments should be prepared ahead of time and be kept secret from the investigators who enter the patients so that their choices are not influenced by the knowledge of the next treatment assignment. This would severely compromise the integrity of the randomization procedure and thus the study.

The number of stratifying factors used should be kept to a minimum. If they are not, there exists a possibility of introducing a serious imbalance in the distributions of the treatment assignments across the strata. For multiinstitution studies, one may wish to include institution as a stratification variable to prevent serious treatment imbalances from occurring within an institution and to ensure that each institution treats approximately the same number of patients with the experimental and the standard programs. Unfortunately, it is virtually impossible to include "institution" in a stratified randomization procedure if the number of participating institutions is large, such as in RTOG. Zelen provided a solution to this problem.[50] At the time of randomization by telephone, a tentative treatment assignment is determined by taking the next assignment from the appropriate stratum as defined by the patient's prognosis. The difference between the number of patients assigned to the treatment with the tentative assignment and the number on the other treatment is calculated within the participating institution. If the difference is less than some prescribed number, then the tentative assignment is the one given to the investigator, and it is marked in the block. However, if the difference exceeds the prescribed number, then the other treatment is assigned, and its next occurrence in the block is marked so that this assignment will not be used at a later date.

QUALITY CONTROL FOR PROTOCOL EXECUTION

For every protocol, it is important to check the eligibility for each possible patient entry before registration. This eliminates the work of tracking ineligible cases and enhances the credibility of any published results, because many exclusions might introduce a bias. The smaller the number of patients excluded from the analysis, the greater the credibility it has. This eligibility check should be carried out by an individual other than the clinician who is immediately responsible for the particular patient.

Because clinical studies provide a prescription of how patients are to be treated, it is critical to ensure that the prescription is successfully implemented. With radiation therapy, the prescription in terms of total dose to specific points and placement of field borders can be checked easily. For the earlier patient entries, the execution of the protocol prescription should be reviewed to identify any problem, ideally before or during initial delivery of the treatment, allowing corrections for the immediate patient and preventing problems for future patients. In RTOG, initial review of the treatment prescription is routinely done for all patients whose treatment takes more than 2 weeks to deliver. For the first 3 years of formalized initial review, RTOG found in their lung and head and neck studies that over 90% of the patients had to have their treatment modified so that it was put in line with the protocol prescription. Since then, the percentage of patients needing modification after initial review has been less than 5% for lung studies and 2% for head and neck studies.[49]

In addition to the initial review of the protocol prescription, there should be a final review once the treatment data are available to evaluate the delivery of the treatment relative to the protocol prescription. If the classification scheme for deviations from it is defined beforehand, the criteria can be applied uniformly. The results of this final review of treatment factors assist in interpreting the findings from the study. For example, if no improvement with a new experimental treatment is observed, it may be the result of the inability to deliver the treatment as prescribed in the protocol or its inherent ineffectiveness.

DATA COLLECTION

Obtaining information on the endpoints to be evaluated is of primary importance in data collection. The frequency of collection should be comparable for all treatment groups under study to avoid systematic bias. For instance, patients being treated with a placebo should be evaluated as often and at approximately the same times as patients receiving an active treatment. If they are not, it may appear that the placebo group is doing better simply because the patients are seen less often.

One method of capturing the desired data is to use specially designed data collection forms that are filled out prospectively. All information pertaining to the endpoints of a study and known prognostic variables must be included on the forms. However, a balance must be struck between the number of data items collected and the simplicity of the form.

ANALYSES DURING THE STUDY

Before a trial is begun, a plan for various types of analyses during its execution should be developed.[16,20] One type of analysis, which occurs while patients are being entered into the study, is commonly referred to as "interim." The analysis done after all the patients are entered and followed for a sufficient time is often designated as "final."

For interim analyses, the first decision is what kind of information should be given to whom. For multicenter trials done by the RTOG, information about patient accrual, types of patients entered, morbidity, and study execution is routinely reported to the entire group membership. However, interim response or survival analyses are reported in a coded fashion to a special monitoring committee that is set up for each study. Limiting the persons with access to the interim results reduces the chances of the investigators prematurely deciding what the trial shows and, as a consequence, discontinuing the entry of more patients.

A major problem associated with interim analyses is the number of significance tests to be performed and their timing. Unless appropriate safeguards are taken, as the number of tests performed increases, the false-positive rate (saying there is a treatment difference when there is not) correspondingly increases.[32] To guard against this, the tests for statistical significance must be done at specific points in the study, and their associated significance levels must be adjusted so that the overall false-positive rate for the study is equal to 0.05. Specific action must be detailed for the situation in which statistical significance is found at the time of interim analysis.

In the RTOG studies, the significance testing of a primary endpoint is done as soon as data on approximately 50% of the required sample size are available. If the experimental arm shows either significant improvement or inferiority compared with the standard arm at $P < 0.005$, patient accrual to the study is discontinued and a detailed analysis of the data is begun to determine if the difference may be the result of something other than the treatment. If the midstudy test of significance does not achieve statistical significance, patient accrual continues until the projected sample size is reached, and then significance testing is repeated. If the resulting significance level is less than 0.006, an analysis of the treatment comparison is undertaken immediately with the intention of publication of the results. Otherwise, the timing of the next analysis is determined by the length of follow-up as specified in the protocol with significance testing at 0.047. These three P levels were selected by RTOG to preserve a false-positive rate (overall significance level) of 0.05 for the trial.[36]

The length of follow-up needed beyond patient accrual is a direct function of the disease under study and probability of survival. Another concern is which patients should be included or excluded from the final analysis. For randomized studies, all patients registered ideally should be included in the analysis. The randomization process guarantees on the average that the treatment groups have the same prognostic profile. However, as patients are dropped from randomized arms, there is no longer any guarantee that the resulting treatment groups used in subsequent analyses have the same prognostic profile. A bias may be introduced such that any treatment difference found is simply a function of patient exclusion, as when patients are excluded when they receive lesser amounts of drugs or irradiation. Any difference found probably is the result of the difference in prognosis between the two patient groups analyzed.

Before the final analysis can begin, all outstanding data problems must be resolved, and the final review of the treatment delivery for each patient must be completed. The following are the usual components of the final analysis:

1. Disposition of all cases entered into the study with respect to their inclusion and exclusion in the analysis;
2. Distribution of the important prognostic pretreatment characteristics for each treatment regimen;
3. The initial response, the tumor control, and the survival rates associated with each treatment regimen;
4. Frequency and severity of the reported toxicities for each treatment regimen;
5. Compliance rates of treatment delivery relative to the protocol prescription;
6. Comparison of the various outcome measures by treatment regimen.

The statistical methods routinely used are summarized. Differences in percentages for categorical data, such as sex and initial complete response rates between two patient groups, are commonly evaluated by the Pearson Chi-square test. Differences in continuous variables, such as age, are evaluated with the Wilcoxon nonparametric test or by comparing the means with the assumption of a normal distribution (*i.e.*, t-test). The differences in timed events, such as survival, are evaluated with the logrank test.[33,39]

Logistic modeling is used to simultaneously evaluate the influence of disease factors and treatment on a binary outcome variable, such as achieving an initial complete response.[6] Cox proportional hazards models are used to evaluate simultaneously the influence of disease factors and treatment on time-related events, such as locoregional control and survival.[7] The Kaplan-Meier method is used to estimate the rates for timed events, such as survival at 1 year.[26] Temporal events are plotted as step functions. Time is measured from the start of randomization until the time of the first failure or the time of the last follow-up if the patient did not fail (censored data). Peto and associates,[41] in a comprehensive practical guide to survival data, provide further details of life tables and logrank tests.

Subset analysis is often undertaken when the analysis of all the patients from the study fails to show a statistically significant difference in the treatments being compared. It is hoped that a particular subgroup of patients can be found for which one of the treatments is markedly superior. However, there are several difficulties associated with subset analysis.[17,47] A common problem, especially if the trial was not designed with any subset analyses in mind, is diminished statistical power to detect a clinically meaningful difference because of a small number of patients in the subset in question. Even a randomized trial does not necessarily ensure the desired balance if only a part of its study population is examined. Careful attention should be paid to the distribution of known prognostic factors among the treatments in each subset examined. A third problem is the increased probability of finding a statistical difference simply by chance because of multiple testing. An adjustment of the α level (false-positive rate), similar to that made for interim analyses, is required to maintain the overall false-positive rate at a specified value for the subset.

Given these problems, subset analysis should be considered a means of hypothesis generation for a particular treatment rather than a means of hypothesis confirmation. Any hypotheses generated requires further studies for confirmation.[19] Ideally, a prospective phase III study should be used to confirm the treatment hypothesis generated by subset analysis. This is possible only if the treatment under study is associated with potential benefit for the patients, not with a potential adverse effect. This point is illustrated in two studies, one of low-dose preoperative irradiation and the other of postoperative adjuvant chemotherapy as adjuvant therapy for rectal cancer. A phase II trial of 500 cGy of preoperative irradiation versus no adjuvant treatment done at Princess Margaret Hospital showed no overall survival difference between the two treatment groups. Subset analysis based on only 22 patients assigned to preoperative radiation therapy and 16 patients to none did suggest a significant difference favoring preoperative irradiation in patients with Duke's Stage C rectal cancer.[43] A phase III trial was conducted by the Medical Research Council in the United Kingdom, which found no difference in overall survival or in patients with Duke's Stage C rectal cancer.[34]

A phase III study of postoperative adjuvant combination chemotherapy with semustine, vincristine, and 5-fluorouracil (MOF regimen) was conducted by the NSABP.[15] It showed significantly improved overall survival for the MOF patients ($P = 0.01$). However, subset analysis revealed a rather conflicting treatment result by sex. The estimated 5-year survival rate for the 119 males treated with MOF was 60% and 37% for 119 males treated without MOF. The 5-year survival for 68 women treated with MOF was 37%, but it was 54% for 65 females treated without MOF. A follow-up trial of postoperative MOF in females to confirm or refute this result is virtually impossible because of ethical considerations.

Acknowledgment

The author wishes to thank Ms. Clare Guse for helping to translate "statistics" into readable English and Ms. Joanne Corish for typing the chapter. The author also wishes to thank the RTOG investigators for ideas and suggestions concerning topics for the chapter.

REFERENCES

1. Armitage P: The role of randomization in clinical trials. Stat Med 1:345, 1982
2. Bernstein D, Lagakos SW: Sample size and power determination for stratified clinical trials. J Stat Comput Simul 8:65, 1978
3. Byar DP, Simon RM, Friedewald WT, et al: Randomised clinical trials. Perspectives on some recent ideas. N Engl J Med 295:74, 1976
4. Casagrande JT, Pike MC, Smith PG: An improved approximate formula for calculating sample sizes for comparing two binomial distributions. Biometrics 34:483, 1978
5. Cooper MR, Pajak TF, Gottlieb AJ, et al: Long-term follow-up of nitrosourea (CCNU) containing 4-drug programs for the treatment of advanced Hodgkin's disease (CALGB). Cancer Treat Rep 66:1062, 1982
6. Cox DR: The Analysis of Binary Data. London, Chapman and Hall, 1970.
7. Cox DR: Regression models and life tables. J R Stat Soc B34 34:187, 1972
8. Cox JD: Fractionation: A paradigm for clinical research in radiation oncology. [Presidential Address] Int J Radiat Oncol Biol Phys 13:1271, 1987
9. Crissman JD, Pajak TF, Zarbo RJ, Marcial VA, Al-Sarraf M: Improved response and survival to combined cisplatin and

radiation in non-keratinizing squamous cell carcinomas of the head and neck: An RTOG study of 114 advanced stage tumors. Cancer 59:1391, 1987

10. Diener-West M, Dobbins T, Phillips TL, Nelson DF: Identification of an optimal subgroup for treatment evaluation of patients with brain metastases using RTOG 7916. Int J Radiat Oncol Biol Phys 16:669, 1989
11. Ellenberg S: Determining sample sizes for clinical trials. Oncology 3:39, 1989
12. Fazekas J, Pajak TF, Wasserman T, et al: Failure of misonidazole-sensitized radiotherapy to impact upon outcome among stage III–IV squamous cancers of the head and neck. Int J Radiat Oncol Biol Phys 13:1155, 1987
13. Fazekas JT, Scott C, Marcial VA, et al: The role of hemoglobin concentration in the outcome of misonidazole-sensitized radiotherapy of head and neck cancers based on RTOG 7915. Int J Radiat Oncol Biol Phys 17:1177, 1989
14. Fisher B, Bauer M, Margolese R, et al: Five-year results from the NSABP trial comparing total mastectomy to segmental mastectomy with and without breast radiation in treatment of breast cancer. N Engl J Med 312:665, 1985
15. Fisher B, Wolmark N, Rockette H, et al: Postoperative adjuvant chemotherapy or radiation therapy for rectal cancer: Results from NSABP Protocol R-01. JNCI 80:21, 1988
16. Fleming TR, Green SJ, Harrington DP: Considerations for monitoring and evaluating treatment effects in clinical trials. Controlled Clin Trials 5:55, 1984
17. Fleming TR, Watelet LF: Approaches to monitoring clinical trails. JNCI 81:188, 1989
18. Freedman LS: Tables of the number of patients required in a clinical trial using the log rank test. Stat Med 1:121, 1982
19. Gail M, Simon R: Testing for qualitative interactions between treatment effects and patient subsets. Biometrics 41:361, 1985
20. Green SJ, Fleming TR, O'Fallon JR: Policies for study monitoring and interim reporting of results. J Clin Oncol 5:1477, 1987
21. Hanks GE, Martz KL, Diamond JJ: The effect of dose on local control of prostate cancer. Int J Radiat Oncol Biol Phys 15:1299, 1988
22. Haselow RE, Adams GL, Oken MM, et al: Cis-platinum (DDP) with radiation therapy (RT) for locally advanced unresectable head and neck cancer. Proceedings of 19th Annual Meeting of American Society of Clinical Oncology 2:160, 1983
23. Haselow RE, Warshaw MG, Oken MM, et al: Radiation alone versus radiation with weekly low dose cis-platinum in unresectable cancer of the head and neck. In Fee WE, Goepfert H, Johns ME, et al (eds): Head and Neck Cancer, vol 2, pp 279–281. Toronto, BC Decker, 1990.
24. Jacobs JR, Pajak TF, Kinzie J, et al: Induction chemotherapy in advanced head and neck: A Radiation Therapy Oncology Group study. Arch Otolaryngol Head Neck Surg 113:193, 1987
25. Jacobs JR, Pajak TF, Snow JB, Lowry LD, Kramer S: Surgical quality control in head and neck cancer: Study 73-03 of the Radiation Therapy Oncology Group. Arch Otolaryngol Head Neck Surg 115:489, 1989
26. Kaplan EL, Meier P: Nonparametric estimation from incomplete observations. J Am Stat Assoc 53:457, 1958
27. Kramer S, Gelber RD, Snow JB, et al: Combined radiation therapy and surgery in the management of advanced head and neck cancer: 73-03 of the Radiation Therapy Oncology Group. Head Neck Surg 10:19, 1987
28. Lachin JM, Foulkes MA: Evaluation of sample size and power for analyses of survival with allowance for nonuniform patient entry, losses to follow-up, noncompliance, and stratification. Biometrics 42:507, 1986
29. Lachin JM: Statistical properties of randomization in clinical trials. Controlled Clin Trials 9:289, 1988
30. Laramore GE, Krall J, Thomas FJ, et al: Fast neutron radiotherapy for locally advanced prostate cancer: Results of an RTOG randomized study. Int J Radiat Oncol Biol Phys 11:1621, 1985
31. McGowan DG: The adverse influence of prior transurethral resection on prognosis is carcinoma of prostate treated by radiation therapy. Int J Radiat Oncol Biol Phys 6:1121, 1980.
32. McPherson K: Interim analysis and stopping rules. In Buyse ME, Staquet MJ, Sylvester RJ (eds): Cancer Clinical Trials: Method and Practice, pp 405. Oxford, Oxford University Press, 1984
33. Mantel N: Evaluation of survival data and two new rank order statistics arising in its consideration. Cancer Chem Rep 5:163, 1966
34. Medical Research Council Working Party. The evaluation of low-dose preoperative x-ray therapy in the management of operable rectal cancer: Results of a randomly controlled trial. Br J Surg 71:21, 1984
35. Moertel CG, Hanley JA: The effect of measuring error on the results of therapeutic trials in advanced cancer. Cancer 38:388, 1976
36. O'Brien PC, Fleming TR: A multiple testing procedure for clinical trials. Biometrics 35:549, 1979
37. Overgaard J, Hansen HS, Andersen AP, et al: Misonidazole combined with split-course radiotherapy in the treatment of invasive carcinoma of larynx and pharynx: Report from the DAHANCA 2 Study. Int J Radiat Oncol Biol Phys 16:1065, 1989
38. Perez CA, Walz BJ, Zivnuska FR, Pilepich M, Prasad K, Bauer W: Irradiation of carcinoma of the prostate localized to the pelvis: Analysis of tumor response and prognosis. Int J Radiat Oncol Biol Phys 6:555, 1980.
39. Peto R, Peto J: Asymptotically efficient rank invariant test procedures. J R Stat Soc [A] 135:185, 1972
40. Peto R, Pike MC, Armitage P, et al: Design and analysis of randomized clinical trial requiring prolonged observation of each patient. I. Introduction and design. Br J Cancer 34:585, 1976
41. Peto R, Pike MC, Armitage P, et al: Design and analysis of randomized clinical trials requiring prolonged observation of each patient: II. Analysis and examples. Br J Cancer 35:1, 1977
42. Pilepich MV, Krall JM, Johnson RJ, et al: Extended field (periaortic) irradiation in carcinoma of the prostate: Analysis of RTOG 75-06. Int J Radiat Oncol Biol Phys 12:345, 1986
43. Rider WD, Palmer JA, Mahoney, LJ, et al: Preoperative irradiation in operable cancer of the rectum: Report of the Toronto Trial. Can J Surg 20:335, 1977
44. Rose G: Bias. Br J Clin Pharmacol 13:157, 1982
45. Sacks H, Chalmers TC, Smith H: Randomized versus historical controls for clinical trials. Am J Med 72:233, 1982
46. Schuller DE, Laramore GE, Al-Sarraf M, Jacobs J, Pajak T: Surgery-chemotherapy-radiation therapy for resectable head and neck cancer: A phase III head and neck intergroup study. Arch Otolaryngol Head Neck Surg 115:364, 1989
47. Simon R: Patient subsets and variation in therapeutic efficacy. Br J Clin Pharmacol 14:473, 1982
48. Van Den Bogaert W, Van Der Schueren E, Horiot JC, et al: Early results of the EORTC randomized clinical trial on multiple fractions per day (MFD) and misonidazole in advanced head and neck cancer. Int J Radiat Oncol Biol Phys 12:587, 1986
49. Wallner PE, Lustig RA, Pajak TF, et al: Impact of initial quality control review on study outcome in lung and head/neck cancer studies—review of the Radiation Therapy Oncology Group experience. Int J Radiat Oncol Biol Phys 17:893, 1989
50. Zelen M: The randomization and stratification of patients to clinical trials. J Chronic Dis 27:365, 1974

8

Principles of Radiologic Physics, Dosimetry, and Treatment Planning

James A. Purdy
Glenn P. Glasgow
David A. Lightfoot

A solid foundation in the principles of radiologic physics, dosimetry, and treatment planning is essential for the practice of radiation oncology. In this chapter, we will consider several topics that lay the foundation for the material covered in Chapter 9. This chapter also discusses basic concepts used in calculating the dose administered to a patient and the standard correction methods used to account for air gaps and tissue inhomogeneities.

ATOMIC AND NUCLEAR STRUCTURE

The atom may be thought of as consisting of a centrally located core, the nucleus, surrounded by small orbiting particles, electrons. The overall dimension of the atom is about 10^{-10}m, and the nucleus, about 10^{-14}m. Most of the mass of the atom is contained in the nucleus, making it extremely dense (10^{15} kg/m^3). The nucleus is composed of two kinds of particles, protons and neutrons, known collectively as nucleons. A proton has a mass (m_p) of 1.673×10^{-27} kg and has a positive electrical charge equal in magnitude to the charge of the electron (1.602×10^{-19} coulomb). Collectively, the protons constitute the electrical charge of the nucleus. A neutron is slightly more massive than a proton ($m_n = 1.675 \times 10^{-27}$ kg) and has no electrical charge. Each negatively charged electron has a rest mass (m_0) of 9.110×10^{-31} kg, contributing very little mass.

In 1913, Niels Bohr formulated a planetary model of the hydrogen atom, consisting of an electron orbiting around a nucleus of equal and opposite charge. In extending his theory to multielectron atoms, Bohr proposed a nucleus surrounded by electrons arranged in concentric shells or energy levels (Fig. 8-1). Energy is released when an electron moves to an orbit closer to the nucleus, and energy is required to move an electron into a higher orbit. Historically, the shells are labeled, from innermost outward, by the letters K, L, M, and so forth. There is a maximum number of electrons that can be accommodated in each shell: two in the first shell, eight in the second, eighteen in the third, and so on.

The maximum number of electrons allowed in each shell is given by the relationship $2n^2$; n is an integer specific to each shell and is called the *principal quantum number.* Other properties of the electron also have discrete values specified by quantum numbers. These include the electron's angular momentum as it orbits the nucleus, denoted by quantum number l (l = 0,1, . . . ,n-1) ; its spin about its axis, denoted by s (s = ± ½); and its magnetic moment, denoted by m_l ($m_l = 0, \pm 1, \ldots, \pm l$). Thus, each electron in an atom has an associated set of quantum numbers (n,l,s,m_l). This is the basis of the *Pauli exclusion principle,* which states no two electrons can have the same set of quantum numbers within a particular atom.

Modern physics has replaced the simplistic orbiting electron model of Bohr with an abstract model of diffuse electron clouds that represent probability functions of the electron's position. However, for understanding of radiologic physics, the simple model of a nucleus composed of protons and neutrons and surrounded by electrons is sufficient.

The atom of an element is specified by its *atomic number,* denoted by the symbol Z, and its *mass number,* denoted by the symbol A. The atomic number is equal to the number of protons in the nucleus, and the mass number is equal to the number of nucleons (protons and neutrons) in the nucleus. Hence, A minus Z is equal to the number of neutrons, denoted by the symbol N, within the nucleus. In addition, each element has an associated chemical symbol. When these definitions are used, the standards notation to specify an atom is ${}^{A}_{Z}X$ is illustrated by ${}^{60}_{27}Co$, which is a radioactive isotope of the element cobalt that has an atomic number 27 (*i.e.,* 27 protons) and a mass number of 60 (*i.e.,* 60 nucleons or 27 protons and 33 neutrons).

Isotopes of an element, such as ${}^{58}_{27}Co$, ${}^{59}_{27}Co$, and ${}^{60}_{27}Co$, have the same atomic number but different numbers of neu-

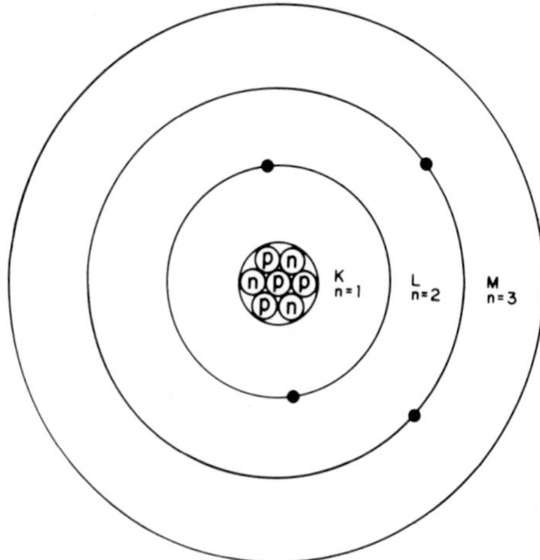

FIGURE 8–1. Schematic drawing of the Bohr model of the atom. The nucleus contains protons and neutrons. Electrons revolve around the nucleus in specific orbits having discrete energy levels. By convention the orbits (energy levels) are assigned either quantum numbers (n = 1,2,3, . . .) or letters (K,L,M, . . .)

trons and therefore different mass numbers. Isotopes have the same chemical properties but different physicial properties. *Isobars* such as $^{60}_{27}$Co and $^{60}_{28}$Ni are atoms having the same mass number but different numbers of protons and neutrons. Atoms such as $^{57}_{27}$Co and $^{56}_{26}$Fe, that have the same number of neutrons but different atomic and mass numbers, are called *isotones*.

To complete the picture of atomic structure, the concept of binding energy of an electron must be considered. An electron in an inner shell of an atom is attracted to the nucleus by a force greater than that which the nucleus exerts on an electron in an outer shell. To move an electron from an inner shell to an outer shell (*excitation*) or to remove it completely from the atom (*ionization*), energy must be supplied. The energy required to remove an electron completely from an atom is called the *binding energy* for the electron. Binding energies are considered negative because energy must be supplied to remove the electron. Atomic shells are often described in terms of binding energy, as shown in Figure 8-2 for the tungsten atom. The binding energies for the K, L, and M shells are −69,500 eV, −11,000 eV, and −2,500 eV, respectively. The electrons in the outermost shells are called *valence* electrons, which have a binding energy of only a few electron volts because they are very loosely bound.

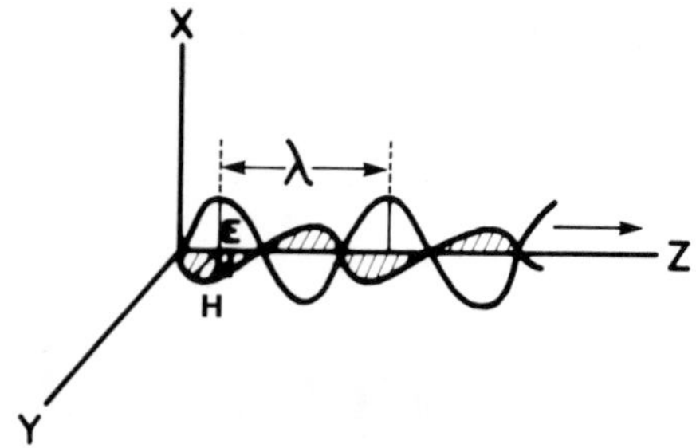

FIGURE 8–3. Classic wave description of electromagnetic radiation showing relationship between wavelength, frequency, and velocity. E and H represent the peak amplitudes of the electric and magnetic fields, which are perpendicular to one another.

ELECTROMAGNETIC RADIATION

Electromagnetic radiation can be represented by a varying electric and magnetic field that is conveniently described using a sine-wave model (Fig. 8-3). The sine wave is characterized by two parameters: the frequency, represented by the Greek letter ν, and the wavelength, represented by the Greek letter λ. The wavelength is the distance from one crest of the sine wave to another; the frequency is the number of complete cycles or oscillations per second and is measured in hertz (Hz). The product of the frequency and wavelength is the speed with which the wave is propagated, which in a vacuum is the speed of light (3×10^8 m/second).

Electromagnetic radiation wavelengths extend from approximately 10^7 m to 10^{-13} m. The frequencies associated with these radiations are approximately 10^1 to 10^{21} Hz. The electromagnetic spectrum shown in Figure 8-4 includes the radio and television bands; radar and microwaves; the infrared, visible, and ultraviolet regions; and x-rays and cosmic rays.

Quantum physics allows these radiations to be represented as particles, called *photons*. The photon energy is directly proportional to the classic wave frequency and is related to it through a constant of proportionality known as *Planck's constant*

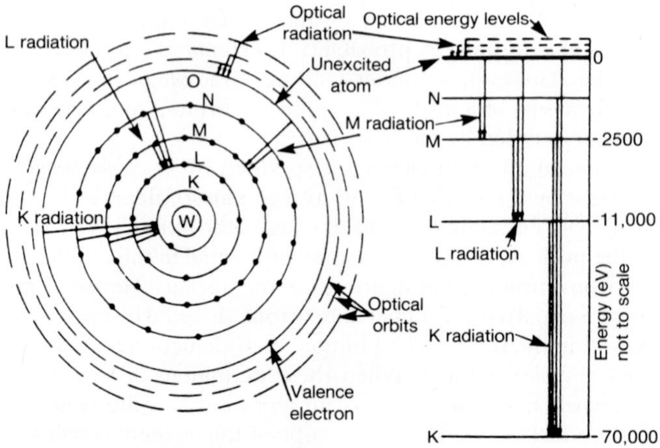

FIGURE 8–2. Schematic drawing of tungsten atom showing electron configuration and energy levels. (Redrawn from Johns HE, Cunningham JR: The Physics of Radiology, 4th ed. Springfield, IL, Charles C Thomas, 1983)

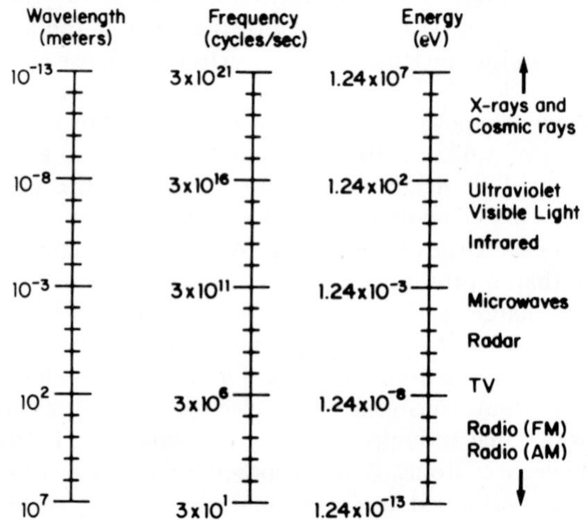

FIGURE 8–4. Electromagnetic spectrum extending over several orders of magnitude and listing values of wavelengths, frequency, and identifying values in some of the more common regions of the spectrum.

($\hbar$), which has a numerical value of 6.625×10^{-27} erg seconds. The relationship between energy, E, and frequency, ν, is given by the following equation:

$$E = h\nu$$

The relationship between photon energy and photon wavelength is given by the following equation:

$$E = hc/\lambda$$

where c is the speed of light in a vacuum.

PRODUCTION OF X-RAYS

The production of x-rays involves energetic electrons that impinge on a target and interact with either the orbital electrons or the nuclei of target atoms. The kinetic energy of the electrons is then converted into thermal energy or electromagnetic energy in the form of x-rays by the interaction of the incoming electron with an outer-shell electron of a target atom. However, there is not sufficient energy transferred to these outer-shell electrons to free or ionize them from the atom. Instead, the excited orbital electrons are raised to higher energy levels. In time, the excited electrons then return to their normal energy levels, emitting low-energy (infrared) electromagnetic radiation (Fig. 8-2).

The second process by which the impinging electron gives up its kinetic energy is in the production of *characteristic x-rays* (Fig. 8-5). If the impinging electron interacts with an inner-orbital electron and the interaction ionizes the electron, characteristic x-rays are produced as an outer-orbital electron moves to the electron vacancy produced in the inner shell. The characteristic x-ray energy is equal to the difference in the binding energies of the orbital electrons involved. Occasionally, this excess energy is transferred directly to an orbital electron that is ejected (*Auger electron*).

The third type of interaction in which the impinging electron can lose its kinetic energy is called *bremsstrahlung* (braking radiation). When the electron interacts with the nucleus of an atom, instead of orbital electrons, the incident electron interacts with the electric field of the nucleus and is deflected; the change of direction indicates a deceleration and therefore a loss of energy by the incoming electron. The lost energy reappears in the form of an x-ray photon. Because the impinging electron can lose any amount of its kinetic energy in the bremsstrahlung process, x radiation is characterized by a continuous range of values, unlike characteristic x-rays, which have specific energies. A bremsstrahlung spectrum (*i.e.*, a graph of x-ray intensity versus energy) is shown in Figure 8-6. Superimposed on the continuous spectrum are the characteristic radiations. The maximum energy of a bremsstrahlung x-ray is numerically equal to the energy of the incident electrons. The direction of emission of the bremsstrahlung x-ray depends on the energy of the incident electron, with higher-energy electrons yielding more forwardly directed x-rays.

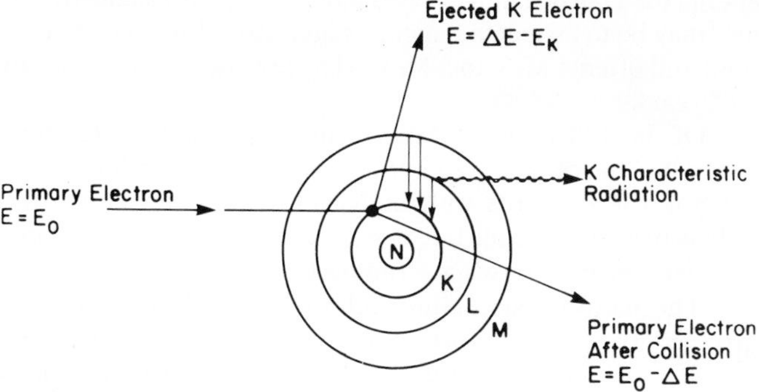

FIGURE 8–5. Schematic diagram illustrating characteristic x-ray production.

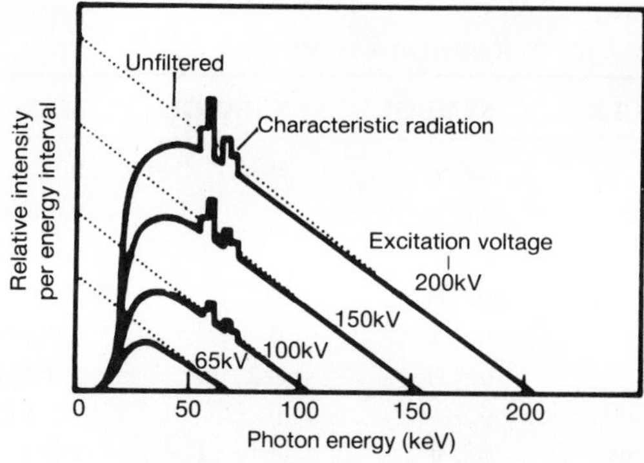

FIGURE 8–6. A bremsstrahlung x-ray spectrum, calculated for a thick tungsten target, extends from zero to the maximum energy of the electron. The dotted lines are for no filtration, and the solid curves are for a filtration of 1 mm of aluminum. Notice the superimposed characteristic x-ray emission spectrum. (Redrawn from Johns HE, Cunningham JR: The Physics of Radiology, 4th ed. Springfield, IL, Charles C Thomas, 1983)

RADIOACTIVITY

The discovery of radioactivity was a result of investigations of x-rays. Roentgen observed that a paper screen coated with fluorescent material glowed when placed in the vicinity of a tube of gas at low pressure through which electricity was being passed. The x-rays were produced where the electron beam struck the anode.

In 1896, the French physicist Henri Becquerel conducted experiments in which he wrapped a photographic plate in black paper to keep out the light and then placed pieces of various elements against the wrapped plate. He correctly postulated that if these materials emitted x-rays, the rays would pass through the paper and blacken the photographic plate. He discovered that the mineral pitchblende did emit x-rays. Other elements, such as thorium, actinium, and two new elements discovered by Pierre and Marie Curie, polonium and radium, also emitted these rays.

The radioactive elements emitted three types of radiation: α particles having a positive electrical charge, β particles having a negative charge, and τ-rays having no charge at all. We now know that an α particle is a helium nucleus, β particles are electrons, and τ-rays are electromagnetic radiation that is similar to x-rays but originate from within the nucleus of the atom.

Other elementary particles have been detected. Properties of the particles relevant to radiation therapy are listed in Table 8-1. Many of these elementary particles are important topics in current physics research, but they are not germane to our discussion of radiation oncology physics.

The radioactive decay processes are related to the forces involved. Huge electrical forces of repulsion exist between the positively charged and closely spaced protons in a nucleus. However, a much stronger nuclear force of attraction exists among the neutrons and protons, binding them together to form the nucleus. The nuclear force is much more complicated than the electrical force and is not completely understood. It is known, however, that the nuclear force between nucleons de-

TABLE 8–1
Particles Used in Radiation Therapy

PARTICLE	SYMBOL	CHARGE	MASS
Photon	$h\nu, \gamma$	0	0
Electron	e, e^-, β^-	−1	0.000549 amu*
Positron	e^+, β^+	+1	0.000549 amu
Proton	$p, {}^1_1H$	+1	1.007277 amu
Neutron	$n, {}^1_0n$	0	1.008665 amu
Alpha	$\alpha, {}^4_2He^{++}$	+2	4.002604 amu
Neutrino	ν	0	<1/2000 m_0†
Pi Mesons	π^+, π^-	+1, −1	273 m_0
	π^0	0	264 m_0
Mu Mesons	μ^+, μ^-	+1, −1	207 m_0
K Mesons	K^+, K^-	+1, −1	967 m_0
	K^0	0	973 m_0

**1 amu = 1.66043×10^{-27} kg.*
† m_0 = rest mass of an electron = 9.1091×10^{-31} kg.

pends on the distance between them and is effective only over a very short distance, whereas the electrical force decreases with the square of the distance. The nuclear force easily overcomes the electrical force of repulsion as long as the protons are very close together. For a large nucleus, however, the attractive nuclear force may be weaker than the electrical force repulsing the protons on opposite sides of the nucleus. Therefore, a large nucleus is not as stable as a smaller nucleus.

Because neutrons interact only through the attractive nuclear force, they can be considered stabilizing particles for the nucleus. For example, in light nuclei, only an equal number of neutrons and protons is required, but in heavier nuclei, the number of neutrons must be about 1.5 times greater than the number of protons to counteract the repulsive electrical forces of the protons. A nuclide having too many more protons than neutrons is said to have an unfavorable N-to-Z ratio, and it decays to reach a stable configuration.

The *decay constant* of a radioactive nucleus is defined as the fraction of the total number of atoms that decay per unit of time and is denoted by the symbol λ. The decay process can be represented mathematically. If N_0 radioactive nuclei are initially present in a particular sample, the number of radioactive nuclei, N, remaining at a particular time, t, is given by the following equation:

$$N = N_0 e^{-\lambda t}$$

Activity, which describes the radioactivity of a sample and is denoted by the symbol A, is defined as the total number of disintegrations per time interval and is given by the following relationship:

$$A = \frac{N}{t} = \lambda N$$

The decay constant equation given above can be expressed in terms of activity:

$$A = A_0 e^{-\lambda t}$$

where A is the activity at time t and A_0 is the initial activity. The *curie* (Ci), a unit of activity, is equal to 3.7×10^{10} disintegrations per second, the approximate number of decays per second by 1 g of ^{226}Ra. The *becquerel* (Bq), a name for the SI unit for activity, is equal to one disintegration per second.

The *half-life* of a radioactive nuclide is the time required for the number of atoms in a particular sample to decrease by one half. The half-life, $T_{1/2}$, is related to the decay constant by the following equation:

$$T_{1/2} = \frac{0.693}{\lambda}$$

The *average life,* T_a, of a radioactive nuclide is related to the decay constant and the half-life by the following equation:

$$T_a = \frac{1}{\lambda} = 1.44\ T_{1/2}$$

The average life represents the period that a hypothetical source would need, if it retained its original activity for that period and then suddenly decayed to zero activity, to produce the same number of disintegrations as produced over an infinite time by the source if it decayed exponentially.

Gamma decay occurs when a nucleus undergoes a transition from a higher to a lower energy level. In this process, a high-energy photon, called a τ-ray, is emitted. These τ-rays are identical to the x-rays emitted by excited atoms, except that τ-rays originate from within the nucleus and x-rays originate from outside the nucleus. Half-lives for τ decay are usually very short, typically 10^{-15} seconds.

Closely related to τ decay is the process called *internal conversion.* Instead of emitting a τ-ray, the excess energy from the excited nucleus is transferred to an electron in one of the inner atomic shells, causing ejection of the electron from the atom with emission of characteristic x-rays. The probability of internal conversion occurring increases as the atomic number increases.

In *β decay,* a neutron within the nucleus is converted into a proton, and an electron and an antineutrino are emitted, or a proton is converted into a neutron, and a positron and a neutrino are emitted. The *positron,* a particle discovered in cosmic-ray experiments in 1932, is a positively charged particle with the same mass and spin as the electron and is considered the antiparticle of the electron. Antiprotons, antineutrons, and many other antiparticles have been experimentally observed. Particle-antiparticle pairs interact by annihilating each other, converting all their mass to electromagnetic energy. In β decay, the emitted particles may vary in the kinetic energy they possess, which is rarely greater than 3 MeV. Half-lives for β decay are long compared with τ-decay half-lives, varying from seconds to years. The forces responsible for the β-decay processes are weak compared with both the strong nuclear forces and the electromagnetic forces among the nucleons. Accordingly, the forces responsible for β decay are referred to as *weak interactions.*

In *α decay,* the ratio of neutrons to protons is low in nuclides with atomic numbers above 82. The emitted particle in α decay is a helium nucleus (two protons and two neutrons). The kinetic energy for a particular α decay is monoenergetic (*i.e.,* the transition may be to an excited energy state with subsequent τ emission) and often 4 MeV to 5 MeV. Half-lives range from 10^{-3} to 10^{10} years.

Of the 103 elements known currently, the first 92 occur naturally. The remaining 11 have been produced artificially. In general, the elements with high atomic number tend to be radioactive; in fact, all but one of the elements with atomic number above 82 (lead) are radioactive; ${}^{209}_{83}Bi$ is stable.

The naturally occurring radioactive elements have been grouped into three *radioactive series* called the *uranium series,* the *actinium series,* and the *thorium series,* all of which terminate with a stable isotope of lead. The uranium series (Fig. 8-7) provides an example of radioactive nuclides undergoing successive trans-

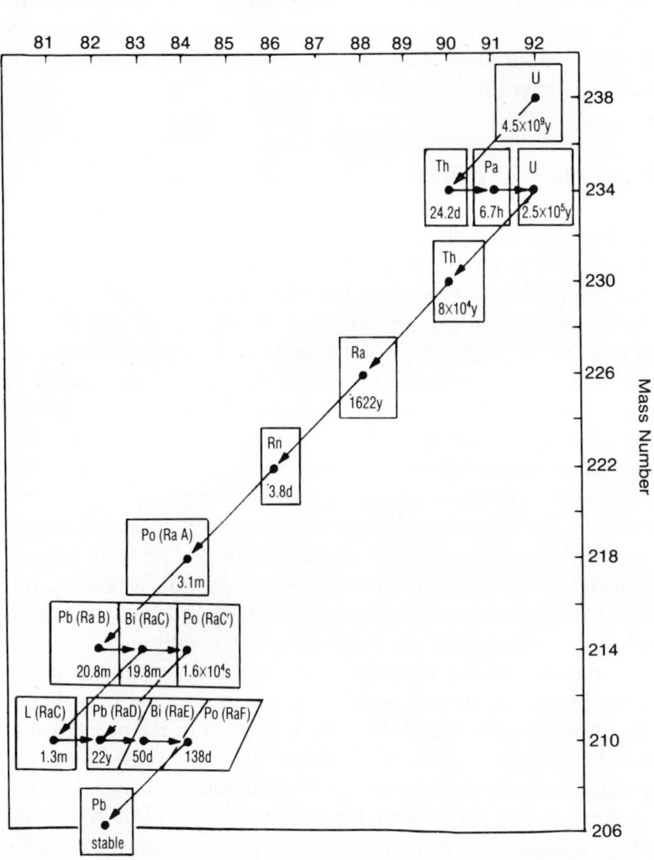

FIGURE 8–7. The uranium series. (Redrawn from Khan FM: The Physics of Radiation Therapy. Baltimore, Williams & Wilkins, 1984)

formations through α and β decay, in which the *parent nuclide* produces a radioactive product called the *daughter nuclide.*

When the half-life of the parent nuclide is longer than the half-life of the daughter nuclide, an equilibrium condition exists. When this occurs, the ratio of the activity of the daughter nuclide to the activity of the parent nuclide becomes constant, and the apparent decay rate of the daughter nuclide is controlled by the parent nuclide's decay rate.

Two types of radioactive equilibria are *transient equilibrium* and *secular equilibrium.* Transient equilibrium is established when the parent nuclide's half-life is not much greater than the daughter nuclide's half-life (Fig. 8-8). In secular equilibrium, the half-life of the parent nuclide is much greater than that of the daughter nuclide (Fig. 8-9).

The two types of equilibria are described mathematically by the following equations, in which A_P and A_D represent the activity of the parent and daughter nuclides, respectively:

$$\text{Transient Equilibrium: } \frac{A_D}{A_P} = \frac{\lambda_D}{\lambda_D - \lambda_P}$$

$$\text{Secular Equilibrium: } A_D = A_P$$

INTERACTION OF X-RAYS WITH MATTER

X-rays and τ-rays may be considered as bundles of energy called *photons.* If an x-ray photon enters a thin layer of matter, it is possible that it will pass through without interaction, or it may interact (usually with the atomic electrons) in one of several ways, including coherent scattering, photoelectric effect,

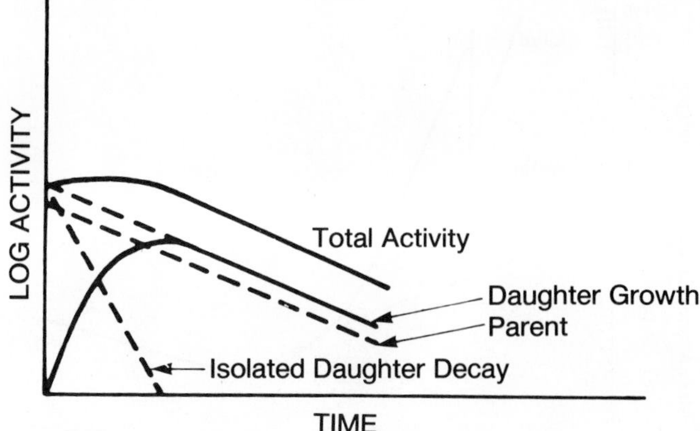

FIGURE 8–8. Semilog plot of activity versus time for parent and daughter radionuclides illustrates the conditions of transient equilibrium that may be achieved when the parent nuclide's half-life is not much greater than the half-life of the daughter nuclide. After equilibrium is established, the daughter activity exceeds the parent activity, and both decay with the half-life of the parent.

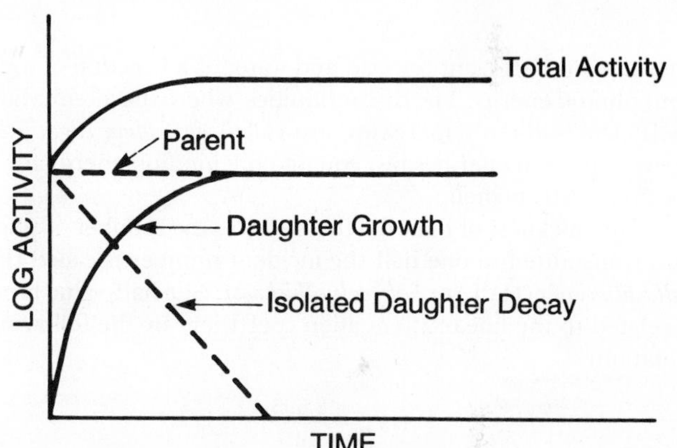

FIGURE 8–9. Semilog plot of activity versus time for parent and daughter radionuclides illustrates the conditions of secular equilibrium that may be achieved when the parent nuclide's half-life is much greater than the half-life of the daughter nuclide. After secular equilibrium is established, the activities of parent and daughter are equal.

Compton scattering, pair production, and photodisintegration. The probability that a photon will interact when it traverses through a given thickness of material is the product of the individual interaction probabilities for each of these five processes. The *attenuation process* can be described mathematically by the following equation:

$$N = N_0 e^{-\mu x}$$

where N_0 is the number of photons in the beam impinging on an absorber of thickness x, e is the base of the natural logarithm, and μ is the linear attenuation coefficient. The quantity μ is actually the sum of the individual attenuation coefficients for the five processes listed above. Its numeric value depends on the energy of the photon and the type of attenuating material.

There are a variety of tabulated *attenuation coefficients,* including the mass attenuation coefficient (μ/ρ), mass energy-transfer coefficient (μ_{tr}/ρ), and mass energy-absorption coefficient (μ_{en}/ρ). Each type of coefficient is intended for use in the solution of different types of attenuation or energy-absorption problems; division by ρ, the physical density of the medium, makes them medium independent. Figure 8-10 shows the mass

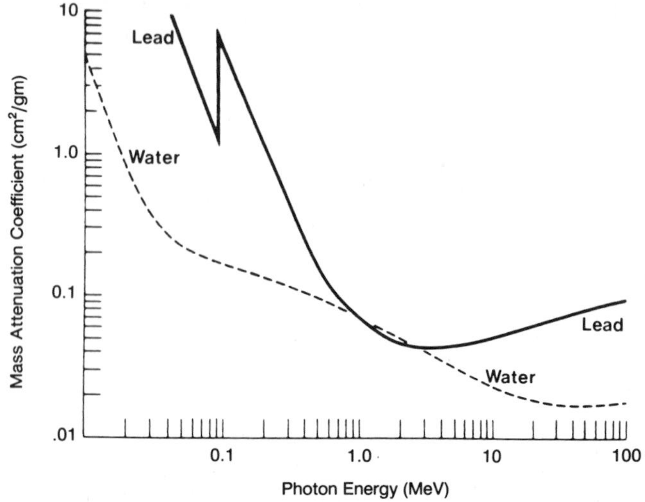

FIGURE 8–10. Mass attenuation coefficient for lead and water. Notice the sharp discontinuities, which are called absorption edges. (Johns HE, Cunningham JR: The Physics of Radiology, 4th ed. Springfield, IL, Charles C Thomas, 1983)

attenuation coefficient for lead and water as a function of incident photon energy. The discontinuities, where the attenuation coefficient suddenly increases, are called *absorption edges* and occur at photon energies just equal to the binding energy for a specific electron shell.

The thickness of material that reduces the number of photons transmitted to one half the incident number is called the *half-value layer* (HVL) or *half-value thickness.* The half-value layer is related to the linear attenuation coefficient by the following equation:

$$\text{HVL} = \frac{0.693}{\mu}$$

This parameter is used to describe the quality or penetrability of the radiation and is discussed further later in this chapter.

Coherent or Classical Scattering

If the photon energy is low enough that the quantum effects of the interaction are unimportant but the electron(s) can still be regarded as free, the interaction corresponds to the "classical" situation, in which the incident electrical field accelerates one or more orbital electrons and causes them to radiate (Fig. 8-11). There are two types of coherent scattering: *Thomson scattering,* in which a single orbital electron is involved, and *Rayleigh scattering,* in which the orbital electrons act as a single group. In coherent scattering, no energy is transferred; only the direction of the incident photon is changed. The coherent mass attenuation coefficient is denoted by σ_{coh}/ρ.

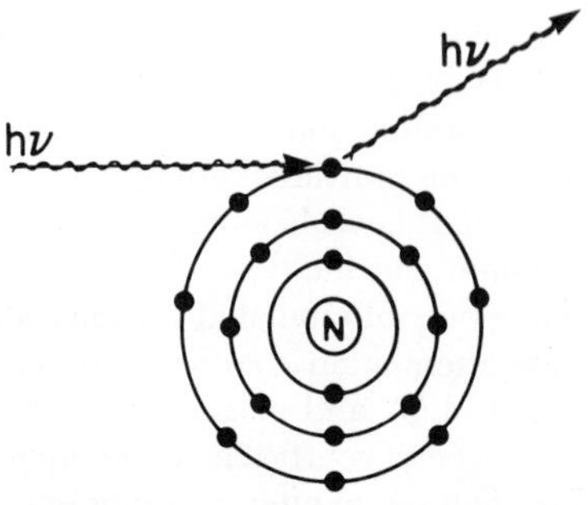

FIGURE 8–11. Schematic drawing illustrates the process of coherent or classic scattering. Notice that the scattered photon has the same energy as the incident photon, but the direction is changed.

Photoelectric Effect

In the photoelectric effect, the total energy of the photon is transferred to an orbital electron, usually close to the nucleus, and the photon disappears. The electron is then ejected from the atom with an energy equal to the energy of the photon minus the binding energy of the electron (Fig. 8-12). The direction in which the electron is emitted depends on the energy of the incident photon. For the low-energy photons (*e.g.,* 50 keV), the photoelectron is ejected at a large angle with respect to the incoming photon's direction, increasing in the forward direction as the photon's energy increases. After ejection of the electron, the neutral atom becomes a positively charged ion with a vacancy in an inner shell that must be filled. The atom returns to a stable condition by filling the vacancy with a nearby, less tightly bound electron farther out from the nucleus, and characteristic radiation or an Auger electron is emitted.

The probability that a given photon will interact by means of the photoelectric process (denoted by τ/ρ) is a function of both the photon's energy and the atomic number of the target atom. For the process to occur, the incident photon must have energy greater than the binding energy of the involved orbital electron. In general, the probability per electron that a photon will undergo a photoelectric interaction is inversely proportional to the third power of the photon's energy and directly proportional to the third power of the atomic number of the target atom.

Compton Effect

The Compton effect is the interaction of a photon with a loosely bound orbital electron in which part of the incident photon's energy is transferred as kinetic energy to the electron and the remaining energy is carried away by another photon, which has less energy than the incident one (Fig. 8-13). The binding energy of the electron is insignificant compared with the incident photon's energy. The energy of the Compton-scattered

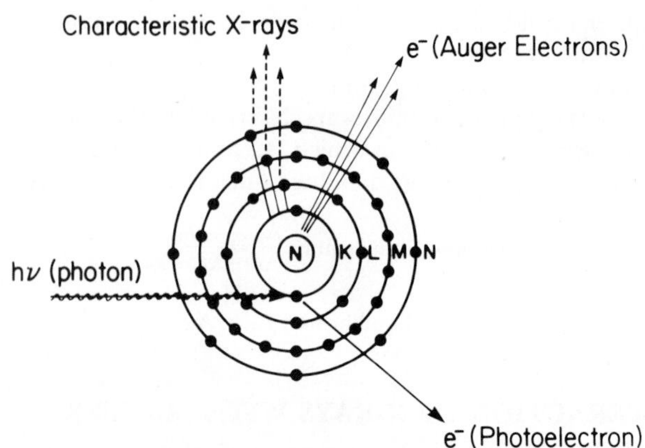

FIGURE 8–12. Schematic drawing illustrates the process of the photoelectric effect. The incident photon disappears, and an electron is ejected with kinetic energy equal to the incident photon's energy minus the binding energy of the electron. Characteristic x-rays and Auger electrons are emitted as the atom's electrons cascade to fill the vacancy created by the ejected electron.

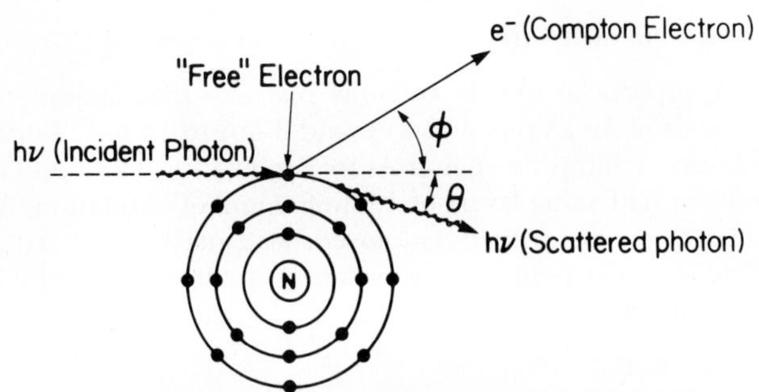

FIGURE 8–13. Schematic drawing illustrates the process of the Compton effect. The incident photon interacts with one of the atom's outer electrons, and the energy is shared between the ejected electron and a scattered photon.

photon is equal to the difference between the energy of the incident photon and the energy transferred to the electron. If the incoming photon's energy is low (*e.g.*, 100 keV), very little energy is transferred to the electron. As the photon's energy increases, a greater proportion of the energy is transferred to the electron, so the scattered photon necessarily retains a smaller proportion of the incident energy. The photon may be scattered at any angle with respect to the direction of the incident photon, but the Compton electron is confined to angles between zero and 90 degrees with respect to the direction of the incident photon. If the incoming photon's energy is low, the distribution of the scattered photons is isotropic, equal in all directions. The scatter angles decrease for photons and electrons as the incident photon's energy increases (*e.g.*, at megavoltage photon energies, both are scattered predominantly in the forward direction).

As a result of conservation of energy and momentum, the energies of the incident photon, hν, the scattered photon, hν′, and the scattered electron, E, are given by the following relationships:

$$E = h\nu_0 \frac{\alpha(1 - \cos\theta)}{1 + \alpha(1 - \cos\theta)}$$

$$h\nu' = h\nu_0 \frac{1}{1 + \alpha(1 - \cos\theta)}$$

$$\cot(\phi) = (1 + \alpha)\tan(\theta/2)$$

where $\alpha = h\nu_0/m_0c^2$, and m_0c^2, is the rest energy of the electron (= 0.511 MeV). If $h\nu_0$ is expressed in MeV, then $\alpha = h\nu_0/0.511$.

The probability that a photon will interact with a target atom via the Compton process (σ_c/ρ) depends on the energy of the incoming photon, generally decreasing as the energy of the photon is increased. The probability of a Compton interaction is nearly independent of the atomic number of the absorber and is directly proportional to the number of electrons per gram.

Pair Production

Pair production (Fig. 8-14) is possible only with photons having energies greater than 1.02 MeV. When such an energetic photon approaches closely enough to the nucleus of the target atom, the incident photon energy may be converted directly into an electron-positron pair. Energy possessed by the photon in excess of 1.02 MeV appears as kinetic energy, which may be distributed in any proportion between the electron and the positron. When the positron comes to rest, it will combine with an electron, and both particles then undergo mutual annihilation, with the appearance of two photons with energy of 0.511 MeV traveling in opposite directions.

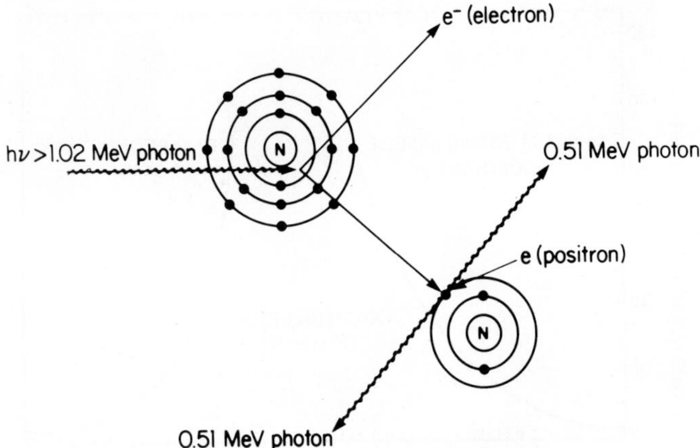

FIGURE 8–14. Schematic drawing illustrates the process of pair production. The incident photon interacts with the electromagnetic field of the nucleus. The photon disappears, and two energetic electrons (a positron and a negatron) are produced. Two annihilation photons of energy 0.511 MeV are produced when the positron interacts with its antiparticle, another electron.

The probability of pair production (π/ρ) occurring increases rapidly with incident photon energy above the 1.02 MeV threshold and is proportional to the second power of the atomic number of the target nuclei.

Photodisintegration

In photodisintegration, a high-energy photon interacts with the nucleus of an atom, totally disrupting the nucleus, with the emission of one or more nucleons (Fig. 8-15). It typically occurs at photon energies much higher than those encountered in radiation therapy.

Relative Importance of Interaction Processes

Figure 8-16 illustrates the relative importance of the photoelectric, Compton, and pair-production processes, three principal modes of interactions pertinent to radiation therapy, as a function of energy and atomic number of the absorber.[14] For example, for an absorber with an atomic number of approximately equal to that of tissue, 7, and for monoenergetic photons, the photoelectric effect is the dominant interaction below about 30 keV. Above 30 keV, the Compton effect becomes dominant and remains so until approximately 24 MeV, at which point pair production becomes the dominant interaction. The total mass attenuation coefficient is given by the sum of the individual coefficients

$$\mu_{en}/\rho = \sigma_{coh}/\rho + \tau/\rho + \sigma_c/\rho + \pi/\rho.$$

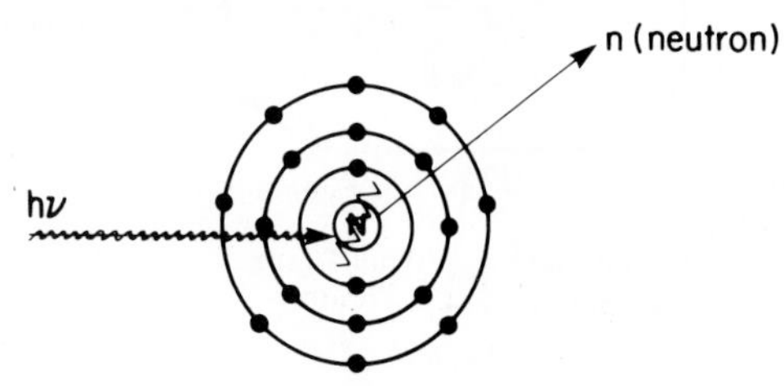

FIGURE 8–15. Schematic drawing illustrates the process of photodisintegration.

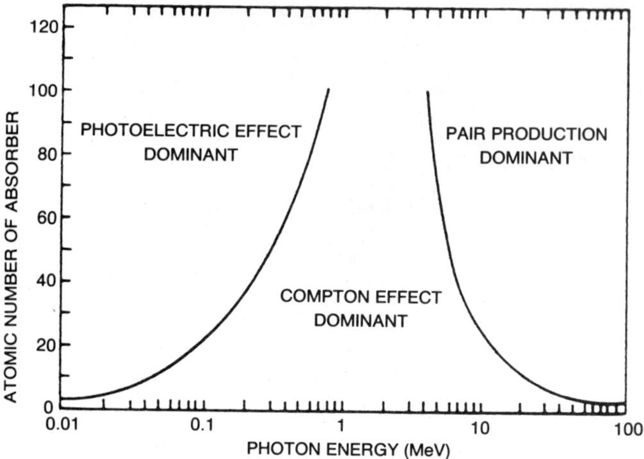

FIGURE 8–16. Relative importance of the three principal modes of interaction as a function of photon energy and atomic number of the medium. (Redrawn from Hendee WR: Medical Radiation Physics, 2nd ed. Chicago, Year Book Medical Publishers, 1979)

RADIATION THERAPY TREATMENT MACHINES

Kilovoltage Units

Before 1951, most radiation treatment units were x-ray machines capable of producing photon beams having only limited penetrability. In these machines, the electrons are accelerated by an electric field produced from a high voltage generated in a transformer that is applied directly between the filament (cathode) and the x-ray target (anode). A schematic diagram of a radiation therapy x-ray tube is shown in Figure 8-17. The potential difference (kVp) is variable on these machines, and metal filters can be added to absorb the lower-energy photons preferentially, changing the penetrability of the beam. The combination of variable kVp and different filtration provides the capability of generating multiple x-ray beams. The degree of penetrability is used to categorize the units as contact, superficial, and orthovoltage (deep-therapy) x-ray machines.

Contact Units

A contact unit is an x-ray machine that operates at potentials of 40 kVp to 50 kVp, typically at a tube current of 2 mA. Attached cones are used for a source-skin distance of typically 2 cm or less. Filters of 0.5 mm to 1.0 mm of aluminum are used to give a typical half-value layer of 0.6 mm of aluminum.

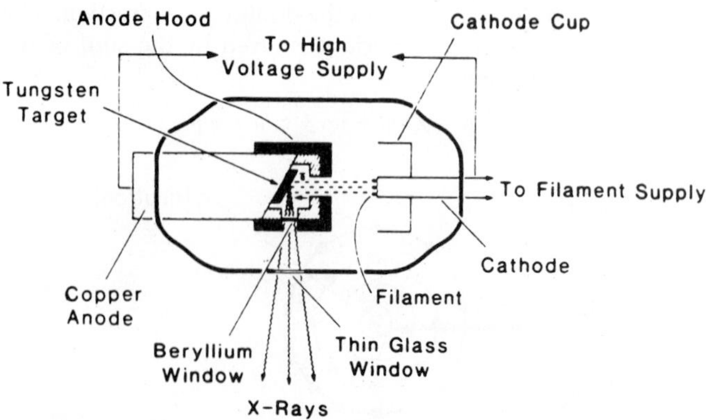

FIGURE 8–17. Schematic diagram of radiation therapy x-ray tube. (Redrawn from Khan FM: The Physics of Radiation Therapy, p 294. Baltimore, Williams & Wilkins, 1984)

Superficial Units

A superficial unit is an x-ray machine that operates at potentials of 50 kVp to 150 kVp and 5 mA to 10 mA. Added thickness of filtration (1 mm Al to 1 mm Al + 0.25 mm Cu) produces half-value layers of 1.0 to 8.0 mm of aluminum. Attached cones are usually employed; lead masks are used to define irregular fields. The skin-source distance is typically 15 cm or 20 cm.

Orthovoltage (Deep-Therapy) Units

An orthovoltage unit is an x-ray machine that operates at potentials of 150 kVp to 500 kVp. Most orthovoltage equipment operates between 200 kVp and 300 kVp with tube currents of 10 mA to 20 mA. Half-value layers of 1 mm to 4 mm of copper are common with the use of added filters, such as the *Thoreaus filter,* a combination of sheets of tin, copper, and aluminum arranged so that highest atomic number is always closest to the x-ray target, ensuring that the higher-energy characteristic x-rays are absorbed by the lower Z metal. Fields are usually defined by detachable cones. The skin-source distance is typically 50 cm.

Supervoltage and Megavoltage Units

The first supervoltage machines were resonant transformer and Van de Graaff generator x-ray units operating at 1 to 2 MV. Only a few of these machines, now considered obsolete, are still in operation. They were quite large and provided only limited flexibility in angulation of the x-ray beam.

^{60}Co Teletherapy Machine

The late 1940s brought the development of nuclear reactors, which allowed the man-made production of radioactive nuclides that emitted high-energy τ-rays in sufficient amounts and at a reasonable price for commercial use in radiation therapy. The first ^{60}Co teletherapy unit was developed in Canada in 1951.[19]

For a radioactive nuclide to be a useful teletherapy source, it must emit high-energy τ-rays to effect adequate penetration, have a high specific activity (*i.e.*, a large number of curies of activity per gram of material) to ensure an adequate dose rate for a small source, and have a long half-life so that the source can be used for a reasonably long time without replacement.

The advantages of any radioactive isotope teletherapy machine are that it has constancy of beam intensity, it allows predictability of decay with a well-defined half-life, and it does not have the day-to-day fluctuations typically found in electrical machines. Most ^{60}Co machines, because they are easily operated and have no need for heavy cables for electrical power, have been installed as isocentric units. Most ^{60}Co machines use a typical source-to-axis distance (SAD) of 80 cm. Newer models provide for 100 cm SAD with higher-activity (10,000 Ci) sources.

The high specific activity of ^{60}Co permits the fabrication of small, high-activity sources, typically 6000 Ci to 7000 Ci in 1.5- to 2.0-cm-diameter sources, giving dose rates of about 150 cGy to 200 cGy per minute at 80 cm when the source is new. Maximum field sizes of 40 cm x 40 cm at the treatment distance of 80 cm are now available on some of the newer machines. The penetration of the 1.17-MeV and 1.33-MeV τ-rays from ^{60}Co is such that the $d_{1/2}$ in tissue (the depth at which the dose has been reduced to 50% of the d_{max} value) is about 10 cm. Disadvantages

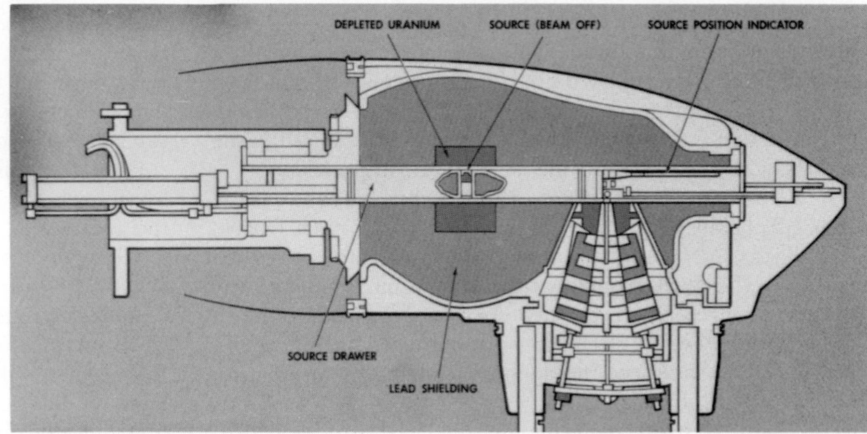

FIGURE 8–18. Schematic cutaway diagram shows ^{60}Co source head. (Courtesy of Atomic Energy Canada, Ltd).

of ^{60}Co units include the need for source replacement approximately every 4 to 5 years and poor field flatness for large fields.

In the design of ^{60}Co teletherapy machines, source movement, beam collimation, and overall radiation shielding are areas of special concern. A typical design is illustrated in Figure 8-18.

Betatron

The first betatron, developed by Kerst in 1941, produced x-rays of 2 MV.[24] Medical betatrons produce x-ray beams with energies of over 40 MV. Figure 8-19 illustrates the basic design and operation of the betatron.[19,28] It resembles a large electric power transformer. Electrons are accelerated by magnetic induction. The accelerating tube is an evacuated circular structure called a doughnut. A magnetic field is produced by passing an alternating current through the primary windings or exciting coils of a large electromagnet. Shown schematically is a vertical section through the betatron. Between the magnet poles is mounted the toroidal evacuated accelerator tube (*doughnut*). The electrons accelerate within the doughnut. A stream of electrons, when injected at the appropriate time in the magnetic

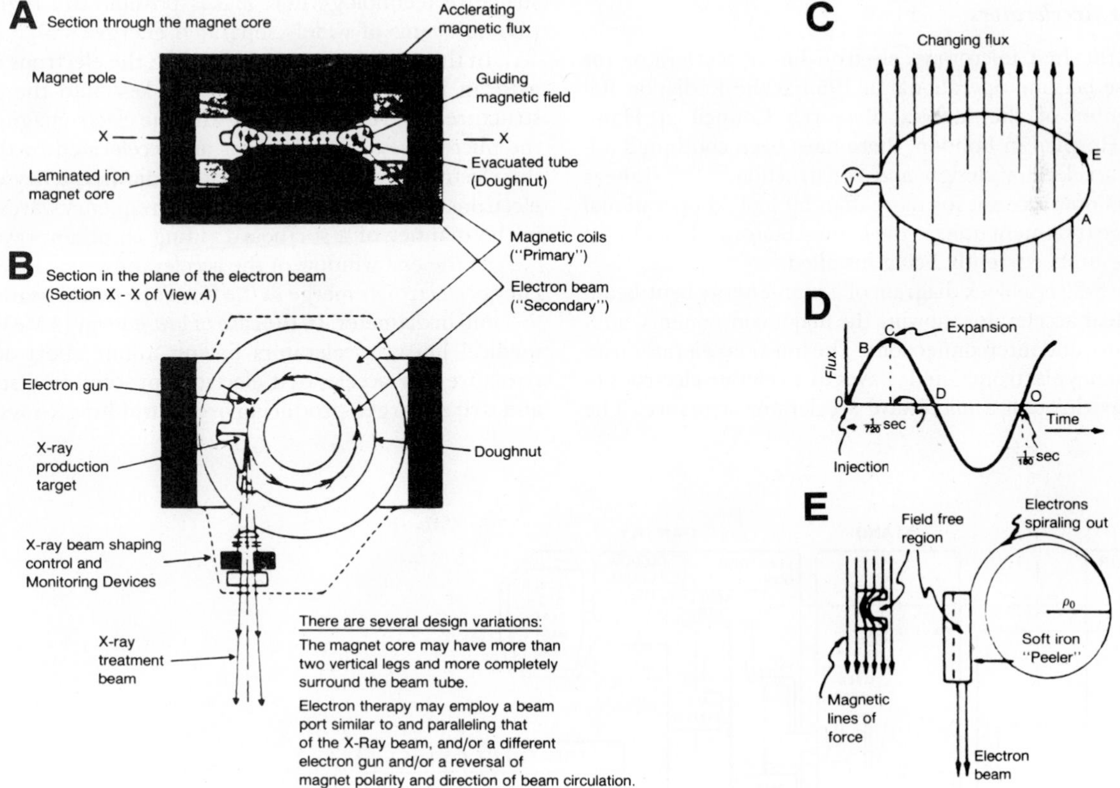

FIGURE 8–19. The construction and operation of the betatron. (**A**) Cross-sectional diagram showing the AC magnet, the poles, the doughnut, and the injector. (**B**) The paths of the electrons within the doughnut and the method of production of the x-rays. (**C**) How an electric field is produced by a changing magnetic flux. (**D**) The cycle of operation of the betatron, showing the time of injection and expansion. (**E**) The operation of the electron "peeler" for obtaining an electron beam. The sketch showing the magnetic lines of force is a cross-sectional view of the peeler device taken at right angles to the diagram through the center of the peeler. (*A* and *B* redrawn from Megavoltage Radiation Therapy Equipment: A Source Document for the February 1981 Blue Book on Criteria for Radiation Oncology in Multidisciplinary Cancer Management, American College of Radiology, 1983; *C, D,* and *E* redrawn from Johns HE, Cunningham JR: The Physics of Radiology, 4th ed. Springfield, IL, Charles C. Thomas, 1983)

induction cycle, follows an orbital path and remains in an equilibrium orbit for hundreds of thousands of revolutions in a fraction of a second. The acquired energy depends primarily on the value of the magnetic induction at the time of the extraction. Only the first one quarter of the induction cycle is used in the acceleration, and the radiation is produced in pulses.[19]

A horizontal cross-section through the doughnut plane shows the details of the production of the clinical beams. Extraction is achieved by applying a contraction pulse to change the path of the electrons from the equilibrium orbit. When an x-ray beam is required, the accelerated electrons are made to strike a target. Otherwise, the electrons can be extracted through a thin metal window built into the doughnut, providing an electron beam for clinical use.

Because of small beam currents and thin target x-ray production, betatrons are low-intensity x-ray machines. The dose rate at 100 cm increases with energy from 25 cGy/minute at approximately 15 MV to 90 cGy/minute at 45 MV. Electron dose rates are typically much higher, ranging from 100 cGy to 300 cGy/minute. Because of the betatron's low-intensity x-ray dose rate, its field size is limited to no greater than about 20 cm x 20 cm at a treatment distance of 100 cm. Betatrons are usually heavy and bulky machines, but some, such as the Brown-Bovari machine, are isocentrically mounted, allowing moving beam therapy and the positioning of the beam at different orientations. The number of medical betatrons in clinical use has decreased significantly, and only a few are still in operation.

Linear Accelerators

Since the first microwave electron linear accelerator for medical use became operational in 1953 at the Radiation Research Center of the Medical Research Council at Hammersmith Hospital in London, there have been continued advances in accelerator design and construction.[23,29,33] Linear accelerators now account for more than 50% of all operational megavoltage treatment units in the United States and for almost 90% of the units currently being installed.[23]

Figure 8-20 is a block diagram of a high-energy bent-beam medical linear accelerator showing the major components, auxiliary systems, and interconnections. The linear accelerator uses high-frequency electromagnetic waves to accelerate electrons to high energy through a microwave accelerator structure. The high-energy electron beam itself can be used for treating superficial tumors or it can be made to strike a target to produce an x-ray beam for treating deep-seated tumors. Modern medical linear accelerators are designed so that the source of radiation can rotate around a horizontal axis (gantry axis). As the gantry rotates, the collimating axis moves in a vertical plane. The isocenter is the point of intersection of the collimator axis and the gantry axis.

The microwave accelerator structure consists of a stack of cylindrical cavities having an axial hole through which the accelerated electrons pass. Medical linear accelerators accelerate electrons by traveling or standing electromagnetic waves of frequencies in the microwave region (3000 MHz). In the standing wave design, the microwave power is coupled into the structure by side-coupling cavities, rather than through the beam aperture. This design tends to be more efficient than the traveling wave design, but it can be more expensive. For further details on this subject and overall linear accelerator operation, refer to the review article by Karzmark and Pering.[23] The accelerator structure in low-energy linear accelerators is typically mounted in the treatment head colinear with the components associated with producing, controlling, and monitoring the x-ray beam. The magnetron or klystron and associated electronics, with the waveguide necessary to transmit the radio frequency power from the magnetron to the accelerator structure, are all situated within the gantry or connecting stand. The high-energy machines use a horizontally mounted accelerator structure with a beam-bending magnet system. Accelerator structure technology now makes possible two high-dose-rate photon beams of widely separated energy.

In the medical linear accelerator, the electrons are ejected with an initial energy of about 50 keV into the accelerator structure, where they interact with the electromagnetic field of the microwaves. The electrons are accelerated by the force of the electrical field associated with radio frequency waves. The electrons are carried along the radio frequency waves somewhat in the manner of a surfboard riding an ocean wave.

At the exit window of the accelerating structure, the high-energy electrons emerge in the form of a pencil beam of about 2 to 3 mm in diameter. In the case of low-energy (4 MeV to 6 MeV) medical linear accelerators having in-line short accelerating structure, the accelerated electrons proceed in a straight line and strike a target, producing bremsstrahlung x-rays. However,

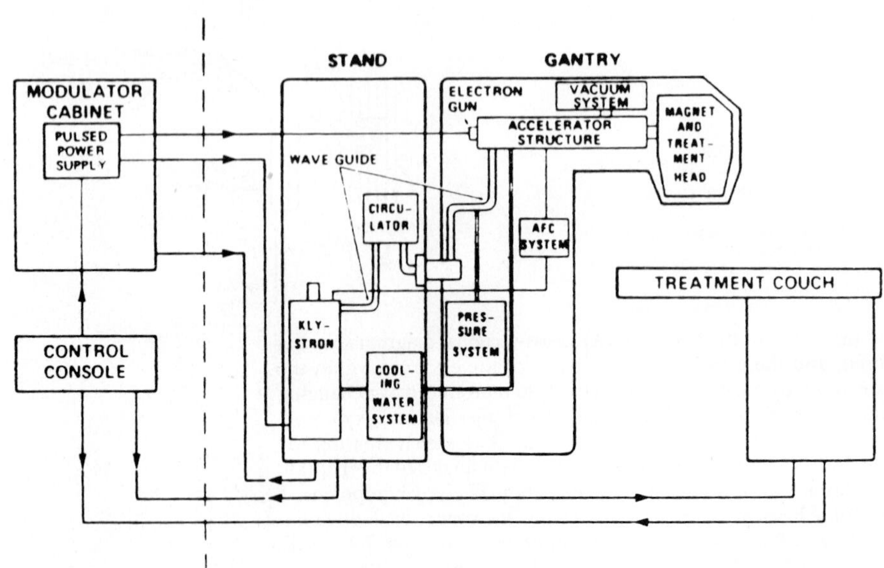

FIGURE 8–20. Schematic block diagram shows the major components of high-energy bent-beam medical linear accelerator. (Courtesy of Varian Associates, Palo Alto, CA)

in high-energy medical linear accelerators, the accelerating structure is much longer and is placed horizontally or at some angle with respect to the horizontal, requiring that the electrons be bent through a suitable angle, usually 90 degrees or 270 degrees between the accelerating structure and the target. This is enabled by the beam transport system, which consists of an achromatic focusing bending magnet and steering and focusing coils.

The angular distribution of x-rays produced by megavoltage electrons incident on a target is forward peaked. To make the x-ray beam intensity uniform across the field, a conical flattening filter is inserted in the beam. Filters have been constructed of lead, tungsten, uranium, steel, and aluminum (or some combination of these), depending on x-ray energy.

The flattened x-ray beam then passes through a monitor ionization chamber. This is typically a monitoring system that consists of several transmission-type parallel-plate ionization chambers, which cover the entire beam. These chambers are used to monitor the integrated dose, the field symmetry, and the dose rate.

After passing through the monitor chamber, the beam can be further collimated by continuously movable x-ray collimators, consisting of two pairs of lead or tungsten blocks (jaws), which provide a rectangular opening from zero to the maximum field size. In the newer units, independent jaw capability is available.

In the electron mode, the x-ray target is retracted and the pencil electron beam strikes an electron-scattering foil to broaden the beam and produce a flat field across the treatment field. The scattering-foil system typically consists of dual lead foils. The thickness of the first foil ensures that most of the electrons are scattered with only a minimum of bremsstrahlung x-rays. The second foil is generally thicker in the central region and is used to flatten the field. The bremsstrahlung produced appears as x-ray contamination of the electron beam and is typically less than 5% of the maximum. In some medical linear accelerators, the electron beam field flatness is accomplished by electromagnetic scanning of the electron pencil beam over the irradiated area rather than the use of scattering foils. A schematic diagram of beam subsystems for both x-ray and electron beams is shown in Figure 8-21.[22]

Microtrons

The microtron, the concept of which is credited to Veksler, is an electron accelerator that combines the basic principles of the electron linear accelerator and the cyclotron.[35,40] The principles of operation are illustrated in Figure 8-22. There are two types of microtrons. In the *circular microtron,* electrons are accelerated as they pass through a microwave cavity and move in a uniform magnetic field, where they describe circular trajectories of increasing radius. Adjustments are made to the cavity voltage, frequency, and magnetic field so that the electrons always encounter the electric field of the microwave cavity in phase. The *racetrack microtron* uses two D-shaped magnet pole pieces that are separated by a fixed distance, between which is a multicavity accelerator structure. This configuration provides much higher energy gains than the circular microtron. It uses a multicavity accelerating structure, rather than a single cavity between the separated pole pieces, and provides energy gains of 5 MeV per orbit. Exit-beam energies ranging from 5 MeV to 50 MeV for electrons and photons are available. The performance characteristics of the microtron are similar to those of a typical medical linac.

Cyclotrons

The cyclotron is used primarily to accelerate protons for proton beam therapy and to generate neutron beams for radiation therapy.[15] The principles of the cyclotron are shown in Figure 8-23.

X-ray Simulator

The x-ray simulator is a machine that duplicates a radiation treatment unit in terms of its geometric, mechanical, and optical properties but uses a diagnostic x-ray tube to simulate the

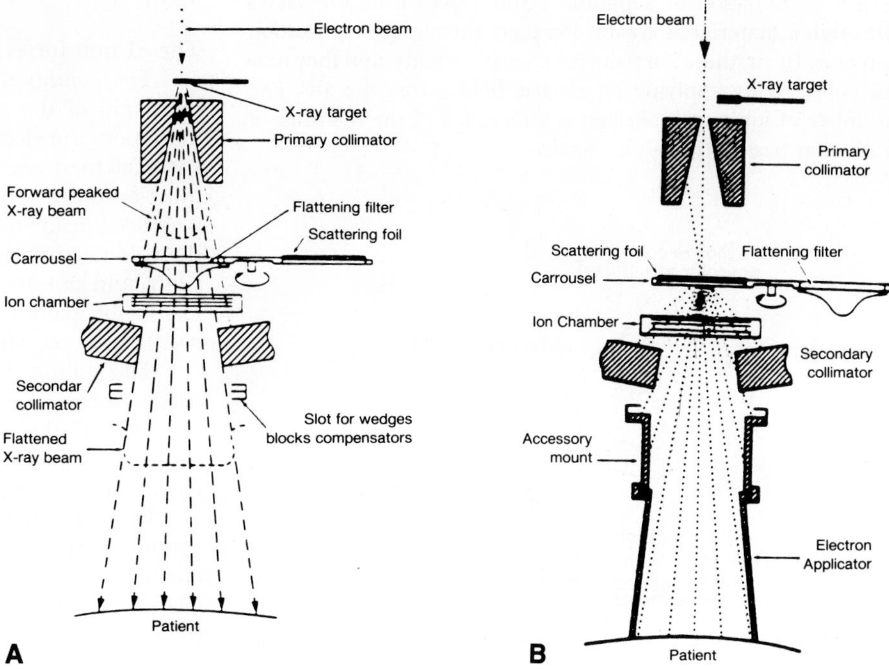

FIGURE 8–21. Schematic diagram of beam subsystems for (**A**) x-ray beam and (**B**) electron-beam therapy. (Redrawn from Karzmark CJ, Morton RJ: A Primer on Theory and Operation of Linear Accelerators in Radiation Therapy. Reprinted with permission of the Department of Health and Human Services, Public Health Service, Food and Drug Administration, Bureau of Radiological Health, Rockville, MD 20857)

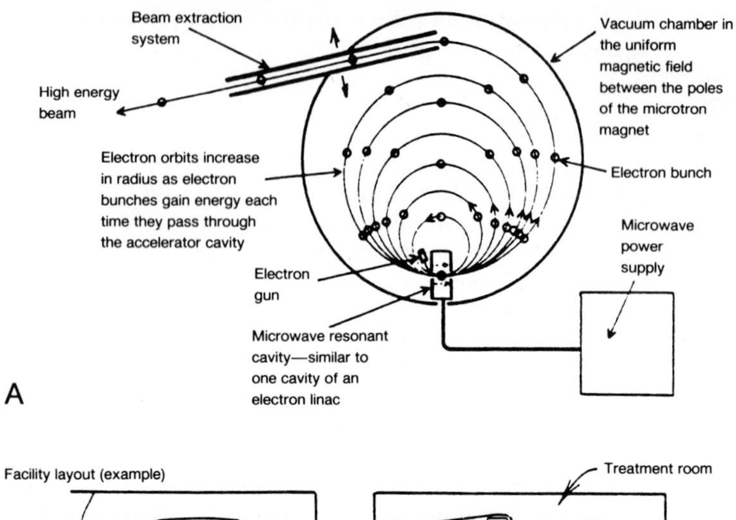

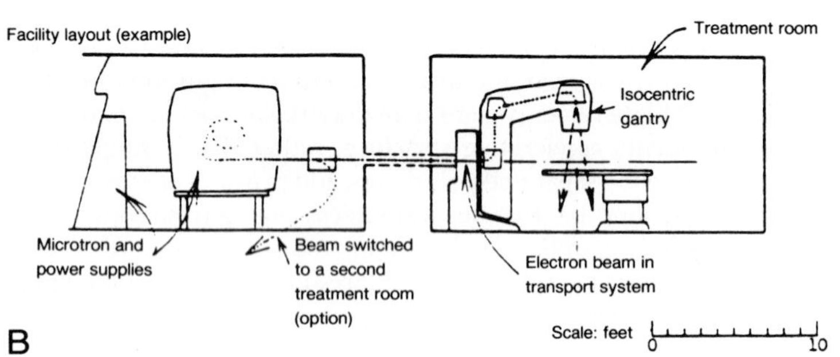

FIGURE 8–22. (**A**) Schematic drawing shows the principles of circular microtron operation. (**B**) Medical characteristics. (Redrawn from Megavoltage Radiation Therapy Equipment: A Source Document for the February 1981 Blue Book on Criteria for Radiation Oncology in Multidisciplinary Cancer Management. American College of Radiology, 1983)

radiation properties of the treatment beam.[5] A simulator allows the beam direction and the treatment fields to be determined to encompass the target volume and to spare normal structures excessive radiation. Radiographic visualization of internal structures in relation to external landmarks allows special shielding devices to be constructed. Most simulators are equipped with x-ray fluoroscopy to expedite field setup and beam angulations.

RADIATION EXPOSURE

In 1928, at the second International Congress of Radiology, the ionization of air, called *exposure,* was adopted as the measurable effect of radiation of a photon beam.[19] As the beam passes through a material, it creates ion pairs through the ionization process. In air, these ion pairs have some mobility, and they may be collected by applying an electric field across the air. The number of ion pairs collected is a measure of the quantity of radiation passing through the air.

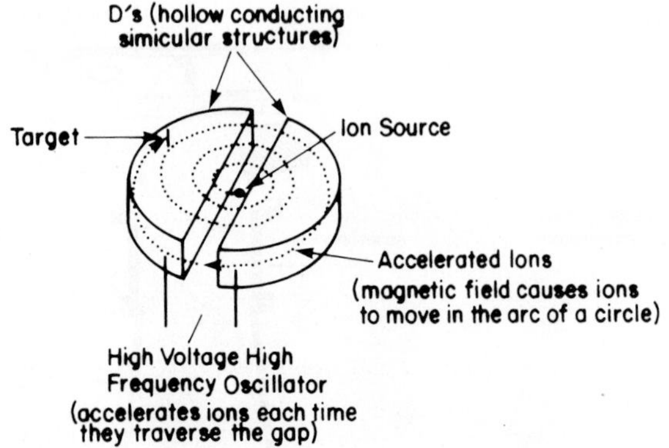

FIGURE 8–23. Schematic drawing shows the principles of cyclotron operation.

The roentgen, the unit for exposure, was defined at the 1928 Congress. The definition has been modified slightly by subsequent Congresses, but the basic concept remains the same. The *roentgen* is that amount of x or gamma radiation that causes the associated corpuscular emission per 0.001293 g of air to produce, in air, ions carrying one electrostatic unit of charge (esu) of either sign.[19] The value 0.001293 g is the mass of 1 cm^3 of air at 0°C and 760 mm Hg pressure; "associated corpuscular emission" refers to the Compton and pair-production electrons set in motion by the interactions between the incident photons and the air molecules. By conversion of units, the roentgen is presently defined as

$$1 \text{ R} = 2.58 \times 10^{-4} \text{ C/kg of air}$$

The SI unit for exposure is C/kg of air.

The condition of *electronic equilibrium* must exist for the definition of the roentgen to be satisfied. According to the definition, the electrons produced in a specified volume must spend all their energies by ionization in air and the total charge must be measured. However, because some of the electrons produced inside the specified volume create ion pairs outside the volume and some electrons produced outside the volume contribute ionization inside the specified volume, the gain and loss of ion pairs must be the same for the definition of the roentgen to be satisfied.

The standard free-air ionization chamber (Fig. 8-24) is used to measure exposure directly in roentgens. It is designed to collect all the ions produced in a defined volume by the radiation beam. Details on the design and limitations of free-air ion chambers can be found in standard texts.[25]

Free-air chambers are bulky and too complicated to use for routine measurements. Instead, small ionization chambers, *thimble chambers,* are typically used to measure exposure. The chambers give a measure of the ionization produced, which is then converted to exposure in roentgens by use of an exposure calibration factor, N_x, assigned to the chamber by a calibration

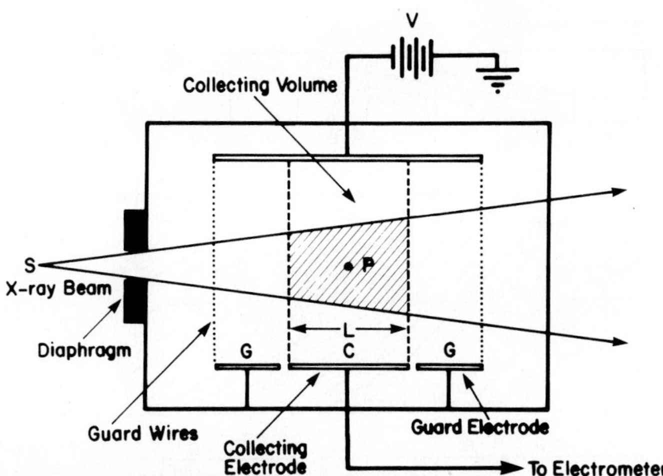

FIGURE 8–24. Schematic diagram of free-air ionization chamber. (Redrawn from Khan FM: The Physics of Radiation Therapy. Baltimore, Williams & WIlkins, 1984)

laboratory, such as the American Association of Physicists in Medicine Accredited Dosimetry Calibration Laboratories. Thimble chambers are designed for use at certain energies; the thickness of the chamber wall is equal to the maximum electron range (electronic equilibrium established). If they are used at higher energies, at which the electron range is greater, an added wall thickness or "build-up" cap must be used.

A standard procedure is currently used to determine the exposure rate from an x-ray or τ-ray machine using an exposure-calibrated thimble chamber. The ionization chamber, with appropriate wall thickness, is placed at beam center, in air, at right angles to the beam's central axis and at the point where the exposure rate is to be specified. The field size for which the exposure rate is to be measured is set, and the radiation machine is turned on for a known time, t, to achieve a reading, M, on the chamber readout instrument. The reading is corrected for temperature and atmospheric pressure, timer error, stem effect, and ion-recombination effects. The therapy machine exposure rate, X, is given in roentgens per minute by the following equation:

$$X = \frac{M \cdot N_x \cdot C_{tp} \cdot C_{st} \cdot C_s}{T + \alpha}$$

where

M = ionization chamber reading

N_x = exposure calibration factor obtained from a standards laboratory

C_{tp} = temperature (t) and pressure (p) correction factors = $\left(\frac{t + 273.16}{295.16}\right)\left(\frac{760}{760 + p}\right)$

C_{st} = stem effect correction factor

C_s = ion recombination correction factor

$T + \alpha$ = timer setting plus timer error

The timer error is given by the following equation:

$$\frac{M_1}{T + \alpha} = \frac{M_2}{T + n\alpha}$$

where M_1 is the instrument reading for a single, long exposure of T, M_2 is the instrument reading for n short exposures of total time, T, and α is the timer or monitor end error for a single exposure.

Beyond 3 MeV, the definition of the roentgen cannot be applied, and calibrations are performed using the calibrated chamber as a Bragg-Gray cavity, and the ionization readings are converted to absorbed dose.

QUALITY OF RADIATION

From the physical standpoint, the *quality* (*i.e.*, penetrability) of any ordinary x-ray beam is completely specified by its spectral distribution curve. The spectral distribution curve is based on the relative intensities of photons of various energies and is a result of fluctuations of tube potential, the bremsstrahlung radiation process, characteristic radiation, and multiple interactions of the incident electrons and the x-ray target.

Figure 8-25 shows a typical spectral distribution curve for a photon beam. The distribution of the photon energies, including the peak photon energy, in the continuous spectrum is governed solely by the x-ray tube potential. However, the energy of the characteristic photons increases with increasing atomic number of the target element. All other factors being equal, the radiation intensity is proportional to the atomic number of the target element.

Spectral distribution of an x-ray beam can be modified by placing absorbing materials of various thickness (*i.e.*, filters) in the beam. In general, a filter removes relatively more low-energy photons than high-energy photons, although photons of all energies are removed to some extent. For radiation in the orthovoltage region (except for the absorption edge effect), the lower the energy of the photons, the larger the total mass attenuation coefficient and therefore the greater the likelihood that the photon will be absorbed. Therefore, the beam emerges from the filter with a larger percentage of high-energy photons than it had on entering the filter. This beam has a greater penetration power and is said to have been "hardened" by the filter. The quality of an x-ray beam improves with increasing tube potential and with increasing thickness and atomic number of the filter.

A specification of beam quality based entirely on a spectral distribution is too cumbersome for radiation therapy. The usual method of specifying beam quality in superficial and orthovoltage therapy is by indicating the half-value layer and the accelerating potential. For megavoltage beams, only the maximum energy of the electrons striking the x-ray target is typically

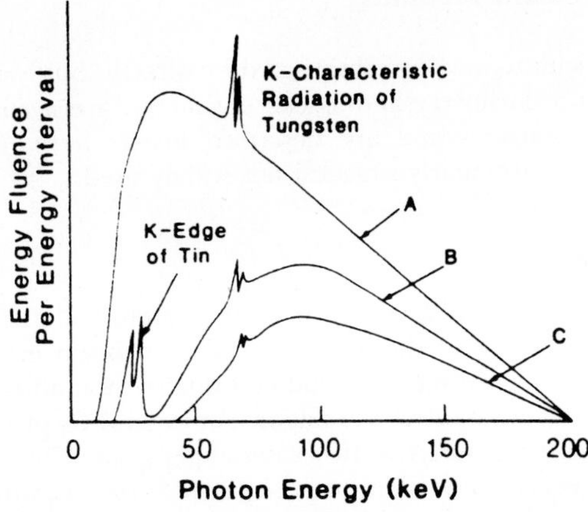

FIGURE 8–25. Schematic graph showing spectral distribution of 200-kVp x-ray beam with different added filters. (Redrawn from Khan FM: The Physics of Radiation Therapy. Baltimore, Williams & Wilkins, 1984)

used. The *homogeneity coefficient* denotes how homogeneous an x-ray beam is with respect to its photon energies. It is defined as the ratio of the first half-value layer to the second. As the filtration is increased, the exposure rate decreases; therefore, there is a practical limit of filter thickness in orthovoltage therapy with a given combination of kilovolts, milliamperes, and distance. In certain situations it is convenient to express the quality of the x-ray beam in terms of an "equivalent energy," which can be derived from knowledge of the half-value layer. The type of x-ray beam that is used in radiation therapy is always heterogeneous, consisting of many different energies; however, the beam can be considered to have a definite equivalent energy if monoenergetic radiation of that energy has the same half-value layer as the radiation in question.

ABSORBED DOSE

In 1953, the International Commission on Radiological Units and Measurements introduced the concept of absorbed dose and defined its unit, the rad.

As a beam of radiation passes through an absorbing medium, it interacts with it in a two-stage process. The first step occurs when energy carried by the photons, the indirectly ionizing particles, is transformed into kinetic energy of high-speed electrons, and the second step occurs as these electrons, the directly ionizing particles, are slowed down and deposit their energy in the medium.

Kerma, an acronym for the *k*inetic *e*nergy *r*eleased in the *m*edium, represents the transfer of energy from the photons to the directly ionizing particles (step 1). The subsequent transfer of energy from the directly ionizing particles to the medium (step 2) is represented by the absorbed dose. The relationship between kerma and absorbed dose is illustrated in Figure 8-26.

Absorbed Dose is defined in terms of the energy deposited by the radiation beam as it passes through the medium of interest. The *rad* represents the absorption of 0.01 joule per kilogram of the medium:

$$1 \text{ rad} = 0.01 \text{ J/kg}$$

The SI unit for absorbed dose is 1 J/kg and called a "Gray." Notice that 100 rad = 1 J/kg = 1 Gy. Therefore, 1 rad = 1 centigray (cGy).

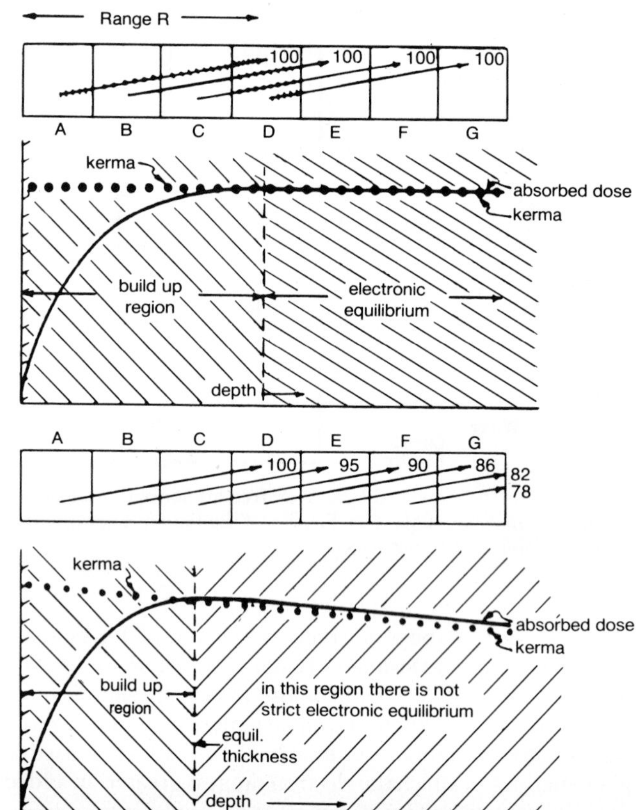

FIGURE 8–26. Schematic relationship of kerma and absorbed dose. (Redrawn from Johns HE, Cunningham JR: The Physics of Radiology, 4th ed. Springfield, IL, Charles C Thomas, 1983)

Measurement Methods

It is difficult to measure absorbed dose directly, but two direct methods, calorimetry and Fricke dosimetry, are available in some laboratories and are described briefly here. Neither method is particularly practical nor widely used.

Calorimetry

Calorimetry is based on the fact that almost all the energy deposited in the medium by the radiation beam eventually appears as heat within the medium. A small temperature rise of the medium occurs after irradiation. For water, 1 Gy produces a temperature rise of 2.4×10^{-4} calories per gram. Thus, a dose of 200 cGy gives a temperature rise of 0.5×10^{-3}°C, which can be measured using sensitive devices called thermistors. The calorimeter, although simple in concept, is technically difficult to implement.

Fricke Dosimetry

Fricke dosimetry is based on chemical changes caused by radiation. The chemical radiation dosimeter most commonly used is the Fricke dosimeter, in which ferrous sulfate is oxidized by radiation to ferric sulfate. The ferric ion concentration is measured by absorption spectrometry at 224 nm and 304 nm. Chemical dosimetry is not a direct measurement in that the chemical yield or G value, which is the number of molecules of ferric ion produced per 100 eV of absorbed energy, must be known. G values are energy dependent for x-rays and range from 15.3 to 15.7 molecules per 100 eV of energy absorbed, with the higher values for electrons.

Exposure Measurement

Because calorimetry and Fricke dosimetry are technically difficult to apply in absorbed dose measurements, their use is not widespread. A simpler, indirect method using ionization chambers is usually employed for absorbed dose determination. If an ionization chamber has been calibrated by a standards laboratory, exposure in air can be determined as described in the section on Radiation Exposure. The energy deposited in a fixed mass of air from a known exposure can be calculated, because it is known that an exposure of 1 R creates a finite number of ion pairs per unit mass of air (*i.e.*, 1.61×10^{15} ion pairs per kilogram of air) and that a fixed amount (*i.e.*, 33.85 eV) of mean energy is required to create an ion pair in air. When these values are used, the relationship between the exposure, X, and the dose "in free space," D_{fs} (*i.e.*, the dose in units of cGy to a small mass of condensed air just large enough to provide electronic equilibrium), can be given by the following expression:

$$D_{fs} = 0.873 \cdot X \cdot A_{eq}$$

where A_{eq} is an attenuation correction factor accounting for the photon attenuation in the condensed air mass. Typical values of A_{eq} are 0.989 and 1.00 for ^{60}Co and 250-kV energies, respectively.

For a small mass of phantom-like material of dimensions similar to those of the condensed air, the equation for the absorbed dose in free space differs only by the ratio of the mass energy absorption coefficients (μ_{en}/ρ) and is given by

$$D_{fs} = \left(0.873 \cdot \frac{(\mu_{en}/\rho)_{med}}{(\mu_{en}/\rho)_{air}}\right) \cdot X \cdot A_{eq}$$

The term in brackets is called the f factor or the *roentgen-to-rad conversion factor.* The previous equation can also be expressed as

$$D_{fs} = f_{med} \cdot X \cdot A_{eq}$$

Values of f are shown in Figure 8-27 over the energy range commonly used in radiation therapy. Notice that the f factor is a function of the medium and the energy of the photon beam.

The calibration procedure has a standard approach. The wall of the ionization chamber (having an exposure calibration factor) should be thick enough to ensure electronic equilibrium. The chamber is placed in air with its sensitive volume on the central axis of the beam and its stem at right angles to the beam direction. The center of the chamber should be at a distance from the source (or target) equal to the nominal source-skin distance of the machine plus the buildup depth. A standard field size is set, usually 10 cm x 10 cm, using either movable collimators or the standard treatment applicator. An exposure is made for a known time. The ionization chamber reading can be converted to units of cGy/min at the depth of the maximum dose within a phantom, d_{med}, using the following equation:

$$\dot{D}_{med} = M \cdot N_x \cdot C_{tp} \cdot C_{st} \cdot C_s \cdot A_{eq} \cdot f_{med} \cdot PSF \times \frac{1}{T + \alpha}$$

where M, N_x, C_{tp}, C_{st}, C_s, A_{eq}, f_{med}, T, and α are used as defined

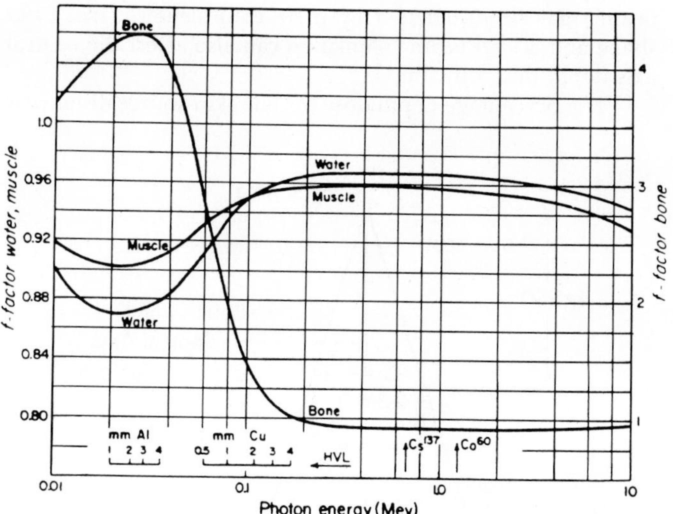

FIGURE 8–27. The roentgen-to-rad conversion factor for bone, muscle, and water as a function of photon energy. (Redrawn from Johns HE, Cunningham JR: The Physics of Radiology, 4th ed. Springfield, IL, Charles C Thomas, 1983)

previously. The term PSF represents the peakscatter factor and converts the dose in free space to the dose in a phantom at the depth of maximum dose. This parameter is discussed further later. The above equation can be rewritten:

$$\dot{D}_{med} = f_{med} \cdot X \cdot A_{eq} \cdot PSF$$

and

$$\dot{D}_{med} = \dot{D}_{fs} \cdot PSF$$

This method is also valid when the measurements are made with the exposure-calibrated ion chamber embedded within a medium, such as a water phantom. In that case, the PSF term is not included in the calculation and the A_{eq} factor is replaced by a displacement factor, A_m. The numerical value of A_m is very close to that of A_{eq}, and for exposure measurements made within a water phantom, the dose rate is given by the following expression:

$$\dot{D}_{med} = f_{med} \cdot \dot{X} \cdot A_m$$

Bragg-Gray Ionization Measurement

The previous expression for absorbed dose includes the standards laboratory's exposure calibration factor. For energies above the level of ^{60}Co, exposure calibration factors are not available. Instead, a quantity known as C_λ has been determined based on the Bragg-Gray theory. Other sources offer the details of this theory and the derivation of C_λ.[19,25] The C_λ factor is used to convert the ionization readings to absorbed dose using an ion chamber in a phantom and the exposure calibration factor for ^{60}Co. This approach assumes that the C_λ factor is independent of chamber design and construction material. Information is available about the corresponding factor, C_E, which is similarly used for electron beams.[17]

For this calibration approach, an ion chamber having a known ^{60}Co exposure calibration factor is placed in a water phantom at the maximum buildup depth or at another known depth (*e.g.*, 5–7 cm, depending on photon energy). The water surface is set at the nominal skin-source distance of the machine, and the calibration field size (10 cm x 10 cm) is set. The machine is set to deliver a given amount of radiation. For medical linear accelerators, this is typically designated in terms of number of monitor units (*e.g.*, 100 MU). The dose rate in units of cGy/MU in water is then given by

$$\dot{D}_{water} = M \cdot N_x \cdot C_{tp} \cdot C_{st} \cdot C_s \cdot C_\lambda \cdot \frac{1}{(MU + \alpha)} \cdot \frac{1}{(P/100)}$$

where C_λ is the overall factor that converts the corrected chamber reading to absorbed dose (cGy) at that energy. P/100 is the percent depth dose factor needed to obtain the dose at the depth of dose maximum; it is discussed later in this chapter.

N_{gas} Method

In 1983, the American Association of Physicists in Medicine introduced a new protocol for the calibration of high-energy photon and electron beams.[39] The protocol updated physical parameters and procedures for calibration and measurement, and it accounted for the different phantom materials (*e.g.*, plastic and water) used for calibration and differences in ion chamber design and construction. A new factor, the cavity-gas calibration factor (N_{gas}), is used in conjunction with restricted stopping-power ratios, $\overline{L}/\rho$, for the radiation beam in question to convert the ionization reading from a ^{60}Co exposure-calibrated chamber to absorbed dose according to the following expression:

$$D_{med} = M \cdot N_{gas} \cdot (\bar{L}/\rho)^{med}_{gas} \cdot P_{ion} \cdot P_{repl} \cdot P_{wall}$$

M = Ionization chamber reading corrected for temperature and pressure
$\bar{L}/\rho$ = Mean restricted collision mass stopping power
P_{ion} = Ion recombination correction factor
P_{repl} = Correction factor for replacement of phantom material by ionization chamber
P_{wall} = Correction factor to account for ionization chamber wall composition

Details of the protocol for this calibration procedure are available elsewhere.[39]

Thermoluminescence Dosimetry

Certain crystalline materials exhibit a phenomenon known as thermoluminescence. When a crystal capable of thermoluminescence is irradiated, a very small portion of the energy absorbed is stored in the structure of the crystal lattice. If the material is heated, the energy is released in the form of visible light. There are several thermoluminescent phosphors available, but lithium fluoride (LiF), with an effective atomic number of 8.2, is the most commonly used.

The physical theory of thermoluminescence dosimetry is elementary. In the individual atom, electrons occupy discrete energy levels. However, in the crystal lattice, the electronic energy levels are perturbed by mutual interactions between atoms, giving rise to energy bands, so-called allowed energy bands and forbidden energy bands. Impurities in the crystal create energy traps in the forbidden bands, allowing metastable states to exist; for example, when the phosphor is irradiated, some of the electrons in the valence band (ground state) receive sufficient energy to be raised to the conduction band. If there is an instantaneous emission of light, the phenomenon is called *fluorescence.* If an electron in the trap requires energy to get out of the trap and return to the valence band, the emission of light is called *phosphorescence.* If the emission of light is slow at room temperature but can be sped up with heating, the process is called *thermoluminescence.*

The thermoluminescence dosimetry response is defined as thermoluminescence output per unit of absorbed dose in the phosphor. Studies of energy response for photons above the energy of ^{60}Co and for high-energy electrons show somewhat conflicting results. If considerable care is used, precision within approximately 3% may be obtained.[25]

Thermoluminescence dosimeters must be calibrated before they can be used for measuring an unknown dose. Because the response of the thermoluminescent material is affected by its radiation history and thermal history, the material must be annealed to remove residual effects. The standard preirradiation annealing procedure for LiF is 1 hour of heating at 400°C and 24 hours at 80°C.

Film Dosimetry

When an x-ray film is exposed to ionizing radiation, the exposed silver bromide crystals form a latent image. In the film development process, the affected crystals cause a darkening of the film, and the unaffected crystals leave the film clear. The degree of blackening of the film is proportional to the energy absorbed and is measured by determining the optical density with a densitometer. The optical density is defined as follows:

$$OD = \log (I_0/I_T)$$

where I_0 is the amount of light detected without the film in place and I_T is the amount of light detected with the film in place. For radiation dosimetry, the net optical density is obtained by subtracting the densitometric reading for the base fog (clear portion of the film) from the measured optical density. Most films are exposed to yield an optical density between 1.3 and 1.7 for optimal viewing.

A plot of net optical density as a function of radiation exposure or dose is called the sensitometric curve or the Hunter-Driffield (H-D) curve. If the curve is nonlinear, appropriate corrections must be applied to convert net optical density to absorbed dose.

The use of film is a relatively straightforward method of dosimetry for electron beams, but it must be done with extreme care in photon dosimetry. The problem is that the photoelectric effect depends on Z^3 (Z_{silver} = 47), and the film emulsion strongly absorbs radiation below 100 kV.

DOSIMETRY PARAMETERS

Percentage Depth Dose

Percentage depth dose may be understood by reference to Figure 8-28. It is the ratio, expressed as a percentage, of the absorbed dose on the central axis at depth d to the absorbed dose at the reference point d_o. Percentage depth dose is given by

$$PDD(d,d_o,S,f,E) = \frac{D_d}{D_{d_o}}(100)$$

The functional symbols have been inserted in the above expression to make it clear that the percentage depth dose is affected by a number of parameters including the d, d_o, the field dimension S, the source-to-surface distance f, and the radiation beam energy (or quality) E. S refers to the side length of a square beam at a specified reference depth. Nonsquare beams may be designated by their equivalent square. Field shape and added beam collimation can also affect the central axis depth dose distribution.

The percentage depth dose for one skin-source distance is

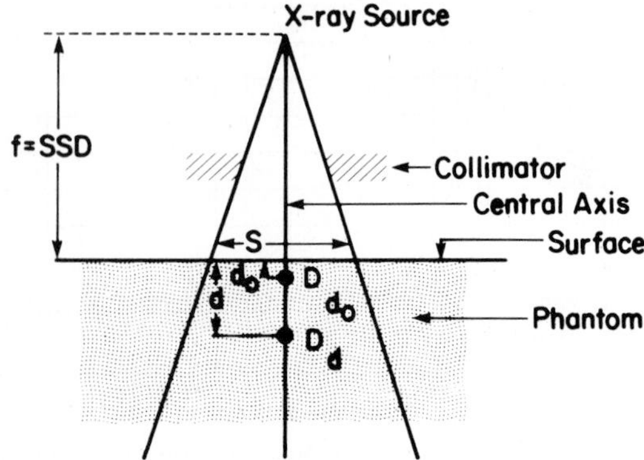

FIGURE 8–28. Schematic drawing illustrates the definition of the percentage depth dose, in which d is any depth and d_l is the reference depth, usually d_{max}.

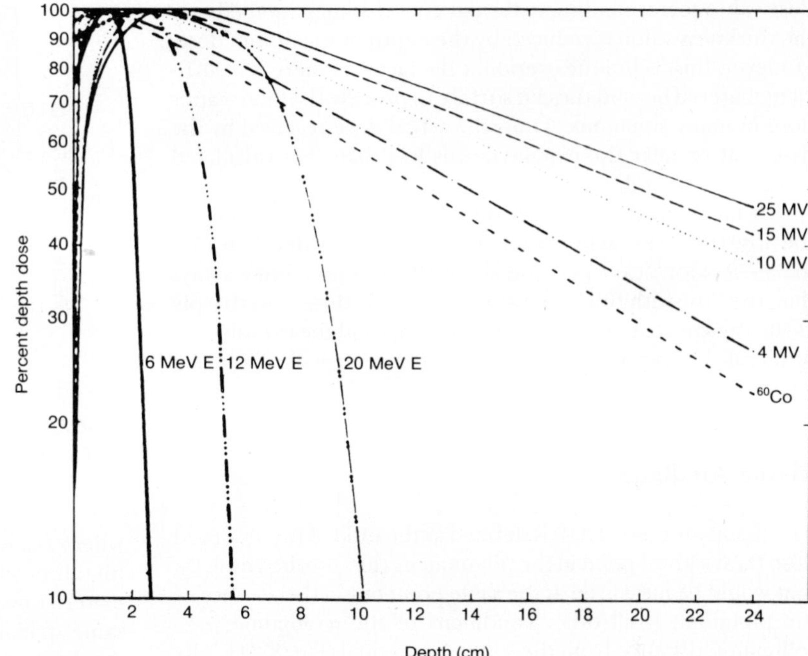

FIGURE 8–29. Examples of central-axis percentage depth doses for megavoltage x-ray beams ranging from ^{60}Co to 25-MV x-rays and 6-MeV to 20-MeV electron beams. (Redrawn from Purdy JA: IEEE Trans Nucl Sci 26:1833, © 1979 IEEE)

related to the percentage depth dose at a second skin-source distance by the following equation:

$$PDD(d,S,f_2) = PDD(d,S,f_1) \cdot \left(\frac{f_1 + d}{f_2 + d} \cdot \frac{f_2 + d_{max}}{f_1 + d_{max}}\right)^2$$

The term in the parentheses is called the Mayneord F factor.[27]

In 1961, the first extensive compilation of central axis depth dose data that included values for high-energy accelerators was presented by the Scientific Sub-committee of the Hospital Physicists' Association.[36] The data were reviewed in 1968 and updated in 1972 and again in 1983.[8,20] These reports indicated that the depth dose characteristics varied for different types of accelerators operating at the same nominal energy. These variations can be attributed to differences in energy of the electrons striking the x-ray target, the type of x-ray target and flattening filter material, and the materials and geometry of the collimating system.

Photon beam percentage depth dose increases with increasing energy, increasing skin-source distance, and increasing field size. Figure 8-29 shows that the depth of the 50th percentile increases from 13.8 cm for 4-MV x-rays to over 22 cm for 25-MV x-rays.[32] The depth of maximum dose varies from 1 cm for 4-MV x-rays to over 3.5 cm for 25-MV x-rays. However, the depth of maximum dose position is not unambiguously defined by the energy of the x-ray beam, but depends on the field size and on the treatment-head design of the particular machine. This shift in dose maximum is principally the result of electron scattering from the x-ray collimator. The specification of x-ray percentage depth dose in terms of the maximum electron energy impinging on the x-ray target is not sufficient to characterize the x-ray beam. An improved specification encompasses the depth of maximum dose and the depth of a particular percentile (*e.g.*, the 50th) for a specific field size or range of field sizes.[34]

The percentage depth dose at the surface and in the buildup region for megavoltage photon beams depends sensitively on the variables of radiation geometry, such as skin-source distance, field size, distance between the skin and the collimator, and the presence or absence of a secondary blocking tray.[41,42] Examples of measured buildup region depth dose data for photon energies ranging from ^{60}Co τ-rays to 25-MV x-rays are presented in Figure 8-30.

In general, the dose to the surface and in the buildup region for megavoltage photon beams increases with an increase in field size, with the introduction of a blocking tray into the beam, and with a decrease in the distance between skin and blocking tray. The surface dose tends to decrease with increasing x-ray beam energy.

Although the central axis dose distribution of megavoltage photon irradiation at the entrance surface has been well documented, the dose at the exit surface has not received adequate consideration. The exit dose is frequently calculated by multiplying the maximum dose by the central axis percentage depth

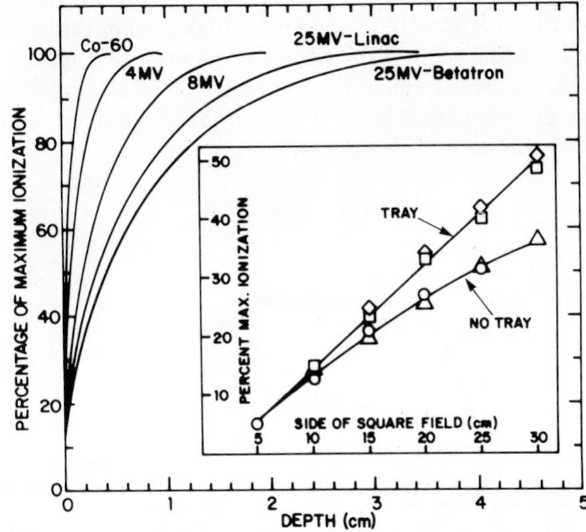

FIGURE 8–30. Examples of percentage depth dose curves in the buildup region for photon energies ranging from ^{60}Co to 25-MV x-rays. (Redrawn from Velkley DE, Manson DJ, Purdy JA, et al: Med Phys 2:14, 1975)

dose value corresponding to the patient's thickness; sometimes, the thickness value is reduced by the depth of maximum dose. However, this technique overlooks the fact that there is insufficient material beyond the exit surface to provide the total scatter dose in many situations. Thus, the actual dose received by the tissues at or near the exit surface is less than that calculated using this method.

It has been shown that if there is no backscatter material, the dose to the skin at the exit surface ($\approx$ 4 mg/cm^2 depth) is 15% to 20% less for ^{60}Co τ-rays and about 10% less for 25-MV x-rays than the dose with full backscatter.[11] The skin dose rises sharply as the thickness of material is increased beyond the exit surface, until full backscatter conditions are obtained with about 0.5 g/cm^2 of added material.

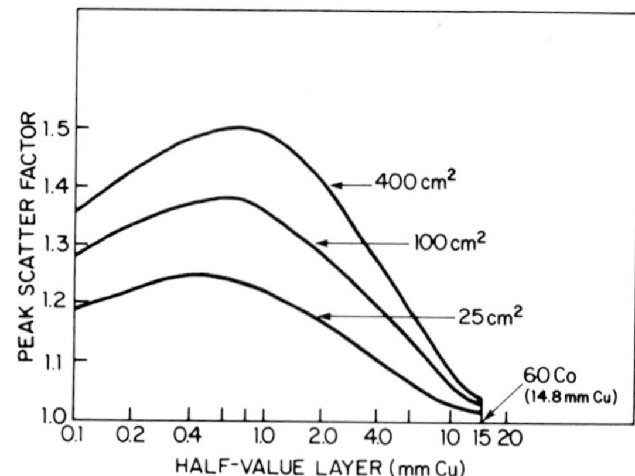

FIGURE 8–32. Variation of peakscatter factor with beam quality (half-value layer). (Redrawn from Johns HE, Cunningham JR: The Physics of Radiology, 4th ed. Springfield, IL, Charles C Thomas, 1983)

Tissue-Air Ratio

The tissue-air ratio (TAR) is defined as the ratio of the absorbed dose D_d at a given point in the phantom by the absorbed dose D_{fs} that would be measured at the same point but in the absence of the phantom, if all other conditions of the irradiation (*e.g.*, collimator, distance from the source) are equal (Fig. 8-31). The TAR is expressed as

$$TAR(d,S_d,E) = \frac{D_d}{D_{fs}}$$

where d is depth, E is radiation beam energy, and S_d is the beam dimension measured at depth d. TAR depends on depth, field size, and beam quality but is assumed to be independent of the distance from the source. Because of this assumption, the measurement of TAR is exact only to within about 2% over the range of distances used clinically.[19]

The TAR at the depth of maximum dose is given the special name *peakscatter factor.* It is perhaps better known as the *backscatter factor,* but because of the finite depth d_o this tends to be misleading. Figure 8-32 shows the peakscatter factors for various field sizes and beam qualities.

Tissue-Phantom Ratio and Tissue-Maximum Ratio

The concepts of tissue-phantom ratio (TPR) and tissue-maximum ratio (TMR) were proposed for high-energy radiation as alternatives to TAR in response to arguments raised against the use of in-air measurement for a photon beam with a maximum energy greater than 3 MeV.[16,21] As originally defined, TPR is given by the ratio of two doses:

$$TPR(d,d_r,S_d,E) = \frac{D_d}{D_{d_r}}$$

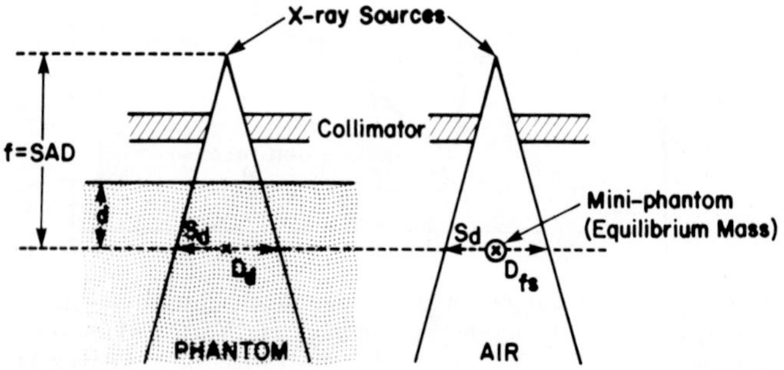

FIGURE 8–31. Schematic drawing illustrates the definition of the tissue-air ratio, in which d is the thickness of overlying material.

where D_{d_r} is the dose at a specified point on the central axis in a phantom with a fixed reference depth, d_r, of tissue-equivalent material overlying the point; D_d is the dose in phantom at the same spatial point as before but with an arbitrary depth, d, of overlying material; and S_d is the beam width at the level of measurement (Fig 8-33). In each instance, there is sufficient underlying material to provide for full backscatter. There is no general agreement about the magnitude of the reference depth to be used for this quantity, particularly for high energies. The TPR is intended to be analogous to the TAR but has an advantage because the reference dose, D_{d_r}, is directly measurable over the entire range of x-rays and τ-rays in use, eliminating problems in obtaining a value for the dose in free space when the depth for electronic buildup is great.

The TMR definition is similar to the definition of TPR, except that the reference depth, d_r, is just large enough to provide maximum dose buildup at that point.[16,31] However, the depth of maximum dose for megavoltage x-ray beams has been found to vary significantly with field size, and it is a function of skin-source distance. Thus, the definition of TMR creates a measurement problem because a variable d_r is required, and the TMR depends on skin-source distance.

Scatter-Air and Scatter-Maximum Ratios

The scatter-air ratio (SAR), the scatter component of the TAR, is defined as follows:[10]

$$SAR(d,S_d,E) = TAR(d,S_d,E) - TAR(d,O,E)$$

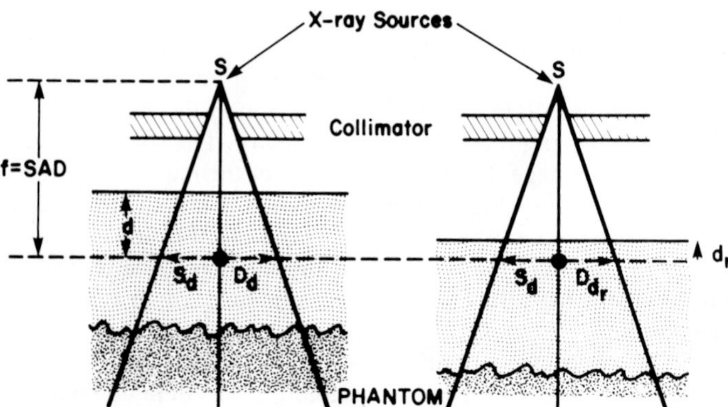

FIGURE 8–33. Schematic drawing illustrates the definition of the tissue-phantom ratio and tissue-maximum ratio, in which d is the thickness of overlying material and d_r is the reference thickness.

SAR is the difference between the TAR for a field of finite area and the TAR for a zero-area field size. The zero-area TAR is a mathematical abstraction obtained by extrapolation of the TAR values measured for finite field sizes.

Similarly, the scatter-maximum ratio (SMR), the scatter component of the TMR, is defined as follows:

$$SMR(d,S_d,E) = TMR(d,S_d,E) \cdot \frac{S_p(S_d,E)}{S_p(O,E)} - TMR(d,O,E)$$

where S_p is a phantom scatter correction factor, which takes into account changes in scatter radiation originating in the phantom at the reference depth as the field size is changed.[25]

Output Factor

For a given field size, the output factor is defined as the ratio of the dose rate at the depth of maximum dose for the given field size to that for the reference field size (usually 10 cm × 10 cm) at its d_{max}. The dose rate for that field is simply the output factor multiplied by the reference field dose rate.

The customary method for specifying output factors for rectangular x-ray fields is to determine an equivalent square field based on data published by the *British Journal of Radiology*[20] or on an area/perimeter calculation. However, for rectangular fields, the value of the output factor depends on the upper or lower collimator settings for the larger dimension. It has been suggested that accelerator users adopt the convention of setting the longer dimension for a rectangular field on one of the two collimators for all treatments, permitting an appropriate output factor to be selected without confusion.

Isodose Curve

An isodose curve represents points of equal dose. A set of these curves, normally given in 10% increments normalized to the dose at the reference depth, can be plotted on a chart (*i.e.*, isodose chart) to give a visual representation of the dose distribution in a single plane (Fig. 8-34). Beam parameters, such as source size, flattening filter, field size, and skin-source distance, play important roles in the shape of the isodose curve.

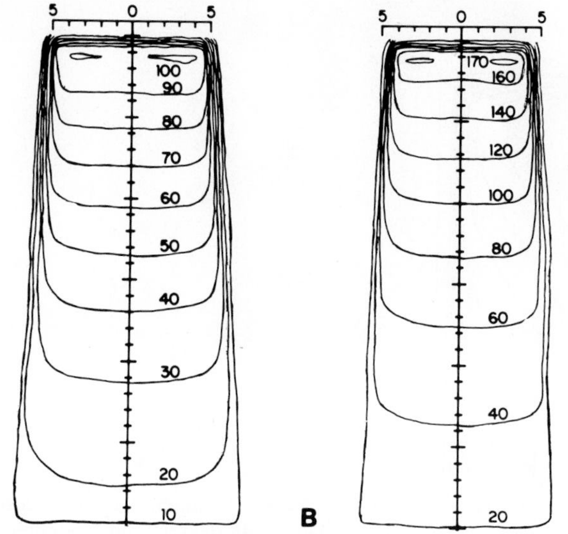

FIGURE 8–34. Example of an isodose chart for a 4-MV x-ray beam. (**A**) SSD type: 80-cm SSD, 10 cm × 10 cm at surface. (**B**) SAD type: 80-cm SAD, 10 cm × 10 cm at isocenter.

Isodose distributions are typically measured with ionization chambers in a water phantom under conditions of idealized geometry. Automated plotter systems are now commercially available.

Dose Profiles

A dose profile is a representation of the dose in an irradiated volume as a function of spatial position along a single line. Dose profiles are particularly well suited to the description of field flatness and penumbra. The data are typically given as ratios of doses normalized to the dose on the central axis (Fig. 8-35). The profiles, called off-axis factors or off-center ratios, may be measured in-air (*i.e.*, with only a buildup cap) or in a phantom at selected depths. The in-air off-axis factor gives only the variation in primary beam intensity; the in-phantom off-center ratio shows the added effect of phantom scatter.

Wedge Filter

Wedge filters are generally constructed of brass, steel, or lead, and when placed in the beam, they progressively decrease intensity across the field, causing the isodose distribution to have a planned asymmetry (Fig 8-36).

The *wedge angle* is defined as the angle the isodose curve subtends with a line perpendicular to the central axis at a specific depth and for a specified field size. Current practice is to use a depth of 10 cm. Past definitions were based on the 50th percentile isodose curve and, more recently, the 80th percentile isodose curve. The wedge angle is a function of field size and depth.

The *wedge factor* is defined as the ratio of the dose measured in a tissue-equivalent phantom at the depth of maximum buildup on the central axis with the wedge in place to the dose at the same point with the wedge removed.

Wedge isodose curves are generally normalized to the D_{max} dose of the unwedged beam, resulting in percentiles greater than 100% under the thin portion of the wedge. However, this normalization is not always used. The normalization and the use of the wedge factor should be clearly understood before they are used clinically.

Beam hardening occurs when a wedge is inserted into the radiation beam. The percentage depth dose, therefore, can be considerably increased at depth. Differences in percentage depth dose of nearly 7% have been reported for a 4-MV x-ray, 60-degree wedge field, compared with the open field at a depth of 12 cm, and there have been reports of as much as a 3% difference between the 60-degree wedge field and the open field for a 25-MV x-ray beam.[1,37]

METER SET AND DOSE CALCULATION TECHNIQUES

Meter set (timer or monitor unit) calculations and dose calculations to a point in a patient are performed using parameters such as output factor, percentage depth dose, and TAR. These parameters are usually measured in a water phantom for idealized geometries. Two situations, fixed skin-source distance and isocentric, are typically encountered in radiation therapy dose calculations.

For the fixed skin-source distance, the patient's skin is

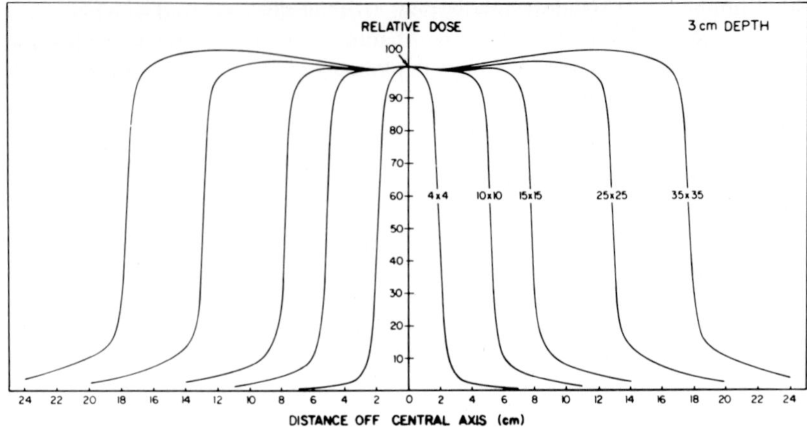

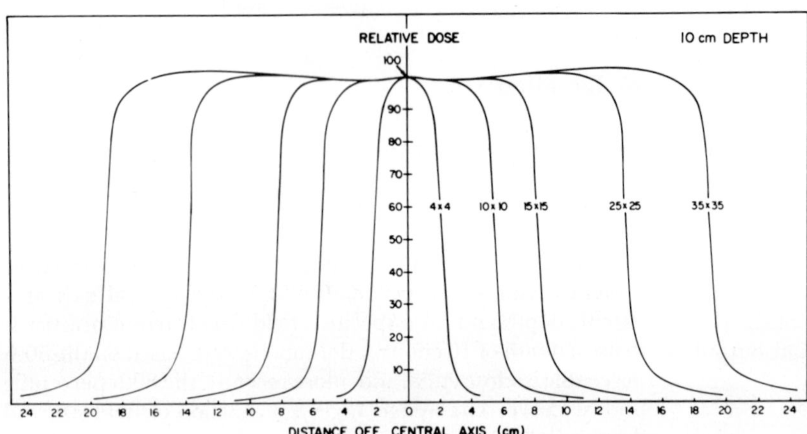

FIGURE 8–35. Example of dose profiles for a 25-MV linear accelerator x-ray beam measured at depths of 3 cm and 10 cm. (Redrawn from Purdy JA, Keys DJ, Abrath FG: Int J Radiat Oncol Biol Phys 4:337, 1978)

positioned at a fixed distance from the radiation source. The field size is defined at this fixed distance and a specified depth below the skin surface, usually representing the depth at which electronic equilibrium is established or at which the maximum dose occurs along the central ray. The relative dose at this point is assigned the value of 100%, and all other doses in the beam are referenced to it.[3,4]

Modern treatment machines are designed to rotate about a fixed point, the isocenter. The reference point for the isocenter is placed at a fixed distance from the source. The beam size is defined there, the relative dose at that point is assigned a 100% value, and all other dose values from the beam are referenced to that point.

The following sections provide guidelines for routine meter set and dose calculation to points in tissue for these two techniques, for rotation therapy, and for irregular fields.

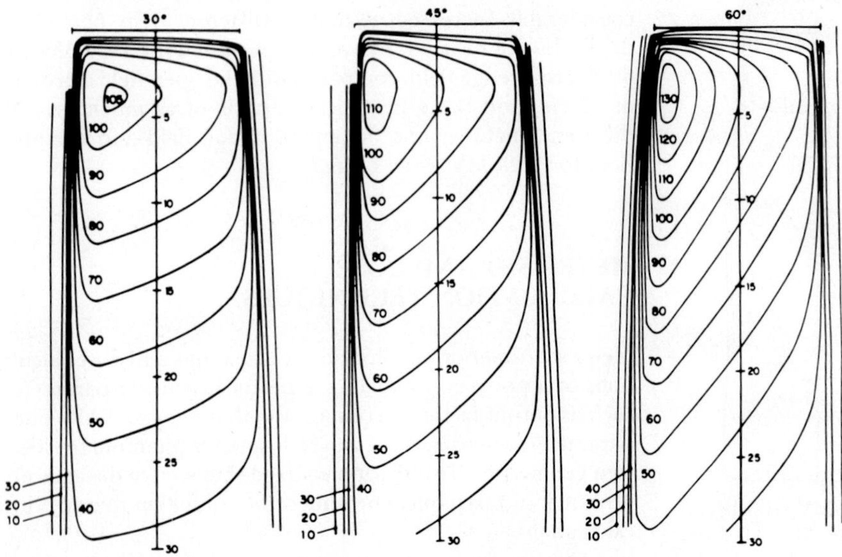

FIGURE 8–36. Example of wedge isodose curves for 30-degree, 45-degree, and 60-degree wedges for a 10 cm × 10 cm field. (Redrawn from Abrath FG, Purdy JA: Radiology 136:757, 1980)

Source-Skin Distance Technique

The timer or monitor setting (in monitor units or MU) to deliver a prescribed dose at some depth may be calculated as follows:

$$MU = \frac{TD \cdot 100}{PDD \cdot D_c \cdot I_{SSD} \cdot RPSF \cdot fsd_{air} \cdot f_{tray} \cdot f_{table} \cdot f_{wedge}}$$

and the dose at the depth of maximum dose, called the given dose (GD), is given by

$$GD = \frac{TD \cdot 100}{PDD}$$

where

MU = monitor units setting on machine console
TD = dose at depth d
GD = dose at reference depth (d_{max})
PDD = PDD for the equivalent square field size at the surface, for SSD used, and for depth d
D_c = dose rate in phantom at d_{max} for calibration field size (10 cm × 10 cm) and source-to-chamber distance

$$I_{SSD} \text{ (inverse square factor)} = \left(\frac{\text{source-to-chamber}}{\text{source-skin distance} + d_{max}}\right)^2$$

$$RPSF = \frac{\text{Peakscatter factor for equivalent square field at surface}}{\text{Peakscatter factor for 10 cm} \times \text{10 cm field}}$$

fsd_{air} = field size dependence factor in air (dose rate in air relative to that for 10 cm × 10 cm field; based on equivalent square of collimator setting)
f_{tray} = transmission factor for block support tray
f_{table} = transmission factor for treatment table
f_{wedge} = wedge factor for wedge on central ray

The equivalent square field at the surface for a blocked field requires an estimate of the effective field size. The equivalent square of the collimator setting may be obtained either from published data[20] or from the following equation:

$$S = \frac{2 \cdot L \cdot W}{L + W}$$

where L is field length and W is field width.

Isocentric Technique

The timer or monitor setting to deliver a prescribed dose at the isocenter may be calculated by the following expression:

$$MU = \frac{TD}{TPR \cdot D_c \cdot I_{SAD} \cdot RPSF \cdot fsd_{air} \cdot f_{tray} \cdot f_{table} \cdot f_{wedge}}$$

and the dose at any other depth d on the central axis by the following expression:

$$D(d) = TD \cdot \frac{TPR(d,S_d)}{TPR(d_I,S_I)} \cdot \left(\frac{SAD}{SAD - d_I + d}\right)^2 \cdot \frac{PSF(S_d)}{PSF(S_I)}$$

where the previously defined symbols have the same meaning and

TD = dose at isocenter with thickness d_I of tissue overlying
TPR = TPR for effective field size at isocenter
PSF = peakscatter factor

$$I_{SAD} \text{ (inverse square factor)} = \left(\frac{SCD}{SAD}\right)^2$$

Determination of S_I and S_d, the equivalent square field sizes at the isocenter and at the depth d for a blocked field needed to determine TPR, RPSF, and PSF, requires an estimate of the effective field size. For the purpose of determining fsd_{air}, the effective field size based on the collimator settings can be determined as before.

Rotation Technique

Calculations using monitor units for rotation therapy may be done using the following expression:

$$MU = \frac{TD}{TPR_{avg} \cdot D_c \cdot I_{SAD} \cdot RPSF \cdot fsd_{air} \cdot f_{tray} \cdot f_{table}}$$

and the monitor unit per degree setting is given by

$$MU/deg = \frac{\text{monitor unit setting}}{\text{degrees of rotation}}$$

where the symbols have the previous meanings and TPR_{avg} is average TPR (averaged over radii at intervals of not less than 20 degrees).

Irregular-Field Technique

For large, irregularly shaped fields and at points off the central axis, it is necessary to take account of the off-axis change in intensity (relative to the central axis) of the beam, the variation of the skin-source distance within the field of treatment, the influence of the primary collimator on the output factor, and the scatter contribution to the dose. Changes in the beam quality as a function of position in the radiation field should also be considered.[12,13]

The general method used for irregular-field calculations consists of summation at each point of interest of the primary and scatter irradiation, with allowance for the off-axis change in intensity (off-axis factor) and skin-source distance.[6] The absorbed dose at an arbitrary point in an irregular field (Fig. 8-37) is calculated as follows:[9]

$$D = D_{fs} \cdot fsd_{air} \cdot \left(\frac{SSD + d_{max}}{SSD + g + d}\right)^2 \cdot OAF \cdot [TAR(d,O) + \overline{SAR}(d)]$$

where

D = absorbed dose to an arbitrary point in the phantom
D_{fs} = absorbed dose in a small mass of tissue, in air, on the central axis at normal SSD + d_{max} for the calibration field size
fsd_{air} = field size dependence factor in air
SSD = nominal skin-source distance for treatment constraints
d_{max} = depth of dose maximum
g = vertical distance between skin surface over point in question and nominal SSD (beam vertical)
d = vertical depth, skin surface to point in question
OAF = in-air off-axis factor
TAR(d,O) = zero field size TAR at depth d
$\overline{SAR}(d)$ = average SAR for point in question at depth d, determined using the Clarkson technique

This method has come under scrutiny, and several modifications to the original method have been suggested. These include using the expanded field size at a depth for the SAR calculation; determining the off-axis factor using the distance

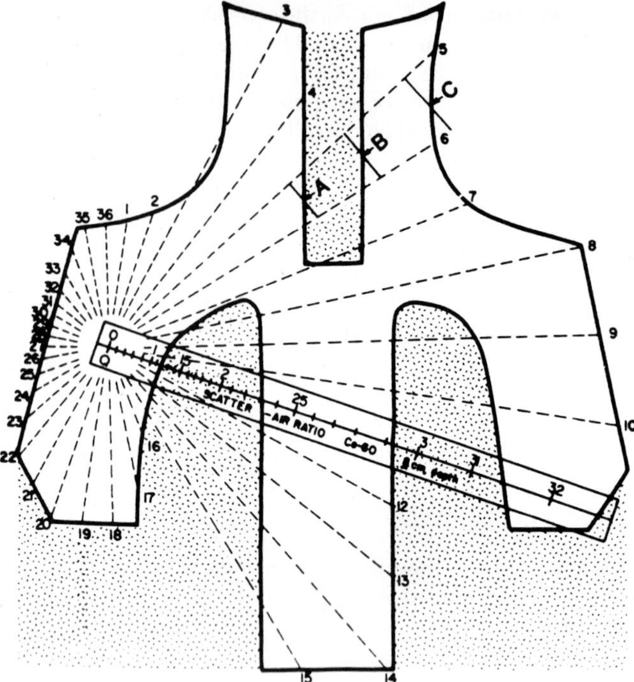

FIGURE 8–37. Outline of mantle field illustrates the method of determining scatter-to-air ratio used for irregular-field dose calculations. (Redrawn from Cundiff JH, Cunningham JR, Golden R, et al: Am J Roentgenol 117:30, 1973 © by American Roentgen Ray Society)

from the central axis to the slant projection of the point of calculation to the skin-source distance plane along a ray from the source; and determining the zero-area TAR using the slant depth along a ray going from the source to the point of calculation. It is generally accepted that the off-axis factor should be multiplied by the sum of the zero-area TAR and the SAR as originally proposed.

Beam quality is a function of position in the field for beams generated by linear accelerators.[12,13] The TAR_0 may be expressed as a function of position in the beam so that changes in beam quality can be incorporated into calculations, and it can be related to the half-value layer of water by the equation:

$$TAR(d,O,r) = e - \frac{0.693(d - d_{max})}{HVL(r)}$$

where d is the depth of the point of reference, d_{max} is the depth of maximum dose, r is the radial distance from the central axis of the beam to the point of calculation, e is the base of the natural logarithm, and HVL(r) is the beam quality expressed as the half-value layer measured in water.

One final point about irregular-field or off-axis dose calculations concerns the off-axis factor. In some computerized treatment planning systems, the calculation of dose to points off the central axis is based on the assumption that the off-axis factor can be represented by a separable function given by

$$OAF(x,y) = OAF(x,O) \cdot OAF(O,y)$$

where x and y are the symmetry axes perpendicular to the beam axis and the functions OAF(x,O) and OAF(O,y) are equal for a square open field. For some accelerator-generated beams, this assumption is invalid because measured values differ from those predicted by the above equation by as much as 20%.[26]

CORRECTION FOR AIR GAPS

Because basic dose distribution data are obtained for idealized geometries (*e.g.*, flat surface, unit density media), corrections are needed to determine the dose distribution in actual patients. Methods have been developed to account for the air gap caused by the patient's varying topography and for internal heterogeneities. In one approach, the dose data calculated for idealized geometry are multiplied by a correction factor to obtain the revised dose distribution.[18] The methods commonly used to correct for the air gap are discussed briefly in the next few sections.

Tissue-Air Ratio or Tissue-Phantom Ratio Method

In the TAR or TPR method, the surface (along a ray line) directly above point P is unaltered, so the primary dose distribution at this point is unchanged (Fig. 8-38). For relatively small changes in surface topography, the scatter component is essentially unchanged. Thus, the dose at point P can be considered as unaltered by patient shape. However, for points where there are considerable variations in the patient's topography, both the primary and scatter components of the radiation beam are altered. The correction factor (CF) may be determined using two TARs or TPRs:

$$CF = \frac{T(d - h, S_d)}{T(d, S_d)}$$

where h = air gap.

Effective Source-Skin Ratio Method

In the effective skin-source distance method, the isodose chart to be used is placed on the contour representation, positioning the central axis at the distance for which the curve was mea-

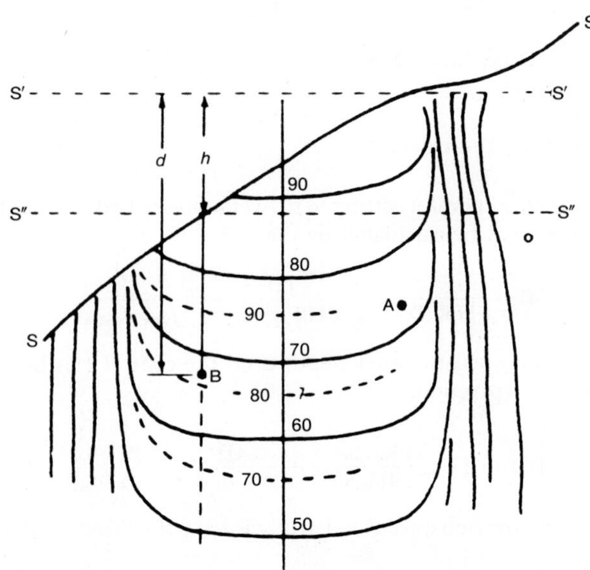

FIGURE 8–38. Schematic drawing illustrates the tissue-air ratio and effective SSD methods for the correction of isodose curves under a sloping surface. (Redrawn from International Commission of Radiation Units and Measurements: Report 24: Determination of absorbed dose in a patient irradiated by beams of x or gamma rays in radiotherapy procedures. Washington, ICRU, 1976)

sured (Fig. 8-38). It is then shifted down along the ray line for the length of the air gap, h. The percentage depth dose value at point P is read and modified by an inverse square calculation to account for the effective change in the peak dose. The CF can be expressed as follows:

$$CF = \frac{P(d - h, d_o, S, f, E)}{P(d, d_o, S, f, E)} \cdot \left(\frac{f + d_o}{f + h + d_o}\right)^2$$

Isodose Shift Method

Manual construction of an entire dose distribution for an actual patient with the previous methods would be time consuming. The isodose shift method (Fig. 8-39), although simplistic, is efficient and gives satisfactory results in most cases. In this method, the isodose chart is moved down along a diverging ray by a fractional amount of the air gap, h. The intersection of the isodose lines with this ray are read off directly. For ^{60}Co radiation, a shift of two thirds of h is used, and for 25-MV x-rays, a shift of one half of h is used.

CORRECTION FOR INHOMOGENEITIES

Patient tissues may differ from water by composition or density, which alters the dose distribution (Fig. 8-40). Four inhomogeneities are usually encountered: air cavities, lung, fat, and bone. To correct fully for these inhomogeneities, it is necessary to know their size, shape, and position and to specify their electron density and atomic number.[18,30] The correction methods for tissue inhomogeneities closely resemble the three methods discussed for correcting for patient topography and are described below.

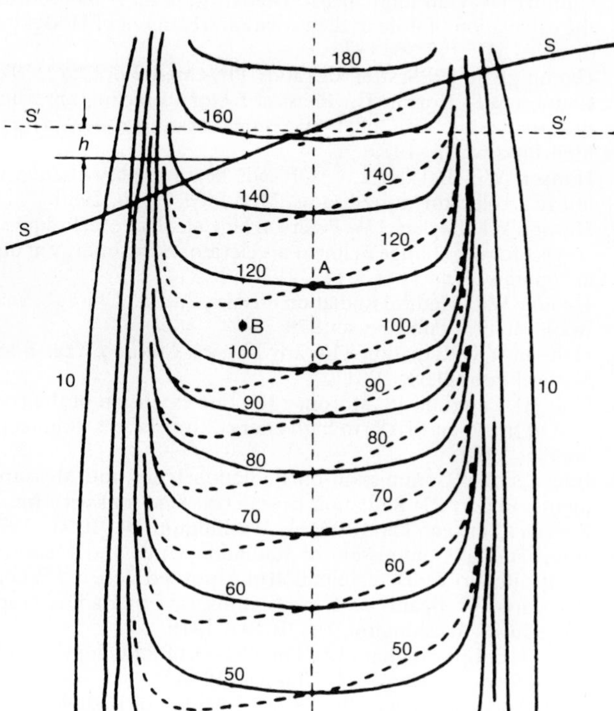

FIGURE 8–39. Schematic diagram illustrates the isodose shift method of correcting isodose curves under a sloping surface. (Redrawn from International Commission of Radiation Units and Measurements: Report 24: Determination of absorbed dose in a patient irradiated by beams of x gamma rays in radiotherapy procedures. Washington, ICRU, 1976)

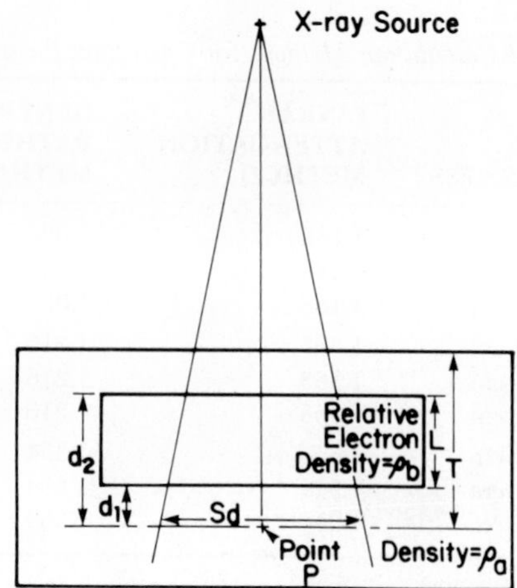

FIGURE 8–40. Schematic diagram showing inhomogeneity of relative density, ρ_b = 0.33, in a water-equivalent phantom. The thickness from the top surface of the phantom to the outermost (lateral) surface of the inhomogeneity is a constant equal to 3.0 cm. The alteration in dose to the inhomogeneity is to be calculated at point P. (Redrawn from Coffey CW, Hines HC: Am Assoc Med Dosimetr J 8:6, 1983)

Tissue-Air Ratio Method

The TAR method of correction for inhomogeneities uses the ratio of two TARs

$$CF = \frac{T(d_{eff}, S_d)}{T(d, S_d)}$$

where the numerator is the TAR for the equivalent water thickness, d_{eff}, and the denominator is the TAR for the actual thickness, d, of tissue between the point of calculation and the surface along a ray passing through the point. S_d is the dimension of the beam cross section at the depth of calculation. The TAR method accounts for the field size and depth of calculation. It does not account for the position of the point of calculation with respect to the heterogeneity. It also does not take into account the shape of the inhomogeneity, but rather assumes that it extends the full width of the beam and has a constant thickness (*i.e.*, a slab-type geometry).

Isodose Shift Method

Isodose lines are shifted by an amount equal to a constant times the thickness of the inhomogeneity as measured along a line parallel to the central axis and passing through the calculation point. Values for the shift constant empirically determined for ^{60}Co and 4-MV x-rays are −0.6 for air cavities, −0.4 for lung, 0.5 for hard bone, and 0.25 for spongy bone. The isodose curves are shifted away from the surface for lung and air cavities and toward the surface for bone.

Power Law Tissue-Air Ratio Method

The power law TAR method was proposed by Batho and generalized by Young and Gaylord.[2,43] This method attempts to

TABLE 8–2
Comparison of Calculation Methods for Correction for a Lung-like Inhomogeneity

LUNG THICKNESS		LINEAR ATTENUATION METHOD	GENERALIZED BATHO METHOD	TAR METHOD*	EFFECTIVE ATTENUATION METHOD	POWER LAW TAR METHOD	EQUIVALENT TAR METHOD†
	D_1 = 2 cm	1.188	1.069	1.189	1.122	1.139	7
5 cm	D_1 = 4 cm	1.188	1.069	1.200	1.137	1.166	2
	D_1 = 6 cm	1.188	1.069	1.203	1.153	1.186	8
	D_1 = 2 cm	1.363	1.216	1.378	1.273	1.309	7
9 cm	D_1 = 4 cm	1.363	1.216	1.390	1.292	1.346	6
	D_1 = 6 cm	1.363	1.216	1.392	1.310	1.373	5
	D_1 = 2 cm	1.511	1.354	1.547	1.406	1.460	5
12 cm	D_1 = 4 cm	1.511	1.354	1.552	1.425	1.506	7
	D_1 = 6 cm	1.511	1.354	1.558	1.444	1.536	0

** TAR, tissue-air ratio.*
† Computer-generated inhomogeneity correction algorithm, AECL Theraplan system.
(Coffey CW, Hines HC: Am Assoc Med Dosimetrists J 8:6, 1983)

account for the nature of the inhomogeneity and its position relative to the point of calculation. However, it does not account for the extent or shape of the inhomogeneity. The correction factor for the point P is given by

$$CF = \left(\frac{T(d_2,S_d)}{T(d_1,S_d)}\right)^{\rho_2 - 1}$$

where d_1 and d_2 refer to the distances from point P to the near and far sides of the non-water-equivalent material, respectively; S_d is the beam dimension at the depth of P; and ρ_2 is the relative electron density of the inhomogeneity with respect to water.

Sontag and Cunningham derived a more general form of this correction factor, which can be applied to a case in which the effective atomic number of the inhomogeneity is different from that of water and the point of interest lies within the inhomogeneity.[38] The correction factor in this situation is given by

$$CF = \frac{T(d_2,S_d)^{(\rho_b - 1)}}{T(d_1,S_d)^{(\rho_b - \rho_a)}} \cdot \frac{(\mu_{en}/\rho)_a}{(\mu_{en}/\rho)_b}$$

where ρ_a is the density of the material in which point P lies at a depth d below the surface and ρ_b is the density of an overlying material of thickness (d_2-d_1); μ_{en}/ρ_a and μ_{en}/ρ_b are the mass energy absorption coefficients for the media a and b.

Experimentally determined correction factors derived by the various correction methods are compared in Table 8-2.[7]

At an interface between two materials of different composition, there is a loss of equilibrium as a result of changes in the electron fluence, that is, the number of electrons generated from the photon interactions. Therefore, the dose over a distance comparable to the range of the electrons is perturbed. For ^{60}Co radiation, the alteration in the dose distribution occurs in only the few millimeters surrounding the interface. However, for high-energy photon beams, the region extends for several centimeters. As yet, no practical method of dose calculation accounts for this effect.[30]

REFERENCES

1. Abrath FG, Purdy JA: Wedge design and dosimetry for 25 MV x-rays. Radiology 136:757, 1980
2. Batho HF: Lung corrections in cobalt 60 beam therapy. J Can Assoc Radiol 15:79, 1964
3. Bentel GC, Nelson CE, Noell KT: Treatment Planning and Dose Calculation in Radiation Oncology, 3rd ed. New York, Pergamon Press, 1982
4. Bleehen NM, Glatstein E, Haybittle JL (eds): Radiation Therapy Planning. New York, Marcel Dekker, 1983
5. Bomford CK, Craig LM, Hanna FA, et al: Treatment Simulators, Special Report No. 10. London, British Institute of Radiology, 1976
6. Clarkson JR: A note on depth doses in fields of irregular shape. Br J Radiol 14:265, 1941
7. Coffey CW, Hines HC: Inhomogeneity corrections in treatment planning of the thorax. American Association of Medical Dosimetrists Journal 8:6, 1983
8. Cohen M, Jones DEA, Greene D: Central axis depth dose data for use in radiotherapy. Br J Radiol [Suppl] 11:1, 1972
9. Cundiff JH, Cunningham JR, Golden R, et al: A method for the calculation of dose in the radiation treatment of Hodgkin's disease. AJR 117:30, 1973
10. Cunningham JR: Scatter-air ratios. Phys Med Biol 17:42, 1972
11. Gagnon WF, Horton JL: Physical factors affecting absorbed dose to the skin from cobalt-60 gamma rays and 25 MeV x-rays. Med Phys 6:285, 1979
12. Hanson WF, Berkley LW: Off-axis beam quality change in linear accelerator x-ray beams. Med Phys 7:145, 1980
13. Hanson WF, Berkley LW, Peterson M: Calculative technique to correct for the change in linear accelerator beam energy at off-axis points. Med Phys 7:147, 1980
14. Hendee WR: Medical Radiation Physics, 2nd ed. Chicago, Year Book Medical Publishers, 1979
15. Hendee WR: Radiation Therapy Physics. Chicago, Year Book Medical Publishers, 1981
16. Holt JD, Laughlin JS, Moroney JP: The extension of the concept of tissue-air (TAR) to high energy x-ray beams. Radiology 96:437, 1970
17. International Commission on Radiation Units and Measurements: Report 21: Radiation Dosimetry: Electrons with Initial Energies Between 1 and 50 MeV. Washington, DC, ICRU, 1972
18. International Commission of Radiation Units and Measurements: Report 24: Determination of Absorbed Dose in a Patient Irradiated by Beams of X or Gamma rays in Radiotherapy Procedures. Washington, DC, ICRU, 1976
19. Johns HE, Cunningham JR: The Physics of Radiology, 4th ed. Springfield, IL, Charles C Thomas, 1983
20. Joint Working Party of the British Institute of Radiology and the Hospital Physicists' Association: Central axis depth dose data for use in radiotherapy. Br J Radiol [Suppl] 17:1, 1983
21. Karzmark CJ, Deubert A, Loevinger R: Tissue-phantom ratios: An aid to treatment planning. Br J Radiol 38:185, 1965
22. Karzmark CJ, Morton RJ: A Primer on Theory and Operation of Linear Accelerators in Radiation Therapy. Rockville, MD, Bureau of Radiological Health, U.S. Department of Health and Human Services, 1981

23. Karzmark CJ, Pering NC: Electron linear accelerators for radiation therapy: History, principles and contemporary developments. Phys Med Biol 18:321, 1973
24. Kerst DW: The betatron. Radiology 40:115, 1943
25. Khan FM: The Physics of Radiation Therapy, p. 294. Baltimore, Williams & Wilkins, 1984
26. Lam WC, Lam KS: Errors in off-axis treatment planning for a 4 MeV machine. Med Phys 10:480, 1983
27. Mayneord WV: The measurement of radiation for medical purposes. Nature 149:600, 1942
28. Megavoltage Radiation Therapy Equipment: A source document for the February 1981 blue book on criteria for radiation oncology in multidisciplinary cancer management. Philadelphia, American College of Radiology, 1983
29. Miller CW: Travelling-wave linear accelerator for x-ray therapy. Nature 171:297, 1953
30. Orton CG: Progress in Medical Radiation Physics, vol 1. New York, Plenum Press, 1982
31. Purdy JA: Relationship between tissue-phantom ratio and percentage depth dose. Med Phys 4:66, 1977
32. Purdy JA: The application of high energy x-rays and electron beams in radiotherapy. IEEE Trans Nucl Sci 26:1833, 1979
33. Purdy JA, Goer DA: Dual energy x-ray beam accelerators in radiation therapy: An overview. Nucl Inst Method Phys Res 10/11:1090, 1985
34. Purdy JA, Keys DJ, Abrath FG: 25 MV x-ray beam characteristics from a 35 MeV linear accelerator. Int J Radiat Oncol Biol Phys 4:337, 1978
35. Reistad D, Brahme A: The microtron, a new accelerator for radiation therapy. In Digest of the Third International Conference of Medical Physics. Gotenborg, Sweden, Third ICMP Executive Committee, Chalmers University of Technology, 1972
36. Scientific Sub-committee of the Hospital Physicists' Association: Depth dose tables for use in radiotherapy. Br J Radiol [Suppl] 10:1, 1961
37. Sewchand W, Khan FM, Williamson J: Radiation in depth dose data between open and wedged fields 4 MV x-rays. Radiology 127:789, 1978
38. Sontag MR, Cunningham JR: Corrections to absorbed dose calculations for tissue inhomogeneities. Med Phys 4:431, 1977
39. Task Group 21, Radiation Therapy Committee, American Association of Physicists in Medicine: A protocol for the determination of absorbed dose from high-energy photon and electron beams. Med Phys 10:741, 1983
40. Veksler VJ: A new method for acceleration of relativistic particles. Dokl Akad Nauk SSSR 43:329, 1944
41. Velkley DE, Manson DJ, Purdy JA, et al: Build-up region of megavoltage photon radiation sources. Med Phys 2:14, 1975
42. Velkley DE, Purdy JA: Variation in depth of maximum dose of megavoltage photon beams. Appl Radiol, January/February, 1980
43. Young MEJ, Gaylord JD: Experimental tests of corrections for tissue inhomogeneities in radiotherapy. Br J Radiol 43:349, 1970

9

○ ○ ○ ∘ • ∘

External Beam Dosimetry and Treatment Planning

Glenn P. Glasgow
James A. Purdy

We can describe the dose distribution from radiation beams of γ-rays, x-rays, electrons, or mixtures of these impinging on regularly shaped, homogeneous, tissue-equivalent phantoms. However, the patient presents an irregularly shaped topography containing many tissues and heterogeneities, and the radiation beams must often be modified to achieve the desired dose distribution.

Although the *plan of therapy* properly refers to all aspects of the patient's treatment course (*e.g.*, surgery, chemotherapy, radiation therapy), the term *treatment planning* in radiation therapy is synonymous with selecting the target dose prescription, daily dose, fractionation schedule, and arrangement of the radiation beams to achieve the desired dose distribution in a target volume. The radiation beams selected and their arrangement depend on the location and three-dimensional shape of the target volume, which consists of the tumor volume with adequate margins.

Several questions arise in treatment planning. Are there critical structures in or near the target volume that require shielding? Are there heterogeneities in the tissue that will alter the dose distribution? Moreover, what technical capabilities are available to the radiation oncologist to achieve an optimal dose distribution? The selection of a particular treatment technique is dictated by the armamentarium available in the treatment facility.

Delineation of the patient's geometry and composition, the target volume, and the critical radiation-sensitive organs in and near this volume constitutes the important initial steps in treatment planning. Additional considerations include the simulation of treatment fields, appropriate positioning of the patient, selection and preparation of patient positioning and immobilization devices, selection of radiation field shapes and beam entry and exit points to encompass the target volume, preparation of organ shielding blocks, measurements of patient topography and anatomic thicknesses, and decisions about the necessity of beam modifiers (*e.g.*, wedges and missing-tissue compensators) and the desirability of heterogeneity corrections.

The dose prescription and isodose computations to determine the suitability of the plan of therapy are the final steps of this process. Ideally, verification of the selected treatment method on the simulator, using all treatment aids, reveals any deficiencies in the proposed plan of therapy and allows modifications before therapy is begun.

In this chapter, we consider most of the factors influencing treatment planning and external beam dosimetry. For those desiring additional material, the references list four excellent monographs on treatment planning in radiation oncology.[5,9,97,142]

TREATMENT SIMULATION

Target Volume Localization

To complement physical examinations, the radiation oncologist has access to a host of imaging modalities for target volume localization. The classic techniques of radiography and fluoroscopy, combined in a radiation therapy simulator that mimics the geometries of actual therapy units, may be augmented with computed tomography (CT), nuclear medicine scanning, sonography, magnetic resonance (MR) imaging, and CT simulators.

Day and Harrison[27] review the historic development of the radiation therapy simulator; Doppke compares the salient features of eight commercial units.[33] The modern simulator mimics the functions and allowed motions of a therapy unit (Fig. 9-1). Gantry arms are rigid enough to support heavy shielding blocks and simulated electron cones; couch widths are similar to therapy unit couch widths; and operating consoles feature digital displays of parameters and programmable settings for source-axis distance, gantry angles, and field sizes. Some units feature automatic exposure control for improved radiographic techniques.

Through traditional radiography (or fluoroscopy) methods using radiopaque rulers placed or projected on the patient's surface, dimensions of treatment areas on films are ascertained, and target volumes are selected. Bentel and colleagues[5] provide excellent site-specific examples of simulation procedures. A radiation therapy simulator is necessary in any facility using state-of-the-art methods of radiation therapy. Simulators are cost effective and allow more efficient use of the therapy units for actual treatment of patients.[94] A special report by the British Institute of Radiology concluded that two simula-

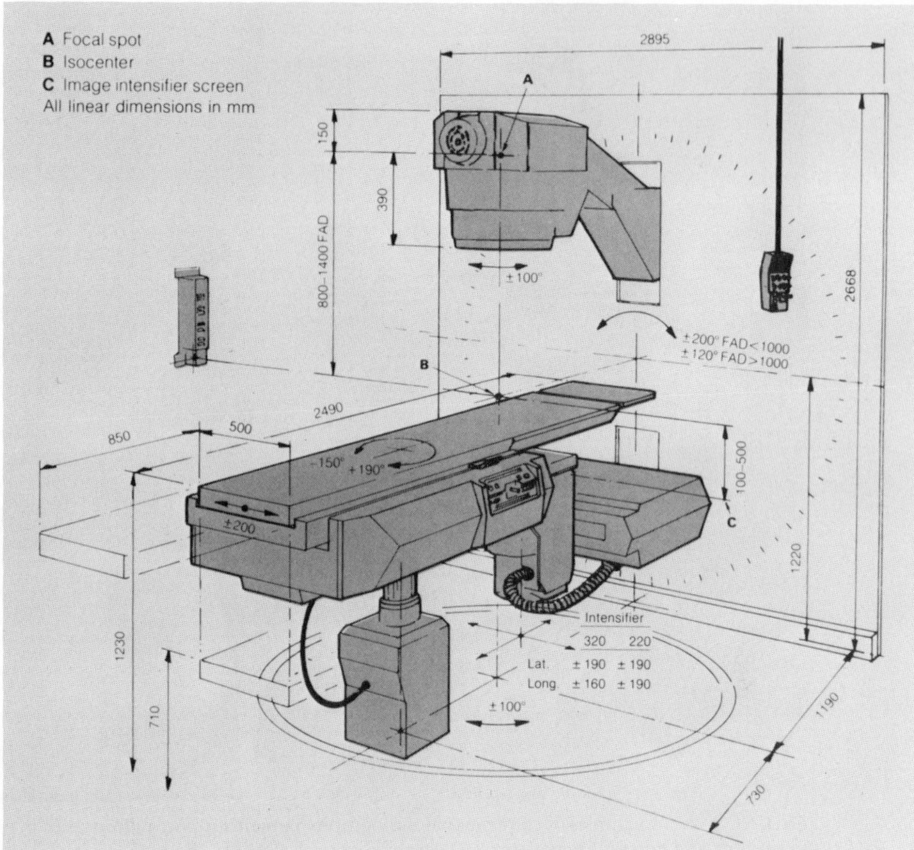

FIGURE 9–1. Basic features of a radiation therapy treatment simulator. (Courtesy of Varian Associates, Palo Alto, CA)

tors can support about five therapy units and allow the therapy units to be used fully for patient treatment.[11]

Multiple off-axis CT images can be obtained, and the target area, critical organs, and heterogeneities can be defined in each plane.[85] Conventional transverse CT images are now supplemented with sagittal or other desired planes reconstructed from the transverse scans. The CT numbers are correlated with the electron densities of the tissues imaged and used for calculating the dose, accounting for heterogeneities. For CT scans used in treatment planning, the patient's position should be identical to the position to be used during radiation therapy. Numerous studies have documented the improvements in target volume localization and dose distributions achieved with the anatomic data obtained from CT scans.[112]

A CT unit with many of the features of a radiation therapy simulator features beam's eye view display, which allows the anatomy to be viewed from the perspective of the radiation beam, allows field shaping electronically at the graphics display station, and allows computer-controlled marking of treatment fields on the patient's skin surface.[49] Dedicated CT simulators integrate a CT scanner designed for radiation therapy with a radiation therapy planning computer and many other advanced image manipulation and viewing advantages.[50,123] Current CT simulators do not allow verification of the actual shielding blocks, an important process in conventional simulation.

Patient Positioning

During tumor localization, the desired position of the patient must be considered relative to the incident beams and the patient's ability to reproduce this position throughout the radiation therapy course. Factors affecting daily positioning of a patient include the patient's age, general health, weight, and anatomic site under treatment; obese patients and small children are the most difficult to position. Haus and Marks[62] observed that about a third of the localization errors achieved treating mantle and pelvic portals were caused by patient movement. Although modern imaging technologies allow the radiation oncologist millimeter precision in tumor localization and target volume definition, the daily positioning of the patient usually depends on less accurate visual alignment techniques, precise to only several millimeters. More accurate and precise positioning is achievable with casting and immobilization techniques, but these methods are relatively expensive, prolong simulation, and usually are employed only for the most difficult cases.

The common devices used to position a patient are the treatment machine field localization light and distance indicator and the lateral and overhead laser alignment lights, which provide transverse, coronal, and sagittal light lines on the patient. Visible skin marks, skin marks visible only under an ultraviolet light, India-ink tattoos, and plastic shells are used for field delineation by most radiation oncologists.[136] A host of positioning pillows and supports are available (Fig. 9-2). These are designed for irradiation of specific anatomic sites and can be used, often with restraining straps, to achieve immobilization during radiation therapy.

Complex positioning methods, such as video subtraction methods and tapes that reflect laser lights, have not gained widespread use because they add expense without proven value and are impractical.

Although all of these devices assist in the daily alignment and immobilization of the patient, they do not permanently register the patient's initial treatment position for subsequent treatments.

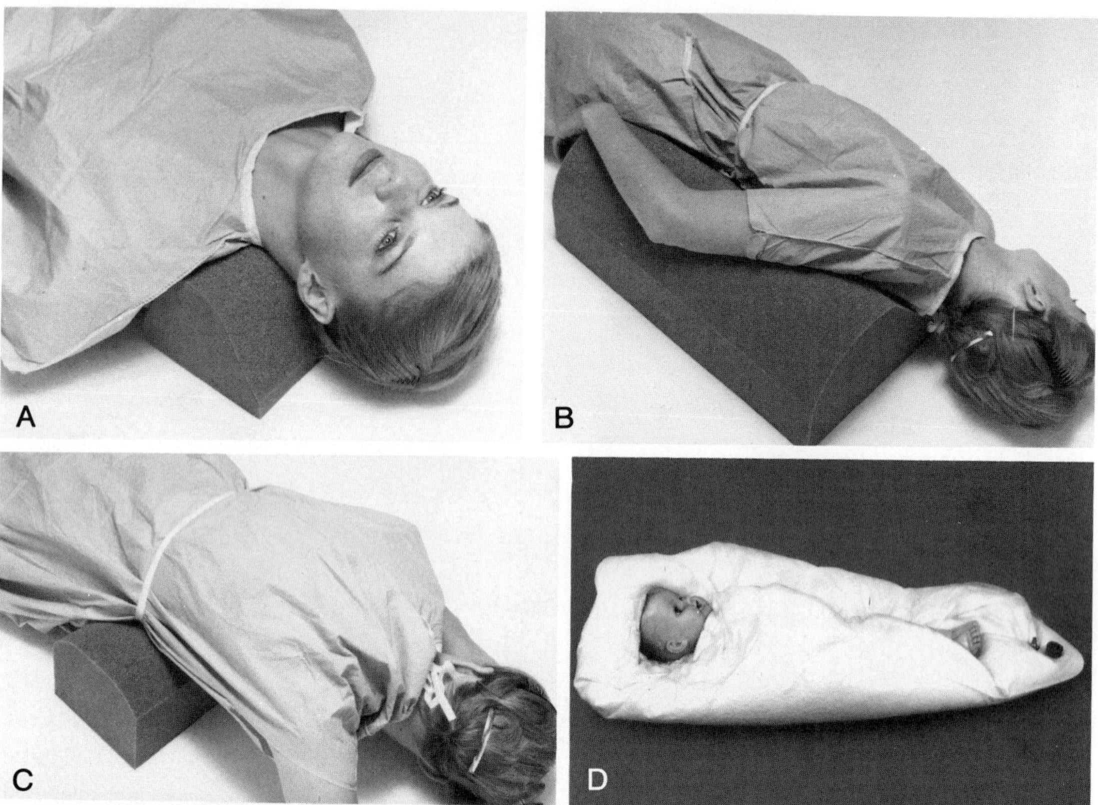

FIGURE 9–2. Examples of conventional radiography patient support pillows used in radiation therapy to support and immobilize patients. (**A**) A head and neck support. (**B**) A 45-degree oblique spinal wedge. (**C**) A bolster. (Courtesy of Contour Fabricators, Inc., Grand Blanc, MI) (**D**) A vacuum device that molds Styrofoam beads around the child. (Courtesy of Nuclear Associates, Inc., Carlyle, NY)

Patient Registration and Immobilization

Some devices are designed to register an initial treatment position to which the patient is returned daily. Many systems have been designed for the head, an anatomic site most difficult to position.[89,101,131] A "lollipop," a bite-block on a stick, is widely used (Fig. 9-3). Once in the treatment position, the patient bites into a prepared impression material (*e.g.*, dental impression compounds) on a fork attached to a supporting device. When the material hardens, it records an impression of the teeth. This bite-block is mounted on an identical support device on the therapy unit and may be used with or without recording scales to identify treatment positions.

Molding techniques may be divided into those that require a cast of the anatomic site to be immobilized and those that use materials that can be formed directly over and around the site without the preparation of a cast. The former include traditional plaster casting techniques, impression compounds (*e.g.*, Jeltrate Plus Type 1 Fast Set), and transparent plastic shells formed over a cast with a vacuum device.[30] Watkins[136,137] gives excellent descriptions of both methods. Plastic shells filled with tissue-equivalent materials can be used to confirm the patient's dosimetry. Shell techniques use thermal plastics that, after being placed in warm water and draped over the site, harden as they cool.[51,96] Polyurethane foams that harden after chemical mixing in a frame surrounding the site are widely used.[96] Vacuum-formed molds for adults are available. The preferences of therapists and technologists influence the acceptance and use of registration and immobilization devices, although cost and ease of preparation are probably the major considerations.

Beam Direction and Shape

The selection of radiation beams, their entry and exit points on the patient, and their shapes in the planes perpendicular and parallel to their incident direction is the crucial step in treatment simulation.

Beam direction on conventional simulators and therapy units is determined by an optical system that projects a light field and cross hair onto the skin surface to indicate the entry point of the beam. The distance to the skin surface is measured with an *optical distance indicator*; mechanical distance indicators are usually reserved for confirming the accuracy of the optical distance indicator. *Beam edges* are outlined with radiopaque markers. Lead beads or wires that project 1 cm apart at 100 cm, with every fifth centimeter marked, are useful on simulation localization radiographs for direct field size measurements and on therapy units.[132] Laser light and back pointers are commonly available to identify the *beam exit point.*

The most common form of *beam modification* is field shaping the beam transversely in the plane at 90 degrees with respect to the direction of the beam. The fixed circular, square, and rectangular cones commonly found on orthovoltage units were replaced on cobalt units and linear accelerators (linacs) by paired variable collimators that move symmetrically toward or

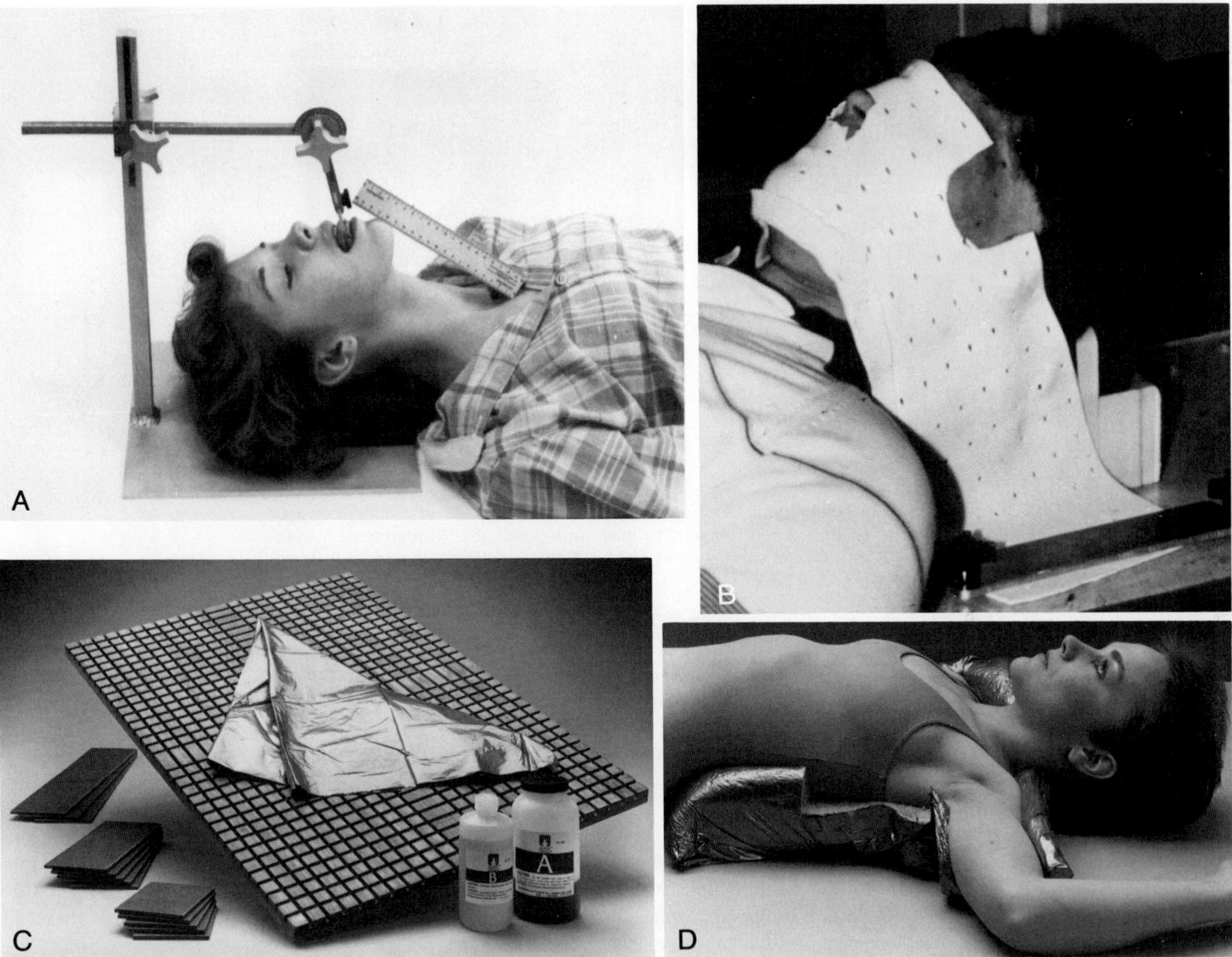

FIGURE 9–3. Examples of registration and immobilization systems for the head. (**A**) Bite block or "lollipop" system. (Courtesy of Radiation Products Design, Inc., Buffalo, MN) (**B**) Thermal plastic. (Courtesy of WFR/Aquaplast Corporation, Ramsey, NJ) (**C**) Complete Alpha Cradle mold-maker kit used for patient repositioning: foaming agents, bag, board, and dividers for constructing device. (Courtesy of Smithers Medical Products, Hudson, OH) (**D**) Example of patient in Alpha Cradle repositioning device. Cutouts allow clear access to the treatment area. (Courtesy of Smithers Medical Products, Hudson, OH)

away from the central axis of the beam. Some modern linacs now allow one pair or both pairs of opposing collimators to operate independently, which permits rectangular fields to be formed off the central axis (Fig. 9-4) and allows primary collimator shielding at midfield and beyond.[76,78,88]

Multivaned collimators that allow true transverse field shaping without adding secondary blocking systems are an expensive option. They are currently being offered on some medical accelerators and may be the collimation method of all linacs by 2000.[14,74] They also allow dynamic conformational therapy[128] (*e.g.*, changes of field shape *during* therapy, often while the gantry rotates). This conformational radiation therapy is ideal for implementing three-dimensional treatment planning.[129]

Secondary beam shaping blocks made from lead sheets or bricks, lead shot in a mold, or low-melting-point bismuth alloys are placed beneath the primary collimators.[79,90,110] Component steps of the procedure are shown in Figure 9-5.[115] Using a radiograph from the simulator, the radiation oncologist outlines the transverse field dimensions of the treatment volume on a film. The film is placed on a view box, and a heated wire cuts the desired shape out of a foam block above the view box to form a mold into which the shielding material is placed. The latest technology allows the desired field shape to be digitized from a film or other computer hard copy into a computer, which operates a numerically controlled milling machine or wire cutter that produces the desired mold. Low-melting-point bismuth alloys currently are the most popular materials for secondary collimation for both x-ray and electron beams.[68,115] After solidification, the completed-block edges are smoothed; the block is mounted on a tray that can be attached beneath the primary collimators of the simulator and therapy unit. After the patient's therapy course is completed, the block is melted for reuse. The bismuth alloys offer greater safety to personnel than similar systems using molten lead.[29,57]

Pseudoblocks constructed from thin lead or foam with the field edges coated with a radiopaque substance and identical in shape to transverse field shaping blocks may be attached di-

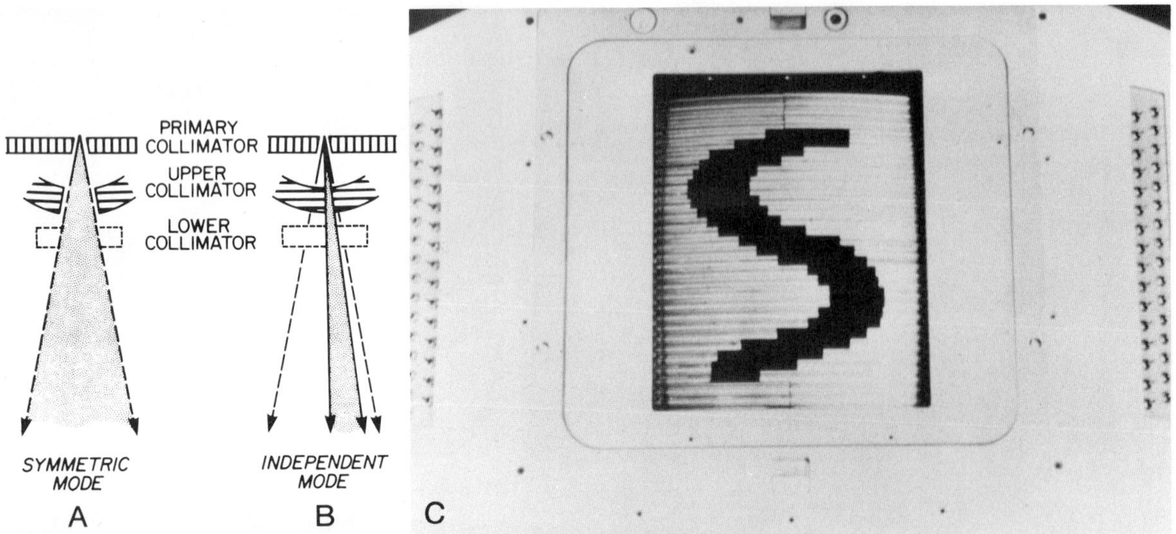

FIGURE 9–4. Methods of beam collimation. (**A**) Conventional symmetric pairs of collimators. (**B**) Symmetric collimators with one collimator pair allowed to move independently. (Courtesy of Varian Associates, Palo Alto, CA) (**C**) A multivaned collimator assembly. (Courtesy of Scanditronix AB, Husbyborg, Uppsala, Sweden)

rectly to the simulator for verification of the desired field shape, if the simulator does not tolerate the weight of the actual treatment blocks.[105]

Topography and Anatomic Measurements

During measurements of topography and anatomic thickness, the patient should be in the desired treatment position, because the patient's position alters the thickness of some anatomic regions. Plaster cast strips, lead (solder) wire, flexible curves, or other devices, combined with anatomic thickness measurements using calipers, are common methods of measuring topography.[27,126,139] Normally, the shape registration device is placed over the anatomic region and transferred to graph paper, onto which the shape is traced. Optical techniques for external topography include stereo shift film, Moire pattern images, and numerous methods employing projected lines or dot patterns recorded by a video camera.[52,126] Newer manual methods include sonic digitizers and a magnetic stylus that traces over the patient to obtain the contour.[3,13,125] Anatomic thicknesses measured are also recorded on the diagram, and the entry and exit points of the beams and their field edges are marked for isodose computations. The outline of the tumor, target volume, and internal organs of interest are added to the diagram from information obtained from orthogonal films, CT scans, and other imaging modalities or from anatomic atlases if other means are not available.

Employing the power of computer work stations and images available from the CT or MR scans, the radiation oncologist can delineate internal and external contours. *Automatic contouring* uses edge detection differences in CT numbers to distinguish tissue or bone from air volumes. Anatomic thickness is obtained from the images. From these procedures, the radia-

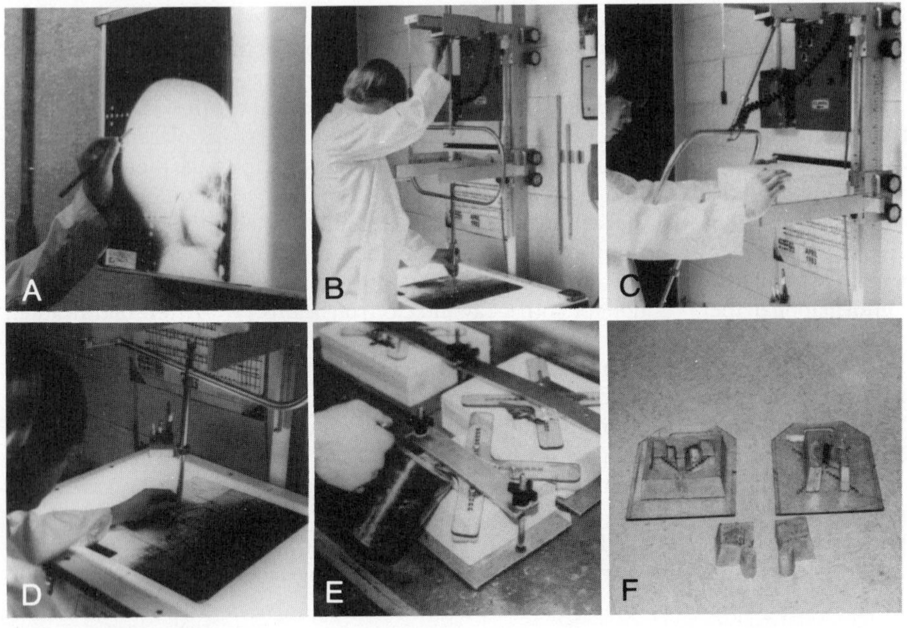

FIGURE 9–5. (**A**) Physician defining the treatment volume on the x-ray simulator radiograph. (**B**) Physics technician adjusting the source-skin distance and skin-film distance of a hot-wire cutter to emulate simulator geometry. (**C**) Proper-thickness foam block aligned to the central axis of the cutter. (**D**) Foam mold cut with hot-wire cutter. (**E**) Foam pieces aligned and held in place using a special clamping device. Molten alloy is poured into the mold and allowed to harden. (**F**) Examples of typical shielding blocks cast using this system.

tion oncologist determines the external topography; tumor, target, treatment, and irradiated volumes; critical organs; and heterogeneities in all three dimensions of the patient.

Nomenclature

The International Commission on Radiation Units and Measurements has recommended definitions of important concepts in treatment planning.[70] The *tumor volume* refers to the actual physical dimensions of the tumor and includes regions of presumed occult spread. *Target volume,* defined arbitrarily by the radiation oncologist, represents the tumor volume, including potential areas of local and regional spread, and *a margin* of surrounding normal tissue, to allow for patient movement and positioning errors (Fig. 9-6). This target volume is to be irradiated to a specified *absorbed dose* in a specified time-dose pattern.[70]

Dose Prescriptions

Methods of dose prescription and dose calculation include specifying the dose at the point in the volume where the central axes of multiple beams intersect, the minimum target absorbed dose in the volume, the maximum target absorbed dose in the volume, the modal target absorbed dose or most frequently occurring dose in the volume, the median target absorbed dose, the average dose, and the dose assigned to the highest-value isodose curves that totally encompass the target volume.[70]

The range of doses within a target volume is determined by the *maximum target absorbed dose* and *minimum target absorbed dose* within the target volume; in a two-dimensional display of isodose curves on a conventional anatomic cross-section, it is conventional to consider the absorbed dose per unit area within the target area (Fig. 9-7).

The *median target absorbed dose* is a dose in which one half of the target volume (area) contains a dose greater than the median, while the other half of the target volume (area) contains a dose less than the median. The most frequently occurring dose, the *modal target absorbed dose,* covers the greatest volume (area), and the *average target absorbed dose,* obtained by averaging all doses within some selected volume (area) dimension over the target volume (area), can also be calculated. For comparing alternate methods of treatments, Ellis and Oliver[41] introduced the parameters of *local efficiency factor* and *nonuniformity factor.*

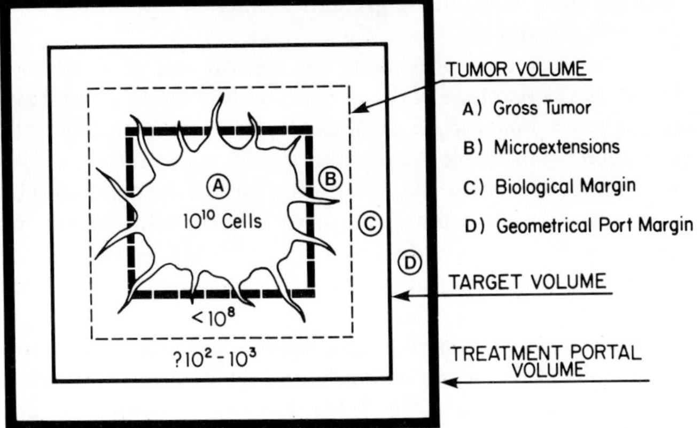

FIGURE 9–6. A schematic representation of the tumor volume and target volume. The treatment volume includes the tumor volume, potential areas of local and regional microscopic disease around the tumor, and a margin of surrounding normal tissue.

These parameters were successfully used in the EXTREP software developed at Memorial Hospital in New York, and they were used for comparing isodose distributions with and without the benefit of CT scans (Fig. 9-7C).[73] The optimal plan with lung corrections has a higher local efficiency factor and lower nonuniformity factor than the other two treatment plans. An ideal local efficiency factor is unity (*i.e.,* a completely uniform dose to the tumor with no dose to surrounding normal tissue); most treatment plans have a local efficiency factor of 20% to 50%.

Generally, it is desirable to have a uniform dose within the target volume, with the ratio of maximum target dose to minimal target dose not exceeding 1.10, a dose variation within the target volume of 10% or less. Three-dimensional treatment plans (Fig. 9-8A) may be evaluated using *dose volume histograms* (Fig. 9-8B). Dose volume histograms simplify comparing the wealth of dosimetry exhibited in a three-dimensional dose display.[95] However, they fail to identify the location of the volume receiving the dose and thus only complement spatial dose distributions.

A common method of dose prescription specifies the dose at some depth in the patient (*e.g.,* target depth, midplane depth, or depth determined by a common intersection point of multiple fields). Normally, the dose at the depth of maximum dose, frequently called the *given dose,* is recorded for each radiation beam because this dose is associated with subcutaneous tissue tolerance. For parallel opposed or other multiple-beam techniques, the total dose at the point of maximum dose (d_{max}) on the exiting side is frequently recorded, including contributions from all beams, to confirm that the total subcutaneous tissue dose is within accepted tolerances. With high-energy electron beams, it may be necessary to distinguish between the true dose on the skin and the dose at d_{max} in the buildup region.

A proper dose prescription states the total absorbed dose, daily total dose, fractionation schedule, and where and how the dose is prescribed, so that ambiguities are avoided. The *dose medium* must be identified (*e.g.,* 5000 cGy *in tissue,* 2500 cGy *in bone*) because *absorbed dose* is medium-specific by definition.

A clear statement of the dose to critical organs and the fraction or volume of a critical organ receiving a specified dose is required. Dose prescriptions must be unambiguous; misunderstanding about whether a prescribed tumor dose is a *point dose* at some convenient point within the target volume or is the *dose to an isodose curve* (*e.g.,* 90%) encompassing the target volume can lead to undertreatment of tumor at the edges of the target volume or overdosing of normal tissues within the target volume, with subsequent complications.

Excellent suggestions, too extensive to include here, on adequate documentation of radiation treatments are given by the International Commission on Radiation Units and Measurements[70] and by Cohen.[22] Figure 9-9 illustrates some suggested notations for isodose charts.[22] The Radiological Society of North America's Standardization Committee has promoted the use of standard radiation therapy charts and diagrams, and more recently, the Radiological Physics Center has suggested parameters to include in a radiation therapy chart.[61,120] An abbreviated checklist of these parameters is presented in Table 9-1.

The *integral dose* is the dose per unit mass of tissue multiplied by the mass of tissue receiving this dose and summed over the target volume to yield the total energy absorbed in the target volume.[91] It has failed to gain widespread use, although a treatment technique that produces a lower integral dose is prefer-

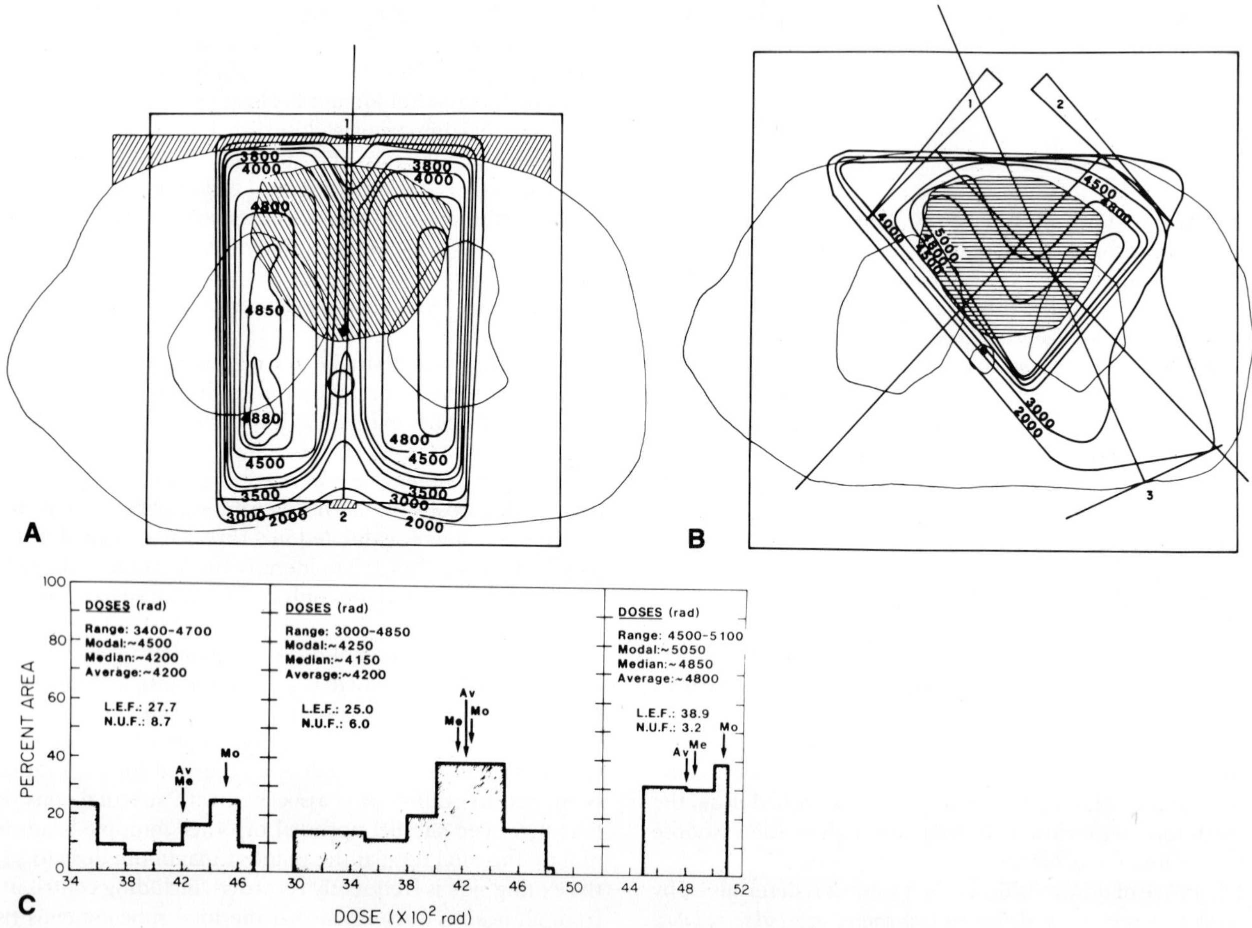

FIGURE 9–7. (**A**) Computed tomographic (CT) unoptimized treatment plan with lung transmission correction. Beam configuration and weights were identical to those in the conventional plan. Hatched area within patient's contour represents the target area as defined by a CT scan. Accurate lung transmission correction could be made because the lung outline and density could be obtained directly from CT scans. Hatched area outside the patient's contour represents the compensating filter and spinal cord block. (**B**) CT optimized plan with lung transmission correction. Wedged beams improved the uniformity of dose and reduced the dose to normal structures. (**C**) Doses and local efficiency and nonuniformity factors for each plan. Notice the decreased mediastinal dose resulting from the posterior spinal cord block. (Prasad S, Pilepich MV, Perez CA: Am J Roentgenol 136:123, 1981)

able to one with a higher integral dose, all other parameters being equal. With three-dimensional dose-calculation software, it is easier to calculate and compare integral doses than with conventional two-dimensional isodose calculations.

By carefully considering the dose at points in the target volume and the dose to adjacent structures, the radiation oncologist hopes to find an optimal beam arrangement. Computer algorithms that assist in these selections are becoming available.[84] The actual selection of a treatment method may be governed by more practical considerations. An "optimal" plan that requires the use of multiple radiation beams available only on separate therapy units and that requires multiple simulations of a very ill patient is probably unacceptable.

X-RAY (PHOTON) BEAMS

Single Photon Beam Dosimetry

^{60}*Co teletherapy units, linacs, betatrons,* and *microtrons* with electron beams from 4 MeV to 50 MeV, capable of generating x-ray beams covering this same energy range, are used for radiation therapy. Treatment techniques employing individual photon beams, multiple photon beams of the same energy, photon beams of different energies, photon beams mixed with electron beams, or electron beams alone allow the radiation therapist with modern equipment great flexibility in optimizing each patient's treatment.

The dose at depths along the central axis of a radiation beam, as a percentage of the maximum dose on the central axis (*e.g.*, the *percentage depth dose*), expresses the penetrability of a radiation beam. Table 9-2 lists the depths at which the dose is a maximum, 80% of the maximum, and 50% of the maximum for the τ-ray and x-ray beams in Figure 9-10 at conventional source-to-skin or focus-to-skin distances.[23,24] A 25-MV x-ray beam has about twice the penetrability of a ^{60}Co beam with an average τ-ray energy of 1.25 MV.

The *isodose curves* show the relative uniformity and nonuniformity of the beams at depths and the dose distributions in the penumbra region (Fig. 9-11). Because of source designs, cobalt units exhibit a large penumbra near the beam edge, and their isodose distributions are rounded toward the source; linac isodose distribution can exhibit "horns" (*i.e.*, greater penetrability away from the central axis, with some portions of the

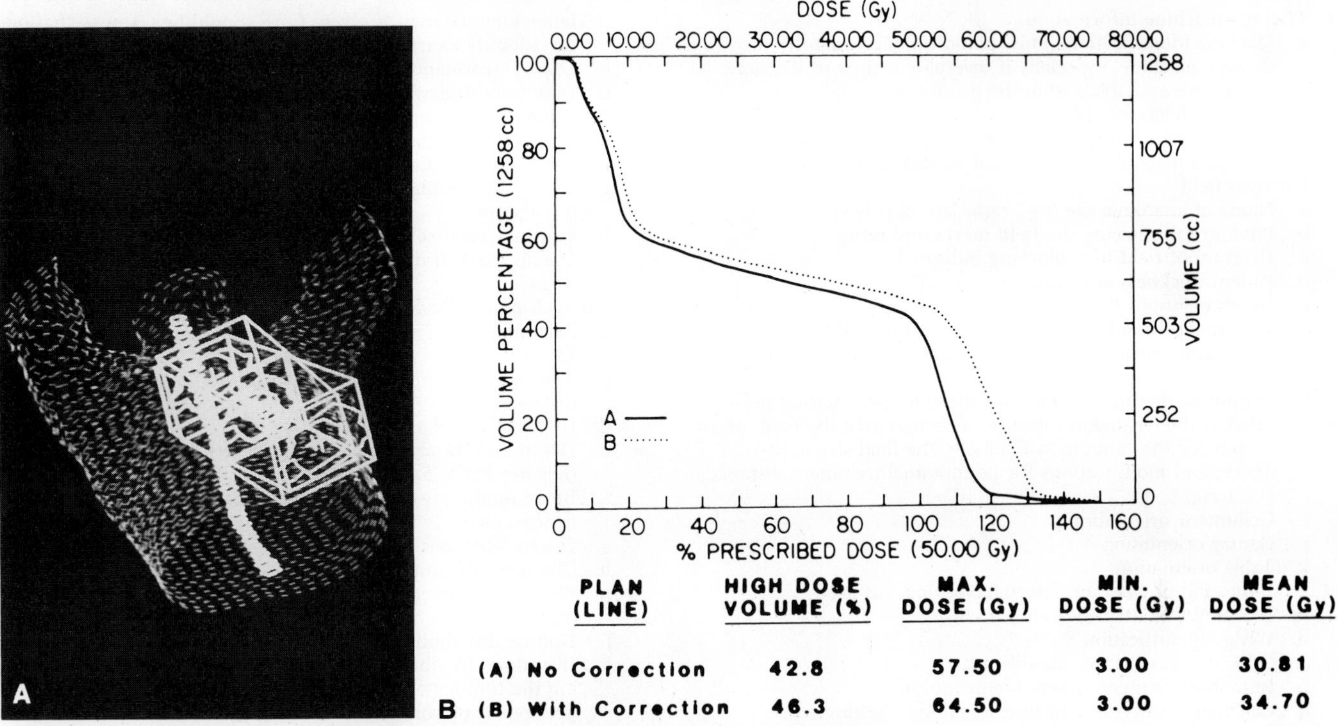

PLAN (LINE)	HIGH DOSE VOLUME (%)	MAX. DOSE (Gy)	MIN. DOSE (Gy)	MEAN DOSE (Gy)
(A) No Correction	42.8	57.50	3.00	30.81
(B) With Correction	46.3	64.50	3.00	34.70

FIGURE 9–8. (**A**) Display on viewing monitor shows the various capabilities of the 3D radiation treatment planning system developed at Mallinckrodt Institute of Radiology: serial computed tomography (CT) section contours and multiradiation beam representation; all contours except those for the external skin surface and the spinal cord have been turned off; and the spinal cord is brightened. (**B**) Cumulative dose-volume histogram for the right lung of a patient with lung cancer. The plan was calculated first without correcting for any heterogeneities (Plan A) and then repeated without changing the beam settings but correcting for heterogeneities (Plan B). The dose-volume histogram provides a tool to quickly assess the impact of the inhomogeneity on dose distribution.

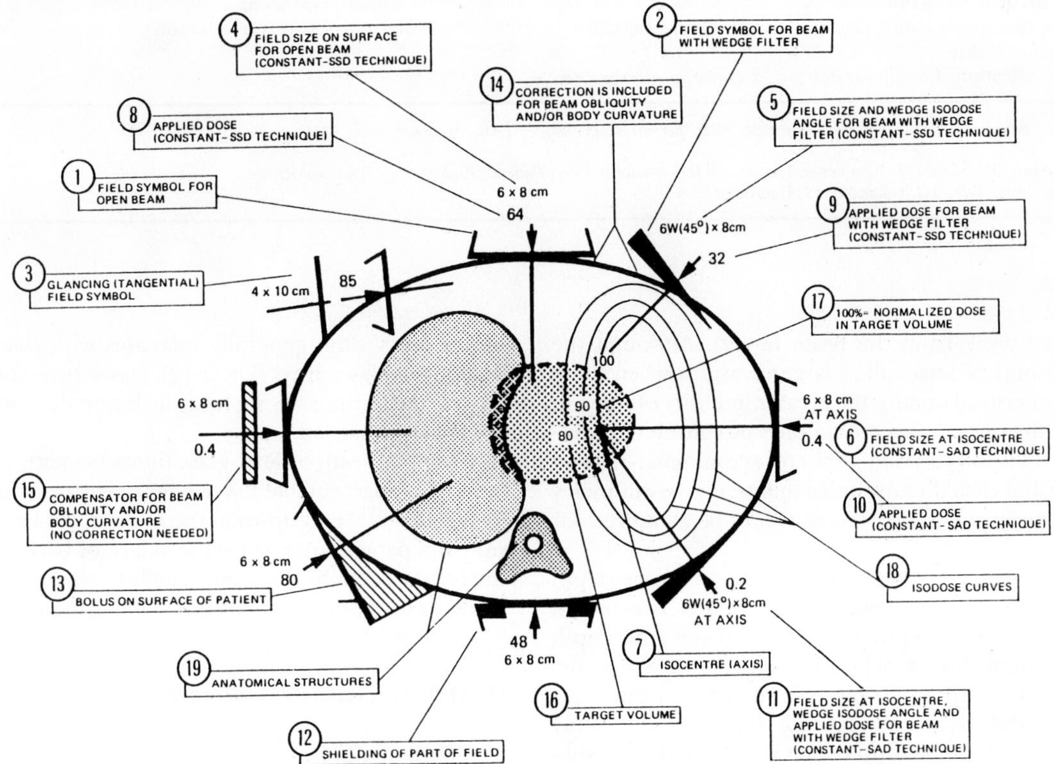

FIGURE 9–9. Isodose chart with the International Atomic Energy Commission's suggested standardized symbols and conventions. (Cohen M, Mitchell JS (eds): Cobalt-60 Teletherapy: A Compendium of International Practice. Vienna, International Atomic Energy Commission, 1984)

TABLE 9–1
Recommended Information to be Included in the Radiation Therapy Treatment Record

1. Therapy machine information
   a. Machine identification. This should uniquely identify the therapy machine, especially if several machines of the same energy are available within the institution.
   b. Modality (electron, photon)
   c. Beam energy. For orthovoltage therapy, the kvp, added filtration, and half-value layer should be included.
2. For each field
   a. Name of anatomic site (*e.g.*, right lateral pelvis)
   b. Photograph showing the field marks and setup
   c. Diagram of field with blocking indicated
   d. Patient thickness at central ray
   e. Depth of tumor (target)
   f. Treatment distance (clearly marked whether SSD or SAD)*
   g. Collimator setting (for electrons, indicate cone used, if applicable)
   h. Output of therapy machine for the collimator setting indicated at the treatment distance. This may take the form of an output for the calibration field size, the field-size dependence, and modifications for nonnominal treatment distance ($1/r^2$), etc.
   i. Collimator orientation
   j. Gantry orientation
   k. Table orientation
   l. Indication of whether external blocking was used
   m. Blocking tray identification
   n. Wedge identification
   o. Other beam modifier identification
   p. Immobilization equipment identification
   q. Calculation of treatment time or monitor setting
   r. For rotation, stop and start angles and dose per degree
   s. For ^{60}Co machines, description of trimmer extension (up, down, 45 cm, 65 cm, etc.)
3. Dose prescription
   a. Technique (AP-PA, four-field box, obliques, etc.)
   b. Number of fields treated per day
   c. Daily tumor dose per field
   d. Total prescribed tumor dose
   e. Dose to critical structures
   f. Clear notes indicating when the patient is to be reevaluated for dose or field reduction
   g. Radiation therapist's name, typed (or printed) and signature
4. Daily treatment record
   a. Field identification. Usually under No. 2 above, a number or letter identification is given. Care should be taken so that one can identify exactly when changes in the field were made.
   b. Day of treatment (*i.e.*, 1, 2, 3, . . .)
   c. Date (month/day/year) of treatment
   d. Time or monitor units set for each field (indicated daily)
   e. Daily and cumulative given (max) dose
   f. Daily and cumulative tumor (target) dose from each field
   g. Daily and cumulative dose from all fields, to every point of calculation
   h. Critical structure dose (cumulative, etc.)
   i. Initials marked daily by the person administering the treatment
5. For each point of calculation
   a. Anatomic site
   b. Effective area of the field on the patient
   c. Treatment distance: variation from the nominal treatment distance
   d. Depth of calculation
   e. Depth dose factors (it should be clearly indicated whether they are PDD, TAR, TMR, etc.)*
   f. Beam-modifying factors (wedge, compensator, tray factors, etc.)
   g. Distance off axis if applicable
   h. Changes of beam intensity at off-axis points
   i. Patient contour at level of the treatment field for complex treatments
   j. Isodose distribution if done
   k. If isodose distributions are used, the isodose line encompassing the tumor (target) volume should be clearly indicated. The point, or volume, to which the prescribed dose is calculated should also be clearly indicated. Critical structures should also be indicated on the plan.
   l. Calculation of the daily and total tumor dose to each point of calculation
   m. Initials of person doing the calculation and initials of person checking the calculation
6. Additional data
   a. Simulator, port, or verification films for every field including every modification of the port margins
   b. Notes on treatment interruptions, reasons for not completing treatment, and so on
   c. Notes on previous irradiation

**SSD, source-to-skin distance; SAD, source-to-axis distance; PDD, percent depth dosage; TAR, tissue-air ratio; TMR, tissue-maximum ratio.*
(After Hansen WF, Shalek RJ, Kirby TH: Information That Should Be Included in Every Patient's Radiotherapy Treatment Record. Radiological Physics Center Technical Report No. 18, Houston, 1985)

curves rounded away from the beam target). Although the narrow penumbras of linacs allow larger margins when these beams pass near critical organs, the greater intensity of some of the beams off the central axis must always be considered carefully. Figure 9-11 illustrates isodose curves at common τ-ray and x-ray energies, but each therapy unit exhibits unique dosimetry features, and such isodose distributions must be measured for each unit.

When a τ-ray or x-ray beam strikes tissue, at some depth beneath the entry surface, maximum ionization is achieved from the surface to that depth; the dose increases with depth until the maximum dose is achieved. Figure 9-12 shows the buildup[134] of dose with depth beneath the entry surface for common τ-ray and x-ray energies. For higher-energy x-ray beams, the depth of the buildup region is increased. The subcutaneous tissue-sparing effects of these higher-energy x-rays, combined with their great penetrability, make them popular for treating deep lesions. For a specific x-ray energy, the magnitude of the entry dose generally increases with field size and the addition of plastic trays (Fig. 9-12). Plastic trays should be at least 20 cm above the skin surface; at lesser distances, entry skin doses are enhanced.

Copper, lead, or lead-glass filters beneath plastic trays remove the unacceptable lower-energy electrons that contribute to skin dose.[118] Exit doses in the build-down region on the exit side of a patient are reduced by a lack of backscatter material; the full dose may be restored, usually by the addition of material equal in thickness to about one half of the d_{max} depth.[48, 114]

Dual X-Ray Beam Dosimetry

The radiation therapist must understand the x-ray beam characteristics as a function of field size, patient thickness, and treatment distance to select the optimal x-ray energy for superior dose distribution.

TABLE 9–2
Depths at Which the Dose Is 100%, 80%, and 50% of the Maximum Dose for Some Common Photon Energies

PHOTON BEAM ENERGY	DEPTH (cm) VERSUS PERCENTAGE OF MAXIMUM DOSE		
	100%	80%	50%
230 kV	0	3.0	6.8
^{60}Co	0.5	4.7	11.6
4 MV	1.0	5.6	13.0
6 MV	1.2	6.8	15.6
10 MV	2.0	7.8	19.0
25 MV	3.0	10.2	21.8

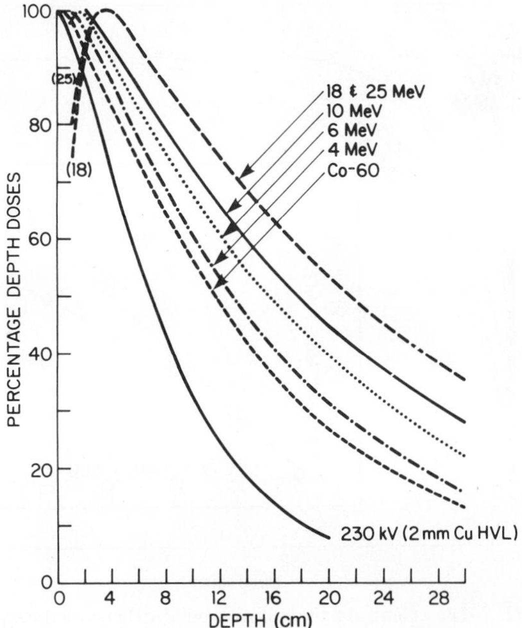

FIGURE 9–10. Typical x-ray or photon beam central-axis percentage depth dose curves for a 10-cm × 10-cm beam for 230 kV (2-mm Cu HVL) at 50-cm SSD, ^{60}Co and 4 MV at 80-cm SSD, and 6 MV, 10 MV, 18 MV, and 25 MV at 100-cm SSD. The latter two beams coincide at most depths but do not coincide in the first few millimeters of the buildup region. The 4-MV, 6-MV, 18-MV, and 25-MV data are for the Varian Clinac 4, 6, 20, and 35 units, respectively, at the Mallinckrodt Institute of Radiology in St. Louis. (Cohen M, Jones DEA, Greene D: Br J Radiol [Suppl] 11:21, 1972)

When only two unmodified x-ray beams are used in radiation therapy, they usually are parallel opposed beams (*i.e.*, directed toward each other from opposite sides of the anatomic site with the central axes coinciding). Figure 9-13 presents the normalized relative-axis dose profiles from parallel opposed photon beams for a 10-cm × 10-cm field at source-to-skin distance of 100 cm and for patient diameters of 15 cm to 30 cm in 5-cm increments. The weight of a beam denotes a numeric value assigned to the beam at some normalization point. The beams in Figure 9-13 are weighted 1 to 1 (*i.e.*, assigned equal value, 100%, at d_{max}), but the dose profiles have been normalized to the cumulative midline percent depth dose.

The maximum-diameter patient who can be easily treated with parallel opposed beams for a midplane tumor requiring 5000 cGy or less with a cobalt unit or 4-MV x-rays is about 18 cm; for thicker patients, higher x-ray energies (10 MV to 20 MV) produce improved dose profiles with less dose variation along the central axis, without resorting to complex multibeam arrangements.

The underdosing achieved near the skin surface with very-high-energy, parallel opposed x-ray beams must be evaluated carefully; in some treatment sites, this is a highly advantageous feature, but in others, it may be desirable to achieve a higher dose near the skin. For example, Figure 9-14 compares ^{60}Co and 25-MV x-ray whole-brain treatments. For uniform irradiation of the cranial contents laterally, the cobalt distribution is superior; for irradiation of a small midline lesion with sparing of

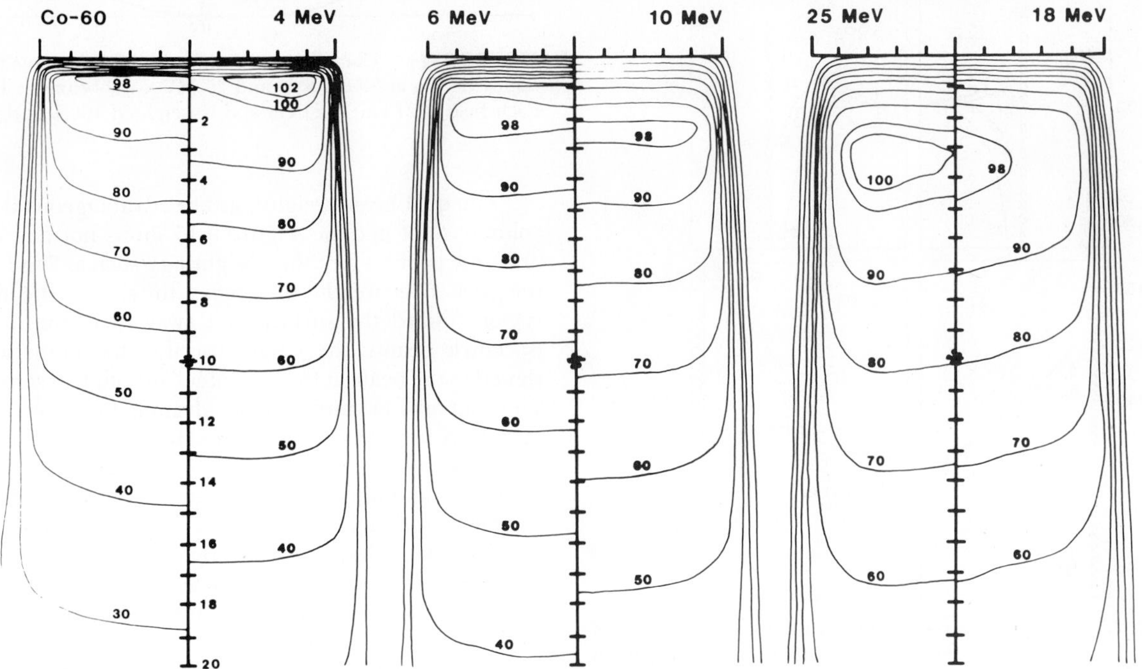

FIGURE 9–11. Typical γ-ray and x-ray beam central-axis isodose curves for a 10-cm × 10-cm field. The ^{60}Co and 4-MV isodose distributions are at 80-cm SSD; all others are at 100-cm SSD.

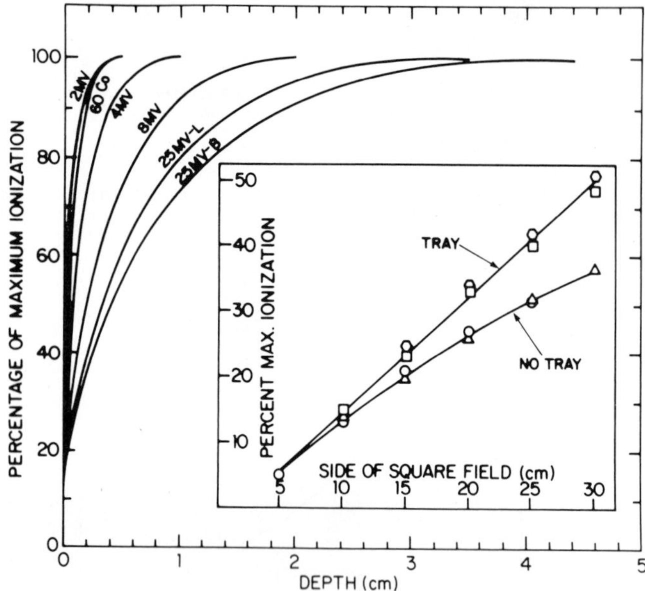

FIGURE 9–12. Central-axis ionization buildup beneath the entry surface for a 10-cm × 10-cm field for typical x-ray beams. All are 100-cm SSD, except the ^{60}Co and 4-MV distributions, which are 80-cm SSD. At 25 MV, data for both a linac (L) and a betatron (B) are shown. The *inset* shows the effects of field size and a plastic tray for 4 MV units. (Gagnon WF, Grant W: Radiology 117:705, 1975; Velkey DE, Manson DJ, Purdy JA, et al: Med Phys 2:14, 1974)

hair, the 25-MV distribution is superior. The lateral extent of disease in the brain dictates optimal beam selection.

With very-high-energy x-ray beams transversing small anatomic thicknesses, the exit dose can exceed the entry dose, and the exact dose distribution in the regions beneath the entry and exit surfaces from parallel opposed high-energy x-ray beams must be carefully evaluated to consider properly the contribution from each beam, including entrance and exit components.

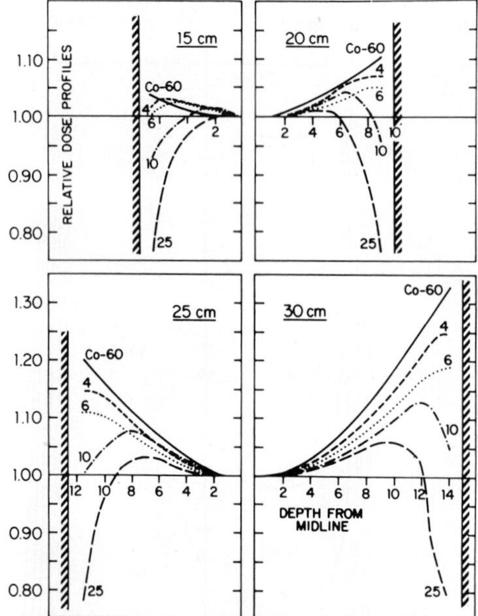

FIGURE 9–13. Relative central-axis dose profiles as a function of x-ray energy (^{60}Co, 4 MV, 6 MV, 10 MV, and 18 MV) and patient thickness (15-cm, 20-cm, 25-cm, and 30-cm). The parallel opposed beams are equally weighted, and the profiles are normalized to unity at midline. Because of symmetry, only half of each profile is shown.

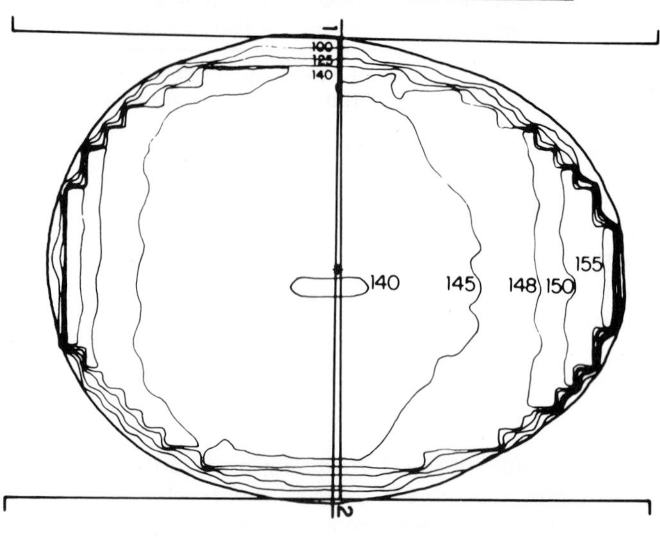

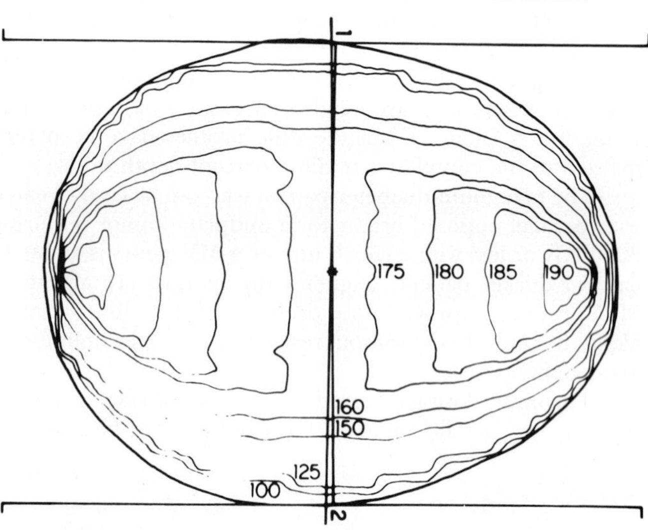

FIGURE 9–14. Comparison of whole-brain treatments with parallel opposed ^{60}Co at 80-cm SSD and 25-MV x-ray beams at 100-cm SSD. Each field is 21 cm × 21 cm and is weighted 100% at d_{max}.

Unequal beam weightings are advantageous if the target volume is not midline. Figure 9-15 shows normalized central-axis dose profiles for other weightings, such as 2 to 1 and 3 to 1; the greater the weight, the greater the shift of the higher-dose region toward the surface and away from the midline. For isocentric beams, the weight specifies the numeric value assigned to the beam at the isocenter. Although in some anatomic sites, unequal loading may be advantageous, special attention must be paid to the doses delivered to anatomic structures in the high-dose volume. Grant and Fletcher[60] reported a higher incidence of mandibular necrosis in tumors of the oropharynx, and a greater incidence of pericarditis has been observed in patients with Hodgkin's disease at Washington University when unequal loadings were used to treat these anatomic sites at high doses.[93]

The dose distribution from unmodified beams directed at, for example, 90 degrees relative to one another exhibits a usually undesirable nonuniform dose distribution (Fig. 9-16). Methods of beam modifications to achieve dose uniformity for these beams are discussed in this chapter.

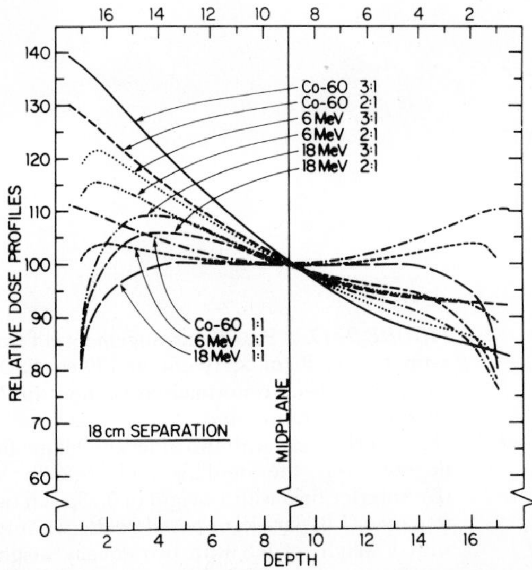

FIGURE 9–15. Dose profiles achieved with various weightings of parallel opposed photon beams; profiles are normalized to unity at midline.

Three-Field X-Ray Beam Dosimetry

There are many ways to combine three radiation fields; Figure 9-17 shows four commonly used coplanar arrangements. A direct anterior field with two anterior oblique fields can be used to generate a high-dose region in which the three fields overlap, with a low-dose region beyond this intersection point. For example, if this arrangement is used for treating the mediastinum, the spinal cord may be included in the anterior beam but spared by the anterior oblique beams.

An anterior field with two symmetrically placed posterior oblique beams yields the generally elongated isodose curves in Figure 9-17C. The degree of elongation is determined by the relative thickness of tissue each beam transverses to the point of intersection and the relative weights of the beams. Two anterior oblique fields with a posterior field is useful in treating the larynx and hypopharynx.[45]

Three-field arrangements often are useful for treating tumors lateral to the midline of a patient (Fig. 9-17D). Three-field noncoplanar arrangements are readily achieved with modern therapy units with rotating tables.

A common technique for treating pituitary tumors employs two lateral fields and a vertex field with the beam entering through the top of the head. Astrocytomas often are treated with parallel opposed lateral fields and a frontal field entering through the forehead. In each case, a 90-degree couch rotation is used laterally with the therapy unit.[42]

Four-Field X-Ray Beam Dosimetry

Four-field techniques often are necessary in sites like the abdomen or the pelvis. Historically, use of multiple, low-energy x-ray beams has allowed the radiation oncologist to deliver a high dose to a central anatomic region. In most instances, the arrangements consist of pairs of parallel opposed fields with a common intersecting point, which yield a box dose distribution.

Figure 9-18 compares the dose distributions achieved with a four-field box technique for ^{60}Co, 6-MV, and 18-MV x-ray beams. The central dose distribution is similar for all beam energies, but the greater penetrability of the higher-energy beams yields a lower dose to the region outside the box. Variations in the dose gradient are achieved by differential weighting of each pair of beams.

Figure 9-19 shows other possible four-beam arrangements. Angulation of the beams yields a diamond-shaped dose distribution; the butterfly distribution is achieved if each pair of beams has a point of intersection lying on a common line but separated by a few centimeters.

Rotational Techniques

Rotational therapy is an infinite, multiple-field technique, and basic techniques described for supervoltage units may be applied to megavoltage units.[135] Rotating an x-ray beam around a small-diameter, centrally located tumor is an excellent method

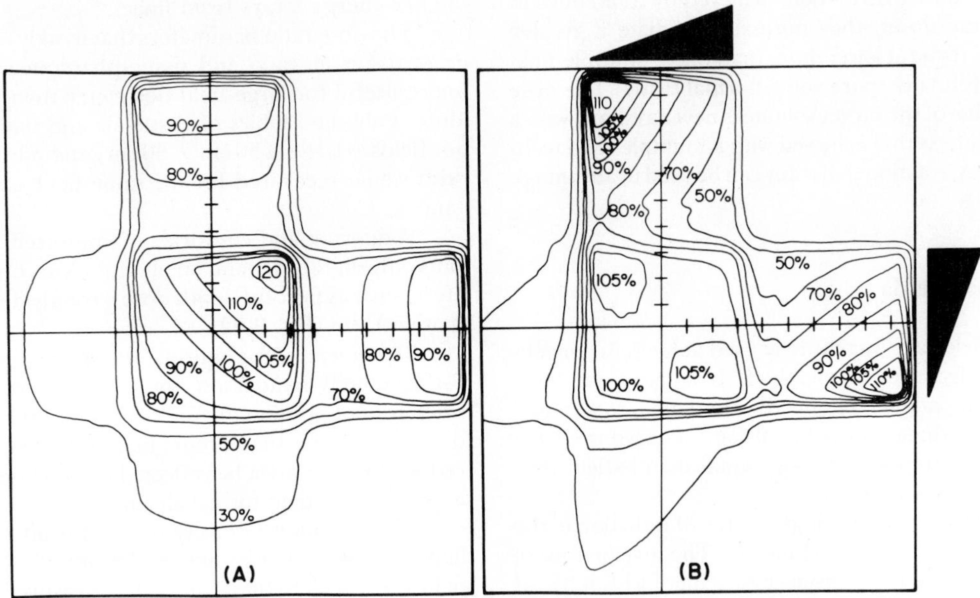

FIGURE 9–16. (**A**) Orthogonal x-ray beams yield highly nonuniform dose distributions with sharp dose gradients where the beams intersect. (**B**) Forty-five-degree wedges added to the fields yield a more uniform dose distribution where the beams intersect.

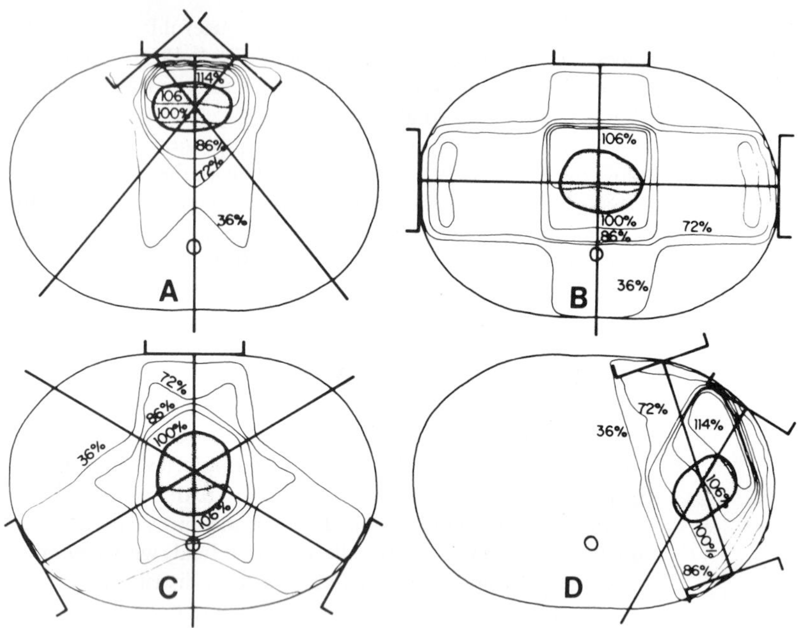

FIGURE 9–17. Possible arrangements of three 6-MV x-ray beams, 8 cm × 10 cm, at 100-cm SSD. Isodose curves have been renormalized to show the 100% line almost encompassing the target volume. (**A**) Anterior field with two anterior oblique fields at 40 degrees off the midline, all equally weighted. (**B**) Anterior field with a weight of 0.75, with two equally weighted (1.0) parallel opposed fields. (**C**) Anterior field with a weight of 0.8 with two equally weighted (1.0) posterior oblique fields separated by 120 degrees. (**D**) Three arbitrary fields to treat an off-axis tumor mass. The anterior beam has a weight of 1.14 relative to the other two equally (1.0) weighted beams.

of treatment that delivers a high dose to the tumor and a low dose to surrounding tissue. The technique usually is limited to fields less than about 10 cm wide for the treatment of lesions that are centrally located (*i.e.*, that have approximately an equal amount of tissue in all directions).

There is only a small difference between the rotational dose distributions achieved using a ^{60}Co and those using a 25-MV x-ray beam, although the latter is superior; there is less elongation in the direction of the shorter dimension of the anatomy for the 25-MV beam, and the dose distribution is more circular (Fig. 9-20).

Other coplanar rotational methods (Fig. 9-21) include the 90-degree, 180-degree, and 270-degree arc distributions and "skip" distributions, bilateral rotations, and arc rotations around points that are separated by a few centimeters to achieve an oval dose distribution.

Although the dose distributions achieved by rotation yield high target volume doses, they normally irradiate a greater volume of normal tissue at lower doses than fixed, multiple-field techniques, which totally spare some normal tissue. The dose gradient at the edge of the target volume is never as sharp with a rotational technique as that achieved with a multiple-field technique. Nonetheless, rotational therapy can be used to advantage in many cases.

Large Radiation Fields

Large radiation fields are increasingly used at long, unconventional treatment distances in total-body irradiation for bone marrow transplant patients, hemibody irradiation, total nodal irradiation, and irradiation of the total central nervous system (*e.g.*, for medulloblastoma).[55] Conventional mantle-field dosimetry is discussed in Chapter 8.

The distance from a fixed, single source of radiation to the treatment plane should be several meters. The inverse-square law requires a 3-m treatment distance to achieve within 5% of uniformity in radiation intensity over a transverse length of 2 m; at 3 m, the percentage depth doses are essentially the same as those obtained from a source infinitely far away. The field size for total-body irradiation should be as large as possible. For example, a therapy unit that projects a 40-cm × 40-cm field at 1 m will project a field only 120 cm × 120 cm at 3 m; the 167-cm diagonal dimension would be too short to treat a 6-foot (182-cm) patient lying on a stretcher. Moreover, the useful treatment field may be substantially smaller than the projected light field.

Hemibody irradiation involves fewer geometric restrictions than total-body irradiation. Usually, the hemibody can be encompassed by the field size projected 2 m from the source. The dose rates (centigray per minute) or the output (centigray per monitor unit) of a teletherapy unit should be measured in the plane of treatment, because dose rates or outputs calculated according to the inverse-square law may be incorrect if they fail to include the backscatter radiation from a nearby wall or floor, an effect more pronounced for cobalt photons than for the higher-energy x-rays from linacs.[80]

The dose ratio parameters that weakly depend on distance (*e.g.*, tissue-air ratio and tissue-phantom ratio) probably are more useful for large-field dosimetry than the percent depth dose. Published tables of tissue-air and tissue-phantom ratios for fields as large as 30 cm × 30 cm generally agree to within 3% with values measured for the same field size at extended distances.

Podgorsak and co-workers[109] reported that machine outputs only slightly depend on phantom size, but that ratio parameters, such as percent depth dose strongly depend on phantom (patient) size (Fig. 9-22).

To determine the equivalent square area a patient presents for total-body irradiation, the radiation oncologist must consider patient position during treatment. Because a patient produces less scatter than occurs in an infinite cubic phantom, the reduced scatter must be reflected in the dose calculations. This is particularly true for cobalt units.

Any radiation intensity nonuniformity is likely to be enhanced in large fields; hence, the uniformity of the radiation field (*i.e.*, field flatness) must be measured at the treatment plane. For cobalt units, underdosing around the periphery[71] of the field is common (Fig. 9-23). For linacs, the opposite is true

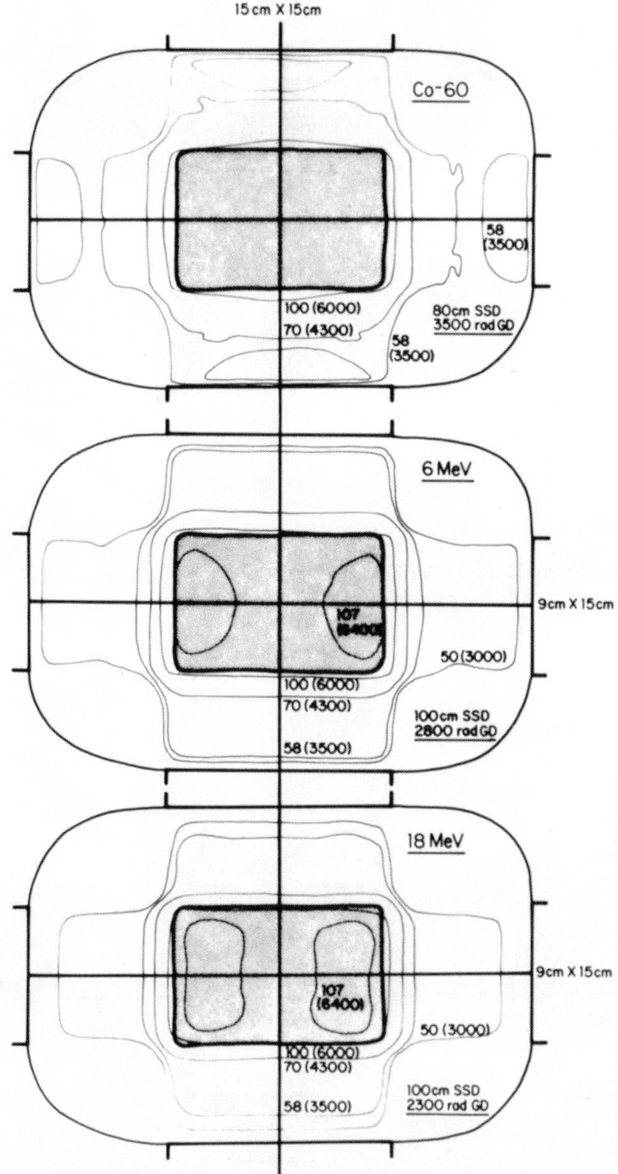

FIGURE 9–18. Box dose distributions using 15-cm × 15-cm fields as a function of x-ray beam energy. All beams are equally weighted at d_{max} to yield 6000 cGy (100%) encompassing the target volume. The highest energy beam at the lowest dose produces the greatest fall-off outside the box.

(*i.e.*, horns are enhanced). The doses to the skin surface and in the region of buildup to maximum dose must be measured for the therapy unit and treatment geometry used for total-body and hemibody irradiation; contribution from treatment aids normally present during total-body or hemibody irradiation should be included in the dosimetry. Generally, skin dose increases as the angle between the beam axis and the normal to the irradiated surface increases; the increase is greatest beyond 45 degrees. The skin and superficial tissue on the side of the patient from which the beam exits receives a reduced dose if little backscattering material is present.[48,114] The depths at which doses have been prescribed in total-body and hemibody irradiation include the midline depth of the head, neck, chest, and abdomen and the half-depth of the maximum width of the body. The dose prescription should consider the limiting doses to the critical organs. Generally, anteroposterior irradiation yields more uniform doses throughout the body than bilateral irradiation, because it presents more uniform anatomic dimensions to the incident beam.

Given the importance of lung dose in large-field therapy, it is imperative that the lung dose, corrected for heterogeneities, be measured or calculated for all patients experiencing irradiation of the lung(s).[35,39]

Total-body and hemibody irradiation doses should be confirmed by dose distribution measurements in the anthropomorphic phantom and *in vivo* measurements in patients. Sites for *in vivo* measurements include the mouth, axilla, inner thighs, and rectum; parallel opposed entry and exit doses at diverse locations estimate the dose midway between the dosimeters. Thermoluminescent dosimeters are excellent for *in vivo* dosimetry; diodes are useful for measuring entry and exit doses.

Craniospinal Irradiation Techniques

Craniospinal irradiation is well established as a standard method of treatment of suprasellar dysgerminoma, pineal tumors, medulloblastomas, and other tumors involving the central nervous system. Treatment of the entire central nervous system uniformly is possible using separate parallel opposed, lateral, whole-brain portals rotated to match their inferior borders with the superior border of the spinal portal, which is treated with one or two fields, depending on the length of spine being treated. Lim[86,87] articulates the dosimetry of optional methods of treating medulloblastoma (Fig. 9-24). The techniques are similar to those described in Chapter 23. Two junctional moves are made at one third and two thirds of the total dose. The spinal-field central axis is shifted away from the brain by 0.5 cm, and the field length is reduced by 0.5 cm, with corresponding increases in the length of the whole-brain field, matching the inferior border of the brain portal and the superior border of the spine portal. The whole-brain portals are rotated by an angle

$$\theta = \tan^{-1}\left(\frac{\frac{1}{2}\text{ spinal field length}}{\text{SSD}}\right)$$

to achieve the match. To eliminate the divergency between the brain portal and spine portal, the table is rotated through a floor angle

$$\alpha = \tan^{-1}\left(\frac{\frac{1}{2}\text{ skull field length}}{\text{SSD}}\right)$$

Van Dyke and colleagues[133] described a sophisticated multiple-field moving-junction treatment; however, the risk of inducing myelopathy with the potentially excessive dose from misaligned overlapping fields is always a concern when central nervous system tumors are treated.

Glasgow and Marks[56] avoid the use of a splice or moving junction required with multiple fields by irradiating the craniospinal axis using a single portal, with the patient lying prone about 2 m from the radiation source; if the collimators are rotated 45 degrees, the maximum diagonal dimension of the field encompasses the entire craniospinal axis of most adults in a single field.

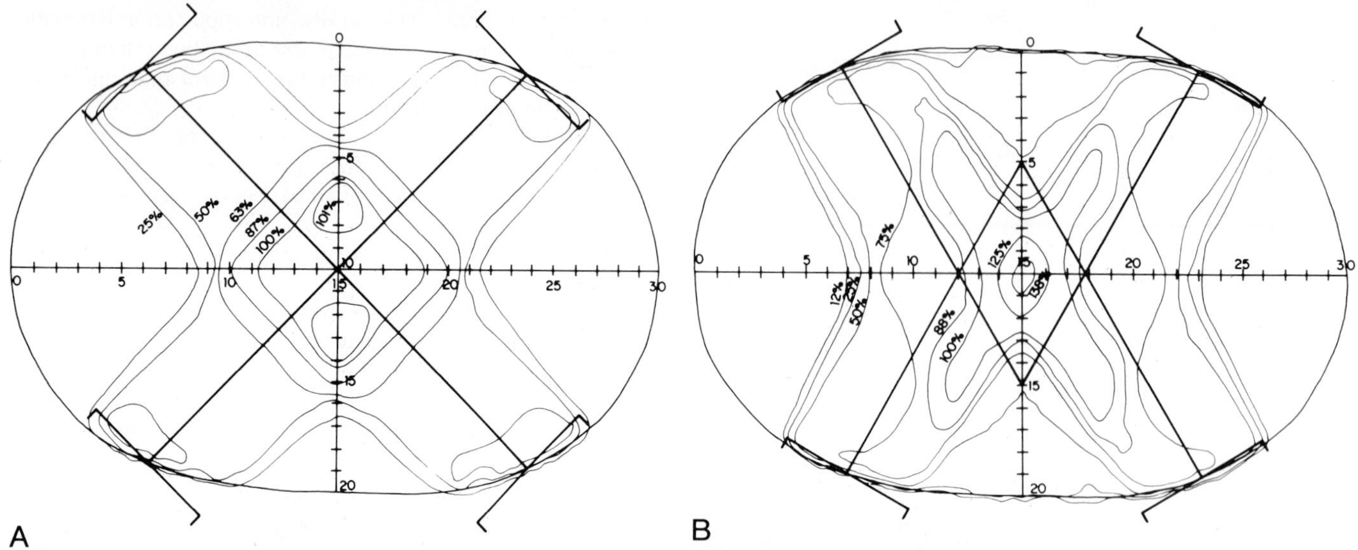

FIGURE 9–19. Isodose distributions (6 MV, 8 cm × 10 cm). The diamond-shaped dose distribution (**A**) is changed to a butterfly distribution (**B**) by allowing each beam pair to intersect at a different point on a common line. All beams are equally weighted.

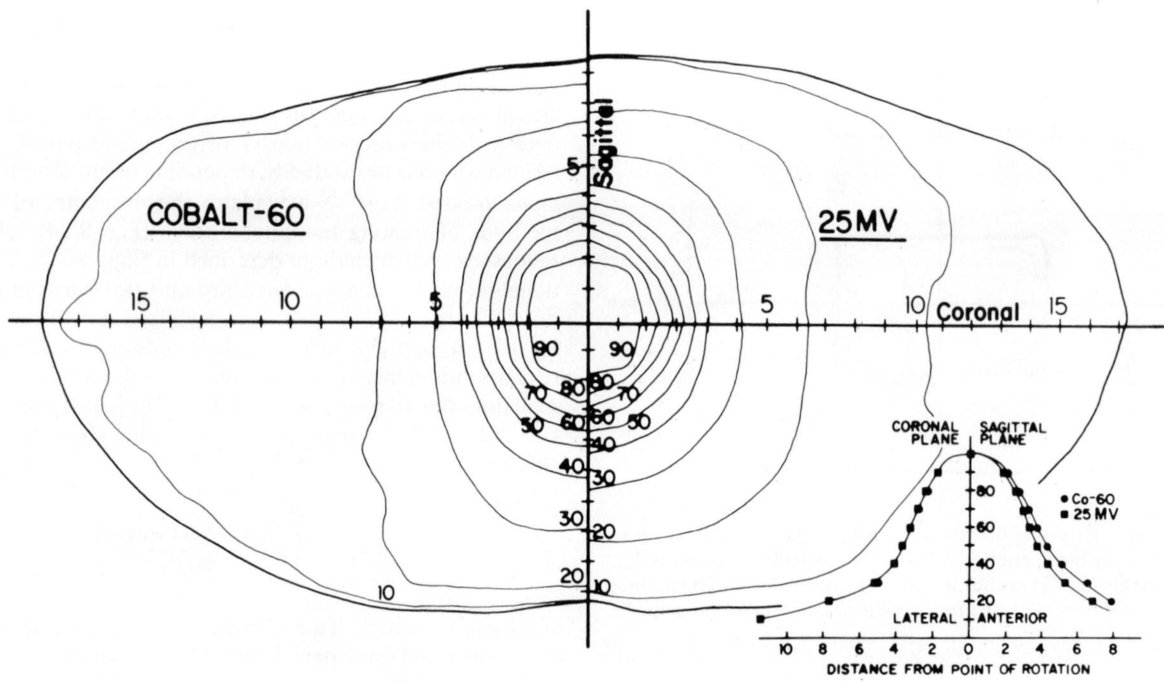

FIGURE 9–20. Comparative 360-degree rotational ^{60}Co and 25-MV dose distributions on an 18-cm × 36-cm abdomen. Dose distributions have similar shapes, but there is a greater degree of elongation of the ^{60}Co isodose curves along the shorter (anteroposterior) dimension. The *inset* shows the dose profiles of the two beams along the two primary axes of the cross-section.

Adjacent X-Ray Fields

The numerous methods of matching adjacent x-ray fields have been reviewed by Hopfan and co-workers,[67] and Dea[28] reviews radiographic methods of confirming gaps. The geometries of adjacent fields, either a single pair or parallel opposed pairs, are illustrated in Figure 9-25. A commonly used method matches adjacent radiation fields at depth d. The necessary separation between adjacent field edges for producing junction doses similar to central axis doses follows from the similar triangles formed by the half-field length and source-to-skin distance in each field. The field edge is defined by the dose at the edge that is 50% of the dose at d_{max}. Consider two contiguous fields of lengths L_1 and L_2; the separation, S, of these two fields at the skin surface follows from these expressions:

$$s_1 = \tfrac{1}{2}L_1\left(\frac{d}{SSD}\right)$$

$$s_2 = \tfrac{1}{2}L_2\left(\frac{d}{SSD}\right)$$

$$S = s_1 + s_2$$

where d is the depth dose specification and s_1 and s_2 are the respective half-field lengths (Fig. 9-25). Table 9-3 lists the half-

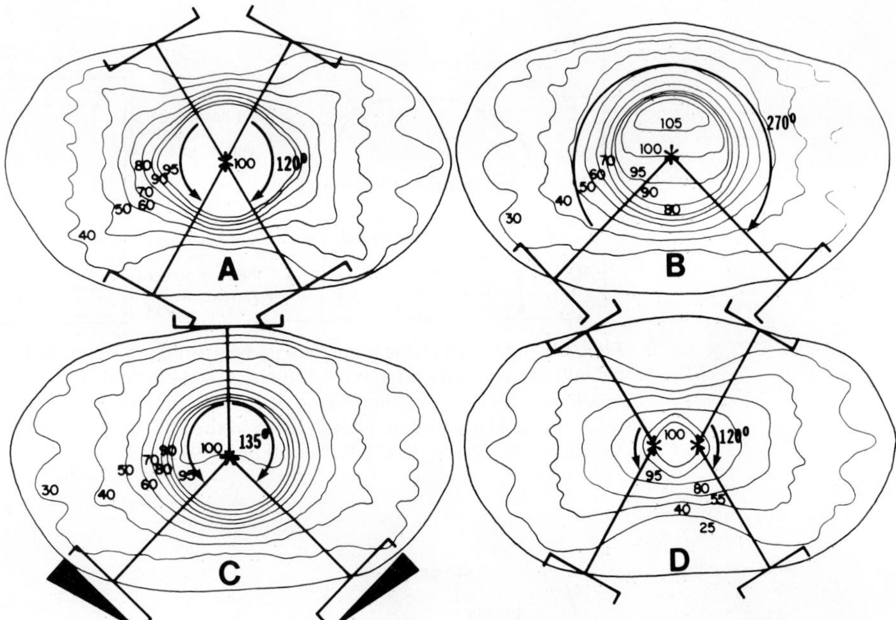

FIGURE 9–21. Some conventional rotational and arc dose distributions with 6-MV x-rays, 8-cm × 8-cm beam. (**A**) 120-degree bilateral arcs. (**B**) A 270-degree anterior arc. (**C**) 135-degree bilateral arcs with 30-degree wedges. (**D**) 120-degree bilateral arcs with isocenters separated by 4 cm, using 20-MV x-rays.

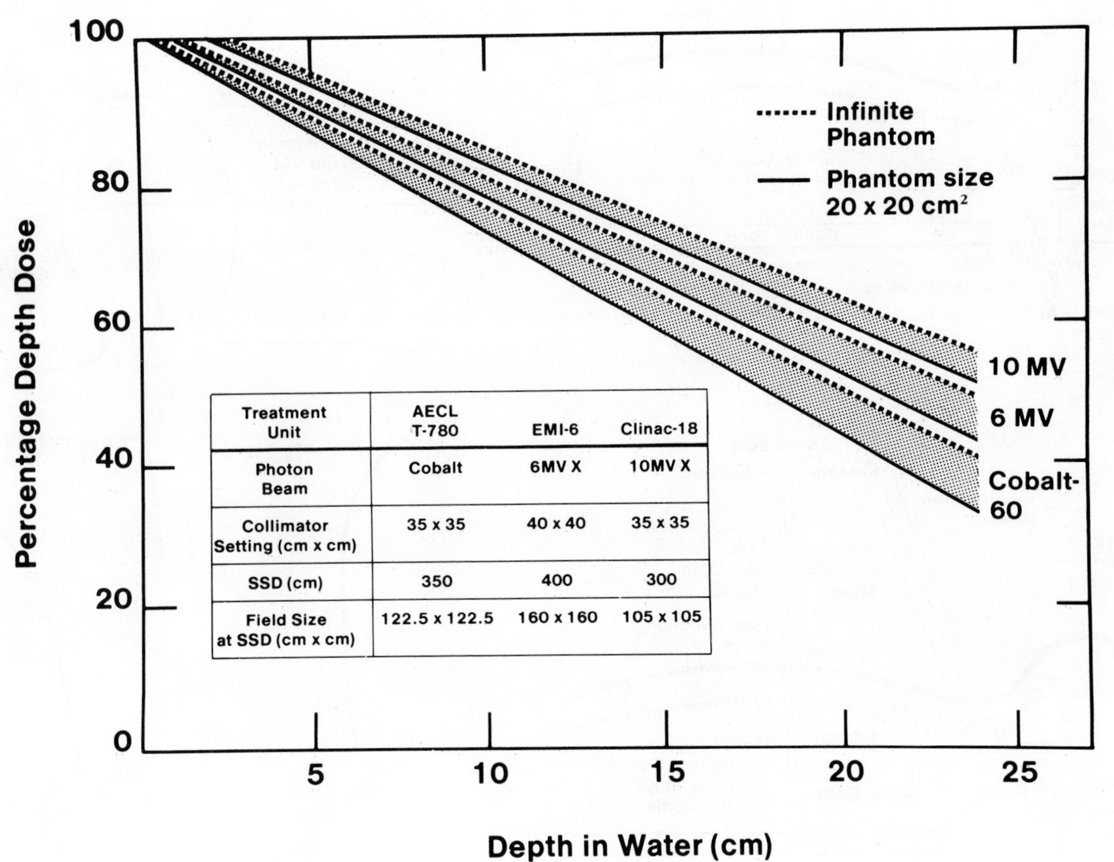

Treatment Unit	AECL T-780	EMI-6	Clinac-18
Photon Beam	Cobalt	6MV X	10MV X
Collimator Setting (cm x cm)	35 x 35	40 x 40	35 x 35
SSD (cm)	350	400	300
Field Size at SSD (cm x cm)	122.5 x 122.5	160 x 160	105 x 105

FIGURE 9–22. Percentage depth dose distributions for a 20 × 20 cm^2 phantom and an infinite phantom for three photon beams: cobalt, 6 MV, and 10 MV. The actual field sizes and SSDs are listed in the *inset.* The shaded areas represent the location of percentage depth dose curves for intermediate phantoms. (Podgorsak EB, Pla C, Evans MDC, Pla M: Med Phys 12:639, 1985)

(A)
(B)
Distance 315cm
Depth 12cm
Relative Dose
100
90
80
70
60
50
40
Parallel to a side
Along a diagonal
100
50
0
50
100cm
140cm
A
80%
90%
95%
•100%
140cm
Y
Field borders at the wall and midplane
Zone located at 20cm from the field border at the wall

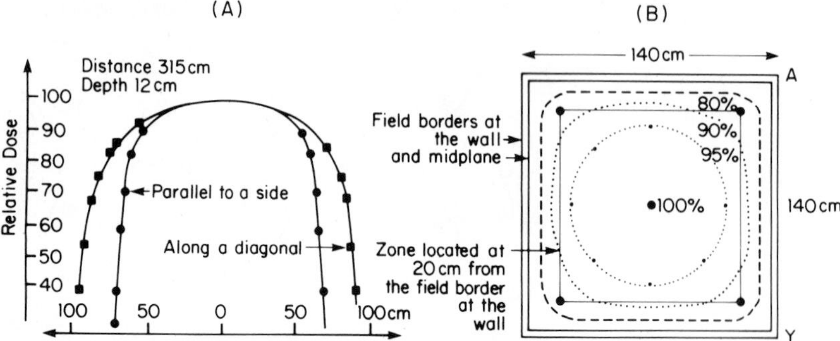

FIGURE 9–23. (**A**) Dose homogeneity measured at a depth of 12 cm along the principal and diagonal axes for about a 140-cm × 140-cm field, 315-cm from a Theratron-80 cobalt unit. (**B**) Dose homogeneity in the treatment plane at a depth of 12 cm. The useful treatment field is approximately defined by the 90% isodose curve. (Jablonski O, Motta-Veyssiere CC, Guerin RA: J Radiol 60:339, 1979)

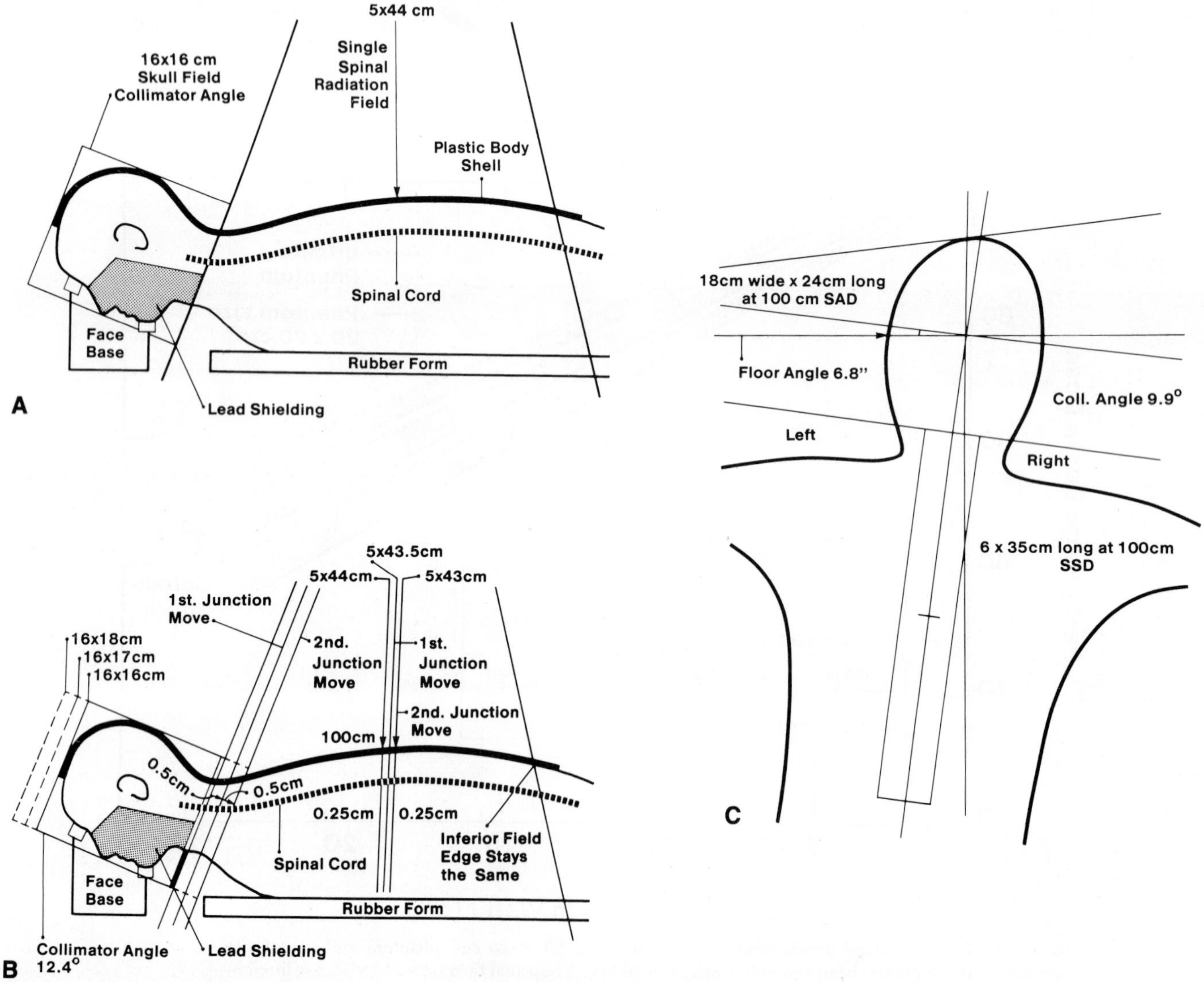

5x44 cm
16x16 cm
Skull Field
Collimator Angle
Single
Spinal
Radiation
Field
Plastic Body
Shell
Spinal Cord
Face
Base
Rubber Form
A
Lead Shielding
5x43.5cm
5x44cm
5x43cm
1st. Junction
Move
16x18cm
16x17cm
16x16cm
2nd.
Junction
Move
1st.
Junction
Move
2nd. Junction
Move
100cm
0.5cm
0.5cm
0.25cm
0.25cm
Inferior Field
Edge Stays
the Same
Spinal Cord
Face
Base
Rubber Form
Collimator Angle
12.4°
Lead Shielding
B
18cm wide x 24cm long
at 100 cm SAD
Floor Angle 6.8"
Coll. Angle 9.9°
Left
Right
6 x 35cm long at 100cm
SSD
C

FIGURE 9–24. (**A**) Treatment of medulloblastoma with lateral and posterior fields. The lateral field collimators are rotated to match the lateral field inferior edge with the superior (caudal) edge of the spinal field. (**B**) Two junctional moves at one third and two thirds of the therapy course. (**C**) The table is rotated to remove the divergency and improve the match. (Lim MLF: Am Assoc Med Dosim J 11:25, 1986)

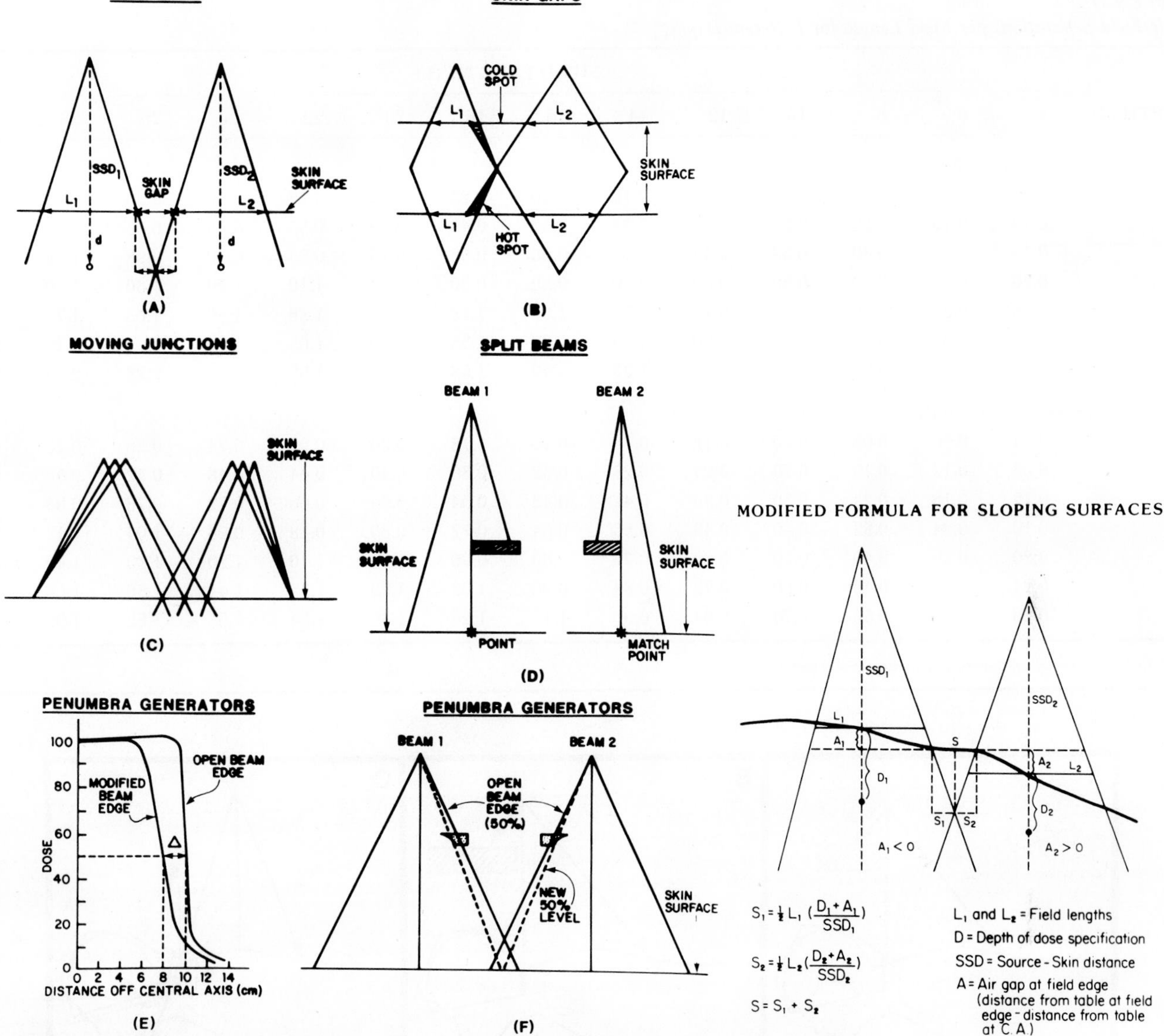

FIGURE 9–25. The geometry of field matching and possible solutions. Panels *A* and *B* illustrate the presence of hot and cold spots commonly encountered at matching field edges. Possible solutions include **(C)** moving junctions, **(D)** split-field blocks, and **(E, F)**, penumbra generators. **(A)** The gap separation S = $s_1 + s_2$, where $s_1 = \frac{1}{2} L_1 (\frac{d}{SSD})$, $s_2 = \frac{1}{2} L_2 (\frac{d}{SSD})$, and L_1 and L_2, are the field length and d is the depth of dose specifications. (Christopherson D, Courtlas GJ, Jette D, et al: Med Phys 3:369, 1984) When the gap separation is calculated if there is a sloping surface, the formula takes into account the additional tissue thickness (A_1) or air gap (A_2) due to sloping surface. The first value is included in the D_1 distance, and A_2 is added to D_2. For isocentric techniqes L (field size) is taken at isocenter. (Courtesy of Richard A. Keyes, Mallinckrodt Institute of Radiology, St. Louis, MO)

field lengths, s, as a function of d and lists L for 80-cm and 100-cm source-to-skin distance treatment geometries. To reduce the hot and cold spots that arise with this technique, the skin gap location is moved frequently, and the adjacent fields must be treated concurrently. The match point can be on the skin surface (Fig. 9-25C) with frequent moves to smear out the hot spots beneath the surface.

Beam divergency may be eliminated by using a "beam splitter," a 5- or 6-half-value-layer (HVL) block over one half of the treatment field.[19] The central axes of the adjacent fields, where there is no divergence, are then matched. This is a useful method on linacs with independent collimators. Match-line wedges or penumbra generators that generate a broad penumbra for linac beams have been used with success as a method of field matching.[46] The intent is to broaden the narrow penumbra of the linacs, facilitating the match to 50% isodose levels. The resulting dose distributions are similar to those obtained with a moving gap technique.

There are numerous reports of edge-matching techniques based on the mathematic relationships between adjacent beams and the allowed angles of the gantry, collimators, and couch. Christopherson and co-workers[20] developed a useful nomograph for field matching in treating cancer of the breast.

Matching abutting orthogonal photon beams is always a challenge, particularly in the head and neck region where the spinal cord can be in area of beam overlap, in treatment of medulloblastoma with multiple spinal portals and lateral brain ports, and in multiple-field treatments of the breast.[122, 133]

TABLE 9–3
*Half-Field Separations per Field Length for Different Depths**

	FIELD LENGTH (L)													
DEPTH (d)	4	6	8	10	12	14	16	18	20	22	24	26	28	30
SSD = 80 cm (s = ½ L [d/80])														
2	0.50	0.80	0.10	0.13	0.15	0.18	0.20	0.23	0.25	0.28	0.30	0.33	0.35	0.38
4	0.10	0.15	0.20	0.25	0.30	0.35	0.40	0.45	0.50	0.55	0.60	0.65	0.70	0.75
6	0.15	0.23	0.30	0.38	0.45	0.53	0.60	0.68	0.75	0.83	0.90	0.98	1.05	1.13
8	0.20	0.30	0.40	0.50	0.60	0.70	0.80	0.90	1.00	1.10	1.20	1.30	1.40	1.50
10	0.25	0.38	0.50	0.63	0.75	0.79	1.00	1.13	1.25	1.38	1.50	1.63	1.75	1.88
12	0.30	0.45	0.60	0.75	0.90	1.05	1.20	1.35	1.50	1.65	1.80	1.95	2.10	2.25
14	0.35	0.53	0.70	0.88	1.05	1.23	1.40	1.58	1.75	1.93	2.10	2.28	2.45	2.63
SSD = 100 cm (s = ½ L [d/100])														
2	0.04	0.06	0.08	0.10	0.12	0.14	0.16	0.18	0.20	0.22	0.24	0.26	0.28	0.30
4	0.08	0.12	0.16	0.20	0.24	0.28	0.32	0.36	0.40	0.44	0.48	0.52	0.56	0.60
6	0.12	0.18	0.24	0.30	0.36	0.42	0.48	0.54	0.60	0.66	0.72	0.78	0.84	0.90
8	0.16	0.24	0.32	0.40	0.48	0.56	0.64	0.72	0.80	0.88	0.96	1.04	1.12	1.20
10	0.20	0.30	0.40	0.50	0.60	0.70	0.80	0.90	1.00	1.10	1.20	1.30	1.40	1.50
12	0.24	0.36	0.48	0.60	0.72	0.84	0.96	1.08	1.20	1.32	1.44	1.56	1.68	1.80
14	0.28	0.42	0.56	0.70	0.84	0.98	1.12	1.26	1.40	1.54	1.68	1.82	1.96	2.10

**All dimensions are in centimeters; SSD, source-to-skin distance.*

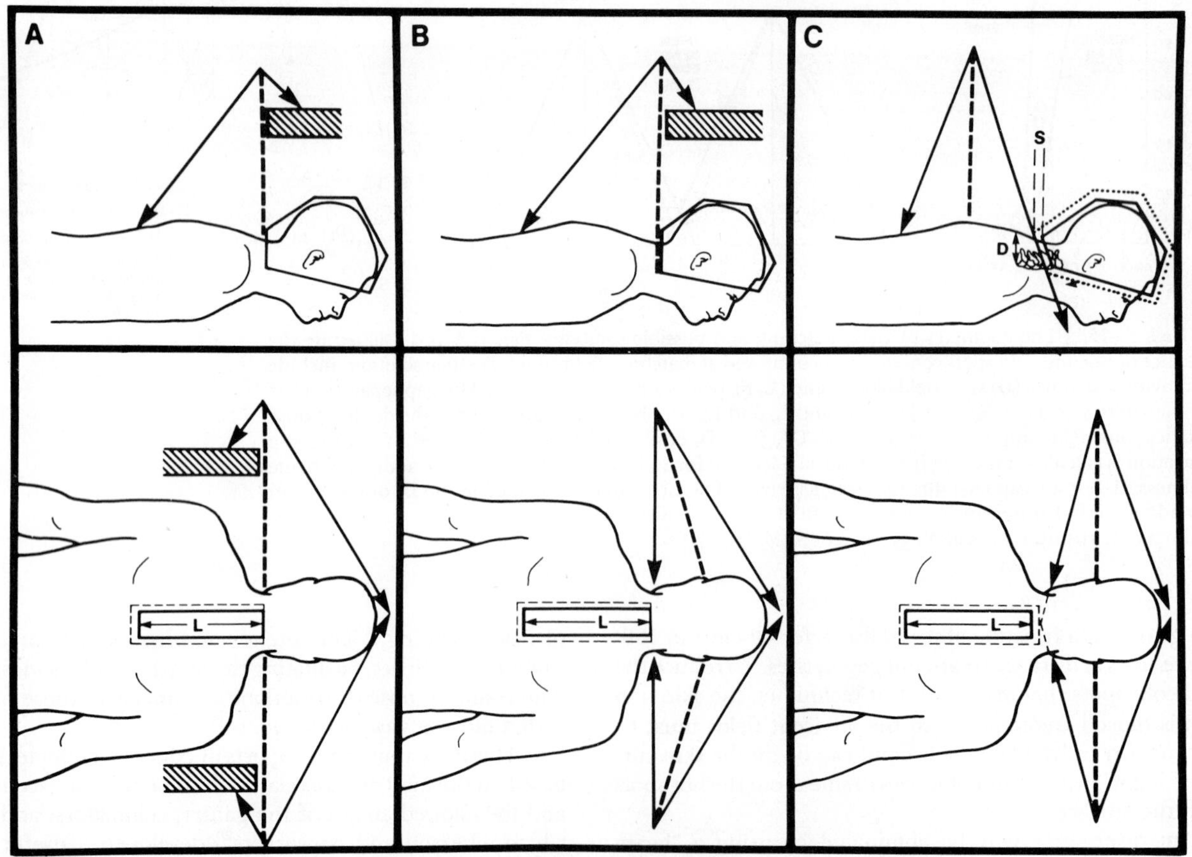

FIGURE 9–26. Some solutions for the problem of overlap for orthogonal fields. (**A**) A beam splitter, a shield that blocks half of the field, is used on the lateral and posterior fields and on the spinal cord portal to match the nondivergent edges of the beams. (**B**) The divergence in the lateral beams may also be removed by angling the lateral beams so that their caudal edges match. Because most therapy units cannot be angled like this, the couch is rotated through small angles in opposite directions to achieve the same effect. (**C**) A gap technique allows the posterior and lateral field to be matched at depth using a gap S on the skin surface. The dashed lines indicate projected field edges at depth D, where the orthogonal fields meet. (Modified from Williamson TJ: Int J Radiat Oncol Biol Phys 5:111, 1979)

Figure 9-26 illustrates the geometry of orthogonal treatments.[75] A common solution to avoid overlap is to use a half-block to ensure that abutting anterior and lateral field edges are perpendicular to the gantry axis; a notch in the posterior corner of lateral oral cavity portals is commonly used to avoid overlap of the spinal cord when midline cord blocks cannot be used on anteroposterior portals when irradiating the lower neck and matched to the oral cavity portals.[75] Other techniques rotate the couch about a vertical axis to compensate for the divergence of the lateral field,[122] with the angle of rotation given by

$$\theta = \tan^{-1}\frac{1}{2}\left(\frac{\frac{1}{2}\text{ field width}}{\text{SAD}}\right)$$

or to leave a gap, S, on the anterior neck surface between the posterior field of length L and lateral field edges,[15,54,77,141] where d is the depth of the spine beneath the posterior field and where

$$S = \frac{1}{2}(L)\left(\frac{d}{\text{SSD}}\right)$$

ELECTRON RADIATION FIELDS

Single Electron Beam Dosimetry

With the increased availability of linacs and microtrons, there is greater use of electron beams to treat superficial lesions. In large therapy centers, about 15% of the patients are treated with electrons at some time during their therapy.

Electron beam dosimetry is remarkably different from megavoltage x-ray dosimetry. As shown in Figure 9-27 and Table 9-4, the central-axis percent depth doses fall off rapidly, particularly at the lower electron energies. The range, in centimeters, of electrons in tissue is approximately one half of their energy, in million electron volts; 12-MeV electrons have a range of about 6 cm. Electrons lose about 2 MeV of energy for each centimeter of tissue transversed, which accounts for their finite ranges. Because electron beams are available on linacs in relatively small energy intervals (3 MeV to 4 MeV), the radiation oncologist must know the lesion depth accurately to select the correct energy. Normally, the 80% or 90% depth isodose curve is used to encompass the target volume; the 80% isodose curve usually lies at a depth (cm) of tissue that is about one third of the electron energy (MeV). Misunderstandings about the target dose at 80% or 90% depth and the given dose at d_{max} are avoided by carefully stating both for the therapy course.

There is usually a significant constriction on the central axis of the 80% isodose line compared with the bulging of the lower percentile isodose curves at the edge of the field, caused by electrons scattering out of the field. Electron-beam dosimetry is unique to each therapy unit, mandating individual dosimetric calculations (Fig. 9-28).

Figure 9-29 shows the electron-beam central-axis doses in the region beneath the entry surfaces. Generally, higher-energy electron beams exhibit a higher surface dose than lower-energy electron beams. There is also less variation in the depth at which the dose reaches its maximum value over the electron beams' energy range than with x-ray beams. With lower-energy electron beams (below 15 MeV) and small field sizes, there is a

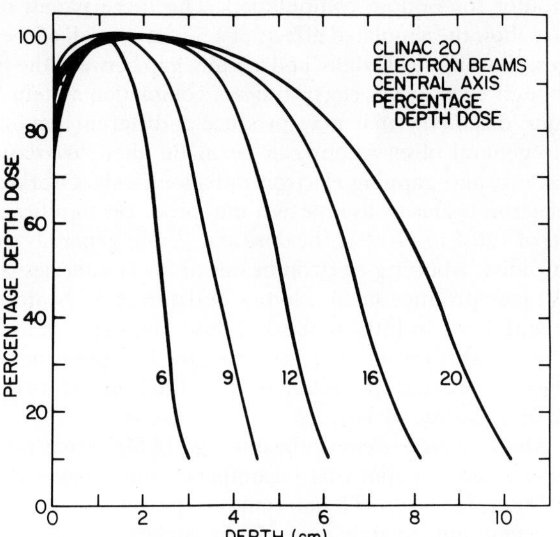

FIGURE 9–27. Electron-beam central axis isodose curves for a 10-cm × 10-cm field at 100-cm SSD. These data are for the Varian Clinac 20 at Mallinckrodt Institute of Radiology, St. Louis, MO.

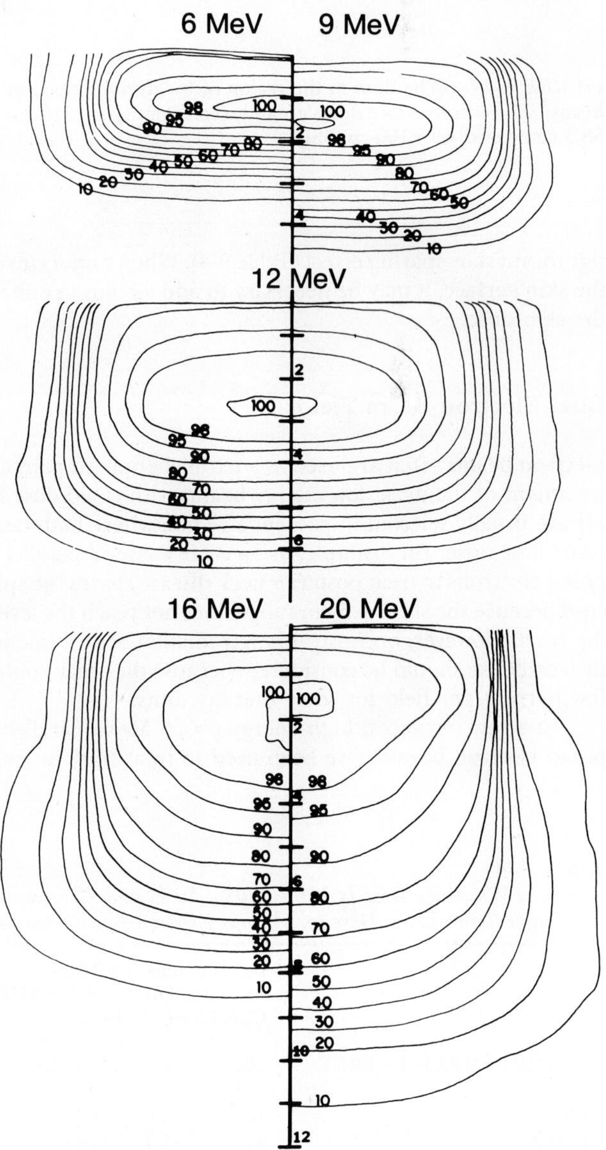

FIGURE 9–28. Typical linac electron beam central axis isodose distributions for a Varian Clinac 20. For comparison, half-field widths are shown in the upper and lower panels.

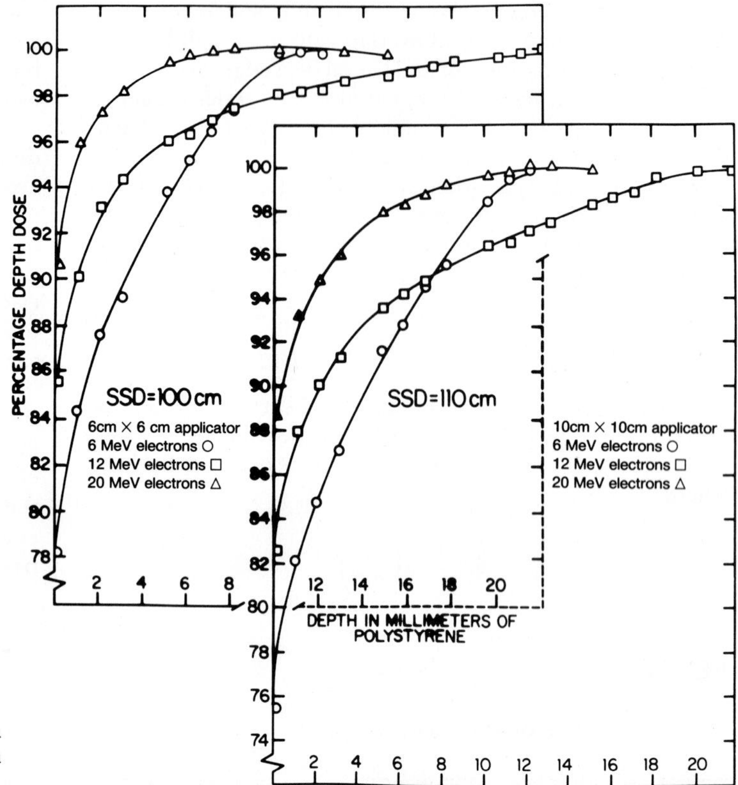

FIGURE 9–29. The dose in the region of buildup for electron beams. The entry-surface doses are reduced somewhat at 110-cm SSD compared with 100-cm SSD.

significant skin-sparing effect (Table 9-4). When tumors involve the skin surface, it may be necessary to add a bolus to enhance the skin dose.

Dual Electron Beam Fields

Electron beams often are used as a parallel opposed pair, as in treatment of the neck; low-energy beams with rapid dose fall-off are usually selected to prevent a region where both beams contribute dose. For example, using 9-MeV lateral parallel opposed electrons to treat posterior neck disease spares the spinal cord because the short 4.5-cm range does not reach the level of the cord. However, bremsstrahlung radiation contributions to the cord dose should be considered, because they may confer a few percent per field for some therapy units.

In a few instances, high-energy (≈ 30 MeV) parallel opposed electron beams have been used to treat thick anatomic areas, but the treatment is not popular because of dosimetry uncertainties, and few machines are capable of producing the high-energy electrons.

TABLE 9–4
Depths at Which the Dose Is 100%, 80%, 50%, and 10% of the Maximum Central-Axis Dose for Various Electron Beam Energies

	DEPTH (cm) VERSUS PERCENTAGE OF MAXIMUM CENTRAL-AXIS DOSE			
ELECTRON BEAM ENERGY	100%	80%	50%	10%
6 MeV	1.4	2.0	2.4	2.9
9 MeV	2.0	3.1	3.6	4.4
16 MeV	3.0	5.7	6.6	7.9
20 MeV	1.9	6.9	8.3	10.1

Adjacent Electron Beam Fields

Electron beams often are used adjacent to one another. Although the problem of matching adjacent electron beams is well documented, the solutions are less evident.

Figure 9-30 displays the isodose curves measured at 7 MeV and 16 MeV and digitized into a radiation therapy planning computer for isodose computation. The three panels of the figure show the simulated effects of a 5-mm overlap of the field edges, abutting field edges, and a 5-mm gap between the fields. Although each linac's electron beam collimation system has a unique dosimetry that may produce a different penumbra, some general observations can be made about overlapping, matching, and gapping electron radiation fields. Overlapping of electron beams by as little as 5 mm produces significant hot spots of 120% to 170% of the dose at d_{max} and generally should be avoided. Abutting electron beams of lower energies (*e.g.*, 7 MeV) may produce small volumes of tissue at the beam edges receiving 110% to 130% of the d_{max} dose. Gaps as large as 5 mm on the skin surface, although reducing the hot spot beneath the surface, leave a cold spot within the first 1 to 2 mm with a dose of 80% of d_{max} dose or less.

Abutting higher-energy beams (*e.g.*, 16 MeV) may produce an elongated hot spot that encompasses more tissue than at lower energies; a gap of 5 mm removes the hot spot but leaves a cold region immediately beneath the surface.

Abutting lower-energy electron fields is the most suitable technique for most clinical situations, particularly for a high skin dose within the first 1 mm of tissue. Abutting 7- or 10-MeV

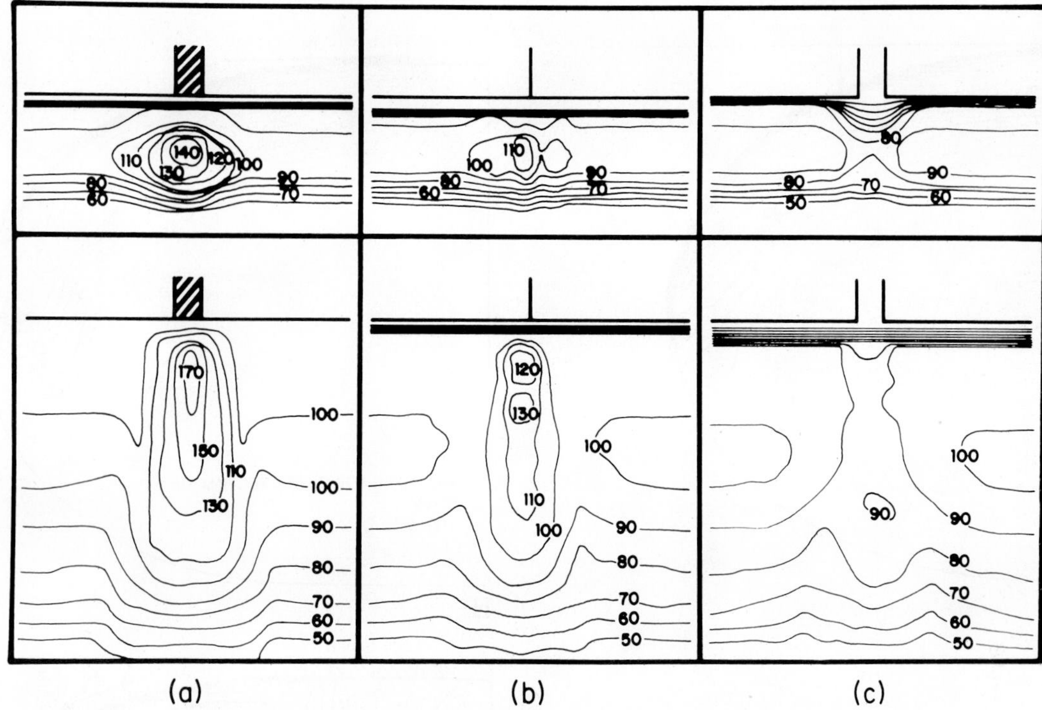

FIGURE 9–30. Adjacent electron fields. For 7-MeV (*upper panels*) and 16-MeV (*lower panels*) electron beams, the dose distributions arise from (**A**) a 5-mm overlap of the fields; (**B**) abutment of the field edges; and (**C**) a 5-mm gap between the field edges.

beams with other 7-, 10-, 13-, or 16-MeV beams on a flat surface, using parallel beams (*i.e.*, no angulation), takes small volumes of tissue at the beam edges to doses that are 110% ± 10% of the given dose. This small overdose can be avoided by gapping the beams no more than 5 mm. However, this takes small volumes of tissues to doses no greater than 80% of the given dose.

Abutting higher-energy electron beams with other high-energy beams (*e.g.*, 13- or 16-MeV beams), produces a somewhat greater hot spot than is produced when abutting lower-energy fields. Substantial volumes of tissue are taken to doses of 120% ± 10%. Moreover, because these higher-energy beams are more penetrating, the hot spot is elongated and encompasses more tissue. Gapping these beams by 5 mm reduces the hot spot to 100% ± 10%. However, this creates a small underdosing in the first few millimeters of tissue. The key point is the clinical need to irradiate the first few millimeters of tissue. Angulation of the beams *away* from one another by

$$\theta = \tan^{-1}\left(\frac{\frac{W}{2}\text{ field width}}{\text{SSD}}\right)$$

where W is the field width, can reduce hot spots.[6] Some clinics have used small junction wedges at beam edges to solve these problems, but very precise dosimetry is required. Angulation of beams *toward* one another increases the magnitude and volume of the hot spots. Angulation frequently occurs when a curved surface is treated, such as the chest wall, and the multiple electron fields produce the hot spots shown in Figure 9-31.

Rotational Electron Beams

Theoretically, rotating an electron beam around a curved surface affords solutions to many of the difficulties encountered in irradiation of curved surfaces with single and multiple electron beams.

The interest in treating with rotational electron beams has spurred various manufacturers of linacs to develop electron arc capabilities for their accelerators. Some systems allow the operator to treat a patient using an electron field in which the dose rate delivered can be varied with the orientation of the gantry. Because the system monitors the gantry position, the operator may enter a predetermined dose rate that is adjusted automatically at the prescribed transition angle. Although electron arc therapy may offer a solution to the problems of abutted or gapped fields and the dose fall-off at the lateral portion of the fields, the technique presents many other technical problems.[104]

Isodose distributions measured in a Lucite chest wall phantom using film dosimetry methods for both fixed-field and arc techniques are shown in Figure 9-31. The single fixed-field technique demonstrates a slightly greater area encompassed by the 80% dose line, although the opposite is true for the 60% dose line. The overall shape of the dose distribution for the arc technique is more clinically acceptable than for the single-field technique. The multiple-field isodose distribution exhibited the same general shape as the arc technique except for the undesirable high-dose areas at the abutted edges. Many aspects of electron arc therapy are under active investigation.[65,82,83]

Large-Field Electron Beams

Certain superficial skin lesions that cover large skin areas, such as mycosis fungoides, can be treated with electron total-body irradiation. Basic requirements are a large field with uniform flatness over a major portion of the field, high dose rates of several tens of centigrays per minute, and low x-ray contamination. Radiation techniques include rotating the patient in fixed electron beams, moving the patient linearly beneath the beam, and multiple fixed-field methods employing from two to eight

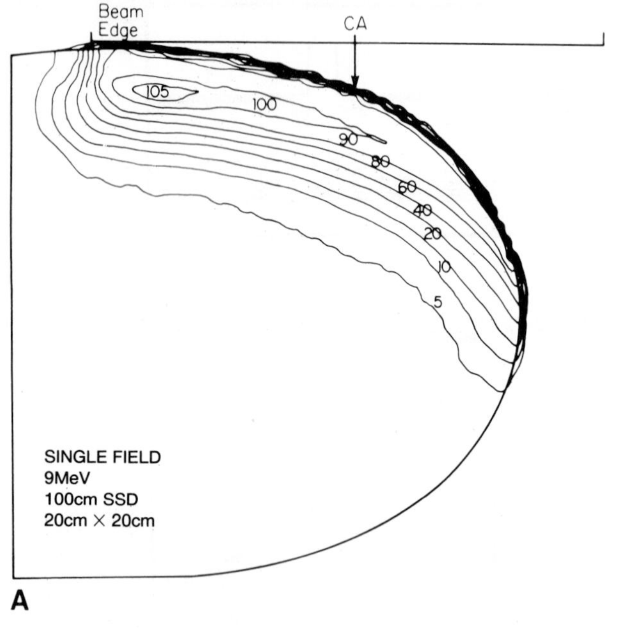

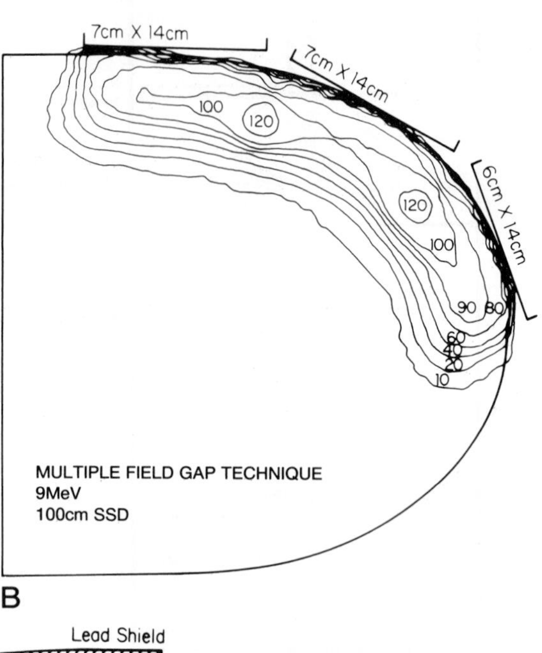

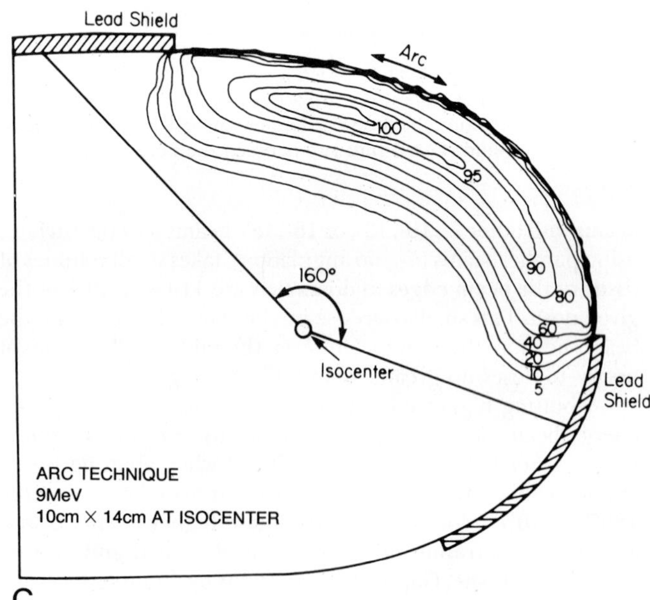

FIGURE 9–31. Electron dose distributions on a curved surface. (**A**) Single fixed-field technique (9 MeV, 100-cm SSD, 20 cm × 20 cm). (**B**) Multiple-field gap technique (9 MeV, 100-cm SSD). (Courtesy of R. Gerber, St. Louis, MO). (**C**) Arc technique (9 MeV, 10 cm × 14 cm at isocenter).

overlapping fields.[25,59,108] The technique used at Mallinckrodt Institute of Radiology was modeled after the Stanford University six-field technique.[103] The dosimetry of numerous techniques has been reviewed by Almond.[2]

For total-body irradiation, a 7-MeV beam with beam degraders gives the most suitable dose distributions (Fig. 9-32). To treat the total skin surface adequately requires a large field size, a uniform dose across the field, suitable combinations of fields to cover the skin, adequate depth dose, and reasonable treatment time. A distance of 300 cm from the electron source was chosen to provide a large field without unduly increasing the treatment time. To achieve a suitable uniformity of dose across the large field, a dual-field arrangement was used (Fig. 9-32 inset).

Figure 9-32 also shows the six treatment fields: anterior, right posterior oblique, left posterior oblique, posterior, right anterior oblique, and left anterior oblique. Three fields at 120 degrees to one another are treated on alternate days; 2 treatment days are required to treat all six fields.

A specially designed treatment stand was constructed to position the patient for total-body irradiation. The stand was equipped with handles for patient support and positioning reproducibility. Each of the six treatment fields is delivered with the gantry angled at 290 degrees for half of the treatment and 250 degrees for the other half. Hands may be shielded with lead gloves, fingernails with lead cutouts, and eyes with lead shields.

THE IRRADIATED MEDIUM

The previous dosimetry of x-ray and electron beams was theoretical; we assumed that the radiation beams were incident on a homogeneous flat tissue-equivalent medium of infinite thickness and semiinfinite extent (Fig. 9-33). Physicists approximate this medium by using large phantoms of nearly tissue-equivalent material (*e.g.*, a large tank of water or a polyethylene phantom) for dosimetry measurements. There must be an adequate margin (usually 5 cm) between the edges of the beam and the

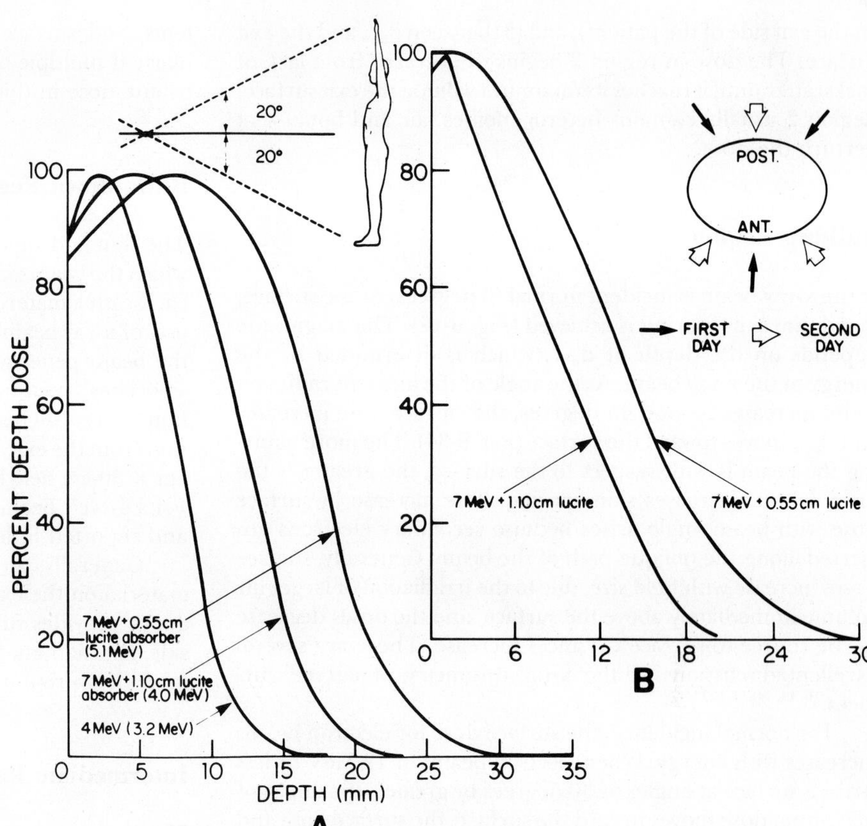

FIGURE 9–32. (**A**) Relative depth dose at the midplane treatment point for a single 20-degree dual-field irradiation with degraded 7-MeV electron beams. (**B**) Beam angulation and treatment sequence for the 6-field electron beams for treating mycosis fungoides.

phantom to provide full scattering of radiation to the central axis of the beam, and the phantoms must be thick enough to provide full backscatter radiation to points of dose measurement at certain depths in the phantom.

A patient is a finite medium, containing tissue and heterogeneities, with an irregularly shaped surface (Figure 9-33). Three distinct dosimetry regions are: (1) between the skin surface and the depth of maximum ionization, frequently called the buildup region because the dose builds to its maximum value in this region; (2) from d_{max} to d_{min}, where d_{min} is the farthest depth from the entry surface that receives full scatter radiation from the surrounding points (d_{min} coincides with d_{max}

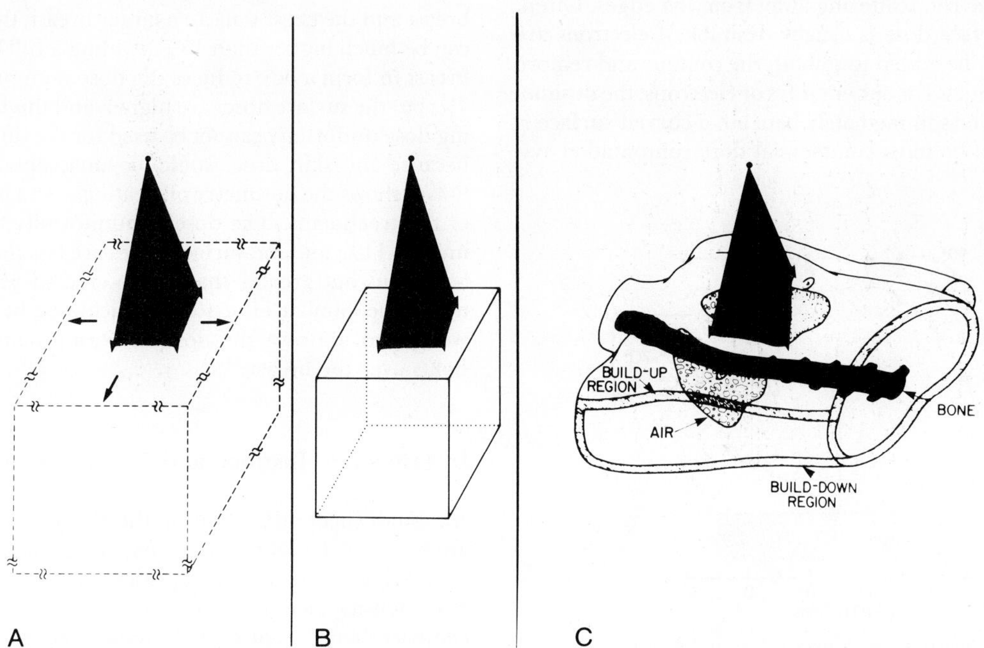

FIGURE 9–33. (**A**) Radiation incident on an infinitely thick tissue-equivalent medium of semi-infinite extent. (**B**) A large, nearly tissue-equivalent phantom used for dosimetry. (**C**) The stylized patient: a finite, thin medium of irregular shape containing heterogeneities.

on the exit side of the patient); and (3) between d_{min} and the exit surface. The dose in region 3 begins to decrease from lack of backscatter until it reaches its minimum value at the exit surface. Region 2 usually contains heterogeneities (air and bone) that perturb the dose.

Buildup Region

If the x-ray beam is incident normal (0 degrees) to the surface, maximum skin sparing is achieved (Fig. 9-12). The magnitude depends on the depth of d_{max}, which is determined by the energy of the x-ray beam. As the angle of the incident radiation beam increases beyond 45 degrees, the surface dose increases and d_{max} moves toward the surface (Fig. 9-34). The more glancing the beam is with respect to the surface, the greater is the dose, which decreases skin sparing. The increase in surface dose with beam angle arises because secondary electrons are ejected along the oblique path of the beam. Generally, surface doses increase with field size, due to the irradiation of larger air volume immediately above the surface, and the doses decrease as the source-to-surface distances increase. There are several excellent discussions of the x-ray dosimetry of curved surfaces.[16,44,54,72,127]

For normal incidence, the surface dose for electron beams increases with energy. When electron beams of 12 MeV or less strike a surface at angles of 30 degrees or greater, the depth of maximum dose moves toward the surface, the surface dose and the dose in the buildup region increase, and the depth of the 90% and 80% isodose curves is decreased (Fig. 9-35).[7,34] Above 12 MeV, there is little increase in surface dose as the angle of incidence increases, and the decrease in the depths of the 90% and 80% isodose curves is less pronounced.[7]

On a smoothly curved surface, such as an arm, these effects generally increase the doses on the lateral surfaces, and substantial overdosing can occur at these points if parallel opposed electrons beams are used. However, a sharp surface irregularity (*e.g.*, protrusion) can cause scattering away from the irregularity, producing a hot spot (Fig. 9-36).[69] Conversely, a depression produces electron scattering away from the edges. Often, because high surface dose is usually desirable if electrons are used, a bolus may be added to smooth the contour and remove surface irregularities. For either x-rays or electrons, the dosimetry a few millimeters immediately beneath a curved surface is not modeled well by most commercial dose computation systems, and surface dose measurements are required, particularly if multiple beams are employed and exiting beams contribute dose in this region.

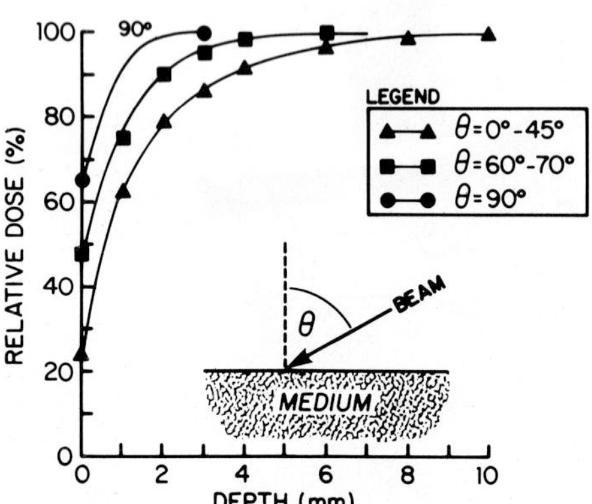

FIGURE 9–34. The variation of surface dose and depth of maximum dose as a function of the angle of incidence of the x-ray beam with the surface (4 MV, 10 cm × 10 cm).

Build-down Region and Exit Doses

The skin and superficial tissue on the side of the patient from which the beam exits receive a reduced dose if there is not much backscatter material. The amount of dose reduction is a function of x-ray beam energy, field size, and the thickness of tissue the beam penetrated reaching the exit surface. Gagnon and associates[47] measured a 16% reduction in dose at a depth of 0.01 mm for a cobalt beam penetrating 7.7 cm or 15 cm of tissue. At 1 mm from the exit surface, the dose was reduced by 8% for a 30-cm × 30-cm field but by only 3% to 4% for a 6-cm × 6-cm field. For a 6-MeV beam, Purdy[114] measured a 15% reduction in dose and reported little dependency on field size.

Generally, the addition of a thickness of tissue-equivalent material on the exit side equal to about two thirds of the d_{max} depth provides full dose to the build-down region on the exit side. For high-energy beams (*e.g.*, 25 MV), the dose reduction is much less pronounced.

Intermediate Region and Surface Curvature

The region between d_{max} and d_{min} contains the target volume. Here the effects of surface irregularities and heterogeneities on the dose distributions are a primary concern.

When x-ray beams strike a curved surface, the isodose curves at depths tend to follow the surface curvature. Methods for correcting isodose curves for air gaps and surface obliquity at depths beyond d_{max} are presented in Chapter 8.

The single-beam isodose curves generally follow the curvature of the surface (Fig. 9-37). When the opposing beam is added, the dose nonuniformity is about 15% between the apex of the breast and the 100% isodose line, which, in this example, was selected at two thirds of the separation between apex of the breast and the chest wall. In a larger breast, the nonuniformity can be much higher than 15%. Adding a full bolus around the breast to form a box reduces the dose nonuniformity to about 7%, but the surface doses are higher, and this method of achieving dose uniformity cannot be used for the duration of therapy because the skin dose would be unacceptably high. Figure 9-37D shows the dosimetry of treating with a bolus for only half of the treatments. The dose nonuniformity becomes approximately 11%, and the surface doses are less than those with the box bolus but greater than those created with an open-field technique. Similar effects can be achieved by using 30-degree wedges to improve the dose uniformity and a thin-contour bolus over the breast.[44]

Intermediate Regions and Patient Heterogeneities

Although small differences in the electron densities of tissues are used in CT to distinguish tissues, for radiation therapy, the human body is adequately represented by a cruder, five-component density model: normal tissue, air, lung, soft bone, and compact bone. Figure 9-38 shows the correlations of CT numbers with the physical and electron densities of materials; both methods have been used in algorithms for dose calcula-

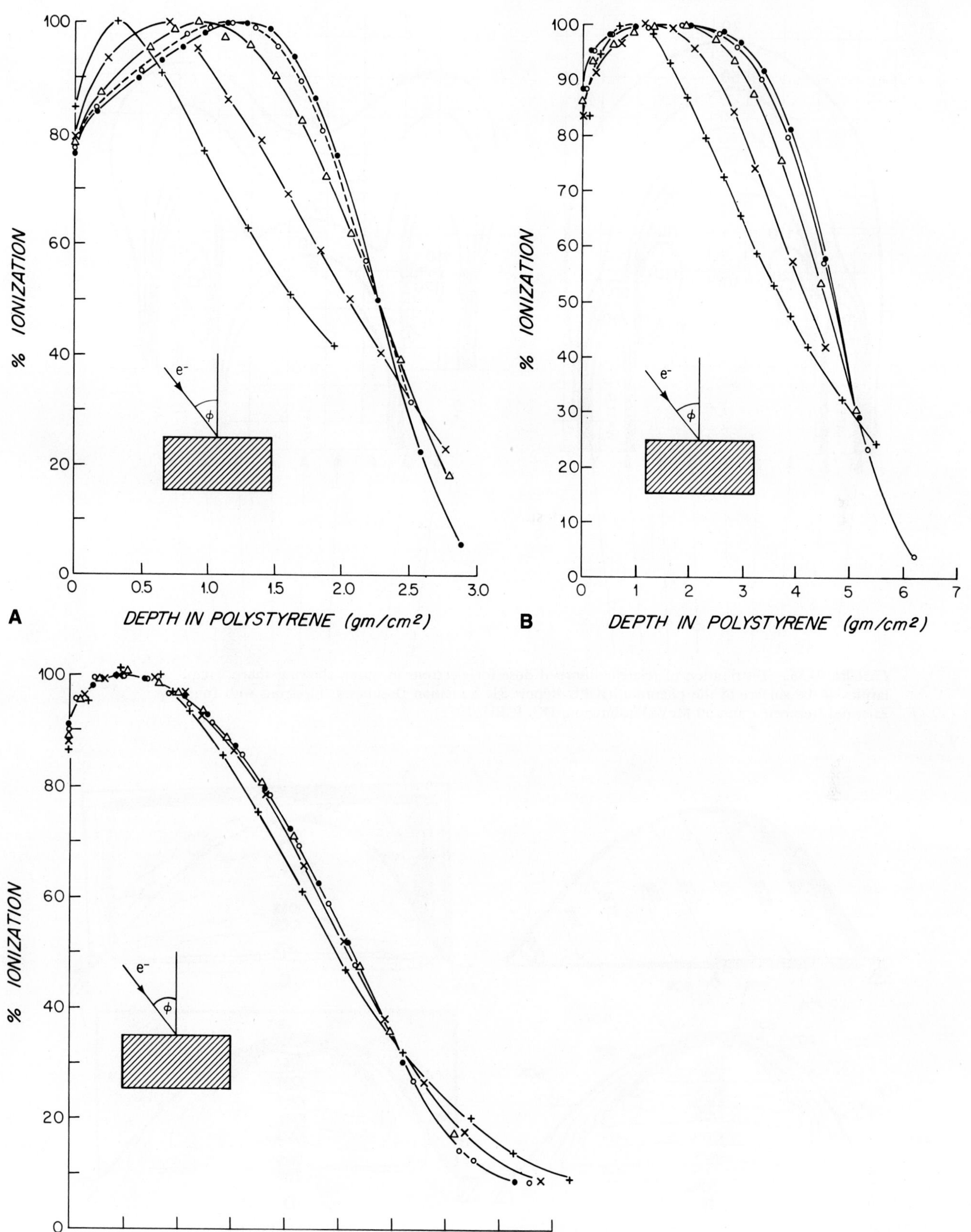

FIGURE 9–35. Curves plotting the percent of ionization for (**A**) 6-MeV electrons, (**B**) 12-MeV electrons, and (**C**) 18-MeV electrons for a 6 × 6 cm^2 field. Notice that the depth is measured along the central axis of the beam. φ = 0° (•), φ = 15° (○), φ = 30° (Δ), φ = 45° (×) and φ = 60° (+). (Biggs PJ: Am Assoc Med Dosim J 9:25, 1984)

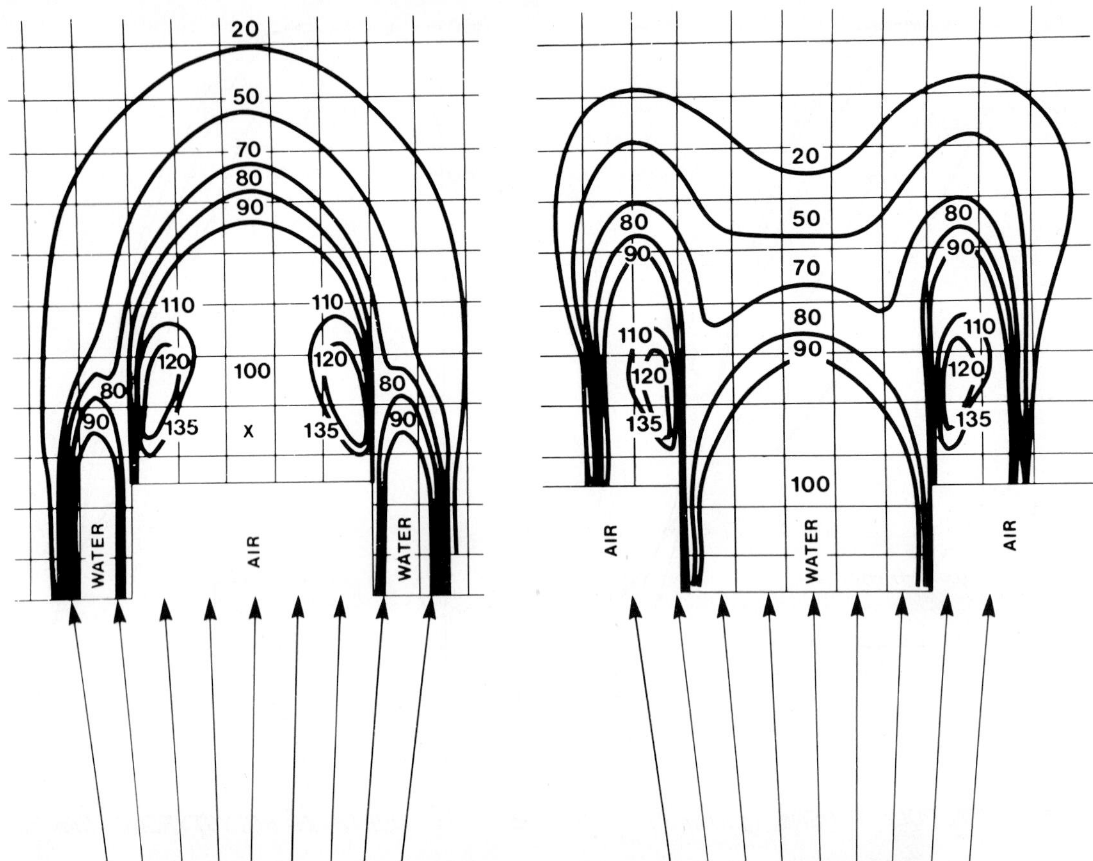

FIGURE 9–36. Distribution of relative absorbed dose for electrons in water, showing sharp irregularities at the surface of the phantom. (ICRU Report 21: Radiation Dosimetry: Electrons with Initial Energies Between 1 and 50 MeV. Washington, DC, ICRU, 1972)

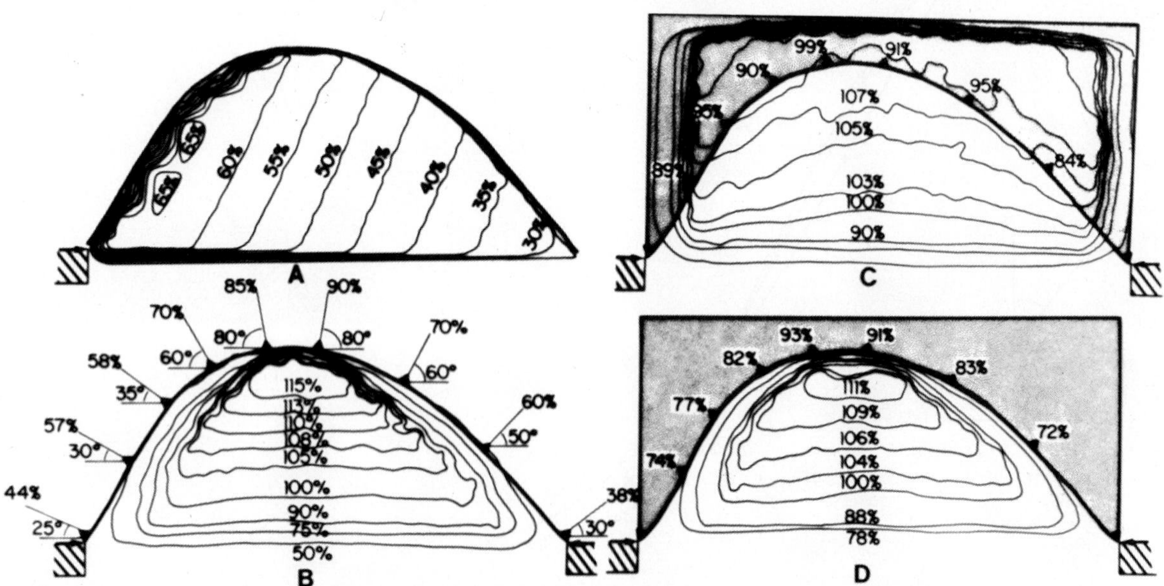

FIGURE 9–37. (**A**) Dose distributions for a single 4-MV x-ray beam, 16 cm × 16 cm, on a curved surface (breast) with a half-field block. (**B**) Composite isodose curves for breast treatment from parallel opposed tangential beams, using a half-field block. The points on the surface depict the angle the beam makes with the surface and the entry dose expressed as a percentage; surface measurements include contributions from both beams. Because of tangential incidence, these doses increase as the angles increase. (**C**) Adding a full-box bolus yields dose uniformity but produces higher skin doses. (**D**) Using a box bolus for only half of the treatments yields an acceptable dose uniformity and intermediate surface doses. All surface doses were measured with thin TLDs; the computer-generated isodose curves were also confirmed by thermoluminescent dosimetry.

tions, but dose calculation corrections using electron densities are more correct.[106,111] The perturbing effects of air, lung, and bone are caused by their different physical and electron densities and by the physical size of the heterogeneities and how they alter the primary and scatter radiations to the normal tissue surrounding the heterogeneities. Several methods of dose corrections are presented in Chapter 8, and the topic is being actively investigated.

Small air cavities (*e.g.*, air passage in the trachea) allow transmission of a higher dose to the region behind the cavity, but surface effects (*e.g.*, loss of buildup at the cavity surfaces) can cause underdosing at the edges of the cavity.[102]

Larger cavities, such as the lung, perturb the dose in several ways, and dose-correction algorithms are being investigated.[37,130] Figure 9-39 compares the transmission measured throughout the lung of an anthropomorphic phantom using a ^{60}Co and a 25-MV, single x-ray beam. There is an increased transmission of radiation through the lower-density lung; at a depth of 17 cm, the ratio of correction to uncorrected ^{60}Co isodose curves in the lung is about 1.54 (57% to 37%), and for 25 MV, the ratio is about 1.24 (62% to 50%) at the same depth. The dose to the mediastinum is altered because there is less scatter to the mediastinum than if the lungs were tissue equivalent. The availability of complete three-dimensional anatomy from multiple CT scans combined with improved three-dimensional computational algorithms will provide more accurate dose heterogeneity correction in the future.

The dose to bone and the dose to tissue beyond bone must be considered separately. Because much of the bone in the body is not compact, corrections again depend on the availability of CT scans to provide electron densities for dose-correction algorithms. Henson and Fox[64] showed that the relative electron density of bone may be estimated within 5% accuracy from measured CT numbers. Although compact bone attenuates the beam, reducing the dose to the normal tissue beyond the bone, the dose to the bone is determined by the f factor for photon energies less than 3 MV; for cobalt, this factor is slightly less than for tissue. Usually, bone is ignored in megavoltage treatment planning.

The influence of air and bone on electron-beam dose distributions are being investigated. The concept of a coefficient of equivalent thickness, introduced by Laughlin,[81] is widely used clinically to estimate the effects of these heterogeneities. Isodose curves are shifted by a thickness, Z × CET, where CET is the coefficient of equivalent thickness, with the values of the shift depending on the energy of the beam. The absorption equivalent thickness method uses the ratios of physical and electron densities to calculate an equivalent thickness of water or tissue to that of the heterogeneity, and Muller-Runkel and Vijayakumar[100] provide an excellent summary of this correction applied to bone. Hogstrom[66] investigated the perturbing effects of small bone and air cavities, and Figure 9-40 shows the general features of the correction for a 17-MeV beam using a "pencil-beam" algorithm. The increased use of CT data for isodose computations will probably create greater interest in making these corrections.

The problem facing the radiation oncologist is a practical decision about the clinical necessity of making heterogeneity corrections. Current correction algorithms for photon- and electron-beam heterogeneities are much improved over earlier correction algorithms, and heterogeneity corrections are being used more frequently by radiation oncologists; these corrections will probably soon become standard practice.

MODIFICATIONS TO THE RADIATION FIELDS

Often the radiation fields must be modified to achieve desired dose distributions and to correct for some of the perturbing influences previously discussed. The five most frequently used

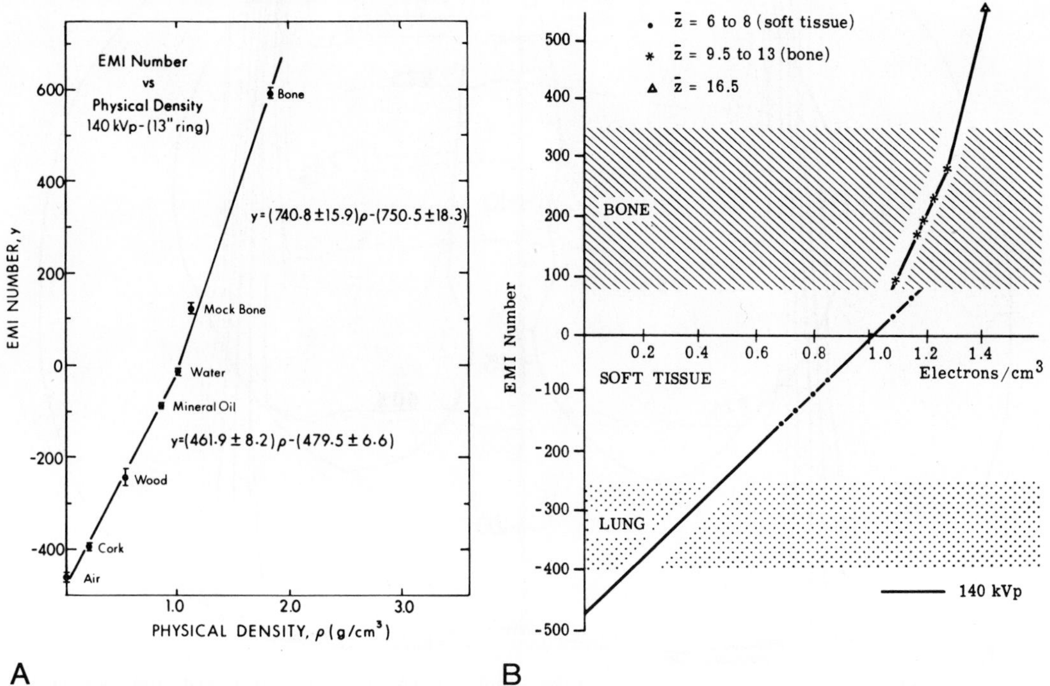

FIGURE 9–38. (**A**) Correlation of computed tomographic (CT) numbers with the physical densities of various materials for a scan at 140 kVp. (Prasad SC, Glasgow GP, Purdy JA: Radiology 13:777, 1979). (**B**) Correlation of CT number with the electron densities of various materials for a scan at 140 kVp. (Parker RP, Hobday PA, Cassell KL: Phys Med Biol 24:802, 1979)

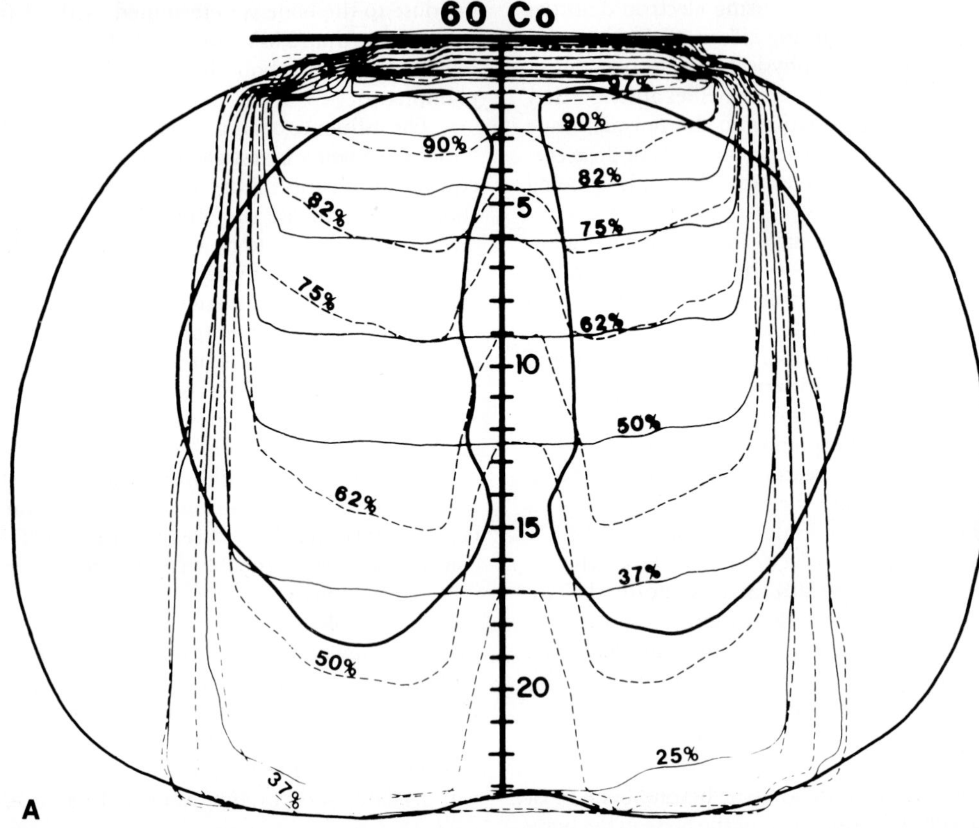

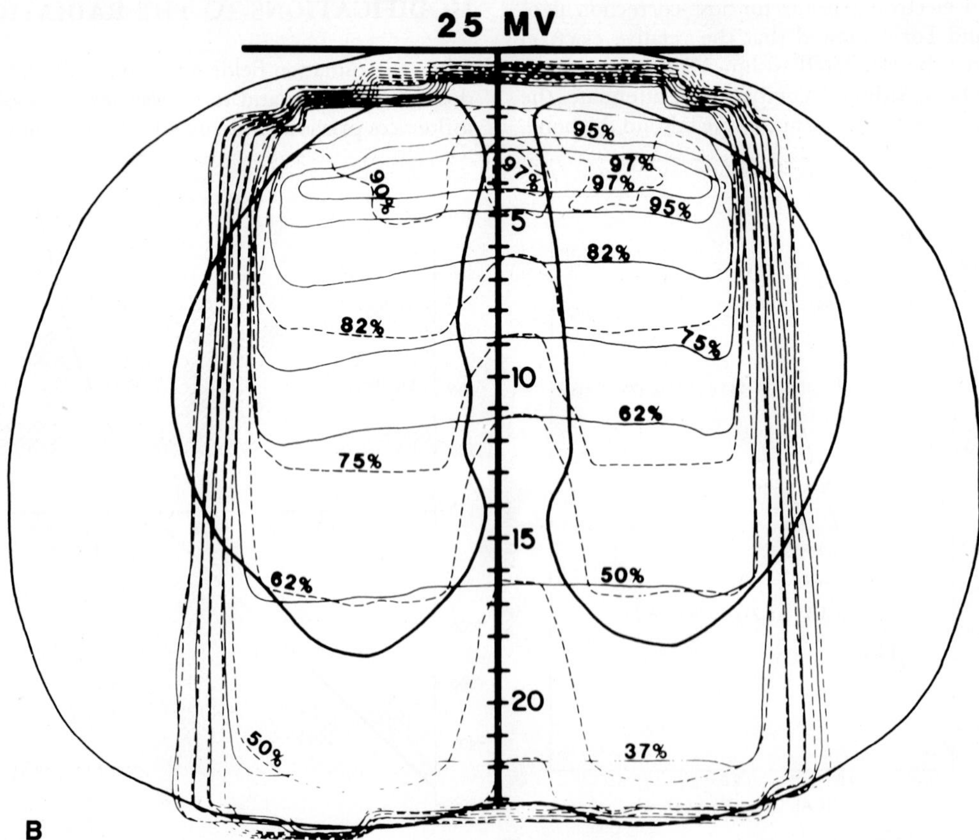

FIGURE 9–39. Dose distributions for single ^{60}Co (80-cm SSD) γ-rays (**A**) and 25-MV (100-cm SSD) x-rays (**B**), 16-cm × 16-cm fields, demonstrating the increased transmission in the lung and the effect of the inhomogeneity corrections in the computed treatment-plan dose distributions. The solid lines are the isodose curves, assuming a homogeneous medium; the dashed lines are the isodose curves including lung heterogeneity.

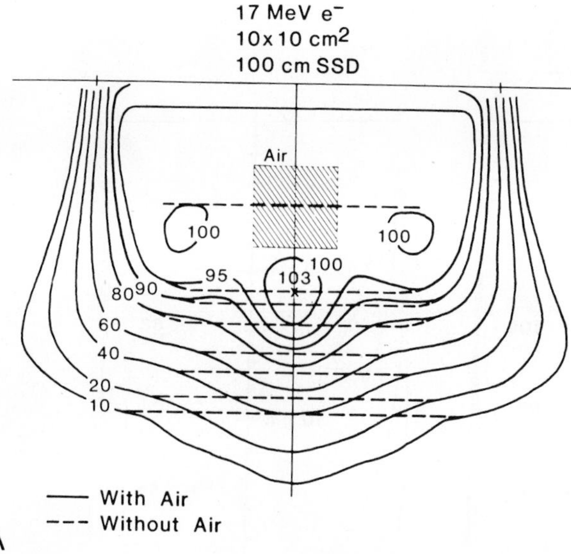

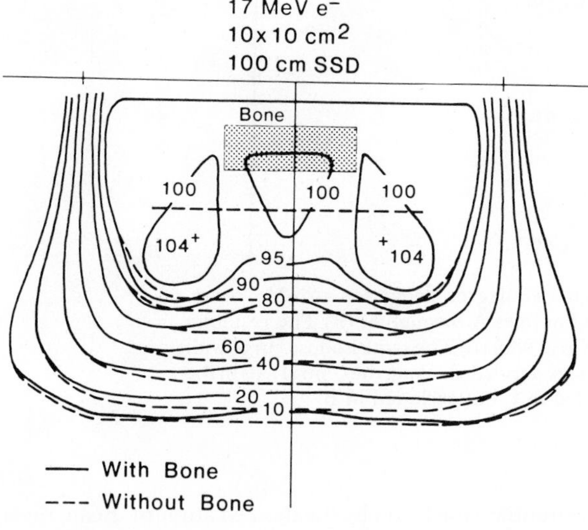

FIGURE 9–40. Perturbation in electron-beam dose distribution by (**A**) air and (**B**) bone. (Hogstrom K: Dosimetry of electron heterogeneities. In Wright AE, Boyer AL (eds): Advances in Radiation Therapy Treatment Planning. New York, American Institute of Physics, 1983)

methods of beam modification are bolus, wedges, missing tissue compensators, heterogeneity compensators, and critical-organ-shielding blocks. All involve changing the radiation beam characteristics in the incident direction of the beam and transverse to this direction, in one or two dimensions.

Bolus

A tissue-equivalent bolus should have electron density, physical density, and atomic number similar to that of tissue or water. Inexpensive, nearly tissue-equivalent materials used as a bolus in radiation therapy include slabs of paraffin wax, rice bags filled with soda, and gauze coated with petrolatum.[140] These forms of bolus are not as equivalent to tissue as some of the newer, synthetic-based substances, such as "Super-Flab," "Super-Stuff," Elastomeric Polymer, and Elasto-Gel.[8,18,98]

Generally, thin slabs of bolus that follow the surface contour increase the dose to the skin beneath the bolus if the bolus thickness is approximately equal to the d_{max} depth for the x-ray beam. For electron beams with higher entry doses, the addition of only a few millimeters of bolus adequately increases the skin dose. Nontissue materials, such as lead, are used as bolus, but the dosimetry is more complex than for a nearly tissue-equivalent bolus.[99]

An irregular surface may be smoothed by adding a bolus to fill the tissue deficit, and an external cavity, such as the ear canal or nasal passage, also can accommodate a bolus. A bolus can be shaped to alter the dose distribution, but normally missing-tissue compensators or wedges are usually employed to alter the dose distribution and retain the skin-sparing effects. Sharp edges on a bolus should be avoided for photons and electrons; outscattering from the sharp edges produces hot spots.[69]

Wedges

A wedge bends the dose distribution at some specified depth to some desired angle relative to the incident beam direction over the entire transverse dimension of the radiation beam. For cobalt units, the depth of the 50% isodose usually is specified for the wedge angle; for higher-energy linacs, higher-percentile isodose curves, such as an 80% curve, or the isodose curves at a specific depth, are used to define the wedge angle (Fig. 9-41). On cobalt units, wedges designed for specific field sizes (nonuniversal wedges) were required to keep the dose rate of the unit within a useful clinical range. On modern linacs, these wedges have been replaced with multiple wedges (universal) that may be used with an allowed range of field sizes. Some newer linacs feature a single wedge (autowedge) with the desired wedge angle obtained by fractional use.

Although wedges can be designed for any desired angle, 15-, 30-, 45-, or 60-degree wedges are most common. The wedged isodose curves can be normalized in two ways. Older ^{60}Co wedge dose distributions had the wedge factor (*i.e.*, the ratio of the measured central axis dose rate without and with the wedge) incorporated into the wedged isodose distribution. The current practice normalizes the wedged isodose curves to 100% at d_{max} and employs a wedge factor to calculate the actual treatment time. McCullough and associates[92] noticed that these wedge factors are correct to 2% to a depth of 10 cm; at greater depths, the wedge factor defined at d_{max} is accurate to 5% or less. Modern linacs have a wedge interlock to prevent mistreatments arising from the use of an incorrect wedge or to prevent treatment without a wedge if one is required.

By the proper combination of wedged and unwedged treatment, an effective wedge angle, Θ_{eff}, may be achieved that is less than the wedge angle being employed Θ_n. $\Theta_{eff} = \Theta_n/F$, where F is the ratio of the dose from the open field, D_{open}, to $D_{open} + D_{wedge}$ (*i.e.*, the sum of doses from the unwedged and wedged fields). This relationship has been verified by several authors for many photon energies and is the basis of single autowedges on some linacs.[1,143] Wedged fields are commonly arranged so that the angle between the beams, the *hinge angle*, ϕ, is related to the *wedge angle*, Θ, by $\Theta = 90$ degrees $- \phi/2$. For example, 45-degree wedges orthogonal to one another yield a uniform dose distribution (Fig. 9-16).

Compensating Filters

Another form of beam modifier is a compensator, so named because its addition to the radiation field is intended to compen-

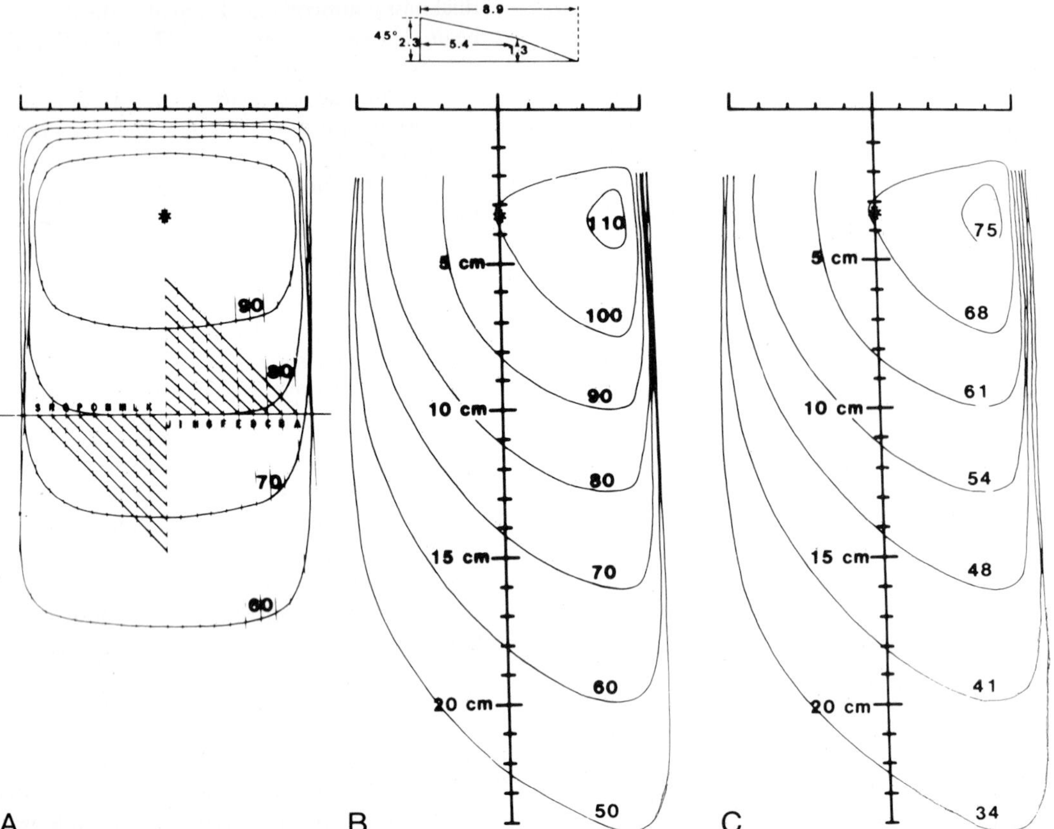

FIGURE 9–41. (**A**) A 10-cm × 10-cm isodose plot to design a 45-degree wedge for a 25-MV beam. Parallel lines at 45 degrees intersect the central axis and the fan lines A through S. (**B**) The resulting wedged isodose curve. (Abrath FG, Purdy JA: Radiology 136:757, 1980) (**C**) The same isodose curve with the wedge factor included. Notice the differences in the percentage depth dose along the central axis in the two wedged isodose curves. The wedge factor, 0.68, is included in C but excluded in B.

sate for some topographic deficit, such as "missing tissue" (Fig. 9-42). A bolus placed in the tissue deficit on the patient is the simplest way to compensate, but because it diminishes the skin-sparing effects, retracted tissue compensators are usually employed. Tissue compensation depends on the field size, x-ray beam energy, depth of target volume, compensator material and thickness, and distance of compensator from the topographic deficit.[12] A nearly tissue-equivalent compensator made of wax, Lucite, or solid water generally must have a thickness less than the missing tissue deficit to correct for the lack of scatter produced with retracted compensators.[26, 117] Compensators are designed to compensate to a specified depth, for a given geometry, and for a specified beam energy. Overcompensation (less dose) usually occurs above and undercompensation (more dose) below the specified compensator depth.[12] Purdy and colleagues[116] developed a one-dimensional compensating system tailored for a patient's chest curvature using Lucite plates. The source-to-skin distance is set to the highest point of the anatomic area (chest) to be irradiated (Fig. 9-43) A sagittal contour of the chest is obtained, and the number of layers of Lucite, each with thickness equivalent to 1 cm of tissue, is obtained. Figure 9-43B shows the degree of compensation achieved.

Ellis and associates[40] developed a practical two-dimensional compensator system that is widely used. A rod-box device, a formulator, is used to measure the tissue deficit in a 1-cm grid over the treatment surface. Aluminum or brass blocks of appropriate thicknesses are then mounted on a tray above the patient to attenuate the beam by the desired amount. Beam divergency may also be incorporated into this system. Clark and Evans[21] describe a standard compensator for ear, nose, and throat therapy fields. Boge and colleagues[10] describe a device that routs a pattern in a mold that can then be filled with a compensator material like wax. Improved designs use low-melting-point bismuth alloys, polyethylene lead, and gypsum mixed with fine particles of steel or iron as attenuating material.[63, 124, 138]

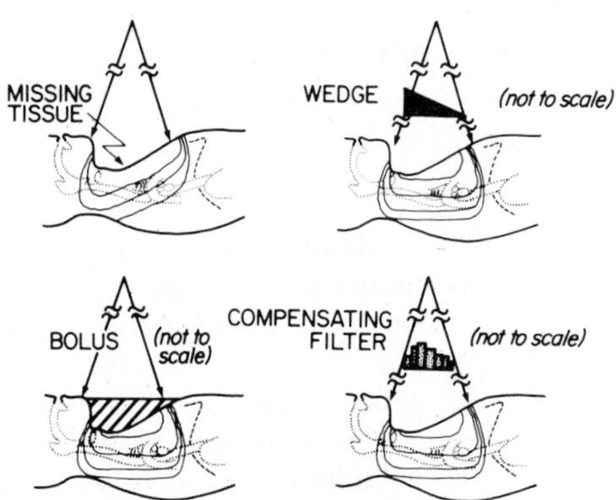

FIGURE 9–42. Schematic diagrams illustrating the principles of compensation for "missing" tissue or tissue deficits with a bolus, wedge, or compensator filter.

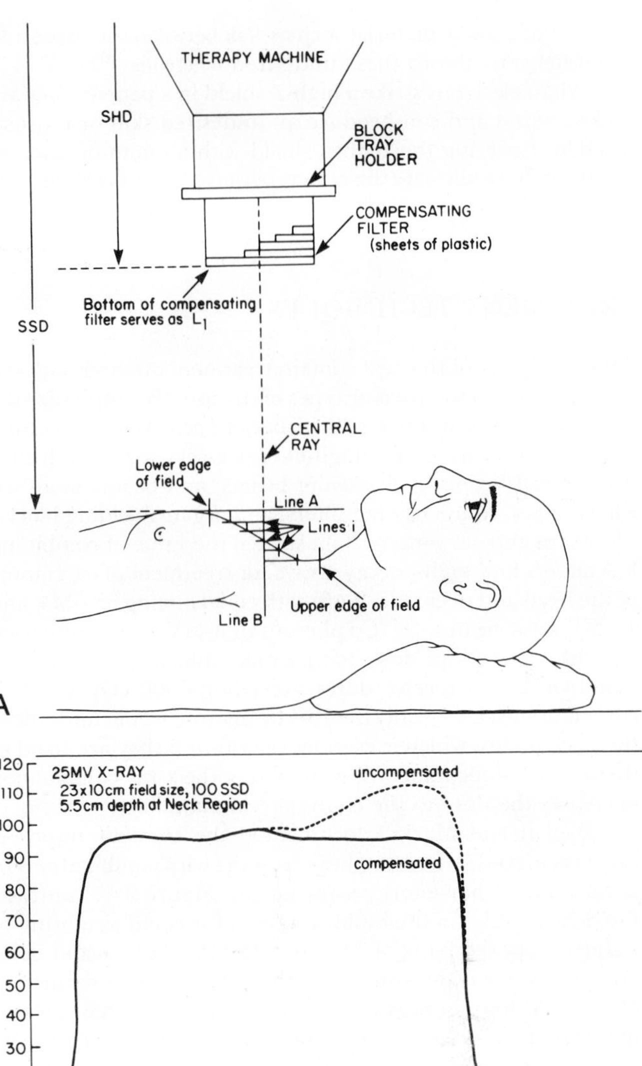

FIGURE 9–43. (A) Design of a one-dimensional chest compensator for a 25-MV x-ray beam using Lucite plates. (**B**) Sagittal dose profile with and without the compensator.

The literature is replete with discussions of manual and optical methods of measuring the patient's topography. Manual techniques include topography tracing, formulators (*i.e.*, contouring gauge or rod boxes), and using a stylus to perturb a magnetic field established around the patient.[3,139] Optical methods include stereoradiography, Moire fringe patterns, video camera recordings of dot patterns, laser lines, or other patterns projected onto the patient.[13,52,126]

The topography obtained is processed, and automatic milling machines are used to prepare the compensator from a suitable material. Compensators need not be limited to compensating for missing tissue. Dixon and colleagues[31] describe a method of film dosimetry used to measure the differential exit doses through the treatment volume. Compensating material is then added to achieve a uniform exit dose, compensating for both topography and heterogeneities. Serial CT scans provide information for designing compensators for heterogeneities within the patient and for topography deficits.

Blocks Shielding Critical Organs

Frequently, the target volume is immediately above, behind, or adjacent to a critical organ, and the radiation therapist faces the difficult task of treating the target volume while maintaining the dose to the critical organ below some tolerance level. Tables 5-13 and 5-15 list some frequently used tolerance doses for these organs, but these doses are not unconditional recommendations; often larger doses may be given to small fractional volumes of these organs.

Doses to critical organs may be limited by using a full shield, usually 5 HVL (3.125% transmission) or 6 HVL (1.562% transmission), or a partial transmission shield, such as a single HVL (50% transmission) of shielding material.

The true percentage dose level is usually greater than the percentage stated because of scatter radiation beneath the blocks from adjacent unshielded portions of the field, and the dose level generally increases with depth as more radiation scatters into the volume beneath the shield. The exact transmission is a function of block material, thickness, and width, field size, and energy. These blocks change the energy characteristics of the beam in a complex manner.[38] Clinically, the radiation oncologist must compare the radiation biology of allowing an organ to reach its full-tolerance dose over a portion of the therapy course and then using a full shield for the remainder of the course to a partial shield designed to allow the organ to reach its tolerance dose over the full therapy course.

Although lead can be used, low-melting-point bismuth alloys that can be easily shaped to cover a critical organ are widely used for construction of organ shields, and Figure 9-44 shows the transmission coefficients for common x-ray energies.[17,68] Mass attenuation, linear attenuation, and mass energy absorption coefficients are now available for these alloys.[36] Most organ shields are static; they are simply placed on the shielding tray attached to the therapy unit. Gravity-oriented spinal shields and eye shields have been developed for rotational therapy.[43,113]

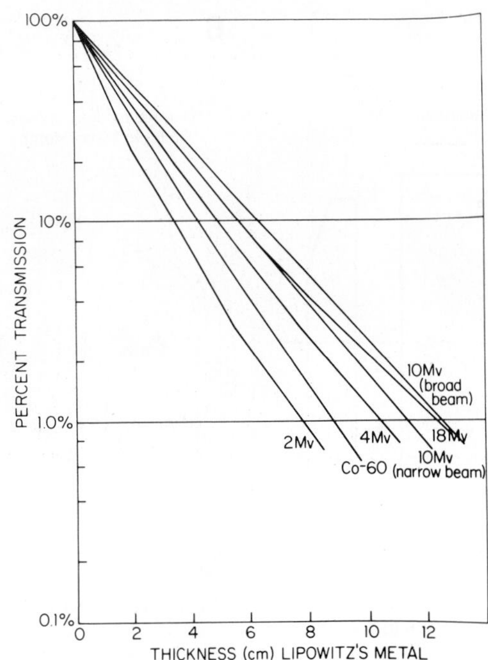

FIGURE 9–44. Beam x-ray transmission of Lipowitz's metal. (Huen A, Findley DO, Skov DD: Med Phys 6:147, 1979)

An organ shield must be properly positioned to cover the organ, and the radiation oncologist must ensure that it is properly constructed. Organ shields do perturb the beam and beam output. Figure 9-45 illustrates how an off-axis spinal shield in a 4-MV treatment portal reduced the dose to the small port generated by the shield. Often, one or two extra treatments to such small ports are required to deliver the desired dose to the entire target volume.

When high-Z shielding blocks are placed in higher-energy electron beams, the electrons produce a very penetrating bremsstrahlung radiation. Therefore, composite shielding blocks with a low-Z material, such as wax or plastic, are placed on the upstream side of the beam followed by a high-Z shield. The wax or plastic degrades the electron beam energy before it strikes the high-Z shield, and less bremsstrahlung radiation is produced.

Although most shields are above the patient, in some instances, it is necessary to place a shield within the patient (*e.g.*, in the oral cavity); x-rays striking metal produce backscattered electrons, which often can produce an enhanced dose and undesired reactions in surfaces in contact with the shield. The addition of a low-Z material such as wax between the tissue and metal helps to absorb these undesired electrons.[121]

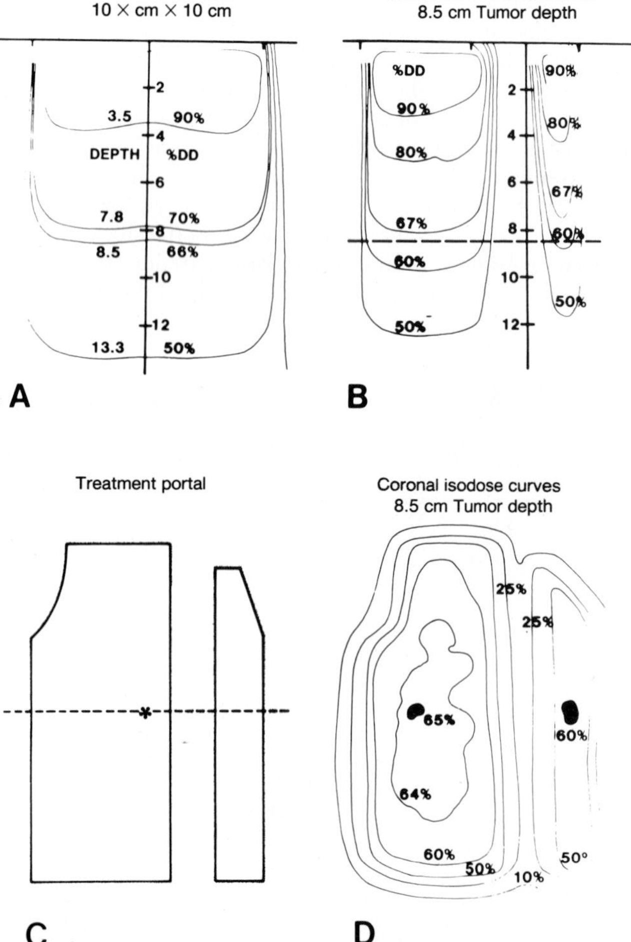

FIGURE 9–45. Dosimetry of a 4-MV treatment with an off-axis 5-HVL spinal shield. (**A**) Transverse isodose curves in the unblocked port and the 66% line at a treatment depth of 8.5 cm. (**B**) Transverse isodose curves, showing the lower isodose curves in the small port. (**C**) The treatment portal. (**D**) Coronal isodose curves at a treatment depth of 8.5 cm, showing the dose reductions introduced by the spinal cord shield.

When electrons strike a high-Z shield in a patient, they are backscattered and can produce an undesired skin or mucosal reaction. Covering the high-Z shield with aluminum, wax, or plastic helps to alleviate the effects because fewer backscattered electrons are produced.[119]

TREATMENT TECHNIQUES

Other chapters of this text contain treatment methods tailored to specific anatomic areas or types of disease. We emphasize the general features of the dose distributions achieved with combinations of low-energy and high-energy x-rays, x-rays with electrons, fixed beams with moving beams, and beams modified with wedges, compensating filters, and organ-shielding blocks.

Perez and co-workers[107] illustrated the value of combining low-energy and high-energy x-rays for treatment of carcinoma of the head and neck (Fig. 9-46) with equal mixing of 4-MV and 18-MV x-ray beams. If ^{60}Co photons or 4-MV x-rays were used to deliver the entire dose, temporomandibular joints and the mandible would receive doses exceeding 7000 cGy, creating complications. Using only the 18-MV photons would underdose the neck nodes, which is even more critical if they are fixed to the skin and subcutaneous tissue. Using the x-ray combination decreases the dose to the contralateral mandible.

Baglan and Marks[4] documented the cosmetic improvements achieved in treating brain tumors with combinations of lower- and higher-energy x-ray beams. Figure 9-47 contrasts the dose profiles in the buildup region for equal weighting of parallel opposed pairs of ^{60}Co and 25-MV photons and demonstrates some two-to-one weightings. Using the combination of low- and high-energy beams yielded improved hair growth in this patient series. Figure 9-48 is the dose distribution from an opposing pair of 20-MeV electron and 18-MV photon beams used to treat a massive lesion extending from the skin surface to the patient's midline. The parallel opposed photon-electron combination produced the lowest dose gradient across the target volume with a photon-to-electron weight ratio of 1.4 to 1.

Fixed fields in combination with moving fields are frequently useful. For example, in treating stage B carcinoma of the prostate, 16.5-cm x 16.5-cm portals at a 100-cm source-to-axis distance, parallel opposed with an 18-MV photon beam and with an additional 120-degree bilateral area yielded an adequate dose distribution.

Wedge fields have many applications in radiation therapy. Parallel opposed 15-degree or 30-degree wedges, as tissue compensators, often are used in treating the larynx or the breast to produce better dose distributions. This keeps the surface dose low while improving the dose distribution throughout the treatment volume. Sixty-degree wedges at a 60-degree angle yield a triangular dose distribution suitable for treating diseases of the eye.

Three-field techniques may employ a wedge on one, two, or all three fields (Fig. 9-49). The use of lateral opposed wedges without an unwedged anterior field can be used to advantage in treating abdominal disease while sparing the kidneys. Multiple-wedge fields frequently are used in treating lung lesions (Fig. 9-49). Rotational wedge fields can also be used. Four-field techniques in the abdomen frequently employ kidney shields, spinal shields, and liver shields to protect these organs during treatment (Fig. 9-50).

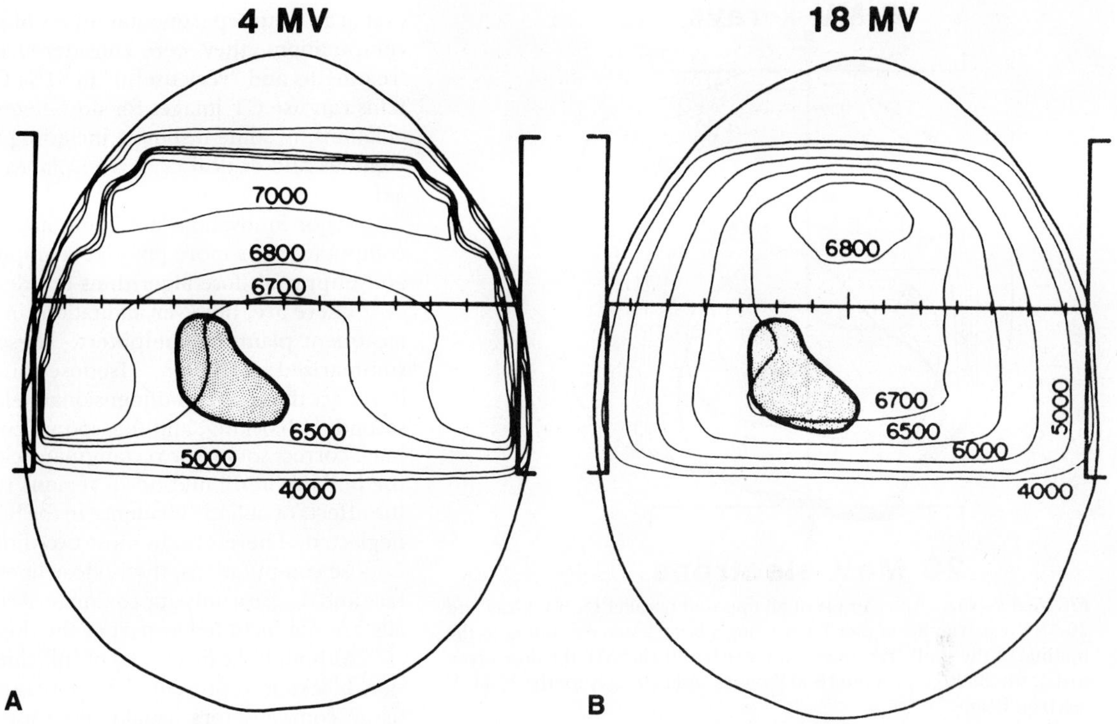

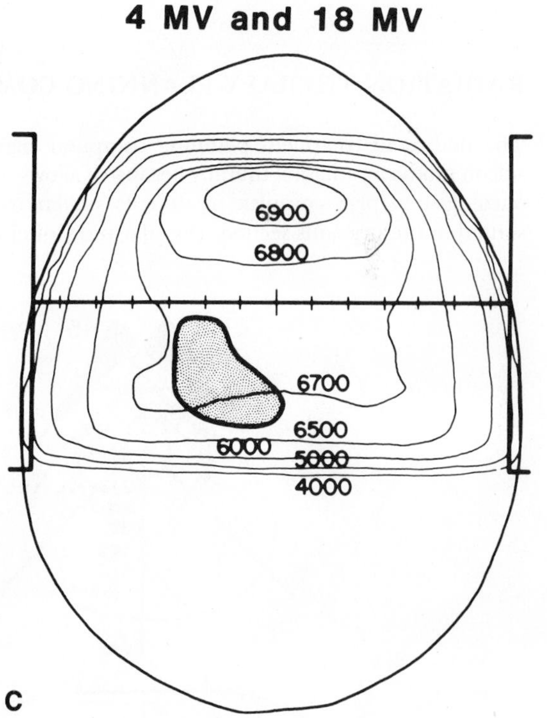

FIGURE 9–46. Examples of treatment plans for a carcinoma of the tonsil using equally weighted beams to deliver 6500 cGy. (**A**) 4 MV x-ray beams. (**B**) 18-MV x-ray beam. (**C**) Treatment with 50% of the 18-MV and 4-MV x-ray beam. The combination of low and high energy adequately covers the tumor but delivers a lower dose to the temporomandibular joint.

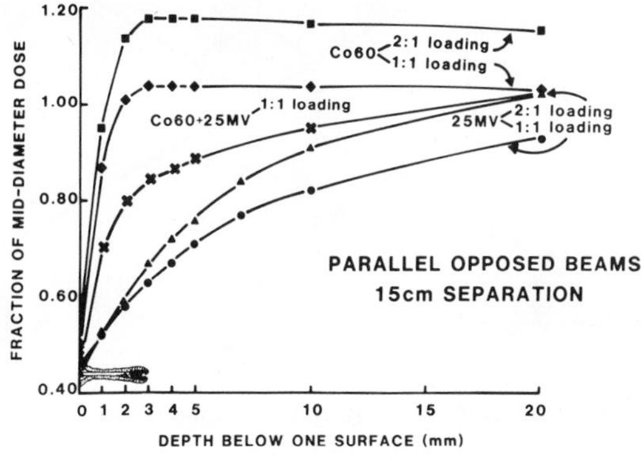

FIGURE 9–47. Dose profile in the first 2 cm below the skin surface for parallel opposed beams separated by 15 cm. Data are shown for equally and unequally loaded ^{60}Co and 25-MV beams and for a combination of ^{60}Co and 25-MV beams, with each beam delivering half of the midplane tumor dose. For unequal loading (2:1), the dose distribution to the surface receiving the highest given dose is shown. A typical hair follicle is shown. (Baglan RJ, Marks JB: Int J Radiat Oncol Biol Phys 7:455, 1984)

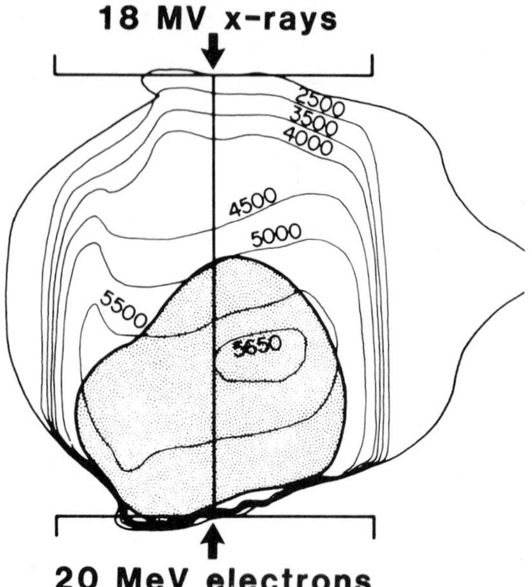

FIGURE 9–48. An example of an opposed parallel 18-MV x-ray and 20-MeV electron beam pair for treating a large lesion extending to the midline of the skull. Treatment distance is 100-cm SSD; the dose given to d_{max} was 3600 cGy for the 18-MV x-rays and 2000 cGy for the 20-MeV electron beams.

RADIATION THERAPY PLANNING COMPUTERS

The dedicated treatment planning computer plays a pivotal role in modern radiation therapy because it allows the radiation oncologist to plan complex treatments similar to those presented in the previous section. Doppke and Goitein[32] reported that in an intradepartmental survey of the usefulness of isodose computations, they were considered essential in 27% of the treatments and "very useful" in 31%. Current commercial systems can use CT images for dose-heterogeneity-corrected calculations, in some instances including the effects of the target volumes and critical organs in planes adjacent to the central axis.

Major innovations are being made in treatment planning computations as more powerful computers become affordable and improved dose algorithms are developed.

There are, however, limitations in current state-of-the-art treatment planning computers. These limitations, have been summarized by Goitein.[58] Isodose computations generally fail to reflect the true two-dimensional field shaping achieved with secondary blocking, and the isodose curves used only approximate correct square or rectangular fields. Dose computation in the buildup and build-down regions is not well modeled, and the effects of oblique incidence in the buildup region are usually neglected. Therefore, in most two-dimensional cross-sectional isodose computations, the isodose lines between the entry surface and d_{max} are only approximate. Actual surface doses generally are not included as part of the dose-calculation algorithm.

Although the dosimetry of full-shield and partial-transmission blocks is represented with reasonable accuracy, missing tissue compensators usually are represented as the patient's surface rather than in their true location away from the patient's surface. Therefore, isodose computations that include these compensators are somewhat approximate, particularly near the surface. Methods of comparing different isodose computations to select the best treatment plan are usually limited to comparing maximum, minimum, and average doses for most systems. Nevertheless, the radiation therapy treatment planning computer is a valuable tool that must be available in all facilities with high-energy linacs with multiple radiation beam capabilities.

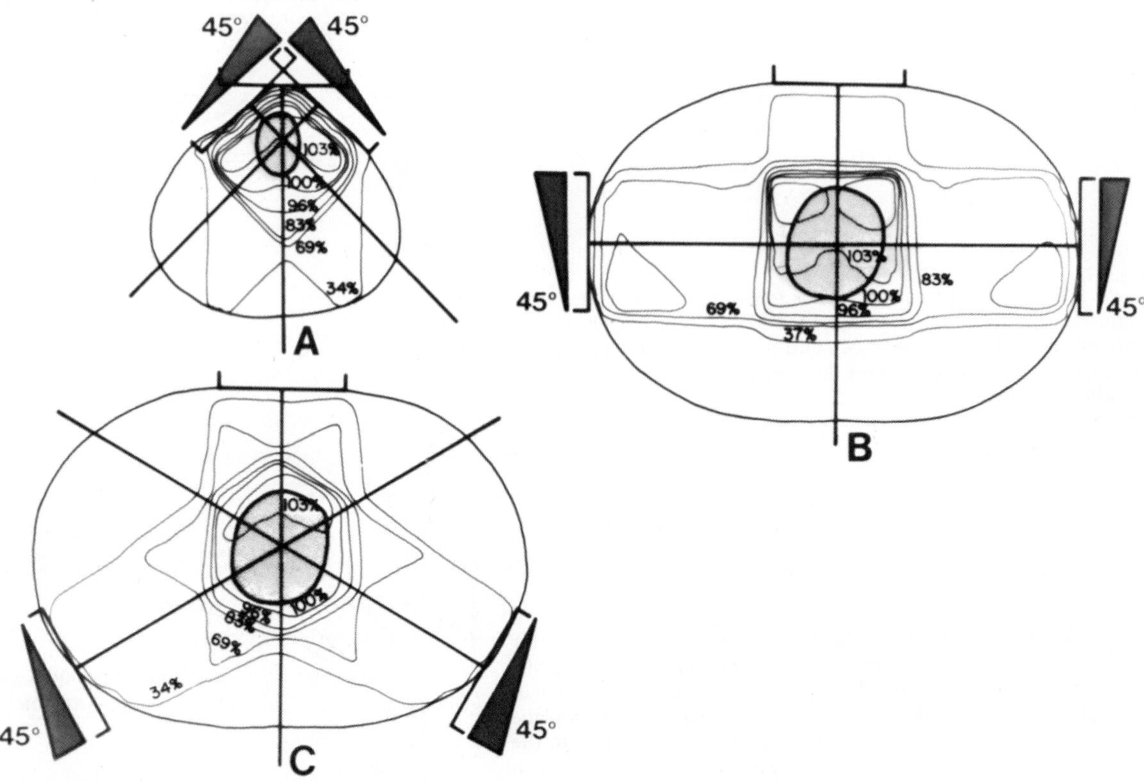

FIGURE 9–49. Three-field techniques with wedges, with 6-MV x-rays at 100-cm SSD and 45-degree wedges on two fields with the other field unwedged and all fields equally weighted.

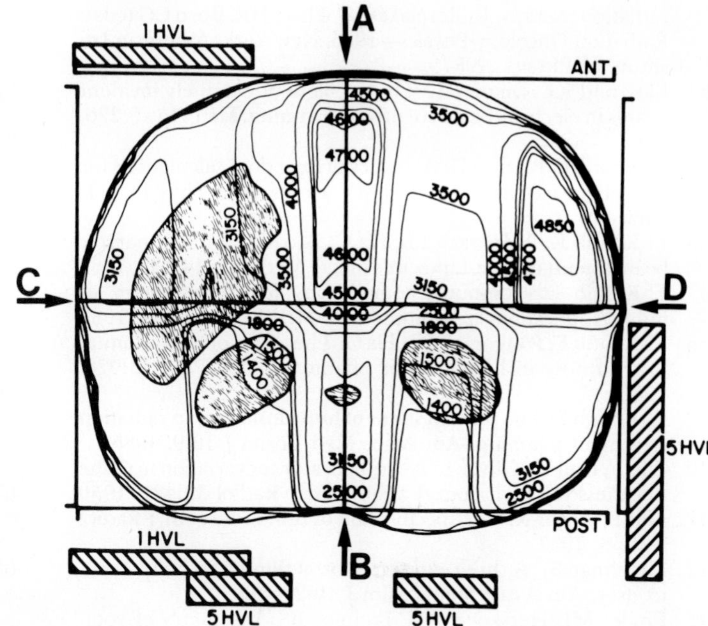

FIGURE 9–50. An 18-MV x-ray four-field technique in the abdomen with 5-HVL kidney shields and 1-HVL liver shields. Beams A and B are equally weighted to give 750-cGy each at midline; beams C and D each yield 1500-cGy at midline for a 4500-cGy midline dose.

REFERENCES

1. Abrath FG, Purdy JA: Wedge design and dosimetry for 25-MV x-rays. Radiology 136:757, 1980
2. Almond P: Total skin/electron irradiation technique and dosimetry. In Kereiakes, JG, Elson HR, Born CG (eds): Radiation Oncology Physics—1986. New York, American Institute of Physics, 1987
3. Amols HI, Reinstein LE, Baldwin BC: A computerized tissue compensator. [Abstract] Phys Med Biol 33:51, 1988
4. Baglan RJ, Marks JE: Soft tissue reactions following irradiation of primary brain and pituitary tumors. Int J Radiat Oncol Biol Phys 7:455, 1981
5. Bentel GC, Nelson CE, Noell KT: Treatment Planning and Dose Calculation in Radiation Oncology, 4th ed. New York, Pergamon Press, 1989
6. Bhaduri D, Choi MC, Weaver J, et al: Matching adjacent electron ports on flat surfaces. Am Assoc Med Dosim J 9:12, 1984
7. Biggs PJ: The change in the percentage depth dose of electrons due to beam angulation. Am Assoc Med Dosim J 9:25, 1984
8. Binder W, Karcher KH: "Super-Stuff" als Bolus in der Strahlentherapie. Strahlentherapie 153:754, 1977
9. Bleehen NM, Glastein E, Haybittle JL (eds): Radiation Therapy Planning. New York, Marcel Dekker, 1983
10. Boge JR, Edland RW, Matthes DC: Tissue compensators for megavoltage radiotherapy fabricated from hollow Styrofoam filled with wax. Radiology 111:193, 1974
11. Bomford CK, Craig LM, Hanna FA, et al: Treatment Simulators. Special Report No. 10. London, British Institute of Radiology, 1976
12. Boyer AL: Compensating filters for high energy x-rays. Med Phys 9:430, 1982
13. Boyer A, Goitein M: Simulator mounted Moiré topography camera for constructing compensator filters. Med Phys 7:19, 1980
14. Brahme A, Eenmma J, Lindback S, et al: Neutron beam characteristics from 50-MeV protons on beryllium using a continuously variable multileaf collimator. Radiother Oncol 1:65, 1983
15. Burkoritz AG, Deutsch M, Slayton R: Orthogonal fields: Variation of dose vs. gap size for treatment of the central nervous system. Radiology 126:795, 1978
16. Bush RS, Johns HE: The measurement of build-up on curved surfaces exposed to ^{60}Co and ^{137}Cs beams. AJR 87:89, 1962
17. Campbell DW, Loyd MD: Correcting for field shaping blocks used with Varian's electron beam applicator system. Am Assoc Med Dosim J 9:6, 1984
18. Chang F, Benson K, Share F: The study of Elasto-Gel pads used as surface bolus material in high energy photon and electron therapy. [Abstract] Med Phys 16:449, 1989
19. Chiang TC, Culbert H, Wyman B, et al: The half field technique of radiation therapy for the cancers of head and neck. Int J Radiat Oncol Biol Phys 5:1899, 1979
20. Christopherson D, Courlas GJ, Jette D, et al: Field matching in radiotherapy. Med Phys 3:369, 1984
21. Clark BG, Evans MDC: Standard compensators for ENT therapy fields. Med Dosim 13:173, 1988
22. Cohen M: Guidelines for the documentation of radiation therapy methods. In Cohen M, Mitchell JS (eds): Cobalt-60 Teletherapy: A Compendium of International Practice. Vienna, International Atomic Energy Agency, 1984
23. Cohen M, Jones DEA, Greene D: Central axis depth dose data for use in radiotherapy. Br J Radiol Suppl 11:21, 1972
24. Conner WG, Hicks JA, Boone MLM, et al: 10 MV x-ray beam characteristics from a new 18-MeV linear accelerator. Int J Radiat Oncol Biol Phys 1:705, 1976
25. Connors S, Scrimger J, Logus W, et al: Development of a translating bed for total body irradiation. Med Dosim 13:195, 1988
26. Constantinou C, Harrington JC: Tissue compensators made of solid water or lead for megavoltage x-ray therapy. Med Dosim 14:41, 1989
27. Day MJ, Harrison RM: Cross sectional information and treatment simulation. In Bleehen NM, Glatstein E, Haybittle JL (eds): Radiation Therapy Planning. New York, Marcel Dekker, 1983
28. Dea D: Dosimetric problems with adjacent fields: Verification of gap size. Am Assoc Med Dosim J 10:37, 1985
29. Demeyer CL, Whitehead LW, Jacobson AP, et al: Potential exposure to metal fumes, particulates, and organic vapors during radiotherapy shielding block fabrication. Med Phys 13:748, 1986
30. DeVereux C. Grundy G, Littman P: Plastic molds for patient immobilization. Int J Radiat Oncol Biol Phys 1:553, 1976
31. Dixon RL, Ekstrand KE, Ferre C: Compensating filter design using megavoltage radiography. Int J Radiat Oncol Biol Phys 5:281, 1979
32. Doppke KP, Goitein M: A survey of the information gained from planning treatment computer. Med Phys 15:258, 1988
33. Doppke KP: X-ray simulator developments and evaluation for

radiation therapy. In Kereiakes JG, Elson HR, Born CG (eds): Radiation Oncology Physics—1986. New York, American Institute of Physics, 1987
34. Ekstrand KE, Dixon RL: The problem of obliquely incident beams in electron-beam treatment planning. Med Phys 9:276, 1982
35. El-Khatib E, Battista JJ: Accuracy of lung dose calculations for large field irradiation with 6-MV x-rays. Med Phys 13:111, 1986
36. El-Khatib E, Podgorsak EB, Pla C: Broad beam and narrow beam attenuation in Lipowitz's metal. Med Phys 14:135, 1987
37. El-Khatib E: Computed tomography for densitometry of lung: Applications in radiotherapy. Med Dosim 12:31, 1987
38. El-Khatib E, Podgorsak EB, Pla C: The effect of lead attenuators on dose in homogenous phantoms. Med Phys 13:928, 1986
39. El-Khatib E: The present status of lung dosimetry in radiation treatment planning. Am Assoc Med Dosim J 10:9, 1985
40. Ellis F, Hall EJ, Oliver R: A compensator for variation in tissue thickness for high energy beams. Br J Radiol 32:421, 1959
41. Ellis F, Oliver R: The specification of tumor dose. Br J Radiol 34:258, 1961
42. Engelman SJ: A three exposure portal filming technique and its uses. Am Assoc Med Dosim J 10:27, 1985
43. Engler MJ, Herskovic AM, Proimos BS: Dosimetry of rotational photon fields with gravity-oriented eye blocks. Int J Radiat Oncol Biol Phys 10:431, 1984
44. Fessenden P, Palow BB, Karzmark CT: Dosimetry for tangential chest. Radiology 128:485, 1978
45. Fields JN, Weller MK, Marks JE: Irradiation of advanced carcinoma of the larynx and hypopharynx: Dosimetry of a three field technique. Med Dosim 12:7, 1987
46. Frass BA, Tepper JE, Glatstein E, et al: Clinical use of a match line wedge for adjacent megavoltage radiation field matching. Int J Radiat Oncol Biol Phys 9:209, 1983
47. Gagnon WF, Grant W: Surface dose from megavoltage therapy machines. Radiology 117:705, 1975
48. Gagnon WF, Horton JL: Physical factors affecting absorbed dose to the skin from cobalt-60 τ-rays and 25-MeV x-rays. Med Phys 6:285, 1979
49. Galvin JM, Heidtman B, Cheng E, et al: The use of a CT scanner specially designed to perform the functions of a radiation therapy treatment unit simulator. Med Phys 9:615, 1982
50. Galvin JM, Turrisi AT, Cheng E: Treatment simulation using a CT unit. In Kereiakes JG, Elson HR, Born CG (eds): Radiation Oncology Physics—1986. New York, American Institute of Physics, 1987
51. Gerber RL, Marks JE, Purdy JA: The use of thermal plastics for immobilization of patients during radiotherapy. Int J Radiat Oncol Biol Phys 8:1461, 1982
52. Gerbi BJ: Compensating filter design using radiographic stereo shift information. Med Phys 12:646, 1985
53. Gerbi BJ, Meigooni A, Khan FM: Dose buildup for obliquely incident photon beams. Med Phys 14:393, 1987
54. Gillin MT, Kline RW: Field separation between lateral and anterior fields on a 6-MV linear accelerator. Int J Radiat Oncol Biol Phys 6:233, 1980
55. Glasgow GP: The dosimetry of fixed, single source hemi-body and total-body irradiators. Med Phys 9:311, 1982
56. Glasgow GP, Marks JE: The dosimetry of a single "hockey stick" portal for treatment of tumors of the cranio-spinal axis. Med Phys 10:672, 1983
57. Glasgow GP, Reeves GI: Safety considerations during the production of radiation therapy shielding blocks from low melting temperature bismuth alloys. Proceedings of the Health Physics Society Mid-Year Symposium on Medical Physics, Hyanis, MA, 1980
58. Goitein M: Limitations of two dimensional treatment planning programs. Med Phys 9:580, 1982
59. Gosselin M, Podgorsak EB: The McGill rotational total skin electron irradiation technique. Am Assoc Med Dosim J 10:29, 1985
60. Grant BP, Fletcher GH: Analysis of complications following megavoltage therapy for squamous cell carcinomas of the tonsillar area. AJR 96:28, 1966
61. Hansen WF, Shalek RJ, Kirby TH: Information that Should be Included in Every Patient's Radiotherapy Treatment Record. Technical Report No. 18. Houston, Radiological Physics Center, 1985
62. Haus AG, Marks JE: Detection and evaluation of localization errors in patient radiation therapy. Invest Radiol 8:384, 1973
63. Henderson SD, Gerber RL, Purdy JA, et al: Evaluation of a new tissue compensator system: Dosimetry and practical aspects. Int J Radiat Oncol Biol Phys 9:162, 1983
64. Henson PW, Fox RA: The electron density of bone for inhomogeneity correction in radiotherapy planning using CT numbers. Phys Med Biol 29:351, 1984
65. Hogstrom KR, Leavitt DD: Dosimetry of arc electron therapy. In Kereiakes JG, Elson HR, Born CG (eds): Radiation Oncology Physics—1986. New York, American Institute of Physics, 1987
66. Hogstrom, K: Dosimetry of electron heterogeneities. In Wright AE, Boyer AL (eds): Advances in Radiation Therapy Treatment Planning. New York, American Institute of Physics, 1983
67. Hopfan S, Reid A, Simpson L, et al: Clinical complications arising from overlapping of adjacent fields. Physical and technical considerations. Int J Radiat Oncol Biol Phys 2:801, 1977
68. Huen A, Findley DO, Skov DD: Attenuation in Lipowitz's metal of x-rays produced at 2, 4, 10, and 18 MV and gamma rays from cobalt-60. Med Phys 6:147, 1979
69. International Commission on Radiation Units and Measurements: Report No. 21: Radiation Dosimetry Electrons with Initial Energies Between 1 and 50 MeV. Washington, DC, International Commission on Radiation Units and Measurements, 1972
70. International Commission on Radiation Units and Measurements: Report No. 29: Dose Specification for Reporting External Beams Therapy with Photons and Electrons. Washington, DC, International Commission on Radiation Units and Measurements, 1978
71. Jablonski O, Motta-Veyssiere CC, Guerin RA: Irradiations corporelles totales-technique d irradiation fractionnee par telecobalt. J Radiol 60:339, 1979
72. Jackson W: Surface effects of high energy x-rays at oblique incidence. Br J Radiol 44:109, 1971
73. Jones D, Washington J: The quantitative description of a radiation therapy plan. Radiology 115:451, 1975
74. Källman P, Lind B, Eklöf A, Brahme A: Shaping of arbitrary dose distributions by dynamic multileaf collimation. Phys Med Biol 33:1291, 1988
75. Karzmark CJ, Huisman PA, Palos BB, et al: Overlap at the cord in abutting orthogonal fields: A perceptual anomaly. Int J Radiat Oncol Biol Phys 6:1366, 1980
76. Khan FM, Gerbi BJ, Deibel FC: Dosimetry of asymmetric x-ray collimators. Med Phys 13:936, 1986
77. Khan FM: The Physics of Radiation Therapy, p 294. Baltimore, Williams & Wilkins, 1984
78. Klemp PFB, Perry AM, Hedland-Thomas B, et al: Commissioning of a linear accelerator with independent jaws: Computerized data collection and transfer to a planning computer. Phys Med Biol 33:865, 1988
79. Kuisk H: New methods to facilitate radiotherapy planning and treatment, including a method for fast production of solid lead blocks with diverging wall for cobalt-60 beam. AJR 117:161, 1973
80. Lam WL, Order SE, Thomas ED: Uniformity and standardization of single and opposing cobalt-60 sources for total body irradiation. Int J Radiat Oncol Biol Phys 6:245, 1980
81. Laughlin JS: High energy electron treatment planning for inhomogeneities. Br J Radiol 38:143, 1965
82. Leavitt DD, Peacock, LM, Gibbs FA, et al: Electron arc therapy: Physical measurement and treatment planning techniques. Int J Radiat Oncol Biol Phys 11:987, 1985
83. Leavitt DD, Stewart JR, Moeller JH, et al: Optimization of electron arc therapy doses by multivane collimator control. Int J Radiat Oncol Biol Phys 16:489, 1989
84. Legras J, Legras B, Lambert JP, et al: The use of a microcomputer for non-linear optimisation of doses in external radiotherapy. Phys Med Biol 31:1353, 1986
85. Lichter AS, Frass BA, Van de Geijn J, et al: An overview of clinical requirements and clinical utility of computer tomog-

raphy based radiotherapy treatment planning. In Ling CC, Rodgers CC, Morton RJ (eds): Computed Tomography in Radiation Therapy. New York, Raven Press, 1983

86. Lim MLF: A study of four methods of junction change in the treatment of medulloblastoma. Am Assoc Med Dosim J 10:17, 1985
87. Lim MLF: Evolution of medulloblastoma treatment techniques. Am Assoc Med Dosim J 11:25, 1986
88. Loshek DD: Applications and physics of the independent collimator feature of the Varian Clinac 2500. 10th Varian Users Meeting, Palm Springs, CA, April 15–17, 1984
89. Mallion WE, White DR: Immobilization of the head in radiotherapy. Br J Radiol 41:236, 1968
90. Maruyama Y, Moore VC, Burns D, et al: Individualized lung shields from lead shot in plastic. Radiology 92:634, 1969
91. Mayneord WV: The measurement of radiation for medical purposes. Proc Phys Soc 54:405, 1942.
92. McCullough EC, Gortney J, Blackwell CR: A depth dependence determination of the wedge transmission factor for 4–10 MV photon beams. Med Phys 15:621, 1988
93. Mill WB, Baglan RJ, Kurichety P, et al: Symptomatic radiation induced pericarditis in Hodgkin's disease. Int J Radiat Oncol Biol Phys 10:2061, 1984
94. Mizer S, Scheller RR, Deye JA: Radiation therapy simulation workbook. New York, Pergamon Press, 1986
95. Mohan R, Brewster LJ, Barest GD: A technique for computing dose volume histograms for structure combinations. Med Phys 14:1048, 1987
96. Mondalek PM, Orton CG: Transmission and build-up characteristics of polyurethane-foam immobilization devices. Treat Plan 7:5, 1982
97. Mould RF: Radiotherapy Treatment Planning. Bristol, Adam Hilger, 1981
98. Moyer RF, McElroy WR, O'Brien JE, et al: A surface bolus material for high energy photon and electron therapy. Radiology 146:531, 1983
99. Moyer RF, King GA, Hauser JF: Lead as surface bolus for high-energy photon and electron therapy. Med Phys 13:263, 1986
100. Muller-Runkel R, Vijayakumar S: Spinal axis irradiation with electrons: Measurements of attenuation by the spinal process. Med Phys 13:539, 1986
101. Nelson TJ, Lindberg RD: Bite block head immobilizer system. Med Dosim 14:147, 1989
102. Nilsson B, Schnell PO: Build-up effects at air cavities measured with thin thermoluminescent dosimeters. Acta Radiol Ther Phys Biol 15:427, 1976
103. Page V, Gardner A, Karzmark CT: Patient dosimetry in the electron treatment of large superficial lesions. Radiology 94:635, 1970
104. Paliwal B (ed): Proceedings of the Symposium on Electron Beam Dosimetry Arc Therapy. New York, American Institute of Physics, 1982
105. Paliwal BR, Asp L: A technique to evaluate styrofoam cutouts used in irregular field shaping. Int J Radiat Oncol Biol Phys 1:791, 1976
106. Parker RP, Hobday PA, Cassell KL: The direct use of CT numbers in radiotherapy dosage calculations for inhomogeneous media. Phys Med Biol 24:802, 1979
107. Perez CA, Purdy JA, Korba A, et al: High energy x-ray beams in the management of head and neck and pelvic cancers. In Kramer S, Suntharalingam N, Zinninger GF (eds): High Energy Photons and Electrons. New York, John Wiley, 1975
108. Podgorsak EB, Pla C, Pla M, et al: Physical aspects of a rotational total skin electron irradiation. Med Phys 10:159, 1983
109. Podgorsak EB, Pla C, Evans MDC, Pla M: The influence of phantom size on output, peakscatter factor, and percentage depth dose in large-field irradiation. Med Phys 12:639, 1985
110. Powers WE, Kinzie JK, Demidecki AJ, et al: A new system of field shaping for external-beam radiation therapy. Radiology 108:407, 1973
111. Prasad SC, Glasgow GP, Purdy JA: Dosimetry evaluation of a computed tomography treatment planning system. Radiology 130:777, 1979
112. Prasad S, Pilepich MV, Perez CA: Contribution of CT to quantitative radiation therapy planning. Am J Radiol 136:123, 1981
113. Promos BS, Goldson AL: Dynamic dose shaping by gravity oriented absorbers for total lymph node irradiation. Int J Radiat Oncol Biol Phys 7:973, 1981
114. Purdy JA: Buildup/surface dose and exit dose measurements for 6-MV linear accelerator. Med Phys 13:259, 1986
115. Purdy JA: Secondary field shaping. In Wright AE, Boyer AL (eds): Advances in Radiation Therapy Treatment Planning. New York, American Institute of Physics, 1983
116. Purdy JA, Keys DJ, Zivnuska F: A compensation filter for chest portals. Int J Radiat Oncol Biol Phys 2:1213, 1977
117. Robinson DM, Scrimger JW: Limitations of retracted missing tissue compensators: an experimental analysis. Med Dosim 14:49, 1989
118. Rustgi SN, Rodgers JE: Improvement in the buildup characteristics of a 10-MV photon beam with electron filters. Phys Med Biol 30:587, 1985
119. Saunders JE, Peters VG: Backscattering from metals in superficial therapy with high energy electron beams. Br J Radiol 47:467, 1974
120. Schulz MD, Hale J: Instructions for use of radiotherapy charts. Radiology 74:843, 1960
121. Scrimger JW: Backscatter from high atomic number materials in high energy photon beams. Radiology 124:815, 1977
122. Siddin RL, Tonnesen GL, Svensson GK: Three-field techniques for breast treatment using a rotatable half-beam block. Int J Radiat Oncol Biol Phys 7:1473, 1981
123. Smith RM, Sanfilippo LJ, Stiedley KD, et al: Clinical patterns of use of a CT-based simulator. Med Dosim 12:17, 1987
124. Spicka J, Fleury K, Powers W: Polyethylene-lead tissue compensators for megavoltage radiotherapy. Med Dosim 13:25, 1988
125. Steidley KD: A three dimensional offset sonic digitizer for patient contouring. Am Assoc Med Dosim J 11:29, 1986
126. Sternick ES: Spherical contouring techniques. In Wright A, Boyer A (eds): Advances in Radiation Therapy Treatment Planning. New York, American Institute of Physics, 1983
127. Svensson GK, Bjarngard BE, Chen GTY, et al: Superficial doses in treatment of breast and tangential fields using 4-MV x-rays. Int J Radiat Oncol Biol Phys 2:705, 1977
128. Takahashi K, Purdy JA, Liu YY: Treatment planning system for conformation radiotherapy. Radiology 147:567, 1983
129. Takahashi S: Conformational radiotherapy. Acta Radiol Suppl (Stockh) 242:1, 1965
130. Tang WL, Khan FM, Gerbi BJ: Validity of lung correction algorithms. Med Phys 13:683, 1986
131. Van Arsdale ED, Greenlaw RH: Formalized immobilization and localization in radiotherapy. Radiology 99:697, 1971
132. Van de Geijn J, Harrington FS, Fraass B: A graticule for evaluation of megavoltage x-ray port films. Int J Radiat Oncol Biol Phys 8:1999, 1982
133. Van Dyk J, Jenkins RDT, Leung PMK, et al: Medulloblastoma: Treatment technique and irradiation dosimetry. Int J Radiat Oncol Biol Phys 2:993, 1977
134. Velkley DE, Manson DJ, Purdy JA, et al: Build-up region of megavoltage photon radiation sources. Med Phys 2:14, 1974
135. Wachsmann F, Barth G: Moving field radiotherapy. Chicago, University of Chicago Press, 1962
136. Watkins DMB: Beam direction shells in the treatment planning of head and neck cancer. Med Dosim 11:45, 1986
137. Watkins DMB: Radiation Therapy Mold Technology. Toronto, Pergamon Press, 1981
138. Weeks KJ, Fraass BA, Hurchins KM: Gypsum mixtures for compensator construction. Med Phy 15:410, 1988
139. Weller MK, Glasgow GP: The flexible curve, a useful contouring device. Treat Plan 7:8, 1982
140. White DR: Tissue substitutes in experimental radiation physics. Med Phys 5:467, 1978
141. Williamson TJ: A technique for matching orthogonal megavoltage fields. Int J Radiat Oncol Biol Phys 5:111, 1979
142. Wright AE, Boyer AL (eds): Advances in Radiation Therapy Treatment Planning. New York, American Institute of Physics, 1983
143. Zwicker RD, Shahabi S, Wu A, et al: Effective wedge angles for 6 MV wedges. Med Phys 11:370, 1984

10

○ ○ ○ ∘ • ∘

Clinical Applications of Electron-Beam Therapy

Luther W. Brady
Larry D. Simpson
John L. Day
Norah duV. Tapley

PHYSICAL CHARACTERISTICS

Electron Interactions

The interactions that occur as a high-energy electron traverses a medium may be classified as either collisional or radiative.[1] In a collision, the incident electron interacts with the Coulomb force field of the atomic electrons, producing excitation or ionization of the atom. The ejected atomic electrons are known as secondary electrons or as δ-rays if they have sufficient energy to cause further ionization. In radiative interactions, the incident electron interacts with the Coulomb force field of the nucleus to produce x-rays, referred to as bremsstrahlung ("braking radiation"). Eventually, the electron loses enough energy to be captured by an atom of the medium.

The rate of energy loss, ΔE, per path length traveled, Δl, divided by the density of the medium, ρ, is known as the total mass stopping power, $(S/\rho)_{tot}$.

$$(S/\rho)_{tot} = (S/\rho)_{col} + (S/\rho)_{rad};\ \frac{\text{MeV cm}^2}{\text{g}}$$

$(S/\rho)_{col}$ is the mass collision stopping power and $(S/\rho)_{rad}$ is the mass radiative stopping power. A plot of $(S/\rho)_{col}$ and $(S/\rho)_{rad}$ for water and lead is given in Figure 10-1.

Energy losses by collisions are higher in materials with a lower atomic number (Z) than in materials with a higher Z because there are more electrons per gram in lower-Z material, and the electrons are more tightly bound in higher-Z materials.[9] For water, the energy loss by collision is approximately 2 MeV/cm in the energy range of 1 to 100 MeV. The radiative loss of electron energy in water is not as uniform as collisional losses. From 1 to 20 MeV, the rate of radiative loss rises from 0.01 to 0.4 MeV/cm.[8] Unlike collisional losses, radiative losses increase for higher-Z materials, because the losses are more proportional to the energy of the electron and to the Z^2 of the material. An approximation of the ratio of radiative to collisional losses is given by

$$\frac{\text{Radiative loss}}{\text{Collisional loss}} \cong E\,(\text{MeV}) \times Z/800$$

where E is the electron energy.[10] For dosimetric calibration of accelerator photon and electron beams using ionization chambers, a modification of $(S/\rho)_{col}$ must be used: the restricted mass collision stopping power, $(L/\rho)_{col,\Delta}$. Given that secondary electrons with an energy Δ or greater are not locally absorbed, the interest is in restricting the S/ρ_{col} to energy losses of less than Δ from the incoming or primary electrons to the secondary electrons.

$$(L/\rho)_{col\,\Delta} = (dE/\rho\Delta l)_{col,\,\Delta}$$

A discussion of this modification may be found in Report No. 35 of the International Commission on Radiation Units and Measurements.[8]

Electron Beam

The energy spectrum changes as an electron beam passes from the accelerator to a depth, z, in a phantom (Fig. 10-2). Before leaving the accelerator, the spectrum is quite narrow and may be considered to be almost monoenergetic with an energy E_a, the accelerator energy. In reaching the surface of the phantom, the electron beam goes through various interactions with the window, scattering foils, and beam monitors. These effect changes in the spectrum. The maximum energy $(E_{max})_0$ is less than E_a and has a broader full width at half maximum, Γ_0. $(Ep)_0$ is defined as the most probable energy and $\overline{E}_0$ as the mean energy. Within the phantom, there is further degradation of the energy spectrum, producing a Γ_Z that is larger than Γ_0 and an $(Ep)_Z$ that is less than $(Ep)_0$.

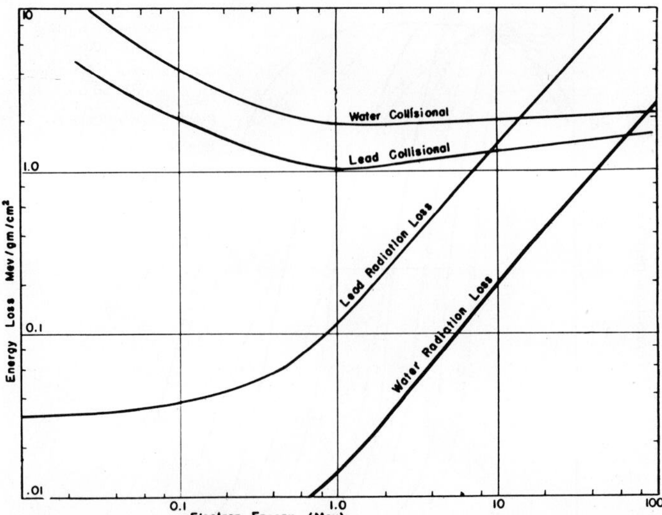

FIGURE 10–1. The mass collision stopping power, $(S/\rho)_{col}$, and the mass radiative stopping power, $(S/\rho)_{rad}$, are shown for water and lead. (Johns HE, Cunningham JR: The Physics of Radiology, 3rd ed, p 47. Springfield, IL, Charles C Thomas, 1974)

There is a decrease in the mean electron energy at increasing depth, and there is an increase in the angular spread of the beam. Because of collisional interactions, the electrons "scatter" away from a straight-line path. The angular spread of the electrons is described by the mass scattering power, T/ρ.[8]

$$\frac{T}{\rho} = \frac{1}{\rho}\frac{\overline{\Delta\theta}^2}{\Delta l}$$

where $\overline{\theta}^2$ is the mean square scattering angle. The dependence of angular spread on atomic number, Z, and energy, E, is approximately Z^2/E. The degree of scattering and the position of the scattering material relative to the phantom surface influence the shapes of the depth dose and the isodose curves within the irradiated material. This is one reason that special consideration is given to the design and calibration of electron collimators.

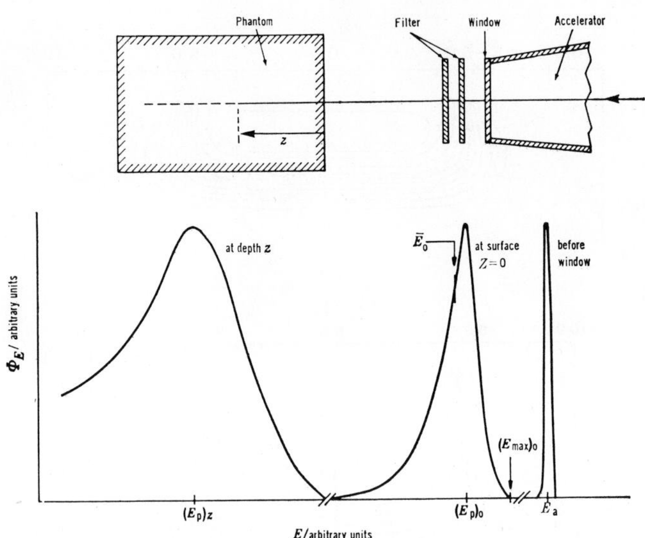

FIGURE 10–2. Changes in the electron-beam spectrum from accelerator into phantom. (International Commission on Radiation Units and Measurements Report No. 21: Radiation dosimetry: Electrons with initial energies between 1 and 50 MeV, p 2. Washington, DC, Washington International Commission on Radiation Units and Measurements, 1972)

One method of spreading the electron beam for large-field, clinical use employs scattering foils. Dual foils of high and intermediate Z are desirable because the amount of energy degradation is lower for the same angular spread than with foils constructed from materials with a lower Z.[15] Another method is to steer or scan the beams with magnetic fields.[15]

The beam is designed to pass through a quadrupole magnet, which has different frequencies applied to each pole pair. These frequencies change the strength of the magnetic field for the pole pairs, which causes the electron beam to travel in a random scan pattern. The advantage of this method over the use of scattering foils is that there is minimal energy degradation and x-ray contamination. Figure 10-3 compares the depth dose curves produced by various systems. Although the depth for the 85% isodose curve is almost the same for all systems, the dual-foil and scanning systems have lower energy and more rapid drop-off than the single-foil systems.

The mean incident energy $\overline{E}_0$ at the surface of an irradiated phantom may be found by plotting the relative ionization readings from a chamber against the depth within the phantom (Fig. 10-4). The $\overline{E}_0$ at the surface may be found by multiplying the depth at which the ionization has fallen to 50% of its maximum value, R_{50} (*e.g.*, by 2.33 MeV/cm^{-1} in water).

$$\overline{E}_0 = 2.33 \times R_{50}$$

The mean energy, $\overline{E}_Z$, at other depths, z, is given by the approximation due to Harder,[6A]

$$\overline{E}_Z = \overline{E}_0 \times (1 - z/R\rho)$$

where R_p is the practical range in centimeters for the electron beam.[5] R_p may be found in the ionization plot at the point where the tangent at the steepest portion of the descending ionization curve intersects with the extrapolated background.

CLINICAL CHARACTERISTICS

The central-axis depth dose of several electron beams is shown in Fig. 10-5. Unlike megavoltage x-ray beams, electron beams exhibit rapid fall-off, especially if the energy is below 15 MeV. This is significant clinically because there is almost no dose other than that from x-ray contamination to tissue lying beyond

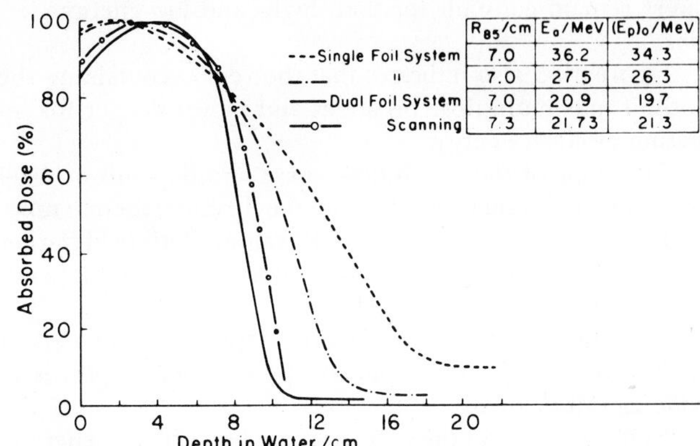

FIGURE 10–3. Comparison of depth dose curves of single-foil, dual-foil, and scanning systems. (Almond PR: Calibration of megavoltage electron radiotherapy beams. In Waggener RG, Kereiakes JG, Shalek RJ [eds]: Handbook of Medical Physics, vol 1. Boca Raton, CRC Press, 1982)

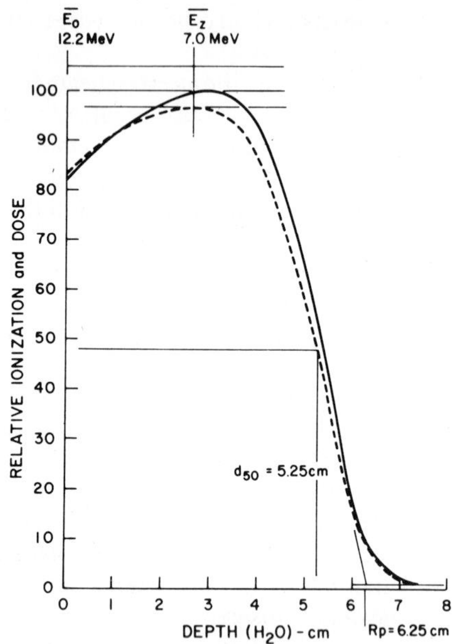

FIGURE 10–4. Depth ionization (*broken*) and depth dose (*solid*) curves for an electron beam. Because electrons lose energy with depth, the ionization and dose curves are slightly different. (Task Group 21, Radiation Therapy Committee, American Association of Physicists in Medicine: Med Phys 11:213, 1984)

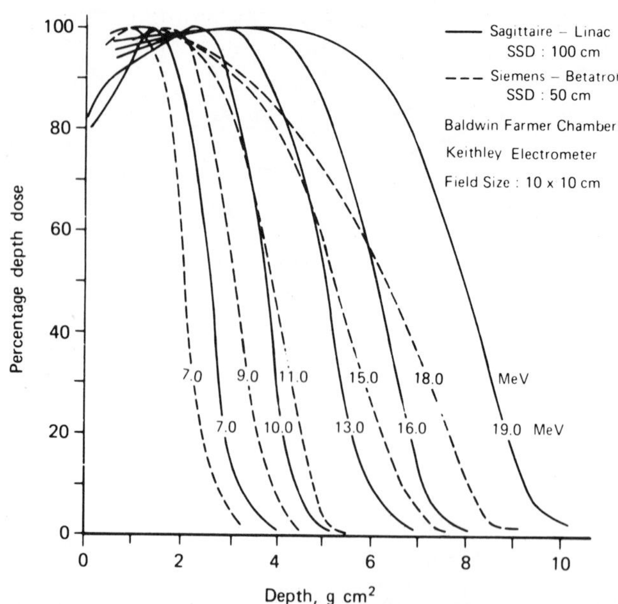

FIGURE 10–5. Comparison of central-axis depth dose curves for a linear accelerator and a betatron for the nominal machine energies. (Tapley N [ed]: Clinical Applications of the Electron Beam, p 46. New York, John Wiley & Sons, 1976)

the practical range, R_p. This sparing, however, decreases the higher energies because the dose gradient diminishes. As a rough rule of thumb, the central-axis depth dose is about 10% or less of the dose at d_{max} at a depth, in centimeters, obtained by dividing the beam energy by a factor of 2. R_p(cm) can be estimated by taking $\bar{E}_0/2$. This rule is derived from the fact that the electron energy loss $(S/\rho)_{col}$ is approximately 2 MeV per centimeter in water.

For most machines, the amount of x-ray contamination caused by bremsstrahlung production is 5% or less of the dose at d_{max}.[2] The amount of x-ray contamination rises with beam energy because $(S/\rho)_{rad}$ increases with higher energies.

With electron beams, skin sparing is less possible than with x-ray beams. As Figure 10-5 indicates, the surface dose is in the range of about 80% to 100% of d_{max}, and in contrast to photon beams, is proportional to electron-beam energy.[4,6] With increased energy, the surface dose rises, because higher-energy electrons are not as easily deflected or pass through angles as large as lower-energy electrons. Also, collisional stopping powers remain constant for both high- and low-energy electrons.

Figure 10-5 also indicates that the region containing the depth of maximum dose broadens and moves deeper for increasing electron energy.

The slope of the depth dose curve also depends on field size. If the field is smaller than twice the R_p value, there is more rapid dose fall-off than for higher R_p values. With fields larger than twice the R_p value, the gradient is less steep and depends less on further increases in field size.

A method for approximating the depth in centimeters of the 80% isodose value (a common prescription depth) is to divide $\bar{E}_0$ (MeV) by 3.

Isodose curves for the same field size but different energies are given in Figure 10-6. All curves exhibit the effect of ballooning at the field edges, caused by electron scattering below the surface. This effect is more prevalent for lower isodose values in all cases. At approximately 15 MeV, the phenomenon of lateral constriction of the higher isodose values, such as at the 80% line, occurs. This constriction is more noticeable with small fields. One must verify that the tumor volume is adequately covered by the 80% isodose value.

A method of describing field uniformity, specified by the Nordic Association of Clinical Physics, is denoted by the symbol $U_{90/50}$.[12] A plane perpendicular to the beam is chosen at a depth

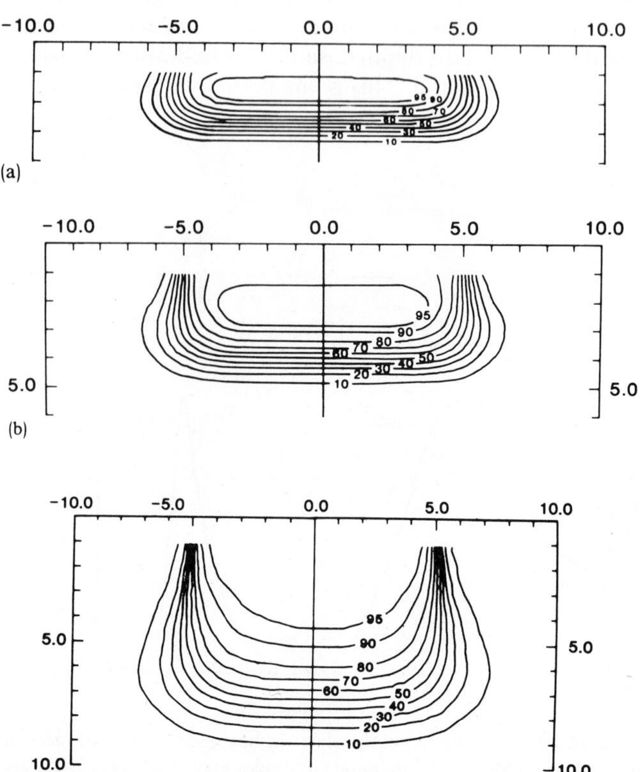

FIGURE 10–6. Isodose measurements for a 10-cm × 10-cm field at (**A**) 7 MeV, (**B**) 12 MeV, and (**C**) 18 MeV. (Meyer JA, Palta JR, Hogstrom KR: Phys Med Biol 11:676, 1984)

equal to one half the depth of the 85% depth dose. At this depth, all values are normalized to the dose at the central axis of the beam, which is designated as 100%. $U_{90/50}$ is the ratio of the area enclosed by the 90% isodose line to the area enclosed by the 50% isodose line. The ratio should be greater than 0.8 for field sizes larger than 10 cm × 10 cm. There should be no portion of the plane with an isodose value greater than 103%. Figure 10-7 is an example of the determination of field uniformity. $P_{80/20}$, the penumbra, is the distance between the 80% and 20% isodose lines. For convenience, measurements of uniformity are usually made with film.

The characteristics of clinical electron beams may depend strongly on each machine design and individual machines of the same design. Some of the parameters that differ among machines are energy, construction, and functioning of the monitoring chamber; use of scanning foils or magnets; and collimator design. Calibration and treatment planning require measurements of unique machine parameters and individualized patient environments (*e.g.*, source-skin distance, air gap, field size, blocking).

For the interested reader, there are descriptions of various methods of dosimetry and treatment planning.[2,3,10,11,13,14,16,18]

CLINICAL APPLICATIONS

Electron beams are particularly useful in the treatment of superficial and subcutaneous volumes of tissue, particularly if the treatment should be limited to a unilateral lesion requiring a low dose to the opposite side of the body. These cases include tumors of the parotid, ear, oral cavity, and oropharynx. Electron beams may be the primary mode of therapy or combined with photon beams.

There are major clinical applications, such as treating a radically dissected neck or areas in which there is a high risk of residual disease. Electron beam therapy can also be used to boost the dose to specific sites, such as the breast or to lymph nodes.

It is mandatory that radiation oncologists be familiar with the idiosyncrasies of their machines. There are many different designs for electron-beam generators, with different design

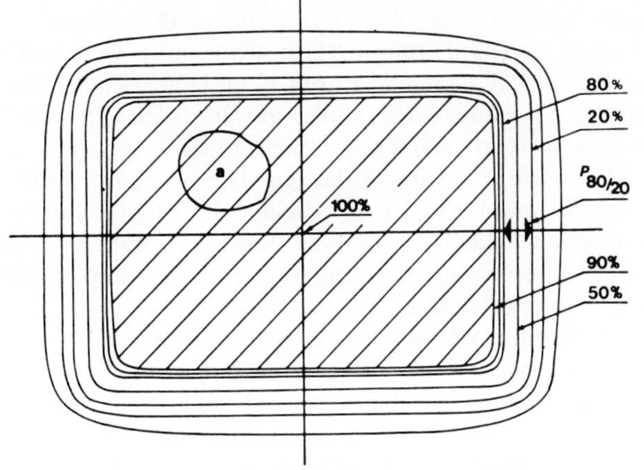

FIGURE 10–7. Dose distribution in a plane perpendicular to the beam. The plane is located at a distance equal to half the depth of the 85% isodose line. The dose in the area marked may be greater than 100%. (International Commission on Radiation Units and Measurements Report No. 35: Radiation dosimetry: Electron beams with energies between 1 and 50 MeV, p 110. Washington, DC, Washington International Commission on Radiation Units and Measurements, 1984)

factors used to scatter the narrow electron stream into a wide and uniform beam for therapy. There are machines that are based primarily on scattering foils to degrade the beam and "smear" its energy profile, which yields an increased surface dose, decreased depth dose gradient, shallower therapeutic depth, and bremsstrahlung produced in the foil, which contributes to the x-ray component. All of these effects are greater at high energies.

Scanning-beam machines rely on electronics and bending magnets to modify a pencil beam to produce a broad beam that theoretically has a more of homogeneous energy profile and a lower, but not zero, x-ray component, with specific attention to scan pattern and frequency when measuring the beam data. These types of machines may cause dangerous overdoses if scanning systems fail, the beam becomes stationary, and interlocks simultaneously fail.

Various measuring techniques must be understood in terms of their potential for accurate definition of the dose being delivered. These can be achieved by the use of ionization chambers, thermoluminescent dosimeters, silicon diodes, film dosimetry, and phantom measurements in water or plastic.

The field can be defined as a geometric field, in which the projection of the collimator from the virtual source onto a plane perpendicular to the central axis is used, or as the radiation field, which is the area within the 50% isodose line in the plane perpendicular to the central axis located at d_{max} depth.

The beam characteristic is determined by the energy being used and varies along the beam path. Scattering foils, collimators, and cones "smear" the beam's energy and direction. Penetration into the patient degrades the energy approximately linearly with depth. There are several ways to specify the energy at the surface, including the most probable energy, the mean energy at the surface, or the mean energy at depth z. In general, as the beam energy increases, the surface dose increases, the dose gradient decreases, and the film edges sharpen at surface but soften at depth. Because of the different depth dose and isodose curves generated by the machines being used, the dose distribution must be measured for each clinical machine, rather than being obtained from standard tables.

Inhomogeneities in the treatment field significantly affect the dose distribution. Compact bone attenuates the beam and reduces the dose behind it. Spongy bone may have little effect. In the lung, the range of the electrons is increased by a factor of 3, with an associated increase in dose to the lung and the tissues beyond the lung. For uniformity, the reference plane is at the depth of the 95% dose deep to the dose maximum. Dose in this plane should not vary more than + 5% within an area defined 2 cm inside the projected field edges for fields greater than 10 cm × 10 cm. An alternate specification is the uniformity index, which is the ratio of areas of the 90% and 50% isodose lines defined at a depth of half that of the 85% dose. This should be a minimum of 0.7 for fields greater than 10 cm × 10 cm.

The dose profiles must be measured for each energy in clinical use, including the surface dose defined at the depth of 0.5 mm, the relative dose due to the x-ray component determined beyond the range of the electrons, the therapeutic range defining the clinically useful part of the beam, the depth in water of the dose maximum, and the depth of the 50% dose; the practical range and the reduced dose gradient are the slope of the steep portion of the depth dose curve. Central-axis depth doses may decrease with small field dimensions. Any field with a short dimension less than the practical range has reduced depth dose and shallower d_{max} depth because of scatter, disequilibrium effects.

The x-ray component is due to the bremsstrahlung interactions along the beam path and is altered by collimation and air gap. It increases with energy to approximately 3% at 10 MeV, but the effect can be as much as 10% at 40 MeV. The bremsstrahlung tail is measured 2 cm beyond the practical range.

The $dose_{max}$ depth increases with increasing energy, decreases with oblique incidence, increases with increasing field size, and changes little with increasing source-skin distances. However, the dose gradient decreases with increasing energy, decreases with oblique incidence, increases with increasing field size, and changes little with increasing source-skin distance.

The variables that influence output are field size, primary collimator opening, applicator, and distance. Output measurements should be made for all standard jaw, cone, and insert combinations in clinical use. The electron output varies with photon collimator settings, even if all other factors are held equal. This effect is greater with lower energies. As a result, most machines have fixed jaw settings for each cone, with the calibrations performed at these settings. The scatter from electron cones is small, but it is a noticeable contribution to output; this effect, decreasing, with increasing energy.

Field size has a significant impact. As depth increases, the higher value isodose curves are constricted, reducing the effective field size (Figs 10-6 and 10-7). At the depth of the 80% isodose line, the area over which the dose distribution is acceptable may be reduced by 0.75 to 1 cm on each side, constricting the isodose curve. However, the effect of field size is small at high energies. It can become significant, however, when large cones are used with inserts to treat very small field sizes at low energies.

The effect of air gap between the cone surface and the area being treated varies for each energy and cone combination. The penumbra increases dramatically with distance from the applicator; this is particularly significant at low energies and for small fields.

Because of the propensity of lower energy electrons to scatter, the ratio of the surface dose to the dose maximum increases with increasing energy. This correlation is opposite to the association for x-rays. With electron energies below 12 MeV, there is a significant skin-sparing effect: the surface dose is 82% to 90% of the maximum, depending on energy. The surface dose increases with high energies, approaching 100% with 18-MeV electrons. In many institutions, a bolus is routinely used with 6- to 12-MeV electrons if the skin is at risk for tumor involvement (Fig. 10-8).

An appropriate admonition is to allow enough margin around the area being treated, remembering that the margin is a three-dimensional concept. Remember that the high-dose lines constrict substantially inside the geometric field. Therefore, allow enough depth of margin to keep the target volume out of the high dose-gradient; choose energies based on the 90% depth, and use a bolus if the clinical problem requires it. Small square blocks of bolus must be avoided, because they behave like large air or tissue inhomogeneities and generate significant hot spots in the shadows of their edges. A bolus should be taken into consideration when choosing the energy level for treatment of the patient's disease; use the total depth, including the bolus thickness to the deep part of the target. At energies above 12 MeV, a bolus may not be necessary with skin doses greater than 90% for scattering-foil machines. However, for energies below 9 MeV, the skin is effectively treated if a bolus is used.

Shielding should be applied carefully with the appropriate thickness to avoid edge effects coating internal, high-Z shielding with low-Z media absorbs backscatter electrons.

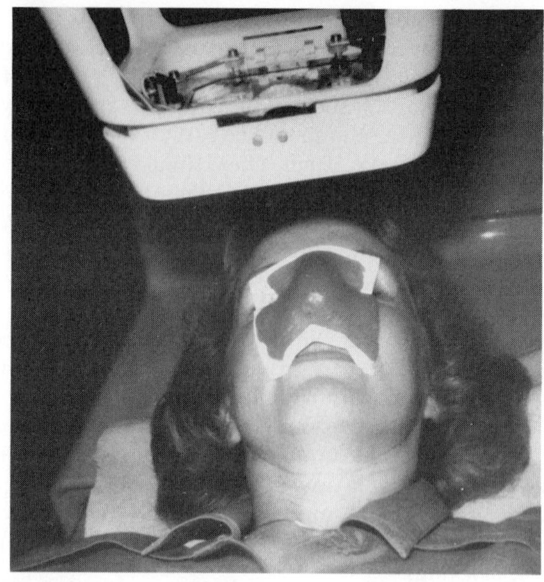

FIGURE 10–8. Photograph of a patient with basal cell carcinoma of the nose treated with 9-MeV electron beams and appositional portal. A 1-cm bolus was used to increase surface dose. A Cerrobend mask delineated treatment volume.

In general, oblique-incidence fields should be avoided, because they significantly alter the dose pattern. The surface dose increases, the d_{max} decreases, the dose gradient decreases, and the practical range increases only slightly.

The radiation oncologist must be aware of tissue inhomogeneities. The dose is altered by changes in electron density and atomic number of the medium. The classical empirical methods, such as coefficient of equivalent thickness, are often used for large, uniform slabs of material, but these results may break down under most common treatment circumstances. The typical coefficient of equivalent thickness for lung is 0.5, 1.5 for compact bone (*e.g.*, mandible), and 1.1 for spongy bone (*e.g.*,sternum). Computed tomography data make accurate calculations possible, even if too complex for routine use. Backscatter causes dosages to increase by 3% to 7% in front of a dense material, such as bone. The dose is similarly decreased in front of a less dense material, such as lung. The greatest effects are in line with the edges of the inhomogeneity. The dose within compact bone may be 10% to 18% higher than within tissue because of increased stopping and scattering powers and the shorter range of electrons within bone. The electron range within lung is much farther than in water, delivering higher doses inadvertently to larger volumes of deep tissues.

The choice of an appropriate gap between abutted fields is critical. The gap may vary with field size, distance, and beam characteristics. Matching for even dose at the surface implies hot spots at depth, and matching for even dose at depth implies cold spots at the surface.

The features of the electron beam that make it a unique therapeutic tool are related to physical qualities rather than biologic effectiveness. Laboratory studies have shown that the biologic effectiveness of the electron beam is nearly equal to that of the megavoltage photon irradiation.

Electron beams can be used in the principal treatment of several malignancies, which are discussed later in this chapter. A variation of combination treatment is that of "additional" or "boost" therapy, using reduced portals to raise the total dose to the initial gross disease. This practice is predicated on the hypothesis that microscopic disease can be permanently controlled with doses on the order of 5000 cGy in 5 weeks (*i.e.*, large

TABLE 10–1
Tolerance Doses for Different Anatomic Locations, Field Sizes, and Electron Energies

ANATOMIC LOCATION	FIELD SIZE (cm^2)	ELECTRON ENERGY (MeV)	DOSE (cGy)	TOTAL TIME (wk)
Lateral face	50	15–18	6500	6–6.5
Neck and chest wall	50	7–11	5000–5500	4

fields, large volumes, photos). Reducing the area receiving the high dose reduces the risk of damage to normal tissue (*i.e.*, small photon fields, interstitial therapy, or electrons).

Normal Tissue Reactions

The higher the electron-beam energy, the greater is the surface buildup dose and the more intense are the skin reactions. There is relatively less skin sparing with electron beams produced by betatrons than with those produced by linear accelerators. The difference between the measured surface doses for the same nominal energies is attributed in part to the method by which the beams are flattened in the different units. Tapley[19] developed skin tolerance tables correlating the factors of dose, time, area, electron energy, and anatomic site, including the lateral face, the upper and lower neck, and the chest wall. The intensity of skin reactions at high energies suggests that electron beams should be used in combination with megavoltage photon beams. Table 10-1 gives the tolerance doses for treating small fields on the lateral face and large fields on the neck and the chest wall with electron beams of the energies routinely used in these areas. The acute mucous membrane reactions seen with electron-beam therapy are similar to those produced by photon beams at the same doses but are sharply localized to the ipsilateral side. Limiting the high dose to one side of the oral cavity ensures less discomfort, improved nutrition, and decreased interference with salivary gland function. If electron-beam therapy is used exclusively in the treatment of lateralized lesions, fibrosis and late radiation sequelae usually become unacceptable. Electron-beam therapy should be combined with other radiation modalities.

Techniques

Shielding electron beams clinically is easily done with high-density materials, such as lead or lead amalgams. One centimeter of lead transmits only 5% of an 18-MeV electron dose. Electrons produced at the 7-MeV level require only 2.3 mm of lead. Added distance alone offered by intervening tissues significantly decreases the dose to deeper structures. For treating lesions of the oral cavity, intraoral stents contain lead, and protection of adjacent tissues is achieved by increasing the distance with tissue-equivalent Lucite.

Because of the easy blocking of the beam by dense materials, lead or Cerrobend is used extensively for defining treatment fields and for actual field shaping. The fields may be defined by lead or Cerrobend cutouts placed on a tray attached to the head of the accelerator. Special electron-beam cones are commercially available (Fig. 10-9).

The area covered to the 80% line of the 18-MeV electron beams is decreased by 0.5 to 0.75 cm at all margins of the field by shielding, requiring a proportionately larger field to ensure coverage of the entire lesion and a satisfactory surrounding margin. Implanting metallic seeds at the gross margins of the lesion permits evaluation of the adequacy of field margins in simulator localization films.

A differential in depth dose may be achieved by plastic energy moderators placed over a portion of the field. With 11-MeV electron beams, the addition of 1 cm of Lucite provides a dose distribution comparable to that of 9-MeV electron beams in the area covered by Lucite. This technique is used when only a portion of the treatment is to be given with the electron beam because all skin sparing is lost by the interposition of this tissue-equivalent material.

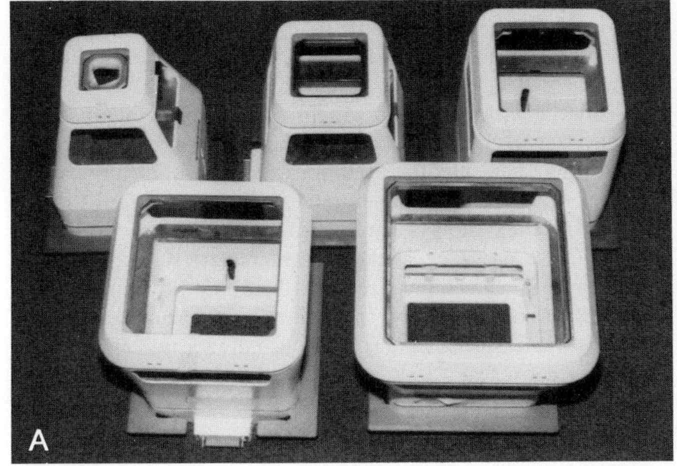

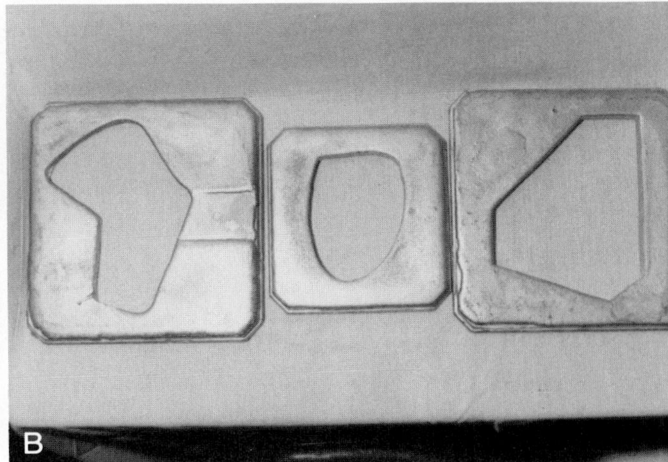

FIGURE 10–9. (**A**) Cones used in electron-beam therapy. (**B**) Cerrobend masks to delineate treatment volume.

Skin and Lip Tumors

Electron-beam therapy is ideal for radiation therapy of all skin and lip cancers and is particularly useful in the treatment of lesions that present problems or are critically located (*e.g.*, lesions involving the eyelid, nose, or ear).

For small superficial basal cell carcinomas, a 1-cm margin surrounding the gross lesion is adequate. In large infiltrative lesions with diffuse induration associated with a surgical scar, 2-cm or 3-cm margins are required, with wide borders of uninvolved tissue. For squamous cell carcinoma, the field usually can be reduced at 5000 cGy.

Most lesions located on the eyelids, external nose, cheeks, or ears are not deeply invasive and are treated with electron beams at energies of 6 MeV to 9 MeV. If the lesion approaches 2 cm in thickness, 9-MeV to 12-MeV electron beams should be used.

Protective devices should be designed to delineate the treatment field and to conform to the irregular shape of a lesion (Fig 10-10). A wax ledge placed around the opening in a lead mask may provide a seating for the treatment portal and enhance precision in directing the beam. To achieve almost complete protection, 2.8 mm of lead, which absorbs almost 98% of 7-MeV electron beams, should be used; for 9-MeV electron beams, 4 mm of lead is required to absorb 98%, and 3.3 mm is required for 95% energy absorption. With 11-MeV electron beams, 8 mm of lead is required for 98% attenuation, and 3.8 mm to 4.3 mm of lead is required for 95% attenuation. Lead is also used for protection of the deeper structures. In treatment of the cheek or the lip, lead in an intraoral stent made for the patient protects the gingiva and tongue (Fig.10-11). For treatment of the eyelid or near the eye, a lead shield is placed under the lid. Because the eye shields must be thin, they are suitable only for 7-MeV electron beams. The eye shields should be wax-coated to decrease backscatter electron dose to the eyelid. Thicker external blocks may be necessary to protect the eye at higher electron energies. Table 10-2 presents the results of treatment of cancers of the skin and lips using the electron beam.[17]

Whenever there is potential skin involvement, an appropriately chosen bolus should be used.

Upper Respiratory and Digestive Tracts

Electron beams alone may be used to treat carcinomas of the upper respiratory tract and digestive passages, frequently combined with external-beam high-energy photons or with interstitial brachytherapy, as in the treatment of well-lateralized lesions of the oral cavity, oropharynx, hypopharynx, or supraglottic larynx.

Electron-beam therapy for lesions of the oral cavity may be used with intraoral cones, which must provide coverage of the lesion with an adequate margin of normal mucous membrane on all sides. An intraoral stent may be necessary to maintain the position of the cone and to reproduce the placement of the cone at each treatment session. The electron energy (6, 9, or 12 MeV) is chosen according to the characteristics of the tumor and the depth of extension of the tumor.

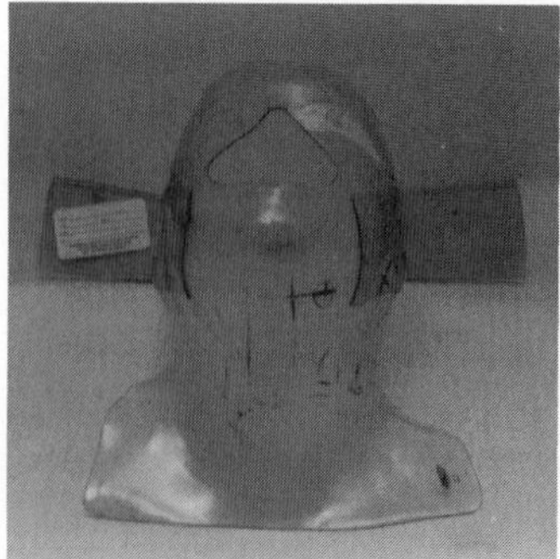
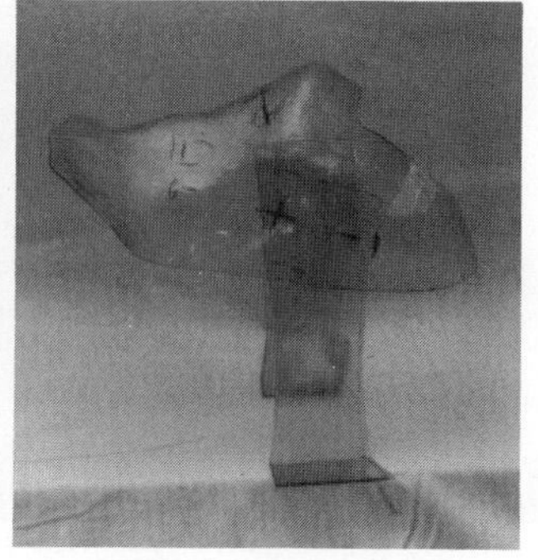

FIGURE 10–10. Plastic masks used with electron-beam therapy.

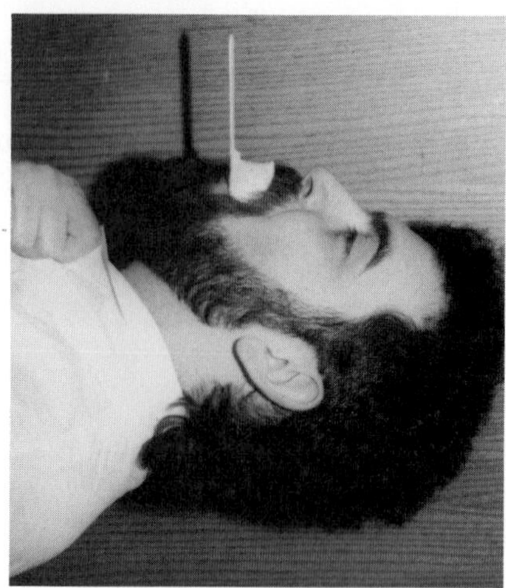

FIGURE 10–11. Intraoral stent used to displace normal structures.

Salivary Gland Tumors

Treatment for salivary gland tumors generally uses electrons (75% to 80% of dose) in combination with photons (20% to 25% of dose). The application of electron-beam therapy alone or with photon beams is most effective after the bulk of the tumor has been removed. The area to be irradiated includes the entire parotid bed and the full extent of the surgical scar. However, special consideration should be given to potential seventh cranial nerve involvement in all patients with adenocystic carcinomas. The temporal bone must be irradiated.

The entire ipsilateral neck may be irradiated in treating the parotid gland area if the primary tumor is a high-grade malignancy, if the tumor is found in connective tissues, if there is extensive invasion of perineural lymphatics, or if there are positive nodes in the operative specimen. The treatment of the entire neck may be given by electron beams (9 MeV).

Cervical Lymphatics

Metastasis to the cervical lymphatics from squamous cell carcinomas of the upper respiratory tract and digestive tract traditionally has been considered a uniquely surgical problem. Irradiation can be administered to both sides of the neck, except if only one side is affected and the contralateral side is at negligible risk for development of metastatic disease.

Patients with clinically evident neck disease or recurrent disease after neck dissection should have the entire neck irradiated, rather than only the area of gross disease. In a review by Fletcher and Evers[5] of patients treated for recurrent disease after surgical excision of carcinomas of the upper respiratory and digestive passages, a higher control rate was observed in patients who received localized irradiation to the area of recurrence. Recurrent disease may present as a small cutaneous nodule or an infiltrative mass. It is usually located close to the neck dissection scar.

Breast Cancer

Electron-beam therapy has been of particular value in the treatment of breast cancer, both for administering an additional

TABLE 10–2
Cancer of Skin and Lips: Results of Treatment With Electron Beam (May 1963 to December 1970)

		HISTORY			TREATMENT RESULTS			
ANATOMIC SITE	**NUMBER OF CASES**	NO PRIOR TREATMENT	EXCISION WITH CLOSE SURGICAL MARGIN	RECURRENCE AFTER SURGERY	PERSISTENT OR RECURRENT	CON-TROLLED	SURGICAL SALVAGE	TOTAL WITH NO EVIDENCE OF DISEASE
Eyelids	41	28	7	6	5	36	2	38
Nose	24	11	6	7	3	21	3	24
Temple and cheek	19	6	6	7	3	16	3	19
Lip	14	7	1	6	1	13	1	14
Miscellaneous	13	3	7	3	3	10	1	11
Total	111	55	27	29	15	96	10	106

(From Tapley N [ed]: Clinical Applications of the Electron Beam. New York, John Wiley & Sons, 1976)

dose to the site of tumor excision in conservation treatment and for treating subclinical disease in patients who have had surgical removal of the primary breast lesion and axillary lymphatics.

During radiation therapy, the supine patient has the arm abducted to 90 degrees and the forearm maintained in an upright position by a hanging bar, which the hand grasps. The head may be turned sharply to the contralateral side. The beam remains vertical. Various manipulations of the machine, collimator, and other factors may be needed to achieve proper placement of the treatment field (Fig. 10-12).

Radiation therapy may also be designed for the chest wall. Because the average chest wall thickness after radical mastectomy is in the range of 1.5 cm to 2.0 cm, low-energy electron beams (6 to 9 MeV) may be appropriate. If the chest wall thickness is greater, electron beams of high energy (12 MeV) may be necessary. Computed tomography offers an excellent means of measuring the thickness of the chest wall and aids in the choice of the appropriate energy level to be used. A 1-cm bolus may be required to increase the surface dose, and as a consequence, the energy may need to be increased to maintain adequate penetration.

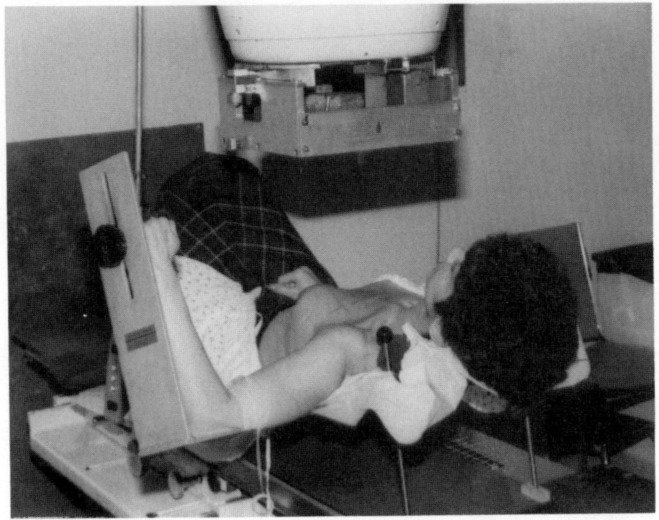

FIGURE 10–12. Setup for electron-beam therapy for breast cancer.

Neoplasms of Other Sites

Certain lymphomas that present as subcutaneous masses or dermal lesions can be treated by electron-beam therapy. In many soft tissue sarcomas, electron-beam therapy can be used as total treatment or as an adjunct to photon-beam treatment, with preservation of function and diminution in the number of late side effects of the treatment. Primary or recurrent carcinomas of the vulva, distal vagina, urethra, suburethral area, or other areas that recur after surgical removal and carcinomas of the cervix that recur in the vagina may be treated with electron beams (6, 9, or 12 MeV), incorporating an appropriate bolus.

Intraoperative electron-beam used as a boost followed by photon-beam treatment represents an innovative regimen, particularly in treating gastric cancer, retroperitoneal sarcomas, head and neck cancers, and genitourinary and gynecologic cancers.

High-Energy Electron-Beam Therapy

Electron-beam therapy in high-energy ranges (18 to 35 MeV) may be used in the treatment of various deep-seated tumors, usually in combination with photon-beam therapy. Techniques have been designed for treatment of bladder cancers (with excellent results), tumors of the head and neck, carcinomas of the esophagus, carcinomas of the lung, and breast cancer in certain situations. Treatment of cancers of the lung, bladder, colon, rectum, and cervix with combinations of photon beams and electron beams has been reported.[5]

FUTURE DEVELOPMENTS

In the treatment of the chest wall, fixed electron portals suffer from field-matching problems because of surface curvature and poor dose distributions along the lateral chest wall, where the electron beam is more nearly parallel to the skin surface. Because of these problems, arc electron techniques have been developed.[8] The ability of the electron beam to penetrate the low-density lung can result in substantial irradiation of the lung. The border between the lung and the mediastinum is long and parallel to the beam, compromising the accuracy of the dose

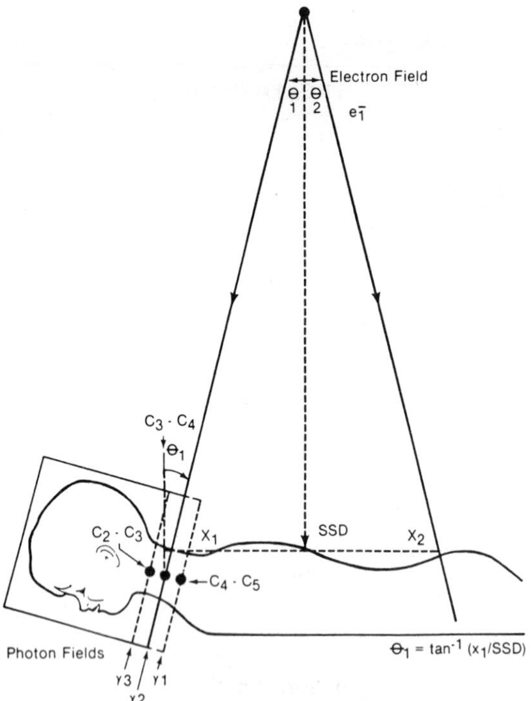

FIGURE 10–13. Craniospinal irradiation field placement.

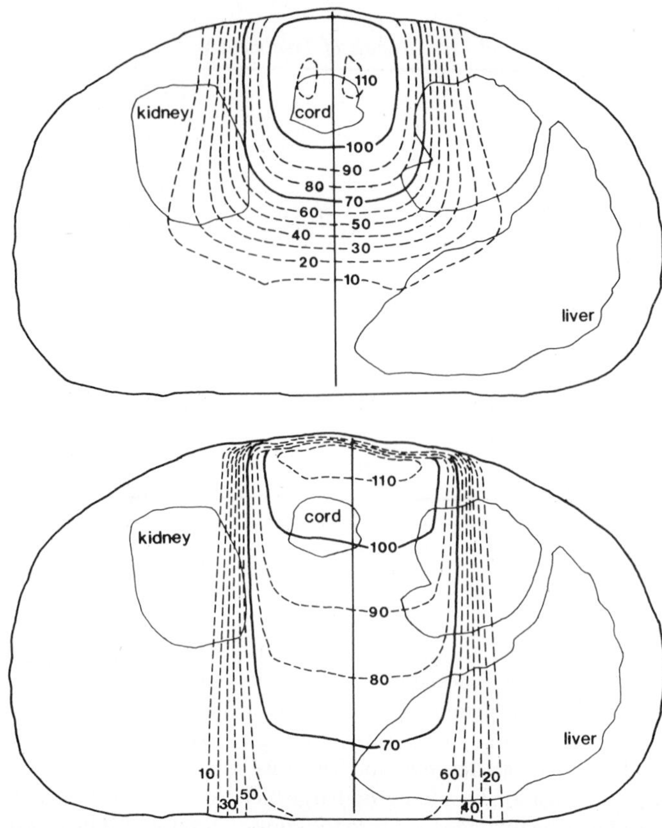

FIGURE 10–14. Craniospinal irradiation technique using 15-MeV electron beams, 110-cm SSD (*top*) and ^{60}Co photon beams, 80-cm SSD (*bottom*).

distribution in that region. Hogstrom and associates[7,8] are in the process of studying the applicability of arc electron techniques to radiation treatment of the chest wall.

Electron-beam treatment techniques for irradiation of the spinal axis have been developed by Hogstrom and co-workers (Figs. 10-13 and 10-14). The treatment plans are designed using existing pencil-beam algorithms. There is some question about the accuracy of the dose in the spinal cord because of the irregular nature of the spinal column in the sagittal dimension, the heterogeneous spinous processes that are parallel to the beam, and the depth of the vertebral column. Although current doses are limited to 3000 cGy for craniospinal irradiation of brain tumors, there may be cases in which tumor extending into the cervical spine requires higher doses, approaching cord tolerance. Increasing tumor doses to 5000 cGy requires a high confidence level in the dose delivered to the spinal cord.

In the treatment of retinoblastoma, the aim is to irradiate the entire retina with minimal dose to the lens of the eye.

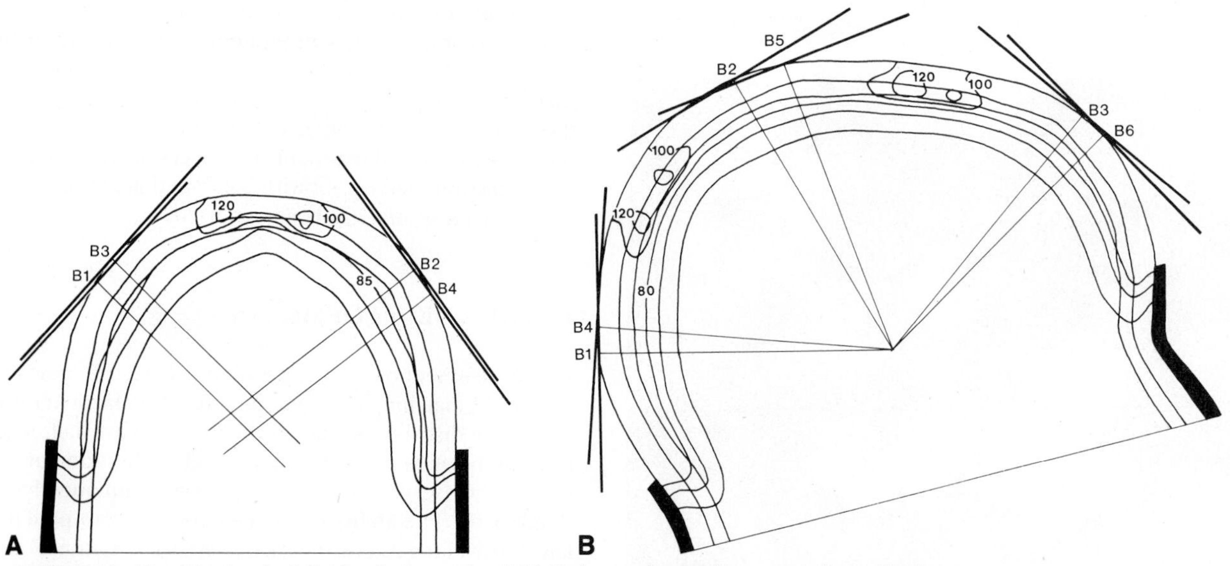

FIGURE 10–15. Total-scalp 6-field technique using 7-MeV electron-beam therapy, performed using a Lucite bolus. Lead on the skin surface defines the field. (**A**) Cross-sectional view. (**B**) Sagittal view.

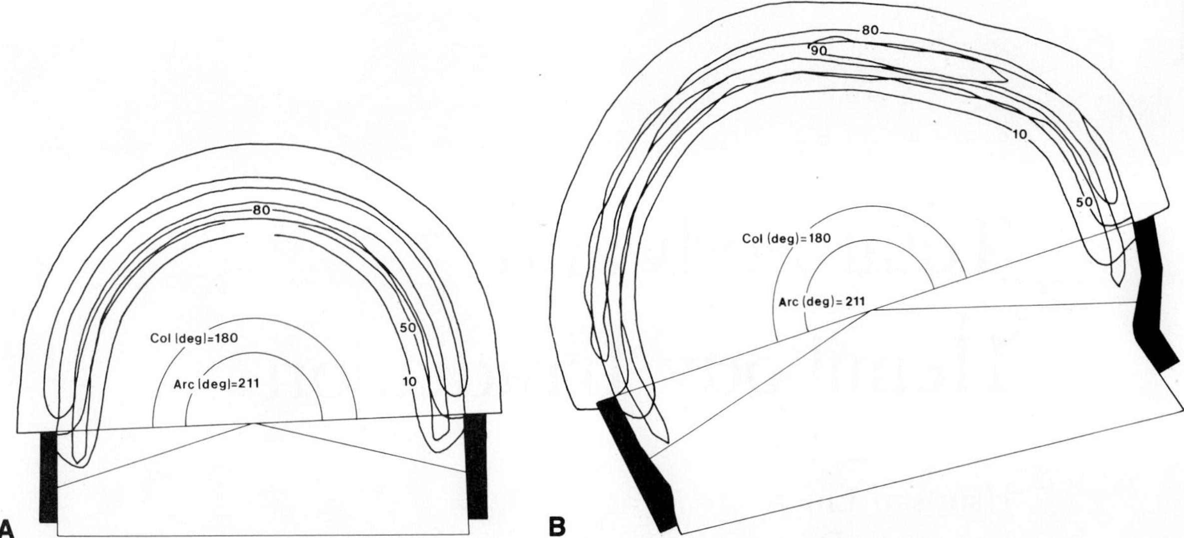

FIGURE 10–16. Total-scalp electron arc technique (7 MeV). (**A**) Cross-sectional view. (**B**) Sagittal view.

Schipper[15] devised a precise technique for localizing the tumor that permits submillimeter accuracy for sparing the lens but that may limit the dose to the most anterior position. Hogstrom and co-workers[7,8] are supplementing this technique with anterior electron-beam irradiation with a central lens block. This technique has been studied by Hogstrom in detail, but the influences of bone and the irregular surfaces of the eye and skin on the dosimetry are still being evaluated.

Irradiation of the whole scalp remains a difficult problem because of the topology of the head. It is currently done by abutting several fixed electron beams (Figs. 10-15 and 10-16). Problems in dosimetry arise at the abutment points and due to the scattering of electrons off the cranial bones laterally and backward. Hogstrom and associates[7,8] are developing an improved technique that can offer both improved dosimetry and more rapid treatment.

REFERENCES

1. Ahix FH: Introduction to Radiological Physics and Dosimetry. New York, John Wiley & Sons, 1986.
2. Almond PR: Characteristics of current medical electron accelerator beams. In Chu F, Laughlin J (eds): Proceedings of the Symposium on Electron Beam Therapy, p 47. New York, Memorial Sloan-Kettering Cancer Center, 1981
3. American Association of Physicists in Medicine, RTC Task Group 21: A protocol for the determination of absorbed dose from high energy photons and electrons. Med Phys 10:752, 1983
4. Dawson, DJ: Percentage depth dose for high energy x-rays. Phys Med Biol 21:228, 1976
5. Fletcher GH, Evers WT: Radiotherapeutic management of surgical recurrences and postoperative residuals in tumors of the head and neck. Radiology 95:185, 1970
6. Gagnon WF, Grant W: Surface dose from megavoltage therapy machines. Radiology 117:707, 1975

6A. Harder D: Energiespektren schneller Elektronen in verdener Tiefe. Symposium on High Energy Electrons. Montreux, 1964:26. Berlin, Springer Verlag, 1965

7. Hogstrom KR, Almond PR: Comparison of experimental and calculated dose distribution: A review of electron beam dose planning at the M.D. Anderson Hospital. Acta Radiol [Suppl] 364:89, 1983
8. Hogstrom KR, Karup RG: Derivation of a pencil-beam algorithm for arc electron therapy. Med Phys 11:378, 1984
9. International Commission on Radiation Units and Measurements: Report No. 35: Radiation Dosimetry: Electron Beams with Energies Between 1 and 50 MeV, p 107. Washington, DC, International Commission on Radiation Units and Measurements, 1984
10. International Commission on Radiation Units and Measurements: Report No. 35: Radiation Dosimetry: Electron Beams with Energies Between 1 and 50 MeV, pp 6,7,12,13. Washington, DC, International Commission on Radiation Units and Measurements, 1984
11. Kahn FM: The Physics of Radiation Therapy, p 301. Baltimore, Williams & Wilkins, 1984
12. Kase KR, Nelson WR: Concepts of Radiation Dosimetry, p 60. New York, Pergamon Press, 1978.
13. Nordic Association of Clinical Physics: Procedures in external radiation therapy dosimetry with electrons and photon beams with maximum energies between 1 and 50 MeV. Acta Radiol 19:64, 1980
14. Orton CG, Bagne F (eds): Practical Aspects of Electron Beam Treatment Planning. New York, American Association of Physicists in Medicine, 1978
15. Schipper J: An accurate and simple method for megavoltage radiation therapy of retinoblastoma. Radiother Oncol 1:31, 1983
16. Svenson H: Electron beam parameters, p 68. Proceedings of the American Association of Physicists in Medicine—1976, Summer School, 1976
17. Tapley N (ed): Clinical Applications of the Electron Beam. New York, John Wiley & Sons, 1976
18. Tapley N: General considerations. In Tapley N (ed): Clinical Applications of the Electron Beam, pp 81–91. New York, John Wiley & Sons, 1976
19. Tapley N: Skin and lips. In Tapley N (ed): Clinical Applications of the Electron Beam, pp 93–122. New York, John Wiley & Sons, 1976

11

○ ○ ○ ● ● ●

Total-Body and Hemibody Irradiation

Hsiu-san Lin
Robert E. Drzymala

TOTAL-BODY IRRADIATION

Total-body irradiation has been used as a form of systemic therapy for various malignant diseases since 1900.[11,31,54] However, the usefulness of total-body irradiation without bone marrow rescue was limited because the median lethal dose of total-body irradiation given as a single fraction is about 300 cGy in humans. It was mainly used for palliating symptoms or obtaining short-term remissions.[11,31,54] This limited role was decreased even further with the advent of cytotoxic chemotherapy in the 1960s.

Interest was revived, primarily because of the pioneering work of Thomas and associates,[89] who showed that a supralethal dose of both total-body irradiation and cytotoxic drugs followed by bone marrow rescue could be used for long-term control of malignancies that had become refractory to conventional treatments. Intensive cytoreductive chemoradiotherapy followed by bone marrow transplantation was once a modality employed as a last resort after multiple relapses of leukemias or lymphomas, but recent studies indicate that it may be the treatment of choice for patients with early-stage chronic myelogenous leukemia, acute leukemia (adult), and high-grade lymphomas.[1,9,86]

Applications

Immunosuppression

All hemopoietic stem cells and lymphoid cells are sensitive to ionizing radiation. Low-dose total-body irradiation, less than 200 cGy given as a single fraction or as 5-cGy to 15-cGy fractions given 2 to 5 times weekly, has been used for patients with autoimmune diseases.[20,37,40] In allogeneic bone marrow transplantation, a higher dose (> 750 cGy) is often required to prevent graft rejection if it is used alone.[89] When patients with aplastic anemia are prepared for bone marrow transplantation, a single dose of 300 cGy is used in conjunction with cyclophosphamide to reduce the probability of graft rejection.[22]

Low-Dose Systemic Therapy for Leukemias and Lymphomas

Low-dose total-body irradiation has been useful in inducing remission in chronic lymphocytic leukemia and low-grade non-Hodgkin's lymphomas in advanced stages.[10,18,32,36,50,53] The patients receive 5-cGy to 15-cGy fractions 2 to 5 times weekly. It is generally recommended that the patient takes 4 to 8 weeks off after each 50 cGy of total-body irradiation to avoid severe thrombocytopenia.[14,35] About 33% of patients with chronic lymphocytic leukemia attained complete remission with low-dose total-body irradiation alone, and 39% had remissions with a combination of total-body irradiation and chemotherapy.[35,36] However, this was not confirmed in another report.[70]

High-Dose Cytoreductive Therapy Before Bone Marrow Transplantation

The role of total-body irradiation used in conjunction with autologous or syngeneic bone marrow transplant is to kill tumor cells.[63,64,88,89] However, when allogeneic bone marrow transplantation is used, an additional role is to kill host lymphohemopoietic stem cells and lymphoid cells to prevent rejection of donor cells.[89] It is also postulated that the elimination of host hemopoietic stem cells may create spaces in bone marrow for donor cells to seed and grow. The Seattle group originally used a single fraction of 1000 cGy of total-body irradiation before bone marrow transplantation because they had found that 950 cGy was required to obtain consistent and sustained engraftment of allogeneic marrow in experimental animals.[89]

Because of the high incidence of idiopathic interstitial pneumonitis, most transplant centers now use a fractionated-dose total-body irradiation regimen.[28,63,64,69,81,87] This has greatly reduced the incidence of interstitial pneumonitis to less than 20% to 30% without increasing the rate of tumor recurrence.[28,64,81,87] The most commonly employed fraction size is 200 cGy, which is given once or twice daily.[28,63,87] With this fractionation, no significant increase in the incidence of interstitial pneumonitis occurs up to a total dose of 1400 cGy.[63] Shank and co-workers[81] used 120 cGy, given three times daily as well as using partial lung blocks to protect the lungs. The use of this hyperfractionation schedule has reduced the incidence of interstitial pneumonitis to 33%, compared with 70% for single-dose total-body irradiation (1000 cGy).

Lowering the dose rate has been proposed as another approach to reduce the incidence of interstitial pneumonitis. Although successful, the use of this approach is limited for medical and logistic reasons.[4] If the dose rate is lowered to 5 cGy/minute, it takes more than 3 hours to deliver 1000 cGy.[4] The patient often develops acute radiation side effects while being irradiated, and the treatment is therefore interrupted. Unless a dedicated unit is available, this long treatment time will certainly cause scheduling problems for treatment centers.

Technique

Implementing Large-Field Technique

Three approaches are available for implementing large-field radiation therapy in the clinic: designing a dedicated unit, developing a special treatment method by modifying existing facilities, or using an unmodified radiation therapy unit within its constraints. Some compromises must be made, thereby departing from the ideal treatment technique. With this in mind, several factors must be considered[93] when designing a large-field technique: dose homogeneity, lung sparing, dose prescription, and accuracy of treatment. Simplicity, reproducibility, and reliability of treatment setup, simplicity of treatment planning, comfort for patient and staff, minimal staff time, and integration of the technique into the daily treatment routine are also desirable goals. Only a limited number of parameters can be manipulated to optimize large-field technique. These include selecting the energy of radiation, treatment distance, and dose rate; enhancing of the surface dose with a bolus or scatter screen (*i.e.*, a plastic sheet in front of the patient that scatters electrons to the patient's surface); compensating for missing and heterogeneous tissue; and choosing between anteroposterior (AP) and posteroanterior (PA) or lateral treatments or a combination of these.

Several rules-of-thumb derived from the physics of large-field radiation beams can serve as guidelines in implementing a sensible technique[93]:

1. Generally, there is lower dose variation in the treated volume with higher-energy photon beams; however, the effects of the buildup region and tissue inhomogeneities must be ignored. If high-energy beams of linear accelerators are used, some consideration should be given to the effects of low dose in the buildup and build-down regions. Although there are no data indicating clinical problems, the buildup effect can be minimized with the prudent use of a bolus or scatter screen.
2. There is lower dose variation with larger treatment distance, because this tends to minimize field aperture and the effects of the inverse-square law.
3. A larger dose variation occurs with larger patient diameter.
4. AP and PA treatments yield a variation not larger than 15% for most megavoltage energies and distances, but lung blocks must be used to achieve this.
5. Lateral opposed beams usually give a greater dose variation compared with AP and PA treatments, especially for adult patients. When pediatric patients are treated with higher energy beams, ± 15% uniformity with bilateral fields may be achieved.

Facilities for Large-Field Photon Irradiation

Because of the diversity of restrictions found in various treatment centers, many different techniques have evolved.[93] Figure 11-1 shows several methods of total land hemibody irradiation.

DEDICATED FACILITIES

A description of one of the first dedicated total-body irradiation facilities in North America appeared in the literature in 1932.[31] It was a lead-lined room with four beds at one end and an x-ray tube at the other end. Four patients could be simultaneously irradiated about 5 to 7 m from the tube. During a treatment, the tube operated continuously for 20 hours at 185 kVp and 3 mA, with 2-mm copper filtration.

Jacobs and Pape[33] report on a device used at the City of Hope Medical Center in the early 1960s. Four rods were housed at each end of a treatment bed, each rod containing two 300-Ci ^{137}Cs sources separated by 2 m from each other. The source rods retracted below the floor in the off position. Lead attenuators were employed to obtain the desired dose rates.

Webster[98] reviewed the physics of designing irradiators that would give a ± 10% total-body dose. He concluded the

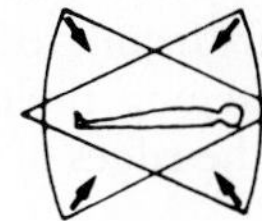

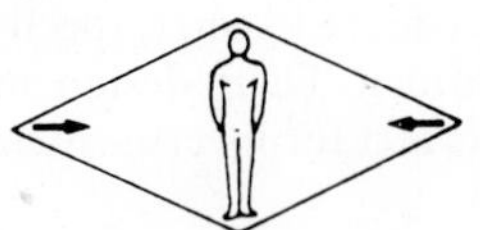

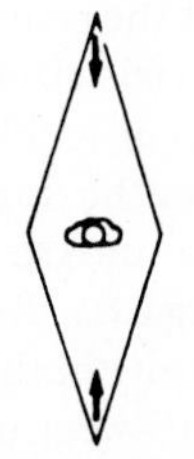

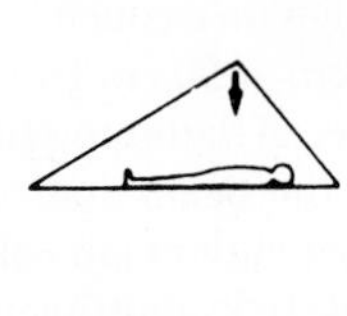

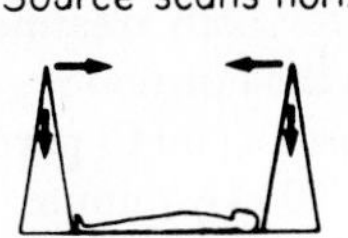

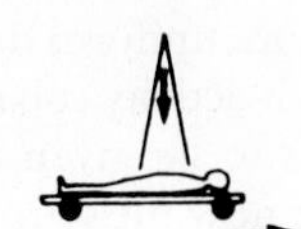

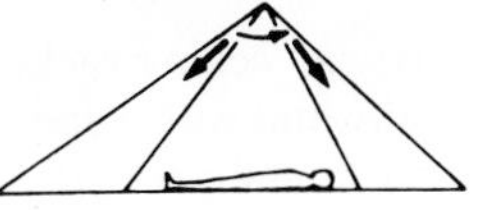

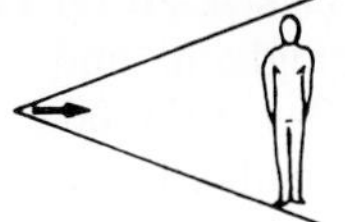

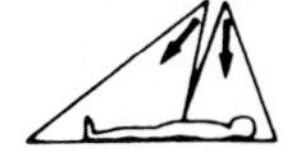

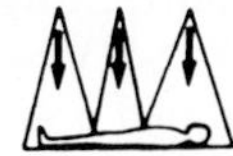

FIGURE 11–1. Different methods of total and hemibody irradiation. (Reprinted with permission from Report No. 17, American Association of Physicists in Medicine)[93]

following characteristics are desirable: a small room size to minimize cost, shielding, and building space; sources distributed above and below the patient; a minimum number of sources to reduce cost and maintenance; and a simple procedure for controlling exposure. He judged that a minimum of four radiation sources were required to uniformly irradiate the entire body. Despite their appeal, dedicated multiple-source irradiation rooms are too expensive for most medical facilities.

In 1959, Sahler[75] developed an irradiator consisting of two cobalt units, one conventional and the other an industrial large-field irradiator. The two units generated a horizontal, parallel opposed field approximately 3 m from the patient that produced low-dose-rate total-body irradiation. The collimators of the conventional cobalt unit had to be removed to obtain a large field.

Surmount and associates[84] performed total-body irradiation at the Institute Gustave Roussy in the 1960s using twin opposed ^{60}Co sources separated by a movable concrete wall. In their bone marrow transplantation program at The Fred Hutchinson Cancer Research Center in Seattle, Washington, Thomas and colleagues[88] used two parallel opposed ^{60}Co sources that moved along a track and had specially designed collimators for total-body irradiation. A similar design was used by the Munich Cooperative Group[43] for bone marrow transplantation studies in dogs. Lutz and co-workers[49] described a dual-source large-field facility using parallel opposed 4-MeV linear accelerators mounted on the ceiling and floor. Each machine moves vertically with the source-to-source distance varying from 240 to 410 cm. The patient lies on a couch between the accelerators. Field size varies, with a maximum width and length of 75 cm and 210 cm, respectively. Dose rates vary from 4 to 225 cGy/minute. Their design incorporates a flattening filter to help correct for inverse-square effects toward the edges of the field.

Princess Margaret Hospital, Toronto, has housed a single-source large-field ^{60}Co irradiator since 1977.[47] The radiation beam projects down from the source located at the ceiling, and the patient lies on a couch beneath the source. Field sizes are 50 cm × 160 cm at 90 cm from the source or 83 cm × 265 cm at 150 cm. Special flattening filters compensate for the dose variation across the beam aperture and for inverse-square effects. Having independent jaw collimation in the long axis, the device allows simple field abutting for patients who receive both upper- and lower-hemibody treatments separated by a 6-week interval. One jaw acts as a beam splitter near the central ray. Therefore, setting the central ray to the umbilicus for both treatments yields a more uniform dose distribution in the junction region. Use of high-activity cobalt sources of almost 10,000 Ci permits treatments to be given at approximately 50 cGy/minute. An attenuator near the source also allows low-dose-rate treatments.

CONVENTIONAL UNITS MODIFIED FOR LARGE-FIELD TREATMENTS

Cunningham and Wright[13] describe a ceiling-rack-mounted Picker C3000 Cobalt-60 Teletherapy unit with a specially designed collimator. The source can horizontally scan the length of a patient lying on the couch and is positioned at a source-to-skin distance of 120 cm. Quast[68] describes a similar method, but the patient is moved on a mobile couch beneath a fixed ^{60}Co source. Engler and associates[21] developed a technique using a 42-MV betatron that arcs over the patient. Pla and others[66] modified a 4-MV linac that scans over a patient. To accomplish this, the source located above the patient rotates with the head of the irradiator from the foot to the head of the patient. A similar technique using an isocentric cobalt unit having an automatic arcing capability and a curved couch was presented by Mulvey and colleagues.[57] Peters and Herer[62] described a quick procedure accomplished by removing the collimators from a standard ^{60}Co unit. The machine could be readied in 15 minutes.

USE OF UNMODIFIED CONVENTIONAL TREATMENT UNITS

Many reports have appeared in the literature describing the use of conventional therapy units for total-body irradiation and hemibody irradiation.[41,42,69,80,93]

To enclose the patient within a single radiation field, patients have been treated laterally while seated or reclining or AP while lying on a side, with arms and legs folded to the trunk in some cases. In the past, a single-fraction, low-dose-rate (*i.e.*, < 10 cGy/minute) treatment has been the standard. However, the high outputs currently available with linacs have encouraged treatments at high dose rates (*i.e.*, 50 cGy/minute) in multiples to reduce lung complications. This approach significantly reduces the treatment time and increases the comfort of the patient.

Use of multiple, adjacent fields is another technique for delivering total-body irradiation on an unmodified conventional treatment unit. However, two significant disadvantages accompany this approach: field junctions are difficult to match, producing hot or cold spots, and target cells circulate out of the treatment field and receive less than the prescribed dose.

In 1983, Shank[80] reviewed treatment methods at several institutions in the United States that had ongoing large-field treatment programs. At the University of California in Los Angeles, no compensators or bolus was employed. The patient lay on a couch with the beam at a 17-degree angle to the patient's sagittal plane. The ^{60}Co machine gave the prescribed dose to the patient's midline at a source-to-axis distance of 325 cm to 330 cm.

At the University of Washington, Seattle, two parallel opposed ^{60}Co sources, 500 cm apart, irradiated the midline of the patient. The sources projected horizontally to the patient. Half the treatment is accomplished with the patient lying on his or her side, and the other half is done with the patient lying supine on the couch.

The Johns Hopkins technique required no compensators or bolus, but used lung blocks. A single ^{60}Co source irradiates at a distance of 340 cm to the midline of the patient, lying on his or her side. Half of the treatment is given PA, and the other half is given AP.

In the City of Hope Hospital technique, blankets provide an 8-mm tissue-equivalent bolus. The patient lies on his or her side at a skin-to-source distance of 370 cm from a 10-MV linear accelerator. Compensators attenuate the beam for the calf, foot, and neck, and a 6-mm Lucite screen scatters electrons AP.

At the University of Minnesota, a compensator covered all except the pelvis. The patient was seated on a stretcher, where a 0.375-in Lucite screen provided scattered electrons to the patient's skin surface.[42] The treatment was given at a skin-to-axis distance of 411 cm. Half of the prescription dose was given on the right side, and half of the prescription dose was given on the left.

The Memorial Sloan-Kettering Cancer Center technique employed no compensators. Treatments were given at a skin-to-axis distance of 420 cm to 575 cm from a 10-MV linear accelerator with the patient in a "tucked" position. A 1-cm Lexan screen between the source and the patient enhanced the patient's surface dose. Lung blocks were used, alternating between the AP and PA fields.

Quast[69] reviewed the various techniques implemented in Europe, where over 70 treatment centers employ large-field radiation treatments.

Comparing Treatment Techniques

Analyzing the results of AP or PA and lateral field treatments for 6 MV x-rays on a humanoid phantom shows that for AP or PA fields the dose variation to the various parts along the axis of the body can range from ± 7% to ± 10%.[93] However, for lateral fields, the dose variation can range up to 50% in the head and neck region and 15% in the remainder of the body. This variation can be decreased to the same level as that in the rest of the body with the appropriate use of compensators in the head and neck region. Alternatively, tissue-equivalent bolus material may be placed directly on the skin if the loss of skin-sparing effects is not a concern; however, it may be quite uncomfortable for the patient during the long treatment times.

If compensators are positioned in the head and neck region, care must be taken not to underdose the shoulders by shifting the compensator too far inferiorly. Total-body irradiation and hemibody irradiation patients are rarely immobilized, and the compensator material is usually mounted at some distance from the patient (*e.g.*, at the head of the machine). Because it is very hard to match the compensator to index marks on the skin under these conditions, a simple one-dimensional compensator constructed of lead, copper, brass, or Cerrobend is adequate.

Compensation for tissue inhomogeneities is important, particularly in the region of the chest, where the lung is a critical structure. For the AP/PA technique, think lung blocks are used to increase the homogeneity of dose throughout the chest. For the lateral technique, the arm can be used to shield the lungs, providing better dose homogeneity. Without such corrections, particularly for AP or PA treatments, dose inhomogeneities can exceed the prescribed dose by 40%.[93]

It may seem that the AP/PA technique is preferred to the lateral technique because it minimizes the patient thickness along the central axis of the beam. Its use may be precluded, however, by the inability to obtain the needed source-to-patient distance. If it were possible to achieve a source-to-patient distance of 375 cm for a treatment machine with a 40 cm × 40 cm collimator setting at a skin-to-axis distance of 110 cm, a 6-foot patient could stand in a diagonal of the field and be covered by one continuous field. At these distances, the dose variation resulting from inverse-square differences from the center to the edge of the field would be no more than 4%.

Comparing Doses Among Institutions

Because there is no standard treatment technique for total-body irradiation, hemibody irradiation, or other large-field treatments, significant differences in the dose distributions exist with different treatment methods. Two institutions can prescribe the same dose at some selected point, but if different techniques are used, the dose to other points can vary considerably. Uncertainties in absolute dosimetry and large variations of dose across the target volume make it difficult to assess clinical effectiveness when results from different treatment centers are compared.

To facilitate comparisons among institutions, various methods for describing the dose from large-field treatments have been reported.[27,41] One reasonable approach uses a single point prescription and specifies limits for the highest and lowest dose acceptable for any point in the body. Dose limits are also set for specific tissues, such as the lungs. A good example of a total-body irradiation prescription is given in American Association of Physicists in Medicine Report No. 17, using the midpoint at the level of the umbilicus as a convenient prescription point.[93] A typical prescription may read the dose to the midpoint at the level of the umbilicus as 800 cGy. A'l points in the body must fall within the limits of 840 cGy and 720 cGy, or +5% and −10%. The dose to more than half the lung volume must not exceed 800 cGy. The dose rate at the prescription point must not exceed 10 cGy/minute.

A good total-body irradiation program includes a program for dose measurement in a phantom, including calibration in a water phantom or other appropriate material at the treatment geometry. If necessary, dose measurements must be converted to dose in water. Percent ionization or tissue-phantom ratio measurements are required. Tissue-phantom ratio and tissue-maximum ratio tables are practical to use for monitoring unit calculations, because these ratios are essentially independent of distance. Checks of beam flatness at the treatment distance are important, especially along the diagonal near the corners of the field. Energies may vary there, too. An ionization chamber is the recommended method for these measurements, but care must be taken to minimize irradiation of the cable. Measurements of build-down and buildup regions can be useful in determining what the surface doses are (Fig. 11-2). A parallel plate ionization chamber in plastic phantom is very useful for these measurements. Ultimately, dose verification should also be done on an anthropomorphic phantom. Thermoluminescent dosimetry measurements can verify point doses, and film can record dose distributions.

For any new technique, *in vivo* verification is required. Changes in patient position can alter dose distributions dramatically. Thermoluminescent dosimeters, ionization chambers, and diodes are typical choices for monitoring the dose to the patient. They may be used at entrance and exit point, but scatter from the room must be carefully considered. Midline doses can usually be measured directly in rectum, mouth, and esophagus and between legs and feet. Multiple diode systems are convenient for these types of measurements.

A bone marrow transplantation protocol imposes strict time constraints on the availability of large-field irradiation treatment, because the patient needs to be irradiated within a certain interval from the time of drug administration. A backup method of treatment should be accessible, particularly if linacs are used for primary treatment, because they tend to have a greater frequency of repair than ^{60}Co units.[93]

Complications

Low-Dose Total-Body Irradiation

Some patients may develop mild nausea and vomiting. However, the major side effect of low-dose total-body irradiation is thrombocytopenia, which usually occurs after doses exceeding 100 to 150 cGy.[36,53] The mechanism responsible for thrombocytosis after ionizing irradiation is unknown.

High-Dose Total-Body Irradiation

High-dose total-body irradiation is primarily used in conjunction with high-dose cytotoxic drugs and bone marrow transplantation.

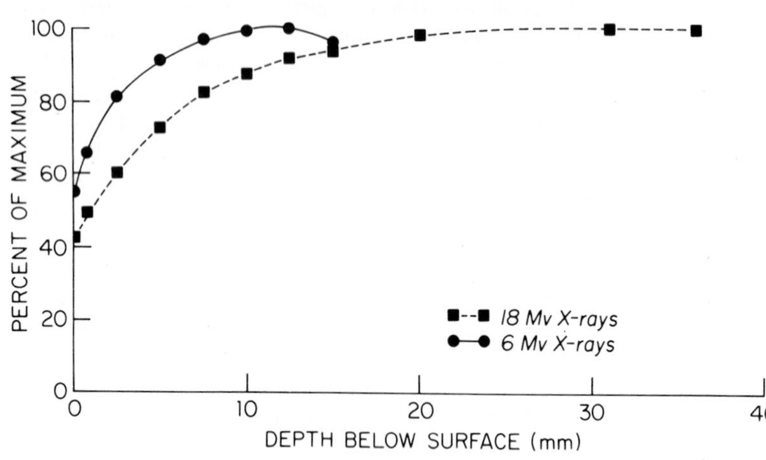

FIGURE 11–2. Ionization along the central axis of the perpendicularly incident beam in a polystyrene phantom. At depths shallower than 10 mm, 6-MV x-rays give significantly greater doses than 18-MV x-rays.

ACUTE TOXICITY

Nausea, vomiting, and diarrhea are the most common early side effects after a single fraction of 800 cGy to 1000 cGy of total-body irradiation is given.[6,14,67,88,89] These side effects can also be caused by cytotoxic drugs, which usually precede the administration of total-body irradiation; the irradiation may or may not exacerbate the side effects. The use of fractionated or low-dose-rate total-body irradiation reduces the incidence and the severity of side effects.[28,87] Patients also develop dry mouth, reduced tear formation, and sore throat within 10 days. One side effect that is unique to total-body irradiation is parotitis, which usually occurs after the first day of irradiation and subsides in 24 to 48 hours.[14,16] Reversible alopecia develops at about 2 weeks in all patients.[89] Veno-occlusive disease of the liver, which is characterized by hepatic enlargement, ascites, jaundice, encephalopathy, and weight gain, can occur in 10% to 20% of the patients.[52,67] Insidious weight gain is the first sign of veno-occlusive disease, occurring a mean of 6 days after transplantation.[52]

DELAYED TOXICITY

For a preparatory regimen containing high-dose total-body irradiation, the lung appears to be the dose-limiting normal tissue. Interstitial pneumonitis occurs in about 50% of bone marrow transplant patients who receive a single, large fraction of total-body irradiation, and about half of them die of this complication.[38,60,89] However, the use of fractionated total-body irradiation or low-dose-rate total-body irradiation has greatly diminished the incidence of interstitial pneumonitis.[3,4,17,28,56,60,63,64,73,87] About 26% of interstitial pneumonitis cases may be attributed directly to total-body irradiation or chemotherapy, and 42% are associated with cytomegalovirus.[80] The median time from cessation of therapy to diagnosis for this complication is about 2 months. Predisposing factors for interstitial pneumonitis are preexisting pulmonary abnormalities, previous chest irradiation, graft-versus-host disease, and advanced age.[6,55,56,60,64,83,92,99]

The incidence of cataracts is also influenced by the way total-body irradiation is given. About 80% of the patients who receive a single, large dose of total-body irradiation develop cataracts within 5 years, but the incidence is reduced to 19% if fractionated doses are used.[15] Approximately 18% of marrow transplant patients who receive chemotherapy alone as a preparatory regimen also develop cataracts.[15] Because cataracts can be corrected surgically, they are no longer a major issue.

Almost all children who undergo bone marrow transplantation after total-body irradiation experience decreased growth velocity.[3,5,14,44]

High-dose total-body irradiation produces primary gonadal failure in almost all patients, but gonadal recovery has occurred in a few.[3,39,79] In children, puberty is usually delayed by treatment, but it can be induced by appropriate hormone replacement.[3,14] Thyroid dysfunction has been observed in about 43% of patients after total-body irradiation.[82] Subclinical hypothyroidism is the most commonly reported condition, with raised thyroid-stimulating hormone and normal T_4 levels.

Deterioration of renal function occurs in most patients undergoing bone marrow transplantation.[7,85] Because these patients receive various nephrotoxic drugs (*i.e.*, VP-16, VM-26, amphotericin B) during and after the intensive cytoreductive therapy, the contribution of total-body irradiation to renal dysfunction is not well established.

The incidence of second tumors after intensive chemoradiotherapy and marrow transplantation appears to be low.[3,14,101] However, the follow-up period for these studies is not long enough for the development of solid tumors, which have a longer latent period than leukemia.

Radiobiologic Considerations

Based on clinical experience with total-body irradiation before marrow transplantation and hemibody irradiation, the most important dose-limiting tissue is the lung.[2,4,56,60,65,83,94,99] A review of experiences at several centers using single-fraction total-body irradiation or hemibody irradiation suggested that the development of interstitial pneumonitis is related to the absorbed radiation dose to lung.[24,26,38,94]

A quantal dose-response curve based on the experience at Toronto using high dose rates of 50 to 400 cGy/minute is quite steep, indicating that the onset of radiation-induced pneumonitis occurs at an absolute dose of 750 cGy (which is 10% to 24% higher than the uncorrected dose), with the 5% actuarial incidence occurring at approximately 820 cGy.[94] One important finding was a "threshold" or "tolerance" dose, below which no or a very low incidence of interstitial pneumonitis was observed. The sigmoidal complication curve rises dramatically, demonstrating a 50% and 95% incidence at 930 cGy and 1060 cGy, respectively.[94] Another report estimated the incidence of radiation-induced pneumonitis to be between 10% to 20% for an 800-cGy uncorrected dose to lung.[78] Interstitial pneumonitis can cause death for about 50% of the patients who develop it.[38,56,60,83] Because of the high mortality, it has generated considerable experimental works.[8,12,16,19,23,43,65,91,96,97]

Although the exact target cells associated with idiopathic interstitial pneumonitis are yet to be identified, they are thought to have a much greater capacity to repair sublethal damage than hemopoietic stem cells or leukemic and lymphomatous cells.[61] If this assumption is correct, the therapeutic ratio could be improved by modifying the way total-body irradiation is administered. The use of fractionated total-body irradiation has significantly reduced the incidence of interstitial pneumonitis despite the fact that a higher total dose of 1200 cGy has been given to compensate for the sparing of leukemic cells, which probably have a small but significant quasi-threshold dose (Dq).[28,87]

The next question studied was whether the killing of tumor cells can be increased even more by escalating the total dose of whole-body irradiation without increasing the incidence of interstitial pneumonitis. A systemic dose-escalating study was carried out by Phillips and co-workers[63] using 200 cGy per fraction for total doses ranging from 1000 cGy to 1600 cGy. No significant increase in the incidence of interstitial pneumonitis was revealed up to 1400 cGy, but both patients who received the next higher dose of 1600 cGy died of pulmonary complications. Compared with single-fraction total-body irradiation, the data suggest that the use of 200-cGy dose fractionation gives a lung-sparing factor of about 1.6, which is lower than the value of 2.0 obtained in mice.[12,58,96] One possible explanation for the discrepancy is the use of high-dose chemotherapy in conjunction with total-body irradiation in humans. Another possibility is that the time interval of 6 to 8 hours between 2 fractions given on the same day is not long enough to repair all sublethal damage.[63]

The use of doses per fraction smaller than 200 cGy has not been adequately investigated. Shank and co-workers[84] used a hyperfractionated regimen of 120-cGy fractions, administered in three fractions per day. However, the use of lung blocks limits the dose to the lung to less than 80 cGy per fraction and to less than 900 cGy for the total lung dose. Animal data from two groups using death from pneumonitis as the endpoint indicated that the doses required to produce 50% mortality (LD_{50}) increase continuously as dose per fraction is decreased from 160 cGy to between 110 cGy and 115 cGy per fraction.[58,96] The LD_{50} value is 4467 cGy if 115 cGy per fraction is used. Because the value is 1343 cGy for the single-fraction group, this fractionation gives a factor of more than 3.3.[96] When even smaller doses per fraction are tested, the lung-sparing continues to increase, probably down to 80 cGy.[59] However, their data are also consistent with no significant repair below 50 cGy per fraction. These results are consistent with the linear-quadratic model having, a α/β value of about 3 to 5 for pneumonitis.[58,95,97] When the radiosensitivity of two important types of lung cells, type II pneumocytes and alveolar macrophages, is determined, the value of Dq for both cell types has been between 100 and 200 cGy.[29,45,46] In sharp contrast to x-rays, negligible differences in the sparing of lungs are observed for the fractionated neutron schedules.[58]

If the data from mice can be extrapolated directly to humans, it may be possible to give more than 3000 cGy to the lung if approximately 100 cGy per fraction is used. An additional advantage of using a fraction size of 110 cGy appears to be associated with a significantly shorter repair time than with the use of larger fraction sizes.[25] Similar data in humans are urgently needed to determine the optimal dose per fraction and time interval between fractions.

Another approach to reduce the incidence of interstitial pneumonitis is the use of low-dose-rate total-body irradiation (< 5 cGy/minute). The efficacy of low-dose-rate total-body irradiation in reducing the incidence of pulmonary complications has been well documented in humans and animals.[4,8,12] The maximal sparing of lung damage has been estimated to be by a factor of 1.7 to 2.1, which is smaller than the 3.5 to 4 obtainable with the use of dose fractionation.[8,12,58,96]

The most important finding appears to be a threshold dose. However, the size of threshold dose is not fixed; it depends on the way in which irradiation is given. The use of dose fractionation or low dose rates increases the value of threshold dose by a factor of 1.5 to 4.0. If fractionated total-body irradiation is used, the ideal cytocidal fraction size for the purpose of minimizing lung damage would be close to the value of Dq of the cells that are associated with the development of interstitial pneumonitis. However, the total time required to deliver total-body irradiation and the number of fractions that can be given in a day must be taken into account. It may not be practical to require more than 7 days to give all total-body irradiation and to use more than three fractions per day.

Many cytotoxic drugs by themselves can cause pneumonitis.[34,100] The proper timing of using chemotherapy and radiation therapy to reduce the incidence of pneumonitis while maximizing tumor cell kill has not been adequately explored.

HEMIBODY IRRADIATION

Hemibody irradiation was developed as a method to treat patients with disseminated tumors involving multiple sites.[24,74] Early attempts to use total-body irradiation were successful only for a few of these patients because the dose of total-body irradiation that could be given without hematologic support was limited to about 300 cGy. Use of subtotal-body irradiation, such as hemibody irradiation, makes it possible to give higher doses without bone marrow transplantation. The pioneering work done at Toronto[24] and in subsequent prospective randomized trials by the Radiation Therapy Oncology Group[24,76,77] has shown that single, high-dose hemibody irradiation is as effective as conventional fractionated radiation therapy in achieving pain control in patients with metastatic diseases.

Application

The pain relief produced by hemibody irradiation for skeletal metastases involving several sites is fast, with nearly 50% of all responding patients doing so within 48 hours and 80% within 1 week from the treatment.[76–78] More than 70% of treated patients can be expected to obtain pain relief. The duration of pain relief is substantial and persists for at least 50% of the patient's remaining life.[24,77] The most effective hemibody irradiation doses found by Radiation Therapy Oncology Group study are 600 cGy for upper-hemibody irradiation and 800 cGy for lower- and middle-hemibody irradiation. Doses beyond these levels do not appear to increase pain relief or duration of relief or give a faster response.[77] When treatment of the other half of the body is indicated, it is advisable to wait 6 to 8 weeks to allow blood cells to recover.[24]

Hemibody irradiation and large-field irradiation appear to be capable of delaying progression of existing asymptomatic metastases and development of new metastases.[30,48,51] Frequently, patients treated with small-field radiation therapy return within a few weeks with other symptomatic sites adjacent to the field. The use of hemibody irradiation may prevent the development of new symptomatic sites within the treated area, which eliminates or reduces the need for patients to spend a substantial portion of their remaining lives commuting to treatment centers.[30,51]

Sequential upper- and lower-hemibody irradiation 6 to 8 weeks apart has been used in treating multiple myeloma, malignant lymphoma, and other widely disseminated tumors.[24,48,51,71] The ability of sequential hemibody irradiation given alone or in conjunction with systemic chemotherapy to eradicate occult metastases in patients with various solid tumors is under investigation.[51,71,72]

Technique

The physical considerations for hemibody irradiation are similar to those delineated for total-body irradiation. The field size required for hemibody irradiation is much smaller than that for total-body irradiation, and hemibody irradiation can usually be given with an unmodified therapy unit.

For convenience, subtotal-body irradiation is usually divided into upper-hemibody irradiation, lower-hemibody irradiation, and middle-hemibody irradiation (Fig. 11-3).[72,76,77] A line passing across the bottom of the L4 vertebra is commonly used as the line to separate upper- and lower-hemibody irradiation.[72] However, the field may be shaped to accommodate the needs of each patient. The patient is commonly treated with AP parallel opposed fields. In the patient setup, a vertical beam covers the half the body, with the treatment table lowered to the appropriate level or to the floor. This facilitates shielding of previously irradiated areas and parotid glands and aids the use of lung blocks. The dose should be delivered to the middle thickness of the patient on the central axis of the beam; half the irradiation is delivered through an AP field and half through a PA field. When upper hemibody irradiation is given, appropriate lung blocks should be used to limit the midline lung dose to less than 700 cGy.[72,77,78] When upper hemibody irradiation is administered, an overnight hospitalization is recommended, although it is not mandatory.[51] The premedication program consists of steroids, antiemetics, and intravenous fluids.[72,76,77]

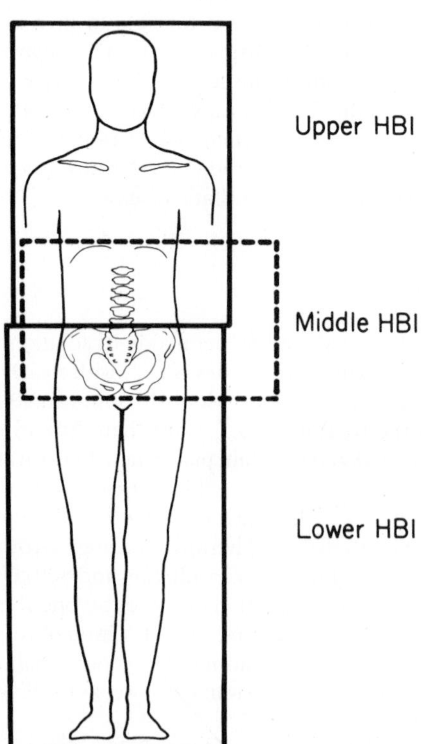

FIGURE 11–3. The most commonly used hemibody irradiation fields.

Complications

The types and degrees of side effects depend greatly on the site and size of the irradiated volumes. The most common toxicities associated with single, high-dose hemibody irradiation are nausea and vomiting.[24,77,78] The toxicities of upper-hemibody irradiation are more severe than those of lower-hemibody irradiation. They occur soon after radiation delivery and last a few hours. Diarrhea occurs after lower- or middle-hemibody irradiation is administered and can last for several days. The severity of diarrhea can be reduced by appropriate premedications.[77] Hematologic toxicity usually disappears in 4 to 6 weeks. The potentially fatal interstitial pneumonitis can be avoided if the dose of upper-hemibody irradiation is limited to 600 cGy.

REFERENCES

1. Armitage JO: Bone marrow transplantation in the treatment of patients with lymphoma. Blood 73:1749, 1989
2. Bamberg M, Beelen DW, Mahmoud HK, et al: The incidence of interstitial pneumonitis: Comparison of total body irradiation schedules for allogeneic bone marrow transplantation. Strahlentherapie 162:218, 1986
3. Barrett AJ: Bone marrow transplantation. Cancer Treat Rev 14:203, 1987
4. Barrett AJ, Depledge MH, Powles RL: Interstitial pneumonitis following bone marrow transplantation after low dose rate total body irradiation. Int J Radiat Oncol Biol Phys 9:1029, 1983
5. Barrett A, Nicholls, J, Gibson B: Late effects of total body irradiation. Radiother Oncol 9:131, 1987
6. Bearman SI, Appelbaum FR, Back A, et al: Regimen-related toxicity and early transplant survival in patients undergoing marrow transplantation for lymphoma. J Clin Oncol 7:1288, 1989
7. Bergstein J, Andreoli SP, Provisor AJ: Radiation nephritis following total-body irradiation and cyclophosphamide in preparation for bone marrow transplantation. Transplantation 41:63, 1986
8. Cardozo BL, Zoetelief H, van Bekkum DW, et al: Lung damage following bone marrow transplantation. I. The contribution of irradiation. Int J Radiat Oncol Biol Phys 11:907, 1985
9. Chadha M, Shank B, Fuks Z, et al: Improved survival of poor prognosis diffuse histiocytic (large cell) lymphoma managed with sequential induction chemotherapy, "boost" radiation therapy, and autologous bone marrow transplantation. Int J Radiat Oncol Biol Phys 14:407, 1988
10. Chaffey JT, Rosenthal DS, Moloney WC, et al: Total body irradiation as treatment for lymphosarcoma. Int J Radiat Oncol Biol Phys 1:399, 1976
11. Chaoul H, Lange K: Uber lymphogranulomatose und ihre Behandlung mit Rontgenstrahlen. Munchen Med Wechmschr 70:725, 1923
12. Collis CH, Down JD: The effect of dose rate and multiple fractions per day on radiation-induced lung damage in mice. Br J Radiol 57:1037, 1984
13. Cunningham JR, Wright DJ: A simple facility for whole body irradiation. Radiology 78:941, 1962

14. Deeg HJ: Acute and delayed toxicities of total body irradiation. Int J Radiat Oncol Biol Phys 9:1933, 1983
15. Deeg HJ, Flournoy N, Sullivan KM, et al: Cataracts after total body irradiation and marrow transplantation: A sparing effect of dose fractionation. Int J Radiat Oncol Biol Phys 10:957, 1984
16. Deeg HJ, Storb R, Longton G, et al: Single dose or fractionated total body irradiation and autologous marrow transplantation in dogs: Effects of exposure rate, fraction size, and fractionation interval on acute and delayed toxicity. Int J Radiat Oncol Biol Phys 15:647, 1988
17. Deeg HJ, Storb R, Thomas ED: Bone marrow transplantation: A review of delayed complications. Br J Haematol 57:185, 1984
18. Del Regato JA: Total body irradiation in the treatment of chronic lymphogenous leukemia. Am J Roentgenol 120:504, 1974
19. Dutreix J, Wambersie A, Loierette M, et al: Time factors in total body irradiation. Pathol Biol 27:365, 1979
20. Engel WK, Lichter AS, Galdi AP: Polymyositis: Remarkable response to total body irradiation. Lancet 1:658, 1981
21. Engler NJ, Feldman MI, Spira J: Arc technique for total body irradiation by a 42 MV betatron. Med Phys 4:524, 1977
22. Feig SA, Champlin R, Arenson E, et al: Improved survival following bone marrow transplantation for aplastic anemia. Br J Haematol 54:509, 1983
23. Field SB, Hornsey S, Kutsutani Y: Effects of fractionated irradiation on mouse lung and a phenomenon of slow repair. Br J Radiol 49:700, 1976
24. Fitzpatrick PJ, Rider WD: Half body radiotherapy. Int J Radiat Oncol Biol Phys 1:197, 1976
25. Fowler JF, Whitsed CA, Joiner MC: Repair Kinetics in mouse lung: A fast component at 1.1 Gy per fraction. Int J Radiat Oncol Biol Phys 56:335, 1989
26. Fryer C, Fitzpatrick P, Rider W, et al: Radiation pneumonitis: Experience following a large single dose of radiation. Int J Radiat Biol 4:931, 1978
27. Galvin JM: Calculation and prescription of dose for total body irradiation. Int J Radiat Oncol Biol Phys 9:1919, 1983
28. Goolden AWG, Goldman JM, Kam CC, et al: Fractionation of whole body irradiation before bone marrow transplantation for patients with leukemia. Br J Radiol 56:245, 1983
29. Guichard M, Deschavanne PJ, Malaise EP: Radiosensitivity of mouse lung cells measured using an *in vitro* colony method. Int J Radiat Oncol Biol Phys 6:441, 1980
30. Hazra TA, Giri S: Prophylactic pelvic girdle irradiation in the treatment of prostatic carcinoma. Int J Radiat Oncol Biol Phys 7:817, 1981
31. Heublein AC: Preliminary report on continuous irradiation of the entire body. Radiology 18:1051, 1932
32. Hoppe RT, Kushlan P, Kaplan HS, et al: The treatment of advanced stage favorable histology non-Hodgkin's lymphoma: A prelimiary report of a randomized trial comparing single agent chemotherapy, combination chemotherapy, and whole body irradiation. Blood 58:592, 1981
33. Jacobs ML, Pape L: A total body irradiation chamber and its uses. Int J Appl Radiat Isotopes 9:141, 1960
34. Jagannath S, Dicke KA, Armitage JO, et al: High dose cyclophosphamide, carmustine, and etoposide and autologous bone marrow transplantation for relapsed Hodgkin's disease. Ann Intern Med 104:163, 1986
35. Johnson RE: Treatment of chronic lymphocytic leukemia by total body irradiation alone and combined with chemotherapy. Int J Radiat Biol Phys 5:159, 1979
36. Johnson RE, Ruhl U: Treatment of chronic lymphocytic leukemia with emphasis on total body irradiation. Int J Radiat Oncol Biol Phys 1:387, 1976
37. Kardamark D, Berry RJ: Low dose total body irradiation in the management of refractory rheumatoid arthritis. Br J Radiol 60:297, 1987
38. Keane TJ, Van Dyk J, Rider WD: Idiopathic interstitial pneumonia following bone marrow transplantation: The relationship with total body irradiation. Int J Radiat Oncol Biol Phys 7:1365, 1981
39. Keiholz U, Korbling M, Fehrentz D, et al: Long term endocrine toxicity of myeloablative treatment followed by autologous bone marrow/blood derived stem cell transplantation in patients with malignant lymphohemopoietic disorders. Cancer 64:641, 1989
40. Kelly JJ, Madoc-Jones H, Adelman LS, et al: Response to total body irradiation in dermatomyositis muscle. Nerve 11:120, 1988
41. Kim TH, Khan FM, Galvin JM: A report of the work party: Comparison of total body irradiation techniques for bone marrow transplantation. Int J Radiat Oncol Biol Phys 6:779, 1980
42. Kim TH, Kersey J, Sewchand W, et al: Total body irradiation with a high-dose-rate linear accelerator for bone-marrow transplantation in aplastic anemia and neoplastic disease. Radiology 122:523, 1977
43. Kolb HJ, Rieder I, Bodenberger U, et al: Dose rate and dose fractionated studies in total body irradiation in dogs. Pathol Biol 27:370, 1979
44. Leiper AD, Stanhope R, Lau T, et al: The effect of total body irradiation and bone marrow transplantation during childhood and adolescence on growth and endocrine function. Br J Haematol 67:419, 1987
45. Lin H-S, Hsu S: Effects of dose rate and dose fractionation of irradiation on pulmonary alveolar macrophage colony-forming cells. Radiat Res 103:260, 1985
46. Lin H-S, Kuhn C, Chen D: Radiosensitivity of pulmonary alveolar macrophage colony-forming cells. Radiat Res 89:283, 1982
47. Leung PMK, Rider WD, Webb HP, et al: Cobalt-60 therapy unit for large-field irradiation. Int J Radiat Oncol Biol Phys 7:705, 1981
48. Lombardi F, Rottolil L, Gianni C, et al: Advanced neuroblastoma: Results of two treatment programs including sequential hemibody irradiation. Int J Radiat Oncol Biol Phys 17:485, 1989
49. Lutz WR, Dougan PW, Bjarngard BE: Design and characteristics of a facility for total body and large field irradiation. Int J Radiat Oncol Biol Phys 15:1035, 1988
50. Lybert MLM, Meerwaldt JH, Deneve W: Long-term results of low dose total body irradiation for advanced non-Hodgkin's lymphoma. Int J Radiat Oncol Biol Phys 13: 1167, 1987
51. MacLennan I, Selim HM, Rubin P: Sequential hemibody radiotherapy in poor prognosis localized adenocarcinoma of the prostate gland: A preliminary study of the RTOG. Int J Radiat Oncol Biol Phys 16:215, 1989
52. McDonald GB, Sharma, P. Matthews DE, et al: The clinical course of 53 patients with venoocclusive disease of the liver after marrow transplantation. Transplantation 39:603, 1985
53. Mendenhall NP, Noyes WD, Million RR: Total body irradiation for stage II–IV non-Hodgkin's lymphoma: Ten-year follow-up. J Clin Oncol 7:67, 1989
54. Medinger FG, Craver LF: Total body irradiation. AJR 48:651, 1942
55. Meyers JD, Flournoy N, Wade JC, et al: Biology of interstitial pneumonia after marrow transplantation. In Gale RP (ed): Recent Advances in Bone Marrow Transplantation, pp 405–423. New York, Alan R Liss, 1983
56. Molls M, Budach V, Bamberg M: Total body irradiation: The lung as critical organ. Strahlentherapie 162:226, 1986
57. Mulvey PJ, Godlee JN: Technique and dosimetry for a TBI at University College Hospital, London. J Eur Radiother 3:241, 1982
58. Parkins CS, Fowler JF: Repair in mouse lung of multifraction x-rays and neutrons: Extension to 40 fractions. Br J Radiol 58:1097, 1985
59. Parkins LS, Fowler JF: The linear quadratic fit for lung function after irradiation with x-rays at smaller doses per fraction than 2 Gy. Br J Cancer 53(suppl 7):320, 1986.
60. Pecego R, Hill R, Appelbaum FR, et al: Interstitial pneumonitis following autologous bone marrow transplantation. Transplantation 42:575, 1986
61. Peters LJ, Withers HR, Cundiff JH, et al: Radiobiological considerations in the use of total-body irradiation for bone-marrow transplantation. Radiology 131:243, 1979
62. Peters VG, Herer AS: Modification of a standard cobalt-60

unit for total body irradiation at 150 cm SSD. Int J Radiat Oncol Biol Phys 10:927, 1983

63. Phillips GL, Herzig RH, Lazarus HM, et al: Treatment of resistant malignant lymphoma with cyclophosphamide, total body irradiation, and transplantation of cryopreserved autologous marrow. N Engl J Med 310:1557, 1984
64. Phillips GL, Wolf SN, Herzig RH, et al: Treatment of progressive Hodgkin's disease with intensive chemoradiotherapy and autologous bone marrow transplantation. Blood 73:2086, 1989
65. Pino y Torres JL, Bross DS, Lam W, et al: Risk factors in interstitial pneumonitis following allogeneic bone marrow transplantation. Int J Radiat Oncol Biol Phys 8:1301, 1982
66. Pla M, Chenery SG, Podgorsak EB: Total body irradiation with a sweeping beam. Int J Radiat Oncol Biol Phys 9:83, 1983
67. Press OW, Schaller RT, Thomas ED: Bone marrow transplant complications. In Toledo-Pereyra LH (ed): Complications of Organ Transplantation. New York, Marcel Dekker, 1987
68. Quast U: Physical treatment planning of total body irradiation: Patient translation and beam zone method. Med Phys 12:567, 1985
69. Quast U: Total body irradiation: Review of treatment techniques in Europe. Radiother Oncol 9:91, 1987
70. Rubin P, Bennett JM, Begg C, et al: The comparison of total body irradiation vs chlorambucil and prednisone for remission irradiation of active chronic lymphocytic leukemia: An ECOG study. I. Total body irradiation: Response and toxicity. Int J Radiat Oncol Biol Phys 7:1623, 1980
71. Rubin P, Heilmann HP: Large-field trials. Int J Radiat Oncol Biol Phys 14(suppl 1):565, 1988
72. Rubin P, Salazar O, Zagars G, et al: Systemic hemibody irradiation for overt and occult metastastes. Cancer 55:2210, 1985
73. Rybka WB, Caplan S, Freeman CR, et al: Experience with single dose and fractionated total body irradiation schedules in bone marrow transplantation. Int J Cell Cloning 4:219, 1986
74. Saenger EL, Silverstein EB, Aron B, et al: Whole body and partial body radiotherapy of advanced cancer. Am J Roentgenol Radium Ther Nucl Med 117:670, 1973
75. Sahler OD: Development of a room specifically designed for total body irradiation. Radiology 72:266, 1959
76. Salazar OM, Rubin P, Hendrickson FR, et al: Single-dose half-body irradiation for the palliation of multiple bone metastasis from solid tumors: A preliminary report. Int J Radiat Oncol Biol Phys 7:773, 1981
77. Salazar OM, Rubin P, Hendrickson FR, et al: Single-dose half-body irradiation for palliation of multiple bone metastases from solid tumors: Final Radiation Therapy Oncology Group report. Cancer 58:29, 1986
78. Salazar OM, Rubin P, Keller B, et al: Systemic (half-body) radiation therapy: Response and toxicity. Int J Radiat Oncol Biol Phys 4:937, 1978
79. Sanders JE, Buckner CD, Leonard JM, et al: Late effects on gonadal functions of cyclophosphamide, total-body irradiation, and marrow transplantation. Transplantation 36:252, 1983
80. Shank B: Techniques of magna-field irradiation. Int J Radiat Oncol Biol Phys 9:1925, 1983
81. Shank B, Hopfan S, Kim JH, et al: Hyperfractionated total body irradiation for bone marrow transplantation. I. Early results in leukemic patients. Int J Radiat Oncol Biol Phys 7:1109, 1981
82. Sklar CA, Kim TH, Ramsay NKC: Thyroid dysfunction among long term survivors of bone marrow transplantation. Am J Med 73:688, 1982
83. Sullivan KM, Meyers JD, Flournoy N, et al: Early and late interstitial pneumonia following human bone marrow transplantation. Int J Cell Cloning 4(suppl 1):107, 1986
84. Surmount J, Dutreix A, Lalanne CM: Les irradiations *in toto* pour greffes de tissu ou transplantation d'organe chez l'homme. Problems techniques. J Radiol Electrol 41:679, 1960
85. Tarbell NJ, Guinan EC, Niemeyer C, et al: Late onset of renal dysfunction in survivors of bone marrow transplantation. Int J Radiat Oncol Biol Phys 15:99, 1988
86. Thomas ED, Cliftt RA: Indications for marrow transplantation in chronic myelogenous leukemia. Blood 73:861, 1989
87. Thomas ED, Clift RA, Hersman J, et al: Marrow transplantation for acute nonlymphoblastic leukemia in first remission using fractionated or single-dose irradiation. Int J Radiat Oncol Biol Phys 8:817, 1982
88. Thomas ED, Storb R, Buckner CD: Total body irradiation in preparation for bone marrow engraftment. Transplant Proc 4:591, 1976
89. Thomas ED, Storb R, Clift RA et al: Bone marrow transplantation. N Engl J Med 292:832, 895, 1975
90. Tobias JS, Richards JDM, Blackman GM, et al: Hemibody irradiation in multiple myeloma. Radiother Oncol 3:11, 1985
91. Travis EL, Down JD, Holmes SJ, et al: Radiation pneumonitis and fibrosis in mouse lung assayed by respiratory frequency and histology. Radiat Res 84:133, 1980
92. Valteau D, Hartmann O, Benhamou E, et al: Nonbacterial nonfungal interstitial pneumonitis following autologous bone marrow transplantation in children treated with high dose chemotherapy without total body irradiation. Transplantation 45:737, 1988
93. Van Dyk J, Galvin JM, Glasgow GP, et al: The physical aspects of total and half body photon irradiation. A report of Task Group 29 Radiation Therapy Committee: AAPM Report No 17. New York, American Association of Physicists in Medicine, June 1986
94. Van Dyk J, Keane TJ, Kau S, et al: Radiation pneumonitis following large single dose irradiation: A re-evaluation based on absolute dose to lung. Int J Radiat Oncol Biol Phys 7:461, 1981
95. Van Dyk J, Mah K, Keane TJ: Radiation-induced lung damage: Dose-time-fractionation considerations. Radiother Oncol 14:55, 1989
96. Vegesna V, Withers HR, Thames HD, et al: Multifraction radiation response of mouse lung. Int J Radiat Biol 47:413, 1985
97. Wara WM, Phillips TL, Margolis LW, et al: Radiation pneumonitis: A new approach to the derivation of time-dose factors. Cancer 32:547, 1973
98. Webster EW: Physics considerations in a design of facilities for the uniform whole body irradiation of man. Radiology 75:19, 1960
99. Weiner RS, Bortin MM, Gale RP, et al: Intertstitial pneumonitis after bone marrow transplantation. Ann Intern Med 104:165, 1986
100. Weiss, RB, Muggia FM: Cytotoxicity-induced pulmonary disease: Update 1980. Am J Med 68:259, 1980
101. Witherspoon RP, Fisher LD, Schoch G, et al: Secondary cancers after bone marrow transplantation for leukemia or aplastic anemia. N Engl J Med 321:784, 1989

12

○ ○ ○ • • •

Physics of Brachytherapy

Glenn P. Glasgow
Carlos A. Perez

In 1901, Pierre Curie loaned Dr. Danlos, a physician, a small quantity of radium, which Danlos used to prepare some surface applicators for treatment of skin lesions.[58] This was the beginning of brachytherapy, the treatment of lesions using radioactive materials at short distances. Hilaris[58] and del Regato[30] present excellent reviews of the development of brachytherapy.

From 1920 to 1950, physicians learned much more about the therapeutic use of radium and radon gas. At the Radiumhemmet in Stockholm, Heyman and others[55] treated cervical cancer using three equal 20- to 24-hour treatments with a 1-week interval between the first and second applications and 2 or 3 weeks before the final application. In Paris, Regaud[126] concluded that therapy that was extended over several days and used low-intensity radium tubes was more effective than using higher-intensity radium tubes and shorter treatment intervals. In Manchester, England, special applicators for gynecologic treatments were developed; Paterson and Parker[112] designed interstitial source distribution rules, still used today, using radium sources with different linear activities. In New York, Quimby[122] studied the radiation dose distributions of radium packs, prepared dosimetry tables for individual sources, and proposed a set of source distribution rules for therapists who had an inventory of radium with only one linear activity.[123,124] During the 1950s and 1960s, radioisotopes made possible during the new atomic age were used as sources, and afterloading methods were developed to protect physicians performing brachytherapy.[16,32,57,109,149]

The advent of ^{60}Co teletherapy units and medical linear accelerators for electron-beam treatment diminished the popularity of brachytherapy during the 1960s and 1970s. In the 1980s, there was a renewed interest in all forms of brachytherapy, alone or in conjunction with other new modalities, such as hyperthermia, to treat a host of diseases. The 1990s offer new radioisotopes, refined dosimetry, and new treatment methods, including greater use of remote afterloading technology.

In this chapter, we present the fundamental concepts and definitions of brachytherapy and an overview of the newest applications and developments in this field. The references list several classical textbooks.[38,58,115] Two important new texts are required reading for the serious brachytherapist.[48,61]

BRACHYTHERAPY DOSIMETRY

Some of the fundamental concepts of radioactivity are presented in Chapter 8. The radioactive decay of a particular radioisotope is characterized by its *decay constant* or *transformation constant.* Each radioisotope exhibits the property that the number of atoms (ΔN) that decay per unit time (Δt) is proportional to the number of atoms (N_0) present with the potential to decay. The fractional decay rate, $\lambda = -(\Delta N/N_o)/\Delta t$, is a constant, where N_o is the number of atoms at any given time, ΔN is the number of transformations that occur during some interval Δt, and λ is the proportionality constant (transformation constant) with units of reciprocal time (*e.g.,* seconds^{-1}, days^{-1}, years^{-1}).

The constant fractional decay of a radionuclide is commonly expressed by stating its radioactive half-life, $T_{1/2}$, expressed in seconds, hours, days, or years, which is the time in which some initial number of atoms, N_o, decays to one-half of that number, $N_o/2$. Hence, $T_{1/2} = 0.693/\lambda$.

The *activity* of a radioisotope is a measure of the magnitude of the rate decay of the material. Historically, a *curie* (Ci) of radon was defined as the number of α-particles emitted by radon in secular equilibrium with 1 g of radium; the value now designated for the curie is 3.7×10^{10} disintegrations per second. In the International System of Units, the unit of activity is a becquerel (Bq), which is 1 disintegration per second. Hence, 1 Bq equals about 2.7×10^{-11} Ci. Thus, a 1-mg ^{226}Ra source has an activity of 3.7×10^7 Bq or 37 MBq. In the remainder of this chapter, we choose to express activity first in millicuries (mCi) or milligram radium equivalents (mg Ra eq) and then, in parenthesis, in megabecquerels (MBq) or gigabecquerels (GBq). In some instances the SI units are omitted to retain clarity.

The *apparent activity* of an encapsulated source states the activity of the source as if it were not encapsulated; because of source self-attenuation, the *true activity,* or *content activity,* within the source is generally greater than the apparent activity of the source. The activity of an encapsulated source can be compared with the activity of a different radioisotope with known encapsulation. For example, a *milligram radium equivalent* of a radioisotope source such as ^{137}Cs is the mass (in mg) of ^{226}Ra, in equilibrium with its decay products and screened by a 0.5 mm thick, 90% platinum, 10% iridium wall, that would yield the same *exposure rate in air* in scatter-free conditions as produced by the encapsulated ^{137}Cs source at the same distance in the same geometry. Platinum, a soft metal, is hardened by the addition of iridium, and the combination is called iridioplatinum. Depending on its design and encapsulation, a source containing about 25 to 27 mCi (925 MBq to 999 MBq) of ^{137}Cs doubly encapsulated in iridioplatinum or stainless steel yields an exposure rate equivalent to a 10-mg (370-MBq) ^{226}Ra source with 0.5-mm iridioplatinum walls.

Another useful concept is the *mean life*, $\overline{T}$, of the radionuclide. Numerically, $\overline{T} = 1.44\ T_{1/2}$. Conceptually, the mean life is particularly useful in understanding the decay process of radioisotopes with very short half-lives. Suppose that the decay rate of a radionuclide was not proportional to the number of atoms présent but was a constant, equal to the initial decay rate of the exponentially decaying radionuclide. If the radionuclide decayed at this constant rate, with a mean life of $1.44\ T_{1/2}$, the total number of decays that occurred during the source's lifetime would be the same as the number of decays from the exponentially decaying source with the variable decay rate and a half-life of $T_{1/2}$. An example appears later to clarify these concepts.

Secular equilibrium is achieved in a sealed radium tube. The half-life (1622 years) of the parent radioisotope (^{226}Ra) is much longer than the half-line (3.82 days) of the daughter radioisotope (^{222}Rn). Secular equilibrium is established after about seven daughter half-lives; then the activity (A_p) of the parent isotope equals the activity (A_d) of the daughter isotope (A_p) = (A_d).

Radioisotopes in *transient equilibrium* are not used in brachytherapy but are widely used in nuclear medicine as radioisotope generators (cows). The half-life of the parent is not much greater than the half-life of the daughter; after transient equilibrium is established, the ratio of the activity of the parent radioisotope to that of the daughter radioisotope is given by

$$A_p/A_d = \frac{(\lambda_d - \lambda_p)}{\lambda_d}$$

The *exposure rate constant*, Γ_δ, is a measure of the inherent radioactive intensity of a radioisotope and is given the quotient of $l^2(\Delta x/\Delta t)$ by A, where $(\Delta x/\Delta t)$ is the exposure rate due to photons of energy greater than δ at a distance, l, from a point source of this nuclide with an activity A.[67] Numerically, Γ_δ is given by

$$\begin{aligned}\Gamma_\delta = &(3.7 \times 10^7/\text{sec/mCi})(3.6 \times 10^3\ \text{sec/h})\\ &\times (10^6\text{eV/MeV})(4.803 \times 10^{-10}\text{esu})\\ &\times (1.293 \times 10^{-3}\text{gcm}^{-3})/(4\pi)/(33.85\ \text{eV})\\ &\times (\text{E,MeV})_i(\text{I},\gamma\text{'s/decay})_i(\mu_{en}/\rho\text{cm}^2/\text{g})_i\end{aligned}$$

where E_i is the energy, in MeV, of the *i*th x-ray or τ-ray; I_i is the ray's intensity, and $(\mu_{en}/\rho)_i$ is its mass energy absorption coefficient in air. In the nomenclature of the 1950s and 1960s, this was called the k constant, and it includes all photon radiations, both nuclear and nonnuclear in origin, with energies greater than δ, where δ depends on the application; often δ is 11.3 keV or higher (*i.e.*, it includes the characteristic x-rays and bremsstrahlung radiation arising from conversion electrons).[66,67] When a radioactive source is encapsulated in metal, some of the soft radiations (*e.g.*, β-particles, low-energy τ-rays, and x-rays) are removed by filtration of the metal. The *specific τ-ray constant* excludes these softer radiations and is a function of source design and the wall thickness of the encapsulating material. Although the International Commission on Radiation Units and Measurements has recommended that the term *specific τ-ray constant* no longer be used, the term and its meaning are widely known.[67] An alternative is the *filtered exposure rate constant.* Table 12-1 lists the exposure rate constants and specific τ-ray (filtered exposure rate) constants and other important physical parameters for many radioisotopes used historically or currently in brachytherapy.

For many years, radium needles with a 0.5-mm-thick iridioplatinum wall were believed to have a specific τ-ray constant of 8.4 R cm^2/h/mCi, and much of the literature and many dosimetry tables are based on this value. The filtered exposure rate constant is now known to be 8.25 R cm^2/h/mCi or 0.825 R m^2/h/Ci; in SI units, the exposure rate constant becomes the *air kerma rate constant,* and 8.25 R cm^2/h/mCi = 7.2 cGy cm^2/h/mCi, assuming that an exposure of 114.5 R is equivalent to an air kerma of 1 Gy.[15,114] This also corresponds to 5.40934×10^{-17} Gy m^2/sec/Bq or 0.19473 μGy m^2/MBqh.

The *exposure rate in air,* $\Delta x/\Delta t$ (R/h), at some distance, l, from a point source radioisotope is given by: $\Delta x/\Delta t = \Gamma_\delta A l^{-2}$ where Γ_δ is the filtered exposure rate constant (R m^2/h/Ci) of the source, A is its apparent activity (Ci), and l is the distance (m) from the source to the point where the exposure rate is stated.

In SI units the *air kerma rate* (μGy/hour) is calculated by multiplying the stated *activity* (MBq) by the *air kerma rate constant* of the radionuclide (μGy m^2/MBqh). To obtain the *absorbed dose* in water, it is necessary to multiply air kerma at the same point by the ratio of the mean mass energy absorption coefficients for water and air.[84] For photon energies between 180 keV and 4 MeV, this ratio is almost constant at 1.11.[15] Most radionuclides used in brachytherapy, except ^{125}I, emit τ-rays with energies within this range.

Specification of Brachytherapy Sources

Brachytherapy sources generally have been specified in terms of an equivalent mass of radium, their apparent activity, or the exposure rate produced at a specific distance from the source. The National Council on Radiation Protection and Measurements[106] Report No. 41 recommends specification in terms of the exposure rate at 1 m from, and perpendicular to, the long axis of the source at its center. The British Commission on Radiation Units and Measurements[15] recommends specification of air kerma rate at 1 m, in micrograys per hour (μGy/h). Commercially, sources purchased from vendors are specified several ways, and users must apply great caution, particularly if they are converting a relatively unfamiliar dose rate unit (μGy/h) into a dose prescription unit (cGy or mg Ra eq). Gooden provides an excellent review of methods of source specification.[48]

Penetrability of Brachytherapy Sources

The penetrability of brachytherapy sources is commonly expressed by stating their half-value layer (HVL) or tenth-value layer (TVL) in lead or tissue. The layers are the thickness of the specified substance that, when introduced into the path of the radiation coming from the source, reduces the exposure rate at some point of measurement by one half or one tenth, respectively. The higher-energy τ-ray sources have higher HVLs and TVLs. For a polyenergetic source, such as ^{192}Ir, which has a spectrum of τ-rays with an average energy of 0.38 MeV, about one third less than the monoenergetic 0.66-MeV τ-rays from

TABLE 12–1
Physical Properties of Radionuclides Historically and Currently Used in Therapy

ELEMENT	ISOTOPE	E_β (MeV)	E_γ (MeV)	$\bar{E}_\gamma$ (MeV)	EXPOSURE RATE CONSTANT* (R cm²/h/mCi)	SPECIFIC γ-RAY CONSTANT* (R cm²/h/mCi)	$T_{1/2}$	HVL† (water; cm)	HVL† (lead; cm)	CURRENT CLINICAL USE	SOURCE FORM
Radium	^{226}Ra	0.017–3.26	0.047–2.44	0.83	10.27 (0.2424)§	8.25‡ (0.1947)§	1622 y	10.6	1.4	Temporary intracavitary, interstitial implants	Tubes, needles
Radon	^{222}Rn	0.017–3.26	0.047–2.44	0.83	10.27 (0.2424)§	8.25‡ (0.1947)§	3.82 d	10.6	1.4	Permanent implants, many sites	Seed
Cobalt	^{60}Co	0.313	1.17,1.33	1.25	13.07 (0.3085)§	13.07 (0.3085)§	5.26 y	10.8	1.1	Eye lesions; temporary intracavitary, interstitial implant	Plaques, RAS¶
Cesium	^{137}Cs	0.514,1.17	0.662	0.662	3.275 (0.0773)§	3.226 (0.0761)§	30 y	8.2	0.65	Temporary intracavitary, interstitial implants	Tubes, needles, RAS¶
Gold	^{198}Au	0.96	0.412–1.088	0.416	2.376 (0.0561)§	2.327 (0.0549)§	2.7 d	7.0	0.33	Permanent implants, prostate and other sites	Seed
Tantalum	^{182}Ta	0.18–0.514	0.043–1.453	0.67	6.87 (0.1621)§	6.71‖ (0.1584)§	115 d	10.0	1.2	Temporary interstitial implants	Wire
Iridium	^{192}Ir	0.24–0.67	0.136–1.062	0.38	4.69 (0.1107)§	4.62‖ (0.1090)§	74.2 d	6.3	0.30	Temporary interstitial implants	Wire, seeds, RAS¶
Iodine	^{125}I	None	0.0355	0.028**	1.403 (0.0331)§	1.208# (0.0285)§	60.25 d	2.0	0.002‡‡	Permanent interstitial implants	Seed
Palladium	^{103}Pd	None	0.02–0.48	0.021	1.48 (0.0349)§		17 d	1.6	0.002‡‡	Permanent implants	Seed
Iodine	^{131}I	0.25–0.61	0.08–0.637	0.364		2.2 (0.0519)	8.06 d	5.8	0.30	"Swallow" for thyroid therapy	Liquid, capsule
Strontium	^{90}Sr, ^{90}Y	0.54, 2.27					28.9 y 64 h	0.15	0.014‡	Temporary application for shallow lesions	Plaque
Phosphorus	^{32}P	1.71					14.3 d	0.1	0.01‡‡	Sodium for bone, blood diseases; Chromic for pleural effusions	Liquid
Ruthenium	^{106}Ru, ^{106}Rh	3.55					367 d	0.3	0.01‡‡	Eye lesions	Plaque

* *For an unfiltered point source with $\delta \geq 11.3$ keV.*
† *Assumes narrow beam geometry, a condition usually not found in practical brachytherapy applications.*
‡ *For a filtered source with a wall thickness equivalent to 0.5 mm of 90% Pt and 10% Ir.*
§ *Air kerma rate constant in μGy m²/h/MBq; 1 R cm²/h/mCi = 1.9371×10^{-19} C m²/kg/second Bq = 2.36×10^{-2} μGy m²/h/MBq.*
‖ *For an unfiltered point source with $\delta \geq 11.3$ keV.*
¶ *Remote afterloading source.*
\# *Includes filtration and anisotropy inherent in commercially available seeds.*
** *Includes x-rays.*
†† *Approximate values.*

^{137}Cs, the HVL in lead is 0.3 cm (the HVL in lead of ^{137}Cs is 0.65 cm). However, the ^{192}Ir TVL in lead (2.0 cm) is approximately the same as for ^{137}Cs (2.1 cm).[44,105] Table 12-1 lists the HVL values in lead and water for many radioisotopes. The narrow beam geometry inherent in the definitions of HVL and TVL do not occur in brachytherapy treatments in which the sources are within and surrounded by the attenuating medium. For β-emitters, the range (in cm) in tissue is about one half of the maximum β-ray energy (in MeV). For example, for ^{32}P, with a 1.71-MeV β-ray, the range in tissue is about 0.8 cm. For β-ray emitters, the HVL in lead is not a commonly used concept, because these β-rays often may be adequately shielded by a few millimeters of tissue or tissue-equivalent materials. The values listed in Table 12-1 for lead are only approximate and are listed to emphasize the extreme differences in penetrability of τ-rays and β-particles in lead.

RADIUM AND RADIUM SUBSTITUTES

Radium and Radon

Although the use of radium is declining, it remains the standard against which therapy and dosimetry with substitute radioisotopes must be compared; Table 12-2 lists the major features of the radium decay scheme.

Radium 226 has a half-life of 1622 years. The 78 τ-rays from radium and its decay products range in energy from 0.05 MeV to 2.4 MeV; the average energy is about 0.8 MeV, but the energy distribution is bimodal.[114] The maximum β-ray energy is about 3.26 MeV.

The ^{226}Ra sources consist of a radium salt (radium sulfate) mixed with filler (usually barium sulfate) and contained in cylindric foil cells; placed in needles or tubes with iridioplatinum walls of thicknesses of 0.5 mm and 1.0 mm, respectively. Radium tubes 22 mm long containing from 5 mg to 25 mg of radium in 15-mm active lengths are used at M. D. Anderson Cancer Center.[137] The *full-intensity needles* popularized in the Manchester System of dosimetry have 0.66 mg Ra/cm; *half-intensity* needles have 0.33 mg Ra/cm, and *quarter-intensity* needles have 0.165 mg Ra/cm.[112] Needles with 1.0 mg Ra/cm and 0.5 mg Ra/cm have also been used. Indian club needles have one "hot" end, and dumbbell needles have two hot ends, usually with 1.0 mg Ra/cm between the ends. In addition to knowing the activity per unit active length of a source, it is necessary to state its total activity, total physical length, active length, source diameter, and wall filtration. Radium sources are still available through a German vendor, Amersham-Buchler GmHt & Company.

Radon 222, with a half-life of 3.82 days, is a gas produced when radium decays; it was the first radioisotope used for permanent implants.[58] The radon gas was extracted and encapsulated in gold seeds, which were used in brachytherapy for many years. Because of extreme hazard to patients and personnel posed by radon from ruptured seeds or from ruptured radium sources, ^{222}Rn seeds and ^{226}Ra needles are no longer manufactured in the United States. As nuclear technology developed after World War II, many other radioisotopes (Table 12-1) were developed as radium or radon substitutes.

Cobalt 60

Cobalt 60 has a high cross-section for thermal neutrons. The neutron capture produces ^{60}Co. The subsequent decay to ^{60}Ni releases two highly energetic τ-rays (1.17 MeV and 1.33 MeV), but ^{60}Co has a relatively short half-life (5.26 years), an undesirable feature for a brachytherapy source. However, ^{60}Co tubes and needles were used for brachytherapy during the 1960s and 1970s, and ^{60}Co eye plaques are still used for treating eye lesions (*e.g.*, melanomas) and as sources in remote afterloading devices.[146]

Cesium 137

Cesium 137, a fission by-product, is a popular radium substitute because of its 30-year half-life; its single τ-ray (0.66 MeV) is less

TABLE 12–2
Characteristics of Radioisotopes in the Radium Series

RADIOISOTOPE*	ELEMENT	HALF-LIFE	PARTICLE ENERGIES† (MeV)	γ-RAY ENERGIES (MeV)
Radium	^{226}Ra	1620 y	α, 4.78 (94.3%) α, 4.59 (5.7%)	0.187 (5.7%)
Radon	^{222}Rn	3.82 d	α, 5.49 (99+%) α, 4.98 (<0.1%)	0.51 (0.07%)
Ra A	^{218}Po	3.05 min	α, 6.00 (99+%)	
Ra B	^{214}Pb	26.8 min	β^-, 0.67–1.03	0.053–0.352
Ra C	^{214}Bi	19.7 min	β^-, (99+%), 0.4–3.18 α, (0.04%), 5.51–5.54	0.61–2.43
Ra C′ (99+%)	^{214}Po	160 μsec	α, 7.68	
Ra C″ (0.04%)	^{210}Tl	1.32 min	β^-, 1.96	0.30–2.36
Ra D	^{210}Pb	21.4 y	β^-, 0.017 (85%) β^-, 0.064 (15%)	0.047 (85%)
Ra E	^{210}Bi	5.0 d	β^-, 1.16 (99+%)	
Ra F (polonium)	^{210}Po	138.4 d	α, 5.30 (99+%)	
Ra G	^{206}Pb	Stable		

** Historical name.*
† Where the β- or γ-spectra contain many lines, only ranges of energy without abundances are given.
(Spiers FW: Radioisotopes in the Human Body: Physical and Biological Effects, p 8. New York, Academic Press, 1968)

penetrating (HVL in lead = 0.65 cm) than the τ-rays from radium (HVL_{Pb} = 1.4 cm) or ^{60}Co (HVL_{Pb} = 1.1 cm). Modern ^{137}Cs sources contain the radioactive material in insoluble microspheres, presenting far less hazard from ruptured sources than the radon in a radium tube. The ^{137}Cs tubes usually have external diameters of approximately 2.65 mm, with lengths of about 21 mm and active lengths between 14 and 20 mm, depending on the vendor's design. They have activities equivalent to 5 to 40 mg of radium (472 MBq to 3.77 GBq ^{137}Cs); miniaturized sources equivalent to 10 mg of radium (370 MBq ^{137}Cs) with external diameters of approximately 1.25 mm attached to the end of a long metal stem are used to treat endometrial cancer. The ^{137}Cs needles with 0.66 mg Ra/cm (62.3 MBq/cm ^{137}Cs) and 0.33 mg Ra/cm (31.1 MBq/cm ^{137}Cs), external diameters of 1.65 mm, and active lengths from 15 mm to 45 mm are commonly used for interstitial implants. Seeds containing ^{137}Cs have been developed, but their use is not widespread.[9] Cesium 137 is also a popular source for remote afterloaders.

Tantalum 182 and Iridium 192

Tantalum 182 yields 41 τ-rays (maximum τ-ray energy, 1.45 MeV) and was used as a seed and wire source for temporary interstitial implants, but ^{192}Ir, which has a 74-day half-life and lower-energy τ-rays (average τ-ray energy, 0.38 MeV), is now widely used for temporary interstitial implants.[42,44] Iridium 192 is available as a wire (Amersham Corp, Chicago, IL; CIS-US, Sylmar, CA) with a core of 25% iridium and 75% platinum, either 0.3 mm or 0.1 mm in diameter, encased in a sheath of pure platinum 0.1 mm thick, to form an outside diameter of 0.5 mm or 0.3 mm. The ^{192}Ir seeds have a 0.3-mm-diameter core of 10% iridium and 90% platinum encased in 0.1 mm of pure platinum to form a seed with a 0.5-mm external diameter that is about 3 mm long (Alpha-Omega Services, Inc., Paramount, CA). In another design, stainless steel is encapsulated around a core of 30% iridium and 70% platinum, forming a seed with an outside diameter of 0.5 mm (Best Industries, Inc., Springfield, VA; RAD-IRID, Inc., Washington, DC). Iridium is insoluble in the body, but sources encapsulated in pure platinum should be handled with care to avoid damage to the encapsulating layer and the subsequent emission of high-energy β-particles normally filtered out by this encapsulating layer of material.[11]

Gold 198, Iodine 125, and Palladium 103

Insoluble ^{198}Au, with a 2.7-day half-life, releases a 0.412-MeV τ-ray, and gold seeds are still used as a radon-seed substitute for permanent implants.[142] However, ^{125}I seeds, emitting τ-rays and x-rays with energies below 0.0355 MeV, are readily shielded against by a few tenths of a millimeter of lead (HVL_{Pb} = 0.002 cm). The encapsulation of ^{125}I in a 0.5-mm external tube about 6 mm long with titanium welds on each end and a metallic (*i.e.*, gold ball or silver rod) radiopaque marker in the middle produces a sealed source with a dose distribution with high anisotrophy (Fig. 12-1).[82,83] Ruptured seeds damaged during the implant procedure can leak the ^{125}I, which follows the iodine metabolic pathway in the body and lodges in the thyroid. Careful inspection and leak tests of ^{125}I seeds before and after the implant procedure are required, particularly when seeds are reused several times.

Palladium 103 is a new alternative to ^{125}I for permanent implants (Theragenics Corp., Atlanta, GA).[95] From thermal neutron capture in ^{102}Pd, ^{103}Pd decays by electron capture to ^{103}Rh, with the subsequent emission of 20- to 23-keV characteristic x-rays. With a 17-day half-life, initial dose rates are higher than with similar ^{125}I seeds. The 4π averaged anisotropy of the dose around the seed is 0.83, with isodoses that exhibit more rapid spatial gradients than those from ^{125}I.[95]

Iodine 131 and Phosphorus 32

Iodine 131 and ^{32}P, with 8.05-day and 14.3-day half-lives, respectively, are used as unsealed radiopharmaceuticals. The ^{131}I treatment of the thyroid uses the energetic β-rays, ranging in mean energy from 69 keV to 192 keV, to deliver about 90% of the dose; only about 10% of the dose comes from the 80- to 637-KeV τ-rays emitted. Phosphorus 32, a pure β-emitter with a maximum β-ray energy of 1.71 MeV, is used as sodium phosphate to treat blood diseases; chromic phosphate is used as a colloidal in intracavitary instillations.

Strontium 90 and Ruthenium 106

Strontium 90, a fission by-product with a half-life of 28.9 years, decays to ^{90}Y, which decays in 64 hours to ^{90}Zr. Yttrium 90, a β-ray emitter with a maximum energy of 2.27-MeV, is widely used as a sealed source to treat shallow lesions of the skin or eye.[144] As powdered yttrium oxide, plastic exchange beads, or glass radiomicrospheres, ^{90}Y is used to treat liver disease.[131] Ruthenium 106, in radioactive equilibrium with ^{106}Rh, with a 1-year half-life and energetic β-rays of 3.5 MeV, has also been used for the treatment of eye lesions.[85,101]

Other Radioisotopes

Radioisotopes under active investigation or development include ^{241}Am, with a 432-year half-life and 60-keV τ-rays, as an appealing alternative for ^{137}Cs; ^{131}Cs, with a 9.7-day half-life and 30- to 35-keV x-rays, for permanent implants; ^{145}Sm, with a 340-day half-life and τ-rays and x-rays with less energy than 61 keV, for eye plaques; and ^{75}Se, with a 118.5-day half-life and τ-rays ranging from 0.136 MeV to 0.401 MeV, for temporary seed implants.[33,104,160]

DOSIMETRY OF SINGLE SOURCES

Large dose gradients over small (mm) dimensions hinder accurate physical dose measurements around brachytherapy sources. Finite volume detectors preclude dose measurements to greater than 2% accuracy within 1 cm of a finite source.[13] Many reported data were taken to determine the equivalency of radium substitutes to radium sources.[14,31,62,73,74] Although recent reports of standard-design source dosimetry are useful, most therapy facilities lack individually measured source isodosimetry.[31,41]

The Ideal Radioactive Source

The ideal brachytherapy source would be a single, infinitely small, encapsulated, monoenergetic-τ-ray point source that would interact with tissue in the same manner as with air. Moreover, the source activity would be known exactly; the *radia-*

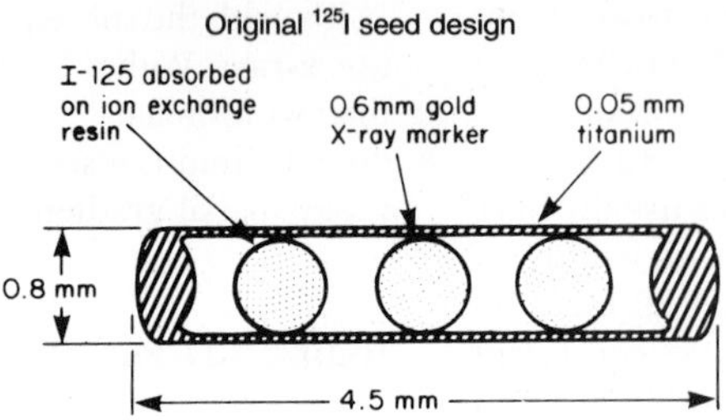

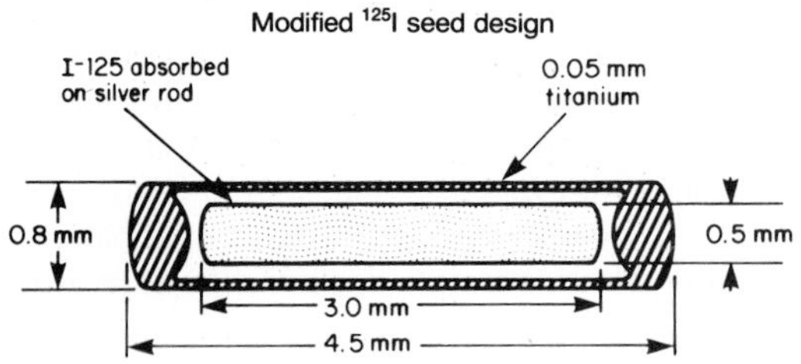

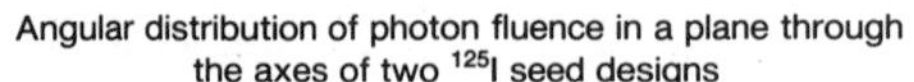

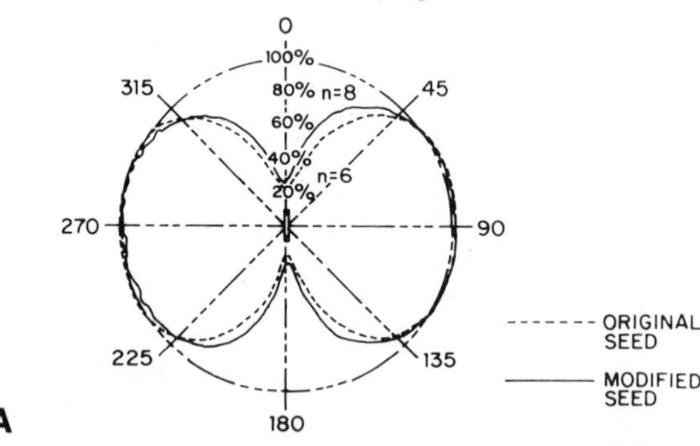

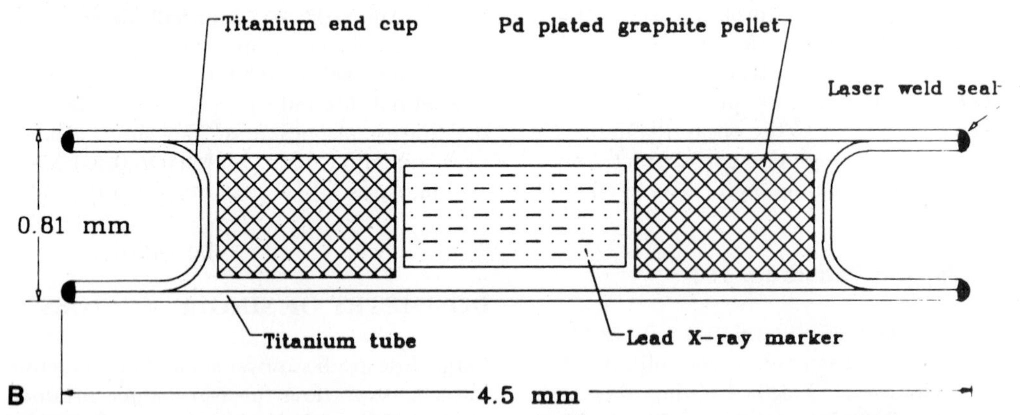

FIGURE 12–1. (**A**) (*Top*) Construction details of the original ^{125}I seed with a gold ball marker (Model No. 6701). (*Middle*) Construction details of the new ^{125}I seed with a silver rod marker (Model No. 6711). (*Bottom*) Angular distribution of photon fluence in a plane through the axes of two ^{125}I seed designs. (Ling CC, Yorke ED, Spiro IJ, et al: Int J Radiat Oncol Biol Phys 9:1747, 1983) (**B**) A Model 2000 ^{103}Pd source. The source has a lead x-ray marker in the center with a palladium-plated graphite pellet on each end. The source's external dimensions are identical to those of a ^{125}I seed; this allows ^{125}I guns to be used to insert ^{103}Pd seeds. (Courtesy of Theragenics Corp., Norcoss, GA)

tion fluence, the number of photons per unit area emanating from the source, would be governed by the *inverse square law,* k/r^2, and would be *isotropic* (*i.e,* of the same magnitude in all directions around the source). No self-attenuation or multiple scattering would occur in the source or in the medium (air) surrounding the source. Monoenergetic photons with an ideal energy of about 200 keV would avoid increased absorption of radiation in bone. This source would be ideal because its radiation fluence distribution could be easily modeled mathematically and the dosimetry would be known exactly at all locations around the source. It is unfortunate that such a source does not exist.

Actual Brachytherapy Sources

Brachytherapy sources are single, finite, encapsulated sources, often emitting β-rays and a spectrum of photons with energies from a few keV to greater than 2 MeV. The source activity is known only approximately; radiation fluence is governed by the inverse square law, k/r^2, far from the source but by more complex functions at distance, r, comparable to the dimensions of the source. The radiation fluence is anisotropic because of the source's finite size, design, and encapsulations. Self-attenuation and multiple scattering occur in the radioactive material, the sheathing around the source, the applicator in which the source is placed, and the tissue around the source.[98] In some instances, the effects of tissue heterogeneities on dose must be considered.[121]

The physics of brachytherapy sources was first elucidated by Rolf Sievert.[141] Sievert's method for calculating the radiation distribution around a finite source is presented in detail by Wood.[166] The source model is a line source of radioactivity in a cylindric container of attenuating material of diameter, 2d, with plane end faces (*i.e.*, no eyelets or trocar points). Exposure rates were found in four zones around the source (Fig. 12-2). In zone I, at point P, such that no line from the source to P passes through an end face, the exposure rate is given by

$$\dot{X} = \frac{M\Gamma}{lb}\int_{\theta_1}^{\theta_2} \exp(-\mu d/\cos\theta)d\theta$$

where M is the source activity (mCi), l is the source active length (cm), Γ is the specific τ-ray constant in R cm²/h/mCi for zero filtration, and b is the geometry parameter shown in the diagram. This yields

$$\dot{X} = \frac{M\Gamma(\theta_2 - \theta_1)}{lb}$$

for an unfiltered line source. In other zones, more complex forms of the integral apply.[166]

Using graphic integration, Sievert tabulated values of the integral and calculated the intensity patterns of single- and multiple-source arrangements and obtained isointensity curves. Using a small ionization chamber, he measured the relative dose distributions and concluded that, near the sources, the effects of the secondary or scatter radiation in tissue could, to a first approximation, be neglected.

Many refinements to these basic solutions have been made by others using improved mathematical methods, representing the integral as a series or polynomial.[18] Developed for radium sources, the solutions apply to radium substitutes if appropriate changes are made in the physical parameters. Monte Carlo calculations have confirmed the validity of the Sievert integral for ^{226}Ra and ^{192}Ir sources.[163,164] Gooden presents the mathematics of ring, circular disk, cylindric, and spheric sources.[48]

Toepfer and Rosen have obtained a solution to the Sievert integral suitable for a small programmable calculator.[153]

$$I(\theta) = \int_0^{\theta} \exp(-\mu d \sec\theta)d\theta$$

where

$$I(\theta) = \theta - 2\mu_0 dA \tan b^{-1}\left(B \tan\frac{\theta}{2}\right)$$

$$A = \frac{1}{[1 - (\mu_0 d)^2]^{1/2}}$$

$$B = \frac{[1 - \mu_0 d]^{1/2}}{[1 + \mu_0 d]^{1/2}}$$

This function can be used to calculate the dose at points near a single linear source using a programmable calculator.

Source Self-Attenuation

The encapsulated radioactive material that constitutes the source absorbs some of the radiation it is producing. Many authors have developed and applied models to correct for source self-attenuation.[10,50,96] For radium, with its complex spectrum, the effective attenuation coefficient, μ, depends on the thickness of the material traversed. Sievert approximated the radium spectrum by using three different photon energies and the attenuating coefficients.[141] Kemp introduced "screenage functions" that accounted for the spectral dependency of the effective linear attenuation coefficients of radium on the

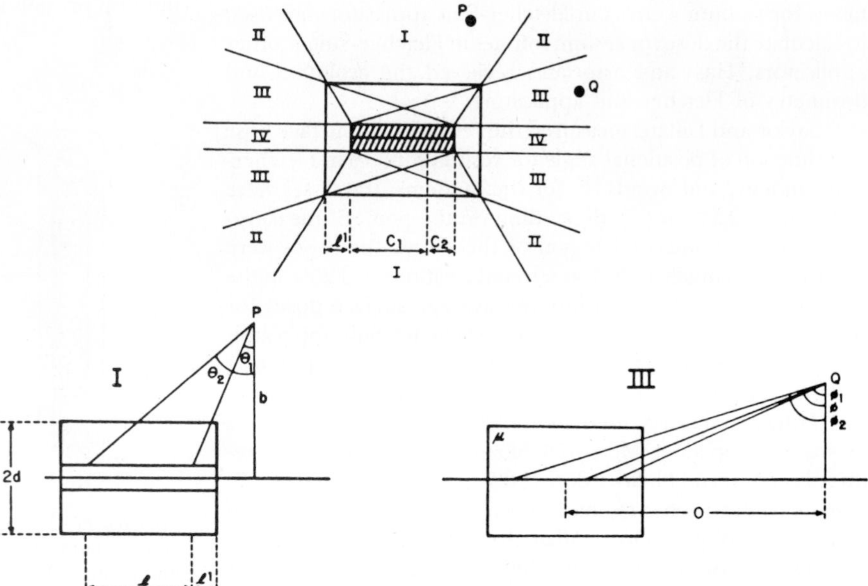

FIGURE 12–2. (*Top*) The four calculational zones around a finite source used in Sievert's original calculations. Modern computations follow the same principles using more zones. (*Bottom*) Geometry in zones I and III. (Courtesy of Butterworth & Co., Scarborough, Ontario)

effective wall thickness of platinum.[72] Whyte measured the linear attenuation coefficients for radium in platinum.[161] Keyser determined the ratio of effective wall thickness to actual wall thickness for radium sources.[73] Shalek and Stovall used 17 mm^{-1} as the effective attenuation coefficient for radium needles with walls of 0.5 mm of iridioplatinum, and one analytic function has been proposed to describe wall attenuation in those needles.[138]

The dramatic effects of source self-attenuation near the ends of sources are more difficult to model. Krishnaswamy, using Monte Carlo calculations, showed that the ratio of ^{137}Cs to ^{226}Ra isodose curves, although 1 to 1 along the transverse axis, was about 1.5 to 1 at points near the ends of the sources, where oblique filtration is most important.[77] Gooden's review of ^{137}Cs sources noted that the pinched isodoses near the ends of ^{137}Cs sources encapsulated in iridioplatinum were less evident in sources encapsulated in stainless steel.[48]

The extremely soft x-rays from ^{125}I are greatly attenuated in the original and current design of seeds (Fig. 12-1).[83] When these dose distributions are averaged over a 4π geometric source, activities are reduced by 14% to account for anisotropy, and the actual spatial dose variation is neglected in dose computations. Similar but less dramatic source and effects on dose distribution have been measured for ^{198}Au and ^{192}Ir seeds.[49] Achieving adequate near isotropic isodosimetry is a major obstacle in designing encapsulated sources of ^{241}Am and other proposed radioisotopes with low energy x-rays and τ-rays.[104]

Applicator Influence on Attenuation

The attenuations from the source holders (applicators), historically neglected in brachytherapy dose calculations, have been included in the clinical dosimetry of a few groups. Applicator corrections usually are made by reducing the activity of the sources by some constant fraction obtained by averaging the dosimetry over 4π geometry rather than accounting for the effects of attenuation as a function of position around the applicators. At the M. D. Anderson Cancer Center, when 1.5-cm active-length radium sources are used in Fletcher-Suit applicators, the source activity is reduced by 6% to account for ovoid attenuation; no correction is made when these sources are placed in a tandem.[36,37] Delclos[29] and colleagues warned that significant dosimetry errors can arise if published time-dose tables for radium sources in Fletcher-Suit applicators are used to calculate the dose for cesium sources in Fletcher-Suit or other applicators. Hass and associates reviewed the evolution and dosimetry of Fletcher-Suit applicators.[53]

Saylor and Dillard measured the reduction in surface dose as a function of positional angle for cesium sources in Fletcher-Suit tandems and ovoids.[133] For the tandems, the doses were reduced by 2.5% to 5%, depending on the point of measurement. In the nonleaded region of the ovoids the doses were reduced by as much as 20% at selected locations and 25% in the leaded region. Table 12-3 lists the average surface doses for some common activities of ^{137}Cs in a Fletcher-Suit applicator. Yorke and colleagues reviewed a method of incorporating Fletcher-Suit dosimetry in isodose computations.[168]

Tungsten inserts used in the 2-cm-diameter Henschke ovoids developed at Memorial Sloan-Kettering Hospital reduced rectum and bladder doses 10% and 15%, respectively.[100] Shields alter dosimetry, and more complex computational methods are required to calculate the dose around the shielded sources.[168] However, including the effects of shields allows far more accurate rectum and bladder dose estimates.

TABLE 12–3
Calculated Surface Dose Rates for a Model 6D6C ^{137}Cs Tube in a 2.0-cm-diameter Ovoid

^{137}Cs ACTIVITY (mg Ra eq)	AVERAGE SURFACE DOSE RATE (cGy/h)
5	30.6
10	61.3
15	92.0
20	122.6

The unit dose rate is 6.13 cGy/h/mg Ra eq; 1 mg Ra eq equals 94.35 MBq of ^{137}Cs. The dose rates calculated by Krishnaswamy[77] and confirmed by measurements by Saylor and Dillard[133] were reduced 10% to reflect the average dose rate reduction produced by the ovoid. These rates neglect any contributions from the adjacent tandem and ovoid.

Attenuation and Multiple Scattering in Tissue

As shown in Figure 12-3, τ-rays in tissue attenuate and multiply scatter. Not all τ-rays traversing toward a point, P, will reach it. Some are attenuated along the path; others scatter away from the point; others not heading toward P are scattered, contributing to the dose at P. Sievert, to a first approximation, suggested that these effects could be neglected for radium sources, because they were compensatory, and within a few centimeters of the source, it was possible to assume that the tissue was not even present.[141] This assumption was used for brachytherapy dosimetry for over 50 years. Many experiments and calculations have been performed to test this assumption for radium and radium substitutes.

Early mathematic models, some of which are listed in Tables 12-4 and 12-5, are used in dose calculational algorithms, normally as the ratio of dose or exposure in water (D_w, X_w) to dose or exposure in air (D_a, X_a) to account for these effects on tissue.[10,62,63,96,143,169] Measurements and Monte Carlo calculations have proven the validity of representing these effects in water by polynomial expressions and have been extended to include tissue, fat, and specific organs.[27,151] Figure 12-4 shows the ratio of X_w to X_a for several radioisotopes. These effects are a function of τ-ray energy; attenuation and multiple scattering in tissue are nearly compensatory for ^{192}Ir and ^{198}Au within about 5 cm from the source; for lower τ-ray energies, source buildup prevails near the source, and for higher τ-ray energies,

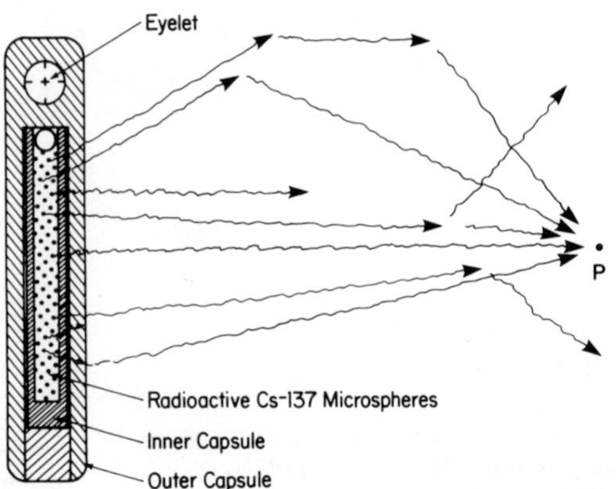

FIGURE 12–3. Schematic representation of the competing processes of attenuation and multiple scattering in a source and in tissue. Compton-scattered photons experience numerous individual scatterings before they ultimately yield all their energy.

TABLE 12–4
Some Mathematical Models Accounting for Attenuation and Multiple Scattering in a Medium Surrounding a Radioactive Source

INVESTIGATORS	MODEL	DEFINITIONS
Hale[50]	$D_W/D_A = (e^{-\mu r})(e^{+0.77E-0.29\mu r})$*	D_W = Dose to water D_A = Dose to air μ = Mass attenuation coefficient for water r = Distance from source E = Average γ-ray energy in MeV
Batho et al[10]	Fractional transmission through water = $1 - 0.0074\ r^{3/4}$	r = Distance (cm) from radium source to point of calculation; applies only approximately for other radioisotopes
Meisberger et al[96]	$X_W/X_A = A + Br + Cr^2 + Dr^3$	X_W = Exposure in water X_A = Exposure in air r = Distance (cm) from source to point of calculation A, B, C, D = 0, 1st, 2nd, 3rd order polynomial fitting coefficients (Table 12-5)
Van Keffens, and Star[156]	$f_2(d, \theta) = (1 + ad^2)/(1 + bd^2)$	d = Distance (in cm) from source to point of calculation θ = angular dependency term

**Model valid for d < 1; 0.25 MeV < E < 2MeV.*

source attenuation prevails near the source because there is less multiple scattering of high-energy photons.[50]

Source Localization

To calculate dose distributions manually or by computer, the positions and orientations of the radioactive sources relative to the target volume and to each other must be known. Orthogonal radiographs[56] yield the geometric relationships for the Pythagorean theorem (Fig. 12-5), from which source lengths can be calculated from the source projections on the two radiographs as

$$\overline{MN} = (\overline{MN}^2 + p^2)^{1/2},$$

after correcting each film for magnification, where point p lies on the baseline common to each film. The beam central axis must be perpendicular to each film, which must be perpendicular to each other. Stereo films, either a double-exposure film obtained with the x-ray beam in two different positions or obtained on separate films, use similar triangles for source localization (Fig. 12-6).[103,110] The height, z, of the source follows from

$$\frac{S_T}{s} = \frac{F - f}{f}$$

$$\frac{S_T}{y_1 + s - y_2} = \frac{F - z}{z}$$

$$z = F[(F - f)(y_2 - y_1) - S_T f][(F - f)(y_2 - y_1) - S_T F]$$

Large shifts of about 60 cm are required to minimize certain errors.[35,64] Practically, such shifts are difficult to achieve, and a shift of 20 cm (± 10 cm from center) with the 100-cm source-to-film distance is common, but not error free.[108,140,156]

Source magnification is commonly determined by placing a 5-cm-diameter ring at the level of the sources; one diameter of the ring is magnified without foreshortening. Placing a ring on each of the four surfaces of the patient yields a highly accurate source reconstruction.[48] Reconstruction errors introduced by patient movement between films can be eliminated by using fiducial markers imaged in both films, as described by several authors.[48,138,140]

TABLE 12–5
Polynomial Fitting Coefficients for the Ratio of Exposure in Water to Exposure in Air

	MEISBERGER ET AL COEFFICIENTS				VAN KLEFFENS & STAR COEFFICIENTS	
ISOTOPE	A ($\times 10^0$)	B ($\times 10^{-3}$)	C ($\times 10^{-3}$)	D ($\times 10^{-5}$)	a	b
^{198}Au	1.0306	−8.134	1.111	−15.970		
^{192}Ir	1.0128	5.019	1.178	−2.008		
^{137}Cs	1.0091	−9.015	−0.3459	−2.817	0.0083	0.0108
^{226}Ra	1.0005	−4.423	−1.707	7.448	0.0068	0.0097
^{60}Co	0.99423	−5.318	−2.610	13.270	0.0100	0.0145

(Data from Meisberger LL, Keller RJ, Shalek RJ: Radiology 90:953, 1968; Van Kleffens HJ, Star WM: Int J Radiat Oncol Biol Phys 2:731, 1979)

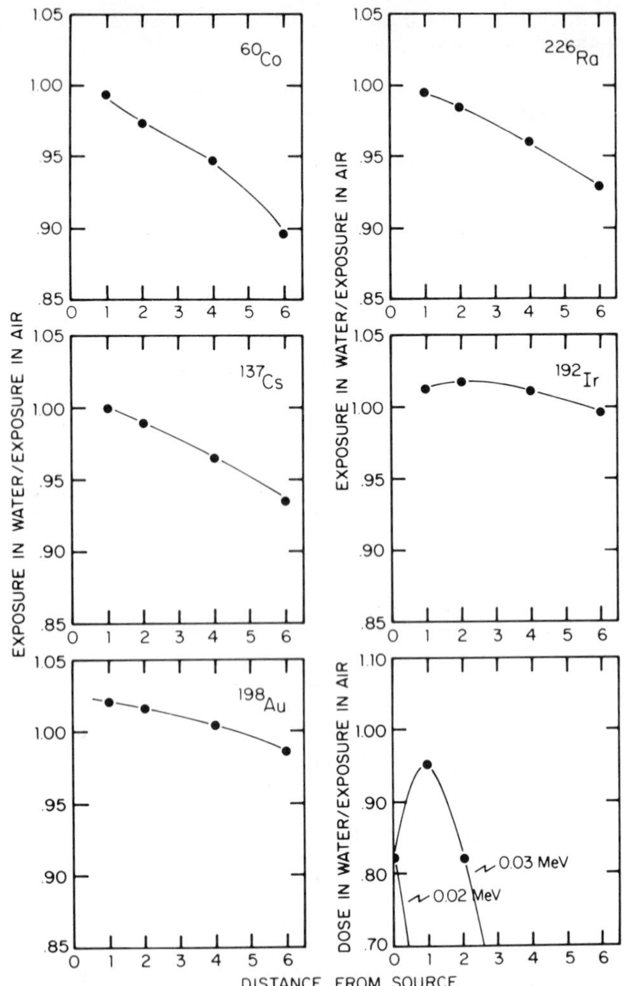

FIGURE 12–4. The ratio of the exposure in water to exposure in air for several radioisotopes. For radioisotopes with an average γ-ray energy of about 0.4 MeV (^{192}Ir, ^{198}Au), attenuation and multiple scattering in tissue are nearly compensatory, and the ratio curve is flat. For those with higher average energies (^{60}Co, ^{226}Ra, ^{137}Cs) within 5 cm of the source, multiple scattering fails to compensate fully for attenuation. The ratio of dose in water to exposure in air is shown for 0.02-MeV and 0.03-MeV x-rays. (*Bottom right*) Most x-ray and γ-ray emissions from ^{125}I are bound by these curves, which exhibit a rapid fall-off with distance as this soft radiation is attenuated in tissue. (Modified from Meisberger LL, Keller RJ, Shalek RJ: Radiology 90:953, 1968)

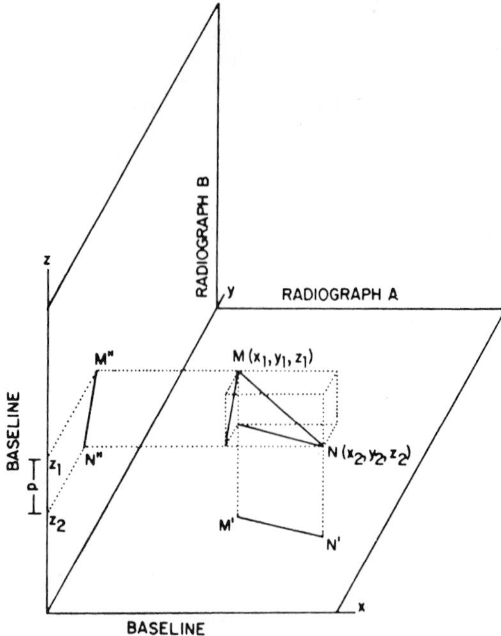

FIGURE 12–5. The Pythagorean theorem is used with orthogonal radiographs to calculate the source length and to determine source positions relative to one another. The source length of $\overline{MN}$ lies between coordinates $M(x_1, y_1, z_1)$ and $N(x_2, y_2, z_2)$ and projects a length $\overline{M'N'}$ on radiograph A and a length $\overline{M''N''}$ on radiograph B. $\overline{M''N''}$ projects a length p onto the z axis orthogonal to radiograph A; hence, $\overline{MN} = p^2 + \overline{M'N'}^2$. (Shalek RJ, Stovall M: The calculation of dose in interstitial implantations. In Friedman M (ed): Radiation Therapy in the Management of Cancer of the Oral Cavity and Oropharynx. Springfield, IL, Charles C Thomas, 1962)

Excellent stereo-shift films are obtained by using a conventional radiation therapy simulator with a rotating gantry.[34] Rotating the gantry 20 degrees from the vertical in either direction effectively achieves a large stereo shift (Fig. 12-7). The film is angled at 20 degrees on the image intensifier table to maintain it parallel to the table, as in a conventional stereo-shift technique. The method of calculating the source position is identical to that for the conventional stereo-shift technique.

Three-film and other radiography methods allow reconstruction of seed implants without identifying the same seed in each film; random seed entry is used, and an algorithm is used to sort out and identify the same seeds in each film.[3] The multiple-slice capability of computed tomography (CT) scanners and their ability to reconstruct in various viewing planes are being investigated by several researchers for brachytherapy source localization.[88]

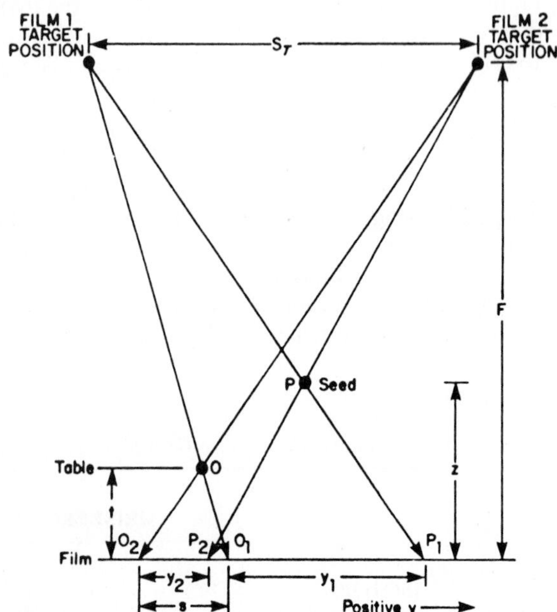

FIGURE 12–6. The geometry of stereo-shift radiographs: y_1 is the distance on the first film between images of a seed at P and a tabletop reference point, which is seen as an origin at 0; y_2 is the distance between images at the same points on the second film, taken from shifting a tube a distance s_t toward the patient's head (*i.e.*, in the positive y direction). The image of the origin shifts a distance s in the opposite direction. From these distances and the target-to-film distances, F, and the tabletop distance, t, the vertical distance, z, of the seed from the film can be calculated. (Courtesy of L. Anderson Memorial-Sloan-Kettering Cancer Center, NY)

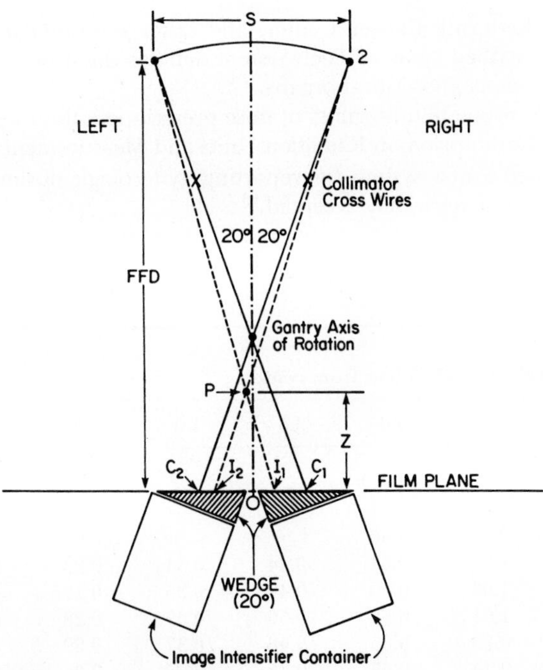

FIGURE 12–7. The geometry or a rotating simulator used to obtain a pair of stereo films. The simulator rotates from 1 to 2 and moves the focal spot through a shift of S. I_1 and I_2 represent the seed images on each film; C_1 and C_2 denote the centers of the two films. From this stereo film pair, the height, Z, of the seed is determined. (Feldman A: Int J Radiat Oncol Biol Phys 5[Suppl 2]:80, 1979)

Computer Dose Calculations

Computers allow rapid calculations of the dose distribution around single and multiple brachytherapy sources. Nelson and Meurk[107] developed an algorithm to sum the doses, using only inverse-square law considerations, at a point from an array of seeds. Stovall and Shalek[147] reviewed the cogent features of 20 computer codes developed worldwide by 1972. Many of these codes (*e.g.*, radcomp, brachy, isodos) were developed at the university hospitals and gained widespread use at other regional hospitals and, with adaptations, are the dose computation algorithms used on commercial computers sold for radiation therapy dose computations.

All computer codes do not make the corrections discussed here or use the same methods of computation; given the same brachytherapy data, their solutions differ. Powers and associates[119] analyzed four popularly used codes and found them to be "clinically acceptable."

Tolbert and Reed[154] used four test cases on four commercial systems and compared the results with the average data from three widely used codes (*i.e.*, brachy, radcomp and isodos). They reported "differences of 11% and 15% for clinical points A and B, around a [single] intracavitary [radium] application." Users must be well versed in the details of these computer computations. Errors arise from using incorrect dosimetry parameters or failing to understand whether a particular correction, such as tissue attenuation, is made in an algorithm. For example, failure to use the correct unfiltered exposure rate constant or using source activity in millicuries when milligram radium equivalents are required can produce major dose errors. Jayaraman and Lanzl[70] reviewed the uncertainties inherent in calculating the exposure rate from linear sources and concluded that, if the terms of exposure rate at a distance from the source are specified, the overall uncertainties in the dosimetry at regions of clinical interest around the sources are limited to about 6%.

From these codes and from measured data, "away" and "along" tables have been obtained for many different linear sources with different design characteristics. Table 12-6 provides data for some of the ^{226}Ra sources used at M. D. Anderson Cancer Center; similar useful tables exist.[54,137] The dosimetry of a single source is shown as a graph of the dose rates along lines bisecting a linear source and cutting through the source in other segments (Fig. 12-8) or "escargot curves," popularized by those using ^{192}Ir wires (Fig. 12-9).[51,116] Gillin and co-workers presented ^{192}Ir wire dosimetry in an "away" and "along" table.[40]

Classical Dose Prescriptions and Distribution Rules

The earliest method of dose prescription stated the amount in milligrams or activity in millicuries of the radioisotope placed in a patient and the duration in hours of treatment, yielding milligram hours (mgh) and millicurie hours (mCih). For example, if a permanent implant involved 10 radon seeds, each of 15 mCi, the duration of the decaying permanent implant is represented by the mean life, $\overline{T}$, of the radon, which is 1.44 $T_{1/2}$ (*i.e.*, as if the implant had constant initial activity A_0 present for a time equal to 1.44 $T_{1/2}$). In this time, the same number of disintegrations would occur if they were calculated on a continual decay basis using the activities present at each moment and the physical half-life. For ^{222}Rn, $T_{1/2}$ = 3.82 days (91.68 hours); hence, $\overline{T}$ = 132.0 hours, and 15 mCi × 132 hours yields 1980 mCih, which corresponds to 2.63711 × 10^{14} disintegrations. Historically, the term *emitted radiation* described this process.

The *destroyed activity* (e.g., 15 mCi in the previous example) in an implant is the difference between the initial and the final activity. If 10 radium sources, each with 1.5 mg of radium, are used, and the source is removed after, for example, 132 hours, the milligram hours will be numerically the same: 1980 mgh. The amount of radium that decays in 132 hours is 0.0001087 mg, which represents the destroyed activity. The emitted radiation, or total number of disintegrations, would be the same as if the destroyed activity, 0.0001087 mg of radium, were available for 1.44 $T_{1/2}$, which for radium is 6.543454 × 10^{10} seconds. The product of 1.087 × 10-^{4} × 6.543454 × 10^{10} seconds × 3.7 × 10^7 disintegrations/sec yields 2.631711 × 10^{14} decays, identical to the figure in the previous example. Hence, the milligram hours concept physically represents the total number of radioactive transformations that occur during the use of a permanent or removable implant. The milligram hours concept is still used in brachytherapy treatment prescriptions, with the activity of substitute radioisotopes expressed in equivalent milligrams of radium, even though the concept contains no information about the dose distribution.

In 1938, Tod and Meredith[152] proposed that the doses for gynecologic treatments be calculated at point A, 2 cm above the mucous membrane of the lateral vaginal fornix and 2 cm lateral to the center of the uterine canal. A dose of 8000 R in 144 hours was delivered at a rate of 55.5 R per hour, using ^{226}Ra sources with 1-mm platinum filtration. Point B was established at the same level as point A but 5 cm from the midline; this point was near the obturator lymph node and gave an indication of the lateral throw-off dose. Because the lower end of the intrauterine tube is commonly level with the lateral fornix, point A is now defined as 2 cm from the lower end of this source and 2 cm lateral from its center. Point A and point B definitions are further described in Chapter 13.

Cunningham and colleagues[26] have shown that there is a strong correlation between the milligram hours prescription and the dose to points A and B (Fig. 12-10), an observation confirmed by Jani and associates.[69]

More detailed point-dose description systems include the lymphatic trapezoid method developed at the M. D. Anderson Cancer Center, the New York System developed at Memorial Sloan-Kettering Cancer Center, and other less-popular, but well-described systems. Each system denotes the dose at specified points and critical organs.[37,61]

To promote uniformity of dose prescription, the International Commission on Radiation Units and Measurements has proposed a new system for reporting gynecologic dosimetry, but it is not yet widely accepted.[68]

TABLE 12–6
Centigrays per Milligram Hour in Tissue Delivered at Various Distances by Linear Sources

PERPENDICULAR DISTANCE FROM SOURCE (cm)	DISTANCE ALONG SOURCE AXIS (cm from center)										
	0	0.5	1.0	1.5	2.0	2.5	3.0	3.5	4.0	4.5	5.0
RADIUM*											
Active Length of 1.5 cm											
0.25	50.67	43.75	11.94	3.34	1.48	0.81	0.50	†	†	†	†
0.5	20.26	16.95	8.18	3.38	1.70	1.00	0.64	0.44	0.31	0.23	0.18
0.75	10.84	9.29	5.67	2.99	1.67	1.03	0.69	0.48	0.35	0.276	0.21
1.0	6.67	5.89	4.10	2.52	1.55	1.01	0.69	0.50	0.37	0.28	0.22
1.5	3.20	2.96	2.38	1.74	1.24	0.89	0.65	0.48	0.37	0.29	0.23
2.0	1.85	1.76	1.52	1.23	0.96	0.74	0.57	0.45	0.35	0.28	0.23
2.5	1.20	1.15	1.04	0.89	0.74	0.60	0.49	0.40	0.32	0.26	0.22
3.0	0.83	0.81	0.75	0.67	0.58	0.49	0.41	0.34	0.29	0.24	0.21
3.5	0.61	0.60	0.57	0.52	0.46	0.40	0.35	0.30	0.26	0.22	0.19
4.0	0.47	0.46	0.44	0.41	0.37	0.33	0.29	0.26	0.23	0.20	0.17
4.5	0.37	0.36	0.35	0.33	0.30	0.28	0.25	0.22	0.20	0.18	0.16
5.0	0.30	0.29	0.28	0.27	0.25	0.23	0.21	0.19	0.17	0.16	0.14
Active Length of 3.0 cm											
0.25	27.93	27.58	25.77	14.50	3.20	1.28	†	†	†	†	†
0.5	12.64	12.32	10.91	6.96	2.97	1.43	0.83	0.53	0.36	0.26	0.20
0.75	7.54	7.28	6.33	4.42	2.47	1.39	0.85	0.57	0.40	0.30	0.23
1.0	5.04	4.85	4.22	3.14	2.03	1.28	0.83	0.57	0.42	0.31	0.24
1.5	2.69	2.59	2.30	1.87	1.40	1.02	0.73	0.54	0.41	0.31	0.25
2.0	1.65	1.60	1.46	1.25	1.01	0.80	0.62	0.48	0.38	0.30	0.24
2.5	1.11	1.08	1.00	0.89	0.76	0.63	0.51	0.42	0.34	0.28	0.23
3.0	0.79	0.77	0.73	0.66	0.58	0.50	0.42	0.36	0.30	0.25	0.21
3.5	0.58	0.58	0.55	0.51	0.46	0.41	0.35	0.31	0.26	0.23	0.19
4.0	0.45	0.44	0.43	0.40	0.37	0.33	0.30	0.26	0.23	0.20	0.18
4.5	0.36	0.35	0.34	0.32	0.30	0.28	0.25	0.23	0.20	0.18	0.16
5.0	0.29	0.29	0.28	0.27	0.25	0.23	0.21	0.19	0.18	0.16	0.14
Active Length of 4.5 cm											
0.25	19.12	19.06	18.83	†	†	†	†	†	†	†	†
0.5	9.01	8.95	8.71	8.09	6.36	3.16	1.42	0.77	0.48	0.33	0.24
0.75	5.60	5.54	5.33	4.84	3.81	2.35	1.31	0.79	0.52	0.36	0.27
1.0	3.90	3.85	3.67	3.29	2.65	1.83	1.16	0.76	0.52	0.37	0.28
1.5	2.23	2.19	2.07	1.86	1.56	1.21	0.89	0.65	0.48	0.36	0.28
2.0	1.44	1.41	1.34	1.22	1.05	0.87	0.69	0.54	0.43	0.34	0.27
2.5	0.99	0.98	0.93	0.86	0.76	0.66	0.55	0.45	0.37	0.30	0.25
3.0	0.72	0.71	0.69	0.64	0.58	0.51	0.44	0.38	0.32	0.27	0.23
3.5	0.55	0.54	0.52	0.49	0.45	0.41	0.36	0.32	0.27	0.24	0.20
4.0	0.43	0.42	0.41	0.39	0.36	0.33	0.30	0.27	0.24	0.21	0.18
4.5	0.34	0.34	0.33	0.32	0.30	0.27	0.25	0.23	0.20	0.18	0.16
5.0	0.28	0.28	0.27	0.26	0.25	0.23	0.21	0.20	0.18	0.16	0.14
CESIUM‡											
Active Length of 1.4 cm											
Stainless Steel Wall Thickness of 1.0 mm											
0.5	21.052	17.445	8.404	3.663	1.943	1.187	0.794	0.566	0.422	0.326	0.258
1.0	6.808	5.997	4.177	2.597	1.639	1.093	0.768	0.564	0.429	0.335	0.268
1.5	3.241	2.996	2.409	1.777	1.275	0.925	0.686	0.522	0.407	0.325	0.263
2.0	1.866	1.773	1.536	1.245	0.975	0.757	0.591	0.466	0.374	0.304	0.250
2.5	1.204	1.162	1.051	0.902	0.750	0.613	0.500	0.408	0.336	0.279	0.233
3.0	0.837	0.816	0.758	0.676	0.585	0.498	0.420	0.353	0.298	0.252	0.214
3.5	0.614	0.602	0.569	0.521	0.464	0.407	0.353	0.304	0.262	0.226	0.195
4.0	0.468	0.461	0.441	0.411	0.375	0.336	0.298	0.262	0.230	0.201	0.177
4.5	0.368	0.364	0.351	0.331	0.307	0.280	0.253	0.226	0.202	0.179	0.159
5.0	0.296	0.293	0.285	0.271	0.255	0.236	0.216	0.196	0.177	0.159	0.143

(continued)

TABLE 12–6
(Continued)

PERPENDICULAR DISTANCE FROM SOURCE (cm)	DISTANCE ALONG SOURCE AXIS (cm from center)										
	0	0.5	1.0	1.5	2.0	2.5	3.0	3.5	4.0	4.5	5.0
Active Length of 3.0 cm											
Stainless Steel Wall Thickness of 0.5 mm											
0.5	12.891	12.572	11.229	7.452	3.371	1.726	1.046	0.704	0.506	0.381	0.296
1.0	5.073	4.890	4.289	3.252	2.150	1.386	0.934	0.664	0.493	0.379	0.300
1.5	2.697	2.603	2.326	1.905	1.448	1.064	0.783	0.588	0.453	0.357	0.288
2.0	1.651	1.603	1.464	1.260	1.031	0.818	0.643	0.507	0.405	0.377	0.268
2.5	1.104	1.078	1.003	0.893	0.765	0.639	0.526	0.432	0.356	0.295	0.246
3.0	0.785	0.770	0.727	0.663	0.587	0.508	0.433	0.367	0.310	0.263	0.224
3.5	0.584	0.575	0.549	0.509	0.461	0.410	0.359	0.312	0.270	0.233	0.202
4.0	0.450	0.444	0.427	0.402	0.370	0.336	0.300	0.266	0.234	0.206	0.181
4.5	0.356	0.352	0.341	0.324	0.303	0.278	0.253	0.228	0.204	0.182	0.162
5.0	0.288	0.285	0.278	0.266	0.251	0.234	0.215	0.197	0.178	0.161	0.145
Active Length of 4.5 cm											
Stainless Steel Wall Thickness of 0.5 mm											
0.5	9.306	9.237	8.991	8.375	6.715	3.527	1.688	0.975	0.642	0.457	0.342
1.0	3.960	3.907	3.731	3.370	2.744	1.936	1.267	0.849	0.599	0.444	0.341
1.5	2.244	2.208	2.095	1.892	1.599	1.257	0.941	0.699	0.526	0.406	0.321
2.0	1.440	1.417	1.346	1.228	1.070	0.891	0.718	0.569	0.452	0.362	0.294
2.5	0.995	0.980	0.936	0.865	0.771	0.667	0.562	0.466	0.385	0.318	0.265
3.0	0.724	0.715	0.686	0.641	0.583	0.517	0.499	0.385	0.328	0.278	0.237
3.5	0.518	0.542	0.523	0.493	0.455	0.412	0.366	0.322	0.280	0.243	0.211
4.0	0.427	0.423	0.410	0.390	0.364	0.335	0.303	0.271	0.240	0.212	0.187
4.5	0.341	0.338	0.330	0.316	0.298	0.277	0.254	0.230	0.208	0.186	0.186
5.0	0.278	0.276	0.270	0.260	0.247	0.232	0.215	0.198	0.180	0.164	0.148

**Filtration = 0.5-mm platinum. Entries are absorbed dose rates (cGy/h) in muscle tissue per milligram of radium and include corrections for source self-attenuation and attenuation and multiple scattering in the muscle tissue around the source. (Shalek RJ, Stovall M: Dosimetry in implant therapy. In Attix FH, Tochlin E [eds]. Radiation Dosimetry, p 776. New York, Academic Press, 1969)*
† Dose rates omitted where γ-rays traverse more than 7-mm platinum.
‡ (Krishnaswamy V: Radiology 105:181, 1972)

Other useful point-dose prescription methods include using the stated surface dose on a gynecologic ovoid applicator to approximate the dose to the tissue surface in contact with the ovoid or at a 0.25-cm depth in tissue surrounding the ovoid. Fletcher included surface dose rate tables for ovoids and vaginal cylinders with and without spacers for use with the ^{226}Ra sources in Fletcher-Suit applicators.[37] A 6% reduction in dose is made to account for the attenuation of radium in the ovoids. When ^{137}Cs sources are used in Fletcher-Suit applicators, 10% dose reductions occur. A 3% dose reduction occurs in the tandem. Tables 12-3 and 12-7 are appropriate for model 6D6C cesium sources in Fletcher-Suit ovoids and Delclos vaginal cylinders. Similar tables can be constructed for other source activities.

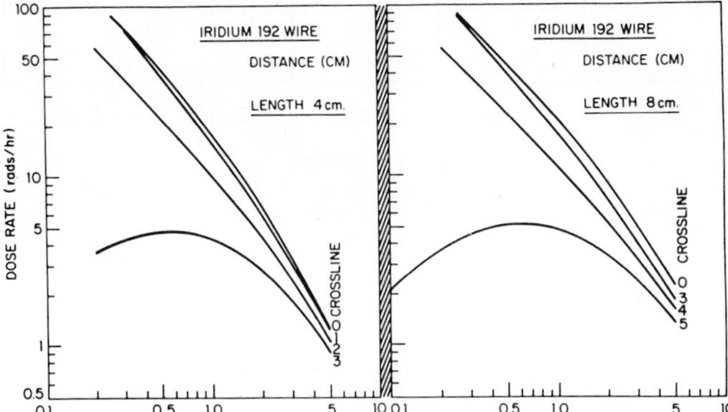

FIGURE 12–8. The dose rates (cGy/hour) along lines perpendicular to 4-cm and 8-cm lengths of ^{192}Ir wire, with a linear activity of 1.0 mg Ra eq/cm (63.3 MBq/cm of ^{192}Ir). The crossline numbers denote the distance (cm) of the crossline from the central crossline. (Hall EJ, Oliver R, Stepstone BJ: Acta Radiol 4:155, 1966)

In interstitial implants, the prescriptions and dose distribution rules developed by Paterson, Parker, Tod, Meredith, Spiers, and Stephenson from 1934 to 1953 (Manchester system) achieve a relatively homogeneous dose distribution using combinations of sources of different linear intensities (*i.e.*, 0.66 mg, 0.50 mg, 0.33 mg Ra/cm).[97] In extending their rules, developed for surface applicators, to interstitial implants, the authors state, "As applied to interstitial work by a homogeneous field or zone of irradiation, we mean an area over which, or a volume throughout the whole of which the irradiation is 'effectively constant' (*i.e.*, does not vary by more than ± 10% *except* for the localized 'hot spots' immediately around implanted τ-ray or sources."[97] Dosage tables assumed 1000 R as the clinical working unit or *effective minimum dose* (10% above the absolute minimum dose) in the plane or volume to be irradiated.[97] Tables 12-8 and 12-9, derived from the original tables, include many correction factors that reflect modern dosimetry concepts.[97]

The distribution rules are extensive, and readers are referred to the original articles. Investigators have provided limited synopses of the rules, most recently Gooden, with excellent examples.[48, 54] Table 12-10 presents a limited summary of the main features of the Manchester system.

The goal is to achieve an effective minimum dose with a dose variation of less than ± 10%. For areas larger than 25 cm^2, two thirds of the activity is distributed on the periphery and the remaining one third in the center. For areas larger than 25 cm^2

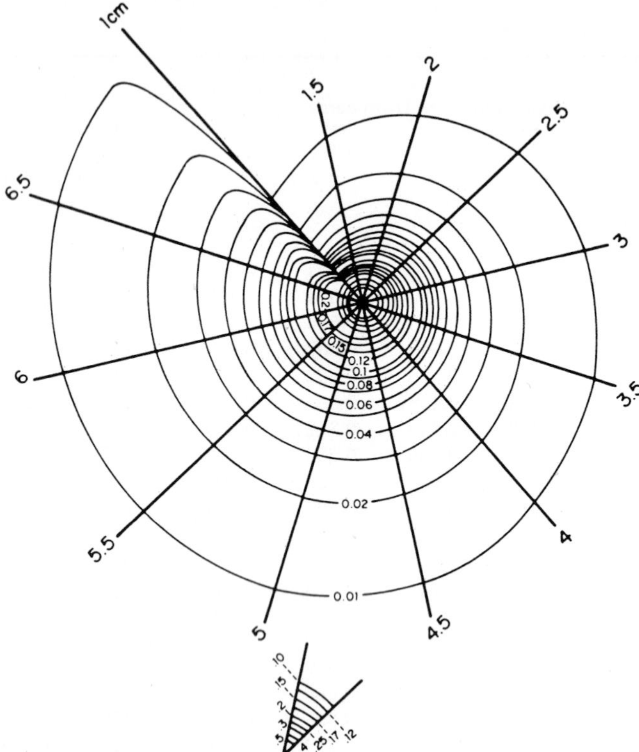

FIGURE 12–9. An "escargot curve" for ^{192}Ir wire. Radial line denotes source lengths (cm). Dose rates (Gy/hour) assume a source linear activity of 1 mCi/cm (37 MBq/cm of ^{192}Ir). If clear sheets are used for commonly used magnifications, the dose at a point near a source array can rapidly be calculated manually by placing the center of the spiral curve on each linear source, noting the dose contributed to the point by each source and, by summation, obtaining the cumulative dose. (*Inset*) Rapid dose gradient near the source.

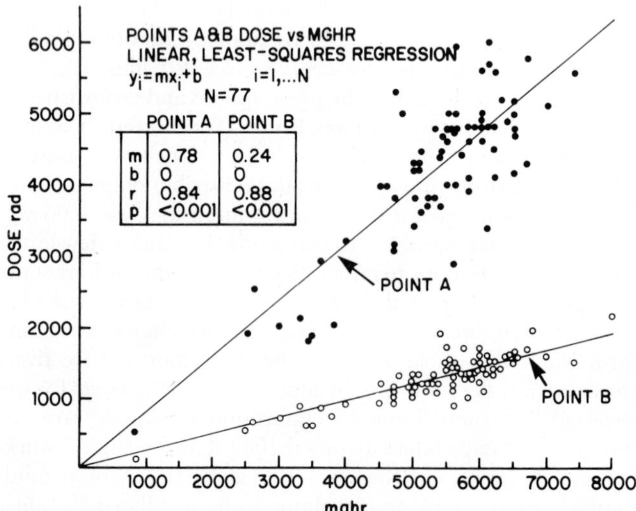

FIGURE 12–10. Correlation between milligram hours (mgh) and doses to points A and B in the treatment of 77 patients with carcinoma of the cervix, using Fletcher-Suit afterloading applicators. For nominal comparisons, the dose at point A was about 0.75 cGy/mgh. (Cunningham DE, Stryker JA, Velkey DE: Int J Radiat Oncol Biol Phys 7:121, 1981)

TABLE 12–7
Calculated Surface Dose Rates for Vaginal Cylinders for Model 6D6C ^{137}Cs Tubes

SOURCE POSITION	DOSE AT POINT LOCATION (cGy/mgh)† A	B	C	D	E
2.0-cm-DIAMETER CYLINDER					
1	6.81	1.64	0.43	0.18	0.10
2	1.64	6.81	1.64	0.43	0.18
3	0.43	1.64	6.81	1.64	0.43
4	0.18	0.43	1.64	6.81	1.64
5	0.10	0.18	0.43	1.64	6.81
2.5-cm-DIAMETER CYLINDER					
1	4.56	1.46	0.42	0.18	0.10
2	1.46	4.56	1.46	0.42	0.18
3	0.42	1.46	4.56	1.46	0.42
4	0.18	0.42	1.46	4.56	1.46
5	0.10	0.18	0.42	1.46	4.56
3.0-cm-DIAMETER CYLINDER					
1	3.25	1.28	0.40	0.18	0.10
2	1.28	3.25	1.28	0.40	0.18
3	0.40	1.28	3.25	1.28	0.40
4	0.18	0.40	1.28	3.25	1.28
5	0.10	0.18	0.40	1.28	3.25
3.5-cm-DIAMETER CYLINDER					
1	2.42	1.11	0.39	0.18	0.10
2	1.11	2.42	1.11	0.39	0.18
3	0.39	1.11	2.42	1.11	0.39
4	0.18	0.39	1.11	2.42	1.11
5	0.10	0.18	0.39	1.11	2.42
4.0-cm-DIAMETER CYLINDER					
1	1.87	0.98	0.39	0.17	0.10
2	0.98	1.87	0.98	0.37	0.17
3	0.37	0.98	1.87	0.98	0.37
4	0.17	0.37	0.98	1.87	0.98
5	0.10	0.17	0.37	0.98	1.87

* *For 20-mm long tubes without any spacers between the sources.*
† *Sum of all doses from all sources within vaginal cylinder.*
(Dose rate data from Krishnaswamy V: Radiology 105:181, 1972)

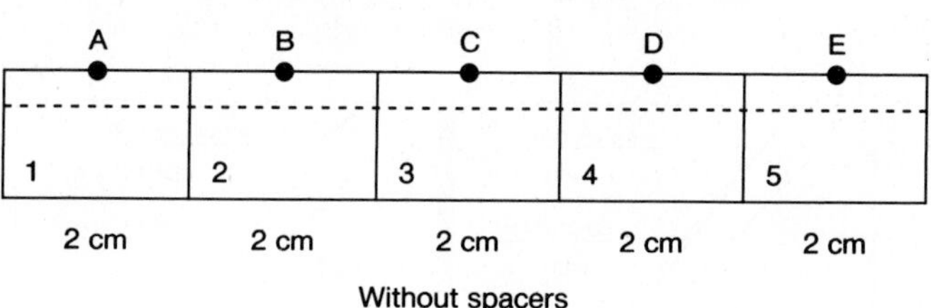

TABLE 12–8
Milligram Hours per 1000 cGy for Various Areas and Treating Distances (Manchester System)

AREA (cm^2)*	TREATING DISTANCE (cm)						AREA (cm^2)*	TREATING DISTANCE (cm)					
	0.5	1.0	1.5	2.0	2.5	3.0		0.5	1.0	1.5	2.0	2.5	3.0
0	32	129	289	514	803	1157	36	603	949	1369	1769	2212	2702
1	73	185	353	585	874	1230	38	627	982	1413	1820	2268	2767
2	105	230	405	646	934	1293	40	651	1009	1453	1870	2324	2830
3	130	267	454	702	993	1353	42	674	1039	1495	1922	2379	2891
4	152	300	499	754	1048	1409	44	695	1069	1534	1971	2435	2952
5	174	330	540	801	1101	1465	46	718	1096	1573	2020	2489	3011
6	191	360	579	844	1151	1517	48	740	1126	1609	2068	2542	3070
7	207	388	614	885	1200	1570	50	761	1158	1644	2115	2594	3129
8	222	415	647	923	1247	1620	52	783	1186	1678	2003	2646	3186
9	239	441	677	960	1290	1668	54	803	1215	1715	2211	2700	3243
10	254	468	707	997	1334	1717	56	823	1244	1747	2259	2752	3299
11	268	492	737	1033	1375	1762	58	843	1271	1782	2308	2805	3354
12	282	518	767	1069	1417	1807	60	864	1302	1816	2354	2853	3413
13	296	542	745	1103	1456	1850	62	883	1328	1849	2400	2907	3469
14	311	566	825	1137	1497	1893	64	904	1361	1879	2443	2955	3522
15	326	590	852	1170	1537	1935	66	923	1388	1910	2486	3004	3575
16	340	611	879	1202	1577	1976	68	943	1418	1942	2592	3054	3629
17	354	632	915	1232	1611	2016	70	961	1447	1973	2570	3105	3683
18	369	653	932	1264	1647	2057	72	981	1476	2005	2614	3156	3737
19	383	673	957	1293	1681	2097	74	1001	1505	2038	2651	3205	3791
20	397	692	983	1323	1715	2137	76	1021	1535	2068	2689	3254	3845
22	424	728	1036	1382	1782	2213	78	1040	1562	2096	2729	3303	3897
24	450	763	1089	1442	1849	2286	80	1059	1591	2123	2767	3351	3949
26	477	796	1140	1499	1909	2363	84	1097	1646	2182	2840	3447	4055
28	503	828	1188	1553	1972	2434	88	1136	1698	2241	2914	3544	4157
30	529	859	1233	1606	2030	2506	92	1174	1750	2300	2986	3641	4258
32	554	889	1280	1660	2091	2570	96	1212	1801	2361	3054	3736	4356
34	580	922	1324	1714	2151	2637	100	1247	1853	2417	3121	3829	4450

**Modified for the 0.957 cGy/R and 1.015 correction for oblique filtration, attenuation, and effective attenuation coefficients for platinum, and using 8.25 R cm²/h/mCi such that "R" (cGy) = 8.4/8.25 × 8.4/8.25 × 1/1015 = 1.08. Filtration = 0.55-mm platinum.*

(Meredith WJ [ed]: Radium Dosage: The Manchester System, 2nd ed, pp 31–136. Baltimore, Williams & Wilkins, 1967. Modified with suggestions from Gibb R, Massey JB: Br J Radiol 53:1100, 1980)

but smaller than 100 cm^2, half of the activity is distributed on the periphery, and other half is in the center. Above 100 cm^2, one third of the activity goes on the periphery and two thirds in the center. Center sources are added parallel to one side, uniformly distributed about 1 cm apart. If a rectangle in which the longer side, b, is twice as long as the shorter side, a, the milligram hours required are increased by 5%, as shown in Table 12-10, under *elongation correction*; larger increases are required for more elongated rectangles.

Consider an idealized implant in a target volume 5 cm long by 4 cm wide by 1 cm thick, which can be uniformly dosed with a single plane implant.[97] Figure 12-11 shows the suggested source arrangement following Manchester distribution rules: Seven parallel sources separated by 1 cm and two crossing sources located just at the active end of the parallel source array. From the data in Table 12-8, for an area of 20 cm^2, 397 mgh is required to deliver 1000 cGy at 0.5 cm. Assuming therapy requires giving 6500 cGy in about 7 days, using sources with 0.5-mm Pt-Ir filtration requires

$$\frac{397 \text{ mgh}}{1000 \text{ cGy}} \times \frac{6500 \text{ cGy}}{7 \times 24 \text{ h}} = 15.4 \text{ mg Ra}$$

Two thirds of this activity (10.3 mg) occurs on the 18-cm-long periphery. Hence, sources with a linear activity of 0.57 mg Ra/cm are suggested. The 5.1 mg of radium in the center (4 cm × 4 cm) requires an activity of 0.32 mg Ra/cm. Actually, the standard sources available in England that would have been used in this implant consisted of B2 needles (2 mg of Ra, 3-cm active length, 4.2-cm physical length), B3 needles (3 mg of Ra, 4.5-cm active length, 5.8-cm total length), and A2 needles (1 mg of Ra, 3.0-cm active length, 4.2-cm physical length). The original example suggests that a B3 needle should be used on each long side, a B2 on each short side, and five A2 needles in the center (Fig. 12-11).[97] A total of 15 mg (2 × 3 mg + 2 × 2 mg + 5 × 1 mg) would be implanted as shown, with a dose rate of 6500 cGy delivered in 163.6 hours (40 cGy/h). A permanent inventory of sources of different physical lengths and active lengths designed to implement these rules was available.[97]

Two planes are required to uniformly dose slabs more than 1.5 cm but less than 2.5 cm thick, with the effective minimum dose stated midway between the planes. The tabular activity obtained from the area must be increased 25%, 40%, and 50%, respectively, for plane separations of 1.5 cm, 2.0 cm, and 2.5 cm.[48]

In the United States, these sources of 0.66 mg Ra/cm and 0.33 mg Ra/cm were not available. Quimby,[124] who had previously developed ^{226}Ra-source "away and along" dose tables useful to U.S. radiation therapists, investigated the dose gradients produced when only one linear activity source of a greater intensity (1.0 mg Ra/cm) than that used in the Manchester system was used in implants.[122] She believed that 5000 R to 6000 R over 3 to 4 days (60–70 R/h) might be biologically equivalent to the Manchester dose schedule (Table 12-10). In 1952, Quimby and Castro concluded that 1.0 mg Ra/cm sources yielded too high a dose rate and that implants of 6000 R in 3 to 4 days could only be achieved with 0.50 mg Ra/cm.[122] Ultimately radium sources of 0.66, 0.33, 0.165, 0.50, and 0.25 mg Ra/cm became available to radiation therapists in the United States. Table 12-11 is a Quimby table for planar implants with corrections for modern dosimetry concepts, and Figure 12-12 shows the source array for the previous example.[46] For an area of 4 cm × 5 cm (20 cm^2), we interpolated linearly from the table, using the area and obtaining 255 mgh per 1000 cGy. To deliver an

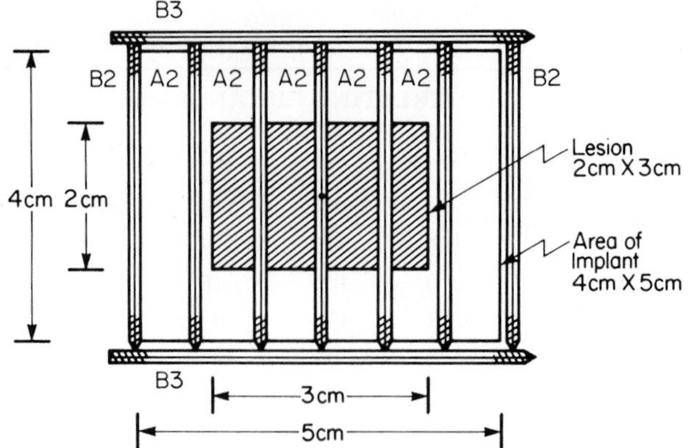

FIGURE 12–11. A Manchester-style interstitial single-plane implant of a target 1 cm thick, 5 cm long, and 4 cm wide. A2, B2, and B3 denote the types of radium needles used. The inactive tips and ends of the needles are denoted by crosshatching.

TABLE 12–9
Milligram Hours per 1000 cGy for Various Active Lengths and Treating Distances (Manchester System)

ACTIVE LENGTH (cm)*	TREATING DISTANCE (cm)						
	0.5	0.75	1.0	1.5	2.0	2.5	3.0
FILTRATION = 0.5-mm PLATINUM							
0.0	32	71	129	289	514	804	1157
0.5	36	76	131	294	516	807	1159
1.0	41	83	137	299	523	813	1169
1.5	51	93	149	310	538	825	1183
2.0	59	106	165	325	554	842	1203
2.5	69	121	181	346	578	864	1228
3.0	80	135	199	370	603	890	1256
3.5	91	151	219	397	630	921	1287
4.0	102	165	238	423	660	957	1320
4.5	113	183	258	450	693	995	1358
5.0	125	198	280	478	729	1034	1398
5.5	137	216	300	508	765	1084	1442
6.0	149	231	321	538	801	1118	1488
6.5	160	248	342	568	839	1162	1538
7.0	172	264	364	597	877	1207	1588
7.5	184	280	387	630	918	1253	1639
8.0	194	296	410	661	958	1300	1693
8.5	205	313	432	693	998	1348	1747
9.0	216	332	455	725	1040	1395	1803
9.5	228	348	477	758	1082	1445	1858
10.0	239	364	500	789	1125	1495	1916
11.0	261	400	544	855	1207	1595	2034
12.0	284	433	590	921	1292	1699	2154
13.0	308	468	635	987	1377	1804	2276
14.0	330	503	681	1054	1463	1911	2398
15.0	353	539	727	1120	1552	2020	2522
16.0	377	575	772	1188	1639	2128	2648
17.0	402	608	820	1255	1729	2235	2773
18.0	426	644	866	1322	1818	2344	2902
19.0	447	680	912	1391	1907	2453	3034
20.0	472	715	958	1460	1997	2561	3164

(continued)

TABLE 12–9
(Continued)

ACTIVE LENGTH (cm)*	TREATING DISTANCE (cm)						
	0.5	0.75	1.0	1.5	2.0	2.5	3.0
FILTRATION = 1.0-mm PLATINUM							
0.0	36	80	143	322	570	891	1283
0.5	42	84	146	326	576	895	1286
1.0	51	92	154	335	584	903	1296
1.5	59	105	168	346	598	917	1312
2.0	70	121	186	367	618	936	1333
2.5	81	138	205	390	643	964	1361
3.0	94	154	228	417	672	998	1393
3.5	108	174	251	448	706	1035	1430
4.0	121	191	274	478	743	1075	1472
4.5	134	210	299	512	781	1117	1517
5.0	148	230	324	544	824	1163	1568
5.5	162	249	349	580	866	1210	1620
6.0	175	269	375	616	912	1260	1676
6.5	188	288	400	652	957	1313	1734
7.0	202	309	427	689	1004	1367	1795
7.5	216	329	449	726	1051	1425	1857
8.0	230	351	480	766	1101	1481	1918
8.5	244	372	507	804	1148	1537	1982
9.0	257	393	535	842	1199	1597	2046
9.5	272	414	562	882	1247	1656	2111
10.0	286	434	590	921	1296	1716	2182
11.0	315	476	644	1001	1399	1836	2322
12.0	342	518	699	1081	1501	1961	2468
13.0	370	559	755	1161	1604	2088	2615
14.0	400	603	810	1243	1709	2214	2765
15.0	427	646	865	1324	1814	2343	2916
16.0	456	688	922	1406	1922	2472	3067
17.0	484	730	978	1490	2029	2603	3222
18.0	513	773	1035	1572	2136	2732	3376
19.0	542	815	1090	1656	2244	2865	3532
20.0	570	859	1145	1739	2352	2998	3688

**Modified for the 0.957 cGy/R and 1.015 correction for oblique filtration, attenuation, and effective attenuation coefficients for platinum, and using 8.25 R cm²/h/mCi such that R (cGy) = 8.4/8.25 × 1/0.957 × 1.015 = 1.08.*
(Meredith WJ [ed]: Radium Dosage: The Manchester System, 2nd ed, pp 135–136. Baltimore, Williams & Wilkins, 1967. Modified with suggestions from Gibb R, Massey JB: Br J Radiol 53:1100, 1980)

assumed (by us) biologically equivalent dose of 5500 cGy in 72 hours would require

$$\frac{255 \text{ mgh}}{1000 \text{ cGy}} \times \frac{5500 \text{ cGy}}{72 \text{ h}} = 19.5 \text{ mg Ra}$$

or, about 20 mg of radium using radium sources with only 0.50 mg Ra/cm and with the commonly available physical lengths of 58 mm and 45 mm, with the 45-mm and 35-mm active lengths, respectively. The implant would appear (Fig. 12-12) similar to the Manchester array, except that all of the sources have the same linear activity of 0.5 mg/cm. The sources would contain 16.8 mg of radium and deliver 5500 cGy on the perpendicular bisector to the implant plane in 84 hours at 65 cGy/h. In the Quimby system for planar implants, the dose is the maximum dose that occurs in the implant plane at the selected distance, b, from the sources.

For volume implants, the dose prescription point in the Quimby system is at the periphery of the implanted region. Although the Quimby tables have been included here for completeness, Shalek and Stovall[138] and Anderson[5] have warned that the tables may contain some original errors and they should be used with caution.

The Paris System was developed for linear iridium wire sources.[116] Iridium wire, technically an unsealed source, has been used in the United States only at medical training facilities possessing a broad-form U.S. Nuclear Regulatory Commission license. In France, ^{192}Ir wire and pins have been the materials of choice for interstitial implants. The Paris System allows a source implant pattern and subsequent dose distributions that can be adjusted as target dimensions change. Table 12-10 summarizes the cogent features of the system, and Figure 12-13 defines the dosimetry parameters. Gooden presents an excellent review.[48]

Uniform linear activity sources are implanted parallel to one another. The separation between the sources is determined by the dimensions of the implant. Crossing sources are not

TABLE 12–10
Features of Three Dose Distributions Systems for Linear Sources

FEATURE	PATERSON AND PARKER (MANCHESTER)	QUIMBY	PARIS
Dose and dose rate	6000 to 8000 R in 6 to 8 days (1000 R/d; 40 R/h)	5000 to 6000 R in 3 to 4 days (60 to 70 R/h is expected to be biologically equivalent to Manchester system)	6000 to 7000 cGy in 3 to 11 days (25 to 90 cGy/h); usually in 3 to 6 days
Dose prescription points	Effective minimum dose is 10% above the absolute minimum dose in a plane or volume	For planar implants, it is on the perpendicular bisector to the plane; for volume implants, it is to the periphery point receiving a minimum dose; minimum is the actual implanted region	Basal dose is the average of the minimum doses in the central plane in the region defined by the source; reference dose is 85% of the basal dose and encompasses the target plane, or volume
Dose gradient	Does not vary by more than ±10%, except for localized hot spots around the source for single-plane implants; for double-plane implants, gradients increased to 20% to 30%, depending on plane separation; separation factors required to select proper mgh from tables	No stated goal; the intent was to determine the increased dose gradients resulting from using sources with the same linear activity; gradient frequently approaches 100% with twice the dose in the center as at the edge of the region	15% between reference dose and basal dose (average minimum) by definition
Linear activity	Variable (0.66 mg Ra/cm, 0.50 mg Ra/cm, 0.33 mg Ra/cm)	Constant (1.0 mg Ra/cm used historically; 0.20 to 0.70 mg Ra eq/cm commonly used.)	Constant (1.8 to 0.6 mg Ra eq/cm commonly used)
Activity distribution: single plane	For areas less than 25 cm^2, $\frac{2}{3}$ activity on periphery, $\frac{1}{3}$ activity in center; for areas less than 100 cm^2, $\frac{1}{2}$ activity in center; for areas greater than 100 cm^2, $\frac{2}{3}$ activity in center, $\frac{1}{3}$ on periphery	Uniform distribution over implant plane	Uniform distribution over implant plane
Activity distribution: volume	Cylinder: 4/8 of the activity in the belt 2/8 of the activity in the core 1/8 of the activity on each end Sphere: 6/8 of the activity in the belt 2/8 of the activity in the core Cube: 1/8 of the activity in each face 2/8 of the activity in the core	Uniform distribution of activity through the volume	For volume, the sources are arranged in planes such that the sources in adjacent planes from either equilateral triangles or squares; spacing between planes is about 0.87 times spacing between sources for equivalent triangles
Source implant pattern and spacing between sources as a function of implant volume	Constant uniform spacing; 1-cm separation between sources recommended	Variable but uniform spacing with up to 2-cm separation allowed between sources; spacing between sources determined by implant target dimensions	Variable but uniform spacing; spacing determined by implant target dimensions; larger source separation in larger volume; 5-mm minimum to 20-mm maximum separation
Crossing needles	Perpendicular to and at the active ends of the plane of sources; if placed beyond the active ends of the needles, should be double strength; crossing needles required; if one end uncrossed, then area of implant for calculation is decreased 10%; 20% area reduction correction (10% each end) for both ends uncrossed	Same as Paterson and Parker	Not used; active sources are 20% to 30% longer than the target volume at *both* ends to compensate for uncrossed ends
Elongation correction factors	Area: Long side/short side ratio and % correction: 2/1(+5%); 3/1(+9%); 4/1(+12%) Volume: Length/diameter ratio and % correction: 1.5/1(+3%); 2/1(+6%); 2.5/1(+10%); 3/1(+15%)	Same as Paterson and Parker	Not used
Relation of source length to target (volume) length	Active length determines target length (or *vise versa*); inner needles (not periphery) determine target width	Same as Paterson and Parker	Active source lengths 20% to 30% longer than the target dimensions at both ends to compensate for uncrossed ends

TABLE 12–11
Milligram Hours Required for an Absorbed Dose of 1000 cGy at Locations Along a Line Perpendicular to the Center of the Applicator or Implant Plane in the Quimby System

Circular Appplicators

DISTANCE (cm)	DIAMETER (cm) 1	2	3	4	5	6
0.5	47	80	110	181	234	319
1.0	145	187	234	319	394	482
1.5	301	345	426	506	598	725
2.0	528	577	646	745	846	977
2.5	782	846	920	1016	1229	1346
3.0	1160	1224	1298	1404	1522	1665

Square Applicators

DISTANCE (cm)	LENGTH OF SIDE (cm) 1	2	3	4	5	6
0.5	49	85	122	210	266	372
1.0	150	200	253	348	431	544
1.5	314	367	442	544	638	782
2.0	532	606	686	795	910	1064
2.5	777	846	952	1075	1213	1458
3.0	1160	1224	1351	1479	1617	1777

Rectangular Applicators

DISTANCE (cm)	DIMENSIONS (cm) 1 × 1.5	2 × 3	3 × 4	4 × 6	6 × 9	8 × 12
0.5	54	110	152	305	606	1016
1.0	157	228	291	453	772	1181
1.5	317	394	496	664	1005	1442
2.0	538	628	761	930	1319	1777
2.5	767	894	1053	1213	1617	2128
3.0	1181	1266	1420	1617	2054	2660

Modified by dividing the original tables by the 0.957 cGy/R factor for muscle and by the ratio of 8.25 to 8.4 to correct for the use of the original specific γ-ray constant for ^{226}Ra. The 0.5-mm Pt (Ir)-radium sources are distributed uniformly across the plane.
(Modified from Glasser O, Quimby EH, Taylor LS, et al: Physical Foundations of Radiology, 2nd ed. New York, Paul B Hoeber, 1952)

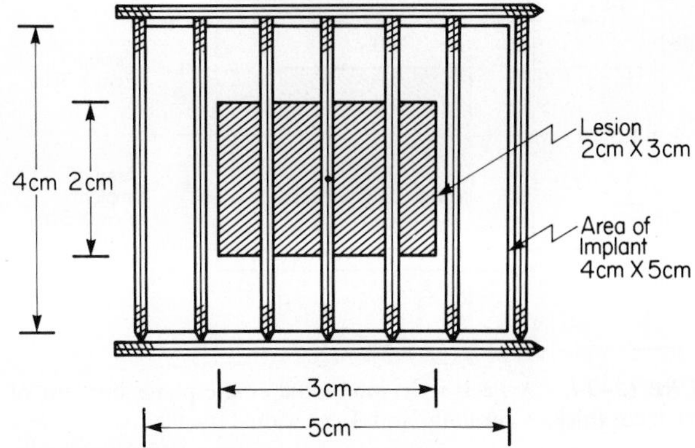

FIGURE 12–12. A Quimby-style interstitial single-plane implant of a target 1 cm thick, 5 cm long, and 4 cm wide. Inactive tips and ends are denoted by crosshatching.

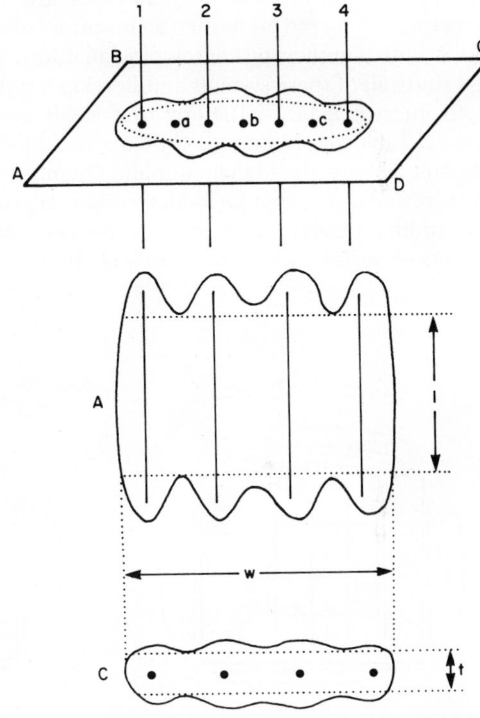

FIGURE 12–13. Some definitions used in the Paris System of interstitial implant. Four lines (1,2,3,4) transect the central plane (A,B,C,D), for which the dose calculation is carried out. The basal dose rate (BD) is the mean of the dose rates at A,B, and C, midway between the sources. The reference dose rate (0.85 BD) has an irregular contour (*wavy line*) and totally encloses the target volume. The length (l) of the treatment volume is the separation between the minimum indentations in the reference isodose curves; the width (w) is determined by the maximum extent of the reference dose rate curve. The reference dose rate and length and width are specified in the plane containing the sources.

allowed, but the active lengths of the implanted sources extend well beyond the implant dimensions. Figure 12-14 shows the Paris System distribution used for a 20-cm^2 single-plane implant.[40] Only three sources are required, with an active length of 7 cm, with 1 cm of the active length extending beyond the implanted dimension. The sources are spaced about 1.7 cm apart. The dose rate depends on the linear activity of the wire selected. If each wire contained 8 mCi, the 24-mCi total content would correspond to 14 mg of Ra, using the 1.71-mCi/mg Ra conversion factor commonly used by the vendor of the wire. This wire would have a uniform linear intensity of 0.67 mg Ra/cm. The *basal dose rate* would be 38 cGy/h, and the *reference dose rate* would be 32 cGy/h in the plane containing the sources. To deliver 5500 cGy to the reference dose rate line would require 203 hours, almost 8.5 days.

For equal implanted activities, the Paris System yields a lower reference dose rate and requires longer treatment times than does the Manchester System. Figure 12-15 shows the dose distributions achieved with the Manchester, Quimby, and Paris Systems in a plane that is 0.5 cm from the radioactive sources. Gillin and associates[40] provide additional comparisons of the Manchester and Paris dosimetry systems.

The ^{137}Cs needles that are substitutes for radium needles

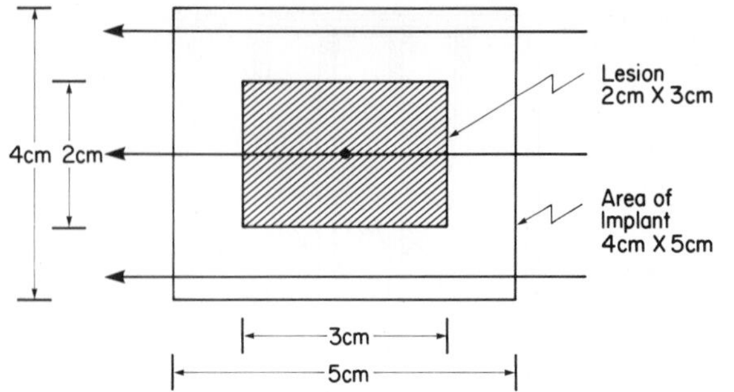

FIGURE 12–14. A Paris-style interstitial single-plane implant of a target 1 cm thick, 5 cm long, and 4 cm wide.

are now generally available only in 0.66 and 0.33 mg Ra/cm activities. Moreover, ^{192}Ir wire and seeds that allow afterloading of the sources are often used even when an inventory of needles is available. A radiation therapist developing an interstitial service should study all of these systems and develop a systematic approach to interstitial brachytherapy that yields consistent clinical results. Tables 12-12 and 12-13, based on the original volume implant tables in the Manchester and Quimby systems, have been corrected to incorporate modern dosimetry concepts and understanding. Readers are referred to the original works for full details of various volumetric implants in each of the systems.[97, 122]

CURRENT DOSE PRESCRIPTION AND DISTRIBUTION RULES

Iridium Seeds

The ^{192}Ir seeds for permanent and temporary interstitial implants were developed at Memorial Sloan-Kettering Cancer Center as a radon seed substitute; iridium wire was used in England and Europe, where ^{222}Rn seeds were not popular. Anderson[7] presents an excellent review of ^{192}Ir dosimetry, and the *Atlas of Brachytherapy* explains current techniques and dosimetry.[61]

Iridium seeds are usually treated as point sources; the dose distribution is described by the inverse square law because attenuation and multiple scattering are compensating effects in tissue for several centimeters from the sources (Fig. 12-4). Shalek and colleagues[139] observed that a regular array of iridium seeds of the same activity in volumes greater than 100 cm^3 yields doses within 5% of those calculated using Manchester dose volume tables; for smaller volumes, greater differences exist between the two systems. Laughlin and co-workers[80] defined the *minimum peripheral dose* and the *maximum reference dose* in a volume implant achieved with a cubic array of seeds (Fig. 12-16). Tables 12-14 and 12-15 list the values for planar and volume implants. For a given geometric array of seeds, the Manchester planar implant tables yield doses that fall between the maximum and minimum doses from Laughlin's tables for uniformly spaced seeds.[80]

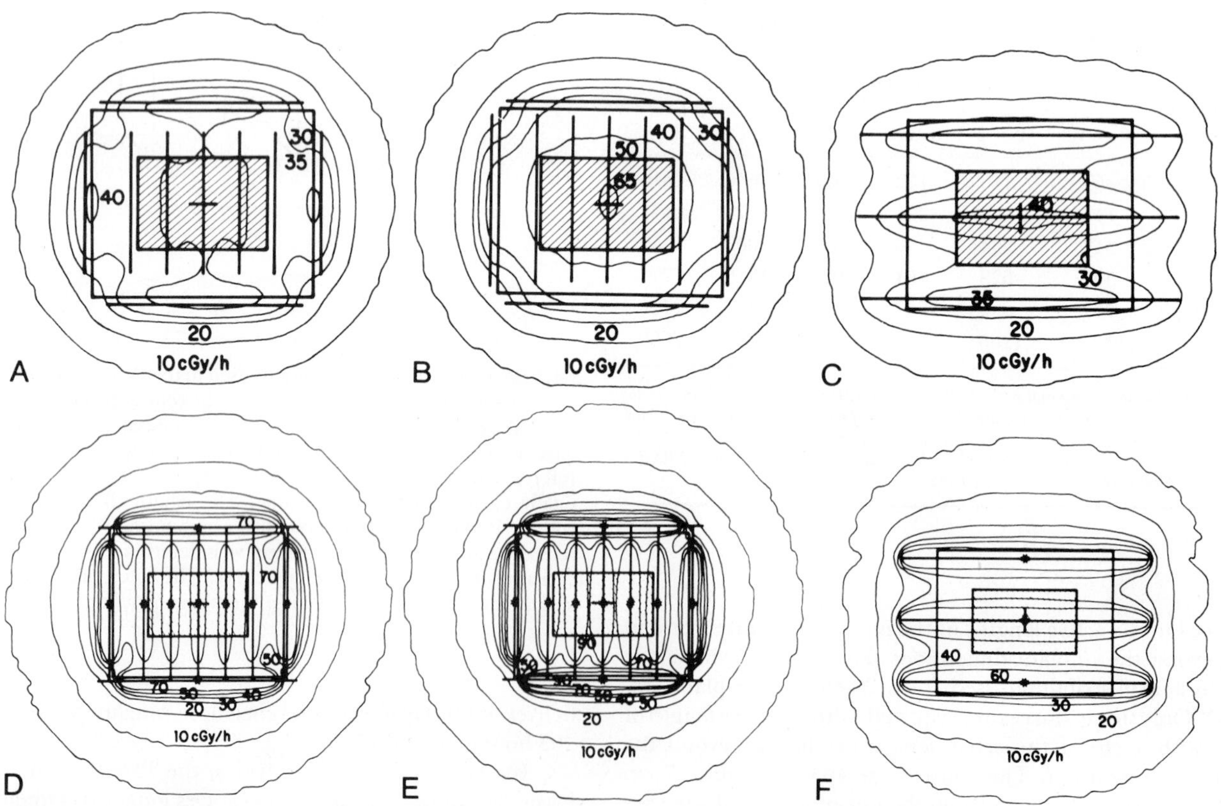

FIGURE 12–15. Computer-generated dose distribution achieved with Manchester (**A, D**), Quimby (**B, E**), and Paris (**C, F**) distribution rules for planar implant of a target 1 cm thick, 5 cm long, and 4 cm wide. The dose distributions are shown in planes parallel to the sources and 0.5 cm away from the sources (**A, B, C**) and in the plane containing the source (**D, E, F**). (**A**) The effective minimum dose ranges between 35 cGy/hour and 40 cGy/hour over most of the implanted area. (**B**) A large dose gradient exists over the implanted area, with dose rates ranging from 65 cGy/hour at the center to about 40 cGy/hour on the perimeter. (**C**) The reference dose rate of 32 cGy/hour is shown approximately by the line 30 at cGy/hour.

TABLE 12–12
Milligram Hours Required for an Absorbed Dose of 1000 cGy Throughout a Volume Implant in the Manchester System

VOLUME (cm^3)	mgh/1000 cGy (0.5 mm Pt [Ir])	LENGTH/ DIAMETER	ELONGATION FACTOR
1	36.8	1.5/1	+3%
3	76.6	2.0/1	+6%
5	107.7	2.5/1	+10%
10	171.0	3.0/1	+15%
15	223.6		
20	271.1		
30	355.3		
40	430.9		
50	500.0		
60	564.8		
80	683.6		
100	793.8		
140	993.6		
180	1174.0		
220	1342.4		
260	1501.2		
300	1651.3		

Modified for the 0.957 cGy/R, and 1.015 correction for oblique filtration, attenuation, and effective attenuation coefficients for platinum, and using 8.25 R cm^2/h/mCi, such that R (cGy) = 8.4/8.25 × 1/0.957 × 1.015 = 1.08.
(Meredith WJ [ed]: Radium Dosage: The Manchester System, 2nd ed, pp 135–136. Baltimore, Williams & Wilkins, 1967. Modified with suggestions from Gibb R, Massey JB: Br J Radiol 53:1100, 1980)

TABLE 12–13
Milligram Hours Required for a Minimum Absorbed Dose of 1000 cGy in a Volume Implant in the Quimby System

VOLUME (cm^3)	mgh/1000 cGy	DIAMETER OF SPHERE (cm)	mgh/1000 cGy
5	213	1.0	43
10	340	1.5	106
15	415	2.0	192
20	468	2.5	298
30	575	3.0	415
40	660	3.5	505
60	798	4.0	612
80	926	4.5	718
100	1064	5.0	841
125	1192	6.0	1138
150	1330	7.0	1490
175	1479		
200	1596		
250	1788		
300	1915		

Modified by dividing the original tables by the 0.957 cGy/R factor for muscle and by the ratio of 8.25 to 8.4 to correct for the use of the original specific γ-ray constant for ^{226}Ra. The 0.5-mm Pt (Ir)-radium sources are distributed uniformly across the plane.
(Modified from Glasser O, Quimby EH, Taylor LS, et al: Physical Foundations of Radiology, 2nd ed. New York, Paul B Hoeber, 1952)

Anderson[7] has developed single- and double-plane nomograms (Fig. 12-17) to allow rapid calculation in the operation room of the number of seeds required to yield a dose rate of approximately 1000 cGy/day to a peripheral reference point (Fig. 12-18). Murphy and associates[102] published nomograms for single-plane implants. Actual implants exhibit geometric irregularities, such as nonuniform needle spacing and curvature along the ribbon containing the seeds. Rosen and coworkers[130], after investigating the dose variations produced by these irregularities and by localization errors, concluded that the peripheral target dose would be accurate to within 5% if all seeds were reconstructed to be within 0.5 mm of their true position.

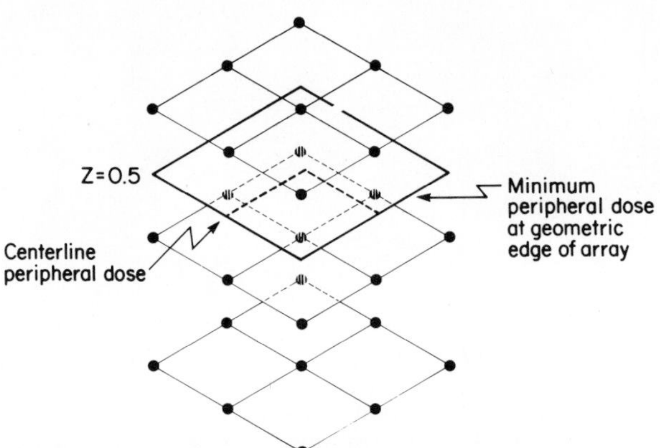

FIGURE 12–16. Minimum peripheral and maximum reference dose points for a cubic array of seeds. (Laughlin JS, Siler MN, Holodny EI, et al: Am J Roentgenol Radiat Ther Nucl Med 89:470, 1963 © by American Roentgen Ray Society)

It is instructive to compare the dosimetry of seed implants for the previous example of the 4-cm × 5-cm × 1-cm planar implant. The Manchester table (Table 12-8) for 20 cm^2 yields 397 mgh.

$$\frac{397 \text{ mgh}}{1000 \text{ cGy}} \times \frac{6500 \text{ cGy}}{168 \text{ h}} = 15.4 \text{ mg}$$

Assuming that iridium seeds of 0.5 mg Ra eq and 0.3 mg Ra eq are available in ribbons with seeds spaced 1 cm apart, the implant requires 30 seeds; about 18 seeds of 0.5 mg Ra eq should be on the periphery; the remaining 12, each with activity of 0.3 mg Ra eq, go in the center. The array in Figure 12-18 is a possible solution using 30 seeds. Using Laughlin's method and Table 12-14, the 6500 cGy prescribed to the minimum peripheral point requires 488 mgh, compared with the 397 mgh from Table 12-9:

$$\frac{488 \text{ mgh}}{1000 \text{ cGy}} \times \frac{6500 \text{ cGy}}{168 \text{ h}} = 19 \text{ mg}$$

Thirty seeds could be implanted as previously shown, but with an activity of 0.63 mg Ra per seed. Some of the difference in the results of the Manchester system arises from the prescription point, for which the net minimum dose is 10% higher than the absolute minimum dose given by definition.

Using the more recent nomogram of Anderson (Fig. 12-17) and 0.5 mg Ra eq seeds yields seven ribbons, which would be implanted as shown in Figure 12-19, with the 6500 cGy peripheral dose point defined at the corner of the implant volume in the plane, 0.5 cm from the source plane, at a point 1.5 spacing units (1.5 cm) inward along the ribbon direction from an end

TABLE 12–14
Planar Implants: Milligram Hours to Deliver 1000 cGy at Designated Point Locations in the Laughlin System

AREA (cm^2)	DOSE AT POINT LOCATION* (mgh/1000 cGy) MINIMUM PERIPHERAL	REFERENCE MAXIMUM	RATIO OF MINIMUM PERIPHERAL TO REFERENCE MAXIMUM DOSE POINT LOCATIONS
1	95	84	1.13/1
2	116	94	1.23/1
3	138	107	1.29/1
4	165	124	1.333/1
5	189	138	1.367/1
6	211	152	1.39/1
7	236	166	1.42/1
8	256	178	1.44/1
9	280	193	1.45/1
10	300	204	1.47/1
12	342	228	1.50/1
14	380	250	1.52/1
16	419	272	1.54/1
18	454	291	1.56/1
20	488	311	1.57/1
25	570	354	1.61/1
30	650	399	1.63/1
35	734	442	1.66/1
40	812	485	1.675/1
45	892	528	1.69/1
50	973	569	1.71/1

**Dose points are defined in a plane 0.5 cm from plane of implant. The sources are assumed uniform in strength and located on a 1-cm grid.*
(Laughlin JS, Siler WM, Holodny EI, et al: Am J Roentgenol Radiat Ther Nucl Med 89:470, 1963 © by American Roentgen Ray Society)

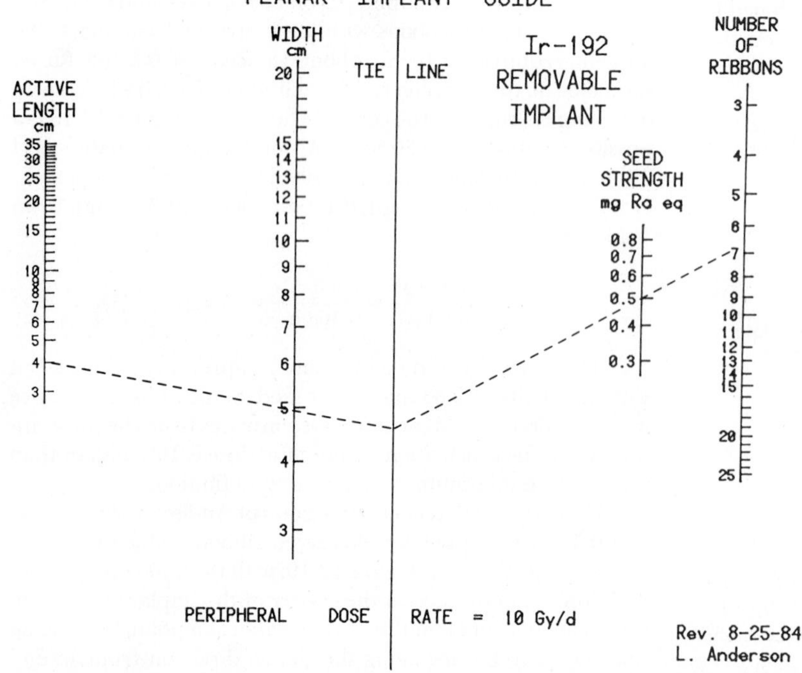

FIGURE 12–17. A nomogram for ^{192}Ir seed implants. For example, with an implant 4 cm long and 5 cm wide, a line is drawn as shown to the tie line, an intermediate variable in the calculation. A second line is drawn through the seed strength to obtain the number of ribbons to the nearest integer. (Anderson LL: Experiences with ^{192}Ir. In Wright AE, Boyer AL (eds): Advances in Radiation Therapy Treatment Planning. New York, American Institute of Physics, 1983)

TABLE 12–15
Volume Implants: Milligram Hours to Deliver 1000 cGy at Designated Point Locations in the Laughlin System

	DOSE AT POINT LOCATION* (mgh/1000 cGy)				
VOLUME (cm^3)	MINIMUM PERIPHERAL	CENTER LINE PERIPHERAL	REFERENCE MAXIMUM	RATIO OF MINIMUM PERIPHERAL TO REFERENCE MAXIMUM DOSE POINT LOCATIONS	RATIO OF CENTER LINE PERIPHERAL TO REFERENCE MAXIMUM DOSE POINT LOCATIONS
1	95	95	84	1.13/1	1.13/1
5	184	165	145	1.27/1	1.14/1
10	254	214	185	1.37/1	1.155/1
15	322	263	225	1.43/1	1.165/1
20	378	301	255	1.48/1	1.18/1
25	433	339	285	1.52/1	1.19/1
30	472	366	305	1.55/1	1.20/1
40	560	424	350	1.60/1	1.21/1
50	640	478	390	1.64/1	1.225/1
60	719	544	430	1.67/1	1.235/1
80	865	625	500	1.73/1	1.25/1
100	1000	715	565	1.77/1	1.265/1
120	1130	800	625	1.81/1	1.28/1
140	1240	875	680	1.83/1	1.285/1
160	1365	952	735	1.86/1	1.295/1
180	1475	1020	785	1.88/1	1.30/1
200	1575	1090	830	1.90/1	1.31/1
250	1840	1250	945	1.95/1	1.32/1
300	2080	1400	1050	1.98/1	1.335/1
350	2310	1550	1155	2.00/1	1.34/1
400	2540	1690	1255	2.20/1	1.35/1

** The sources are assumed uniform in strength and located on a 1-cm grid.*
(Laughlin JS, Siler WM, Holodny EI, et al: Am J Roentgenol Radiat Ther Nucl Med 89:470, 1963 © by American Roentgen Ray Society)

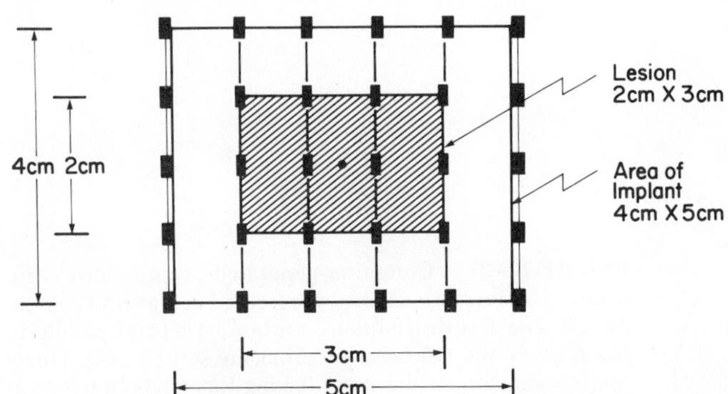

FIGURE 12–18. A 30-seed array for interstitial implant of a 1-cm thick, 5-cm long, and 4-cm wide block of tissue, following Manchester System rules or using planar implant tables of Laughlin and co-workers. (Laughlin JS, Siler WM, Holodny EI, et al: Am J Roentgenol Radiat Ther Nucl Med 89:470, 1963 © by American Roentgen Ray Society)

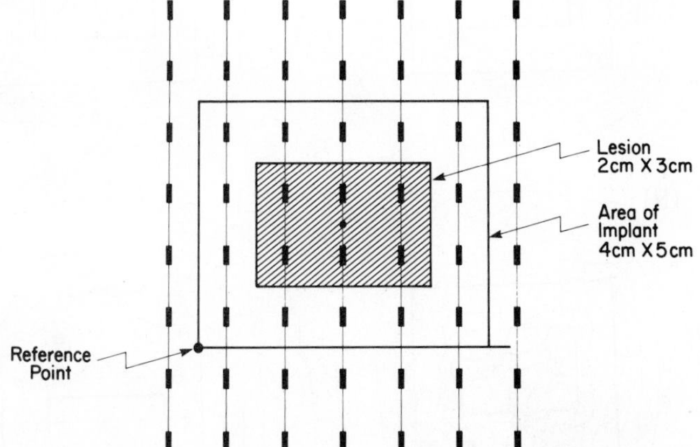

FIGURE 12–19. A 56-seed array for interstitially implanting a 1-cm × 5-cm × 4-cm target, following Memorial Sloan-Kettering (Anderson's) system rules. The reference point is defined as a "peripheral" point 1.5 spaces inward from the end sources and 0.5 spaces inward from the edge of the ribbon; a space is the separation, outer to center, between two seeds along a ribbon.

source and 0.5 cm spacing units inward transversely from the edge ribbon.[7] Using 0.5 mg Ra per seed, the 56 seeds would have a total activity of 28 mg of radium.

The planar implant tables of the Manchester system and Laughlin and associates and the nomograms of Anderson are based on the concept of a minimum dose at some well-defined point on or near the geometric periphery. Quimby's planar implant table, on the other hand, specifies the dose at specific distances perpendicular to the center of the implant plane.

Using the Quimby table for the same dose prescription of 6500 cGy in 7 days yields

$$\frac{255 \text{ mgh}}{1000 \text{ cGy}} \times \frac{6500 \text{ cGy}}{168 \text{ h}} = 9.9 \simeq 10 \text{ mg}$$

If 0.5-cm seeds were available, only 20 seeds would be

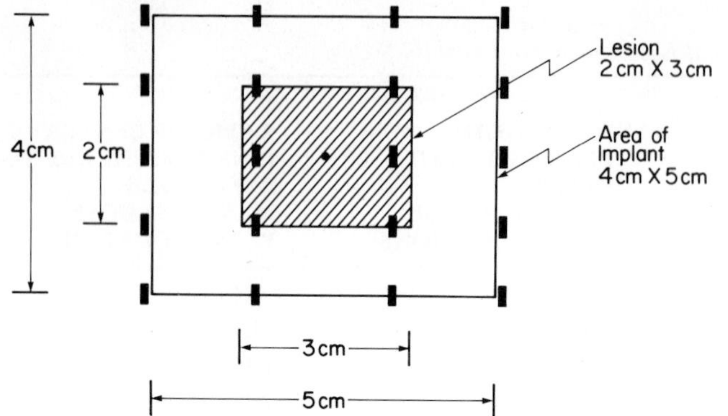

FIGURE 12–20. A 20-seed array for interstitial implant of a 1-cm × 5-cm × 4-cm target, following Quimby rules for planar implant. This spacing was arbitrarily selected because the rules require only a uniform spacing over the lesion. The 30-seed array in Figure 12–18 also satisfies the rules.

required, and they could be spaced as shown in Figure 12-20, actually using 21 seeds for symmetry. The dose at the periphery is not stated in Quimby planar implant tables. Figure 12-21 compares the isodose curves for these three arrays of seed implants. Dosimetry from the Paris System is not included because it applies to linear sources. The equivalency of a strand of ^{192}Ir seeds as a substitute for ^{192}Ir wire has been investigated by Williamson[163] and Marinello and associates,[91] who advised against using the "Paris System" rules with seeds.

Numerous recent publications have offered refinements or have further elucidated implant dosimetry, emphasizing methods to improve or report dose uniformity.[113,132] For example, Kwan and associates suggested that a 1.5-cm spacing between both the seeds and the planes was best for a double-plane implant.[79] In using any of the established dosimetry tables or more recent dosimetry systems, it is imperative that the radiation therapist have a clear understanding of the *points of dose prescription* and the *dose variations* likely to be produced within the target plane or volume by use of a system, particularly when comparing the dosimetries produced by different methods.

Iodine 125 Seeds

Iodine 125 seeds were developed at Memorial Sloan-Kettering Cancer Center as a radon substitute for permanent implants.[60] Some radiologists have used these for temporary implants.[23,82] With their low energy (< 0.035 MeV), they are easily shielded; radiation exposure to personnel is reduced dramatically. The Memorial clinical dosimetry system appears in many articles, and those unfamiliar with its evolution must pay careful attention because it has been modified several times.[6,8,52,61]

The original *dimension-averaging method* involved implanting a number of millicuries of ^{125}I seeds numerically equal to five times the average of the three perpendicular measured dimensions of the target volume to be implanted. As explained by Anderson and co-workers, "The dose would vary approximately as the negative one sixth power of volume [$V^{-1/6}$] since classical activity per unit dose is roughly proportional to the

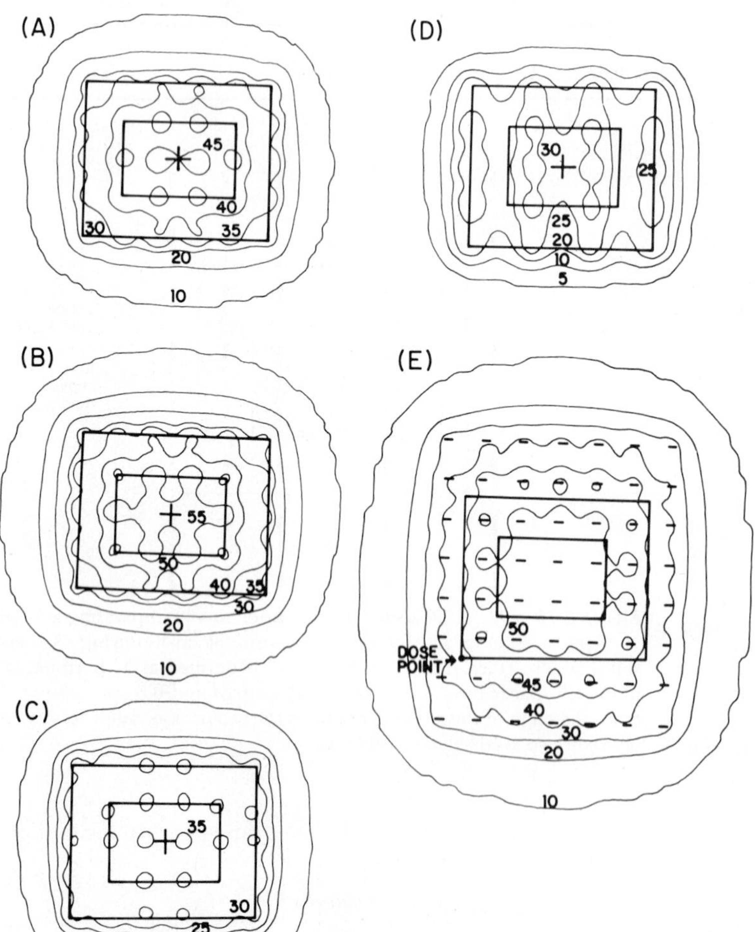

FIGURE 12–21. Computer-generated comparative isodose curves for the seed arrays presented in Figures 12–18 to 12–20. The dose distributions are shown in a plane parallel to the sources and 0.5 cm away from the sources. (**A**) Thirty seeds, each with an activity of 0.5 mg Ra eq (about 0.9 mCi) and uniformly distributed, yield a minimum peripheral dose rate of about 35 cGy/hour and a higher dose rate of 45 cGy/hour near the center, with 15 mg Ra eq of total activity. (**B**) Thirty seeds of 0.63 mg Ra eq each, with a total of 19 mg Ra eq, yield a minimum peripheral dose rate of about 40 cGy/hour, consistent with the values in Table 12–14 and over 10% greater than in (**A**). (**C**) To achieve the net minimum dose variation of ± 10% in the Manchester System, the activity of the inner 12 seeds has been reduced to 0,33 mg Ra eq per seed, with 4 mg Ra eq of total activity. The 18 seeds on the perimeter have a total activity of 9 mg Ra eq, so that about 30% of the activity is in the center, consistent with the Manchester System rules. This is difficult to implement clinically. (**D**) Twenty seeds of 0,50 mg Ra eq each, with an activity of 10 mg Ra eq yield between 25 and 30 cGy/hour, which is consistent with the values calculated from Table 12–11. (**E**) Fifty-six seeds of 0.50 mg Ra eq each, with a total activity of 28 mg Ra eq, yield 40 to 45 cGy/hour (about 1000 cGy/day) as desired by Memorial Sloan-Kettering distribution rules.

TABLE 12–16
Activity of ^{125}I Seed Implantation Correlated with Average Tumor Dimension

AVERAGE TUMOR DIMENSION (d_a)* (cm)	ACTIVITY REQUIRED (mCi compensated)
≤2.4	5 d_a
≤3.24	3.87 $d_a^{1.293}$
>3.24	2.76 $d_a^{1.581}$

* $d_a = \left(\frac{A + B + C}{3}\right)$ *cm, where A, B, and C are the three mutually perpendicular dimensions of the tumor.*
(Anderson LL, Kuan HM, Ding IY: Clinical dosimetry with I-125. In George FW [ed]: Modern Interstitial and Intracavitary Radiation Cancer Management. New York, Masson Publishing, 1981)

square root of the volume and the average dimension is roughly proportional to the cube root volume."[8] However, it was observed that the peripheral implant dose fell off more rapidly than $V^{-1/6}$ because of the lower energy of the ^{125}I seeds than the radon seeds for which they were substituted. The modified relationship shown in Table 12-16 was introduced in 1977 to adjust the implanted activity to the volume. A nomogram was developed for these equations.[6] Since July 1978, the specific dose rate factors listed in Table 12-17 have been used to describe the dose distribution around a source. More recently, the treatment area has been arbitrarily increased 1 cm in each direction after the initial measurements of the area to be implanted are made. This larger average dimension is used to select the total recommended activity and number of seeds, while the original 1-cm average dimension is used on the right-hand side of the nomogram to obtain the spacing information. We refer the reader to the articles that describe the original and modified clinical dosimetry and nomographs.[6,8,61,83,120]

Several excellent articles report the calculation of the

TABLE 12–17
Specific Dose Rate Factor for ^{125}I Seeds

DISTANCE FROM SOURCE (cm)	Λ (cGy/cm²/mCih)*
0.057	1.10
0.5	1.11
1.0	1.10
1.5	1.04
2.0	0.95
2.5	0.86
3.0	0.77
4.0	0.59
5.0	0.44
6.0	0.33
7.0	0.24
8.0	0.18
10.0	0.10
12.0	0.057

**Specific dose rate $\Lambda = D/GA$, where D is the dose rate, A is the activity, and G is the geometric attenuation factor ($1/l^2$ for point sources, if l is distance from the source).*
(Anderson LL, Kuan HM, Ding IY: Clinical dosimetry with I-125. In George FW [ed]: Modern Interstitial and Intracavitary Radiation Cancer Management. New York, Masson Publishing, 1981)

dose distribution around ^{125}I seeds by Monte Carlo techniques[17,78,134,162,165] and Wu and colleagues' analysis following Manchester System definitions using net minimum doses.[167] Wu stresses that the shape of the implant volume is an important factor in determining total implant activity, a point originally made by Anderson[6] when he developed the ^{125}I nomogram based on an average elliptic elongation, $\epsilon = 1.5$. Tables 12-18 and 12-19 emphasize the variation in activity and seed strength with implant volume. Based on animal tumor studies, it is believed that the relative biologic effectiveness of ^{125}I is greater than 1.0 and less than 1.5.[170]

UNIQUE BRACHYTHERAPY SOURCES

Ophthalmic Applicators

Ophthalmic applicators are used for treating choroidal melanoma and other intraocular lesions. In 1948, ^{60}Co eye plaques were developed at St. Bartholomew's Hospital. They replaced radon seed implants for treatment of eye lesions.[146] The disks and crescents were designed to the average radius of curvature of an infant's sclera (radius = 11 mm, diameter = 22 mm) to treat retinoblastoma, for which the height of the neo-

TABLE 12–18
Activity Required to Deliver a Net Minimum ^{125}I Dose of 1 Gy to Implants of Various Volumes

IMPLANT VOLUME (cm³)	ACTIVITY/UNIT DOSE (MBq/Gy)*
0.5-cm SPACING ALONG SEEDS	
10	1.628
20	2.85
30	3.85
40	4.81
50	5.74
60	6.59
80	8.21
100	9.73
150	13.10
200	16.43
250	19.80
300	23.16
1.0-cm SPACING ALONG SEEDS	
10	1.406
20	2.55
30	3.59
40	4.51
50	5.37
60	6.14
80	7.59
100	8.99
150	12.17
200	15.24
250	18.39
300	21.46

**Divide by 3.7 to convert to mCi/10 Gy.*
(Wu A, Zwicker RD, Sternick ES: Med Phys 12:27, 1985)

TABLE 12–19
Seed Strength Required to Deliver a Net Minimum ^{125}I Dose of 10 Gy to Implants of Various Volumes

IMPLANT VOLUME (cm^3)	SEED STRENGTH (MBq/10 Gy)
0.5-cm SPACING ALONG SEEDS	
10	0.763
20	0.668
30	0.601
40	0.563
50	0.538
60	0.515
80	0.481
100	0.456
150	0.409
200	0.385
250	0.371
300	0.362
1.0-cm SPACING ALONG SEEDS	
10	1.406
20	1.275
30	1.197
40	1.128
50	1.074
60	1.023
80	1.949
100	1.899
150	1.811
200	1.762
250	1.736
300	1.715

(Wu A, Zwicker RD, Sternick ES: Med Phys 12:27, 1985)

plasms was about two thirds of the diameter of the base. Each applicator has a design depth d = 1.5 + ⅔ diameter, where the average choroid thickness is 1.5 mm. The activity in each applicator was selected to give 4000 R in 6 days to the design depth. The plaques have a platinum casing 0.5 mm thick and a central well 0.3 mm deep, into which radioactive cobalt wire, in the form of concentric rings, is placed. Eleven different plaques of various dimensions are available.

These applicators were used to treat melanomas of the choroid in adults, delivering 7000 to 14,000 R at the design depth with high doses of 18,000 to 36,000 R at the surface of the plaque. For these lesions, the ratio of height to diameter was between one third and one half to one.[146]

Innes[65] first reported the design depths and activities of the ^{60}Co plaques in 1964. Subsequent articles by Mangus and colleagues,[86,87] Casebow,[20] and Chan and associates[21] contained additional dosimetry information. The calculated isodose curves (corrected to cGy) of Chan and associates[21] agreed with the isodose curves measured by Casebow.[20]

The ^{125}I seeds are now being used to construct individual eye plaques.[75,128,159] For distances from 1 to 20 mm, the dose distribution for a point source of ^{125}I is within 10% of the dose distribution from higher-energy isotopes. However, from about 2 cm and beyond, the dose fall-off is more rapid for high-energy isotopes, such as ^{60}Co, because the low-energy x-rays and τ-rays are attenuated more than the higher-energy τ-rays. The low energy (<35 keV) allows gold foil or stainless steel foil to be used at the plaque edge to shield adjacent structures (retina). Sealy and colleagues[136] describe individually designed ^{125}I applicators in detail. The relative biologic effectiveness of ^{125}I, possibly from 1.2 to 1.4 compared with 250-keV x-rays, may be important for a radioresistant tumor like melanoma.[89]

Standard-design ^{125}I eye plaques are available in five sizes.[75] The seed carrier, a medical-grade silicone rubber, holds seeds in preselected locations to yield desired shapes of dose distributions. The carriers fit into gold plaques of 12- to 18-mm diameters, with tabs to suture to the eye. A template aids in plaque placement. However, the seeds are expensive and have a short shelf life ($T_{1/2}$ of 60 days), there is the hazard of broken seeds and absorption of ^{125}I into the body, and those preparing the plaques receive some radiation exposure.

β-ray applicators employing ^{106}Ru or ^{106}Rh are predominantly used to treat shallow lesions, because the 50% isodose curve is at about 3 mm; they are not used for lesions over 5 mm deep.[85] Tumor base doses are very high, above 50,000 cGy. Because these plaques are similar in design to ^{60}Co eye plaques, they have many of the same advantages, but they have a shorter shelf life ($T_{1/2}$ of 1 year). Doses to adjacent structures should be limited because of rapid dose fall-off at the edges of the plaques.

Eye plaques incorporating ^{90}Sr are available for treating very shallow eye lesions. Figure 12-22 shows the dose distribution measured using several methods of dosimetry. Improvements in methods of absolute calibration of ^{90}Sr plaques are being investigated.[24]

Californium 252

In the early 1950s, scientists identified a radioisotope that decays mostly by α-emission, with an occasional decay by spontaneous fission. The decaying ^{252}Cf produces charged particles,

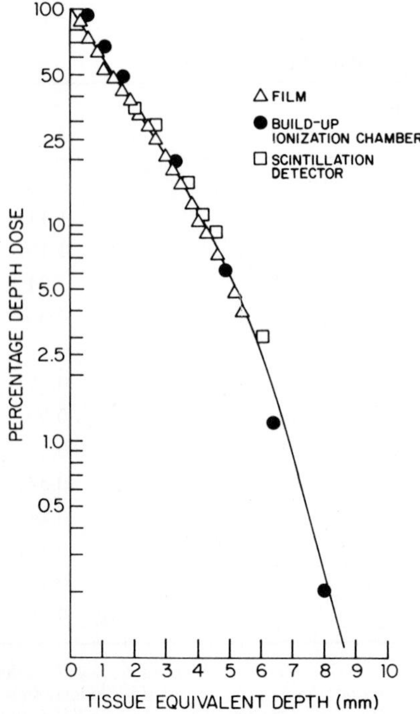

FIGURE 12–22. Central-axis percentage depth dose curves measured for a ^{90}Sr eye applicator using various methods of dosimetry. (Coffey C, Sayeg J, Beach L, et al: Med Phys 8:558, 1981)

τ-rays, and neutrons for which the neutron fission spectrum has an average energy between 2.1 MeV and 2.3 MeV, and most of the τ-rays have energies between 0.5 MeV and 1.0 MeV. Very near the source, the ratio of the dose from neutrons to the dose from τ-rays is about 2 to 1; at 5 to 10 cm from the source, the τ-rays and neutrons contribute about equally to the tissue dose.

Californium 252 has a 2.65-year half-life; a typical source contains about 0.25 μg to 0.45 μg of the isotope. Each microgram emits 2.34×10^6 neutrons/sec. The sources contain a core of californium oxide mixed with palladium, placed in a double-encapsulated iridioplatinum sheath; seeds have an external diameter of 0.8 mm and a physical length of 6 mm, of which 4 mm is active length. Seeds are available in linear ribbon arrays, with three to seven seeds per ribbon. Tubes that are 1.05 mm in diameter are also available.

Dosimetry measurements of the radiation fields around this mixed neutron and τ-ray emitter are difficult; the isodose distributions reported by Krishnaswamy[76] and Colvett and colleagues[25] are commonly used. Anderson[4] did an excellent review of ^{252}Cf dosimetry, and Maruyama and co-workers[93] reported the clinical experience at Lexington, KY, and reviewed the published literature.

Californium 252 exhibits a high relative biologic effectiveness for hypoxic cells compared with oxic cells and a lower oxygen enhancement ratio than conventional radioisotopes emitting only τ-rays. Although early clinical experiences with ^{252}Cf in brachytherapy were discouraging, clinical studies continue.[93]

AFTERLOADING SYSTEMS AND INTERSTITIAL APPLICATORS

Remote Afterloading Systems

Low-activity and high-activity remote afterloading devices are becoming more common in brachytherapy.[1, 19, 81, 118, 135, 155] Almond[2] reviewed the systems commercially available, some of which are listed in Table 12-20. Remote afterloading techniques eliminate or reduce radiation exposure to attending medical personnel, increase treatment capacity using high-dose-rate methods, and improve therapy by providing more consistent treatments than with manual applicators.[118] Remote afterloading devices are most useful in facilities with high patient loads, although fifty brachytherapy patients per year justify remote afterloading.

Remote afterloading devices represent a new technology, the reliability of which must be established; high-dose-rate techniques represent a deviation from the accepted radiobiologic principles established over many years by the classic methods of

TABLE 12–20
Features of Remote Afterloading Systems

NAME	MANUFACTURER OR VENDOR	NUMBER OF SOURCES	NUMBER OF CHANNELS	RADIOISOTOPES AND NOMINAL ACTIVITIES	LOW DOSE RATE	HIGH DOSE RATE	INTRA-CAVITARY APPLI-CATOR	INTER-STITIARY APPLI-CATOR
Afterloading Buchler	Buchler GmbH (West Germany)	1 (oscillating)	3 (uses 2 additional stationary sources)	0.1 Ci ^{137}Cs 4.0 Ci ^{137}Cs 10.0 Ci ^{192}Ir 1.2 Ci ^{60}Co	yes	yes	yes	yes
Curietron	CIS-US (France)	6	6	0.05 Ci ^{137}Cs 0.50 Ci ^{137}Cs	yes	yes	yes	yes
Curieton-192	CIS-US (France)	20-LDR 2-HDR	20	0.001 Ci ^{192}Ir* 10.0 Ci ^{192}Ir	yes	yes	yes	yes
Gamma Med II	Isotopen-Technik Dr. Sauerwein GmbH (West Germany)	1 (stepping)	2	10.0 Ci ^{192}Ir	no	yes	yes	no
Gamma Med IIi	Isotopen-Technik Dr. Sauerwein GmbH (West Germany)	1 (stepping)	12	10.0 Ci ^{192}Ir	no	yes	yes	yes
Gamma Med I2i	Isotopen-Technik Dr. Sauerwein GmbH (West Germany)	1 (stepping)	24	10.0 Ci ^{192}Ir	no	yes	yes	yes
Selectron (low dose rate)	Nucletron Engineering BV (Netherlands)	48 pellet sources per channel	3 or 6	0.01 to 0.04 Ci* per pellet; 2.2 Ci ^{137}Cs	yes	no	yes	no
Selectron (high dose rate)	Nucletron Engineering BV (Netherlands)	20	3	0.01 to 0.05 Ci per source; 12 Ci ^{60}Co	no	yes	yes	no
MicroSelectron (low dose rate)	Nucletron Engineering BV (Netherlands)	45 ribbons	15	0.001 Ci ^{192}Ir* 0.001 Ci ^{137}Cs*	yes	no	yes	yes
MicroSelectron (high dose rate)	Nucletron Engineering BV (Netherlands)	1	18	10.0 Ci ^{192}Ir	no	yes	yes	yes

**Nominal activity; user selects desired activity.*

treatment with lower activity sources and dose rates. Clinical results with high-dose-rate units are encouraging.[135,155] The early developmental work by Walstam[157] resulted in the development of two commercial machines that were precursors of the Curietron and the low-dose-rate Selectron.

The original low-dose-rate Selectron was designed for 48 ^{137}Cs sources with activities from 0.01 Ci to 0.04 Ci. They contained three channels for moving the gynecologic tubes into position. The current Selectron features advanced pneumatic engineering and is microprocessor controlled for source pellet arrangements. The current device is available with three or six channels; six channels allow treatment of two patients simultaneously. A high-dose-rate unit contains 20 ^{60}Co pellets, with a total activity of 10 Ci.

The Gamma Med II features a 10-Ci ^{192}Ir source that is moved by a stepping motor over the length of the applicator; the desired dose distribution is achieved by allowing different dwell times at each location. Model IIi of this unit features 12 channels into which the single source can be moved sequentially for interstitial implants; a new unit contains 24 channels. The smaller external diameter of the 10-Ci ^{192}Ir source allows interstitial implants to be remotely afterloaded. With a half-life of 74.2 days, three source changes each year are usually required. The Curietron-192 and MicroSelectron-HDR are similar units designed for high-dose-rate interstitial implants.

Another afterloading system is marketed by Buchler and is available as a low-, medium-, or high-dose-rate system. The user may request ^{60}Co, ^{137}Cs, or ^{192}Ir as a source. All of these devices features numerous safety and fail-safe systems to ensure safe operation and feature many popular applicators adapted for remote operation.

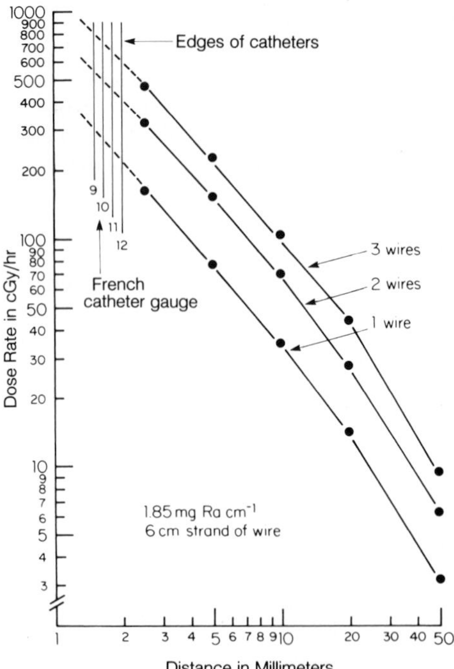

FIGURE 12–23. Dose rates along the perpendicular bisector of multiple strands of 6-cm ^{192}Ir wires containing 1.85 mg Ra eq/cm. Dose rates at the catheter surfaces are much higher than the dose rates 1 cm from the catheter.

Molds and Interstitial Applicators

Molds are still of value in treating anatomic sites that are difficult to access with a superficial cone or electron beam applicator.[122,129] Sources embedded in a wax carrier are easily and cheaply made; tissue-equivalent materials, such as superflab or silicone, are readily implanted with radioactive sources to form a carrier that conforms to surface curvature and that can be held in place with conventional medical dressings.[71] A new visible-light-curing resin is available for brachytherapy prosthetics.[99]

Intraoral molds are made from dental impression compounds.[22] The radiation carrier is usually attached to a dental plate that can be secured to the teeth to hold it in position in the oral cavity. Wire made with ^{192}Ir is a useful radioactive source for such carriers; the fine wire, with a 0.3-mm external diameter, can be inserted into very small holes drilled into the mold. By using multiple strands of wire, the radiologist can use classic Manchester System distribution rules to achieve good dose uniformity at the desired dose rate.

Glasgow and Marks[45] used an endolaryngeal mold to treat a carcinoma of the larynx that recurred after surgery and irradiation. Excellent tumor control was achieved.

Bile duct lesions may be treated with single or multiple strands of ^{192}Ir wire or seeds.[158] The radioactive sources are introduced into the site through a drainage catheter. The dose distribution around a single linear source generally is not desirable for therapy. The dose gradients from the surface of the linear source to 1 cm away from the source, where doses are often prescribed, vary markedly. Figure 12-23 shows the dose rates from one, two, and three strands of 6-cm wires of ^{192}Ir with an activity equivalent to 1.85 mg Ra/cm. The high activity is required to treat quickly at high dose rates to avoid medical problems of blockage and infection.

Afterloading interstitial techniques have reduced the use of radioactive needles for temporary interstitial implants. Specific methods and techniques developed at Memorial Hospital have been described by Hilaris and Henschke.[59] Delclos[28] reviewed the methods popular at M. D. Anderson Cancer Center, and Paine[111] offers an excellent description of the single and double hairpin needle guides, sources, and methods of afterloading as developed in France. Syed and Feder[148] review these techniques and the use of templates to improve the control of needle spacing and alignment. Table 12-21 provides a limited overview of the important features of interstitial implant instruments. Chapter 13 contains further descriptions of interstitial techniques.

Plastic templates are frequently used with one-sided techniques in the vagina and perineum to ensure that the needles and sources remain parallel to each other during the insertion.[92] Significant improvements have been reported in securing radioactive sources in needle guides.[12] Zwicker and associates[171] developed an improved locking mechanism.

The use of interstitial implants in conjunction with hyperthermia necessitates the use of nonmetallic fasteners to secure sources in plastic guides. We developed a technique in which a plastic hub is glued to a plastic stylet (Flexi Guide) protruding from the implant site. A disposable Leur lock handle that carries the radioactive source attaches securely to the hub with a firm twist of the wrist. Later, the source can be easily removed when necessary for other medical treatments, after which they are reinserted and refastened.[43]

Modern interstitial applicators include a variety of "guns" of different designs. The seeds are placed in cartridges that are loaded into the site during an operation, and seeds are inserted one at a time into the lesion. Figure 12-24 shows the Mick applicator, widely used to implant ^{125}I seeds in sites such as the

TABLE 12–21
Features of Interstitial Implant Instruments

TYPE OF DEVICE	FEATURES	SITES
Hypodermic needle	Usually 3 cm to 8 cm long; 19 or 20 gauge	Particularly useful in implanting projecting structures (ear, lower lip, penis): small gauge minimizes surgical trauma; can accept smallest-diameter iridium wire
Stainless steel afterloading needle (opened end)	Available in 10-, 15-, and 20-cm lengths; 17 to 14 gauge commonly used, depending on external diameter of radioactive source	Breast, base of tongue, and rectal implants
Single- or double-cutter guides	Available in 3-cm and 4-cm lengths, straight or curved	Mobile tongue implants, epiglottis, and other sites of limited access; double needle guide yields a loop or crossed-end effect
Stainless steel afterloading stylettes (closed end)	Fabricated from stainless steel tubing, the sharp end is crimped above the point to prevent the sources from protruding; blunt end contains a metal suture button attached to the stylette	Useful in one-sided sites, such as head and neck, vagina. Stylettes remain in place for the duration of the implant
Spears	A solid, sharp needle with the blunt end reduced in size to accept the plastic tubing that has same external diameter as spear	Used in sites where clearance is limited; pin vise is placed over the tubing and spear to provide a firm grip during insertion
Plastic stylettes	About 20-cm long and 14-gauge flexible plastic guides feature a sharp end to penetrate most tissue sites	An alternative to methods using metal needle guides and plastic tubing; generally retains its linear shape after implanting and does not bend as easily as plastic tubing; very useful in conjunction with hyperthermia
Plastic tubing	Smallest gauges used as carriers for iridium wire or seeds; larger gauges used in afterloading needles to accept radioactive sources	Particularly useful in oral sites, for loop technique for which flexibility is desirable; in other sites its flexibility is a disadvantage because it conforms to lesion shape, producing nonlinear sources
Plastic buttons	About 1-cm diameter with a lumen to accept plastic tubing; can be heat sealed to some types of plastic tubing	Secured to one end of a plastic tube before the implant; prevents the tube from being pulled through the implant site; a second plastic button is usually placed between the skin surface and metal securing button
Hemispherical and spherical balls	About 1-cm in diameter with a lumen to accept plastic tubing	Used between the skin surface and the securing button in sites subject to swelling to reduce pressure and subsequent skin irradiation and trauma
Stainless steel buttons and lead buttons	Stainless steel buttons are similar to plastic buttons, but have suture holes; lead buttons serve the same function; both can be crimped to secure radioactive sources in the plastic tubing and the tubing in the site	Almost all sites, except the oral cavity where the looping technique is used
Gold buttons	Similar to stainless steel buttons, the more dense gold provides some shielding near source ends	Useful in sites where a degree of shielding is needed, such as oral cavity
Inactive or "dummy" sources	Lengths of solid radiopaque wire or wire segments in small-gauge plastic tubing with specific spacing between the segments	Used for localization films and in some instances to determine the exact length of wire or number of seeds needed in a particular afterloading tube
Templates	Metal or plastic devices with preselected holes spaced in a regular array to achieve a desired distribution of sources	Breast, cervix, urethra, rectum, brain
Crimping tool	Usually long-handled pliers with parallel closing jaws that allow maximum pressure to be exerted on the metal or lead fastener	Used to crimp stainless steel or lead fasteners
Cutting tool	Special jaws that provide an angled cut	Used to cut tubing smoothly without deforming the end of the tubing
Stripping tool	Ability to cut through the outer tubing without cutting through the radioactive source	Used where conventional wire strippers serve the purpose

prostate and lung. Other applicators for ^{125}I seeds use dissolvable sutures as spacers between the seeds; the seeds are spaced as desired, and with one motion, a linear array of seeds is implanted in the site. The ^{125}I seeds in a flexible dissolvable suture are also popular in certain neck implants, as described by Goffinet and associates.[47] The ^{125}I seeds, spaced on 1-cm centers, are contained in a braided, synthetic, absorbable carrier and are marketed in a sterile pack. Marchese and co-workers[90] used a gel foam for similar implants.

THERAPY WITH UNSEALED RADIOISOTOPES

The major uses of unsealed radioisotopes for therapy include the treatment of diseases of the thyroid (*i.e.*, hyperthyroidism, thyroid ablation for which surgery is not possible, and thyroid carcinoma) with ^{131}I; treatment of hematologic diseases (polycythemia vera and leukemia); treatment of malignant bone lesions with ^{32}P; and treatment of malignant disease in serosal cavities by intracavitary therapy with radioisotopes ^{198}Au, ^{90}Sr,

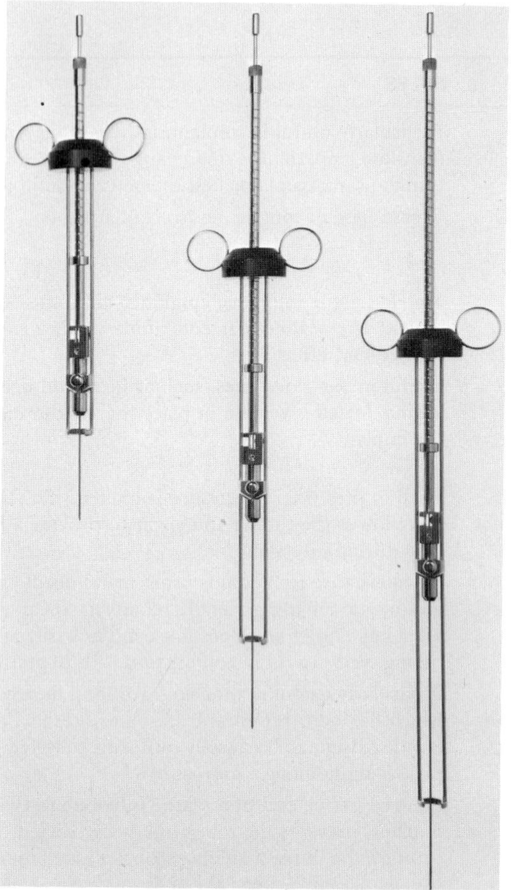

FIGURE 12–24. Mick applicators. For prostrate implants, 15-cm needles are used. Applicators using 9-cm needles for superficial lesions and 20-cm needles for perineal implants are also available.

and colloidal ^{32}P. An excellent text addresses these therapies and other nuclear medicine therapies using less common radioisotopes.[144]

Iodine 131

Iodine 131 has a high production cross-section (> 1000 barns) as a fission by-product and follows the metabolic pathways of stable ^{127}I. Its 8.06-day half-life makes it highly useful for a host of medical applications in diagnosis, labeling, and imaging. Iodine 123, with a 13.1-hour half-life, is a pure τ-ray emitter that has been used instead of ^{131}I in some facilities with cyclotrons capable of producing it.

The biokinetics of ^{131}I in the euthyroid individual have received much attention because of the importance of ^{131}I as an imaging agent in nuclear medicine and because ^{131}I is produced in nuclear fallout and is a carcinogen if ingested in sufficient amounts and deposited in the thyroid.

The normal adult is in "iodine balance" if an adequate supply of natural iodine is available; the body ingests about 150 μg of iodine daily and excretes the same amount. If, as an inorganic salt, NaI is injected intravenously, it distributes in a short time throughout the "iodide space," which consists of the bloodstream and body fluids, with a concentration of 3 μg/L. The iodide space comprises about 30% of body weight. As the blood circulates through the thyroid, the gland concentrates the iodide and converts it to protein-bound iodine, with a normal value of 3.5 to 7.5 μg/dL. About 20% of plasma-bound iodide is removed by the thyroid during each pass; depending on the individual, 0.5% to 6.8% of the iodide in the circulating pool is extracted each hour. In a normal adult, as much as 30% of the injected or ingested NaI can be accumulated. The normal adult contains 8 mg of iodine, but there are wide individual variations. The thyroid releases about 1% of its iodine content daily. The amount of protein-bound iodine in the thyroid determines whether an individual is hyperthyroid or hypothyroid. Iodine also concentrates in the gastric mucosa and salivary glands.

The amount of protein-bound iodine released by the thyroid is controlled by enzymatic action of the pituitary gland. The protein-bound iodine is degraded in the body and returns to the iodide pool. Excretion of ^{131}I is almost entirely by the kidney.

In a normal adult, the biologic half-life (T_{bio}) of iodine varies from 20 to 200 days; because both are much longer than physical half-life (T_{phy}) of 8.06 days, the effective half-life (T_{eff}) is between 5.74 and 7.74 days as

$$T_{eff} = \frac{T_{phy} \times T_{bio}}{T_{phy} + T_{bio}}$$

Although numerous compartmental models have been developed to explain the biokinetics of iodine in the euthyroid individual, the literature is less clear on adequate models in the individual with thyroid disease.[127]

We limit our discussion to review of quantitative data in an excellent article by Pochin and Kermode.[117] Their compartment model is shown in Figure 12-25, and Table 12-22 lists other important parameters of the model, designed to account for therapy for hyperthyroidism, ablation of normal thyroid, and thyroid cancer. For orally administered radioiodine, the model uses mean retention times before absorption from the gut while circulating in inorganic form (iodide) in the iodide pool; while present in the thyroid, tumor, or residual thyroid tissue, while circulating in organic form after being released but before breakdown to iodine, and before excretion or recycling (Fig 12-25).

Moreover, the model assumes the following:

1. Thirty minutes is required for uptake from the gut into the blood.
2. The thyroid exponentially accumulates radioiodine at a constant rate, a.
3. A constant fraction, b, of the radioiodine in the thyroid or tumor is discharged in organic form per unit time.
4. A constant fraction, c, of the circulating organically bound radionuclide, r, is reduced to iodine per unit time.
5. This circulating radioiodide, s, is excreted at a constant rate, g, without significant recirculation through the thyroid or tumor.

The rate of change of activity in each compartment is obtained by adding the uptake (or incoming) rate with the decay (or outgoing) rate. For example, if a dose, D, is administered to the individual, in the inorganic iodide pool the activity, p, is

$$\frac{\Delta p}{\Delta t} = -(a + e)p$$

so that

$$\int_0^t p\Delta t = D/(a + e)$$

Although space prohibits discussing all the rates for each compartment, they are shown in Figure 12-25.

The total activity-time integral of millicurie days (mCid) per millicurie from all phases is the mean retention time of the

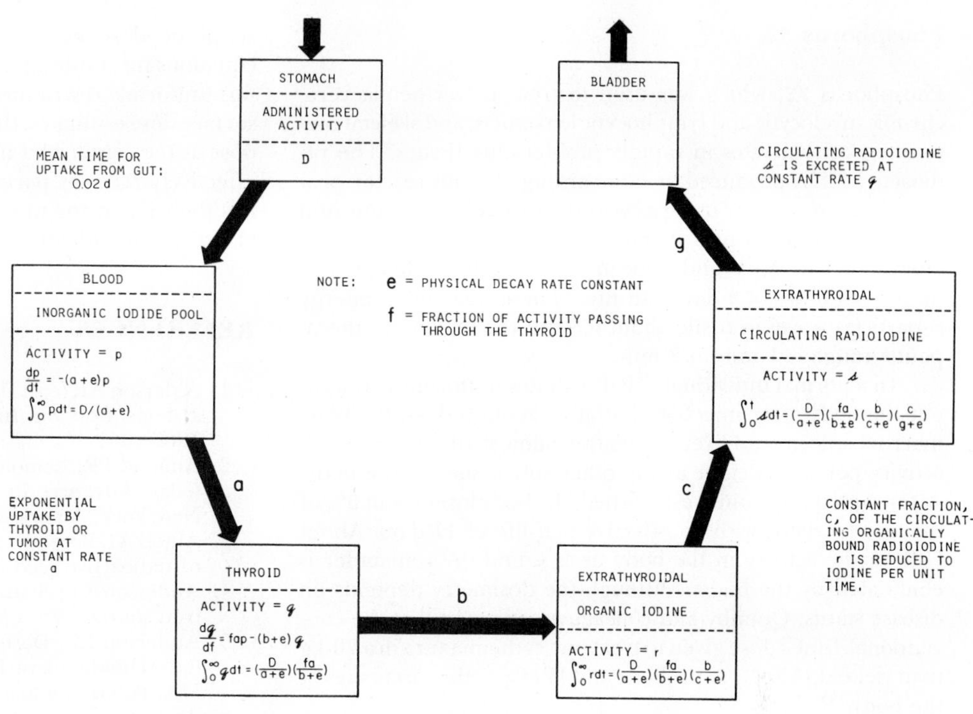

FIGURE 12–25. A compartment model for estimating the mean retention time of administered activity during treatment of hyperthyroidism, ablation of normal thyroid, and treatment of thyroid cancer. (Pochin EE, Kermode JC: Br J Radiol 48:299, 1975)

administered activity. Table 12-22 lists the values quoted by Pochin and Kermode[117] for these and other parameters of the model for patients treated for hyperthyroidism, thyroid ablation, and thyroid cancer.

The 3.6% uptake in the average patient with thyroid cancer is much lower than in the other two categories, as is the fraction, f, of the administered dose passing through the thyroid or tumor. The mean retention time is also the shortest in the thyroid and in the body. The product of the administered activity (mCi) and mean retention time (mCid/mCi) yields the total millicurie days (mCid), which is greatest for the cancer patient because of the large dose (150 mCi) administered. Pochin and Kermode[117] provide many tables that further aid in understanding the biokinetics of ^{131}I in the thyroid or tumor.

The dose to the thyroid is hard to estimate because of the difficulty in knowing the concentration of ^{131}I in the thyroid. Conventional nuclear medicine scans yield qualitative distribution data but give no quantitative estimate of the amount of ^{131}I in the thyroid or tumor.

Use of conjugate views and a calibrated τ-camera allowed Mason and associates[94] and Thomas and co-workers[150] to make reasonable estimates of the thyroid dose in treating 76 patients with adenocarcinoma. They concluded that at least 30,000 cGy was required to ablate the thyroid, and 8000 cGy was required to obtain a therapeutic response in patients with metastatic disease. However, in most thyroid therapies, dose estimates are not made because of inadequate knowledge about the concentration and duration of ^{131}I in the tissue.

TABLE 12–22
Synopsis of Iodine Biokinetics Model Parameters for Treating Hyperthyroidism, Thyroid Ablation, and Treatment of Thyroid Carcinoma

MODEL PARAMETER OR END POINT	HYPERTHYROIDISM	THYROID ABLATION	THYROID CANCER
24-hour uptake (%)	68	29.5	3.6
Percentage of administered dose passing through thyroid or tumor	0.72		0.055
Discharge rate (%/d)	6.4		
Activity administered (mCi)	5.3	80	150
Mean retention time in thyroid (mCid/mCi)	4.7	1.2	0.17
Mean retention time in body (mCid/mCi)	5.61	1.77	0.97
Total mCid	30	142	145
Cumulative exposure (R at 1 m)	0.1	0.49	0.5

(Pochin EE, Kermode JC: Br J Radiol 48:299, 1975)

Phosphorus 32

Phosphorus 32, which was used to treat polycythemia vera, chronic myelocytic and lymphocytic leukemias, and skeletal metastases, concentrates in rapidly proliferating tissues. The radioactive ^{32}P is produced by bombarding ^{32}S with reactor-produced neutrons or by using a cyclotron to accelerate deuterium into ^{32}S. The resulting ^{32}P emits a β-particle with a maximum energy of 1.71 MeV and a mean energy of 0.69 MeV, which decays with a 14.3-day half-life. These maximum-energy β-particles travel in tissue about 0.8 cm; the maximum therapeutic range is 1 mm to 2 mm.

In a normal individual, ^{32}P distributes uniformly throughout the body after injection, but after about 3 days, the bone marrow, spleen, and liver concentrate almost 10 times as much activity per unit weight as the other soft tissues in the body. After this equilibrium is established, the body loses about 6% of the activity daily, with an effective half-life of 11 days. About 70% of the activity in the body decays, and the remainder is eliminated by the body. Although the dosimetry depends on disease status, Quimby and colleagues estimated that the conventional 4-mCi dose given to treat polycythemia vera in a 70-kg man yielded 115 cGy to the bone and 17 cGy to the soft tissues of the body.[125]

In a given organ tissue in which the concentration of ^{32}P is C μCi per gram of tissue, the dose rate D is given by

$$D(\text{cGy/day}) = 2.13C \times \overline{E}_\beta$$

where $\overline{E}$ is the average energy (0.69 MeV) per decay of the radioisotope. The total dose to the organ or tissue is

$$D(\text{cGy}) = 73.8C_{max} \times \overline{E}_\beta T_{eff}(1 - e^{T_{eff} \times t})$$

C_{max} is the maximum concentration in microcuries per gram of the radioisotope that occurs in the tissue, T_{eff} is the effective half-life in days, and t is the total elapsed time that the radioisotope is present in the organ or tissue. Both equations include an assumption that the radioisotope is uniformly distributed in the tissue. The dosimetry of β-emitters is explained in detail by Spiers.[145]

Chromic Phosphate in Colloidal Suspension

Chromic phosphate is a radiocolloid used to treat malignant diseases in which dissemination results in exudation of fluid in serosal cavities, such as metastatic carcinoma of the lung, disseminated lymphoma, and some cases of gastrointestinal cancer. The short range of the ^{32}P β-particles gives a high dose to tissue surfaces in contact with the radioisotope while sparing healthy tissue. Other radioisotopes used for similar therapy include ^{198}Au and ^{90}Y. Although the short half-life of ^{198} is an advantage, its penetrating 0.412-MeV τ-rays are not, and it is not often used for intracavitary therapy. Although ^{90}Y, with its 2.2-MeV β-particles with a 2.7-day half-life, is well suited to such therapies, it requires a stable carrier in concentrations that are almost toxic.

The colloid particles of chromic phosphate are 0.05 to 1 μm in diameter in a glucose suspension, and the greatest difficulty with this therapy is achieving a uniform distribution of particles on the surface to be treated. The ^{32}P particles plate out fairly rapidly onto the surface. For treating the pleura, usually 10 mCi to 15 mCi is administered, and the peritoneum requires 15 mCi to 20 mCi.

Knowledge of the dose to the surface is usually based on simplistic dose estimates, yielding large uncertainties. The equations for sodium phosphate assumed that the radioisotope was uniformly distributed in the tissue receiving the dose. For surface dose estimates, the dose is estimated to be one half of the dose at the center of a uniform distribution, because the edge effectively receives particles from only one direction. Usually less than 1% of the injected radioisotope is transmitted to the bloodstream and subsequently excreted by the body.

REFERENCES

1. Alderson AR (ed): Dosimetry and clinical uses of afterloading systems. London, Institute of Physical Sciences in Medicine, 1986
2. Almond PR: Remote afterloading. In Wright AE, Boyer AL (eds): Advances in radiation therapy treatment planning. New York, American Institute of Physics, 1983
3. Amols AI, Rosen II: A three film technique for reconstruction of radioactive seed implants. Med Phys 9:210, 1981
4. Anderson LL: Status of dosimetry for Cf-252 medical neutron sources. Phys Med Biol 18:779, 1973
5. Anderson LL: Dosimetry in implant therapy. In Hilaris BS (ed): Handbook of Interstitial Brachytherapy, p 101. Acton, MA, Publishing Sciences Group, 1975
6. Anderson LL: Spacing nomograph for interstitial implants of I-125 seeds. Med Phys 3:48, 1976
7. Anderson LL: Experiences with ^{192}Ir. In Wright AE, Boyer AL (eds): Advances in Radiation Therapy Treatment Planning. New York, American Institute of Physics, 1983
8. Anderson LL, Kuan HM, Ding IY: Clinical dosimetry with I-125. In George FW (ed): Modern Interstitial and Intracavitary Radiation Cancer Management. New York, Masson, 1981
9. Aristizabal SA, Herezi JM, Seminoff J: Cesium-137 microspheres as a substitute for iridium 92 in interstitial implants. Third Annual Mid-Winter Meeting, American Endocurietherapy Society, Lake Tahoe, Nevada, 1981
10. Batho HR, Young NET: Tissue absorption corrections for linear radium source. Br J Radiol 37:689, 1964
11. Bello J, Oyarzun C, Abrath FG: Characteristics of Ir-192 shielding. Radiology 145:224, 1982
12. Bourland JD, Reynolds KL, Chaney EL, et al: An integrated system for interstitial ^{192}Ir implants. Int J Radiat Oncol Biol Phys 13:45, 1987
13. Boyer AL: A fundamental accuracy limitation of measurements of brachytherapy sources. Med Phys 6:454, 1979
14. Breitman KE: Dose rate tables for clinical ^{137}Cs sources sheathed in platinum. Br J Radiol 47:657, 1974
15. British Committee on Radiation Units and Measurements: Specification of brachytherapy sources. Br J Radiol 57:941, 1984
16. Burnett AW: A vaginal radium applicator. Radiology 84: 859,1965
17. Burns GS, Raeside DE: Monte Carlo simulation of the dose distribution around ^{125}I seeds. Med Phys 14:296, 1987
18. Busch M: Role of computers in radiotherapy. Vienna, International Atomic Energy Agency, 1968
19. Bush M, Alberti W: High dose rate afterloading therapy of uterine cancer. Essen, Radiologisches Zentrum, Universitätsklinikum Essen, 1985
20. Casebow MP: The calculation and measurement of exposure distribution from Co-60 ophthalmic applicators. Br J Radiol 44:618, 1971
21. Chan B, Rotman M, Randall GJ: Computerized dosimetry of Co-60 ophthalmic applicators. Radiology 103:705, 1972
22. Cheng STV, Oral K, Aramamy MS: The use of acrylic resin oral prosthesis in radiation therapy of oral cavity and paranasal sinus cancer. Int J Radiat Oncol Biol Phys 7:1245, 1982
23. Clarke DH, Edmundson GK, Martinez A, Matter RC, Warmelink C: Utilization of I-125 seeds as a substitute for Ir-192 seeds in temporary implants: An overview and description of the William Beaumont Hospital technique. Int J Radiat Oncol Biol Phys 15:1027, 1988

24. Coffey C, Sayeg J, Beach L, et al: Calibration of surface dose rate for Sr-90 beta applicator: Comparison of experimental, theoretical, and biological methods. Med Phys 8:558, 1981
25. Colvett RD, Rossi HH, Krishnaswamy V: Dose distributions around a californium-252 needle. Phys Med Biol 17:356, 1972
26. Cunningham DE, Stryker JA, Velkley DE, et al: Intracavitary dosimetry: A comparison of mg hr prescription to doses at points A and B in cervical cancer. Int J Radiat Oncol Biol Phys 7:121, 1981
27. Dale RG: Some theoretical deviations relating to the tissue dosimetry of brachytherapy nuclides, with particular reference to iodine. Med Phys 10:176, 1983
28. Delclos L: Interstitial irradiation techniques. In Levitt SH, Tapley N (eds): Technological Basis of Radiotherapy: Practical Clinical Applications. Philadelphia, Lea & Febiger, 1984
29. Delclos L, Fletcher GH, Sampiere V, et al: Can the Fletcher gamma ray colpostat system be extrapolated to other systems. Cancer 41:970, 1978
30. Del Regato JA: Foreword. In Pierquin B, Chassagne DJ, Chahbazian CM, et al (eds): Brachytherapy. St Louis, Warren H Green, 1978
31. Diffey BL, Klevenhagen SC: An experimental and calculated dose distribution in water around CDC-K type cesium-137 sources. Phys Med Biol 20:446, 1975
32. Ellis F, Taylor GBG: The Amersham Cesium-137 Afterloading System for Gynecological Brachytherapy. Amersham, England, Amersham International Publications, 1982
33. Fairchield RG, Kalef-Ezra J, Packer S, et al: Samarium-145: A new brachytherapy source. Phys Med Biol 32:847, 1987
34. Feldman A: Brachytherapy implant coordinates from stereoradiographs: A modified technique giving high accuracy. Int J Radiat Oncol Biol Phys 5(suppl 2):80, 1979
35. Fitzgerald LT, Manderil W: Analysis of errors in three-dimensional reconstruction of radium implants from stereo radiographs. Radiology 115:455, 1975
36. Fletcher GH: Cervical radium applicators with screening in the direction of bladder and rectum. Radiology 60:77, 1953.
37. Fletcher GH: Textbook of Radiotherapy, p 768. Philadelphia, Lea & Febiger, 1973
38. George FN (ed): Modern Interstitial and Intracavitary Radiation Cancer Management. Chicago, Masson, 1981
39. Gibb R. Massey JB: Radium dosage: SI units and the Manchester system. Br J Radiol 53:1100, 1980
40. Gillin MT, Kline RW, Wilson JF, et al: Single and double plane implants: A comparison of the Manchester system with the Paris system. Int J Radial Oncol Biol Phys 10:921, 1984
41. Gillin MT, Lopez F, Kline RW, et al: Comparison of measured and calculated dose distributions around iridium-192 wire. Med Phys 15:915, 1988
42. Glasgow GP: The specific τ-ray constant and exposure rate constant of ^{182}Ta. Med Phys 9:250, 1982
43. Glasgow GP, Budreau LA, Emami B: A disposable Leur lock afterloading catheter for interstitial hyperthermia. Endocuriether Hypertherm Oncol 2:189, 1986
44. Glasgow GP, Dillman LT: Specific τ-ray constant and exposure rate constant of ^{192}Ir. Med Phys 6:49, 1979
45. Glasgow GP, Marks JE: An endolaryngeal brachytherapy mould for carcinoma of the larynx recurrent after surgery and radiation. Laryngoscope 93:111, 1983
46. Glasser O, Quimby EH, Taylor LS, et al: Physical Foundations of Radiology, 2nd ed. New York, Paul B. Hoeber, 1952.
47. Goffinet DR, Martinez A, Poller D, et al: Perineal brachytherapy. Front Radiat Ther Oncol 12:72, 1978
48. Gooden TJ: Physical Aspects of Brachytherapy (Medical Physical Handbook 19). Bristol, Adam Hilger, 1988
49. Gromadzki Z, Ling CC, Rustig S, et al: Radiation fluence anisotropy of ^{192}Ir and ^{198}Au seeds. Med Phys 8:570, 1981
50. Hale J: The use of interstitial dose rate tables for other radioactive isotopes. AJR 79:49, 1958.
51. Hall EJ, Oliver R, Shepstone BJ: Routine dosimetry with tantalum 182 and iridium-192 wires. Acta Radiol 4:155, 1966
52. Hashemi AM, Mills MD, Hogstrom KR, Almond PR: The exposure rate constant for a silver wire ^{125}I seed. Med Phys 15:228, 1988
53. Hass JS, Dean RD, Mansfield Cm: Dosimetry comparison of the Fletcher family of gynecologic colpostats 1950–1980. Int J Radiat Oncol Biol Phys 11:1317, 1985
54. Hendee WR: Medical Radiation Physics. Chicago, Year Book Medical Publishers, 1970
55. Heyman J: The so-called Stockholm Method and the results of treatment of the uterine cancer of the Radiumhemmet. Acta Radiol 16:129, 1935
56. Hidalgo BS, Spear VD, Garcia M, et al: The precision reconstruction of radium implants. AJR 100:852, 1967
57. Hilaris BS (ed): Afterloading: 20 Years of Experience, 1955–1975: Memorial Sloan-Kettering Cancer Center. New York, Robert C. Gold & Associates, 1975
58. Hilaris BS (ed): Handbook of Interstitial Brachytherapy, p xiii. Acton, MA, Publishing Sciences Group, 1975
59. Hilaris BS, Henschke UK: General principles and techniques of interstitial therapy. In Hilaris BS (ed): Handbook of Interstitial Brachytherapy. Acton, MA, Publishing Sciences Group, 1975
60. Hilaris BS, Holt GJ, St. Germain J: The Use of Iodine-125 for Interstitial Implants. Publication (FDA) 76–8022. Rockville, MD, Department of Health, Education and Welfare, 1975
61. Hilaris BS, Nori D, Anderson LL: Atlas of Brachytherapy. New York, MacMillan, 1988
62. Hine GJ, Friedman M: Isodose measurements of linear radium sources in air and water by means of an automatic isodose plotter. AJR 64:989, 1950
63. Horsler AFC, Jones JC, Stacey AJ: Cesium-137 sources for use in intracavitary and interstitial radiotherapy. Br J Radiol 37:385, 1964
64. Hughes HA: Accuracy of foreign body localization from "tube-shift" radiographs. Br J Radiol 29:116, 1956.
65. Innes GS: The application of physics in the treatment of ocular neoplasms. In Boniuk M (ed): Ocular and Adnexal Tumors: New and Controversial Aspects, pp 142–157. St. Louis, CV Mosby, 1964
66. International Commission of Radiation Units and Measurements: Report 10(e): Radiobiology Dosimetry. Washington, DC, U.S. Government Printing Office, 1963
67. International Commission on Radiation Units and Measurements: Report 19, Radiation Quantities and Units, p 11. Washington, DC, ICRU Publications, 1971
68. International Commission on Radiation Units and Measurements: Report 38, Dose and Volume Specification for Reporting Intracavitary Therapy in Gynecology. Bethesda,, 1985
69. Jani SK, Pennington EC, Wach JE, et al: Correlation of point doses with total activity in intracavitary cesium-137 applicators for treating gynecologic cancers. Endocuriether Hypertherm Oncol 4:107, 1988
70. Jayaraman S, Lanzl LH: An overview of errors in line source dosimetry for τ-ray brachytherapy. Med Phys 10:871, 1983
71. Karolis C, Reay-Young PS, Chir M, et al: Silicone plesiotherapy molds. Int J Radiat Oncol Biol Phys 9:569, 1983
72. Kemp LAW: Calculator circuit for tandems of screened linear radium sources. Br J Radiol 18:5, 1945.
73. Keyser GM: Absorption corrections for radium standardization. Can J Phys 29:301, 1951.
74. Klevenhagen SL: An experimental study of dose distribution in water around ^{137}Cs tubes used in brachytherapy. Br J Radiol 46:1073, 1973
75. Kline RW, Yeakel PD: Ocular melanoma I-125 plaques. [Abstract] Med Phys 14:475, 1987
76. Krishnaswamy V: Calculation of the dose distribution about californium-252 needles in tissue. Radiology 98:155, 1971
77. Krishnaswamy V: Dose distribution about ^{137}Cs sources in tissue. Radiology 105:181, 1972
78. Krishnaswamy V: Dose distribution around an I-125 seed source in tissue. Radiology 126:489, 1978
79. Kwan DK, Kagan AR, Olch AJ, et al: Single and double plane iridium-192 interstitial implants: Implantation guidelines and dosimetry. Med Phys 10:456, 1983
80. Laughlin JS, Siler WM, Holodny EI, et al: A dose description system for interstitial radiation therapy. Am J Roentgenol Radiat Ther Nucl Med 89:470, 1963
81. Leung PMK: Experience with remote afterloading technique

in intracavitary therapy. Int J Radiat Oncol Biol Phys 10:157, 1984
82. Ling CC, Huang DY, Barnett C, et al: Improved dose distributions with customized I-125 source loading in temporary interstitial implants. Int J Radiat Oncol Biol Phys 15:769, 1988
83. Ling CC, Yorke Ed, Spiro IJ, et al: Physical dosimetry of I-125 seeds of a new design for interstitial implant. Int J Radiat Oncol Biol Phys 9:1747, 1983
84. Loevinger R: Absorbed dose from interstitial and intracavitary sources. In Simon N (ed): Afterloading in Radiotherapy (Proceedings of a Conference, New York, 1971). FDA Publication No. 72–8024. Rockville, MD, Department of Health, Education and Welfare Publications, 1971
85. Lommatzch PK: Beta irradiation of choroidal melanoma with ^{106}Ru/^{106}Rh applicators. Arch Ophthalmol 101:713, 1983
86. Magnus L: Tiefendosisberechnung fur die Co-60 augennapplikatoren. Strahlentherapie 120:379, 1952.
87. Magnus L, Gobbeler T, Strotges W: Tiefendosisberechnung fur die Co augenapplikatoren. Strahlentherapie 136:170, 1968
88. Mansfield CM, Kyo RL, Dwyer S, et al: Computed tomography in brachytherapy. In Ling CC, Rodgers CC, Morton RJ (eds): Computed Tomography in Radiation Therapy. New York, Raven Press, 1983
89. Marchese MJ, Hall EJ: Clinical, physical, and radiobiological aspects of encapsulated I-125 in radiation oncology. Endocuriether Hypertherm Oncol 2:67, 1985
90. Marchese MJ, Nori D, Anderson LL, Hilaris BS: A versatile permanent planar implant technique utilizing iodine-125 seeds embedded in gel foam. Int J Radiat Oncol Biol Phys 10:747, 1984
91. Marinello G, Valero M, Levng S, Pierquin B: Comparative dosimetry between iridium wire and seed ribbons. Int J Radiat Oncol Biol Phys 11:1733, 1985
92. Martinez A, Cox RS, Edmundson GK: A multiple-site perineal applicator for treatment of prostatic, anorectal, and gynecologic malignancies. Int J Radiat Oncol Biol Phys 10:297, 1984
93. Maruyama Y, van Nagell JR, Yoneda J, et al: Dose response for californium-252 neutron brachytherapy by histological eradications and bulky state 1B cervical tumors. Endocuriether Hypertherm Oncol 5:111, 1989
94. Mason HR, Thomas SR, Hertzberg VS, et al: Relation between effective radiation dose and outcome of radioiodine therapy for thyroid cancer. N Engl J Med 309:937, 1983
95. Meigooni AS, Nath R: Measurements of dose distribution around a Pd-103 model 2000 source. [Abstract] Med Phys 16:458, 1989
96. Meisberger LL, Keller RJ, Shalek RJ: The effective attenuation in water of the τ-rays of gold-198, iridium-192, cesium-137, radium-226, and cobalt-60. Radiology 90:953, 1968
97. Meredith WJ (ed): Radium Dosage: The Manchester System, 2nd ed, pp 31–136. Baltimore, Williams & Wilkins, 1967
98. Meredith WJ, Greene D, Kawashima K: The attenuation and scattering in a phantom of τ-rays from some radionuclides used in mould and interstitial τ-ray therapy. Br J Radiol 39:280, 1966
99. Minsley GE, Rosenman J, Varia MA: Use of a new visible light curing resin system for radiation brachytherapy prosthetics. Endocuriether Hypertherm Oncol 4:23, 1988
100. Mohan R, Ding IY, Martel MK, et al: Measurement of radiation dose distribution of shielded cervical applicators. Int J Radiat Biol Phys 11:861, 1985
101. Müller RP, Busse H, Pötter R, et al: Results of high dose 106-ruthenium irradiation of choroidal melanomas. Int J Radiat Oncol Biol Phys 12:2203, 1986
102. Murphy DJ, Memula N, Doss LL: A ^{192}Ir nomogram system for single plane implants. Int J Radiat Oncol Biol Phys 12:267, 1986
103. Mussel LE: The rapid reconstruction of radium implants: A new technique. Br J Radiol 29:402, 1956.
104. Nath R, Gray L: Dosimetric studies on a prototype ^{241}Am source for brachytherapy. Int J Radiat Oncol Biol Phys 13:897, 1987
105. National Council on Radiation Protection and Measurements: Report No 40, Protection Against Radiation From Brachytherapy Sources. Washington, DC, NCRP Publications, 1972
106. National Council on Radiation Protection and Measurements: Report No. 41, Specification of Gamma Ray Brachytherapy Sources. Washington, DC, NCRP Publications, 1974
107. Nelson RF, Meurk ML: The use of automatic computing machines for implant dosimetry. Radiology 70:90, 1958.
108. Niroomand-Rad A, Thomadsen BR, Vainio P: Evaluation of the reconstruction of brachytherapy implants in three-dimensions from stereo radiographs. Radiother Oncol 8:337, 1987
109. Nolan JF, Anson JH, Stewart M: A radium applicator for use in the treatment of cancer of the uterine cervix. Am J Roentgenol Radiat Ther Nucl Med 79:36:1958.
110. Nuttal JR, Spiers FW: Dosage control in interstitial radium therapy. Br J Radiol 19:133, 1946.
111. Paine CH: Modern afterloading methods for interstitial radiotherapy. Clin Radiol 23:263, 1972
112. Paterson R, Parker AM: A dosage system for τ-ray therapy. Br J Radiol 7:592, 1934.
113. Paul JM, Koch RF, Phillips PC, Khan FR: Uniformity of dose distribution in interstitial implants. Endocuriether Hypertherm Oncol 2:107, 1986
114. Payne WH, Waggener RG: A theoretical calculation of the exposure rate constant for radium-226. Med Phys 1:210, 1974
115. Pierquin B, Chassange DJ, Chahbazian CM, et al: Brachytherapy, p v. St Louis, Warren H Green, 1978
116. Pierquin B, Dutreix A, Paine CH, et al: The Paris System in interstitial radiation therapy. Acta Radiol Oncol 17:33, 1978
117. Pochin EE, Kermode JC: Protection problems in radionuclide therapy: The patient as a τ-ray source. Br J Radiol 48:299, 1975
118. Porter AJ, Scrimger JW, Pocha JS: Remote interstitial afterloading in cancer of the prostate: Preliminary experience with the microselectron. Int J Radiat Oncol Biol Phys 14:571, 1985
119. Powers WE, Schneider AK, Shumate K, et al: Evaluation of methods of computer estimation of interstitial and intracavitary dosimetry. AJR 96:59, 1966
120. Prasad SC, Bassano DA, Fuet PI: Dose distributions for ^{125}I implants due to anisotropic radiation emission and unknown seed orientation. Med Phys 14:296, 1987
121. Prasad SC, Bassano DA, Peng JG: Lung density effect on ^{125}I dose distribution. Med Phys 12:99, 1985
122. Quimby EH: The grouping of radium tubes in packs on plaques to produce the desired dose distribution. AJR 27:18, 1932
123. Quimby EH: Dosage tables for linear radium sources. Radiology 43:572, 1944
124. Quimby EH, Castro V: The calculation of dosage in interstitial radium therapy. AJR 70:739, 1953
125. Quimby EH, Feitelberg S, Silver S: Radioisotopes in Clinical Practice, p 352. Philadelphia, Lea & Febiger, 1958
126. Regaud C: Quelques fondements radiobiologiques de la radiotherapie des meoplasmes malins. Paris Med 15:113, 1925
127. Riggs DS: Quantitative aspect of iodine metabolism in man. Pharmacol Rev 4:284, 1952
128. Robertson DM, Earle J, Kline RW: Brachytherapy for choroidal melanoma. In Ryan SJ, Ogden TE, Schachat AP (eds): Retina. St. Louis, CV Mosby, 1989
129. Rosen II, Gorden W, Loyd M: A surface mold using iridium-192 seeds. Int J Radiat Oncol Biol Phys 12:2203, 1986
130. Rosen II, Khan KM, Lane RG, et al: The effects of geometry errors in the reconstruction of iridium-192 seed implants. Med Phys 9:220, 1982
131. Russell JL, Carden JL, Herron HL: Dosimetry calculations for yttrium-90 used in the treatment of liver cancer. Endocuriether Hypertherm Oncol 4:171, 1988
132. Saw CB, Suntharalingam N: Reference dose rates for single and double plane ^{192}Ir implants. Med Phys 15:391, 1988
133. Saylor WL, Dillard M: Dosimetry of ^{137}Cs sources with the Fletcher/Suit gynecological applicator. Med Phys 3:117, 1976
134. Schell MC, Ling CC, Gromadzki ZC, Working KR: Dose distributions of model 6702 I-125 seeds in water. Int J Radiat Oncol Biol Phys 13:795, 1987
135. Schulz U, Busch M, Bormann U: Interstitial high-dose-rate brachytherapy: Principles, practice and first clinical experi-

ences with a new remote-controlled afterloading system using Ir-192. Int J Radiat Oncol Biol Phys 10:915, 1984

136. Sealy R, Buret E, Cleminshaw A, et al: Progress in the use of iodine therapy for tumors of the eye. Br J Radiol 53:1052, 1980
137. Shalek RJ, Stovall M: Implant Dosimetry, p 4. Houston, MD Anderson Hospital and Tumor Institute, 1967
138. Shalek RJ, Stovall M: Dosimetry in implant therapy. In Attix FH, Tochlin E (eds): Radiation Dosimetry, pp 776–798. New York, Academic Press, 1969
139. Shalek RJ, Stovall M, Sampiere VA: The radiation distribution and dose specification in volume implants of radioactive seeds. Am J Roentgenol Radiat Ther Nucl Med 77:863, 1956
140. Sharma SC, Williamson JF, Cytacki E: Dosimetry analysis of stereo and orthogonal reconstruction of interstitial implants. Int J Radiat Oncol Biol Phys 8:1803, 1982
141. Sievert RM: Eine methods zur messung von röntgen, radium und ultrastrahlung nebst einique untersuchungen uber die answendbarkeil derselben in der physik und der medizin. Acta Radiol Suppl [Stockh] 14:, 1932
142. Slanina J, Wannenmacher M: Interstitial radiotherapy with ^{198}Au seeds in the primary management of carcinoma of the oral tongue. Int J Radiol Biol Phys 8:1683, 1982
143. Smocovitis D, Young NEJ, Batho HR: Apparent absorption of the τ-rays of radium in water. Br J Radiol 40:771, 1967
144. Spencer RP (ed): Therapy in Nuclear Medicine. New York, Grune & Stratton, 1978
145. Spiers FW: Radioisotopes in the Human Body: Physical and Biological Effects, p 8. New York, Academic Press, 1968
146. Stallard HB: Malignant melanoma of the choroid treated with radioactive applicators. Ann R Coll Surg Engl 29:170, 1961
147. Stovall M, Shalek RJ: A review of computer techniques for dosimetry of interstitial and intracavitary radiotherapy. Comput Programs Biomed 2:125, 1972
148. Syed AM, Feder BH: Technique of afterloading interstitial implants. Radiol Clin 46:458, 1977
149. Ter-Pogossian M, Sherman AI, Arneson AN: An expanding fixed tandemovoid colpostat for the treatment of carcinoma of the cervix. Am J Obstet Gynecol 64:937, 1952
150. Thomas SR, Maxon HR, Kereiakes JG: *In vivo* quantitation of lesion radioactivity using external counting methods. Med Phys 3:253, 1976
151. Thomason C, Higgins P: Radial dose distributions of ^{192}Ir and ^{137}Cs seed sources. Med Phys 16:254, 1989
152. Tod MC, Meredith WJ: A dosage system for use in the treatment of cancer of the uterine cervix. Br J Radiol 11:809, 1938
153. Toepfer KD, Rosenow U: A simple function describing the absorption in platinum for dose rate calculations around radium applicators. Br J Radiol 53:1078, 1980
154. Tolbert DD, Reed SA: An examination of the consistency and accuracy of computerized brachytherapy dose predictions. Int J Radiat Oncol Biol Phys 7:675, 1981
155. Utley JF, Von Essen CF, Horn RA, Moeller JH: High dose rate after-loading brachytherapy in carcinoma of the uterine cervix. Int J Radiat Oncol Biol Phys 10:2259, 1984
156. Van Kleffens HJ, Star WM: Application of stereo x-ray photogrammetry (SRM) in the determination of absorbed dose values during intracavitary radiation therapy. Int J Radiat Oncol Biol Phys 5:557, 1979
157. Walstam R: Remotely controlled afterloading radiotherapy apparatus. Phys Med Biol 7:225, 1962
158. Wang JYC, Vora NL, Chou CK, et al: Intracatheter hyperthermia and iridium-192 radiotherapy in the treatment of bile duct carcinoma. Int J Radiat Oncol Biol Phys 14:353, 1988
159. Weaver KA: The dosimetry of ^{125}I seed eye plaques. Med Phys 13:78, 1986
160. Weeks KJ, Schulz RJ: Selenium-75: A potential source for use in high activity brachytherapy irradiators. Med Phys 13:728, 1986
161. Whyte GH: Attenuation of τ radiation in cylindrical geometry. Br J Radiol 28:635, 1955.
162. Williamson JF: Monte Carlo evaluation of specific dose constants in water for ^{125}I seeds. Med Phys 15:686, 1988
163. Williamson JF: The accuracy of the line and point dose approximation in Ir-192 dosimetry. Int J Radiat Oncol Biol Phys 12:409, 1986
164. Williamson JF, Morin RL, Khan FM: Dose calibrator response to brachytherapy sources: A Monte Carlo and analytic evaluation. Med Phys 10:135, 1983
165. Williamson JF, Qusintero FJ: Theoretical evaluation of dose distribution in water about models 6711 and 6702 ^{125}I seeds. Med Phys 15:891, 1988
166. Wood RG: Isodose curves around sealed sources. In Wood RG (ed): Computers in Radiotherapy: Physical Aspects, p 48. London, Butterworth, 1974
167. Wu A, Zwicker RD, Sternick ES: Tumor dose specification of I-125 seed implants. Med Phys 12:27, 1985
168. Yorke ED, Schell MC, Gaskill JW, et al: Using measurement dose distribution data for the Fletcher-Suit-Delclos colpostat in brachytherapy treatment planning. Int J Radiat Oncol Biol Phys 13:1413, 1987
169. Young MEJ, Batho HF: Dose tables for linear radium sources calculated by an electronic computer. Br J Radiol 37:38, 1964
170. Zeitz L, Kim SH, Kim JH, et al: Determination of relative biological effectiveness (RBE) of soft x-rays. Radiat Res 70:552, 1977
171. Zwicker RD, Schmidt-Ullrick R, Schiller B: Planning of Ir-192 seed implants for boost irradiation to the breast. Int J Radiat Oncol Biol Phys 11:2163, 1985

13

○ ○ ○ ● ● ●

Clinical Applications of Brachytherapy

Carlos A. Perez
Delia M. Garcia
Perry W. Grigsby
Jeffrey F. Williamson

The chapter was written with the collaboration of Luis Delclos in sections on general aspects of brachytherapy and special techniques for head and neck, gynecologic, male genital, and breast; and Karen Fu on remote control afterloading.

Brachytherapy was rapidly applied to the treatment of malignant tumors shortly after the discovery of radium by Marie Curie and Becquerel. In 1960, Henschke[85] published the first paper on afterloading brachytherapy in gynecologic malignancies and later in other tumors, followed shortly by a publication describing the Fletcher-Suit afterloading applicators.[41,229] New isotopes were also available for brachytherapy, including ^{198}Au, ^{60}Co, ^{137}Cs, ^{192}Ir, and a few years later, ^{125}I, ^{252}Cf, ^{241}Am, and ^{103}Pd.

Computers have enhanced the ability to carry out more precise dosimetric calculations. The combined administration of superficial and interstitial thermoradiation therapy in a variety of lesions has gained considerable popularity.[50] Eric Hall published excellent reviews of the biologic basis of brachytherapy and clinical implications of dose rate.[78] The distribution of dose around radioactive sources depends on the physical properties of the isotopes, including the encapsulation and activity of the sources, and on the inverse square law. At distances greater than three times the physical length of a source, the inverse square law applies within practical approximation; at closer distances the dosimetry is more complex.

SELECTION OF RADIOACTIVE MATERIAL

To meet all clinical situations, a variety of radioisotopes must be available in addition to the standard ^{137}Cs or radium sources.[43] Afterloaded ^{192}Ir wires or seeds in nylon strands are used in many sites (Fig 13-1). Because iridium has a relatively short half-life, the wires must be calibrated often, which involves a fairly elaborate bookkeeping system. Gold 198 grains or ^{125}I seeds are used occasionally for permanent implants in less-accessible tumor sites that require exposure at laparotomy or thoracotomy, such as the pancreas or the prostate. Newer isotopes introduced into the armamentarium of the radiation oncologist include palladium 103 (^{103}Pd), americium 241 (^{241}Am), and californium 152 (^{152}Cf).

The dose distribution within an ^{192}Ir implant is influenced by the assumed distribution of radioactivity within each source and oblique filtration of τ-rays by the active core and filter of the seed. Dose-volume histograms are used to calculate dose distribution data.[259]

The dosimetry with continuous ^{192}Ir wires or seed ribbons was compared using computer-generated dose distributions by Marinello and associates.[136] They concluded that seed ribbons yielded greater inhomogeneity in dose distribution with less flexibility and simplicity. However, if the seed ribbons are chosen so that the length of the seed is not too short compared with the distance separating the seeds (*i.e.*, ratio between the distances separated in the center of the seeds and length of seeds $\leq$1.5), the dosimetry of the Paris system remains valid. The authors did not advise the use of the seed ribbons with the Paris system. With continuous wire, the basal dose rates are defined geometrically and uniquely in the central plane, which can be calculated simply even with manual methods, but use of ^{192}Ir seeds requires a complex computer program for dose computations.

Anderson and associates[7] developed a nomographic planning guide to be used for planar implants of ^{192}Ir seeds in ribbons (Fig. 13-2). A graph was also generated for elongation correction factors, which is implicit in the use of the nomogram (Fig. 13-3).

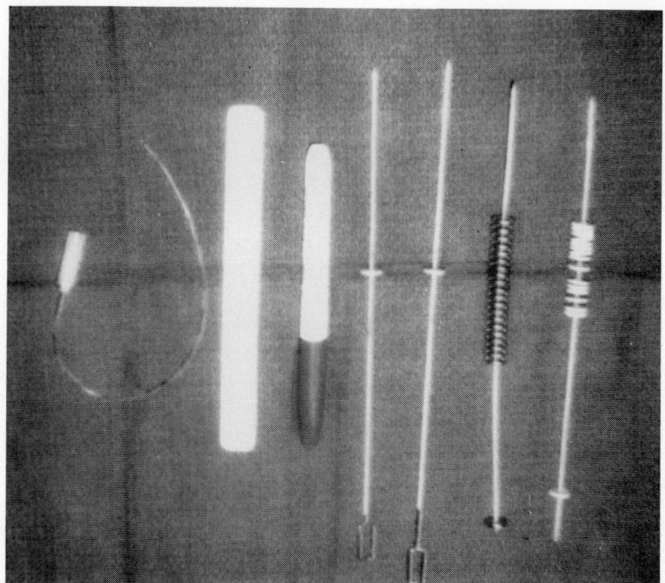

FIGURE 13–1. Operating room tray showing items used for interstitial implants (left to right): nylon tubing with dummy sources, metallic ruler, marking pencil, four plastic catheters with metallic guides and plastic buttons.

A simplified dosimetry system for ^{192}Ir volume implants was designed by Olch and co-workers.[161] Dose parameters of ^{192}Ir and ^{125}I seeds have been reported by Weaver and colleagues.[253]

As longer iridium wires have become available in many countries, the necessity for crossing one or both ends of the implant has almost disappeared, and Dumbbell and Indian Club rigid needles are seldom used. Sources of 0.66 mCi Ra eq/cm ("full intensity") or 0.5 mCi Ra eq/cm linear intensity are used for single-plane arrangements, and sources of 0.33 mCi Ra eq/cm ("half intensity") or 0.25 mCi Ra/cm linear intensity are used for multiple-plane or volume implants. The two intensities are combined for complex implants.[43]

AFTERLOADING INTERSTITIAL BRACHYTHERAPY

The flexible carrier method was first used with radon seeds by Hames in 1937[79] and later by Morton and associates,[154] who used cobalt sources. Afterloading was systematized by Henschke and colleagues[87] and Suit and Fletcher.[41]

Except for small and medium-sized tumors of the tongue and floor of the mouth, for which ^{137}Cs or ^{226}Ra needles have been used, afterloaded iridium is the more popular isotope for interstitial brachytherapy. Since the early 1960s, Pierquin and Chassagne[181] have popularized the Henschke techniques with personal modifications and have contributed the use of "hairpins" for afterloading with thicker iridium wires (0.5-mm diameter), mainly for lesions of the oral cavity and oropharynx. There are several other reports describing techniques and instrumentation for the use of afterloading interstitial therapy modalities employing radium and other isotopes, such as tantalum wires and ^{125}I seeds.[3,21,39,83,84,87,90,153,156,166]

Afterloading Iridium 192 Wires or Ribbons

Removable implants in the form of ^{192}Ir wires or ribbons are performed with stainless steel needles or flexible Teflon or nylon catheters with metallic guides (Fig. 13-4).

Stainless Steel Guides

Stainless steel or Teflon tubing of gauge 16 (1.6 mm in outer diameter) is cut into the desired length. The distal end of the tubing is beveled at a 30-degree or 45-degree angle and is crimped but not closed to hold the afterloaded iridium insert in place, allowing repositioning if necessary. A nylon or Teflon ball or a

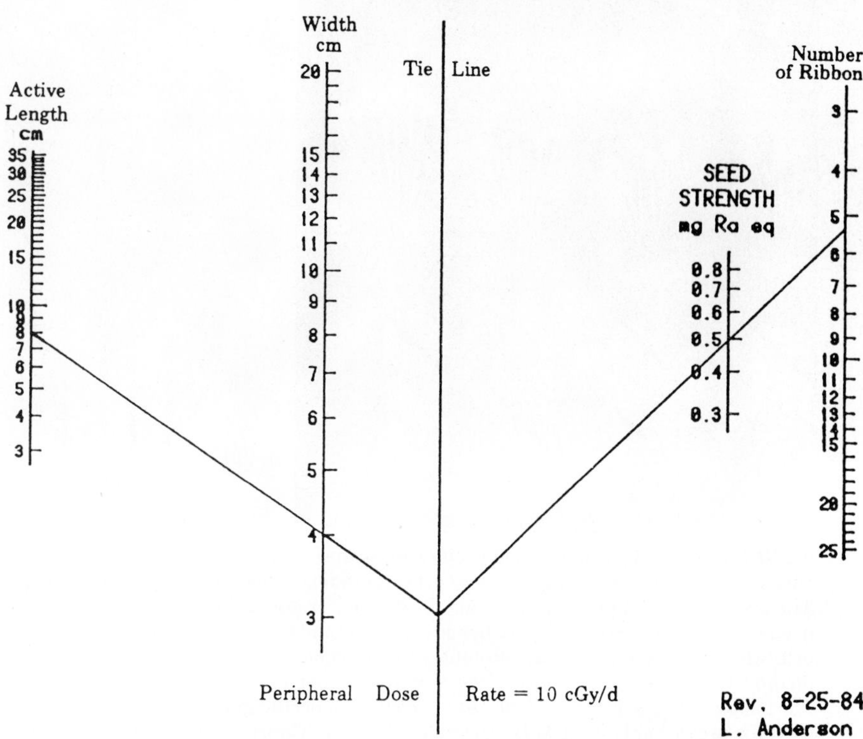

FIGURE 13–2. Planar implant nomograph expressing the relationships among length, width, seed strength, and the number of ribbons (of seeds at 1-cm intervals) to produce a peripheral reference dose-rate of 10 cGy/d. The added lines illustrate its use for L = 8 cm, W = 4 cm, and S = 0.5 mg Ra, indicating five ribbons. (Anderson LL, Hilaris BS, Wagner LK: Endocuriether Hypertherm Oncol 1:9, 1985)

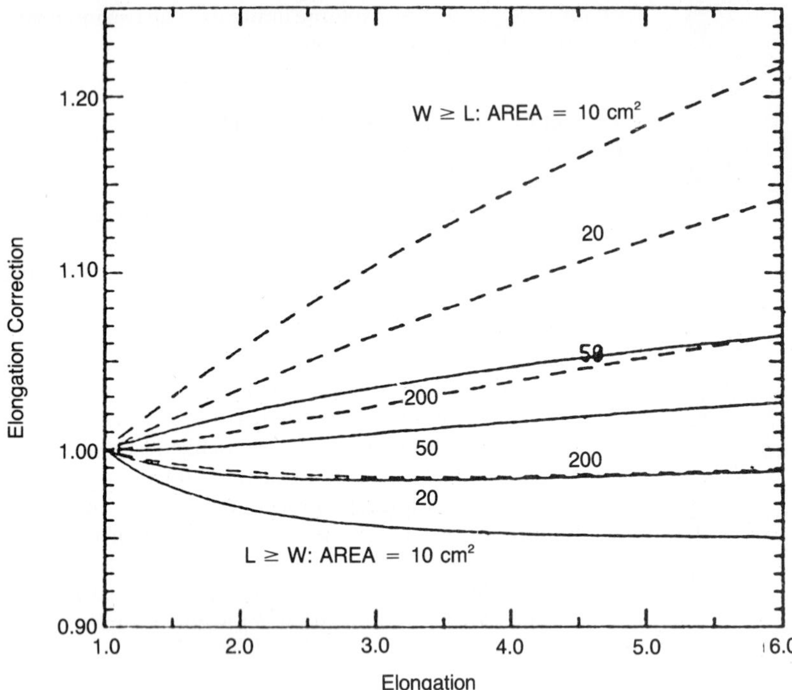

FIGURE 13–3. Elongation correction factor implicit in the use of the revised planar implant nomograph. (Anderson LL, Hilaris BS, Wagner LK: Endocuriether Hypertherm Oncol 1:9, 1985)

metallic button is fitted snugly at the proximal end (Fig. 13-5). In this Teflon ball or metallic button, there is a hole for threading the suture, and a lead bead is added for x-ray localization.[79, 166] Figure 13-6 shows the procedures followed for insertion and afterloading of the iridium guides. This type of rigid guide is used in tumors approachable from one side only (*e.g.*, tumors of the collumnela and nasal septum, base of the tongue, female urethra, and anal margin). This technique can also be used to treat involved lymph nodes in the neck and the parotid gland and for a boost dose to primary breast cancer.

Through-and-Through Plastic Tubing Technique

The through-and-through technique is used if a tumor can be transfixed from either of two sides (*e.g.*, lower and upper lip, buccal mucosa, breast, or neck masses). In locations in which the

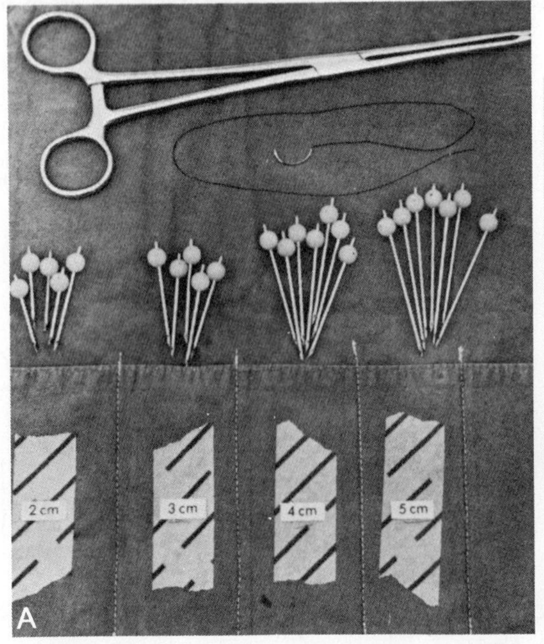

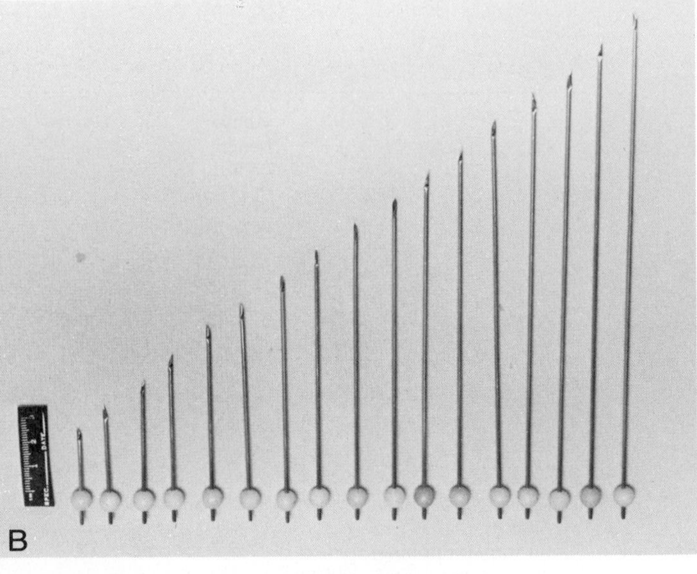

FIGURE 13–4. (**A**) Stainless steel needles are manufactured to any desired length; a Teflon or nylon button with a hole for suturing and a lead pellet for radiographic identification are incorporated at the ball. The distal end is crimped to position and holds the ^{192}Ir insert. The needles are inserted with a standard needle-inserting forceps (Radium Chemical Co., NY) and sutured into place with a C-0 suture. The Teflon ball, which causes less trauma, substitutes for the metal flange used earlier. (Delclos L: Afterloading method for interstitial gamma-ray therapy. In Fletcher GH [ed]: Textbook of Radiotherapy, 3rd ed. Philadelphia, Lea & Febiger, 1980) (**B**) Stainless steel needle guides of various lengths with Teflon balls used for breast implants at M.D. Anderson Hospital. (Courtesy of Luis Delclos, M.D.)

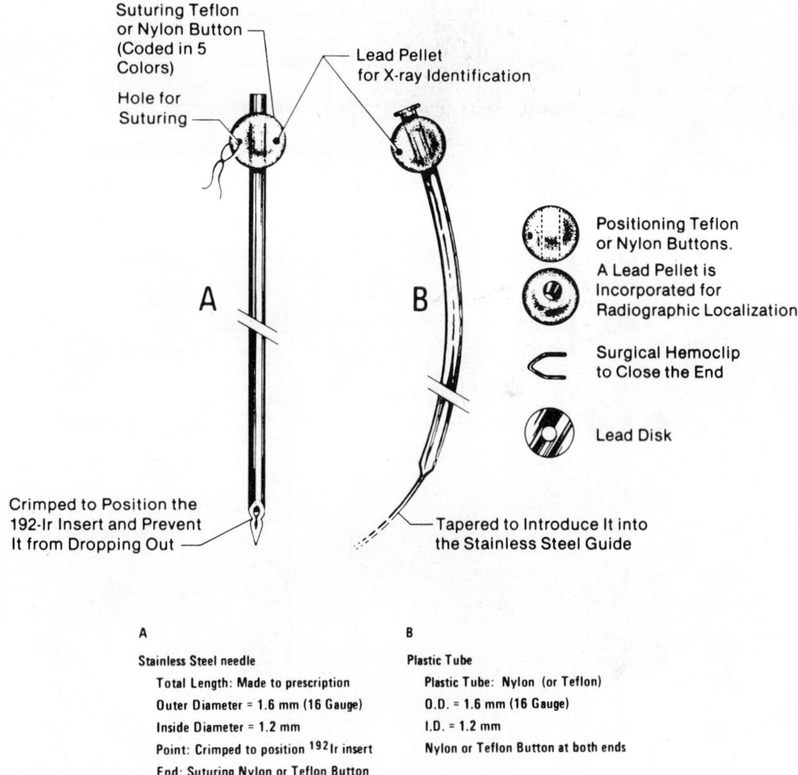

FIGURE 13–5. (**A**) Stainless steel afterloadable needle with plastic, Teflon, or nylon buttons. The needles are made to any desired length. (**B**) Teflon or nylon tube, closed-end variety, used for the through-and-through technique. A stainless steel guide of the same outside diameter is inserted first. (Delclos L: In Johnson DE, Boileau A [eds]: Genitourinary Tumors: Fundamental Principles and Surgical Techniques. New York, Grune & Stratton, 1982)

guide can be placed through the tumor or normal tissues, the 16-gauge metallic guides are inserted at the appropriate distances to achieve the desired distribution (Fig. 13-7). The lead of the nylon tube that will contain the ^{192}Ir nylon thread is inserted through the metallic guide and is progressively pushed all the way through, along with the nylon tube. When the nylon tube is in place, a metallic button is crimped or a Teflon ball is placed at the distal end to secure it. When all the nylon tubing has been implanted, the desired length of the active wire is measured by using a "dummy" wire (to 0.5 cm below the skin at the opposite end) and cut a few centimeters longer, so it will protrude beyond the skin and will be easier to manipulate. After localization x-ray films are taken, with inactive wires or seeds used to determine the length and position of the tubes, the ^{192}Ir active sources are prepared and inserted, and the proximal end of the tubing is crimped with a metallic button. We specify each dummy and corresponding active source wire with different color threads and buttons and specific radiopaque patterns to identify each tube or loading on the patient or the implant radiographs.

If thermoradiation therapy is planned, the technique is modified, using Teflon catheters, a B-D lock, and a special plastic insert to secure the catheter to the skin. An adapter that locks in the Teflon catheter holds the nylon tubing with the ^{192}Ir in place.

Afterloading of the active sources with stainless steel needles or flexible guides can be done after the patient is back in the hospital room, avoiding radiation exposure within the operating and recovery rooms.

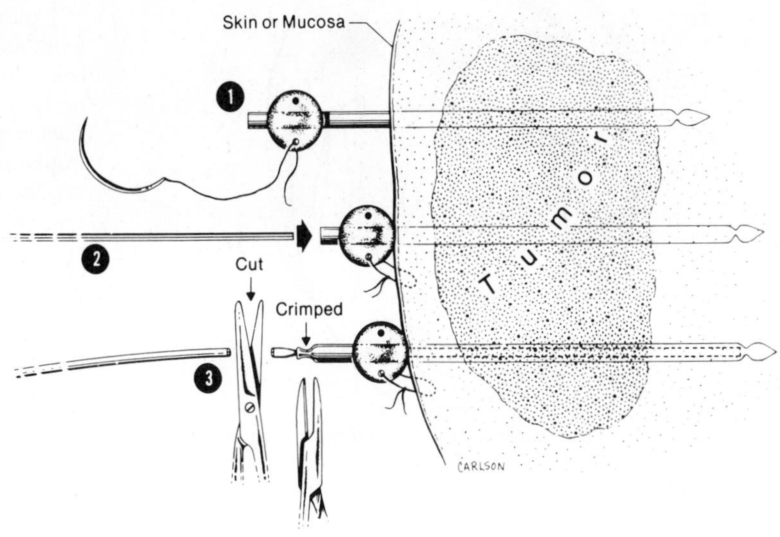

FIGURE 13–6. One-end implant technique for tumors approached from one side: (1) insertion of an empty stainless steel needle with a nylon button. The needle is sutured to the skin or mucosa through a hole in the nylon button; (2) the iridium wire mounted in a plastic tube carrier is introduced into the stainless steel needle; and (3) the open end is crimped to close it. The plastic tube carrier is cut, leaving about 0.5 cm protruding to facilitate removal of the iridium wire later. For removal, cut the suture, remove the needle with the iridium inside, and deposit the iridium in the leaded carrier for transportation and further manipulation in the laboratory or uncrimp the end of the stainless steel needle with a specially designed uncrimper and pull out the plastic tube carrier with the iridium insert inside. (Delclos L: Afterloading method for interstitial gamma-ray therapy. In Fletcher GH [ed]: Textbook of Radiotherapy, 3rd ed. Philadelphia, Lea & Febiger, 1980)

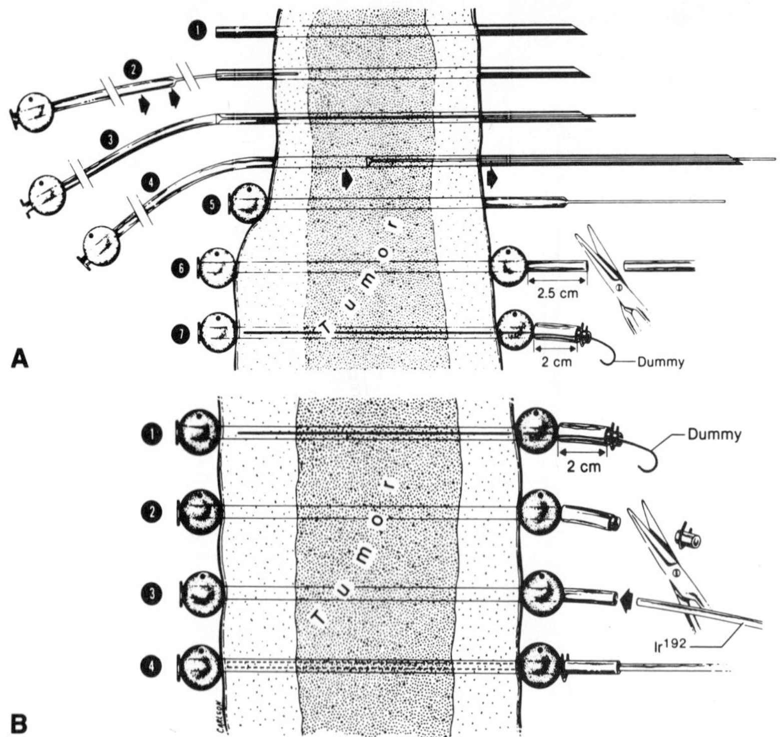

FIGURE 13–7. Through-and-through implant technique for tumors approachable from two sides. (**A**) To insert (1) through the stainless steel guide, (2) the leader (tapered end) of the nylon implant tube is introduced and (3) passed down the guide until the plastic tube is in contact with the end of the stainless steel guide; (4) both the stainless steel guide and the tapered end (leader) of the nylon implant tube are pulled through the other end; (5) after the stainless steel guide is out, the nylon tube is pulled until the closed-end nylon implant tube with the nylon button is in contact with the surface; (6) another nylon button is inserted at the opposite end of the nylon implant tube and the nylon tube is cut at about 2.5 cm from the nylon button surface; and (7) a larger nylon tube 2 cm long is placed on top of the protruding end of the nylon tube. A dummy wire is placed inside, protruding 1 cm, for localization. A hemoclip is placed at the end to prevent the nylon tube from slipping out during manipulation. (**B**) To load, (1) the dummy wire is removed; (2) the nylon end of the implant tube is cut with the hemoclip; (3) the ^{192}Ir wire in plastic tube carrier (insert) is inserted into the nylon implant tube; and (4) a hemoclip is placed near the nylon button to close the nylon tube. (Modified from Delclos L: Afterloading method for interstitial gamma-ray therapy. In Fletcher GH [ed]: Textbook of Radiotherapy, 3rd ed. Philadelphia, Lea & Febiger, 1980)

Suturing of Needles or Guides and Plastic Buttons

The needles or guides are sutured to the implanted tissues in various ways (Fig. 13-8). Separate 2-0 silk or cotton sutures permanently attached to a half-circle taperpoint needle, which is threaded through the loop of the color-coded silk before insertion, are preferred.

Color-coded silk threads are used to identify the different lengths and strengths of the radioactive sources. This facilitates selection of sources at the time of the implant and the orderly removal of the implant.

Needles or buttons holding the catheters should be sutured systematically. For a double-plane implant, all suturing is done outside the needle rows to simplify removal.

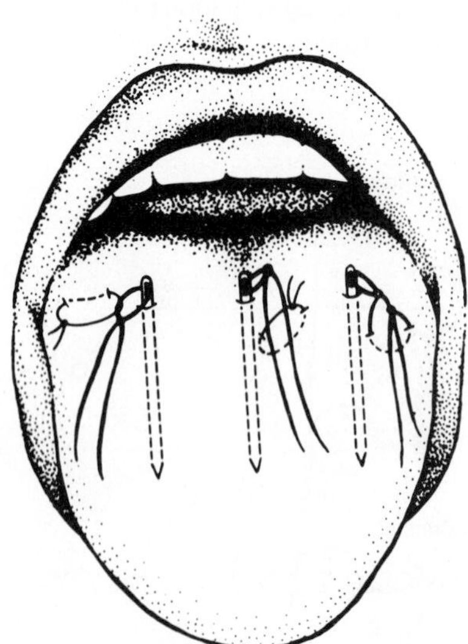

FIGURE 13–8. Three ways of suturing radium or cesium needles in place. (Fletcher GH, MacComb WS: Radiation Therapy in the Management of Cancers of the Oral Cavity and Oropharynx. Springfield, IL, Charles C Thomas, 1962)

Removable Iridium 192 Hairpin Technique

The physical characteristics of the removable hairpin or Paris technique have been described.[180] Metallic gutter guides have been constructed to facilitate insertion of the iridium wires (Fig. 13-9). The usual separation of the legs is 1.2 cm, although 0.9 or 1.5 cm can be used. The standard gutter lengths are 2.5, 3, 4, or 5 cm. Iridium wire ends are inserted along the gutters and held in place with a fine-tip clamp while the gutter guide is removed (Fig. 13-10). Gutter guides allow predictable insertion of the hairpin, which yields an acceptable geometry and homogeneous dose distribution of the implant (Fig. 13-11). The gutter guide technique is used primarily in smaller tumors of the oral cavity and in the anal region.

Removable Iodine 125 Plastic Tube Implants

Clarke and co-workers[32,33] described a temporary removable ^{125}I plastic tube implant technique. The seeds were 4.5 mm long, and the interseed spacing within the ribbons (from seed center to seed center) ranged from 4.5 mm (seeds back to back) to 12.5 mm (8-mm spacers). The operative technique using hollow, stainless steel, 17-gauge trocars is identical to the ^{192}Ir implant procedure. Dosimetric considerations for both isotopes are similar. However, the ^{125}I tubes must have a greater diameter to house the ^{125}I seed ribbons, which are larger than the ^{192}Ir ribbons. The seed ribbons are prepared by loading loose seeds into the hollow ribbons; the seeds are separated by spacers and held in position by a "pusher." The open end of the seed ribbon is heated for sealing. The seed separation depends on the activity, the geometry of the implant, and the desired dose rate, which is individualized for each patient and determined after the procedure in the operating room is completed.

Compared with the ^{192}Ir implants, use of the ^{125}I seed ribbons requires additional time by the physicist or dosimetrist to assemble and disassemble the ribbons. However, this is offset

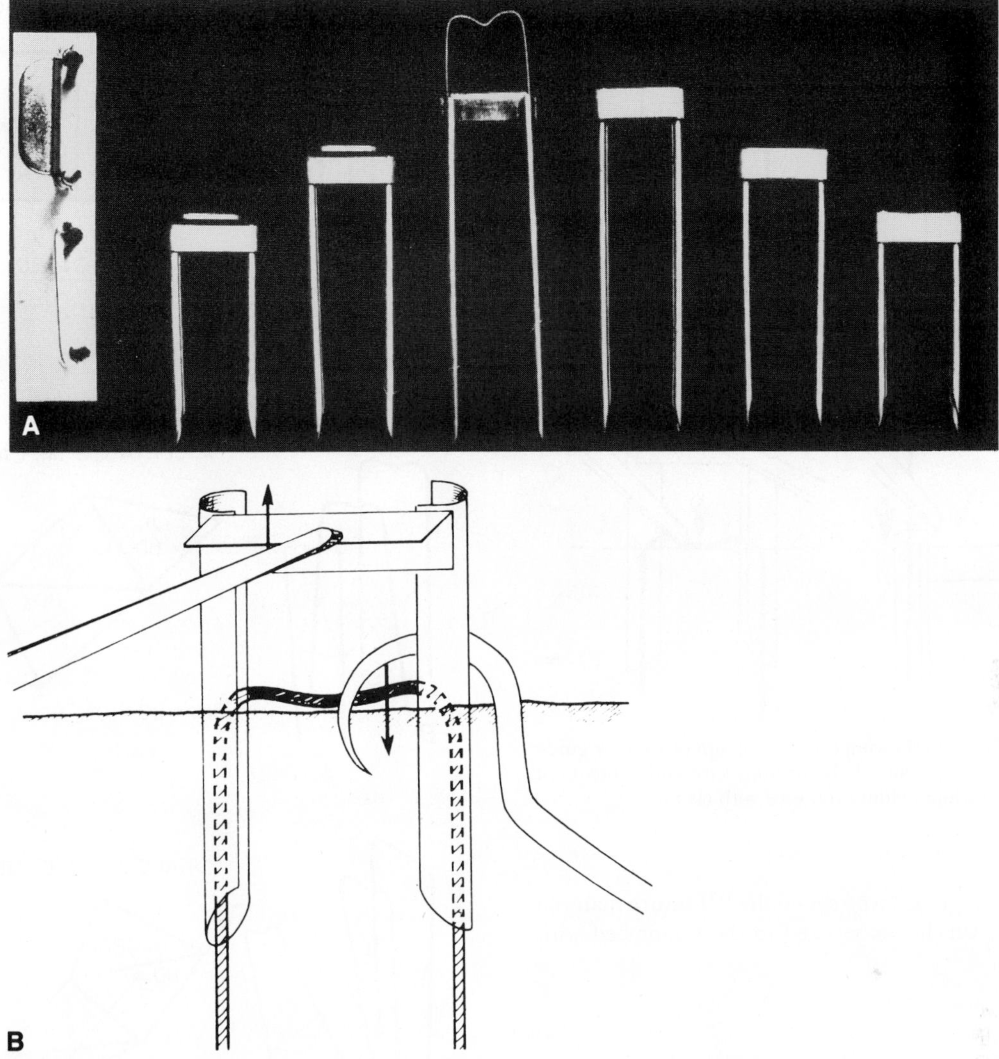

FIGURE 13–9. (**A**) Hairpins of different sizes and iridium wire (center). (**B**) Diagram of gutter guide used by Pierquin and small hook to hold the iridium wire in place while the guide is being removed with a clamp. (Pierquin B, Wilson J-F, Chassagne D: Modern Brachytherapy. New York, Masson, 1987)

by a compensatory decrease in other tasks that are required for preparing ^{192}Ir seeds or wires. Because of the lower energy of the ^{125}I, shielding is easily accomplished, which enhances safety during the operation and for the nurses caring for the patient.

Permanent Interstitial Iodine 125 Implants

A system with ten ^{125}I seeds contained within a braided synthetic absorbable carrier has been developed for implants in a shallow plane of tissue or for a tumor site that is inaccessible to standard implant devices.[81,212] The ^{125}I seeds are spaced at 1.0 cm, center to center. The carrier retains a half-circle, taper-point surgical needle. Each strand of 10 seeds is contained within a stainless steel tubular ring, which effectively shields radiation. The unopened package has a surface dose rate of less than 0.2 mR/hour for a loading of ten 0.5-mCi seeds. It can be handled and stored without additional shielding.

In circumstances in which the supplied surgical needle is unsuitable, it can be replaced by a tie-on needle (*e.g.*, a French spring-eye needle). The placement of the strands and spacing of the seeds should follow appropriate dosimetric considerations (Fig. 13-12A). The absorbable carrier material and ^{125}I seeds are implanted in the tumor tissues by successively advancing the needle and gently pulling the carrier, as illustrated in Figure 13-12B.

The carrier material is absorbed by body tissue; the rate depends on the nature of the implanted tissue. Intramuscular implantation studies in rats showed that the absorption of the carrier is minimal until day 40 after surgery, and it is essentially complete between days 60 and 90.

Goffinet and co-workers[68] reported 64 intraoperative ^{125}I implants with absorbable Vicryl suture carriers performed in 53 patients with head and neck cancer, many of them with recurrent disease after initial, definitive radiation therapy. Among 14 patients who had received no prior therapy, local control was achieved in ten (71%), and five (40%) of them were alive between 2 and 45 months after therapy. Among 34 patients who had received prior therapy, local control was achieved in 20 (59%), and no recurrences developed in any head and neck sites in 13 (38%). Complications occurred in seven (50%) of 14 patients treated definitively, including skin ulceration and intraoral and intrapharyngeal ulceration, which usually healed. Of 34 patients who had ^{125}I implants after prior therapy, seven (20%) had complications.

A variation of this technique was described in detail by

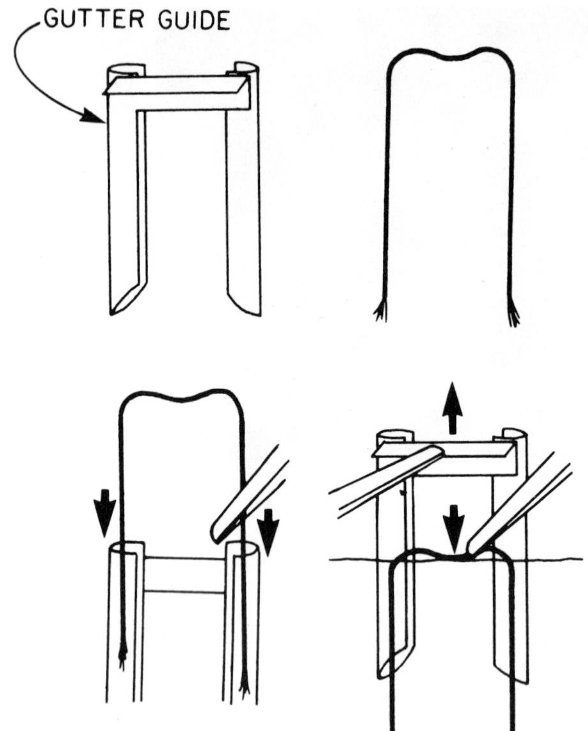

FIGURE 13–10. Diagram showing the basic design of a gutter guide and the technique for insertion of the iridium wire and subsequent removal of the guide while holding the wire with clamp.

Greenblatt and colleagues,[70] who sewed the ^{125}I suture material through Gelfoam, which was secured to the tumor bed with special clips.

TEMPLATES

A variety of templates have been designed to more easily place the interstitial sources and obtain more homogeneous doses with implants.

Syed-Neblett Templates

Several Syed-Neblett templates have been devised and are marketed by Alpha Omega Services, Inc. The template is primarily used for gynecologic tumors. It consists of two Lucite plates joined by six screws that tighten to grasp as many as 38 afterloading, hollow, stainless steel needles. An additional six needles fit into grooves of a 2-cm-diameter plastic vaginal cylinder that is placed inside an opening in the middle of the template. These needles are arranged in concentric circles or arcs with a spacing of 1 cm between adjacent needles (Fig. 13-13). A 4-cm × 10-cm area can be implanted in a butterfly distribution. The 17-gauge needles supplied with the templates are 20 cm long, but they can be shortened to treat more shallow areas. The vaginal cylinder has a central opening for placement of a tandem if desired.

A rectal template is similar to the one just described, but the two plates contain three concentric circular rings with a total of 36 needles with 1-cm spacing. Cylindric volumes with diameters of 2, 4, or 6 cm can be implanted. A rectal tube can be placed in the central hole if necessary, but this hole can be left open if the template is placed in an area not covering the anus, such as the vulva.

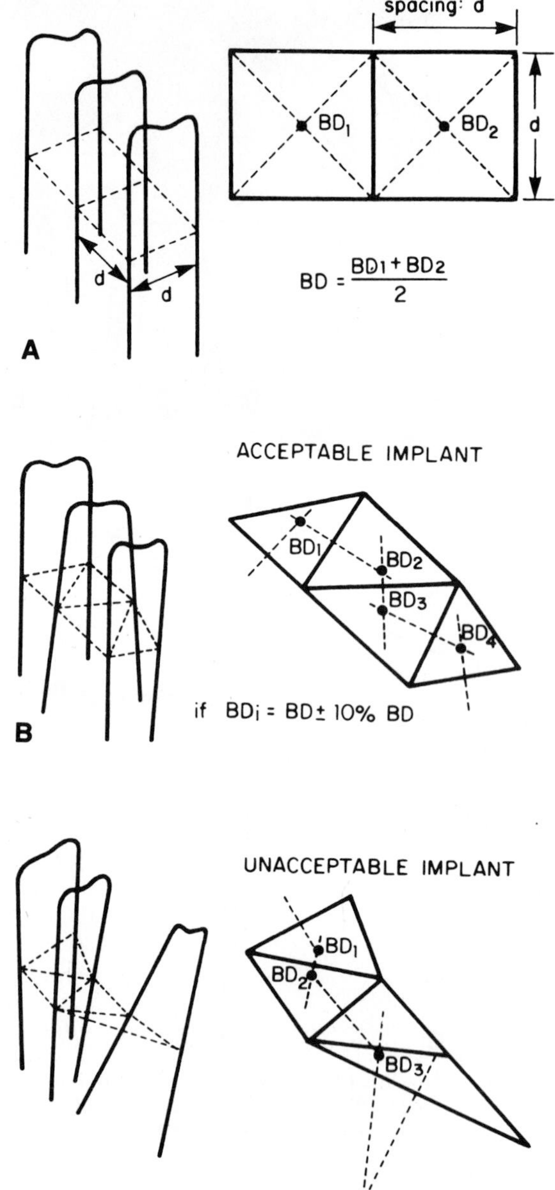

FIGURE 13–11. Diagrams illustrating dosimetry principles of the Paris system. (**A**) For implants containing more than one plane, equidistant radioactive lines imply that the intersections of the lines with the central plane will be arranged as the apices of equilateral triangles or as the corners of squares. Calculation of the basal dose rate (BD) is made at various points. Dose is specified along an isodose surface defined as a given proportion of the basal dose rate calculated inside the implant volume (reference isodose, which should encompass target volume as closely as possible). In practice, the value of the reference isodose is fixed at 85% of the basal dose rate. (**B**) Geometry of acceptable implant. (**C**) Geometry of unacceptable implant.

Syed and associates[231] described a prostate template used to guide the insertion of metallic source guides transperineally. The template consists of two concentric rings with radii of 1 cm and 2 cm, containing 6 and 12 guide holes, respectively (Fig 13-14). As many as 18 metallic source guides (17-gauge, 20-cm-long needles) are inserted transperineally through the prostate and seminal vesicles as indicated. The tips of the guides are usually 1 cm above the level of the bladder neck. The template is fixed to the perineum by "00" silk sutures, and the space between the perineum and the template is filled with a gauze soaked in antibiotic cream.

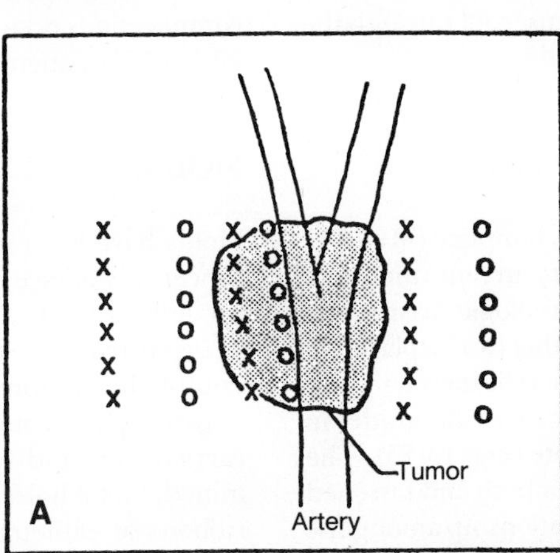

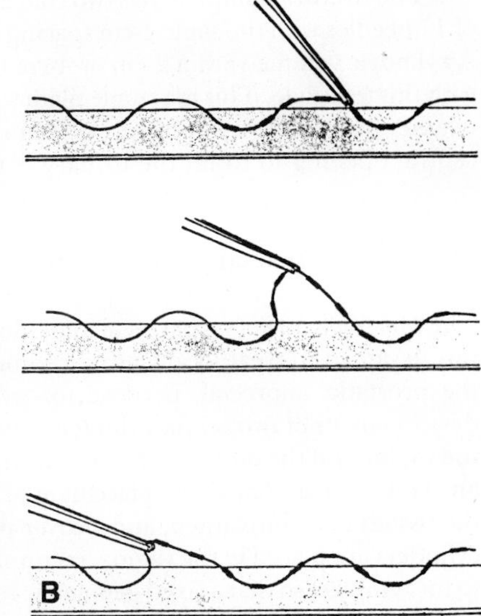

FIGURE 13–12. (**A**) Preimplant plan. The area is determined, allowing adequate margins. A pattern that sharply bends the carrier must be avoided because the seeds are unable to follow the implant pathway. (**B**) Method to pull the leader at the needle end for implantation of the absorbable carrier. In one pull parallel to the plane of the simulated tissue, a few seeds are advanced through the first bite and out of the simulated tissue to form a small loop. Grasping the carrier material with forceps advances the loop containing seeds through the second and subsequent bites. (Courtesy of Minnesota Mining and Manufacturing Co., St. Paul, MN)

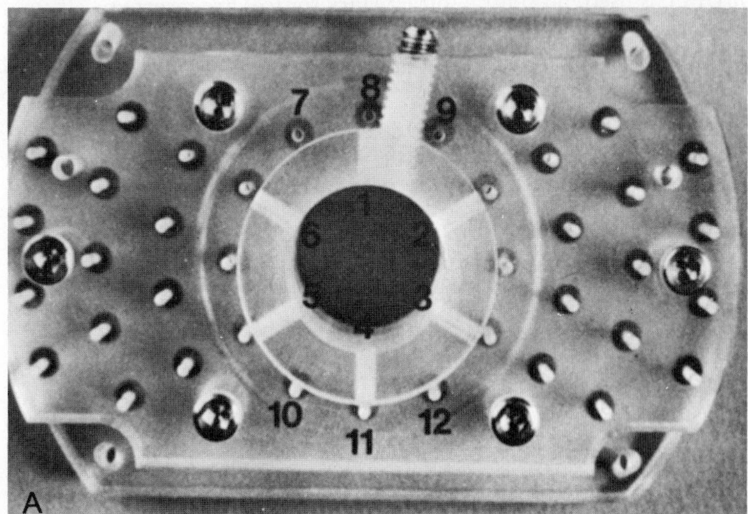

FIGURE 13–13. Syed-type perineal template used for interstitial parametrial irradiation. (Aristizabal SA, Valencia A, Ocampo G, et al: Endocuriether Hypertherm Oncol 1:41, 1985)

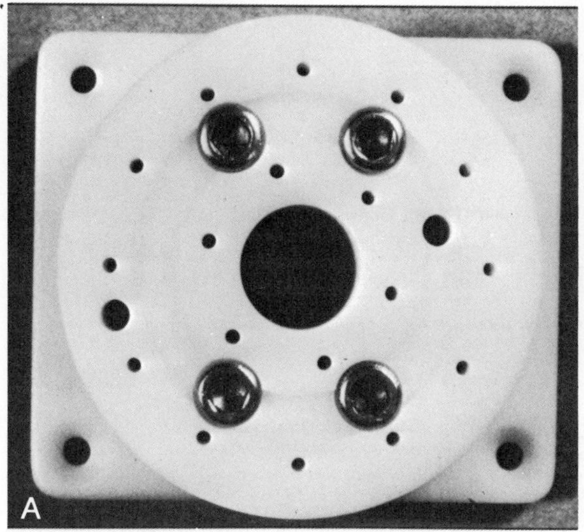

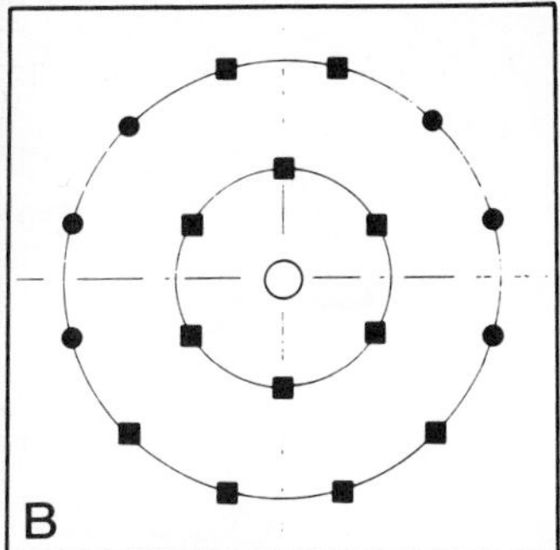

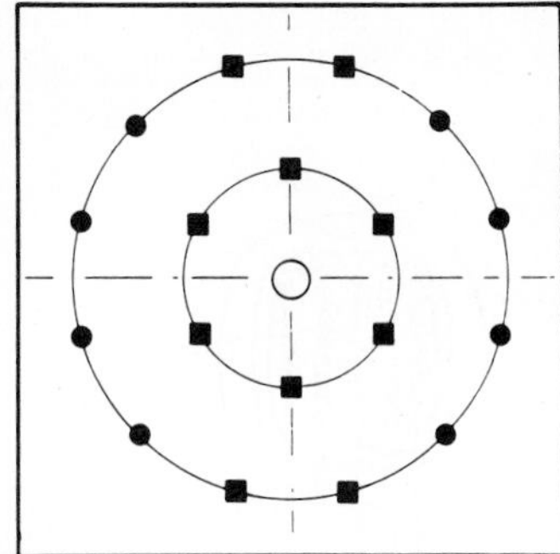

FIGURE 13–14. (**A**) Syed/Neblett prostate template. (Syed AMN, Puthawala AA, Tansey LA, et al: Temporary iridium-192 implantation in the management of carcinoma of the prostate. In Hilaris BS, Batata MA [eds]: Brachytherapy Oncology—1983, p 83. New York, Memorial Sloan-Kettering Cancer Center, 1983) (**B**) Example of different intensity sources used with Syed template to decrease doses to urethra, bladder, and rectum. (Puthawala AA, Syed AM, Tansey LA, et al: Endocuriether Hypertherm Oncol 1:25, 1985)

The urethral template has two concentric rings with a total of 17 needles with the same 1-cm spacing as the rectal template. A cylindric volume with a 2-cm or 4-cm diameter is implanted with this template. This is a single plate with no machine screws to other plates. A Foley urethral catheter is inserted through the central opening to drain the urinary bladder.

Martinez Universal Perineal Interstitial Template

The Martinez universal perineal interstitial template (MUPIT) was designed to treat locally advanced or recurrent tumors in the prostatic, anorectal, perineal, or gynecologic areas. The device consists of two acrylic cylinders, one that can be placed in the vagina and the other in the rectum, an acrylic template with an array of holes that allows placement of the metallic guides in the tissues to be implanted, and a cover plate (Fig. 13-15). The cylinders are placed in the vagina, rectum, or both and fastened to the template so that a fixed geometric relationship among the tumor volume, normal structures, and source placement is preserved throughout the course of the implantation. When the MUPIT is used, no central intracavitary sources are inserted, except in some patients requiring an intrauterine tandem beyond the volume treated with the interstitial sources.

Gaddis and associates[62] reported their experience with perineal interstitial implants in 75 women with squamous cell carcinoma of the cervix. Follow-up ranged from 3 to 60 months, with a median of 17 months. The recurrence rate in the pelvis was 46.2% (12 of 26) for patients with Stage IIIB and 20% (five of 25) for patients with Stage IIB tumors. The non-tumor-associated fistula rate was 13.3%. Severe (grade 3) nonfistula complications occurred in an additional six patients; thus 16 of 75 (21.3%) patients had severe morbidity.

MOLDS

Molds have been used for the treatment of patients with skin cancer of the face or hands or other anatomic locations[170] and for lesions of the lip and oral cavity. The mold can be constructed from plastic or acrylic, after obtaining the configuration of the anatomic area with a liquid plaster cast to form a negative plaster mold. Computations for the dose desired are carried out, and optimal placement of the sources is determined. Small holes are drilled in the mold to contain the nylon ribbons or catheters with the radioactive sources or the rigid radium (or cesium) needles. These techniques have been extensively used by Paterson[170] and Fletcher.[56]

Marchese and associates[134] described a technique using ^{125}I or ^{192}Ir sources embedded in Gelfoam to permanently implant small residual tumors or tumor margins in anatomic locations where standard implant techniques may not be feasible (*e.g.*, tissues adjacent to major blood vessels, the vertebral column, or the brain). The technique consists of preparing an adequate size

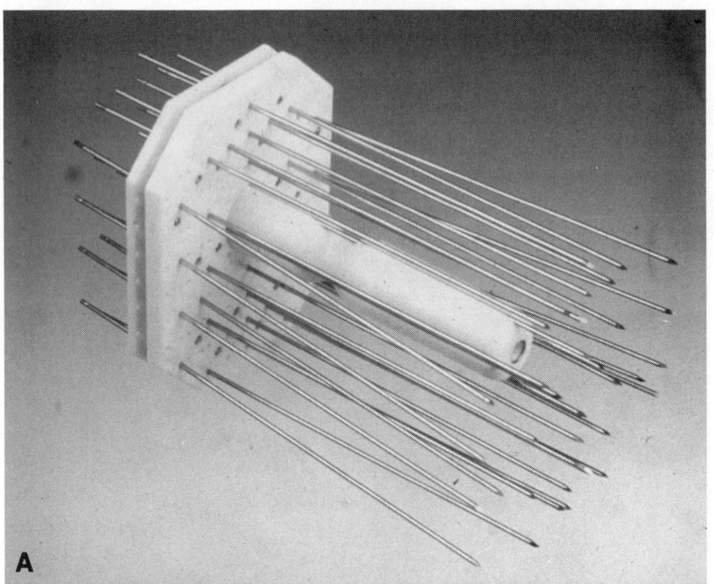

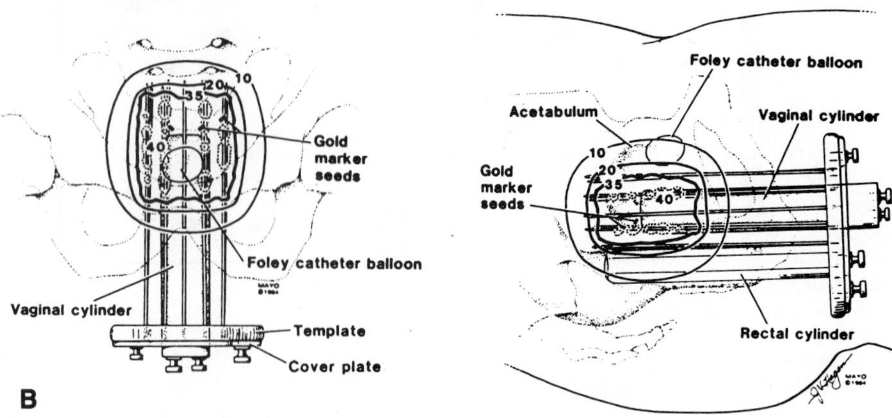

FIGURE 13–15. (**A**) Martinez Universal Perineal Interstitial Template. (Courtesy of Dr. Alvaro Martinez, William Beaumont Hospital, Detroit, MI) (**B**) Diagrammatic representation in coronal and sagittal planes of the same template. (Martinez A, Edmundson GK, Cox RS, et al: Int J Radiat Oncol Biol Phys 11:391, 1985)

and thickness of Gelfoam and fixing it to the implant site. When the nomogram for ^{125}I seeds or dose calculations for ^{192}Ir seeds are used, the number, configuration of the planes, and intensity of the radioactive sources are determined according to the dose to be delivered. Catheters with ^{125}I seeds inserted into the Gelfoam are placed at 1-cm intervals. The absorbable Gelfoam mesh is sutured with catgut absorbable material, and both are absorbed over 6 weeks. With ^{192}Ir, provision must be made for removal of the catheters.

Acrylic molds have been used for the treatment of vaginal or uterine cervical lesions. Lichter and colleagues[127] described the use of thermoplastic vaginal molds. The locations of the channels for insertion of the sources and for the central tandem (if desired) are determined by the topography of the tumor. The central tandem can be placed in the uterus or the vagina, through the vaginal mold, and locked into position.

High-Dose-Rate Surface Molds

Use of surface molds is being revived with high-dose-rate remote-control afterloading devices. This modality can effectively treat cutaneous neoplasias, particularly in the head and neck (Fig. 13-16), trunk, dorsum of the hand, or lower extremities. Doses ranging from 1500 cGy to 2000 cGy in one or two fractions to 4500 cGy to 5000 cGy in ten to 15 fractions are delivered, depending on the size of the tumor and expected cosmetic results.[115]

IMPLANTATION TECHNIQUES

Anesthesia

Although small implants can sometimes be done under local anesthesia, general anesthesia is better for good visualization, palpation of the tumor, and the patient's comfort.

General anesthesia is administered by nasotracheal intubation for implants of the oral cavity and lips. A tracheostomy is initially performed in patients with extensive oral cavity lesions requiring large implants and for all tumors of the glossopalatine sulcus, base of the tongue, or vallecula, because the associated edema may cause serious breathing difficulties.[43]

Breast implants can be done with local or general anesthesia. For brachytherapy procedures in the pelvis, patients are placed in the lithotomy position, and general or spinal anesthesia is administered. Occasionally a pudendal nerve block may be used.

Preoperative and Postoperative Orders

The radiation oncologist must assess the condition of the patient the day before the brachytherapy procedure is performed and log in the chart the detailed instructions for the nursing personnel, including tests results to be obtained, medications to be administered, preparation procedures for the operating room, and radiation safety measures. After the procedure is completed, a description of it should be recorded in the chart, including a diagram illustrating the exact location and pattern of placement and the characteristics of the sources (*e.g.*, length, strength). Unambiguous postoperative orders are necessary, including the time of removal of radioactive sources, appropriate medications, and special precautions.

RADIATION SAFETY IN THE OPERATING ROOM

If radioactive sources are prepared in the operating room, a workbench with shielding should be placed in one corner of the room to protect everyone except the brachytherapy technician from radiation exposure. The workbench is designed with a frontal working area with an L-shaped lead screen to protect the trunk, lower extremities, and medial aspect of the technician's arms. In addition, a leaded-glass screen reduces exposure to the eyes.

Behind the barrier, there should be a lead well to store the remaining radioactive material while the individual needles, wires, grains, or seeds are being prepared for insertion into the patient. The bench is covered with sterile drapes.

Sterilization of the radioactive sources is done by soaking the radium or cesium needles in a germicidal solution like Cydex. Gold-grain magazines and iridium wires are sterilized by gas.

When using radioactive sources, the operating surgeon, assistants, and anesthesiologists should work behind individual lead barriers. Exposure to the eyes and hands can be reduced only by distance and by dexterity gained through experience. All radioactive sources should be handled with long instruments. Because most procedures are performed with afterloading techniques, exposure to the fingers during manipulation is minimal.

The details of protective procedures used during the preparation and transportation of radioactive materials and the regulations governing them were described in detail by Pierquin and associates[185] and Van Roosenbeek and Delclos.[244]

Feeding the Patient with an Implant

Although some patients undergoing head and neck implants can be allowed to sip a liquid formula through a straw, most are fed through a nasogastric tube. This is mandatory if the lips have been sutured together for implants involving the buccal commissure.

Removal of Implants

Small implants of the anterior oral cavity can be removed in a treatment room and should not be removed in the patient's room. For patients with standard needles directly implanted in the posterior tongue and for less-than-cooperative patients, it is better to remove the implant in the operating room with adequate lighting, suction, and assistants and with the patient under general anesthesia. Bleeding at the time of needle removal is infrequent, but when it occurs, it may cause the patient or the assisting staff to panic. Firm and steady pressure with a finger on a compress over the bleeding point for several minutes usually provides adequate treatment; occasionally, suturing with absorbable catgut may be necessary. It is not uncommon for the needle thread to be accidentally cut instead of the suture, and trying to find the needle requires an optimal surgical environment because the task is complex and time consuming. Radiographic localization of the needle may be required before the needle base can be surgically exposed.

The afterloading nylon tubing is more easily removed. For the sake of radiation protection, it is advisable to uncrimp the metallic buttons and carefully remove the radioactive sources, which are accounted for and immediately placed in a portable

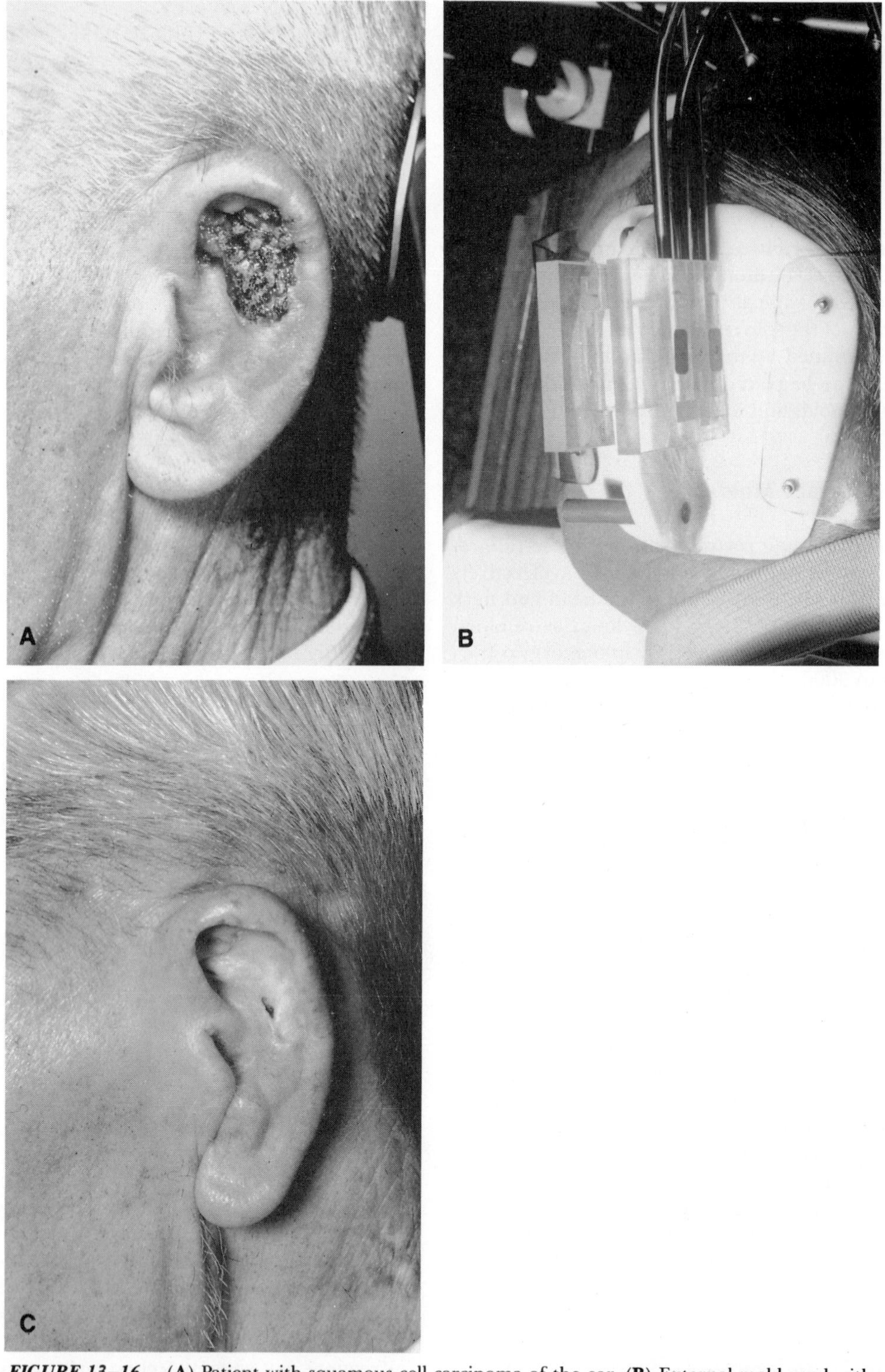

FIGURE 13–16. (**A**) Patient with squamous cell carcinoma of the ear. (**B**) External mold used with a high-dose-rate remote-control afterloading device. (**C**) Posttreatment photograph showing complete tumor regression and satisfactory cosmetic results. (Courtesy of C.A. Joslin, University of Leeds, Regional Radiotherapy Centre, Cookridge Hospital, Leeds, UK)

safe or shielded cart. Then each tube is removed by freeing one end. For oral cavity or oropharynx implants, we prefer to cut the two ends of the tubing at the skin and pull it out through the oral cavity. A previously tied silk thread inside the cavity on the nylon tube loop helps in this maneuver.

After all needles or tubes are removed, the implanted site may be gently palpated to verify that all implant materials have been removed. After the radioactive sources are taken out of the room, the patient and the room should be surveyed with a Geiger counter or other radiation detector to make sure there is no residual radioactivity.

Appropriate notes on the patient's chart, isotope form, and radiation survey form should be completed to record all procedures performed.

BRACHYTHERAPY TECHNIQUES FOR SPECIFIC SITES

Interstitial Brain Implants

Brachytherapy may allow delivery of interstitial radiation boosts to primary brain tumors after conventional external radiation therapy or for recurrent brain tumors.

Patients with primary malignant brain tumors who received initial doses of more than 5000 cGy of radiation to the whole brain survived 20.5 weeks longer than patients treated by surgery.[246] Walker and colleagues,[247] analyzing the Brain Tumor Study Group data, showed stepwise increments in survival in patients receiving 5000, 5500, or 6000 cGy. However, higher irradiation doses may significantly increase the risk of brain necrosis.

At some institutions, permanent implants have been used, but removable implants tend to be more popular. In our opinion, the advantages of the removable implants include greater control of the dose of irradiation because the source placement can be rearranged to improve dose distribution and the time of the implant is controlled by the operator, decreased possibility of migration of the radioactive sources by necrosis or fibrosis, easy removal of the sources if emergency decompressive surgery is required, less exposure to the patient's family and others in close proximity after hospital discharge, and provision of dose rates greater than 30 cGy/hour, which are necessary to treat fast-growing malignant brain tumors as suggested by some data.[74]

Several techniques have been used for interstitial irradiation of the brain, some using multiple planar implants and ^{192}Ir wires or seeds and others with a few higher-intensity ^{125}I sources. Although experience with these techniques is limited, stereotactic techniques have been used to implant radioactive sources into brain tumors.[232]

Saw and associates[208] evaluated the differences in dose distribution among various interstitial implant stereotactic techniques used at four institutions on an idealized tumor phantom that was 5 cm in diameter and 5 cm long. Either 4 or 6 sources of ^{125}I or 9 or 24 ^{192}Ir catheters were used with different numbers of sources (Table 13-1). Quantitative evaluation of dose homogeneity using three volumetric irradiation indexes indicated that the dose homogeneity improved as the number of catheters and number of sources increased (Fig. 13-17). Dose-volume histograms demonstrated inhomogeneous irradiation; the area under the histogram is the target volume. Institution A's technique (4 catheters and 20 ^{125}I seeds) showed a highly inhomogeneous dose distribution compared with a more homogeneous irradiation obtained with the technique from institution B (24 catheters and 140 ^{192}Ir seeds). The dose homogeneity of the implants from institutions B and C were between the other values.

Irradiation of the surrounding normal tissues should be given special consideration. The dose gradient outside the target volume was believed to depend more on the geometry of the implant than on the type of radioisotope. At distances beyond the first centimeter, the dose rate falls off at a lower rate for implants using ^{192}Ir sources than with ^{125}I.

TABLE 13–1
Characteristics of Brain Implants From Four Institutions

CHARACTERISTICS	INSTITUTION A	B	C	D
Source type	^{125}I	^{125}I	^{192}Ir	^{192}Ir
No. of catheters used	4	6	9	24
No. of seeds used	20	42	36	140/28*
Seed spacing (cm)	0.95	1.0	1.5	1.0
Activity (mCi/seed)	30	12	2	0.79/0.54*

**The implant consists of 140 and 28 seeds with seed activity of 0.79 mCi and 0.54 mCi, respectively.*
(Saw CB, Suntharalingam N, Ayyangar KM, Tupchong L: Int J Radiat Oncol Biol Phys 17:887, 1989)

Technique with Multiple Iridium 192 Sources

The technique described here was developed at Washington University using radioactive sources placed in Teflon catheters inserted into the brain under direct computed tomography (CT) monitoring.

A radiolucent ring frame immobilizes the patient's head on the CT table top (Fig. 13-18A). Multiple burr holes are made in the brain at 1-cm intervals with the patient under local anesthesia. The location of the burr holes is determined by a template, which is attached to a stereotactic frame and to the patient's head. The template used is a thick acrylic block containing a 7-cm × 7-cm array of holes spaced at 1-cm intervals. The holes along the diagonal axis of the template have slightly larger diameters to provide a method for orienting each CT slice. The tumor is outlined on the CT screen with the aid of intravenously administered contrast material. Following the grid pattern, under CT observation, the Teflon angiocath catheters with a metallic stylette are inserted through the burr holes into the brain substance to ensure straight and parallel insertion (Fig. 13-18B).

After the tumor volume is implanted, the length of the radioactive sources is determined, and films, with the distribution of the catheters, are obtained for dosimetry calculations. Dummy seeds and ribbons are loaded in each of the catheters. After the catheters are secured, the patient is transferred to the intensive care unit, where the dummy sources are replaced by ribbons of active ^{192}Ir seeds with a specific activity of about 0.6 mCi per seed. Metal buttons are attached to the catheters to fasten them to the scalp (Fig. 13-18C). Careful records are maintained of the position and length of all the catheters.

Paterson-Parker's computer calculations are used to determine the dose and distribution in the implant volume (Fig. 13-18D). The dose rate ranges from 50 to 80 cGy/hour. In general, the implant duration is 70 to 100 hours, delivering 6000 cGy to 7000 cGy total dose to the entire tumor. Verification dosimetry with thermoluminescent dosimeters placed in catheters disclosed an agreement of ± 5% to 10% between the computer calculations and the actual doses at any point within the irradiated volume.[1] This method has been used in more than 60 patients at Washington University, most of them with glioblastoma multiforme, sometimes recurrent after external irradiation, and in a few patients for solitary brain metastases. Fatal intracranial bleeding has been rare (<5%), and edema is not severe enough to represent a significant management problem; brain necrosis has been observed in about 25% of the patients.

Technique with High-Intensity Iodine 125 Sources

Gutin and others[74,75] reported a technique implanting a few high-activity ^{125}I or ^{192}Ir sources into the tumor. Sources are

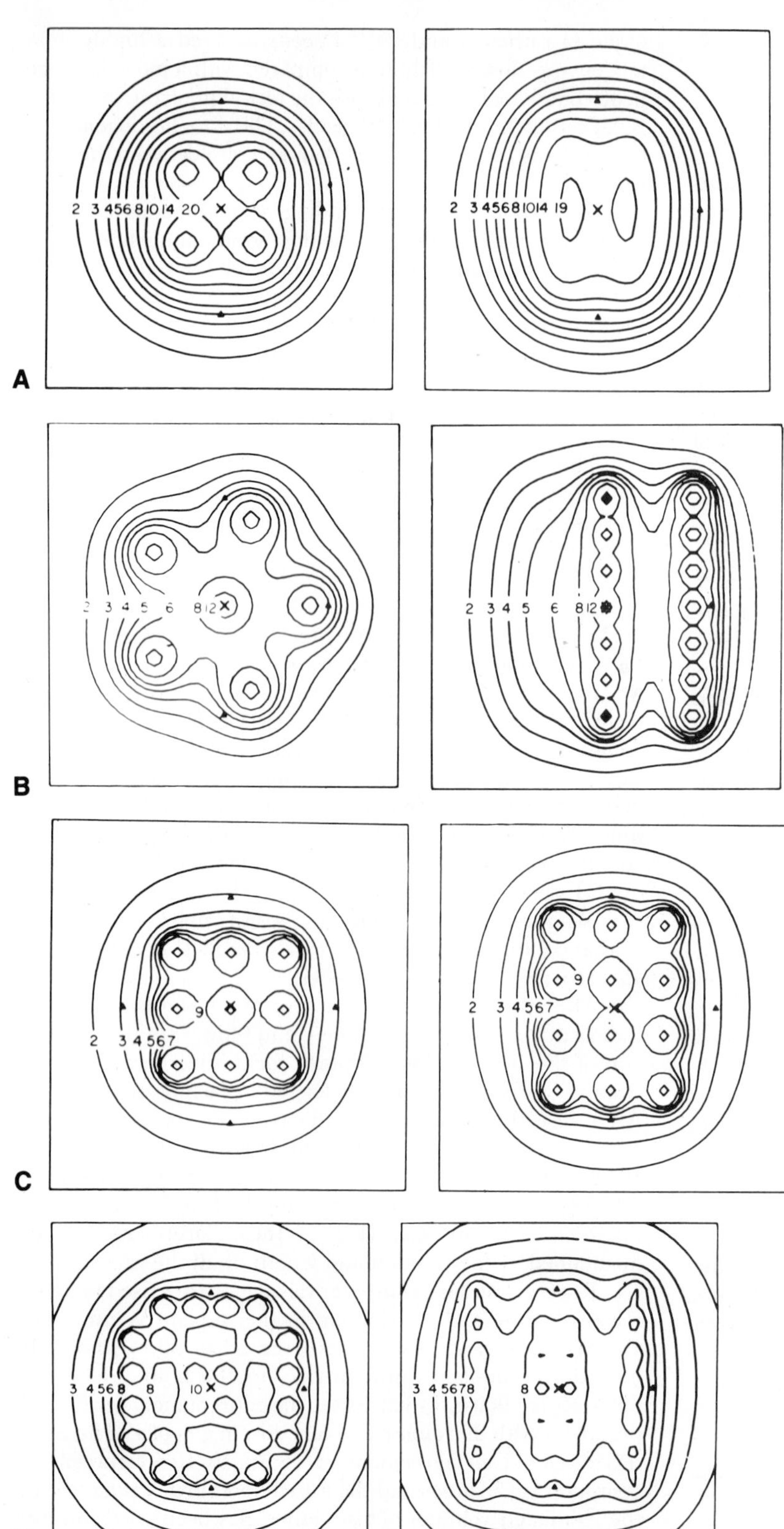

FIGURE 13–17. (**A**) Dose distributions of a brain implant by Institution A in two orthogonal planes: (a) the transverse plane and (b) the longitudinal plane, both bisecting the implant. Isodose rates in units of 10 cGy/hour are labeled. (**B**) Dose distributions of the implant by Institution B in two orthogonal planes: (a) the transverse plane, taken 0.5 cm above the central plane, and (b) the longitudinal plane. Isodose rates in 10 cGy/hour are labeled. (**C**) Dose distributions of the implant by Institution C in two orthogonal planes: (a) the transverse plane, bisecting the implant, and (b) the longitudinal plane. Isodose rates are given in units of 10 cGy/hour. (**D**) Dose distributions of the implant by Institution D in two orthogonal planes: (a) transverse plane and (b) the longitudinal plane, both bisecting the implant. Isodose rates in units of 10 cGy/hour are labeled. (Saw CB, Suntharalingam N, Ayyangar KM, Tupchong L: Int J Radiat Oncol Biol Phys 17:887, 1989)

implanted in the tumor site under local anesthesia using the Leksell stereotactic system. Most implants require two separate stereotactic procedures. At the first operation, one or more nonradioactive (dummy) soft copper seeds, 1 mm to 2 mm long, are placed under CT scan guidance through a burr hole in a location as near as possible to the tumor's center. A CT scan then localizes the dummy seeds and relates them to the target sites for radioactive sources, which are determined by the tumor's geometry and the isotope's physical characteristics. In a separate procedure performed later, the radioactive sources are placed at the target sites, using the dummy seeds as stereotactic reference points.

The Leksell stereotactic system was modified for use with a General Electric CT scanner.[132] A base plate is fixed at four points to the skull's outer table, and a CT scan is performed with a plastic replica of the conventional metal stereotactic frame

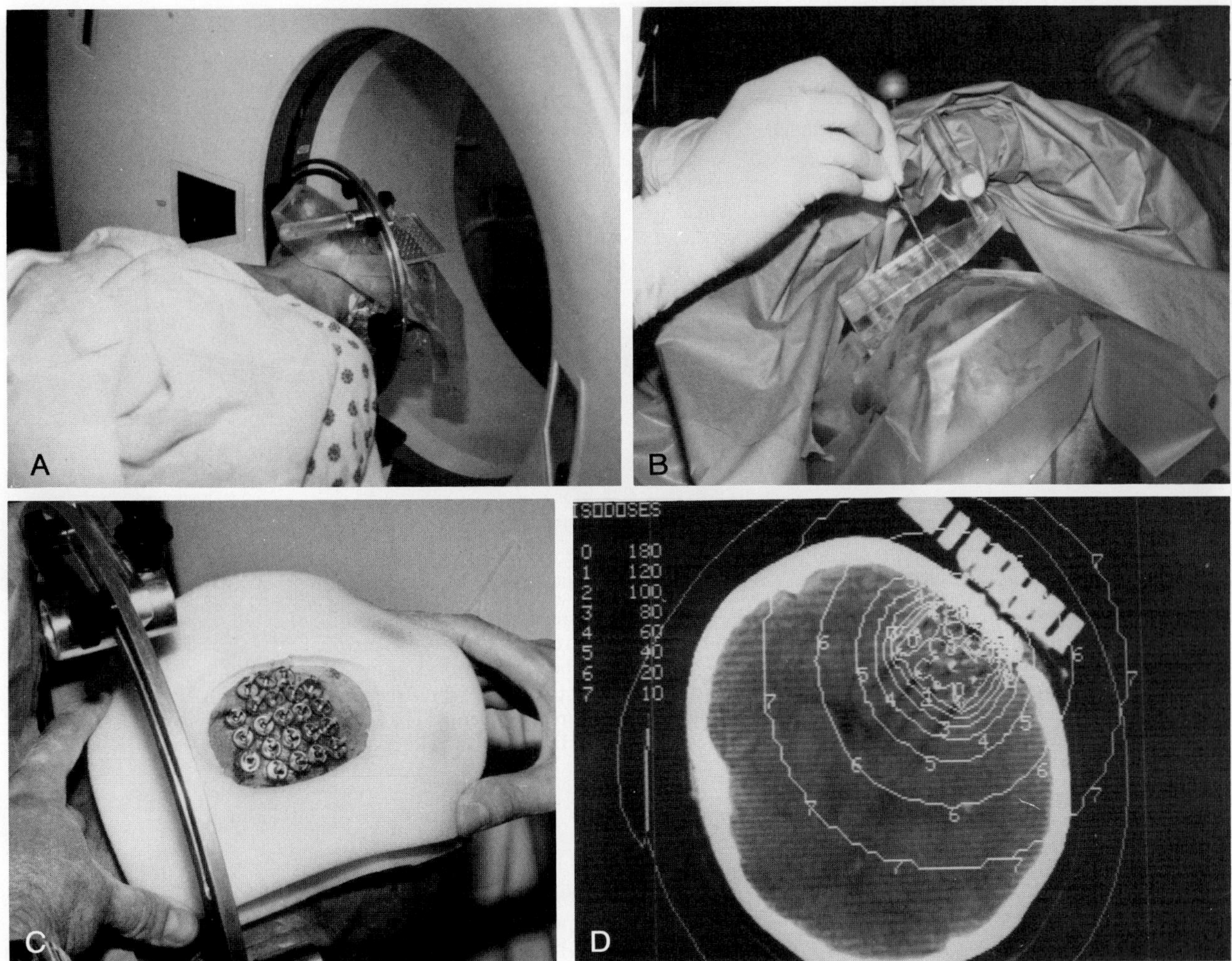

FIGURE 13–18. (**A**) Patient in the computed tomographic (CT) scanner, in position for ^{192}Ir brain implant, showing the stereotactic ring and plastic template used to direct placement of catheters. (**B**) Insertion of afterloading plastic catheter with metallic guide into the brain through small burr holes in the skull. A plastic template is used to determine exact positioning of catheters. (**C**) Patient after implant is finished, demonstrating metallic buttons sewn to scalp to secure the catheters in place. (**D**) CT scan of skull with ^{192}Ir sources in place and isodose curves.

attached to the base plate. With the plastic frame in position, scan artifacts are avoided, and the tumor target(s) can be visualized and related precisely to the frame's center by the computer program intrinsic to the scanner (Fig. 13-19A). The coordinates for the target sites are calculated; the patient is taken to the operating room, and with the metal frame in position, the radioactive sources are implanted. This method enables precise positioning of the sources in a single operation.

Implants can be permanent, or the ^{125}I sources can be mounted in plastic catheters and removed later. For the removable implants, one or more sources are sealed at the tips of the implant catheters and passed to the target, with a stylet used to push the catheter through the guides of the stereotactic frame and through the interposed brain. The stylet is removed, and the catheter is cut and fixed to the burr hole with a plastic plug fashioned for this purpose. The wound edges are then reapproximated, covering the catheter(s) and burr hole plug(s).

Several high-activity ^{125}I implants have been done with an afterloaded Silastic implant catheter developed in cooperation with a commercial supplier (American Heyer-Schyulte Corporation, Goelta, CA). This catheter affords greater accuracy of placement and allows radiographic position verification before the radioactive sources are loaded. An outer cannula is passed to the target, and after radiographic verification of its position, it is afterloaded with a coaxial inner cannula containing the ^{125}I source(s).

A CT scan is used for treatment planning. For spheroidal tumors, all sources are positioned at the tumor's center. In ellipsoidal tumors, the sources are positioned along the long axis to make the dose more uniform. After stereotactic placement of the sources, orthogonal radiographs are taken to determine the source relationships, and a computer program converts position data, source strengths, and implant duration into total-dose contours in any plane. The resulting dose plot is scaled to match the magnification of the radiographs, which allows superimposition of the isodoses on the tumor (Fig. 13-19B).

Doses are calculated by assuming each source to be a point source of isotropic radiation. The ^{192}Ir and ^{198}Au sources were assumed to produce the same dose distributions as ^{226}Ra of the same equivalency. For ^{125}I, a dose rate constant of 1.2 cGy cm^2/hour mCi at 0.5 cm is assumed.

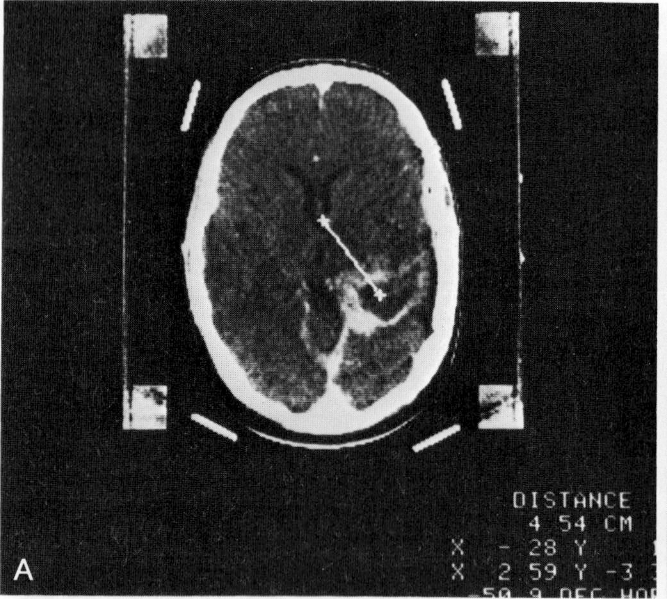

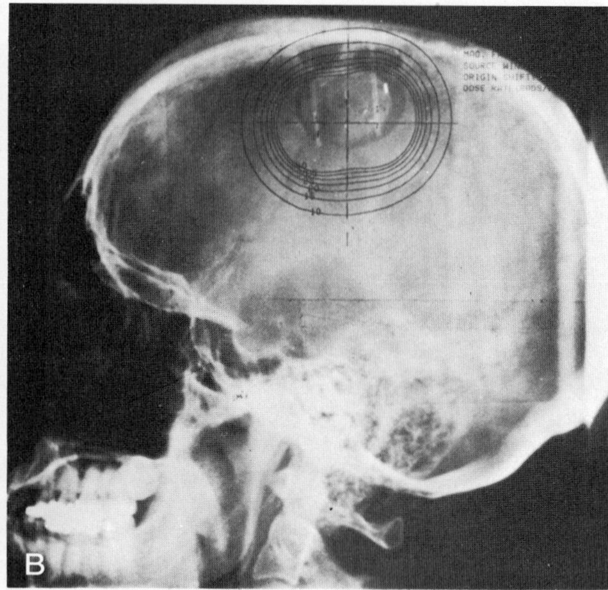

FIGURE 13–19. (**A**) Computed tomographic scan taken with the plastic stereotactic frame in position for ^{125}I brain implant. The four vertical (*square*) posts of the frame are visible. The geometric center of the frame (*small cross*) is related to the target for ^{125}I placement in the tumor by the scanner's computer. The coordinates of the frame's center and the target are seen at the lower right. (**B**) Plain radiograph showing two catheters, each containing two high-activity ^{125}I sources, implanted in a right parietal anaplastic astrocytoma. Isodose curves are superimposed. (Gutin PH, Phillips TL, Hosobuchi Y, et al: Int J Radiat Oncol Biol Phys 7:1371, 1981)

Eye

Episcleral Plaque

Episcleral plaque therapy is a cost-effective approach for treating localized intraocular malignancies like retinoblastoma and choroidal melanoma. The technique consists of fabricating a small, spherically curved plaque containing radioactive sources, immobilizing the patient's eye, and suturing the plaque onto the sclera opposite the tumor, where it remains for 3 to 10 days. Because of the proximity of the radioactive sources to the tumor, a highly localized and intense dose of irradiation is delivered to the tumor, which spares more normal tissue than is possible by conventional external-beam techniques and is competitive with the precision of heavy particle therapy. An interinstitutional randomized clinical trial through the Collaborative Ocular Melanoma Study (COMS) compared eye plaque therapy to enucleation using survival and preservation of vision as end points.

Historically, plaque therapy has been delivered using the ^{60}Co plaque system originally developed by Stallard[227] for treatment of retinoblastoma. These plaques (Fig. 13-20) are available in a limited range of sizes (8–12 mm in diameter). Both circular and semicircular notched plaques are available for treatment of posterior lesions abutting the optic nerve. Although easy to prepare and use, ^{60}Co plaques do not allow customization of the dose distribution, shielding of critical structures, or treatment of eye tumors on an outpatient basis.

Packer and Rotman[165] used ^{125}I seeds as a substitute for ^{60}Co plaques in the treatment of ocular melanoma. Within the COMS clinical trial, ^{125}I seeds are being used in conjunction with standardized gold-alloy plaques ranging from 12 mm to 20 mm in diameter. Each plaque is accompanied by a Silastic insert with precut channels for reproducibly positioning the seeds in concentric circles (Fig. 13-21). After the seeds are positioned in the insert, it is securely glued to the plaque so that the seeds are "sandwiched" between a 1-mm-thick layer of plastic and the gold backing of the plaque. A COMS plaque can be assembled within 30 minutes, almost entirely eliminates the possibility of seed loss during treatment, fixes the seeds in a rigid geometry, and retains a high degree of individualization. Notched or noncircular plaques can be fabricated using dental casting techniques.

Luxton[129] and Chiu-Tsao[29] demonstrated that ^{125}I plaques give relative dose distributions very similar to those of ^{60}Co plaques.The ^{125}I plaque therapy delivers retinal surface doses of 27,000 cGy to 40,000 cGy for a prescribed dose of 10,000 cGy to the tumor apex (Fig. 13-22). The ^{125}I plaques offer several dosimetric advantages over the ^{60}Co plaques. The 0.5-mm-thick gold plaque almost completely attenuates ^{125}I primary x-rays, providing a high degree of protection (95%) to tissue posterior to the eye. The 2.5- to 3.3-mm-high lip of the COMS plaque produces limited collimation of the ^{125}I x-rays, which reduces the area of the retina treated to a high dose. Moreover, a thin lead foil (0.2 mm thick) placed over the patient's eye affords substantial radiation protection, making possible treatment with plaques on an outpatient basis.

When using ^{125}I plaques, physicists and clinicians should be aware that currently used dosimetry data significantly overestimate the dose received by the patient. Williamson[260] and Weaver[252] showed that conventional ^{125}I data overestimate the dose rate to water at 1 cm from a model 6711 seed by 13% to 20%. Weaver[252] demonstrated that the gold backing of the plaque, which significantly reduces the volume of tissue contributing scatter dose to tissue anterior to the plaque, may reduce doses to points on the plaque axis by an additional 5% to 8%. Chiu-Tsao[30] has shown that the 1-mm-thick Silastic insert, which has an effective atomic number (11.2) higher than that of tissue, may reduce doses on the central axis of the plaque by

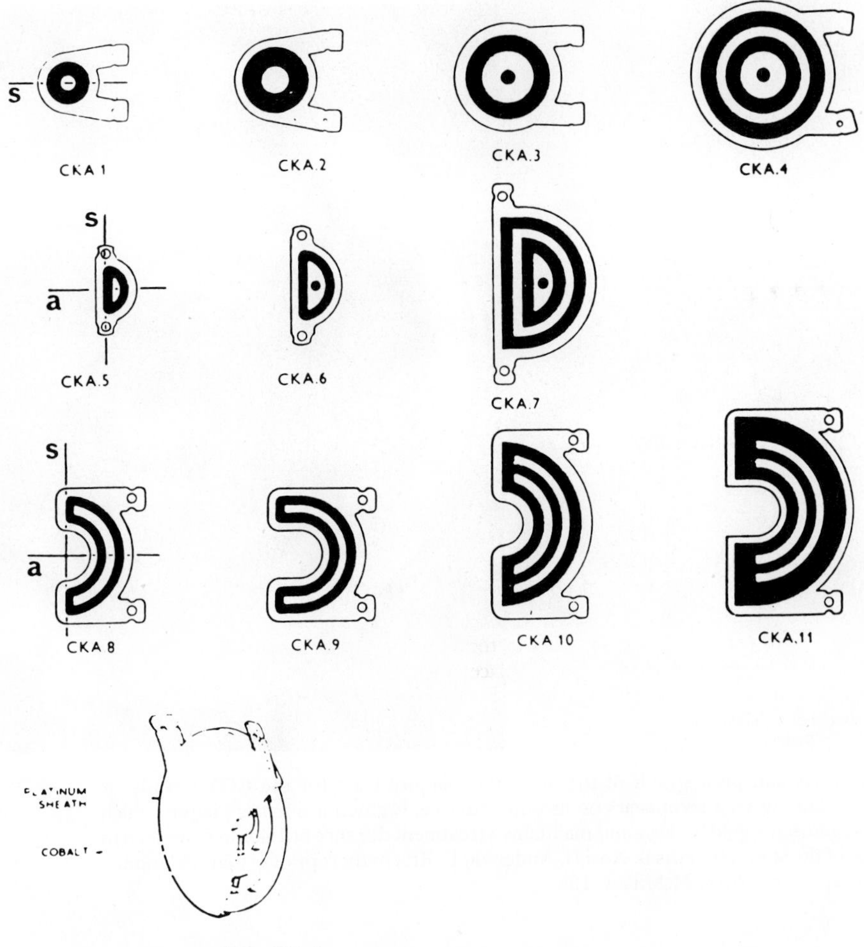

FIGURE 13–20. Axial views of the standard Stallard plaques used for treatment of intraocular malignancies. The ^{60}Co, distributed evenly over the blackened rings, is encapsulated in a platinum sheath. (Stallard HB: Ann R Coll Surg Engl 29:170, 1961)

10%. Because currently used dosimetry algorithms and data take none of these effects into account, minimum tumor doses delivered by COMS plaques are probably no greater than 75% of the normally prescribed values.

Before plaque fabrication, all relevant imaging studies should be examined to define the basal dimensions of the tumor and its location. A-mode ultrasound studies are used to define the maximum height of the tumor. Fluorescein angiograms are often helpful in determining the posterior boundary of the tumor. The fundus view diagram, used by the ophthalmologist to record clinical impressions, represents a polar plot of the surface anatomy of the retina with its origin at the macula. When the anterior margin of the tumor is anterior to the equator, every attempt should be made to localize this margin relative to the ora serrata using transillumination. After the basal diameters, height, and location of the tumor are defined, a plaque is fabricated with its diameter 4 mm to 8 mm larger than the assumed diameter of the tumor. With a dummy plaque of identical size, the plaque position is defined in the operating room using transillumination as the definitive guide to tumor localization and size. A small caliper should be available for measuring the orthogonal dimensions and location of the tumor relative to the ora serrata. These data should be used as the basis for the final treatment plan. The fundus view isodose curves, which give the dose distribution on the retinal surface, and conventional transverse view are useful.

Pterygium

After surgical resection of the pterygium, it is common practice to administer radiation therapy because of the high recurrence rate (20%–69%).[24,35,242,262] In most institutions a ^{90}Sr β-ray applicator is used for the treatment of these patients. The overall diameter of the applicator is 12.7 mm; the center is a circular radioactive disk 5 mm in diameter containing the isotope. The dose rate is generally about 500 cGy/minute. In some models, a Lucite disk on the shaft of the applicator shields the operator's hands (Fig. 13-23A). Irradiation is begun within 24 hours after resection, because failure increases with greater time delays.[242]

The patient is placed in a comfortable supine position, with the head slightly tilted for optimal positioning of the medial portion of the eye. A lid retractor is inserted to hold the eye open. The cornea and conjunctiva are anesthetized with a few drops of 0.5% to 1% lidocaine. After the anesthetic takes effect for 30 seconds to 1 minute, the applicator is carefully applied on the surface of the resected sclera (Fig.13-23B). Doses of about 1000 cGy are delivered. The application is repeated in three consecutive weekly fractions for a total of 3000 cGy. If a larger area of resection is to be irradiated, it may require application to two contiguous areas, each receiving the same dose. The lens, which is located at the depth of 3.5 mm to 5 mm from the surface, receives less than 5% of the dose.[69]

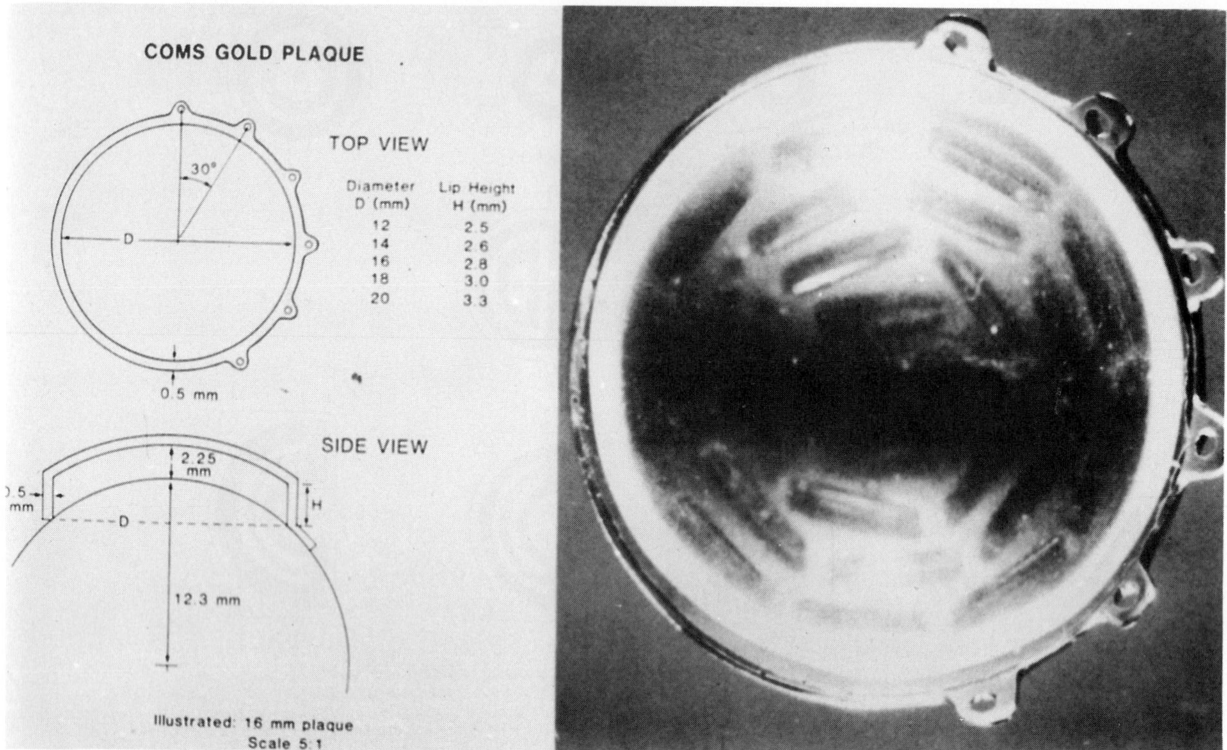

FIGURE 13–21. Drawings and photograph of the gold-alloy plaques used for the COMS study. A Silastic plastic insert, containing seed receptacles on its outer surface, is glued inside the plaque, which positions the ^{125}I seeds against the gold backing and maintains a treatment distance of 1.4 mm from seed to center to outer surface of the sclera. (Hilaris B, Nori D, Anderson L: Brachytherapy of ocular melanoma. In Atlas of Brachytherapy. New York, McMillan, 1988)

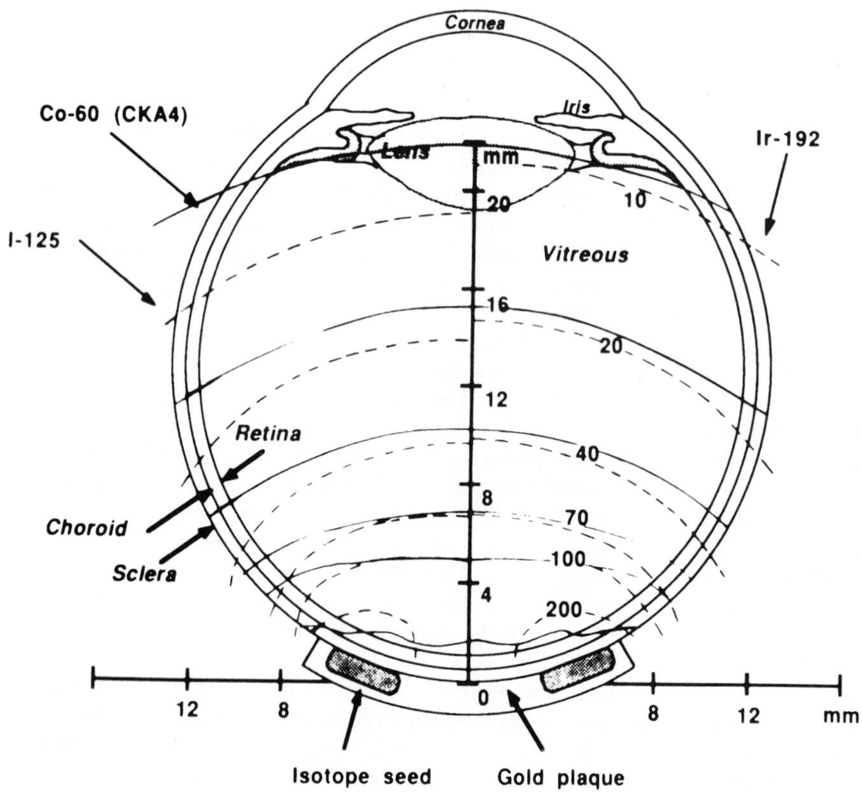

FIGURE 13–22. Isodose curves in the transverse plane of the eye for a 12-mm-diameter plaque. The solid lines indicate isodoses arising from the CKA-4 ^{60}Co plaque; the broken lines on the right and left denote isodose curves arising from ^{192}Ir and ^{125}I seeds, respectively. All isodoses are normalized to 100% on the central axis 5 mm from the plaque surface. (Luxton G, Astrahan MA, Liggett PE, et al: Int J Radiat Oncol Biol Phys 15:167, 1988)

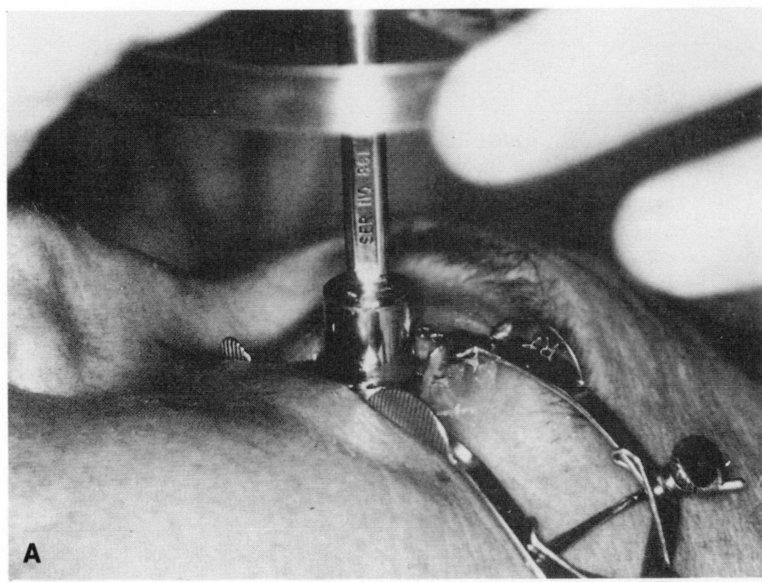

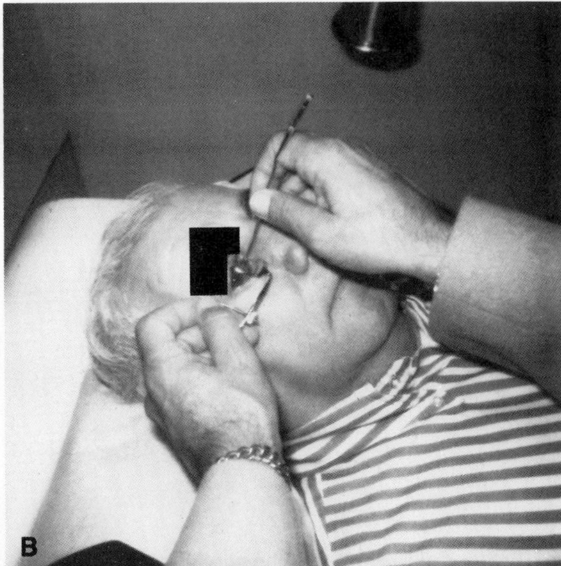

FIGURE 13–23. (**A**) Patient undergoing ^{90}Sr application with eyelids retracted. Applicator has plastic shielding to protect operator's hands. (Pierquin B, Wilson J-F, Chassagne D: Modern Brachytherapy. New York, Masson, 1987) (**B**) Similar ^{90}Sr application without shielding on applicator.

Head and Neck

The role of brachytherapy and the philosophy of management for primary tumors in various anatomic locations and for different stages are analyzed in detail throughout this book and will not be discussed in this chapter. A recent review on the management principles, brachytherapy techniques, and treatment results for various tumors of the head and neck is also available.[145]

Brachytherapy may provide a useful method for the retreatment of patients with recurrent, persistent, or second primary head and neck malignant tumors in a previously irradiated region. Fontanesi and associates[60] recommended a dose rate of 42 cGy/hour or less to deliver total doses of 5000 cGy to 6000 cGy to these lesions.

Nasopharynx

Wang[249] described the use of intracavitary brachytherapy alone or combined with external irradiation to boost the dose to the nasopharynx, in conjunction with external-beam irradiation. Briefly, two pediatric endotracheal tubes with inner and outer diameters of 5 mm and 6.9 mm, respectively, each loaded with two 20-mg Ra eq ^{137}Cs sources are used. Local anesthesia of the nasal cavity is achieved with cocaine. The endotracheal tubes are introduced through the nares into the nasopharynx with the head hyperextended. Under fluoroscopic control on the simulator, the tips of the cesium sources are placed at the free edge of the soft palate posteriorly and behind the posterior wall of the maxillary sinus anteriorly. A 5-cc balloon, which is attached to the distal end of the endotracheal tube, is inflated for anchoring purposes and to improve the dose to the nasopharynx by increasing the distance from the source. The dose reference point is 0.5 cm below the mucosa of the nasopharyngeal vault; the dose rate is approximately 120 cGy/hour.

Denham and associates[47] described remote afterloading techniques for intracavitary irradiation of patients with carcinoma of the nasopharynx. This is accomplished by the introduction of afterloading catheters of different curvatures that are readily introduced into the nasopharynx by way of the nasal cavity, with appropriate anesthesia. The major difficulty with this technique is the successful rigid anchoring of the catheters to prevent movements that could be potentially injurious to the nasal cavity or nasopharynx. A special plastic face mask was constructed with adjustable universal joint fittings for rigid attachment of the catheters with minimal discomfort to the patient. Because of asymmetry of the nasopharynx, different angle catheters can be used (22.5, 40, or 50 degrees).

Oral Cavity

The oral cavity should be kept dry with adequate preanesthesia medication, including scopolamine, and suction. It is desirable to outline the tumor with gentian violet, Castellani's paint, or one of the available surgical markers. A metric ruler should always be on the implant tray. If rigid needles are being implanted in the oral cavity, one assistant retracts the patient's lips and another pulls or depresses the tongue while the operating radiation therapist performs the implant.

The anterolateral needles of an implant of the oral cavity should be kept away from the thin mucous membrane that covers the bone in the upper and lower gum, as well as from the periosteum, teeth, and bone. To increase and maintain the distance, a regular fluoride carrier is thickened on the inside by one to four layers (one layer = 2 mm) to increase the distance and keep the unavoidable "hot spot" around each needle away from the adjacent normal mucosa.

Tongue and Floor of Mouth

Lesions beneath the tongue or in the floor of the mouth, if standard needles or substitutes are used, usually are implanted through the dorsum of the tongue. The anterolateral needles emerge from the undersurface of the tongue and are reinserted

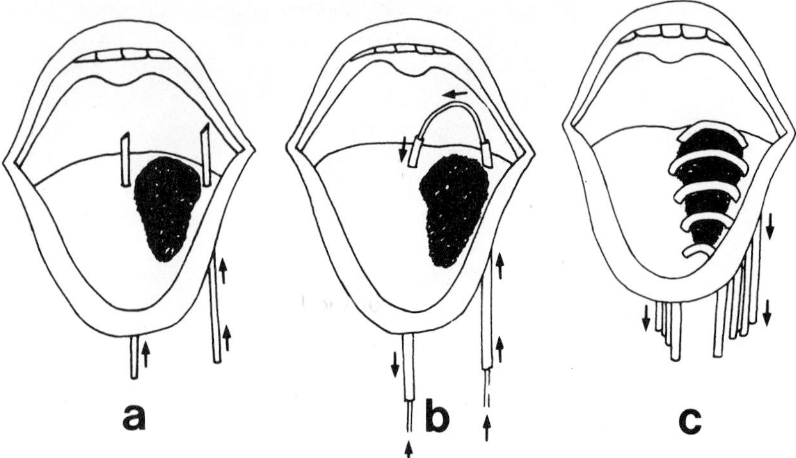

FIGURE 13–24. Diagram illustrating submental or submaxillary approach for insertion of Teflon catheters with metallic guides into the oral cavity for lesions on the floor of the mouth or lateral border of the tongue. (**A**) Metallic guides are introduced, with one hand positioning the guide inside the oral cavity. (**B**) Introduction of nylon strand for placement of the ^{192}Ir wire or seeds, looped over dorsum of the tongue. (**C**) Various nylon tubes in position on dorsum of the tongue. At this point the metallic guides have been withdrawn from the submaxillary region. After position of the radioactive sources is radiographically determined using dummy sources, active sources are inserted, and the ends of the plastic tubes are crimped with metallic buttons.

into the floor of the mouth. The implants should extend beyond the visible or palpable tumor by at least 1 cm in all directions. A popular technique of interstitial implants with nylon tubing and ^{192}Ir sources for lesions of the oral tongue or floor of the mouth uses a submental or submaxillary approach for the insertion of metallic guides into the oral cavity with one hand. The exit points of the guides in the oral cavity are carefully verified with the index finger of the other hand (through-and-through technique).

The major nylon tubing is threaded through the metallic guides, looped around the dorsum of the tongue, and exits through a parallel metallic guide. The metallic guides are pulled out externally, and the nylon thread is secured by crimping with a metallic button at one end. The procedure continues as described previously, leaving the other end open for insertion of the radioactive sources. To facilitate removal, we prefer to tie a silk thread on the loop of each nylon tube inside the oral cavity.

After position of the sources is verified on x-ray films using radiopaque inactive dummy sources, the appropriate ^{192}Ir wires (or seeds in nylon tubing) are inserted, and the other end of the larger nylon tube is crimped. The sequence of needle implantation for lesions involving the oral tongue and the anterior floor of the mouth is illustrated in Figure 13-24.

Mendenhall and associates[145] described an implant template for the floor of the mouth that is made of aluminum, stainless steel, or nylon and individually customized to fit the lesion of each patient (Fig. 13–25). The device is inserted into the floor of the mouth of the patient under general anesthesia and is secured by one suture through the submental area, which is tied to a cotton cigarette roll. The active ends of the radium

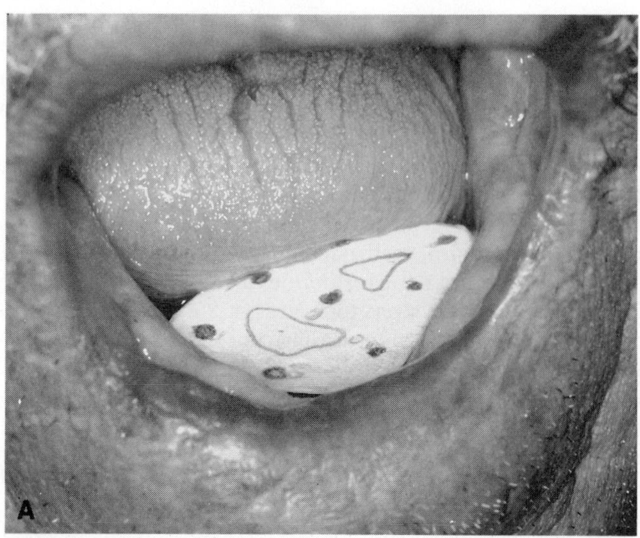

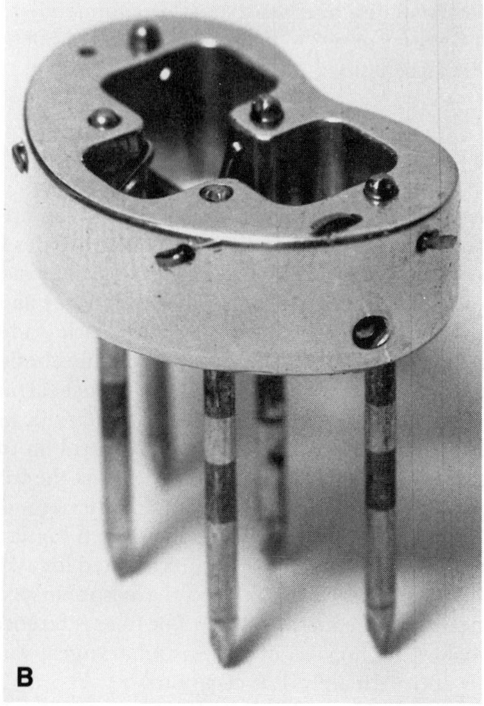

FIGURE 13–25. (**A**) Cardboard template is cut to fit the lesion in the floor of the mouth. (**B**) Customized floor-of-mouth implant device. Needles are secured to the implant device with stainless steel wire passed through the needle eyes. A crossing needle can be mounted through the device if desired. (Marcus RB Jr, Million RR, Mitchell TP: Int J Radiat Oncol Biol Phys 6:111, 1980)

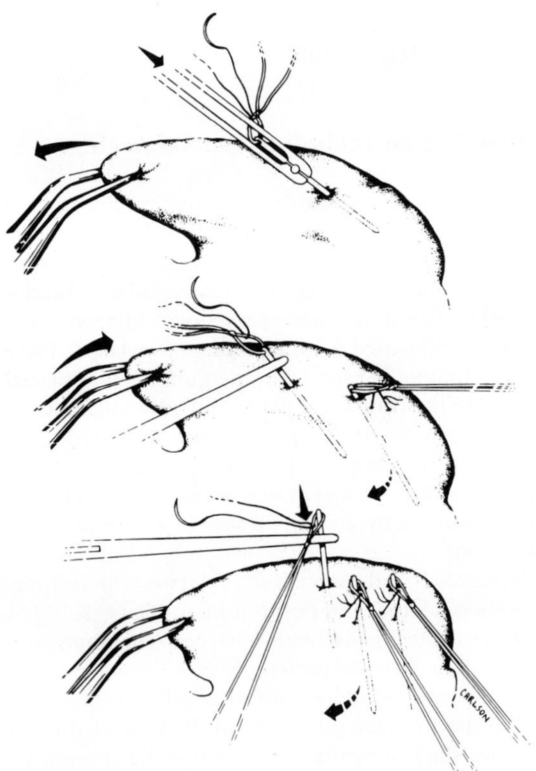

FIGURE 13–26. Recommended technique for implants of the posterolateral border of the tongue with rigid needles. (Delclos L: Interstitial irradiation techniques. In Levitt SH, Tapley NduV [eds]: Technological Basis of Radiation Therapy: Practical Clinical Applications. Philadelphia, Lea & Febiger, 1984)

needles may be positioned above the level of the mucosa to ensure an adequate surface dose. Crossing is accomplished by placing a needle parallel to the mucosal surface on the implant device. The system is not afterloaded, but the procedure can be performed rapidly with predictable geometry, ensuring that the radiation exposure to the operating staff is lower than with the hairpin technique.

The advantage of this technique over use of iridium hairpins is that all of the needles with the template are rigidly fixed in relationship to one another, and the isodose distributions can be calculated before the procedure or can be modified if necessary by adjusting the arrangement of the needles.

Implantation with rigid needles of the posterolateral border of the tongue via the oral cavity requires pulling the tongue forward to start the implant at the base of the tongue (Fig. 13-26). The first needle is inserted pointing posteriorly and inferiorly at about 45 degrees; a lesser angle is used for successive needles. At the end of the implant, when the tongue returns to its normal position, the implant needles adopt a vertical position.

At the University of Florida, a technique has been employed using radium or cesium needles mounted on rigid bars made of stainless steel or nylon.[145] The number of needles depends on the diameter of the lesion. A crossing needle is usually added to one or both bars to ensure adequate irradiation dose to the dorsal muscosal surface of the tongue.

Another technique described by Baillet and co-workers[13] uses the ^{192}Ir hairpin technique. Inactive gutter guides are placed into the tongue, and under fluoroscopic control, it is verified that the gutter guides are parallel. The iridium hairpins are afterloaded into the guides, which are removed at that time. A suture is used to secure each hairpin to the tongue. A cotton roll sutured between the tongue and the mandible with either technique displaces the tongue medially and decreases the irradiation given to the mandible.

The advantage of the iridium hairpin technique over the radium or cesium rigid needles is that the overall source length is shorter for the same active length because of the 6-mm inactive tips at either end of the rigid needles. Furthermore, there are only two vertical sources per hairpin, instead of the three or four radium or cesium needles on each bar, making it easier to position the hairpins in the tongue (Fig 13-27). This is particularly helpful in patients with small mouths, trismus, or full dentition, where it is very difficult to adequately position the rigid needles.

Base of Tongue

Because of the possibility of airway obstruction, it is imperative to perform an elective temporary tracheostomy before the implant procedure is initiated.

Implantation of the base of the tongue (and sometimes the posterolateral border of the oral tongue) is best accomplished by using long metallic or Teflon catheters with guides inserted through the submaxillary or subdigastric region, with the index finger of the other hand in the oropharynx to verify the position of the guide at the exit point, the base of the tongue. The nylon thread is inserted through the tubing into the oropharynx, looped around, and brought out through the opposite guide,

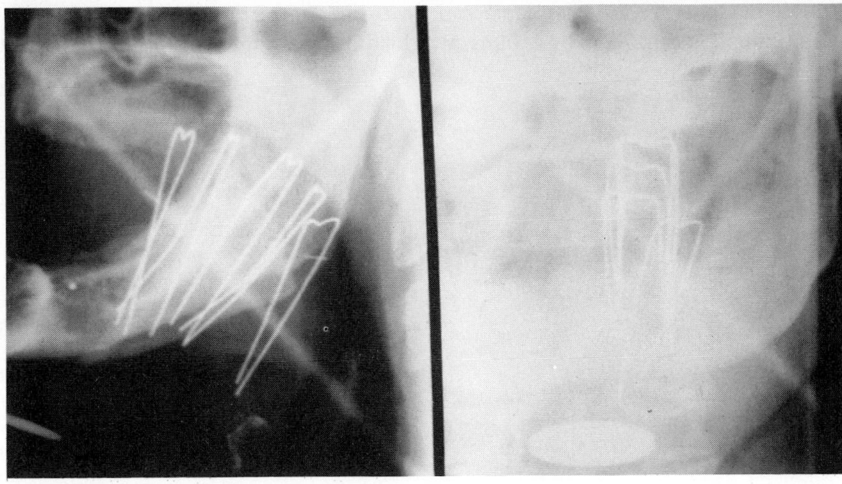

FIGURE 13–27. Roentgenograms of an ^{192}Ir hairpin implant for carcinoma of the left side of the oral tongue, stage T2NO, measuring 3.5 cm × 2.0 cm × 2.0 cm, with submucosal extension to within 0.5 cm of the midline of the tongue. Treatment consisted of 3000 cGy in ten fractions, followed by an ^{192}Ir implant using the gutter-guide technique with the patient sitting. A gauze pack was secured onto the lateral floor of the mouth to displace the tongue medially away from the mandible. The implant delivered 4000 cGy tumor dose to the area of gross disease (55 cGy/hour). The patient remained free of disease at 36 months. (Parsons JT, Mendenhall WM, Bova FJ, Million RR: Irradiation techniques for head and neck cancer. In Levitt SL: Technological Basis of Radiation Therapy: Practical Clinical Applications. Philadelphia, Lea & Febiger, in press)

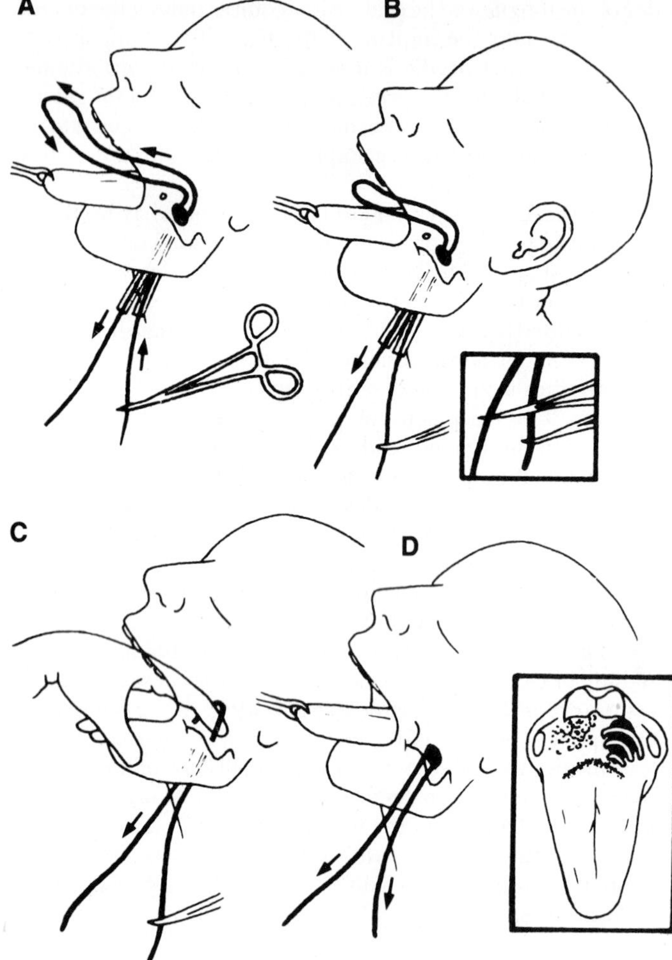

FIGURE 13–28. Diagram illustrating the use of stainless steel guides inserted through the submaxillary region for patients with carcinoma of the left base of the tongue (**A, B**). As described in Figure 13–24, the nylon tubing is looped around the dorsum of the tongue (**C**), the stainless steel guides are removed, and dummy and later radioactive sources are inserted and secured with metallic buttons (**D**).

providing the equivalent of a crossing needle in the cephalad end of the implant (Fig. 13-28A). The metallic guides are withdrawn from the submental region (Fig. 13-28B–D), and the nylon tubes are secured externally with metallic buttons as described before. If it is not possible to open the oral cavity adequately, the only recourse is to perform a submandibular implant with metallic guides and afterloading ^{192}Ir (Fig. 13-29). Double-plane or volume implants can be easily performed. After implant localization x-ray films, afterloading ^{192}Ir wire or seeds in nylon threads are inserted into the nylon tubing or metallic guides (Fig 13-30).

Tonsillar Region Including Faucial Arch

Fletcher[57] described a double-plane pterygomaxillary implant with radium needles to boost the dose in patients with carcinoma of the faucial arch or tonsillar region with extension into the tongue. The ^{192}Ir hairpin or plastic tube techniques have been used by Pierquin[182] and Mazeron.[140] The nylon tube technique may also be used to implant the soft palate.[52] The iridium hairpin technique is used with one gutter guide placed in the soft palate in the transverse plane and additional gutter guides placed vertically into the anterior tonsillar pillars, depending on the extent of the lesion. Iridium hairpins are afterloaded into the gutter guides, which are removed as described before. If the uvula is involved by tumor, it should be amputated before implantation.[52]

Mendenhall and associates[145] reviewed the techniques for implantation of the anterior tonsillar pillars, soft palate, or tonsillar region using two nylon bars, each containing three full-intensity, 2- to 3-cm active-length radium or cesium needles implanted into the anterior tonsillar pillar and another 1 cm medial to the tonsillar pillar bar, in the base of the tongue. A crossing needle is sometimes included in the anterior pillar bar to ensure adequate mucosal dose.

Nasal Vestibule

Small lesions of the nasal vestibule can be adequately treated with external or interstitial irradiation, but more advanced lesions require a combination of both modalities. Irradiation is an excellent alternative to surgery in the treatment of these tumors, because tumor control can be very good, and cosmetic results are better than with surgery.[143, 144] These tumors are implanted with single- or double-plane techniques using rigid radium or cesium needles or ^{192}Ir nylon tubing techniques. According to Mendenhall and associates,[145] the distal vertical needles (perpendicular to the dorsum of the nose) in each plane may be mounted in a nylon bar to stabilize the distal needles and adequately cover a tumor involving the opening of the nasal vestibule (Fig. 13-31).

Skin and Lip

Brachytherapy for the treatment of skin and lip tumors was popular before the advent of external irradiation techniques.

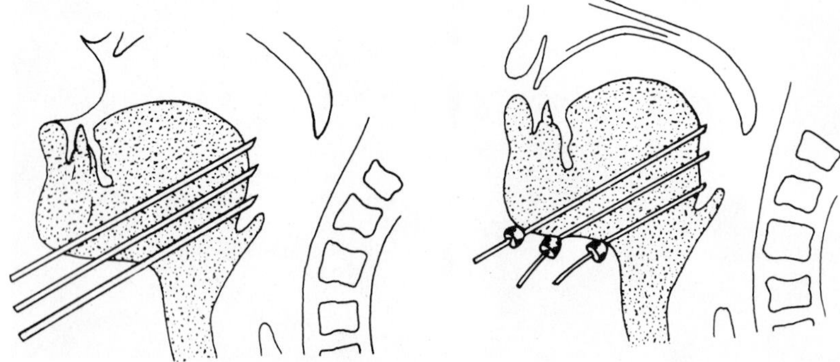

FIGURE 13–29. Illustration of submandibular implant with metallic guides in which it was not possible to loop nylon strands over the base of the tongue (one-end technique). The nylon tubing is cut to fit the tumor volume to be implanted, and metallic buttons are used to secure the nylon tubes and guides in position. The buttons are sutured to the skin to ensure the placement of the stainless steel guides.

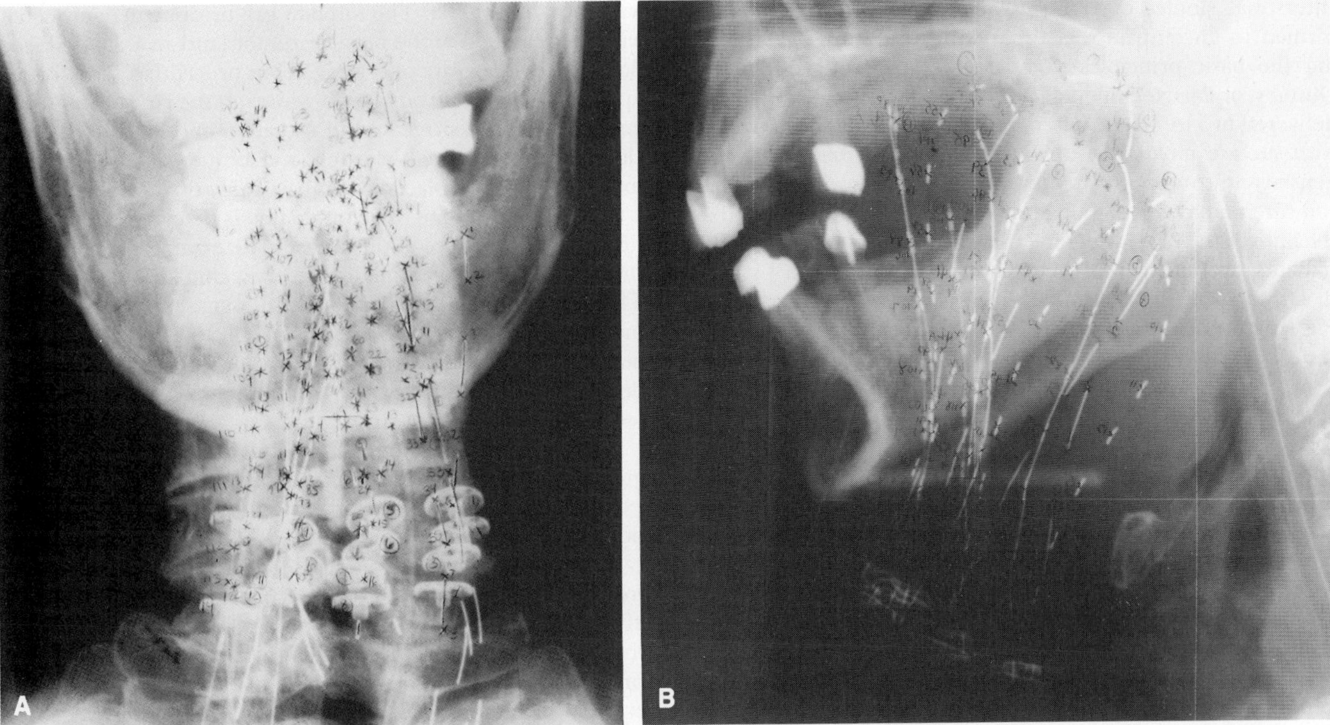

FIGURE 13–30. Position of stainless steel guides for implantation of a large T3 epidermoid carcinoma of the base of the tongue to deliver 3000 cGy in approximately 65 hours. Patient received 4500 cGy with external-beam irradiation before the ^{192}Ir implant. (**A**) Anteroposterior and (**B**) lateral radiographs illustrate the positions of the dummy sources in base of the tongue.

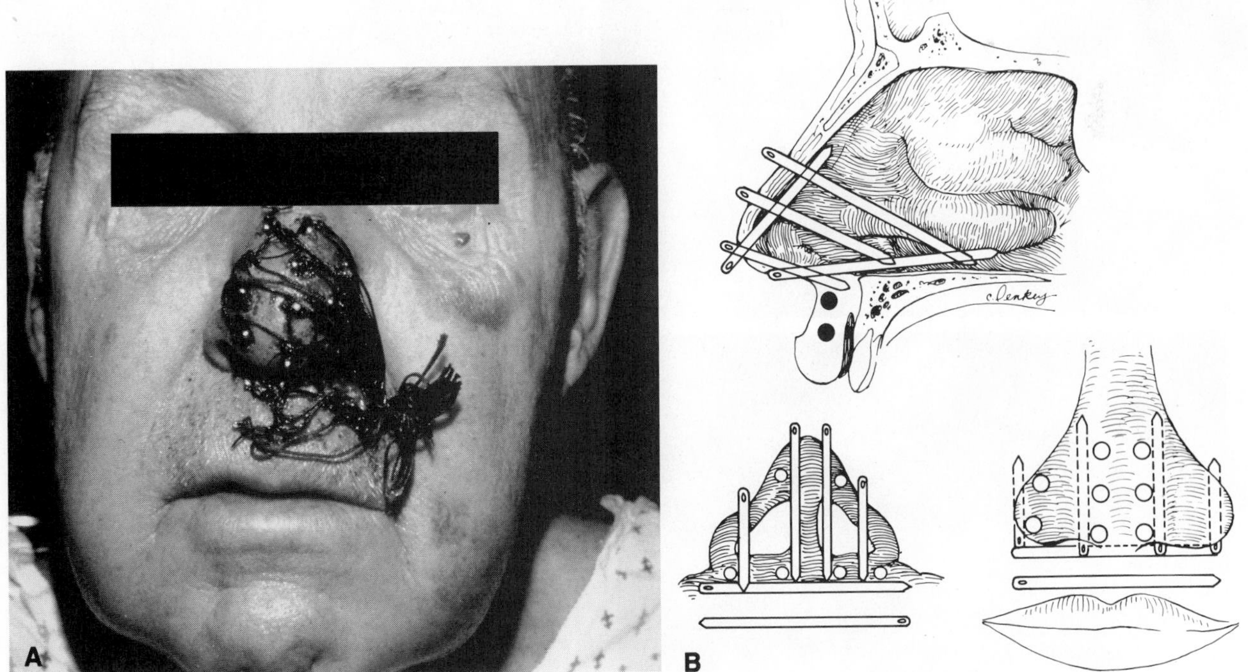

FIGURE 13–31. (**A**) The basic interstitial treatment plan for nasal septum tumors consists of multiple planes of needles (usually two to four) inserted through the skin and cartilage of the nose perpendicular to the nasal bridge. Crossing needles parallel to the floor of the vestibule or bridge of the nose are necessary to ensure homogeneous irradiation of the tumor volume. One or two needles are also implanted in the upper lip, even if it is clinically uninvolved. (Million RR, Cassisi NJ, Clark JR: Cancer of the head and neck. In DeVita VT Jr, Hellman S, Rosenberg SA [eds]: Cancer: Principles and Practice of Oncology, 3rd ed, p 565. Philadelphia, JB Lippincott, 1989) (**B**) Treatment consisted of a radium needle implant with three planes of needles perpendicular to the nasal bridge plus two crossing needles in the upper lip and one needle in the floor of the nose; the dose was calculated to be 6500 cGy in 130 hours. (Million RR, Cassisi NJ, Hamlin DJ: Nasal vestibule, nasal cavity, and paranasal sinuses. In Management of Head and Neck Cancer: A Multidisciplinary Approach, p 432. Philadelphia, JB Lippincott, 1984)

Interstitial single- or double-plane implants could be performed to encompass the tumor with a safe margin, following the basic principles of brachytherapy (Paterson-Parker, Quimby, or Paris technique). Doses of 5000 cGy to 7000 cGy are delivered in 5 to 7 days. Carcinoma of the skin has been treated with surface molds or with interstitial brachytherapy.[170] Jorgensen and co-workers[112] reported 869 patients with squamous cell carcinoma of the lip, 844 of whom received irradiation as the initial form of treatment. Radium implants were used in 766 patients, producing local tumor control rates of 93% in T1, 87% in T2, and 75% in T3 tumors. Similar results were described by Pigneux and co-workers.[186]

Breast

Interstitial irradiation of the breast has been used as a boost after the whole organ is given external irradiation (4500–5000 cGy) in conjunction with conservation surgery.[14] Selection of patients for this technique is limited to those with an adequate breast volume and lesions <4 cm in diameter (see Chap. 42). Only the interstitial implant, which is done with ^{192}Ir wires or seeds, is described in this chapter.

The procedure usually is performed with the patient under general anesthesia, although at some institutions it is performed with local anesthesia. The implant can be done in conjunction with the resection of the primary tumor (and an axillary dissection) or as a separate operating room procedure. The former approach has the advantage of reducing the cost of treatment and allowing the surgeon and radiation oncologist to interact closely in determining the extent and location of the tumor and to better plan the placement of the interstitial implant.

After the volume to be implanted is determined, lines are drawn on the surface of the breast to determine the position of the single- or (usually) the double-plane implant (Fig. 13-32A). The implant planes are drawn with 1.5-cm separation, and the metallic or plastic guides are set 1.2 cm to 1.5 cm from each other (Fig. 13-32B). Depending on the configuration of the breast and the location of the tumor, the needles may be inserted on a coronal or a transverse plane.

Rigid metallic guides or Teflon catheters with metallic guides are inserted into the breast, passing through the tumor excision site until the end of the guide reaches the opposite portion of the breast. In general, if a double-plane implant is carried out, the guides for the deep plane are inserted first, followed by those for the superficial plane. The nylon tubing for afterloading insertion of the ^{192}Ir wire or seed nylon thread is then inserted through the metallic guides, which are withdrawn progressively. The distal end of the nylon tubing is secured by crimping metallic buttons at the level of the skin surface (Fig.

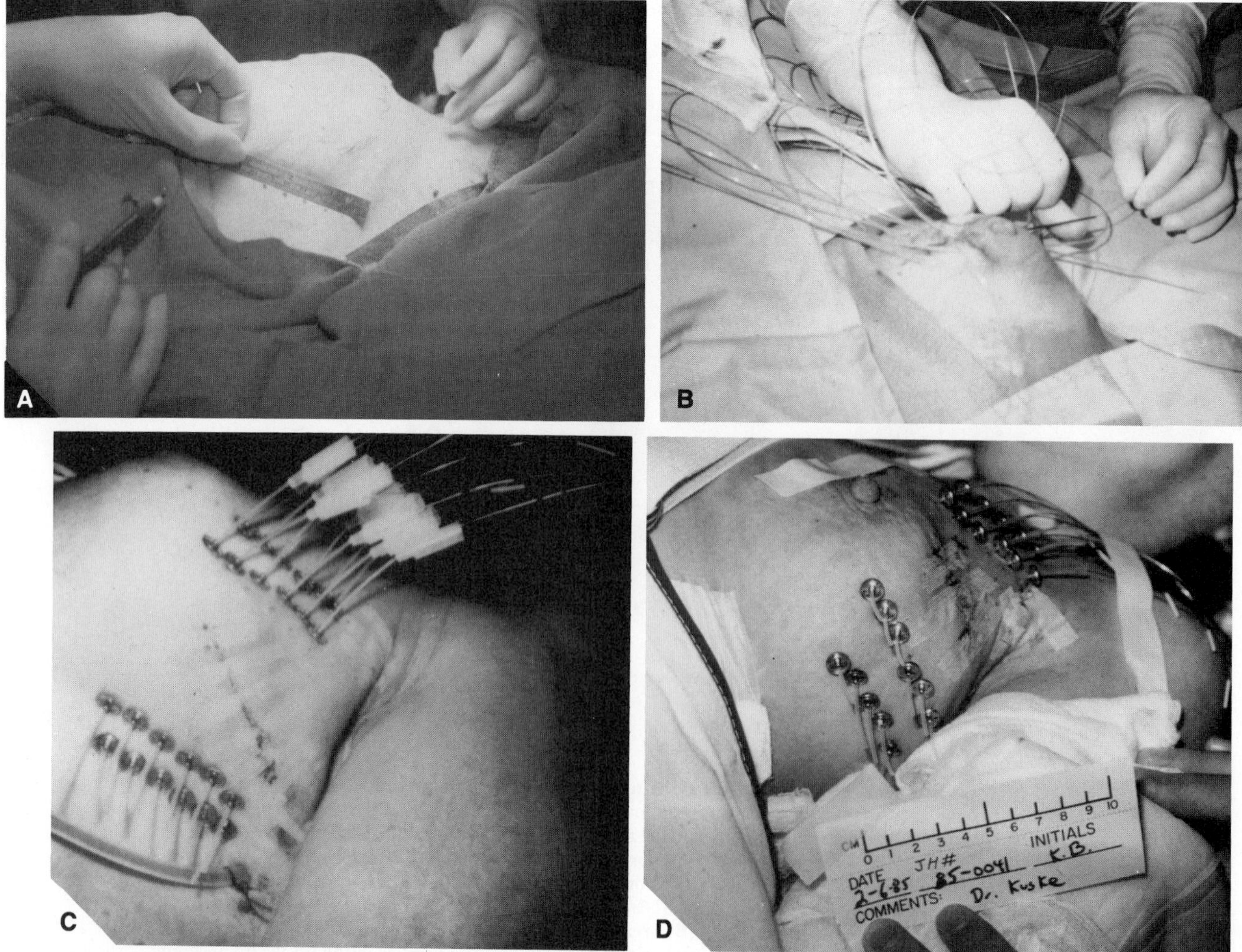

FIGURE 13–32. (**A**) Drawing lines on the surface of a breast for a source implant. (**B**) Placement of metallic or plastic guides for a breast implant. (**C**) Plastic tubes are secured at the skin surface using metallic buttons. (**D**) Sources are inserted in the proximal end of the tubing.

13-32C). The length of the ^{192}Ir wire or seed nylon thread is determined by inserting dummy sources and measuring the depth of penetration, which should be 0.5 cm to 1 cm from the skin surface at both ends to prevent excessive skin reaction. Radiopaque dummy sources are inserted into the nylon tubing with appropriate identification (colored) tags. The proximal end of the tubing is left open for future removal of the dummy sources and insertion of the radioactive wires (seeds) (Fig. 13-32D).

The patient is allowed to recover from the anesthesia, and x-ray films (anteroposterior and lateral) of the breast are obtained (Fig. 13-33). The patient is then taken to her hospital room, and the radioactive sources of appropriate length (*i.e.*, active ends are 0.5 cm under the skin) and strength are inserted

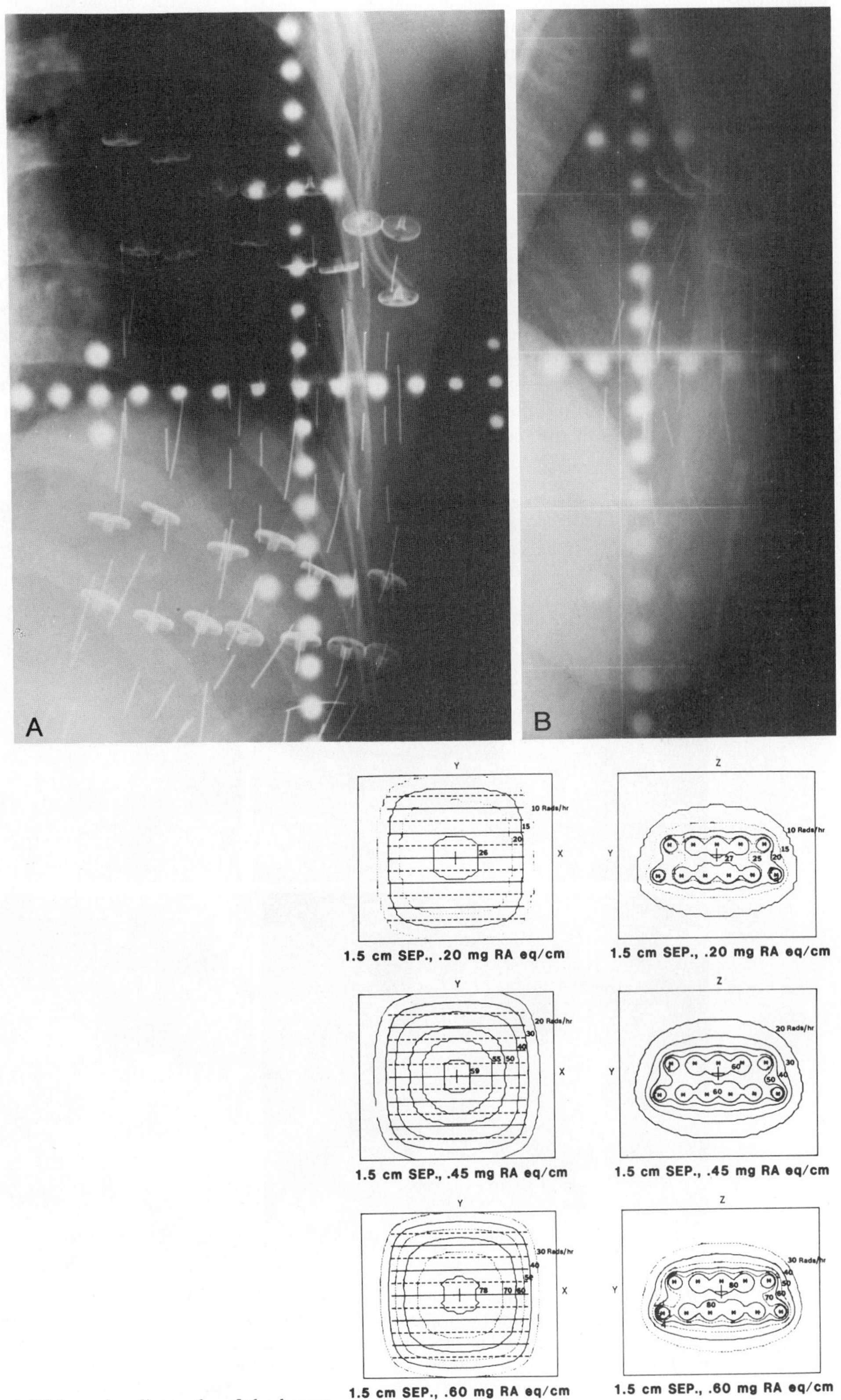

FIGURE 13–33. (**A**) Anteroposterior and (**B**) lateral radiographs of the breast obtained for dosimetry purposes. (**C**) Dose distribution for the breast implant.

into the plastic tubing, which is cut about 2 cm from the skin surface. Metallic buttons are crimped at the level of the skin to secure the plastic tubes in place.

The minimal desired dose rate is 50 to 60 cGy/hour. The usual strength of the wire is 0.4 mCi ^{226}Ra eq/cm (or per seed). In general, doses of 1000 cGy to 2000 cGy are delivered to the volume. Optimally, the maximal dose distribution throughout the implant volume should be within 10% to 15% of the minimal tumor dose.

A variation in the interstitial implantation of the breast with stainless steel guides using only one point of entrance to improve cosmetic results has been used by Delclos at M.D. Anderson Cancer Center. Examples of this technique are illustrated in Figure 13-34.

Lung and Mediastinum

The group at Memorial Sloan-Kettering Cancer Center has published several reports[92,93,139] on the use of ^{125}I seeds and ^{198}Au grains for permanent perioperative brachytherapy in patients with persistent or recurrent bronchogenic carcinoma after external irradiation or for residual disease after surgical resection. The radioactive seeds or grains are directly implanted in the tumor at the time of thoracotomy under general anesthesia. Temporary implants of the mediastinum with or without resection followed by a moderate dose of postoperative external irradiation (3500–4000 cGy) have been used alone or combined with ^{125}I implantation of the primary known tumor. Several reports described local tumor control in 78% of the patients with stage I and II tumors and control in 67% of those with stage III lesions.[92] Patients with microscopic residual tumor have significantly better tumor control and survival than those with gross residual disease.

Intrabronchial insertion of medium- or high-dose-rate radioactive sources has gained popularity for the treatment of patients with symptoms related to bronchial obstruction or hemoptysis. The technique is described further later in this chapter.

Pancreas

Interstitial irradiation, most frequently using ^{125}I permanent implants, has been used in patients with locally advanced unresectable carcinoma of the pancreas.[48,96,218,230] With the patient under general anesthesia, after the tumor is exposed by the surgeon and biopsies are performed, tumor volume is evaluated and biliary or gastric bypasses are performed as required. Multiple seeds are implanted in the pancreas with ^{125}I implantation techniques and a device like the Mick applicator, usually at 0.5-cm or 1-cm intervals, depending on the volume to be implanted

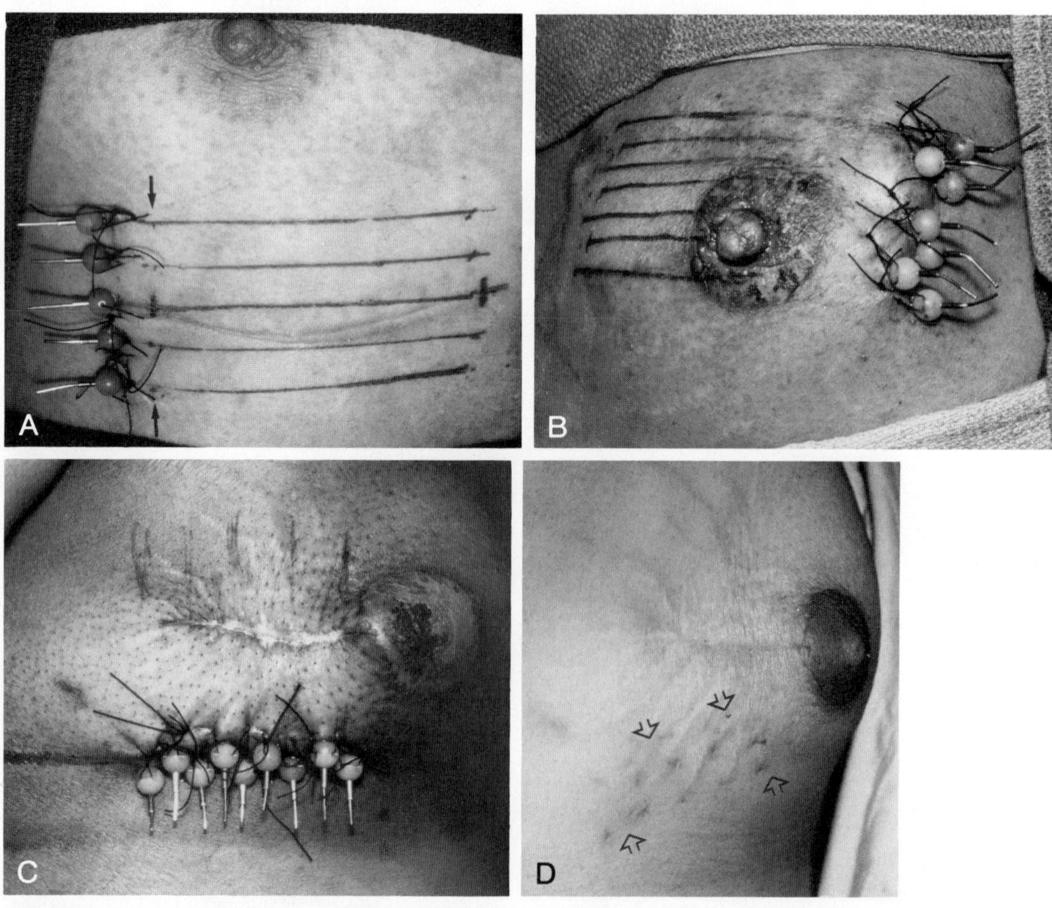

FIGURE 13–34. (**A**) Single-plane implant (inferior half of the breast). Needles are parallel to the scar. The active end (*arrows*) of the iridium wires are 1 cm inside the tissues. (**B**) Staggered, double-plane implant under the nipple. The superficial plane is shorter than the deep plane to follow contour of breast. (**C**) Double plane from the lateral and inferior breast (no exit). (**D**) Entrance points marked on skin (*arrows*). The breast also could have been implanted with needles parallel to the scar, entering the breast from the axillary side rather than from below the breast, still preserving cosmesis in the areas most exposed when the patient wears a low-cut dress. (Courtesy of Luis Delclos, M.D., Houston, Texas)

and intensity of the sources. After localization x-ray films are obtained by the stereoshift or orthogonal technique, computer dose calculations to determine the minimal peripheral dose are obtained.[94]

In a group of 98 patients described by Peretz and associates,[171] the mean matched peripheral dose (MPD) dose was 13,660 cGy. The mean activity of the implant was 35 mCi, and the mean volume was 53 cm^3. Ten patients (10%) survived more than 18 months, and three patients are long-term survivors (18, 19, and 45 months). Twenty-eight (45%) of 68 patients who had one or more follow-up radiographic studies to assess tumor response showed 30% or more reduction in tumor size. Significant pain relief was observed in 37 (65%) of 57 patients. Nineteen patients (20%) experienced postoperative complications: one patient died of a pancreatic fistula and generalized sepsis, and 8 patients (8%) experienced major complications that included fistula formation, gastrointestinal bleeding, gastrointestinal obstruction, and intraabdominal abscess. Similar survival results in groups of 12 to 18 patients have been reported by Mohiuddin and associates,[151] Shipley and co-workers,[218] and Syed and colleagues.[230]

Because of putative potential biologic disadvantages of ^{125}I (*i.e.,* long half-life and low dose rate), Peretz and associates[171] introduced palladium 103 (half-life of 17 days and 20–23 keV) as a new isotope for pancreatic implants.

Biliary Tree

An increasingly popular technique is the insertion of radioactive sources in Teflon catheters placed in the biliary tree under fluoroscopic conditions. The main objective is to drain bile and palliate obstructive jaundice. Because these tumors have a tendency to spread to the periductal tissues and the regional lymph nodes, intracatheter irradiation is considered a boost, administered as a supplement to external irradiation to a larger volume.[54, 106, 121]

A transhepatic cholangiogram is performed; in patients who have undergone a surgical procedure, the cholangiogram can be performed through the T-tube. In patients not treated surgically, a percutaneous cholangiogram is carried out under fluoroscopic control.

After the site of obstruction is identified, flexible catheters are inserted into the biliary tree to appropriate depths, under fluoroscopic control. A dual-lumen catheter or two separate catheters should be inserted, one for lodging the radioactive sources and the other for bile drainage. The patency of the biliary tree is monitored with injection of radioactive material under fluoroscopic control. Special care must be taken to maintain biliary drainage. Otherwise, the patient will develop pain and fever as a result of obstructive cholangitis.[54] The catheter is sutured to the skin.

Radiographs are obtained to determine the length of active radioactive sources to be inserted and the exact position of the catheter for dosimetric purposes (Fig. 13-35). Doses of 2000 cGy to 3000 cGy are delivered at 1 cm from the catheter. This is combined with external irradiation (4500–5000 cGy) to encompass the periductal tissues and regional lymph nodes. If only intracavitary irradiation is prescribed, the doses with this modality are 6000 cGy to 6500 cGy at 1 cm.

Meerwaldt and associates[141] reported 42 patients with bile duct tumors treated with one or two brachytherapy sessions and external irradiation. A dose of 1500 cGy was delivered at each of two sessions or 2500 cGy in one session, calculated at 1 cm from the wire, combined with external irradiation (4000 cGy in 16 fractions). Fourteen percent of the patients survived for 2 years or more. Fever occurred shortly after the insertion of the ^{192}Ir wire in 6 of 38 brachytherapy sessions; it was usually controlled with antibiotics.

Herskovic and colleagues[88] reported ten patients in whom ^{192}Ir sources were inserted into intrabiliary tree catheters to deliver doses of approximately 5000 cGy. Fields and Emami[54] reported eight patients with extrahepatic biliary duct carcinomas treated with intracavitary ^{192}Ir implants, usually combined with external irradiation. Total doses ranged from 6000 cGy to 7600 cGy at 1 cm from the sources. Median survival was

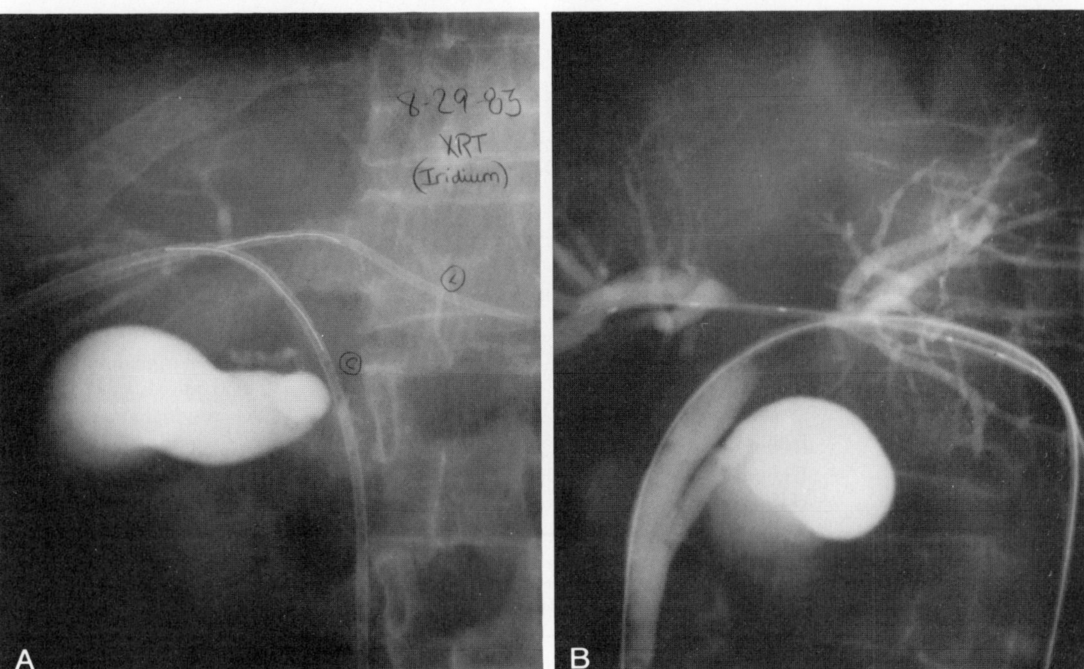

FIGURE 13–35. (**A**) Radiograph of ^{192}Ir afterloading implant in common bile duct. (**B**) Biliary tree with contrast material.

15 months, and only one patient survived as long as 3 years. Two patients developed fatal cholangitis: one during the implant and another later on; two patients developed symptomatic duodenal ulcers, one of them complicated with small bowel obstruction. Others, including Kopelson[122] and Conroy and associates,[34] have reported their results with similar techniques (Table 13-2).

Uterine Cervix

Fletcher[55] illustrated the importance of selecting the appropriate diameter for cylinders or colpostats and the length for intrauterine tandems. The use of a colpostat or vaginal cylinder with the largest clinically indicated diameter yields the highest tumor dose at the depth for a given mucosal dose. Keep in mind the surface dose because excessive irradiation to the vaginal mucosa (maximum 15,000 cGy total dose to the proximal and 10,000 cGy total dose to the distal vagina) may cause severe mucosal atrophy, fibrosis, and vaginal stenosis or necrosis.[100] Similarly, longer tandems improve the doses delivered to the lateral parametrium and the pelvic lymph nodes.

Brachytherapy Systems

Initially, three systems for brachytherapy in carcinoma of the uterine cervix were developed: the Paris, the Swedish, and the Manchester systems[155] (Fig. 13-36). The systems differed in the type of applicator used, strength of the source, and time of administration.[155] In the United States, most of the systems used are derivations of the Manchester technique.

It has always been difficult to express the radiation dose in the treatment of gynecologic tumors. The Manchester intracavitary system, introduced by Tod and Meredith[237] in 1938, was the first applicator and loading system designed to meet certain dosimetric specifications, and it used a dosimetric field quantity, total exposure at point A, to prescribe treatment, rather than milligram hours. Point A was defined as being 2 cm above the mucous membrane of the lateral vaginal fornix and 2 cm lateral to the center of the uterine canal. Allegedly, this area corresponded to the paracervical triangle, in the medial edge of the broad ligament, where the uterine vessels cross the ureter. A subsequent arbitrary convention defined point A as being 2 cm above the external cervical os and 2 cm lateral to the midline. Yet another definition located point A 2 cm above the distal end of the lowest source in the cervical canal and 2 cm lateral to the tandem. Batley and Constable[15] illustrated how these modifications to the basic conventions affected the dose to point A because of the different definitions (Fig. 13-37).

The two most vulnerable points in the pelvis were thought to be the vaginal mucosa and the rectovaginal septum, opposite the cervix. No more than 40% of total dose at point A could be delivered safety through the vaginal mucosa. The rectal dose should be 80% or less of the dose at point A; this rectal dose can usually be achieved by careful packing.

Point B was established at the same level as point A, 5 cm from the midline; this point was near the obturator lymph nodes and gave an indication of the lateral throw-off dose.

Applicators for Treatment of Cervical Carcinoma

Applicators used to insert intracavitary sources in the uterus and vagina include rubber catheters and ovoids developed by French researchers, metallic tandems and plaques designed in Sweden, and the plastic tandems and ovoids of the Manchester system. Fletcher[55] designed a preloadable colpostat, which Suit[229] modified and made afterloadable.

Plastic caps placed posteriorly over the 2.0-cm ovoids increase the diameter to 2.5 cm or 3 cm. At Washington University, the 2-cm diameter ovoids have a surface dose of 6.3 cGy/mgh and are loaded with 20-mg sources. If plastic caps are used with the regular ovoids, the surface dose with 2.5-cm ovoids is 4.2 cGy/mgh and 3.0 cGy/mgh with 3-cm ovoids. Therefore, 25-mg or 30-mg sources are inserted.

The tandems, about 6 mm in diameter, are available in three curvatures. A flange or stopper is used to keep the uterine tandem in the selected position; a keeled flange can be used to avoid rotation of the tandem. Recently, a special yoke was de-

TABLE 13–2
*Intraluminal Radiation Therapy in Biliary Tract Cancer**

INVESTIGATIONS	NO. OF PATIENTS	ISOTOPE	RADIATION DOSE (cGy)	PATIENTS WITH EXTERNAL BEAM ALSO	PATIENTS WITH LOCAL FAILURE	ALIVE ≥2 YEARS
Shahbazian et al[215]	6	Radium	20,000	1/6	4	0
Conroy et al[34]	8	Iridium	4000 to 4800	0/8	3	0†
Fletcher et al[58]	8					
Herskovic et al[88] Chitwood et al[28] Heaston et al[82]	15	Iridium	5000	11/18	2 marginal misses; 1 microscopic residual at autopsy	0‡
Meerwaldt et al[141]	35	Iridium	6500	35/35		14%
Fields an Emami[54]	8	Iridium	6000 to 7500	8/8	6	1 patient
Druy et al[49]	7	Iridium	1950 to 4669	6/7	5§	0

* *The series of Shahbazian et al and Conroy et al include patients with primary bile duct carcinomas and patients with other lesions in this area (pancreatic carcinoma or metastases to the porta hepatis); the data from Duke University[28,82,88] include only primary bile duct cases. The data of Druy et al include five extrahepatic biliary duct primary tumors and two local recurrences of adenocarcinoma of the ampulla of Vater.*
† *Two alive at 22+ and 23+ months.*
‡ *One alive at 18+ months.*
§ *Including local persistence and local recurrence.*
(Kopelson G, Gunderson LL: J Clin Gastroenterol 5:43, 1983)

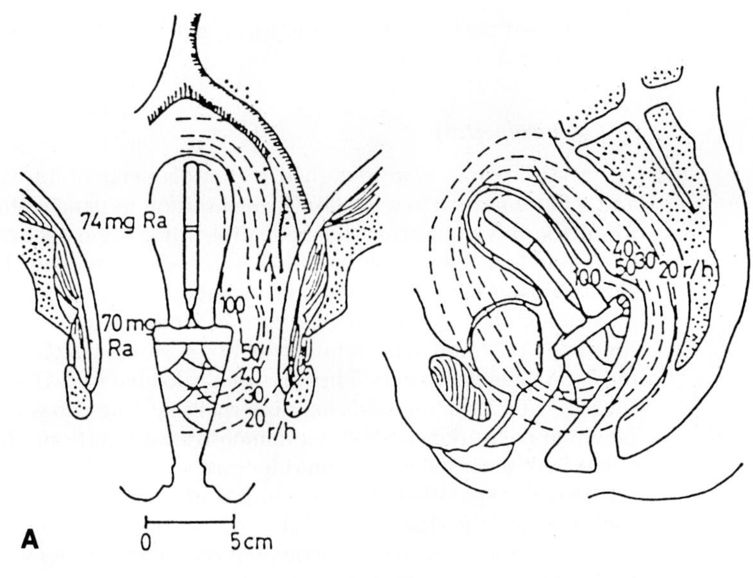

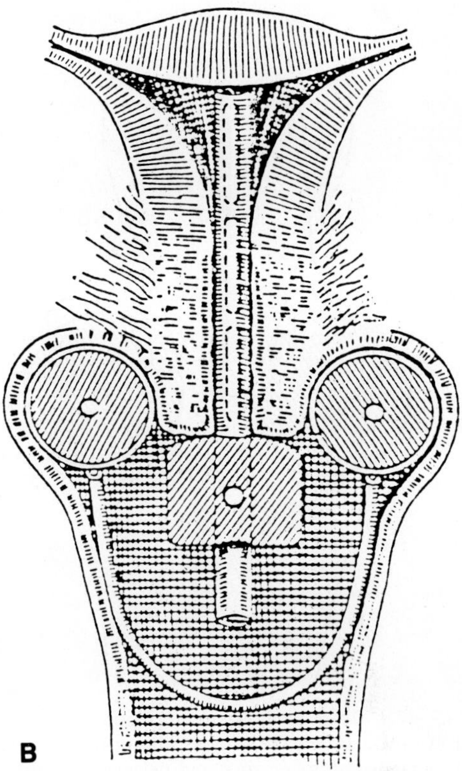

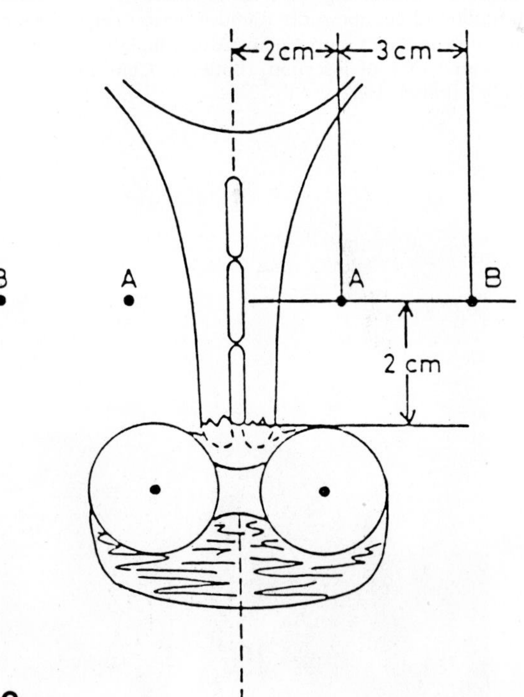

FIGURE 13–36. (**A**) The Stockholm system. The intrauterine rod-shaped applicator is loaded with 53 to 88 mg of radium (74 mg in the example shown). The vaginal applicator usually consists of a flat box containing 60 to 80 mg of radium (70 mg in the example shown), but in special cases, other forms of vaginal applicators may be used. Classically, the two applicators are not fixed to each other, but fixed or semifixed combinations have been developed. The vaginal applicator is held against the cervix and lateral fornices by careful and systematic gauze packing. Typically, 2 or 3 applications are given with 3-week intervals, each application lasting for 27 to 30 hours. (Walstam R: Acta Radiol 42:237, 1954) (**B**) The Paris system. Typical radium application for treatment of cervix carcinoma consisting of three individualized vaginal sources (one in each lateral fornix and one in front of the cervical os), one intrauterine source made of three radium tubes (in so-called tandem position). The active length of the sources is usually 16 mm, with linear activity between 6 and 10 mg/cm and strength between 10 and 15 mg of radium. The total activity is one of the lowest used for such treatments and implies a typical application duration of 6 to 8 days. Typically, the ratio of the total activity of the vaginal sources to the total activity of the uterine sources should be 1 (with variations between 0.66 and 1.5). (Pierquin B: Precis de Curietherapie, Endocurietherapie et Plesiocurietherapie. Paris, Masson, 1964) (**C**) The Manchester system. Definitions of points A and B in the classical Manchester system are found in the text. In a typical application, the loading of intrauterine applicators varied between 20 and 35 mg of radium and between 15 and 25 mg of radium for each vaginal ovoid. The resultant treatment time to get 8000 R at point A was 140 hours. (Meredith WJ: Radium Dosage: The Manchester system. Edinburgh, Livingston, 1967).

signed to maintain the position between the intrauterine tandem and the colpostats.[43] In general, the loading in the tandem is with 20–10–10 mg Ra eq ^{137}Cs sources.

It is extremely important when applicators are purchased to examine the design, obtain radiographs to identify the position of the shielding,[45] and take dosimetric measurements after determining the diameter and thickness of the walls of the applicator to determine the exact dose distribution around the applicators.[76,77,209]

If ideally inserted in the patient, the tandem should be in the midline or nearly equidistant from the lateral pelvic wall, and the vaginal colpostats should be symmetrically positioned against the cervix in relation to the tandem (Fig. 13-38A). The tandem should be kept along the sagittal axis of the pelvis, equidistant from the pubis, sacral promontory, and lateral pelvic wall (Fig. 13-38B) as allowed by the geometry of the patient and the tumor to avoid overdosage to the bladder, rectosigmoid, or either ureter.

The total number of milligram hours prescribed depends on the total dose (cGy) desired at point A according to tumor stage or volume, the number and strength of sources inserted in the tandem and vaginal colpostats, the number of insertions

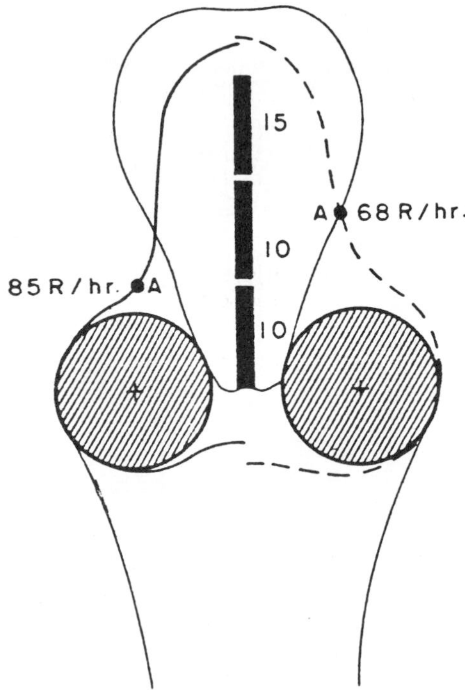

FIGURE 13–37. Diagram showing the position of point A when the cervix protrudes between the ovoids. The position of point A is no longer the same using the original and newer definitions. The newer definition (2 cm above distal end of lowest cervical source and 2 cm lateral to midline) moves point A to a higher dose level, resulting in decreased time of insertion. (Batley F, Constable WC: J Can Assoc Radiol 18:396, 1967)

(one or two) performed, and the whole-pelvis dose delivered with external irradiation.

Minicolpostats

Minicolpostats were designed with a diameter of 1.6 cm and a flat inner surface to allow their insertion in patients for whom the only alternative would be a protruding vaginal source in the tandem.[44] Some miniovoids have no shielding, and the surface dose is significantly higher than with the regular ovoids; at Washington University, with cesium 3M sources, the surface dose is 9.8 cGy/mgh in the miniovoids, in contrast to 6.3 cGy for the 2-cm diameter ovoids. They are usually loaded with 10-mg sources. The 3M miniovoids have internal shielding. However, phantom measurements did not demonstrate a significant decrease in dose for the newer minicolpostats with rectal shielding for a source separation of 3 cm, which could allow undue user confidence in the doses delivered.

Kuske and associates[126] carried out dosimetry studies with thermoluminescent dosimeters in phantoms and compared them with computer-calculated doses to point A, bladder, and rectum. The calculated or computed doses for the minicolpostats or regular colpostats were in close agreement. The measured dose to point A, bladder, and rectum with the minicolpostats is approximately 10% higher than with the regular ovoids. Because of the decreased capacity of the vaginal vault, packing may be more difficult, which results in the bladder and rectum being closer to the cesium sources. Despite using 10 mg Ra eq sources in the miniovoids, the tandem in the minicolpostat system contributes a 6% to 8% higher dose to point A and the surrounding structures than with the regular colpostats.

Evaluating the results of therapy in 99 patients with carcinoma of the cervix on whom miniovoids were used, Kuske and colleagues[126] reported a 15% incidence of grade 3 complications

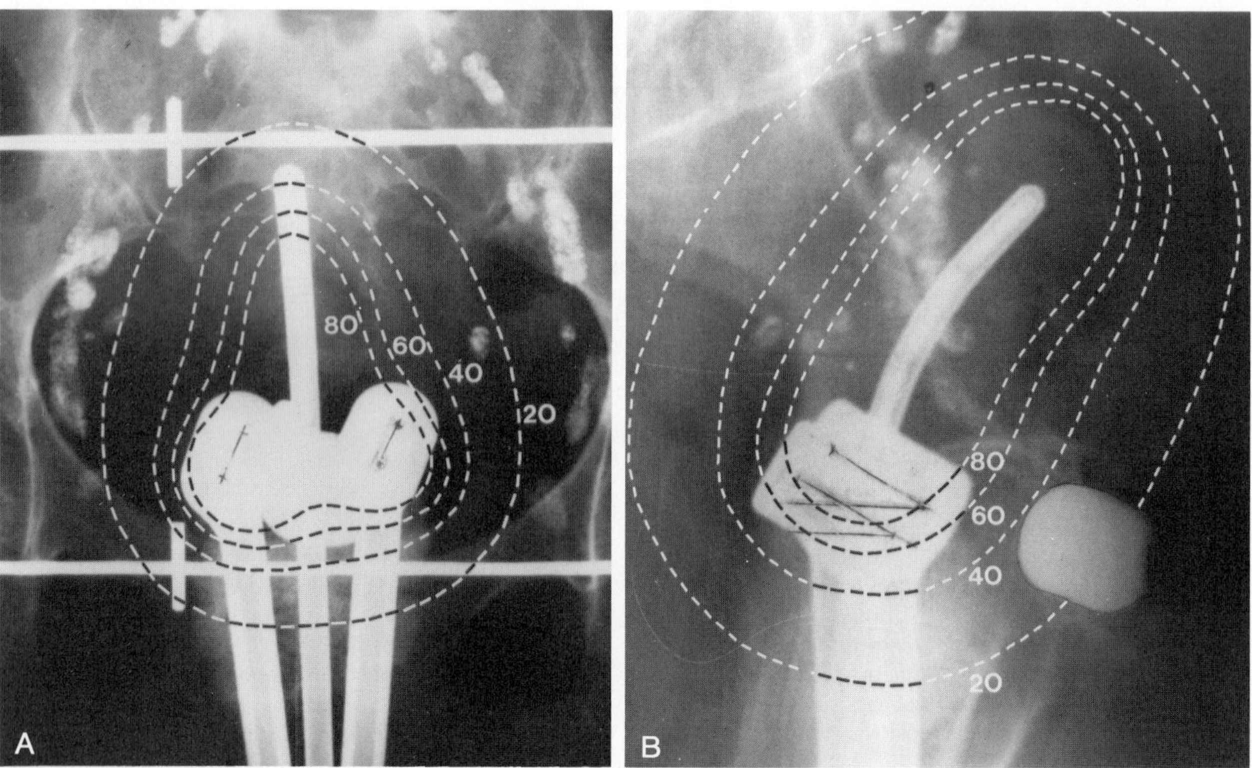

FIGURE 13–38. **(A)** Anteroposterior view of intracavitary insertion for carcinoma of the uterine cervix. **(B)** Lateral view of same implant. Isodose curves (cGy/hour) are superimposed.

compared with 8% observed in a group of 194 patients treated concurrently with regular (2-cm) colpostats ($P=0.08$).

Henschke Applicator

The Henschke[45] and other applicators are commercially available. The hemispheric ovoids are inserted parallel to the lateral wall of the vaginal vault and the intrauterine tandem. Three ovoid diameters and various tandems are available. Although this applicator's configuration conforms better to a narrow vaginal vault, the radioactive sources are placed parallel to the long axis of the bladder and the rectum and do not have any shielding, potentially delivering a higher dose to these organs. Delclos and colleagues[45] emphasized that the dosimetry with the Fletcher colpostats is unique and that treatment techniques and tables derived for this applicator should not be used with other applicators to avoid significantly higher doses to the vagina, bladder, or rectum. Figure 13-39 illustrates the differences in dose delivered with the Fletcher or the Henschke applicator to the bladder or rectum for a normalized dose of 7000 cGy to point A.

Interstitial Implants for Cervical Carcinoma

Metallic needles containing ^{226}Ra, ^{60}Co, or ^{137}Cs and, more recently, afterloading metallic guides or Teflon catheters for insertion of ^{192}Ir wires or seeds have been implanted in the parametrium or in the cervix, using a transvaginal or transperineal approach, sometimes instead of intracavitary insertions if the cervical canal could not be identified.[194]

The procedure is similar to that followed in intracavitary insertions. The cervix should always be held firmly with a tenaculum. For implants in the cervix itself, the needles or nylon catheters with metallic guides (5–6 cm long) are inserted straight, about 1.2 cm apart, following the position of the uterus, which can be verified with a finger in the rectum, in a single- or double-circle arrangement. If a single circle is used, full-intensity sources are required. If a double circle is implanted, the central one should have half-intensity sources (usually four), and the periphery should have full-intensity sources. At Washington University, the parametrial Teflon catheters with metallic guides, usually 12 to 15 cm long, are inserted through the vaginal fornices. A double-plane or volume-type implant usually can be placed in each parametrium. The catheters are implanted starting at 1 o'clock on the patient's left side and at 11 o'clock on the right, directed parallel to the coronal plane of the patient and 5 to 10 degrees lateral toward the pelvic wall. The peripheral plane should be placed 1.2 to 1.5 cm lateral to the medial plane, and the catheters should be inserted in the same fashion, about 10 degrees lateral from the midline.

Avoid insertion of the needles into the bladder, unless it is necessary to cover the tumor volume. The operator should keep in mind the expected anatomic location of the major pelvic vessels, especially veins, because arteries are more difficult to pierce.

If the uterosacral ligament area is to be implanted, the catheters are directed 5 to 10 degrees posteriorly. In general, six to ten catheters can easily be implanted in each parametrium. We prefer to implant the interstitial catheters alone, without vaginal colpostats or cylinders, to prevent displacement or enhanced penetration of the needles (Fig. 13-40). Gentle packing with iodoform gauze keeps the needles in place. Cystoscopy and a careful rectal examination at the completion of the procedure help identify any misplaced needles, which should be withdrawn or replaced immediately.

Aristizabal and co-workers,[12] Martinez and associates,[138] and Syed and colleagues[231] popularized the use of interstitial implants, using perineal templates, with introduction of long metallic guides through the perineum into the parametrial tissues (Fig. 13-41). The ^{192}Ir seeds or ^{137}Cs microspheres in nylon tubes are inserted in an afterloading fashion after x-ray films are obtained with dummy sources for dosimetry computations. Aristizabal and colleagues[12] modified their technique by deleting three anteriorly and three posteriorly placed needles in the central row; the central tandem also was omitted to decrease the initially high incidence of vesicovaginal or rectovaginal fistula. The authors reported about 75% pelvic tumor control in 118 patients with stage IIB and III carcinoma of the uterine cervix. The major complication rate was 6% with less than 4500 mgh, 16% with 4500 mgh to 4999 mgh, 28% with 5500 mgh, and 87% with higher intracavitary doses, combined with 4500 cGy to 5000 cGy to the whole pelvis.

Martinez and others[138] reported the results of treating 104 patients with locally advanced or recurrent pelvic tumor using a MUPIT combined with external irradiation of 3600 cGy to the whole pelvis and 1400 cGy to the pelvic sidewall with a midline

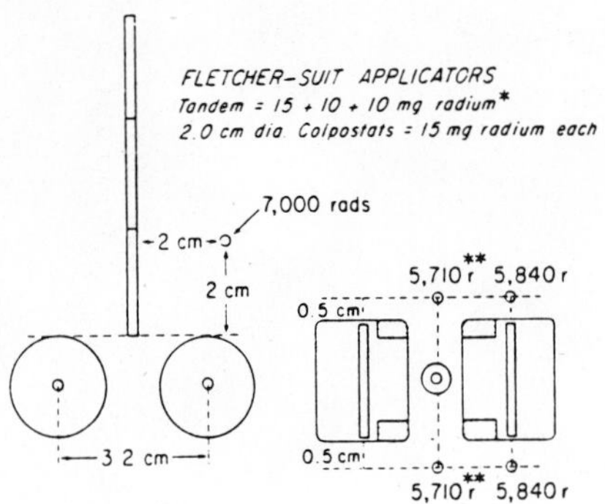

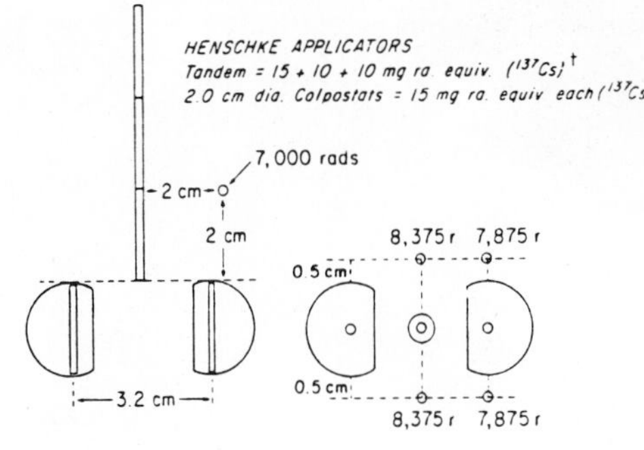

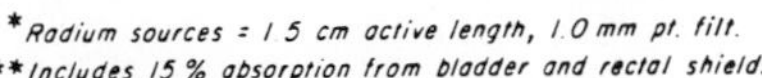

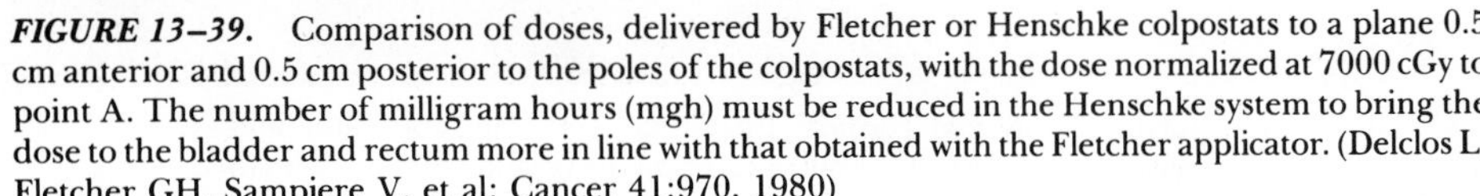
FIGURE 13–39. Comparison of doses, delivered by Fletcher or Henschke colpostats to a plane 0.5 cm anterior and 0.5 cm posterior to the poles of the colpostats, with the dose normalized at 7000 cGy to point A. The number of milligram hours (mgh) must be reduced in the Henschke system to bring the dose to the bladder and rectum more in line with that obtained with the Fletcher applicator. (Delclos L, Fletcher GH, Sampiere V, et al: Cancer 41:970, 1980)

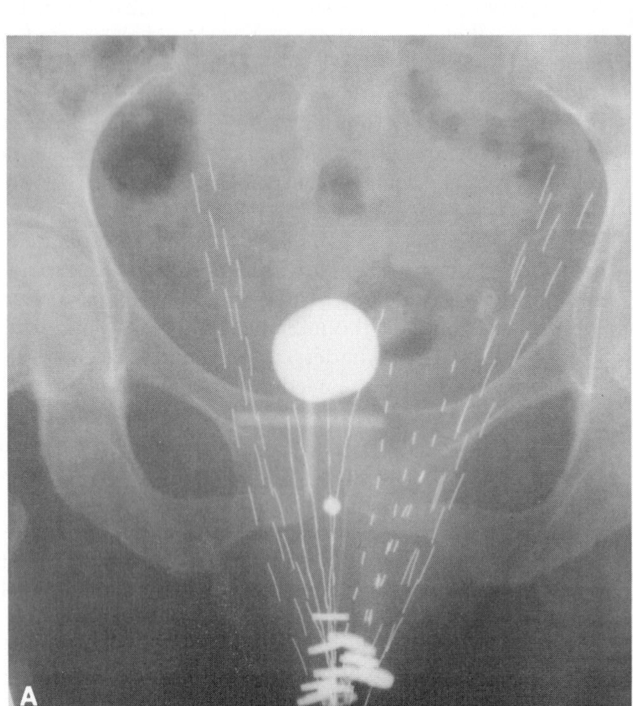

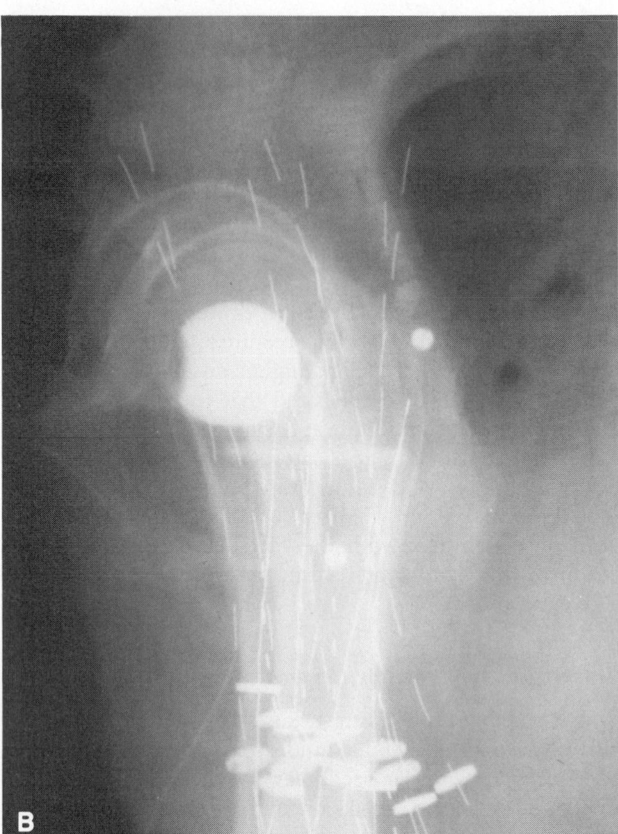

FIGURE 13–40. (**A**) Anteroposterior and (**B**) lateral radiographs of the pelvis illustrating bilateral parametrial implants (with sources extending into vaginal walls) for extensive carcinoma of the uterine cervix. Upper radiopaque marker indicates the position of the cervix. Lower radiopaque marker denotes the distal margin of the vaginal tumor extension.

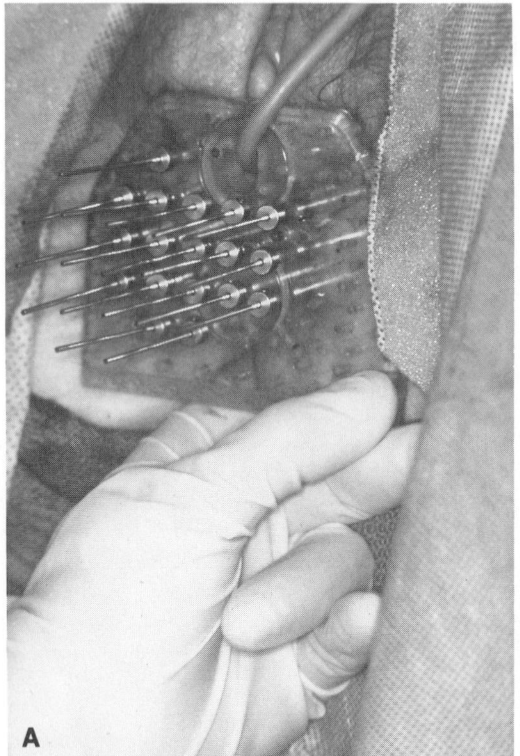

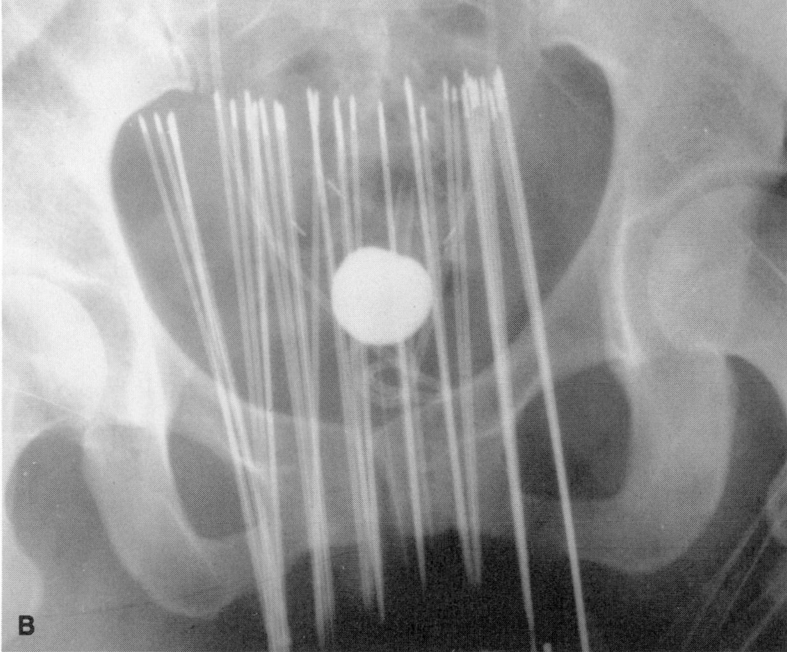

FIGURE 13–41. (**A**) Patient with Martinez Universal Perineal Interstitial Template applicator and metallic guides in place. (**B**) Anteroposterior radiograph of the pelvis showing the position of the guides in the parametrium.

TABLE 13–3
Results of External Beam and Template for Locally Advanced (IIB, IIIB) Cervical Cancer

INVESTIGATIONS	PATIENTS IN SERIES	LOCAL RECURRENCE (No./%)	COMPLICATIONS (No./%)
Feder et al[53]	35	14 (40)	3 (9)
Aristizabal et al[12]	118	30 (25)	25 (21)
Martinez et al[138]	37	37 (17)	2 (5.4)
Gaddis et al[62]	51	17 (33)	8 (16)
Ampuero et al[4]	24	9 (38)	7 (29)
Total of series	230	62 (27)	42 (18)

block using four-field techniques and 4-MV or 10-MV photons. Local tumor control was obtained in 82% of 63 patients with gynecologic lesions. The major complication rate was 3.2%.

Results reported by several authors using templates in locally advanced uterine carcinoma are shown in Table 13-3.

Endometrium

Carcinoma of the endometrium may grow irregularly into the uterine cavity and produce deformity of the lumen from exophytic tumor, thickening of the uterine wall caused by myometrial infiltration, or uterine enlargement. It is important to determine the size and shape of the uterus; this can be accomplished by rotating the uterine sound and measuring the width and depth of the uterine cavity and by bimanual palpation or hysterogram. Special care should be taken to avoid a perforation, but if one occurs, packing with Heyman capsules should not be performed at that time. However, a carefully inserted tandem may be used, avoiding the site of perforation. Ultrasound may help in ascertaining the exact position of the tandem. Rutledge and Delclos[205] also caution against rupture (splitting) of the cervix, which may be caused by excessive, careless dilatation.

Uterine packing with capsules was originally described by Heyman in 1934.[89] The practice of introducing as many capsules as possible to stretch the wall of the uterus has several advantages, as outlined by Rutledge and others[205]: a bulky tumor can be flattened out, allowing the base of the lesion to be more effectively irradiated; stretching of the uterine wall to make it thinner permits higher doses to be delivered to the serosa of the organ; and a more uniform distribution of the radiation is delivered to the entire myometrium.

In addition to the metallic and plastic standard Heyman capsules, afterloading Heyman-Simon capsules have become commercially available in diameters of 6 mm, 8 mm, and 10 mm and lengths of 2 cm to 3 cm. Inactive metallic guides and later ^{137}Cs sources are inserted.

If capsules are used, it is convenient to insert an afterloading tandem to cover the lower uterine segment. This permits more flexibility in the loading and improves coverage of this portion of the uterus and the cervical canal. Afterloading colpostats should be used to irradiate the vaginal cuff (Fig. 13-42). A technical problem with the afterloading Heyman-Simon capsules is the relatively large thickness of the stems, requiring continued dilatation of the cervical canal (Hegar dilators) after a few capsules have been inserted.

It is critical to record the order of insertion of the capsules (by numbers that are printed on each capsule), so that the removal is done in the reverse order of insertion. Otherwise, the capsules may become jammed, making removal more difficult. Ideally, a minimum of four capsules should be inserted. If fewer are allowed by the size of the endometrial cavity, it may be better to insert an afterloading tandem.

The dose of irradiation delivered with this system is somewhat empirically derived. In preoperative insertions, we use 3500 mgh in the uterine cavity; however, cavities larger than 8 cm receive doses of approximately 4000 mgh. Doses of 6000 cGy to 6500 cGy to the mucosal surface of the vagina are delivered (1900–2000 mgh) with 2-cm diameter vaginal ovoids. Grigsby and colleagues[72] reported higher survival and fewer pelvic recurrences and distant metastases in patients with stage I poorly differentiated endometrial carcinoma after doses higher than 3500 mgh were delivered in the uterus. Less benefit was derived in treating moderately differentiated tumors.

In patients treated with radiation therapy alone, higher intracavitary doses (in the range of 8000 mgh) are given in two or three insertions. This is combined with 2000-cGy whole-pelvis external irradiation and an additional 3000 cGy to the parametria with midline shielding.

For postoperative irradiation in endometrial carcinoma, if no preoperative irradiation was delivered, we use afterloading colpostats to deliver 6000 to 7000 cGy to the vaginal mucosa (1800–2000 mgh) in patients with moderately or poorly differentiated tumors, even if there is no myometrial invasion. If there is deep myometrial invasion (>50%), regardless of the histologic features, the intracavitary therapy is combined with 2000-cGy whole-pelvis external irradiation and 3000 cGy to parametria with midline shielding. If a preoperative implant was performed, only external irradiation is administered.

Vagina, Vulva, and Female Urethra

The indications for and techniques of interstitial therapy for carcinomas of the vagina, vulva, and urethra have been described.[172,174,175] These areas are potentially vulnerable to severe complications because of the reported lower tolerance of the surrounding tissues to irradiation and because they are exposed to the irritation of perspiration, urine, and feces. It is important to minimize irradiation to the surrounding normal areas.

The use of interstitial implants ideally should be limited to a volume encompassing 75% or less of the circumference of the vagina, particularly if the lesion involves the posterior wall and rectovaginal septum. The remaining normal tissues should be kept away from the implanted area as much as possible with the judicious use of gauze packing or cylinders or templates. Two

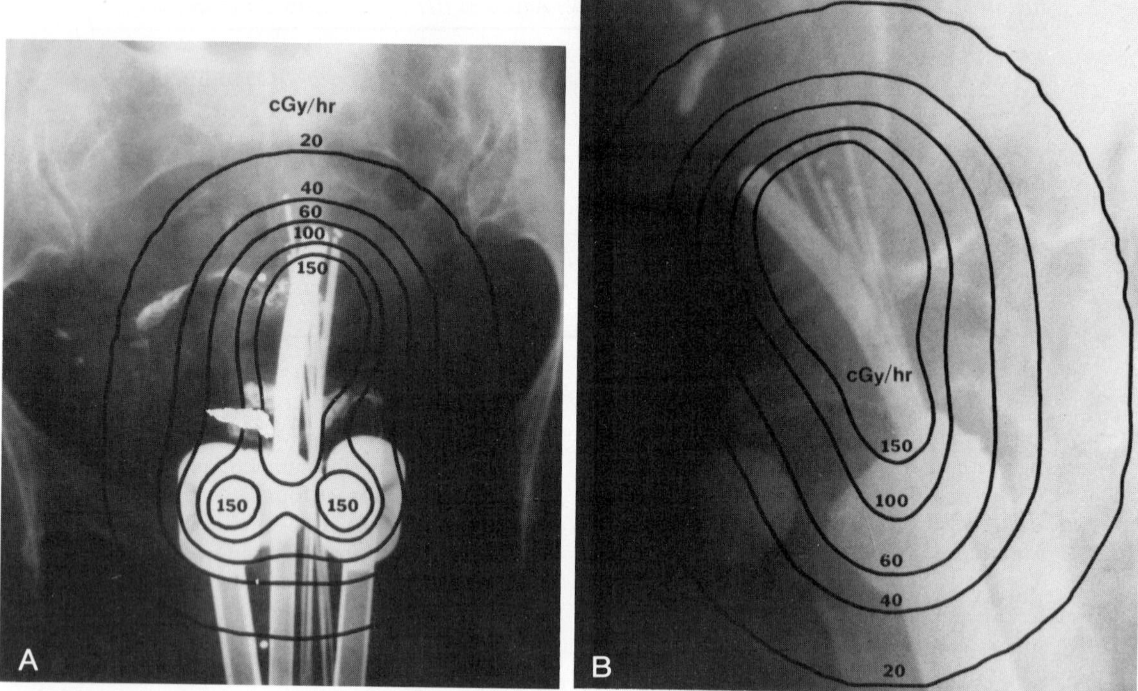

FIGURE 13–42. (**A**) Anteroposterior and (**B**) lateral views of an implant for treatment of carcinoma of the endometrium using Heyman-Simon capsules, afterloading tandem, and vaginal colpostats. Isodose curves (cGy/hour) are superimposed.

rolls of gauze are placed on top of and between the thighs, so that when the legs are brought down from the lithotomy position after implantation, the inside surfaces of the thighs are separated as much as possible from the radioactive sources.

Vaginal Cylinders

Afterloading vaginal cylinders have a central, hollow metallic cylinder, in which the sources are placed, and 2.5-cm-long plastic rings of various diameters, which are inserted over the cylinder. Domed cylinders are used to irradiate the vaginal cuff homogeneously (Fig. 13-43A). Delclos recommends a short cesium source at the top to obtain a uniform dose around the dome, because a lower dose occurs at the end of the linear cesium sources.[44] Some cylinders have lead shielding to protect selected portions of the vagina (Fig. 13-43B). A flange with a keel is placed over the tandem after the last plastic cylinder has been inserted to secure the system in place and avoid rotation.

The Bloedorn applicator incorporated a configuration of vaginal colpostats or a single midline ovoid and vaginal cylinder. Although extensively used, it was never described in detail; the Bloedorn applicator was later adapted for afterloading.[44]

Perez and co-workers[176] designed a vaginal applicator that incorporates two ovoid sources and a central tandem to treat the entire vagina, alone or in combination with the uterine cervix. The applicator has vaginal apex caps and additional cylinder sleeves that allow increased dimensions (Fig. 13-44). The average surface dose rate around the 2-cm ovoids is about 120 cGy/hour, and in the 2.5-cm diameter vaginal cylinder the dose rate is 100 cGy/hour with loading of 20 mg Ra eq ^{137}Cs sources in the ovoids and 10 mg to 15 mg Ra eq ^{137}Cs sources in the cylinder (Fig. 13-45). The tandem in the uterus can be used with standard loadings, depending on the depth of the uterus (20–10–10 or 20–10 mg Ra eq). When the tandem and vaginal cylinder are used, the strength of the sources in the ovoids should always be 15 mg Ra eq. The vaginal cylinder or uterine tandem never carry an active source at the level of the ovoids.

Because there is substantial individualization in the management of patients with vaginal carcinoma, the policies at Mallinckrodt Institute of Radiology for each stage are summarized here.

Carcinoma in Situ

An intracavitary application with a vaginal cylinder or similar applicator (*i.e.,* Bloedorn, Burnett, Delclos, MIRALVA) delivering about 7000 cGy to 8000 cGy to the mucosa is adequate to control all carcinomas *in situ.* Higher doses of irradiation may cause significant vaginal fibrosis and stenosis. Because of the multicentric nature of this tumor, the entire vaginal mucosa must be treated.

Stage I Tumors

The most superficial tumors are treated with an intracavitary insertion alone, usually with a cylinder 2.5 cm to 3 cm in diameter, covering the entire vagina. If the lesion is thicker, a single-plane needle implant is used in addition to the intracavitary cylinder. This has the advantage of increasing the tumor depth dose without delivering excessive irradiation to the uninvolved vaginal mucosa, which receives 6000 cGy to 6500 cGy. The gross tumor is treated with 6500 cGy to 7000 cGy calculated 0.5 cm beyond the plane of the implant; the vaginal mucosa in this area receives an estimated 8000 cGy to 12,000 cGy, depending on the size of lesion and prescribed tumor dose (Fig. 13-46).

At Washington University, more extensive tumors are treated with intracavitary and interstitial therapy supplemented with external-beam irradiation, administering a whole-pelvis dose of 1000 cGy or 2000 cGy, with an additional parame-

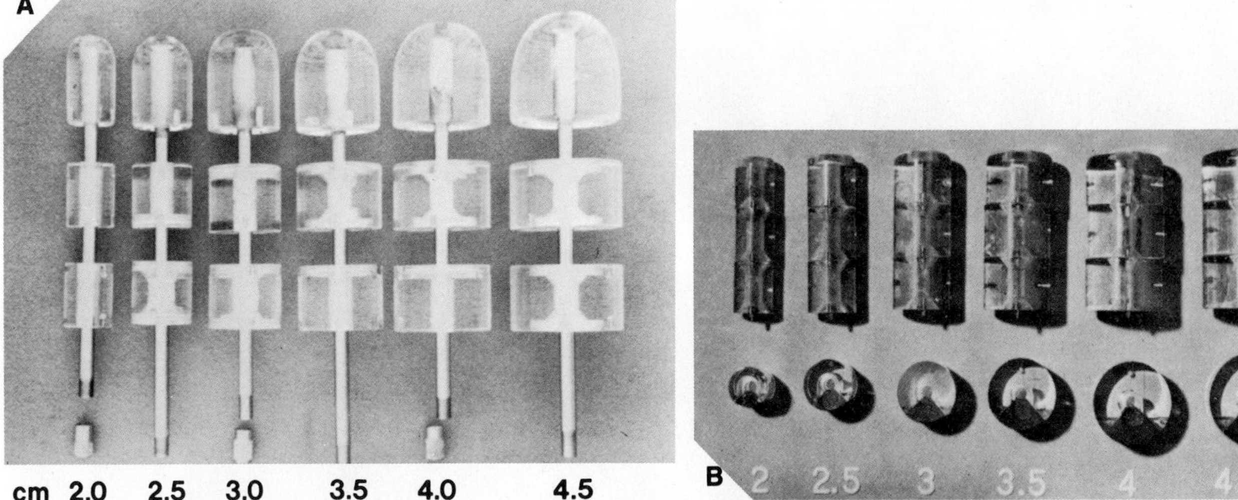

FIGURE 13–43. (**A**) Dome colpostats to treat vaginal cuff alone or vaginal cuff and any selected vaginal length in a patient who had a hysterectomy. The curvature of each dome cylinder follows an isodose of a ^{137}Cs minisource placed at an adequate distance from the dome in the afterloading stem. Vaginal cylinders can be added to the dome cylinders, as shown. Any length of vaginal surface can be treated by combining a ^{137}Cs minisource with radium tubes or cesium sources. (Delclos L, Wharton JT, Rutledge FN: Tumors of the vagina and female urethra. In Fletcher GH [ed]: Textbook of Radiotherapy. Philadelphia, Lea & Febiger, 1980) (**B**) Cylinders with a segment of lead incorporated to shield part of the vaginal wall, rectum, bladder, or urethra. (Delclos L, Fletcher GH, Moore EB, et al: Int J Radiat Oncol Biol Phys 6:1195, 1980)

trial dose with a midline block, to deliver a total of 4500 cGy to 5000 cGy to the lateral pelvic wall.

Stage II Tumors

Patients with more advanced paravaginal tumors without extensive parametrial infiltration (stage II lesions) are always treated with a greater external irradiation dose (2000 cGy to 4000 cGy to the whole pelvis) and an additional parametrial dose with a midline block, to deliver a total of 5000 cGy to 6000 cGy to the lateral pelvic wall. In these patients, intracavitary therapy should also be used to deliver a total of 6500 cGy to the entire vaginal mucosa and an interstitial implant to administer about 7000 cGy to a volume 0.5 cm to 1 cm around the palpable tumor; the dose includes the whole-pelvis external-beam contribution. Because of the extent of the tumor, double-plane or volume implants are frequently necessary.

Stage III and IV Tumors

For stage III and IV tumors, 4000 cGy to the whole pelvis and a total of 5500 cGy to 6000 to cGy parametrial dose with a midline block are administered. As in stage IIA tumors, a vaginal cylinder and an interstitial implant are used to complete total doses of 7500 cGy to 8000 cGy to the tumor volume and 6500 cGy to 7000 cGy to the uninvolved vaginal mucosa. If the

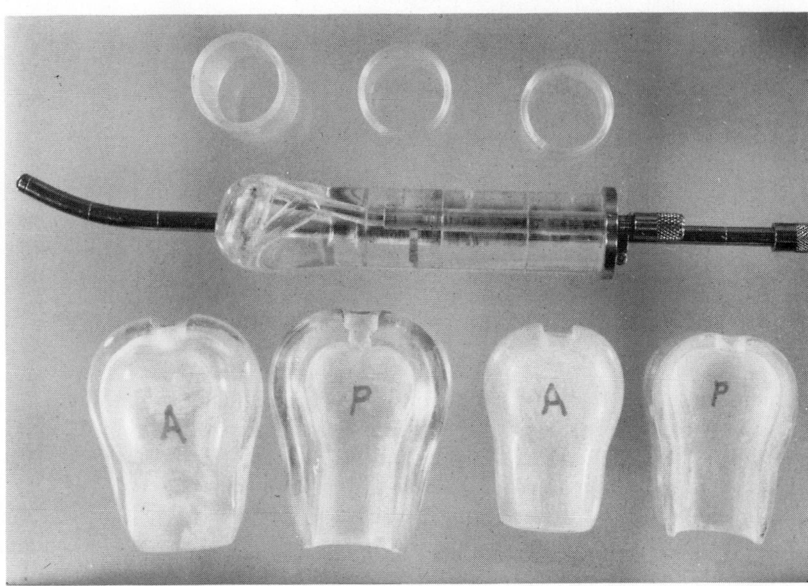

FIGURE 13–44. MIRALVA applicator with plastic sleeves to increase the diameter of the vaginal cylinder, afterloading tandem, and plastic caps (A-P) of different sizes to increase diameter of vaginal cuff portion of applicator.

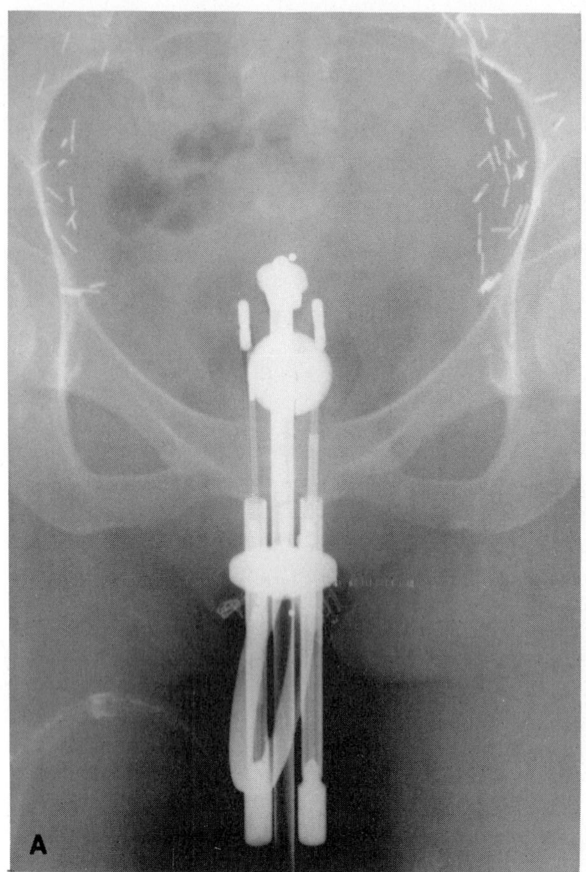

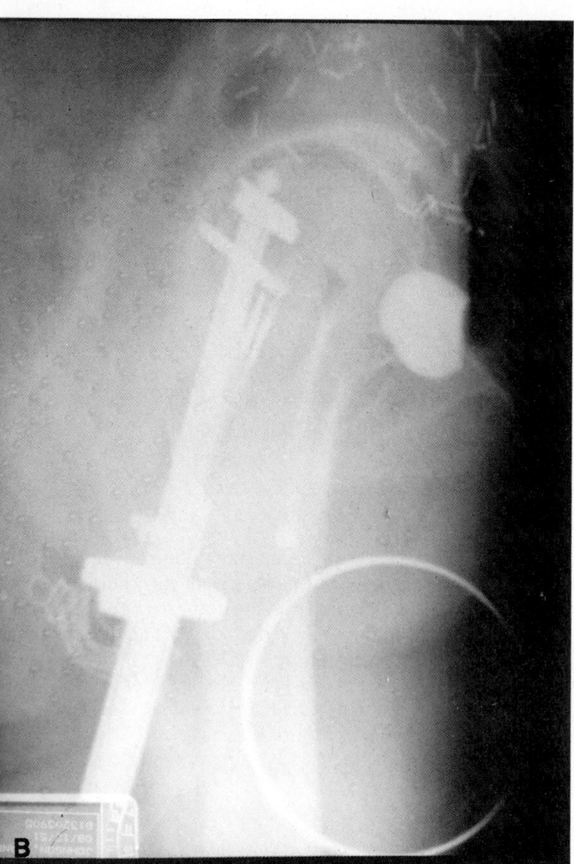

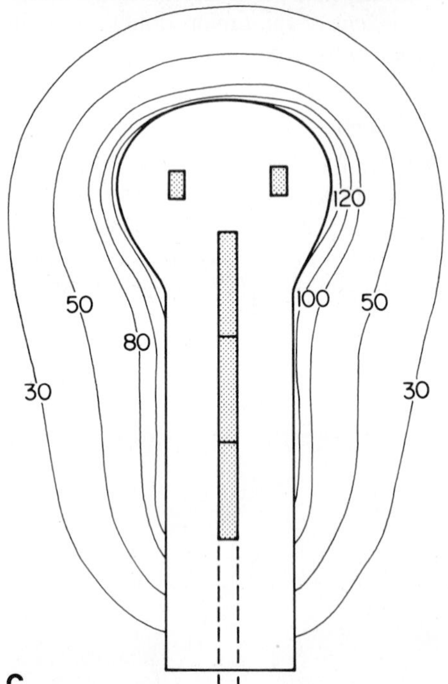

FIGURE 13–45. (**A**) Anteroposterior and (**B**) lateral radiographs depicting position of the MIRALVA applicator for treatment of a patient with vaginal recurrence of a carcinoma of the uterine cervix, previously treated with a radical hysterectomy. (**C**) Isodose curves of the MIRALVA applicator.

tumor is located in the middle or lower third of the vagina, it is possible to combine in one procedure the insertion of a cylinder with the ^{192}Ir implant along the vaginal walls. However, if the tumor is in the upper third or involves the parametrium, we prefer to perform two procedures, because the cylinder may displace the interstitial catheters and distort the geometry of the implant. In patients with parametrial infiltration, in addition to the standard doses, it is advisable to deliver additional 1500 cGy to 2000 cGy with an interstitial implant (Fig. 13-47).

Tumors of the Rectovaginal Septum

When needles or stainless steel guides are being implanted for tumors of the posterior vaginal wall, the rectal ampulla is

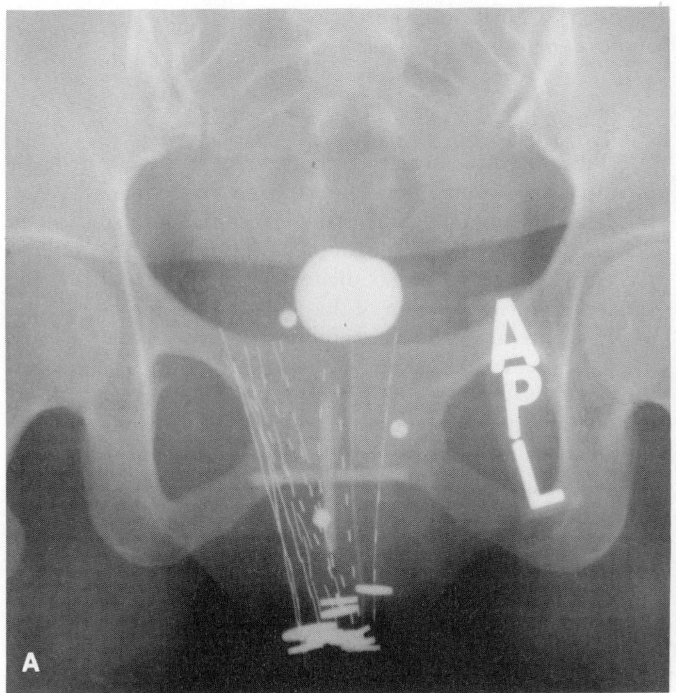

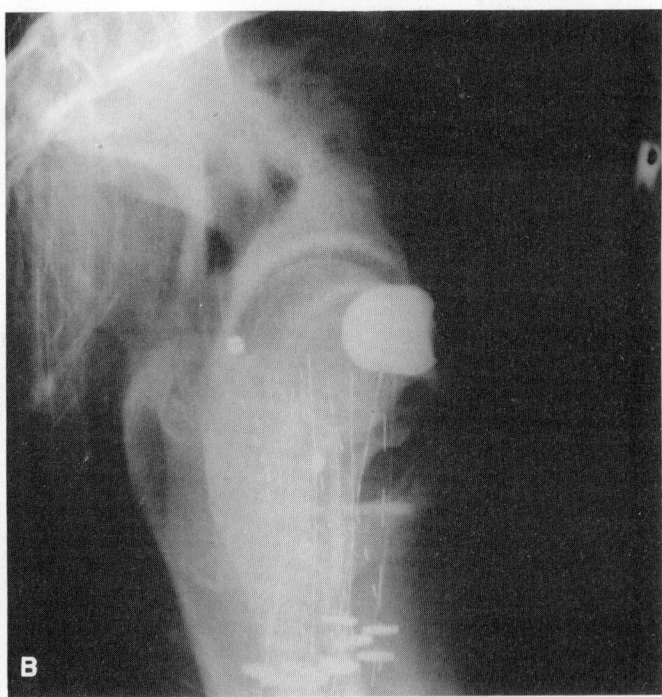

FIGURE 13–46. (**A**) Anteroposterior and (**B**) lateral radiographs of the pelvis illustrating an interstitial implant in a patient with carcinoma of right vaginal wall (intracavitary cylinder omitted).

kept distended with a 30-ml Foley catheter to minimize radiation to the opposite rectal wall.

While the catheters are being inserted in the thin rectovaginal septum, one finger (covered with a second glove) should be inserted in the rectum to ensure that the catheters do not protrude beyond the rectal mucosa. If this occurs, the catheters should be withdrawn and reinserted in a satisfactory position.

Lesions of the Bladder or Proximal Female Urethra

An open-bladder implant may be necessary for lesions of the bladder or tumors of the proximal portion of the female urethra that extend into the bladder neck. This procedure also allows direct visualization of tumor extension into the bladder (Fig. 13-48). If the tumor has extended beyond the vesical wall, the implant procedure is stopped, and external irradiation is used.

Van der Werf-Messing popularized bladder implants with radium or cesium needles.[243] In addition to surgery and general anesthesia, the disadvantages of this technique were radiation safety, impaired wound healing because of acute side effects, and some difficulty in removing the radioactive sources. In a series of 160 patients, the mean hospitalization was 36 days after the operation. In 10% of the patients, the abdomen had to be reopened to remove one or more needles.[16,19]

A different method using iridium wires was designed in

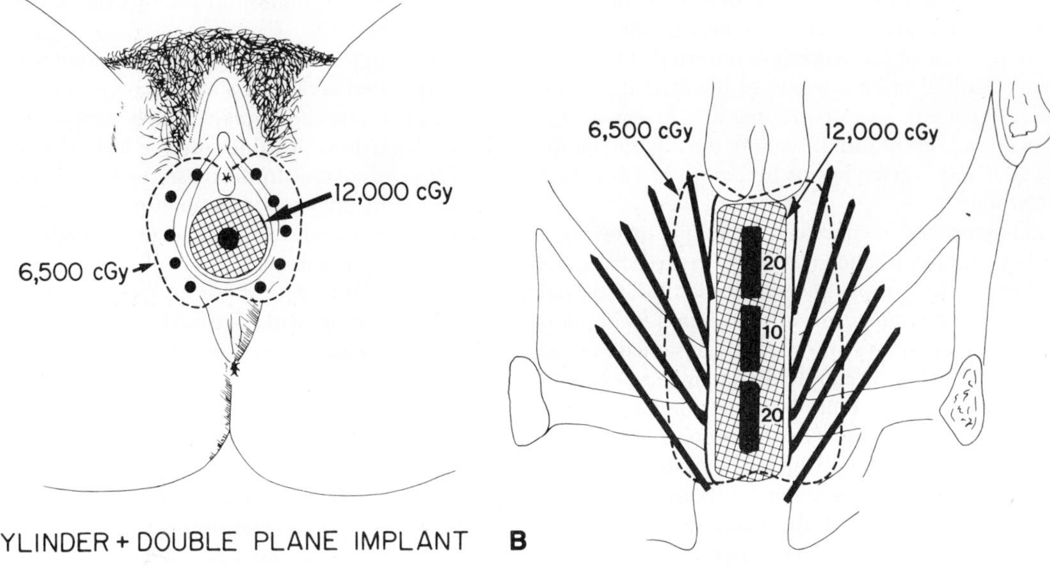

FIGURE 13–47. (**A**) Cross-section (perineal) view of source arrangement for interstitial and intracavitary implant in a patient with involvement of the right and left lateral vaginal walls and paravaginal tissues. (**B**) Coronal illustration of interstitial and intracavitary implant for the same patient.

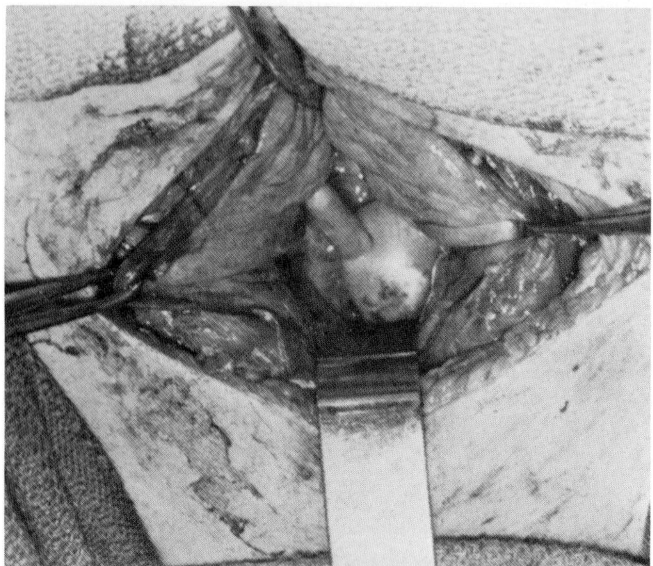

FIGURE 13–48. A suprapubic cystostomy allows the placement of index and middle fingers around the balloon of the Foley catheter to position the stainless steel guides or needles along the vesicovaginal septum and bladder trigone, which minimizes the possibility of a needle entering the urinary bladder. (Delclos L: In Deeley TJ [ed]: Topical Reviews in Radiotherapy and Oncology—2. London, John Wright & Sons, 1982)

France; it was modified by Batterman[16,17] to overcome most of the disadvantages of the rigid needle technique. After a lower abdominal incision, the bladder is opened to visualize the tumor area. Plastic carriers, consisting of a hollow part and a thinner leading end, are inserted 1.5 cm apart. The tubes penetrate the abdominal wall, are tunneled in the bladder muscle, and penetrate the abdominal wall again. The catheters should be placed in such a way that removal is feasible without a second laparotomy, although this may be necessary in more complex cases. Dummy sources are introduced in the carriers to visualize the length of the source to be used while the bladder is still open. After the bladder is closed, the positions of the sources are checked, and the abdomen is closed. A Foley catheter is placed for drainage. After film localization, the dose distribution is determined. The carriers are connected to the MicroSelectron, and the radioactive phase of the procedure is started. The tubes are well tolerated and, after completion of irradiation, can be removed easily. All patients receive preoperative external irradiation (3000 cGy) to prevent tumor seeding during the operation. A dose of 4000 cGy is given by brachytherapy at a dose rate of 30 to 50 cGy/hour.

Gerard and associates[65] reported a technique involving a combination of external irradiation (1050 cGy in three fractions in 3 days), external iliac lymph node dissection, and partial cystectomy to remove the tumor, in addition to an ^{192}Ir implant using a nylon thread technique or a specially designed curved needle to implant the nylon thread. Radiopaque markers help to position the ^{192}Ir wires, which are 5 cm to 9 cm long, with a linear activity of 1.2 to 2 mCi/cm. The thickness of the treated volume depends on the spacing of the wires (6–10 mm). The dose is calculated using the Paris system: 4000 cGy to 5000 cGy specified on the 85% isodose of the basal dose. The brachytherapy application lasts 2 to 5 days, depending on the dose desired, and removal is accomplished by pulling the plastic tubes. Somewhat comparable brachytherapy techniques for treatment of carcinoma of the bladder have been described by Moonen,[152] Maat and Venselaar,[130] Battermann and Boon,[17] and Wijnmaalen and associates.[257]

Tumors of the Vulva or Distal Urethra

Vulvar or distal urethral tumors can be treated with similar brachytherapy techniques. The patient is placed in a lithotomy position, and single, double-plane, or volume implants can be designed around the urethra or in the vulvar labia. We prefer to place a No. 8 or 10 Hegar dilator in the urethra during the procedure for orientation of the planes of the implant. If the proximal urethra is involved, the radioactive sources must be inserted reaching the bladder. After the procedure is completed, the Hegar dilator is withdrawn; cystoscopy is performed to ascer-to ascertain the position of the catheters in the bladder, and an indwelling catheter is inserted. If there is intravesical bleeding, periodic irrigation of the bladder is necessary every 4 hours while the implant is in place, and it is preferable to leave the catheter in place for 3 to 7 days to avoid clot formation and bladder neck obstruction. If the vulva is involved, the sources must protrude into the perineum. If the tumor extends into the vagina, an intravaginal cylinder with some sources may be necessary to increase the dose to the vaginal mucosa (Fig. 13-49).

The design of the implant, placement of the radioactive sources, and tumor doses are similar to those for comparable lesions in the vagina.

Anal Canal and Rectum

Interstitial or intracavitary techniques have been used for many years to treat anorectal carcinoma. Ideally, implants should be restricted to lesions that require implantation of no more than half the circumference of the anal canal for preservation of sphincter function. Single-plane, double-plane, or volume implants may be necessary, depending on the extent of the tumor.

The catheters are inserted through the perianal area in the central plane 0.5 cm away from the anal or rectal mucosa, with one double-gloved finger in the rectum to verify placement. Peripheral planes are placed with 1-cm to 1.5-cm spacing. The anal canal is kept distended with a custom-designed rectal plug, which reduces the dose to the opposite side of the canal to less than 15% of the minimum tumor dose at the implanted area (Fig. 13-50).

Although a colostomy may be avoided with diligent care of the implanted area, this is not always practical. It may be necessary to precede the implant with a temporary diverting colostomy, regardless of tumor size or lack of bowel constriction.

It is important to decrease the irradiation of the adjacent buttock and thighs as described in the section on treating tumors of the vagina, vulva, and urethra. Ivalon or gauze is placed in the intergluteal space.

The MUPIT applicator has been used in the treatment of anorectal tumors with satisfactory results.[138]

Kin and associates[119] used a template for insertion of hollow, steel needles to place the ^{192}Ir and a rubber drain for treatment of patients with carcinoma of the anal canal, combined with external-beam irradiation in some patients. A ring-shaped template with the appropriate number and length of radioactive hollow, steel needles was placed over the anus, and the needles were successfully implanted into the corresponding holes (about 1 cm apart) into the anal or rectal wall. The template and rubber drain were carefully withdrawn while maintaining the needles in place. The needles were secured, and the whole applicator was held in place by suturing the drain and the

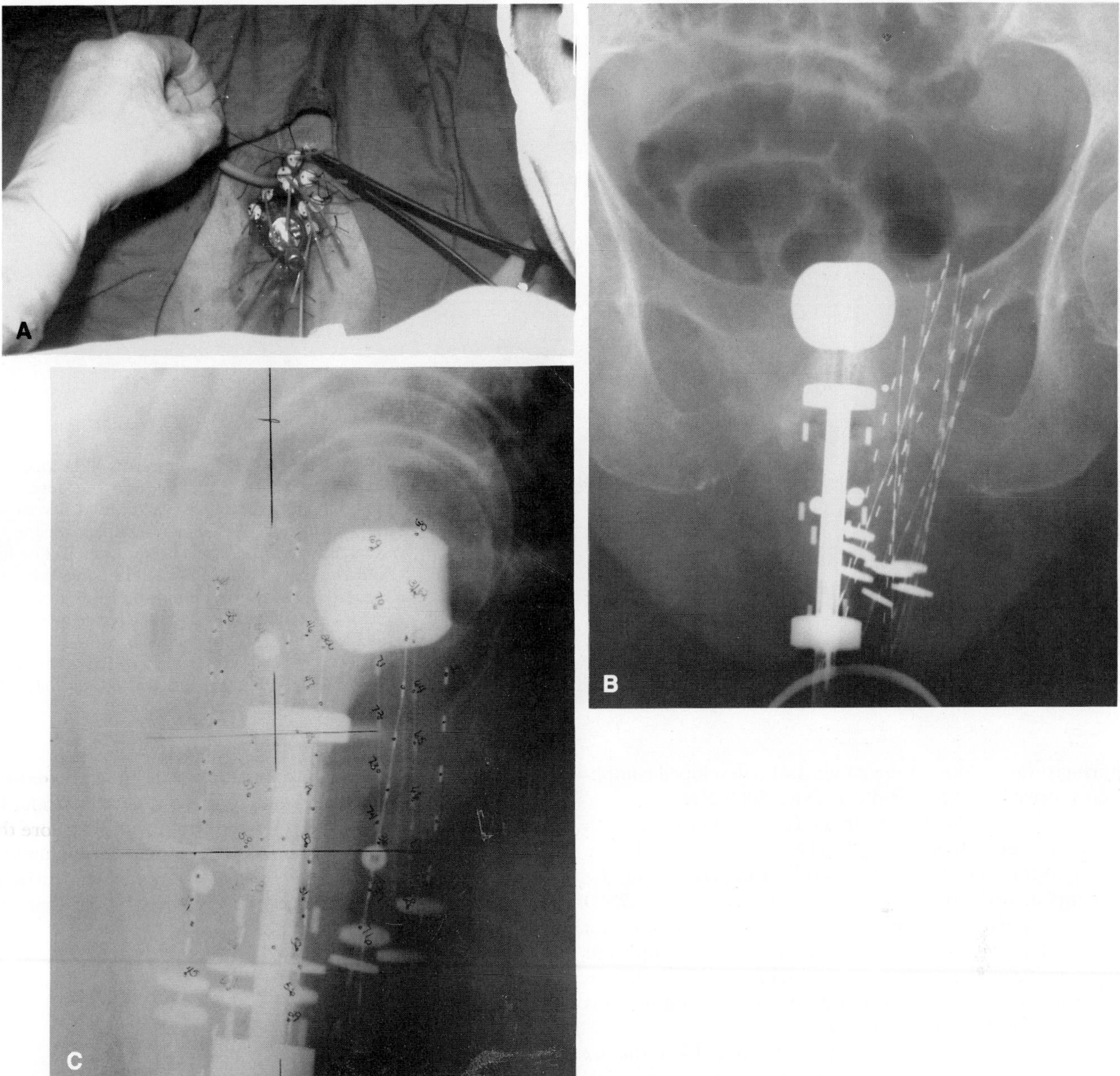

FIGURE 13–49. (**A**) Patient at completion of interstitial implant and intracavitary insertion with stainless steel guides for ^{192}Ir tubing and Delclos vaginal cylinder. The bladder catheter is in place. The metallic buttons on the plastic catheters are being sutured to the skin to secure the position of the implant. (**B**) Anteroposterior and (**C**) lateral radiographs of an implant for a urethral tumor with left paraurethral extension.

template to the perianal skin. Later orthogonal x-ray films were obtained, and dose calculations were performed. The total tumor dose from the external-beam and interstitial irradiation ranged from 5400 cGy to 8000 cGy (mean, 6420 cGy).

Of 32 patients treated, 24 (74%) had tumor control. Four patients had severe complications: two had radionecrosis, one had atony of the sphincter, and one had severe rectitis; one of these patients required colostomy and another an abdomioperineal resection. Fourteen other patients had less severe complications. The probability of preserving good or acceptable anal function was 69% (22 of 32).

Papillon[167] described two techniques for treating anorectal carcinoma with irradiation. Small, mobile, well-differentiated tumors were irradiated with endocavitary irradiation using 50 kVp x-rays (see Chap. 47). In patients unsuitable for this treatment, external irradiation (3000 cGy in ten fractions) was given, followed by an interstitial ^{192}Ir implant. The ^{192}Ir sources were implanted with the aid of a small metallic template, and an additional 3000 cGy to 4000 cGy was administered. Local control was achieved in 28 (84.8%) of 33 patients.

Price and associates[195] described the treatment of 44 patients with inoperable anorectal carcinoma treated with interstitial implants using ^{226}Ra or ^{137}Cs needles to administer doses of 5000 cGy to 6000 cGy (preceded by external irradiation in five patients). They recommend a dose of 6000 cGy at 0.5 cm if external irradiation is not used. Local control was achieved in 16 (52%) of 31 patients assessed for tumor response. Late morbidity was observed in 12 patients: four had occasional bleeding or diarrhea; one had intermittent rectal bleeding; three developed stricture requiring surgery, and three developed necrosis

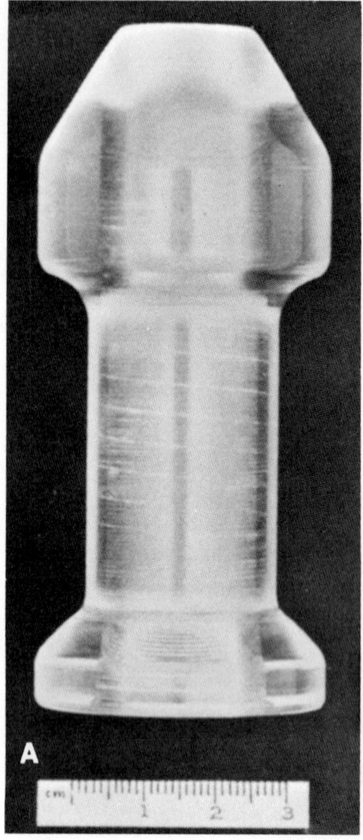

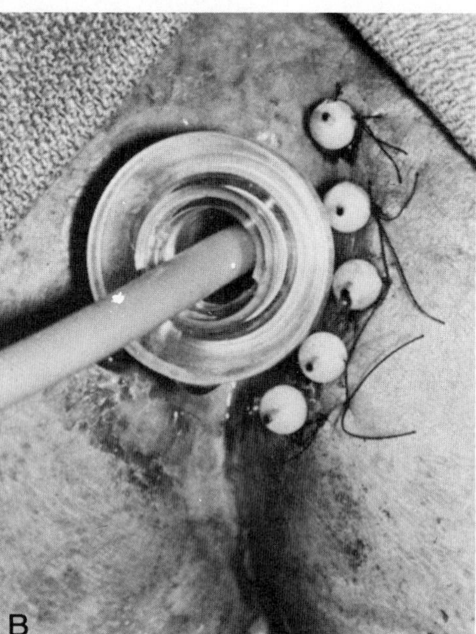

FIGURE 13–50. (**A**) For implants of the anal canal, a hollow rectal plug that reduces the dose to the opposite side of the implant can be used. Several sizes are available. (**B**) Single-plane implant of the anal canal, using stainless steel needles with Teflon balls. Notice the rectal plug in place. The patient also has a Foley catheter inserted into the rectum to keep the rectum distended. The catheter retractor is recommended only for implants performed with long guides. (Delclos L: In Deeley TJ [ed]: Topical Reviews in Radiotherapy and Oncology—2. London, John Wright & Sons, 1982)

requiring surgery. Most of the patients who developed complications received total tumor doses above 8000 cGy.

Puthawala and associates[196] treated each of 40 patients with anorectal cancer with 4000 to 5000 cGy of external irradiation in 25 to 30 fractions, followed by two ^{192}Ir implants using the Syed template to deliver a total tumor dose of 6500 cGy to 7500 cGy. Local control was achieved in 70% of the tumors, with a 20% rate of major morbidity. James and associates[110] updated the experience in 74 tumors treated with interstitial irradiation at Manchester. The local control rate was 47.3%, and necrosis was observed in 8.1% of the patients.

Interstitial implants with 10-cm to 15-cm nylon catheters for ^{192}Ir ribbons are used in the treatment of patients with recurrent carcinoma of the rectum in the perineal and presacral fossa after abdominoperineal resection. Care should be exercised to direct the metallic guides or catheters posteriorly, 5 to 10 degrees from the horizontal plane. In many instances, the needles encounter resistance from the sacrum; occasionally, the sources are inadvertently placed in the bladder. We have performed intraoperative implants at the time of resection of the recurrent tumor, which allows better identification of the volume to be treated and placement of the catheters (Fig. 13-51).

Penis and Male Urethra

Carcinoma of the penis is rare in the United States, and therefore experience in the treatment of these tumors is scarce. For small lesions of the glans or distal penis, interstitial therapy has been used in the form of single- or double-plane implants (Fig. 13-52). Doses of 6000 cGy to 7000 cGy are delivered in 6 to 7 days with a dose rate of 45 to 50 cGy/hour. Molds have been used, particularly in earlier years in Europe, but tumor control and functional results were not as satisfactory as with other irradiation techniques.[108]

Small tumors of the proximal urethra can be treated with an intraurethral catheter containing radioactive sources, but distal urethral lesions are irradiated with techniques similar to those for penile tumors. Tumors larger than 2 cm should be treated with a combination of external irradiation and intracavitary or interstitial techniques or with surgery (see Chap. 53).

Prostate

Permanent Iodine 125 Implants

Hilaris and Whitmore[97] popularized the use of ^{125}I seeds for the treatment of prostatic carcinoma for patients in relatively good general condition. Tumors treated are stage A, B, or early C, with a size not exceeding 5 cm to 6 cm in average dimension. In patients with stage C tumors implants with ^{125}I seeds are discouraged because of the difficulty in adequately irradiating periprostatic extension of tumor.

The ^{125}I seeds are implanted permanently in the prostate through an open retropubic laparotomy incision. The patient is placed in a modified lithotomy position and prepared with O'Connor's drape to facilitate sterile rectal examination during retropubic exploration. A Foley catheter is placed in the bladder. After this, through a midline suprapubic abdominal incision from the umbilicus to the pubic symphysis, an extraperitoneal bilateral pelvic lymphadenectomy is performed. The prevesical space is exposed, but the peritoneum is not opened. The bladder is moved posteriorly away from the pubic symphysis and superior pubic rami to the area of the femoral canal. The peritoneal envelope is retracted superiorly and medially on either side. The ureter is identified at the level of the common iliac artery bifurcation. Lymph node dissection is carried out along the medial aspect of the external iliac artery, below the external iliac vein, down to Poupart's ligament, the obturator

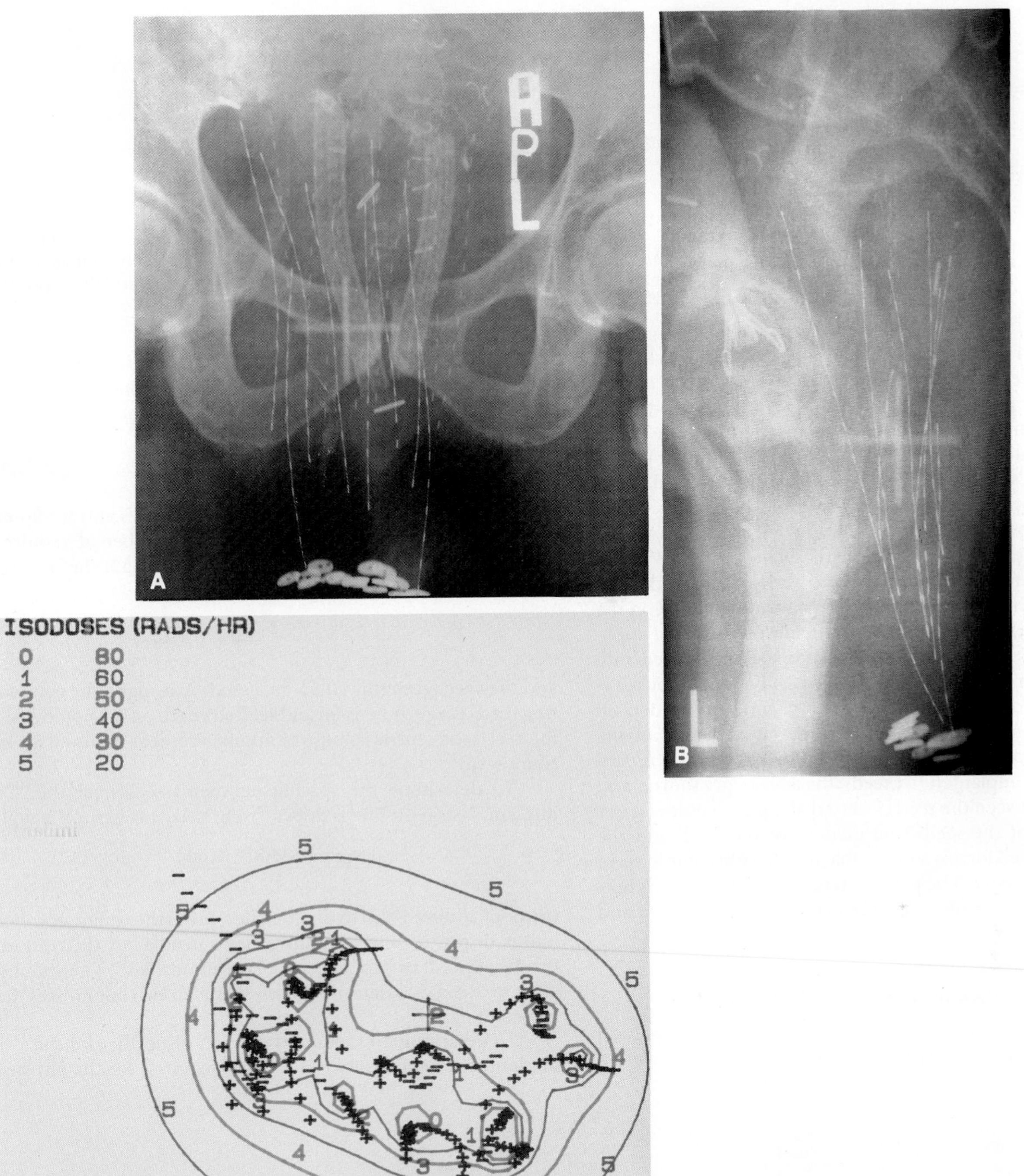

FIGURE 13–51. (**A**) Anteroposterior and (**B**) lateral radiographs of an interstitial implant performed intraoperatively with plastic catheters and ^{192}Ir sources in patient with recurrent carcinoma of the rectum in the posterior pelvis. The patient had received 4500 cGy preoperatively a year earlier. (**C**) Cross-section isodose curves of the implant showing a dose rate of approximately 40 cGy/hour. An additional 5000 cGy was administered with the interstitial implant.

fossa, and along the lateral aspect of the hypogastric vessels.[223] If the lymph nodes are negative, the endopelvic fascia is opened anteriorly and laterally to facilitate mobilization of the prostate, which is exposed anteriorly and laterally. It is palpated from above and from the rectum.

Hilaris and Batata[91] described the implant technique in detail. Small surgical clips are placed on the prostate capsule at the midline, superiorly, inferiorly, and laterally, to outline the prostatic gland and the urethral tract. The entire prostate is measured in three diameters with a specially designed caliper to determine the volume to be implanted. The depth is measured by introducing a 15-cm metallic guide (needle) into the prostate, feeling it through the rectum, and subtracting the protruding length of the needle from the total length. Hollow, 16- or 17-gauge metallic guides are inserted into the prostate approximately 1 cm apart, although the spacing is determined by a

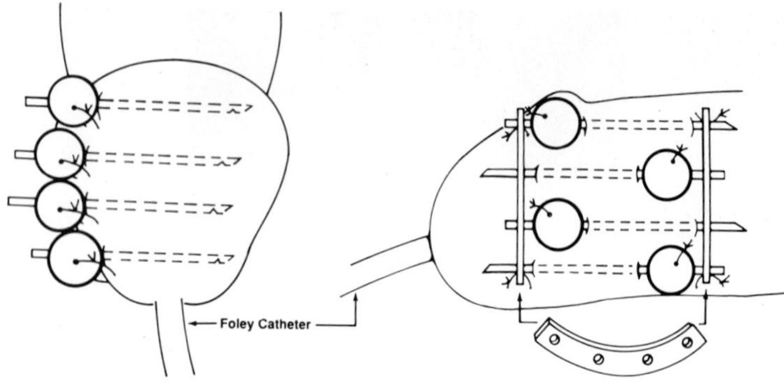

FIGURE 13–52. Diagram illustrating a one-end interstitial implant (*left*) or through-and-through interstitial implant with crossing needles and plate to secure the position of the implant in a carcinoma of the penis.

special nomogram designed at Memorial Hospital (Fig.13-53). Insertion of the guides is usually started at the superior medial margin of the prostate, near the bladder base, lateral to and avoiding the urethra. The guides are inserted into the gland until the operator can feel their tips with an index finger placed in the patient's rectum. Each guide is then retracted for a distance of approximately 0.5 cm to avoid placement of the sources too close to the rectum (Fig. 13-54A).

Multiple guides are placed in the gland until the entire volume is covered. The exact number and spacing of the ^{125}I seeds are determined using the nomogram and depend on the strength of the sources. With the Henschke or Mick seed applicator attached to each guide, the seeds are introduced into prostatic tissue at appropriate distances. The applicator is retracted the predetermined distance (0.5–1 cm) after the deposit of each seed into the prostate until the entire length of the needle has been covered. It is important to diagram and record the number of implanted ^{125}I seeds, the activity per source, and the spacing between the seeds inserted along each guide. After the insertion of the seeds, the guides are removed, and the patient is checked for any sources that may have become loose in the peritoneal cavity. The patient should be told that seeds may be excreted in the urine and instructed to look for them and dispose of them appropriately.

Dose Calculation for Iodine 125 Implants

A description of the dose nomogram used at Memorial Hospital, as outlined by Hilaris and Batata,[91] is given here. To calculate the number of ^{125}I sources required for the prostate implant, a straight line is drawn from the "average dimension," given by

$$\frac{(\text{length} + \text{width} + \text{depth})}{3} + 1$$

to "seed strength" (mCi). This line intersects the central column of "number of seeds" and indicates the number of required sources. In the example shown in Figure 13-53, the average dimension is

$$\frac{l + w + d}{3} = \frac{3 + 3 + 3}{3} + 1 = 4 \text{ cm}$$

and the seed strength is 0.55 mCi/seed. A straight line connecting the average dimension and seed strength on the nomogram intersects the central column of number of seeds required (at 46 sources of ^{125}I).

To determine the spacing between needles for the ^{125}I implant, a straight line is drawn from "seed strength" through

$$\frac{(\text{length} + \text{width} + \text{depth})}{3}$$

(without adding 1 cm) to the "tie line." From the tie line another line is drawn through "spacing along needle" of the sources (preferably 1.0 cm) to "spacing between needles." The spacing between needles is determined where the drawn line crosses the last column.

To determine the required number of needles for the ^{125}I implant, the total number of sources required for the implant

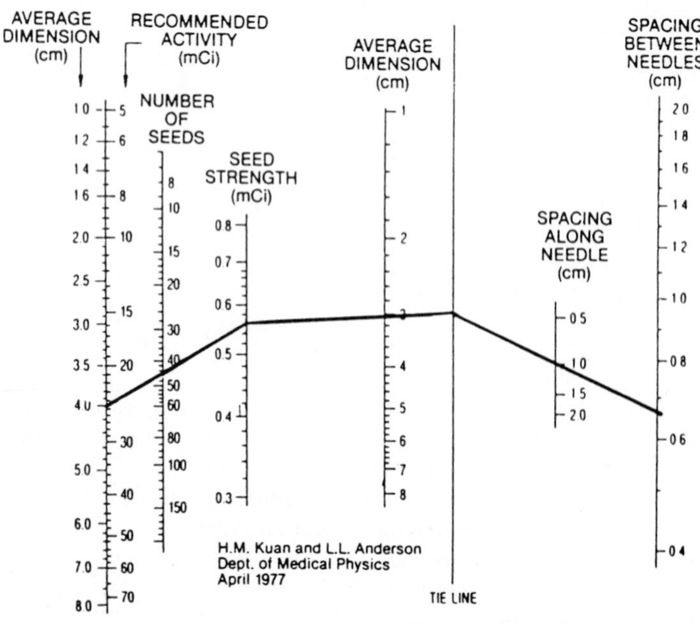

FIGURE 13–53. ^{125}I nomogram for determining seed placement. (Hilaris BS, Batata MA [eds]: Brachytherapy Oncology—1983, p 41. New York, Memorial Sloan-Kettering Cancer Center, 1983)

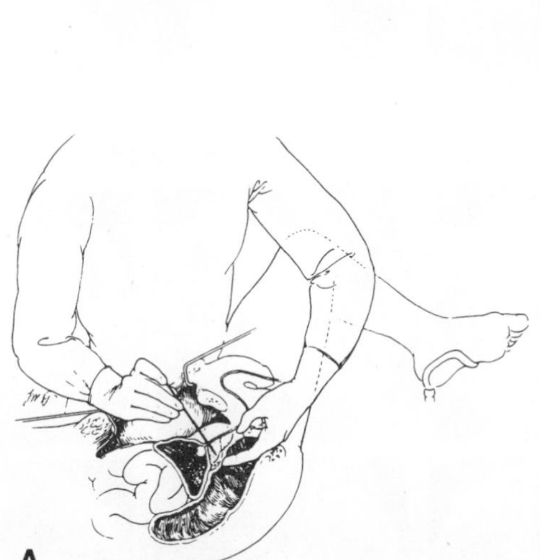
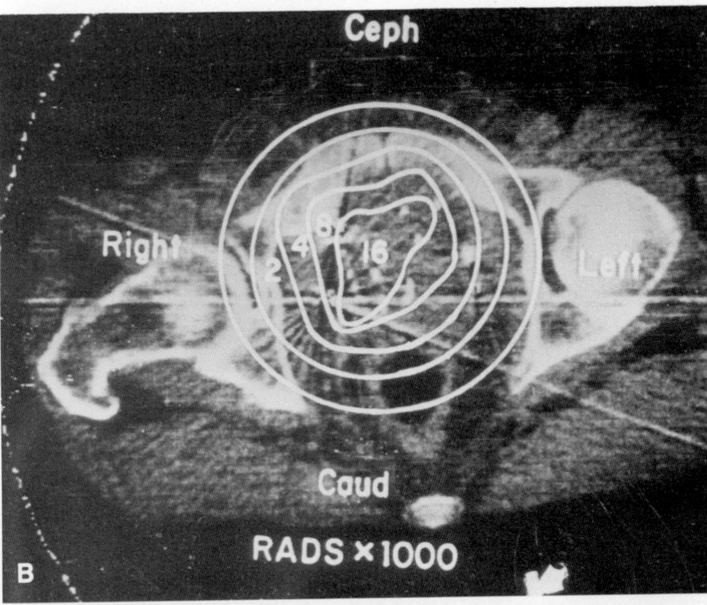

FIGURE 13–54. (**A**) Diagram illustrating insertion of metallic guides in the prostate with a finger in the rectum to assess the relationship of the guides to the anterior rectal wall. (Hilaris BS, Batata MA [eds]: Brachytherapy Oncology—1983, p 41. New York, Memorial Sloan-Kettering Cancer Center, 1983) (**B**) Radiograph showing location of ^{125}I sources in an implant for carcinoma of the prostate.

(in this example, 46 ^{125}I sources) is calculated. Then, the number of sources per needle is determined by deciding spacing along needle (H-II) and the average depth of the implant:

$$\text{Estimated number of sources per needle} = \frac{\text{Depth}}{\text{Spacing along needle}}$$

Then

$$\frac{\text{Total } ^{125}\text{I sources required for implant}}{\text{Number of sources per needle}} = \text{Number of 15-cm, 17-gauge needles for the implant}$$

After the patient is completely recovered from the immediate postoperative period, posterior and lateral or a stereoshift pair of films is obtained for a computer calculation of the implant. It is important to identify the location of all of the sources on the implant (Fig. 13-54B).

The methods for calculating the dose administered by the seeds have been described by Anderson and Aubrey.[6] The matched peripheral dose (MPD) and the integral dose within the MPD contour are identified. For 208 implants performed at Memorial Hospital during 1981 and 1982, the average volume (ellipsoidal approximation) was 39 cm^3, with a standard deviation of 14 cm^3. The average MPD was 14,500 cGy, with a standard deviation of 1300 cGy.

Palladium 103 Implants

Palladium 103 is currently available in seed form for use in permanent implants. The ^{103}Pd seed is physically similar to ^{125}I, and therefore techniques for ^{125}I implantation are applicable to ^{103}Pd. However, ^{103}Pd differs from ^{125}I in possessing a slightly lower energy (21 keV versus 27 keV) and a significantly shorter half-life (17 days versus 60 days). These differences in energy and half-life require a change in guidelines.

The lower energy of ^{103}Pd produces a minor reduction of tissue penetration compared with ^{125}I. The dose distribution effect of this difference is insignificant for seed-to-seed distances of 1.7 cm or less, and linear, planar, biplanar, and cubic configurations are similar for both sources, provided proper spacing requirements are met.[157] Because of the more rapid fall-off of dose beyond 1.7 cm, Blasko and Schumaker[22] strongly recommend a maximum 1-cm spacing seed-to-seed and needle-to-needle to decrease the rectal volume receiving a high dose.

A typical ^{125}I prostate implant is targeted to a matched peripheral dose of 16,000 cGy, which yields an initial dose rate of 8 to 10 cGy/hour (Fig. 13-55). Although the initial dose rate in the center of the implant may be double this value, the peripheral dose rate is considered the determining factor. The substantially larger amounts of total activity implanted with ^{103}Pd (*i.e.*, typically 110 mCi to 130 mCi compared with 30 mCi to 35 mCi for ^{125}I) produces an initial dose rate two- to threefold greater than ^{125}I. However, because of the half-life difference, the dose rate of ^{103}Pd decreases much more rapidly with time than the dose rate of ^{125}I. At 5 weeks after implantation, the dose rates of the two sources is approximately equal, but thereafter, ^{125}I delivers a somewhat higher dose rate to full decay. At 5 weeks, the ^{103}Pd has delivered approximately 76% of its 11,500 cGy dose and the ^{125}I implant has delivered only 33% of its 16,000 cGy.

Because tissue tolerance is a function of total dose and dose rate, some adjustment of target dose must be made when considering ^{103}Pd rather than ^{125}I for implantation. Orton[162,164] mathematically quantified clinical observations of the effects of permanent implant on normal tissue into "biologic" dosimetric terms of time-dose factor (TDF). Russell (unpublished data) used Orton's equations to correlate the biologic effect of 17-day half-life ^{103}Pd seeds to 60-day half-life ^{125}I seeds. The calculations showed that a biologically equivalent total dose from ^{103}Pd may be achieved by multiplying the customary ^{125}I dose by 0.72. The customary dose for ^{125}I as a sole treatment modality is 16,000 cGy; therefore, the equivalent ^{103}Pd target dose is 11,500 cGy. The initial dose rate for this target dose is 18 to 20 cGy/hour, substantially higher than for ^{125}I.

Based on previous experience with a combined approach of 4500 cGy of external-beam irradiation (pelvis/prostate, four-field technique, 180 cGy/fraction) and a 1200 cGy ^{125}I boost for

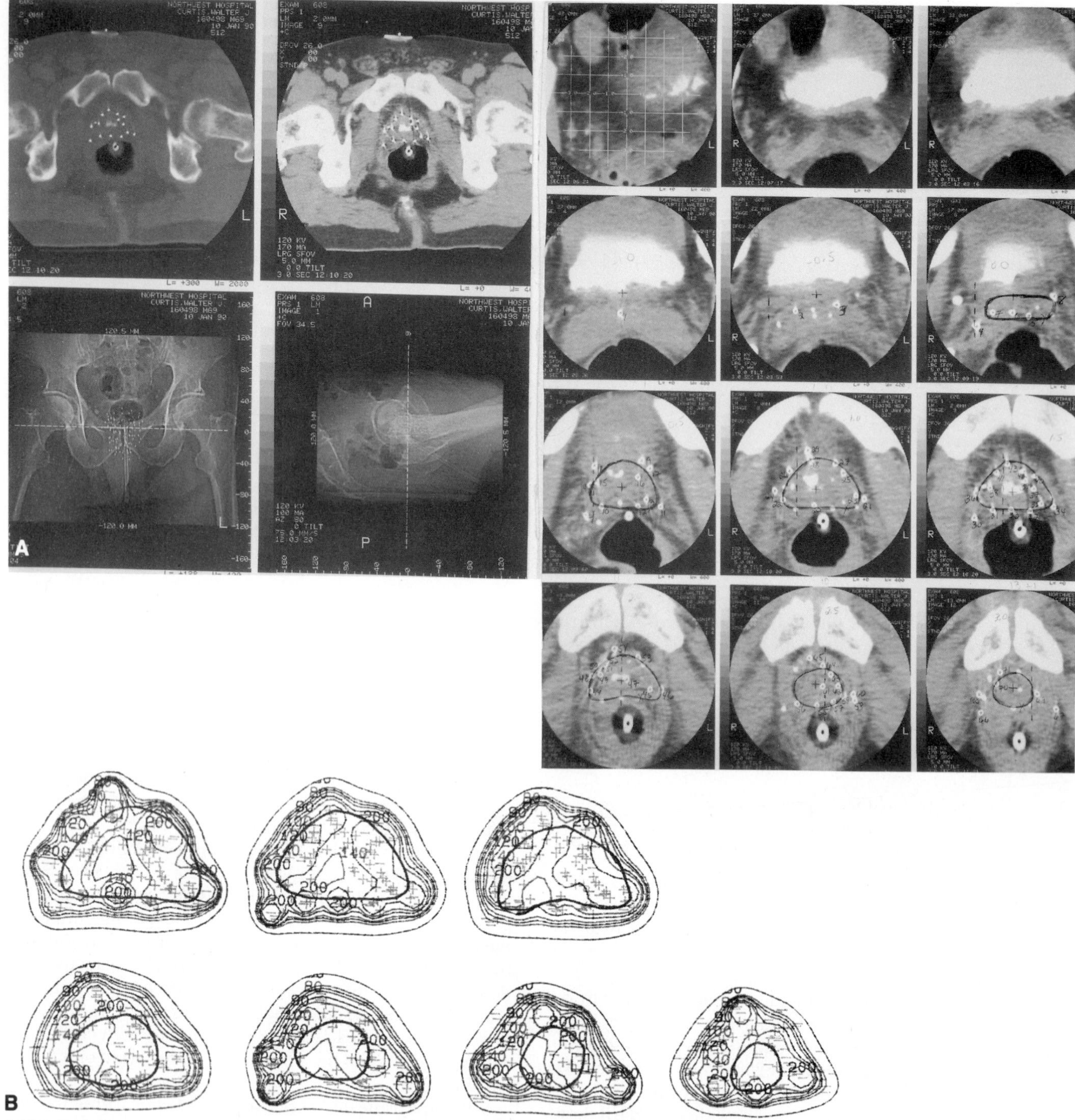

FIGURE 13–55. (**A**) Multiple computed tomographic scan transverse sections and anteroposterior and lateral radiographs of the pelvis illustrating the position of ^{103}Pd sources in the prostate. (**B**) Multiple cross-section isodose curves of the implant. (Courtesy of John C. Blasko, M.D., Northwest Tumor Institute, Seattle, WA)

selected patients, Blasko and Schumaker[22] have chosen 9000 cGy (12,000 × 0.72) as a ^{103}Pd boost dose after 4500 cGy of external-beam irradiation for appropriate patients.

Gold Grain Permanent Implants

Carlton and others[25] described a technique to implant a smaller number of radioactive colloidal gold grains in the prostate to deliver approximately 3500 cGy to the gland. This is combined with 4000 cGy of external irradiation.

Removable Interstitial Implants with Iridium 192

Charyulu[26] and Syed and colleagues[231] developed an interstitial implant technique using removable ^{192}Ir sources with a transperineal template for the treatment of carcinoma of the prostate.

In Syed's technique, a bilateral pelvic lymphadenectomy is carried out without mobilization of the prostate. With the patient in a semilithotomy position, a bladder catheter with a Foley bag containing 10 ml of Hypaque solution is inserted. The prostate template is placed in the perineum, and metallic guides are inserted transperineally through the prostate and, if indicated, seminal vesicles. The tip of the source guide is usually 1 cm above the level of the bladder neck. The template is fixed to the perineum by 2-0 silk sutures. The hollow guides are loaded with inactive dummy sources for x-ray localization films, which are taken in anteroposterior and lateral orthogonal projections. Usually seven seeds of radioactive ^{192}Ir, spaced 1 cm apart in either ribbon, are loaded into each of 18 guides placed through the template. Activity of the iridium sources in the central guides is about 0.25 mg Ra eq to 0.3 mg Ra eq, and in the outer 12 guides, 0.4 mg Ra eq to 0.5 mg Ra eq per seed. The dose rate per hour is 70 cGy to 90 cGy, with the bladder neck and rectum receiving only 30 to 40 cGy/hour. The implant is removed after 3000 cGy to 3500 cGy is delivered (40–45 hours).

After the interstitial irradiation is completed, the radioactive sources are withdrawn with long forceps, and the template is removed with all guides in place, after the perineal sutures are transected. The Foley catheter is removed 1 day later. This interstitial therapy is combined with 4000 cGy of external irradiation to the pelvis. Some modification of this technique was done by Puthawala and associates.[197]

Garcia and co-workers[63] modified this technique using a template to insert hollow, 20-cm, 17-gauge metallic guides (Alpha Omega Co.) in the prostate by a perineal route under ultrasound control. A transrectal ultrasound scan of the prostate is initially obtained in the transverse and sagittal planes to identify the tumor and the position and volume of the prostate. The metallic guides are successively inserted under sagittal ultrasound visualization. After insertion of each guide, a transverse scan is performed to determine the position of the next guide in relation to those already implanted. The guides are advanced 1 to 1.5 cm beyond the superior aspect of the prostate, avoiding piercing of the bladder or urethra. After all guides inserted, the template is sutured to the perineal skin.

After the patient has recovered from anesthesia, anteroposterior and lateral x-ray films of the pelvis are obtained for dose computations (Fig. 13-56). Later, about eight ^{192}Ir seeds per ribbon with 0.3 mCi Ra eq are inserted in the guides; the dose rate is 70 to 80 cGy/hour to the periphery of gland. Minimum tumor doses of 3000 cGy to 3500 cGy are delivered. This is combined with 4000 cGy (200 cGy per fraction) to the prostate or the whole pelvis, as required.

Martinez and colleagues[137] and Brindle and associates[23] described implantation of the prostate with a MUPIT. A bilateral, staging pelvic lymphadenectomy is performed; the length of metallic guides is determined by palpation, and palpable tumor margins are identified with inactive gold seeds. In a modification of the technique, the first needle is placed with the guidance of a finger in the rectum to prevent piercing of that organ. A rectal tube is inserted to help position the template for proper spacing of the remainder of the needles. The template is carefully aligned parallel to the floor of the pelvis, not conforming to the perineal slope, to avoid posterior angling of the needles. The needles are differentially loaded with nylon ribbons containing ^{192}Ir seeds of various activities and number of seeds, using ribbon spacers. The posterior needles, which are primarily directed to the seminal vesicles, are loaded only in the superior half. The implant dose is 3300 cGy, which is combined with external irradiation of 500 cGy in one dose before the implant and 3000 cGy in 17 fractions after the implant. Local

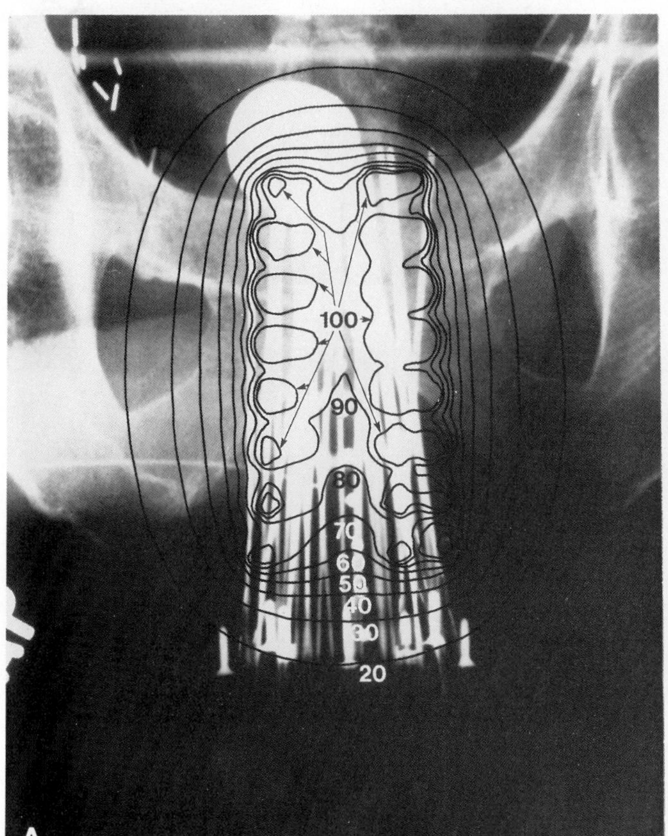

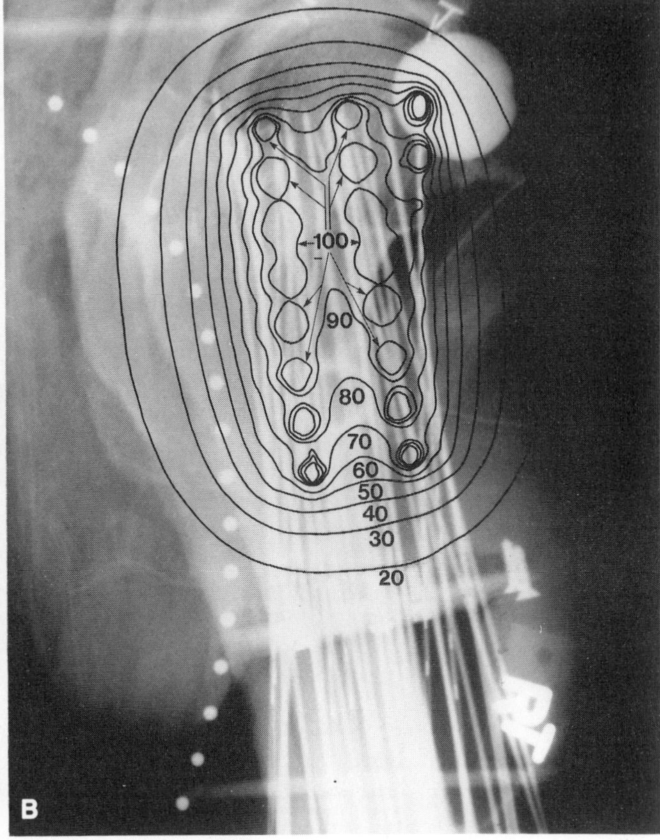

FIGURE 13–56. (**A**) Anteroposterior and (**B**) lateral radiographs of the pelvis showing the position of metallic guides inserted through the perineum under ultrasound control for a patient with localized carcinoma of the prostate. Isodose curves are superimposed on the films.

control rates of 100% determined by clinical examination and 84.5% by biopsy have been reported, with an 89% actuarial rate of disease-free survival.[23]

REMOTE-CONTROL AFTERLOADING BRACHYTHERAPY

Remote-control afterloading brachytherapy for interstitial and intracavitary applications is being used with increasing frequency for low and high-dose-rate implants. According to the International Commission on Radiation Units (ICRU),[105] dose rates in the range of 400 to 2000 cGy/hour are referred to as low dose rates; those in the range of 2000 to 12000 cGy/hour are medium dose rates; and those greater than 12000 cGy/hour are high dose rates. Anderson[5] reviewed the developmental aspects of remote afterloading and described the characteristics of several commercially available systems (Table 12-20).

Low-Dose-Rate Remote-Control Afterloading

The advantages of low-dose-rate remote-control afterloading[1] include

1. Reduced radiation exposure to hospital personnel
2. Improved control of isodose distributions
3. Low probability of misplacing or losing sources
4. Less source preparation work for the source curator
5. Medical and nursing staff not rushed; no fear of exposure while caring for the patient
6. Source loading, unloading, and recording performed automatically

Low-dose-rate units employ ^{137}Cs or ^{192}Ir, and high-dose-rate systems are built for ^{60}Co or ^{192}Ir sources. Low-dose-rate applications do not require shielded rooms, but specially shielded rooms are necessary for ^{60}Co high-dose-rate procedures.

After the unloaded applicators are placed in the patient, the sources are loaded under pneumatic or mechanical control through hollow tubes connected with the applicators by a remotely activated system. A sorting and selection device and transport train for the sources are available. Safety mechanisms for checking correct connection of the applicator and the position of the sources are integral components of the system.[106] Most units produce a hardcopy of the treatment at completion of the procedure. Equipment for remote-control afterloading brachytherapy is available for multiple anatomic sites and applications (Fig.13-57).

A special problem with remote afterloading equipment for gynecologic use is reproduction of the isodose distributions obtained with standard 2-cm cesium tubes and the Fletcher-Suit-Delclos tandem, ovoids, and vaginal cylinders. A fixed source train decreases flexibility unless several source trains are in inventory. A system of active and inactive pellets (Selectron) required the compilation of a dose distribution atlas to duplicate the standard 2-cm cesium-tube dose distribution of the Fletcher-Suit applicators (Appendices 13-1 through 13-3).

Wilkinson and associates[258] and Jones and colleagues[111] described the use of Selectron afterloading equipment to simulate the Manchester system for intracavitary therapy, and Dean and co-workers[38] described its use with the Newcastle system.

Results of therapy with low-dose-rate remote-control afterloading implants are generally not compared with the results obtained with manual afterloading systems because there are

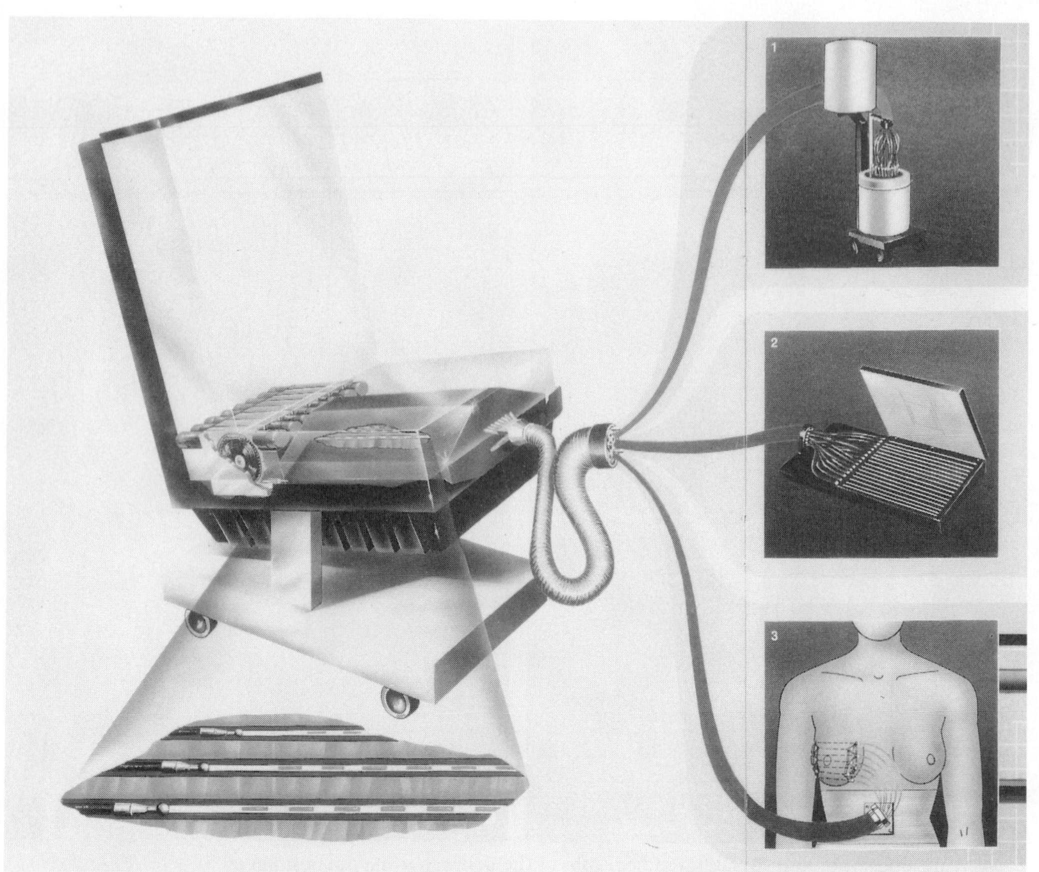

FIGURE 13–57. Artist's rendition of Microselectron remote-control afterloading for interstitial implants in multiple anatomic sites. (Courtesy of Nucletron Engineering BV, The Netherlands)

no significant changes in isotopes or dose rates. Battermann and Szabol[18] replaced their traditional manual afterloading system with the Selectron afterloading machine for patients with cancer of the cervix but used the same treatment policy. Local tumor control and complications were the same for remote-control afterloading and the previously used manual afterloading.

High-Dose-Rate Remote-Control Afterloading

There are several advantages in using high-dose-rate remote-control afterloading techniques:

1. Radiation exposure of medical and nursing personnel is virtually eliminated.
2. Patient immobilization time is short; therefore, complications resulting from prolonged bed rest, such as pulmonary emboli, and patient discomfort is decreased.
3. The use of external applicator fixation devices allows more constant and reproducible geometry of source positioning.
4. Treatment planning and dosimetry are more exact.
5. Treatment can be performed on an outpatient basis, reducing health care costs.

Fractionation and adjustment of total dose are crucial factors in lowering the frequency of complications without compromising the results of therapy with high-dose-rate systems.[47,73,104,199,236] Orton[163] suggests that total doses with high-dose-rate therapy be reduced 20% to 50% from those of low-dose-rate therapy, although several dose-time relationship calculations (TDF, cumulative radiation effect [CRE]) require higher doses than are currently prescribed with high dose rates.

Warmelink and associates,[251] using the extrapolative response dose model, proposed fractionation schemes for high dose rates, based on experience derived from low-dose-rate brachytherapy (Table 13-4). Dose distributions around Selectron applicators have been previously reported.[187,188]

High-dose-rate remote-control afterloading brachytherapy is increasingly used in the treatment of patients with curative intent.[99,204,245] It is currently applied to gynecologic malignancies[20,109,200] and intrabronchial lung cancer.[211,214,226]

Joslin[114] published an interesting historic review of the evolution of remote afterloading techniques and the results in the treatment of gynecologic tumors. Remote-control high-dose-rate afterloading techniques have been widely used in Europe and Asia since the late 1960s.[160,240]

TABLE 13–4
Minimum Number of High-Dose-Rate Fractions for Equivalent Biologic Response to Low-Dose-Rate Interstitial Treatment

EQUIVALENT LOW DOSE RATE (cGy)*	MINIMUM NUMBER OF FRACTIONS	HIGH-DOSE-RATE DOSE/FRACTION
1000	2.9	286
2000	5.3	308
3000	7.8	314
4000	10.3	316
5000	12.8	318
6000	15.2	321

**It is assumed that the dose rate at the normal tissues and at the tumor is 50 cGy/h. (Warmelink C, Ezzell G, Orton C: Use of a time-dose-fractionation model to design high dose-rate fractionation schemes. In Mould RF [ed]: Brachytherapy 2, pp 41–48. Netherlands, Nucletron International BV, 1989)*

Randomized Studies

There have been two randomized studies comparing high- and low-dose-rate brachytherapy for carcinoma of the cervix.[73,107] Trial results were reported by Shigematsu and co-workers.[217] Although patients with stage IIB or III disease treated with the high-dose-rate technique had higher 1-year local control (90% with high dose rates; 77% with low dose rates), the rectal complication rate was also greater than in the low-dose-rate group. The 5-year survival rate was 55% for both groups.

Results of another trial including patients with stages IB, IIA, IIB, and III disease was presented by Gupta and associates.[73] The local control rate was similar for the high-dose-rate (80%) and low-dose-rate (85%) groups. However, the stage distribution in each group, the survival, and complication rates were not described.

Nonrandomized Studies

There are at least 11 nonrandomized studies in which the results of high dose rates were compared with those of historic or concurrent low-dose-rate controls in the same institution.[10,11,31,61,66,98,108,111,202,210,217,234,241] As shown in Table 13-5, the dose fractionation schedules are quite variable. Most studies use point A as a reference point, although the definition of point A may differ from center to center. The dose per fraction at point A varied from 300 cGy to 1000 cGy; the number of fractions varied from two to 13, and the number of fractions per week varied from one to three. However, most centers used a schedule of 700 cGy to 800 cGy per fraction per week for three to six fractions. The external-beam dose depended on the stage of disease.

Table 13-6 illustrates the 5-year survival rates of patients who received high- and low-dose-rate brachytherapy combined with external-beam irradiation for carcinoma of the cervix. Stage for stage, 5-year survival rates of patients treated with the high-dose-rate technique were comparable with those of the historic or concurrent nonrandomized low-dose-rate controls treated in the same institution. Two studies from Germany[67,241] showed significantly better survival for the high-dose-rate group. In the series by Glaser,[67] the difference in relapse-free survival was seen primarily in patients with stage III disease. In the series by Vahrson,[241] the difference in survival was significant for stages II ($P<0.05$) and III ($P<0.001$) but not for stage I disease. In a series by Shigematsu and co-workers,[217] patients with stages IIB or III disease treated with the high-dose-rate technique had significantly better local control rates, although survival was similar to that of the low-dose-rate group. In the 1987 International Federation of Gynecology and Obstetrics (FIGO) annual report, similar 5-year survival rates were recorded for high- and low-dose-rate intracavitary brachytherapy for cervical carcinoma.[8]

Local control rates were available for three studies.[2,125,217] Stage-for-stage results with high dose rates appear to be equal to those with low dose rates in two series.[2,128] However, Shigematsu[217] reported 90% tumor control with high dose rates and 77% control with low dose rates in patients with stages IIB or III disease ($P = 0.01$).

Table 13-7 shows rectal complication rates, which are comparable for high- and low-dose-rate techniques. However, in the

TABLE 13–5
High-Dose-Rate Brachytherapy for Carcinoma of the Cervix: Dose Fractionation Schedules

INVESTIGATION (Country)	DOSE/ FRACTION AT POINT A (cGy)	NO. OF FRACTIONS	FRACTIONS/WEEK	EXTERNAL BEAM	
				DOSE (cGy)	TIMING
Glaser [67] (Germany)	600–700	5–6	1	4000–5000	A*
Vahrson[241] (Germany)	600–1400†	3–7	0.5–1	4500–4600	C
Cikaric[31] (Yugoslavia)	900–1000	4	1	4500–4600	C
Akine[2] (Japan)	300–500	5–6	2–3	2900–6700	B
Himmelman[98]	850‡	5	1	50000–6000	A
Kuipers[124,125] (Netherlands)	850	2	2	4600	B
Sato[206] (Japan)	600	5	1	5000–6000	B
Shigematsu[217] (Japan)	800–1000	3	1	4000	C
Taina[234] (Finland)	750–1000	3–5	1	5000	A
Arai[10] (Japan)	300–700	4–13	1–3	4500–6005	C

** A, after; B, before; C, concurrent with brachytherapy.*
† Dose maximum on the A line (or A plane) 2 cm lateral from the central axis of the applicator.
‡ Dose at the surface of the target volume.
(FU KK, Phillips TL: Int J Radiat Oncol Biol Phys 19:791, 1990)

series by Cikaric,[31] the rectal complication rate was significantly higher in the low-dose-rate group. Table 13-8 depicts bladder complication rates, which are lower than rectal complication rates. Except for the series by Cikaric[31] showing a higher complication rate with the low-dose-rate technique, there was no significant difference between the two techniques.

In addition to these same-institution studies, there were six other large series that examined the results of high-dose-rate remote-control afterloading intracavitary brachytherapy for carcinoma of the cervix.[107,114,150,235,239] In most centers, brachytherapy was carried out concurrently with external-beam irradiation. Results of treatment according to stage are shown in Table 13-9; they are comparable to those reported around the world in the 1987 FIGO annual report[8] and in the Patterns of Care Study in the United States.[80] The rectal complication rate varied from 1.4% to 10% for major or severe effects and from

TABLE 13–6
Survival After High- and Low-Dose-Rate Brachytherapy for Carcinoma of the Cervix

INVESTIGATION (YEAR)	STAGE	NO. OF PATIENTS (HIGH/LOW DOSE RATES)	5-YEAR SURVIVAL (%)	
			HIGH DOSE RATE	LOW DOSE RATE
Glaser[67] (1988)	I–III	493/288	59*	33*(P = .001)
Vahrson[241] (1988)	I	24/206	71	74
	II	37/213	76	53 ($P < .05$)
	III	29/138	62	24 ($P < .001$)
Cikaric[31] (1988)	II	85/66	54	70
	III	52/120	37	43
Akine[2] (1988)	IIB	20/83	60	56
	IIIB	37/212	54	38
Kupiers[125] (1984)	I	21/32	76	80
	II	54/71	74	68
	III	36/42	36	48
Sato[206] (1984)	II	31/40	55	55
	III	44/85	57	49
Shigematsu[217] (1983)	IIB & III	143/106	55	55
Taina[234] (1981)	I & II	40/30	90†	73†
Rotte[202] (1980)	I	42/28	83	89
	II	59/121	75	76
Arai[10] (1980)	I	86/31	83	87
	II	173/125	71	75
	III	212/253	51	49
	IV	46/80	24	16

** Relapse-free survival.*
† 3-year survival.
(FU KK, Phillips TL: Int J Radiat Oncol Biol Phys 19:791, 1990)

TABLE 13–7
Rectal Complications After High- and Low-Dose-Rate Brachytherapy for Carcinoma of the Cervix

INVESTIGATION	NO. OF PATIENTS (HIGH/LOW DOSE RATES)	COMPLICATION RATE (%) HIGH DOSE RATE	COMPLICATION RATE (%) LOW DOSE RATE
Vahrson[241]	147/835	3.0 (late, severe)	2.0 (late, severe)
Cikaric[31]	140/187	7.1	16.6 ($P < .01$)
Akine[2]	84/372	24.0 (moderate) 2.4 (severe)	36.0 (moderate) 4.0 (severe)
Kupiers[124]	111/145	7.0 (grade 3)	6.6 (grade 3)
Sato[207]	87/147	14.9	13.6
Shigematsu[217]	143/106	36.0*	25.0*
Rotte[202]	112/237	2.6	10.5

**Rectal bleeding.*
(FU KK, Phillips TL: Int J Radiat Oncol Biol Phys 19:791, 1990)

0.7% to 24% for minor to moderate complications. The bladder complication rate was low, from 0.3% to 4.0%.

Dose Fractionation in Treating Carcinoma of Cervix

Available clinical data suggest that, in addition to total dose, the most important factors determining late complications are the dose per fraction and the number of fractions.

The association between dose and fractionation for high- and low-dose-rate intracavitary irradiation of stage I and II carcinoma of the cervix was examined by Arai and colleagues.[10,119] The dose rate at point A was 200 to 300 cGy/minute (12,000–18,000 cGy/hour) for high-dose-rate therapy and 1 to 1.5 cGy/minute (60–90 cGy/hour) for low-dose-rate irradiation. The overall time was 28.9 ± 6 to 36.6 ± 4.9 days for high dose rates and 24.8 ± 7.4 to 44.8 ± 10.2 days for low dose rates in most cases. Concurrent external-beam irradiation of 4500 cGy to 5000 cGy in 5 weeks was given to the parametria with a central shield. From these data, they determined the optimal dose fractionation schedules for intracavitary irradiation:

1. For high dose rate: 2800 ± 300 cGy in four or five fractions; 3400 ± 400 cGy in eight to ten fractions; or 4000 ± 500 cGy in 12 to 14 fractions at point A.
2. For low dose rate: 5100 ± 500 cGy in three or four fractions at point A.

The dose at point A with the low-dose-rate technique appeared low compared with European and American practice. Not all cases treated were included in their graph.[10]

With high-dose-rate intracavitary brachytherapy, the complication rate increases with higher dose per fraction and decreased number of fractions. The optimal time/dose/fractionation scheme and the technique for remote-control afterloading intracavitary brachytherapy for cervical cancer have yet to be established through systematic clinical trials.

High-Dose-Rate Brachytherapy for Endometrial Carcinoma

Nori and associates[158] noted that for dose rates between 100 to 200 cGy/minute to point A, there is a linear relationship between total dose and fractionation dose. This relationship correlates the total dose to point A and fractionation with local tumor control and complications for high- and low-dose-rate brachytherapy.[9]

Nori and associates[159] and Mandell and colleagues[133] reported 330 patients treated postoperatively with high-dose-rate remote-control afterloading brachytherapy to the vaginal vault for stage I or II endometrial carcinoma who were at high risk for pelvic recurrence (*i.e.*, deep myometrial invasion, high histologic grade, extrauterine tumor extension). The total vaginal vault dose was 2100 cGy to a depth of 0.5 cm given in three fractions at 2-week intervals. Additional external-beam pelvic

TABLE 13–8
Bladder Complications After High- and Low-Dose-Rate Brachytherapy for Carcinoma of the Cervix

INVESTIGATION	NO. OF PATIENTS (HIGH/LOW DOSE RATES)	COMPLICATION RATE (%) HIGH DOSE RATE	COMPLICATION RATE (%) LOW DOSE RATE
Vahrson[241]	147/835	3.0 (late, severe)	2.0 (late, severe)
Cikaric[31]	140/187	5.0	9.6 ($P < .01$)
Akine[2]	84/372	1.2 (moderate) 0 (severe)	11 (moderate) 0.5 (severe)
Kupiers[124]	111/145	3.5 (grade 3)	3.3 (grade 3)
Sato[206]	87/147	9.2	7.5
Shigematsu[217]	143/106	2.0	7.0
Rotte[202]	112/237	0.8	2.5

(Fu KK, Phillips TL: Int J Radiat Oncol Biol Phys 19:791, 1990)

TABLE 13–9
High-Dose-Rate Brachytherapy for Carcinoma of the Cervix

INVESTIGATION	EXTERNAL IRRADIATION (cGy)	HDR BRACHYTHERAPY (cGy)*	RESULTS (SURVIVAL)	COMPLICATIONS
Joslin[116]	3200/12 Fx with step wedge (12 × 200 cGy point A)	4000/4 Fx	89% stage I 52% stage II 31% stage III	22% small bowel 6% severe (laparotomy)
Joslin[113]	4000/16 Fx with step wedge (16 × 150 cGy point A)	4250/5 Fx	75% stage IB	9.4% late small bowel 3.6% severe (laparotomy)
	4500/20 Fx without wedge	Rest 7 d between 1700/2 Fx	56% stage IIB 32% stage IIIB	3.6% late small bowel
Ward[250]	3150 (10 Fx, 1–3x/wk)	2850/3 Fx (Cathetron)	40% stage II–III	10/82 (12%) (1 urethra, 6 small bowel, 1 bladder, 2 RV fistula)
Rotte[202]	4000/15–20 Fx	4000/4 Fx (^{192}Ir)	83% stage I 75% stage II 37% stage II	4/112 (3.4%) (1 bladder, 3 rectal, only ulceration or bullous)
Snelling[222]	5500 (Fx ?)	1500/2 Fx (Brachytron)	80% stage I 72% stage II 47% stage III–IV	3% (2/66) (1 rectovaginal fistula, 1 radiation cystitis)
Glaser[66]	4000–5000/20 Fx point B, 2600–3250/20–25 Fx point A (given after HDRB)	3000–3600/5–6 Fx (600 or 700 cGy/Fx)	93% NED stage I–II	6% (3/43) (1 bladder ulcer, 2 hemorrhagic proctitis)
Kauppila[118]	3500/10 Fx (split course, 350 cGy/Fx 2x/wk)	3000/6 Fx (Cathetron)	92% stage I 79% stage II 43% stage III	4% (12/310) (includes cancer endometrium)
Arai[9, 10]	4500–5000/25 Fx (MLB) for nonbulky tumors initially; MLB after 2000–3000 for bulky tumors	2800–4000/4–14 Fx some twice weekly (10–13 Fx) (Ralstron)	83% stage I 70% stage II 51% stage III	3% (15/517)
Newman[158]	2400/6 Fx (nonbulky); 4320/24 Fx (bulky + additional boost 1000–1200 to involved parametrium); advanced 6300/35 Fx	4250/5 Fx (nonbulky) 3500/5 Fx (bulky) 1700/2 Fx (advanced) (Cathetron)	81% stage I 74% stage IIA 40% stage IIB 27% stage III	3% (severe)
Shigematsu[217]	2000/10 Fx + 2000/20 Fx parametria (MLB)	2500–3000/3 Fx	60% stage IIB 57% local control Stage III (90% cervical control for all patients)	2% ileus
Sato[206]	4000/20 Fx + 1000–2000 parametrial boost	3000/5 Fx (RALS—^{60}Co) point A	97% stage I 55% stage II 57% stage III 29% stage IV	20%–25% (however, includes moderate)
Utley[239]	2000/10 Fx + 3000/12 Fx MLB on M-W-F	3996/6 Fx biweekly initially; 4000–5000/8–10 Fx biweekly subsequently (Brachytron)	89% stage I 58% stage II 33% stage III	10% severe (earlier) 4% severe (current) 2/5 stage IV
Himmelmann[98]	4000–5000/17–23 Fx with midline block after HDR brachytherapy	4250/5 Fx	88% stage IB–IIA	0%
Teshima[235]	4000–4600/20–23 Fx with MLB after: 1400 stage IB, 2800 stage IIB–III, 6000/30 Fx (MLB after 4000 cGy) for stage IV	3750–4500/5–6 Fx stage IA,B–IIA; 3000/4 Fx stage IIB–III; 2250/3 Fx stage IV (RALS)	86%–100% stage I 65%–72% stage II 41% stage III 20% stage IV	Among 200 patients: 7% rectum, 3% bladder, 1% sigmoid colon, 2% small bowel (only 4% of all patients required surgery for grade 3 sequelae)
Koga[120]	4000/20 Fx + 2000/10 Fx to parametria with MLB stages IIB–III	1800–3000/3–5 Fx (RALS)	85% stage I 68% stage II 51% stage III	5% grade 3 rectosigmoid (among 79 patients)
Akine[2]	5000/25 Fx; MLB in 3/84 patients from start	1500–3000/3–6 Fx (twice weekly, mean 2190 cGy) (RALS)	60% stage IIB 54% stage IIIB (64%–71% local control)	2.4% rectosigmoid (of 84 patients)
Streeter[228]	4000/20 Fx	3000/4 Fx (RALS)	100% stage I 70% stage II 60% stage III 42% stage IV	8% (8/104) (? severity)

(continued)

TABLE 13–9
(Continued)

INVESTIGATION	EXTERNAL IRRADIATION (cGy)	HDR BRACHYTHERAPY (cGy)*	RESULTS (SURVIVAL)	COMPLICATIONS
Shu-Mo[219]	4000–5500/16–22 Fx	6000–6500/11–12 Fx (2 Fx/wk) (Ralstron)	100% stage I 82% stage II 74% stage III 0% stage IV	11.8% moderate rectal 1.6% severe rectal 7.1% moderate bladder
Roman[201]	4600/18 Fx	8000–10000/1–3 Fx (Selectron)	82% stage IIA 67% stage IIB 33% stage IIIB	Grade 2 cystitis (1/81), grade 2–3 proctitis (6/81), fistula (3/81), bowel obstruction (6/81)

**Once weekly HDR brachytherapy unless otherwise stated. All HDR doses are prescribed to point A.*
MLB, midline block. Fx, fraction; NED, no evidence of disease.

irradiation was given to higher-risk patients at doses of 4000 cGy to the midplane of the pelvis with the four-field technique. The total pelvic or vaginal recurrence rate was 2.7%, with a 3.7% incidence of vaginal complications, none requiring surgical correction. The 5-year survival rate was 92% for stage I and 82% for stage II. A nonrandomized comparison of their results with surgery alone or combined with irradiation is shown in Table 13-10.

Sorbe and colleagues[224] treated 366 patients for stage I endometrial carcinoma with preoperative high-dose-rate remote-control afterloading brachytherapy (275 patients) or irradiation alone (91 patients). All patients received six intracavitary fractions in 8 days, with 500 cGy to 1200 cGy per fraction. External irradiation was given to all medically inoperable patients and to operable patients found to have high-risk factors at the time of surgery. The dose per fraction of high-dose-rate intracavitary irradiation was the most important factor in the development of complications, local tumor control, and residual disease in the uterus. Their recommendation was to deliver six fractions of 500 cGy to 800 cGy per fraction for preoperative and medically inoperable patients with stage I endometrial cancer.

Pettersson and associates[179] employed low-dose-rate remote-control afterloading for postoperative prophylactic vaginal cuff irradiation in 258 patients with endometrial cancer, and only two patients developed severe (grade 3) complications.

Peschel and associates[177] reported their experience with 103 patients with stage I carcinoma of the endometrium treated with high-dose-rate remote-control afterloading techniques in addition to surgery. Tumor control in the vaginal apex was 99%. Severe complications were seen in 6% of the patients treated with external irradiation and remote afterloading brachytherapy.

High-Dose-Rate Brachytherapy for Lung Disease

Although most of the experience in treating lung disease with remote-control afterloading brachytherapy has been with a single linear source, the use of more than one catheter allows better dose distribution and coverage of a larger volume. The ^{192}Ir can be encapsulated in very small sources of high activity, allowing passage through catheters with internal diameters of 1.5 mm. Although the short half-life of 74 days is a drawback, treating several patients with a supply of sources and keeping the relative source strength within a high-dose-rate range with periodic replacements make it a practical isotope. Schray and associates[210] initially reported the use of YAG laser resection and brachytherapy in 14 patients who underwent a total of 21 insertions for treatment of malignant airway obstruction. A flexible, blunt-ended nylon catheter was placed through a fiberoptic bronchoscope 2 cm beyond the distal end of the tumor; it was afterloaded with ^{192}Ir. The sources delivered approximately 50 cGy/hour at 1 cm. A minimum dose of 3000 cGy at 1 cm was initially delivered to the trachea and bronchi. This was later modified to administer 3000 cGy in the trachea at 1 cm and in the bronchi at 1.5 cm. No acute morbidity was reported.

Schray and co-workers[211] later reported the results of treating 65 patients (93 placements). Forty of the 65 patients received YAG laser treatment before brachytherapy. Forty pa-

TABLE 13–10
Carcinoma of Endometrium: Comparative Survival and Recurrences

REVIEW PERIOD	STAGE	TYPE OF TREATMENT	TOTAL NUMBER	5-YEAR NED SURVIVAL	PELVIC RECURRENCES
1949–1965*	I	S	536	70%	22%
	II	S	24	46%	
1969–1976†	I	S + RT	247	92%	2.7%
	II	S + RT	22	82%	

**Mainly surgery alone.*
† Radiation therapy and surgery.
NED, no evidence of disease.
(Nori D, Hilaris BS, Batata M, et al: Remote afterloading in cancer management. II. Clinical applications of remote afterloaders. In Hilaris BS, Batata MA (eds): Brachytherapy Oncology—1983, pp 101–118. New York, Memorial Sloan-Kettering Cancer Center, 1983)

tients had bronchoscopic follow-up, and 60% demonstrated tumor regression. Eleven patients (17%) developed fistula or hemorrhage, seven cases of which were believed to be interrelated.

Seagren and co-workers[214] reported the use of high-dose-rate endobronchial brachytherapy for patients who had previously received a minimum of 5000 cGy of external irradiation. Twenty symptomatic patients with bronchoscopically documented endobronchial tumors were treated with a remote afterloading (Brachytron) unit using 3-mm-diameter ^{60}Co with an average strength of 0.7 Ci. The unit oscillated the source up to 16 cm. A single catheter was inserted, and a dose of 1000 cGy in a single fraction was delivered to 1 cm in 12 to 27 minutes. Complete palliation of symptoms was described in 25% of the patients and partial and complete palliation in 94%. Seagren[213] updated this experience in 1988, describing 50 patients who received doses of 2000 cGy in three weekly fractions if they resided locally or one fraction of 1000 cGy if they lived at a distance.

Joyner and associates[117] reported the use of ^{192}Ir solid wire in endobronchial afterloading therapy in combination with YAG photoresection and external irradiation in a group of 14 patients with previously untreated stage III non-oat-cell bronchogenic carcinoma. Doses of 3000 cGy at 0.5 cm were delivered in 8 to 20 hours.

Weiner and associates[256] reported 80 patients treated with the Gamma Med unit for primary bronchogenic carcinoma in 56 and recurrent carcinoma in 24 patients. A dose of 500 cGy per fraction was delivered at 1 cm, for a total of four to six endobronchial treatments given concomitantly with external irradiation.

Speiser and Spratling[225] initially reported 45 patients treated with medium-dose-rate remote-control afterloading intraluminal brachytherapy, delivering 200 to 1000 cGy/hour at 0.5 cm or 100 to 500 cGy/hour at 1 cm. External irradiation consisted of 6000 cGy in 200 cGy/day fractions for stage T3 non-oat-cell carcinoma and 3750 cGy in 250 cGy/day fractions for T4 or M1 categories. Patients with large airway obstructions or respiratory distress and patients with metastatic endobronchial carcinoma were treated on weeks 1, 2, and 3 without concomitant external irradiation. In the medium-dose-rate group, the minimum dose per fraction was 1000 cGy to 0.5 cm, and in the high-dose-rate patients, the minimum dose per fraction was 1000 cGy at 1 cm. The total dose was 3000 cGy delivered in three treatments. In the medium-dose-rate group, most patients had two catheters, but in the high-dose-rate group, two or three catheters were used. The medium-dose-rate group had an overall improvement of obstruction of 70%, and the high-dose-rate group had an improvement rate of 65%. Complications in 3.1% of the patients consisted mostly of arrhythmia, pneumothorax, hemoptysis, pneumonia, and bronchospasm (usually one per group). The survival in these patients was approximately 10% to 15% at 1 year, with no difference between the two groups.

Garcia and colleagues (unpublished data) have treated 26 patients at our institution with high-dose-rate remote-control afterloading for recurrent or newly diagnosed bronchogenic carcinoma causing endobronchial obstruction. The technique is carried out in close collaboration with a pulmonologist. The patient is sedated, and antisialogogue medication is administered. Topical anesthetic with 4% lidocaine is given. A fiberoptic bronchoscope is introduced nasally and advanced to define the location and extent of tumor. If there is significant airway obstruction, laser photocoagulation therapy is performed to aid in opening the airway and form a channel for an endobronchial catheter. A flexible, closed-ended nylon catheter is advanced through the biopsy channel of the bronchoscope approximately 5 cm beyond the distal extent of disease. The catheter position is verified fluoroscopically, and the catheter is advanced as the bronchoscope is withdrawn over it. To document or, if necessary, to adjust the catheter's position, the bronchoscope may be reintroduced. After the catheter is satisfactorily positioned, it is secured with tape at the nasal vestibule.

A dummy source line is placed in the catheter, and x-ray films in anteroposterior and lateral projections are obtained for documentation and computerized treatment planning. Treatment margins of 2 cm to 3 cm beyond the distal end of the tumor are required. After the dose and volume have been prescribed and the isodose curves generated and reviewed by the radiation oncologist, the patient is taken to the treatment room. The catheter is connected to the Nucletron high-dose-rate remote-control afterloading unit, and the treatment is delivered in 10 to 20 minutes. The dose prescribed is 1000 cGy to 1500 cGy at 1 cm; two fractions are given 7 to 14 days apart, for a total of 2000 cGy to 3000 cGy. Figure 13-58 illustrates the catheter position and isodose curves for an endobronchial insertion. At the completion of the therapy, the catheter is disconnected from the Nucletron unit and then removed from the patient. The patient is able to leave the hospital shortly thereafter.

Summary of results with endobronchial irradiation are shown in Table 13-11.

High-Dose-Rate Brachytherapy for Esophageal Carcinoma

Intraesophageal medium- and high-dose-rate brachytherapy have been used for treating patients with esophageal carcinoma. Tumor extent is assessed by the usual methods of gastrointestinal endoscopy, barium swallow, and CT scan. The sources are inserted in the esophagus, covering 3 cm to 5 cm beyond the distal end of the tumor (Fig.13-59).

Flores and associates[59] have delivered 1500 cGy at 1 cm

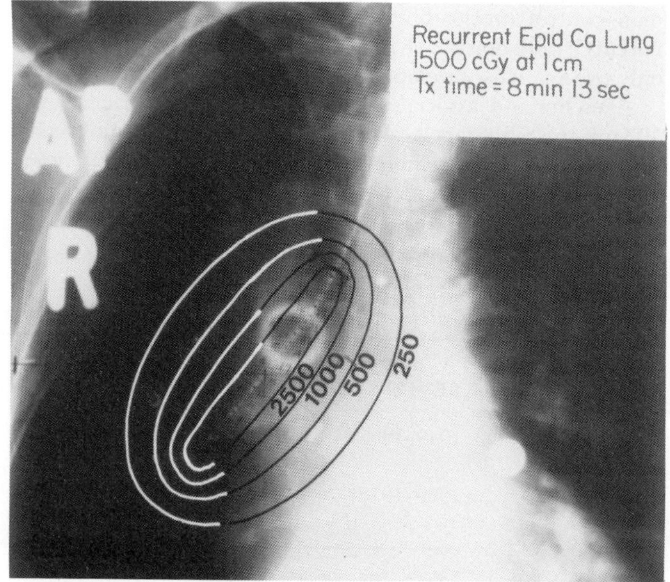

FIGURE 13–58. Radiograph of the thorax demonstrating the position of an intrabronchial catheter with radioactive sources inserted with a high-dose-rate remote-control afterloading device. Isodose curves (cGy/hour) are superimposed.

TABLE 13–11
Selected Results of Endobronchial Irradiation in Carcinoma of the Lung

INVESTIGATION	NO. OF PATIENTS	RECEIVING EXTERNAL BEAM (%)	DOSE AT 1 CM (cGy)	FRACTIONS	LASER (%)	COMPLICATIONS (%)	X-RAY IMPROVED (%)	BRONCHIAL OBSTRUCTION IMPROVED (%)	SYMPTOMS IMPROVED (%)
LOW DOSE RATE									
Schray[211]	40	100	3000	1	65	10		74	
Mehta[142]	38	41	5240	1	27	10	70	86	80
Speiser[226]	45		3000–4500	2–3		3		69	
HIGH DOSE RATE									
Macha[131]	171		1800	3		5		65	
Korba[123]	160	100	1800	3		4	60		
Seagren[214]	50	100	1000–2000	1–3	34				80
Speiser[226]	45		2000–3000	2–3		3		85	

over 1.5 hours combined with external irradiation of 4000 cGy given in five fractions to 171 patients. Thirty (33%) of 90 patients were alive at 1 year, 14 (26%) of 55 at 2 years, and five (19%) of 26 at 3 years. The survival was higher with intracavitary irradiation, and only one third of patients died of aspiration pneumonia secondary to persistent tumor, compared with 82% of 483 patients treated with external irradiation alone.

Hishakawa and associates[101,102] treated 119 patients with external irradiation or external irradiation plus high-dose-rate intracavitary irradiation for carcinoma of the esophagus. Patients received from 600 cGy to 2400 cGy given in one to four fractions from the intracavitary therapy. Total doses ranged from 5200 cGy to 9000 cGy from combined intracavitary and external irradiation. The 3-year actuarial survival rates for those receiving combined therapy were 42% for stage I and 18% for stage II disease. These results were better than for patients receiving external irradiation alone. Ten (19%) of 53 patients developed esophageal fistula between 3 and 14 months after completing irradiation.[103]

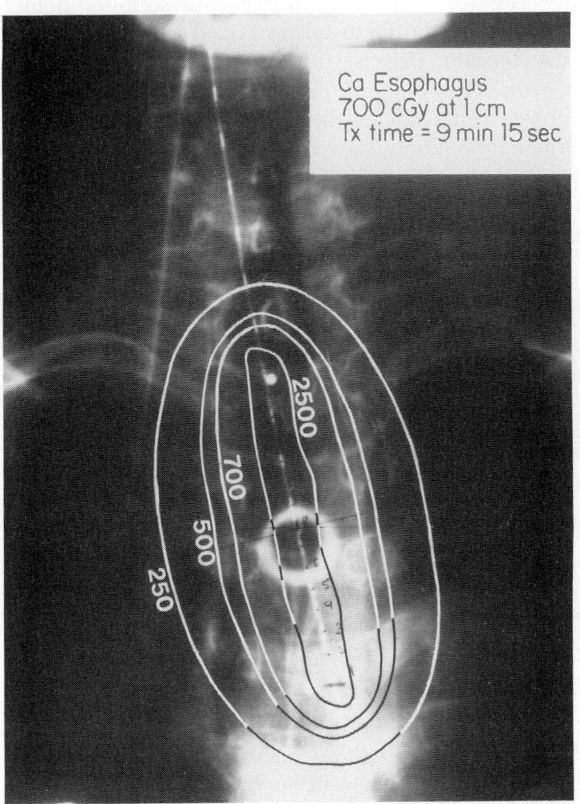

FIGURE 13–59. Radiograph of the thorax showing the position of a catheter and ^{192}Ir sources in the cervical and proximal thoracic esophagus. Isodose curves (cGy/hour) are superimposed.

Rowland[203] reported 22 patients with inoperable carcinoma of the esophagus treated with external irradiation and intracavitary therapy with a high-dose-rate system. He used a flexible applicator with external diameter of 8 mm, containing 48 ^{137}Cs sources of 40 mCi each; doses in the range of 1250 cGy at 1 cm from the center of the tube were administered in about 1 hour to a 15-cm segment of esophagus.

Garcia and colleagues (unpublished data) treated 12 patients with esophageal carcinoma at Washington University with doses of 700 cGy at 1 cm delivered over 5 to 10 minutes for a total of 2100 cGy given in three fractions. Patients also received external irradiation of 5000 cGy in 25 fractions. Fifty-five percent of the patients had complete restoration of their ability to swallow solid food. Complications of endocavitary high-dose-rate brachytherapy include esophagitis, ulceration, tracheoesophageal fistula, and stricture requiring intermittent dilatation.

Syed and colleagues[230] described a technique for irradiation of esophageal lesions combining external (4500–5000 cGy) and intraluminal irradiation to deliver an additional 3000 cGy to 4000 cGy at 0.5 cm from the surface of the applicator in two insertions in 2 weeks. The Syed-Puthawala-Hedger esophageal applicator consists of a specially designed tube with an outer diameter of 1.0 cm and a central nasogastric tube with six longitudinally placed afterloading catheters, each equally spaced to accommodate radioactive sources (*i.e.*, ^{192}Ir, ^{125}I, or ^{137}Cs microspheres). The nasogastric tube in the center can be used for feeding and suction. The proximal ends of the afterloading catheters are funnel-shaped, allowing easy loading of the radioactive source ribbons. Insertion of the applicator can be accomplished with deep sedation or general anesthesia for high-risk patients.

Petrovich and associates[178] reported an 11% 5-year survival rate among 46 patients with carcinoma of the esophagus treated with a combination of external irradiation and intraluminal brachytherapy; the survival rate was 2% among 137 patients treated with external irradiation alone.

High-Dose-Rate Brachytherapy for Breast Carcinoma

Rowland and associates[204] reported 24 patients with carcinoma of the breast using conservation surgery and irradiation with external-beam and high-dose-rate brachytherapy. Based on the linear quadratic equation, an α/β ratio of 10 Gy for early effects and 2.5 Gy for late effects was used.[37] Patients with clinically negative lymph nodes and well-differentiated or moderately differentiated tumors less than 3 cm in diameter received a primary implant of 2800 cGy in four fractions or 2000 cGy in two fractions. No recurrences or significant reactions have been reported.

DOSIMETRY AND DOSE PRESCRIPTION IN GYNECOLOGIC BRACHYTHERAPY

Principles of Applicator Design

Manchester System

The Manchester applicators consisted of a rubber intrauterine tandem and two ellipsoid "ovoids" that conformed to the isodose curves from ^{226}Ra tubes positioned on the long axis of the applicator. The applicators were intended to be used with ^{226}Ra tubes 2.2 cm long, with 1-mm platinum filtration and an active length between 1 and 1.5 cm. The small, medium, and large ovoid diameters were 2, 2.5, and 3 cm, respectively, and are the same as Fletcher's small, medium, and large colpostats. The preloaded ovoids contained no shielding and relied on extensive anterior and posterior packing (1–1.5 cm thick) to spare bladder and rectal tissue. The ovoid dimensions and applicator loadings were designed to ensure that the point A dose rate, about 53 cGy/hour in modern units, remained constant for all allowed applicator loadings and combinations. The design also ensured that the vaginal contribution to point A was limited to 40% of the total dose.

Small, medium, and large ovoids were loaded with 17.5 mg, 20 mg, and 22.5 mg of radium, respectively, to compensate for the greater source-to-point A treatment distances with the larger ovoids. The point B dose, determined largely by the inverse square law, was calculated assuming 900 cGy to point B for every 400 mgh administered.

Without external-beam treatment, a total point A exposure of 8000 R (7280 cGy) given in 144 hours split between two applications was traditionally prescribed. Because the point A dose rate is constant, whether the application contains 60 mg or 80 mg of ^{226}Ra, point A prescription amounts to using time, not mgh, as the factor that quantifies treatment. In contrast to the Paris and Stockholm systems, which prescribed a fixed number of mgh, equivalent Manchester treatment regimens could deliver from 8400 mgh to 11,200 mgh.[237,238]

Fletcher Applicator System

The Fletcher applicators[55] adhered to the basic Manchester design with many improvements, including internal shielding consisting of 3- to 5-mm-thick tungsten screens located on the medial, anterior, and posterior faces of the colpostat. The shielding allowed sparing of the bladder and rectum without use of the extensive vaginal packing characteristic of Manchester insertions. Afterloading capability was incorporated into the Fletcher applicator by Suit.[229] The Fletcher colpostat has a diameter of 2 cm and can be increased to 2.5 cm and 3 cm by use of small and large slip-on plastic caps so that the dose to the vaginal mucosa relative to doses delivered at larger distances can be minimized (Fig. 13-60).

The Fletcher loadings of 15 mg, 20 mg, and 25 mg in small, medium, and large colpostats, respectively, are similar to those of the Manchester system. By increasing the source strength to compensate for increasing source-to-prescription-point distance, the time required to deliver a fixed dose remains approximately constant. Because the radioactive sources are distributed over the longest possible tandem, penetration is maximized and a smaller dose is delivered to the uterine mucosa than doses administered at distances on the order of 2 cm. Because of the similarity of Fletcher loadings (55–85 mg) to the Manchester loadings, point A dose rates are nearly independent of the loading.

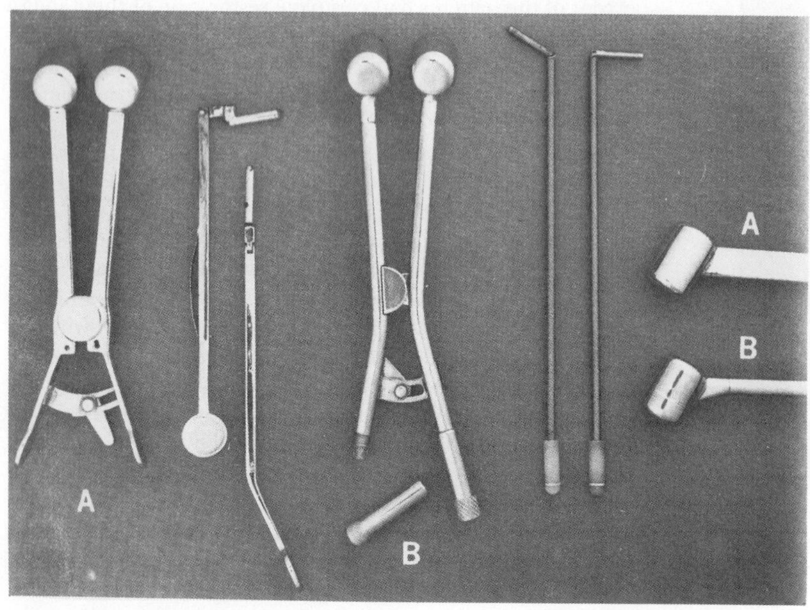

FIGURE 13–60. Fletcher afterloading colpostats: (**A**) Fletcher-Suit rectangular-handle model; (**B**) current round-handle, lighter model. Both models are acceptable. The round-handle model, however, is less bulky and the source inserter (radium holder) is simpler. (Delclos L, Fletcher GH, Sampiere V, Grant WH III: Cancer 41:970, 1978)

The internal structure of the 3M Fletcher-Suit-Delclos (FSD) colpostat and the traditional Fletcher-Suit rectangular-handled (FSRH) applicator have been described.[261] These two applicators have shields of significantly different shape, thickness, and position that decrease the dose to the bladder trigone and the anterior rectal wall without decreasing the irradiation to the uterosacral and broad ligaments. The rectal shield subtends 180 degrees, and the bladder shield subtends 150 degrees (Fig. 13-61). The design of the handle (square or round) influenced slightly how the shielding was placed. If the effects of the intrauterine tandem and the contralateral colpostat are included, applicator shielding reduces midline rectal and bladder doses by 10% to 20% over conventional treatment planning calculations, which ignore shielding and include only the effects of source encapsulation.

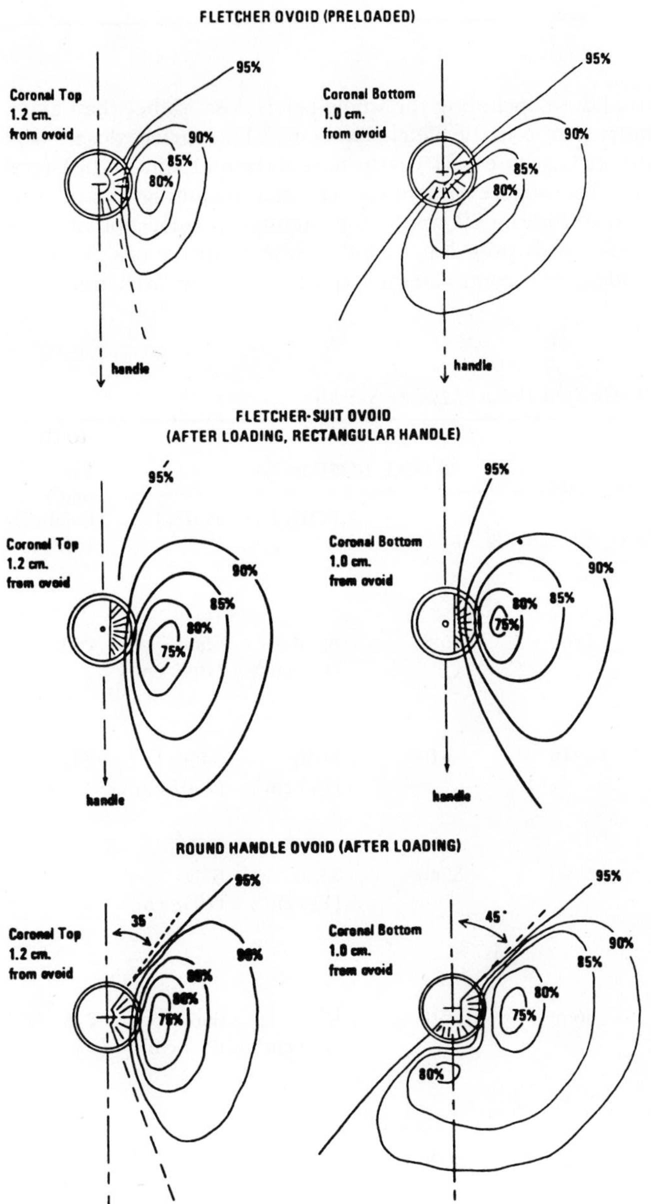

FIGURE 13–61. Transmission in vaginal colpostats of Fletcher-Suit application through the tungsten shielding was determined by measurement. The tungsten sectors, or half buttons, provide screening for the anterior rectal wall and trigone of the bladder. (Delclos L, Fletcher GH, Sampiere V, Grant WH III: Cancer 41:970, 1978)

By adopting an applicator-source combination that differs from that on which the radiation oncologist's clinical experience is based, critical structures can be overdosed and the tumor can be undertreated. For example, FSRH applicators loaded with ^{226}Ra tubes give rise to midline rectal and bladder doses 7% to 15% smaller than those of the FSD or FSRH systems loaded with ^{137}Cs for equivalent doses to point A. Corrections should also be made for internal applicator shielding, because dose rates vary from 10% to 25% as a result of differential absorption in the colpostats.[209]

Weeks and associates[254, 255] described specially constructed plastic afterloading Fletcher-Suit colpostats that can be used for CT-guided treatment planning in gynecologic tumors. This eliminates the artifacts that are produced by metallic applicators on CT scans. The dose output of the loaded colpostat is 2% higher than the standard metallic applicators. In the direction of maximum shielding, the transmission rate is approximately 50%, compared with 70% for the standard applicator. The plastic applicator has been used on several patients with satisfactory results.

The dosimetric features and dose prescription for the Fletcher system have been described in detail; pertinent data about dose prescription are summarized in Table 13-12.[56, 76, 77, 125]

Mallinckrodt Institute System for Treatment of Cancer of the Cervix

Treatment techniques for gynecologic malignancies, including cancer of the cervix, have rapidly evolved. The Manchester applicators in conjunction with ^{226}Ra or ^{60}Co tubes were initially used through the late 1950s when the Ter-Pogossian applicator was introduced. Newer concepts emerged with the introduction of high-energy x-ray external-beam therapy in 1958, the adoption of the Fletcher-Suit applicator in 1965, and the acquisition of ^{137}Cs tubes in 1971.[173]

The applicator loadings and the prescribed doses for standard external-beam and intracavitary components of treatment are listed in Table 13-13. Small, medium, and large Fletcher colpostats are loaded with 20-, 25-, and 30-mg Ra eq sources, respectively, and the standard tandem is loaded 20–10–10.

The isodose curves passing through point A for the standard 80-mg Ra eq loading consisting of small (2-cm diameter) colpostats and a regular tandem are illustrated in Figure 13-62A. Use of small, medium, or large colpostats loaded according to Table 13-13 gives a constant 65 cGy/hour point A dose, assuming average colpostat source separation (3–4 cm). At the Mallinckrodt Institute of Radiology (MIR), the classic location of point A is used, and dose to the pelvic lymph nodes is calculated at point P, located 2 cm superior to the lateral fornix and 6 cm lateral to the center of the uterine canal. Bladder and rectal reference points are defined according to Chassagne and Horiot.[27] Dose contributions from the tandem or colpostats to these points are illustrated.

Like the Fletcher system, MIR intracavitary therapy is also prescribed in terms of mgh except that Ra eq of ^{226}Ra filtered by 1 mm of platinum is used. The prescribed quantity of Ra eq mgh is thought of as a target, rather than as a fixed prescription, because it is delivered exactly only in the case of the standard 80-mg Ra eq application and is modified according to Figure 13-62B,C for other loadings using miniovoids or 3-cm-diameter colpostats. Unlike in the Fletcher system, the uterine and vaginal components (each contributing 50% for the standard load-

TABLE 13–12
Dosimetric Characteristics of Fletcher Intracavitary System

TREATMENT COMBINATION	WHOLE PELVIS (cGy)	PARAMETRIA* (cGy)	MGH (HOURS)		POINT A DOSE (cGy)†		POINT B DOSE (cGy)		6000 cGy VOLUME (cm³)‡	
			55 MG	85 MG	55 MG	85 MG	55 MG	85 MG	55 MG	85 MG
A	0	0	6600 (120)	10,000 (118)	5870 (100)	6270 (162)	1680	2210	97	174
B	0	4000	6600 (120)	9000 (106)	5870 (100)	5630 (163)	5680	5980	97	147
C	2000	2000	5500 (100)	7500 (88)	6890 (100)	6690 (162)	5400	5650	137	209
D	4000	1000	5280 (96)	6500 (76)	8990 (100)	8060 (163)	6340	6420	350	474

**Midline shield.*
†Numbers in parentheses indicate volume in cm³.
‡Neglecting parametrial doses.

ing) are calculated independently. For example, when a small or medium tandem is used, the uterine Ra eq mgh correspond to the fraction of standard loading delivered by the sources present in the tandem. For a shorter tandem (20–10 loading), only 3000 Ra eq mgh in two applications is actually delivered to the uterus.

Intracavitary treatment is constrained by the vaginal mucosal dose, including the whole-pelvis dose, rather than maximum time as in the Fletcher system.[56] This surface dose, called rad surface dose (RSD), is the dose at the midpoint of the lateral cylindric surface of a single colpostat, including its cap. The RSD includes a 6% applicator attenuation correction and any whole-pelvis dose but excludes dose contributions from the tandem and contralateral colpostat. Current MIR treatment

TABLE 13–13
MIR Cancer of the Cervix: 8000 mgh, 2000 cGy Whole Pelvis and 3000 cGy Split Pelvis (Midline Shield)

APPLICATION	TIME Mg Ra Eq-HOUR		VAGINAL SURFACE DOSE (RSD) (cGy) SINGLE COLPOSTAT	ALL SOURCES	TOTAL DOSE (cGy) BLADDER	RECTUM	POINT A*	POINT P*	VOLUME (cm³) 6000 cGy Isodose
20 10 10 20 20 (2-cm ovoids)	× 100 hours = 4000 × 100 hours = 4000 8000	Ratio 1:0 1:1	14960	19280	7260	5520	8550 (133 cm³)	6560 (1095 cm³)	283
20 10 20 20 (2-cm ovoids)	× 100 hours = 3000 × 100 hours = 4000 7000	1:1.33	14960	19480	7340	5510	8940 (103 cm³)	6430 (1007 cm³)	234
20 10 10 30 30 (3-cm ovoids)	× 100 hours = 4000 × 80 hours = 4800 8800	1:1.2	9410	11980	6500	5240	8160 (154 cm³)	6790 (1058 cm³)	322
20 10 30 30 (3-cm ovoids)	× 100 hours = 3000 × 80 hours = 4800 7800	1:1.6	9460	11960	6650	5210	8510 (120 cm³)	6660 (989 cm³)	273
20 10 10 10 10 (miniovoids)	× 100 hours = 4000 × 128 hours = 2560 6560	1:0.64	15000	17730	6740	5020	7980 (114 cm³)	6240 (1140 cm³)	209
20 10 10 10 (miniovoids)	× 100 hours = 3000 × 100 hours = 2560 5560	1:0.85	15000	19840	6780	4990	8330 (84 cm³)	6170 (959 cm³)	165

** Volume is in parentheses.*

STANDARD 2 cm OVOID		Point A cGy/hr	Point B cGy/hr	Pelvic Nodes cGy/hr	Rectum	Bladder
20 10 10 20 20		11.6 15.3 }65% 15.4 6.6 16.4 {35%	4.3 2.9 }50% 2.9 2.7 7.5 {50%	3.2 2.0 }50% 2.0 2.1 5.4 {50%	2.7 2.7 5.3 11.7 11.7	3.0 2.8 6.2 17.4 17.4
	Single Ovoid Surface					
Dose Rate cGy/hr	126.6	65	20.2	14.6	34.1	46.8
Dose/1000 mgh cGy	1582.5	818	253	183	426	585

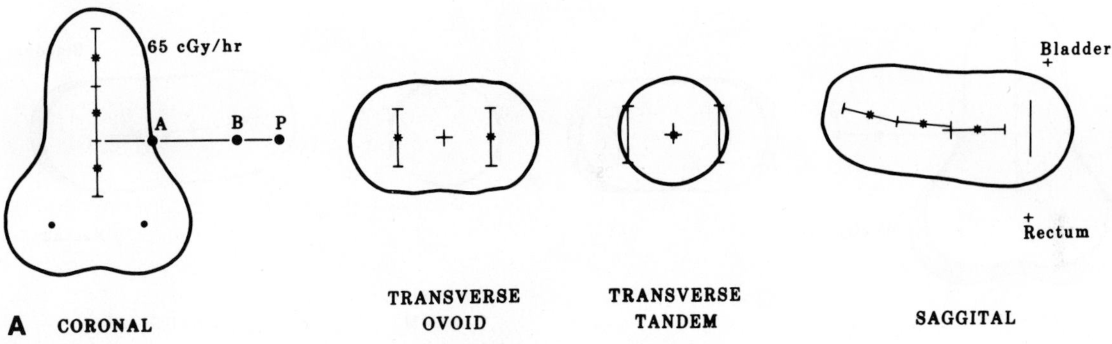

Mini Ovoid		Point A cGy/hr	Point B cGy/hr	Pelvic Nodes cGy/hr	Rectum	Bladder
20 10 10 10 10*		11.6 15.3 } 71% 15.4 5.2 11.8 {29%	4.3 2.9 } 61% 2.9 2.0 4.5 {39%	3.2 2.0 }61% 2.0 1.5 3.2 {39%	3.2 3.6 8.6 13.8 13.8	4.8 5.0 10.7 13.1 13.1
	Single Ovoid Surface					
Dose Rate cGy/hr	99.3	60	16.5	11.8	43	46.7
Dose/1000 mgh cGy	1956	899	250	179	652	708

*Weight to 13

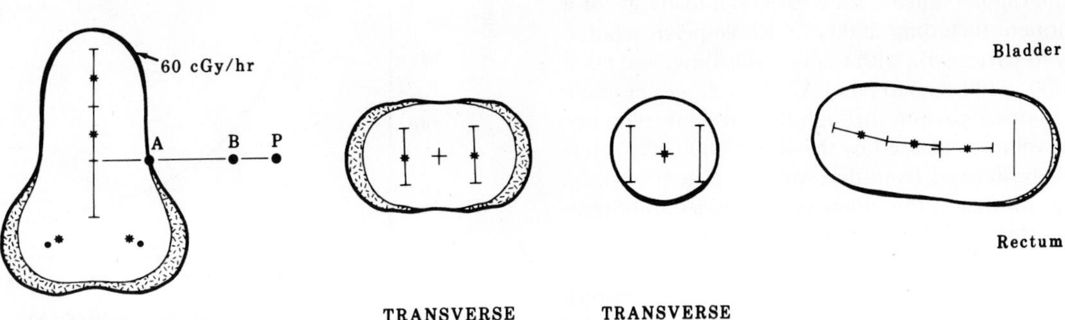

FIGURE 13–62. (**A**) Isodose curves in various planes and proportional dose contributions from the tandem or the vaginal colpostats to various points of interest in the pelvis using 2-cm diameter ovoids. (**B**) Isodose curves and dose contributions with miniovoids. Notice the smaller effective volume being covered at the 60 cGy/hour isodose line. (**C**) Isodose curves and dose contributions at various points in the pelvis from tandem and 3-cm colpostats. Notice the larger volume receiving 65 cGy/hour around the vaginal ovoids.

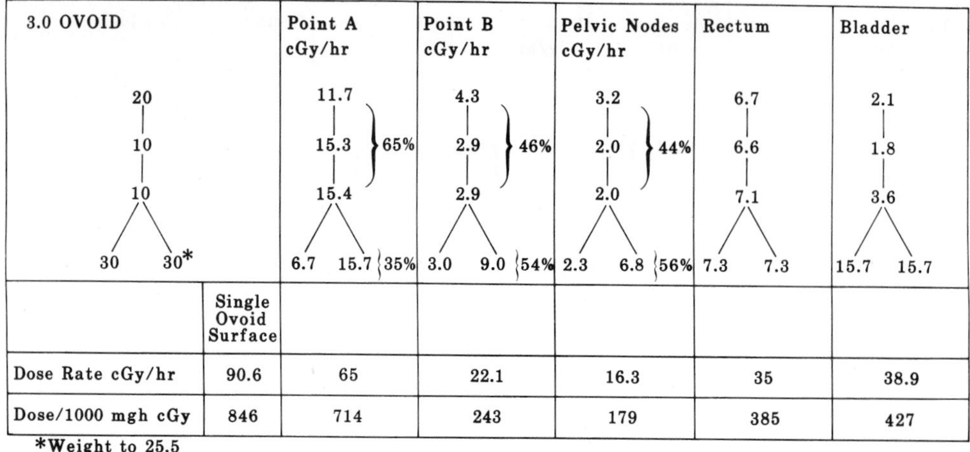

3.0 OVOID		Point A cGy/hr	Point B cGy/hr	Pelvic Nodes cGy/hr	Rectum	Bladder
20 10 10 30 30*		11.7 15.3 } 65% 15.4 6.7 15.7 } 35%	4.3 2.9 } 46% 2.9 3.0 9.0 } 54%	3.2 2.0 } 44% 2.0 2.3 6.8 } 56%	6.7 6.6 7.1 7.3 7.3	2.1 1.8 3.6 15.7 15.7
	Single Ovoid Surface					
Dose Rate cGy/hr	90.6	65	22.1	16.3	35	38.9
Dose/1000 mgh cGy	846	714	243	179	385	427

*Weight to 25.5

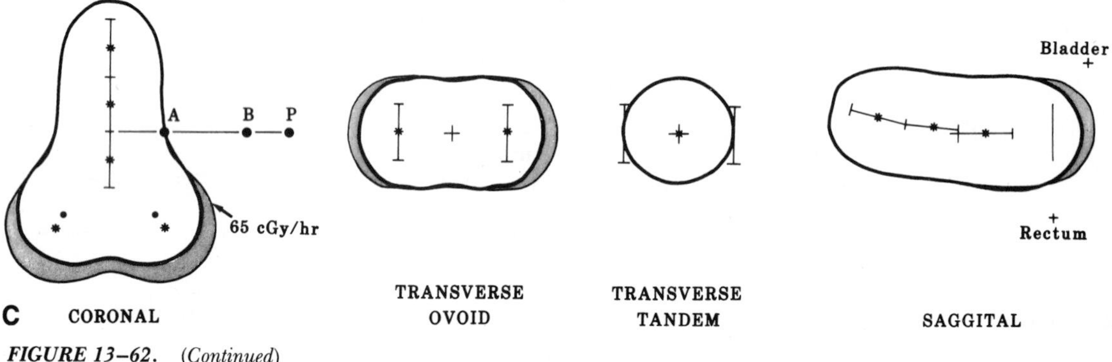

FIGURE 13–62. (*Continued*)

policies limit this dose to approximately 15,000 cGy to the upper vagina and 10,000 cGy to the distal vagina.

The total Ra eq mgh delivered can range from 5600 to 9100, depending on the applicator size and loading. For some patients, the intrauterine and vaginal sources must be unloaded at different times. The Selectron remote afterloading device, with its six independently programmable channels, makes implementation of the MIR prescription system convenient and logistically practical. The isodose curves in Figure 13-62 and dose-volume histograms, which are plots of volume enclosed by an isodose surface as a function of the corresponding dose (Fig. 13-63), assume the relative source loadings characteristic of an entire course of schema C treatment and are normalized to 1000 Ra eq mgh.

Table 13-13 lists total doses for bladder, rectum, point A, point P, and the vaginal mucosa for a variety of loadings for a course of treatment including 2000-cGy whole-pelvis irradiation, 3000 cGy to parametria with midline shielding, and 8000 Ra eq mgh (7000–7200 cGy) to point A. The volumes of tissue enclosing the isodoses passing through the cardinal reference points and the volume enclosed by the ICRU 6000-cGy reference isodose were derived from dose-volume histograms.

The data show that as the tumor size increases and therapeutic emphasis shifts from intracavitary insertions to external-beam irradiation, total point A doses increase from 6500 cGy for small IB lesions to 9000 cGy for IIB, III, and IV lesions. Despite use of mgh as the basis of prescription, the loading rules yield approximately constant treatment times and total point A doses independent of loading, similar to the defining features of the Manchester system. As a result, the tissue volumes enclosed by the point A and 6000-cGy isodose surfaces may vary by as much as a factor of 2 from one another in the same treatment group.

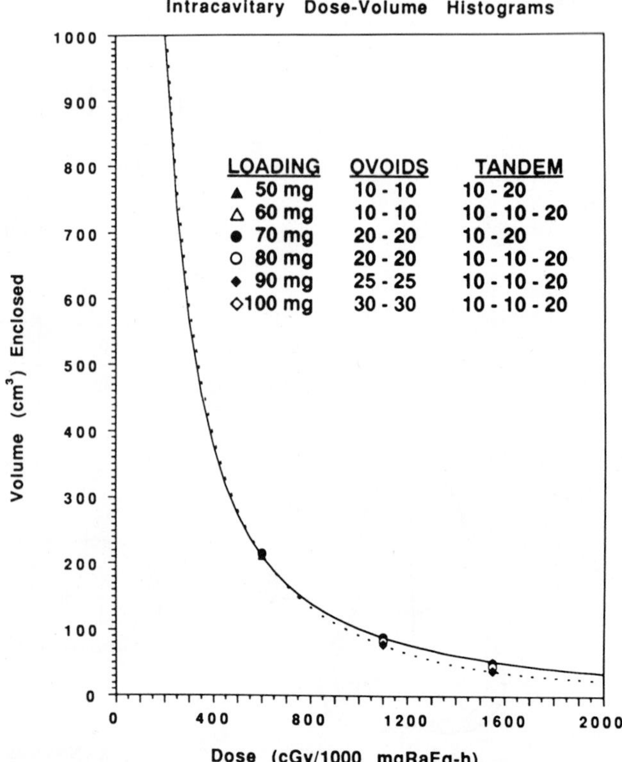

FIGURE 13–63. Dose-volume histograms for seven Mallinckrodt Institute of Radiology (MIR) intracavitary insertions using 1.4-cm active length ^{137}Cs sources. The strength of each source was determined by the loading rules for MIR schema C (2000 cGy whole pelvis plus 8000 mgh) and was then scaled down to 1000 mgh. Notice that as the size of the insertion increases, the volume of tissue encompassed by the high-dose isosurfaces decreases. Point A doses ranged from 828 to 1135 cGy.

As the stage and extent of the disease increase, the treatment system delivers 6000 cGy to an ever-larger volume of tissue. Compared with the Fletcher system, the MIR system treats point A to higher doses and treats larger volumes of tissue to a minimum dose of 6000 cGy. Because the Fletcher system uses ^{226}Ra tubes filtered by 1 mm of platinum, each mgh delivers 7% less radiation to the patient than the Ra eq mgh used at MIR, which quantifies source strength relative to ^{226}Ra sources filtered by 0.5 mm of platinum.

Dose Specification in Gynecologic Intracavitary Therapy

The physical relationships between point A dose and mgh prescriptions are important determinants for gynecologic intracavitary therapy.[190] Although a minimum dose to a predefined target volume could be used as the basis of treatment prescription, it is difficult to define. The lack of accurate dose computation algorithms that account for applicator shielding is another factor mitigating against use of minimum tumor dose as a prescription criterion. Knowledge of tumor control and complication rates in terms of mgh and dose at fixed reference points relative to the applicator remains the basis of intracavitary treatment prescription.[56,105,237]

The conceptual significance of point A has been obscured by the widespread current practice of defining point A to be 2 cm superior to the cervical os rather than 2 cm superior to the lateral vaginal fornix, as originally specified by Tod and Meredith.[237] In practice, the os is radiographically demarcated by the tandem collar or the most inferior aspect of the caudal intrauterine source, and the lateral fornix is indicated by the colpostat surface. Because the vertical position of the colpostat relative to the caudal aspect of the tandem varies significantly from patient to patient, the distance between the "revised" point A and the vaginal sources varies, creating large fluctuations in the dose rate. This phenomenon is illustrated by Potish's study[191] of 90 Fletcher intracavitary applications, in which he compared dose rates calculated on the basis of the classic and revised point A definitions. Revised point A dose rates are higher and much more varied than their classic counterparts. The classic values are nearly independent of the applicator loading and have a mean value ($52\ cGy \cdot h^{-1}$) very close to that predicted by the Manchester system.

Recently, the ICRU[105] introduced the concept of reference volume (isodose surface) to report and compare intracavitary treatments. *Reference volume* describes the tissue encompassed by a reference isodose surface. This reference volume (Fig. 13-64) is defined by three dimensions: the height (d_h), which is the maximum dimension along the intrauterine source and is measured in the oblique frontal plane containing that source; the width (d_w), which is the maximum dimension perpendicular to the intrauterine source measured in the same plane; and thickness (d_t), which is the maximum dimension perpendicular to the intrauterine source and is measured in the oblique sagittal plane containing that source.[105] An absorbed dose level of 6000 cGy (external and intracavitary) is widely accepted as the reference level for low-dose-rate therapy.

Potish[189] analyzed the effect of applicator geometry on classic dose specification parameters in 90 Fletcher-Suit intracavitary applications for cervical cancer. He identified five significant factors: mg in colpostats, mg in tandems, lateral displacement of colpostats in frontal plane, vertical separation between the colpostats and tandem sources, and anteroposterior displacement of the colpostats relative to the tandem. Applicator or source geometry had little effect on the product of ICRU volume specification, but it greatly influenced the individual ICRU components and "traditional" dose calculation points.

In contrast to point A dose and mgh, the ICRU proposal is only a means of describing or reporting treatment, not a formal prescription. No insight is given into how to load an applicator, how long it should remain in the patient, or how to divide treatment between intracavitary and external-beam irradiation. It is not obvious whether ICRU reference isodose measurements are correlated with clinical outcome or how they are to be used to differentiate good from bad treatment plans.[192] Crook and associates[36] and Esche with the same group,[51] using computerized dosimetry, correlated the parameters described in ICRU Report 38 with the mgh and external irradiation using the Fletcher system. The reference volume dose was directly proportional to mgh and doses of external irradiation to the pelvis over 3000 cGy, but it did not depend appreciably on moderate changes in source geometry.[51] The authors described a close correlation between treatment sequelae and reference doses to various critical organs.[36]

Some points of dose calculation (*e.g.*, lymphatic trapezoid and pelvic wall reference points) in ICRU Report 38 are not used in everyday practice.[105] Although it is logical that the dose rates and volumetric distribution between external and intratherapy may give rise to different biologic effects in tumor and normal tissues, there are not sufficient data to introduce correction factors into dose prescription systems to account for these effects. However, it is important to state the duration of each application and the time interval between brachytherapy procedures when multiple insertions are performed. Similarly, when external-beam and intracavitary therapy are combined, the time-dose schedule of the entire treatment should be reported.

Reference Points Related to Organs at Risk

In addition to prescription of intracavitary therapy to achieve local tumor control, a means of quantifying absorbed dose delivered to therapy-limiting normal structures, such as the bladder and rectum, is needed. Many different reference points have been proposed. The bladder and rectal reference points proposed by Chassagne and Horiot[27] are illustrated in Figure 13-65. The bladder reference point is outlined by a Foley catheter with 7 ml of radiopaque fluid in the balloon. The catheter is pulled downward to bring the balloon against the bladder neck and urethra. On lateral radiographs the reference point is obtained by drawing an anteroposterior line through the center of the balloon and projecting it to where it crosses the posterior surface of the balloon. The point of reference for the rectal dose is obtained on the lateral radiograph at a point where an anteroposterior line drawn from the lower end of the intrauterine source (or from the middle of the intravaginal sources) crosses the rectal wall, which is arbitrarily displaced 5 mm posterior to the vaginal wall. The vaginal wall is identified by an intravaginal mold or by opacification with the packing gauze soaked in radiopaque (40% iodine) material.

DOSE PRESCRIPTION AND SPECIFICATION IN INTERSTITIAL BRACHYTHERAPY

The ability to compare different interstitial implants according to geometric accuracy of dose delivery, normal tissue sparing, and dose homogeneity depends on dose specification. Proper

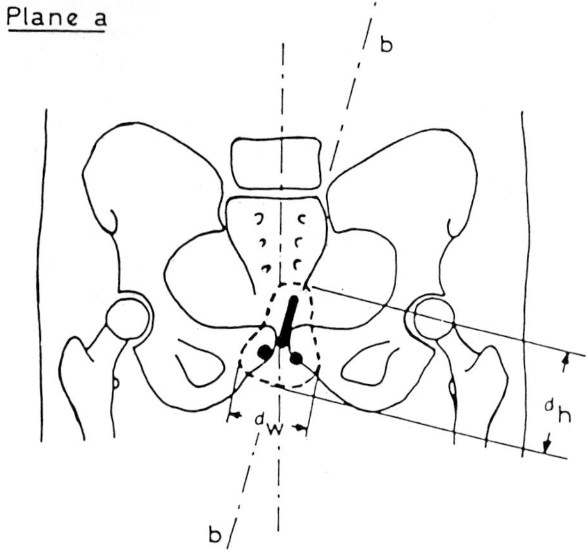

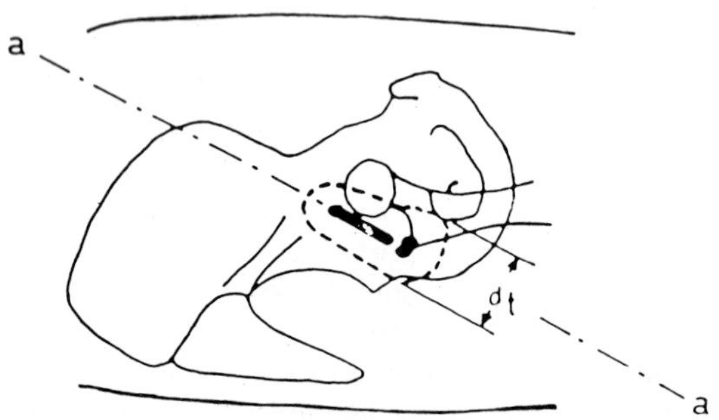

FIGURE 13–64. Geometry for measurement of the size of the pear-shaped ICRU reference isodose surface (*broken line*) in a typical treatment of cervix carcinoma using one rod-shaped uterine applicator and two vaginal applicators. *Plane a* is the "oblique" frontal plane that contains the intrauterine device. The oblique frontal plane is obtained by rotation of the frontal plane around a transverse axis. *Plane b* is the "oblique" sagittal plane that contains the intrauterine device. The oblique sagittal plane is obtained by rotation of the sagittal plane around the anteroposterior axis. The height (d_h) and the width (d_w) of the reference volume are measured in *plane a* as the maximal sizes parallel and perpendicular to the uterine applicator, respectively. The thickness (d_t) of the reference volume is measured in *plane b* as the maximal size perpendicular to the uterine applicator. (International Commission on Radiation Units and Measurements: Report 38: Dose and Volume Specification for Reporting Intracavitary Therapy in Gynecology. Bethesda, MD, ICRU, 1985)

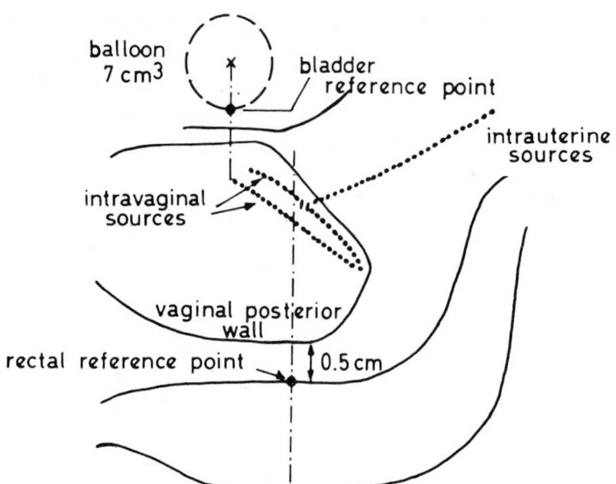

FIGURE 13–65. Reference points for bladder and rectal brachytherapy doses proposed by the ICRU. (International Commission on Radiation Units and Measurements: Report 38: Dose and Volume Specification for Reporting Intracavitary Therapy in Gynecology. Bethesda, MD, ICRU, 1985)

selection of the reference dose rate to deliver a homogeneous dose throughout the target volume is critical in interstitial brachytherapy.[207]

Specifications of prescribed dose and evaluation of "implant quality" in interstitial brachytherapy are more elusive than in external-beam irradiation. The adequacy of an implant could be evaluated in terms of three volumetric irradiation indices:[207]

1. The coverage index represents the percent of the target volume receiving dose rates equal to or greater than the reference dose rate.
2. The relative dose homogeneity index represents the percent of the target volume receiving dose rates between 100% and 150% of the reference dose rate.
3. The external volume index represents the percent volume outside the target volume, normalized to the target volume, receiving dose rates equal to or greater than the reference dose rate.

The reference dose rate at which the relative dose homogeneity index is maximum is expected to appear as an isodose rate contour that has a width larger than the thickness of the target volume in the central plane.

Because the peripheral sources are inserted near or on the boundary of the target volume, the dose is prescribed in a region of high dose gradients, making the choice of prescription isodose quite variable and subjective. In addition, the dose distribution depends greatly on the location of the calculation plane relative to the implant. Because implant dose distributions are intrinsically three dimensional (3D), the conventional 2D treatment planning approximations have less validity than in external-beam therapy.

Other methods have been proposed to quantitate prescribed dose and implant quality. *Minimum target dose* is difficult to implement clinically. In general, no 3D geometric description of the target volume relative to the implanted volume is available. As in intracavitary therapy, the interstitial surgical procedure is guided by palpation, visualization, and the experience and dexterity of the radiation oncologist. Only in stereotactic interstitial therapy of intracranial lesions is a 3D geometric description of the target volume derived from CT or MR images available for preplanning an implant and mechanisms for accurately implanting the sources and objectively verifying their location relative to the target volume.

Clinical implant dosimetry is based on 3D reconstruction of radioactive source positions from planar radiographs. This procedure yields accurate doses relative to the sources at various planes but not relative to anatomic structures. Thus it is natural to prescribe treatment to a point or surface that has a fixed relationship to the peripheral sources, which collectively define the implanted volume. This is perhaps the most widely used prescription philosophy and is the basis of the historic Manchester,[168] Paris,[184] and Quimby[198] systems. Because the boundary of the implanted volume is in a region of high dose gradients, the producible and objective selection of *minimum peripheral dose* from 2D isodose distributions remains a problem.

Using a *mean central dose* approach to dose specification employs a generalization of the Paris system basal dose, the 2D isodose distribution in a central transverse plane, which is perpendicular to and bisecting the needle or catheter axis. Specifically, mean central dose is defined as the arithmetic mean of the local minimum doses at points equidistant from each group of three adjacent needles forming acute triangles in the central transverse plane.

Without an objective definition of target or implanted volume, *3D dose-volume histograms* in themselves do not solve the problem of objective dose prescription. However, they can be used to objectively quantify dose homogeneity, like the amount of tissue treated to doses greater than a fixed fraction of the prescribed dose (*e.g.*, 150%) and the volume of tissue treated and volume of tissue outside the prescription isodose treated to a specified fraction (*e.g.*, 75%) of the prescribed dose.

QUALITY ASSURANCE AND RADIATION SAFETY IN BRACHYTHERAPY

It is extremely important in the use of brachytherapy to formulate and strictly observe radiation safety procedures at each institution, in full compliance with Nuclear Regulatory Commission (NRC) regulations.

The safety of personnel, patients, and visitors is based on three basic factors: *time* of radiation exposure should be as short as possible; *distance* should be as great as practically allowed between the radioactive sources and the operator; and *shielding* should be employed to diminish radiation exposure to all concerned.

Careful quality control procedures should be followed in the prescription and calculation of doses, in preparing, calibrating, and handling radioactive sources, and in verifying treatment parameters. If promptly discovered, an error in brachytherapy can be corrected, but it is more difficult to do than in external-beam irradiation.

At the Radiation Oncology Center of Washington University's Mallinckrodt Institute of Radiology, formal procedures for brachytherapy have been established to minimize treatment errors. For temporary implants, source loadings are usually prescribed after the physician has reviewed the orthogonal dummy source localization radiographs. The prescription is written on a form that is given to the brachytherapy source curator (Fig. 13-66) specifying the configuration of source strengths for intracavitary treatment or the array of active lengths and linear activity if iridium wires or seed ribbons are

RADIATION ONCOLOGY CENTER TO BE PLACED ON FRONT OF HOSP. CHART
MALLINCKRODT INSTITUTE OF RADIOLOGY
WASHINGTON UNIVERSITY SCHOOL OF MEDICINE
CAUTION
GYN BRACHYTHERAPY

NAME: ______ BIRTHDATE: ______ RAD. ONC. NO.: ______
PRIMARY SITE: ______ REF. PHYSICIANS: ______
STAGE: ______ HISTOPATHOLOGY: ______
IMPLANT NO.: ______ DATE OF IMPLANT: ______ RADIOTHERAPISTS: ______
REMOTE AFTERLOADER: ______
APPLICATORS: ______
ISOTOPE: ______
SOUNDING: ______ CM

	IN	OUT	
TIME			
DAY			
DATE			
TOTAL TIME		HRS.	HRS.

RAD. ONC. RESIDENT ______
GYN. ONC. SURGEON: ______
GYN. ONC. RESIDENT: ______

AFTERLOADING SOURCE CONFIGURATION	REMOTE AFTERLOADING SOURCE CONFIGURATION (PHYSICIAN INDICATE RADIOACTIVE PELLETS •)		
	CHANNEL 1	CHANNEL 2	CHANNEL 3
	1.–48. ○	1.–48. ○	1.–48. ○
TOTAL (mg Ra eq) / TOTAL (mg-hrs)	TOTAL (mg Ra eq)	TOTAL (mg-hrs)	

ORDER OF HEYMAN CAPSULE INSERTION	
CAPSULES	CHANNEL/LOADING
1	
2	
3	
4	
5	
6	
7	
8	
9	
10	
11	
12	
13	
14	
15	
16	
17	
18	
19	
20	
TOTAL (mg Ra eq)	TOTAL (mg-hrs)

SPECIAL INSTRUCTIONS ______
IMPLANT REMOVED AT: TIME: ______ DATE: ______ ACTUAL TOTAL TIME: ______ HR
SIGNATURE: X ______
SIGNATURE OF RAD. ONC. M.D. OR CESIUM CURATOR RECEIVING ISOTOPE: ______
RADIOACTIVE MATERIAL
MIR-RO # 53 (3-87)

FIGURE 13–66. Example of a brachytherapy prescription sheet used at Mallinckrodt Institute of Radiology. The configuration of the source loading in the various channels of remote-control afterloading applications can be indicated in the appropriate section.

used for interstitial techniques. Treatment duration is usually determined after reviewing the computer planar isodose rate distributions and is double-checked with hand calculations. The source curator documents the preparation of sources in a treatment log book, on a source inventory sheet that is posted on the patient's door, and also on a magnetic source inventory board in the radioactive source room. If iridium is used, the vendor's lot identification code is also documented. A well-type dose calibrator (Berkley) is used to verify the source activity.

If manual intracavitary afterloading is used, for the sake of prompt patient loading, the various cesium tubes are color coded. The attending physician or resident (after verifying the source loading) and the source curator load the applicator in the patient. The loading time is documented by the physician, and the curator or physicist measures the radiation exposure levels around the patient and arranges lead shields appropriately. The nursing division is also actively involved in checking every 3 to 4 hours that applicators or sources do not become dislodged over the course of treatment.

The physician's orders sheet contains the home telephone number and the beeper number of at least two physicians who can be contacted in an emergency if source removal is required. The attending physician or resident is responsible for the unloading of the implant. The physician counts the sources as they are removed and places them in a lead carrier.

After removal of the sources, the patient is surveyed to ensure that no sources remain in the patient or in the patient's room. The time of unloading is documented, and all radiation warning signs are removed from the patient's door. The source curator checks that all sources have been recovered and returns the sources to their designated storage area. The magnetic inventory board is revised to reflect that the sources have been returned to their storage area. Source recovery is also documented in the source logbook.

REFERENCES

1. Abrath FG, Henderson SD, Simpson JR, et al: Dosimetry of CT-guided volumetric Ir-192 brain implant. Int J Radiat Oncol Biol Phys 12:539, 1986
2. Akine Y, Arimoto H, Ogino T, et al: High-dose-rate intracavitary irradiation in the treatment of carcinoma of the uterine cervix: Early experience with 84 patients. Int J Radiat Oncol Biol Phys 14:893, 1988
3. Allt WEC, Hunt JW: Experience with radioactive tantalum wire as a source for interstitial therapy. Radiology 80:581, 1963
4. Ampuero F, Doss LL, Khan LM, et al: The Syed-Neblett interstitial template in locally advanced gynecological malignancies. Int J Radiat Oncol Biol Phys 9:1897, 1983
5. Anderson LL: Remote afterloading in cancer management. I. Afterloader design and optimization potential. In Hilaris BS, Batata MA (eds): Brachytherapy Oncology—1983, pp 93–100. New York, Memorial Sloan-Kettering Cancer Center, 1983
6. Anderson LL, Aubrey RF: Computerized dosimetry for ^{125}I prostate implants. In Hilaris BS, Batata MA (eds): Brachytherapy Oncology—1983, pp 57–63. New York, Memorial Sloan-Kettering Cancer Center, 1983
7. Anderson LL, Hilaris BS, Wagner LK: A nomograph for planar implant planning. Endocuriether Hypertherm Oncol 1:9, 1985
8. Annual Report on the Results of Treatment of Gynecological Cancer. In Pettersson F (ed): Twentieth Volume Statements of Results Obtained in Patients Treated in 1979–1981: Inclusive 5-Year Survival up to 1985, Stockholm, Sweden, pp 20–52. Stockholm, Sweden, International Federation of Gynecology and Obstetrics, 1987
9. Arai T: Relationship between total isoeffect dose and number of fractions for the treatment of uterine cervical carcinoma by high dose rate intracavitary irradiation: Working party on the use of radionuclides and afterloading techniques in the treatment of cancer of the uterus. London, High Dose Workshop, 1978
10. Arai T, Morita S, Kutsutani Y, et al: Relationship between total iso-effect dose and number of fractions for the treatment of uterine cervical carcinoma by high dose rate intracavitary irradiation. In Bates TD, Berry RJ (eds): High Dose Rate Afterloading in the Treatment of Cancer of the Uterus, Special Report 17, pp 89–92. London, British Institute of Radiology, 1980
11. Arai T, Morita S, Linuma TK, et al: Radiation treatment of cervix cancer using the high dose rate remote afterloading intracavitary irradiation: An analysis of the correlation between optimal dose range and fractionation. Jpn J Cancer Clin 25:605, 1979
12. Aristizabal SA, Valencia A, Ocampo G, et al: Interstitial parametrial irradiation in cancer of the cervix stage IIB–IIIB. Endocuriether Hypertherm Oncol 1:41, 1985
13. Baillet F, Decroix Y, Mazeron JJ: Oral tongue. In Pierquin B, Wilson J-F, Chassagne D (eds): Modern Brachytherapy, pp 107–118. New York, Masson, 1987
14. Bartelink H, Borger JH: Breast conservation therapy: Current and future role of interstitial boost irradiation. In Mould RF (ed): Brachytherapy 2, pp 497–502. Netherlands, Nucletron International BV, 1989
15. Batley F, Constable WC: The use of the "Manchester system" for treatment of cancer of the uterine cervix with modern after-loading radium applicators. J Can Assoc Radiol 18:396, 1967
16. Battermann JJ, Boon TA: Interstitial therapy in the management of T2 bladder tumors. Endocuriether Hypertherm Oncol 4:1, 1988
17. Battermann JJ, Boon TA: Treatment of T2 bladder tumours with interstitial therapy: The role of lymph node dissection. In Mould RF (ed): Brachytherapy 2, pp 187–191. Netherlands, Nucletron International BV, 1989
18. Battermann JJ, Szabol B: Preliminary results of radiation therapy for carcinoma of the uterine cervix, using the Selectron afterloading machine. In Mould RF (ed): Brachytherapy 2, pp 229–234. Netherlands, Nucletron International BV, 1989
19. Battermann JJ, Tierie AH: Results of implantation for T1 and T2 bladder tumours. Radiother Oncol 5:85, 1986
20. Bekerus M, Durbaba M, Frim O, et al: Comparison of HDR and LDR results in endometrium cancer. In Vahrson H, Rauthe G (eds): High Dose Rate Afterloading in the Treatment of Cancer of the Uterus, Breast and Rectum, p 222. Baltimore, Urban & Schwarzenberg, 1988
21. Bier R, Small RC, Leake DL, et al: An afterloading technique for radium needles in the treatment of carcinoma of the oral cavity. Radiology 108:711, 1973
22. Blasko JC, Schumacher D: Palladium-103 Implantation for Prostate Carcinoma: Dose Rationale (personal communication)
23. Brindle JS, Martinez A, Schray M, et al: Pelvic lymphadenectomy and transperineal interstitial implantation of ^{192}Ir combined with external-beam radiotherapy for bulky stage C prostatic carcinoma. Int J Radiat Oncol Biol Phys 17:1063, 1989
24. Cameron ME: Pterygium Throughout the World. Springfield, IL, Charles C Thomas, 1965
25. Carlton CE Jr, Dawoud F, Hudgins PT, et al: Irradiation treatment of carcinoma of the prostate: A preliminary report based on 8 years of experience. J Urol 108:924, 1972
26. Charyulu KKN: Transperineal interstitial implantation of prostate cancer: A new method. Int J Radiat Oncol Biol Phys 6:1261, 1980
27. Chassagne D, Horiot JC: Propositions pour une definition commune des points de reference en curietherapie gynecologique. J Radiol Electrol 58:371, 1977
28. Chitwood WR Jr: Diagnosis and treatment of primary extrahepatic bile duct tumors. Am J Surg 143:99, 1982

29. Chiu-Tsao ST, Anderson LL, Stabile L: TLD dosimetry for ^{125}I eye plaque. Phys Med Biol 33:28, 1988
30. Chiu-Tsao ST, Tsao HS, Vialotti C, et al: Monte Carlo dosimetry for ^{125}I and ^{60}Co in eye plaque therapy. Med Phys 13:678, 1986
31. Cikaric S: Radiation therapy of cervical carcinoma using either HDR or LDR afterloading: Comparison of 5-year results and complications. Strahlenther Onkol [Suppl] 82:119, 1988
32. Clarke DH, Edmundson GK, Martinez A, et al: The utilization of I-125 seeds as a substitute for Ir-192 seeds in temporary interstitial implants: An overview and a description of the William Beaumont Hospital technique. Int J Radiat Oncol Biol Phys 15:1027, 1988
33. Clarke DH, Edmundson GK, Martinez A, et al: The clinical advantages of I-125 seeds as a substitute for Ir-192 seeds in temporary plastic tube implants. Int J Radiat Oncol Biol Phys 17:859, 1989
34. Conroy RM, Shahbazian AA, Edwards KC, et al: A new method for treating carcinomatous biliary obstruction with intracatheter radium. Cancer 49:1321, 1982
35. Cooper FS: Postoperative irradiation of pterygia: Ten more years of experience. Radiology 128:753, 1978
36. Crook JM, Esche BA, Chaplain G, et al: Dose-volume analysis and the prevention of radiation sequelae in cervical cancer. Radiother Oncol 8:321, 1987
37. Dale RG: The application of the linear quadratic dose effect equation to fractionated and protracted radiation therapy. Br J Radiol 58:515, 1985
38. Dean E, Lambert G, Dawes P: Gynaecological treatments using the Selectron remote afterloading system. Br J Radiol 61:1053, 1988
39. Delclos L: Are interstitial radium applications passe? Front Radiat Ther Oncol 12:42, 1978
40. Delclos L: Afterloading method for interstitial gamma-ray therapy. In Fletcher GH (ed): Textbook of Radiotherapy, 3rd ed. Philadelphia, Lea & Febiger, 1980
41. Delclos L: In Deeley TJ (ed): Topical Reviews in Radiotherapy and Oncology—2. London, John Wright & Sons, 1982
42. Delclos L: Interstitial irradiation of the penis. In Johnson DE, Boileau MA (eds): Genitourinary Tumors: Fundamental Principles and Surgical Techniques. New York, Grune & Stratton, 1982
43. Delclos L: Interstitial irradiation techniques. In Levitt SH, Tapley NduV (eds): Technological Basis of Radiation Therapy: Practical Clinical Applications, pp 55–84. Philadelphia, Lea & Febiger, 1984
44. Delclos L, Fletcher GH, Moore EB, et al: Minicolpostats, dome cylinders, other additions and improvements of the Fletcher-Suit after-loadable system: Indications and limitations of their use. Int J Radiat Oncol Biol Phys 6:1195, 1980
45. Delclos L, Fletcher GH, Sampiere V, Grant WH III: Can the Fletcher gamma ray colpostat system be extrapolated to other systems? Cancer 41:970, 1978
46. Delclos L, Wharton JT, Rutledge FN: Tumors of the vagina and female urethra. In Fletcher GH (ed): Textbook of Radiotherapy, 3rd ed. Philadelphia, Lea & Febiger, 1980
47. Denham, JW: The radiation dose-response relationship for control of primary breast cancer. Radiother Oncol 7:107, 1986
48. Dobelbower RR, Merrick HW, Ahuja RK, et al: I-125 interstitial implant, precision high-dose external-beam therapy, and 5-FU for unresectable adenocarcinoma of pancreas and extrahepatic biliary tree. Cancer 58:2185, 1986
49. Druy EM, Carabell SC, Ling CC: Treatment of bile duct tumors with ^{192}Ir. Presented at the 67th Annual Meeting of the Radiological Society of North America, Chicago, November 19, 1981
50. Emami B, Perez CA: Interstitial thermoradiotherapy in the treatment of malignant tumors. In Sauer R (ed): Interventional Radiation Therapy Techniques—Brachytherapy. Springer-Verlag (in press)
51. Esche BA, Crook JM, Isturiz J, et al: Reference volume, milligram-hours and external irradiation for the Fletcher applicator. Radiother Oncol 9:255, 1987
52. Esche BA, Haie CM, Gerbaulet AP, et al: Interstitial and external radiotherapy in carcinoma of the soft palate and uvula. Int J Radiat Oncol Biol Phys 15:619, 1988
53. Feder BH, Syed AMN, Neblett D: Treatment of extensive carcinoma of the cervix with the "transperineal parametrial butterfly": A preliminary report on the revival of Waterman's approach. Int J Radiat Oncol Biol Phys 4:735, 1978
54. Fields JN, Emami B: Carcinoma of the extrahepatic biliary system: Results of primary and adjuvant radiotherapy. Int J Radiat Oncol Biol Phys 13:331, 1987
55. Fletcher GH: Cervical radium applicators with screening in the direction of bladder and rectum. Radiology 60:77, 1953
56. Fletcher GH: In Fletcher GH (ed): Textbook of Radiotherapy, 3rd ed. Philadelphia, Lea & Febiger, 1980
57. Fletcher GH, MacComb WS: Radiation Therapy in the Management of Cancers of the Oral Cavity and Oropharynx. Springfield, IL, Charles C Thomas, 1962
58. Fletcher MS: Treatment of high bile duct carcinoma by internal radiotherapy with ^{192}Ir wire. Lancet 2:172, 1981
59. Flores AD, Nelems B, Evans K, et al: Impact of new radiotherapy modalities on the surgical management of cancer of the esophagus and cardia. Int J Radiat Oncol Biol Phys 17:937, 1989
60. Fontanesi J, Hetzler D, Ross J: Effect of dose rate on local control and complications in the reirradiation of head and neck tumors with interstitial Iridium-192. Int J Radiat Oncol Biol Phys 17:365, 1989
61. Fu KK, Phillips TL: High-dose-rate versus low-dose-rate intracavitary brachytherapy for carcinoma of the cervix. Int J Radiat Oncol Biol Phys 19:791, 1990
62. Gaddis O Jr, Morrow, CP, Klement V, et al: Treatment of cervical carcinoma employing a template for transperineal interstitial ^{192}Ir brachytherapy. Int J Radiat Oncol Biol Phys 9:819, 1983
63. Garcia D, Fathman A, Drzymala R, et al: Localized carcinoma of the prostate: Preliminary results of transperineal interstitial ^{192}Ir implantation and external irradiation. (unpublished data)
64. Gelb AF, Epstein JD: Lasers and endocurietherapy in lung cancer. Endocuriether Hypertherm Oncol 2:153, 1986
65. Gerard JP, Rozan R, Mazeron JJ, et al: Iridium-192 brachytherapy in urinary bladder cancer: The French experience. In Mould RF (ed): Brachytherapy 2, pp 179–182. Netherlands, Nucletron International BV, 1989
66. Glaser FM: Decatron remote afterloading therapy with high activity sources. In Bates TD, Berry RJ (eds): High Dose Rate Afterloading in the Treatment of Cancer of the Uterus, Special Report No. 17, pp 51–58. London, British Institute of Radiology, 1980
67. Glaser FH: Comparison of HDR afterloading with ^{192}Ir versus conventional radium therapy in cervix cancer: 5-year results and complications. Strahlenther Onkol [suppl] 82:106, 1988
68. Goffinet DR, Martinez A, Fee WE Jr: ^{125}I Vicryl suture implants as a surgical adjuvant in cancer of the head and neck. Int J Radiat Oncol Biol Phys 11:399, 1985
69. Greenberg M: Eye: Choroidal melanomas and pterygium. In Pierquin B, Wilson J-F, Chassagne D (eds): Modern Brachytherapy, pp 301–314. New York, Masson, 1987
70. Greenblatt DR, Nori D, Tankenbaum A, et al: New brachytherapy techniques using iodine-125 seeds for tumor bed implants. Endocuriether Hypertherm Oncol 3:73, 1987
71. Grigsby PW, Perez CA, Eichling J, et al: Reduction in radiation exposure to nursing personnel with the use of remote afterloading brachytherapy devices. Int J Radiat Oncol Biol Phys 20:627, 1991
72. Grigsby PW, Perez CA, Kuten A, et al: Clinical stage I endometrial cancer: Results of adjuvant irradiation and patterns of failure. Int J Radiat Oncol Biol Phys (in press)
73. Gupta BD, Ayyagari S, Sharma SC, et al: Carcinoma of the cervix: Optimal time-dose fractionation of HDR brachytherapy and comparison with conventional dose-rate brachytherapy. In Mould RF (ed): Brachytherapy 2, pp 307–308. Netherlands, Nucletron International BV, 1989
74. Gutin PH, Phillips TL, Hosobuchi Y, et al: Permanent and

removable implants for the brachytherapy of brain tumors. Int J Radiat Oncol Biol Phys 7:1371, 1981
75. Gutin PH, Phillips TL, Wara WM, et al: Brachytherapy of recurrent malignant brain tumors with removable high-activity iodine-125 sources. J Neurosurg 60:1, 1984
76. Haas JS, Dean D, Mansfield CM: Evaluation of a new Fletcher applicator using ^{137}Cs. Int J Radiat Oncol Biol Phys 6:1589, 1980
77. Haas JS, Dean RD, Mansfield CM: Dosimetric comparison of the Fletcher family of gynecologic colpostats, 1950–1980. Int J Radiat Oncol Biol Phys 11:1317, 1985
78. Hall E: The biological basis of endocurietherapy. Endocuriether Hypertherm Oncol 1:141, 1985
79. Hames F: A new method in the use of radon gold seeds. Am J Surg 38:235, 1937.
80. Hanks GE, Herring DF, Kramer S: Patterns of care outcome studies. Cancer 51:959, 1983
81. Harter DJ, Delclos L: Sealed sources in synthetic absorbable suture. Radiology 116:727, 1975
82. Heaston DK, Herskovic AM, Engler MJ, et al: Intrabiliary irradiation of primary and metastatic bile duct carcinoma (personal communication)
83. Henschke UK: Interstitial implantation with radioisotopes. In Hahan PF (ed): Therapeutic Use of Artificial Radioisotopes. New York, John Wiley, 1956
84. Henschke UK: Artificial radioisotopes in nylon ribbons for implantation in neoplasms. International Conferences on the Peaceful Uses of Atomic Energy. New York, United Nations, 1956
85. Henschke UK: Afterloading applicator for radiation therapy of carcinoma of the uterus. Radiology 74:834, 1960
86. Henschke UK, Hilaris BS, Mahan DG: Remote afterloading with intracavitary applicators. Radiology 83:344, 1964
87. Henschke UK, James AG, Myers WG: Radiogold seeds for cancer therapy. Nucleonics 11:45, 1953
88. Herskovic A, Heaston D, Engler MJ, et al: Irradiation of biliary carcinoma. Radiology 139:219, 1981
89. Heyman J, Reuterwall O, Benner S: The Radiumhemmet experience with radiotherapy in cancer of the corpus of the uterus: Classification, method of treatment and results. Acta Radiol 11:11, 1941
90. Hilaris BS: Handbook of Interstitial Brachytherapy. Acton, MA, Acton Publishing Science Group, 1975
91. Hilaris BS, Batata MA: Brachytherapy techniques. In Hilaris BS, Batata MA (eds): Brachytherapy Oncology—1983, pp 41–56. New York, Memorial Sloan-Kettering Cancer Center, 1983
92. Hilaris BS, Gomez J, Nori D, et al: Combined surgery, intraoperative brachytherapy, and postoperative external radiation in stage III non-small-cell lung cancer. Cancer 55:1226, 1985
93. Hilaris BS, Martini N: The current state of intraoperative interstitial brachytherapy in lung cancer. Int J Radiat Oncol Biol Phys 15:1347, 1988
94. Hilaris BS, Nori D, Anderson LL: Interstitial brachytherapy planning and evaluation. In Hilaris BS, Nori D, Anderson LL (eds): Atlas of Brachytherapy, pp 70–95. New York, McMillan, 1988
95. Hilaris BS, Nori D, Anderson L: Brachytherapy of ocular melanoma. In Hilaris BS, Nori D, Anderson LL (eds): Atlas of Brachytherapy. New York, McMillan, 1988
96. Hilaris BS, Rousssi K: Cancer of the pancreas. In Hilaris BS (ed): Handbook of Interstitial Brachytherapy, pp 251–262. Acton, MA, Acton Publishing Science Group, 1975
97. Hilaris BS, Whitmore WF, Batata MA, et al: Behavioral patterns of prostate adenocarcinoma following an I-125 implant and pelvic node dissection. Int J Radiat Oncol Biol Phys 2:631, 1977
98. Himmelmann A, Holmberg E, Oden A, et al: Intracavitary irradiation of carcinoma of the cervix stage IB and IIA: A clinical comparison between a remote high dose-rate afterloading system and a low dose-rate manual system. Acta Radiol Oncol 24;139, 1985
99. Himmelmann A, Ragnhult I: High dose rate afterloading treatment in carcinoma of the uterine cervix using an individual planning and reconstruction system. Acta Radiol Oncol 22:263, 1983
100. Hintz BL, Kagan AR, Chan P, et al: Radiation tolerance of the vaginal mucosa. Int J Radiat Oncol Biol Phys 6:711, 1980
101. Hishikawa Y, Kamikonya N, Tanaka S, et al: Radiotherapy of esophageal carcinoma: Role of high-dose-rate intracavitary irradiation. Radiother Oncol 9:13, 1987
102. Hishikawa Y, Tanaka S, Miura T: Early esophageal carcinoma treated with intracavitary irradiation. Radiology 156:519, 1985
103. Hishikawa Y, Tanaka S, Miura T: Esophageal fistula associated with intracavitary irradiation for esophageal carcinoma. Radiology 159:549, 1986
104. Huilgol N, Ashok R, Mehta MD, et al: Hypofractionated external radiation with high and low dose rates in the treatment of advanced cancer of the cervix. Int J Radiat Oncol Biol Phys 14:577, 1988
105. ICRU Report No. 38: Dose and Volume Specification for Reporting Intracavitary Therapy in Gynecology, pp 1–16. Bethesda, MD, International Commission on Radiation Units and Measurements, 1985
106. Ikeda H: Intraluminal irradiation with ^{192}Ir wires for extrahepatic bile duct carcinoma. Nippon Igaku Hoshasen Gakkai Zasshi 39:1356, 1979
107. Ilic S, Ristic B: 5-year results with HDR afterloading cervix cancer: Dependence on fractionation and dose. Strahlenther Onkol [Suppl] 82:139, 1988
108. Jackson SM: The treatment of carcinoma of the penis. Br J Surg 53:33, 1966
109. Jacobs H: Experiences with interstitial HDR afterloading therapy in genital and breast cancer. In Vahrson H, Rauthe G (eds): High Dose Rate Afterloading in the Treatment of Cancer of the Uterus, Breat and Rectum, p 258. Baltimore, Urban & Schwarzenberg, 1988
110. James RD, Pointon RS, Martin S: Local radiotherapy in the management of squamous carcinoma of the anus. Br J Surg 72:282, 1985
111. Jones D, Notley H, Hunterk R: Geometry adopted by Manchester radium applicators and Selectron afterloading applicators in intracavitary treatment for carcinoma cervix uteri. Br J Radiol 60:481, 1987
112. Jorgensen K. Elbrond O, Andersen AP: Carcinoma of the lip: A series of 869 cases. Acta Radiol Ther Phys Biol 12:177, 1973
113. Joslin CAF: The Catherton as part of the radical management of cervix cancer. In Bates TD, Berry RJ (eds): High Dose Rate Afterloading in the Treatment of Cancer of the Uterus, Special Report No. 17, pp 11–16. London, British Institute of Radiology, 1980
114. Joslin CAF: High-activity source afterloading in gynecologic cancer and its future prospect. Endocuriether Hypertherm Oncol 5:69, 1989
115. Joslin CAF: Moulds for high dose afterloading devices for carcinoma of skin. (Personal communication, 1990)
116. Joslin CAF, Smith CW, Mallik A: The treatment of cervix cancer using high activity Co sources. Br J Radiol 45:257, 1972
117. Joyner LR: A new simple handloading technique for intrabronchial radiation with iridium-192. (unpublished data, 1986)
118. Kauppila A, Kiviniity K: High dose rate intracavitary irradiation in the treatment of cervical and endometrial carcinomas: Preliminary observations. In Bates TD, Berry RJ (eds): High Dose Rate Afterloading in the Treatment of Cancer of the Uterus, Special Report No. 17, pp 59–64. London, British Institute of Radiology, 1980
119. Kin NYK, Pigneux J, Auvray H, et al: Our experience of conservative treatment of anal canal carcinoma combining external irradiation and interstitial implant: 32 cases treated between 1973 and 1982. Int J Radiat Oncol Biol Phys 14:253, 1988
120. Koga K, Watanabe K, Kawano M, et al: Radiotherapy for carcinoma of the uterine cervix by remotely controlled afterloading intracavitary system with high dose rate. Int J Radiat Oncol Biol Phys 13:615, 1987
121. Kopelson G, Gunderson LL: Primary and adjuvant radiation

therapy in gallbladder and extrahepatic biliary tract carcinoma. J Clin Gastroenterol 5:43, 1983
122. Kopelson G, Harisiadis L, Tretter P, et al: The role of radiation therapy in cancer of the extrahepatic biliary system: An analysis of 13 patients and a review of the literature of the effectiveness of surgery, chemotherapy and radiotherapy. Int J Radiat Oncol Biol Phys 2:883, 1977
123. Korba AL, Spear RK, Howard D, et al: High dose fraction intrabronchial radiation therapy for non-small cell carcinoma of the lung. (unpublished data, 1986)
124. Kuipers T: Dosimetry and complication rate in the treatment of cervix carcinoma with external irradiation and brachytherapy. Strahlenther Onkol [Suppl] 82:127, 1980
125. Kuipers T: High dose-rate intracavitary irradiation: Results of treatment. In Mould RF (ed): Brachytherapy, pp 169–1975. Netherlands, Nucletron International BV, 1984
126. Kuske RR, Perez CA, Jacobs AJ, et al: Mini-colpostats in the treatment of carcinoma of the uterine cervix. Int J Radiat Oncol Biol Phys 14:899, 1988
127. Lichter AS, Dillon MB, Rosenshein NB, et al: The use of custom molds for intracavitary treatment of carcinoma of the cervix. Int J Radiat Oncol Biol Phys 4:876, 1978
128. Ling CC, Spiro IJ: Measurement of dose distribution around Fletcher-Suit-Delclos colpostats using a Therados radiation field analyzer (RFA-3). Med Phys 11:326, 1984
129. Luxton G, Astrahan MA, Liggett PE, et al: Dosimetric calculations and measurements of gold plaque ophthalmic irradiators using ^{192}Ir and ^{125}I seeds. Int J Radiat Oncol Biol Phys 15:167, 1988
130. Maat B, Venselaar JLM: Improved afterloading technique for interstitial brachytherapy of bladder cancer. In Mould RF (ed): Brachytherapy 2, pp 183–186. Netherlands, Nucletron International BV, 1989
131. Macha HN, Koch K, Stadler M, et al: New technique for treating occlusive and stenosing tumours of the trachea and main bronchi: Endobronchial irradiation by high dose iridium-192 combined with laser canalisation. Thorax 42:511, 1987
132. MacKay A, Gutin P, Hosobuchi Y, et al: CT stereotaxis and interstitial radiation for brain tumor. In Moss AA, Goldberg HI (eds): Interventional Radiologic Techniques: Computerized Tomography and Ultrasonography, pp 93–99. Berkeley, University of California, 1981
133. Mandell L, Dattatreyudu N, Anderson L, et al: Postoperative vaginal radiation in endometrial cancer using a remote afterloading technique. Int J Radiat Oncol Biol Phys 11:473, 1985
134. Marchese MJ, Nori D, Anderson LL, et al: A versatile permanent planar implant technique utilizing iodine-125 seeds embedded in Gelfoam. Int J Radiat Oncol Biol Phys 10(5):747, 1984
135. Marcus RB Jr, Million RR, Mitchell TP: A preloaded, custom-designed implantation device for stage T1–T2 carcinoma of the floor of mouth. Int J Radiat Oncol Biol Phys 6:111, 1980
136. Marinello G, Valero M, Leung S, et al: Comparative dosimetry between iridium wires and seed ribbons. Int J Radiat Oncol Biol Phys 11:1733, 1985
137. Martinez AM, Benson RC, Edmundson GE, Brindle JS: Pelvic lymphadenectomy combined with transperineal interstitial implantation of Iridium-192 and external beam radiation for locally advanced prostatic carcinoma: Technical description. Int J Radiat Oncol Biol Phys 11:841, 1985
138. Martinez AM, Edmundson GK, Cox RS, et al: Combination of external beam irradiation and multiple-site perineal applicator (MUPIT) for treatment of locally advanced or recurrent prostatic, anorectal, and gynecologic malignancies. Int J Radiat Oncol Biol Phys 11:391, 1985
139. Martini N: Clinical application of interstitial implantation in carcinoma of the lung. In Hilaris B, Nori D (eds): Brachytherapy, pp 23–27. New York, Memorial Sloan-Kettering Cancer Center, 1984
140. Mazeron JJ, Lusichini A, Marinello G, et al: Interstitial radiation therapy for squamous cell carcinoma of the tonsillar region: The Creteil experience (1971–1981). Int J Radiat Oncol Biol Phys 12:895, 1986
141. Meerwaldt JH, Veeze-Kuijpers B, Visser AG, et al: Combined modality radiotherapy in the treatment of bile duct carcinoma. In Mould RF (ed): Brachytherapy 2, pp 577–583. Netherlands, Nucletron International BV, 1989
142. Mehta MP, Shahabi S, Jarjour NN, Kinsella TJ: Endobronchial irradiation for malignant airway obstruction. Int J Radiat Oncol Biol Phys 17:847, 1989
143. Mendenhall NP, Parsons JT, Cassisi NJ, et al: Carcinoma of the nasal vestibule. Int J Radiat Oncol Biol Phys 10:627, 1984
144. Mendenhall NP, Parsons JT, Cassisi NJ, et al: Carcinoma of the nasal vestibule treated with radiation therapy. Laryngoscope 97:626, 1987
145. Mendenhall WM, Parsons JT, Mendenhall JP, Million RR: Brachytherapy in head and neck cancer. Oncology 5:44–54, 87–93, 1991
146. Meredith WJ: Radium Dosage: The Manchester System. Edinburgh, Livingstone, 1967
147. Million RR, Cassisi NJ: Oral cavity. In Management of Head and Neck Cancer: A Multidisciplinary Approach, p 273. Philadelphia, JB Lippincott, 1984
148. Million RR, Cassisi NJ, Clark JR: Cancer of the head and neck. In DeVita VT Jr, Hellman S, Rosenberg SA (eds): Cancer: Principles and Practice of Oncology, 3rd ed, p 565. Philadelphia, JB Lippincott, 1989
149. Million RR, Cassisi NJ, Hamlin DJ: Nasal vestibule, nasal cavity, and paranasal sinuses. In Management of Head and Neck Cancer: A Multidisciplinary Approach, p 432. Philadelphia, JB Lippincott, 1984
150. Mizoe J, Tsujii T, Kamada T, et al: Five-year results and complications with HDR afterloading in cervix cancer using a linear arrangement of source. Sonderb Strahlenther Onkol 82:114, 1988
151. Mohiuddin M, Canton RJ, Bierman W, et al: Combined modality treatment of localized unresectable adenocarcinoma of the pancreas. Int J Radiat Oncol Biol Phys 14:79, 1988
152. Moonen L: Brachytherapy in the management of bladder cancer. In Mould RF (ed): Brachytherapy 2, pp 174–178. Netherlands, Nucletron International BV, 1989
153. Morphis OL: Teflon tube method of radium implantation. AJR 83:455, 1960
154. Morton JL, Callendine GW Jr, Myers WG: Radioactive cobalt-60 in plastic tubing for interstitial radiation therapy. Radiology 56:553, 1951
155. Moss WT, Brand WN, Battifora H (eds): Radiation Oncology: Rationale, Technique, Results, 5th ed. St. Louis, CV Mosby, 1979
156. Mowatt KS, Stevens KA: Afterloading: A contribution to the protection problem. J Fac Radiol 8:28, 1956
157. Nath R, Meigooni AS: Some treatment planning considerations for palladium-103 and iodine-125 permanent interstitial implants. [Abstract] Endocuriether Hypertherm Oncol 5:244, 1989
158. Newman H, James KW, Smith CW: Treatment of cancer of the cervix with a high-dose-rate afterloading machine (the Cathetron). Int J Radiat Oncol Biol Phys 9:931, 1983
159. Nori D, Hilaris BS, Batata MA, et al: Remote afterloading in cancer management. II. Clinical applications of remote afterloaders. In Hilaris BS, Batata MA (eds): Brachytherapy Oncology, pp 101–118. New York, Memorial Sloan-Kettering Cancer Center, 1983
160. O'Connell D, Howard N, Joslin AF, et al: A new remotely controlled unit for the treatment of uterine carcinoma. Lancet 2:570, 1965
161. Olch AJ, Kagan AR, Wollin M, et al: A simple volume iridium implant dosimetry system. Endocuriether Hypertherm Oncol 3:183, 1987
162. Orton CG: Time-dose factors (TDFs) in brachytherapy. Br J Radiol 47:603, 1974
163. Orton CG: Radiobiological dose rate considerations with remote afterloading. In Shearer DR (ed): Recent Advances in Brachytherapy Physics, pp 190–200. New York, American Institute of Physics, 1981
164. Orton CG, Webber BM: Time-dose factor (TDF) analysis of dose rate effects in permanent implant dosimetry. Int J Radiat Oncol Biol Phys 2:55, 1977
165. Packer S, Rotman M, Salanitro P: Iodine-125 irradiation of

choroidal melanoma: Clinical experience. Ophthalmology 91:1700, 1984
166. Paine CH: Modern afterloading methods for interstitial radiotherapy. Clin Radiol 23:263, 1972
167. Papillon J: New prospects in the treatment of rectal cancer. Dis Colon Rectum 27:695, 1984
168. Parker HM: A dosage system for interstitial radium therapy. II. Physical aspects. Br J Radiol 11:313, 1938.
169. Parsons JT, Mendenhall WM, Bova FJ, Million RR: Irradiation techniques for head and neck cancer. In Levitt SL: Technological Basis of Radiation Therapy: Practical Clinical Applications. Philadelphia, Lea & Febiger (in press)
170. Paterson R: The Treatment of Malignant Disease by Radiotherapy, 2nd ed. Baltimore, Williams & Wilkins, 1963
171. Peretz T, Nori D, Hilaris B, et al: Treatment of primary unresectable carcinoma of the pancreas with I-125 implantation. Int J Radiat Oncol Biol Phys 17:931, 1989
172. Perez CA, Camel HM, Galakatos AE, et al: Definitive irradiation in carcinoma of the vagina: Long-term evaluation of results. Int J Radiat Oncol Biol Phys 15:1283, 1988
173. Perez CA, Camel HM, Kuske RR, et al: Radiation therapy alone in treatment of the uterine cervix: A 20 year experience. Gynecol Oncol 23:127, 1986
174. Perez CA, Korba A, Sharma S: Dosimetric considerations in irradiation of carcinoma of the vagina. Int J Radiat Oncol Biol Phys 2:639, 1977
175. Perez CA, Kuske R, Glasgow GP: Review of brachytherapy for gynecologic tumors. Endocuriether Hypertherm Oncol 1:153, 1985
176. Perez CA, Slessinger E, Grigsby PW: Design of an afterloading vaginal applicator (MIRALVA). Int J Radiat Oncol Biol Phys 18:1503, 1990
177. Peschel RE, Healey GA, Smith RJ, et al: High dose rate remote afterloading for endometrial cancer. Endocuriether Hypertherm Oncol 5:209, 1989
178. Petrovich Z, Langholz B, Formenti S, et al: The importance of brachytherapy in the treatment of unresectable carcinoma of the esophagus. Endocuriether Hypertherm Oncol 5:201, 1989
179. Pettersson B, Jansson H, Nilsson A, et al: Prophylactic vaginal irradiation with low dose rate afterloading technique in women with endometrial cancer. In Mould RF (ed): Brachytherapy 2, pp 240–244. Netherlands, Nucletron International BV, 1989
180. Pierquin B: Precis de Curietherapie, Endocurietherapie et Plesiocurietherapie. Paris, Masson, 1964
181. Pierquin B, Chassagne D, Baillet F, et al: The place of implantation in tongue and floor of mouth cancer. JAMA 215:961, 1971
182. Pierquin B, Pernot M, Baillet F: Tonsillar region. In Pierquin B, Wilson J-F, Chassagne D (eds): Modern Brachytherapy, pp 141–145. New York, Masson, 1987
183. Pierquin B, Wilson J-F, Chassagne D (eds): Modern Brachytherapy. New York, Masson, 1987
184. Pierquin B, Wilson J-F, Chassagne D: The Paris system: In 6Pierquin B, Wilson J-F, Chassagne D (eds): Modern Brachytherapy, pp 25–42. New York, Masson, 1987
185. Pierquin B, Wilson J-F, Chassagne D: Radiation protection and the organizational plan of a brachytherapy department. In Pierquin B, Wilson J-F, Chassagne D (eds): Modern Brachytherapy, pp 43–59. New York, Masson, 1987
186. Pigneux J, Richaud PM, Largade C: The place of interstitial therapy using ^{192}Ir in the management of carcinoma of the lip. Cancer 43:1073, 1979
187. Pla C, Evans MDC, Podgorsak EB: Dose distributions around Selectron applicators. Int J Radiat Oncol Biol Phys 13:1761, 1987
188. Pla C, Evans MDC, Podgorsak EB, Roman TN: The measurement of dose distributions around Selectron applicators. In Mould RF (ed): Brachytherapy 2, pp 147–155. Netherlands, Nucletron International BV, 1989
189. Potish RA: The effect of applicator geometry on dose specification in cervical cancer. Int J Radiat Oncol Biol Phys 18:1513, 1990
190. Potish RA, Deibel FC, Khan FM: The relationship between milligram-hours and dose to point A in carcinoma of the cervix. Radiology 145:478, 1982
191. Potish RA, Gerbi BJ: Role of point A in the era of computerized dosimetry. Radiology 158:827, 1986
192. Potish RA, Gerbi BJ: Cervical cancer intracavitary dose specification and prescription. Radiology 165:555, 1987
193. Pourquier H, Dubois JB, Delard R: Cancer of the uterine cervix: Dosimetric guidelines for prevention of late rectal and rectosigmoid complications as a result of radiotherapeutic treatment. Int J Radiat Oncol Biol Phys 8:1887, 1982
194. Prempree T: Parametrial implant in stage IIIB cancer of the cervix. III. A five-year study. Cancer 52:748, 1983
195. Price A, Kerr GR, Arnott SJ: Radioactive needle implants in the treatment of anorectal cancer. Clin Radiol 39:186, 1988
196. Puthawala AA, Syed AMN, Gates TC, et al: Definitive treatment of extensive anorectal cancer by external and interstitial irradiation. Cancer 50:1746, 1982
197. Puthawala AA, Syed AM, Tansey LA, et al: Temporary iridium-192 implant in the management of carcinoma of the prostate. Endocuriether Hypertherm Oncol 1:25, 1985
198. Quimby EH, Castro V: The calculation of dosage in interstitial radium therapy. Am J Roentgenol Rad Ther Nucl Med 70:789, 1953
199. Rattka P: Experience in the treatment of cancer of the cervix using HDR brachytherapy in Gliwice. In Mould RF (ed): Brachytherapy 2, pp 296–300. Netherlands, Nucletron International BV, 1989
200. Rauthe G, Vahrson H, Giers G: Five-year results and complications in endometrium cancer: HDR afterloading versus conventional radium therapy. In Vahrson H, Rauthe G (eds): High Dose Rate Afterloading in the Treatment of Cancer of the Uterus, Breast and Rectum, p 240. Baltimore, Urban & Schwarzenberg, 1988
201. Roman T, Souhami L, Freeman C, et al: High dose rate remote afterloading intracavitary therapy in carcinoma of the cervix. Int J Radiat Oncol Biol Phys 17:199, 1989
202. Rotte K: A randomized clinical trial comparing a high dose rate with a conventional dose-rate technique. In Bates TD, Berry RJ (eds): High Dose Rate Afterloading in the Treatment of Cancer of the Uterus, Special Report No. 17, pp 75–79. London, British Institute of Radiology, 1980
203. Rowland CG: Treatment of carcinoma of the esophagus with a new Selectron applicator. In Mould RF (ed): Brachytherapy 1984, pp 248–250. Netherlands, Nucletron International BV, 1985
204. Rowland CG, Ingham D, Cook S, et al: HDR implants as the sole treatment of early breast cancer. In Mould RF (ed): Brachytherapy 2, pp 512–515. Netherlands, Nucletron International BV, 1989
205. Rutledge FN, Delclos L: Adenocarcinoma of the uterus. In Fletcher GH (ed): Textbook of Radiotherapy, 3rd ed, pp 798–808. Philadelphia, Lea & Febiger, 1980
206. Sato S, Yajima A, Suzuki M: Therapeutic results using high-dose-rate intracavitary irradiation in cases of cervical cancer. Gynecol Oncol 19:143, 1984
207. Saw CB, Suntharalingam S: Reference dose rates for single- and double-plane ^{192}Ir implants. Med Phys 15(3):391, 1988
208. Saw CB, Suntharalingham N, Ayyangar K, et al: Dosimetric considerations of stereotactic brain implants. Int J Radiat Oncol Biol Phys 17:887, 1989
209. Saylor WL, Dillard M: Dosimetry of ^{137}Cs sources with Fletcher-Suit gynecological applicator. Med Phys 3:117, 1976
210. Schray MF, McDougall JC, Martinez A, et al: Management of malignant airway obstruction: Clinical and dosimetric considerations using an iridium-192 afterloading technique with the neodynium-YAG laser. Int J Radiat Oncol Biol Phys 11:403, 1985
211. Schray MF, McDougall JC, Martinez A, et al: Management of malignant airway compromise with laser and low dose rate brachytherapy. Chest 93:264, 1988
212. Scott WP: Simplified interstitial therapy technique (Vicyrl) for unresectable lung cancer. Radiology 117:734, 1975
213. Seagren SL: Endobronchial irradiation with or without preirradiation laser in treatment of symptomatic recurrent endobronchial malignancy. Proceedings of 2nd Annual Interna-

tional HDR Remote Afterloading Symposium, pp 3–11. San Diego, CA, 1987

214. Seagren SL, Harrell JH, Horn RA: High-dose-rate intraluminal irradiation in recurrent endobronchial carcinoma. Chest 88:810, 1985
215. Shabazian H, Conroy R: A new method for treating carcinomatous biliary obstruction with intracatheter radium. [Abstract] Int J Radiat Oncol Biol Phys 7:72, 1981
216. Sharma S, Williamson JF, Kahn FM, Jones TK: Dosimetric consequences of asymmetric positioning of active source in ^{137}Cs and ^{226}Ra intracavitary tubes. Int J Radiat Oncol Biol Phys 7:555, 1981
217. Shigematsu Y, Nishiyama K, Masaki N, et al: Treatment of carcinoma of the uterine cervix by remotely controlled afterloading intracavitary radiotherapy with high-dose rate: A comparative study with a low-dose rate system. Int J Radiat Oncol Biol Phys 9:351, 1983
218. Shipley WU, Nardi GL, Cohen AM, Ling CC: Iodine-125 implant and external beam irradiation in patients with localized pancreatic carcinoma. Cancer 45:709, 1980
219. Shu-MO C, Xiang EW, Qi W: High dose rate afterloading in the treatment of cervical cancer of the uterus. Int J Radiat Oncol Biol Phys 16:335, 1989
220. Simon N, Silverstone SM: Intracavitary radiotherapy of endometrial cancer by afterloading. J Gynecol Oncol 1:13, 1972
221. Slessinger E, Grigsby PW, Williams J: Improvements in brachytherapy quality assurance. Int J Radiat Oncol Biol Phys 16:497, 1989
222. Snelling MD, Lambert ME, Yarnold J: Clinical results and complications following treatment of carcinoma of the cervix and endometrium using the Cathetron at the Middlesex Hospital. In Bates TD, Berry RJ (eds): High Dose Rate Afterloading in the Treatment of Cancer of the Uterus, pp 32–37. London, British Institute of Radiology Special Report #17, 1980
223. Sogani PC: Pelvic lymphadenectomy: Techniques and complications. In Hilaris BS, Batata MA (eds): Brachytherapy Oncology—1983, pp 79–82. New York, Memorial Sloan-Kettering Cancer Center, 1983
224. Sorbe B, Frankendal B, Risberg B: Intracavitary irradiation of endometrial carcinoma stage I by a high dose rate afterloading technique. Int J Radiat Oncol Biol Phys 33:135, 1989
225. Speiser B, Spratling L: Comparison of intermediate versus high dose-rate remote afterloading brachytherapy in the control of endobronchial carcinoma. In Mould RF (ed): Brachytherapy 2, pp 469–480. Netherlands, Nucletron International BV, 1989
226. Speiser B, Spratling L: Intermediate dose rate remote afterloading brachytherapy for intraluminal control of bronchogenic carcinoma. Int J Radiat Oncol Biol Phys 18:1443, 1990
227. Stallard HB: Malignant melanoma of the choroid treated with radioactive applicators. Ann R Coll Surg Engl 29:170, 1961
228. Streeter OE Jr, Goldson AL, Chevallier C, et al: High dose rate remote afterloading irradiation in cancer of the cervix in Haiti, 1977–1984. Int J Radiat Oncol Biol Phys 14:1159, 1988
229. Suit HD, Moore EB, Fletcher GH, et al: Modifications of Fletcher ovoid system for afterloading using standard sized radium tubes (milligram and microgram). Radiology 81:126, 1963
230. Syed AMN, Puthawala AA, Neblett DL: Interstitial Iodine-125 implant in the management of unresectable pancreatic carcinoma. Cancer 52:808, 1983
231. Syed AMN, Puthawala AA, Tansey LA, et al: Temporary iridium-192 implantation in the management of carcinoma of the prostate. In Hilaris BS, Batata MA (eds): Brachytherapy Oncology—1983, pp 83–91. New York, Memorial Sloan-Kettering Cancer Center, 1983
232. Szikla G (ed): Stereotactic Cerebral Irradiation. Amsterdam, Elsevier/North-Holland Biomedical Press, 1979
233. Taina E: Complications following high and low dose-rate intracavitary radiotherapy for stages I–II cervical carcinoma: A comparison of remotely afterloaded ^{60}Co (Cathetron) and conventional radium therapy. Acta Obstet Gynecol Scand [Suppl] 103:39, 1981
234. Taina E, Gropnroos LM: A comparison of clinical results following high dose-rate intracavitary afterloading irradiation with ^{60}Co (Cathetron) and conventional radium therapy for stage I–II cervical carcinoma. Acta Obstet Gynecol Scand [Suppl] 103:31, 1981
235. Teshima T, Chatani M, Hata K, et al: High-dose rate intracavitary therapy for carcinoma of the uterine cervix. I. General figures of survival and complication. Int J Radiat Oncol Biol Phys 13:1035, 1987
236. Teshima T, Chatani M, Hata K, et al: High-dose rate intracavitary therapy for carcinoma of the uterine cervix. II. Risk factors for rectal complication. Int J Radiat Oncol Biol Phys 14:281, 1988
237. Tod MC, Meredith WJ: A dosage system for use in the treatment of cancer of the uterine cervix. Br J Radiol 11:809, 1938.
238. Tod M, Meredith WJ: Treatment of cancer of the cervix uteri: A revised "Manchester method." Br J Radiol 26:252, 1953
239. Utley JF, von Essen CF, Horn RA, et al: High-dose-rate afterloading brachytherapy in carcinoma of the uterine cervix. Int J Radiat Oncol Biol Phys 10:2259, 1984
240. Vahrson H, Glaser FH: History of HDR afterloading in brachytherapy. Strahlenther Onkol [Suppl] 82:2, 1988
241. Vahrson G, Romer G: Five-year results with HDR afterloading in cervix cancer: Dependence on fractionation and dose. Strahlenther Onkol [Suppl] 82:139, 1988
242. van den Brenk HAS: Results of prophylactic postoperative irradiation in 1300 cases of pterygium. AJR 103:723, 1968
243. van der Werf-Messing B: Interstitial radium therapy of superficial bladder cancer (category T1NXMO and T2NXMO). In Smith PH, Prout GB Jr (eds): Urology 1, Bladder Cancer, pp 191–202. London, Butterworths, 1984
244. Van Roosenbeek E, Delclos L: The Radioactive Patient: Care, Precautions, and Procedures in Diagnosis and Therapy. Flushing, NY, Medical Examination Publishing Co, 1975
245. Von Essen CF, Seary DG, Moeller MS, et al: Fractionated intracavitary radiation therapy with the Brachytron: General techniques and preliminary results in the treatment of cervix cancer. AJR 120:101, 1974
246. Walker MD: Chemotherapy: Adjuvant to surgery and radiation therapy. Semin Oncol 2:69, 1975
247. Walker MD, Strike TA, Sheline GE: An analysis of dose-effect relationship in the radiotherapy of malignant gliomas. Int J Radiat Oncol Biol Phys 5:1733, 1979
248. Walstam R: The dosage distribution in the pelvis in radium treatment of carcinoma of the cervix. Acta Radiol 42:237, 1954
249. Wang CC: Re-irradiation of recurrent nasopharyngeal carcinoma: Treatment techniques and results. Int J Radiat Oncol Biol Phys 13:953, 1987
250. Ward AJ, Stubbs B, Dixon B, et al: A schedule of radiotherapy, including the use of the Cathetron for advanced carcinoma of the cervix. In Bates TD, Berry RJ (eds): High Dose Rate Afterloading in the Treatment of Cancer of the Uterus, Special Report No. 17, pp 17–23. London, British Institute of Radiology, 1980
251. Warmelink C, Ezzell G, Orton C: Use of a time-dose-fractionation model to design high dose-rate fractionation schemes. In Mould RF (ed): Brachytherapy 2, pp 41–48. Netherlands, Nucletron International BV, 1989
252. Weaver K: The dosimetry of ^{125}I seed eye plaques. Med Phys 13:78, 1986
253. Weaver K, Smith V, Huang D, et al: Dose parameters of ^{125}I and ^{192}Ir seed sources. Med Phys 16:636, 1989
254. Weeks KJ, Dennett MS: Dose calculation and measurements for a CT compatible version of the Fletcher applicator. Int J Radiat Oncol Biol Phys 18:1191, 1990
255. Weeks KJ, Schoeppel SL, Pruss K, et al: A computed tomography-compatible afterloading Fletcher-Suit-Delclos colpostat with adjustable shielding. Endocuriether Hypertherm Oncol 5:169, 1989
256. Weiner S: Remote high-dose afterloading treatment in non-small cell carcinoma of the lung. In Proceedings of the 2nd Annual International High Dose Rate Remote Afterloading Symposium, p 17, San Diego, CA, 1987
257. Wijnmaalen AJ, Helle PA, Koper PCM, et al: Combined exter-

nal beam and interstitial radiation for bladder cancer. In Mould RF (ed): Brachytherapy 2, pp 192–195. Netherlands, Nucletron International BV, 1989
258. Wilkinson J, Moore C, Notley H, et al: The use of Selectron afterloading equipment to simulate and extend the Manchester system for intracavitary therapy of the cervix uteri. Br J Radiol 56:409, 1983
259. Williamson JF: The accuracy of the line and point source approximations in ^{192}Ir dosimetry. Int J Radiat Oncol Biol Phys 12:409, 1986
260. Williamson JF: Monte Carlo evaluation of specific dose constants in water for ^{125}I seeds. Med Phys 15:686, 1988
261. Williamson JF: Dose calculations about shielded gynecological colpostats. Int J Radiat Oncol Biol Phys 19:167, 1990
262. Zolli CI: Experience with the avulsion technique in pterygium surgery. Ann Ophthalmol 11:1569, 1979

APPENDIX 13–1
Selectron LDR-6 Fletcher-Suit Ovoid Surface Dose Rates at the Center of the Ovoid†

SURFACE CONFIGURATION	SURFACE DOSE RATE (cGy) at the OVOID CENTER PER TOTAL mgh IN THE OVOID†			
	1.6 cm	2.0 cm	2.4 cm	3.0 cm
Standard	10.04	6.41	4.28	3.05
1******	7.76	5.41	3.84	2.82
*2****	10.24	6.58	4.40	3.12
3*	12.20	7.41	4.74	3.31
***4**	12.20	7.41	4.74	3.31
****5*	10.24	6.58	4.40	3.12
*****6	7.76	5.41	3.84	2.82
34	12.20	7.41	4.76	3.31
*2**5*	10.24	6.58	4.40	3.14
1****6	7.76	5.40	3.84	2.84
**345*	11.55	7.13	4.64	3.25
*2*4*6	10.07	6.47	4.34	3.10
1*3*5*	10.07	6.47	4.34	3.10
*234**	11.55	7.13	4.64	3.25
1**4*6	9.24	6.07	4.15	3.00
1*3**6	9.24	6.07	4.15	3.00
12**56	9.00	6.00	4.13	2.98
2345	11.23	6.99	4.58	3.22
1*34*6	9.98	6.40	4.30	3.07
1234**	10.60	6.69	4.44	3.15
**3456	10.60	6.69	4.44	3.15
12345*	10.54	6.68	4.43	3.14
1234*6	10.03	6.44	4.32	3.08
123*56	9.64	6.27	4.25	3.05
12*456	9.64	6.27	4.25	3.05
1*3456	10.03	6.44	4.32	3.08
*23456	10.54	6.68	4.43	3.14
123456	10.07	6.46	4.33	3.09

† Miniovoids; no shielding; no attenuation factor; 2.0-, 2.5-, 3.0-cm ovoids with shielding and 0.94 attentuation factor; 3M, 6D6C/CA source, 2.0-cm overall length and 1.4-cm active length is the standard source for comparison.
**: inactive pellet position.*

APPENDIX 13–2
Selectron LDR-6 Tandem Source Positions

TANDEM LENGTH (cm)	NOMINAL SOURCE LOADING	SELECTRON ACTIVE PELLET POSITIONS†
2	20	*2*45*7*
2	10	*2****7*
4	20–10	*2*45*7**10****15*
4	10–10	*2****7**10****15*
6	20–10–10	*2*45*7***11***15***19***23*
6	10–10–10	*2****7***11***15***19***23*
6	10–20–10	*2****7**10*1213*15**18****23*
8	10–20–10–10	*2****7**10*1213*15***19***23***27***31*
8	10–10–10–10	*2****7***11***15***19***23***27***31*

† * = *inactive pellet position; active pellets are 5 mg Ra eq.*

APPENDIX 13–3
Surface Dose for Vaginal Cylinders

CYLINDER DIAMETER (cm)	CYLINDER LENGTH (cm)	RSD cGy/hr FACTOR	ACTIVE PELLET POSITION
2.0	2.5	26.4	1-3-5-8-10
	5.0	21.1	1-2-6-10-14-19-20
	7.5	23	1-2-6-10-14-18-22-26-29-30
	10.0	22.1	1-2-6-10-14-18-22-26-30-34-39-40
2.5	2.5	20.6	1-2-3-8-9-10
	5.0	20.8	1-2-3-7-11-15-18-19-20
	7.5	23	1-2-3-6-9-12-15-18-21-24-28-29-30
	10.0	22.9	1-2-3-6-9-12-15-18-21-24-27-30-34-38-39-40
3.0	2.5	22.5	1-2-3-4-7-8-9-10
	5.0	24.7	1-2-3-4-5-8-11-14-16-17-18-19-20
	7.5	22.6	1-2-3-4-5-10-11-15-16-20-21-26-27-28-29-30
	10.0	24.2	1-2-3-4-5-9-10-14-15-19-2023-26-27-31-32-36-37-38-39-40
3.5	2.5	22.6	1-2-3-4-5-6-7-8-9-10
	5.0	21.3	1-2-3-4-5-6-9-12-15-16-17-18-19-20
	7.5	23.5	1-2-3-4-5-6-7-11-12-15-16-19-20-24-25-26-27-28-29-30
	10.0	22.8	1-2-3-4-5-6-7-11-12-17-20-21-24-25-29-30-34-35-36-37-38-39-40

14

○ ○ ○ ● ● ●

Particle-Beam Radiation Therapy

Thomas W. Griffin

Over the last two decades, advances in the field of radiation oncology have substantially improved the outlook for patients with various malignancies. Nevertheless, there are still many patients in whom failure to control local disease contributes materially to death. Heavy-particle-beam radiation therapy may offer a therapeutic gain over conventional photon- and electron-beam therapy.

Several heavy particle beams are being clinically tested: fast neutrons, protons, helium ions, heavy ions (*e.g.*, carbon, neon, argon), and negative pions.[40, 84, 89] Fast neutrons are being investigated because they have radiobiologic properties that potentially are superior to those of conventional x-rays and τ-rays. Protons and helium ions are being studied because the dose distributions that may be achieved with these particles are superior in many clinical situations to those obtainable with photons or electrons. Heavy ions and pions have potential biologic and dose distribution advantages.

BIOLOGIC EFFECTS OF PARTICLE BEAMS

The biologic effects of a radiation beam depend on the spatial distribution of the ionizing events produced in tissue. The rate at which charged particles deposit energy per unit distance is known as the *linear energy transfer* (LET), expressed in keV/μm. Protons, helium ions, electrons, and photons are sparsely ionizing, characterized by a low LET. Conversely, fast neutrons, heavy ions, and pions are densely ionizing and are referred to as high-LET radiations. Review of the possible causes of cancer treatment failure with conventional radiation therapy suggests that there are major areas in which neutrons and other high-LET radiations may offer a biologic advantage.

Tumor Cell Hypoxia

The *oxygen enhancement ratio* is defined as the ratio of the dose of radiation required to produce a specified biologic effect under anoxic conditions to the dose required to produce the same effect under well-oxygenated conditions. With photons, the oxygen enhancement ratio for most mammalian cells is 2.5 to 3.0. With neutrons, heavy charged particles, or pions, the oxygen enhancement ratio is significantly smaller (1.4 to 1.7), and the protection conferred on tumor cells by hypoxia is diminished. Figure 14-1 illustrates survival curves for Chinese hamster ovary cells irradiated with ^{60}Co τ-rays or 50-MeV neutrons (*i.e.*, from deuteron-on-beryllium reactions). The oxygen enhancement ratio for neutrons is 1.4, appreciably improved over the value of 2.4 for ^{60}Co τ-rays.

In practice, the clinical advantage of high-LET radiation may be less than that suggested by the differences in oxygen enhancement ratios. Not all tumor cells are severely hypoxic, and reoxygenation may occur during intervals between dose fractions, diminishing the influence of hypoxic cells on tumor recurrence.[37]

Relative Biologic Effectiveness

The relative biologic effectiveness of an ionizing radiation is the ratio of the dose of that radiation compared with the dose of a reference radiation required to produce a specific end point in a specific tissue. A potential area of therapeutic gain from high-LET radiation exists if tumor cells are relatively radioresistant because of their increased capacity to accumulate sublethal radiation injury. This situation is reflected in a wide shoulder for the tumor-cell-survival curve. With neutrons and other high-LET radiation, most cell killing results from single lethal events, producing survival curves that are almost exponential in the range of clinical relevance (Fig. 14-2). Tumors characterized by a large capacity to accumulate and repair sublethal radiation injury should have a higher value of relative biologic effectiveness for neutrons than for normal tissue.[88] However, Howlett and others[50] have shown that the values for the relative biologic effectiveness of neutrons for different experimental tumors vary considerably, and no general statement about which types of tumors are best treated with high-LET radiation can be made.

Tumor Cell Kinetics

The cell-cycle-dependent variation of radiosensitivity is similar for neutrons and τ-rays, but the magnitude of the difference is

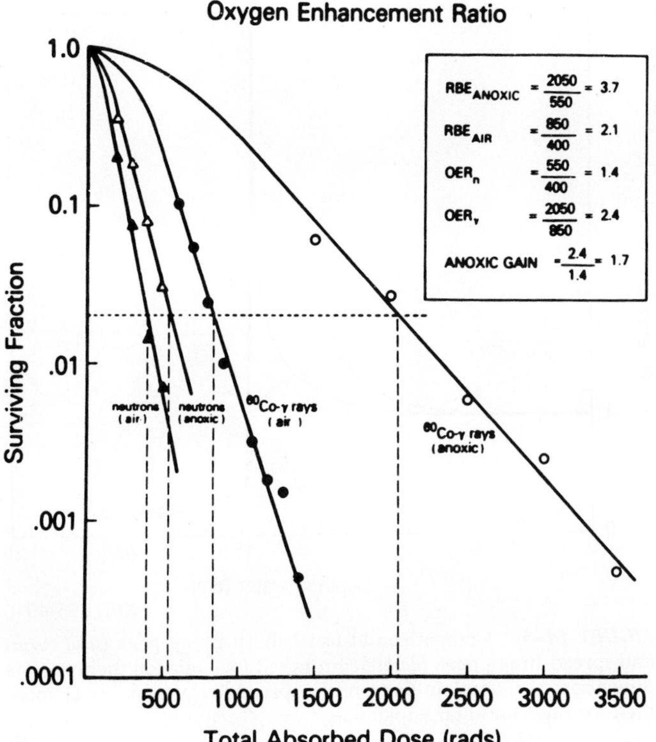

FIGURE 14–1. Survival curves for Chinese hamster ovary (CHO) cells irradiated with ^{60}Co gamma rays or 50 MeV d⇒Be fast neutrons under aerated and anoxic conditions. At the survival level illustrated, the oxygen enhancement ratio for neutrons is 1.4, compared with 2.4 for ^{60}Co γ-rays.

smaller for neutrons (Fig. 14-3).[36] Whether this property constitutes a therapeutic advantage for high-LET radiation cannot be predicted. Tumors in which cell stages redistribute poorly or in which the spectrum is demonstrated by cells in resistant phases are more effectively treated with high-LET radiation.

Repair of Potentially Lethal Damage

Repair of potentially lethal damage occurs following x-irradiation and τ-irradiation, but it is observed less frequently after neutron irradiation (Fig. 14-4).[35] If, as has been suggested by Hall and Kraljevic,[47] potentially lethal damage repair after x-irradiation and τ-irradiation occurs in nutritionally deprived tumor cells but not in normal tissue cells, then the use of the high-LET beams would be therapeutically advantageous.

PHYSICAL EFFECTS OF PARTICLE BEAMS

Fast neutron beams can be generated for radiation therapy either by bombarding a target containing tritium (T) with accelerated deuterium (D) ions in a dT generator or by bombarding a suitable target, such as beryllium (Be), with protons (p) or deuterons (d) accelerated in a cyclotron or linear accelerator. The dT generator produces a monoenergetic 14-MeV neutron beam, and the proton-on-beryllium (p→ Be) reactions produce neutron beams with a spectrum of energies. High-energy particle accelerators are required to produce medically useful beams of heavy charged particles.

Neutrons have no dose distribution advantages over pho-

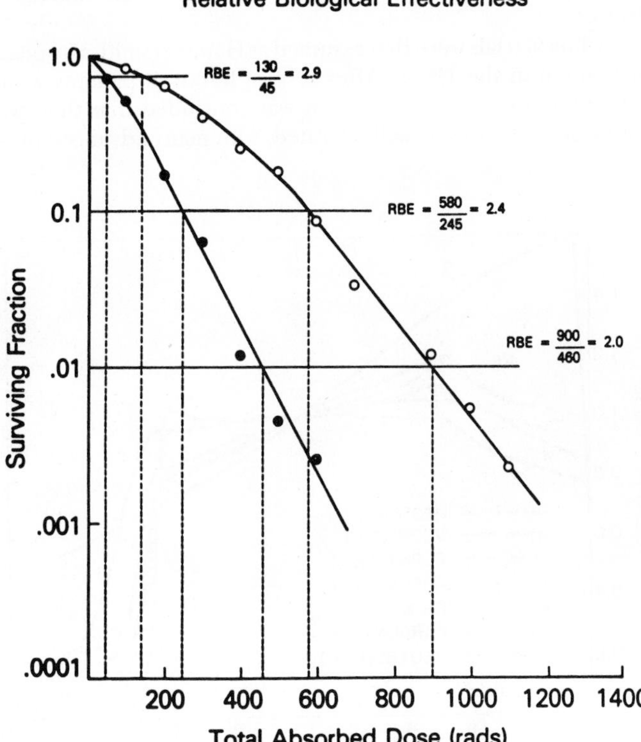

FIGURE 14–2. Survival curves for CHO cells exposed to ^{60}Co gamma rays or 50 MeV d⇒Be fast neutrons, illustrating the increase in relative biologic effectiveness with decreasing dose per fraction. With fast neutron irradiation, most cell killing results from single-hit lethal events, producing survival curves with little or no shoulder.

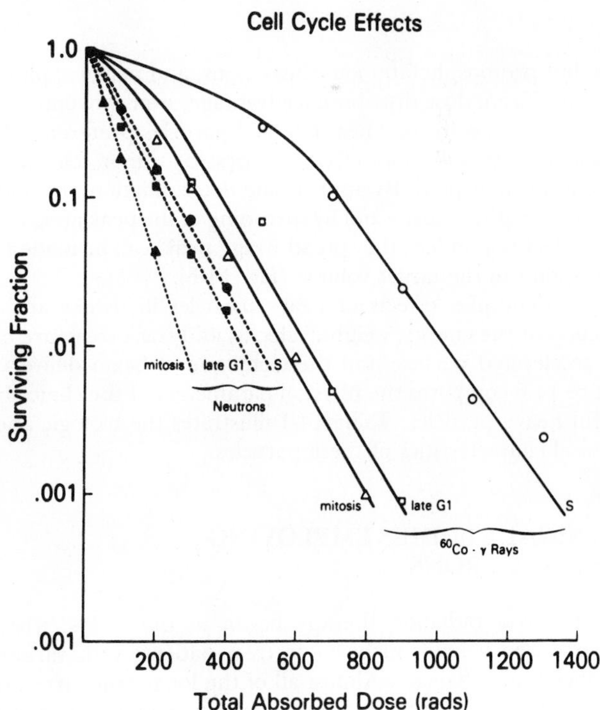

FIGURE 14–3. Survival curve for synchronized CHO cells irradiated with ^{60}Co gamma rays or 50 MeV d⇒Be fast neutrons illustrating the variation in radiosensitivity with the position in the cell cycle. The cells were irradiated in three different positions in the cell cycle: mitosis, late G1/early S, and mid-to-late S phase. The cell-cycle-dependent variation in radiation sensitivity is qualitatively similar for neutrons and gamma rays, but the magnitude of the variation is reduced by a factor of 4 for neutrons.

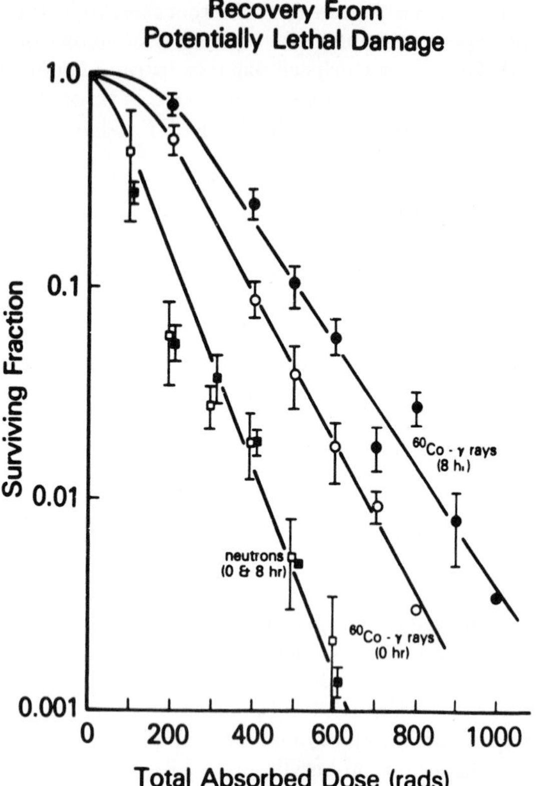

FIGURE 14–4. Potentially lethal damage: survival curves for plateau-phase CHO cells irradiated with ^{60}Co gamma rays (*circles*) or 50 MeV d⇒Be fast neutrons (*squares*) and plated either immediately (*open symbols*) or 8 hours after irradiation (*solid symbols*). Repair of potentially lethal damage occurs after irradiation with gamma rays but is not observed after neutron irradiation.

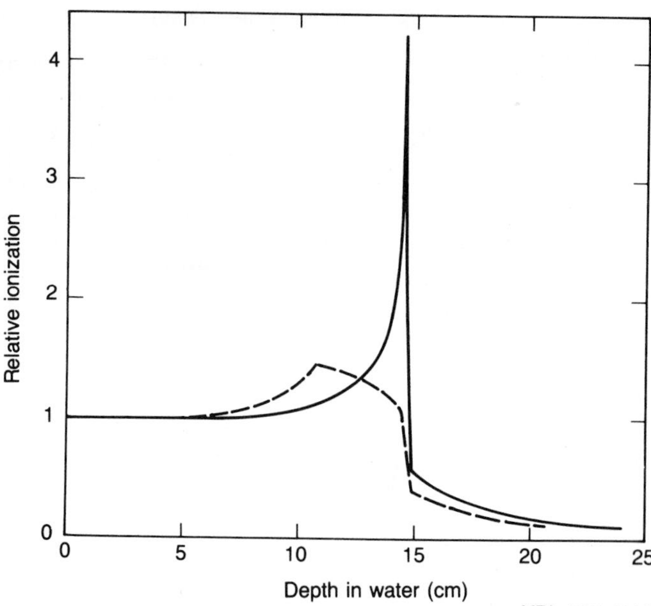

FIGURE 14–5. Comparison of usual sharp Bragg peak (*solid curve*) and spread Bragg peak (*dashed curve*) used for radiation therapy. The dimensions and depth in tissue of the spread Bragg peak can be modified for the clinical target volume.

tons, but protons, helium ions, heavy ions, and negative pions have significant dose distribution advantages over conventional photons and electrons. These charged particles preferentially deposit energy and more effectively destroy tumor cells near the end of their path. By appropriate determination of range (or path length) in tissue and by spreading of the peak area, the high effect region (*i.e.*, the spread Bragg peak) can be made to correspond to the target volume (Fig. 14-5).

The complex effects of heavy particles in tissues are a function of the energy, weight, velocity, and track structure of the accelerated particle and the technique of beam delivery. Figure 14-6 compares the physical parameters of the clinically useful heavy particles. Table 14-1 illustrates the biologic and physical characteristics of these particles.

CLINICAL STUDIES EMPLOYING FAST NEUTRONS

Fast neutron radiation therapy began in the 1930s, when Stone[79] used a neutron beam to treat patients with various advanced malignancies. Almost all of the long-term survivors from that clinical trial had severe radiation sequelae in the normal tissue surrounding the tumor sites. This effect was initially interpreted as being a result of increased relative biologic effectiveness values influencing the late effects, and it deterred further clinical investigation of high-LET radiation for approximately 20 years.[7] In the 1950s, mammalian cell culture techniques were developed, and it became apparent that the shapes of postirradiation cell-survival curves were very different for high-energy photons and fast neutrons. This difference demonstrated that the clinically used neutron fraction sizes corresponded to much higher values for relative biologic effectiveness than were extrapolated from the large-dose-increment animal model studies done before Stone's clinical work.[46,92] Therefore, most of Stone's patients with serious radiation sequelae had inadvertently received extremely high radiation doses.

Clinical trials were first resumed at Hammersmith Hospital in London in the 1960s. After several hundred patients with extensive cancer were treated, it was concluded that therapy with fast neutrons was well tolerated, with many advanced ma-

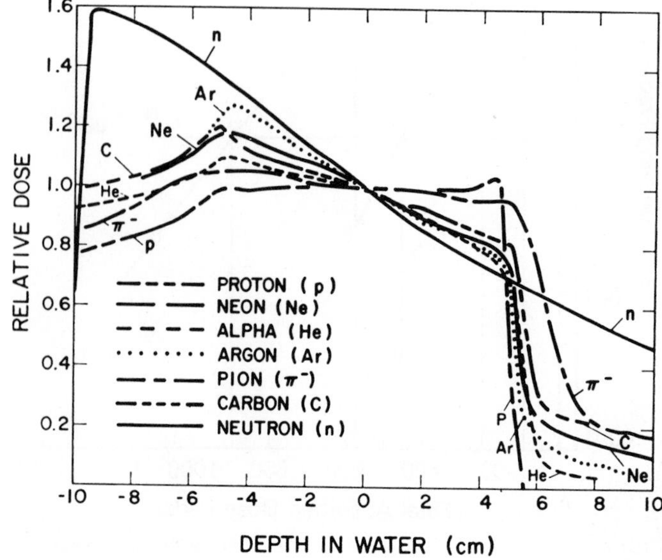

FIGURE 14–6. Comparison of depth dose (spread peak curves) for various charged particles of clinical interest.

TABLE 14–1
Comparison of Relative Physical and Biologic Parameters of Particles in Clinical Use

					HEAVY IONS			
HIGH-LET ADVANTAGE	PROTONS	HELIUM	PIONS	NEUTRONS	C	Ne	Si	Ar
Physical depth dose	+++	+++	+++	no	+++	+++	++	+
Relative biologic effectivness	no	+	+	++	++	++	+++	+++
Oxygen enhancement ratio	no	+	+	+++	+	++	+++	+++

+: *slight advantage.*
++: *moderate advantage.*
+++: *very significant advantage.*

lignancies responding dramatically.[15,16] On the basis of these encouraging results, various centers throughout the world again began clinical trials with fast neutrons.[27] In the United States, patient treatments were started in 1972 at the M.D. Anderson Hospital, using the Texas A & M University variable energy cyclotron (50-MeV d→Be reaction). Clinical trials were instituted in 1973 at the University of Washington, using a fixed energy cyclotron (22-MeV d→Be reaction). Additional patients were treated on physics-laboratory-based machines at the MANTA facility (35-MeV d→Be reaction) at George Washington University in Washington DC, at the GLANTA facility (25-MeV d→Be reaction) in Cleveland, OH, and at the Fermi Laboratory facility (66-MeV p→Be reaction) in Batavia, IL. Initially, phase I clinical trials were carried out on patients with advanced tumors who were estimated to have less than a 10% 5-year survival with conventional forms of treatment. This work yielded considerable information about the different values of relative biologic effectiveness for different tissues and the variation of the neutron values from facility to facility.

From the late 1970s to the mid-1980s, patients receiving fast-neutron radiation therapy were entered into randomized, prospective clinical trials using these physics-laboratory-based machines. These trials were hampered by the physical limitations of this relatively unsophisticated equipment:

Poor depth dose characteristics
Poor skin sparing
Fixed horizontal treatment beams
Inadequate collimation
Inadequate beam film capabilities
Inadequate treatment simulation
Difficult logistics
Frequent accelerator breakdown

The clinical results presented in this chapter were obtained on these laboratory-based machines. Beginning in the mid-1980s, high-energy, isocentric, hospital-based neutron therapy systems became available for patient treatment. These new-generation accelerators are capable of physical dose distributions comparable to those of conventional megavoltage radiation therapy equipment. Currently, patients treated in the United States, the United Kingdom, and Korea are treated on these types of machines. Approximately 10,000 patients have been treated with neutrons worldwide, resulting in a fairly extensive patient database.

Brain

There has been considerable experience in using fast neutrons in the treatment of malignant gliomas. Laramore and associates[57] were the first to report that fast neutrons had the potential for eradicating this disease. A total of 36 patients received whole-brain irradiation using fast neutrons, alone or in combination with megavoltage photons as part of a "mixed-beam" regimen. There was no difference in survival compared with historic photon controls for grade IV lesions, but the survival was substantially less for those patients with grade III lesions (Kernohan schema).[52] Autopsies were performed on 15 patients, and the tumor had been eradicated in 14 instances. The patients' brains exhibited a coagulation necrosis replacing the gross tumor volume; some sparsely scattered abnormal cells (probably reactive astrocytes) were intermixed with the coagulation necrosis, but these were not expansively growing. A diffuse gliosis and white matter demyelination were found in regions of the brain far from the tumor, and this presumably was related to the ultimate cause of death.

Another report by Catterall[15] described 16 patients treated with fast neutrons to the entire brain who had posttreatment assessment of disease status either at a second-look craniotomy or at autopsy. There was no improvement in survival compared with historic controls. In 69% of the cases, no tumor was found or only microscopic foci of abnormal cells were discovered. These results contrast with those for photon-treated patients using x-rays alone or in combination with chemotherapeutic agents or radiosensitizers. It appeared that fast neutrons had the potential for eradicating this disease, but that the concomitant side effects to normal brain tissue were too severe.

Based on this information, the Radiation Therapy Oncology Group designed a study that confined the neutron radiation to a boost volume around the primary tumor mass that was determined by computed tomography scans. After receiving 5000-cGy whole-brain irradiation, the patients were randomized to receive either a 1500-cGy photon boost or an equivalent boost with fast neutrons, with the physical dose scaled by the relative biologic effectiveness of the particular neutron treatment facility in question. A total of 158 evaluable patients were entered on the study, and the results were reported by Griffin and colleagues.[44] For those patients with glioblastoma multiforme, the median survival was 9.6 months for the neutron-boost group and 8.5 months for the photon-boost group (no statistical significance). For those patients with anaplastic astrocytoma, the median survival was 15.8 months for the neutron-boost group and 26.3 months for the photon-boost group.[65] Although highly suggestive, this difference was not statistically significant because of the small patient numbers in this disease category.

Postmortem neuropathologic studies on 12 neutron-boost patients and 12 photon-treated patients were carried out at the University of Washington (Seattle). In nine of 12 of the neutron-boost patients, there was significant necrosis of the primary tumor with only a few, sparsely scattered, bizarre cells present. No proliferating, infiltrating tumor was found. This was in sharp contrast to the photon-treated patients, all of whose autopsy specimens revealed proliferating, infiltrating, viable tumor masses with actively proliferating vascular components around necrotic central cores. Death in the photon-treated patients was caused by progressing tumor, but death in most of the neutron-treated patients was related to the side effects of the treatment.

Based on these early results, a subsequent study opened in 1980, and a total of 203 patients were entered. Of these, 190 were analyzable. Patients received 150-cGy whole-brain photon irradiation given 5 days each week, for a total dose of 4500 cGy. Concomitantly, patients received neutron irradiation to a boost field defined by the primary tumor volume plus a 1.5-cm margin. The neutron irradiation was given before and within 3 hours of the photon treatment for that day.[66] Four neutron institutions participated in the study: Seattle (University of Washington), GLANTA (Cleveland Clinic), University of Chicago, and Fermi (Fermi National Accelerator Laboratories). Because each of these facilities used a somewhat different nuclear reaction to produce the neutron beam, the neutron doses were specified for the Seattle facility, and the doses for the other facilities scaled by the factors shown in Table 14-2. Dose definition was further complicated because the GLANTA facility changed the reaction used to produce their neutron beam midway through the study. These institutional scale factors were determined by both radiobiologic data and clinical experience on other tumor systems. Neutron doses are specified for the Seattle facility and include the τ-ray contaminant.

To assess late and acute effects, the dose levels were randomly assigned rather than sequentially searched. Initially, patients were randomized among three total doses of neutrons: 360 cGy, 420 cGy, and 480 cGy. In November 1981, these arms were closed, and three other dose levels of neutrons opened: 520 cGy, 550 cGy, and 600 cGy. The 600-cGy neutron arm was closed April 1983, because of observed toxicity. To maintain three open treatment arms, the 480-cGy neutron arm was reopened in December 1983. Figure 14-7 shows survival by neutron dose for the six treatment arms. Median survival ranged from 8.6 months for the 520-cGy neutron arm to 13.9 months for the 360-cGy neutron arm, with no significant differences among the six arms. Comparing the three lower doses with the three higher doses in the subgroup of patients with the diagnosis of glioblastoma multiforme, again no significant difference was seen. Figure 14-8 shows survival by dose for the patient subgroup with the diagnosis of anaplastic astrocytoma, comparing the three lower doses with the three higher doses. The appearance of the plot is highly suggestive of the deleterious effect of the higher-neutron doses, but because there were only 30 patients with this diagnosis (six on the lower-dose arms and 24 on the higher-dose arms), the apparent difference is not statistically significant.

TABLE 14–2
Participating Neutron Treatment Facilities and Relative Scaling Factors for the Neutron Dose

FACILITY	REACTION	INSTITUTIONAL SCALING FACTOR
Seattle	22-Mev d⇒Be	1.0
GLANTA	25-MeV d⇒Be	1.0
GLANTA	42-MeV p⇒Be	1.24
U. Chicago (gaseous target)	d⇒d	1.0
Fermi	66-MeV p⇒Be	1.24

(From Griffin TW, Wambersie A, Laramore GE, et al: Int J Radiat Oncol Biol Phys 14:583, 1988)

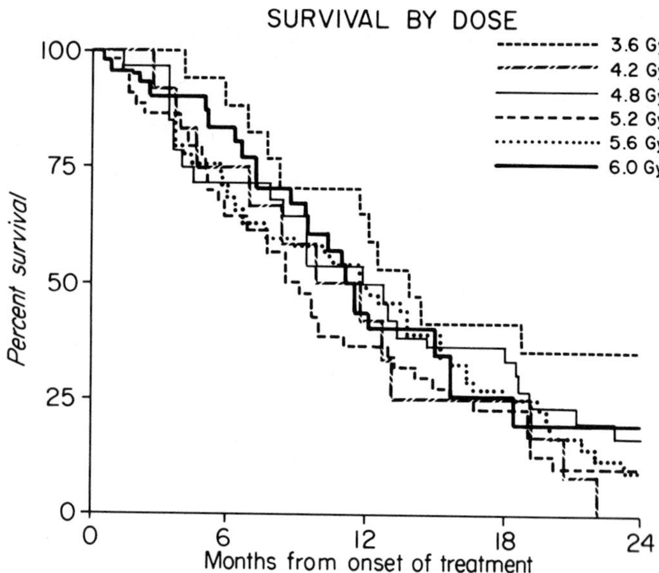

FIGURE 14–7. Patient survival as a function of neutron boost dose for the six treatment arms.

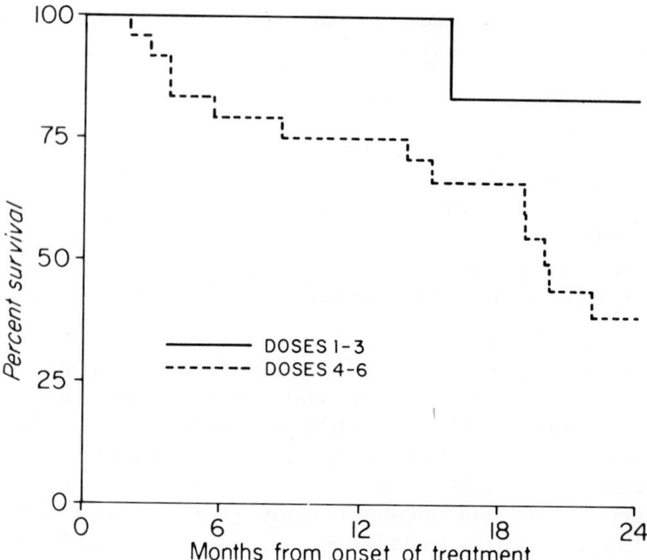

FIGURE 14–8. Patient survival as a function of neutron boost dose for the subgroup having the diagnosis of anaplastic astrocytoma. The lower three doses are compared with the higher three doses.

An attempt was made to correlate radiation dose with autopsy findings. At neutron doses lower than 447 cGy, all seven patients who went to autopsy had evidence of viable tumor, and in three cases, there was evidence of concomitant radiation damage. At the doses higher than 578 cGy, there was viable tumor in 13 (72%) of 18 cases and concomitant radiation damage in 8 (44%) of 18 cases. Although there were some instances of pathologic tumor sterilization, there continued to be a high incidence of associated radiation injury. Radiation damage occurred at all of the dose levels, and even at the doses higher than 578 cGy, there was pathologic evidence of tumor sterilization in only five (28%) of 18 autopsied cases. Higher neutron doses may increase the tumor sterilization rate, but the expected incidence of concomitant radiation damage would be no lower.

Head and Neck

The use of fast neutrons for the treatment of patients with squamous cell head and neck cancer has been studied intermittently for four decades.[2,59,61] Following Stone's early work, Catterall and co-workers[17] conducted a randomized study in the 1960s at Hammersmith Hospital in London, reporting a significant advantage for neutrons over conventional photon treatment for this group of tumors. Using the low-energy MRC cyclotron, they observed a 76% (53 of 70) local control rate for neutrons, compared with a 19% (12 of 63) local control rate for photons in a group of patients with advanced disease. The survival rates were poor in both treatment groups. Their early work led to many follow-up studies in Europe, Japan, and the United States.[25,42,84]

A second randomized study of fast neutrons for treating earlier stage head and neck cancer was later reported by Duncan and colleagues.[24] They reported the results of a randomized, cooperative study conducted at the Antoni van Leeuwenhoek Ziekenhuis in Amsterdam, the Department of Clinical Oncology in Edinburgh, and Universitatsklinikun in Essen. No significant advantage for neutrons over photons could be demonstrated. The complete response rate for neutrons was 70% (70 of 100), and the complete response rate for photons was 66% (63 of 95). The ultimate local control rates were 44% (44 of 100) for neutrons and 40% (38 of 95) for photons. There was no significant difference in the overall survival rates between the two groups. These results stand in contrast to the results obtained at Hammersmith Hospital.

A third major study of neutrons for squamous cell carcinomas of the head and neck was carried out in the United States; 327 patients with inoperable squamous cell carcinomas of the head and neck region were entered on a cooperative, randomized study comparing mixed-beam radiation therapy with conventional photon radiation therapy.[38] Patients with previously untreated, histologically proven, inoperable squamous cell carcinomas of T-stage T2, T3, or T4 and any N-stage originating in the oral cavity, oropharynx, supraglottic larynx, or hypopharynx were eligible. Five neutron facilities participated in this study: The University of Washington with a 22-MeV d→Be cyclotron, GLANTA with a 25-MeV d→Be cyclotron, MANTA with a 35-MeV d→Be cyclotron, TAMVEC with a 50-MeV d→Be cyclotron, and the Fermilab with a 66-MeV p→Be linear accelerator. Patients randomized to photons received 6600 cGy to 7400 cGy delivered in 180-cGy to 200-cGy daily fractions, five fractions each week. Patients randomized to mixed-beam irradiation received 4000-cGy to 4400-cGy photons plus 750-cGy to 1000-cGy neutrons. Three fractions of photons plus two fractions of neutrons were given each week. Photons were given in 180-cGy to 200-cGy fractions, and neutrons were given in fractions equivalent to 180 cGy to 200 cGy of photon irradiation. The actual neutron doses given were based on the relative biologic effectiveness values for each facility.

The decision to make the experimental arm a neutron and photon mix rather than neutrons alone arose from the poor depth dose characteristics of the neutron beams available at the time of the study. All neutron beams were produced by accelerators located in nuclear physics laboratories. All of the neutron facilities shared the additional handicap of primitive beam delivery systems. Patients were generally treated in the sitting position through a fixed cone collimator with an immobile horizontal beam. External blocking was primitive or nonexistent. Figure 14-9 illustrates a typical patient setup on one of these machines, and Figure 14-10 illustrates a typical acute reaction seen after treatment with neutrons alone with a low-energy beam.

The initial complete response rates were 56% for mixed-beam-treated patients and 58% for photon-treated patients.[38] The initial complete primary tumor clearance rates were 63% with mixed beam and 64% with photons. The initial complete nodal clearance rates were 68% with mixed beam and 55% with photons. The overall locoregional tumor control rates were 31% for mixed-beam-treated patients and 34% for photon-treated patients. This difference is not statistically significant ($P = 0.77$).[38]

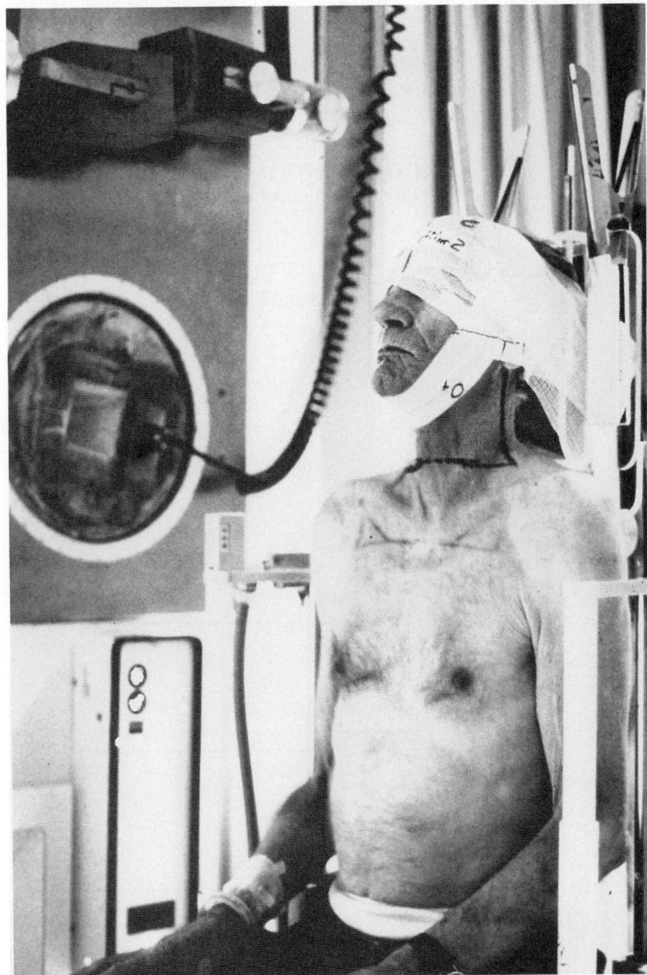

FIGURE 14–9. Patient setup on a physics-laboratory-based fixed horizontal-beam treatment system.

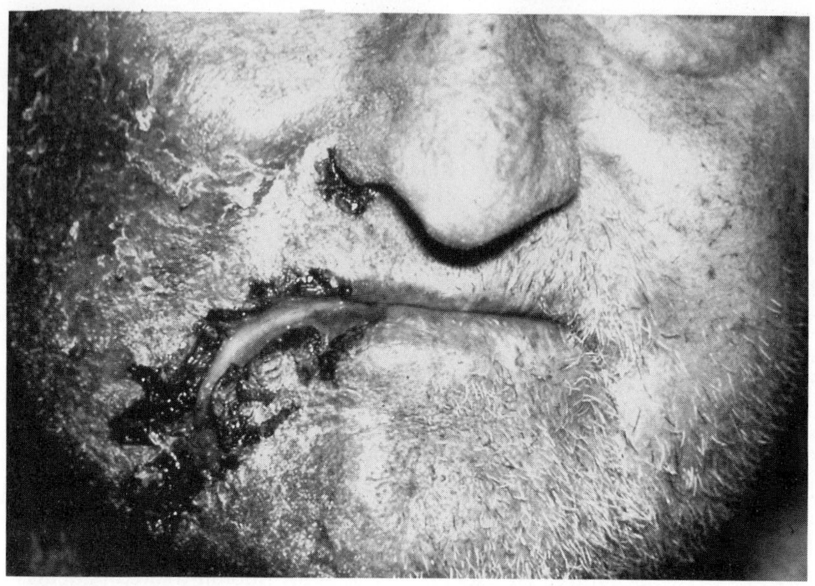

FIGURE 14–10. Moist desquamation typical of acute reactions seen after treatment with low-energy neutrons.

The overall primary tumor control rates of 41% for mixed-beam-treated patients and 46% for photon-treated patients are not significantly different ($P = 0.43$). However, a significant advantage for mixed-beam treatment was demonstrated in the local control of tumor in lymph nodes. The nodal tumor control rates were 49% for mixed-beam-treated patients and 29% for photon-treated patients. The differences in nodal control rates are illustrated in Figure 14-11 and are significant at the $P = 0.004$ level.

The primary tumor control rates as a function of nodal status and treatment are illustrated in Figures 14-12 and 14-13. Locoregional tumor control rates for patients presenting with positive lymph nodes are 30% for mixed-beam-treated patients and 18% for photon-treated patients ($P = 0.05$). Locoregional tumor control rates for patients presenting without positive lymph nodes are 64% for photon-treated patients and 33% for mixed-beam-treated patients ($P = 0.004$).

Figure 14-14 illustrates survival rates by treatment. The difference is not statistically significant ($P = 0.32$). Analyzing survival as a function of nodal status and treatment, there was no significant difference in survival rates for patients present-

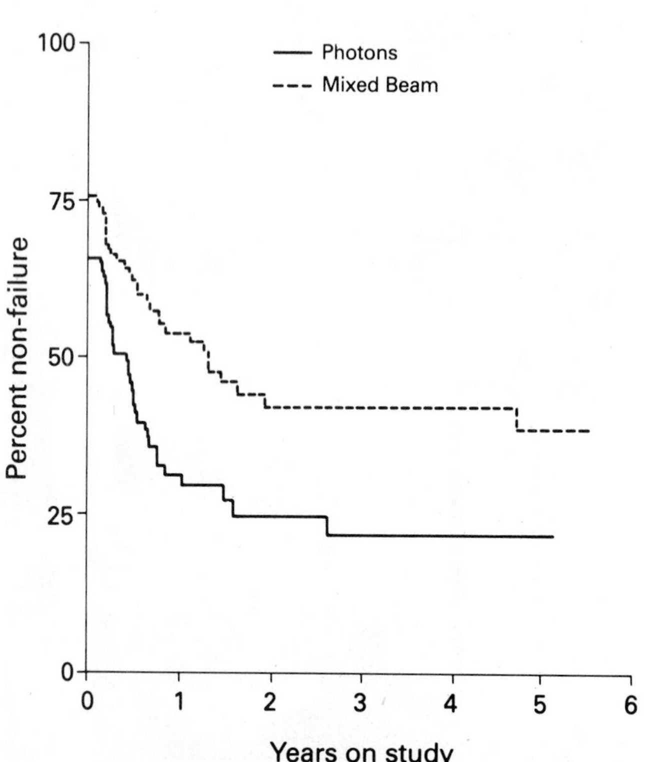

FIGURE 14–11. Tumor control rates for the lymph nodes as a function of treatment. The difference is significant at the $P = 0.004$ level.

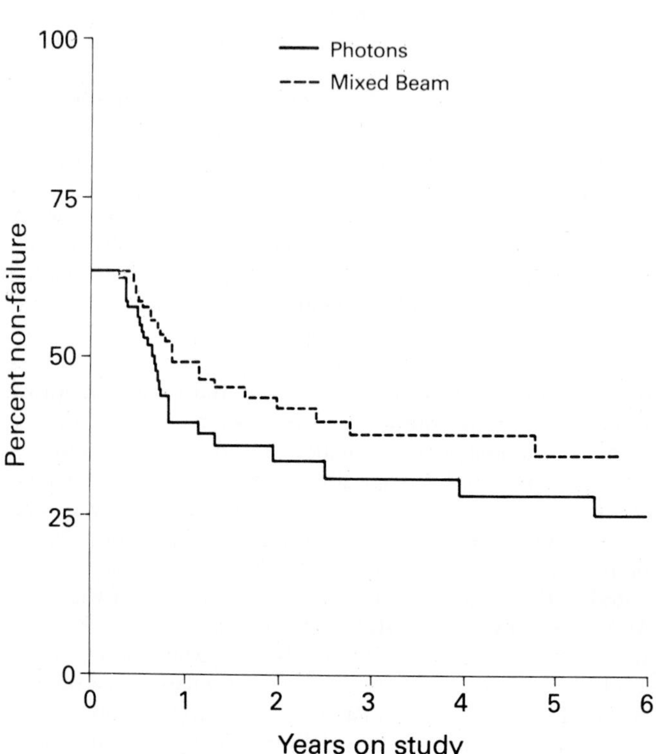

FIGURE 14–12. Primary tumor control rates for patients presenting with positive lymph nodes as a function of treatment. The trend is not statistically significant ($P = 0.22$).

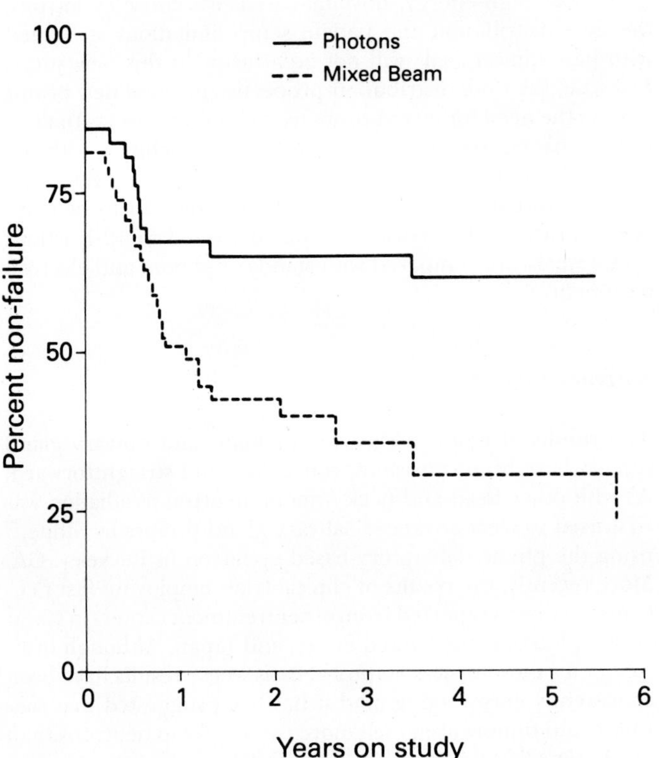

FIGURE 14–13. Primary tumor control rates for patients presenting with negative lymph nodes as a function of treatment. The difference is significant at the $P = 0.009$ level.

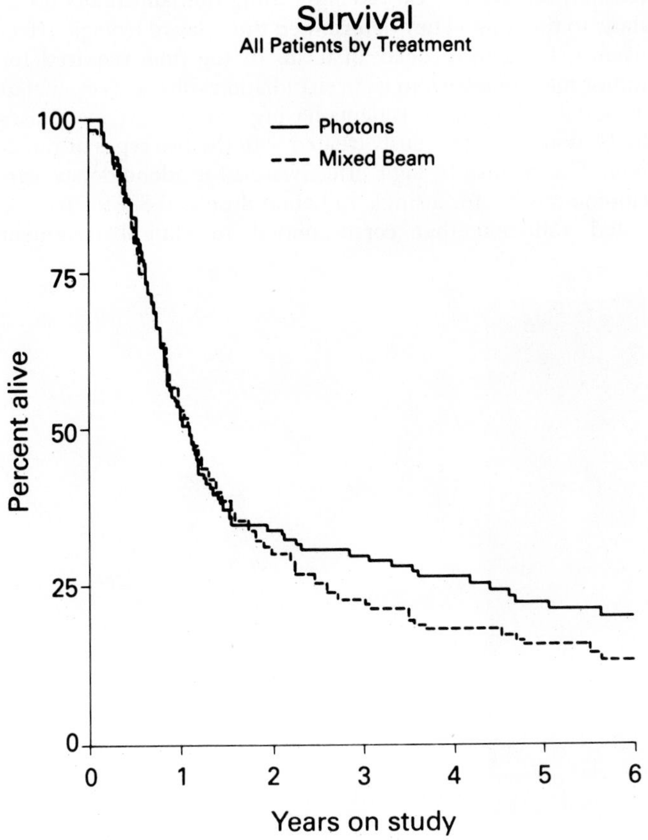

Survival
All Patients by Treatment
Photons
Mixed Beam
Percent alive
100
75
50
25
0
0 1 2 3 4 5 6
Years on study

FIGURE 14–14. Overall survival rates as a function of treatment. The difference is not statistically significant.

ing with positive lymph nodes ($P = 0.55$). Figure 14-15 shows an advantage for photon-treated patients presenting with negative lymph nodes ($P = 0.01$). There were no significant differences in late normal tissue toxicities or the occurrence of second primary malignant tumors between the two treatment groups.

The differences in the patient populations in these three randomized studies were evidenced by differences in photon local control rates and the percentage of patients with neck node involvement: 83% in the U.S. cooperative study; 66% in the Hammersmith study; approximately 50% in the Edinburgh study.[17,24,42] Although the overall results of the U.S. cooperative study fail to demonstrate a significant difference between the two treatment groups, subgroup analysis reveals major differences between results for patients presenting with positive lymph nodes and those presenting with negative lymph nodes.[38,43] The reasons for these differences are not understood.

Guichard and associates[45] were able to demonstrate that lymph nodes with metastatic lesions from an experimental mouse tumor contained an increased population of hypoxic cells compared with equivalent-sized primary tumors. Because neutrons have a reduced oxygen enhancement ratio compared with photons and electrons, neutrons and other high-LET treatments could be expected to achieve better results in a tumor system with an increased population of hypoxic cells. However, if the differences between treatments observed in this study in patients presenting with positive and negative nodes were due to this effect, there should have been a consistent response at the primary tumor site that was independent of nodal status, not the observed association of response between primary and nodal sites.

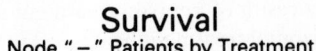

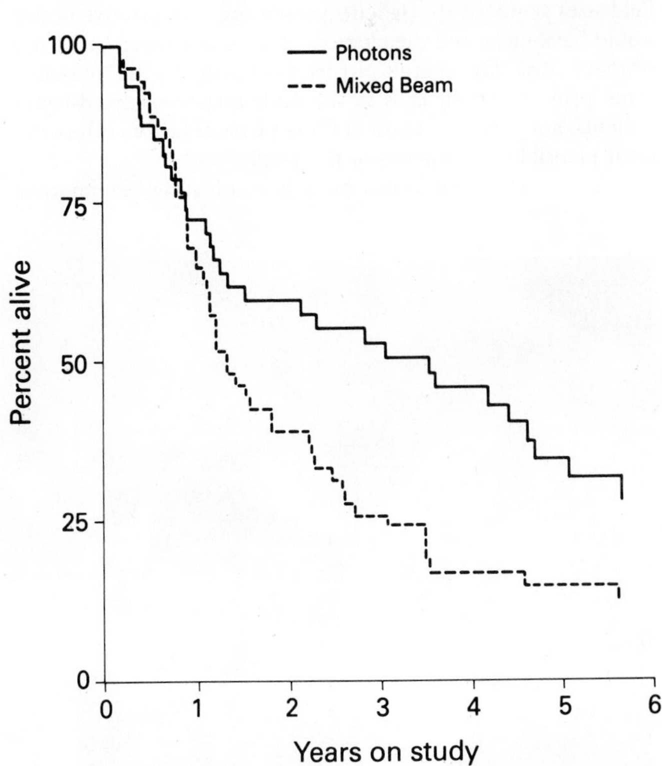

FIGURE 14–15. Survival rates of patients presenting with negative lymph nodes as a function of treatment. The difference is significant at the $P = 0.01$ level.

In a large retrospective analysis of the Radiation Therapy Oncology Group database, lymph node positivity served as a predictor of response, identifying tumors with biologic characteristics leading to radioresistance to low-LET radiations. The same characteristics could make these tumors relatively more sensitive to high-LET radiations. Incorporating this type of selection criteria into clinical trials has been suggested by Withers.[88] Although this hypothesis could explain the improved results observed in mixed-beam-treated patients presenting with positive nodes, it does not explain the unexpected finding of significantly improved results in photon-treated patients compared with neutron-treated patients presenting without positive lymph nodes.

Although a biologic explanation of the results of the U.S. cooperative trial is plausible and possible, it is not likely. However, there are several explanations based on the physical distribution of radiation dose. The poor depth dose characteristics of the neutron beams available for the study would have delivered an increased radiation dose to the neck compared with the deeper primary sites. In addition, the proportion of neutrons and photons as a percentage of total dose would have been increased in the neck because of increasing τ-ray contamination of the neutron beams at depth.

The physical characteristics of the neutron beams could explain an increased rate of nodal tumor control versus primary tumor control, but they do not account for the differences in primary tumor control rates observed in patients presenting with and without positive lymph nodes. Underdosage of a portion of the primary tumors could have occurred as a consequence of the exaggerated "hour glass effect" associated with low-energy neutron isodose curves at depth. Likewise, a geographic miss of a portion of the primary tumors could have occurred as a result of neutron treatment restrictions imposed by fixed horizontal treatment beams lacking adequate methods of portal verification (Fig. 12-9). In both instances, the large field sizes required for patients presenting with positive nodes would have increased the chances of adequate coverage of the primary sites. The overall picture is consistent with "missing" some primary tumor cells in the node-negative, mixed-beam patients, and a combination of these physical factors offers the most plausible explanation of the results.

An international consortium is conducting yet another study of radiation therapy with fast neutrons for advanced squamous cell carcinomas of the head and neck. With the introduction of high-energy, hospital-based, isocentric cyclotrons, the dose distribution and patient setup limitations associated with past clinical trials will not be a factor in this new study. Likewise, the dose distribution properties of these new beams obviate the need for mixed-beam treatment. Figure 14-16 illustrates a patient setup on one of these new machines, with the multileaf collimation system shown in Figure 14-17. Based on current accrual rates, the new study is projected to be completed in the early 1990s. Neutrons delivered in 12 fractions over 4 weeks are compared with standard photon and electron treatment.

Salivary Gland

The results of neutron therapy for malignant salivary gland tumors have been consistent, conclusive, and straightforward. As with other head and neck tumors, neutron irradiation was first used to treat advanced salivary gland tumors by Stone,[79] using the physics-laboratory-based cyclotron in Berkeley, CA. More recently, the results of clinical trials employing fast neutrons have been reported from other treatment centers in Great Britain, Europe, the United States, and Japan. Although instituted on a more-or-less empirical basis, these results have been consistently encouraging, and it has been suggested that salivary gland tumors are much more responsive to neutrons than to photons.[51]

The first radiobiologic evidence that neutrons could be particularly effective in the treatment of salivary gland tumors came from Battermann and co-workers.[4] They measured the relative biologic effectiveness of neutrons produced by a d→T reaction relative to ^{60}Co radiation using human tumors metastatic to the lung. They determined the relative biologic effectiveness for growth delay in terms of the time required for tumor mass to return to its preirradiation volume as evaluated on serial radiographs. Patients having two or more metastases had lesions simultaneously treated with the two types of radiation. The relative biologic effectiveness for adenoidcystic carcinoma was 5.7 for a single radiation dose and 8.0 for fractionated radiation that corresponded to clinical treatment

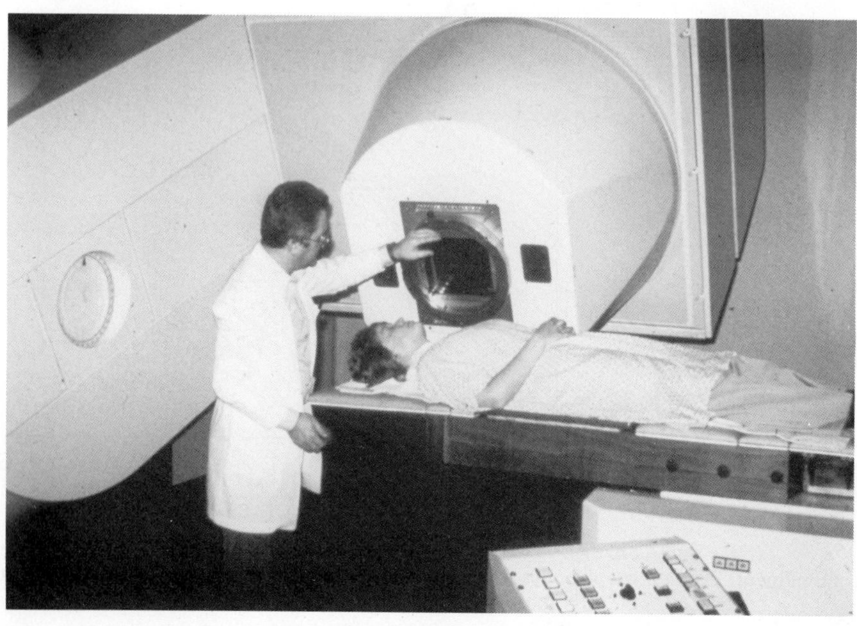

FIGURE 14–16. Patient setup on a hospital-based isocentric treatment system.

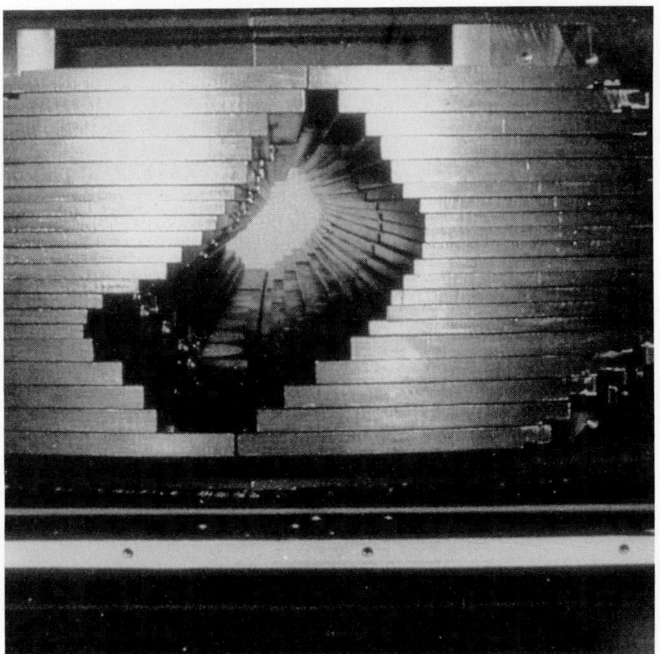

FIGURE 14–17. Multileaf collimation system from a hospital-based neutron treatment facility.

schemes. The relative biologic effectiveness values for most other tumors were in the range of 2.5 to 4.0.

Based on encouraging results from earlier nonrandom clinical trials and the strong supporting evidence from Battermann's radiobiology studies, the Radiation Therapy Oncology Group in the United States and the Medical Research Council of Great Britain sponsored a prospective, randomized study comparing the effects of fast neutrons with low-LET photons with or without electrons for the treatment of inoperable, malignant salivary gland tumors.[39] A total of 32 patients were entered on this study. Twenty-five were entered from the United States and seven from Scotland. Seventeen patients were randomized to receive neutrons, and 15 were randomized to receive standard radiation therapy of photons with or without electrons. Sixty-one percent of the neutron-treated patients and 75% of the photon-treated patients presented with inoperable or unresectable primary tumors, and 39% of the neutron-treated and 25% of the photon-treated patients presented with unresectable recurrent disease.

At a minimum follow-up period of 2 years, the complete tumor clearance rates at the primary site were 85% for neutrons and 33% for photons after protocol treatment ($P = 0.01$). The complete tumor clearance rates in the cervical lymph nodes were 86% for neutrons and 25% for photons. The overall locoregional complete tumor response rates were 85% and 33% for neutrons and photons, respectively (Fig. 14-18A). The locoregional control rates at 2 years (Fig. 14-18B) for the two groups are 67% for neutrons and 17% for photons ($P < 0.005$). The 2-year survival rates are 62% and 25% for neutrons and photons, respectively ($P = 0.10$) (Figure 14-19). There was no significant difference between the normal tissue complication rates of the two groups.

Before this study, the results of neutron treatment of 289 patients with inoperable salivary gland tumors had been reported.[39] This number excludes patients who were treated for presumed residual disease after surgery. Some of these patients received mixed-beam treatment (40% neutrons, 60% photons); others were treated with neutrons alone. Treatment was delivered in 12 to 38 fractions over 4 to 7 weeks. Despite this variability, the results are remarkably consistent. Table 14-3 lists the reported experiences in achieving local control of malignant salivary gland tumors with neutron therapy. The composite local control rate was 67% (194 of 289).

Local tumor control rates after irradiation with low-LET photons with or without electrons for inoperable salivary gland carcinomas are less satisfactory (Table 14-4). The composite local control rate after photons in these series was 24% (61 of 254).

Table 14-5 compares the randomized study results with the historic results. Taken as a whole, the data from the radiobiologic studies, the nonrandom clinical studies, and the prospective randomized clinical trial overwhelmingly support the contention that therapy with fast neutrons offers a significant

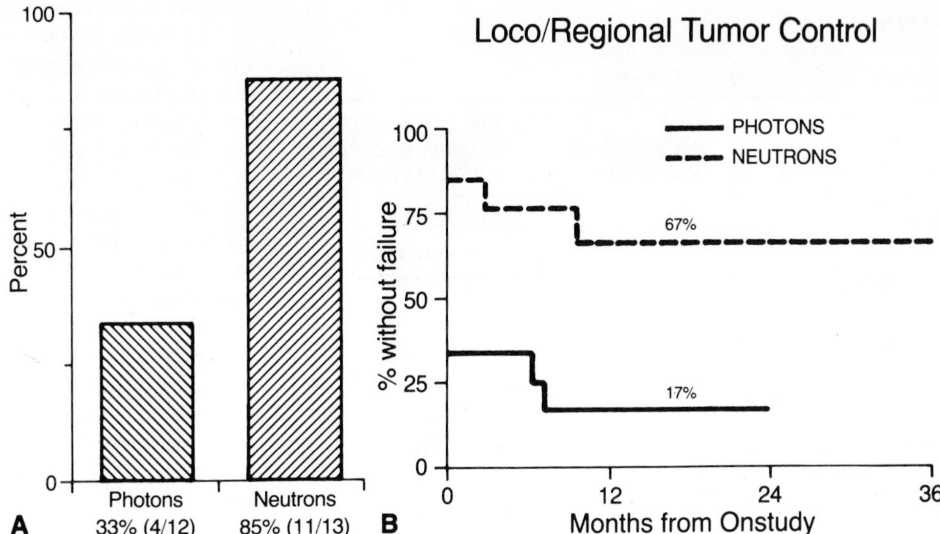

FIGURE 14–18. (**A**) Complete response rates for neutron-treated and photon-treated patients. The difference is statistically significant at the $P = 0.01$ level. (**B**) Locoregional tumor control rates for neutron-treated and photon-treated patients. The difference is statistically significant at the $P < 0.005$ level.

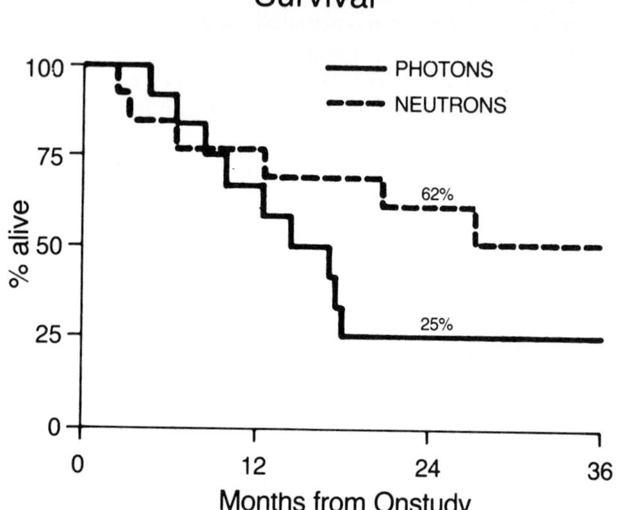

FIGURE 14–19. Survival rates for neutron-treated and photon-treated patients. The difference is significant at the $P = 0.10$ level.

advance in the treatment of inoperable and unresectable primary and recurrent malignant salivary gland tumors. There was no observable difference in tumor response to neutron therapy according to histologic subtypes.

Lung

Therapy employing fast neutrons was first investigated as a treatment for lung cancer by Eichhorn and colleagues[26] at the Central Institute for Cancer Research of the Academy of Sciences of the German Democratic Republic. Using a Soviet cyclotron generating a low-energy neutron beam with a mean energy of 6.2 MeV, Eichhorn investigated the treatment of locally advanced lung cancer with various combinations of neutron and photon radiation. Using histologic examination of surgical and autopsy specimens as an end point for local tumor control, the investigators compared the results of their neutron and photon treatment with historic control treatment using only photons. Pathologic examinations revealed that a substantially higher fraction of neutron-treated patients had complete sterilization of their tumors than the control patients treated with photons alone.[27] The tumor sterilization rates were 33% in the photon-only treated patients, 48% in patients receiving 20% of their total dose with neutrons, and 57% in patients receiving 37% of their total dose with neutrons. Despite this local control advantage, no overall survival advantage was noted in this group of advanced patients. The low energy of the neutron beam produced by the Soviet cyclotron precluded investigation of treatment with neutrons alone.

TABLE 14–3
Neutron Locoregional Tumor Control Rates for Malignant Salivary Gland Tumors

INVESTIGATOR	NUMBER OF PATIENTS	LOCOREGIONAL TUMOR CONTROL RATE (PATIENTS)
Saroja[73]	113	63% (71/113)
Caterall[14]	65	77% (50/65)
Battermann[1]	32	66% (21/32)
Griffin[41]	32	81% (26/32)
Duncan[22]	22	55% (12/22)
Maor[61]	9	67% (6/9)
Ornitz[67]	8	38% (3/8)
Eichhorn[28]	5	60% (3/5)
Skolyszewski[78]	3	67% (2/3)
Total	289	67% (194/289)

TABLE 14–4
Low-LET (Photon/Electron) Locoregional Tumor Control Rates for Malignant Salivary Gland Tumors

INVESTIGATOR	NUMBER OF PATIENTS	LOCOREGIONAL TUMOR CONTROL RATE (PATIENTS)
Fitzpatrick[30]	50	12% (6/50)
Vikram[88]	49	4% (2/49)
Borthne[6]	35	23% (8/35)
Rafla[68]	25	36% (9/25)
Fu[34]	19	32% (6/19)
Stewart[79]	19	47% (9/19)
Dobrowsky[20]	17	41% (7/17)
Shidnia[77]	16	38% (6/16)
Elkon[29]	13	15% (2/13)
Rossman[71]	11	54% (6/11)
Total	254	24% (61/254)

Schnabel and associates[75] reported a series of patients with bronchogenic cancer treated with a neutron beam from a dT generator. Although low in intensity, this neutron beam had high enough energy to allow treatment with neutrons alone. A prospective, randomized study compared a neutron treatment regimen consisting of 1800-cGy neutrons delivered in 20 fractions over 5 weeks to a treatment regimen consisting of 5400-cGy photons delivered in 20 fractions over 4 weeks. Many patients had prior surgery with or without chemotherapy and were entered on the study with persistent or recurrent disease. A total of 115 patients were entered on the study; however, only 30 of 48 neutron-randomized patients and only 46 of 67 photon-randomized patients were able to complete treatment according to protocol guidelines, primarily because of equipment failure. Analysis of results revealed no significant differences in locoregional tumor control, survival, or complication rates. Survival at 1 year was approximately 37% on both treatment arms.

In 1985, Breteau and co-workers[8] described 26 patients with inoperable non-small-cell lung cancer treated with a mixture of photons and neutrons in Orleans, France. The patients first received 4000-cGy photons over 4 weeks through anterior and posterior (AP/PA) portals followed by 670-cGy neutrons delivered in eight fractions over 2 weeks through lateral portals. The neutrons were generated by a 34-MeV proton-on-beryllium (p→ Be) reaction. With follow-up times ranging from 6 to 26 months, local control was achieved in 21 of 26 patients. Six cases became operable, and in three of them, examination revealed no residual tumor. Side effects included two cases of infection in the irradiated volume and one treatment-related death. In an additional 11 patients with Pancoast tumors treated with the same regimen of 4000-cGy photons and 670-cGy neutrons, Breteau and colleagues reported complete pain relief in ten, with a median survival of 9 months.[8] No long-term survival results were published for either series of patients.

Neutron treatment of Pancoast tumors of the lung has been

TABLE 14–5
Comparison of the RTOG-MRC Study Results with Historic Results

INVESTIGATION	NUMBER OF PATIENTS	LOCOREGIONAL TUMOR CONTROL RATE
LOW LET		
Low LET historic experience	254	24%
RTOG/MRC photon controls	12	17%
NEUTRON		
Historic neutron experience	289	67%
RTOG/MRC neutron results	13	67%

(From Griffin TW, Pajak TF, Laramore GE, et al: Int J Radiat Oncol Biol Phys 15:1085, 1988)

investigated by seven other groups. Sawada and associates[74] reported treatment of 23 patients using the 30-MeV d→Be reaction at the NIRS facility in Chiba, Japan. The mean survival for this group of patients was 11.5 months. Locoregional tumor control rates were not reported. Komaki and others[54] reported a 100% (10 patients) locoregional tumor control rate for Pancoast tumors treated with the 50-MeV d→Be and the 42-MeV p→Be neutron beams available at M.D. Anderson Hospital in Houston. This result is significantly better than the locoregional tumor control rates reported for photon treatment at the same institution.

In 1986, Laramore and colleagues[56] published the results of a Radiation Therapy Oncology Group prospective study that randomly assigned 102 patients to one of three treatment arms. The control arm consisted of 6000-cGy photons in 30 fractions over 6 to 7 weeks. The second arm consisted of 1800-cGy neutrons in 12 to 24 fractions over 6 to 7 weeks. The third arm used a mixed beam consisting of two neutron and three photon treatments each week in daily doses of an approximately equal relative biologic effectiveness to a total dose of 6000-cGy photon-equivalent. The participating neutron facilities all used horizontal fixed beams, and patients received the neutron portions of their treatments in a sitting or a standing position. Fixed collimators with external iron or tungsten blocks were used for beam shaping.

Analysis revealed no difference in median survival among the three treatment arms: 7.5 months on the neutron arm, 8.1 months on the mixed-beam arm, and 6.9 months on the photon arm. Early failure tended to be dominated by distant metastases. To estimate the impact of improved locoregional control on patients without early metastatic spread of their cancers, a separate analysis was performed on the subgroup of patients exhibiting complete or partial response at 6 months after initiation of therapy (Fig. 14-20). The 3-year survival was better on the neutron and mixed-beam arms than on the photon arm, but because of small patient numbers at the longer follow-up times, these differences were not statistically significant.

A third-generation protocol using the high-energy, isocentric, hospital-based neutron beams is currently accruing patients. Patients are randomized to receive either 2040-cGy neutrons in 12 fractions over 4 weeks or 6000-cGy photons in 30 fractions over 6 weeks.

Prostate

Clinical investigations of neutron therapy in prostate cancer have been reported from the United States, Europe, and Japan. The largest group of patients has been treated in the United States, under the auspices of the Radiation Therapy Oncology Group. This trial is also the only randomized prospective trial that has been carried out comparing neutron therapy directly with conventional megavoltage photon therapy. Details of the study design and execution have been fully reported.[58] Patients with clinical Stage C and D1 disease were randomized to treatment employing photon irradiation or treatment employing a combination of neutrons and photons (mixed beam). A major reservation in using lower-energy neutron beams available at some institutions stemmed from the lack of skin sparing with these units relative to that achievable with higher-energy cyclotron beams or megavoltage photon irradiation. The lack of skin sparing and the poor penetration of these beams raised the possibility of producing unacceptably high rates of normal tissue complications, similar to those from orthovoltage-era pho-

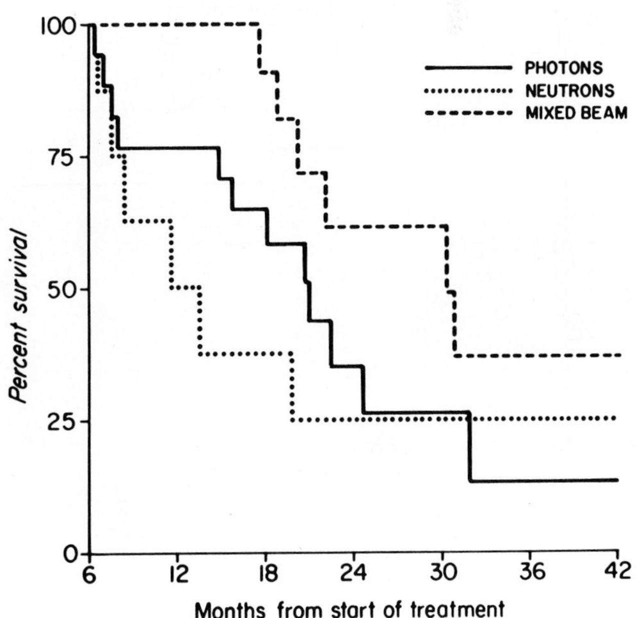

FIGURE 14–20. Actuarial curves showing patient survival as a function of treatment options for the subgroup of patients exhibiting complete or partial tumor responses at 6 months after initiation of therapy. The median survival is 20.8 months on the photon arm, 13.4 months on the neutron arm, and 30.2 months on the mixed-beam arm. The survival at 3 years is approximately 12% on the photon arm, 25% on the neutron arm, and 37% on the mixed-beam arm.

ton units, if neutrons alone were used to treat the large volumes required to incorporate pelvic lymph node chains.

The mixed-beam approach involved twice-weekly treatment with neutrons and 3-times-weekly treatment with photons. Because the relative biologic effectiveness of neutrons varied with the facility, the daily neutron dose was adjusted (*i.e.*, neutron dose + a percentage of cyclotron output containing photon contamination × individual institutional value of relative biologic effectiveness) to give equivalent biologic doses of neutrons or photons each day.

Between 1977 and 1983, 91 patients were enrolled on the study, with a purposely skewed randomization leading to 55 patients assigned to the mixed-beam arm and 36 to the conventional photon arm. Seventy-four patients were staged as C, and 17 were staged as D1. Prior hormonal treatment had been given in 25% of the patients randomized to receive photons and in 11% of patients randomized to mixed-beam therapy.

Patients randomized to photons received 5000 cGy in 180-cGy to 200-cGy fractions to the prostate and regional pelvic lymph nodes. A subsequent boost of 2000 cGy was given to the prostate and periprostatic tissues. Patients treated with mixed-beam irradiation received a dose of 5000-cGy "photon equivalent," followed by a similar 2000-cGy photon-equivalent boost, using the alternating schedule of neutrons and photons outlined earlier.

With a median follow-up time approaching 10 years, 91% of the neutron-treated patients remained clinically free of local tumor recurrence compared with 78% of the patients treated with photons alone (Fig. 14-21). This difference is statistically significant ($P<0.01$). Although no standard approach to routine posttreatment biopsy was mandated in this study, 16 patients had second prostate biopsies a minimum of 2 years after treatment while in clinical remission. Combining the pathologic criterion of a positive biopsy with the clinical criteria, 79% of the neutron-treated patients and 62% of the photon-treated patients remained free of local disease. These differences remain statistically significant ($P=0.02$), and the positive biopsy rate for photon-treated patients is consistent with other reports in the literature (Fig. 14-22).

Survival data are graphically displayed in Figure 14-23: 71% of the neutron-treated group were alive at 5 years but only 55% of the photon-treated cohort were alive, and 46% of the neutron-treated group were alive at 10 years, compared with 32% of the photon-treated cohort ($P=0.06$). There were a large number of intercurrent deaths on this study, presumably because of the advanced average age of the patients entered. If intercurrent deaths from causes other than prostate cancer are excluded, the corresponding disease-specific survival data for the neutron-treated group of patients is 82%, compared with 54% for the photon-treated group. The difference remains statistically significant ($P=0.02$).

A stepwise Cox analysis showed that the most significant factor associated with patient survival was type of treatment (mixed beam versus photons, $P<0.01$). The second most significant factor was patient age ($P<0.05$). No significant differences were noted for acute or late normal tissue toxicities.

In Europe, prostate clinical trials involving irradiation with fast neutrons have been carried out primarily in the cyclotron facilities at Louvain-la-Neuve, Belgium, and at Hamburg, Germany. In the Belgian experience,[70] a neutron regimen similar to the Radiation Therapy Oncology Group mixed-beam approach was employed, but combining photons with high-energy 65-MeV p→Be neutrons allowed better delivery of a neutron dose to greater tissue depths. Accordingly, three treatments a week

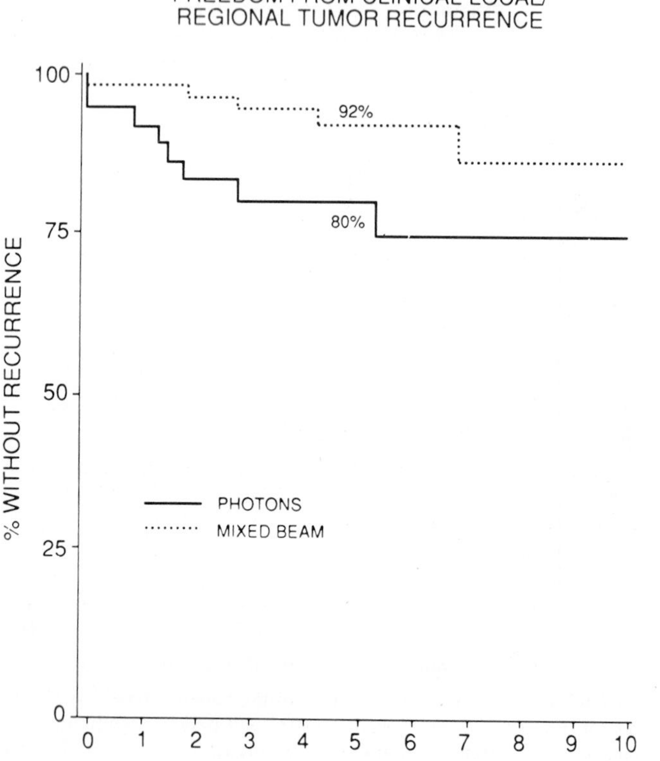

FIGURE 14–21. Freedom from clinical locoregional tumor recurrence as a function of treatment. The two curves are different at the $P < 0.01$ level.

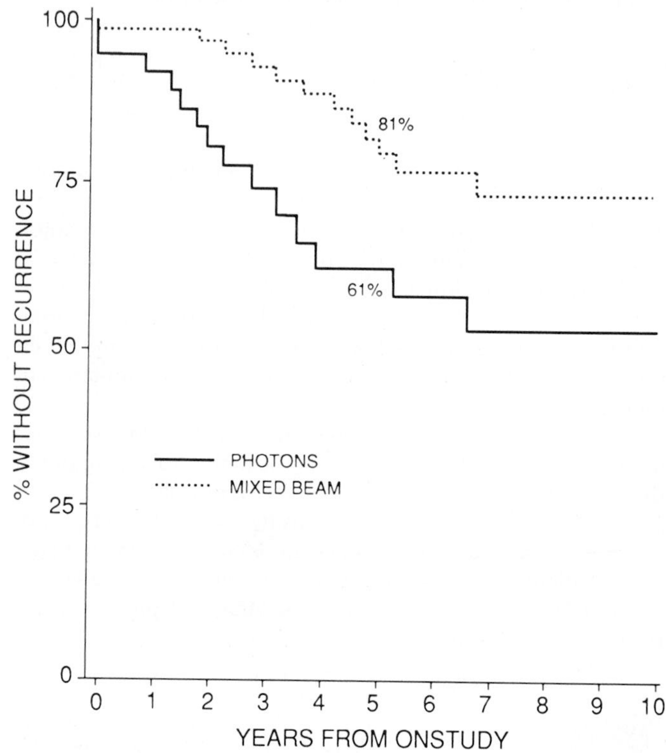

FIGURE 14–22. Freedom from locoregional tumor recurrence or persistence, including results of posttreatment biopsies as a function of treatment. The two curves are different at the $P = 0.02$ level.

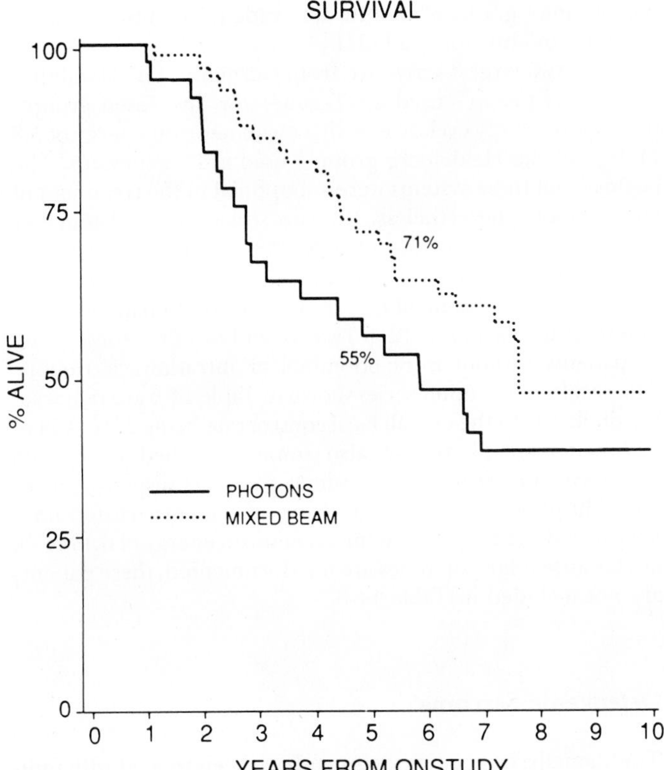

FIGURE 14–23. Patient survival as a function of treatment. The two curves are different at the $P = 0.06$ level.

(or 60% of the total treatment) were composed of neutrons, a prominent alteration from the 40% neutron contribution in the mixed-beam treatment used in the Radiation Therapy Oncology Group trial. Treatment to the pelvis was carried to a total dose of 5000-cGy photon equivalent, and the prostate received an additional 1600-cGy photon equivalent boost. Patients were treated in a phase II setting without any intended randomization. At the time of last analysis, treated patients numbered 50, with a distribution of 14 Stage A, 130 Stage C, and 6 Stage D2 patients. Twenty-eight of the Stage C patients had been followed up for a minimum of 1 year. Local control rates of 93% and 90% were reported at 1 and 3 years, respectively, in the Stage C patients, with 28 and ten patients available for analysis at these times. Seven of the ten patients followed for 3 years are alive and without evidence of disease. Complications in this group of patients have been minimal, with only one patient having a urethral stricture.

The group in Hamburg reported similarly encouraging results.[33] Originally, a mixed-beam schedule was employed, combining 14-MeV (deuterium-tritium) neutrons and megavoltage photons. Pelvic nodes were treated with photons alone, to a total of 3000 cGy to 4500 cGy over 3 to 4.5 weeks at conventional 200-cGy/day fractions. The boost dose to the prostate was carried out with neutrons alone, treating eight isocentrically centered fields a day, for three treatments each week, for a total neutron boost of 390 cGy to 840 cGy (approximately 1200-cGy to 2600-cGy photon equivalent). The treatment of 13 Stage C (UICC Stage T3NX-2MX-0 and T4NX-2MX-0) tumors was well tolerated, with all patients achieving complete tumor regression, and with no patient suffering adverse long-term reactions. An update of this experience reported 5-year survival figures for the 12 evaluable patients, with seven (85%) of the patients with T3 tumors alive and five (20%) of the patients with T4 disease alive.[31] No adverse sequelae of neutron treatment in the form of bowel, bladder, or intestinal complications were observed in these patients.

At Chiba University in Japan, 26 patients received primary radiation therapy consisting of fast neutrons alone (15 patients) or mixed-beam radiation (11 patients).[62] Treatment fields encompassed the pelvic nodes, with a subsequent boost to the prostate (16 patients) or were limited to the prostate alone (ten patients). A number of radiation doses were employed, reported as time-dose-fractionation values, in the range of 98 to 124. For the 14 patients with Stage C tumors, a 77% 3-year survival rate was reported.

A successor study to the U.S. cooperative mixed-beam study was initiated with patients with stages B2 (Gleason pattern score >6), C, and D1 adenocarcinomas of the prostate. Surgical staging of pelvic lymph nodes is encouraged, and patients are subjected to routine biopsies 2 years after treatment. Patients randomized to neutrons receive treatments three times weekly, 10 cGy per fraction, for a total dose of 1360 cGy to the pelvis and 2040 cGy to the prostate. These neutron doses were chosen as maximally tolerated safe doses based on data previously collected in phase I dose-searching protocols investigating tolerance of pelvic tissues to high-energy fast neutrons. Neutron treatments are therefore completed in 12 fractions over 4 weeks, compared with the 35 fractions in 7 weeks required to complete photon irradiation.

As of October 1989, 167 patients were entered into this collaborative trial. As of 1990, acute reactions among the patients treated with high-energy neutrons have been reasonable, and patient acceptance of the rapid treatment course has been high.

Soft Tissue Sarcomas

Currently surgery is the main form of treatment for soft tissue sarcomas, with radiation therapy and chemotherapy being relegated to "adjuvant" status. The local recurrence rate after conservation surgery alone is about 50%, and the use of radiation therapy either preoperatively or postoperatively reduces the recurrence to approximately 10%.

The effectiveness of chemotherapy in preventing or eradicating distant metastases is less clear. For adjuvant photon or electron irradiation to be effective, it is generally thought that all gross tumor must be excised. The problem with this approach is that most types of soft tissue sarcomas tend to infiltrate along tissue planes or beyond obvious tumor margins and become quite extensive before discovery. This is especially true for lesions of the trunk, retroperitoneum, or proximal thigh.

Reported series of inoperable tumors treated definitively with radiation therapy tend to be rather small and contain many histologic subtypes, grades, and stages. The focus is local tumor control rather than survival. The results of definitive radiation therapy for soft tissue sarcomas are summarized in Table 14-6. The neutron experience is summarized in the upper portion of the table and photon and electron experience in the lower portion.

The photon experience in the treatment of this disease dates back to Windeyer and others[79] in 1966. They treated 11 patients *de novo* and 11 with high-dose irradiation after a postsurgical recurrence. All patients had fibrosarcomas. Their overall control rate was 59%. McNeer and colleagues[64] treated 25 patients with mixed histologies and found an overall local control rate of 56%. Duncan and Dewar reported 25 patients with

TABLE 14–6
Local Control Rates for Soft-Tissue Sarcomas Treated Definitively with Radiation Therapy

INVESTIGATION*	LOCAL CONTROL (PATIENTS)	LOCAL CONTROL (RATE)
NEUTRONS		
Hammersmith[15]	26/50	52%
NIRS[86]	7/12	58%
Fermi Laboratory[18]	13/26	50%
MANTA[67]	4/10	40%
TAMVEC[72]	18/29	62%
Edinburgh[23]	5/12	42%
Hamberg/Eppendorf[32]	27/45	60%
Heidelberg/Essen[75]	31/60	52%
Louvain[90]	4/19	21%
Amsterdam[3]	8/13	61%
Seattle[55]†	15/21	71%
Total	158/297	53%
PHOTONS/ELECTRONS		
McNeer[64]	14/25	56%
Windeyer[91]	13/22	59%
Duncan[23]	5/25	20%
Tepper[84]	17/51	33%
Leibel[60]	0/5	0%
Total	49/128	38%

* *Patients treated* de novo *or for gross disease after surgery are included but not patients treated postoperatively for microscopic residual disease or for limited macroscopic residual disease.*
† *Two-year actuarial data.*

very extensive tumors treated with low-LET irradiation in whom the overall local control rate was 20%.[23] They remarked that an amputation was the only alternative form of treatment. The most recent report is by Tepper and Suit,[83] who found a 33% local control rate at 5 years in a group of 51 patients treated with irradiation alone. For patients receiving >6400 cGy, the local control rate was 43.5%. The local control rate varied as a function of the lesion size: 87.5% for lesions <5 cm, 53% for lesions 5 cm to 10 cm, and 30% for lesions >10 cm. This underscores the importance of using adequate radiation doses and the difficulty of comparing series dealing with different patient populations. The summed local control rate for all the series was 38% (49 of 128).

Paradoxically, although fast-neutron irradiation is a newer form of radiation therapy practiced at a relatively small number of centers throughout the world, the number of definitively treated patients was about 2.5 times that of patients treated with photons with or without electrons. If neutrons alone were used, doses ranged from 1560 cGy to 2600 cGy, and fields were in general designed to cover the tumor volume plus a reasonable margin. The time at which the local control rate was quoted varied from series to series, but in general it was for periods greater than 2 years.

The most recently published series is from Hammersmith.[13] It reports a local control rate of 52% (26 of 50 patients). Twenty patients were treated for recurrent tumors after previous surgery or radiation therapy, and 62% of the tumors were >10 cm in diameter. The main cause of death was metastatic disease, and the median survival was strongly a function of tumor grade: 63 months for grade I, 7 months for grade II, and 9 months for grade III.

The two largest series are from Germany. The Hamburg-Eppendorf group[26] used a dT generator, the Essen group[25] used a low-energy cyclotron with a mean neutron energy of 5.8 MeV, and the Heidelberg group[65] used a dT generator. The beams from these systems were suboptimal in the treatment of large tumors; nevertheless, the two series summed together show a local control rate of 55% (58 of 105 patients). The highest-energy neutron beam was used at Fermi Laboratory,[18] producing a local control rate of 50% (13 of 26 patients). The lowest local control rate (21%) was from Louvain[79] for a group of patients without intraabdominal or intrathoracic tumors. The results of the other series shown in Table 14-6 are remarkably similar, with the overall local control rate being 53% (158 of 297 patients). There are also some published data from Eichhorn and colleagues[23] showing a complete response rate of 48% (39 of 82 patients) in a group of patients treated on a Soviet-made 4120 cyclotron (mean neutron energy of 6.1 MeV), but because follow-up times are not documented, these patients are not included in Table 14-6.

Osteogenic Sarcoma

Traditionally, osteogenic sarcomas have been treated with radical surgery, often an amputative procedure. Chemotherapy is currently being used to forestall metastatic dissemination. However, for tumors arising in the axial skeleton, radical surgery may not be possible. In patients with distant metastases at diagnosis, radical radiation therapy would be an acceptable alternate form of treatment if local control could be achieved with reasonable morbidity. Unfortunately, conventional radiation therapy for these lesions requires quite high radiation doses.

DeMoor[19] described a series of 43 patients treated with 6600 cGy to 7700 cGy over 6 to 8 weeks. All patients with lower extremity lesions who were followed for more than 1 year had pronounced subcutaneous fibrosis and partial flexion ankylosis of the knee. Eleven required an amputation, and no tumor was present in the operative specimens of three patients. In another three patients, there were significant radiation-induced changes, and tumor cells of questionable viability were seen during pathologic examination. The net local control rate was 33% (nine of 43 patients).

Beck and associates[5] reported a series of 21 patients treated at the University of California at San Francisco. They had only one long-term survivor with local control. This patient had a lesion of the mandible and received 5200-cGy external-beam therapy and an additional 5600 cGy by means of an implant. Tudway[76] reported nine patients treated with orthovoltage radiation to doses of 5500 cGy to 8000 cGy. The local control rate was 56% (five of nine patients), but three patients had sequelae that restricted motion of the involved extremities. The photon data are summarized in the lower half of Table 14-7. The overall local control rate in the photon-treated patients was 21% (15 of 73 patients).

A total of 73 patients have received high-dose neutron therapy for osteogenic sarcomas. These data are summarized in the upper half of Table 14-7. The largest series is from the NIRS facility in Japan.[49] These patients were treated with chemotherapy (*i.e.*, doxorubicin, vincristine sulfate, and high-dose methotrexate) and with irradiation. Seventeen patients later underwent an amputation or a second-look incisional biopsy. Fifteen (88%) of the 17 patients were found to be histologically

TABLE 14–7
Local Control Rates for Osteogenic Sarcomas Treated Definitively with Radiation Therapy

INVESTIGATION*	LOCAL CONTROL (PATIENTS)	LOCAL CONTROL (RATE)
NEUTRONS		
MANTA[67]	1/1	100%
TAMVEC[72]	0/1	0%
Fermi Laboratory[18]	2/9	22%
Amsterdam[3]	0/3	0%†
Edinburgh[21]	1/5	20%†
NIRS[49]	33/41	80%
Seattle[55]‡	3/13	23%
Total	40/73	55%
PHOTONS		
DeMoor[19]	9/43	33%
Beck[5]	1/21	5%
Tudway[87]	5/9	56%
Total	15/73	21%

** Patients treated postoperatively for microscopic residual disease or for limited macroscopic residual disease are not included.*
† Persistent mass and calcification treated as failure; local control rates may be underestimated.
‡ Two-year actuarial data.

free of viable tumor. The three failures in the Amsterdam series[2] and the four failures in the Edinburgh series[22] were classified as such because of persistent mass and calcification. Because it is doubtful that the osteoid matrix left behind would resolve even if the tumor cells were sterilized, these reports may have underestimated the local control rates. The one treatment "success" in the Edinburgh series died of metastatic disease; an autopsy confirmed tumor control in the two treated regions.

An updated report from Japan does not discuss local control at all, but instead focuses on survival.[83] Forty-eight patients who were treated with fast neutrons had a 5-year survival rate of 67%, compared with 19% in a group of 17 patients treated with photon irradiation. However, it was not a randomized trial. The incidence of late skin reactions was found to be equivalent in the two groups. The overall local control rate for the summed series of patients was 55% (40 of 73 patients).

Chondrosarcoma

The literature on the results of radical photon irradiation for chondrosarcomas is rather sparse. McNaney and associates[63] reported ten patients who were definitively treated at M.D. Anderson. They determined treatment failure by progressing symptoms or increasing size of the lesion. The local control rate was 30% (three of ten patients). The same group reported a local control rate of 100% for four patients treated with fast neutrons at the TAMVEC facility.[63] Three of the photon failures occurred at quite long times after treatment: 42 months, 132 months, and 156 months. The neutron-treated patients have not been at risk for these long periods.

Harwood and colleagues[48] reported local control in seven (35%) of 20 patients who were definitively treated with megavoltage photon therapy at Princess Margaret Hospital. They noted that the clinical response of the tumors took many months to complete. Radiographically, the affected bone never returned to normal. They concluded that chondrosarcomas should not be classified as radioresistant and that radical irradiation has a definite role in selected cases. The data on photon irradiation for this tumor are summarized in the lower portion of Table 14-8. The overall photon local control rate is 33% (ten of 30 patients).

The neutron experience for chondrosarcoma is summarized in the upper portion of Table 14-8. The overall local control rate is 49% (25 of 51 patients) despite two series showing no local control in any of the treated patients. Both of these groups counted persistent mass and calcification as failures, when this may not be the case. A chondroid matrix is elaborated by these tumors and is left behind after radiation therapy regardless of whether the tumor cells are sterilized. Therefore, the overall figure of 49% is probably an underestimate of the effectiveness of fast-neutron irradiation for this class of tumor.

Other Tumor Sites

Neutron studies have been carried out for tumors of the esophagus, breast, pancreas, bladder, and cervix.[80] Although some of the early results from these studies look promising, no definitive advantages have yet been demonstrated for neutrons in these sites.

CLINICAL STUDIES EMPLOYING HEAVY CHARGED PARTICLES

Neutrons (uncharged particles) were introduced into clinical therapy at the Radiation Laboratory of the University of California shortly after the development of the cyclotron by Ernest Lawrence. Radiation therapy with charged particles was also first suggested by physicists. However, despite two decades of small-volume treatment of pituitary diseases, study of large-

TABLE 14–8
Local Control Rates for Chondrosarcomas Treated Definitively with Radiation Therapy

INVESTIGATION*	LOCAL CONTROL (PATIENTS)	LOCAL CONTROL (RATE)
NEUTRONS		
MANTA[67]	7/9	78%
TAMVEC[72]	4/4	100%
Fermi Laboratory[18]	9/16	56%
Amsterdam[3]	0/6	0%†
Edinburgh[21]	0/5	0%†
NIRS[49]	1/2	50%
Seattle[55]‡	4/9	44%
Total	25/51	49%
PHOTONS		
McNanny[63]	3/10	30%
Harwood[48]	7/20	35%
Total	10/30	33%

** Patients treated postoperatively for microscopic residual disease or for limited macroscopic residual disease are not included.*
† Persistent mass and calcification treated as failure. Hence, local control rates may be underestimated.
‡ Two-year actuarial data.

TABLE 14–9
Proton and Helium Ion Therapy of Choroidal Melanoma

TUMOR SIZE	TOTAL NUMBER OF PATIENTS	PATIENT STATUS*	
		LOCAL CONTROL	DISTANT METASTASIS
Small (<10 × 2 mm)			
Protons	24	23	0
Helium ions	2	2	1
Medium (10–15 × 2–5 mm)			
Protons	198	195	4
Helium ions	65	61	1
Large (>15 × >5 mm)			
Protons	244	242	22
Helium	123	116	16
Total	656	639	44

** Minimum 1-year follow-up.*
(From Castro JR, Chen GTY, Pitluck S, et al: Am J Clin Oncol 6:629, 1983; Richard F, Renard L, Wambersie A: Bull Cancer [Paris] 73:562, 1986)

field, charged-particle cancer therapy did not begin until the mid-1970s.

American clinical trials began in 1975 with helium ions (α-particles) at the University of California Lawrence Berkeley Laboratory and at the Harvard cyclotron using protons (hydrogen nuclei).[81] Introduced in 1976 were pi mesons (subatomic particles) at the Los Alamos Scientific Laboratory and, from 1977 to 1981, heavier nuclei, such as carbon, neon, and silicon at the Lawrence Berkeley Laboratory.[17,37]

The U.S. experience with protons and helium ions has now reached over 1000 patients, while pions and heavier ions have each been used in about 250 patients.[9–13,86] Because of limitations on beam availability and the need to develop new pioneering treatment techniques, accumulation of clinical data has been slow.

Precision High-Dose Charged-Particle Therapy

The results of precision high-dose proton and helium treatment of selected malignant tumors, such as melanoma of the uveal tract of the eye and tumors lying close to the spinal cord or base of the brain, are shown in Tables 14-9 and 14-10.

These patients had chordomas, low-grade chondrosarcomas, or meningiomas lying at the base of the brain or near the spinal cord that could not have complete surgical extirpation, and conventional radiation therapy could not deliver a sufficiently high tumor dose without serious risk of severe complications. With charged-particle therapy, tumor doses of 6000 to 7500 ^{60}Co-equivalent cGy (particle cGy equivalent to low-LET cobalt or x-ray treatment) have been given in 25 to 35 fractions over 6 to 8 weeks (Fig. 14-24). Local control rates have been high; however, many patients have had low-grade malignancies with slow growth patterns, and many years of follow-up are needed to evaluate tumor control and complications.

Many patients have been treated with protons and helium ions for arteriovenous malformations in phase II studies. Although more follow-up is needed, the early results have been highly encouraging.[53] Other studies are ongoing for carcinomas of the brain, head and neck, lung, retroperitoneum, and prostate and for sarcomas in selected anatomic sites.

TABLE 14–10
Proton and Helium Ion Therapy for Tumors of Base of Skull or Cervical Spine Abutting CNS

HISTOLOGY	TOTAL NUMBER OF PATIENTS	MEAN FOLLOW-UP (MONTHS)	PATIENT STATUS*		
			LOCAL CONTROL	MARGINAL FAILURE	DISTANT METASTASIS
PROTONS					
Chordoma, chondrosarcoma	88	26	78	4	2
Meningioma, craniopharyngioma	19	23	18		
Total	107	25	96	4	2
HELIUM IONS					
Chordoma, chondrosarcoma	24	24	16		3
Meningioma, craniopharyngioma	10	27	9		
Total	38	25	25		3

** Follow-up of 6 to 98 months.*
(From Castro JR, Chen GTY, Pitluck S, et al: Am J Clin Oncol 6:629, 1983; Richard F, Renard L, Wambersie A: Bull Cancer [Paris] 73:562, 1986)

TABLE 14–11
Results of Fast Neutron Clinical Trials

SITE/HISTOLOGY	NUMBER OF PATIENTS	RESULTS*
Salivary gland	280	++++ positive
Prostate cancer	285	+++ positive
Bone sarcomas	75	++ positive
Soft tissue sarcomas	350	++ positive
Squamous cell head and neck cancer	>2000	equivocal
Lung	425	equivocal
Bladder	160	equivocal
Cervix	260	equivocal
Brain	>600	negative
Esophagus	120	negative
Pancreas	>100	negative

** Patients were treated with physics-laboratory-based fixed beam machines.*

High-LET Charged Particles

Phase I and II studies have been carried out with negative pions and carbon, neon, and silicon ions.[82] At the present time, studies are centered on neon ions in the United States and negative pions in Canada and Switzerland. Carcinomas of the brain, head and neck, esophagus, lung, pancreas, stomach, and biliary tract and sarcomas of various sites have been studied.[9] The impression is that promising results have been observed in patients with sarcoma of soft tissue and bone, tumors of the head and neck, unresectable carcinoma of the lung, and locally advanced carcinoma of the prostate.[13] However, these impressions are based on small numbers of patients. Phase III trials are in progress.

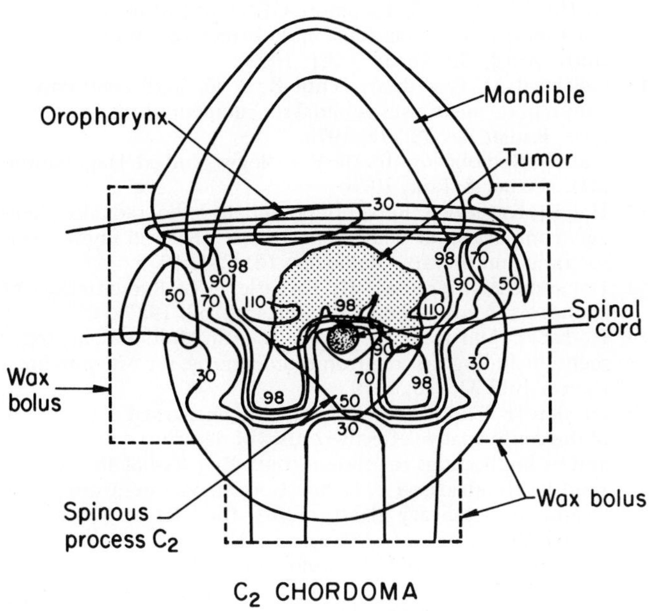

FIGURE 14–24. Composite treatment plan for precision high-dose helium irradiation of a chordoma of the upper cervical spine.

FUTURE DIRECTIONS

The biologic advantages of high-LET radiations, compared with low-LET radiations, can be summarized as a decreased oxygen enhancement ratio, a diminished capacity for cellular sublethal damage repair, a diminished capacity for potentially lethal damage repair, and diminished variability of radiosensitivity of cells in different stages of the cell cycle. These advantages led to the neutron and high-LET charged particle trials outlined in the preceding pages. A summary of these and other neutron trials is given in Table 14-11. Dose distribution advantages led to the low-LET charged particle trials.

Until recently, heavy-particle radiation research has been limited by equipment availability and versatility. Laboratory-based, fixed-horizontal-beam machines placed a severe handicap on the development of these treatment modalities.[67] The installation of hospital-based, high-energy cyclotrons capable of isocentric beam delivery for neutrons and the development of a hospital-based synchrotron capable of isocentric proton therapy have greatly improved the situation; however, cost and size considerations still make these machines impractical for most hospital settings. New developments in superconducting technology suggest a future of small, relatively inexpensive particle accelerators suitable for heavy-particle radiation therapy. If this promise is realized, therapy with protons, neutrons, and heavy ions may become practical for a large number of treatment centers.[93]

REFERENCES

1. Battermann JJ, Mijnheer BJ: The Amsterdam fast neutron radiotherapy project: A final report. Int J Radiat Oncol Biol Phys 12:2093, 1986
2. Battermann JJ, Breur K: Results of fast neutron teletherapy for locally advanced head and neck tumors. Int J Radiat Oncol Biol Phys 7:1045, 1981
3. Battermann JJ, Breur K: Fast neutron therapy for locally advanced sarcomas. Int J Radiat Oncol Biol Phys 7:1051, 1981
4. Battermann JJ, Breur K, Hart BAM, et al: Observations on pulmonary metastases in patients after single doses and multiple fractions of fast neutrons and cobalt-60 gamma rays. Eur J Cancer 17:539, 1981
5. Beck JC, Wara WM, Bovill Jr EG, et al: The role of radiation therapy in the treatment of osteosarcoma. Radiology 120:163, 1976

6. Borthne A, Kjellevold K, Kaalhus O, et al: Salivary gland malignant neoplasms: treatment and prognosis. Int J Radiat Oncol Biol Phys 12:747, 1986
7. Brennan JT, Phillips TL: Evaluation of past experience with fast neutron teletherapy and its implications for future applications. Eur J Cancer 7:219, 1971
8. Breteau N, Distembert B, Sabattier R, et al: An interim assessment of the experience of fast neutron boost in glioblastomas, rectal and bronchus carcinomas in Orleans. Strahlentherapie 161:787, 1985
9. Castro JR: Heavy charged particle irradiation of human cancers. In Radiation Medicine, vol 1, pp 70–75. Tokyo, Japan, Radiation Medicine Association, University of Tokyo, 1983
10. Castro JR, Chen GTY, Pitluck S, et al: Helium charged particle radiotherapy of locally advanced carcinoma of the esophagus, stomach and biliary tract. Am J Clin Oncol 6:629, 1983
11. Castro JR, Saunders WM, Quivey JM, et al: Clinical problems in radiotherapy of carcinoma of the pancreas. Am J Clin Oncol 5:579, 1982
12. Castro JR, Saunders WM, Tobias CA, et al: Treatment of cancer with heavy charged particles. Int J Radiat Oncol Biol Phys 8:2191, 1982
13. Castro JR, Quivey JM, Lyman JT, et al: Current status of clinical particle radiotherapy at Lawrence Berkeley Laboratory. Cancer 46:633, 1980
14. Catterall M: The treatment of malignant salivary gland tumors with fast neutrons. Int J Radiat Oncol Biol Phys 7:1737, 1981
15. Catterall M: The treatment of advanced cancer by fast neutrons from the Medical Research Council's cyclotron at Hammersmith Hospital, London. Eur J Cancer 10:343, 1974
16. Catterall M, Bewley DK: Fast Neutrons in the Treatment of Cancer, pp 14–27. London, Academic Press, 1973
17. Catterall M, Bewley DK, Sutherland I: Second report on a randomized clinical trial of fast neutrons with x or gamma rays in the treatment of advanced cancers of the head and neck. Br Med J 1:1942, 1977
18. Cohen L, Hendrickson F, Mansell J, et al: Response of sarcomas of bone and soft tissue to neutron beam therapy. Int J Radiat Oncol Biol Phys 10:821, 1984
19. deMoor NG: Osteosarcoma: A review of 72 cases treated by megavoltage radiation therapy with or without surgery. S Afr J Surg 13:137, 1975
20. Dobrowsky W, Schlappack O, Karcher KH, et al: Electron beam therapy in treatment of parotid neoplasm. Radiother Oncol 6:293, 1986
21. Duncan W, Arnott SJ, Jack WJL: The Edinburgh experience of treating sarcomas of soft tissue and bone with neutron irradiation. Clin Radiol 37:317, 1986
22. Duncan W, Orr JA, Arnott SJ, et al: Neutron therapy for malignant tumors of the salivary gland. A report of the Edinburgh experience. Radiother Oncol 8:97, 1987
23. Duncan W, Dewar JA: A retrospective study of the role of radiotherapy in the treatment of soft-tissue sarcoma. Clin Radiol 36:629, 1985
24. Duncan W, Arnott SJ, Batterman JJ, et al: Fast neutrons in the treatment of advanced head and neck cancers: The results of a multi-centre randomly controlled trial. Radiother Oncol 2:293, 1984
25. Duncan W, Arnott SJ, Orr JA, et al: The Edinburgh experience of fast neutron therapy. Int J Radiat Oncol Biol Phys 8:2155, 1982
26. Eichhorn HJ, Lessel A, Matschke S: Comparison between neutron therapy and ^{60}Co gamma ray therapy of bronchial, gastric and oesophagus carcinomata. Eur J Cancer 10:361, 1974
27. Eichhorn HJ: Results of a pilot study on neutron therapy with 600 patients. Int J Radiat Oncol Biol Phys 8:1561, 1982
28. Eichhorn HJ: Pilot study on the applicability of neutron radiotherapy. Radiobiol Radiother 3:262, 1981
29. Elkon D, Colman J, Hendrickson FR: Radiation therapy in the treatment of malignant salivary gland tumors. Cancer 41:502, 1978
30. Fitzpatrick PJ, Theriault C: Malignant salivary gland tumors. Int J Radiat Oncol Biol Phys 12:1743, 1986
31. Franke HD, Schmidt R: Clinical results with fast neutrons (DT, 14 MeV). Radiat Med 3:151, 1985
32. Franke HD, Hess A, Brassow F, et al: Clinical results after irradiation of intracranial tumors, soft tissue sarcomas, and thyroid cancers with fast neutrons at Hamburg-Eppendorf. In Karcher KH (ed): Progress in Radio-Oncology II, pp 123–137. New York, Raven Press, 1982
33. Franke HD, Hess A, Langendorff G, et al: The combined treatment of prostate cancer (stage C) with definitive megavoltage irradiation and fast neutrons (DT, 14 MeV). Urologe 19:341, 1980
34. Fu KK, Leibel SA, Levine MG, et al: Carcinoma of the major and minor salivary glands: Analysis of treatment results and sites and causes of failure. Cancer 40:2882, 1977
35. Gragg RL, Humphrey RM, Meyn RE; The response of Chinese hamster ovary cells to fast neutron radiotherapy beams. II. Sublethal and potentially lethal damage recovery capabilities. Radiat Res 71:461, 1977
36. Gragg RL, Humphrey RM, Thomas HT, et al: The response of Chinese hamster ovary cells to fast neutron radiotherapy beams. I. Variations in relative biologic effectiveness with position in the cell cycle. Radiat Res 76:283, 1978
37. Gray LH, Conger AE, Ebert M, et al: Concentration of oxygen dissolved in tissues at time of irradiation as factor in radiotherapy. Br J Radiol 26:638, 1953
38. Griffin TW, Pajak TF, Maor MH, et al: Mixed neutron/photon irradiation of unresectable squamous cell carcinomas of the head and neck: The final report of a randomized cooperative trial. Int J Radiat Oncol Biol Phys 17:959, 1989
39. Griffin TW, Pajak TF, Laramore GE, et al: Neutron vs photon irradiation of inoperable salivary gland tumors: Results of an RTOG-MRC cooperative randomized study. Int J Radiat Oncol Biol Phys 15:1085, 1988
40. Griffin TW, Wambersie A, Laramore GE, et al: High LET: Heavy particle trials. Int J Radiat Oncol Biol Phys 14:583, 1988
41. Griffin BR, Laramore GE, Russell KJ, et al: Fast neutron radiotherapy for advanced malignant salivary gland tumors. Radiother Oncol 12:105, 1988
42. Griffin TW, Davis R, Hendrickson FR: Fast neutron radiation therapy for unresectable squamous cell carcinomas of the head and neck: The results of a randomized RTOG study. Int J Radiat Oncol Biol Phys 10:2217, 1984
43. Griffin TW, Davis R, Laramore GE, et al: Fast neutron irradiation of metastatic cervical adenopathy: the results of a randomized RTOG study. Int J Radiat Oncol Biol Phys 9:1267, 1983
44. Griffin TW, Davis R, Laramore GE, et al: Fast neutron radiation therapy for glioblastoma multiforme: Results of an RTOG study. Am J Clin Oncol 6:661, 1983
45. Guichard M, Courdi A, Fentil B, et al: Radiosensitivity of lymph node metastases vs initial subcutaneous tumors in nude mice. Radiat Res 78:278, 1979
46. Hall EJ: Radiobiology for the Radiologist, 2nd ed. Hagerstown, MD, Harper & Row, 1978
47. Hall EJ, Kraljevic J: Repair of potentially lethal radiation damage: comparison of neutron and x-ray RBE and implications for radiation therapy. Radiology 121:731, 1976
48. Harwood AR, Krajbich JI, Fornasier VL: Radiotherapy of chondrosarcoma of bone. Cancer 45:2769, 1980
49. Hodaka E, Maruyama K, Takada N, et al: Multimodality treatment, including fast neutron radiotherapy, for osteosarcoma. Cancer Bull 31:216, 1979
50. Howlett JF, Thomlinson RH, Alper T: A marked dependence of the conformative effective causes of neutrons on tumor line and its implications for clinical trials. Br J Radiol 48:40, 1975
51. Kaul R, Hendrickson F, Cohen L, et al: Fast neutrons in the treatment of salivary gland tumors. Int J Radiat Oncol Biol Phys 7:1667, 1981
52. Kernohan JW, Sayre GP: Tumors of the central nervous system. In Atlas of Tumor Pathology, sec. 10, fasc. 35 and 37, pp 17–42. Washington DC, Armed Forces Institute of Pathology, 1952
53. Kjellberg R, Hanamura T, Davis K, et al: Bragg peak proton beam therapy for arteriovenous malformations of the brain. New Engl J Med 309:269, 1983
54. Komaki R, Mountain LF, Holbert JM, et al: Superior sulcus tumors: Treatment selection and results in 85 patients without

distant metastasis (M_0) at presentation. Int J Radiat Oncol Biol Phys 17:157, 1989
55. Laramore GE, Griffeth JT, Boespflug M, et al: Fast neutron radiotherapy for sarcomas of soft tissue, bone, and cartilage. Am J Clin Oncol 12:320, 1989
56. Laramore GE, Bauer M, Griffin TW, et al: Fast neutron and mixed beam radiotherapy for inoperable non-small cell carcinoma of the lung: results of an RTOG randomized study. Am J Clin Oncol 9:233, 1986
57. Laramore GE, Griffin TW, Gerdes AJ, et al: Fast neutron and mixed (neutron/photon) beam teletherapy for grades III and IV astrocytomas. Cancer 42:96, 1978
58. Laramore GE, Griffin TW, Maor MH: Mixed beam radiation therapy for carcinoma of the prostate: The results of a randomized RTOG study. Int J Radiat Oncol Biol Phys 112:1621, 1985
59. Laramore GE, Griffin TW, Tesh DW, et al: Phase I pilot study on fast neutron teletherapy for advanced carcinoma of the head and neck region: Final report on local control rate and survival. Cancer 51:192, 1983
60. Leibel SA, Tranbaugh RF, Ware WM, et al: Soft tissue sarcomas of the extremities: Survival and patterns of failure with conservative surgery with postoperative irradiation compared to surgery alone. Cancer 56:475, 1985
61. Maor MH, Hussey DH, Fletcher GH, et al: Fast neutron therapy for locally advanced head and neck tumors. Int J Radiat Oncol Biol Phys 7:155, 1981
62. Maruoka M, Ando K, Nozumi K, et al: Fast neutron therapy of prostatic cancer (Japanese). Nippon Hinyokika Gakkai Zasshi 74:409, 1983
63. McNaney D, Lindberg RD, Ayala AG, et al: Fifteen-year radiotherapy experience with chondrosarcoma of bone. Int J Radiat Oncol Biol Phys 8:187, 1982
64. McNeer GP, Cantin J, Chu F, et al: Effectiveness of radiation therapy in the management of sarcoma of the soft somatic tissues. Cancer 22:391, 1968
65. Nelson JS, Schoenfeld D, Tsukada Y, et al: Necrosis as a prognostic criterion in malignant, supratentorial astrocytic gliomas. Cancer 52:550, 1983
66. Ngo FQH, Blakely EA, Tobias CA: Sequential exposures of mammalian cells to low and high-LET radiation. I. Lethal effects following x-ray and neon ion irradiation. Radiat Res 87:59, 1981
67. Ornitz R, Herskovic A, Bradley E: Clinical observations of early and late normal tissue injury and tumor control in patients receiving fast neutron irradiation. In Barendsen GW, Broerse J, Breur K (eds): High LET Radiations in Clinical Radiotherapy, pp 44–50. New York, Pergamon Press, 1979
68. Rafla S: Malignant parotid tumors: Natural history and treatment. Cancer 40:136, 1977
69. Reddy EK, Mansfield CM, Hartman GV, et al: Malignant salivary gland tumors: role of radiation therapy. JAMA 71:959, 1979
70. Richard F, Renard L, Wambersie A: Current results of neutron therapy at the UCL for soft tissue sarcomas and prostatic adenocarcinomas. Bull Cancer (Paris) 73:562, 1986
71. Rossman KJ: The role of radiation therapy in the treatment of parotid carcinomas. Am J Radiol 123:492, 1975
72. Salinas R, Hussey DH, Fletcher GH: Experience with fast neutron therapy for locally advanced sarcomas. Int J Radiat Oncol Biol Phys 6:267, 1980
73. Saroja KR, Mansell J, Hendrickson F, et al: An update on malignant salivary gland tumors treated with neutrons at Fermilab. Int J Radiat Oncol Biol Phys 13:1319, 1987
74. Sawada K, Fukuma S, Seki Y, et al: Clinical experience in patients with Pancoast's tumor treated by fast neutron radiotherapy. Gan No Rinsho A7:111, 1983
75. Schmitt G, Schnabel K, Sauerwein W, et al: Neutron and neutron-boost irradiation of soft tissue sarcomas: A 4.5 year analysis of 139 patients. Radiother Oncol 1:23, 1983
76. Schnabel K, Dari S, Hover KH, et al: Radiation therapy of bronchogenic carcinoma with a neutron generator. In Karcher KH, Kogelnik H, Reinartz G (eds): Progress in Radio-Oncology II, pp 139–144. New York, Raven Press, 1982
77. Shidnia H, Hornback NB, Hamaker R, et al: Carcinoma of major salivary glands. Cancer 45:693, 1980
78. Skolyszewski J, Byrski E, Chrzanowska A, et al: A preliminary report on the clinical application of fast neutrons in Krakow. Int J Radiat Oncol Biol Phys 8:1781, 1982
79. Stewart JG, Jackson AW, Chew MK: The role of radiation therapy in the management of malignant tumor of salivary glands. AJR 102:100, 1968
80. Stone RS: Neutron therapy and specific ionization. AJR 59:771, 1940
81. Suit HD, Griffin TW, Castro JR, et al: Particle radiation therapy research plan. Am J Clin Oncol 11:330, 1988
82. Suit H, Munzenrider GJ, Verhey L, et al: Evaluation of the clinical applicability of proton beams in definitive fractionated radiation therapy. Int J Radiat Oncol Biol Phys 8:2199, 1982
83. Tenforde TJ, Azal SM, Parr SS, et al: Cell survival in rat rhabdomyosarcoma tumors irradiated in vivo with extended peak silicon ions. Radiat Res 92:208, 1982
84. Tepper JE, Suit HD: Radiation therapy alone for sarcoma of soft tissue. Cancer 56:475, 1985
85. Tsunemoto H, Morita S, Sato S, et al: Present status of fast neutron therapy in Asian countries. Strahlenther Onkol (in press)
86. Tsunemoto H, Morita S, Arai T, et al: Results of clinical trial with 30-MeV d-Be neutrons at NIRS. In Sakamoto MAK, Phillips TL (eds): Treatment of Radioresistant Cancers. Amsterdam, Elsevier-North Holland, 1979
87. Tudway RC: Radiotherapy for osteogenic sarcoma. J Bone Joint Surg [B] 43:61, 1961
88. Vikram B, Strong E, Shah JP, et al: Radiation therapy in adenoid-cystic carcinoma. Int J Radiat Oncol Biol Phys 10:221, 1984
89. Von Essen CF, Blattman H, Crawford JF, et al: The piotron: Initial experience, preparation and experience with pion therapy. Int J Radiat Oncol Biol Phys 8:1499, 1982
90. Wambersie A: The European experience in neutron therapy at the end of 1981. Int J Radiat Oncol Biol Phys 8:2145, 1982
91. Windeyer W, Dische S, Mansfield CM: The place of radiotherapy in the management of fibrosarcoma of the soft tissues. Clin Radiol 17:32, 1966
92. Withers HR, Thames HD, Peters LJ: Biological bases for high RBE values for late effects of neutron irradiation. Int J Radiat Oncol Biol Phys 8:2071, 1982
93. Withers HR: Neutrons and other clinical trials: Impossible dreams? Int J Radiat Oncol Biol Phys 13:1967, 1987

15

○ ○ ○ ● ● ●

Intraoperative Radiation Therapy

Joel E. Tepper
Felipe A. Calvo

There is evidence indicating that for most tumor types local tumor control increases with higher doses of radiation. The use of intraoperative radiation therapy (IORT) is a direct extension of standard techniques to improve the dose distribution. By irradiating during the operative procedure, the physician is able to visualize directly the tumor volume and areas at risk for microscopic spread of disease and to confine the radiation to these tissues. Because the irradiated volume is directly visible, it is not necessary to allow any tissue margin for patient motion or inaccuracy of field placement, although it is still mandatory to irradiate tissues at risk for tumor involvement that may extend beyond visible tumor masses. By delivering the radiation during surgery, normal structures, such as stomach or small intestine, can be moved out of the way of the radiation beam. It is also possible to shield tissues underneath the tumor volume or to adjust the electron energy to spare structures located beneath the tumor mass. For all these reasons it is possible to deliver a very high dose to the tumor while minimizing the dose to the normal tissue.

RADIATION BIOLOGY

Because most of the clinical data on normal tissue tolerance to radiation have been based on the use of fractionated external-beam radiation therapy, it was necessary to preface the therapeutic assessment of IORT by generating information on the sensitivity of various normal structures receiving single, high doses of radiation. Some information has been garnered from the work of Abe and associates[1–3] in Kyoto, Japan. These studies demonstrated good tolerance of various retroperitoneal structures to single, high doses of radiation. Laboratory investigations also have been performed at the National Cancer Institute[5,27,31–33,36] and at Colorado State University.[4,10,11,20,22,24] The National Cancer Institute studies were designed to evaluate normal retroperitoneal structures, including the aorta, vena cava, kidney, ureters, bile duct, and retroperitoneal soft tissues, including vascular and intestinal anastomoses. Dogs were irradiated with single doses of electrons ranging between 2000 cGy and 4500 cGy to 5000 cGy; evaluation of long-term tolerance extended to 3 years.

These studies demonstrated that normal vascular structures generally tolerate IORT well. There was no evidence of loss of structural integrity in the large abdominal blood vessels, and histologic abnormalities in the vasculature at 2 years after therapy were mild. The retroperitoneal structures showed some fibrosis and scarring, but this was minimal considering the high doses employed.[31,32]

In contrast to the excellent tolerance of the vasculature and soft tissues, functioning organ systems tolerated the irradiation quite poorly. Marked kidney damage was seen at the lowest dose levels of 2000 cGy, with atrophic changes in the kidney and glomerular hyalinization. Structures with narrow lumina (*e.g.*, bile duct and ureters) were quite sensitive to irradiation. At doses greater than 2000 cGy, marked ureteral and biliary ductal fibrosis led to ureteral stenosis with hydronephrosis and biliary stricture with secondary biliary cirrhosis. McChesney and associates[22] from Colorado State have estimated a tolerance dose for 50% complications of 2900 cGy for IORT to the ureter. In evaluating the tolerance of the intestine, the NCI investigators found that functional bowel developed evidence of perforation at doses greater than 2000 cGy, but there were few complications after irradiation of a bypassed loop of intestine. This has significant implications for irradiating patients with pancreatic carcinoma, in whom the duodenal C-loop would almost always be within the radiation portal. Table 15-1 summarizes the experience at the National Cancer Institute on normal tissue tolerance to intraoperative radiation in dogs.

There also have been studies performed evaluating the tolerance of surgically manipulated tissues.[36] Experiments evaluated the tolerance of an aortic anastomosis and a blind loop of jejunum at the 4500-cGy level, with fibrosis and stricture of the aortic anastomosis being observed at doses greater than 2000 cGy. However, the demonstrated ability of an anastomosis to heal in the face of high-dose irradiation, without anastomotic disruption, is important for many of the clinical studies in progress.

These radiobiologic experiments have served as guidelines

TABLE 15–1
Normal Tissue Tolerance to Intraoperative Radiation Therapy

ANATOMIC SITE	EFFECTS (DOSE)
Large blood vessels	Fibrosis of vessel wall (>3000 cGy); aneurysms and thrombi (>3000 cGy IORT or 5000 cGy EBRT + 2000 cGy IORT)*
Kidney	Atrophy and fibrosis (<2000 cGy)
Ureter	Fibrosis, stenosis (2000 cGy)
Bile duct	Fibrosis, stenosis (2000 cGy)
Peripheral nerves	Neuropathy, loss of axon and myelin; increase in connective tissue (IORT > 3500 cGy or 5000 cGy EBRT + 1500 cGy IORT)
Bone necrosis	50% empty lacunae (3820 cGy IORT or 3250 cGy IORT + 5000 cGy EBRT)
Small intestine (functional)	Ulceration, fibrosis, stenosis (≥2000 cGy); obstruction, perforation (≥3000 cGy)
Colon	Ulceration, fibrosis, stenosis (≥4500 cGy); perforation (>5000 cGy)

**IORT, intraoperative radiation therapy; EBRT, external-beam radiation therapy.*

for subsequent clinical work. The poor tolerance of the ureters and bile duct was not expected, but ureteral stenosis has occurred in clinical studies after the ureter received high-dose irradiation, corroborating the laboratory findings.

Gillette and colleagues[10,11] at Colorado State University evaluated the long-term effects of IORT combined with external-beam irradiation in various abdominal structures and compared the effects of external-beam irradiation and IORT, which had not been done in earlier radiobiologic studies. In evaluating the tolerance of the abdominal aorta, they found that 2000 cGy of IORT combined with 5000 cGy of external-beam irradiation or 3000 cGy of IORT alone was associated with significant risks of aneurysms or large thrombi at 4 to 5 years after irradiation. They estimated that, for late tissue injury, an IORT dose of 1000 to 1500 cGy had an effect of five times or greater than that amount given in 200-cGy fractions.

LeCouteur and co-workers[20] from Colorado State have evaluated the effect of IORT on peripheral nerves after data from clinical studies suggested that nerves might be a dose-limiting normal tissue. Peripheral neuropathy arose as early as 6 months after IORT doses of 3500 cGy or greater, whether or not the animals had received external-beam irradiation (5000 cGy), and neuropathy (at any time) was seen after IORT doses as low as 1500 cGy. Most of the clinical neuropathy occurred 6 to 18 months after treatment and was associated with a histologically verified loss of myelin and axons and an increase in endoneurial, perineurial, and epineurial connective tissue. No neuropathy was seen after external-beam therapy alone using doses as high as 8000 cGy.

Of greater concern is the report by Powers and associates[24] analyzing dogs with long-term follow-up after IORT doses of 1500 cGy to 5500 cGy and external-beam doses of 5000 cGy to 8000 cGy. Of 26 dogs, receiving IORT alone one developed an osteosarcoma after 4 to 5 years (ten of the 26 dogs received doses of 4000 cGy or more). However, seven of 27 dogs developed osteosarcoma after IORT plus 5000 cGy of external-beam irradiation (six of 13 dogs developed osteosarcomas after receiving IORT doses of 3250 cGy and above). No osteosarcomas were seen in another group of 14 animals receiving external-beam irradiation alone to doses of 6000 cGy to 8000 cGy.

FACILITIES AND EQUIPMENT

Machines

Although a definition of the ideal facility for use of IORT is not established, some information is available from the experience of centers that have used this technique.[18] Electrons of various energies are the preferred method of irradiation. Selection of the optimal energy depends on the thickness (depth) of tissues to be irradiated. For a dedicated intraoperative machine, maximum flexibility can be obtained with at least a 6-cm depth of penetration at the 90% isodose line. This can be accomplished with a 20-MeV linear accelerator with a specially designed treatment head.

Some investigators use IORT with orthovoltage x-rays, but most view this as suboptimal and prefer treatment with high-energy electrons from a linear accelerator. However, cost and relative ease of installation are significant advantages in using an orthovoltage machine. There are also disadvantages. Because low-energy x-rays have poor penetration through tissue, the superficial dose is at least twice that given with high energies to tissues at depth when irradiating a thick tumor (≥5 cm). Orthovoltage radiation also has an increased absorption in bone, an effect related to a predominance of the photoelectric process. This higher bone dose could cause excessive long-term osseous complications and possibly radiation-induced carcinogenesis. These problems can be ameliorated by using a highly filtered x-ray beam and avoiding irradiating patients in whom the underlying bone is damaged. However, this still remains a substantial drawback to the use of orthovoltage radiation for IORT. Preliminary clinical trials have not yet encountered major difficulties with the use of orthovoltage irradiation.

Location of Installation

Most current IORT installations are in radiation therapy departments, requiring transportation of the patient from the operating room to the department. Alternatives that have been employed include designing a room in the radiation therapy department where the whole operation can be performed with ready access to the radiation therapy section or having a dedicated IORT machine placed in the operating room. Moving the patient from the operating room to the radiation therapy department is the most cost-efficient technique in the short term. The primary disadvantage is that the patient, who is under general anesthesia, must be moved into areas of the hospital not designed for sterile surgical procedures. The experience at several institutions indicates that this is feasible, but only with very careful planning involving many people, and the possibility of complications caused by the transportation does exist.

Radiation therapy department installations also require planning the use of IORT well ahead of time. There are many situations in which likelihood of delivering IORT is low, forcing the physician to weigh the small possibility that IORT will be appropriate against the necessity of idling a radiation machine room during routine treatment hours. Having a dedicated machine in the operating room avoids these problems. It ensures availability of the technique to patients who may benefit and causes the fewest logistical problems, but at substantial cost for the machine and room modifications for a unit that may have relatively little use.

Technical Procedures

Specifically designed treatment applicators must be available to be attached to the machine head. There must be no gap between the collimating system on the machine and the tumor volume, because the applicator acts as a normal tissue retractor as well as a radiation-beam collimator. The radiation oncologist cannot be certain of the accuracy of placement of the radiation field if the applicator is not directly touching the tumor volume. Normal tissues, such as small bowel, can slide under the applicator and into the treatment field if there is a gap.

Typical applicators are circular with internal diameters from 4 cm to 9 cm, but the 6-cm and 7-cm applicators are most commonly used. Cones have also been built with beveled edges, allowing direct apposition of the applicator to the tumor volume in sloping areas. These are essential for treating masses in the pelvis. Rectangular and elliptical cones for treating paraaortic lymph nodes or large retroperitoneal surfaces are very helpful, although the sharp corners on a rectangular cone can make it difficult to use. Applicators should be made of a clear plastic material that permits viewing through the applicator directly onto the tumor volume. Many institutions have designed applicators that slide into the head of the radiation therapy machine. This allows pressure to be removed from retroperitoneal structures while still ensuring proper alignment of the applicator with the electron beam. A disadvantage of the sliding system is that the applicator may slide up and away from the tumor volume (*e.g.*, with respiration), but will not slide down, thereby allowing normal tissues to slip under the cone. It may be necessary to jam the sliding mechanism to prevent this from happening. Newer applicators have physically separated the final collimation, which is in the patient from the machine, and have maintained alignment with a laser system.

A hole in the applicator, allowing instruments to be inserted into the radiation field when the patient is positioned, is valuable, as is a side-mounted periscope inserted into the machine head to confirm the proper treatment after the setup has been completed but before delivering radiation.

Standard physics evaluation of the machine must be performed.[6] There must be a good definition of the depth dose distribution and the lateral distribution across the beam at depth. It is important to evaluate specifically the effect of the bevel on the total depth of penetration, remembering that tissues immediately under the base of a beveled cone do not receive the full radiation dose and the applicator must be placed accordingly.

As is true for all electron beams, it is best to have the sharpest possible distal dose fall-off. One should be able to design an electron machine with a sharper distal dose fall-off than is available in many conventional accelerators, because the total field size required is relatively small. A field size greater than 15 cm × 12 cm is rarely required, because it is often impossible to put a treatment applicator larger than this into the abdominal cavity. It may be possible to change the design of the filters in the machine head to optimize the depth dose distribution.

Wherever the IORT machine is located, there must be full facilities available for any surgical contingency, including a complete set of surgical instruments for use in the radiation therapy department. There must be adequate operating room lighting and accessibility to operating room supplies and blood products.

TECHNIQUE

Although there are differences in the details of delivering IORT at various institutions, a typical technique is offered here to illustrate the general approach. Most patients are currently treated with a combination of high-dose external-beam radiation therapy and surgical resection, if feasible, in addition to IORT. Often, a preoperative dose of 4500 cGy to 5000 cGy is given with conventional fractionation to a volume encompassing the gross tumor with an appropriate margin. The patient is then given approximately a 4-week rest, followed by surgery. Resection is done if possible, after which the surgeon and the radiation therapist identify sites of gross or microscopic residual disease for treatment with IORT. It is often necessary to take frozen-section biopsies of areas in the tumor bed to confirm whether residual disease remains and to determine its extent. Metastatic disease outside the radiation portal is cause for excluding patients from treatment in many protocols, but patients with regional metastatic nodal disease can be irradiated.

The area that needs to be irradiated intraoperatively is defined. An applicator is selected that can best include the whole tumor volume in the field while excluding normal tissues. Occasionally it is necessary to perform additional surgery to move normal tissues from the radiation beam or to insert specially designed lead cutouts to block tissues that cannot be moved physically. It is also necessary to define the thickness of the tissues requiring irradiation for selecting the appropriate electron energy.

The patient must often be transported from the operating room to the radiation therapy department. The room in the radiation therapy department is cleaned and supplied to function as an operating room. After adequate patient hemostasis is obtained, the incision is closed loosely with a few stay sutures, and the wound is covered with a plastic adhesive dressing and layers of sterile drapes. The patient is placed on a Surgi-Lift stretcher and, while under portable anesthesia, is transported to the radiation therapy department. Despite problems that could arise from the transportation, none have been described. On arrival in the radiation therapy department, the patient is placed on the radiation therapy couch, the original drapes are removed, and the patient is reprepped and redraped for the IORT. The treatment volume is again exposed, and a cylinder of the same dimension as that used in the operating room is placed over the tumor volume. Great care is taken to ensure that normal structures are out of the radiation field. Very often it is necessary to put a suction catheter near the base of the field to avoid any buildup of blood. This is especially important in dependent portions of the abdomen or in the pelvis, where fluid buildup is likely, which could markedly decrease the penetration of the electrons. Occasionally, when low-energy electrons are used, it is necessary to place bolus material over the field to get full surface dose.

The treatment cylinder is then attached to the head of the radiation therapy machine, and the position of the treatment applicator is confirmed by a periscope. Confirmation is important, because it is possible that the position of the applicator could be altered while the applicator is being attached to the machine or that normal tissue (*e.g.*, small bowel) could slip underneath the applicator and into the radiation field. At times it is quite easy to attach the applicator to the machine head, but if

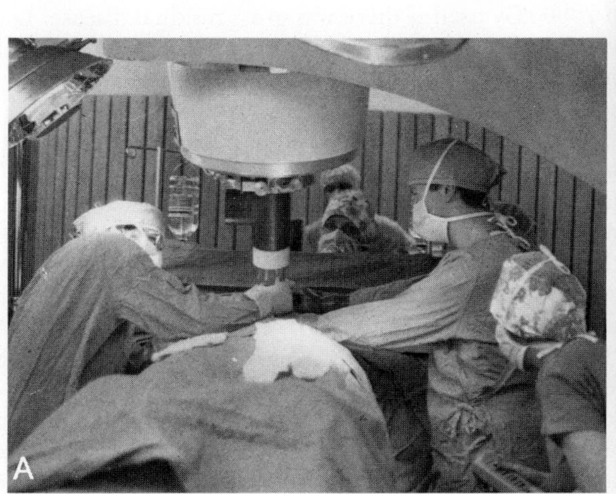

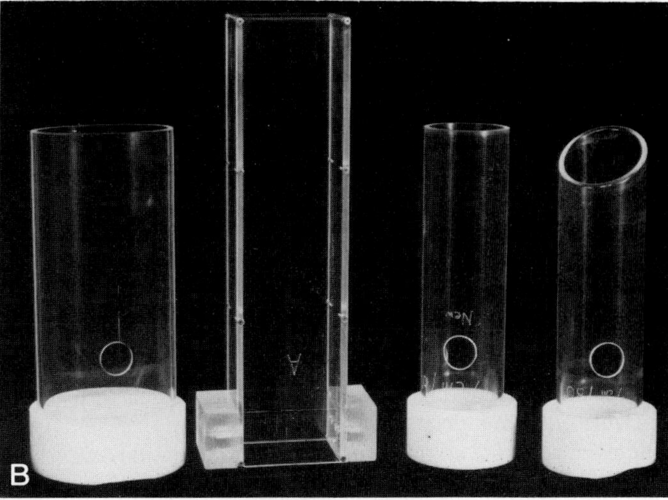

FIGURE 15–1. (**A**) Setup for intraoperative radiation therapy (IORT). The field is designed to treat residual tumor on the pelvic sidewall. (**B**) Different types of cones with flat or beveled end used for IORT.

the applicator is placed at a steep angle off to the side, as is often done for pelvic fields, the attachment can be difficult and can require three-dimensional table motions combined with gantry angulation. A typical treatment setup is shown in Figure 15-1.

While the patient is monitored by closed-circuit television, the radiation is delivered. The IORT dose ranges from 1000 cGy to 2000 cGy. Typically, a dose of 1500 cGy is used for patients with microscopic residual disease, and a dose of 2000 cGy is administered for those with gross residual tumor after incomplete resection or with no resection. Patients can be placed on 100% O_2 before the IORT to maximize tumor oxygenation.

At the completion of the radiation therapy, the surgeon and radiation therapist reenter the room, and before the applicator is removed from the patient, its position on the tumor and away from normal tissue is reconfirmed. If only closure is needed, this can be done in the radiation therapy department. If additional surgery needs to be performed, such as anastomoses that have been deferred because they would have been in the IORT portal, the patient is transported back to the operating room for completion of the operative procedure.

RESULTS

The various institutions using IORT have emphasized different disease sites, and techniques have varied among institutions. A summary of reported results at various sites is given here.

Adenocarcinoma of the Pancreas

Most institutions using IORT in the United States and Japan have had an interest in the treatment of adenocarcinoma of the pancreas. Abe and colleagues have reported data from a combined Japanese series.[1,3] Most patients were treated with IORT alone, without any external-beam radiation therapy. The survival in this series was poor, with the longest being 3 years and 7 months. The initial experience in the United States was from Howard University, where IORT alone was used on 19 patients in a pilot study.[12,13] Ten of these patients had evidence of metastatic disease at the time of treatment. The overall survival was 5.5 months.

The Massachusetts General Hospital[35] and the Mayo Clinic[25] reported their results using similar treatment regimens. Patients have typically received 1000 cGy in five fractions preoperatively through anteroposterior portals (500 cGy at the Mayo Clinic). The patient then has surgery with the delivery of IORT to a dose of 2000 cGy with high-energy electrons to the tumor mass. Generally no surgical resection is performed. Postoperatively, the patients receive 4000 cGy (4500 cGy at the Mayo Clinic) through a four-field box technique given in 22 fractions. Although the regional lymphatic glands are included in the radiation therapy portal, no attempt is made to cover the entire pancreas or to treat distal pancreatic or splenic hilar lymph nodes for tumors in the pancreatic head. The external-beam radiation is given in conjunction with 3 days of 5-fluorouracil at a dose of 500 mg/m^2, and patients are considered for chemotherapy postoperatively with 5-fluorouracil, doxorubicin (Adriamycin), and mitomycin-C. The results are shown in Table 15-2. At the Massachusetts General Hospital only three patients had surgical resection; the results were poor, with all three patients experiencing local failure. Most patients had no resection because of tumor extension onto superior mesenteric vessels or the portal vein, which made a Whipple's resection or a total pancreatectomy infeasible; regional pancreatectomies were not attempted. Resection was technically possible in only one patient, and it was not performed because of medical contraindications.

In patients with unresected disease or with partial resec-

TABLE 15–2
Intraoperative Radiation Therapy for Carcinoma of the Pancreas

TREATMENT RESULTS	MASSACHUSETTS GENERAL HOSPITAL	MAYO CLINIC
Number of patients	73	52
Local failure	26 (36%)	
Distance metastases	42 (58%)	
Alive, no evidence of disease	23 (32%)	11 (21%)
Median survival	13 months	12.2 months
2-Year survival	17%	8%

tion, the median survival was 13 months at the Massachusetts General Hospital and 12 months at the Mayo Clinic. The failure patterns are analyzed in Table 15-2. The median survival of 13 months compared favorably with the median survival of 10.5 months that was obtained with surgical resection in patients treated at the Massachusetts General Hospital between 1961 and 1971 for resectable adenocarcinoma of the pancreas. The early data from the Massachusetts General Hospital suggested better local control with the use of misonidazole as a hypoxic cell sensitizer than for an earlier group of patients treated with IORT but without the use of misonidazole. However, this trend was not supported by follow-up data, which showed no advantage to the use of misonidazole.[35] Median survival without mis6onidazole (15.7 months) was actually superior to that with misonidazole (12.5 months).

Sindelar[29] reported on the results of two randomized trials of IORT in pancreatic cancer from the National Cancer Institute. The first trial evaluated conventional external-beam versus IORT alone given after surgical resection. Operative mortality was high (28%), and median survival (12 months) was the same in the two groups, but local control and the disease-free interval in patients surviving the surgery were improved with the use of IORT. The second trial tested external-beam radiation therapy plus 5-fluorouracil versus external-beam irradiation plus 5-fluorouracil and IORT in patients with unresectable tumors.[28] Median survival in both arms was 8 months.

A number of other series have shown similar results with IORT, with median survival not being substantially improved over that obtained in patients from historic trials of external-beam radiation therapy, either alone or combined with 5-fluorouracil. This is supported by a subsequent Mayo Clinic analysis that compared treatment for localized tumors with external-beam irradiation alone versus external-beam irradiation plus IORT (plus 5-fluorouracil in some of the patients).[25] Although local control at 2 years was obtained in 66% of the patients treated with IORT but in only 20% of those treated with external-beam irradiation alone, this success was not translated into an improved survival; median survivals were 13.4 and 12.6 months, respectively.

Good pain palliation has been obtained in a number of studies. Calvo reported 14 of 16 patients who had relief of abdominal pain with IORT. The Massachusetts General Hospital data showed pain relief in 75% of patients, with pain being controlled for the duration of the patients' lives for half of the patients.[39] Nonetheless, the survival statistics have been disappointing and indicate that distant metastases determine survival in these patients. Although local control appears to be improved compared with historic data, local recurrence is still a significant problem.

Rectal Carcinoma

There has been significant interest in using IORT for patients presenting with locally advanced carcinomas of the rectum.[15] These patients present with tumors that are fixed, most commonly to sacrum or pelvic sidewall, and their surgeons believe that surgical resection alone could not produce local control. Several previous studies have demonstrated that high-dose, preoperative, external-beam radiation therapy can allow a resection to be performed in 50% to 75% of these patients, but local failure still occurs in 35% to 45%.[9,23] Because of this, IORT has been added to the area of tumor fixation after a dose of 5000 cGy to the pelvis.

IORT has been used if there is clinical evidence of fixation, with a dose of 1500 cGy used after grossly complete resection, and 2000 cGy used if there was gross residual disease. Locally advanced primary tumors and locally advanced recurrent tumors (*i.e.*, after previous low anterior resection or abdominoperineal resection) have been treated with IORT.

Similar treatment protocols have been carried out at the Massachusetts General Hospital[37] and the Mayo Clinic.[16] The data demonstrate that local control has been excellent in patients who presented with locally advanced primary disease, and survival results have been substantially improved over historic controls. The Massachusetts General Hospital has demonstrated an 86% actuarial local disease control rate and a 54% survival rate at 4 years for this group. In patients with recurrent disease, neither local control nor survival was as good, with 4-year actuarial rates of 32% and 26%, respectively. The higher local failure rate in patients with recurrent tumors is probably related to the fact that these patients have more diffuse pelvic involvement, with tumor extending to multiple adjacent structures; it is difficult to obtain adequate surgical resection, and the IORT coverage may not be sufficient in these patients. Similar data have been generated from the Mayo Clinic and are summarized in Tables 15-3 and 15-4.

These encouraging results suggest an advantage in both local control and survival in patients with locally advanced tumors. Even if there were no major survival advantage, the improvement in local control would be of value because of the morbidity experienced by patients who develop a local recurrence.

Gastric Carcinoma

The best information on IORT treatments of patients with gastric carcinoma has been provided by Abe and colleagues,[1–3] who performed a prospective, nonrandomized study comparing gastrectomy alone with gastrectomy with the addition of IORT. The IORT was given in a dose of 2800 cGy to 4000 cGy to a pentagonal field that encompassed areas of posterior tumor spread onto the pancreas and major vessels. The results of this study are summarized in Table 15-5. A moderate increase in survival among patients with Stage II and Stage III disease was revealed. The survival rate increased from 62% to 84% in Stage II disease patients and from 37% to 62% in Stage III patients. For patients with Stage IV tumors (Japanese staging: tumor invading adjacent structures without evidence of distant metastases), the survival rate improved from zero with surgery alone to 15% with the addition of IORT. This is the group of patients in whom a survival improvement would be most likely with the use of adjuvant radiation therapy. It is possible, however, that a similar improvement in survival could be obtained by the use of

TABLE 15–3
Intraoperative Radiation Therapy for Locally Advanced Primary Rectal Carcinoma

TREATMENT RESULTS	MASSACHUSETTS GENERAL HOSPITAL	MAYO CLINIC
Number of patients	36	15
Local failure	3 (8%)	2/12 (17%)
Distant failure	14 (39%)	4/12 (33%)
Alive, no evidence of disease	19 (53%)	8 (53%)
4-Year actuarial survival rate	54%	53%

TABLE 15–4
Intraoperative Radiation Therapy for Locally Advanced Recurrent Rectal Carcinoma

TREATMENT RESULTS	MASSACHUSETTS GENERAL HOSPITAL	MAYO CLINIC
Number of patients	22	36
Local failure	12 (57%)	6/32 (19%)
Distant failure	12 (55%)	14/32 (44%)
Alive, no evidence of disease	5 (23%)	14 (39%)
4-Year actuarial survival rate	26%	23%

external-beam irradiation therapy. This question has not been addressed in Japanese trials.

The National Cancer Institute conducted a small, randomized trial of IORT for patients with gastric carcinoma.[30] The trial compared gastrectomy plus postoperative external-beam radiation therapy to gastrectomy plus IORT to the tumor bed. In the 10 patients who received IORT, median survival was 20.8 months with a disease-free interval of 14.2 months, compared with 10.2 months and 6.9 months, respectively, in the 18 patients receiving external-beam irradiation. These values did not have a statistically significant difference. Other investigators have been interested in accruing patients for a trial of preoperative external-beam radiation therapy to a maximum dose of 4500 cGy followed by surgical resection and IORT to the tumor bed for patients with locally extensive disease.

Calvo treated 22 patients with resectable gastric cancer with surgical resection followed by IORT (1500 cGy) to the tumor bed and external-beam irradiation to a maximum of 4600 cGy. Patient tolerance to the therapy was good, and early data showed a median survival of more than 13 months. Despite the aggressive local therapy, the upper abdominal failure rate was at least 22%, although tumor progression in the IORT field occurred in only two patients.

Tumors of Other Sites

Calvo investigated the use of IORT in patients with gynecologic tumors. Twenty-four patients, primarily with carcinoma of the cervix, were treated with a combination of surgical resection, IORT, and external-beam irradiation (if not previously irradiated). Although follow-up is limited, local control has been in the range of 80% to 85%, with the primary complication being pelvic pain. Goldson and associates[14] treated patients to the paraaortic nodes with IORT, sometimes combined with external-beam, but there are no data available on efficacy.

Matsumoto and associates[21] investigated the use of IORT for patients with early-stage bladder carcinoma using 3000 cGy to 4000 cGy intraoperatively. The recurrence rate was 9.4% at 2 years, with a local recurrence rate of 5.7% in patients with solitary tumors and 23.1% in those with multiple tumors. The 5-year survival rate for patients with T1 lesions was 96%, compared with 62% for those with T2 tumors, with good bladder function maintained.

Calvo treated 18 patients with advanced-stage bladder cancers with urinary diversion and lymphadenectomy, IORT (1500 cGy), and external-beam irradiation (4600 cGy), followed by cystectomy. Eleven of 18 patients had no residual tumor, but follow-up is too limited to assess efficacy. Shipley and coworkers[26] have also discussed the use of IORT in patients with locally advanced bladder cancer, using IORT to sites of local adherence or tumor invasion.

There has been some use of IORT for soft tissue sarcomas, predominantly in the retroperitoneum. At the Massachusetts General Hospital, patients were treated with 4500 cGy to 5000 cGy preoperatively, followed by surgical resection and doses of 1500 cGy to 2000 cGy to the tumor bed intraoperatively. Preliminary data have shown local failure in only two of 20 patients, with ten of 20 remaining alive without evidence of disease. The Mayo Clinic had three of 20 patients with local failure (only one in the IORT field), and 11 of 20 patients are alive without evidence of disease.[17] The National Cancer Institute conducted a randomized trial of resection followed by 2000 cGy of IORT plus 4000 cGy to 4500 cGy of external-beam radiation therapy compared with the same surgical resection followed by 5000 cGy to 5500 cGy of external-beam therapy.[19] No significant difference has been found in median survival, although there is a suggestion of an advantage in local control. These trials indicate that the tolerance of the normal retroperitoneum is good, even when extremely large IORT fields are employed, as is necessary with retroperitoneal sarcomas.

Other studies have evaluated biliary or gallbladder carcinoma, glioblastomas, various thoracic malignancies, and many pediatric tumors.[8,38] Although these trials suggest the feasibility of this approach in many sites, they do not allow for conclusions about treatment efficacy.

SEQUELAE OF INTRAOPERATIVE RADIATION THERAPY

In studies evaluating toxicity of IORT, it has been found that the tolerance of retroperitoneal structures is good, although the tissues that were found to be sensitive to single, high-dose irradiation in animal experiments, such as ureter, bile duct, and functioning organ systems, have indeed not tolerated high

TABLE 15–5
Intraoperative Radiation Therapy at Kyoto University for Gastric Carcinoma

DISEASE STAGE	RESECTION ALONE: NUMBER OF PATIENTS	RESECTION ALONE: 5-YEAR SURVIVAL RATE (%)	RESECTION + RADIATION: NUMBER OF PATIENTS	RESECTION + RADIATION: 5-YEAR SURVIVAL RATE (%)
Stage I	43	93	24	87
Stage II	11	62	20	84
Stage III	38	37	30	62
Stage IV	18	0	27	15

doses in humans. There has not been a significant incidence of acute complications related to the radiation therapy itself or to the transportation of patients from the operating room to the radiation therapy department.

A detailed analysis of the complications of IORT in patients with locally advanced rectal carcinomas has been done at the Massachusetts General Hospital.[34] For patients with locally advanced primary tumors, there were no more complications than for patients in a historic group who were treated with external-beam radiation therapy and resection without IORT. However, in patients with recurrent tumors, there was a high incidence of complications, generally occurring in the soft tissues of the pelvis. It is impossible to tell whether the increase in complications was related to the advanced stage of the tumors, the difficulty in surgical resection, or the IORT itself, in part because no similar historic group is available for comparison.

Pelvic pain syndrome was reported for three patients in the Massachusetts General Hospital series. This may be secondary to nerve entrapment and may be a limiting factor in tolerance of pelvic structures to IORT. Pelvic pain syndrome has been noticed by other investigators and seems to be related to the combination of an extensive surgical procedure and IORT, often in patients with locally recurrent tumors. Calvo reported a 29% incidence of pelvic pain in a group of patients with locally advanced rectal cancer, with the pain typically arising 2 to 3 months after IORT.[7] It occurred in two of 11 patients with locally advanced primary tumors, four of 11 with locally advanced recurrent tumors, and two of five who had prior radiation therapy. Gunderson and colleagues[16] reported an incidence of 32% (12 of 37) of pelvic pain syndrome in patients with locally advanced rectal cancer; the pain resolved in five patients. Sensory and motor abnormalities were seen in eight and seven patients, respectively; all 15 had pain. Neuropathy has also been reported by Calvo[7] in patients treated for extremity sarcomas, gynecologic tumors, and locally advanced rectal cancer.

Ureteral obstruction, predicted from the animal studies, has been seen in humans. At the Mayo Clinic, nine patients had irradiated ureters that were unobstructed before the IORT, and 4 (44%) of these patients developed subsequent hydronephrosis.[16] Resolution of the hydronephrosis occurred in two of three ureters that were initially obstructed. Duodenal bleeding has been observed in patients treated for pancreatic cancer, in whom the C-loop of the duodenum was in the radiation field. Most of these patients also received high-dose external-beam irradiation, often with chemotherapy. Other complications of IORT have been relatively infrequent, but they have been primarily related to difficulties with soft tissue healing or fibrosis.

CRITIQUE OF INTRAOPERATIVE RADIATION THERAPY AND FUTURE DIRECTIONS

Many of the advances in radiation therapy in the last few decades have been based on the ability to improve the dose distribution between the tumor and the normal tissue. Because it appears likely that IORT will extend this differential in dose delivery between tumor and normal tissue, it has the potential to make a significant impact on the local control of certain tumors. In particular, the data presented for locally advanced rectal tumors indicate a substantial improvement in survival by the addition of IORT to conventional radiation therapy and surgical resection. However, the ultimate value of IORT will be determined after tumor and normal tissue conditions have been defined in which the addition of a direct dose delivery system allows a higher dose to be delivered to the tumor without producing undue normal tissue sequelae.

IORT can improve survival only if local failure alone is a major impediment to survival. Unfortunately, for tumors such as pancreatic carcinoma and retroperitoneal soft tissue sarcomas, the lack of an effective adjuvant chemotherapy regimen and the high incidence of distant metastases may preclude a major improvement in long-term survival rates through the use of IORT. However, the impact of local control with IORT may be greater when treatments for metastatic disease are available. It also seems likely that IORT will be most effective for treating defined areas at high risk for local recurrence, rather than wide areas of potential tumor contamination. The sensitivity of nearby healthy tissues may preclude the use of IORT in certain clinical situations because these tissues cannot safely be removed from the radiation field despite surgical exposure.

Although there are indications of benefit from IORT in the treatment of certain pancreatic, rectal, and gastric carcinomas, the work that has been done does not allow explication of many other situations for which IORT may offer substantial advantages. The use of this modality for gynecologic tumors has been explored only minimally. Gynecologic tumors often adhere to the pelvic sidewall, where the use of IORT with surgical resection may substantial benefit these patients. IORT can be used for paraaortic nodal irradiation, but this use also demands full evaluation. Some Japanese investigators have reported very encouraging results in the treatment of early-stage bladder carcinomas with IORT, but this research has not been pursued elsewhere. Some patients with locally extensive bladder carcinomas may benefit from IORT to areas of tumor adherence or fixation after preoperative irradiation and resection.

Although there has been minimal use of IORT for thoracic or brain tumors, the approach is worthy of investigation. It is important that these studies are implemented in a way that maximizes the likelihood of detecting an advantage to IORT if one exists. It is essential that IORT be used to supplement high-dose external-beam radiation therapy and surgical resection for controlling local tumors.

REFERENCES

1. Abe M, Takahashi M: Intraoperative radiotherapy: The Japanese experience. Int J Radiat Oncol Biol Phys 7:863, 1981
2. Abe M, Takahashi M, Ono K, et al: Japan gastric trials in intraoperative radiation therapy. Int J Radiat Oncol Biol Phys 15:1431, 1988
3. Abe M, Takahashi M, Yobumoto E, et al: Clinical experiences with intraoperative radiotherapy of locally advanced cancers. Cancer 45:40, 1980
4. Ahmadu-Suka F, Gillette EL, Withrow SJ, et al: Pathologic response of the pancreas and duodenum to experimental intraoperative irradiation. Int J Radiat Oncol Biol Phys 14:1197, 1988
5. Barnes M, Pass H, DeLuca A, et al: Response of the mediastinal and thoracic viscera of the dog to intraoperative radiation therapy (IORT). Int J Radiat Oncol Biol Phys 13:371, 1987
6. Biggs PJ, Epp ER, Ling CC, et al: Dosimetry, field shaping and other considerations for intraoperative electron therapy. Int J Radiat Oncol Biol Phys 7:875, 1981
7. Calvo FA, Algarra SM, Azinovic I, et al: Intraoperative radiotherapy for recurrent and/or residual colorectal cancer. Radiother Oncol 15:133, 1989
8. Calvo FA, Sierrasesumaga L, Martin I, et al: Intraoperative radiotherapy in the multidisciplinary treatment of pediatric tumors. Acta Oncol 28:257, 1989
9. Dosoretz D, Gunderson LL, Hoskins B, et al: Preoperative

irradiation for unresectable rectal and rectosigmoid carcinomas. Cancer 52:814, 1983

10. Gillette EL, Powers BE, McChesney SL, Withrow SJ: Aortic wall injury following intraoperative irradiation. Int J Radiat Oncol Biol Phys 15:1401, 1988
11. Gillette EL, Powers BE, McChesney SL, Withrow SJ: Response of aorta and branch arteries to experimental intraoperative irradiation. Int J Radiat Oncol Biol Phys 15:202, 1988
12. Goldson AL: Past, present and prospects of intraoperative radiotherapy (IOR). Semin Oncol 8:59, 1981
13. Goldson AL, Ashaveri E, Espinosa MC, et al: Single high dose intraoperative electrons for advanced stage pancreatic cancer: Phase 1 pilot study. Int J Radiat Oncol Biol Phys 7:869, 1981
14. Goldson A, Delgado G, Hill L: Intraoperative radiation of the para-aortic nodes in cancer of the uterine cervix. Obstet Gynecol 52:713, 1978
15. Gunderson LL, Cohen AM, Dosoretz DD, et al: Residual, unresectable or recurrent colorectal cancer: External beam irradiation and intraoperative electron beam boost resection. Int J Radiat Oncol Biol Phys 9:1597, 1983
16. Gunderson LL, Martin JK, Beart RW, et al: Intraoperative and external-beam irradiation ± 5FU for locally advanced colorectal cancer. Ann Surg 27:52, 1988
17. Gunderson LL, Nagorney DM, McIlrath DC, et al: External beam and intraoperative irradiation of soft tissue sarcomas. Int J Radiat Oncol Biol Phys 15:184, 1988
18. Gunderson LL, Tepper JE, Biggs PJ, et al: Intraoperative ± external beam irradiation. Curr Probl Cancer 7:11, 1983
19. Kinsella TJ, Sindelar WF, Glatstein EJ, Rosenberg SA: Preliminary results of a phase III study of adjuvant radiotherapy in resectable adult retroperitoneal soft tissue sarcomas: High dose external beam radiotherapy (HEBT) versus intraoperative and low dose external beam radiotherapy (IORT + LEBT). Proc Am Soc Clin Oncol 6:136, 1987
20. LeCouteur RA, Gillette EL, Powers BE, et al: Response of peripheral nerves to experimental intraoperative radiotherapy. Int J Radiat Oncol Biol Phys 15:203, 1988
21. Matsumoto K, Kakizoe T, Shuichi M, et al: Clinical evaluation of intraoperative radiotherapy for carcinoma of the urinary bladder. Cancer 47:509, 1981
22. McChesney SL, Gillette EL, Powers BE, Withrow SJ: Ureteral injury following experimental intraoperative radiation. Int J Radiat Oncol Biol Phys 15:204, 1988
23. Pilepich MV, Munzenrider JE, Tak WK, et al: Preoperative irradiation of primarily unresectable colorectal carcinoma. Cancer 42:1077, 1978
24. Powers BE, Gillette EL, McChesney SL, Withrow SJ: Bone necrosis and tumor induction following experimental intraoperative irradiation. Int J Radiat Oncol Biol Phys 15:204, 1988
25. Roldan GE, Gunderson LL, Nagorney DM, et al: External beam versus intraoperative and external beam irradiation for locally advanced pancreatic cancer. Cancer 61:1110, 1988
26. Shipley WU, Kaufman SD, Prout GR: Intraoperative radiation therapy in patients with bladder cancer. Cancer 60:1485, 1987
27. Sindelar WF, Hoekstra HJ, Kinsella TJ, et al: Response of canine esophagus to intraoperative electron beam radiotherapy. Int J Radiat Oncol Biol Phys 15:663, 1988
28. Sindelar WF, Kinsella TJ: Randomized trial of intraoperative radiotherapy in unresectable carcinoma of the pancreas. Int J Radiat Oncol Biol Phys 12(Suppl):148, 1986
29. Sindelar WF, Kinsella TJ: Randomized trial of intraoperative radiotherapy in resected carcinoma of the pancreas. Int J Radiat Oncol Biol Phys 12(Suppl):148, 1986
30. Sindelar WF, Kinsella TJ: Randomized trial of resection and intraoperative radiotherapy in locally advanced gastric cancer. Proc Am Soc Clin Oncol 6:91, 1987
31. Sindelar WF, Morrow BM, Travis EL, et al: Effects of intraoperative electron irradiation in the dog on cell turnover in intact and surgically anastomosed aorta and intestine. Int J Radiat Oncol Biol Phys 9:523, 1983
32. Sindelar WF, Tepper JE, Travis EL, et al: Tolerance of retroperitoneal structures to intraoperative radiation. Ann Surg 196:601, 1982
33. Sindelar WF, Tepper JE, Travis EL: Tolerance of bile duct to intraoperative irradiation. Surgery 92:533, 1982
34. Tepper JE, Gunderson LL, Orlow E, et al: Complications of intraoperative radiation therapy. Int J Radiat Oncol Biol Phys 10:1831, 1984
35. Tepper JE, Shipley WU, Warshaw AL, et al: The role of misonidazole combined with intraoperative radiation therapy in the treatment of pancreatic carcinoma. J Clin Oncol 5:579, 1987
36. Tepper JE, Sindelar WF, Travis E, et al: Tolerance of canine anastomoses to intraoperative radiation therapy. Int J Radiat Oncol Biol Phys 9:987, 1983
37. Tepper JE, Wood WC, Cohen AM: Treatment of locally advanced rectal cancer with external beam radiation, surgical resection, and intraoperative radiation therapy. Int J Radiat Oncol Biol Phys 16:1437, 1989
38. Todoroki T, Iwasaki Y, Okamura T, et al: Intraoperative radiotherapy for advanced carcinoma of the biliary system. Cancer 46:2179, 1980
39. Wood CW, Shipley WU, Gunderson LL, et al: Intraoperative irradiation for unresectable pancreatic carcinoma. Cancer 49:1272, 1982

16

○ ○ ○ ○ ● ○

Hyperthermia

Carlos A. Perez
Bahman Emami
Robert J. Myerson
Joseph L. Roti Roti

RATIONALE FOR CLINICAL USE OF HEAT

The effect of heat on malignant tumors was first mentioned by Hippocrates. In 1866 Busch[31] described the disappearance of a soft tissue sarcoma following high fever in a patient with erysipelas. Later, Coley[44] induced fever by injecting bacterial toxins; Warren[464] and Westermark[475] used localized hyperthermia to produce tumor regression in patients.

In the past 20 years interest has been rekindled in the clinical application of heat, encouraged by biologic reports that there may be a significant advantage in the use of heat combined with radiation and cytotoxic drugs to enhance the killing of tumor cells.[63,64,72,107,399] The clinical use of heat has been hampered by a lack of adequate equipment to effectively deliver heat in deep-seated and even large superficial lesions and of thermometry techniques that provide reliable information on heat distribution in the target tissues. However, significant progress has been made.[180,256,307]

In vitro and *in vivo* biologic experiments suggest that heat may be more damaging to tumors than to normal tissues for several reasons: chronically hypoxic cells may have an increased sensitivity to heat[64] (they are at least as thermosensitive as oxygenated cells); cells with a low pH (<6.8) that are metabolically deprived (as in a tumor) are more heat-sensitive; heat affects cells in S phase, which are known to be resistant to irradiation[385,425]; and blood flow in the tumor is reduced.[63,64,219] Heat causes a greater degree of mitotic delay than radiation, and this factor may affect the distribution of cells in the cell cycle after exposure to heat or radiation.[65,180] The sensitivity of hypoxic cells to heat is complicated by the possible association of low oxygen tension with nutrient deficiency or reduced pH. As Dewey and associates[64] pointed out, the response of the tumor may be affected by physiologic changes associated with lowering of the blood flow and oxygen tension produced by hyperthermia. The differential heat sensitivity of tumors is a consequence of tumor physiology, with nutrient deprivation[96,191,332] and lower pH[119] being the main contributing factors and not a consequence of the intrinsic state of malignancy of the cells.[124,125,136,217,283,301]

The biologic rationale for combining hyperthermia and irradiation in the treatment of cancer rests in two biologic mechanisms: radiosensitization and direct hyperthermia cytotoxicity. It can be hypothesized that hypoxic cells in the center of a tumor are relatively radioresistant but thermosensitive, whereas well-vascularized peripheral portions of the tumor are more sensitive to irradiation.[293,299] This supports the use of combined radiation and heat; hyperthermia is especially effective against centrally located hypoxic cells and irradiation eliminates the tumor cells in the periphery of the tumor, where heat would be less effective. In experiments on a transplanted mammary carcinoma, Overgaard[286] reported no cures with 1600 cGy (single dose), 22% with heat alone (43°C, 60 minutes) and 77% when the two modalities with the same parameters were applied.

An area in which hyperthermia may be useful, perhaps alone at high temperatures (45°C) or at 43°C combined with moderate doses of radiation (about 4000 cGy), is in the treatment of patients with recurrences following definitive radiation therapy (6000 cGy to 7000 cGy). Likewise, large epithelial tumors or specific histologic lesions (melanomas, soft tissue sarcomas, neurogenic tumors) that are not usually controlled by irradiation alone because of tolerance of surrounding normal tissues potentially could be more efficaciously treated with definitive doses of radiation (6500 cGy to 7500 cGy) and heat. Hypothetically this combination would enhance the biologic effects of irradiation on the tumor without increasing morbidity in the normal tissues. Because growing tissues are more sensitive to irradiation than are mature organs, it may be possible that a combination of hyperthermia with cytotoxic agents or the combination of these two modalities with low doses of irradiation may be effective in the treatment of pediatric neoplasias.

Hahn[135] has demonstrated *in vitro* the additive or supra-additive cell killing effects of heat combined with a variety of chemotherapeutic agents. Further, the effects of hypoxic sensitizers combined with irradiation or cytotoxic drugs can be enhanced by the administration of heat.[19,126]

Whole-body hyperthermia has been used for the treatment of disseminated disease, alone or with chemotherapeutic agents.[323] It may have potential value not only in the treatment of overt metastatic disease but also as an adjuvant, combined with chemotherapy, for the treatment of micrometastasis.

BIOLOGIC ASPECTS OF HYPERTHERMIA

Despite the publication of numerous observations of heat-induced alterations of subcellular structures and systems,[342] no consensus concerning the molecular mechanisms of cell kill has emerged. Most commonly postulated mechanisms involve damage to three major cellular structures:

Plasma Membrane. Hyperthermia produces numerous alterations in the plasma membrane including effects on membrane (*e.g.,* receptor proteins and transport proteins),[34,205,234,331,386,398,452] extensive bleeding,[22,51] and regions of altered cholesterol content.[335] The involvement of damage to the plasma membrane in the lethal event is supported by the observation that membrane-active agents (local anesthetics)[487] and aliphatic alcohols[226] act synergistically with heat, and cell kill by the action of these agents alone is strikingly similar to the action of heat by itself.[227] In addition, several studies suggest a relationship between membrane lipid composition and cell kill.[133,161,201,202,263,487]

Cytoskeleton/Cytosol. In tissue, culture cells contain stress fibers resulting from bundling of actin-containing microfilaments. Within 5 minutes of exposure of Chinese hamster ovary (CHO) cells to 45°C, 90% of cells do not contain observable stress fibers.[122] Spindle microtubules are disorganized and disassociated (15 minutes) on exposure of CHO cells to 45°C,[51] suggesting that this effect may be responsible for the increased thermal sensitivity of mitotic cells. The vimentin-containing intermediate filaments collapse on heat exposure to form a pernicular cap.[103,427,474] Most of the effects of heat on the cytoskeleton are reversible with postheat incubation at 37°C. Hyperthermia induces alterations in both the structure and function of numerous cytoplasm elements: mitochondria,[474] lysosomes,[172,299] and protein synthesis apparatus.[152,252] Hyperthermia induces disruption of respiration and glycolysis,[41,75,262] which appears to be related to morphologic changes in mitochrondria. Polysomes are destroyed,[146,474] and protein synthesis is inhibited at the incubation step[82,152,302] and may be mediated by phosphorylation of initiation factors.[59,275] The association of polysomes and initiation factors with cytoskeletal structures is altered,[171] indicating the possibility of a functional correlate between heat-induced cytoskeletal changes and protein synthesis.

Nucleus. In addition to inducing a number of structural changes, hyperthermia alters or disrupts many nuclear functions.[342] One of the distinct substructures within the nucleus is the nucleolus, a heat-sensitive organelle, which undergoes marked changes at heat exposure that leave cytoplasmic organelles largely unaffected.[384] An increase in the overall median protein content is observed in nuclei isolated from cells exposed to hyperthermia.[344,428] The increased nuclear protein content is a large and rapid effect[344] and appears to result from the heat-induced association of specific proteins (including heat shock protein 70) with the nuclear matrix[469] and the nucleus.[276] When cell kill, as surviving fraction, is plotted as a function of excess nuclear protein content immediately following hyperthermia, a linear quadratic type correlation curve is obtained, which holds even when cells are thermal-sensitized or thermal-protected by chemical modifiers.[370] When time of association between these proteins and the nucleus is included, the correlation becomes a simple exponential (linear on the semilog plot) and applies for all conditions tested.[181] Additional studies implicate the association of excess proteins in the nucleus with inhibition of DNA replication[468,482] and DNA repair.[43,258,465] DNA replication is inhibited at all defined steps in the process: initiation, elongation, and assembly of replicated DNA into mature chromatin structure. However, these steps have different thermal sensitivities.[342]

A model for the mechanism of heat-induced cell kill based on the foregoing considerations proposed by a number of investigators[62,342,343,483] is as follows: disruption of critical plasma membrane structures (*e.g.,* plasma membrane-cytoskeleton attachment points and protein channels); collapse of the cytoskeleton toward the nucleus; absorption of protein onto the nuclear matrix; disruption of nuclear functions, possibly involving inhibition of DNA supercoiling changes; and damage to critical nuclear structures.

When mechanisms of cell kill are considered, it is important to note that at least two and possibly three modes of cell death are distinguished by cell-cycle progression (or lack thereof) before the death process. In the quiescent mode no cell progression occurs.[452] The other two modes appear to be after either at least one S-phase transit (not necessarily complete)[241] or at least one mitosis.[51] Regardless of the different modes, cell kill resulting from heat exposure can be represented typically as surviving fraction plotted as a function of heating time (Fig. 16-1). The resulting survival curves can be analyzed by either the target theory equation, $S/So = 1-(1-e^{D/Do})^n$, or the linear quadratic equation, $S/So = e^{\alpha D-\beta D2}$. The former relationship has formed the basis of the current concept of thermal dose.[190]

Thermal Dose

The concept of thermal dose has arisen from attempts to convert heat exposures at various temperatures to equivalent time at a reference temperature (usually 43°C) based on the biologic effectiveness of the actual temperature.[153] Sapareto and Dewey[354] developed a thermal dose concept that converts a thermal exposure to an equivalent exposure at an arbitrarily chosen reference temperature of 43°C. This phenomenon has been observed *in vitro* and *in vivo.*[46,64,106,108,354]

These time-temperature conversions have been shown to be good prognostic indicators by Dewhirst and associates[73] for

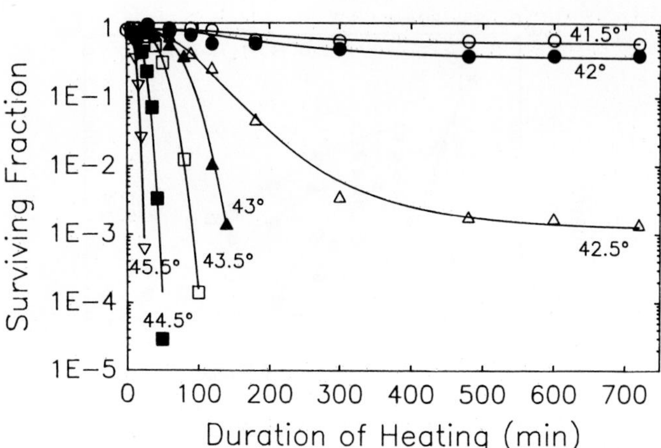

FIGURE 16–1. Cell kill as a function of time and temperature in G_1 Chinese hamster ovary cells. (Redrawn from Mackey M, Roti Roti JL: J Theor Biol, in press)

spontaneous tumor treatment in dogs and cats when the thermal dose calculated for the coolest part of the treated tumor is used. These results indicated that equivalent minutes of exposure was the best predictor of long-term tumor response. However, Dewhirst and colleagues[74] stressed the importance of three-dimensional (3D) dose mapping. A recent workshop on thermal dose demonstrated that a number of factors must still be evaluated and their importance resolved before this concept is generally accepted. These factors include the temperature of the transition or breakpoint, the R value below the breakpoint, the effect of step-down heating, the effect of thermotolerance, the effect of the interaction and radiation on equation 1, and the importance of blood flow and other physiologic factors. The workshop concluded that "any attempt to plan thermal treatments based on any of these dose concepts or to predict clinical response from a calculated dose is very inappropriate and premature."[351,352] However, Sapareto and Dewey's model is the most practical method available for the comparison of clinical treatments. Therefore the method should be clinically tested to fully determine its potential usefulness.

THERMOTOLERANCE AND STEP-DOWN HEATING

It has been frequently reported that mammalian cells are substantially more resistant to heat following prior heat exposure.[149] Henle and Leeper[151] noted that cells initially exposed to 45°C became resistant to subsequent exposure to 45°C if allowed a 10- to 20-hour period at 37°C between treatments (Fig. 16-2). Thermotolerance is a transient phenomenon and thus does not represent a selection of genetically resistant cells, which occurs at too low a frequency to account for this phenomenon.[144,143] The mechanism for thermotolerance is not known; however, protein or RNA synthesis must occur before thermotolerance can develop.[212,358]

Both Henle[148] and Li and associates[225] have indicated that prior exposure to temperatures above 43°C sensitizes cells to lower temperatures. This phenomenon has been termed step-down heating. Also, Li and colleagues[225] have shown that thermotolerance is inhibited for several hours immediately following exposure to 45°C.

Recent studies indicate that thermotolerance is accompanied by enhanced ability to repair (restore) certain types of

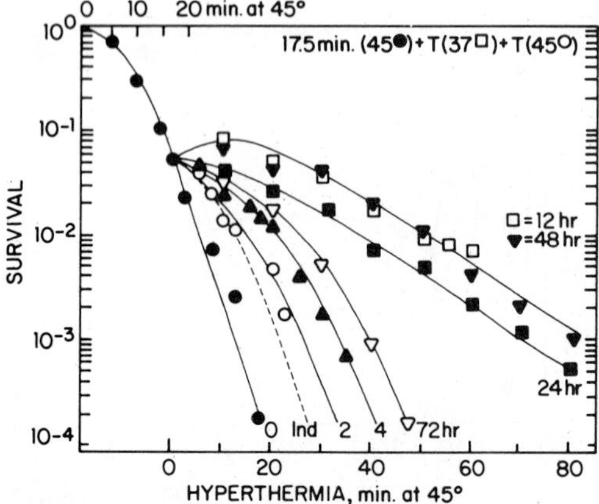

FIGURE 16–2. Development of thermotolerance in asynchronous CHO (Chinese hamster ovary) cells at various times after an initial heat dose of 45°C for 17.5 minutes. Top abscissa shows the scale for the initial heat treatment; bottom abscissa shows the duration of the second heat dose at 45°C. (Henle KJ, Leeper DB: Radiat Res 66:505–518, 1976)

heat-induced cellular alterations. The following effects are repaired more rapidly in thermotolerant cells: nuclear localization of heat shock protein (hsp70),[276] disassembly of the cytoskeleton,[201] increased nuclear protein binding,[181] and inhibition of certain types of DNA repair.[484] Further studies may show that enhanced ability to repair heat-induced damage contributes more significantly to heat-resistance than does protection from damage.

HEAT SHOCK PROTEINS

Thermotolerance appears to be closely related to the induction of a class of protein polypeptides of molecular weights of 25 kd to 110 kd.[208,230,416] These "heat shock proteins" (hsp) have been well characterized and occur as a result of gene transcription induced by thermal stress in *Drosophila melanogaster*[259] and most other living systems[370]; however, their function is unknown. A good correlation exists between the increased induction and degradation of these constitutive proteins and the induction and decay of thermotolerance (Fig. 16-3), whether induced by heat shock or other toxic stress phenomena.[231] Particular interest has been generated by hsp70,[229] which migrates to the nucleus during heat shock.[276,473] Different types of thermotolerance appear to be associated with a period of enhanced synthesis of hsp70 and the period during which cells have elevated levels of hsp70.[209] Although it appears that increased levels of hsp70 are sufficient to cause increased heat resistance, it is becoming clear that they are not necessary. A series of heat-resistant cell lines from RIF1 tumors do not express increased levels of hsp70.[4] Also transfection of cells with genes for hsp27 leads to increased heat resistance.[38] Although the cellular response to thermal stress appears to be one of the most conserved biologic mechanisms in nature,[370] the function of the various heat shock proteins remains by and large a mystery despite numerous eloquent studies.

HEAT INTERACTION WITH RADIATIONS

Several good reviews are available on this subject.[64,72,287,417] The first and most generally observed phenomenon is that heat radiosensitizes cells.[64,357,401] Most reports note that the maximum increase in the slope of the radiation survival rate curves is 25% and that cells in S phase are more radiosensitized by heat than are cells in G_1.[355]

The cause of this radiosensitization has not been firmly established; however, it is believed that the accumulation of proteins in the nucleus, which bind to the nuclear matrix following heat treatment, prevents the cell from repairing radiation damage.[43,258,466] The ability for enzymatic excision of radiation-induced thymine damage is inhibited in chromatin isolated from heated cells even when the repair enzymes are obtained from control cells, whereas the repair enzymes from heated cells were able to excise damage in chromatin from control cells.[466] A correlation exists between the amount of excess nuclear protein and the inhibition of exogenous nucleases[467] and digestion of DNA in chromatin, which suggests that access to the DNA damage is blocked, thereby inhibiting repair.[182,467]

Another factor of possible clinical relevance is that cells in G_1 are less sensitive to heat than cells in S phase, whereas the opposite is true for cellular sensitivity to radiation (Fig. 16-4). This effect has often been cited as one of the principal factors contributing to the "biologic rationale" for the clinical use of

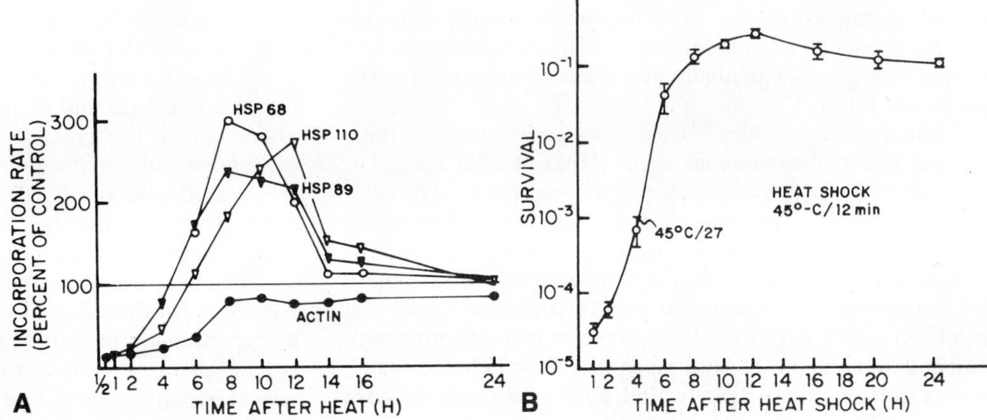

FIGURE 16–3. Correlation between heat shock protein synthesis (**A**) and thermotolerance (**B**) for Chinese hamster ovary cells. (Subjeck JR, Sciandra JJ, Chao CF, et al: Br J Cancer 45:127–131, 1982)

hyperthermia. In fact, a marked complementary synergism across the cell cycle was observed when heat (45°C for 30 minutes) and radiation (400 cGy) were combined.[199] It can be argued that in a tumor the proliferating cells are likely be a small fraction of quiescent cells that are nutrient-deprived[191] or at low pH[118] and are heat-sensitive, and that the heat sensitivity is not affected by acute hypoxia.[117]

Enhanced cell kill by irradiation and heat has been defined as the thermal enhancement ratio (TER), expressed as follows:

$$\text{TER} = \frac{\text{Dose of irradiation alone}}{\text{Dose of irradiation + heat}} \rightarrow \text{Same biological effect}$$

The relationship of the TER in the tumor and the normal tissues is called the therapeutic gain factor (TGF):

$$\text{TGF} = \frac{\text{TER in tumor}}{\text{TER in normal tissues}}$$

Both TER and TGF should have values greater than 1 to have a positive therapeutic implication.

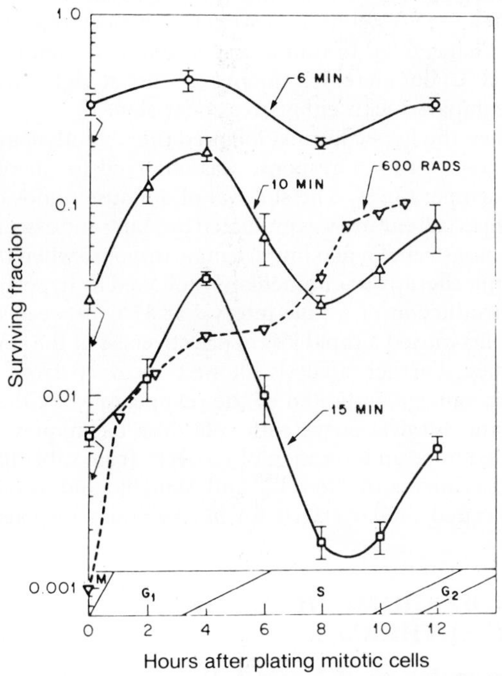

FIGURE 16–4. Variation in the survival of Chinese hamster ovary cells following exposures to either heat (45.5°C for 6, 10, or 15 minutes) or radiation (600 cGy). (Westra A, Dewey WC: Int J Radiat Oncol Biol Phys 19:467–477, 1971)

Urano and associates[435] and Stone[401] have reported a greater enhancement of early damage than late damage with a combination of irradiation and heat in mice.

Timing of Irradiation and Heat Administration

To combine heat and radiation effectively, carefully consider the sequence of application. Dewey and co-workers[64] have hypothesized that if heat is delivered 3 hours before radiation, cells with a low pH will have minimal ability to repair heat damage and therefore may be greatly sensitized to the effects of subsequent radiation. Hill and Denekamp,[162] Field,[105] and Overgaard[285] strongly suggest that when preferential (selective) heating of the tumor exists in relation to normal tissues, it is best to administer the two modalities *simultaneously.*[65,112,217,228,286,356,358,400] However, when the temperature in the tumor and in the normal tissues is the same, a therapeutic gain occurs only when the heat is delivered 4 hours or more after exposure to radiation (Fig. 16-5). In some tumors in humans treated with radiation and heat, the impact of timing of both modalities has been shown to have varying influence on the effects of the treatment on the tumor or the normal tissues.[5,6,295]

The interaction between heat and radiation does not exhibit the same time-temperature relationship as does heat alone. This is proven by both *in vitro* and *in vivo* studies.[211,357] A

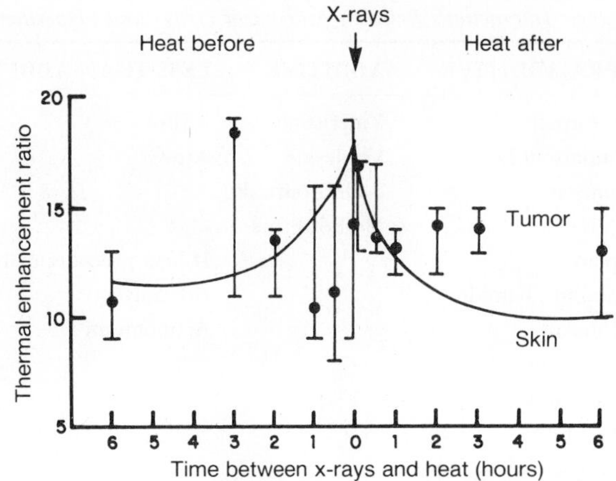

FIGURE 16–5. Thermal enhancement ratio (TER) as a function of the time interval between heat and irradiation. Solid line represents skin data of Stewart and Denekamp.[399] TER values are for fibrosarcoma at 20 days' regrowth delay (*i.e.,* at the same x-ray dose as used for skin). (Stewart FA, Denekamp J: Radiology 51:307–316, 1978)

maximum effectiveness is seen near 43°C for simultaneous treatment, suggesting that there may be an optimal temperature for combined modality treatment. However, when the modalities were given sequentially, little effect of temperature variations was found.[287]

Mittal and co-workers[260] carried out experiments in transplanted RIF-1 fibrosarcomas in the flanks of C3H mice. Tumors were treated with fractionated x-rays (400 cGy twice weekly × 10) alone or in combination with heat (RF currents, 43°C, twice weekly). Animals treated with radiation alone or with heat and radiation delivered with sequential fractionation (all heat sessions given before or after the radiation exposures) exhibited a 20% cure rate. In the animals treated with simultaneous combination of both modalities (heat delivered same day as radiation, immediately after x-ray exposure), the cure rate was 70%.

Interaction of Heat with Chemotherapeutic Agents

Hahn and associates[135,138] and other clinicians[155,270] have reported on the interaction of heat with a variety of cytotoxic agents. The type of drug, dose, temperature, and time of administration of the agents are important factors in determining cell kill by combination of these agents.[23,136,247] The interaction of heat and drugs in patients is not completely understood. Since Hahn's original work,[135] there have been numerous reports on this subject, and some excellent reviews have been published.[56,99,136,159]

Enhanced cytotoxicity of drugs at elevated temperatures is not a predictable process. The vinca alkaloids and most antimetabolites have only additive cytotoxicity with hyperthermia.[136,159] In two anticancer agents, AMSA and Ara-C, cell kill was actually inhibited at elevated temperatures[155] (BE Magum, personal communication). Doxorubicin (Adriamycin) and dactinomycin (Actinomycin D) exhibit complex interactions with hyperthermia, and both increased killing and protection have been observed with these agents, depending on the scheduling of drugs and heat.[78,139]

A summary of interactions between anticancer drugs and hyperthermia is shown in Table 16-1. In addition, a category of agents not normally considered to be of therapeutic value at 37°C shows significant killing ability at elevated temperatures. These agents include alcohols, amphotericin-B, cysteine, cysteamine, and AET (2-amino-ethyl-isothiourea).

TABLE 16–1
Cytotoxic Interactions Between Anticancer Drugs and Hyperthermia

SUPRA-ADDITIVE	ADDITIVE	LESS THAN ADDITIVE
Adriamycin	Vincristine	AMSA
Actinomycin D	Vindesine	Ara-C
Bleomycin	5-Fluorouracil	
BCNU	Methotrexate	
Cisplatin		If heat precedes drug:
Cyclophosphamide		Adriamycin
Melphalan		Actinomycin D
Mitoxantrone		
Mitomycin C		
Thio-TEPA		
Misonidazole*		
5-thio-D-glucose*		

** In hypoxic cells*
(Modified from Donaldson et al[78]; Kim et al[198]; Hahn[135]; Marmor[247]; Teicher et al[424]; Adams et al[2]; Herman [155]; Goldfeder and Newport[127].

The wide variety in mechanisms of drug cell kill precludes the idea that heat and drug interaction is a simple unilateral phenomenon. In fact, heat can enhance drug resistance in the case of doxorubicin[135] and dactinomycin.[78] As heating duration is increased, cells in culture become highly resistant to killing by either drug. This may be caused by heat-induced alteration in drug transport into the cell.[107]

The sensitizing effects of heat in combination with cisplatin have been confirmed *in vivo*.[80,270] Herman[157,158] demonstrated in experimental models (murine RIF tumor) the substantial enhancement of antitumor effect obtained with the combination of radiation, heat, and cytotoxic agents (cisplatin). This hypothesis is being evaluated in prospective clinical trials.[158,159]

Hyperthermia and Photodynamic Therapy

Earlier investigations with hematoporphyrin derivatives suggested that at least some of the results attributed to phototherapy were partially caused by a hyperthermic effect.[160] Studies by Svaasand[421] demonstrated that tumor response may originate from either pure photodynamic effect or pure hyperthermic effect as well as from a combination of both. Later other investigators[40,147,243,254,460,461] reported increased effectiveness of photodynamic therapy when combined with hyperthermia.

The cellular target, the effect of these photodynamic agents, and the optimal way to combine them are not completely understood. A report by Star and associates[394] noted that tumor cells treated with photodynamic therapy and subsequently transplanted were still viable and growing a new tumor. This observation, as well as the demonstration that vascular damage is the major effect of photodynamic therapy, led these investigators to conclude that this modality destroys the vascular bed of the tumor. Experiments by Waldow and associates[459,460] delivering a combination of heat and photodynamic therapy to an implanted SMT-F mammary carcinoma demonstrated minimal or no enhancement in tumor response at lower temperatures (below 40°C) but increased tumor response at higher temperatures, compared with either treatment alone.

When the hyperthermia followed the photodynamic therapy, a greater tumor response was observed for increasingly higher temperatures. The survival of a mouse tumor cell line (EMT-6) in cell culture was evaluated by Mang and associates,[243] who demonstrated a maximum tumor response when the photodynamic therapy was immediately followed by hyperthermia. The introduction of a time interval at 37°C between the two treatments caused a rapid loss of effectiveness of the combined modalities. Further analysis showed recovery from photodynamic damage, indicated by the reappearance of the shoulder in the survival curve with split-dose techniques. This is presumed to be an indication of recovery from sublethal damage. Experiments by Hetzel[160] and Mattiello and associates[250] demonstrated similar effects for *in vivo* tumor response.

PHYSIOLOGIC MECHANISMS IN HYPERTHERMIA

Microvasculature of Normal Tissue

There is great variation in the microcirculation of different tissues such as striated muscle, skin, and so on. Nevertheless, there is regularity in distribution within a specific tissue.[203] In a typical "model," all exchanges between blood and parenchymal cells take place at the capillary level (microcirculation). True capillaries in normal tissues have a diameter close to that of an erythrocyte (7 μ to 10 μ).

Microvasculature of Tumors

At an early stage of tumor development the tumor cells probably proliferate by using energy and nutrients supplied through the host's blood vessels. As the tumor grows, host vessels are occasionally incorporated into the tumor mass. As the demand for nutrients and oxygen exceeds the supply capacity of the host vessels, a new vascularization in the tumor begins (formation of "buds" and, by confluence, "sprouts"). It has been suggested that certain humoral factors are important for the initiation of this process (*e.g.,* tumor angiogenesis factor [TAF] and endothelial proliferating factor [EPF]). The capillaries formed by random fusion of sprouts are tortuous, elongated, and dilated, and they lack basement membranes.[84] A large proportion of tumor blood does not exchange with blood in the general circulation (stasis). This intermittent circulation–periods of stasis followed by resumption of blood flow–is probably a normal feature of the intravascular transport system of neoplastic tissues.[134, 448] The histologic patterns and functional status of vascular networks in malignant tumors vary, depending on the type, age, and size of the tumor.[453]

Tannock[423] has suggested that the longer turnover time of endothelial cells (their slower proliferation relative to that of neoplastic cells) accounts for the decline in vascular density. Reduced vascular density together with the sluggish perfusion of blood through the capillaries may account for the decrease in total blood flow.[390, 448] In general, tumor blood flow is vigorous in the periphery and sluggish in the center.[332, 389]

Hyperthermia and Normal Tissue Microcirculation

Song and associates[391] observed that the blood flow of skin overlying the tumor and of muscle *near* the tumor is more than twice that of the skin and muscle *far* from the tumor. They attribute this phenomenon to inflammatory processes near the tumors. A significant increase in the blood flow occurred in skin and muscle both near and far from the tumor when heated to 43°C for 1 hour.[388] It should be noted that the magnitude of increase was higher in the normal tissues adjacent to the tumor than in the tissues far from the tumor.

The dynamic changes of skin and muscle blood flow are both time- and temperature-dependent. Peak blood flows are different for various times and temperatures; similar trends have been observed in muscle blood flow. Blood vessels in mouse gut were particularly sensitive to heat: A temperature of 41°C for 1 hour to the lower body resulted in a sizable reduction in the visible venous tree.[102] The microcirculation of connective tissue was investigated in rats[68] and in rabbit ear chambers.[81]

Hyperthermia and Tumor Microcirculation

Several excellent reviews have been published on the subject of hyperthermia and tumor microcirculation.[85, 96, 332, 405] The complex relationship between temperature, exposure time, and physiologic response for tumors and for normal tissue has been depicted in a simplified diagram in Figure 16-6. The data are based almost entirely on rodent studies (mostly murine models). Tumor vasculature seems to be less able to show vasodilation to elevated temperature and is also more heat-labile than the vasculature of normal tissue. Both tumor and normal tissues increase their blood flow as a result of hyperthermia exposure. However, the vasodilatory effect in normal tissue may

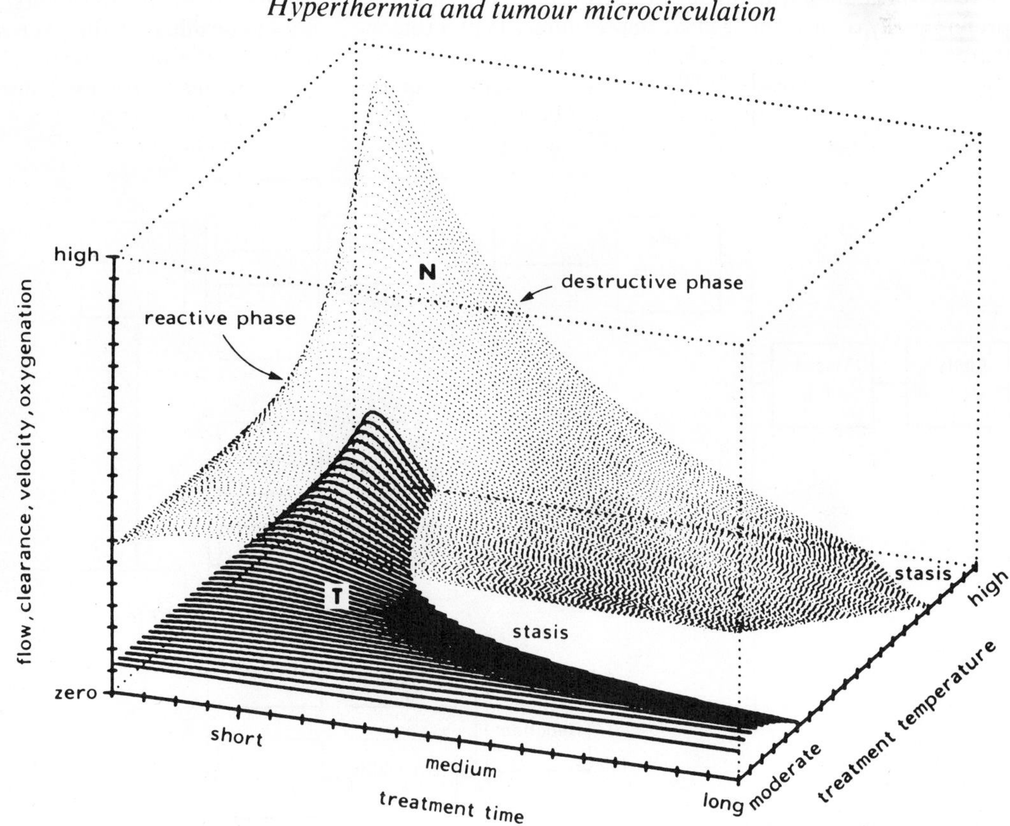

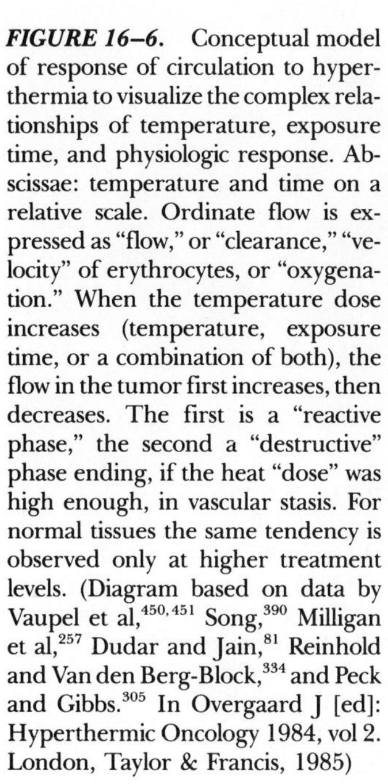
FIGURE 16–6. Conceptual model of response of circulation to hyperthermia to visualize the complex relationships of temperature, exposure time, and physiologic response. Abscissae: temperature and time on a relative scale. Ordinate flow is expressed as "flow," or "clearance," "velocity" of erythrocytes, or "oxygenation." When the temperature dose increases (temperature, exposure time, or a combination of both), the flow in the tumor first increases, then decreases. The first is a "reactive phase," the second a "destructive" phase ending, if the heat "dose" was high enough, in vascular stasis. For normal tissues the same tendency is observed only at higher treatment levels. (Diagram based on data by Vaupel et al,[450, 451] Song,[390] Milligan et al,[257] Dudar and Jain,[81] Reinhold and Van den Berg-Block,[334] and Peck and Gibbs.[305] In Overgaard J [ed]: Hyperthermic Oncology 1984, vol 2. London, Taylor & Francis, 1985)

be greater. Even in normal tissues, however, if the temperature exceeds 46°C for a few minutes, vascular destruction occurs, and this leads to direct tissue damage due to ischemia. The temperature threshold for this type of vascular destruction in tumors (rodent models) is lower than in normal tissues (40°C to 43.5°C).[14,76,84,91,98,333,388,419,451,454] Confirmatory data for a similar effect in human tumors are yet to be provided. Song and associates[392] noted that vascular damage after hyperthermia is progressive even after the heating is completed. This damage makes the tissue highly sensitive to a second heat treatment given a few hours after the first. Extremely important information was recently provided by Reinhold and van den Berg-Block,[333] who studied the response of microcirculation to hyperthermia in five different tumors, growing in "sandwich" observation chambers in the back of the rat. Their conclusions were as follows:

1. The various tumors required significantly different exposure times for inducing 50% stoppage of the tumor microcirculation (ST_{50}). This seems to indicate that differences in the characteristics of the tumor cells were more important for causing microcirculatory stoppage than in the sensitivity of the cells of the blood vessels.
2. An increase in surface (volume) was observed in all four tumors examined; the rate of increase was, however, significantly different among various tumors.
3. The relative velocity of the erythrocytes in selected capillaries in the tumors decreased as a result of hyperthermic treatment and was probably related to the tumor specific ST_{50}.

Several different mechanisms have been proposed to explain the vascular events occurring in tumors during hyperthermia (Fig. 16-7).[81] However, none of the proposed single causative factors has been fully explained.

The previously mentioned observations led to the speculation that the manipulation of tumor blood flow could be used to increase intratumoral temperature during hyperthermia (to preferentially reduce tumor blood flow to induce higher tumor temperatures). This approach has been studied in both murine and canine tumor models.[332,455] Vorhees and Babbs[48,55] demonstrated that hydralazine, a peripheral vasodilator, could achieve this effect. This agent, however, is difficult to use clinically because of the risk for postural hypotension in normotensive patients with doses that are typically used for the treatment of hypertension. Effects of hydralazine are long-lasting, thereby making use of this agent for outpatients impossible. It is well known that 25% of the dose used clinically for hypertension can cause thermal effects in canine muscle.[341] Dewhirst[66] subsequently studied this reduced dose of hydralazine for modification of tumor temperatures in both canine and human subjects. Unfortunately, the results showed that doses in this range are insufficient to induce a blood pressure drop, which appears to be necessary to cause temperature elevation during heating. From current information, clinical trials using hydralazine appear unlikely.

Hyperglycemia has also been studied as a modifier of tumor blood flow.[462] Administration of glucose has been shown to reduce both human and murine tumor pH.[426] The mechanisms of this effect are thought to be partially related to microvascular effects.[463] The increase in the acidity of tumor tissue that enhances the therapeutic effect of hyperthermic treatment is based on results of *in vitro* investigations using cell cultures.[33,34,405,449,478] No such study has been done involving experimental or human tumors *in situ*.[442]

Hyperthermia and Intratumor pH

The pH of arterial blood is 7.4 and that of venous blood and interstitial fluid is 7.35. Intracellular pH usually ranges from 6.0 to 7.4 in different cells, averaging about 7.0. Studies have shown that no significant difference exists between the intracellular pH of normal cell lines and that of their malignant counterparts.[176]

Song and co-workers[391] and Bicher and associates[16] have shown that hyperthermia triggers an immediate and significant decrease in the pH of tumors. Bicher reported that when heating was terminated, the pH rose to 6.78 but decreased to 6.5 to 6.6 when the tumors were reheated.

Ryu and associates[346] observed that the lactic acid content

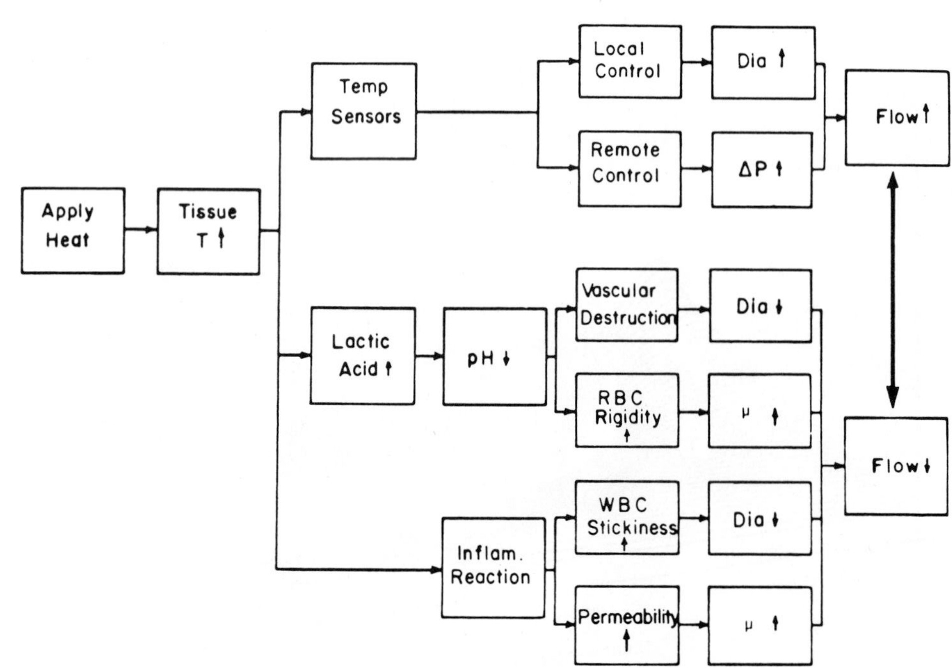

FIGURE 16–7. Theoretical framework for blood flow regulation during hyperthermia. Physiologic mechanisms, different in normal and in neoplastic tissues, are thought to be responsible. Note that some factors increase flow, whereas others decrease flow. The overall response is the result of these opposing factors. (Dudar TE, Jain RK: Cancer Res 44:605–612, 1984)

TABLE 16–2
Physical Agents and Techniques for Local Hyperthermia

	MICROWAVES		RF ELECTRIC AND MAGNETIC FIELDS		
	EXTERNAL (WAVE-GUIDE CAVITIES)	INTERSTITIAL (COAXIAL ANTENNAS)	EXTERNAL (PLATES, COILS)	INTERSTITIAL (NEEDLE ARRAYS)	ULTRASOUND EXTERNAL (PIEZO-ELECTRIC CRYSTAL TRANSDUCERS)
Frequency range	300–2450 MHz	300–1000 MHz	0.1–27 MHz	0.1–1.0 MHz	0.3–3.0 MHz
Area coverage	10–400 cm²*	Implant volume (20–1000 cm³)	10–200 cm²*	Implant volume (20–1000 cm³)	5–75 cm²*
Therapeutic depth	Up to 3 cm (muscle)	—	Up to 8 cm (muscle)	—	Up to 6 cm (muscle)
Power required	20–300 W*	10–200 W	20–400 W*	10–200 W	10–100 W*
Suitable for heating	Tumors in superficial muscle; in muscle behind fat or bone	Tumors in any volume that can be implanted	Tumors in superficial muscle or muscle behind fat (coils)	Tumors in any volume that can be implanted	Tumors in muscle; in muscle behind fat; deep-seated tumors (multiple beams)
Unsuitable for heating	Deep-seated tumors	Tumor in volumes that cannot be surgically invaded	Tumors in muscle behind fat (plates)	Tumors in volumes that cannot be surgically invaded	Tumors behind (or near) bone or air cavities

** Single applicator or pair of plates*
(Perez C, Emami B, Nussbaum GH: Front Radiat Ther Oncol 18:83, 1984)

in mouse tumors significantly increased with heating. Streffer and colleagues[405] also reported that hyperthermia caused an increase in the amount of both lactic acid and β-hydroxybutyric acid in mouse tumors. The pH of human tumors is significantly lower than that of normal tissue[479]; there is no significant difference among different types of human tumors in this respect.[480] Also, human tumor pH appears to consistently increase after treatment with a combination of localized hyperthermia and radiation therapy.[442,480]

BASIC PRINCIPLES OF PHYSICS AND INSTRUMENTATION

Power Deposition

The physical agents employed for power deposition in local clinical hyperthermia are electromagnetic fields at very high microwave frequencies (300 MHz to 2450 MHz), "low frequency" microwaves (60 MHz to 120 MHz), electromagnetic fields at radiofrequencies (0.1 MHz to 27 MHz), and ultrasound at frequencies of 0.3 MHz to 3 MHz. The main characteristics of these modalities are summarized in Table 16-2.

Temperature elevations with radiofrequency (RF) electric fields may be produced through conductive, dielectric, or inductive heating of the tissue (Fig. 16-8). Conductive or resistive heating refers specifically to heating with RF currents driven between pairs of external electrodes. The resulting power deposition is effected through collisions of moving ions with tissue molecules. With dielectric or capacitive heating the power is deposited in tissue through the interaction of the electric fields produced by electrodes with a dielectric medium (polarization charges) (Fig. 16-9).[218] Inductive heating refers to tissue heating with RF "eddy current" induced by the RF magnetic fields produced in the tissue by an external coil applicator surrounding the tissue.

The mechanical waves of frequencies above the audible range are called ultrasound (US). Ultrasound is generated by conversion of electric voltage charges into mechanical forces in motion in the piezoelectric crystal (Fig. 16-10). At present, however, most ultrasonic transducers have ceramic crystals, which have the advantage of low cost and the possibility of manufacturing crystals of practically any shape. For further study of physical characteristics and basic principles of electromagnetic energy absorption, excellent reviews by Paliwal and Buchler[300] and Hand and James[141] are highly recommended. Similarly, further in-depth knowledge of physical characteristics and properties of ultrasound can be found in excellent reviews by Fry and Dunn,[113] Goss and associates,[132] and Hynynen.[173]

Heat transfer may be mediated by conduction through vibrational and rotational interaction of adjacent molecules or by convection of heat through blood flow. In muscle tissue an absorbed power density of 0.060 watts/g produces an initial rate

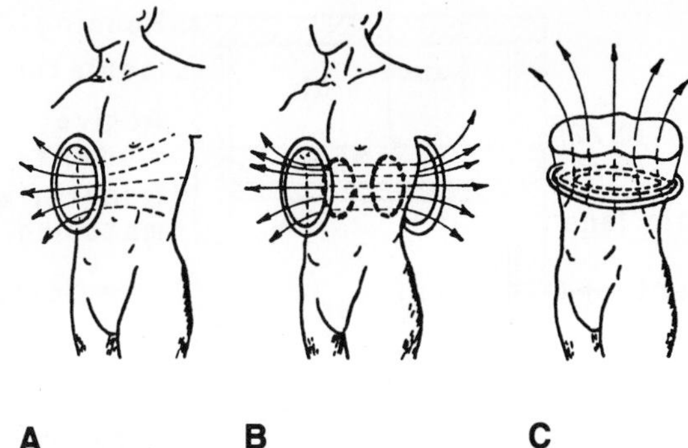

FIGURE 16–8. Radiofrequency heating. Three arrangements of current loops and the corresponding directions of magnetic field lines. Eddy currents are also shown: (**A**) resistive, (**B**) capacitive, and (**C**) inductive. (Cheung AY, Neyzari A: Cancer Res 44(Suppl): 4736S–4744S, 1984)

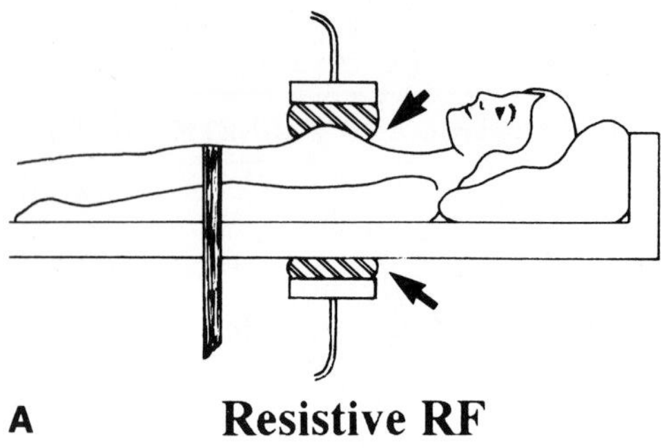

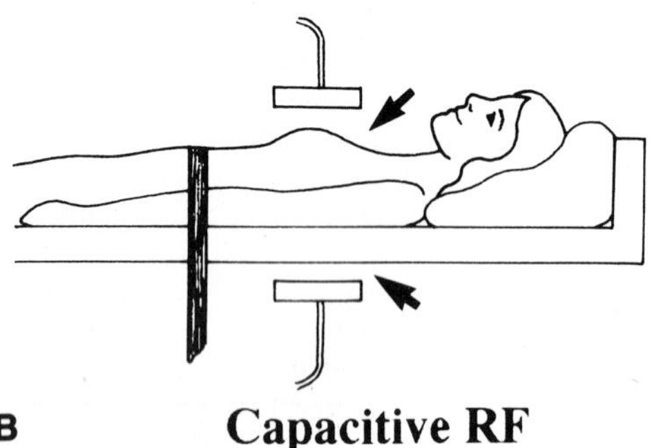

FIGURE 16–9. Position of electrodes in (**A**) resistive radiofrequency and (**B**) capacitive radiofrequency.

of temperature rise of 1°C per minute. During later stages of the hyperthermia session, the rate of temperature rise gradually decreases as the heat transfer process such as conduction and blood flow becomes more dominant.

Local External Heating (Superficial)

Microwaves

PENETRATION DEPTH. Several important factors affect the performance of waveguide applicators that must be taken into consideration in their design. The basic characteristics of microwave penetration in muscle for externally beamed "plane waves" (approximated only when applicator aperture size is significantly greater than the wavelength of microwaves in muscle) or various applicator apertures are presented in Figure 16-11. At all frequencies, microwaves are far more penetrating in fat than in muscle. At 915 MHz, for example, the penetration depth in fat is 17.7 cm compared with only 3.0 cm in muscle. Penetration depth increases with decreasing frequency. Thus the plane wave penetration depth in muscle, for example, increases from 3.0 cm at 915 MHz to 3.9 cm at 300 MHz to 6.7 cm at 100 MHz.

For waveguide applicators of clinically practical dimensions the increase in penetration with decreasing frequency is far less pronounced than is suggested by the plane wave analysis shown earlier. A detailed theoretical analysis of the problem by Turner and Kumar[430] has shown that over the frequency range of 300 MHz to 1000 MHz, the change in penetration depth is very modest. Measurements of power deposition from a variety of applicators used for local hyperthermia suggest that the increase in penetration (*e.g.*, in muscle) that occurs at 300 MHz over that which occurs at 915 MHz is minimal for all but the largest applicators.[222]

The term *penetration depth* (13.5%), widely used in engineering, has no clinical use. A more reliable indicator of clinically useful penetration depth is probably 50% of the surface value. When this definition is used, the increase in penetration with decreasing frequency is even less (Fig. 16-12). Intersection of the curves in the figure with the horizontal broken lines yields the depths at which the specific absorption rate (SAR) falls to 50% and 13.5%, respectively, of its value at the surface. The penetration depth is tabulated for a number of different frequencies for both high (muscle, skin) and low (fat, bone) water content tissues in Table 16-3. None of the commonly available microwave waveguide applicators has clinically useful penetration depth (50%) of over 3 cm. This important factor for quality assurance has been one of the major limitations in clinical use of hyperthermia. Decreasing the frequency of microwaves enhances the depth of penetration of the beam. However, because an inverse relationship exists between frequency and wavelength, the size of the applicator becomes impractically larger for clinical use.[110]

THERMAL FIELD. From fundamental considerations, it is unlikely that useful therapeutic heating at a given depth can be

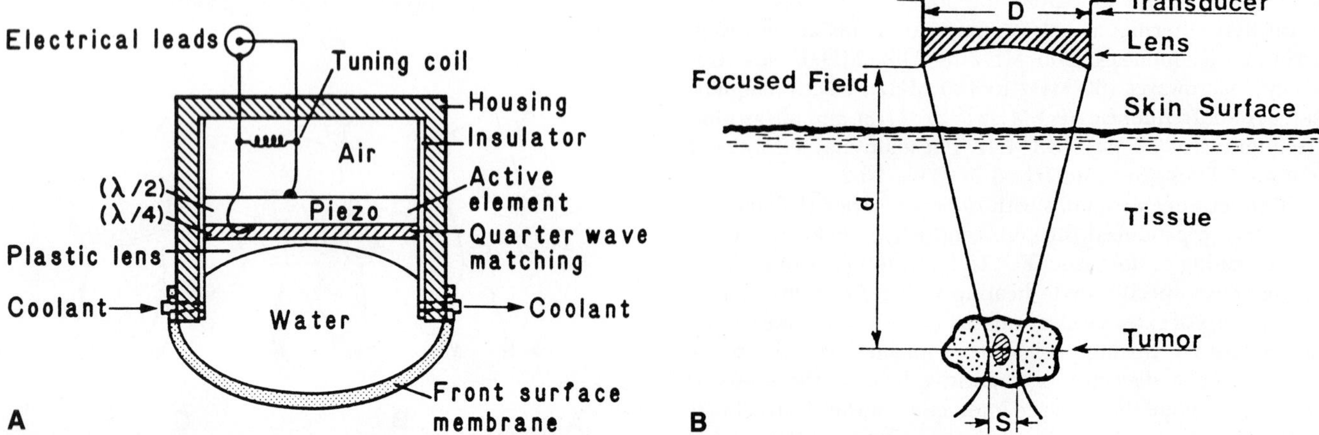

FIGURE 16–10. (**A**) High power tranducer design. (Barber FE, Friffice CP: Power deposition for ultrasound hyperthermia. In Nussbaum GH [ed]: Physical Aspects of Hyperthermia, pp 209–230. New York, American Association of Physicists in Medicine, 1982) (**B**) Schematic representation of energy deposition from a focusing transducer into the tumor. (Lele PP: Radiat Environ Biophys 17:205–217, 1980)

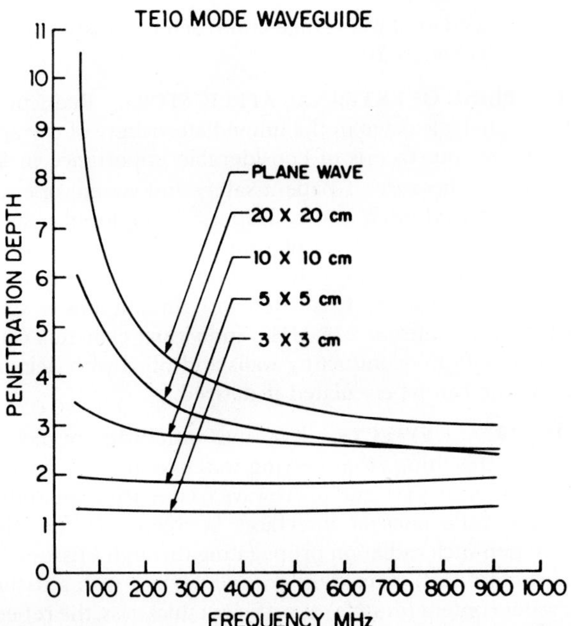

FIGURE 16–11. Penetration depth for various microwave frequencies (TE10 mode waveguide).

TABLE 16–3
Plane Wave Penetration of Microwaves in Homogeneous Media of High and Lower Water Content

	PENETRATION DEPTH (cm)	
FREQUENCY (MHz)	d_p^{H*}	$d_p^{L\dagger}$
2450	1.7	11.2
915	3.0	17.7
433	3.6	26.2
300	3.9	32.1
100	6.7	60.4

**H: high water content (muscle, skin)*
†L: low water content (fat, bone)

extended to regions in which the absorbed power density is less than 25% to 50% of the maximum at that depth. For some microwave applicators used in clinical hyperthermia, the thermotherapeutic field size is considerably smaller than the area of the applicator aperture. This is illustrated in Figure 16-13 for an 8-cm × 8-cm applicator operating at 915 MHz; according to the 50% criterion, the therapeutically useful area is only 23% of the geometric area of 64 cm^2. New applicators have larger therapeutic fields because they have more than one antenna and antenna modifications designed to improve the area heated.[222] Figure 16-13 shows the isopower density curves (at 1 cm depth) for the same 8-cm × 8-cm applicator, fitted with three antennas (placed as shown) driven 180 degrees out of phase. The therapeutically useful heating area has been more than doubled (Eg = 0.51).[222]

Various approaches have been tried in an effort to improve the performance and versatility of external applicators. Fessenden and associates,[104] in cooperation with Varian Associates, have successfully designed and clinically used a spiral microstrip applicator operated at 915 MHz or 433 MHz (Fig. 16-14). The antennas are packaged with an integral 1 cm or 2 cm thick circulating water bolus with a flexible front end. These applicators have resulted in good coupling, a broad band width in clinically useful frequency ranges, and a symmetrically circular thermal field.

A device with two mechanical scanning applicators has been constructed to reduce potential "cold spots" between the spiral units. Another approach has been the incorporation of several microspiral applicators in an array that will cover a larger area (Fig. 16-15). These devices have improved versatility of application, but penetration depth is still limited.

Leybovich and co-workers[220] reported a significant increase in depth of penetration with a novel design of dual-antenna applicators operated at 80 MHz to 100 MHz that have

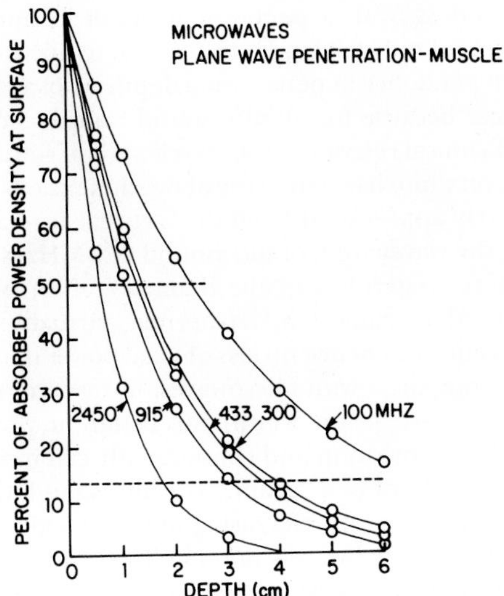

FIGURE 16–12. Variation of axial absorbed power density (watts/cm^3) with depth in a muscle-like medium for incident plane waves at a number of different frequencies. Values at depth are expressed as percentage of value at surface. Intersection of curves with lower broken line yields "penetration depths" for the respective frequencies (see Table 16-3).

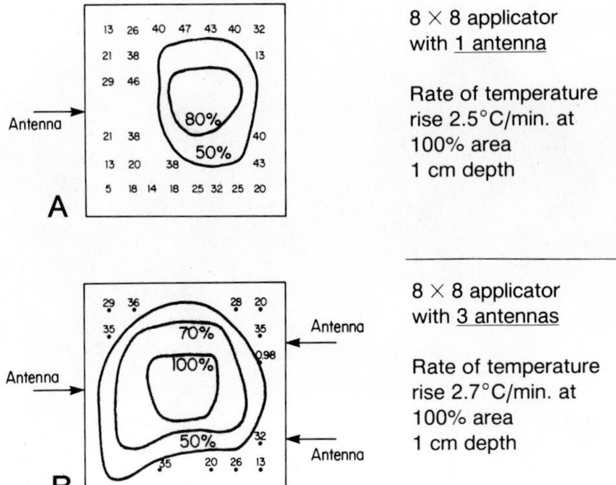

FIGURE 16–13. (**A**) Relative isopower density curves for 8 × 8 cm^2 applicator with a single antenna. (**B**) Relative isopower density curves for 8 × 8 cm^2 applicator with three antennas, driven 180 degrees out of phase, under same experimental conditions as in (**A**). The applicator is fully loaded with ε = 6 dielectric powder and operates at 915 MHz. Applicator-phantom coupling is through 1 cm deionized water. Measurements are made at depth of 1 cm in muscle phantom.

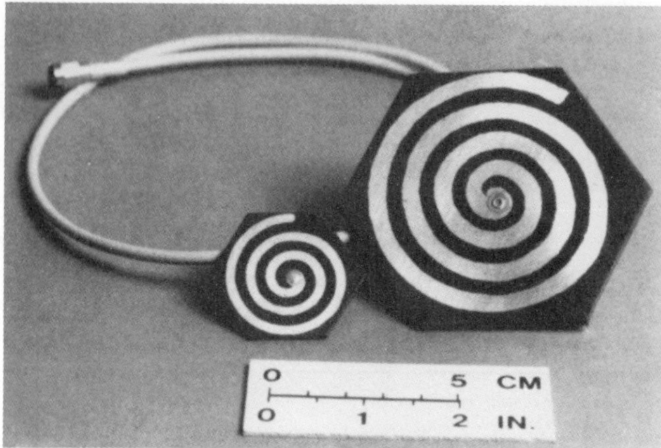

FIGURE 16–14. Two spiral microstrip antennas that operate over broad frequency ranges near 915 MHz (*left*) and 433 MHz (*right*). (Fessenden P, et al: Clinical microwave applicator design. In Paliwal BR, Hetzel FW, Dewhirst MW [eds]: Biological, Physical and Clinical Aspects of Hyperthermia, pp 123–131. New York, American Association of Physicists in Medicine, 1989)

permitted the applicators to have acceptable dimensions (21 cm × 26 cm; Fig. 16-16).

It is important to point out that as depth increases, the volume receiving the 25% or 50% SAR decreases. Straube and associates[404] determined the SAR distribution in a muscle-equivalent phantom with various size 915 MHz microwave applicators at different depths. Table 16-4 and Figure 16-17 illustrate the significant reduction in the 50% and 25% SAR values at 2 cm or 3 cm depth. Only small volumes receive 25% of the SAR at 3 cm depth. Myerson and colleagues[267] correlated the tumor control probability with the temperature obtained (minimum temperature 40°C for 30 minutes) and the 25% SAR of the applicator; a lower incidence of tumor control was noted in lesions with inadequate 25% SAR coverage compared with those having adequate coverage and reaching satisfactory temperatures (Table 16-5).

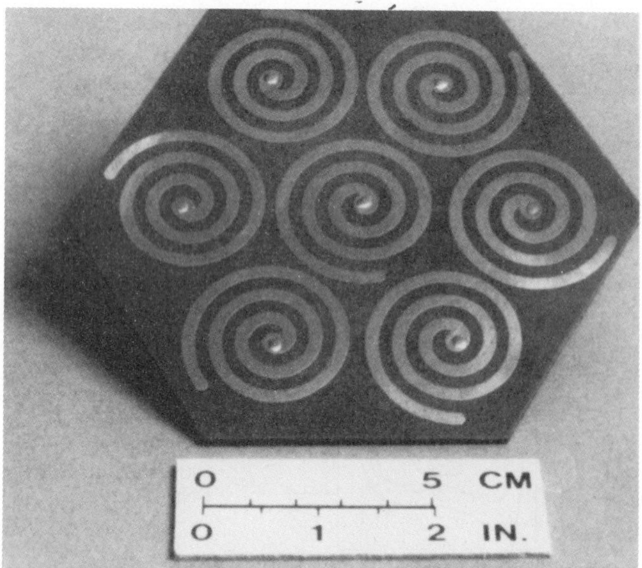

FIGURE 16–15. Seven of the small 915 MHz spirals etched on a rigid substrate. This was mounted in an applicator with circulating water bolus. (Fessenden P, et al: Clinical microwave applicator design. In Paliwal BR, Hetzel FW, Dewhirst MW [eds]: Biological, Physical and Clinical Aspects of Hyperthermia, pp 123–131. New York, American Association of Physicists in Medicine, 1989)

COUPLING OF EXTERNAL APPLICATORS. Reduction of electromagnetic leakage in the immediate vicinity of the applicator-patient interface is of considerable importance in local hyperthermia because of patient safety and system operating efficiency.[272] Leybovich and colleagues[223] employed a six-element conformable "soft" applicator for applications of local microwave hyperthermia to the lateral chest wall, an area of pronounced curvature. It is fitted with an antenna of special design and operates at 915 MHz; individual elements can be fabricated with nonconducting walls and filled with deionized water, which can be circulated if desired.

INTERFACE EFFECTS. In tissues with different dielectric properties (resulting from varying water content) electromagnetic radiation at VHF and microwave frequencies can undergo significant reflections at interfaces between different tissue types. When such radiation propagating through a tissue of low water content (fat) is incident on an interface with a tissue of high water content (muscle) of sufficient thickness, the reflected wave is nearly 180 degrees out of phase with the incident wave, thereby producing a standing wave with an intensity minimum (a cold spot) near the interface. If the wave is propagating in a tissue of high water content (muscle) and is incident on a tissue of low water content (bone), the reflected wave is in phase with the incident wave, thereby producing a standing wave with an intensity maximum (a hot spot) near the interface. The significant reflections indicated at tissue interfaces of clinical interest establish cold spots in the vicinity of fat-muscle interfaces and hot spots in the immediate region of muscle-bone and especially muscle-air interfaces.

Ultrasound Heating

PENETRATION DEPTH

For a given frequency, ultrasound is significantly more penetrating in fat than in muscle and far more penetrating in water than in fat. For example, at 1 MHz penetration depths are 3.8 cm in skeletal muscle, 10 cm in fat, and 2000 cm in degassed, distilled water. Also, the penetration of ultrasound in bone is extremely modest, with a penetration depth in human skull bone at 1 MHz of only 0.3 cm.[132] In contrast to microwaves, the frequency dependence of penetration depth is not a function of applicator size because for all ultrasound transducers with dimensions of clinical relevance, the wavelength of sound in clinical media is very much less than the above dimensions. This can be immediately appreciated from the fact that for water, muscle, and fat, the wavelength of ultrasound at 1 MHz is only 0.16 cm. Therefore, regardless of the diameter of an ultrasound applicator used in clinical hyperthermia, virtually no beam spreading occurs and hence no loss of axial power density from dispersion. Compared with microwaves, ultrasound retains its collimation (surface beam width) far better in propagating through a clinical medium and consequently can more appropriately be thought of as a "beam." For ultrasound, the reduction of power density with increasing depth in a given tissue is caused predominantly by absorption in the tissue medium and reflection at interfaces between different tissues.

COUPLING

The major objective of coupling in ultrasound hyperthermia is the elimination of air interface between the applicator and the area to be heated, which would cause total reflection of the ultrasound at that point. Usually the applicator is coupled to

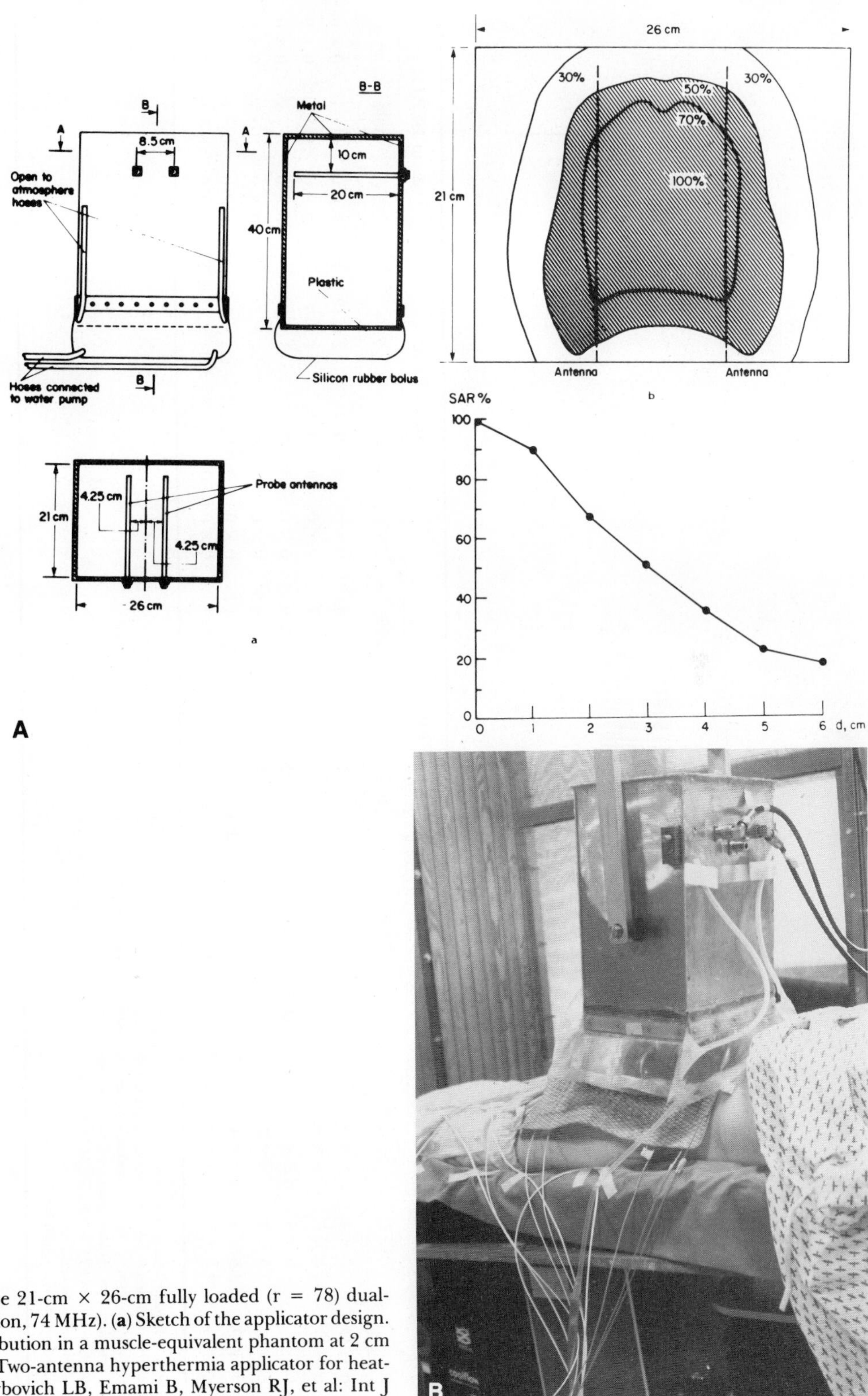

FIGURE 16–16. (**A**) Clinical prototype 21-cm × 26-cm fully loaded (r = 78) dual-antenna applicator (frequency of operation, 74 MHz). (**a**) Sketch of the applicator design. (**b**) Specific absorption rate (SAR) distribution in a muscle-equivalent phantom at 2 cm depth. (**c**) Depth SAR distribution. (**B**) Two-antenna hyperthermia applicator for heating tumors at intermediate depth. (Leybovich LB, Emami B, Myerson RJ, et al: Int J Hyperthermia, in press)

a degassed water column that is contained at the patient's surface by a soft plastic membrane conformable to the patient. It is of critical importance that the water be sufficiently degassed; otherwise the dissolved air in the water could cavitate out of the solution during the application of ultrasonic power, causing areas with no ultrasonic transmission. The plastic membrane can usually be coupled to the patient with most of the ultrasonic coupling gels used in diagnostic ultrasound. If the wet bond between the patient and the membrane dries during hyperthermia treatment, air pockets can form causing reflection of ultrasonic radiation at that point. After the applicator is coupled to the patient properly, there is little possibility of leakage of ultrasonic power.

THERMAL FIELD. For single beam applications, ultrasound frequencies of 0.3 MHz to 3 MHz are typically used; thus the heated region is in the near field (Fig. 16-18). The typical diameter of a transducer is 3 cm to 10 cm. Therapeutic heating

TABLE 16–4
Rectangular Contours in cm²

SIZE OF APPLICATOR (cm^2)	COUPLING	1 cm DEPTH			2 cm DEPTH			3 cm DEPTH			4 cm DEPTH		
		75%	50%	25%	75%	50%	25%	75%	50%	25%	75%	50%	25%
8 × 8	1 cm deionized H_2O	3 × 4	5 × 5	7 × 6	0 × 0	3 × 2	6 × 4	0 × 0	0 × 0	2 × (2 ± 1)	0 × 0	0 × 0	0 × 0
10 × 10	1 cm deionized H_2O	4 × 6	8 × 8	9.5 × 9	0 × 0	2 × 2	7 × 7	0 × 0	0 × 0	4 × 4	0 × 0	0 × 0	0 × 0
15 × 15	2 cm mineral oil	6 × 5	8.5 × 7.5	10 × 10.5	0 × 0	3 × 2	9 × 9	0 × 0	0 × 0	3 × 2	0 × 0	0 × 0	0 × 0
10 × 10	2 cm mineral oil	5 × 5	6 × 7	9 × 9	0 × 0	2 × 1	7.5 × 6.5	0 × 0	0 × 0	4 × 3	0 × 0	0 × 0	0 × 0
5.5 × 9	1 cm deionized H_2O	2.5 × 3	3.5 × 4	5 × 6	0 × 0	(2.5 ± 1) × (1.5 ± 1)	4 × 4.5	0 × 0	0 × 0	(2) × 1.5	0 × 0	0 × 0	0 × 0
(MA150) 10 × 13	1 cm deionized H_2O	6.5 × 4	8.5 × 6	9 × 7	0 × 0	4 × 4	7.5 × 9	0 × 0	0 × 0	(2 ± 1) × (2 ± 1)	0 × 0	0 × 0	0 × 0

NOTE: Rectangles approximating iso-SAR contours. SAR distributions in a uniform muscle equivalent phantom were determined from rate of rise measurements at every point on a 1 cm grid. One hundred percent was normalized to the point of maximum SAR at a depth of 1 cm. Rectangles were constructed that represented the area of iso-SAR contours without overestimating the area and without overshooting any one dimension of the contour by more than 1 cm. Applicators include two in-house applicators (with apertures of 8 × 8 cm² and 5 × 9 cm²) and three commercial applicators (CTCM1 15 × 15, CTCM2 10 × 10, MA150 10 × 13). Coupling medium (deionized water or mineral oil) as used in our clinic was studied.
(Straube WL, Myerson RJ, Emami B, et al: Int J Hyperthermia 6:665–670, 1990)

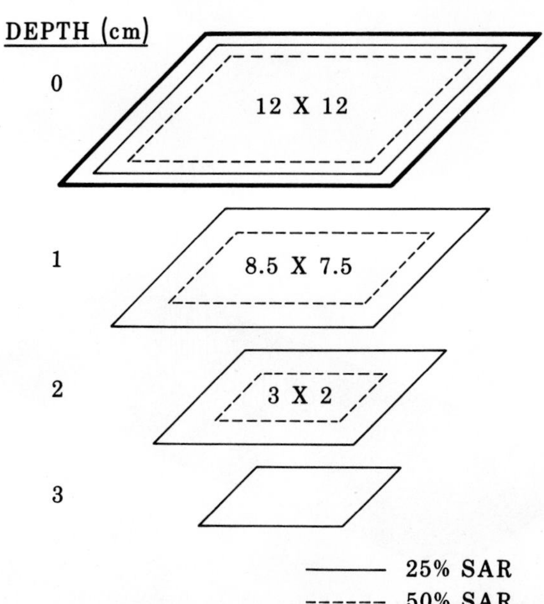

FIGURE 16–17. Reduction in the 50% and 25% specific absorption rate (SAR) values at 2 cm or 3 cm depth with 915 MHz microwaves. (Straube W, Leybovich L, Myerson RJ, et al: Volumetric characterization of SAR patterns of 915 MHz hyperthermia applicators, in preparation)

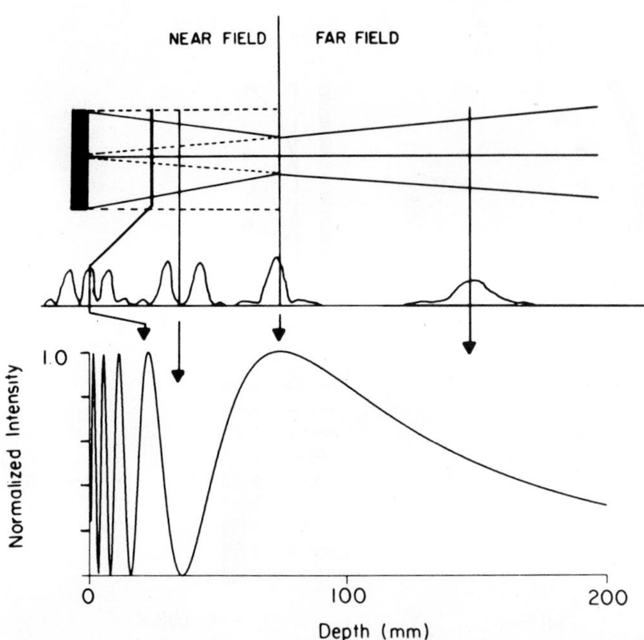

FIGURE 16–18. Normalized intensity distribution along the axis of a plane ultrasonic transducer (*bottom*). Outline of ultrasonic field (*top*) and intensity distributions across the axis at various locations (*middle*) are also illustrated. (Hynynen K: Induction of local hyperthermia using ultrasound. In Paliwal BR, Hetzel FW, Dewhirst MW [eds]: Biological, Physical and Clinical Aspects of Hyperthermia, pp 152–166. New York, American Association of Physicists in Medicine, 1988)

to depths of 6 cm in muscle is sometimes attainable, and power required ranges from 1 watt to 100 watts. Transducers can be focused or unfocused. The shape and direction of ultrasound beams can be modified by focusing, which is accomplished by optical or electrical means (Fig. 16-19*A*). The focused acoustic field is very complex between the acoustic focus and the transducer, resembling the near field of a plane transducer (Fig. 16-19*B*). Beyond the focus the field behaves in a fashion similar to that of the far field of a plane transducer, except that the divergence of the beam is dominated by the geometric divergence angle of the transducer beyond the focus.[145,173]

Heating to larger tissue volumes as well as at greater depths may be obtained by using a multiplicity of overlapping (or intersecting) ultrasound beams. For multiple beam ultrasound, typical operating parameters are frequency, 0.3 MHz to 1.0 MHz; volume coverage, 20 cm^3 to 500 cm^3; therapeutic depth, up to 10 cm; and power required, 30 watts to 200 watts. Several scanning, focused multitransducer apparatuses have been constructed or are in various phases of testing at a few institutions.[173,214,377] Generally, the temperature elevation appears to be limited to the scanned area[174,215,216] and extends in front of the focal zone.[173] In an effort to increase volume and depth of heating, a device with elaborate computer interfacing to optimize position and frequency of 32 focused transducers was designed by engineers at Varian Associates (Fig. 16-20).[377] Lele[213,216] and Hynynen[174] have reported on the design of similar devices. By tailoring the scanning pattern to cover large volumes (Fig. 16-21), it may be possible to heat deep-seated tumors. However, this is often limited by the window available for the propagation of the ultrasound from the surface into the treatment volume because of interposing gas or bone extension, temperature measurements, and accurate scanning of the ultrasound systems in clinical practice.

TABLE 16–5
Tumor Control Rate as a Function of SAR Coverage and Min t_{43}

	SAR < 25%	SAR ≥ 25%
Min t_{43} < 30	1/11 (9%)	3/8 (38%)
Min t_{43} ≥ 30	3/8 (38%)	19/26 (73%)

The difference between the group satisfying both SAR ≥ 25% and Min_{43} ≥ 30 and the group satisfying only one but not both criteria is significant at the P = 0.02 level. (Myerson RJ, Perez CA, Emami B, et al: Int J Radiat Oncol Biol Phys 18:1123–1129, 1990)

INTERFACE EFFECTS. Reflections of ultrasound at tissue interfaces can result in cold or hot spots in the vicinity of the interfaces, depending on whether the reflected wave is 180 degrees out of phase or in phase with the incident wave. At a muscle-bone interface, undesirable cold spots could well be produced in the muscle tissue upstream of the interface, and a hot spot is likely to be produced in the first few millimeters of bone itself.

Ultrasound-induced hyperthermia is well suited to therapeutic heating in homogeneous muscle and in muscle behind fat. However, because of its extremely high absorption rate in bone surface and its virtually total reflection at tissue-air interfaces, ultrasound-induced hyperthermia is unsuited for therapeutic heating of lesions with either bone or air in the path.[48]

External Local Deep (Intermediate Depth) Hyperthermia

Several different technical approaches to deep local hyperthermia that are still in the early developmental stages show promise.

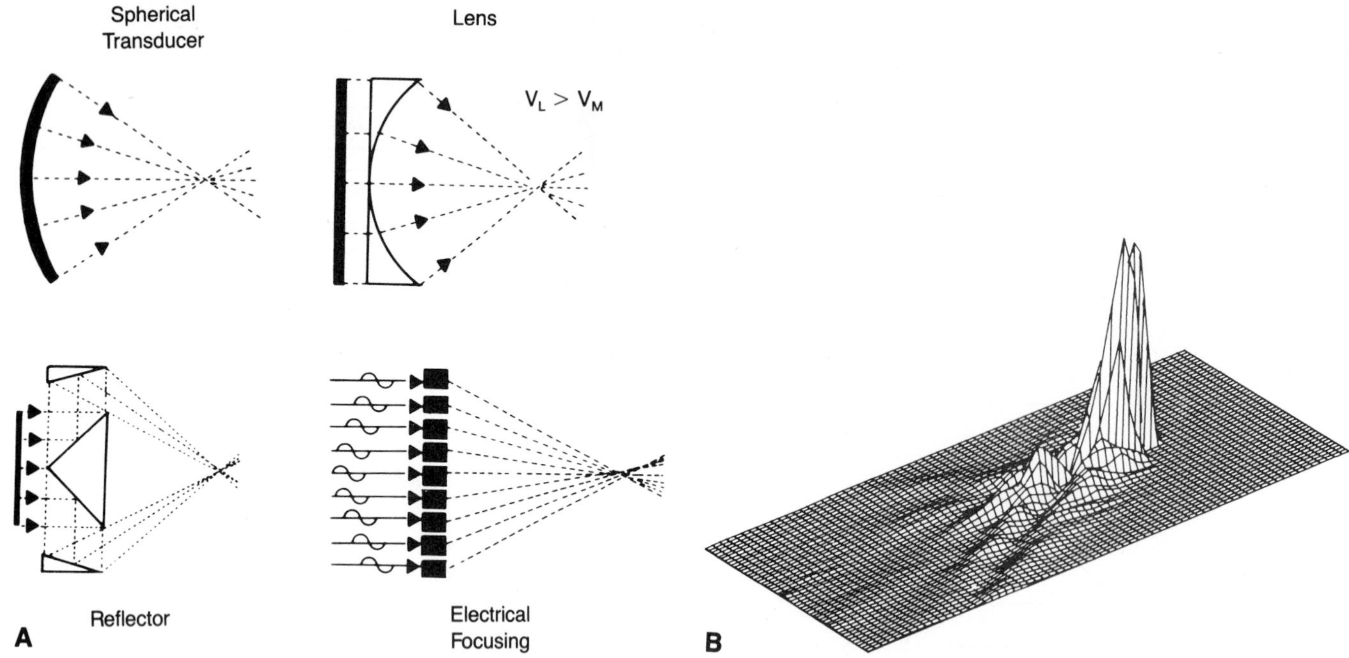

FIGURE 16–19. (**A**) Ultrasonic focusing systems. (**B**) Intensity distribution on axial plane from focused ultrasonic transducer (diameter 75 mm, radius of curvature 70 mm, frequency 1.15 MHz). The measurement was done in castor oil (attenuation 9.6 Np m^{-1}). The transducer is located on the left. (Hynynen K: Induction of local hyperthermia using ultrasound. In Paliwal BR, Hetzel FW, Dewhirst MW [eds]: Biological, Physical and Clinical Aspects of Hyperthermia, pp 152–166. New York, American Association of Physicists in Medicine, 1988)

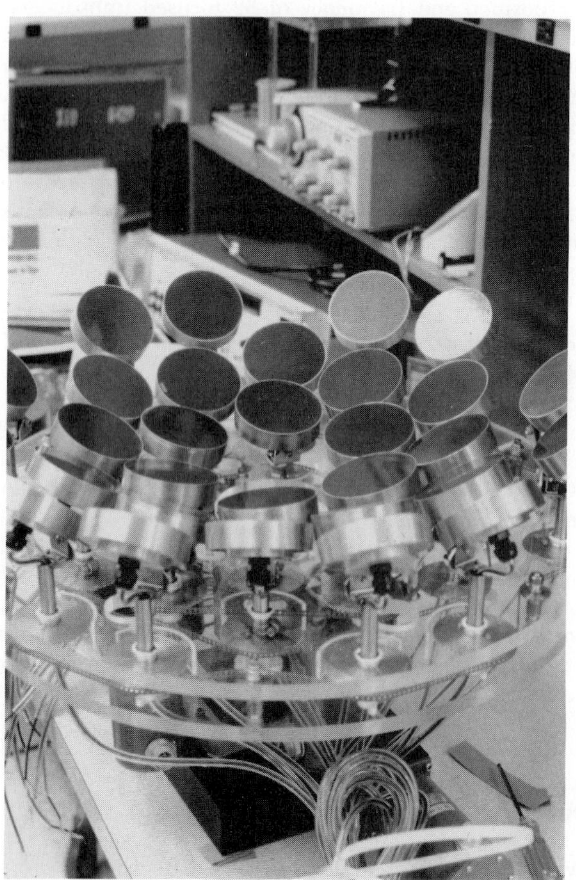

FIGURE 16–20. Top view of transducer array distributed over four rings of Varian Helios ultrasonic hyperthermia system.

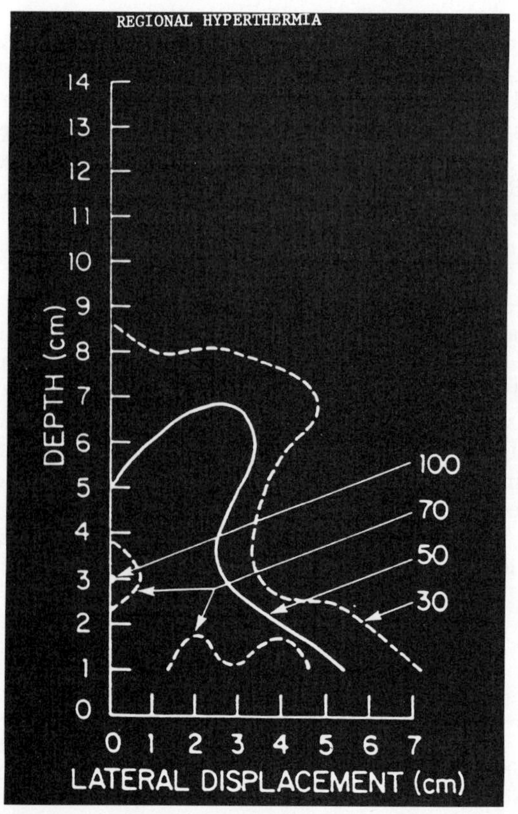

FIGURE 16–21. Example of relative initial heat array distribution *versus* depth in phantom and displacement from central axis of transducer array. (Nussbaum GH, Straube WL, Drage MD, et al: Potential for localized, adjustable deep heating in soft tissue environments with a thirty-beam ultrasonic hyperthermia system. Int J Hyperthermia, 7(2):279–299, 1991)

Microwave

Leybovich and associates[220] have developed a series of low-frequency microwave applicators of several different sizes operated at 80 MHz to 120 MHz for deep local heating for various anatomic locations. The 50% SAR depth is about 4 cm and the 25% SAR is about 7 cm. The preliminary clinical experience with these devices has been technically satisfactory. Although patient tolerance for skin heating up to 42°C to 43°C is good with superficial devices, skin tolerance with devices intended to heat tissues at intermediate depth may present a problem, perhaps because larger areas are heated. For such patients, it is often necessary to use circulating cold water to cool the most superficial 1 cm of the skin and subcutaneous tissue. If there is tumor at these depths, additional sessions with a superficial hyperthermia device are necessary.

Radiofrequency

Kato and co-workers[188, 189] developed a magnetic induction device that operates at frequencies less than or equal to 20 MHz, which has been used primarily for heating head and neck tumors. The SAR at a depth of about 5 cm to 6 cm is 50% of its peak value. As with other magnetic induction devices, this device operates at a high wattage (several thousand watts), and considerable caution must be taken to avoid direct contact between the patient and any current-carrying elements to avoid a severe thermal burn. Preliminary clinical results have been encouraging.[114]

Ultrasound

The use of multiple-applicator ultrasound devices in anatomic sites where there are no bone and muscle interfaces has been discussed elsewhere in this chapter.

Interstitial Hyperthermia

Interstitial hyperthermia can be administered by means of coaxial microwave antennas, radiofrequency electric current, or "hot source" techniques (inductively heated ferromagnetic seeds or resistant wires).

Microwave

Interstitial microwave hyperthermia may be produced through the use of coaxial microwave antennas inserted in Teflon catheters (tubes) implanted in the tissue volume of interest with a spacing of 1 cm to 2 cm, depending on the volume heated.[395] Generally, the frequency required is 300 MHz to 915 MHz. A cross-sectional view of one type of antenna is shown in Figure 16-22. As discussed by Strohbehn and Mechling,[412] this antenna is made from either standard or custom-made braided 50 ohm coaxial cable. At the junction, the inner conductor is soldered to the outer conductor of an extension section with a length of h_A. At an operating frequency of 915 MHz, h_A is approximately 3.5 cm. As shown in Figure 16-22, the antenna is inserted into an insulating nylon catheter so that the distance from the tissue-air interface to the junction is h_B, with the value of h_B dictated by the depth of the insertion.

The heating pattern of a coaxial antenna operating at microwave frequencies is ellipsoidal, coincident with the antenna axis (Fig. 16-23).

Both longitudinal and transverse extent of the therapeutically significant power absorption, and therefore heating from a given antenna, depend on the depth of insertion, the length of the exposed inner conductor, and the frequency of operation. For a given microwave antenna currently commercially available, the therapeutically useful volume of heating is approximately 3.0 cm to 4.5 cm (longitudinally) and 1.0 cm to 1.5 cm (transverse section). The greatest absorbed power density and therefore the greatest amount of heating occurs in the immediate vicinity of the antenna and specifically at the junction of the antenna and the connector.

The therapeutic heating potential of an array of four, single-junction coaxial antennas operating at 915 MHz, placed parallel and intersecting the corners of a 2 cm square, is shown in Figure 16-24. The distribution is normalized to its maximum value at the center of the array. Nearly 85% of the 4 cm^2 area bounded by the antennas lies within the 50% SAR curve. The longitudinal heating pattern depends on depth of insertion.

A major problem with the design of microwave antennas is the so-called dead space at the distal end of the antenna. The physical significance of this process is that when attempts have been made to increase the length of the antenna by increasing the length of the exposed inner conductor, the dead space becomes proportionally longer. The clinical significance is that in certain situations (such as the treatment of brain tumors with interstitial thermal radiation therapy), the volume of implant has to be significantly longer than tumor volume at the expense of normal tissue. Some modifications of basic antenna design have been carried out, as illustrated by Hamnerius, to eliminate this dead space and to improve the thermal distribution. A

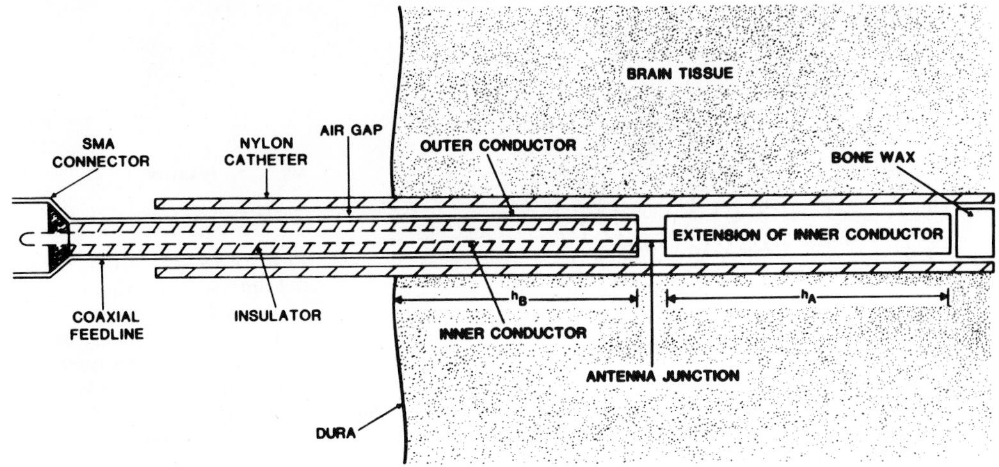

FIGURE 16–22. Basic design of interstitial microwave antenna. (Lyons BE, Britt RH, Strohnbehn JW: IEEE Trans BME 31:53–62, 1984)

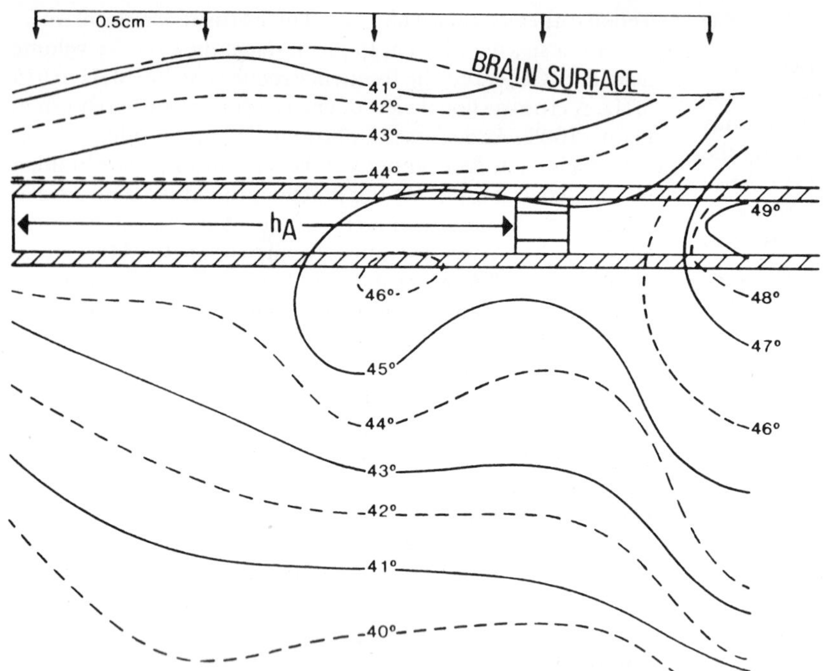

FIGURE 16–23. Isotherms from a single antenna in dog brain. (Lyons BE, Britt RH, Strohnbehn JW: IEEE Trans BME 31:53–62, 1984)

comparison of the SAR for a modified and a conventional antenna is shown in Figure 16-25.

The tissue heated by an application of interstitial hyperthermia is usually the implanted volume (*e.g.*, 20 cm^3 to 1000 cm^3). Measurement of SAR (W/kg) distributions produced in phantoms by a variety of antenna arrays and operating conditions has provided valuable insight into methods for producing improved therapeutic heating across the entire treatment volume. To this end we have employed bolus material, independent control of power to component subvolumes, and repositioning of antennas within respective catheters in clinical applications of interstitial hyperthermia.

INTRACAVITARY MICROWAVE ANTENNAS. Intracavitary microwave antennas are used to deliver local hyperthermia to tumor sites in and adjacent to hollow viscera or cavities, such as in gastrointestinal (esophagus, rectum), female reproductive (vagina, cervix, uterus), and genitourinary (prostate, bladder) systems. Intracavitary antennas have been used recently, inserted transurethrally, for the treatment of benign prostatic hypertrophy and carcinoma of the prostate.[360] Temperatures of 42°C were achieved for lengths of about 5 cm with effective penetration of about 0.5 cm around the applicator.

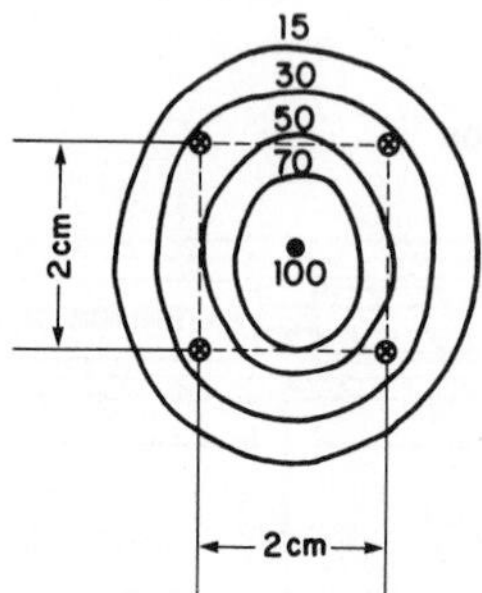

FIGURE 16–24. Relative distribution of specific absorption rate (SAR, W/kg) for an array of four coaxial antennas operating at 915 MHz, through a plane containing the antenna junctions.

Radiofrequency

Interstitial heating with radiofrequency electric fields is essentially resistive heating, produced by currents driven between electrically connected arrays of metallic needles (or between an intracavitary electrode and a needle array; Fig. 16-26). The connected respective needle arrays constitute flat or curved electrodes *in vivo*. The slabs of tissue between respective pairs of adjacent arrays all can be heated simultaneously, either by connecting alternate arrays to form a circuit with two "multiplane" electrodes (arrays 1, 3, 5 . . . , as one electrode; arrays 2, 4, 6 . . . , as the second electrode) or by heating only one slab at any instant but sweeping rapidly back and forth (by electronic switching) through successive pairs of "single plane" electrodes. The optimal spacing of the electrodes is 1 cm to 2 cm with gradual decline in heating effectiveness with increasing array size.[395] The frequencies used in such applications are usually in

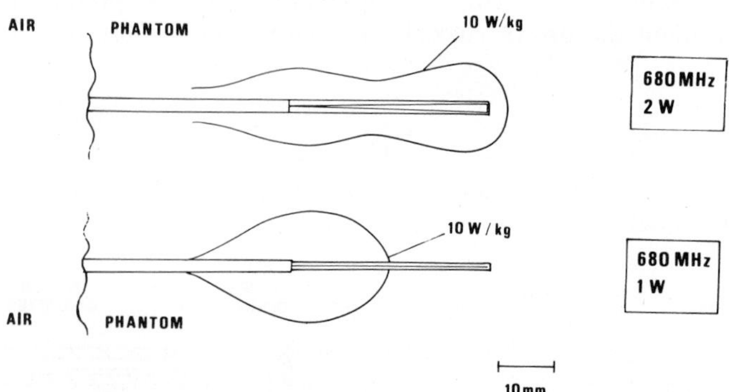

FIGURE 16–25. Comparison of conventional (*bottom*) with improved (*top*) interstitial microwave applicator developed at Chalmers University of Technology. The specific absorption rate (SAR) lines were measured by temperature probing using Bowman-type thermistors in the initial phase of heating. Measurements were performed at 680 MHz with a delivered power of 20 W for the improved and 10 W for the conventional applicator. The SAR values were recalculated to the therapeutic levels of 2 W and 1 W, respectively. (Courtesy of Yngue Hamnerius, PhD)

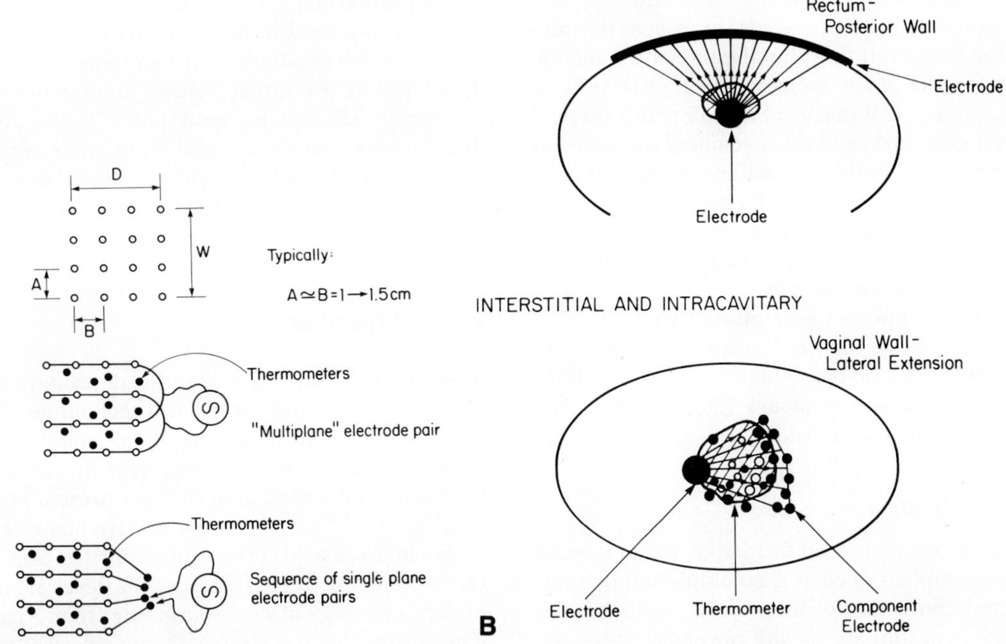

FIGURE 16–26. Radiofrequency current heating: (**A**) interstitial and (**B**) intracavitary techniques.

the range 0.1 MHz to 1.0 MHz. The power required typically ranges from 10 watts to 200 watts.

Electric fields between pairs of subarrays become increasingly nonuniform over the distance between the electrode pairs as the electrode width is reduced, leading to increasingly nonuniform heating across the slab. In general, heating of a given slab is most satisfactory when the ratio of the electrode width to the electrode separation is kept as large as possible. Stauffer and colleagues[395] demonstrated, in dog muscle, more uniform heating in depth along the RF-LCF electrodes and more consistent heating within the array boundaries than with dipole MW (915 MHz) antennas of comparable spatial configuration.

It has been proposed that hollow stainless-steel guides (needles) be used for implantation. Similar to old-fashioned preloaded radium needles, they can be used for both radiofrequency heating and interstitial radiation therapy. This procedure requires rigid metallic needles to be in place (in the tumor) for about 6 to 8 days. Patient discomfort and misarrangement of needles from patient motion during these several days, resulting in unsatisfactory thermal radiation therapy, are of great concern. There is a newly developed material (polyethylene carbon-impregnated material) that conducts radiofrequency currents. These catheters can be used with both radiofrequency and microwave antennas; however, their availability is limited.

Hot Source Technique

With this technique no power is deposited directly in the tissue. Rather, the tissue is heated by thermal redistribution within the implanted arrays of essentially equal temperature hot sources.

Inductively Heated Ferromagnetic Seeds

With the technique of inductively heated ferromagnetic seeds, the tissue is heated by thermal conduction and convection (by blood perfusion) of heat radially away from the implanted seeds. The ferromagnetic material is heated by inducing large eddy currents on the surface of the metal by means of an externally generated magnetic field (Fig. 16-27). These "ferroseeds" can be constructed of any desired length and do not require externalized connections. It should be noted that distribution of tissue temperature along with implanted length is not uniform, even for equal temperature sources. In spite of good temperature at the middle of the implant, there is little heating near the ends at larger distances. This problem has been dealt with in two ways: either the tumor volume has been overimplanted by seeds so that the centrally heated zone corresponds with tumor boundaries, or, preferably, the metal ferroseeds are broken into short segments and inserted as multiseed strings. With proper seed length and interseed spacing, the overall heating characteristics of this seed string can be adjusted to achieve uniform heating patterns.

Special alloys have been used (*e.g.*, Ni + 4% Si or Ni +

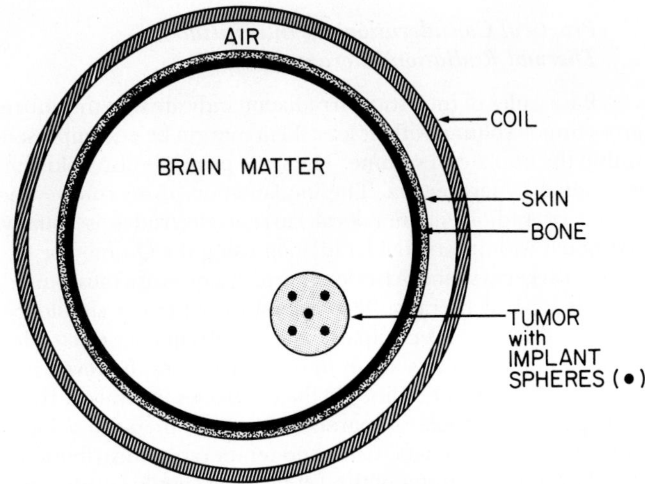

FIGURE 16–27. Schematic representation of technique of magnetic induction heating by ferromagnetic seeds.

palladium) that pass from a ferromagnetic state at low temperatures to a Curie transition near therapeutic temperatures (Curie point) to a nonmagnetic state. These seeds function as thermostats to regulate the temperature within the implanted region. The Curie point for the above mentioned alloys is 40°C to 50°C.[28] Power deposition with this technique depends on seed properties, implant geometry, and relationship of the access of the implant with the access of the external magnetic field. The tissue temperatures within an array of ferromagnetic seeds reach a "pseudo" thermal equilibrium that is primarily dependent on the blood perfusion pattern and, to a lesser degree, on the intrinsic tissue thermal conductivity.

Au and associates[10] reported on a phase I trial involving four patients with tumors of the head and neck heated with ferromagnetic seeds with Curie points between 55°C and 67°C. They were heated with a low-frequency (86.5 to 92.5 kHz) externally applied axial magnetic field.

Resistance Wire Heaters

As with the ferromagnetic seed technique, tissue heating with high-resistance implant needles is accomplished by thermal conduction and convection of heat energy radially away from the cylindrical heat sources. As with previous techniques, these wires are less likely to have a uniform surface temperature. This is because the basic heating mechanism of the needles is an ohmic loss from the electric current flowing through the high-resistance implant material. The resistance is normally distributed uniformly along the needle so that for any given needle current, there is a correspondingly uniform power deposition per unit length of the needle. Because of this cooling temperature may be nonuniform. It is extremely important to note that proper insulation of all low-frequency implant tubes and electrical wire connections from the body is essential to avoid electrical shock. Although plastic catheters could provide adequate electrical insulation, care must be taken in maintaining the integrity of the catheter wall and in the handling of electrical wire connections. A variant of this technique is the so-called hot water technique, which is currently being explored in a few centers. With the latter, tumors are implanted with tubes through which circulating hot water is maintained at a fixed temperature. A temperature distribution with arrays of hot tubes reaches a "pseudo" thermal equilibrium (slowly varying in time with changes in blood flow) as the position of individual patterns of temperature rise from each implant.

Practical Considerations in Interstitial Thermal Radiation Therapy

Basic rules of interstitial irradiation indicate that the entire gross tumor volume with at least 1 cm margin be encompassed within the implanted volume. The same principle also holds for interstitial hyperthermia. The implantation of microwave antennas or radiofrequency local current electrodes is usually combined with interstitial irradiation using the Quimby or Paterson-Parker systems. Afterloading techniques are most suited for this type of therapy. The microwave antennas should be implanted 1 cm to 1.5 cm apart. The radiofrequency electrodes must be implanted at similar, uniform distances; however, it is extremely important to line up the electrodes in straight rows, each plane being exactly parallel with the others, to achieve uniform electromagnetic fields and temperature distributions.

The inner diameter of the Teflon tubes should be adequate for placement of ^{192}Ir radioactive sources (ribbons) and microwave coaxial antennas. The Teflon catheters prevent the conduction of radiofrequency current and therefore are not useful for hyperthermia with this modality (unless E–M conducting materials are used to manufacture catheters).

Attention to minimum tumor temperature (T_{min}; 42.5°C to 43°C) within the target volume is extremely critical. In the University of Arizona experience[281] the average T_{min} was 40.7°C, which resulted in 38% complete response (CR) rate, whereas in the series reported from the Institut Gustav-Roussy,[53] using similar technique, T_{min} was 44°C, which resulted in 83% CR rate.

Deep Hyperthermia

Two basic modalities are used for depositing energy at depth: electromagnetic and ultrasound techniques. The electromagnetic devices used for heating deep-seated tumors all use low-frequency (≤ 100 MHz) electromagnetic radiation to overcome problems with attenuation that are present at higher frequencies.[121,140,141,266,273,367] In the low-frequency range, the wavelength in tissue is 30 cm to 50 cm, which implies, in turn, that the electromagnetic deep hyperthermia devices cannot be expected to deposit energy in a volume greater than 5 cm with precision. This means that the electromagnetic devices used for external deep-seated hyperthermia should be able to heat a quadrant of the patient's cross section and should not be expected to confine their energy distribution with the precision of an external radiation therapy device. Ultrasound devices use much shorter wavelengths (≤ 1 cm) and therefore, in principle, could be more precisely defined than external electromagnetic devices. However, they often are rendered useless for heating deep-seated tumors because of problems with reflections at interfaces and coupling.

Magnetic Induction Hyperthermia

Radiofrequency range magnetic fields can penetrate biologic tissues essentially without attenuation. Magnetic induction devices have an additional advantage in that the current coils that generate the magnetic fields do not need a bolus medium to couple them to the patient. The electromagnetic energy, however, is not a direct result of the magnetic fields but is generated by electric fields that are induced (by Faraday's law) by the time-varying magnetic fields. The local electromagnetic energy deposited is proportional to the conductivity of the tissue multiplied by the electric field squared. Unfortunately, the geometry of most magnetic induction devices is such that the electric field is identically zero at the center of a patient, which means that magnetic induction devices have been used more effectively for deep local hyperthermia than for true regional hyperthermia. Magnetic induction devices also tend to require greater power than the other electromagnetic approaches, and the large voltages present in the current-carrying elements require that electric insulation be carefully applied to avoid any patient contact.

Capacitive Devices

Capacitive devices also use frequencies in the radiofrequency range. The devices consist of parallel opposed plates on opposite sides of the patient. A dielectric coupling medium is required. A displacement current (polarization current) runs between the plates through the patient. The dimensions of the plates must be comparable to the separation. If equal-sized plates are used, the volume heated will be approximately uniform. Some degree of steering of the power distribution, either anteriorly or posteriorly, can be achieved by using a smaller plate on the side on which one wishes to achieve greater concentration of electric field and therefore greater local energy deposition per unit mass (SAR). The capacitive devices do not have the problem of zero electromagnetic energy at the core of the patient in contradistinction to inductive devices. Unlike both inductive and low-frequency microwave devices, however, capacitive devices generate an electric field oriented perpendicularly to the long axis of the patient. The local SAR in the subcutaneous fat is increased (by a factor of 3 or greater) relative to that in the deeper tissues. This problem can be overcome with surface cooling only when the subcutaneous fat is less than approximately 1 cm thick.

Low-Frequency Microwave Devices

Low-frequency microwave devices use microwave radiators operating in the 60 MHz to 100 MHz range; a single applicator can heat tumors to a depth of about 5 cm to 6 cm. Coupling with a dielectric bolus medium is required, which can be uncomfortable to the patient. If arrays of microwave applicators are arranged around the circumference of the patient and driven coherently to interface positively at depth within the patient, true regional hyperthermia can be obtained. The most recently developed microwave array device (the BSD-2000 with Sigma 60 applicator) uses eight antennas. If the electric fields from the eight antennas interfere constructively at a point at depth, the resultant power is increased by a factor of $8^2 = 64$. This can more than compensate for effects of attenuation on the power from individual applicators. "Steering" of the SAR distribution (producing a distribution that spares portions of the patient's cross section) can be achieved by adjusting the relative phases and amplitudes between the applicators. As with other electromagnetic devices, the volume in which energy is deposited cannot be defined with the same precision as with external beam irradiation. It is not realistic to expect the SAR to drop from peak values to low values over distances of less than about 3 cm to 5 cm.

Ultrasound Devices

Arrays of ultrasound applicators designed to interfere constructively at depth offer, in principle, the same advantages as arrays of microwave applicators with the additional advantage of a low wavelength and therefore the theoretic possibility of precisely defining the volume in which heat is deposited. Unfortunately, ultrasound applicators are more sensitive to problems with incomplete coupling and, more important, are unable to penetrate across major interfaces such as air/tissue and bone/tissue. The problems with interfaces limit the utility of ultrasound for regional hyperthermia, although some institutions have had experience with ultrasound devices for deep local hyperthermia.

Regional Hyperthermia Devices

The sites most amenable to regional hyperthermia are the pelvis, extremities, and abdominal or lower chest wall areas.[121, 140, 184] Although recent technical developments permit a fair degree of confidence in determining beforehand where heat will be deposited,[221, 368, 410] the actual temperatures also depend on a given patient's ability to dissipate the heat in areas of poor perfusion. In fact, cases of fat necrosis,[325] myonecrosis,[366] and transient peripheral neuropathy[325] lasting several weeks to months have been reported in the literature. For this reason, it is necessary that a patient receiving regional hyperthermia be given minimal or no sedatives and analgesics. The treating physician and physicist must assume that any severe complaints that the patient has during a hyperthermia session reflect excessive temperatures at unmonitored locations. Hyperthermia sessions are often limited by local pain, anxiety, or discomfort. Perhaps, in many cases, problems could be alleviated with higher doses of sedatives if there were a way to rule out excessive temperatures at unmonitored locations. Currently, this cannot be done.

Several commercially available approaches to the delivery of regional hyperthermia exist. The Thermotron is a capacitive device that consists of parallel opposed plates that deposit electromagnetic energy across a cross section of the patient.[393] A potential drawback of this device is that it deposits more than three times the SAR in the superficial fat layers than in the deeper muscle equivalent layers. This does not pose an obstacle when a patient is sufficiently lean (about 1 cm of subcutaneous fat at most) to permit surface cooling of these superficial layers. Hiraoka and co-workers[163] report 53% complete responses in 36 patients treated in Japan. It is possible that these results would be difficult to reproduce in a more obese population group. An investigational device reported in preliminary data by Nussbaum and associates[321] uses multiple capacitor plates. No clinical results have been reported to date.

The Magnetrode is a commercially available device for regional hyperthermia by magnetic induction.[301] It has the geometry of a solenoid with multiple electric current carrying coils wrapped around the long axis of the patient. Such geometry deposits identically zero power at the center of the patient.[367] The SAR scales with distance from the center of the patient (r) as r^2.[367] Any temperature elevation at the patient's core must, therefore, be the consequence of thermal conduction from the outer layers of the patient. Thus it is not surprising that, in a comparison of the Magnetrode with the Annular Phased Array System, Sapozink and colleagues[367] found that the Magnetrode consistently had poorer heating at depth and more sessions were limited by severe pain in the outer layers of the patient.

The principal experience in the United States in regional hyperthermia has been with the Annular Phased Array System (APAS or BSD 1000).[88, 121, 261, 265, 320, 322, 324, 363, 364, 433] This device consisted of 16 microwave sources operating in the 70 MHz to 110 MHz range and was designed to interfere constructively at the patient's center.[429] If operated in this manner, the APAS would deposit electromagnetic energy uniformly throughout a cross section of the patient. A certain measure of skill was required of the treating physicist because the power deposition pattern was very sensitive to choice of frequency and patient positioning. Nonetheless, sufficient heating could be obtained to demonstrate superiority to the Magnetrode in Sapozink's study.[367] Furthermore, several authors including Samulski and associates[349] and Sathiaseelan and co-workers[369] demonstrated that, with various "steering techniques," uninvolved portions of the patient's cross section could be relatively spared. Samulski and colleagues[349] showed that the use of steering techniques produced better rates of temperature rise during early portions of hyperthermia sessions with less systemic cardiovascular stress than did nonsteered distributions. However, because of multiple clinical difficulties, they were not able to demonstrate an improvement in achieving the overall temperature/time objectives.

The successor to the BSD 1000 was the BSD 2000 (Fig. 16-28).[431] This device consists of four quadrants composed of two antennas each. The relative phase and amplitude of the quadrants can be varied, which allows control over where,

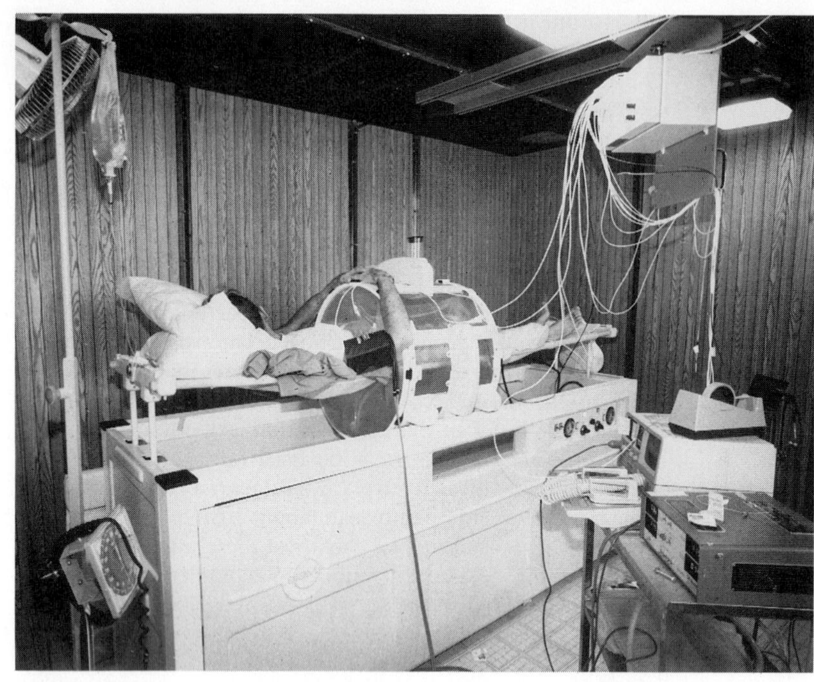

FIGURE 16–28. The BSD 2000 device for regional hyperthermia. (B.S.D. Corporation, Salt Lake City, UT)

within a patient's cross section, the electromagnetic radiation interferes constructively. This allows for much more reliable steering of the power distribution and permits sparing of large portions of a patient's cross section. Also a preplanning capability makes several approximations to keep computing time acceptable and allows a qualitative estimate of SAR distributions. It is possible to choose an arrangement of phases and amplitudes that optimizes sparing of uninvolved tissues. At Washington University, the first seven patients treated with the BSD 2000 were treated with steering techniques similar to those shown in Figure 16-29. The cardiovascular stress to six of seven patients was minimal, with pulse rates remaining under 120/minute during the sessions. Sixty-five percent of the sessions achieved 42°C for at least 30 minutes in contrast to only 25% of the sessions reaching this goal with the BSD 1000.[266]

Whole-Body Hyperthermia

Whole-body hyperthermia results from directly or indirectly heating the circulating blood to temperatures of 41°C to 42°C for about 2 hours. Major clinical experience in the United States has been at the University of Texas[29] and the University of Wisconsin—Madison.[338] As no externally applied energy is deposited deep within the patient, any temperature elevation at depth must be the result of thermal conduction or heat transfer by the circulating blood, which means that no point in the body will be at a higher temperature than that of the circulating blood. Therefore the physician may use whatever medications are necessary to keep a patient comfortable during the session.

Whole-body hyperthermia has been administered using radiant heat,[338] a "space suit" with circulating hot water,[29] or extracorporeal temperature elevation employing a heat exchanger through which the blood is circulated (after shunting it with an arteriovenous femoral bypass). Temperatures of 40.5°C to 41.5°C have been delivered to patients with distant metastases for several hours, sometimes in combination with cytotoxic drugs.

Whole-body hyperthermia does produce significant cardiovascular stress; Robins[338] reports doubling of the heart rate and cardiac output during a session. Prophylaxis against arrhythmia and seizures is necessary.[338] In many instances general anesthesia is required, and careful monitoring of body temperature and multiple physiologic functions is mandatory (cardiovascular, respiratory, neurologic, fluids, electrolytes). Sudden development of myelopathy after whole-body hyperthermia was reported in three patients previously irradiated to the thorax.[79]

Trials are in progress investigating whole-body hyperthermia in conjunction with systemic agents or irradiation or both.[337]

Preliminary reports by Barlogie and co-workers,[12] Bull and associates,[29] Kubota,[204] and Robbins[338] suggest that there may be definite therapeutic efficacy in the combination of these agents for treatment of advanced or disseminated neoplasms in humans.

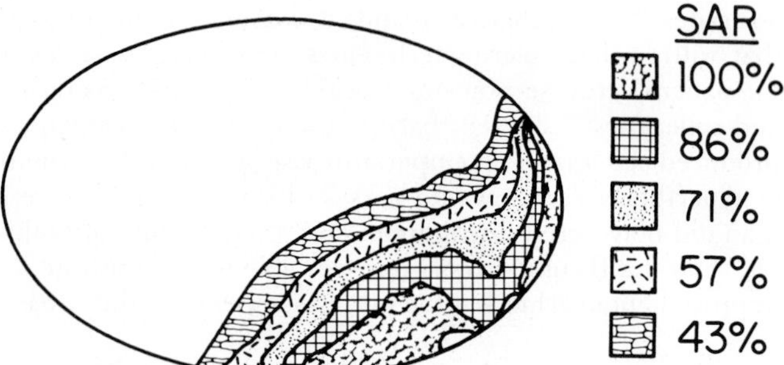

FIGURE 16–29. Computer preplan for "steering" the specific absorption rate (SAR) distribution with the BSD 2000. The patient was treated for abdominal wall recurrence of colon carcinoma.

THERMOMETRY

Currently, direct and continuous monitoring of temperatures in clinical hyperthermia with invasive probes constitutes the only reliable method of thermal treatment verification.[132] Clinical temperature probes should be able to measure temperature to both an accuracy and precision of 0.1°C in phantoms for calibration and 0.2°C when used *in vivo.*[382] Reference thermometers and other devices used for calibration should be able to establish temperature to within 0.02°C by National Bureau of Standards (NBS) calibrated mercury-in-glass thermometers, by NBS traceable highly stable thermistor probes, and by use of a variety of hydrated salt solutions to establish several physicochemical thermometric fixed points in the range of 30°C to 50°C. It is desirable for clinical probes to function accurately in intense electromagnetic or ultrasound fields.[348] The performance goals of clinical thermometers are summarized in Table 16-6.

Thermometers (probes) used in clinical practice should be calibrated in relation to NBS-calibrated mercury-in-glass thermometers and other traceable standard thermometers (stable thermistors) in stable temperature reference sources (high flow circulating water bath, ice, melting points, and so on). Samulski[348] recently reviewed the basic principles of thermometry.

Invasive thermometers fall into three basic categories: electrically conducting, minimally conducting, and nonconducting (optical) probes. They are typically designed to fit in 20- to 29-gauge plastic tubes or hypodermic needles.

Conducting probes include standard thermistor and thermocouple sensors with metallic leads. The standard thermistor has a sensor that is a semiconductor, the resistance of which decreases with increasing temperature. The temperature-dependent parameter is the resistivity of the semiconductor material. Thermal couple sensors use the junction between these two similar metals; redistribution of charge across the junction leads to the establishment of a potential difference of known temperature dependence.

An example of a *minimally conducting probe* is the high resistivity thermistor with carbon-impregnated plastic leads developed by Bowman,[24] which is encased in a Teflon tube that can be inserted into a 16-gauge catheter.

Nonconducting "optical" probes use sensors composed of gallium arsenide (GaAs) or a mixture of two rare earth phosphors. The "leads" of both optical probes are optical fibers. The GaAs sensor, designed by Christensen,[39] is a semiconductor for which the "band gap" (the energy separation of electrons in the conduction and valence bands) is a known function of temperature. The fraction of an incident beam of light (of a given wavelength) reflected or scattered by the GaAs sensor depends on the width of the band gap compared with the energy of photons in the beam. In the rare earth biphosphor probe developed by Wickersheim,[477] a pulse of incident light excites both phosphor materials, using them to subsequently fluoresce. The ratio of the intensities of a pair of fluorescence emission lines—one from each phosphor—is a known function of temperature. Both the GaAs and rare earth biphosphor probes are encased in Teflon tubing and can be inserted into 16- to 20-gauge catheters.

TABLE 16–6
Thermometry Performance Goals

PARAMETER	MINIMUM PERFORMANCE GOALS
Calibration accuracy	≤ ± 0.2°C over hyperthermia range (30°–60°C; *e.g.*, comparison with standard immediately following calibration)
Resolution	≤ ± 0.2°C
Drift	≤ ± 0.1° hour
Recalibration period	≥24 hours
Response time	≤4 second
Bend artifact	≤0.1° for 5 mm bend radius
EM and/or US artifact	≤0.1°
EM interference	≤0.1° for 10 mW/cm² EM exposure
Durability	Suitable for multiple implantations and mechanical mapping
Thermal smearing	Smearing length ≤1.5 mm when tested in 10°C step thermal gradient
Date acquisition I/O	≤10 second update

EM: electromagnetic; US: ultrasound
(Reproduced with permission from Samulski TV: Current technologies for invasive thermometry. In Paliwal BR, Hetzel FW, Dewhirst MW [eds]: Biological, Physical and Clinical Aspects of Hyperthermia, pp 168–181. New York, American Association of Physicists in Medicine, 1988)

Thermometry Artifacts

Incorrect high temperature readings can be produced by direct heating of either the probe or the catheter. The presence of such artifacts is indicated by rapid decay of temperature with time for a short period immediately following power shut-off followed by a slower decay commensurate with the surrounding tissues (Fig. 16-30). Such artifacts may be effectively eliminated for electromagnetic systems by using either high-resistive thermistors or optical probes. For ultrasound, however, artifacts pose a more significant problem. Through the direct absorption of ultrasound by plastic or Teflon probe sheaths or catheters, temperature artifacts of several degrees can easily be produced. The magnitude of ultrasound-induced temperature artifacts present in measurements with a Teflon-coated, GaAs "optical" probe increases with increasing diameter (decreasing gauge) of the Teflon or plastic catheters used to house the thermometry probe. Inaccuracies caused by such artifacts can be reduced by using "bare" thermocouple probes or placed in hypodermic needles, as is demonstrated by the lowest temperature decay curve (0.2°C artifact) in Figure 16-31.

Because the absence of catheters makes mapping along the probe track relatively difficult to effect, multisensor probes are recommended for acquisition of the multiple-point temperature data desired. Measurement errors can also be significantly reduced by sampling temperatures with power off.[311] Recent publications[471,472] have examined in detail these artifacts for bare thermocouples or for those placed inside catheters.

Noninvasive thermometry is currently the subject of considerable research and will not be commercially available in the near future. Techniques being evaluated are infrared thermography, microwave thermography (radiometry), and ultrasound reconstruction (to provide mappings of temperature-dependent ultrasound velocity or absorption). Infrared thermography is commercially available but provides information on surface temperatures only.

Thermal Treatment Planning

Planning of hyperthermia treatment may be carried out as in radiation therapy through measurements in phantoms and calculations with models of tissue heating. The fabrication of phantoms that are "patient-equivalent" is far more difficult to achieve in hyperthermia than in radiation therapy; phantoms must be equivalent to the tissue of interest in both power deposition and heat transfer *in vivo*. This is usually impossible to

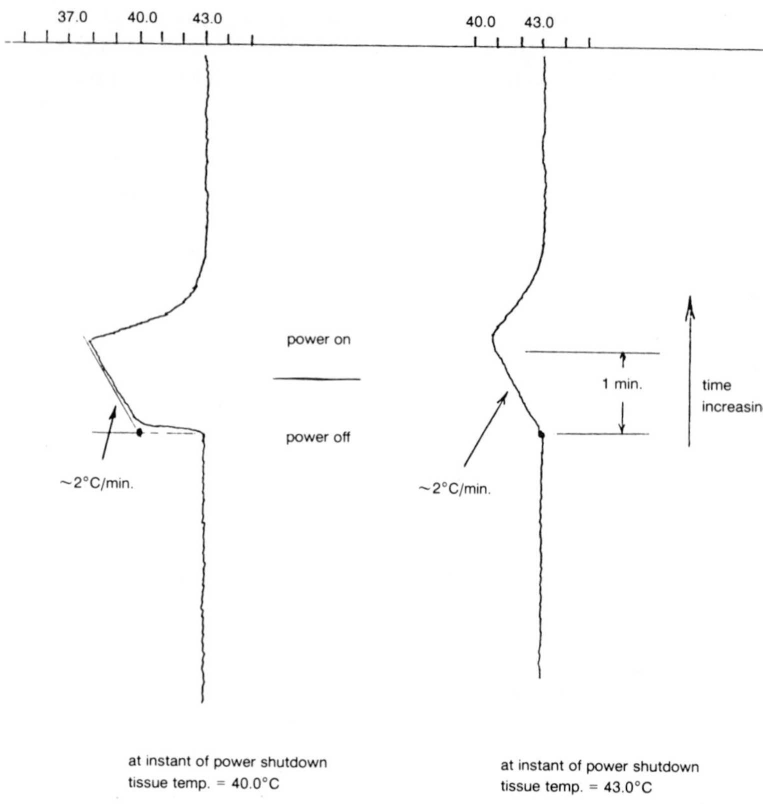

FIGURE 16–30. Representative temperature-time plots, expressed as strip chart recorder output curves, for two different conducting probes (*e.g.*, thermistors) in a microwave of radiofrequency field. With the power on, the indicated temperatures at the locations of the respective probe sensors in the given medium are identical at 43°C. Analysis of the decay of temperature with time for both probes, after the power is shut off, identifies the actual temperatures at the two points in the medium to be 40°C (*left curve*) and 43°C (*right curve*).

achieve because of the inability to satisfactorily simulate and reliably predict convective heat transfer due to blood flow. For electromagnetic energies (microwaves and RF fields), phantom material of value includes dielectric liquids; sponges soaked in saline solution; mixtures of "superstuff," polyethylene powder, salt, and water; saline-formaldehyde gels; beef; and live animal tissue.

Table 16-7 illustrates various phantom compositions used to simulate a variety of organs. In liquid phantoms mappings of electric (or acoustic) fields can be readily made because of the ease with which the appropriate probes can be scanned across the phantom volume. Absorbed power density distributions may be obtained from measurements of the initial slopes of temperature-time curves at chosen points in solid or gel phantoms. Measurement of absorbed power density distributions (watts/kg) in such phantoms with site-specific or patient-specific geometries can yield valuable information about the types, sizes, number, and placement of applicators well suited to a specific, proposed application of clinical hyperthermia. Information can also be used to improve the coupling of the applicators to the patient's surface, thereby reducing (*e.g.*, for microwaves) both leakage and field spreading across air gaps.

Finally, absorbed power density distributions obtained from measurements in patient-appropriate phantoms can be used as input data for calculation of temperature distributions using thermal models. It should be noted that the distribution of static state temperatures obtained from measurements in solid and gel phantoms cannot be taken as accurate indications of the three-dimensional temperature distributions produced in the corresponding living tissues, because of the absence of heat dissipation related to blood flow in the phantoms.

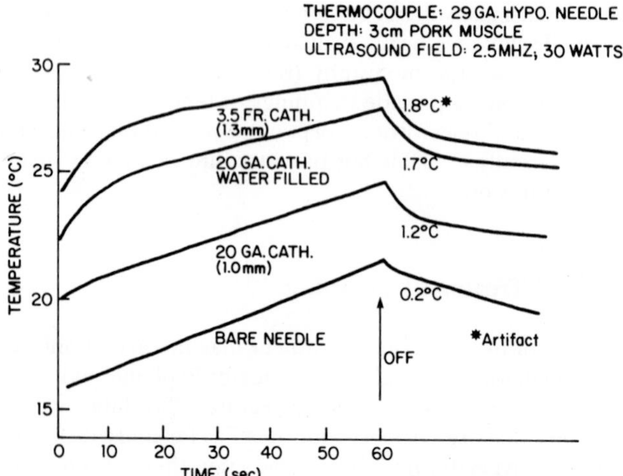

FIGURE 16–31. Reduction of artifact using thermocouple probes in hypodermic needles.

Thermal Dosimetry in Clinical Practice

A great deal of controversy exists among hyperthermia investigators concerning the best way to define a "thermal dose" that incorporates temperature and time factors.[61, 116, 292, 354] Currently it is impossible to determine an exact thermal dose in the clinical setting because of the inability to continuously establish the values for such physiologic factors involved in cell kill as blood flow, pH, and oxygen tension. Major obstacles to the reliable monitoring of temperatures in clinical hyperthermia are related to the invasive techniques and paucity of probes that can practically be placed in a patient; the nonhomogeneous power deposition yielded by most external applicators or interstitial sources; and the effect of blood flow on heat dissipation.[413]

Temperature inhomogeneity is illustrated in 83 patients with chest wall recurrences from carcinoma of the breast on

TABLE 16–7
Compositions of Some Phantom Materials

TISSUE	f(MHz)	ε′	σ(S/m)	COMPOSITION
Skin	2450	43	—	60% H_2O, 1% NaCl, 39% cellulose paper
Muscle	10	65.8	1.17	75.5% H_2O, 0.9% NaCl, 15.2% PEP, 8.4% TX150
	50	44.1	1.20	
	100	44.8	1.43	
	13.56		0.69	90% H_2O, 0.5% NaCl, 9.5% TX150
	30	110	0.65	76.57% H_2O, 0.153% NaCl, 13.78% Al powder, 9.495% TX150
	2450	50	2.18	69% H_2O, 30% gelatin, 1% NaCl
	8500	34–48	4.5–7.1	H_2O, NaCl, PEP, TX150
	10000	30–45	5.6–8.3	For formulas see original reference
Brain	2450	42	2.59	59% H_2O, 1% NaCl, 40% gelatin
Viscera	13.56		0.43	90% H_2O, 0.26% NaCl, 9.7% TX150
Lung	13.56		0.12	81.15% polyester resin, 16.65% Al powder, 1.19% acetylene black, MEK catalyst
Fat and bone	13.56		0.23	83.71% polyester resin, 14.9% Al powder, 1.37% acetylene black, MEK catalyst
	30	19	0.28	79% Laminac 4110, 20.72% Al powder, 0.28% acetylene black, MEK catalyst
Fat and bone	451	7.3	0.038	66.67% flour, 30% oil, 3.33% of 0.9% NaCl solution

(Data from Cetas TC[35]; Langedijk JJW, Nilsson P[206]; Stuchly MA, Stuchly SS[415]; Chou C-K[37])

whom detailed information on thermometry was available[309] (Fig. 16-32). Furthermore, the number of probes reaching 42.5°C in relation to the entire expected time (60 minutes at prescribed temperature at each session) was only 54% if the probe was at or less than 1 cm in depth, 35% at 1.1 cm to 2 cm, 7% at 3 cm, and 2.8% at depths greater than 3 cm. This is a reflection of the decreasing power deposition at increasing depth of the lesion.

The definition of parameters used to express thermal dose should be properly defined.[183] T_{ave} is defined as the average temperature of all intratumoral measurements made during a treatment session. It includes both spatial and temporal averages. This frequently involves taking multiple thermal or temperature measurements at 0.5 cm intervals along each catheter track throughout the entire hyperthermia session. The T_{ave} of each session can be added and a total T_{ave} may be obtained. For a given point, the T_{ave} can be obtained by averaging the measurements at that specific point throughout every session and in all treatment sessions.

T_{min} represents the minimum temperature that is observed at any time at any specific point during a session or after a series of sessions.

T_{max} represents the maximum intratumoral (or in the normal tissues) temperature measured at a site during a session or for a total after all treatment sessions.

T_{90} is a term proposed by Oleson[280] to indicate the ability of a heating device to obtain a given temperature in 90% of the points measured throughout the heated volume, for example, $T_{90} \geq 41°C$, $T_{90} \geq 42°C$, and $T_{90} \geq 43°C$.

Valdagni and associates[440] summarized the prognostically significant thermal parameters that correlate with response rate in trials of irradiation and hyperthermia; in some studies it was

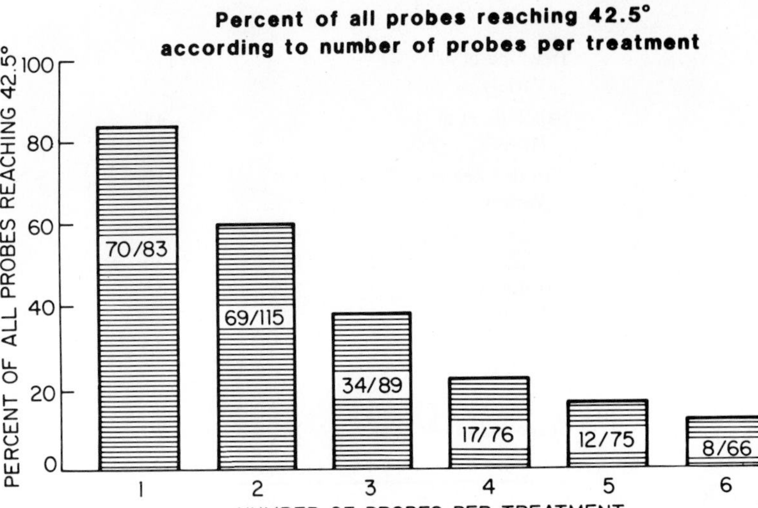

FIGURE 16–32. Percent of all probes reaching 42.5°C according to number of probes per treatment in 83 patients with chest wall recurrence. (Perez CA, et al: Irradiation and hyperthermia in the treatment of recurrent carcinoma of the breast in the chest wall: MIR and RTOG experience. In Sugahara T, Saito M [eds]: Hyperthermic Oncology 1988, vol 2, pp 422–424. London, Taylor & Francis, 1989)

the average temperature and, in others, the minimum temperature (mean or total; Table 16-8).

Dewhirst and associates[67] reported in pet animals a good correlation between the minimum tumor temperature and tumor control and between the maximum temperature and morbidity in normal tissues. Sapareto and co-workers[359] evaluated the temperatures recorded in 21 patients with superficial measurable tumors treated according to the Radiation Therapy Oncology Group (RTOG) (81-04) with radiation and heat. When patients are divided into complete responders and partial or nonresponders, in the former group longer periods at Eq 43°C temperature during the first treatment and a minimum average temperature were noted, in comparison with the findings of the nonresponders. These trends are strong, but not statistically significant because of the small number of patients.

To accommodate variation in temperature during a heating session or in different treatments, Sapareto and Dewey[354] have recommended a thermal dose expressed in 43°C equivalent time (T_{equiv} 43°C), using a biologically derived equation based on the Arrhenius plot and observations in animal and human skin.[154,354] Although there is no good clinical basis for the use of such a formula, some studies suggest that in selected clinical settings thermal doses have a positive correlation with the probability of tumor control and maximum doses with incidence of complications.[93,291] Several institutions have devised mathematical models using the bioheat equation for expression of thermal dose in a volume, sometimes using computed tomography information.[340,408] In the future a combination of this mathematical modeling with some real time measurements, such as temperature, blood flow, and pH, may allow for a reliable three-dimensional presentation of thermal dose.[24,339,409,470]

One of the most significant obstacles to accurate representation of thermal dose by the proposed methods is that the data do not represent the temperatures reached throughout the heated tumor.[74] Until such three-dimensional temperature and

TABLE 16–8
Thermal Parameters that Correlate with Response Rate

AUTHOR/TYPE OF TUMOR	NO. OF LESIONS	THERMAL PARAMETER
Dewhirst et al[73] Variety of animal tumors	59	Minimum Eq43 at first treatment
Dewhirst and Sim[71] Variety of animal tumors	116	Average minimum Eq43
Hiraoka et al[163] Variety	40	Average tumor center temperature
Luk et al[238] Variety	133	Lowest daily average temperature
Oleson et al[282] Variety	161	Minimum tumor temperature averaged over all treatments
Sim et al[383] Variety of animal and human tumors	109	Estimated treated volume (ETV) obtaining >42.5°C
Van der Zee et al[446] Breast	82	Mean temperature Mean of maximum temperature
Arcangeli et al[5] Neck nodes	38	Average overall Eq42.5
Kapp et al[187] Breast	31	% temperature <40.0°C First % temperature ≥42.5°C treatment Minimum temperature Average temperature % temperature ≤40.0°C Average % temperature ≥42.5°C all treatments
Dewhirst et al[69] Variety	115	Minimum Eq43
Sapozink et al[363] Pelvis	43	Number of treatments with any tumor temperature ≥42°C at some time
Van der Zee et al[445] Variety	112	Mean minimum T_{mean} Mean minimum T_{max} Total minimum DMEqT43 Total minimum EqT43
Arcangeli et al[6] Melanoma	38	Eq42.5
Storm et al[402] Variety	100	Lowest tumor temperature—first treatment Eq43—first treatment Cumulative Eq43 for all treatments
Seegenschmiedt et al[376] Breast	27	Total/mean minimum Eq43

(Valdagni R, Liu FF, Kapp DS: Int J Radiat Oncol Biol Phys 15:959–972, 1988)

thermal dose fields can be represented accurately, methods that correlate the various temperatures with the fraction of tumor volume greater than the T_{index} must be developed. An alternative suggested by Oleson and associates[279] is to express the relationship between the tumor edge temperature and the temperature gradient extending toward the center of the tumor.

In a recent issue of the *International Journal of Hyperthermia,* several authors[74] presented interesting theoretical and experimental observations in an attempt to clarify thermal dose concepts. Dewey[61] strongly advocated that the actual time and temperature values used in the treatment of patients be recorded and reported while at the same time models to express biologic isoeffect relationships are developed and tested. Separeto and Corry[353] published a proposed standard data file format for hyperthermia treatments. Clinical studies are needed to evaluate these parameters.[306] RTOG completed a phase I study of 41 patients which demonstrated that only 16 (40%) tolerated temperatures of 45°C for at least 15 minutes in one session, only four patients tolerated that temperature for two sessions, and three patients for four or more sessions, suggesting that this temperature is not feasible under typical clinical conditions.[308]

Oleson[277] underscored the present difficulties in prescribing and defining temperature distributions in a clinical setting. However, major efforts should be directed to phase II studies that may improve our knowledge of thermal distribution and the technical parameters required to achieve it.

Thermal Modeling

Several authors have designed mathematical models to simulate thermal dosimetry in clinical situations.[340,406]

For hyperthermia, the applications of thermal dosimetry simulations can be divided into four main categories (comparative, prospective, concurrent, and retrospective) according to the time they are performed relative to the patient's treatment.[339] The goal of *comparative thermal dosimetry* is to assess the abilities of different heating modalities and configurations to properly heat general classes of patients and tumors in standardized patient models that contain anatomic and physiologic features of a typical patient and characteristics of the power deposition patterns. In *prospective thermal dosimetry,* detailed information is needed regarding specific patient anatomy and expected blood flow for individual patient treatment planning. *Concurrent thermal dosimetry* (feedback control during treatment) involves calculating complete temperature fields during a treatment and adjusting power deposition parameters and other variables to optimize the actual treatment. *Retrospective thermal dosimetry* calculates the complete temperature fields and thermal dose obtained during the treatment based on knowledge of temperatures at specific measurement locations. A practical approach to simulated thermal dosimetry involves a numerical model of the bioheat transfer equation to calculate temperature distributions, using known power deposition patterns of the various heating systems with respect to the region of interest, and measured temperature, blood flow, oxygen tension, pH, and other environmental parameters (Fig. 16-33). With multiple temperature sensors and the microprobes described by Bowman[24,25] to obtain many of these values using all of this information, computations can be performed to determine actual thermal dose distributions. Comparative evaluation using this technique was performed for the Magnetrode and BSD Annular Phase Array System.[364] Two-dimensional analyses have been performed for complex models of the patient's anatomy[304] and for various interstitial techniques.[26,249,253,407] This analysis can be used to measure the percentage of the tumor volume that reaches a therapeutic temperature and to calculate a hyperthermia equipment performance (HEP) rating.[337] Whereas comparative evaluation of heating devices has made some practical contributions to hyperthermia, the use of computer models in individual treatment planning is not practical at the present time because of the large amount of real time patient information needed.[337]

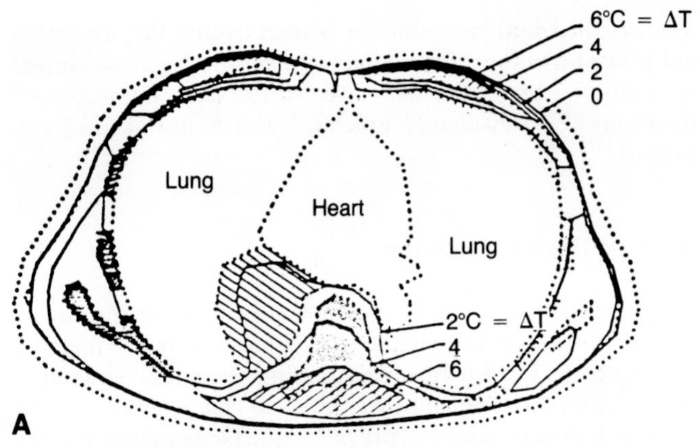

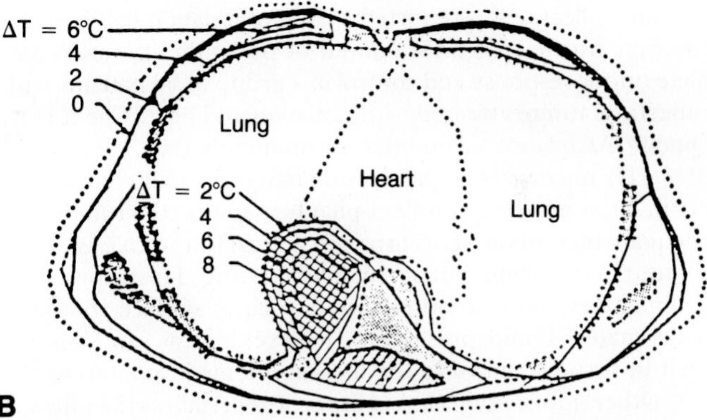

FIGURE 16–33. Correlation between the ratio of tumor blood perfusion to that of surrounding muscle, fat, and bone, and therapeutic heating in thoracic model. (**A**) Tumor/muscle blood perfusion ratio = 1.0; tumor/fat = 90; tumor/bone ∞. (**B**) Tumor/muscle = 0.18; tumor/fat = 0.54; tumor/bone = 0.54. Isotherms represent 2°C increments. The therapeutically heated region of the tumor is indicated. All other normal tissues have basal perfusion rates. (Paulsen KD, Strohbehn JW, Lynch DR: Int J Radiat Oncol Biol Phys 11:1659–1671, 1985)

QUALITY ASSURANCE IN CLINICAL HYPERTHERMIA

The delivery of adequate uniform heating to the tumor volume must be the main goal of a program of quality assurance in hyperthermia. The temperature specification must be sufficiently quantitative and comprehensive to unambiguously define the thermal state of the heated tissue. In general, both absorbed power density (watts/kg) and local heat transfer (cal/sec/cm^3) will vary considerably over tissue volumes of clinical interest, making it extremely difficult to produce uniform temperature distributions within the heated tissues. Requirements and procedures for effective quality assurance and assessment in clinical hyperthermia are discussed by Corry,[49] Shrivastava,[380] Dewhirst,[70] Emami,[97] and Sapozink and colleagues.[362]

Heating Device Selection

It is important to have an accurate assessment of the tumor extent, which can be obtained by clinical or other imaging techniques (CT, radionuclide scanning, magnetic resonance imaging), and to determine the physical characteristics of the heating devices required to provide a satisfactory energy deposition in the volume of interest.[70,142,145,361,381]

Guidelines for clinical trials stress that there is no scientific evidence proving that a predictable relationship exists between relative SAR measurements in phantoms and temperatures achieved in heterogeneously diffused tissues.[70] However, Myerson and colleagues[267] reported a close correlation between the coverage by the 25% SAR contour of the applicator and complete tumor response and control in a group of 60 patients with superficial tumors treated with radiation and heat. The RTOG Quality Assurance Committee recommends that selection of 915 MHz microwave applicators be based on SAR characteristics in a flat muscle-equivalent phantom so that the tumor and adequate margins are encompassed at least by the 25% iso-SAR contour as determined from phantom testing. This approach is rudimentary, because other factors such as surface contours, bolus material, and presence of intervening fat can alter the SAR in tissues relative to the measurements in phantoms.[74]

Other information should be recorded, such as the physical agent employed to heat the tissue (microwaves, 915 MHz; ultrasound, 2 MHz); the nature, size, shape, number, and placement of the applicators; and the method of coupling the applicator to the tissue. The total net power delivered to the applicators and to the tissue load should be estimated and recorded. If skin cooling is used, it should be clearly noted. Finally, problems encountered and adjustments made during the course of treatment should be noted.

Tumor Thermometry Factors

Multiple thermometry catheters should be placed in the tumor in such a way that temperature profiles are obtained across a major axis of the tumor, at the greatest possible depth, at the periphery of the tumor, and in tumor/normal tissue interfaces. The thermometry catheters in general can remain in place between treatments, because only about 10% of them either show evidence of infection or become dislodged. Figure 16-34 illustrates the recommended location of catheters for superficial tumors, and Figure 16-35 for deep tumors. Thermometry catheters may be inserted under local anesthesia, usually 1% lidocaine (Xylocaine). Use of a buffered solution[42,326] is highly recommended to decrease the pain and burning associated with the anesthetic injection.

Several devices are available that have been designed for and allow for more accurate recording of multiple point temperatures.[100,120] Dewhirst and associates[70] recommend a 0.5 cm step size for catheter tracts less than 5 cm in length and 1 cm step size for tracts longer than 5 cm, with a minimum of four positions along each catheter tract. Mapping must be done on a routine basis throughout the treatment, about once every 10 minutes, to capture temporal variations in temperature measurements that occur from vasodilatation or technical factors during the treatment. The location of the temperature probes on superficial tumors should be documented with Polaroid photographs and in deep tumors with radiographic techniques, including computed tomography or magnetic resonance scanning. The Radiation Therapy Oncology Group has published a detailed document on quality assurance guidelines for clinical trials using hyperthermia.[70]

Interstitial hyperthermia, because of the possible occurrence of steep thermal gradients, increases the demand for accurate thermometry. When microwave and local radiofrequency are used, interstitial heating fiberoptic probes have been reported to provide the most reliable and artifact-free thermometry, showing minimal interaction between the lower thermal mass and nonmetallic probes with the electromagnetic and thermal fields.[70] RF-shielded thermocouples or thermistors have been used, by sampling during brief interruptions of microwave power to reduce errors from the electrical artifact as described previously. The use of small metallic sensors mounted directly on the microwave antenna may be acceptable for source temperature measurements to balance power between individual antennas.[70] Recommendations for placement of thermometry catheters for microwave antenna heating are shown in Figure 16-36.

For hot source interstitial techniques the following are requirements for thermometry: to verify source surface temperatures and to obtain measurements at the greatest distance from the implants as possible. These techniques include the thermoregulating ferromagnetic seeds in which seed temperatures (Curie point) should be constant along the entire implanted length so that knowledge of a single source temperature for each seed should be sufficient. This direct measurement is necessary until it is further verified that thermal regulation indeed is adequate. In addition, temperature mapping along the central axis of each four-source square array is recommended to get an indication of the spread of minimum temperatures within the array.

With hot water tubes, thermometric considerations are basically the same as discussed earlier, except for the source temperature measurements. Temperatures near the tissue-catheter interface should be monitored at the entrance points, in low perfusion normal tissues, and in the tumor volume at depth. In addition, the temperature of the circulating water in each catheter should be measured before it enters and as it exits the temperature volume so that water flow rate can be adjusted to ensure uniform temperatures along the catheters. Proper flow rate and water temperature are required for each catheter. For DC-resistance wire heaters, more detailed measurement of surface temperature along the implants is required. Special attention should be given to the temperatures of lower perfusion tissues such as subcutaneous fat, where undesirable accumulation of heat may result.[70]

Normal Tissue Thermometry

Multiple points of normal tissue temperature should be obtained throughout every treatment session. Temperatures should be measured along each thermometric catheter track as well as at the surface. Dewhirst and associates[70] emphasized that skin surface measurements are not true indicators of the skin temperatures because they represent an average between the conditions above the skin or tumor surface and the skin or

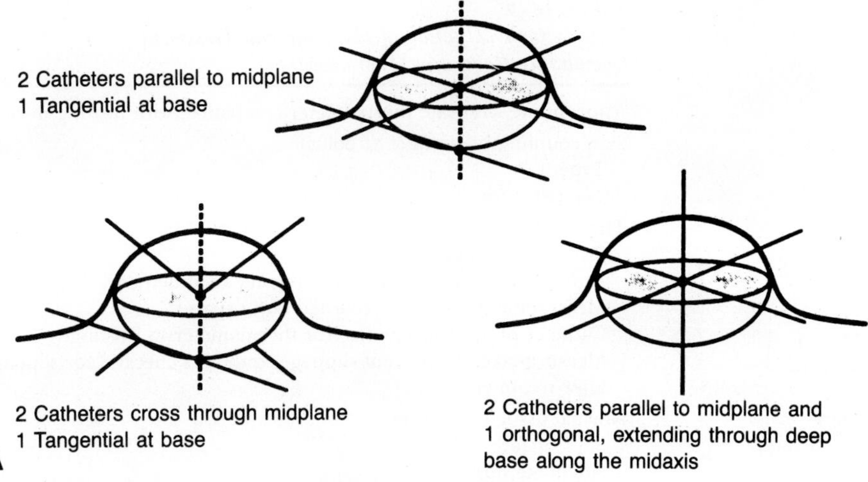

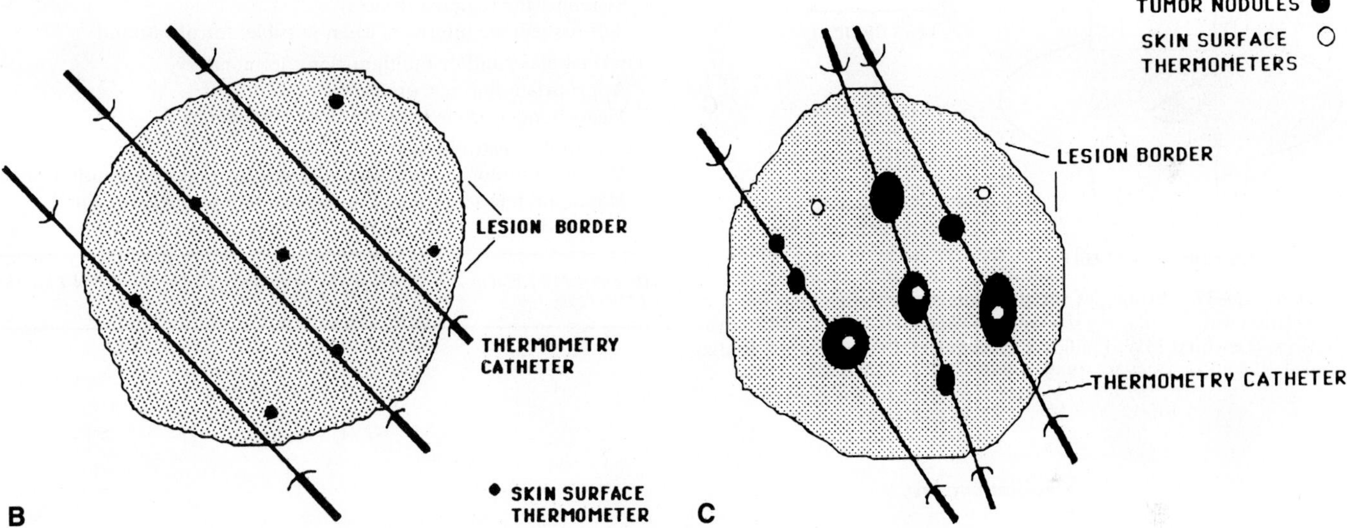

FIGURE 16–34. (**A**) Optimal strategies for thermometry locations in superficial bulky malignancies. Note: Catheters extend beyond margin of tumor when possible, allowing for measurement of normal tissue temperature. (**B**) Placement of thermometry catheter and surface probes for diffuse pattern or plaque of breast carcinoma on the chest wall. (**C**) Catheter fields involving multiple small nodules.

tumor surface itself. Skin measurements are particularly important in expected high SAR areas such as scars with fibrosis. In the case of ultrasound, soft tissue/bone interfaces should be monitored, if possible.

Treatment Prescription

Currently there is no accurate and realistic method to prescribe hyperthermia treatments. However, as a minimum, all prescriptions should define the target temperature distributions in the volume of interest for a fixed time (*e.g.,* 42.5°C for 60 minutes). Minimal and average temperatures and T_{90} (temperature exceeded by 90% of monitored intratumoral points)[280] have been correlated with tumor response. Maximum temperatures have correlated with frequency of thermal injury.[71,315] These various temperatures should be included as part of the treatment prescription.

A diagram or photographs of the setup of each treatment should be made, indicating clearly the anatomic location of the treatment site; the location and extent of tumor (dimensions) should be given, and the physical characteristics and location of applicators and thermometers (or thermometry catheters) within and around the tumor volume should be noted.

Patient Monitoring

The tolerance of the patient to the administration of heat should be assessed carefully and documented. Intolerant reactions should be monitored closely. Periodically (at least once weekly) tumor measurements should be taken to document regression, and the effect of therapy on the normal tissues should be recorded. Table 16-9 lists the criteria for evaluation of hyperthermia treatment.

CLINICAL APPLICATIONS OF HYPERTHERMIA

Depending on the volume treated, hyperthermia is classified as local, regional (deep), or systemic (whole-body). A complete

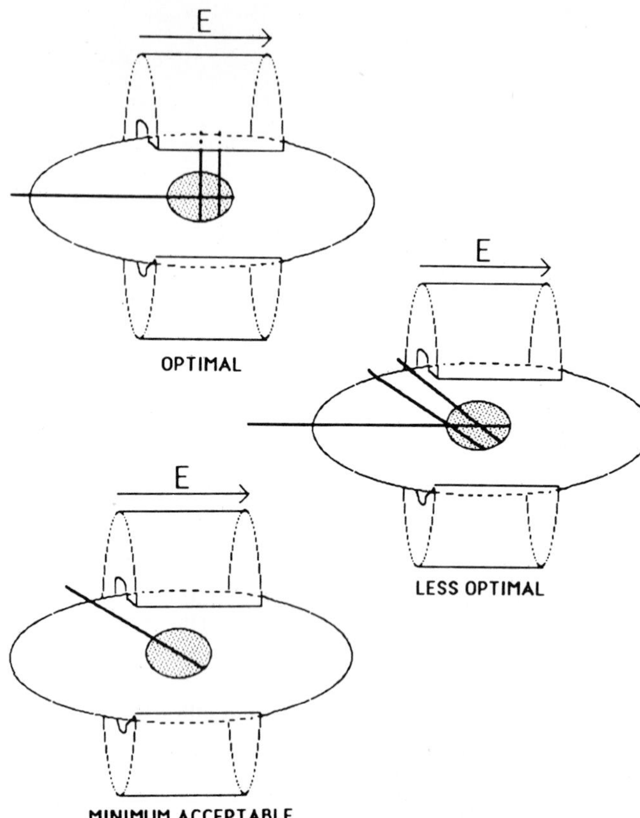

FIGURE 16–35. Strategies for thermometry catheter placement in association with annular microwave (MW) or radiofrequency (RF) array devices. (Dewhirst MW, Phillips TL, Samulski TV, et al: Int J Radiat Oncol Biol Phys 18:1249–1259, 1990)

TABLE 16–9
Criteria for Evaluation of Hyperthermia Treatment: Compliance Regarding Thermometry

Appropriate, accurate thermometer compatible with heating device
Skin coupling medium (*e.g.*, bolus)
Type
Temperature
Thermometry catheters
Prescribed number used
Path through tumor and normal tissue documented
Measurement positions recorded (x,y,z space)
Catheter of appropriate size for thermometer to fit snugly
Measure taken to prevent slippage; catheters checked for slippage after treatment
Normal tissue measurement
Skin surface
Adequate number
Critical positions monitored (scars, high SAR)
Tumor/normal tissue interface
Systemic (for regional devices)
Soft tissue/bone interface, when possible, for ultrasound
Thermal maps and/or multijunction thermometry
Appropriate step size or spacing
Measurements done with prescribed frequency
Temperature distributions
Minimum tumor temperature achieved for required length of time
Maximum temperatures in tumor and/or normal tissue not exceeded

(Dewhirst MW, Phillips TL, Samulski TV, et al: Int J Radiat Oncol Biol Phys 18: 1249–1259, 1990)

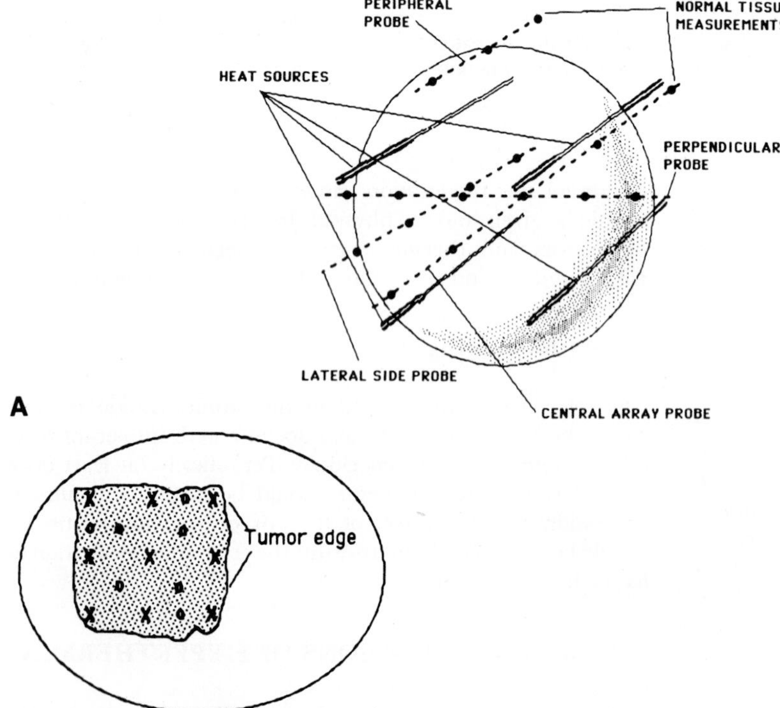

FIGURE 16–36. (**A**) Thermometry placement for interstitial heating methods relative to heat sources. (**B**) When more than one set of four sources is used, a central array probe should be used for each set. Thermometry catheters should be placed in the center of each set of four heat sources and at the tumor edge. (Dewhirst MW, Phillips TL, Samulski TV, et al: Int J Radiat Oncol Biol Phys 18:1249–1259, 1990)

hyperthermia clinical service requires the availability of several heating modalities and clinical thermometry systems.

A typical hyperthermia clinical setup is composed of the following basic elements:

Variable power supply with stabilizing electronic circuitry
Applicators, transducers, or antennas for the delivery of the heat in the tissues
Coupling devices (surface applicators), when necessary, to improve heat deposition in the tissues and decrease leakage
Thermometry system (thermistors, thermocouples, optical thermometers) and appropriate devices to record temperature
Feedback mechanisms, usually controlled by electronic circuits and microprocessors to vary power supply to maintain reference tissue temperature at constant level

Several models are commercially available for a variety of clinical applications.

If pretreatment studies in patient-specific phantoms indicate that electromagnetic leakage intensities in critical "nontarget" areas of the patient (*e.g.*, the eye) are likely to exceed 10 mW/cm^2, these areas should be shielded.

Prognostic Factors in Clinical Hyperthermia

A number of interrelated factors can influence the response of neoplastic lesions to the combined effects of ionizing radiation and hyperthermia. Recognition of these factors is important for developing guidelines for patient and tumor selection for hyperthermia clinical trials, or outlining quality assurance procedures, and for documenting the optimal conditions under which irradiation and hyperthermia can be delivered. The following is a brief overview of these factors.

The Patient

Following a given therapy, it is necessary that the patient survive for a period of time to exhibit a complete response and tumor control. One of the pretreatment eligibility criteria in the RTOG 81-04 protocol was a minimum life expectancy of 3 months.[315] Analysis of this study showed that about 30% of the patients died within the first 3 months and only 20% survived 1 year after therapy. Patients in poor general condition also are less likely to tolerate intensive hyperthermia treatment sessions. A beneficial therapeutic impact of hyperthermia was more clearly demonstrated in long-term tumor control than in early tumor response.[92,315] For tumors less than 3 cm in diameter no significant difference in complete response within the first 3 months was observed with radiation alone or radiation combined with heat. At 12 months, however, there was an 80% probability of local tumor control for combined treatment in contrast to 15% with irradiation alone ($P = 0.02$).

Tumor Characteristics

TUMOR SIZE. The impact of tumor size on the outcome of hyperthermia clinical trials has been the subject of much debate and analysis.[92,180,256,307,312,319,382,440] In an analysis of the experience at Washington University, Perez and coworkers[307] reported 70% of tumors less than 3 cm in depth achieved temperatures over 42°C, whereas tumors over 3 cm in depth achieved this "therapeutic temperature" in only 20% of the lesions. The complete response rate for tumors less than 3 cm in diameter was 77.6% compared with 63.6% for tumors over 3 cm in diameter. Similar observations were reported by Kapp and colleagues[186] and Valdagni and associates.[439] In RTOG protocol 81-04, 78% of lesions in both arms were over 3 cm in diameter.[315] This is considered a major contributing factor to the negative overall results of that study. Figure 16-37 illustrates the probability of remaining in response for tumors

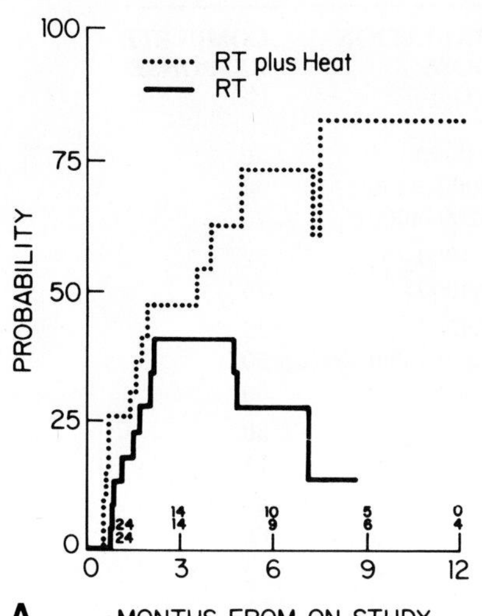

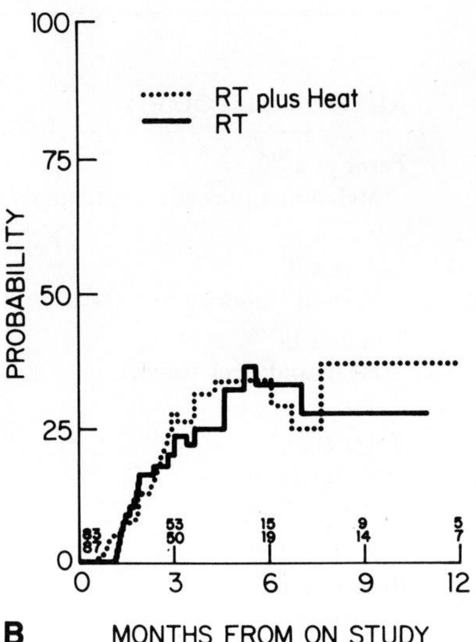

FIGURE 16–37. The Radiation Therapy Oncology Group (RTOG) randomized protocol comparing irradiation alone or combined with heat. Probability of remaining in response by size of tumor: (**A**) Tumors < 3 cm in diameter. (**B**) Tumors ≥ 3 cm in diameter. (Perez CA, et al: Int J Radiat Oncol Biol Phys 16:551–565, 1989)

TABLE 16–10
Tumor Control Versus *SAR Coverage (Patients with Measurable Disease Only)*

SAR COVERAGE	TUMOR CONTROL RATE
$0 \leq SAR < 25\%$	4/19 (21%) ($P < 0.01$)
$25\% \leq SAR \leq 50\%$	9/15 (60%)
$50\% \leq SAR$	13/19 (65%)

SAR: specific absorption dose
(Myerson RJ, Perez CA, Emami B, et al: Int J Radiat Oncol Biol Phys 118:1123–1129, 1990)

less than 3 cm in diameter or greater than 3 cm. Thus, large tumor size is currently a significant adverse factor in the response of lesions to thermal radiation therapy, as a result of our inability to heat larger tumors with current hyperthermia technology. Myerson and colleagues[267] reported better tumor control in long-term survivors following superficial hyperthermia when the tumors were covered with at least 25% SAR than that found in tumors not covered by 25% SAR, regardless of tumor size (Table 16-10).

TUMOR LOCATION. Anatomic sites such as chest wall, which can be heated easily with current hyperthermia technology, have demonstrated better therapeutic outcomes than sites such as head and neck, which are more difficult to heat[256,267,315,372] because of the complex contours of the head and neck anatomy. More detailed analysis of RTOG 81-04 showed that even for tumors smaller than 3 cm in diameter, complete response rates for chest wall lesions and head and neck lesions were 62% and 38%, respectively. In another report from RTOG (81-13) by Scott and co-workers[372] complete response rates for chest wall and head and neck tumors were 85% and 51%, respectively.

TUMOR HISTOLOGY. Although it is generally assumed that melanomas and sarcomas have better complete response rates after themoradiotherapy than epidermoid carcinoma and adenocarcinoma,[318] review of the literature shows that no histologic subtype is particularly sensitive to the effects of combined radiation therapy and hyperthermia.[69,256,307,440]

Treatment Parameters

RADIATION THERAPY-RELATED FACTORS. Two important factors with potential impact on the outcome of trials with radiation therapy are *total tumor dose* and *dose per fraction.* Some reports on tumor response as a function of total radiation dose are shown in Table 16-11. A strong correlation exists between the total radiation dose and complete response and the tumor control rate. Perez and associates[312] reported a 40% complete response rate in patients who received less than 3200 cGy compared with 67% for patients who received 3200 cGy to 4000 cGy. Valdagni and colleagues[441] reported no complete responses with doses of 1000 cGy to 2900 cGy, a 50% complete response rate with 3000 cGy to 3900 cGy, and 67% for doses of 4400 cGy to 4900 cGy.

Impact of dose per fraction on the outcome of thermal radiation therapy trials is less well defined. In the RTOG and Washington University experiences,[312] no difference in tumor control rate occurred with fraction sizes less than 400 cGy and over 400 cGy for either head and neck lesions or chest wall recurrences. Similar results were reported by Luk and co-workers.[237] Results of treatment of malignant melanomas are controversial. Many radiation oncologists believe that high dose per fraction will result in higher tumor control.[291] Results of thermal radiation therapy trials are similarly conflicting. Although Kim and co-workers[189] and Gonzales Gonzales and associates[130] demonstrated higher tumor control rates with higher dose per fraction, this was not confirmed by Emami and co-workers.[93]

THERMAL DOSE-RELATED FACTORS. Although it is anticipated that adequate heating will enhance the effects of irradiation,[383] it is difficult to determine which thermal parameter is most predictive of tumor control. Because of its inherent

TABLE 16–11
Tumor Response as a Function of Total Radiation Dose

AUTHOR/HISTOLOGY	NO. OF PATIENTS OR LESIONS	RADIATION DOSE (cGy)	COMPLETE RESPONSE (%)
Perez et al[318]		<2000	36
Melanoma plus adenocarcinoma	52	2000–3100	50
		3200–4000	76
Luk et al[238]	133	<4000	32
Various tumors		>4000	75
Tan and Li[422]		<4500	33
Head and neck tumors	50	4500–6000	50
		>6000	66
Kapp et al[185]		<2340	50
Various tumors	43	3600–6000	71
van der Zee et al[445]		<3900	27
Various tumors	111	≥3900	62
Bicher et al[17]		2000	42
Various tumors	111	4000	65
Valdagni et al[438]		<6000	50
Neck lymph nodes (squamous carcinoma)	54	≥6000	78

(Valdagni R, Liu FF, Kapp DS: Int J Radiat Oncol Biol Phys 15:959–972, 1988)

problems, thermal dose has yet to be used in clinical practice, as discussed by Valdagni and associates.[440] Several authors, however, have tried to correlate some thermal parameters with response rate (see Table 16-8). Overall, it appears that minimum tumor temperature has some correlation with tumor control in more tightly controlled studies. However, Oleson and co-workers[280] reported that when a univariate analysis was performed, the average minimum temperature for all hyperthermia treatments was statistically significant for response prediction ($P < 0.005$). A multivariate analysis of the same material showed that this parameter no longer remains significant because of the greater influence of other factors such as treatment technique, radiation dose, and tumor volume.

Currently tumor and normal tissue temperatures are measured in only one or a few catheter tracks at several points along each track, either automatically or manually; these are hardly representative of a 3D temperature distribution within the tumor during a course of a 30- to 60-minute hyperthermia session. It appears reasonable to make an attempt to rely on alternative methods to study temperature- or time-related factors. Three pathways are currently being investigated:

Refinement of computational methods and models that can predict three-dimensional tumor temperature profiles from a few measured points was studied by Roemer[339] and Strohbehn and co-workers.[440] Although most attractive, this appears to be a difficult task, with many technologic difficulties to overcome.

Myerson and colleagues[267] recently reported on a study of physically measurable parameters (SAR, specific absorption rate) and correlation of measured temperature with therapeutic outcome. This approach does not take into consideration physiologic events during heating.

Oleson and co-workers[278,280] have used a model involving a time-averaged temperature achieved at >90% and >50% of sites of temperature monitoring as descriptors of the temperature distribution. This approach appears to be attractive, and further investigation may confirm its usefulness.

Other treatment-related parameters that can potentially affect the therapeutic outcome are duration of the hyperthermia session, frequency of the hyperthermia sessions (per week), and total number of hyperthermia treatments. Review of the literature suggests that heating session durations of 30 to 45 minutes and 60 minutes produce similar results.[256] This factor, however, has never been studied prospectively. Many reported series have used two hyperthermia sessions per week for a total of eight to ten sessions. The concept of twice-weekly hyperthermia sessions was initially based on biologic considerations for thermotolerance.[149] In a prospective randomized study of 150 lesions at Washington University, patients were treated with once-weekly (total of four) hyperthermia sessions *versus* twice-weekly (total of eight) hyperthermia sessions and irradiation (3200 cGy in eight fractions delivered twice weekly).[178] No difference was found in any study end points (tumor control) between the two treatment arms. Similarly, Kapp and associates[185] and Valdagni and co-workers[441] reported no difference in tumor response using two or six hyperthermia sessions per course of treatment. Different results were reached by Alexander and colleagues,[3] who found superior complete response rate (42%) for one hyperthermia session per week compared with 21% for two hyperthermia sessions per week combined with comparable radiation doses. The number of patients was small, and the analysis was preliminary. Arcangeli and colleagues[6] reported a superior complete response rate for ten *versus* five hyperthermia treatments (78% and 64%, respectively). Further investigation to settle this issue is warranted.

Sequencing of Heat and Radiation Therapy

Biologic reports indicate that the maximum therapeutic ratio is achieved when irradiation is followed by hyperthermia.[432] It is further stated that physiologic changes after hyperthermia (blood flow) would make tumor cells more hypoxic and therefore more resistant to subsequent irradiation. In clinical practice, however, neither sequence has proven to be superior (Table 16-12). Experimental work suggests that more therapeutic gain can be achieved if the hyperthermia is delayed for 4 hours after completion of irradiation.[286] Arcangeli and co-workers[7] and Overgaard and Overgaard[295] suggest that although slightly better tumor control could be achieved by irradiation followed immediately by hyperthermia, skin reaction (percentage of moist desquamation) was less when hyperthermia was delayed for 4 hours after radiation therapy.

Finally, review of the literature reveals that no specific format has been followed in reporting the details of hyperther-

TABLE 16–12
External Radiation Therapy Plus Heat Clinical Trials:
"Unconventional" Sequence of Heat Plus External Radiation Therapy

AUTHOR	NO. OF LESIONS	SEQUENCE	COMPLETE RESPONSE (%)
Corry et al[50]	21	Ht-XRT	62
Kim et al[194]	28	Ht-XRT	64
	22	XRT-Ht	68
Arcangeli et al[8]	13	XRT-Ht (immediate)	77
	12	XRT-Ht (4 hours' delay)	67
Overgaard and Overgaard[295]	65	XRT-Ht (immediate)	TER = 1.5*
		XRT-Ht (3 to 4 hours' delay)	TER = 1.3*
Lauche et al[210]	22	Ht-XRT	41
Cosset et al[54]	57	Ht-XRT (interstitial)	79

** TER: thermal enhancement ratio based on 50% tumor control dose*
(Valdagni R, Liu FF, Kapp DS: Int J Radiat Oncol Biol Phys 15:959–972, 1988)

mia trials. Considering the multiplicity of factors affecting outcome, it is essential that a standard format for documentation and reporting of hyperthermia trials be devised and followed. The Radiation Therapy Oncology Group has adapted the format proposed by Sapareto and Corry.[353] From the preceding discussion, it appears that certain prognostic factors (Table 16-13) are important and should be considered in the design of clinical protocols and the evaluation of results of clinical trials.

CLINICAL RESULTS WITH HYPERTHERMIA

Heat Alone

Summary of results reporting use of hyperthermia alone in the treatment of recurrent superficial tumors is shown in Table 16-14. Of 131 patients, 19 (15%) had complete responses and 42 (32%) had partial responses. The duration of these responses was short, and no long-term tumor control was available.

TABLE 16–13
Important Factors to be Considered in Protocol Design and Analysis of Hyperthermia Clinical Trials

- Treatment aim
  - Definitive
  - Palliative
- Patient characteristics
  - Performance status (life expectancy)
- Tumor characteristics
  - Anatomic site
  - Tumor volume (including geometric description)
  - Tumor histology
- Treatment
  - Radiation therapy
    - Modality
      - External
      - Interstitial
    - Dose/fractionation
    - Total time
  - Hyperthermia
    - Technique
      - External (radiofrequency *versus* microwave *versus* ultrasound)
      - Interstitial (radiofrequency *versus* microwave *versus* ferromagnetic seeds)
    - Applicator description (design, size, volumetric SAR characteristics)
    - Treatment setup information (applicator position, hyperthermia field size, coupling, skin cooling)
    - Thermometry
      - Probe type
      - Probe(s) location
    - Temperature monitoring method (manual, automatic, interval)
    - Time-temperature parameters
      - Thermal dose or other methods
      - Min/max/average temperatures (includes method of calculation)
      - Sequencing of two modalities and interval additional modalities (*i.e.*, chemotherapy) and their related factors (drug type, dose, rate of delivery, and so on)
- Posttreatment assessment
  - Tumor response
  - Tumor control
  - Survival
  - Normal tissue effects
- Standardized methods of documentation and reporting
- Statistical methods in analysis of results

Local External Hyperthermia and Irradiation

Patients receiving radiation and hyperthermia have been treated with daily doses ranging from 200 cGy to 300 cGy or with two to three fractions per week of 300 cGy to 600 cGy. Total doses of radiation have varied from 1800 cGy to 6000 cGy. It is not certain whether, as reported by Hornback and associates[167] and Scott and colleagues,[371] higher doses of irradiation will yield greater tumor control over that observed with moderate doses (3000 cGy to 4000 cGy). In general, temperatures of 42°C to 44°C have been used for 30 to 60 minutes after irradiation, one, two, three, or even five times per week. In most instances skin cooling has been used when no evidence of superficial tumor involvement exists. External microwaves (usually 915 MHz) have been used more frequently, although a few institutions such as the M. D. Anderson Cancer Center[47] and Stanford University[248,255] have published their experiences with ultrasound.

Several reports, summarized in Table 16-15, compare results in matched comparable lesions or by randomized allocation to results in treatment with irradiation alone or irradiation and hyperthermia. The complete response rate with irradiation alone ranges from 0% to 86%, with an average of 33%. With irradiation and hyperthermia the complete response rate has ranged from 7% to 100%, with an average of 60%; the TER ranged from 1 to 6.14.[239]

Egawa and associates[86] reported on a prospectively controlled, multi-institutional randomized trial in which patients with superficial tumors were randomized to irradiation alone or irradiation combined with hyperthermia. Of 113 patients accrued to this study, analysis was done on 92 patients. Forty-four patients were treated with combined modality (group A) and 48 patients were treated with radiation alone (group B). Complete response (CR) rate and complete response plus partial response rates were 45.5% and 81.8% in group A compared with 37.5% and 62.5% in group B. The authors indicated that the difference in complete response plus partial response rate between the two groups was statistically significant ($P < 0.05$). No difference in CR rate was found between the two arms in patients with head and neck carcinoma (44.8% compared with 44.4%), whereas in patients with chest wall recurrences the CR rate with combined modality was twice as high as in the irradiation alone group (66.6% and 33.3%). In contrast, in a randomized trial reported by RTOG,[315] in which 236 superficial tumors were treated with eight fractions of 400 cGy delivered twice weekly or the same dose of radiation combined with hyperthermia (42.5°C, 60 minutes), there was no significant difference in overall complete response rate or tumor control between the two treatment arms (30% with radiation therapy and 33% with radiation therapy and heat).

In the head and neck the tumor response and control rates were the same (approximately 30%) regardless of tumor size. Tumor control with irradiation and heat in recurrent chest wall lesions less than 3 cm in diameter was substantially superior to irradiation alone (85% *versus* 15%; $P = 0.02$), whereas no difference was noted in lesions larger than 3 cm. Problems encountered in correlating tumor response with quality of heat in clinical trials include less than optimal power deposition in larger lesions because of poor penetrability of the microwave equipment used, inadequate SAR deposition because of applicator not covering larger surface lesions, and the limited ability to determine volumetric temperature distributions in a tumor with current thermometry techniques.[315] Despite the fact that some thought this protocol was a premature phase III study in clinical hyperthermia,[277] it was the first time that a cooperative

TABLE 16–14
Responses of Superficial Tumors to Hyperthermia Alone

STUDY	HYPERTHERMIA METHOD (MHz)	PRESCRIBED TEMPERATURE × TIME	NUMBER OF TREATMENTS	EVALUABLE PATIENTS	CR	PR
Manning et al[244]	MW (915,2450) RF Capacitive (0.5–3.3)	42.5°–44°C × 40 min	2–22	11	2	3
Luk[239]	MW(915,2450)	42.5°C × 60 min	5–12	11	2	2
U et al[432]	MW (915,2450)	42°–44°C × 40–50 min	2–9	6	0	3
Abe et al[1]	RF Capacitive (13.56)	41°–46°C × 30–60 min	4–9	6	0	1
Corry et al[50]	US (1–3)	43°–50°C × 60 min	6–12	28	5(18%)	11(39%)
Kim and Hahn[192]	RF Inductive (27.12)	41°–43.5°C × 30–40 min	2–9	19	4(21%)	6(32%)
Marmor[246]	US (1–3)	43°–45°C × 30 min	6	44	5(11%)	14(32%)
Perez et al[318]	MW (915)	41°–43°C × 60–90 min	NS	6	1	2
Total				131	19(15%)	42(32%)

CR: complete response; PR: partial response
(Modified from Meyer JL: Cancer Res 47[Suppl]:4745S–4751S, 1984; Meyer JL, Kapp DS, Fessenden P, et al: Pharmacol Ther 42:251–288, 1989)

TABLE 16–15
Effect of Adjuvant Hyperthermia on Tumor Radiation Response

		COMPLETE RESPONSE		
STUDY	NO. OF TUMORS	IRRADIATION ALONE (%)	IRRADIATION AND HEAT (%)	ISODOSE TER
Arcangeli et al[8]	163	38	74	1.95
Perez et al[317]	154	41	69	1.68
Overgaard et al[287, 296]*	101	39	62	1.59
U et al[432]	14	14	86	6.14
Gonzalez et al[130]	46	33	50	1.52
Kim et al[192, 193, 195]	238	39	72	1.85
Valdagni et al[438, 439]	78	36	73	2.03
Bide et al[18]	76	0	7	>1
van der Zee et al[445]*	71	5	27	5.40
Corry et al[50]	34	0	62	≫1
Scott et al[374]	62	39	87	2.23
Lindholm et al[236]	85	25	46	1.84
Li et al[232, 233]	124	29	54	1.86
Steeves et al[396]	90	31	65	2.10
Dunlop et al[83]	86	50	60	1.20
Goldobenko et al[128]	65	86	100	1.16
Muratkhodzhaev[264]	313	25	63	2.52
Hiraoka et al[163]	33	25	71	2.84
Bey et al[13]	45	9	42	4.67
Shidna et al[378]	185	33	64	1.94
Datta et al[58]	65	46	66	1.43
Uozumi et al[434]	16	63	88	1.40
Hornback et al[168]	66	35	72	2.06
Fuwa et al[115]	24	63	83	1.32

** Plus unpublished data*
(Overgaard J: Int J Radiat Oncol Biol Phys 16:535–549, 1989)

group definitely demonstrated the impact of tumor size on the outcome of irradiation and heat clinical trials and the technical difficulties in heat delivery and monitoring of temperatures.

Clinical Results in Specific Anatomic Sites

Head and Neck Tumors

Of 131 measurable epithelial tumors in the head and neck (except for nine melanomas and three sarcomas) reported by Perez and co-workers,[313] 91 (69.5%) exhibited a complete response (CR) and 25 (19.1%) a partial response (PR), defined as more than 50% regression in all diameters. Approximately 75% of the epidermoid carcinomas, 92% of the adenocarcinomas, 57% of the melanomas, and 33% of sarcomas that had a CR went on to exhibit control of the tumor (no recurrence) in the volume treated with irradiation and hyperthermia. In a nonrandomized comparison with a group of patients with recurrent head and neck lesions treated with irradiation alone reported by Emami and Marks,[87] better tumor control was observed with irradiation and hyperthermia.

Arcangeli and co-workers[7] described their experience in four separate randomized trials using various doses and fractionation schedules of irradiation, ranging from 4000 cGy to 6000 cGy, with two or five daily fractions per week, and hyperthermia at 42.5°C for 45 minutes or 45°C for 30 minutes applied before or after irradiation. Tumor control was 75% with irradiation and hyperthermia compared with about 40% with irradiation alone. In 1985, Arcangeli and colleagues[5] updated their experience in 38 patients with 81 multiple neck lymph node metastases from squamous cell carcinoma of the head and neck. The complete response rate was 79% (30 of 38) with irradiation and hyperthermia compared with 42% (18 of 43) with irradiation alone.

Valdagni and associates[437] treated 85 metastatic squamous cell carcinoma neck nodes in 82 patients with a combination of 3222 cGy (mean dose) of radiation for palliation and 6576 cGy for definitive radiation therapy and heat (42.5°C for 30 minutes delivered within 20 to 30 minutes after irradiation). In lymph nodes less than 70 cc, the CR rate with definitive irradiation and heat ranged from 77% to 100%, whereas in the larger lymph nodes it was 50% or less ($P = 0.0005$). Higher doses of radiation were correlated with better tumor control.

Sannazzari and associates[350] observed three complete responses in 31 patients (9.7%) with recurrent or persistent head and neck cancer treated with hyperthermia alone (434 MHz and 915 MHz, 42.5°C to 44°C, 30 minutes twice a week for a total of six to ten sessions during 3 to 5 weeks). This was contrasted to 12 of 36 complete responses (33.3%) observed with radiation and heat. RTOG reported on 60 patients with superficial tumors in the head and neck treated in a randomized study (81-04) with radiation alone (3200 cGy in eight fractions delivered twice weekly) and 53 patients receiving the same dose of radiation followed by two weekly sessions of external hyperthermia (42.5°C, 60 minutes). No difference was seen in the complete tumor response rate (35% and 34%) or tumor control in the two treatment arms.

Advanced Primary Breast Cancer

Fuwa and co-workers[115] reported on nine patients with inoperable advanced carcinoma of the breast treated with radiation (5000 cGy to 5500 cGy) to the breast and 1500 cGy to 2000 cGy electron beam boost with reduced portal in addition to 5000 cGy to 6000 cGy to the regional lymph nodes in combination with hyperthermia delivered once or twice weekly (2 hours after irradiation, 40°C to 42°C, 40 to 60 minutes) delivered with the Thermotron RF-8. Six patients achieved a complete response and three a partial response. The most common limiting symptoms are pain and skin burning around the ribs, sternum, and clavicle, which disappear completely within 3 weeks after conservative treatment.[309,444]

Recurrent Carcinoma of the Breast in the Chest Wall

At the Mallinckrodt Institute of Radiology varying doses of radiation (between 2000 cGy and 5000 cGy in fractions of 200 cGy daily or 400 cGy every 72 hours) followed by external microwave hyperthermia (915 MHz, 41°C to 43°C, 30 to 60 minutes) were given to a group of 99 patients; results were compared with historic controls (116 patients) with similar recurrent carcinoma of the breast treated with radiation alone (2000 cGy to 6000 cGy, usually in 200 cGy to 300 cGy TD daily fractions). For 1 cm to 3 cm lesions, higher rates of complete tumor regression and control were found in those receiving over 3000 cGy to 4000 cGy (Fig. 16-38*A*). This difference is statistically significant. For lesions greater than 3 cm in diameter or depth, no significant difference was found between those treated with radiation alone or with radiation and heat (Fig. 16-38*B*).[309]

van der Zee and associates[443] noted higher response rates (82%) in 17 chest wall recurrences from carcinoma of the breast less than 15 mm^3 treated with higher doses of radiation (3200 cGy) compared with 33% response rate in 30 receiving lower doses. In larger lesions, the differences in response were less striking (28% and 16%, respectively). In a previous publication,[447] they reported a correlation of better tumor control with increasing thermal doses in the same group of patients. Similar results were described by Seegnschmiedt and associates.[376]

Kjellen and associates[200] observed a 68% complete response rate in 22 patients treated with radiation and heat compared with 27% in 22 patients treated with radiation alone for chest wall recurrences of carcinoma of the breast. The difference was statistically significant ($P = 0.0027$).

Overgaard[293] summarized various reports comparing radiation alone or combined with heat in the treatment of chest wall recurrence from carcinoma of the breast, with superior complete responses in the latter group (Table 16-16).

In the RTOG study,[319] a total of 81 patients with single lesions in the chest wall were randomized; 38 were treated with radiation alone, and 43 received radiation combined with hyperthermia. In lesions less than 3 cm in diameter, the complete response rate was 62% and 40%, respectively. In tumors larger than 3 cm, complete response rate was 21% with radiation and heat and 29% with radiation alone. In lesions less than 3 cm in diameter, tumor control was significantly superior with radiation and heat (80% *versus* 15%; $P = 0.02$), but no difference was noted in tumors larger than 3 cm in comparison with radiation alone.

Melanoma

Emami and associates[93] reported on 49 superficial recurrent primary or metastatic malignant melanomas in 18 patients treated with a combination of radiation therapy and hyperthermia. Dose of radiation varied from less than 400 cGy to 800 cGy per fraction, and total dose ranged from 2000 cGy to over 6000 cGy. Of 30 patients who received dose fractions of 400 cGy or less, 19 had complete tumor responses (63.3%). Of 19 patients

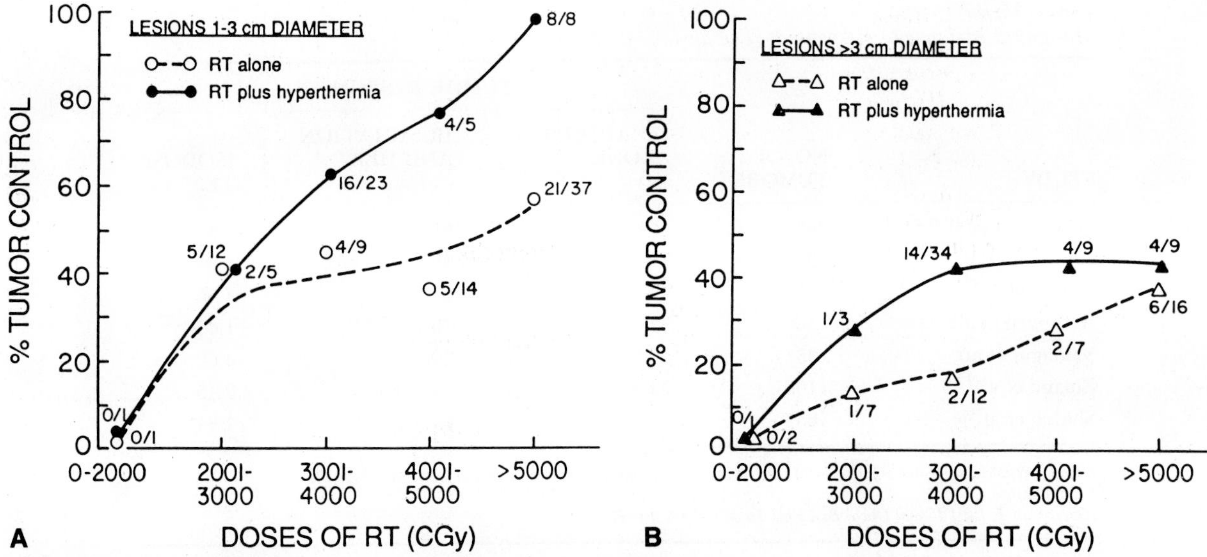

FIGURE 16–38. Probability of tumor control in chest wall recurrence of breast carcinoma. (**A**) Lesions 1 cm to 3 cm in diameter. (**B**) Lesions > 3 cm in diameter. (Perez CA, Emami B: Radiol Clin North Am 27:525–542, 1989)

treated with dose per fraction greater than 400 cGy, ten had complete responses (52.6%). Complete response rates for total doses of less than 3000 cGy, 3000 cGy to 4000 cGy, and over 4000 cGy were 38.1%, 76.2%, and 76%, respectively. These differences are not statistically significant.

Kim and associates[196] described their experience with four different dose fractionations ranging from 300 cGy per fraction to 660 cGy per fraction and hyperthermia once or twice per week. Complete response rates for radiation alone and radiation plus hyperthermia for two different dose levels per fraction were 50% to 55% and 72% to 75%, respectively. Smaller lesions treated with *lower* dose per fraction had higher complete response rates when hyperthermia was added compared with that which occurred with irradiation alone. However, smaller tumors treated with *high* dose per fraction had no beneficial effect from the addition of hyperthermia. For larger lesions the addition of hyperthermia resulted in an increased complete response rate for both low and high dose per fraction.

Scott and co-workers[373] reported complete response in eight of 12 patients treated with 500 cGy per fraction for a total of six treatments in combination with hyperthermia. They described a thermal enhancement ratio (TER) of 2.2. In a report by Overgaard and co-workers[298] on the treatment of malignant melanomas with radiation therapy alone *versus* radiation plus hyperthermia, the observed TER was 1.6, similar to that noted by Kim and associates.[193] In an updated report Overgaard[288] notes a TER of 2.0.

Overgaard,[294] in an analysis of 110 tumors treated with radiation alone or combined with heat, observed a local control rate of 80% with radiation and heat compared with 49% with radiation alone ($P < 0.05$). In a review of over 800 patients, he showed an isoeffect TER of approximately 1.5.[293, 296]

Gonzalez and associates[130] in 38 malignant melanoma lesions treated with a combination of radiation therapy and hyperthermia noted a complete response rate of 50%.

Overgaard[293] summarized various reports comparing radi-

TABLE 16–16
Breast-Chest Wall Recurrence: Isodose TER

AUTHOR	NO. OF TUMORS	TUMOR RESPONSE*: IRRADIATION ALONE (%)	TUMOR RESPONSE*: IRRADIATION AND HEAT (%)	ISODOSE TER
Perez et al[317]	35	43	86	2.00
van der Zee et al[447]†	40	0	24	>>1
Scott et al[374]	34	47	94	2.00
Gonzalez et al[131]	18	33	78	2.36
Lindholm et al[236]†	66	35	70	2.00
Li et al[233]	42	36	73	2.03
Dunlop et al[83]	32	67	82	1.22
Overgaard et al†	14	40	78	1.94

* *Tumor response after treatment with the same radiation dose given either alone or combined with hyperthermia*
† *Unpublished*
(Overgaard J: Int J Radiat Oncol Biol Phys 16:535–549, 1989)

TABLE 16–17
Malignant Melanoma: Response to Therapy

STUDY	NO. OF TUMORS	TUMOR RESPONSE* IRRADIATION ALONE (%)	IRRADIATION AND HEAT (%)	ISODOSE TER
Overgaard et al[287, 296]	63	57	90	1.58
Gonzalez et al[130]	24	17	83	4.88
Kim et al[192–197]	149	43	67	1.56
Arcangeli et al[6]	38	53	76	1.43
Valdagni et al†	35	20	80	4.00
Emami et al[93]	116	24	59	2.45
Shidna et al[378]	185	33	64	1.94

* *Tumor response after treatment with the same radiation dose given either alone or combined with hyperthermia*
† *Unpublished*
(Overgaard J: Int J Radiat Oncol Biol Phys 16:535–549, 1989)

ation alone or combined with heat in the treatment of malignant melanoma, with superior complete responses in the latter group (Table 16-17).

With radiation alone, dose per fraction and larger tumor volume both have negative influences on the outcome or therapy.[297] Unlike that which occurs with radiation alone, thermal radiation therapy results in higher response rates for larger tumors. Thermal dose appears to be an important factor in hyperthermic treatment of these tumors, as demonstrated by a 100% complete response rate at thermal doses above 500 equivalent minutes at 43°C.[93]

Clinical Results with Deep (Regional) Hyperthermia

The experience with the first generation of regional hyperthermia devices reported in single-institution studies and a recently completed RTOG phase I/II study indicates that, although temperatures exceeding 42°C could be obtained in 10% to 20% of patients, in only a minority of the sessions could the temperature be maintained long enough to achieve the desired goal of heating the tumor to at least 42°C (72% of the sessions for 0 to 20 minutes, 24% for 21 to 40 minutes, and only 4% for over 41 minutes). Incomplete duration was usually the result of local pain and discomfort (reported incidence of 30% to 70%) or systemic stress (10% to 25%).[88, 90, 164, 261, 265, 320, 322, 324, 363, 364, 433] Tumors in the upper abdomen were more likely to be associated with systemic cardiovascular stress. However, pelvic heating was limited by local pain (28% to 68% of sessions), discomfort or anxiety (6% to 23%), or cardiac symptoms (5% to 13%).[123, 266, 322, 363] Complications of treatment are unusual. In a series of 105 patients treated at the University of Utah, Sapozink and associates[364] reported six cases of local soft tissue breakdown and three complications attributable to invasive temperature probes. In an RTOG study (84-01) four grade 4 toxicities occurred out of 54 patients, three of which were attributable to the catheter used for temperature monitoring and one resulted from unrecommended surgery following maximum-dose irradiation.[90] No grade 4 complications were directly attributable to the regional hyperthermia itself. Response rates in single-institution and multi-institution studies ranged from 20% to 53%, with response showing better correlation with radiation dose than with hyperthermia delivery indicators.[88, 90, 164, 261, 265, 320, 322, 324, 363, 464] Toxicity was acceptable and desired temperatures could be achieved, but duration was limited because of patient discomfort (Table 16-18).

Oleson used a scaled-down version of the Annular Phased Array System (mini-APAS) to heat lower extremity sarcomas.[280] He was able to achieve better duration at desired temperatures. All lesions in the sarcoma series received 5000 cGy and hyperthermia preoperatively. Histologic response was graded by a scale proposed by Suit and co-workers[418] with 63% of the tumors showing grade 2 or grade 3 responses (complete necrosis or rare isolated intact cells).

Petrovich and associates[322] recently summarized the results in 353 patients treated with regional hyperthermia for a variety of pelvic and abdominal tumors at several institutions. Complete response was observed in 35 of the patients (10%) and partial response in 59 (17%). Complete response was noted in 12% of patients receiving radiation in addition to heat compared with 2% of those treated with heat alone. Treatment tolerance was good in 149 (42%) of the patients, fair in 112 (32%), poor in 62 (18%), and not recorded in 30 (8%). Pain during the heat session was observed in 123 patients (35%). Cardiovascular symptoms were experienced by ten patients (3%), anxiety reaction by six (2%), and claustrophobia by four (1%). Ten patients (3%) developed blisters in the hyperthermia-treated areas.

TABLE 16–18
Complete Response Rate in Patients with Deep-Seated Tumors with Radiation Therapy and Hyperthermia

AUTHOR	HEATING MODALITY	COMPLETE RESPONSE	TUMOR CONTROL
Sapozink[365]	MW	4/23 (17%)	3/23 (13%)
Yanagawa[486]	MW	5/13 (38%)	5/13 (38%)
Hiraoka[163]	RF	21/40* (53%)	20/40* (50%)
Howard[170]	MW	1/20 (5%)	—
Shimm[380]	MW	6/44 (14%)	—
Nishimura[269]	RF	4/33 (12%)	—
Petrovich[322]	MW	35/353 (10%)	—
Emami[90]	MW/RF	17/44 (39%)	14/44 (32%)

* *Forty tumors in 36 patients*
(Emami B, Meyerson RJ, Scott C, et al: Int J Radiat Oncol Biol Phys, submitted for publication)

TABLE 16–19
Clinical Results with Interstitial Thermal Radiation Therapy

AUTHOR	NO. OF EVALUABLE PATIENTS	CR	PR	NR	FOLLOW-UP (months)
Bicher et al[15] (1984)	8	5	2	1	—
Cosett et al[53] (1985)	57	45	7	5	2
Emami et al[94] (1987)	44	26	12	6	6–60
Linares et al[235] (1986)	10	5	5	—	Short
Oleson et al[281] (1984)	52	20	22	10	3–18
Petrovich et al[321] (1988)	44	28	15	1	6–30
Puthawala et al[327] (1985)	43	37	6	—	6
Strohbehn et al[411] (1984)	6	3	2	1	Short
Vora et al[456] (1982)	15	11	1	3	1–13
Yabumoto et al[485] (1984)	7	1	2	4	2–13
Total	286	181 (63.3%)	74 (25.9%)	31 (10.8%)	

CR: complete response; PR: partial response (over 50% regression of tumor volume); NR: less than 50% regression of tumor volume

Clinical Results with Interstitial Hyperthermia

The experience with interstitial hyperthermia has been more limited than with external applicators. Emami and colleagues[94] reported on 48 recurrent/persistent tumors in 46 patients treated with interstitial thermal radiation therapy. Of 44 tumors available for evaluation of response, there were 26 (59%) complete and 12 (27%) partial responses with follow-up periods of 6 to 60 months. These results are in general agreement with other reported series (Table 16-19); of the total 286 lesions, 181 (63.3%) had complete tumor response and 74 (25.9%) had partial response. The response rate has been analyzed as a function of quality of heating in three reported series.[94] The two criteria for satisfactory hyperthermia were encompassment of the entire gross tumor volume (with margins) within implanted volume and measured temperatures above 42°C for a minimum of 30 minutes. Of the 96 evaluable lesions with at least one satisfactory hyperthermia session, 77 (80%) had complete response, whereas in 14 lesions with no satisfactory hyperthermia session no complete responses occurred. The difference is statistically significant ($P \geq 0.01$; Table 16-20). The overall complication rate varied from 19% to 40%, and severe complication rates were from 6% to 17%.

The Radiation Therapy Oncology Group currently is conducting a prospective randomized trial (RTOG 84-19) to evaluate the efficacy of interstitial radiation alone *versus* interstitial thermal radiation therapy.[330]

Interstitial thermal radiation therapy has been used in several specific tumor sites.[20,21,207,281,347,375,387] Interstitial hyperthermia in the brain has been used by several authors,[336] starting with Sutton,[420] who treated seven patients with recurrent malignant glioma with a heating probe inserted in the brain. Salcman and Samaras[347] used a single 2450 MHz microwave antenna following partial resection of recurrent malignant gliomas in a few patients. Winter and colleagues[481] and Borok and associates[20,21] described results in 20 patients receiving from one to 12 60-minute heat sessions (45°C delivered with one to six probes); 80% of the patients experienced symptomatic improvement and objective tumor response. Marchosky and associates[245] used a hot source in patients with recurrent glioblastoma and a few metastatic tumors. Over 80% of the patients reportedly had good tumor regression and lack of regrowth for several months.

Recurrent or persistent head and neck tumors have also been treated with this technique.[52,95,207,321,328] Of a total of 158 patients in three series, 77.2% had complete response rate. The

TABLE 16–20
Interstitial Thermal Radiation Therapy: Comparison of Complete Response Rates

	TOTAL NO. OF PATIENTS	COMPLETE RESPONSE (%)
Total number of lesions with satisfactory heating from three institutions* (evaluable lesions)	96	77(80)
Total number of lesions with unsatisfactory heating from three institutions (evaluable lesions)	14	0(0)
Total number of lesions reported from three institutions	120†	77(64)
Total number of patients from selected published series	201	112(55.7)

**Results from series reported from Washington University, Memorial Medical Center, and Institut Gustave-Roussy in which information regarding quality of hyperthermia and tumor response was available*
† Results of treatment of ten lesions were not evaluable

reported complication rate ranged from 2% to 12%. Gynecologic and breast tumors have also been treated with interstitial thermal radiation therapy.[457,458] In 14 patients with Stage III and Stage IV cervix carcinoma reported on by Vora and co-workers,[457] eight had complete response and one had partial responses. Five of eight complete responders were alive without any tumor at follow-up, which ranged from 6 to 47 months. Vora and associates[458] have also reported on the treatment of 11 patients with inoperable advanced and inflammatory carcinoma of the breast; ten had complete responses and one had partial response. Interstitial hyperthermia has also been used intraoperatively,[32,55,111,129] and it has been shown that this approach is safe and feasible.

Interstitial thermal radiation therapy using thermally regulated ferromagnetic seeds has been used in several laboratories with exciting prospects.[27,28,60,303] Clinical results, however, are preliminary.[379]

In a somewhat different application of thermal radiation therapy, Finger[109] reported tumor reduction in 11 to 14 cloroidal melanomas (78.6%) treated with a plaque-like intraocular device containing ^{125}I seeds and an ingeniously designed microwave applicator.

Clinical Results with Intracavitary Hyperthermia

A few reports have been published regarding clinical experience with intracavitary applicators. Yerushalmi[488] reported on the results of an intracavitary coaxial antenna operated at 915 MHz or 2450 MHz inserted in the rectum to heat the prostate. Hyperthermia was combined with radiation (5000 cGy to the pelvis and 1000 cGy boost to the prostate) in patients with adenocarcinoma. For benign prostate hyperplasia, 12 to 16 sessions of heat alone (43°C) lasting 1 hour each were delivered twice weekly. Symptomatic relief was achieved and maintained in 65% to 70% of the benign prostatic hyperplasia patients. The results in carcinoma of the prostate are more difficult to assess.

Preliminary reports on 20 patients with adenocarcinoma of the prostate treated with transrectal hyperthermia (915 MHz MW skirt-type antenna) were reported by Strohmaier and associates.[414] Four hyperthermia sessions (twice a week, 41°C to 43°C for 60 minutes) were delivered. Histologic material obtained at TURP, radical prostatectomy, or needle biopsy showed diffuse edema of the stroma and interstitial inflammation and swelling of the wall and damage of major blood vessels. Definite signs of tumor cell destruction were not observed in any of the patients.

Li and colleagues[224] described the design and heating patterns of 915 MHz and 2450 MHz applicators for intracavitary therapy of carcinoma of the uterine cervix. The applicator consists of a helical coil on one end and a dielectric rod at the other. The uterine applicator is made of a coaxial cable with its outer conductor connected to a 6 cm and 6-turn spiral. Vaginal heating and cervical heating were done separately, one to three times, to temperatures of 43.5°C to 45°C. The applicators were used in 30 patients with Stage IIB and Stage IIIB cervical carcinoma, who were treated with radiation therapy. Results of therapy were not reported.

Colvin and co-workers[45] described a small radiofrequency (RF) intracavitary applicator that can be inserted through a fiberbronchoscope to treat lung lesions. The unit is battery-powered and provides temperature feedback control from 35°C to 60°C. Monopole electrodes can be used for larger lesions, and bipolar probes can straddle small tumors. Current is generated by 2 MHz RF.

Clinical Results with Thermochemotherapy

Experience with thermochemotherapy in the treatment of human malignancies is limited.[7,57,89,175,397,489,490] Arcangeli and associates[7] reported on 43 neck nodes treated with chemotherapy with or without hyperthermia. The overall response rate for thermochemotherapy was 95% compared with 45% for chemotherapy alone ($P = < 0.01$). Steindorfer and co-workers[397] described the treatment of ten patients with heat and radiation therapy and 12 patients treated with heat and bleomycin and cisplatin. Although they achieved eight of 11 overall responses with irradiation and heat, they had only one to 12 partial responses in the heat and chemotherapy group. In contrast, Emami and colleagues[89] treated 24 recurrent superficial lesions (previously heavily irradiated) with hyperthermia and bleomycin (15 units/m^2). Of the 21 evaluable lesions with minimum follow-up of 3 months, there were ten complete responses (49%) and four partial responses, with an overall response rate of 67%.

The difference in the two latter small series might be in the method of treatment delivery and the pharmacokinetics of bleomycin. In Steindorfer's study, bleomycin was given intramuscularly 4 to 6 hours before heating, whereas in the study by Emami, bleomycin was given intravenously within 60 minutes before hyperthermia. Perfusion hyperthermia in combination with chemotherapy (mitomycin C plus cisplatin) has been reported in the treatment of bladder carcinoma by Zhang and co-workers.[490] In their series of 28 patients, 11 achieved complete and 12 had partial responses.

Trimodality Trials

Herman and associates[156] reported on the treatment of 24 patients with hyperthermia, radiation, and cisplatin. The results, despite a small number of patients, are impressive (25% to 67% CR, depending on cisplatin dose). Zeung and colleagues (personal communication) reported on the treatment of 34 patients with esophageal carcinoma with cisplatin, radiation therapy, and intracavitary hyperthermia. Of 26 patients who had trimodality therapy as the primary management, a 1-year survival rate of 85% and 2-year survival rate of 50% were noted. In eight patients in whom treatment was delivered for recurrent disease, a 2-year survival rate of 25% was observed. Matsufuji and associates[251] reported on preoperative hyperthermia combined with radiation therapy and chemotherapy in three groups of patients with esophageal carcinoma: 16 patients were treated with surgery alone; 38 patients were treated with surgery, radiation therapy, and chemotherapy; and ten patients had trimodality treatment followed by surgery. Median survival for the three groups was 6 months, 7.5 months, and 11 months, respectively.

Bull and colleagues[30] reported on whole-body hyperthermia and cisplatin in the treatment of disseminated malignant melanoma; of seven patients, two had partial responses and one had complete response. Neumann and co-workers[268] reported on moderate whole-body hyperthermia in combination with chemotherapy in the treatment of oat cell carcinoma of the lung; of 18 patients, nine had complete and seven had partial responses, with an overall response rate of 90%.

TOLERANCE AND SIDE EFFECTS OF HYPERTHERMIA

Treatment with local hyperthermia and irradiation has been described as well tolerated, with side effects similar to those observed with irradiation alone, except for some local pain noted in 20% to 25% of the patients and superficial burns or ulceration reported in 10% to 20%. The incidence of local burns is related to the temperature used, the coupling of the applicators on irregular surfaces of the body, and the use or not of skin cooling.

The development of rapid tumor necrosis sometimes obscures the determination of complications related to heating. In most cases, after complete débridement of the necrotic tissue, no clinical tumor was identified. The long delay in healing is most likely a result of poor blood supply to the tumor bed, which is the result of extensive prior treatment such as surgery or radiation therapy or both. These necrotic craters require many weeks of careful nursing care to heal; occasionally surgical intervention (skin grafting) is necessary.

The Radiation Therapy Oncology Group conducted a study in which 236 evaluable superficial tumors were randomized to receive radiation alone (400 cGy twice weekly for a total of 3200 cGy) or followed by hyperthermia (42.5°C for 60 minutes twice weekly). The side effects of this therapy were comparable in both arms, except for a 23% incidence of thermal burns in patients treated with radiation and hyperthermia (Table 16-21).

FUTURE CLINICAL RESEARCH IN LOCAL HYPERTHERMIA

When protocols for clinical hyperthermia are designed, it is pertinent to emphasize the features of an adequate clinical trial, including criteria for patient and tumor selection, technical and quality assurance parameters for heating and temperature monitoring, and definition of quantitative and realistic end points to assess the results of the trial.[9] The significance of any findings must be thoroughly evaluated with appropriate statistical tests.[436] Many of these published reports fail to adhere to these criteria, making the evaluation of results more difficult.

Another significant obstacle to the optimal application of hyperthermia to cancer therapy resides in the currently available coarse invasive thermometry techniques and the complexities in the application of thermal dose concepts in clinical practice.

A Consensus Conference on Clinical Hyperthermia (Trento, Italy 1989) organized by Ricardo Valdagni[436] summarized the state of the art on the biologic, physics, instrumentation, and clinical aspects of hyperthermia and concluded that the design and conduct of phase I/II clinical trials remained of highest importance for defining temperatures that safely enhance response to radiation or chemotherapy and that phase III trials could subsequently be defined for sites and therapeutic combinations in which the necessary thermal parameters could be safely and routinely achieved. This requires, as stressed by Overgaard,[290] the organization of multicenter studies, because single institutions will be unable to accumulate enough patients to complete a study in a reasonable period of time.

TABLE 16–21
*Most Severe Acute Complications of Irradiation (RT) and Irradiation Plus Hyperthermia (RT + HT) in Patients with Single Superficial Tumors**

	RATE IN ALL PATIENTS ANALYZED	
COMPLICATION	RT	RT + HT
No visible reaction	25%	23%
Erythema	34%	27%
Dry desquamation	16%	11%
Moist desquamation	8%	3%
Ulceration	7%	7%
Necrosis	7%	6%
Thermal blister	—	23%

**Acute complications are those reported within 6 months of start of therapy.*
(Perez CA, Emami B: Radiol Clin North Am 27:525–542, 1989)

REFERENCES

1. Abe M, Hiraoka M, Takahashi M, et al: Clinical experience with microwave and radiofrequency thermotherapy in the treatment of advanced cancer. Natl Cancer Inst Monogr 61:411–414, 1982
2. Adams GE, Stratford IJ, Rajaratnam S: Interaction of the cytotoxic and sensitizing effects of electron-affinic drugs and hyperthermia. Natl Cancer Inst Monogr 61:27–35, 1982
3. Alexander GA, Moylan DJ, Waterman FM, et al: Randomized trial of 1 vs 2 adjuvant hyperthermia treatments in patients with superficial metastases. Presented at the 7th Annual Meeting of the North American Hyperthermia Group, Atlanta, Georgia, February 21–26, 1987
4. Anderson RL, van Kersen I, Kraft P, et al: The use of heat resistant mutant to explore the involvement of heat shock proteins in thermal protection. In Sugahara T, Saito M (eds): Hyperthermic Oncology 1988, vol 2, pp 119–122. London, Taylor & Francis, 1989
5. Arcangeli G, Arcangeli G, Guerra A, et al: Tumor response to heat and radiation: Prognostic variables in the treatment of neck node metastases from head and neck cancer. Int J Hyperthermia 1:207–217, 1985
6. Arcangeli G, Benassi M, Cividalli A, et al: Radiotherapy and hyperthermia: Analysis of clinical results and identification of prognostic variables. Cancer 60:950–956, 1987
7. Arcangeli G, Cividalli A, Nervi C, et al: Tumor control and therapeutic gain with different schedules of combined radiotherapy and local external hyperthermia in human cancer. Int J Radiat Oncol Biol Phys 9:1125–1134, 1983
8. Arcangeli G, Nervi C, Cividalli A, et al: Problem of sequence and fractionation in the clinical application of combined heat and radiation. Cancer Res 44(Suppl):4857S–4863S, 1984
9. Arcangeli G, Overgaard J, Gonzalez Gonzalez D, et al: Hyperthermia trials. Int J Radiat Oncol Biol Phys 14:S93–S109, 1988
10. Au KS, Cetas TC, Shimm DS, et al: Interstitial ferromagnetic hyperthermia and brachytherapy: Preliminary report of a phase I clinical trial. Endocurie Hypertherm Oncol 5:127–136, 1989
11. Barber FE, Griffice CP: Power deposition for ultrasound hyperthermia. In Nussbaum GH (ed): Physical Aspects of Hyperthermia, pp 209–230. New York, American Association of Physicists in Medicine, 1982
12. Barlogie B, Corry PM, Yip E, et al: Total body hyperthermia

with and without chemotherapy for advanced human neoplasms. Cancer Res 39:1482–1489, 1979

13. Bey P, Marchal C, Forchard JJ, et al: Potentialisation de la radiotherapie locale. A propos de 90 tumeurs superficielles comparables (Abstract). Bull Cancer 71:263, 1984
14. Bicher HI, Hetzel FW, Sandhu TS, et al: Effects of hyperthermia on normal and tumor microenvironment. Radiology 137:523–530, 1980
15. Bicher HI, Moore DW, Wolfstein RW: A method for interstitial thermo-radiotherapy. In Overgaard J (ed): Hyperthermic Oncology 1984, vol 1. London, Taylor & Francis, 1984
16. Bicher HI, Sandhu TS, Hetzel FW: Hyperthermia and radiation in combination: A clinical fractionation regime. Int J Radiat Oncol Biol Phys 6:867–870, 1980
17. Bicher HI, Wolfstein RS, Lewsinsky BS: Microwave hyperthermia as an adjunct to radiation therapy: Summary experience of 256 multifraction treatment cases. Int J Radiat Oncol Biol Phys 12:1667–1671, 1986
18. Bide Z, Xiaoxiong W, Diven Z, et al: Hyperthermia in combination with radiotherapy for middle and late stage bladder carcinoma. In Overgaard J (ed): Hyperthermic Oncology 1984, vol 1, pp 783–784. London, Taylor & Francis, 1984
19. Bleehen NM, Honess DJ, Morgan JE: The combined effects of hyperthermia and hypoxic cell sensitizers. In Streffer C, van Bereningen D, Dietzel F, et al (eds): Cancer Therapy by Hyperthermia and Radiation, p 62. Baltimore, Urban & Schwarzenberg, 1978
20. Borok TL, Winter A, Laing J, et al: Microwave hyperthermia radiosensitized iridium-192 for recurrent brain malignacy (Abstract). Int J Radiant Oncol Biol Phys 12(Suppl 1):146, 1986
21. Borok TL, Winter A, Laing J, et al: Microwave hyperthermia radiosensitized iridium-192 for recurrent brain malignancy. Med Dosim 13:29–36, 1988
22. Borrelli MJ, Wong RSL, Dewey WC: A direct correlation between hyperthermia-induced membrane bleeding and survival in synchronous G1 CHO cells. J Cell Physiol 126:181–190, 1986
23. Bowden GT, Kasunic M, Sim D: Sequence dependence for the hyperthermic potentiation of cis-diamine-dichloroplatinum(II) induced cytotoxicity and DNA damage. Proceedings of the Radiation Research Society, 31st Annual Meeting, San Antonio, Texas, Feb 27–March 3, 1983
24. Bowman HF: Invasive method for monitoring tumor physiology. In Paliwal BR Hetzel FW, Dewhirst MD (eds): Biological, Physical and Clinical Aspects of Hyperthermia, pp 244–278. New York, American Association of Physicists in Medicine, 1988
25. Bowman HF: Thermodynamics of tissue heating: Modeling and measurements for temperature distributions. In Nussbaum GH (ed): Physical Aspects of Hyperthermia, pp 511–548. New York, American Association of Physicists in Medicine, 1982
26. Brezovich IA, Atkinson WJ, Chakraborty DP: Temperature distributions in tumor models heated by self-regulating nickel-copper alloy thermoseeds. Med Phys 11:145–152, 1984
27. Brezovich IA, Atkinson WJ, Lilly MB: Local hyperthermia with interstitial techniques. Cancer Res 44(Suppl):4752S–4756S, 1984
28. Brezovich IA, Meredith RF: Practical aspects of ferromagnetic thermoseed hyperthermia. Radiol Clin North Am 27:589–602, 1989
29. Bull JM, Lees D, Schyuette W, et al: Whole body hyperthermia: A phase I trial of potential adjuvant chemotherapy. Ann Intern Med 90:317, 1979
30. Bull JM, Mansfield B, Cronau L: Whole body hyperthermia and cisplatin in the treatment of malignant melanoma. Abstracts of papers from the 36th Annual Meeting of the Radiation Research Society, p 31, Philadelphia, Pennsylvania, April 16–21, 1988
31. Busch W: Uber den Einfluss Welchen heftigere Erysipelen zuweilen auf Organsierte Neubildungen Amiben. Verh Naturh: Preuss Rheinl 23:28–30, 1866
32. Byiou G: Clinical study on surgical treatment of hepatocarcinoma with implantable microwave radiation apparatus: 32 case reports. In Sugahara T, Saito M (eds): Hyperthermic Oncology 1988, vol 2. London, Taylor & Francis, 1989
33. Calderwood SK, Dickson JA: Effect of hyperglycemia on blood flow, pH and response to hyperthermia (42) of the Yoshid sarcoma in the rat. Cancer Res 40:4728–4733, 1980
34. Calderwood SK, Hahn GM: Thermal sensitivity and resistance of insulin receptor binding. Biochem Biophys Acta 756:1–8, 1983
35. Cetas TC: The philosophy and use of tissue-equivalent electromagnetic phantoms. In Nussbaum GH (ed): Physical Aspects of Hyperthermia, pp 441–461. New York, American Association of Physicists in Medicine, 1982
36. Cheung AY, Neyzari A: Deep local hyperthermia for cancer therapy: External electromagnetic and ultrasound techniques. Cancer Res 44(Suppl):4736S–4744S, 1984
37. Chou C-K: Electromagnetic energy deposition patterns in phantoms. In Paliwal BR, Hetzel FW, Dewhirst MW (eds): Biological, Physical and Clinical Aspects of Hyperthermia, Medical Physics Monograph No. 16, pp 132–151. New York, American Association of Physicists in Medicine, 1988
38. Chretien P, Landry J: Enhanced constitutine expression of the 27-kDa heat shock proteins in heat-resistant variants from Chinese hamster cells. J Cell Physiol 137:157–166, 1988
39. Christensen DA: A new non-perturbing temperature probe using semiconductor band edge shift. J Bioeng 1:541–545, 1977
40. Christensen T, Wahl A, Smedshammer L: Effects of hematoporphyrin derivative and light in combination with hyperthermia on cells in culture. Br J Cancer 50:85–89, 1984
41. Christensen EN, Kvamme E: Effects of thermal treatment on mitochondria of brain, liver and ascites cells. Acta Physiol Scand 76:472–484, 1969
42. Christoph R: Pain reduction in local anesthetic administration through pH buffering. Ann Emerg Med 17:117–120, 1988
43. Clark EP, Dewey WC, Lett JT: Recovery of CHO cells from hyperthermia potentiation to x-rays: Repair of DNA and chromatin. Radiat Res 85:302–313, 1981
44. Coley WB: The treatment of malignant tumors by repeated inoculations of erysipelas: With a report of 10 original cases. Am J Med Sci 105:487–511, 1893
45. Colvin DP, March BR, Gravely BT, et al: Endoscopic interstitial localized RF hyperthermia system for deep tumors. In Sugahara T, Saito M (eds): Hyperthermic Oncology 1988, vol 1, pp 881–883. London, Taylor & Francis, 1989
46. Connor WG, Gerner EW, Miller RC, et al: Prospects for hyperthermia in human cancer therapy. II. Implications of biological and physical data for applications of hyperthermia to man. Radiology 123:497–503, 1977
47. Corry PM, Barlogie B, Tilchen EJ, et al: Ultrasound-induced hyperthermia for the treatment of human superficial tumors. Int J Radiat Oncol Biol Phys 8:1225–1229, 1982
48. Corry PM, Jabboury K, Armour EP: Clinical ultrasound. In Paliwal BR, Hetzel FW, Dewhirst MW (eds): Biological, Physical and Clinical Aspects of Hyperthermia, Medical Physics Monograph No. 16, pp 315–329. New York, American Association of Physicists in Medicine, 1988
49. Corry PM, Jabboury K, Kong JS, et al: Evaluation of equipment for hyperthermia treatment of cancer. Int J Hyperthermia 4:53, 1988
50. Corry PM, Spanos WJ, Tilchen EJ, et al: Combined ultrasound and radiation therapy treatment of human superficial tumors. Radiology 145:165–169, 1982
51. Coss RA, Dewey, WC, Bamburg JR: Effects of hyperthermia on dividing Chinese hamster ovary cells and on microtubules *in vitro*. Cancer Res 42:1059–1071, 1982
52. Cosset JM, Dutreix J, Dufour J, et al: Combined interstitial hyperthermia and brachytherapy: Institut Gustave-Roussy technique and preliminary results. Int J Radiat Oncol Biol Phys 10:307–312, 1984
53. Cosset JM, Dutreix J, Haie C, et al: Interstitial thermoradiotheraphy: A technical and clinical study of 29 implantations performed at the Institut Gustave-Roussy. Int J Hyperthermia 1:3–13, 1985

54. Cosset JM, Gerard JP, Janoray P, et al: Advances in interstitial thermoradiotherapy (Abstract). Int J Hyperthermia (in press)
55. Coughlin CT, Wong TZ, Strohbehn JW, et al: Intraoperative interstitial microwave-induced hyperthermia and brachytherapy. Int J Radiat Oncol Biol Phys 11:1673–1678, 1985
56. Dahl O: Hyperthermia and drugs. In Wathmong DJ, Ross WM (eds): Hyperthermia, pp 121–153. Glasgow, Blackie, 1986
57. Dahl O, Mella O, Mehus A, et al: Clinical hyperthermia combined with drugs and radiation: A phase I/II study. Strahlenther Onkol 163:446–448, 1987
58. Datta NR, Bose AK, Kapoor HK: Thermoradiotherapy in the management of carcinoma cervix (IIIB): A controlled clinical study. Indian Med Gazette 121:68–71, 1987
59. DeBenedetti A, Baglioni C: Activation of hemin-regulated initiation factor-2 kinase in heat-shocked HeLa cells. J Biol Chem 261:338–342, 1986
60. Deshmukh R, Damento M, Demer L, et al: Ferromagnetic alloys with Curie temperatures near 50°C for use in hyperthermic therapy. In Overgaard J (ed): Hyperthermic Oncology 1984, vol 1. London, Taylor & Francis, 1984
61. Dewey WC: Editorial. Int J Hyperthermia 3:287–288, 1987
62. Dewey WC, Freeman ML, Raaphorst GP, et al: Cell biology of hyperthermia and radiation. In Meyn RE, Withers HR (eds): Radiation Biology in Cancer Research, pp 589–621. New York, Raven Press, 1980
63. Dewey WC, Highfield DP, Freeman ML, et al: Cell biology of hyperthermia and radiation. Proceedings 6th International Congress of Radiation Research, pp 832–840, Tokyo, Japan, 1979
64. Dewey WC, Hopwood LE, Sapareto SA, et al: Cellular responses to combinations of hyperthermia and radiation. Radiology 123:463–474, 1977
65. Dewey WC, Westra A, Miller HH, et al: Heat-induced lethality and chromosomal damage in synchronized Chinese hamster cells treated with 5-bromodeoxyuridine. Int J Radiat Oncol Biol Phys 20:505–520, 1971
66. Dewhirst MW: Physiological effects of hyperthermia. In Paliwal BR, Hetzel FW, Dewhirst MW (eds): Biological, Physical and Clinical Aspects of Hyperthermia, Medical Physics Monograph No. 16, pp 16–29. New York, American Association of Physicists in Medicine, 1988
67. Dewhirst MW: Thermal dose: conclusions from animal studies. In Sugahara T, Saito M (eds): Hyperthermic Oncology 1988, vol 2, pp 306–307. London, Taylor & Francis, 1989
68. Dewhirst MW, Gross JF, Sim D, et al: The effect of rate of heating or cooling prior to heating on tumor and normal tissue microcirculatory blood flow. Biorheology 21:539–558, 1984
69. Dewhirst MW, Lindley J, Vaguine V: Variables influencing the palliative treatment of malignant lesions with hyperthermia and radiation (Abstract). Thirty-Third Annual Meeting of the Radiation Research Society, p 27, Los Angeles, CA, May 5–9, 1985
70. Dewhirst MW, Phillips TL, Samulski TV, et al: RTOG quality assurance guidelines for clinical trials using hyperthermia. Int J Radiat Oncol Biol Phys 18:1249–1259, 1990
71. Dewhirst MW, Sim DA: The utility of thermal dose as a predictor of tumor and normal tissue responses to combined radiation and hyperthermia. Cancer Res 44:4772S–4780S, 1984
72. Dewhirst MW, Sim DA: Estimation of therapeutic gain in clinical trials involving hyperthermia and radiotherapy. Int J Hyperthermia 2:165–178, 1986
73. Dewhirst MW, Sim DA, Sapareto SA, Connor WG: Importance of minimum tumor temperature in determining early and long-term response of spontaneous canine and feline tumors to heat and radiation. Cancer Res 44:43–50, 1984
74. Dewhirst DW, Winget JM, Edelstein-Keshet L, et al: Clinical application of thermal isoeffect dose. Int J Hyperthermia 3:307–318, 1987
75. Dickson JA, Calderwood SK: Effects of hyperglycemia and hyperthermia on the pH, glycolysis and respiration of the Yoshida sarcoma *in vivo*. J Natl Cancer Inst 63:1371–1375, 1979
76. Dickson JA, Shah DM: The effects of hyperthermia (43C) on the biochemistry and growth of a malignant cell line. Eur J Cancer 8:561–571, 1972
77. Dike PG, Machler RC: Thermometry. In Licht S (ed): Therapeutic Heat and Cold, 2nd ed, pp 36–39. New Haven, Elizabeth Licht, 1965
78. Donaldson SS, Gordon LF, Hahn GM: Protective effect of hyperthermia against the cytotoxicity of actinomycin D in Chinese hamster cells. Cancer Treat Rep 62:1489–1495, 1978
79. Douglas MA, Parks LC, Bebin J: Sudden myelopathy secondary to therapeutic total-body hyperthermia after spinal cord irradiation. N Engl J Med 304:583–585, 1981
80. Douple EB, Jones EL, Kellogg KC, et al: Treatment sequence effects of combined cisplatin and hyperthermia in a murine tumor system. In Sugahara T, Saito M (eds): Hyperthermic Oncology 1988, vol 1, pp 221–222. London, Taylor & Francis, 1989
81. Dudar TE, Jain RK: Differential response of normal and tumor microcirculation to hyperthermia. Cancer Res 44:605–612, 1984
82. Duncan R, Hershey JWB: Heat shock-induced translational alterations in HeLa cells: Initiation factor modifications and the inhibition of translation. J Biol Chem 259:1182–1189, 1984
83. Dunlop PRC, Hand JW, Dickinson RJ, et al: An assessment of local hyperthermia in clinical practice. Int J Hyperthermia 2:39–50, 1986
84. Eddy HA: Microangiographic techniques in the study of normal and tumor tissue vascular systems. Microvasc Res 11:391–413, 1976
85. Eddy HA: Alterations in tumor microvasculature during hyperthermia. Radiology 137:515–521, 1980
86. Egawa S, Tsukiyama I, Watanabe S, et al: A randomized clinical trial of hyperthermia and radiation versus radiation alone for superfically located cancers. J Jpn Soc Ther Radiol Oncol 1:135–140, 1989
87. Emami B, Marks JE: Retreatment of recurrent carcinoma of the head and neck by afterloading interstitial ^{192}Ir implants. Laryngoscope 93:1345–1347, 1983
88. Emami B, Myerson RJ, Pilepich MV, et al: Regional hyperthermia in the treatment of recurrent deep-seated tumors: preliminary analysis of phase I trial. Strahlenther Onkol 165(10):709, 1989
89. Emami B, Myerson RJ, Pilepich MV, et al: Treatment of recurrent superficial tumors with hyperthermia and bleomycin. Presented at the 9th Annual Meeting of the North American Hyperthermia Group, Seattle, Washington, March 19–21, 1989
90. Emami B, Myerson RJ, Scott C, et al: Phase I/II study, combination of radiotherapy and hyperthermia in patients with deep-seated malignant tumors: Report of a pilot study by the Radiation Therapy Oncology Group. Int J Radiat Oncol Biol Phys 20:73–79, 1991
91. Emami B, Nussbaum GH, Ten Haken RK, et al: Physiological effects of hyperthermia: Response of capillary blood flow and structure to local tumor heating. Radiology 137:805–809, 1980
92. Emami B, Perez CA, Bignardi M, et al: Non-randomized, comparative study of radiation alone versus radiation + hyperthermia in recurrent head and neck cancer (in preparation)
93. Emami B, Perez CA, Konefal J, et al: Thermoradiotherapy of malignant melanoma. Int J Hyperthermia 4:373–381, 1988
94. Emami B, Perez CA, Leybovich L, et al: Interstitial thermoradiotherapy in treatment of malignant tumors. Int J Hyperthermia 3:107–118, 1987
95. Emami B, Perez CA, Myerson RJ, et al: Interstitial hyperthermia and brachytherapy in the treatment of head and neck cancer. In Sugahara T, Sito M (eds): Hyperthermic Oncology 1988, vol 2, pp 442–445. London, Taylor & Francis, 1989
96. Emami B, Song CW: Physiological mechanisms in hyperthermia: A review. Int J Radiat Oncol Biol Phys 10:289–295, 1984
97. Emami B, Stauffer B, Prionas S, et al: RTOG Quality assurance guidelines for interstitial hyperthermia. Int J Radiat Oncol Biol Phys 20(5):1117–1124, 1991

98. Endrich B, Zweifach BW, Reinhold HS, et al: Quantitative studies of microcirculatory function in malignant tissue: Influence of temperature on microvascular hemodynamics during the early growth of the BA-1112 rat sarcoma. Int J radiat Oncol Biol Phys 5:2021–2030, 1979
99. Englehardt R: Hyperthermia and drugs. Rec Res Cancer Res 104:133–203, 1987
100. Engler MJ, Dewhirst MW, Oleson JR: Stability of temperatures during thermotherapy. Int J Hyperthermia 5:59–67, 1989
101. Fajardo LF, Egbert B, Marmor J, et al: Effects of hyperthermia in a malignant tumor. Cancer 45:613–623, 1980
102. Falk P: The effect of elevated temperature on the vasculature of mouse jejunum. Br J Radiol 56:41–49, 1983
103. Falkner FG, Saumweber H, Biessman H: Two *Drosophila melanogaster* proteins related to intermediate filament proteins of vertebrate cells. J Cell Biol 91:175–183, 1981
104. Fessenden P, Kapp DS, Lee ER, et al: Clinical microwave applicator design. In Paliwal BR, Hetzel FW, Dewhirst MW (eds): Biological, Physical and Clinical Aspects of Hyperthermia, pp 123–131. New York, American Association of Physicists in Medicine, 1988
105. Field SB: Cancer Therapy by Hyperthermia, Drugs and Radiation (Abstract) The Third International Symposium, p 83. Fort Collins, Colorado, June 22–26, 1980
106. Field SB: Studies relevant to a means of quantifying the effects of hyperthermia. Int J Hyperthermia 3:291–296, 1987
107. Field SB, Bleehen NM: Hyperthermia in the treatment of cancer. Cancer Treat Rev 6:63–94, 1979
108. Field SB, Morris CC: The relationship between heating time and temperature: Its relevance to clinical hyperthermia. Radiother Oncol 1:179–186, 1983
109. Finger PT, Parker S, Paglione RW, et al: Thermal radiotherapy of choroidal melanoma. Ophthalmology 96:1384–1388, 1989
110. Franconi C, Tiberio CA, Raganell L, et al: Low-frequency RF twin-dipole applicator for intermediate depth hyperthermia. IEEE Trans Microwave Energy 34:612–619, 1986
111. Frazier OH, Corry PM: Induction of hyperthermia using implanted electrodes. Cancer Res 44(Suppl):4864S–4866S, 1983
112. Freeman ML, Holahan EV, Highfield DP, et al: The effect of pH on hyperthermia and x-ray induced cell killing. Int J Radiat Oncol Biol Phys 7:211–216, 1981
113. Fry WJ, Dunn F: Ultrasound: Analysis and experimental methods in biological research. In Physical Techniques in Biological Research, vol 4. New York, Academic Press, 1962
114. Furukawa M, Kato H, Uchia N, et al: Clinical results of RF inductive hyperthermia treatment with an inductive aperture-type applicator (Abstract presented to RSNA)
115. Fuwa N, Mortiz K, Kimura C, et al: Combined treatment of radiotherapy and local hyperthermia using 8 MHz RF-wave for advanced carcinoma of the breast. In Sugahara T, Saito M (eds): Hyperthermic Oncology 1988, vol 2, pp 414–417. London, Taylor & Francis, 1989
116. Gerner EW: Thermal dose and time-temperature factors for biological responses to heat shock. Int J Hyperthermia 3:319–327, 1987
117. Gerweck LE: Effects of microenvironmental factors on the response of cells to single and fractionated heat treatments. Natl Cancer Inst Monogr 61:19–26, 1982
118. Gerweck LE: Modifiers of thermal effects: Environmental factors. In Urano M, Douple E (eds): Hyperthermia and Oncology, pp 83–98. The Netherlands, VSP BV Publishers, 1988
119. Gerweck LE, Steele EL: Metabolic indices for hyperthermia in cancer therapy. In Paliwal BR, Hetzel FW, Dewhirst NW (eds): Biological, Physical and Clinical Aspects of Hyperthermia, Medical Physics Monograph No. 16, pp 2–15. New York, American Association of Physicists in Medicine, 1988
120. Gibbs FA Jr: "Thermal mapping" in experimental cancer treatment with hyperthermia: description and use of a semiautomatic system. Int J Radiat Oncol Biol Phys 9:1057–1063, 1983
121. Gibbs FA Jr: Non-invasive electromagnetic heating techniques and the operational characteristics of the annular phased array. Front Radiat Ther Oncol 18:56–61, 1984
122. Gibbs FA Jr: Regional hyperthermia: A clinical appraisal of noninvasive deep-heating methods. Cancer Res 44(Suppl): 4765S–4770S, 1984
123. Gibbs FA Jr: Regional hyperthermia in the treatment of cancer. In Paliwal BR, Hetzel FW, Dewhirst MW (eds): Biological, Physical and Clinical Aspects of Hyperthermia, Medical Physics Monograph No. 16, pp 330–344. New York, American Association of Physicists in Medicine, 1988
124. Giovanella BC, Morgan AC, Stehlin JS, at al: Selective lethal effect of supranormal temperatures on mouse sarcoma cells. Cancer Res 33:2588–2578, 1973
125. Giovanella BC, Stehlin JS, Morgan AC: Selective lethal effect of supranormal temperatures on human neoplastic cells. Cancer Res 36:3944–3950, 1976
126. Goldfeder A, Brown DM, Berger A: Enchancement of radioresponse of a mouse mammary carcinoma to combined treatment with hyperthermia and radiosensitizer misonidazole. Cancer Res 39:2966–2970, 1979
127. Goldfeder A, Newbort S: Thermally enhanced tumor regression in mice treated with melphalan. Anticancer Res 4:19–22, 1984
128. Goldobenko GV, Durnov LA, Knysh VI, et al: Experience in the use of thermoradiotherapy of malignant tumors (in Russian). Med Radiol 32:36–37, 1987
129. Goldson AL, Smyles JM, Ashayeri E, et al: Simultaneous intraoperative radiation therapy and intraoperative interstitial hyperthermia for unresectable adenocarcinoma of the pancreas. Endocuriether Hypertherm Oncol 3:201–208, 1987
130. Gonzalez Gonzalez D, van Dijk JDP, Blank LECM, et al: Combined treatment with radiation and hyperthermia in metastatic malignant melanoma. Radiother Oncol 6:105–113, 1986
131. Gonzalez Gonzalez D, van Dijk JDP. Blank LECM, et al: Chest wall recurrences of breast cancer: Results of combined treatment with radiation and hyperthermia. Radiother Oncol 12:95–103, 1988
132. Goss SA, Johnson RL, Dunn F: Comprehensive compilation of empirical ultrasonic properties of mammalian tissues. J Acoust Soc Am 64:423–457, 1978
133. Guffy MM, Rosenberger JA, Simon I, et al: Effect of cellular fatty acid alteration on hyperthermic sensitivity in cultured LK1210 murine leukemia cells. Cancer Res 42:3625–3630, 1982
134. Gullino PM: Extracellular compartments of solid tumors. Cancer 3:317–354, 1975
135. Hahn GM: Potential for therapy of drugs and hyperthermia. Cancer Res 39:2264–2268, 1979
136. Hahn GM: Hyperthermia and Cancer, pp 1–285. New York, Plenum Press, 1982
137. Hahn GM, Braun J, Har-Kedar I: Thermochemotherapy: Synergism between hyperthermia (42°–43°C) and Adriamycin (or bleomycin) in mammalian cell inactivation. Proc Natl Acad Sci USA 79:937–940, 1975
138. Hahn GM, Li GC, Shiu E: Interaction of amphotericin B and 43° hyperthermia. Cancer Res 37:761–764, 1977
139. Hahn GM, Strande DP: Cytotoxic effect of hyperthermia and Adriamycin on Chinese hamster cells. J Natl Cancer Inst 37:1063–1067, 1976
140. Hand JW: Invasive hyperthermia for deep seated tumors: Lower body. In Sugahara T, Saito M (eds): Hyperthermic Oncology 1988, vol 2, pp 398–401. London, Taylor & Francis, 1989
141. Hand JW, James JR (eds): Physical Techniques in Clinical Hyperthermia. New York, John Wiley & Sons, 1986
142. Hand JW, Lagendijk JJW, Bach Anderson J, et al: Quality assurance for ESHO protocols. Int J Hyperthermia 5:421, 1989
143. Harris M: Stable heat-resistant variants in populations of Chinese hamster cells. J Natl Cancer Inst 64:1495–1501, 1980
144. Harris M: Temperature-resistant variants in clonal populations of pig kidney cells. Exp Cell Res 46:301–314, 1967
145. Harrison GH: Ultrasound hyperthermia applicators: Inten-

sity distributions and quality assurance. Int J Hyperthermia 6:169–174, 1990

146. Heine U, Severak L, Kondratick J, Bonar RA: The behavior of HeLa-S_3 cells under the influence of supranormal temperatures. J Ultrastruct Res 75:396, 1971
147. Henderson BW, Waldow SM, Potter WR, et al: Interaction of photodynamic therapy and hyperthermia: Tumor response and cell survival studies after treatment of mice *in vivo*. Cancer Res 45:6071–6077, 1980
148. Henle KJ: Sensitization to hyperthermia below 43C induced in Chinese hamster ovary cells by step-down heating. J Natl Cancer Inst 64:1479–1483, 1980
149. Henle KJ, Dethlefsen LA: Heat fractionation and thermotolerance: A review. Cancer Res 38:1843–1851, 1978
150. Henle KJ, Dethlefsen LA: Time-temperature relationships for heat-induced killing of mammalian cells. Ann NY Acad Sci 335:234–253, 1980
151. Henle KJ, Leeper DB: Interaction of hyperthermia and radiation in CHO cells: Recovery kinetics. Radiat Res 66:505–518, 1976
152. Henle KJ, Leeper DB: Effects of hyperthermia (45°) on macromolecular synthesis in Chinese hamster ovary cells. Cancer Res 39:2665–2674, 1979
153. Henle KJ, Roti Roti JL: Time-temperature conversions in biological applications of hyperthermia. Radiat Res 82:138–145, 1980
154. Henriques FC: Studies of thermal injury. V. The predictability and the significance of thermally induced rate processes leading to irreversible epidermal injury. Arch Pathol 43:489–502, 1947
155. Herman TS: Effect of temperature of exposure on the cytotoxicity of three new anticancer drugs. Cancer Treat Rep 67:1019–1022, 1983
156. Herman TS, Jochelson MS, Teicher BA, et al: A phase I–II trial of cisplatin, hyperthermia and radiation in patients with locally advanced malignancies. Int J Radiat Oncol Biol Phys 17:1273–1279, 1989
157. Herman TS, Sweets CC, White DM, et al: Effect of heating on lethality due to hyperthermia and selected chemotherapeutic drugs. J Natl Cancer Inst 68:487–491, 1982
158. Herman TS, Teicher BA: Sequencing of trimodality therapy (cis-Diamminedichloroplatinum (II)/hyperthermia/radiation) as determined by tumor growth delay and tumor cell survival in the FSaIIC fibrosarcoma. Cancer Res 48:2693–2697, 1988
159. Herman TS, Teicher BA, Jochelson M, et al: Rationale for use of local hyperthermia with radiation therapy and selected anticancer drugs in locally advanced human malignancies. Int J Hyperthermia 4:143–158, 1988
160. Hetzel FW, Mattiello J: Interactions of hyperthermia with other modalities. In Paliwal BR, Hetzel FW, Dewhirst MW (eds): Biological, Physical and Clinical Aspects of Hyperthermia, Medical Physics Monograph No. 16, pp 30–56. New York, American Association of Physicists in Medicine, 1988
161. Hidvegi EG, Yatvin MB, Dennis WH, Hidvegi A: Effect of altered membrane lipid composition and procaine on hyperthermic killing of ascites tumor cells. Oncology (Basel) 37:360–363, 1980
162. Hill SA, Denekamp J: The Third International Symposium, Cancer Therapy by Hyperthermia, Drugs and Radiation (Abstract), p 91. Fort Collins, Colorado, June 22–26, 1980
163. Hiraoka M, Jo S, Dodo Y, et al: Clinical results of radiofrequency hyperthermia combined with radiation in the treatment of radioresistant cancers. Cancer 54:2898–2904, 1984
164. Hiraoka M, Jo S, Takahashi M, et al: Clinical application of RF capacitive heating for deep-seated tumors. In Matsuda T, Kikuchi M (eds): Hyperthermic Oncology. Proceedings of the Sixth Annual Meeting of Hyperthermia Group of Japan, pp 190–191. Tokyo, Japanese Society of Hyperthermic Oncology, 1984
165. Hofman P: Clinical hyperthermia: Medical aspects. Thesis, Utrecht, 1987
166. Hofman P, Lagendijk JJW, Schipper J: The combination of radiotherapy with hyperthermia in protocolized clinical studies. In Overgaard J (ed): Hyperthermic Oncology, vol 1, pp 379–382. London, Francis & Taylor, 1984
167. Hornback NB, Shupe RE, Shidnia H, et al: Preliminary clinical results of combined 433 megahertz microwave therapy and radiation therapy on patients with advanced cancer. Cancer 40:2854–2863, 1977
168. Hornback NB, Shupe RE, Shidnia H, et al: Advanced stage IIIB cancer of the cervix treatment by hyperthermia and radiation. Gynecol Oncol 23:160–167, 1986
169. Howard GCW, Sathiaseelan V, Freedman L, et al: Hyperthermia and radiation in the treatment of superficial malignancy: An analysis of treatment parameters, response and toxicity. Int J Hyperthermia 3:1–8, 1987
170. Howard GCM, Sathiaseelan V, King GA, et al: Regional hyperthermia for extensive pelvic tumours using an annular phased array applicator: A feasibility study. Br J Radiol 59:1195–1201, 1986
171. Howe JG, Hershey JWB: Translational initiation factor and ribosome association with the cytoskeletal framework fraction from HeLa cells. Cell 37:85–93, 1984
172. Hume PS, Field SB: Acid phosphatase activity following hyperthermia of mouse spleen and its implication in heat potentiation of x-ray damage. Radiat Res 72:145–153, 1977
173. Hynynen K: Induction of local hyperthermia using ultrasound. In Paliwal BR, Hetzel FW, Dewhirst MW (eds): Biological, Physical and Clinical Aspects of Hyperthermia, pp 152–166. New York, American Association of Physicists in Medicine, 1988
174. Hynynen K, Roemer R, Anhalt D, et al: A scanned, focused, multiple transducer ultrasonic system for localized hyperthermia treatments. Int J Hyperthermia 3:21–35, 1987
175. Ishiwata J, Kamisawa T, Egawa N, et al: RF Capacitive heating in combination with chemotherapy for abdominal tumors. In Sugahara T, Saito M (eds): Hyperthermic Oncology 1988, vol 2, pp 559–562 105. London, Taylor & Francis, 1989
176. Jahde E, Rajewsky MF, Baumgartl H: pH distributions in transplanted neural tumors and normal tissues of BDIX-rats as measured with pH microelectrodes. Cancer Res 42:1505–1512, 1982
177. Johnson RJR, Sandhu TS, Hetzel FW, et al: A pilot study to investigate skin and tumor thermal enhancement ratios of 41.5–42.0°C hyperthermia with radiation. Int J Radiat Oncol Biol Phys 5:947–953, 1979
178. Jones Paris KG, Emami B, et al: Preliminary clinical results with ultrasound (in preparation)
179. Kai H, Matsufuji H, Okudaira Y, et al: Heat, drugs and radiation given in combination is palliative for unresectable esophageal cancer. Int J Radiat Oncol Biol Phys 14:1147–1152, 1988
180. Kal HB, Hatfield M, Hahn GM: Cell cycle progression of murine sarcoma cells after irradiation or heat shock. Radiology 117:215–217, 1975
181. Kampinga HH, Turkel-Uygur N, Roti Roti JL, et al: The relationship of increased nuclear protein content induced by hyperthermia to killing of HeLa S3 cells. Radiat Res 117:511–522, 1989
182. Kampinga, HH, Wright WD, Konings AW, et al: The interaction of heat and radiation affecting the ability of nuclear DNA to undergo supercoiling change. Radiat Res 116:114–123, 1988
183. Kapp DS: Areas of need for continued phase II testing in human patients. In Paliwal BR, Hetzel FW, Dewhirst DW (eds): Biological, Physical and Clinical Aspects of Hyperthermia, pp 424–443. New York, American Association of Physicists in Medicine, 1988
184. Kapp DS: Indications for the clinical use of deep local and regional hyperthermia in conjunction with radiation therapy. Strahlenther Onkol 165:724, 1989
185. Kapp DS, Bagshaw MA, Meyer JL, et al: Optimization of hyperthermia and low dose irradiation in the treatment of superficial tumors: a prospective randomized trial of 2 vs 6 heat treatments. Presented at the Thirty-third Annual Meeting of the Radiation Research Society, Los Angeles, California, May 5–9, 1985
186. Kapp DS, Samulski TV, Fessenden P, et al: Prognostic signifi-

cance of tumor volume on response following local-regional hyperthermia (HT) and radiation therapy (XRT) (Abstract). Presented at the Thirty-Fifth Annual Meeting of the Radiation Research Society, p 17, Atlanta, Georgia, February 21–26, 1987

187. Kapp DS, Samulski TV, Meyer JL, et al: Metastatic breast cancer with chest wall recurrences in previously irradiated areas: Management with low-moderate dose irradiation therapy and hyperthermia (Abstract). Presented at the Thirty-Third Annual Meeting of the Radiation Research Society, p 29, Los Angeles, California, May 5–9, 1985
188. Kato H, Ishida I: Studies of a deep heating apparatus. In Kano E (ed) Curr Res Hyperthermia pp. 3–18, Tokyo, Academic Press. 1988
189. Kato H, Ishida T: A new inductive applicator for hyperthermia. J Microwave Power 18:331, 1983
190. Kato H, Ishida T: Dose concepts derived from theoretical physics. In Sugahara T, Saito M (eds): Hyperthermic Oncology 1988, vol 2, pp 302–303. London, Taylor & Francis, 1989
191. Kim JH: Modification of thermal effects: Chemical modifiers. In Urano M, Douple E (eds): Hyperthermia and Oncology, pp 99–120. The Netherlands, VSP BV Publisher, 1988
192. Kim JH, Hahn EW: Clinical and biological studies of localized hyperthermia. Cancer Res 39:2258–2261, 1979
193. Kim JD, Hahn EW, Ahmed SA: Combination hyperthermia and radiation therapy for malignant melanoma. Cancer 50:478–482, 1982
194. Kim JH, Hahn EW, Ahmed SA, et al: Clinical study of the sequence of combined hyperthermia and radiation therapy of malignant melanoma. In Overgaard J (ed): Hyperthermic Oncology, vol 1, pp 387–390. London, Taylor & Francis, 1984
195. Kim JH, Hahn EW, Antich PP: Radiofrequency hyperthermia for clinical cancer therapy. Natl Cancer Inst Monogr 61:339–342, 1982
196. Kim JH, Hahn EW, Tokita N: A combination hyperthermia and radiation therapy for cutaneous malignant melanoma. Cancer 41:2143–2148, 1978
197. Kim JH, Hahn EW, Tokita N, et al: Local tumor hyperthermia in combination with radiation therapy. I. Malignant cutaneous lesions. Cancer 40:161–169, 1977
198. Kim JH, Kim SH, Hahn SW: 5-Thio-d-glucose selectively potentiates hyperthermic killing of hypoxic tumor cells. Science 200:206–207, 1978
199. Kim SH, Kim JH, Hahn EW: The enhanced killing of irradiated HeLa cells in synchronous culture by hyperthermia. Radiat Res 66:337–345, 1967
200. Kjellen E, Lindholm C-E, Nilsson P: Radiotherapy in combination with hyperthermia in recurrent or metastatic mammary carcinomas. In Sughara T, Saito M (eds): Hyperthermic Oncology 1988, vol 2, pp 426–429. London, Taylor & Francis, 1989
201. Konings AWT: Development of thermotolerance in mouse fibroblast LM cells with modified membranes and after procaine treatment. Cancer Res 45:2016–2019, 1985
202. Konings AWT, Ruifrok ACC: Role of membrane lipids and membrane fluidity in thermosensitivity and thermotolerance of mammalian cells. Radiat Res 102:86–98, 1985
203. Krogh A: The Anatomy Physiology of Capillaries. New Haven, Conn, Yale University Press, 1922
204. Kubota Y: Hyperthermic therapy of the bladder cancer. III. Clinical studies. Nippon Hinyokika Gakkai Zasshi 72:742–751, 1981
205. Kwock L, Lin P-S, Hefter K, et al: Impairment of Na+-dependent amino acid transport in a cultured human T-cell line by hyperthermia and irradiation. Cancer Res 38:83–87, 1978
206. Lagendijk JJW, Nilsson P: Hyperthermia dough: A fat and bone equivalent phantom to test microwave/radiofrequency hyperthermia heating systems. Phys Med Biol 30:709–712, 1985
207. Lam K, Astraham M, Langholz B, et al: Interstitial thermoradiotherapy for recurrent or persistent tumors. Int J Hyperthermia 4:259–266, 1988
208. Landry J, Bernier D, Chretien P, et al: Synthesis and degradation of heat shock proteins during development and decay of thermotolerance. Cancer Res 42:2457–2461, 1982
209. Laszlo A: Evidence for two states of thermotolerance in mammalian cells. Int J Hyperthermia 4:513–526, 1987
210. Lauche HM, Jung GM, Kotewicz A, et al: Critical review of phase II-therapeutic trials of radiofrequency hyperthermia (13 MHz) alone or combined with radiotherapy with special reference to head-and-neck tumors (Abstract). Seventh Meeting of the European Society for Hyperthermic Oncology, September 16–18, 1985. Strahlentherapie 161:541, 1985
211. Law MP, Ahier RG, Field SB: The response of the mouse ear to heat applied alone or combined with x-rays. Br J Radiol 51:132–138, 1978
212. Leeper DB, Karamuz JE, Henle KJ: Effect of inhibition of macromolecular synthesis on the induction of thermotolerance. Proc Am Assoc Cancer Res 18:139, 1977
213. Lele PP: Induction of deep, local hyperthermia by ultrasound and electromagnetic field. Radiat Environ Biophys 17:215–216, 1980
214. Lele PP: Local hyperthermia by ultrasound. In Nussbaum GH (ed): Physical Aspects of Hyperthermia, AAPM Monograph No 8, pp 393–440. New York, American Institute of Physics, 1982
215. Lele PP: Physical aspects and clinical studies with ultrasound hyperthermia. In Storm FC (ed): Hyperthermia in Cancer Therapy, pp 333–367. Boston, Hall Medical Publishers, 1983
216. Lele PP: Physical aspects and clinical studies with ultrasound hyperthermia. In Overgaard J (ed): Hyperthermic Oncology 1984, vol 2, pp 129–154. London, Taylor & Francis, 1984
217. Lepoc JR, Massicotte-Nolan P, Rule GS, et al: Lack of correlation between hyperthermic cell-killing thermotolerance, and membrane lipid fluidity. Radiat Res 87:300–313, 1981
218. LeVeen HH, Obrien P, Wallace KM: Radiofrequency thermotherapy for cancer. JSC Med Assoc 76:5–9, 1980
219. LeVeen HH, Wapnick W, Piccone V, et al: Tumor eradication by radio-frequency therapy. JAMA 235:2198–2200, 1976
220. Leybovich LL, Emami BE, Myerson RJ, et al: Dual antenna applicator for hyperthermia of tumors of intermediate depth. Int J Hyperthermia (in press)
221. Leybovich LB, Myerson RJ, Emami BN, et al: Evaluation of the BSD 200 Sigma 60 applicator in terms of scattering parameters (submitted for publication)
222. Leybovich L, Nussbaum GH: Multiple antenna applicators for microwave-induced local hyperthermia (submitted for publication)
223. Leybovich L, Nussbaum GH, Straube W, et al: Multi-element, conformable applicators for local microwave hyperthermia (submitted for publication)
224. Li DJ, Chou CK, Luk KH, et al: Design of intracavitary microwave applicators for the treatment of uterine cervix carcinoma and its preliminary clinical applications. In Sugahara T, Saito M (eds): Hyperthermic Oncology 1988, vol 1, pp 604–605. London, Taylor & Francis, 1989
225. Li GC, Cameron RB, Sapareto SA, et al: Reinterpretation of Arrhenius analysis of cell inactivation of heat. Natl Cancer Inst Monogr 61:111–113, 1982
226. Li GC, Hahn GM: Ethanol-induced tolerance to heat and Adriamycin. Nature 274:699–701, 1978
227. Li GC, Hahn GM: Adaptation of different growth temperatures modifies some mammalian cell survival responses. Exp Cell Res 128:475–485, 1980
228. Li GC, Kal HB: Effect of hyperthermia on the radiation response of two mammalian cell lines. Eur J Cancer 13:65–69, 1977
229. Li GC, Laszlo A: Thermotolerance in mammalian cells: A role for heat shock proteins? In Atkinson BG, Walden DB (eds): Changes in Gene Expression in Response to Environmental Stress. New York, Academic Press, 1985
230. Li GC, Petersen NS, Mitchell HK: Induced thermal tolerance and heat shock synthesis in Chinese hamster ovary cells. Br J Cancer 45:132–136, 1982
231. Li GC, Shrieve DC, Werb Z: Correlations between synthesis of heat shock proteins and development of tolerance to heat and to Adriamycin in Chinese hamster fibroblasts: Heat shock

and other inducers. In Schlesinger M (ed): Heat Shock: From Bacteria to Man. Cold Springs Harbor, New York, Cold Spring Harbor Laboratory, 1982

232. Li RY, Shazng TZ, Lin SY, et al: Effect of hyperthermia combined with radiation in the treatment of superficial malignant lesions in 90 patients. In Overgaard J (ed): Hyperthermic Oncology 1984, vol 1, pp 395–397. London, Taylor & Francis, 1984
233. Li RY, Wang H-P, Lin S-Y, et al: Clinical evaluation of combined radiotherapy and thermotherapy on carcinoma of the breast (in Chinese). Clin Oncol 12:73–76, 1985
234. Lin P-S, Kwock L, Hefter K, et al: Modification of rat thymocyte membrane properties by hyperthermia and ionizing radiation. Int J Radiat Biol 33:371–382, 1978
235. Linares LA, Nori D, Brenner H, et al: Interstitial hyperthermia and brachytherapy: A preliminary report. Endocuriether Hypertherm Oncol 2:S39–S44, 1986
236. Lindholm CE, Kjellen E, Nilsson P, et al: Microwave-induced hyperthermia and radiotherapy in human superficial tumours: Clinical results with a comparative study of combined treatment *versus* radiotherapy alone. Int J Hyperthermia 3:393–411, 1987
237. Luk KH, Francis ME, Perez CA, et al: Combined radiation and hyperthermia: Comparison of two treatment schedules based on data from a registry established by the Radiation Therapy Oncology Group (RTOG). Int J Radiat Oncol Biol Phys 10(6):801–809, 1984
238. Luk K. Pajak T, Perez C, et al: Prognostic factors in tumor response after hyperthermia and radiation. In Overgaard J (ed): Hyperthermic Oncology 1984, vol 1, pp 353–356. London, Taylor & Francis, 1984
239. Luk KH, Purser PR, Castro JR, et al: Clinical experiences with local microwave hyperthermia. Int J Radiat Oncol Biol Phys 7:615–619, 1981
240. Lyons BE, Britt RH, Strohbehn JW: Localized hyperthermia in the treatment of malignant brain tumors using an interstitial microwave antennae array. IEEE Transactions BME 31:62, 1984
241. Mackey MA, Dewey WC: Cell cycle progression during chronic hyperthermia in S phase CHO cells. Int J Hyperthermia 5:405–415, 1989
242. Mackey M, Roti Roti JL: A thermal dynamic model of heat-induced cell-killing. J Theor Biol (in press)
243. Mang TS: Time and sequence dependent influence of *in vitro* photodynamic therapy: Survival by hyperthermia. Photochem Photobiol 42:533–540, 1985
244. Manning MR, Cetas TC, Miller RC, et al: Clinical hyperthermia: Results of a phase I trial employing hyperthermia alone or in combination with external beam or interstitial radiotherapy. Cancer 49:205–216, 1982
245. Marchosky JA, Moran C, Fearnot N: Volumetric interstitial hyperthermia: Phase I clinical study (Abstract). Presented at the 8th Annual Meeting of the North American Hyperthermia Group, Philadelphia, Pennsylvania, 1988
246. Marmor JB: Clinical use of localized hyperthermia. In Williams CJ, Whitehouse JMA (eds): Recent Advances in Clinical Oncology, pp 35–44. Edinburgh, Churchill-Livingstone, 1982
247. Marmor J: Reactions of hyperthermia and chemotherapy in animals. Cancer Res 39:2269–2276, 1979
248. Marmor JB, Pounds D, Hahn GM: Clinical studies with ultrasound induced hyperthermia. Natl Cancer Inst Monogr 61:333–337, 1982
249. Matloubieh AY, Roemer RB, Cetas TC: Numerical simulation of magnetic induction heating of tumors with ferromagnetic seed implants. IEEE Trans Biomed Eng BME 31:227, 1984
250. Mattiello J, Vandenheede L, Hennig T, et al: Tumor growth delay and TCD_{50} curves for combined photodynamic therapy and hyperthermia. Presented at the 35th Annual Meeting of the Radiation Research Society, Atlanta, Georgia, February 21–26, 1987
251. Matsufuji H, Kuwano H, Kai H, et al: Preoperative hyperthermia combined with radiotherapy and chemotherapy for patients with incompletely resected carcinoma of the esophagus. Cancer 62:889–894, 1988
252. McCormick W, Penman S: Regulation of protein synthesis in HeLa cells: Translation at elevated temperatures. J Mol Biol 39:315–333, 1969
253. Mechling JA, Strohbehn JW: A theoretical comparison of the temperature distributions produced by three interstitial hyperthermia systems. Int J Radiat Oncol Biol Phys 12:2137–2149, 1986
254. Melloni E: Hyperthermal effects in phototherapy with mematoporphyrin derivative sensitization. Tumori 70:321–325, 1984
255. Meyer JL: The clinical efficacy of localized hyperthermia. Cancer Res 44 7(Suppl):4745S–4751S, 1984
256. Meyer JL, Kapp DS, Fessenden P, et al: Hyperthermic oncology: Current biology, physics and clinical results. Pharmacol Ther 42:251–288, 1989
257. Milligan AJ, Conran PB, Ropar MA, et al: Predictions of blood flow from thermal clearance during regional hyperthermia. Int J Radiat Oncol Biol Phys 9:1335–1343, 1983
258. Mills MD, Meyn RE: Effects of hyperthermia on repair of radiation-induced DNA strand breaks. Radiat Res 87:314–328, 1981
259. Mitchell HK, Moller G, Petersen NS, et al: Specific protection from phenoscopy induction by heat shock. Dev Genet 1:181–192, 1979
260. Mittal B, Emami B, Sapareto S, et al: Effects of sequencing of the total course of combined hyperthermia and radiation on the RIF-1 murine tumor. Cancer 54:2889–2897, 1984
261. Molls M, Feldmann, HJ, Adler S, et al: Regional hyperthermia: A feasibility study. Strahlenther Onkol 165(10):717:1989
262. Mondovi B, Strom R, Rotillio G, et al: The biochemical mechanism of selective heat sensitivity of cancer cells. I. Studies on cellular respiration. Eur J Cancer 5:129–136, 1969
263. Mulcahy RT, Gould MN, Hidvegi E, et al: Hyperthermia and surface morphology of P388 ascites tumour M.B. cells: Effects of membrane modifications. Int J Radiat Biol 39:95–106, 1981
264. Muratkhodzhaev NK, Svetitsky PV, Kochegarov AA, et al: Hyperthermia in therapy of cancer patients (in Russian). Med Radiol 32:30–36, 1987
265. Myerson RJ, Emami BN, Pilepich MV, et al: Physical predictors of adequate hyperthermia with the Annular Phased Array. Int J Hyperthermia 5:749, 1989
266. Myerson RJ, Leybovich L, Emami BN, et al: Phantom studies and preliminary clinical experience with the BSD 2000 Int J Hyperthermia, in press
267. Myerson RJ, Perez CA, Emami BN, et al: Tumor control in long-term survivors following superficial hyperthermia. Int J Radiat Oncol Biol Phys 18:1123–1129, 1990
268. Neumann H, Fabricius H-A, Engelhardt R: Moderate whole-body hyperthermia in combination with chemotherapy in the treatment of small cell carcinoma of the lung: A pilot study. Natl Cancer Inst Monogr 61:427–429, 1982
269. Nishimura Y, Hiraoka lM, Jo S, et al: Radiofrequency (RF) capacitive hyperthermia combined with radiotherapy in the treatment of abdominal and pelvic deep-seated tumors. Radiother Oncol 16:139–149, 1989
270. Nishiue T, Kojima O, Majima T, et al: Studies on combination of hyperthermia and chemotherapy for cancer. In Sugahara T, Saito M (eds): Hyperthermic Oncology 1988, vol 1, pp 204–206. London, Taylor & Francis, 1989
271. Nussbaum GH: Quality assessment and assurance in clinical hyperthermia: Requirements and procedures. Cancer Res 44(Suppl):4811S–4817S, 1984
272. Nussbaum GH, Goodman RE, Bruce AA: Improved applicator-patient coupling in microwave-induced hyperthermia. Med Phys 10:897–898 1983
273. Nussbaum GH, Sidi J, Rouhanizadeh N, et al: Manipulation of central axis heating patterns with a prototype, three-electrode capacitive device for deep-tumor hyperthermia. IEEE Trans Microwave Theory Tech MTT 34(5):620, 1986
274. Nussbaum GH, Straube WL, Drag MD, et al: Potential for

localized, adjustable deep heating in soft tissue environments with a thirty-beam ultrasonic hyperthermic system. Int J Hyperthermia 7(2):279–299, 1991

275. Ochoa S: Regulation of protein synthesis initiation in eucaryotes. Arch Biochem Biophys 223:325–349, 1983
276. Ohtsuka K, Laszlo A: Expression of heat shock proteins after hyperthermia. Cell Technol 7:71–81, 1988
277. Oleson JR: Editorial: If we can't define the quality, can we assure it? Int J Radiat Oncol Biol Phys 16:879, 1989
278. Oleson JR: Combined preoperative radiation and hyperthermia treatment for soft tissue sarcoma. Presented at the Consensus Meeting on Clinical Hyperthermia in Cancer Treatment, Trento, Italy, May 1989
279. Oleson JR, Calderwood SR, Coughlin CT, et al: Biological and clinical aspects of hyperthermia in cancer therapy. Am J Clin Oncol 11:368–380, 1988
280. Oleson JR, Dewhirst MW, Harrelson JM, et al: Tumor temperature distributions predict hyperthermia effect. Int J Radiat Oncol Biol Phys 16:559–570, 1989
281. Oleson JR, Manning MR, Sim DA, et al: A review of the University of Arizona human clinical experience. Front Radiat Ther Oncol 18:136–143, 1984
282. Oleson JR, Sim DA, Manning MR: Analysis of prognostic variables in hyperthermia of 163 patients. Int J Radiat Oncol Biol Phys 10:2231–2239, 1984
283. Overgaard J: Effect of hyperthermia on malignant cells *in vivo.* Cancer 39:2637–2646, 1977
284. Overgaard J: The effect of local hyperthermia alone, and in combination with radiation, on solid tumors. In Streffer C (ed): Cancer Therapy by Hyperthermia and Radiation, pp 49–61. Munich, Urban & Schwarzenberg, 1978
285. Overgaard J: Fractionated hyperthermia and radiation *in vivo.* Natl Cancer Inst Monogr 61:287–289, 1982
286. Overgaard J: Simultaneous and sequential hyperthermia and radiation treatment of an experimental tumor and its surrounding normal tissue *in vivo.* Int J Radiat Oncol Biol Phys 6:1507–1517, 1980
287. Overgaard J: Fractionated radiation and hyperthermia: Experimental and clinical studies. Cancer 48:1116–1123, 1981
288. Overgaard J (ed): Hyperthermic Oncology 1984, vol 1. London, Taylor & Francis, 1984
289. Overgaard J (ed): Hyperthermic Oncology 1984, vol 2. London, Taylor & Francis, 1985
290. Overgaard J: Rationale and problems in the design of clinical studies. In Overgaard J (ed): Hyperthermic Oncology 1984, vol 2, pp 325–338. London, Taylor & Francis, 1985
291. Overgaard J. The role of radiotherapy in recurrent and metastatic malignant melanoma: A clinical radiobiological study. Int J Radiat Oncol Biol Phys 12:867–872, 1986
292. Overgaard J: Some problems related to the clinical use of thermal isoeffect doses. Int J Hyperthermia 3:329–336, 1987
293. Overgaard J: The current and potential role of hyperthermia in radiotherapy. Int J Radiat Oncol Biol Phys 16:535–549, 1989
294. Overgaard J: Combined hyperthermia and radiation treatment of malignant melanoma. In Sugahara T, Saito M (eds): Hyperthermic Oncology 1988, vol 2, pp 464–467. London, Taylor & Francis, 1989,
295. Overgaard J, Overgaard M: A clinical trial evaluating the effect of simultaneous or sequential radiation and hyperthermia in the treatment of malignant melanoma. In Overgaard J (ed): Hyperthermic Oncology, vol 1, pp 383–386. London, Francis & Taylor, 1984
296. Overgaard J, Overgaard M: Hyperthermia as an adjuvant to radiotherapy in the treatment of malignant melanoma. Int J Hyperthermia 3:483–501, 1987
297. Overgaard J, Overgaard M, Hansen PV, et al: Some factors of importance in the radiation treatment of malignant melanoma. Radiother Oncol 5:183–192, 1986
298. Overgaard J, von der Maase H, Overgaard M: A randomized study comparing two high-dose per fraction radiation schedules in recurrent or metastatic malignant melanoma. Int J Radiat Oncol Biol Phys 11:1137–1839, 1985
299. Overgaard K, Overgaard J: Investigations on the possibility of a thermic tumor therapy. I. Short wave treatment of a transplanted isologous mouse mammary carcinoma. Eur J Cancer 8:65–78, 1972
300. Paliwal BR, Buechler DN: Basics of physical parameters in hyperthermia. In Paliwal BR, Hetzel FW, Dewhirst MW (eds): Biological, Physical and Clinical Aspects of Hyperthermia, pp 72–81. New York, American Association of Physicists in Medicine, 1988
301. Paliwal BR, Gibbs FA Jr, Wiley AL Jr: Heating patterns induced by a 13.56 MHz radiofrequency generator in large phantoms and pig abdomen and thorax. Int J Radiat Oncol Biol Phys 8:857–864, 1982
302. Panniers R, Henshaw EC: Mechanism of inhibition of polypeptide chain initiation in heat-shocked Ehrlich ascites tumour cells. Eur J Biochem 140:209–214, 1984
303. Partington BP, Steeves RA, Su SL, et al: Temperature distributions, microangiographic and histopathologic correlations in normal tissue heated by ferromagnetic needles. Int J Hyperthermia 5:319–327, 1989
304. Paulsen KD, Strohbehn JW, Lynch DR: Comparative theoretical performance for two types of regional hyperthermia systems. Int J Radiat Oncol Biol Phys 11:1659–1671, 1985
305. Peck JW, Gibbs FA: Capillary blood flow in murine tumors, feet and intestines during localized hyperthermia. Radiat Res 96:65–81, 1983
306. Perez CA, Emami B: A review of current clinical experience with irradiation and hyperthermia. Endocuriether Hypertherm Oncol 1:265–277, 1985
307. Perez CA, Emami B: Clinical trials with local (external and interstitial) irradiation and hyperthermia: Current and future perspectives. Radiol Clin North Am 27:525–542, 1989
308. Perez CA, Emami B, Hornback NB, et al: A non-randomized phase I–II study of the efficacy of radiation and hyperthermia (45°C for 15 minutes) in the treatment of some measurable superficial human tumors (in preparation)
309. Perez CA, Emami B, Kuske RR, et al: Irradiation and hyperthermia in the treatment of recurrent carcinoma of the breast in the chest wall: MIR and RTOG experience. In Sugahara T, Saito M (eds): Hyperthermic Oncology 1988, vol 2, pp 422–425. London, Taylor & Francis, 1989
310. Perez CA, Emami B, Nussbaum GH: Clinical experience with external local hyperthermia in treatment of superficial malignant tumors. Front Radiat Ther Oncol 18:83–102, 1984
311. Perez CA, Emami B, Nussbaum GH: Hyperthermia. In Perez CA, Brady L (eds): Principles and Practice of Radiation Oncology, p 317. Philadelphia, JB Lippincott, 1987
312. Perez CA, Emami B, Pajak TJ, et al: Prognostic factors in clinical application of irradiation and heat: MIR and RTOG experience. Relevance of irradiation dose and fractionation. In Sugahara T, Saito M (eds): Hyperthermic Oncology 1988, vol 2, pp 615–617. London, Taylor & Francis, 1989
313. Perez CA, Emami B, Straube W, et al: Irradiation and external hyperthermia in treatment of head and neck cancer. In Sugahara T, Saito M (eds): Hyperthermic Oncology 1988, vol 2, pp 446–449. London, Taylor & Francis, 1989
314. Perez CA, Emami B, VonGerichten D: Clinical results with irradiation and local hyperthermia in cancer therapy. In Overgaard J (ed): Hyperthermic Oncology, vol I, pp 398–402. London, Taylor & Francis, 1984
315. Perez CA, Gillespie B, Pajak T, et al: Quality assurance problems in clinical hyperthermia and its impact on therapeutic outcome: A report by the Radiation Therapy Oncology Group. Int J Radiat Oncol Biol Phys 16:551–558, 1989
316. Perez CA, Kopecky W, Rao DV, et al: Local microwave hyperthermia and irradiation in cancer therapy: Preliminary observations and directions for future clinical trials. Int J Radiat Oncol Biol Phys 7:765–772, 1981
317. Perez CA, Kuske RR, Emami B, Fineberg B: Irradiation alone or combined with hyperthermia in the treatment of recurrent carcinoma of the breast in the chest wall: A nonrandomized comparison. Int J Hyperthermia 2:179–187, 1986
318. Perez CA, Nussbaum G, Emami B, et al: Clinical results of irradiation combined with local hyperthermia. Cancer 52:1597–1603, 1983
319. Perez CA, Pajak T, Emami B, et al: Randomized phase III

study comparing irradiation and hyperthermia with irradiation alone in superficial measurable tumors: Final report by the Radiation Therapy Oncology Group. Am J Clin Oncol 14:133–141, 1991

320. Petrovich Z, Emami B, Astrahan M, et al: Regional hyperthermia with the BSD-1000 annular phased array in the management of recurrent deep seated malignant tumor. Strahlenther Onkol 163:430, 1987
321. Petrovich Z, Lam K, Langholz B, et al: Interstitial thermoradiotherapy for recurrent head and neck cancer. Am J Otolaryngol 10:257–260, 1989
322. Petrovich Z, Langholtz B, Gibbs FA Jr, et al: Regional hyperthermia for advanced tumors: A clinical study of 353 patients. Int J Radiat Oncol Biol Phys 16:601–607, 1989
323. Pettigrew RT, Galt JM, Ludgate CM, et al: Clinical effects of whole-body hyperthermia in advanced malignancy. Br Med J 4:679–682, 1974
324. Pilepich MV, Myerson RJ, Emami BN, et al: Regional hyperthermia: A feasibility analysis. Int J Hyperthermia 3:347, 1987
325. Pilepich MV, Myerson RJ, Emami BN, et al: Regional hyperthermia: Assessment of tolerance to treatment. Int J Radiat Oncol Biol Phys 14:347, 1988
326. Pontasch MJ, Brodell RT: pH buffering of local anesthetic solutions: Marked reduction in pain with local infiltration of anesthetic solutions (Letter). J Dermatol Surg Oncol 14:672, 1988
327. Puthawala AA, Nisar AM, Sheikh Khalid MA, et al: Interstitial hyperthermia for recurrent malignancies. Endocuriether Hypertherm Oncol 1:125–131, 1985
328. Puthawala AA, Syed AMN, Sheikh KMA, et al: Thermoendocurietherapy for recurrent and/or persistent head and neck cancers. Int J Radiat Oncol Biol Phys 12:110, 1986
329. Raaphorst GP, Romano SL, Mitchell JB, et al: Intrinsic differences in heat and/or x-ray sensitivity of seven mammalian cell lines cultured and treated under identical conditions. Cancer Res 39:396–401, 1979
330. Radiation Therapy Oncology Group, Bahman Emami, Chairman: Protocol 84–19: A randomized phase II study of interstitial thermoradiotherapy (43°C) compared with interstitial radiotherapy alone in the treatment of recurrent or persistent human tumors
331. Reeves OR: Mechanisms of acquired resistance to acute heat shock in cultured mammalian cells. J Cell Physiol 79:157–170, 1972
332. Reinhold HS, Endrich B: Tumor microcirculation as a target for hyperthermia: A review. Int J Hyperthermia 2:111–137, 1986
333. Reinhold HS, van den Berg-Block A: Enhancement of thermal damage to the microcirculation of "sandwich" tumors by additional treatment. Eur J Cancer Clin Oncol 17:781–795, 1981
334. Reinhold HS, van den Berg-Block AE: Hyperthermia-induced alteration in erythrocyte velocity in tumors. Int J Microcirc Clin Exp 2:285–295, 1983
335. Rice GC, Fiher G, Devlin M, et al: Use of N-Σ-dansyl-L-lysine and flow cytometry to identify heat-killed mammalian cells. Int J Hyperthermia 1:186–191, 1985
336. Roberts DW: Interstitial hyperthermia of the brain. In Paliwal BR, Hetzel FW, Dewhirst MW (eds): Biological, Physical and Clinical Aspects of Hyperthermia, Medical Physics Monograph No. 16, pp 300–314. New York, American Association of Physicists in Medicine, 1988
337. Robins HI: Whole body hyperthermia: The University of Wisconsin Clinical Cancer Center experience. In Paliwal BR, Hetzel FW, Dewhirst MW (eds): Biological, Physical and Clinical Aspects of Hyperthermia, Medical Physics Monograph No. 16, pp 345–355. New York, American Association of Physicists in Medicine, 1988
338. Robins HI: The role of whole body hyperthermia in the treatment of neoplastic disease: Its current status and future prospects. Cancer Res 44:4878S, 1984
339. Roemer RB: Heat transfer in hyperthermia treatments: Basic principles and applications. In Paliwal BR, Hetzel FW, Dewhirst MW (eds): Biological, Physical and Clinical Aspects of Hyperthermia, pp 210–242. New York, American Association of Physicists in Medicine, 1988
340. Roemer RB, Cetas TC: Applications of bioheat transfer simulations in hyperthermia. Cancer Res 44(Suppl):4788S–4798S, 1984
341. Roemer RB, Forsyth K, Oleson JR, et al: The effect of hydralazine dose on blood perfusion changes during hyperthermia. Int J Hyperthermia 4:401–415, 1988
342. Roti Roti JL: Heat-induced cell death and radiosensitization: Molecular mechanisms. Natl Cancer Inst Monogr 61:3–10, 1982
343. Roti Roti JL, Laszlo A: The effects of hyperthermia on cellular macromolecules. In Urano M, Douple E (eds): Hyperthermia and Oncology, pp 13–56. The Netherlands, VSP BV Publisher, 1988
344. Roti Roti JL, Winward RT: The effects of hyperthermia on the protein-to-DNA ratio of isolated HeLa cell chromatin. Radiat Res 74:159–169, 1978
345. Roti Roti JL, Wright WD, Higashikubo R: DNase I sensitivity of nuclear DNA measured by flow cytometry. Cytometry 6:191-208, 1985
346. Ryu KH, Kang MS, Levitt SH, et al: Effect of hyperthermia on the lactic acid content in tumor and muscle. (Radiat Res)
347. Salcman M, Samaras GM: Interstitial microwave hyperthermia for brain tumors: Results of a phase-I clinical trial. J Neurol Oncol 1:225–236, 1983
348. Samulski TV: Current technologies for invasive thermometry. In Paliwal BR, Hetzel FW, Dewhirst MW (eds): Biological, Physical and Clinical Aspects of Hyperthermia, pp 168–181. New York, American Association of Physicists in Medicine, 1988
349. Samulski TV, Kapp DS, Fessenden P, Lohrbach A: Heating deep seated eccentrically located tumors with an Annular Phased Array System: A comparative clinical study using two annular array operating configurations. Int J Radiat Oncol Biol Phys 13:83, 1987
350. Sannazzari GL, Gabriele P, Orecchia R, et al: Head and neck tumors: Hyperthermia alone. In Sugahara T, Saito M (eds): Hyperthermic Oncology 1988, vol 2, pp 438–441. London, Taylor & Francis, 1989
351. Sapareto SA: A workshop on thermal dose in cancer therapy: Introduction. Int J Hyperthermia 3:289–290, 1987
352. Sapareto SA: Thermal isoeffect dose: Addressing the problem of thermotolerance. Int J Hyperthermia 3:297–305, 1987
353. Sapareto SA, Corry PM: A proposed standard data file format for hyperthermia treatments. Int J Radiat Oncol Biol Phys 16:613–627, 1989
354. Sapareto SA, Dewey WC: Thermal dose determination in cancer therapy. Int J Radiat Oncol Biol Phys 10:787–800, 1984
355. Sapareto SA, Hopwood LE, Dewey WC: Combined effects of x irradiation and hyperthermia in CHO cells for various temperatures and orders of application. Radiat Res 73:221–233, 1978
356. Sapareto SA, Hopwood LE, Dewey WC: Part D: Effects on survival of cells. In Streffer C, et al (eds): Cancer Therapy by Hyperthermia and Radiation, p 199. Munich, Urban & Schwarzenberg, 1978
357. Sapareto SA, Hopwood LE, Dewey WC, et al: Effects of hyperthermia on survival and progression of Chinese hamster ovary cells. Cancer Res 38:393–400, 1978
358. Sapareto SA, Raaphorst GP, Dewey WC: Cell killing and the sequencing of hyperthermia and radiation. Int J Radiat Oncol Biol Phys 5:343–347, 1979
359. Sapareto SA, Seegenschmidt H, Shrivastava P, et al: Thermal dose: Basic concepts of clinical analysis. In Sugahara T, Saito M (eds): Hyperthermic Oncology 1988, vol 2, pp 299–301. London, Taylor & Francis, 1989
360. Sapozink MD, Boyd SD, Astrahan MA, et al: Transurethral hyperthermia for benign prostatic hyperplasia: Preliminary clinical results. J Urol 143:944, 1990
361. Sapozink MD, Cetas T, Corry PM, et al: Introduction to hyperthermia device evaluation. Int J Hyperthermia 1:1–15, 1988

362. Sapozink MD, Corry PM, Kapp DS, et al: RTOG quality assurance guidelines for clinical trials using hyperthermia for deep-seated malignancy. Int J Radiat Oncol Biol Phys 20(5):1109–1115, 1991
363. Sapozink MD, Gibbs FA, Egger MJ, et al: Regional hyperthermia for clinically advanced deep-seated pelvic malignancy. Am J Clin Oncol 9:162–169, 1986
364. Sapozink MD, Gibbs FA, Egger MJ, Stewart JR: Abdominal regional hyperthermia with an annular phased array. J Clin Oncol 4:775, 1986
365. Sapozink MD, Gibbs, FA Jr, Gates KS, et al: Regional hyperthermia in the treatment of clinically advanced, deep seated malignancy: Results of a pilot study employing an annular array applicator. Int J Radiat Oncol Biol Phys 10:775–786, 1984
366. Sapozink MD, Gibbs FA, Gibbs P, et al: Myonecrosis following deep pelvic hyperthermia. Int J Hyperthermia 4:251, 1988
367. Sapozink MD, Gibbs FA, Thomson JW, et al: A comparison of deep regional hyperthermia from an annular array and a concentric coil in the same patients. Int J Radiat Oncol Biol Phys 11:179, 1985
368. Sathiaseelan V: Potential for patient-specific optimization of deep heating patterns through manipulation of amplitude and phase. Strahlenther Onkol 165:743–745, 1989
369. Sathiaseelan V, Iskander MF, Howard GCW, et al: Theoretical analysis and clinical demonstration of the effect of power pattern control using the annular phased-array hyperthermia system. IEEE Trans Microwave Theory Tech MTT 34(5):514, 1986
370. Schlesinger MJ, Ashburner M, Tissieres A (eds): Heat Shock from Bacteria to Man. Cold Spring Harbor, NY, Cold Spring Harbor Laboratory Press, 1982
371. Scott RS, Chou CK, McCumber M, et al: Complications resulting from spurious fields produced by a microwave applicator used for hyperthermia. Int J Radiat Oncol Biol Phys 12:1883–1886, 1986
372. Scott R, Gillespie B, Perez CA, et al: Hyperthermia in combination with definitive radiation therapy: Results of a phase I/II RTOG study. Int J Radiat Oncol Biol Phys 15:711,716, 1988
373. Scott RS, Johnson RJR, Kowal H, et al: Hyperthermia in combination with radiotherapy: A review of 5 years' experience in the treatment of superficial tumors. Int J Radiat Oncol Biol Phys 9:1327–1333, 1983
374. Scott RS, Johnson RJR, Story KV, et al: Local hyperthermia in combination with definitive radiotherapy: Increased tumor clearance, reduced recurrence rate in extended follow-up. Int J Radiat Oncol Biol Phys 10:2119–2123, 1984
375. Seegenschmiedt MH, Brady LW, Karlsson UL, et al: A critical review of interstitial thermoradiotherapy for recurrent malignant astrocytoma: Problems and promises. Int J Hyperthermia 3:589, 1987
376. Seegenschmiedt MH, Brady LW, Rossmeissl G: External microwave hyperthermia combined with radiation therapy for extensive superficial chest wall recurrences (Abstract), p 32. Hyperthermia Meeting 1987–Second European BSD Users' Meeting, Muchen, West Germany, April 2–4, 1987
377. Seppi E, Shapiro E, Zitelli L, et al: A large aperture ultrasonic array system for hyperthermia of deep-seated tumors. Proc IEE Ultrasonic Symposium, pp 942–948, 1985
378. Shidnia H, Hornback NB, Shupe R, et al: Correlation between hyperthermia and large dose per fraction in treatment of malignant melanoma. Presented at the Annual Meeting of the International Clinical Hyperthermia Society, Lund, Sweden, 1987
379. Shim D, Cetas T, Buechler D, et al: Interstitially placed, thermoregulating ferromagnetic seeds: Initial clinical results. Presented at the 36th Annual Meeting of the Radiation Research Society and 8th Annual Meeting of the North American Hyperthermia Group, Philadelphia, Pennsylvania, April 16–21, 1988
380. Shimm DS, Cetas TC, Oleson JR, et al: Regional hyperthermia for deep-seated malignancies using the BSD annular array. Int J Hyperthermia 4:159–170, 1988
381. Shrivastava P, Luk K, Oleson J, et al: Hyperthermia quality assurance guidelines. Int J Radiat Oncol Biol Phys 16:571–587, 1988
382. Shrivastava PN, Taylor IK, Matloubich AY, et al: Hyperthermia thermometry evaluation: Criteria and guidelines. Int J Radiat Oncol Biol Phys 14:327, 1988
383. Sim DA, Dewhirst MW, Oleson JR, et al: Estimating the therapeutic advantage of adequate heat. In Overgaard J (ed): Hyperthermic Oncology 1984, vol 1, pp 367–371. London, Taylor & Francis, 1984
384. Simard R, Bernhard W: A heat-sensitive cellular function located in the nucleolus. J Cell Biol 34:61–76, 1967
385. Sinclair WK: Dependence of radiosensitivities upon cell age. In Time and Dose Relationships in Radiation Biology as Applied to Radiotherapy, p 97. Brookhaven National Lab Report 50203 (C-57), 1969
386. Slusser H, Hopwood LER, Kapiszewska M: Inhibition of membrane transport by hyperthermia. Natl Cancer Inst Monogr 61:85–87, 1982
387. Sneed PK, Matsumoto K, Stauffer P, et al: Interstitial microwave hyperthermia in canine brain model. Int J Radiat Oncol Biol Phys 12:1887–1897, 1986
388. Song CW: Effect of hyperthermia on vascular function of normal tissue and experimental tumors. J Natl Cancer Inst 60:711–713, 1978
389. Song CW: Hyperthermia in Cancer Therapy, pp 187–296. Boston, GK Hall Medical Publishing, 1983
390. Song CW: Effect of local hyperthermia on blood flow and microenvironment: A review. Cancer Res 44(Suppl):4721S–4730S, 1984
391. Song CW, Kang MS, Rhee JG, et al: Effect of hyperthermia on vascular function, pH and cell survival. Radiology 137:795–803, 1980
392. Song CW, Lokshina A, Rhee JG, et al: Implication of blood flow in hyperthermic treatment of tumors. IEEE Trans Biomed Eng BME 31:9–16, 1984
393. Song CW, Rhee JG, Lee CKK, Levitt SH: Capacitive heating of phantom and human tumors with an 8 MHz radiofrequency applicator (Thermotron RF-8*). Int J Radiat Oncol Biol Phy 12:365, 1986
394. Star WM, Marijnissen HPA, van den Berg-Block AE, et al: Destruction of rat mammary tumor and normal tissue microcirculation by hematoporphyrin derivative photoradiation observed *in vivo* in sandwich observation chambers. Cancer Res 46:2532–2540, 1984
395. Stauffer PR, Sneed, PK, Suen SA, et al: Comparative thermal dosimetry of interstitial microwave and radiofrequency—LCF hyperthermia. Int J Hyperthermia 5:307–318, 1989
396. Steeves RA, Severson SB, Paliwal BR, et al: Matched-pair analysis of response to local hyperthermia and megavoltage electron therapy for superficial human tumours. Endocuriether Hypertherm Oncol 2:163–170, 1986
397. Steindorfer P, Jakse R, Germann R, et al: Hyperthermia as an adjuvant to radiation and/or chemotherapy in far advanced recurrences of the head and neck region. Strahlenther Onkol 163:449–452, 1987
398. Stevenson AP, Galey WR, Tobey RA: Hyperthermia-induced increase in potassium transport in Chinese hamster cells. J Cell Physiol 115:75–86, 1983
399. Stewart FA, Denekamp J: Sensitization of mouse skin to X-irradiation by moderate heating. Radiology 123:195–200, 1977
400. Stewart FA, Denekamp J: The therapeutic advantage of combined heat and x-rays on a mouse fibrosarcoma. Br J Radiol 51:307–316, 1978
401. Stone HB: Hyperthermia enhances early radiation damage in normal tissues more than late damage. In Sugahara T, Saito M (eds): Hyperthermic Oncology 1988, vol 1, pp 171–172. London, Taylor & Francis, 1989
402. Storm FK, Roe D, Drury B, et al: Analysis of thermal dose response to heat (Abstract), p 16. Thirty-fifth Annual Meeting of the Radiation Research Society, February 21–26, 1987
403. Straube W, Leybovich L, Myerson RJ, et al: Volumetric characterization of SAR patterns of 915 MHz hyperthermia applicators (in preparation)
404. Straube WL, Myerson RJ, Emami B, et al: SAR patterns of

external 915 MHz microwave applicators. Int J Hyperthermia 6(3):665–670, 1990
405. Streffer C, van Beuningen D: The biological basis for tumor therapy by hyperthermia and radiation. Rec Res Cancer Res 104:24–70, 1987
406. Strohbehn JW: Theoretical temperature distributions for solenoidal-type hyperthermia systems. Med Phys 9:673–682, 1982
407. Strohbehn JW: Temperature distributions from interstitial RF electrode hyperthermia systems: Theoretical predictions. Int J Radiat Oncol Biol Phys 9:1655–1667, 1983
408. Strohbehn JW: Calculation of absorbed power in tissue for various hyperthermia devices. Cancer Res 44(Suppl):4781S–4887S, 1984
409. Strohbehn JW: Numerical techniques for modeling electromagnetic applicators. Presented at 1987 Hyperthermia School, Physical Aspects of Hyperthermia, Durham, North Carolina, April 27–May 1, 1987
410. Strohbehn JW, Curtis EH, Paulsen KD, et al: Optimization of the absorbed power distribution for an annular phased array hyperthermia system. Int J Radiat Oncol Biol Phys 16:589–599, 1989
411. Strohbehn JW, Douple EB, Coughlin C: Interstitial microwave antenna array system for hyperthermia. Front Radiat Ther Oncol 18:70–74, 1984
412. Strohbehn JW, Mechling JA: Interstitial techniques for clinical hyperthermia. In Hand JW, James JR (eds): Physical techniques in Clinical Hyperthermia, pp 210–287. Letchworth, England, Research Studies Press, 1986
413. Strohbehn JW, Trembly BS, Douple EB: Blood flow effects on the temperature distributions from an invasive microwave antenna array used in cancer therapy. IEEE Trans Biomed Eng 29:649–661, 1982
414. Strohmaier WL, Bichler K-H, Fluchter SH, et al: Histological findings in prostatic cancer treated by local hyperthermia. In Sugahara T, Saito M (eds): Hyperthermic Oncology 1988, vol 1, pp 548–550. London, Taylor & Francis, 1989
415. Stuchly MA, Stuchly SS: Dielectric properties of biological substances tabulated. J Microwave Power 15:19–26, 1980
416. Subjeck JR, Sciandra JJ, Chao CF, et al: Heat shock proteins and biological response to hyperthermia. Br J Cancer 45:127–131, 1982
417. Suit HD, Gerweck LE: Potential for hyperthermia and radiation therapy. Cancer Res 39:2290–2298, 1979
418. Suit HD, Proppe KH, Mankin HJ, et al: Preoperative radiation therapy for sarcoma of soft tissue. Cancer 47:2269, 1981
419. Sutton CH: Necrosis and altered blood flow produced by microwave-induced tumor hyperthermia in a murine glioma (Abstract). American Association for Cancer Research, 1976
420. Sutton CH: Tumor hyperthermia in the treatment of malignant gliomas of the brain. Trans Am Neurol Assoc 96:195, 1971
421. Svaasand LO: Photodynamic and photohyperthermic response of malignant tumors. Med Phys 10:455–461, 1985
422. Tan W, Li Q: Clinical effects of microwave combined with radiation in 50 head and neck malignant tumor patients. In Overgaard J (ed): Hyperthermic Oncology 1984, vol 1, pp 357–358. London, Taylor & Francis, 1984
423. Tannock IF: The relation between cell proliferation and the vascular system in transplanted mouse mammary tumor. Cancer Res 30:2470–2474, 1970
424. Teicher BA, Kowal CD, Kennedy KA, et al: Enhancement by hyperthermia of the *in vitro* cytotoxicity of mitomycin C toward hypoxic tumor cells. Cancer Res 41:1096–1099, 1981.
425. Terasima T, Tolmach LJ: Variations in several responses of HeLa cells to x-irradiation during the division cycle. Biophys J 3:11, 1963
426. Thistlethwaite AJ, Alexander GA, Moylan DJ, et al: Modification of human tumor pH by elevation of blood glucose. Int J Radiat Oncol Biol Phys 13:603–610, 1987
427. Thomas GP, Welch WJ, Matthews MB, et al: Molecular and cellular effects of heat shock and related treatments of mammalian tissue-culture cells. Cold Spring Harbor Symp Quant Biol 46:985–996, 1982
428. Tomasovic SP, Turner GN, Dewey WC: Effect of hyperthermia on nonhistone proteins isolated with DNA. Radiat Res 73:535–552, 1978
429. Turner PF: Regional hyperthermia with an annular phased array. IEEE Trans Biomed Eng BME 31:106, 1984
430. Turner PF, Kumar L: Computer solution for applicator heating patterns. Natl Cancer Inst Monogr 61:521–523, 1982
431. Turner PF, et al: Future trends in heating technology of deep seated tumors. Appl Hyperthermia Treat Cancer 107:249, 1988
432. U L, Noell KT, Woodward KF, et al: Microwave induced local hyperthermia in combination with radiotherapy of human malignant tumors. Cancer 45:638–646, 1980
433. Uehara S, Omagari J: Deep local and regional hyperthermia with annular phased array. Strahlenther Onkol 165:715, 1989
434. Uozumi H, Baba Y, Yasunaga T, et al: Clinical evaluation of combined hyperthermia and radiation therapy of superficial malignant tumors. In Onoyama Y (ed): Hyperthermic Oncology, pp 311–312. Proceedings of the 3rd Annual Meeting of the Japanese Society of Hyperthermic Oncology, Japan, 1986
435. Urano M, Kenton LA, Kahn J: The effect of hyperthermia on the early and late appearing mouse foot reactions and on radiation carcinogenesis: Effect on the early and late appearing reactions. Int J Radiat Oncol Biol Phys 15:159–166, 1988
436. Valdagni R (ed): International Consensus Meeting on Hyperthermia: Final Report. Int J Hyperthermia 6:839–877; discussion 879–880, 1990
437. Valdagni R, Amichetti M, Graiff C, et al: Parameters influencing outcome of combined radiation therapy and hyperthermia in neck node metastases. In Sugahara T, Saito M (eds): Hyperthermic Oncology 1988, vol 2, pp 458–461. London, Taylor & Francis, 1989
438. Valdagni R, Amichetti M, Pani G: Radical radiation alone versus radical radiation plus microwave hyperthermia for N3 (TNM-UICC) neck nodes: A prospective randomized clinical trial. Int J Radiat Oncol Biol Phys 15:13–24, 1988
439. Valdagni R, Kapp DS, Valdagni C: N3 (TNM-UICC) metastatic neck nodes managed by combined radiation therapy and hyperthermia: Clinical results and analysis of treatment parameters. Int J Hyperthermia 2(2):189–200, 1986
440. Valdagni R, Samulski TV, Cox RS, et al: Local and regional hyperthermia treatment of superficial and deep tumors: Analysis of thermal washouts (Abstract). Strahlentherapie 161:552, 1985
441. Valdagni R, Liu FF, Kapp DS. Important prognostic factors influencing outcome of combined radiation and hyperthermia. Int J Radiat Oncol Biol Phys 15:959–972, 1988
442. van den Berg AP, Wike-Hooley JL, van den Berg-Block, et al: Tumour pH in human mammary carcinoma. Eur J Cancer Clin Oncol 18:457–462, 1982
443. van der Zee J, van den Berg AP, Treurniet-Donker AD, et al: Hyperthermia in combination with radiotherapy: A palliative treatment for patients with breast cancer recurring in previously irradiated areas. In Sugahara T, Saito M (eds): Hyperthermic Oncology 1988, vol 1, pp 475–477. London, Taylor & Francis, 1989
444. van der Zee J, van den Berg AP, Treurniet-Donker AD, et al: Results of hyperthermia in combination with reirradiation in patients with breast cancer. In Sugahara T, Saito M (eds): Hyperthermic Oncology 1988, vol 2, pp 418–421. London, Taylor & Francis, 1989
445. van der Zee J, van Putten WLJ, van den Berg AP, et al: Retrospective analysis of the response of tumours in patients treated with a combination of radiotherapy and hyperthermia. Int J Hyperthermia 2:337–349, 1986
446. van der Zee J, van Rhoon GC, Wike-Hooley JL, et al: Thermal enhancement of radiotherapy in breast carcinoma. In Overgaard J (ed): Hyperthermic Oncology, vol 1, pp 345–349. London, Francis & Taylor, 1984
447. van der Zee J, van Rhoon GC, Wike-Hooley JL, et al: Clinically derived dose effect relationship for hyperthermia with low dose radiotherapy. Br J Radiol 58:243–250, 1985
448. Vaupel P: Hypoxia in neoplastic tissue. Microvasc Res 13:399–408, 1977
449. Vaupel P, Kallinowski F: Physiological effects of hyperthermia. Rec Res Cancer Res 104:71–109, 1987

450. Vaupel P, Muller-Klieser W, Otte J, et al: Blood flow, tissue oxygenation, and pH distribution in malignant tumors upon localized hyperthermia. Basic pathophysiological aspects and the role of various thermal doses. Strahlentherapie 159:73–81, 1983
451. Vaupel P, Ostheimer K, Muller-Klieser W: Circulatory and metabolic responses of malignant tumors during localized hyperthermia. J Cancer Res Clin Oncol 98:15–29, 1980
452. Vidair CA, Dewey WC: Evaluation of a role of intracellular Na+, K+, CA2+, and MG2+ in hyperthermic cell killing. Radiat Res 105:187–200, 1986
453. Von Ardenne M: Selective multiphase cancer therapy: Conceptual aspects and experimental basis. Adv Pharmacol Chemother 10:339–380, 1982
454. VonArdenne M, Lippmann HG, Reitmauer PG, Justus J: Histological proof for selective stop of microcirculation in tumor tissue at pH-6.1 and 41C. Naturwissenschaften 66:59, 1979
455. Voorhees WE III, Babbs CF: Hydralazine-enhanced selective heating of transmissible venereal tumor implants in dogs. Eur J Cancer Clin Oncol 18:1027–1033, 1982
456. Vora N, Forell B, Joseph C, et al: Interstitial implant with intertitial hyperthermia. Cancer 50:2518–2523, 1982
457. Vora NL, Luk KH, Forell B, et al: Interstitial local current field hyperthermia for advanced cancers of the cervix. Endocuriether Hypertherm Oncol 4:97–106, 1988
458. Vora N, Shaw S, Forell B, et al: Primary radiation combined with hyperthermia for advanced (stage III–IV) and inflammatory carcinoma of breast. Endocuriether Hypertherm Oncol 2:101–106, 1986
459. Waldow SM: Enhanced tumor control following sequential treatments of photodynamic therapy (PDT) and localized microwave hyperthermia *in vivo.* Lasers Surg Med 4:79–85, 1984
460. Waldow SM, Dougherty TJ: Interaction of hyperthermia and photoradiation therapy. Radiat Res 97:380–385, 1984
461. Waldow SM, Henderson BW, Dougherty TJ: Potentiation of photodynamic therapy by heat: Effect of sequence and time interval between treatments *in vivo.* Lasers Surg Med 5:83–94, 1984
462. Ward KA, Jain RK: Response of tumours to hyperglycemia: Characterization significance and role of hyperthermia. Int J Hyperthermia 4:223–250, 1988
463. Ward-Hartley KA, Jain RK: Effect of glucose and galactose on microcirculatory flow in normal and neoplastic tissues in rabbits. Cancer Res 47:371–377, 1987
464. Warren SL: Preliminary study of the effect of artificial fever upon hopeless tumor cases. Am J Roentgenol 33:75–87, 1935
465. Warters RL, Roti Roti JL: Excision of X-ray-induced thymine damage in chromatin from heated cells. Radiat Res 70:113–121, 1979
466. Warters RL, Roti Roti JL: Nucleosome structure in chromatin from heated cells. Radiat Res 84:504–513, 1980
467. Warters RL, Roti Roti JL, Winward RT: Production and excision of 5′,6′-dihydroxydihydrothymine type products in the DNA of preheated cells. Int J Radiat Oncol Biol Phys 3:381–384, 1978
468. Warters RL, Stone OL: The effects of hyperthermia on DNA replication in HeLa cells. Radiat Res 93:71–84, 1983
469. Warters RL, Yasui LS, Sharma R, et al: Heat shock (45°C) results in an increase of nuclear matrix protein mass in HeLa cells. Int J Radiat Biol 50:253–268, 1986
470. Waterman FM: Measurement of perfusion in human tumors. In Paliwal BR, Hetzel FW, Dewhirst MW (eds): Biological, Physical and Clinical Aspects of Hyperthermia, Medical Physics Monograph No. 16, pp 182–207. New York, American Association of Physicists in Medicine, 1988
471. Waterman FM, Leeper JB: Temperature artifacts produced by thermocouples used in conjunction with 1 and 3 MHz ultrasound. Int J Hyperthermia 6:383–399, 1990
472. Waterman FM, Nerlinger RE, Leeper JB: Catheter induced artifacts in ultrasound hyperthermia. Int J Hyperthermia 6:371–381, 1990
473. Welch WJ, Feramisco JR: Nuclear and nucleolar localization of the 72000-dalton heat shock protein in heat-shocked mammalian cells. J Biol Chem 259:4501–4513, 1984
474. Welch WJ, Suhan JP: Morphological study of the mammalian stress response: Characterization of changes in cytoplasmic organelles, cytoskeleton and nucleoli and appearance of intranuclear actin filaments in rat fibroblasts after heat-shock treatment. J Cell Biol 101:1198–1211, 1985
475. Westermark F: Uber die Behandlung des Ulcerirended Cerixacarcinoms. Mittle Konstanter Warme. Zentralbl Gynakol 22:1335–1339, 1898
476. Westra A, Dewey WC: Variation in sensitivity to heat shock during the cell-cycle of Chinese hamster cells *in vitro.* Int J Radiat Oncol Biol Phys 19:467–477, 1971
477. Wickersheim KA: A new fiberoptic thermometry system for use in medical hyperthermia. SPIE Proc, vol 713, Sept 14, 1986
478. Wike-Hooley JL, Haveman J, Reinhold HS: The relevance of tumour pH to the treatment of malignant disease. Radiother Oncol 2:343–366, 1984
479. Wike-Hooley JL, van den Berg AP, van der Zee J, et al: Human tumour pH and its variation. Eur J Cancer Clin Oncol 21:785–795, 1985
480. Wike-Hooley JL, van der Zee J, van Rhoon GC, et al: Human tumour pH changes following hyperthermia and radiation therapy. Eur J Cancer Clin Oncol 20:619–623, 1984
481. Winter A, Laing J, Paglione R, et al: Microwave hyperthermia for brain tumors. Neurosurgery 17:387–399, 1985
482. Wong RL, Dewey WC: Molecular studies on the hyperthermic inhibition of DNA synthesis in Chinese hamster ovary cells. Radiat Res 92:370–395, 1982
483. Wong RSL, Dewey WC: Effect of hyperthermia on DNA synthesis. In Anghileri LJ, Anghileri RJ (eds): Hyperthermia in Cancer Treatment, pp 80–91. Boca Raton, FL, CRC Press, 1986
484. Wynstra JH, Wright WD, Roti Roti JL: Repair of radiation-induced DNA damage in thermotolerant and nonthermotolerant HeLa cells. Radiat Res 124:85–89, 1990
485. Yabumoto E, Suyama S: Interstitial radiofrequency hyperthermia combined with electron beam radiotherapy. In Overgaard J (ed): Hyperthermic Oncology, vol 1, pp 579–582. London, Taylor & Francis, 1984
486. Yanagawa S, Tsukiyama I, Watai K, et al: Regional hyperthermia combined with radiation for locally advanced deep-seated malignancy (submitted for publication)
487. Yatvin MB: The influence of membrane lipid composition and proteins on hyperthermia death of cells. Int J Radiat Oncol Biol Phys 32:513–521, 1977
488. Yerushalmi A: Non-invasive hyperthermia for treatment of prostatic tumors: Benign and malignant. In Sugahara T, Saito M (eds): Hyperthermic Oncology 1988, vol 2, pp 406–409. London, Taylor & Francis, 1989
489. Yonemura Y, Fujimura T, Urade M, et al: Continuous hyperthermic peritoneal perfusion with cisplatin and mitomycin C for peritoneal dissemination in gastric carcinoma. In Sugahara T, Saito M (eds): Hyperthermic Oncology 1988, vol 2, p 163. London, Taylor & Francis, 1989
490. Zhang Z, et al: The effect of hyperthermia-chemotherapy on bladder carcinoma: Experimental and clinical studies. Abstracts of the satellite meeting of the International Congress on Hyperthermic Oncology, Beijing, China, September 1988

17

Radioimmunoglobulins in Cancer Therapy

Stanley E. Order

All disciplines engaged in oncologic therapy share a fundamental concern for selective tumor cytotoxicity with limited normal tissue damage. The use of immunoglobulins as radiation carriers depends on their specificity to achieve biologic selectivity by the attraction of specific antibodies against tumor-associated antigens. Delivery of isotopes by radiolabeled antibodies achieves tumor cytotoxicity by continuous radiation.

Studies on tumor localization suggest that radiolabeling of appropriate antibodies with ^{131}I and ^{125}I can yield both diagnostic images of cancer and possible therapeutic results.[2,42,43,54] A few investigators pursued such leads, originally with polyclonal antibodies sometimes purified by column techniques (affinity chromatography) and derived by immunization of intact animals.[9–11,12–14,27,28,42,43,54] The results of techniques such as subtraction scanning, single photon emission tomographic scans (SPECT), and scanning of transplanted human tumors in immune privileged sites (hamster cheek pouch, nude mice) further demonstrated the potential of radioimmunoglobulins for cancer therapy.[3,13,14,28,42,43] Advances in monoclonal antibody production, after the discovery by Nobel laureates Kohler and Milstein, promised to accelerate the use of these agents for possible therapeutic application in the rapid production of high titer, high specific activity monoclonal antibody without the requirement of antigen isolation.[20,21] The use of such monoclonal antibodies has not yet been explored fully, nor has their full potential been realized.[20,21,35]

TUMOR BIOLOGY

Recently attention has been drawn to the innate biology of cancer.[19,50] Using ^{131}I antiferritin, it has been shown that small ferritin-bearing tumors have a better vascular-to-tumor mass ratio and are therefore more ideally targeted by radiolabeled antibody.[46–48] As tumors enlarge, the vascular ratio decreases and reduces tumor targeting. Further tumor enlargement leads to central hypoxia and a lack of central tumor targeting because of decreased vascularity and reduced central ferritin production.[46–48] Tumors with equivalent ferritin content are targeted by radiolabeled antibody directly proportional to vascular content.[46–48] Small doses of external radiation increase vascular permeability and allow for greater accumulation of radiolabeled antibody.[26,33]

The vascular dependency of radiolabeled antibody tumor targeting is also linked with the fundamental hydrodynamics of tumors, which include hydraulic conductivity, large interstitial diffusion, interstitial convection, high interstitial flow, hydrophilic attraction, and absence of lymphatics.[19,50] Opposed to these forces and to radiolabeled antibody targeting are low microvascular pressure and high interstitial pressure.[19,50]

A classic example of these anatomic, metabolic, and physiologic factors is the relative hypovascularity of colorectal metastases, which produce carcinoembryonic antigen (CEA) and do not target with ^{131}I anti-CEA intact IgG, whereas in the same patient pulmonary metastases (more vascular) take up the radiolabeled antibody.[1] Fab^2 fragments target liver metastasis due to the lower molecular weight and increased vascular permeability but with a reduced tumor effective half-life.[2,22,35,36] Finally, primary intrahepatic cholangiocarcinoma (CEA+ in the tissue) targets with ^{131}I anti-CEA IgG whole IgG and leads to remission, which has not been the case with colorectal cancer that is metastatic to the liver.[56] Intrahepatic cholangiocarcinomas, however, are hypervascular in contrast to metastatic colorectal cancer.

ANTIBODIES

Historically, the conventional method of producing antibodies has been the immunization of a wide variety of animal species.[34–41] In medical applications, the early tradition was to produce antitoxins and antibacterial antibodies.[34] Rebirth of interest in radiolabeled antibodies was kindled when Pressman and colleagues examined double-labeling techniques with ^{131}I and ^{125}I and treated patients with ^{131}I anti-fibrin antibodies.[4,42,54] The antigen was not tumor-specific, the dosimetry was not determined, and a clinical team did not initiate defined phase I and phase II protocols.

Meanwhile, fundamental studies of immunology increased understanding of the cellular interaction leading to antibody production.[45] The T lymphocyte derived from thymus anlage was recognized as central to the immune reaction. After macrophage processing of antigenic material, T lymphocytes communicate with B lymphocytes (marrow or bursal derived) and lead to antibody production by mature B lymphocytes.[45] Various antibody classes could be produced (IgA, IgE, IgM, IgG), but the classic sequence of interest proved to be IgM early in the primary response and IgG in the late humoral immune response.[45] It had been clear that antibodies possessed the unique quality of specific antigen recognition and that biologic "cell factories" achieved antigen recognition far beyond the capability of laboratory synthesis. Studies identified the fragment antigen binding (Fab) ends of the IgG molecule as the recognition end, and the fragment crystallizable (Fc) end was characterized by its interplay in immune reactions, such as complement fixation and macrophage cytotoxicity.[35,37,38]

IGG AND AFFINITY-PURIFIED ANTIBODIES

For the clinician interested in the diagnostic and therapeutic use of radiolabeled antibodies, the IgG molecule (molecular weight, 150,000 daltons) was of paramount interest. When crystallized antigen of high purity was used, immunization of an intact animal led to polyclonal (multiple lymphocyte-derived) antibodies with 20% maximum specificity, which could then be isolated from the serum.[39–41] These antibodies recognized all major and minor components of a given antigen. The antibodies could be increased in specific activity by affinity purification, a process whereby the antigen was bound to a sepharose (sugar) column and the specific antibody allowed to bind. Cleansing of the column followed by chemical manipulation increased specific activity up to at least 70%.[35,36]

These affinity-purified polyclonal antibodies became the first immunoglobulins to be radiolabeled and to demonstrate a wide variety of tumor targets available for diagnostic scanning techniques.[12,27,43] In later therapeutic trials, ^{131}I affinity-purified antibodies had a reduced persistence at the tumor-bearing site (a reduced tumor effective half-life), thus lowering the tumor dose and being less effective than the non-affinity-treated same antibody with ^{131}I as the radiolabel.[24,35]

THE FRAGMENTS: FAB, FAB^2

Papain and pepsin were shown to cleave the antigen-binding end or ends from the IgG molecule.[45] This allowed the use of specific immunoglobulin fragments to smaller molecular weights of 50,000 and 100,000 daltons.[45] The Fab fragment accomplished the treatment of digoxin intoxication, both experimentally and clinically, and the Fab^2 fragment the scanning of malignant melanoma.[2,22] Fab^2 proved ideal for scanning, producing rapid uptake in tumor and rapid reduction of background counts, although the requirements for therapy (high concentration and prolonged tumor saturation) were not satisfied according to criteria for assessing tumor effective half-life.

$$T_{1/2}\,\text{eff} = \frac{T_{1/2}P \times T_{1/2}B}{T_{1/2}P + T_{1/2}B}$$

$T_{1/2}$ = half-life; P = physical; B = biologic

Perhaps the newest and most exciting application seeking the advantage of reduced molecular weight (IgG—150,000 daltons, Fab^2—100,000 daltons) and increased vascular permeability, while minimizing the negative aspect of reduced effective half-life, has been the "bifunctional antibody."[55] In this instance an Fab^2 fragment has one end directed toward tumor-associated antigen and the other toward a haptenic chelate. The patient is infused with Fab^2, and 24 hours later when normal tissue has cleaned the fragment and the tumor concentration is good, the isotope-labeled chelate is infused, binding the other end of the Fab^2 fragment.[55] The potential for higher dose rates and higher total tumors doses could bring this technology into the 3000 cGy to 5000 cGy total tumor dose type of application.

MONOCLONAL ANTIBODIES

The fusion of a mature, antibody-producing B lymphocyte with a nonsecretory myeloma cell, both derived from a syngeneic mouse strain, led to the formation of the *hybridoma cell,* which could be grown in tissue culture or transplanted into a mouse peritoneal cavity.[20,21] In both situations the hybridoma cellular growth led to the production of high specific activity antibody, originally derived from the first antibody-producing cell, thus the term *monoclonal antibody* (Fig. 17-1). A mere 10 years after this discovery, monoclonal antibodies capable of recognizing antigens for many malignancies were produced in institutions throughout the world. Antibodies have in essence developed into reagents.[18] Simple diagnostic tests flourish on the commercial market for *in vitro* evaluation of pregnancy, hormones, biomarkers, and so on, and diagnostic cancer studies have been accomplished with ^{131}I, ^{99}Tc, and ^{111}In labels.[43,49]

Initially, therapeutic approaches with monoclonal antibodies were limited because intravenous infusions led to the dehalogenation of the ^{131}I isotope from the murine antibodies.[35] New and interesting results in intraperitoneal and intrapleural applications have been reported and require further study.[6,7,16]

In these applications, ^{131}I has not dehalogenated because the enzymes available in the circulation are not present in the third space cavities.[6,7,16] Although remissions were recorded in early ovarian cancer, more powerful isotopes and higher tumor doses were sought. Chelated yttrium-90 (^{90}Y) was then bound to three monoclonal antibodies: anti-HMFG (human milk fat globulin), AUA (glycoprotein), and PLAP (placental alkaline phosphatase). In an important elucidation of monoclonal antibody application by immunoperoxidase, antigenic profiles were developed for each patient, and the appropriate blend of the radioactive ^{90}Y antibodies were administered. However, the chelation of the ^{90}Y was not sufficient to prevent free ^{90}Y from occurring in the circulation and leading to significant hematologic toxicity. Thus, the investigators are now considering EDTA intravenous infusion timed after the intraperitoneal treatment. The loss of ^{90}Y from the chelate has not been the case in other preparations to be discussed.[41]

Repeated administrations of monoclonal antibodies are plagued by the production of human anti-murine antibodies (HAMA), which will be discussed later in this chapter.[51] A development to avoid anti-antibody production has been the genetic engineering of human-murine chimeric antibodies in which the available region is murine and the constant regions human.[52] In the first ten patients treated with a nonlabeled antibody, the serum half-life was 3 to 6 days, and immunogenicity occurred in one patient.[52] In addition, a totally human *in vitro* synthesized antibody created by the fusion of a murine-nonsecreting tumor B cell and a human antibody-producing cell has been radiolabeled; it took 6 days to deposit its full content at the tumor target and had a half-life of 10 to 12 days.[17]

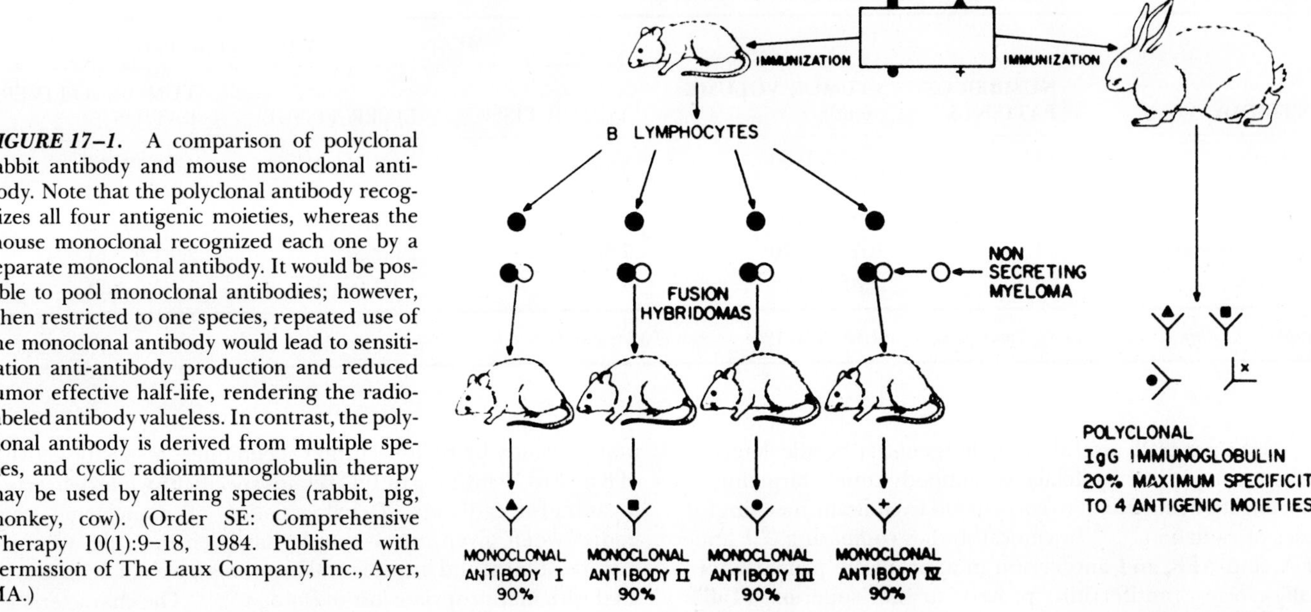

FIGURE 17–1. A comparison of polyclonal rabbit antibody and mouse monoclonal antibody. Note that the polyclonal antibody recognizes all four antigenic moieties, whereas the mouse monoclonal recognized each one by a separate monoclonal antibody. It would be possible to pool monoclonal antibodies; however, when restricted to one species, repeated use of the monoclonal antibody would lead to sensitization anti-antibody production and reduced tumor effective half-life, rendering the radiolabeled antibody valueless. In contrast, the polyclonal antibody is derived from multiple species, and cyclic radioimmunoglobulin therapy may be used by altering species (rabbit, pig, monkey, cow). (Order SE: Comprehensive Therapy 10(1):9–18, 1984. Published with permission of The Laux Company, Inc., Ayer, MA.)

ANTIBODIES (IGG) AS CARRIERS FOR RADIOACTIVITY

The specificity of the Fab ends of the antibody (IgG) molecule provide the basis for selective tumor targeting. Therefore, a discussion of antibody as a carrier must include considerations of the antigenic target, molecular structure and state of the antibody, method of chemical isotopic linkage, concentration and tumor-effective half-life (persistence of the radiolabeled antibody), and anti-antibodies or host response.

Antigenic Target

Past research directed toward the therapeutic use of radiolabeled antibody sought antigenic uniqueness or tumor-specific antigens.[31] Most of the early successes, however, have been with tumor-associated antigens present in a variety of disorders and in normal tissue (*e.g.,* CEA, chorionic gonadotropin, α-fetoprotein [AFP], and ferritin). In particular, ferritin has been used successfully in radiolabeled antibody therapy, and fundamental answers have been elucidated concerning the uptake of radiolabeled antiferritin by experimental and clinical hepatomas.[39,40,46–48]

Ferritin is synthesized and secreted by a number of cancers, including Hodgkin's disease and hepatomas.[39,40,57] It has now been demonstrated that T4 lymphocyte ribosomes synthesize and secrete ferritin, which binds T8 lymphocytes and leads to immunosuppression in Hodgkin's disease and AIDS.[32] Ferritin has also been described for its immunosuppressive quality in head and neck cancer. Normal tissues such as spleen, lymph nodes, and bone marrow store iron in ferritin, yet there is preferential selection of the tumor by the radiolabeled antiferritin, a phenomenon called the *biologic window.*[36] The window results from tumor ferritin synthesis and tumor neovasculature, although the slow blood flow in tumors may also contribute to tumor antibody binding.[36] Our laboratory has shown in the H42E hepatoma that ferritin synthesis is greatest in small tumors and decreases as the tumors enlarge parallel with a decrease in radiolabeled ^{131}I antiferritin concentrations.[46–48]

In addition, tumor neovasculature is more dense in smaller tumors and diminishes as tumors enlarge. Regions within large tumors exist when ferritin is either maximal (at the periphery) or minimal (at the center). Actual excision of the tumor has shown parallel ferritin content and ^{131}I antiferritin localization.[33,46–48]

Perhaps the most fascinating observation has been that the hepatomas that lack significant neovascularity and synthesize ferritin do not "target" with radiolabeled antiferritin.[33] That is, such hepatomas fail to accumulate significantly high concentrations of ^{131}I antiferritin, unlike tumors that both synthesize and secrete ferritin and also have significant neovasculature.[33] Thus, both ferritin synthesis and neovascularization are necessary for tumor targeting.

Antigenic weight, distribution, presence in the circulation, access to the neovasculature, concentration, and antibody kinetics are some of the variables affecting radiolabeled antibody targeting and concentration. Possibly the most specific application of tumor antibody has occurred without radioactivity, that is, therapeutic applications in which unique specificity is used for tumor treatment. B-cell lymphomas themselves produce abnormal tumor-derived monoclonal antibodies as part of tumor cell proliferation. In an interesting series of biologic maneuvers, a monoclonal anti-idiotype antibody (antibody that recognizes the Fab end of another antibody molecule and is the specific abnormality of the B-cell lymphoma) was produced, which targeted the tumor with a reported complete remission of disease.[31] The patient in this study, following a traumatic incident beyond the sixth year of remission, had a recurrence within a site of trauma with the same clinical B-cell idiotype (clonal-specific recurrence), and remission was achieved with external radiation. Since then a second patient has achieved complete remission. However, it is clear that for more general applications linkage to a cytotoxic isotope is needed. Cytotoxic agents were not attached to the antibody in that case. Specific targeting of similar highly restricted antigenic moieties is not available to date in other solid tumors.

TABLE 17–1
Mean Activities per Gram in Tumor and Liver Tissues and Tumor-to-Liver Ratios

			MEAN ACTIVITY (Range) (μCi/g)		
ANTIBODY	NUMBER OF PATIENTS	TUMOR VOLUME (cm^3)	TUMOR TISSUE	LIVER TISSUE	TUMOR-TO-LIVER RATIOS
Antiferritin	18	200–1700	8.4(6.2–12)	1.8(1.1–3.4)	4.8(0.19–7.0)
	4	2290–3020	2.6(1.7–3.6)	1.6(1.1–2.3)	1.6(1.1–2.2)
Anti-AFP	5	145–2705	2.7(1.0–4.8)	2.7(1.1–4.7)	1.0(0.83–1.3)
Antiferritin + anti-AFP	3	780–1326	7.3(5.0–9.8)	2.6(2.3–2.7)	2.9(1.9–3.6)
Anti-CEA	5	467–1275	4.7(3.9–5.7)	1.1(1.0–1.1)	4.4(3.5–5.2)

(Leichner PK, Klein JL, Fish EK, et al: Cancer Drug Deliv 1:321–328, 1984; courtesy of Mary Ann Liebert, Inc)

To be generally useful as single agents, antigenic determinants must provide radiolabeled antibody tumor targeting at concentrations sufficient to correspond to clinically meaningful doses of radiation.[23–26] In clinical studies comparing ^{131}I anti-CEA, anti-AFP, and antiferritin in appropriate primary liver malignancies, antiferritin proved to be superior (Table 17-1).[8,23] The molecular weight of AFP is 70,000 daltons; that of ferritin is 400,000 daltons. In addition, ferritin is bound in the stroma, the stroma apparently sheds the AFP antigen, and a significant ^{131}I anti-AFP concentration could not be achieved. In the case of CEA in intrahepatic biliary cancers, the tumor fails to establish a CEA blood titer; the CEA can be detected only by direct immunoperoxidase staining of the malignant tissue. Tumor remissions thus have occurred with both ^{131}I antiferritin and ^{131}I anti-CEA when significant deposition of radiolabeled antibody has occurred (6 μCi to 12 μCi/g).[25,26] Similar attempts to use the same ^{131}I anti-CEA in colorectal metastasis to the liver were not successful. In colorectal metastasis CEA circulates, the tumor is hypovascular; although tumor targeting occurs, significant tumor concentrations of ^{131}I radiolabeled anti-CEA IgG for therapeutic purposes has not occurred.

The Radiation Therapy Oncology Group (RTOG) carried out a randomized prospective study comparing chemotherapy with radiolabeled antibody in nonresectable hepatoma (RTOG 83-19), which demonstrated that all long-term survivors with AFP-hepatoma had radiolabeled antibody therapy. In addition, patients (AFP−) assigned to chemotherapy treatment that failed responded to ^{131}I antiferritin and could even be converted to surgical resectability. Conversion to surgical resectability occurred only in antibody-treated patients and occurred in the AFP+ and AFP− group (Fig. 17-2).[53]

Trials with radiolabeled antibodies directed toward remission in non-Hodgkin's lymphoma, chronic lymphatic leukemia, ovarian cancers, and gliomas have also been initiated (Table 17-2).[1,5,6,7,15,16,44] In some of these trials unique principles are being tested, such as the use of ^{131}I iodinated antibodies as a method of whole-body irradiation and tumor cytotoxicity[44] and the use of ^{125}I anti-EGF (epidermal growth factor) for antibody internalization and auger electron irradiation.[1,30] Thus, isotopes and their range of cytotoxicity as well as their linkage are important for tumor cell cytotoxicity.

ISOTOPES AND LINKAGE TO ANTIBODY

The classic and initial approach to radiolabeled antibodies was with ^{131}I labeled by chloramine T, later lactoperoxidase, and more recently by Bolton-Hunter techniques. A specific activity of 8 mCi to 10 mCi/mg of IgG retains specificity while delivering meaningful radiation. Dehalogenation of monoclonal antibodies when given intravenously has been the rule, whereas intraperitoneal and intrapleural infusions have not been associated with inappropriate loss of isotope.[6,7,16] The characteristics and range of ^{131}I and other isotopes being used are given in Table 17-3. Similar linkage is accomplished with ^{125}I and antibody. However, cytotoxicity depends on close opposition of the isotope to nuclear DNA for auger electron irradiation. Clinical evaluation is being carried out in gliomas and colorectal cancers.[1]

^{90}Y, because of its more powerful β-irradiation, is attractive.[41,57,58] Its metallic nature requires chelation to the antibody. Currently, safe chelation without isotope release has required all sites to be chelated. To determine tumor targeting, similarly chelated indium-111 (^{111}In) antibodies are used first so that appropriate tumor localization is proven. This is seen by some as a disadvantage due to insecurity in parallelism between the two isotope chelates (^{111}In and ^{90}Y), whereas others see it as a major safety factor because, if inappropriate distribution of the ^{111}In antibody occurs, the ^{90}Y antibody is not given. It must be appreciated that all chelated ^{90}Y antibodies are not equivalent. The best conjugated material to date does not release free ^{90}Y; however, it is also not excreted and yields nondesirable normal liver and spleen irradiation. In a dose escalation study, it was determined that 30 mCi was the hematologic limiting toxic dose for grade 3 and grade 4 toxicity.[41] The issue is made even more complex because the same ^{90}Y antiferritin, when administered in advanced Hodgkin's disease, was effective, whereas in hepatocellular cancer the chelate was overly attracted to the normal liver, thereby dominating the Fab end attraction to the tumor which has been described as "chelate domination."[41]

Rhenium-186 (^{186}Re) is of interest because it is somewhat similar to ^{90}Y. However, because of the τ-emission of rhenium targeting and treatment would be carried out with the same isotope, which is a distinct advantage. Clinical trials have not yet been reported.

Bismuth-212 (^{212}Bi) and astatine-211 (^{211}At), both α-emitters, have been evaluated in the laboratory to some extent but not as yet in clinical applications.[29]

As discussed with chelation, different biodistribution patterns occur with different linkages of isotope to antibody, and this field of linkage chemistry is still in early investigative efforts. A chelate that would tightly bind the metallic isotope while allowing non-tumor-bound antibody excretion should increase the therapeutic ratio by increasing tumor irradiation and decreasing normal tissue irradiation.

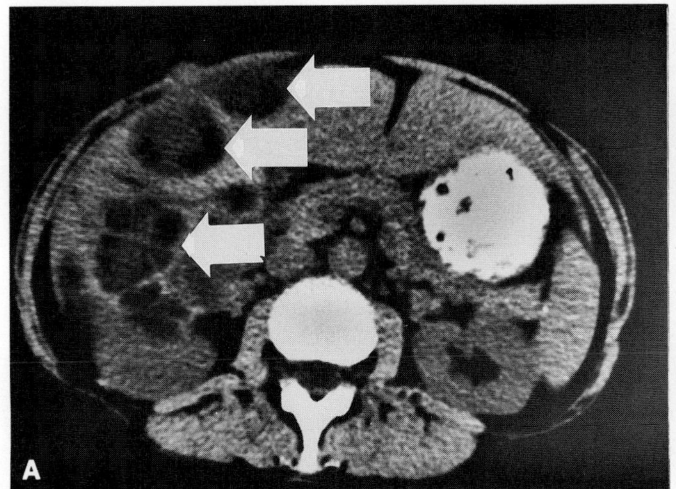

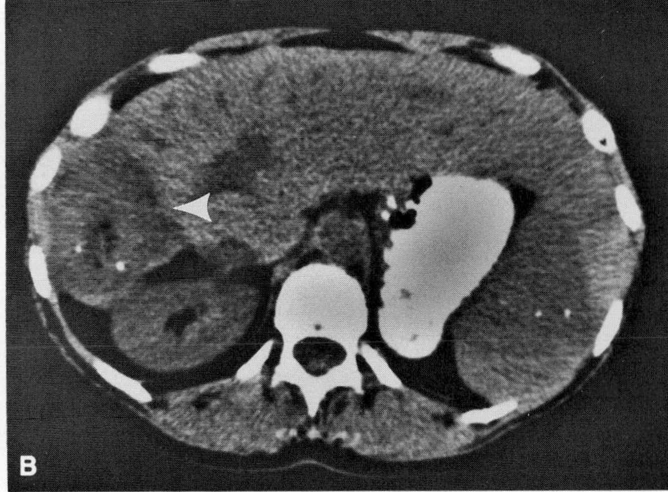

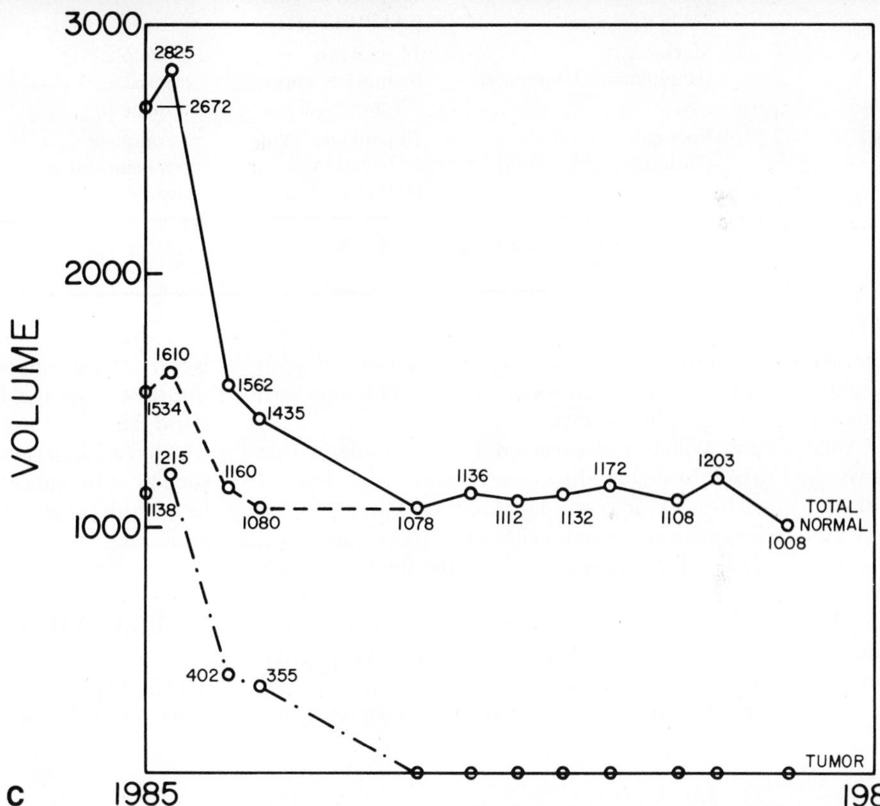

FIGURE 17–2. (**A**) Multifocal nodular lesions throughout the right and middle lobe with extension into the abdominal wall. Arrows demonstrate several lesions. (**B**) Following ^{131}I antiferritin therapy, the tumor is reduced to a single mass in the right pole before resection. (**C**) Tumor volumetrics demonstrating reduction in tumor volume, retention of normal volume, and total liver volume and prolonged disease-free remission, which is continuing.

TOXICITY

From the presently applied radiolabeled antibodies, hematologic toxicity remains as the single major toxicity. There are already protocols using marrow transplant and escalating radiolabeled antibodies in Hodgkin's and non-Hodgkin's lymphomas.[44,57] Marrow replacement has unequivocally allowed for dose escalation.[44,57] The second organ for toxicity has not as yet been identified.

PHYSICS

The approaches to measuring dose distribution have varied from the historical and useful Medical Internal Radiation Dosimetry (MIRD) committee calculations to computed tomography (CT) reconstruction and dose deposition, by scan in combination, to quantitative single photon emission computed tomography (SPECT) and, finally microthermoluminescent dosimeters (TLDs).[23,26,57] It is generally agreed that tumor dose rates are presently low and total doses are low as well. Thus, why do the tumors remit?

TUMOR RESPONSE AND RADIOBIOLOGY

Classically it has been taught that external radiation of 4000 cGy in 4 weeks for Hodgkin's disease, 5000 cGy in 5 weeks for microscopic foci in the neck, and 6000 cGy to 7000 cGy for early head and neck lesions are the dose requirements for conventional cancers. Yet there are remarkable differences between external radiation and the radiation of radioimmunoglobulin

TABLE 17–2
*Clinical Results of Radioimmunoglobulin Trials**

INVESTIGATOR	PATIENTS	RESULTS	SPECIAL FEATURES
DeNardo (University of California—Davis)	18 patients; non-Hodgkin's ^{131}I Lym-1 5 patients; chronic lymphatic leukemia	80% partial remission	60 mCi (2–3 wk) 6 treatments
Bernstein (University of Washington—Seattle)	4 patients; non-Hodgkin's ^{131}I Pan-B	4 complete remissions	Dose escalation 480 mCi; 2 relapses
Royston (University of California—San Diego)	2 patients	1 partial remission	1 anti-ID bond in circulation
Hale† (University of Cambridge)	2 patients; IgG, human chimera, CAMPATH-IH	2 partial remissions	Response to genetic-engineered antibody
Markoe (Hahnemann University)	14 patients; high-grade glioma, ^{125}I anti-e.g.f.	1 complete remission; 1 partial remission	Intraarterial antibody internalized
Epenetos (University of London)	25 patients; ^{90}Y PALP, AUA-1 HMFG-1	2 complete remissions; 3 ascites, cleared	Free ^{90}Y occurs

**Recent references in text data, updated as of 7/89.*
**Nonradioactive.*

treatment. The continuous depreciating low dose rate radiation without a period of no ionization is a new form of radiation with its own radiobiologic phenomena.

Dillehay and Williams constructed a ^{137}Cs irradiator that allows water to be infused to reduce dose rates and total doses of radiation, much like the radioimmunoglobulins. These preliminary studies demonstrate not only cell kill but, more important, a shift in the cell cycle to G_2 and M where the final doses of a protracted radiation actually led to tumor cell destruction. To date the use of doxorubicin (Adriamycin) also enhances the cellular shift to G_2 and M, thus amplifying the cellular population that is sensitized.

As the technology of radiolabeled antibodies presently exists, there are antibodies with powerful β-emitters (^{90}Y) in which the dose response is sufficient to anticipate tumor remission (Hodgkin's and non-Hodgkin's disease) and other tumors in which combination therapy will enhance tumor destructiveness such as in hepatocellular cancer. The next problem that needs to be addressed is how to treat sequentially with radiolabeled antibodies.

ANTI-ANTIBODIES

The first approach to solving the need for repeated administrations of radiolabeled antibodies was to use polyclonal antibodies

TABLE 17–3
Isotopes for Radioimmunoglobulin Treatment

ISOTOPE	ENERGY	HALF-LIFE	ADVANTAGES	DISADVANTAGES
^{131}I*	0.183 MeV	192 h	Scan, treat 0.9 mm range	Dehalogenation; monoclonal, short range
^{90}Y*	0.937 MeV	64 h	5.9 mm range	Need ^{111}In pretreatment evaluation
^{186}Re*	0.35 MeV	91 h	Scan, treat 1.6 mm range	Purification
^{67}Cu†	0.39 MeV	62 h	Scan, treat 2 mm range	Purification
^{212}Bi†	0.6 MeV	60 min	Compartmental treatment: perianal or peritoneal	Short range, 40–80 μ

** Used in clinical trials.*
† Restricted to laboratory studies.

derived from different species, thereby avoiding specific antibody problems (rabbit, pig, baboon, and horse antibodies) (Fig. 17-2).[39,40] All antibodies chosen had at least 3-day tumor effect half-lives. Thus, if patients developed anti-rabbit antibodies, administering porcine antibodies posed no problem. It was even possible to administer or recycle the same antibody if a radioimmunoassay showed no anti-antibody when ^{131}I was the isotope because of the lack of significant danger from free ^{131}I.

In certain patients such as those with Hodgkin's disease and some with non-Hodgkin's lymphoma, malignancy-induced immunosuppression also allowed several antibody administrations. However, in general oncology a solution is needed for patient produced human anti-mouse immunoglobulin (HAMA), resulting from radiolabeled monoclonal antibodies.[51] One of the more promising approaches to the HAMA problem is to use genetic engineering to create the human-murine chimeric antibodies that may not be immunogenic when injected into the human patient.[15,17,52] Already, clinical testing has begun, and two remissions have been reported using CAMPATH-IH, a human-murine engineered antibody that induces antibody-dependent cytotoxicity.[15] Whether anti-idiotypic antibodies will form against the Fab ends or just anti-antibody will occur requires further evaluation. However, with the work of these and other investigators chimeric antibodies have entered the clinical picture. None of the genetically engineered antibodies to date has been reported for use by treatment as a radiolabeled immunoconjugate. Another approach to the HAMA problem has been chemical modification of murine monoclonal antibodies. Experimental studies have indicated that this technique may have clinical feasibility. Chemical modification as a means to overcome HAMA is now being considered by RTOG.

CLINICAL RESULTS

RTOG was the first cooperative group to report clinical remissions in phase I and phase II studies in hepatoma (RTOG 79-28; 83-01), and Hodgkin' disease (RTOG 83-09).[40,57] In hepatoma, 41% partial remission and 7% complete remission with a median survival of 5 months in α-fetoprotein-positive (AFP+) patients, and 10 months in α-fetoprotein-negative (AFP−)patients was noted.[40] More recently, in a randomized phase III trial (RTOG 83-19), remission after failing the chemotherapy arm (AFP−), conversion to surgical resectability (AFP+, AFP−), and survival beyond 6 months (AFP−) have been restricted to patients treated with ^{131}I antiferritin.[39] No difference in survival between chemotherapy and ^{131}I antiferritin occurred in the AFP+ patients.

In Hodgkin's disease, the ^{131}I antiferritin in 37 patients that failed MOPP-ABVD or other chemotherapy led to a 40% partial remission rate with one complete remission. However, with a new ^{90}Y antiferritin, four of eight patients had complete remissions in the newest study.[57]

In intrahepatic cholangiocarcinoma, a 26.7% partial remission rate was recorded in 37 patients with ^{131}I anti-CEA.[56]

Partial remission in chronic lymphatic leukemia and non-Hodgkin's lymphoma has been reported in three patients using ^{131}Lym-I by DeNardo and associates.[5] Four complete remissions using very high doses of ^{131}I Pan B antibodies has been reported by Press and colleagues,[44] and dose escalation is continuing in an attempt to replace total-body irradiation.

Intraperitoneal iodinated and, more recently, ^{90}Y-labeled monoclonal antibodies have led to remission in ovarian cancer patients with minimal residual disease, as described by Epenetos and others.[6,7,16]

SUMMARY

Radiation oncologists, because of their specialized training in oncology and their knowledge of radiobiology and physics, have a unique opportunity to participate in systemic radiation therapy. Such participation requires knowledge of immunology, biology, cancer physiology, oncology, nuclear medicine, physics, radiobiology, and the integration of different cytotoxic agents. There seems to be little question that radiolabeled antibodies are even more realistically entrenched in oncology today and should be an active part of radiation oncology training.

Radiolabeled antibodies have had demonstrable efficacy in clinical applications. In most clinical applications, administration of radiolabeled antibodies does not require hospitalization and normally does not cause acute side effects. From previous studies some of the tumor physiologic and biologic restrictions that reduce radiolabeled antibody deposition are being overcome. Appreciation of dosimetry, chemical linkage of isotopes, isotopes of choice, genetic engineering or modification of antibodies, new systems of antibody isotope delivery, and new radiobiologic studies indicate the broad range of investigative and clinical opportunities for improved cancer therapy that currently exist.

REFERENCES

1. Brady LW, Markoe AM, Woo DV, et al: ^{125}I labeled anti-epidermal growth factor receptor-425 in the treatment of glioblastoma multiforme: A pilot study. In Frontiers in Radiation Therapy and Oncology, vol 24. Basel, S Karger, 24: 151–165, 1990
2. Butler VE Jr. Watson JF, Schmidt DR, et al: Reversal of the pharmacological and toxic effects of cardiac glycosides by specific antibodies. Pharmacol Rev 25:239, 1973
3. Davis DAL, O'Neil GJ: In vivo and in vitro effects of tumor specific antibodies with chlorambucil. Br J Cancer 28:285, 1983
4. Day ED, Planisek SA, Pressman D: Localization of radioiodinated rat fibrinogen in transplanted rat tumors. J Natl Cancer Inst 23:799, 1959
5. DeNardo SJ, DeNardo GL, O'Grady LF, et al: Pilot studies of radioimmunotherapy of B cell lymphoma and leukemia using I-131 lym-1 monoclonal antibody. Antib Immunoconjug Radiopharm 1:17, 1988
6. Epenetos AA, Britton KE, Mather S, et al: Targeting of iodine123 labelled tumor associated monoclonal antibodies to ovarian, breast, and gastrointestinal tumors. Lancet ii:999, 1982
7. Epenetos AA, Munro AJ, Stewart S et al: Antibody guided irradiation of ovarian cancer with imtraperitoneally administered radiolabeled monoclonal antibodies. J Clin Oncol 5:1890, 1987
8. Ettinger DS, Order SE, Wharam MD, et al: Phase I-II study of isotopic immunoglobulin therapy for primary liver cancer. Cancer Treat Rep 66:289, 1982
9. Ghose T, Blair AA: Antibody linked cytotoxic agents in the treatment of cancer: Current status and future projects. J Natl Cancer Inst 61:651, 1978
10. Ghose T, Norvell ST, Guclu A, et al: Immunotherapy of cancer with chlorambucil carrying antibody. Br Med J 3:495, 1972
11. Goldenberg DM: Targeting of cancer with radiolabeled antibodies: Prospects for imaging and therapy. Arch Pathol Lab Med 112:580, 1988
12. Goldenberg DM, Deland F, Kim, E, et al: Use of radiolabeled

antibodies to carcinoembryonic antigen for detection and localization of diverse cancers by external photoscanning. N Engl J Med 298:1384, 1978

13. Goldenberg DM, Gaffar SA, Bennett SS, et al: Experimental radioimmunotherapy of xenografted human colonic tumor (GW-39) producing carcinoembryonic antigen. Cancer Res 41:4354, 1981
14. Goldenberg DM, Preston DF, Primus FJ, et al: Photoscan localization of GW-39 tumors in hamsters using radiolabeled anticarcinoembryonic antigen immunoglobulin G. Cancer Res 34:1, 1974
15. Hale G, Clark MR, Marcus R, et al: Remission induction in nonHodgkin's lymphoma with reshaped human monoclonal antibody CAMPATH-IH. Lancet i:1394, 1988
16. Hammersmith Oncology Group and Imperial Cancer Research Fund: Antibody guided irradiation of malignant lesions: Three cases illustrating a new method of treatment. Lancet ii:1441, 1984
17. Hanna M: Presented at the 24th Annual San Francisco Cancer Symposium: Clinical experience with human monoclonal antibodies. San Diego, California, 1989
18. Jackson AP, Siddle K, Thompson RJ: Two site monoclonal antibody assays for human heart and brain type creatine kinase. Clin Chem 30:1157, 1984
19. Jain RK: Transport of molecules in the tumor interstitium: A review. Cancer Res 47:3039, 1987
20. Kohler G, Howe SC, Milstein C: Infusion between immunoglobulin nonsecreting myeloma cell lines. Eur J Immunol 6:292, 1976
21. Kohler G, Milstein C: Derivation of specific antibody producing tissue culture and tumor lines by cell fusion. Eur J Immunol 6:511, 1976
22. Larson SN, Carasquillo HJ, Krohn K, et al: Localization of 131-I labeled p^{97} specific Fab fragments in human melanoma as a basis for radiotherapy. J Clin Invest 72:2101, 1983
23. Leichner PK, Klein JL, Fishman EK, et al: Comparative tumor dose from 131-labeled polyclonal antiferritin, anti-AFP and anti-CEA in primary liver cancer. Cancer Drug Deliv 1:321, 1984
24. Leichner PK, Klein JL, Garrison JB, et al: Dosimetry of I-131 labeled antiferritin in hepatoma: A model for radioimmunoglobulin dosimetry. Int J Radiat Oncol Biol Phys 7:323, 1981
25. Leichner PK, Klein JL, Siegelman S, et al: Dosimetry of I-131 labeled antiferritin in hepatoma: Specific activities in the tumor and liver. Cancer Treat Rep 67:647, 1983
26. Leichner PK, Yang NC, Frenkel TL, et al: Dosimetry and treatment planning for ^{90}Y labeled antiferritin in hepatoma. Int Radiat Oncol Biol Phys 14:1033, 1988
27. Mach JP, Carrel S, Forni M, et al: Tumor localization of radiolabeled antibodies against carcinoembryonic antigen in patients with carcinoma. N Engl J Med 303:5, 1980
28. Mach JP, Carrel S, Merenda C, et al: In vivo localization of radiolabelled antibodies to carcionembryonic antigen in human colon carcinoma grafted into nude mice. Nature 248:704, 1974
29. Macklis RM, Kinsey B., Kassis A, et al: Alpha particle radioimmunotherapy: Animal models and clinical prospects. Int J Radiat Oncol Biol Phys, 16:1377–1387, 1989
30. Mendelsohn J: Anti-epidermal growth factor in oat cell carcinoma. Proc NCI-EORTC, Amsterdam, The Netherlands, 1988
31. Miller RA, Maloney DG, Wamke R, et al: Treatment of B-cell lymphoma with monoclonal anti-idiotype antibody. N Engl J Med 306:517, 1982
32. Moroz C, Bessler H, Lurie Y, et al: New monoclonal antibody enzymoassay for specific measurement of placental ferritin isotope in hematologic malignancies. Exp Hematol 15:258, 1987
33. Msirikale JS, Klein JL, Schroeder J, et al: Radiation enhancement of radiolabeled antibody deposition in tumors. Int Radiat Oncol Biol Phys 13:1839, 1987
34. Order SE: The history and progress of serologic immunotherapy and radiodiagnosis. Radiology 2:219, 1976
35. Order SE: Monoclonal antibodies: Potential role in radiation therapy and oncology. Int J Radiat Oncol Biol Phys 8:1193, 1981
36. Order SE: Radioimmunoglobulin therapy of cancer. Compr Ther 10:9, 1984
37. Order SE, Donahue V, Knapp R: Immunotherapy of ovarian carcinoma: An experimental model. Cancer 3:573, 1973
38. Order SE, Kirkman R, Knapp R: Serologic immunotherapy: Results and probable mechanism of action. Cancer 34:175, 1974
39. Order SE, Pajak T, Klein JL, et al: A randomized prospective trial in nonresectable hepatoma comparing adriamycin and 5-fluorouracil + 131-I antiferritin: An RTOG study. Int J Radiat Oncol Biol Phys 21:953–964, 1991
40. Order SE, Stillwagon GB, Klein JL, et al, Iodine 131 antiferritin, a new treatment modality in hepatoma: A Radiation Therapy Oncology Group Study. J Clin Oncol 3:1573, 1985
41. Order SE, Vriesendorp HM, Klein JL, et al: A phase I study of ^{90}Yttrium antiferritin: Dose escalation and tumor dose. Antib Immunoconjug Radiopharm 1:163, 1988
42. Ott RJ, Grey LJ, Zivanovic MA, et al: The limitations of the dual radionuclide subtraction technique of tumors by radioiodine labelled antibodies. Br J Radiol 56:101, 1983
43. Pettit WA, Deland FH, Bennet SJ, et al: Radiolabeling of affinity purified goat anticarcinoembryonic antigen immunoglobulin G with technetium-99M. Cancer Res 40:3043, 1980
44. Press O, Eary J, Badger C, et al: High dose radioimmunotherapy of B-cell lymphomas. In Frontiers in Radiation Therapy and Oncology, vol 24. Basel, S Karger, 24:204–213, 1990
45. Roitt I: Essential Immunology, 3rd ed. Oxford, Blackwell Scientific Publications, 1977
46. Rostock RA, Klein JL, Kopher K, et al: Variables affecting the tumor localization of I-131 antiferritin in experimental hepatoma. Am J Clin Oncol 6:9, 1984
47. Rostock RA, Klein JL, Leichner PK, et al: Selective tumor localization in experimental hepatoma by radiolabeled antiferritin antibody. Int J Radiat Oncol Biol Phys 9:1345, 1983
48. Rostock RA, Klein JL, Leichner PK, et al: Distribution of and physiologic facts that effect I-131 antiferritin tumor localization in experimental hepatoma. Int J Radiat Oncol Biol Phys 10:1135, 1984
49. Royston I, Halpren SE, Dillman RD, et al: Radiolabeling of monoclonal antitumor antibodies: Comparison of ^{125}I and ^{111}In anti-CEA with GA-^{67}in a nude mouse human colon tumor model. Cancer Res 23:953, 1982
50. Sands H: Radioimmunoconjugates: An overview of problems and promises. Antib Immunoconjug Radiopharm 1:213, 1988
51. Schroff RW, Beatty SM, Foon KA: Human anti-murine immunoglobulin responses in patients receiving monoclonal antibody therapy. Cancer Res 45:879, 1985
52. Shaw DR, Kazaeli MB, LoBuglio AF: Mouse/human chimeric antibodies to a tumor associated antigen: Biologic activity of the four human IgG subclasses. J Natl Cancer Inst 80:1553, 1988
53. Sitzmann JV, Order SE, Klein JL, et al: Conversion by new treatment modalities of nonresectable hepatocellular cancer. J Clin Oncol 5:1655, 1987
54. Spar IL, Bale WF, Marrack D, et al: ^{131}I labeled antibodies to human fibrinogen: Diagnostic studies and therapeutic trials. Cancer 30:865, 1967
55. Stickney DR, Slater JB, Kirk GA, et al: Bifunctional antibody: ZCE/CHH Indium^{111} BLEDTA-IV clinical imaging in colorectal cancer. Antib Immunoconjug Radiopharm, 2:1–13, 1989
56. Stillwagon GB, Order SE, Klein JL, et al: Multimodality treatment of primary nonresectable cholangiocarcinoma with ^{131}I anti-CEA: A Radiation Therapy Oncology Group Study. Int Radiat Oncol Biol Phys 13:687, 1987
57. Vriesendorp HM, Herpst JM, Leichner PK, et al: Polyclonal ^{90}Y labeled antiferritin for refractory Hodgkin's disease. Int J Radiat Oncol Biol Phys, 17:815–821, 1989
58. Wesels BE, Griffith MH: Miniature thermoluminscent dosimeter absorbed dose measurements in tumor phantom models. J Nucl Med 27:1308, 1986

18

○ ○ ○ • • •

Chemical Modifiers of Radiation

Todd H. Wasserman
Morton M. Kligerman

Irradiation is a physical event that damages cells through biochemical mechanisms. The physical effects of radiation are independent of pharmacology and physiology and modifiable through electronics and physics, but they are nonselective regarding tumor and normal tissue. The biochemical effects depend on cellular physiology (oxygen, cell cycle), may be modifiable through biochemical additives (sensitizers, protectors), and may be selective regarding tumor and normal tissue.

Because an understanding of radiation biochemistry has developed, it has been possible to study drug compounds that may modify the initial radiochemical event. Also, certain physiologic means such as hyperbaric oxygen or blood flow restriction were also developed to modify radiation response through radiochemical processes.

Following the partial success of certain hyperbaric oxygen clinical trials, an effort was made to develop chemical agents that would mimic oxygen in their sensitization of hypoxic cells.[1,76] A large series of compounds was identified with such properties, and several of these have entered clinical trials.[6,7,18,98]

Misonidazole, the first compound to receive widespread clinical testing, proved to be too toxic to be used in adequate doses for clinically relevant sensitization. Newer nitroimidazole analogues that are excluded from the central nervous system promise to allow higher drug doses and potentially useful sensitization. Other newer nonnitroimidazole compounds are also under development.

Other methods of differential chemical sensitization, such as incorporation of pyrimidine analogues into DNA in rapidly dividing tumors, modification of naturally occurring radioprotectors, and interference with repair of certain kinds of radiation injury, also are receiving extensive laboratory evaluation and may enter clinical evaluation.

Differential radioprotection (rather than sensitization) also appears to be promising because of the further understanding of radiochemical events and because of the development of highly hydrophilic protective compounds that are now in clinical testing. Radioprotection can be achieved through various methods, including restriction of blood flow and the use of sulfhydryl-containing compounds that modify the initial radiochemical events. To be successful in tumor therapy, such compounds must be selective in protecting normal tissues. One class of compounds, the thiophosphates, shows differential protection of tumor tissue compared with normal tissue. After extensive animal testing, one of these compounds, WR-2721, is in clinical trials.

RADIOSENSITIZERS

Rationale for the Development of Chemical Modifiers of Radiation

Local tumor failure is the cause of 40% to 60% of cancer deaths and may be present in 60% to 80% of other cancer patients at the time of death. If adjuvant chemotherapy or other systemic therapy increases overall survival, greater local tumor control will be required. As future treatments involve less disfiguring and radical surgery, local tumor control must also improve.

The following is the rationale for clinical trials of hypoxic cell sensitizers:

Clinical need for improved local tumor control
Presence of hypoxic portions of clinical tumors
Radiobiologic knowledge of the oxygen effect
Radiochemical knowledge of compounds with electron affinity
Radiobiologic proof of efficacy *in vitro* and *in vivo* of hypoxic cell sensitizers
Clinical results of improved tumor control with hyperbaric oxygen (cervix,lung, head, and neck) and blood transfusions (cervix, head, and neck)

Use of an effective radiosensitizer or protector would be expected to improve local control probability without a parallel increase in treatment morbidity. Because there are data on many tumors for which higher radiation doses increase the probability of local control due to more killing of malignant cells, any process that enhances tumor cell kill for a given radiation dose (sensitization) or decreases the relative amount of normal tissue injury (protection) could have a significant therapeutic benefit.

The presence of hypoxic portions in human tumors has been shown.[104] Extensive radiobiologic knowledge has been achieved of the oxygen effect and of compounds, including the nitroimidazoles, with high electron affinity mimicking oxygen in the radiobiologic effect. There is radiobiologic proof of the efficacy of the nitroimidazoles, specifically misonidazole, *in vitro* and *in vivo* under multiple experimental conditions.[6,7,18,98] The clinical results of improved local tumor control with hyperbaric oxygen in cervix, lung, and head and neck cancers[47,48] and the improved local tumor control with blood transfusions and maintaining of hemoglobin levels in patients with cervical and head and neck cancer lend indirect evidence to the problem of hypoxia in clinical cancer radiation treatments.[34,49,80]

The Oxygen Effect

The recognition that oxygen has a major effect on radiosensitivity has led to extensive biologic investigations of the potential relevance of this phenomenon in tumor therapy.[43] Numerous pathologic studies revealed the presence of necrotic zones in human tumors, and extensive animal testing has proven the presence of 1% to 30% hypoxic cells in most solid tumors.[28] Cells in rapidly growing tumors become deprived of oxygen through abnormal tumor blood supply and rapid tumor cell growth as opposed to capillary proliferation. Limitations in oxygen diffusion compound this problem and lead to the presence of hypoxic cells. The survival curves for oxygenated and hypoxic cells *in vitro* and *in vivo* yield a slope ratio, with an oxygen enhancement ratio (OER) for most tissues of 2.5 to 3.0. The postulated mechanism for radioresistance of hypoxic cells is that free radical formation (caused by the ionization effect of radiation) is less effective in inducing DNA damage, because without oxygen the free radical forms are very unstable. Cells that are sufficiently anoxic as to not be clonogenic are not of concern. Cells that are relatively hypoxic so as to be radioresistent, however, may continue to be clonogenic and lead to tumor repopulation.

Current hypoxic cell radiosensitizers are designed to replace oxygen in hypoxic cells at the time of radiation to yield increased cell kill. Because hypoxic cell sensitizers diffuse readily through the tumor and are not consumed by cells closer to the vascular support system, they reach the central tumor cells that are usually hypoxic.

If the tumor or cells that started out hypoxic remained so throughout treatment, after the first log of cells was killed the remaining 10% of the initial cell population would be hypoxic and resistant to irradiation. Animal studies have shown that within a few hours of a single radiation dose the percentage of hypoxic cells is similar to that before irradiation.[46] Because reoxygenation occurs after each fraction of radiation, radiation would be best exploited using a treatment scheme with more, rather than fewer, fractions. It may be that reoxygenation with fractionated radiation therapy overcomes the hypoxic cell problem of radioresistance.[36] However, if this is not so, hypoxic cell radiosensitizers are needed.

Many clinical trials using hyperbaric oxygen or radiosensitizers used few radiation fractions. Thus the benefit of reoxygenation is decreased. It is therefore not possible to compare accurately the efficacy of sensitized radiation therapy with standard fractionated radiation when the treatment scheme used with the sensitizer used different fractionation.

Hyperbaric Oxygen

Oxygen was the first radiation sensitizer used. The addition of oxygen in the form of increased ambient pressure causes further oxygen solution in the blood and potential penetration into the tumor. The sensitization of animal and most human tumors is variable because of the physiologic changes that exposure to hyperbaric oxygen causes in tumor blood flow. The clinical trials of hyperbaric oxygen were cumbersome, and in most trials only a few fractions of radiation were used. Yet these randomized clinical trials (radiation ± hyperbaric oxygen) showed positive results in head and neck, cervix, and lung cancer.[48,118] Henk[47] summarized the difficulties with interpretation of the results of the hyperbaric oxygen trials. The end point of the trials should emphasize local control and not survival because the purpose was to augment the efficacy of radiation therapy (local treatment). Normal tissue injury appeared to be increased.

Hypoxic Cell Radiosensitizer Compounds

Currently at least five classes of compounds have potential for differential sensitization of tumor rather than normal tissue. The first group of hypoxic cell sensitizers sufficiently nontoxic for use *in vivo* which sensitized hypoxic mammalian cells were the nitroimidazoles.

In 1974, the first of these compounds, metronidazole, entered clinical trial. In its phase I trial, metronidazole, a 5-nitroimidazole, produced nausea and vomiting in patients as its dose-limiting toxicity.[106] Later studies showed that neurologic toxicity reactions, particularly central neuropathy, could occur.[38] This drug was tested in a randomized trial for treatment of malignant gliomas.[105] Because of dose-limiting neurotoxicity, metronidazole was used only in nine doses in a hypofractionation radiation schema. Patients who received metronidazole had a statistically superior median survival compared with those not receiving the drug. However, the group receiving sensitizer plus radiation had a survival rate equivalent to that of patients given standard fractionated radiation; thus the clinical value of this effect was not established. The therapeutic benefit of a sensitizer must be evaluated using standard radiation fractionation so that it can be shown that hypoxia *per se* is a cause of tumor resistance during conventionally fractionated radiation treatment.

Other nitroimidazoles, particularly misonidazole, have received extensive clinical testing throughout the world.[76] Because the earlier compounds clinically tested were highly toxic to the peripheral nervous system and even the central nervous system, intensive synthesis work has been done in the laboratory and clinical testing has been carried out to develop less neurotoxic compounds.

Extensive chemical, biologic, toxicologic, and pharmacologic data have preceded the clinical trials to be described.[6,7,18,98] They have involved principally, the four 2-nitroimidazole compounds shown in Figure 18-1.

In the United States, evaluation of misonidazole was begun in 1977; phase III evaluation was completed 7 years later. Subsequent assessment of two analogues in phase I trial, desmethylmisonidazole and SR-2508, has occurred. The phase I trials were designed to study the pharmacology and short-term toxicity, both qualitative and quantitative, and give some information about tumor clearance. Efficacy was not a goal of these trials.[82] The phase II trials were designed to established more

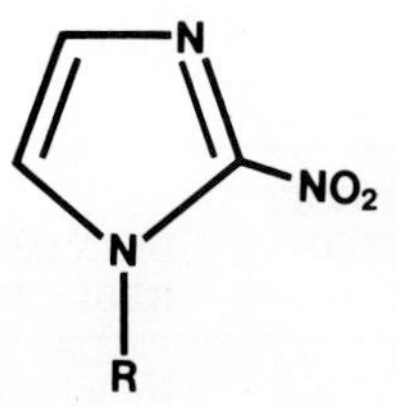

Compound	R	Mol Wt	Partition Coeff (P)
MISO	$CH_2CH(OH)CH_2OMe$	201	0.43
DMM	$CH_2CH(OH)CH_2OH$	187	0.13
Etanidazole (SR-2508)	$CH_2CONHCH_2CH_2OH$	214	0.046
Pimonidazole (RO-03-8799)	$CH_2CH(OH)CH_2N$ (piperidine ring)	291	8.5

FIGURE 18–1. Structure of four nitroimidazole drugs tested in clinical trials and the partition coefficient of each. The partition coefficient is a reflection of lipid solubility.

information regarding toxicity, tumor clearance, and tumor-free interval. Because of the already moderate to high level of effectiveness of irradiation with regard to these end points, it is necessary for randomized phase III trials that are controlled for various prognostic factors by stratification and large numbers of patients to determine the efficacy of the hypoxic cell sensitizer in terms of tumor clearance rate, tumor-free interval, and overall effect on survival.[116,117]

The nitroimidazoles are also undergoing increasing laboratory and early clinical investigation as chemotherapy sensitizers[93]; this trend is discussed briefly in the following text, but more information is available elsewhere.[6,7,18,98] The problem of dose-limiting neurotoxicity of misonidazole is not a factor in its intermittent use as a chemosensitizer.

Misonidazole Phase I Trials

It has been demonstrated in the laboratory that 2-nitroimidazoles are more efficient than 5-nitroimidazoles.[2] The change in position of the nitro group increases the electron affinity of the compound, an important determinant in its ability to act as a hypoxic cell sensitizer.[2]

Misonidazole first underwent phase I trials in the United States and England.[8,33,77,89,114] It was used as an oral preparation, given 4 hours before radiation therapy. The general findings of these trials are as follows:

1. The single-dose maximum tolerated dose (MTD) was 4 g to 5 g/m^2 because of nausea and vomiting.
2. The multiple-dose MTD was approximately 10 g to 12 g/m^2. Peripheral neuropathy occurred in approximately 40% to 50% of patients at this dose, and was characterized by sensory dysesthesia and paresthesia with very occasional motor weakness. This could be debilitating and long-lasting, particularly with a higher grade of toxicity.[77,103] Central neuropathy characterized by confusion occurred in approximately 10% of patients as well as ototoxicity with mild hearing loss. The MTD was not dependent on dose schedule, and various dose sizes were given over schedules ranging from 3 to 7 weeks.[114]
3. Misonidazole was well absorbed orally. The estimated bioavailability was 80% to 100%.[89]
4. The drug penetrated well into tumors. The tumor concentration near the necrotic center was approximately 70% to 80% that of the plasma level.[3,29]
5. Misonidazole had a prolonged terminal half-life of 13 hours after oral administration and 8 to 9 hours after intravenous administration. A patient's drug exposure per dose of drug could be defined by calculating the area under the curve of plasma concentration over time. Patients with neurotoxicity generally had a higher area under the curve.[33,103]
6. Approximately 10% of the parent compound was excreted unchanged in the urine. An additional 20% of the drug was excreted as the demethylated compound, desmethylmisonidazole (DMM). This metabolite was found in the plasma when high-performance liquid chromatography was used.[114] Because it is more water-soluble than misonidazole, DMM was more rapidly cleared, producing a lower drug exposure for a given dose, which led to its use in later clinical trials.
7. Phenytoin (Dilantin) and dexamethasone decreased the incidence of neuropathy.[40,109,115] It is believed that the phenytoin effect was a result of induction of hepatic enzymes that facilitated misonidazole metabolism to DMM. The mechanism of action of dexamethasone is not known, but it is not pharmacologic. It appears that higher doses of misonidazole can be given if concomitant dexamethasone is used.[99]

Misonidazole Phase III Trials

Before the conduct of phase III trials with misonidazole, the RTOG did a series of limited phase II trials, which will not be discussed but have been reported elsewhere.[78,116]

The mean 4- to 6-hour serum levels varied with the dose in grams per square meter. A dose of 2.5 g/m^2 was required to achieve between 80 μg and 90 μg/ml. With tumor concentrations of 50% to 70% of this, the tumor sensitizer levels were probably 45 μg to 60 μg/g at the maximal dose used in these trials. Most of the trials were carried out at doses below 2.5 g/m^2.

The seven sites studied in the phase III trials are given in Table 18-1. Two of the trials (gliomas and head and neck cancers) used misonidazole with only some of the fractions. The follow-up in the glioma trial[69,70] is longer than in the other trials and the survival time is short, concluding that the treatments were equal and the results were null. The trial for head and neck cancers[35] showed no significant difference in the initial complete response rate, although a trend exists toward a slightly higher duration of complete response in the misonidazole arm. The trials in advanced lung cancer[94,95] show no significant differences (a null result), and the same is true in cervical cancer.[60,73]

Between 1979 and 1985, the Danish Head and Neck Cancer Study (DAHANCA) did a double-blind randomized study evaluating the effect of misonidazole given in two drug schedules with split-course radiation in the treatment of carcinoma of the larynx and pharynx. Patients were stratified according to tumor site (larynx *versus* pharynx), nodal status, and institution. The total misonidazole dose was 11 g/m^2. The study was carried out on 626 patients. Overall, the misonidazole-treated group did not have significantly better local control than the placebo group. Statistically better locoregional control was found in females than in males and in pharynx carcinomas in the misonidazole group *versus* the placebo group. The pretreatment

TABLE 18–1
RTOG Phase III Misonidazole Trials

STUDY NO.	SITE	DATES OPENED	DATES CLOSED	TOTAL CASE ACCESSION*	MISO DOSE/ FRACTION g/m²	PRELIMINARY RESULTS	REFERENCE
79–15	Head and neck	8/79	3/83	304	2.0	No advantage	35
79–16	Brain metastasis	8/79	7/83	848	1 OR 2	No advantage	75
79–17	Lung-definitive Rx	9/79	2/83	268	0.4	No advantage	94
79–18	Glioma	10/79	1/83	312	2.5	No advantage	69,70
79–25	Lung-palliative	1/80	7/83	116	1.75	No advantage	95
80–03	Hepatic metastasis	5/80	7/83	214	1.5	No advantage	61
80–05	Cervix	8/80	11/84	119	0.4	No advantage	60
Total				2181			

** Only 50% of the patients received misonidazole.*

hemoglobin level was a prognostic parameter, and its effect was apparently independent of tumor size, which was also a prognostic parameter. The hemoglobin level plus misonidazole had apparent additive prognostic effects; patients with high hemoglobin level who received misonidazole did best overall with a 40% 5-year locoregional control rate. The peripheral neuropathy rate for misonidazole was 26%, consistent with the RTOG studies. The current DAHANCA protocol is testing nimorazole and blood transfusions in the same population looking for even greater improvements in locoregional control.[74]

The phase III trials with misonidazole have generally yielded only minimal toxicities because of control of total drug dose. Most of the drug-related neuropathies were grade 1 or grade 2, with the overall incidence of serious toxicity reactions being very low. Some trials were carried out with very low doses of misonidazole given with each radiation fraction, a small number of radiation fractions given with higher misonidazole doses, or, in the two trials mentioned, with moderately high misonidazole doses given with only a small proportion of the radiation fractions. At best, the misonidazole effect was too diluted or the dose was too low in most of these trials. In the few trials using higher doses of misonidazole, a small number of fractions were involved, and probably insufficient reoxygenation occurred for optimal response in conjunction with the sensitizer.

Use of misonidazole has not produced any therapeutic advantage. The problem with using an unusual fractionation schema has been discussed. The *oxygen enhancement ratio* is the ratio of the dose of radiation necessary to produce a given level of cell kill without oxygen compared with the dose of radiation needed to produce the same level of cell kill with oxygen. A *sensitizer enhancement ratio* (SER) is a similar ratio using a sensitizer rather than oxygen and can be calculated. Although initial predictions were that misonidazole doses of 1 g and 2 g/m² would yield an SER of 1.3 to 1.7, more recent animal data suggest that these predictions were too high.[8,9] Because tumor concentration is probably only 50% to 70% of plasma levels and SER is probably a linear function of concentration, the maximal doses used in these trials will give a ratio of 1.2 to 1.3.[9,68] The misonidazole doses and the expected SER based on more recent animal data from Brown[9] are shown in Figure 18-2. Even if misonidazole is effective, it would be very unlikely to yield a statistically significant improvement, in a limited-size clinical trial, because of the small gain provided by the dose used.

The lack of positive clinical results with misonidazole does not mean that hypoxic cells are not important in the local control of advanced cancers treated with radiation or that a therapeutic gain could not be expected with an improved radiosensitizer. The 1.1 to 1.3 SER achieved with misonidazole is probably not measurable clinically in terms of benefit when one considers that tumors contain anywhere from 1% to 30% hypoxic cells. It is also likely that some of these tumor sites or histologies may not fail conventional radiation therapy because of hypoxic cells.

Desmethylmisonidazole Phase I Trial

Because neuropathy was the dose-limiting toxicity reaction with misonidazole, it became desirable to produce a drug that would not cross into the neural tissue. Also, because a higher total drug exposure as measured by the area under the plasma curve correlated with toxicity, it was desired to have a drug with more rapid excretion after reaching a rapid peak level. A less lipid-soluble drug would achieve this and, because of its higher water

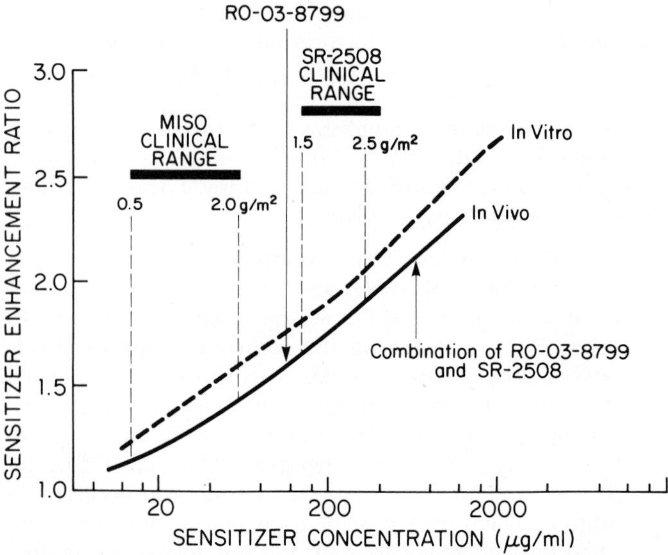

FIGURE 18–2. Graph showing the expected sensitizer enhancement ratio (SER) relative to the sensitizer in concentration of μg/ml. It is on a linear log scale. The clinical range of misonidazole from 0.5 g to 2.0 g/m² results in an SER of 1.1 to 1.3. The clinical range of SR-2508 from 1.5 g to 2.5 g/m² results in an SER of 1.5 to 2.0. (Modified from Brown JM: Int J Radiat Oncol Biol Phys 10:425, 1984)

solubility, would also provide for an intravenous preparation and eliminate the variables of oral absorption. Figure 18-1 shows the two principal analogues that were developed: desmethylmisonidazole (DMM) and SR-2508. Both have a lower partition coefficient and thus less lipid solubility.[8,9]

DMM, an endogenous metabolite of misonidazole and the principal product excreted in human urine, was the next compound to enter clinical trial. The phase I trial of intravenous DMM gave the following results[26,112]:

Peripheral neurotoxicity was the dose-limiting toxicity and was qualitatively similar to that of misonidazole. Serial nerve biopsies established qualitative pathologic changes and quantitative grading.[113] Unlike misonidazole, no documented cases of central neuropathy were found.

The total dose of DMM that produced 30% to 50% incidence of neuropathy was 13.5 g to 15.0 g/m^2. Assuming a bioavailability of 80% to 90% for oral misonidazole compared with 100% for intravenous DMM, the total dose of DMM delivered to produce an incidence of neuropathy similar to that of misonidazole was about 1.5 times that of misonidazole, close to the prediction in animals.

The pharmacokinetic parameters were as predicted (Table 18-2). Being more hydrophilic, DMM is excreted more rapidly than is misonidazole, and more of the parent compound is excreted unchanged in the urine. DMM achieved a reasonable tumor-plasma ratio of approximately 85%.

DMM was not sufficiently better than misonidazole, so further trials were not planned.

SR-2508 (Etanidazole) Clinical Trials

After preclinical chemical, biologic, toxicologic, and pharmacologic data were obtained, a rationally synthesized sensitizer with less lipid solubility and equal radiosensitizing efficiency, SR-2508, a 2-nitroimidazole analogue of misonidazole (see Fig. 18-1), entered into clinical trial. Animal data predicted less neurotoxicity than with misonidazole or DMM.[8,110] This phase I trial was done at five medical centers under the auspices of the Radiation Therapy Oncology Group (RTOG).[23,25] SR-2508 was given intravenously for 10 minutes in incremental doses three times per week for 3 weeks (or nine doses) on the short schedule,[25] and for three to four times per week for 5 to 6 weeks (or 15 to 24 doses) on the long schedule.[23] Radiation was given 30 minutes after drug administration. The highest single dose given, 3.7 g/m^2, was not dose-limiting.

As predicted, pharmacologic comparison (see Table 18-2) shows a significant increase in the percentage of urine excretion and a decrease in the β-half-life while maintaining a high plasma level. Blood levels obtained at 30 minutes for 2 g/m^2 have a mean of 100 μg/ml and for 3 g/m^2 a mean of 191 μg/ml. Tumor levels were generally 65% of plasma levels at 20 to 30 minutes postinfusion. Higher tumor levels have been seen in the bladder. The principal dose-limiting toxicity reaction is a transient, peripheral sensory neuropathy with no central neuropathy, ototoxicity, or myopathy. The total drug dose of SR-2508 is not significantly predictive for toxicity at doses above 21 g/m^2. However, the total area under the plasma pharmacology curve is very predictive: no toxicity reactions with area under curve below 38 mM × hr in 23 patients; 100% toxicity reactions in nine patients with area under curve above 39 mM × hr; and in four patients above 50 mM × hr, all having grade 2 neurotoxicity reactions. By monitoring the total area under curve and lengthening the time of drug administration, some amelioration of the incidence and grade of toxicity has been possible.

On the long dose schedule, total doses of SR-2508 as high as 40.8 g/m^2 have been achieved. Table 18-3 compares the incidence of neurotoxicity for the two SR-2508 dose schedules with those in the phase I DMM and misonidazole studies. SR-2508 has improved therapeutic ratio with 30 g/m^2 total dose tolerated in 5 weeks and 36 g to 40 g/m^2 in 6 weeks. A drug dose of 2 g/m^2 yields an SER of 1.5 to 1.7[9] (see Fig. 18-2), which could be achieved with 15 to 20 doses of drug and radiation, using an every-other-day drug schedule. SR-2508 is better than misonidazole for testing the efficacy of radiosensitizers with fractionated radiation therapy.

Following the completion of the phase I trial of SR-2508, the RTOG began a phase II/III trial in head and neck cancer (85-27).[59] In the phase II part of the trial, 33 patients were entered receiving conventional irradiation plus SR-2508 (2 g/m^2, three times per week, for a total of 17 doses). Patients received radiation therapy in a conventional manner (6600 cGy to 7400 cGy at 200 cGy/fraction, five fractions/week). Patients had unresectable stage III and IV head and neck cancers. The incidence of drug toxicity reactions in the first 33 patients was as expected, with a 24% grade I peripheral neuropathy, 6% grade II peripheral neuropathy, 21% grade I or grade II nausea and vomiting, 15% allergic reaction, and 9% reversible neutropenia.

Patients were then entered into the phase III part of the study and randomized to receive radiation with or without SR-2508. From June 1988 to August 1989, 224 patients were entered into the protocol, which continues patient entry to date. The drug toxicity continues to be as expected, with 22% grade I or II peripheral neuropathy (see Table 18-3), 26% nausea and vomiting, 14% allergy, and 13% reversible neutropenia. Serum pharmacology measured on 99 patients to date shows an average single dose area under the curve (AUC) of 2.56 ± 0.9 mm/hour.

Efficacy analysis has not yet been done on the study because patients are still being entered. Efficacy analysis in the phase II study[59] indicated a 58% initial complete response rate in 33 patients. Patients had advanced head and neck cancer with 61% Stage T4 and 49% Stage N3. The complete efficacy analysis for

TABLE 18–2
Pharmacokinetic Comparison of SR-2508, DMM, and Misonidazole (Normalized for a Dose of 1.0 g/m^2 [Mean Values])

	SR-2508	DMM	IV MISONIDAZOLE	ORAL MISONIDAZOLE
1-hr Blood-level (μg/ml)	45	41	48	30 (at 4–6 hr)
β-Half-life (hr)	5.4	6	9.3	13.8
Percentage urine recovery in 24 hr	71	62	23 (2/3 as DMM)	30 (2/3 as DMM)

TABLE 18–3
Incidence of Neuropathy Following Radiosensitizer Doses Greater than 9 g/m²

RADIOSENSITIZER	NO.	% PERIPHERAL NEUROPATHY	% PERIPHERAL NEUROPATHY GREATER THAN GRADE 1	% CENTRAL NEUROPATHY	% OTOTOXITY	DOSE RANGE (g/m^2)	MEAN TOTAL DOSE (g/m^2)
MISONIDAZOLE							
Phase I study	65	62	51	12	12	9–21	12
Phase II studies	559	25	13	4	5	11–15	12
Phase III studies	967	14	4	3	1	11–15	12
DESMETHYLMISONIDAZOLE							
Phase I study	90	47	16	0	4	9–19	12
SR-2508							
Phase I 3-wk schedule	31	29	13	0	0	22–32	27
Phase I 5- to 6-wk schedule	50	60	6	0	0	14–41	34
Phase III study	110	22	5	0	0	—	34

the phase III part of the study should be completed at the beginning of 1992.

Coleman and associates[24] have reported on the initial results of phase I trials with continuous infusion SR-2508 to take advantage of the oxygen-mimetic and preincubation effects of the drug. Patients were treated with brachytherapy and received a loading of 2 g/m^2 and continued drug dose for up to 48 hours. Patients have received a total of up to 15 g/m^2 in 48 hours with no toxicity. The steady state plasma concentration has been 50 μg to 70 μg/ml.

Other New Hypoxic Cell Radiosensitizers

The biologic studies of chemical manipulation of tissue oxygenation for therapeutic benefit involve the hypoxic cell radiosensitizers just discussed, oxygen carriers, calcium antagonists, drugs that shift the oxygen hemoglobin curve to the right and improve oxygen release in the tumors, and drugs that shift the oxygen hemoglobin disassociation curve to the left by using vasodilators.[15,45]

RO-03-8799

Another 2-nitroimidazole, RO-03-8799, has entered into phase I clinical trials in England. This compound is equal in radiosensitization to misonidazole in *in vitro* and *in vivo* experiments. It has a greater electron affinity than misonidazole, and its basic side chain leads to higher concentrations in areas of low pH, as may be found in tumors. Results from the clinical phase I pharmacology-toxicology studies show a short half-life of 5.1 hours and a peak plasma concentration equal to that of misonidazole, but a higher tumor-to-plasma ratio of 3.4 to 1. Unfortunately, toxicity reactions of malaise, disorientation, and other generalized symptoms limit the dose to 750 mg/m^2 given intravenously daily, up to 20 doses.[28] The dose-limiting toxicity of this compound is not apparently similar to the dose-limiting peripheral neurotoxicity for misonidazole. The clinical and preclinical advantages of R0-03-8799 over misonidazole are somewhat controversial.[82,97,120] R0-03-8799 is not available in the United States for clinical testing. In England, clinical trials evaluated the combination of SR-2508 and R0-03-8799.[5,32,51,71,72] It is possible that the clinical use of both compounds in an alternate daily schedule will allow high individual doses of each compound, without achieving the dose-limiting toxicity of either. The use of two compounds with similar efficacy, but non-cross-resistant toxicity, is a cornerstone of combination chemotherapy.

Pyrimidine Analogues

The initial clinical trials of the halogenated pyrimidine analogue, BUdR, when used intraarterially, yielded mixed results.[4,14,53] Currently, there has been a revival of interest in the use of halogenated pyrimidine analogues in sites where the normal tissue uptake is low and a relatively rapid tumor growth occurs. A phase I study of intravenous BUdR was carried out at the National Cancer Institute, and pharmacologic data suggested good bioavailability.[55,56] It is believed that high concentrations to prolong drug exposure of the tumor cells so that there will be a high incorporation into the DNA are necessary. This phase I study of BUdR led to two phase II trials in patients with malignant glioma.[79,85] Systemic toxicity reactions were limited to the bone marrow, and skin toxicity reactions were limited the duration of intravenous infusions of BUdR. Attention therefore turned to IUdR, particularly at the National Cancer Institute (NCI). A phase I study of intravenous IUdR shows less toxicity, especially to the skin, and higher drug levels with comparable incorporation into the tumor cells.[57] Clinical evaluation of IUdR will continue in several cooperative group trials and other trials including those at NCI.[54,108]

Perfluorochemicals

Perfluorocarbons are able to absorb a large amount of oxygen in high-oxygen environs and release oxygen when environmental oxygen is low. A mixture of perfluorochemicals, fluosol, has been used as an oxygen transport fluid clinically and preclinically. It acts not only to transport oxygen to tissues but to carry carbon dioxide away. It has been used clinically as an oxygen transport fluid after surgery in Japan and the United States. Limited single-dose clinical evaluations have been done. Because the perfluorochemical particles are small, they enhance circulation of poorly vascularized tumors as well as oxygen distribution. This may provide for improved effectiveness of irradiation and chemotherapy by increasing the local concentration of oxygen in the tumor. Animal studies have shown somewhat enhanced radiation effects of fluosol similar to that of increased oxygen.[37,96,101,102]

Early clinical evaluation of fluosol in head and neck cancer in conjunction with radiation therapy is in progress and has been reported.[84] A report of fluosol as an adjuvant to irradiation in the treatment of advanced tumors of the head and neck has recently been published.[62] The study accrued 46 patients in 4 years; 37 were evaluable. The patients were infused weekly with fluosol, breathing 100% oxygen for a minimum of 30 minutes before irradiation. Radiation doses ranged from 6600 cGy to 7500 cGy in daily fractions of 200 cGy. Patients received fluosol at 8 ml/kg, with a total dose of 40 ml/kg initially, and an escalation of the dose to a maximum of 56 ml/kg. Initial complete response rate was 76%, which is believed to be an improvement over historical controls. Fluosol toxicity reactions included allergic reaction to the test dose, elevated liver enzymes, and other minor reactions. A proposed phase III trial to test the effectiveness of fluosol in advanced head and neck cancer is under consideration.

Some authors have combined the effects of nitroimidazole hypoxic cell sensitizers with fluosol-DA/carbogen, hyperthermia, and radiation.[100] This area should develop over the next several years with compounds better designed for antitumor use, rather than as artificial blood.[42]

Thiol Depletors

The oxygen effect on radiation sensitivity is modulated by the cellular nonprotein thiol pool. Glutathione (GSH) is the major intracellular non-protein-bound sulfhydryl in most mammalian cells. It thus plays an important role in determining the intrinsic radiosensitivity of cells. Glutathione participates as an electron donor in a wide range of cellular reactions and can protect against radiation damage by donating a proton to radiation-induced radicals, thus competing with oxygen or oxygen-mimetic compounds, such as misonidazole, for fixation or repair of intracellular lesions. There has been recent experimental interest in increasing the efficiency of radiosensitizers by depleting the intracellular glutathione pool before irradiation. With greater knowledge of glutathione metabolism, several compounds have been identified that could influence glutathione pools. Diethylmaleate (DEM) is a compound that binds intracellular nonprotein sulfhydryl. Buthionine sulfoximine (BSO) is a specific inhibitor of glutathione synthesis which binds to the generating enzyme, preventing the formation of new glutathione. Increasing experimental data are developing with both compounds, effecting sensitizer efficacy and toxicity.[12,58,83,121]

It has not yet been established that nontoxic doses of buthionine sulfoximine can be given at a level at which glutathione depletion can produce a consistent and clinically significant enhancement of the radiosensitizing efficacy of sensitizers. More laboratory studies of combinations of thiol depleters and sensitizers are desirable.

Glutathione pools are also important in determining chemosensitivity.[44,86] Clinical trials of BSO plus melphalan chemotherapy have begun.

More laboratory evidence is needed of a differential effect of potentially lethal damage repair inhibitors between tumor and normal tissues before these compounds can enter clinical trials.[67,76]

Bioreductive Alkylating Agents

A new class of compounds is being developed as hypoxic cell toxins. SR-4233 (3-amino-1,2,4-benzotriazine 1,4-dioxide) is the lead compound in a series of benzotriazine di-*N*-oxides that exhibit high selective killing of hypoxic mammalian cells *in vitro*. The hypoxic specific cytotoxicity of SR-4233 apparently results from the bioreductive metabolism. This can enhance radiation-induced tumor cell kill when the drug is administered before or shortly after radiation.[122]

Use of bioreductive alkylating agents in conjunction with radiation therapy is based on the principle of enzymatic reduction to form an active alkylating species. The drug is preferentially metabolized and selectively toxic to hypoxic cells.[37,87] A group at Yale University[119] reported a randomized clinical trial of mitomycin-C in conjunction with radiation in head and neck cancer; 120 patients were entered and randomly assigned to receive or not receive mitomycin-C. There was an apparent increase in the actuarial disease-free survival rate at 5 years from 49% to 75% with mitomycin-C and in the local recurrence-free survival rate from 66% to 87%. No increased normal tissue reactions were seen.

Another alkylating compound, porfiromycin, may have greater differential effects.[87]

Other Techniques of Drug Delivery

Because of the known *in vivo* activity of misonidazole and other sensitizers and the clinical limitation of their usefulness when given orally or intravenously, other modes of more direct administration are being tried preclinically. The actions of misonidazole as a hypoxic cell sensitizer are concentration-dependent. Sealy and associates[90,91] injected solid misonidazole directly into tumors at high concentrations without evidence of significant local toxicity. Japanese researchers[52] have studied the role of local tumor injections of liquid misonidazole in conjunction with radiation. They also achieved high local tumors levels without apparent local toxicity.

Intraperitoneal administration of sensitizers has also been studied[41]; more work is needed before widespread clinical trials are possible.

Other Uses of Sensitizers

Chemosensitization

Use of hypoxic cell radiosensitizers with chemotherapeutic agents, primarily alkylating agents, has been studied extensively in the laboratory and is now in clinical trials.[13,93] Use of misonidazole with CCNU was evaluated in phase I and phase II trials in patients with glioma.[39] Other groups are engaged in sensititizer-chemotherapy clinical trials.[22,27] A randomized phase II trial by the Northern California Oncology Group[22] with melphalan *versus* melphalan and oral misonidazole in 85 patients with advanced lung cancer is reported. The melphalan-misonidazole group had a superior response rate with equivalent hematologic toxicity and a plasma concentration that was 25% higher than the group treated with melphalan alone. The concept of clinical chemosensitization needs further clinical evaluation.

Hypoxic Cell Markers

Metabolism selectively binds radiosensitizer compounds to the molecules of viable hypoxic cells. Sensitizers form adducts with cellular macromolecules that may be a specific marker or index of viable hypoxic cells.[16] With effective radiolabeling with ^{14}C (in the 2-carbon position), it is possible to confirm the presence of hypoxic cells in animal tumor systems with quantitative autoradiography. Work is under way on development of τ-emitter radioisotopes of the sensitizer adducts and imaging with single-photon emission tomography; use of sensitizers labeled with positron emitters in conjunction with positron emission tomography; and use of other radiolabels with other scanning techniques. Some early clinical data have been generated.[107] The implications of these scanning techniques for staging and evaluation for recurrence of cancer, provided that the techniques are sensitive and specific for hypoxic cells, are enormous.

An exciting by-product of the scientific development of hypoxic sensitizers is their use as markers of hypoxic tissue. The work at Washington University in St. Louis and the University of Washington in Seattle has confirmed fluoromisonidazole as a useful marker for hypoxic myocardium.[65,92] Binding of a hypoxic tracer would also be useful in cerebral ischemia and potential earlier tumor detection.[17,50,66,81]

Concluding Remarks About Radiosensitizers

The RTOG's clinical trials of radiosensitizers have met several objectives. RTOG has developed the methodology to test any drug from phase I to phase III trials. Three phase I trials have been conducted, and good pharmacology data have developed with the technique of high-performance liquid chromatography. All phase II and phase III misonidazole trials met their objectives with completed accrual and full toxicity and efficacy analyses completed and published. Although all the phase III trials seem to have null results, there were no negative results; that is, misonidazole did not adversely affect the end points compared with irradiation alone. The phase III trials with misonidazole established a framework and baseline data for analysis of future trials. These trials developed important data bases for defining the best subpopulations of patients to use in future clinical trials and established important factors regarding the end points of toxicity, pharmacology, and efficacy.

The misonidazole clinical trials promoted increased experimental interest in radiosensitizers, which has led to considerable growth of biologic data and knowledge.[11,76] They also promoted clinical investigation of the drug as a chemosensitizer without the problem of dose-limiting neurotoxicity and have led to development of use of these compounds as markers of hypoxic cells for scanning research.[16]

The clinical trials of the analogues have exploited pharmacologic differences with some improvements in toxicity reactions (see Table 18-3). If a good sensitizer can be found that could achieve desirable drug doses, then a series of efficacy trials for such a sensitizer would ensue. A good sensitizer is defined as one with an individual drug dose in g/m^2 that would yield a blood level in μg/ml and a tumor level in μg/ml (which, based on animal data, would yield a sensitizer enhancement ratio greater than or equal to 1.5) and a total drug dose in g/m^2 that yields minimal clinical significant toxicity after 15 or more doses. Data suggest that this is possible with SR-2508.

Phase II and phase III trials are ongoing in advanced cancers of the head and neck, bladder, and prostate. Further efficacy trials depend on analysis of these proposed trials. If SR-2508 cannot achieve adequate drug doses as just defined, attempts to modify toxicity reactions with dexamethasone, glutathione depletion, or other means could be studied.[11] Other drugs also will be developed for possible phase I clinical trials, including analysis of the British data on R0-03-8799. Possible combinations of sensitizers with nonoverlapping toxicities could be developed.[5,51,71] Other clinical trials will study different routes of administration, different classes of sensitizers, use with chemotherapy, and use as hypoxic cell markers. Potential use of markers to choose the patients or tumors with hypoxic cells, may yield more specific use.

The final chapter on the evaluation of hypoxic cell radiosensitizers has not been written.[10,19,20,21,30,31,63,64,76,110,111]

RADIOPROTECTORS

A strategy to increase the effectiveness of irradiation is to use compounds that are absorbed by normal tissue cells and to reduce their response to radiation without a significant or comparable reduction of the cytotoxic effect on tumor cells. The ideal radiation protector would be a stable, orally or intravenously administered compound without life-threatening or permanent tissue toxicity reactions. One radiation protector is 5-hydroxytryptamine (serotonin), which acts directly on the central nervous system in the hypothalamic region to inhibit corticosteroid production. This inhibition was found by Streffer[149] to reduce sensitivity to ionizing radiation. This chemical mediator also causes a reduction in intracellular oxygen, the most potent radiosensitizer.

Vitamin E,[143,146] vitamin C,[143] and β-carotene[142] protect cellular membrane lipids from the action of radiation-produced peroxy radicals by scavenging these radicals. The scavenging of the free hydroxy radical (OH •) is a common property of many radioprotectors, including alcohols[132] such as *N*-butinol and ethanol, sulfur-containing compounds such as dithiocarbamate and thiourea, and a class of compounds known as aminothiols. Aminothiols are the most promising clinical radioprotectors and are the main subject of this section.

In 1949, Patt[144] observed that rats given cysteine immediately before 800 cGy of whole-body radiation were significantly more resistant to the effects of radiation; lethality was reduced from 90% to 20%. Cysteine also reduced the degree of splenic atrophy and leukopenia. Cysteine pretreatment also decreases the cytotoxic effect of nitrogen mustard. Under the auspices of the US Army Medical Research and Development Command (Walter Reed = WR), a series of analogues of the aminothiol mercaptoethylamine (cysteamine) has been synthesized. Clinically, the most attractive of these is *S*-2-(3-aminopropylamino)-ethylphosphorothioic acid, or WR-2721.

Direct and Indirect Effects of Ionizing Radiation

The excitation and ionization of intracellular critical molecules occur as the initial event of the interaction of ionizing radiation with cells. This effect takes place between 10^{-17} and 10^{-10} seconds after exposure. An estimated 30% cellular inactivation results from the direct effect of radiation on macromolecules such as DNA and enzymes.[124] This direct action converts a critical molecule into a free radical that is inactivated by oxidation, which takes place in 10^{-9} to 10^{-8} seconds.

The direct action of ionizing radiation on intracellular water yields a series of highly reactive products. Cellular inactivation by indirect effect results from the interaction of these products with critical molecules. Chapman and Reuvers[124] point out that 60% of the effect of ionizing radiation results from the action of the free hydroxy radical, OH•, on target molecules, designated R. The free radicals of the critical molecules are rendered inoperative by oxidation by dissolved molecular oxygen.

Ward[156] indicated that strand breaks in DNA are caused by the elimination of a hydrogen atom from the C4 position on deoxyribose by the free hydroxy radical. The loss of the phosphate linkage results in the strand break.

Mechanism of Radiation Protection by Sulfhydryl Compounds

Sulfhydryl compounds protect cells from radiation damage by scavenging the products of irradiated water (equations 1 and 2), repairing critical molecules to their active form (equation 2) by the donation of a hydrogen atom to the free radical. Intracellular glutathione (GSH) is the naturally occurring radioprotector.

$$\cdot OH + GSH \rightarrow H_2O + GS\cdot \quad (1)$$

$$R\cdot + GSH \rightarrow RH + GS\cdot \quad (2)$$

(RH represents the reconstituted critical molecule.)

GSH is reduced to glutathione by hydrogen transfer from reduced nicotinamide adenine dinucleotide in the reversible reactions:

$$NADH \rightarrow NAD\cdot + H \quad (3)$$

$$GS\cdot + H \rightarrow GSH \quad (4)$$

The competition between glutathione and oxygen for combining with the free radical critical molecules overwhelmingly favors oxygen. Ward[156] believes that 10 μM of oxygen is reactively equal to the total intracellular concentration of 1 mM glutathione. He points out that the intracellular concentration of oxygen under normal atmospheric conditions is equal to 200 μM. Thus to have complete protection, sulfhydryl donors must be present in considerable excess of the intracellular oxygen concentration.

Within the cell, enzymatic removal of the more slowly reacting radiation products of water takes place.[124] Superoxide dismutase catalyzes the combination of negatively charged oxygen-free radicals and hydrogen to form hydrogen peroxide and oxygen. The hydrogen peroxide generated is reduced to water by the enzyme catalase or by intracellular peroxidases.

The Radioprotector WR-2721

The analogues of cysteamine vary in the length of the carbon chain between the sulfhydryl group and the active amino group. Doherty and co-workers[127] believed that the most effective structure was one in which the functional amino group was separated from the available sulfhydryl moiety by a 3-carbon chain. Recently, however, it has been found that in some compounds, a 2-carbon chain may be ideal.[123]

Of the analogues of mercaptoethylamine (cysteamine) that have been prepared, *S*-2-(3-aminopropylamino)-ethylphosphorothioic acid (WR-2721) was found by Yuhas and Storer[161] to protect mice against lethality with a dose-reduction factor (DRF) of 2.6 to 2.72. They also found that mammary tumors in mice irradiated 15 minutes after the intraperitoneal injection of WR-2721 were only slightly more resistant to irradiation, whereas skin reactions of the mice were reduced. This represented a therapeutic gain in these experimental animals because differential protection was achieved. All normal tissues, except the brain and spinal cord, concentrate this radiation protector. Utley and colleagues[154] and Washburn and associates[157] confirmed the localization of WR-2721 in high concentration in normal tissues relative to experimental tumors. Only two experimental tumors tested concentrated WR-2721.[141]

Using labeled WR-2721, Yuhas[159] demonstrated the facilitated absorption of WR-2721 by normal tissues, whereas tumor tissue passively absorbed the protector and never exceeded serum levels. The maximum normal tissue concentration in mice occurred between 15 and 30 minutes and was sustained for 90 minutes. Because of this, patients are treated with radiation or chemotherapeutic agents 15 to 30 minutes after intravenous infusion of WR-2721. The following is the rationale for clinical trials of radioprotectors:

Dose-limiting local toxicity from radiation

Radiobiologic data for selective normal tissue *versus* tumor protection owing to differential absorption and less protection of hypoxic cells

Potential for increased radiation dose with increased tumor effect and equal toxicity

Phase I Clinical Trials

The first clinical cancer trial with WR-2721 was carried out by Tanaka and Sugahara[152] with daily doses of approximately 60 mg/m^2. Irradiation was given 30 minutes after the intravenous administration. Nausea and vomiting occurred in 15% of patients. Using the time of onset of first- and second-degree mucosal reactions as criteria, a DRF of 1.7 and 1.3, respectively, was observed.

In the United States, phase I trials with WR-2721 were initiated at the University of New Mexico[136] and later transferred to the University of Pennsylvania. The maximum tolerated dose (MTD) of single doses of WR-2721 has been established with therapeutic doses of radiation therapy and chemotherapy. The MTD of WR-2721 before therapeutic doses of fractionated radiation therapy has been determined. This multiple-dose study was carried out in five cooperating institutions under the auspices of RTOG.

WR-2721 is designated NSC-296,961 by the National Cancer Institute, which supplied the material in 500 mg vials containing an equal amount of mannitol. To prevent dephosphorylation by hydrolysis, the drug was reconstituted in 5% dextrose-lactated Ringer's solution and buffered with sodium bicarbonate to a pH of 7.20. It was infused 15 to 30 minutes before radiation therapy or chemotherapy. The drug was given in 5 minutes when the doses were 25 mg/m^2 to 300 mg/m^2 and in 7 minutes in those patients receiving 340 mg/m^2. With doses of 450 mg/m^2 and higher, the infusion rate was between 14 mg and 20 mg/m^2/minute, designated as "long infusion time." Later doses of 450 mg/m^2 and greater were delivered in 15 minutes and designated as "short infusion time."

In the single-dose toxicity study of WR-2721, 201 patients

were entered.[130, 153] Patients with advanced malignancies received WR-2721 before palliative radiation therapy or before cyclophosphamide, cisplatin, or nitrogen mustard. Single doses between 25 mg/m^2 and 1330 mg/m^2 were escalated according to a modified Fibonacci schedule. Blood pressure was monitored for 1 hour before the first injection to establish baseline readings. This monitoring was continued during the injection and for an appropriate time after infusion. Toxicity reactions in the single-dose study included hypotension, emesis, somnolence, sneezing, metallic taste, and hypocalcemia. The two major toxicity reactions were emesis and hypotension. The incidence increased with dose. Of 39 patients who received WR-2721 in the long infusion time, 21 (54%) vomited after administration of 450 mg/m^2. At 740 mg/m^2, 18 of 22 patients (82%) suffered emesis (P = 0.3). However, when patients were infused in 15 minutes, only 42% of patients receiving 740 mg/m^2 vomited compared with 82% with the long infusion time (P = 0.002).

Significant hypotension is defined as a drop in systolic blood pressure by 20 mm Hg sustained for a minimum of 5 minutes. Hypotension occurred in 15% of the 201 patients. However, a highly significant decrease in hypotension occurred when patients were infused with WR-2721 within 15 minutes (6% in 107 patients) as opposed to the long infusion time (24% in 115 patients; P = 0.0001). A strong correlation exists between hypotension and tumor site in that 25 of the 34 instances of hypotension occurred in patients with head and neck and lung cancers. In 18 patients (8%), hypotension was deep and sustained, requiring termination of WR-2721 administration. In all these patients blood pressure rapidly returned to normal when the protector was stopped, and the patient was continued on intravenous fluids while supine.

One patient who received WR-2721 before chemotherapy was observed with carpopedal spasm and distal paresthesia that disappeared spontaneously. The clinical diagnosis of hypocalcemia was confirmed by serum calcium determination.[124] Subsequent studies revealed nonclinically relevant reactions in serum calcium. No other changes in the chemical enzymatic studies were observed in the 12 months following administration of WR-2721. It was concluded that the dose-limiting toxicity for single doses of WR-2721 is emesis and that 740 mg/m^2 delivered in 15 minutes represents the maximum tolerated dose. However, because of the observation relating toxicity reaction to site (*i.e.*, lower tolerance of the drug in patients treated for thoracic or head and neck malignancies), Glover and associates[134] again tested higher doses of the protector before single doses of cisplatin. It was determined that the MTD with infusion time of 15 minutes for single doses of WR-2721 for tumors in the head and neck and thoracic areas was 740 mg/m^2, but that patients with tumors of other sites could tolerate 910 mg/m^2.

No clinical evidence of tumor protection was seen in any of these patients. No drug-related deaths occurred.

Multiple Doses of WR-2721 Before Fractionated Radiation Therapy

Eighty-four patients were entered into a multiple-dose trial.[138] Doses were escalated from 100 mg/m^2 once a week to 450 mg/m^2 four times a week for 5 weeks. In one group of six patients at the 250 mg/m^2 level, the drug was delivered four times a week for 6 weeks.

Seventeen patients did not complete treatment for reasons not related to drug toxicity. Withdrawal of patients from the protocol was either physician- or patient-related. Physicians withdrew patients because of cancellation of radiation therapy or cardiac arrhythmia. Patients withdrew themselves from the program because of discomfort from nausea with mucus (not true vomiting) or because they feared injury by the drug.

Fifteen of the 84 patients failed to complete treatment because of varying severity of drug toxicity reactions. This was a five-institution study, and the interpretation of unacceptable toxicity reactions varied among the physicians involved. Four of the 84 patients developed drug reactions that included symptoms and signs of fever, chills, rash, and hypotension. Seven patients were withdrawn because of sustained lowered blood pressure. Two patients were cancelled because of persistent vomiting. After 2 or more weeks of treatment, seven of the 39 patients receiving daily doses of 250 mg/m^2 and more developed symptoms designated as "malaise," which was characterized as a feeling of generalized discomfort, uneasiness, and asthenia.

To evaluate the toxicity reactions for the determination of the MTD, the observed toxicity at the highest doses delivered was examined (Table 18-4). Fifteen patients who received 340 mg/m^2 four times per week for 3, 4, and 5 weeks developed toxicity reactions in only two instances. One who received the treatment over 3 weeks developed malaise, and one who received 4 weeks of treatment was withdrawn because of excessive vomiting. Of the five patients receiving four treatments per week for 5 weeks, none developed toxicity reactions, although one patient withdrew because it was inconvenient for him to wait the hour each day for observation. On the other hand, of four patients in whom the next higher dose was attempted (450 mg/m^2, four times per week for 4 weeks) only one patient completed treatment. However, this patient was clearly toxic with seven episodes of systolic blood pressures below 90 mm Hg.

It was concluded that 340 mg/m^2 four times per week for 5 weeks before therapeutic doses of radiation therapy was the maximum tolerated dose. This dose is now being tested in a

TABLE 18–4
WR-2721 Dose and Schedule Related to Limiting Toxicity

mg/m^2	NO. OF DOSES/ WK × NO. OF WK	NO. OF PATIENTS	COMPLETED	COMPLETED W/TOXICITY	INCOMPLETE TOLERATED	DRUG-LIMITING TOXICITY		
						EMESIS	<BP	MALAISE
340	4 × 3	5	4	1				1
	4 × 4	5	4	2		1		
	4 × 5	5	4		1			
450	4 × 5	4	1	1			3*	1

** One completed treatment but with seven episodes of severe hypotension.*

phase II/III study. If appropriate conversion adjustments are made, the dose of 340 mg/m^2 in humans corresponds to a dose level in mice at which effective radioprotection has been observed.

No long-term chemical, hematologic, or enzymatic changes were observed in any patients treated with WR-2721. There have been no drug-related deaths.

Pharmacokinetics

Several groups are investigating newly developed techniques of WR-2721 pharmacokinetics[128, 140, 147, 150, 151] in an attempt to measure the pharmacokinetic parameters in humans, in order to optimize the drug dose and schedule of WR-2721 to enhance its protective effects. Shaw and associates[147, 148] have measured WR-2721 and its free sulfhydryl metabolite (WR-1065) in plasma, using a specific electrochemical high-pressure liquid chromatography procedure.[147] Patients received 150 mg/m^2 of WR-2721 as an intravenous bolus. Most of the WR-2721 disappeared from the plasma within 10 minutes. Renal excretion of either WR-2721 or WR-1065 was minimal (less than 10%). The short α-half-life (0.87 ± 0.17 minutes), the small volume of distribution (Vd) (0.10 ± 0.05 L/kg), and the low urinary excretion (4.42 ± 2.21 L/hr/kg) suggested to Shaw and associates[147] that WR-2721 rapidly leaves the plasma, enters the cells, and is converted to metabolites. The β-half-life is also short at 9.46 ± 2.04 minutes. These authors are currently studying patients at higher WR-2721 doses and at longer infusion times.

The preliminary human pharmacokinetic data just mentioned are consistent with published rat pharmacokinetic data using a different method of analysis.[128, 155] The animal data also show rapid disappearance of the WR-2721 from the blood (more than 94% disappearing within 5 minutes) with a short α-half-life of 1 minute and a β-half-life of 10 to 30 minutes. Most of the WR-2721 again seems to be rapidly converted to WR-1065 in tissue.

Phase II and Phase III Trials

A study was initiated[137] to see whether a dose of 740 mg/m^2 WR-2721 before three large doses of radiation (800 cGy × 3) given on days 0, 7, and 14 would offer palliation without later normal tissue changes. Rapid and successful palliation occurred in seven of eight patients presenting with 15 masses. One patient with two masses was not palliated, nor were other metastases palliated in this patient using conventional treatment of 2000 cGy in 5 days and 3000 cGy in 12 days. No gross evidence of tumor protection was seen.

Coia and co-workers[126] reported a therapeutic gain in combining the radioprotector with total-body irradiation in a murine lymphoma. The gain of 2.5 for five-fraction treatment suggested a combination of marrow protection and a tumor-cytotoxic effect mediated by WR-2721 pretreatment. Based on these data, Coia[125] established a clinical protocol to establish the MTD of WR-2721 given twice weekly before total-body irradiation (TBI) and to establish the MTD of TBI given twice per week with the radioprotector MTD. Patients with advanced lymphoproliferative diseases are eligible. These include Stages II to IV non-Hodgkin's lymphoma with favorable histology; Stages III to IV non-Hodgkin's lymphoma with intermediate histology for whom TBI could be palliative; and refractory chronic lymphocytic leukemia. This study is underway.

In January 1989, a phase II/III trial of WR-2721 administered before curative radiation therapy[135] was initiated at the Cancer Hospital of Shanghai Medical University in cooperation with the University of Pennsylvania. The test site is the rectum, and patients are stratified for randomization into inoperable, unresectable, or postoperative recurrent tumors. The radioprotector (340 mg/m^2) and radiation are given 4 days a week (except Wednesday) for 5 weeks to the entire pelvis followed by cone-downs without WR-2721. The protocol calls for three levels of radiation in combination with the radioprotector: level 1 = 4500 cGy; level 2 = 4920 cGy; and level 3 = 5300 cGy. Each of these total doses is divided into 20 fractions. The isoeffective doses, if given five times per week, would approximate 4950 cGy, 5412 cGy, and 5830 cGy, respectively. Patients with recurrent disease following abdominoperineal resection then receive a single cone down through a portal not exceeding 144 cm^2. The total dose is 720 cGy in four fractions.

Patients with inoperable and nonresectable disease receive a second cone-down of 64 cm^2 with a total dose of 720 cGy in four fractions. WR-272 is not given with the cone-down treatments. The total equivalent doses for levels one, two, and three with the two cones are 6390 cGy, 6852 cGy, and 7270 cGy, respectively. One hundred patients will be randomized at the first level. From those data a measure of the acute and late effects of irradiation will be ascertained. This will permit calculation of the size of the groups needed to demonstrate statistical significance at subsequent levels of irradiation. Ninety-three of the 100 patients at level one have been accessed to date. Details of acute toxicity reactions to WR-2721, which has been acceptable, are in preparation.[139]

WR-2721 and Chemotherapeutic Agents

Yuhas and associates[160] and Phillips and Wasserman[76, 145, 158] found that WR-2721 protected selected normal animal tissues against the cytotoxicity of cyclophosphamide and cisplatin. At the University of Pennsylvania in a trial of 25 patients,[130] cyclophosphamide was given alone on the first injection, followed 4 weeks later by cyclophosphamide and WR-2721 pretreatment. The doses of cyclophosphamide were between 1200 mg and 1800 mg/m^2. With 450 mg to 1100 mg/m^2 of WR-2721 pretreatment, 12 of 25 patients had white blood cell counts with a higher nadir. The mean of 1550 cells/mm^3 with cyclophosphamide alone increased to 1850 cells/mm^3 with WR-2721 followed by cyclophosphamide ($P = 0.02$). Moreover, when the mean nadir granulocyte counts were compared, it increased from a mean of 449 cells/mm^3 for patients receiving cyclophosphamide alone to 844 cells/mm^3 for those who received WR-2721 before cyclophosphamide ($P = 0.001$).

Clinical data on a variety of tumors show WR-2721 protection of cisplatin nephrotoxicity, ototoxicity, and neurotoxicity.[131] During this trial, objective evidence of partial response of metastatic melanoma was observed. Thirty-six patients received WR-2721 before 60 mg to 150 mg/m^2 of cisplatin. Partial responses occurred in 53% of the patients.[133] These data suggest that WR-2721 may have antitumor properties; this finding has led to the establishment of an Eastern Cooperative Oncology Group study to test administration of the protector before cisplatin in metastatic melanoma.

No clinical evidence of tumor protection from WR-2721 has been found. Preclinical and clinical scientific studies now in progress should establish the role of radioprotectors and the use of WR-2721 in clinical practice. Further drug development in search of analogues with improved clinical usefulness is necessary and ongoing.[11, 76]

REFERENCES

Radiosensitizers

1. Adams GE: Hypoxia-mediated drugs for radiation and chemotherapy. Cancer 48:696, 1981
2. Adams GE, Clarke ED, Flockhart IR, et al: Structure-activity relationships in the development of hypoxic cell radiosensitizers. I. Sensitization efficiency. Int J Radiat Oncol Biol Phys 35:133, 1979
3. Ash DV, Smith MR, Bugden RD: Distribution of misonidazole in human tumours and normal tissues. Br J Cancer 39:503, 1979
4. Bagshaw MA, Doggett RLS, Smith KC, et al: Intra-arterial 5-bromodeoxyuridine and x-ray therapy. Radiology 99:886, 1967
5. Bleehen NM, Newman HFV, Maughan TS, Workman P: A multiple dose study of the combined radiosentisizers Ro 03-8799 (pimonidazole) and SR 2508 (etanidazole). Int J Radiat Oncol Biol Phys 16(4):1093–1096, 1989
6. Brady LW (ed): Radiation Sensitizers. New York, Masson, 1980
7. Breccia A, Fowler JF: New Chemo and Radiosensitizing Drugs. Bologna, Italy, Lo Scarabeo, 1985
8. Brown JM: Clinical perspectives for the use of new hypoxic cell sensitizers. Int J Radiat Oncol Biol Phys 8:1491, 1982
9. Brown JM: Clinical trials of radiosensitizers: What should we expect? Int J Radiat Oncol Biol Phys 10:425, 1984
10. Brown JM: Keynote address: Hypoxic cell radiosensitizers: Where next? Int J Radiat Oncol Biol Phys 16(4):987–993, 1989
11. Brown JM, Biaglow JE, Hall EJ, et al: Sensitizers and protectors to radiation and chemotherapeutic drugs. Cancer Treat Symp 1:85, 1984
12. Bump EA, Yu NY, Brown JM: Radiosensitization of hypoxic tumor cells by depletion of intracellular glutathione. Science 217:544, 1982
13. Busutti L, Breccia A, Stagni C, et al: Clinical trials with cyclophosphamide and misonidazole combination for maintaining treatment after radiation therapy of lung carcinoma. Int J Radiat Oncol Biol Phys 10:1739, 1984
14. Calabresi P, Cardoso SS, Finch SC, et al: Initial clinical studies with 5-iodo-2'deoxyuridine. Cancer Res 21:550, 1961
15. Chaplin DJ: Hydralazine-induced tumor hypoxia: A potential target for cancer chemotherapy. J Natl Cancer Inst 81:618–622, 1989
16. Chapman JD: The detection and measurement of hypoxic cells in solid tumors. Cancer 54:2441, 1984
17. Chapman JD, Lee J, Meeker BE: Keynote address: Cellular reduction of nitroimidazole drugs: Potential for selective chemotherapy and diagnosis of hypoxic cells. Int J Radiat Oncol Biol Phys 16(4):911–917, 1989
18. Chapman JD, Whitmore GF (eds): Chemical modifiers of cancer treatment. Int J Radiat Oncol Biol Phys 10:1161, 1984
19. Coleman CN: Hypoxic cell radiosensitizers: Expectations and progress in drug development. Int J Radiat Oncol Biol Phys 11:323, 1985
20. Coleman CN: Newer methods of cancer treatment. In DeVita VT Jr, Hellman S, Rosenberg SA (eds.): Cancer: Principles and Practice of Oncology, 3rd ed, pp 2436–2449. Philadelphia, JB Lippincott, 1989
21. Coleman CN, Bump EA, Kramer RA: Chemical modifiers of cancer therapy. J Clin Oncol 6:709–733, 1988
22. Coleman CN, Carlson RW, Halsey J, et al: Enhancement of the clinical activities of melphalan by the hypoxic cell sensitizer misonidazole. Cancer Res 48:3528, 1988
23. Coleman CN, Halsey J, Cox RS, et al: Relationship between the neurotoxicity of the hypoxic cell radiosensitizer SR-2508 and the pharmacokinetic profile. Cancer Res 47:319, 1987
24. Coleman CN, Noll L, Howes AE, et al: Initial results of a phase I trial of continuous infusion SR 2508 (etanidazole): A Radiation Therapy Oncology Group study. Int J Radiat Oncol Biol Phys 16(4):1085–1087, 1989
25. Coleman CN, Urtasun RC, Wasserman TH, et al: Initial report of the phase I trial of the hypoxic cell radiosensitizer SR-2508. Int J Radiat Oncol Biol Phys 10:1749, 1984
26. Coleman CN, Wasserman TH, Phillips TL, et al: Initial pharmacology and toxicology of intravenous desmethylmisonidazole. Int J Radiat Oncol Biol Phys 8:371, 1982
27. Davila E, Klein L, Vogel CL, et al: Phase I trial of metronidazole (NSC #261037) plus cyclophosphamide in solid tumors. J Clin Oncol 3:121, 1985
28. Denekamp J, Hirst DG, Stewart FA: Is tumor radiosensitization by misonidazole a general phenomenon? Br J Cancer 41:1, 1980
29. Dische S: Hypoxic cell sensitizers in radiotherapy. Int J Radiat Oncol Biol Phys 4:157, 1978
30. Dische S: Chemical sensitizers for hypoxic cells: A decade of experience in clinical radiotherapy. Radiother Oncol 3:97, 1985
31. Dische S: Keynote address: Hypoxic cell sensitizers: Clinical developments. Int J Radiat Oncol Biol Phys 16(4):1057–1060, 1989
32. Dische S, Saunders MI, Dunphy EP, et al: Concentrations achieved in human tumors after administration of misonidazole, SR-2508, and RO-03-8799. Int J Radiat Oncol Biol Phys 12:1109, 1986
33. Dische S, Saunders MI, Flockhart IR, et al: Misonidazole—a drug for trial in radiotherapy and oncology. Int J Radiat Oncol Biol Phys 5:851, 1979
34. Dunphy EP, Petersen IA, Cox RS, Bagshaw MA: The influence of initial hemoglobin and blood pressure levels on results of radiation therapy for carcinoma of the prostate. Int J Radiat Oncol Biol Phys 16(5):1173–1178, 1989
35. Fazekas J, Pajak TF, Wasserman TH, et al: Failure of misonidazole-sensitized radiotherapy to impact upon outcome among stage III–IV squamous cancers of the head and neck. Int J Radiat Oncol Biol Phys 13:1155, 1987
36. Finkelstein E, Glatstein E: Seduced by oxygen. Int J Radiat Oncol Biol Phys 14:205–207, 1988
37. Fischer JJ, Rockwell S, Martin DF: Perfluorochemicals and hyperbaric oxygen in radiation therapy. Int J Radiat Oncol Biol Phys 12:95–102, 1986
38. Frytak S, Moertel CG, Childs DS, et al: Neurologic toxicity associated with high-dose metronidazole therapy. Ann Intern Med 88:361, 1978
39. Fulton DS, Urtasun RC, et al: Misonidazole and CCNU chemotherapy for recurrent primary malignant brain tumors. J Neurooncol 4:383, 1987
40. Gangji D, Schwade JG, Strong JM: Phenytoin-misonidazole: Possible metabolic interaction. Cancer Treat Rep 64:155, 1980
41. Gianni L, Jenkins JF, Greene RF, et al: Pharmacokinetics of the hypoxic radiosensitizers misonidazole and desmethylmisonidazole after intraperitoneal administration in humans. Cancer Res 43:913, 1983
42. Goodman RL, Moore RE, Davis ME, et al: Perfluorocarbon emulsions in cancer therapy: Preliminary observations of presently available formulations. Int J Radiat Oncol Biol Phys 10:1421, 1984
43. Gray LH, Conger AD, Ebert M, et al: The concentration of oxygen dissolved in tissues at the time of irradiation as a factor in radiotherapy. Br J Radiol 26:638, 1953
44. Green JA, Zistica DT, Young RC, et al: Potentiation of melphalan cytotoxicity in human ovarian cancer cell lines by glutathione depletion. Cancer Res 44:5427, 1984
45. Guichard M: Keynote address: Chemical manipulations of tissue oxygenation for therapeutic benefit. Int J Radiat Oncol Biol Phys 16(5):1125–1130, 1989
46. Hall EJ: Radiobiology for the Radiologist, 2nd ed, pp 3;79. New York, Harper & Row, 1978
47. Henk JM: Does hyperbaric oxygen have a future in radiation therapy? Int J Radiat Oncol Biol Phys 7:1125, 1981
48. Henk JM, Smith CW: Radiotherapy and hyperbaric oxygen in head and neck cancer. Lancet 2:104, 1977
49. Hirst DG: Anemia: A problem or an opportunity in radiotherapy? Int J Radiat Oncol Biol Phys 12:2009–2017, 1986
50. Hoffman JM, Rasey JS, Spence AM, et al: Binding of the hypoxia tracer [^{3}H] misonidazole in cerebral ischemia. Stroke 18:168–176, 1987

51. Honess DJ, Wasserman TH, Workman P, et al: Additivity of radiosensitization by the combination of SR 2508 (etanidazole) and Ro 03-8799 (pimonidazole) in a murine tumour system. Int J Radiat Oncol Biol Phys 15:671–675, 1988
52. Hong SS, Abe Y, Kaneta K, et al: Combined treatment of radiation and local injections of misonidazole. Int J Radiat Oncol Biol Phys 10:2369, 1984
53. Hoshino T, Sano K: Radiosensitization of malignant brain tumors with bromouridine (thymidine analogue). Acta Radiol Ther Phys Biol 8:15, 1969
54. Kinsella TJ, Glatstein E: Clinical experience with intravenous radiosensitizers in unresectable sarcomas. Cancer 59:908–915, 1987
55. Kinsella TJ, Mitchell JB, Russo A, et al: Continuous intravenous infusions of bromodeoxyuridine as a clinical radiosensitizer. J Clin Oncol 2:1144, 1984
56. Kinsella TJ, Russo A, Mitchell JB, et al: A phase I study of intermittent intravenous bromodeoxyuridine (BUdR) with conventional fractionated irradiation. Int J Radiat Oncol Biol Phys 10:69, 1984
57. Kinsella TJ, Russo A, Mitchell JB, et al: A phase I study of intravenous iododeoxyuridine as a clinical radiosensitizer. Int J Radiat Oncol Biol Phys 11:1941, 1985
58. Kramer RA, Soble M, Howes AE, Montoya VP: The effect of glutathione (GSH) depletion in vivo by buthionine sulfoximine (BSO) on the radiosensitization of SR 2508. Int J Radiat Oncol Biol Phys 16(5):1325–1329, 1989
59. Wasserman TH, Lee DJ, Cosmatos D, et al: Clinical trials with etanidazole (SR-2508) by the Radiation Therapy Oncology Group (RTOG). Radiother Oncol 20(Suppl 1):129–135, 1991
60. Leibel S, Bauer M, Wasserman TH, et al: Radiotherapy with or without misonidazole for patients with stage IIIB or stage IVA squamous cell carcinoma of the uterine cervix: Preliminary report of a Radiation Therapy Oncology Group randomized trial. Int J Radiat Oncol Biol Phys 13:541–549, 1987
61. Leibel SA, Pajak TF, Massullo V, et al: A comparison of misonidazole sensitized radiation therapy to radiation therapy alone for palliation of hepatic metastases: Results of a Radiation Therapy Oncology Group randomized prospective trial. Int J Radiat Oncol Biol Phys 13:1057, 1987
62. Lustig R, McIntosh-Lowe N, Rose C, et al: Phase I/II study of fluosol-DA and 100% oxygen as an adjuvant to radiation in the treatment of advanced squamous cell tumors of the head and neck. Int J Radiat Oncol Biol Phys 16:1587, 1989
63. Malaise EP, Guichard M, Siemann DW: Chemical Modifiers of Cancer Treatment (part 1), Paris, France, March 21–25, 1988. Int J Radiat Oncol Biol Phys 16(4):885–1122, 1989
64. Malaise EP, Guichard M, Siemann DW: Chemical Modifiers of Cancer Treatment (part 2), Paris, France, March 21–25, 1988. Int J Radiat Oncol Biol Phys 16(5):1125–1345, 1989
65. Martin GV, Caldwell JH, Rasey JS, et al: Enhanced binding of the hypoxic cell market [^{3}H]Fluoromisonidazole in ischemic myocardium. J Nucl Med 30:194, 1989
66. Mathias CJ, Welch MJ, Kilbourn MR, et al: Radiolabeled hypoxic cell sensitizers: Tracers for assessment of ischemia. Life Sci 41:199, 1987
67. Mitchell JB, Cook JA, DeGraff W, et al: Keynote address: Glutathione modulation in cancer treatment: Will it work? Int J Radiat Oncol Biol Phys 16(5):1289, 1989
68. Moulder JE: Dependence of misonidazole radiosensitization on drug and radiation schedules. Int J Radiat Oncol Biol Phys 8:75, 1982
69. Nelson DF, Gillespie BW, Diener MD, et al: Is misonidazole neurotoxicity altered by the use of phenytoin and/or dexamethasone in RTOG 79-18 and RTOG 79-16? Int J Radiat Oncol Biol Phys 10:1731, 1984
70. Nelson DF, Schoenfeld D, Weinstein AS, et al: A randomized comparison of misonidazole sensitized radiotherapy plus BCNU and radiotherapy plus BCNU for treatment of malignant glioma after surgery: Preliminary results of an RTOG study. Int J Radiat Oncol Biol Phys 9:1143, 1983
71. Newman HFV, Bleehen NM, Ward R, Workman P: Hypoxic cell radiosensitizers in the treatment of high grade gliomas: A new direction using combined Ro-03-8799 (pimonidazole) and SR-2508 (etanidazole). Int J Radiat Oncol Biol Phys 15:677–684, 1988
72. Newman HF, Bleehen NM, Workman P: A phase I study of the combination of two hypoxic cell radiosensitizers, RO-03-8799 and SR-25: Toxicity and pharmacokinetics. Int J Radiat Oncol Biol Phys 12:1113, 1986
73. Overgaard J, Bentzen SM, Kolstad P, et al: Misonidazole combined with radiotherapy in the treatment of carcinoma of the uterine cervix. Int J Radiat Oncol Biol Phys 16(4):1069–1072, 1989
74. Overgaard J, Hansen HS, Anderson AP, et al: Misonidazole combined with split-course radiotherapy in the treatment of invasive carcinoma of larynx and pharynx: Report from the DAHANCA 2 study. Int J Radiat Oncol Biol Phys 16(4):1065–1068, 1989
75. Phillips TL, Diener MD, Wasserman TH, et al: Hypofractionated radiotherapy with or without misonidazole for the treatment of brain metastases. Int J Radiat Oncol Biol Phys 10(2):145, 1984
76. Phillips TL, Wasserman TH: Promise of radiosensitizers and radioprotectors in the treatment of human cancer. Cancer Treat Rep 68(1):291, 1984
77. Phillips TL, Wasserman TH, Johnson RJ, et al: Final report on the United States phase I clinical trial of the hypoxic cell radiosensitizer, misonidazole (RO-07-0582 NSC #261037). Cancer 48:1697, 1981
78. Phillips TL, Wasserman TH, Stetz J, et al: Keynote address: Clinical trials of hypoxic cell sensitizers. Int J Radiat Oncol Biol Phys 8:327, 1982
79. Phuphanich S, Levin EM, Levin VA: Phase I study of intravenous bromodeoxyuridine used concomitantly with radiation therapy in patients with primary malignant brain tumors. Int J Radiat Oncol Biol Phys 10:1769, 1984
80. Quilty PM, Duncan W: The influence of hemoglobin level on the regression and long term local control of transitional cell carcinoma of the bladder following photon irradiation. Int J Radiat Oncol Biol Phys 12:1735–1742, 1986
81. Rasey JS, Grunbaum Z, Magee S, et al: Characterization of radiolabeled fluoromisonidazole as a probe for hypoxic cells. Radiat Res 111:292–297, 1987
82. Roberts JT, Bleehen NM, Workman P, et al: A phase I study of the hypoxic cell radiosensitizer RO-03-8799. Int J Radiat Oncol Biol Phys 10:1755, 1984
83. Rojas A, Smith KA, Soranson JA, et al: Enhancement of misonidazole radiosensitization by buthionine sulphoximine. Radiother Oncol 2:325, 1984
84. Rose C, Lustig R, McIntosh M, et al: A clinical trial of fluosol-DA 20% in advanced squamous cell carcinoma of the head and neck. Int J Radiat Oncol Biol Phys 12:1325, 1986
85. Russo A, Gianni L, Kinsella TJ, et al: A pharmacologic evaluation of intravenous delivery of BUdR to patients with brain tumors. Cancer Res 44:1702, 1984
86. Russo A, Mitchell JB, McPherson S, et al: Alteration of bleomycin cytotoxicity by glutathione depletion or elevation. Int J Radiat Oncol Biol Phys 10:1675, 1984
87. Sartorelli AC: Therapeutic attack of hypoxic cells of solid tumors. Cancer Res 48(4):775–778, 1988
88. Saunders MI, Anderson PJ, Bennett MH, et al: The clinical testing of RO-03-8799—pharmacokinetics, toxicology, tissue and tumor concentrations. Int J Radiat Oncol Biol Phys 10:1759, 1984
89. Schwade JG, Strong JM, Gangji D: IV misonidazole (NSC 261037). Report of initial clinical experience. In Brady LW (ed): Radiation Sensitizers, p 414. New York, Masson, 1980
90. Sealy R, Cridland S, Blekkenhorst G, et al: Interstitial misonidazole: Clinical experience in advanced mouth cancer. Proceedings of the Conference on Chemical Modifies of Cancer Treatment, p 1. Clearwater, FL, October 1985
91. Sealy R, Korrubel J, Cridland S, et al: Interstitial misonidazole. A preliminary report on a new perspective in clinical radiation sensitization and hypoxic cell chemotherapy. Cancer 54:1535, 1984
92. Shelton ME, Dence CS, Hwang D-R, et al: Myocardial kinetics of fluorine-18 misonidazole: A marker of hypoxic myocardium. J Nucl Med 30:351–358, 1989

93. Siemann DW: Modification of chemotherapy by nitroimidazoles. Int J Radiat Oncol Biol Phys 10:1585, 1984
94. Simpson JR, Bauer M, Perez CA, et al: Radiation therapy alone or combined with misonidazole in the treatment of locally advanced non-oat cell lung cancer: Report of an RTOG prospective randomized trial. Int J Radiat Oncol Biol Phys 16:1483–1491, 1989
95. Simpson JR, Bauer M, Wasserman TH, et al: Large fraction irradiation with or without misonidazole in advanced non-oat cell carcinoma of the lung: A phase III randomized trial of the Radiation Therapy Oncology Group. Int J Radiat Oncol Biol Phys 13:861, 1987
96. Song CW, Zhang WL, Pence DM, et al: Increased radiosensitivity of tumors by perfluorochemicals and carbogen. Int J Radiat Oncol Biol Phys 11:1833, 1985
97. Stratford MRL, Minchinton AI, Hill SA, et al: Pharmacokinetic studies using multiple administration of RO-03-8799, a 2-nitroimidazole radiosensitizer. Int J Radiat Oncol Biol Phys 8:469, 1982
98. Sutherland RM: Chemical modification: Radiation and cytotoxic drugs. Int J Radiat Oncol Biol Phys 8(3,4):323, 1982
99. Tanasichuk H, Urtasun RC, Fulton DS, et al: Misonidazole with dexamethasone rescue: An escalating dose toxicity study. Int J Radiat Oncol Biol Phys 10:1735, 1984
100. Teicher BA, Herman TS, Holden SA, Jones SM: Addition of misonidazole, etanidazole, or hyperthermia to treatment with fluosol-DA/carbogen/radiation. J Natl Cancer Inst 81:929–934, 1989
101. Teicher BA, Rose CM: Oxygen-carrying perfluorochemical emulsion as an adjuvant to radiation therapy in mice. Cancer Res 44:4285, 1984
102. Teicher BA, Rose CM: Perfluorochemical emulsion can increase tumor radiosensitivity. Science 223:934, 1984
103. Thomas GM, Rauth AM, Black RE, et al: A phase I study of misonidazole and pelvic irradiation in patients with carcinoma of cervix. Br J Cancer 45:860, 1982
104. Thomlinson RH, Gray LH: The histological structure of some human lung cancers and the possible implications for radiotherapy. Br J Cancer 9:539, 1955
105. Urtasun R, Band P, Chapman JD, et al: Radiation and high-dose metronidazole in supratentorial glioblastomas. N Engl J Med 294:1364, 1976
106. Urtasun RC, Chapman JD, Band P, et al: Phase I study of high-dose metronidazole: A specific in vivo and in vitro radiosensitizer of hypoxic cells. Radiology 117:129, 1975
107. Urtasun RC, Chapman JD, Raleigh JA, et al: Binding of 3H misonidazole to solid human tumors as a measure of tumor hypoxia. Int J Radiat Oncol Biol Phys 12:1263, 1986
108. Urtasun RC, Fulton DS, Lester SG, et al: A phase I RTOG study of idodeoxyuridine (IUdR) and radiotherapy in the treatment of primary malignant brain tumors. Int J Radiat Oncol Biol Phys 17(Suppl 1):221, 1989
109. Walker MD, Strike TA: Misonidazole peripheral neuropathy. Its relationship to plasma concentration and other drugs. Am J Clin Oncol 3:105, 1980
110. Wasserman TH: Hypoxic cell radiosensitizers—present and future (Editorial). Int J Radiat Oncol Biol Phys 7:849, 1981
111. Wasserman TH: Hypoxic cell radiosensitizers: Illusion or elusion? (Editorial) Int J Radiat Oncol Biol Phys 15:779–784, 1988
112. Wasserman TH, Coleman CN, Urtasun R, et al: Final report: Phase I trial of desmethylmisonidazole (DMM)—an hypoxic cell sensitizer. Int J Radiat Oncol Biol Phys 8(1):76, 1982
113. Wasserman TH, Nelson JS, VonGerichten D: Neuropathy of nitroimidazole radiosensitizers: Clinical and pathological description. Int J Radiat Oncol Biol Phys 10:1725, 1984
114. Wasserman TH, Phillips TL, Johnson RJ, et al: Initial clinical and pharmacologic evaluation of misonidazole (R1-07-0582) an hypoxic cell radiosensitizer. Int J Radiat Oncol Biol Phys 5:775, 1979
115. Wasserman TH, Phillips TL, Van Raalte G, et al: The neurotoxicity of misonidazole: Potential modifying role of phenytoin sodium and dexamethasone. Br J Radiol 53:172, 1980
116. Wasserman TH, Stetz JA, Phillips TL: Radiation Therapy Oncology Group clinical trials with misonidazole. Cancer 47:2382, 1981
117. Wasserman TH, Stetz JA, Phillips TL: Misonidazole clinical trials in the United States Radiation Therapy Oncology Group. In Breccia A, Rimondi C, Adams GE (eds.): Advanced Topics on Radiosensitizers of Hypoxic Cells, p 211. New York, Plenum Press, 1982
118. Watson ER, Halnan KE, Dische S, et al: Hyperbaric oxygen and radiotherapy: A medical research council trial in carcinoma of the cervix. Br J Radiol 51:879, 1978
119. Weissberg JB, Son YH, Papac RJ, et al: Randomized clinical trial of mitomycin C as an adjunct to radiotherapy in head and neck cancer. Int J Radiat Oncol Biol Phys 17:3, 1989
120. Williams MV, Denekamp J, Minchinton AI, et al: In vivo testing of a 2-nitroimidazole radiosensitizer (RO-03-8799) using repeated administration. Int J Radiat Oncol Biol Phys 8:477, 1982
121. Yu NY, Brown JM: Depletion of glutathione in vivo as a method of improving the therapeutic ratio of misonidazole and SR 2508. Int J Radiat Oncol Biol Phys 10:1265, 1984
122. Zeman EM, Hirst VK, Lemmon MJ, Brown JM: Enhancement of radiation-induced tumor cell killing by the hypoxic cell toxin SR 4233. Radiother Oncol 12:209–218, 1988

Radioprotectors

123. Brown DQ, Pittock JW, Rubinstein JS: Early results of the screening program for radioprotectors. Int J Radiat Oncol Biol Phys 8:565, 1982
124. Chapman JD, Reuvers AP: The time-scale of radioprotection in mammalian cells. In Locker A, Flemming K (eds): Radioprotection, p 9. Verlag, Basel and Stuttgart, Birkhauser, 1977
125. Coia L: NCI protocol #88-999, phase I study of WR-2721 in combination with total body irradiation (TBI) in patients with refractory lymphoid malignancies
126. Coia LR, Brown DQ, Hardiman J: WR-2721 as cytotoxic and radioprotective agent in treatment of murine lymphoma with total body irradiation. NCI Monogr 6:235–239, 1988
127. Doherty DG, Burnett WT Jr, Shapira R: Chemical protection against ionizing radiation. II. Mercaptoalkylamines and related compounds with protective activity. Radiat Res 7:13, 1957
128. Fahey RC, Newton GL: The measurement of WR-2721, WR-1065, and WR-33278 in plasma. Int J Radiat Oncol Biol Phys 11:1193, 1985
129. Glick JH, Glover DJ, Turrisi A, et al: Clinical trials of WR-2721 with chemotherapy. In Nygaard OF, Simic MG (eds): Radioprotectors and Anticarcinogens, p 719. New York, Academic Press, 1983
130. Glick JH, Glover DJ, Weiler C, et al: Phase I controlled trials of WR-2721 and cyclophosphamide. Int J Radiat Oncol Biol Phys 10:1777, 1984
131. Glover D, Glick J, Weiler C: Phase I trials of WR-2721 and cis-platinum. Int J Radiat Oncol Biol Phys 10:1781, 1984
132. Glover D, Riley L, Carmichael K, et al: Hypocalcemia and inhibition of parathyroid hormone secretion after administration of WR-2721 (a radioprotective and chemoprotective agent). N Engl J Med 309:1137, 1983
133. Glover D, Glick JH, Weiler C, et al: WR-2721 and high dose cis-platinum: An active combination in the treatment of metastatic melanoma. J Clin Oncol 5:574–578, 1987
134. Glover D, Grabelsky S, Fox K, et al: Clinical trials of WR-2721 and cis-platinum. Int J Radiat Oncol Biol Phys 16:1201–1204, 1989
135. Kligerman MM: NCI protocol #T87-0232, University of Pennsylvania protocol #00-A-0465 phase II/III trial of WR-2721 before protracted fractionated radiotherapy. December 1988
136. Kligerman MM, Shaw MT, Slavik M, et al: Phase I clinical studies with WR-2721. Cancer Clin Trials 3:217, 1980
137. Kligerman MM, Turrisi AT, Norfleet AL: Palliative radiotherapy by three large weekly fractions and WR-2721 pre-

treatment (Abstract). Proceedings VI International meeting on Chemical Modifiers of Cancer Treatment, Section 5, p 6. Paris, March 21–25, 1988

138. Kligerman MM, Turrisi AT, Urtasun RC, et al: Final report on phase I trial of WR-2721 before protracted fractionated radiation therapy. Int J Radiat Oncol Biol Phys 14:1119, 1988
139. Liu TF, Zhang ZY, Kligerman MM: Multiple dose WR-2721 and radiotherapy: Patient acceptance and lack of toxicity. Unpublished
140. McGovern EP, Swynnerton NF, Steele PD, et al: HPLC assay for 2-(3-aminopropylamino)ethanethiol (WR-2721) in plasma. Int J Radiat Oncol Biol Phys 10:1517, 1984
141. Milas L, Hunter M, Reid BO, et al: Protective effects of S-2-(3-aminoprophylamino)ethylphosphorothoic acid against radiation damage of normal tissues and a fibrosarcoma in mice. Cancer Res 42:1888, 1982
142. Packer JE, Mahood JS, Mora-Arellano VA, et al: Free radicals and singlet oxygen scavengers. Biochem Biophys Res Commun 98:901, 1981
143. Packer JE, Slater TF, Willson RL: Direct observation of a free radical interaction between vitamin E and vitamin C. Nature 278:737, 1979
144. Patt HN, Tyree, Straube RL, et al: Cysteine protection against irradiation. Science 110:213, 1949
145. Phillips TL, Yuhas JM, Wasserman TH: Differential protection against alkylating agent injury in tumors and normal tissues. In Nygaard OF, Simic MG (eds): Radioprotectors and Anticarcinogens, p 735. New York, Academic Press, 1983
146. Raleigh JA, Shum FY: Radioprotection in model lipid membranes by hydroxyl radical scavengers: Supplementary role for α-tocopherol in scavenging secondary peroxy radicals. In Nygaard OF, Simic MG (eds): Radioprotectors and Anticarcinogens, p 87. New York, Academic Press, 1983
147. Shaw LM, Bonner H, Turrisi A, et al: A liquid chromatographic electrochemical assay for S-2-(3-aminopropylamino)ethylphosphorothioate (WR-2721) in human plasma. J Chromat 7:2447, 1984
148. Shaw LM, Turrisi A, Glover D, et al: Human pharmacokinetics of WR-2721 Int J Radiat Oncol Biol Phys 12:1501, 1986
149. Streffer C: Studies on the mechanism of 5-hydroxytryptamine in radioprotection of mammals. In Locker A, Flemming K (eds): Radioprotection, p 71. Basel and Stuttgart, Birkhauser, Verlag, 1977
150. Swynnerton NF, McGovern EP, Mangold DJ, et al: HPLC assay for S-2-(3-aminopropylamino)ethylphosphorothioate (WR-2721) in plasma. J Liq Chromat 6:1523, 1983
151. Swynnerton NF, McGovern EP, Nino JA, et al: An improved HPLC assay for S-2-(3-aminopropylamino)ethylphosphorothioate (WR-2721) in plasma. Int J Radiat Oncol Biol Phys 10:1521, 1984
152. Tanaka Y, Sugahara T: Clinical experiences of chemical radiation protection in tumor radiotherapy in Japan. In Brady LW (ed): Radiation Sensitizers, p 421. New York, Masson, 1980
153. Turrisi AT, Glover DJ, Glick JH, et al: The final report of the Phase I trial of single dose WR-2721, S-2-(3-aminopropylamino)ethylphosphorothioic acid. Cancer Treat Rep 70:1389, 1986
154. Utley JF, Marlowe C, Waddell WJ: Distribution of 35 S-labelled WR-2721 in normal and malignant tissues of the mouse. Radiat Res 68:284, 1976
155. Utley JF, Seaver N, Newton GL, et al: Pharmacokinetics of WR-1065 in mouse tissue following treatment with WR-2721. Int J Radiat Oncol Biol Phys 10:1525, 1984
156. Ward JF: Chemical aspects of DNA radioprotection. In Nygaard OF, Simic MG (eds): Radioprotectors and Anticarcinogens, p 73. New York, Academic Press, 1983
157. Washburn LC, Carlton JE, Hayes RI: Distribution of WR-2721 in normal and malignant tissues of rats and mice. Dependence on tumor type, drug dose, species. Radiat Res 59:475, 1974
158. Wasserman TH, Phillips TL, Rose G, et al: Differential protection against cytotoxic chemotherapeutic effects on bone marrow CFU's by WR-2721. Am J Clin Oncol 4:3, 1981
159. Yuhas JM: Active versus passive absorption kinetics as the basis for selective normal tissue protection by S-2-(3-aminopropylamino) ethylphosphorothioic acid. Cancer Res 40:1519, 1980
160. Yuhas JM, Spellman JM, Jordan SW: Treatment of tumors with the combination of WR-2721 and cis-dichlorodiammine platinum or cyclophosphamide. Br J Cancer 42:574, 1980
161. Yuhas JM, Storer JB: Differential chemoprotection of normal and malignant tissues. J Natl Cancer Inst 42:331, 1969

19

○ ○ ○ • • •

Continuous Infusion Chemotherapy and Irradiation

Marvin Rotman
Hassan Aziz

In vitro investigations into the pharmacokinetics of cytotoxic agents showed that an alternative method of delivery by concomitant intravenous continuous infusion (CCIC) might prove equally effective without the accompanying toxicity associated with the more concentrated methods of delivery. Clinical investigations are confirming the effectiveness of this approach.[12, 14, 22, 26, 40, 41, 53, 69, 92]

MECHANISM OF ACTION

The use of infusion chemotherapy increases the duration of exposure of tumor cells to the drug. Another advantage of this method of delivery is reduction in systemic toxicity[84] because peak concentrations of the drug associated with bolus delivery are avoided.

A number of chemotherapeutic agents, such as bleomycin, etoposide (VP16), 5-fluorouracil (5-FU), cisplatin, and doxorubicin (Adriamycin), have been administered by intravenous infusion. However, the last three drugs have been used most often with concomitant irradiation.

5-FLUOROURACIL

5-Fluorouracil (5-FU) has been known to be a radiosensitizing agent for more than three decades.[2, 39, 97] The reason for the enhanced effectiveness of combination therapy is not fully understood. The most likely explanation is that 5-FU, a pyrimidine analogue, inhibits the *de novo* synthesis of DNA by binding thymidylate synthetase. In addition, the presence of 5-FU may lead to defective synthesis of RNA, as it may also be taken up as an RNA precursor nucleotide. Vietti and co-workers,[98] in *in vitro* experiments on the mouse leukemia AKR cell system, suggested that the radiosensitizing effect of 5-FU may be due to its interference with the repair of sublethal damage produced by x-irradiation.

Data produced by Vietti and co-workers[98] and Byfield and associates[11] suggest that optimal scheduling of therapy plays a major part in its effectiveness. The suggestion is that a synergistic effect occurs between 5-FU and radiation if the cells are continuously exposed to 5-FU for 8 hours or more following irradiation. Because 5-FU has a short biologic life of 10 minutes, bolus administration does not allow for continuous exposure of the cells; 120 hours of continuous infusion is required to cover five daily exposures. An additional advantage of prolonged continuous intravenous infusion of 5-FU compared with bolus administration is a reduction in myelotoxicity; however, stomatitis and diarrhea can increase.

CISPLATIN

The radiosensitizing effect of cisplatin when used together with radiation on experimental tumors was first demonstrated by Wodinsky and colleagues[103] in 1974. Further work by Douple and associates[23] in 1978 on *Escherichia coli* bacteria and V79 Chinese hamster cells showed that cisplatin radiosensitizes tissues by inhibiting the repair of potentially lethal damage. Kyriazis and co-workers[49] again demonstrated the radiosensitizing effect of cisplatin on human bladder carcinoma cells implanted in nude mice. Experimental data suggest that the antitumor effects are greater if cisplatin is administered by continuous infusion because it may be a phase-cycle nonspecific drug with preferential action on the G_1 phase of the cell cycle. In addition, with continuous infusion, triphasic decay of the drug occurs with a terminal half-life of 24 hours.

Important benefits of continuous infusion of cisplatin are a reduction in systemic toxicity and a lower incidence of severe nausea and renal toxicity. Salem and associates,[82] after infusing cisplatin, 20 mg/m^2/24 hours, for 5 days with irradiation, found a nephrotoxicity rate of 5%, with 7% of patients developing grade 3 nausea and vomiting.

It is noteworthy that the radiosensitizing effect of cisplatin appears to increase if the accompanying radiation therapy is given in multiple daily fractions. Dritschillo and colleagues[24] showed a significant increase in destruction of V79 Chinese hamster cells when radiation therapy was given twice daily with cisplatin. This increase was attributed to inhibition of repair of sublethal damage. With single fractions, the destruction was considerably less because the inhibition of repair affected only potentially lethally damaged cells. This experimental work has been proven by clinical work at SUNY–Health Science Center at Brooklyn (HSCB).[16,74] In a group of patients with advanced carcinoma of the head and neck who received hyperfractionated irradiation with continuous cisplatin infusion, the complete response rate was 87% compared with 37% in patients who received only single-fraction radiation therapy.

DOXORUBICIN

Doxorubicin (Adriamycin) inhibits mitochondrial and tumor cell respiration.[25] Reduced oxygen consumption by cells in the outer layers of the tumor may lead to improved oxygenation and hence radiosensitization of the usually hypoxic central tumor cells. Doxorubicin has also been shown by Watering, Byfield, and co-workers[8,9,100] to inhibit the enzymatic repair of radiation-induced single-strand breaks in DNA.

The radiosensitizing effect of doxorubicin can be maximized by giving the drug during or just after radiation therapy.[86] Studies by Rosenthal and associates[73] of the kinetics of doxorubicin given by intravenous bolus at 60 mg/m^2 revealed a rapid rise of the plasma level of the drug to 500 ng/ml within 5 to 10 minutes. Plasma levels then decline to 10% within 48 hours and to 5% in 120 hours. In contrast, if the drug is given by continuous intravenous infusion, an equal dose results in a steady plasma level of 60 ng/ml for 100 hours. The amount of drug excreted is also greater when given by continuous infusion. Thus continuous infusion of doxorubicin, by avoiding peak plasma concentrations and achieving higher rates of excretion, reduces the risk of cardiac toxicity without compromising antitumor activity.[4,50]

CLINICAL EXPERIENCE

Most clinical experience in continuous drug infusion has been with treatment of advanced tumors of the gastrointestinal tract, head and neck, and urinary bladder. Despite the lack of controlled trials, substantial gains appear to have been made in the treatment of these advanced carcinomas, especially in the area of locoregional control and possibly survival. Experience with the treatment of advanced, inoperable soft tissue sarcomas, to date, is limited and largely anecdotal.

Anus

In 1974, the observation by Nigro and associates[63] and later by others[58] that a small preoperative dose of radiation (3000 cGy) given concomitantly with intravenous infusion of 5-FU and bolus mitomycin produced a 74% rate of tumor sterilization in patients with squamous cell carcinoma of the anus, led the way for the use of modified techniques in this difficult area.

Sischy,[89] Cummings and co-workers,[19,20] and John and associates,[45] following up with increased amounts of both chemotherapy and radiation, obtained even better results. Sischy[89] administered 4500 cGy in 4.5 weeks to the whole pelvis and anal area, followed by a perineal boost of 1500 cGy delivered either by external beam or interstitial technique, concomitantly with an infusion of 1000 mg/m^2 of 5-FU for 96 hours during the first and fourth weeks. The regimen included one intravenous bolus of mitomycin C, 10 mg on the first day of irradiation. The local control and survival rates at 5 years were 89.6% and 86%, respectively. Initially, Cummings and co-workers[19,20] used a fraction of 250 cGy per treatment, giving a total dose of 5000 cGy in a continuous course of radiation therapy. One course of concomitant infusion of 5-FU and one bolus injection of mitomycin were also given. This treatment resulted in a rather high complication rate of 13%, however, and led to a reduction of the daily fraction to 200 cGy. Using a split-course technique, only 2400 cGy was delivered to the pelvic, inguinal, and anal area in 2.5 weeks. Four weeks later, in the second half of the course, another 2400 cGy was delivered, but to the anal area alone. On the first 4 days of each course of radiation therapy, a concomitant infusion of 5-FU at 1000 mg/m^2 was given and one bolus injection of mitomycin at 10 mg/m^2. The complete local control rate achieved for tumors more than 5 cm in size was 90%, and the survival rate was 74%.

To further minimize the complication rate while still delivering a cancericidal dose to the anal area, John and associates[45] described a shrinking field technique. Only 3060 cGy was delivered to the upper pelvis at the rate of 180 cGy per fraction; the lower pelvis received 4140 cGy to 4500 cGy, and a boost of 900 cGy to 1000 cGy was given to the tumor if required. The complete local response rate for T3 and T4 staged tumors (Union Internationale Contre le Cancer [UICC]) was 86%. Using 3000 cGy as external therapy and concomitant infusion of 5-FU at 600 mg/m^2/day on the third through fifth days, plus mitomycin, 12 mg/m^2 on the first day, followed by a boost delivered by implants, Papillon and Montbarbow[66] obtained a complete local response rate of 84%.

Rectum

Haghbin and associates[36] treated a series of 64 patients with advanced rectal carcinoma with preoperative 5-FU infusion and irradiation. All tumors were at least 4 cm or larger, ulcerated, and located in the lower third of the rectum; 25% of the tumors were completely fixed, whereas 47% were partially fixed.

Patients received 4000 cGy in 4.5 weeks along with two courses of 5-FU infusion of 96 hours each, beginning on the 2nd and the 28th days of radiation therapy. Mitomycin C was also given at 10 mg/m^2 as bolus on the second day. Six to eight weeks later, at surgery, 12.5% of patients had no residual tumor and only 26.5% had positive nodes. This is in contrast to the 40% incidence of lymph nodes usually found in patients with advanced rectal cancer treated by surgery only. Thirty-seven of 64 patients from this series are alive without disease; 18 have died with disease; three are alive with disease, and six patients have died of intercurrent disease. The overall 5-year survival rate is 64%.

Several studies have shown the benefit of combining radiation with concomitant bolus chemotherapy. In the Gastrointestinal Tumor Study Group (GITSG)[32] four-arm trial postoperative adjuvant therapy for Stages B2 and C rectal carcinomas consisted of 4000 cGy to 4400 cGy delivered in 4.5 to 5.5 weeks to the pelvis and perineum with an intravenous bolus of 5-FU at 500 mg/m^2 during the first and last 3 days of therapy. Sequential 5-FU and methyl-CCNU (lomustine) were also administered for 18 months. Only 33% of patients in the group receiving combined treatment had disease recurrence, compared with 55% in the surgery-only control group, 48% in the radiation therapy group, and 46% in the chemotherapy-alone group.

The North Central Cancer Treatment Group reports similar findings to the GITSG in the Rectal Surgical Adjuvant protocol for Stages B and C.[64] Patients in these trials received either radiation alone to a total dose of 5040 cGy in 5.5 weeks or radiation combined with bolus 5-FU and methyl-CCNU chemotherapy. Patients receiving combined treatment showed a local recurrence rate of 11% compared with 23% in the radiation-alone group. The disease-free survival rate at 3 years and the rate of distant metastases in the combined treatment group were 60% and 17%, respectively. Comparable rates in the radiation-alone group were 45% and 32%.

NSABP reports[27] on a postoperative rectal trial for Stages B2 and C comparing the results of using either postoperative radiation or chemotherapy alone. In the chemotherapy group, there was a greater benefit for younger males whose 5-year survival rate was 60% with adjuvant chemotherapy compared with 37% in the control group. The radiation group, however, was most effective in reducing the local recurrence rate from 25% to 16%. The radiation delivered was 4600 cGy to 4700 cGy in 26 or 27 fractions. The Radiation Therapy Oncology Group has started a four-arm protocol to clarify this issue. Two arms will test the effectiveness of 5-FU given as bolus against its use in protracted infusion; two other arms will evaluate methyl-CCNU.

Esophagus

To improve locoregional control, Byfield and colleagues[7] first used irradiation combined with 5-FU delivered by concomitant continuous infusion on six patients with unresectable carcinoma of the esophagus (Table 19-1). A complete local response rate of 83% was achieved. Leichman and associates[52] reported a trial at Wayne State University in which 55 patients received 3000 cGy as preoperative irradiation together with 5-FU concomitant continuous infusion chemotherapy (CCIC) and bolus cisplatin or mitomycin C; 25% of the patients showed a complete response at surgery with a 2-year survival rate of 60%.

A larger series of 140 patients was treated by the Southwest Oncology Group and the Radiation Therapy Oncology Group (RTOG)[52]; 3000 cGy was given in 3 weeks as preoperative treatment together with 75 mg/m^2 of cisplatin given as bolus and 1000 mg/m^2 of 5-FU as infusion during the first 4 days of radiation. Twenty-two percent of patients were free from cancer at surgery. An important feature of these three trials is that when residual tumor was present at surgery, the prognosis was poor; 80% of patients who had residual cancer in the esophageal specimen after preoperative treatment died of metastases. On the other hand, 60% of patients without residual tumor survived for at least 2 years. Other studies, using a preoperative radiation dose of 3000 cGy and two courses of concomitant 5-FU infusion with or without cisplatin and mitomycin intravenous push,[29,47] have similarly demonstrated the importance of sterilization of tumor.

The value of surgery in patients with residual tumor is doubtful.[71] These results prompted several authors, including John and colleagues,[46] to remove surgery from their treatment plan and to incorporate instead higher doses of radiation and CCIC to achieve better results. In a series of 35 patients, 4140 cGy to 5040 cGy was used in 4.5 to 8 weeks, together with three courses of infusion 5-FU (800 mg to 1000 mg/day) with bolus mitomycin or cisplatin. Maintenance chemotherapy was methotrexate (200 mg/m^2 IV), leucovorin (10 mg/m^2 orally every 6 hours for 5 days), and 5-FU (600 mg/m^2 in weeks 10, 12 and 14). The complete response rate has increased to 77% with a median survival time of 15 months, compared with only 8 months in the irradiation-alone group.

In other trials, Coia[17] treated 30 patients with Stage I and Stage II disease with 6000 cGy in 6 to 7 weeks, together with two courses of 5-FU infusion with mitomycin bolus. The reported

TABLE 19–1
Treatment of Carcinoma of Esophagus With CCIC and Radiation Therapy

AUTHORS	NO. OF PATIENTS	CHEMOTHERAPY	RADIATION THERAPY	COMPLETE RESPONSE RATE	2-YEAR SURVIVAL RATE
Byfield et al[7]	6	Infusion 5-FU at 20 mg/kg/day for 5 days; repeat on 6 alternate weeks	1000 cGy in 4 fractions/wk	83%	30%
Wayne State University,[52] (preop study)	55	Infusion 5-FU at 1000 mg/m^2 daily for 4 days/wk for 2 weeks. Mitomycin at 15 mg/m^2 on day 1 or cisplatin bolus at 100 mg/m^2 on days 1 and 29	3000 cGy in 3 wk	25%	60%
SWOG and RTOG[52] (preop study)	140	Infusion 5-FU at 1000 mg/m^2/plus cisplatin bolus at 75 mg/m^2 on days 1 and 29	3000 cGy in 3 wk	22%	60%
Keane et al[47]	45	Infusion 5-FU at 1000 mg/m^2/day plus mitomycin bolus at 10 mg/m^2 on day 1	6000 cGy in 6 wks or split course	48%	28%
Coia et al[17]	30	Infusion 5-FU at 1000 mg/m^2/day and mitomycin bolus at 10 mg/m^2 on day 2	6000 cGy in 6 wk	—	Median 24 mo
John et al[46]	21	Infusion 5-FU at 1000 mg/m^2/Dx4D on weeks 1, 4, 12. Mitomycin bolus at 10 mg/m^2 on weeks 1 and 8; cisplatin 75 mg/m^2 on weeks 4 and 12	3000–5040 cGy in 3.5–5.5 wk	77%	Median 15 mo

CCIC: concomitant continuous infusion chemotherapy

median survival was 24 months. Keane and associates[47] reported on a series of 35 patients with esophageal carcinoma who were treated, again, with infusion chemotherapy and irradiation, but without surgery. At 2 years the survival rate was 28%, with a local control rate of 48%.

Pancreas

Childs and colleagues,[15] in 1965, first described the beneficial effect of irradiation and 5-FU and showed a doubling of the survival time. The Gastrointestinal Tumor Study Group (GITSG)[59] reported on the results of a three-arm trial for unresectable carcinoma of the pancreas. In the first arm, patients received a split course of radiation delivering a total dose of 6000 cGy. In the second and third arms of split-course therapy, 4000 cGy and 6000 cGy, respectively, were delivered with intravenous bolus 5-FU. In addition, the patients randomized to the second and third arms continued to receive 5-FU on a weekly basis for up to 2 years. The median survival time for patients with radiation therapy alone was 20 weeks, compared with 36 weeks for those who received 5-FU and 4000 cGy in the split-course arm.

Later the GITSG,[94] in phase II trials, showed that the multidrug combination of 5-FU, streptozocin, and mitomycin gave better results than radiation therapy alone and similar results to the combination of 5-FU and radiation. The GITSG[30] conducted further trials on the treatment of unresectable carcinoma of the pancreas. The combination of 5-FU and radiation followed by streptozocin, 5-FU, and mitomycin was compared with that of multidrug chemotherapy only. The median survival time in the combined group was 42 weeks, compared with 32 weeks for the multidrug chemotherapy-only group. One-year survival rate was 41% for the group receiving radiation and 19% for the multidrug chemotherapy group.

Hepatic Metastases

In 1981, the RTOG[6] studied palliative treatment of liver metastases and compared the results of 2100 cGy of radiation at 300 cGy per fraction with those at 3000 cGy at 200 cGy per fraction. In both groups, the response and the tissue tolerance were similar. In another RTOG study,[51] adding misonidazole to radiation therapy in the treatment of liver metastases only slightly improved the therapeutic response. The median survival time of the group receiving misonidazole was 29 weeks compared with 25 weeks without misonidazole.

In 1959, Sullivan[93] used a hepatic artery infusion of FUDR (deoxyriboside) for the treatment of metastases from colorectal cancer and obtained a 59% response rate. A series of 27 patients at SUNY-HSCB[77] with liver metastases secondary to colorectal cancer received 2700 cGy to 3200 cGy to the whole liver in five daily fractions of 150 cGy to 200 cGy, along with concomitant intravenous 5-FU infusion for 5 days in the first, third, and fifth weeks. No treatment was given in the second and fourth weeks. Response to treatment was judged by pretreatment and post-treatment liver scans and liver function tests. In 56% of patients, partial responses were obtained. The median survival of responders and nonresponders was 45 weeks and 17 weeks, respectively. Patients whose disease was confined to the liver, with a Karnofsky performance status better than 60, had a median survival of 49 weeks compared with 27 weeks in patients whose performance was below 60.

Head and Neck

In the treatment of advanced carcinoma of the paranasal sinuses, oral cavity, and oropharynx with infusion intraarterial chemotherapy, Carter[12] reported a response rate of 53%. Auresberg and associates,[1] with the use of sequential intra-arterial chemotherapy and irradiation, obtained a 100% response rate.

Using two 96-hour infusions of 5-FU in the treatment of advanced carcinoma of the head and neck, Kish and colleagues[48] reported an overall response rate of 88% and a complete response rate of 19.2%. As demonstrated by Byfield and co-workers,[10] the complete response rate, however, increased to 75% with a 70% survival rate at 2 years with the concomitant use of 5-FU infusion and irradiation. Squamous cell carcinoma of the head and neck has been treated with cisplatin with a reported response rate of 20% to 30%[48,72]; combining infusion 5-FU and bolus cisplatin increased the complete response rate to 54%. With the addition of radiation, the response rates increased still further.

Forty-four patients with advanced cancer of the head and neck were treated by Murthy and associates[60] using CCIC and radiation therapy (Table 19-2). Cisplatin was delivered on the first day as bolus at 60 mg/m^2 and 5-FU infusion at 800 mg/m^2/day for 5 days with concomitant radiation at 200 cGy per fraction. The treatment was repeated every 2 weeks for seven cycles. A complete response rate of 87% and a 2-year survival rate of 60% were obtained. Similar results were reported by Showell and colleagues,[88] who treated their 27 patients with infusion of 5-FU, radiation therapy, and bolus cisplatin; results were a complete response rate of 60% and a 2-year survival rate of 70%. Hahn and co-workers[37] reported on a series of 44 patients with advanced carcinoma of the head and neck, treated preoperatively with mitomycin C bolus on the first day (10 mg/m^2), 5-FU infusion on the first through fourth days (1000 mg/m^2), and two split-course radiation treatments of 3000 cGy each. Sixty-two percent of these patients had complete resolution of their primary tumors at surgery, and 33% of the neck nodes removed were negative for tumor.

In an effort to minimize the toxicity of CCIC and radiation therapy and to increase tumor clearance, Choi[16] and Rotman and colleagues[74] used low-dose cisplatin in continuous infusion over 2 weeks with concomitant hyperfractionated radiation. Cisplatin infusion was given at 5.7 mg/m^2/day for 2 weeks, with 125 cGy of radiation given concomitantly twice a day, followed by a rest period of 1 or 2 weeks. In three such cycles, a total dose of 6000 cGy to 7200 cGy was given for curative treatment, whereas 5000 cGy in two cycles of chemotherapy was delivered for palliative treatments. Fourteen patients with either locally advanced or recurrent carcinoma of the nasopharynx or paranasal sinuses were treated. In 11 of 12 patients (91.6%) who received curative treatment, complete response was obtained. In one of two patients who received palliative treatment only, a complete response was achieved, but the patient died of other causes. A total of eight patients (66.7%) who received curative treatment have survived for 22 to 57 months without severe late sequelae.

Bladder

Deren and Wilson[21] in 1960 and later Glen and colleagues[33] in 1963 showed that 5-FU was active against bladder carcinoma. Woodruff and co-workers[105] in 1963 and Stein and Kaufman[91]

TABLE 19–2
Treatment for Advanced Carcinoma of Head and Neck With CCIC and Radiation Therapy

AUTHORS	NO. OF PATIENTS	CHEMOTHERAPY	RADIATION THERAPY	COMPLETE RESPONSE RATE	2-YEAR SURVIVAL RATE
Showell et al[87]	27	Infusion 5-FU at 1000 mg/m^2 day for 5 days and cisplatin bolus	6000 cGy in 6 wk	60%	70%
Hahn et al[37]	44	Infusion 5-FU at 1000 mg/m^2 daily for 4 days; mitomycin at 10 mg/m^2	3000 cGy in 3 wk for two 3-wk courses (split course)	60%	—
Byfield et al[10]	18	Infusion 5-FU at 20–25 mg/kg/day for 5 days/cycle	1250 cGy/wk	75%	70%
Rotman et al[73]	Paranasal sinus 3	Infusion of cisplatin at 5–7 mg/m^2/day (low dose rate) for 2-wk cycles	Hyperfractionated 125 cGy dose/twice daily; total dose 6000—7200 cGy	100%	—
Murthy et al[60]	44	Infusion 5-FU at 800 mg/m^2/day for 5 days and cisplatin bolus at 60 mg/m^2 on day 1	1000 cGy/wk for 6–9 wk	87%	60%
Choi et al[16]	Advanced paranasal sinus and nasopharynx 14	Infusion cisplatin at 5–7 mg/m^2/day (low dose rate) for 2-wk cycles	Hyperfractionated 125 cGy/twice daily; total dose 5000–7200 cGy	91%	66.7%

CCIC: concomitant continuous infusion chemotherapy

in 1968 suggested the use of 5-FU as a radiosensitizer in the treatment of bladder carcinoma.

Rotman and co-workers[76] treated 25 patients with advanced bladder carcinoma with 5-FU CCIC and radiation and mitomycin intravenous bolus.[76,77] With the Jewett-Marshall staging system, one patient had Stage A disease, seven patients had Stage B1, nine had Stage B2, six had Stage C, and two patients had Stage D disease. In 26% of the patients, more than 50% of the bladder was involved with tumor. On intravenous pyelogram (IVP), hydronephrosis was present in eight of 25 patients, whereas 63% had residual tumor present at the beginning of therapy. Therapy consisted of continuous infusion of 5-FU given over 120 hours at the rate of 25 mg/kg/day concomitantly with radiation therapy on weeks 1, 4, and 7 or 2, 5, and 8. In addition, five patients received mitomycin as intravenous bolus at 10 mg/m^2 on the first day of radiation therapy. All patients received 4000 cGy to 4500 cGy to the whole pelvis with "box technique" plus a boost dose using rotation arc, for a total dose of 6000 cGy to 6500 cGy in 33 to 35 fractions of 180 cGy each.

Response was evaluated in 22 of 25 patients. A complete response (cystoscopy and biopsies) was obtained in 63.6% of patients within a period of 6 months. Patients who had either persistent abnormal cytologic findings or frank residual tumors underwent further treatment with intravesical mitomycin C or BCG vaccine, with or without additional transurethral resection. The complete response rate then rose to 86%. After a complete response was attained, local failure was very rare: only one patient came into this category. Two of three patients who failed to achieve a complete response had salvage cystectomy and are alive and well. The adjusted 5-year survival rate is 54%, which is superior to that achieved with radiation therapy or surgery alone or with preoperative irradiation and surgery. An additional advantage of this approach is the preservation of the bladder in the majority of patients. Late complications from this treatment have been moderate: only three patients developed irritable bladder and one patient had chronic diarrhea.

Results of similar treatment were reported by Russell and co-workers.[81] A series of 28 patients with invasive transitional cell bladder carcinoma were initially treated with 4000 cGy in 5 weeks, along with two 96-hour infusions of 5-FU in the first and third weeks of radiation therapy. At 3 weeks, 57% of the patients achieved complete response as determined by cystoscopy and biopsy. These patients were allowed to complete a curative dose of radiation, receiving a total dose of 6000 cGy including the boost dose and additional chemotherapy. Patients who did not achieve complete response with the 4000 cGy given initially underwent cystectomy. Two of these patients did not show tumor in the surgical specimen, taking the final complete response rate to 71%. The studies by both Rotman[78] and Russell[81] and their associates (Table 19-3) demonstrate the possibility of late complete response, which may take up to 6 months or more; thus the decision to undertake cystectomy should wait until the completion of this period.

Cervix

5-FU, cisplatin, and mitomycin are active against cervical cancer, with response rates ranging from 20% to 50%. Using 5-FU and mitomycin, together with radiation in advanced stages, investigators at Princess Margaret Hospital[95] reported a complete response rate of 74%, with 59% of the patients remaining disease-free at 15 months. John and associates[44] at Fresno Community Hospital, using 5-FU CCIC and radiation and cisplatin in advanced cervical carcinoma, reported a 100% complete response rate in a small series of patients. At a median follow-up of 28 months, 80% were alive and free from disease. Recently, clinicians at Washington University[80] reported on a series of advanced cervical carcinoma patients similarly treated with 5-FU CCIC and radiation and cisplatin; 64% of patients were disease-free at 6 to 30 months.

The most recent series of advanced cervical carcinoma patients treated with CCIC and radiation has been reported by

TABLE 19–3
Treatment of Carcinoma of the Bladder With CCIC and Radiation Therapy

AUTHORS	NO. OF PATIENTS	CHEMOTHERAPY	RADIATION THERAPY	COMPLETE RESPONSE RATE	2-YEAR SURVIVAL RATE
Rotman et al[76]	22	Infusion 5-FU at 25 mg/kg/day for 5 days on weeks 1, 4, and 7 or on weeks 2, 5, and 8; mitomycin bolus on day 1	4000–4500 cGy in 4.5–5 wk to whole pelvis followed by 2000–2500 cGy as boost dose to bladder	89%	53.6%
Russel et al[81]	14	Infusion 5-FU at 1000 mg/m²/day for 4 days on weeks 1 and 3	4000 cGy in 5 wks if complete response; dose to 6000 cGy, otherwise cystectomy	57% No tumor found in additional 2 patients at cystectomy—CR, 71%	Median follow-up 7 mo; NED 93%
Sauer et al[83]	41	Infusion cisplatin (short duration) at 25 mg/m²/day on weeks 1 and 5	4140 cGy in 4.5 wk to whole pelvis + 1000 cGy boost to bladder	85%	Short follow-up

CCIC: concomitant continuous infusion chemotherapy
CR: complete response

Ludgate and colleagues[54]; 38 patients with bulky Stage IIB, Stage III, and Stage IVA squamous cell carcinoma of the cervix were included. These patients received mitomycin C at 10 mg/m² on the first day and two courses of 5-FU infusion at 1000 mg/m²/day on days 2 through 5 and 21 through 24 of external irradiation. Complete response was achieved in 76% of these patients 3 months after completion of therapy, with 55% surviving at 3 years. The 3-year survival rate of 79% for Stage IIB bulky disease was significantly better than the 36% obtained with conventional treatment. A phase II study has been started by RTOG to determine survival rates and tolerance using 5-FU CCIC with irradiation, mitomycin, and cisplatin in the treatment of advanced cervical cancer.

Soft Tissue

In 1982, Sordillo and co-workers[90] used low-dose doxorubicin together with radiation to treat a variety of soft tissue sarcomas. Although doxorubicin (Adriamycin) was administered 90 minutes before radiation, radiosensitization still appeared to have an important impact on results. Of 29 patients, six obtained a complete response, whereas 12 had a partial response. No response was observed in tumor-containing areas outside the radiation portal. Irradiation of these lesions without doxorubicin produced almost no regression, emphasizing the importance of radiosensitization.

A phase II study was started at SUNY-HSCB and SUNY-LICH[73] in which eight patients with locally advanced soft tissue sarcoma were treated with doxorubicin CCIC and radiation therapy. Doxorubicin was administered by continuous 5-day infusion at a dose of 12 mg/m²/day. Patients received concomitant radiation therapy. A 3- to 4-week rest period to overcome bone marrow toxicity followed. All patients received three or four cycles. Complete response was obtained in three patients, whereas the rest had partial responses.

Doxorubicin infusion with concomitant irradiation must be used with caution; 200 cGy fractions encompassing a large area, especially in the retroperitoneal or thoracic area, should be avoided. If these areas must be treated, dose per fraction should be limited to 150 cGy. In extreme cases, dose per fraction may be increased to 180 cGy.

REFERENCES

1. Auersberg M, Furlan L, Marlot F, Jereb B: Intra-arterial chemotherapy and radiotherapy in locally advanced cancer of the oral cavity and oropharynx. Int J Radiat Oncol Biol Phys 4:273–277, 1978
2. Bagshaw MA. Possible role of potentiators in radiation therapy. Am J Roentgol 85:822–833, 1961
3. Beahrs OH: Management of squamous cell carcinoma of anus and adenocarcinoma of lower rectum (Editorial). Int J Radiat Oncol Biol Phys 11:1741–1742, 1985
4. Benjamin RS, Riggs CE Jr, Bachur NR: Pharmacokinetics and metabolism of Adriamycin in man. Clin Pharmacol Ther 14:591–600, 1973
5. Bengmark S, Hafston L: The natural history of primary and secondary malignant tumors of the liver. Cancer 20:198–202, 1969
6. Borgelt BB, Gelber R, Brady LW, et al: The palliation of hepatic metastases: Results of the Radiation Therapy Oncology Group pilot study. Int J Radiat Oncol Biol Phys 7:587–591, 1981
7. Byfield JE, Barone R, Mendelsohn J, et al: Infusional 5-fluorouracil and x-ray therapy for nonresectable esophageal cancer. Cancer 45:703–708, 1980
8. Byfield JE, Lee YC, Tu L: Molecular interactions between Adriamycin and x-ray damage in mammalian tumor cells. Cancer 19:186–193, 1977
9. Byfield JE, Lynch M, Kulhaman F, Chan PYM: Cellular effects of combined Adriamycin and x-rays in human tumor cells. Int J Radiat Oncol Biol Phys 19:194–204, 1977
10. Byfield J, Sharp T, Tang S, et al: Phase I and II trial of cyclical 5 day infused 5-fluorouracil and concomitant radiation in advanced cancer of the head and neck. J Clin Oncol 2:406–413, 1984
11. Byfield JE, Frankel SS, Hornback CL, et al: Phase I and pharmacological study of 72 hour infused and hyperfractionated cyclical radiation. Int J Radiat Oncol Biol Phys 11:791–800, 1985
12. Carter SK: The chemotherapy of head and neck cancer. Semin Oncol 4:413–424, 1977
13. Case TJ, Warthin AS: The occurrence of hepatic lesions in

patients treated by intensive deep Roentgen irradiation. Am J Roentgenol 12:27–46, 1924
14. Chabner B: Pharmacologic Principles of Cancer Treatment. Philadelphia, WB Saunders, 1982
15. Childs DS Jr, Moertel CG, Holbrook MA, et al: Treatment of malignant neoplasms of the gastrointestinal tract with a combination of 5-fluorouracil and radiation therapy: A randomized, double blind study. Radiology 84:843–848, 1965
16. Choi K, Aziz K, Rotman M: Concomitant radiation and infusion cisplatinum in advanced cancers of the head and neck: Influence of radiation fractionation. ASCO Abstract, 1988
17. Coia LR: Esophageal cancer: Is esophagectomy necessary? Oncology 3:101–110, 1989
18. Coppa GF, Eng K, Ranson JHC, et al: Hepatic resection for metastatic colon and rectal cancer. Ann Surg 202:203–208, 1985
19. Cummings BJ, Harwood AR, Keane TJ: Anal canal carcinoma: Improving the therapeutic ratio with combined radiation and chemotherapy. Int J Radiat Oncol Biol Phys 9(1):110, 1983
20. Cummings B, Keane T, Harwood A, Thomas G: Combined modality therapy with 5-fluorouracil, mitomycin C, and radiation therapy for squamous cell cancers. In Rosenthal JC, Rotman M (eds): Clinical Applications of Continuous Infusion Chemotherapy and Concomitant Radiation Therapy, pp 133–147, New York, Plenum Press, 1986
21. Deren TL, Wilson WL: Use of 5-fluorouracil in treatment of bladder carcinomas. J Urol 8:390–393, 1960
22. DeVita VT, Lippman M, Hubbard SM, et al: The effect of combined modality therapy on local control and survival. Int J Radiat Oncol Biol Phys 12:487–501, 1986
23. Douple EB, Richmond RC: Platinum complexes as radiosensitizer of hypoxic mammalian cells. Br J Cancer 37:98–102, 1978
24. Dritschillo A, Pizo A, Kellman A: The effect of cisplatinum on the repair of radiation damage in plateau phase Chinese hamster (V-79) cells. Int J Radiat Oncol Biol Phys 5:1345–1349, 1979
25. Durand R: Adriamycin: A possible indirect radiosensitizer of hypoxic tumor cells. Radiology 119:217–222, 1976
26. Fazekas JT, Pajak TF, Marcial VA, Davis LW: The RTOG randomized trial 79–15: Misonidazole adjuvant to radiation therapy in advanced head and neck squamous cancers. Proc Soc Clin Oncol 3:185, 1984
27. Fisher B, Wolmark N, Rockette H, et al: Postoperative adjuvant chemotherapy or radiation therapy for rectal cancer: Results from NSABP Protocol R-01. J Natl Cancer Inst 80:21–29, 1988
28. Fletcher GH, Lindberg RD, Caderao JB, et al: Hyperbaric oxygen as a radiotherapeutic adjuvant in advanced carcinoma of the uterine cervix: Preliminary results of a randomized trial. Cancer 39:617, 1977
29. Franklin R, Steiger Z, Vaishampayan G: Combined modality therapy for esophageal carcinoma. Cancer 51:1062–1071, 1983
30. Gastrointestinal Tumor Study Group: Treatment of locally unresectable carcinoma of the pancreas. J Natl Cancer Inst 80:751–755, 1988
31. Gastrointestinal Study Group: Pancreatic cancer. Adjuvant combined radiation and chemotherapy following potentially curative resection. ASCO, 2:122, 1983
32. Gastrointestinal Tumor Study Group: Prolongation of the disease-free interval in surgically treated rectal carcinoma. N Engl J Med 23:1465–1472, 1985
33. Glen JF, Hunt LD, Latham JE: Chemotherapy of bladder carcinoma with 5-fluorouracil. Cancer Chemother Rep 27:67–69, 1963
34. Goffinet DR, Schneider MJ, Glatstein EJ: Bladder cancer results of radiation therapy in 384 patients. Radiology 153:771–782, 1972
35. Goodman MS, Wickham R: Venous access devices: An overview. Oncol Nurs Forum 11(5):16–23, 1984
36. Haghbin M, Sischy B, Hinson J: Combined modality preoperative therapy in poor prognostic rectal adenocarcinoma. Radiother Oncol 13:75–81, 1988
37. Hahn SS, Kim JA, Constable WC: Concomitant chemotherapy and radiotherapy for advanced squamous cell carcinoma of head and neck. Int J Radiat Oncol Biol Phys 10(2):191, 1984
38. Hamberger AD: Squamous cell carcinoma of the cervix. In Fletcher G (ed): Textbook of Radiotherapy, pp 720–722. Philadelphia, Lea & Febiger, 1980
39. Heidelberger C, Greisbach L, Montag BJ, Cruz D, Schnitzner RJ, Grunberg E: Studies in fluorinated pyrimidines. II. Effects of transplanted tumor. Cancer Res 18:305–317, 1958
40. Henk JM, Kunkler PB, Smith CW: Radiotherapy and hyperbaric oxygen in head and neck cancer: Final report of the first clinical trial. Lancet 2:104–105, 1977
41. Henk JM, Smith CW: Radiotherapy and hyperbaric oxygen in head and neck cancer: Interim report of the second clinical trial. Lancet 2:104–105, 1977
42. Hornback NB, Shidnia H, Shupe RE, et al: Results comparing hyperthermia and radiation versus radiation alone in treatment of 79 patients with stage IIIB carcinoma of cervix (Abstract). Int J Radiat Oncol Biol Phys 6:1384, 1980
43. Ingold JA, Reed GB, Kaplan HS, Bagshaw MA: Radiation hepatitis. Am J Roentgenol 93:200–208, 1965
44. John M, Cooke K, Flam M, et al: Preliminary results of concomitant radiotherapy and chemotherapy in advanced cervical carcinoma. Gynecol Oncol 28:101–110, 1987
45. John M, Flam M, Lovalvo L, et al: Feasibility of nonsurgical definitive management of anal canal carcinoma. Int J Radiat Oncol Biol Phys 13:299–303, 1987
46. John MJ, Flam MS, Mowry PA, et al: Radiotherapy alone and chemoradiation for nonmetastatic esophageal carcinoma. Cancer 63:2397–2403, 1989
47. Keane TJ, Harwood AR, Rider WD, et al: Concomitant radiation and chemotherapy for squamous cell carcinoma of esophagus (Abstract). Int J Radiat Oncol Biol Phys 10(2):89, 1984
48. Kish J, Drelichman A, Jacobs J: Clinical trial of cisplatinum and 5FU infusion as initial treatment for advanced squamous carcinoma of the head and neck. Cancer Treat Rep 66:471–474, 1982
49. Kyriazis AP, Yagoda A, Kereiaskes JG, et al: Experimental studies on the radiation modifying effect of cis-diamminedichloroplatinum II (BDP) in human bladder transitional cell carcinomas grown in nude mice. Cancer 52:452–457, 1983
50. Legha S, Benjamin R, Mackay B, et al: Reduction of doxorubicin cardiotoxicity by prolonged continuous intravenous infusion. Ann Int Med 96:133–139, 1982
51. Leibel SA, Pajak TF, Order SE, et al: Hepatic metastases: Results of treatment and identification of prognostic factors. Radiation Therapy Oncology Group report (Abstract). Int J Radiat Oncol Biol Phys 11(1):116–117, 1985
52. Leichman L, Steiger Z, Sydel HG, Vaitkevicus VK: Combined preoperative chemotherapy and radiation therapy for cancer of the esophagus: The Wayne State University, South West Oncology Group and Radiation Therapy Oncology Group experience. Semin Oncol 11(2):178–185, 1984
53. Lokich J, Zipoli T: Phase I study of protracted infusion of cisplatinum. Cancer Drug Deliv 1:247–250, 1984
54. Ludgate SM, Crandon AJ, Hudson CN, et al: Synchronous 5-fluorouracil, mitomycin C and radiation therapy in the treatment of locally advanced carcinoma of the cervix. Int J Radiat Oncol Biol Phys 15:893–899, 1988
55. Marks RD, Scruggo HJ, Wallace KM: Preoperative radiation therapy for carcinoma of esophagus. Cancer 38:84–89, 1976
56. Maruyama Y, Muir W: Human cervical clearance after ^{252}Cf neutron brachytherapy versus conventional photons brachytherapy. Am J Clin Oncol 7:347,1984
57. Meoz RT, Spanos WJ, Doss L, et al: Misonidazole combined with large fraction pelvic radiation in the treatment of patients with advanced pelvic malignancies: Preliminary report of an ongoing RTOG phase I, II study. Am J Clin Oncol 6:417, 1983
58. Michaelson R, Magell G, Quan S, et al: Preoperative chemotherapy and radiation therapy in the management of anal canal epidermoid carcinoma. Cancer 51:390–395, 1983

59. Moertel CG, Frytak S, Harhn RG, et al: Therapy of locally unresectable pancreatic cancer: A randomized comparison of high dose (6000 R) radiation alone, moderate dose radiation (4000 R plus 5-fluorouracil) and high dose radiation plus 5-fluorouracil: The Gastrointestinal Tumor Study Group. Cancer 48:1705–1710, 1981
60. Murthy, AK, Taylor WSG, Showel J, et al: Treatment of advanced head and neck cancer with concomitant radiation and chemotherapy. Int J Radiat Oncol Biol Phys 13:1807–1813, 1987
61. Nakayama K, Yanagisawa F: Concentrated preoperative radiation therapy. Arch Surg 87:1003–1018, 1963
62. Newaishy GA, Read GA, Duncan W, Kerr GR: Results of radical radiotherapy of squamous cell carcinoma of the esophagus. Clin Radiol 33:347–352, 1982
63. Nigro ND, Vaitkevicius VK, Considine B: Combined therapy for cancer of the anal canal: A preliminary report. Dis Colon Rectum 17:354–356, 1974
64. North Central Cancer Treatment Group: Unpublished data
65. Ogata K, Hizawa K, Yoshida M, et al: Hepatic injury following irradiation: A morphologic study. Tukushima J Exp Med 9:240–251, 1963
66. Papillon J, Montbarbow JF: Epidermoid carcinoma of the anal canal: A series of 276 cases. Dis Colon Rectum 30:324–333, 1987
67. Perez CA, Camel HM: Radiation therapy alone in the treatment of carcinoma of cervix: A 20-year experience. Gynecol Oncol 23:127, 1986
68. Perez CA, Breaux S, Madoc-Jones H: Radiation therapy alone in the treatment of carcinoma of cervix. II. Analysis of complications. Cancer 54:235, 1984
69. Phillips T, Wasserman TH, Stetz J, Brady L: Clinical trials of hypoxic cell sensitizers. Int J Radiat Oncol Biol Phys 8:327–334, 1982
70. Rich T, Byrd M: Protracted 5FU infusion in gastrointestinal tumors. Neoadjuvant Chemother 137:683–689, 1986
71. Richmond J, Seydel HG, Bae Y, et al: Comparison of three strategies for esophageal cancer within a single institution. Int J Radiat Oncol Biol Phys 13:1617–1620, 1987
72. Rooney M, Kish J, Jacobs J, et al: Improved complete response rate and survival in advanced head and neck cancer after three course induction therapy with 120 hour 5FU infusion and cisplatin. Cancer 55:1123–1128, 1985
73. Rosenthal CJ, Rotman M, Bhutiani I: Concomitant radiation therapy and doxorubicin by continuous infusion in advanced malignancy—a phase I, II study: Evidence of synergistic effect in soft tissue sarcomas and hepatomas. In Rosenthal CJ, Rotman M (eds): Clinical Applications of Continuous Infusion Chemotherapy and Concomitant Radiation Therapy, pp 159–176. New York, Plenum Press, 1986
74. Rotman M, Choi K, Isaacson S, et al: Treatment of recurrent carcinoma of the paranasal sinuses using concomitant infusion cisplatinum and radiation therapy. In Rosenthal CJ, Rotman M (eds): Clinical Applications of Continuous Infusion Chemotherapy and Concomitant Radiation Therapy, pp 189–193. New York, Plenum Press, 1986
75. Rotman M, Aziz H: Carcinoma of the anus (Editorial). Int J Radiat Oncol Biol Phys 13:465–466, 1987
76. Rotman M, Aziz H, Porrazzo M, et al: Treatment of advanced transitional cell carcinoma of the bladder with irradiation and concomitant 5-fluorouracil infusion. Int J Radiat Oncol Biol Phys 18:1131–1137, 1990
77. Rotman M, Kuruvilla A, Choi K, et al: Response of colorectal hepatic metastases to concomitant radiotherapy and intravenous infusion of 5FU. Int J Radiat Oncol Biol Phys 12:2179–2187, 1987
78. Rotman M, Macchia R, Silverstein M, et al: Treatment of advanced bladder carcinoma with irradiation and concomitant 5FU infusion. Cancer 59:710–714, 1987
79. Rowley R, Bacharach M, Hopkins HA, et al: Adriamycin and irradiation effects upon an experimental solid tumor resistant to therapy. Int J Radiat Oncol Biol Phys 5:1291–1295, 1979
80. RTOG Protocol No. 85-15, Phase II nonrandomised study using chemotherapy and radiation for advanced carcinoma of the cervix. pp 1–13, 1985
81. Russell KJ, Boileau MA, Ireton R, et al: Transitional cell carcinoma of the urinary bladder: Histologic clearance with combined 5FU chemotherapy and radiation therapy. Preliminary results of a bladder-preservation study. Radiology 167(3):845–840, 1988
82. Salem P, Khalyl M, Jabboury K, Hashimi L: Cis-diamminedichloroplatinum II by 5 day continuous infusion. Cancer 53:837, 1984
83. Sauer R, Schrott KM, Dunst J, et al: Preliminary result of treatment of invasive bladder carcinoma with radiotherapy and cisplatinum. Int J Radiat Oncol Biol Phys 15:817–875, 1988
84. Seifert P, Baker LH, Reed ML: Comparison of continuously infused 5FU with bolus injection in treatment of patients with colorectal carcinoma. Cancer 36:123–128, 1975
85. Seydel H, Leichman L, Byhardt R, et al: Preoperative radiation and chemotherapy for localized squamous cell carcinoma of the esophagus: RTOG Study. Int J Radiat Oncol Biol Phys 14:33–35, 1988
86. Shaefer J, Al-Mahdi A: Combination Adriamycin and radiation treatment in pulmonary tumors in mice. Oncology 38:35–38, 1981
87. Shipley WU, Coombs LJ, Einstein AB Jr: Cisplatin and full dose irradiation for patients with invasive bladder carcinoma: A preliminary report of tolerance and local response. J Urol 132:899–903, 1984
88. Showell, JL, Murthy AK, Hutchinson LD, et al: Synchronous radiation therapy and cisplatin-5FU chemotherapy in advanced head and neck carcinoma. Proc 2nd Europ Conf Clin Oncol (Abstract) 162, 1983
89. Sischy B: The use of radiation therapy combined with chemotherapy in the management of squamous cell carcinoma of the anus and marginally resectable adenocarcinoma of the rectum. Int J Radiat Oncol Biol Phys 11:1587–1593, 1985
90. Sordillo P, Magill G, Schauer P, et al: Preliminary trial of combination therapy with Adriamycin and radiation in sarcomas and other malignant tumors. J Surg Oncol 21:23–26, 1982
91. Stein JJ, Kaufman JJ: Treatment of carcinoma of bladder with special reference to use of preoperative radiation therapy combined with 5-fluorouracil. Am J Roentgenol Radium Ther Nucl Med 102:519–529, 1968
92. Suit HD: The scope of the problem of primary tumor control. Cancer 61:2141–2147, 1988
93. Sullivan R: Systemic and arterial infusion chemotherapy for metastatic liver cancer. Int J Radiat Oncol Biol Phys 1:973–976, 1976
94. The Gastrointestinal Tumor Study Group Phase II studies of drug combinations in advanced pancreatic carcinoma: Fluorouracil plus doxorubicin plus mitomycin C and two regimens of streptozotocin plus mitomycin C plus fluorouracil. J Clin Oncol 4:1794–1798, 1986
95. Thomas G, Dembo A, Beale F, et al: Concurrent radiation mitomycin C and 5-fluorouracil in poor prognosis carcinoma of cervix: Preliminary result of phase I, II study. Int J Radiat Oncol Biol Phys 10:1785–1790, 1984
96. Turner S, Shetty R, Gandhi H, et al: Combination of radiation with concomitant continuous Adriamycin infusion in a patient with partially excised pleomorphic soft tissue sarcoma of the lower extremity. In Rosenthal CJ, Rotman M (eds): Clinical Applications of Continuous Infusion Chemotherapy and Concomitant Radiation Therapy, pp 183–188. New York, Plenum Press, 1986
97. Vermund H, Hodgett J, Ansfield FJ: Effects of combined radiation and chemotherapy on transplanted tumors in mice. Am J Roentgenol 85:559–567, 1961
98. Vietti J, Eggerding F, Valeriote F: Combined effect of x-radiation and 5-fluorouracil on survival of transplanted leukemic cells. J Natl Cancer Inst 47:865–870, 1971
99. Volterrani F, Lambardi F: Long term results of radium therapy in cervical cancer. Int J Radiat Oncol Biol Phys 6:565, 1980
100. Watering W, Byfield J, Lagasse L, et al: Combination Adriamycin and radiation therapy in gynecologic cancer. Gynecol Oncol 2:518–526, 1974

101. Watson ER, Halnan KE, Dische S, et al: Hyperbaric oxygen and radiotherapy: A Medical Research Council Trial in carcinoma of cervix. Br J Radiol 51:879, 178
102. Whitmore WF Jr, Batata MA, Hilaris BS: A comparative study of two pre-operative radiation regimens with cystectomy for bladder cancer. Cancer 40:10775 1977
103. Wodinsky I, Swinarski J, Kensher CI, Venditi, JM: Combination radiotherapy and chemotherapy for P388 for lymphocytic leukemia *in vivo*. Cancer Chemother Rep 4:73–97, 1974
104. Wood CR, Gillis CO, Blumgart LH: A retrospective study of the natural history of patients with liver metastasis from colorectal cancer. Clin Oncol 2:285–288, 1976
105. Woodruff MW, Murphy WT, Hopson JM: Further observation on use of combination 5-fluorouracil and supervoltage irradiation therapy in treatment of advanced carcinoma of bladder. J Urol 90:747–758, 1963

20

Skin

Merrill J. Solan
Luther W. Brady
Steven A. Binnick
Peter J. Fitzpatrick

ANATOMY

The integumentary system comprises the skin and the appendageal structures traversing the skin.[4] Both benign and malignant tumors may present as palpable or visible (nodular, ulcerative, infiltrating) lesions in the skin. The basic structure of the skin consists of the following components[48] (Fig. 20-1).

Epidermis

The outer layer of the skin varies in depth from 0.3 mm on the eyelids and flexural areas to 1.5 mm on the palms of the hand and soles of the feet. The major function of the epidermis is the synthesis of keratin, which provides the skin with much of its protective properties. The outermost layer of the epidermis is the stratum corneum, composed of completely keratinized epithelial cells. The thickness of the stratum corneum varies greatly on various parts of the body; it is thickest on the palms and soles and totally absent on the oral mucosa. The basal layer rests on the basement membrane separating the epidermis from the dermis; these basal cells are the only epidermal cells that proliferate. Melanocytes, located between the basal cells of the epidermis, are the pigment-producing cells of the skin.

Dermis

The dermis consists of spindle-shaped fibroblasts, which produce collagen, giving the skin much of its strength. Other fibrillar proteins, reticulum and elastin, are also found in the dermis. The space between the fibrillar proteins of the dermis is occupied by the ground substance consisting of mucopolysaccharides, hyaluronic acid, water, and various nutrients.

Vessels, Nerves, and Lymphatics

The epidermis contains no blood vessels or nerves. Its nourishment and perceptive qualities must be obtained from the dermis. Two vascular plexuses are found in the dermis: one located at the junction of the dermis and the subcutaneous tissue and one located within the upper part of the dermis. Both sensory and autonomic nerves supply the dermis. Sensory nerves either terminate as free nerve endings in the upper dermis or enter special nerve end-organs, mediating pressure, touch, heat, and cold. The autonomic nerves derive from the sympathetic nervous system and supply the blood vessels, musculi arrectores pilorum, and the eccrine and apocrine glands.

Muscles of the Skin

The skin contains smooth muscle in the form of the musculi arrectores pilorum, the tunica dartos of the external genitalia, and in the areola of the breast. The musculi arrectores pilorum arise in the dermis and attach to the hair shaft; here they are responsive to cold and sweat, giving rise to the characteristic "goose flesh." Striated muscles are located in the neck as the platysma and in the muscles of facial expression.

Appendageal Structures of the Skin

The appendageal structures of the skin include the sebaceous glands found throughout the skin except on the palms and soles; they are most numerous on the face and upper portions of the chest and back. Eccrine glands are present in the skin except in the nail beds and certain mucosal surfaces. The release of eccrine sweat is a response to either thermal or emotional stimuli. The apocrine glands are found mainly in the axillae and to a lesser degree in the anal and genital areas. Modified apocrine glands may be found in the breast, ear canal, and eyelids. The apocrine glands are adrenergic and appear to be stimulated by stress.

EPIDEMIOLOGY

Carcinomas of the skin are the most common of all cancers, with over 500,000 new cases estimated each year in the United States.[53] Most occur on the head and neck; they may be disfiguring but are rarely fatal (Fig. 20-2).

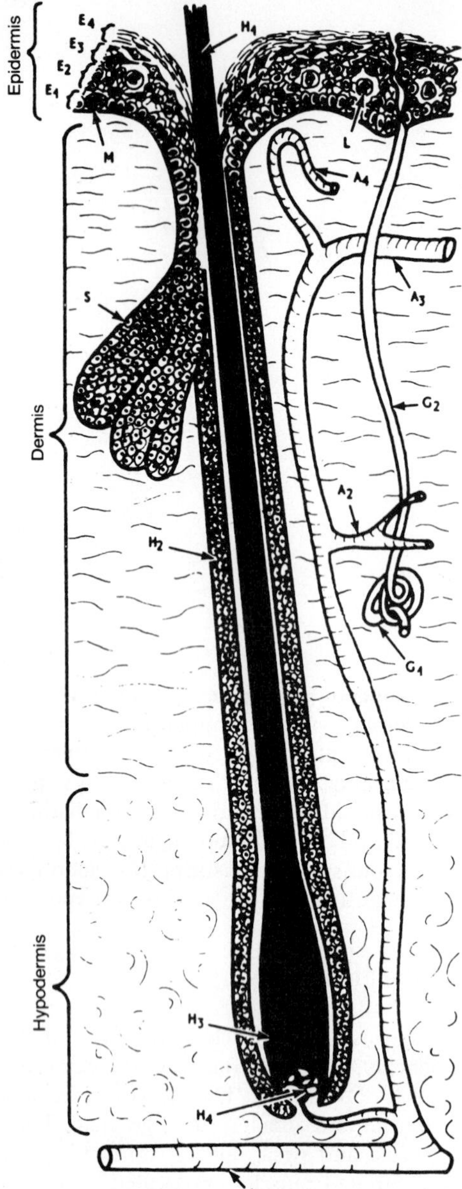

FIGURE 20–1. Diagram of structure of normal skin. E_1, basal cell layer; E_2, prickle cell layer; E_3, granular cell layer; E_4, horny cell layer; L, Langerhans' cell; M, melanocyte; S, sebaceous gland; H_1, hair shaft; H_2, inner and outer hair root sheaths; H_3, hair matrix; H_4, dermal papillae; A_1, subcutaneous vessel; A_2, deep vascular plexus; A_3, superficial vascular plexus.

Exposure to solar radiation is the single most common cause of skin cancer as well as the most preventable.[33] Carcinogenesis results from somatic mutations caused by unrepaired damage. About 95% of squamous cell carcinomas and 70% of basal cell carcinomas in North America occur in blue-eyed blondes, among whom multiple lesions are common. Farmers, fishermen, golfers, sun worshippers, and others whose occupations or hobbies involve frequent sun exposure are at high risk.

Genetic relationships also are important in the development of skin cancers. Xeroderma pigmentosa, albinism, phenylketonuria, autosomal recessive disorders, and Gorlin syndrome, an autosomal dominant disorder, are associated with an increased incidence of skin cancer.

Repeated exposure to ionizing radiation can give rise to dermatitis, with subsequent development of skin cancers within the involved areas.[2] Among those treated for acne, hirsutism, or other benign skin disorders by radiation and among diagnostic radiologists working without adequate protection, skin cancers and other malignant tumors are commonly seen.[57]

Skin cancers also can develop as a result of long-term chronic ulcerations seen in syphilis or burns. Exposure to various chemicals such as arsenic trioxide (AS203), soot, and tar also can give rise to skin cancers. More recently, exposure to oncoviruses has been suggested as another epidemiologic agent, particularly in cases of keratoacanthoma.

DIAGNOSTIC WORKUP

The diagnosis of a malignant skin lesion requires a careful history and an appreciation of subtle changes in the normal appearance of the skin. Age, race, ethnic background, occupation, geographic factors, and gender are important. A specific history should include the time of onset of the skin lesion, the site of onset, and the dates of exacerbation and recurrence as well as its extension into adjacent areas; symptoms associated with the lesion should be documented. The patient should be asked about topical treatment used in the past, history of chemical exposure, or prior irradiation to the involved area.

Various tools to assess the skin should be used, including the Wood's light and potassium hydroxide preparations (to diagnose superficial fungus infections), fungal cultures, skin biopsies, Tzanck smears, and patch testing.[17] It is important to define the tumor precisely with respect to size, diameter, degree of invasion, and multifocality. Regional lymph nodes must be evaluated carefully and biopsy or excision performed when malignancy is suspected. Correlation between the clinical presentation and the pathologic examination is important, and any evidence of previous treatment must be noted.[48] Depth of invasion and the presence of bone or cartilage invasion should be documented with the aid of plain radiographs, computed tomography, or magnetic resonance imaging.

The staging system for skin cancer is summarized in Table 20-1.

CLINICOPATHOLOGIC MANIFESTATIONS

Most skin tumors arise from damaged skin from existing lesions. Basal cell and squamous cell carcinomas are the most common, and melanomas the most serious. Some keratoacanthomas, or the so-called self-healing epitheliomas, undoubtedly undergo malignant transformation, behaving as aggressive squamous cell carcinomas. Examples of premalignant lesions are the following:

- epithelial hyperplasia
- keratoses
- leukoplakia
- nevi

Adnexal and connective tissue tumors, malignant lymphomas, and metastases are other important tumors that occur within the skin. Malignant tumors of the skin frequently are multiple.

Examples of malignant lesions are the following:

- basal cell carcinoma
- intraepithelial carcinoma (Bowen's)
- squamous cell carcinoma
- keratoacanthoma (acute epithelial cancer)
- melanoma

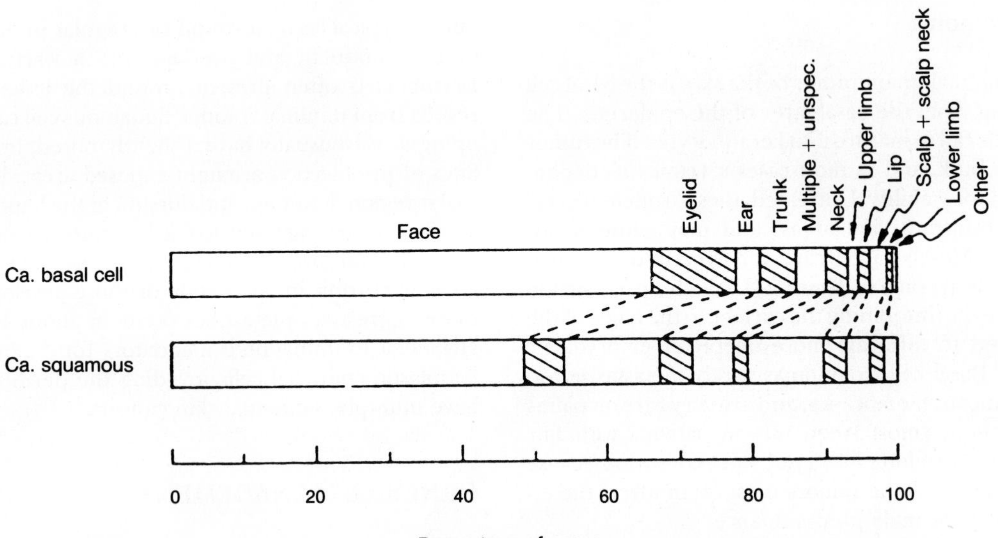

FIGURE 20–2. Sites of occurrence for basal and squamous cell skin cancers. Most skin cancers develop on the exposed areas of the head and neck. They arise from hair-bearing skin and are exceptionally rare on the palms and soles.

- Merkel cell carcinoma
- adnexal tumors
- connective tissue tumors
- malignant lymphomas
- mycosis fungoides
- Kaposi's sarcoma
- metastases

Bowen's Disease

Bowen's disease is a nonfamilial precancerous dermatosis characterized by a velvety, keratotic plaque occurring anywhere on the body.[4] Lesions may be single or multiple and are typically reddish-brown, sharply demarcated plaques covered by a scale of variable thickness. Ulcerated areas or crusting may occur, although this is unusual. Mild pruritus is usually the only symptom. Growth is slow, and the lesion may be present for several years before undergoing transformation into an invasive squamous cell carcinoma. Chronic arsenic ingestion may predispose to multiple bowenoid lesions. Typical treatment is surgical excision, although desiccation and curettage or cryotherapy may be used. Topical 5-fluorouracil (5-FU) therapy also may be effective. Radiation therapy has been used to treat Bowen's disease with excellent control.[5]

TABLE 20–1
AJC Staging System for Skin Cancer

PRIMARY TUMOR (T)

TX	Primary tumor cannot be assessed
T0	No evidence of primary tumor
Tis	Carcinoma *in situ*
T1	Tumor 2 cm or less in greatest dimension
T2	Tumor more than 2 cm but not more than 5 cm in greatest dimension
T3	Tumor more than 5 cm in greatest dimension
T4	Tumor invades deep extradermal structures (*i.e.*, cartilage, skeletal muscle, or bone)

REGIONAL LYMPH NODES (N)

NX	Regional lymph nodes cannot be assessed
N0	No regional lymph node metastasis
N1	Regional lymph node metastasis

DISTANT METASTASIS (M)

MX	Presence of distant metastasis cannot be assessed
M0	No distant metastasis
M1	Distant metastasis

AJC: American Joint Committee
(Beahrs OH, Henson DE, Hutter RVP, Myers MH [eds]: Manual for Staging of Cancer, 3rd ed. Philadelphia, JB Lippincott, 1988)

Lentigo Maligna

Lentigo maligna is a pigmented patch containing abnormal melanocytes, which may progress to malignant melanoma. It is commonly found in elderly people, almost always on exposed surfaces of the body, particularly the face. Lentigo maligna begins as a tan, nonpalpable patch, gradually enlarging and developing into various shades of brown. Typical treatment is surgical excision or cryotherapy. However, conventional radiation therapy with doses of 4500 cGy to 5000 cGy in ten to 20 fractions can be highly effective in controlling the disease. Because it progresses over a long period—often 10 to 15 years—before developing into a melanoma, cautious observation with biopsies of elevated areas may be indicated, depending on the patient's age and general health.

Keratoacanthoma

Keratoacanthomas are benign lesions in general and usually are self-healing. They have the ability, however, to destroy large volumes of tissue and are on occasion associated with squamous cell carcinomas. Fortunately, they tend to be extremely radiation-sensitive and can be irradiated, particularly when there is evidence of coexisting squamous cell carcinoma on biopsy. Doses of 3500 cGy in 12 to 14 fractions to 4500 cGy in 15 to 20 fractions have been used. Surgical excision also is a very effective means of management.

Basal Cell Carcinoma

The most common malignant tumor of the skin is the basal cell carcinoma, arising from the basal layer of the epidermis. The involved basal cells fail to mature into keratinocytes. The tumor steadily grows in bulk, and in most cases it retains its dependency on the skin for viability. Untreated, these "rodent ulcers" burrow deeply, infiltrate vital areas, and may cause major marked deformity. Most basal cell carcinomas occur on the head and neck, nearly always on hair-bearing skin with a predilection for the head above the line joining the earlobe to the angle of the mouth. They tend to infiltrate more deeply at embryologic junctional areas. Basal cell carcinomas rarely metastasize, do not develop on mucous membranes, and are very rare on palms and soles. They occur most frequently in patients with fair complexions who have a long history of sun exposure. Because sun exposure is additive, the tumors most often affect the elderly. There is a slight male predominance.

The typical basal cell carcinoma is that of a smooth, small nodule, usually on the face. A characteristic central depression secondary to necrosis is surrounded by raised, pearly, or translucent borders. Telangiectatic vessels are usually present in or around the lesion. A history of bleeding with minor trauma may be diagnostically important. Generally, lesions double in size about every 6 to 12 months, and tumors of several centimeters are most often the result of neglect.

Superficial basal cell carcinomas may present as well-demarcated erythematous plaques with slightly raised borders. These tumors generally appear on the covered areas of the body. The sclerosing basal cell carcinoma, morphea subtype, is characterized by deep infiltration of the skin with sparing of the skin surface. It is associated with an increased recurrence rate after initial treatment, possibly because of difficulty in adequately assessing tumor borders. Basal cell epitheliomas may be pigmented. Histologic examination reveals nests of basaloid cells extending beyond the dermal-epidermal junction.

Squamous Cell Carcinoma

Squamous cell carcinoma is a dysplastic tumor of keratinizing cells of the epidermis which have invaded beyond the dermal-epidermal junction. Such tumors are preceded by premalignant lesions, the most common of which is the actinic keratosis. Squamous cell carcinomas also may arise in old burn scars, areas of chronic radiation dermatitis, or other areas of long-standing inflammation. They are variable in their clinical presentation, but the typical lesion is round to irregular in shape, plaque-like or even nodular, and overlaid with a warty keratotic scale. Erythema is often present around the lesion, and bleeding results from minimal trauma. Squamous cell carcinomas developing *de novo* usually have a slightly raised, indurated border. Sites of predilection are light-exposed areas, in particular the malar region, lower lip, and dorsum of the hand. Squamous cell carcinomas arising from actinic keratoses are slow-growing and rarely metastasize. Lesions arising from old burn scars and areas of chronic inflammation or those developing *de novo* are more aggressive; metastases occur in about 10% of all cases. Histologic examination is mandatory for diagnosis and reveals neoplastic epithelial cells invading the dermis. Patients often have multiple sequential skin cancers.[3]

GENERAL MANAGEMENT

Together basal cell carcinoma and squamous cell carcinoma make up approximately 95% of all primary malignant skin lesions. For most lesions, surgical excision or radiation therapy offers equivalent excellent cure rates. The treatment modality selected should offer the greatest potential for cure with acceptable cosmetic and functional results. Factors to be considered in treatment selection include the size and anatomic location of the lesion, involvement of adjacent cartilage or bone, depth of invasion, tumor grade, previous treatment, and the general medical condition of the patient. Table 20-2 outlines various malignant and premalignant conditions of the skin for which ionizing radiation may be indicated.[8]

The treatment technique used by dermatologists is electrodesiccation and curettage. With the patient under local anesthesia, the tumor is scooped out with a sharp curet and electrodesiccated. Often the dermatologist may do a second curettage and desiccation to increase the possibility of total tumor removal. With this procedure, the cure rate is approximately 90% to 95%. Recurrent tumors can be identified early and removed by surgery or treated by radiation therapy.

Another method used in the treatment of skin tumors is Mohs chemosurgery (microscopically controlled surgery).[55] The tumor and the adjacent scar are fixed in zinc chloride, mapped, and surgically excised. Frozen-section samples are taken to locate areas still containing tumor; these areas are further excised until there is no microscopic evidence of residual disease. In recent years, the fresh-tissue technique (omitting the usually painful zinc chloride) has become popular. It is generally reserved for advanced tumors, recurrent lesions, or

TABLE 20–2
Malignant Conditions of the Skin for Which Radiation Therapy is Indicated

HIGHLY INDICATED AND OF UNIQUE ADVANTAGE	OFTEN INDICATED AND COMPETITIVE WITH OTHER TREATMENT METHODS	RARELY INDICATED
Kaposi's sarcoma	Basal cell and squamous cell carcinoma of head and trunk, vulva, and perineum	Fibrosarcoma
Mycosis fungoides	Keratoacanthoma	Basal cell and squamous cell carcinoma of scrotum, soles, and palms
Lymphoma cutis	Bowen's disease	
	Erythroplasia	
	Angiosarcoma	
	Melanoma	
	Merkel cell carcinoma	

tumors located near the orbit. With this method, the 5-year cure rate should be 95% or better. The disadvantages of the fresh-tissue technique are the expense and the fact that the patient's cosmetic appearance is usually poor following the procedure, although appearance improves with time.

Cryotherapy with liquid nitrogen also has been used to treat basal cell and squamous cell carcinomas; this treatment technique requires experience in the use of thermocouples and should be performed only by clinicians experienced in the technique.

Basal cell and squamous cell carcinomas may be surgically excised. Excision is more time-consuming than electrodesiccation and curettage and is difficult if the tumor is located on the nose or ear or adjacent to the eyelid, areas in which radiation therapy techniques may be preferable. Surgery often is the preferred treatment for lesions of the scalp because of the resultant hair loss following irradiation. Surgical excision, curettage, electrodesiccation, or cryotherapy is usually the treatment of choice over irradiation for small lesions under 3 cm that are amenable to removal with little cosmetic or functional deficit. These methods offer the advantage of expediency of treatment. For small lesions of the lip, eyelid, ear, or nose, radiation therapy may offer an advantage over surgical techniques in terms of cosmesis and function.[45]

Larger lesions with deep fixation or involvement of adjacent structures often are better treated with radiation therapy because adequate surgical margins may be difficult to obtain without the need for extensive cosmetic reconstruction. Contrary to the early belief that bone or cartilage involvement was a contraindication to radiotherapeutic management of skin cancers, excellent control rates with good cosmesis, function preservation, and rare complications are seen.[46] Radiation therapy has the advantage in the treatment of multiple lesions or when the inclusion of regional lymph nodes is warranted. Although lymph node metastases are rare for basal cell carcinomas, 5% to 10% of squamous cell carcinomas metastasize to regional nodes. The location of the involved lymph nodes is determined by the site of the primary lesion. Parotid area nodal involvement is seen in squamous cell carcinomas of the face, scalp, and ear and is particularly suited to treatment with radiation therapy.[38]

At times it is necessary to irradiate a patient who has had an incomplete resection.[8] In such an instance, biopsy reveals evidence of recurrence or persistence, or a pathologic examination of the surgical specimen shows transected tumor tissue in the margin. In the treatment of such patients, the extent of the original tumor must be adequately defined. Treatment is often predicated on that definition and includes the entire scar as well as all evidence of tumor present before the operation.

Because irradiation results in poorly vascularized skin and subcutaneous tissue, the treatment site usually does not tolerate additional radiation therapy.[8] For this reason, it is best to implement some type of surgery to eradicate a persistent tumor in an irradiated site. Re-irradiation of skin cancer is seldom attempted and then only when the involved tissue bed appears to have an even chance of surviving further treatment or when surgery might cause greater emotional and economic loss.

Chemotherapy has been used with some success in the treatment of advanced, metastatic basal cell and squamous cell carcinomas. The most active agents have been cisplatin and doxorubicin, with reports on significant long-term palliation.[23,62]

Retinoids, vitamin A derivatives, are emerging as a potential new treatment modality in refractory advanced squamous cell carcinoma of the skin.[34] The presumed mode of action lies in an effective increase in the number of receptors to epidermal growth factor, because epidermal growth-factor binding capacity has been directly related to growth inhibition of squamous cell carcinoma. Early studies show encouraging responses; however, because these series are based on very small numbers of patients, further investigation is needed.

RADIATION THERAPY TECHNIQUES

Many radiation sources are available for the treatment of skin cancer. Orthovoltage and supervoltage x-rays and electron beams are most often applied. The technique chosen is determined by the size, depth, and anatomic location of the lesion. The quality of radiation should be chosen on the basis of the best ratio between surface dose and the ideal depth dose (Table 20-3; Fig. 20-3). Similarly, the time-dose fractionation schedule selected depends on cosmetic and functional considerations balanced against the desire for expedient, less costly treatment.

Tolerance to irradiation appears to increase with protraction of dose and reduction of the irradiated volume. The problems of the relationship between radiation energy, volume, dose, time, tumor size, normal tissue volume, and limiting adjacent tissue tolerances have been explored by many investigators, including Strandquist,[54] Cohen,[13] and von Essen.[58,59]

Practically all skin cancers can be irradiated successfully by x-ray beams ranging from one half-value layer (HVL) of 0.6 mm of aluminum up to 1.0 mm of copper, depending on the area and thickness of the lesion. Most of the lesions are irradiated with half-value layers of 1.2 mm to 4.25 mm of aluminum using x-ray generators operating between 100 kV and 120 kV or with half-value layers of 1.0 mm of copper using 200 kV x-rays.

The focal skin distance (FSD) should be short, consistent with the best ratio between surface dose and maximal depth dose. As illustrated in Figure 20-4, irregular body contours may significantly alter the surface dose when short treatment distances are used. The underlying normal tissues should be spared to the greatest degree possible.

Electron beams (3.75 MeV to 16 MeV) are increasingly used in the treatment of skin cancers as dual-energy treatment machines with electron capability gradually replace orthovoltage units. Electron beams offer the advantage of rapid falloff of depth dose and therefore greater ease of sparing under-

TABLE 20–3
*Percentage Depth Doses for Various Radiation Sources Used in Treatment of Skin Cancers**

SOURCE	d90% (cm)	d50% (cm)	d10% (cm)
Surface applicators (^{90}Sr)	≃0.03	≃0.1	≃0.25
Radium mold 10^2 cm			
0.5 cm		≃1.0	≃4.0
1.0 cm		≃2.0	≃7.0
Electron beam 10^2 cm			
5 MeV	1.45	2.1	2.5
10 MeV	0.8	4.2	5.1
20 MeV	6.1	8.3	10.0
X-rays 10^2 cm			
100 kV	≃0.2	≃0.9	≃4.0
125 kV	≃1.0	≃4.0	≃15.0
250 kV	≃2.5	≃7.0	≃18.0

**At Princess Margaret Hospital, Toronto, Canada*

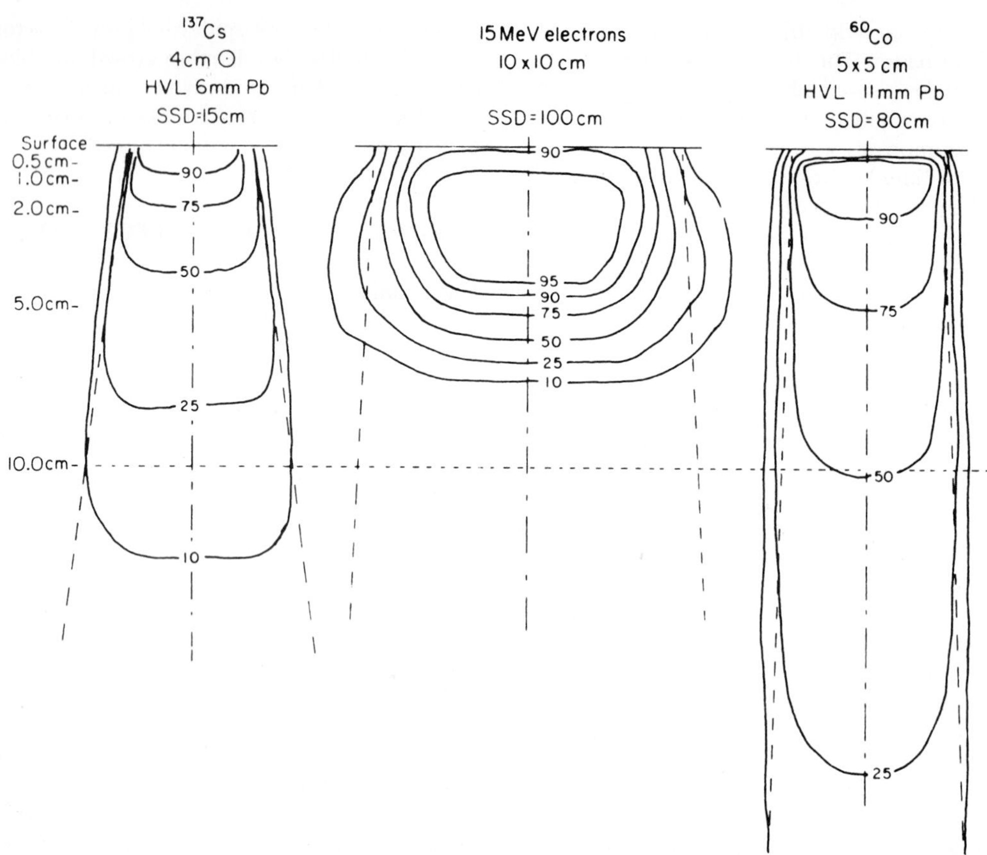

FIGURE 20–3. Isodose curves from units used to treat skin cancers.

lying normal structures. For most tumors, the electron-beam energy selected puts the 80% or 90% isodose line at the desired treatment depth. The 80% isodose depth in centimeters is approximately one third the beam energy expressed in million electron volts (MeV). When electrons below 18 MeV are used, there is a significant skin-sparing effect, and bolus (usually 1 cm to 1.5 cm) should be applied to increase the skin surface dose (Fig. 20-5).

Supervoltage irradiation (with surface bolus) is used for more advanced lesions with deep penetration and involvement of bone or cartilage. Special treatment techniques may be necessary so that larger volumes can be irradiated to higher total doses.

Field sizes depend not only on the size of the lesion, but also on the site treated and the quality of radiation used. The irradiated area must include at least a 1.0 cm border of normal tissue in small lesions and a larger margin (2.0 cm) in larger lesions. When a lesion is treated with low-energy electron-beam irradiation, allowance must be made for constriction of the isodose lines at depth, and therefore a relatively wider margin of normal tissue must be included at the surface. The field size should be carefully delineated. Treatment aids such as lead cutouts are used to define more carefully the borders of the lesions, and protective shields are used if necessary (Fig. 20-6). The anatomic part should be immobilized for treatment accuracy. This may require the preparation of a plastic mask or immobilization device to achieve stability during the treatment itself (Fig. 20-7).

The definitive radiation doses recommended vary with the histologic type, size, and depth of the lesion, size of the treatment field, dose fractionation, and overall time of delivery. In general, daily treatment fractions may range from 200 cGy to 500 cGy with total tumor doses of 3000 cGy to 5000 cGy in six to 20 fractions for most basal cell carcinomas and 5000 cGy to 6000 cGy in six to 30 fractions over a period of 10 to 35 elapsed days (Fig. 20-8; Table 20-4) for squamous cell carcinomas. Large basal cell carcinomas (>5 cm in diameter or >0.5 cm thick) should be treated with doses similar to squamous cell carcinoma. Radiation therapy techniques are particularly suitable for treatment of lesions located about the eyelids,[19,21,37] in the periorbital areas, in the medial triangle of the cheek, and in the ear[15,27,44] and nose.[15,39] The incidence of treatment failure should be very low, and with proper follow-up patients in whom irradiation has failed can be identified early for surgical salvage. Most patients have excellent functional and cosmetic results. Scarring persists more and changes relative to the radiation therapy are more pronounced in lesions that were large or infected when first seen.

RESULTS OF IRRADIATION

Lovett and associates[35] reported on 339 biopsy-proven squamous cell and basal cell skin carcinomas (92 squamous cell, 242 basal cell, and five variants of squamous cell carcinoma in various locations). Radiation therapy was the initial treatment modality in 212 patients; 127 were treated after failing initial surgical excision. Overall local tumor control was achieved in 292 of 339 patients (86%): 220 of 242 patients (91%) with basal cell and 73 of 97 (75%) with squamous cell carcinoma. Tumor control was closely related to the size of the primary lesion. For lesions less than 1 cm, tumor control was 97% (86 of 89) for basal cell carcinoma and 91% (21 of 23) for squamous cell carcinoma. For lesions 1 cm to 5 cm, tumor control was 87% (116 of 133) for basal cell and 76% (39 of 51) for squamous cell tumors, and for

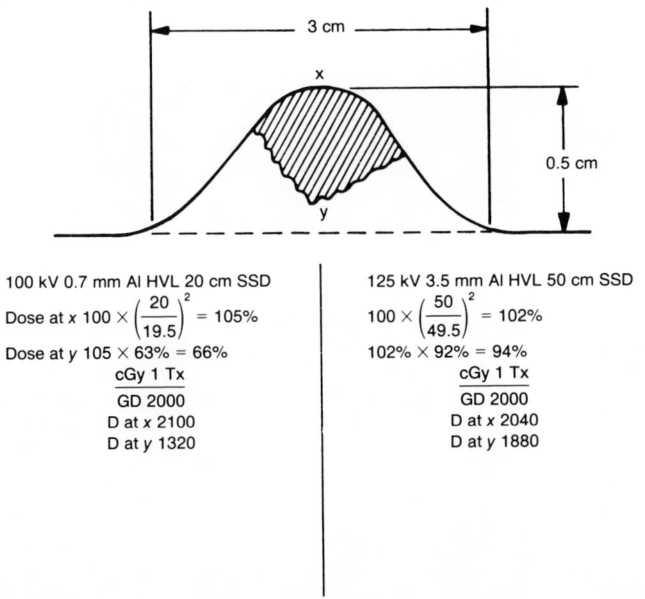

FIGURE 20–4. Treatment of convex surfaces. For convex surfaces and in cases in which any significant invasion of the deeper tissues is present, there is an advantage in increasing the beam energy and surface-source distance (SSD). The given dose (GD) is measured where the cone touches the skin. In the example shown, increasing the SSD from 20 cm to 50 cm, the beam energy from 100 kV to 125 kV, and the half-value layer (HVL) from 0.7 mm Al to 3.5 mm Al results in a greater homogeneity of the radiation dose to the tumor.

lesions greater than 5 cm, tumor control was 87% (13 of 15) and 56% (nine of 16), respectively. Tumor control was related to the modality used to treat the patient despite stratification by primary lesion size. When superficial x-rays were used, tumor control was 98% (81 of 83) for lesions less than 1 cm, 93% (94 of 101) for lesions 1 cm to 5 cm, and 100% (five of five) for lesions greater than 5 cm. With electrons, tumor control was 88% (14 of 16), 72% (23 of 32), and 78% (seven of nine) for the three groups, respectively. For mixed beams, tumor control was 90% (nine of ten), 76% (32 of 42), and 64% (nine of 14), respectively. Tumor control was 100% (three of three), 67% (six of nine), and 33% (one of three), respectively, when ^{60}Co, 4 MV x-rays were used.

Table 20-5 shows the experience at Hahnemann University with radiation therapy as a means of treating malignant lesions of the skin. Fitzpatrick and colleagues[21] have reviewed the results from the Princess Margaret Hospital for basal cell and squamous cell carcinomas in various sites. Many of their findings are summarized in the following sections.

TREATMENT BY SPECIFIC ANATOMIC SITE

Carcinoma of the Lip

In carcinoma of the lip there is a marked male predominance. Fitzpatrick and associates[21] report regional nodal involvement in up to 7% of cases and a 3% tumor-related mortality rate. The majority of tumors involve the lower lip, and large lesions of the upper lip commonly extend up to the ala nasi and columella nasi. Basal cell carcinomas arise from the skin and cross the vermilion border to invade the lip. Squamous cell carcinomas most frequently develop at the vermilion margin, an embryologic junctional area.

Techniques used to treat carcinomas of the lip commonly include interstitial implant or external-beam irradiation or both, with orthovoltage or low-energy electron beams. Figure 20-9 illustrates the successful treatment of squamous cell carcinoma of the lip with radiation therapy. Because of the low incidence of regional node involvement, prophylactic neck irradiation generally is not used.

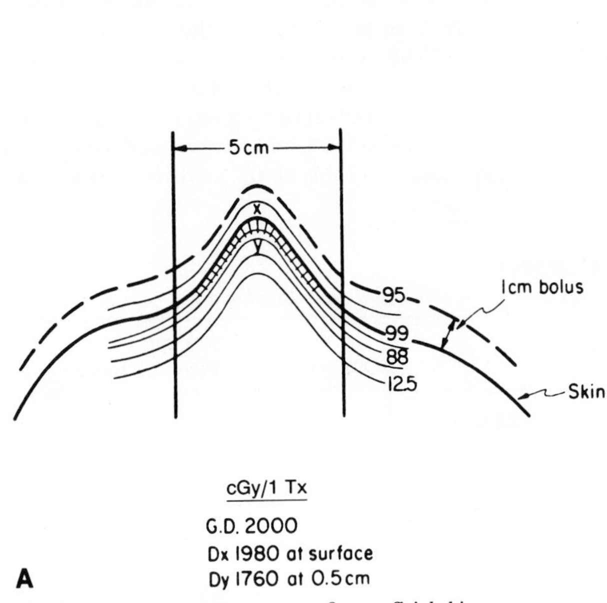

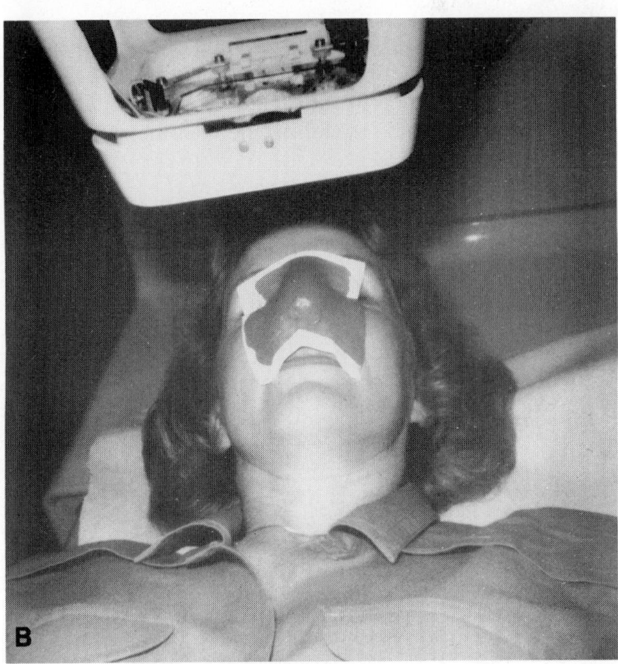

FIGURE 20–5. (**A**) Treatment of superficial skin cancer on curved surface using 5 MeV electron beam with 1 cm tissue equivalent bolus. Because of the initial buildup before the maximal absorbed dose is reached, bolus is used in such cancers to maximize the surface dose and reduce the depth dose. (**B**) A 36-year-old woman with extensive basal cell carcinoma of the nose treated with 6 MeV electron beam (5000 cGy in 25 fractions). She is tumor-free and has excellent cosmetic results 6 years later.

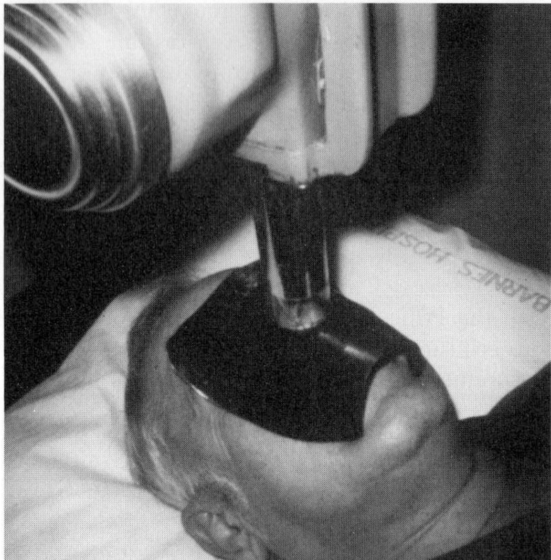

FIGURE 20–6. Patient in treatment position for small basal cell carcinoma in the nasolabial fold. Lead mask with port cut-out is used to protect adjacent structures.

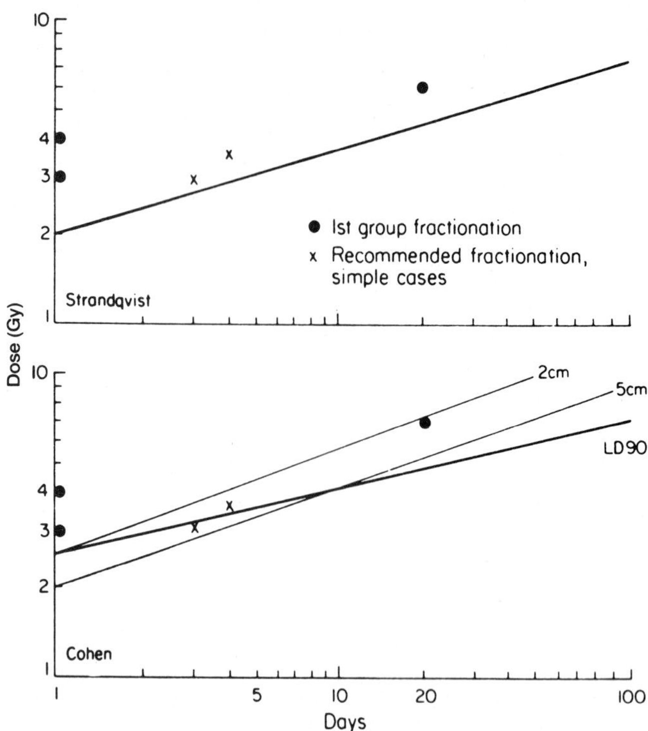

FIGURE 20–8. Two studies showing relationship between total radiation dose and total treatment time for simple skin cancer.

Carcinoma of the Eyelid

Surgery is usually the preferred treatment for eyelid tumors under 0.5 cm or for salvage of radiation therapy failures. Because of the difficulty associated with achieving adequate surgical excision, most larger carcinomas of the eyelids and canthi are treated with either orthovoltage or electron-beam irradiation (Fig. 20-10). Meticulous attention to treatment technique is essential to spare the radiovulnerable anterior segment of the eye. Many eyelid tumors may appear small and superficial on preliminary inspection but actually penetrate deep into the globe. Computed tomography is an essential diagnostic test for accurate determination of tumor extent prior to treatment planning.

The most common technique for treating eyelid tumors by irradiation is shown in Figure 20-11. A lead cutout, the thickness of which is determined by the quality of radiation used, is fashioned for each patient to define the treatment field, to shield surrounding normal tissue, and to allow accurate daily reproducibility. A lead eye shield is inserted into the conjunctival sac daily (using a local anesthetic) for protection of the anterior segment when orthovoltage or electron-beam irradiation is employed. An alternative method of protection involves rotation of the lens and cornea out of the beam by asking the patient to turn his or her eyes away from the beam source during treatment.

Fitzpatrick and colleagues[21] reviewed the Princess Margaret Hospital experience in the treatment of basal cell and squamous cell carcinomas of the eyelid. Most tumors treated by radiation therapy arose at the inner canthus or on the lower lid, reflecting the difficulties associated with surgical excision. Of 1166 tumors, a recurrence rate of 5% for basal cell carcinoma and 6.7% for squamous cell carcinoma was seen. Significant late effects were acceptable at 9.6% and were related to both tumor and irradiation damage (Table 20-6). No difference was found

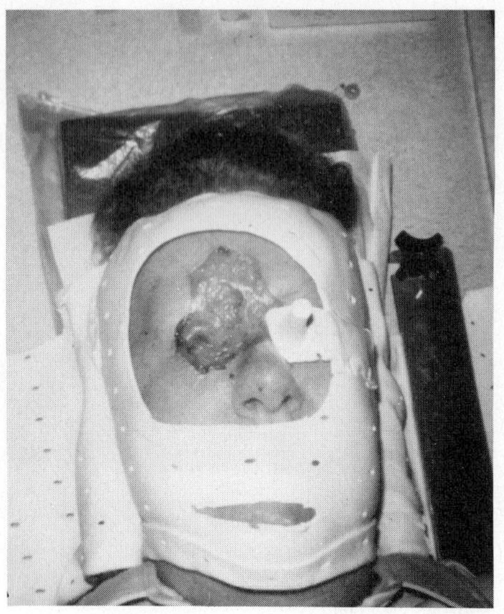

FIGURE 20–7. Mask and eye shield used for treatment of patient with extensive squamous cell carcinoma of the face.

TABLE 20–4
Skin Cancer: Recommended Dose/Fractionation

	DOSE (cGy)	NO. OF FRACTIONS	DAYS
SMALL AREA			
(less than 5 cm^2)	2000*	1–2	1–2
	3000*	5	5–7
	4000	10–16	16–28
LARGER AREA			
	4500	15–18	21–30
	5000	20–25	28–35
	6000	20–30	28–40

**Less satisfactory cosmetic results*

TABLE 20–5
*Control of Malignant Skin Lesions With Radiation Therapy**

DIAGNOSIS	NO. IRRADIATED	NO. OF TREATMENT FAILURES	NO. OF RECURRENCES CONTROLLED BY REIRRADIATION	NO EVIDENCE OF DISEASE 4 YEARS OR LONGER
Basal cell carcinoma	444	20	2	426/444 (95.9%)
Squamous cell carcinoma	156	12	—	144/156 (92.3%)
Keratoacanthoma	12	0	—	12/12 (100%)

**Hahnemann University experience, 1960–1980*

in radiation sensitivity between the two tumor histologies; however, squamous cell carcinoma showed a 6% rate of regional node metastases.

In selected patients with small lesions, Fitzpatrick and associates[21] reported excellent cosmetic and functional results with a single dose of 2000 cGy. Overall, for most tumors of an average size of 12 mm, a dose of 3500 cGy in five fractions over 5 days was found to be optimal. Because the dermis of the eyelid is extremely thin, protracted fractionation schemes at relatively small daily doses usually give the best cosmetic and functional results, especially for larger, more infiltrative lesions. When radiation therapy fails to control a tumor, recurrences are nearly always seen within 1 year of treatment.

Carcinoma of the Nose and Ear

Lesions of the nose[15,39,41] and ear[15,27,41,44] are successfully treated with irradiation. In most instances, electron-beam irradiation offers advantages over orthovoltage and surgical techniques.[27,41] The more extensive, deeply infiltrating tumors with bone or cartilage involvement require supervoltage techniques and more protracted fractionation schemes, and lymphatic irradiation may be warranted. Lesions of the nasal vestibule may be particularly suitable for interstitial techniques for all or a portion of the treatment.[39]

When orthovoltage or electron beams are used to treat nasal carcinomas, a wax-coated lead strip inserted into the nasal cavity helps to shield normal tissue. A lead face mask outlines the treatment field and minimizes the potential for overirradiation of normal tissue secondary to patient movement. Bolus should be used to raise the surface skin dose when low-energy electrons or supervoltage beams are used. Figures 20-12 to 20-14 illustrate various techniques used in treating tumors in these locations.

Carcinoma of the Dorsum of the Hand

The most common tumor involving the dorsum of the hand is squamous cell carcinoma. In general, tumors in this location are best treated by surgical excision. The most common method of treatment by radiation therapy is with radioactive molds of radium, gold, or radon seeds. Primary tumor control rates of over

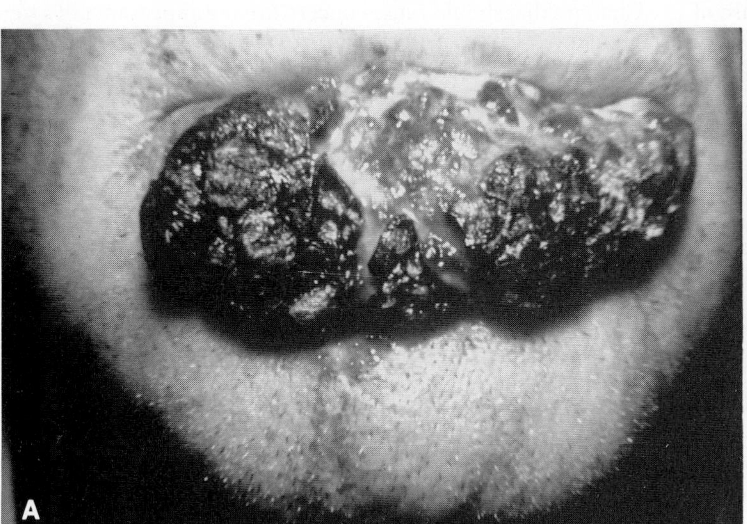

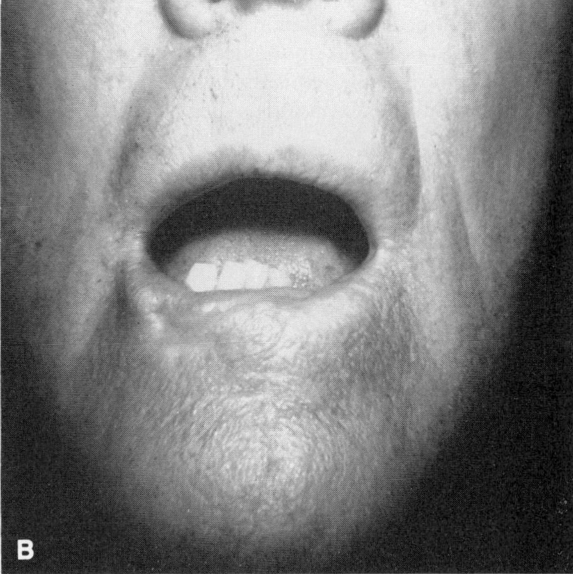

FIGURE 20–9. A 64-year-old man (**A**) before and (**B**) 5 years after irradiation for a squamous cell carcinoma of the lower lip. He received 6000 cGy in 30 fractions given over 6 weeks. The radiation beam was 250 kV, HVL 1.5 mm Cu.

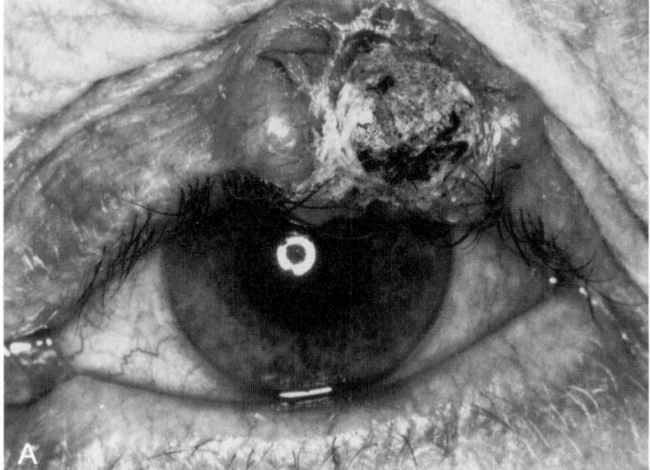

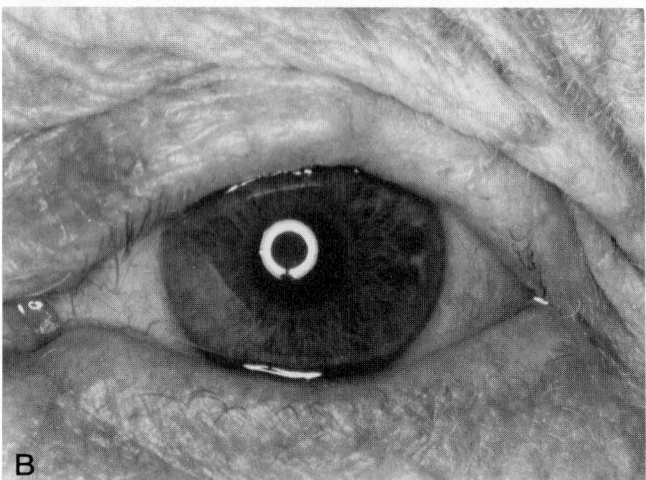

FIGURE 20–10. Basal cell carcinoma of the upper eyelid before and 4 years after treatment with 3500 cGy in five daily fractions (100 kV; HVL 0.7 mm Cu).

TABLE 20–6
*Incidence of Side Effects of Radiation Therapy for Eyelid Carcinoma Among 1166 Patients**

SIDE EFFECT†	INCIDENCE (%)
Skin atrophy	64
Ectropion	36‡
Entropion	6
Epiphora	27‡
Keratinization	21
Keratitis	5
Cataract	11
Perforated globe	3

** Treated at Princess Margaret Hospital, Toronto, Canada*
† Moderate skin changes and epilation are considered equivalent to a surgical scar and are not listed as complications.
‡ Often present before treatment

90% are reported. Lesions in the thumb web space, interdigital clefts, or proximal phalanges often are aggressive tumors prone to recurrence, lymph node metastases, and radionecrosis.[51]

External-beam irradiation techniques are discouraged in the treatment of lesions on the dorsum of the hand because of the paucity of subcutaneous tissue and the high incidence of radiation-induced complications such as radionecrosis and loss of function.

MELANOMA

Melanoma is a malignant tumor of the skin arising in the epidermis. The cell of origin is the melanocyte, which is present in all areas of the skin as well as in parts of the eye and upper respiratory, gastrointestinal, and genitourinary tracts.

Melanoma accounts for about 1.5% of all skin cancers; however, its incidence has more than doubled over the past 10 years and continues to increase at an alarming rate.[52] Increased leisure time with more exposure to sunlight has been implicated as the cause. In the United States, melanoma occurs most frequently in white adults. It is rare in darked-skinned races and, when found, occurs mostly on the palms of the hand and the soles of the feet. Incidence is equal in men and women, with a peak incidence in the fourth and fifth decades. Melanoma tends to involve the extremities in women and the head and neck and trunk in men; women have an apparent advantage in survival rate.[6]

Although most malignant melanomas are believed to arise *de novo,* they also commonly develop from preexisting benign nevi, especially those subject to repeated trauma and irritation. Changes that should cause concern are the appearance of a new pigmented lesion, a change in size or color of an existing pigmented spot, the appearance of satellite spots around an existing mole or freckle, and crusting, bleeding, or persistent itching

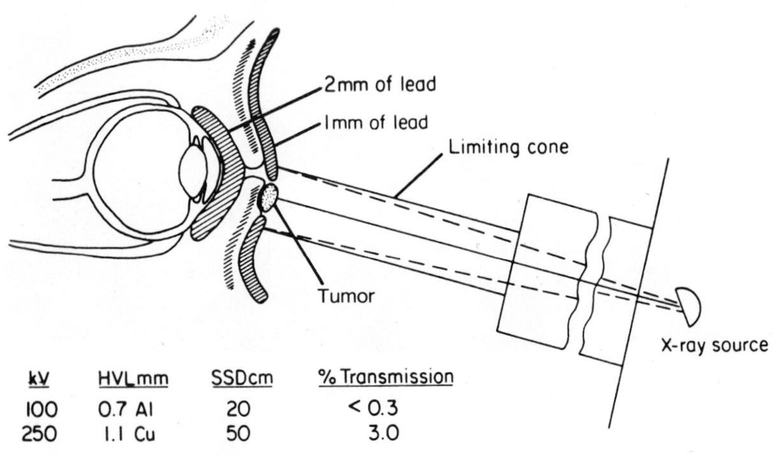

FIGURE 20–11. The most common way to treat eyelid tumors by radiation therapy. The radiovulnerable anterior segment of the eye gets less than 0.3% of the prescribed dose at 100 kV and only 3% at 250 kV.

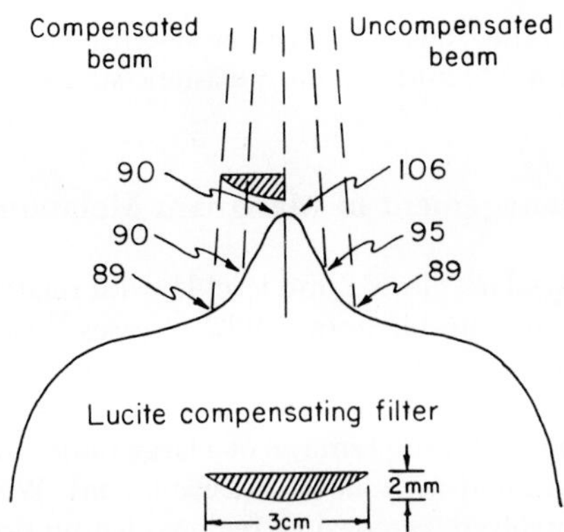

FIGURE 20–12. Compensating filter used in treating tumor on the bridge and dorsum of the nose (100 kV; HVL 0.7 mm Al; SSD 20 cm). The simplest way to treat tumors on the nose is to flatten the surface. However, too much pressure renders the tissues anoxic. If the surface cannot be flattened, a compensator should be used.

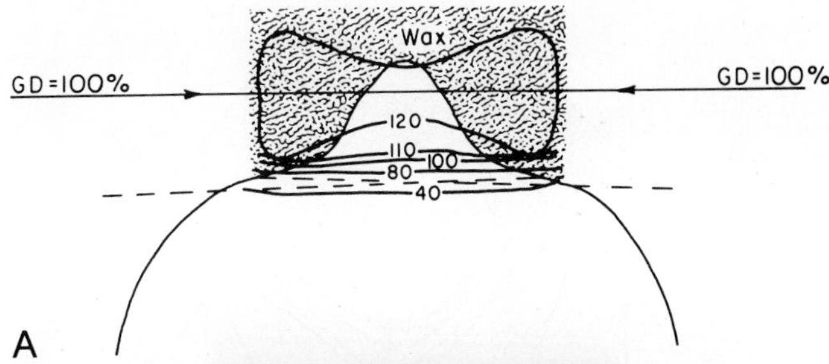

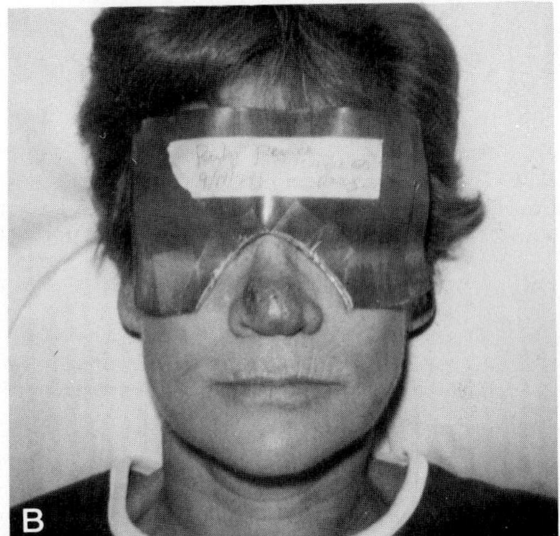

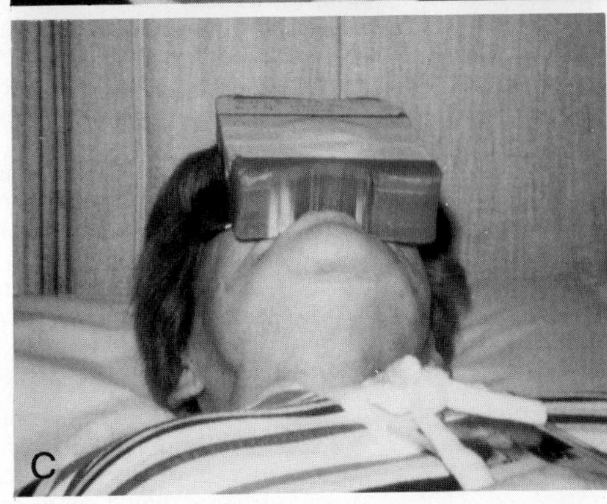

FIGURE 20–13. (**A**) A wax or tissue equivalent block ensures homogeneous irradiation in treating extensive, superficial, or invasive nasal skin tumors. This plan, delivering a dose of 4000 cGy in 10 treatments in 2 weeks, was successful in curing a superficial tumor involving all the skin of the lower half of the nose. (**B**) Patient with a squamous cell carcinoma of the nose showing lead cut-out to shield eyes from scattered radiation. (**C**) Patient with wax bolus in position.

of a pigmented spot. Persons with dysplastic nevus syndrome are at high risk for developing malignant melanoma.

Three main forms of malignant melanoma are described.[1] Superficial spreading melanoma (SSM) accounts for 60% to 70% of cases and displays a horizontal growth pattern within the epidermis with invasion into the papillary dermis. Nodular melanoma (NM) is characterized by vertical growth and makes up about 30% of all cases. Lentigo maligna melanoma (LMM) is a disease of the elderly with a mean patient age of about 70 years and characteristic plaque-like radial growth within the basilar regions of the epidermis. The variant acral lentiginous melanoma involves the palms and soles or the subungual regions and grows in both radial and vertical phases.

Complete excision is the best method for diagnosis of cutaneous melanoma because precise depth of various portions of the lesion within the skin layers can be evaluated.

Staging of Malignant Melanoma

Three staging systems have been described for malignant melanoma based on the known prognostic factors of depth of invasion,[12] tumor thickness,[9] and Tumor Nodal Metastasis (TNM) staging.

As outlined by Clark[12] tumors can be classified according to the depth of invasion;

Level I: melanoma *in situ* (also called atypical melanocytic hyperplasia)
Level II: invading the papillary dermis
Level III: invading and filling the papillary dermis and abutting the junction between the papillary dermis and the deeper reticular dermis
Level IV: invading the reticular dermis
Level V: penetrating the subcutis

Cure rate decreases with increasing Clark's level, dropping most significantly for level IV and level V lesions. However, the risk of each lesion also depends on careful evaluation of the individual tumor characteristics, ulcerations, evidence of regression, mitotic rate, and lymphatic invasion as well as patient age, sex, and family history.[40]

Breslow[9] described the actual thickness in millimeters of the lesion from the surface of the skin to the base of the tumor:

- ≤ 0.75 mm
- 0.76–1.50 mm
- 1.51–4.0 mm
- > 4.0 mm

A melanoma is generally considered thin if it is less than 0.76 mm in depth, intermediate if between 0.76 mm and 1.50 mm, and thick if greater than 1.50 mm. Melanomas greater than 2.25 mm thick have a high incidence of concurrent metastases.

The American Joint Committee (AJC) staging system (Table 20-7) for malignant melanoma is more comprehensive and

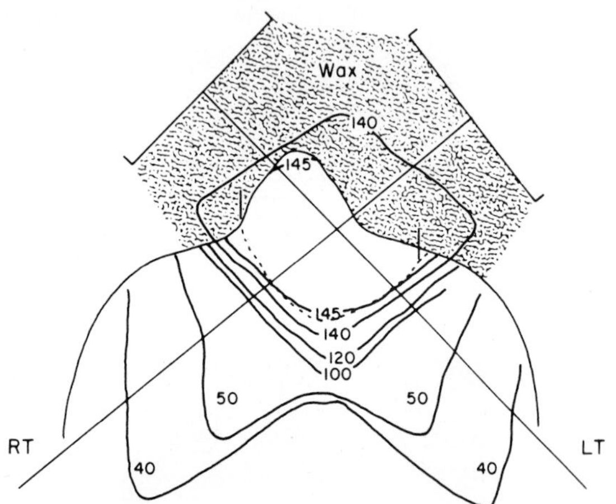

FIGURE 20–14. This treatment plan, using supervoltage irradiation and delivering a dose of 5000 cGy in 15 treatments in 3 weeks, controlled a squamous cell carcinoma that deeply invaded the nasal tissues.

employs both the Clark and Breslow systems while adding descriptions of nodal and distant metastatic status.

General Management of Malignant Melanoma

Early lesions, Clark's level I and level II, with relatively little or no invasion, are curable in over 95% of cases.[33] Clark's level I and thin level II lesions are best treated by a surgical excision wide enough to remove the lesion and a safe border around it. Wide excision, including removal of a large radius of surrounding skin, is needed with more invasive lesions. Where thicker lesions are involved, removal of regional lymph nodes should also be considered because elimination of tumor-bearing lymph nodes may cure some patients.

When a metastasis has occurred, treatment must be tailored to the type and location of disease spread. Localized disease confined to the skin or subcutaneous tissue may be amenable to additional surgery. Regional or distant spread of tumor may require surgery, radiation therapy, chemotherapy, immunotherapy, or a combination of these modalities.

TABLE 20–7
AJC Staging System for Melanoma of the Skin (Excluding Eyelid)

PRIMARY TUMOR (pT)

pTX Primary tumor cannot be assessed
pT0 No evidence of primary tumor
pTis Melanoma *in situ* (atypical melanocytic hyperplasia, severe melanocytic dysplasia), not an invasive lesion (Clark's level I)
pT1 Tumor 0.75 mm or less in thickness and invades the papillary dermis (Clark's level II)
pT2 Tumor more than 0.75 mm but not more than 1.5 mm in thickness and/or invades to papillary-reticular dermal interface (Clark's level III)
pT3 Tumor more than 1.5 mm but not more than 4 mm in thickness and/or invades the reticular dermis (Clark's level IV)
- pT3a Tumor more than 1.5 mm but not more than 3 mm in thickness
- pT3b Tumor more than 3 mm but not more than 4 mm in thickness

pT4 Tumor more than 4 mm in thickness and/or invades the subcutaneous tissue (Clark's level V) and/or satellite(s) within 2 cm of the primary tumor
- pT4a Tumor more than 4 mm in thickness and/or invades the subcutaneous tissue
- pT4b Satellite(s) within 2 cm of the primary tumor

REGIONAL LYMPH NODES (N)

NX Regional lymph nodes cannot be assessed
N0 No regional lymph node metastasis
N1 Metastasis 3 cm or less in greatest dimension in any regional lymph node(s)
N2 Metastasis more than 3 cm in greatest dimension in any regional lymph node(s) and/or in-transit metastasis
- N2a Metastasis more than 3 cm in greatest dimension in any regional lymph node(s)
- N2b In-transit metastasis
- N2c Both (N2a and N2b)

DISTANT METASTASIS (M)

MX Presence of distant metastasis cannot be assessed
M0 No distant metastasis
M1 Distant metastasis
- M1a Metastasis in skin or subcutaneous tissue or lymph node(s) beyond the regional lymph nodes
- M1b Visceral metastasis

STAGE GROUPING

Stage I	pT1	N0	M0
	pT2	N0	M0
Stage II	pT3	N0	M0
Stage III	pT4	N0	M0
	Any pT	N1, N2	M0
Stage IV	Any pT	Any N	M1

(Beahrs OH, Henson DE, Hutter RVP, Myers MH [eds]: Manual for Staging of Cancer, 3rd ed. Philadelphia, JB Lippincott, 1988)

Chemotherapy for metastatic melanoma has not been particularly successful. The most successful regimens have included imidazole carboxamide (DTIC) alone or in combination with vincristine, lomustine, and bleomycin. Efforts have also focused on the development of immunotherapeutic techniques that might be used as adjunctive treatment to surgery in high-risk patients. The use of interferon, tumor cell vaccines, and tumor-specific monoclonal antibodies is under investigation. Immunologic treatments generally involve periodic vaccinations with a preparation (BCG, interferon, tumor cell vaccine, or transfer factor) intended to stimulate increased immune activity and prevent disease recurrence.

Radiation Therapy Techniques

In vitro studies of malignant melanoma cells have shown a wide shoulder on the cell survival curve, suggesting a large capacity for repair of sublethal damage. This information has prompted the application of higher-than-conventional doses per fraction to enhance cell kill[24,26,42] and therapy to overcome apparent radioresistance of malignant melanoma cells.

Overgaard[42] used varying dose fractionation regimens to treat cutaneous melanoma lesions and lymph node metastases. He showed a marked correlation between increasing fraction size and tumor response and found no relationship between response and total given dose or nominal standard dose (NSD). His preferred treatment regimen consisted of three fractions of 900 cGy each over 8 days, and he concluded that radioresponsiveness of malignant melanoma was enhanced by large doses per fraction. Konefal and associates[32] similarly reported a strong correlation between increased fraction size (≥500 cGy) and response rate in patients with cutaneous extremity lesions.

Katz[29] reviewed the data from the American Oncologic Hospital and supported Overgaard's observations of improved control of cutaneous lesions and lymph node metastases with high doses per fraction (≥400 cGy). He further reported benefit of high-dose fractionation in the control of non-CNS visceral metastases. Although he showed no such advantage in the treatment of bone metastases, Katz established an overall 77% palliative response rate and found an apparent advantage to higher total doses for longer duration of response in metastatic melanoma to bone. Konefal and colleagues[31] found no benefit to high dose fractionation for visceral melanoma metastases. They reported improved palliation of appendicular (88%) over axial (60%) bone metastases.

Regarding central nervous system (CNS) metastases from malignant melanoma, Katz[28] and Pate and associates[50] found an advantage to large doses per fraction only in patients with solitary brain metastases and longer duration of response in patients treated first by surgical excision. No advantage was seen using high-dose fractionation in patients with multiple brain metastases; unexpectedly, an adverse effect of chemotherapy was found.[50]

In a report from Roswell Park Memorial Institute,[36] surgical excision of a solitary brain lesion resulted in a median survival of 26 weeks. However, 73% of these patients had multiple brain metastases and were not suitable for this approach. These patients had a significant survival advantage, as demonstrated with the use of cranial irradiation and intraarterial chemotherapy.

Choi and colleagues[11] reported the M. D. Anderson Cancer Center results with accelerated fractionation in 194 patients with malignant melanoma metastatic to brain. Although they showed no overall advantage to accelerated fractionation, a benefit was seen in the subgroups of patients treated after complete resection of a solitary lesion and those without detectable extracranial disease at the time of treatment.

Experience is accumulating in the treatment of malignant melanoma with radiation therapy and hyperthermia. Emami and associates[18] reported on 49 recurrent primary and metastatic lesions treated with this combined approach and show improved complete response rates (59%) over those achieved with radiation therapy alone (24%). The addition of hyperthermia to irradiation improved response rates in larger tumors and resulted in response rates with conventional fractionation that were comparable to those previously achieved only with high-dose fractionation schedules.

MERKEL CELL CARCINOMA (TRABECULAR CARCINOMA, CUTANEOUS NEUROENDOCRINE CARCINOMA)

Merkel cell carcinoma is a rare primary skin tumor first described in 1972[56]; it occurs most frequently in the seventh and eighth decades. Tumors are characterized by a high rate of local recurrence after surgical excision (25% to 60%) and by frequent involvement of regional lymph nodes (45% to 79%).[10,22,25,43,47,49,62] Distant metastatic failure is common (22% to 48%).[25]

The cell of origin has been the subject of controversy but is believed to be similar to the Merkel cell described in the basal layers of the epidermis. Merkel cells, located predominantly around hair follicles, have been implicated in the sensation of tactile stimuli.[47,60,61]

The neuroectodermal derivation of Merkel cell tumors is suggested by ultrastructural and immunochemical similarity to the well-described small cell carcinoma of the lung and malignant carcinoid. Characteristic of these neuroendocrine tumor cells are dense core membrane-bound cytoplasmic granules identified by electron microscopy. Cytoplasmic extensions are common, and the mitotic index is usually high.

Multiple immunohistochemical markers have been reported in Merkel cell tumors. Most consistently, these cells have demonstrated cytoplasmic staining with polyclonal antisera to neuron-specific enolase (NSE) and calcitonin, neurofilament monoclonal antibody and cytokeratin (CAM 5.2).[7,16,43] The epithelial origin of the tumor cells is suggested by the presence of epithelial membrane antigen, keratin, by desmosomes and cytoplasmic filaments.

Light and electron microscopy and immunohistochemical studies help to differentiate Merkel cell tumors from malignant lymphoma, small cell sarcoma, melanoma, metastatic undifferentiated carcinoma, and anaplastic adnexal tumors.

Merkel cell tumors usually involve the reticular dermis and subcutaneous tissue with only occasional extension to the papillary dermis and sparing of the overlying dermis. Vascular and lymphatic permeation are common. Three histologic variants of Merkel cell carcinoma have been described: trabecular, solid, and diffuse. The solid type appears to be the most prevalent and the diffuse type prognostically the most unfavorable.[47] Regardless of the histologic type, the most important prognostic factor appears to be the extent of tumor at initial diagnosis (localized, regional, or distant disease).

The gross appearance is most often that of a firm, nontender, pink-red nodular lesion with an intact epidermis. Most tumors measure under 3 cm at diagnosis and may be only a few millimeters when first discovered. In spite of a relatively benign appearance and small primary tumor size, these lesions can behave aggressively with early regional nodal and distant metastatic spread.[10,14]

Tumors occur with greatest frequency in the head and neck region (50%).[25] Less often, they are reported to involve the extremities, but rarely the trunk.[49] For head and neck sites, although palpable adenopathy is present at initial diagnosis in about 45% of patients, contralateral neck disease is unusual and tends to occur only with midline lesions or where extensive ipsilateral neck involvement is present.[22]

General Management of Merkel Cell Carcinoma

The initial treatment approach for Merkel cell tumors is usually surgical, with wide excision of the primary tumor. Plastic reconstruction with skin grafting is often necessary, and with a preponderance of head and neck sites, adequate surgical margins may be difficult to obtain. Recurrences requiring multiple excisions are common, and failure to control the primary site has shown the strongest correlation with the development of distant and regional nodal metastases.[22]

Because of the poor control obtained with local excision alone, most recent series have abandoned the recommendation of Wick and associates[61] for wide local excision and "strict postoperative observation" in favor of a more aggressive initial approach. Raaf and colleagues[49] suggest the addition of prophylactic regional node dissection, but they only briefly mention a possible palliative benefit of radiation therapy or chemotherapy.

Reports of sensitivity of Merkel cell carcinoma to multiagent chemotherapy are emerging.[20,63] Doxorubicin (Adriamycin), cyclophosphamide, and vincristine are among the most active agents. Responses often have been dramatic but short-lived. The use of chemotherapy has been suggested in a population believed to be at high risk: patients with tumors composed of smaller cells or with nodal involvement at the time of diagnosis, patients with over 30% replacement of resected nodal tissue, and patients with advanced metastatic disease.[20]

Radiation Therapy Techniques

The radiation therapy experience in the treatment of Merkel cell carcinoma is still relatively sparse; however, a few series have shown promising results when radiation therapy is added to the initial surgical management. In a series of Merkel cell tumors involving only head and neck sites from the M. D. Anderson Cancer Center, Goepfert and associates[22] documented improved locoregional control with initial aggressive combined modality management of primary excision and neck dissection followed by postoperative irradiation. They found a 50% incidence of subclinical disease in elective neck dissections and a 75% failure rate in untreated necks. In contrast, 83% (ten of 12) of patients treated with surgery and radiation therapy for palpable neck disease showed disease control.

Cotlar and associates[14] and Brown and colleagues[10] recommend postoperative radiation therapy to the primary site and to regional lymphatics in all patients. They suggest 5000 cGy in 25 fractions over 5 weeks for control of subclinical disease and boost doses up to 6000 cGy to 6500 cGy for known residual microscopic disease. Therapeutic lymph node dissection before irradiation is recommended when the suspicion of nodal involvement is high, but lympathic irradiation without dissection might be adequate for very small lesions without clinical evidence of nodal involvement. Routine postoperative radiation therapy might therefore obviate the need for extensive surgical procedures in early lesions.

Further evidence of the radiosensitivity of Merkel cell tumors is found in the report by Pacella and associates.[43] In their series of 20 patients, they attained a 96% complete response rate in patients irradiated in the presence of known residual disease; there was only one recurrence in an irradiated site in a patient who had received a single 800 cGy fraction of radiation. Furthermore, they saw no locoregional recurrence in 13 sites given prophylactic irradiation to the primary site or regional lymph nodes after complete surgical excision.

Hyperthermia is emerging as a promising treatment modality when used in conjunction with conventional external-beam irradiation in the treatment of Merkel cell carcinoma.[30]

Therapeutic lymph node dissection is warranted for all cases of suspected lymphatic involvement, followed by postoperative irradiation. When the first echelon lymph nodes lie in close proximity to the primary tumor, they may be excised electively with the primary lesion. Otherwise, prophylactic nodal irradiation is indicated. For head and neck primary sites, bilateral lymph node irradiation is warranted for midline lesions or when ipsilateral nodal involvement is extensive.

Radiation therapy portals should be designed to encompass the original tumor volume with an appropriate wide margin of normal tissue (about 5 cm) as well as the entire surgical bed and scar. Doses of 5000 cGy at conventional fractionation appear adequate for the treatment of subclinical disease, but where microscopic or gross residual disease is known to exist, boost doses to 6000 cGy to 7000 cGy are indicated.

SEQUELAE OF SKIN IRRADIATION

In general, treatment of most skin cancers requires doses and fractionation schemes that destroy the basal layers of the epidermis but spare the underlying dermis.

Erythema of the skin is usually the earliest noticeable radiation effect. Its appearance is dependent on dose, field size, fractionation regimen, and beam quality. Dry desquamation, or peeling, occurs at intermediate dose levels. Moist desquamation occurs with doses required to control skin cancers. The eradication of all basal cells of the epidermis results in exposure of the dermis and serous oozing from the surface. Epidermal regrowth occurs from the field periphery and from the more radioresistant epithelial cells around hair follicles within the field.

Treatment of acute radiation reactions involves avoidance of trauma to the skin such as shaving, scratching, or sun exposure. The skin should be cleansed with a mild soap and patted dry. Application of creams, cosmetics, or harsh cleansers, especially those containing alcohol, should be avoided. A mild steroid cream such as 1% hydrocortisone or 0.025% triamcinolone treats skin erythema and dry desquamation and relieves pruritus. Moist reactions may be treated with dilute hydrogen peroxide or 1% aqueous gentian violet to dry the lesion and guard against infection. Silvadene cream also is commonly used to treat moist desquamation and promote healing.

The new skin formed after a course of irradiation is thin and atrophic and is easily injured by mechanical trauma, chemical or sun exposure, or re-irradiation. Capillaries are reduced in number and dilated, resulting in telangiectasia. Whereas radiation therapy initially may cause hyperpigmentation by melanocyte stimulation, cancerocidal doses result in permanent hypopigmentation secondary to melanocyte destruction. Permanent hair loss also is dose-dependent and usually follows radiation

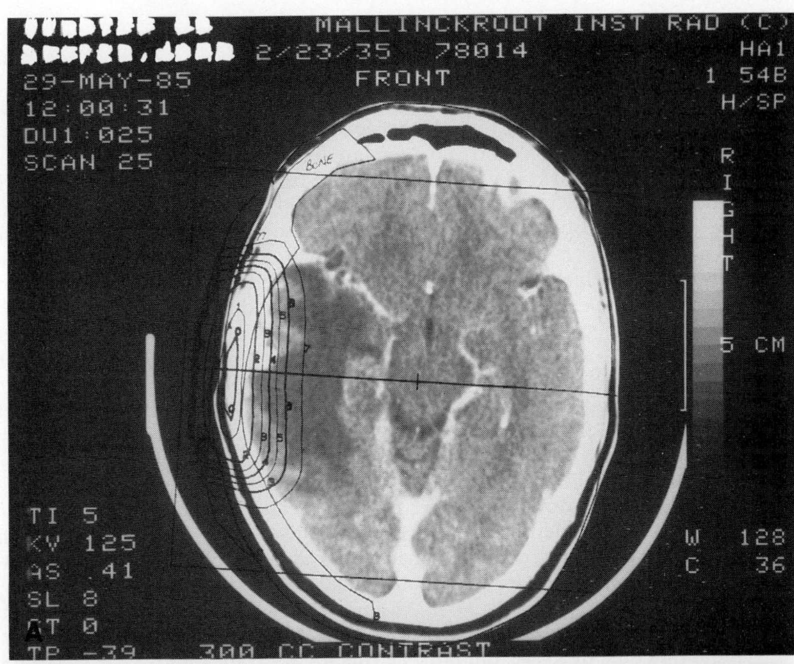

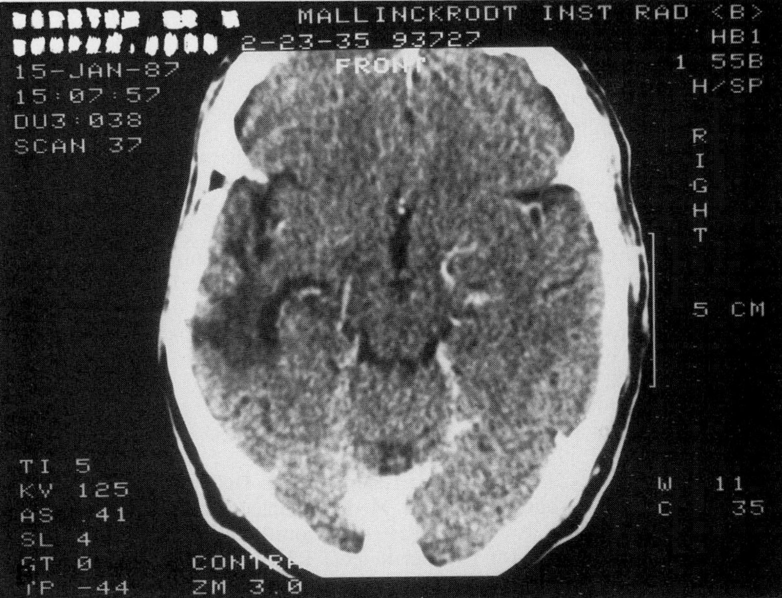

FIGURE 20–15. (**A**) Computed tomography scan with superimposed isodose curves showing an area of necrosis in the parietal lobe in a 48-year-old patient who received 6160 cGy for an extensive basal cell carcinoma in the left tragal area extending to the pinna. Radiation dose of 4560 cGy was delivered with 10 MeV electrons (0.75 cm bolus) and ^{60}Co (0.5 cm bolus), 240 cGy per fraction. Dose was calculated at 2 cm (4:1 ratio). Additional 1600 cGy was delivered with 10 MeV electrons (0.75 cm bolus), 200 cGy per fraction. The patient developed decreased hearing and tinnitus. Six years later same patient presented with neurologic symptoms and was treated by partial removal of temporal and parietal lobe, with minimal neurologic deficit. (**B**) Brain scan performed 2 years later showing disappearance of necrosis and edema of the brain. The patient had excellent functional recovery.

therapy for skin cancer. Deeper penetrating, skin-sparing megavoltage radiation often results in subcutaneous fibrosis. Both sebaceous and sweat glands are sensitive to radiation and show decreased or absent function within the treated area after radiation therapy for skin cancer.

Radiation necrosis may occur at any time after radiation therapy but is more likely in patients receiving large increment techniques in the treatment for skin cancers (Fig. 20-15). If more protracted techniques are used with smaller fields, the incidence of necrosis should not exceed 3%. Certain anatomic sites are more likely than others to develop radiation necrosis, such as the canthi, the alae of the nose, and the ears. Generally, radiation necrosis is preceded by an inflammatory episode, trauma, or prolonged sun exposure. Most radiation necroses heal with patience, local care, avoidance of trauma, and use of topical antibiotics and steroids. Surgery should be the last resort. In the Hahnemann University experience, only seven instances of radiation necrosis have been encountered in patients irradiated definitively by previously described techniques.[8]

Lovett and colleagues[35] observed an overall complication rate of 5.3% in 339 patients, which was directly related to primary lesion size. For lesions 1 cm or less, the complication rate was 0.9% (one of 112); for lesions 1 cm to 5 cm, it was 6.5% (12 of 184); and for lesions larger than 5 cm, it was 13% (four of 31). An excellent or good cosmetic result was found in 88% (244 of 276) of the patients, and was related to treatment modality. Excellent or good cosmesis was seen in 161 of 169 (95%) patients treated with superficial x-rays, 37 of 46 (80%) patients treated with electrons, 39 of 51 (76%) patients treated with mixed beams, and seven of ten (70%) patients treated with photons.

REFERENCES

1. American Joint Committee on Cancer: Melanoma of the skin. In Beahrs OH, Myers MH (eds): Manual for Staging of Cancer, 2nd ed, p 117. Philadelphia, JB Lippincott, 1983

2. Becquerel AH: Sur les radiation emises par phosphorscences. CR Acad Sci (Paris) 122:420, 1896
3. Bergstresser PR, Halprin KM: Multiple sequential skin cancers. Arch Dermatol 111:995, 1975
4. Binnick SA: Introduction to dermatology. In Binnick SA (ed): Skin Diseases: Diagnosis and Management in Clinical Practice, pp 1–12. Menlo Park, CA, Addison-Wesley, 1982
5. Blank AA, Schnyder UW: Soft x-ray therapy in Bowen's disease and erythroplasia of Queyrat. Dermatologica 171:89, 1985
6. Blois MS, Sagebiel RW, Abarbanel RM, et al: Malignant melanoma of the skin. The association of tumor depth and type, and patient sex, age, and site with survival. Cancer 52:1330, 1983
7. Bonfiglio TA: Neuroendocrine carcinoma of the skin: Diagnostic and management considerations. Int J Radiat Oncol Biol Phys 14:1321, 1988
8. Brady LW, Faust DS, Kazem I, et al: Principles of radiation treatment of carcinomas of the skin. In Proceedings of Special Graduate Course on Cancer for Latin American Physicians, pp 617–630. Philadelphia, JB Lippincott, 1967
9. Breslow A: Thickness, cross-sectional areas and depth of invasion in the prognosis of cutaneous melanoma. Ann Surg 172:902, 1970
10. Brown PE, Pinkston JA, Blackmon JA, et al: Merkel cell carcinoma: Report of a case and possible role for adjuvant radiotherapy. J Surg Oncol 34:136, 1987
11. Choi KM, Withers HR, Rotman M: Intracranial metastases from melanoma. Clinical features and treatment by accelerated fractionation. Cancer 56:1, 1985
12. Clark WH Jr, Mihm MC Jr: Lentigo maligna and lentigo-maligna melanoma. Am J Pathol 55:39, 1969
13. Cohen L: The statistical prognosis in radiation therapy: A study of optimal dosage in relation to physical and biological parameters for epidermoid cancer. Am J Roentgenol 84:741, 1960
14. Cotlar AM, Gates JO, Gibbs FA Jr: Merkel cell carcinoma: Combination surgery and radiation therapy. Am Surg 52:159, 1986
15. del Regato JA, Vuksanovic M: Radiotherapy of carcinoma of the skin overlying the cartilages of the nose and ear. Radiology 79:203, 1962
16. Drijkoningen M, De Wolf-Peeters C, Van Limbergen E, et al: Merkel cell tumor of the skin: An immunohistochemical study. Hum Pathol 17:301, 1986
17. Eaglstein WH, Pariser DM: Office Techniques for Diagnosing Skin Disease. Chicago, Year Book Medical Publishers, 1978
18. Emami B, Perez CA, Konefal J, et al: Thermoradiotherapy of malignant melanoma. Int J Hyperthermia 4:373, 1988
19. Fayos JU, Wildermuth O: Carcinoma of the skin of the eyelids. Arch Ophthalmol 67:298, 1962
20. Feun LG, Savaraj N, Legha SS, et al: Chemotherapy for metastatic Merkel cell carcinoma. Review of the M. D. Anderson Hospital's Experience. Cancer 62:683, 1988
21. Fitspatrick PJ, Thompson GA, Easterbrook WM, et al: Basal and squamous cell carcinoma of the eyelids and their treatment by radiotherapy. Int J Radiat Oncol Biol Phys 10:449, 1984
22. Goepfert H, Remmier D, Silva E, et al: Merkel cell carcinoma (endocrine carcinoma of the skin) of the head and neck. Arch Otolaryngol 110:707, 1984
23. Guthrie TH, McElveen LJ, Porubsky ES, et al: Cisplatin and doxorubicin: an effective chemotherapy combination in the treatment of advanced basal cell and squamous cell carcinoma of the skin. Cancer 55:1629, 1985
24. Habermalz HJ, Fischer JJ: Radiation therapy of malignant melanoma: Experience with high individual treatment doses. Cancer 38:2258, 1976
25. Hitchcock C, Bland K, Laney R, et al: Neuroendocrine (Merkel cell) carcinoma of the skin: Its natural history, diagnosis, and treatment. Ann Surg 207:201, 1988
26. Hornsey S: The relationship between total dose, number of fractions and fraction size in the response of malignant melanoma in patients. Br J Radiol 51:905, 1978
27. Hunter RD, Pereira DT, Pointon RC: Megavoltage electron beam therapy in the treatment of basal and squamous cell carcinomata of the pinna. Clin Radiol 33:341, 1982
28. Katz HP: The relative effectiveness of radiation therapy, corticosteroids and surgery in the management of melanoma metastatic to the central nervous system. Int J Radiat Oncol Biol Phys 7:897, 1981
29. Katz HP: The results of different fractionation schemes in the palliative irradiation of metastatic melanoma. Int J Radiat Oncol Biol Phys 7:907, 1981
30. Knox SJ, Kapp DS: Hyperthermia and radiation therapy in the treatment of recurrent Merkel cell tumors. Cancer 62:1479, 1988
31. Konefal JB, Emami B, Pilepich MV: Analysis of dose fractionation in the palliation of metastases from malignant melanoma. Cancer 61:243, 1988
32. Konefal JB, Emami B, Pilepich MV: Malignant melanoma: Analysis of dose fractionation in radiation therapy. Radiology 164:607, 1988
33. Kopf AW: Prevention and early detection of skin cancer: Melanoma. Cancer 62:1791, 1988
34. Lippman SM, Meyskens FL Jr: Treatment of advanced squamous cell carcinoma of the skin with isotretinoin. Ann Intern Med 107:499, 1987
35. Lovett RD, Perez CA, Shapiro SJ, Garcia DM: External irradiation of epithelial skin cancer. Int J Radiat Oncol Biol Phys 19:235–242, 1990
36. Madajewicz S, Karadousis C, West CR, et al: Malignant melanoma brain metastases: Review of Roswell Park Memorial Institute experience. Cancer 58:2550, 1984
37. McKenna RJ, MacDonald I: Carcinoma of the eyelid treated by irradiation. Analysis of 157 primary and 22 recurrent cases. Calif Med 96:184, 1962
38. Mendennall NP, Million RR, Cassisi NJ: Parotid area lymph node metastases from carcinoma of the skin. Int J Radiat Oncol Biol Phys 11:707, 1985
39. Mendenhall NP, Parsons JT, Cassisi NJ, et al: Carcinoma of the nasal vestibule treated with radiation therapy. Laryngoscope 97:626, 1987
40. Meyskens FL Jr, Berdeaus DH, Parks B, et al: Cutaneous malignant melanoma (Arizona Cancer Center experience): Natural history and prognostic factors influencing survival in patients with stage I disease. Cancer 62:1207, 1988
41. Miller RA, Spittle MF: Electron beam therapy for difficult cutaneous basal and squamous cell carcinoma. Br J Dermatol 106:429, 1982
42. Overgaard J: Radiation treatment of malignant melanoma. Int J Radiat Oncol Phys 6:41, 1980
43. Pacella J, Ashby M, Ainslie J, Minty C: The role of radiotherapy in the management of primary cutaneous neuroendocrine tumors (Merkel cell or trabecular carcinoma): Experience at the Peter MacCallum Cancer Institute (Melbourne, Australia). Int J Radiat Oncol Biol Phys 14:1077, 1988
44. Parker RG, Wildermuth O: Radiation therapy of lesions overlying cartilage: Carcinoma of the pinna. Cancer 15:57, 1962
45. Petrovich Z, Parker R, Luxton G, et al: Carcinoma of the lip and selected sites of head and neck skin: A clinical study of 896 patients. Radiother Oncol 8:11, 1987
46. Petrovich Z, Kuisk H, Langholz B et al: Treatment of carcinoma of the skin with bone and/or cartilage involvement. Am J Clin Oncol 11:110, 1988
47. Pilotti S, Rilke F, Bartoli C, Grisotti A: Clinicopathologic correlations of cutaneous neuroendocrine Merkel cell carcinoma. J Clin Oncol 6:1863, 1988
48. Pinkus H, Mehregan AH: A Guide to Dermatohistopathology, 2nd ed. New York, Appleton-Century-Crofts, 1976
49. Raaf JH, Urmacher C, Knapper WK, et al: Trabecular (Merkel cell) carcinoma of the skin. Cancer 57:178, 1986
50. Rate WR, Solin LJ, Turrisi AT: Palliative radiotherapy for metastatic malignant melanoma: Brain metastases, bone metastases, and spinal cord compression. Int J Radiat Oncol Biol Phys 15:859, 1988
51. Rayner CR: The results of treatment of 273 carcinomas of the hand. Hand 13:183, 1981
52. Rigel DS, Kopf AW, Friedman RJ: The rate of malignant

melanoma in the United States: Are we making an impact? J Am Acad Dermatol 17:1050, 1987
53. Silverberg E, Lubera JA: Cancer statistics, 1989. CA 39:3, 1989
54. Strandquist M: Studieu uber die rumulative wirkung der Pontgenstrohlenbel Fraktionierung Erfanrungen aus dem Radium-hemmet on 280—und Lippenkarzinomen. Arch Dermatol Syph 72:442, 1955
55. Swanson NA: Mohs' surgery: Technique, indications, applications and the future. Arch Dermatol 119:761, 1983
56. Toker C: Trabecular carcinoma of the skin. Arch Dermatol 105:107, 1972
57. van Vloten WA, Hermans J, van Daal WAJ: Radiation-induced skin cancer and radiodermatitis of the head and neck. Cancer 59:411, 1987
58. von Essen CF: Roentgen therapy of skin and lip carcinoma: Factors influencing success and failure. Am J Roentgenol 83:556, 1960
59. von Essen CF: Indications for radiation therapy of skin cancer. In Tumors of the Skin. Chicago, Year Book Medical Publishers, 1964
60. Warner TFCS, Uno H, Hafez GR, et al: Merkel cells and Merkel cell tumors: Ultrastructure, immunocytochemistry and review of the literature. Cancer 52:238, 1983
61. Wick MR, Goellner JR, Scheithauer BW, et al: Primary neuroendocrine carcinomas of the skin (Merkel cell tumors): A clinical, histologic and ultrastructural study of thirteen cases. Am J Clin Pathol 79:6, 1983
62. Wieman TJ, Shively EH, Woodcock TM: Responsiveness of metastatic basal cell carcinoma to chemotherapy: A case report. Cancer 52:1583, 1983
63. Wynne CJ, Kearsley JH: Merkel cell tumor: A chemosensitive skin cancer. Cancer 62:28, 1988

21

○ ○ ○ ∘ • ∘

Classic and Acquired Immunodeficiency Syndrome (AIDS)-Related Kaposi's Sarcoma

Jay S. Cooper

In 1872, Kaposi described five patients who had red-brown lesions he called "idiopathisches multiples Pigmentsarkom der Haut,"[28] and in 1912, Sternberg suggested the eponym Kaposi's sarcoma (KS).[15] Despite Kaposi's accurate description of the tumor, few cases were identified in the first half of this century. However, the description in 1981 of young homosexual men who developed KS proved to be the world's introduction to the acquired immunodeficiency syndrome (AIDS) and the start of an explosion in the incidence and recognition of KS.

NON-AIDS-ASSOCIATED KAPOSI'S SARCOMA

Epidemiology and Risk Factors

In the United States, non-AIDS-related Kaposi's sarcoma ("classic KS": CKS) constitutes only a small fraction of 1% of all cancers.[16] Although commonly perceived as a disease that affects persons of Mediterranean origin (Ashkenazi Jews and northern Italians), the greatest concentration of non-AIDS-associated KS occurs in the rain forests of Central Africa where KS ("endemic KS") accounts for more than 5% of all tumors.[42] In the United States most victims are more than 60 years old. Men are several times more likely to be affected.

Patterns of Disease

In the typical American patient, a violaceous macule, generally in the region of the ankle (see Color Fig. 21-1 after p. 510), heralds the onset of disease. In 75% of cases the first site of clinical involvement is the lower extremities (see Color Fig. 21-2 after p. 510). The next most common site is the arms, particularly the hands (see Color Fig. 21-3 after p. 510). Involvement of other cutaneous sites, mucosal orifices, or the conjunctivae is rare. The tumor probably does not metastasize; instead, new lesions develop in a multicentric fashion over time. Ackerman and Gottlieb[1] note that the disease progresses through the same stages of formation in virtually every lesion—an evolution that does not occur in metastases.

Macules grow by local extension, forming larger macules, plaques, or nodules. The patterns frequently coexist.

Lesions coalesce as they grow, forming irregular-shaped clusters. As the disease progresses, it tends to obstruct deep lymphatic flow, producing edema (which can be striking in its extent; see Color Fig. 21-4 after p. 510) that may involve parts of the legs with no visible lesions or associated regional lymph node enlargement.

Classic Kaposi's sarcoma sometimes involves internal organs, where lesions easily go undetected. The gastrointestinal (GI) tract is the most common visceral site; autopsies of patients who die of widespread Kaposi's sarcoma nearly always demonstrate involvement in the GI tract. Enlargement of regional lymph nodes typically reflects a reactive change rather than a direct involvement by tumor. Bone lesions are rare. In general, the disease follows a chronic course, and most patients with classic Kaposi's sarcoma die of unrelated causes years later.

Diagnostic Workup

The typical Kaposi's sarcoma lesion presents little diagnostic difficulty. However, biopsy confirmation is essential.[21] If the lesion is very small, excisional biopsy establishes the diagnosis and provides therapy at the same time. Physical examination should include all skin and mucosal surfaces. In patients under 60 years old, classic Kaposi's sarcoma is so unusual that the presence of AIDS should be suspected and a human immunodeficiency virus (HIV) titer should be drawn. Suggested diagnostic procedures are listed in Table 21-1.

TABLE 21–1
Diagnostic Workup of Kaposi's Sarcoma

I. All patients
- A. History
  1. Age
  2. Ancestry
  3. Behavior (sexual, drug use)
  4. Receipt of blood products
  5. Prior opportunistic infections
  6. Visceral symptoms (*e.g.,* gastrointestinal, central nervous system)
  7. Constitutional symptoms (fever, weight loss)
- B. Physical examination
  1. All cutaneous surfaces
  2. Visible mucosal surfaces
  3. Lymph nodes
  4. Body temperature
  5. Body weight
- C. Biopsy of suspected lesion

II. Obtain HIV titer if
- A. Patient <60 years old *or*
- B. High-risk factors present
  1. Homosexual or bisexual behavior
  2. Intravenous drug use
  3. Receipt of blood products
- C. Extracutaneous disease present

III. Endoscopic examination if HIV-positive and visceral symptoms co-exist

Pathology

Although it is generally agreed that Kaposi's sarcoma is a neoplasm, the proof of this is by no means conclusive. Several aspects of its behavior are suggestive of a reactive lesion: the course of the lesion is somewhat unpredictable; it can remain quiescent for long periods of time or evolve rapidly; spontaneous regression is uncommon but does occur; survival for many years after diagnosis is typical; the patient can feel and look well despite widespread evidence of disease; and the precise cell of origin remains controversial.

To compound the confusion, viral material is associated with Kaposi's sarcoma. Elevated antiviral antibody levels,[20] herpesvirus fragments,[52] and cytomegalovirus (CMV) DNA and RNA[2] have been found in patients who have Kaposi's sarcoma.

Whatever the true nature of the lesion, the histologic diagnosis of Kaposi's sarcoma requires the identification of both spindle cell and vascular elements within the lesion. The spindle-shaped cells are nondistinctive and look much like fibroblasts. Despite electron microscopy and the use of special immunocytochemical stains (a factor VIII-related antigen called FVIII-RA that is present in normal or neoplastic endothelial cells of blood vessel origin but is inconsistently present in KS), there is no proof of the spindle cell's ancestry. However, the general consensus is that the spindle cell is is endothelial in origin. The vascular component is the more distinctive part of the lesion. The overall appearance often is suggestive of slit-like embryonic vascular channels filled with red blood cells; red cells characteristically are also found mixed within the spindle cell framework of the tumor.

Prognostic Factors

There are no quantitative aspects of individual lesions that provide prognostic information, and the multifocal nature of the disease limits the value of the usual TNM staging. In 1983, Krigel and co-workers[29] proposed a staging system for KS (see Table 21-2*A*). Virtually all classic KS falls into Stage I.

General Management

Because classic Kaposi's sarcoma tends to be a slowly progressive disease confined to the legs, locoregional therapy can provide long-term disease-free survival. In CKS it is reasonable to think in terms of "cure" of disease, at least in the sense of allowing the typically elderly patient to die of other causes, clinically free of KS.

Small lesions can be surgically excised, vaporized by laser, or frozen off with liquid nitrogen. However, radiation therapy generally is considered the treatment of choice for localized or regionalized disease.

When disease is overtly widespread, systemic treatment should be considered. For totally asymptomatic disease that poses no risk to critical structures, a policy of "watch and wait" is prudent. For mild to moderately symptomatic disease, treatment with single-agent chemotherapy often strikes an appropriate balance between benefit and risk. Vinblastine and dactinomycin (actinomycin D) each have been reported to produce response rates of about 90%.[51] For rapidly progressing or life-threatening disease, combinations such as vincristine and dactinomycin (with or without dacarbazine [DTIC]) produce response rates that border on 100%.

Radiation Therapy

There are two philosophical approaches to irradiation of limited classic Kaposi's sarcoma: local (involved field) treatment and elective regional treatment.

Local irradiation of Kaposi's sarcoma includes the lesion plus a normal tissue border of approximately 1.5 cm to 2.0 cm. Thin, cutaneous lesions can be effectively treated either by superficial quality x-ray beams (*e.g.,* 100 kV) or relatively low-energy electron beams (*e.g.,* 4 MeV or 6 MeV), covering the lesions with bolus material when an electron beam is used. Thick plaques or nodules are best treated by electron beams that encompass the entire lesion homogeneously, but spare underlying normal tissues. Lesions on the eyelids can be treated with either superficial x-rays or electrons, making sure that appropriate protective shields are used to protect the optic lens. When substantial edema is present (in CKS, edema is nearly always limited to the legs), it is usually necessary to use parallel opposed portals and megavoltage therapy to treat the deep tissues. Treatment within a water bath[55] provides both bolus and homogeneity of dose, but it is not mandatory.

Although Kaposi's sarcoma is a radioresponsive disease, the optimal dose is in question. Previous practice[3] was to give total doses of only 1000 R. With this, 35% of lesions regressed completely, but local recurrence often ensued. Some authors[7] have recommended using the "smallest amount of radiation that will cause involution of lesions" so that additional treatment can be given in the future.

The modern era of radiation therapy for KS was begun by Cohen's 1962 analysis[8] of 58 cases, which indicated that lesions frequently could be "cured" with doses ranging from 1000 cGy in a single exposure to 2500 cGy over 1 month. However, issues remained: Cohen's patients were African; their average age was 40; approximately one third had no follow-up; and, although follow-up ranged from 2 to 12 years in the other two thirds, no information about mean or median follow-up was provided.

Later reports agree with Cohen's findings, but tend to be anecdotal. By 1985, Harris and Reed[23] could find only three other series[18,24,34] that contained sufficient detail to permit quantitative dose/time/failure analysis. Doses equivalent to single fractions of at least 800 cGy controlled the irradiated lesions 80% of the time.

Our own data,[9] published after Harris and Reed's analysis, yield a similar conclusion. Doses of 1200 ret (the equivalent of 2750 cGy in ten fractions over 2 weeks) or more were associated with an 85% likelihood of local freedom from disease, compared with approximately 30% following lesser doses. Single fractions of 800 cGy yielded results statistically indistinguishable from fractionated courses of 1200 ret or more. Consequently, sufficient dose (3000 cGy in ten fractions over 2 weeks or 800 cGy in one fraction) should be used when CKS is irradiated.

Wide-field irradiation provides an alternative approach because Kaposi's sarcoma is a multifocal disease. In addition, the variable tempo of the disease makes it difficult, if not impossible, to predict when or if new lesions will appear in adjacent tissues. Based on the experience observed in the patient population seen at the Princess Margaret Hospital in Toronto, Canada, the appearance of Kaposi's sarcoma in tissues adjacent to those treated by local radiation therapy was a sufficiently common problem to prompt the elective use, since 1965, of wide-field, megavoltage τ-ray or x-ray irradiation with overlying bolus for localized lesions. Ten of the first 12 patients with KS (83%) treated by 800 cGy in one fraction[26] to at least half a limb (proximal margin at least 15 cm from the closest lesion) had their lesions respond completely. A 1986 update of this experience[22] described complete remission in 38 of 56 patients (68%) treated by wide-field techniques (usually 800 cGy in one session), with 24 remaining disease-free (median follow-up of 3 years). In comparison, 17 of 26 patients (65%) attained complete remission following local field irradiation (300 cGy to 800 cGy in one fraction to 3500 cGy in five fractions), but only six patients remained completely disease-free.

Nisce and colleagues[40] used elective subtotal skin electron-beam therapy (when disease was not above the knees, the irradiated area covered from umbilicus to soles) in nine patients and total skin electron-beam therapy in 11 patients. Once-weekly doses of 400 cGy to 500 cGy for 6 to 8 weeks, depending on response, were delivered with 2.5 MeV to 3.5 MeV electron beams. Seventeen patients (85%) exhibited complete response (defined as complete regression of the lesions within the irradiated volume for at least 6 months); two subsequently suffered recurrence of disease.

KAPOSI'S SARCOMA IN IMMUNOSUPPRESSED STATES

In contrast to its overall rarity in the pre-AIDS era, KS occurs not infrequently in patients who receive kidney transplants. Harwood and colleagues[25] tabulated a 400- to 500-fold increase over a matched-control population; Penn[43] observed that KS accounted for approximately 5% of all malignancies in the Denver Transplant Tumor Registry. The development of Kaposi's sarcoma also has been linked to the immune system by other evidence. Kaposi's sarcoma and lymphomas arise in concert more often than would be anticipated by chance, and the disease often regresses in iatrogenically immunosuppressed patients if the immunosuppressive agent is discontinued.

However, Kaposi's sarcoma does not develop as a direct consequence of all forms of immunosuppression. Several hereditary diseases that place their host at increased risk of malignancy do not appear to facilitate the development of Kaposi's sarcoma.[44]

Interestingly, based on the results of radiation therapy for KS in the first few patients who were kidney transplant recipients, Harwood and colleagues[25] suspected that the sensitivity of such disease was less than in nonimmunosuppressed circumstances. However, with additional follow-up and more patients, the group reversed its thinking and concluded that this was not so.[22]

EPIDEMIC KAPOSI'S SARCOMA

Epidemiology and Risk Factors

As part of the acquired immunodeficiency syndrome (AIDS), Kaposi's sarcoma has been dubbed "epidemic" (EKS). The entire syndrome is now known to result from infection by the human immunodeficiency virus (HIV), a retrovirus of the lentivirus family.

Kaposi's sarcoma is the most common neoplastic manifestation of the acquired immunodeficiency syndrome; however, its incidence varies among subgroups. Of the initial AIDS cases documented in the New York City Department of Health files, 46% of the homosexual/bisexual males had KS, compared with 4% of the heterosexual intravenous (IV) drug users.[14] Also, homosexual/bisexual males represented a four times larger group of AIDS victims than heterosexual IV drug users. Over time, this has changed. As the many diverse opportunistic infections that are a part of AIDS have been documented, the criteria for its diagnosis have expanded[4] and the relative incidence of Kaposi's sarcoma *as the presenting evidence* of AIDS has decreased. In addition, Drew and associates[17] have chronicled a parallel decrease in KS as the presenting sign of AIDS and a decrease in the seroconversion of cohorts of initially CMV antibody-negative homosexual males in San Francisco from 1981 through 1985. In their study group the prevalence of KS dropped from 63% to 24%, while the seroconversion rate fell from 71% to 4%.

Levy and Ziegler[33] have postulated that KS develops as a result of enhanced secretion of immunomodulating factors with angiogenesis-promoting activity by cells attempting to compensate for the HIV-induced immunodeficiency. Some data[37] implicate the use of nitrite inhalants in the development of Kaposi's sarcoma, whereas other data[45] imply a genetic susceptibility related to the HLA-DR5 genotype.

The male : female ratio is far greater for epidemic Kaposi's sarcoma than for classic Kaposi's sarcoma. EKS in females is extremely rare, although 10% of AIDS victims are women. The typical patient is 30 to 40 years old.

Patterns of Disease

The legs are the most common site of involvement in epidemic Kaposi's sarcoma (see Color Fig. 21-5 after p. 510). Facial lesions are common, particularly on the tip of the nose and around the eyes (see Color Fig. 21-6 after p. 510) and ears. The size and shape of individual lesions vary, and their color ranges from light pink to dark purple-black. Edema secondary to deep disease can be striking and frequently involves not only the legs but the face and less frequently the arms. Lesions of the palate (see Color Fig. 21-7 after p. 510) and penis are common, as are lesions of the conjunctivae. Visceral lesions occur in the majority of patients.

TABLE 21–2A
Comparison of Staging Systems

STAGE	KRIGEL ET AL[29]	MITSUYASU ET AL[38]
I	Cutaneous, locally indolent	Limited cutaneous (<10 lesions or one anatomic area)
II	Cutaneous, locally aggressive, +/− regional lymph node involvement	Disseminated cutaneous (>10 lesions or more than one anatomic area)
III	Generalized mucocutaneous, +/− lymph node involvement	Visceral only (gastrointestinal, lymph node)
IV	Visceral	Cutaneous and visceral
SUBTYPES OF BOTH SYSTEMS		
A—no systemic signs or symptoms		
B—temperature >100°F (Krigel) or >37.8°C (Mitsuyasu), unrelated to an identifiable source of infection lasting >2 weeks, or 10% loss of body weight		

Diagnostic Workup

In addition to inspection of all visible skin and mucosal surfaces and because the likelihood of visceral KS is sufficiently high, endoscopic evaluation of the gastrointestinal tract is required for any patient with even slight GI symptoms (see Table 21-1). Any signs or symptoms that might herald the occurrence of an opportunistic infection should be aggressively investigated.

Pathology

Despite the major differences in behavior between epidemic and other forms of KS, the microscopic findings are identical.

Prognostic Factors

In contrast to classic/endemic KS, approximately 85% of patients who have epidemic KS have Stage III or Stage IV disease by the Krigel[29] system (Table 21-2*A*). Mitsuyasu and associates[38] used a somewhat different system that essentially compresses Krigel's Stage I and Stage II into Stage I and classifies disseminated cutaneous disease as Stage II. By this system, approximately 75% of their patients who had EKS had Stage II to Stage IV disease. However, the resulting survival patterns violate the usual concepts of a staging system; patients who had Stage I or Stage III disease lived longer than patients who had Stage II or Stage IV disease. Far better predictors were measures of the patient's immune status (*e.g.*, prior opportunistic infections, constitutional symptoms, total T4 lymphocyte count, T4 : T8 ratio). This implies that even widespread Kaposi's sarcoma is less life-threatening than the opportunistic infections that are also part of AIDS. Because of this reality, Krown and coworkers[30] developed a system that groups patients into good risk and poor risk categories based on the status of their tumors, immune systems, and associated illnesses (Table 21-2*B*). In support of this concept, Rothenberg and colleagues[48] found a 1-year survival rate of more than 80% in white males, ages 30 to 34, whose AIDS was diagnosed solely on the basis of EKS.

General Management

The far greater likelihood of systemic, rather than regionalized, disease in EKS and the uniformly fatal outcome of AIDS thus far (typically from opportunistic infections rather than tumor) limit the intent of current treatments for epidemic Kaposi's sarcoma to palliation (Table 21-3).

A systemic approach to treatment is logical; unfortunately, cytotoxic chemotherapy is immunosuppressive. Vinblastine was reported to "control" EKS in approximately 30% of patients and to arrest tumor progression temporarily in another 50%.[50] Vincristine produced a 61% partial response rate plus amelioration of preexistent thrombocytopenia in one series.[36] In patients who had "early" stage disease, etoposide (VP-16) yielded a 30% complete remission and 46% partial remission rate.[32]

Combination therapy potentially offers increased response rates and toxicity. Vinblastine/methotrexate/leukovorin,[35] vinblastine/bleomycin,[54] vinblastine/vincristine,[27] or vinblastine/bleomycin/doxorubicin[32] produce some degree of response in approximately 75% of patients treated.

An alternative approach to the management of widespread symptomatic Kaposi's sarcoma is the use of a biologic response modifier (interferons, interleukins, ampligen) in hopes of improving the host's immune system to a level that will combat either the inciting cause (AIDS), the tumor, or both. Recombinant leukocyte A interferon (in doses that sometimes exceeded the maximum tolerated dose) produced a 15% (five of 34) complete and 26% (nine of 34) partial response rate which lasted more than 9 months from the initiation of treatment in one early trial.[31] More recent work has demonstrated a dose/

TABLE 21–2B
Tumor, Immune System, Systemic Illness (TIS) Staging System

	TUMOR	IMMUNE	SYSTEMIC
GOOD RISK			
	Confined to skin +/or lymph nodes +/or minimal oral disease	CD cells ≥ 200 per microliter	No history of OI or thrush No "B" symptoms Karnofsky ≥ 70
POOR RISK			
	Tumor-associated edema or ulceration Extensive oral KS Visceral involvement (non-nodal) including GI tract	CD4 cells <200 per microliter	History of OI or thrush Karnofsky <70 Other HIV-related illness (*e.g.*, lymphoma, neurologic disease)

TABLE 21–3
Philosophic Approach to Treatment of Epidemic Kaposi's Sarcoma

SYMPTOMS	TREATMENT
Asymptomatic, several lesions	Observation
Individual lesion, symptomatic site	Radiation therapy
Disseminated, slow-glowing, A-type	Gentle chemotherapy; interferon
Systemic signs, rapid progression	Aggressive chemotherapy

response relationship: at high doses (*e.g.,* 36 × 10^6 units intramuscularly daily) response was observed in 38% of patients, whereas at low doses (*e.g.,* 3 × 10^6 units intramuscularly daily) responses were seen in only 3%.[46] Based on response rates of 30% to 50% in a variety of trials totaling more than 350 patients, α-interferon was approved for the treatment of EKS in late 1988[49] for patients who have not had prior opportunistic infections and who have no constitutional symptoms.

A third approach is the use of antiviral therapy such as zidovudine (*i.e.,* Azidothymidine, AZT), acyclovir, or foscarnet. AZT, a thymidine analogue that inhibits HIV replication *in vitro,* has become a standard therapy for AIDS and its precursor ARC (AIDS-related complex).[19] Unfortunately, these results come only at the cost of toxicity: Nausea, anemia, leukopenia and neutropenia are common and are frequently severe.[47] Although AZT clearly is beneficial for AIDS, a prospective trial at the National Institute of Health[31A] has shown no significant effect of the drug on the progression of epidemic Kaposi's sarcoma.

Radiation Therapy

In 1984, we published our initial observations of the effect of radiation therapy on epidemic Kaposi's sarcoma[12] based on 17 lesions in our first 15 patients, all of whom had been followed up for a minimum of 3 months. We described complete objective regression in nine patients, clearance of the mass but persistence of pigmentation in three, and partial regression in the remaining three (see Color Figs. 21-8 and 21-9 after p. 510). We commented that lesions often took weeks to months to regress maximally and reported one local recurrence of disease 7 months after therapy. Within months, similar data from other centers appeared. Harris and Reed[23] compared the dose/time parameters of 15 patients whose EKS was controlled by radiation therapy for 3 to 18 months with those of patients who had classic KS as reported in the literature. No difference was evident. They also observed that lesions may take 3 to 4 months to resolve and that radiation-induced edema of the foot and face, as well as symptomatic mucositis, was more severe in AIDS victims than in other patients.

Nisce and Safai[39] described the care of 38 patients who had EKS. In contrast to their standard use of total or subtotal skin electron-beam therapy for classic KS, less than 30% of their patients who had EKS could be treated by this method. Following doses of 750 cGy to 3000 cGy, three of the five patients who survived for more than 5 months had local recurrence 4 to 6 months after therapy. A general inability to deliver effective radiation therapy to mucosal lesions because of severe mucositis at relatively low dose levels was also reported.

As time passed, we began to recommend[10] that radiation therapy be reserved for specific indications: pain, functional impairment, or improvement of the appearance of cosmetically disfiguring lesions.

Irradiated regions sometimes are left with a purple hemosiderin stain, reminiscent of the color of the original tumor, but with no tumor mass. This fact limits the cosmetic benefit of radiation therapy. However, the residual pigmentation has no prognostic implications.[13] Interestingly, complete response (without residual pigmentation) occurred more often in patients who had higher Karnofsky scores at the time of treatment.

Our preferred dose-fractionation scheme for most lesions in patients with good general condition is 3000 cGy in ten fractions over 2 weeks. Large lesions that cover most of the legs, particularly in patients whose condition is limited, are best treated with a single midplane single-fraction dose of 800 cGy. Data from the University of California at San Francisco[1A] suggest that a single fraction of 800 cGy is as likely to induce regression of disease as more prolonged fractionated regimens and can be used for a wide variety of lesions. However, NYU data[13A] indicate that the response of Kaposi's sarcoma to radiotherapy is a complex function of tumor and host-related factors (treatment intention [cosmesis, pain relief, and so forth], anatomic location, Karnofsky performance status). Patients in good condition who are treated because of cosmetically disfiguring facial lesions have a greater likelihood of tumor response than patients in poor general condition who are treated because of a painful lesion on their feet. There may not be one fractionation regimen that is ideal for all patients. It is clear, however, that when lesions are treated, sufficient dose should be used. Chak and associates[6] reported that six of 22 (27%) patients had to be retreated in less than 4 months average follow-up following doses of up to 2000 cGy in ten fractions.

It is difficult to measure the precise value of radiation therapy for EKS. Nearly all patients receive at least one other type of treatment before, during, or after radiation therapy. Based on our most recent analysis, approximately 73% of lesions flatten completely, although residual pigmentation remains in approximately one third of these cases. Local recurrence of tumor has not been a substantial problem; less than 7% of such lesions subsequently demand attention.[13] Complete relief of pain occurs in two thirds of treated patients (Table 21-4). Response in one site does not accurately predict response to treatment of another site.

Treatment generally is well tolerated. However, two anatomic sites—the soles of the feet and the oral cavity—can exhibit unique behavior. Patients who have lesions of the soles often develop moderate to severe pain and fluid-containing blisters in the irradiated site approximately 1 week after treatment (see Color Fig. 21-10 after p. 510). Although the pain generally subsides if the fluid is aspirated from the blister, healing typically requires several weeks. The oral cavity also is associated with toxicity from radiation therapy. Our group[11] and Watkins and colleagues[53] have reported a consistent inability to deliver conventional radiation therapy to oral cavity lesions without inducing intolerable mucositis after only a few gray (Gy), even if the daily dose rate is substantially decreased or the patient is electively pretreated with antifungal medication.

One possible explanation for enhanced mucosal sensitivity is suggested by the data of Chak and co-workers,[6] who cultured diploid fibroblast cells that they obtained from the "normal skin" biopsy specimens from patients with AIDS. They irradiated the cells and observed a steeper slope of the radiation survival curve than expected (D_0 about 95 cGy compared with the expected D_0 of 140 cGy). Yet, it must be remembered that

TABLE 21–4
Reported Response of Epidemic Kaposi's Sarcoma to Radiation Therapy

	PAIN		COSMESIS		FUNCTION		MASS/EDEMA	
STUDY	CR	PR	CR	PR	CR	PR	CR	PR
Chak[5]	17/27	8/27	0/22	11/22	6/8	2/8	7/30	18/30
Cooper[10]*	14/21	3/21	1/9	8/9	5/5	0/5	6/7	1/7
Nobler[41]			6/12	6/12			6/11	5/11
Weighted average	65%	23%	16%	58%	85%	15%	40%	50%

CR: complete response; PR: partial response
**For this analysis residual pigment was ignored for assessment of function or mass, but rendered the response partial (at best) for cosmesis.*

the typical skin reactions in patients who have AIDS are indistinguishable from those seen in non-AIDS patients. Therefore, it must be concluded that the explanation for the enhanced mucosal sensitivity remains unknown at present.

REFERENCES

1. Ackerman AB, Gottlieb GJ: Atlas of the gross and microscopic features. In Ackerman AB, Gottlieb GJ (eds): Kaposi's Sarcoma: A Text and Atlas, p 33. Philadelphia, Lea & Febiger, 1988

1A. Berson AM, Quivey JM, Harris JW, et al: Radiation therapy for AIDS-related Kaposi's sarcoma. Int J Radiat Oncol Biol Phys 19:569–575, 1990

2. Boldogh I, Beth E, Huang ES, et al: Kaposi's sarcoma. IV. Detection of CMV DNA, CMV RNA and CMNA in tumor biopsies. Int J Cancer 28:469, 1981

3. Braun-Falco O, Lukacs S, Goldschmidt H: Dermatologic Radiotherapy, p 107. New York, Springer-Verlag, 1976

4. Centers for Disease Control. Revision of the CDC surveillance case definition for acquired immunodeficiency syndrome. MMWR 36(Suppl 1S):1S–6S, 1987

5. Chak LY, Gill PS, Levine AM, et al: Radiation therapy for acquired immunodeficiency syndrome-related Kaposi's sarcoma. J Clin Oncol 6:863–867, 1988

6. Chak LY, Hill CK, Gill PS, et al: Radiation therapy for Kaposi's sarcoma (KS) in patients (Pts) with acquired immune deficiency syndrome (AIDS) (Abstract-9). Proc ASCO 6:3, 1987

7. Cipollaro AC, Crossland PM: X-ray and Radium in the Treatment of Diseases of the Skin, p 636. Philadelphia, Lea & Febiger, 1967

8. Cohen L: Dose, time and volume parameters in irradiation therapy of Kaposi's sarcoma. Br J Radiol 35:485–488, 1962

9. Cooper JS: The influence of dose on the long-term control of classic (non-AIDS associated) Kaposi's sarcoma by radiotherapy. Int J Radiat Oncol Biol Phys 15:1141–1146, 1988

10. Cooper JS, Fried PR: Defining the role of radiation therapy for epidemic Kaposi's sarcoma. Int J Radiat Oncol Biol Phys 13:35–39, 1987

11. Cooper JS, Fried PR: Treatment of aggressive epidemic Kaposi's sarcomas of the conjunctiva by radiotherapy. Arch Ophthalmol 106(1):20–21, 1988

12. Cooper JS, Fried PR, Laubenstein LJ: Initial observations of the effect of radiotherapy on epidemic Kaposi's sarcoma. JAMA 252:934–935, 1984

13. Cooper JS, Steinfeld AS, Lerch IA: The prognostic significance of residual pigmentation following radiotherapy of epidemic Kaposi's sarcoma. J Clin Oncol 7:619–621, 1989

13A. Cooper JS, Steinfeld AD, Lerch I: Intentions and outcomes in the radiotherapeutic management of epidemic Kaposi's sarcoma. Int J Radiat Oncol Biol Phys 20:419–422, 1991

14. De Jarlais DC, Marmor M, Thomas P, et al: Kaposi's sarcoma among four different AIDS risk groups. N Engl J Med 310:1119, 1984

15. Dirckx JH: On the name Kaposi. In Gottlieb J, Ackerman AB (eds): Kaposi's Sarcoma: A Text and Atlas, pp 25–26. Philadelphia, Lea & Febiger, 1988

16. Dorn HF, Cutler SJ: Morbidity from cancer in the United States. I. Variation and incidence by age, sex, marital status and geographic region, p 121. Washington, DC, Public Health Monograph No. 29, 1955

17. Drew WL, Mills J, Hauer LB, et al: Declining prevalence of Kaposi's sarcoma in homosexual AIDS patients paralleled by fall in cytomegalovirus transmission Lancet 1(8575/6):66, 1988

18. Duncan JTK: Radiotherapy in the management of Kaposi's sarcoma in Nigeria. Clin Radiol 28:503–509, 1977

19. Fischl MA, Richman D, Grieco MH, et al: The efficacy of azidothymidine (AZT) in the treatment of patients with AIDS and AIDS-related complex. N Engl J Med 317:185–191, 1987

20. Giraldo G, Beth E, Henle G, et al: Antibody patterns to herpesvirus in Kaposi's sarcoma. II. Serological association of American Kaposi's sarcoma with cytomegalovirus. Int J Cancer 22:126, 1978

21. Gottlieb GJ, Ackerman AB: Atlas of the gross and microscopic features of simulators. In Ackerman AB, Gottlieb GJ (eds): Kaposi's Sarcoma: A Text and Atlas, pp 73–76. Philadelphia, Lea & Febiger, 1988

22. Hamilton C, Cummings BJ, Harwood AR: Radiotherapy of Kaposi's sarcoma. Int J Radiat Oncol Biol Phys 12:1931–1935, 1986

23. Harris JW, Reed TA: Kaposi's sarcoma in AIDS: the role of radiation therapy. Front Radiat Ther Oncol 19:126–132, 1985

24. Harwood AR: Kaposi's sarcoma: An update on the results of extended field radiotherapy. Arch Dermatol 117:5–778, 1981

25. Harwood AR, Osaba D, Hofstader SL, et al: Kaposi's sarcoma in recipients of renal transplants. Am J Med 67:759–765, 1979

26. Holecek MJ, Harwood A: Radiotherapy of Kaposi's sarcoma. Cancer 41:1733–1738, 1978

27. Kaplan L, Abrams D, Volberding P: Treatment of Kaposi's sarcoma in acquired immunodeficiency syndrome with an alternating vincristine-vinblastine regimen. Cancer Treat Rep 70:1121–1122, 1986

28. Kaposi M: Idiopathisches multiples Pigmentsarkom der Haut. Arch Dermatol Syphilol 4:265, 1872

29. Krigel RL, Laubenstein LJ, Muggia FM: Kaposi's sarcoma: A new staging classification. Cancer Treat Rep 67:531–534, 1983

30. Krown SE, Metroka C, Wernz J: Kaposi's sarcoma in the acquired immune deficiency syndrome: A proposal for uniform evaluation, response, and staging criteria. J Clin Oncol 7:1201–1207, 1989

31. Krown SE, Real FX, Cunningham-Rundles S, et al: Interferon in the treatment of Kaposi's sarcoma. N Engl J Med 309:923–924, 1983

31A. Lane HC, Falloon J, Walker RE, et al: Zidovudine in patients with human immunodeficiency virus (HIV) infection and Kaposi sarcoma. Ann Intern Med 111:41, 1989

32. Laubenstein L, Krigel RL, Odajnyk CM, et al: Treatment of

epidemic Kaposi's sarcoma with etoposide or a combination of doxorubicin, bleomycin, and vinblastine. J Clin Oncol 2(10):1115–1120, 1984
33. Levy JA, Ziegler JL: Acquired immunodeficiency syndrome is an opportunistic infection and Kaposi's sarcoma results from secondary immune stimulation. Lancet 2(8341):78–81, 1983
34. Mann SD: Kaposi's sarcoma: Experience with ten cases. Am J Roentgenol Ther Nucl Med 121:793–800, 1974
35. Minor DR, Brayer T: Velban and methotrexate (MTX) combination chemotherapy for epidemic Kaposi's sarcoma (Abstract). Proc ASCO 5:1, 1986
36. Mintzer DM, Real FX, Jovino L, et al: Treatment of Kaposi's sarcoma and thrombocytopenia with vincristine in patients with the acquired immunodeficiency syndrome. Ann Intern Med 102:200–202, 1985
37. Mirvish SS, Haverkos HW: Butyl nitrite in the induction of Kaposi's sarcoma in AIDS. N Engl J Med 317:1603, 1987
38. Mitsuyasu RT, Taylor JMG, Glaspy J, et al: Heterogenicity of epidemic Kaposi's sarcoma. Cancer 57:1657–1661, 1986
39. Nisce L, Safai B: Radiation therapy of Kaposi's sarcoma in AIDS. Front Radiat Ther Oncol 19:133–137, 1985
40. Nisce L, Safai B, Poussin-Rosillo H: Once weekly total and subtotal skin electron beam therapy for Kaposi's sarcoma cancer 47:640–644, 1981
41. Nobler MP, Leddy ME, Huh SH: The impact of palliative irradiation on the management of patients with acquired immune deficiency syndrome. J Clin Oncol 5:107–112, 1987
42. Oettlé AG: Geographic and racial differences in the frequency of Kaposi sarcoma as evidence of environmental or genetic causes. Acta Un Int Cancr 18:330, 1962
43. Penn I: Kaposi's sarcoma in organ transplant recipients. Transplantation 27:8–11, 1979
44. Penn I: Cancer as a complication of severe immunosuppression. Surg Gynecol Obstet 162:603–610, 1986
45. Pollack MS, Safai B, Dupont B: HLA-DR5 and DR2 and susceptibility factors for acquired immunodeficiency syndrome with Kaposi's sarcoma in different ethnic subpopulations. Dis Markers 1:135–139, 1983
46. Real FX, Oettgen HF, Krown S: Kaposi's sarcoma and the acquired immunodeficiency syndrome: Treatment with high and low doses of recombinant leukocyte A interferon. J Clin Oncol 4:544–551, 1986
47. Richman D, Fischl MA, Grieco MH, et al: The toxicity of azidothymidine (AZT) in the treatment of patients with AIDS and AIDS-related complex. N Engl J Med 317:192–197, 1987
48. Rothenberg R, Woelfel M, Stoneburner R, et al: Survival with the acquired immunodeficiency syndrome. N Engl J Med 317:1297–1302, 1987
49. Stockwell S: Alpha interferon approved for AIDS-related Kaposi's sarcoma. Oncol Times 11(1):1, 1989
50. Volberding P: The role of chemotherapy for epidemic Kaposi's sarcoma. Semin Oncol 14(2):23–26, 1987
51. Volberding P, Conant MA, Strickler RB, et al: Chemotherapy in advanced Kaposi's sarcoma. Am J Med 74:652–656, 1983
52. Walter PR, Philippe E, Nguemby-Mbina C, et al: Kaposi's sarcoma: Presence of herpes virus particles in a tumor specimen. Hum Pathol 15:1145, 1984
53. Watkins EB, Findlay P, Gelmann E, et al: Enchanced mucosal reactions in AIDS patients receiving oropharyngeal irradiation. Int J Radiat Oncol Biol Phys 13:1403–1408, 1987
54. Wernz J, Laubenstein L, Hymes K, et al: Chemotherapy and assessment of response in epidemic Kaposi's sarcoma (EKS) with bleomycin(B)/velban(V) (Abstract). Proc ASCO 5:4, 1986
55. Weshler Z, Loewinger E, Loewenthal E, et al: Megavoltage radiotherapy using water bolus in the treatment of Kaposi's sarcoma. Int J Radiat Oncol Biol Phys 12:2029–2032, 1986

22

Cutaneous T-Cell Lymphoma

Eric C. Vonderheid
Bizhan Micaily

Cutaneous T-cell lymphoma (CTCL) refers to a spectrum of closely related malignant T-cell lymphoproliferative disorders in which the predominant clinical manifestations involve the skin.[73,140] There are two major subgroups within the CTCL spectrum: mycosis fungoides (MF) and Sézary syndrome, in which the malignant cells have an immunophenotype characteristic of mature T cells, usually with CD4 positivity and show a propensity to infiltrate the epidermis (epidermotropism).[11,18,19,27,55,57,65,79,85,95,102,137,142] The malignant nature of CTCL has been established by autopsy findings showing widespread infiltration of almost every organ system by malignant T cells in advanced disease[37,72,96,115] and by DNA cytophotometric and cytogenetic studies of the abnormal cells.[17,23,31,52,74,88,137]

The etiology of CTCL is still unknown. Its relation to occupational or environmental factors has been stressed in several studies.[28,40] Cohen and colleagues compared patients with age- and sex-matched controls and found a statistically significant correlation between industrial exposure and mycosis fungoides.[28] Genetic factors are implicated by reports of MF occurring in families[46,100,107] and an increased incidence of HLA-antigens Aw31 and Aw32[33] or DR5[98] in MF and B8 and Bw35 in Sézary syndrome.[97] Finally, a viral etiology has been suggested because of clinical similarities between CTCL and adult T-cell lymphoma, a disease caused by a type C retrovirus, designated human T-cell lymphoma virus type 1 (HTLV-1),[15] and the demonstration of type C virus-like particles in skin and lymph node biopsies from patients with MF.[108,122] However, screening of blood samples for antibodies against HTLV-1 antigens[44] and molecular studies on DNA extracted from cells of CTCL patients for HTLV-1 viral sequences[41] argue against a pathologic role for HTLV-1 in classic CTCL. The possibility that a different virus may be the cause has not been excluded by these studies.[76]

EPIDEMIOLOGY

According to recent data from the Surveillance, Epidemiology and End Results (SEER) Program of the National Cancer Institute,[134] the incidence of cutaneous T-cell lymphoma in the United States has increased 3.2 times over the last 14 years and currently exceeds 0.4 new cases per 100,000 population. CTCL occurs more frequently in men than in women by about a 2-to-1 ratio, and blacks are twice as likely to be afflicted as whites. As with other lymphomas, the incidence of CTCL rises sharply with age.

NATURAL HISTORY

Mycosis Fungoides

In 1806, Alibert provided the first description of mycosis fungoides (MF), naming it *pian fungoide* because of a suspected etiologic relationship to yaws.[2] In 1832, Alibert renamed the same case *mycosis fungoide* because of the mushroom-like qualities of the cutaneous tumors.[3] In 1870, Bazin extended these initial observations by dividing the course of the disease into three clinical phases based on the appearance of the skin: *période erythemateuse* (erythematous patch or premycotic phase), *période lichenoide* (infiltrated plaque or mycotic phase), and the *période fungoidique* (tumor or fungoid phase).[5] Most cases of MF evolve slowly and progressively through these three clinical phases, and this typical evolution is referred to as the classic or Alibert–Bazin form.

The patch phase of classic MF is the most variable in clinical appearance and duration. These early lesions are frequently mistaken for other dermatoses, particularly eczema, superficial fungal infections, pityriasis rosea, psoriasis, parapsoriasis en plaques, or skin eruption caused by a drug. In some patients the patch phase of MF manifests as chronic poikilodermatous patches that traditionally have been diagnosed as poikiloderma atrophicans vasculare, retiform parapsoriasis (parakeratosis variegata, parapsoriasis lichenoides), or prereticulotic parapsoriasis (Fig. 22-1). After many years these lesions ultimately can develop superimposed infiltrative plaques or tumors more typical of MF.[99]

The plaque and tumor phases of classic MF are characterized by clinically perceptible accumulations of atypical lymphoid cells within the skin to produce palpable lesions. Individual lesions tend to regress spontaneously in areas and merge with adjacent lesions to form lesions with irregular shapes. The magnitude of infiltration varies from lesion to lesion, which, with the characteristic configurations, produces a virtually diagnostic clinical appearance (Fig. 22-2). Tumorous lesions may develop gradually from preexisting plaques or may appear suddenly in an eruptive manner, indicating a biologically more aggressive clone of malignant cells. Cutaneous ulceration and secondary infections are frequently encountered in this phase.[93]

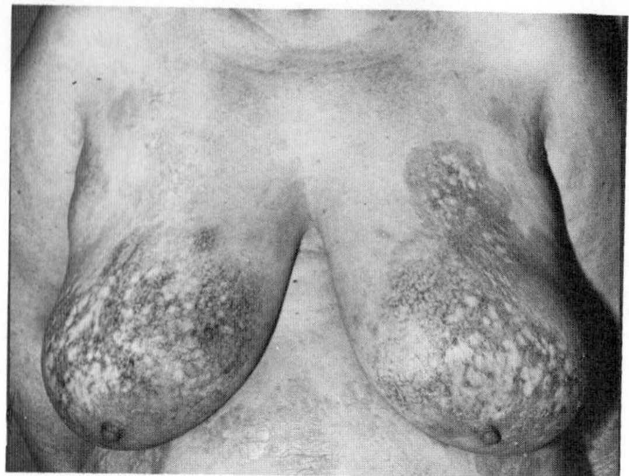

FIGURE 22–1. Classic mycosis fungoides, premycotic phase, presenting as poikiloderma.

In 1885, Vidal and Brocq described several patients with MF on whom cutaneous tumors appeared *de novo* without being preceded by patch or plaque lesions.[128] This sequence of evolution is referred to as *MF tumeurs d'emblée* (*d'emblée* means "at the very onset"). This variant is controversial because many cases described as *MF tumeurs d'emblée* in the past were examples of other lymphomas with secondary involvement of the skin.[9] The histopathologic diagnosis of MF in this circumstance may be more difficult to establish on a skin biopsy specimen because the malignant T cells may not invade the epidermis (nonepidermotropic form of CTCL). In our experience, only about 1% of patients with CTCL present with *MF tumeurs d'emblée.*

Erythrodermic CTCL Including Sézary Syndrome

In 1892, Besnier and Hallopeau described cases of mycosis fungoides in which erythroderma developed during the course of disease, either before or after the appearance of tumors (erythrodermic MF).[7] Later, from 1938 to 1949, Sézary[106] observed the presence of large mononuclear cells with peculiar cerebriform nuclei (Sézary cells) in the skin and peripheral blood of four patients with chronic pruritic erythroderma. Lutzner and co-workers[74] subsequently extended the definition of Sézary syndrome to include erythrodermas and other extensive dermatoses with small hyperconvoluted mononuclear cells in the blood (small cell variant). Because of its histopathologic and cytologic similarities to MF, most investigators consider Sézary syndrome to be an erythrodermic and leukemic expression of CTCL.[101] The MF distinction between Sézary syndrome and erythroderma is based solely on the presence or absence of malignant T cells in the peripheral blood.[16,129] In our experience, about 17% of patients with CTCL present with generalized erythroderma, and about 50% of these have clear-cut Sézary syndrome.

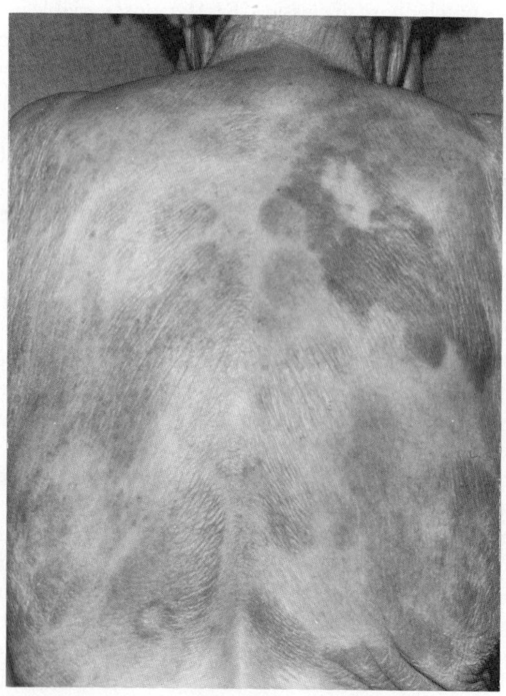

FIGURE 22–2. Classic mycosis fungoides, plaque phase.

Course of Disease

The median duration from the onset of skin lesions to histologic diagnosis of CTCL is about 8 to 10 years with considerable variation from patient to patient. After the histologic diagnosis is established, the median survival for all patients has been reported to be less than 5 years.[28,37,43] However, more recent series record a median survival after histopathologic confirmation of about 10 years, which may reflect earlier diagnosis or improvement in treatment approaches.[60,132]

Extracutaneous involvement is present in over 80% of cases of CTCL at autopsy.[37,72,96] Skin-associated peripheral lymph nodes are involved preferentially, if not initially, during the process of dissemination[116] and are considered a poor barrier against further spread. Any organ system can be infiltrated by malignant lymphocytes in advanced CTCL, but the most common extracutaneous sites at autopsy are the lymph nodes (68%), spleen (56%), liver (49%), lungs (50%), and bone marrow (42%).[37,72,96] The median survival time of patients with histopathologically confirmed lymph node involvement is less than 2 years. Patients with visceral disease have a more ominous prognosis, with median survival of less than 1 year.[21,28,37,60,132]

DIAGNOSTIC WORKUP

With clinical data alone, the physician has considerable information about the likely stage, biologic aggressiveness of disease, and prognosis of the patient.[66] Several punch biopsy specimens should be taken from the most infiltrated lesions for routine and immunopathologic processing to establish the diagnosis and to define the characteristics of the malignant infiltrate.

Additional procedures commonly used in the staging evaluation of patients are outlined in Table 22-1. Of primary importance is the status of lymph nodes in cervical, axillary, and inguinal regions. If lymph nodes are palpable, a biopsy should be obtained. If the nodes are nonpalpable, it is less certain that a lymph node biopsy should be performed at random. In practice, we perform a biopsy of a nonpalpable lymph node only when the patient presents with extensive cutaneous involvement or when radiographic or laboratory evidence of systemic disease is present.

If abnormalities are detected clinically or by tests, an effort should be made to confirm the presence of extracutaneous involvement by histopathologic means. Staging laparotomies have been performed in patients with CTCL, but their usefulness relative to the morbidity of the procedure is uncertain at present.[34,48]

TABLE 22–1
Evaluation of Cutaneous T-Cell Lymphoma

GENERAL
History (attention to pace of disease evolution)
Dermatologic examination to assess degree of lesion infiltration and surface involvement
Routine physical examination including palpation for lymphadenopathy, hepatosplenomegaly, other visceral abnormalities

RADIOGRAPHIC STUDIES
Chest radiograph
Computed tomography of abdomen and pelvis
Isotope scans of liver and spleen or bone (when clinically indicated)

LABORATORY STUDIES
CBC, blood chemistry
Blood smear for presence and quantitation of atypical mononuclear (Sézary) cells
Biopsy studies
- Punch biopsies from most infiltrated lesions
- Biopsy of palpable lymph nodes
- Bone marrow biopsy

STAGING SYSTEMS

The staging system proposed originally by Fuks and associates has particular significance to the radiation oncologist because it concerns data generated from patients treated with total-skin electron-beam irradiation (Table 22-2).[43] More recently, a unifying staging system based on the tumor-node-metastasis (TNM) format was proposed at a Mycosis Fungoides Cooperative Group workshop on CTCL[22] at the National Cancer Institute (NCI; Tables 22-3 and 22-4). Both the Stanford and MF Cooperative Group staging systems recognize the prognostic importance of cutaneous tumors. lymphadenopathy, and extracutaneous involvement.

TABLE 22–2
Stanford Staging System

STAGE	DESCRIPTION
Stage I	Mycosis fungoides limited to the skin. No tumors, ulcers, significant adenopathy, or visceral involvement (clinical or pathologic)
Stage Ia	Eczematous or limited plaque disease with involvement of less than 25% of the total skin surface
Stage Ib	Involvement of more than 25% of the total skin surface. Includes the generalized plaque, lichenoid, and generalized erythroderma variants
Stage II	The presence of skin tumors or biopsy-proven dermatopathic lymphadenopathy. No extracutaneous involvement
Stage III	Mycosis fungoides involving the skin with biopsy-proven involvement of the lymph nodes or spleen. No other visceral involvement
Stage IV	Cutaneous and extracutaneous mycosis fungoides with documented visceral involvement

(Hoppe RT, Fuks Z, Bagshaw MA: Int J Radiat Oncol Biol Phys 2:843–851, 1977)

TABLE 22–3
Proposed TNM Classification of Cutaneous T-Cell Lymphoma

MAGNITUDE OF SKIN INVOLVEMENT (T)*

T0	Clinically or pathologically suspicious lesions
T1	Premycotic lesions, papules, or plaques involving less than 10% of the skin
T2	Premycotic lesions, papules, or plaques involving more than 10% of the skin
T3	One or more tumors on the skin
T4	Extensive, often generalized erythroderma

STATUS OF PERIPHERAL LYMPH NODES (N)†

N0	Clinically normal; pathologically not involved
N1	Clinically abnormal; pathologically not involved
N2	Clinically normal; pathologically involved
N3	Clinically abnormal; pathologically involved

STATUS OF PERIPHERAL BLOOD (B)‡

B0	Atypical circulating cells not present
B1	Atypical circulating cells present

STATUS OF VISCERAL ORGANS (M)

M0	Pathologically not involved
M1	Pathologically involved

**T1–T4 require pathologic confirmation. When more than one classification applies, indicate both ratings and use highest for staging* (e.g., *T3 [T2]).*
† Record sites of abnormal nodes (e.g., *axillary [L + R]).*
‡ Record total WBC, total lymphocyte count, and number of atypical cells per 100 lymphocytes. (Note: *the criterion for blood involvement based on blood smears has not been agreed on and therefore is not used in staging.)*

PATHOLOGIC CLASSIFICATION

The cellular infiltrate of CTCL consists of malignant T cells admixed with varying numbers of normal lymphocytes, histiocytes, eosinophils, plasma cells, and other cells (a polymorphous cellular infiltrate).[68] If cellular atypism is not pronounced, the diagnosis of CTCL often cannot be established definitively by histopathologic means. The cytomorphology of the atypical lymphoid cells varies from small cells with hyperchromatic, convoluted nuclei (referred to as *cerebriform cells*) to large cells with pale-staining vesicular nuclei and prominent nucleoli.[14,130] Many intermediary cellular forms with pleomorphic nuclei may occur, including the so-called mycosis cell, a mononuclear cell with a large hyperchromatic nucleus. In some instances, lymphocytoid or histiocytoid lymphoma cells may predominate in the infiltrate to such an extent that a diagnosis of a monomorphous lymphoma is suggested.

TABLE 22–4
Mycosis Fungoides Cooperative Group Staging System for Cutaneous T-Cell Lymphomas

STAGE	T	N	M
Ia	T1	N0	M0
Ib	T2	N0	M0
IIa	T1–2	N1	M0
IIb	T3	N0–1	M0
III	T4	N0–1	M0
IVa	T1–4	N2–3	M0
IVb	T1–4	N0–3	M1

In patch, plaque, and erythrodermic lesions of CTCL, the cellular infiltrate is located predominantly in the superficial part of the dermis, often arranged in a band-like distribution immediately beneath the epidermis. However, it may extend into deeper regions around hair follicles and eccrine glands. With tumor formation, the infiltrate penetrates between the collagen bundles of the reticular dermis and into the subcutaneous fat; the depth may range from a few millimeters to several centimeters, an important factor in treatment planning. Characteristically, atypical lymphoid cells in classic MF and Sézary syndrome invade the epidermis and follicular epithelium to form small groups surrounded by a halo-like clear space (Pautrier's microabscesses). The appreciation of functional interactions between keratinocytes, Langerhans cells, and normal T lymphocytes provides the rationale that accounts for the observed homing properties of malignant T cells.[91,103]

The histopathologic appearance of CTCL in organ systems other than the skin may be confused with that of other lymphomas. The presence of clusters and sheets of mononuclear cells with convoluted nuclei is highly suggestive of CTCL.[96]

Lymph node involvement is underestimated by routine methods because early nodal involvement cannot be easily differentiated from dermatopathic lymphadenitis or other nonspecific changes. Malignant T cells frequently can be demonstrated in lymph nodes, otherwise diagnosed as dermatopathic lymphadenitis, using special techniques such as quantitative morphometry of nuclear shapes,[121] DNA cytophotometry,[23,127] cytogenetic analysis,[38,136] demonstration of tumor-associated antigens on the cell membrane with monoclonal antibodies,[6] and molecular studies to show clonal rearrangement of T-cell receptor genes.[135] The T-cell characteristics of the malignant cells explain the early localization of the infiltrate in the paracortical regions of lymph nodes and periarteriolar regions of the spleen.

PROGNOSTIC FACTORS

Age of Patient

Several studies have implicated age to be a prognostic variable in CTCL.[37,47,53,118] On average, patients over 60 years at the time of diagnosis have a significantly shortened survival rate compared with that of younger patients, even when the survival data are corrected for deaths related to CTCL only. When subjected to multivariate analysis in the presence of staging information, age no longer retains its prognostic significance,[47] which indicates that older patients more often present with advanced disease.

Stage of Disease

Several clinical parameters have been identified as having prognostic implications for patients with CTCL. These include the type and extent of skin involvement, lymph node enlargement, and overt visceral organ involvement. The probability of survival for 5 years is approximately 90% for patients with limited patch–plaque disease (T1), 67% for extensive patch–plaque disease (T2), 35% for tumorous disease (T3), and 40% for erythrodermic disease (T4).[25,66,140]

Likewise, lymph node enlargement *per se* connotes an unfavorable prognosis for patients with CTCL. Histopathologic documentation of lymph node involvement (effacement of nodal architecture by malignant T cells) is associated with a median survival of less than 2 years.[21,29,37] Moreover, in the National MF Cooperative Group study, the 3-year survival rates were 85% for patients without nodal enlargement, 68% for patients with enlarged nodes located in only one region, and 60% for patients with enlarged nodes in more than one region.[66] Multivariate analysis indicates that although skin and lymph node parameters are highly correlated findings, more prognostic information is provided when both variables are used independently in staging.[47]

Clinical evidence of visceral involvement by CTCL (liver, spleen, or lung abnormalities) is associated with median survival of less than 1 year.[21,28,37,131] These prognostic variables have been incorporated into the Mycosis Fungoides Cooperative Group staging system based on the TNM format (see Tables 23-3 and 23-4).

Laboratory Studies

The demonstration of malignant T cells (Sézary cells) in the peripheral blood is associated with an unfavorable prognosis.[28,37,84,87,121,131] Median survival intervals have ranged from less than 1 year to about 3 years, depending on the criteria used for the definition of blood involvement.[129] The presence of markedly aneuploid cells by DNA cytophotometry or cytogenetic studies signifies an even shorter survival interval in this situation.[23,88,136] This observation may explain why the presence of Sézary cells with diameters greater than 14 μm on blood smears from patients with Sézary syndrome was found to correlate more significantly with survival patterns than did absolute numbers of Sézary cells.[129]

Other laboratory studies that may have prognostic importance include immunopathologic findings (loss of maturation antigens or expression of antigens of activation by malignant T cells),[18,58,65] responsiveness of peripheral lymphocytes to various mitogens and antigens,[82] and proliferation kinetics of the malignant T cells.[13,35,105,114]

General Management

Staging procedures define two general situations based on the localization of CTCL: patients with disease apparently limited to the skin and those with pathologic evidence of extracutaneous involvement. Current evidence indicates that malignant cells readily circulate between the skin and extracutaneous tissues, particularly the so-called skin-associated lymph nodes and spleen[116,117]; therefore, separation of CTCL into these two groups is arbitrary.

Because CTCL may originate in the skin, intensive therapy directed at the skin alone seems to offer the possibility of cure mostly for patients with early, limited involvement (Stage Ia). Frequent remissions and sustained long-term disease-free intervals have occurred in such patients treated with total-skin electron-beam irradiation,[60,61,81,118] topically applied solutions of mechlorethamine,[132] and photochemotherapy using oral methoxsalen (8-methoxypsoralen) followed by intensive exposure to long-wave ultraviolet light.[59] The determination of "cure" requires considerable follow-up intervals because of the characteristically indolent time course of early MF. At the present time, sufficient numbers of patients have been followed up after treatment with total-skin electron-beam irradiation, topical mechlorethamine chemotherapy, and methoxsalen photochemotherapy, indicating a cure rate approaching 40%, largely in patients with limited intracutaneous CTCL.

For patients with widespread intracutaneous CTCL, particularly in the presence of cutaneous tumors, long-lasting complete remissions are uncommon following therapies with cutaneous effects only, regardless of the treatment modality. The current trend is to administer therapy with systemic effects for these unapparent foci of extracutaneous disease.[140] For patients treated with total-skin electron-beam irradiation, this treatment may consist of administering concomitant multiagent systemic chemotherapy[20,49] or total lymph node irradiation[82] if the treatment is being provided with curative intent. However, if treatment is being administered for palliation alone, patients should be placed on maintenance therapy with topical mechlorethamine chemotherapy or well-tolerated systemic drugs after a course of total-skin electron-beam irradiation.

Pathologically confirmed extracutaneous involvement usually means that systemic chemotherapy must be provided to control cutaneous T-cell lymphoma. Several single agents produce beneficial, albeit temporary, responses in most patients treated. These include several alkylating agents (mechlorethamine,[37,64,124] cyclophosphamide,[1,37,73,123] and chlorambucil[24,37,139,144]), antimetabolites (methotrexate[37,56,143,144]), and antitumor antibiotics (bleomycin[32,39,112,126,145] and doxorubicin[69]). More recently, attention has been given to combinations of several drugs, and preliminary results have been encouraging.[26,37,50,51,67,75,77,83,119,146] However, cytotoxic chemotherapy with either single or multiple drugs results in complete responses in only 20% to 25% of patients with advanced CTCL, and there are no long-term disease-free survivors with chemotherapy alone.[140]

Failure of systemic drugs to control advanced CTCL usually is the result of incomplete responses of cutaneous lesions, whereas extracutaneous foci of disease often respond completely. For this reason, additional treatment for cutaneous lesions (*e.g.*, topical mechlorethamine chemotherapy) would be expected to have additive beneficial effects for patients treated primarily with systemic drugs and should be considered for every patient.

Development of autologous bone marrow transplantation as an adjunct to systemic therapy promises to improve the outlook for patients with advanced CTCL.[92] We believe that radiation in the form of total-skin electron-beam irradiation combined with ablative total photon irradiation will prove to be an important contribution to treatment administered with curative intent. Systemic drugs and serotherapy with murine monoclonal anti-T-cell antibodies are potential additional therapeutic measures that can be used in advanced CTCL to further ensure that such radiation therapy will eradicate the malignant T-cell population.

RADIATION THERAPY TECHNIQUES

The overall thickness of normal skin varies from less than 0.5 mm (eyelids) to 5 mm or more (back), the average thickness being 2 mm to 3 mm. The cellular infiltration of CTCL tends to localize primarily in the superficial portion of the skin but often extends into deeper regions around hair follicles and eccrine glands, even in minimally infiltrated lesions.[68,96] The cellular infiltration associated with tumor formation usually extends into the subcutaneous tissue to a depth of 15 mm or more. The quality of radiation must be chosen to provide an adequate dose to the lowest margins of the lesion. Several types of ionizing radiation are used in the treatment of CTCL. Grenz-ray radiation is no longer recommended because of poor penetration. Soft radiation from beryllium-windowed tubes in the 40 kV to 60 kV range[45,141] and β-rays emitted from ^{90}Sr sources[12] are suitable for very superficial lesions and have been used successfully for treatment of extensive skin involvement, primarily in Europe. In the United States, the major radiotherapeutic approach for extensive CTCL is total-skin electron-beam irradiation. Superficial, orthovoltage, or supervoltage x-irradiation also may be used for individual infiltrated lesions.

Conventional Radiation Therapy

Superficial radiation (80 kVp to 140 kVp) with a half-value layer (HVL) of 0.7 mm to 1.0 mm Al and a target-to-skin distance of 15 cm to 30 cm can be used for most infiltrated plaques. For markedly infiltrated plaques and tumors, higher energy orthovoltage radiation (200 kVp to 280 kVp) or local-field electron-beam (10 MeV to 15 MeV) radiation is recommended. Discrete lesions may be treated satisfactorily with a variety of protraction-fractionation schedules, ranging from 1000 cGy to 1200 cGy in three to four treatment fractions over a 3- to 4-day period, up to 2000 cGy to 3000 cGy in ten to 15 fractions over a 2- to 3-week period. Generous portals should be used to cover defined anatomic areas. Because of the possible need for subsequent treatment in adjacent areas, it is important to document the treated areas with Polaroid photographs, accurate portal drawings, and (if feasible) tattooing of the corners of the fields with India ink.

Cotter and co-workers reported on 20 patients (110 lesions) who underwent palliative radiation therapy for cutaneous MF.[30] The modalities for treatment included superficial x-rays, ^{60}Co, and electron-beam irradiation. The total tumor doses ranged from 600 cGy to 4000 cGy. Fifty-three percent of the lesions were classified as plaques, 20% as tumors up to 3 cm in diameter, and 27% as tumors greater than 3 cm in diameter. Complete response (CR) to treatment was observed in 95% of plaque lesions, 95% of tumors up to 3 cm in diameter, and 93% of tumors greater than 3 cm in diameter. A complete response to treatment was noted in all lesions receiving more than 2000 cGy. In the total population of lesions having a CR, a local in-field recurrence rate of 42% was noted in the group receiving up to 1000 cGy, 32% in those receiving 1001 cGy to 2000 cGy, 21% in those receiving 2001 cGy to 3000 cGy, and 0% in the group receiving more than 3000 cGy (Tables 22-5 and 22-6). Eighty-three percent of the 30 recurrences were seen within 1 year of treatment; all recurrences occurred within 2 years of treatment (Fig. 22-3). The data from this study indicate that tumor doses equivalent to at least 3000 cGy, 200 cGy per fraction, five fractions per week (total dose fraction [TDF] ≥49), are needed for adequate local control of cutaneous MF lesions.

Total-Skin Electron-Beam Therapy

The advantages and application of high-energy electrons for cutaneous radiation therapy are discussed in Chapter 10. Adoption of electron beam for treatment of the total skin surface involves placing the patient in various positions to allow a fairly uniform dose distribution to the exposed surfaces. Verification of delivered doses should be carried out periodically using thermoluminescent dosimeters placed on skin surfaces.

Various treatment techniques have been used since the introduction of total-skin electron-beam therapy in the early 1950s. Initially treatment was administered to the anterior and posterior skin surfaces by passing patients on a moving couch under a narrow radiation beam.[120] Subsequent techniques have used stationary two- and four-field positions, but at this time the

TABLE 22–5
Local Response to Treatment as a Function of Radiation Dose: 110 Total Lesions

	≤1000 cGy	1001 cGy–2000 cGy	2001 cGy–3000 cGy	3001 cGy–4000 cGy
No. lesions	27	46	28	9
Complete response	26 (96%)	41 (89%)	28	9
Partial response	1	5	0	0
Recurrence after complete response	11/26 (42%)	13/41 (32%)	6/28 (21%)	0/9
Mean time to recurrence	5 months	10 months	16 months	No failures
Treatment failures (persistent or recurrent lesions)	12/27 (44%)	18/46 (39%)	6/28 (21%)	0/9

(Cotter GW, Baglan RJ, Wasserman TH, et al: Int J Radiat Oncol Biol Phys 9:1477–1480, 1983)

optimal technique with maximum uniformity of dose appears to be a six-field technique, described originally by Karzmark and later refined by Page (Fig. 22-4).[8,89] The electron beam with an effective central axis energy of 3 MeV to 4 MeV is used to treat three anterior and three posterior stationary treatment fields, each having a superior and inferior portal with beam angulation 20 degrees above and 20 degrees below the horizontal axis. The patient is placed in front of the beam in six positions during treatment (see Fig. 22-4). The straight anterior, right posterior oblique (RPO), and left posterior oblique (LPO) fields are treated on the first day of each treatment cycle, and the straight posterior, right anterior oblique (RAO), and left anterior oblique (LAO) fields are treated on the second day of each cycle. A dose fraction of 32.8 cGy is administered to each field per day. The entire wide-field skin surface would receive 200 cGy each 2-day cycle. Radiation generally is administered on a 4-day-per-week dose schedule, with total dose levels of 3000 cGy to 4000 cGy delivered over an 8- to 10-week interval. Figure 22-5 depicts the current method of total-skin electron-beam therapy used at Hahnemann University.

The average skin dose is calculated as the product of the dose delivered to the center of the treatment plane for one of the dual fields multiplied by a correction factor (F). Factor F represents the fact that any given point on the surface receives some radiation from at least two of the six dual-exposure fields and is calculated from phantom measurements. The percentage of photon contamination for a single dual-field cycle should not exceed 0.3%. Machine calibration is performed daily, as are point-of-dose prescription and side-to-side flatness.

During wide-field skin irradiation, internal eye shields are used routinely to protect the cornea and lens. Occasional shielding of the digits and lateral surfaces of the hands or feet may be necessary because of local skin reaction from overlapping treatment fields in these areas. Areas not directly exposed to the path of the electron beam (soles of feet, perineum, medial upper thighs, axillae, posterior auricular and inframammary regions, and vertex of scalp) are treated with separate 3 MeV to 4 MeV electron-beam fields, generally at a rate of 100 cGy daily to a total dose of 2000 cGy (Fig. 22-6). Markedly infiltrated tumors may be treated with supplemental orthovoltage radiation or higher energy electrons (additional 2000 cGy in ten fractions).

RESULTS OF RADIATION THERAPY

Historical Aspects

Scholtz was the first to use ionizing radiation in the treatment of mycosis fungoides.[104] Although a few hundred centigrays usually promotes complete regression of an individual lesion, the disease invariably continues to progress because of the multifocal and widespread nature of the disorder. In 1939 Sommerville suggested an "x-ray bath" to large cutaneous areas, but this technique was limited by adverse side effects, particularly bone marrow suppression.[110,111] Likewise, other investigators reported severe bone marrow suppression in patients treated with superficial radiation therapy to many treatment fields.[90]

Total-Skin Electron-Beam Irradiation

In 1951 Trump and associates[120] used a modified Van de Graaff accelerator to treat disseminated MF with a beam of 2.5 MeV electrons to a total dose of 600 cGy to 800 cGy over an 8- to 10-

TABLE 22–6
Local Response to Treatment as a Function of Radiation Dose for Recurrent Mycosis Fungoides Lesions (n = 28)

	≤1000 cGy	1001 cGy–2000 cGy	2001 cGy–3000 cGy	3001 cGy–4000 cGy
No. lesions	7	16	5	0
Complete response	7 (100%)	13 (81%)	5	0
Partial response	0	3	0	0
Recurrence after complete response	3/7 (43%)	7/13 (54%)	1/5	0
Treatment failures (persistent or recurrent lesions)	3/7 (43%)	10/16 (63%)	1/5	0

(Cotter GW, Baglan RJ, Wasserman TH, et al: Int J Radiat Oncol Biol Phys 9:1477–1480, 1983)

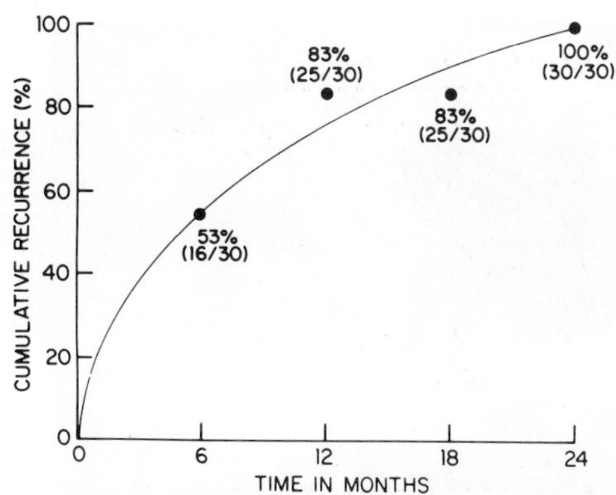

FIGURE 22–3. Cumulative percentage of recurrences as a function of time after complete response to radiation therapy. (Cotter GW, Baglan RJ, Wasserman TH, et al: Int J Radiat Oncol Biol Phys 9:1477, 1983)

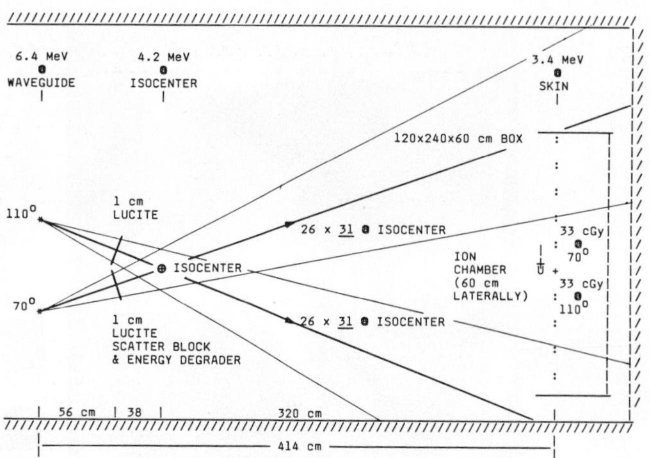

FIGURE 22–5. The portal geometry of total-skin electron beam therapy, as administered at Hahnemann University.

day interval, and then repeated the treatment course as needed for recurrent disease. Of 220 patients with MF (50% in the tumoroulcerative phase) treated in this fashion during the next 10 years,[109] 89 (40%) were reported to survive 2 to 7 years, but detailed actuarial survival rates are unavailable. In 1971, Fuks and Bagshaw presented therapeutic results on 107 patients treated with 2.5 MeV electrons at Stanford University.[42] These investigators increased the total dose to 3000 cGy and presented evidence indicating that the posttreatment disease-free intervals justified a more aggressive therapeutic approach than that used previously, particularly in patients with early manifestations of disease.

The Stanford University experience with total-skin electron-beam irradiation was updated by Hoppe and associates.[60,61] Since 1972, patients have been treated with 4 MeV electrons to doses up to 4000 cGy. Initial clearance of disease was found to depend primarily on the initial dose of electrons administered and the clinical status of the patient. A complete response occurred in 47%, 67%, and 94% of patients treated with low dosage (800 cGy to 1999 cGy), moderate dosage (2000 cGy to 2999 cGy), and high dosage (3000 cGy to 4000 cGy), respectively. With initial doses exceeding 2000 cGy, 118 of 140 (84%) patients achieved a complete remission of disease overall, with clearance rates of 96%, 87%, 72%, and 71% for patients with limited plaque, generalized plaque, tumors, or erythrodermic disease, respectively. The actuarial 5-year survival rates for these patients were about 96% for those with limited plaque disease, 75% for those with generalized plaque disease, 28% for those with tumorous disease, and 54% those with for erythrodermic disease.

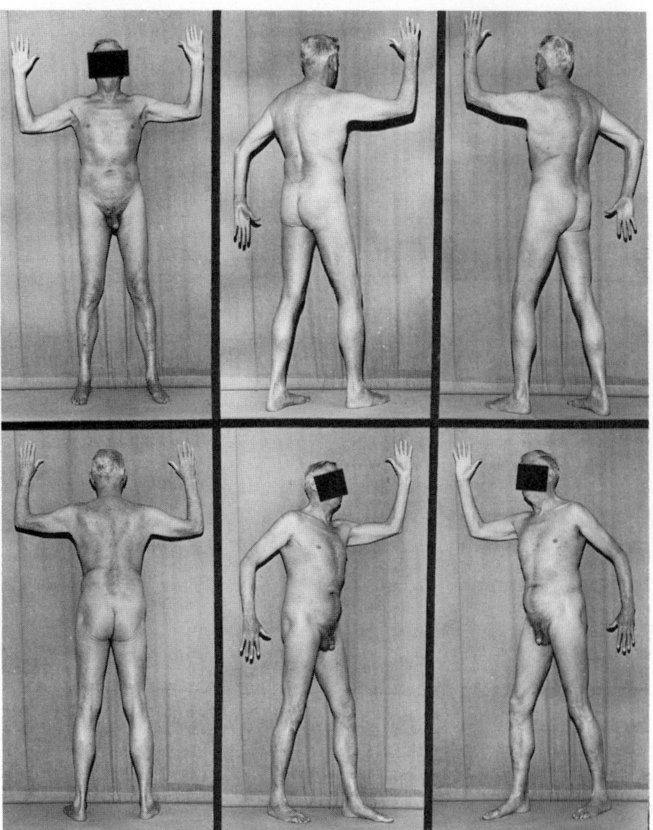

FIGURE 22–4. Positions assumed by the patient for total-skin electron beam radiation, six-field technique.

Of particular interest to the radiation oncologist was the demonstration by the Stanford group that up to 40% of patients with early CTCL (Stages Ia and Ib) who are treated with high-dose, total-skin electron-beam irradiation remain relapse-free for long intervals after treatment, a strong argument for the administration of total-skin electron-beam irradiation for cure rather than for palliation in the management of early CTCL.

The high frequency of initial clearing after high-dose electron beam irradiation has been confirmed by other groups,[10,81,87,118,125,133,138] but most have reported a somewhat lower continuous disease-free survival rate for early CTCL—up to 30% in some series.[81,118] Moreover, not all investigators agree that administration of high-dose, total-skin electron-beam irradiation is the method of choice.[71,113] For example, Lo and coworkers at the Leahy Clinic found that the prognosis of patients with widespread CTCL who were treated with high-dose, total-skin electron-beam irradiation was not significantly different from that of patients treated with lower doses in their experience,[71] and that long-term disease-free survival can be achieved with small-field megavoltage irradiation in patients with localized disease.[70]

Several radiation oncology groups have used more aggressive radiotherapeutic approaches for advanced CTCL. At Hahnemann University, Micaily and associates[82] treated 19 patients with rapidly progressing plaque- or tumor-phase MF with high-dose, total-skin electron-beam irradiation (3600 cGy to 4000 cGy over 8 to 10 weeks) and total nodal irradiation (2500 cGy to 3000 cGy in 4 to 5 weeks). Fourteen patients had disease apparently confined to the skin (Stages Ib, IIa, and IIb), and five patients had proven lymph node involvement (Stage IVa).

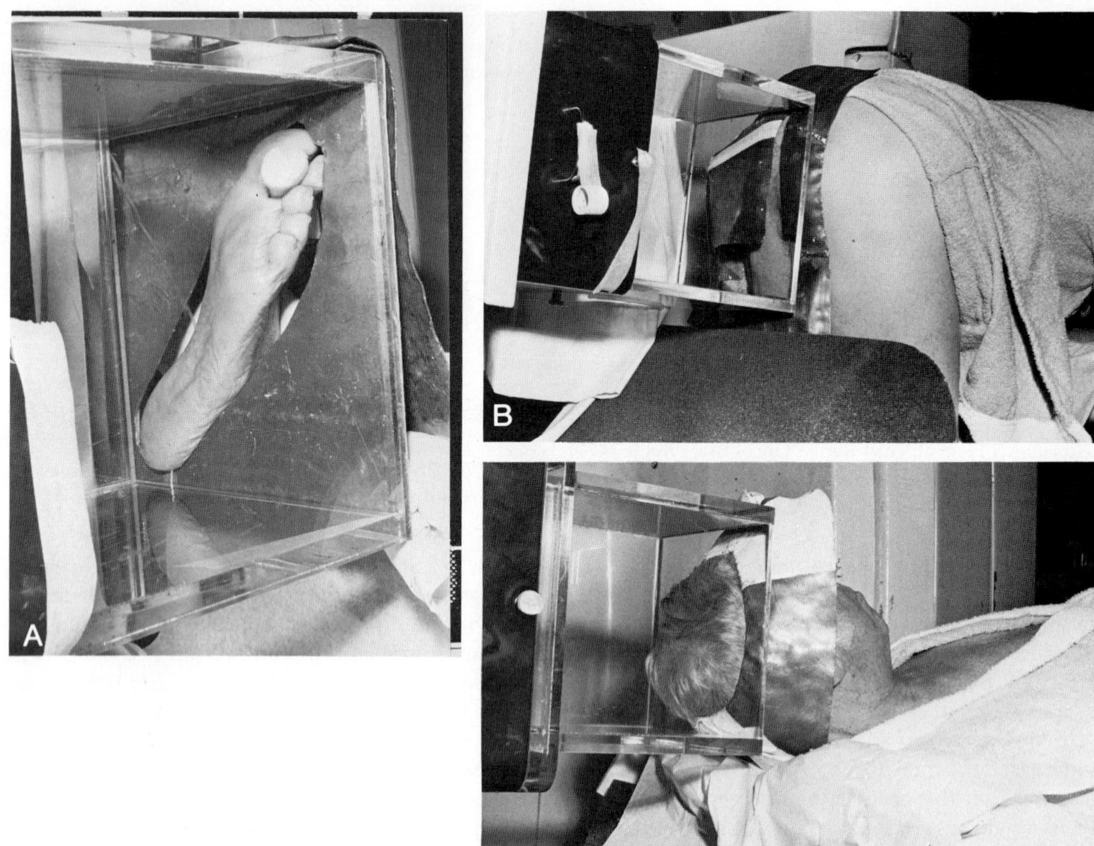

FIGURE 22–6. Supplemental radiation is administered to treatment fields not directly exposed to the electron beam. (**A**) Soles of feet. (**B**) Perineum. (**C**) Vertex of scalp.

Although a complete response was recorded in nearly all instances, sustained disease-free intervals were recorded primarily for patients with Stage Ib and Stage IIa disease. These patients had an overall survival rate of 100% and a disease-free survival rate of 44% at 6 years. The acute effects of this treatment approach were well tolerated, but three patients developed second malignancy and one patient developed myelodysplasia, possibly the result of radiation therapy.

Total-body photon irradiation may play an important role in the management of advanced CTCL. Horriot and co-workers have had promising results with low-dose, total-body fractionated photon irradiation.[62] Five of ten patients with extracutaneous CTCL have remained disease-free more than 12 to 56 months after treatment.

SEQUELAE OF TREATMENT

The cutaneous complications of total-skin radiation therapy for cutaneous T-cell lymphoma depend primarily on the total dose of radiation administered. These complications may be divided into short-term and long-term sequelae.

Short-Term Radiation Therapy Sequelae

The skin of patients treated with total-skin electron-beam irradiation at doses in excess of 1000 cGy usually develops mild erythema and dry desquamation that may become uncomfortably symptomatic. Lesions frequently become more erythematous than clinically normal areas during the early phase of treatment and may later become hyperpigmented. At higher doses (>2500 cGy), some patients develop transient swelling of the hands, edema of the ankles, and occasionally large blisters that may necessitate local shielding or temporary discontinuation of therapy.

Unless hair and nails are shielded, loss of these skin appendages invariably occurs by the end of treatment, but they regenerate within 4 to 6 months (unless previously destroyed by the disease process). Gynecomastia may also develop; the mechanism for this is unknown.

With current methods, patients treated with total-skin electron-beam irradiation may develop a mild leukopenia during treatment, but they no longer are subject to severe bone marrow suppression from contaminating radiation. Other reported systemic sequelae such as arthralgias and nausea have not been observed in our patients.

Long-Term Radiation Therapy Sequelae

Chronic cutaneous damage from total-skin electron-beam irradiation is unusual at doses of less than 1000 cGy and is acceptably mild through 2500 cGy.[94] Superficial atrophy with wrinkling, telangiectasias, xerosis, and uneven pigmentation are the most common changes. With higher total dosages, frank poikiloderma, permanent alopecia, skin fragility, and subcutaneous fibrosis are more likely to occur but are uncommon. An increased incidence of radiation-induced cutaneous neo-

COLOR FIGURES

Classic and Acquired Immunodeficiency Syndrome (AIDS)-Related Kaposi's Sarcoma

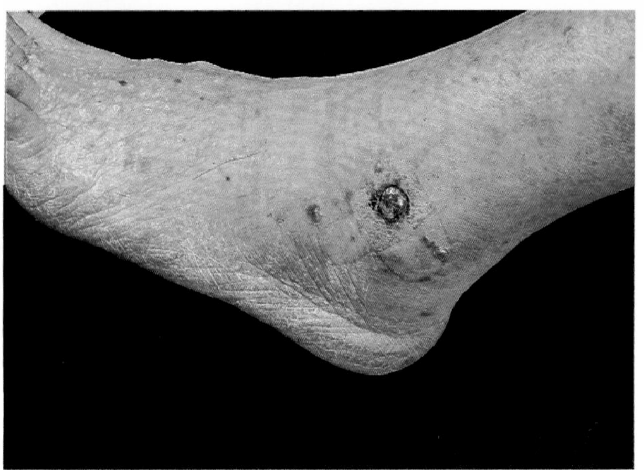

COLOR FIGURE 21–1

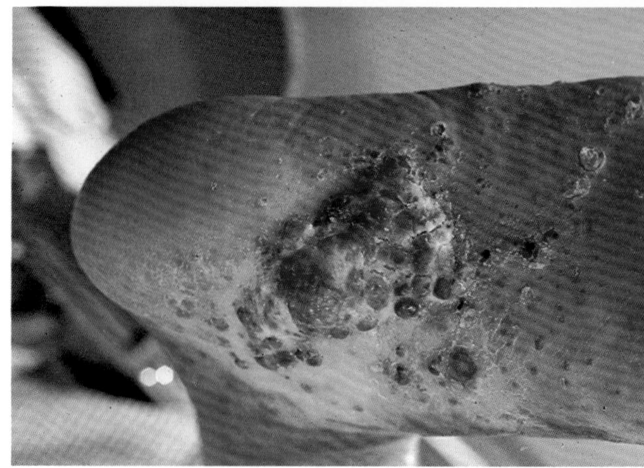

COLOR FIGURE 21–2

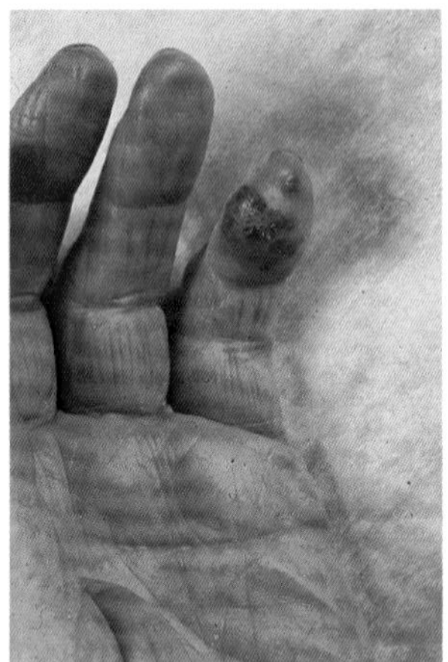

COLOR FIGURE 21–3

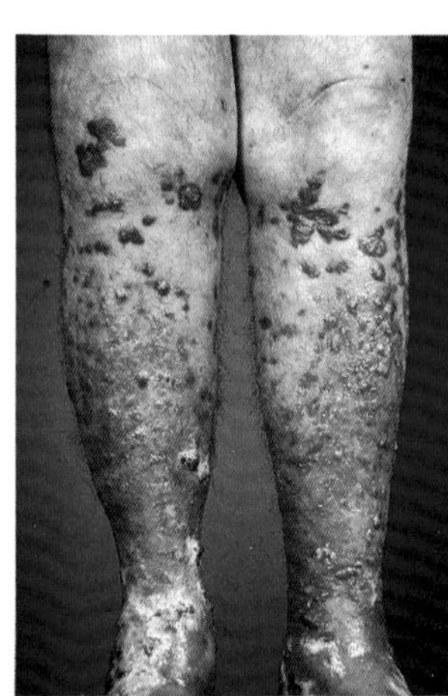

COLOR FIGURE 21–4

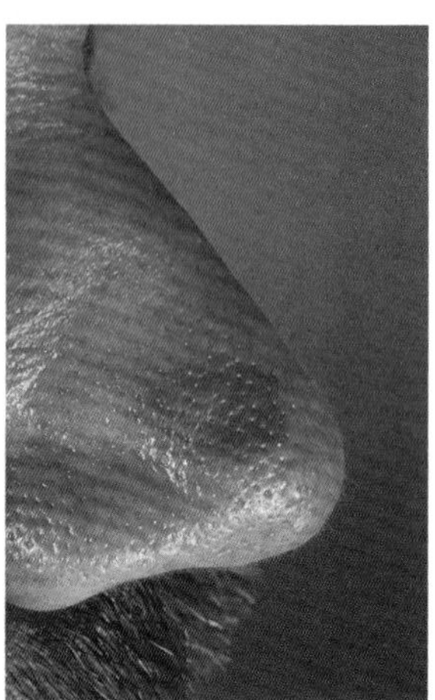

COLOR FIGURE 21–5

COLOR FIGURE 21–1. Purple, 1.5 cm nodular classic Kaposi's sarcoma on ankle of an elderly man. (Krigel RL, Friedman-Kien AE: Kaposi's sarcoma in AIDS: diagnosis and treatment. In DeVita VT Jr, Hellman S, Rosenberg SA [eds]: AIDS: Etiology, Diagnosis, Treatment, and Prevention, ed 2. Philadelphia, JB Lippincott, 1988)

COLOR FIGURE 21–2. Classic Kaposi's sarcoma. Multiple red to purple papules on sole of foot. (Krigel RL, Friedman-Kien AE: Kaposi's sarcoma in AIDS: diagnosis and treatment. In DeVita VT Jr, Hellman S, Rosenberg SA [eds]: AIDS: Etiology, Diagnosis, Treatment, and Prevention, ed 2. Philadelphia, JB Lippincott, 1988)

COLOR FIGURE 21–3. Nodular purple classic Kaposi's sarcoma near the tip of patient's fifth finger. (Krigel RL, Friedman-Kien AE: Kaposi's sarcoma in AIDS: diagnosis and treatment. In DeVita VT Jr, Hellman S, Rosenberg SA [eds]: AIDS: Etiology, Diagnosis, Treatment, and Prevention, ed 2. Philadelphia, JB Lippincott, 1988)

COLOR FIGURE 21–4. Extensive superficial and deep Kaposi's sarcoma producing lymphedema. (Krigel RL, Friedman-Kien AE: Kaposi's sarcoma in AIDS: diagnosis and treatment. In DeVita VT Jr, Hellman S, Rosenberg SA [eds]: AIDS: Etiology, Diagnosis, Treatment, and Prevention, ed 2. Philadelphia, JB Lippincott, 1988)

COLOR FIGURE 21–5. Epidemic Kaposi's sarcoma. Red-purple macule near tip of patient's nose. (Krigel RL, Friedman-Kien AE: Kaposi's sarcoma in AIDS: diagnosis and treatment. In DeVita VT Jr, Hellman S, Rosenberg SA [eds]: AIDS: Etiology, Diagnosis, Treatment, and Prevention, ed 2. Philadelphia, JB Lippincott, 1988)

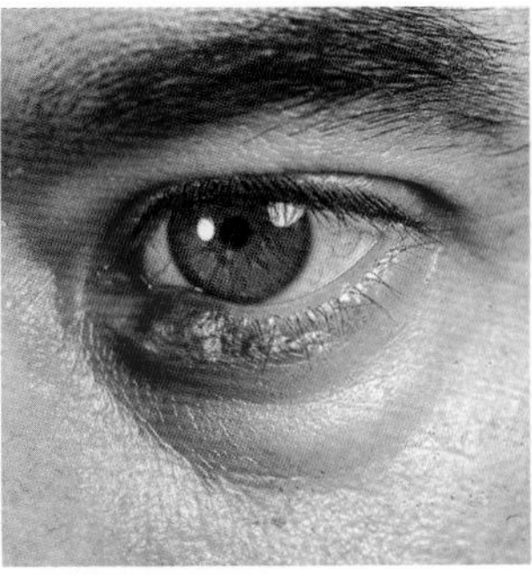

COLOR FIGURE 21–6

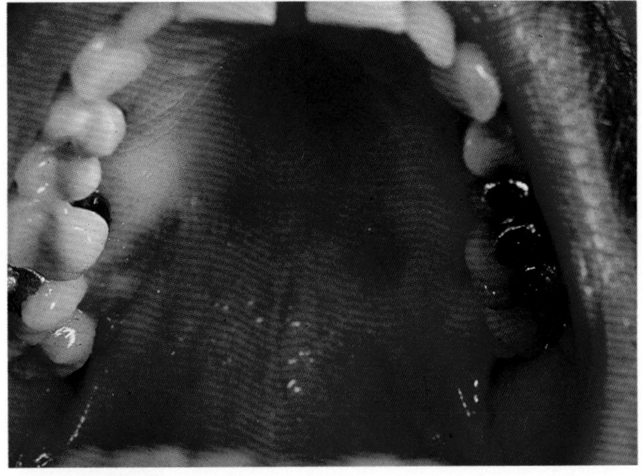

COLOR FIGURE 21–7

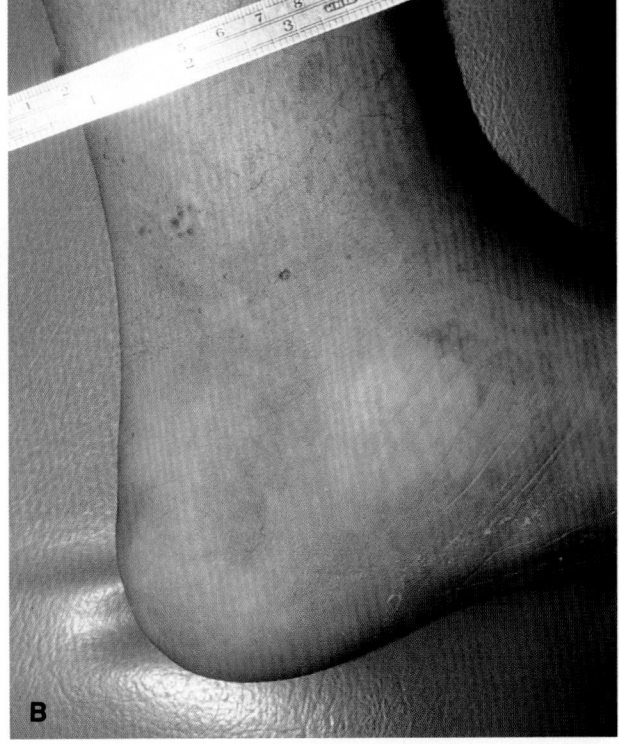

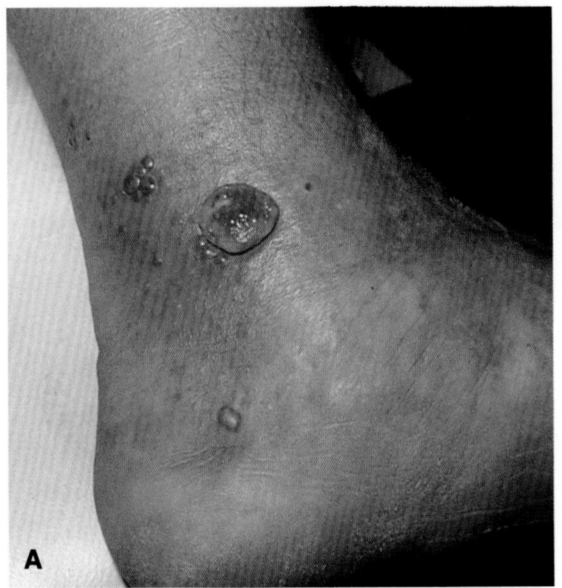

B

COLOR FIGURE 21–8

COLOR FIGURE 21–6. Nodular purple epidemic Kaposi's sarcoma on patient's lower eyelid. (Krigel RL, Friedman-Kien AE: Kaposi's sarcoma in AIDS: diagnosis and treatment. In DeVita VT Jr, Hellman S, Rosenberg SA [eds]: AIDS: Etiology, Diagnosis, Treatment, and Prevention, ed 2. Philadelphia, JB Lippincott, 1988)

COLOR FIGURE 21–7. Epidemic Kaposi's sarcoma. Red-purple papules on hard palate. (Krigel RL, Friedman-Kien AE: Kaposi's sarcoma in AIDS: diagnosis and treatment. In DeVita VT Jr, Hellman S, Rosenberg SA [eds]: AIDS: Etiology, Diagnosis, Treatment, and Prevention, ed 2. Philadelphia, JB Lippincott, 1988)

COLOR FIGURE 21–8. (**A**) Epidemic Kaposi's sarcoma of the foot before treatment. (**B**) Same patient approximately 1.5 years after 3000 cGy was delivered in ten fractions over 2 weeks by 6 MeV electron beam therapy (with bolus).

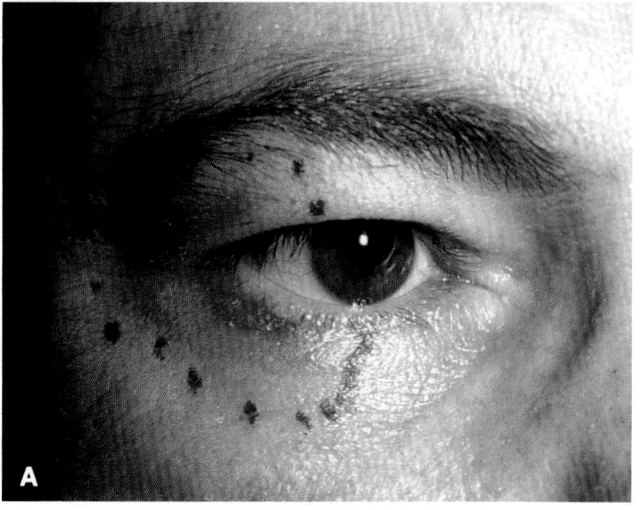

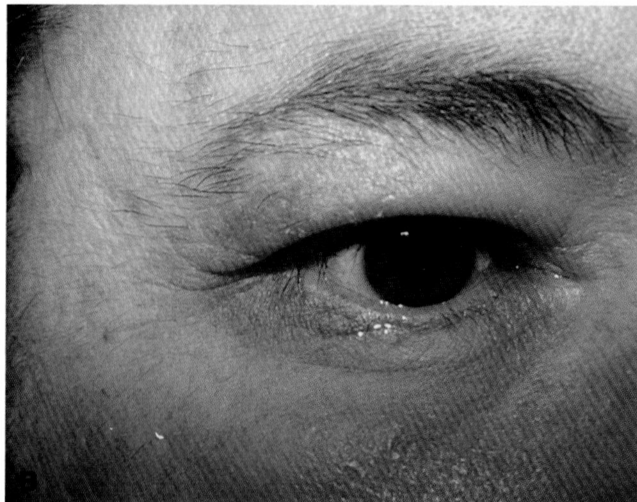

COLOR FIGURE 21–9

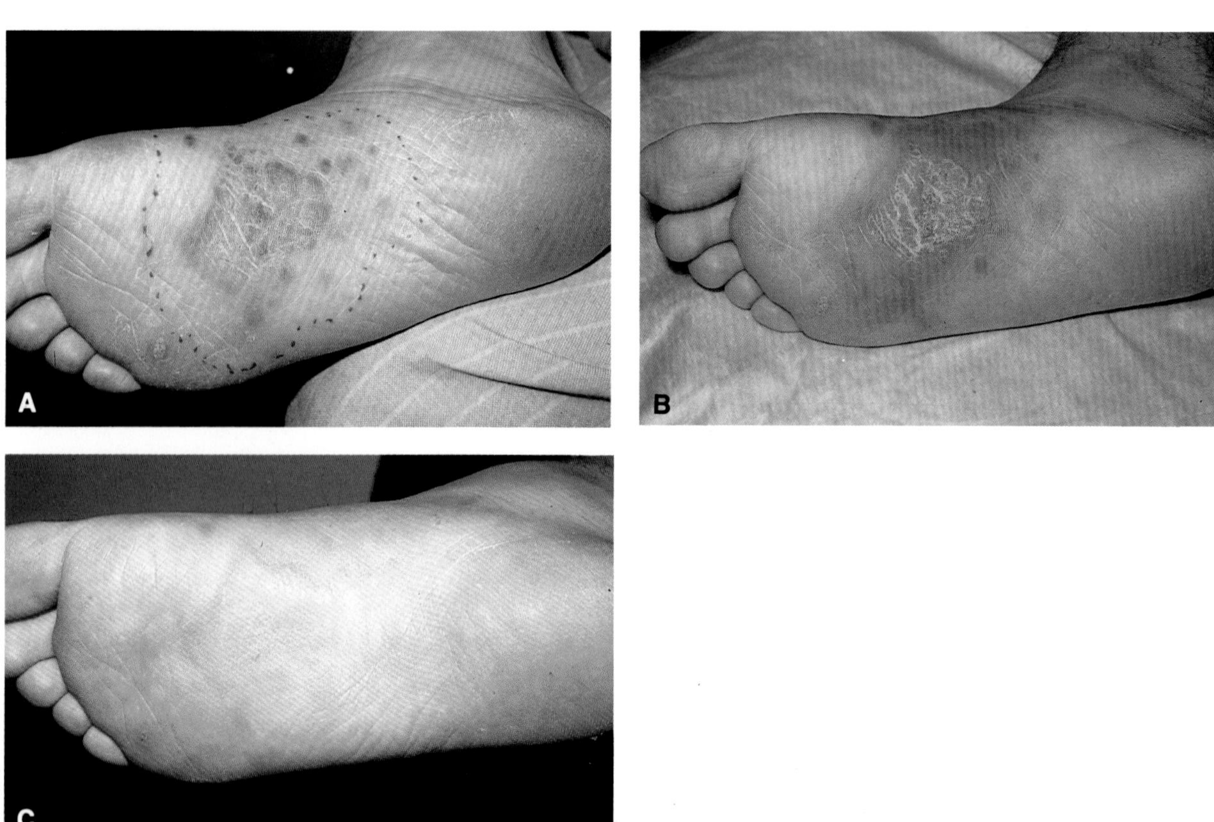

COLOR FIGURE 21–10

COLOR FIGURE 21–9. (**A**) Epidemic Kaposi's sarcoma of the upper and lower lateral eyelids before treatment. (**B**) Same patient approximately 1 month after 3000 cGy was delivered in ten fractions over 2 weeks by kilovoltage x-rays. An eye shield was used to protect the lens of the eye. Residual pigmentation is visible.

COLOR FIGURE 21–10. (**A**) Epidemic Kaposi's sarcoma of the sole before treatment. (**B**) Same patient approximately 2 weeks after 3000 cGy was delivered in ten fractions over 2 weeks by 6 MeV electron beam therapy (with bolus). An intense reaction is visible including the residua of a blister. (**C**) Same patient 5 weeks after treatment showing resolution of the reaction and clearing of his disease.

plasia has not yet become apparent, but this may require additional follow-up.

SUMMARY OF CLINICAL TRIALS

Total-Skin Electron-Beam Irradiation *Versus* Topical Mechlorethamine Chemotherapy

In 1975, a multi-institutional Mycosis Fungoides Cooperative Group was organized to evaluate uniformly patients with MF and to compare therapeutic results in patients randomly selected for total-skin electron-beam irradiation, topically applied mechlorethamine, or a combination of both.[36] However, the number of patients registered was insufficient to show statistically meaningful results. It is worth noting, however, that one randomized prospective study[54] and one retrospective study[131] compared total-skin electron-beam irradiation and mechlorethamine chemotherapy and found no difference in overall survival patterns.

Aggressive *Versus* Conservative Treatment of CTCL

Several groups have reported on the feasibility of combining total-skin electron-beam irradiation with some cutaneous or sequential administration of cytotoxic chemotherapy for CTCL.[20, 49] The response rates generally exceed 90%, with complete responses occurring in most patients. At the National Cancer Institute a randomized study was conducted to compare the "aggressive" combined modality approach with traditional "conservative" management, consisting of various topical treatments and single-agent systemic drugs administered sequentially as needed. The results indicate no significant differences in survival patterns between the two groups.[63] The median duration of complete responses after combined modality therapy for advanced disease was less than 2 years.

REFERENCES

1. Abele DC, Dobson RL: The treatment of mycosis fungoides with a new agent, cyclophosphamide (Cytoxan). Arch Dermatol 82:725, 1960
2. Alibert JLM: Description des Maladies de la Peau: Observées a l'Hôpital Saint-Louis, et Exposition des Meilleures Méthodes Suives pour Leur Traitment, p 157. Paris, Barrois l'Aine et Fils, 1806
3. Alibert JLM: Monographie des Dermatoses ou Précis Théorique et Pratique des Maladies de la Peau. Paris, Daynac, 1832
4. Bast RC Jr, Ritz J, Lipton JM, et al: Elimination of leukemia cells from human bone marrow using monoclonal antibody and complement. Cancer Res 43:1389, 1983
5. Bazin PAE: Lçons sur le Traitment des Maladies Chroniques en General, Affections de la Peau en Particulier, par l'emploi Compaté des Eaux Minerales de l'Hydrothérapie et des Moyens Pharmaceutiques, p 425. Paris, Adrien Delahaye, 1870
6. Berger CL, Morrison S, Chu A, et al: Diagnosis of cutaneous T-cell lymphoma by use of monoclonal antibodies reactive with tumor-associated antigens. J Clin Invest 70:1205, 1982
7. Besnier E, Hallopeau H: On the erythroderma of mycosis fungoides. J Cutan GU Dis 10:453, 1892
8. Bjarngard BE, Chen GTY, Piontek RW, et al: Analysis of dose distributions in whole body superficial electron therapy. Int J Radiat Oncol Biol Phys 2:319, 1977
9. Blasik LG, Newkirk RE, Dimond RL, et al: Mycosis fungoides d'emblée: A rare presentation of cutaneous T-cell lymphoma. Cancer 49:742, 1982
10. Blasko J, Becker L, Griffin TW, et al: Electron beam therapy of mycosis fungoides. Acta Radiol Oncol 18:321, 1979
11. Boumsell L, Bernard A, Reinherz EL, et al: Surface antigens on malignant Sézary and T-CLL cells correspond to those mature T-cells. Blood 57:526, 1982
12. Bratherton DG: Strontium beam therapy. Mod Trends Radiother 2:176, 1982
13. Braylan RC, Fowlkes BJ, Jaffe ES, et al: Cell volumes and DNA distributions of normal and neoplastic human lymphoid cells. Cancer 41:201, 1987
14. Brehmer-Andersson E: Mycosis fungoides and its relation to Sézary's syndrome, lymphomatoid papulosis, and primary cutaneous Hodgkin's disease. Acta Derm-Venereol (Stockh) 57(Suppl):75, 1976
15. Broder S, Bunn PA Jr, Jaffe ES, et al: T-cell lymphoproliferative syndrome associated with human T-cell leukemia/lymphoma virus. Ann Intern Med 100:543, 1984
16. Broder S, Edelson RL, Lutzner MA, et al: The Sézary syndrome: A malignant proliferation of helper T-cells. J Clin Invest 58:1297, 1976
17. Brouet JC, Flandrin G, Seligmann M: Indications of the thymus-derived nature of the proliferating cells in six patients with Sézary's syndrome. N Engl J Med 289:341, 1973
18. Buechner SA, Winkelmann RK, Banks PM: T cells in cutaneous lesions of Sézary's syndrome and T-cell leukemia. Arch Dermatol 119:895, 1983
19. Buechner SA, Winkelmann RK, Banks PM: T-cells and T-cell subsets in mycosis fungoides and parapsoriasis. Arch Dermatol 120:897, 1984
20. Bunn PA Jr, Fischmann AB, Schechter GP, et al: Combined modality therapy with electron beam irradiation and systemic chemotherapy for cutaneous T-cell lymphomas. Cancer Treat Rep 63:713, 1979
21. Bunn PA Jr, Huberman MS, Whang-Peng J, et al: Prospective staging evaluation of patients with cutaneous T-cell lymphoma. Ann Intern Med 93:223, 1980
22. Bunn PA Jr, Lamberg SI: Report of the committee on staging and classification of cutaneous T-cell lymphomas. Cancer Treat Rep 63:725, 1979
23. Bunn PA, Whang-Peng J, Carney DN, et al: DNA content analysis by flow cytometry and cytogenetic analysis in mycosis fungoides and Sézary syndrome. J Clin Invest 65:1440, 1980
24. Campbell EW, Fromer JL: Adjunct chemotherapy in the treatment of cutaneous malignancies. Surg Clin North Am 39:585, 1959
25. Carney DN, Bunn PA Jr: Manifestations of cutaneous T-cell lymphomas. J Dermatol Surg Oncol 6:369, 1980
26. Case DC Jr: Combination chemotherapy for mycosis fungoides with cyclophosphamide, vincristine, methotrexate, and prednisone. Am J Clin Oncol 7:453, 1984
27. Chu A, Patterson J, Berger C, et al: *In situ* study of T-cell subpopulations in cutaneous T-cell lymphoma. Cancer 54:2414, 1984
28. Cohen SR, Stenn KS, Braverman IM, et al: Mycosis fungoides: Clinicopathologic relationships, survival, and therapy in 59 patients with observations on occupation as a new prognostic factor.
29. Colby TV, Burke JS, Hoppe RT: Lymph node biopsy in mycosis fungoides. Cancer 47:351, 1981
30. Cotter GW, Baglan RJ, Wasserman TH, et al: Palliative radiation treatment of cutaneous mycosis fungoides: A dose response. Int J Radiat Oncol Biol Phys 9:1477, 1983
31. Crossen PE, Mellor JEL, Finley AG, et al: The Sézary syndrome: Cytogenetic studies and identification of the Sézary cell as an abnormal lymphocyte. Am J Med 50:24, 1971
32. de Bast C, Moriame N, Wanet J, et al: Bleomycin in mycosis fungoides and reticulum cell lymphoma. Arch Dermatol 104:508, 1971
33. Dick HM, Mackie R: Distribution of HLA antigens in patients with mycosis fungoides. Dermatologica 155:275, 1977
34. Doyle JA, Winkelmann RK: Staging laparotomy in cutaneous T-cell disease. Arch Dermatol 117:543, 1981
35. Edelson RL: Efficacy of leukopheresis procedures in the man-

agement of cutaneous "T" cell lymphoma: Leukemic phase. Proc Adv Blood Components Semin 4:1, 1977
36. Editorial: The Mycosis Fungoides Cooperative Study Group Steering Committee: Mycosis Fungoides Cooperative Study. Arch Dermatol 111:457, 1975
37. Epstein EH Jr, Levin DL, Croft JD, et al: Mycosis fungoides: Survival, prognostic features, response to therapy and autopsy fundings. Medicine 15:61, 1972
38. Erkman-Balis B. Rappaport H: Cytogenetic studies in mycosis fungoides. Cancer 34:626, 1974
39. European Organization for Research on the Treatment of Cancer: Co-operative Group for Leukaemia and Reticulocytoses: Bleomycin in the Reticuloses. Br Med J 285:1972
40. Fischmann AB, Bunn PA Jr, Guccion JG, et al: Exposure to chemicals, physical agents, and biologic agents in mycosis fungoides and the Sézary syndrome. Cancer Treat Rep 63:591, 1979
41. Franchini G, Wong-Staal F, Gallo RC: Molecular studies of human T-cell leukemia virus and adult T-cell leukemia. J Invest Dermatol 83:635, 1984
42. Fuks Z, Bagshaw MA: Total-skin electron treatment of mycosis fungoides. Radiology 100:145, 1971
43. Fuks ZY, Bagshaw MA, Farber EM: Prognostic signs and the management of the mycosis fungoides. Cancer 32:1385, 1973
44. Gallo RC, Kalyanaraman VS, Sarngadharan MG, et al: Association of the human type C retrovirus with a subset of adult T-cell cancers. Cancer Res 43:3892, 1983
45. Goldschmidt H, Lukacs S, Schoefinius HH: Teleroentgentherapy for mycosis fungoides. J Dermatol Surg Oncol 4:600, 1978
46. Greene MH, Pinto HA, Kant JA, et al: Lymphomas and leukemias in the relatives of patients with mycosis fungoides. Cancer 49:737, 1982
47. Green SB, Byar DP, Lamberg SI: Prognostic variables in mycosis fungoides. Cancer 47:2671, 1981
48. Griem ML, Moran EM, Ferguson DJ, et al: Staging procedures in mycosis fungoides. Br J Cancer 31(Suppl II):362, 1975
49. Griem ML, Tokars RP, Petras V, et al: Combined therapy for patients with mycosis fungoides. Cancer Treat Rep 63:655, 1979
50. Groth O, Molin L, Thomsen K, et al: Tumour stage of mycosis fungoides treated by bleomycin and methotrexate: Report from Scandanavian Mycosis Fungoides Study Group. Acta Derm Venereol (Stockh) 59:59, 1979
51. Grozea PN, Jones SE, McKelvey EM, et al: Combination chemotherapy for mycosis fungoides: A Southwest Oncology Group study. Cancer Treat Rep 63:647, 1979
52. Hagedorn M, Kiefer G: DNA content of mycosis fungoides cells. Arch Dermatol Res 258:127, 1977
53. Hamminga L, Hermans J, Noordijk EM, et al: Cutaneous T-cell lymphoma: Clinicopathologic relationships, therapy, and survival in 92 patients. Br J Dermatol 107:145, 1982
54. Hamminga B, Noordijk Em, van Vloten WA: Treatment of mycosis fungoides: Total-skin electron-beam irradiation versus topical mechlorethamine therapy. Arch Dermatol 118:150, 1982
55. Haynes BF, Metzgar RS, Minna JD, et al: Phenotype characterization of cutaneous T-cell lymphoma: Use of monoclonal antibodies to compare with other malignant T-cells. N Engl J Med 304:1319, 1981
56. Haynes HA, Van Scott EJ: Therapy of mycosis fungoides. Prog Dermatol 3:1, 1968
57. Holden CA, Morgan EW, MacDonald DM; The cell population in the cutaneous infiltrate of mycosis fungoides: *In situ* studies using monoclonal antisera. Br J Dermatol 106:385, 1982
58. Holden CA, Staughton RCD, Campbell M-A, et al: Differential loss of T-cell lymphocyte marker in advanced cutaneous T-cell lymphoma. J Am Acad Dermatol 6:507, 1982
59. Honigsmann H, Brenner W, Rauschmeier W, et al: Photochemotherapy for cutaneous T-cell lymphoma. J Am Acad Dermatol 10:238, 1984
60. Hoppe RT, Cox RS, Fuks Z, et al: Electron-beam therapy for mycosis fungoides: The Stanford experience. Cancer Treat Rep 63:691, 1979
61. Hoppe RT, Fuks Z, Bagshaw MA: The rationale for curative radiotherapy in mycosis fungoides. Int J Radiat Oncol Biol Phys 2:843, 1977
62. Horriot JC: Personal communication, December 1983
63. Kaye F, Bunn PA Jr, Steinberg SM, et al: A randomized trial comparing combination electron-beam radiation and chemotherapy with topical therapy in the initial treatment of mycosis fungoides. N Engl J Med 321:1784, 1989
64. Kierland RR, Watkins CH, Shullenberger CC: The use of nitrogen mustard in the treatment of mycosis fungoides. J Invest Dermatol 9:195, 1947
65. Kung PC, Berger CL, Goldstein G, et al: Cutaneous T-cell lymphoma: Characterization by monoclonal antibodies. Blood 57:261, 1981
66. Lamberg SI, Green SB, Byar DP, et al: Clinical staging for cutaneous T-cell lymphoma. Ann Intern Med 100:187, 1984
67. Leavell UW Jr, DeSimone P: Combined chemotherapy (COP) in treatment of mycosis fungoides: Report of four cases. South Med J 69:915, 1976
68. Lever WF, Schaubburg-Lever G: Histopathology of the Skin, 5th ed, p 696. Philadelphia, JB Lippincott, 1975
69. Levi JA, Diggs CH, Wiernik PH: Adriamycin therapy in advanced mycosis fungoides. Cancer 39:1967, 1977
70. Lo TCM, Salzman FA, Costey GE, et al: Megavolt electron irradiation for localized mycosis fungoides. Acta Radiol Oncol 20:71, 1981
71. Lo TCM, Salzman FA, Moschella SL, et al: Whole body surface electron irradiation in the treatment of mycosis fungoides. Radiology 130:453, 1979
72. Long JC, Mihm MC: Mycosis fungoides with extracutaneous dissemination: A distinct clinopathologic entity. Cancer 34:1745, 1974
73. Lutzner M, Edelson R, Schein P, et al: Cutaneous T-cell lymphomas: The Sézary syndrome, mycosis fungoides, and related disorders. Ann Intern Med 83:534, 1975
74. Lutzner MA, Emerit I, Durepaire R, et al: Cytogenetic, cytophotometric, and ultrastructural study of large cerebriform cells of the Sézary syndrome and description of a small-cell variant. JNCI 50:1145, 1973
75. Maguire A: Treatment of mycosis fungoides with cyclophosphamide and chlorpromazine. Br J Dermatol 80:54, 1968
76. Manzari V. Gismondi A, Barillari G, et al: A new human retrovirus isolated in a Tac-negative T cell lymphoma/leukemia. Science 238:1581, 1987
77. McDonald CJ, Bertino JR: Treatment of mycosis fungoides lymphoma: Effectiveness of infusion of methotrexate followed by oral citrovorum factor. Cancer Treat Rep 62:1009, 1978
78. McMillan EM, Wasik R, Everett MA: HLA DR-positive cells in large plaque (atrophic) parapsoriasis. J Am Acad Dermatol 5:444, 1981
79. McMillan EM, Wasik R, Beeman K, et al: *In situ* immunologic phenotyping of mycosis fungoides. J Am Acad Dermatol 6:888, 1982
80. McMillan EM, Wasik R, Peters S, et al: OKT 9, reactivity in mycosis fungoides and large plaque (atrophic) parapsoriasis. Cancer 51:403, 1983
81. Meyler TS, Blumberg AL, Purser P: Total skin electron beam therapy in mycosis fungoides. Cancer 42:1171, 1978
82. Micaily B, Campbell O, Moser C, et al: Total-skin electron beam and total nodal irradiation of cutaneous T-cell lymphoma. Int J Radiat Oncol Biol Phys 20:809, 1991
83. Molin L, Thomsen K, Volden G, et al: Combination chemotherapy in the tumour stage of mycosis fungoides with cyclophosphamide, vincristine, VP-16, adriamycin and prednisone (COP, CHOP, CAVOP): A report from the Scandanavian Mycosis Fungoides Study Group. Acta Derm Venereol (Stockh) 60:542, 1980
84. Moran EM, Walther JR, Aronson IK, et al: Clinical significance of circulating Sézary cells in mycosis fungoides. Proc Am Soc Clin Oncol 18:276, 1977

85. Nasu K, Said J, Vonderheid EC, et al: Immunopathology of cutaneous T cell lymphomas. Am J Pathol 119:436, 1985
86. Nickoloff BJ: Role of interferon-gamma in cutaneous trafficking of lymphocytes with emphasis on molecular and cellular adhesion events. Arch Dermatol 124:1835, 1988
87. Nisce IZ, Safai B, Kim JH: Effectiveness of once-weekly total skin electron beam therapy in mycosis fungoides and Sézary syndrome. Cancer 47:870, 1981
88. Nowell PC, Finan JB, Vonderheid EC: Clonal characteristics of cutaneous T cell lymphomas: Cytogenetic evidence from blood, lymph nodes, and skin. J Invest Dermatol 78:69, 1982
89. Page V, Gardner A, Karzmark CJ: Patient dosimetry in the electron treatment of large superficial lesions. Radiology 94:635, 1970
90. Pascher F, Kanee B: Reactions of the hemopoietic system to agents used in the treatment of dermatoses. Effects of low-voltage roentgen ray therapy. Arch Dermatol 53:1, 1946
91. Patterson JAK, Edelson RL: Interactions of T cells with the epidermis. Br J Dermatol 107:117, 1982
92. Phillips GL, Herzig RH, Lazarus HM, et al: Treatment of resistant malignant lymphoma with cyclophosphamide, total body irradiation, and transplantation of cryopreserved autologous marrow. N Engl J Med 310:1557, 1984
93. Posner LE, Fossieck BE Jr, Eddy JL, et al: Septicemic complications of the cutaneous T-cell lymphomas. Am J Med 71:210, 1981
94. Price NM: Radiation dermatitis following electron beam therapy. Arch Dermatol 114:63, 1978
95. Ralfkiaer E, Lange Wantzin G, Mason DY, et al: Phenotypic characterization of lymphocyte subsets in mycosis fungoides. Am J Clin Pathol 84:610, 1985
96. Rappaport H, Thomas LB: Mycosis fungoides: The pathology of extracutaneous involvement. Cancer 34:1198, 1974
97. Rosen ST, Radvany R, Roenigk J Jr, et al: Human leukocyte antigens in cutaneous T-cell lymphomas. J Am Acad Dermatol 12:531, 1985
98. Safai B, Myskowski PL, Dupont B, et al: Association of HLA-DR5 with mycosis fungoides. J Invest Dermatol 80:395, 1983
99. Samman PD: Mycosis fungoides and other cutaneous reticuloses. Clin Exp Dermatol 1:197, 1976
100. Sandbank M, Katzenellenbogen I: Mycosis fungoides of prolonged duration in siblings. Arch Dermatol 98:620, 1968
101. Schein PS, MacDonald JS, Edelson R: Cutaneous T-cell lymphoma. Cancer 38:1859, 1976
102. Schmitt D, Souteyrand P, Brochier J, et al: Phenotype of cells involved in mycosis fungoides and Sézary syndrome (blood and skin lesions): Immunomorphological study with monoclonal antibodies. Acta Derm Venereol (Stockh) 62:193, 1982
103. Schmitt D, Thivolet J: Lymphocyte-epidermis interactions in malignant epidermotrophic lymphomas. I. Ultrastructural aspects. Acta Derm Venereol (Stockh) 60:1, 1980
104. Scholtz W: Ueber den einfluee der roentgenstrahlen auf die haut in gesunden und krankein zustande. Arch Dermatol Syph (Berlin) 59:421, 1902
105. Schwarzmeier JD, Paietta E, Radaszkiewicz T, et al: Proliferation kinetics of Sézary cells. Blood 57:1049, 1981
106. Sézary A: Une nouvelle réticulose cutanée. La réticulose maligne leucémique a histiomonocytes monstreux et a forme d'érythrodermie oedémateuse et pigmentée. Ann Dermatol Venereol (Paris) 9:5, 1949
107. Shelley WB: Familial mycosis fungoides revisited. Arch Dermatol 116:1177, 1980
108. Slater D, Bleehan S, Rooney N, et al: Type C retrovirus-like particles in mycosis fungoides. Br J Dermatol 109:120, 1983
109. Smedal MI, Johnston DO, Salzman FA, et al: Ten-year experience with low megavolt electron therapy. Am J Roentgenol 88:215, 1962
110. Sommerville J: Mycosis fungoides treated with general x-ray bath. Br J Dermatol 51:323, 1939
111. Sommerville J: General x-ray baths in generalized dermatoses. Br J Dermatol 54:234, 1942
112. Spigel SC, Coltman CA Jr: Therapy of mycosis fungoides with bleomycin. Cancer 32:767, 1973
113. Spittle MF: Electron-beam therapy in England. Cancer Treat Rep 63:639, 1979
114. Sterry W, Pullmann H, Steigleder G-K: Proliferation kinetics of the dermal infiltrate in cutaneous malignant lymphomas. Arch Dermatol Res 270:285, 1981
115. Stokar LM, Vonderheid EC, Abell MB, et al: The antemorten clinical manifestations of intrathoracic cutaneous T-cell lymphoma. Cancer 56:2694, 1985
116. Streilein JW: Lymphocyte traffic, T-cell malignancies and the skin. J Invest Dermatol 71:167, 1978
117. Streilein JW: Skin-associated lymphoid tissues (SALT): Origins and functions. J Invest Dermatol 80:125, 1983
118. Tadros AAM, Tepperman BS, Hryniuk WM, et al: Total skin electron irradiation for mycosis fungoides: Failure analysis and prognostic factors. Int J Radiat Oncol Biol Phys 9:1279, 1981
119. Tirelli U, Carbone A, Veronesi A, et al: Combination chemotherapy with cyclophosphamide, vincristine and prednisone (CVP) in TNM-classified stage IV mycosis fungoides. Cancer Treat Rep 66:167, 1982
120. Trump JG, Wright KA, Evans WW, et al: High energy electrons for the treatment of extensive superficial malignant lesions. Am J Roentgenol 69:623, 1953
121. van der Loo EM, Meijer CJLM, Scheffer E, et al: The prognostic value of membrane markers and morphometric characteristics of lymphoid cells in blood and lymph nodes from patients with mycosis fungoides. Cancer 48:738, 1981
122. van der Loo EM, van Muijen GNP, van Vloten WA, et al: C-type virus-like particles specifically localized in Langerhans cells and related cells of skin and lymph nodes of patients with mycosis fungoides and Sézary syndrome. Virchows Arch B Cell Path 31:193, 1979
123. Van Scott EJ, Auerbach R, Clendenning WE: Treatment of mycosis fungoides with cyclophosphamide. Arch Dermatol 85:499, 1962
124. Van Scott EJ, Grekin DA, Kalmanson JD, et al: Frequent low doses of intravenous mechlorethamine for late-stage mycosis fungoides lymphoma. Cancer 36:1613, 1975
125. van Vloten WA, de Vroome H, Noordijk FM: Total skin electron beam irradiation for cutaneous T-cell lymphoma (mycosis fungoides). Br J Dermatol 112:697, 1985
126. van Vloten WA, Polano MK: Bleomycin therapy in mycosis fungoides. Dermatologica 150:50, 1975
127. van Vloten WA, Scheffer E, Meijer CJLM: DNA cytophotometry of lymph node imprints from patients with mycosis fungoides. J Invest Dermatol 73:275, 1979
128. Vidal E, Brocq L: Étude sur le mycosis fungoide. La France Medical 2:946, 957, 969, 983, 993, 1005, 1019, 1775
129. Vonderheid EC, Sobel EL, Nowell PC, et al: Diagnostic and prognostic significance of Sézary cells in peripheral blood smears from patients with cutaneous T-cell lymphoma. Blood 66:358, 1985
130. Vonderheid EC, Tam DW, Johnson WC, et al: Prognostic significance of cytomorphology in cutaneous T-cell lymphomas. Cancer 47:119, 1981
131. Vonderheid EC, Van Scott EJ, Wallner PE, et al: A 10-year experience with topical mechlorethamine for mycosis fungoides: Comparison with patients treated by total-skin electron beam radiation therapy. Cancer Treat Rep 63:681, 1979
132. Vonderheid EC, Tan ET, Kantor AF, et al: Long-term efficacy, curative potential, and carcinogenicity of topical mechlorethamine chemotherapy in cutaneous T-cell lymphoma. J Am Acad Dermatol 20:416, 1989
133. Wallner PE, Vonderheid EC, Brady LW, et al: Evaluation and recommendations for therapy of advanced mycosis fungoides lymphoma. Int J Radiat Oncol Biol Phys 5:23, 1979
134. Weinstock MA, Horm JW: Mycosis fungoides in the United States. JAMA 260:42, 1988
135. Weiss LM, Hu E, Wood GS, et al: Clonal rearrangements of T-cell receptor genes in mycosis fungoides and dermatopathic lymphadenopathy. N Engl J Med 313:539, 1985
136. Whang-Peng J, Bunn PA Jr, Knutsen T, et al: Clinical implications of cytogenitic studies in cutaneous T-cell lymphoma (CTCL). Cancer 50:1539, 1982

137. Willemze R, De Graaff-Reitsma CB, Cnossen J, et al: Characterization of T-cell subpopulations in skin and peripheral blood of patients with cutaneous T-cell lymphomas and benign inflammatory dermatoses. J Invest Dermatol 80:60, 1983
138. Williams PC, Hunter RD, Jackson SM: Whole body electron therapy in mycosis fungoides: A successful translational technique achieved by modification of an established linear accelerator. Br J Radiol 52:302, 1979
139. Winkelmann RK, Diaz-Perez JL, Buechner SA: The treatment of Sézary syndrome. J Am Acad Dermatol 10:1000, 1984
140. Winkler CF, Bunn PA Jr: Cutaneous T-cell lymphoma: A review. CRC Crit Rev Oncol Hematol 1:49, 1983
141. Wiskemann A, Buck C: Radiotherapy of mycosis fungoides: Twenty years of experience with teleroentgen and low voltage x-ray therapy. J Dermatol Surg Oncol 4:606, 1978
142. Wood GS, Deneau DG, Miller RA, et al: Subtypes of cutaneous T-cell lymphoma defined by expression of Leu-1 and la. Blood 59:876, 1982
143. Wright JC, Gumport SL, Golomb FM: Remissions produced with the use of methotrexate in patients with mycosis fungoides. Cancer Chemother Rep 9:11, 1960
144. Wright JC, Lyons MM, Walker DG, et al: Observations on the use of cancer chemotherapeutic agents in patients with mycosis fungoides. Cancer 17:1045, 1964
145. Yagoda A, Mukherji B, Young C, et al: Bleomycin: An antitumor antibiotic. Ann Intern Med 77:861, 1972
146. Zachariae H, Grunnet E, Thestrup-Pederson K, et al: Oral retinoid in combination with bleomycin, cyclophosphamide, prednisone, and transfer factor in mycosis fungoides. Acta Derm Venereol (Stockh) 62:162, 1982

23

○ ○ ○ • • •

Brain

Ulf L. Karlsson
Steven A. Leibel
Kent Wallner
Lawrence W. Davis
Luther W. Brady

With a special section on
STEREOTACTIC EXTERNAL BEAM IRRADIATION

David A. Larson, Todd H. Wasserman,
Robert E. Drzymala, Joseph R. Simpson

Over the last 30 years, radiation therapy for neoplasms in the central nervous system (CNS) has attained a respected role,[157] providing the opportunity for prolonged survival, regression of neurologic deficits, and improved quality of life. Lindgren[145] reviewed the earlier literature on primary malignant lesions, which are discussed in this chapter, and secondary malignant and some histologically benign lesions. Much clinical information in this chapter is summarized within five tables (Tables 23-1, 23-2, 23-4 to 23-6). All five tables present a similar organization of lesions that provides a concise reference structure for data often used in the field. The chapter is composed of a general part followed by sections analyzing each of several common tumor types. Immediately following is a special section on the new stereotactic external-beam irradiation technique.

CLASSIFICATION OF INTRACRANIAL TUMORS

Primary intracranial tumors arise from the brain, cranial nerves, meninges, pituitary, and vessels. They derive from ectoderm (brain) and mesoderm (vessels, meninges, blood components). Malignant lesions of the eye bulb (retinoblastoma, melanoma, astrocytoma) and pituitary and children's tumors are described elsewhere (see Chaps. 24, 26, and 69). Optic nerve glioma is included in the primary group because the optic nerve is an outgrowth of the central nervous system. Lymphoma is included as a primary tumor. Medulloblastoma and craniopharyngioma are included because they also occur in adult patients.

The nomenclature of brain tumors has changed over time. Table 23-1 includes commonly used synonyms for most of the tumor types listed. The term *glioma*[8] is not used by some (except optic nerve glioma) because it is too broad. Also, the Kernohan grade classification of astrocytomas is controversial because it does not readily serve a prognostic purpose.

Overall frequencies of brain tumors and possible benefits from radiation therapy are listed in Table 23-2. Astrocytomas are predominant; pituitary tumors (see Chap. 24) and meningiomas are relatively common. Other listed primary tumors are less common. Rare tumors requiring radiation therapy are listed in a separate section.

ANATOMIC AND FUNCTIONAL CONSIDERATIONS

The brain is situated in the cranial cavity, with the cerebellum and brain stem occupying the posterior fossa (Fig. 3-1). Apart from the bony calvaria for the brain and the spinal column for the spinal cord, the central nervous system is enveloped by meninges. The dura mater covers the outside. The soft pia mater is innermost and folds into the sulci, indentations, and irregularities of the CNS surface. Between them is the arachnoid mater, which is separated from the pia mater by the subarachnoid space filled with cerebrospinal fluid.

The developing central nervous system folds into a groove on the dorsal aspect of the embryonal ectoderm. With midline fusion the cranial and caudal tube openings (neural pores) grow superiorly and inferiorly with the embryo and close.[134] The cells lining the neural tube are therefore derived from ectoderm, as are most primary brain tumors. Astrocytes differentiate around the neurons, ingrown vessels, and pathways, and on the surface abutting the pia mater. The glial cells outnumber the neurons by a factor of 10 and are assumed to form a structural, func-

TABLE 23–1
Symptoms, Signs, and Diagnostic Characteristics of Various Intracranial Tumors

TUMOR	COMMON SYMPTOMS	COMMON SIGNS	DIAGNOSTIC CHARACTERISTICS*
PRIMARY			
Malignant astrocytoma	Headache, seizure, unilateral weakness, mental changes	Focal presentation related to tumor location	Enhancing CT lesion, tumor blush on angiography
Glioblastoma multiforme (GM)			Hypodense interior of enhanced CT lesion
Astrocytoma with anaplastic foci (AAF)			No hypodense interior portion of enhanced CT lesion
Brain stem or thalamus	Nausea, vomiting, ataxia	Increased intracranial pressure (papilledema), abducens and oculomotor nerve defects	May not enhance on CT scan; biopsy may not be appropriate
Meningioma (B, M)	Localized headache, seizure	Focal presentation related to tumor location	Enhancing CT lesion associated with dura
Astrocytoma (B, M)	Headache, seizure, unilateral weakness, mental changes	Focal presentation related to tumor location	May not enhance on CT
Cerebral	Headache, seizure, unilateral weakness, mental changes	Focal presentation related to tumor location	
Cerebellar	Occipital headache	Increased intracranial pressure (papilledema), abducens and oculomotor nerve defects; coordination	
Brain stem or thalamus	Nausea, vomiting, ataxia	Increased intracranial pressure (papilledema), abducens and oculomotor nerve defects; coordination	May be seen only on MR imaging; biopsy may not be appropriate
Optic nerve	Ocular changes	Ocular changes	Detailed CT scan
Pituitary (B, M)	Vertex headache, ocular changes	Ocular, endocrine abnormalities	Hormone analysis; resection gives histopathology
Medulloblastoma (M)	Morning headaches, nausea, vomiting	Coordination, increased intracranial pressure (papilledema), abducens and oculomotor nerve defects	CT scan, careful lumbar puncture recommended
Ependymoma (B, M)	Morning headaches, nausea, vomiting	Coordination, increased intracranial pressure (papilledema), abducens and oculomotor nerve defects	CT scan, careful lumbar puncture recommended
Hemangioma, arteriovenous malformation (B, M)	"Migrainous" headache	Focal presentation related to tumor location	Angiography; biopsy may not be appropriate
Neurilemoma, schwannoma, neurinoma (B, M)	Unilateral deafness, vertigo	Ipsilateral acoustic and facial or trigeminal nerve defects	CT scan; resection gives histopathology
Oligodendroglioma (B, M)	Insidious headache, mental changes	Focal presentation related to tumor location	Radiographic calcification
Sarcoma (M), neurofibroma (B)	Focal presentation related to tumor location	Focal presentation related to tumor location	
Pinealoma (B, M), dysgerminoma	Various (ocular, vestibular, endocrine)	Parinaud's syndrome, endocrine changes, ocular changes. Increased intracranial pressure (papilledema), abducens and oculomotor nerve defects	Biopsy or resection may not be obtained; markers in CSF may be informative
Lymphoma (M), reticulum cell sarcoma, microglioma	Focal presentation related to tumor location	Focal presentation related to tumor location	"Soft" CT enhancement
Unspecified (B, M)	Focal presentation related to tumor location	Focal presentation related to tumor location	
OTHER			
Craniopharyngioma	Headache, mental changes, hemiplegia, seizure, vomiting (and ocular changes)	Cranial nerve defects (II–VII)	Bone erosion, mass effect from base of skull
Syringomyelia, syringobulbia	Pain, weakness	Sensory level, paresis	MR imaging, CT scan; myelogram; biopsy not appropriate
Midline granuloma syndrome, lymphoid granulomatosis	Various (ocular, vestibular, endocrine)	Various (ocular, vestibular, endocrine)	Diagnosis presumed
Arachnoiditis		Fasciculations	

** Unless noted, biopsy is assumed.*
B: benign; M: malignant; CT: Computed tomography; MR: Magnetic resonance.

TABLE 23–2
Intracranial Tumors: Approximate Frequency, Metastatic Potential, Age Relation, and Potential Benefit from Radiation Therapy, in Order of Decreasing Frequency

TUMOR	INCIDENCE			METASTATIC POTENTIAL (%)	POTENTIAL BENEFIT FROM RADIATION THERAPY
	OVERALL	ADULT	CHILD		
PRIMARY					
Overall	<20*	<95	>5	Few	Majority
Malignant astrocytoma	40	35 ± 15	20 ± 10	<10†	Majority
Brain stem and thalamus	Few	<1	<5	NA	All
Glioblastoma multiforme	30	30±10	<20	<12	Majority
Astrocytoma with anaplastic foci	<10	<10	<1	<6	Majority
Meningioma (B, M)	15–20	>15	<5	Rare (M)	Unresectable, M
Astrocytoma (B, M)	15–20	15 ± 10	30–50	Rare (M)	Majority
Cerebral			Most		
Cerebellar			Most		Unresectable, M
Brain stem		<1	>5		
Pituitary (B, M)	<10	10	<1	Rare	Unresectable
Medulloblastoma (M)	4–8	<1	25	≥10†	Majority
Ependymoma (B, M)	1–8	<5	10 ± 5	<10 (M)†	Majority
Hemangioma, arteriovenous malformation (B, M)	3	3	3	Rare	Unresectable
Neurilemoma, schwannoma, neurinoma (B, M)	6	6–10	<1	Rare	Unresectable, M
Oligodendroglioma (B, M)	<2	1–5	<1	Rare	Majority
Sarcoma (M), neurofibroma (B)	<2	2	2	Some	Unresectable, M
Optic nerve glioma	1	Rare	<5	Rare	Unresectable
Pinealoma (B, M), dysgerminoma	1	<1	>2	All M	All
Lymphoma (M), reticulum cell sarcoma, microglioma	~1	<1	—	All	All
Unspecified (B, M)	3	3	<10	NA	Unresectable, M
OTHER					
Overall	<1	<1	—	NA	Unresectable progressive
Craniopharyngioma	Few	—	—	NA	All
Syringomyelia, syringobulbia	—	—	—	NA	Unresectable progressive
Midline granuloma syndrome, lymphoid granulomatosis	—	—	—	NA	Unresectable progressive
Arachnoiditis	—	—	—	NA	Unresectable progressive

* *Of primary and metastatic. All other figures refer to primary only.*
† *Rare outside the central nervous system.*
B: histologically benign; M: malignant; NA: not applicable.
All are primary neoplasms unless otherwise noted.

tional, metabolic, and protective framework for the functioning neuron circuits.[85, 185]

Intracranial Nervous System: Oncologically Relevant Facts

The brain dimensions are about 16 cm anteroposteriorly, 14 cm transversely, and 12 cm superoinferiorly. Brain volume is approximately 1300 cm^3, its surface area is approximately 2000 cm^2, and it weighs approximately 1300 g (range 800 g to 2000 g). The average thickness of the cerebral cortex is 2.5 mm.[205] The central nervous system is composed of 40% gray matter and 60% white matter.

The gray matter is composed of nondividing neurons (after a few years of life), astrocytes (which surround and support the neuronal functions), and relatively few oligodendroglia (in the form of myelin for entering and exiting neuronal axons). The white matter is almost exclusively composed of nerve fibers with axons, oligodendroglia, and supporting astrocytes. Both astrocytes and oligodendroglia are dividing cell populations, presumably dividing at a moderate rate compared with other cell populations in the body.[213]

The major parts of intracranial central nervous system anatomy are depicted in Figures 23-1 through 23-5. The tentorium, consisting of dense fibrous tissue, separates the supratentorial and infratentorial compartments. The notch of the "tent" is located approximately at the horizontal level of the pineal body. Anteriorly, the "slit" slopes anteriorly down to the petrosal ridges bilaterally. Posteriorly, the median part of the tentorium slopes inferiorly to the posteriorly located internal occipital tuberosity. Laterally from the median, the tent also slopes inferiorly down to the transverse sinus on both sides.

In the supratentorial cerebrum both primary motor and

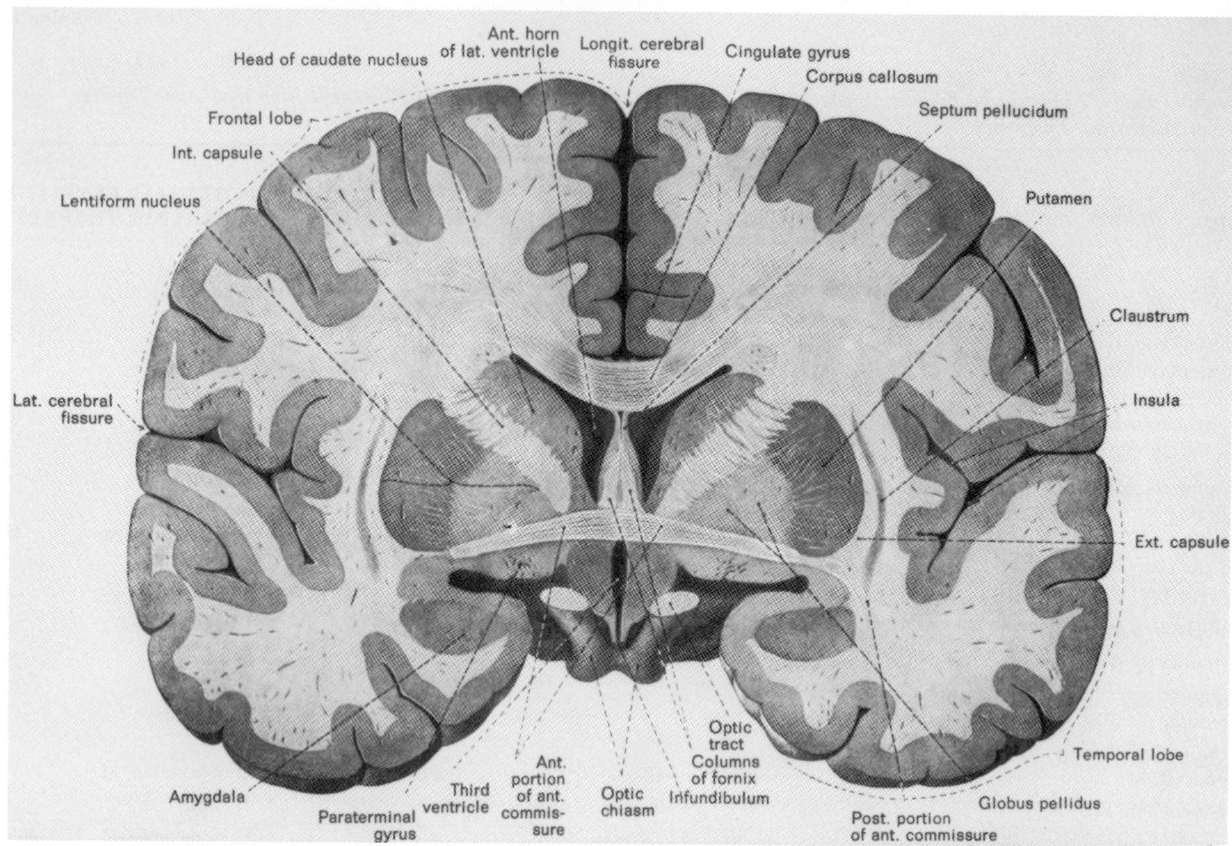

FIGURE 23–1. Frontal section through the telencephalon at the plane of the anterior commissure. (Sobotta/Figge Atlas of Human Anatomy, vol 2, ed 9. Munich, Urban & Schwartzenberg, 1977)

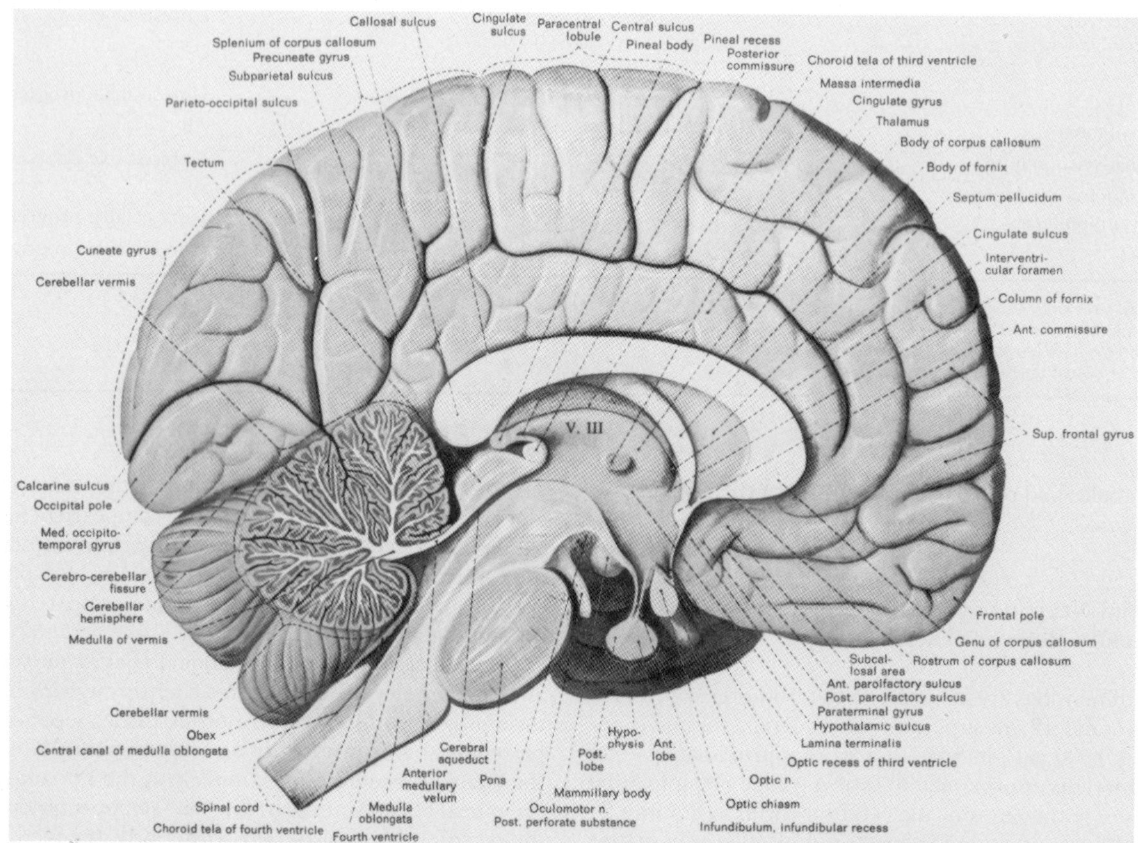

FIGURE 23–2. The supratentorial parts of the central nervous system (CNS) include the telencephalon (cerebral hemispheres with frontal, parietal, occipital, and temporal lobes) and the diencephalon, with the dominant thalamus nucleus, the hypothalamus, the pituitary stalk, and the neurohypophysis infero-anteriorly and the pineal body posteriorly, which represents the midline central structures of the supratentorial CNS. (Sobotta/Figge Atlas of Human Anatomy, vol 2, 9th ed. Munich, Urban & Schwartzenberg, 1977)

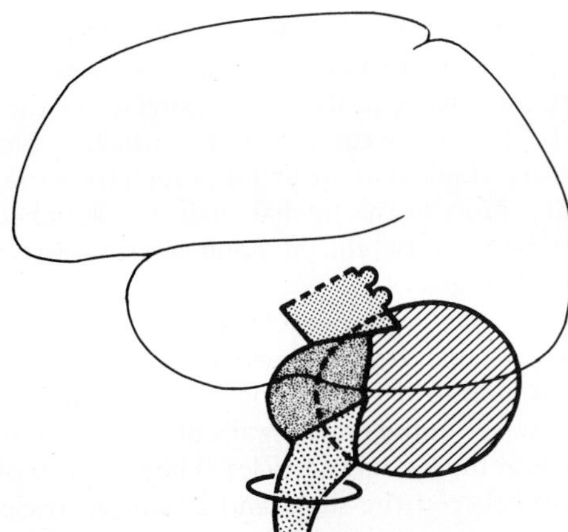

FIGURE 23–3. The mesencephalon (*medium stipple*) connects the brain stem with the diencephalon above the tentorium. Below the mesencephalon are the pons (*fine stipple*) and the medulla oblongata (*coarse stipple*). Posteriorly the cerebellum (*striped area*) is attached to posterior parts of the pons and the medulla oblongata. The functional medulla oblongata continues below the foramen magnum into the spinal canal; its anatomic border is at the level of the foramen.

sensory areas at the central sulcus control the body from the knees to the feet in the medial cortex and the trunk, arms, and head laterally (the representation is called *homunculus*). The motor-speech area of Broca is located in the dominant frontal lobe just above the lateral sulcus. Damage to this area causes expressive aphasia. Sensory aphasia (Wernicke's) results from damage to the dominant temporal lobe at the posterior end of the lateral sulcus. The anterior part of the temporal lobe is partially associated with short-term memory. Most of the primary visual cortex is represented on the medial and inferior surface at the occipital pole.

The central nervous system exits and the functions of the cranial nerves are illustrated in Figure 23-6 and tabulated in Table 23-3, together with their entry ports into the bony cranium.

The diencephalon consists of the thalamus (the major sensory synaptic station for all stimuli in ascending spinocortical and cranial nerve pathways), the hypothalamus (a major center for endocrine and autonomic functions), the subthalamus (primarily a path from the diencephalon to the brain stem), and the pineal region (oncologically important but with obscure function).

At the tentorial notch the mesencephalon rides on the upper part of the clivus. Its interior, the tectum, is partially occupied by cranial nerve nuclei (for the oculomotor, trochlear, and proprioceptive portion of trigeminal nerves). The oculomotor and trochlear nerves are sensitive to increased intracranial pressure. The dorsal plate houses the superior and inferior colliculi, which regulate eye movements and hearing impulses, respectively. The trochlear nerve is the only cranial nerve that exits from this dorsal location.

The pons relays information between the two cerebellar hemispheres, carries the major pathways from the mesencephalon down to the medulla oblongata, and houses the major motor and tactile sensory nuclei for the trigeminal nerve, which emerges from its lateral surface.

The border between the pons and the medulla oblongata is noteworthy for the emergence of abducens, facial, and vestibulocochlear (acoustic) cranial nerves. The nuclei for these nerves are more or less shared between these two brain parts.

The cerebellum develops laterally and posteriorly from the pons region and differentiates into the median vermis cerebelli (from which medulloblastomas are believed to originate) and the bilateral hemispheres. The vermis cerebelli is the most medial part of the cerebellum, with both lateral hemispheres

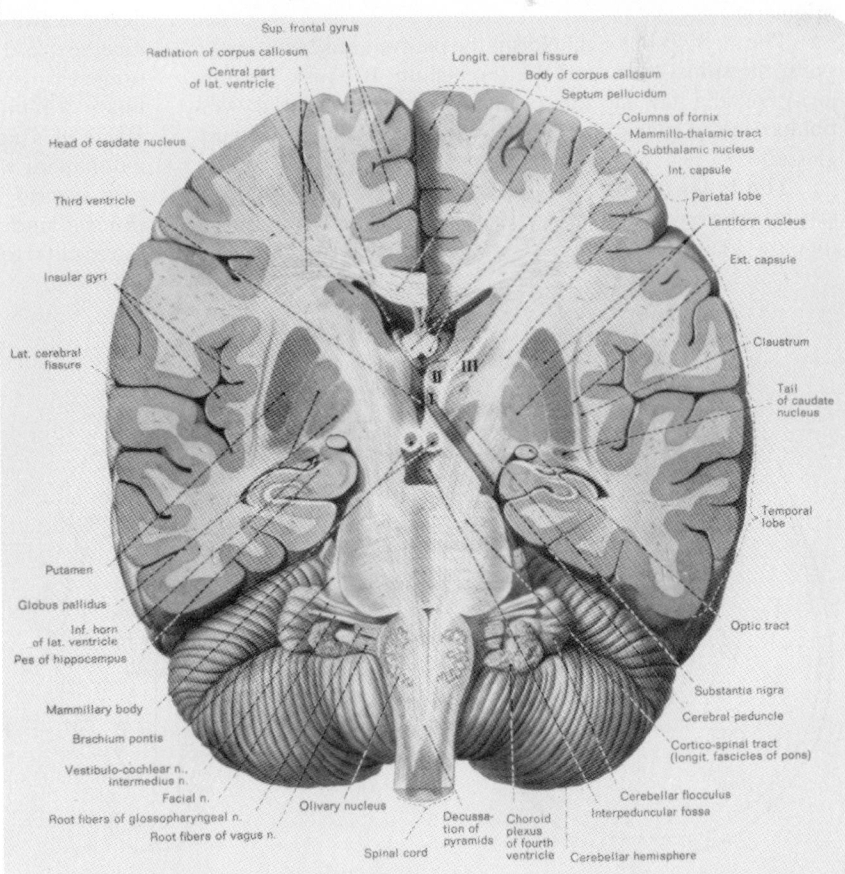

FIGURE 23–4. Section through telencephalon and brain stem parallel with the cerebral peduncles. View of the posterior surface of the plane of sectioning. On right side of figure the section reaches back to about the middle of the cerebral peduncle (*oblique section*). I to III indicate thalamic nuclei. I, medial nucleus; II, anterior nucleus; III, lateral nucleus. (Sobotta/Figge Atlas of Human Anatomy, vol 2, 9th ed. Munich, Urban & Schwartzenberg, 1977)

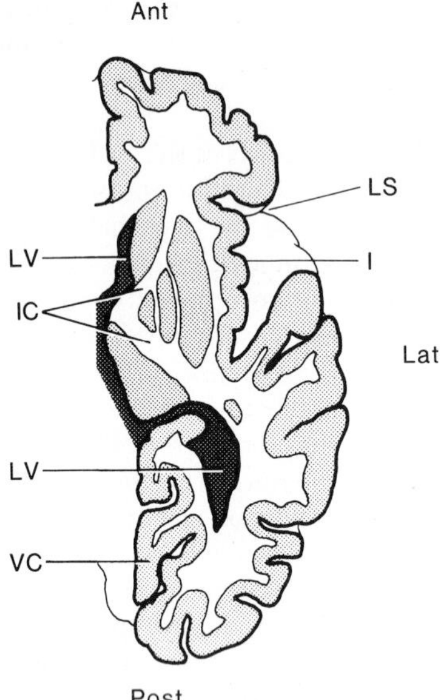

FIGURE 23–5. This section displays the structures from the depth of the insula in the lateral sulcus (LS) to the midline. Parts of the lateral ventricles (LV), the corpus anteriorly and the posterior horn posteriorly, and the primary visual cortex (VC) can be seen at the midline. Laterally from the head of the caudate nucleus anteriorly (lateral to anterior LV), the thalamus (posterior to IC lines), and the cauda just lateral to the posterior horn of the LV are the clinically important internal capsule (IC), putamen, and globus pallidus (lateral to IC), which make up most of the bulge of the insula (I).

being flattened by the sloping tentorium on both sides. Anteriorly, the cerebellum faces the dorsal aspects of the pons and the medulla oblongata (in the form of the floor of the fourth ventricle from which many ependymomas are believed to originate).

The medulla oblongata forms the pathway link between the pons, the spinal cord, and the cerebellum. It houses the majority of the cranial nerve nuclei (abducens, facial, vestibulocochlear, glossopharyngeal, vagal, accessory, and hypoglossal).

The brain receives its arterial supply from the internal carotid arteries (supratentorial parts) and the vertebral vessels (mainly the infratentorial parts). Midline crossover communicating vessels (circle of Willis) allow for bilaterally uninterrupted oxygen supply in case of local vascular obstruction.

The arterial supply to the convex surface of the brain is dominated by the middle cerebral artery, which emerges anteriorly in the lateral sulcus as the major branch from the internal carotid artery. Most of the medial surface is supplied by the anterior cerebral artery; the occipital lobe is served by the posterior cerebral artery.

The ventricular system develops by ballooning from the primitive neural canal. It is lined with ependyma and produces cerebrospinal fluid (CSF) in the roofs of the fourth and third ventricles as well as in the medial walls of the central body and inferior horns of the lateral ventricles. The foramina of Monro transmit CSF between the third and lateral ventricles at the superolateral corners of the third ventricle. The aqueduct of Sylvius in the midbrain is the narrowest canal of the intracranial nervous system and is therefore the most common location of obstruction of flow by compression, which causes noncommunicating hydrocephalus and headache.

Cerebrospinal fluid escapes the ventricular system through the median foramen of Magendie and the two lateral foramina of Luschka to the subarachnoid space. All three foramina are located in the roof and lateral corners of the fourth ventricle at the level of the medulla oblongata. The subarachnoid space widens into several cisterns, the largest of which are cisterna magna (posterior to the medulla oblongata just at the foramen magnum), the cistern of the lateral sulcus bilaterally at the base of the brain, and the ambient cistern posterior to the midbrain.

EPIDEMIOLOGY

About 15,000 new cases of primary brain tumors are diagnosed in the United States each year.[6] Brain tumors account for about 1.5% of all malignancies in the United States. The overall incidence is five in 100,000 of the population[300] and varies with race, sex, and age. In the United States, the incidence of brain tumors is considerably higher for whites than for blacks (5.6 *versus* 3.4 in 100,000).[248] The incidence for males (6.3 in 100,000) is higher than that for females (4.4 in 100,000). Age is a dominant variable; the incidence is above 20 in 100,000 for men around 70 years of age and less than two in 100,000 for children under 15 years of age. Most cases are found in the age range of 50 to 80 years. A small but significant peak occurs at 5

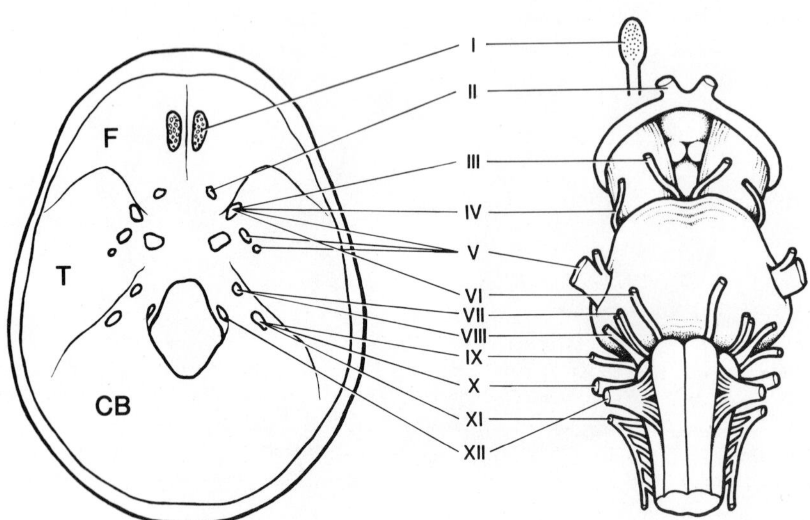

FIGURE 23–6. Schematic representation of the locations of the cranial nerve exits (*right*) from the anterior CNS to the subarachnoid space and their entries into the skull (*left*) at different locations relative to cranial fossae (*F,* anterior; *T,* middle; *CB,* posterior). See Table 23-3 for names.

TABLE 23–3
Cranial Nerve Topography and Functions

NUMBER	NAME	EXIT FROM CNS	ENTRY IN SKULL	MAIN FUNCTION	ACCESSORY FUNCTIONS
I	Olfactory	Olfactory bulb	Cribriform plate	Smell	
II	Optic	Optic disk	Optic canal	Vision	
III	Oculomotor	Interpeduncular fossa	Superior orbital fissure	Motor to most orbital muscles, including superior levator palpebrae	Autonomic to the pupillary sphincter
IV	Trochlear	Inferior colliculus	Superior orbital fissure	Motor to oblique superior muscle	
V	Trigeminal	Pons	Ophthalmic nerve, superior orbital fissure; maxillary nerve, foramen rotundum; mandibular nerve, foramen ovale	Sensory to most skin, mucous membranes on and in the head	Motor to masticatory muscles
VI	Abducens	Medially between pons and medulla oblongata	Superior orbital fissure	Motor to lateral rectus muscle	
VII	Facial	Intermediary between pons and medulla oblongata	Internal acoustic meatus	Motor to all facial muscles	Secretory to lacrimal, submandibular, nasal, oral, and sublingual glands; taste to anterior two-thirds of tongue; motor to stapedius muscle
VIII	Acoustic	Laterally between pons and medulla oblongata	Internal acoustic meatus	Hearing through cochlear nerve Posture through vestibular nerve	
IX	Glossopharyngeal	Superiorly behind olive	Jugular foramen	Motor to stylopharyngeus muscle only	Taste to posterior one-third of the tongue; secretory to parotid gland
X	Vagus	Intermediary behind olive	Jugular foramen	Autonomic to most thoracic and abdominal viscera	Motor to pharyngeal, laryngeal, and esophageal muscles; sensory to external auditory meatus
XI	Accessory	Inferiorly behind olive	Jugular foramen	Motor to upper parts of trapezius and sternocleidomastoid muscles	
XII	Hypoglossal	Anterior to olive	Hypoglossal canal	Motor to tongue	

to 10 years, when the rate reaches about two in 100,000.[248] Incidence of brain tumors also varies with geography.[60]

In absolute numbers, brain tumors rank among the five leading causes of death in children and young adults. In relative terms, these tumors are a leading cause of death because of the patient's poor prognosis after diagnosis.[248] Five to ten percent of all brain tumors occur in children under 15 years of age. About 20% of all pediatric malignancies are brain tumors. An estimated 50% of affected children with brain tumors reach tertiary or university hospitals.[70]

Table 23-2 shows the incidence of various tumor types according to age. Posterior fossa tumors (cerebellar and brain stem astrocytomas, medulloblastomas, and ependymomas) and those in juxtaposition to but not in the sellar location (optic gliomas, craniopharyngiomas, and choroid plexus papillomas) predominate among children and young adults. Most other tumors occur predominantly in those 20 years of age and older. Occurrence of ependymoma ranges from childhood up to the age of 50 years. There is preponderance among males for most tumor types except neurinomas, for which the ratio approximates 2 to 1 in favor of females. Meningiomas are almost equally distributed between the sexes.[164]

ETIOLOGY

Epidemiologic and animal research studies have implicated genetic factors (tuberous sclerosis, von Recklinghausen's, and von Hippel-Lindau diseases,[234] environmental factors (aromatic hydrocarbons,[125] occupational exposure),[235] viruses,[16,76] and postnatal irradiation[171] as plausible causes of CNS tumors.

Irradiation is reputed to be potentially carcinogenic.[143] A search of the literature from 1978 to 1984 unearthed fewer than 30 published articles that reported cerebral malignancies in patients with previous radiation therapy to the head. In all, about 100 tumor cases were found (70% meningiomas, 15% astrocytomas, 6% sarcomas, and 9% miscellaneous). Sixteen cases reported in recent literature were calculated to a latency range of 14 ± 9 years. An incidence of about 1% was found in analyses by Spallone,[254] Danoff,[57] and Potish and co-workers.[199]

Cahan's criteria[40] must be applied for credibility (*i.e.*, a new tumor in a previously normal tumor site, a tumor site with prior irradiation, a dose range of 2000 cGy to 10,000 cGy, and appropriate latency [several years]). The oncogene theory is still unvalidated in terms of intracranial tumors.[132]

NATURAL HISTORY

Primary intrabrain neoplasms generally spread invasively without formation of a natural capsule to impede tumor growth. First presentation of symptoms depends mainly on available expansion volume for the tumor and edema in different locations.

Intracranial primary neoplasms are unique because they do not metastasize through a lymphatic drainage system. Extracranial true metastases from primary brain tumors through vascular channels are rare but can occur with high-grade medulloblastomas, dysgerminomas, sarcomas, and astrocytomas. These hematogenous metastases often appear in the lung. Medulloblastomas have an affinity for bone and lymph nodes.

The high-grade neoplasms in brain and meninges can metastasize by "seeding" into the subarachnoid and ventricular spaces and, by gravity or flow, cause metastatic deposits in the spinal canal. Because of this tendency, some tumor treatment regimens require coverage of the spinal axis as well as of the entire cranial contents. Causes for metastatic seeding are lack of intercellular cohesiveness (a condition for other poorly differentiated neoplasms) and proximity to CSF channels (meningeal, intraventricular, or subependymal growth).

Intracranial tumors exert their effects in different fashions. For example, a cerebellopontine-angle neurinoma causes pressure degeneration in both nervous structures and bone tissue in the vicinity. Conversely, a low-grade astrocytoma may infiltrate extensively in the white matter and thus destroy the functional pathways by crowding or metabolic effects.[38]

The question of multiplicity of primary brain tumors in patients is pertinent to the radiation therapy approach. Early literature (through 1967) indicates an average incidence of about 10% for astrocytomas.[299] This figure is comparable to that found in recent literature.[33,104] In von Recklinghausen's and von Hippel-Lindau diseases, multiple neoplasms are more common.

Astrocytomas arise in the white matter, preferentially in one hemisphere. A few display bilateral presentation through the corpus callosum ("butterfly astrocytoma") or the thalamus. Local spread usually occurs in the white matter in a sagittal direction, following vessels and nerve pathways. Oligodendrogliomas follow the same pattern.

Meningiomas commonly are locally malignant (by mechanical pressure), but invasion of bone is not uncommon. A minority, usually the histopathologically malignant varieties, may spread through CSF channels, and even fewer may spread to sites outside the bony confines of the central nervous system, especially to lung. Incompletely resected meningiomas recur.[169]

Medulloblastomas, ependymomas, and dysgerminomas are essentially midline tumors that spread infiltratively and may show metastatic seeding in the CSF space. Neurinomas exert pressure mainly on nerves, bone, and brain stem.

Brain tumors exhibit variable growth kinetics with small growth fractions.[109] Clinical tumor volume doubling time for malignant astrocytomas has been estimated to be as short as 20 days.[297] Hypoxic cell populations are presumed to be present in at least the more malignant tumor types.[37,66]

Edema and Tumor Type

Edema may be vasogenic, ischemic, or cytotoxic.[79,111,124] It is commonly seen in computed tomography (CT) scans of brain tumor patients and is believed to cause at least part of the clinical symptoms and signs. The edema is considered to be a consequence of altered blood-brain barrier permeability,[12] and vasogenic edema is considered to be a major component. Different tumors cause varying amounts of edema. In descending order, these tumors are metastases, astrocytomas, meningiomas, and oligodendrogliomas. Tumor infiltration does not appear to be directly related to the amount of edema.[36]

CLINICAL PRESENTATION

Commonly encountered symptoms and signs of different tumor types are listed in Table 23-1. The most common initial symptoms are headache, seizure, mental change, and sensorimotor defects, any of which can eventually be found in more than 50% of the patient population.[164] Increased intracranial pressure is a sign that may be related to many of these symptoms.[126]

Focal signs related to tumor localization encompass unilateral signs (which usually derive from contralateral lesions except for nuclear-type cranial nerve lesions, in which the midline crossing of nerve pathways has already occurred) and lobar signs (aphasia, agnosia, cortical apraxia, hemiplegia, or paresis from parietal tumors; short-term memory loss and psychic seizures with aura and hallucinations from temporal tumors; anosmia, personality changes, and olfactory hallucinations from frontal tumors; and contralateral homonymous visual field defects and alexia from occipital tumors).

Headache location may at times give information about the location of the tumor.

Seizures indicate irritation of the central nervous tissue, believed to result from transient local changes followed by spreading discharge patterns in the gray matter. Grand mal and focal siezures are the most common types encountered with tumor patients. They are less common with tumors affecting white matter (small astrocytomas and oligodendrogliomas).

Mental changes are most common in patients with frontal and temporal lobe tumors, either primary or metastic in origin.

Hemiparesis indicates side and to some degree site of lesion; it may be caused by brain edema.

Dysphasia may be expressive (Broca's type, in which the patient understands and knows but cannot express), sensory (Wernicke's type, in which the patient does not understand and therefore communicates nonsensically), or mixed. The expressive type indicates that the tumor is located in the lateroposterior portion of the frontal lobe (opercular area) on the dominant side or is compromising pathways to this area in deeper regions. The sensory type of aphasia indicates that the lesion is in the region of the end of the lateral sulcus, also in the dominant hemisphere.

Ocular symptoms include diffuse or focal decrease in visual acuity, ophthalmic defects, oculomotor defects, paresis or paralysis, and proptosis.

Sensory loss usually signifies parietal lobe tumor or, more

infrequently, thalamic or brain stem compromise of synapse stations or spinothalamic pathways, respectively.

Increased intracranial pressure is usually caused by obstruction of CSF flow and results in headaches, papilledema, mental changes, lethargy, and difficulty of locomotion. Nausea and vomiting are often associated with midline and posterior fossa tumors. The latter may also cause ataxia and vertigo. Hydrocephalus (seen on CT) is often the result of tumor interference with CSF flow and production. Endocrine defects (*e.g.*, acromegaly) and hormonal changes (*e.g.*, elevations in growth hormone, adrenocorticotropic hormone, thyroid-stimulating hormone, luteinizing hormone, follicle stimulating hormone, melanocyte-stimulating hormone, and prolactin) lead the diagnosis toward pituitary tumors.

DIAGNOSTIC WORKUP

History and Physical Examination

The basic initial workup of patients with brain tumors must include a complete history and general physical examination. Data obtained from relatives and friends are often more helpful than those given by the patient because many tumors cause mental changes that are not appreciated or perceived correctly by the patient. Previous medical, social, and family histories are important. Inherited diseases associated with brain tumors, exposure to chemicals, and history of infections may be indicators of etiology.

The neurologic examination includes assessment of mental condition (behavior, mood, sensorium, intelligence, thought content, language, insight into own disease), coordination (walking, balance, alternating movement), sensation (pain, touch, vibration, position sense, stereognosis, point discrimination), reflexes (deep, superficial, clonus), motor (strength, tonus, resistance to passive movement), and cranial nerves. Another routine test is ophthalmoscopy to check for papilledema as a sign of increased intracranial pressure.

Laboratory Tests

The present "gold standards" in laboratory diagnosis of brain tumors are evaluations of the CSF and the histopathology of the tumor. The best method of obtaining the histologic specimen is by stereotactic biopsy,[24,27,142] which allows the pathologist to correlate the histopathologic findings with the CT scan details. Metabolic profiles (liver enzyme, uric acid, and electrolyte levels; kidney function tests) are important because most brain tumors are metastic from other primary sites (*e.g.*, liver, kidney, lung, breast).

Radiographic Findings

Skull radiographs may show calcifications of tumors (*e.g.*, meningioma, craniopharyngioma, oligodendroglioma), deviation of a calcified pineal body, or erosion of the posterior clinoid process because of chronically increased intracranial pressure, which may also cause a "hammered" effect in the inner table of the skull.

The computed tomography scan enables anatomic description of areas that have lower (necrosis, edema) or higher (calcification, accumulation of contrast) x-ray scattering power than the normal brain. Contrast-enhanced CT scan of the brain not only offers the opportunity to localize a tumor but also provides information about tumor extension (at least as far as blood-brain barrier disruption is concerned), tumor grade (combinations of hypodense areas with enhancing periphery indicate a fast-growing tumor), and mode of growth (seeding, multicentricity, bilaterality).[92] Although a central hypodense area of enhancement in a CT scan often denotes necrosis, this interpretation may not be assured.

Tumor is usually associated with a contrast-enhanced volume; malignant astrocytomas also have a tendency to infiltrate irregularly a few centimeters beyond the border of enhancement[36] or even farther (Fig. 23-7).[118]

Magnetic resonance imaging (MRI) reveals changes in the

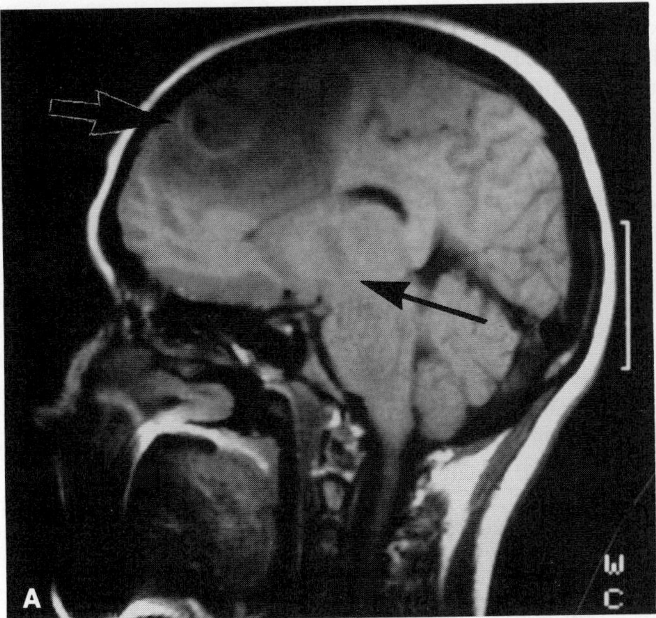

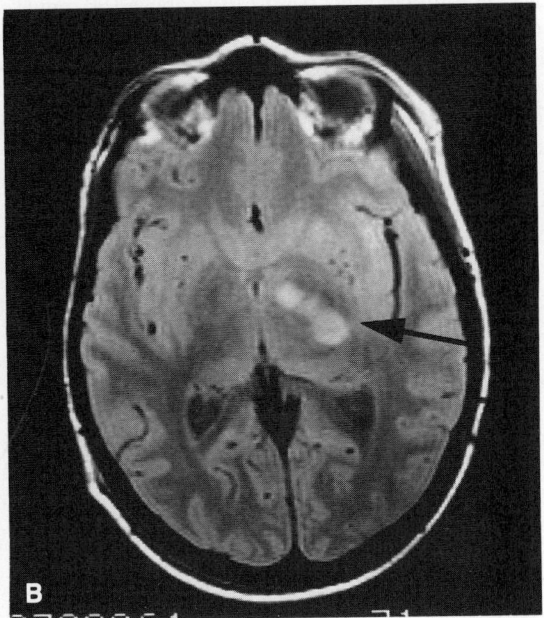

FIGURE 23–7. (**A**) Sagittal MRI of the head demonstrating a large frontal astrocytoma, grade 3 (*large arrow*) with extensive surrounding edema. A second smaller lesion is noted in the thalamus (*small arrow*). (**B**) Axial MRI of the head outlining the tumor in the left thalamic area.

brain parenchyma with great detail[261] and provides good resolution of normal anatomic structures. The physical basis for the MRI technique is the capability of electromagnetic forces to align atomic spins.

Cerebral angiography gives typical vascular anatomy patterns for some tumors (*e.g.*, arteriovenous malformation or glioblastoma tumor blush). Myelography and MRI are useful for the demonstration of seeded brain tumors.[65] Nuclear scanning of the brain after ^{99m}Tc injection is now used for lesions causing a compromised blood-brain barrier or for vascular lesions or for the purpose of obtaining blood flow data.

Ancillary Studies

Positron emission tomography (PET) may be helpful in determining tissue viability. This technique may therefore enable the differentiation of area of high metabolism (malignancy growth) from brain necrosis.[191] For example, a fluorinated glucose is injected and the localized emission of the radionuclide ^{18}F is detected. It has been suggested that ^{11}C-methionine PET scans are even more specific for tumor.[14]

Electroencephalography is a relatively good method for discovering abnormal electric fields caused by brain tumors, but it is not reliable for tumor localization unless the patient presents with seizure symptoms. Visual field testing is useful when the tumor is medially located in areas affecting optic nerve pathways at the anterior base of the brain or in the occipital lobe (calcarine fissure area). Caloric testing (temperature stimulation of the external acoustic canal) can reveal brain stem or corticopontine-angle lesions through analysis of nystagmus. Audiometry results suggest corticopontine-angle tumors when unilateral low frequency and discrimination loss are present.

Lumbar puncture is relatively contraindicated in patients suspected of having increased intracranial pressure. Patients with signs or symptoms of increased intracranial pressure (papilledema, lethargy) and those with cerebellar or temporal lobe tumors are more likely to have tentorial or foramen magnum herniation. Cerebrospinal fluid examination reveals effects or spread of tumor including CSF pressure above 150 mm H_2O at the lumbar level in a laterally positioned patient, protein level between 20 and 40 mg/dl, sugar level below 50 mg/ml, and color or viscosity changes. CSF cytology and marker content are being used for diagnosis of some brain tumors. Cytology mainly indicates metastatic spread. Medulloblastoma is suggested if the polyamines, putrescine or spermidine, are found in the CSF.[70] Enolase, which is specific for neuronal tissue, is being evaluated as a screening marker. α-Fetoprotein (AFP) and human chorionic gonadotropin (HCG) levels may be of value in special situations.

STAGING SYSTEMS

The American Joint Committee on Cancer (AJCC) has published a staging system for brain tumors[13] as described by McDonald.[162] An individual system for medulloblastoma staging has been proposed by Chang.[48] No system has as yet gained widespread use.

The AJCC system is built on a GTM classification (G: grade; T: size and location; M: metastasis); the T stage is divided into supratentorial and infratentorial locations. It is also separated into five staging groups (clinical-diagnostic, surgical-evaluative, postsurgical resection-pathologic, retreatment, and autopsy). N (lymph node metastic) staging is irrelevant because the brain does not contain classic lymphatic drainage channels.

The G classification has prognostic significance.[206] G1 through G3 represent stages from well-differentiated to poorly cytology. G4 adds features of pleomorphism and necrosis. G4 tumors correspond to the histopathologic picture of glioblastoma multiforme.

The T stage is similar for both infratentorial and supratentorial locations, except that size limits differ; these are 3 cm and 5 cm, respectively. T1 denotes less than 3 (or 5) cm with unilateral extension, T2 denotes more than 3 (or 5) cm with unilateral extension, T3 denotes ventricular encroachment, and T4 denotes crossing of midline and extension beyond the tentorium for supratentorial tumors.

Stage groupings I through IV follow the G classification, with subgroups A (for T1) and B (for T2 to T3) within Stages I to III. Chang's staging system for medulloblastoma[49] is similar to the infratentorial AJCC system. However, the unilaterality condition need not be fulfilled, and the origin of tumor and metastatic spread are further specified.

PATHOLOGIC CLASSIFICATION

Table 23-4 summarizes, and the sections on individual tumors present details about typical anatomic locations and histopathologic characteristics of the various types of brain tumors that have relevance to radiation therapy. Comparison of these details with the information given in Table 23-5 indicates the effect of pathology on prognosis. Lack of capsule is an important characteristic of most primary brain tumors.

The distinction between benign and malignant tumors in Tables 23-1, 23-2, and 23-4 to 23-6 denotes only the histopathologic appearance. All intracranial tumors are regarded as locally malignant because of their volume restrictions on spread within the cranium. The histopathologic degree of malignancy is important in radiation therapy because benign lesions have a better prognosis and may be cured by surgery alone or radiation therapy below tolerance-dose levels.[206] Also, some histopathologically malignant lesions may necessitate treatment of the neuraxis because of risk of metastatic seeding.

The histopathologic diagnosis is the most important factor in prognosis. It should, however, be remembered that biopsies and partial resections may not represent the structure of the entire tumor. For example, biopsy may not show necrotic areas in a tumor erroneously diagnosed as an anaplastic astrocytoma.

PROGNOSTIC FACTORS

The following factors have been identified as being of prognostic value for brain tumor patients: age, tumor type, tumor grade, tumor friability, seizure symptoms, duration of symptoms, hypovascularity, performance status, type of surgery performed, radiation therapy, corticosteroid medication, and chemotherapy.[22,23,274,275]

For malignant astrocytomas, before radiation therapy has been given, the strongest prognostic factors (in order) are age, tumor type, performance status, and extent of surgery.[39,181,182]

Higher age is associated with worse prognosis,[230] presumably due to the increasing incidence of malignant astrocytomas and the lack of general adaptability of aging central nervous system functions. However, a patient under 15 years carries a worse prognosis for malignant astrocytoma.[188]

TABLE 23–4
Common Pathologic Characteristics of Intracranial Tumors

TUMOR	LOCATION OR ORIGIN	HISTOLOGIC CHARACTERISTICS
PRIMARY		
Malignant astrocytoma	Supratentorial (adults mostly)	(M) Small cells dominate, cellularity, mitoses, pleomorphism, invasion, vascular proliferation
Brain stem or thalamus	Brain stem (more frequently) or thalamus	50% low grade, but locally malignant
Glioblastoma multiforme	Frontal, temporal white matter	M with necrosis
Astrocytoma with anaplastic foci	Frontal, temporal white matter	M without necrosis
Meningioma (B, M)	Supratentorial, parasagittal, sphenoid wing, falx cerebri	(B) Psammoma bodies, whorls, circumscribed tumor; (M) Sarcomatous or angioblastic
Astrocytoma (B, M)	Supratentorial (adults mostly)	(B) Cellularity, diffuse; (M) B plus mitoses
Cerebral	White matter	Majority low grade
Cerebellar	Hemispheres	Majority low grade but (M) necrosis, calcification, or high cell density
Brain stem or thalamus	Supratentorial: mesencephalon (thalamus); infratentorial: pons and medulla oblongata	Almost 50% high grade, all locally malignant
Optic nerve glioma	At optic canal, orbit, or chiasm	Mostly low grade, but all locally malignant
Pituitary (B, M)	Anterior, glandular portion, sellar and suprasellar	80% chromophobe (most with hormones); acidophilic (GH, prolactin); basophilic, often intrasellar
Medulloblastoma (M)	Vermis cerebelli in children	Uniform, cytoplasm-poor cells, some in rosettes
Ependymoma (B, M)	Ventricular ependyma, 70% infratentorial	Rosetted cell groups with cell processes Pleomorphism (M)
Hemangioma, hemangioblastoma	Infratentorial, cystic	Vascular
Arteriovenous malformation	Anywhere	Vascular
Neurilemoma, schwannoma, neurinoma (B, M)	Cerebellopontine angle, cranial nerve VIII	Palisading or stellar bipolar cells, Verocay bodies, Antoni patterns
Oligodendroglioma (B, M)	Frontal white matter	Uniform, vascular, cellular, calcification
Sarcoma (M), neurofibroma (B)	Rare inside cranium	(M) pleomorphic, (B) fibroblastic
Pinealoma (B, M), dysgerminoma, embryonal carcinoma	Midline from suprasellar to pineal regions; a few cases in both locations	Seminomatous, hemorrhagic, pleomorphic varieties
Lymphoma (M), reticulum cell sarcoma, microglioma	Cerebrum	Diffuse histiocytic, large lymphocytes, various differentiation, perivascular infiltrate
OTHER		
Craniopharyngioma	Suprasellar and intrasellar	Solid, columnar cells, cystic, calcification
Syringomyelia, syringobulbia	White matter in spinal cord and medulla oblongata	Cystic, gliotic
Midline granuloma syndrome, lymphoid granulomatosis	Anywhere, often in the midline structures	Lymphomatous and/or plasmocytoid cells
Arachnoiditis	Anywhere in the subarachnoid space	Proliferating meningeal tissues

B: histologically benign; M: malignant; GH: growth hormone

Seizure symptoms and signs of normal vascularity appear to be associated with a better prognosis.[89] Performance status is of prognostic value[276] by virtue of its dependence on the quantity and quality of neurologic defects. Long duration of symptoms lengthens survival,[276] possibly because of slower tumor growth.

Tumor types are highly correlated with prognosis (see Table 23-5 and sections on individual tumors). Tumor grade is one of the main factors. Necrosis is a critical parameter in the diagnosis of glioblastoma. Location of tumor is a natural prognostic factor in survival as well as neurologic deficit. For example, posterior optic gliomas have a worse prognosis than those in anterior locations. Friable tumors are associated with worse prognosis, presumably because they represent tumors with higher histologic grades.

Biopsy alone appears to carry a worse prognosis than partial or total resection.[89,285] This may also be related to patient selection. Resection, as a debulking treatment, is clearly justified when iatrogenic neurologic defects can be avoided. Subtotal resection with postoperative irradiation appears historically to be the optimal treatment modality for many brain tumors.[285] Brain stem tumors may have to be irradiated without biopsy.[270]

GENERAL MANAGEMENT

Patients with primary brain tumors benefit from multidisciplinary treatment planning before the histopathologic diagnosis has been obtained. Detailed three-dimensional analysis of CT or MRI scans by the diagnostic neuroradiologist enables the neurosurgeon and radiation oncologist to comment on biopsy approaches, preferably stereotactic. Stereotactic biopsy has an ad-

TABLE 23–5
Documented Results of Radiation Therapy to Intracranial Tumors (With Resection or Biopsy)

TUMOR	PRIMARY RESULTS (5-YEAR SURVIVAL*)	DOSAGE	COMMENTS
PRIMARY			
Malignant astrocytoma	<10%	<6000 cGy/7 wk	>50% improved; (M) local and/or histologic
Brain stem (M)	Few	<5500 cGy/6 wk	
Glioblastoma multiforme	<5% 2-year survival; 8-month median survival	<6000 cGy/7 wk	Age, general performance status, and extent of surgery are prognostic factors
Astrocytoma with anaplastic foci	<20% survival; 27-month median survival	<6000 cGy/7 wk	
Meningioma (B, M)	75 ± 5%	>5000 cGy/6 wk	Partial resection; benign histology
Astrocytoma			Partial resection; (M) local and/or histologic
Cerebral	35 ± 15%	<5500 cGy/6 wk	Children
	45 ± 5%		Children and adults
Cerebellar	65 ± 15%	<5500 cGy/6 wk	Children
Brain stem	25 ± 5%	<5500 cGy/6 wk	Children (pons, medulla)
	50 ± 20%	<5500 cGy/6 wk	Children (midbrain and thalamus)
Optic nerve	75 ± 25%	<5500 cGy/6 wk	Children
Pituitary (B, M)	85 ± 10%	<5000 cGy/>5 wk	Adults
Medulloblastoma (B, M)	40–80% (40–50% 10-year survival)	<5500 cGy/<7 wk	Children, Collin's rule; adults, higher incidence of extracranial metastases
Ependymoma (B, M)	50 ± 30%	<5500 cGy/<7 wk	Children
	75% 10-year survival		Low grade
	67% 10-year survival		High grade
Hemangioma, arteriovenous malformation	NA	<5000 cGy/>5 wk	Recurrent
Neurilemoma, schwannoma, neurinoma (B, M)	NA	>5000 cGy/>5 wk	
Oligodendroglioma (B, M)	60 ± 20% 35 ± 20% 10-year survival	<6000 cGy/>7 wk	
Sarcoma (M), neurofibroma (B)	Few	<5500 cGy/>6 wk	Children and young adults
Pinealoma (B, M), dysgerminoma	60 ± 15%	<5500 cGy/>6 wk	Children and young adults
Embryonal carcinoma	<5%	<5500 cGy/>6 wk	Children
Lymphoma (M), reticulum cell sarcoma, microglioma	<5%	5500 cGy/>6 wk	Controversial
OTHER			
Craniopharyngioma	90% 10-year survival (80% children; 60% adults)	<6000 cGy/7 wk	Controversial
Syringomyelia, syringobulbia	60% improve	<2000 cGy/3 wk	Progressive
Midline granuloma syndrome, lymphoid granulomatosis	NA	<55000 cGy/6 wk	
Arachnoiditis	NA	<2000 cGy/3 wk	

** Unless otherwise noted.*
B: histologically benign; M: malignant; NA: not available.

vantage over open surgery biopsy because deep tumor regions and borders may be analyzed before tumor deformation has occurred during surgery. Whenever edema and increased intracranial pressure are verified or suspected, steroid medications are indicated unless specific contraindications exist.

Debulking surgery is generally indicated when the tumor is in an accessible region or exhibits a large volume. Postoperative irradiation is frequently indicated after partial tumor resection. Small tumors may be considered for primary interstitial brachytherapy if unresectable. Tumors in surgically inaccessible regions (diencephalon, brain stem, cortical motor regions) may have to be considered for primary external-beam radiation therapy after stereotactic biopsy or, exceptionally, without definitive diagnosis. Chronic phenytoin medication schedules are often prescribed to prevent seizures.

Steroids (*e.g.*, dexamethasone) are believed to reduce the risk for radiation-induced edema or cerebritis, especially in the beginning of the treatment regimen.[99] Slow tapering of steroid schedules (25% reduction/week) is advisable with close monitoring for withdrawal side effects if the medication has been prescribed for a few weeks.

During the treatment period, frequent attention must be paid to acute side effects that may influence the patient's quality of life. Medications, performance and neurologic status, blood values, and the patient's social situation must be monitored frequently to optimize his or her ability to accept and receive the appropriate treatment.

First, the function of the follow-up schedule for the brain tumor patient must be to check on side effects and to properly taper any steroid medications shortly after the treatment regimen has ended. Second, the physician must ensure that recuperation and neurologic improvement are proceeding optimally, and third, tumor recurrence must be detected before the patient presents with symptoms. The latter requires periodic CT or MRI scans. This policy optimizes the effectiveness of further therapy.

It is most important that the brain tumor patient has adequate social support, both from the treatment personnel and from the family and environment. This requires the attending physician to provide constant and compassionate attention as well as communication regarding all these factors in the patient's environment.

RADIATION THERAPY TECHNIQUES

Pertinent Anatomic Reference Points

The skull contains some radiographic and surface topographic reference points for appreciation of beam-to-head projection geometry. The external acoustic meatus are bilaterally symmetric; they participate in the definition of anatomic reference planes in the head (*e.g.*, Reid's baseline and the Frankfort horizontal plane, connecting points in the two external acoustic meatus and one anterior infraorbital edge). Unless marked at simulation, the external acoustic meatus may be difficult to see on lateral projections because of the overlying temporal bone structures. The two lateral parts of the anterior cranial fossa, the two anterior parts of the middle cranial fossa floors, and the two mandibular angle points represent appropriate reference points because they are all laterally located.

In a lateral projection radiograph, the sella turcica is centrally located and marks the lower border of the median telencephalon and diencephalon. The hypothalamic structures are located an additional 1 cm superior to the sellar floor, and the optic canal runs at the most 1 cm superior and 1 cm anterior to that point. The pineal body (or the tentorial notch) usually sits 1 cm posterior and 3 cm superior to the external acoustic meatus.

The cribriform plate is the most inferior part of the anterior cranial fossa. It is an important reference point for the inferior border of whole-brain irradiation fields. In most patients little distance is found between the lateral projections of the lens and the most inferior part of the cribriform plate. Without a good head fixation device, it may not be possible to both block out the lens and include the cribriform plate for a prescribed dose in both locations.

The temporal lobes are situated in the middle cranial fossae; the floor of the latter is easily identified in lateral radiographs. In "slant brain" fields (with a straight inferior border of the whole brain lateral port), there is a tendency to either exclude the tip of the middle fossa or irradiate much of the nasopharynx and the cervical spine if the field is properly placed in relation to the cribriform plate and the lens. Whole-brain fields therefore should always be applied with individualized blocks for the inferior field border.

On an anteroposterior radiograph with a Frankfort horizontal plane (ear markers and one inferior orbital edge in a horizontal plane), the temporal bones (pyramids) project in the orbits. This implies that the ethmoid sinuses and the sphenoid sinus will project between the orbits, the sella just above these air cavities, and the foramen magnum just below the connection line between the inferior orbital edges. The frontal and occipital lobes therefore project above the orbits, the temporal lobes in and the cerebellum in as well as somewhat below the orbits.

Treatment Setup

The head is difficult to align so that its major axes are parallel and perpendicular to the incident beam. In addition, daily variations in head position create smeared border regions with uncontrolled dose distributions. The errors encountered are rotation of the head and longitudinal axis deviation (tilting). In both cases the deviation may inadvertently amount to about 5 degrees.

These errors may be countered by a simple simulation technique. A measurable round coin (dime) taped medial to each tragus provides a symmetric marker that satisfies the anatomic condition of one transverse line in the head. The simulator's central ray can be fluoroscopically adapted to pass through both coin centers by adjustment of the head. This represents an ideal lateral projection.

The desired treatment field may now be applied to the lesion by adjustment of field size and central ray location. This results in a measurable and documentable distortion of the coins.

Reproducibility of head positioning can be achieved by using a fixation device. The Fixster stereotactic device[93,94] (table-fixed reference plate attached to a plastic turban plus mouthpiece) enables both treatment and diagnostic precision. It has 1 mm precision frontally and approximately 2 mm precision nuchally and allows for 5 mm safety margins of field with megavoltage linear accelerators. Other devices include the individually made mouthpiece attached to a table frame and the table-fixed plastic net mask.

Neuraxis Irradiation

Several brain tumors may require irradiation of both the central nervous system and the entire subarachnoid space (neuraxis). Such tumors are medulloblastoma, high-grade posterior fossa ependymoma, and reticulum cell sarcoma (diffuse histiocytic lymphoma). Each patient is simulated and may be irradiated with "boost," "helmet," and "spine" fields, in that order. The helmet and spine radiation may be delivered separately (which may be preferred because of bone marrow exposure) or simultaneously.

The boost is an individual portal arrangement that depends on tumor size and localization. We always attempt to provide a ≥ 2 cm three-dimensional margin around the presurgical (CT-enhanced tumor) volume. Wedges and angles as well as multiple portals or rotational fields may be used.

The helmet field simulation is prepared first by manufacture of a fixation device (a combination of trunk and head fixation devices). The patient is fixed in a prone position with the head ideally aligned and the neck as straight as possible. Eyelid markers are necessary.

Parallel opposed large lateral fields are simulated with the central ray in the pineal region. The inferior field border is allowed to reach the most inferior cervical vertebra without traversing the ipsilateral shoulder. When the junctions are moved, this field can be conveniently decreased without a change in the position of the isocenter.

The gantry may be angled up from the horizontal position so that the eyelid markers coincide. This allows the ocular bulb behind the lens to reach full dose levels because the field is no longer allowed to diverge from either direction. The collimator should be angled to accommodate the superior diverging spine field. By abutment, this avoids gap junctions in the cervical spinal cord.

Blocks are drawn on the radiograph (Fig. 23-8*A*) so that the irradiated volume includes the olfactory groove (cribriform plate), the orbits 3 cm posterior to the eyelid markers (2 cm if gantry is angled), the middle cranial fossa plus > 1 cm margin, and the posterior halves of the odontoid process and the included cervical vertebral bodies (Fig. 23-8*A*). A posterior block is optional; if used, it should project through the tips of the cervical spinous processes and follow the external contour of the occipital bone but not be allowed to turn anteriorly with the skull contour.

The superoinferior dimension of the helmet field is decreased by 2 cm for every 1000 cGy of tumor dose to allow for a 1 cm movement of the junction in the cervical region. Because the central ray is placed so high in the head, splaying of the cranial vault by the superior field border continues, even with decreased field sizes.

The spine fields are usually one superior and one inferior field in the adult patient. The superior field has a stationary central ray location. The moving junction at each 1000 cGy of additional radiation dose therefore moves with the superior spine field (Fig. 23-8*B*)

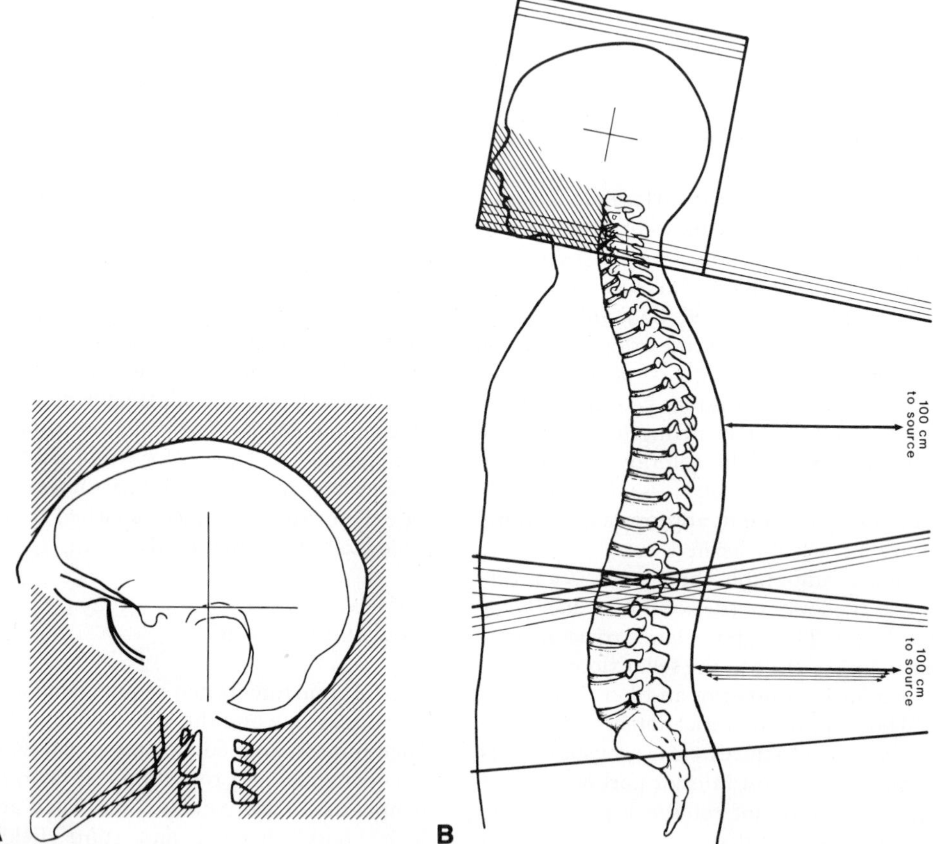

FIGURE 23–8. (**A**) A *helmet field* with Cerrobend blocking (*striped area*) is displayed. (**B**) *Craniospinal* field set-up. The central ray of the helmet field is stationary such that the superior field border splays the cranial vault at least 5 cm superior to the vertex. The inferior field border traverses the lowest possible cervical vertebra but not the ipsilateral shoulder. This allows a moving junction of 1 cm for each 1000 cGy tumor dose. Abutment adaptation to the superior spine field border is achieved by rotating the helmet field 9 or 11 degrees (100 cm or 80 cm SAD with 30 cm superior plane field height) against the transverse plane through the body. With ideal head fixation, the anterior block (*striped area*) border is about 0.5 cm inferior to the projections of the cribriform plate, 3 cm posterior to the ipsilateral eyelid surface (1.5 cm between eyelid and posterior lens surface + 1 cm to protect the contralateral lens from the diverging beam + 0.5 cm safety margin) and 0.5 cm inferior to the middle cranial fossa floor, and it approximately bisects the cervical vertebral bodies. The posterior block courses through the spinous process tips and follows the external lamina of the cranium to the anterior field border. Spine beams for neuraxis irradiation are displayed. The superior spine beam has a stationary central ray in a transverse plane of the body. This enables optimal reproducibility of simultaneous movement of superior and inferior junctions after each 1000 cGy. If possible, the superior beam should reach to the L1–L2 space to avoid junctions over the inferior part of the spinal cord. The inferior beam has a stationary inferior border at S3 because the dural sac ends at S2. The central ray and superior border have to move with the step junctions unless the beam is angled. For optimal junction abutment, the inferior beam may be angled 18 or 22 degrees (100 cm or 80 cm SAD with 30 cm field height) against the transverse plane through the body. Without angling, the junctions have to be gapped according to junction dose summations. Note that the central ray is stationary for helmet and superior spine fields, with the moving junction steps obtained through field size changes.

The field width should be adjusted so that the lateral field borders are at least 1 cm lateral to the lateral edge of each ipsilateral pedicle. For scoliotic patients it may be necessary to cut tailored blocks. Unless angled (or with a block below S3), the central ray for the inferior field must be moved with the moving junction because the inferior border of that field must stay at the S3 level (the dural sac and subarachnoid space end at S2).

If helmet field rotation and inferior spine beam angling are not used, the junction must be "gapped." The dimensions of the gaps between adjoining fields must be determined individually by dose calculation summations. This is helped by measurements from lateral radiographs on which the patient's midsagittal plane is marked. When the field borders are placed to optimize the gap conditions, consideration must also be given to divergence angles and the individual attenuation characteristics of each treatment machine. All simulation radiographs must be indicated for midplane magnification, field size, and SSD (SAD) setup parameters (SSD: source-skin distance; SAD: source-axis distance).

Irradiation of the Entire Intracranial Contents

Treatment of the entire intracranial contents (commonly referred to as whole-brain irradiation) is executed through parallel opposed lateral portals. The inferior field border should be inferior to the cribriform plate, the middle cranial fossa, and the foramen magnum, all of which should be distinguishable on simulation radiographs. The safety margin depends on penumbra width, head fixation, and anatomic factors but should be at least 1 cm, even under optimal conditions. A special problem arises anteriorly because sparing of the ocular lenses may require blocking with less than 5 mm margins to the cribriform plate. Ideal head fixation is a necessity. Many practitioners prefer to have a few centimeters fall-off of the beam over the calvarium because this provides a more homogeneous dose distribution to the superomedial structures.

The anterior block border must be distanced 3 cm posterior to the ipsilateral eyelid for the diverging beam to exclude the contralateral lens. However, this supplies the posterior ocular bulbs with only about 40% of the prescribed dose. The better alternative is to angle the beam about 5 degrees or 7 degrees (100 cm or 80 cm SAD midline but also field size-dependent) against the frontal plane so that the anterior beam border traverses the head in a frontal plane about 0.5 cm posterior to the lenses (2 cm posterior to eyelid markers). This arrangement provides full dose to the posterior parts of the ocular bulbs.

Treatment Volume

Brain tumors may be irradiated with small portals when risk of spread is low or when the purpose is boost treatment.

Exact volume to be irradiated in malignant brain astrocytomas has been the subject of several publications. Thirty years ago, Bull and Rovit[30] and later Kramer,[128] based on autopsy studies of patients irradiated for glioblastoma multiforme, recommended that because of the diffuse nature of the tumors the entire intracranial contents or larger volumes should be irradiated for better results. With the advent of computed tomography, Hochberg and Pruitt[104] reported that in 35 patients who had had a CT scan within 2 months of an autopsy, 78% of recurrences of glioblastoma multiforme were within 2 cm of the margin of the initial tumor bed and 56% were within 1 cm or less of the volume outlined by the CT scan. These findings were confirmed by Wallner and associates.[278] Large tumors were generally not more likely to recur farther from the initial tumor margin than smaller tumors. Furthermore, no unifocal tumor recurred as a multifocal lesion.

In a correlative study, Halperin and colleagues[97] reviewed CT scans and multiple pathologic sections of 15 brains of patients with glioblastoma multiforme who received minimal or no radiation therapy. They noted that if radiation treatment portals had been designed to cover the contrast-enhancing volume along with the peritumoral edema with a 1 cm margin, the portals would have covered histologically identified tumor in only six of 11 cases. On the other hand, treatment of the contrast-enhancing area and all surrounding edema with a 3 cm margin around the edema would cover all histologically identified tumor in all cases.

Kelly and colleagues[118] reported on 40 patients with intracranial glial neoplasms who underwent stereotactic serial biopsies assisted by computed tomography and magnetic resonance imaging. Histologic analysis of 195 biopsy specimens obtained from various locations within the volumes defined by CT and MRI revealed the following: contrast enhancement most often corresponded to tumor tissue without intervening parenchyma; hypodensity corresponded to parenchyma infiltrated by isolated tumor cells or in some instances to tumor tissue in low-grade gliomas or to simple edema; and isolated tumor cell infiltration extended at least as far as T2 prolongation on magnetic resonance images. The study indicated that the zone of low attentuation surrounding a mass or ring of contrast enhancement on CT scan corresponded to edematous parenchyma, which is usually infiltrated by isolated tumor cells. Prolongation of T2 on MRI revealed much larger volumes of infiltrated parenchyma than did low attenuation on CT scans.

In an autopsy study of 100 high-grade brain tumors, Matsukado and associates[160] found that these lesions infiltrated significant distances along major white matter pathways in the majority of cases. Therefore, relatively generous margins and inclusion of all radiographic evidence of tumor and associated edema must be the rule in the design of the treatment portals. Figure 23-9 illustrates the initial portal used for the treatment of a grade III multifocal malignant astrocytoma with some brain edema (*solid line*) to deliver 4500 cGy and the reduced portal (*dotted line*) to deliver additional 1500 cGy.

Local Irradiation

With a precise head fixation device, it is advisable to plan for a 3 cm margin outside the tumor border, and surrounding edema. All bilateral or medial cerebral hemispheric tumors are best treated with parallel opposed portals, with unequal weighting of beams if the tumor location is asymmetric.

Treatment of unilateral hemispheric tumors is planned and carried out according to location. Frontal lesions encompassing only the anterior parts of the lobe can be treated with anterior and lateral isocentric perpendicular beams, and the dose distribution may be optimized with or without wedges in either or both beams (Fig. 23-10). Midcerebral tumors (either posterior frontal or anterior parietal) are best treated with parallel opposed anterior and posterior portals as well as with lateral portals, again all isocentric and with or without wedges. Posterior parietal or occipital lesions can be treated with posterior and lateral isocentric beams, both suitably wedged for dose homogenization.

Superficial tumor lesions (*e.g.*, superior sagittal sinus meningiomas) can be adequately treated with parallel opposed

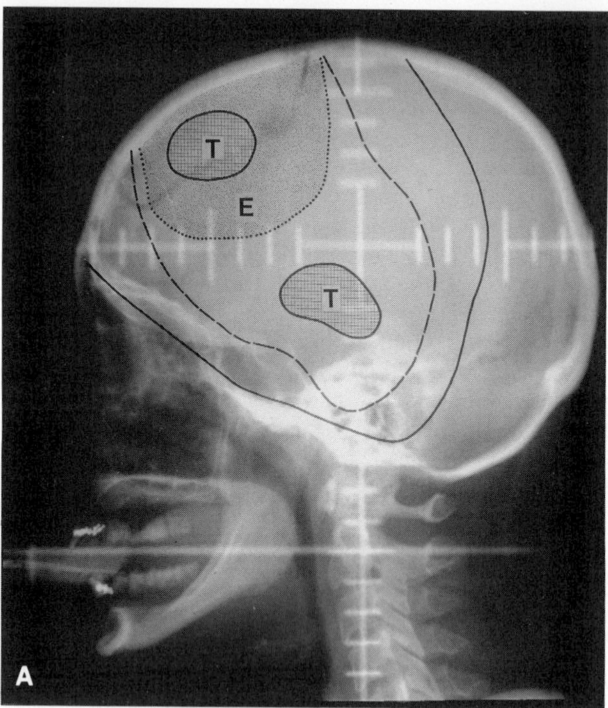

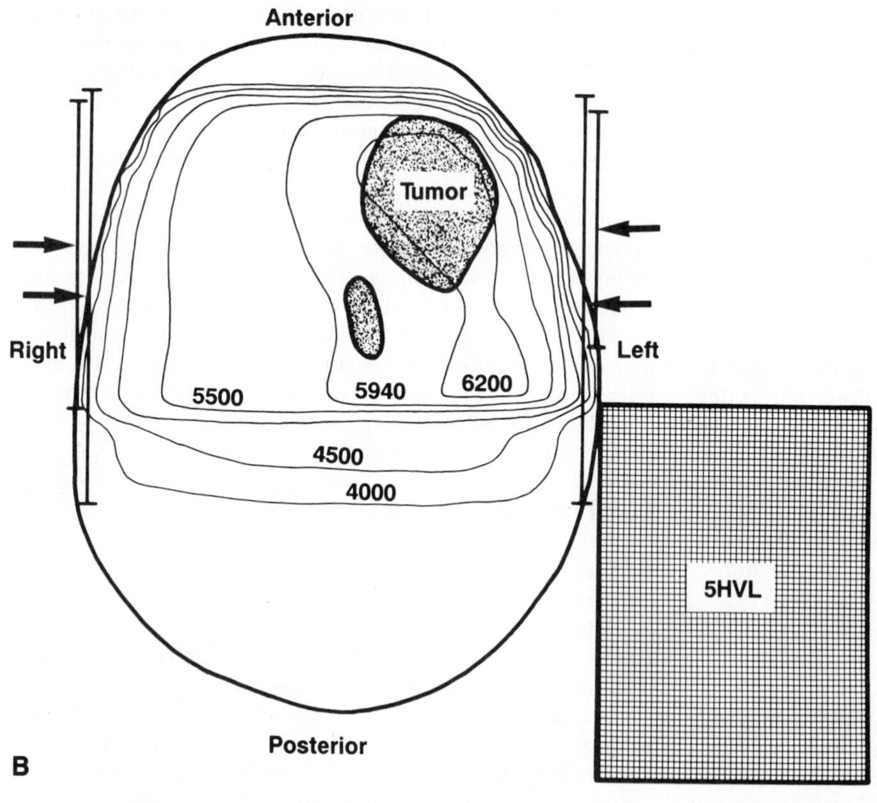

FIGURE 23–9. (**A**) Simulation film of the head outlining the frontal and thalamic tumors with associated edema previously illustrated in Figure 23-7. Solid line depicts the initial portal used to deliver 4500 cGy to the brain with opposing lateral fields (combination of 6 and 18 MV photons). The broken line outlines a reduced volume irradiated through a left lateral portal to deliver additional 1400 cGy radiation to the midplane of the brain with 6 MV photons. (**B**) Isodose curves demonstrating dose distributions.

isocentric tangential fields or with half-beam block to avoid the divergence of beams to the normal brain.

Lesions in the temporal lobe tip are difficult to treat with other than lateral ports (Fig. 23-11) unless the patient is flexible enough to tuck chin against chest (Fig. 23-12) such that a sagittal beam does not traverse the lens. In that case an added lateral portal may result in an acceptable local dose distribution, which could be further improved by a posterior parallel opposed field.

Pituitary, optic nerve, hypothalamic, and brain stem tumors and craniopharyngiomas are deep and centrally located. Depending on extent, these lesions may be treated with isocentric three-portal, four-portal, rotation, or arc-rotation treatment techniques. Stationary beams give adequate dose homogeneity in and around the sella turcica. The three-field box technique consists of parallel opposed lateral portals and an anterior portal. The lateral portals may be wedged to compensate for the declining anteroposterior dose gradient from the anterior portal. The four-field box technique uses both lateral and sagittal parallel opposed portals. A 360-degree rotation technique can be used if fixation is adequate to avoid geo-

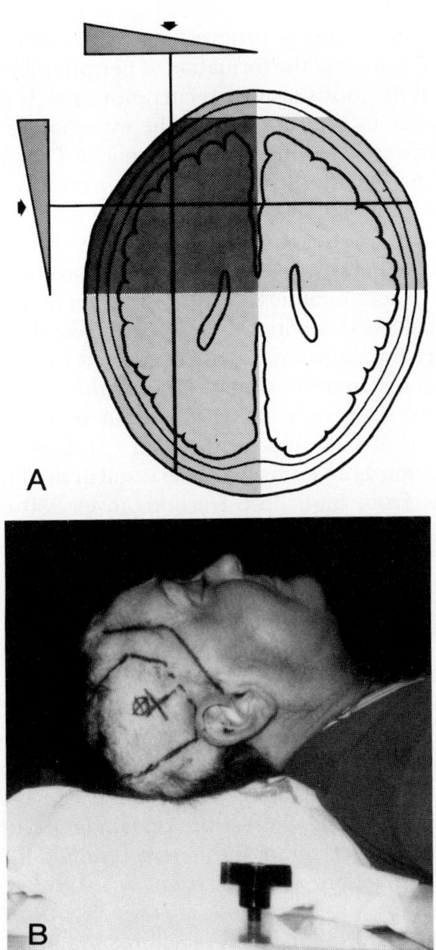

FIGURE 23–10. (A) Anterior frontal lesions may be boosted with anterior and lateral wedged portals to homogenize the dose distribution. Wedging allows compensations for sloping surfaces as well as differences in depth dose. (B) Example of portals used for treatment of intermediate-grade astrocytoma in the right temporoparietal region: 5000 cGy was given in 6 weeks with unequal weighting, using a combination of 6 MV and 18 MV photons. An additional 480 cGy was delivered in three fractions through smaller right side of field.

graphic misses. Because of the shorter distance from the anterior surface, the cylindrical dose distribution becomes flattened posteriorly. The 50% isodose line occurs about halfway toward the lateral surfaces of the head. Arc rotation with reversed edges is an elegant technique that enables an elliptoid dose distribution.[19]

Brain stem lesions are adequately treated with parallel opposed lateral portals combined with a posterior midline portal. Unilateral cerebellar lesions can also be covered by posterior and lateral portals, appropriately wedged. It is essential to make certain that the ocular lenses are not in the irradiated volume. Pineal lesions are often treated with parallel opposed sagittal (and lateral) portals. (Fig. 23-13).

Table 23-6 represents our general choice of treatment plans for the different tumors. It should be noted that most recommended doses are close to tolerance; therefore, increasing the dose to improve cure or survival figures is always accompanied by a higher complication risk.

TREATMENT SEQUELAE

The sensitivity of the normal brain to irradiation is a central issue for the radiation oncologist.[133] Histopathologic aspects have been reviewed in the literature.[75] Radiation necrosis is the classic complication. Other late complications are optic nerve-chiasmal injury, intellectual deficit, and pituitary-hypothalamic dysfunction. In addition, attention is now being paid to delayed reactions (somnolence, transient worsening of symptoms, and leukoencephalopathy). The radiation oncologist also needs to be aware of acute reactions to irradiation, particularly edema. It must be remembered that all other tissues in the irradiated volume may exhibit side effects and complications. Complications of the scalp, ears, bone, and temporomandibular joints are noted in the literature.[155] The mechanism of radiation injury has been theorized to encompass vascular intima proliferation, demyelinization due to oligodendroglia vulnerability, and possible immunologic factors.

Tolerance of the central nervous system to irradiation has

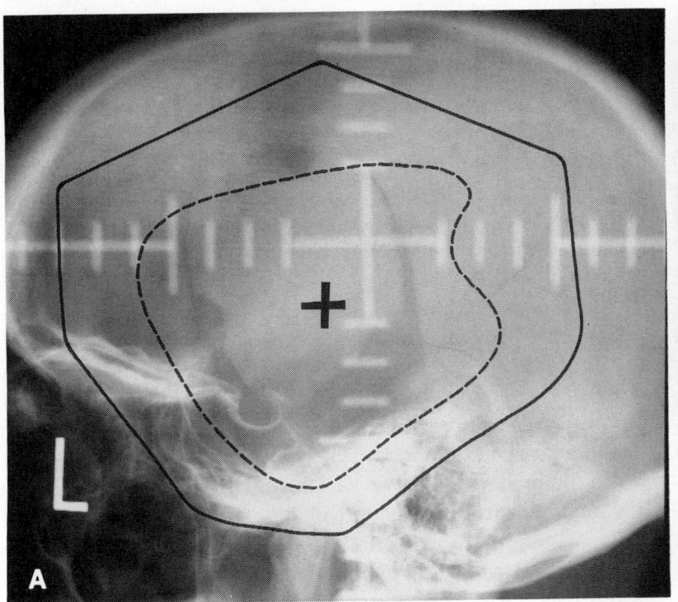

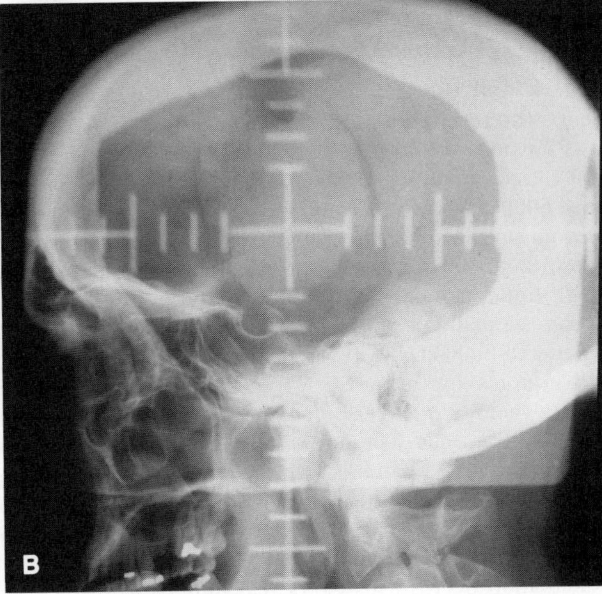

FIGURE 23–11. (A) Lateral simulation film demonstrating a large portal used to deliver 4500 cGy of radiation and reduced field for additional 1400 cGy to treat a patient with large recurrent oligodendroglioma in the left temporoparietal area. (B) Block check film outlining initial portal on same patient.

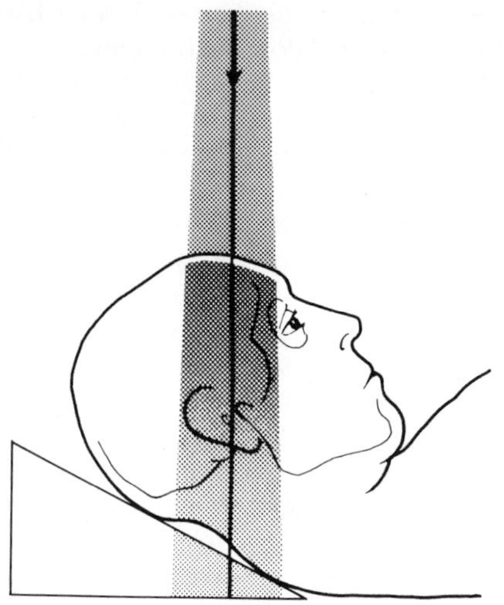

FIGURE 23–12. The anteroposterior beam enables temporal lobe irradiation without inclusion of the ocular bulb or midline structures in the irradiated volume. This setup requires either a patient with a flexible neck or the convenience of angling the beam in a sagittal plane of the body (*e.g.*, by rotating the table 90 degrees and then angling the beam). Parallel opposed anterior and posterior portals, with or without a lateral portal, are suitable for boosting the dose to temporal lobe lesions when the lobe tip needs to be included. Be aware of beam divergence.

been extensively researched[71]. Animal studies have been conducted by Caveness.[45] Sheline discussed the published human patient material up to that time.[243] His conclusion is that the tolerance of the central nervous system is very dependent on the number of fractions and less dependent on overall treatment time. The Ellis formula,[243] NSD (RET) $= D \times N^{-0.24} \times T^{-0.11}$, does not apply but has been modified in several versions to NSD (NEURET) $= D \times N^{-0.44} \times T^{-0.06}$ or ED $= D \times N^{-0.377} \times T^{-0.058}$. This implies that TDF values need recalculation.[54]

NSD = nominal standard dose
RET = rad equivalent dose
ED = equivalent dose
NEURET = neurad equivalent therapy
D = dose in cGy
N = number of fractions
T = number of elapsed days of treatment

Marks and associates[156] found 5% of radiation necrosis in patients who received a total megavoltage dose of above 5500 cGy at fractions ≥ 200 cGy. They also found no risk for 5400 cGy at 180 cGy per fraction. Sheline regards a total megavoltage dose of 6000 cGy with the same fractionation but without other compromising factors as reasonably safe.[241] Rubin's group[214] suggests that 5000 cGy to the whole brain imposes a 5% risk of necrosis under standard conditions. The upper dose limit for the brain stem and posterior fossa has been suggested to be at 5500 cGy to 6000 cGy in fractions below 200 cGy.[129]

Symptoms appearing a few weeks to a few months after radiation therapy include somnolence and worsening of pretreatment symptoms. These reactions have been attributed to demyelination. Histopathologic terms include necrotizing leukoencephalopathy and microangiopathy. Necrotizing leukoencephalopathy has a gradual presentation from 4 to 12 months after treatment.[200]

Radiation necrosis may appear 6 months to many years (peak at 3 years) after the irradiation. Radiation necrosis can mimic recurrent tumor by progressive reappearance of initial symptoms and signs; a progressive, irreversible, enhancing mass on CT scan; and the formation of peripheral brain edema. Differential diagnosis against recurrent tumor is difficult but may be easier in the future with the evolution of PET scanning,[92] nuclear scanning, and dynamic CT scanning procedures.[78] So far, the best treatment approach is surgical debulking in combination with steroid treatment.[73]

In children treated with combinations of chemotherapy and radiation therapy, several late sequelae have been observed, such as endocrinopathies,[69,70,236] optic nerve injury,[190] impaired intellectual abilities,[69,70,174] and secondary tumors.[58] Danoff[58] has summarized the risk conditions for appearance of necrotizing leukoencephalopathy in children, indicating less than 1% risk from irradiation alone but over 5% risk from combinations of radiation therapy and intrathecal methotrexate. Irradiation as an exclusive cause is still in doubt. Visual loss may follow from high dose fractions (over 250 cGy) to the chiasm and optic nerve.[98]

ASTROCYTOMAS

Low-Grade Astrocytomas

The "differentiated" or "low-grade" astrocytomas make up 15% to 20% of all intracranial gliomas[8] and 30% to 48% of childhood gliomas.[23,215] Approximately 75% of astrocytomas arise in the supratentorial region, whereas the remainder occur below the tentorium. The cerebellum is the most common infratentorial site.[26] Cerebral lesions are more common in adults in the third to fifth decades, whereas lesions at other sites (third ventricle, hypothalamus, optic chiasm, cerebellum, and brain stem) typically occur during the first 3 decades.[35,140,158,220]

Astrocytomas arise from and are composed of astrocytes that vary in morphologic appearance and display different degrees of cytologic maturation.[215] They are variously classified under the term "astrocytoma" or grouped according to grade or histologic subtype. Grading systems classify gliomas by ascending order of malignancy with low-grade tumors grouped within grades 1 and 2. In the Kernohan classification,[119] the distinction between grade 1 and grade 2 is of variable prognostic significance[21,77,135,140,166,230] because of sampling errors and the absence of explicit criteria for the assignment of lesions into different grades.[215] Daumas-Duport and co-workers[59] recently described a grading scheme using more objective criteria that appears to better differentiate grade 1 from grade 2 lesions than does the Kernohan system. Astrocytomas are also classified according to histology. The World Health Organization (WHO) system[302,306] divides astrocytic tumors into pilocytic astrocytomas (including the midline and hemispheric juvenile pilocytic and cystic as well as solid cerebellar astrocytomas), which occur predominantly in children and young adults, and astrocytomas (including the fibrillary, protoplasmic, and gemistocytic subtypes), which most commonly arise in the cerebral hemispheres in adults. Pilocytic astrocytomas are locally infiltrating, well-demarcated lesions. They have a long natural history and rarely de-differentiate into anaplastic astrocytomas.[238,302] Within the favorable group are the benign astrocytic variants including the subependymal giant cell astrocytomas and pleomorphic xanthoastrocytomas. The remaining astrocytomas are less favorable and frequently evolve into anaplastic gliomas.[135,215] Although classified among the low-grade lesions, gemistocytic astrocytomas behave as if they are anaplastic, and 80% transform into glioblastoma multiforme.[220] Representative survival rates for patients with astro-

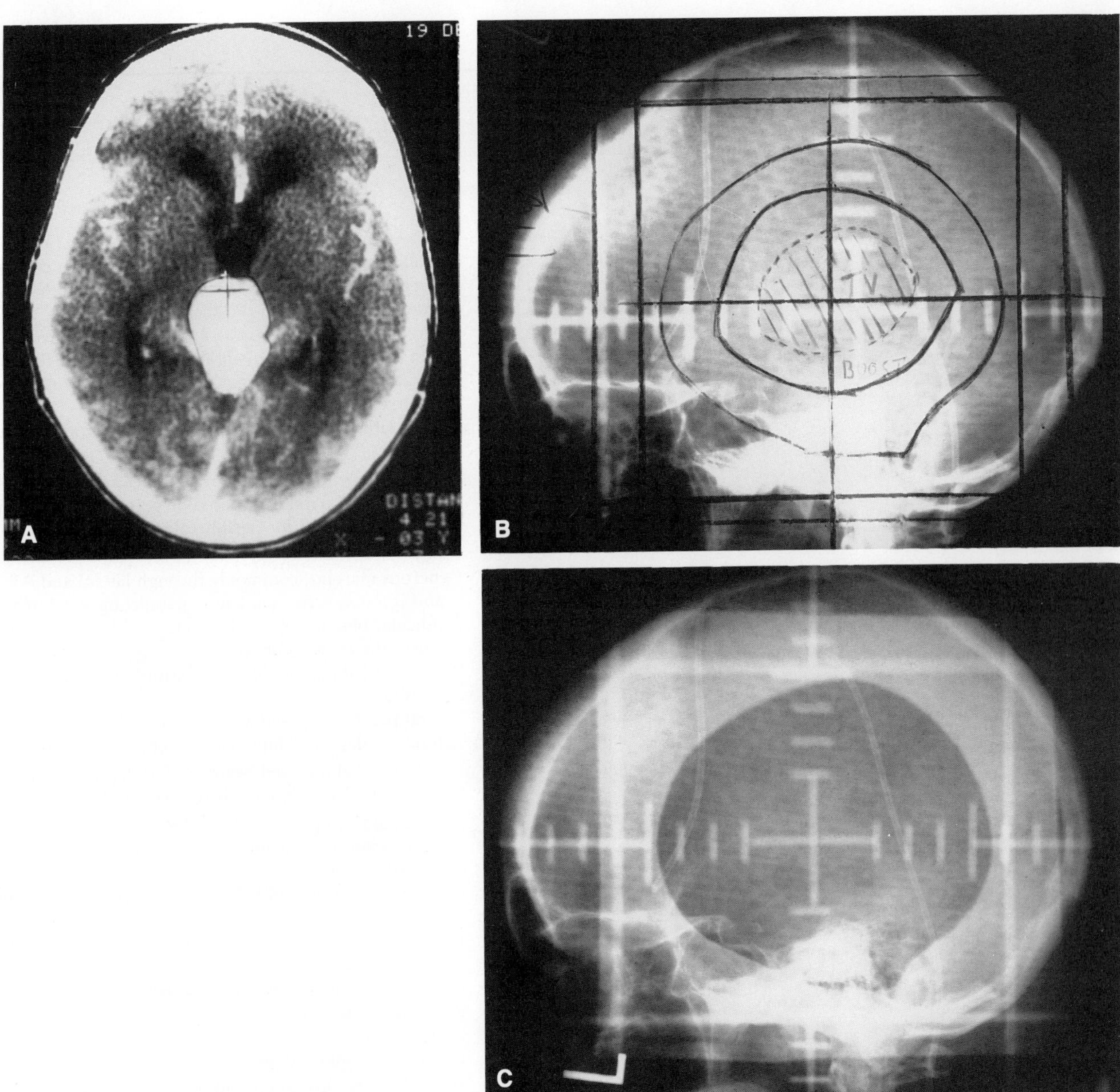

FIGURE 23–13. (**A**) Computed tomographic scan of the head with contrast enhancement outlining large pineal germinoma in a 45-year-old woman. (**B**) Simulation film illustrating the tumor volume (TV), the initial portal used to treat the patient up to 4500 cGy, and reduced fields for a boost of 900 cGy. Parallel opposed fields and 18 MV photons were used. (**C**) Block check film for same patient.

cytomas are shown in Table 23-7. In a review of 461 patients with supratentorial low-grade gliomas, Laws and co-workers[135] reported a 5-year survival rate of only 36.5%, or nearly one third of that estimated for a comparable normal population; by 15 years it was reduced to 16%, or more than one fifth of that expected.[244]

One of the most important determinants of prognosis is age; younger patients have a better prognosis than older patients.[135, 140, 158, 166, 196, 238] This is closely related to histology; patients with pilocytic astrocytomas are younger than patients with nonpilocytic tumors.[238]

Survival is significantly longer in patients with no postoperative performance deficit, no alteration of consciousness, and no personality change than when any of these features are present.[135] The extent of surgical resection is of variable prognostic significance; survival is directly related to the completeness of resection in pilocytic astrocytomas, but prognosis appears to be independent of the degree of resection for the more unfavorable, diffuse astrocytomas.[238]

Considerable controversy exists regarding the use of radiation therapy for the treatment of low-grade astrocytomas. There are no randomized studies comparing the outcome of patients treated by surgery alone or with surgery and radiation therapy. To make a meaningful comparison between treatment groups, the criteria for selection of a particular treatment, patient characteristics, tumor pathology, location of lesion, extent of resection, and radiation therapy technique must be taken into consideration. Studies limited to the era of advanced neuroimaging are difficult to compare with earlier studies.

Only 10% to 35% of astrocytomas are amenable to total surgical resection.[77, 135, 140, 166, 196, 238] Postoperative irradiation is usually not recommended after a macroscopically complete

TABLE 23–6
*Suggested Photon Irradiation Technique and Doses (1 MV–10 MV)**

TUMOR	DOSE (cGy) LARGE FIELDS	DOSE (cGy) SMALL FIELDS	TECHNICAL ASPECTS
PRIMARY			
High-grade astrocytoma			
Glioblastoma multiforme	about 4000	about 2000–3000 BO	Tolerance 5000–6000 cGy/5–7 wk; often large fields lateral opposing or "whole brain"; smaller fields depend on location of tumor margin, usually ≥2 cm from tumor or edema; dose fraction ≤200 cGy
Astrocytoma with anaplastic foci	about 4000	about 2000–3000 BO	Tolerance 5000–6000 cGy/5–7 wk; often large fields lateral opposing or "whole brain"; smaller fields depend on location of tumor margin, usually ≥3 cm from tumor or edema; dose fraction ≤200 cGy
Brain stem or thalamus		5500	Usually lateral parallel opposing fields, sometimes with PA field
Meningioma (B, M)		5500	Field size dependent on tumor size, location, and histology; tangential parallel opposed or perpendicular oblique beams may be used for peripheral lesions
Astrocytoma (B, M)			
Cerebral	5500		Generous margins, commonly through lateral and AP beams if lesion is frontal, lateral parallel opposed or perpendicular oblique beams if parietal and lateral, and PA beams if the lesion is occipital
Cerebellar		5500	Usually lateral parallel opposed beams, but three fields or arc desirable
Brain stem or thalamus		5500	Lateral parallel opposed and PA beams
Optic nerve		5000	Lateral, 15-degree oblique parallel opposed beams
Pituitary (B, M)		5000	Lateral parallel opposed beams *or* 360-degree rotation *or* 220-degree rotation arcs with reversed wedges
Medulloblastoma (B, M) or high-grade intracranial ependymoma		1000 BO	Lateral parallel opposed and wedged or perpendicular wedged beams to remaining tumor location at 200 cGy per fraction *and*
	4500		lateral parallel opposed helmet fields, 180 cGy fractions *and*
	<4000		PA beam(s) to spinal axis with 150 cGy fractions *and* moving gap junctions *and*
		1000 BO	to gross remaining tumor *or* if patient is <3 years old
	3500		to cranial contents *and*
	<3000		to spinal canal *and*
		1000 BO	to gross remaining tumor
Low-grade ependymoma		5500	Small fields for low-grade tumor
Hemangioma, arteriovenous malformation (B, M)		5000	Small fields with preferentially multibeam geometry
Neurilemoma, schwannoma, neurinoma (B, M)		5000	Small fields with preferentially multibeam geometry
Oligodendroglioma (B, M)		5500	AP and lateral beams if lesion is frontal
Sarcoma (M)	5000	1000 BO	If malignant, neuraxis irradiation may be necessary (as for medulloblastoma above)
Neurofibroma (B)	5000 or	5000	Large field if multiple; small field if solitary
Pinealoma, dysgerminoma, embryonal carcinoma		2000 3500	AP–PA parallel opposed beams, *then* CT scan; *add* three-beam "box" technique if unchanged or benign histology
	3500		*or* if decreased on CT or malignant histopathology *add* lateral parallel opposed helmet fields *plus*
	3500		PA beam(s) to spinal axis with gapped and moving junctions (as for medulloblastoma above)
Lymphoma (M), reticulum cell sarcoma, microglioma	5000		Lateral parallel opposing helmet beams
Unspecified (B, M)	Variable		Beam geometry depends on tumor location
OTHER			
Craniopharyngioma		5000 1000–2000 BO 5500	"Large" local field, often lateral parallel opposing beams *and* small multibeam *or* rotation ports *except* in children, multibeam

(continued)

TABLE 23–6
(Continued)

TUMOR	DOSE (cGy) LARGE FIELDS	SMALL FIELDS	TECHNICAL ASPECTS
Syringomyelia, syringobulbia	2000		PA narrow beams or perpendicular oblique PA beams
Midline granuloma syndrome, lymphoid granulomatosis		5000	Lateral parallel opposing helmet fields
Arachnoiditis	2000		Smallest possible fields encompassing involved areas

** 80–100 cm SSD (source-skin distance) or SAD (source-axis distance), 100 to 300 cGy/minute, 180–200 cGy/fraction, 5 times/wk unless otherwise noted.*
AP: arteroposterior beam direction; B: benign; BO: boost; M: malignant; PA: posteroanterior beam direction.

resection. For cerebellar astrocytomas in children, local control with complete resection alone approaches 100%.[77,140] Similarly, for patients with juvenile pilocytic astrocytomas, survival rates of 5 and 10 years are close to 100% after completion of "radical subtotal" resection.[88,238,280] In contrast, Shaw and associates[238] found that patients (including children) with supratentorial nonpilocytic ("ordinary") astrocytomas or mixed oligoastrocytomas who underwent total or radical subtotal resection did not do as well as those with juvenile pilocytic astrocytomas. The 5- and 10-year survival rates were 52% and 21%, respectively, even though 14 of the 23 patients also received postoperative irradiation. These results were similar to those observed in patients with the same histology undergoing subtotal resection or biopsy. Most single-institution studies comparing the outcome of patients with incompletely resected astrocytomas receiving postoperative irradiation with that of nonirradiated patients treated over the same period show a survival advantage for the irradiated group (Table 23-8).[77,88,140,255]

In the series reported by Leibel and colleagues,[140] 108 patients had incompletely resected tumors; 71 patients received postoperative irradiation, and 37 patients did not. The extent of resection, age distributions, and performance status of the patients in the two groups were similar. Radiation therapy was administered to doses of 5000 cGy to 5500 cGy. The 5-year recurrence-free survival rate after incomplete resection alone was 19% compared with 46% for incomplete resection and irradiation. The 10-year survival rates were 11% and 35%, respectively. For adults, the 5-year survival rate was 10% after surgery alone and 32% when radiation therapy was added. By 20 years, all nonirradiated patients had died, whereas 23% of irradiated patients were alive and free of recurrence. When the data were analyzed according to the Kernohan classification,[119] the 5-year survival rates were 58% for grade 1 and 25% for grade 2 lesions in patients who received postoperative irradiation compared with survival rates of 25% for grade 1 and 0% for grade 2 lesions in nonirradiated patients.

Similarly, Fazekas,[77] compared 32 patients who had incomplete resection and postoperative irradiation with 15 patients who had incomplete resection only. Although, prognostically, the nonirradiated patients represented a more favorable subgroup, the 5-year survival was 41% for those with radiation therapy and only 13% for those with surgery alone.

In their series of 126 patients with supratentorial "ordinary" astrocytomas and mixed oligoastrocytomas, Shaw and colleagues[240] found that the patients receiving high-dose postoperative radiation therapy had a significantly higher survival rate than patients receiving low-dose radiation therapy or surgery alone. The 5- and 10-year survival rates were 68% and

TABLE 23–7
Astrocytoma: Overall 5- and 10-Year Survival Rates

AUTHOR	NO. OF CASES	TREATMENT	SURVIVAL RATE (%) 5-YEAR	10-YEAR
Leibel et al[140]	51	S	41	33
	40*	S	25	17
	71	S + RT	46	35
Marsa et al[158]	40	S + RT	41	20
Fazekas[77]	23	S	32	32
Laws et al[135]	461	S, S + RT	36	20
Garcia et al[88]	23	S	21	10
	57	S + RT	50	25
Medbery et al[166]	50	S + RT	45	32
Shaw et al[238]	41†	S, S + RT	85§	79
	126‡	S, S + RT	51§	23

S: surgery alone, includes gross total and subtotal resection; RT: radiation therapy.
** Excludes children with completely resected cerebellar tumors*
† Pilocytic astrocytomas
‡ Nonpilocytic astrocytomas and mixed oligoastrocytomas
§ Difference significant, $P < 0.001$

TABLE 23–8
Astrocytoma: 5-Year Survival After Subtotal Resection Alone Compared With Subtotal Resection and Radiation Therapy

AUTHOR	YEAR	NO. OF PATIENTS (S/S + RT)	5-YEAR SURVIVAL (%)	
			S ALONE	S + RT
Leibel et al[140]	1975	108 (37/71)	19	46
Fazekas[77]	1977	47 (32/15)	13	41
Garcia et al[88]	1985	80 (23/57)*	21	50
Shaw et al[238]	1989	126 (19/107)†	32	68 (≥5300 cGy) (<5300 cGy)

S: surgery; RT: radiation therapy.
**Includes 6 patients with total resection.*
†Includes 23 patients with total resection.

39%, respectively, for patients receiving postoperative irradiation to doses of 5300 cGy or higher, 47% and 21% for those treated with less than 5300 cGy, and 32% and 11% for nonirradiated patients ($P = 0.04$). As observed by others,[88, 135] these differences were most pronounced in older patients. Patients 35 years of age or older who received adjunctive radiation had 5- and 10-year survival rates of 67% and 45%, whereas patients treated with low-dose irradiation or surgery alone had survival rates of 37% and 5% at the same time intervals ($P = 0.008$). In contrast, although the survival rate of younger patients was improved by irradiation, the magnitude of improvement was not statistically significant.

Patients with incompletely resected pilocytic astrocytomas have a better prognosis than patients with subtotally removed nonpilocytic tumors. The 10- and 20-year progression-free survival rates for patients with incompletely resected juvenile pilocytic astrocytomas receiving postoperative radiation reported by Wallner and associates[280] were 74% and 41%, respectively. A control group of patients with incompletely resected, nonirradiated pilocytic astrocytomas was not available for comparison. Shaw and co-workers[238] found that patients with supratentorial pilocytic astrocytomas who underwent subtotal resection or biopsy and postoperative irradiation survived longer than nonirradiated patients, although the number of patients treated by surgery alone was small. The 5-year survival rate of patients treated by subtotal resection or biopsy alone was 50% compared with 85% for those who received postoperative radiation ($P = 0.08$).

Although it is generally agreed that patients with neurologic impairment, evidence of tumor progression, or malignant transformation should undergo radiation therapy, there is a trend among some practitioners to defer treatment in asymptomatic patients or those with seizures only. Proponents of this approach argue that it is not certain whether early irradiation has an advantage over delayed irradiation or whether radiation therapy has an impact at all on the natural history of the disease.[41] Available information suggests that except for selected cases, most astrocytomas are highly lethal tumors and more effective therapeutic strategies are needed.[244] For pilocytic astrocytomas, postoperative irradiation is not indicated when a complete or near-complete surgical excision has been performed. After subtotal surgical removal, either immediate radiation therapy or close follow-up, with treatment reserved for disease progression, may be recommended.

Postoperative irradiation appears to be beneficial for patients with incompletely resected unfavorable astrocytomas. Because of their diffuse pattern of growth and poor prognosis, postoperative irradiation has also been recommended for patients with totally resected unfavorable astrocytomas. With conventionally fractionated radiation therapy (180 cGy to 200 cGy per fraction), doses of 5500 cGy are recommended. Limited radiation fields are used[158, 166, 238] with a 2 cm to 3 cm margin around the lesion defined by CT scan and at least 1 cm to 2 cm beyond the T2-weighted MR image, whichever volume is larger. The dose is reduced to 5000 cGy for children under 5 years of age.

Properly designed prospective studies are needed to better define the natural history of astrocytomas, the impact of the extent of surgery on prognosis, and the response of these tumors to radiation therapy. Two such studies are now being conducted in the United States. An intergroup study by the Brain Tumor Cooperative Group (BTCG), the Radiation Therapy Oncology Group (RTOG), and the Southwest Oncology Group compares the effect of radiation therapy in asymptomatic patients immediately after pathologic diagnosis with the effect of radiation administered at the time of clinical and CT/MRI progression in adult patients with supratentorial, nonpilocytic astrocytomas. Patients with symptomatic neurologic impairment receive immediate irradiation. A randomized study is being conducted by the North Central Cancer Treatment and the Mayo Clinic comparing 5040 cGy in 28 fractions with 6480 cGy in 36 fractions to determine whether higher radiation doses improve the therapeutic results. Eligible for randomization are patients with pilocytic astrocytomas who have had a biopsy only and all patients with "ordinary" astrocytomas.[238]

High-Grade Astrocytomas

High-grade (malignant) astrocytomas represent approximately 40% of all intracranial primary tumors and about two thirds of all astrocytic tumors. The overall 5-year survival rate is less than 10%.

The pathologic classification of astrocytomas has varied in published reports and at institutions. A widely used system is that of Kernohan,[120] which grades astrocytomas from 1 to 4 with malignant lesions being 3 or 4.

Nelson[178, 183] emphasized that patients with grade 3 tumors according to the Kernohan classification do not consistently have a superior prognosis compared with those with grade 4 tumors. He proposed that malignant astrocytomas be divided into anaplastic astrocytomas, which are those with multifocal or diffuse cellularity or with nuclear pleomorphism; and glioblastoma multiforme, which has the same features with the addition of necrosis involving neoplastic astrocytes. Five-hundred fifty-six patients were entered into RTOG glioma studies and classified by this system. Those with anaplastic astrocytoma showed a median survival of 36.2 months and those with glioblastoma multiforme showed only 8.6 months.

Several reports have attempted to identify the major prognostic factors in patients with malignant gliomas. Nelson[178,180] identified three prognostic factors in addition to histology: age, extent of surgery, and performance status. In that analysis, younger patients, those with procedures more extensive than a biopsy, and those with a Karnofsky performance status of 80 or greater were in the most favorable group.

Using the Brain Tumor Study Group data on 225 patients, Gehan and Walker[89] reported six prognostic factors. The favorable factors included a younger age, the presence of seizures, cranial nerve deficits, and an encapsulated tumor, whereas the unfavorable factors were surgery limited to biopsy only and a tumor in the parietal region.

In 1986, Shapiro[237] reported further on these data. He identified eight unfavorable prognostic factors: age greater than 64 years, histology of glioblastoma, performance status less than 50, symptoms of less than 6 months' duration, abnormal level of consciousness, blood type A or AB, pretreatment white blood count greater than 8500, and pretreatment platelet count less than 300,000.

With regard to irradiation techniques in 1960, Concannon[55] published a study on the adequacy of treatment fields in 21 patients treated using two lateral 8-cm × 10-cm fields and a superior 6-cm × 10-cm field. In that study, only two patients (< 10%) had adequate tumor coverage. In 1969, Kramer[128] published more on these data and, in view of the large proportion of missed tumors using limited fields, concluded that the entire intracranial contents should be irradiated in patients with glioblastomas. Salazar and Rubin,[226] in a study of 43 patients with an autopsy within 1 month of treatment, found that only six (14%) patients had an accurate assessment of tumor extent and 35 (82%) had contiguous spread as a component of the discrepancy between clinical and pathologic assessment. They further identified the frontal lobe at the corpus callosum and the thalamus as two sites of midline crossing for brain tumors, which supported the conclusion that malignant gliomas required treatment of the entire intracranial contents.

However, CT[32,33] and MRI have provided new tools to assess the extent of the tumor. In 1980, Hochberg and Pruitt[104] concluded that CT is sufficiently sensitive for defining the tumor volume, and irradiation of the entire brain is not necessary. In comparing MRI with CT to evaluate tumor extent, Halperin and colleagues[97] noted that the region identified by the prolongation of T2 in the T2-weighted magnetic resonance image may be larger than the abnormal zone on CT. They reported autopsy studies that showed a significant proportion of patients to have tumor more than 2 cm beyond the CT contrast-enhancing region, thus, challenging the concept of a localized malignant glioma. Also, Kelly and associates[118] found "tumor" cells in stereotactic biopsies from normal brain distant from the enhancement.

Nonetheless, with a tumor in which the primary site of failure is within the contrast-enhancing region on CT, it seems reasonable to consider the target volume to be the contrast-enhancing region with a 3 cm to 4 cm margin.[63,278]

Conflicting reports have been published concerning the optimal radiation dose to use in the treatment of malignant gliomas. In 1979, Walker[277] reported a dose-response analysis using data from 420 patients treated on several Brain Tumor Cooperative Group protocols. Doses ranged from less than 4500 cGy to 6000 cGy using daily fractions of 170 cGy to 200 cGy. No reason was given for the use of the lower doses, and only one third of the patients received less than 6000 cGy. Median survival increased from 13.5 to 42 weeks in the total group and from 28 to 42 weeks in the group treated with doses of 5000 cGy to 6000 cGy (Fig. 23-14*A*). On the other hand, in a randomized study reported by Chang and associates,[49] no significant difference was found in survival or tumor control in over 600 patients entered on the study who were treated with 6000 cGy alone or

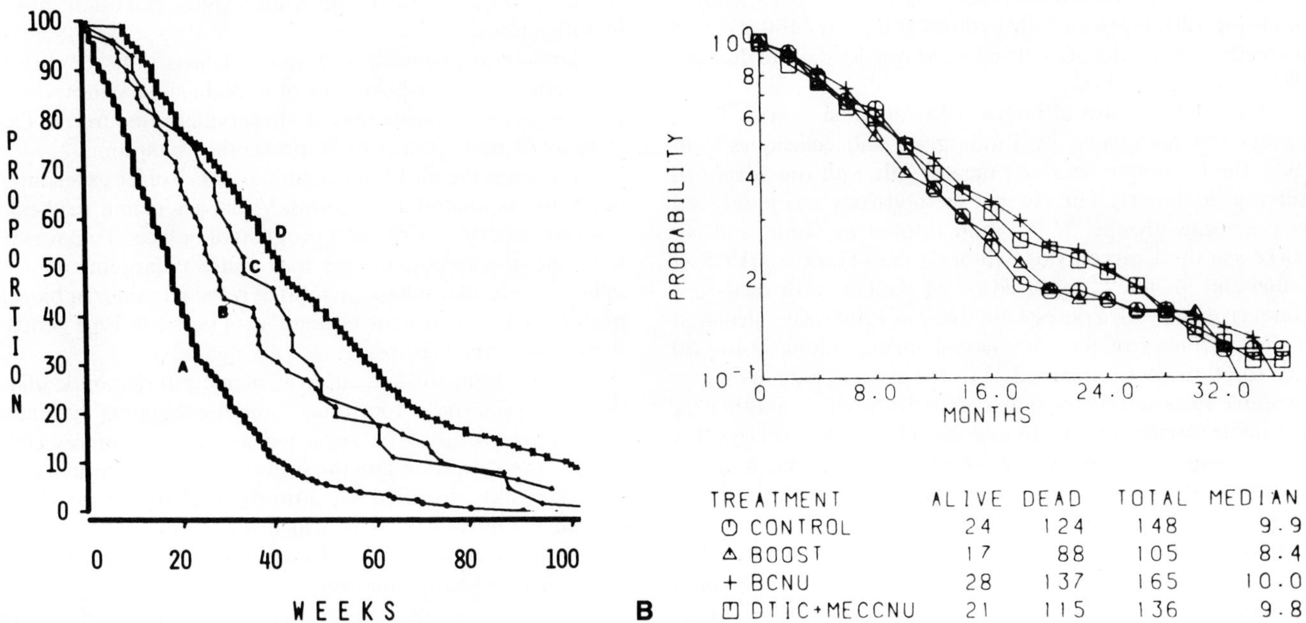

TREATMENT	ALIVE	DEAD	TOTAL	MEDIAN
⊙ CONTROL	24	124	148	9.9
△ BOOST	17	88	105	8.4
+ BCNU	28	137	165	10.0
⊡ DTIC+MECCNU	21	115	136	9.8

FIGURE 23–14. (**A**) Survival curves of all patients with malignant glioma who received no radiation therapy (A), 5000 cGy (B), 5500 cGy (C), or 6000 cGy (D). (Walker MD, Strike TA, Sheline GE: Int J Radiat Oncol Biol Phys 5:1725, 1979) (**B**) Survival rates by treatment options for all ages and tissue groups (astrocytoma with foci of anaplasia and glioblastoma) plotted according to the life-table method. (Chang CH, Horton J, Schoenfeld D, et al: Cancer 52:997, 1983)

combined with BCNU or methyl-CCNU and DTIC or with 6000 cGy to the brain plus 1000 cGy boost to the tumor volume (Fig. 23-14*B*).

In a study reported by Salazar[227] in 1979, 28 patients were treated with doses between 7000 cGy and 8200 cGy. Although median survival was improved in patients treated with these very high doses, at the last report, 26 (93%) had tumor recurrence and 11 had tumor documented either at autopsy or reoperation.

The RTOG conducted a randomized study in which two of the treatment options were 6000 cGy given in 6 to 7 weeks to the entire brain or 6000 cGy plus a 1000 cGy boost to a limited volume given in 7 to 8 weeks[177]; 253 patients were evaluable on these two arms. There was no statistically significant benefit for the higher radiation dose. Median survival was 9.3 months for those receiving 6000 cGy and 8.2 for those receiving 7000 cGy.

In view of these data, with daily fractions of 180 cGy to 200 cGy, a total dose of 6000 cGy should be adequate to treat most patients with malignant gliomas.

The use of multiple daily fractions for the treatment of malignant gliomas is under investigation, because accelerated fractionation may be indicated for rapidly growing tumors. Randomized reports using multiple daily fractions have been published by Simpson,[249] Payne,[192] Shin,[246,247] and Deutsch,[64] and their co-workers. These studies include one using twice-daily fractionation, three using three daily fractions, and one using four daily fractions.

Only one of these studies—that of Shin and colleagues[247]—reported an improvement in survival using multiple daily fractionation. In their study, 69 patients were randomized to either 89 cGy whole-brain irradiation given three times daily followed by five 200 cGy fractions on consecutive days to a limited volume to a total dose of 6000 cGy or conventional fractionation given as 4000 cGy to the entire brain followed by a 2000 cGy boost. They reported an improvement in median survival from 27 to 49 weeks and an increase of 1-year survival rate from 20% to 45%. However, other studies have failed to confirm the results of Shin and colleagues.

The RTOG conducted a phase II study of hyperfractionation using 120 cGy twice daily to doses as high as 8160 cGy and of accelerated fractionation using 160cGy twice daily to doses of 4800 cGy and 5440 cGy.

Although the use of interstitial irradiation to treat brain tumors was mentioned by Pendergrass and colleagues[193] in 1922, the technique became practical only with the advent of stereotactic devices. The current methodology was pioneered by European groups[141,175,264] and refined by Gutin and co-workers at the University of California–San Francisco (UCSF). Leibel and Sheline[139] reported on 41 patients with recurrent tumors treated with a dose of 8000 cGy to 12000 cGy calculated at the periphery of the contrast-enhancing volume using 30 mCi to 50 mCi of implanted ^{125}I. Twenty-one patients had a favorable response lasting 5 to 53 months, whereas another six had stable disease for 4 to 48 months. The median survival for patients with recurrent glioblastoma was 35 weeks, and the median survival had not been reached for those with recurrent anaplastic astrocytomas.

Studies have been conducted using radiation modifiers in conjunction with radiation therapy to overcome the presumed hypoxia present in malignant gliomas. Hyperbaric oxygen therapy usually required the use of hypofractionated treatment schedules. Chang[47] reported a study of 38 patients treated with hyperbaric oxygen and radiation using fractionation schedules ranging from 3600 cGy given in 3 weeks to 6000 cGy given in 6 to 7 weeks. This was compared with 42 concurrent, historic controls treated in a similar fashion. Chang reported an improvement in 18-month survival rate from 10% to 28% and an increase of median survival from 31 to 38 weeks.

Randomized studies reported by Bleehen,[20] Urtasun,[271] and Nelson for the RTOG[178] and Deutsch for the BTCG[64] failed to show a significant improvement with the addition of misonidasole. The RTOG is continuing to investigate radiation modifiers in the treatment of malignant gliomas and is currently conducting a study with the halogenated pyrimidine IUDR.

Adjuvant Chemotherapy

The Brain Tumor Cooperative Group, Radiation Therapy Oncology Group, and Scandanavian Glioblastoma Study Group (SGSG)[131] investigated the use of adjuvant chemotherapy in conjunction with irradiation in the treatment of malignant gliomas. Such studies included BCNU, CCNU, procarbazine, bleomycin, and streptozotocin. Although early BTCG studies confirmed a significant increase in survival when radiation therapy was combined with surgery, only modest advantage has been documented for the addition of the nitrosourea, BCNU.[64] The RTOG has confirmed this advantage in patients under 60 years of age. In patients 40 to 60 years, 2-year survival rate increased from 8% to 23% with the addition of BCNU.[177] Other agents have not proved to be superior to BCNU as an adjuvant.

OPTIC GLIOMAS

Optic (nerve) glioma is less common in persons over 15 years of age(~15%)[298] than in children. The name is justified by the mixture of astrocytic-dominant[218] and oligodendroglial cell lines. The incidence is about 1% of all CNS tumors[218] A significant number of neurofibromatosis patients contract this tumor. A slight female preponderance has been noted. A genetic factor has been implicated.[113]

Optic glioma grows slowly. Symptoms often predate diagnosis by about 2 years.[17] The tumor often engages the optic chiasm (>50% of cases), and some exhibit extension into the hypothalamus.

Unilateral proptosis and vision defects indicate chiasmal involvement and the possibility of hypothalamic symptoms (endocrine defects and increased intracranial pressure).[116] Optic atrophy or nystagmus can be presenting symptoms.[7]

CT scanning and MRI examinations[149] offer excellent evidence for an anatomic diagnosis. Visual acuity and field examinations indicate severity and progress of defects. Tumor extension into the hypothalamus may cause enlargement of the sella.[116] A histopathologic analysis of resected tumor or biopsy is preferred for treatment evaluation. The adult type tends to show malignant features.[5]

In children, the similarity of many anterior optic glioma tumors to pilocytic astrocytoma[284] and meningioma[4] has caused this tumor group to be regarded as benign and resectable. Progressive symptoms and the prevalence of intracranial tumor extension have justified an attitudinal change toward postoperative adjuvant therapy, which is assuming a more prominent role in management. Chemotherapy is evolving as an alternative in young children.[212]

Completeness of surgical excision correlates with survival, but intracranial lesion surgery alone exhibits low survival figures.[216,267] Radiation therapy is indicated when intracranial or progressive symptoms are evident.[108,228] Bilateral temporal or multiportal beam geometries are preferred for intracranial lesions. A wedged-beam pair could be appropriate for intraorbital lesions. A dose of 5000 cGy in 180 cGy to 200 cGy fractions five times per week is generally recommended for adults.

The literature is clear about the positive value of modern radiation therapy for patients with optic glioma.[3,29,81,95,108,172,197,208,273,288] Long-term survival rates range from 80% to 100%. Improvement or stabilization of symptoms can be expected in a majority of patients. Recurrences are rare. Radiation therapy complications (calcification,[136] necrosis, and chiasmal damage) are rare except for endocrine disorders in children.[197,204] Reirradiation for recurrent disease may be advantageous.[80,288]

OLIGODENDROGLIOMAS

Oligodendrogliomas are relatively rare neoplasms, accounting for 1% to 5% of primary intracranial tumors in adults. Approximately 10% of oliogodendrogliomas occur in pediatric patients. Nearly all of the tumors are supratentorial, most frequently arising in the frontal cortex. Forty to seventy percent of tumors contain calcifications, visible on plain x-ray film or CT scan.[279]

Oligodendrogliomas frequently have a long natural history. Before the introduction of CT or MRI, patients commonly had neurologic symptoms for several years before diagnosis.[31] There is wide variation in histologic features, including the degree of cellularity, vascular proliferation, number of mitoses per high-power field, endothelial proliferation, and necrosis. Although the degree of tumor anaplasia is commonly remarked on in practice, it is unclear whether pathologic features can reliably predict prognosis. Several investigators have retrospectively reviewed histologic features and have shown some correlation with survival.[34,144,251] Focal necrosis correlated with poor prognosis in the series by Burger and colleagues.[34] Unfortunately, the grading systems have not been verified among different investigators. The A, B, C, and D system proposed by Smith and colleagues[251] was not useful in a recent series reviewed by Wallner and associates,[279] for whom most of the cases were clustered in grades B and C.

Oligodendrogliomas frequently appear as a minor component in predominantly astrocytic tumors. Similarly, tumors that are predominantly oligodendroglial commonly have a minor component of astrocytoma. Mixed tumors seem to carry the same prognosis as pure tumors of the predominant cell type.[251,279]

Recurrent oligodendrogliomas frequently show histologic progression to high-grade astrocytomas. In the series by Wallner and associates,[279] 60% (six of ten) of recurrent tumors were composed wholly or in part of anaplastic astrocytoma or glioblastoma multiforme.[279] It is unknown whether the astrocytic components were present but not detected in the original tumor or whether they arose by metaplasia during the course of tumor recurrence.

As in low-grade astrocytomas, oligodendrogliomas are usually poorly demarcated from surrounding neural tissue. Total excision is not usually possible,[144,279] suggesting that effective adjuvant therapy is needed. Table 23-9 summarizes three recent retrospective patient series. Median survival increased from 23 to 60 months in those without adjuvant irradiation to 38 to 132 months in those with irradiation[31,144,279]; some studies are highly suggestive of a beneficial effect of postoperative irradiation.

Patterns of failure for oligodendrogliomas have not been well studied. Four of five autopsies at the University of California–San Francisco showed failure only in the immediate vicinity of the primary site.[279]

In general, patients should receive partial-brain irradiation, treating the original tumor bed and surrounding edema plus a 3 cm to 4 cm margin, identified by CT or MRI scan. If the tumor is not well visualized on constrast-enhanced CT scan, an MRI with gadolinium enhancement should be obtained to better define the target volume. A wedged-beam pair field arrangement is preferable over bilateral opposed portals, to spare as much normal brain parenchyma as possible from high-dose irradiation. The target volume should be treated at 180 cGy to 200 cGy daily to a total dose of 5500 cGy to 6000 cGy. The field may be reduced to a 1 cm to 2 cm margin around the tumor volume after 4500 cGy to 5000 cGy.

Spinal seeding by oligodendrogliomas is unusual, even with high-grade tumors. Only one of 40 patients in the UCSF series developed seeding following partial-brain irradiation, and that patient had failure at the primary site also. Prophylactic spinal irradiation is unnecessary.[279]

Data are limited on the efficacy of chemotherapy for treatment of oligodendrogliomas. Investigators at the University of Western Ontario reported a partial or complete response in eight of eight patients treated with chemotherapy, six of whom received a combination of procarbazine, CCNU, and vincristine.[42]

MENINGIOMAS

Meningiomas represent 15% to 20% of primary intracranial neoplasms.[25,56,202] They arise from the arachnoidal cells, dural fibroblasts, and pial cells that form the meninges.[215] The most common sites of presentation are the parasagittal-falx region, cerebral convexities, and the sphenoid ridge.[287] The majority of meningiomas are benign, slow-growing, well-circumscribed neoplasms, but they may invade surrounding dura, bone, and

TABLE 23–9
Summary of Recent Reports on the Value of Postoperative Irradiation for Oligodendroglioma

		MEDIAN SURVIVAL		
AUTHOR	TREATMENT DATES	SURGERY ALONE	SURGERY + RADIATION THERAPY	*P* VALUE
Lindegaard[144]	1953–1977	23 mo (62 pts)	38 mo (107 pts)	0.039
Bullard[31]	1940–1983	52 mo (35 pts)	62 mo (36 pts)	0.67
Wallner[279]	1940–1983	60 mo (11 pts)	132 mo (14 pts)	0.092

pts: patients

extracranial soft tissues. They compress rather than infiltrate adjacent brain.[161,215] Meningiomas are occasionally multicentric, especially when associated with von Recklinghausen's disease.[215] They are uncommon in children (see Table 23-2).

Although benign meningiomas exhibit a variety of histologic appearances, there is little relation among histology, biologic behavior, and prognosis.[161,287] The syncytial, transitional, and fibroblastic subtypes account for over 90% of meningiomas.[161] Approximately 8% of meningiomas are malignant.[287] Clinical and pathologic criteria for malignancy include rapid recurrence after initial surgical resection, local invasiveness of the brain, atypical histologic features, high mitotic index, and metastases to extracranial sites.[150,268,292] Included within the classification of malignant meningiomas are the hemangiopericytic variant of angioblastic meningioma, anaplastic meningiomas, and papillary meningiomas.[292]

Meningiomas grow at a slow rate. After initial surgery, the average interval to recurrence is approximately 4 years.[123,167,194,265] Consequently, survival and recurrence rates are difficult to assess without long-term follow-up.[10] The location of the lesion, extent of surgical resection, and histopathologic features of the tumor (benign or malignant) are the most important determinants of prognosis.[82]

Complete surgical extirpation offers the highest probability of tumor control. However, the size and location of the tumor often limit the neurosurgeon's ability to perform a complete resection.[265] Lesions of the convexity and parasagittal-falx regions are most amenable to total resection.[10] In contrast, it may be difficult to excise tumors along the base of the skull because of their poor surgical access and their proximity to critical neurovascular structures.[96] The percentage with which a total resection can be achieved varies from 38% to 83% in reported series.[2,10,46,167,169,265,296] The wide variation in these figures probably reflects differences in referral patterns, operative technique, and surgical aggressiveness. In the series reported by Barbaro and colleagues,[10] only two of 51 patients with completely excised meningiomas followed up for 5 to 15 years had recurrences, and neither patient died of tumor. Mirimanoff and colleagues[169] found that the actuarial risk of recurrence after total resection was 7% at 5 years and 32% at 15 years. Because of the low risk of recurrence after complete resection, further adjunctive therapy is not recommended.

The risk of recurrence is substantially greater after subtotal resection without adjuvant therapy and varies from 30% to 60%.[2,10,167,169,265] In the series reported by Luk and coworkers,[150] the 5-year survival rate for those after complete excision was 88% compared with 48% for those after incomplete excision.

Several recent reports suggest that the addition of postoperative radiation after partial resection may prolong the interval to recurrence, prevent tumor regrowth in some cases, and improve survival rate.[10,21,82,150,194,265] Barbaro and coworkers[10] retrospectively compared 54 patients who underwent subtotal resection and radiation therapy with a control group of 30 patients who underwent subtotal resection alone. Sixty percent of nonirradiated patients developed recurrence, whereas 32% of patients who received radiation therapy had recurrences. The recurrence-free interval was significantly longer in the irradiated group; their median time to recurrence was 125 months compared with 66 months in the nonirradiated group ($P < 0.05$). Taylor and associates[265] also found that recurrence of meningioma was significantly reduced by the addition of radiation therapy: 15% of patients treated with subtotal excision and postoperative irradiation had recurrences, whereas 69% relapsed after subtotal excision alone ($P = 0.01$). The 10-year survival rate was 81% for patients who received combined treatment and 49% for nonirradiated patients. The actuarial probability of local control achieved by the use of radiation therapy after subtotal resection was similar to that observed for total excision.

An area of controversy is whether to treat patients with radiation therapy immediately after initial subtotal resection or when signs of disease progression appear. Some investigators suggest that patients with benign meningiomas do equally well with either option.[82,253] Others have found that initial postoperative irradiation is the preferable treatment approach because recurrence has an adverse influence on outcome and because many patients who have recurrence after initial subtotal excision alone may not be salvaged at the time of recurrence.[44,265,287,296]

In cases in which only a biopsy can be performed and in which more aggressive surgery is not an option, radiation therapy may relieve symptoms and substantially decrease the rate of tumor progression.[21,44,82,250] In the elderly or in patients whose overall medical condition is poor, postoperative irradiation or even initial surgery may be deferred until there is evidence of symptomatic progression.[265]

The target volume for radiation therapy is generally restricted to a 2 cm margin beyond the tumor volume defined by CT or MRI scan and modified by the neurosurgeon's description of the site of residual tumor. More generous margins may be necessary for extensive skull base meningiomas.[194] Multiple fields with wedge filters or rotational fields are used to maximally spare normal brain tissue. A dose of 5500 cGy in daily fractions of 180 cGy to 200 cGy, 5 days per week, is generally recommended. The target volume for malignant meningiomas is more generous (3 cm to 4 cm margin) than that used for benign lesions, and the dose is increased to 600 cGy.

The few reports that describe the outcome of patients with malignant meningiomas suggest that these tumors behave in an aggressive fashion.[44,46,82,87,123,150,253,268,296] Chan and Thompson[47] found that the mean survival of six patients treated with surgery alone was 7.2 months compared with 5.1 years for 12 patients treated with surgery and postoperative irradiation. In the series reported by Solan and Kramer,[253] only two of seven patients with malignant tumors treated by surgery and radiation therapy remained alive; four of the five deaths occurred within 9 months of treatment. Table 23-10 summarizes the results of six series reported in the literature according to extent of resection and records whether postoperative irradiation was given.[44,82,87,150,253,287] Overall, 26 (49%) of the 53 patients had recurrences. The results of these small series indicate that complete resection and postoperative

TABLE 23–10
Malignant Meningioma: Results According to Treatment

TREATMENT	NO. OF PATIENTS	NO. OF RECURRENCES
CR alone	12	4
CR + RT	8	1
SR alone	6	6
SR + RT	27	15
Total	53	26

Data from references 44, 82, 87, 150, 253, and 287
CR: complete resection; SR; subtotal resection; RT: radiation therapy.

irradiation afford the best opportunity for tumor control and that patients with malignant meningiomas should be offered postoperative irradiation regardless of the extent of resection.[44,150]

Preliminary data suggest a role for interstitial brachytherapy in patients with meningiomas who develop localized recurrences after surgery and radiation therapy. Gutin and colleagues[96,138] intraoperatively implanted low-activity ^{125}I sources into 11 patients with recurrent benign or malignant tumors that were primarily located at the base of the skull. Nine of the 11 patients remained locally controlled for 2 to 77 months after implantation.

EPENDYMOMAS

Ependymomas account for 1% to 8% of primary intracranial tumors. Two thirds of ependymomas occur in children. Approximately 50% of ependymomas occur in the posterior fossa, arising in the midline of the fourth ventricle.[173] Supratentorial tumors are generally paraventricular. The lesions are easily visualized on CT scan and commonly exhibit calcifications and inhomogeneous contrast enhancements.[263]

Histologic classification of ependymomas has been an area of controversy for several decades. The first widely accepted grading system was proposed by Kernohan,[121] with the degree of malignancy increasing from grade I to grade IV. Because the tumors are so uncommon, it has been practical to maintain four separate grades. Investigators have generally combined grade I and grade II tumors as "low grade" and grade III and grade IV tumors as "high grade." Although the prognosis is generally better for low-grade tumors, marked variability is seen from series to series in the percentage of high-grade tumors and the prognosis by grade.[11,122,173,283] The variability probably reflects the lack of uniformity in applying a grading system for these tumors. In 1983, WHO[209] published a simplified grading system, with less malignant-appearing tumors termed "ependymoma." The WHO criteria for anaplastic ependymoma are subjective (nuclear atypia, increased mitoses, and so on). Therefore, considerable disagreement will probably still exist among pathologists. Reproducible histologic grading is important because higher-grade lesions generally have a poorer prognosis[23,51,122,225,242] and disseminate more frequently through the CNS, possibly requiring more generous radiation fields.

Earlier surgical series showed that about 25% of patients are cured with surgical resection alone, without adjuvant therapy.[207] Despite the fact that some patients may be cured with surgery alone, virtually all patients currently receive postoperative irradiation. In patients who receive postoperative irradiation, the extent of surgical resection has not consistently influenced survival, so that aggressive debulking may not be justified.[11,137,225,239]

Special attention should be directed to the upper cervical spinal cord for posterior fossa tumors, because 10% to 30% of such tumors extend down through the foramen magnum to the upper cervical spine.[239,283] All patients with posterior fossa tumors should have a myelogram. CSF cytology should be obtained, although the significance of a positive result is uncertain.

It is well established from retrospective series that irradiation prolongs survival for patients with ependymoma.[11,195] Phillips and associates[195] showed a 5-year survival rate of 87% in patients treated with surgery and postoperative irradiation compared with 10% for those patients given low-dose or no postoperative irradiation. A dose response is evident; tumor doses of 4500 cGy or more are more likely to control disease.[122,195]

The major controversies in treatment of ependymomas involve the use of elective spinal irradiation and the use of whole-brain *versus* partial-brain irradiation. The rationale for spinal irradiation dates back to an autopsy series published in 1949 by Svien and colleagues,[262] which showed a 32% incidence of tumor failure (six of 19) in the spine. However, all patients studied had died of tumor, and the autopsy findings represented the end stage of recurrent disease. Subsequent reports have shown a much lower incidence of spinal failures.[130,239,283] In general, tumors that show a propensity for failure in the spine are high-grade lesions and those in the posterior fossa.[23,122,242,262] Several recent series with adequate follow-up show an incidence of spinal failure of as high as 20% for high-grade posterior fossa lesions to 2% for low-grade supratentorial lesions.[23,122,242,262] The importance of spinal seeding is further obscured by the fact that patients who develop spinal seeding nearly always also have tumor recurrence in the primary site.[154,225,239,283] One important study has substantially influenced the treatment policies of ependymomas over the last several years.[225] Patients with low-grade tumors survived longer when prophylactic spinal irradiation was added to whole-brain irradiation. There are several potential problems in the study's conclusions due to the retrospective nature of the work:

Patients treated with limited field irradiation tended to be treated in the early part of the studies, before introduction of CT or MRI imaging. A portion of their tumors could have been missed when partial brain fields were designed.

Patients who developed spinal seeding almost always also had failure at the primary site, so that it is unclear whether prevention of spinal seeding with prophylactic irradiation would have improved their overall prognosis.[239,283]

The number of patients reported on was small; there were only 17 patients with low-grade tumors (eight and nine in the partial- and whole-brain therapy groups, respectively).

A number of other investigators have shown that whole-brain irradiation is not superior to partial-brain irradiation for high-grade or low-grade tumors.[239,283] Furthermore, these recent series have shown comparable long-term survival rates without using prophylactic spinal irradiation.

Treatment recommendations for ependymoma have varied widely. Most investigators agree that patients with low-grade tumors should be treated with partial-brain irradiation only, because substantial evidence exists that these tumors are far more likely to fail at the primary site than in other areas of the brain.[225,239,283] If possible, wedged-beam pair field arrangements should be used, to spare as much cerebral cortex as possible from full-dose irradiation. Whether the entire ventricular system should be included in the treatment field is not certain. It seems reasonable to do so in cases in which the tumor has invaded the ventricular system. High-grade supratentorial tumors should be treated with cranial irradiation only, because the incidence of spinal seeding seems low. Either high-grade or low-grade tumors could be treated with partial- or whole-brain irradiation; little strong data exist either way.

Partial-brain irradiation for ependymomas may be preferable to whole-brain irradiation, because the survival advantage for those treated with whole-brain irradiation is probably small or nonexistent, and the long-term morbidity of whole-brain irradiation is probably large. Partial-brain doses of 5500 cGy to 6000 cGy should be used for adults, and 4500 cGy to 5000 cGy for children. Prophylactic spinal irradiation should be considered in high-grade infratentorial tumors, although its contribution to survival is unclear. Areas of gross spinal disease should be boosted with an additional 1000 cGy.

The role of chemotherapy in treatment of ependymoma is unclear. Partial responses to various agents have been reported. A recent randomized trial conducted by the Children's Cancer Study Group studied the effect of chemotherapy (CCNU, vincristine, and prednisone) added to conventional irradiation. No survival advantage was seen.[137]

CRANIOPHARYNGIOMAS

A craniopharyngioma (and/or suprasellar epidermoid cyst) is an intrasellar or suprasellar tumor that grows slowly and causes mechanical pressure on the surrounding brain structures. It makes up only a small percentage of all intracranial tumors.[217]

When it is intrasellar, craniopharyngioma has been associated with Rathke's cleft cyst (between the adenohypophysis and the neurohypophysis), a remnant from the developing posterior part of the oral cavity or its duct to the pituitary. The tumor is therefore more related to jaw or oral cavity than to brain. Its intracranial growth in adults justifies its inclusion in this chapter.

Suprasellar extension gives rise to symptoms from the tumor. Pressure anteriorly compromises the optic chiasm, inferiorly compromises the pituitary, and superiorly compromises the third ventricle and the interventricular foramina. Respectively, visual, hormone, and cerebrospinal fluid circulation abnormalities may lead to the diagnosis.

Histologically, craniopharyngioma can be solid and cystic, with cyst fluid rich in cholesterol crystals.[217] Usually it presents a capsule to surrounding brain but can infiltrate together with gliotic elements. The cysts are lined with squamous stratified epithelium, the solid parts with columnar cells. Calcifications are common.

Craniopharyngiomas exhibit a small growth fraction, similar to dermoids and chordomas.[52] They are more common in the younger population and show a small male preponderance.[304] Mechanical effects on the sella and calcification make it possible to diagnose from plain radiographs.

Radical surgery is considered by some[165] as the therapy of choice, but tumor control is not ensured. Recurrence indicates a worse prognosis.[290] Radiation therapy[152] after limited surgery is suggested to give a better 5-year survival rate (75% to 100%)[223] and tumor control with fewer complications.[290] Radiation therapy alone is an acceptable alternative for inoperable patients.[43]

The recommended dose is 5000 cGy to 5500 cGy in 180 cGy fractions with limited fields, preferably multiportals. Surgery can be used for salvage. No data are available on chemotherapy. Complications include visual defects, but they are rare. Hormonal deficiencies arising after therapy can be supplemented.

PINEAL TUMORS

The WHO classification subdivides pineal tumors into pineocytomas, pineoblastomas, and germinomas. The two former tumors are rare, and the incidence of germinoma is <1% of all intracranial tumors.[305]

There has been controversy about the histologic relationship between pineal and other tumors. For example, the pineocytoma resembles the pilocytic astrocytoma, and the pineoblastoma is identical with the medulloblastoma. The germinoma resembles the seminoma of the testis[86] and is sometimes referred to as *pinealoma.*

Little is known about the *pineocytoma* in relation to radiation therapy. The tumor is a so-called one-celled tumor histologically; it can exist as a grade I to grade III tumor; and it may be mixed with germinoma in older literature. A recent small series from UCSF indicates that pineocytoma can recur and disseminate after radiation therapy.[67]

Pineoblastoma is rare, soft, and poorly differentiated (grade IV) and looks like medulloblastoma. It may infiltrate inferiorly in the brain stem and anteriorly to the foramina of Monro. It can seed into the ventricular system and is reported to be sensitive to radiation therapy.

The *germinoma,* formerly called the pinealoma, resembles the seminoma, and is a two-celled pattern tumor because of infiltrating lymphocytes. Zulch[305] argues for pinealoma as a separate entity. This tumor is usually found in young patients and exhibits a male preponderance.The tumor displaces the normal brain and exerts pressure that causes the symptoms. It is known to grow anteriorly to the suprasellar region and sometimes only in that location, thereby the name *suprasellar germinoma.*[86] Like seminoma, it is radiosensitive.

Common symptoms of pineal tumors are visual disturbances because of the pressure on the superior colliculi and the posterior parts of the lateral geniculate nuclei, endocrinologic signs (especially diabetes insipidus), and third ventricle obstruction. Parinaud's ophthalmoplegia (paralysis of conjugate upward movement of the eyes without paralysis of convergence) is a characteristic sign.

Affected patients are typically treated with biopsy, shunt if necessary, and radiation therapy. In general, the neurosurgeon is currently more likely to perform a biopsy or resection[256] compared with an earlier time,[305] when techniques were less developed and significant risks of complications were encountered.

As a group, pineal tumors are regarded as radiosensitive,[223] but some controversy exists about how to treat them with radiation therapy,[50, 146, 245] because of varying opinions regarding seeding incidence (8% to 37%).[260, 286]

Some authors (Lindstadt and associates[146]) favor local irradiation because of low incidence of seeding. They recommend craniospinal irradiation when tumor is spilled at surgery, when CSF is positive for tumor cytology, or when subependymal or subarachnoid metastasis signs are present. Others favor craniospinal irradiation up front even in cytology-negative patients when the tumor presents along ventricular walls or in suprasellar locations.[106, 127, 260]

One approach[127] for undiagnosed lesions is to irradiate locally the known lesion to 2000 cGy and to verify the effect with CT scanning. If lesser enhancement is evident, this is interpreted to mean that the tumor is more malignant and radiosensitive, therefore justifying craniospinal irradiation up to tolerance dose.

There is a consensus on total dose requirements because lower doses have been found to compromise tumor control.[260] Thus, the tumor dose should approximate 4500 cGy to 5000 cGy in 180 cGy fractions for adults with dose reduction in children. If large fields or craniospinal irradiation is also used, a total dose of at least 4000 cGy should be given to the brain with subarachnoid space and 2500 cGy to 3000 cGy to the spinal axis. These doses are believed to eradicate microscopic disease, although valid data are lacking.[127]

Survival and tumor control figures for pineal tumors in adults are scarce. Most recurrences are local,[28] indicating that minimal necessary dose levels have not been reached, at least not for some of these tumor cases. A few cases recur with seeding outside the original tumor volume.

A 5-year survival rate of up to 60% has been reported for pineal tumors as a group.[127] Higher figures have been given for the suprasellar germinoma type.[260,286] Adjuvant chemotherapy may have justification but has not been tried sufficiently to warrant an opinion.

Finally, the pineal body also can harbor astrocytomas of all grades, teratomas (for which the pineal is the most common intracranial site), and, more rarely, cysts, meningiomas, and melanomas.[221] The treatment naturally has to be adjusted according to the tumor type.

PRIMARY CENTRAL NERVOUS SYSTEM LYMPHOMAS

Primary lymphoma of the central nervous system accounts for 0.3% to 1.5% of intracranial neoplasms.[114,301] A variety of terms have been applied to these tumors, including microglioma, perithelial sarcoma, and perivascular sarcoma. This reflects the controversy regarding their histogenesis.[292] It is now recognized that these tumors are of lymphoid origin and that the neoplastic cells are similar to those in non-Hodgkins's lymphoma arising outside the CNS.[110,114,252] The majority of CNS lymphomas are classified as diffuse histiocytic and diffuse undifferentiated lymphomas in the Rappaport System or immunoblastic, small noncleaved and large noncleaved lymphomas according to the Working Formulation System.[100] CNS lymphomas are predominantly of B-cell origin,[266,272] and only a few cases of T-cell lymphoma (mostly primary leptomeningeal tumors) have been reported.[91,232]

The incidence of CNS lymphoma appears to be increasing.[72] This, in part, reflects the association of primary CNS lymphomas with inherited and acquired immunodeficiency syndrome (AIDS). However, the incidence is also increasing within the immunologically normal population.[72] CNS lymphoma is found at autopsy in 5.5% of patients with AIDS and represents 50% of all lymphomas affecting both AIDS patients and renal transplant recipients.[18,289] An etiologic association between CNS lymphoma and the Epstein-Barr virus has been suggested both in immunocompromised and nonimmunodeficient patients.[103,211]

Central nervous system lymphomas occur most frequently in adults, with a peak incidence in the sixth decade[176]; the age of onset is lower in the immunosuppressed population.[233,252] CNS lymphomas most frequently arise in the paraventricular supratentorial region, but they may also occur in the cerebellum and the brain stem. Rarely, they present only in the leptomeninges[151,170] or spinal cord. The tumor is multicentric at diagnosis in 16% to 60% of patients[139]; multiple diffusely enhancing paraventricular masses are characteristic findings on CT or MRI studies.[61] CNS lymphomas tend to infiltrate extensively along the corpus callosum or other deep white matter tracts. Leptomeningeal seeding or subependymal spread is present in approximately 30% of patients at diagnosis and in nearly all patients at autopsy.[62,231] Malignant cells are found in the CSF in at least 20% of patients. [62,100,114,203] Extraneural involvement is rare.[101,114,176].

Ocular lymphoma is found in association with CNS lymphoma in 15% to 20% of patients.[61,198] Ocular involvement either results from direct extension from the brain or reflects the multicentricity of this tumor.[201] Of patients with ocular lymphoma, 50% to 67% already have or will subsequently develop CNS lymphoma.[62,153,210] The time from onset of ocular symptoms to the appearance of CNS disease ranges from 2 to 94 months (median 9 months).[62,210] Because of this association, a thorough ophthalmologic evaluation should be performed on all patients with CNS lymphoma.

Primary CNS lymphomas are clinically aggressive. Although limited to one "extranodal" site, their biologic behavior is comparable to that of disseminated high-grade systemic lymphomas.[62] The prognosis for patients receiving supportive care alone is poor. Survival time from the onset of symptoms to death ranges from 1.8 to 3.3 months.[101,114] Corticosteroids may cause transient shrinkage or complete disappearance of tumor masses on neuroimaging studies in a significant proportion of patients.[62] Corticosteroid administration has been used as a "diagnostic test" in patients who are not candidates for biopsy. A biopsy performed after cortisoteroid treatment may reveal nondiagnostic tissue.[62]

Survival after surgical resection (without adjunctive therapy) ranges from 0.9 to 4.6 months.[101,114] Because of the multifocal and infiltrative nature of this tumor, the extent of resection does not influence survival. This observation has led to the use of stereotactic needle biopsy combined with immunochemical analysis as the initial diagnostic procedure when CNS lymphoma is suspected.[176]

Radiation therapy usually results in prompt clinical and radiographic improvement. However, the duration of response is short, lasting for an average of 12 to 24 months,[90] and local recurrence generally ensues.[139] The median survival after treatment with radiation therapy is from 10 to 18 months[15,61,84,101,114,147,168,176,179,203,224,294] with a 5-year disease-free survival rate of only about 3%.[139] Thus, although radiation therapy prolongs survival, its curative potential is limited. Because of the multifocal nature of CNS lymphomas, their predilection to infiltrate the leptomeninges, and their tendency to be more widespread than indicated by neuroimaging studies, the entire intracranial contents are encompassed within the treatment fields.

Several reports suggest that a direct relationship exists between radiation dose and tumor control. Pollack and colleagues[198] observed that patients treated with doses of 4000 cGy to 5000 cGy to the whole brain survived significantly longer than patients who received smaller doses to the whole brain. Furthermore, Murray and associates[176] found that patients who received 5000 cGy or more to the primary tumor site survived significantly longer than those treated with less than 5000 cGy. The RTOG recently completed a prospective phase II study in which patients were given 4000 cGy to the whole brain followed by an additional 2000 cGy to the primary lesion. The median survival of 41 evaluable patients was 11.6 months. Forty-eight percent of patients survived 1 year, and 28% survived 2 years. Age and Karnofsky performance status were important predictors of outcome; patients who were 60 years or older or who had a performance status of less than 70 had an especially poor prognosis.[179] The survival rates according to age and performance status are shown in Table 23-11. These results provide convincing evidence that more aggressive therapeutic regimens are needed.

Based on available data, it is generally recommended that patients with solitary lesions receive 4000 cGy to 5000 cGy to the whole brain supplemented by an additional 1000 cGy to 1500 cGy to the primary tumor site. Because of the high incidence of ocular involvement and the efficacy of orbital irradiation in affected patients, inclusion of the posterior orbits within the

TABLE 23–11
CNS Lymphomas: Survival by Age and Performance Status

SIGNIFICANCE FACTOR	1-YEAR SURVIVAL (%)	SURVIVAL MEDIAN (MONTHS)	P VALUE
Age			
<60 yr	23.1	70	0.001
≥60 yr	7.6	36	
Karnofsky performance status			
70–100	21.1	69	<0.001
40–60	5.6	25	

(Data from Nelson DF, Martz KL, Bonner H, et al: J Neurosurg, submitted for publication)[179]

field of whole-brain irradiation to minimize the risk of ocular recurrence has been recommended.[198] In patients with ocular involvement, 4000 cGy in 4.5 weeks frequently results in improved visual acuity unless extensive retinal damage has occurred.

Although craniospinal axis (CSA) irradiation may be of value in patients with spinal cord or primary leptomeningeal lymphoma, data are insufficient to evaluate the efficacy of this approach in other patients.[168,203] Because most patients, including those who develop spinal seeding, fail at the primary site, it is unlikely that prophylactic CSA irradiation will improve survival. Some investigators have used CSF cytology as a basis for selection for CSA irradiation. However, the clinical significance of positive or negative cytology has not been established.[139] Moreover, in this situation spinal irradiation has been replaced by intrathecal chemotherapy.

There has been considerable enthusiasm regarding the use of chemotherapy for CNS lymphomas. This interest has been generated by the demonstration of complete or partial responses in several small series of patients with recurrent disease and the suggestion that CNS lymphomas are disseminated throughout the nervous system at the time of initial diagnosis.[61] High-dose intravenous methotrexate with leucovorin rescue,[1,74] high-dose intravenous cytosine arabinoside,[85] intrathecal methotrexate[1,102] and multiagent chemotherapy alone[117,259] or with osmotic blood-brain barrier modifications[184] have produced objective responses. Although experience with any single regimen is limited, the data suggest that the combination of chemotherapy and irradiation is more effective than radiation therapy alone.

Loeffler and colleagues[148] reported a median survival of 44 months for five patients treated with combined therapy, whereas the median survival of five patients treated with radiation therapy alone was 14 months. Although different chemotherapeutic regimens were used, four of the five patients who were alive at the time of reporting received intrathecal methotrexate as part of their treatment program. Stewart and coworkers[258] reported on a patient receiving a combination of cyclophosphamide, doxorubicin, vincristine, and dexamethasone (CHOD) together with radiation therapy. Kawakami and associates[117] found that a similar regimen was superior to other combinations.

Yahalom and DeAngelis[295] treated 15 patients on a protocol of intravenous and intra-Ommaya methotrexate followed by whole-brain irradiation to 4000 cGy in 4 weeks with an additional 1500 cGy boost to the tumor area and postirradiation intravenous cytosine arabinoside (cytarabine). Fourteen patients achieved a complete response, whereas only one patient progressed in the brain. At the time of reporting, 12 (80%) patients were alive with a median follow-up of 24 months (range, 9 to 36 months), and ten (67%) were free of recurrence. The 3-year actuarial survival rate was 71%.

Several cooperative groups are conducting prospective phase I/II studies integrating chemotherapy into the radiotherapeutic treatment of non-AIDS patients with primary CNS lymphoma. In the RTOG trial, patients initially receive two cycles of CHOD chemotherapy. Patients who respond or have stable disease on CT scan receive a third cycle of chemotherapy before cranial irradiation. If disease progresses after the second cycle, radiation therapy is begun without further chemotherapy. Patients with tumor cells in the CSF at the time of diagnosis also receive intrathecal methotrexate. The North Central Cancer Treatment Group and the Mayo Clinic are conducting a similar study except that patients receive intravenous cytarabine after cranial irradiation. In the CALGB trial, high-dose methotrexate and leucovorin rescue are given with CHOD before radiation therapy. These and other studies[61] will more clearly define the role of chemotherapy in the treatment of CNS lymphoma.

The prognosis of AIDS patients with CNS lymphoma is much poorer than in non-AIDS-related CNS lymphoma. The median survival time is as short as 2 months in some series, and patients frequently die of other causes.[68,83,252] A dose of 4000 cGy in 3 to 4 weeks to the whole brain results in tumor regression and symptomatic palliation. Intrathecal methotrexate may be used when tumor cells are found in the cerebrospinal fluid. These patients are generally unable to tolerate systemic chemotherapy.

MEDULLOBLASTOMAS

By definition medulloblastoma is located in the posterior fossa and originates in the cerebellar vermis (roof of the fourth ventricle). Older patients may exhibit the tumor in the cerebellar hemispheres. It is often referred to as *cerebellar medulloblastoma.* WHO recognizes two variants: desmoplastic medulloblastoma and medullomyoblastoma, incorporating fibrous and striated muscle components, respectively. Medulloblastoma is part of the undifferentiated PNET (primitive neuroectodermal tumor) group of tumors. A special variant is medulloepithelioma, which is rare, supratentorial, and highly malignant with necrosis and hemorrhage.

The tumor arises out of abnormal persistence of the fetal granular layer of the cerebellum.[219]

Medulloblastoma represents 4% to 8%[219,303] of all primary

brain tumors and 25% of the intracranial tumors in children. The peak incidence occurs when the child is between 5 and 10 years of age,[9] with fewer cases in adolescence. It is rarely encountered in adulthood. The literature contains suggestions of correlations of medulloblastoma with polio vaccination and family history of brain tumors as well as other tumors.[219]

The histology of medulloblastoma is characteristically very cellular, with carrot-shaped cells, high nucleus/cytoplasm ratio, antigenic features similar to pineoblastoma, chromosome features similar to retinoblastoma, and high labeling index (10% to 30%).[219]

Presenting symptoms of those with medulloblastoma are related to cerebellum and CSF obstruction. The diagnosis of a midline CT-enhanced lesion in the posterior fossa is almost pathognomonic.

Surgery and postoperative megavoltage radiation therapy both are the only primary treatment modalities with prognostic significance.[139,163] Survival for adults is dependent on optimal surgical tumor removal and at least 5000 cGy of radiation therapy to the primary tumor location, 4000 cGy to intracranial contents, and 2500 cGy to 3000 cGy to the spinal cord. Lower doses may be advisable for younger children.[22] Chemotherapy may improve survival.

The cribriform plate in the anterior fossa is an important location to include in the radiation volume because recurrences have been noted there, probably because of inappropriate concern for blocking the ocular lens out of the field.[115]

Recurrence of medulloblastoma usually is local and fatal. The diagnosis of spread into the CSF space may be aided by the finding of elevated spermidine or putrescine in CSF.[159] The cerebrospinal fluid spread incidence is 10% to 15% at diagnosis,[189] but metastatic disease has been noted in more than 50% of autopsies of patients who have died of recurrent disease.[219] Systemic metastatic incidence is about 5%, especially to lymph nodes and bone. Shunt procedures have been suggested as a cause.

Improved survival for patients with medulloblastoma coincides with the implementation of postsurgical megavoltage radiation therapy.[187] Survival depends on extent of tumor removal and radiation dose given. A 5-year survival rate of 40% to 80% and a 10-year survival rate of 40% to 50% have been reported.[139] Removal in excess of 75% and at least 5000 cGy gross tumor dose is said to yield a 5- and 10-year survival rate of 75%.[219]

NEURILEMOMAS

Neurilemomas arise from Schwann cells of the myelin sheath of peripheral nerves, most frequently of the eighth cranial nerve as it enters the internal acoustic meatus. These tumors are histologically distinct from neurofibromas. Neurilemomas occasionally arise from other cranial nerves.[281] The tumors have been referred to variously as acoustic neuroma, schwannoma, neurinoma, and perineural fibroblastoma. They are relatively common, accounting for 6% to 10% of primary brain tumors in adults. The only known predisposing factor is hereditary neurofibromatosis, although the majority of patients with neurilemoma do not have neurofibromatosis.

Histologically, neurilemomas are composed of intermixed areas of tightly packed Schwann cells (Antoni A pattern), alternating with areas of loosely packed pleomorphic cells (Antoni B pattern). Most tumors appear to be histologically benign. In the series by Wallner and colleagues,[282] approximately 5% of cases were more densely cellular and pleomorphic. The more malignant-appearing tumors did not tend to recur more frequently (unpublished observation).

Acoustic neurilemomas arise in the cerebellar pontine angle and can be technically difficult to excise, but advances in imaging and microsurgery have increased the resectability rate. At the University of California–San Francisco, the percentage of tumors that were totally resected has increased from 50% to over 80% over the last 3 decades.[282] In this series, only two of 63 patients who had total resection (described in the operative note) had recurrences.[282] Patients who have an aggressive debulking of tumor also remain free of disease progression for a prolonged time. The patients operated on at UCSF were subclassified as having (1) near-total resection (NTR), defined as removal of 90% to 99% of the tumor, as judged by the surgeon at the time of operation (patients with NTR had only a 7% recurrence rate without adjuvant irradiation) or (2) subtotal resection (STR) when less than 90% of their tumor was resected and had a far higher recurrence rate. Six of thirteen patients (46%) with STR and no postoperative irradiation had recurrences, with an actuarial recurrence rate of 59% at 15 years. Patients who received postoperative radiation following subtotal resection had an actuarial recurrence rate of only 6% at 15 years ($P = 0.01$). Three patients treated with radiation after biopsy alone were without disease progression at 7 to 14 years after therapy. All tumor recurrences were in the immediate area of the tumor bed.

Patients with subtotal resection should be considered for postoperative irradiation with fields to cover the tumor bed plus a 2 cm margin and doses of 5000 cGy to 5500 cGy, delivered at 180 cGy to 200 cGy per day.

Preoperative irradiation has been used effectively to diminish excessive vascularity of large tumors, facilitating total resection.[112,282] Stereotactic radiosurgery has been used in some cases for these lesions.[186]

Acoustic neurilemomas are frequently slow-growing and often occur in elderly patients. Some patients may remain neurologically stable for long periods of time with therapy.[53] When total excision is not possible, radiation may be given immediately or the patient may be evaluated at regular intervals with CT scanning and irradiated only if tumor progression is demonstrated. Although this policy spares some patients the expense and side effects of irradiation, it could be detrimental to others, because tumors that progress may be less likely to respond to irradiation than if the treatment had been instituted earlier.

VASCULAR MALFORMATIONS

Tumors of vascular origin (see also Chap. 74) in the nervous system constitute a variety of malformations.[222]

Arteriovenous malformation (AVM) is a mass of abnormal arteries and veins,[304] characterized by hemorrhage as a symptom, and is best diagnosed by angiography, where feeding and draining vessels can be located. Surgical excision is the preferred treatment; embolization is sometimes indicated. For surgically inaccessible lesions, radiation therapy is a good therapeutic option[269] because of the cumulative risk of rebleeding, which is estimated to be 3% per year.[291]

Arteriovenous malformation may be irradiated with local fractionated regimens up to about 5000 cGy in conventional 180 cGy to 200 cGy fractions,[107,293] with radiosurgery (small volume, multiportal, 1500 cGy to 2500 cGy in single or few fractions, linear accelerator[229]) or with Leksell's "gamma-knife" (ste-

TABLE 23–12
Rare Primary Brain Tumors That May Require Radiation Therapy if Incompletely Resected

ANGIOSARCOMA
Extremely rare, identical with peripheral tumor

ASTROBLASTOMAS
Form of astrocytoma in cerebral hemispheres of young adults with intermediate malignancy potential

CHOROID PLEXUS PAPILLOMA AND CARCINOMA
Childhood tumors, the latter with anaplasia and seeding tendency

EPENDYMOBLASTOMA
Type of primitive neuroectodermal tumor (PNET)

GANGLIOGLIOMA
Rare childhood tumor, supratentorial, midline location, slow-growing with good prognosis; anaplastic variant exists

GANGLIONEUROBLASTOMA
Type of PNET

GANGLIONEUROMA (CYTOMA)
Differentiated ganglioneuroblastoma with reasonable prognosis

HEMANGIOBLASTOMA
Vascular local tumor seen at all ages, most often with good prognosis; may spread and show anaplastic features

HEMANGIOPERICYTOMA
Vascular meningioma variant

LIPOMA
Most often benign tumors above the corpus callosum, often asymptomatic, possibly arising from arachnoid mater

MEDULLOEPITHELIOMA
Rare childhood tumor in posterior fossa with variation of mixed differentiation, tendency for CSF spread, and poor prognosis

NEUROBLASTOMA
Type of PNET

NEUROPITUITARY TUMORS
Rare astrocytic and granular cell tumors of varying prognosis

PITUITARY CARCINOMA
Rare anterior pituitary lobe anaplastic tumor with tendency for bone invasion and cerebrospinal fluid spread

POLAR SPONGIOBLASTOMA
Rare ventricular (especially third) wall tumor with palisading cells, seeding tendency, and poor prognosis

PRIMITIVE NEUROECTODERMAL TUMORS (PNET)
A group of tumors from embryonal cells showing no (medulloblastoma, pineoblastoma) or little (primitive gliomas, ependymoblastoma, neuroblastoma, choroid plexus tumor, ganglioneuroma, melanin-containing tumors) differentiation. These tumors are often found in the midline in children and exhibit poor prognosis because of anaplasia and tendency toward cerebrospinal fluid spread.

XANTHOSARCOMA (ASTROCYTOMA)
Rare childhood astrocytic tumor with lipid inclusions

reotactic focused cobalt sources, > 1500 cGy in single or a few fractions).[257] Small lesions are more easily controlled, but all lesions involute slowly, requiring long follow-up. Up to 85% lesion control has been claimed for small lesions.[257] No apparent side effects or complications have been reported.

RARE PRIMARY BRAIN TUMORS

Rare primary brain tumors that may require radiation therapy are listed in Table 23-12.

REFERENCES

1. Abelson HT, Kufe DW, Skarin AT, et al: Treatment of central nervous system tumors with methotrexate. Cancer Treat Rep 650(Suppl 1):137–140, 1981
2. Adegbite AB, Khan MI, Paine KWE, Tan LK: The recurrence of intracranial meningiomas after surgical treatment. J Neurosurg 58:51–56, 1983
3. Albers GW, Hoyt WF, Forno LS, Shratter LA: Treatment response in malignant optic glioma of adulthood. Neurology 38:1071, 1988
4. Alper MG: Management of optic nerve meningiomas: Current status—therapy in controversy. J Clin Neur Ophthalmol 1:101, 1981
5. Alvord EC, Lofton S: Gliomas of the optic nerve and chiasm: Outcome by patient's age, tumor site, and treatment. J Neurosurg 68:85, 1988
6. American Cancer Society: Cancer Facts and Figures. Atlanta, American Cancer Society, 1991
7. Appleton RE, Jan JE: Delayed diagnosis of optic nerve glioma: A preventable cause of visual loss. Pediatr Neurol 5(4):226–228, 1989
8. Bailey P, Cushing H: A classification of the tumors of the glioma group on a histogenic basis with a correlated study of prognosis. Philadelphia, JB Lippincott, 1926
9. Bailey P, Cushing H: Medulloblastoma cerebelli: A common type of midcerebellar glioma of childhood. Arch Neurol Psychiatr 43:1041, 1925
10. Barbaro NM, Gutin PH, Wilson CB, et al: Radiation therapy in the treatment of partially resected meningiomas. Neurosurgery 20:525–528, 1987
11. Barone BM, Elridge AR: Ependymomas: A clinical survey. J Neurosurg 33(4):428–438, 1970
12. Bartkowski HM: Peritumoral edema. In Rosenblum ML, Wilson CB (eds): Brain Tumor Biology. Basel, S. Karger, pp 179–190, 1984
13. Beahrs OH, Myers MH (eds): Manual for Staging of Cancer, 2nd ed, American Joint Committee on Cancer. Philadelphia, JB Lippincott, pp 249–254, 1983
14. Bergstrom M, Collins VP, Ehrin E, et al: Discrepancies in brain tumor extent as shown by computer tomography and positron emission tomography using ^{68}Ga-EDTA, 11-C-glucose and 11-C-methionine: Case report. J Comput Assist Tomogr 7:1062, 1983
15. Berry MP, Simpson WJ. Radiation therapy in the management of primary malignant lymphoma of the brain. Int J Radiat Oncol Biol Phys 7:55–59, 1981
16. Bigner DD: Role of viruses in the causation of neural neoplasia. In Laerum OD, Bigner DD, Rajansky MF (eds): Biology of Brain Tumors, pp 85–111. Geneva, International Union Against Cancer, 1978
17. Bilgic S, Erbengi A, Tinaztepe B, Onol B: Optic glioma of childhood: Clinical, histopathological, and histochemical observations. Br J Ophthalmol 73(10):832–837, 1989
18. Birkeland SA: Malignant tumors in renal transplant patients: The Scandia transplant material. Cancer 51:1571–1575, 1983
19. Bleehen NM: The central nervous system. In Bleehen NM,

Glatstein E, Haybittle JL (eds): Radiation Therapy Planning, pp 607–615. New York, Marcel Dekker, 1983

20. Bleehen NM, Wiltshire DR, Plowman PN, et al: A randomized study of misonidazole and radiotherapy for grade 3 and 4 cerebral astrocytoma. Br J Cancer 43:436–441, 1981
21. Bloom HJG: Intracranial tumors: Response and resistance to therapeutic endeavors, 1970–1980. Int J Radiat Oncol Biol Phys 8:1083–1113, 1982
22. Bloom HJG, Wallace ENK, Henk JM: The treatment and prognosis of medulloblastoma in children. AJR 105:43, 1969
23. Bloom HJG, Walsh LS: Tumors of the central nervous system. In Bloom HJG (ed): Cancer in Children: Clinical Management, pp 93–119. New York, Springer-Verlag, 1975
24. Boethius J, Collins VP, Edner G, et al: Stereotactic biopsies and computerized tomography in gliomas. Acta Neurochir 40:223, 1980
25. Boldrey E: The meningiomas. In Minckler J (ed): Pathology of the Nervous System, vol 2, pp 2125–2144. New York, McGraw-Hill, 1971
26. Bouchard J: Central nervous system. In Fletcher GH (ed): Textbook of Radiotherapy, 3rd ed, pp 444–498. Philadelphia, Lea & Febiger, 1980
27. Bouzaglou A: Radiotherapy of brain tumors. In Stereotactic Biopsy and Brachytherapy of Brain Tumors, pp 87–141. Baltimore, University Park Press, 1984
28. Bradfield JS, Perez CA, Schwartz H: Pineal tumors and ectopic pinealomas: An analysis of treatment and failures. Radiology 103:399, 1972
29. Brand WN, Hoover SV: Optic glioma in children: Review of 16 cases given megavoltage radiation therapy. Child's Brain 5(5):459–466, 1979
30. Bull JWD, Rovit RL: The radiographic localization of intracerebral gliomata. J Fac Radiol Lond 8:147–157, 1957
31. Bullard DE, Rawlings CE, Phillips B, et al: Oligodendroglioma: An analysis of the value of radiation therapy. Cancer 60:2179–2188, 1987
32. Burger PC: Pathological anatomy and CT correlations in the glioblastoma multiforme. Appl Neurophysiol 46:180, 1983
33. Burger PC, DuBois PJ, Schoid C Jr, et al: Computerized tomographic and pathologic studies of the untreated quiescent and recurrent glioblastoma multiforme. J Neurosurg 58:159, 1983
34. Burger PC, Rawlings CE, Cox EB, et al: Clinicopathologic correlations in the oligodendroglioma. Cancer 59:1345–1352, 1987
35. Burger PC, Vogel FS: Surgical Pathology of the Nervous System and Its Coverings. New York, John Wiley & Sons, 1976
36. Burger PC, Vollmer RT: Histologic factors of prognostic significance in glioblastoma multiforme. Cancer 46:1179, 1980
37. Bush RS, Jenkin RDR, Allt WEC, et al: Definitive evidence for hypoxic cells influencing cure in cancer therapy. Br J Cancer 37(Suppl 111):302, 1978
38. Butler, AB, Netsky MG: Classification and biology of brain tumors. In Youmans JR (ed): Neurological Surgery, 2nd ed, pp 2659–2701. Philadelphia, WB Saunders, 1982
39. Byar DP, Green SB, Strike TA: Prognostic factors for malignant glioma. In Walker MD (ed): Oncology of the Nervous System, pp 379–395. Boston, Martinus Nijhoff, 1983
40. Cahan WG, Woodard HQ, Higinbotham NL, et al: Sarcoma arising in irradiated bone: Report of eleven cases. Cancer 1:3, 1948
41. Cairncross JG, Laperriere NJ: Low-grade glioma: To treat or not to treat? Arch Neurol 46:1238–1239, 1989
42. Cairncross JG, Macdonald DR: Successful chemotherapy for recurrent malignant oligodendroglioma. Ann Neurol 23:360–364, 1988
43. Calvo FA, Hornedo J, Arellano A, et al: Radiation therapy in craniopharyngiomas. Int J Radiat Oncol Biol Phys 9:493, 1983
44. Carella RJ, Ransohoff J, Newall J: Role of radiation therapy in the management of meningioma. Nuerosurgery 10:332–339, 1982
45. Caveness WF: Experimental observations: Delayed necrosis in normal monkey brain. In Gilbert H, Kagan R (eds): Radiation Damage to the Nervous System: A Delayed Therapeutic Hazard, pp 1–38. New York, Raven Press, 1980
46. Chan RC, Thompson GB: Morbidity, mortality, and quality of life following surgery for intracranial meningiomas. J Neurosurg 60:52–60, 1984
47. Chang CH: Hyperbaric oxygen and radiation therapy in the management of glioblastoma. Natl Cancer Inst Monogr 46:163–169, 1977
48. Chang CH, Housepian EM, Herbert C Jr: An operative staging system and a megavoltage radiotherapeutic technique for cerebellar medulloblastomas. Radiology 93:1351, 1969
49. Chang CH, Horton J, Schoenfeld D, et al: Comparison of postoperative radiotherapy and combined postoperative radiotherapy and chemotherapy in the multidisciplinary management of malignant gliomas. Cancer 52:997, 1983
50. Chapman PH, Linggood RM: The management of pineal area tumors: A recent reappraisal. Cancer 46:1253, 1980
51. Chin HW, Maruyama Y, Markesbery W, et al: Intracranial ependymoma: Results of radiotherapy at the University of Kentucky. Cancer 49:2276–2280, 1982
52. Cho KG, Armond SJ de, Barnwell S, et al: Proliferative characteristics of intracranial and spinal tumors of developmental origin. Cancer 62:740–748, 1988
53. Clark WC, Moretz WH, Acker JD, et al: Nonsurgical management of small and intracanalicular acoustic tumors. Neurosurgery 16:801–803, 1985
54. Cohen L, Creditor M: An iso-effect table for radiation tolerance of the human spinal cord. Int J Radiat Oncol Biol Phys 7:961, 1981
55. Concannon JP, Kramer S, Berry, R: The extent of intracranial gliomata at autopsy and its relationship to techniques used in radiation therapy of brain tumors. AJR 84:99–107, 1960
56. Cushing H, Eisenhardt L: Meningiomas: Their Classification Regional Behavior, Life History, and Surgical End Results. Springfield, IL, Charles C Thomas, 1938
57. Danoff BF: Brain tumors in children. In Mansfield C (ed): Therapeutic Radiology, pp 109–126. Garden City, NY, Medical Examination Publishing, 1983
58. Danoff BF: Complications and late effects of irradiation for brain tumors. Course 718A in therapy of CNS tumors. In Marks JE, Griem ML (eds): Radiological Society of North America, 69th Annual Meeting, 1983
59. Daumas-Duport C, Scheithauer B, O'Fallon J, et al: Grading of astrocytomas: A simple and reproducible method. Cancer 62:2152–2165, 1988
60. Davies JNP: Some variations in childhood cancer throughout the world. In Marsden HB, Steward JK (eds): Recent Results in Cancer Research, vol 13, pp 13–33. Berlin, Springer-Verlag, 1968
61. DeAngelis LM, Yahalom J, Heinemann MH, et al: Primary central nervous system lymphoma: Combined treatment with chemotherapy and radiotherapy. Neurology 40(1), 80–86, 1990
62. DeAngelis LM, Yahalom J, Rosenblum M, Posner JB: Primary CNS lymphoma: Managing patients with spontaneous and AIDS-related disease. Oncology 1:52–59, 1987
63. DeSchryver A, Greitz T, Forsby N: Localized shaped field radiotherapy of malignant glioblastoma multiforme. Int J Radiat Oncol Biol Phys 1:713, 1976
64. Deutsh M, Green SB, Strike TA, et al: Results of a randomized trial comparing BCNU plus radiotherapy, streptozotocin plus radiotherapy, BCNU plus hyperfractionated radiotherapy, and BCNU following misonidazole plus radiotherapy in the postoperative treatment of malignant glioma. Int J Radiat Oncol Biol Phys 16:1389–1396, 1989
65. Deutsch M, Riegel DH: The value of myelography in the management of childhood medulloblastoma. Cancer 45: 2197, 1980
66. Dische S: Role of hypoxic cells and local failures of irradiation. In Plenary Session Proceedings, pp 165–170. Hawaii, XVI International Congress of Radiology, July 1985
67. Disclafani A, Hudgins RJ, Edwards MSB, et al: Pineocytomas. Cancer 63:302, 1989
68. Donahue B, Cooper J, Newall J, Rush S: Results of empiric

radiotherapy for HIV associated primary CNS lymphomas. Int J Radiat Oncol Biol Phys 17(Suppl 1):223, 1989

69. Duffner PK, Cohen ME, Anderson S, et al: Long-term effects of treatment on endocrine function in children with brain tumors. Ann Neurol 14:528, 1983
70. Duffner PK, Cohen ME, Freeman AI: Pediatric brain tumors. CA 35:287, 1985
71. Duffner PK, Cohen ME, Thomas PRM, et al: The long-term effects of cranial irradiation on the central nervous system. Cancer 56:1841, 1985
72. Eby NL, Grufferman S, Flannelly CM, et al: Increasing incidence of primary brain lymphoma in the US. Cancer 62:2461–2465. 1988
73. Edwards MS, Wilson CB: Treatment of radiation necrosis. In Gilbert H, Kagan R (eds): Radiation Damage to the Nervous System: A Delayed Therapeutic Hazard, pp 129–144. New York, Raven Press, 1980
74. Ervin T, Canellos GP: Successful treatment of recurrent primary central nervous system lymphoma with high-dose methotrexate. Cancer 45:1556–1557, 1980
75. Fajardo LF: Nervous system. In Pathology of Radiation Injury, pp 216–230. New York, Masson, 1982
76. Farwell JR, Dohrmann GJ, Flannery JT: Medulloblastoma in childhood: An epidemiological study. J Neurosurg 61:657, 1984
77. Fazekas JT: Treatment of grades I and II brain astrocytomas: The role of radiotherapy. Int J Radiat Oncol Biol Phys 2:661–666, 1977
78. Fike JR, Sheline GE, Cann CE, et al: Radiation necrosis. In Rosenblum ML, Wilson CB (eds): Progress in Experimental Tumor Research, Brain Tumor Therapy, vol 28, pp 136–151. Basel, S Karger, 1984
79. Fischman RA: Brain edema. N Engl J Med 293:706, 1975
80. Flickinger JC, Deutsch M, Lunsford LD: Repeat megavoltage irradiation of pituitary and suprasellar tumors. Int J Radiat Oncol Biol Phys 17(1):171–175, 1989
81. Flickinger JC, Deutsch M, Torres C, Deutsch M: Management of low-grade gliomas of the optic nerve and chiasm. Cancer 61(4):635–642, 1988
82. Forbes AR, Goldberg ID: Radiation therapy in the treatment of meningioma: The Joint Center for Radiation Therapy experience, 1970 to 1982. J Clin Oncol 2:1139–1143, 1984
83. Formenti SC, Gill PS, Lean E, et al: Primary central nervous system lymphoma in AIDS: Results of radiation therapy. Cancer 63(1):158–163, 1989
84. Freeman CR, Shustik C, Brisson ML, et al: Primary malignant lymphoma of the central nervous system. Cancer 58:1106–1111, 1986
85. Frick JC, Hansen RM, Anderson T, et al: Successful high-dose intravenous cytarabine treatment of parenchymal brain involvement from malignant lymphoma. Arch Intern Med 146:791–792, 1986
86. Friedman NB: Germinoma of the pineal: Its identity with germinoma (seminoma) of the testis. Cancer Res 7:363, 1947
87. Fukui M, Kitamura K, Nakagaki H, et al: Irradiated meningiomas: A clinical evaluation. Acta Neurochir 54:33–43, 1980
88. Garcia DM Fulling KH, Marks JE: The value of radiation therapy in addition to surgery for astrocytomas of the adult cerebrum. Cancer 55:919–927, 1985
89. Gehan EA, Walker MD: Prognostic factors for patients with brain tumors. Natl Cancer Inst Monogr 46:189–195, 1977
90. Gonzales DG, Schuster-Uitterhoeve ALJ: Primary non-Hodgkin's lymphoma of the central nervous system: Results of radiotherapy in 15 cases. Cancer 51:2048–2052, 1983
91. Grant JW, Gallagher PJ, Jones DB: Primary cerebral lymphoma: A histologic and immunohistochemical study of six cases. Arch Pathol Lab Med 110:897–901, 1986
92. Greitz TVB: Combined and selective use of modern imaging methods of neuroradiology. In Plenary Session Proceedings. Hawaii, XVI International Congress of Radiology, July 1985
93. Greitz T, Bergstrom M, Boethius J, et al: Head fixation system for integration of radiodiagnostic and therapeutic procedures. Neuroradiology 19:1, 1980
94. Greitz T, Lax I, Bergstrom M, et al: Stereotactic radiotherapy of intracranial lesions: Methodological aspects. Acta Radiol (Oncol) 25:81, 1986
95. Gunnesson-Nordin V, Blennow G, Garwicz S, et al: Gliomas of the anterior visual pathway in children: Tumour behavior and effect of treatment. Neuropediatrics 13(2):82–87, 1982
96. Gutin PH, Leibel SA, Hosobuchi Y, et al: Brachytherapy of recurrent tumors of the skull base and spine with iodine-125 sources. Neurosurgery 20:938–945, 1987
97. Halperin EC, Burger PC, Bullard DE: The fallacy of the localized supratentorial malignant glioma. Int J Radiat Oncol Biol Phys 15:505–509, 1988
98. Harris JR, Levene MP: Visual complications following irradiation for pituitary adenomas and craniopharyngiomas. Radiology 120:167, 1976
99. Hatam A, Yu Z-Y, Bergstrom M, et al: Effect of dexamethasone treatment on peritumoral brain edema: Evaluation by computed tomography. J Comput Assist Tomogr 6:586, 1982
100. Helle TL, Britt RH, Colby TV: Primary lymphoma of the central nervous system: Clinicopathological study of experience at Stanford. J Neurosurg 60:94–103, 1984
101. Henry JM, Heffner RR Jr, Dillard SH, et al: Primary malignant lymphomas of the central nervous system. Cancer 34:1293–1302, 1974
102. Herbst KD, Corder MP, Justile GR: Successful therapy with methotrexate of a multicentric mixed lymphoma of the central nervous system. Cancer 38:1476–1478, 1976
103. Hochberg FH, Miller G, Schooley RT, et al: Central nervous system lymphoma related to Epstein-Barr virus. N Engl J Med 309:745–748, 1983
104. Hochberg FH, Pruitt A: Assumptions in the radiotherapy of glioblastoma. Neurology 30:907–911, 1980
105. Hoogenhout J, Otten BJ, Kazem J, et al: Surgery and radiation therapy in the management of craniopharyngiomas. Int J Radiat Oncol Biol Phys 10:2293, 1984
106. Hope-Stone HF: Pineal and third ventricle tumors. In Hope-Stone HF (ed): Radiotherapy in Clinical Practice, pp 345–346. London, Butterworth & Co, 1986
107. Hope-Stone HF: Vascular tumours. In Hope-Stone HF (ed): Radiotherapy in Clinical Practice, p 355. London, Butterworth & Co, 1986
108. Horwich A, Bloom HJ: Optic gliomas: Radiation therapy and prognosis. Int J Radiat Oncol Biol Phys 11(6):1067–1079, 1985
109. Hoshino T, Barker M, Wilson CB, et al: Cell kinetics of human glioma. J Neurosurg 37:15, 1972
110. Houthoff HJ, Poppema S, Ebels EJ, et al: Intracranial malignant lymphomas: A morphologic and immunocytologic study of twenty cases. Acta Neuropathol 44:203–210, 1978
111. Ignelzi RJ: Cerebral edema: Present perspectives. Neurosurgery 4:338, 1979
112. Ikeda K, Ito H, Kasihara K, et al: Effective preoperative irradiation of highly vascular cerebellopontine angle neurinomas. Neurosurgery 22:566–573, 1988
113. Janisch JW, Schneider M, Gerlach H: Role of genetic factors in the pathogenesis of optic nerve glioma. Neurochirurgie 37(3):169–176, 1976
114. Jellinger K, Radaskiewicz TH, Slowik F: Primary malignant lymphomas of the central nervous system in man. Acta Neuropathol (Berlin) 95–102, 1975
115. Jereb B, Krishnaswamis S, Reid A, Allen JC: Radiation for medulloblastoma adjusted to prevent recurrence to the cribriform plate region. Cancer 54:602, 1984
116. Kalifa C, Ernest C, Rodary C, et al: Optic glioma in children: A retrospective study of 57 cases treated by irradiation. Arch Franc Pediatr 38(5):309–313. 1981
117. Kawakami Y, Tabuchi K, Ohnishi R, et al: Primary central nervous system lymphoma. J Neurosurg 62:522–527, 1985
118. Kelly PJ, Daumas-Duport C, Scheithauer BW, et al: Stereotaxic histologic correlations of computed tomography and magnetic resonance imaging defined abnormalities in patients with glial neoplasms. Mayo Clin Proc 62:450–459, 1987

119. Kernohan JW, Mabon RF, Svien HJ, Adson AW: A simplified classification of the gliomas. Proc Staff Meet Mayo Clin 24:71–75, 1949
120. Kernohan JW, Sayre GP: Astrocytomas. In Tumors of the Central Nervous System, Fascicle 35, pp 22–42. Washington, DC, Armed Forces Institute of Pathology, 1952
121. Kernohan JW, Sayre GP: Tumors of the central nervous system. In Atlas of Tumor Pathology, Section 10, Fascicle 35 pp 43–59. Washington, DC, Armed Forces Institute of Pathology, 1952
122. Kim YH, Fayos JV: Intracranial ependymomas. Radiology 124:805, 1977
123. King DL, Chang CH, Pool JL: Radiotherapy in the management of meningiomas. Acta Radiol Ther Phys Biol 5:26–33, 1966
124. Klatzo I: Neuropathological aspects of brain edema. J Neuropathol Exp Neurol 261:1, 1967
125. Kleihues P: Chemical carcinogens in the nervous system. In Laerum OD, Bigner DD, Rajansky MF (eds): Biology of Brain Tumors, pp 113–128. Geneva, International Union Against Cancer, 1978
126. Kornblith PL: Increased intracranial pressure. In DeVita VT, Hellman S, Rosenberg SA (eds): Cancer: Principles and Practice of Oncology, pp 1586–1588. Philadelphia, JB Lippincott, 1982
127. Kornblith PL, Walker MD, Cassady JR: Treatment of tumors of the pineal area. In Kovinblith PL, Walker MD, Cassady JR (eds): Neurological Oncology, pp 199–201. Philadelphia, JB Lippincott, 1987
128. Kramer S: Tumor extent as a determining factor in radiotherapy of glioblastomas. Acta Radiol (Oncol) 8:11–117, 1969
129. Kramer S, Lee KF: Complications of radiation therapy. The central nervous system. Semin Roentgenol IX:75, 1974
130. Krischeff IL, Becker M, Schneck SA, et al: Intracranial ependymomas: A study of survival in 65 cases treated by surgery and irradiation. AJR 91:167, 1964
131. Kristiansen K, Hagen S, Kollevoid T, et al: Combined modality therapy of operated astrocytomas grade III and IV. Confirmation of the value of postoperative irradiation and lack of potentiation of bleomycin on survival time: A prospective trial of the Scandanavian Glioblastoma Study Group. Cancer 47:649, 1981
132. Laerum OD, Mork SJ, DeRidder L: The transformation process. In Rosenblum ML, Wilson CB (eds): Brain Tumor Biology: Progress in Experimental Tumor Research, pp 17–31. Basel, S Karger, 1984
133. Lampert PW, Davis RL: Delayed effects of radiation on the human central nervous system. "Early" and "late" delayed reactions. Neurology 14:912, 1964
134. Langman J: Medical Embryology, 3rd ed, pp 318–367. Baltimore, Williams & Wilkins, 1975
135. Laws ER, Taylor WF, Clifton MB, Okazaki H: Neurosurgical management of low-grade astrocytoma of the cerebral hemispheres. J Neurosurg 61:665–673, 1984
136. Lee KF, Suh JH: CT evidence of grey matter calcification secondary to radiation therapy. Comput Tomogr 1(1):103–110, 1977
137. Lefkowitz I, Evans A, Sposto R, et al: Adjuvant chemotherapy of childhood posterior fossa ependymoma: Craniospinal radiation with or without CCNU, vincristine and prednisone. Proc ASCO 8:87, 1989
138. Leibel SA, Gutin PH, Sneed PK, et al: Interstitial irradiation for the treatment of primary and metastatic brain tumors. Prin Pract Oncol 3:1–11, 1989
139. Leibel SA, Sheline GA: Radiation therapy for neoplasms of the brain. J Neurosurg 66:1–22, 1987
140. Leibel SA, Sheline GE, Wara WM, et al: The role of radiation therapy in the treatment of astrocytomas. Cancer 34:1551, 1975
141. Leksell: A stereotaxic apparatus for intracerebral surgery. Acta Chir Scand 99:209–233, 1949
142. Lewander R, Bergstrom M, Boethius J, et al: Stereotactic computer tomography for biopsy of gliomas. Acta Radiol (Diagn) 19:867, 1978
143. Li FP, Cassady JR, Jaffe N: Risk of second tumors in survivors of childhood cancer. Cancer 35:1230, 1975
144. Lindegaard K, Mork SJ, Eide GE, et al: Statistical analysis of clinicopathological features, radiotherapy, and survival in 170 cases of oligodendroglioma. J Neurosurg 67:224–230, 1987
145. Lindgren M: Roentgen treatment of gliomata. Acta Radiol 40:325, 1953
146. Lindstadt D, Wara WM, Edwards MSB et al: Radiotherapy of primary intracranial germinomas: The case against routine craniospinal irradiation, UCSE. Int J Radiat Oncol Biol Phys 15:291–297, 1988
147. Littman P, Wang CC: Reticulum cell sarcoma of the brain: A review of the literature and a study of 19 cases. Cancer 35:1412–1420, 1975
148. Loeffler JS, Ervin TJ, Mauch P, et al: Primary lymphomas of the central nervous system: Patterns of failure and factors that influence survival. J Clin Oncol 3:490–494, 1985
149. Lufkin R, Flannigan BD, Bentson JR, et al: Magnetic resonance imaging of the brainstem and cranial nerves. Surg Radiol Anat 8(1):49–66, 1986
150. Luk KH, Caderao JB, Leavens ME: Radiotherapy for treatment of meningioma and meningiosarcoma. Cancer Bull 31:220–225, 1979
151. Macdonald DR, Jaeckle K, Posner JB: Primary leptomeningeal lymphoma. Ann Neurol 12:100, 1982
152. Manaka S, Teramoto, Takakura K: The efficacy of radiotherapy for craniopharyngioma. J Neurosurg 62:648, 1985
153. Margolis L, Fraser R, Lichter A, Char DH: The role of radiation therapy in the management of ocular reticulum cell sarcoma. Cancer 45:688–692, 1980
154. Marks JE, Adler SJ: A comparative study of ependymoma by site of origin. Int J Radiat Oncol Biol Phys 8:37:43–43, 1982
155. Marks JE, Baglan RJ: Cerebral radionecrosis and the effects on radiation on cranial soft tissues. Course 718B in Therapy of CNS tumors: A categorical course in radiation therapy. The Radiological Society of North America, 69th Annual Meeting, 1983
156. Marks JE, Baglan RJ, Prassad SC, et al: Cerebral necrosis: Incidence and risk in relation to dose, time, fractionation and volume. Int J Radiat Oncol Biol Phys 7:243, 1981
157. Marks JE, Sheline GE: The value of radiation for brain tumors. Course 418A pp 1–30. In Syllabus: Therapy of CNS tumors. The Radiological Society of North America, 69th Scientific Assembly and Annual Meeting, 1983
158. Marsa GW, Goffinet DR, Rubinstein LJ, Bagshaw MA: Megavoltage irradiation in the treatment of gliomas of the brain and spinal cord. Cancer 36:1781–1789, 1975
159. Marton LJ, Edwards MS, Levin VA, et al: Polyamines: A new and important means of monitoring patients with medulloblastoma. Cancer 47:757, 1981
160. Matsukado Y, MacCarty CS, Kernohan JW: The growth of glioblastoma multiforme (astrocytomas, grades 3 and 4) in neurosurgical practice. J Neurosurg 18:636, 1961
161. McComb RD, Burger PC: Pathologic analysis of primary brain tumors. Neurol Clin 3:711–728, 1985
162. McDonald JV, Salazar OM, Rubin P, et al: Central nervous system tumors. In Rubin P (ed): Clinical Oncology: A Multidisciplinary Approach, 6th ed, pp 262–278. New York, American Cancer Society, 1983
163. McFarland DR, Horwitz H, Saenger EL, et al: Medulloblastoma: A review of prognosis and survival. Br J Radiol 42:198, 1969
164. McKeran RO, Thomas DGT: The clinical study of gliomas. In Thomas DGT, Graham DI (eds): Brain Tumors: Scientific Basis. Clinical Investigation and Current Therapy, p 197. London, Butterworth & Co, 1980
165. McKissack W, Ford RK: Results of treatment of the craniopharyngioma. J Neurol Neurosurg Psychiatry 29:475, 1975
166. Medbery CA III, Straus KL, Steinberg SM, et al: Low-grade astrocytomas: Treatment results and prognostic variables. Int J Radiat Oncol Biol Phys 15:837–841, 1988
167. Melamed SH, Sahar A, Bellar AJ: The recurrence of intracranial meningiomas. Neurochirurgia (Stuttg) 22:45–51, 1979

168. Mendenhall NP, Thar TL, Agee OF, et al: Primary lymphoma of the central nervous system: Computerized tomography scan characteristics and treatment results for 12 cases. Cancer 52:1993–2000, 1983
169. Mirimanoff RO, Dosoretz DE, Linggood RM, et al: Meningioma: Analysis of recurrence and progression following neurosurgical resection. J Neurosurg 62:18–24, 1985
170. Mitsumoto H, Breuer AC, Lederman RJ: Malignant lymphoma of the central nervous system: A case of primary spinal intramedullary involvement. Cancer 46:1258–1262, 1980
171. Modan B, Baidatz D, Mart H, et al: Radiation-induced head and neck tumors. Lancet 1:277, 1974
172. Montgomery AB, Griffin T, Parker RG, Gerdes AJ: Optic nerve glioma: The role of radiation therapy. Cancer 40(5):2079–2080, 1977
173. Mork SJ, Loken AC: Ependymoma: A follow-up study of 101 cases. Cancer 40:907–915, 1977
174. Mulhern RK, Horowitz ME, Kovnar EH, et al: Neurodevelopmental status of infants and young children treated for brain tumors with preirradiation chemotherapy. J Clin Oncol 7:1660–1666, 1989
175. Mundiger F: Stereotactic biopsy and technique of implantation (instillation) of radionuclides, pp 134–187. In Jellinger K (ed): Therapy of Malignant Brain Tumors. New York, Springer-Verlag, 1987
176. Murray K, Kun L, Cox J: Primary malignant lymphoma of the central nervous system: Results of treatment of 11 cases and review of the literature. J Neurosurg 65:600–607, 1986
177. Nelson DF, Diener-West M, Horton J, et al: Combined modality approach to treatment of malignant gliomas—re-evaluation of RTOG 7401/ECOG 1374 with long-term follow-up: A joint study of the Radiation Therapy Oncology Group and the Eastern Cooperative Oncology Group. Natl Cancer Inst Monogr 6:279–284, 1988
178. Nelson DF, Diener-West M, Weinstein AS, et al: A randomized comparison of misonidazole sensitized radiotherapy plus BCNU and radiotherapy plus BCNU for treatment of malignant glioma after surgery: Final report of an RTOG study. Int J Radiat Oncol Biol Phys 12:1793–1800, 1986
179. Nelson DF, Martz KL, Bonner H, et al: Definitive radiation therapy in the treatment of primary non-Hodgkin's lymphoma of the central nervous system, non-AIDS related: Report of RTOG study 8315. J Neurosurg (submitted)
180. Nelson DF, Nelson JS, Davis DR, et al: Survival and prognosis of patients with astrocytoma with atypical or anaplastic features. J Neurooncol 3:99–103, 1985
181. Nelson DF, Nelson JS, Davis DR, et al: Survival and prognosis of patients with astrocytoma with atypical and anaplastic features. J Neurooncol 3(2), 99–103, 1985
182. Nelson JS, Schoenfeld D, Tsukada Y, et al: Histological criteria with prognostic significance for malignant glioma. In Change CH, Housepian E (eds): Tumors of the Central Nervous System: Modern Radiotherapy in Multidisciplinary Management. New York, Masson, 1984
183. Nelson, JS, Tsukada Y, Schoenfeld D, et al: Necrosis as a prognostic criterion in malignant supratentorial, astrocytic gliomas. Cancer 52(3):550–554, 1983
184. Neuwelt EA, Frenkel EP, Gumerlock MK, et al: Developments in the diagnosis and treatment of primary CNS lymphoma: A prospective series. Cancer 58:1609–1620, 1986
185. Noback CR: The Human Nervous System: Basic Elements of Structure and Function. New York, McGraw-Hill, 1967
186. Noren G, Arndt J, Hindmarsh T: Stereotactic radiosurgery in cases of acoustic neurinoma: Further experiences. Neurosurgery 13:12–22, 1983
187. Norris DG, Bruce DA, Byrd RL, et al: Improved relapse-free survival in medulloblastoma utilizing modern techniques. Neurosurgery 9:661, 1981
188. Onoyama Y, Abe M, Yabumoto E, et al: Radiation therapy in the treatment of glioblastoma. AJR 126:481, 1976
189. Park TS, Hoffman HJ, Hendrick EB, et al: Clinical presentation and management. Experience at the Hospital for Sick Children, Toronto, 1950–1980. J Neurosurg 58:543, 1983
190. Parsons JE, Fitzgerald CR, Hood CI, et al: The effects of irradiation on the eye and optic nerve. Int J Radiat Oncol Biol Phys 9:609, 1983
191. Patronas NJ, Di-Chiro E, Brooks RA, et al: Work in progress: (18F) fluorodeoxyglucose and positron emission tomography in the evaluation of radiation necrosis of the brain. Radiology 144:885, 1982
192. Payne DG, Simpson WJ, Keen C, Platts ME: Malignant astrocytoma: Hyperfractionated and standard radiotherapy with chemotherapy in a randomized prospective clinical trial. Cancer 50:2301–2306, 1982
193. Pendergrass EP, Hayman M Jr, Houser KM, Rambo VC: The effect of radium on the normal tissues of the brain and spinal cord of dogs, and its therapeutic application. AJR 9:553–569, 1922
194. Petty AM, Kun LE, Meyer GA: Radiation therapy for incompletely resected meningiomas. J Neurosurg 62:502–507, 1985
195. Phillips TL, Sheline GE, Bodrey E: Therapeutic considerations in tumors affecting the central nervous system: Ependymomas. Radiology 83:98–105, 1964
196. Piepmeier JM: Observations on the current treatment of low-grade astrocytic tumors of the cerebral hemispheres. J Neurosurg 67:177–181, 1987
197. Pierce SM, Barnes PD, Loeffler JS, et al: Definitive radiation therapy in the management of symptomatic patients with optic glioma: Survival and long-term effects. Cancer 65(1): 45–52, 1990
198. Pollack IF, Lunsford ID, Flickinger JC, Dameshek HL: Prognostic factors in the diagnosis and treatment of primary central nervous system lymphoma. Cancer 63:939–947, 1989
199. Potish RA, Dehner LP, Haselow RE, et al: The incidence of second neoplasms following megavoltage radiation for pediatric tumors. Cancer 56:1534, 1985
200. Price RA, Jamieson PA: The nervous system in childhood leukemia. II. Subacute leukoencephalopathy. Cancer 42:306, 1978
201. Qualman SJ, Mendelsohn G, Mann RB, Green WR: Intraocular lymphomas: Natural history based on a clinicopathologic study of eight cases and review of the literature. Cancer 52:878–886, 1983
202. Quest DO: Meningiomas: An update. Neurosurgery 3:219–225, 1978
203. Rampen FHJ, van Andel JG, Sizoo W, et al: Radiation therapy in primary non-Hodgkin's lymphomas of the CNS. Eur J Cancer 16:177–184, 1980
204. Rappaport R, Brauner R: Growth and endocrine disorders secondary to cranial irradiation (Review). Pediatr Res 25(6):561–567, 1989
205. Rauber, Kopsch: Lehrbuch und Atlas der Anatomie des Menschen, 19th ed, vol II, pp 323–324. Stuttgart, Georg Thieme-Verlag, 1955
206. Ringertz N: "Grading" of gliomas. Acta Microbiol Scand 27:51, 1950
207. Ringertz N, Reymond A: Ependymomas and choroid plexus papillomas. J Neuropathol Exp Neurol 8:355–380, 1949
208. Robertson AG, Brewin TB: Optic nerve glioma. Clin Radiol 31(4):471–474, 1980
209. Rorke LB, Gilles FH, Davis RL, et al: Revision of the World Health Organization classification of brain tumor for childhood brain tumors. Cancer 56:1869–1886, 1985
210. Rosenbaum TJ, MacCarty CS, Buettner H: Uveitis and cerebral reticulum-cell sarcoma (large-cell lymphoma): Case report. J Neurosurg 50:660–664, 1979
211. Rosenberg NL, Hochberg FH, Miller G, et al: Primary central nervous system lymphoma related to Epstein-Barr virus in a patient with acquired immune deficiency syndrome. Ann Neurol 20:98–102, 1986
212. Rosenstock JG, Packer RJ, Bilaniuk L, et al: Chiasmatic optic glioma treated with chemotherapy: A preliminary report. J Neurosurg 63(6):862–866, 1985
213. Rubin P, Casarett GW: Clinical Radiation Pathology, vols 1–2. Philadelphia, WB Saunders, 1968
214. Rubin P, Cooper R, Phillips TL (eds): Radiation Biology and

Radiation Pathology Syllabus. Chicago, American College of Radiology, 1975

215. Rubinstein LJ: Tumors of the central nervous system. Atlas of Tumor Pathology, Series 2, Fascicle 6. Washington, DC, Armed Forces Institute of Pathology, 1972
216. Rush JA, Younge BR, Campbell RJ, MacCarty CS: Optic glioma: Long-term follow-up of 85 histopathologically verified cases. Ophthalmology 89(11):1213–1219, 1982
217. Russell DS, Rubinstein LJ: Craniopharyngiomas and suprasellar epidermoid cysts. In Russell DS, Rubinstein LJ (eds): Pathology of Tumors of the Nervous System, 5th ed, pp 695–704. Baltimore, Williams & Wilkins, 1989
218. Russell DS, Rubinstein LJ: Gliomas of the optic nerve and chiasm. In Russell DS, Rubinstein LJ (eds): Pathology of Tumors of the Nervous System, 5th ed, pp 370–376. Baltimore, Williams & Wilkins, 1989
219. Russell DS, Rubinstein LJ: Medulloblastomas. In Russell DS, Rubinstein LJ (eds): Pathology of Tumors of the Nervous System, 5th ed, pp 251–254. Baltimore, Williams & Wilkins, 1989
220. Russell DS, Rubinstein LJ (eds): Pathology of Tumors of the Nervous System, 4th ed. Baltimore, Williams & Wilkins, 1977
221. Russell DS, Rubinstein LJ: Tumors of pineal parenchymal and glial cells. In Russell DS, Rubinstein LJ (eds): Pathology of Tumors of the Nervous System, 5th ed, p 380. Baltimore, Williams & Wilkins, 1989
222. Russell DS, Rubinstein LJ: Tumors of vascular origin. In Russell DS, Rubinstein LJ (eds): Pathology of Tumors of the Nervous System, 5th ed, p 639. Baltimore, Williams & Wilkins, 1989
223. Sach H: Radiation therapy of brain tumors. In Grundmann E (ed): Cancer Campaign, vol 10: Experimental Neurooncology, Brain Tumor and Pain Therapy, pp 255–263. Stuttgart, Gustav Fischer, 1987
224. Sagerman RH, Collier CH, King GA: Radiation therapy of microgliomas. Radiology 149:567–570. 1983
225. Salazar OM, Castro-Vita H, VanHoutte P, et al: Improved survival in cases of intracranial ependymoma after radiation therapy. J Neurosurg 59:652–659, 1983
226. Salazar OM, Rubin P: The spread of glioblastoma multiforme as a determining factor in the radiation treated volume. Int J Radiat Oncol Biol Phys 1:627–637, 1976
227. Salazar OM, Rubin P, Feldstein ML, et al: High dose radiation therapy in the treatment of malignant gliomas: Final report. Int J Radiat Oncol Biol Phys 5:1733, 1979
228. Sauer R: Optic gliomas. In Jellinger K (ed): Therapy of Malignant Brain Tumors, pp 242–245. Wien, Springer-Verlag, 1987
229. Saunders WM, Winston KR, Siddon RL, et al: Radiosurgery for arteriovenous malformations of the brain using a standard linear accelerator: Rationale and technique. Int J Radiat Oncol Biol Phys 15:441–447, 1988
230. Scanlon PW, Taylor WR: Radiotherapy of intracranial astrocytomas: Analysis of 417 cases treated from 1960 through 1969. Neurosurgery 5:301–308, 1979
231. Schaumberg HH, Plank CR, Adams RD: The reticulum cell sarcoma-microglioma group of brain tumors: A consideration of their clinical features and therapy. Brain 95:199–212, 1972
232. Schmitt-Graff A, Pfitzer P: Cytology of the cerebrospinal fluid in primary malignant lymphomas of the central nervous system. Acta Cytol 27:267–272, 1983
233. Schneck SA, Penn I: De-novo brain tumours in renal-transplant recipients. Lancet i:983–986, 1971
234. Schoenberg BS: The epidemiology of central nervous system tumors. In McGuire WL (ed): Cancer Treatment and Research. Boston, Martinus Nijhoff, 1983
235. Selikoff IJ, Hammond EC: Brain tumors in the chemical industry. Ann NY Acad Sci 3:81, 1982
236. Shalet SM, Price DA, Beardwell CG, et al: Normal growth despite abnormalities of growth hormone secretions in children treated for acute leukemia. J Pediatr 94:719, 1979
237. Shapiro WR: Therapy of adult malignant brain tumors. What have the clinical trials taught us? Semin Oncol 13:38–45, 1986
238. Shaw EG, Duamas-Duport C, Scheithauer BW, et al: Radiation therapy in the management of low-grade supratentorial astrocytomas. J Neurosurg 70:853–861, 1989
239. Shaw EG, Evans RG, Scheithauer BW, et al: Postoperative radiotherapy of intracranial ependymoma in pediatric and adult patients. Int J Radiat Oncol Biol Phys 13:1457–1462, 1987
240. Shaw EG, Scheithauer BW, Gilbertson DT: Postoperative radiotherapy of supratentorial low-grade gliomas. Int J Radiat Oncol Biol Phys 16:663–668, 1989
241. Sheline GE: Radiation therapy of brain tumors. Cancer 39:873, 1977
242. Sheline GE: Radiation therapy of tumors of the central nervous system in childhood. Cancer 35:957, 1975
243. Sheline GE: Radiotherapy of adult primary cerebral neoplasms. In Walker MD (ed): Oncology of the Nervous System, pp 223–245. Boston, Martinus Nijhoff, 1983
244. Sheline GE: The role of radiation therapy in the treatment of low-grade gliomas. Clin Neurosurg 33:563–574, 1986
245. Shibamoto Y, Abe M, Yamashita J, et al: Treatment results of intracranial germinoma as a function of the irradiated volume. Int J Radiat Oncol Biol Phys 15:285–290, 1988
246. Shin KH, Muller PJ, Geggie PHS: Superfractionation radiation therapy in the treatment of malignant astrocytoma. Cancer 52:2040–2043, 1983
247. Shin KH, Urtasun RC, Fulton D, et al: Multiple daily fractionated radiation therapy and misonidazole in the management of malignant astrocytoma: A preliminary report. Cancer 56:758–760, 1985
248. Silverberg E: Cancer statistics. CA 32:1, 1982
249. Simpson WJ, Platts ME: Fractionation study in the treatment of glioblastoma multiforme. Int J Radiat Oncol Biol Phys 1:639–644, 1976
250. Smith JL, Vuksanovic MM, Yates BM, et al: Radiation therapy for primary optic nerve meningiomas. J Clin Neuro Ophthalmol 1:85, 1981
251. Smith MT, Ludwig CL, Godrey AD, et al: Grading of oligodendrogliomas. Cancer 52:2107–2114, 1983
252. So YT, Beckstead JH, Davis RL: Primary central nervous system lymphoma in acquired immune deficiency syndrome: A clinical and pathological study. Ann Neurol 20:566–572, 1986
253. Solan MJ, Kramer S: The role of radiation therapy in the management of intracranial meningiomas. Int J Radiat Oncol Biol Phys 11:675–677, 1985
254. Spallone A: Meningioma as a sequel of radiotherapy for pituitary adenoma. Neurochirurgia (Stuttg) 25(2):68, 1982
255. Stage W, Stein J: Treatment of malignant astrocytomas. AJR 120:7–18, 1974
256. Stein BM: Supracerebellar-infratentorial approach to pineal tumors. Surg Neurol 11:331–337 1979
257. Steiner L: Radiosurgery in cerebral arteriovenous malformations. In Fein JM, Flamm E (eds): Textbook of Cerebro-vascular Surgery, p 1161. New York, Springer-Verlag, 1985
258. Stewart DJ, Russell N, Atack EA, et al: Cyclophosphamide, doxorubicin, vincristine, and dexamethasone in primary lymphoma of the brain: A case report. Cancer Treat Rep 67:287–291, 1983
259. Stewart DJ, Russell N, Dennery J, et al: Cyclophosphamide, Adriamycin, vincristine and dexamethasone in the treatment of bulky central nervous system lymphomas. J Neurooncol 2:289, 1984
260. Sung DH, Harisiadis L, Chang CH: Midline pineal tumors and suprasellar dysgerminomas highly curable by irradiation. Radiology 128:749, 1978
261. Sutcliffe SB, Henkelman RM, Poon PY: MRI in clinical radiation oncology. Plenary Session Proceedings. Hawaii, XVI International Congress of Radiology, July 1985
262. Svien HJ, Gates EM, Kernohan JW: Spinal subarachnoid implantation associated with ependymoma. Arch Neurol Psychiatr 62:847–856, 1949
263. Swartz JD, Zimmerman RA, Bilaniuk LT: Computed tomography of intracranial ependymomas. Radiology 143:97–101, 1982
264. Szikla G: Stereotactic cerebral irradiation. Proceedings of the

Inserm Symposium on Stereotactic Irradiations, Paris 1979. Amsterdam, Elsevier/North Holland Biomedical Press, 1979
265. Taylor BW, Marcus RB Jr, Friedman WA, et al: The meningioma controversy: Postoperative radiation therapy. Int J Radiat Oncol Biol Phys 15:299–304, 1988
266. Taylor CR, Russell R, Lukes RJ, et al: An immunohistological study of immunoglobulin content of primary central nervous system lymphomas. Cancer 41:2197–2205, 1978
267. Tenny RT, Laws ER, Younge BR, et al: The neurosurgical management of optic gliomas: Results in 104 patients. J Neurosurg 57:452–458, 1982
268. Thomas HG, Dolman CL, Berry K: Malignant meningioma: Clinical and pathological features. J Neurosurg 55:929–934, 1981
269. Tognetti F, Andreoli A, Cuscini A, et al: Successful management of an intra-cranial arteriovenous malformation by conventional irradiation. J Neurosurg 63:193, 1985
270. Tomita T, LeLone DG, Naidich TP: Brain stem gliomas in childhood: Rational approach and treatment. J Neurooncol 2:117, 1984
271. Urtasun R, Feldstein ML, Partington J, et al: Radiation and nitroimidazoles in supratentorial high grade gliomas: A second clinical trial. Br J Cancer 46:101–108, 1982
272. Varadachari C, Palutke M, Climie ARW, et al: Immunoblastic sarcoma (histiocytic lymphoma) of the brain with B cell markers: Case report. J Neurosurg 49:887–892, 1978
273. Visot A, Rougerie J, Derome PJ, Evrard E: Optic chiasmic gliomas. Neurochirurgie 26(3):181–192, 1980
274. Walker MD: Brain and peripheral system tumors. In Holland JF, Frei E (eds): Cancer Medicine, pp 1385–1407. Philadelphia, Lea & Febiger, 1973
275. Walker MD: Tumors of the central nervous system. In Levine AS (ed): Cancer in the Young. Part VI. The Malignant Diseases, pp 695–706. New York, Masson, 1982
276. Walker MD, Green SB, Byar DP, et al: Randomized comparison of radiotherapy and nitrosureas for the treatment of malignant gliomas after surgery. N Engl J Med 303:1323, 1980
277. Walker MD, Strike TA, Sheline GE: An analysis of dose-effect relationship in the radiotherapy of malignant gliomas. Int J Radiat Oncol Biol Phys 5:1725–1731, 1979
278. Wallner KE, Galicich JH, Krol G, et al: Patterns of failure following treatment for glioblastoma multiforme and anaplastic astrocytoma. Int J Radiat Oncol Biol Phys 16:1405–1409, 1989
279. Wallner KE, Gonzales M, Sheline GE: Treatment of oligodendrogliomas with or without postoperative irradiation. J Neurosurg 68:684–688, 1988
280. Wallner KE, Gonzales MF, Sheline GE, et al: Treatment results of juvenile pilocytic astrocytoma. J Neurosurg 69:171–176, 1988
281. Wallner KE, Pitts LH, Davis RL, et al: Radiation therapy for the treatment of non-eighth nerve intracranial neurilenoma. Int J Radiat Oncol Biol Phys 14:287–290, 1988
282. Wallner KE, Sheline GE, Pitts LH, et al: Efficacy of irradiation for incompletely excised acoustic neurilemomas. J Neurosurg 67:858–863, 1987
283. Wallner KE, Wara WM, Sheline GE, et al: Intracranial ependymomas: Results of treatment with partial or whole brain irradiation without spinal irradiation. Int J Radiat Oncol Biol Phys 12:1937–1941, 1986
284. Walter GF: Cerebellar astrocytoma and optic glioma: A comparative ultra-structural study. Virch Arch (A) 380(1):59–79, 1978
285. Wara WM: Radiation therapy of brain tumors. Cancer 55(Suppl):2291, 1985
286. Wara WM, Jenkins RDT, Evans A, et al: Tumors of the pineal and suprasellar region: Children's Cancer Study Group treatment results, 1960–1975. Cancer 43:698, 1979
287. Wara WM, Sheline GE, Newman H, et al: Radiation therapy of meningiomas. AJR 123:453–458, 1975
288. Weiss L, Sagerman RH, King GA, et al: Controversy in the management of optic nerve glioma. Cancer 59(5):1000–1004, 1987
289. Welch K, Finkbeiner W, Alpers CE, et al: Autopsy findings in the acquired immune deficiency syndrome. JAMA 252:1152–1159, 1984
290. Wen BC, Hussey DH, Staples J, et al: A comparison of the roles of surgery and radiation therapy in the management of craniopharyngiomas. Int J Radiat Oncol Biol Phys 16:17–24, 1989
291. Wilkins RH: Natural history of intracranial vascular malformations: A review. Neurosurgery 16:421, 1985
292. Wilson CB, Liu HC, Davis RL, et al: Sarcomas of the nervous system. In Eilber FR, Morton DL, Sondak VK, Economou JS (eds): The Soft Tissue Sarcomas, pp 111–139. Orlando, FL, Grune & Stratton, 1978
293. Wolkov HB, Bagshaw M: Conventional radiation therapy in the management of arteriovenous malformations of the central nervous system. Int J Radiat Oncol Biol Phys 15:1461–1464, 1988
294. Woodman R, Shin K, Pineo G: Primary non-Hodgkin's lymphoma of the brain: A review. Medicine 64:425–430, 1985
295. Yahalom J, DeAngelis LM: Primary CNS lymphoma: Improved survival with an intensive combined modality treatment approach. Int J Radiat Oncol Biol Phys 17(Suppl 1):135, 1989
296. Yamashita J, Handa H, Iwaki K, Abe M: Recurrence of intracranial meningiomas, with special reference to radiotherapy. Surg Neurol 14:33–40, 1980
297. Yamashita T, Kuwabara T: Estimation of rate of growth of malignant brain tumors by computed tomography scanning. Surg Neurol 20:464, 1983
298. Yanoff M, Davis RL, Zimmerman LE: Juvenile pilocytic astrocytoma ("glioma") of optic nerve: Clinicopathological study of 63 cases. In Jakobiek FA (ed): Ocular and Adnexas Tumors, p 685. Birmingham, Alabama, Aesculapius, 1978
299. Youmans JR: Neurological Surgery. Philadelphia, WB Saunders, 1982
300. Young JL, Percy CL, Asire AJ (eds): Surveillance, Epidemiology and End Results: Incidence and Mortality Data 1973–1977. National Cancer Institute Monograph 57. Washington, DC, US Government Printing Office, 1981
301. Zimmerman HM: Malignant lymphomas of the central nervous system. Acta Neuropathol (Berl) (Suppl. 6) 69–74, 1975
302. Zulch KJ: Histological typing of tumors of the central nervous system. Geneva, World Health Organization, 1979
303. Zulch KJ: Medulloblastomas. In Zulch KJ (ed): Brain Tumors, 3rd ed, pp 324–325. Berlin, Springer-Verlag, 1986
304. Zulch KJ: Other malformative tumors and tumor-like lesions. In Zulch KJ (ed): Brain Tumors, 3rd ed, pp 426–432. Berlin, Springer-Verlag, 1986
305. Zulch KJ: Pineal cell tumors. In Zulch KJ (ed): Brain Tumors, 3rd ed, pp 283–292. Berlin, Springer-Verlag, 1986
306. Zulch KJ: Principles of the New World Health Organization (WHO) classification of brain tumors. Neuroradiology 19:59, 1980

Stereotactic External-Beam Irradiation

David A. Larson
Todd H. Wasserman
Robert E. Drzymala
Joseph R. Simpson

Radiosurgery is a term originally used to describe a procedure that allowed for three-dimensional stereotactic irradiation of small intracranial targets with orthovoltage x-rays.[44] It is now applied to varying techniques, including gamma-units using ^{60}Co; proton, helium ion, and neutron beams; and modified cobalt or linac radiation therapy units. These techniques all aim to deliver a large single fraction of radiation to a small intracranial target with great accuracy. Several thousand patients with arteriovenous malformation (AVM) and several hundred patients with benign and malignant lesions have been treated. Only a fraction of treated patients are adequately followed up and reported on, and standards for indications, techniques, and doses of radiosurgery are evolving.

An intracranial target can be irradiated through a large number of small, stationary portals by fixing a semicircular stereotactic frame at different angles and moving a collimator and x-ray tube circumferentially along the frame, resulting in a three-dimensional distribution of beams about an isocenter.[44] Improved methods involve the use of Bragg peak or intersecting non-Bragg peak proton beams from a synchrotron[23,40] or the use of a linear accelerator. During the 1950s, Bragg peak studies with charged particles were carried out in Berkeley[93] and in Boston.[38] In 1968, Leksell began clinical studies with a device producing multiple, intersecting, static, ^{60}Co beams called a gamma-unit or gamma-knife.[43] In the early 1980s, clinical studies involving linear accelerators and standard ^{60}Co units began.[4,10,71] In 1980, Bragg peak radiosurgery using helium ion beams was developed in Berkeley.[18,56]

At the present time, numerous groups have developed or are developing radiosurgery units associated with conventional linear accelerators, and several are planning gamma-unit installations.

GENERAL TECHNIQUES

A stereotactic apparatus fixed to the patient's skull is used during target localization studies (magnetic resonance imaging [MRI], computed tomography [CT], angiography) such that the location and extent of the target can be determined in a coordinate system established with respect to the stereotactic apparatus. A known relationship between this coordinate system and the radiation source allows subsequent accurate delivery of radiation to the target. Radiosurgery thus differs from conventional external-beam radiation therapy in several important respects:

Small volumes are treated, in the range of 1 cm^3 to 30 cm^3.

Usually a single fraction of radiation is used. A single fraction can be effective in producing localized necrosis, depending on target dose and volume, which may or may not be desirable. Use of a single fraction avoids potential practical difficulties associated with multiple stereotactic radiations.

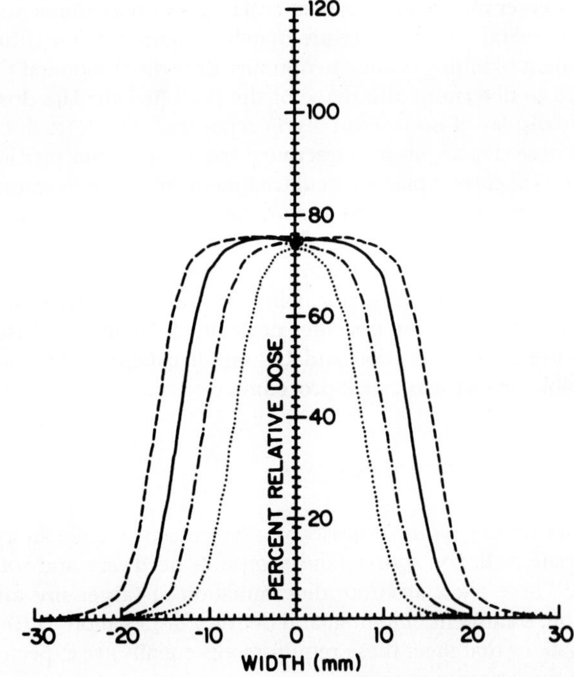

FIGURE 23–15. Representative static beam dose profiles in water from Jewish Hospital of St. Louis. Varian Clinac 6/100 beams modified by divergent secondary circular collimators.[55] Curves correspond to apertures with 15 mm (*dotted line*), 20 mm (*dash-dot line*), 25 mm (*solid line*), and 30 mm (*broken line*) diameters. The dose gradient is typically about 15% per mm at the field edge.

Extra precision with target localization and treatment geometries is required.

Dose gradients at field edges are high to minimize dose deposition outside the target volume (Fig. 23-15). The volume of tissue beyond the target that receives significant dose is strongly dependent on target size.

Beams intersect at a common point within the skull after entering through points distributed over the surface of the skull. This three-dimensional distribution of beams reduces the volume of normal tissue receiving moderate or high doses of radiation.

Table 23-13 outlines steps in a typical linac radiosurgery procedure. Completion of all the steps for an AVM requiring single-vessel injection at angiography and treatment with a sin-

TABLE 23–13
Typical Linac Radiosurgery Procedure

OUTSIDE RADIATION ONCOLOGY	IN RADIATION ONCOLOGY
Anesthesia (if needed)	Linac setup/alignment and output checks
Stereotactic frame attachment	
CT scanning, MRI, or other studies	Obtain patient coordinates Patient-specific quality assurance
Patient transport to radiation oncology	Treat patient on linear accelerator
	Remove stereotactic frame/ release patient or observe overnight (elsewhere)

gle isocenter may require only several hours with a gamma unit. Up to several additional hours may be required if individual treatment planning is done to optimize dose distribution, if CT is used to determine the shape of the skull (to calculate dose) and to display of isodose curves on arbitrary CT cuts (to document dose deposition in intracranial tissue), and film verification tests of correct placement of treatment volume with respect to isocenter are performed to eliminate accidental target malpositioning. The gamma-unit dose calculation uses a mechanical determination of skull shape and does not require CT in addition to angiography, nor is film verification of treatment volume with respect to isocenter performed. Some linac-based units use film verification and CT on all patients, which are desirable quality assurance procedures.

RADIOSURGERY SYSTEMS

A radiosurgery system consists of a stereotactic frame, an appropriate radiation source, and computer hardware and software. These allow accurate determination of target size and location, treatment planning, and delivery of radiation. Different systems that meet these requirements equally are expected to produce similar outcomes in similar groups of patients.[24,39] Existing systems may differ from one another in various ways, such as accuracy of beam alignment with a target, accuracy of localization of an intracranial target, overall accuracy of placement of dose, accuracy of dose calculated and delivered, number of points in the target and surrounding tissues where dose is calculated, treatment verification capability, ability to compare alternative treatment plans, ease of operation, support staff requirements, cost, and safety.[72] Some persons argue that only the gamma-unit (gamma-knife) fulfills the name "radiosurgery," whereas others argue against this restriction.[30,42,97] Lack of published documentation of various systems prevents detailed comparisons.

The gamma-knife system requires a large capital purchase of about $3.5 million with construction of new space. It produces a target size of about 3 mm to 25 mm with a target accuracy of 0.1 mm. The gamma-knife has no other known uses beyond stereotactic radiosurgery. A linear accelerator (linac) can be modified to perform stereotactic radiation at a cost of $50,000 to $300,000, depending on whether any external treatment planning devices need be purchased. The linear accelerator can give a target size of 10 mm to 50 mm with a target accuracy of 0.1 mm to 1 mm. The resolutional accuracy of radiologic studies is about 0.5 mm to 1 mm. Clearly more quality assurance is required in the use of a linac, and the possible choices for dose delivery are greater than for those with the gamma-knife. The linac also has additional uses for treating other patients with other cancers. If a linac is purchased and a new installation has to be made, the total cost could approach $1.75 million.

Detailed descriptions of one linac-based radiosurgery system have been published.[55,78,80,82,98] In particular, extensive measurements and analysis of errors in the treatment process were performed. The total alignment error in the treatment process was separated into contributions resulting from mechanical alignment error (0.48 ± 0.16 mm) and those from lesion localization error (the dominant error). It was concluded that further refinements in the treatment delivery apparatus could lead to only very small gains in overall treatment accuracy.

Dose distributions produced by one radiosurgical apparatus may differ from those produced by a different apparatus, although demonstrations of this difference are difficult and may be misleading. For example, the dose distribution obtained by plotting dose *versus* distance from the isocenter depends on whether the radius along which dose is calculated points directly toward a source position or not. Podgorsak and associates[74,75] have discussed this in detail and demonstrated differences among systems based on worst-case and best-case choice of radial direction along which dose is calculated. Differences between systems are manifested mainly in dose distributions away from the target involving low doses. Comparisons of alternative treatment techniques can also be examined with the aid of dose-volume histograms.[72]

Specialized radiation sources used for radiosurgery include gamma-units (gamma-knife) containing 5500 Ci to 6000 Ci of cobalt distributed in 201 sources over a portion of a hemisphere, such that circular beams from collimators of 4 mm to 18 mm diameter enter the skull through a large number of points distributed relatively uniformly over the convexity[41,53,54,57,96,100]; proton beams, as used in Boston[34–38]; and helium ion beams, as used in Berkeley,[17,18,56] where shaped beams of various sizes enter the skull through a small number of portals.

The gamma-knife consists of a permanent 18,000 kg shield surrounding a hemispheric array of cobalt sources. Four interchangeable outer collimator helmets with beam diameters from 4 mm to 18 mm are used to vary the target volume.[53,57,100]

Linear accelerators are used for radiosurgery in different ways. The group in Vicenza[9,10,12] uses a Varian Clinac 4 (4 MV) without major modifications. Both the stereotactic frame and the patient are supported by the patient support assembly. No additional collimator is used; the internal collimators are adjusted to produce square or rectangular fields of 5 mm to 35 mm. During treatment, the gantry rotates through an arc for each of several stationary couch angles; the resulting points of beam entry on the convexity are analogous to the seams on a football, with the ends of the football at the nose and occiput. Up to 17 arcs are used.

The group in Heidelberg[26,70,91] uses a Mevatron 88 (15 MV) in a manner similar to that of the Vicenza group, and using 11 arcs. However, an additional circular collimator is placed in the block tray to reduce the penumbra. Collimator diameters of 6 mm to 54 mm are available.

The group in Montreal[73] uses a Varian Clinac 18 (10 MV). Both the stereotactic frame and the patient are supported by the treatment couch, and additional circular collimators of diameter 5 mm to 30 mm are placed in the block tray. During treatment, gantry and couch move simultaneously, and the resulting points of beam entry on the convexity of the skull resemble the seam on a baseball. The technique has been termed "dynamic stereotactic radiosurgery." Beam entrance and exit doses do not overlap. One advantage of this technique is that treatment proceeds quickly.

The group in Buenos Aires[7] uses a Varian Clinac 18 (10 MV) with additional circular collimators of 5 mm to 20 mm diameter. The patient sits on a chair mounted on circular rails and the gantry rotates through an arc for each of several stationary chair positions. The resulting points of beam entry on the surface of the skull trace out a series of diadems (like football seams, with the ends of the football at the ears). Beam entrance and exit doses do not overlap.

Numerous groups, including those in Boston, San Francisco, and St. Louis, use the Varian Clinac 6/100 (6 MV). Neither the couch nor the lasers are used to precisely position the lesion at the isocenter.[49,50,51,55,80,98] To improve treatment accuracy, the stereotactic frame is supported by and positioned with a rigid, adjustable support stand fixed to the plate over the couch

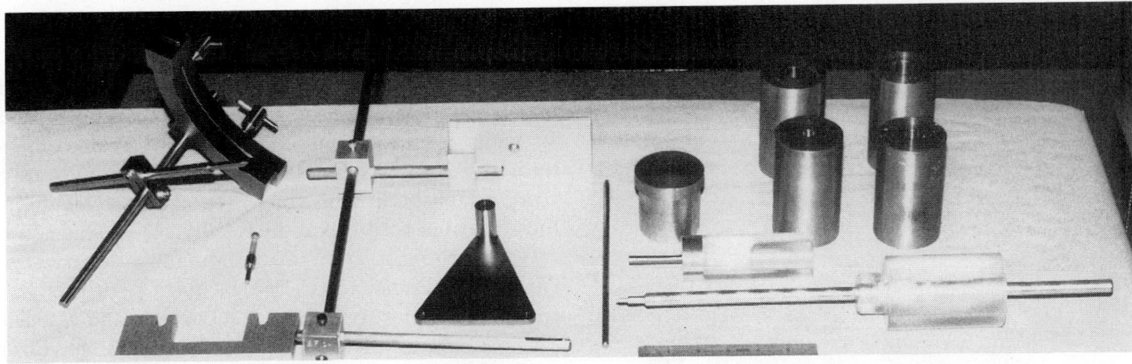

FIGURE 23–16. Display of the apparatus fabricated at Jewish Hospital of St. Louis to perform radiosurgery with a Varian Clinac 6/100: dosimetry devices, measurement devices, and circular collimators. (Adapted from Lutz W, Winston KR, Maleki N: Int J Radiat Oncol Biol Phys 14:373–381, 1988)

rotation bearing, while the patient's torso is supported by the couch. Circular collimators of 12.5 mm to 40 mm diameter are placed reproducibly on dowel pins on the gantry rather than being slid into the block tray (Figs. 23-16 to 23-18).

A film technique allows verification of all positioning adjustments after the coordinates of the isocenter are determined. The points of beam entry trace out a football-seam pattern on the convexity of the skull, similar to that of the Vicenza and Heidelberg groups. In most cases four or five arcs per isocenter are used. Beam entrance and exit doses may but need not overlap. Essentially identical systems have been developed (or are under development) at several dozen facilities, all closely following the original design of Lutz and colleagues.[55]

A different technique has been developed at the University of Florida[21] to produce a similar pattern of noncoplanar arcs, but with a separate bearing to support the collimator to avoid small positional errors introduced by the gantry bearing.

Developmental approaches include the use of electrons with a multiportal machined helmet[6] and fractionated treatments with a noninvasive stereotactic frame with multiple arcs.[25]

Various linac-based radiosurgery systems and their dose fall-off variability are listed in Table 23-14. Table 23-15 demonstrates how irradiation of normal tissue volume is dependent on target size.

TARGET VOLUME DETERMINATION

The technique used to determine target geometry depends on the type of target. For arteriovenous malformation (AVM), the target volume should include the entire nidus as visualized by angiography. Siddon and Barth[82] developed a method for determining the center and maximum dimensions of an AVM nidus, whereby most constraints on source-frame-film geometry are relaxed. The technique allows determination of magnification factors as well as distance between anteroposterior and lateral angiogram treatment volume. Orthogonal angiograms are not sufficient to determine dimensions of that portion of the nidus which is visualized at angiography; they do not allow determination of its three-dimensional structure. If the nidus is irregular-shaped, a spherical isodose surface that encloses it may needlessly enclose a substantial amount of normal tissue. In principle, treatment volume can be reduced somewhat by obtaining multiple stereoscopic angiographic pairs,[22] possibly by using MRI,[65,83] or by using an asymmetric distribution of collimators/arcs.

A second difficulty associated with target volume determination is related to the arterial supply of AVMs. In many cases AVMs are fed by several arteries, and injections of contrast into different vessels may be necessary. Orthogonal angiographic views of each injection must be obtained. Because the apparent nidus volumes obtained from separate injections may differ, the true nidus volume is considered to be that volume which encloses all separate nidus volumes. The process of overlaying these separate volumes may introduce errors in the treatment volume. Determination of the nidus volume is dependent on resolution and contrast and on subjective variables of interpretation. For example, small outlying AVM vessels may not be

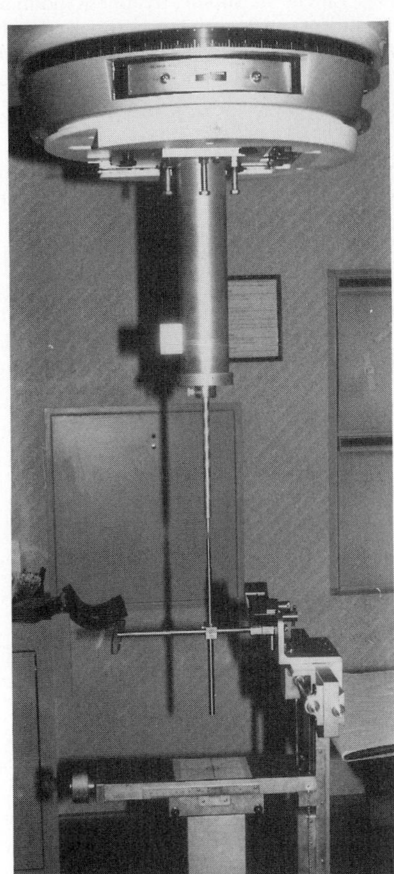

FIGURE 23–17. Setup of the circular collimators attached to the block tray as used at Jewish Hospital of St. Louis and the head frame attached to the base stand and with a physical pointer test system to ensure physical reproducibility.

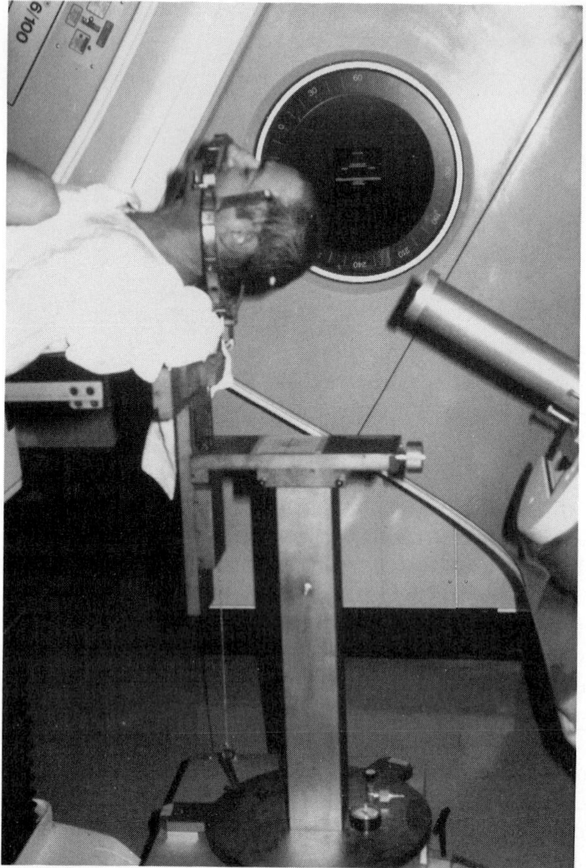

FIGURE 23–18. Patient in supine treatment position, body supported by the treatment couch, with head supported in the stereotactic frame and stand fixed to the turntable of the treatment couch, and the gantry of the machine rotated with the circular collimator attached.

readily detected and may therefore not be treated, but could eventually hemorrhage. Interpretation may be difficult if a large artery or draining vein—not part of the nidus—overlies the nidus.

Magnetic resonance imaging and computed tomography can be used to determine treatment volumes for lesions other than vascular malformations. The main limitations involve errors of localization and lack of knowledge of the actual (rather than apparent) extent of the lesion, especially for infiltrative lesions. Newer techniques of multiple-image correlation should prove useful.[102]

INDICATIONS FOR RADIOSURGERY

Radiosurgery has been used to treat a variety of benign and malignant lesions and some functional disorders (Table 23-16). In many instances, only a small number of cases have been treated; results have not been reported, and indications are far from established. Kihlstrom[33] reported 1311 gamma-unit radiosurgical procedures at the Karolinska Hospital from 1968 to 1986. The most common treatment categories were arteriovenous malformation (41%), acoustic neurinoma (14%), and functional radiosurgery (14%). Chierego and associates[9] listed 150 patients treated with a linac-based system; the most frequent categories were AVM (44%) and malignancy (33%). Lunsford and co-workers[53] reported their experience with AVMs, as the majority of lesions treated (Table 23-17).

Evidence suggests that the natural history[31] of inoperable AVMs may be favorably influenced following radiosurgery, as discussed in the following text. For many other lesions the indications for treatment have not been clearly established; for some, radiosurgery must be regarded as investigational.[55, 79, 92]

Ideal target volumes for radiosurgery are nearly spherical and small, up to about 3 cm in maximum dimension. Irregular volumes may require treatment to multiple isocenters to shape a selected isodose surface to conform to the target volume. Larger treatment volumes appear to be associated with lower response rates for AVMs.

ARTERIOVENOUS MALFORMATIONS

Treatment Options

Standard therapeutic intervention is craniotomy and surgical excision for small circumscribed arteriovenous malformations (AVMs) located on or near a polar region of the brain's surface. Modern surgical results and complications have been reviewed.[8, 13, 19, 28, 86] For large AVMs with a major subcortical portion fed by deep and superficial vessels, treatment options are nonintervention, irradiation, multiple embolization, and staged resection. The main treatment goal is to eliminate the risk of hemorrhage. In some cases, the AVM may be inaccessible, especially if centrally located, in the speech area or in the brain stem. Patients with such AVMs may be candidates for radiosurgery.[67] Other candidates are patients with concomitant medical problems that preclude craniotomy or embolization and patients who refuse these approaches.

Radiosurgical principles applicable to the treatment of AVMs are evolving but may be similar to established surgical

TABLE 23–14
Dose Falloffs Outside the Target for Various Radiosurgical Techniques

	MIN/MAX DISTANCE IN MM FOR DOSE TO FALL FROM		
RADIOSURGICAL TECHNIQUE*	90% TO 50%	90% TO 20%	90% TO 10%
Gamma unit	2/4	4/12	5/22
Single plane rotation	1/4	1/14	2/32
Multiple converging arcs (4 arcs)	2/3	4/8	8/19
Dynamic rotation (McGill)	2/2	3/8	5/17

** The 90% isodose surface coincides with a 1 cm diameter spherical target volume.*
(Modified from Podgorsak EB, Pike GB, Oliver A, et al: Int J Radiat Oncol Biol Phys 16:857–865, 1989)[74]

TABLE 23–15
Volume of Normal Tissue Receiving Significant Radiosurgery Dose

TARGET DIAMETER (cm)*	GRADIENT THICKNESS (cm)†	TARGET VOLUME (cm^3)	NORMAL TISSUE VOLUME (cm^3)‡
1	1	0.5	13.6
2	1	4.2	29.3
3	1	14.1	51.3
4	1	33.5	79.6

**Diameter of 80% isodose surface*
†Approximate difference between 20% and 80% isodose surface radii
‡Volume between 20% and 80% isodose surfaces

principles[69]: within the nidus of the AVM, the physician may be rather destructive because usually little normally functioning tissue is found therein; feeding arteries or draining veins should not be pursued beyond their points of attachment to the nidus to avoid unnecessary normal tissue damage; obliteration of a final feeding artery only improves tissue nutrition, and obliteration of any other artery only worsens tissue nutrition; total obliteration is of vastly greater benefit than is partial obliteration.

Pathologic Changes After Irradiation

In 1928, neurosurgeon Harvey Cushing recognized that irradiation of AVMs could lead to intimal proliferation and vascular occlusion.[14] It has since been recognized that small vessels are occluded more easily than large, in part because small vessels have less latitude for endothelial changes to occur before patency is compromised. Radiosurgery of AVMs may lead to an intense gliosis around the malformation, possibly producing an endarteritis obliterans.[3,61,64] Kjellberg and co-workers[36] observed an endotheliitis within small vessels of AVMs irradiated with protons with associated subendothelial deposition of collagen and hyaline. Recently Colombo[12] and Pozza and associates[77] published informative sample photomicrographs of operative specimens following radiosurgery, confirming Kjellberg's observations.

Usually, obliteration of AVMs after radiosurgery is not complete for 1 to 2 years. The exact mechanism of damage to AVMs, or to normal brain tissue, following high-dose, small-volume irradiation is not yet completely understood.

TABLE 23–16
Reported Uses of Radiosurgery

Acoustic neurinoma	Glioblastoma
Astrocytoma, anaplastic	Glomus
Astrocytoma, low grade	Lymphoma
Arterial aneurysm	Medulloblastoma
Arteriovenous malformation	Meningioma
Carotid-cavernous fistula	Metastasis
Cavernous angioma	Oligodendroglioma
Choroid plexus papilloma	Pinealoma
Craniopharyngioma	Pineoblastoma
Ependymoma	Pineocytoma
Functional radiosurgery	Pituitary
Germinoma	Venous Angioma

TABLE 23–17
*Uses of Stereotactic Gamma Radiosurgery at the University of Pittsburgh**

	NUMBER	%
Arteriovenous malformation	113	55
Acoustic neurinoma	39	19
Meningioma	22	11
Pituitary adenoma	11	5
Glial tumor	9	4
Anaplastic astrocytoma	3	—
Glioblastoma	3	—
Ependymoma	2	—
Astrocytoma	1	—
Chordoma	1	1
Total	207	100

**August 1987 through December 1988*
(Modified from Lunsford LD, Flickinger J, Coffey RJ, et al: Arch Neurol 47:169–175, 1990)[53]

Fractionated Radiation Treatment Results

Early reports on the use of radiation for AVMs frequently failed to provide important information necessary for interpretation of results, such as minimum and maximum radiation dose, size of AVM, fractionation scheme, long-term angiographic or clinical follow-up, number of patients lost to follow-up, and availability of techniques for simulation and verification. When modern external radiation therapy equipment and techniques are used, fractionated radiation is unlikely to result in complete AVM obliteration in a large percentage of cases.[47,76,99,101] Lindqvist and colleagues[47] reported patients with large AVMs treated with fractionated irradiation using individually shaped plastic helmets during planning, angiography, and treatment. AVM sizes were 7 cm^3 to 107 cm^3 (mean 43 cm^3). Patients received 4200 cGy in 6 weeks (350 cGy twice weekly). Of 26 AVMs evaluated at 18 months, angiography demonstrated one complete response and one subtotal response (76% to 99% obliteration). Of five AVMs evaluated at 5 years, there was one complete response. Four patients in the series hemorrhaged (two fatally).

Radiosurgery Treatment Results

Several factors make comparison of the results of treatments among various radiosurgery series difficult: grading systems for AVMs are not used, although their use has been suggested[81,85]; patient selection factors vary; AVM location within the brain varies; concomitant medical problems may play a role; and brain exposed to prior injury (stroke, open excision) may have decreased tolerance to therapy. AVMs pretreated with partial embolization may have an altered radiosurgical response. Criteria for judging a complete response may vary. Lindqvist and Steiner[46] suggest that a complete angiographic response should not be declared without demonstration of a normal circulation time, complete absence of pathologic vessels in the former nidus, and normalization or disappearance of draining veins. Radiosurgery outcomes may vary for technical reasons: no established minimum volume beyond the nidus that should be treated or established minimum dose required in whatever volume is selected; difficulty in determination of the treatment volume; and the presence of small outlying AVM vessels that are beyond the resolution and detection of current angiography and could eventually hemorrhage despite completely normal follow-up angiography. The likelihood of hemorrhage may depend on how generously the treatment volume was selected. Finally, the number of patients treated has often been substantially larger than the number followed up and reported on.

To maximize the possibility of obtaining a complete response, it appears necessary to include the entire nidus in the treatment volume. Steiner[89] reported 2-year complete and partial angiographic response rates of 87% and 11%, respectively, in 104 patients in whom the radiation field completely covered the nidus; corresponding numbers in 19 patients in whom only partial coverage of the nidus was possible were no complete responses and seven partial responses. Valentino[94] reported complete response in ten of 11 patients in whom the entire nidus was covered, and in none of 12 patients in whom the nidus was uncovered.

Fabrikant and co-workers[16] treated more than 300 AVMs using helium ions. The complete response rate for patients in whom the entire arterial phase of the AVM was covered was 90% to 95% for volumes no larger than 4 cm^3, 80% to 85% for volumes in the range of 4 cm^3 to 14 cm^3, and 65% to 70% for volumes larger than 14 cm^3. The overall complete response rate for volumes up to 60 cm^3 was 80%. They have reported a hemorrhage rate in treated patients well below that in a population of untreated patients.[16] Hosobuchi and co-workers[29] reported results of treatment for AVMs with helium ions. With minimum follow-up of 26 months, 56% of patients demonstrated complete angiographic response.

Kjellberg and associates[35,36] reported results for 439 AVMs treated with protons. A complete angiographic response at 2 years was obtained in 22% of patients studied. The lower complete response rates obtained with protons compared with other techniques may be related to patient selection or other factors such as AVM size. (The mean size of AVMs treated by Kjellberg and associates was 4.3 cm—larger than in other series.) The rate of fatal hemorrhage within 18 months of treatment was thought to be consistent with that in untreated patients. Two years following treatment, patients who initially presented with hemorrhage bled at a significantly reduced rate (2% per year compared with 7% per year), implying protection against hemorrhage after a 2-year latent period.

Betti,[7] using a linac-based system, treated 66 AVMs and reported a 66% complete response rate in 41 patients followed up for 2 years. In several patients, the entire nidus was not treated. The 1- and 2-year complete response rates were 23% and 93% in patients in whom the entire nidus was treated. Smaller AVMs responded better. Five patients rebled. Seizures were reduced in six of ten patients who had seizures before radiosurgery.

Colombo and colleagues,[12] using a linac system without additional collimation, treated 97 AVMs and reported an overall complete response rate of 52% in 50 patients who underwent angiography at 1 year and 75% in 20 patients who underwent angiography at 2 years. The response rate at 1 year was dependent on AVM size: 76% if less than 15 mm, 37.5% if between 15 mm and 25 mm, and 11% if larger than 25 mm. The corresponding rates at 2 years were 90%, 80%, and 40%, respectively. No effects on frequency of seizure were seen.

Kemeny and co-workers[32] described the 1-year results in 52 patients treated with a gamma-unit in Sheffield. The complete response rate was 31%. Lateral AVMs responded better than midline AVMs. Lesions fed by more than one large vessel were less likely to respond. Interestingly, the chance of response at 1 year was not dependent on AVM size. In patients already suffering from seizures, no change in the nature or frequency of seizures was seen.

Souhami and associates[84] reported results in 33 patients treated with the dynamic radiosurgery technique; 14 underwent angiography at 1 year, with a complete response rate of 43%.

Barcia-Salorio,[4] using a standard cobalt therapy unit, treated 42 patients with AVMs and reported a complete response in 41% of patients at 1 year and 85% at 2 years.

To determine the relative importance of confounding variables, multivariate analysis of clinical and technical parameters must be performed. This has not yet been done.

Dose-Volume Relationships

Considering radiobiologic effects, one would expect the therapeutic ratio to get worse, not better, as one proceeds from multifractionated to single-fraction irradiation. If a target volume contains little normally functioning tissue and if an almost negligible dose of radiation is deposited in the surrounding normal tissue volume, this expectation may be less compelling. The available response and complication rate data on the treatment of AVMs with radiosurgery appear to favor single fractionation.

Kjellberg and co-workers[37] attempted to summarize information on dose-volume relationships for single-fraction treatments by plotting brain necrosis data from various animal and human studies on a log-log plot with dose on the vertical axis and radius of the treatment volume on the horizontal axis. They incorporated data on the development of necrosis in mice following irradiation with proton microbeams, data from monkeys following treatment with protons, data from humans treated with protons, and historical data from humans treated with x-rays. The data thus plotted follow a curve, which may be approximated over small ranges of log dose and log radius by a straight line. The absolute position and slope of the line are considerably uncertain.

Kjellberg and co-workers[37] estimated the location on the plot of separate lines representing low and high risks for ionizing necrosis of the human brain.[35,36] These lines are called the 1% and 99% necrosis lines, and treatment doses that tended to lie around the 1% necrosis line were selected. Some groups select doses such that the dose at the 80% isodose surface, which encloses the target volume, lies near the 1% necrosis line. Although this line can be considered no more than a rough guide, because it is not based on complications following radiosurgery for AVM, it does emphasize that the risk of complications following radiosurgery is based on a presumed relationship between prescribed dose and treatment volume. Additional variables that are probably related to risk include patient age, location of target volume, and concomitant medical problems.

Various radiosurgery dose schemes are used. Steiner and co-workers[90] initially treated AVMs with a gamma-unit with doses of 3000 cGy to 12,500 cGy, sometimes with multiple overlapping fields. More recently the edge of the nidus has received about 2000 cGy to 2500 cGy[46,87]; brain stem lesions receive somewhat less. Doses in children and adults are similar. For small lesions, treated with a single isocenter, the dose at the periphery, about 2500 cGy, corresponds to the 80% to 90% isodose surface. For somewhat larger lesions (collimator sizes are no larger than 18 mm), more than one isocenter is used. In this case the dose at the periphery, about 2000 cGy to 2500 cGy, corresponds to the 50% to 60% isodose surface. Kemeny and associates,[32] also using a gamma-unit, treated all patients to 2500 cGy, prescribed at the 50% isodose surface that surrounded the nidus.

Fabrikant and co-workers[16] initially treated to a maximum dose of 4500 cGyE; currently they deliver 1500 cGyE to 2500 cGyE prescribed at the 90% isodose surface.

Betti,[7] using a linac system, treated AVMs with maximum doses of 2000 cGy to 7000 cGy (mostly 3000 cGy to 5000 cGy); the prescription at the periphery was 70% to 75%. Colombo and colleagues,[12] using a linac system, prescribed 1500 cGy to 3000 cGy at the 60% to 90% isodose surface. The Montreal group[73] has treated AVMs with a linac system, prescribing 4000 cGy to 5000 cGy at the 90% isodose surface, which encloses the target volume. Barcia-Salorio,[4] using a standard cobalt therapy system, delivers 2000 cGy to 5000 cGy to the center of the target. The Heidelberg group, using a linac system, prescribes single doses of 1000 cGy to 5000 cGy at the 80% isodose surface, depending on lesion size; doses generally follow the 1% necrosis line.

In summation, various doses and normalizations have been used. To increase understanding of dose-volume relationships in normal tissue as well as in AVMs, it is recommended that clinical response and complication rates be subcategorized, if possible, according to AVM size and dose. Radiosurgery groups are encouraged to describe completely the doses used, including both peripheral and maximal tumor doses, especially when multiple isocenters are used.

Side Effects and Complications

Depending on the type of stereotactic frame used, some degree of discomfort may be caused by radiosurgery. To minimize the risk of vomiting with the patient in a fixed position, the patient is instructed to take nothing by mouth before the procedure. It is necessary to minimize the length of time that the patient is immobilized and to instruct all participants on the rapid separation of patient and apparatus. Some groups observe patients overnight following radiosurgery. Occasional acute reactions have been reported, including headache, elevated temperature, and increased risk of seizure.[36] Nausea and vomiting may be associated with radiosurgery near the area postrema in the floor of the fourth ventricle, unless patients are premedicated.[2,32,52]

Steiner[87] reported new neurologic deficits in four (3%) of 135 AVM patients treated with a gamma-unit. He subsequently reported seven cases (2%)[88] of delayed radionecrosis in 300 AVM patients. Recently Steiner reported 20 cases of radiation-induced changes following radiosurgery, typically manifesting clinically after a 3- to 8-month latency.[89] Of the 20, eight had moderate to marked symptoms, six had slight to moderate transitory or permanent deficits, and six were asymptomatic.

Fabrikant and co-workers[17,18] saw no neurologic complications in the first 55 AVM patients treated with helium ions but subsequently reported neurologic deterioration in five (8%) of 66 patients. Hosobuchi and associates[29] described seven (9%) complications in 76 AVM patients treated with helium ions. Marks and colleagues[59,60] reported new symptoms and corresponding radiologic abnormalities in five (25%) of 20 AVM patients 11 to 22 months after treatment with helium ions; two of six patients with small lesions (less than 8 cm^3) compared with three of 14 with larger lesions were affected. No significant differences in doses were seen among the patients who developed symptoms and those who did not; maximum doses were 2800 cGy to 4500 cGy. Most recently Fabrikant and associates[16] reported serious permanent neurologic damage occurring within 2 years in 5% to 6% of patients, including those treated earlier with higher doses. Permanent neurologic damage is thought to occur in 2% to 3% of patients with currently used doses.

Kjellberg and co-workers[35,36] described neurologic complications in four (15%) of their first 27 AVM patients treated with protons, in eight (11%) of the first 74 patients treated, and in nine (2%) of the first 444 patients, with improvements in complication rates attributed to changes in doses and field sizes.

Betti[7] reported that two of 66 AVM patients developed neurologic deficits. Colombo and associates[12] reported clinical or radiologic complications in seven of 97 AVM patients. Kemeny and co-workers[32] reported no clinical or radiologic complications of radiosurgery in 52 AVM patients other than nausea and vomiting immediately following treatment in some patients treated to the posterior fossa. Souhami and co-workers[84] reported three late side effects in 33 AVM patients. Barcia-Salorio[4] reported no complications in 42 AVM patients.

No complications attributable to dose deposition external to the brain during radiosurgery are likely, with the exception of alopecia adjacent to a treatment volume near the inner table of the skull.

Complication rates are difficult to compare because often neither the population at risk for complication at a given time point nor the population actually followed up to a given time point is clearly defined. In addition, some reported complication rates represent clinical complications, some represent radiologic complications, and some incorporate both.

ASTROCYTOMAS

It might be argued that radiosurgery, with its dose localization characteristics, is contraindicated in the treatment of malignant intracranial lesions, in which tumor cells are known to infiltrate beyond the borders of abnormalities seen on CT or MRI. Nevertheless, most groups have treated small numbers of such patients; whether treatment enhances survival or local control is uncertain.

Colombo and colleagues[11] reported nine low-grade astrocytomas of apparent 7 mm to 25 mm diameters treated with a linac radiosurgery system. Patients were followed up by CT for 18 to 43 months. Radiologic response was noted in seven cases, and six patients improved clinically. An almost complete shrinkage of abnormality on CT was noted within 2 to 4 weeks in several patients with malignant radiation-sensitive tumors (medulloblastoma, germinoma, lymphoma).

Pozza and co-workers,[77] reporting on the same group, described 14 patients with low-grade astrocytoma who were followed up for 18 to 48 months after treatment. These patients received 1600 cGy to 5000 cGy in one or two fractions at the 80% to 90% isodose surface, which encompassed CT evidence of tumor. Field sizes ranged from 0.5 mm^2 by 0.5 mm^2 to 3.5 mm^2 by 3.5 mm^2, as defined by the linac jaws (no additional collimation was used). Patients were selected according to the following criteria: nonoperable; lesion not larger than 30 mm diameter; biopsy-proven grade 1 or grade 2 astrocytoma; clear margins confirmed by multiple stereotactic biopsies; spherical shape. Tumor volumes ranged from 180 mm^3 to 8200 mm^3. In ten of 14 patients Karnofsky performance scores improved following radiosurgery. Although marked shrinkage of the tumor was seen eventually in 11 of 14 patients, clinical and CT responses usually did not occur within the first 6 months following treatment.

Serial contrast-enhanced CT scans demonstrated a gradual increase in apparent tumor size over a period of up to 6 to 9 months. Also noted was the simultaneous development of a dense central core that evolved into a contrast-enhanced ring over the same 6- to 9-month period, roughly corresponding to the border of the apparent target volume. From this time until 12 to 24 months after radiosurgery, progressive shrinkage of the glioma was noted. Similar radiologic responses have been described in patients undergoing interstitial implants[63,68] and may represent radiation-induced modification of capillary permeability.

BRAIN METASTASES

The behavior of metastatic lesions following radiosurgical treatment may be different from that following treatment for astrocytomas. Sturm and colleagues[91] described 12 patients with a solitary 10 mm to 35 mm brain metastasis treated with a linac radiosurgery system. Most patients were treated in a single fraction to 2000 cGy to 3000 cGy, delivered to the 80% isodose surface, which surrounded the apparent tumor margin on CT. Seven patients were followed up for at least 3 months. Of these, two had complete response by CT, all improved clinically, and three recuperated fully from their neurological dysfunction.

Marin-Gomez and associates[58] of the same group reported 40 patients with solitary brain metastases from lung cancer, hypernephroma, and colorectal tumors, 26 of whom were followed up for a mean of 8 months. Partial or complete responses on CT were seen in 11 patients. No response was seen in 13 patients. Two patients demonstrated tumor progression. Clinical responses reflected the CT responses and often commenced within a few days. Mean survival measured from the time of the radiosurgery was 9 months, similar to that seen in patients treated surgically or with fractionated radiation therapy. Radiosurgical treatment resulted in greatly reduced hospitalization days and hospital visits.

Patil[71] reported seven patients with primary or metastatic brain tumors treated with radiosurgery (average dose 5500 cGy, plus 3000 cGy conventional external-beam irradiation in standard fractions). In all cases but one, progressive decrease in tumor size was seen over a period of 4 to 5 weeks following treatment. Reduction in CT contrast enhancement, without evidence of significant swelling, was seen within 24 hours. Two patients with primary brain tumors progressed locally at 8 and 12 months. In the remaining cases, patients died of their primary lesions outside the brain without increased intracranial tumor progression.

Loeffler and associates[51] treated 18 patients with 21 persistent or recurrent lesions. Patients had prior external radiation therapy. Single doses of 900 cGy to 2500 cGy were given to small volumes ($<27 cm^3$) using a linac system. With a median follow-up of 9 months (1 to 39 months), local control was achieved in all treated sites.

ACOUSTIC NEURINOMAS

Acoustic neurinomas are usually approached microsurgically with a goal of preserving facial nerve function and hearing, and cure is defined as total removal of the tumor. Wallner and colleagues[95] have demonstrated that standard radiation therapy is effective following biopsy. With radiosurgery, response is defined as lack of further tumor growth. Noren and co-workers[66] reported radiosurgical treatment of 115 acoustic neurinomas (110 patients) treated with a gamma-knife and followed up adequately. Most tumors were smaller than 30 mm in diameter. In 44% of cases tumor size decreased, and growth was arrested in 42%, for a response rate of 86%. Patients with unilateral tumors responded better than those with neurofibromatosis. Temporary facial weakness was seen in 15% of cases and was dose-related; no patient developed permanent facial weakness or facial paralysis. Preoperative hearing was preserved in 26% of cases. A mild facial hypesthesia developed in 18% of patients. For most patients the peripheral tumor dose was 1800 cGy to 2500 cGy, depending on lesion size and patient age, and the maximum tumor dose was 2200 cGy to 5000 cGy. The Pittsburgh group[48] reported 26 patients with a median follow-up of 13 months and a tumor response in 42%.

IMAGING STUDIES FOLLOWING RADIOSURGERY

Various imaging studies following radiosurgery may help elucidate the nature and time course of changes in lesions and surrounding brain tissue.[27] Mindus and associates[62] obtained MRI and CT scans in seven patients several years after treatment with high-dose functional radiosurgery. T2-weighted images were more accurate than CT in detecting and defining the size and configuration of the lesions. Leksell and colleagues[45] reported that MRI changes can be almost immediate. They presented a patient who underwent radiosurgical internal capsulotomy on the right and left sides, 1 month apart. The dose to the right side was 10,000 cGy and to the left, 12,000 cGy. One day following the second treatment MR images were obtained, demonstrating a small lesion in each internal capsule. Following treatment with lower radiosurgical doses the latent period before MR changes are seen is longer. These results suggest that radiosurgery produces focal regions of noninflammatory demyelination, edema, and necrosis, all having similar appearance on T2-weighted images, and suggests that gadolinium may be useful in defining the presence or absence of necrosis. Marks and co-workers[59,60] described CT and MRI changes in seven patients who developed complications following treatment of intracranial vascular malformations with helium ion radiosurgery.

Beginning at about 6 months after radiosurgery, MRI is useful for monitoring the possible development of edema or signs of radiation damage. For patients with AVM, angiography should be performed to determine level of response after no evidence of the AVM is visible on MRI.

Positron emission tomography (PET) has recently emerged as a useful way to differentiate tumor from necrosis in previously irradiated patients. It may also be a potential way of evaluating recurrent brain tumors for malignant degeneration[20] and of predicting prognosis after therapy.[1] PET scans using 18FDG (fluorodeoxyglucose) reveal hypermetabolic states associated with tumors compared with the hypometabolic foci associated with necrosis.[15] Serial scanning with PET scans of patients who have undergone stereotactic external-beam irradiation may allow better evaluation of the time course and efficacy of this modality in controlling small malignant tumors. We have seen marked diminution of metabolic activity in 1-month follow-up PET scans.

REFERENCES

1. Alavi JB, Alavi A, Chawluk J, et al: Positron emission tomography in patients with glioma. A predictor of prognosis. Cancer 62:1074–1078, 1988
2. Alexander E, Siddon RL, Loeffler JS: The acute onset of nausea and vomiting following stereotactic radiosurgery: Correlation with total dose to area postrema. Surg Neurol 32:40–44, 1989
3. Andersson B, Larsson B, Leksell L, et al: Histopathology of late radio lesions in the goat brain. Acta Radiol 9:385–394, 1940
4. Barcia-Salorio JL: Special stereotactic techniques: Single-beam photon radiotherapy. In Heilbrun M (ed.): Stereotactic Neurosurgery, vol 2, pp 211–217. Baltimore, Williams & Wilkins, 1988
5. Barcia-Salorio JL, Hernandez G, Broseta J, et al: Radiosurgical treatment of carotid-cavernous fistula. Appl Neurophysiol 45:520–522, 1982
6. Barish RJ, Barish SV: A new stereotactic knife. Int J Radiat Oncol Biol Phys 14:1295–1298, 1988
7. Betti O: Treatment of arteriovenous malformations with the linear accelerator. Appl Neurophysiol 50:262, 1987
8. Brown RD, Wiebers DO, Forbes G, et al: The natural history of unruptured intracranial arteriovenous malformations. J Neurosurg 68:352–357, 1988
9. Chierego G, Marchetti M, Avanzo RC, et al: Dosimetric considerations on multiple arc stereotaxic radiotherapy. Radiother Oncol 12:141–152, 1988
10. Colombo F, Benedetti A, Pozza F, et al: External stereotactic irradiation by linear accelerator. Neurosurgery 16:154–159, 1985
11. Colombo F, Benedetti A, Pozza F, et al: Radiosurgery using a 4 MV linear accelerator. Acta Radiol 369(Suppl):603–307, 1986
12. Colombo F, Benedetti A, Pozza F, et al: Linear accelerator radiosurgery of cerebral arteriovenous malformations. Neurosurgery 24:833–840, 1989
13. Crawford PM, West CR, Chadwick DW, et al: Arteriovenous malformations of the brain: Natural history in unoperated patients. J Neurol Neurosurg Psychol 49:1–10, 1986
14. Cushing H, Bailey P: Tumors arising from the blood vessels of the brain. Springfield, IL, Charles C Thomas, 1928
15. DiChiro G, Oldfield E, Wright DC, et al: Cerebral necrosis after radiotherapy and/or intraarterial chemotherapy for brain tumors: PET and neuropathologic studies. Am J Neuroradiol 8:1083–1091, 1987
16. Fabrikant JI, Levy RP, Frankel KA, et al: Stereotactic helium-ion radiosurgery for the treatment of intracranial arteriovenous malformations. In Heikkinen E, Kiviniitty K (eds): Proceedings of the International Workshop on Proton and Narrow Photon Beam Therapy, pp 33–37. Oulu, University of Oulu Press, 1989
17. Fabrikant JI, Lyman J, Frankel KA: Heavy charged-particle Bragg peak radiosurgery for intracranial vascular disorders. Radiat Res 104:S244–S258, 1985
18. Fabrikant JI, Lyman J, Hosobuchi Y: Stereotactic heavy-ion Bragg peak radiosurgery for intra-cranial vascular disorders: Method for treatment of deep arteriovenous malformations. Br J Radiol 57:479–490, 1984
19. Foerster DM, Steiner L, Hakanson S: Arteriovenous malformations of the brain: A long term clinical study. J Neurosurg 37:562–570, 1972
20. Francavilla TL, Miletich RS, DiChiro G, et al: Positron emission tomography in the detection of malignant degeneration of low-grade gliomas. Neurosurgery 24:1–5, 1989
21. Friedman WA, Bova FJ: The University of Florida radiosurgery system. Surg Neurol 32:334–342, 1989
22. Giorgi C, Cerchiari U, Broggi G, et al: 3-D reconstruction of cerebral angiography in stereotactic neurosurgery. Acta Neurochir 39(Suppl):13–14, 1987
23. Graffman S, Brahme A, Larsson B: Proton radiotherapy with the Uppsala cyclotron: Experience and plans. Strahlentherapie 161:764–770, 1985
24. Gutin PH, Wilson CB: Radiosurgery for malignant brain tumors. J Clin Oncol 8(4):571–573, 1990
25. Hariz MI, Henriksson R, Löfroth P-O, et al: A non-invasive method for fractionated stereotactic irradiation of brain tumors with linear accelerator. Radiother Oncol 17:57–72, 1990
26. Hartmann GH, Schlegel W, Sturm V, et al: Cerebral radiation surgery using moving field irradiation at a linear accelerator facility. Int J Radiat Oncol Biol Phys 11:1185–1192, 1985
27. Hecht-Leavitt C, Grossman RI, Curran WJ, et al: MR of brain radiation injury: Experimental studies in cats. Am J Neuroradiol 8:427–430, 1987
28. Heros RC, Tu Y-K: Is surgical therapy needed for unruptured arteriovenous malformations? Neurology 37:279–286, 1987
29. Hosobuchi Y, Fabrikant J, Lyman J: Stereotactic heavy-particle irradiation of intracranial arteriovenous malformations. Appl Neurophysiol 50:248–252, 1987
30. Hudgins WR: What is radiosurgery? Neurosurgery 23(2):272, 1988
31. Jane JA, Kassell NF, Torner JC, et al: The natural history of aneurysms and arteriovenous malformations. J Neurosurg 62:321–323, 1985
32. Kemeny A, Dias PS, Forster DMC: Results of stereotactic radiosurgery of arteriovenous malformations: An analysis of 52 cases. J Neurol Neurosurg Psychol 52:554–558, 1989
33. Kihlstrom L: Stereotactic radiosurgery—epidemiologic considerations. Karolinska Hospital, Stockholm, personal communication
34. Kirn TJ: Proton radiotherapy: Some perspectives. JAMA 259:787–788, 1988
35. Kjellberg RN: Stereotactic Bragg peak proton beam radiosurgery for cerebral arteriovenous malformations. Ann Clin Res 47(Suppl):S17–S19, 1986
36. Kjellberg RN, Davis KR, Lyons S, et al: Bragg peak proton beam therapy for arteriovenous malformation of the brain. Clin Neurosurg 31:248–290, 1983
37. Kjellberg RN, Hanamura T, Davis KR, et al: Bragg-peak proton-beam therapy for arteriovenous malformations of the brain. N Engl J Med 309:269–274, 1983
38. Kjellberg RN, Preston WM: The use of the Bragg peak of a proton beam for intracerebral lesions. In Second International Congress of Neurological Surgery. Excerpta Medica 36:E103, 1961
39. Larson DA, Gutin PH, Leibel SA, et al: Stereotaxic irradiation of brain tumors. Cancer 65:792–799, 1990
40. Larsson B, Leksell L, Rexed B: The use of high energy protons for cerebral surgery in man. Acta Chir Scand 125:1–7, 1963
41. Larsson B, Linden K, Sarby B: Irradiation of small structures through the intact skull. Acta Radiol Ther Phys Biol 13:512–534, 1974
42. Leksell D: Radiosurgery. Neurosurgery 24(2):297–298, 1989
43. Leksell DG: Stereotactic radiosurgery: Present status and future trends. Neurolog Res 9:60–68, 1987
44. Leksell L: A stereotaxic apparatus for intracerebral surgery. Acta Chir Scand 99:231, 1949
45. Leksell L, Herner T, Leksell D, et al: Visualization of stereotactic radiolesions by nuclear magnetic resonance. J Neurol Neurosurg Psychol 48:19–20, 1985
46. Lindqvist C, Steiner L: Stereotactic radiosurgical treatment of arteriovenous malformations. In Lunsford LD (ed): Modern Stereotactic Neurosurgery, pp 488–505. Boston, Martinus Nijhoff, 1988
47. Lindqvist M, Steiner L, Blomgren H, et al: Stereotactic radiation therapy of intracranial arteriovenous malformations. Acta Radiol 369(Suppl):610–613, 1986
48. Linskey ME, Lunsford LD, Flickinger JC: Radiosurgery for acoustic neurinomas: Early experience. Neurosurgery 26: 736–745, 1990
49. Loeffler JS, Alexander E: The role of stereotactic radiosurgery in the management of intracranial tumors. Oncology 4(3):21–31, 1990
50. Loeffler JS, Alexander E, Eben A, et al: Stereotactic radiosurgery for intracranial arteriovenous malformations using a

standard linear accelerator. Int J Radiat Oncol Biol Phys 17:673–677, 1989

51. Loeffler JS, Kooy HM, Wen PY, et al: The treatment of recurrent brain metastases with stereotactic radiosurgery. J Clin Oncol 8(4):576–582, 1990
52. Loeffler JS, Siddon RL, Wen PY, et al: Stereotactic radiosurgery of the brain using a standard linear accelerator: A study of early and late effects. Radiother Oncol 17:311–321, 1990
53. Lunsford LD, Flickinger J, Coffey RJ, et al: Stereotactic gamma knife radiosurgery: Initial North American experience in 207 patients. Arch Neurol 47:169–175, 1990
54. Lunsford LD, Flickinger J, Lindner G, et al: Stereotactic radiosurgery of the brain using the first United States 201 Cobalt-60 source gamma knife. Neurosurgery 24:151–159, 1989
55. Lutz W, Winston KR, Maleki N: A system for stereotactic radiosurgery with a linear accelerator. Int J Radiat Oncol Biol Phys 14:373–381, 1988
56. Lyman JT, Kanstein L, Yeater F, et al: A helium-ion beam for stereotactic radiosurgery of central nervous system disorders. Med Phys 13:695–699, 1986
57. Maitz AH, Lunsford LD, Wu A, et al: Shielding requirements for on-site loading and acceptance testing of the Leksell gamma knife. Int J Radiat Oncol Biol Phys 18:469–476, 1990
58. Marin-Gomez M, Kimmig B, Engenhart R, et al: High dose percutaneous stereotactic irradiation of solitary brain metastases using a 15 MeV linear accelerator (Abstract). Int J Radiat Oncol Biol Phys 15(Suppl I):231, 1988
59. Marks MP, Delapaz RL, Fabrikant JI, et al: Intracranial vascular malformations: Imaging of charged-particle radiosurgery. I. Results of therapy. Radiology 168:447–455, 1988
60. Marks MP, Delapaz RL, Fabrikant JI, et al: Intracranial vascular malformations: Imaging of charged-particle radiosurgery. II. Complications. Radiology 168:457–462, 1988
61. McCormick WF: Pathology of vascular malformations of the brain. In Wilson CB, Stein BM (eds): Intracranial Arteriovenous Malformations, pp 44–64. Baltimore, Williams & Wilkins, 1984
62. Mindus P, Bergstrom K, Thomas KA, et al: Magnetic resonance imaging of stereotactic radiosurgical lesions in the internal capsule. Acta Radiol 369:S614–S617, 1986
63. Mundinger F: Stereotactic biopsy and technique of implantation of radionuclides. In Jellinger K (ed): Therapy of Malignant Brain Tumors, pp 134–194. Vienna, Springer-Verlag, 1985
64. Nielsen SL, Kjellberg RN, Asbury AK, et al: Neuropathologic effects of proton beam irradiation in man. Acta Neuropathol 20:348–356, 1972
65. Noorbehesht B, Fabrikant JI, Enzmann DR: Size determination of supratentorial arteriovenous malformations by MR, CT and angio. Neuroradiology 29:512–518, 1987
66. Noren G, Arndt J, Hindmarsh T, et al: Stereotactic radiosurgical treatment of acoustic neurinomas. In Lunsford LD (ed): Modern Stereotactic Neurosurgery, pp 481–489. Boston, Martinus Nijhoff, 1988
67. Ogilvy CS: Radiation therapy for arteriovenous malformations: A review. Neurosurgery 26(5):725–735, 1990
68. Ostertag CB, Weigel K, Birg W: CT-changes after long-term interstitial iridium-192-irradiation of cerebral gliomas. In Szikla G (ed): Stereotactic Cerebral Irradiation, pp 149–155. Amsterdam, Elsevier, 1979
69. Parkinson D: Arteriovenous malformations. Neurol Res 4:163–175, 1982
70. Patil A: Isocentric placement of target in the linear accelerator using CT stereotaxis. Acta Neurochir (Wien) 78:168, 1985
71. Patil A: Adaptation of linear accelerators to stereotactic systems. In Lunsford LD (ed): Modern Stereotactic Neurosurgery, pp 471–480. Boston, Martinus Nijhoff, 1988
72. Phillips MH, Frankel KA, Lyman JT, et al: Comparison of different radiation types and irradiation geometries in stereotactic radiosurgery. Int J Radiat Oncol Biol Phys 18:211–220, 1990
73. Podgorsak EB, Olivier A, Pla M, et al: Dynamic stereotactic radiosurgery. Int J Radiat Oncol Biol Phys 14:115–126, 1988
74. Podgorsak EB, Pike GB, Olivier A, et al: Radiosurgery with high energy photon beams: A comparison among techniques. Int J Radiat Oncol Biol Phys 16:857–865, 1989
75. Podgorsak EB, Pike GB, Pla M, et al: Radiosurgery with photon beams: Physical aspects and adequacy of linear accelerators. Radiother Oncol 17:349–358, 1990
76. Poulsen M. Arteriovenous malformation: A summary of 6 cases treated with radiation therapy. Int J Radiat Oncol Biol Phys 13:1553–1557, 1987
77. Pozza F, Colombo F, Chierego G, et al: Low-grade astrocytomas: Treatment with unconventionally fractionated external beam stereotactic radiation therapy. Radiology 171:565–569, 1989
78. Rice RK, Hansen JL, Svensson GK, et al: Measurements of dose distributions in small beams of 6 MV x-rays. Phys Med Biol 32:1087–1099, 1987
79. Salorio JLB, Roldan P, Hernandez G, Gomez LL: Radiosurgical treatment of epilepsy. Appl Neurophysiol 48:400–403, 1985
80. Saunders WM, Winston KR, Siddon RL, et al: Radiosurgery for arteriovenous malformations of the brain using a standard linear accelerator: Rationale and technique. Int J Radiat Oncol Biol Phys 15:441–447, 1988
81. Shi YQ, Chen XC: A proposed scheme for grading intracranial arteriovenous malformations. J Neurosurg 65:484–489, 1986
82. Siddon RL, Barth NH: Stereotaxic localization of intracranial targets. Int J Radiat Oncol Biol Phys 13:1241–1246, 1987
83. Smith HJ, Strother CM, Kikuchi Y, et al: MR imaging in the management of supratentorial intracranial AVM's. Am J Radiol 150:1143–1153, 1988
84. Souhami L, Olivier A, Podgorsak E, et al: Dynamic stereotactic radiosurgery: Treatment results on 33 patients with AVM. In Heikkinen E, Kiviniitty K (eds): Proceedings of the International Workshop on Proton and Narrow Photon Beam Therapy, pp 72–76. Oulu, University of Oulu Press, 1989
85. Spetzler RF, Martin NA: A proposed grading system for arteriovenous malformation. J Neurosurg 65:476–483, 1986
86. Stein BM, Mohr JP: Vascular malformations of the brain. N Engl J Med 319:368–370, 1988
87. Steiner L: Treatment of arteriovenous malformations by radiosurgery. In Wilson CB, Stein BM (eds): Intracranial Arteriovenous Malformations, pp 295–314. Baltimore, Williams & Wilkins, 1984
88. Steiner L: Radiosurgery in cerebral arteriovenous malformations. In Flam E, Fein J (eds): Textbook of Cerebrovascular Surgery, pp 1161–1215. New York, Springer-Verlag, 1986
89. Steiner L: Stereotactic radiosurgery with the cobalt 60 gamma unit in the surgical treatment of intracranial tumors and arteriovenous malformations. In Schmidek HH, Sweet WH (eds): Operative Neurosurgical Techniques, vol I, pp 515–529. Philadelphia, WB Saunders, 1988
90. Steiner L, Backlund EO, Greitz T, et al: Radiosurgery in intracranial arteriovenous malformations. Int Congr Neurol Surg 433:168, 1978
91. Sturm V, Kober, Hover KH, et al: Stereotactic percutaneous single dose irradiation of brain metastases with a linear accelerator. Int J Radiat Oncol Biol Phys 13:279–282, 1987
92. Thoren M, Rahn T, Hallengren B, et al: Treatment of Cushing's disease in childhood and adolescence by stereotactic pituitary irradiation. Acta Paediatr Scand 75:388–394, 1986
93. Lawrence JH, Tobias CA, Born JL, et al: Pituitary irradiation with high energy proton beams: A preliminary report. Cancer Res 18:121–134, 1958
94. Valentino V: Radiosurgery in cerebral tumors and AVM. Acta Neurochir 42(Suppl):193–197, 1988
95. Wallner KE, Sheline GE, Pitts LH, et al: Efficacy of irradiation for incompletely excised acoustic neurilemomas. J Neurosurg 67:858–863, 1987
96. Walton L, Bomford CK, Phil M, et al: The Sheffield stereotactic radiosurgery unit: Physical characteristics and principles of operation. Br J Radiol 60:897–906, 1987
97. Winston KR, Lutz W: What is radiosurgery (Reply). Neurosurgery 23(2):272–273, 1988

98. Winston KR, Lutz W: Linear accelerator as a neurosurgical tool for stereotactic radiosurgery. Neurosurgery 22:454–464, 1988
99. Wolkov HB, Bagshaw M: Conventional radiation therapy in the management of arteriovenous malformations of the central nervous system. Int J Radiat Oncol Biol Phys 15:1461–1464, 1988
100. Wu A, Lindner MS, Maitz AH, et al: Physics of gamma knife approach on convergent beams in stereotactic radiosurgery. Int J Radiat Oncol Biol Phys 18:941–949, 1990
101. Zeilstra DJ, Makoski H-B, Nocken U, et al: Semi-stereotactic irradiation of inoperable intracranial arteriovenous malformations. Preliminary results. Eighth International Congress of Neurological Surgery. Toronto, Canada, 1985
102. Zhang J, Levesque MF, Wilson CL: Multimodality imaging of brain structures for stereotactic surgery. Radiology 175:435–441. 1990

24

Pituitary

Perry W. Grigsby
Glenn E. Sheline

ANATOMY OF THE PITUITARY GLAND

The pituitary gland is a midline structure situated in the sella turcica in the body of the sphenoid bone (Fig. 24-1). Superior to the pituitary, the diaphragma sellae separates the pituitary from the chiasmatic cisterns and the floor of the anterior portion of the third ventricle. The optic chiasm overlies the diaphragma sellae and the pituitary in most cases but is over the tuberculum sellae (prefixed) in 10% and over the dorsum sellae (postfixed) in 15%.[76] The anterior cerebral arteries are superior, and the cavernous sinuses, containing the internal carotid arteries and multiple cranial nerves, are lateral to the sella turcica. The sphenoid sinus and nasopharynx are inferior. The pituitary normally weighs about 0.6 g.[53,76]

Posterior Lobe

The posterior lobe of the pituitary arises as an evagination from the floor of the third ventricle[27] with the infundibular recess representing an outpocketing of the anterior floor into the pituitary stalk. Many nerve fibers originating in the supraoptic and paraventricular nuclei of the hypothalamus (which forms the lower lateral walls and floor of the third ventricle) terminate either in the pituitary stalk or in the posterior lobe. Tumors intrinsic to the posterior lobe are virtually unknown.

Anterior and Intermediate Lobes

The anterior and intermediate lobes of the pituitary arise from Rathke's pouch as an evagination from the roof of the nasopharynx.[27] In adults the intermediate lobe is attached to the posterior lobe and separated from the anterior lobe by a narrow cleft, a remnant of Rathke's pouch.

Control of Hormone Output

Secretion of anterior pituitary hormones is controlled largely by hypothalamic hormones carried by the portal system. Presently there are eight known releasing or inhibiting hormones:

- corticotropin releasing hormone (CRH)
- thyrotropin releasing hormone (TRH)
- growth hormone releasing hormone (GH-RH)
- growth hormone release inhibiting hormone (GH-RIH), or somatostatin
- follicle-stimulating hormone releasing hormone (FSH-RH)
- luteinizing hormone releasing hormone (LH-RH)
- prolactin releasing hormone (PRH)
- prolactin inhibiting hormone (PIH)

These hypothalamic hormones in turn control the production and release of six anterior pituitary hormones:

- adrenocorticotropic hormone (ACTH)
- thyroid-stimulating hormone (TSH)
- growth hormone (GH)
- follicle-stimulating hormone (FSH)
- luteinizing hormone (LH)
- prolactin

The output of hypothalamic hormones is controlled primarily by a combination of feedback of endocrine products and direct neural impulses.[28] However, some hormones (*e.g.*, thyroid hormone) are thought to act directly on the pituitary.

EPIDEMIOLOGY

In surgical specimens at the Mayo Clinic,[52] 12% of all intracranial tumors arose in the pituitary gland. About 20% to 25% of presumably normal pituitary glands removed at autopsy and examined by serial section contain adenoma.

The etiology of pituitary adenomas is unknown.[38,69,99] Hardy and co-workers[43] found that 75% of women undergoing surgery for galactorrhea–amenorrhea syndrome had taken oral contraceptives. Other researchers have made similar observations. A recent review of the literature reports a 4% incidence of intracranial aneurysms in patients with pituitary adenomas.[1] Environmental factors are generally not considered to affect the incidence of pituitary adenomas. However, Mirabelli and co-workers[68] have reported three cases of acromegaly occurring in cosmetic factory workers.

NATURAL HISTORY OF PITUITARY TUMORS

Pituitary adenomas vary greatly in size and direction of spread. When small, they tend to be smooth, round tumors, but as size

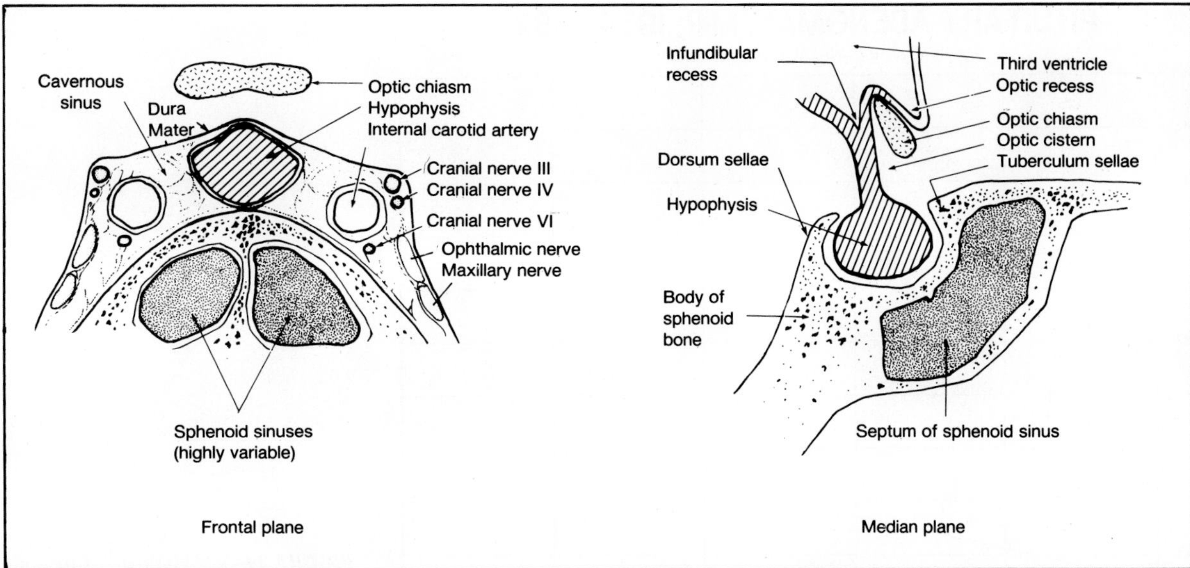

FIGURE 24–1. Frontal and median planes of the pituitary fossa region.

increases, they often become irregular, with nodules extending in various directions (Fig. 24-2). Microadenomas (less than 1 cm in diameter) do not cause gross enlargement of the sella turcica but may cause focal anterior bulging, asymmetry, or sloping of the sella floor. The local invasive properties of pituitary adenomas are well known. Rarely, separate subdural nodules appear; generally these are associated with recurrent tumors.[81] Implants in the subarachnoid space of the spinal cord, dura of the cerebrum, and even metastasis outside the central nervous system have been reported for pituitary tumors associated with Cushing's syndrome.[5,84]

Pituitary tumors generally have a long natural history. The onset of symptoms and signs tends to be insidious. In a group of 95 previously untreated patients, the elicitable duration of symptoms ranged from a few days to over 10 years.[89] In 20% of patients, visual symptoms had been recognized for less than 2 months, but in 10% they had been present for 4 years or longer. Evidence of endocrine deficiency tended to be of even longer duration.

Sheline[86] reported on 16 patients with a presumptive diagnosis of chromophobe adenoma observed several years without treatment. Although two patients showed no evidence of growth over periods of 4 and 20 years, 14 ultimately demonstrated an increase in visual field deficit or size of the sella. The increases became evident after 6 months to 15 years (average 4 years).

Grigsby and co-workers[34] demonstrated the long time to recurrence for patients treated with surgery and postoperative irradiation in a hazard functions analysis of 121 patients followed up for up to 30 years. The risk of developing recurrent disease was less than 0.5% during the first 5 years after treatment, but it progressively increased to a maximum risk factor of 4.4% during the 25- to 30-year follow-up interval (Fig. 24-3).

Asymptomatic Pituitary Adenomas

Kernohan and Sayre[52] reported a 22% autopsy incidence of previously undiagnosed adenomas in presumably normal pituitary glands; most were microscopic adenomas, but a few were large enough to displace optic nerves. If an asymptomatic pituitary tumor (*e.g.*, diagnosed from an incidental skull roentgenogram) is not treated, it must be evaluated periodically for the duration of the patient's life so that growth may be detected before irreversible damage occurs.

Hyperfunctional Adenomas

Hyperfunctional adenomas also progress slowly. In one reported series of 50 acromegalic patients,[61] the mean duration of symptoms was 9.6 years. Roth and co-workers[80] followed up seven untreated acromegalic patients; five showed an increase in plasma growth hormone level, ranging from 35% to 55%, over a period of 1 to 4 years.

CLINICAL PRESENTATION AND DIAGNOSTIC WORKUP

Pituitary adenomas are the most common cause of pituitary dysfunction in adults. Their presentation may be a consequence of malfunction or of local tumor growth with pressure effects. The procedures used for diagnosis are outlined in Table 24-1.

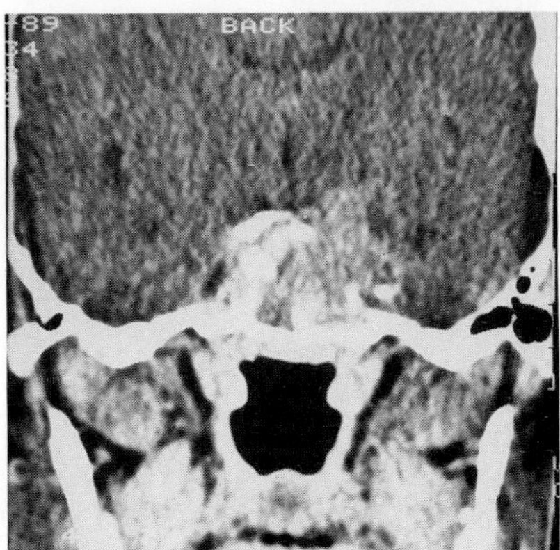

FIGURE 24–2. Large pituitary macroadenoma with suprasellar extension, compression of the medial temporal lobe, and extension into the cavernous sinus.

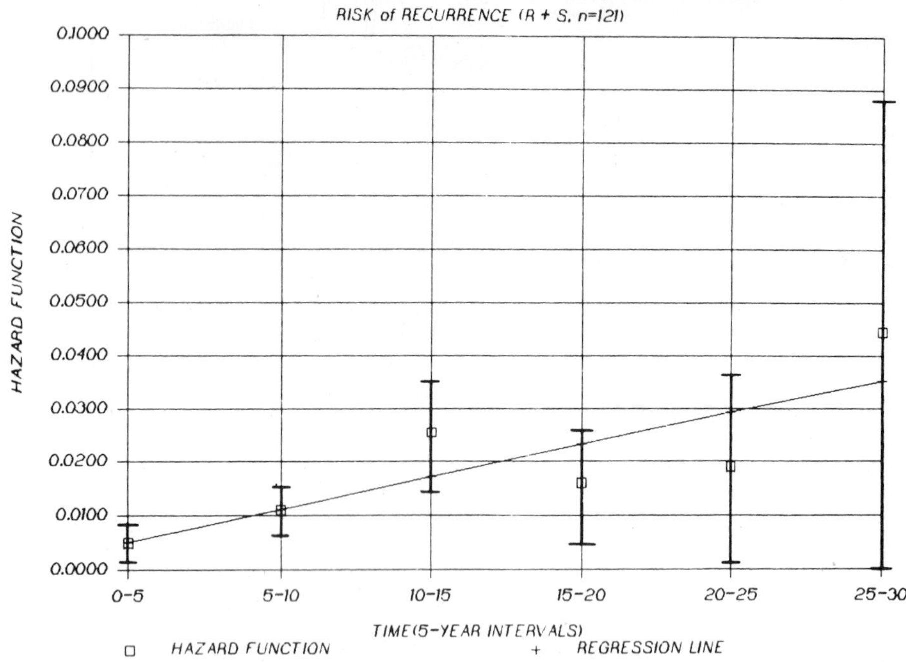

FIGURE 24–3. Hazard functions over 5-year intervals for surgery plus irradiation. The solid line is the regression line. Error bars denote the standard deviation for each point. (Grigsby PW, et al: Cancer 63:1308–1323, 1989)

Decreased visual acuity, papilledema, ophthalmoplegia, and ocular motor abnormalities can occur. The most common visual field defects are bitemporal hemianopic and superior temporal defects (Fig. 24-4). Other visual field defects are homonymous hemianopia, central scotoma, and inferior temporal field cuts.[67,94]

Endocrine abnormalities are often the earliest manifestation of pituitary tumors and may be a consequence of either hypersecretion or hyposecretion of one or more of the anterior pituitary hormones. Endocrine manifestations of pituitary tumors are summarized in Table 24-2.

Endocrine evaluation before and after therapy permits assessment of response to treatment and determines the necessity for hormonal replacement therapy. Such endocrine evaluation should include tests of gonadal, thyroid, and adrenal function. Immunoassays are available for each of the major anterior pituitary hormones.

TABLE 24–1
Diagnostic Workup for Pituitary Tumors

General
- History
- Physical examination

Special Tests
- Neurologic examination with special attention to cranial mass
- Funduscopic examination; tests of visual field

Radiologic Studies
- Standard
  - Chest radiographs
  - Skull film
  - Magnetic resonance imaging
- Complementary
  - Skeletal survey (for acromegaly)
  - Pneumoencephalogram (rarely used)
  - Carotid arteriogram or cavernous sinus venograph (rarely used)
  - Computed tomography (if MRI unavailable)

Laboratory Studies
- Complete blood count, blood chemistry, urinalysis
- Endocrine evaluation
  - Gonadal function: follicle-stimulating hormone, luteinizing hormone, plasma estradiol, testosterone
  - Thyroid function: thyroxine, triiodothyronine, serum thyroid-stimulating hormone
  - Adrenal function: basal plasma or urinary steroids; cortisol response to insulin hypoglycemia and plasma ACTH response to metyrapone administration

STAGING

Pituitary tumors should be considered according to both endocrine function and anatomic staging. TSH, GH, ACTH, and prolactin-secreting tumors and the nonfunctional adenomas differ in clinical presentation, required workup, disease sequelae, treatment, and prognosis. Interpretation of the literature is confounded by the frequent failure to report results according to function and by the lack of a commonly accepted staging system.

Hardy and Vezine[41,45] developed a classification system that has gained partial acceptance, particularly by neurosurgeons. They classified pituitary tumors into four grades according to the extent of expansion or erosion of the sella:

Grade I: Normal-sized sella with asymmetry of the floor
Grade II: Enlarged sella with an intact floor
Grade III: Localized erosion or destruction of the sellar floor
Grade IV: Diffusely eroded floor

It is assumed that grades I and II represent enclosed adenomas and that grades III and IV are invasive adenomas. Suprasellar extension requires the secondary designation by type:

Type A: Tumor bulges into the chiasmatic cistern.
Type B: Tumor reaches the floor of the third ventricle.
Type C: Tumor is more voluminous with extension into the third ventricle up to the foramen of Monroe.
Type D: Tumor extends into temporal or frontal fossa.

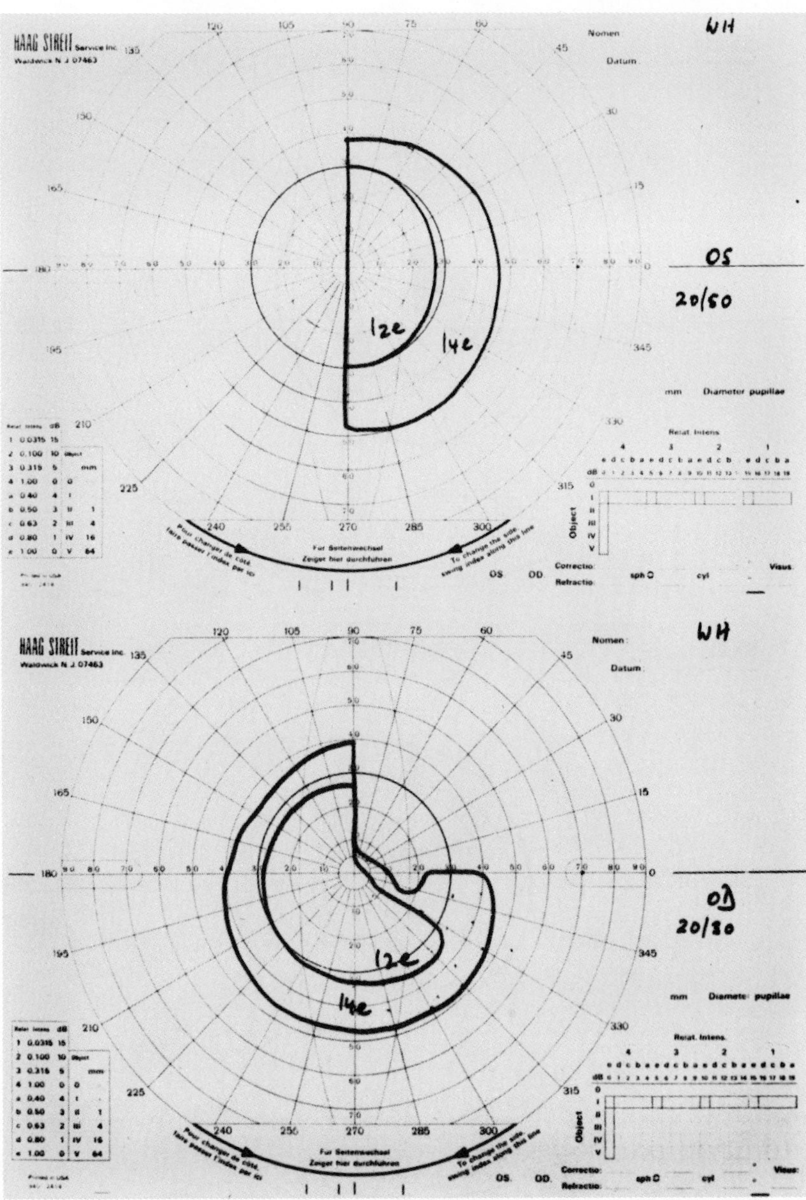

FIGURE 24–4. (**A**) Complete temporal field cut in left eye. Right eye shows only a superior temporal defect. (Melen O: Endocrinol Metab Clin North Am 16:585–608, 1987)

This system is based primarily on radiologic evidence and tends to emphasize inferior extensions. It assigns a lesser degree of importance to extension or invasion other than through the floor of the sella. Involvement of brain, cavernous sinus, optic apparatus, and other areas, however, has a serious impact on both selection and effectiveness of therapy and is at least as important as extension into or through the sphenoidal sinus.

PATHOLOGIC CLASSIFICATION

The typical pathologic classification into benign or malignant tumors has little significance for lesions arising within the pituitary. Local invasion of bone or soft tissues is common with benign adenomas. The presence of cellular pleomorphism, nuclear hyperchromatism, and venous permeation does not correlate with clinical malignancy.

Historically, when classic fixation, staining, and light microscopy were used, pituitary tumors were designated as chromophobic, basophilic, acidophilic, or mixed. Clinically, acidophilic tumors were generally thought to be associated with acromegaly, basophilic tumors with Cushing's disease, and chromophobic tumors with nonfunction. Using the classic techniques, Costello[15] reported that of asymptomatic adenomas found at autopsy, 52.8% were chromophobic, 27.2% were basophilic, 7.5% were eosinophilic, and 12.5% were mixed. At the Mayo Clinic, where most patients with acromegaly were irradiated and those with Cushing's disease received adrenalectomy, 93.4% of resected pituitary tumors were chromophobe adenomas and 6.6% were eosinophilic adenomas. No basophilic tumors were found.[52]

Newer methods of fixation and staining, electron microscopy, and immunohistologic procedures have been shown that GH, ACTH, TSH, and prolactin are secreted by specific pituitary cells.[10] There is a question whether two different gonadotropic cells exist or whether LH and FSH are secreted by the same cell.[58] Growth hormone and prolactin are derived from subtypes of acidophilic cells, whereas ACTH, TSH, LH, and FSH are secreted by different basophilic cells. With the exception of the follicular cells, granules are present in virtually all pituitary cells, including those considered chromophobic by classic staining and light microscopy.[58] According to Landolt,[58] the amount of hormone that reaches the peripheral circulation from a pituitary tumor is dependent on production rate, de-

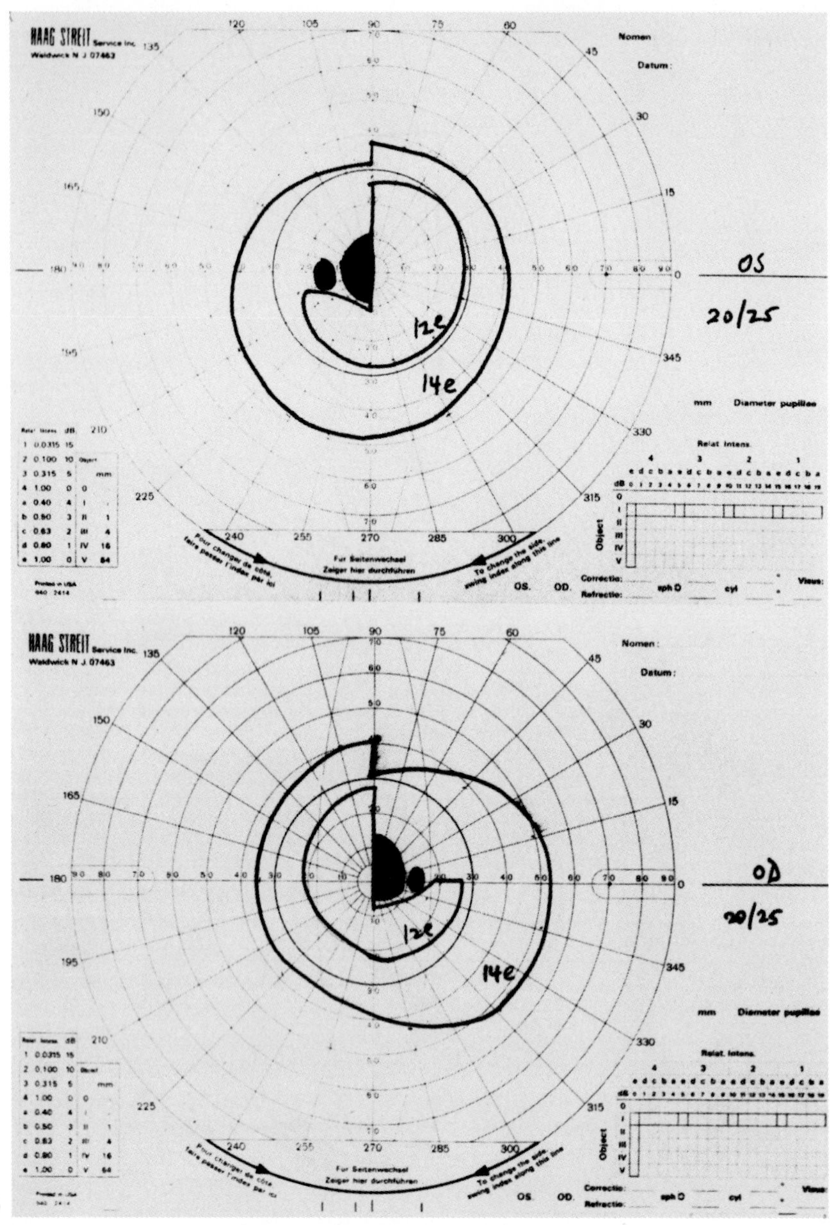

FIGURE 24–4. (*Continued*) (**B**) Bitemporal hemianopic scotoma with peripheral bitemporal field loss due to compression of the chiasm from behind.

struction by lysosomes, and retention by cell membrane. McCormick and Halmi[66] found no unequivocal chromophobic adenoma in 145 asymptomatic pituitary adenomas examined at autopsy or in 25 symptomatic adenomas removed surgically. A close correlation exists between Cushing's disease and the presence of corticotropic adenomas. Probably all functioning adenomas are composed primarily of cells that secrete the particular hormone.

Kovacs and co-workers[54] advocate the following morphologic classification of adenomas: growth hormone cell, prolactin cell, mixed growth hormone prolactin cell, acidophilic stem cell, corticotropic cell, thyrotropic cell, gonadotropic cell, and undifferentiated cell adenomas.

PROGNOSTIC FACTORS

Prognosis varies with type of adenoma and depends on a combination of factors[33,36]: the extent of the abnormality (secondary to either mass or endocrine effect) present at time of diagnosis; the degree to which the injury is reversible; the success of therapy in normalizing endocrine activity or relieving pressure effects; and the permanency of response to treatment (freedom from recurrence).

GENERAL MANAGEMENT OF PITUITARY TUMORS

The management of pituitary tumors is complex and should not be undertaken unless the full range of complementary skills is available. These are neuroradiology, neuro-ophthalmology, endocrinology, neurosurgery, radiation oncology, and a reliable laboratory. The goals are to accomplish the following without producing hypopituitarism or injury to adjacent structures: define the extent of tumor, evaluate hormone deficits or excesses, remove or destroy tumor masses, control hypersecretion, and correct endocrine deficiencies.

Medical Management

Over the past few years medical management has assumed a more important role in suppression of pituitary hyperfunction.

TABLE 24–2
Endocrine Manifestations of Pituitary Tumor

DISEASE	CAUSE	CLINICAL MANIFESTATIONS	DIAGNOSIS	COMMENTS
Acromegaly	Growth hormone hypersecretion causing overgrowth of soft tissue, cartilage, and bone, with acral enlargement	Changes in skull, facial features, jaws, hands, feet; hyperhidrosis; heat intolerance; fatigue; weight gain; paresthesias; arthralgias; headache; enlargement of sella; visual impairment (20% of patients); glucose intolerance (50% of patients); hypogonadism (>50% of patients); rarely, hypoadrenalism or hypothyroidism	Elevated basal state serum growth hormone (in excess of 10 ng/ml in 90% of patients); if normal or borderline, nonsuppressibility with hyperglycemia establishes diagnosis. Elevated somatomedin C	Adenomas may have associated mass effects, which are less likely than with endocrine inactive tumors or prolactinomas in males.
Hyperprolactinemia	Prolactin hypersecretion	Amenorrhea, oligomenorrhea or infertility in females; decreased libido or impotence in males Galactorrhea (mild, transient, if present) Hypopituitarism; more common with large tumors and sellar enlargement	Basal serum prolactin level >100 ng/ml (normal, 5–20 ng/ml); range of 30–100 mg/ml may indicate microadenoma. If hyperprolactinemia is present, demonstration of abnormal sella confirms diagnosis.	Most common type of pituitary adenoma; majority of tumors thought to be nonfunctioning "chromophobe adenomas" have been shown to hypersecrete prolactin. Tumor may be large with resulting mass effects.
Cushing's disease	ACTH hypersecretion leading to bilateral adrenal hyperplasia and hypercortisolism; majority of patients have ACTH-secreting pituitary microadenomas	Obesity (central distribution); hypertension; glucose intolerance; hirsutism; easy bruising; striae; osteoporosis; psychologic changes; hypogonadism; rarely hypopituitarism	Elevated plasma and urine corticosteroids nonsuppressible with low-dose dexamethasone, partially suppressed with high-dose dexamethasone. Plasma cortisol > 10 μg/ml 8–9 h after 1.0 mg dexamethasone is diagnostic in 95% of cases. Confirmed by urinary free cortisol of >10 μg/24 h. Plasma ACTH is normal to moderately elevated.	Must be differentiated from other causes of Cushing's syndrome (primary adrenal tumors, ectopic ACTH syndrome). With adrenal tumors ACTH level is depressed to <20 pg/ml. ACTH level associated with ectopic ACTH syndrome is usually markedly elevated.
Endocrine inactive pituitary tumor	Tumor growth	Hypogonadism secondary to gonadotropin deficiency (early); hypothyroidism and hypoadrenalism as tumor enlarges; headache; visual disturbances; panhypopituitarism if tumor is large; enlarged sella	Anterior pituitary function tests; radiologic examination of sella turcica and parasellar region Ophthalmologic examination	Mass effects are usually present. Rule out other possible diagnoses: craniopharyngioma, primary CNS neoplasm, metastatic tumor, cyst, carotid aneurysm, inflammatory lesion, and empty sella (if enlarged sella but normal anterior pituitary function).

The drugs used are bromocriptine (a dopamine agonist), cyproheptadine, mitotane, and somatostatin. These drugs may have distressing side effects, and relapse uniformly follows discontinuation. They have been used as primary therapy and also to provide temporary control or remission while awaiting the slower but permanent response of irradiation. Other drugs, especially longer-acting dopamine agonists, for controlling anterior pituitary secretions are under investigation and in the future may play a more significant role in the management of these disorders.[14,30,32,49,51,57,62,85,97,98,100,104]

Surgical Management

The role of surgery has changed markedly in the past 10 to 15 years. This has resulted from improved techniques for diagnosing hyperfunctioning adenomas, while they are still small enough for selective adenomectomy, and for performing transsphenoidal microsurgery. At University of California–San Francisco (UCSF), for example, 15 to 20 years ago, more than 95% of pituitary surgery was conducted by means of craniotomy. Currently, more than 95% of surgery is transsphenoidal. Transsphenoidal microsurgery is particularly effective in selective removal of microadenomas, but it is also used for adenomas that extend outside the sella.[8,9,40,79] According to Wilson and Dempsey,[103] contraindications to the transsphenoidal approach include dumbbell-shaped adenomas with constriction at the diaphragma sellae, lateral suprasellar extension, massive suprasellar tumor, and an incompletely pneumatized sphenoid. Poor results have been reported when inexperienced surgical teams have been used.[6]

Because transsphenoidal selective resection of functioning

microadenomas is a relatively new surgical procedure, the ultimate results achievable with this technique are uncertain. If these adenomas are comparable to hyperfunctioning adenomas of the parathyroid or thyroid glands, perhaps the favorable experience with parathyroid or thyroid adenomectomy can be extrapolated to the pituitary. With larger tumors, recurrence may be delayed many years, but following surgery alone, the recurrence rate is high.

Radiation Therapy

Radiation therapy is often effective in control of hypersecretion and of the neoplastic or mass effects of large tumors. External radiation therapy controls hypersecretion in about 80% of patients with acromegaly, in 50% to 80% of those with Cushing's disease, and in about one third of those with hyperprolactinemia. Normalization of circulating hormone levels requires from a few months to several years for those with acromegaly and from about 3 months to 1 year for those with Cushing's disease. Primary radiation therapy is often effective for control of mass effects of larger tumors; in general, however, it is preferable to perform a biopsy and decompress the optic chiasm, and then irradiate postoperatively to prevent recurrence. In contrast to conventional radiation therapy, proton and α-particle irradiation and implantation of radioactive sources (^{90}Y or ^{198}Au) as presently practiced are techniques based on delivery of very large doses to highly restricted volumes within the pituitary gland; thus their application is limited to small, essentially intrasellar tumors.

Fraser and colleagues[26] used ^{90}Y and ^{198}Au implants in over 200 patients with pituitary tumors. Their stated doses were up to 50,000 cGy, but the dose distribution through the adenoma or pituitary gland is unclear. In patients with Cushing's disease, a 60% remission rate was achieved. The best results in patients with acromegaly were in those with "mild disease" without "greatly expanded" sellae. About 20% gained normal growth hormone levels, but at the expense of a 50% complication rate (cerebrospinal fluid leaks requiring plugging, 9%; visual loss or paresis, 4%; hypopituitarism requiring replacement therapy, 33%; diabetes insipidus, 2%; and mortality, 2%); only 51% were free of complication. Their data for functionless tumors are difficult to interpret; however, the authors state that ^{90}Y "is a good treatment for functionless pituitary tumors which have not extended too far beyond the sella."

Posttherapy Evaluations

In acromegaly, posttreatment GH values of less than 10 ng/ml indicate a successful response to therapy. Subsequently, GH levels should be followed to predict tumor recurrence. In prolactin-secreting tumors, the therapeutic objective is to lower the prolactin level into the normal range. Evaluation of the response to therapy in Cushing's disease can be accomplished by measurement of plasma and urine steroids and plasma ACTH levels. For all patients treated for pituitary tumors, periodic assessment of gonadal, thyroid, and adrenal function is necessary because hypopituitarism may occur as a result of radiation or surgical treatment. Patients treated with radiation therapy may develop hypopituitarism a number of years after treatment.

RADIATION THERAPY TECHNIQUES

Acceptable techniques include bilateral coaxial wedge fields plus a coronal field, moving arc fields, and 360-degree rotational fields. Occasionally with very large tumors, two bilateral coaxial fields may be used, but in general this technique is to be discouraged as delivering an unnecessarily high radiation dose to the temporal lobes.

All diagnostic evidence, including that from tomograms, arteriograms, and CT scanning as well as clinical and surgical findings, should be combined to define the tumor volume. The treatment volume should be slightly larger to include a margin for error in estimating tumor volume and for variation in day-to-day setup. For well-defined adenomas, the uncertainty of margin is small. With invasive tumors there is greater uncertainty, which, whether the extension is into the sphenoid or into intracranial structures, must be considered in determining the volume to be included. Variability of setup should be no more than 2 mm or 3 mm.

To ensure accuracy and reproducibility, the patient's head must be fixed. The use of three localizing light or laser beams permits easy repositioning. Both lateral and sagittal beam check films must be obtained at the beginning of therapy and periodically thereafter. The technique should be designed to restrict the high-dose region to the treatment volume. Special care must be taken to avoid exposure to the eyes; this requires observation of the actual setup on the treatment machine by the radiation oncologist. Radiopaque markers, placed on the contralateral eye when field verification films are taken, documents the location of the eye with respect to the radiation beam. It should be kept in mind that the eye is approximately 25 mm in length and the lens lies in the anterior 1 cm. The lens is particularly sensitive to radiation cataractogenesis. Doses of 4500 cGy to 5000 cGy approach retinal tolerance.

The volume treated includes the pituitary fossa and adjacent tissues, as determined by evaluation of extent of the adenoma. In general, portals 5 cm x 5 cm to 6 cm x 6 cm or shaped fields 5 cm to 6 cm in diameter are used. Parallel opposed lateral portals, which are easily localized, are used. Fifteen-degree wedges with the heel placed anteriorly assist in obtaining a more homogeneous dose distribution and decreasing the dose delivered to the optic chiasma. With energies below 10 MV photons it is strongly recommended that a vertex field be used to decrease the radiation dose to the temporal lobes. To localize this portal the patient is placed in the supine position, with head flexed and chin close to the lower neck. A beam entering through the vertex of the head, at approximately the midline of the hairline, is directed posteriorly to pass about 1 cm behind the posterior clinoid processes (Fig. 24-5). Even with higher energy photons the vertex portal is recommended to optimize the dose distribution.

A different technique is shown in Figure 24-6. It was chosen for illustration because it meets the desired criteria, and the 4 MV linear accelerator is widely available. Generally, treatment is given with bilateral 110-degree arc rotation using a reversing, moving 30-degree wedge. The head is positioned on a rigid board angled so that the plane of rotation of the treatment beam is posterior to the eyes. The target or tumor volume is enclosed in the 95% isodose line; the dose decreases rapidly outside this volume. Both arcing fields are treated daily. This illustration assumes a 5-cm diameter tumor centered in the sella. For tumors of different size or those eccentrically located, axis of rotation, size of fields, length of arcs, and thickness of wedges are altered correspondingly.

A variation on the basic technique is shown in Figure 24-7. It was designed to spare the temporal lobes in a patient with a recurrent adenoma; previous radiation therapy (with a 50-cm ^{60}Co machine and small bilateral fixed temporal fields) had given a high dose to the temporal lobes. Sixty-degree arcs and wedges are used.

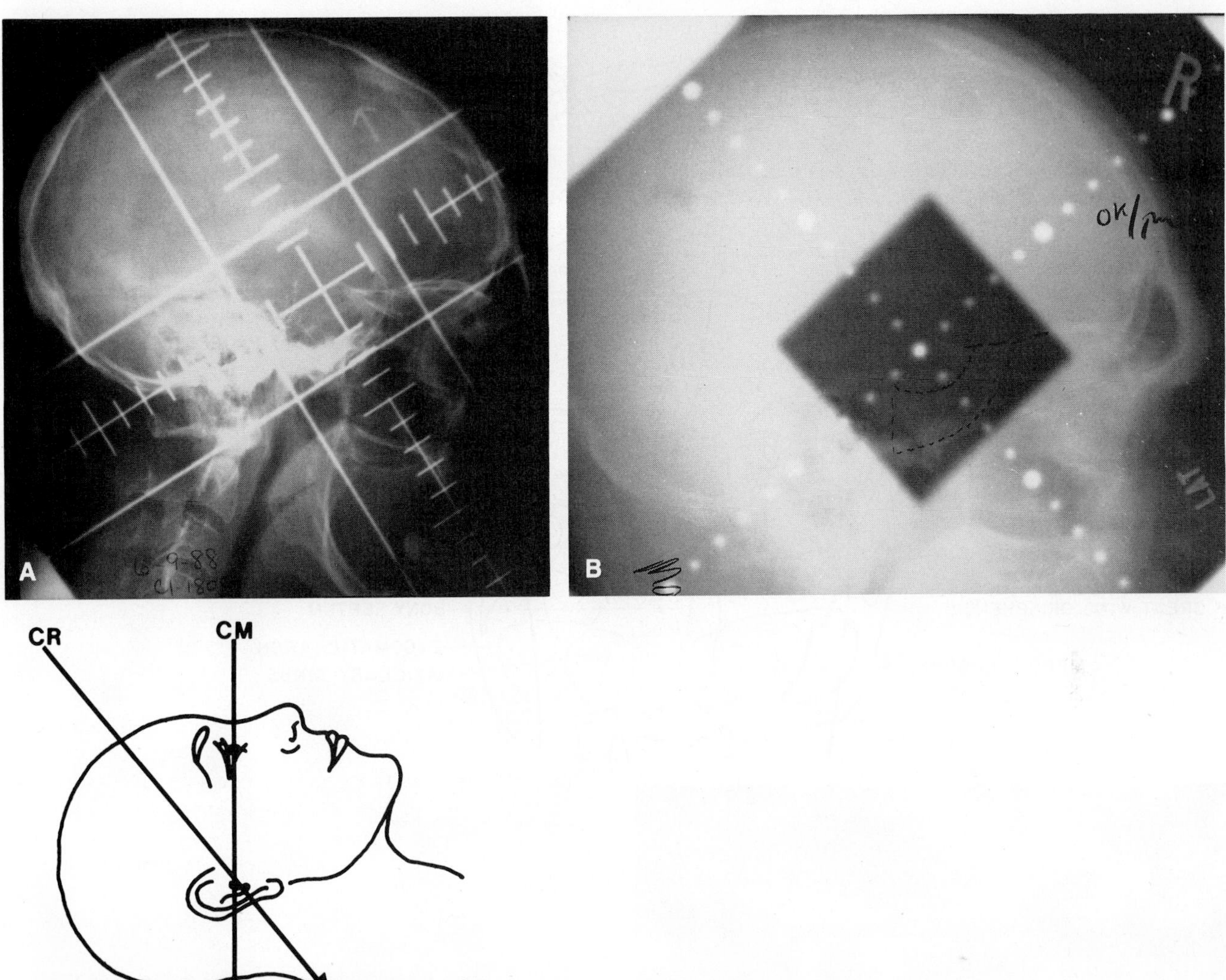

FIGURE 24–5. (**A**) Lateral simulation film illustrating portal used for external irradiation of pituitary adenoma. Black arrow indicates plane of rotation. White arrow shows radiopaque marker on contralateral eyelid. (**B**) Localization film on therapy machine. (**C**) Lateral view of head illustrating position and angle of beam for frontovertex portal, similar to radiographic Towne's projection. (Paris DQ: Craniographic Positioning with Comparison Studies. Philadelphia: FA Davis, 1983).

As calculated at the 95% isodose line, the daily dose is 180 cGy to 200 cGy, and the total dose is 4500 cGy to 5000 cGy with any of the techniques described. In patients with masses larger than 2 cm, we administered 5400 cGy.

Isodose curves for 4 MV and 18 MV photons using bilateral fixed wedged and a vertex field are shown in Figure 24-8. The isodose curves for 4 MV and 18 MV photons using two fixed parallel opposed fields are shown in Figure 24-9. The latter arrangements yield poor isodose distributions and should be avoided.

ACROMEGALY

Radiation Therapy

Before the GH assay, results of therapy were judged on parameters such as soft tissue overgrowth, visual field deficits, headaches, abnormal glucose metabolism, elevated basal metabolic rate, and other indirect measurements of pituitary endocrine activity. Grigsby and associates[36] demonstrated a 90% 5-year control rate and a 69% 10-year control rate in 22 patients. Others have reported control rates ranging from 25% to 90%.[17,18,55,59,74,90] These data suggest that radiation doses ranging from 4500 cGy to 5500 cGy are needed to control these tumors. Results from UCSF, Stanford, and Thomas Jefferson University Hospital based on these parameters are given in Table 24-3. Control of endocrine hyperfunction was achieved in 80% to 90% of patients.

After the GH assay became available, it was found that plasma GH levels remain high in the early months following radiation therapy. This caused a shift to other methods of therapy, and it became difficult to obtain enough patients to evaluate GH response to radiation therapy. Table 24-4 summarizes pooled data[92] on 40 patients from UCSF and other institutions, showing fasting plasma GH concentrations as a function of time after irradiation. Response was slow, but by 3 years, the fasting GH concentration was less than 10 ng/ml in 92% of the cases. The control rate was higher for those with preirradiation fasting GH concentrations less than or equal to 45 ng/ml, but, because of the small numbers, the difference is of uncertain significance.

Eastman and associates[18] treated 47 patients, 16 of whom were observed for at least 10 years, with conventional radiation

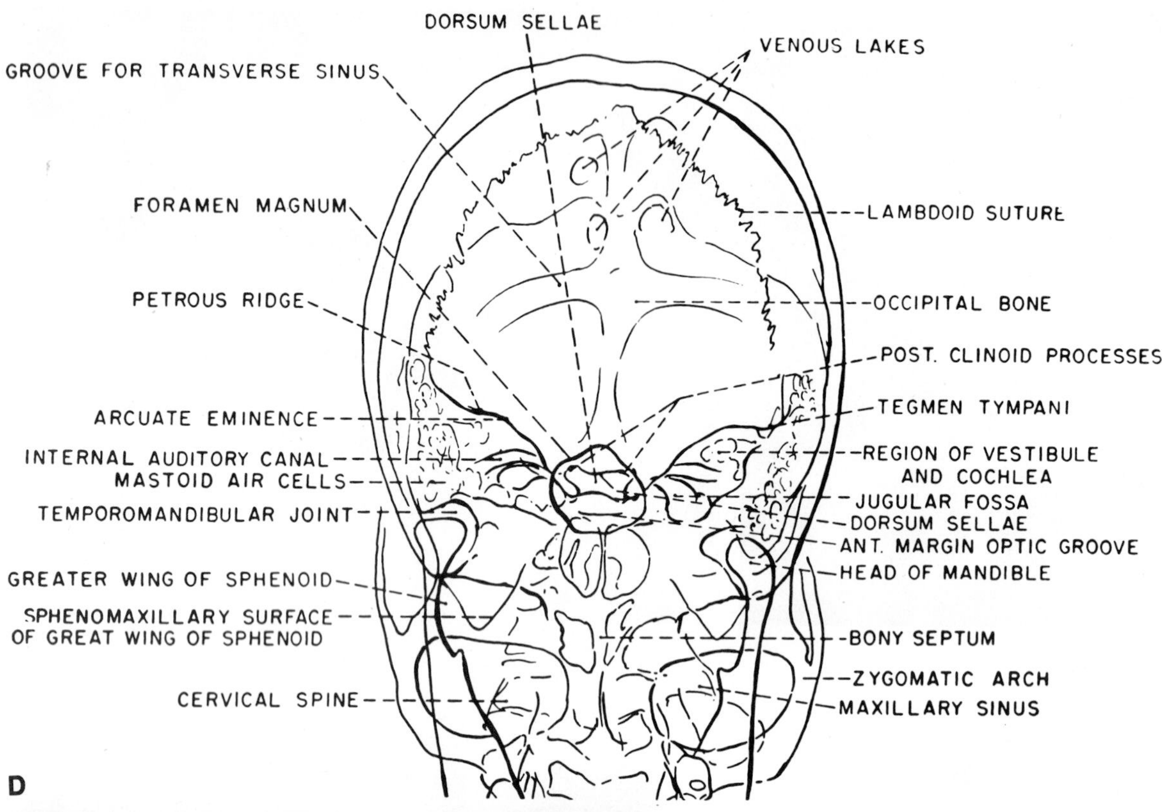

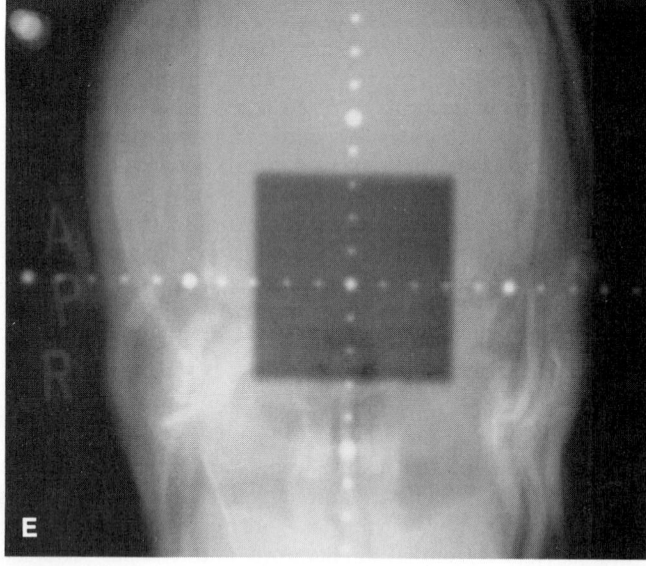

FIGURE 24–5. (*Continued*) (**D**) Line drawing depicting anatomy of skull seen on Towne's projection. (Meschan I: Radiographic Positioning and Related Anatomy, ed 2. Philadelphia, WB Saunders, 1978). (**E**) Simulation film of anteroposterior vertex portal (similar to Towne's projection in diagnostic radiology) that can be used to deliver a portion of the dose without irradiating temporal lobes.

TABLE 24–3
Acromegaly: Results of Radiation Therapy

STUDY	PATIENTS TREATED	VISUAL FIELD DEFECTS	DOSE (cGy)	CONTROLLED	INDUCED HYPOPITUITARISM
Sheline et al[90]	37	15 (41%)*	≤3500	5/19 (26%)	None
			>3500	14/18 (78%)	None
Pistenmaa et al[73]	19	6 (32%)	5800 (avg)	17 (90%)	1/11
Kramer[55]	29	Not known	4400–5000	25 (86%)	Not known
Grigsby et al[36]	22	Not known	400–5600	17/22 (77%)	None

** Ten patients recovered normal vision after irradiation.*
(Sheline GE, Tyrrell JB: Pituitary adenomas. In Phillips TL, Pistenmaa DA [eds]: Radiation Oncology Annual, pp 1–35. New York, Raven Press, 1983)

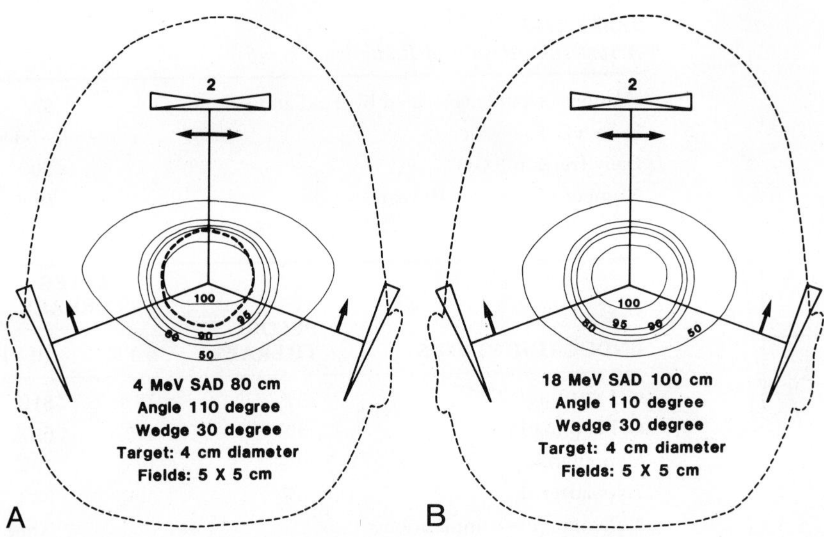

FIGURE 24–6. (**A**) Isodose curves for 4 cm (diameter) tumor volume (*broken line circle*) centered in the sella, using a 4 MV linear accelerator, bilateral coronal arc (110-degree) fields with moving wedge (30-degree) filters. (**B**) Dose distribution for similar beam arrangement using 18 MV photons.

therapy. Results are reported in Table 24-5. Only four of the patients with hypoadrenalism allocated to the postirradiation period required steroid replacement therapy.

Transsphenoidal Resection

Results of transsphenoidal microsurgery for growth hormone-secreting pituitary adenoma in a series in 214 patients showed 54% with GH levels less than 5 ng/ml and 74% with levels below 10 ng/ml immediately after surgery. Only 10.6% of patients with an immediate postoperative GH level of less than 5 ng/ml had a recurrence of elevated GH levels and required additional therapy, whereas 21.2% of those with postoperative levels between 5 and 10 ng/ml required subsequent therapy. Severe complications of the surgery were meningitis in four patients(1.8%) and cerebrospinal fluid leak requiring surgical repair in five (2.2%).[79]

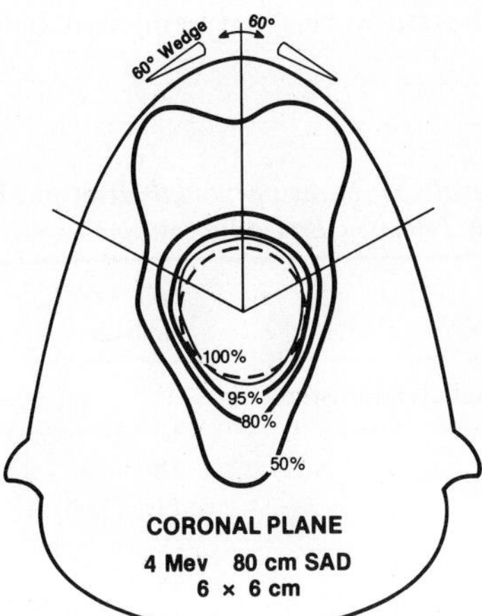

FIGURE 24–7. Isodose curves for 5 cm (diameter) tumor volume in the sella, using a 4 MV linear accelerator, bilateral coronal arc (60-degree) fields with moving wedge (60-degree) filters. This technique shifts the 50% isodose line away from the temporal lobes and toward the frontoparietal region. (Sheline GE: Role of conventional radiation therapy in the treatment of functional pituitary tumors. In Linfoot JA [ed]: Recent Advances in the Diagnosis and Treatment of Pituitary Tumors. New York, Raven Press, 1979)

Hardy and co-workers[44] reported similar results for transsphenoidal resection using the operating microscope with televised radiofluoroscopic control (Table 24-6).

In summation, radiation therapy and transsphenoidal resection are equally effective for primary therapy of acromegaly. When selective resection is possible, the surgical procedure has the advantage of a rapid response and a low rate of hypopituitarism. Popularization of the selective adenomectomy is recent, and permanency of surgical cure cannot yet be assessed.

Postoperative Radiation Therapy

Immediate postoperative radiation was administered to 121 patients by Grigsby and co-workers[33] and resulted in a 76% control rate at 10 years following therapy. Results of patients treated with radiation for a postoperative recurrence at UCSF[88] by Eastman and co-workers,[18] by Williams and colleagues,[102] and by Werner and associates[101] are given in Table 24-7. Seven patients initially treated by cryohypophysectomy at UCSF were irradiated several months after surgery because fasting GH levels remained elevated (17 to 48 ng/ml). The 20 patients with transsphenoidal surgery at UCSF were known to have had

TABLE 24–4
Acromegaly: Fasting Growth Hormone Response to Radiation Therapy

PREIRRADIATION	POSTIRRADIATION	
FASTING GH (ng/ml)	INTERVAL (YEARS)	FASTING GH (<10 ng/ml)
≤45	1	8/21*
	2	19/23
	3	17/17
≥50	1	5/10
	2	5/9
	3	5/7

**Number of patients controlled/number of patients at risk*
(Sheline GE, Tyrrell JB: Pituitary adenomas. In Phillips TL, Pistenmaa DA [eds]: Radiation Oncology Annual, pp 1–35. New York, Raven Press, 1983)

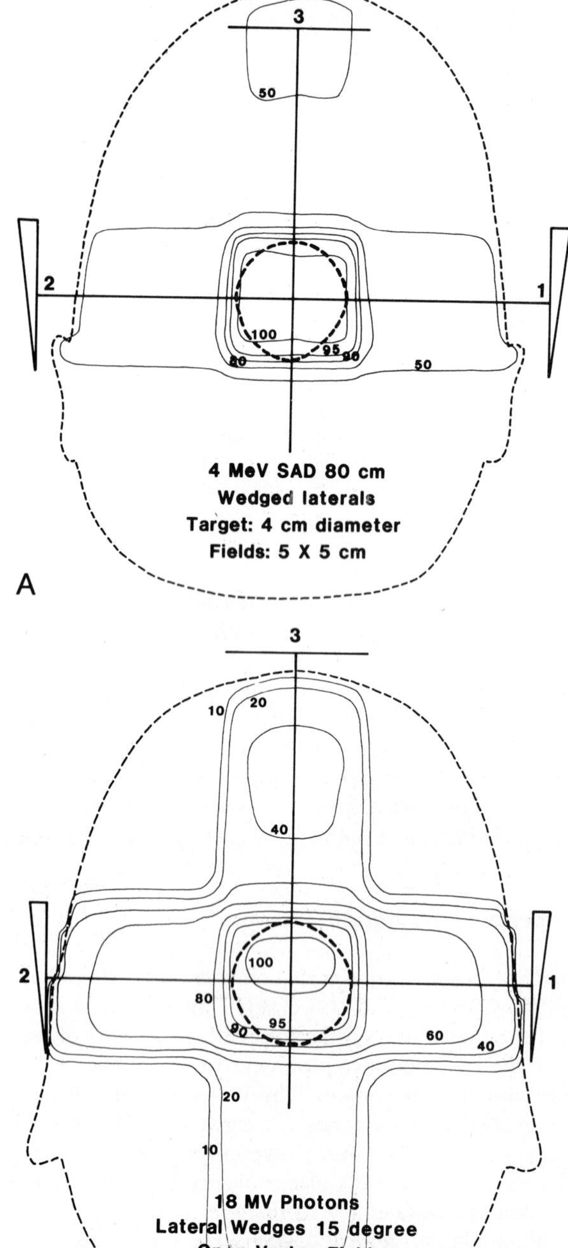

FIGURE 24–8. Three-portal arrangement with open vertex and two lateral 15-degree wedged fields using (**A**) 4 MV or (**B**) 18 MV photons.

incomplete resections and postoperatively were referred for radiation. Of the 61 patients included in Table 2-7, 50 (82%) achieved normal GH levels. Radiation therapy appears to be as successful in treatment of surgical failures as it is in primary therapy for acromegaly.

CUSHING'S DISEASE

Radiation Therapy

Results of several reports on pituitary irradiation for Cushing's disease are summarized in Table 24-8. With doses of 3500 cGy to 5000 cGy, control rates varied from approximately 50% for Orth and Liddle[72] to 100% for Grigsby and co-workers.[35] Dohan and colleagues[16] treated another six patients, not included in Table 24-8, with less than 1600 cGy and failed in each instance to control the disease. The reported control rates varied according to the stringency of the criteria applied. Orth and Liddle,[72] who used the most strict criteria, found that 23 of 44 patients were either normalized or improved to the point that further therapy was unnecessary. In ten patients, the 24-hour 17-hydroxycorticosteroid excretion was reduced to less than 7 mg/g creatinine and the mean plasma cortisol to less than 10 μg/dl. Another 13 patients achieved values of less than or equal to 10 mg/g and 13 μg/dl, respectively.

Using similar criteria, Jennings and co-workers[50] had an 80% cure rate without complication in 15 children with Cushing's disease. They concluded that megavoltage irradiation of the pituitary (4000 cGy to 4500 cGy; 200 cGy per fraction) is safe and effective treatment for childhood Cushing's disease. Time to remission was generally less than 9 months, but two of the children in the study reached remission between 9 and 18

TABLE 24–5
Acromegaly: Results of Radiation Therapy

Number of patients treated by irradiation alone	47
Dose (cGy)	4000–5000
Daily fraction (cGy)	≤200
Number observed ≥10 years	16
Mean decrease in plasma GH 5 years after therapy	77%

ENDOCRINE STATUS	BEFORE THERAPY	AFTER THERAPY 5 YR	AFTER THERAPY 10 YR
GH ≤ 10 ng/ml	13%	73%	81%
GH ≥ 5 mg/ml	2%	42%	69%
Hypothyroid	9%	12%	19%
Hypoadrenal	6%	30%	38%
Nonendocrine complications			None

(Eastman RC, Gorden P, Roth J: J Clin Endocrinol Metab 48:931, 1979, © The Endocrine Society, 1979)

TABLE 24–6
Acromegaly: Results of Transsphenoidal Resection Using Operating Microscope with Televised Radiofluoroscopic Control

ACROMEGALY	NO. OF CASES	CURED (GH ≤ 5 ng/ml)
Without Suprasellar Extension		
Grade I	13	12 (92%)
Grade II	18	15 (83%)
Grade III	11	10 (91%)
Grade IV	2	0
Total	44	37 (84%)
With Suprasellar Extension	13	9 (69%)
Total	57	46 (81%)
Hypopituitarism	7 (12%)*	

**In five cases, selective adenomectomy was not possible, and a total hypophysectomy was done.*
(Hardy J, Somma M, Vezina JL: Treatment of acromegaly: Radiation or surgery. In Morley GP [ed]: Current Controversies in Neurosurgery, p 377. Philadelphia, WB Saunders. 1976)

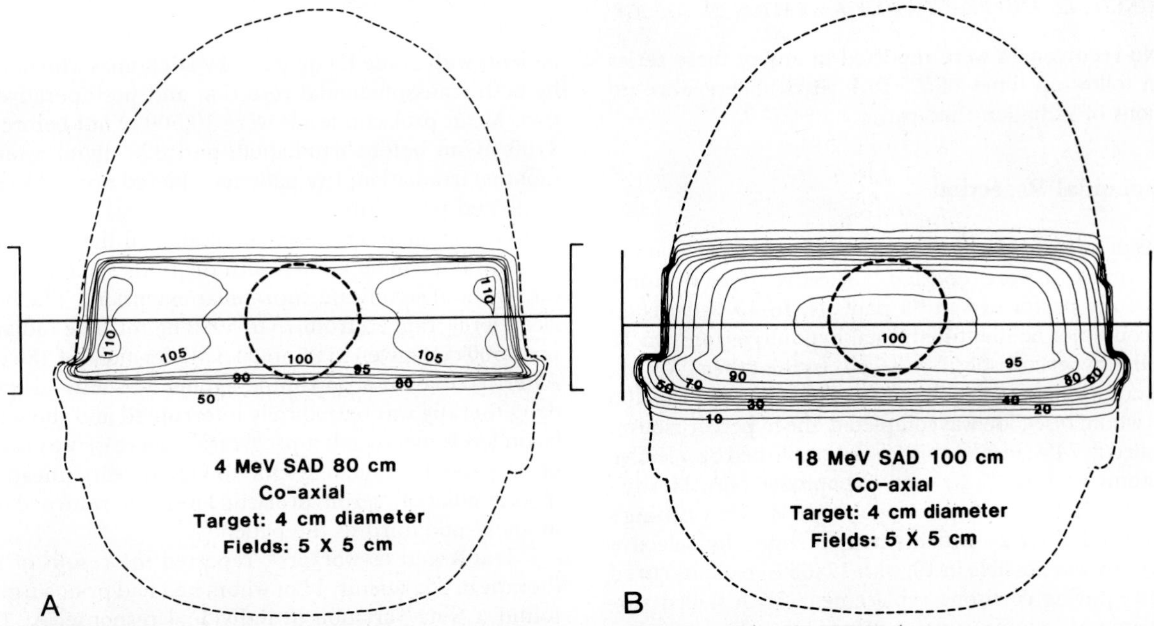

FIGURE 24–9. Isodose curves for parallel opposed open portals using (**A**) 4 MV or (**B**) 18 MV photons. Neither isodose distribution is optimal compared with those shown in Figures 24-6 through 24-8 because of the large dose delivered to the adjacent temporal lobes. Even greater doses are delivered to those normal structures with the 4 MV photons.

TABLE 24–7
Acromegaly: Results of Radiation Therapy for Failure of Resection to Control Activity

STUDY	HYPOPHYSECTOMY	GH (ng/ml) POSTSURGERY AND PREIRRADIATION	POSTIRRADIATION INTERVAL (YEARS)	POSTIRRADIATION NO. OF PATIENTS WITH NORMAL GH
Sheline[88]	Cryohypophysectomy	17–48	2	4/7
	Transfrontal		2	3/4
	Transsphenoidal		1–10	16/16
Eastman et al[18]	Transfrontal	12–70	2	4/5
Williams et al[102]	Transsphenoidal			4/6
Werner et al[101]	Transsphenoidal		2–10	16/19
Grigsby[35]	Transfrontal		3–30	3/4
Total				50/61 (82%)

GH: growth hormone
(Modified from Sheline GE, Tyrrell JB: Pituitary adenomas. In Phillips TL, Pistenmaa DA [eds]: Radiation Oncology Annual, pp 1–35. New York, Raven Press, 1983)

TABLE 24–8
Cushing's Disease: Results of Radiation Therapy

	DOBAN ET AL[16]	HEUSCHELE AND LAMPE[47]	ORTH AND LIDDLE[72]	EDMONDS ET AL[19]	JENNINGS ET AL[50]	GRIGSBY ET AL[35]
No. of patients	6	16	44	15	15 (children)	6
Pituitary dose (cGy)	3800–5200 in 5–7 wk	4000 in 4–5 wk	4000–5000 in 1 mo	3500–5000 in 3–5 wk	4000–5000*	4500–5000 in 5–6 wk
No. of pts. cured	5	10	23	9	12	6
Time to remission	3–6 mo	5–7 mo		1–6 mo	≤18 mo†	
Complications	0		0	0	0	0
Recurrences	0		0	0	0	0
Follow-up (years)						
Range	5–7.5	3–7	1–14	.25–10	1–19	6–29
Mean	6		9	2.5	8	16

** 150 cGy to 200 cGy per fraction, 5 times per week*
† Ten patients were in remission in 9 months.
(Modified from Sheline GE, Tyrrell JB: Pituitary adenomas. In Phillips TL, Pistenmaa DA [eds]: Radiation Oncology Annual, pp 1–35. New York, Raven Press, 1983)

months. No recurrences were reported in any of these series with mean follow-up times of 2.5 to 9 years. There were no complications of radiation therapy.

Transsphenoidal Resection

The results of attempted selective transsphenoidal resection in 104 patients at UCSF were reported.[11] Selective adenomectomy was successfully performed in 85 patients. In 15 patients an adenoma could not be identified; total hypophysectomy in 12 corrected the hypercortisolism in seven. In the other four patients surgery was incomplete because of bleeding. Of the 100 patients in whom resection was completed, the hypercortisolism was controlled in 74%; in 67% this was accomplished by selective adenomectomy and in 7% by total hypophysectomy. Hardy's results[42] with selective transsphenoidal resection for Cushing's disease are similar. Of 25 patients treated surgically, selective adenomectomy was possible in 19, with 17 (68%) patients cured and three requiring cortisone replacement. With skilled surgery, if a microadenoma can be identified, selective transsphenoidal resection yields a comparable control rate with rapid response. If an adenoma cannot be identified or resection fails to correct the hypercortisolism, radiation therapy may be tried before resorting to total hypophysectomy or adrenalectomy. The main arguments against radiation therapy are the delay before response is obtained.

PROLACTIN-SECRETING ADENOMAS

The prolactin assay is of recent origin, and reported experience with radiation therapy alone for prolactin-secreting tumors is limited. Results of Grigsby and associates,[33,35] Kleinberg and colleagues,[53] Gomez and co-workers,[31] and Sheline[88] are reported in Table 24-9. The mean prolactin levels after irradiation ranged from 25% to 50% of the pretreatment levels, but at the time of reporting few patients had achieved normal values.

Antunes and associates[2] presented data (Table 24-10) for 30 patients, some of whom were treated by surgery alone,[30] surgery and radiation therapy,[16] or radiation therapy alone.[13] As indicated by decrease in mean prolactin, cessation of galactorrhea, and return of menses, responses were similar for the three treatment groups. Normalization of prolactin levels, however, occurred more frequently (seven of 16) in patients treated by transsphenoidal resection. Sheline[88] presented results for 14 patients with grade III or grade IV adenomas who were treated by both transsphenoidal resection and postoperative irradiation. Mean prolactin levels were 10,500 ng/ml before surgery, 4700 ng/ml before irradiation, and 820 ng/ml after (3 to 6 months) irradiation; five patients achieved normal levels by the combined procedure.

Grossman and colleagues[39] evaluated the use of radiation therapy alone in 36 women with relatively small prolactinomas (*i.e.*, without significant suprasellar extension). The initial prolactin levels ranged from 75 to 5000 ng/ml. The radiation dose was 4500 cGy, given in 25 equal daily fractions of 180 cGy each. After irradiation a dopamine agonist was administered. The drug therapy was periodically interrupted and the serum prolactin levels measured; a progressive decrease was found in 26 of 27 patients evaluated. One to eleven years (mean, 4 years) after irradiation, serum prolactin levels had returned to normal in about one third of the patients.

Frantz and co-workers[25] reported the results of radiation therapy in 26 patients, 11 of whom had had prior surgery. They found a wide variation in individual response. At 1 year an average prolactin decrease of 60% was found. In ten patients followed up for 3 years or longer, the mean prolactin level had decreased by about 90%. These patients had relatively large tumors (grade II to grade IV) and relatively high initial serum prolactin levels (up to 10,000 ng/ml).

The results of Hardy and colleagues[43] for transsphenoidal resection in 80 females with galactorrhea or amenorrhea were published, from a group of 180 with surgically treated prolactin-secreting pituitary adenomas; males and recently treated females were excluded for obvious reasons, but the reason why other female patients were excluded is not clear. The control rate was much better for small tumors than for larger ones: 90% for grade I *versus* 53% for grade II. A similar inverse relationship was found between prolactin concentration and cure rate.

Rush and Newall[82] treated 29 patients with irradiation alone for pituitary adenomas. Of ten patients with hyperprolactinemia, seven achieved normalization of prolactin levels over a period of 3 to 8 years, and three had elevated levels between 4 and 9 years after radiation therapy.

The value of primary radiation therapy is less certain. It appears to be of value and should be used for large, incompletely resected tumors and for patients desiring resumption of menses who have not had a satisfactory result with surgery. It also may be used as an alternative to resection, but the response is slow and, at least to date, less certain than with resection.

TABLE 24–9
Results of Irradiation for Prolactin-Secreting Adenomas

PARAMETER	KLEINBERG AND CO-WORKERS[53]	GOMEZ AND CO-WORKERS[31]	SHELINE[88]	GRIGSBY[36]	GRIGSBY[33]
Number of patients	8	8	4	17	28
Treatment	Irradiation	Irradiation	Transsphenoidal or transcranial plus irradiation	Irradiation	Transsphenoidal or transcranial plus irradiation
Mean prolactin level (ng/ml)					
Before treatment*	195 (61–10,000)	168 (38–480)	387 (937–1300)		
After treatment*	50 (32–1000)	64 (12–200)	192 (28–450)		
Galactorrhea ceased	3/8	2/8	1/2	4/8	7/13
Menses resumed	2/6	4/?	0/2	5/9	8/15
Follow-up (years)		.5–5	0–1.5	6–29	3–30

* *Range of values in parentheses*

TABLE 24–10
Prolactin-Secreting Pituitary Tumors: Pretreatment and Posttreatment Prolactin Determinations

	TREATMENT*		
	T	T OR C + R	R
RADIOGRAPHIC GRADE OF TUMOR†			
I	8	2	0
II	3	0	2
IIA	4	0	1
IIB	1	4	0
IIIB	0	2	1
IV	0	0	2
TOTAL	16	8	6
MEAN PROLACTIN LEVEL (ng/ml)‡			
Pretreatment	381 (27–900)	1070 (21–3600)	2500 (1100–10,000)
Posttreatment	80 (6–361)	144 (3–490)	165 (32–560)
MEAN DECREASE PROLACTIN (Posttreatment)	80%	59%	87%
PROLACTIN RETURNED TO NORMAL	7	2	0
MENSES RETURNED TO NORMAL	3/13	0/3	1/3
GALACTORRHEA CEASED	4/12	1/3	2/3
MEAN FOLLOW-UP (MONTH)‡	6 (1–28)	18 (3–39)	32 (13–72)

** T: transsphenoidal resection; C: transcranial resection; R: radiation therapy (4500 cGy over 5-week period). There was a tendency to use irradiation alone for patients with larger tumors and higher prolactin concentrations.*
† Hardy's staging system used
‡ Ranges appear in parentheses.
(Antunes JL, Housepian EM, Frantz AG, et al: Ann Neurol 2:148, 1977)

ADENOMAS WITH MASS EFFECT

This section deals with mass effects from pituitary tumors, except those associated with acromegaly or Nelson's syndrome. Patients with pituitary tumors usually present with decreased visual acuity or visual field deficits; hypopituitarism caused by pressure-induced pituitary atrophy also is common. Previously such tumors were thought to be nonfunctioning chromophobe adenomas. In light of present information the majority of pituitary tumors probably secrete prolactin. Landolt[58] has suggested that those without evidence of excess hormone secretion should be termed endocrine-inactive adenomas.

At UCSF between 1934 and 1968,[87] 23 patients, predominantly those with minimal visual field deficits or those who were elderly and thought to be poor surgical risks, were treated by radiation therapy alone. Thirty-seven had resection only and 80 had resection and postoperative radiation therapy; 115 of the 117 operations were transcranial. Response to treatment according to extent of pretreatment visual field loss is shown in Table 24-11. This analysis credits surgery with posttreatment visual field changes, whether or not radiation therapy was given. When the visual field loss was limited to approximately one quadrant, improvement was similar for radiation therapy and for surgery (two thirds regained normal fields). With larger

TABLE 24–11
Adenomas with Mass Effect: Visual Field Change After Therapy (UCSF 1934–1968)

		VISUAL FIELDS AFTER TREATMENT			
APPROXIMATE FIELD LOSS BEFORE THERAPY	**TREATMENT**	NORMAL (%)	IMPROVED (%)	UNCHANGED (%)	WORSE (%)
≤1 quadrant	R (17)	65	12	24	0
	S (42)	67	7	17	9
1 to 2 quadrants	R (10)	0	60	40	0
	S (109)	32	28	29	11
≥2 quadrants	S (17)	6	29	59	6

R: radiation therapy; S: surgical resection (with or without radiation therapy); number of eyes at risk indicated in parentheses.
(Sheline GE, Tyrrell JB: Pituitary adenomas. In Phillips TL, Pistenmaa DA [eds]: Radiation Oncology Annual, pp 1–35. New York, Raven Press, 1983)

TABLE 24–12
Adenomas with Mass Effect: Determinate Recurrence-Free Survival Rates

	RECURRENCE-FREE SURVIVAL RATES*		
INTERVAL (YEARS)	RADIATION THERAPY	SURGERY	SURGERY PLUS RADIATION THERAPY
2	100% (18)	70% (26)	98% (79)
5	93% (15)	38% (24)	96% (68)
10	100% (5)†	14% (21)	86% (43)
20		0 (14)	73% (15)

**Number of patients at risk indicated in parentheses.*
† These five patients were known to be alive and well at 15 years after radiation therapy.
(Sheline GE, Tyrrell JB: Pituitary adenomas. In Phillips TL, Pistenmaa DA [eds]: Radiation Oncology Annual, pp 1–35. New York, Raven Press, 1983)

defects surgery had the advantage. If the deficit involved more than 25% but not more than 50% of the visual field, normalization of visual fields was achieved in one third of surgical patients but in none treated by radiation therapy alone. Surgical complications included a 7% mortality (4% after 1945), major increase in visual field deficit in 6%, and severe brain damage in 1%. Other authors have reported similar poor results with invasive tumors.[64,71,73]

Long-term recurrence-free survival rates are presented in Table 24-12. Patients who died during the postoperative period or who died of unrelated causes and were relapse-free have been excluded. Because a number of patients irradiated earlier in the study period received doses less than 4000 cGy and because response is dose-dependent, it is anticipated that the long-term control rates with current techniques will be superior to those indicated.

Grigsby and co-workers[33,35] treated 100 patients with nonfunctioning adenomas between 1954 and 1982. Radiation therapy alone was used in 19, and 81 received postoperative irradiation. Improvement in visual field deficits occurred in 95% of all patients (including other syndromes) treated with radiation alone. There was also a trend for increased control rates for radiation doses greater than 4500 cGy ($P = 0.15$). Improvement in vision for those receiving surgery and postoperative radiation (all syndromes) occurred in 48% of those with pretreatment visual field deficits (Table 24-13). A significant dose response was observed for those with nonfunctioning adenomas. Local regrowth significantly decreased with higher doses (Table 24-14 and Fig. 24-10).

Flickinger and co-workers[22] irradiated 112 patients with nonfunctioning adenomas. A multivariate analysis showed decreased tumor control to be significantly associated with increasing field size ($P = 0.036$). No dose response was observed.

In summation, the treatment of choice for large tumors presenting with mass effects generally is surgical resection followed by radiation therapy. Although radiation therapy alone is effective in selected cases, surgical decompression plus postoperative radiation provides better results, particularly in patients with moderately advanced visual field deficits. With very large invasive tumors, reliance should be primarily on radiation therapy, because complete resection is usually not possible and because attempted radical removal is associated with a high mortality and morbidity.

PITUITARY ADENOMAS IN CHILDREN AND ADOLESCENTS

Primary central nervous system (CNS) neoplasms are common in the pediatric population, representing approximately 20% of all childhood tumors. However, pituitary adenomas are rare in children. Brain tumors in this age group are 100 times more common than pituitary tumors.[48] Cushing's disease is the most common pediatric pituitary disorder.[24,65]

Grigsby and co-workers[37] reported the results of surgery and postoperative irradiation or irradiation alone in 11 children and adolescents (< 19 years of age). Patients' conditions at diagnosis were acromegaly (1), Nelson's syndrome (1), prolactinemia (3), chromophobe adenoma (3), and Cushing's disease (3). With a median follow-up of 15.6 years, only two patients

TABLE 24–13
Correlation of Vision Improvement and Dose of Irradiation in 121 Pituitary Adenomas Treated with Surgery and Irradiation (Radiation Oncology Center, MIR, 1954–1982)

		FAILURES AND DOSE (cGy)				
VISUAL STATUS	NUMBER OF PATIENTS	<3000	3000–3999	4000–4999	5000–5400	>5400
Improved*	44	1	7	8	28	0
No Change	47	6	17	11	12	1
Total	91	7	24	19	40	1
Percent Improved	48.4	14.3	29.2	42.1	70	0

**$P = 0.003$*
(Grigsby PW, Simpson JR, Emami BN, et al: Int J Radiat Oncol Biol Phys 16:1411–1417, 1989)

TABLE 24–14
Correlation of Clinical Syndrome and Dose of Irradiation in 121 Pituitary Adenomas Treated With Surgery plus Irradiation (Radiation Oncology Center, MIR, 1954–1982)

		FAILURES AND DOSE (cGy)					
SYNDROME	**NUMBER OF PATIENTS**	<3000	3000–3999	4000–4999	5000–5400	>5400	TOTAL
Nonfunctioning*	81	3/4	3/13	1/13	2/49	0/3	9/81
Amenorrhea/galactorrhea†	28	2/3	2/8	0/3	1/14	0/2	5/28
Acromegaly‡	12	0	1/3	2/4	1/5	0	4/12
Total§	121	5/7	6/24	3/20	4/68	0/5	18/121
Percent Failures		71.4	25.0	15.0	5.9	0	14.9

**P = 0.0003*
†P = 0.07
‡P = 0.64
§P = 0.000059
(Grigsby PW, Simpson JR, Emami BN, et al: Int J Radiat Oncol Biol Phys 16:1411–1417, 1989)

have failed. No long-term visual complications were found; all returned to work or school, and three of eight females have borne children.

Other authors have reported similar excellent results in the treatment of children. Jennings and colleagues[50] reported tumor control in 12 of 15 patients (80%) with Cushing's disease. Cassar and co-workers[12] irradiated nine children with Cushing's disease, and all had local control. Styne[95] controlled disease in 14 of 15 patients (93%) with transsphenoidal microadenomectomy. Control of nonfunctioning adenomas, prolactinomas, and acromegaly is also excellent in children.[4,60,63,70,78]

SEQUELAE OF RADIATION TREATMENT

Complications of modern conventional radiation therapy for pituitary tumors include epilation, scalp swelling, and otitis and are essentially the only side effects during or immediately after irradiation.[7]

Until a few years ago, function of the normal pituitary was thought to be unaffected by conventional radiation therapy. It is now known that irradiation-induced hypofunction can and does occur. Its incidence as a function of radiation dose, however, has not been clearly established. Repeated courses of therapy, occasionally necessary for tumor recurrence, carry an increased risk. AT UCSF, with pituitary doses of 4000 cGy to 5200 cGy (180 cGy per fraction), late hypopituitarism manifesting primarily as GH deficiency[77] has occurred in children treated for brain stem tumors, but its incidence is unknown. Samaan and associates[83] reported both hypothalamic dysfunction and primary hypopituitarism after irradiation for extracranial neoplasms. The hypothalamic pituitary axis received doses ranging from 3000 cGy to 8500 cGy, with 92% of doses being at least 4500 cGy. When evaluated 3 to 20 years after irradiation, 54 of 65 patients showed evidence of hypothalamic pituitary impairment and 25 had primary hypopituitarism. Thirteen young adults had growth failure with delayed bone age. Other patients displayed signs and symptoms of adrenal insufficiency that responded to cortisol administration. In 36 women with prolactinomas treated by radiation therapy and dopamine agonist therapy and observed 2 to 10 years after irradiation, the only deficiency found was that of GH.[91] Twenty-one patients developed GH deficiency, but this is of no clinical relevance in the adult. No patient developed TSH or ACTH deficiency, and no change was found in LH or FSH response to LH-RH. In 15 children with Cushing's disease treated with radiation, subse-

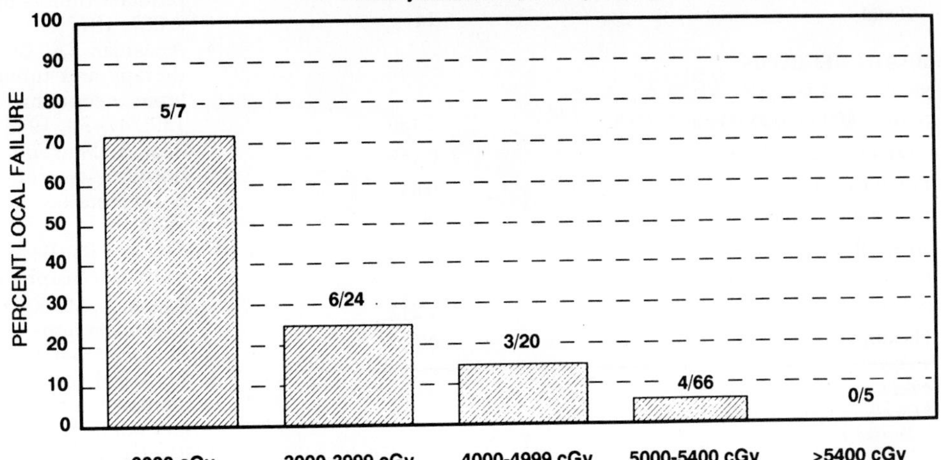

FIGURE 24–10. Correlation of dose of radiation and tumor control in 121 pituitary adenomas treated with surgery and irradiation at the Radiation Oncology Center, Mallinckrodt Institute of Radiology, 1954–1982.

TABLE 24–15
Complications of Radiation Therapy: Optic Nerve or Chiasmal Injury

STUDY	INCIDENCE OF INJURY
Aristizabal et al[3]	4/122
Daily fraction (cGy)	
<200	0/7
200–220	2/99
>220	2/16
Total dose (cGy)	
≤4600	0/96
>4600	4/26
Harris and Levene[46]	5/55*
Sheline[88]	
Daily dose (cGy)	
≤200	0/180
225	1/1
Grigsby et al[35]	
Daily dose (cGy)	
≤200	2/212
Flickinger et al[22]	
Daily dose (cGy)	
≤238	1/112

**Daily dose ≥ 250 cGy in all patients developing optic injury*
(Modified from Sheline GE, Tyrrell JB: Pituitary adenomas. In Phillips TL, Pistenmaa DA [eds]: Radiation Oncology Annual, pp 1–35. New York, Raven Press, 1983)

quent development of sexual characteristics, sexual function, and intellect was normal in all cases.[52]

Goldfine and Lawrence[29] reported three instances of hypopituitarism in 12 patients irradiated for acromegaly. Ten years after treatment for acromegaly, Eastman and colleagues[18] found a 10% increase in hypothyroidism and a 32% increase in hypoadrenalism. It is important to keep in mind that hypopituitarism can occur after many years; endocrine replacement therapy can then be instituted as needed.

Injuries to optic nerves or chiasm are rare but have been reported in patients treated for pituitary tumors (Table 24-15) Except for cases of acromegaly, most cases reported have had either doses in excess of 5000 cGy or daily fractions greater than 200 cGy, or both.

Although radiation-induced neoplasia may occur with a single course of radiation therapy, the incidence is exceedingly small (Table 24-16). The same is true for brain necrosis in patients irradiated for pituitary tumors.

TABLE 24–16
Complications of Radiation Therapy for Pituitary Adenomas

COMPLICATION	NO. OF CASES
SARCOMA	
Waltz and Brownell[96] (literature to 1966)	12*
Multiple courses of radiation†	(7)
Dose unknown	(3)
3500 to 4500 cGy in 3.5–4 wk	(2)
Rubinstein and Garg[81] (AFIP), dose unknown	1
Powell and co-workers,[75] 5000 cGy/? fractionation	1
Total	14
BRAIN NECROSIS	
Sheline and Wara‡[93] (mostly 4000–5000 cGy in 5–6 wk)	0/180
Kramer[56] (4500 cGy in 4.5 wk)	0/169
Pistenmaa et al[73,74] (av 5750 cGy/6 wk)	0/84
Emmanuel[20] (4000 cGy in 4 wk)	0/96
Aristizabal et al[3] (4900 cGy)	1/122
Grigsby et al[35] (mostly 4500–5500 cGy in 5–6 wk)	1/212
Flickinger et al[23] (3500–6300 cGy in 5–6 wk)	0/112

**Ten fibrosarcomas and two osteosarcomas*
† Usually very large total dose
‡ Observed 10 to 35 years
(Modified from Sheline GE, Tyrrell JB: Pituitary adenomas. In Phillips TL, Pistenmaa DA [eds]: Radiation Oncology Annual, pp 1–35. New York, Raven Press, 1983)

TABLE 24–17
Policies of Treatment at Radiation Oncology Center, Mallinckrodt Institute of Radiology

RADIATION ALONE*	
Cushing's disease	4500–5000 cGy
Microadenomas	5000 cGy (or transsphenoidal resection)
Macroadenomas	5000–5400 cGy (medically inoperable)
POSTOPERATIVE IRRADIATION*	
Invasive disease	5000 cGy
Incomplete resection	5400 cGy

**180 cGy per day*

CLINICAL TRIALS

At present there are no clinical trials available evaluating optimal therapy for patients with pituitary adenomas.

The policies of treatment at the Radiation Oncology Center, Mallinckrodt Institute of Radiology, are shown in Table 24-17.

REFERENCES

1. Acqui A, Ferrante L, Fraioli, et al: Association between intracranial aneurysms and pituitary adenomas. Neurochirurgia 30:177–181, 1987
2. Antunes JL, Housepian EM, Frantz AG, et al: Prolactin-secreting pituitary tumors. Ann Neurol 2:148, 1977
3. Aristizabal S, Caldwell WL, Avila J: The relationship of time-dose fractionation factors to complications in the treatment of pituitary tumors by irradiation. Int J Radiat Oncol Biol Phys 2:667, 1977
4. Arslanian SA, Becker DJ, Lee PA, et al: Growth hormone therapy and tumor recurrence: Findings in children with brain neoplasms and hypopituitarism. Am J Dis Child 139:347–50, 1985
5. Asai A. Matsutani M, Funada N, et al: Malignant growth hormone-secreting pituitary adenoma with hematogenous dural metastasis: Case report. Neurosurgery 22:1091–1094, 1988
6. Atkinson RL, Becker DP, Martins AN, et al: Acromegaly: Treatment by transsphenoidal microsurgery. JAMA 233:1279, 1975
7. Baglan R, Marks J: Soft-tissue reactions following irradiation of primary brain and pituitary tumors. Int J Radiat Oncol Biol Phys 7:455–459, 1981
8. Black PM, Zervas NT, Candia GI: Incidence and management of complications of transsphenoidal operation for pituitary adenomas. Neurosurgery 20:920–924, 1987
9. Black PM, Zervas NT, Candia G: Management of large pituitary adenomas by transsphenoidal surgery. Surg Neurol 29:443–7, 1988

10. Bloodworth JMB Jr, Kovacs K, Horvath E: Light and electron microscopy of pituitary tumors. In Linfoot JA (ed): Recent Advances in the Diagnosis and Treatment of Pituitary Tumors, pp 141–159. New York, Raven Press, 1979
11. Boggan JE, Tyrrell JB, Wilson CB: Transsphenoidal microsurgical management of Cushing's disease: Report of 100 cases. J Neurosurg 59:195, 1983
12. Cassar J, Doyle FM, Mashite RK, et al: Treatment of Cushing's disease in juveniles with interstitial pituitary irradiation. Clin Endocrinol 11:313–21, 1979
13. Chang RJ, Jeye WR Jr, Young Jr, et al: Detection, evaluation, and treatment of pituitary microadenomas in patients with galactorrhea and amenorrhea. Am J Obstet Gynecol 128:356, 1977
14. Comi R, Gesundheit N, Murray L, et al: Response of thyrotropin-secreting pituitary adenomas to a long-acting somatostatin analogue. N Engl J Med 317:12–17, 1987
15. Costello RT: Subclinical adenoma of the pituitary gland. Am J Pathol 12:205, 1936
16. Dohan FC, Raventos A, Boucot N, et al: Roentgen therapy in Cushing syndrome without adrenocortical tumor. J Clin Endocrinol Metab 17:8, 1957
17. Dons RF, Reith KG, Gorden P, et al: Size and erosive features of the sella turcica in acromegaly as predictors of therapeutic response to supervoltage irradiation. Am J Med 74:69–72, 1983
18. Eastman RC, Gorden P, Roth J: Conventional supervoltage irradiation is an effective treatment of acromegaly. J Clin Endocrinol Metab 48:931, 1979
19. Edmonds MW, Simpton WJK, Meakin JW: External irradiation of the hypophysis for Cushing's disease. Calif Med Assoc J 107:860, 1972
20. Emmanuel IG: Symposium on pituitary tumors: IV. Historical aspects of radiotherapy, present treatment technique and results. Clin Radiol 17:154, 1966
21. Flickinger JC, Deutsch M, Lunsford LD: Repeat megavoltage irradiation of pituitary and suprasellar tumors. Int J Radiat Oncol Biol Phys 17:171–175, 1989
22. Flickinger JC, Nelson PB, Martinez AJ, et al: Radiotherapy of nonfunctional adenomas of the pituitary gland. Cancer 63:2409–2413, 1989
23. Flickinger JC, Nelson PB, Taylor FH, et al: Incidence of cerebral infarction after radiotherapy for pituitary adenoma. Cancer 63:2404–2408, 1989
24. Fraioli B, Ferrante L, Celli P, et al: Pituitary adenomas with onset during puberty: Features and treatment. J Neurosurg 59:590–5, 1983
25. Frantz AG, Cogen PH, Chang CH, et al: Long-term evaluation of the results of transsphenoidal surgery and radiotherapy in patients with prolactinoma. In Crosignani PG, Rubin BL (eds): Endocrinology of Human Infertility: New Aspects, pp 161–170. New York, Grune & Stratton, 1981
26. Fraser R, Doyle F, Joplin GF, et al: The assessment of the endocrine effect and the effectiveness of ablative pituitary treatment by ^{90}Y and ^{198}Au implantation. In Kohler PO, Ross GT (eds): Diagnosis and Treatment of Pituitary Tumors, pp 35–46. New York, Excerpta Medica, 1973
27. Ganong WF: Neural centers regulating visceral function. In Ganong WF (ed): Review of Medical Physiology, 8th ed, p 158. Los Altos, CA, Lange Medical Publications, 1977
28. Ganong WF: Regulation of the secretion of hypothalamic hormones. Presented at the International Symposium on Recent Advances in the Diagnosis and Treatment of Pituitary Tumors, San Francisco, May 31–June 4, 1978
29. Goldfine ID, Lawrence AM: Hypopituitarism in acromegaly. Arch Intern Med 130:720, 1972
30. Goldfine ID, Vigneri R: Pharmacologic therapy of acromegaly. In Linfoot JA (ed): Recent Advances in the Diagnosis and Treatment of Pituitary Tumors, pp 341–346. New York, Raven Press, 1979
31. Gomez F, Reyes FI, Faiman C: Nonpuerperal galactorrhea and hyperprolactinemia: Clinical findings, endocrine features and therapeutic responses in 56 cases. Am J Med 62:648, 1977
32. Gorden P (moderator): Somatostatin and somatostatin analog (SMS 201–995) in treatment of hormone-secreting tumors of the pituitary and gastrointestinal tract and non-neoplastic diseases of the gut. Ann Intern Med 110:35–50, 1989
33. Grigsby PW, Simpson JR, Emami BN, et al: Prognostic factors and results of surgery and postoperative irradiation in the management of pituitary adenomas. Int J Radiat Oncol Biol Phys 16:1411–1417, 1989
34. Grigsby PW, Simpson JR, Fineberg B: Late regrowth of pituitary adenomas after irradiation and/or surgery. Cancer 63:1308–1312, 1989
35. Grigsby PW, Simpson JR, Stokes S, et al: Results of surgery and irradiation or irradiation alone for pituitary adenomas. J Neurooncol 6:129–134, 1988
36. Grigsby PW, Stokes S, Marks JE, et al: Prognostic factors and results of radiotherapy alone in the management of pituitary adenomas. Int J Radiat Oncol Biol Phys 15:1103–1110, 1988
37. Grigsby PW, Thomas PR, Simpson JR, et al: Long-term results of radiotherapy in the treatment of pituitary adenomas in children and adolescents. Am J Clin Oncol 11:607–611, 1988
38. Gross CJ, Harris RD, Seljeskog EL, et al: Pyridine nucleotide synthesis in normal and neoplastic human pituitary cells in culture. Cancer 52:2100–2106, 1983
39. Grossman A, Cohen BL, Charlesworth M, et al: Treatment of prolactinomas with megavoltage radiotherapy. Br Med J 288:1105–1109, 1984
40. Guidetti B, Fraioli B, Cantore GP: Results of surgical management of 319 pituitary adenomas. Acta Neurochir 85:117–124, 1987
41. Hardy J: Transsphenoidal surgery of hypersecreting pituitary tumors. In Koyhler PO, Ross GT (eds): Diagnosis and Treatment of Pituitary Tumors, p 179. New York, Excerpta Medica, 1973
42. Hardy J: Transsphenoidal microsurgical treatment of pituitary tumors. In Linfoot JA (ed): Recent Advances in the Diagnosis and Treatment of Pituitary Tumors, pp 375–388. New York, Raven Press, 1979
43. Hardy J, Beauregard H, Robert F: Prolactin-secreting pituitary adenomas: Transsphenoidal microsurgical treatment. In Robyn C, Harter M (eds): Progress in Prolactin Physiology and Pathology, p 361. Amsterdam, Elsevier/North Holland Biomedical Press, 1978
44. Hardy J, Somma M, Vezina JL: Treatment of acromegaly: Radiation or surgery? In Morley GP (ed): Current Controversies in Neurosurgery, p 377. Philadelphia, WB Saunders, 1976
45. Hardy J, Vezine JL: Transsphenoidal neurosurgery of intracranial neoplasm. Adv Neurol 15:261, 1976
46. Harris JR, Levene MB: Visual complications following irradiation for pituitary adenomas and craniopharyngiomas. Radiology 120:167, 1976
47. Heuschele R, Lampe I: Pituitary irradiation for Cushing's syndrome. Radiol Clin Biol 36:27, 1967
48. Hoffman HJ: Pituitary adenomas. In American Association of Neurological Surgeons (ed): Pediatric Neurosurgery: Surgery of the Developing Nervous System, pp 493–499. New York, Grune & Stratton, 1982
49. Imura H, Kato Y, Motohashi T, et al: Pharmacologic treatment of hyperprolactinemia. In Linfoot JA (ed): Recent Advances in the Diagnosis and Treatment of Pituitary Tumors, pp 375–388. New York, Raven Press, 1979
50. Jennings AS, Liddle GW, Orth DN: Results of treating childhood Cushing disease with pituitary irradiation. N Engl J Med 297:957, 1977
51. Johnston D, Hall K, Kendall-Taylor, et al: Effect of dopamine agonist withdrawal after long-term therapy in prolactinomas: Studies with high-definition computerized tomography. Lancet July 28:187–192, 1984
52. Kernohan JW, Sayre GP: Tumors of the pituitary gland and infundibulum, section X, fascicle 26, p 7. Washington, DC, Armed Forces Institute of Pathology, 1956
53. Kleinberg DL, Noel GL, Frantz AG: Galactorrhea: A study of 235 cases, including 48 with pituitary tumors. N Engl J Med 296:589, 1977
54. Kovacs K, Horvath E, Ezrin C: Pituitary adenomas. In Sommers SC (ed): Pathology Annual 1977. Norwalk, CT, Appleton-Century-Crofts, 1977

55. Kramer S: Indications for, and results of, treatment of pituitary tumors by external radiation. In Kohler PO, Ross GT (eds): Diagnosis and Treatment of Pituitary Tumors, p 217. New York, Excerpta Medica, 1973
56. Kramer S: Personal communication, 1978. In Sheline GE, Tyrrell JB: Pituitary tumors. In Perez CA, Brady LW (eds): Principles and Practice of Radiation Oncology, pp 1108–1125. Philadelphia, JB Lippincott, 1987
57. Krieger DT: Pharmacological therapy of Cushing's disease and Nelson's syndrome. In Linfoot JA (ed): Recent Advances in the Diagnosis and Treatment of Pituitary Tumors, pp 375–388. New York, Raven Press, 1979
58. Landolt AM: Ultrastructure of human sella tumors: Correlations of clinical findings and morphology. Acta Neurochir 22:1, 1975
59. Lawrence AM, Pinsky SM, Goldfine ID: Conventional radiation therapy in acromegaly: A review and reassessment. Arch Intern Med 128:369–377, 1971
60. Laws ER, Scheithauer BW, Groover RV: Pituitary adenomas in childhood and adolescence. Prog Exp Tumor Res 30:359–361, 1987
61. Levin S: Manifestations and treatment of acromegaly. Calif Med 116:57, 1972
62. Liuzzi A, Dallabonzana D, Oppizzi G, et al: Low doses of dopamine agonists in the long-term treatment of macroprolactinomas. N Engl J Med 313:656–659, 1985
63. Ludecke DK, Herrman HD, Sculte FJ: Special problems with neurosurgical treatment of hormone-secreting pituitary adenomas in children. Prog Exp Tumor Res 30:362–370, 1987
64. Martins AN, Hayes GH, Kempe LG: Invasive pituitary adenomas. J Neurosurg 22:268, 1965
65. McArthur RG, Cloutier MD, Hayles AB, et al: Cushing's disease in children: Findings in 13 cases. Mayo Clin Proc 47:318–26, 1972
66. McCormick WF, Halmi NS: Absence of chromophobe adenomas from a large series of pituitary tumors. Arch Pathol 92:231, 1971
67. Melen O: Neuro-opthalmologic features of pituitary tumors. Endocrinol Metab Clin North Am 16(3):585–608, 1987
68. Mirabelli D, Ciccarelli E, Merletti F: Pituitary adenomas in a cosmetics factory. Br J Industr Med 44:845, 1987
69. Molitch ME: Pathogenesis of pituitary tumors. Endocrinol Metab Clin 16:503–527, 1987
70. Newman CB, Levine LS, New MI: Endocrine function in children with intrasellar and suprasellar neoplasms before and after therapy. Am J Dis Child 135:347–50, 1985
71. Ogilvy KM, Jakubowski J: Intracranial dissemination of pituitary adenomas. J Neurol Neurosurg Psychiatry 36:199, 1973
72. Orth DN, Liddle GW: Results of treatment in 108 patients with Cushing syndrome. N Engl J Med 285:243, 1971
73. Pistenmaa DA, Goffinet DR, Bagshaw MA, et al: Treatment of chromophobe adenomas with megavoltage irradiation. Cancer 35:1574, 1975
74. Pistenmaa DA, Goffinet DR, Bagshaw MA, et al: Treatment of acromegaly with megavoltage radiation therapy. Int J Radiat Oncol Biol Phys 1:885, 1976
75. Powell HC, Marshall LF, Igneizi RJ: Post-irradiation pituitary sarcoma. Acta Neuropathol 39:165, 1977
76. Renn WH, Rhoton AL Jr: Microsurgical anatomy of the sellar region. J Neurosurg 43:288, 1975
77. Richards GE, Wara WM, Grumbach MM, et al: Delayed onset of hypopituitarism: Sequelae of therapeutic irradiation of central nervous system, eye, and middle ear tumors. J Pediatr 89:553, 1976
78. Richmond IL, Wilson CB: Pituitary adenomas in childhood and adolescence. J Neurosurg 49:163–168, 1978
79. Ross DA, Wilson CB: Results of transsphenoidal microsurgery for growth hormone-secreting pituitary adenoma in a series of 214 patients. J Neurosurg 68:854–867, 1988
80. Roth J, Gorden P, Brace K: Efficacy of conventional pituitary irradiation in acromegaly. N Engl J Med 282:1386, 1970
81. Rubinstein LJ, Garg UK: Secondary tumors of the central nervous system. In Tumors of the Central Nervous System, pp 313–314. Bethesda, MD, Armed Forces Institute of Pathology, 1972
82. Rush SC, Newall J: Pituitary adenoma: The efficacy of radiotherapy as the sole treatment. Int J Radiat Oncol Biol Phys 17:165–169, 1989
83. Samaan N, Maor M, Sampiere VA, et al: Hypopituitarism after external irradiation of nasopharyngeal cancer. In Linfoot JA (ed): Recent Advances in the Diagnosis and Treatment of Pituitary Tumors, pp 315–330. New York, Raven Press, 1979
84. Scholz DA, Gastineau CF, Harrison EG Jr: Cushing's syndrome with malignant chromophobe tumor of the pituitary and extracranial metastasis: Report of a case. Proc Mayo Clin 37:31, 1962
85. Schteingart DE, Tsao HS, Taylor CI, et al: Sustained remission of Cushing's disease with mitotane and pituitary irradiation. Ann Intern Med 92:613–619, 1980
86. Sheline GE: Treatment of chromophobe adenomas of the pituitary gland and acromegaly. In Kohler PO, Ross GT (eds): Diagnosis and Treatment of Pituitary Tumors, pp 201–216. Amsterdam, Excerpta Medica, 1973
87. Sheline GE: Treatment of nonfunctioning chromophobe adenomas of the pituitary gland. AJR 120:553, 1974
88. Sheline GE: The role of conventional radiation therapy in the treatment of functional pituitary tumors. In Linfoot JA (ed): Recent Advances in the Diagnosis and Treatment of Pituitary Tumors, pp 289–313. New York, Raven Press, 1979
89. Sheline GE, Boldrey EB, Phillips TL: Chromophobe adenomas of the pituitary gland. AJR 92:160, 1964
90. Sheline GE, Goldberg MB, Feldman R: Pituitary irradiation for acromegaly. Radiology 76:70, 82, 1961
91. Sheline GE, Grossman A, Jones AE, et al: Radiation therapy for prolactinomas. In Black PM, Zervas NT, Ridgway ED, et al (eds): Secretory Tumors of the Pituitary Gland, pp 93–108. New York, Raven Press, 1984
92. Sheline GE, Tyrell JB: Pituitary adenomas. In Phillips TL, Pistenmaa DA (eds): Radiation Oncology Annual, pp 1–35. New York, Raven Press, 1983
93. Sheline GE, Wara WM: Radiation therapy of acromegaly and nonsecretory chromophobe adenomas of the pituitary. In Seydel HG (ed): Tumors of the Central Nervous System, pp 119–131. New York, John Wiley & Sons, 1975
94. Steiner E, Imhof H, Knosp E: Gd-DTPA enhanced high resolution MR imaging of pituitary adenomas. RadioGraphics 9:587–598, 1989
95. Styne DM, Grumbach MM, Kaplan SL, et al: Treatment of Cushing's disease in childhood and adolescence by transsphenoidal microadenomectomy. N Engl J Med 310:889–93, 1984
96. Waltz TA, Brownell B: Sarcoma: A possible late result of effective radiation therapy for pituitary adenoma: Report of two cases. J Neurosurg 24:901, 1966
97. Wass J, Thorner M, Morris D: Long-term treatment of acromegaly with bromocriptine. Br Med J 1:875–878, 1977
98. Wass JAH, Besser GM: The medical management of hormone-secreting tumors of the pituitary. Ann Rev Med 34:283–294, 1983
99. Weber T, Saeger W, Ludecke D: Light microscopical morphometry, immunocytochemistry, and clinical correlations of pituitary adenomas at various stages of oncocytic transformation. Acta Endocrinol 116:489–496, 1987
100. Wemeau JL, Dewailly D, Leroy R: Long term treatment with the somatostatin analog SMS 201–995 in a patient with a thyrotropin- and growth hormone-secreting pituitary adenoma. J Clin Endocrinol Metab 66:636–639, 1987
101. Werner S, Trampe E, Palacios P, et al: Growth hormone producing pituitary adenomas with concomitant hypersecretion of prolactin are particularly sensitive to photon irradiation. Int J Radiat Oncol Biol Phys 11:1713, 1985
102. Williams RA, Jacobs HS, Kurtz AB, et al: The treatment of acromegaly with special reference to transsphenoidal hypophysectomy. Q J Med 44:79, 1975
103. Wilson CB, Dempsey LC: Transsphenoidal microsurgical removal of 250 pituitary adenomas. J Neurosurg 48:13, 1978
104. Youssen DM, Arrington JA, Zinreich SJ, et al: Pituitary adenomas: Possible role of bromocriptine in intratumoral hemorrhage. Radiology 170:239–243, 1989

25

○ ○ ○ • • •

Spinal Canal

Delia M. Garcia
Ulf L. Karlsson

Few physicians have the opportunity to treat patients with primary tumors of the spinal canal because these tumors are quite rare. Ependymomas, astrocytomas, and oligodendrogliomas are tumors of the spinal cord. Ependymomas and neurolemmomas affect the nerves of the canal. Meningiomas are neoplasms of the meninges, hemangiomas are lesions of the vessels, and lipomas are neoplasms of the connective tissue. These spinal canal tumors are commonly characterized as intramedullary (*i.e.,* cord, vessels), intradural-extramedullary (*i.e.,* meninges, nerves, vessels), and extradural or epidural (*i.e.,* meninges).

Radiation therapy has proved important in the management of primary spinal canal tumors, especially for those incompletely excised.

ANATOMY

The Spinal Cord

The spinal cord contains about 35 segments, with a corresponding number of spinal nerves and cord exits. The spinal cord develops as an ectodermal plate that forms a groove and fuses into a tube, temporarily open inferiorly and superiorly (*i.e.,* neuropores). The spinal cord gray matter develops by proliferation of the inner lining of the neural tube and differentiates into neurons, astrocytes, oligodendroglia, and ependymal cells. The neurons send processes into and superficial to this layer to form the white matter of the cord with the glial cells. These processes form the pathways of the central nervous system (CNS) when the pathways to and from the brain are added to the system.

The developmental process produces somatotopically distinct regions of the cord (*i.e.,* the bilateral posterior sensory and anterior motor horns of the gray matter). The sensory and motor regions are separated by the autonomic nuclei on each side. Lateral to the gray matter run several crossed pathways: the corticospinal tract that controls voluntary movements and the spinothalamic tract that conveys pain impulses and, posteriorly, the posterior spinocerebellar tracts for proprioceptive and touch impulses. The spinal cord proper ends at about the first lumbar vertebra.

The Spinal Canal

The spinal canal is formed by the posterior body surfaces and arches of the stacked vertebrae. It is triangular in the lumbar and cervical regions, where most of the mobility resides, and is round in the thoracic region.

The spinal canal is lined with ligaments, including the posterior longitudinal ligament on its anterior wall, the flava (yellow) ligmenta between adjacent arches, and the interspinous ligaments between the spinous processes.

The cord is surrounded by the meninges, the innermost of which is the pia mater that houses the vessels of the cord. This layer condenses laterally into about 20 pairs of dentate ligaments, which suspend the cord laterally to the dura mater. Meningiomas are commonly attached to these ligaments.

The dura mater forms a dense, fibrous barrier between the spinal canal and the cord. The dura ends inferiorly at the level of the second sacral vertebra but continues with the filum terminale down to the coccyx. The filum terminale is the vestige of the original neural tube, extending from the cord to the coccyx. Between the dura mater and the pia mater resides the arachnoid mater (*i.e.,* spider web meninx).

The arachnoid encloses the subarachnoid space, with cerebrospinal fluid (CSF). The subarachnoid space follows the arachnoid down to the end of the dural sac. At each spinal ganglion and nerve, there is a subarachnoid space sleeve. It is not known if the subarachnoid space ends at the dorsal ganglion or follows the nerves to the periphery.

CSF pressure depends on body position. With a person in a horizontal position, CSF pressure is 70 to 200 mm H_2O, increasing to 100 to 300 mm H_2O in an erect position (measured in the lumbar region), in which the CSF pressure can be negative in the lateral ventricles.[67] The amount of CSF is normally 150 ml, with a turnover of 300 ml each 24 hours.

Spinal Canal Vessels

The spinal cord is supplied by two posterolateral arteries and one anterior longitudinal artery, formed by radicular arteries through the intervertebral foramina. The vertebral artery supplies the cervical and upper thoracic segments. The midthoracic region is supplied from the radicular artery at about T7, and the thoracolumbar region is supplied from the lower thoracic radicular artery. The venous supply for the cord and the spine is more extensive. Intradural and extradural venous plexa communicate with each other and with intervertebral veins through the foramina.[67]

Topography of the Spine

The relationship between vertebral levels, spinal cord levels, and palpable spine parts is important for a radiation oncologist because the spinal defect levels do not correspond to the signs indicating spinal cord levels. The reason for this is that the cord is shorter than the spine. Many cord levels are located superior to corresponding vertebral body levels. When spinous process levels are related to vertebral levels or cord levels, the situation becomes more complicated because the palpable spinous process tips slant differently in the various parts of the spine.

EPIDEMIOLOGY

Primary tumors of the spinal canal are rare, occurring far less often than those of the brain. The ratio of intraspinal to intracranial neoplasms ranges from 1 : 5 to 1 : 10 in adults and to 1 : 20 in children.[19,30,41,42] According to estimates from the National Cancer Institute SEER program, approximately 1500 new primary spinal canal neoplasms were diagnosed in the United States in 1989.[62]

The incidences of different histologies vary according to age and sex, but the approximate frequencies are as follows: neurolemmoma, 30%; meningioma, 25%; ependymoma, 15%; astrocytoma, 10%; oligodendroglioma, 5%; and lipoma, hemangioma, dermoid, and epidermoid combined, 15%.[71] Frequencies according to anatomic location are given in Table 25-1.

At least 50% of all spinal canal tumors are extradural, and most are metastatic. Thus, almost all primary tumors of the spinal canal are intradural; approximately one third are intramedullary, and the remaining two thirds are extramedullary (Table 25-1). Ependymomas belong in both intradural-extramedullary and intramedullary groups.

Primary tumors of the spinal canal affect a young population.[23,72] Almost 50% of the pediatric patients are younger than 5 years of age.[15,34] In children, 50% of primary spinal canal neoplasms are astrocytomas, and approximately 25% are ependymomas.[19] Meningiomas and neurolemmomas are extremely rare, but congenital tumors, such as epidermoids, dermoids, teratomas, and lipomas, balance the overall distribution of tumor types. In adults, neurolemmoma represents the most common primary tumor of the spinal cord, followed by meningioma and the group of astrocytoma, ependymoma, and oligodendroglioma.

Although most spinal cord neoplasms are distributed equally between men and women, certain histologic types have gender predilections; these differences are discussed later.

NATURAL HISTORY

Although many primary tumors of the spinal canal are histologically benign, they must be regarded as malignant because of their propensity to compress or invade the spinal cord and interfere with neurologic function. Intramedullary tumors produce neurologic damage by local invasion, and extramedullary lesions produce pressure and displacement of the spinal cord.

The CNS has no lymphatics, obviating direct spread to lymph nodes. Hematogenous spread is uncommon, as is seeding to the CSF.[23,33,46,69] The inability to control tumor locally is

TABLE 25–1
Primary Spinal Canal Tumors: Locations, Types, and Frequencies

LOCATION	LOCATION FREQUENCY (%)	TYPES	COMMENTS
Extradural	Few	Meningioma	~10% of spinal meningiomas
Intradural-extramedullary	70	Neurolemmoma (neurofibroma, schwannoma)	45% of primary tumors in this location, thoracic preference
		Meningioma	<40% of primary tumors at this location, thoracic preference
		Ependymoma in cauda	60% of all spinal canal ependymomas, lumbosacral preference
		Vascular malformations	<10% of primary tumors at this location
		Teratoma, dermoid, squamous cell neoplasia	<10% of primary tumors at this location, sacrococcygeal preference
		Lipoma	Few, subpial
Intradural-intramedullary	30	Ependymoma in cord	40% of all spinal canal ependymomas
		Astrocytoma	<45% of primary tumors at this location
		Vascular maformations	Few
		Oligodendroglioma	~15% of primary tumors at this location
		Teratoma	Few
		Hemangioma	Few

the major reason these patients die prematurely, although complications of paraplegia or quadriplegia (*i.e.*, infection and respiratory compromise) may also contribute to a shorter survival.

Primary spinal cord tumors may be focal or relatively localized in some patients, but the entire cord can be involved in other patients. As many as 60% of affected children present with widening of the entire spinal cord from the medulla or cervicomedullary junction to the conus; these lesions are known as holocord astrocytomas.[17] Tumors originating in the cauda equina tend to be less extensive than those of the spinal cord.[23]

CLINICAL PRESENTATION OF SPINAL TUMORS

Pain is the presenting symptom in 75% of patients with primary neoplasms of the spinal canal. Often the pain is localized to the region of involvement and may be present for a long time before the patient manifests localizing neurologic signs. Radicular pain, a result of pressure on nerve roots, reflects the distribution of the involved root and indicates that conduction is intact. Distention of the dura causes pain that is characteristically aggravated by recumbency because of venous congestion. Thus, pain is often worse at night.[17] Pain may also be worsened by movement and the Valsalva maneuver, and it is most severe in the region of the tumor. Less commonly, pain is characterized as a burning sensation in one or more extremities. The painful dysesthesia is often bilateral, is not distributed along a nerve root, and is not influenced by the Valsalva maneuver. Numbness replacing pain is a more advanced sign that indicates compromise of nerve or pathway conduction.

Other symptoms of CNS involvement include weakness (75% of patients), sensory changes (65%), and sphincter dysfunction (15%).[23] Bladder and bowel dysfunction as presenting symptoms are relatively uncommon and are usually seen in extradural tumors of the conus medullaris and cauda equina.

Lower-extremity weakness often manifests as a disturbance in gait. In young children, there may be a history of failure to achieve milestones, such as ambulation and control of bladder and bowel, or of regression of already acquired skills. With tumors of the cervical region, torticollis may occur in children, but adult patients may complain of neck pain and stiffness.

DIAGNOSTIC WORKUP

History and Physical Findings

The diagnostic workup for primary tumors of the spinal cord is given in Table 25-2. Meticulous and accurate patient history and physical examination cannot be overemphasized. The neurologic examination should concentrate on testing motor and sensory functions and reflexes.

A cutaneous sensory level may be definable, although the level of cord compression is a few segments higher than the superior level of sensory loss because of pathway crossing characteristics. Loss of pain, heat, and cold sensation below a specific dermatomal level indicates compromise of the spinothalamic pathway in the lateral column. Impaired posture, gait, and coordination and loss of vibration sense indicate compromise of the posterior spinocerebellar pathways in the posterior columns.

At the level of the lesion, there may be flaccid weakness and loss of tendon reflexes. Below the lesion, the same signs are noticed in acute stages, but spastic plegia and hyperactive tendon reflexes plus an upward Babinski's toe sign ensue in subacute and chronic stages. These findings are consistent with the phenomena experienced and observed with lower and upper motor neuron disease, respectively.

TABLE 25–2
Diagnostic Workup for Primary Spinal Cord Tumors

General
History
Physical examination
Complete neurologic examination
Radiographic studies
Plain radiography
Myelography
Magnetic resonance imaging
Computed tomography
Laboratory
Cerebrospinal fluid analysis
Complete blood count
Urinalysis

Autonomic reflexes (*e.g.*, sweating) frequently are increased below the level of the lesion and may encompass the whole body if the lesion is cervical.[4] Sweating disappears at the level of the compressed cord. Disruption of urinary and bowel function usually occurs later than sensory and motor dysfunction. Early loss of bladder function, saddle anesthesia, and late pain characterize neoplasms of the conus medullaris and filum terminale. With tumors of the cauda equina, pain is usually the presenting symptom, and bladder and bowel dysfunction occur late.[29] With tumors involving higher levels of the spinal cord, sphincter disturbance occurs late, usually long after other signs and symptoms have manifested.

Laboratory Data

A patient suspected of having a spinal canal neoplasm should not be subjected to a lumbar puncture before myelography or magnetic resonance imaging (MRI). Symptoms may be exacerbated after a spinal tap because of shifting of the cord and incarceration before the tumor can be localized adequately.[10] The CSF usually has increased protein levels and may exhibit xanthochromia, especially with extradural compression conditions, but lower values are found in cases of intramedullary disease and with compression in the cervical region.[4]

Radiographic Studies

Primary neoplasms of the spinal cord and canal have been categorized by anatomic location: intramedullary, intradural-extramedullary, and extradural. This classification of intraspinal neoplasms according to anatomic compartment is extremely useful in evaluating the patient radiographically (Fig. 25-1).

Plain X-ray Films

Abnormalities detected on plain films that are caused by increased intracanalar pressure include erosion of vertebral pedicles, enlargement of the anteroposterior diameter of the bony canal, or scalloping of the posterior wall of the vertebral bodies.

Calcification may be seen in extramedullary tumors, especially meningiomas, and less frequently in neurolemmomas. Spinal canal tumors may also be associated with scoliosis or kyphoscoliosis, especially in children.[3]

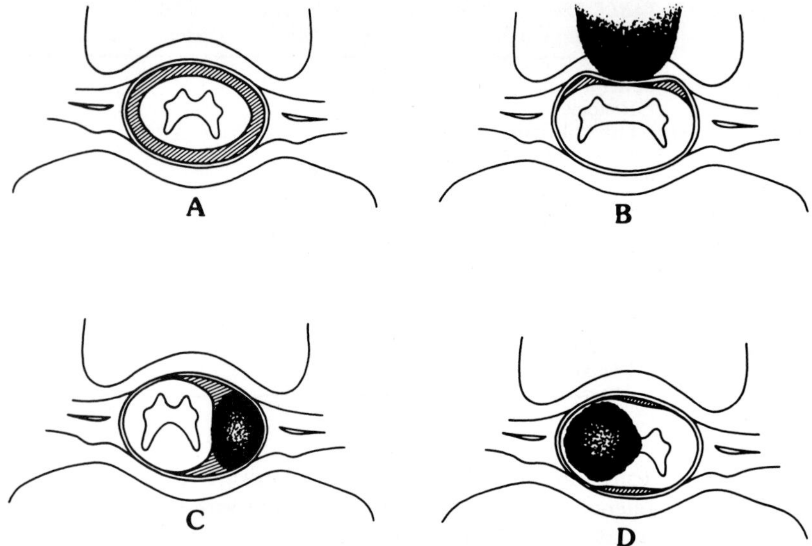

FIGURE 25–1. Neoplasms affecting the spinal cord. (**A**) Normal transverse spine. The spinal cord is enveloped by the pia mater, arachnoid, and dura mater, which are housed in the spinal canal and surrounded by ligaments supporting the vertebral bony structures. The subarachnoid space contains cerebrospinal fluid (*striped*). (**B**) Transverse spine with extradural mass. An extradural mass (*e.g.*, metastasis) from the vertebral body is compressing the dural sac and the spinal cord from the anterior direction. The subarachnoid space becomes obliterated at that level, causing a myelographic block. (**C**) Transverse spine with intradural-extramedullary mass. The mass, a meningioma or neurolemmoma, is compressing the spinal cord and roots in the dural sac, causing a myelographic block with a laterally displaced cord and, at times, producing a capping contour of contrast border. (**D**) Transverse spine with intramedullary mass. An intramedullary mass (astrocytoma or ependymoma) is infiltrating and expanding the spinal cord within the dural sac, causing a myelographic block.

Overall, plain x-ray films of the spine show abnormalities in approximately 50% of the patients with primary spinal canal neoplasms.[5,25,56,65] Changes are more likely to be detected on plain x-ray films for children than adults.[15,29,34]

Myelography

Myelography with water-soluble contrast medium has long been the examination of choice if a spinal canal neoplasm is suspected. This procedure is now often combined with or replaced by computed tomography (CT) scanning or MRI. An intramedullary tumor appears as an expansible lesion that attenuates contrast medium in the subarachnoid space by displacing it peripherally (Fig. 25-2). An intradural-extramedullary tumor displaces the spinal cord to the contralateral side and enlarges the subarachnoid space above and below the tumor (Fig. 25-3). An extradural tumor manifests as a mass extrinsic to the subarachnoid space, with compression of the cord and narrowing of the subarachnoid space ipsilaterally (Fig. 25-4). With myelography alone, a widened spinal cord may be attributed to syringomyelia or hydromyelia, making it necessary to augment the data with CT or MRI.[3]

Spinal Angiography

If myelography suggests a vascular malformation, selective spinal angiography is performed when experienced support staff are available. The procedure defines the extent of an arteriovenous malformation and its relationship to the spinal cord. Unlike infiltration of the spinal cord by tumor, angiomas do not commonly produce total obstruction.[3]

Computed Tomography

CT scanning is often combined with myelography, because intrathecal administration of water-soluble contrast medium is often required for visualizing intradural structures.[22] CT with bolus injection of intravenous contrast medium has limited usefulness in the spine; however, vascular lesions (*e.g.*, hemangioblastomas and arteriovenous malformations) may be enhanced with intravenous contrast injection.[3,22]

Some intramedullary tumors and cavities can be identified on CT scans because of a lower or higher density compared with surrounding normal tissues. However, it is sometimes impossible to differentiate between tumors associated with cysts and simple syringomyelia or hydromyelia.[22]

Intradural-extramedullary tumors are usually indistinguishable by CT. However, the sex, age, location, and number of lesions may provide clues about the histology. Neurolemmomas often enlarge the intervertebral foramen or canal and cause a smooth erosion of bone, and meningiomas may

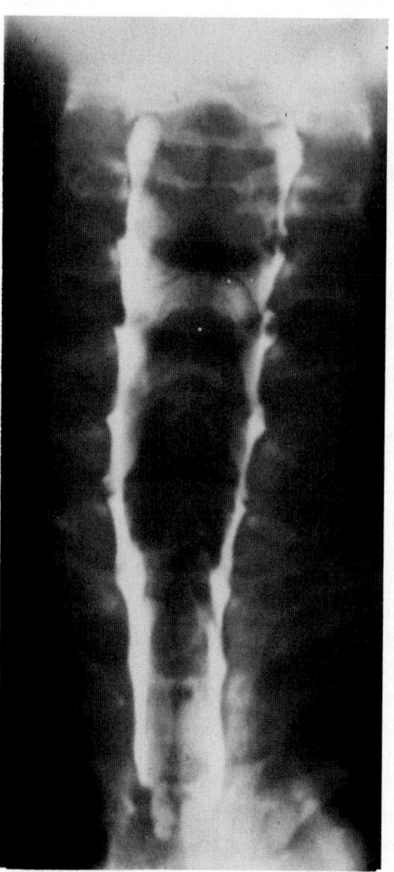

FIGURE 25–2. Myelogram with intramedullary mass. Abnormal widening of the cord silhouette is the typical myelographic feature. Widened interpedicular distances or enlarged intervertebral foramina may verify the diagnosis on plain radiographs. (Courtesy of Mokhtar Gado, M.D., Mallinckrodt Institute of Radiology, St. Louis, MO)

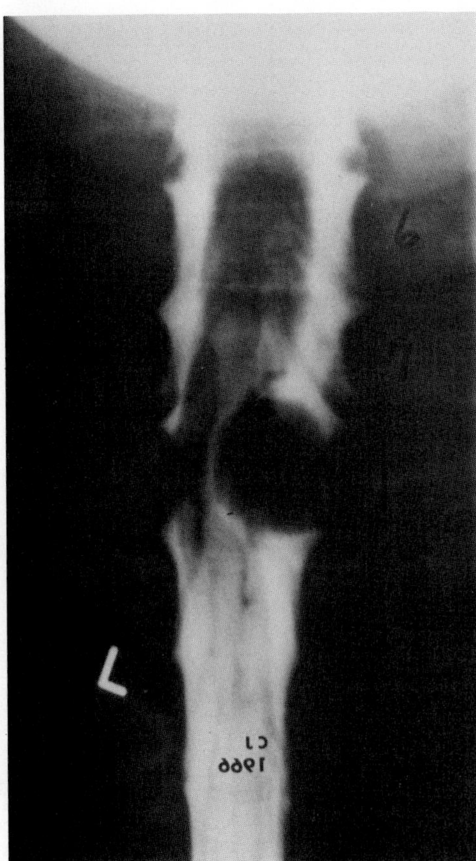

FIGURE 25–3. Myelogram with intradural but extramedullary mass. The tumor may be visualized as a capping silhouette because the mass is in the subarachnoid space with the contrast material. The cord is displaced toward the contralateral side. Both borders can be visualized if contrast is injected from above and below. This image is typically caused by neurolemmomas or meningiomas. (Courtesy of Mokhtar Gado, M.D., Mallinckrodt Institute of Radiology, St. Louis, MO)

calcify. Both of these neoplasms are partially outlined by CSF and produce an extramedullary deformity or displacement of the spinal cord.[22]

Metastatic tumors and lymphomas deform or compress the extradural compartment, although the tissues in this region can give rise to any number of rare primary neoplasms.

Magnetic Resonance Imaging

MRI is often the study of choice if a primary spinal canal tumor is suspected. Unlike CT and myelography, intrathecal contrast medium is not needed. The most beneficial view is the midline sagittal or lateral examination, although coronal and axial views are easily obtained. Even without intravenous gadolinium, MRI will demonstrate most tumors and cysts.[22]

Although lipomas are extremely rare and are usually easily seen on CT scans, MRI is superior in identifying them. Calcification is better detected by CT, but enlarged blood vessels are better detected by MRI. CT better demonstrates bone involvement, but MRI more dramatically depicts tumor that replaces normal fat or the marrow of the vertebra. Abnormalities of epidural soft tissues are better assessed by MRI, and CT scanning requires intrathecal injection of contrast medium to demonstrate the relationship of neoplasm to spinal cord.[22] Figures 25-5 and 25-6 are examples of spinal canal tumors diagnosed by MRI.

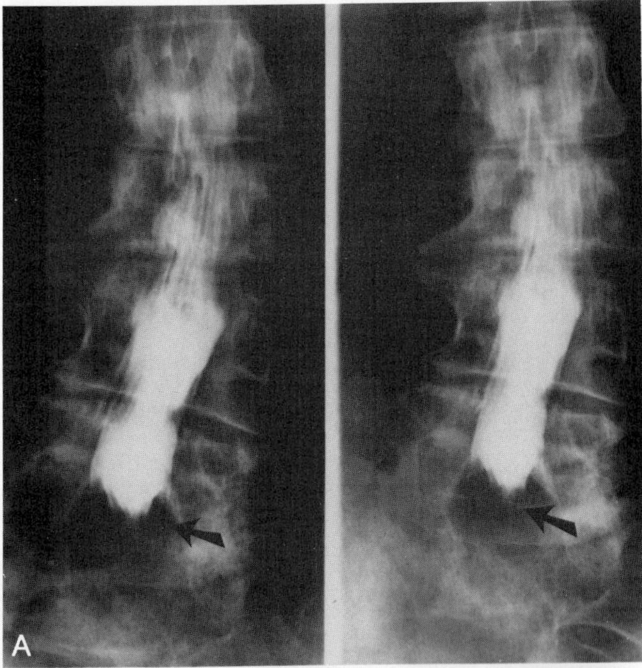

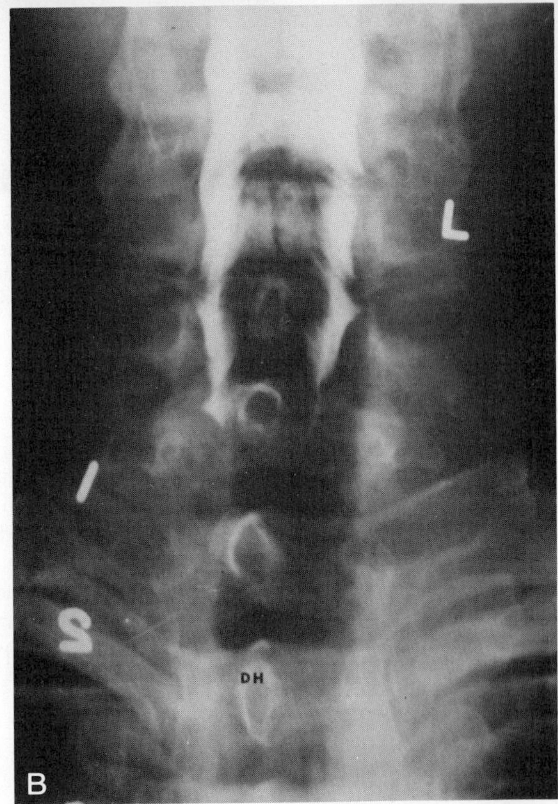

FIGURE 25–4. (**A**) Myelogram with extradural mass behind the L4 body. Extradural compression causes a "paintbrush" silhouette of the contrast border in the myelogram. This pattern presumably indicates contrast penetration between cords of the cauda equina or longitudinal wrinkling of the dura in response to the pressure from the tumor. Contrast medium injection at L2–L3 precludes visualization of the inferior block border. (**B**) Myelogram with extradural mass in the thoracic region. In this region the paintbrush border is often replaced by a straight blockage border of the contrast medium. Both block borders can be visualized if contrast medium is injected from above and below or if the incomplete block allows contrast medium to trickle past the blocked region. (Courtesy of Mokhtar Gado, M.D., Mallinckrodt Institute of Radiology, St. Louis, MO)

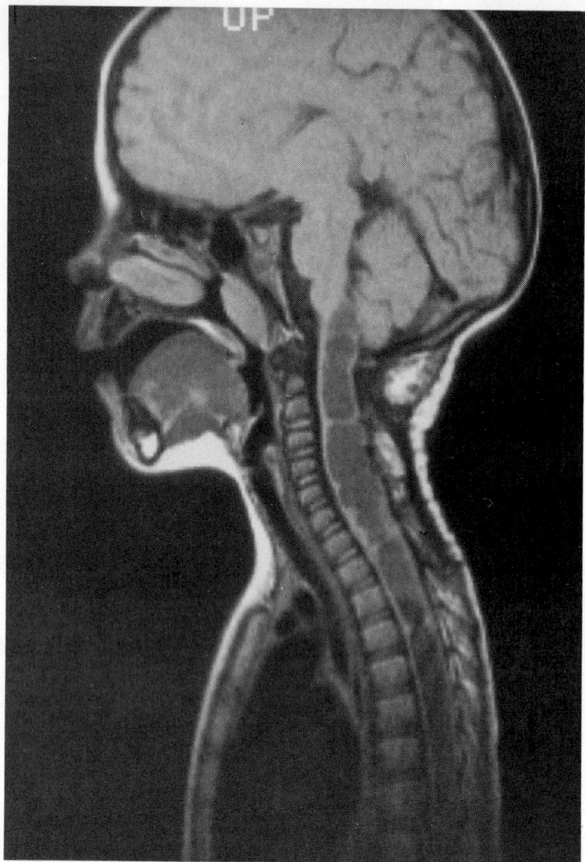

FIGURE 25–5. Sagittal MR scan of a 4-year-old child with an extensive cystic astrocytoma involving the cervical spinal cord and extending into the thoracic cord. (Gado M: The spine. In Lee JK, Sagel SS, Stanley RJ [eds]: Computed Body Tomography with MRI Correlation, 2nd ed, p. 1049. New York, Raven Press, 1989)

Intraoperative Ultrasonography

Intraoperative ultrasonography of the spine can be invaluable in evaluating lesions of the spinal cord, dural sac, and ventral surface of the vertebra. After the bone has been removed by laminectomy, real-time ultrasonography is used to localize the lesion, define its extent, and characterize the tumor as cystic or solid.[54] It can be used repeatedly during the course of surgery to evaluate the progress and expected end result of the operation.[57]

Tissue Diagnosis

Tumors of the spinal cord and spinal canal should be confirmed surgically whenever possible.

Extradural tumors, primarily metastatic in origin, are usually subjected only to a biopsy. Percutaneous needle biopsy under CT guidance often avoids the need for a more invasive procedure. However, in patients presenting with spinal cord compression, a laminectomy for decompression may be indicated, depending on the histologic type.

PATHOLOGIC CLASSIFICATION

Primary tumors of the spinal cord are histopathologically similar to those found intracranially, but the distribution of the various tumor types depends on the relationship of the neoplasm to the spinal cord and dura.

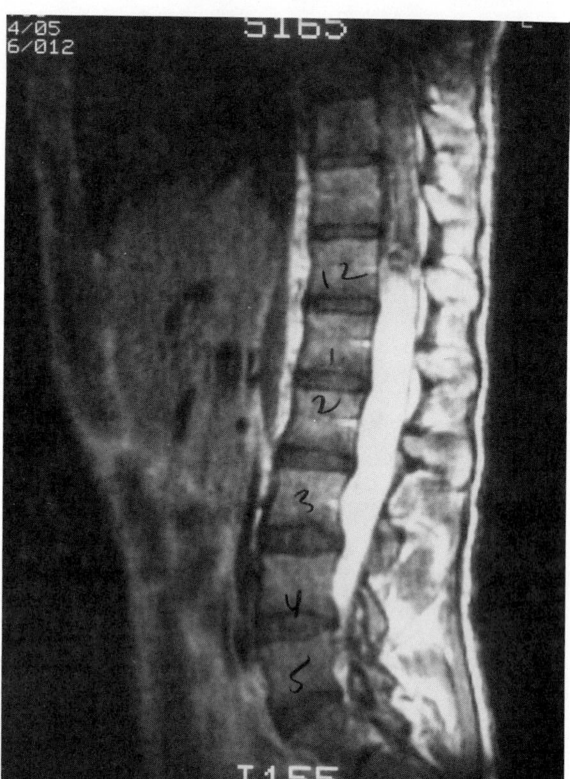

FIGURE 25–6. Sagittal MR scan of a 21-year-old man with a contrast-enhanced intramedullary myxopapillary ependymoma obliterating the conus medullaris and nerve roots of the cauda equina. Posterior scalloping of L1, L2, and L3 is demonstrated.

Intramedullary Tumors

Intramedullary neoplasms of the spinal cord comprise approximately one third of all primary spinal canal tumors. As many as 95% of the tumors in this anatomic location are ependymomas and astrocytomas. Vascular malformations, lipomas, dermoids, and teratomas may also originate within the cord.

Astrocytomas

Astrocytomas are derived from glial cells that make up most of the intraparenchymal cells. The histologic differentiation varies from benign, with a well-defined margin between tumor and normal spinal cord tissue, to the malignant glioblastoma multiforme. High-grade tumors are relatively rare within the spinal cord and are more commonly well-differentiated cystic lesions. The clinical course can therefore vary from extremely indolent to rapid neurologic deterioration and eventual death.

Astrocytomas and ependymomas occur with equal frequency, but astrocytomas are most commonly located in the cervical and thoracic regions. No sex predilection is evident.[34,42] Although astrocytomas are more common in adults than in children, a greater proportion of intramedullary astrocytomas are seen in children.[19] Pediatric astrocytomas are often holocord, associated with huge cysts rostrally and caudally and with the solid component spanning several segments.[17]

Ependymomas

Ependymomas are derived from glial cells similar to those lining the ventricular system and are classified as cellular or myxopapillary. They are often histologically benign and follow an indolent clinical course. Poorly differentiated ependymomas are rare. Approximately two thirds occur in the region of the cauda; these are discussed under intradural-extramedullary tumors. Ependymomas are more common in adults than in children, and there is no recognized sex predominance.

Vascular Malformations

A variety of vascular neoplasms can arise within the spinal canal, including arteriovenous malformations and hemangiomas.[63] Intramedullary vascular neoplasms are rare and may occur in all age groups from infants to older adults. They are seen more often in patients with evidence of vascular tumor formation in other organs.[12,63]

Intradural-Extramedullary Tumors

Most intradural-extramedullary neoplasms are meningiomas, neurolemmomas, or myxopapillary ependymomas, which are usually amenable to complete surgical excision. Ependymomas arising in the region of the conus medullaris and filum terminale are not truly intramedullary and are therefore described here.

Meningiomas

Meningiomas are usually benign, well-encapsulated neoplasms that are easily separated from the spinal cord; most can be completely excised and rarely recur. They may arise anywhere within the intradural space, but they are found in the thoracic region in approximately 80% of the patients.[45,63] Meningiomas are quite uncommon in the lumbar region and rare in the sacrum. At least 80% of meningiomas occur in women 40 years of age or older.[45,52]

Neurolemmomas

Neurolemmomas arise from the sheath of Schwann, which envelops the extramedullary axons of the nerve roots. Several names are used interchangeably, including schwannoma, neuroma, neurinoma, neurilemoma, and neurofibroma. Neurolemmomas occur in all sections of the spinal canal and are almost evenly distributed in the cervical, thoracic, and lumbar regions; they are less common in the sacral region. They occur twice as often in females as males, and they are rarely seen in patients over the age of 20.[60] These tumors are benign, well-encapsulated neoplasms and are often amenable to total surgical excision. Local recurrences after complete excision are rare. The lesions are usually solitary, but if they are part of a neurofibromatosis syndrome, multiple tumors may be present. Because neurolemmomas are always attached to a nerve root, dumbbell-type lesions may be present in the intradural-extramedullary and extradural compartments.

Ependymomas

About two thirds of all ependymomas occur in the lumbosacral region. These tumors are derived from the filum terminale or detached neuroectodermal cells when the cord "ascended" in the spine during development. Such ependymomas are most often of myxopapillary type and may be completely excised without compromise of neurologic function. Biologically, these tumors are less aggressive than the cellular ependymomas and are known to have a better prognosis.[51]

Rare Neoplasms

Unusual intradural-extramedullary tumors include lipomas, dermoids, and epidermoid tumors.

Dermoids are so rare that their incidence is not easily assessed. There is a slight male predominance, and most occur in the lumbosacral region.[59] If incompletely excised, dermoids recur. However, their growth is slow and clinical signs of recurrence may not be evident for many years.

Epidermoid tumors are more common in males than in females, and they are usually discovered in patients between the ages of 20 and 50 years.[59] They can be seen anywhere along the spinal canal and are usually benign. If incompletely excised, recurrences are usually slow.

Lipomas may be intramedullary or extramedullary, and they account for approximately 1% of spinal canal primary neoplasms. They occur more commonly in men than in women.[2] Some patients with lipomas have congenital anomalies. Small tumors are often amenable to complete removal with excellent neurologic results.[14]

Extradural Tumors

Almost all extradural tumors are metastatic. They are discussed in Chapter 76.

PROGNOSTIC FACTORS

The major prognostic factors in patients with primary neoplasms of the spinal canal include tumor type, histologic grade, extent of disease, anatomic location or relation of the tumor to the spinal cord and its coverings, feasibility of complete surgical excision, and presenting neurologic function. Many of these factors are interdependent.

The preoperative neurologic status of the patient determines the outcome after radical surgical resection of primary tumors of the spinal canal. Patients with severe neurologic deficit at presentation rarely improve after surgery even if the entire tumor can be excised, although the downhill course is often abated.[65] In contrast, patients with mild to moderate neurologic deficit often experience excellent recovery of neurologic function after excision. Although a transient increase in motor and sensory deficit is common in the postoperative period, neurologic improvement usually occurs over several weeks in patients who were able to walk preoperatively. Even with tumor that can only be subtotally removed, patients may improve neurologically or stabilize for many years. Patients with high-grade tumors, especially astrocytomas, tend to follow a rapid downhill course regardless of treatment.

Neurologic function is better for patients with tumors of the conus medullaris and filum terminale than those of the spinal cord. Explanations for this observation include greater concentration of function per unit volume of spinal cord than cauda equina and an earlier presentation of cauda equina tumors, resulting in smaller tumors at presentation.[23]

Poor neurologic function in patients with primary spinal

cord tumors is attributable to the disease process and prolonged delay in diagnosis rather than to the effects of surgery or irradiation.[15,17,20,47] Unfortunately, far too many patients are diagnosed after their neurologic deficit has become severe, and there is little opportunity for recovery.

SURGICAL MANAGEMENT

Intradural-Extramedullary Tumors

The treatment of choice is complete surgical excision with preservation of neurologic function. Most of these tumors are meningiomas, neurolemmomas, and myxopapillary ependymomas, most of which can be completely excised. Even patients with severe neurologic deficit may improve dramatically after surgery. If complete excision could cause unacceptable neurologic deficit, the most complete excision possible is performed. Regrowth of nonexcised tumor is often slow, and symptoms may not recur for many years.

Intramedullary Tumors

Intramedullary tumors, 95% of which are astrocytomas and ependymomas, present a challenge. Complete surgical excision is the treatment of choice if it can be achieved without compromise of neurologic function. Complete excision of intramedullary tumors with preservation of neurologic function was not possible until 1940, when Greenwood[29] introduced the bipolar coagulation forceps. Radical total gross resection of intramedullary tumors has been facilitated by microsurgical techniques and, more recently, use of the Cavitron ultrasonic surgical aspirator (CUSA), intraoperative ultrasound imaging, the CO_2 laser, and the development of MRI.

With modern surgical techniques, ependymomas are relatively easy to excise completely.[28,31,51] However, astrocytomas are infiltrating tumors with ill-defined margins, often limiting surgical removal. Removal must begin from within the tumor and proceed until the interface between tumor and normal spinal cord is evident by changes in color and consistency.[18] The CUSA allows aspiration of tissue fragments within 1 mm of the vibrating tip, permitting dissection immediately adjacent to vital neural tissue. The CO_2 laser is used to vaporize remaining fragments with minimal risk of injury.[17]

Table 25-3 shows the incidence of complete surgical excision in various series. The greatest success with total excision is achieved in tumors of the cauda equina, followed by intramedullary ependymomas; astrocytomas are the most difficult to excise.

If complete excision of spinal cord tumors is feasible, no further treatment is necessary because the local recurrence rate is low and prognosis excellent.

If complete surgical excision is not feasible without sacrificing neurologic function, subtotal excision should be performed, followed by irradiation. Postoperative irradiation can sterilize remaining tumor cells after surgery and improve survival.

CHEMOTHERAPY

The use of chemotherapy for gliomas of the spinal cord is still in an experimental stage. Chemotherapy is reserved for patients with tumor progression despite surgery and radiation therapy.

STEROID THERAPY

Dexamethasone has proved invaluable in decreasing surgical complications. Steroid therapy is started before surgery and continued for approximately 1 week.[10] Steroids are continued for several weeks after the operation if neurologic function deteriorates.[17]

TABLE 25–3
Primary Spinal Cord Tumors: Incidence of Total Gross Excision

YEAR	INVESTIGATION	ASTROCYTOMA	EPENDYMOMA
1963	Greenwood[27]		9/9 (100)‡
1970	Barone[5]		16/27 (59)
1977	Mork[51]		15/51 (29)
1978	Fearnside[20]		13/30 (43)
1978	Malis[47]	4/21 (19)‡	18/19 (95)
1978	Schwade[61]	0/7 (0)	1/12 (8)
1979*	DeSousa[15]	0/11 (0)	2/7 (29)
1980	Kopelson[41]	0/10 (0)	2/12 (17)
1981	Guidetti[32]	2/53 (4)	36/48 (75)
1983	Stein[65]	5/10 (50)	
1985†	Cooper[11]	8/11 (73)	12/14 (86)
1985	Garcia[24]	1/17 (6)	0/15 (0)
1985†	Reimer[56]	2/32 (6)	
1986†	Epstein[17]	120/120 (100)	
1988	Herrmann[37]	2/3 (67)	3/4 (75)
Total		144/295 (49)	127/248 (51)

* *Pediatric series.*
† *Adult series.*
‡ *Data provided as number of patients with total gross excision/total patients in the series (% of patients with total excision).*

RADIATION THERAPY

Radiation therapy has been used as an adjunct to surgery in the treatment of intramedullary astrocytomas and ependymomas. For tumors that are completely excised, no irradiation is indicated. In our opinion, lesions that are subtotally excised should be irradiated, because radiation therapy maximizes the opportunity for local control and survival in these typically young adults and children in whom uncontrolled local tumor is the major cause of death. However, there are advocates of careful follow-up after surgery only, reserving radiation therapy until after the second operation for clinical recurrence.

Postoperative irradiation is beneficial in prolonging survival for patients with astrocytomas of the cerebrum, and it is reasonable to assume that the response to irradiation would be similar in the spinal cord.[24] Older reports in the literature, which do not convincingly show the benefit of irradiation, were published before development of modern radiation therapy techniques. The equipment was poor by today's standards, and the doses employed were unlikely to sterilize tumor. Unfortunately, even the newer reports on spinal canal tumors subjected to radiation therapy span several decades, resulting in a heterogeneously treated group of patients. However, control of tumor was found to be superior if adequate doses of radiation were delivered.[23]

We believe that the patient with a high-recurrence-rate tumor and microscopic residual disease should be considered for radiation therapy up to tolerance dose levels. This view is substantiated by the potential mortality and morbidity risks of neurosurgical procedures, the fact that the neurologic deficit at recurrence is never more advantageous than at the time of the first diagnosis, and that modern knowledge about irradiation techniques and tolerance allows us to predict better the outcome of a treatment regimen.

RADIATION THERAPY TECHNIQUES

Primary tumors of the spinal canal are usually treated through a direct posterior field, although lesions of the cauda equina may be more appropriately treated by opposed anteroposterior and posteroanterior portals because of the lumbar lordosis and location of the vertebral bodies near the middle of the trunk.

The width of the fields for treatment typically is 7 cm or 8 cm. The superior and inferior borders should include at least two vertebral bodies in either direction from the gross tumor determined by myelogram, CT scan, and MRI scan to ensure an adequate margin. The field width should encompass the intervertebral foramina if tumor extension is suspected. The vertebral bodies may be partially spared from irradiation by using two oblique-wedged posterior-field half-beam arcs or parallel opposed lateral fields. These techniques may be considered as part of the treatment regimen if short segments are irradiated in children in an attempt to spare the developing epiphyseal plates.

For small treated segments of the spinal cord, the depth of the cord beneath the skin surface can be determined from CT or MRI scans, and this depth used for the dose prescription. The depth can also be determined by obtaining a lateral radiograph of the spine on the simulator, using a wire on the skin surface and then calculating the spinal cord depth by employing the magnification factor used for the film (Fig. 25-7).

If large segments of the spinal cord are irradiated, it is necessary to compute the spinal cord dose at multiple points because of the variation in curvature and depth of spinal cord and the different source-to-skin distances above and below the central axis of the beam. A transverse treatment plan and a sagittal treatment plan using the CT or MRI scan should be performed (Fig. 25-8). A sagittal treatment plan can be discerned from a lateral radiograph of the spine with the midline skin wired and documentation of the magnification factor of the film.

Intramedullary ependymomas and astrocytomas should be irradiated to a total dose of 5000 cGy, given in 180-cGy daily fractions. If more than half of the spinal cord is irradiated, the total tumor dose should probably not exceed 4500 cGy, but small segments may safely tolerate 5400 cGy. Long, narrow fields may give increased doses at the short borders (*i.e.*, dog-ear effect), especially at low megavoltage energies. Ependymomas of the cauda equina should be irradiated to between 4500 cGy and 5000 cGy in 180-cGy fractions, with field widths adapted to the intervertebral foramina and meningeal sleeves. In children,

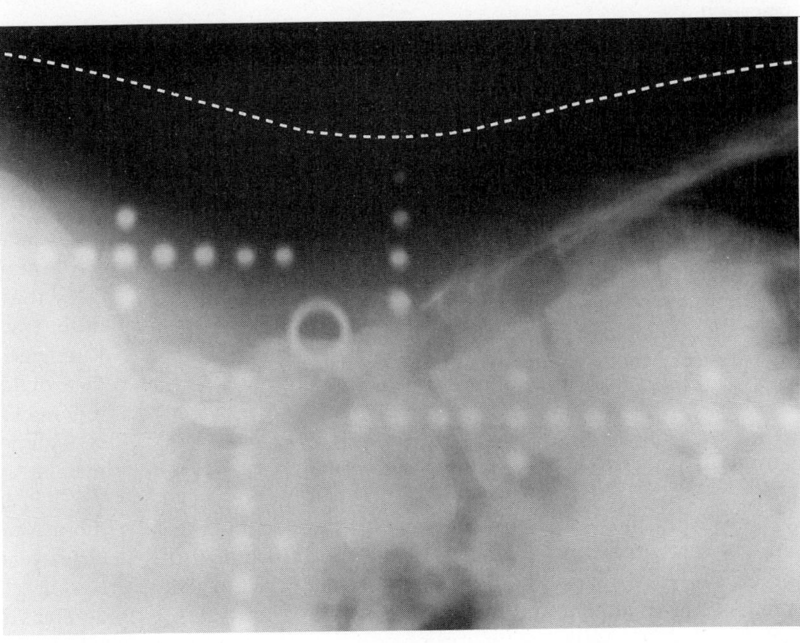

FIGURE 25–7. Lateral simulation film of the lumbar spine with a wire on the skin surface to determine the depth of the spinal cord.

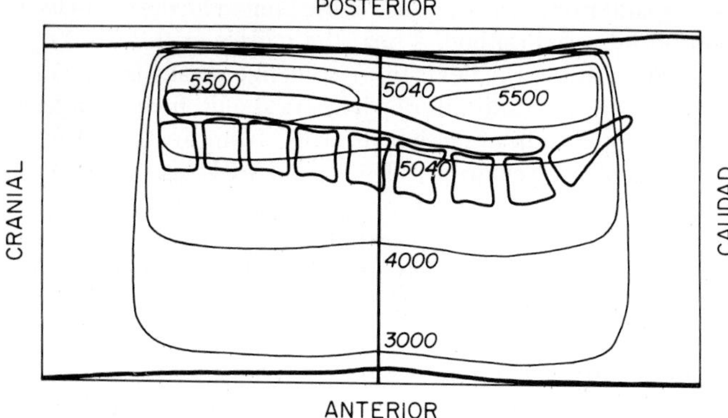

FIGURE 25–8. Sagittal computerized treatment plan obtained from an MR scan of the lower thoracic and lumbar spine. The 5040 cGy isodose line completely encompasses the spinal cord. The optimized treatment was obtained by combining 6-MV photons (10 fractions, 180 cGy/fraction) and 18-MV photons (18 fractions, 180 cGy/fraction).

the dose to the spinal cord should be limited to between 4000 cGy and 4500 cGy in 150-cGy to 160-cGy daily fractions on the assumption that the developing cord has a lower tolerance to irradiation.

The treatment plan should reflect a homogeneous dose distribution. For small lesions of the cervical spinal cord, opposed lateral fields may be employed, especially in the patient with a long neck in whom the shoulders can be retracted downward. With lateral fields, use of 4-MV to 6-MV photons achieves a homogeneous dose distribution. However, lesions involving the thoracic and lumbar spine often require a combination of low-energy (4–6 MV) and high-energy (18–25 MV) photons to achieve a homogeneous dose distribution (Fig. 25-8). In children, because the spinal cord is situated more superficially, a combination of electrons and low-energy photons may be employed.

RESULTS OF RADIATION THERAPY

The results of treatment depend on the neurologic function of the patient, the type of tumor and its differentiation, the anatomic compartment occupied by the tumor, and the extent of resection.

A summary of the results of therapy for primary tumors of the spinal canal are equivocal for many reasons. The tumors are rare, and the reports often span many decades, treatment philosophies, and diagnostic and therapeutic modalities. Results from heterogeneous radiation therapy techniques are almost impossible to compare. Because of the rarity of these tumors, series include children and adults, and studies rarely correlate treatment with histologic types. Moreover, there has been a lack of information about the extent of surgical excision in treating the various types of spinal cord tumors. Pathologic review has been almost nonexistent, and there has been inadequate follow-up because of the indolent nature of many primary spinal canal tumors.

Survival

Patients with spinal canal tumors generally have better 5-year and 10-year survival rates than patients with intracranial tumors. The exception is malignant astrocytoma, which usually recurs after treatment and causes death within a few years.[46] With time and improved therapeutic techniques, survival figures appear to have improved for most of these tumors.[7,23,26,41,51,69]

Most ependymoma patients are now cured if treated appropriately; survival figures range from 85% to 100%.[46,64,69] Intramedullary tumors have a lower survival rate than the lumbosacral type.[23,26,51] However the tumors may recur after many years, and a few cases have been reported to metastasize.[23,46,69]

Astrocytoma patients generally have intermediate survival periods, with 10-year survival rates as low as 50%.[23,26,40,46] Many of these patients may live with mild to severe neurologic deficits.[23]

Meningiomas, neurolemmomas, vascular malformations, lipomas, hemangiomas, oligodendrogliomas, teratomas, and dermoids are so rare that valid survival figures are difficult to obtain.

Intradural-Extramedullary Tumors

The prognosis is excellent for most patients with intradural-extramedullary tumors, and the tumors rarely recur after total excision. If only subtotal excision was performed, postoperative irradiation has been administered. However, good data regarding the efficacy of radiation therapy are rare. Recent data attest to the benefits of radiation therapy for ependymomas.[44,46,64,69]

Intramedullary Tumors

Control of the primary tumor and survival are best for cauda equina ependymomas, intermediate for intramedullary ependymomas, and worst for astrocytomas.[23]

Regardless of the histology, most authors agree that if complete surgical excision of a primary spinal cord tumor is feasible, no further treatment is necessary.[20,27,28,31,47,69] With total removal, local recurrence rates are low, and survival is excellent. Compared with ependymomas, a smaller proportion of astrocytomas can be completely removed.[17,65]

Postoperative irradiation is beneficial in patients with biopsy and subtotally excised primary tumors of the spinal cord.[5,20,51,61,69]

SEQUELAE OF RADIATION THERAPY

Tolerance

Excessive radiation to the spinal cord may produce demyelination and necrosis.[68] A clinically acceptable tolerance dose level carries less than a 5% risk of unacceptable sequelae. Higher doses increase the risk disproportionately.

Animal experiments and empirical patient data have indicated that the tolerance depends on the region irradiated, total dose, fraction size, and volume irradiated.[1,9,16,39,43,53,58,70] A widely accepted regimen for treating 10 cm of cord is a total dose of 4500 cGy given in 180-cGy to 200-cGy fractions for 4.5 to 5 weeks.[6,9,53] For the cervical cord, the total dose may be 500 cGy higher with the same fractionation, because the tolerance may be somewhat greater.[66]

The latency period for radiation myelopathy ranges from 6 months to at least 3 years.[43] Clinically, radiation myelopathy is characterized by progressive weakness or paralysis with variable sensory changes and sometimes the later development of bowel and bladder dysfunction. These permanent signs are caused by presumed vascular damage and damage to oligodendrocytes, resulting in white matter necrosis and demyelination.

Transient myelitis is a rare syndrome (*i.e.*, Lhermitte's syndrome) that appears about 6 weeks after treatment and may last up to 5 months.[8,21,35,38]

Late Effects in Children

Children diagnosed and treated for primary tumors of the spinal canal present special prognostic concerns and apprehensions about the increased potential for treatment-induced morbidity. The CNS is thought to complete its development in humans between 20 and 25 years of age, and the spinal cord in children and adolescents may have a lower tolerance to irradiation; the recommended total tumor doses range from 4000 cGy to 4500 cGy administered in 150-cGy to 160-cGy daily fractions.

Irradiation of the spine in a child may produce a spinal deformity (*i.e.*, scoliosis or kyphosis) because of retardation of bone growth from damage to epiphyseal plates of the vertebral bodies and soft tissue fibrosis and contracture.[48] Children are at risk for second malignancies within the radiation field due to the susceptibility of developing cells to radiation.[55] The risk is in the realm of 1%.

Children are at greater risk than adults of developing complications after surgery. Extensive laminectomy can produce severe kyphosis and scoliosis, which are typically accentuated during the adolescent growth spurt. Reconstructive procedures, such as Harrington rod or Cotrel-Dubousset system placement, may be necessary to prevent significant damage, and children must be followed very closely by the neurosurgeon and by a pediatric orthopedist to ensure early treatment of skeletal abnormalities.[17] Treatment with body braces during the patient's waking hours for a few years after surgery may prevent spinal growth problems.[18]

REFERENCES

1. Abbatucci JS, Delozier T, Quint R, et al: Radiation myelopathy of the cervical spinal cord: Time, dose and volume factors. Int J Radiat Oncol Biol Phys 4:239, 1978
2. Ammerman BJ, Henry JM, DeGirolami U, et al: Intradural lipomas of the spinal cord: A clinicopathological correlation. J Neurosurg 44:331, 1976
3. Baleriaux D: Spinal cord tumors. In Jeanmart L (ed): Tumors, p 39. Berlin, Springer-Verlag, 1986
4. Bannister R: Disorders of the spinal cord. In Brain's Clinical Neurology, 6th ed, p 358. London, Oxford University, 1985
5. Barone BM, Elvidge AR: Ependymomas: A clinical survey. J Neurosurg 33:428, 1970
6. Bleehen NM: The central nervous system: In Bleehen NM, Glatstein E, Haybittle JL (eds): Radiation Therapy Planning, pp 607–615. New York, Marcel Dekker, 1983
7. Bouchard J: Central nervous system. In Fletcher GH (ed): Textbook of Radiotherapy, 3rd ed, pp 444–498. Philadelphia, Lea & Febiger, 1980
8. Castaigne P, Cambier J, Escourolle R: Post-radiotherapy myelopathies during Hodgkin's disease. Rev Neurol (Paris) 123:369, 1970
9. Chang CH, Hilal SK: Brain tumor localization: Determination of extent and volume for radiation treatment. In Levitt SH, Tapley ND (eds): Technological Basis of Radiation Therapy, pp 172–192. Philadelphia, Lea & Febiger, 1984
10. Connolly ES: Spinal cord tumors in adults. In Youman JR (ed): Neurological Surgery, 2nd ed, p 3196. Philadelphia, WB Saunders, 1982
11. Cooper PR, Epstein F: Radical resection of intramedullary spinal cord tumors in adults: Recent experience in 29 patients. J Neurosurg 63:492, 1985
12. Cosgrove GR, Bertrand G, Fontaine S, et al: Cavernous angiomas of the spinal cord. J Neurosurg 68:31, 1988
13. D'Angio GJ, Fuller LGA, Kim TW, et al: Intrathecal radiogold for medulloblastoma and ependymoblastoma: Survival rate and complications. In Hilaris BS (ed): Afterloading, 20 Years of Experience, 1955–1975, p 83. New York, Memorial Sloan-Kettering Cancer Center, 1975
14. deDivitiis E, Cerillo A, Carlomagno S: Subpial spinal lipomas. Neurochirurgia (Stuttg) 25:14, 1982
15. DeSousa AL, Kalsbeck JE, Mealey J Jr, et al: Intraspinal tumors in children. J Neurosurg 51:437, 1979
16. Dynes JB, Smedel MI: Radiation myelitis. AJR 83:78, 1960
17. Epstein F: Spinal cord astrocytomas of childhood. Adv Tech Stand Neurosurg 13:135, 1986
18. Epstein F, Epstein N: Surgical treatment of spinal cord astrocytomas of childhood. J Neurosurg 57:685, 1982
19. Farwell JR, Dohrmann GJ: Intraspinal neoplasms in children. Paraplegia 15:262, 1977
20. Fearnside MR, Adams CBT: Tumours of the cauda equina. J Neurol Neurosurg Psychiatry 41:24, 1978
21. Fishman RA: Reactions to radiation therapy. N Engl J Med 293;669, 1975
22. Gado M, Sartor K, Hodges F III: The spine. In Lee JK, Sagel SS, Stanley RJ (eds): Computed Body Tomography, 2nd ed, p 991. New York, Raven Press, 1989
23. Garcia DM: Primary spinal cord tumors treated with surgery and postoperative irradiation. Int J Radiat Oncol Biol Phys 11:1933, 1985
24. Garcia DM, Fulling KH, Marks JE: The value of radiation therapy in addition to surgery for astrocytomas of the adult cerebrum. Cancer 59:919, 1985
25. Giuffre R, DiLorenzo N, Fortuna A: Primary spinal tumors in infancy and childhood. Zentralbl Neurochir 42:87, 1981
26. Glanzmann C: Radiation therapy in the treatment of intraspinal gliomas. Strahlenther Onkol 156:616, 1980
27. Greenwood J Jr: Intramedullary tumors of the spinal cord: A follow-up study after total surgical removal. J Neurosurg 20:665, 1963
28. Greenwood J: Surgical removal of intramedullary tumors. J Neurosurg 26:276, 1967
29. Greenwood J Jr: Spinal cord tumors. In Youman JR (ed): Neurological Surgery, 2nd ed, p 1514. Philadelphia, WB Saunders, 1982
30. Gudmundsson KR: A survey of tumours of the central nervous system in Iceland during the 10-year period 1954–1963. Acta Neurol Scand 46:538, 1970
31. Guidetti B: Intramedullary tumours of the spinal cord. Acta Neurochir (Wien) 17:7, 1967
32. Guidetti B, Mercuri S, Vagnozzi R: Long-term results of the surgical treatment of 129 intramedullary spinal gliomas. J Neurosurg 54:323, 1981
33. Hely M, Fryer J, Selby G: Intramedullary spinal cord glioma with intracranial seeding. J Neurol Neurosurg Psychiatry 48:302, 1985
34. Hendrick EB: Spinal cord tumors in children. In Youman JR (ed): Neurological Surgery, 2nd ed, p 3215. Philadelphia, WB Saunders, 1982
35. Henson RA, Urich H: Involvement of the vertebral column and the spinal cord. In Cancer and the Nervous System, pp 120–154. Oxford, Blackwell, 1982
36. Heppner F, Ascher P, Holzer P, et al: CO_2 laser surgery of intramedullary spinal cord tumors. Lasers Surg Med 7:180, 1987
37. Herrmann HD, Neuss M, Winkler D: Intramedullary spinal cord tumors resected with CO_2 laser microsurgical technique: Recent experience in fifteen patients. Neurosurgery 22:518, 1988
38. Jones A: Transient radiation myelopathy (with reference to Lhermitte's sign of electrical paraesthesia). Br J Radiol 37:727, 1964
39. Kagan AR, Wollin M, Gilbert HA, et al: Comparison of the tolerance of brain and spinal cord to injury by radiation. In

Gilbert HA, Kagan AR (eds): Radiation Damage to the Nervous System, pp 183–190. New York, Raven, 1980

40. Karlsson UL, Ravalese J, Brady LW: Cervical cord astrocytoma: Radiation therapy results. (unpublished data)
41. Kopelson G, Linggood RM, Kleinman GM, et al: Management of intramedullary spinal cord tumors. Radiology 135:473, 1980
42. Kurland LT: The frequency of intracranial and intraspinal neoplasms in the resident population of Rochester, Minnesota. J Neurosurg 15:627, 1958
43. Lambert P: Radiation myelopathy of the thoracic spinal cord in long term survivors treated with radical radiotherapy using conventional fractionation. Cancer 41:1751, 1978
44. Lemberger A, Stein M, Dorin J, et al: Sacrococcygeal extradural ependymoma. Cancer 64:1156, 1989
45. Levy W, Bay J, Dohn D: Spinal cord meningioma. J Neurosurg 57:804, 1982
46. Lindstadt DE, Wara W, Leibel S, et al: Postoperative radiotherapy of primary spinal cord tumors. Int J Radiat Oncol Biol Phys 16:1397, 1989
47. Malis LI: Intramedullary spinal cord tumors. Clin Neurosurg 25:512, 1978
48. Mayfield JK: Postradiation spinal deformity. Orthop Clin North Am 10:829, 1979
49. McCunniff AJ, Liang MJ: Radiation tolerance of the cervical spinal cord. Int J Radiat Oncol Biol Phys 16:675, 1989
50. McLone D, Naidich T: Laser resection of fifty spinal lipomas. Neurosurgery 18:611, 1986
51. Mork SJ, Loken AC: Ependymoma: A follow-up study of 101 cases. Cancer 40:907, 1977
52. Onofrio BM: Intradural extramedullary spinal cord tumors. Clin Neuorsurg 25:540, 1978
53. Phillips TL, Buschke F: Radiation tolerance of the thoracic spinal cord. AJR 105:659, 1969
54. Platt JF, Rubin JM, Chandler WF, et al: Intraoperative spinal sonography in the evaluation of intramedullary tumors. J Ultrasound Med 7:317, 1988
55. Potish RA, Dener LP, Haselow RE, et al: The incidence of second neoplasms following megavoltage radiation for pediatric tumors. Cancer 56:1534, 1985
56. Reimer R, Onofrio B: Astrocytomas of the spinal cord in children and adolescents. J Neurosurg 63:669, 1985
57. Rubin JM, Chandler WF: The use of ultrasound during spinal cord surgery. World J Surg 11:570, 1987
58. Rubin P, Cooper R, Phillips TL: Radiation oncology. In Rubin P, Cooper R, Phillips TL (ed): Radiation Biology and Radiation Pathology Syllabus. Chicago, American College of Radiology, 1975
59. Russell DC, Rubenstein LJ (eds): Pathology of tumors of the nervous system, 4th ed. Baltimore, Williams & Wilkins, 1977
60. Sandt G, Kaiser MC, Capesius P: Spinal neurinomas. In Jeanmart L (ed): Tumors, p 56. Berlin, Springer-Verlag, 1986
61. Schwade J, Wara W, Sheline G, et al: Management of primary spinal cord tumors. Int J Radiat Oncol Biol Phys 4:389, 1978
62. Silverberg E, Lubera J: Cancer statistics, 1989. CA 39:3, 1989
63. Simeone FA, Lawner PM: Intraspinal neoplasms. In Rothman, Simeone FA (eds): The Spine, 2nd ed, vol II, p 1041. Philadelphia, WB Saunders, 1982
64. Sonneland PRL, Sheithauer BS, Onofrio BM: Myxopapillary ependymoma: A clinicopathological and immunocytochemical study of 77 cases. Cancer 56:883, 1985
65. Stein BM: Intramedullary spinal cord tumors. Clin Neurosurg 30:717, 1983
66. Vaeth J: Radiation-induced myelitis. In Buschke F (ed): Progress in Radiation Therapy. New York, Grune & Stratton, 1965
67. Vakili H (ed): Spinal Cord. New York, Intercontinental Medical Book Corp, 1967
68. Van der Kugel AJ: Mechanisms of late radiation injury in the spinal cord. In Meyn RE, Withers HR (eds): Radiation Biology in Cancer Research, pp 461–470. New York, Raven, 1980
69. Wen BC, Hussey DH, Hitchon PW, et al: The role of radiation therapy in the management of ependymomas of the spinal cord. Int J Radiat Oncol Biol Phys 20:781–786, 1991
70. Wollin M, Kagan AR: Modification of biological dose to normal tissue by daily fractionation. Acta Radiol 15:481, 1976
71. Woltman HW: Tumors of spinal cord and gliomas of intradural portion of filum terminalis. Arch N Psychiatr 65:378, 1951
72. Wood EH, Berne AS, Taveras JM: The value of radiation therapy in the management of intrinsic tumors of the spinal cord. Radiology 63:11, 1954

26

Eye

Arnold M. Markoe
Luther W. Brady
Ulf L. Karlsson
Jerry A. Shields
James J. Augsburger

Primary tumors of the globe and ocular adnexae are uncommon, but innovative therapeutic techniques and improved understanding of ocular anatomy are being applied by radiation oncologists to advance the role of irradiation in managing tumors of the eye.

ANATOMY

The ocular adnexae consist of structures such as the eyelids, cilia, lacrimal glands, drainage apparatus, and conjunctiva. The eyeball, or globe (Fig. 26-1), is composed of three tunicae. The outer coat consists of the clear cornea and the opaque sclera. The six ocular muscles controlling eye movement insert upon the sclera. The uvea, or middle coat, is formed by the choroid, ciliary body, and iris. The inner layer, consisting of the retina and its analogues, is the sensory layer. This coat extends from the ora serrata retinae anteriorly to the optic nerve posteriorly. The vascular supply to the posterior half of the retina derives from the central retinal artery that enters the globe through the optic nerve. The anterior half of the retina derives its blood supply from the ciliary system. The lens is suspended from the ciliary body and is posterior to the iris. The orbit is composed of seven bones (Fig. 26-2). The bony orbit encloses the ocular globe, vessels, nerves, orbital fat, and ocular muscles.

BENIGN OCULAR DISEASES

There are a variety of diseases that are categorized as benign or malignant ophthalmic tumors (Table 26-1).[51] Radiation therapy of nonmalignant ocular disease is, for the most part, of historic interest, although it may still be employed to treat certain benign ocular conditions.

Pterygium

The most common benign ocular condition for which irradiation is beneficial is the pterygium. Although the primary therapy for this condition is surgical removal of the growth, the recurrence rate is high, ranging up to 67%.[41] Recurrence rates are higher in females than in males and higher in patients under age 40. Postoperative irradiation using a $^{90}Sr/^{90}Y$ β-emitting contact applicator significantly reduces recurrence rates to 20% or less.[1,41,61,66,88] Postexcision β-irradiation doses and application schemes reported in the literature vary widely.[6,13,35,53,74-79,81,155] Our protocol calls for weekly application of 1000 R surface dose for 3 to 5 weeks, depending on the size of the surgical defect. The bare sclera surgical excision technique appears to be associated with a higher risk for recurrence without adjuvant irradiation than the newer lamellar keratoplasty technique after excision.[22,77]

Capillary Hemangioma

Although capillary hemangiomas usually occur elsewhere in the body, they present unique problems when they occur on the eyelids. The natural history of the lesion is a spontaneous regression over 3 to 4 years. A conservative approach of observation, therefore, is the treatment of choice.[97] Occasionally, however, the lesion may be large enough to obstruct the child's vision, and amblyopia may occur. The lid may ulcerate because of tumor compression of the vascular supply. Intervention is then accomplished by the cautious use of steroids or low-energy x-ray or electron-beam therapy, delivering 500 cGy to 750 cGy in two or three fractions.[42,67] Radiation therapy is usually reserved until after other treatment methods fail.

Orbital Pseudolymphoma

Benign primary lymphoreticular tumors, if localized to the orbit, have a good prognosis with a 5-year survival rate of 70%.[55] Approximately 20% to 25% of cases of apparent pseudolymphoma may convert to malignant lymphoma.[105,121] However, it is often difficult to differentiate between the pseudolymphoma and true lymphoma by biopsy specimens.[71]

Steroids can be effective, but radiation therapy appears to

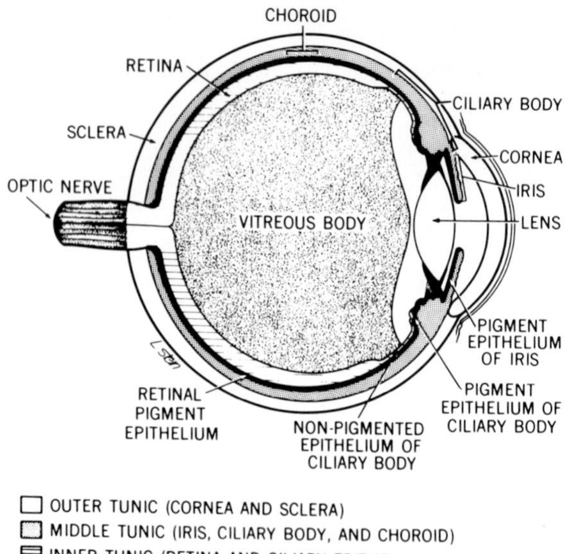

FIGURE 26–1. Various ocular interrelationships.

be more effective and can control cases that have been refractory to steroids.[9] In our experience, surgical excision of localized pseudolymphomas has been associated with the least chance of control. Radiation therapy may consist of a single exposure of 800 cGy directed through an anterior portal.[55,61,62] However, we elect to treat with 2000 cGy to 2500 cGy given in ten to 14 fractions, which can cause the condition to dramatically resolve.[7,9,75] Anterior, lateral, or oblique portals similar to those employed in the therapy of malignant lymphoma of the orbit, ^{60}Co, 4-MV to 6-MV photons, or 15-MeV to 16-MeV electron beams are used for treatment of these lesions. Orbital pseudolymphoma associated with a histologic picture of angiitis is refractory to this therapy, but inflammatory lymphocytic infiltration responds dramatically.[7]

Graves' Ophthalmopathy

In some patients with hyperthyroidism (thyrotoxicosis), exophthalmos may occur. The primary tissues involved are the intraocular muscles. Indications for therapy include corneal exposure secondary to proptosis and optic nerve compression, which may cause permanent visual loss. The diagnosis is aided by computed tomography (CT), which may demonstrate thickened muscles. Steroid therapy is the first-line treatment, but radiation therapy can be beneficial if steroids fail. Treatment can be given by a single lateral portal excluding the ipsilateral lens. A dose of 1500 cGy to 2000 cGy in ten fractions is usually sufficient to alleviate symptoms.[11,14,44,75,123,132] Electrons, usually 12 MeV to 15 MeV, are ideal for the treatment of these patients. In a series of 35 patients with thyroid ophthalmopathy, Sandler and associates[132] reported that 71% of patients receiving 2000 cGy in 200-cGy fractions required no further steroid therapy or surgical decompression. Of the failures, seven (33%) of 21 patients had failed prior steroid therapy; two (28%) of the seven patients had failed prior surgical decompression; and only one (14%) of the seven patients had no prior treatment. The main prognostic factor for failure was an interval of less than 6 months between eye disease and radiation therapy. In a series of over 300 patients, Peterson and colleagues[115] showed that 2000 cGy in ten fractions gave identical results to 3000 cGy in 15 fractions and that as many as 76% of treated patients responded positively to treatment. Corneal involvement and visual loss were more likely to improve after radiation therapy than proptosis or ocular muscle impairment.

OCULAR MALIGNANCIES

Basal and Squamous Cell Carcinomas

In the treatment of basal cell and squamous cell carcinomas of the eyelids, radiation therapy can achieve an overall 90% to 95% cure rate. After the diagnosis is confirmed by biopsy, 4500 cGy to 6000 cGy (depending on histology and size of the tumor) can be delivered by photon or electron-beam techniques. The globe may be protected by an internal eye shield. Radiation therapy may be able to provide acceptable cosmesis better than surgery while providing similar cure rates.

Meibomian Gland Carcinoma

Meibomian gland (sebaceous) carcinomas are uncommon and have a mortality rate of 30%.[26] These tumors may be multicentric, which may lead to local recurrences. Radiation therapy may be used for the treatment of these tumors in selected cases, particularly if surgery would not provide acceptable cosmesis or the disease recurs after surgery. In our experience, high doses of irradiation (6000–6500 cGy in 6–7 weeks) are required. Recently, Pardo and others[114] reported a series of 30 patients with this tumor, ten of whom received radiation therapy. Four were treated with curative intent, and the remaining six were treated postoperatively for parotid metastases after initial surgery. Doses ranged from 4500 cGy to 6300 cGy, but the irradiation schema varied from 4500 cGy in four fractions over 5 days to 6000 cGy delivered in 200-cGy fractions over 51 days. The four patients treated definitively all are free of disease at 36 to 117 months, and the patients treated adjuvantly after surgery for metastatic disease are all free of disease at 24 to 84 months.

Uveal Tumors

Metastatic Carcinoma of the Posterior Uvea

Tumor metastases to the uvea were once considered rare events.[57,147] However, it is now recognized that metastatic carcinoma is probably the most common malignant disease involving the eye.[48] Metastatic uveal lesions arise as precocious metastases in approximately 15% of cases, as synchronous metastases in approximately 4% of cases, and as metachronous metastases in most of the remaining cases, except in 8% for which the appropriate parameters cannot be established.[20] The most common primary sites for uveal metastases are the lung in males and the breast in females.[20,153] In an autopsy series of breast cancer patients, a third of the cases included uveal metastases.[15] Uveal metastases are most often unifocal but may be multifocal within the eye or may be bilateral.[144]

The aim of therapy is to return visual function to the patient, although survival time may be limited to an average of 3 to 6 months after the diagnosis of uveal metastases. Observation for small lesions may be appropriate if the patient is on an effective regimen of systemic management, which can stabilize or regress metastatic intraocular tumors.

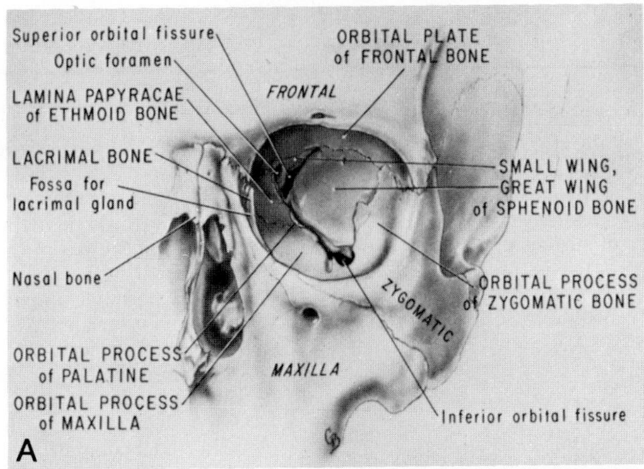

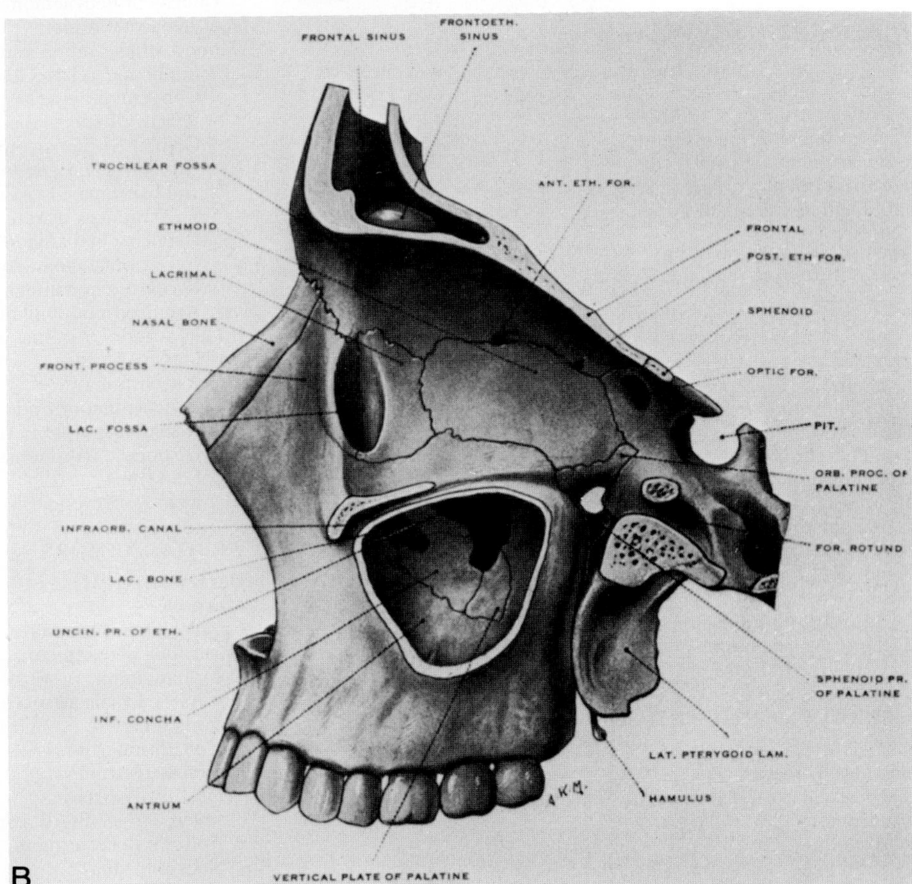

FIGURE 26–2. (**A**) Orbital cavity: boundaries, sutures, and fissures of left side, seen from the front. The walls of the orbital cavity go over and into one another with rounded angles. It is convenient to regard the space as having four walls. The medial wall is composed of the lacrimal bone, the lamina papyracea of the ethmoid bone, and the lateral surface of the body of the sphenoid bone. The lateral wall is composed of the orbital surface of the zygomatic bone, the orbital surface of the greater wing of the sphenoid bone, and the medial surface of the zygomatic process of the frontal bone. The inferior wall consists of the orbital surface of the body of the maxilla, the orbital surface of the zygomatic bone, and the orbital process of the palatine. The superior wall is formed by the orbital part of the frontal bone and the lesser wing of the sphenoid bone. (Anson B, McVay CB: Surgical Anatomy, vol 1, p 57. Philadelphia, WB Saunders, 1971) (**B**) Roof and medial wall of the orbit. The roof of the orbit is formed by the orbital process of the frontal bone and the sphenoid. The medial or inner wall is composed of the frontal process of the maxilla, the lacrimal bone, and the lamina papyracea of the ethmoid bone. (Last RJ: Wolff's Anatomy of the Eye and Orbit. London, HR Lewis, 1968)

If the patient has visual symptoms, we recommend prompt initiation of radiation therapy. Almost 90% of patients have positive, objective responses to their therapy.[20] For patients with uveal metastases and active systemic disease, we palliate by delivering 3000 cGy to 3500 cGy tumor dose over 3 weeks to the entire ocular structure on the affected side. In the absence of active systemic disease, in the case of precocious metastases and in patients with breast or colon cancer, in whom the potential for long-term survival is greater, a more aggressive approach is taken. We treat the affected globe to 4500 cGy to 5000 cGy over 4.5 to 5.5 weeks.

Lateral portals are usually employed. Shielding of the lens and cornea may be attempted, but it may produce underdosing of anteriorly located metastases. Electrons in the range of 15 MeV to 18 MeV may be employed, but equally satisfactory results may be obtained with ^{60}Co or 4-MV to 6-MV photons. In these cases, lateral fields should be tilted posteriorly 5 to 10 degrees, to avoid irradiating the contralateral lens and cornea.

Malignant Melanoma of the Posterior Uvea

Of the approximately 1800 new cases of primary malignant tumors of the eye in 1989, almost 75% were malignant melanoma.[20] The ophthalmologic community has long been familiar with the problems of uveal melanomas, but there remains considerable controversy about the optimal management of this disease. Most data have come from small series. Even the larger series have been performed in a nonprospective or nonrandomized fashion, relying on statistical matching of populations for evaluations and conclusions.

TABLE 26–1
Categories of Ophthalmic Tumors

EYELIDS AND LACRIMAL DRAINAGE SYSTEMS

Benign tumors of the surface epithelium of eyelids
- Papilloma
- Keratoacanthoma
- Seborrheic keratosis

Premalignant and malignant tumors of surface epithelium of eyelids
- Senile (actinic) keratosis
- Basal cell epithelioma
- Nevoid basal cell carcinoma syndrome
- Squamous cell carcinoma

Glandular and adnexal tumors of eyelids
- Sebaceous gland carcinoma
- Sweat gland and hair follicle tumors

Melanocytic tumors of eyelids
- Nevus
- Malignant melanoma
- Congenital melanocytosis

Neurogenic tumors of eyelids
- Neurofibroma
- Neurilemoma

Vascular tumors of eyelids
- Capillary hemangiomas
- Port-wine stain

Xanthomatous tumors of eyelids
- Xanthelasma
- Metastatic tumors to eyelids
- Tumors of lacrimal drainage system

CONJUNCTIVA

Congenital tumors
- Dermoid

Benign tumors of surface epithelium
- Papilloma
- Benign hereditary intraepithelial dyskeratosis

Premalignant/malignant lesions of surface epithelium
- Dysplasia
- Carcinoma *in situ*
- Invasive squamous cell carcinoma

Melanocytic tumors
- Nevus
- Benign acquired melanomas
- Malignant melanoma

Other conjunctival tumors

SYSTEMIC HAMARTOMATOSES

Tuberous sclerosis
Neurofibromatosis
Retinocerebellar capillary hemangiomatosis (von Hippel-Lindau syndrome)
Encephalofacial cavernous hemangiomatosis (Sturge-Weber syndrome)
Racemose hemangiomatosis (Wyburn-Mason syndrome)
Retinal cavernous hemangiomatosis with cutaneous and CNS involvement

INTRAOCULAR TUMORS

Melanocytic tumors of the iris
- Nevus
- Malignant melanoma
- Tumors of iris pigment epithelium

Melanocytic tumors of the posterior uvea
- Choroidal nevus
- Ciliary body melanoma
- Choroidal melanoma

Other uveal tumors
- Circumscribed choroidal hemangioma
- Metastatic carcinoma
- Medulloepithelioma (diktyoma)
- Choroidal osteoma
- Choroidal neurilemoma
- Other uveal tumors

Tumors of the retina and optic disc
- Tumors and related lesions of the retinal pigmented epithelium
  - Congenital hypertrophy
  - Reactive hyperplasia
  - Combined hamartoma
  - Adenoma and adenocarcinoma
- Retinoblastoma
- Vacular tumors of retina and optic disc
  - Capillary hemangioma
  - Cavernous hemangioma
  - Racemose hemangioma
  - Acquired nonfamilial retinal hemangioma
- Glial tumors of retina and optic disc
  - Massive gliosis
  - Astrocytoma
- Melanocytoma of optic nerve
- Intraocular lymphoid tumors and leukemias
  - Histiocytic lymphoma (reticulum cell sarcoma)
  - Leukemias
  - Reactive lymphoid hyperplasia of uvea

ORBITAL TUMORS

Dermoid cyst
Mucocele
Capillary hemangioma
Cavernous hemangioma
Lymphangioma
Juvenile pilocytic astrocytoma
Meningioma
Fibrous histiocytoma
Fibro-osseus tumors
- Fibrous dysplasia
- Juvenile ossifying fibroma

Peripheral nerve tumors
- Neurofibroma
- Neurilemoma

Rhabdomyosarcoma
Lymphoid tumors
Leukemia
Metastatic tumors to orbit
Lacrimal gland tumors

The diagnosis of malignant uveal melanoma has been made more precise with a variety of techniques, reducing the risk of an error that can prompt unnecessary enucleation.[143] Indirect ophthalmoscopy is now combined with fluorescent angiography and ultrasonography in a standard assessment battery. The use of CT and magnetic resonance imaging studies have also influenced assessment of uveal melanomas.

Melanomas of the anterior uvea are usually detected earlier than those located posteriorly and may be surgically removed by iridectomy or iridocyclectomy.[158,159] However, lesions of the posterior uvea are not readily accessible to a biopsy, although fine-needle aspiration biopsy is possible if the diagnosis is in doubt, and the clinical diagnosis may occasionally be difficult. If there remains a degree of uncertainty about the diagnosis or if the lesion is small and relatively flat, a conservative approach of careful, sequential observation may be indicated.

Posterior uveal melanoma has traditionally been treated by enucleation of the affected eyeball. Recently the concept of enucleation has been questioned.[161] In assessing the outcome of enucleation by actuarial survival tables, Zimmerman and associates[161] suggested that the prognosis after enucleation may be worse than for an untreated patient. Some authors have postulated that tumor seeding is effected by the manipulation of the globe during the surgical procedure, and they advocate a "no-touch" approach to enucleation.[56] Another suggestion is that radical reduction of tumor burden by enucleation alters the immune surveillance capacity, and extant micrometastases begin to grow.[47] As stated by Curtin and Cavender,[36] "The overall death rate of 50% does little to inspire confidence in our present management of the disease." Other treatment modalities, such as photocoagulation, cryotherapy, diathermy, and local resection, have been evaluated.[38, 54, 84, 91, 101, 116, 134, 151, 156]

Radiation therapy has been widely employed in the treatment of choroidal melanoma. A variety of approaches have been followed.[112] External-beam techniques use ^{60}Co, most recently with the γ-knife technique, and therapy with the proton beam or the helium ion beam.[28, 29, 34, 40, 58, 60, 73, 85, 108, 109, 120, 133, 138] Brachytherapeutic techniques have employed a variety of sources as ophthalmic applicators, including ^{60}Co, ^{106}Ru/^{106}Rh, radon seeds, radon gas, ^{125}I, ^{198}Au seeds, and ^{182}Ta.[10, 18, 19, 31, 39, 86, 87, 89, 90, 92, 94, 96, 107, 113, 149, 150, 152]

Recently, a uniform staging system (Table 26-2) was introduced for clinical and pathologic staging of uveal melanomas.[3] However, it is not in general use in this country. The problems associated with nonrandomzied studies are being addressed by a multi-institutional national Cooperative Ocular Melanoma Study, which is comparing enucleation with radioiodine plaque brachytherapy in a randomized, prospective manner.

When similar populations are compared, conservative therapy of ocular melanomas with the various techniques of radiation therapy produces survival rates similar to those after enucleation. Moreover, there does not appear to be a major difference in local control rates among the various brachytherapy techniques. However, there can be up to a 15% local recurrence rate over many years, and these patients require retreatment by conservative means or by enucleation. Such retreatment can salvage 58% of these patients. Therefore, there is an overall local control rate of nearly 95%. The fact that local control is excellent and that survival after plaque brachytherapy appears not to be different than after enucleation does not justify the preferential use of enucleation as some have suggested.[70]

TABLE 26–2
AJC Staging of Choroidal Melanomas

TUMOR (T)	
TX	Primary tumor cannot be assessed
T0	No evidence of primary tumor
T1	Tumor greatest dimension ≤10 mm with elevation ≤3 mm
T1a	Tumor ≤7 mm in greatest dimension with elevation ≤2 mm
T1b	Tumor >7 mm but ≤10 mm in greatest dimension with >2 mm but ≤3 mm elevation
T2	Tumor >10 mm but ≤15 mm in greatest dimension with >3 mm but ≤5 mm elevation
T3	Tumor greatest dimension of >15 mm *or* elevation of >5 mm
T4	Tumor with extraocular extension
REGIONAL LYMPH NODES (N)	
NX	Regional lymph nodes cannot be assessed
N0	No regional lymph node metastasis
N1	Regional lymph node metastasis
DISTANT METASTASES (M)	
MX	Cannot be assessed
M0	No distant metastases
M1	Distant metastases present

More than 85% of locally controlled brachytherapy patients may retain useful binocular vision for prolonged periods.[83, 113] Analysis of our patients treated primarily by ^{60}Co plaque brachytherapy shows the trend for visual and ocular survival (Fig. 26-3). Cox proportional hazards analysis indicates that the two major prognostic factors for severe visual loss and ocular death are the size of the tumor and the proximity of the tumor to the optic nerve.

The results with particle-beam therapy have been reported to yield higher local control rates than with common brachytherapy techniques. The Harvard group reported an estimated 5-year probability of local tumor control of 96.3%.[10] The absolute local recurrence after helium ion therapy in patients observed for more than 5 years after treatment is given as only 2.4%.[73] However, it was unclear whether all tumors were included or only those of the posterior uvea. The more anterior tumors, especially ciliary body tumors, are associated with high enucleation.[40] There does not appear to be any dose-response correlation for helium ion therapy from 5000 cGyE to 8000 cGyE (*i.e.*, centigray equivalent, which is equal to the physical dose in cGy multiplied by the relative biological effectiveness factor of 1.3). A similar result with proton-beam therapy, which employed a relative biologic effectiveness factor of 1.1, has not been reported. Survival, complications, and visual acuity also did not show any dose-response association for helium ion therapy.[21, 73]

It is generally agreed that very large ocular melanomas and cases of extrascleral extension of tumor at diagnosis are not readily amenable to radiation treatment. These eyes should be enucleated. However, the arguments of Zimmerman and coworkers[161] that the process of enucleation may worsen the prognosis of these patients and the fact that the survival of patients with very large intraocular tumors has been only about 50% in classic series have led to the investigation of preoperative radiation therapy as a means of improving survival in these patients. The adopted schema has been 2000 cGy delivered to the globe and proximal optic nerve (including the major draining vessels from the posterior uveal tract) in five fractions over 5 to 7 days, with enucleation within 24 to 48 hours of the last treatment fraction. Eyes thus treated have been enucleated and cells harvested for tissue culture analysis. The irradiated cells did not grow and did not attach to culture vessels, demonstrating that irradiation can alter the *in vitro* growth of human ocular melanomas.[72] Unfortunately, the initial clinical report, using nonrandomized techniques, has suggested a significantly lower survival in 41 patients receiving preoperative irradiation compared with the survival of 31 patients treated by enucleation alone.[30] However, there were significant differences between the two groups, and the results must be interpreted cautiously. We have conducted a prospective, statistically matched study with 29 patients in each group and have shown no survival differences between preoperative radiation therapy and enucleation alone over a 5-year follow-up interval.

Retinal Tumors

Retinoblastoma

Retinoblastoma is the most common intraocular malignancy of childhood. The incidence is approximately one in 15,000 to 18,000 live births, and it is seen infrequently in routine ophthalmologic practice.[8, 45, 68, 111, 141] The disease is bilateral in 20% to 30% of the patients.[43] Of newly diagnosed children, 10% have a family history of retinoblastoma, and

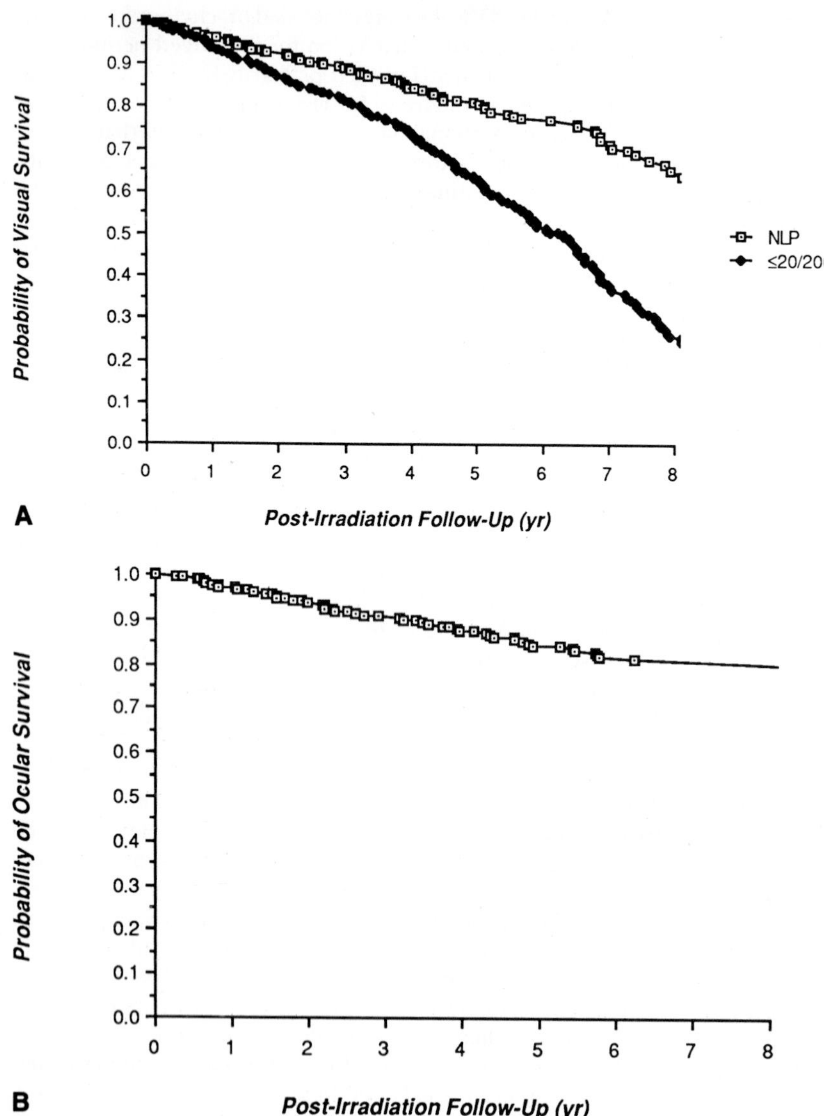

FIGURE 26–3. (**A**) Time course for visual changes after radioactive plaque brachytherapy. Visual acuity (VA) and no light perception (NLP) are both represented. (**B**) Ocular survival in patients treated by radioactive plaque brachytherapy. This curve is based on the end point of enucleation for tumor regrowth or treatment complication without tumor regrowth. Enucleation equals ocular death.

these are always heritable cases.[43,45] The remaining 90% of cases are sporadic, of which 20% to 30% are bilateral, and these are heritable cases. Of the remaining 70% to 80% of apparent unilateral, sporadic cases, 10% to 12% are heritable.[43] Therefore, of all cases diagnosed in the United States annually, approximately 40% to 50% are heritable.

Retinoblastoma can arise in hereditary, nonhereditary, and chromosome deletion forms, the latter occurring on the long arm of chromosome 13.[43,45] In general, the hereditary form is diagnosed earlier than the nonhereditary form of the disease, carries a risk of other malignancies, and can affect the offspring of the affected individual. The disease may be bilateral or unilateral. The chromosomal abnormality can result from a germinal mutation or may be inherited.

The nonhereditary form is unilateral; the children of the affected individual are normal, and this form of the disease is not associated with an increased risk of other malignancies.[43,45] The chromosomal abnormality is from a somatic mutation.[45]

As a result of newly emerging molecular genetic studies, it is now understood that the gene mutated on the long arm of chromosome 13 is a tumor suppressor gene termed the RB gene. It is a large gene of about 200,000 base pairs that encodes a protein whose inhibitory function is thought to be on cell growth. When the function is lost, there is increased cellular growth unopposed by any inhibitory signal. Loss of the entire RB gene, a portion of it, or a point mutation within it leading to a subtle change in the encoded protein may lead to a lack of inhibitory function. Because there are two copies of each gene, one on each of the paternally- and maternally-derived chromosome, if one copy is defective or missing, the other copy is still capable of producing sufficient regulatory protein to prevent uncontrolled growth.

In the hereditary form of retinoblastoma, the mutation is thought to be in the germ cell and, therefore, every cell in the body of the offspring will contain the defective gene copy. Either through spontaneous mutation or under the influence of some event (biological, physical, chemical) that increases the probability of mutation, the normal gene copy may be sufficently damaged in the offspring during retinal development to allow for the complete inhibition of the regulatory protein, leading to the development of retinoblastoma. Whether the defective allele is, in fact, inherited from an affected parent or arises as a new mutation in a parental germ cell, the end result will be identical. There is a high possibility in this inherited form of the disease for bilaterality as well as multifocality. Because the child has inherited only one defective allele in the germ cell, there is a 50% probability of transmission of this allele to any offspring.

The true sporadic disease is postulated to arise from two separate mutations, each in a separate copy of the RB gene within the same somatic cell. This form of the disease is not heritable, because the germ cells are not involved, and not all cells in the body are affected. Therefore, there is a low probability for multifocality and bilaterality.

The conventional wisdom in the molecular genetics of cancer is that, besides inactivation of suppressor genes, such as RB, activation of at least one oncogene may be required. The oncogene for retinoblastoma has not been identified, but it is known that the growth promotion of the myc oncogene can be modulated by the protein encoded by the RB gene.[156A]

Most children with retinoblastoma are diagnosed before age 3 or 4 (although the disease may be present at birth) and rarely beyond the age of 6 years.[43] The most common presenting signs and symptoms are leukocoria (white pupillary reflex), strabismus (squint), or a mass in the fundus noticed during ocular examination.[141] Accurate diagnosis is paramount because several nonmalignant conditions can present similarly. In a series of 136 children referred for evaluation, only 44% had retinoblastoma, and the remainder had pseudoretinoblastoma.[140]

Evaluation begins with an accurate history that emphasizes prenatal and parturition information, prematurity, oxygen therapy, whether leukocoria was present at birth or was noticed later, whether the child has had contact with puppies or other animals, and whether anyone in the family has had retinoblastoma. Children with retinoblastoma rarely have leukocoria or strabismus at birth, but this sign is usually noticed at 6 to 24 months of age.

A careful ophthalmologic examination of the child must be performed to rule out other diagnoses compatible with pseudoretinoblastoma. Slit-lamp biomicroscopy with the pupils dilated may reveal congenital cataract or a retrolental membrane, suggesting diagnoses other than retinoblastoma in which the lens and anterior chamber usually remain clear. Binocular indirect ophthalmoscopy seeking characteristic ophthalmic features of retinoblastoma or spontaneously regressed retinoblastoma remains the most important diagnostic tool.[144]

Ultrasonography has supplanted orbital radiography in detection of retinoblastoma.[141] These tumors exhibit typical, but not pathognomonic, sonographic features. CT scanning can detect intraocular tumors and, more importantly, the rare cases of optic nerve enlargement secondary to posterior tumor extension. It can also demonstrate brain metastases, especially in the pineal region (*i.e.*, trilateral retinoblastoma).

The final ophthalmologic procedure is accurate mapping and sizing of tumor deposits in both eyes, which is best accomplished by indirect bilateral ophthalmoscopy with the child under general anesthesia. Mapping and sizing permit visual prognostic classification using the system of Reese and Ellsworth[125] (Table 26-3). Final staging studies, usually performed by the pediatric oncologist, consist of lumbar puncture with cytospin analysis of the cerebrospinal fluid for malignant cells and a bone scan. The siblings of the affected child and the child's parents should also undergo bilateral indirect ophthalmoscopy to detect disease or regressed disease.

Enucleation of the involved globe has been the traditional method of therapy for unilateral disease, and early enucleation after diagnosis has been given as the major reason for the marked improvement in survival during the past half century.[140] The fellow eye, although apparently normal at diagnosis, remains at risk and must be examined at frequent intervals until the child is at least of school age.

TABLE 26–3
Reese-Ellsworth Classification System for Retinoblastoma

GROUP I

Very favorable
- Solitary tumor, less than 4 dd* in size, at or behind the equator
- Mutiple tumors, none over 4 dd in size, all at or behind the equator

GROUP II

Favorable
- Solitary lesion 4 to 10 dd in size, at or behind the equator
- Multiple tumors, 4 to 10 dd in size, behind the equator

GROUP III

Doubtful
- Any lesion anterior to the equator
- Solitary tumors larger than 10 dd behind the equator

GROUP IV

Unfavorable
- Multiple tumors, some larger than 10 dd
- Any lesion extending anteriorly to the ora

GROUP V

Very unfavorable
- Massive tumors involving over half the retina
- Vitreous seeding

**dd, optic disc diameter of 1.6 mm.*
(Reese AB, Ellsworth RM: Trans Am Acad Ophthalmol Otolaryngol 67:164, 1963)

The therapy of bilateral disease is more complex and traditionally has consisted of enucleation of the eye with more advanced disease and radiation therapy for the lesser-involved eye. Tragically, in some cases, both eyes contain advanced tumors, and there is no hope of retaining useful vision. In such cases, bilateral enucleation has been traditionally recommended. Fortunately, there is often asymmetric development of the disease, and one of the two eyes may be salvageable by radiation therapy. Even if the most advanced eye has more than half of the retina spared or a potential for retention of useful vision, an attempt may be made to salvage both eyes by radiation therapy, reserving enucleation for salvage of failures.[140]

If the eye contains group I or II tumors, external-beam radiation therapy may be employed. An alternative to radiation therapy is ablation by cryopexy or radioactive eye plaque therapy. Group III and IV tumors can be treated by external-beam radiation therapy or complex plaque techniques. Because of the severe nature of the disease in group V, there is frequent failure of radiation therapy, and enucleation may be the final outcome.

EXTERNAL-BEAM TECHNIQUES FOR RETINOBLASTOMA

The first successful treatment of retinoblastoma by x-rays was reported by Hilgartner in 1903.[65] External-beam radiation therapy is applied if preservation of sight is possible and the tumor is not thought to be life-threatening. Armstrong[5] and Weiss and colleagues[157] described various techniques, including the classic single temporal portal (Fig. 26-4) and modifications, that allowed retinal irradiation and shielding of the lens and anterior chamber to minimize the development of new tumors near the ora serrata and minimize the development of radiation-induced cataracts. The modified technique uses a lateral portal with the anterior beam edge at the equator of the globe and an anterior portal containing a 7-mm-diameter central

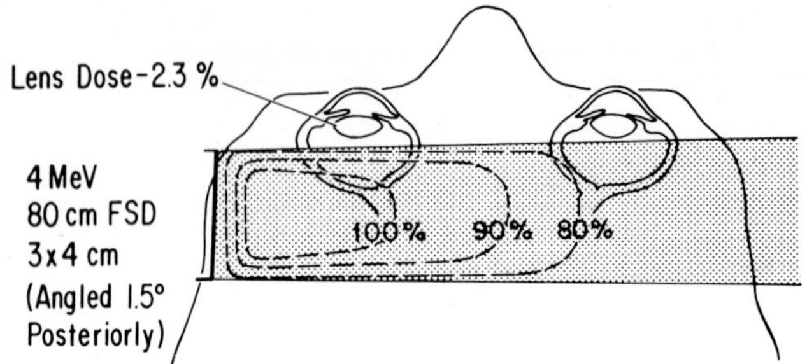

FIGURE 26–4. Computer-calculated isodose distribution for a single 3-cm × 4-cm lateral field using a 4-MeV Varian linear accelerator. The anterior beam edge is placed at the bony canthus and the beam is angled 1.5 degrees posteriorly if the contralateral eye remains in place. The ipsilateral lens dose is estimated using an Li_2BO_4 thermoluminescent dosimeter. (Weiss DR, Cassady JR, Petersen R: Radiology 114:705, 1975)

divergent block hung in a pendulum fashion along the central axis of the beam (Fig. 26-5) to protect the lens.[157] Donaldson and Egbert[43] have recommended that the initial portal setup be done with the ophthalmologist and radiation oncologist working together to establish the posterior border of the lens, the position of the ora serrata, and other key landmarks. They have advised using a Comberg contact lens at setup to delineate the cornea. For tumors located posterior to the equator, the portals can be moved posteriorly to reduce lenticular dose. Anterior portals are not necessary with this technique. Recurrences in this area, however, may seed into the recess of the ciliary body and iris and be difficult to control.

In the past, we discouraged lens-sparing techniques for external-beam irradiation of retinoblastoma. We attempted uniform treatment of the entire retina using a hinged wedge technique, accepting the potential for ultimate cataract formation. This philosophy has recently been confirmed by other radiation oncologists. McCormick and colleagues[99] compared a lens-sparing technique with a modified lateral technique designed to reduce the lens dose to 50% of the volume dose to the globe. The lens-sparing technique was associated with relapse in about two thirds of the treated eyes compared with 17% with the more elegant modified lateral technique. Chin and co-workers[32] have used three pairs of noncoplanar arcs to treat the globe and expose the lens to 30% to 35% of the target dose. No patient data were given. Foote and others[50] reported that treatment of retinoblastoma by anterior segment-sparing techniques resulted in ten of 14 treated eyes requiring further treatment. When an anterior approach with no attempt at lens sparing was used, only four of 11 treated eyes required further treatment. Three of these four eyes required additional treatment for tumors in the posterior pole.

Schipper[135] described various techniques for the treatment of retinoblastoma with lateral or oblique portals, depending on whether the contralateral eye was to be spared (Fig. 26-6). With associates, he reported the results of several therapeutic approaches, including irradiation, with 100% (14 of 14 patients),

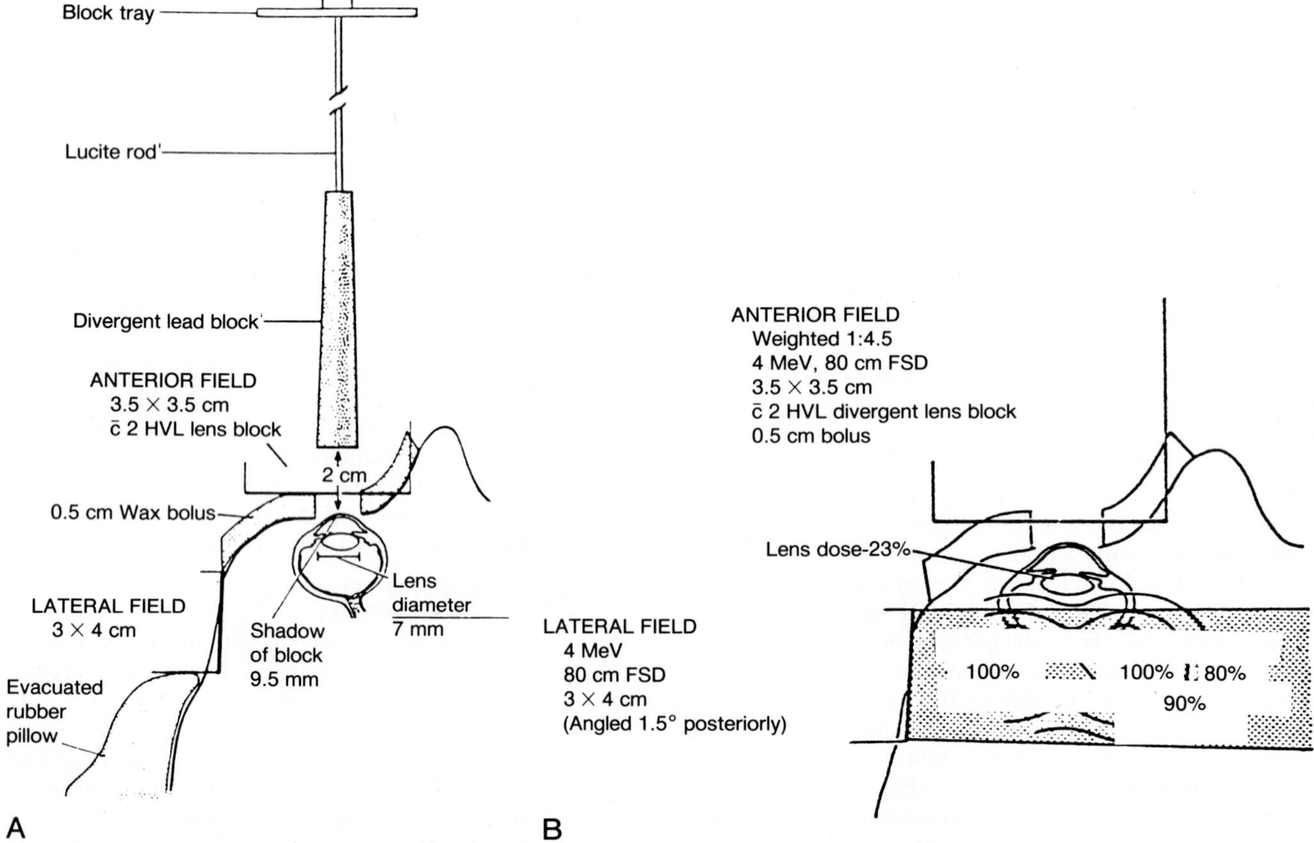

FIGURE 26–5. (**A**) Clinical setup of the two-field technique employing a conventional 3-cm × 4-cm lateral field and a 3.5-cm × 3.5-cm anterior field with a divergent lens block equal to two half-value layers. A 0.5-cm bolus is used anteriorly. The lateral field is angled 1.5 degrees posteriorly if the contralateral eye remains in place. (**B**) Computer-calculated isodose distribution for the two-field technique using a 4-MeV Varian accelerator. Fields are weighted 1 to 4.5 (anterior to lateral). Ipsilateral lens dose is estimated using Li_2BO_4 thermoluminescent dosimetry. (Weiss DR, Cassady JR, Petersen R: Radiology 114:705, 1975)

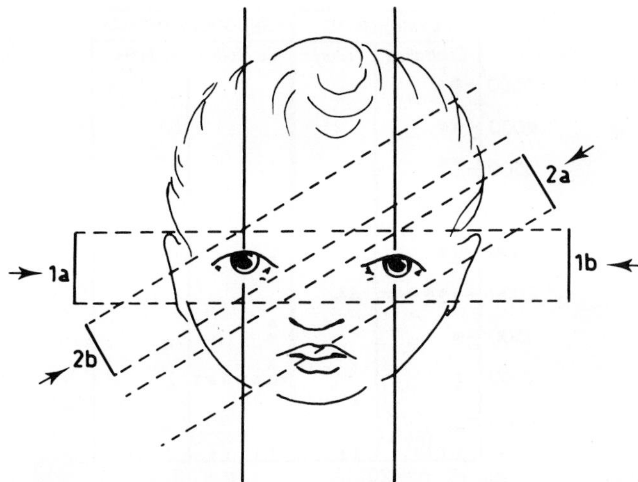

FIGURE 26–6. Schematic representation of unilateral or bilateral treatment of retinoblastoma. If the left eye is affected and the contralateral eye is to be spared, treatment can be carried out with the oblique lateral field (2a). If the right eye later becomes affected, a field (2b) parallel to but not overlapping the oblique lateral field is applied. Simultaneous irradiation in bilateral disease is carried out by alternately treating the opposing fields (1a and 1b).

100% (nine of nine), 83% (ten of 12), 79% (11 of 14), and 0% (zero of five) cure rates in group I through group V eyes, respectively.[136] Of the eyes preserved, 95% retained useful vision.

Cassady and associates[25] reported on 230 patients treated with tumor doses of 3250 cGy to 4500 cGy administered in fractions ranging from 333 cGy to 400 cGy given three times weekly. Local control was achieved in 109 (49%) of the 223 treated eyes. Doses of 4000 cGy to 4500 cGy appeared as effective in achieving local control as those of 3250 to 3500 cGy. Combination chemotherapy was used as well, but it was not shown to improve the overall outcome.

BRACHYTHERAPY FOR RETINOBLASTOMA

In 1929, Foster-Moore and Scott[53] reported their experience with radon seed implantation of retinoblastoma. Stallard[148] described his development of the radium applicator in 1948, which was subsequently replaced by the ^{60}Co plaque. Our past technique using cobalt episcleral applicators consisted of delivering 4000 cGy to the tumor apex, with the tumor base receiving 10,000 cGy to 20,000 cGy. We reserved this technique with cobalt plaques for single, recurring tumors in a potentially salvageable eye.

We recently extended our use of episcleral applicator brachytherapy to other isotopes and employed ^{192}Ir, ^{106}Ru, and ^{125}I plaques. We also extended the use of brachytherapy to previously untreated patients. We treated 20 patients with brachytherapy as a boost after external-beam therapy for very large tumors or for locally recurring tumors. Sixteen (80%) of the 20 patients had favorable responses; the remaining four patients required enucleation for failure.[2]

Another 16 patients were treated primarily and definitively by scleral plaque brachytherapy without antecedent treatment. Three of 14 patients required replaquing, and only one patient ultimately required enucleation. Cataracts formed in only two of these patients. This was the first report of our use of the sequential paired opposed plaque technique (SPOP).[2]

Shields and associates[142] updated this report. In selected retinoblastoma patients, they administered 97 plaque applications to 51 eyes in 50 children. Each SPOP application is the equivalent of four single plaque applications. Plaque therapy was primary treatment in 15 eyes and salvage treatment after failure of external-beam radiation therapy, photocoagulation, or cryotherapy in 36 eyes. In 49 of the 51 eyes, viable vitreous seeding was present. In 18 patients, the contralateral eye had been enucleated, and the remaining eye was being considered for enucleation because all prior therapy had failed. In two of these patients, the remaining eye was salvaged with preservation of some vision. In the 33 eyes with less-advanced tumors (31 of 33 with vitreous seeding), the brachytherapy technique enabled retention of all treated eyes and preservation of useful vision in most. However, these results are quite preliminary and must be regarded cautiously. Although it would seem reasonable to consider brachytherapy techniques for salvage of an eye that has failed the more conventional modes of conservative treatment, use of such techniques for primary therapy cannot be recommended until there is more data available.

SECOND MALIGNANCIES IN RETINOBLASTOMA

There has been extensive evaluation of second malignancies in retinoblastoma. Smith and co-workers[145] reviewed 55 patients seen at Stanford University Medical Center between 1954 and 1986. Of 53 available patients, eight developed 11 second primary tumors. All occurred in the group of patients having the hereditary form of the disease. Three of the 11 second primary tumors were outside the area treated for the primary retinoblastoma. The actuarial incidence for development of second primary malignancies was 4.4% to 6% at 10 years after treatment for retinoblastoma, and the rate increased to 26% to 38% at 30 years.[127,145] The latent period from primary therapy to development of the second primary tumor ranged from 5.2 to 36.2 years, with a median of 16 years. Aggressive multimodal treatment of the second primary disease in five of eight patients was associated with 80% survival without evidence of disease at 22 to 72 months after treatment. Seven of the 11 second primary tumors were osteogenic sarcomas.

Loss or mutation of both copies of the growth-control genes on chromosome 13 that causes retinoblastoma is also associated with the development of osteogenic sarcoma and other types of mesenchymal tumors.[137] Schwarz and others[137] report that the second malignant tumors arising after treatment for retinoblastoma consist of osteogenic sarcoma (58%), fibrosarcoma (21%), and other sarcomas (21%). They propose a strong role for radiation induction based on the increased number of sarcomas arising in the previously irradiated field and prolonged latency periods (12.4 years) and that the predominant sites for these secondary sarcomas are not characteristic for spontaneously occurring primary sarcomas.

Hawkins and colleagues[64] reported observing 30-fold more second primary tumors and over 400-fold more osteogenic sarcomas than would be expected in the general population after the diagnosis of retinoblastoma. In the absence of radiation therapy or chemotherapy, the inherent risk of second primary tumors after primary genetic retinoblastoma was 13-fold greater than the expected number and over 200-fold greater than the expected number of osteogenic sarcomas.

Leukemic Retinopathy

Retinal hemorrhage and infiltration of the optic nerve and retina are both manifestations of childhood leukemia, which may cause permanent visual damage. Treatment consists of low-dose irradiation of 1000 cGy to 1500 cGy fractionated over 4 to 5 days to the eye and retrobulbar region.[126]

Intraocular Lymphomas

By virtue of its rarity, malignant lymphoma of the retina is a diagnostic challenge. The initial manifestation is usually blurred vision resulting from a cellular infiltration of the vitreous cavity. In many cases, there appears to be no systemic manifestation, and the diagnosis is made either by enucleation or by vitreous biopsy.[104] Michels and co-workers[102] treated two cases of intraocular lymphoma with 3000 cGy external-beam irradiation directed through lateral ports. We advocate treating the entire globe by a hinged wedge technique, delivering a minimum tumor dose of 3500 cGy to 4000 cGy in 150-cGy fractions over approximately 5 weeks.[9]

Orbital Tumors

Primary malignant tumors of the orbit are rare. Malignant lymphoma, rhabdomyosarcoma, and lacrimal gland tumors account for most cases.[80] Of these, rhabdomyosarcoma has generated the most interest.

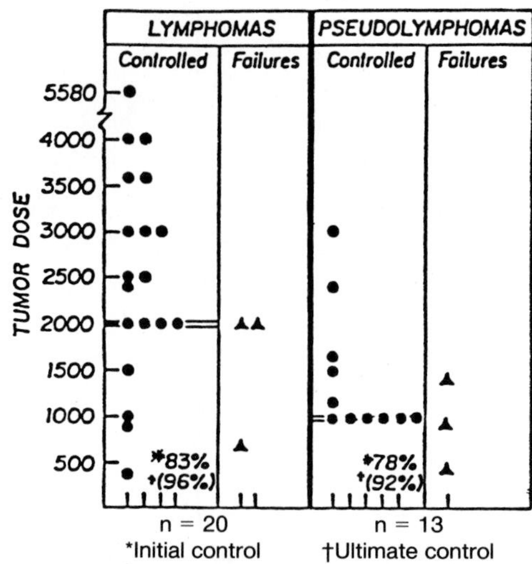

FIGURE 26–7. Radiation dose and local control in treatment of malignant lymphomas and pseudolymphomas of the orbit. (Rao DV, Smith M, Griffith R, et al: Int J Radiat Oncol Biol Phys 8:114, 1982)

Rhabdomyosarcoma

Rhabdomyosarcoma of the orbit is most often seen in young children. It has a rapid onset with marked proptosis and swelling of the adnexal tissue. There is no entirely satisfactory staging system.[117] The Intergroup Rhabdomyosarcoma Study Group clinical staging system is presented in Table 72-2.[98] Previously, the recommended treatment was orbital exenteration, because many ophthalmologists thought that the tumor was radioresistant.[23,69,118] The current recommendations are for combined radiation therapy and chemotherapy as the initial management, limiting surgical intervention to biopsy or local excision.[80,82,129]

Lederman[78] provided the foundations for integrated management with surgery and radiation therapy and developed guidelines for the radiation therapeutic technique and dosage. Sagerman and associates[131] suggested the necessity of higher radiation doses. A minimum tumor dose of 4500 cGy to 5000 cGy should be delivered by megavoltage equipment over 5 to 7 weeks with some protection of sensitive ocular structures. All long-term survivors exhibit late radiation effects ranging from minimal change to phthisis bulbi, requiring enucleation.

Malignant Lymphoma of the Orbit

Although there are clear pathologic criteria for malignant lymphomas of the orbit that differentiate them from pseudolymphomas, the diagnosis is not always clear.[71,122] Malignant lymphomas are characterized by diffuse or nodular lymphoid infiltrates and frequently exhibit atypical cells, mitoses, and invasion of adjacent tissues in contrast to the pseudotumors, which are characterized by a polymorphic admixture of cells including mature lymphocytes organized in reactive germinal centers with inflammatory changes. Surface markers may indicate a specific cell type.

Rao and colleagues[121] and Mittal and co-workers[105] reported 23 and 22 patients, respectively, treated for malignant or indeterminate lymphomas of the orbit. Treatment was given with anterior or lateral portals covering the entire orbit and using ^{60}Co, 4-MV to 6-MV photons, or 15-MeV to 16-MeV electrons. Control of the orbital tumor was achieved in 20 of 23 of Rao's patients with doses of 3000 cGy to 4000 cGy. The few patients who failed to respond received doses below 2000 cGy (Fig. 26-7).

Fitzpatrick and Macko[49] observed tumor control in 100% of 19 patients with malignant lymphoma confined to the orbit after delivery of doses ranging from 2500 cGy in ten fractions to 4500 cGy in 15 fractions. Austin-Seymour and associates[7] had comparable results in 24 patients with benign lymphomatous conditions and eight patients with malignant lymphomas of the orbit treated with mean doses of 2360 cGy and 3625 cGy, respectively. Their techniques are illustrated in Figures 26-8 and 26-9.

Reddy and colleagues[124] reported 17 patients with primary orbital lymphoma. Fourteen of these had 18 eyes treated by radiation therapy, and four patients were treated for local recurrence after surgery. Local control was achieved in 100%. Three of the 17 patients died of systemic progression of lymphoma; 11 died of unrelated causes, and three patients remain alive without evidence of disease.

In a smaller series of patients with primary lymphoma of the orbit, Makepeace and associates[95] reported 100% local re-

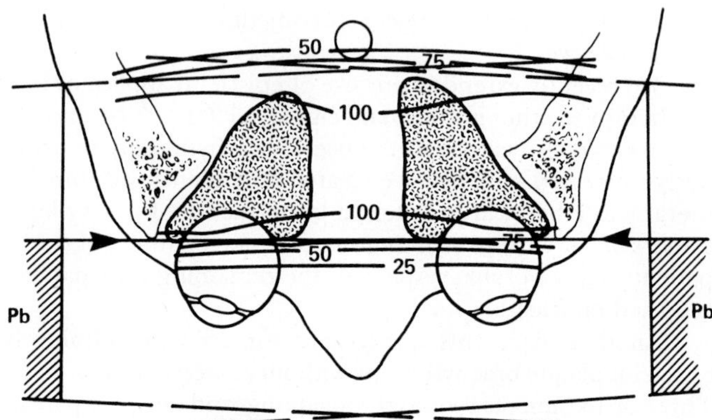

FIGURE 26–8. Isodose distribution for the split-beam technique on an outline through the orbit demonstrating the central axis of the treatment beam at the anterior border of the effective treatment area, here located at the anterior border of the lateral orbital rim. (Austin-Seymour MM, Donaldson SS, Egberg PR, et al: Int J Radiat Oncol Biol Phys 1:371, 1985)

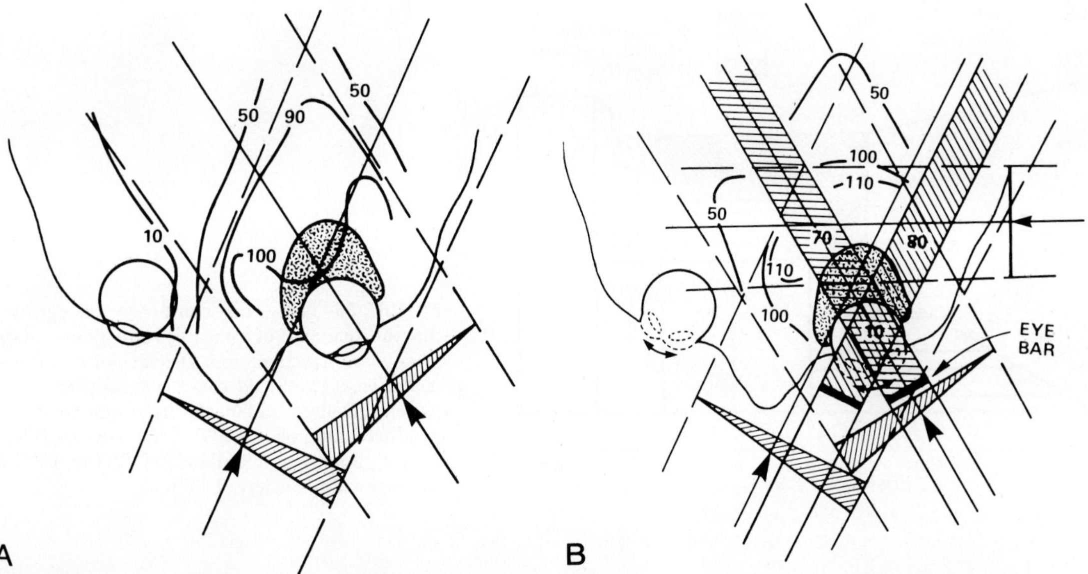

FIGURE 26–9. (**A**) Isodose distribution using the isocentric technique for a unilateral treatment volume (*stippled area*). Numbers indicate percentages of the absorbed dose at the isocenter. Two wedged oblique fields are used to optimize the 90% isodose contour to the treatment volume. (**B**) At the level of the lens, an eye bar is inserted in both oblique fields with the patient looking at the eye bar for each oblique treatment field. (Austin-Seymour MM, Donaldson SS, Egbert PR, et al: Int J Radiat Oncol Biol Phys 1:371, 1985)

gression after radiation therapy. However, a third of their patients developed recurrent disease. The 5-year overall survival rate was 89%.

Bessell and others[12] treated 115 patients with orbital lymphoid tumors. Eighteen patients had high-grade malignant lymphomas; 43 of 115 had low-grade malignant lymphomas; and the remainder (47%) were considered to have indeterminate lymphocytic lesions. The authors report that the survival of patients presenting with Stage I low-grade malignant lymphoma and indeterminate lymphocytic lesions was similar to that of a normal population of the same age characteristics. However, the clinical features and dissemination pattern of the indeterminate lymphoid lesions were identical to those for low-grade malignant lesions. This suggested to them that most, if not all, lymphoid masses presenting in the orbit are neoplastic rather than reactive.The indication is that all cases of primary orbital lymphoma should be evaluated for systemic component and should be as completely staged as lymphomas arising in other primary sites.

Radiation therapy is now considered the treatment of choice for localized primary orbital lymphomas.[124] The suggested radiation dose is 3500 cGy to 4500 cGy administered in conventional fractionation schedules.

Lacrimal Gland Tumors

The high mortality rate of lacrimal gland tumors is partially caused by the difficulty of the surgical approach and the tendency of these tumors to invade the surrounding orbital bone. Although relatively radioresistant, lacrimal gland tumors should routinely be irradiated following surgery to reduce postoperative recurrences.[55] Tumor doses of 5000 cGy to 6000 cGy are necessary, depending on the size of the lesion (Fig. 26-10).

Metastatic Orbital Tumors

Metastatic tumors to the orbit may be treated with 3500 cGy to 4500 cGy fractionated over 3 weeks. The treatment design depends on the location and extent of tumor within the orbit. The techniques are similar to those described for ocular metastases.

COMPLICATIONS OF THERAPY

Skin and Adnexae

Skin changes resulting from radiation therapy may include erythema, depigmentation, atrophy, telangiectasia, and ectropion or entropion of the eyelid. Although conjunctival changes are usually insignificant, a corneal abrasion may result from the formation of a keratotic plaque in a radiation-injured conjunctiva.

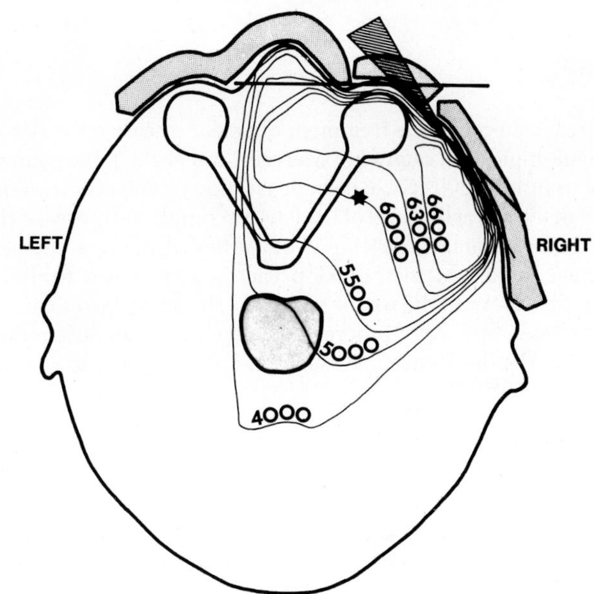

FIGURE 26–10. Example of isodose distribution for anteroposterior and oblique portals with 4-MV photons (including wedges) for treatment of orbital tumors.

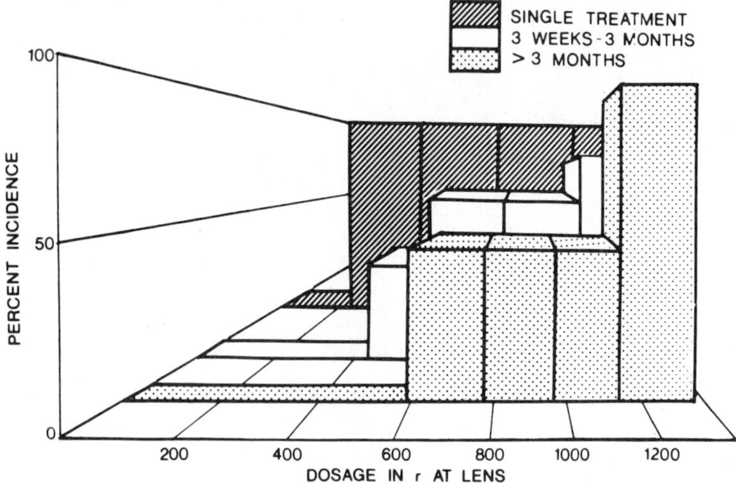

FIGURE 26–11. This composite histogram demonstrates that the incidence of cataract production is related to both total dosage and fractionation. Delivery of 600 cGy over 3 months (*dotted bars*) produced cataract in approximately 50% of the patients. Delivery of 600 cGy in a single treatment (*hatched bars*) produced cataract in 100% of the patients. (Merriam Gr, Focht E: Am J Roentgenol Radiat Ther 77:759, 1957, © by American Roentgen Ray Society, 1957)

Loss of the cilia from the scalp, eyebrow, or eyelid may occur after radiation therapy to the ocular area.[80] Hair loss from the scalp may occur at the exit area of an external-beam portal if a direct anterior or oblique portal is employed. Eyebrow loss occasionally occurs when a ^{60}Co plaque has been used anteriorly and superiorly to treat choroidal malignant melanoma.[10] The loss of eyelashes that may accompany the use of x-ray therapy in the treatment of basal cell carcinoma is usually permanent. Similar lash loss may follow radioactive plaque therapy of ciliochoroidal melanomas.

Cornea

Direct corneal injury may result from irradiation of ocular and adjacent structures.[16,17] Blodi[16] classified this damage as pure epithelial with a good prognosis for recovery or stromal with a poor prognosis. Experiments indicate that 7200 cGy fractionated over 8 days leads to corneal perforation, but 4800 cGy fractionated over the same time produces mostly reversible epithelial changes with minimal stromal damage.

Lens

A great concern in the treatment of ocular disease is the risk of radiation-induced cataract.[33] Merriam and Focht[100] have shown that as little as 200 cGy in a single fraction or 800 cGy fractionated delivered at the level of the lens can significantly elevate the incidence of cataract development. At higher dosages, the percentage of lenses that develop cataracts increases to 100% (Fig. 26-11). With the use of improved shielding, beam-control techniques, and more inherently sharp beams, an 80% reduction in the incidence of radiation-induced cataracts is expected.[57,63,65,100]

Retina and Choroid

Changes in the retina and choroid are observed after doses of 4500 cGy to 6000 cGy.[93] Vascular damage leads to infarction of tissue with the formation of exudates and hemorrhages. Decreased visual acuity may result from damage to the retinal tissue or from atrophy of the optic nerve.[128] Because of the extreme radioresistance of the sclera, which may tolerate doses to 75,000 cGy or more, only a few cases of scleral necrosis have been reported.[24]

Lacrimal Gland and Bony Orbit

Radiation damage to the lacrimal gland may decrease tear production and produce irreversible corneal changes. A particularly distinctive and disfiguring orbital change that sometimes occurs in children irradiated for ocular or orbital tumors is the arrested development of the lateral orbital wall growth center, leading to a subsequent temporal osteomalacia. Another rare, but disastrous, complication is the development of osteogenic sarcoma of the orbit. This complication has been fatal in 100% of reported cases.[52,119,130,139,146,154,160] However, Smith and associates[145] report two of four patients with malignant osteogenic sarcoma surviving without disease more than 3 years after aggressive multimodal therapy.

REFERENCES

1. Alaniz-Camino F: The use of postoperative beta radiation in the treatment of pterygia. Ophthalmic Surg 13:1022, 1982
2. Amendola BE, Markoe AM, Augsburger JJ, et al: Analysis of treatment results in 36 children with retinoblastoma treated by scleral plaque irradiation. Int J Radiat Oncol Biol Phys 17:63, 1989
3. American Joint Committee on Cancer: Manual for Staging of Cancer, 3rd ed. Philadelphia, JB Lippincott, 1988
4. Anson B, McVay CB: Surgical Anatomy. Philadelphia, WB Saunders, 1971
5. Armstrong DI: The use of 4–6 MeV electrons for the conservative treatment of retinoblastoma. Br J Radiol 47:326, 1974
6. Assegadoo ER: Surgery, thio-tepa and corticosteroids in the treatment of pterygium. Am J Ophthalmol 74:960, 1972
7. Austin-Seymour MM, Donaldson SS, Egbert PR, et al: Radiotherapy of lymphoid diseases of the orbit. Int J Radiat Oncol Biol Phys 1:371, 1985
8. Banks CN: Inheritance of retinoblastoma. Br J Ophthalmol 53:212, 1969
9. Barthold HJ, Harvey A, Markoe AM, et al: Treatment of orbital pseudo tumor and lymphoma. Am J Clin Oncol 9:527, 1986
10. Bedford MA, Bedotto C, MacFaul PA: Radiation retinopathy after application of a cobalt plaque: Report of three cases. Br J Ophthalmol 54:505, 1970
11. Beierwaltes WH: X-ray treatment of malignant exophthalmos. J Clin Endocrinol Metab 13:1090, 1953
12. Bessell EM, Henk JM, Wright JE, et al: Orbital and con-

junctival lymphoma treatment and prognosis. Radiother Oncol 13:237, 1988

13. Beyer DC: Single fraction postoperative beta irradiation for pterygia. Presented at 31st Annual ASTRO Meeting, San Francisco, 1989
14. Blahut RJ, Beierwaltes WH, Lampe I: Exophthalmos response during roentgen therapy. Am J Roentgenol Radium Ther Nucl Med 90:261, 1963
15. Bloch RS, Gartner S: The incidence of ocular metastatic carcinoma. Arch Ophthalmol 85:673, 1971
16. Blodi FC: The late effects of x-irradiation on the cornea. Trans Am Ophthalmol Soc 56:413, 1958
17. Blodi FC: The effects of experimental x-radiation on the cornea. Arch Ophthalmol 63:44, 1960
18. Boniuk M, Girard L: Malignant melanomas of the choroid treated with photocoagulation, transscleral diathermy and radon seed implant. Am J Ophthalmol 59:212, 1965
19. Bosworth JL, Packer S, Rotman M, et al: Choroidal melanoma: I-125 plaque therapy. Radiology 169:249, 1988
20. Brady LW, Shields JA, Augsburger JJ, et al: Malignant intraocular tumors. Cancer 49:578, 1982
21. Brady LW, Shields JA, Augusburger JJ, et al: Posterior uveal melanomas. In Phillips TL, Pistenmaa DA (eds): Radiation Oncology Annual, vol 1, pp 233–245. New York, Raven Press, 1984
22. Busin M, Holliday BL, Arffa RC, et al: Precarved lyophilized tissue for lamellar keratoplasty in recurrent pterygium. Am J Ophthalmol 102:222, 1986
23. Calhoun FP, Reese AB: Rhabdomyosarcoma of the orbit. Arch Ophthalmol 27:558, 1982
24. Cappin JM: Radiation scleral necrosis simulating early scleromalacia perforans. Br J Ophthalmol 57:4525, 1973
25. Cassady JR, Sagerman RH, Tretter P, et al: Radiation therapy in retinoblastoma: An analysis of 230 cases. Radiology 93:405, 1969
26. Cavanagh HO, Gren WR, Goldberg HK: Multicentric sebaceous adenocarcinomas of the melbomian gland. Am J Ophthalmol 77:326, 1974
27. Chang CH, Wood EH: The value of radiation therapy for gliomas of anterior visual pathway. In Brockhurst R, Boruchoff S, Hutchinson B (eds): Ophthalmology, pp 878–886. Philadelphia, WB Saunders, 1977
28. Char DH, Castro JR: Helium ion therapy for choroidal melanoma. Arch Ophthalmol 100:935, 1982
29. Char DH, Castro JR, Quivey JM: Helium ion charged particle therapy for choroidal melanoma. Ophthalmology 87:565, 1982
30. Char DH, Phillips TL, Andejeski Y, et al: Failure of preenucleation radiation to decrease uveal melanoma mortality. Am J Ophthalmol 106:21, 1988
31. Chenery SG, Fitzpatrick PJ, Japp B, et al: Treatment of choroidal melanoma with radioisotopes. Presented at the American Society of Therapeutic Radiology, Los Angeles, 1978
32. Chin LM, Harter KW, Svansson GK, et al: An external-beam treatment technique for retinoblastoma. Int J Radiat Oncol Biol Phys 15:455, 1988
33. Cogan DG, Donaldson DD, Reese AB: Clinical and pathological characteristics of radiation cataract. Arch Ophthalmol 47:55, 1952
34. Constable IJ: Proton irradiation therapy for ocular melanoma. Trans Ophthalmol Soc UK 97:430, 1977
35. Cooper JS: Postoperative irradiation of pterygia: 10 more years of experience. Radiology 128:753, 1978
36. Curtin VT, Cavender JC: The natural course of selected malignant melanomas of the choroid and ciliary body. Mod Probl Ophthalmol 12:523, 1974
37. Danoff BF, Kramer S, Thompson N: The radiotherapeutic management of optic nerve gliomas in children. Int J Radiat Oncol Biol Phys. 6:45, 1980
38. Davidorf FH, Newman GH, Havener WH, et al: Conservative management of malignant melanoma. II. Transcleral diatherapy. Arch Ophthalmol 82:273, 1970
39. Davidorf FH, Pajka JT, Makley T, et al: Radiotherapy for choroidal melanoma: An 18-year experience with radon. Arch Ophthalmol 105:352, 1987
40. Decker MM, Castro JR, Linstadt DE, et al: Ciliary body melanoma treated with helium particle irradiation. Presented at 31st Annual ASTRO Meeting, San Francisco, 1989
41. de Keizer RJ, Swart-van-den-Berg M, Baartse WJ: Results of pterygium excision with Sr-90 irradiation, lamellar keratoplasty and conjunctival flaps. [Abstract] Doc Ophthalmol 67:33, 1987
42. de Venecia G, Lobek CC: Successful treatment of eyelid hemangioma with prednisone. Arch Ophthalmol 84:98, 1970
43. Donaldson SS, Egbert PR: Retinoblastoma. In Pizzo P, Poplack D (eds): Principles and Practices of Pediatric Oncology. Philadelphia, JB Lippincott, 1989
44. Donaldson SS, McDougall IR, Egbert PR, et al: Treatment of orbital pseudotumor (idiopathic orbital inflammation) by radiation therapy. Int J Radiat Oncol Biol Phys 6:79, 1980
45. Donaldson SS, Smith LA: Retinoblastoma: Biology, presentation and current management. Oncology 3:45, 1989
46. Dosoretz DE, Blitzer PH, Wang CC: Management of glioma of the optic nerve and/or chiasm: An analysis of 20 cases. Cancer 45:1467, 1980
47. Federman JL, Lewis MG, Clark WH, et al: Tumor-associated antibodies in the serum of ocular melanoma patients. Trans Am Acad Ophthalmol Otolaryngol 78:784, 1974
48. Ferry AP, Font RL: Carcinoma metastatic to the eye and orbit. I. A clinicopathologic study of 227 cases. Arch Ophthalmol 92:276, 1974
49. Fitzpatrick PJ, Macko S: Lymphoreticular tumors of the orbit. Int J Radiat Oncol Biol Phys 10:333, 1984
50. Foote RL, Garretson BR, Schomberg PJ, et al: External-beam irradiation for retinoblastoma: Patterns of failure and dose-response analysis. Int J Radiat Oncol Biol Phys 16:823, 1989
51. Forrest AW: Radiotherapy of ocular lesions by x-rays and gamma rays. Trans Am Acad Ophthalmol 63:455, 1959
52. Forrest AW: Tumors following radiation about the eye. Trans Am Acad Ophthalmol Otolaryngol 65:694, 1961
53. Foster-Moore R, Scott RS: Clinical and pathological report of bilateral glioma retinae. Proc R Soc Med 22:951, 1929
54. Foulds WS: Local excision of choroidal melanomas. Trans Ophthalmol Soc UK 93:343, 1974
55. Franklin CIV: Primary lymphoreticular tumors in the orbit. Clin Radiol 26:137, 1975
56. Fraunfelder FT, Boozman FW III, Wilson DS, et al: "No-touch" technique for intraocular malignant melanomas. Arch Ophthalmol 95:1616, 1977
57. Gotfredsen E: On the frequency of secondary carcinoma of the choroid. Acta Ophthalmol (Copenh) 22:394, 1944
58. Gragoudas ES, Goiten M, Verhey L, et al: Proton beam irradiation of uveal melanomas. Arch Opthalmol 100:928, 1982
59. Gragoudas ES, Goitein M, Koehler A, et al: Proton irradiation of choroidal melanomas: Preliminary results. Arch Ophthalmol 96:1583, 1978
60. Grogoudas ES, Seddon JM, Egan K, et al: Long-term results of proton beam irradiated uveal melanomas. Ophthalmology 94:349, 1987
61. Grayson M: Degenerations, dystrophies and edema of the cornea. In Duane TD (ed): Clinical Opthalmology, pp 4–5. Hagerstown, MD, Harper & Row, 1976
62. Halnan KS: Tumors of the eye treated by radiotherapy. Clin Radiol 13:19, 1962
63. Ham WT: Radiation cataract. Arch Ophthalmol 50:618, 1953
64. Hawkins MM, Draper GJ, Kingston JE: Incidence of second primary tumors among childhood cancer survivors. Br J Cancer 56:339, 1987
65. Hilgartner HL: Report of a case of double glioma treated with x-ray. Texas Med J 18:322, 1903
66. Hilgers JHC: Strontium-90 beta-irradiation, cataractongenicity and pterygium recurrence. Arch Ophthalmol 76:329, 1966
67. Jacobiec FA, Jones IS: Vascular tumors, malformations and degenerations. In Duane TD (ed): Clinical Ophthalmology, vol 2, Ch 37, pp 1–40. Hagerstown, MD, Harper & Row, 1976
68. Jereb B, Koch E, Asard PE: Prognosis of retinoblastoma treated at Radiumhemmet 1926–1963. Acta Radiol 6:369, 1967
69. Jones IS, Reese AB, Krout J: Orbital rhabdomyosarcoma: An

analysis of 62 cases. Trans Am Ophthalmol Soc 63:223, 1965
70. Karlsson UL, Augusburger JJ, Shields JA, et al: Recurrence of posterior uveal melanoma after ^{60}Co episcleral plaque therapy. Ophthalmology 96:382, 1989
71. Kelly AG, Rosas-Uribe A, Kraus ST: Orbital lymphomas and pseudolymphomas: A clinicopathologic study of 11 cases. Am J Ophthalmol 76:371, 1973
72. Kenneally CL, Farber MG, Smith ME, et al: *In vitro* melanoma cell growth after preenucleation radiation therapy. Arch Ophthalmol 106:223, 1988
73. Kindy-Degnan NA, Char DH, Castro JR, et al: Effect of various doses of radiation for uveal melanoma on regression, visual acuity, complications, and survival. Am J Ophthalmol 107:114, 1989
74. Kleis W, Pico G: Thio-tepa therapy to prevent post-operative pterygium occurrence and neovascularization. Am J Ophthalmol 76:371, 1973
75. Knowles DM, Jacobiec FA: Orbital lymphoid neoplasms. Cancer 46:576, 1980
76. Last RJ: Wolff's Anatomy of the Eye and Orbit. London, HK Lewis, 1968
77. Laughrea PA, Arentsen JJ: Lamellar keratoplasty in the management of recurrent pterygium. Ophthalmology 17:106, 1986
78. Lederman M: Radiotherapy in treatment of orbital tumors. Br J Ophthalmol 40:592, 1956
79. Lederman M: Radiotherapy of non-malignant diseases of the eye. In Bushke F (ed): Progress in Radiation Therapy, pp 256–271. New York, Grune & Stratton, 1958
80. Lederman M: Radiotherapy of primary malignant tumors of the orbit. Mod Probl Ophthalmol 14:170, 1975
81. Lentino W, Zaret MM, Rossignol B, et al: Treatment of pterygium by surgery followed by beta irradiation. Am J Roentgenol Radium Ther 81:93, 1949
82. Liebner EJ: Embryonal rhabdomyosarcoma of head and neck in children: Correlation of stage, radiation dose, local control and survival. Cancer 37:2777, 1976
83. Linett PE: Discussion of article: Recurrence of posterior uveal melanoma after ^{60}Co episcleral plaque therapy. Ophthalmology 96:387, 1989
84. Lincoff H, McLean J, Lang R: The cryosurgical treatment of intraocular tumors. Am J Ophthalmol 63:389, 1967
85. Lunstadt D, Char DH, Castro JR, et al: Vision following helium ion radiotherapy of uveal melanoma: A Northern California Oncology Group study. Int J Radiat Oncol Biol Phys 15:347, 1988
86. Lommatzsch P: Treatment of choroidal melanomas with ^{106}Rh beta-ray applicators. Surv Ophthalmol 19:85, 1974
87. Lommatzsch P: Beta-irradiation of retinoblastoma with ^{106}Ru/^{106}Rh applicators. Mod Probl Ophthalmol 18:128, 1977
88. Lommatzsch P: Treatment of choroidal melanomas with ^{106}Ru/^{106}Rh beta-ray applicators. Trans Ophthalmol Soc UK 97:428, 1977
89. Lommatzsch PK: Beta irradiation with ^{106}Ru/^{106}Rh applicators of choroidal melanomas: Sixteen years' experience. In Lommatzsch PK, Blodi FC (eds): Intraocular Tumors, pp 290–301. Berlin, Academie-Verlag, 1983
90. Lommatzsch PK, Kirsch IH: ^{106}Ru/^{106}Rh plaque radiotherapy for malignant melanomas of the choroid: With follow-up results more than 5 years. [Abstract] Doc Ophthalmol 68:255, 1988
91. Long RS, Galin MA, Rotman M: Conservative treatment of intraocular melanomas. Trans Am Acad Ophthalmol Otolaryngol 75:84, 1971
92. MacFaul PA: Local radiotherapy in the treatment of maligant melanoma of the choroid. Trans Ophthalmol Soc UK 97:421, 1977
93. MacFaul PA: Bedford MA: Ocular complications after therapeutic irradiation. Br J Ophthalmol 54:237, 1970
94. MacFaul PA, Morgan G: Histopathological changes in malignant melanomas of the choroid after cobalt plaque therapy. Br J Ophthalmol 61:221, 1977
95. Makepeace AR, Fermont DC, Bennett MH: Primary non-Hodgkin's lymphoma of the orbit. J R Soc Med 81:640, 1988
96. Markoe AM, Brady LW, Shields JA, et al: Radioactive eye-plaque therapy versus enucleation for the treatment of posterior uveal malignant melanoma. Radiology 156:801, 1985
97. Marquileth A, Museles M: Cutaneous hemangiomas in children: Diagnosis and conservative management. JAMA 1974:523, 1965
98. Maurer HM, Moon TE, Donaldson M, et al: The Intergroup Rhabdomyosarcoma Study. Cancer 40:2015, 1977
99. McCormick B, Ellsworth R, Abramson D, et al: Radiation therapy for retinoblastoma: Comparison of results with lens-sparing versus lateral beam techniques. Int J Radiat Oncol Biol Phys 15:567, 1988
100. Merriam GR, Focht E: A clinical study of radiation cataracts and their relationship to dose. Am J Roentgenol Radium Ther Nucl Med 77:759, 1957
101. Meyer-Schwickerath G: Further progress in the field of light coagulation. Trans Ophthalmol Soc UK 77:421, 1957
102. Michels RC, Knox DL, Erozan YS, et al: Intraocular reticulum cell sarcoma: Diagnosis by pars plana vitrectomy. Arch Ophthalmol 93:1331, 1975
103. Miller NR, Iliff WJ, Green WR: Evaluation and management of gliomas of the anterior visual pathways. Brain 97:743, 1973
104. Minckler DS, Font RL, Zimmerman LE: Uveitis and reticulum cell sarcoma of brain with bilateral neoplastic seeding of vitreous without retinal or uveal involvement. Am J Ophthalmol 80:433, 1975
105. Mittal B, Deutsch M, Kennerdell J, et al: Paraocular lymphoid tumors. Radiology 159:793, 1986
106. Montgomery AB, Griffin T, Parker RG: Optic nerve glioma: The role of radiation therapy. Cancer 40:2079, 1977
107. Muller RP, Busse H, Potter R, et al; Results of high dose ^{106}ruthenium irradiation of choroidal melanomas. Int J Radiat Oncol Biol Phys 12:1749, 1986
108. Munzenrider JE, Gragoudas ES, Seddon JM, et al: Conservative treatment of uveal melanoma: Probability of eye retention after proton treatment. Int J Radiat Oncol Biol Phys 15:553, 1988
109. Munzenrider JE, Verhey LS, Gragoudas ES, et al: Conservative treatment of uveal melanoma: Local recurrence after proton beam therapy. Int J Radiat Oncol Biol Phys 17:493, 1989
110. Myles ST, Murphy SB: Gliomas of the optic nerve and chiasm. Can J Ophthalmol 8:508, 1973
111. Neilson M, Goldschmidt E: Retinoblastomas among offspring of adult survivors in Denmark. Acta Ophthalmol (Copenh) 46:736, 1968
112. Newman GH, Davidorf FH, Havener WH, et al: Conservative management of malignant melanoma. I. Irradiation as a method of treatment for malignant melanoma of the choroid. Arch Ophthalmol 83:21, 1970
113. Packer S: Iodine^{125} radiation of posterior uveal melanoma. Ophthalmology 94:1621, 1987
114. Pardo FS, Wang CC, Albert D, et al: Sebaceous carcinoma of the ocular adnexa: Radiotherapeutic management. Int J Radiat Oncol Biol Phys 17:643, 1989
115. Peterson IA, Donaldson SS, McDougall MB, et al: Prognostic factors in the radiotherapy of Grave's ophthalmopathy. Presented at 31st Annual ASTRO Meeting, San Francisco, 1989
116. Peyman GA, Apple DJ: Local excision of a choroidal malignant melanoma: Full thickness eye wall resection. Arch Ophthalmol 92:216, 1974
117. Pizzo PA, Miser JS, Cassady JR, et al: Solid tumors of childhood. In Devita VT Jr, Hellman S, Rosenberg SA (eds): Cancer: Principles and Practice of Oncology, 2nd ed, pp 1511–1589. Philadelphia, JB Lippincott, 1985
118. Porterfield JF, Zimmerman LE: Rhabdomyosarcoma of the orbit: A clinicopathologic study of 55 cases. Virchows Arch [A]. 335:329, 1962
119. Raivio I, Tarkkanen A: Sarcoma following radiation for retinoblastoma. Acta Ophthalmol (Copenh) 43:428, 1965
120. Rand RW, Khonsary A, Brown WJ, et al: Leksell stereotactic radiosurgery in the treatment of eye melanoma. Neurol Res 9:142, 1987
121. Rao DV, Smith M, Griffith R, et al: Orbital lymphomas and pseudolymphomas. Int J Radiat Oncol Biol Phys 8:114, 1982

122. Rappaport H, Winter WJ, Hicks EB: Follicular lymphoma: Based on a survery of 253 cases. Cancer 9:792, 1956
123. Ravin JG, Sisson JC, Knapp WT: Orbital radiation for the ocular changes of Graves' disease. Am J Ophthalmol 79:285, 1975
124. Reddy BK, Bhatia P, Evans RG: Primary orbital lymphomas. Int J Radiat Oncol Biol Phys 15:1239, 1988
125. Reese AB, Ellsworth RM: The evaluation and current concept of retinoblastoma therapy. Trans Am Acad Ophthalmol Otolaryngol 67:164, 1963
126. Ridgeway WE, Jaffe N, Walton DS: Leukemic ophthalmopathy in children. Cancer 38:1744, 1976
127. Roarty JD, McLean IW, Zimmerman CE: Incidence of second neoplasms in patients with bilateral retinoblastoma. Ophthalmology 95:1583, 1988
128. Ross H, Rosenberg S, Friedman AH: Delayed radiation necrosis of the optic nerve. Am J Ophthalmol 76:683, 1973
129. Sagerman RH, Cassady JR, Tretter P: Radiation therapy for rhabdomyosarcoma of the orbit. Trans Am Acad Ophthalmol Otolaryngol 72:849, 1968
130. Sagerman RH, Cassady JR, Tretter P, et al: Radiation-induced neoplasm following external beam therapy for children with retinoblastoma. Am J Roentgenol Radium Ther Nucl Med 105:529, 1969
131. Sagerman RH, Tretter P, Ellsworth RM: The treatment of orbital rhabdomyosarcoma of children with primary radiation therapy. Am J Roentgenol Radium Ther Nucl Med 114:31, 1972
132. Sandler HM, Rubenstein JH, Fowble BL, et al: Results of radiotherapy for thyroid ophthalmopathy. Int J Radiat Oncol Biol Phys 17:823, 1989
133. Saunders WM, Char DH, Quivey JM, et al: Precision high dose radiotherapy: Helium ion treatment of uveal melanoma. Int J Radiat Oncol Biol Phys 11:227, 1985
134. Sautter H, Naumann G: Full thickness scleral resection in iridocyclectomy and choroidectomy for anterior uveal tumors. Ophthalmic Surg 4:25, 1973
135. Schipper J: An accurate and simple method for megavoltage radiation therapy of retinoblastoma. Radiother Oncol 1:31, 1983
136. Schipper J, Tan KEWP, van Peperzeel HA: Treatment of retinoblastoma by precision megavoltage radiation therapy. Radiother Oncol 3:117, 1985
137. Schwarz MB, Burgess LP, Fee WE Jr, et al: Postirradiation sarcoma in retinoblastoma: Induction or predisposition. Arch Otolaryngol Head Neck Surg 114:640, 1988
138. Seddon JM, Gragoudas ES, Egan KA, et al: Uveal melanomas near the optic disc or fovea: Visual results after proton beam irradiation. Ophthalmology 94:354, 1987
139. Shah IC, Arlen M, Miller T: Osteogenic sarcoma developing after radiotherapy for retinoblastoma. Am Surg 40:485, 1974
140. Shields JA: Modern techniques in the management of retinoblastoma. Trans Pacific Coast Otolaryngol Ophthalmol Soc 60:235, 1979
141. Shields JA, Augsburger JJ: Current approaches to the diagnosis and management of retinoblastoma. Surv Ophthalmol 25:347, 1981
142. Shields JA, Giblin ME, Shields CL, et al: Episcleral plaque radiotherapy for retinoblastoma. Ophthalmology 96:530, 1989
143. Shields JA, McDonald PR: Improvement in the diagnosis of posterior uveal melanomas. Arch Ophthalmol 91:259, 1974
144. Shields JA, Stephens RA, Augsburger JJ: Metastatic tumor to the uveal tract. In Lommatzsch PK, Blodi FC (eds): Intraocular Tumors, pp 433–444. Berlin, Akademie-Verlag, 1983
145. Smith LM, Donaldson SS, Egbert PR, et al: Aggressive management of second primary tumors in survivors of hereditary retinoblastoma. Int J Radiat Oncol Biol Phys 17:499, 1989
146. Soloway HB: Radiation-induced neoplasms following curative therapy for retinoblastoma. Cancer 19:1984, 1966
147. Stallard HB: Six cases of metastatic carcinoma of the choroid. Proc R Soc Med 26:1042, 1933
148. Stallard HB: Radiotherapy of malignant intraocular neoplasms. Br J Ophthalmol 32:618, 1948
149. Stallard HB: Malignant melanoma of the choroid treated with radioactive applicators. Trans Ophthalmol Soc UK 79:373, 1959
150. Stallard HB: The conservative treatment of retinoblastoma. Trans Ophthalmol Soc UK 82:473, 1962
151. Stallard HB: Radiotherapy for malignant melanoma of the choroid. Br J Ophthalmol 50:174, 1966
152. Stallard HB: Partial choroidectomy. Br J Ophthalmol 50:660, 1966
153. Stephens RF, Shields JA: Diagnosis and management of cancer metastatic to the uvea:. A study of 70 cases. Ophthalmology 86:1336, 1979
154. Tebbet RD, Vickery RD: Osteogenic sarcoma following irradiation for retinoblastoma. Am J Ophthalmol 3:811, 1952
155. Van Den Brenk HAA: Results of prophylactic postoperative irradiation in 1300 cases of pterygium. Am J Roentgenol Radiat Ther Nucl Med 103:723, 1968
156. Vogel MH: Treatment of malignant choroidal melanoma with photocoagulation: Evaluation of 10-year follow-up data. Am J Ophthalmol 74:1, 1972

156A. Weinberg RA: Integration of molecular genetics into cancer management. Keynote presentation at National Conference on Integration of Molecular Genetics Into Cancer Management, Miami, FL, April 10–12, 1991

157. Weiss DR, Cassady JR, Petersen R: Retinoblastoma: A modification in radiation therapy technique. Radiology 114:705, 1975
158. Winter FC: Surgical excision of tumors of the ciliary body and iris. Arch Ophthalmol 70:19, 1963
159. Winter FC: Iridocyclectomy for malignant melanoma of the iris and ciliary body. In Boniuk M (ed): Ocular and Adnexal Tumors: New and Controversial Aspects, pp 341–352. St. Louis, CV Mosby, 1964
160. Yoneyama T, Greenlaw RH: Osteogenic sarcoma following radiotherapy for retinoblastoma. Radiology 93:1185, 1969
161. Zimmerman LE, McLean IW: Changing concepts concerning the malignancy of ocular tumors. Arch Ophthalmol 78:487, 1975

27

○ ○ ○ • ● •

Ear

V. Rao Devineni

ANATOMY

The external, middle, and inner components of the ear develop from the three embryonic layers: ectoderm, mesoderm, and endoderm.

The external ear consists of the auricle or pinna, the external auditory meatus (canal), and the tympanic membrane (Fig. 27-1). The auricle is composed of elastic cartilage covered with skin. The external auditory meatus connects the tympanic membrane to the exterior and is approximately 2.4 cm long. The outer third is cartilaginous, and the inner two thirds is bony and slightly narrower. The external auditory canal is related anteriorly to the parotid gland at the temporomandibular joint. Inferiorly, it lies near the jugular bulb and the facial nerve as it descends through the stylomastoid foramen. The skin lining the auditory canal is continuous with that of the auricle, and in the outer third of the canal, it contains hair follicles and sebaceous and ceruminous glands. The tympanic membrane, which is made of multiple layers of squamous epithelium, separates the auditory canal from the middle ear.

The tympanic, or middle ear, cavity houses the auditory ossicles and opens into the eustachian tube to communicate with the pharynx. The middle ear cavity is lined with a mucoperiosteal membrane, and the eustachian tube is lined with stratified columnar epithelium and has numerous mucous glands in the two thirds of the tube closer to the pharynx. The overall length of the eustachian tube is 3.5 cm.[17]

The inner or internal ear lies in the petrous portion of the temporal bone and consists of the bony labyrinth and the membranous labyrinth. The membranous labyrinth, which holds the organ of hearing, is housed in the bony labyrinth.

Blood supply to the auricle and the external auditory canal is from branches of the posterior auricular artery and the superficial temporal artery, which arise from the external carotid artery. Blood is supplied to the middle ear region from branches of ascending pharyngeal and middle meningeal arteries and from the artery of the pterygoid canal. The inner ear is supplied by the internal auditory artery, which is a branch of the basilar artery, and from the anterior inferior cerebellar artery.

The nerves innervating the ear include the fifth, eighth, ninth, and tenth cranial nerves. The eighth or acoustic nerve, which arises at the lateral termination of the internal acoustic meatus and ends in the brain stem between the pons and the medulla, is responsible for auditory and vestibular function.

Lymphatic vessels of the tragus and anterior external portion of the auricle drain into the superficial parotid lymph nodes. Those of the posterior external and whole cranial aspect of the auricle drain into the retroauricular lymph nodes, and those of the lobule drain into the superficial cervical group of lymph nodes. Lymphatics from the middle ear and the mastoid antrum pass into the parotid nodes and into the upper deep cervical lymph nodes. The lymphatics in the middle ear and eustachian tube are rather sparse, and the inner ear has no lymphatics.

EPIDEMIOLOGY OF EAR MALIGNANCIES

Malignant diseases of the ear are rare.[17] Chronic otitis media was a predisposing factor in the past, but it is now an infrequent catalyst.[6,16] Tumors of the external ear are most often cutaneous malignancies and may have some correlation to solar exposure. Other predisposing factors described, although their significance is in question, are otorrhea, chronic eczema, chronic dermatologic conditions, and chronic ulcerations from trauma.[24]

Tumors of the external ear most commonly occur in patients between 50 and 80 years of age; tumors of the middle ear and the mastoid are more common in patients between the ages of 40 to 60. More women than men develop middle ear tumors, but more men have tumors of the external ear.[16,28]

CLINICAL PRESENTATION

External Ear

Basal cell carcinomas are more common than squamous cell carcinomas in the external ear. They present as small ulcerations, mostly on the helix.[1,3] Although metastasis to the lymphatics is possible, it is seen in fewer than 15% of the patients.[26,28]

External Auditory Canal

Most patients present with symptomatic lesions of the external canal. Pruritus and pain are very common. Swelling behind the ear, decreased hearing, and facial paralysis are seen in advanced cases. Spread of the tumor into the lymphatic areas is more common than to other areas of the ear. Tumors arising in the cartilaginous portion of the canal invade the cartilaginous walls and spread into the bony canal area. However, those aris-

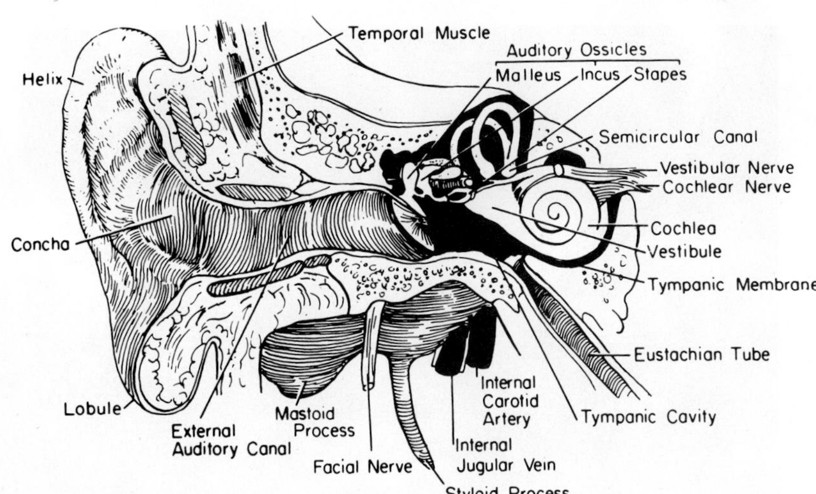

FIGURE 27–1. Anatomy of the ear. (Modified from Million RR, Cassisi NJ [eds]: Management of Head and Neck Cancer: A Multidisciplinary Approach. Philadelphia, JB Lippincott, 1984)

ing in the bony canal have a more effective barrier preventing spread and therefore progress predominantly along the main axis of the canal, eventually invading the middle ear or the cartilaginous part of the canal. Distant metastases are rarely seen with these tumors.

DIAGNOSTIC WORKUP

Table 27-1 summarizes diagnostic procedures. Plain radiography and computed tomography (CT) have now been replaced by high-resolution CT (Fig. 27-2).[5,24,34] The CT scan shows abnormal soft tissue, soft tissue enhancement, distortion of the normal tissue planes, and bone destruction. All areas of the temporal bone, infratemporal fossa, and base of the skull can be adequately evaluated using CT.[4] High-resolution CT scanning can help in determining the operability of tumors.[21] Except in selected cases, angiography and jugular venography have also been abandoned in favor of CT.

Diagnosis is always established by biopsy and occasionally by aspiration of the exudative material or by surgical exploration. A bone scan may be done to determine the changes in the temporal bone around the tumor, but this is very nonspecific information and is not a recommended method of evaluation.

PATHOLOGIC CLASSIFICATION

About 85% of the tumors involving the auditory canal, middle ear, and mastoid area are squamous cell carcinomas. Infrequently, basal cell carcinomas, adenocarcinomas, adenoid cystic carcinomas, and melanomas are seen.[14] Even rarer are sarcomas, specifically embryonic rhabdomyosarcomas. Ceruminous gland tumors and papillomas rarely arise in the auditory canal.[14,20,24,25] Only five cases of carcinoid tumor of the middle ear have been reported.[32] Certain groups of benign adenomas of the middle ear are now called "aggressive papillary middle ear tumors." They are distinct clinicopathologically and are characterized by slow growth but extensive local invasion and bone destruction.[9]

PROGNOSTIC FACTORS

Lesions of the external ear are usually more easily controlled than are lesions of the middle ear or mastoid. External ear lesions are usually diagnosed earlier, they are mostly cutaneous, and adequate surgery or radiation therapy is usually effective.[3] Large lesions involving the middle ear and those with extension into the temporal bone are usually the most difficult to treat. There does not appear to be a correlation between degree of tumor differentiation and survival.[13] Spread of tumors to the lymph nodes usually indicates a poor prognosis, because this is often a late event in the natural history of the disease.[26]

STAGING

Neither the American Joint Committee (AJC) nor the International Union Against Cancer (UICC) has a staging system for tumors of the ear. Stell and McCormick[33] have proposed a staging system using the UICC guidelines. In their study of 47 patients, they were able to correlate significant predictors with the proposed staging system (Table 27-2).

GENERAL MANAGEMENT

External Ear

Tumors of the external ear are most often treated with limited surgery or external radiation therapy. Treatment in early stages with irradiation is usually in the form of orthovoltage or electron-beam therapy.[12] Most techniques have been fairly successful in the treatment of lesions in this area. Surgery is beneficial if

TABLE 27–1
Diagnostic Evaluation for Carcinoma of the Ear

General
History
Physical examination
Otoscopy
Careful assessment of regional lymph nodes
Laboratory Tests
Complete blood count
Blood chemistry
Radiographic Studies
High-resolution computed tomography (standard)
Arteriography (optional)
Biopsy
Other Studies
Audiology testing

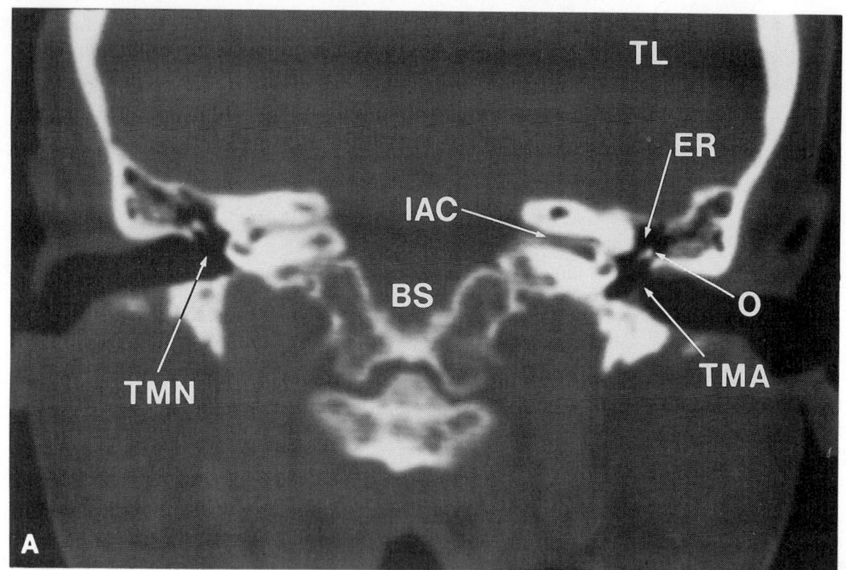
TL
ER
IAC
BS
O
TMN
TMA
A

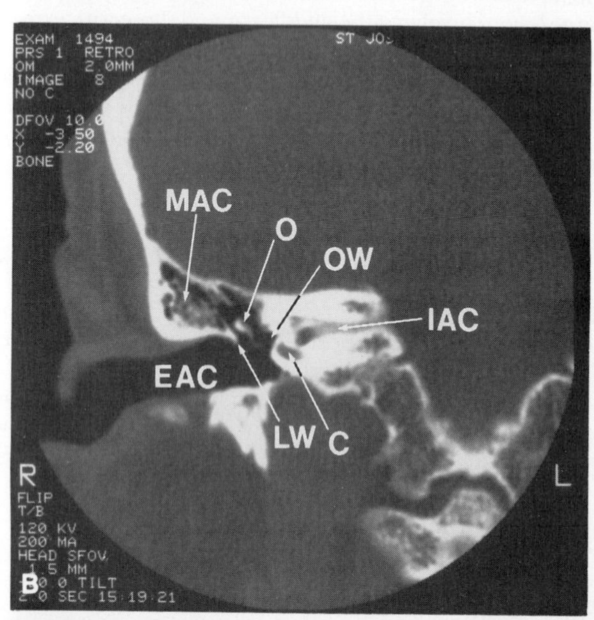
MAC
O
OW
IAC
EAC
LW
C
R
L
B

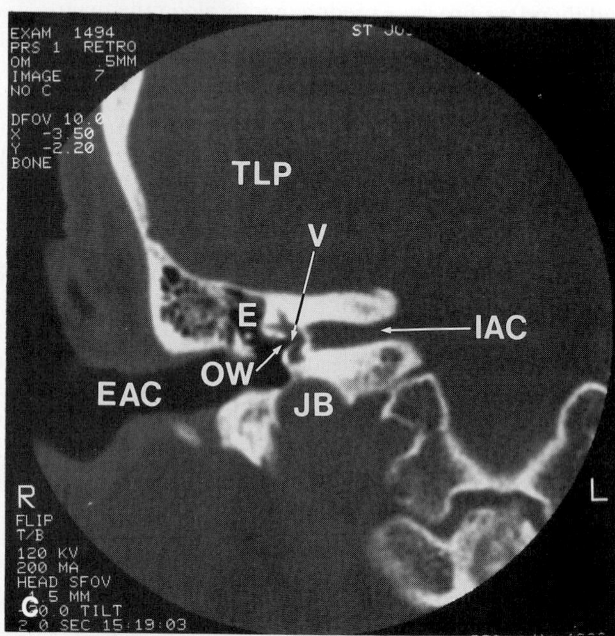
TLP
V
E
IAC
OW
EAC
JB
R
L
C

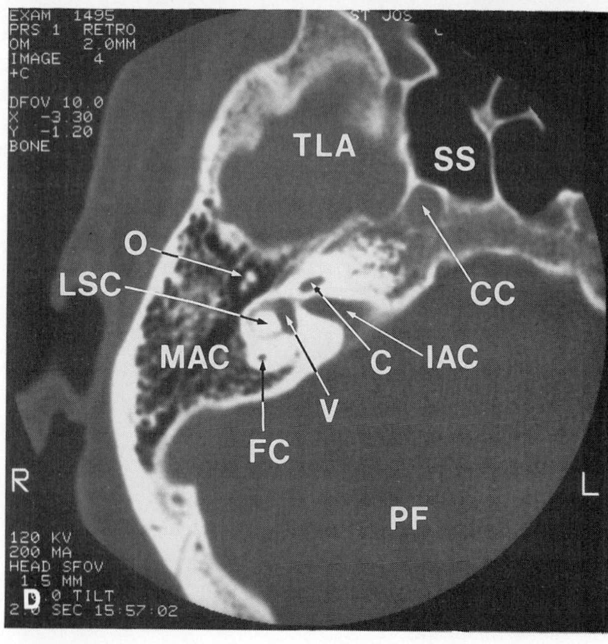
TLA
SS
O
LSC
CC
MAC
C
IAC
V
FC
PF
R
L
D

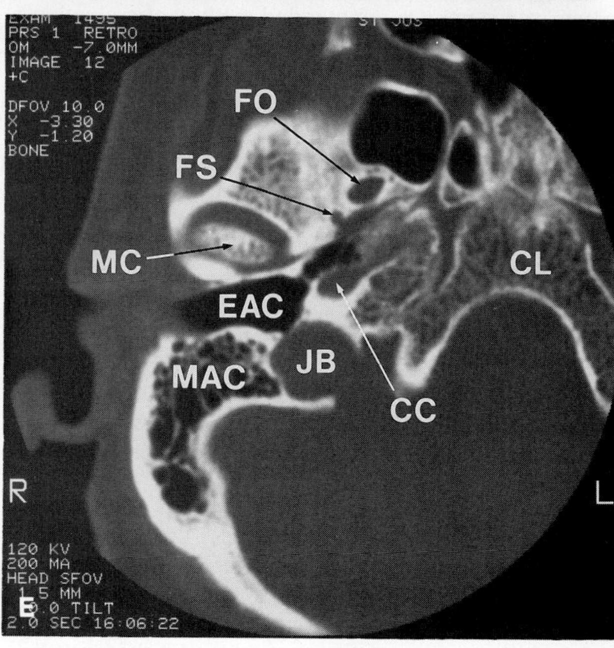
FO
FS
MC
CL
EAC
MAC
JB
CC
R
L
E

TABLE 27–2
Proposed Staging System for Tumors of the Ear

T1	Tumor limited to site of origin, with no facial nerve paralysis and no bone destruction detected radiographically
T2	Tumor extending beyond the site of origin indicated by facial paralysis or radiologic evidence of bone destruction, but no extension beyond the organ of origin
T3	Clinical or radiologic evidence of extension to surrounding structures (*e.g.*, dura, base of the skull, parotid gland, temporomandibular joint)
TX	Insufficient data for classification, including patients previously seen and treated elsewhere

(Stell PM, McCormick MS: J Laryngol Otol 99:847, 1985)

TABLE 27–3
Treatment of Carcinoma of the External Ear

	MODALITY	
RESULT*	SURGERY	IRRADIATION
Local control[3]	49/50 (98)†	42/45 (93)
Cure at 3 yr[26]	330/358 (92)	141/174 (81)
Local control at 2 yr[12]		35/43 (81)
Local control at 4 yr[19]		60/61 (99)

* *Reference to study indicated by superscript.*
† *Results given as number of successful outcomes/patient population (% response).*

the lesion has invaded the cartilage of the ear or extends medially into the auditory canal. If squamous cell carcinoma of the external ear is treated with surgery alone, there is a recurrence rate of 19%.[29] Advanced lesions involving a significant portion of the ear canal are managed with a combination of irradiation and surgery. Palmer and Snell[23] describe the use of radical soft tissue and subtotal temporal bone excision with deltopectoral flap coverage for extensive tumors of the auricular area.

Treatment of draining lymphatics is normally not required for early stages of external ear tumors.[3] Afzelius and associates[1] indicate that lesions over 4 cm and those with cartilage invasion have an increased risk of nodal spread; they recommend prophylactic neck dissection.[2] Most authors do not agree with this approach because the overall chance of lymph node involvement in tumors of the external ear is only 16%.

Interstitial irradiation using afterloading ^{192}Ir, particularly for tumors smaller than 4 cm, is also an effective method of treatment, affording excellent local control with good cosmesis (Table 27-3).[19]

Radical surgery and postoperative radiation therapy are the accepted methods of treatment for more advanced lesions of the external auditory canal and lesions in the middle ear and mastoid.[7,11,13,36] Except in tumors that are detected early, neither modality is considered optimal, and a combination of the two produces the best results.

Lesions of the outer part of the auditory canal require local excision with at least a 1-cm margin between the lesion and the tympanic membrane if there is no radiographic evidence of invasion of the mastoid. Surgery for tumors of the auditory canal is carried out through a U-shaped incision with elevation of the flap from below. A split-thickness skin graft is usually required to cover the deficit along the auditory canal.

When the tumor involves the bony auditory canal and impinges on the tympanic membrane but does not involve the middle ear or the mastoid, a partial temporal bone resection may be necessary; in this procedure the auditory canal, tympanic membrane, malleus, and incus are removed along with the temporomandibular joint, and the defect is grafted with a split-thickness skin graft.

Middle Ear

If the tumor involves the petrous process of the temporal bone, as happens with tumors involving the middle ear and mastoid area, a subtotal resection of the temporal bone is necessary.[2,8] In advanced tumors, a radical temporal bone resection with a combination intracranial-extracranial surgical approach is necessary.[2,8,10] All lesions that require temporal bone resection, either partial or complete, also require postoperative radiation therapy to improve the chances of local control.[7,11,30,35] The British literature seems to contradict the need for subtotal or radical temporal bone resection and contends that a radical mastoidectomy and postoperative radiation therapy may suffice.[27] Chemotherapy has not been beneficial in tumors involving the ear.

Palliative Radiation Therapy

Radiation therapy offers significant palliation in recurrent or advanced disease. Pain relief is reported in 61% of the patients with tumors of the auditory canal and middle ear.[22]

RADIATION THERAPY TECHNIQUES

Tumors involving the pinna can be treated with electrons or with superficial or orthovoltage irradiation. The fields can be round or polygonal, drawn around the tumor to spare surrounding normal tissues. For small superficial tumors, margins of 1 cm are adequate. However, more extensive lesions require larger portals, which may encompass the entire pinna or external canal and require 2-cm to 3-cm margins around the clinically apparent tumor (Fig. 27-3). Lesions involving the pinna must be treated with slow fractionation (180–200 cGy daily) to prevent cartilage necrosis. Doses of 6500 cGy are required over a period of 6.5 weeks to achieve adequate tumor control.

Large lesions of the external auditory canal are treated with

◀ *FIGURE 27–2.* Normal anatomy of the ear. (**A, B, C**) Coronal sections. (**D, E**) Transverse sections. BS, brain stem; c, cochlea; cc, carotid canal; CL, clivus; E, epitympanum; EAC, external auditory canal; ER, epitympanic recess; FC, facial canal; FO, foramen ovale; FS, foramen spinosum; IAC, internal auditory canal, JB, jugular bulb; LSC, lateral semicircular canal; LW, lateral wall, epitympanic recess (scutum); MAC, mastoid air cells; MC, mandibular condyle; OS, ossicles; OW, oval window; PF, posterior fossa; TLA, temporal lobe, anterior portion; TLP, temporal lobe, posterior portion; TMN, tympanic membrane, normal appearance; TMA, tympanic membrane, abnormally thickened; SS, sphenoid sinus; V, vestibule. (CT scans and text courtesy of Robert Gresick, M.D., DePaul Health Center, St. Louis, MO)

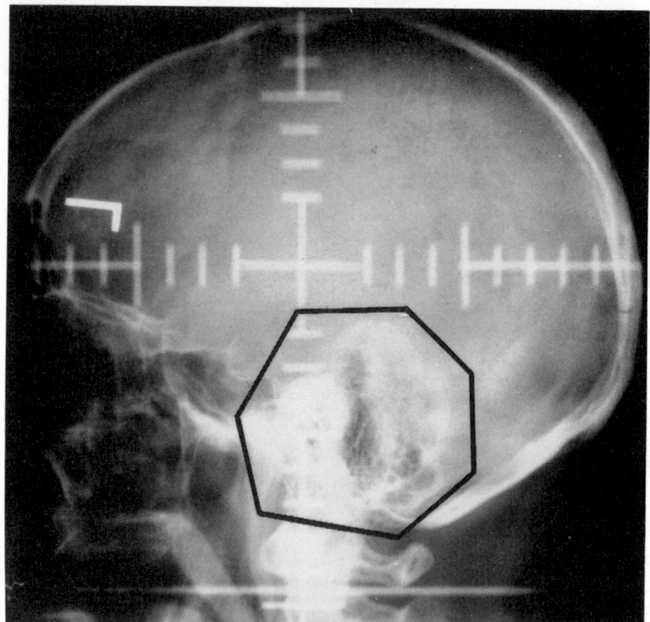

FIGURE 27–3. Example of treatment portal for tumor of the middle ear involving the petrous bone. The mastoid is included in irradiated volume.

irradiation alone or combined with surgery; the portals should encompass the entire ear and temporal bone with an adequate margin (3 cm). The volume treated should include the ipsilateral preauricular, postauricular, and subdigastric lymph nodes. Treating lymphatics beyond the jugulodigastric area is usually not necessary.

Extremely advanced tumors that are unresectable should be treated with high-energy ipsilateral electron-beam therapy (16–20 MeV) alone or mixed with photons (4–6 MV) or with wedge pair (superior inferiorly angled beams) techniques using low-energy photons. Doses of 6000 cGy to 7000 cGy over 6 to 7 weeks are required. Doses higher than this may produce osteoradionecrosis of the temporal bone. If access to various types of radiation therapy beams is available, individualized treatment plans should be devised (Fig. 27-4). Most patients receiving

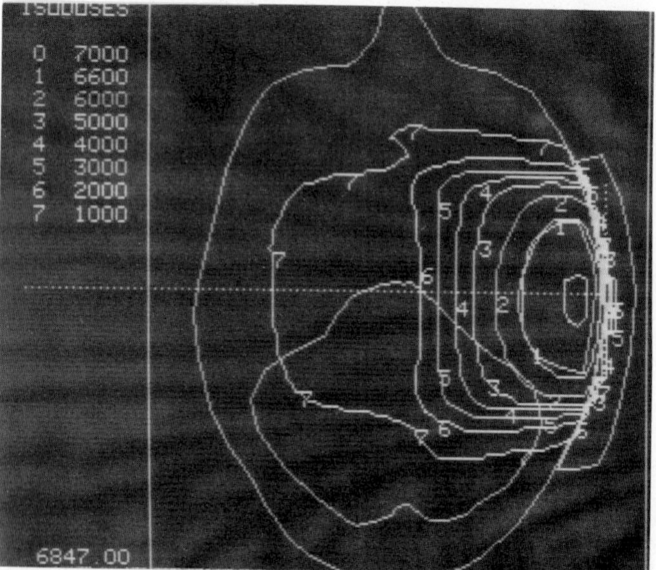

FIGURE 27–4. Computerized isodose distribution for treatment of a middle ear tumor using a combination of 4-MV photons (20%) and 16-MeV electrons (80%).

radiation therapy to the pinna or to the middle ear and temporal bone region do not require immobilization devices unless they are uncooperative, in which case an Aquaplast system or cast should be useful.

RESULTS AND COMPLICATIONS OF THERAPY

The series of patients reported from several institutions are small. Results of treatment with various modalities are shown in Tables 27-3 to 27-5. In more extensive lesions, combinations of surgery and irradiation have yielded satisfactory results. Overall 5-year survival rates with combination therapy for tumors involving the middle ear and external auditory canal range from 40% to 60%, with tumors in the earlier stages achieving a 70% survival rate at 5 years with no evidence of disease.

Data from Washington University (Fig. 27-5). suggest that the main determinant of survival is extent of disease at diagnosis.

Possible sequelae with surgery are hemorrhage, infection, loss of facial nerve function, and, rarely, carotid artery thrombosis. Occasionally, vertigo is reported after temporal bone resection. Vertigo may last for 2 weeks, and a period of unsteadiness may last for a few months. Permanent deafness usually occurs on the operated side.

Radiation therapy sequelae include cartilage necrosis of the external auditory canal and osteoradionecrosis of temporal bone.[3,37] Very rarely, secondary infection and meningitis are reported.[16] Because of the proximity of the brain stem and medulla oblongata, it is extremely difficult to deliver a high dose of radiation to the temporal bone without a significant risk of injury to these structures. An overall incidence of 10% bone necrosis could be expected after administration of 6000 cGy to 6500 cGy. After external ear lesions are treated with interstitial irradiation, there is a 4% incidence of late cutaneous and cartilage necrosis. Risk of necrosis increases for lesions over 4 cm.[19]

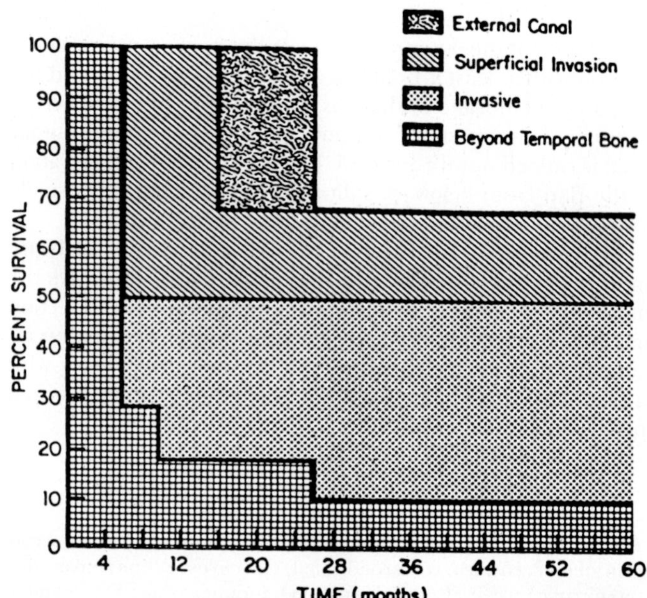

FIGURE 27–5. Data from 24 patients with tumors of middle ear and external auditory canal from Washington University demonstrate the association between survival with no evidence of disease and original extent of disease. (Lesser RW, Spector GJ, Devineni VR: Otolaryngol Head Neck Surg 96:43, 1987)

TABLE 27–4
Treatment of Carcinoma of the Middle Ear

	MODALITY		
INVESTIGATOR	SURGERY	RADIATION THERAPY	SURGERY AND RADIATION THERAPY
Sinha and Aziz[30]		1/7 (14)	6/15 (40)
Lewis[18]	8/28 (28.5)*		18/73 (25) preoperative 11/31 (35.5) postoperative
Lederman[14]		12/39 (31)	
Wang[36]			11/23 (48)
Sorensen[31]			5/11 (45)
Hahn and associates[11]			6/14 (43)†

** Results given as patients surviving 5 years/patient population (% response).*
† The rate of response becomes 55.6% if petrous bone was not involved.

TABLE 27–5
Treatment of Carcinoma of the External Auditory Canal

		MODALITY		
INVESTIGATOR	SURVIVAL (YR)	SURGERY	RADIATION THERAPY	SURGERY AND RADIATION THERAPY
Crabtree and associates[7]	5			9/21 (43%) E 2/14 (14%) A
Johns and Headington[13]	5			5/10 (50%) E 1/10 (10%) A
Hahn and colleagues[11]	5	3/4 (75%) E*		1/1 (100%) E
Lewis[16]	3	5/6 (83%) E 11/13 (85%) A		
Lederman[14]	5		6/25 (24%)	
Million and Cassisi[20]	2		4/5 (80%)	

** Results are given as patients surviving/patient population (% response).*
E, early stage; A, advanced stage.

REFERENCES

1. Afzelius L-E, Gunnarsson M, Nordgren H: Guidelines for prophylactic radical lymph node dissection in cases of carcinoma of the external ear. Arch Otolaryngol Head Neck Surg 2:361, 1980
2. Ariyan S, Sasaki CT, Spencer D: Radical en bloc resection of the temporal bone. Am J Surg 142:443, 1981
3. Avila J, Bosch A, Aristizabal S, et al: Carcinoma of the pinna. Cancer 40:2891, 1977
4. Bird CR, Hasso AN, Stewart CE, et al: Malignant primary neoplasms of the ear and temporal bone studies by high-resolution computed tomography. Radiology 149:171, 1983
5. Chakeres DW, Spiegel PK: A systematic technique for comprehensive evaluation of the temporal bone by computed tomography. Radiology 146:97, 1983
6. Conley J, Schuller DE: Malignancies of the ear. Laryngoscope 86:1147, 1976
7. Crabtree JA, Britton BH, Pierce MK: Carcinoma of the external auditory canal. Laryngoscope 86:405, 1976
8. Gacek RR, Goodman M: Management of malignancy of the temporal bone. Laryngoscope 87:1622, 1977
9. Gaffey MJ, Mills SE, Fechner RE, et al: Aggressive papillary middle-ear tumor. A clinicopathologic entity distinct from middle-ear adenoma. Am J Surg Pathol 12:790, 1988
10. Graham MD, Sataloff RT, Kemink JL, et al: Total en bloc resection of the temporal bone and carotid artery for malignant tumors of the ear and temporal bone. Laryngoscope 94:528, 1984
11. Hahn SS, Kim JA, Goodchild N, et al: Carcinoma of the middle ear and external auditory canal. Int J Radiat Oncol Biol Phys 9:1003, 1983
12. Hunter RD, Pereira DTM, Pointon RCS: Megavoltage electron beam therapy in the treatment of basal and squamous cell carcinomata of the pinna. Clin Radiol 33:341, 1982
13. Johns ME, Headington JT: Squamous cell carcinoma of the external auditory canal. A clinicopathologic study of 20 cases. Arch Otolaryngol 100:45, 1974
14. Lederman M: Malignant tumors of the ear. J Laryngol Otol 79:85, 1965
15. Lesser RW, Spector GJ, Devineni VR: Malignant tumors of the middle ear and external auditory canal: A 20-year review. Arch Otolaryngol Head Neck Surg 96:43, 1987
16. Lewis JS: A guide to cancer of the ear. CA 27:42, 1977
17. Lewis JS: Cancer of the external auditory canal, middle ear, and mastoid. In Suen JY, Myers EN (eds): Cancer of the Head and Neck, pp 557–575. New York, Churchill Livingstone, 1981
18. Lewis JS: Surgical management of tumors of the middle ear and mastoid. J Laryngol Otol 97:299, 1983
19. Mazeron J-J, Ghalie R, Zeller J, et al: Radiation therapy for carcinoma of the pinna using Iridium 192 wires: A series of 70 patients. Int J Radiat Oncol Biol Phys 12:1757, 1986
20. Million RR, Cassisi NJ (eds): Management of Head and Neck Cancer: A Multidisciplinary Approach. Philadelphia, JB Lippincott, 1984

21. Olsen KD, DeSanto LW, Forbes GS: Radiographic assessment of squamous cell carcinoma of the temporal bone. Laryngoscope 93:1162, 1983
22. Paaske PB, Witten J, Schwer S, Hansen HS: Results in treatment of carcinoma of the external auditory canal and middle ear. Cancer 59:156, 1987
23. Palmer JA, Snell GED: Surgical treatment of extensive tumors of the lateral face and auricular area by radical soft tissue and subtotal temporal bone excision with deltopectoral flap coverage. J Otolaryngol 8:531, 1979
24. Pulec JL: Glandular tumors of the external auditory canal. Laryngoscope 87:1601, 1977
25. Rogers KA Jr, Snow JB Jr: Squamous cell papilloma of the external auditory canal and middle ear treated with radiation therapy. Laryngoscope 78:2183, 1968
26. Schewe EJ Jr, Pappalardo C: Cancer of the external ear. Am J Surg 104:753, 1962
27. Shaheen OH: The management of tumours of the middle ear. J Laryngol Otol 97:313, 1983
28. Shiffman N: Squamous cell carcinomas of the skin of the pinna. Can J Surg 18:279, 1975
29. Shockley WW, Stucker FJ: Squamous cell carcinoma of the external ear: A review of 75 cases. Arch Otolaryngol Head Neck Surg 97:308, 1987
30. Sinha PP, Aziz HI: Treatment of carcinoma of the middle ear. Radiology 126:485, 1978
31. Sorensen H: Cancer of the middle ear and mastoid. Acta Radiol 54:460, 1960
32. Stanley MW, Horwitz CA, Levinson RM, Sibley RK: Carcinoid tumors of the middle ear. Am J Clin Pathol 87:592, 1987
33. Stell PM, McCormick MS: Carcinoma of the external auditory meatus and middle ear. Prognostic factors and a suggested staging system. J Laryngol Otol 99:847, 1985
34. Valvassori GE, Mafee MM, Dobben GD: Computerized tomography of the temporal bone. *Laryngoscope* 92:562–565, 1982
35. Wagenfeld DJH, Keane T, van Nostrand AWP, et al: Primary carcinoma involving the temporal bone. Analysis of twenty-five cases. Laryngoscope 90:912, 1980
36. Wang CC: Radiation therapy in the management of carcinoma of the external auditory canal, middle ear, or mastoid. Radiology 116:713, 1975
37. Wang CC, Doppke K: Osteoradionecrosis of the temporal bone: Consideration of nominal standard dose. Int J Radiat Oncol Biol Phys 1:881, 1976

28

○ ○ ○ • ● •

Nasopharynx

Carlos A. Perez

ANATOMY

The nasopharynx is roughly cuboidal, and its borders are the posterior choanae anteriorly, the body of the sphenoid superiorly, the clivus and the first two cervical vertebrae posteriorly, and the soft palate inferiorly (Fig. 28-1*A*). It is open to the nasal fossa anteriorly and to the oropharynx inferiorly but enclosed on all other sides. The lateral and posterior walls are composed of the pharyngeal fascia, which descends from its attachment at the base of the skull, located posteriorly at the pharyngeal tubercle of the basioccipital process and extending outward bilaterally along the undersurface of the apex of the petrous pyramid just medial to the carotid canal. The nasopharynx extends forward to the posterior surface of the medial pterygoid plate.[35]

The roof of the nasopharynx slopes downward and is continuous with the posterior wall. In this area, particularly in children, abundant lymphoid tissues underlie the mucosa and constitute the pharyngeal tonsil or adenoids.

The eustachian tube opens into the lateral wall of the nasopharynx. The posterior portion of the eustachian tube is cartilaginous and protrudes into the nasopharynx, making a ridge just posterior to the orifice called the torus tubarius. Just posterior to the torus is a recess called Rosenmüller's fossa (Fig. 28-1*B*).

The foramen lacerum, which opens directly into the middle cranial fossa, lies wholly within the boundaries of the nasopharynx. It is an important route by which nasopharyngeal cancer can spread into the middle cranial fossa. Many important foramina and fissures are located in the base of the skull, through which several structures pass (Fig. 28-2, Table 28-1); some provide routes of spread of nasopharyngeal carcinoma.

The lymphatics of the nasopharyngeal mucosa run in an anteroposterior direction to meet in the midline. From there they drain into a small group of nodes lying near the base of the skull in the space lateral and posterior to the pharynx, called the parapharyngeal or retropharyngeal space. The uppermost node of this group is called the node of Rouviere. The nodal group lies in close proximity to cranial nerves IX, X, XI, and XII, which run through the parapharyngeal space (Fig. 28-3*A*).

Another lymphatic pathway from the nasopharynx leads to the deep posterior cervical node at the confluence of the spinal accessory and jugular lymph node chains. Involvement of this node, which lies beneath the sternocleidomastoid muscle at the mastoid tip, is so characteristic of nasopharyngeal cancer that a mass in this region, even without other symptoms, should immediately lead the clinician to suspect cancer of the nasopharynx.[35]

A third pathway includes the jugulodigastric node, which according to Lederman[61] is as frequently involved in nasopharyngeal carcinoma as the upper deep cervical node (Fig. 28-3*B*).

EPIDEMIOLOGY

The incidence of carcinoma of the nasopharynx in the United States is 0.8 per 100,000 males and 0.3 per 100,000 females.[17] The male-to-female ratio is 2.4 : 1, and the peak incidence falls between ages 50 and 59, although at the Mallinckrodt Institute of Radiology, 30% of the patients were younger than 50 years.

The incidence of carcinoma of the nasopharynx is very high in southern China. In the provinces of Kwangtung, Kwangsi, and Fukien, rates as high as 20 per 100,000 have been reported.[29] The incidence remains high for descendants of southern Chinese living in other countries, suggesting a genetic predisposition to the disease.[11,84] A correlation between certain genetically determined human lymphocyte antigens (HLAs) and nasopharynx cancer supports this view.[93] On the other hand, two pieces of evidence speak for an environmental factor: among Chinese in the United States, the American-born second generation has a lower risk than the Asian-born first generation, and California whites born in southeast Asia have an increased risk compared with their American-born counterparts.[12,58] Dickson and Flores,[29] reporting 134 patients, noted that the annual incidence of nasopharyngeal carcinoma among Chinese born in Asia is 20.5 per 100,000 persons compared with 1.32 per 100,000 Canadian-born Chinese and 0.19 per 100,000 white Canadians.

Henderson and associates[40] synthesized the epidemiologic evidence by theorizing that there may be an environmental etiologic agent, but that the risk of cancer induction by this agent is modified by certain genetic determinants. They suggested that the environmental agent may be in the smoke from the wood fires used by the south Chinese for cooking. Ho[45] postulates that a more likely agent is a traditional southern Chinese food, salt-preserved fish, which has been shown to produce nasal and paranasal carcinomas in rats.[51] It has been suggested as a contributing factor in the increased incidence of nasopharyngeal carcinoma among Chinese, Icelanders, and Eskimos.[1,21,44,60] Occupations involving exposure to dust, smoke, and other inhalants have also been implicated.[62,63]

Levine and associates[63] examined the geographic distribu-

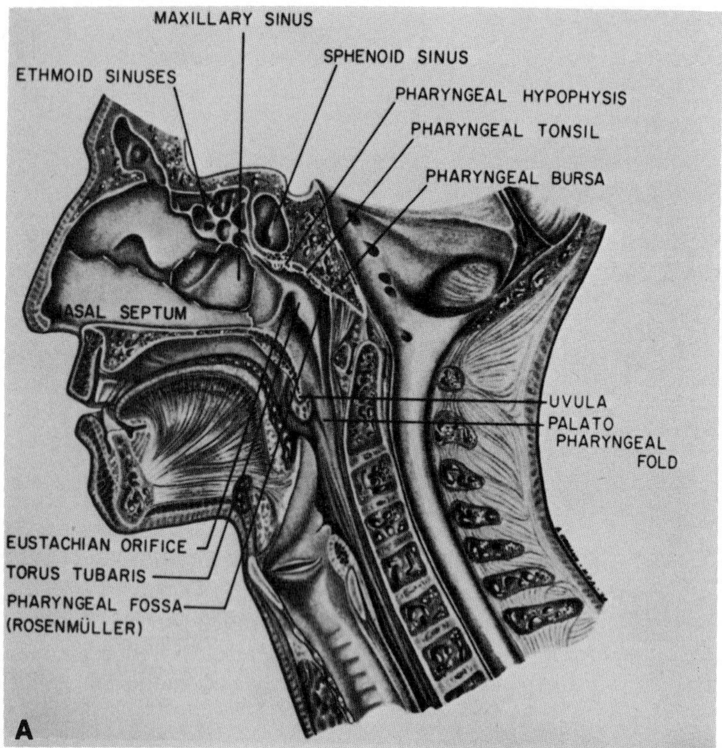

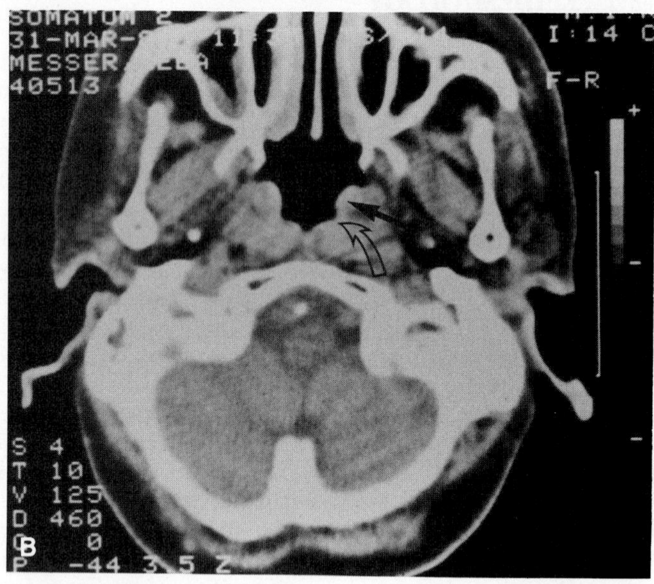

FIGURE 28–1. (**A**) Midsagittal section of the head, showing the nasopharynx and related structures. (Fletcher GH, Healey JR Jr, McGraw JP, Million RR: Nasopharynx. In MacComb WS, Fletcher GH [eds]: Cancer of the Head and Neck. Baltimore, Williams & Wilkins, 1967) (**B**) CT scan of base of skull demonstrating soft tissues of nasopharynx. The torus tubarius (*solid arrow*) and fossa of Rosenmüller (*open arrow*) are indicated on the scan. (Courtesy of Fred J. Hodges III, M.D.)

tion of persons dying of nasopharyngeal carcinoma in the United States based on 15,145 death certificates collected from 1950 through 1979. They observed a greater mortality among white males on the southeast Atlantic and Gulf Coasts. Comparing deaths from 1950 through 1969 and 1970 through 1979, they found no appreciable change in mortality rate for whites or blacks, but the incidence decreased among Chinese males, although the incidence in this group remains six times higher than that for any other ethnic group.

Complicating the epidemiologic picture are antibodies to the Epstein-Barr virus in the serum of patients with nasopharyngeal carcinoma but not in the serum of patients with other head and neck carcinomas.[42] There is also evidence that the epithelial cells of nasopharyngeal carcinoma harbor the Epstein-Barr virus genome.[50] Whether the Epstein-Barr virus is independently associated with nasopharyngeal carcinoma or whether it acts as a carcinogen or cocarcinogen is an unresolved issue.

NATURAL HISTORY

Carcinoma of the nasopharynx frequently arises from the lateral wall, with a predilection for the fossa of Rosenmüller; another common area of origin is the roof of the nasopharynx. The tumor may involve the mucosa or grow predominantly in the submucosa, invading adjacent tissues including the nasal cavity. In more advanced stages, the tumor may involve the oropharynx, particularly the lateral or posterior wall.

The upward extension of the tumor through the basilar foramen involves cranial nerves and destroys the middle fossa. The floor of the sphenoid may occasionally show radiographic

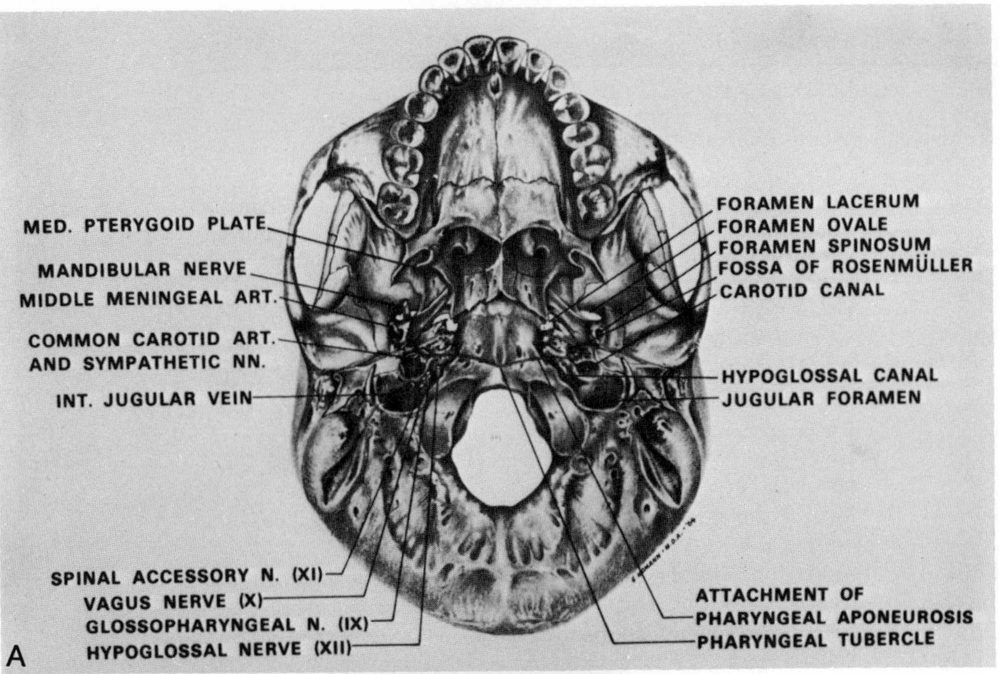

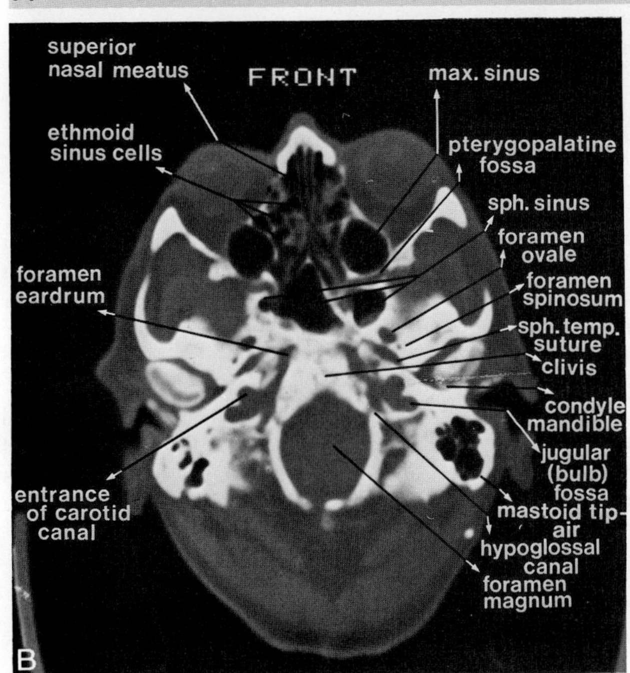

FIGURE 28–2. (**A**) Basal view of skull illustrating the foramina of the base of the skull on the right and the structures occupying these foramina on the left. (Fletcher GH, Healey JR Jr, McGraw JP, Million RR: Nasopharynx. In MacComb WS, Fletcher GH [eds]: Cancer of the Head and Neck. Baltimore, Williams & Wilkins, 1967) (**B**) CT scan of the base of the skull illustrating bony anatomy. (Courtesy of Fred J. Hodges III, M.D.)

evidence of destruction or sclerotic appearance. In approximately 5% of patients, the lesion may extend into the posterior or medial walls of the maxillary antrum and the ethmoids.[2,78]

The nasopharynx has a rich submucosal lymphatic network, and cervical lymph node involvement occurs early in the course of the disease. Approximately 90% of the patients develop lymphadenopathy, which is present in about 60% at the time of initial diagnosis.[64] Mesic and co-workers[68] reported cervical lymphadenopathy at presentation in 213 (85%) of 251 patients; of those, 103 (48%) had bilateral lymph node involvement. Involvement of a lymph node at the tip of the mastoid is quite frequent in nasopharyngeal carcinoma, followed by involvement of the upper, midcervical, and posterior cervical lymph nodes (Fig. 28-4).[79]

The incidence of distant metastases has no relationship to the stage of the primary tumor but correlates strongly with the degree of cervical lymph node involvement, ranging from 25% to 50% for patients with advanced cervical lymph node disease (Table 28-2).[7,15,46] Petrovich and associates[81] reported that 11 (17%) of 193 patients with N0 necks developed metastatic disease compared with 69 (74%) of 93 patients with N3 cervical lymphandenopathy. The most frequent site of distant metastases is bone, followed closely by lung and liver.[56,103]

CLINICAL PRESENTATION

Tumor growing into the posterior nasal fossa can produce symptoms of nasal stuffiness, discharge, or epistaxis. Sometimes the voice takes on a nasal quality (nasal twang) from loss of normal nasal and nasopharyngeal resonance. The orifice of the eustachian tube can be obstructed by a relatively small tumor;

TABLE 28–1
Foramina of the Base of Skull and Associated Anatomic Structures

FORAMEN	STRUCTURES
Cribriform plate (ethmoid)	Olfactory nerve and anterior ethmoidal nerve
Optic foramen	Optic nerve and ophthalmic artery
Superior orbital fissure	Third (oculomotor), fourth (trochlear) and sixth (abducent) cranial nerves, and ophthalmic division of fifth (trigeminal) nerve; ophthalmic vein; orbital branch of middle meningeal and recurrent branch of lacrimal arteries; sympathetic plexus, some filaments from carotid plexus
Foramen rotundum	Maxillary division of trigeminal nerve to pterygopalatine fossa
Foramen ovale	Mandibular division of trigeminal nerve; accessory meningeal artery; lesser superficial petrosal nerve
Foramen lacerum	Upper portion: internal carotid; sympathetic carotid plexus Lower portion: vidian nerve; meningeal branch of ascending pharyngeal artery; emissary vein
Foramen spinosum	Middle meningeal artery and vein; recurrent branch of mandibular nerve
Internal acoustic meatus	Seventh (facial) and eighth (auditory) nerves; internal auditory artery from basilar artery
Jugular foramen	Anterior portion: inferior petrosal sinus Posterior portion: Transverse sinus; meningeal branches from occipital and ascending pharyngeal arteries Intermediate portion: ninth (glossopharyngeal), tenth (vagus), and eleventh (spinal accessory) nerves
Hypoglossal canal	Hypoglossal nerve; meningeal branch of ascending pharyngeal artery
Foramen magnum	Spinal cord; spinal accessory nerve; vertebral vessels; anterior and posterior spinal vessels

hence ear pain or a unilateral decrease in hearing can occur early in the course of the disease. Blockage of the eustachian tube can produce a middle ear transudate, and fluid in the ear for any length of time should prompt a thorough investigation for a primary nasopharyngeal tumor. The association of decreased hearing, impaired movement of the soft palate, and mandibular neuralgia sometimes seen in these patients is called Trotter's triad. The presenting symptoms of nasopharyngeal carcinoma are given in Table 28-3.

Headache or pain in the temporal or occipital region can be caused by destruction of the base of the skull. Proptosis is sometimes the result of direct extension of tumor into the orbit from the posterior nasal fossa by way of the ethmoid air cells or from the cavernous sinus through the superior orbital fissure. Sore throat can occur when the tumor extends downward to involve the oropharynx.

Although a neck mass is the symptom that elicits medical attention in only 18% to 44% of the cases (Table 28-3), clinical involvement of cervical lymph nodes at presentation ranges from 62% to 87%.[7,36,47,61,106]

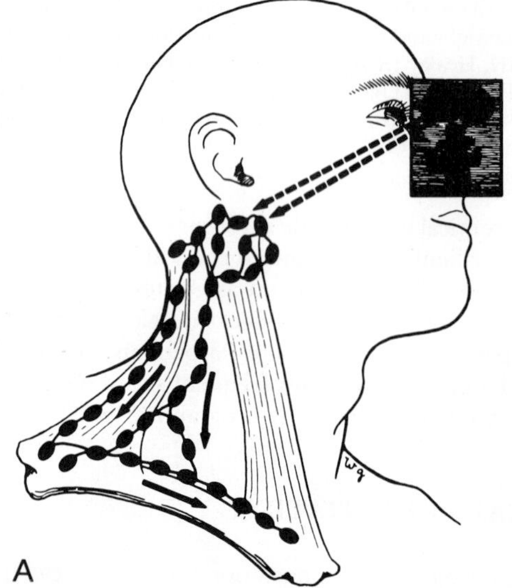

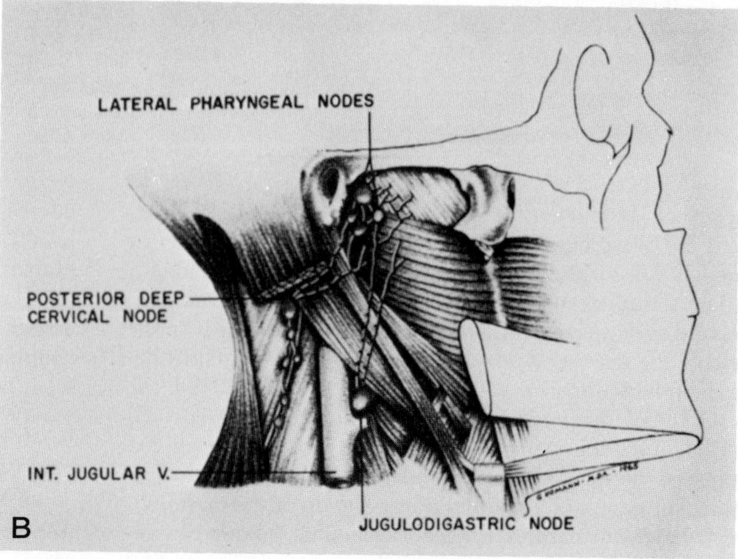

FIGURE 28–3. (**A**) Pathways for the lymphatic spread of carcinoma of the nasopharynx. (Batsakis JG: Tumors of the Head and Neck, 2nd ed. Baltimore, Williams & Wilkins, 1979) (**B**) Major lymphatic drainage of the nasopharynx illustrating drainage to subdigastric and posterior cervical lymph nodes. (Fletcher GH, Healey JR Jr, McGraw JP, Million RR: Nasopharynx. In MacComb WS, Fletcher GH [eds]: Cancer of the Head and Neck. Baltimore, Williams & Wilkins, 1967)

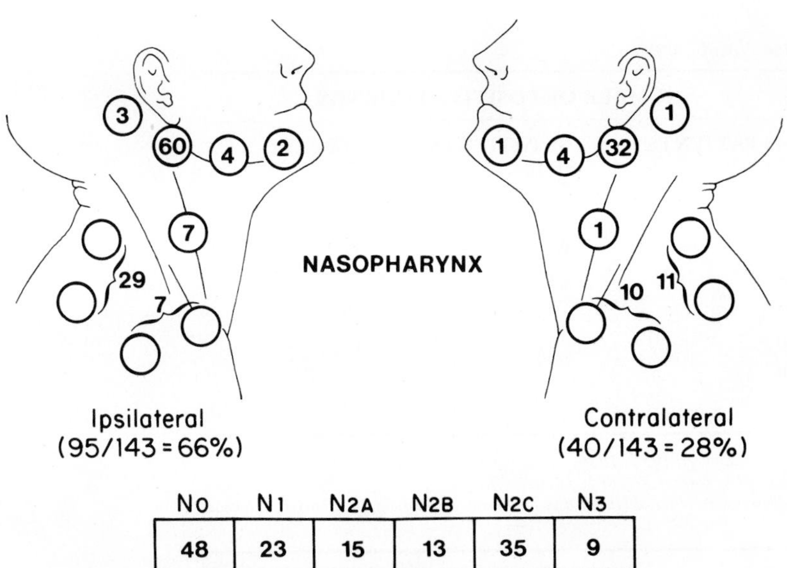

FIGURE 28–4. Distribution of clinically positive nodes and N stage on admission for patients with carcinoma of nasopharynx treated at Mallinckrodt Institute of Radiology. (Perez CA, Devineni, VR, Marcial-Vega V, Simpson JR: Int J Radiat Oncol Biol Phys, submitted for publication)

Cranial Nerve Involvement

Some patients with nasopharyngeal carcinoma may present with cranial nerve involvement (Table 28-4).

In Lederman's series of 218 patients, 26% had cranial nerve involvement, but in only 3% was this involvement the cause of the presenting symptoms.[61] Examination of the relative frequency of cranial nerve involvement in this series showed a preponderance of involvement of cranial nerves III through VI and IX through XII. In 15% of the patients reported in later series, the fifth cranial nerve was most frequently impaired, followed by the sixth cranial nerve (Table 28-4).[2,73,102] Mesic and associates[68] described cranial nerve involvement in 22 (8.8%) of 251 patients with epithelial nasopharyngeal tumors.

Cranial nerves III through VI are involved by tumor extension through the foramen lacerum to the cavernous sinus. The foramen ovale and carotid canal also provide access to these nerves. Involvement of cranial nerves III through VI is sometimes referred to as the *petrosphenoidal syndrome* because the foramina leading to these nerves are in the region of the junction of the petrous and sphenoid portions of the temporal bone (Fig. 28-2). The first nerve to be involved is the sixth cranial nerve, followed by the third, the first and second division of the fifth, and the fourth. A deficit of the third division of cranial nerve V may also be seen if the involvement is at the level of the gasserian ganglion. The clinical manifestations are unilateral ptosis from paralysis of cranial nerve III and complete ophthalmoplegia from the loss of cranial nerves III, IV, and VI. Unilateral pain followed by anesthesia in the supraorbital and superior maxillary regions occurs after the involvement of the first and second divisions of cranial nerve V. Unilateral amaurosis may be caused by ophthalmoplegia or direct involvement of the optic nerve.

Cranial nerves IX, X, XI, and XII, as they emerge from the base of the skull into the parapharyngeal space, can be compressed by involved parapharyngeal nodes. Compression can also result from direct extension of a primary tumor in Rosenmüller's fossa, which is near the parapharyngeal space (Fig. 28-1). Involvement of these nerves is sometimes called *syndrome of the retroparotid space* (Villaret's syndrome). Its clinical manifestations include swallowing difficulty from hemiparesis of the superior constrictor muscle (cranial nerve IX) and soft palate (cranial nerve X); hypoesthesia or anesthesia of the mucous membranes in the soft palate, pharynx, and larynx (cranial nerve X); aberrant sense of taste (cranial nerve IX); paralysis of the trapezius and sternocleidomastoid muscles (cranial nerve XI); and paralysis and atrophy of one side of the tongue (cranial nerve XII). There may also be unilateral Horner's syndrome caused by compression of the cervical sympathetic nerve.

Cranial nerves I, VII, and VIII are rarely involved. The first cranial nerve is a great distance from the nasopharynx, and cranial nerves VII and VIII are protected by the temporal bone throughout their intracranial course. For easy reference, the functions of the cranial nerves are described in Table 28-5.

DIAGNOSTIC WORKUP

In addition to a complete history and physical examination, the workup of a patient suspected of having a neoplasm of the pharynx should include a detailed evaluation of the extent of disease in the pharynx, an assessment of the extent of neck node metastases, a search for distant metastases, and biopsies of the nasopharynx and adjacent suspicious areas. Table 28-6 lists the diagnostic procedures included in this workup.

Visual assessment of tumor extent can be obtained by indirect nasopharyngoscopy. In many patients adequate visualization by the indirect method is not possible unless the soft palate is retracted forward by means of a rubber catheter inserted in the nose and retrieved through the mouth.[23] Evaluation of the extent of the tumor in the nasopharynx should include digital examination of the oropharynx and hypopharynx, a thorough testing of all cranial nerves, and inspection of the tympanic membranes. Blind biopsies with a special curved biopsy forceps can be accomplished with topical anesthesia.[72,98]

TABLE 28–2
Distant Metastasis and Cervical Lymph Node Involvement in Nasopharyngeal Carcinoma

	DISTANT METASTASIS (%)			
INVESTIGATION	N0	N1	N2	N3
Bedwinek[7]	17	25	38	55
Mesic[68]	7	9.6	30	40
Petrovich[81]	17	18	33	74
Perez et al[79]	17	17	37	30.7

TABLE 28–3
Presenting Symptoms in Carcinoma of the Nasopharynx

	NUMBER OF POSITIVE FINDINGS		
PRESENTING SYMPTOM	143 PATIENTS* (%)	82 PATIENTS† (%)	218 PATIENTS‡ (%)
Nasal discharge or obstruction	37	27	38
Ear pain or hearing loss	43	29	17
Neck mess	35	44	18
Cranial nerve deficit	24		3
Pain or headache	40		12
Bleeding	29		
Other	31		12

** Series from Perez CA et al: Mallinckrodt Institute of Radiology, 1956–1986.*
† Series reported in Hoppe RT, Goffinet DR, Bagshaw MA: Cancer 37:2605, 1976.
‡ Series reported in Lederman M: Cancer of the Nasopharynx: Its Natural History and Treatment. Springfield, IL, Charles C Thomas, 1961.

Inspection of the nasopharynx and visually directed biopsies can be performed on patients under general anesthesia by means of fixed or flexible endoscopy.

Because hearing can be affected by the primary tumor and by its radiotherapeutic treatment, baseline audiologic testing is desirable.

A thorough radiographic evaluation of the extent of the primary tumor must be carried out. Because determination of bone destruction is crucial to staging, treatment planning, and prognosis, tomographic techniques should be used instead of plain films, because tomography is more likely to reveal bone destruction or the presence of a soft tissue mass.[113] High-resolution computed tomography (CT) with contiguous cuts is superior to conventional tomography (Table 28-7).[38] Yamashita and associates[116] reported that ten of 17 patients with previously staged T1 or T2 tumors had the lesions upstaged by the CT findings.

Dillon and co-workers[30] analyzed radiographic studies of 12 patients with nasopharyngeal abnormalities and 30 patients with normal nasopharyngeal anatomy. They concluded that magnetic resonance imaging (MRI) was superior to CT in displaying both superficial and deep nasopharyngeal soft tissues, in distinguishing tumor from surrounding normal soft tissues, and in permitting more detailed analysis of the retropharyngeal and deep cervical lymph nodes. Bones, subtle abnormalities of the base of the skull, and calcification were better shown by CT.

Evaluation of Neck Metastases

In addition to palpating both sides of the entire neck, carefully palpate beneath the sternocleidomastoid muscle just below the mastoid tip and above the head of the clavicle, because lymph nodes in these areas can be easily missed. The size and location of each palpable lymph node should be recorded with a judgment about whether it is fixed or mobile. Because the determination of fixation is subjective, the degree of fixation as a staging determinant has been replaced by nodal size in the new American Joint Committee (AJC) staging system.[5]

TABLE 28–4
Incidence of Cranial Nerve Involvement at Initial Presentation of Nasopharyngeal Carcinoma

CRANIAL NERVE	214 PATIENTS* (%)	58 PATIENTS† (%)	143 PATIENTS‡ (%)
I		0.5	
II	3.3	4	1.3
III	10.7	9	3.5
IV	7	8	2.8
V	64	16	7.7
VI	57.9	14	15.4
VII	3.7	3	4.2
VIII	0.9	1	5.6
IX	7	6	2.1
X	8.9	9	5.6
XI	3.3	8	1.3
XII	18.7	6	5.6

** Series from Hsu MM, Tu SM: Cancer 62:362, 1983.*
† Series from Lederman M: Cancer of the Nasopharynx: Its Natural History and Treatment. Springfield, IL, Charles C Thomas, 1961.
‡ Series from Perez CA, et al: Mallinckrodt Institute of Radiology, 1956–1986.

TABLE 28-5
Functions of the Cranial Nerves

CRANIAL NERVE	TYPE OF NERVE	FUNCTIONS
I. Olfactory	Sensory	Smell
II. Optic	Sensory	Vision
III. Oculomotor	Motor	Eye movements: innervates all extraocular muscles except the superior oblique and lateral rectus muscles (see N. IV and VI) Innervates the striated muscle of the eyelid Contains autonomic fibers that mediate pupillary constriction and accommodation of lens for near vision
IV. Trochlear	Motor	Eye movements: innervates superior oblique muscle
V. Trigeminal	Mixed	Sensory: mediates cutaneous and proprioceptive sensations from skin, muscles, and joints in the face and mouth, and sensory innervation of the teeth Motor: innervates muscles of mastication
VI. Abducens	Motor	Eye movements: innervates lateral rectus muscle
VII. Facial	Mixed	Motor: innervates muscles of facial expression Sensory: mediates taste sensation from the anterior ⅔ of the tongue
VIII. Vestibulocochlear	Sensory	Audition Equilibrium, postural reflexes, orientation of the head in space
IX. Glossopharyngeal	Mixed	Contains autonomic axons that innervate the parotid gland Swallowing: mediates visceral sensations from the palate and posterior third of the tongue Innervates the carotid body Innervates taste buds in posterior third of the tongue
X. Vagus	Mixed	Contains autonomic fibers that innervate smooth muscle in heart, blood vessels, trachea, bronchi, esophagus, stomach, and intestine Innervates striated muscles in the larynx and pharynx and controls speech Mediates visceral sensation from the pharynx, larynx, thorax, and abdomen Innervates taste buds in the epiglottis
XI. Spinal accessory	Motor	Motor innervation of trapezius and sternocleidomastoid muscles
XII. Hypoglossal	Motor	Motor innervation of intrinsic muscles of the tongue

(Kandel ER, Schwartz JH [eds]: Principles of Neural Science, 2nd ed. New York, Elsevier Science Publishing, 1985)

Search for Distant Metastases

Before beginning a definitive course of treatment, carry out a reasonable search for distant metastases, intelligently guided by a careful history and physical examination and by two essential screening procedures: a chest radiograph and liver function chemistries. A bone scan should be performed only if bone pain or tenderness is present or if there is an elevation of the heat-labile fraction of alkaline phosphatase. Radiographs of any "hot" areas on the bone scan may help to clarify their significance. A liver scan is prompted by right upper quadrant abdominal pain, an enlarged liver on palpation, or elevation of any of the liver chemistries. A brain scan is not indicated unless there are neurologic signs and symptoms that cannot be attributed to the known extent of the primary tumor.

In 21 of 56 patients with undifferentiated carcinoma of the nasopharynx, Micheau and associates[70] found evidence of metastases in transiliac bone marrow biopsies. Radioisotope bone scans were abnormal for all 56 patients, even those with normal bone biopsy results. Eight of the patients had osteolytic bony metastases; three had osteosclerotic, and ten had mixed type. Most primary lesions were staged as T2, T3, or T4N3 tumors. Eighteen of the patients also had visceral metastases (three in liver and 15 in lung).

TUMOR ASSESSMENT AND PROGNOSIS

Staging

Many staging systems have been applied to carcinoma of the nasopharynx (Table 28-8). This multiplicity of staging systems makes comparing results from different institutions extremely difficult. The latest staging system and the one used widely is the AJC TNM system (Table 28-9 and Fig. 28-5).

TABLE 28–6
Diagnostic Workup for Nasopharyngeal Cancer

GENERAL

History
Physical examination: careful palpation to determine extent of primary tumor and neck node metastases, testing of cranial nerves, and inspection of tympanic membranes

SPECIAL TESTS

Indirect and direct nasopharyngoscopy
Biopsies
Baseline audiologic testing (as clinically indicated)

RADIOGRAPHIC STUDIES

Standard
- Chest radiograph
- Computed tomography (CT) or magnetic resonance scans

Complementary
- CT scan of paranasal sinuses can show involvement of nasal fossa or paranasal sinuses
- Bone scan, only if indicated by pain or tenderness or elevation of heat-labile fraction of alkaline phosphatase
- Bone radiographs, only if indicated by abnormal bone scan or symptoms
- Liver scan, only if indicated by right upper quadrant pain, enlarged liver by palpation, or elevation of liver chemistries

LABORATORY STUDIES

Blood counts
Blood chemistry profile
Liver function studies

Pathologic Classification

Approximately 90% of malignant tumors arising in the nasopharynx are epidermoid or undifferentiated carcinomas. The other 10% are mainly lymphomas but also include plasmacytomas, tumors of minor salivary gland origin, melanomas, rhabdomyosarcomas, and chordomas.[25,78,98]

Because investigators have used different classification systems that recognize some of these entities but not others and because the criteria for designating each of these entities may differ, the histologic classification of carcinoma of the nasopharynx is imprecise. For instance, some reports discriminate only two varieties, squamous cell carcinoma and lymphoepithelioma; others recognize three varieties.[15,78] Within the category of epidermoid and undifferentiated carcinoma, four morphologic entities have been described: squamous cell carcinoma, transitional cell carcinoma, lymphoepithelioma, and undifferentiated carcinoma. Bauer[4] suggested that carcinoma of all head and neck sites be divided into keratinizing and nonkeratinizing types, the former characterized by the formation of keratin pearls or intracellular keratin and the latter by the total absence of keratin formation. Squamous cell carcinoma is classified as a keratinizing carcinoma, and transitional cell carcinoma, lymphoepithelioma, and undifferentiated carcinoma fall under the heading of nonkeratinizing carcinoma. Table 28-10 outlines this classification scheme and shows histologic distribution according to different authors.

Hsu and associates[48] proposed a slight modification of the World Health Organization classification, separating the nonkeratinizing and undifferentiated carcinomas from the spindle cell variant, the round cell form, and mixed cell carcinoma. They found a better prognostic correlation using this classification; however, this subtyping of tumors is not customarily done.

Lymphoepithelioma, originally described by Schmincke,[91] consists of poorly differentiated cells with large nuclei, large nucleoli, and poorly defined cytoplasmic borders, causing the formation of syncytial masses. Interspersed are many small lymphocytes. Bauer[4] pointed out that a tumor in one area may fit perfectly the classical pattern of lymphoepithelioma, but that in another area, the same tumor may have a histologic picture closer to that of a poorly differentiated, nonkeratinizing carcinoma. Some reports indicate that lymphoepithelioma confers a higher local control rate and overall better prognosis than squamous cell carcinoma.[15,47,100] Other reviews, however, indicate that the prog-

TABLE 28–7
Radiographic Findings in Carcinoma of the Nasopharynx

	NUMBER OF POSITIVE FINDINGS		
FINDINGS	PLAIN FILMS (96 PATIENTS)	LINEAR TOMOGRAPHY (70 PATIENTS)	COMPUTED TOMOGRAPHY (40 PATIENTS)
Soft tissue mass	66 (69%)	59 (84%)	36 (90%)
Opacification of sphenoid sinus	18 (19%)	30 (43%)	10 (25%)
Bone destruction, base of skull	13 (14%)	28 (40%)	9 (23%)
Destruction of floor of sphenoid	7 (7%)	18 (26%)	8 (20%)
Opacification of nasal cavity/paranasal sinus	11 (11%)	22 (31%)	6 (15%)
Maxillary sinus involvement	12 (13%)	11 (16%)	4 (10%)
Oropharyngeal involvement	11 (11%)	9 (13%)	5 (13%)
Abnormality of foramina of base of skull	4 (4%)	3 (4%)	2 (5%)
Parapharyngeal lymph nodes	0	0	2 (5%)
Cervical lymph nodes	0	0	7 (18%)
Clivus abnormalities	5 (5%)	12 (17%)	7 (18%)
Pterygoid fossa involvement	3 (3%)	5 (7%)	3 (8%)
Nasal involvement	2 (2%)	6 (9%)	1 (3%)

(Unpublished data from Perez CA: Mallinckrodt Institute of Radiology, 1956–1986)

TABLE 28–8
Staging Systems Used for Primary Tumors of the Nasopharynx

	STAGE			
SYSTEM	T1	T2	T3	T4
UICC, 1968[101]	Tumor limited to one site within the nasopharynx	Tumor extending into two sites within the nasopharynx	Tumor extending beyond the nasopharynx without bone destruction	Tumor extending beyond the nasopharynx with bone involvement including the eustachian tube
AJC, 1988[5]	Tumor limited to one site within the nasopharynx	Tumor extending into two sites within the nasopharynx	Tumor extending into nasal fossa or oropharynx	Bone destruction or cranial nerve involvement
M.D. Anderson[36]	Tumor less than 1 cm in diameter	Tumor greater than 1 cm but confined to nasopharynx	Tumor extending beyond nasopharynx without base of skull or cranial nerve involvement	Tumor involving base of skull or cranial nerves
Ho[45]	Tumor confined to the nasopharynx	Tumor extending into nasal fossa or oropharynx or involvement below the base of the skull	Bone involvement; cranial nerve involvement; or involvement of orbits, hypopharynx, or infratemporal fossa	
Perez[78] modification of the UICC system	Tumor confined to the nasopharynx	Tumor extending into nasal fossa or oropharynx or radiographic involvement of the sphenoid sinus	Tumor extending below the oropharynx, cranial nerve involvement, or bone destruction	Massive tumor with two or more of the characteristics of a T3 lesion

nosis of lymphoepithelioma is no better than that of undifferentiated carcinoma or squamous carcinoma.[91,97,119]

Transitional cell carcinoma is an archaic term used to describe a nonkeratinizing carcinoma that resembles a lymphoepithelioma without the lymphocytic infiltrate.

TABLE 28–9
American Joint Committee TNM Staging System for Nasopharyngeal Carcinoma

PRIMARY TUMOR	
T1	Tumor limited to one subsite of nasopharynx
T2	Tumor invades more than one subsite of nasopharynx
T3	Tumor invades nasal cavity and/or oropharynx
T4	Tumor invades skull and/or cranial nerve(s)
NECK NODES	
NX	Regional lymph nodes cannot be assessed
N0	No regional lymph node metastasis
N1	Metastasis in a single ipsilateral lymph node, 3 cm or less in greatest dimension
N2	Metastasis in a single ipsilateral lymph node, more than 3 cm but not more than 6 cm in greatest dimension, or in multiple ipsilateral lymph nodes, none more than 6 cm in greatest dimension, or in bilateral or contralateral lymph nodes, none more than 6 cm in greatest dimension
N2a	Metastasis in a single ipsilateral lymph node more than 3 cm but not more than 6 cm in greatest dimension
N2b	Metastasis in multiple ipsilateral lymph nodes, none more than 6 cm in greatest dimension
N2c	Metastasis in bilateral or contralateral lymph nodes, none more than 6 cm in greatest dimension
N3	Metastasis in a lymph node more than 6 cm in greatest dimension
METASTASES	
MX	Presence of distant metastasis cannot be assessed
M0	No distant metastasis
M1	Distant metastasis

(Beahrs OH, Henson DE, Hutter RVP, Myers MH [eds]: Manual for Staging of Cancer, 3rd ed, pp 33–35. Philadelphia, JB Lippincott, 1988)

Adenoid cystic carcinoma of the nasopharynx is extremely rare. Conley and Dingman[20] reported 134 adenoid cystic carcinomas in the head and neck; only five (3.7%) arose in the nasopharynx. Yin and associates[120] discovered this histologic type in seven (0.5%) of 1379 patients with nasopharyngeal carcinoma. This tumor is characterized by slow growth, and it has a tendency to infiltrate along the peripheral nerves.[120] Six (85%) of seven patients treated with definitive radiation therapy survived 5 years without evidence of tumor, and three (50%) of six survived 10 years.[120] Metastases to cervical lymph nodes developed in two (20%) of ten patients, and the lymph nodes responded to radiation therapy. Because of this, Yin and associates[120] recommend radiation therapy but not prophylactic neck irradiation.

Most lymphomas of the nasopharynx are large cell types. A few other sarcomas arising from embryonal, vascular, or connective tissue may be observed.[25]

Prognostic Factors

Race, age, and gender frequently do not convey prognostic significance.[2,18,105] However, Perez and co-workers[78] reported a 45% 5-year survival rate in patients younger than 50 years and a 25% to 27% rate in older patients. In Qin's experience, younger patients (< 50 years) and women had better survival rates than men.[83] Moreover, Dickson and Flores[29] showed a better 5-year survival rate for females (61.5%) than for males (30.9%) in a group of 132 patients ($P = 0.006$). This difference was not the result of lower staging of tumors in women, who had a slightly higher percentage of T4 lesions.

Qin and associates[83] reported better survival rates in patients with earlier stages (*i.e.*, 86% for Stage I, 59% for Stage II) than in patients with more advanced lesions (*i.e.*, 45% for Stage III, 29.2% for Stage IV). Survival decreased as cervical lymph node involvement progressed from the upper to the middle and lower nodes.[2] The presence of bilateral cervical lymph node involvement has an ominous prognostic connotation (*i.e.*, 10% 5-year survival rate).

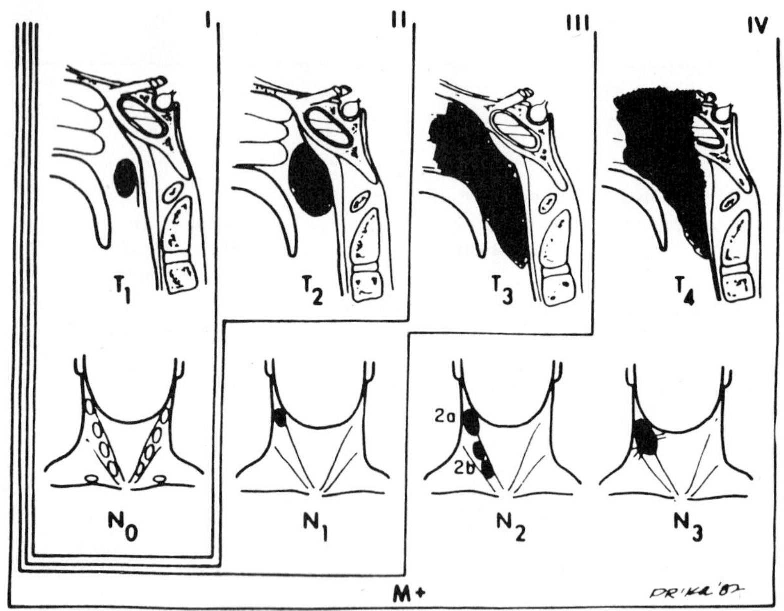

FIGURE 28–5. Anatomic staging for cancer of the nasopharynx. T categories: The number of sites, rather than size, is the crucial factor. Sites are listed as vault (posterosuperior or roof) or lateral walls. One site is T1, two sites are listed as T2, an anterior extension is T3, and deep invasion into base of skull and nerves is T4. Node (N) categories: The size of the node, mobility, and the number and locations are factors in staging cervical nodes. The diameters ≤ 3 cm, 3 cm to 6 cm, and >6 cm were chosen because these are determined more objectively than fixation. (Modified from AJC, UICC, Rubin P [ed]: Clinical Oncology: A Multidisciplinary Approach, 6th ed. Atlanta, American Cancer Society; 1983; courtesy of Philip Rubin, M.D.)

Cranial nerve involvement is not significantly associated with decreased survival.[3, 18, 78]

Histologic type may influence tumor control and survival. Chen and Fletcher[15] and Hoppe and associates[47] reported a 31% to 33% local recurrence rate for squamous cell carcinoma and 10% to 12% for lymphoepithelioma. In contrast, Meyer and Wang[69] found no difference in local failures for the various histologic types. A substantially higher incidence of distant metastases (*i.e.*, 35% to 40% in 113 patients) has been observed in lymphoepithelioma and unclassified carcinoma (30%) than in squamous cell carcinoma (23%).

Dickson and Flores[29] found no significant difference in survival or incidence of distant metastases between keratinizing and nonkeratinizing squamous cell carcinomas. Patients with lymphoepithelioma had a higher (50%; not statistically significant) 5-year survival rate, and none of them developed metastases below the clavicle. Mesic and others[68] reported better survival in patients with lymphoepithelioma than for patients with other epithelial tumors.

RADIATION THERAPY

Because the nasopharynx borders the base of the skull, surgical resection of the neoplasm with an acceptable margin is impossible. Radiation therapy has been the sole treatment for carcinoma of the nasopharynx.

Radical neck dissection has been performed rarely for the treatment of neck node metastasis, but this has not proved superior to irradiation alone. Ho and colleagues[43] point out that radical neck dissection in previously irradiated tissue carries low morbidity and mortality and is preferred in the treatment of residual or recurrent carcinoma from the nasopharynx, because further irradiation may cause more severe complications.

Volume and Doses of Irradiation

The volume (portals) to be irradiated in these patients should include the nasopharynx and adjacent tissues, parapharyngeal lymphatics, and all of the cervical lymphatics (*i.e.*, the jugular, spinal accessory, and supraclavicular nodes) with a 1-cm to 2-cm margin. The standard fields used at the Mallinckrodt Institute of Radiology include the posterior ethmoid cells, the posterior one third of the maxillary antrum, and the nasal cavity but usually not the orbit (Fig. 28-6). We have not observed orbital recurrences. Fletcher[36] and Million and Cassisi[71] include the posterior one fourth of the orbit in the initial treatment volume (Fig. 28-7).

Opposing lateral fields including the upper neck and pri-

TABLE 28–10
Histologic Distribution of Epidermoid Carcinoma of the Nasopharynx

	INVESTIGATION				
HISTOLOGIC TYPE	LEDERMAN[61]	PEREZ[79]*	WANG ET AL[110]	MOENCH AND PHILLIPS[73]	HOPPE ET AL[47]
Keratinizing (squamous cell)	78 (51.6%)	97 (67.8%)	60 (35.2%)	12 (8.2%)	12 (14.3%)
Nonkeratinizing					
Lymphoepithelioma	8 (5.3%)	16 (11.2%)	39 (22.9%)	36 (25%)	44 (52.5%)
Transitional cell	2 (1.3%)	1 (.7%)	48 (28.2%)		
Nonkeratinizing (Nos) or undifferentiated	63 (41.7%)	25 (17.5%)	23 (13.5%)	98 (67%)	28 (33.3%)
Total patients in series	151	139	170	146	84

* *Unpublished data; four patients had other histology or no pathologic diagnosis.*

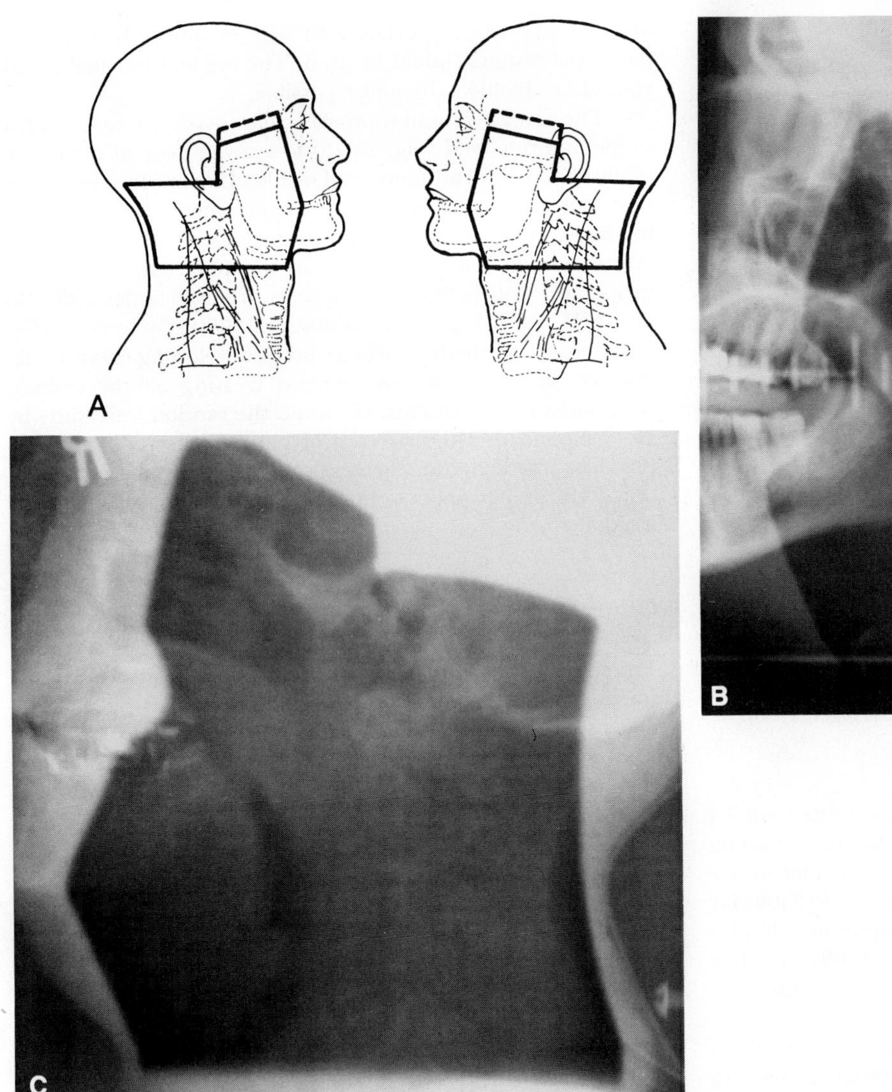

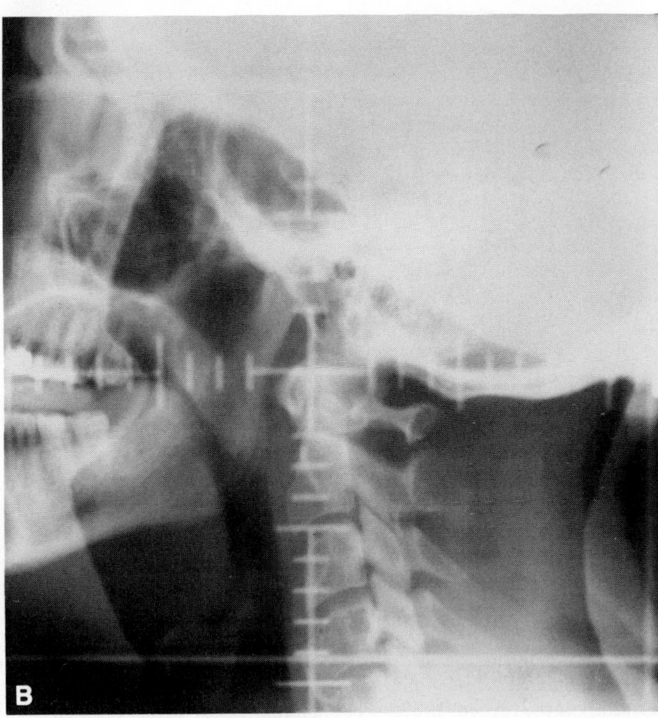

FIGURE 28–6. (**A**) Diagrams of external portals used at Mallinckrodt Institute of Radiology. The upper dotted line indicates the volume treated in patients with involvement of the sphenoid sinus. (**B**) Simulation film illustrates the boundaries of upper lateral portals used to irradiate the nasopharynx, adjacent structures, and upper cervical lymphatics. (**C**) Localization film of upper lateral portal shows modification to shield the posterior portion of the oral cavity.

mary tumor volumes are used to irradiate the nasopharynx and adjacent posterior ethmoid cells, sphenoid sinus and basosphenoid, base of skull, posterior nasal cavity and maxillary antrum, and lateral and posterior pharyngeal wall to the lower pole of the tonsil in addition to the retropharyngeal, upper cervical, mastoid, and posterior cervical lymph nodes. The lateral fields are angled posteriorly 5 degrees to ensure adequate coverage of the posterior wall of the nasopharynx while avoiding direct ipsilateral irradiation to the external and middle ear. This posterior tilt also reduces the irradiation to the contralateral lens.[36]

Several landmarks are used to design the upper lateral treatment portals. The *superior border* of the lateral field splits the pituitary fossa and extends anteriorly along the sphenoidal plate. Externally, this boundary corresponds to a line traced from the lateral canthus of the eye to the upper portion of the helix (above the zygomatic arch). The *anterior border* encompasses the posterior 2 cm of the nasal cavity and the maxillary antrum, and posteriorly the clivus is included with a 1-cm margin. For a lesion involving the base of the skull, the superior border should be at least 1 cm above the pituitary fossa. For a lesion with anterior extension, the anterior border is moved forward 2 cm to cover the extension into the ethmoids or maxillary sinuses with adequate margin. The upper margin must generously cover the mastoid and occipital lymph nodes up to the external occipital prominence. The posterior cervical lymph nodes are included in the upper lateral portals, with a small margin to prevent beam fall-off if there are no enlarged posterior cervical nodes (Fig. 28-7*A*). If lymphadenopathy affects the posterior cervical triangle, it is safer to leave the portals open posteriorly. The *lower margin* is usually placed at the thyroid notch. However, this may be modified, depending on the lower extent of the parapharyngeal tumor or the location of enlarged cervical lymph nodes, to avoid field abutment in the middle of a lymph node or tumor extension.

After administering a tumor dose of approximately 4300 cGy, the posterior border of the lateral field is displaced anteriorly to shield the spinal cord. Through the reduced upper lateral fields, an additional 2200 cGy to 2700 cGy is delivered to the nasopharynx, and if there are palpable lymph nodes, to the

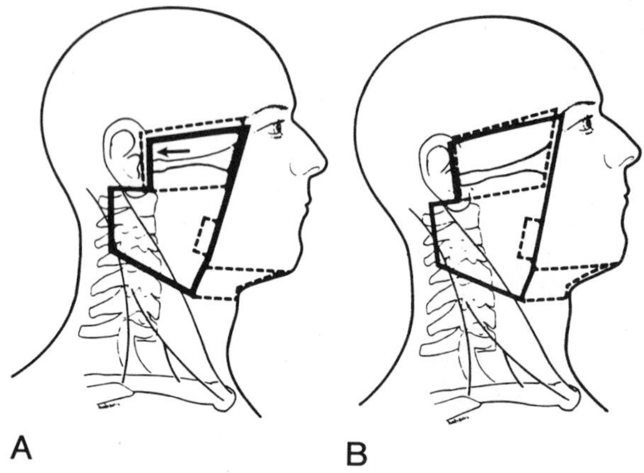

FIGURE 28–7. Portals for irradiation of the primary tumor used at the M.D. Anderson Cancer Center in Houston, TX. (**A**) Lateral portal for T1, T2, and early T3 lesions. (**B**) Lateral portal used for late T3 and T4 lesions. The upper margin of the lateral portal is 1 to 2 cm higher than in (**A**), and it usually extends 1 cm above the pituitary fossa on the verification film. The posterior margin of the portal is the same as in (**A**) with beam tilt or may be located just behind the external auditory canal, in which case no tilt of the beam is necessary. The base of the skull portal boundary is located according to individual requirements. (Fletcher GH, Million RR: Nasopharynx. In Fletcher GH [ed]: Textbook of Radiotherapy, 3rd ed, p 372. Philadelphia, Lea & Febiger, 1980)

upper neck (Fig. 28-8). If a boost is desired, as in treating T4 tumors, 500 cGy to 1000 cGy is delivered to the nasopharynx through reduced lateral portals (Fig. 28-9). We prefer to use high-energy photons (18 MV) for the last 2000 cGy to 2500 cGy to diminish the dose to the mandible and temporomandibular joints. The usual daily fractionation is 180 cGy to 200 cGy in five weekly fractions. Isodose distribution through the nasopharynx is illustrated in Figure 28-10.

Anterior (so-called antral) fields may be added to irradiate anterior tumor extension or if ^{60}Co 4-MV photons are used to avoid excessive dose to the temporomandibular joints (Fig. 28-11). If the nasal cavity or the paranasal sinuses are involved, anterior and lateral portals with wedges similar to those for paranasal tumors should be used. The eye and lacrimal gland should be shielded whenever possible.

The lower neck and supraclavicular fossa are treated with a single anterior field (Fig. 28-12) to a given dose of 5000 cGy (4500 cGy at 3 cm) administered in 200-cGy daily fractions. The posterior neck lymph node dose is supplemented with 500 cGy to 1500 cGy with 9-MeV electrons through small lateral fields. Posterior tangential portals blocking the spinal cord can be used to boost the dose to the posterior cervical lymph nodes with ^{60}Co or 4-MV to 6-MV photons to doses of 5000 cGy to 6000 cGy.

Because of the high likelihood of developing cervical metastases, most authors recommend treating all the cervical lymphatics in N0 patients. However, the randomized study by Ho[45] showed that the survival of N0 patients receiving prophylactic irradiation of the cervical lymphatics was not better than that of N0 patients not receiving prophylactic cervical irradiation.

Other Dose Prescription Considerations

The spinal cord should not receive more than 4500 cGy in daily fractions of 180 cGy to 200 cGy. The reduced upper lateral fields are used to boost the nasopharynx tumor dose to a total of 6500 cGy for T1 and T2 lesions or 7000 cGy to 7500 cGy for T3 and T4 lesions. Justification for the choice of these doses is based on dose-response analyses for tumor control at the primary site (Fig. 28-13). If a high-energy x-ray beam is not available, the nasopharynx can be boosted, sparing the superficial structures, by use of antral fields angled 20 to 30 degrees medially as shown in Figure 28-11. This technique must not be used if there is involvement of the oropharynx or the base of the skull.

Any nodes that were palpable before initiation of radiation therapy should be boosted with posterior glancing or lateral electron beam fields to a total dose of 6500 cGy to 7000 cGy. Because palpable lymph nodes usually regress after 5000 cGy, the margins should be tattooed or accurate anatomic drawings

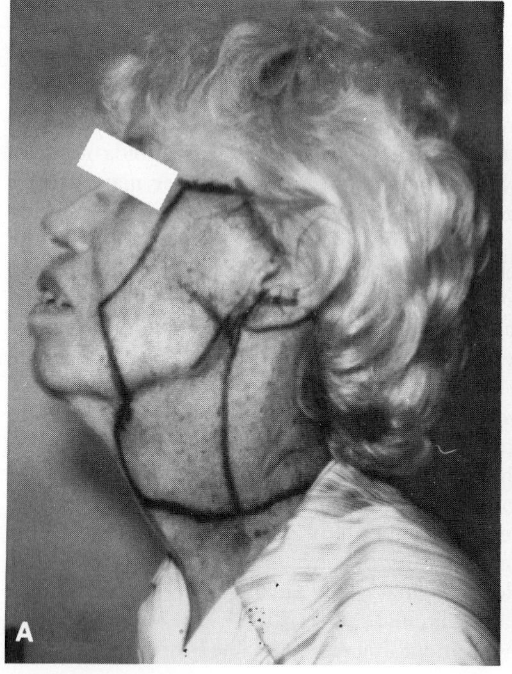

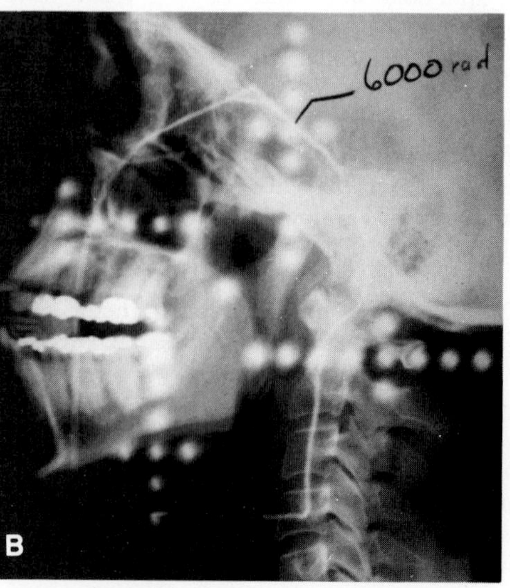

FIGURE 28–8. (**A**) Portal reduction to exclude spinal cord from photon beam portals. Posterior neck is treated with 9-MeV electrons if there are no palpable lymph nodes. (**B**) Simulation film demonstrating exclusion of spinal cord from irradiated volume after 4000 cGy to 4500 cGy midline tumor dose.

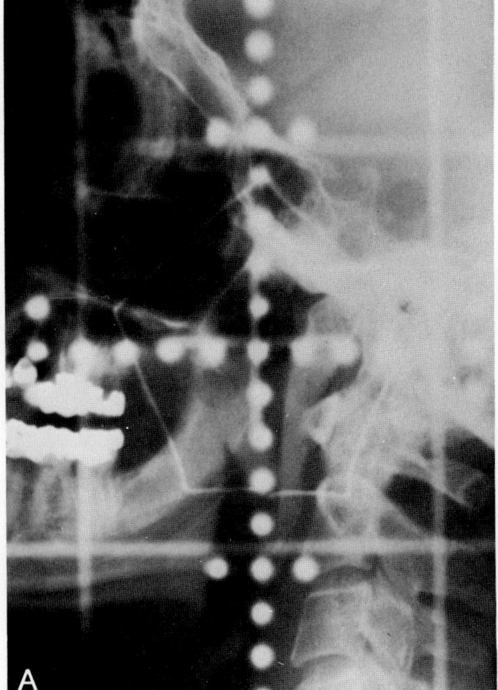

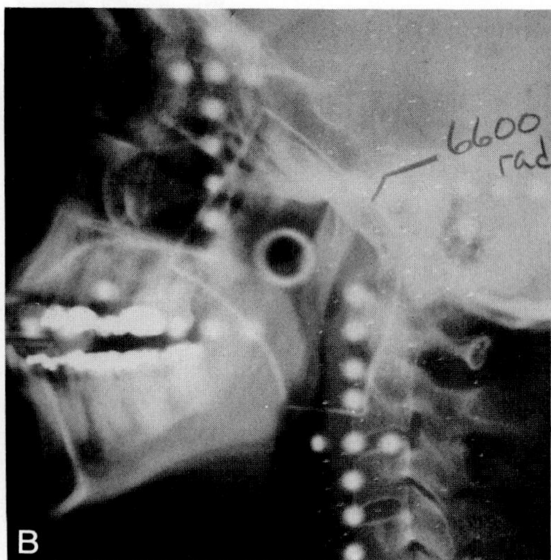

FIGURE 28–9. (**A, B**) Simulation films of small lateral portals used to deliver additional dose (500–1000 cGy boost) to residual tumor in nasopharynx.

should be made before initiation of radiation therapy to ensure accurate placement of these boost fields.

Brown and colleagues,[10] using MRI to define target volume and normal structures for three-dimensional treatment planning, compared the dose distributions of 4-MV x-rays, 4-MV x-rays and protons in a mixed beam, and protons alone. They concluded that using proton beams added complexity to the therapy without improving coverage of the neck lymph nodes; however, the dose to the spinal cord, brain stem, temporal lobe, and parotid gland could be reduced by at least 2000 cGy with proton therapy.

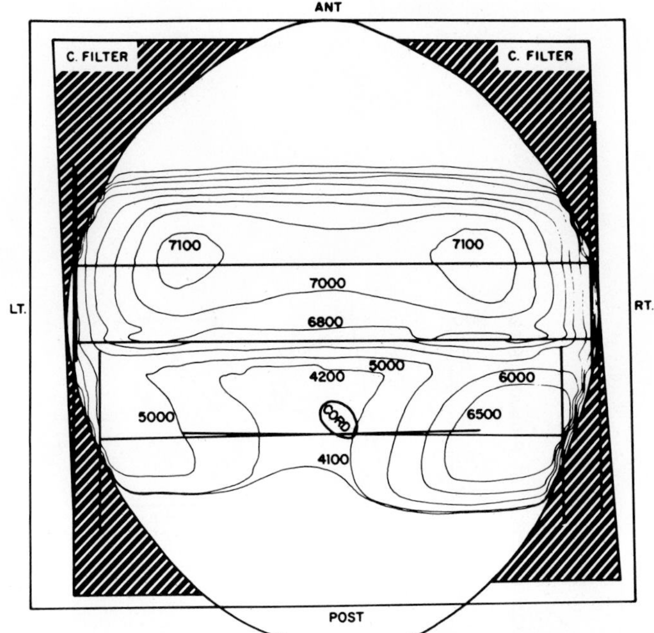

FIGURE 28–10. Isodose distribution through the nasopharynx shows relative sparing of superficial structures by the use of an 18-MV x-ray beam for the nasopharynx boost. Tumor dose of 4000 cGy to 4500 cGy is delivered to the midplane with 4-MV to 6-MV x-rays; the nasopharynx dose is boosted to 6600 cGy to 7000 cGy in the midplane with 18-MV x-rays.

Brachytherapy

Brachytherapy has been used to deliver a higher dose to a limited volume of the nasopharynx. Doses of 500 cGy to 2500 cGy calculated at 0.5 cm to 1 cm combined with external irradiation are usually delivered (Fig. 28-14). Rosenstein and associates[86] described a technique using a silicone direct-impression applicator to carry the radioactive sources. Denham and associates[24] described a technique for intracavitary irradiation of the nasopharynx using remote-controlled afterloading devices. Wang[108] combined intracavitary and external irradiation for the treatment of extensive primary or recurrent carcinoma of the nasopharynx (Fig. 28-15). The techniques for these procedures are presented in detail in Chapter 13.

RESULTS OF TREATMENT

Survival

Reported 5-year survival figures for carcinoma of the nasopharynx range from 35% to 57% and average about 40% (Table 28-11).[15,46,73,78,90,110] Survival is affected by different stages of disease, and the analysis should be made as a function of integrated T and N categories, rather than as a function of T stage or N stage independently, because there is no correlation between T and N stage in carcinoma of the nasopharynx (Fig. 28-16). Relapse-free survival figures for four integrated T and N categories from different series are shown in Table 28-11. Although different staging systems were used in each of these series, reorganization of the patients into comparable categories showed fairly similar results within each category. Survival is good only for patients who have both early primary tumors (AJC T1 and T2) and minimal neck disease (AJC N0 and N1)

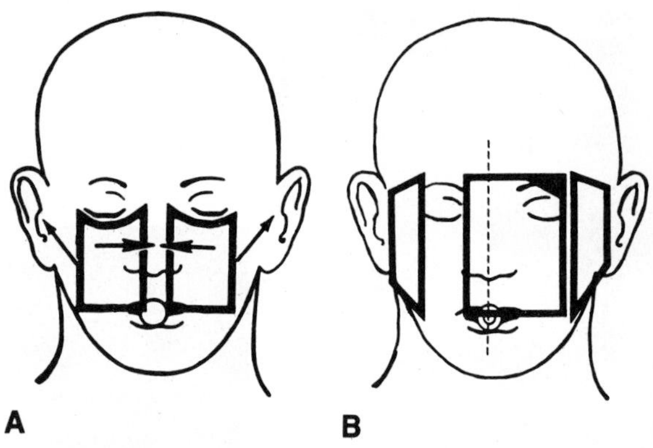

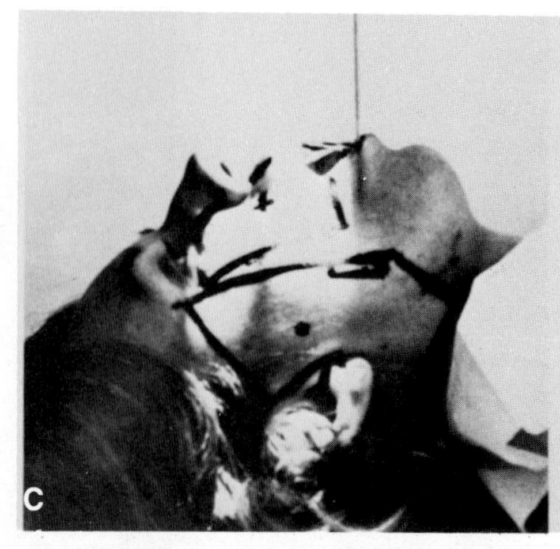

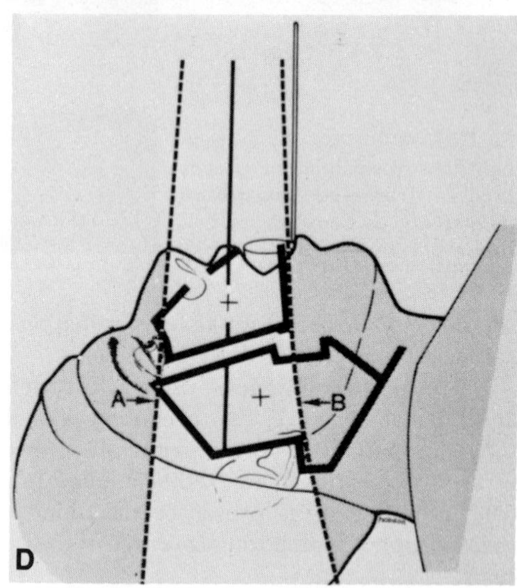

FIGURE 28–11. (**A**) Anterior portals used at M.D. Anderson Hospital and at the University of Florida. The beam is tilted medially an average of 20 degrees to 30 degrees. (**B**) Example of a three-field (AP and lateral) arrangement for anterior spread of tumor into the left orbit, ethmoid sinus, and posterior nose. The anterior field projects 2 cm across the midline and spares one eye. A lacrimal gland shield is used if possible. Wedges are used to produce the required dose distribution in the target volume. (Fletcher GH, Million RR: Nasopharynx. In Fletcher GH [ed]: Textbook of Radiotherapy, 3rd ed, p 372. Philadelphia, Lea & Febiger, 1980) (**C**) The collimator light is used to adjust the beam tilt for the facial fields. The collimator light is adjusted to the superior and inferior margins of the fields, and the collimator is opened laterally to allow the light beam to glance along the lateral aspect of the face. The head position is adjusted so that the beam encloses all of the superior margin of the lateral portal. The head is fixed in position by an immobilization device. The inferior margin usually projects across the angle of the mandible, indicating coverage to about the midtonsillar fossa. (**D**) Schematic drawing of aiming the beam superiorly with the aid of the collimator light. (Fletcher GH, Million RR: Nasopharynx. In Fletcher GH [ed]: Textbook of Radiotherapy, 3rd ed. Philadelphia, Lea & Febiger, 1980)

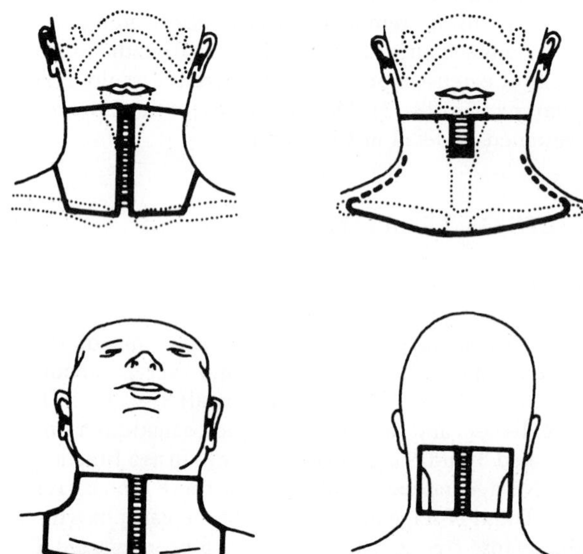

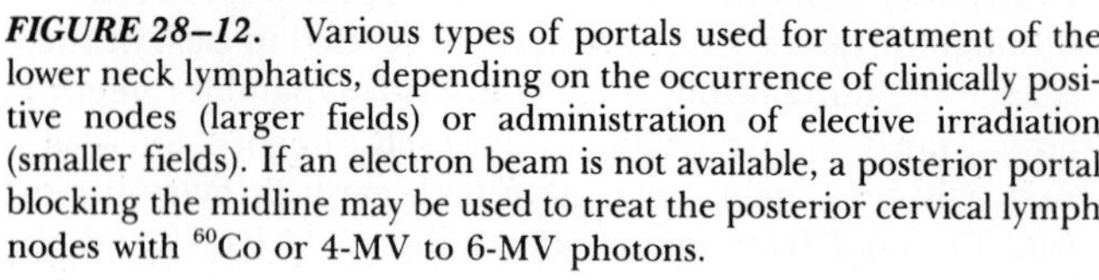

FIGURE 28–12. Various types of portals used for treatment of the lower neck lymphatics, depending on the occurrence of clinically positive nodes (larger fields) or administration of elective irradiation (smaller fields). If an electron beam is not available, a posterior portal blocking the midline may be used to treat the posterior cervical lymph nodes with ^{60}Co or 4-MV to 6-MV photons.

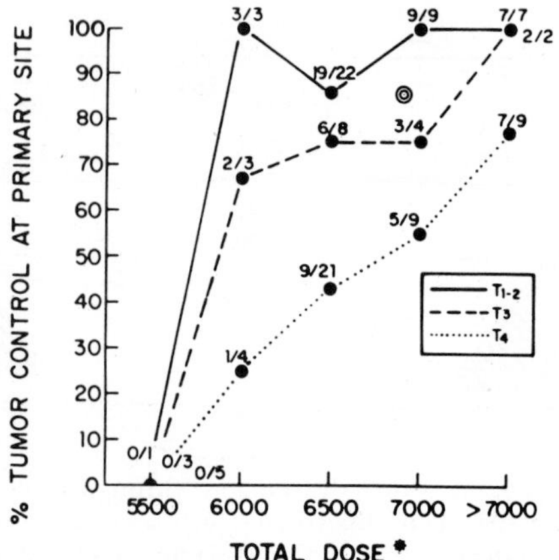

FIGURE 28–13. Dose-response curves for control at the primary site in nasopharyngeal carcinoma. (Bedwinek JM, Perez CA, Keys DJ: Cancer 45:2725, 1980)

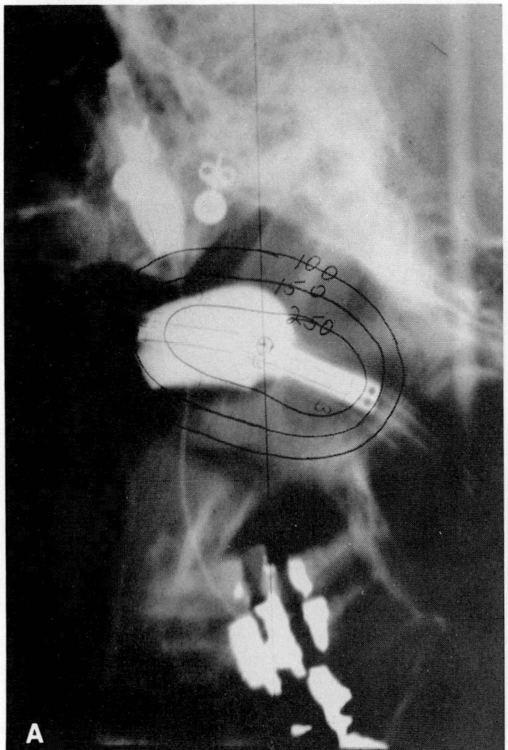

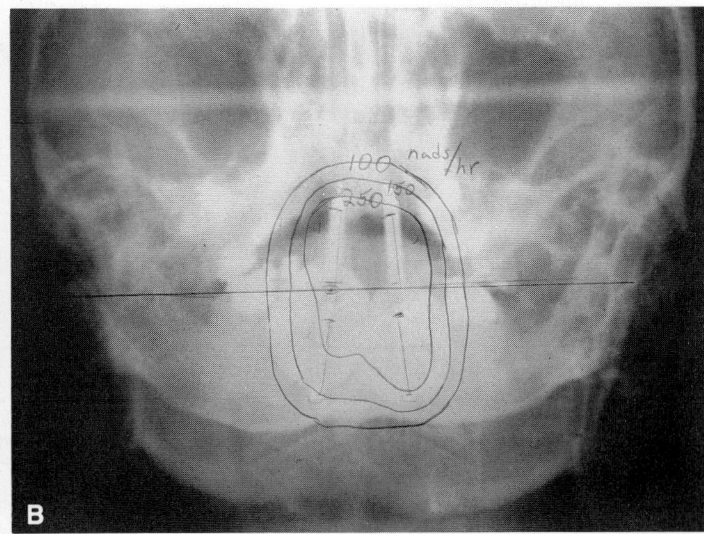

FIGURE 28–14. (**A, B**) Radiographs illustrate an intracavitary application in the nasopharynx with a cesium source. Superimposed is the isodose curve showing dose rate (cGy/h). (Courtesy of C.C. Wang, M.D., Massachusetts General Hospital, Boston, MA)

		SAD	FS	Tumor dose (rad)
Beam 1	^{60}CO	80	11.5 × 8.5	2250 Opposed
Beam 2	^{60}CO	80	11.5 × 8.5	2250 Opposed
Beam 3	^{60}CO	80	6 × 6	2000 Rotation

and nasopharynx implant-500 rad to mucosa

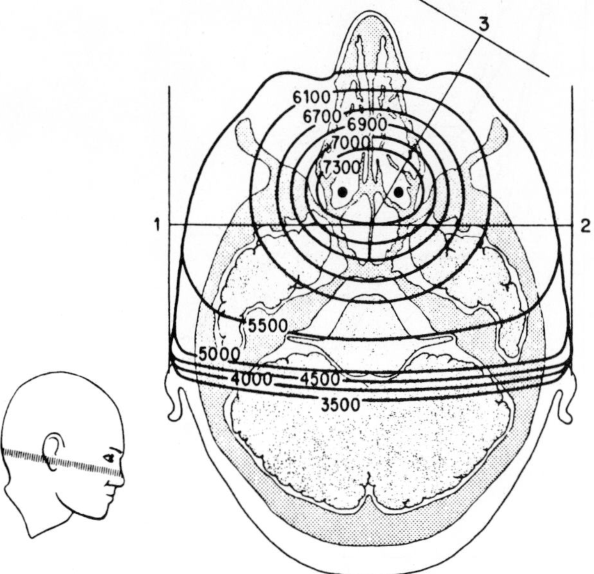

FIGURE 28–15. Composite isodose curves for external-beam and intracavitary implant for carcinoma of nasopharynx. (Wang CC: Otol Clin North Am 13:477, 1980)

and is poor for the other three categories. Wang and colleagues[112] reported a 33% survival rate in 237 patients with Stage III and a 12% rate in 450 patients with Stage IV disease treated with definitive radiation therapy (*i.e.,* doses over 4000 cGy).

Sites of Failure

Many assessments of the sites of failure after irradiation have been published. Figure 28-17 shows the sites of failure for each category in the series reported by Perez and colleagues.[79] For the T1 to T2, N0 to N1 categories, the failure rate is low in all three sites, and survival is very good. Poor survival in the T4, N0 to N1 category is chiefly the result of the high local recurrence rate (63.8%), but for the T1 to T2, N2 to N3 categories, it is the result of the high distant metastases rate, which is approximately 50%. Similar results have been reported by other authors, with increasing rates of failure with more advanced stages of the primary tumor (*i.e.,* T1 or T2 *versus* T3 or T4) or cervical lymph nodes (Tables 28-12 and 28-13). Mesic and associates[68] analyzed the primary recurrences in 251 patients at the M. D. Anderson Cancer Center according to T stage, histology, and two treatment periods. They observed better tumor control in the T1 and T2 tumors with 7000 cGy (94%) than with 6000 cGy (76%). No significant impact of greater doses or larger fields was reported for the T3 and T4 tumors; many of the failures in these advanced tumors were related to widespread disease extending into areas such as the nasal cavity, oropharynx, and base of the skull.

The local failure rate in patients with squamous cell carcinoma was about 40%, in contrast to 10% for lymphoepitheliomas. Of 34 patients with lymphoepithelioma who died of the tumor, 28 had distant metastases only. The overall 5-year

TABLE 28–11
Five-Year Disease-Free Survival Rates for Carcinoma of the Nasopharynx

INVESTIGATION*	T1–T2, N0–N1† (%)	T1–T2, N2–N3‡ (%)	T3–T4, N0–N1§ (%)	T3–T4, N2–N3‖ (%)
Wang and Meyer[110]				
170 patients¶	45	9.5	18	13
Moench and Phillips[73]				
146 patients	61	35	9	7
Bedwinek et al[7]				
111 patients	69	19	18	27
Tokars and Friend[99]				
131 patients	50			10
Chu et al[17]				
80 patients#	45			42
Mesic et al[68]				
251 patients#	60			50
Perez[79]				
143 patients	53	53	42	33

* *TNM staging based on 1977 AJC staging system.*[5]
† *Tumor confined to nasopharynx; negative neck or a single node less than 3 cm.*
‡ *Tumor confined to nasopharynx; single node greater than 3 cm, multiple ipsilateral nodes, or bilateral nodes.*
§ *Tumor beyond nasopharynx, cranial nerve involvement, or base of skull destruction; negative neck or single node greater than 3 cm.*
‖ *Tumor beyond nasopharynx, cranial nerve involvement or base of skull destruction; single node greater than 3 cm, multiple ipsilateral nodes, or bilateral nodes.*
¶ *May include some patients with a single mobile node less than 3 cm or with multiple mobile ipsilateral nodes.*
\# *Estimated survival rates, according to T or N survival reported by authors.*

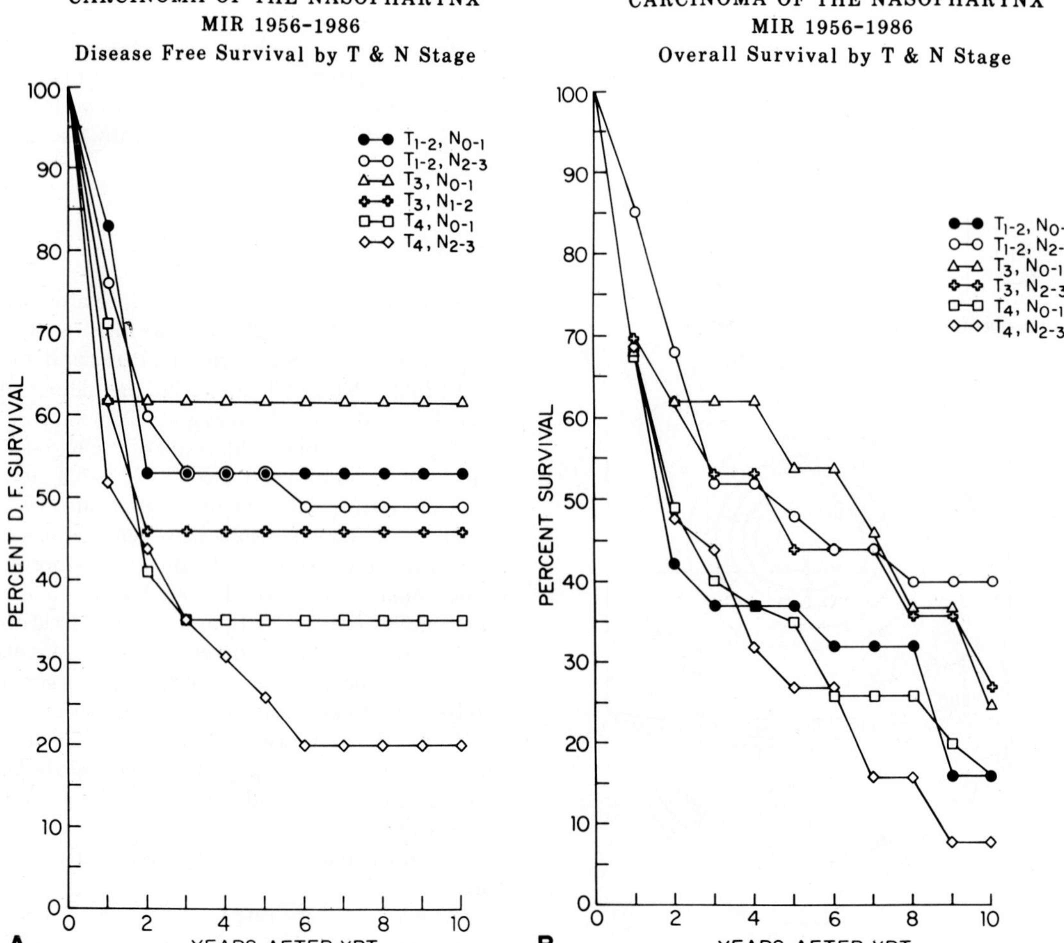

FIGURE 28–16. (**A**) Disease-free and (**B**) overall survival for patients with carcinoma of the nasopharynx treated at the Mallinckrodt Institute of Radiology from 1956 through 1986.

CARCINOMA OF THE NASOPHARYNX
MIR 1956-1986

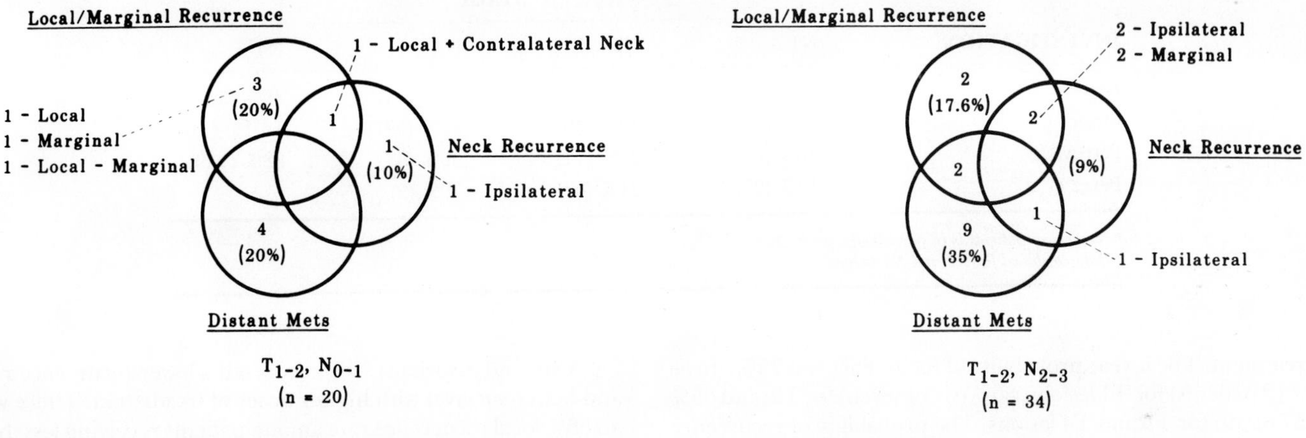

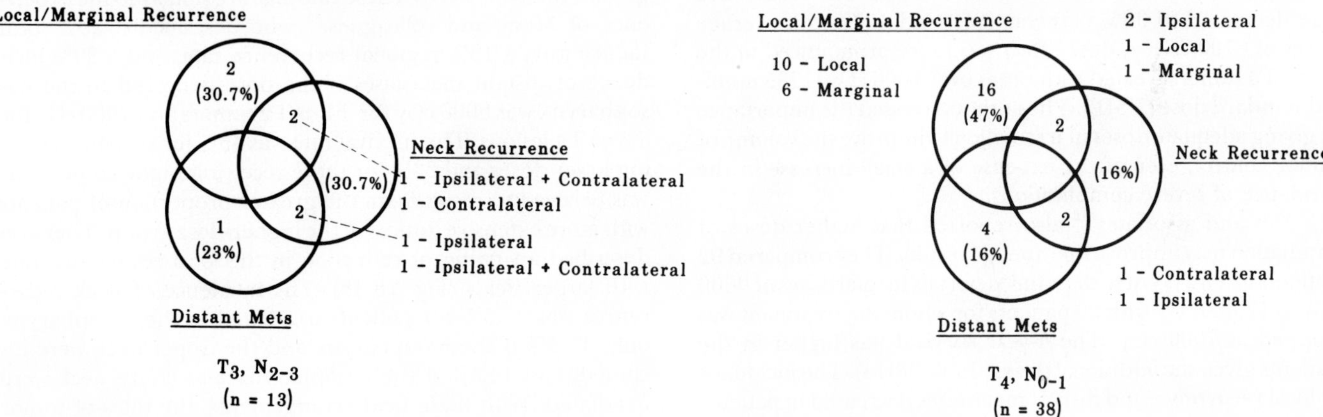

FIGURE 28–17. Anatomic sites of failure for each T and N stage for patients treated at the Mallinckrodt Institute of Radiology.

survival rate for the 251 patients was 52%: 42% for patients with squamous cell carcinoma, 65% for those with lympho-epithelioma, and 14% for those with unclassified carcinoma.

Chu and others[18] reported a 39.5% local failure rate, 28.5% in the cervical lymph nodes, and 18% distant metastases in 80 patients. Petrovich and colleagues[81] described a 15% 5-year survival rate in 256 patients, 82% of whom had Stage IV disease. Most patients received 6000 cGy to 7000 cGy. Failure at the primary site was related to stage of disease: 20% for T1, 32% for T2, 54% for T3, and 88% for T4 lesions. Lack of control at the primary site and the cervical lymph nodes was the cause of failure in 215 (84%) of the patients.

Tokars and Griem,[99] in treating 96 patients treated with definitive radiation therapy (*i.e.,* 4000 cGy to 7500 cGy to the primary tumor and cervical lymph nodes), found increasing evidence of recurrences as a function of stage and time of

TABLE 28–12
Nasopharyngeal Carcinoma: Incidence of Failure at Primary Site by AJC Stage

	STAGE			
INVESTIGATION	T1	T2	T3	T4
Mesic[68]	3% (34)*	15% (102)	26% (35)	28% (70)
Bedwinek[4]	9.5% (42)‡		38% (21)	54% (48)
Chu[18]	24% (25)	21% (14)	63% (19)	45% (22)
Perez et al[79]	14% (12)	21% (33)	31% (26)	52% (63)
Petrovich[81]	20% (15)	32% (34)	54% (100)	88% (107)
Tokars and Griem[99]	25% (12)	86% (7)	95% (39)†	

* *The number of patients is in parentheses.*
† *Data combined for T3 and T4 tumors.*
‡ *Data combined for T1 and T2 tumors.*

TABLE 28–13
Nasopharyngeal Carcinoma: Incidence of Failure in the Neck by AJC Stage

INVESTIGATION	STAGE N1	N2	N3	N4
Bedwinek[7]	2% (54)*†		29% (21)	36% (36)
Mesic[68]	0% (35)	10% (30)	11% (59)	18.4% (114)
Petrovich[81]	16% (65)	27% (11)	30% (33)	83% (149)
Perez et al[79]	13% (23)	21% (63)	30% (9)	

*Number of patients is in parentheses.
†Data combined for N1 and N2 tumors.

treatment. The 5-year probability of recurrence was 25% (three of 12 patients) for T1 lesions, 86% (six of seven) for T2, and 95% (37 of 39) for T3 and T4 lesions. The probability of recurrence was 56% to 72% at various periods between 1950 and 1969 with average tumor doses of 5600 cGy to 6500 cGy. The recurrence rate decreased to 39% between 1970 and 1977 with average doses of 6700 cGy. A dose effect was more pronounced in the T1 to T3 tumors treated with doses over 6000 cGy (1785 nominal standard dose [NSD]). The authors stressed the importance of giving adequate doses of irradiation to improve the volume of tumor control, even at the expense of a small increase in the incidence of severe complications.

Yan and associates[118] also reported that higher doses of irradiation may improve therapeutic results. They compared 92 patients given a boost with reduced portals to total doses of 9000 cGy to 12,000 cGy with 90 patients for whom the treatment was stopped at 7000 cGy. The 5-year survival was higher in the patients given the additional doses (Table 28-14). The incidence of local recurrence and distant metastases decreased in patients receiving the boost doses (Table 28-15). The benefit of boost doses was more apparent in the patients with T1 or T2 tumors. However, the risk of radiation myelopathy was increased from 5.5% to 17.5% with the additional doses.

Valentine and associates[103] discovered that patients with T3 and T4 tumors had significantly reduced recurrence rates after treatment with doses higher than 7000 cGy. No difference was found for the T1 and T2 lesions treated with doses of 6000 cGy to 7000 cGy.

Qin and associates[83] described 5-year survival rates of 46% for patients receiving less than 4900 cGy, 54.1% for patients treated with 7000 cGy to 7900 cGy, and 64% for patients receiving 9000 cGy or more.

Chu and associates[18] also reported a lower recurrence rate and better survival with higher doses of irradiation. There was an 86% local recurrence rate among patients receiving less than 4000 cGy and a 27% rate among those treated with doses greater than 6000 cGy. These findings are similar to the experience of Mesic and colleagues,[68] who described a 20% local failure rate, a 13% regional recurrence rate, and a 39% incidence of distant metastases if the dose delivered to the nasopharynx was 6000 cGy for T1 or T2 tumors and 7000 cGy for T3 or T4 lesions. The survival rate was 45% for patients receiving lower doses and 33% for those receiving higher doses; this was believed to result from the greater proportion of patients with more extensive tumors in the higher-dose group. They also described a significant reduction in the local recurrence rate with larger fields (Fig. 28-18). The incidence of neck recurrences was 37.5% for patients irradiated to the nasopharynx only, 17.5% if the nasopharynx and the upper neck were included, and 14.3% if the nasopharynx and entire neck were irradiated. With these field arrangements, the rates of tumor recurrence in the nasopharynx were 44%, 36%, and 17%, respectively.

Vikram and co-workers[104] found better local tumor control in patients treated with doses between 6700 cGy and 7700 cGy than with lower doses. They also noted decreased local control (34%) in 20 patients for whom radiation therapy was interrupted for periods of 21 days or longer, compared with 67% local tumor control for 87 patients without long interruptions. This detrimental effect was observed regardless of the tumor dose administered (Fig. 28-19). For patients with advanced neck disease (AJC N2 or N3), improvement in locoregional tumor control does not improve survival substantially because approximately 60% of these patients develop distant metastases. Ta-

TABLE 28–14
Influence of Boost Dose on 5-year Survival Rate in Residual Primary Lesion of Nasopharyngeal Carcinoma

STAGE	OBSERVATION GROUP PATIENTS	%	BOOST GROUP PATIENTS	%	P VALUE
I	0	0	3/3	(100)	
II	6/12	(50)*	17/25	68	
III	12/33	36	26/48	54	
IV	1/45	2	4/16	25	
Total	19/90	21	50/92	54	<0.01

*Parentheses denote insufficient number of patients.
(Yan J-H, Qin D-X, Hu Y-H, et al: Int J Radiat Oncol Biol Phys 16:1465, 1989)

TABLE 28–15
Influence of Boost Dose on Local Recurrence and Distant Metastasis of Resistant Primary Lesion

TUMOR STAGE	GROUP	LOCAL RECURRENCE PATIENTS	%	P VALUE	DISTANT METASTASIS PATIENTS	%	P VALUE
T1–T2	Observation	15/33	45		16/33	48	
	Boost	8/48	17	<0.01	9/48	19	<0.01
T3–T4	Observation	38/57	67		23/57	40	
	Boost	23/44	52	>0.05	9/44	20	>0.05
Total	Observation	52/90	58		39/90	43	
	Boost	32/92	35	<0.01	18/92	20	<0.01

(From Yan J-H, Qin D-X, Hu Y-H, et al: Int J Radiat Oncol Biol Phys 16:1465, 1989)

ble 28-16 illustrates a few examples of the influence of primary tumor stage and doses of irradiation on the probability of tumor control.

Wang[109] reported 60 patients treated with hyperfractionated irradiation who were compared with 58 historic controls treated with one daily fraction; for T1 or T2 lesions, the 5-year actuarial tumor control rates were 89% and 55% ($P = 0.002$) and for the T3 or T4 tumors, 77% and 45%, respectively ($P = 0.02$).

Increased local tumor control can be achieved by a thorough evaluation of the extent of the primary tumor, use of large fields to cover all known and suspected tumor extensions, and by delivering doses of at least 7000 cGy to the nasopharynx with adequate techniques.

Marks and others,[66] in a retrospective review of technical factors influencing the treatment of 118 patients, demonstrated that better coverage of the nasopharynx and a decrease in the frequency of inadequate coverage, usually resulting from faulty positioning of blocks to shield the ear, were accomplished with growing sophistication of treatment techniques, such as simulation, Cerrobend blocking, and greater doses of irradiation (Table 28-17).

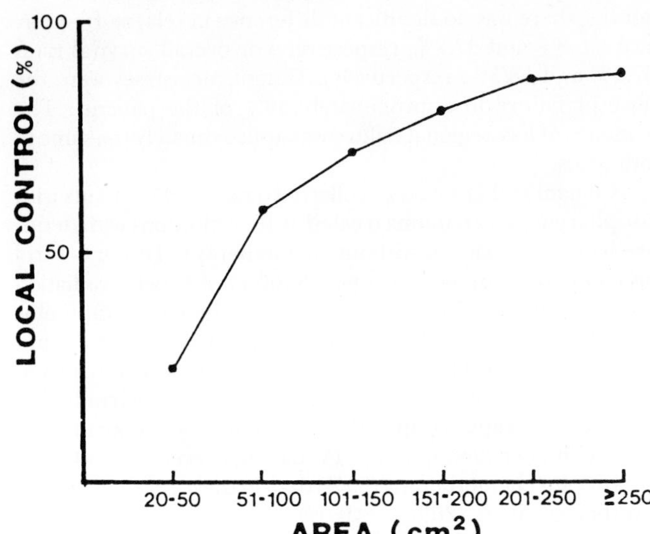

FIGURE 28–18. Influence of field size on local control in patients irradiated for nasopharyngeal carcinoma. (Chu AM, Flynn MB, Achino E, et al: Int J Radiat Oncol Biol Phys 10:2241, 1984)

Valentini and associates[103] reported a 75% neck recurrence rate among 83 patients treated with irradiation alone and a rate of 44% among 26 patients with neck lymph node dissections in addition to irradiation. The 5-year survival rate was 37% with radiation therapy alone and 62% with irradiation and lymph node dissection, but the difference was not statistically significant. Qin and associates[83] described a 5-year survival rate of 53.8% among 1379 patients if the necks were irradiated compared with 23% if prophylactic neck irradiation was not performed. Few investigators have performed a neck dissection after irradiation.

Some patients have excellent palliative results with relatively high doses of irradiation (6000–7000 cGy). Stillwagon and associates[95] observed complete recovery of cranial nerve deficit in 62% and partial recovery in 32% of 18 patients who initially had cranial nerve abnormalities, including four patients with Horner's syndrome. Complete responses were not obtained when cranial nerve deficits had existed longer than 2 months. The 5-year actuarial survival rate for the 18 patients was 31%.

CHEMOTHERAPY

There are varied reports about the use of cytotoxic agents in the management of nasopharyngeal carcinoma, with a wide range

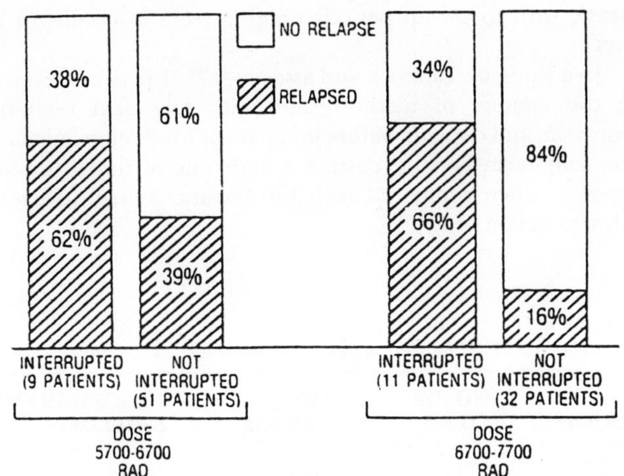

FIGURE 28–19. Proportion of patients remaining free of recurrence at the primary site, analyzed according to dose and whether radiation therapy was interrupted for a total of 3 weeks or longer. (Vikram B, Mishra VB, Strong EW, et al: Int J Radiat Oncol Biol Phys 11:1455, 1985)

TABLE 28–16
Local Tumor Control Correlated with Doses of Irradiation

INVESTIGATION	TUMOR STAGE	TUMOR DOSE (cGy) <5000	5000–6000	6001–6750	>6750
Chu et al[18]	T1	0/1*	13/17 (76%)	6/7 (86%)	
	T2		6/8 (75%)	5/6 (83%)	
	T3	1/2 (50%)	3/11 (27%)	2/5 (40%)	
	T4	0/4	6/10 (60%)	6/8 (75%)	
Tokars and Griem[99]	T1–T2		0/2	4/8 (50%)	7/10 (70%)
	T3–T4		3/12 (25%)	14/43 (32.6%)	3/7 (42.9%)
Chatani et al[14] (RT or RT + CT)	T1		2/3 (66%)	4/6 (66%)	5/5 (100%)
	T2		5/7 (71%)	16/18 (88.9%)	4/8 (50%)
	T3	1/2 (50%)	2/6 (33%)	3/4 (75%)	1/2 (50%)
	T4	0/2	4/5 (80%)	5/10 (50%)	7/10 (70%)
Perez et al[79]	T1		8/9 (89%)	7/8 (88%)	3/4 (75%)
	T2		8/11 (73%)	5/6 (83%)	11/16 (81%)
	T3		7/8 (88%)	4/9 (44%)	7/9 (78%)
	T4	0/2	5/16 (31%)	9/19 (47%)	16/26 (62%)

**Number of patients with local tumor control/total number of patients.*

of results, making it impossible to elucidate the value of chemotherapy in the management of these patients. Huang and colleagues[52] described improved 5-year survival rates among patients entered in several nonrandomized studies using 6000 cGy to 7000 cGy to nasopharynx and 5000 cGy to 6000 cGy to cervical lymph nodes and several cytotoxic drugs. The local recurrence rate decreased from 15.7% to 8.4%, and distant metastases occurred less frequently with combined therapy. According to the authors, acute toxicity was acceptable in most patients.

A controlled study using the same protocols was initiated in 1984. Clark and associates[19] reported a 29% complete response rate and a 46% partial regression rate in 24 patients with Stage IV previously untreated nasopharyngeal carcinoma who were treated with 2 to 4 monthly cycles of combination chemotherapy (*i.e.*, cisplatin, bleomycin, 5-fluorouracil, and methotrexate with leucovorin rescue). After chemotherapy, each patient received 6000 cGy in 30 fractions to the nasopharynx and neck with appropriate spinal cord shielding. Eighteen (75%) of the 24 patients were alive, although 6 had recurrent or persistent disease, with follow-up periods ranging from 6 months to 7 years.

In a study by Tannock and associates,[96] 51 patients receiving two courses of methotrexate (with folic acid rescue), bleomycin, and cisplatin before initiation of irradiation failed to show long-term benefit, despite a high rate of initial tumor response, when compared with 140 historic controls treated with irradiation only.[14,85]

TABLE 28–17
Technical Accuracy by Period for Nasopharyngeal Carcinoma

PERIOD	NO. OF FILMS	INADEQUATE COVERAGE	NASOPHARYNX SHIELDED
1950–1968	271	94 (35%)	34 (14%)
1968–1974	309	89 (29%)	45 (15%)
1974–1978	219	18 (8%)	10 (5%)

(Marks JE, et al: Cancer 50:1042, 1982)

Yamashita and associates[115] reported improved local tumor control (49%) at 5 years and disease-free survival rate (20%) for 42 patients receiving adjuvant chemotherapy in addition to irradiation, compared with 37 patients treated with irradiation alone, who had a 22% recurrence rate and an 11% disease-free survival rate. These differences are statistically significant. However, the overall 5-year survival rates were 24% and 22%, respectively.

Khoury and Paterson[57] determined a 35% 3-year survival rate for 52 patients with nasopharyngeal carcinoma treated with radiation therapy alone and 86% for 14 patients treated with a combination of chemotherapy containing cisplatin followed by a variety of treatments with radiation.

Rossi and colleagues[87] reported on a randomized study of 229 patients with nasopharyngeal carcinoma; 116 were treated with 6000 cGy to 7000 cGy to involved areas and 5000 cGy to clinically negative lymph nodes, and 113 were treated with a combination of irradiation and 6 monthly cycles of vincristine, cyclophosphamide, and doxorubicin (Adriamycin). At 48 months, there was no significant difference in relapse-free survival (55.8% and 57.7%, respectively) or overall survival rates (67.3% and 58.5%, respectively). Distant metastases were the cause of failure in approximately 50% of the patients. The incidence of locoregional failure was approximately the same in both arms.

Chatani and associates[14] collected data on 105 patients with nasopharyngeal carcinoma treated at 16 institutions with definitive irradiation with or without chemotherapy. Tumor control was comparable in both groups: 35 (66%) of 53 with radiation therapy alone and 23 (74%) of 31 with radiation therapy plus chemotherapy. Control of cervical lymph nodes was 80% and 74%, respectively. However, the radiation therapy only group had a higher incidence of metastases (35%) than the irradiation plus chemotherapy group (14%) ($P<0.05$). The 5-year survival rate was higher among Stage IV patients receiving radiation therapy plus chemotherapy (53%) than in those receiving radiation therapy alone (26%) ($P<0.05$).

Dimery and colleagues[31] treated 34 patients with Stage IV nasopharyngeal carcinoma with combined chemotherapy (cisplatin and other drugs) and sequential irradiation. Seventeen (81%) of 21 patients who received chemotherapy followed by irradiation achieved complete responses, and 11 (85%) of 13 patients who received radiation therapy followed by chemotherapy achieved complete responses. Patients treated with irradiation alone had a 91% complete response rate. However, the combined treatment yielded a relapse-free survival rate of 78%, significantly higher than the 44% for the irradiation only group ($P = 0.001$). The recurrence rate at the primary site and in the regional lymph nodes was 7% in the combined therapy group and 36% in the radiation therapy patients ($P = 0.004$). The incidence of distant metastases was similar in both groups. A later report on the same patients by Peters and associates[80] disclosed a 5-year disease-free survival rate of 63% in the combined modality group and a rate of 44% in the radiation only group ($P = 0.15$). Although the Dimery[31] paper mentioned only soft tissue fibrosis as the most significant long-term toxic effect of therapy, Peters and associates[80] reported a rate of 50% (ten of 20 patients) for severe acute toxicity and 45% (15 of 33) for severe, late injury of normal tissue in the combined modality group. There was a rate of 13% (nine of 71 patients) for acute effects and 7% (five of 71) for late morbidity for the group receiving only radiation therapy (Table 28-18). The probability of remaining both disease free and complication free at 5 years was 40% in the irradiation group and 22% in the combined modality group ($P = 0.08$).

The subject of chemotherapy is still highly controversial. The Southwest Oncology Group is conducting a randomized study to evaluate the efficacy of adjuvant chemotherapy.[94]

SEQUELAE OF TREATMENT

Optimal irradiation of carcinoma of the nasopharynx involves large fields and high doses; therefore significant sequelae and side effects are to be expected. Table 28-19 shows the major and minor complications occurring in patients treated with definitive radiation therapy at the Mallinckrodt Institute of Radiology, Washington University, with various treatment techniques in three separate periods, and Table 28-20 summarizes the sequelae reported in selected series.

Mesic and associates[68] reported radiation myelitis in eight (3%) of 251 patients; some of these complications were correlated with a high dose to the spinal cord at the junction of lateral wedge portals and upper neck fields. This sequela could be avoided with adequate portal design and with the delivery of a 4500-cGy maximum dose in 5 weeks to the spinal cord (180–200 cGy daily). Tokars and Griem[99] described four of 96 patients who developed cervical myelopathy: one had received approximately 5600 cGy; one received 5900 cGy, and two received 6500 cGy. Qin and colleagues[83] reported a 4% (two of 48 patients) incidence of myelopathy in patients treated with less than 5000 cGy and 17% to 22% in 1331 patients treated to higher doses up to 9000 cGy to the nasopharynx. However, no dose-response association was observed at these higher dose levels.

Persistent xerostomia was reported in 40% of the patients treated at Washington University,[7] but the effect to some degree has been observed in virtually all patients treated.[15,61]

Trismus occurs to a significant degree in approximately 5% to 15% of patients and is caused by fibrosis of the temporomandibular joints and the muscles of mastication. Keeping the dose to these structures low by using high-energy x-rays (>18 MeV) or an anterior field for the nasopharynx boost may reduce the severity and incidence of this complication.

Osteonecrosis of the mandible or maxilla can be kept to a minimum by avoiding unnecessarily high doses to these structures. Equally important in reducing this potentially debilitating complication is avoidance of elective dental extractions before radiation therapy, a vigorous program of oral hygiene and fluoride applications, and a working alliance between radiation oncologist and dentist.[6,22] Dental decay is occurs, but Mesic and others[68] and Bedwinek and colleagues[6] reported a reduction in dental caries with the prophylactic use of fluorides.

Fibrosis of the subcutaneous tissues of the neck can be minimized by keeping the dose to the neck below 5000 cGy in electively irradiated areas and by using reduced fields to deliver a dose boost to gross neck disease.

Hypopituitarism causing significant clinical signs and symptoms is not commonly reported as a complication in most series of adult nasopharyngeal carcinoma, but it has been described after treatment of nasopharyngeal carcinoma in children.[26,33] However, Samaan and co-workers[89] reported clinical symptoms of hypopituitarism in adults treated for carcinoma of the nasopharynx, particularly symptoms related to deficiency of adrenocorticotropic hormone and thyroid-stimulating hormone. In addition, 14 of 15 patients had some degree of pituitary hormone deficiency as determined by serum hormone levels.

Lam and associates[59] reported a significant decrease in the integrated serum growth hormone response to insulin-induced hypoglycemia in 31 patients receiving radiation therapy for

TABLE 28–18
Grade III Late Sequelae after Irradiation Alone or Combined with Chemotherapy

		CHEMOTHERAPY + RADIATION THERAPY (33 PATIENTS)	
COMPLICATION	**RADIATION THERAPY ONLY (71 PATIENTS)**	PRERADIATION THERAPY + POSTRADIATION THERAPY	POSTRADIATION THERAPY ONLY
Soft tissue neck fibrosis	2	4	6
Trismus	2	1	2
Bone fracture and necrosis	0	2	0
Soft tissue necrosis	1	0	0
Total severe complications	5 (7%)	15 (45%)	

(Peters LJ, Harrison ML, Dimery IW, et al: Int J Radiat Oncol Biol Phys 14:623, 1988)

TABLE 28–19
Carcinoma of Nasopharynx: Irradiation Sequelae by Treatment Periods

	1956–1965 n = 30		1966–1975 n = 54		1976–1986 n = 59	
	NO.	(%)	NO.	(%)	NO.	(%)
SEVERE (GRADE 3–GRADE 4)						
Dysphagia	1*	(3)	0	(0)	3	(5)
Osteonecrosis of mandible	1	(3)	1	(2)	0	(0)
Soft tissue necrosis	0	(0)	1	(2)	1†	(2)
Pharynx stricture/stenosis	0	(0)	2	(4)	1	(2)
Osteomyelitis of cervical spine	1	(3)	0	(0)	0	(0)
Hemorrhage	0	(0)	2†	(4)	0	(0)
Carotid rupture	1†	(3)	0	(0)	0	(0)
Radionecrosis of brain	0	(0)	1†	(2)	1	(2)
Delayed wound healing	0	(0)	1	(2)	0	(0)
Oropharyngeal fistula	1	(3)	0	(0)	0	(0)
Laryngeal edema	0	(0)	1	(2)	0	(0)
Total‡	5	(17)	10	(19)	6	(10)
MODERATE (GRADE 2)						
Xerostomia	0	(0)	3	(6)	4	(7)
Neck fibrosis	1	(3)	3	(6)	2	(3)
Dental decay	2	(7)	10	(19)	1	(2)
Laryngeal edema	0	(0)	1	(2)	0	(0)
Dysphagia	0	(0)	2	(4)	2	(3)
Bone exposure	3	(10)	1	(2)	1	(2)
Other	3	(10)	4	(7)	0	(0)

** Death secondary to cranial nerve XII damage.*
† Includes one fatality each.
‡ Some patients had more than one complicaton.
(Perez CA, Devineni VR, Marcial-Vega V, et al: Int J Radiat Oncol Biol Phys, submitted for publication)

nasopharyngeal carcinoma; the mean dose to the hypothalamus was 3800 cGy, and the dose to the pituitary was 6200 cGy. In males, follicle-stimulating hormone levels increased without significant change in serum leutinizing hormone and testosterone levels. The mean T_4 level remained normal in 16 patients receiving only cranial irradiation, but it decreased in 15 patients who also received irradiation to the cervical lymph nodes. Two women developed oligomenorrhea, four women continued to have regular menstruation, but three who were also hyperprolactinemic at 2 years developed oligomenorrhea 12 to 18 months after irradiation. Four (19%) of 21 patients had evidence of hypopituitarism affecting one or more anterior pituitary functions 2 years after cranial irradiation. All patients had normal endocrine function before radiation therapy, and the abnormal changes could be demonstrated as early as 1 year after irradiation. The authors concluded that the endocrine

TABLE 28–20
Complications of Therapy for Nasopharyngeal Carcinoma

COMPLICATION	82 PATIENTS*	251 PATIENTS†	143 PATIENTS‡
Xerostomia	47%	62%	45%
Otitis	15%	18%	
Dental caries	14%	10%	
Trismus (temporomandibular joint)	8%	14%	2%
Neck fibrosis	11%	39%	14%
Soft tissue/bone necrosis	4%	39%	6%
Transverse myelitis	1%	8%	
Cranial nerve palsy	5%	3%	1%

** Series data from Hoppe RT, Goffinet DR, Bagshaw MA: Cancer 37:2605, 1976.*
† Series data from Mesic JB, Fletcher GH, Goepfert H: Int J Radiat Oncol Biol Phys 7:447, 1981.
‡ Series from Perez CA et al: Mallinckrodt Institute of Radiology, 1956–1986 (unpublished data).

changes are consistent with alteration in the secretion of hypothalamic releasing hormones, caused by radiation-induced damage to the hypothalamus.

deSchryver and co-workers[27] analyzed the ophthalmologic side effects in 80 long-term survivors with nasopharyngeal carcinoma treated with tumor doses between 5000 cGy and 6000 cGy delivered with 190-kV x-rays through lateral and anteroposterior antral portals over 20 to 40 days. Of 30 patients who received radiation therapy 7 to 30 years before evaluation, 25 developed opacities in the lens; in 19 patients, the characteristics of the opacities were similar to those of radiation-induced cataract. Choroidoretinal changes were evident in one of the six patients for whom the estimated absorbed dose was less than 2500 cGy over 3 to 5 weeks and in 11 of the 14 patients in whom the dose was higher. None of the patients sustained obvious damage to the optic nerve.

Midena and associates[71] reported that 4 (36.3%) of 11 patients with nasopharyngeal carcinoma treated with 7000 cGy developed retinopathy 24 to 108 months after treatment. The posterior pole was usually affected, and microaneurysms, intraretinal hemorrhage, cotton wool spots, and exudates existed. Fluorescein angiography demonstrated widespread areas of retinal ischemia; neovascularization was observed in two patients. One patient developed vitreous hemorrhage, one developed ischemic optic neuropathy, and two developed bilateral macular edema, causing loss of vision. Dosimetry analysis showed that the posterior third of both eyes received progressively increasing doses, from 5000 cGy to 6500 cGy. None of the patients had lens opacities or other anterior segment abnormalities.

External otitis, which was observed in 18 (31%) of 57 patients evaluated by Wei and associates,[114] can be avoided by carefully blocking the ear. If clinically significant complaints occur, myringotomy and insertion of middle ear ventilation tubes may be required to relieve symptoms.[114]

Chowdhury and colleagues[16] carried out a randomized comparison of 58 patients irradiated for nasopharyngeal carcinoma who developed decreased hearing, earache, or tinnitus and were treated with insertion of ventilation tubes and of 57 similar patients allocated to an observation group. At 6 months, the patients with middle ear tubes had less conductive hearing loss and tinnitus than the control group. The authors recommend routine insertion of ventilation tubes before initiation of irradiation in these patients. Because this practice does not totally protect the middle and inner ear, some degree of hearing loss should be anticipated.

RETREATMENT OF RECURRENT NASOPHARYNGEAL CARCINOMA

If regular radiation therapy is not feasible, surgical salvage can be attempted for a few patients.[34] Fee and associates[32] reported nine patients with recurrent nasopharyngeal carcinoma treated surgically, seven of them with curative intent. All patients had extensive resection of the tumor; two were fitted with a soft palate obturator, and one required a hard palate obturator. At the time of the report, five of the patients were living without tumor for a median interval of 22.2 months after salvage resection. Two of the seven had recurrent disease. The author emphasized the value of MRI scans to ascertain soft tissue extension and CT scanning to determine bone invasion. A few patients with T4 recurrent tumors treated surgically by Fisch[34] survived, and only one of eight treated in the same manner by Panje and Gross[75] was living 38 months after surgery.

The radiation oncologist often treats patients previously irradiated. Several techniques have been used, including brachytherapy (mold), external irradiation, or combinations of both. The total dose to be delivered depends on the initial dose of irradiation given and the volume of central nervous system included in the portals. It is extremely important to determine the full extent of the recurrent tumor and the possibility of extension into the base of the skull.

Because involvement of the base of the skull or intracranial extension may be a factor, retreatment should be primarily given with external irradiation rather than with brachytherapy. However, the brachytherapy can be used to deliver a portion of the dose (2000–5000 cGy); because of the inverse square law, the effective volume treated is limited.

For retreatment with external beams, relatively small fields must be used. If there is no tumor extension outside the nasopharynx, portals of approximately 6 cm × 6 cm are generally adequate. If there is radiographic evidence of tumor destruction at the base of the skull, somewhat larger fields are required (*i.e.*, 8 cm × 8 cm or 10 cm × 10 cm). The use of higher-energy photon beams (>15 MV) is recommended to decrease the probability of severe normal tissue effects. Depending on the initial dose, the retreatment doses that can be delivered with external irradiation range from 4000 cGy to 6000 cGy administered in 180-cGy to 200-cGy daily fractions.

Many of these patients may survive for several years (Table 28-21), and most experience substantial palliative benefit, which justifies an aggressive approach, even though therapy-induced morbidity is relatively high.

McNeese and Fletcher[67] reported 30 patients reirradiated for recurrent primary nasopharyngeal carcinoma who were initially treated with doses below 4000 cGy. Seven patients had received about 5000 cGy, and five initially received doses higher than 6000 cGy. With megavoltage external irradiation, 12 patients were retreated with 5000 cGy, three with 5500 cGy, five with 6000 cGy, and one with 6500 cGy. In nine patients with localized recurrence, three had no tumor control in the nasopharynx, and two failed because of central nervous system involvement. Two patients died of intercurrent disease, one of

TABLE 28–21
Retreatment of Carcinoma of Nasopharynx

INVESTIGATION	NO. OF PATIENTS	DOSE (cGy)	TUMOR CONTROL	5-YEAR SURVIVAL*
Fu[37]	42	1200–6300	5 (12%)	41%†
McNeese and Fletcher[67]	30	4000–6500	10 (33%)	Not stated
Wang[107]	51	5000–7000	Not stated	30%†
Yan[117]	162	5000–7000	23 (14%)	39 (18%)

* *After first recurrence.*
† *Actuarial.*

complications, and one of distant metastases. However, of six patients with more extensive recurrences involving the base of the skull, five failed because of central nervous system involvement. Of nine patients with more extensive recurrences, seven failed after retreatment because of central nervous system involvement, and two died with distant metastases. According to McNeese and Fletcher,[67] sclerosis of the floor of the sphenoid was not considered a significant prognostic indicator, because it is often observed after irradiation. Fu and others[37] reported a 41% 5-year survival rate and a 25% 10-year survival rate for patients with localized recurrent tumors retreated with external irradiation.

Among 35 patients for whom doses below 5000 cGy were used for retreatment, Wang and Schulz[111] noted that only three of 20 patients survived with no evidence of disease for 5 years or more; however, six of 15 patients receiving higher doses survived for 5 years or more. Wang[107, 108] reported a 5-year survival rate of 45% and a 10-year rate of 39% for 51 patients, 38 of whom received high-dose irradiation (6000 cGy or higher) with external beam, with or without intracavitary brachytherapy. Of 13 patients treated with less than 6000 cGy, the actuarial 3-year survival rate was 15%; none survived more than 5 years. The author did not specify the criteria for selection of doses, although the more advanced tumors probably received lower doses. The initial stage of tumor was a significant factor affecting the 5-year survival rate: 38% of 32 patients with T1 or T2 recurrent tumors and 15% of 6 patients with T3 and T4 lesions.

Complications after retreatment are common, consisting of soft tissue necrosis in the nasopharynx, osteonecrosis of the sphenoid sinus, severe trismus, and even hypopituitarism.

Yan and associates[117] reported 162 patients with recurrent nasopharyngeal carcinoma confined to the head and neck region. There were 74 nasopharyngeal and 68 lymph node recurrences, most of which were confirmed by histologic or cytologic examination; included were 18 patients with clinically diagnosed recurrences. All patients received tumor doses of 5000 cGy to 7000 cGy using multiple and small converging beams to avoid excessive irradiation of normal tissues, especially brain stem and spinal cord. These authors used preauricular, postauricular, infraorbital, or supraorbital fields, in addition to lateral portals, to obtain an optimal dose distribution. Of the 162 patients, 37 (23%) survived 5 years, 23 (14%) without evidence of disease.

The complications of treatment were similar to those observed in 210 patients who received only one course of irradiation and survived for more than 5 years. The most serious sequela, radiation myelitis, occurred in 12% of the retreated patients but in only 9% of those receiving one course of irradiation. Radiation encephalopathy occurred in 8% of the retreated patients and 9% of the patients receiving one course of irradiation. Subcutaneous fibrosis, otitis media, and trismus occurred more frequently in the retreatment patients (9% to 29%), but without significant difference in the two treatment groups. Isolated cervical lymph node recurrences and an interval longer than 3 years from the initial treatment to the development of recurrences were the most important prognostic factors.

NASOPHARYNGEAL CARCINOMA IN PATIENTS YOUNGER THAN 30 YEARS OF AGE

A bimodal age distribution for nasopharyngeal carcinoma has been reported, with a first peak incidence occurring between 15 and 25 years.[39] It is possible that in this age group the tumor may be associated with prior infection with an Esptein-Barr virus.[41]

Children or young adults with nasopharyngeal carcinoma should be treated as adults, with irradiation alone. The volume to be irradiated should include the nasopharynx and adjacent tissues as already outlined and all of the cervical lymph nodes.

Doses of irradiation should be in the range of 5000 cGy to 6000 cGy, depending on the age of the patient and the tumor stage. For children older than 15 years with T3 or T4 tumors in whom skull growth in completed, a dose of 5000 cGy to the nasopharynx and both neck sites is recommended, with an additional boost of 1500 cGy to the nasopharynx and 1000 cGy delivered through reduced fields for residual lymph nodes. Unfortunately, data reported by Jenkin and associates[53] are not adequate to judge the efficacy of treating the lower neck. Lower necks were not usually irradiated in children who had no palpable neck disease initially, but treatment was given if there were palpable cervical lymph nodes.

Jenkin and associates[53] described 119 patients younger than 30 years of age retrospectively reported by the Children's Cancer Study Group. The male-to-female ratio was 5 : 3. There was no significant difference in survival according to age or gender. Lymphoepithelioma was reported in 54 patients, epidermoid carcinoma in 38 patients, transitional cell carcinoma in 15, and anaplastic carcinoma in 12. There was no significant difference in survival according to histologic type. The tumors were retrospectively staged. The 5-year survival rates were 75% for T1 and T2 tumors (41 patients), 37% for T3 (19 patients), 37% for T4 (43 patients), and 44% for TX (16 patients). Nodal stage had no significant influence on survival, nor was there any correlation between doses of irradiation and control of the primary tumor, although analysis was not done according to T stage.

Adjuvant chemotherapy was delivered in addition to irradiation to six (15%) of 39 patients with T4 tumors and six (11%) of 57 patients with non-T4 tumors. Drugs usually administered were vincristine, doxorubicin (Adriamycin), cyclophosphamide, actinomycin D, 5-fluorouracil, bleomycin, methotrexate, and cisplatin. Only five of the patients received chemotherapy for 6 months or longer. There was no significant difference in survival with or without adjuvant chemotherapy. After retreatment, the survival rate was 70% among 76 patients with relapses, indicating that some of these patients may be salvaged by aggressive additional therapy. In fact, 37% of 21 patients with local or regional relapse survived 5 years after recurrence. No major toxicity was reported for the patients treated.

Pao and associates[76] described 29 patients younger than 19 years, all of whom had lymphoepithelioma. Four patients were treated with radiation therapy alone, but most received a combination of irradiation and chemotherapy with cyclophosphamide. More recently, four patients were treated with a combination of irradiation and cisplatin, bleomycin, and vinblastine. Fourteen of the patients are alive without tumor, with a median follow-up of 11 years. Four patients failed locally, and 13 had distant metastasis. The most important prognostic factor was local extent of the tumor.

Morales and colleagues[74] reported 17 patients with nasopharyngeal carcinoma who were younger than 30 years of age at diagnosis. Fourteen had T2 or T3 tumors, and 16 (94%) had clinically detectable cervical encephalopathy at initial examination. Fourteen tumors were lymphoepitheliomas. Patients were treated with doses of 5500 cGy to 7000 cGy to the primary tumor, excluding the spinal cord after 4500 cGy to 5000 cGy, and approximately 5500 cGy to 6600 cGy to the cervical lymph

TABLE 28–22
Carcinoma of Nasopharynx in Young: Results in the Medical Literature

INVESTIGATION	NO. OF PATIENTS	MAXIMUM AGE (YEARS)	5-YEAR ACTUARIAL SURVIVAL RATE (%)
Berry et al[8]	25	30	0
Fernandez et al[33]	10	15	0
Castro-Vita et al[13]	27	20	64
Pick et al[82]	9	18	58
Lombardi et al[65]	20	15	55
Jenkin et al[53]	119	30	51
Papavasiliou et al[77]	26	30	50
Shu-Chen[92]	119	30	45*
Deutsch et al[28]	7	18	19
Jereb et al[54]	16	17	14
Morales et al[74]	17	30	14
Bohorquez[9]	29	30	10*
Pao[76]	29	19	50

**Crude survival rate.*
(Modified from Morales P, Bosch A, Salaverry S, et al: J Surg Oncol 27:181, 1984)

nodes. Primary tumor control was 100% for two patients with T1 tumors, 80% for patients with T2 tumors, and 39% for patients with T3 tumors. Twelve patients (71%) developed distant metastases, and the overall 5-year survival rate was 14%.

Lombardi and colleagues[65] reported a high incidence of undifferentiated carcinoma with prominent lymphocytic infiltration and a high incidence of metastatic lymph nodes (26 of 27 children). The patients were treated with definitive radiation therapy of 5500 cGy to 7700 cGy to the nasopharynx and 4000 cGy to 6000 cGy to the regional lymph nodes. Fourteen of the patients received adjuvant chemotherapy (cyclophosphamide). The 4-year actuarial survival rate was 55%, and the overall survival rate was 40%. Control of primary tumor was achieved in 85% of the patients. However, 45% developed distant metastases as the first treatment failure.

Several of the series reported no significant difference in survival between younger and older patients (Table 28-22).

REFERENCES

1. Armstrong RW, Armstrong MJ, Yu MC, Hendrson BE: Salted fish and inhalants as risk factors for nasopharyngeal carcinoma in Malaysian Chinese. Cancer Res 43:2967, 1983
2. Baker SR, Wolfe RA: Prognostic factors of nasopharyngeal malignancy. Cancer 49:163, 1982
3. Batsakis JG: Tumors of the Head and Neck, 2nd ed. Baltimore, Williams & Wilkins, 1979
4. Bauer W: Varieties of squamous carcinoma: Biologic behavior. Front Radiat Ther Oncol 9:164, 1974
5. Beahrs OH, Henson DE, Hutter RVP, Myers MH (eds): Manual for Staging of Cancer, 3rd ed, pp 33–35. Philadelphia, JB Lippincott, 1988
6. Bedwinek J, Fletcher G, Day T: Osteonecrosis in patients treated with definitive radiotherapy for squamous carcinoma of the oral cavity and naso- and oropharynx. Radiology 119:665, 1976
7. Bedwinek JM, Perez CA, Keys DJ: Analysis of failure after definitive irradiation for epidermoid carcinoma of the nasopharynx. Cancer 45:2725, 1980
8. Berry MP, Smith CHR, Brown TC, et al: Nasopharyngeal carcinoma in the young. Int J Radiat Oncol Biol Phys 6:415, 1980
9. Bohorquez J: Factors that modify the radio-response of cancer of the nasopharynx. Am J Roentgenol Radiat Ther Nucl Med 126:863, 1976
10. Brown AP, Urie MM, Chisin R, Suit HD: Proton therapy for carcinoma of the nasopharynx: A study in comparative treatment planning. Int J Radiat Oncol Biol Phys 16:1607, 1989
11. Buell P: Nasopharyngeal cancer in Chinese of California. Br J Cancer 19:459, 1965
12. Buell P: Race and place in the etiology of nasopharyngeal cancer: A study based on California death certificates. Int J Cancer 11:268, 1973
13. Castro-Vita H, Mendiondo OA, Shaw DL, et al: Nasopharyngeal carcinoma in the second decade of life. Radiology 148:253, 1983
14. Chatani M, Teshima T, Inoue T, et al: Radiation therapy for nasopharyngeal carcinoma: Retrospective review of 105 patients based on a survey of Kansai Cancer Therapist Group. Cancer 57:2267, 1986
15. Chen KY, Fletcher GH: Malignant tumors of the nasopharynx. Radiology 99:165, 1971
16. Chowdhury CR, Ho JHC, Wright A, et al: Prospective study of the effects of ventilation tubes on hearing after radiotherapy for carcinoma of nasopharynx. Ann Otol Rhinol Laryngol 97:142, 1988
17. Chu AM, Cutler SJ, Young JL: Third National Cancer Survey: Incidence data. NCI Monogr 41:1, 1975
18. Chu AM, Flynn MB, Achino E, Mendoza EF, et al: Irradiation of nasopharyngeal carcinoma: Correlations with treatment factors and stage. Int J Radiat Oncol Biol Phys 10:2241, 1984
19. Clark JR, Norris CM Jr, Dreyfuss AI, et al: Nasopharyngeal carcinoma: The Dana-Farber Cancer Institute experience with 24 patients treated with induction chemotherapy and radiotherapy. Ann Otol Rhinol Laryngol 96:608, 1987
20. Conley J, Dingman DL: Adenoid cystic carcinoma in the head and neck. Arch Otol 100:81, 1974
21. Cooper MA, Hallgrimsson J: Tumors in Iceland. IV. Tumors of the upper resperatory tract and ear: A histological classification and some etiological and epidemiological considerations. Acta Pathol Microbiol Scand 89:377, 1981
22. Daly T: Dental care in the irradiated patient. In Fletcher GH (ed): Textbook of Radiotherapy, 3rd ed. Philadelphia, Lea & Febiger, 1980
23. del Regato JA, Spjut HJ: Nasopharynx. In del Regato JA, Spjut HJ, Ackerman LV (eds): Cancer: Diagnosis, Treatment, and Prognosis, 5th ed, p 310. St. Louis, CV Mosby, 1977
24. Denham JW, Baldacchino AC, Gutte J, et al: Remote after

loading techniques for the treatment of nasopharyngeal and endometrial cancer. Int J Radiat Oncol Biol Phys 14:191, 1988
25. deSchryver A: Sarcomas of the nasopharynx. Acta Radiol 13:1, 1974
26. deSchryver A, Ljunggren J-G, Baryd I: Pituitary function in long-term survival after radiation therapy of nasopharyngeal tumours. Acta Radiol 12:497, 1973
27. deSchryver A, Wachtmeister L, Baryd I: Ophthalmologic observations on long-term survivors after radiotherapy for nasopharyngeal tumours. Acta Radiol 10:193, 1971
28. Deutsch M, Mercado R Jr, Parsons JA: Cancer of the nasopharynx in children. Cancer 41:1128, 1978
29. Dickson RI, Flores AD: Nasopharyngeal carcinoma: An evaluation of 134 patients treated between 1971–1980. Laryngoscope 95:276, 1985
30. Dillon WP, Mills CM, Kjos B, et al: Magnetic resonance imaging of the nasopharynx. Radiology 152:731, 1984
31. Dimery IW, Legha SS, Peters LJ, et al: Adjuvant chemotherapy for advanced nasopharyngeal carcinoma. Cancer 60:943, 1987
32. Fee WE Jr, Gilmer PA, Goffinet DR: Surgical management of recurrent nasopharyngeal carcinoma after radiation failure at the primary site. Laryngoscope 98:1220, 1988
33. Fernandez CH, Cangir A, Samaan NA, Rivera R: Nasopharyngeal carcinoma in children. Cancer 37:2787, 1976
34. Fisch U: The infratemporal fossa approach for nasopharyngeal tumors. Laryngoscope 93:36, 1983
35. Fletcher GH, Healey JR Jr, McGraw JP, Million RR: Nasopharynx. In MacComb WS, Fletcher GH (eds): Cancer of the Head and Neck, pp 152–178. Baltimore, Williams & Wilkins, 1967
36. Fletcher GH, Million RR: Nasopharynx. In Fletcher GH (ed): Textbook of Radiotherapy, 3rd ed, pp 364–383. Philadelphia, Lea & Febiger, 1980
37. Fu KK, Newman H, Phillips TL: Treatment of locally recurrent carcinoma of the nasopharynx. Radiology 117:425, 1975
38. Gado M: Personal communication, 1990
39. Greene MH, Fraumeni JF Jr, Hoover R: Nasopharyngeal cancer among young people in the United States: Racial variations by cell type. JNCI 58:1267, 1977
40. Henderson BE, Louie E, Jing JS-H, et al: Risk factors associated with nasopharyngeal carcinoma. N Engl J Med 295:1101, 1976
41. Henle W, Henle G: Evidence for an etiologic relation of the Epstein-Barr virus to human malignancies. Laryngoscope 87:467, 1977
42. Henle W, Henle G, Ho H-C, et al: Antibodies to Epstein-Barr virus in nasopharyngeal carcinoma, other head and neck neoplasms and control groups. JNCI 44:225, 1970
43. Ho JH, Chan M, Tsao SY, Li AKC: Treatment of residual and recurrent cervical metastasis from nasopharyngeal carcinoma. Ann Acad Med 17:22, 1988
44. Ho JHC: Nasopharyngeal carcinoma. In Klein G, Weinhouse S, Haddow A (eds): Advances in Cancer Research, pp 57–92. New York, Academic Press, 1972
45. Ho JHC: An epidemiologic and clinical study of nasopharyngeal carcinoma. Int J Radiat Oncol Biol Phys 4:183, 1978
46. Hoppe RT, Goffinet DR, Bagshaw MA: Carcinoma of the nasopharynx: Eighteen years' experience with megavoltage radiation therapy. Cancer 37:2605, 1976
47. Hoppe RT, Williams J, Warnke R, et al: Carcinoma of the nasopharynx: The significance of histology. Int J Radiat Oncol Biol Phys 4:199, 1978
48. Hsu H-C, Chen C-L, Hsu M-M, et al: Pathology of nasopharyngeal carcinoma: Proposal of a new histologic classification correlated with prognosis. Cancer 59:945, 1987
49. Hsu MM, Tu SM: Nasopharyngeal carcinoma in Taiwan: Clinical manifestations and results of therapy. Cancer 52:362, 1983
50. Huang DP, Ho JHC, Henle W, Henle G: Demonstration of Epstein-Barr virus-associated nuclear antigen in nasopharyngeal carcinoma cells from fresh biopsies. Int J Cancer 14:580, 1974
51. Huang DP, Saw D, Teoh TB, et al: Carcinomas in nasal and paranasal regions in rats fed with Cantonese salted marine fish. Presented at the International Symposium on Etiology and Control of Nasopharyngeal Carcinoma, Kyoto, Japan, 1977
52. Huang S-C, Lui LT, Lynn T-C: Nasopharyngeal cancer: Study III. A review of 1206 patients treated with combined modalities. Int J Radiat Oncol Biol Phys 11:1789, 1985
53. Jenkin RDT, Anderson JR, Jereb B, et al: Nasopharyngeal carcinoma—A retrospective review of patients less than 30 years of age: A report from Children's Cancer Study Group. Cancer 47:360, 1981
54. Jereb B, Huvos AG, Steinherz P, Unal A: Nasopharyngeal carcinoma in children. Review of 16 cases. Int J Radiat Oncol Biol Phys 6:487, 1980
55. Kandel ER, Schwartz JH (eds): Principles of Neural Science, 2nd ed. New York, Elsevier Science Publishing, 1985
56. Khor TH, Tan BC, Chua EJ, Chia KB: Distant metastases in nasopharyngeal carcinoma. Clin Radiol 29:27, 1978
57. Khoury GG, Paterson ICM: Nasopharyngeal carcinoma: A review of cases treated by radiotherapy and chemotherapy. Clin Radiol 38:17, 1987
58. King H, Haenszel K: Cancer mortality among foreign and native born Chinese in the United States. J Chronic Dis 26:623, 1972
59. Lam KSL, Tse VKC, Wang C, et al: Early effects of cranial irradiation on hypothalamic-pituitary function. J Clin Endocrinol Metab 64:418, 1987
60. Lanier A, Bender T, Talbot M, et al: Nasopharyngeal carcinoma in Alaskan Eskimos, Indians and Aleuts: A review of cases and study of Epstein-Barr virus, HLA, and environmental risk factors. Cancer 46:2100, 1980
61. Lederman M: Cancer of the Nasopharynx: Its Natural History and Treatment. Springfield, IL, Charles C Thomas, 1961
62. Levine PH, Connelly RR: Epidemiology of nasopharyngeal cancer. In Wittes RE (ed): Head and Neck Cancer pp 13–34. Chichester, UK, John Wiley & Sons, 1985
63. Levine PH, McKay FW, Connelly RR: Patterns of nasopharyngeal cancer mortality in the United States. Int J Cancer 39:133, 1987
64. Lindberg RD: Distribution of cervical lymph node metastases from squamous cell carcinoma of the upper respiratory and digestive tracts. Cancer 29:1446, 1972
65. Lombardi F, Gasparini M, Cianni C, et al: Nasopharyngeal carcinoma in childhood. Med Pediatr Oncol 10:243, 1982
66. Marks JE, Bedwinek JM, Lee F, et al: Dose-response analysis for nasopharyngeal carcinoma. Cancer 50:1042, 1982
67. McNeese MD, Fletcher GH: Retreatment of recurrent nasopharyngeal carcinoma. Radiology 138:191, 1981
68. Mesic JB, Fletcher GH, Goepfert H: Megavoltage irradiation of epithelial tumors of the nasopharynx. Int J Radiat Oncol Biol Phys 7:447, 1981
69. Meyer JE, Wang CC: Carcinoma of the nasopharynx: Factors influencing results of therapy. Radiology 100:385, 1971
70. Micheau C, Boussen H, Klijanienko J, et al: Bone marrow biopsies in patients with undifferentiated carcinoma of the nasopharyngeal type. Cancer 60:2459, 1987
71. Midena E, Segato T, Piermarocchi S, et al: Retinopathy following radiation therapy of paranasal sinus and nasopharyngeal carcinoma. Retina 7:142, 1987
72. Million RR, Cassisi NJ: Nasopharynx. In Million RR, Cassisi NJ (eds): Management of Head and Neck Cancer: A Multidisciplinary Approach, pp 445–466. Philadelphia, JB Lippincott, 1984
73. Moench HC, Phillips TL: Carcinoma of the nasopharynx: Review of 146 patients with emphasis on radiation dose and time factors. Am J Surg 124:515, 1972
74. Morales P, Bosch A, Salaverry S, et al: Cancer of nasopharynx in young patients. J Surg Oncol 27:181, 1984
75. Panje WR, Gross CE: Treatment of tumors of the nasopharynx: Surgical therapy. In Thawley SE, Panje WR (eds): Comprehensive Management of Head and Neck Tumors, vol 1, pp 662–683. Philadelphia, WB Saunders, 1987
76. Pao WJ, Hustu HO, Douglass EC, et al: Pediatric na-

sopharyngeal carcinoma: Long-term follow-up of 29 patients. Int J Radiat Oncol Biol Phys 17:299, 1989

77. Papavasiliou C, Paulatou M, Pappas J: Nasopharyngeal cancer in patients under the age of thirty years. Cancer 40:2312, 1977
78. Perez CA, Ackerman LV, Mill WB, et al: Cancer of the nasopharynx: Factors influencing prognosis. Cancer 24:1, 1969
79. Perez CA, Devineni VR, Marcial Vega V, Simpson JR: Int J Radiat Oncol Biol Phys (submitted)
80. Peters LJ, Harrison ML, Dimery IW, et al: Acute and late toxicity associated with sequential bleomycin-containing chemotherapy regimens and radiation therapy in the treatment of carcinoma of the nasopharynx. Int J Radiat Oncol Biol Phys 14:623, 1988
81. Petrovich Z, Cox JD, Middleton R, et al: Advanced carcinoma of the nasopharynx. II. Pattern of failure in 256 patients. Radiother Oncol 4:15, 1985
82. Pick T, Maurer HM, McWilliams NB: Lymphoepithelioma in childhood. J Pediatr 84:96, 1974
83. Qin D, Hu Y, Yan J, et al: Analysis of 1379 patients with nasopharyngeal carcinoma treated with radiation. Cancer 61:1117, 1988
84. Quisenberry W, Reimann-Jasinski D: Ethnic differences in nasopharyngeal cancer in Hawaii. In Muin CS, Shaumugaratnam K (eds): Cancer of the Nasopharynx, UICC Monograph Series, no. 1, pp 77–81. Copenhagen, Munksgaard, 1967
85. Rahima M, Rakowsky E, Barzilay J. Sidi J: Carcinoma of the nasopharynx: An analysis of 91 cases and a comparison of differing treatment approaches. Cancer 58:843, 1986
86. Rosenstein HE, DeMasi VM, Fine L, Fattore D: Radiation carrier for treatment of nasopharyngeal carcinomas. J Prosthet Dent 58:617, 1987
87. Rossi A, Molinari R, Boracchi P, et al: Adjuvant chemotherapy with vincristine, cyclophosphamide, and doxorubicin after radiotherapy in local-regional nasopharyngeal cancer: Results of a 4-year multicenter randomized study. J Clin Oncol 6:1401, 1988
88. Rubin P (ed): Clinical Oncology: A Multidisciplinary Approach, 6th ed. American Cancer Society, 1983
89. Samaan NA, Bakdash MM, Caderao JB, et al: Hypopituitarism after external irradiation. Evidence for both hypothalamic and pituitary origin. Ann Intern Med 83:771, 1975
90. Scanlon PW, Rhodes RE Jr, Woolner LB, et al: Cancer of the nasopharynx: 142 patients treated in the 11 year period 1950–1960. AJR 99:313, 1967
91. Schmincke A: Uber lymphoepitheliale Geschevulste. Beitr Pathol Anat 68:161, 1921.
92. Shu-Chen H: Nasopharyngeal cancer: A review of 1605 patients treated radically with ^{60}Co. Int J Radiat Oncol Biol Phys 6:401, 1980
93. Simons MJ, Wee GB, Day NE, et al: Immuno-genetic aspects of nasopharyngeal carcinoma. I. Difference in HL-A antigen profiles between patients and comparison groups. Int J Cancer 13:122, 1974
94. Southwest Oncology Group Protocol 8892: A phase III study of radiotherapy with or without concurrent cisplatin in patients with nasopharyngeal cancer. San Antonio: Southwest Oncology Group, 1988
95. Stillwagon GB, Lee D-J, Moses H, et al: Response of cranial nerve abnormalities in nasopharyngeal carcinoma to radiation therapy. Cancer 57:2272, 1986
96. Tannock I, Payne D, Cummings B, et al: Sequential chemotherapy and radiation for nasopharyngeal cancer: Absence of long-term benefit despite a high rate of tumor response to chemotherapy. J Clin Oncol 5(4):629, 1987
97. Teoh TB: Epidermoid carcinoma of the nasopharynx among Chinese: A study of 31 necropsies. J Pathol Bacteriol 73:451, 1957
98. Thawley SE, Panje WR: Comprehensive Management of Head and Neck Tumors, vol 1. Philadelphia, WB Saunders, 1987
99. Tokars RP, Griem ML: Carcinoma of the nasopharynx: An optimization of radiotherapeutic management for tumor control and spinal cord injury. Int J Radiat Oncol Biol Phys 5:1741, 1979
100. Turgman J, Modan B, Shilon M, et al: Nasopharyngeal cancer in a total population: Selected clinical and epidemiological aspects. Br J Cancer 36:783, 1977
101. Union Internationale Contre le Cancer: TNM Classification of Malignant Tumours. Geneva, UICC, 1968
102. Urdaneta N, Fischer JJ, Vera R, Gutierrez E: Cancer of the nasopharynx: Review of 43 cases treated with supervoltage radiation therapy. Cancer 37:1707, 1976
103. Valentini V, Balducci M, Ciarniello V, et al: Tumors of the nasopharynx: Review of 132 cases. Rays 12:77, 1987
104. Vikram B, Mishra UB, Strong EW, Manolatos S: Patterns of failure in carcinoma of the nasopharynx. I. Failure at the primary site. Int J Radiat Oncol Biol Phys 11:1455, 1985
105. Vikram B, Strong EW, Manolatos S, Mishra UB: Improved survival in carcinoma of the nasopharynx. Head Neck 7:123, 1984
106. Wang CC: Treatment of malignant tumors of the nasopharynx. Otol Clin North Am 13:477, 1980
107. Wang CC: Re-irradiation of recurrent nasopharyngeal carcinoma: Treatment techniques and results. Int J Radiat Oncol Biol Phys 13:953, 1987
108. Wang CC: Local control of nasopharyngeal carcinoma after intracavitary implant: Technique and results. (Abstract). Int J Radiat Oncol Biol Phys 17:172, 1989
109. Wang CC: Accelerated hyperfractionation radiation therapy for carcinoma of the nasopharynx: Techniques and results. Cancer 63:2461, 1989
110. Wang CC, Meyer JE: Radiotherapeutic management of carcinoma of the nasopharynx: An analysis of 170 patients. Cancer 28:566, 1971
111. Wang CC, Schulz MD: Management of locally recurrent carcinoma of the nasopharynx. Radiology 86:900, 1966
112. Wang DC, Cai WM, Hu YH, Zhi X: Long-term survival of 1035 cases of nasopharyngeal carcinoma. Cancer 61:2338, 1988
113. Wastie ML: The value of tomography in carcinoma of the nasopharynx. Br J Radiol 45:570, 1972
114. Wei WI, Lund VJ, Howard DJ: Serous otitis media in malignancies of the nasopharynx and maxilla. J Laryngol Otol 102:129, 1988
115. Yamashita S, Kondo M, Hashimoto S: Squamous cell carcinoma of the nasopharynx: An analysis of failure patterns after radiation therapy. Acta Radiol (Oncol) 24:315, 1985
116. Yamashita S, Kondo M, Inuyama Y, Hashimoto S: Improved survival of patients with nasopharyngeal squamous cell carcinoma. Int J Radiat Oncol Biol Phys 12:307, 1986
117. Yan J-H, Hu Y-H, Gu X-Z: Radiation therapy of recurrent nasopharyngeal carcinoma: Report on 219 patients. Acta Radiol (Oncol) 22:23, 1983
118. Yan J-H, Qin D-X, Hu Y-H, et al: Management of local residual primary lesion of nasopharyngeal carcinoma (NPC): Are higher doses beneficial? Int J Radiat Oncol Biol Phys 16:1465, 1989
119. Yeh S: A histological classification of carcinoma of the nasopharynx with a critical review as to the existence of lymphoepitheliomas. Cancer 15:895, 1962
120. Yin ZY, Wu XL, Hu YH, Gu XZ: Cylindroma of the nasopharynx: A chronic disease. Int J Radiat Oncol Biol Phys 12:25, 1986

29

○ ○ ○ ∘ • ∘

Nasal Cavity and Paranasal Sinuses

James T. Parsons
William M. Mendenhall
Scott P. Stringer
Nicholas J. Cassisi
Rodney R. Million

Primary tumors arising in the nasal cavity and paranasal sinuses are usually considered together. For purposes of treatment planning and reporting results, cancers of the nasal vestibule are usually considered separately because they have a natural history characteristic of skin cancer.

ANATOMY

The bony partitions between the nasal cavity, sinuses, orbits, and cranial vault are quite thin and offer little resistance to cancer spread (Fig. 29-1).[9]

The lamina papyracea between the orbit and the middle and posterior ethmoid air cells is thin, porous, and often incomplete. The ethmoid air cells extend far anteriorly, within 1 cm of the anterior skin surface in the medial canthal region. The right and left sphenoid sinuses, although divided by a septum, are considered as one in treatment planning because the septum is often incomplete or, at best, very thin.

The floor of the maxillary sinus is usually caudad to the floor of the nasal cavity, especially in edentulous patients.[9] The lower border of the radiation portal should extend to the level of the lip commissure to ensure adequate inferior coverage. Tumors that extend through the posterior wall of the maxillary sinus into the pterygoid area, apex of the orbit, or paranasopharyngeal area may be inoperable for technical reasons, because cancer readily extends from these sites to the base of skull (Fig. 29-2).[9]

The orbits are conical. If viewed in a straight anteroposterior projection, the roof of the maxillary sinus (*i.e.*, the floor of the orbit) rises above the level of the orbital rim as palpated anteriorly. The lateral walls of the ethmoid sinuses are parallel in their upper portions, but posteriorly and inferiorly, the walls diverge laterally to form the medial floor of the orbit. Too-tight treatment planning around the eye produces a geographic miss.

If it is necessary to treat a portion of the orbit, the patient is usually instructed to keep the eyes open and gaze straight ahead; lateral or upward gaze often rotates more of the posterior pole of the eye into the high-dose field. The accessory lacrimal glands, which are responsible for the basal flow of tears, are most plentiful in the upper eyelid. Cephalad displacement of the upper lid with a retractor often enables sparing of some of these glands. The major lacrimal gland in the superolateral orbit can often be shielded.

The optic nerves lie at about the same level as the roof of the ethmoid sinuses (Figs. 29-1 and 29-2).[9] It is not possible to irradiate the ethmoid and sphenoid sinuses without irradiating the optic nerves.

The capillary lymphatic plexus of the nasal cavity is well developed over the middle and inferior turbinates, in the olfactory region, and around the choanae; there are few lymphatics over the lower septum. The lymphatics of the paranasal sinuses are delicate and sparse, contributing to the low incidence of metastasis from tumors confined to the sinuses.

EPIDEMIOLOGY

Nasal cavity and paranasal sinus cancers are twice as common in males as in females and usually appear after the age of 40, except for an occasional tumor of minor salivary gland origin, lymphoma, or esthesioneuroblastoma, which may appear before the age of 20. For esthesioneuroblastoma, a bimodal age distribution (10–20 and 50–60 years of age) has been recognized.[11,29,35,36]

Nasal cavity and ethmoid sinus adenocarcinomas have been linked to occupations associated with wood dust (*e.g.*,

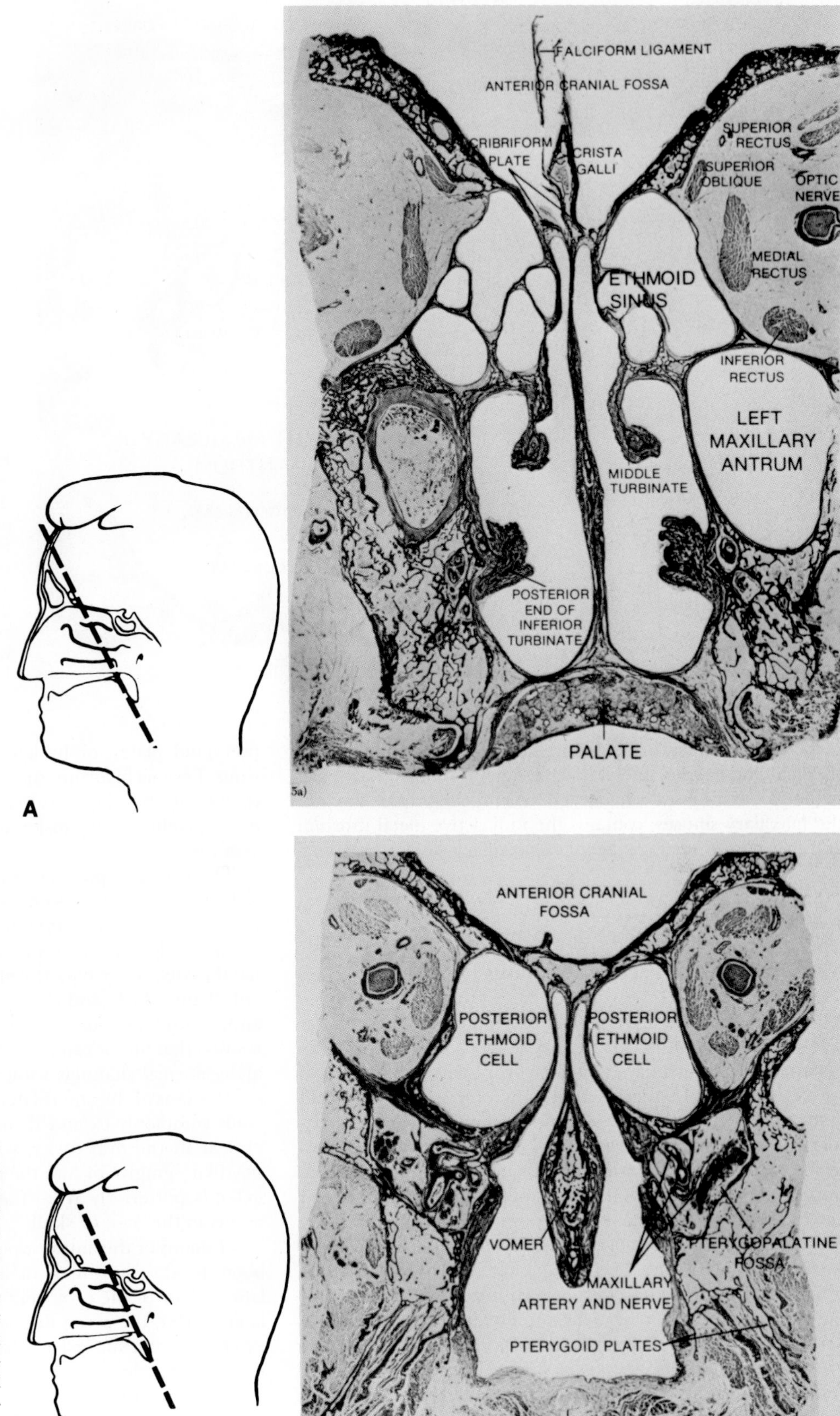

FIGURE 29–1. (**A**) Coronal section (*broken line*) through the cribriform plate, middle ethmoids, and posterior inferior turbinates. Notice the thin walls separating the sinuses from the orbits and nasal cavity. The right and left ethmoids are completely separated at all levels by the septum. The ethmoid cells may extend laterally above the orbits. (**B**) Coronal section (*broken line*) behind the maxillary antrum and anterior to the sphenoid sinus and nasopharynx. Notice relationships in the pterygopalatine fossa. (Bridger WM, van Nostrand P: J Otolaryngol 7:1, 1978)

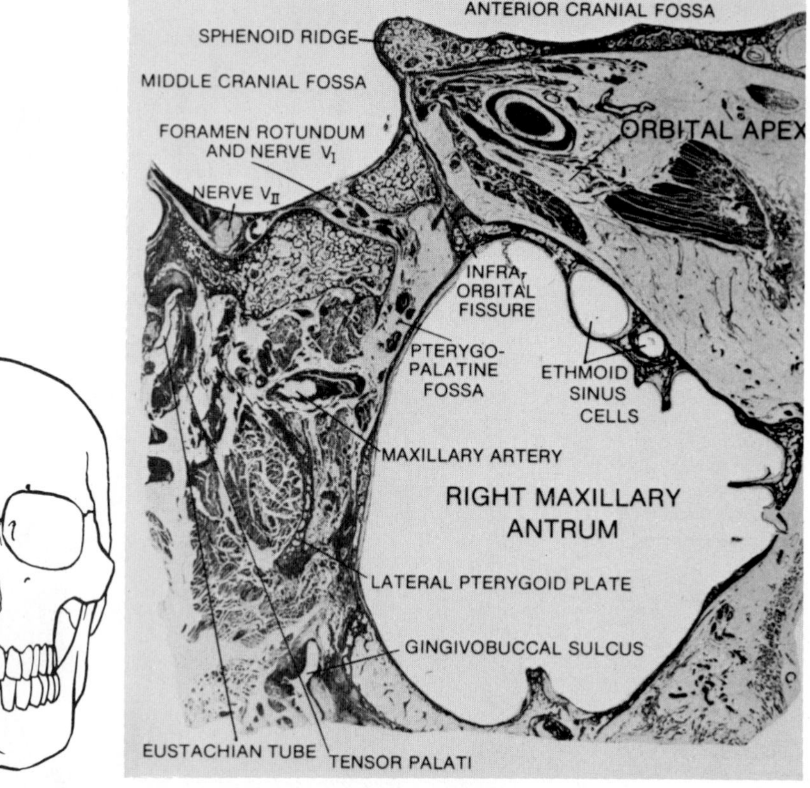

FIGURE 29–2. Sagittal section (*broken line*) through antrum and apex of the orbit. The apex of the orbit communicates with the pterygopalatine fossa by the infraorbital fissure. Extension of tumor through the posterior wall of the antrum provides access to the middle cranial fossa by the neural and vascular foramina. (Bridger WM, van Nostrand P: J Otolaryngol 7:1, 1978)

carpentry, the furniture industry, sawmill work), bootmaking, shoemaking, baking, and flour milling.[1–3, 18] Thorotrast, used in the past as a contrast medium for roentgenographic study of the maxillary sinuses, contains the radioactive metal thorium and is a known etiologic agent in maxillary sinus carcinoma.

NATURAL HISTORY

Nasal Cavity and Paranasal Sinuses

The routes of spread are essentially the same for all nasal cavity and paranasal tumors, with the exception of minor salivary gland tumors, which have a greater propensity for perineural spread. Perineural extension most commonly occurs in adenoid cystic carcinoma, but it may occur with other histologies, particularly those that recur after surgery. Commonly observed patterns of spread include extension through the cribriform plate into the anterior cranial fossa by way of the olfactory nerves and extension into the middle cranial fossa or cavernous sinus by way of the infraorbital nerve or nerves that run through the superior orbital fissure. The pterygomaxillary fossa and infraorbital fissure should be carefully scrutinized with 3-mm computed tomography (CT) sections, preferably in the coronal and axial planes. The region of the cribriform plate and olfactory groove region should always be studied coronally; magnetic resonance imaging (MRI) is probably a better choice than CT for detecting early invasion at this site.

Most lesions are advanced and commonly involve several adjacent sinuses, the nasal cavity, and often the nasopharynx. There is often orbital invasion from maxillary sinus or ethmoid sinus cancers; orbital invasion from nasal cavity tumors occurs late. The anterior cranial fossa is invaded by way of the cribriform plate and roof of the ethmoid sinuses. The middle cranial fossa is invaded by way of the infratemporal fossa, pterygoid plates, or by lateral extension from the sphenoid sinus. Lesions involving the olfactory region of the nasal cavity tend to destroy the septum and may invade through the nasal bone, producing expansion of the nasal bridge and eventually skin invasion.

Inverting papilloma usually arises from the lateral nasal wall. Extension to adjacent paranasal sinuses, orbit, and anterior cranial fossa is common.

Esthesioneuroblastomas originate in the upper (olfactory) nasal cavity. They may traverse the cribriform plate, which is only 1 mm thick, and dura and then invade the frontal lobes and, on rare occasions, seed the cerebrospinal fluid. Harrison[14] showed that tumor can pass from the nose to the olfactory bulb along normal channels without destroying bone.

Lesions of the anterolateral infrastructure of the maxillary sinus commonly extend through the lateral inferior wall and appear in the oral cavity, where tumor erodes through the maxillary gingiva or into the gingivobuccal sulcus. Tumor that extends posteriorly from the maxillary sinus has immediate access to the base of skull.

Lesions of the antral superstructure may invade the malar bone, producing a mass or antrocutaneous fistula below the lateral floor of the orbit (Fig. 29-3).[25] If tumor extends to the lateral orbit, the eye is displaced inward and upward. Medial extension from superstructure cancers leads to invasion of the nasal cavity, ethmoids, lacrimal apparatus, and medial inferior orbit. When multiple anatomic sites are involved, assignment of a primary site is an educated guess: The site that has the greatest tumor bulk is usually designated as the site of origin.

Primary carcinomas of the sphenoid sinus are rare. They mimic nasopharyngeal carcinoma and are most often diagnosed after they break through the floor of the sphenoid sinus into the nasopharynx. Frontal sinus neoplasms are also rare.

Lymph node metastases generally do not occur until tumor has extended to areas that contain abundant capillary lymphat-

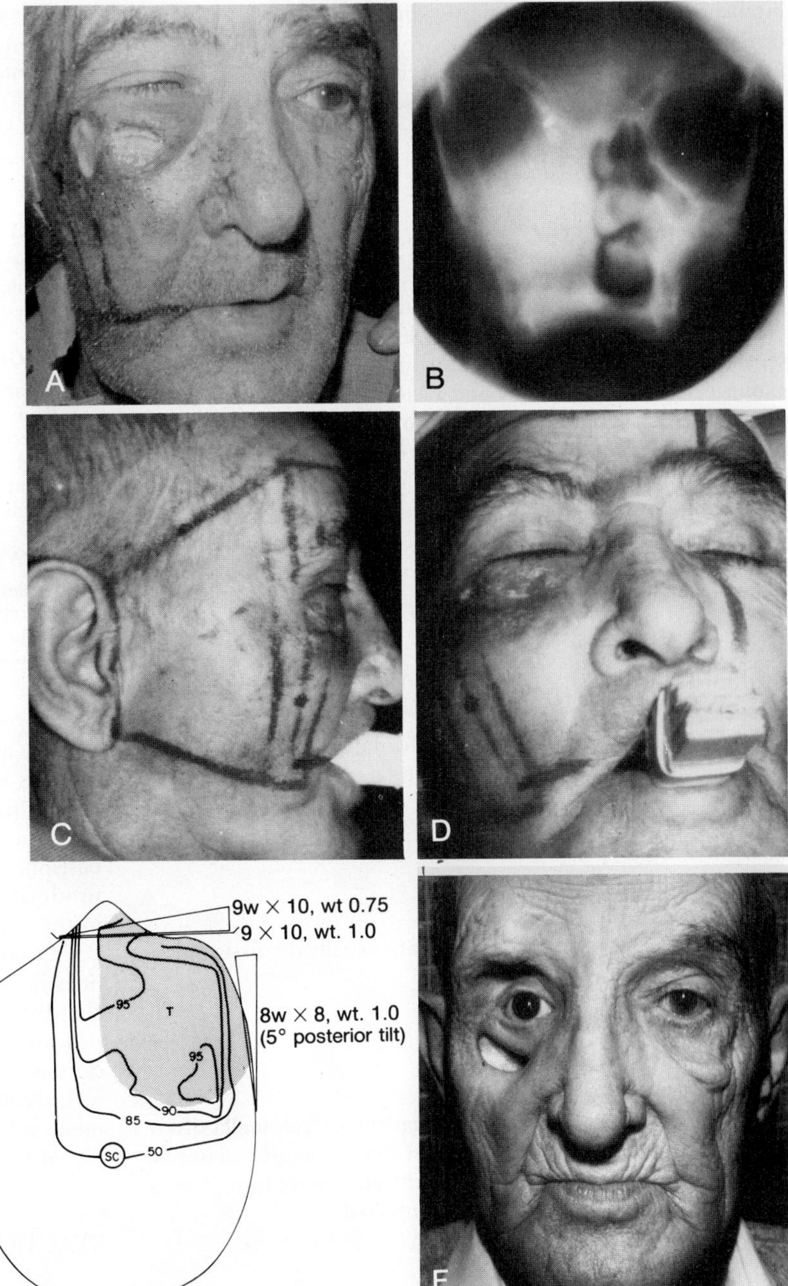

FIGURE 29–3. A 71-year-old man with a long history of sinusitis was treated by polypectomy and bilateral ethmoidectomies. He had a mass below the right lateral eyelid. There was recent onset of diplopia. (**A**) Pus was draining from the right cheek mass. The orbit was filled with a rock-hard mass. The nasal cavity was occluded by tumor, but the nasopharynx was normal (T4N0). The biopsy revealed squamous cell carcinoma. (**B**) Tomography and CT scans showed an opacified right maxillary antrum, right ethmoid and sphenoid sinuses, and right nasal cavity with destruction of the medial and inferior orbital walls. There was no intracranial extension. The patient refused surgery and received radiation treatment using ^{60}Co. (**C**) Right lateral portal. (**D**) Anterior portal. A stack of tongue blades was used to depress the tongue beyond the irradiation portals. Anterior and lateral portals overlapped approximately 2 cm on the skin surface. (**E**) The minimum tumor dose was 7000 cGy given in 40 fractions, specified at 85% of the maximum isodose line and administered by continuous-course irradiation. There was complete regression of obvious tumor after 5000 cGy. Diplopia disappeared, and vision returned to normal. Blurry vision developed at 14 months because of a superficial keratitis caused by dry eye and a cataract. The right cornea perforated and was repaired with a corneal transplant that failed; the right eye was enucleated. (**F**) At 5 years, an artificial eye was inserted but caused intermittent discomfort. The antrocutaneous fistula persists but is asymptomatic and provides a porthole for antrum examination. (Million RR, Cassisi NJ, Hamlin DJ: Nasal vestibule, nasal cavity, and paranasal sinuses. In Million RR, Cassisi NJ [eds]: Management of Head and Neck Cancer: A Multidisciplinary Approach, p 407. Philadelphia, JB Lippincott, 1984)

ics. The submandibular and subdigastric lymph nodes are most commonly involved.

Nasal Vestibule

Vestibule lesions invade the alar and septal cartilages and occasionally grow through to the skin surface. The upper lip is frequently invaded. Posterior extension into the nasal cavity occurs late or after recurrence. Nasal vestibule lesions are quite deceptive because they are more extensive than predicted from the physical findings. This observation is borne out by the number of patients seen with positive margins or recurrence after attempted excision.

Lymph node spread from vestibule cancers is usually to a solitary ipsilateral submandibular node, although bilateral spread is occasionally seen. The facial, preauricular, and submental nodes are at small risk. About 5% of patients have clinically positive lymph nodes on admission, and 15% develop lymph node metastases after treatment has controlled the primary tumor.

CLINICAL PRESENTATION

Nasal Cavity

The patient often describes a history of chronic nasal obstruction and "sinusitis" that has slowly worsened. Many have undergone nasal polypectomy or sinus surgery for inflammatory disease. Nasal discharge and minor epistaxis are common. Epiphora caused by obstruction of the nasal lacrimal system may be a presenting complaint, with the patient initially treated for dacryocystitis. Extension through the ethmoid sinuses to the medial orbit may cause proptosis, diplopia, paralysis of extraocular movements, or blindness. We have treated one patient with esthesioneuroblastoma whose only presenting problem was hyponatremia, presumably caused by a tumor-associated vasopressor-like substance.[35,37,39] Rarely, patients present with olfaction disturbances.

Maxillary Sinus

Maxillary sinus cancers tend to remain silent until they extend outside the sinus. Nasal obstruction, epistaxis, sinus pain, and a sensation of fullness over the antrum are common. Posterior extension produces trismus and headache secondary to invasion of the pterygoid muscles and the base of the skull. Cranial nerve deficits result from invasion of the base of skull or infraorbital nerve in the orbital floor. Inferior tumor extension leads to painful or loose teeth, sometimes leading to dental extractions. Edentulous patients may complain of an ill-fitting denture. An oral-antral fistula may eventually occur. Proptosis is obvious in some patients.

Ethmoid Sinus

Tumor may appear initially as a subcutaneous nodule in the inner canthus. Diplopia, proptosis, and a palpable orbital mass are common.

Sphenoid Sinus

Cranial nerve palsies and headaches are usually the first clinical evidence of sphenoid sinus cancer.

Nasal Vestibule

Early cancers of the membranous septum or columella often appear as little more than a crust or scab with occasional minor bleeding. More advanced lesions perforate the septum. Pain is usually modest unless the lesion is infected.

DIAGNOSTIC WORKUP

The diagnostic workup is presented in Table 29-1. Biopsy is usually made from tumor in the nasopharynx, nasal cavity, or medial canthal area or performed through a Caldwell-Luc incision.

On physical examination, close attention should be paid to signs of orbital invasion, cranial nerve involvement, and soft tissue extensions over the face or temporal fossa. Early orbital invasion is detected by palpating both orbits simultaneously with the tips of the index fingers inserted between the bony rim and eyeball. Anterior and posterior rhinoscopy, after thorough shrinkage and anesthesia of the nasal mucosa with a topically applied cocaine solution, is best accomplished with a straightforward (0-degree) or forward-oblique (30-degree) Hopkins nasal endoscope. A 90-degree Hopkins laryngopharyngoscope provides a better view of the nasopharynx than does a mirror.

CT and MRI have replaced conventional imaging.[21] CT is ordered first. Thin sections are obtained in both axial and coronal projections. If there are specific questions not answered by CT, an MR scan is obtained. Approximately half of the patients require both tests.

TABLE 29–1
Diagnostic Workup for Tumors of the Nasal Cavity and Paranasal Sinuses

GENERAL
- History
- Physical examination

SPECIAL TESTS
- Rhinoscopy with nasal endoscope
- Nasopharyngoscopy with laryngopharyngoscope
- Biopsy of primary tumor

RADIOGRAPHIC STUDIES
- Standard
  - Plain film sinus series
  - Chest radiographs
- Complementary
  - Computed tomography scan
  - Magnetic resonance imaging scan

LABORATORY STUDIES
- Complete blood count on admission
- Blood chemistry
- Urinalysis

In patients with suspected skull base erosion, there is a significant advantage for using MRI at the cribriform plate, basisphenoid, and floor of the middle cranial fossa.[41] MRI can produce consistently high-quality images of the cavernous sinus in the coronal projection.

Obstruction of normal drainage channels is common. CT does not completely answer the question of whether a sinus is cloudy because of tumor or obstructed ostia, although it often provides valuable clues; MRI is more helpful. If the question cannot be answered radiographically, surgical exploration may be indicated if the results will dictate a major change in treatment volume. The infratemporal fossa is usually clearly depicted by CT.

STAGING

The staging system of the American Joint Committee (AJC) on cancer applies only to maxillary sinus tumors (Table 29-2).[4] This staging system was devised at the University of Florida for tumors of the nasal cavity and ethmoid and sphenoid sinuses:

Stage I: Limited to site of origin
Stage II: Extension to adjacent sites (*e.g.*, orbit, nasopharynx, paranasal sinuses, skin, pterygomaxillary fossa)
Stage III: Base of skull or pterygoid plate destruction; intracranial extension

The AJC skin cancer staging scheme (Table 29-3) is appropriate for tumors of the nasal vestibule.[4] The staging system used in this chapter is the 1983 AJC system.

PATHOLOGIC CLASSIFICATION

Squamous cell carcinoma or one of its variants is most common. About 10% to 15% of neoplasms in this region are minor salivary gland tumors. Malignant melanoma accounts for 10% to

TABLE 29–2
TNM Classification for Cancer of the Maxillary Sinus

PRIMARY TUMOR (T)	
TX	Minimum requirements to assess the primary tumor cannot be met
T0	No evidence of primary tumor
T1	Tumor confined to the antral mucosa of the infrastructure, with no bone erosion or destruction
T2	Tumor confined to the superstructure mucosa without bone destruction or to the infrastructure, with destruction of medial or inferior bony walls only
T3	More extensive tumor invading skin of cheek, orbit, anterior ethmoid sinuses, or pterygoid muscle
T4	Massive tumor with invasion of cribriform plate, posterior ethmoids, sphenoid, nasopharynx, pterygoid plates, or base of skull
NODAL INVOLVEMENT (N)	
NX	Minimum requirements to assess the regional nodes cannot be met
N0	No clinically positive node
N1	Single clinically positive homolateral node ≤3 cm in diameter
N2	Single clinically positive homolateral node >3 cm but ≤6 cm in diameter, or multiple clinically positive homolateral nodes, none >6 cm in diameter
N2a	Single clinically positive homolateral node >3 cm but ≤6 cm in diameter
N2b	Multiple clinically positive homolateral nodes, none >6 cm in diameter
N3	Massive homolateral node(s), bilateral nodes, or contralateral node(s)
N3a	Clinically positive homolateral node(s), one >6 cm in diameter
N3b	Bilateral clinically positive nodes; in this situation, each side of the neck should be staged separately
N3c	Contralateral clinically positive node(s) only
DISTANT METASTASIS (M)	
MX	Minimum requirements to assess the presence of distant metastasis cannot be met
M0	No evidence of distant metastasis
M1	Distant metastasis

(American Joint Committee on Cancer: Manual for Staging of Cancer, 2nd ed, p 44. Philadelphia, JB Lippincott, 1983)

15% of cancers of the nasal cavity. Melanomas of the paranasal sinuses are rare.[15,19,34] Other histologic types are lymphoma (usually histiocytic), esthesioneuroblastoma, sarcoma, and inverting papilloma. The histologic picture of an inverting papilloma is that of a papilloma growing into, rather than out of, the stroma. Inverting papilloma, although usually histologically benign, it is best considered as "grade ½" carcinoma because of its 10% to 15% association with squamous cell carcinoma and its often aggressive clinical course, even in the absence of malignancy.

Almost all nasal vestibule cancers are squamous in origin.

PROGNOSTIC FACTORS

The histology, location, extent of tumor, and the patient's age and condition are important in making treatment decisions. Most surgeons regard tumor extension to the base of skull, nasopharynx, or sphenoid sinus as indicators of unresectability. Tumor extension into the orbit usually requires sacrifice of the eye. Surgery causes immediate loss of vision. If irradiation is selected as the primary mode of treatment, visual loss is usually delayed for 1 to 3 years.

TABLE 29–3
TNM Classification for Skin Cancer

PRIMARY TUMOR (T)*	
TX	Minimum requirements to assess the primary tumor cannot be met
Tis	Preinvasive carcinoma (carcinoma *in situ*)
T0	No primary tumor
T1	Tumor ≤2 cm in its largest dimension, strictly superficial or exophytic
T2	Tumor >2 cm but ≤5 cm in its largest dimension or with minimal infiltration of the dermis, regardless of size
T3	Tumor >5 cm in its largest dimension or with deep infiltration of the dermis, regardless of size
T4	Tumor involving other structures, such as cartilage, muscle, or bone

** The authors prefer to code nodal involvement and metastases from nasal vestibule primary lesions according to the standard head and neck 1983 AJC staging system (Table 29-2). (American Joint Committee on Cancer: Manual for Staging of Cancer, 2nd ed, p 124. Philadelphia, JB Lippincott, 1983)*

GENERAL MANAGEMENT

Nasal Cavity

Inverting papilloma without carcinoma is initially treated by surgery. Intranasal excision, Caldwell-Luc procedure, and ethmoidectomy result in a high recurrence rate. After lateral rhinotomy or midface degloving approaches, en bloc removal of the lateral nasal wall and resection of involved mucosa in adjacent sinuses produces a low rate of recurrence.[28,40] If inverting papilloma becomes aggressive (*e.g.*, rapid recurrences or invasion of sinuses, orbit, and cribriform plate), it is managed as a low-grade cancer by more radical en bloc removal or irradiation. Although experience with irradiation is limited, it has proven valuable in several University of Florida patients.[24] Inverting papilloma associated with carcinoma is treated as other nasal carcinomas.

Although surgery or irradiation produce high rates of cure for early nasal cavity cancers, in the last several years there has been a shift toward primary surgery at our institution, followed in most instances by postoperative irradiation to a lesser dose than employed for radiation-only therapy. The shift away from high-dose irradiation alone has been to reduce the risk of unilateral or bilateral optic nerve injury. In most instances, postoperative doses do not exceed 6000 cGy to 6500 cGy (180-cGy fractions); in the past, doses of approximately 7000 cGy were often delivered for radiation-only therapy. Currently, treatment is generally administered twice daily as 110 to 120 cGy per fraction, with 6 hours between fractions. For unresectable lesions, high-dose irradiation remains the only alternative; the current University of Florida approach uses twice daily treatment in an attempt to reduce the risk of optic nerve injury. It is too early to tell if this approach will be successful. A more homogeneous dose throughout the treatment volume can be usually achieved with 6-MV or 8-MV x-rays than with ^{60}Co.

Neither we nor Harwood[15] have found mucosal melanoma to be radioresistant. In three patients at the University of Florida, the tumor disappeared after conventionally fractionated treatment of 180 cGy to 200 cGy a day in five fractions each week. One patient remained free of disease for 8 years, after which distant metastases occurred; the other two developed local recurrences, one in-field tumor and one geographic miss.[24] Adenocarcinomas are also radiosensitive. Klintenberg[18] reported that six of 19 patients who were treated with preoperative irradiation (usually 4500 cGy) had negative tumor specimens.

No clear role for chemotherapy has been defined. At the University of Virginia, Spaulding and co-workers[38] reported one Stage B and five Stage C patients who received two to three cycles of cyclophosphamide and vincristine, followed by preoperative irradiation (5000 cGy) and craniofacial resection, for esthesioneuroblastoma. Five of the six patients subsequently relapsed. Wade and co-workers[42] reviewed the world literature on chemotherapy for esthesioneuroblastoma and noted that, although responses frequently occurred, they were generally incomplete and brief.

Ethmoid Sinus

At the University of Florida, the treatment philosophy for ethmoid sinus tumors is the same as for nasal cavity tumors. If resectable, operation is usually performed first; postoperative irradiation of 6000 cGy to 6500 cGy in 180-cGy fractions is advised, even if resection margins are negative. En bloc removal requires craniofacial resection.

If only a single modality of treatment is selected, irradiation produces better results than surgery alone. Patients with unresectable lesions are offered high-dose irradiation twice daily.

Maxillary Sinus

Resection gives the best results. Early infrastructure lesions are often cured by surgery alone, but in most cases of maxillary sinus cancer, irradiation is given postoperatively, even if the margins are clear. Massive tumor extension to the base of the skull, nasopharynx, or sphenoid sinus usually contraindicates surgery. Borderline resectable lesions are sometimes treated with full-dose external-beam irradiation, followed by operation if technically feasible. Many patients refuse surgery because of the defect imposed by maxillectomy and possible orbital exenteration.

Sphenoid Sinus

Irradiation is usually the treatment by default. Treatment planning is similar to that for advanced carcinoma of the nasopharynx.

Nasal Vestibule

Both surgical and radiation therapy produce a high degree of success in experienced hands. Radiation therapy is the preferred treatment in our clinic, because excision almost always produces deformity, except if the lesion is small and located favorably. Although locally advanced lesions may be considered for resection followed by radiation therapy, the cosmetic loss from rhinectomy is severe, and our approach is generally radical irradiation, with surgery reserved for failure.[25]

Although cartilage that has been compromised by tumor invasion, infection, or prior surgery is theoretically more vulnerable to radiation injury, the risk of necrosis is low with properly fractionated external-beam therapy (with or without radium), even at substantial doses. The probability of tumor control correlates better with tumor volume than with the extent of cartilage invasion.[27]

Neck

Elective neck treatment is generally not prescribed. However, patients with recurrent or poorly differentiated cancers and those that extend to an area with dense capillary lymphatics (*e.g.*, nasopharynx, oropharynx, oral cavity) have a higher risk of metastasis and are often given elective neck irradiation of 5000 cGy in 5 weeks, administered in 200-cGy fractions daily.

Elective neck irradiation is usually not prescribed in patients with nasal vestibule cancers for several reasons. A large volume of tissue would need to be irradiated (*e.g.*, intercalated, submandibular, and jugular nodes), leading to considerable acute morbidity and xerostomia. Because of the technical difficulty of matching these fields to the primary portals, xerostomia and some risk of necrosis due to field junctions would occur. Moreover, the rate of successful surgical salvage (neck dissection) of a solitary submandibular lymph node metastasis is very high.

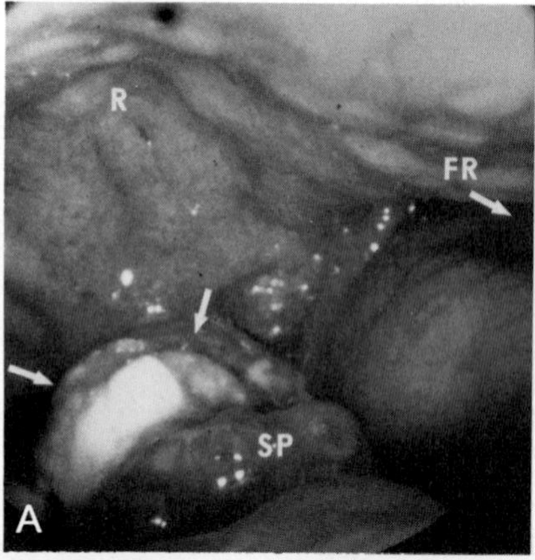

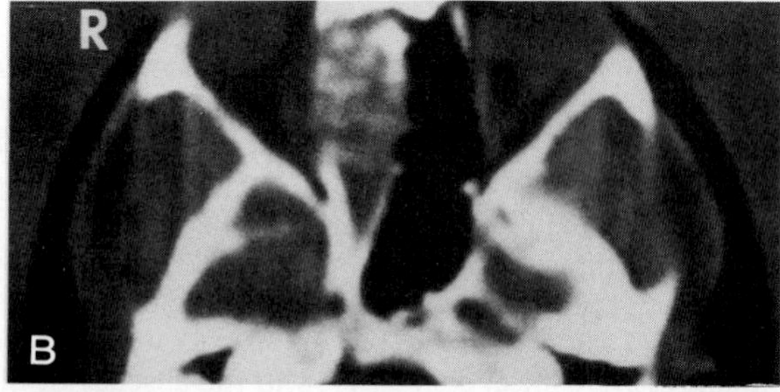

FIGURE 29–4. A 33-year-old black man had a 1-year history of left nasal congestion and frontal headaches, a 6-month history of epistaxis, and a 3-month history of left eye tearing. A granular lesion filled the entire nasal cavity and extended into the nasopharynx. (**A**) Tumor mass extending into nasopharynx (*arrows*). R, roof; SP, soft palate; FR, right fossa of Rosenmuller. (**B**) CT scan at the level of the orbit and ethmoids. There is opacification of the right ethmoid sinus and nasal cavity. The mass bulges into the medial aspect of the left orbit. Diagnosis was squamous cell carcinoma of the ethmoid sinus with invasion of maxillary sinus, sphenoid sinus, nasal cavity, and nasopharynx. The tumor was thought to be unresectable because of nasopharynx involvement and possible sphenoid sinus invasion. (Million RR, Cassisi NJ, Hamlin DJ: Nasal vestibule, nasal cavity, and paranasal sinuses. In Million RR, Cassisi NJ [eds]: Management of Head and Neck Cancer: A Multidisciplinary Approach, p 407. Philadelphia, JB Lippincott, 1984)

In patients with palpable neck lymph nodes on admission, neck dissection is usually added; for patients whose primary site is being treated with irradiation alone, the neck operation follows the irradiation. If the primary tumor is to be treated with surgery, the neck dissection is performed at that time, followed by postoperative irradiation of 6000 cGy over 6 weeks to the primary site and to the neck if there are multiple lymph nodes or extracapsular tumor spread.

RADIATION THERAPY TECHNIQUES

The external-beam techniques for nasal cavity, ethmoid sinus, and maxillary sinus cancers are similar. Treatment emphasizes an anterior portal with one or two posteriorly tilted lateral portals, frequently using wedges. Even if the lesion is apparently localized, we prefer to treat a large initial volume rather than rely too greatly on imaging and physical examination. Fields may be reduced to the initial gross disease, with a margin, after 4500 cGy to 5000 cGy. For limited cancers of the nasal cavity, the initial treatment volume includes the medial maxillary sinus, ethmoid sinus, medial portion of the orbit, nasopharynx, sphenoid sinus, and base of skull.[25,33]

Ethmoid sinus and advanced nasal cavity cancers are similarly managed (Figs. 29-4 and 29-5). The given doses (D_{max}) to the anterior and lateral fields are usually weighted 2 to 1 or 3 to 1 in favor of the anterior portal to avoid excessive irradiation of the contralateral eye. Wedges are used to achieve a satisfactory dose distribution. A reduced anterior open portal is often incorporated into the treatment plan to concentrate the dose to the

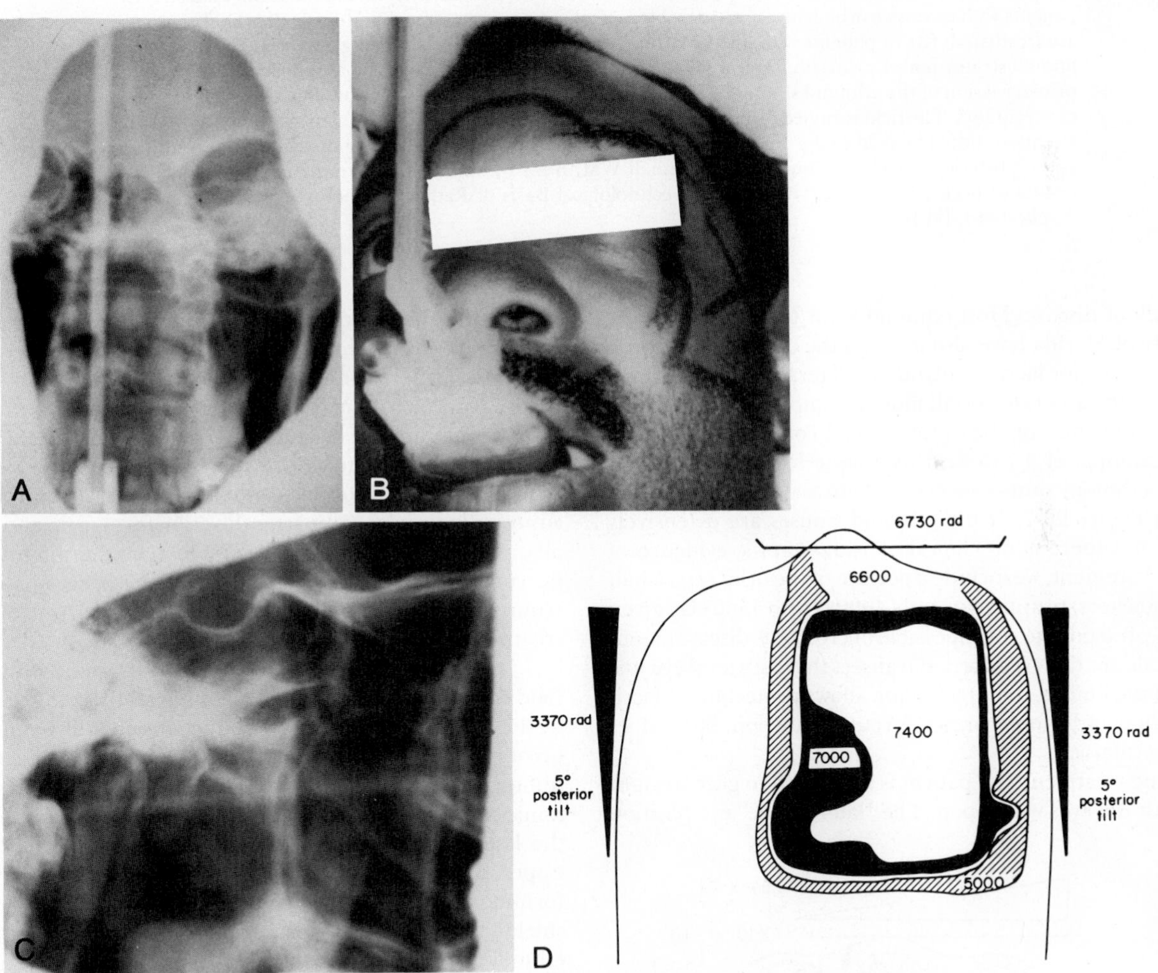

FIGURE 29–5. Treatment techniques for the patient in Figure 29–4. (**A**) Simulation film of the anterior portal. Straight white line is aluminum support for bite-block. (Ellingwood KE, Million RR: Cancer 43:1517, 1979) (**B**) Radiation therapy treatment portals were anterior and left and right laterals. Upper lateral eyelid and lacrimal gland were shielded because only the medial orbit was involved by tumor. (Million RR, Cassisi NJ, Hamlin DJ: Nasal vestibule, nasal cavity, and paranasal sinuses. In Million RR, Cassisi NJ [eds]: Management of Head and Neck Cancer: A Multidisciplinary Approach, p 407. Philadelphia, JB Lippincott, 1984) (**C**) Simulation film of the lateral portal (5-degree posterior tilt). The portal encompasses the base of skull, posterior ethmoid and maxillary sinuses, posterior nasal cavity, sphenoid sinus, nasopharynx, posterior one third of both orbits, pterygoid plates, infratemporal fossa, and parapharyngeal lymph nodes. The posterior border is just anterior to the external auditory canal, excluding the cervical spinal cord and brain stem. (Ellingwood KE, Million RR: Cancer 43:1517, 1979) (**D**) The treatment plan was 7000 cGy minimum (7700 cGy maximum) tumor dose in 7 weeks. The given doses were weighted 2 to 1 in favor of the anterior portal. The right and left upper neck received 4050 cGy in 3 weeks through an anterior portal with midline shielding. Visible tumor disappeared during therapy. The patient returned to full-time work as a truck driver at 4 months after diagnosis. A cataract developed in the left eye at 36 months; after its extraction, visual acuity was only "counts fingers at 2 feet" because of radiation retinopathy. The patient was disease free at 8.5 years.

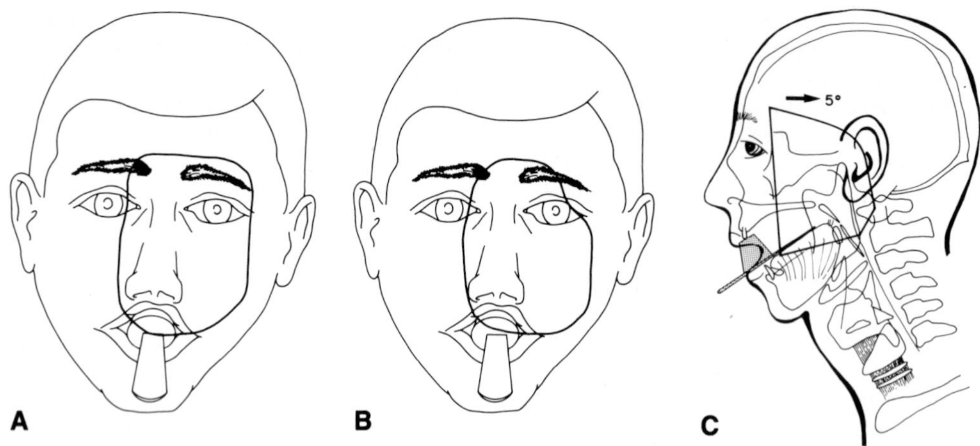

FIGURE 29–6. Portals used to treat patients with tumors of the nasal cavity and paranasal sinuses. (**A**) In patients with extensive orbital invasion (palpable orbital mass, proptosis, or blindness), all orbital contents are irradiated. (**B**) In patients with limited orbital invasion, the major lacrimal gland is shielded. Dotted line illustrates portal primarily used for limited lesions of the nasal cavity or as a reduced field for a primary lesion of the ethmoid sinus. (**C**) Typical lateral portal for treatment of paranasal sinus and nasal cavity tumors. The field is angled 5 degrees posteriorly to avoid exit irradiation to contralateral eye. Special attention should be paid to the dose to the brain stem and spinal cord, including the contribution for the anteroposterior portal. (Parsons JT, Mendenhall WM, Bova FJ, Million RR: Irradiation techniques for head and neck cancer. In Levitt SH [ed]: Technological Basis of Radiation Therapy: Practical Clinical Applications. [in press])

major bulk of disease. Most ethmoid sinus tumors seen at the University of Florida have also invaded the orbit. If invasion is minimal, the major lacrimal gland and lateral upper eyelid are shielded on the anterior portal; more advanced orbital invasion requires irradiation of the entire orbital contents (Fig. 29-6).

An example of a two-field technique for advanced nasal cavity or ethmoid sinus cancers with invasion of the orbits is shown in Figure 29-7. If the ethmoid sinuses are extensively involved, but there is no clinical or radiographic evidence of orbital involvement, we include a portion of the orbit (*e.g.*, a half to three quarters) to approximately 4000 cGy to 4500 cGy given in 180-cGy fractions to cover possible microscopic disease extension. Portals are then reduced to transect the ipsilateral eye just medial to the limbus. This technique allows protection of lacrimal function and should preserve retinal function, but it does produce a cataract.

During treatment, the patient is instructed to gaze straight ahead with the eyes wide open. The "lateral gaze" eye position was discontinued because it rotates the posterior pole of the eye and retina into the treatment portal. An eyelid retractor is useful to displace some of the upper lateral lid from the treatment field. Narrow margins around the eye commonly produce treatment failures. The anterior portal extends 1.5 cm to 2.0 cm across the midline to encompass the entire nasal cavity and ethmoid-sphenoid complex and medial contralateral orbit. The superior margin encompasses the cribriform plate and includes all or part of the frontal sinus. The inferior margin (usually the lip commissure) includes the floor of the nose, maxillary antrum, and alveolar ridge; the tongue is displaced out of the treatment portal by a tongue blade and cork.[12,25,26,33]

In lesions of the nasal cavity without orbital invasion, the field edge is placed at the medial limbus. If there is gross disease in the ethmoid sinuses, field reductions should be made with great caution because of both the high incidence of subclinical tumor extension through the lamina papyracea and the anatomic configuration of the sinus relative to the orbit. Although the lateral walls of the ethmoid sinuses are parallel in their upper portions, inferiorly and posteriorly they diverge, conforming to the cone-shaped orbit. If the eyeball is totally shielded from the anterior portal, some of the posteroinferior ethmoid air cells are also shielded. The same principle applies to the roof of the maxillary sinus. In some patients, the anterior portal is tilted cephalad slightly (*e.g.*, 10 to 12 degrees) so that the beam parallels the inferomedial and inferior orbital walls, allowing greater coverage of the sinuses while irradiating a lesser volume of the orbital contents.

The anterior portal for maxillary sinus cancers resembles that used for nasal cavity and ethmoid sinus lesions. The inferior border must be shaped to cover the lowest extent of disease (*e.g.*, tumor tracking down the buccal mucosa from the gingivobuccal sulcus or tumor in the low parapharyngeal or tonsillar regions must be recognized). If the temporal fossa is grossly invaded, the lateral border of the anterior portal is usually allowed to fall off for all or part of the treatment (Fig. 29-6).[32]

The lateral portals for nasal cavity, ethmoid, and maxillary sinus lesions are all similar (Figs. 29-5 and 29-6*C*). The anterior

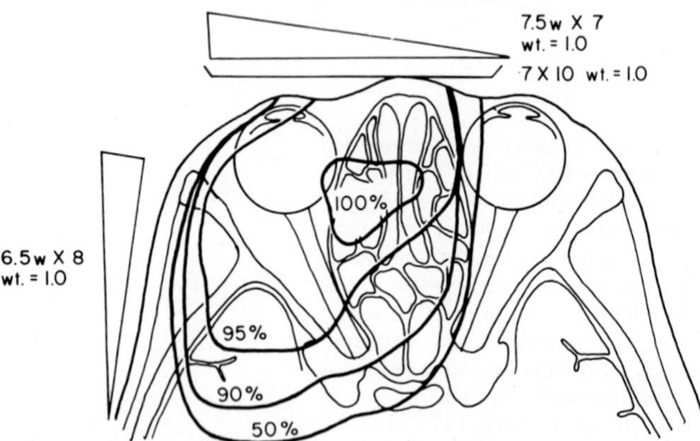

FIGURE 29–7. Isodose distribution for carcinoma of the ethmoid sinus with orbital invasion. The lateral portal is angled 5 degrees posteriorly. (Million RR, Cassisi NJ, Clark JR: Cancer of the head and neck. In DeVita VT, Hellman S, Rosenberg SA [eds]: Cancer: Principles and Practice of Oncology, 3rd ed. Philadelphia, JB Lippincott, 1989)

border of the lateral portals is at the lateral bony canthus, which means that a portion of the posterior pole of the ipsilateral eyeball is included within the lateral fields; the contralateral globe is missed because of the posterior angulation of the lateral portals. The superior border of the lateral field is adjusted according to the extent of disease. It is usually 1.0 cm above the roof of the ethmoid sinuses, but it may be raised 2 cm to 3 cm to cover known or suspected intracranial extension. The inferior border is usually at the level of the lip commissure to generously cover the floor of the antrum, which lies below the floor of the nasal cavity. A cork and tongue blade depress the tongue out of the field. The posterior border and the posterosuperior borders are shaped to exclude the spinal cord and brain stem, respectively. Usually the posterior border is at or near the tragus and bisects the vertebral bodies. The posterosuperior border is usually drawn 2 mm to 3 mm posterior to the clivus.

If the spinal cord and brain stem are encompassed by the lateral portal(s) for the initial 5000 cGy, the total dose to these structures will exceed 5000 cGy at the completion of a typical course of irradiation (*e.g.*, 6000–7000 cGy). This is because it is not possible to shield the cord and brain stem from the reduced anterior field after 5000 cGy. As an example, assume that we plan to deliver 7000 cGy tumor dose with a combination of one anterior and two lateral portals, with the given doses (at D_{max}) weighted 2 to 1 in favor of the anterior field. If the brain stem has already received 5000 cGy at this point, it will receive another substantial contribution from the remaining 2000 cGy given dose to be delivered to the anterior field, even though it is eliminated from the lateral fields. The brain stem and spinal cord are encompassed within the lateral portals only in the rare circumstance of tumor extension posterior to the plane of the cord. In this setting, the patient must be advised of the increased risk of neurologic sequelae.

Radiation therapy to the nasal vestibule may be delivered by external-beam therapy (Figs. 29-8 and 29-9), interstitial therapy, or a combination of the two techniques.[23,25,26] The highest control rates are obtained in patients whose treatment consists of implant alone or implant and external-beam irradiation.

FOLLOW-UP AND RECURRENCES

Nasal Cavity and Paranasal Sinuses

Diagnosis of recurrence is important because salvage may be possible. If a maxillectomy has been done, follow-up is simplified by the ease of physical examination; it is more difficult to assess the patient who was treated by irradiation alone, and exploration of the sinuses may be necessary. Baseline CT or MR scans are obtained about 3 months after treatment. Localized recurrence after surgery may be managed by irradiation alone or by resection and postoperative radiation therapy. Radiation therapy failures are sometimes successfully treated by craniofacial resection.

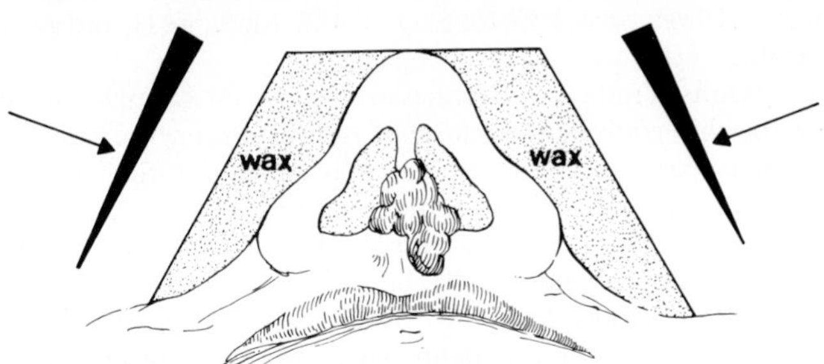

FIGURE 29–8. Treatment plan for external-beam irradiation of nasal vestibule carcinoma. (Million RR, Cassisi, NJ, Clark JR: Cancer of the head and neck. In DeVita VT Jr, Hellman S, Rosenberg SA [eds]: Cancer: Principles and Practice of Oncology, 3rd ed. Philadelphia, JB Lippincott, 1989)

Nasal Vestibule

Salvage surgery for radiation therapy failures is frequently no more extensive than that necessary for the original lesion, if the patient has been observed closely. Irradiation can control many postsurgical recurrences; we usually administer 5000 cGy to 6000 cGy by external beam, followed by a radium implant.[23]

Neck

Neck dissection is frequently successful in salvaging patients whose disease recurs in a submandibular or jugulodigastric node after primary treatment, provided the metastasis is detected early and the primary lesion remains controlled. Postoperative irradiation may be indicated.

RESULTS OF THERAPY

Nasal Cavity, Ethmoid Sinus, and Sphenoid Sinus

Except with mucosal melanomas, distant metastases are unusual; locoregional control is usually tantamount to cure. It is difficult to compare results of various therapies because no standardized staging system has been applied.

Mendenhall and co-workers[24] reported results of irradiation in five patients with advanced or recurrent inverted papilloma. Three were irradiated preoperatively or postoperatively, and two received irradiation alone for unresectable disease. All five remained free of disease for between 3 and 11 years.

Frazell and Lewis[13] reported a 5-year cure rate of 56% for 68 nasal cavity cancers treated surgically. The 5-year cure rate by radiation therapy was 18% for 28 patients treated. The authors reported a 5-year cure rate of 40% for ethmoid sinus patients treated by radiation therapy and a rate of 19% for those treated by surgery; they concluded, however, that surgery was the treatment of choice.

Bosch and associates[8] reported a 5-year survival rate of 56% for patients with tumors of the nasal cavity; 85% were treated by radiation therapy alone. Their series included an unspecified number of nasal vestibule lesions. The series by Hawkins and co-workers[16] reports a 52% 5-year survival rate, but it also includes patients with nasal vestibule cancers. Boone and co-workers[7] reported an absolute 5-year cure rate of 63% for the nasal cavity, but the number of patients treated by surgery and the number receiving radiation therapy were not given.

Between October 1964 and December 1983, 48 patients with malignant tumors of the nasal cavity (31 patients), ethmoid sinus, or sphenoid sinus were treated with definitive irradiation at the University of Florida.[33] There were 21 squamous cell carcinomas, 14 minor salivary gland tumors (*i.e.*, adenocarcinoma, adenoid cystic carcinoma, and mucoepidermoid carcinoma), three malignant melanomas, two soft tissue sarcomas,

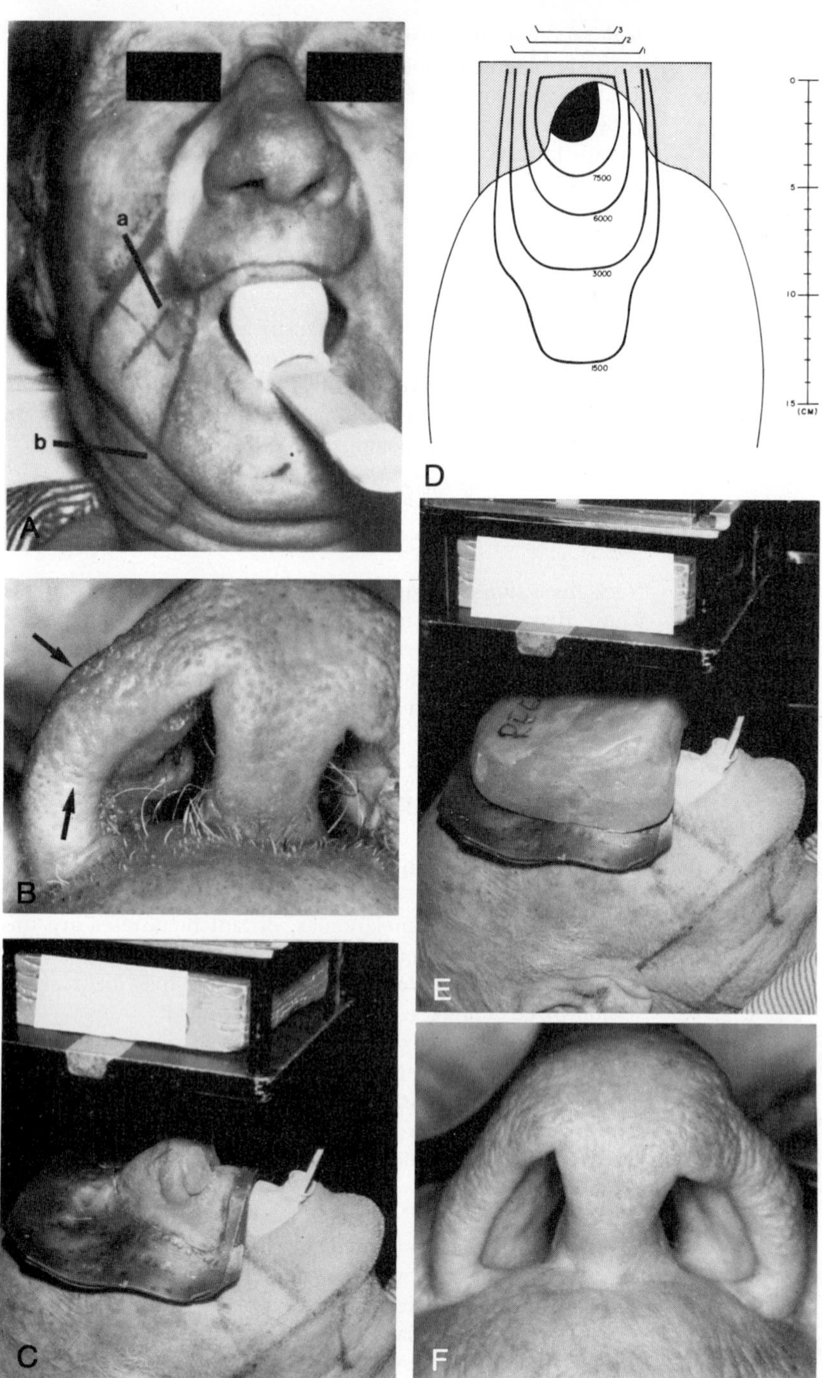

FIGURE 29–9. An 84-year-old man presented with a 3-month history of nosebleeds. (**A**) Squamous cell carcinoma (1.5 cm) on the right lateral wall of the nasal vestibule (*arrows*). Erythema and induration extended to the tip and ala of the nose and just into the lip. There was probably invasion of the lateral alar cartilage. He also had a squamous cell carcinoma of the vocal cord (T1N0). (**B**) Outline of treatment portals. The transit lymphatics and facial lymph nodes (a) were treated with electrons, and the submandibular lymph nodes (b) were electively treated because of the significant dermal extension and the undesirability of doing a neck dissection in this 84-year-old patient. (**C**) Treatment setup with lead shield, wax plugs in nose, and tongue depressor. (**D**) Isodose distribution. Stippled area represents the beeswax bolus or compensator. (**E**) Wax bolus in place. Electron beam was collimated by a Lipowitz's metal block on a tray. The treatment plan was 7500 cGy over 8 weeks using a combination of photons and electrons. (**F**) No evidence of disease at 2 years. (Million RR, Cassisi NJ, Hamlin DJ: Nasal vestibule, nasal cavity, and paranasal sinuses. In Million RR, Cassisi NJ [eds]: Management of Head and Neck Cancer: A Multidisciplinary Approach, p 407. Philadelphia, JB Lippincott, 1984)

and eight esthesioneuroblastomas. Forty-two patients were treated with irradiation alone and six with planned combined irradiation and surgery. The 10-year actuarial local control rate for Stage I (seven patients) was 100%; for Stage II (19 patients), 53%; and for Stage III (22 patients), 30%.[10] Of 24 failures at the primary site, 10 occurred more than 24 months after completion of irradiation. With the exception of adenoid cystic carcinoma, which had a 17% local control rate at 15 years, the ultimate local control rates for all histologies were in the range of 40% to 60% (Fig. 29-10). Although adenoid cystic carcinomas were initially quite responsive, five of six patients developed late primary recurrence at 40, 48, 60, 60, and 148 months. Of seven patients with documented intracranial extension, three (43%) remained free from local recurrence 3.5, 4, and 9 years after treatment. The 5-, 10-, 15-, and 20-year uncorrected actuarial survival rates for all 48 patients were 52%, 30%, 22%, and 22%, respectively. Continuous disease-free survival according to stage at 10 years was 86% for Stage I, 42% for Stage II, and 22% for Stage III.

Results of radical radiation therapy for mucosal melanomas are roughly equivalent to those of radical surgery for equivalent-stage patients; neither treatment is usually curative because of local recurrence or distant metastasis.[15]

After surgery for esthesioneuroblastoma, the 5-year survival rate is approximately 50%, but the continuous disease-free survival rate is much lower.[29,36] Olsen[29] reported that only four (21%) of 19 Mayo Clinic patients remained continuously free of disease 5 years after resection; Shah and Feghali[36] reported 5-year continuous disease-free survival for only two (6%) of 31 Memorial Hospital patients. Twenty-three of the 31 patients required two or more surgical resections, and some required as many as 10 to 17. In both the Memorial and Mayo Clinic series,

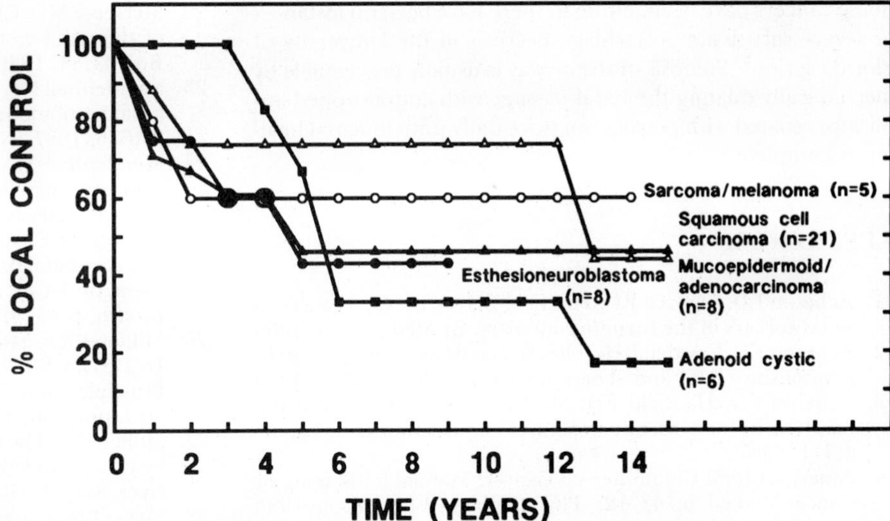

FIGURE 29–10. Local control (life-table method) for cancers of the nasal cavity, ethmoid sinus, or sphenoid sinus according to histologic type (all stages combined, University of Florida data, October 1964 to December 1983). (Parsons JT, Mendenhall WM, Mancuso AA, et al: Int J Radiat Oncol Biol Phys 14:11, 1988)

patients tended to develop a series of increasingly grave local recurrences, which predisposed them to the development of unresectable intracranial extension, lymph node metastasis, and distant metastasis. Late failures 5 to 10 or more years after treatment are not rare.[5,29,36] Eventual development of distant metastases is observed in 25% to 30% of patients.[29,35] In a review of world literature, local recurrence accounted for almost 70% of observed failures.[11] Single modality was as effective as combined treatment in early-stage disease because some failures can be salvaged, but the lowest recurrence rates were noticed after initial combined therapy. We recommend combined-modality treatment because some recurrences are not resectable and others lead to metastasis.

Maxillary Sinus

Jesse[17] reviewed 63 patients with squamous cell carcinoma of the maxillary antrum who received treatment with curative intent. The 3-year survival rate was 44%. The 3-year survival rate after surgery alone for selected lesions was 45% (nine of 20 patients). Patients selected for combined treatment had preoperative or postoperative irradiation, and the results were similar for both techniques. The local recurrence rate with combined therapy was 38%. Patients with infrastructure lesions and superolateral lesions had a 3-year survival rate of 68% (13 of 19 patients), and those with superomedial or superoposterior lesions had a survival rate of only 29%.

Bataini and Ennuyer[6] reported results obtained at the Curie Foundation for 31 patients with carcinoma of the maxillary antrum treated by supervoltage radiation therapy between 1959 and 1965. Only three patients had limited primary disease; 30% had clinically positive lymph nodes. The 3- and 5-year survival rates free of disease were 39% and 32%, respectively.

Nasal Vestibule

For 19 of 22 patients with *de novo* or recurrent cancers of the nasal vestibule, the disease was locally controlled by irradiation (*i.e.,* one of one TX, six of six T1, two of two T2, two of two T3, eight of 11 T4 tumors) at the University of Florida. Twenty patients had clinically negative neck nodes on admission. Two of 17 patients in whom no elective lymph node treatment was administered developed submandibular lymph node metastases; both were salvaged by neck dissection. No neck failures occurred in three N0 patients in whom elective treatment was administered or in two patients with N1 disease after irradiation alone. Five-year absolute and cause-specific survival rates were 75% and 95%, respectively.[23]

McNeese and co-workers reported control in 11 of 11 previously untreated patients who received treatment by interstitial implant alone (*i.e.,* 6000–7500 cGy in 5–7 days) and in 20 of 21 patients who received electron-beam irradiation of 6000 cGy in 4 weeks to 7000 cGy in 6 to 7 weeks.[22]

The series by Mak and co-workers emphasizes the importance of adequate dose; following external-beam irradiation, the recurrence rate after less than 5400 cGy was 63%, but it was 18% at doses equal to or greater than 5400 cGy.[20] Similarly, Wong and co-workers[43] recorded a significant dose-response effect.

SEQUELAE OF TREATMENT

Surgery

Complications of ethmoid sinus surgery include total blindness, loss of ocular motility, hemorrhage, meningitis, cerebrospinal fluid leak, cellulitis and pansinusitis, brain abscess, stroke, fistula between the cavernous sinus and internal carotid artery, and damage to the frontal lobe. Complications of maxillectomy include failure of the split-thickness graft to heal, trismus, cerebrospinal fluid leak, and hemorrhage.

Radiation Therapy

Complications of irradiation of nasal cavity or paranasal sinus tumors include central nervous system damage, unilateral or bilateral loss of vision, serous otitis media, and chronic sinusitis.[30,31,33] Osteoradionecrosis of the maxilla occurs infrequently. Transverse myelitis and brain necrosis have not been observed in the University of Florida series.

Long-term complications after irradiation of nasal vestibule cancers have been minimal; there have been no instances of severe soft tissue or cartilage necrosis in the University of Florida series.[23] Stenosis of the airway is usually preventable by mechanically dilating the nasal passage with cotton-tipped applicators coated with petrolatum twice daily until mucosal healing is complete.

REFERENCES

1. Acheson ED, Cowdell RH, Hadfield EH, et al: Nasal cancer in woodworkers in the furniture industry. Br Med J 2:587, 1968
2. Acheson ED, Cowdell RH, Jolles B: Nasal cancer in the Northamptonshire boot and shoe industry. Br Med J 1:385, 1970
3. Acheson ED, Hadfield EH, Macbeth RG: Carcinoma of the nasal cavity and accessory sinuses in woodworkers. Lancet 1:311, 1967
4. American Joint Committee on Cancer: Manual for Staging of Cancer, 2nd ed, pp 43, 123. Philadelphia, JB Lippincott, 1983
5. Appelblatt NH, McClatchey KD: Olfactory neuroblastoma: A retrospective clinicopathologic study. Head Neck Surg 5:108, 1982
6. Bataini J-P, Ennuyer A: Advanced carcinoma of the maxillary antrum treated by cobalt teletherapy and electron beam irradiation. Br J Radiol 44:590, 1971
7. Boone ML, Harle TS, Higholt HW, et al: Malignant disease of the paranasal sinuses and nasal cavity: Importance of precise localization of extent of disease. Am J Roentgenol Radium Ther Nucl Med 102:627, 1968
8. Bosch IL, Vallecillo L, Frias Z: Cancer of the nasal cavity. Cancer 37:1458, 1976
9. Bridger MWM, van Nostrand AWP: The nose and paranasal sinuses—applied surgical anatomy: A histologic study of whole organ sections in three planes. J Otolaryngol 7:1, 1978
10. Cutler SJ, Ederer F: Maximum utilization of the life table method in analyzing survival. J Chronic Dis 8:699, 1958
11. Elkon D, Hightower SI, Lim ML, Cantrell RW, Constable WC: Esthesioneuroblastoma. Cancer 44:1087, 1979
12. Ellingwood KE, Million RR: Cancer of the nasal cavity and ethmoid/sphenoid sinuses. Cancer 43:1517, 1979
13. Frazell EL, Lewis JS: Cancer of the nasal cavity and accessory sinuses: A report of the management of 416 patients. Cancer 16:1293, 1963
14. Harrison D: Surgical pathology of olfactory neuroblastoma. Head Neck Surg 7:60, 1984
15. Harwood AR: Melanoma of the head and neck. In Million RR, Cassisi NJ (eds): Management of Head and Neck Cancer: A Multidisciplinary Approach, p 513. Philadelphia, JB Lippincott, 1984
16. Hawkins RB, Wynstra JH, Pilepich MV, Fields JN: Carcinoma of the nasal cavity: Results of primary and adjuvant radiotherapy. Int J Radiat Oncol Biol Phys 15:1129, 1988
17. Jesse RH: Preoperative versus postoperative radiation in the treatment of squamous carcinoma of the paranasal sinuses. Am J Surg 110:552, 1965
18. Klintenberg C, Olofsson J, Hellquist H, Sokjer H: Adenocarcinoma of the ethmoid sinuses: A review of 28 cases with special reference to wood dust exposure. Cancer 54:482, 1984
19. Lederman M, Busby ER, Mould RF: The treatment of tumours of the upper jaw. Br J Radiol 42:561, 1969
20. Mak AC, van Andel JG, van Woerkom-Eijkenboom WM: Radiation therapy of carcinoma of the nasal vestibule. Eur J Cancer 16:81, 1980
21. Mancuso AA, Hanafee WN: Computed Tomography of the Head and Neck, p 203. Baltimore, Williams & Wilkins, 1982
22. McNeese MD, Chobe R, Weber RS, Hogstrom KR: Carcinoma of the nasal vestibule: Treatment with radiotherapy. Cancer Bull 41:84, 1989
23. Mendenhall NP, Parson JT, Cassisi NJ, et al: Carcinoma of the nasal vestibule treated with radiation therapy. Laryngoscope 97:626, 1987
24. Mendenhall WM, Million RR, Cassisi NJ, et al: Biologically aggressive papillomas of the nasal cavity: The role of radiation therapy. Laryngoscope 95:344, 1985
25. Million RR, Cassisi NJ, Hamlin DJ: Nasal vestibule, nasal cavity, and paranasal sinuses. In Million RR, Cassisi NJ (eds): Management of Head and Neck Cancer: A Multidisciplinary Approach, p 407. Philadelphia, JB Lippincott, 1984
26. Million RR, Cassisi NJ, Clark JR: Cancer of the head and neck. In DeVita VT Jr, Hellman S, Rosenberg SA (eds): Cancer: Principles and Practice of Oncology, 3rd ed. Philadelphia, JB Lippincott, 1989
27. Million RR: The myth regarding bone or cartilage involvement by cancer and the likelihood of cure by radiotherapy. Head Neck Surg 11:30, 1989
28. Myers EN, Schramm VL, Barnes EL: Management of inverted papilloma of the nose and paranasal sinuses. Laryngoscope 91:2071, 1981
29. Olsen KD, DeSanto LW: Olfactory neuroblastoma: Biologic and clinical behavior. Arch Otolaryngol 109:797, 1983
30. Parsons JT: The effect of radiation on normal tissues of the head and neck. In Million RR, Cassisi NJ (eds): Management of Head and Neck Cancer: A Multidisciplinary Approach, p 173. Philadelphia, JB Lippincott, 1984
31. Parsons JT, Fitzgerald CR, Hood Cl, et al: The effects of irradiation on the eye and optic nerve. Int J Radiat Oncol Biol Phys 9:609, 1983
32. Parsons JT, Mendenhall WM, Bova FJ, Million RR: Irradiation techniques for head and neck cancer. In Levitt SH (ed): Technological Basis of Radiation Therapy: Practical Clinical Applications, 2nd ed. Philadelphia, Lea & Febiger (in press)
33. Parsons JT, Mendenhall WM, Mancuso AA, et al: Malignant tumors of the nasal cavity and ethmoid and sphenoid sinuses. Int J Radiat Oncol Biol Phys 14:11, 1988
34. Robin PE, Powell DJ, Stansbie JM: Carcinoma of the nasal cavity and paranasal sinuses: Incidence and presentation of different histological types. Clin Otolaryngol 4:431, 1979
35. Schwaab G, Micheau C, Le Guillou C, Pacheco L, Marandas P, Domenge C, Richard JM, Wibault P: Olfactory esthesioneuroma: A report of 40 cases. Laryngoscope 98:872, 1988
36. Shah JP, Feghali J: Esthesioneuroblastoma. Am J Surg 142:456, 1981
37. Singh W, Ramage C, Best P, Angus B: Nasal neuroblastoma secreting vasopressin: A case report. Cancer 45:961, 1980
38. Spaulding CA, Kranyak MS, Constable WC, Stewart FM: Esthesioneuroblastoma: A comparison of two treatment eras. Int J Radiat Oncol Biol Phys 15:581, 1988
39. Suh KW, Facer GW, Devine KD, et al: Inverting papilloma of the nose and paranasal sinuses. Laryngoscope 87:35, 1977
40. Srigley JR, Dayal VS, Gregor RT, Love R, van Nostrand AWP: Hyponatremia secondary to olfactory neuroblastoma. Arch Otolaryngol 109:559, 1983
41. Virapongse C, Mancuso A, Fitzsimmons J: Value of magnetic resonance imaging in assessing bone destruction in head and neck lesions. Laryngoscope 96:284, 1986
42. Wade PM, Smith RE, Johns ME: Response of esthesioneuroblastoma to chemotherapy: Report of five cases and review of the literature. Cancer 53:1036, 1984
43. Wong CS, Cummings BJ, Elhakim T, Briant TD: External irradiation for squamous cell carcinoma of the nasal vestibule. Int J Radiat Oncol Biol Phys 12:1943, 1986

30

Salivary Glands

Joseph R. Simpson

The salivary glands consist of three large, paired major glands, the parotid, submandibular, and sublingual (Fig. 30-1), and many smaller minor glands located in the upper aerodigestive tract.

MAJOR SALIVARY GLANDS

Anatomy

Parotid Gland

The largest salivary gland and the most frequently involved with benign and malignant disease is the parotid, which weighs about 30 g. It lies just below the zygomatic arch, below and in front of the external acoustic meatus and the mastoid process, on top of the masseter muscle. The lateral or superficial lobe contains lymph nodes embedded in the gland, is enveloped by an extension of the cervical fascia, and is covered by skin. The medial border of the gland lies next to the internal carotid artery and touches the lateral wall of the pharynx.[30]

Lying partly within the parotid gland is the facial nerve, which enters the posterior surface of the gland and forms the parotid plexus within it. The superficial and deep layers of the gland are connected by one or more isthmi and wrap around the branches of the facial nerve.

The parotid gland contains a rich lymphatic capillary plexus, many aggregates of lymphocytic cells, and numerous intraglandular lymph nodes. Superficial parotid lymph nodes, located in the lateral aspect of the gland, receive afferent vessels from the skin and subcutaneous tissues of the face and from the auricle, external auditory canal, and middle ear.[30] The lymphatic network largely follows the course of blood vessels and ducts; the deep parotid lymphatics course along the external carotid artery, draining portions of the external auditory canal, eustachian tube, and the gland itself, emptying into retrovascular submaxillary lymph nodes at the angle of the mandible, the upper posterior cervical area, or the jugulodigastric node group (Fig. 30-2). The deep internal jugular chain runs from the base of the skull to the midjugular position and receives afferents from the parotid; the spinal accessory chain originates from the apex formed by its upper aspect.

Haagensen and associates[35] reported 33 radical neck dissections performed in 30 patients with parotid cancers; 14 (42%) specimens contained positive lymph nodes. The distribution of nodal metastases was upper jugular, 42%; midjugular, 14%; low jugular, 8%; submandibular, 18%; and posterior triangle, 18%. If the upper and midjugular nodes were involved and blocked with tumor, retrograde flow toward the posterior triangle nodes along the spinal accessory nerve and to the submandibular nodes seemed to occur.

Submandibular Gland

The submandibular gland lies medial to the mandible, located in and below the digastric triangle. Weighing 10 g to 20 g, it has a larger superficial part, or body, and a smaller deep process. The two parts are continuous around the posterior border of the mylohyoid. Bimanual palpation with one finger in the floor of the mouth and one under the edge of the mandible facilitates clinical detection of masses in the gland. The inferior surface is adjacent to the submandibular lymph nodes. The deep process of the submandibular gland lies between the mylohyoid laterally and the hypoglossus medially, and between the lingual nerve above and the hypoglossal nerve below.[3]

A fairly extensive lymphatic capillary network lies in the interstitial spaces of this gland. Lymph flows toward the capsule, and there are usually four collecting pathways. From the lateral and superior portions of the gland, lymph flows to the prevascular or preglandular submandibular lymph nodes. The posterior portion of the gland gives rise to one or two lymphatic trunks, which follow the facial artery and go directly to the anterior subdigastric nodes of the internal jugular chain.[30,35]

The nodes overlying the submandibular gland, followed by the subdigastric and high midjugular lymph nodes, are involved in nodal metastases. In the M. D. Anderson Cancer Center series of previously untreated malignant submandibular gland tumors, 44% of the patients had nodal metastases at presentation.[10]

Sublingual Gland

The smallest of the major salivary glands is the sublingual gland, which lies beneath the mucous membrane (sublingual fold) of the floor of the mouth, above the mylohyoid, and is adjacent anteriorly to the gland of the opposite side. It lies posteriorly close to the deep process of the submandibular gland, laterally to the sublingual fovea on the medial surface of the mandible, and medially to the genioglossus, from which it is separated by the lingual nerve and the submandibular duct (see Fig. 30-1). This is a rare site for malignant neoplasms, occurring

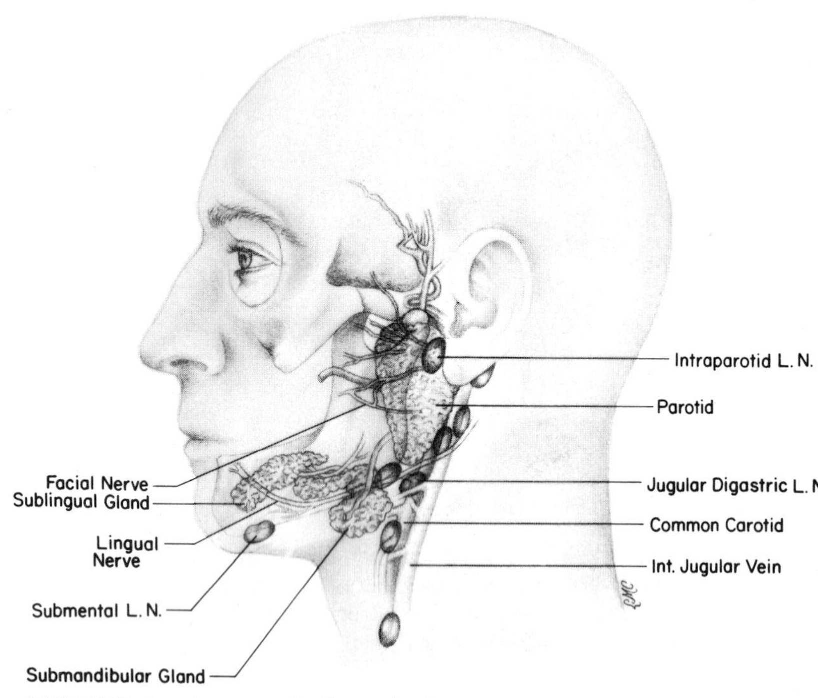

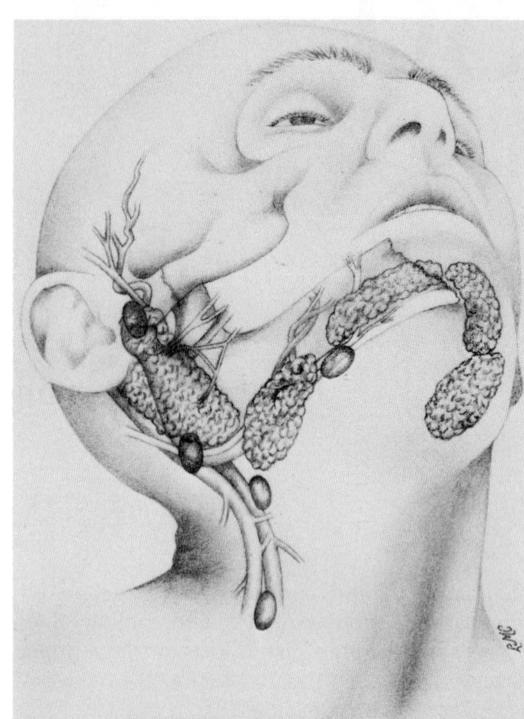

FIGURE 30–1. Anatomy of salivary glands.

in fewer than 5% of all reported cases of salivary gland tumors.[49]

The sublingual glands and many minor salivary glands are contained in loose, deep connective tissue in the floor of the mouth. The duct of the submandibular salivary gland, the lingual nerve, and the collecting lymphatic vessels and trunks of the gum and tongue pass through this area. Because the lymphatics of the floor of the mouth are intimately related to those of the sublingual salivary gland, it is often difficult to identify the site of origin of nodal metastases in the submandibular or submental areas. Sublingual gland tumors are often combined with minor salivary gland tumors originating in the floor of mouth.[74] The sublingual gland drains either to the submandibular lymph nodes or more posteriorly into the deep internal jugular chain between the digastric and omohyoid muscles. Rarely, the lymphatics of the sublingual gland empty into a submental node or supraomohyoid jugular node.[30]

FIGURE 30–2. Lymph node distribution in and around the parotid gland.

Epidemiology

Malignant tumors of the major salivary glands make up only about 0.4% of all cancers and 3% to 4% of head and neck neoplasms. The age-adjusted incidence for all salivary gland tumors gives a male-to-female ratio of 1.3 : 1. There is a preponderance of benign tumors in females; malignant tumors exhibit an equal sex distribution. The proportion of malignant tumors increases from parotid to submandibular to sublingual gland locations, but only a few dozen cases of the latter have been reported.[1,41,45] Two percent to 3% of neoplasms occur in children, in whom 57% of parotid gland tumors are malignant, compared with 15% to 25% in adults.[13,62]

Etiologic factors are not clearly defined. Nutrition may be a factor. Eskimos in the Arctic who have low intake of vitamins A and C have a high incidence.[39] Irradiation also may be a cause, as evidenced by the increased incidence in survivors of the atomic bombs dropped on Hiroshima and Nagasaki and in those irradiated during childhood to the head and neck for benign conditions.[9,49,61,62,65] A correlation of incidence with ultraviolet exposure in the southern surveillance, epidemiology and end results (SEER) district has been reported.[75] Radiation-induced malignant salivary gland neoplasms may occur with higher frequency in the minor salivary glands.[65]

Classification and Histogenesis

The histologic varieties of salivary gland neoplasia are shown in Table 30-1. Usually neoplasms result from transformation of

TABLE 30–1
Classification of Epithelial Salivary Gland Tumors

TYPE OF LESION	VARIATIONS
Benign	Mixed tumor (pleomorphic adenoma)
	Papillary cystadenoma lymphomatosum (Warthin's tumor)
	Oncocytoma-oncocytosis
	Monomorphic tumors
	Basal-cell adenoma
	Glycogen-rich adenoma (?)
	Clear-cell adenoma (?)
	Membranous adenoma
	Myoepithelioma
	Sebaceous tumors
	Adenoma
	Lymphadenoma
	Papillary ductal adenoma (papilloma)
	Benign lymphoepithelial lesion
	Unclassified
Malignant	Carcinoma ex-pleomorphic adenoma (carcinoma arising in a mixed tumor)
	Malignant mixed tumor (biphasic malignancy)
	Mucoepidermoid carcinoma
	Low-grade
	Intermediate-grade
	High-grade
	Adenoid cystic carcinoma
	Acinous-cell (acinic) carcinoma
	Adenocarcinoma
	Mucus-producing adenopapillary and nonpapillary carcinoma
	Salivary duct carcinoma (ductal carcinoma)
	Other adenocarcinomas
	Oncocytic-cell carcinoma (malignant oncocytoma)
	Clear-cell carcinoma (nonmucinous and glycogen-containing or nonglycogen-containing)
	Primary squamous-cell carcinoma
	Hybrid basal-cell adenoma/adenoid cystic carcinoma
	Undifferentiated carcinoma
	Epithelial-myoepithelial carcinoma of intercalated ducts
	Miscellaneous (includes sebaceous lesions, Stensen's duct lesions, melanoma, and carcinoma ex-lymphoepithelial lesions)
	Metastatic
	Unclassified

(Batsakis JG, Regezi JA: Head Neck Surg 1:60, 1978)

more than one cell type or from action of neoplastic stimuli at different stages of differentiation. Pleomorphic adenomas, certain adenocarcinomas, and the rare myoepitheliomas are formed in part from neoplastically transformed myoepithelial cells.[3,4] Electron microscopy studies suggest that these cells may form a significant component in monomorphic adenomas, adenoid cystic carcinomas, and mucoepidermoid carcinomas.[21] The reserve cell system of the intercalated and excretory duct is thought to be the site of origin of most neoplasms (Fig. 30-3).

Natural History

Local invasion is the initial route of spread of malignant tumors of the major salivary glands. As many as 25% of patients with parotid tumors present with lymph node metastases. A similar number present with facial palsy from local nerve invasion. As many as 33% of tumors that arise in the submandibular gland invade the lower jaw.[10,56,71] Nodal metastases usually occur in the parotid, submandibular, and upper cervical regions.

Distant metastases are rare overall, but they are fairly common with adenoid cystic, adenocarcinoma, and undifferentiated carcinomas, and in adenoid cystic carcinoma, they may occur quite late in the course of the disease, even without recurrence of the primary tumor.[17,19,38] Distant metastases are primarily to lung and occasionally to bone; the prognosis for patients with bone metastases is poorer than that for those with pulmonary metastases.[54] Local, regional, and distant spread depend on the size and the histologic type of the primary tumor.[3,10,18,27]

Clinical Presentation

Most parotid masses are benign. Byrne and Spector[11] found that 21% of the 231 parotid masses seen at Washington University between 1982 and 1986 were malignant. Patients most often have a painless, rapidly enlarging mass. Often a mass has been present for years before a sudden change in its indolent growth pattern prompts the patient to seek medical attention.

Although as many as a third of parotid cancers may have facial nerve involvement, only 10% of patients complain of pain. Pain may appear with involvement of deeper structures. Cellular tumors of the parotid can form a large, hemorrhagic, necrotic mass and may invade the sternocleidomastoid, masseter, temporal, and pterygoid muscles.[23,33] Tumors of the parotid

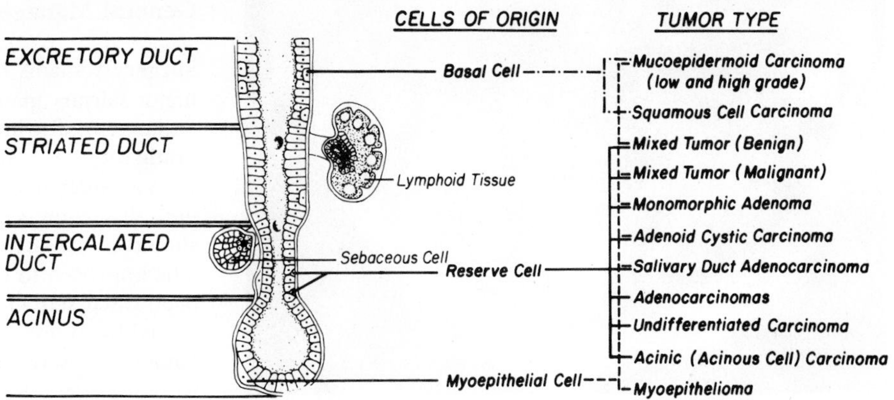

FIGURE 30–3. Reserve cell system of intercalated and excretory duct.[4–6]

rarely involve the base of the skull and cause intractable pain and paralysis of various cranial nerves.

Skin fixation or ulceration occurs in about 10%; cervical adenopathy clinically suggestive of malignancy occurs in 20% to 25%. Clinical features suggesting malignant salivary tumors are rapid growth rate, pain, facial nerve palsy, childhood occurrence, and cervical adenopathy.

Diagnostic Workup

The diagnostic workup of major salivary gland tumors includes a careful history and physical examination with particular attention to signs of local fixation or regional adenopathy. Bone x-rays may be indicated if bone erosion is suspected, and bone scans may be useful if plain films are normal. Computed tomography (CT) scans have been useful in evaluating the extent of lesions involving the parotid gland, especially the deep lobe (Fig. 30-4). Magnetic resonance imaging (MRI) scans can give excellent anatomic detail, but they are not as good as CT scans in cases of inflammatory or diffuse disease.[12]

Some physicians have favored fine-needle aspiration in the diagnosis of masses in the head and neck region, but the heterogeneity of malignant salivary gland tumors has led to a preference for open biopsy technique if a malignant diagnosis is anticipated, with definitive surgery performed if the diagnosis is confirmed.[37] Frozen-section diagnoses, however, have been quite accurate for benign salivary gland tumors.[3,31] Table 30-2 summarizes the diagnostic evaluation procedures for patients with salivary gland neoplasia.

Staging

Many investigators have proposed staging systems for salivary gland malignancies.[29,48,68] Currently, the American Joint Committee on Cancer (AJC) has a staging system for major (parotid and submandibular) salivary gland sites (Table 30-3) based on size, extension, and nodal involvement.[4] It is derived largely from an extensive review of Levitt and colleagues (Fig. 30-5).[48]

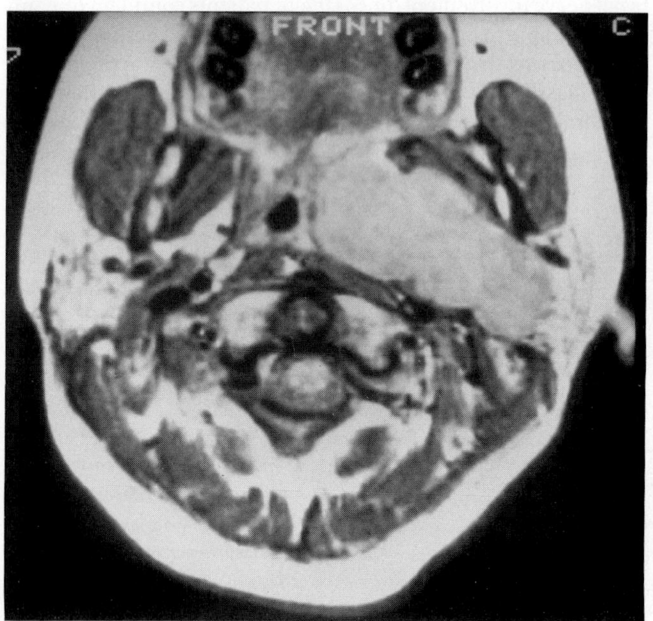

FIGURE 30–4. CT scan of a lesion of the deep lobe of parotid gland.

TABLE 30–2
Diagnostic Workup for Tumors of the Salivary Glands

GENERAL
- History
- Physical examination

RADIOGRAPHIC STUDIES
- Standard
  - Radiographs of chest
  - Craniofacial CT scan
  - Bone scan
- Specific
  - Sialogram
  - Sinus series (minor salivary glands)
  - Panorex of mandible

LABORATORY STUDIES
- Complete blood count
- SMA 12/18

Classification and Prognostic Factors

Foote and Frazell[28] classified salivary gland cancer into subtypes that were further divided into two groups based on prognosis. Low-grade mucoepidermoid and acinic cell carcinomas comprise a group of low or moderate malignancy; high-grade mucoepidermoid, malignant mixed, adenoid cystic (cylindroma), adenocarcinoma, squamous, and undifferentiated carcinomas represent high-grade malignancies.

The percentage of these subtypes varies from series to series (Fig. 30-6). In parotid tumors in children, the most common malignant type is the mucoepidermoid, accounting for almost 50% of the cases.[13,62] The predominance of this cell type appears true also for adult parotid cancer.[66,72] Acinic cell carcinomas usually occur in the parotid gland.[67,70] In the submaxillary gland and in minor salivary glands, the adenoid cystic carcinoma is the most common cancer (Fig. 30-7).[67,69,73] For some cell types (*e.g.*, mucoepidermoid, adenocarcinoma, and adenoid cystic carcinoma), further subdivision has been attempted on the basis of histologic appearance. The adenoid cystic variety has a tubular pattern that has been associated with the best prognosis, a cribriform pattern with an intermediate prognosis, and a solid pattern with the worst prognosis.[52,53,55,64] Spiro[74] reported no significant correlation between grade and survival for adenoid cystic carcinoma but a significant correlation of grade with survival for adenocarcinoma, mucoepidermoid, and squamous carcinoma.

General Management

Surgery remains the primary therapy for carcinomas of the major salivary glands. Surgical technique depends on location and extent of primary disease and regional adenopathy. Low-grade tumors of the parotid are usually treated with a superficial parotidectomy unless the lesion begins in the deep lobe. A neck dissection is not electively done for low-grade tumors but should always be done for clinically palpable neck lymph nodes. The approach to the facial nerve in parotid malignancies has been discussed widely.[8,16,33,39,40] If the facial nerve is not involved by tumor, a nerve-sparing operation is generally done. Patients presenting with facial nerve weakness clinically or whose tumor is found to involve the facial nerve intimately at surgery require facial nerve sacrifice in the course of the total

TABLE 30–3
Proposed AJC Staging System for Major Salivary Gland Cancer (Parotid and Submondibular)

PRIMARY TUMOR (T)*

TX	Primary tumor cannot be assessed
T0	No evidence of primary tumor
T1	Tumor ≤2.0 cm in greatest diameter
T2	Tumor >2.0 cm but <4.0 cm in greatest diameter
T3	Tumor >4.0 cm but <6.0 cm in greatest diameter
T4	Tumor >6.0 cm in greatest diameter
T4b	Tumor of any size with significant local extension

REGIONAL LYMPH NODES (N)

NX	Regional lymph nodes cannot be assessed
N0	No regional lymph node metastasis
N1	Metastasis in a single ipsilateral lymph node, ≤3 cm in greatest dimension
N2	Metastasis in a single ipsilateral lymph node, >3 cm but <6 cm in greatest dimension, or in multiple ipsilateral lymph nodes, none >6 cm in greatest dimension
N2a	Metastasis in a single ipsilateral lymph node >3 cm but <6 cm in greatest dimension
N2b	Metastasis in multiple ipsilateral lymph nodes, none >6 cm in great dimension
N2c	Metastasis in bilateral or contralateral lymph nodes, none >6 cm in greatest dimension
N3	Metastasis in a lymph node >6 cm in greatest dimension

DISTANT METASTASES (M)

MX	Presence of distant metastasis cannot be assessed
M0	No distant metastasis
M1	Distant metastases

STAGE GROUPING

Stage I	TIa	N0	M0
	T2a	N0	M0
Stage II	T1b	N0	M0
	T2b	N0	M0
	T3a	N0	M0
Stage III	T3b	N0	M0
	T4a	N0	M0
	Any T	N1	
Stage IV	T4b	Any N	M0
	Any T	N2, N3	M0
	Any T	Any N	M1

* *All categories are subdivided: (a) no local extension; (b) local extension.*
(Beahrs OH, Henson DE, Hutter RVP, Myers MH [eds]: American Joint Committee of Cancer: Manual for Staging of Cancer, 3rd ed, p 52. Philadelphia, JB Lippincott, 1988)

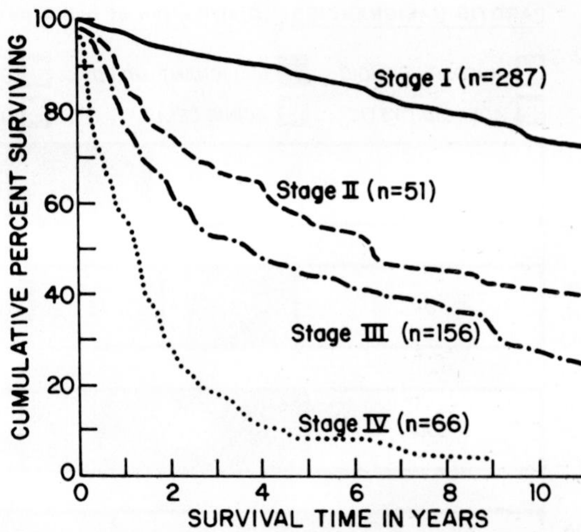

FIGURE 30–5. Survival according to stage of parotid gland cancer. (Levitt SH, McHugh RB, Gomez-Marin O: Cancer 47:2712, 1981)

parotidectomy.[18] Reconstruction of the facial nerve trunk by a cable or sural nerve graft decreases the incidence of facial palsy postoperatively.[33,39]

Patients with disease-free surgical margins and a tumor cell type that is of low or intermediate malignancy have usually not been given adjuvant radiation therapy postoperatively, particularly in the initial treatment program. Patients with recurrent lesions, residual disease left at surgery, and high-grade lesions have increasingly been given postoperative radiation therapy to decrease recurrence.[25,36,51,77] Those who refuse surgery, have medical conditions precluding radical surgical treatment, or demonstrate obviously unresectable local lesions or distant spread at diagnosis are generally referred for radiation therapy alone, with either palliative or, occasionally, curative intent. The large size and slow rate of regression of many of these lesions treated with conventional photon therapy have led to trials with higher doses or with other radiation modalities, such as high-energy neutrons. Several analyses emphasize the beneficial role of routine postoperative irradiation combined with surgery in high-grade malignancies of the major salivary glands.[29,33,50,63,64] Preoperative irradiation is rarely employed if the lesion is resectable.

Radiation Therapy Techniques

Parotid Gland

Two basic radiation therapeutic approaches are used, depending on available equipment. One employs unilateral wedge pair fields using ^{60}Co or 4-MV to 6-MV photons from a linear accelerator. The other technique uses homolateral fields with 12-MeV to 16 MeV electrons or a combination of electrons and photons (Figs. 30-8 through 30-10).[34,66,75,76] In general, 80% of the dose is delivered with electrons and 20% with ^{60}Co or 4-MV to 6-MV photons to spare the opposite salivary gland and decrease the skin reaction produced by electrons.

With the wedged pair technique, slight inferior angulation of beams helps to avoid an exit dose through the contralateral eye (see Fig. 30-8).

In the postsurgical patient with minimal residual disease, 5500 cGy to 6000 cGy at a 5-cm depth is given in daily fractions of 200 cGy over 6 weeks. The primary treatment volume includes the ipsilateral subdigastric nodal areas because the inferior pole of the parotid lies in this region.

The volume of irradiation is determined by pathologic findings, such as perineural invasion. In these cases, more generous irradiation portals may be indicated. Care must be taken to ensure adequate superior and posterior coverage of the entire parotid gland and the surgical bed.

The entire surgical scar(s) with a 2-cm margin should be included in the irradiated volume with a bolus over the scar itself. In tumors with a propensity for perineural invasion (*e.g.*, adenoid cystic carcinoma), it is important to cover the cranial nerve pathways located around the parotid up to the base of the skull. The ipsilateral neck is treated after a neck dissection has been done for clinical disease and in cases of recurrent, high-grade tumors, even without palpable adenopathy. Elective irradiation of the neck should also be considered for tumors that have been incompletely excised and for any high-grade lesions even after complete local excision, with the exception of the adenoid cystic cell type, which has only a 5% to 10% frequency of occult nodal metastasis. A 5000-cGy tumor dose at a depth of

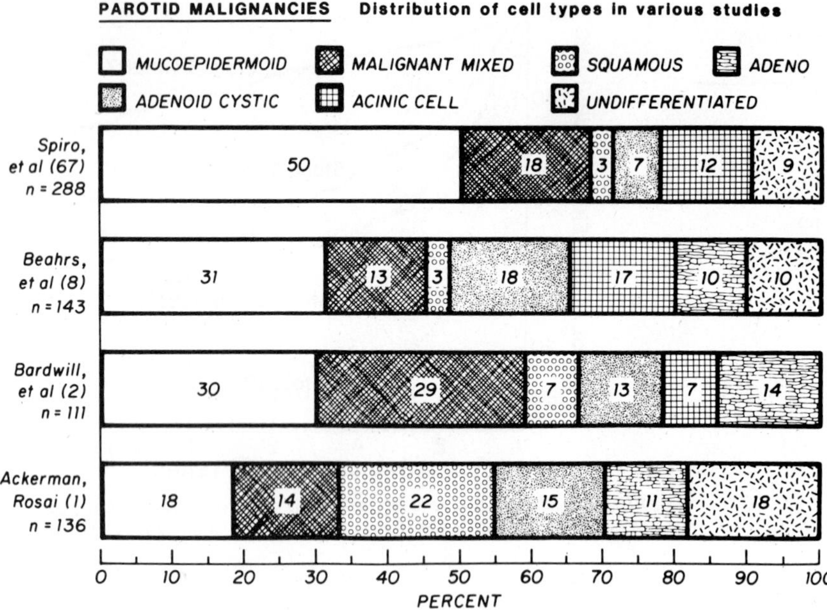

FIGURE 30–6. Parotid malignancies: Distribution of cell types in various studies.

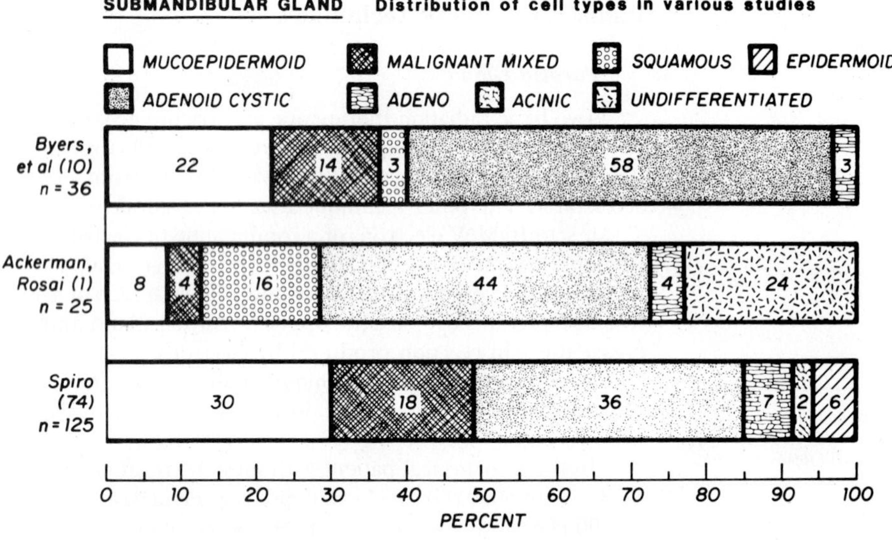

FIGURE 30–7. Submandibular malignancies: Distribution of cell types in three series.

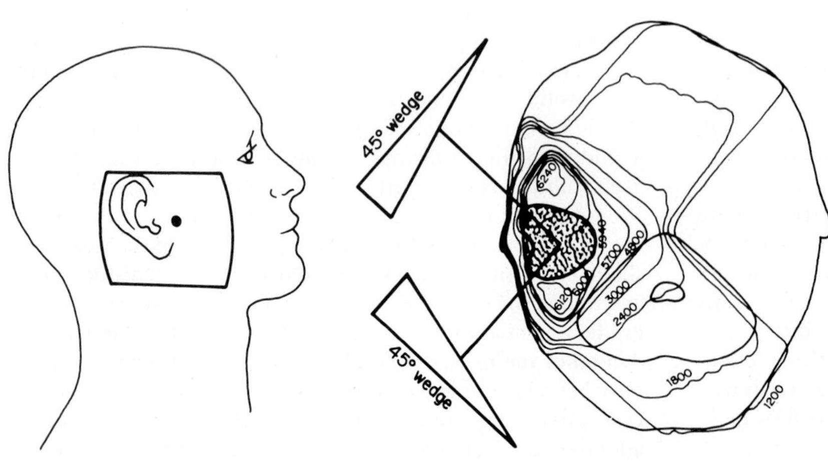

FIGURE 30–8. Unilateral wedge arrangement for parotid treatment and isodose distribution using wedged pair.

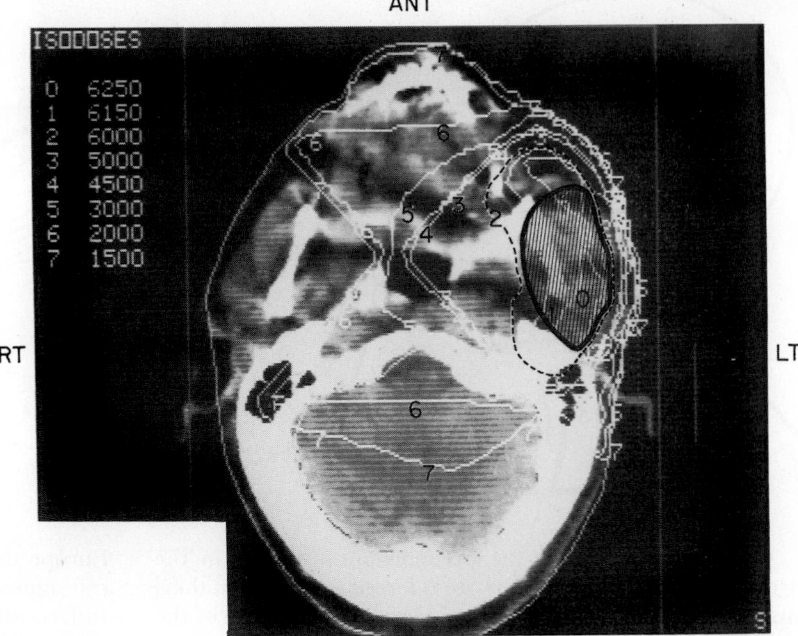

FIGURE 30–9. Wedged pair technique isodoses superimposed on CT scan.

3 cm delivered over 5 weeks is usually adequate for elective neck irradiation. Electron-beam (9–12 MeV) and tangential photon fields are effective techniques for sparing the underlying spinal cord and the opposite parotid gland in elective neck irradiation. In low-grade lesions, elective neck irradiation is not indicated because of the low frequency of unsuspected lymph node involvement.

Submandibular Gland

The entire ipsilateral neck and submandibular area should be irradiated (Fig. 30-11) following the indications outlined for parotid tumors, and the technical considerations are similar. Bilateral fields may be required in the case of tumor extension toward the midline. If there is no gross residual tumor or perineural invasion, 5000 cGy administered in 5 weeks should be adequate for presumed microscopic disease. If there is perineural invasion, a tumor dose of 6000 cGy to 6500 cGy given in 6 to 6.5 weeks is indicated; the nerve pathways to the base of skull also should be treated. Restraint is indicated in the use of electrons for high-grade tumors in this area because bone invasion is not uncommon, and an adequate tumor dose to the base of the skull with electrons may not be achieved or cause excessive morbidity.

Pleomorphic Adenoma

This tumor (benign mixed tumor) is histologically benign, occurs frequently in a relatively young population, and comprises 65% to 75% of all parotid epithelial tumors.[22,74,81] Standard therapy has been conservative (superficial) parotidectomy, with recurrence rates ranging up to 22%. At some institutions, local excision and radiation therapy have been used to lower the frequency of facial nerve injury and Frey's syndrome.[22]

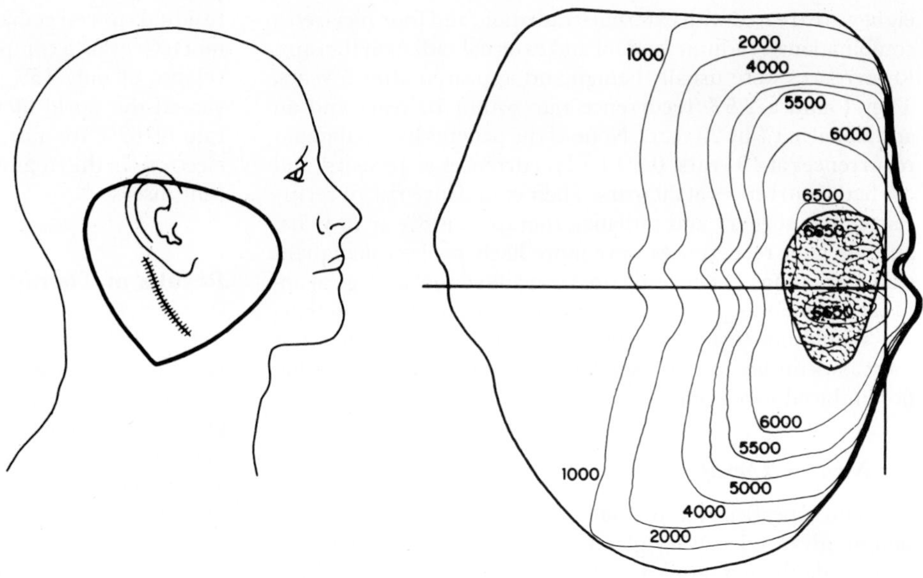

FIGURE 30–10. Ipsilateral 16-MeV electrons plus ^{60}Co (5:1) electron-beam field for postoperative treatment of parotid and neck.

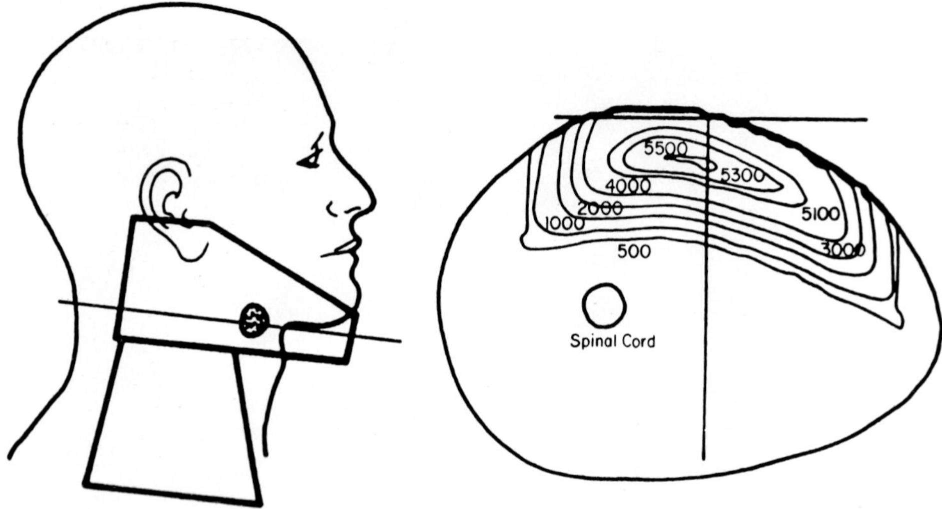

FIGURE 30–11. Unilateral electron-beam technique for submandibular gland and ipsilateral neck treatment.

Although surgery is the predominant approach in the United States, certain patients are referred for radiation therapy. The primary treatment should be surgery because of the patient's young age, the benign histology, and the remote possibility of subsequent radiation-induced malignancy. Nevertheless, there are definite indications for considering radiation therapy:

1. Involvement of the deep lobe of the parotid, which would require sacrificing the facial nerve
2. More than three histologically benign recurrences, with deeper infiltration in successive presentations
3. Large (>5 cm) lesions, which may not allow complete surgical excision with adequate margins
4. Microscopically positive margins after surgical resection
5. Malignant transformation within a predominantly benign tumor

The entire parotid area should be irradiated. Except for the few patients with malignant transformation, it is not necessary to include the subdigastric or retroparotid (mastoid) lymphatics. Doses of 5000 cGy to 6000 cGy given in 5 to 6 weeks calculated at a depth of 4 cm to 5 cm usually control the tumor. Dawson and Orr[22] reported results for 311 patients, 279 of whom were treated with a single-plane radium needle implant delivering 5500 cGy to 6000 cGy at 0.5 cm in 6 days. Twenty-eight were treated with external irradiation, and four received a combination of radium implant and external radiation therapy. Recurrences were usually benign and appeared after 5 years. They found a 2.5% recurrence rate within 10 years and an additional 5.5% by 20 years. None of the patients had malignant recurrences at 10 years, 0.5% had recurrences at 15 years, and 3% had recurrences at 20 years. Their cumulative risk of recurrence after surgery and radiation therapy was 8% at 20 years, and the later recurrences were more likely to show malignant transformation. The investigators concluded that a surgical approach alone was preferable and that adjuvant radiation therapy should not customarily be used in the initial treatment of these patients because of a small risk of developing a late radiation-induced carcinoma.

Neutron Therapy

The superficial location and generally slow rate of regression of advanced salivary gland tumors involving the parotid, have made them a target for alternative radiation therapy approaches, such as fast neutrons. A number of trials from both Europe and the United States have been carried out. Saroja and colleagues[59] reported their experience in treating 113 patients with recurrent or unresectable malignant salivary gland tumors at Fermilab neutron therapy. Local control rates of 67% for major and 50% for minor salivary gland tumors were achieved. Poorer local control was associated with larger size (>5 cm in diameter), which characterized most lesions in the paranasal sinuses. Neutron therapy was administered 3 days a week to a total dose of 2400 cGy to 2600 cGy was achieved over 4 to 6 weeks. Fifty-two patients received between 2000 cGy and 2200 cGy. A sharp rise in complications was seen with doses above 2400 cGy. No dose response for tumor control between the doses of 2000 cGy and 2400 cGy was seen. The investigators concluded that neutron-beam therapy was the treatment of choice for unresectable, residual, or recurrent salivary gland tumors.

Similar conclusions were reached by Catterall and Errington[14] from Hammersmith Hospital. They observed 5-year local control and survival rates of 72% and 50%, respectively, for advanced or recurrent tumors, 89% of which were Stage IV. They reported no facial nerve damage from neutron therapy; 77% regained or maintained facial nerve function; 32% remained normal and 45% regained or improved function.

Griffin and colleagues[32] from Seattle also reported improved local control using fast neutrons in patients with gross residual, unresectable primary, or unresectable recurrent tumors. Overall, a complete response rate of 94% and subsequent relapse of only 13% were observed. Recently, this group reviewed the world literature and found a locoregional control rate of 67% for fast neutrons and only 25% for photons or electrons in the treatment of inoperable, unresectable, or recurrent disease.[46]

Results of Therapy

Tables 30-4 and 30-5 list local control rates and 5- and 10-year survival rates for several series reporting the surgical, radiation, and combination treatment of carcinomas of the major salivary glands. Recurrent tumors generally are more difficult to control than are primary ones, and facial nerve palsy or lymph node metastases worsen the prognosis. Prognosis depends on stage (Fig. 30-5) and histopathologic status (Table 30-6).[2,16,19,29,68]

The Memorial Hospital series of 288 patients with parotid cancer reported by Spiro and associates,[67] in which 90% of the patients were treated with surgery alone, had a 54% determi-

TABLE 30–4
Results of Standard Therapy for Cancer of the Parotid

INVESTIGATOR	NUMBER OF PATIENTS	TREATMENT	5-YEAR SURVIVAL RATE	10-YEAR SURVIVAL RATE	LOCAL CONTROL RATE
Beahrs[8]	162	S	38% to 85%		28% to 50%
Spiro[67]	288	S	62%	54%	73%
King & Fletcher[44]*	93	R and S + R	34% (NED)	62%	75%
Guillamondegui[33]	120	S (104) S + R (10) R (6)	33% to 92% (depends on histology)		74%
Guillamondegui[33]	29	S + R			80% (4 yr)
Kagan[42]†	130	S			49%
Rafla[57]†	62	S ± R	21% (NED)		34%
Fu[29]	63	S S + R R	68%	54%	73%
McNaney[50]	77	S + R			87%
Matsuba[51]	21	S	52%		33%
	26	S + R	65%		73%
Spiro[74]	623	S	55%	47%	

S: surgery; R: irradiation; NED: no evidence of disease.
** Parotid, 88%; submandibular, 12%*
† Malignant.

TABLE 30–5
Results of Standard Therapy for Cancer of the Submaxillary Glands

INVESTIGATOR	NUMBER OF PATIENTS	TREATMENT	5-YEAR SURVIVAL RATE	10-YEAR SURVIVAL RATE	LOCAL CONTROL RATE
Rafla[56]	22	S S + R R	33%		28%
Byers[10]	22	S	50% S + R		64%
McGregor[49]	15	S	53% S + R	33%	40%
Spiro[68]	121	S	26%	17%	50%
Spiro[74]	129	S	31%	22%	

S: surgery; R: irradiation.

TABLE 30–6
Collected Series 5- and 10-Year Survival Rates with Salivary Gland Tumors

TUMOR TYPE	NUMBER OF PATIENTS	5-YEAR SURVIVAL RATE	10-YEAR SURVIVAL RATE
Acinic cell	101	81.0%	67.6%
Mucoepidermoid	749	70.7%	50.0%
Adenoid cystic	1065	62.4%	38.9%
Malignant mixed	383	55.7% (recurrence free)	31.0% (recurrence free)
Pleomorphic adenoma	804	96.9%	93.2%

(Hickman RE, et al: Cancer 54:1620, 1984)

nant cure rate at 10 years and 47% rate at 15 years. Local treatment failure occurred in 27% of patients with a considerable range: only 10% of their Stage I patients had recurrences after surgery, but 60% of Stage III lesions recurred. Local recurrence predicted incurable disease. Eighty percent of patients who did not have local recurrence within 5 years were free of disease at that end point, but only 21% of patients who experienced a local recurrence were free of disease. Distant metastases occurred in 16% of cases overall, ranging from 2% in Stage I to almost 40% in Stage III. King and Fletcher[44] reported a local control rate of 93.5% if postoperative radiation therapy of 6000 cGy in 5 to 6 weeks was given for residual disease after surgery or electively. Similar treatment produced an 81% local control rate for primary inoperable tumors or for postoperative recurrences. Their "cure rate," however, was only 31%, with 46% of the patients dying of intercurrent disease or of distant metastases.

The data reported by Fu and co-workers[29] also demonstrated a stage-dependent survival rate, ranging from 49% to 88% at 5 years and 32% to 83% at 10 years. The best prognosis was associated with the mucoepidermoid or acinic cell variety. There was a precipitous drop in survival between 5 and 10 years for patients with the adenoid cystic cell type, which is known for late recurrences.[42,47,55,63,64] Ultimate local control was achieved in 73% of patients with major salivary gland cancers.

The efficacy of radiation therapy for residual disease after surgery was illustrated in a subset analysis of 35 patients who had microscopic tumor at or close to margins after "curative" surgery.[34] Three (14%) of 22 patients who received postoperative radiation therapy had recurrences, but seven (54%) of 13 unirradiated patients had recurrences. This result was significant ($P \leq 0.05$). Distant metastases occurred in 26 patients, with the highest frequency in the adenoid cystic and undifferentiated cell types. McNaney[50] reported an 87% local control rate for parotid cancers treated with postoperative radiation therapy at M. D. Anderson Cancer Center. At Washington University, we have observed significant improvement in local control for adenoid cystic and adenocarcinomas of the parotid with combined surgery and irradiation.[63,64]

Chemotherapy

The relative rarity of these neoplasms and their localized nature have obviated most opportunities for trials with chemotherapy. Treatment regimens have been both adjuvant and palliative. Adjuvant treatments have usually been administered before definitive local therapy. Dreyfuss and associates[24] reported a 46% response rate in 13 patients with adenoid cystic or adenocarcinomas to a combination of cyclophosphamide (Cytoxan), doxorubicin, and cisplatin. Median response duration in palliative cases was only 5 months.

Kaplan and associates,[43] after reviewing 116 cases of evaluable salivary gland cancer from the literature and their own experience, found a 42% overall response rate, with complete responses in 10% of patients with recurrent, metastatic, or inoperable patients. They suggested that the glandular tumors, such as adenoid cystic, adenocarcinoma, acinous cell, and malignant mixed type, seemed to respond to regimens containing doxorubicin (Adriamycin) and to cisplatin and 5-fluorouracil. Mucoepidermoid carcinoma, on the other hand, seemed not to respond to doxorubicin but rather to cisplatin, methotrexate, and possibly 5-fluorouracil, suggesting a sensitivity similar to squamous cell carcinoma.

Creagan and colleagues[20] evaluated 34 patients with recurrent or disseminated salivary gland neoplasms. A 38% response rate was found with platinum-based chemotherapy. They concluded that, although selected patients might have useful palliation, the impact of chemotherapy on survival was negligible.

In another study reported by Venook and co-workers[79] from the Northern California Oncology Group demonstrating no survival advantage for combination chemotherapy, 17 patients were treated with cisplatin, doxorubicin, and 5-fluorouracil, with an overall response rate of 35%. Six of nine patients who received this as neoadjuvant chemotherapy did not respond, mimicking the nonresponse rate of patients treated for recurrent disease. Adenocarcinomas appeared to be more responsive than other cell types.

Sequelae of Treatment

The most notable complication of treatment of parotid malignancies is facial nerve paralysis, which may result from tumor involvement in 25% to 30% of patients. It is more often caused by the primary or repeated surgical procedures. Various series have shown, however, that nerve sacrifice is rarely necessary, unless a nerve is directly involved by tumor, particularly when postoperative radiation therapy is given.[8,16,25,29] Several surgical series have emphasized that it is the extent of primary tumor rather than the extent of surgery that determines the control rate.[2,8,10,15,16,25,33,44,57] Other postoperative sequelae, such as salivary fistulae and neuromas of the greater auricular nerve, are sometimes seen. Frey's syndrome (*i.e.*, gustatory sweating) may occur in a few patients after parotid surgery, but it is rarely bothersome.[8]

Partial xerostomia, is frequently observed and may be permanent. Elkon and associates[25] reported one case of mucosal necrosis in the oropharynx, two cases of transient moist desquamation, and four cases of severe pharyngeomucositis in a series of 40 patients treated with doses of up to 7500 cGy. Trismus may result from radiation-induced fibrosis of the temporomandibular joint or the masseter muscles. It usually occurs when there is extensive tumor infiltration of the masseter muscle and high doses are given with unilateral technique. Ear complications are also possible and may be troublesome. A serious otitis externa or media associated with partial hearing loss and pain is the most disturbing complication. Fortunately, this is rare.

Treatment of Recurrence

In the retreatment of parotid neoplasms, most series show that preserving facial nerve function and obtaining local control are more difficult than for the primary tumor. Therapy consisting of surgery with postoperative irradiation has demonstrated enhanced local control, and facial nerve sacrifice may be necessary less often if this combination is used.[58] Retreatment usually involves additional surgery, if feasible, and postoperative irradiation in previously unirradiated patients. Significant local control is possible. In certain histologic subtypes (*e.g.*, adenoid cystic carcinoma), retreatment of locally recurrent disease yield prolonged survival.[47,52,63,73] Aggressive local therapy for recurrent disease is indicated if the probability of long-term survival is high.

Chemotherapy has been used for recurrent disease. In view of its significant toxicity in a population that may have recurrent yet indolently progressing disease, aggressive cytotoxic therapy should be used on carefully drafted protocols.

MINOR SALIVARY GLANDS

Anatomy

Minor salivary glands are widely distributed in the upper aerodigestive tract, in the palate, buccal mucosa, base of tongue, pharynx, trachea, cheek, lip, gingiva, floor of mouth, tonsil, paranasal sinuses, nasal cavity, and nasopharynx. Tumors in these sites account for about 23% of all salivary gland neoplasms, and 88% of them are malignant.[49] Adenoid cystic carcinoma is the most common malignant cell type, and the palate is the most common single site, followed by the paranasal sinuses, tongue, and nasal cavity.[3,67]

Epidemiology

In the Memorial Hospital series, the age of patients ranged from 7 to 86 years, with a median of 53 years.[67] The overall incidence of tumors was the same for both sexes, but a slightly higher incidence of malignant tumors was found in males. Fifty percent of the benign lesions occurred in females.

In addition to the roles of irradiation and nutrition mentioned earlier, two reports from England and Scandinavia on the high incidence of adenocarcinoma of the ethmoid sinuses in furniture workers suggest that chronic occupational exposure to fine dust from certain hardwoods is a causative factor.[36,45]

Natural History

The patterns of spread of minor salivary gland carcinomas are diverse, depending on location and histology. Because the most common cell type is the adenoid cystic variety, extensive local, perineural, and vascular invasion and distant metastases may be seen with higher frequency than with malignant neoplasms of the major salivary glands.[80]

Spread to cervical lymph nodes also varies according to histologic cell type and primary location. Adenoid cystic carcinoma has the lowest frequency of cervical node metastases, only about 7.5% at diagnosis, and appearing later in another 5% to 6% of the patients.[47,63,73] On the other hand, malignant mixed tumors have cervical node metastases in 38% of patients, mucoepidermoid carcinoma in 30%, and adenocarcinomas in about 27%.

By anatomic site, tumors arising in the tonsil or nasopharynx show the highest incidence of cervical node metastases, occurring in as many as two thirds of the cases. Tongue or floor of mouth sites are associated with cervical node metastases in about 40%, tumors of the gingiva metastasize in 20% and tumors of the palate, paranasal sinuses, nasal cavity, buccal mucosa, or lips metastasize in about 15% of cases.[64,78] A more favorable prognosis of tumors arising in the hard palate may be related to a decreased tendency for metastases to the cervical nodes or to smaller size at diagnosis.[27]

Clinical Presentation

The signs and symptoms associated with tumors of the minor salivary glands may be quite varied because of their diverse locations. Most are intraoral, and a painless lump is the most common presenting symptom. For tumors arising in the nasal cavity or sinuses, facial pain is the most common presenting symptom, followed by nasal obstruction. Laryngeal primary tumors most frequently cause hoarseness or voice change.

Diagnostic Workup and Staging

Various radiographic studies may be employed, including plain films or tomograms, to ascertain bone erosion in advanced lesions and CT and MRI scanning to evaluate depth and contiguous involvement. The definitive diagnostic procedure, however, is an excisional biopsy, particularly if malignancy is clinically expected. Unplanned incisional biopsies should be avoided, and fine-needle biopsies are impractical because of the pleomorphism of most malignant salivary gland tumors.[37] A formal staging system has not been developed for minor gland tumors, but significant local extension or lymph node metastases confer a poor prognosis. Spiro[74] has used the same staging system for minor salivary glands as for squamous cell carcinoma in sites other than the parotid or submandibular glands.

Classification and Prognostic Factors

The distribution of histologic types among minor salivary gland tumors in several series is shown in Figure 30-12. In the largest series, two cell types not routinely reported were seen: an oat

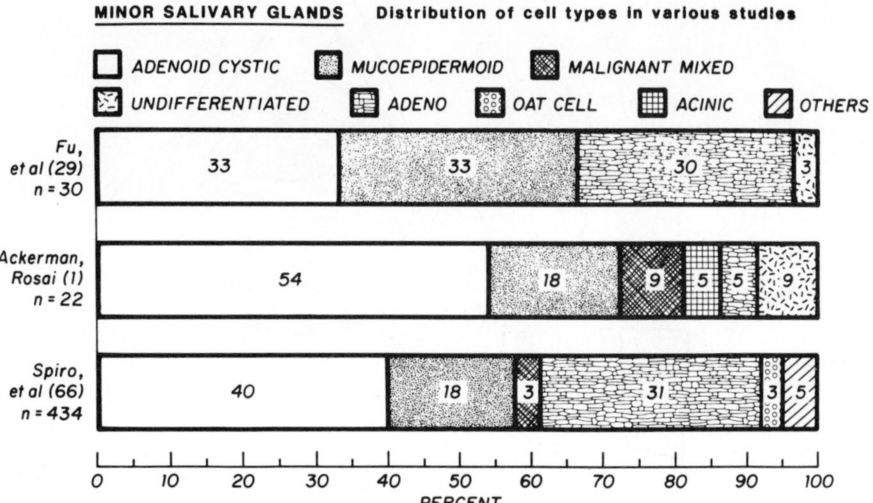

FIGURE 30–12. Minor salivary gland malignancies: Distribution of cell types in various series.

TABLE 30–7
Distribution of Presenting Sites

SITE	NUMBER OF PATIENTS	PERCENT
Palate	228	37.5
Cheek or lips	73	12.0
Antrum	72	11.8
Tongue	63	10.4
Nasal cavity	60	9.8
Gingivae	34	5.6
Floor of mouth	22	3.6
Larynx	21	3.5
Tonsil	13	2.0
Nasopharynx	9	1.4
Ethmoid	9	1.4
Oropharynx	3	1.0
Total	607	100.0

(Spiro RH: Head Neck Surg 8:177, 1986)

cell variety and a colonic-type tumor.[67] The latter resembled the usual colon carcinoma histologically in every way and occasionally even contained Kulchitsky cells. There were, however, only 12 of 492 patients with this histology. Patients with oat cell carcinomas had the highest incidence (50%) of neck nodes and a somewhat better prognosis than is usually found with oat cell carcinoma of the lung; four of 14 patients survived longer than 5 years. The poorest prognosis was associated with the adenoid cystic or malignant mixed cell types, with the adenocarcinoma patients doing somewhat better; the best prognosis was associated with the mucoepidermoid carcinomas. Adenoid cystic cancer in the Memorial Hospital series accounted for 62% of all documented distant metastases, which occurred in 40% of these patients.

General Management

The treatment of minor salivary gland tumors varies with location but generally first involves an attempt at adequate surgical excision. For tumors arising in the palate, tongue, floor of the mouth, oral cavity, or pharynx, surgical exposure is readily available, and resection usually can be accomplished with acceptable morbidity. Tumors arising in the posterior nasal cavity, nasopharynx, or sphenoid region, however, are relatively inaccessible and are treated with radiation therapy. Because the incidence of occult neck metastases from most of these sites is quite low, elective neck dissection is not usually indicated.[16,39] The distribution of presenting sites for almost 500 cases of minor salivary gland tumors, 88% of which were malignant, is shown in Table 30-7.[67] Wide local excision was accomplished in less than 10% of patients with sinus or nasal tumors, essentially those few with polypoid lesions arising in the nasal cavity. Irradiation has been used in surgically inaccessible sites and with surgery in many cases because of locally aggressive behavior and the common occurrence of incomplete resection.[67,73]

The role of irradiation in the palliative treatment of patients with inoperable recurrent and metastatic cancer is well recognized. There is little evidence to support the use of chemotherapy in either primary or secondary management of these tumors.

Radiation Therapy Techniques

The radiation therapy technique for treating minor salivary gland tumors depends on the area involved and is similar to the treatment for squamous cell carcinomas in these areas. There are two significant exceptions to this doctrine. In the case of adenoid cystic carcinomas, which have a high propensity for perineural invasion and local spread for considerable distances, coverage to the base of skull is emphasized, especially for palate lesions. Also, because the incidence of lymph node metastases is generally less than that for squamous cell carcinomas of similar size, the radiation therapy fields are rarely extended to cover areas like the oropharynx if there is no palpable lymph node metastases. The types of radiation therapy portals used in lesions in various minor salivary gland sites are illustrated in Figures 30-13 and 30-14

Results of Therapy

The Memorial Hospital study of minor salivary gland tumors conducted by Spiro and co-workers[67] investigated surgical therapy in almost 500 patients. The initial treatment gave local

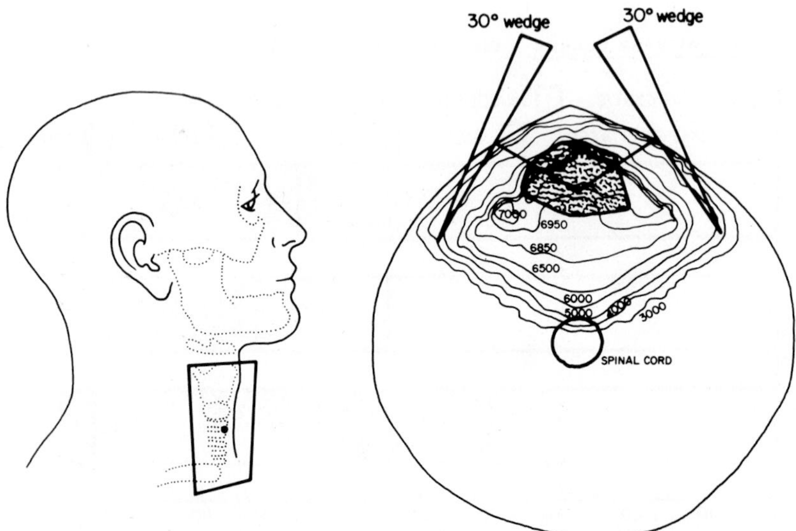

FIGURE 30–13. Example of portals for treatment of adenoid cystic cancer originating in the trachea.

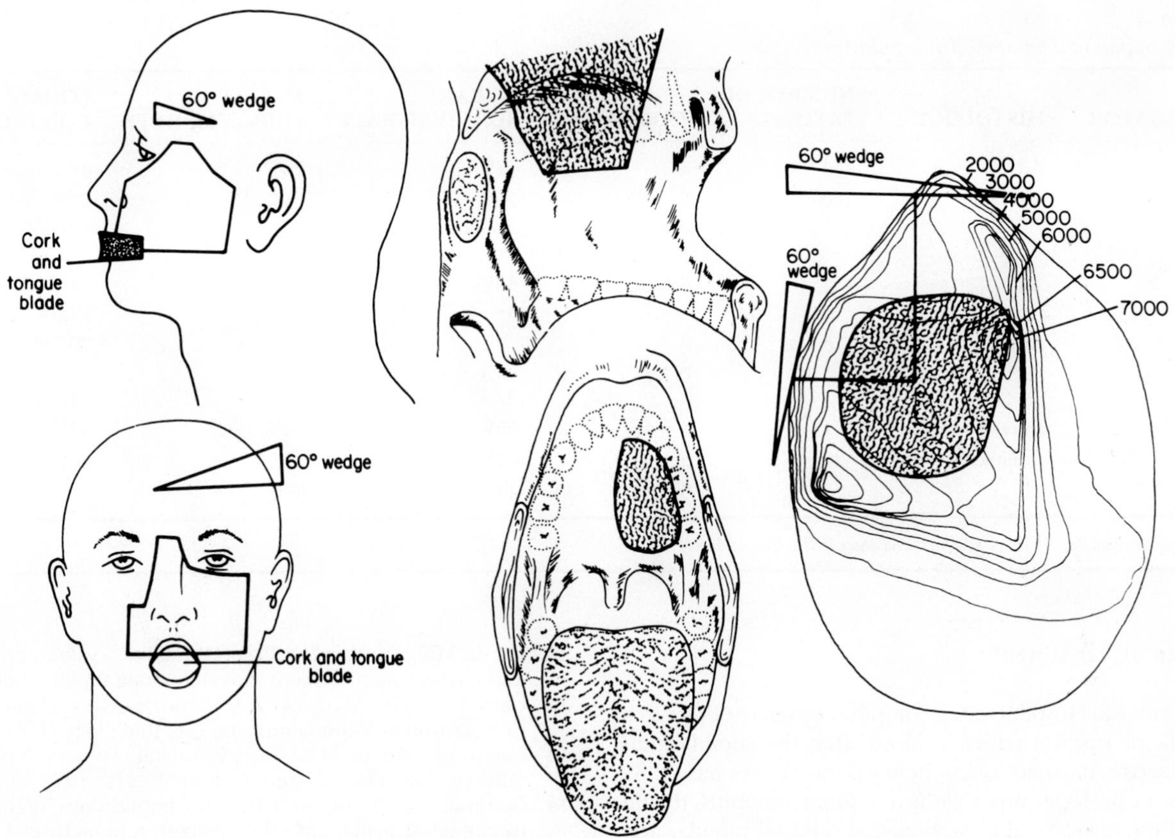

FIGURE 30–14. Portals for treatment of adenoid cystic cancer of the hard palate.

control in only 53% of the patients, and patients also failed at distant or regional sites (*e.g.*, uncontrolled tumor in the neck). This usually was a reflection of the failure to control the primary site, because it occurred twice as frequently in patients with primary site failures as in those with successful treatment of primary tumors. In this series, the 5-year absolute cure rate was only 42%; the 10-year rate was 29%, and the 15-year rate was 17.5%. The determinate cure rates were 44%, 33%, and 21%, respectively.

Local control of disease appears to be improved by the combination of irradiation and surgery, although randomized controlled trials have not been carried out (Fig. 30-15). This improved control rate has been demonstrated particularly for high-grade adenoid cystic carcinomas and adenocarcinomas.[63,67] Anticipated local control rates with combined-modality therapy for these tumors approach 80% at 5+ years.[54,63,64] The results of therapy of minor salivary gland cancer are shown in Table 30-8.

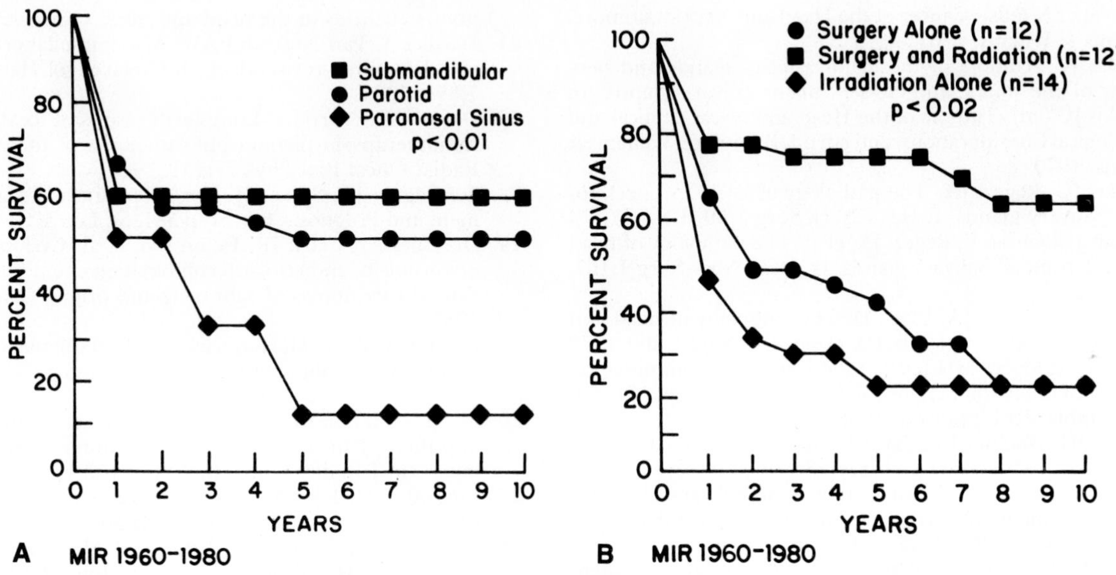

FIGURE 30–15. Local control or survival with no evidence of disease (**A**) according to site and (**B**) treatment for salivary adenocarcinoma.

TABLE 30–8
Results of Standard Therapy: Minor Salivary Glands

INVESTIGATOR	HISTOLOGY	NUMBER OF PATIENTS	TREATMENT	5-YEAR SURVIVAL RATE	10-YEAR SURVIVAL RATE	LOCAL CONTROL RATE
Spiro[66]	All	434	S	42%	29%	47%
Fu[29]	All	30	S S + R R	70% Actuarial	61% Actuarial	63%
Bardwil[2]	All	87	S	38% 3+ yrs NED		47% DOD
Schell[60]	All	118	S S + R R	9% 58% 32%		79%
Simpson[63]	Adenoid cystic	71	S + R	65%	36%	83%
Simpson[64]	Adenocarcinoma	23	S + R	47%	25%	60%
Spiro[74]	All	526	S	48%	37%	

S: surgery; R: irradiation; NED: no evidence of disease; DOD: dead of disease.

Sequelae of Treatment

In the Memorial Hospital series, complications were observed in about 9% of surgical patients. Most often the complications involved sepsis, flap necrosis, or hemorrhage. There was a 2.8% incidence of postoperative deaths due to pneumonitis, thromboembolism, myocardial infarction, and cerebral vascular accident. The addition of irradiation to radical surgery can cause problems in wound healing. Delayed necrosis has not been observed in our experience with irradiation and radical surgery.[63,64] Visual complications were reported by Ellis and associates[26] in nine patients with minor gland tumors; seven of the nine had unresectable disease in close proximity to or with invasion of the orbit.

REFERENCES

1. Ackerman LV, Rosai J: Major and minor salivary glands. In Ackerman LV, Rosai J (eds): Surgical Pathology, 5th ed, p 515. St. Louis, CV Mosby, 1974
2. Bardwil JM, Luna MA, Healey JE Jr: Salivary glands. In Suen JY, Myers EN (eds): Cancer of the Head and Neck. Baltimore, Williams & Wilkins, 1967
3. Batsakis JC: Tumors of the major salivary glands and neoplasms of the minor and "lesser" major salivary glands. In Batsakis JC (ed): Tumors of the Head and Neck: Clinical and Pathological Considerations, 2nd ed, p 1. Baltimore, Williams & Wilkins, 1979
4. Batsakis JG, Regezi JA: The pathology of head and neck tumors: Salivary glands. I. Head Neck Surg 1:59, 1978
5. Batsakis JG, Chinn E, Regezi JA, et al: The pathology of head and neck tumors: Salivary glands. II. Head Neck Surg 1:167, 1978
6. Batsakis JG, Regezi JA, Bloch D: The pathology of head and neck tumors: Salivary glands. III. Head Neck Surg 1:260, 1979
7. Beahrs OH, Myers MH (eds): American Joint Committee on Cancer: Manual for Staging of Cancer, 3rd ed, pp 51–53. Philadelphia, JB Lippincott, 1988
8. Beahrs OH, Woolner LB, Carveth SW, et al: Surgical management of parotid lesions. Arch Surg 80:890, 1980
9. Belsky JL, Tachikawa K, Cihak KW, et al: Salivary gland tumors in atomic bomb survivors, Hiroshima-Nagasaki, 1957–1970. JAMA 219:864, 1972
10. Byers RN, Jesse RH, Guillamondegui OM, et al: Malignant tumors of the submaxillary gland. Am J Surg 126:458, 1973
11. Byrne MN, Spector JG: Parotid masses: Evaluation, analysis and current management. Laryngoscope 98:99, 1988
12. Casselman JW, Mancuso AA: Major salivary gland masses: Comparison of MR imaging and CT. Radiology 165:183, 1987
13. Castro EB, Huvos AG, Strong EW, et al: Tumors of the major salivary glands in children. Cancer 29:312, 1972
14. Catterall M, Errington RD: The implications of improved treatment of malignant salivary gland tumors by fast neutron radiotherapy. Int J Radiat Oncol Biol Phys 13:1313, 1987
15. Chong GC, Beahrs OH, Woner LB: Surgical management of acinic cell carcinoma of the parotid gland. Surg Gynecol Obstet 138:64, 1974
16. Conley J, Baker DC: Cancer of the salivary glands. In Suen JY, Myers EN (eds): Cancer of the Head and Neck, pp 524–556. New York, Churchill Livingstone, 1981
17. Conley J, Dingman DL: Adenoid cystic carcinoma in the head and neck (cylindroma). Arch Otolaryngol Head Neck Surg 100:81, 1974
18. Conley J, Hamaker RC: Prognosis of malignant tumors of the parotid gland with facial paralysis. Arch Otolaryngol Head Neck Surg 101:39, 1975
19. Cowie VJ, Pointon RCS: Adenoid cystic carcinoma of the salivary glands. Clin Radiol 35:331, 1984
20. Creagan ET, Woods JE, Rubin J, et al: Cisplatin-based chemotherapy for neoplasms arising from salivary glands and contiguous structures in the head and neck. Cancer 62:2313, 1988
21. Dardick I, Van Nostrand AW: Myoepithelial cells in salivary gland tumors—revisited. Arch Otolaryngol Head Neck Surg 7:395, 1985
22. Dawson AK, Orr JA: Long-term results of local excision and radiotherapy in pleomorphic adenoma of the parotid. Int J Radiat Oncol Biol Phys 11:451, 1985
23. del Regato JA, Spjut HJ, Cox JD: Cancer: Diagnosis, Treatment and Prognosis, 6th ed, p 581. St. Louis, CV Mosby, 1985
24. Dreyfuss AI, Clark JR, Fallon BG, et al: Cyclophosphamide, doxorubicin, and cisplatin combination chemotherapy for advanced carcinomas of salivary gland origin. Cancer 60:2869, 1987
25. Elkon D, Colman M, Hendrickson FR: Radiation therapy in the treatment of malignant salivary gland tumors. Cancer 41:502, 1978
26. Ellis ER, Million RR, Mendenhall WM, et al: The use of radiation therapy in the management of minor salivary gland tumors. Int J Radiat Oncol Biol Phys 15:613, 1988
27. Eneroth CM, Hjertman L, Moberger G: Adenoid cystic carcinoma of the palate. Acta Otolaryngol (Stockh) 66:248, 1968
28. Foote FW Jr, Frazell EL: Tumors of Major Salivary Glands. Washington DC, Armed Forces Institute of Pathology, 1954
29. Fu KK, Leibel SA, Levine ML, et al: Carcinoma of the major

and minor salivary glands: Analysis of treatment results and sites and causes of failures. Cancer 40:2882, 1977
30. Gardner E, Gray DJ, O'Rahily R (eds): Anatomy: A Regional Study of Human Structure, 3rd ed. Philadelphia, WB Saunders, 1969
31. Granick MS, Erickson ER, Hanna DC: Accuracy of frozen-section diagnosis in salivary gland lesions. Arch Otolaryngol Head Neck Surg 7:465, 1985
32. Griffin TW, Pajak TF, Laramore GE, et al: Neutron vs photon irradiation of inoperable salivary gland tumors: Results of an RTOG-MRC cooperative randomized study. Int J Radiat Oncol Biol Phys 15:1085, 1988
33. Guillamondegui OM, Byers RM, Luna MA, et al: Aggressive surgery in treatment for parotid cancer: The role of adjunctive postoperative radiotherapy. AJR 123:49, 1975
34. Guillamondegui O, Byers RM, Tapley NdV: Malignant tumors of salivary glands. In Fletcher GH (ed): Textbook of Radiotherapy, 3rd ed, p 438. Philadelphia, Lea & Febiger, 1980
35. Haagensen CD, Feind CR, Herter FP: The Lymphatics in Cancer. Philadelphia, WB Saunders, 1972
36. Hadfield EH, MacBeth RG: Adenocarcinoma of ethmoids in furniture workers. Ann Otol Rhinol Laryngol 80:699, 1971
37. Harker LE: Limitations of pathologic diagnosis in salivary gland tumors. Laryngoscope 87:1899, 1977
38. Hickman RE, Cawson RA, Duffy SW: The prognosis of specific types of salivary gland tumors. Cancer 54:1620, 1984
39. Johns ME, Kaplan MJ: Surgical therapy of tumors of the salivary glands. In Thawley SE, Panje W, Batsakis J, et al (eds): Comprehensive Management of Head and Neck Tumors. Philadelphia, WB Saunders, 1986
40. Johns ME, Goldsmith MM: Current management of salivary gland tumors. Oncology 3:85, 1989
41. Johns ME, Goldsmith MM: Incidence, diagnosis, and classification of salivary gland tumors. Oncology 3:47, 1989
42. Kagan AR, Nussbaum H, Handler S, et al: Recurrences from malignant parotid salivary gland tumors. Cancer 37:2600, 1976
43. Kaplan MJ, Johns ME, Cantrell RW, et al: Chemotherapy for salivary gland cancer. Arch Otolaryngol Head Neck Surg 95:165, 1986
44. King JJ, Fletcher GH: Malignant tumors of the major salivary glands. Radiology 100:381, 1971
45. Klintenberg C, Olofsson J, Hellquist H, et al: Adenocarcinoma of the ethmoid sinuses: A review of 28 cases with special reference to wood dust exposure. Cancer 54:482, 1984
46. Koh W, Laramore G, Griffin T, et al: Fast neutron radiation for inoperable and recurrent salivary gland caners. Am J Clin Oncol 12:316, 1989
47. Leafstedt SW, Gaeta JF, Sako K, et al: Adenoid cystic carcinoma of major and minor salivary glands. Am J Surg 122:756, 1971
48. Levitt SH, McHugh RB, Gomez-Marin O: Clinical staging system for cancer of the salivary gland: A retrospective study. Cancer 57:2712, 1981
49. McGregor GI, Robins RE: Submandibular and minor salivary gland carcinoma: A 15-year review. Am J Surg 43:737, 1977
50. McNaney D, McNeese MD, Guillamondegui OM, et al: Postoperative irradiation in malignant epithelial tumors of the parotid. Int J Radiat Oncol Biol Phys 9:1289, 1983
51. Matsuba HM, Thawley SE, Devineni VR, et al: High-grade malignancies of the parotid gland: Effective use of planned combined surgery and irradiation. Laryngoscope 95:1059, 1985
52. Matsuba HM, Spector GJ, Thawley SE, et al: Adenoid cystic salivary gland carcinoma: A histopathologic review of treatment failure patterns. Cancer 57:519, 1986
53. Matsuba HM, Simpson JR, Mauney M, et al: Adenoid cystic salivary gland carcinoma: A clinicopathologic correlation. Arch Otolaryngol Head Neck Surg 8:200, 1986
54. Million RR, Cassissi JN(eds): Management of Head and Neck Cancer: A Multidisciplinary Approach. Philadelphia, JB Lippincott, 1984
55. Perzin KH, Gullane P, Clairmont AC: Adenoid cystic carcinomas arising in salivary glands: A correlation of histologic features and clinical course. Cancer 42:265, 1978
56. Rafla S: Submaxillary gland tumors. Cancer 26:821, 1970
57. Rafla S: Malignant parotid tumors: Natural history and treatment. Cancer 40:136, 1977
58. Reddy SP, Marks JE: Treatment of locally advanced, high-grade, malignant tumors of major salivary glands. Laryngoscope 98:450, 1988
59. Saroja KR, Mansell J, Hendrickson, et al: An update on malignant salivary gland tumors treated with neutrons at Fermilab. Int J Radiat Oncol Biol Phys 13:1319, 1987
60. Schell SR: Malignant Tumors of minor salivary glands. Presented at the annual American Radium Society meeting, Philadelphia, PA, 1979
61. Schneider AB, Favus MJ, Stachura ME, et al: Salivary gland neoplasms as a late consequence of head and neck irradiation. Ann Intern Med 87:160, 1977
62. Schuller DE, McCabe BF: The firm salivary mass in children. Laryngoscope 87:1891, 1977
63. Simpson JR, Thawley SE, Matsuba HM: Adenoid cystic salivary gland carcinoma: Treatment with irradiation and surgery. Radiology 151:509, 1984
64. Simpson JR, Matsuba HM, Thawley SE, et al: Improved treatment of salivary adenocarcinomas: Planned combined surgery and irradiation. Laryngoscope 96:904, 1986
65. Smith SA: Radiation-induced salivary gland tumors. Arch Otolaryngol Head Neck Surg 102:561, 1976
66. Soni SC, Kahn FR, Paul JM. et al: Electron beam treatment of malignant tumors of salivary glands. J Radiol Electrol 48:677, 1977
67. Spiro RH, Koss LG, Hajdu SI, et al: Tumors of minor salivary origin: A clinicopathologic study of 492 cases. Cancer 31:117, 1973
68. Spiro RH, Huvos AG, Strong EW: Cancer of the parotid gland: A clinicopathologic study of 288 primary cases. Am J Surg 130:452, 1975
69. Spiro RH, Hajdu SI, Strong EW: Tumors of the submaxillary gland. Am J Surg 132:463, 1976
70. Spiro RH, Huvos, Strong EW: Acinic cell carcinoma of salivary origin: A clinicopathologic study of 67 cases. Cancer 41:924, 1978
71. Spiro RH, Huvos AG, Strong EW: Adenocarcinoma of salivary origin. Am J Surg 144:423, 1981
72. Spiro RH, Huvos AG, Strong EW, et al: Mucoepidermoid carcinomas of salivary gland origin. Am J Surg 136:461, 1978
73. Spiro RH, Huvos AG, Strong EW: Adenoid cystic carcinoma of salivary origin. Am J Surg 128:512, 1974
74. Spiro RH: Salivary neoplasms: Overview of a 35-year experience with 2,807 patients. Arch Otolaryngol Head Neck Surg 8:177, 1986
75. Spitz MR: Risk factors for salivary gland cancer: A review. Cancer Bull 37:153, 1985
76. Tapley NdV: Clinical Applications of the Electron Beam. New York, John Wiley, 1976
77. Tapley NdV: Irradiation treatment of malignant tumors of the salivary glands. Ear Nose Throat J 56:39, 1977
78. van der Wall JE, Snow GB, Karim A, et al: Intraoral adenoid cystic carcinoma: The role of postoperative radiotherapy in local control. Arch Otolaryngol Head Neck Surg 11:497, 1989
79. Venook AP, Tseng A Jr, Meyers FJ, et al: Cisplatin, doxorubicin, and 5-fluorouracil chemotherapy for salivary gland malignancies: A pilot study of the Northern California Oncology Group. J Clin Oncol 5:951, 1987
80. Vrielinck LJG, Ostyn F, VanDamme B, et al: The significance of perineural spread in adenoid cystic carcinoma of the major and minor salivary glands. Int J Oral Maxillofac Surg 17:190, 1988
81. Woods JE, Weiland LH, Chong GC, et al: Pathology and surgery of primary tumors of the parotid. Surg Clin North Am 57:565, 1977

31

Oral Cavity

C. C. Wang

ANATOMY OF THE ORAL CAVITY

The exterior oral cavity is composed of the upper and lower lips; interiorly, it comprises the gingivobuccal sulcus, the buccal mucosa, the upper and lower gingiva (including the alveolar ridge), the hard palate, the floor of the mouth, and the anterior two thirds of the mobile tongue.

Although some authors include the retromolar trigone, anterior pillar, and soft palate in the oral cavity, for the sake of a uniform presentation, these anatomic structures are grouped together as tumors of the faucial arch and are discussed in Chapter 32.[33,45]

Lips

The lips are composed mostly of the orbicularis muscle, which is covered by skin externally and by mucous membrane covered with stratified squamous epithelium on the inner surface. The transitional area between skin and mucous membrane, where the muscle is covered by a thin layer of squamous epithelium, is called the vermilion border. A lip tumor arises from that portion of the vermilion surface that comes in contact with the opposite lip.

The blood supply comes from the labial artery, a branch of the facial artery. The motor nerve branches come from the facial nerve. The sensory nerve to the upper lip is the infraorbital branch of the maxillary nerve, and to the lower lip are branches of the mental nerve, which originates in the inferior alveolar nerve. The commissure is partially supplied by the buccal branch of the mandibular nerve.

Gingiva

The upper gingiva is formed by the alveolar ridge of the maxilla, which is covered by mucosa and the teeth and continues with the hard palate. The lower gingiva covers the mandible from the gingivobuccal sulcus to the mucosa of the floor of the mouth. It continues posteriorly with the retromolar trigone and above with the maxillary tuberosity. There are no minor salivary glands in the mucous membrane over the alveolar ridges.[30]

Buccal Mucosa

The buccal mucosa is made up of the mucous membrane covering the internal surface of the lips and cheeks (buccinator muscle) extending from the line of attachment of the upper and lower alveolar ridges to the point of contact of the lips posteriorly and the orbicularis anteriorly. The masseter muscle lies posterior and lateral to the buccinator muscle. The blood supply of the buccal mucosa comes from the facial artery. Sensory fibers are supplied by the buccal nerve, a branch of the mandibular nerve. The motor nerve to the buccinator muscle is derived from the facial nerve.

Floor of Mouth

The floor of the mouth extends from the anterior inner aspect of the lower gingiva laterally to the insertion of the anterior tonsillar pillar into the tongue. Anteriorly, it is divided into halves by the lingual frenulum. The floor of the mouth is covered by a mucous membrane with stratified squamous epithelium. Laterally, the sublingual glands are separated by the midline genioglossus and the geniohyoid muscles. The genial tubercles are bony protuberances that occur at the point of insertion of these two muscle groups on the symphysis.[30] The floor of the mouth contains several muscles, including the mylohyoid and, under it, the digastric muscle. The submaxillary glands are located on the external surface of the mylohyoid muscle, between its insertion to the mandible. The submaxillary duct (Wharton's duct) is about 5 cm long and courses between the sublingual gland and the genioglossus muscle; its orifice is in the anterior floor of the mouth, near the midline.

The lingual nerve, a branch of the submaxillary nerve, provides sensation to the floor of the mouth. The arterial supply comes from the lingual artery, a branch of the external carotid.

Oral Tongue

The tongue is a muscular organ composed of the styloglossus, hyoglossus, and hyoid muscles (Fig. 31-1). The tongue is covered by a mucous membrane with stratified squamous epithelium. The circumvallate papillae, situated posteriorly with a

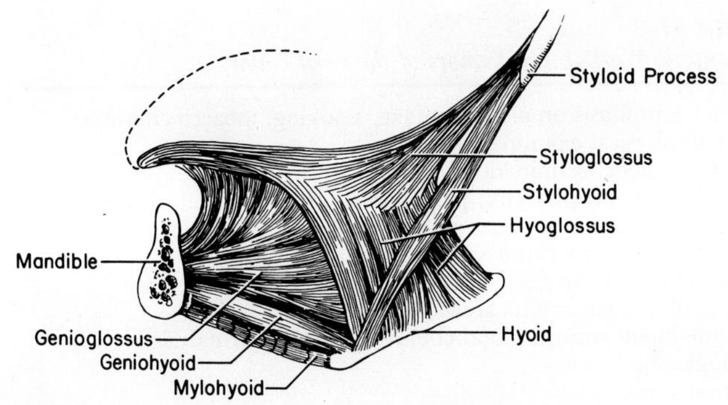

FIGURE 31–1. Musculature of the tongue and floor of the oral cavity. (Redrawn from Clemente CD: Anatomy: A Regional Atlas of the Human Body. Baltimore, Urban & Schwarzenberg, 1987)

V-shaped configuration directed posteriorly toward the foramen cecum, separate the base of the tongue from the mobile tongue. The oral tongue consists of the tip, dorsum, lateral borders, and undersurface. The blood supply is the lingual artery, a branch of the external carotid artery.[33] The sensory branches of the tongue are supplied by the lingual nerve, a branch of the maxillary nerve; the hypoglossal nerve is the motor nerve. The taste buds are innervated by the chorda tympani branch of the sensory root of the facial nerve.

Lymphatics

The lymphatics of the upper lip drain mostly to the submaxillary lymph nodes; the periauricular and parotid lymph nodes occasionally receive lymphatic channels from the upper lip. The lower lip lymphatics drain to the submaxillary and posteriorly to the subdigastric lymph nodes. Lesions located near the midline may drain to the submental nodes or to either side of the submaxillary lymph nodes.

Lymph node involvement in lesions of the lip is relatively rare, although 5% to 10% of the patients with clinically negative necks subsequently develop lymph node metastases.[27]

The lymphatic drainage and incidence of lymph node metastases of the upper gingiva are about 15% to 20% on admission, and there is about the same incidence of subsequent development of clinical cervical lymph node metastasis in initially clinically negative necks.[25] The lymphatics of the lower gingiva drain to the submaxillary and subdigastric lymph nodes. The incidence of clinically positive nodes on admission for gingival tumors depends on the stage, ranging from 15% to 50%. Clinically positive nodes subsequently develop in approximately 20% of the patients who present with N0 necks. Contralateral lymph node metastases are extremely rare.[7]

The first echelon of the lymph node drainage of the floor of the mouth is to the submaxillary and subdigastric lymph nodes. Submental lymph nodes are involved in fewer than 5% of the patients.[25] The incidence of bilateral lymph node involvement is relatively high because many lesions are near or cross the midline.

Primary lymphatic drainage in the oral tongue is to the subdigastric and submaxillary lymph nodes. Rouviere[39] described the lymphatic trunks that bypass this primary lymphatic drainage and go directly to the midjugular lymph nodes, which probably accounts for the relative frequency of metastatic lymph nodes in these locations (Fig. 31-2). About 35% of patients with tumors of the oral tongue have clinically positive lymph nodes, 5% to 10% of them bilateral (Fig. 31-3). Among patients with initially clinically negative nodes, approximately 30% eventually develop metastatic disease in the lymph nodes, the exact incidence depending on the initial stage of the disease.[25]

The lymphatic drainage of the buccal mucosa is primarily to the submaxillary and subdigastric lymph nodes. The incidence of positive cervical lymph nodes on admission is 10% to 30%. The risk of subsequent development of clinical metastases or pathologically positive lymph nodes in the neck that was negative for disease on examination is about 15%.

CANCER OF THE ORAL CAVITY

Epidemiology

In 1990, the estimated number of oral cancers in the United States was 21,900, an incidence of 9.5 per 100,000 population; 4850 persons died of the disease, with a mortality rate of 2.2 per 100,000.[8] This cancer is predominantly a disease of men and of middle age and is often associated with poor oral hygiene and abuse of tobacco and alcohol. In recent years, there has been an increase in oral cancer among relatively young females who apparently never drink alcohol or smoke. The cause of this increase is unclear.

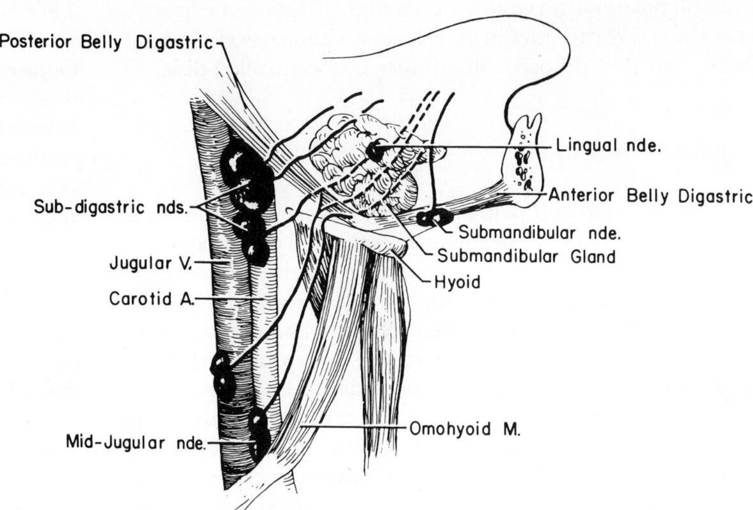

FIGURE 31–2. Lymphatics of the tongue. (Modified from Rouviere H: Anatomy of the Human Lymphatic System, p 44. Ann Arbor, Edwards Brothers, 1938)

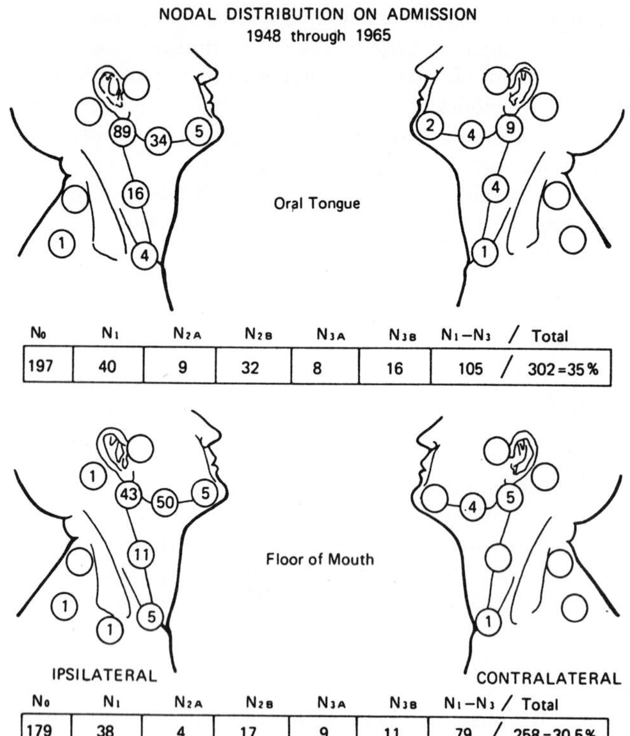

FIGURE 31–3. Incidence of metastatic lymph nodes in patients with carcinoma of the floor of the mouth or anterior two thirds of the tongue. (Lindberg R: Cancer 29:1446, 1972)

Natural History

The early mucosal lesion may appear as an indurated nodule or as a shallow ulcer with poorly defined margins. Because these areas are poorly endowed with pain fibers, pain is not an early symptom. Most patients present with a "canker sore" or a lump in the mouth, frequently of several weeks' duration, as the only symptom of the disease. These tumors may be exophytic or infiltrative and may extend rapidly into the underlying muscle and cause fixation with resultant difficulty in speech or eating. In the advanced stage, trismus of the jaw with pain radiating to the ear may occur. Occasionally, earache may be the only initial presenting symptom of the disease.

Except for lesions arising from the tip of the tongue or extending across the midline, metastatic disease usually occurs in the homolateral cervical lymph nodes.[25] Distant metastases below the clavicle are rare in early lesions without cervical nodal disease, but they do occur in advanced, uncontrolled disease.

Diagnostic Workup

Careful inspection and palpation of the primary site and neck areas are mandatory for an adequate evaluation of the extent of the lesion (Table 31-1). Indirect laryngoscopy is extremely informative in evaluating the oropharyngeal extension of the lesion and the possibility of a second lesion at another anatomic site. Appropriate x-ray examinations (*e.g.*, soft tissue films of the lateral base of the tongue, Panorex or intraoral dental films, and polytomes of the jaw) are indicated to assess the dental condition and bone invasion. Computed tomography (CT) scans of the mandible are used to assess bone involvement in carcinoma of the floor of the mouth, alveolar ridge, and retromolar trigone area. Chest radiographs, and basic blood and liver profiles are

TABLE 31–1
Diagnostic Workup for Tumors of the Oral Cavity

History (emphasis on alcohol intake, smoking, tobacco chewing)
General physical examination
Head and neck examination
- Oral cavity, oropharynx; palpation is important
- Nasopharynx (mirror examination)
- Laryngopharynx (indirect laryngoscopy)

Examination of the neck for lymph nodes
Biopsy of any suspicious areas
Routine blood counts, blood chemistry profile, urinalysis
Radiographic studies
- Chest x-ray films
- Plain radiographs of mandible (Panorex)
- Computed tomography or magnetic resonance imaging scans (optional)

necessary to assess the condition of the patient. Anemia should be corrected because the hemoglobin level may affect the outcome of radiation therapy.[5]

Staging

In 1988, the American Joint Committee on Cancer adopted the system for the classification of oral squamous cell carcinomas shown in Table 31-2.[3]

Pathologic Classification

Carcinomas arising from the mucous membrane of the oral cavity are predominantly squamous cell carcinomas and account for approximately 90% of the cases seen in clinical practice. Pathologically, the lesions may vary in degree of differentiation, ranging from *in situ* to verrucous to poorly differentiated carcinoma.[2] Uncommon nonsquamous cell cancers include malignant tumors of the minor salivary gland, such as adenoid cystic carcinoma, mucoepidermoid carcinoma, and adenocarcinoma, which are found most often in the palate, cheek mucosa, and lips. Rarely, lymphoma, melanoma, or sarcoma can arise in the oral cavity; these lesions comprise approximately 10% of cases. Metastatic carcinomas to the oral structures are infrequent.

THERAPEUTIC OPTIONS

General Management

A variety of therapeutic measures are available for managing localized carcinomas of the oral cavity, including surgical excision, radiation therapy, electrodesiccation, laser-beam excision, and combinations of these methods.[34] The individualized treatment choice depends on the anatomic site and the size of the primary lesion, presence or absence of metastatic disease in the neck, patient's age and general medical health, morbidity associated with the treatment program, experience and skill of both the surgeon and the radiation oncologist and, last but not least, the wishes of the patient.

With few exceptions, irradiation is applicable as the first treatment for all sites regardless of tumor size. In certain instances, surgical removal is as effective for the treatment of small, localized lesions of the oral cavity as radiation therapy (Fig. 31-4). Generally, aged and frail patients tolerate surgical

TABLE 31–2
Classification of Oral Cavity Carcinoma

CLASSIFICATION	CHARACTERISTICS
T1	Tumor ≤2 cm in greatest dimension
T2	Tumor >2 cm but <4 cm in greatest dimension
T3	Tumor >4 cm in greatest dimension
T4 (lip)	Tumor invades adjacent structures (*e.g.*, cortical bone, tongue, skin of neck)
T4 (oral cavity)	Tumor invades adjacent structures (*e.g.*, cortical bone, into deep [extrinsic] muscle of tongue, maxillary sinus, skin)
N0	No regional lymph node metastases
N1	Metastasis in a single ipsilateral lymph node, ≤3 cm in greatest dimension
N2	Metastasis in a single ipsilateral lymph node, >3 cm but <6 cm in greatest dimension; in multiple ipsilateral lymph nodes, none >6 cm in greatest dimension; in bilateral or contralateral lymph nodes, none >6 cm in greatest dimension
N2a	Metastasis in a single ipsilateral lymph node >3 cm but <6 cm in greatest dimension
N2b	Metastasis in multiple ipsilateral lymph nodes, none >6 cm in greatest dimension
N2c	Metastasis in bilateral or contralateral lymph nodes, none >6 cm in greatest dimension
N3	Metastasis in a lymph node, >6 cm in greatest dimension
M0	No distant metastasis
M1	Distant metastasis

(Beahrs OH, Henson DE, Hutter RVP, Myers MH [eds]: Manual for Staging of Cancer, 3rd ed. Philadelphia, JB Lippincott, 1988)

excision much better than high-dose external-beam therapy or interstitial implant in the mouth or intraoral cone therapy. Radical surgery, however, with total or hemiglossectomy and partial mandibulectomy and radical neck dissection (so-called composite resection), although technically feasible, should not be used for treatment of early cancer of the oral cavity but reserved for advanced carcinomas and combined with preoperative or postoperative radiation therapy or for recurrent tumors previously treated by radiation therapy. Laser-beam excision and electrodesiccation may be used as a primary method of managing superficial carcinomas of the oral cavity, but these modalities are usually reserved for treatment of leukoplakia, removal of a small residual nidus of tumor, or areas of marginal recurrence after high-dose radiation therapy.

Radiation Therapy Techniques

The radiation therapy modalities used for treating primary lesions and the lymphatics of the oral cavity are chiefly low-megavoltage radiations, such as ^{60}Co or 4-MV to 6-MV x-ray accelerators. A common technique is to use opposing upper lateral portals for the initial 4500 cGy; the portals are reduced to spare the spinal cord and to bring the dose to the primary site up to a total of 6500 cGy to 7000 cGy through progressively reduced fields. For the lateral portal, the inferior border of the field usually lies at the thyroid notch, and the low neck fields abut the laterals with a 0.5-cm gap and midline spinal cord and pharyngeal block. For lesions of the anterior floor of the mouth, the parotid glands should not be included to avoid excessive

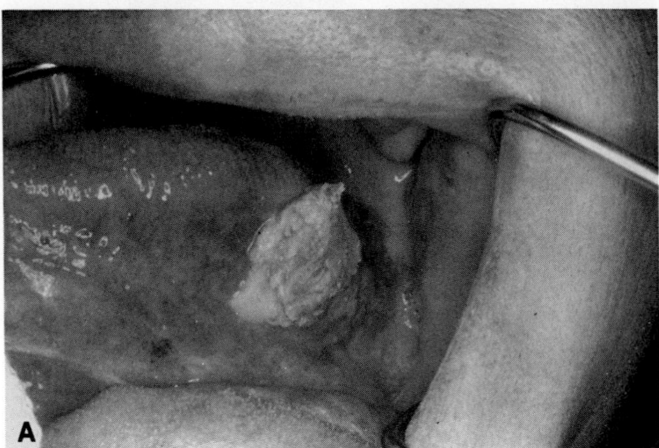

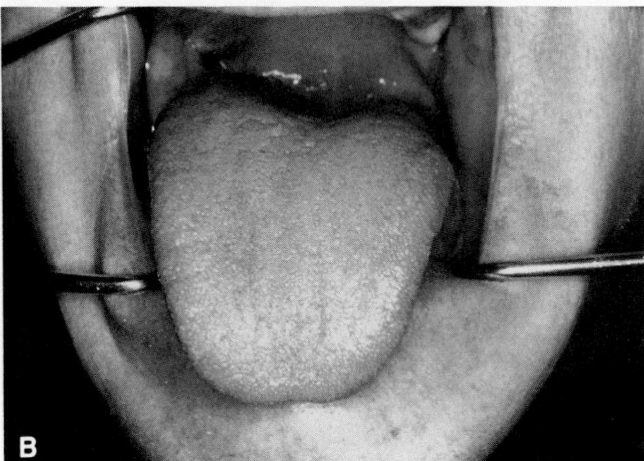

FIGURE 31–4. Excision of carcinoma of the tongue with minimal morbidity. (**A**) Preoperative and (**B**) postoperative pictures.

xerostomia. Another approach is to use ipsilateral wedge pair portals to boost the primary site and the first echelon of lymph nodes to the desired dose, if the primary lesion is lateralized, sparing the contralateral salivary gland.

Electron beam with ipsilateral appositional approach is used to irradiate both metastatic lesions in the neck nodes and eccentrically situated lesions of the oral cavity, such as carcinomas of the buccal mucosa or gingival ridge, often as a boost after comprehensive external-beam radiation therapy. The radiation oncologist must recognize that the width of the electron-beam dose is constricted at depth like the bottom of a saucer when delineating the portal.

When external beam irradiation is used, the oral tongue must be immobilized. This can be achieved by employing a "cork and tongue blade" in the mouth, commonly seen in many radiation therapy centers. I have been using the special tongue bite-block shown in Figure 31-5, which can minimize irradiation to the upper gingiva and palate while the tongue or the floor of mouth is irradiated.

Other boost techniques to the primary lesion consist of interstitial implant and intraoral electron cone. Boost procedures are used to deliver a higher dose to the primary lesion, achieving higher local control, and to spare high-dose effects to the mandible, avoiding osteoradionecrosis.

Interstitial Irradiation

Single, double, or even volume implants can be used to cover an appropriate volume with at least a 0.5 cm to 1 cm margin beyond any palpable tumor. Percutaneous afterloading techniques using angiocath and ^{192}Ir[48] have been used with good results (Fig. 31-6). In patients in whom a surgical resection is done and microscopic tumor is known to be present at the margin of resection, an interstitial implant to add 1500 cGy to 2000 cGy to the external-beam dose may be delivered after 5000 cGy to 5500 cGy to the midplane of the oral cavity.

Intraoral Cone Irradiation

Intraoral cone or peroral irradiation has been used for the past few decades. Originally, it was carried out using an orthovoltage x-ray machine with a poor localization and visualizing device; the results were understandably unsatisfactory. Local control of 50% to 60% of early carcinomas of the oral cavity was achieved. With the advent of linear accelerators with electron-beam capabilities and an improved optic device for localization and visualization, local control of selected oral carcinomas has been greatly improved with reduction of severe radiation complications.[4,46,49] Electron-beam energies of 9 MeV to 12 MeV are commonly used (Fig. 31-7).

Radiation Doses

Radiation dosage is determined by tumor site and volume, irradiated volume, number of treatment fractions, total time of treatment course, various techniques of delivery, tolerance of the patient, and response of the tumor. As shown in Table 31-3, in general, the musculature of the tongue, the buccal mucosa, and the lips have a high tolerance to radiation, and this indicates a high therapeutic ratio. A dose of 7000 cGy to 8000 cGy is well tolerated. On the other hand, the alveolar ridge and mandible have the lowest tolerance and a somewhat lower therapeutic ratio. The floor of the mouth has intermediate tolerance. With these parameters of normal tissue tolerance, a dose level can be formed (*i.e.,* various doses at different tumor sites).[49] In daily practice, the total dose of irradiation is also determined by the size of the tumor, with the final dose capped by the tolerance of the anatomic tumor site.

In conventional radiation therapy, a dose of 5000 cGy to 5500 cGy in 5 to 6 weeks is considered to be adequate for sterilization of microscopic, TX, or occult disease, and 6500 cGy to 7000 cGy in 7 weeks is administered for control of T1 and T2 squamous cell carcinomas.[18] For T3 and T4 tumors, a dose of 7500 cGy to 8000 cGy is required. Unfortunately, this high dose is not well tolerated by normal tissues, such as mandible, gum, and floor of mouth, but lesions may be favorably eradicated if situated at the tongue or buccal mucosa. Advanced tumors, considered difficult to cure by conventional, once-a-day radiation therapy alone, are currently managed by combined radiation therapy and surgery or are treated with altered fractionation schedules, producing some improvement in cure rates.[32,47]

Accelerated Fractionation

In the past decade, twice-a-day (b.i.d.) radiation therapy using 160-cGy fractions, two fractions a day, with a minimum of

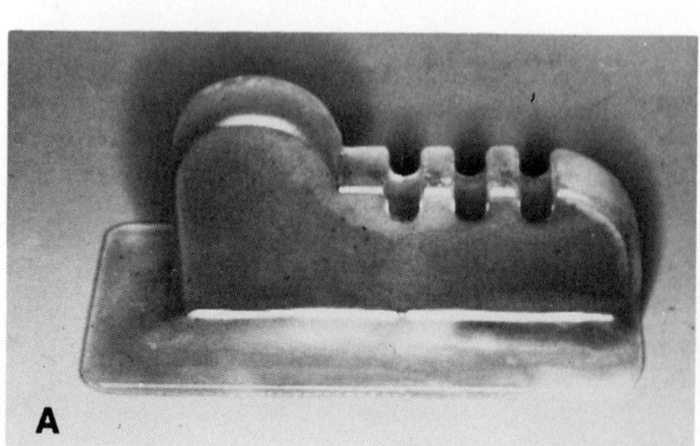

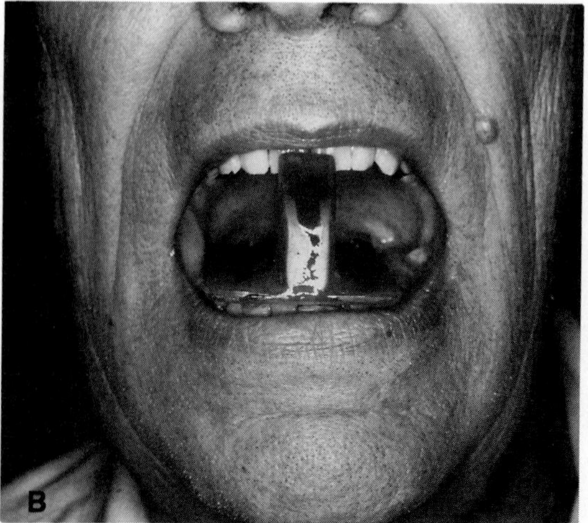

FIGURE 31–5. (**A**) Tongue depressor or bite-block. (**B**) Bite-block in patient's mouth for external beam irradiation of oral cavity carcinoma. The bottom surface sits on the tongue. The notches on the top border allow positioning of incisors for setup.

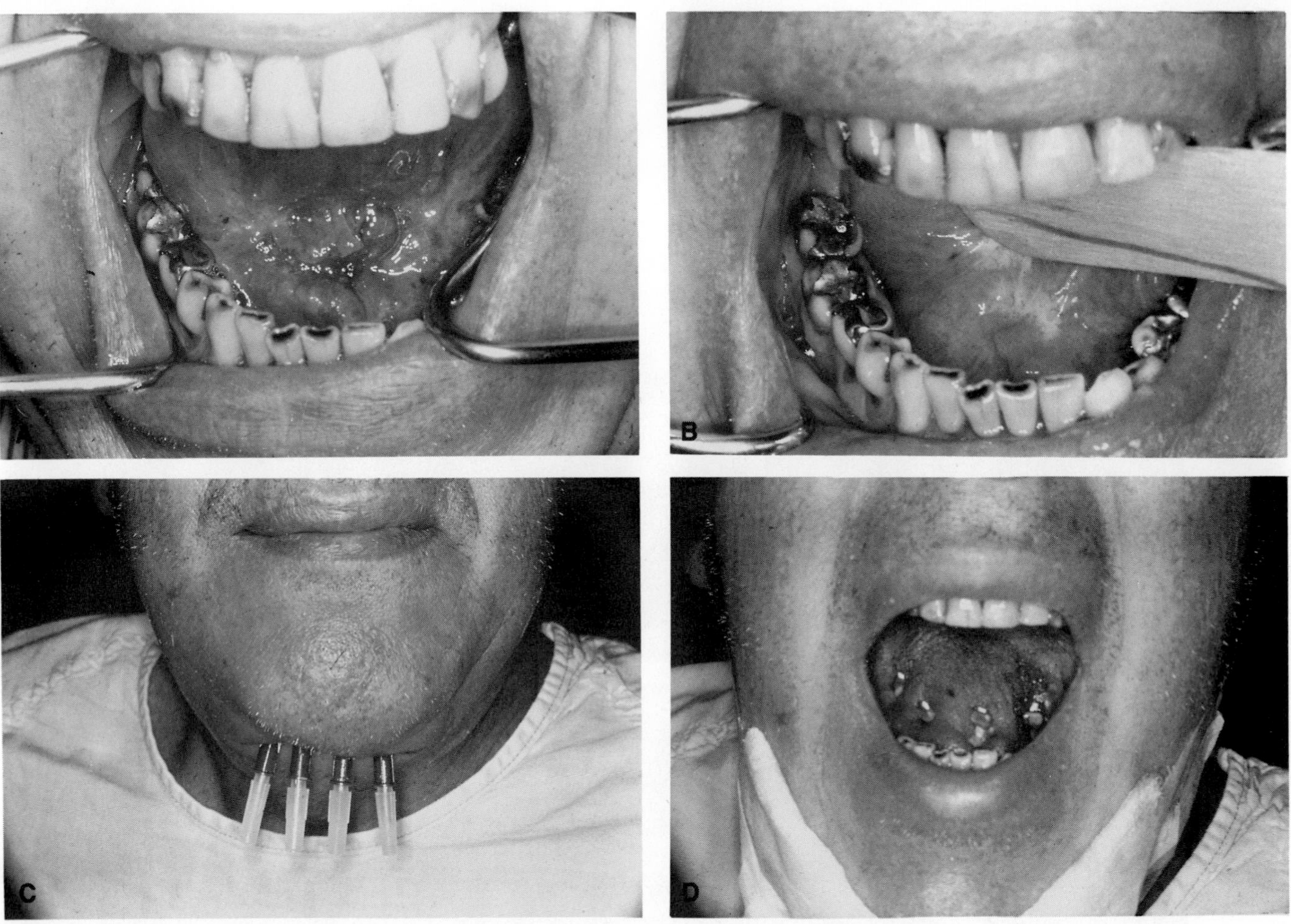

FIGURE 31–6. Percutaneous interstitial implant employing ^{192}Ir angiocath technique for carcinoma of the floor of mouth. (**A**) Before radiation therapy. (**B**) After radiation therapy. (**C**) Percutaneous implant. (**D**) Interstitial plane secured by individual lead shot.

4 hours between fractions and with a 2-week break after 3840 cGy up to a total of 6720 cGy in 6 weeks, has been used for treatment of head and neck carcinomas.[46] The results show significant improvement in local control, particularly for the advanced T2 and T3 lesions.[47] The spinal cord dose is limited to 3840 cGy in 2.5 weeks. Follow-up has indicated no inordinate skin or subcutaneous fibrosis at 8 or more years after twice-daily radiation therapy. Another hyperfractinated radiation therapy program consisting of 120-cGy fractions twice a day, for a total of 7000 cGy to 8000 cGy, has produced some improvement in local control for advanced tumors of the head and neck.[32] However, other series using similar schemes show little or no improvement in a randomized trial.[28]

Combined Surgery and Radiation Therapy

The cure rates for T1 and T2 carcinomas of the oral cavity are quite good.[26,29] However, the cure rates for T3 and T4 tumors, whether treated by radiation therapy or by surgery alone, are less than satisfactory. In these extensive lesions, failures from radiation therapy are primarily caused by an inability to control the radioresistant nidus at the primary site or the nodal disease. Because of this, a program of combined radiation therapy and surgery frequently has been carried out. The planned use of combined radiation therapy and surgery permits surgical resection of gross disease, even if the resection margins are inadequate by previous standards, followed by irradiation for subclinical or occult disease. This approach allows effective palliation and some cures for many patients who are not otherwise salvageable or are faced with functionally and cosmetically unacceptable alternatives.

Two conceptual approaches to combined radiation therapy and surgery have emerged: preoperative and postoperative radiation therapy.[38,43,44]

Preoperative Radiation Therapy

CONVENTIONAL PREOPERATIVE RADIATION THERAPY

Conventional preoperative radiation therapy decreases local recurrence and the incidence of distant metastases. The disadvantages of preoperative radiation therapy are that the exact tumor extent is unknown at the time of surgery, surgery is delayed, and there is an increase in postoperative complications. The dosage employed in this conventional preoperative radiation therapy is 4500 cGy given in 4.5 to 5 weeks. This is followed 1 month later by radical surgery encompassing all possible areas of disease as though radiation therapy had not been given. It is not commonly associated with significant postoperative functional morbidity.

HIGH-DOSE PREOPERATIVE RADIATION THERAPY OR SEQUENTIAL POSTIRRADIATION RESECTION

The dosage used in high-dose preoperative radiation therapy is 6000 cGy to 6500 cGy given in 6 to 7 weeks and delivered homogeneously to the primary site and to the first echelon of lymph nodes. The treatment portal must be progressively re-

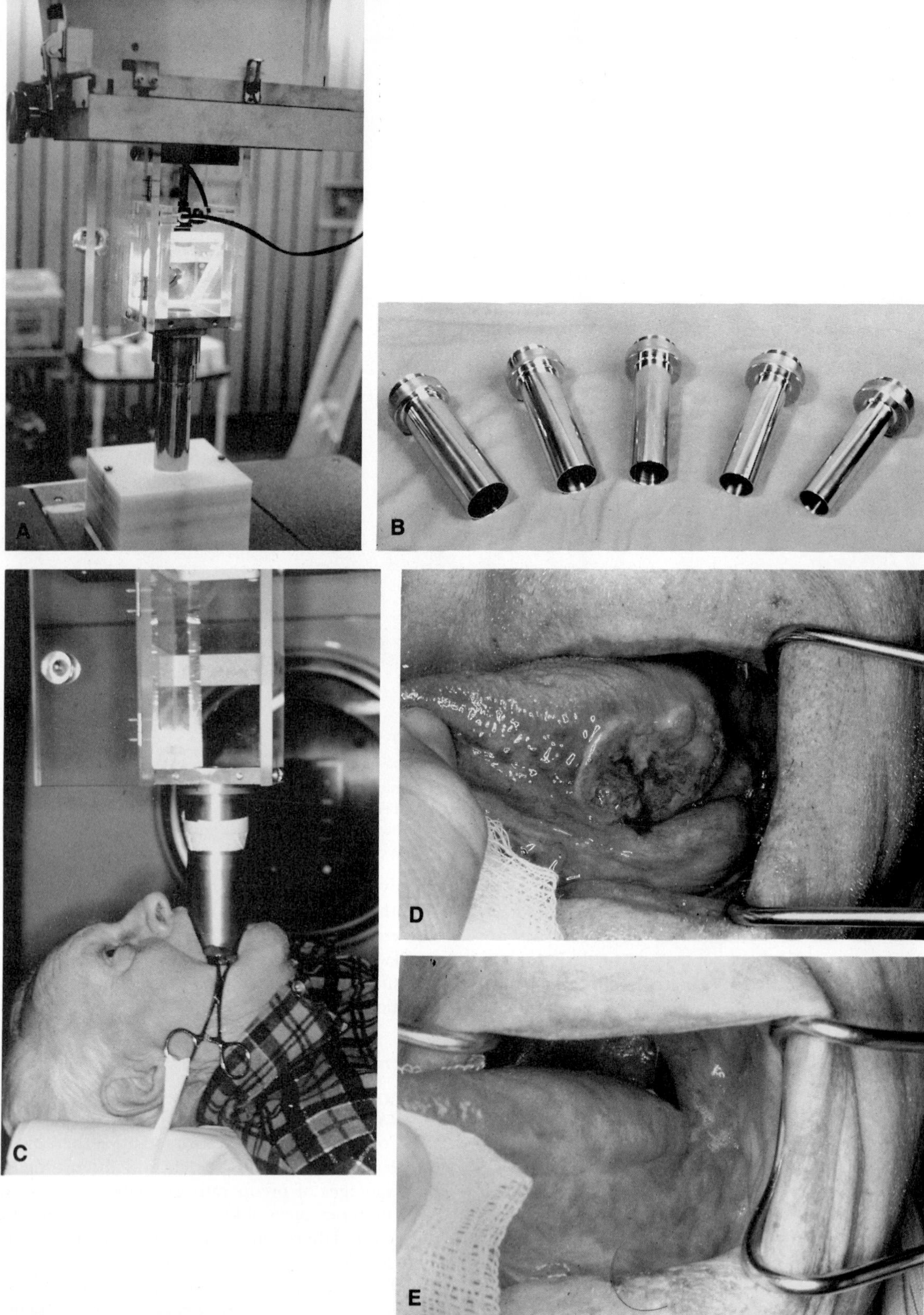

FIGURE 31–7. (**A**) Mechanical setup of IOC apparatus attached to a Clinac 18 linear accelerator currently used at the Massachusetts General Hospital. Notice the detachable telescopic mirror sitting on top of the cone for good visualization of lesion during setup. (**B**) Cones of various sizes and shapes to fit the lesions. (**C**) Intraoral cone in place on patient's tumor; telescopic mirror has been removed. (**D**) Pretreatment photo shows carcinoma of the oral tongue. (**E**) Posttreatment photo shows excellent local tumor control.

TABLE 31–3
Radiation Ulceration and TDF Values for Controlled Tumors

TDF VALUES	APPROXIMATE TOTAL DOSE (cGy)*	ORAL TONGUE	FLOOR OF MOUTH	SOFT PALATE†	RETROMOLAR TRIGONE†	BUCCAL MUCOSA	ALVEOLAR RIDGE	TOTAL‡	
−100	6000	0/4	1/5		0/1			1/10	6/74 (8%)
101–110	6400	0/4	3/12§	0/5	0/2	0/1		3/24§	
111–120	7000	0/8	0/7	0/3	0/2	0/2	1/3§	1/25	
121–130	7600	0/4	0/3	0/1		1/1		1/9	
131–140	8100	0/2	0/1	0/1	0/1	0/1		0/6	
141–150	8700	0/2	3/3§	0/1				3/6§	6/12 (50%)
>150	9000	0/2		2/3	1/1			3/6	
Total		0/26 (0%)	7/31 (23%)	2/14 (14%)	1/7 (14%)	1/5 (20%)	1/3 (33%)	12/86 (14%)	

TDF: time dose factor.
** In 200-cGy daily fractions, 5 days each week.*
† Considered a part of the oropharynx in this book.
‡ All values reflect a minimum follow-up of 24 months.
§ One case with osteonecrosis.
(Wang CC, Doppke KP, Biggs PJ: Int J Radiat Oncol Biol Phys 9:1185, 1983)

duced after 5000 cGy. In this program, unlike in a conventional moderate-dose preoperative program, radiation therapy is followed by limited surgical resection. Only the residual nidus of the primary lesion, mostly in the muscles or bone, is excised, on the assumption that the peripheral, superficial disease has been controlled by high-dose radiation therapy. This approach is intended to avoid excessive functional and cosmetic mutilation by radical surgery and has been useful in managing advanced lesions arising from the posterior oral tongue or alveolar ridge with tumor involvement of the adjacent soft palate or base or tongue. Any attempt at radical surgery would probably yield a high rate of postoperative complications and is therefore ill advised.

Postoperative Radiation Therapy

The advantage of postoperative radiation therapy is that a high dose of radiation can be delivered to known sites of residual disease, and the extent of pathologic involvement is understood. The procedure usually is carried out approximately 3 to 4 weeks after surgery, after the wound is healed. A dose of 5500 cGy in 6 weeks should not be exceeded if the surgery is radical. If the surgery is primarily a debulking procedure, high-dose radiation therapy (6500 cGy in 7 weeks) for gross residual disease must be given through a shrinking-field technique to the area of known disease.

Whether radiation therapy should be used preoperatively or postoperatively has been the subject of debate. Although no major differences have been found between these two approaches in terms of local control of primary lesions or patient survival, in certain tumor sites with exophytic tumors, good tumor response after preoperative irradiation has encouraged additional irradiation to curative levels, eliminating the need for a mutilating surgical procedure. Although preoperative radiation therapy is often preferred at our institution, postoperative radiation therapy has been used lately more frequently for advanced tumors.

Lip

Squamous cell carcinoma of the lip usually is situated in the lower lip (90%), is well differentiated (90%), and occurs predominantly in males (90%). It is more commonly seen in patients with outdoor occupations who have a heavy exposure to sunshine. Pipe smokers have a high predilection, as do persons whose lower lips protrude forward with direct exposure to the sun (Fig. 31-8). Basal cell carcinoma does not occur in the skin but may occur in the skin adjacent and secondarily invade the lip.

Therapeutic Options

Because radiation therapy or surgery yields equally high cure rates for small limited cancers (*i.e.*, 90% 3-year disease-free survival), the selection of treatment modality must depend on the cosmetic result following the procedure. Radiation therapy is best suited for the management of superficial lesions involving more than one third of the entire lip, tumor that involves the commissure and upper and lower lips, and recurrent tumor after surgery.

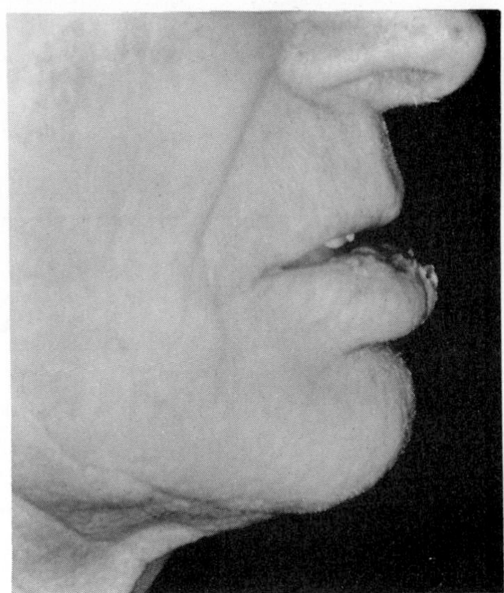

FIGURE 31–8. Everted lower lip, increasing sun exposure and risk of carcinoma.

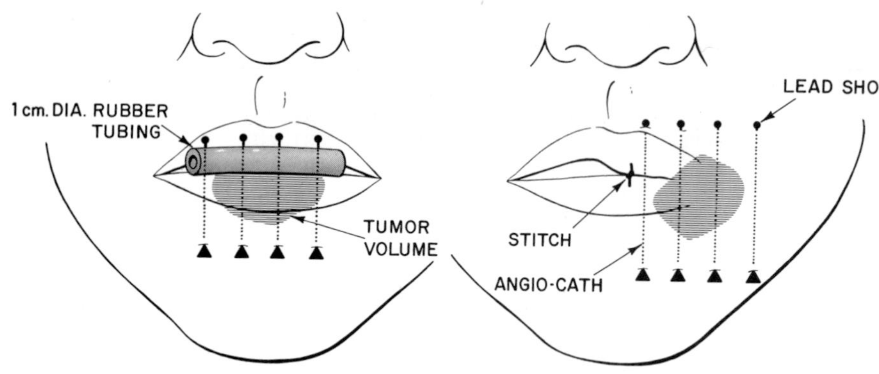

FIGURE 31–9. Technique for interstitial implant for carcinoma of the lower lip. Rubber tubing extends the implant to irradiate the lip surface. For lesions of commissure, suture the lips together.

Radiation Therapy Techniques

As a rule, therapy is directed to the primary lesion if there are no palpable nodes or if the primary lesion is well differentiated. Radiation therapy for superficial T1 tumors consists of low-energy x-rays or megavoltage electron beams (6–9 MeV). The underlying gum and mandible are protected with a lead shield. A dose of 4500 cGy to 5000 cGy in 3 to 3.5 weeks or 6000 cGy in 5 or 6 weeks should suffice.

If the tumor is extensive, spreading below the buccogingival sulcus, lead shield protection of the jaw is not possible, and the best approach is a combination of electron beam and interstitial implant (Fig. 31-9).

Radiation Therapy Results

Control of lip lesions by radiation therapy or surgery is extremely good, with 3-year disease-free survival rates of 80% to 90%, but radiation therapy produces better cosmetic and functional results, depending on the size of the primary lesion and the status of the nodes. Our results with radiation therapy are shown in Tables 31-4 and 31-5.

Oral Tongue

Squamous cell carcinoma of the oral tongue (*i.e.*, the anterior two thirds or mobile portion of the tongue) is a common type of oral cancer and includes lesions arising from the mobile portion of the tongue anterior to the circumvallate papillae. Approximately 20% to 30% of T1 and T2 tongue carcinomas and 70% to 80% of T3 and T4 lesions have nodal metastases when initial diagnosis is made, and of these, 15% to 20% have bilateral involvement.[2,25]

Therapeutic Options

The management of carcinoma of the oral tongue is difficult and controversial and depends on size, location, and growth pattern of the primary lesion and the nodal status in the neck.

T1 and T2 Tongue Lesions

Although surgery or radiation therapy are effective in controlling small cancers, it is not unreasonable to consider transoral surgical resection for small, well-defined lesions involving the tip and anterolateral border of the tongue.[40] These lesions can be cured by resection without risk of functional morbidity, particularly in aged and feeble patients. Radiation therapy is preferred for small, posteriorly situated, ill-defined lesions that are inaccessible for surgical excision through the peroral route.

Large, superficial, exophytic T1 and T2 lesions with little muscle involvement are amenable to successful treatment by radiation therapy. For moderately advanced, medium-sized T2 tumors involving the adjacent floor of the mouth, surgical treatment must include partial glossectomy, partial mandibulectomy, and radical neck dissection. For these lesions, comprehensive radiation therapy to the primary site and neck nodes is preferred, and surgery is reserved for salvage of residual or recurrent disease.

TABLE 31–4
Three-year Disease-free Survival Rates After Irradiation of the Lower Lip

TUMOR GRADE	N0	N1	N2 AND N3	NED AFTER RADIATION THERAPY*	SURGICAL SALVAGE (NED/ ATTEMPTED)	OVERALL NED (INCLUDING SALVAGE)
T1†	18/18 (100%)			18/18 (100%)		18/18 (100%)
T2	63/67 (94%)		0/3	63/70 (90%)	2/2	65/70 (93%)
T3	13/13 (100%)	0/1	1/3	14/17 (82%)		14/17 (82%)
Total	94/88 (96%)	0/1	1/6 (17%)	95/105 (90%)	2/2	97/105 (92%)

**NED: no evidence of disease.*
† Schulz MD, Ketcham AS, Sellers AH, et al: Staging cancer of the lip. In American Joint Committee for Cancer Staging and End Results Reporting Manual for Staging of Cancer. Chicago, American Joint Committee, 1976.
(Wang CC: Radiation Therapy for Head and Neck Neoplasms: Indications, Techniques and Results, 2nd ed. Chicago, Year Book Medical Publishers, 1990)

TABLE 31–5
Three-year Disease-free Survival Rates After Irradiation of the Upper Lip and Commissure

TUMOR GRADE	N0	N1	N2 AND N3	NED AFTER RADIATION THERAPY*	OVERALL NED (INCLUDING SALVAGE)
T1†	1/1	0/1		1/2	1/2
T2	3/6		0/1	3/7	3/7
T3	1/3		0/1	1/4	1/4
Total	5/10 (50%)	0/1	0/2	5/13 (38%)	5/13 (38%)

**NED: no evidence of disease.*
† Schulz MD, Ketcham AS, Sellers AH, et al: Staging cancer of the lip. In American Joint Committee for Cancer Staging and End Results Reporting Manual for Staging of Cancer. Chicago, American Joint Committee, 1976.
(Wang CC: Radiation Therapy for Head and Neck Neoplasms: Indications, Techniques and Results, 2nd ed. Chicago, Year Book Medical Publishers, 1990)

T3 and T4 Tongue Lesions

Advanced disease with deep muscle invasion often associated with cervical lymph node metastases is unlikely to be cured by irradiation alone. It is best managed by planned combined radiation therapy and surgery.

Management of Neck Nodes

With the exception of small, exophytic mucosal lesions, treatment of carcinoma of the oral tongue must include treatment of primary lesions and regional nodes because of the high incidence of occult metastases, even in patients with N0 necks.

Among patients with T1 and T2 lesions of the oral tongue in whom the neck is not treated if clinically negative, approximately 25% to 30% develop nodal metastases during the course of the disease.[45] Therefore, if these lesions are treated by peroral excision or irradiation alone, the neck must be considered at risk for occult metastases and should be followed regularly or irradiated electively to prevent nodal recurrence.[24] The so-called prophylactic neck dissection, however, has not been found necessary or rewarding.

Combination radiation therapy and therapeutic neck dissection is the procedure of choice for the residual N1, N2, or N3 neck after the primary lesion is controlled.

Radiation Therapy Management

In general, the smaller, more anteriorly situated primary lesion in an edentulous jaw is most suitable for interstitial implant or intraoral cone radiation therapy as a boost procedure.

For interstitial implants for treating carcinoma of the oral tongue, single or double planes are used to irradiate a slab of tissue 1 cm or 2 cm thick, respectively.[14] Except in the treatment of tumor arising from the dorsum of the tongue, a volume implant is rarely used. To avoid high doses to the mandible and to prevent possible osteoradionecrosis, rubber tubing or a dental roll may be sutured between the gum and the implant. An afterloading technique using angiocaths and administering ^{192}Ir percutaneously through the submental route facilitates good geometric distribution of the implant.[49]

The edentulous jaw accommodates the intraoral cone smoothly and easily; it may be necessary to sacrifice a few anterior teeth to facilitate insertion of the cone, even if they are in good repair.

Peroral or intraoral cone radiation therapy generally is carried out in the early phase of the treatment program as a boost technique. In an anteriorly situated carcinoma that does not involve the adjacent floor of the mouth or the gingival ridge, a boost dose of 2500 cGy to 3000 cGy in 10 daily fractions, five fractions a week by intraoral cone, can be given. In addition to the comprehensive radiation therapy of 4500 cGy to 5000 cGy, this technique can deliver a very high dose to the primary lesion, producing in high cure rates;[17,23,46,49] It has replaced the interstitial implant for treatment of early carcinoma of the oral tongue in some institutions.[49]

Radiation Therapy Results

Results of radiation therapy for carcinoma of the oral tongue are related to the size of the primary lesion and the presence of metastatic nodes and are comparable to those achieved with surgery.[14,16,19,29,37] Survival rates are twice as good in patients without metastatic nodes as in patients with nodal involvement.[42]

Small mucosal tumors can be successfully treated by radiation therapy or surgical excision, with similar results. The reported series indicated a 5-year survival rate of approximately 80% for T1 lesions and 50% for T2 lesions.[14,36,41,42] Local control for advanced T3 and T4 lesions was poor with surgery or radiation therapy, with 5-year survival rates of approximately 25% to 30%.[14,16,31,45]

Extensive nodal disease (N2 or N3 neck) is rarely salvageable by radiation therapy or surgery and currently is managed by combined modalities, including chemotherapy. Unfortunately, the chemotherapeutic response is usually measured in terms of weeks or months. Chemotherapy given before surgery does not appear to increase the morbidity of subsequent therapies, but it may exaggerate the acute mucosal reaction during radiation therapy.

The experience with radiation therapy for carcinoma of the oral tongue is summarized in Table 31-6. Results are good for those patients in whom intraoral cone radiation therapy is suitable, in the neighborhood of 90% for T1 and T2 lesions (Table 31-7).[49] Combined radiation therapy and surgery was carried out in a small group of patients. The results are shown in Table 31-8.

Floor of the Mouth

Carcinoma of the floor of the mouth is often located in the anterior portion of the floor adjacent to Wharton's duct orifice; it often spreads along the directional course of the submaxillary

TABLE 31–6
Three-year Disease-free Survival Rates After Irradiation of the Oral Tongue

TUMOR GRADE	N0	N1	N2 AND N3	NED AFTER RADIATION THERAPY*	SURGICAL SALVAGE (NED/ ATTEMPTED)	OVERALL NED (INCLUDING SALVAGE)
T1	17/29 (59%)	4/5 (80%)	2/2	23/36 (64%)	5/9	28/36 (78%)
T2	25/63 (40%)	2/13 (15%)	2/4	29/80 (36%)	7/24	36/80 (45%)
T3	6/19 (32%)	2/16 (13%)	1/12	9/47 (19%)	6/9	15/47 (32%)
T4	0/6	1/8	1/26	2/40 (5%)	2/4	4/40 (10%)
Total	48/117 (41%)	9/42 (21%)	6/44 (14%)	63/203 (31%)	20/46 (43%)	83/203 (41%)

**NED: no evidence of disease.*
(Wang CC: Radiation Therapy for Head and Neck Neoplasms: Indications, Techniques and Results. Bristol, UK, John Wright, 1983)

duct. Far-advanced lesions may invade the neighboring mandible.

Incidence of lymph node metastases is less than 10% for T1 lesions.[45] In extensive T3 and T4 tumors, the incidence is higher, ranging from 50% to 75%, and of these, 20% are bilateral.[25]

Therapeutic Options

When the tumor is small or limited to the mucosa, it is highly curable by irradiation alone; therefore, radiation therapy should be the treatment of choice. For moderately advanced T2 or exophytic T3 lesions, a trial course of radiation therapy may be given first, and salvage surgery is used for any residual disease at the primary site or neck nodes. For infiltrative lesions with fixation or tethering to the adjacent mandible, although the surface size is still small or categorized as T1, surgical excision of the tumor with a rim of adjacent normal inner table of the mandible should be followed by postoperative irradiation to sterilize any microscopic disease at the tumor site. For extensive, infiltrative T3 and T4 lesions with marked involvement of the adjacent muscle of the tongue and mandible, radical surgery followed by plastic closure and postoperative radiation therapy is the procedure of choice.

Radiation Therapy Management

Because of its proximity to the gingival ridge, which is vulnerable to high-dose radiation-induced soft tissue ulceration and osteoradionecrosis, the floor of the mouth has a much lower radiation tolerance than the tongue. These facts must be taken into consideration in selecting radiation treatment modalities.

Radiation therapy for T1 and T2 lesions consists of external-beam therapy with various boost techniques (*i.e.*, interstitial implant or intraoral cone). For small, well-defined lesions, intraoral cone therapy may be given at the outset. Otherwise, large-field radiation therapy in the form of a "mouth bath" with 2000 cGy is delivered to the lesion for better delineation of the margins by the development of tumoritis; this is followed by intraoral cone radiation therapy for approximately 2400 cGy in eight daily fractions. Additional external radiation therapy is given to bring the total dose to the primary site to 6500 cGy to 7000 cGy in 7 weeks or its biologic equivalent. Localized boost to the primary lesion by interstitial implant accounts for many cases of localized soft tissue ulceration and osteoradionecrosis of the mandible, and it is not recommended for lesions involving the gingiva.[45] In the patient with an edentulous jaw in whom boost treatment by means of intraoral cone or interstitial implant is not feasible, further irradiation with 2000 cGy in 2 weeks may be given to the primary site with external-beam therapy with anterior and lateral wedge pair reduced portals or with an electron-beam boost through the submental route after 4500 cGy opposed lateral portal treatment. Figure 31-10 illustrates the placement of radiation therapy portal for treatment of early carcinoma of the anterior floor of the mouth.

In T1N0 and early T2N0 lesions, because of the low incidence of occult metastases or developing sequential nodal disease, elective neck irradiation or radical neck dissection is not indicated.

TABLE 31–7
Two-year Disease-free Survival Rates After Radiation Therapy with External Beam or Intraoral Cone

ANATOMIC SITE	T1	T2	T1 + T2*
Oral tongue	20/22 (91%)	10/11 (91%)	30/33 (91%)
Floor of mouth	13/13 (100%)	19/20 (95%)	32/33 (97%)
Soft palate	8/9	6/8	14/17 (82%)
Retromolar trigone	2/3	5/6	7/9 (78%)
Buccal mucosa		4/5	4/5 (80%)
Alveolar ridge	2/3	0/1	2/4 (50%)
Total	45/50 (90%)	44/51 (88%)	89/101 (88%)

**Results include successful salvage surgery for three patients.*
(Wang CC, Doppke KP, Biggs PJ: Int J Radiat Oncol Biol Phys 9:1185, 1983)

TABLE 31–8
Three-year Disease-free Survival Rates After Surgery and Irradiation of the Oral Tongue (1960–1978)

TUMOR GRADE	N0	N1	N2 AND N3	NED AFTER TREATMENT*
T1	1/3			1/3
T2	10/19	5/7	0/3	15/29
T3	1/5	3/4	3/6	7/15
T4		1/1	2/2	3/3
Total	12/27 (44%)	9/12 (75%)	5/11 (45%)	26/50 (52%)

**Of 10 patients receiving postoperative radiation therapy, four had no evidence of disease (NED).*
(Wang CC: Radiation Therapy for Head and Neck Neoplasms: Indications, Techniques and Results. Bristol, UK, John Wright, 1983)

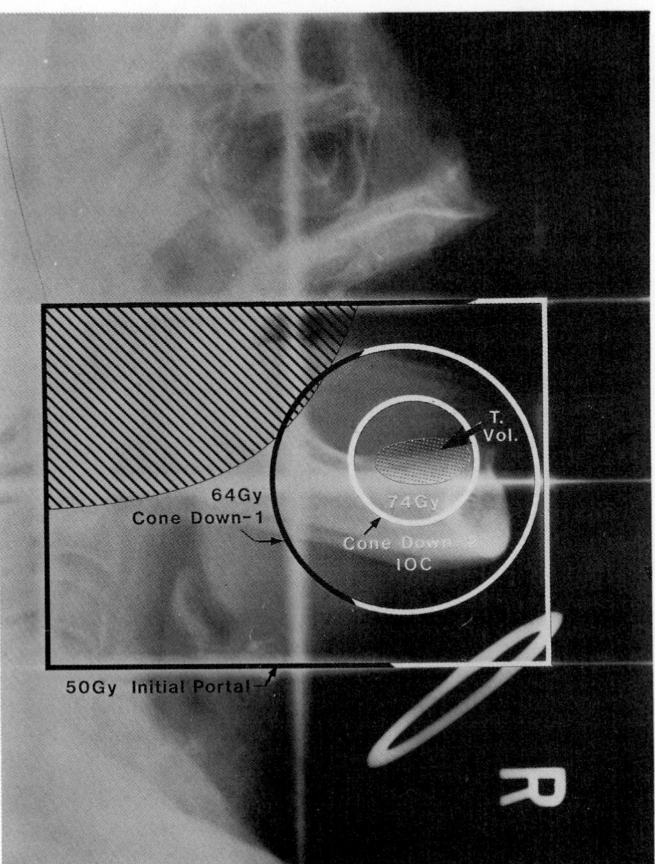

FIGURE 31–10. Portal arrangements for radiation therapy of carcinoma of the anterior floor of the mouth and dose levels with Cerrobend cutout to spare the parotid glands and avoid excessive xerostomia. Initial lateral comprehensive fields received 5000 cGy; first field reduction to 6400 cGy. The primary site was boosted for 1000 cGy through an intraoral cone.

For T3 and T4 lesions, external-beam therapy is given through large opposing lateral portals with equal loading covering the primary lesion and the nodal areas for a dose of approximately 4500 cGy in 5 weeks as a preoperative procedure or 5500 cGy to 6000 cGy in 6 weeks as a postoperative approach. When radiation therapy of 4500 cGy is given before surgery, the margins of the tumor are tattooed first to define the extent of the surgery needed.

Management of nodal disease is similar to that for carcinoma of the oral cavity. For N1, N2, and N3 disease, comprehensive neck irradiation is given with a total dose of approximately 5000 cGy to 5500 cGy in 5 weeks to the whole neck and supraclavicular area, and the residual nodes are dealt with by radical neck dissection or limited nodal resection, depending on the extent of the disease.

Radiation Therapy Results

The results of treatment by radiation therapy of carcinoma of the floor of the mouth vary with the stage of the disease. In the reported series, the 3- and 5-year disease-free survival rates are approximately 80% for T1 lesions and 50% to 60% for T2 lesions.[10,20,33] Advanced disease is rarely curable by radiation therapy alone: cure rates are less than 25%.[30,45] Compared with elective neck dissection for N0 necks, therapeutic neck dissection for nodal metastases does not jeopardize survival. Our results of radiation therapy for carcinoma of the floor of the mouth are shown in Table 31-9. Planned combined radiation therapy and surgery yielded higher local control, particularly for T3 and T4 lesions (Table 31-10).

Buccal Mucosa

The buccal mucosa is composed of the inner lining of the cheeks. Under the mucosa lies the buccinator muscle, which is covered on the outside by the skin of the face. Squamous cell carcinomas arising in this area are usually well differentiated and are frequently associated with areas of leukoplakia. Papillary, verrucous, and exophytic mucosal growths are usually well differentiated with a low incidence of lymph node metastases (*i.e.,* 10% to 20% for T1 and T2 lesions). Ulcerative, advanced tumors, which are often associated with muscle invasion, have a higher propensity (60%) for lymph node metastases.[6,12]

Therapeutic Options

Primary surgery is effective for small, superficial T1 lesions with well-defined margins. The procedure removes the malignancy and eradicates any adjacent leukoplakia. For intermediate T2 lesions, radiation therapy may produce a high cure rate with good functional and cosmetic results, and it is therefore preferred. For T3 and T4 tumors with deep muscular invasion, cure rates after radiation therapy are extremely poor. Preoperative radiation therapy and en bloc excision of the primary lesion and its regional lymph node metastases followed by plastic closure is the treatment of choice.[12]

TABLE 31–9
Three-year Disease-free Survival Rates After Irradiation of the Floor of the Mouth

TUMOR GRADE	N0	N1	N2 AND N3	NED AFTER RADIATION THERAPY*	SURGICAL SALVAGE (NED/ ATTEMPTED)	OVERALL NED (INCLUDING SALVAGE)
T1	60/68 (88%)	2/5 (40%)		62/73 (85%)	3/7	65/73 (89%)
T2	49/76 (64%)	9/19 (47%)	1/6	59/101 (58%)	4/13	63/101 (62%)
T3	1/8 (30%)	0/7	1/14	2/29 (7%)	3/7	5/29 (17%)
T4	3/10 (30%)	1/4	0/18	4/32 (13%)	1/3	5/32 (16%)
Total	113/162 (70%)	12/35 (34%)	2/38 (5%)	127/235 (54%)	11/30 (37%)	138/235 (59%)

**Nine patients died of intercurrent disease with no evidence of recurrence before the 3-year mark.*
NED: no evidence of disease.
(Wang CC: Radiation Therapy for Head and Neck Neoplasms: Indications, Techniques and Results. Bristol, UK, John Wright, 1983)

TABLE 31–10
Three-year Disease-free Survival Rates After Preoperative Irradiation of the Floor of the Mouth

TUMOR GRADE	N0	N1	N2 AND N3	NED AFTER PRE-OPERATIVE THERAPY*
T1		0/1		0/1
T2	10/12 (83%)	2/5	0/1	12/18 (67%)
T3	4/4	1/3	0/3	5/10 (50%)
T4	1/1	2/2		3/3
Total	15/17 (88%)	5/11 (45%)	0/4	20/32 (63%)

**NED: no evidence of disease.*
(Wang CC: Radiation Therapy for Head and Neck Neoplasms: Indications, Techniques and Results. Bristol, UK, John Wright, 1983)

The management of verrucous carcinoma of the buccal mucosa is often controversial. The concept of potential malignant transformation after radiation therapy as reported in the literature is debatable. It is true that the well-differentiated lesions are difficult to control with homeopathic doses of radiation and that recurrences may be more aggressive and hard to manage.[35] Some cases of so-called verrucous carcinoma that are diagnosed by small biopsy and undergo malignant changes after radiation therapy may be diagnosed because of sampling errors, because the entire specimen is not available for pathologic examination before radiation therapy. A few patients with the diagnosis of verrucous carcinoma were treated by radiation therapy and have had no evidence of disease for 10 years or more.[45]

Radiation Therapy Management

Any tumor extension to the gingiva or retromolar trigone probably precludes the use of an interstitial implant as a major treatment modality because of its insufficient coverage and attendant risk of osteoradionecrosis. External-beam therapy is therefore the prime modality.

In T1 and most T2 lesions without nodal involvement, the results of radiation therapy are best when photon or electron-beam therapy is combined with an interstitial implant or intraoral cone therapy. For the interstitial implant, the needles must be inserted percutaneously through the cheek along the base of the lesion, rather than intraorally (Fig. 31-11). Small mucosal lesions are occasionally suitable for intraoral cone radiation therapy in edentulous patients.

In moderately advanced lesions, whether nodes are positive or not, appropriate radiation therapy must include treatment of the primary site and the regional lymph nodes. This is best achieved with external-beam radiation therapy through ipsilateral and anterior wedge pair fields for a tumor dose of 5500 cGy to 6000 cGy in 6 weeks. This is followed by boost radiation therapy, sparing the mandible, by interstitial implant, intraoral cone, or electron beam for an additional 2000 cGy (Fig. 31-12). Fortunately, the tissues of the buccal cheek can tolerate

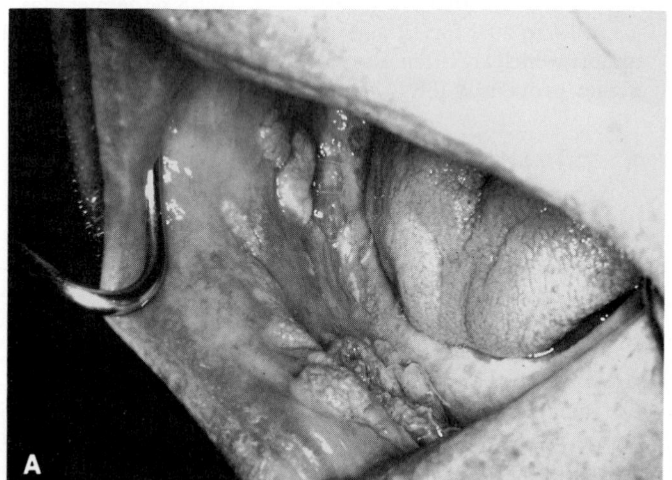

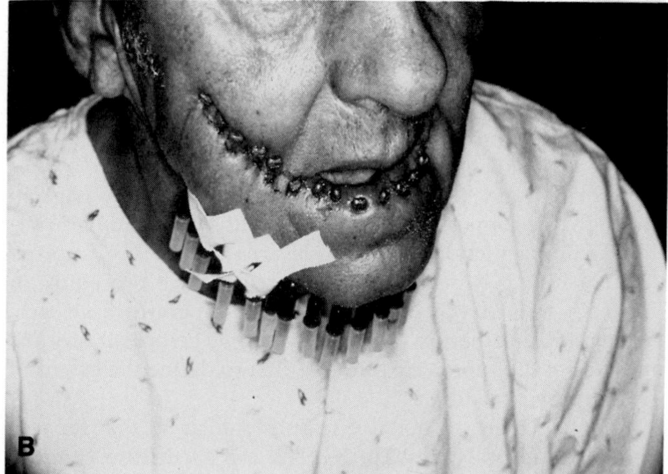

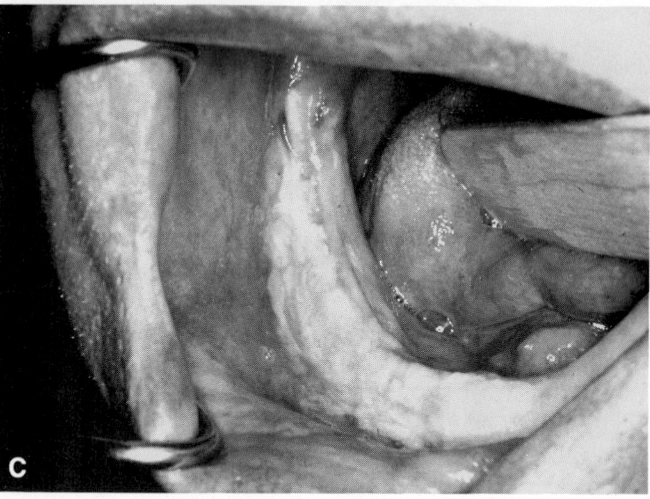

FIGURE 31–11. (**A**) Preimplant photograph shows multiple, small squamous cell carcinomas of the buccal mucosa. (**B**) Percutaneous interstitial brachytherapy in place. (**C**) Postimplant photograph shows complete resolution of the tumors with excellent cosmesis. The patient was free of disease for 10 years.

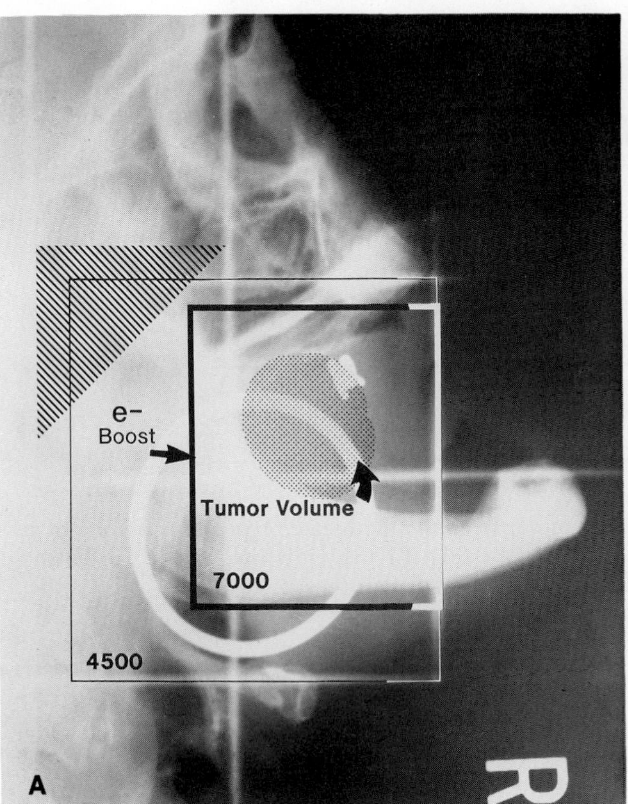

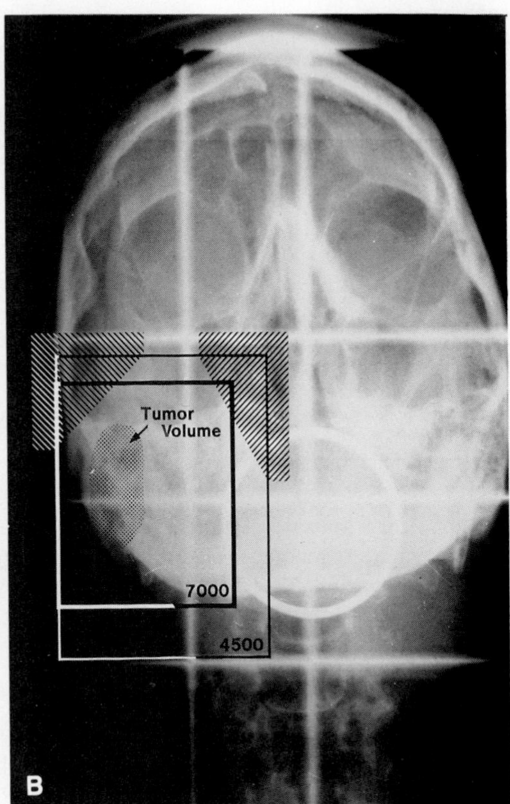

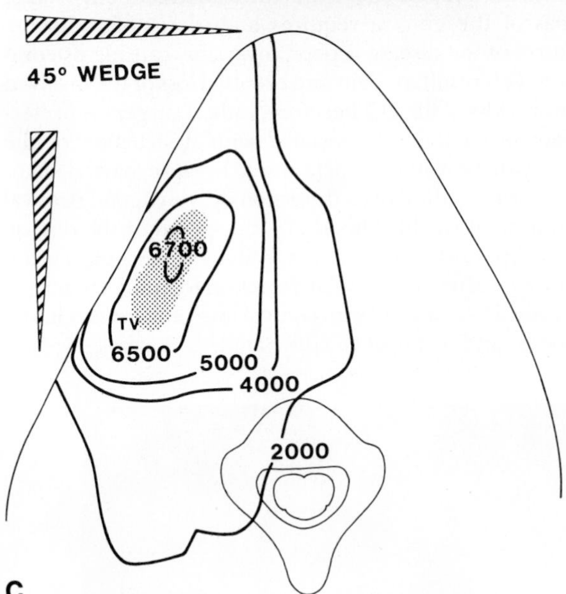

FIGURE 31–12. Portal arrangement for treating carcinoma of the buccal mucosa with initial anteroposterior (AP) and ipsilateral wedge pair approaches for 4500 cGy, followed by field reduction for an additional 1000 cGy. The primary lesion was boosted by 9-MeV electrons for a total of 1500 cGy in 5 days. (**A**) Lateral view. (**B**) AP view. (**C**) Composite isodoses of the treatments.

high-dose radiation therapy. Elective neck radiation therapy generally is not indicated for early lesions with well-differentiated histology. Ipsilateral nodal coverage by elective radiation therapy is advised for large tumors with or without positive nodes. Any residual positive nodes are dealt with by neck dissection.

Radiation Therapy Results

Results for treating carcinoma of the buccal mucosa are sparse. Three series report that the 5-year disease-free survival rates after radiation therapy ranged from 50% to 66%, depending on the stage of the primary lesion and the existence of nodal metastases.[1,6,45] For small and intermediate lesions, surgical salvage for radiation therapy failures has generally been satisfactory. Large, advanced carcinomas are rarely curable by radiation therapy, and 5-year disease-free rates are approximately 25%. Our experience in treating carcinoma of the buccal mucosa is summarized in Table 31-11.

Gingiva

Squamous cell carcinoma of the gingiva usually arises in the posterior portion of the lower dental arch and is associated with leukoplakia. Because the mucous membrane adheres directly to the periosteum of the mandible, tumor arising from the gingiva

TABLE 31–11
Three-year Disease-free Survival Rates After Irradiation of the Buccal Mucosa

TUMOR GRADE	N0	N1	N2 AND N3	NED AFTER RADIATION THERAPY*	SURGICAL SALVAGE (NED ATTEMPTED)	OVERALL NED/ (INCLUDING SALVAGE)
T1	3/6			3/6 (50%)		3/6 (50%)
T2	15/31	3/6		18/37 (49%)	5/5	23/37 (62%)
T3	4/8	1/2	1/2	6/12 (50%)	1/1	7/12 (58%)
T4	0/5			0/5 (0%)		0/5 (0%)
Total	22/50 (44%)	4/8 (50%)	1/2	27/60 (45%)	6/6	33/60 (50%)

**NED: no evidence of disease.*
(Wang CC: Radiation Therapy for Head and Neck Neoplasms: Indications, Techniques and Results, 2nd ed. Chicago, Year Book Medical Publishers, 1990)

may invade underlying bone early in its development. Most of these tumors are well-differentiated squamous cell carcinomas. A primary maxillary antrum tumor involving the gingiva should be excluded by CT scans and other radiographic studies.

Approximately 80% of the gingival carcinomas arise from the lower gingiva, and of these, 60% develop posterior to the bicuspid. Lymphatic spread depends on whether the lesion arises from the buccal or lingual surface of the alveolar ridge. From the buccal side, metastases occur in the submandibular, submental, and subdigastric nodes. From the lingual side, metastases occur in the subdigastric, deep superior jugular, and retropharyngeal nodes. Upper and lower gingival lesions follow similar patterns of spread.[33]

Nodal metastases are found in approximately one third of the patients at diagnosis. The incidence is slightly higher in lower gingival lesions than in the upper lesions. Because bony involvement by carcinoma compromises the results of radiation therapy, careful radiographic examination of the mandible, including Panorex and polytomes of the mandible, is essential as a minimal pretreatment workup. Intraoral dental radiographs or CT scans may better reveal minimal bony involvement of the mandible. Care should be taken to differentiate the smooth, saucer-shaped pressure defect caused by a slowly growing, pushing tumor from the moth-eaten type of infiltration of an aggressive tumor (Fig. 31-13). Only the former can be successfully treated by radiation therapy.

Therapeutic Options

Treatment of carcinoma of the gingiva depends on the extent of the lesion, the status of the cervical lymph nodes, and especially on the presence of bony involvement. Small T1 exophytic lesions without bony involvement can be managed by external-beam therapy alone. Unfortunately, treatment of large carcinomas of the gingiva requires high doses of radiation. Local control of the disease is poor, invariably causing osteoradionecrosis with resultant pain and eventual loss of the involved mandible and loss of life.[35] Therefore, radical surgery is preferred for advanced lesions associated with destruction of the mandible, with or without metastases, because partial mandibulectomy with radical neck dissection provides good survival rates.[9] Because of the likelihood of local spread of the disease along the subperiosteal lymphatics, radiation therapy is often given before or after mandibular resection to eradicate microscopic disease at the margins, to control micrometastases in the lymph nodes, and to improve cure rates.

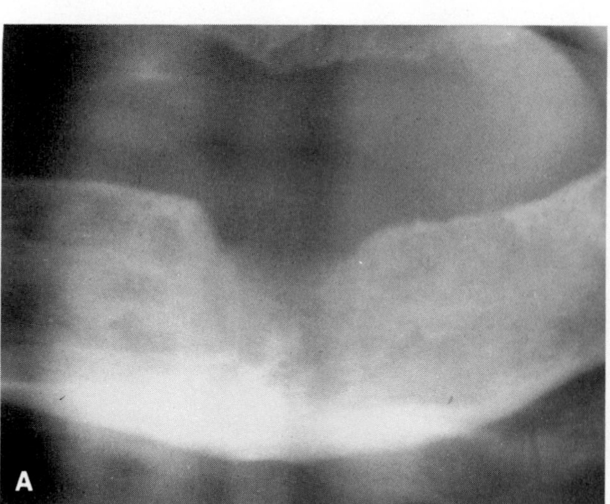

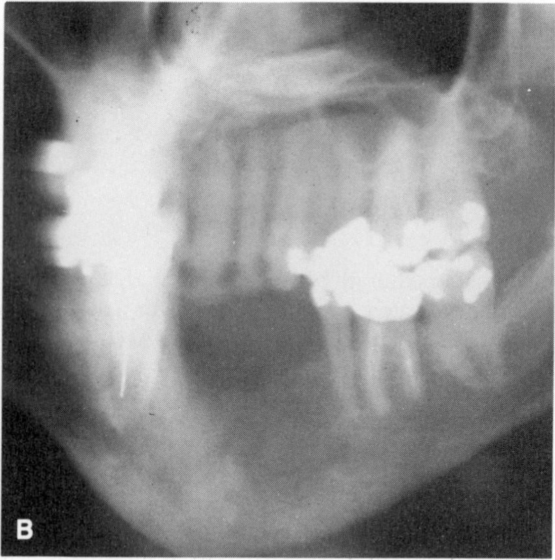

FIGURE 31–13. (**A**) Radiograph showing saucer-shaped pressure defect of the mandible from an adjacent, slowly growing tumor. This condition is treatable and curable by radiation therapy. (**B**) Radiograph showing moth-eaten bone destruction of the mandible from a rapidly growing, aggressive tumor. This condition is rarely curable by radiation therapy alone and should be managed by combined therapy.

Radiation Therapy Management

Because of the eccentric location of the primary lesion and its regional nodes, radiation therapy is delivered by external beam with anteroposterior and lateral wedge pair or electron-beam technique. Small mucosal tumors can be satisfactorily treated by combined external radiation therapy and an intra-oral cone boost if administration is technically feasible. The radium mold has been replaced by modern megavoltage irradiation. The interstitial implant has no place in the management of this disease because of the proximity of bone to tumors and the high risk of osteoradionecrosis.

Radiation portals must include the entire segment of the hemimandible from the mental symphysis to the temporomandibular joint. The ipsilateral neck is irradiated if nodes are present or if lesions are advanced. A dose of 4500 cGy is given in 5 weeks as a preoperative procedure. If postoperative radiation therapy is given, the doses may be increased to 5500 cGy to 6000 cGy without risk of complications (Fig. 31-14). If feasible, an ipsilateral electron beam is used to boost the dose to the high-

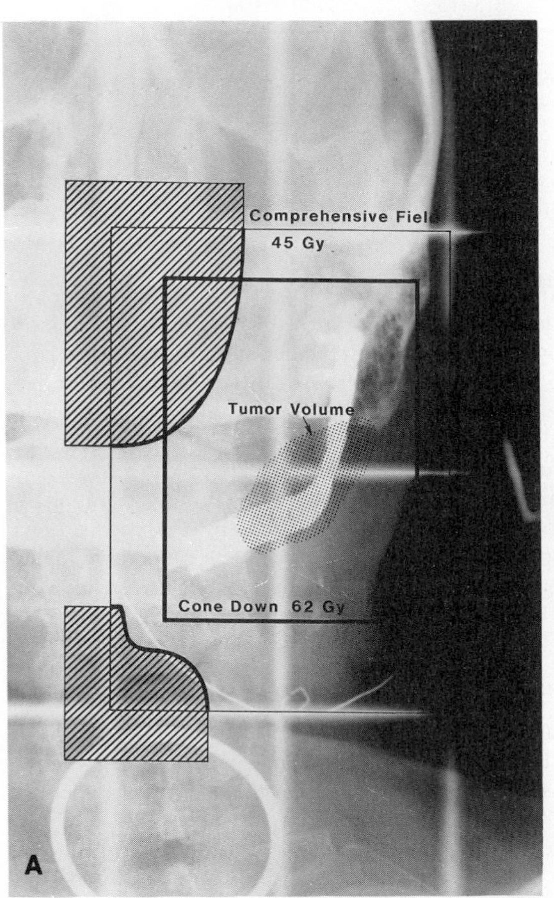

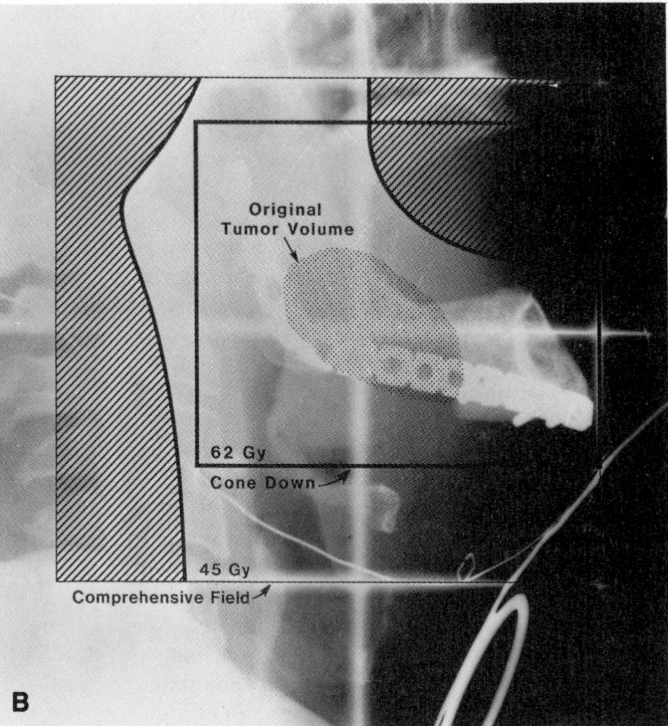

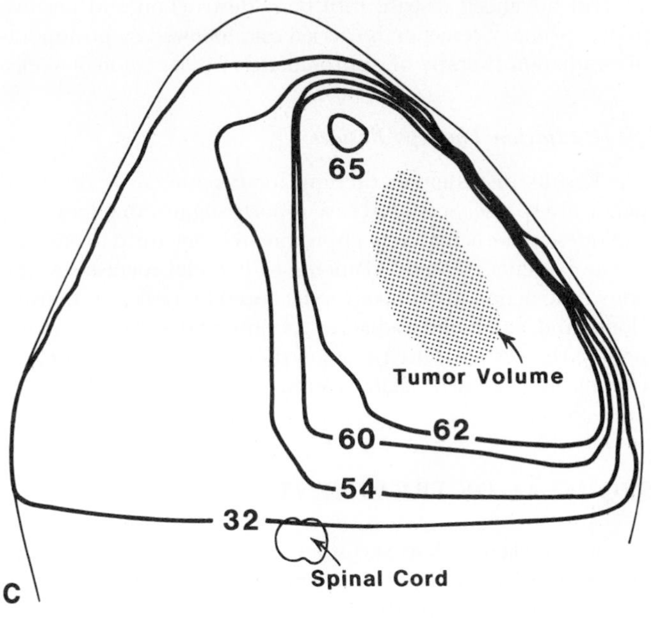

FIGURE 31–14. Portal arrangement after hemimandibulectomy for treating carcinoma of the alveolar ridge consists of opposing laterals with 3840 cGy and field reduction with an additional 640 cGy followed by anteroposterior (AP) and ipsilateral wedge pair approaches for 1800 cGy. Metal prosthesis will replace missing mandible. (**A**) AP view. (**B**) Lateral view. (**C**) Composite isodoses of the treatments.

TABLE 31–12
Three-year Disease-free Survival Rates After Irradiation of the Gingival Ridge

TUMOR GRADE	N0	N1	N2 AND N3	NED AFTER RADIATION THERAPY*	SURGICAL SALVAGE (NED/ ATTEMPTED)	OVERALL NED/ (INCLUDING SALVAGE)
T1	7/9 (78%)	0/2		7/11 (64%)	1/3	8/11 (73%)
T2	4/15 (27%)	0/1		4/16 (25%)	1/6	5/16 (31%)
T3	1/6			1/6 (17%)	0/2	1/6 (17%)
T4	0/3	0/1	0/4	0/8 (0%)	0/2	0/8 (0%)
Total	12/33 (36%)	0/4	0/4	12/41 (29%)	2/13 (15%)	14/41 (34%)

**NED: no evidence of disease.*
(Wang CC: Radiation Therapy for Head and Neck Neoplasms: Indications, Techniques and Results. Bristol, UK, John Wright, 1983)

risk area. Radiation therapy should be started approximately 3 to 4 weeks after surgery.

Radiation Therapy Results

Results of treatment by radiation therapy alone generally are not entirely satisfactory, particularly for T3 and T4 lesions. For most reported series, the 5-year survival rates range from 30% to 50%.[7,22,26] Patients with clinically positive nodes generally carry a poor prognosis and may benefit from surgery as part of the treatment of nodal disease. Our results of radiation therapy for carcinoma of the gingival ridge are shown in Table 31-12; the results following planned combined radiation therapy and surgery are shown in Table 31-13.

HARD PALATE

The hard palate is the most common site of minor salivary gland tumors in the oral cavity. Squamous cell carcinomas arising from the hard palate are rare and are usually ulcerative and invade the underlying bone in the early stage of disease. Most carcinomas are well differentiated with a 15% to 20% incidence of lymph node metastases. Verrucous and *in situ* carcinomas also may occur in this region. The submandibular, upper jugular, and subdigastric nodes are commonly involved.

Painless irregularity or swelling with ill-fitting dentures is usually the only complaint of early carcinoma of the hard palate. Appropriate x-ray films should be obtained before making a decision about management. Examination should include polytomes and CT scans of the palatal bone, maxillary antrum, and floor of the nasal cavity.

TABLE 31–13
Three-year Disease-free Survival Rates After Surgery and Irradiation of the Gingival Ridge

TUMOR GRADE	N0	N1	NED AFTER TREATMENT*
T1	2/2	1/1	3/3 (100%)
T2	5/6	1/2	6/8 (75%)
T3	2/3		2/3 (67%)
T4	0/1	0/2	0/3 (0%)
Total	9/12 (75%)	2/5 (40%)	11/17 (65%)

**NED: no evidence of disease.*
(Wang CC: Radiation Therapy for Head and Neck Neoplasms: Indications, Techniques and Results. Bristol, UK, John Wright, 1983)

Therapeutic Options

Early lesions without bony involvement can be treated satisfactorily by radiation therapy alone; surgery is reserved for salvage of irradiation failures. Advanced, deeply ulcerative, infiltrative lesions with bone destruction are rarely curable by radiation therapy and are better treated by combined radiation therapy and surgery; the resulting bone defect can be corrected by an obturator. Malignant salivary gland tumors, traditionally treated by surgery, are now often treated by combined surgery and postoperative radiation therapy. Some inoperable malignant minor salivary gland tumors have been successfully controlled by high-dose radiation therapy.[15]

Radiation Therapy Management

Radiation therapy for early carcinoma of the hard palate is generally directed to treating the primary site, if the neck is free of metastases. Parallel opposing lateral portals cover the entire palate for delivering doses of approximately 6000 cGy in 6 weeks. The primary lesion may be boosted with intraoral electron-beam therapy, if possible, to bring the total dose to 7000 cGy in 7 weeks.

For advanced disease with bony destruction and positive nodes, primary resection is carried out, followed by postoperative radiation therapy of approximately 6000 cGy in 7 weeks.

Radiation Therapy Results

Results of radiation therapy for carcinoma of the hard palate are sparse. Scattered case reports suggest that local control rates can be achieved in approximately one third to one half of the patients treated.[45] Patients with nodal metastases and bony destruction are unlikely to be cured by radiation therapy alone, and combined radiation therapy and surgery has improved the results. Our radiation therapy experience for carcinomas of the hard palate is summarized in Table 31-14.

SEQUELAE OF TREATMENT

Minor sequelae, such as xerostomia, loss of sense of taste, and dental caries, may follow curative radiation therapy. Major complications include soft tissue ulceration, orocutaneous fistula,

TABLE 31–14
Three-year Disease-free Survival Rates After Irradiation of the Hard Palate

TUMOR GRADE	N0	N1	N2 AND N3	NED AFTER RADIATION THERAPY*
T1	2/2			2/2
T2	3/4			3/4
T3	2/4			2/4
T4		0/1	0/1	0/2
Total	7/10 (70%)	0/1	0/1	7/12 (58%)

**NED: no evidence of disease.*
(Wang CC: Radiation Therapy for Head and Neck Neoplasms: Indications, Techniques and Results. Bristol, UK, John Wright, 1983)

and osteoradionecrosis of the mandible. Osteoradionecrosis may be affected by the proximity of growth, recent dental extractions, health and integrity of the mucous membrane, and radiation dosage. It may also occur in the edentulous jaw from an excessively high dose of radiation.[11] Once osteoradionecrosis of the mandible develops, removal of the devitalized, infected bone by surgery, including sequestrectomy or partial mandibulectomy, may be indicated. Radiation-induced dental caries can be avoided with meticulous dental care with fluoride treatment after radiation therapy.

Although complications are undesirable, they should be accepted as a risk in the treatment of malignant tumors of the oral cavity. They may be minimized by careful radiotherapeutic and surgical techniques.

DENTAL CARE AND RADIATION THERAPY

Dental care by dentists and oral surgeons should constitute a comprehensive part of the overall management of carcinoma of the oral cavity.[13,21] Evaluation before irradiation should include an examination of the soft tissues and teeth. Any tooth that cannot be restored because of severe periodontal disease or dental caries should be extracted before radiation therapy is begun. In general, radiation therapy should not be started until the tooth socket has healed adequately, which usually takes about 2 weeks. Sound teeth or teeth in good repair need not be sacrificed if radiation dosages are kept within the tolerance of the mandible, if the major portion of the salivary gland is spared, or if combined external megavoltage beams and interstitial implant or intraoral cone approach is used.[11]

Postirradiation dental extraction may be possible. If the tooth lies within the previous volume of high-dose irradiation, extraction must be covered by antibiotic therapy before and after the dental procedure.

REFERENCES

1. Ash CL: Oral cancer: A twenty-five year study [Janeway Lecture]. AJR 87:417, 1961
2. Batsakis JG: Tumors of the Head and Neck. Clinical and Pathological Considerations, 2nd ed. Baltimore, Williams & Wilkins, 1979
3. Beahrs OH, Henson DE, Hutter RV, Myers, MH (eds): Manual for Staging of Cancer, 3rd ed. Philadelphia, JB Lippincott, 1988
4. Biggs PJ, Wang CC: An intra-oral cone for 18 MeV linear accelerator. Int J Radiat Oncol Biol Phys 8:1251, 1982
5. Blitzer PH, Wang CC, Suit HD: Blood pressure and hemoglobin concentration: Multivariate analysis of local control after radiation for head and neck cancer. Presented at the annual meeting of ASTRO, Washington DC, October 1984
6. Bloom ND, Spiro RH: Carcinoma of the cheek mucosa. A retrospective analysis. Am J Surg 149:556, 1980
7. Byers RM, Newman R, Russell N, et al: Results of treatment of squamous cell carcinoma of the lower gum. Cancer 47:2236, 1981
8. Cancer statistics: Ca—A Cancer Journal for Clinicians. American Cancer Society: Cancer Statistics, 40(1):9, 1990
9. Cady B, Catlin D: Epidermoid carcinoma of the gum. Cancer 23:551, 1969
10. Campos JL, Lampe I, Fayos JV: Radiotherapy of carcinoma of the floor of the mouth. Radiology 99:677, 1971
11. Cheng VS, Wang CC: osteoradionecrosis of the mandible resulting from external megavoltage radiation therapy. Radiology 12:685, 1974
12. Conley J, Sadoyama JA: Squamous cell cancer of the buccal mucosa. Arch Otolaryngol Head Neck Surg 94:330, 1973
13. Daley TE, Drane JB: Dental care for irradiated patients. In Neoplasia of Head and Neck, p. 225, Chicago, Year Book Medical Publishers, 1974
14. Decroix Y, Ghossein NA: Experience of the Curie Institute in treatment of cancer of the mobile tongue. I. Treatment policies and results. Cancer 47:496, 1981
15. Ellis ER, Million RR, Mendenhall WM, Parsons JT; Cassisi NJ: The use of radiation therapy in the management of minor salivary gland tumors. Int J Radiat Oncol Biol Phys 97:613, 1988
16. Fayos JV, Lampe I: Peroral irradiation of carcinoma of the oral tongue. Radiology 93:387, 1969
17. Fayos JV, Lampe I: Treatment of squamous cell carcinoma of the oral cavity. Am J Surg 124:493, 1972
18. Fletcher GH: Elective irradiation of subclinical disease in cancers of the head and neck. Cancer 29:1450, 1972
19. Frazell EL: A review of the treatment of cancer of the mobile portion of the tongue. Cancer 28:1178, 1978
20. Harold CC: Management of cancer of the floor of the mouth. Am J Surg 122:487, 1971
21. Hinds EC: Dental care and oral hygiene before and after treatment. JAMA 215:964, 1971
22. Lampe I: Radiation therapy of cancer of the buccal mucosa and lower gingiva. Am J Ronetgenol 73:628, 1955
23. Lampe I: Radiotherapeutic experience with squamous cell carcinoma of the oral part of the tongue. Univ Mich Med Center J 33:215, 1967
24. LeBorgne F, Leborgne H, Barlocci LU et al: Elective neck irradiation in the treatment of cancer of the oral tongue. Int J Radiat Oncol Biol Phys 13:1149, 1987
25. Lindberg R: Distribution of cervical lymph node metastases from squamous cell carcinoma of the upper respiratory and digestive tracts. Cancer 29:1446, 1972
26. MacComb WS, Fletcher GH: Cancer of the Head and Neck, p 147. Baltimore, Williams & Wilkins, 1967
27. McKay EN, Sellers AH: A statistical review of carcinoma of the lip. Can Med Assoc J 90:670, 1964
28. Marcial VA, Pajak TF, Chang et al: Hyperfractionated photon radiation therapy in the treatment of advanced squamous cell carcinoma of the oral cavity, pharynx, larynx and sinuses, using radiation therapy as the only planned modality: (preliminary report) by the Radiation Therapy Oncology Group (RTOG). Int J Radiat Oncol Biol Phys 13:41, 1987
29. Marks JE, Lee F, Freeman RB, et al: Carcinoma of the oral tongue. A study of pertinent selections and treatment results. Larygnoscope 91:1548, 1981
30. Marks JE, Lee F, Smith, PG, et al: Floor of mouth cancer: Patient selection and treatment results. Laryngoscope 93:475, 1983
31. Mendelson BC, Hodgkinson DJ, Woods, JE: Cancer of the oral cavity. Surg Clin North Am 57:585, 1977
32. Million RR: The 1989 Franz Buschke Lecture: Hyperfractionation in Cancer Therapy: An Overview. Presented at the Ninth

Annual Current Approaches to Radiation Oncology, Biology and Physics at the University of California at San Francisco, March 1989

33. Million RR, Cassisi NJ: Oral Cavity. In Million RR, Cassisi NJ (eds): Management of Head and Neck Cancer. A Multidisciplinary Approach, p 239. Philadelphia, JB Lippincott, 1984
34. Nagorsky MJ, Sessions DG: Laser resection for early oral cavity cancer. Results and complications. Ann Otol Rhinol Laryngol 96:556, 1987
35. Nair MK, Sankaranarayanan R, Padmanabhan RK, et al: Oral verrucous carcinoma. Treatment with radiotherapy. Cancer 61:458, 1988
36. Phillips TL: Peroral roentgen therapy. Radiology 90:525, 1968
37. Pierquin B, Chassagne D, Baillet F, et al: The placement of implantation in tongue and floor of mouth cancer. JAMA 215:961, 1971
38. Robertson AG, McGreegor IA, Soutar DS, et al: Postoperative radiotherapy in the management of advanced intra-oral cancers. Clin Radiol 37:173, 1986
39. Rouveiere H: Anatomy of the Human Lymphatic System, p 44. Ann Arbor, Edwards Bros, 1938
40. Sprio RH, Spiro JD, Strong EW: Surgical approach to squamous carcinoma confined to the tongue and the floor of the mouth. Arch Otolaryngol Head Neck Surg 9:27, 1986
41. Strong EW: Carcinoma of the tongue. Otolaryngol Clin North Am 12:107, 1979
42. Suen JY, Myers EW: Cancer of the head and neck. New York, Churchill-Livingstone, 1981
43. Thomlinson RH, Gray LH: The histological structure of some human lung cancers and the possible implications for radiotherapy. Br J Cancer 9:539, 1955
44. Wang CC: Radiation Therapy for head and neck cancers. Cancer 36:748, 1975
45. Wang CC: Radiation Therapy for Head and Neck Neoplasms: Indications, Techniques and Results. Littleton, MA, Wright-PSG, 1983
46. Wang CC: Radiotherapeutic management and results of T1N0, T2N0 carcinoma of the oral tongue: Evaluation of boost techniques. Int J Radiat Oncol Biol Phys 17:287, 1989
47. Wang CC, Blitzer PH, Suit HD: Twice-a-day radiation therapy for cancer of the head and neck. Cancer 55:2100, 1985
48. Wang CC, Boyer AL, Mendiondo O: Afterloading interstitial radiation therapy. Int J Radiat Oncol Biol Phys 1:365, 1976
49. Wang CC, Doppke KP, Biggs PJ: Intra-oral cone radiation therapy for selected carcinomas of the oral cavity. Int J Radiat Oncol Biol Phys 9:1185, 1983

32

Tonsillar Fossa and Faucial Arch

Carlos A. Perez

ANATOMY

The tonsillar fossa, posterior faucial pillars, and the base of the tongue are embryologically derived from the oropharyngeal brachial arches. The anterior faucial pillar and the retromolar trigone are embryologically connected to the oral cavity.[26] Although tumors that originate in the palatine arch share biologic behavior with lesions of the oral cavity and some of the oropharynx, it is preferable to classify the tumors of the soft palate, anterior faucial arch, and retromolar trigone with oropharyngeal malignancies.[26] In the faucial arch, there are several well-defined structures: anterior tonsillar pillar, retromolar trigone, soft palate and uvula, glossopalatine (glossopharyngeal sulcus), and posterior tonsillar pillar.

The oropharynx can be subdivided into the palatine (faucial) arch and the oropharynx proper. The oropharynx is the posterior continuation of the oral cavity, which communicates with the nasopharynx above and the laryngopharynx below (Fig. 32-1). The palatine arch is a junctional area between the oral cavity and the laryngopharynx. It is formed by the soft palate and the uvula above, the anterior tonsillar pillar and glossopalatine sulcus laterally, and the glossopharyngeal sulcus and the base of the tongue inferiorly.[10]

The retromolar trigone may be included in the structures of the faucial arch (Fig. 32-2), although it is actually located within the oral cavity, its apex in line with the tuberosity of the maxilla (behind the last upper molar). The lateral border extends upward into the buccal mucosa, and it blends medially with the anterior tonsillar pillar, its base formed by the distal surface of the last lower molar and the adjacent gingivolingual sulcus.[47]

The lateral walls of the oropharynx are limited posteriorly by the tonsillar fossa and the posterior tonsillar pillar (pharyngopalatine folds). These pillars are folds of mucous membrane that cover the underlying glossopalatine and pharyngopalatine muscles.[47] Deep to the lateral wall of the tonsillar fossa are the superior constrictor muscle of the pharynx, the upper fibers of the middle constrictor, the pharyngeus and stylopharyngeus muscles, and the glossopalatine and pharyngopalatine muscles (Fig. 32-3). The tonsillar fossa continues into the lateral and posterior pharyngeal walls. Stratified squamous epithelium covers all these structures. The tonsil has a profuse lymphoid structure.

The tonsillar fossa and faucial arch have a rich submucosal lymphatic network that is laterally grouped in four to six lymphatic ducts that drain into the subdigastric, upper cervical, and parapharyngeal lymph nodes. Submaxillary lymph nodes may be involved in lesions involving the retromolar trigone, the buccal mucosa, or the base of the tongue. If the upper cervical lymph nodes contain metastatic tumor, approximately 25% of the patients have metastases in the midcervical lymph nodes and about 5% to 10% have metastases in the posterior cervical lymph nodes. Metastases in the low cervical chain may appear in about 5% to 15% of patients with upper cervical lymph node involvement. Lymphatic drainage into the contralateral neck is observed occasionally in tumors that extend toward the midline.

EPIDEMIOLOGY

Carcinoma of the tonsil and faucial arch is relatively rare, comprising less than 0.5% of all cancers in men in the United States. According to the Surveillance, Epidemiology, and End Results (SEER) study of the National Cancer Institute, the age-adjusted incidence in 1984 was 0.5 per 100,000 white men and 2.7 per 100,000 black men.[84] Carcinoma of the tonsil is three to four times as frequent in men as in women, and the incidence increases with age; these tumors are most frequently diagnosed in the sixth and seventh decades of life. Malignant lymphomas in this location usually appear in patients who are between 40 and 60 years of age.[8]

No specific predisposing factors have been identified in patients with orophayngeal cancer, but it is believed that excessive consumption of alcohol and a long history of smoking contribute to an increased risk of oropharyngeal tumors.[83]

NATURAL HISTORY

In general, tumors of the anterior tonsillar pillar and soft palate are better differentiated and biologically less aggressive than those of the tonsillar fossa. Their growth is usually slower, and

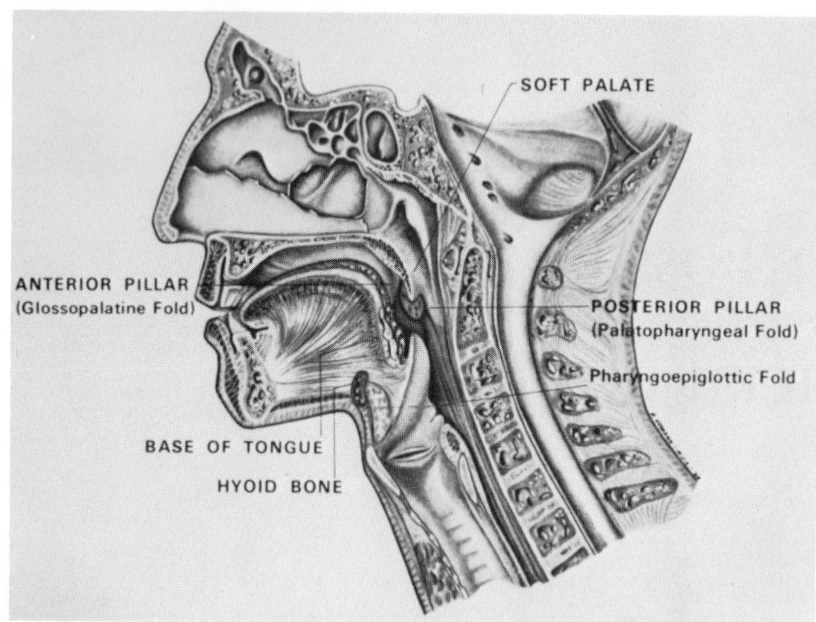

FIGURE 32–1. Sagittal section through the oropharynx. Because there is no anatomic landmark demarcating oropharynx from laryngopharynx on the posterior pharyngeal wall, a line drawn from the hyoid bone to the posterior wall may be used. (MacComb WS, Fletcher GH [eds]: Cancer of the Head and Neck, p 179. Baltimore, Williams & Wilkins, 1967)

they metastasize less frequently to the regional lymph nodes. In a series of 269 patients, only 40% of the palatine arch lesions were larger than 5 cm in diameter, compared with 60% of other oropharyngeal lesions.[36] Moreover, 50% to 60% of the patients with primary tumors in the anterior tonsillar pillar, retromolar trigone, and soft palate had clinically negative necks, in contrast to only 24% of those with tonsillar fossa primary tumors.[36]

Lesions of the tonsillar fossa tend to be infiltrative, often involving the adjacent retromolar trigone, soft palate, and base of the tongue. Perez and associates[63] found that in only 5.4% of 296 patients was the primary tumor confined to the tonsillar fossa; in 65.9%, there was involvement of the soft palate, and 41% had extension into the base of the tongue. Spread to adjacent structures is illustrated in Table 32-1.

Tumors limited to the posterior tonsillar pillar are extremely rare; Million and Cassisi[56] reported only 2 in 99 patients with tonsillar carcinoma. These tumors tend to spread inferiorly along the palatinopharyngeal muscle; the lymph nodes most likely to be involved are the spinal accessory group.

Tumors of the faucial arch can be superficially spreading, exophytic, ulcerative, or infiltrative. The latter two types are frequently combined. They may become extensive and involve the adjacent hard palate or buccal mucosa in less than 20% of patients.

Byers and co-workers[15] described mandibular involvement in 14% of 110 patients with primary retromolar trigone carcinomas; four of these patients had normal-appearing preoperative x-ray films. In 6 of 17 patients, mandibular involvement reported on radiographs was not confirmed on pathologic examinations.

Lymphatic Drainage

Lindberg[44] described the distribution of nodal metastases in various locations. Retromolar trigone, tonsillar pillar, and soft

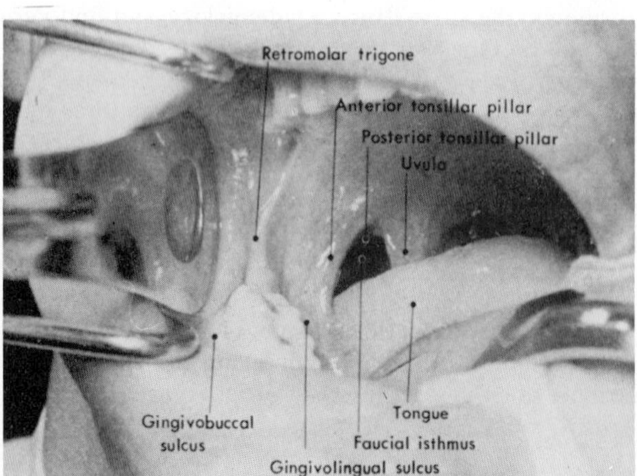

FIGURE 32–2. Photograph shows the areas defined as the palatine arch, including the soft palate (uvula), anterior tonsillar pillar, and retromolar trigone. Only the right side of the arch is illustrated. (MacComb WS, Fletcher GH [eds]: Cancer of the Head and Neck, p 179. Baltimore, Williams & Wilkins, 1967)

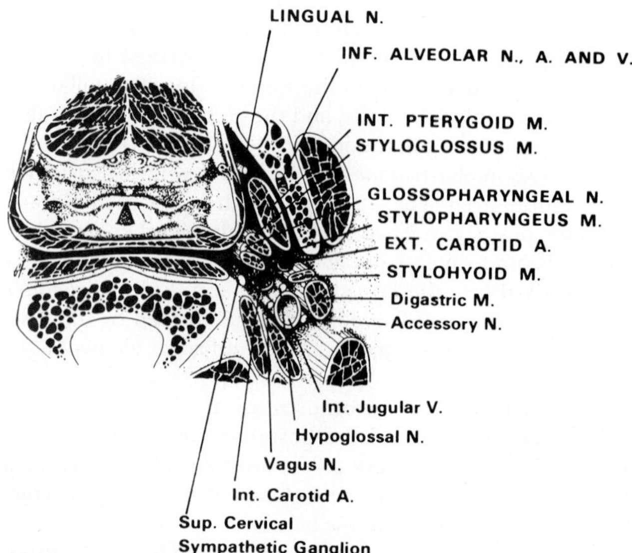

FIGURE 32–3. Lateral pharyngeal space as shown on transverse section through the oropharynx. Structures related to the prestyloid portion of the space are identified in capital letters; those in the poststyloid portion are in lower case. (MacComb WS, Fletcher GH [eds]: Cancer of the Head and Neck, p 179. Baltimore, Williams & Wilkins, 1967)

TABLE 32–1
Sites of Primary Tumor Extension in 296 Patients with Carcinoma of the Tonsil

EXTENSION SITE	NO. OF PATIENTS* (%)
Soft palate	195 (65.9)
Posterior tonsillar pillar	130 (43.9)
Base of tongue	122 (41.2)
Pharyngeal wall	83 (28)
Retromolar trigone	75 (25.3)
Uvula	45 (15.2)
Floor of mouth, anterior tongue	27 (9.1)
Nasopharynx	23 (7.8)
Lower gingiva	19 (6.4)
Hard palate	18 (6.1)
Buccal mucosa	15 (5.1)
Pharyngoepiglottic fold	13 (4.4)
Vallecula	12 (4.1)
Base of skull	5 (1.7)
Glossoepiglottic fold	4 (1.4)
Upper gingiva	3 (1)
Mandible	3 (1)
Other	17 (5.7)

** Patients may have multiple extension sites.*
(Perez CA, Carmichael T, Devineni VR, et al: Head Neck [in press])

palate lesions have an overall metastatic rate of approximately 45%. Initially, the most frequent site of nodal involvement is the jugulodigastric lymph node of the upper cervical chain (Fig. 32-4). About 10% of the patients have submaxillary lymph node involvement. Contralateral spread is infrequent (10%) and is usually confined to the internal jugular chain. The risk of occult disease in the clinically negative neck is 10% to 15%.

Tumors of the tonsillar fossa have a higher incidence (76%) of lymph node metastases; most metastatic lesions are in the subdigastric lymph nodes, midjugular chain, and submaxillary lymph nodes in lesions extending anteriorly. The incidence of occult disease after preoperative irradiation was estimated to be 22%, although the actual risk is probably closer to 50% to 60%.[56,72] Tumors of the retromolar trigone, anterior faucial pillar, and soft palate rarely metastasize to the posterior cervical lymph nodes. However, this location is the site of nodal metastases in 5% to 10% of the patients with tumors of the tonsillar fossa with anterior cervical metastasis. The lower neck is infrequently involved, although metastases in these lymph nodes can be observed in 5% to 15% of patients with upper or midjugular lymphadenopathy. Contralateral lymphadenopathy in tonsillar tumors occurs in 10% to 15% of patients with positive ipsilateral lymph nodes.

The incidence of metastatic involvement of lymph nodes in the neck increases with T stage. In general, less than 10% of the T1 lesions, 30% of the T2 lesions, and 65% to 70% of the T3 and T4 lesions metastasize to cervical lymph nodes.

Distant Metastases

Merino and colleagues[55] reported on 5019 untreated patients with squamous cell carcinoma of the upper respiratory and digestive tracts; 546 developed clinical evidence of distant me-

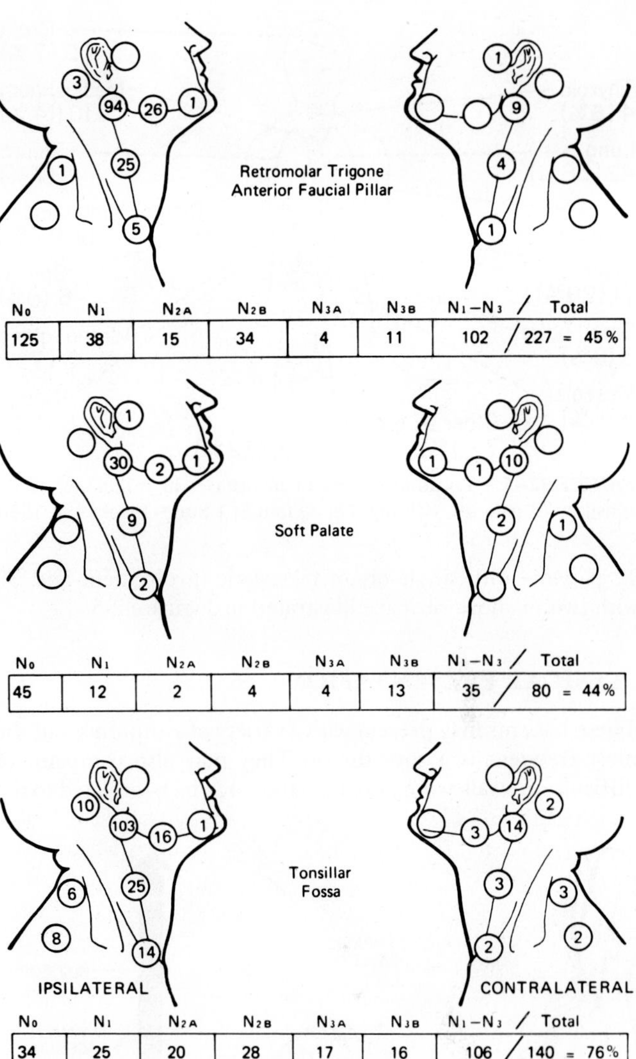

FIGURE 32–4. Nodal distribution on admission of patients with carcinoma of the tonsil and faucial arch. (Lindberg RD: Cancer 29:1446, 1972)

tastases. Of 550 patients with faucial arch primary lesions, 37 (6.7%) developed distant metastases. Eighty percent of metastases appeared within 2 years of treatment. The lungs were the most common site (>50%) of metastases, followed by bone (20%), liver (6%), and mediastinum (2.9%). Overall, for tumors in the oropharynx, the incidence of distant metastases increased with tumor stage: 5.2% for T1, 9.6% for T2, 12.7% for T3, and 16.1% for T4 tumors. There also was an overall correlation between the incidence of nodal metastases and metastatic spread; patients with N0 or N1 cervical lymph nodes had a 5% to 12% incidence of distant metastases, but the rate was 21.8% for N2 and 27.1% for N3 lesions.

Chung and Stefani[19] reported that 72 (15%) of 471 patients with carcinoma of the tonsillar region developed distant metastases. In a subgroup of 115 who underwent autopsy, the incidence was 29%. Although squamous cell carcinoma was the most frequent tumor type, only 58 (14%) of 416 of the patients with tonsillar carcinoma developed distant spread, in contrast to seven (54%) of 13 of those with lymphoepithelioma and five (26%) of 19 of those diagnosed as "transitional" cell carcinoma. Forty-six (16%) of 288 patients with lesions originating in the tonsillar fossa developed metastases, compared with ten (9%) of 111 with lesions originating in the tonsillar pillars. The sites in

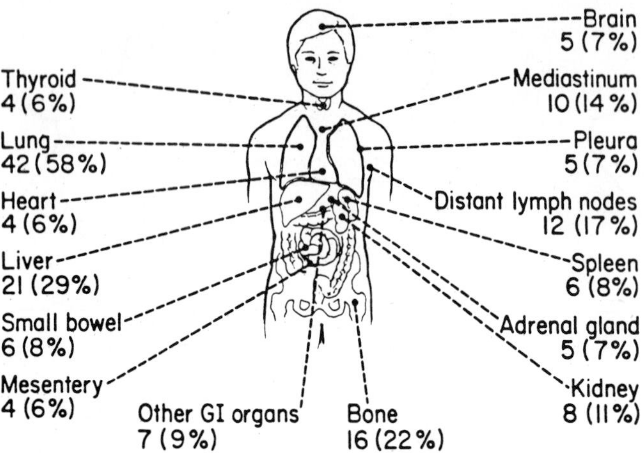

FIGURE 32–5. Location of distant metastases in carcinoma of the tonsil in 72 patients. (Chung TS, Stefani S: J Surg Oncol 14:5, 1980)

42 patients with single-organ metastatic involvement and 30 with two or more sites are illustrated in Figure 32-5.

CLINICAL PRESENTATION

These patients may present with a variety of symptoms, but the most frequent is a sore throat. They may also complain of difficulty in swallowing or pain in the ear, which is related to the anastomotic-tympanic nerve of Jacobson (Fig. 32-6). Trismus may be a late manifestation of the disease if the masseter or pterygoid muscles are involved. It is not uncommon for patients with tonsillar lesions to notice a mass in the cervical region, usually jugulodigastric, as the first manifestation of disease. Initially, distant metastases are extremely rare.

DIAGNOSTIC WORKUP

A complete history and physical examination always begin the evaluation of these patients (Table 32-2). The next step is a complete examination of the head and neck, including oral cavity, oropharynx, nasopharynx, hypopharynx, and larynx, with particular emphasis on detecting abnormalities in the anterior faucial pillar, buccal mucosa, retromolar trigone, soft palate, or uvula. Mirror examination of the nasopharynx, hypopharynx, and larynx should be performed to detect any tumor extension or associated pathology.

After indirect laryngoscopy, careful digital examination with a gloved finger should always be done to detect submucosal involvement of the glossopalatine sulcus, base of the tongue, buccal mucosa, or lateral pharyngeal wall. Direct laryngoscopy under anesthesia is seldom required for carcinoma of the faucial arch, but it is useful to evaluate patients with larger tonsillar lesions.

Physical examination should include a thorough evaluation

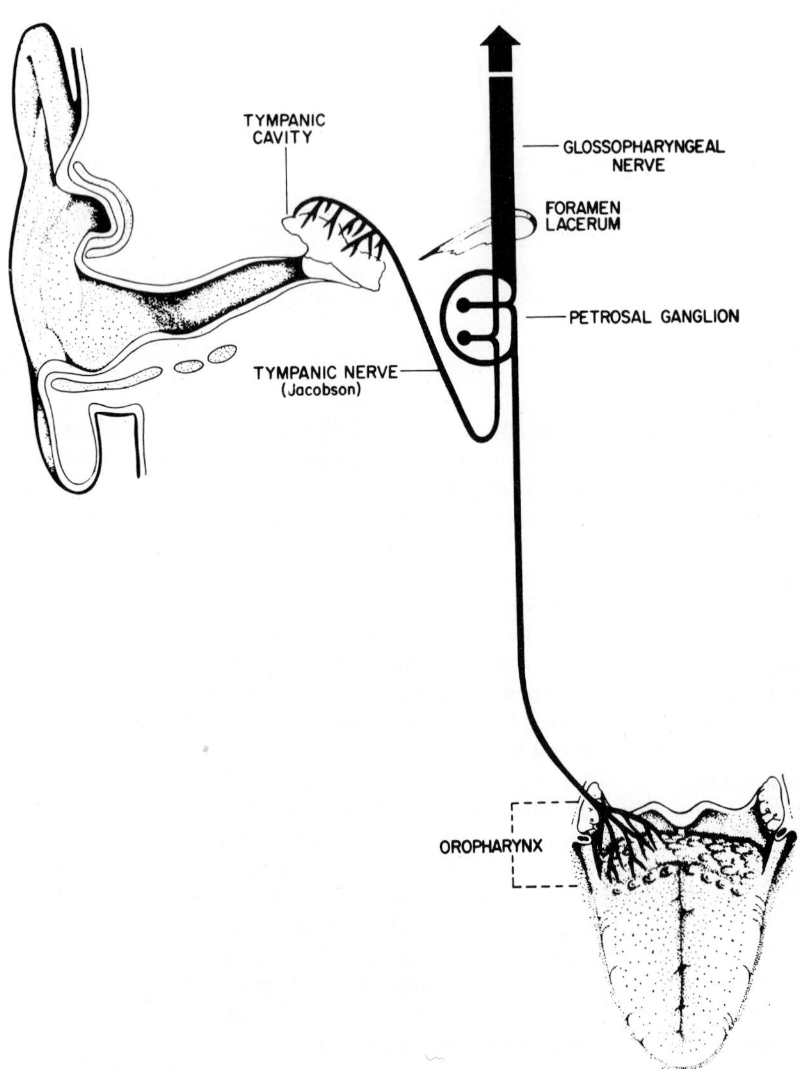

FIGURE 32–6. Nerve paths by which cancer in the oropharynx produces pain in the ear. (MacComb WS, Fletcher GH [eds]: Cancer of the Head and Neck, p 179. Baltimore, Williams & Wilkins, 1967)

TABLE 32–2
Diagnostic Workup for Tumors of the Tonsil and Faucial Arch

GENERAL

History, with emphasis on alcohol intake, smoking, tobacco chewing
General physical examination

HEAD AND NECK EXAMINATION

Oral cavity, oropharynx (palpation is very important)
Nasopharynx (mirror examination)
Laryngopharynx (indirect laryngoscopy)
Examination of the neck for lymph nodes
Direct laryngoscopy
Biopsy (of tumor and any suspicious areas)

LABORATORY STUDIES

Complete blood count
Blood chemistry profile
Urinalysis

RADIOGRAPHIC STUDIES

Chest x-ray films
Plain radiographs of mandible
Computed tomography (or magnetic resonance) scans
Radionuclide bone scan (optional)

SPECIAL STUDIES FOR PATIENTS WITH MALIGNANT LYMPHOMA

Immunological typing of tumor
Electron microscopy
Computed tomography of chest and abdomen
Lymphangiogram
Bone marrow aspiration biopsy (iliac crest)

of the neck for involved lymph nodes and for distant metastases. Examinations of the neck should be done with the physician standing behind the seated patient. Anatomic position, size, consistency, tenderness, and mobility of the cervical lymph nodes should be recorded.

Histologic confirmation of a clinically suspicious malignant lesion must always be done, and multiple biopsies should be performed, preferably at the margins of the tumor. Incisional or punch forceps biopsies can be performed with local anesthesia on an outpatient basis. When a lymphoma is suspected, a large amount of tissue may be required for electron microscopy and immunologic typing of the tumor.

Complete blood counts, chemistry profiles, and urinalysis should be obtained.

Plain films of the soft tissues of the neck or mandible may be taken if involvement of soft tissues or bony structures is suspected. Lateral soft tissue films of the neck may show extension into the posterior pharyngeal wall. Computed tomography is particularly helpful in delineating the tumor and excluding involvement of the mandible or extension into the base of the skull (Fig. 32-7). Chest x-ray films should be routine. Bone scans should be requested only if bone involvement is suspected. X-ray films of the skeleton may be required for patients with positive bone scans or clinical suspicion of bony lesions.

STAGING

In staging these tumors, it is extremely important to include both the ulcerated and infiltrating components of the tumor and all its submucosal extensions. Because of a tendency to overestimate the size of oropharyngeal tumors, a ruler or caliper must be used to measure the diameter of the lesion.[56] Visual, palpatory, and radiographic findings are critical in accurate staging. The usual staging classification for carcinoma of the oropharynx, including lymph node involvement, by the American Joint Committee is shown in Table 32-3 and Figure 32-8.

PATHOLOGIC CLASSIFICATION

The tumors have characteristic features, including keratin in many cases, although occasionally they can be nonkeratinizing. The tumors can be graded I to IV, depending on the degree of differentiation. Carcinomas that arise in the faucial arch, usually of the squamous cell type, tend to be kerantinizing and

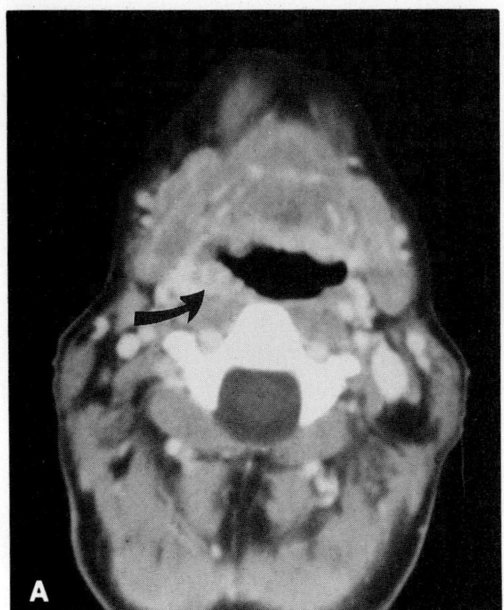

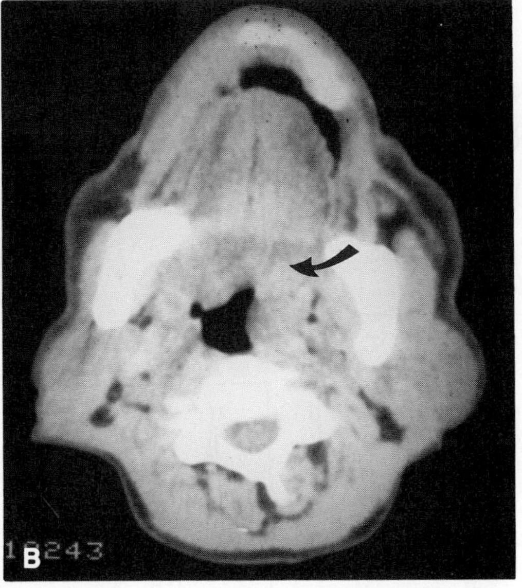

FIGURE 32–7. (**A**) CT scan of the neck shows soft tissue asymmetry produced by a T2 epidermoid carcinoma of the right tonsillar fossa (*arrow*). (**B**) CT scan of the oropharynx demonstrates a large carcinoma of the left tonsil extending to the midline and into the base of the tongue (*arrow*).

TABLE 32–3
TNM Classification for Carcinoma of Oropharynx

PRIMARY TUMOR (T)

TX	Primary tumor cannot be assessed
T0	No evidence of primary tumor
Tis	Carcinoma *in situ*
T1	Tumor ≤2 cm in greatest dimension
T2	Tumor >2 cm but <4 cm in greatest dimension
T3	Tumor >4 cm in greatest dimension
T4	Tumor invades adjacent structures (*e.g.*, cortical bone, soft tissues of neck, deep [extrinsic] muscle of tongue)

REGIONAL LYMPH NODE (N)

NX	Regional lymph nodes cannot assessed
N0	No regional lymph node metastasis
N1	Metastasis in a single ipsilateral lymph node, ≤3 cm in greatest dimension
N2	Metastasis in a single ipsilateral lymph node, >3 cm but <6 cm in greatest dimension; in multiple ipsilateral lymph nodes, none >6 cm in greatest dimension; or in bilateral or contralateral lymph nodes, none >6 cm in greatest dimension
N2a	Metastasis in a single ipsilateral lymph node >3 cm but <6 cm in greatest dimension
N2b	Metastasis in multiple ipsilateral lymph nodes, none >6 cm in greatest dimension
N2c	Metastasis in bilateral or contralateral lymph nodes, none >6 cm in greatest dimension
N3	Metastasis in a lymph node >6 cm in greatest dimension

DISTANT METASTASIS (M)

MX	Presence of distant metastasis cannot be assessed
M0	No distant metastasis
M1	Distant metastasis

(Beahrs OH, Henson DE, Hutter RVP, Myers MH [eds]: Manual for Staging of Cancer, 3rd ed, pp 34–35. Philadelphia, JB Lippincott, 1988)

more differentiated than tumors that arise from the tonsillar fossa.

Carcinomas of the tonsil are usually ulcerated and sometimes exophytic (Fig. 32-9*A*). They infiltrate the glossopharyngeal sulcus and base of the tongue, many times with little or no mucosal involvement. Carcinomas of the tonsil usually are well-differentiated or moderately differentiated (approximately 50% of the patients) squamous cell types, but the proportion of patients with less-differentiated tumors is greater than that for tumors of the faucial arch. Although it has been suggested that kerantinizing, more-differentiated tumors have a somewhat better prognosis than others, no definite correlation between histologic type and pattern of behavior or response to therapy has been reported.[62, 66, 70] Transitional cell carcinoma is an archaic term that formerly was used to describe poorly differentiated, nonkeratinizing squamous cell carcinomas.

As pointed out by MacComb and Fletcher[47] and Perez and associates,[62] lymphoepithelioma is much rarer in the tonsil (<1.5%) than in the nasopharynx. Most pathologists now agree that lymphoepithelioma represents a poorly differentiated, nonkeratinizing squamous cell carcinoma with a profuse lymphoid infiltration. The classic appearance of the tumor is represented by cores and nests of moderately large, sometimes clear epithelial cells, the nuclei of which often contain one or more large nucleoli. Scattered among these masses are multitudes of lymphocytes, which probably are interspersed with the epithelial component of the tumor.[4, 47]

Malignant lymphomas constitute 10% to 15% of malignant tumors of the tonsil. According to the Rappaport classification, they may be equally divided between small and large cell types. They tend to grow submucosally and may reach large sizes without significant mucosal ulceration (Fig. 32-9*B*). The surface of the tumor is covered by the same mucous membrane that covers the soft palate.[2] Primary Hodgkin's disease in the tonsil is extremely rare.[62]

Tumors of the salivary gland type are uncommon in the tonsil or faucial arch. Spiro and associates[78] found only 11 of 345 tumors of the minor salivary glands of the oral cavity in this location. Malignant melanomas of the tonsillar fossa constituted 6% of melanomas in the upper passages found by Conley and Pack.[20]

Koss and associates[39] and Abedi and Sismanis[1] reported a few patients with primary small cell carcinoma of the tonsil, with neurosecretory granules demonstrated by electron microscopy. As in other locations, this tumor has a high propensity for regional, nodal, and distant metastatic spread and has a poor prognosis.

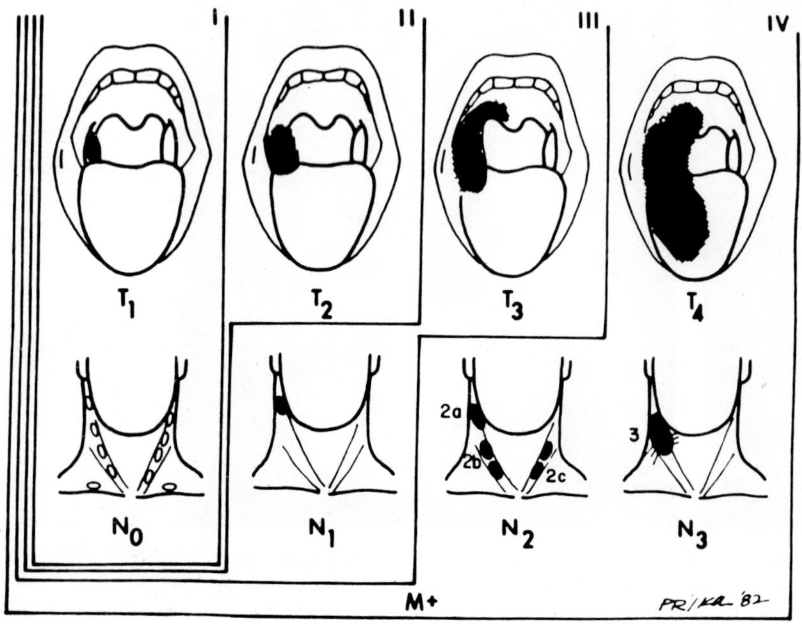

FIGURE 32–8. Diagram of anatomic staging for cancer of the oropharynx. (Modified from AJC, UICC, and Rubin P: Clinical Oncology: A Multidisciplinary Approach, 6th ed. New York, American Cancer Society, 1983; courtesy of Philip Rubin, M.D.)

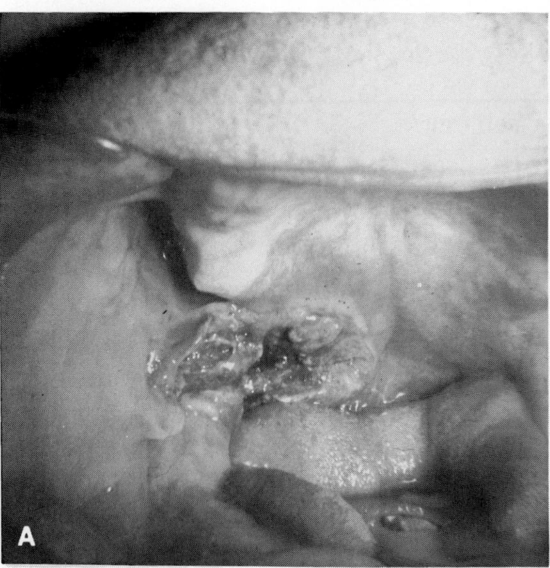

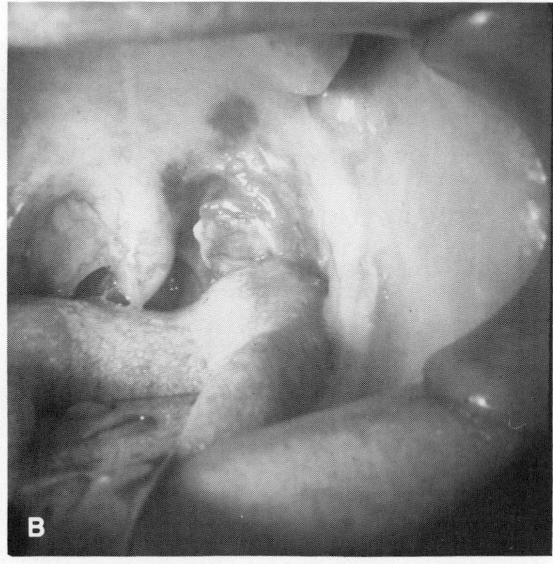

FIGURE 32–9. (**A**) Patient with T3 epidermoid carcinoma of the soft palate extending into the adjacent retromolar trigone and tonsillar area. The ulcerated, somewhat exophytic nature of the tumor is evident. (**B**) Large cell lymphoma of the tonsil, demonstrating the submucosal nature of the lesion and relatively intact mucosa.

PROGNOSTIC FACTORS

Several prognostic factors have been described. Gender may play a role in outcome. Tapley and associates[80] reported a 5-year actuarial survival rate of 63% in 17 women, compared with a 28% rate in 64 men with carcinoma of the tonsillar area. Oreggia and colleagues,[61] reporting the 5-year survival rates among 769 patients with carcinoma of the tonsil, found that women (40%) had a better prognosis than men (9%). In contrast, Perez and co-workers[62] and Vallis and associates[85] observed no significant survival difference between the genders.

There was no appreciable difference in survival rates for patients younger or older than 40 years at the time of diagnosis.[62,64] Johnston and Byers[37] reported a 5-year survival of 14% (significantly below the overall adult rate) in 11 patients under 40 years. Ninety-one percent of the patients had neck node metastasis, 55% of them Stage N3. Five (45%) of the 11 patients had T3 or T4 primary tumors, and all of these died, four with regional failures. Five of six patients with N3 cervical lymph nodes died, all but one with regional failure.

There is a significant correlation between the stage of the primary tumor, the presence of cervical lymph nodes, and 5-year survival rate.[32,63] Tumor extension into the base of the tongue has been associated with a decreased survival rate (Table 32-4).[70,71,88]

There is no definite correlation between histologic type or degree of tumor differentiation and patient survival.[62,70,85]

In patients treated surgically after irradiation, more than 90% of patients with negative histologic specimens survived for 5 years, compared with 30% of patients with persistent tumor.[65]

Patterns of Failure

Lindberg,[43] Strong,[79] and Perez and associates[63] have reported failure rates after irradiation of the tonsillar area of 5% to 30% in Stage T1, 10% to 40% in Stage T2, and 27% to 50% in Stages T3 and T4 (Table 32-5). In approximately half of the patients, primary failure was combined with nodal metastases. The incidence of recurrences in the neck has been 10% for Stage N0 and N1, 25% for Stage N2, and 35% to 40% for Stage N3. Figure 32-10 illustrates the incidence of neck failure after combined surgery and irradiation or irradiation alone in 296 patients.[63] Merino and associates[55] reported a 17.4% (four of 23 patients) incidence of distant metastases in the oropharynx proper after preoperative irradiation and a 27.8% (five of 18) incidence in patients treated with postoperative irradiation.

In the faucial arch, the incidence of distant metastases has been 5% to 7% in more than 500 patients treated with irradiation or surgery and 8% to 14% in patients treated with preoperative or postoperative radiation therapy. Distant metastases correlated with the stage of the primary tumor and lymph node metastases (Table 32-6). Overall incidence of metastases is approximately 15% for patients treated with irradiation or surgery.[43,55,63,79]

More than 85% to 90% of the locoregional recurrences and distant metastases take place within the first 3 years after therapy[30,63]

GENERAL MANAGEMENT

Tumors of the Tonsil

Patients with T1 or T2 tumors of the tonsil can be treated with irradiation or surgery alone. In general, the surgical procedure requires a radical tonsillectomy, with partial removal of the

TABLE 32–4
Tumor Control or Recurrence-Free Survival Correlated with Base of Tongue Involvement by Carcinoma of the Tonsil

INVESTIGATOR	BASE OF TONGUE NOT INVOLVED	BASE OF TONGUE INVOLVED
Remmler et al[70] (tumor control)	15/21 (71%)	8/18 (44%)
Rider[71] (tumor control)	71/84 (85%)	90/148 (61%)
Wang[88] (survival)	17/46 (37%)	12/42 (29%)

TABLE 32–5
Patterns of Failure in Primary Squamous Cell Carcinoma of the Oropharynx Treated by Radiation Therapy

		SITE OF FIRST FAILURE*				
STAGE	**TOTAL**	P	N	P+N	DM	**RELAPSE-FREE**
PRIMARY STAGE						
T1	100	8	10	5	6	71
T2	277	34	28	15	19	181
T3	272	51	22	19	23	157
T4	102	40	6	10	10	36
NODAL STAGE						
N0	311	51	28	21	5	206
N1	123	26	7	6	6	78
N2a	64	11	6	3	4	40
N2b	107	26	8	11	13	49
N3a	53	4	10	3	8	28
N3b	93	15	7	5	22	44
STAGE GROUP						
I	56	5	8	3		40
II	141	15	12	11	3	100
III	205	40	14	10	7	134
IV	349	73	32	25	48	171
Total	751	133 (17.7%)	66 (8.8%)	49 (6.5%)	58 (7.7%)	445 (59.3%)

* *Unless otherwise indicated, values equal number of patients. P, primary; N, neck; DM, distant metastasis.*
(Lindberg RD: Cancer Treat Symp 2:21, 1983)

mandible and ipsilateral neck dissection. Jesse and associates[36] stated that in patients with N0 necks it may not be necessary to carry out elective neck dissection because of the low incidence of metastases to cervical lymph nodes in T1 and even T2 lesions (10% and 25%, respectively). Because of comparable tumor control at the primary site and in the neck, irradiation is the preferred treatment in many institutions.[26,56]

With surgery alone, Whicker and associates[90] reported failure rates as low as 20%, but others have described local failure rates as high as 41%.[82] Maltz and associates[48] reported an absolute survival rate of 56% and a determinate survival rate of 67% in 36 patients with carcinoma of the tonsil treated by preoperative irradiation (4000–4500 cGy) and en bloc resection of the primary tumor and neck dissection. The survival rate was 80% for patients with T1 lesions, 68% for T2 lesions, and 33% for T3 lesions.

In T3 and T4 tumors, a combination of irradiation and surgery has been advocated because of the higher incidence of recurrences with either modality alone.[32,63] To ensure adequate surgical margins in patients who receive preoperative irradiation, it is imperative to define the scope of the operation with accurate anatomic drawings of the lesion and with tattooing of the initial tumor extent.

Preoperative doses of 3000 cGy to 5000 cGy in 3 to 5.5 weeks have been administered to the primary tumor and ipsilateral (or both) neck areas.[63] At Washington University, the current treatment policy for extensive lesions is to carry out a surgical procedure (*e.g.*, radical tonsillectomy with ipsilateral neck dissection) followed by postoperative radiation therapy of 5000 cGy to 6000 cGy, depending on the status of the surgical margins and extent of cervical lymph node involvement.

Tumors of Faucial Arch

Early T1 lesions (< 1 cm in diameter) can be treated with wide surgical resection or irradiation alone in doses of 6000 cGy to 6500 cGy in 6 to 7 weeks. T2 tumors require more extensive surgical procedures, including partial resection of the mandible, if indicated. Because of the tendency of the tumors to extend to the midline, the site of lymph node metastases is less predictable. Therefore, neck dissection should be done only in patients with palpable cervical lymph nodes. These tumors can also be treated with a total dose of 6500 cGy to 7000 cGy; radiation therapy has the advantage of treating subclinical disease in the neck (5000-cGy total dose).

In more extensive lesions, preoperative or postoperative irradiation can be used. Preoperative irradiation doses have varied between 3000 cGy and 4500 cGy in 3 to 5 weeks; postoperative irradiation is usually delivered in higher doses of 5000 cGy to 6000 cGy in 5 to 6.5 weeks, depending on the status of the surgical margins and the cervical lymph nodes. Million and Cassisi[56] observed that combined therapy for lesions of the soft palate is rarely used because of the success rate with radiation therapy alone and the morbidity associated with resection of the soft palate.

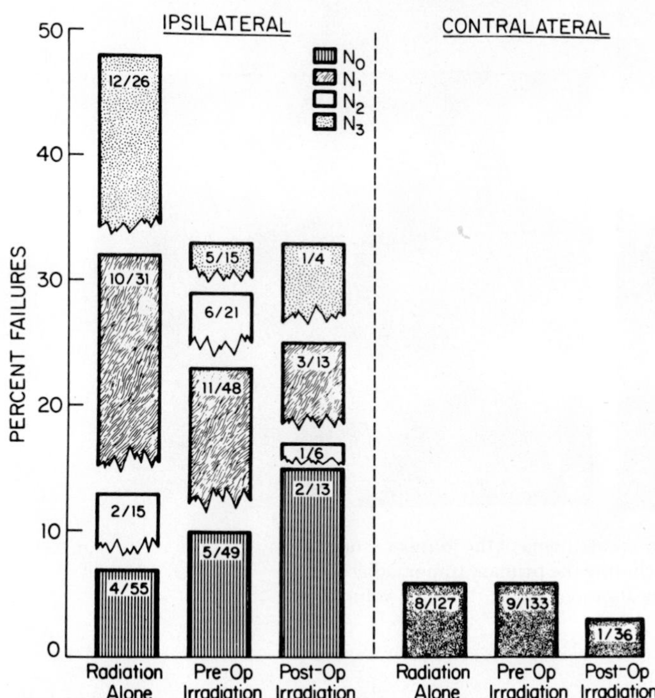

FIGURE 32–10. Incidence of ipsilateral and contralateral neck recurrences in 296 patients treated with irradiation alone or combined with surgery. (Perez CA, Carmichael T, Devineni VR, et al: Head Neck [in press])

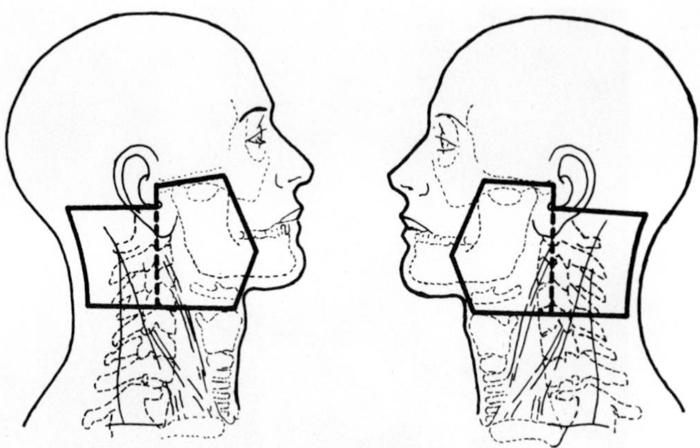

FIGURE 32–11. Outline of lateral portals for treating the primary tumor and the upper neck in patients with carcinoma of the tonsil. After a total dose of 4300 cGy, delivered with 4-MV to 6-MV photons, the portals are reduced to exclude the spinal cord (*dashed line*). The anterior portal can be treated with photons (10–18 MV) and posterior cervical lymph nodes with electrons (9 MeV).

RADIATION THERAPY TECHNIQUES

Volume Treated

In general, the same portals and doses of irradiation can be used for the treatment of tumors of the tonsillar region or the faucial arch, depending on the stage of the primary tumor and status of the lymph nodes. The standard arrangement consists of opposing lateral portals that include the primary tumor, adjacent tissues (*i.e.,* buccal mucosa, gingiva, base of the tongue, distal nasopharynx, and lateroposterior pharyngeal wall), and the upper and posterior cervical lymph nodes (Fig. 32-11).

The external landmark for the *upper margin* is the zygomatic arch. The middle and internal ear should be carefully shielded posteriorly, ensuring that tumor volume is not covered. The portal extends posteriorly around the external auditory canal to a line joining the tip of the mastoid to about 1 cm above the foramen magnum. The *anterior margin* should be set up by clinical examination (inspection and palpation of the buccal mucosa and base of the tongue) with at least a 2-cm margin, confirmed on localization films, beyond any clinical evidence of disease. This margin should project 2 cm to 3 cm forward of the anterior cortex of the ascending ramus of the mandible, depending on tumor extent. The portal should also include the submandibular nodes if there is buccal mucosal involvement. *Inferiorly,* the portal extends to the thyroid notch, except in patients who have downward tumor extension with pharyngeal wall involvement, in which case the margin must be placed below that level (Fig. 32-12). *Posteriorly,* the posterior cervical lymph nodes should be covered; a small amount of subcutaneous tissue should be spared to avoid fall-off, except in patients with palpable posterior cervical lymph nodes.

After a tumor dose of approximately 4300 cGy, the posterior margin of the lateral port is brought anteriorly to the midportion of the vertebral bodies to spare the spinal cord. Examples of simulation and localization films for reduced portals (excluding the spinal cord) are illustrated in Figure 32-13. If desired, doses higher than 4500 cGy may be delivered to the posterior neck sites with lateral electron-beam portals (9 MeV) or, if using photons, with posterior appositional fields, shielding the spinal cord with a midline block. After a minimum total tumor dose of 6000 cGy has been delivered to the oropharynx,

TABLE 32–6
*Incidence of Distant Metastasis by Stage of Carcinoma of Tonsil**

T	N0	N1	N2	N3	TOTAL
T1	0/14 (0%)	0/5 (0%)	0/1 (9%)	0/3 (0%)	0/23 (0%)
T2	0/30 (0%)	1/8 (12.5%)	1/6 (16.7%)	1/6 (16.7%)	3/50 (6%)
T3	0/27 (0%)	2/16 (12.5%)	3/18 (16.7%)	5/25 (20.8%)	10/86 (11.6%)
T4	0/5 (0%)	0/4 (0%)	3/15 (20%)	1/2 (50%)	4/26 (15.4%)
Total	0/76 (0%)	3/33 (9%)	7/40 (17.5%)	7/36 (19.4%)	17/185 (9.2%)

**Results from University of Maryland series, 1956 to 1977.*
(Amornmarn R, et al: Cancer 54:1293, 1984)

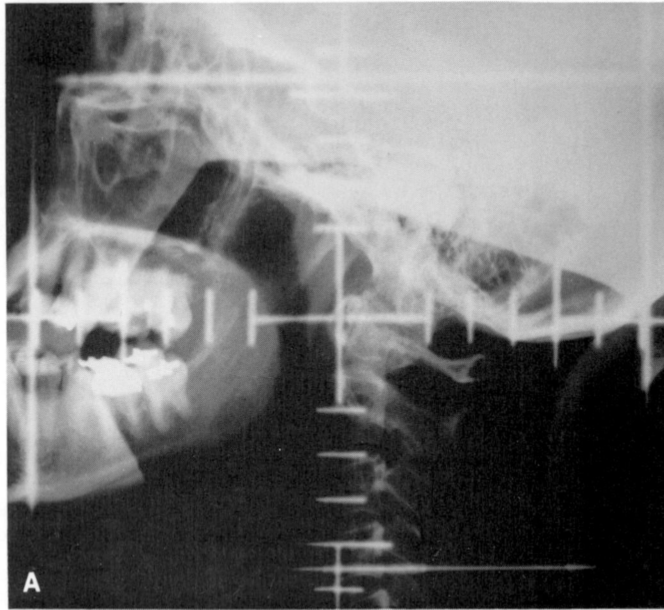

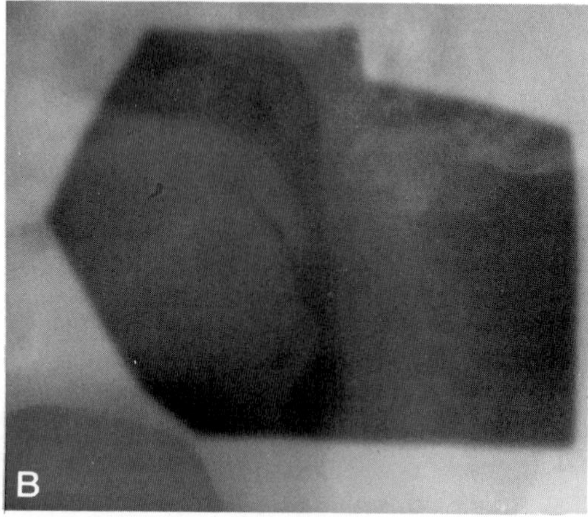

FIGURE 32–12. (**A**) Simulation film shows the volume to be treated in carcinoma of the tonsil or faucial arch and landmarks used in the design of the initial lateral potals, including the primary tumor, adjacent oropharynx, and upper cervical and posterior lymph nodes. (**B**) Localization film of the same volume.

depending on the stage of the tumor, the portals may be concentrically reduced by 1 cm to 2 cm, and an additional dose is delivered to complete the 6500 cGy to 7500 cGy total dose (Fig. 32-14).

At our institution, after the port reduction for shielding of the spinal cord, the Cerrobend block is filled posteriorly and the central axis remains unchanged, allowing the compensating filters initially constructed to be used for the latter part of the treatment.

Compensating filters (Ellis type) designed with the central axis of the field as the point of reference are used with the upper neck lateral portals to compensate for various contours and thicknesses of the neck in the superior-inferior and lateral directions.

It is not necessary to treat the posterior cervical chain or the lower cervical lymph nodes in T1N0 tumors; smaller portals are adequate (Fig. 32-15). Murthy and Hendrickson[58] pointed out that the probability of contralateral lymph node failure is less than 10% in patients with N0 and N1 tonsillar tumors with controlled primary tumor and ipsilateral neck disease, questioning the need for irradiation of the contralateral cervical lymph nodes in these patients. Limiting irradiation to the primary tumor and ipsilateral neck reduces the probability of xerostomia.

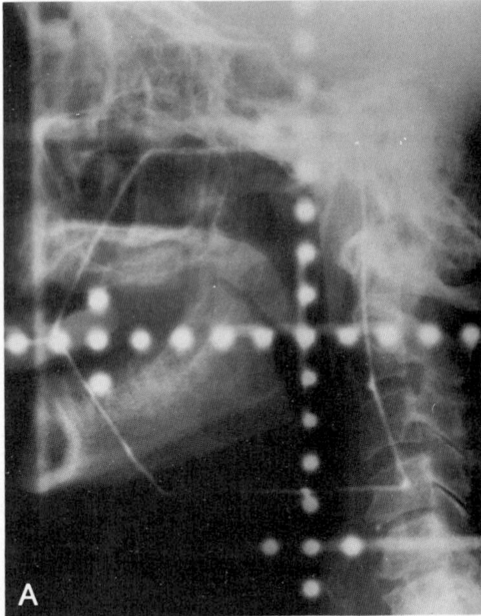

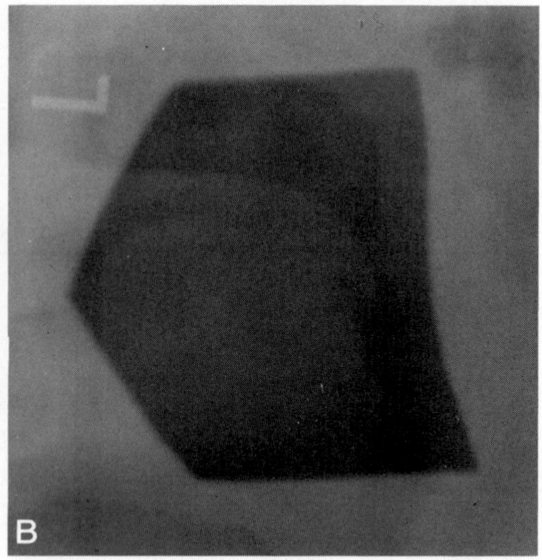

FIGURE 32–13. (**A**) Simulation film of reduced upper-neck lateral portal, excluding the spinal cord. (**B**) Localization film of the same portal.

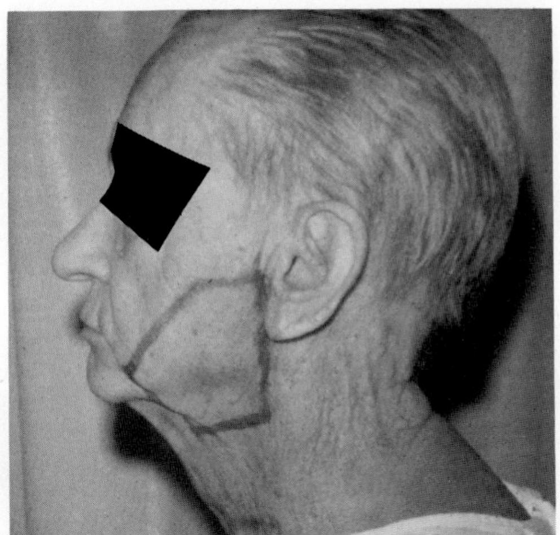

FIGURE 32–14. Example of a reduced field used for an additional boost to a tumor in the tonsil or retromolar trigone.

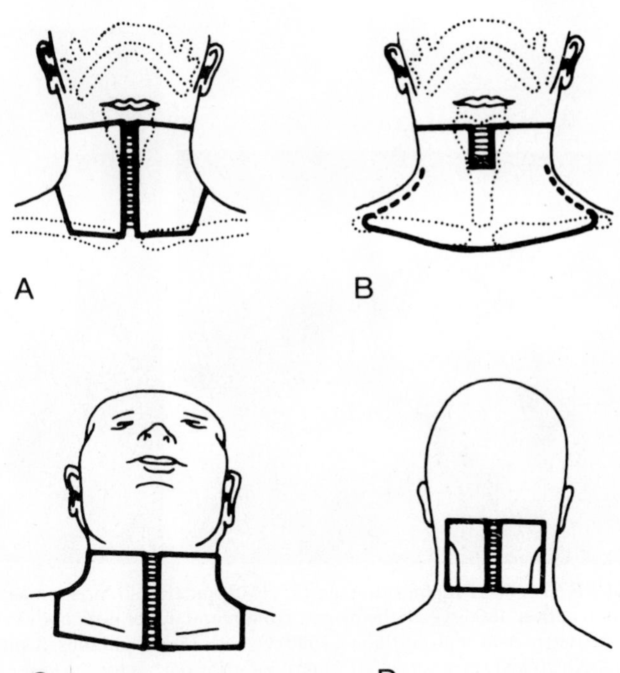

FIGURE 32–16. Portals used for the treatment of cervical lymph nodes, depending on the extent of the lymphadenopathy and the design of the upper neck portals. (**A**) Portal used if there are no palpable lymph nodes in the lower neck. (**B**) Portal used for patients with palpable lymph nodes in the lower neck or supraclavicular regions. (**C**) Portal used if it is necessary to give higher doses to the lower neck and some blocking of the spinal cord is necessary for a portion of the treatment. (**D**) This portal can be used for a posterior cervical boost with photons if electrons are not available.

The lower neck is treated with a standard anteroposterior portal. If there are no palpable lymph nodes, a 5 half-value layer (HVL) 1.5-cm to 2-cm midline block can be used to shield the larynx and spinal cord. However, if lymph node involvement is suspected, only a small block is used to shield the larynx and a portion of the spinal cord (to avoid overlap with the lateral portals) (Fig. 32-16). Figure 32-17 summarizes the various portals used in the treatment of a patient with a T2N1M0 epidermoid carcinoma of the left tonsil.

A technique described by Fletcher[26] for treatment of small tumors of the tonsillar fossa, anterior tonsillar pillar, and retromolar trigone used ipsilateral wedged-angle anterior and posterior fields that irradiated a triangular volume with the base on the neck and the apex in the uvula (Fig. 32-18). With this technique, the dose to the mandible is high, and as with un-

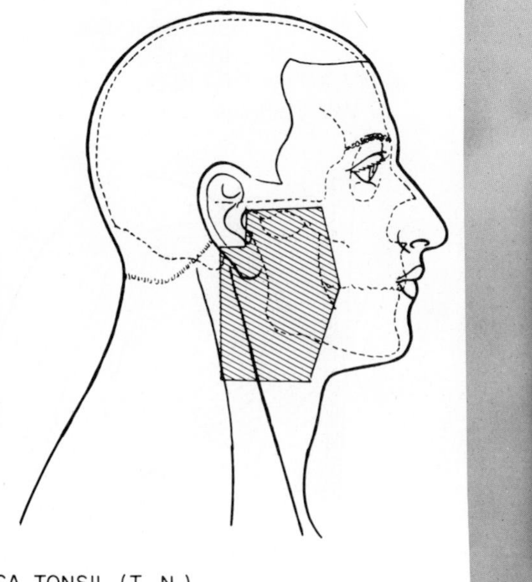

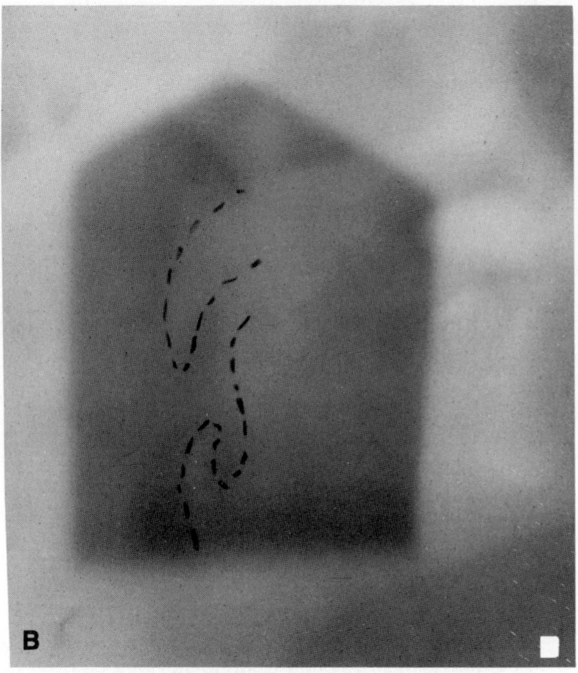

FIGURE 32–15. (**A**) Line diagram of a portal and (**B**) localization film of a small field used for irradiation of a patient with a small tumor of the oropharynx (T1N0M0). The subdigastric lymph nodes are included in this volume, but other cervical lymph nodes are not irradiated.

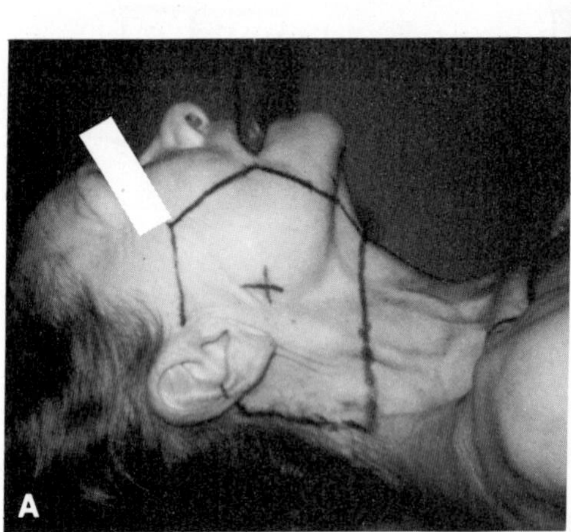

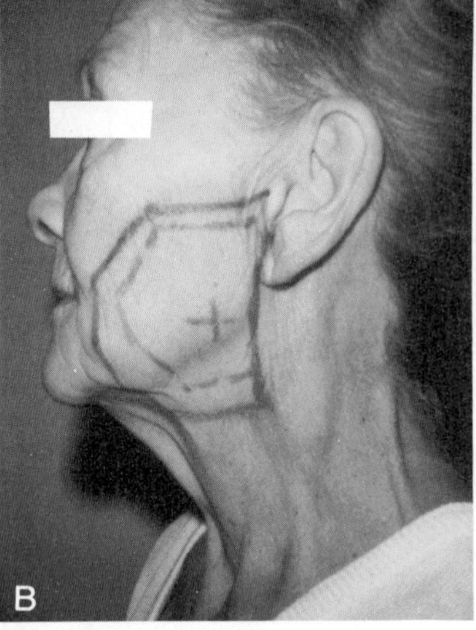

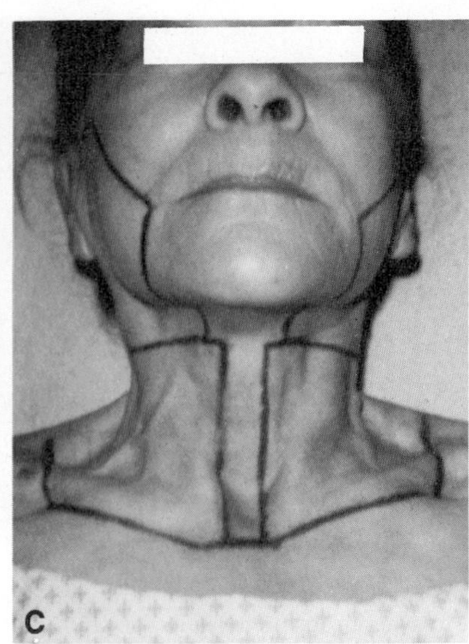

FIGURE 32–17. Patient with stage T2N1M0 epidermoid carcinoma of the left tonsil. (**A**) Lateral portals used to deliver 4500 cGy to the primary tumor and upper neck nodes (4–6-MV photons). (**B**) Left lateral portal used to deliver an additional 1500 cGy with 18-MV photons. A smaller field indicates the volume for a 500 cGy to 1000 cGy boost. (**C**) Anteroposterior portals for the lower neck (4600 cGy calculated at 3-cm depth).

equally loaded fields with low-energy photons, a greater incidence of complications (*e.g.*, soft tissue necrosis and osteonecrosis of the mandible) has been observed.[33]

Doses of Irradiation Alone

Tumor doses are usually calculated at the midline of the upper necks. For T1 tumors, minimal doses of 6000 cGy to 6500 cGy should provide local control in more than 90% of these patients. For T2 tumors, 6500 cGy to 7000 cGy is necessary; for T3 and T4 tumors, doses between 7000 cGy and 7500 cGy are needed to improve the probability of local tumor control. Shrinking fields must be used with doses beyond 6000 cGy to decrease the incidence of complications. Because of the limited tolerance of the normal tissues (*e.g.*, mandible, salivary glands, and even the subcutaneous tissues), it is not advisable to administer tumor doses over 7500 cGy with external megavoltage beams.

The upper neck should receive 4500 cGy to 5000 cGy for N0 nodes (subclinical disease), 6500 cGy for N1 and N2 nodal tumors, and up to 7000 cGy to 7500 cGy for N3 lymph nodes. This can be accomplished by reducing fields and boosting doses with 12-MeV to 16-MeV electrons (Fig. 32-19).

If there are no palpable lymph nodes, the minimal tumor dose delivered to the posterior and lower necks is 4500 cGy (calculated at 3 cm).

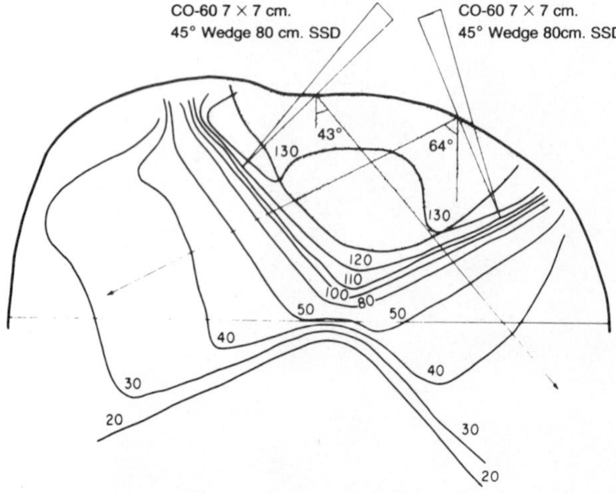

FIGURE 32–18. Dose distribution resulting from use of two 45-degree wedges for treatment of a small tumor in the tonsil, tonsillar pillar, or retromolar trigone. (Fletcher GH: Textbook of Radiotherapy, 3rd ed. Philadelphia, Lea & Febiger, 1980)

4 MV X-Rays – 12 x 14 cm
RT – 2800 CGy
LT – 1000 CGy
18 MV X-Rays – 8 x 10 cm – R/L Lat – 1200 CGy
20 MeV Electrons – 8 x 10 cm – RT – 2700 CGy

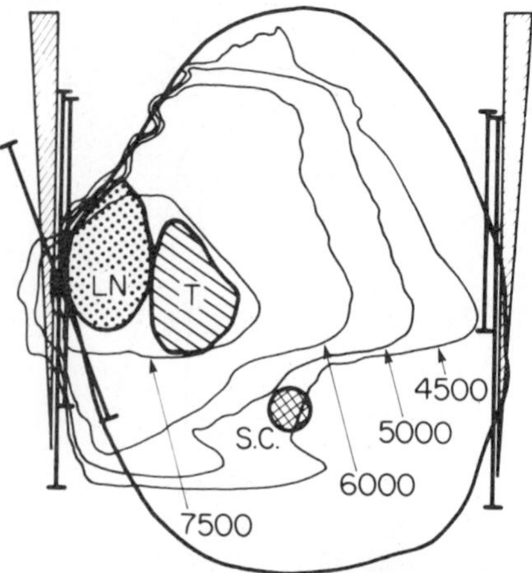

FIGURE 32–19. Composite isodose distribution resulting from various beam combinations, including 20-MeV electrons to deliver definitive irradiation to a patient with T3N3 ipsilateral upper-neck lymph node tumor. A total dose of 7500 cGy can be given to the target volume with reducing fields.

Standard fractionation is 180 cGy to 200 cGy daily, 5 days per week.

Preoperative Irradiation

If preoperative irradiation is employed for large primary tumors with involved cervical lymph nodes, doses of approximately 4000 cGy to 4500 cGy in 4 to 5 weeks are delivered. If possible, a radical surgical resection with neck dissection is carried out. Otherwise, additional irradiation is given to achieve a total tumor dose of 7000 cGy to 7500 cGy.

Postoperative Irradiation

In the past decade, postoperative irradiation has gained popularity. For T2N0 tumors with negative surgical margins, tumor doses of 5000 cGy administered in 5 to 6 weeks to the primary site and both neck sites should suffice. For more extensive primary tumors or for cervical lymph node involvement, 6000 cGy is administered in 6 to 7 weeks. If positive surgical margins, extracapsular nodal extension, or more than three involved lymph nodes exist, an additional 500 cGy to 1000 cGy is given with reduced portals, using 12-MeV to 16-MeV electrons. Interstitial brachytherapy can be used for this purpose.

The policies of treatment are summarized in Table 32-7.

Altered Fractionation

Marcial and colleagues[50] and Scanlon and associates[73] used split-course irradiation for treating patients with tonsillar tumors and for other head and neck malignancies. Each patient received a total dose of 300 cGy daily given in ten fractions in 2 weeks, 2 weeks of rest, and an additional dose of 3000 cGy in 200-cGy daily fractions, 5 days per week. The results are similar to those reported with "conventional" fractionation.

Mendenhall and colleagues[54] and Wang[86,87] used multiple daily fractionation in an attempt to increase the overall dose of radiation without enhancing morbidity. Wang[87] described higher tumor control and survival rates in 52 patients with tumors of the tonsil and 47 with base of the tongue carcinoma treated with twice-daily fractionation to total doses of 6720 cGy than in 71 historic controls with similar tumors treated with one daily fraction of 180 cGy to doses of 6500 cGy. The Radiation Therapy Oncology Group is conducting a randomized trial comparing conventional and hyperfractionation schedules in the treatment of advanced head and neck tumors.[69]

TABLE 32–7
Policies of Treatment for Carcinoma of the Tonsil and Faucial Arch

STAGE	DOSE (cGy)
PRIMARY TUMOR	
T1	6000–6500
T2	6500–7000
T3–T4	7000–7500
LYMPH NODES IN THE NECK	
N0	5000
N1	6500
N2a, b	6500–7000 (reduce fields after 5000)
	7000–7500 (reduce fields after 5000 and 6000)
PREOPERATIVE IRRADIATION	4500 to primary tumor and ipsilateral or both neck sites
POSTOPERATIVE IRRADIATION	
Negative-margin specimen	5000
T3–T4 or N2b, N3, or positive margins	5000 to primary site and both neck sites plus boost to selected volumes to total dose of 6000–6500 cGy
DAILY DOSE FRACTIONATION	180–200

Beam Energy

An optimal energy for the treatment of the cervical lymph nodes is ^{60}Co, 4-MV or 6-MV photons. These beams can also be used for irradiation of tonsillar faucial arch primary lesions and extensions, including the base of the tongue. However, with a 6000-cGy midline dose, the mandible receives 6500 cGy to 7000 cGy total dose. At the Mallinckrodt Institute of Radiology, after a tumor dose of 4300 cGy, high-energy photons (18 MV) are frequently employed for treating patients without palpable neck nodes to achieve a high midline dose while sparing the superficial tissues, the temporomandibular joint, and the mandible. Figure 32-20 illustrates the difference in dose at the level of the mandible using low- or high-energy photons for the last 2000 cGy of the course of therapy.

Electrons with energies ranging from 12 MeV to 20 MeV can be used to boost the dose to the primary tumor or large cervical lymph nodes. If necessary, the posterior cervical nodes are irradiated with 9-MeV electrons. The lower neck is treated with ^{60}Co, 4-MV or 6-MV photons without any difficulty.

Intraoral Cones

The intraoral cone technique, using orthovoltage or electrons, has been selectively used in the treatment of patients with small lesions.[37,70]

Brachytherapy

Fletcher and associates[28] and Bloedorn and colleagues[14] advocated the use of a single- or double-plane "pterygopalatine" implant for the treatment of patients with carcinoma of the tonsil or the palatine arch when external irradiation was not satisfactory. Later, Seydel and Scholl,[75] Beiler,[13] and Amornmarn and associates[4] described similar techniques. This approach can be used to treat recurrent tumors (Fig. 32-21).

RESULTS OF THERAPY

Some of the modern clinical concepts of radiation biology are based on Coutard's[21] study of patients irradiated for tumors of the tonsillar region. He made landmark observations on the effects of radiation on normal tissues, the correlations between radiation doses and probabilities of tumor control, and the importance of the dose-time relationship in the prevention of treatment complications.

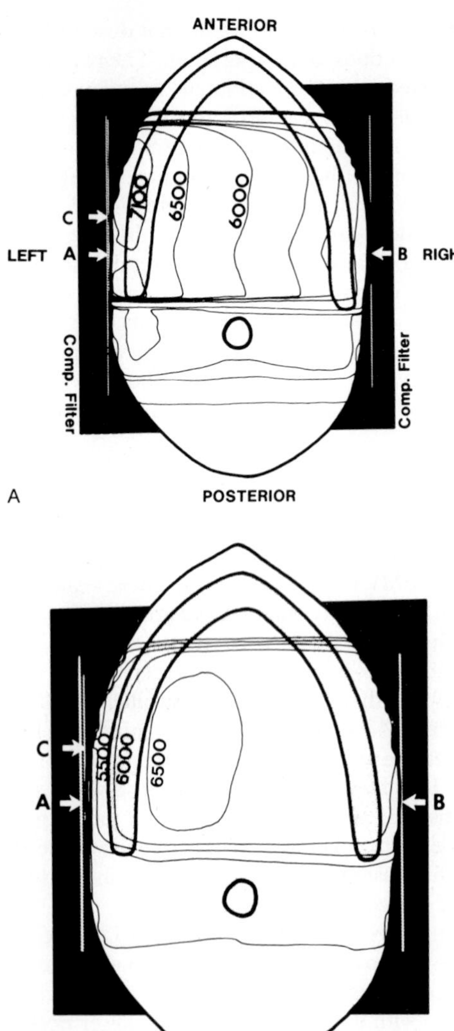

FIGURE 32–20. (**A**) Dose distribution for lateral upper-neck portals treated with 6-MV photons to 4500 cGy to the midline (beams A and B) and an additional 1500 cGy to the midline, delivered with a small left lateral portal using 6-MV photons (beam C). The dose to the mandible is over 7000 cGy. (**B**) Dose distribution with the same portal arrangement, delivering 4500 cGy with 6-MV photons and an additional 1500 cGy to the midline with 18-MV photons. The dose to the mandible is reduced to approximately 6000 cGy, demonstrating the advantage of higher-energy photons for a portion of the treatment to reduce the maximum dose to the mandible and the soft tissues.

Tonsillar Fossa

Radiation therapy yields a high probability of tumor control for T1 (85% to 90%) and T2 tumors (70% to 80%). In T3 and T4 lesions, tumor control rates are 60% and 40%, respectively (Table 32-8).[5,60]

Million and Cassisi[56] reported the results of treating 99 patients with irradiation (6000–7000 cGy) and surgery for salvage of failures; the determinate 5-year survival rates were 100% for Stage I, 90% for Stage II, 75% for Stage III, and approximately 26% for Stage IV. Shukovsky and Fletcher[79] found 2-year disease-free survival rates of 86% for T1, 54% for T2, 43% for T3, and 19% for T4 tumors. These results were updated by Remmler and colleagues'[70] report of 160 patients and by Wong and associates'[91] study of 150 patients. In a recent report, irradiation alone gave excellent tumor control in T1 (94%), T2 (74%), and T3 (58%) lesions.[90] The determinate 5-year survival rates were 100% for Stage I, 80% for Stage II, 74% for Stage III, and 60% for Stage IV. The incidence of severe complications was 4% among 137 patients treated with conventional fractionation and a total dose of less than 6750 cGy, and among 86 patients receiving higher total doses; the complication rate was 18.6%.

Mantravadi and collaborators[49] described the results with radiation therapy alone (6500–7000 cGy) for 94 patients and a combination of surgery and irradiation (2000–5000 cGy) for 23 patients. Survival and tumor control at the primary site or in the necks for both treatment groups were similar to those seen at Washington University.

Mendenhall and associates[54] reported their experience with 104 patients who received irradiation alone and with 32 treated with a combination of irradiation and neck dissection. With a minimum 2-year follow-up, the tumor control rates were 83% (ten of 12 patients) for T1, 78% (36 of 46) for T2, 72% (28 of 39) for T3, and 31% (five of 16) for T4 lesions. A few patients with early tumors could be salvaged surgically. Tumor control in patients with T4 lesions was somewhat improved by the combination of external and interstitial irradiation. Severe complications were reported in four (17%) of 23 patients with T3 lesions.

Comparable results have been described by Fayos and Lampe,[25] Nussbaum and associates,[59] Wang,[88] and Mizono and colleagues.[57] Mendenhall and associates[54] and Perez and colleagues[65] reported that doses of 6000 cGy to 6500 cGy adequately control T1 lesions, and for most T2 tumors 7000 cGy is sufficient if delivered in 180-cGy to 200-cGy daily fractions over 7 weeks. T3 and T4 tumors are controlled locally in 50% to 60% of the patients receiving between 7000 cGy and 7500 cGy.

The lack of dose response in effecting tumor control for the primary tumor or the lymph nodes in some of our patients (Fig. 32-22) does not contradict reports showing a correlation between dose and tumor control, because it is common practice to deliver higher doses of irradiation to those tumors that exhibit a reduced response toward the end of the prescribed therapy.[77] Other authors confirm our experience; Cardinale and Fischer[16] achieved 100% tumor control in 13 T1 lesions with doses of 5000 cGy to 6500 cGy and in two instances with doses as low as 4200 cGy. Most T2 lesions were controlled with doses of 6000 cGy to 7000 cGy, although several failures occurred at these dose levels, and only two of 16 T3 lesions were controlled with similar doses.

Garrett and colleagues[30] did not observe a significant correlation of tumor control in 372 patients treated with irradiation doses ranging from 5000 cGy (delivered in daily fractions of 200 cGy or 250 cGy) to 6000 cGy (200-cGy fractions), but there was a statistically significant improvement in local control and survival if areas greater than 80 cm^2 were treated in T1 or T2 tumors. Among 215 patients with tonsillar region carcinoma, Dubois and associates[22] found a correlation of tumor control with larger volumes treated but not with increasing nominal standard dose. Similarly, Gelinas and Fletcher,[31] in an analysis of 155 patients with tonsillar carcinoma, demonstrated that the failure to control the tumor was related to geographic misses in five patients and lower doses in seven patients, although they found no obvious reason for 11 failures. Another report indicated that inadequate doses of irradiation correlated with the inability to control the tumor in approximately 10% of the patients with T1 and T2 tumors and 20% of those with T3 and T4 lesions.[65] A combination of inadequate portals with geographic misses and lower doses of radiation encumbered another 10% of the patients with small lesions and 20% of those with T3 and T4 tumors.

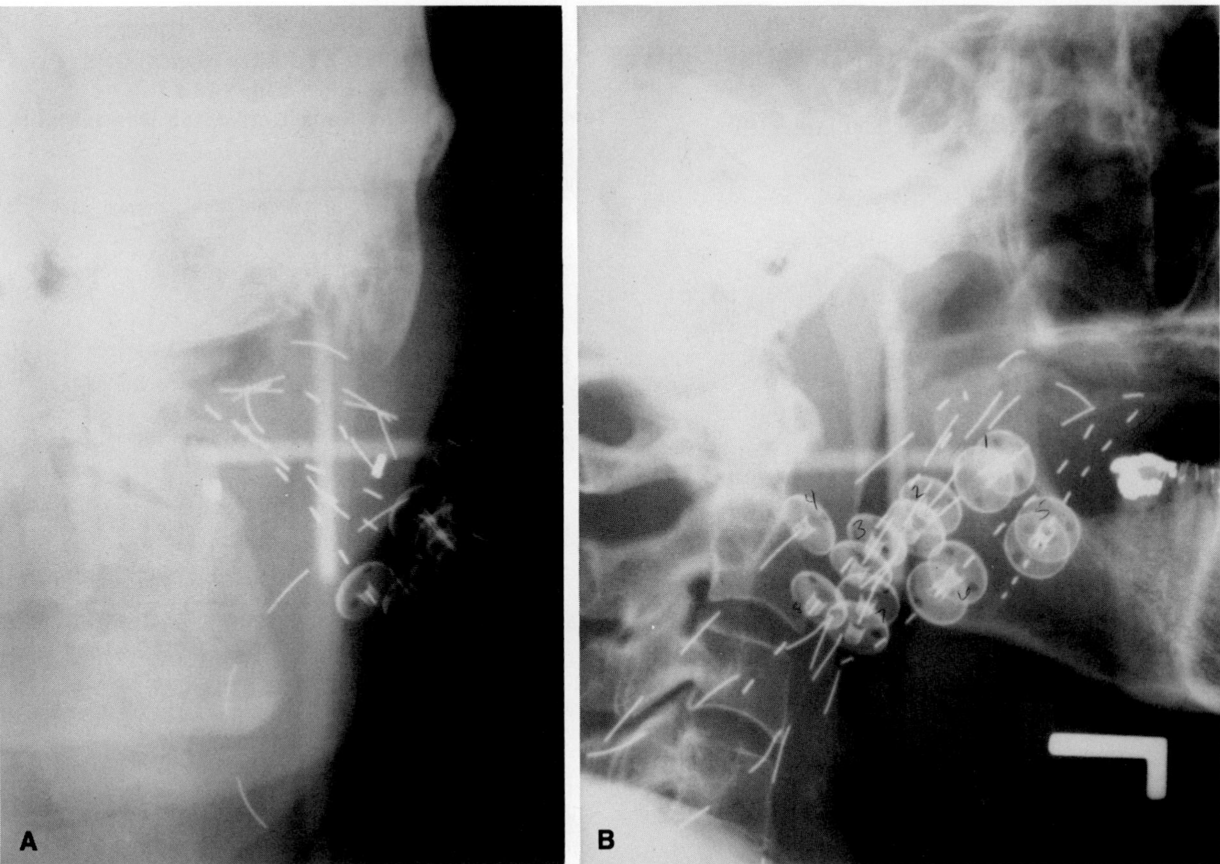

FIGURE 32–21. (**A**) Anteroposterior radiograph of an ^{192}Ir implant in patient with recurrent carcinoma of the tonsil. (**B**) Lateral radiograph shows the position of the dummy wires used to determine the location of the ^{192}Ir sources when inserted. A minimal tumor dose of 6000 cGy can be delivered with this modality.

TABLE 32–8
Initial Local Tumor Control of Carcinoma of the Tonsil with Irradiation Alone

INVESTIGATOR	MINIMAL FOLLOW-UP (YEARS)	T1	T2	T3	T4
Amornmarn et al[4]	5	4/4 (100%)	7/8 (88%)	21/38 (55%)	5/20 (25%)
Bataini et al[9]*	3	32/36 (90%)	78/93 (84%)	111/173 (37%)	77/163 (47%)
Beiler[13]†	3	5/5 (100%)	7/7 (100%)	6/10 (60%)	
Dubois et al[22]	5	34/49 (69.5%)	39/84 (46.4%)	7/82 (8.5%)	
Fayos and Lampe[25]*	5	8/10 (80%)	36/47 (76.6%)	12/31 (38.7%)	4/14 (28.6%)
Lusinchi et al[46]	2	42/48 (88%)	114/145 (79%)		
Mantravadi et al[49]	5	3/3 (100%)	16/21 (76%)	20/61 (33%)	1/9 (11%)
Mendenhall et al[54]	2	4/4 (100%)	17/18 (94%)	23/31 (74%)	5/12 (41.7%)
Million and Cassisi[56]	2	11/13 (85%)	18/23 (78%)	6/13 (46%)	1/4 (25%)
Mizono et al[57]*	3	5/10 (50%)	25/41 (61%)	17/55 (31%)	3/25 (12%)
Perez et al[63]	3	12/14 (86%)	26/41 (63%)	31/41 (76%)	19/31 (61%)
Puthawala et al[67]‡	2	3/3 (100%)	14/15 (93%)	32/43 (74%)	11/19 (58%)
Remmler et al[70]†	2	14/14 (100%)	31/35 (89%)	34/50 (68%)	4/17 (24%)
Wong et al[91]	2	15/16 (94%)	41/52 (79%)	30/52 (58%)	3/6 (50%)
Total		192/229 (83%)	469/630 (74%)	350/680 (51%)	131/320 (41%)

* *Tonsillar region.*
† *Irradiation plus node dissection.*
‡ *Interstitial implant and external radiation therapy.*

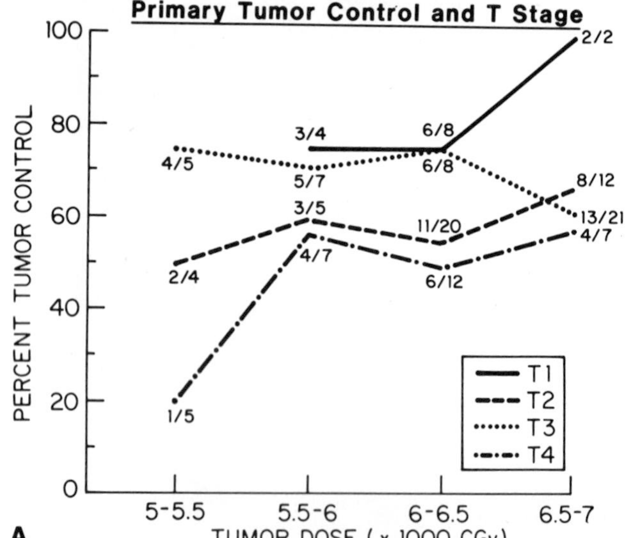

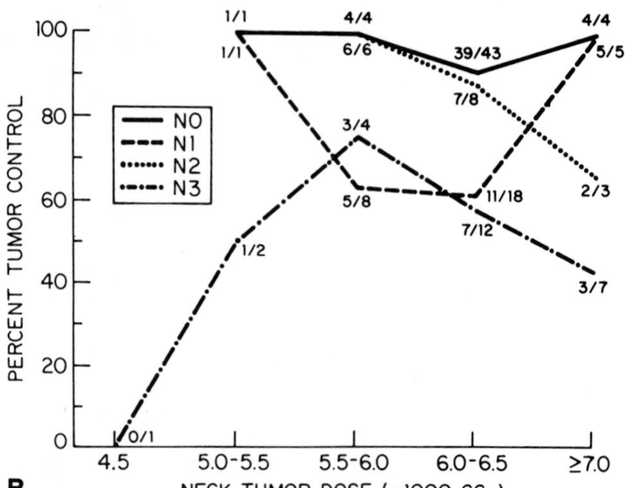

FIGURE 32–22. Irradiation dose-response curves for primary tumor control of (**A**) various T stages and (**B**) initial N stage in carcinoma of the tonsil treated with radiation therapy alone.

Brachytherapy irradiates a localized volume. Among 24 patients treated with external and interstitial irradiation (^{60}Co or 4-MV photons), local tumor control rates of 100% were achieved for 12 T1 and T2 tumors and of 60% for ten T3 tumors.[13] No patient developed bone necrosis. Amornmarn and colleagues[4] reported local tumor control rates of 94% for 16 T1 lesions, 88% for 36 T2 lesions, 62% for 42 T3 lesions, and 19% for six T4 lesions in 100 patients with tonsillar carcinoma treated in a similar fashion. Puthawala and associates[67] reported 80 patients with squamous cell carcinoma of the tonsillar fossa, 65 with locally advanced tumors treated with external irradiation (4500–5000 cGy) followed by interstitial ^{192}Ir implant (2000–2500 cGy for T1 and T2 and 3000–4000 cGy for T3 and T4 lesions). Neck masses were separately implanted to receive an additional 2000 cGy to 4000 cGy. With a minimum 2-year follow-up, the overall tumor control rate was 84%, with almost 100% control of T1 and T2 tumors and 65% to 70% control rates for T3 and T4 tumors. Leborgne and associates[42] achieved a 60% tumor control rate in 15 patients with tongue extension treated with external irradiation and brachytherapy, much improved over the 38% control rate among 39 patients receiving external irradiation alone. Mazeron and colleagues[53] observed 100% local and 94% neck tumor control in 33 patients with T1 and T2 tonsillar carcinoma treated with external radiation therapy and interstitial ^{192}Ir. On the other hand, Garrett and associates[30] found no improvement in local tumor control among 68 patients with tonsillar carcinoma extending into the glossotonsillar sulcus or base of the tongue in whom an interstitial implant was added to external irradiation. At 5 years, the 57% local control rate with implants was not significantly better than the 52% rate achieved without implants.

At Washington University, the results of treating 296 patients with a combination of surgery and irradiation were comparable to those obtained with irradiation alone, except for a suggestion of improved tumor control and survival in T3 and T4 tumors treated with surgery and postoperative irradiation (Table 32-9).[63]

Barrs and colleagues[7] reported 119 patients with carcinoma of the tonsil and base of the tongue treated primarily with a surgical procedure alone (67 patients, most with T1 or T2 tumors), combined operation and irradiation (25 patients), or irradiation alone (remainder of patients). In the surgical group,

TABLE 32–9
Three-Year Disease-Free Survival for Carcinoma of the Tonsil

STAGE	RADIATION THERAPY ALONE	PREOPERATIVE RADIATION THERAPY	POSTOPERATIVE RADIATION THERAPY
T1N0	8/10 (80%)	3/5 (60%)	
T2N0	14/29 (48%)	14/22 (64%)	3/4 (75%)
T3N0	7/11 (64%)	8/18 (44%)	4/6 (66%)
T1–2N1–2	4/11 (36%)	13/18 (72%)	2/4 (50%)
T3N1–2	12/22 (55%)	12/45 (27%)	7/12 (58%)
T1–3N3	3/13 (23%)	3/11 (27%)	2/3 (66%)
T4N1–3	4/31 (13%)	4/14 (29%)	4/7 (57%)

Data given are for patients treated between 1955 and 1984. (Perez CA, Carmichael T, Devineni VR, et al: Head Neck [in press])

the 3-year survival rate for patients with T1 lesions was 63%; for those with T2 lesions, it was 56%; and in the T3 and T4 group, it was 31%. With irradiation alone, the 3-year survival rate was 68% for Stage T1 patients, 52% for Stage T2 patients, and 38% for the Stage T3 group. The differences are not statistically significant.

Quenelle and associates[68] described their experience with 58 patients treated with preoperative irradiation (5000 cGy) followed by complete radical resection of the tumors. As in the previous series, the survival and tumor control rates are similar to those reported for other patients who were treated with irradiation alone.[16,22,25,31,54,66]

Combined therapy was more effective in patients with more extensive tumors (T3 and T4 or clinically palpable neck nodes) who have a lower probability of tumor control with irradiation alone or for patients with persistent tumor after initial definitive irradiation. To improve tumor control in these selected patients, higher doses of irradiation (4500 cGy delivered preoperatively or 6000 cGy postoperatively) combined with surgery should be given. Postoperative and preoperative irradiation are equally effective approaches.

The Radiation Therapy Oncology Group conducted a study of 354 patients with advanced carcinoma of the oral cavity, oropharynx, supraglottic larynx, and hypopharynx, who were randomized to receive preoperative irradiation (5000 cGy, 200-cGy fractions, five times weekly) or postoperative irradiation (6000 cGy to the primary tumor and 5000 cGy to both necks). The overall tumor control rate was slightly better in the postoperative group (65%) than in the preoperative group (48%) ($P = 0.81$). In the oropharynx the 4-year survival rates were 26% with preoperative irradiation and 38% with postoperative radiation therapy. Complications of therapy were approximately the same: 10% to 11% in the surgical group and 11% to 14% in the irradiation group.[40]

At Washington University, the incidence of complications was somewhat higher in patients treated with combined therapy than in those treated with irradiation alone.[63] The observed morbidity with combined therapy is comparable to that reported in patients with tumors of the larynx and pharynx treated at our institution with a surgical procedure alone.[29]

Faucial Arch

In general, tumors of the faucial arch have a better tumor control rate and prognosis than those of the tonsillar fossa. Fletcher and Lindberg[27] reported a failure rate of 10% or less in retromolar trigone and soft palate T1 lesions, 18% in T2 tumors, and 16% in T3 tumors. There was a slightly higher absolute 5-year survival rate among 173 patients with tumors of the faucial arch than for those with tumors of the tonsillar fossa. The 2-year tumor-free survival rate was also correlated with the stage of the cervical lymph nodes.

Barker and Fletcher[6] reported 204 patients with epidermoid carcinoma of the retromolar trigone and anterior tonsillar pillar treated with definitive radiation therapy. Initially, ^{60}Co was used, and 6000 cGy in 4 to 5 weeks was delivered through small fields for early stages. After 1963, 18-MV photons were combined with 18-MeV electrons for the entire treatment or as a boost after administration of 5000 cGy. Control of the primary tumor and survival rates were best for T1 and T2 lesions, with less satisfactory results in more advanced stages (Table 32-10). For T1 lesions, doses of 6000 cGy to 6500 cGy in 6 to 6.5 weeks controlled over 95% of the tumors; for T2 and T3 lesions, a control rate of over 90% was obtained with 7000 cGy given in 7 weeks. Higher doses are required for T4 tumors.

In a study of 110 patients who had squamous cell carcinoma of the retromolar trigone treated with various modalities, depending on tumor stage, Byers and associates[15] reported a local or regional (neck) control rate of 84% with irradiation alone. Regardless of the method of therapy, the primary tumor control rates were 92% for T1, 88% for T2, 90% for T3, and 75% for T4 tumors. The cervical lymph node control rates were 89% for N0, 86% for N1, 83% for N2, and 66% for N3 lesions.

Cheng and co-workers[17] published results of treating with definitive radiation therapy 21 patients with carcinoma of the anterior tonsillar pillar and 45 with tumors of the soft palate and uvula. They employed external irradiation (6500–7500 cGy); external irradiation (4000–4500 cGy) followed by a radon seed implant to deliver 2000 cGy to 4000 cGy, depending on the stage of the lesion; or split-course external irradiation to deliver 6000 cGy to 7500 cGy in 10 to 13 weeks. The 5-year absolute survival rate was 46% to 57% for 23 T1 lesions, 35% to 75% for 24 T2 tumors, and 22% for 11 T3 lesions with the various techniques. The recurrence rate in the neck for T1 and T2 tumors was 7.4% (two of 27) among patients treated with external irradiation to doses of 6000 cGy to 7500 cGy, compared with 33% (three of nine) for patients treated with 4000 cGy to 4500 cGy external irradiation and a radon seed implant in the soft palate.

Lo and associates[45] reported 159 patients with previously untreated squamous cell carcinoma of the anterior faucial pillar or retromolar trigone who received external irradiation, includ-

TABLE 32–10
Control of Primary Squamous Cell Carcinoma of the Faucial Arch Correlated with T Stage

STAGE	TOTAL PATIENTS	PRIMARY FAILURE	DEFINITE ULTIMATE FAILURE AFTER SURGICAL SALVAGE	UNDERDOSE OR GEOGRAPHIC MISS	NED >2 YR	NED LOCALLY, EXPIRED <2 YR OTHER CAUSES (DM, ID, UNK)*	ANALYZABLE CASES
T1	26	4/26 (15%)	1/26 (4%)	2	18	4	20
T2	103	20/103 (19%)	7/103 (7%)	5	66	17	81
T3	61	9/61 (15%)	2/61 (3%)	5	36	16	40
T4	14	5/14 (36%)	3/14 (21%)	2	2	7	5

**DM, distant metastasis; ID, intercurrent disease; UNK, unknown causes; NED, no evidence of disease.*
(Barker JL, Fletcher GH: Int J Radiat Oncol Biol Phys 2:407, 1977)

ing combinations of electron beams with high-energy photons or ^{60}Co to doses ranging from 6000 cGy to 7500 cGy (except 11 patients). In the N0 patients, as a rule, only the ipsilateral subdigastric nodes were treated electively to a dose of 5000 cGy. The 5-year determinate survival rate for the whole group was 83%. The failure rate for the evaluable patients was 29% for T1 lesions, 30% for T2 lesions, 24% for T3 lesions, and 40% for T4 lesions. After salvage surgery, which consisted of intraoral resection in a third of the patients or a composite operation in the other two thirds, the ultimate failure rate was 0% for T1 lesions, 6% for T2 lesions, 8% for T3 lesions, and 20% for T4 lesions (Table 32-11). Of the whole group, 16 patients (10%) experienced neck failures, with eight ultimate failures after salvage surgery. There was a significantly higher failure rate for infiltrative and ulcerated lesions (35%) than for exophytic and superficial lesions (15%), but histologic grade had no prognostic significance. After radiation therapy, 30% of the patients developed some degree of bone exposure, but only 5.5% (nine patients) required a segmental mandibular resection. The probability of bone exposure was not dose related and more likely reflected tumor location on the mucoperiosteum.

Keus and associates[38] reported 235 patients with tumors of the soft palate treated at the Institut Curie; results of definitive radiation therapy were evaluated in 146 cases. Megavoltage x-ray therapy was employed for 103 patients, and a combination of megavoltage and intraoral orthovoltage x-rays was used for 43 patients with small or moderately advanced tumors. The crude 3- and 5-year survival rates were 52% and 40%, respectively, and the disease-free survival rates were 59% and 53%. The local control rate at 3 years was 92% for T1, 70% for T2, 58% for T3, and 49% for T4 lesions. Nodal failure was seen in 19 patients: in nine patients, it was not associated with failure at the primary site, and in seven of nine, it occurred marginally or outside the treatment portals. Complications were observed in 16 patients, with seven requiring surgery.

Among 41 patients with previously untreated soft palate malignancies, Seydel and Scholl[74] reported a local recurrence rate of 32% (10 of 31 patients) with doses of 6000 cGy to 7000 cGy.

Bataini and associates,[9] in a multivariate analysis of 465 patients with tumors of the tonsillar region (including the pillars and glossopalatine sulcus) treated with irradiation alone (6500–6800 cGy in 6–7 weeks), noted that the stage and site of the primary tumor were the only significant prognostic factors influencing tumor control. The length of overall treatment time was the only technical variable associated with local control. Patients with tumors of the tonsil and anterior or posterior tonsillar pillar had better 3-year tumor control (72% and 66%, respectively) than those with tumors in the glossopalatine sulcus (48%).

According to Shukovsky and associates,[76] tumors of the glossopalatine sulcus are believed to arise in the tonsillar fossa, base of the tongue, or anterior tonsillar pillar. In 81 patients with squamous cell carcinoma of the glossopalatine sulcus who were identified from a total group of 662 patients with tumors in the base of the tongue, tonsillar fossa, or faucial arch, 79 were followed up for more than 3 years. The failure rate at the primary site was 0% for five T1, 25% for 20 T2, 25% for 44 T3, and 41.5% for 12 T4 lesions. The 2-year relapse-free survival rate was 80% for T1 (four of five patients), 65% for T2 (13 of 20), 38.5% for T3 (17 of 44), and 16.5% for T4 tumors (two of 12). There was a significant correlation between the dose of irradiation and control of the primary tumor, and complications were associated with increased radiation doses.

Neutrons alone or in combination with photons (mixed beams) have been used in the treatment of advanced head and neck cancer. Hussey and associates[35] summarized the results of four trials at M. D. Anderson Cancer Center involving 142 patients treated on pilot studies and 95 in a randomized clinical trial. Nineteen patients with oropharyngeal tumors were included in the pilot study and 32 in the randomized trial. Nine percent of the patients in the neutrons-only and 26% in the mixed-beam study developed recurrent tumors. The results for faucial arch and pharyngeal wall cancers were slightly better in the neutrons-only and mixed-beam group than with conventional treatment. However, the results for tonsillar fossa lesions were slightly better with conventional photon irradiation. The results suggested that neutron or mixed-beam therapy may be more effective than conventional irradiation in the management of regional lymph node metastasis. In the overall analysis, a significant dose-response relationship was found with neutrons, and the range of acceptable dose was narrow.

TABLE 32–11
Local Control of Carcinoma of the Anterior Tonsillar Pillar and Retromolar Trigone

		EVALUABLE PATIENTS*			
STAGE	**LOCAL CONTROL IN ALL PATIENTS**	LOCAL CONTROL	TREATMENT OF PRIMARY FAILURE	PATIENTS SALVAGED	ULTIMATE CONTROL RATE
T1	15/20 (75%)	12/17 (71%)	Surgery (5)†	5/5	100%
T2	69/93 (74%)	57/81 (70%)	No treatment (2) Surgery (21) Surgery + Irradiation (1)	19/24‡	94%
T3	30/36 (83%)	19/25 (76%)	Surgery (5) Surgery + Chemo (1)	4/6‡	92%
T4	8/10 (80%)	3/5 (60%)	Surgery (1) Chemo (1)	1/2‡	

** Thirty-one patients who died in less than 2 years with no evidence of local disease are not evaluable.*
† Numbers in parentheses indicate number of patients.
‡ Five T2, one T3, and one T4 patients died in less than 2 years with no evidence of local disease.
(Lo K, Fletcher GH, Byers RM, et al: Int J Radiat Oncol Biol Phys 13:969, 1987)

MANAGEMENT OF RECURRENCES

Patients with recurrences after surgery or moderate irradiation doses should receive definitive doses of radiation to the primary tumor and the cervical lymph nodes. Portals are the same as those described previously for primary management.

In patients who initially received full-course radiation therapy, a radical tonsillectomy and ipsilateral neck dissection should be performed if the lesion is resectable. For failures in the neck without primary recurrence, a neck dissection is the treatment of choice.

Palliative doses (4000–4500 cGy in 4–5 weeks) of irradiation with external beam or brachytherapy should be administered to patients with advanced, recurrent disease. The volume treated should encompass the tumor with a 2-cm to 3-cm margin. The risk of soft tissue necrosis or osteonecrosis increases markedly. Survival is poor after a recurrence, and only a few patients can be salvaged, except for localized recurrences in T1 and T2 tumors or N1 cervical lymphadenopathy.

Mazeron and associates[52] described their experience in treating 70 patients with ^{192}Ir afterloading implants who had new or recurrent oropharyngeal cancers arising in previously irradiated tissues. The actuarial local control rates were 72% at 2 years and 69% at 5 years. Tumor control was strongly related to tumor size: 86% for tumors less than 2 cm, 71% for tumors 2.1 cm to 4 cm, and 58% for tumors 4.1 cm to 6 cm. Although local tumor control was achieved in most of these patients, only 10 (14%) patients remained alive at 5 years. Local control was achieved in 100% of the patients with lesions of the faucial arch or posterior pharyngeal wall. Patients with lesions of the base of the tongue and the glossotonsillar sulcus had poorer results; local control was achieved in 61%.

CHEMOTHERAPY

Although there are no specific reports on the use of neoadjuvant or palliative chemotherapy for carcinoma of the oropharynx, the results obtained in treating head and neck tumors can be applied to these patients. Drugs of choice include cisplatin, alone or combined with 5-fluorouracil, and high-dose methotrexate with leucovorin rescue.[23, 81] Bleomycin and nitrosoureas also have been used.[3] Recent reports describe complete responses in 40% of the patients given three cycles of chemotherapy before irradiation or surgery and an additional 30% partial responses, yielding an overall response rate of 75% or higher. Disease-free survival time has been prolonged by a few months, but after 3 years, no appreciable enhancement of overall survival has been demonstrated.

The potential benefit of adjuvant chemotherapy combined with irradiation and surgery in the treatment of these advanced lesions should be further evaluated; its long-term benefit has not been documented.[24] Agents that selectively enhance the effects of irradiation in the tumor are under investigation, such as hypoxic cell sensitizers, chemical modifiers (*i.e.*, cytotoxic agents, halogenated pyrimidines), hyperthermia, and high-LET radiation.[34, 64, 89]

SEQUELAE OF TREATMENT

The most common acute sequelae after irradiation are oropharyngeal mucositis and moderate to severe dysphagia, which may cause malnutrition and jeopardize the patient's survival if drastic support measures, such as gastrostomy or hyperalimentation, are not taken. Severe nutritional problems occur in 5% to 10% of the patients. Temporary xerostomia and loss of taste may last for several months. Marks and colleagues[51] demonstrated a significant reduction in parotid gland salivary flow with doses over 3000 cGy. Other complications include laryngeal edema, fibrosis, hearing loss, and occasional trismus (Table 32-12).

The incidence of osteonecrosis of the mandible depends on tumor stage, dose of irradiation delivered to the mandible, use of prophylactic dental care, trauma (including dental extractions), and the technique of irradiation used. Grant and Fletcher[33] reported severe necrosis requiring mandibulectomy in six (6.8%) of 88 patients with T1 and T2 carcinoma of the tonsillar fossa and in 13 (14.8%) of 88 patients with T3 and T4 tumors. The percent of patients in these two groups with bone exposure was 29.5% and 45.4%, respectively. The incidence of osteonecrosis was greater with single homolateral fields, unilateral wedge filter arrangements, or a combination of external irradiation and interstitial implants (Table 32-13). Cheng and Wang[18] reported osteonecrosis in 13 patients who received between 2000 and 2900 ret (*i.e.*, time-dose factor of 126 to 212); this complication was rarely seen if doses below 2000 ret to the mandible were delivered. Shukovsky and co-workers[76] reported a greater incidence of mandibular necrosis with higher doses of irradiation.

Bedwinek and associates[12] found a significant difference in the incidence of necrosis between tumors sited over or adjacent to the mandible (about 6%) or not (0%). They also described a 5.9% incidence of osteonecrosis requiring mandibular resection in 12 (4%) of 303 patients treated before 1969, when elective dental extractions were performed, and 4.5% (eight of 178) in patients for whom dental conservation was practiced.

Barker and Fletcher[6] reported a 10% incidence of spontaneous necrosis among 112 patients with T1 or T2 tumors of the retromolar trigone and anterior tonsillar pillar after doses of 6000 cGy to 6500 cGy given in 6 to 6.5 weeks and a 16% incidence of necrosis among 57 patients with T3 tumors treated with 7000 cGy (six of these required mandibulectomy). The M. D. Anderson Cancer Center experience was updated by Larson and associates.[41] Of an initial population of 569 patients, 148 were analyzed for complications; only patients free of disease for more than 5 years were evaluated. Twelve of 30 patients with faucial arch tumors and 13 of 26 with tonsillar fossa primary tumors developed osteonecrosis of the mandible, ulceration of the soft tissues, or both. Of these, five from the first group and six from the second group required mandibulectomy for treatment.

Lo and associates[45] observed a lower incidence of complications in patients with anterior faucial pillar or retromolar trigone lesions treated with unilateral electron-beam and photon portals compared with parallel opposed portals delivering 5000 cGy or higher doses (Table 32-14).

Carotid artery rupture was reported in 3% of patients in the Grant and Fletcher series[33] and in 1% of patients analyzed by Perez and co-workers.[63] This complication was discovered in patients undergoing surgery after failure of radiation therapy.

In a study of 133 patients treated with combined preoperative irradiation and surgery, Perez and colleagues[63] reported three patients who died of carotid rupture, two of postoperative pneumonia, one of postoperative pulmonary embolus, and one of postoperative cerbrovascular accident, yielding a 5.3% total complication rate. Other major complications included 18 cases of oropharyngocutaneous fistula, seven patients with osteonecrosis of the mandible, eight with severe dysphagia and malnutrition, two with carotid rupture, and one with laryngeal edema (Table 32-12).

TABLE 32–12
Sequelae of Therapy for Carcinoma of the Tonsil

COMPLICATION*	RADIATION THERAPY ALONE	PREOPERATIVE RADIATION THERAPY AND SURGERY	POSTOPERATIVE RADIATION THERAPY AND SURGERY
NONFATAL			
Oropharyngocutaneous fistula	2	18	1
Osteonecrosis of mandible	6	7	0
Severe dysphagia	4	8	4
Delayed wound healing	0	5	0
Laryngeal edema	3	1	1
Dental decay	2	1	0
Carotid rupture	1	2	0
Cranial nerve neuropathy	2	0	0
Soft tissue necrosis	1	1	1
Postoperative pneumonia	0	1	1
Xerostomia	1	1	0
Esophageal stricture	1	0	0
Total	23 (18%)	45 (33.8%)	8 (22%)
FATAL			
Carotid rupture	1†	3	1
Postoperative pneumonia	0	2	0
Oropharyngeal hemorrhage	0	0	1
Postoperative cerebrovascular accident	0	1	0
Postoperative pulmonary embolus	0	1	0
Malnutrition from dysphagia	1	0	0
Total	2 (1.5%)	7 (5.3%)	2 (5.6%)

* *Unlimited time for determining sequelae. All data are for patients treated at the Mallinckrodt Institute of Radiology.*
† *After surgery for recurrent tumor.*

CONTROVERSIAL ISSUES

There is still controversy about the preferred method of treatment for T1 and T2 tumors, particularly with clinically negative neck nodes. However, because of the lower sequelae and better functional and cosmetic results, definitive radiation therapy should be employed, reserving surgery for recurrences.

T3 and T4 primary tumors are better managed with combined therapy. Postoperative irradiation may be more advantageous because of its ability to deliver higher doses to the tumor with less morbidity. However, a study by the Radiation Therapy Oncology Group[40] disclosed no significant difference between preoperative and postoperative radiation therapy in the treatment of oral cavity and oropharyngeal tumors.

TABLE 32–13
Incidence of Bone Exposure and Osteonecrosis by Technique

TECHNIQUE	NO. OF PATIENTS	NO. OF PATIENTS WITH BONE EXPOSURE	NO. OF PATIENTS WITH NECROSIS REQUIRING MANDIBULECTOMY
Single homolateral field	50	24 (48.0%)	9 (18.0%)
Unequally loaded parallel opposing fields	64	22 (34.4%)	4 (6.25%)
Equally loaded parallel opposing fields	14	2 (13.2%)	0
Paired wedge filter fields	22	10 (45.5%)	3 (13.6%)
External irradiation plus interstitial implantation of radioactive sources	12	4 (33.3%)	2 (16.7%)
Single homolateral field plus intraoral cone	14	4 (28.6%)	1 (7.1%)

(Grant BP, Fletcher GH: Am J Roentgenol 96:28, 1966)

TABLE 32–14
Complications after Irradiation of Carcinoma of Tonsillar Pillar and Retromolar Trigone

	T1, T2, T3		T4
COMPLICATION*	≥5000 cGy PARALLEL OPPOSED PORTALS (25 PATIENTS)	UNILATERAL PORTALS ELECTRON BEAM + PHOTONS (72 PATIENTS)	≥5000 cGy PARALLEL OPPOSED PORTALS (3 PATIENTS)
Trismus	24% (6)†	15% (11)	0
Dental problems	16% (4)	4% (3)	0
Xerostomia	56% (14)	25% (18)	100% (3)
Persistent pain	8% (2)	6% (4)	0
Self-healing bone exposure	40% (10)	25% (18)	0
Mandibular resection	8% (2)	3% (2)	0
Other	(0)	1.4% (1)	67% (2)

* *Complications were analyzed in January 1986 for 100 evaluable patients seen between January 1966 and August 1981. Bone exposure and mandibular resection were always recorded, but other complications and their severity were not always listed in the charts.*
† *The number of patients with complications are in parentheses.*
(Lo K, Fletcher GH, Byers RM, et al: Int J Radiat Oncol Biol Phys 13:969, 1987)

In patients with clinically negative necks, a lymph node dissection is not warranted, because elective irradiation of the neck (5000 cGy) controls subclinical disease in more than 95% of the patients. In patients with small, mobile lymph nodes, it is possible to control the tumor with radiation therapy alone, although a radical neck dissection is equally effective. For multiple lymph nodes larger than 5 cm in diameter or fixed to the soft tissues, the preferred method of treatment is radical neck dissection and postoperative irradiation. In many instances, a composite resection of the primary tumor and a neck dissection can be carried out and followed by radiation therapy. The high rate of deaths from intercurrent disease (25% at 5 years) in these patients precludes having a major impact on overall survival with improvement in locoregional tumor control.[54]

The role of adjuvant chemotherapy in patients with advanced tumors has not been elucidated.

REFERENCES

1. Abedi E, Sismanis A: Extrapulmonary oat-cell carcinoma of the tonsil. Ear Nose Throat J 66:112, 1987
2. Ackerman LV, del Regato JA: Cancer: Diagnosis, Treatment and Prognosis, 6th ed. St. Louis, CV Mosby, 1985
3. Al-Sarraf M: Head and neck cancer: Chemotherapy concepts. Semin Oncol 15:70, 1988
4. Amornmarn R, Prempree T, Jaiwatana J, Wizenberg MJ: Radiation management of carcinoma of the tonsillar region. Cancer 54:1293, 1984
5. Baker RR, Weiner S: The management of tonsillar carcinoma. Surg Gynecol Obstet 121:1035, 1967
6. Barker JL, Fletcher GH: Time, dose, tumor volume relationships in megavoltage irradiation of squamous cell carcinomas of the RMT and AFP. Int J Radiat Oncol Biol Phys 2:407, 1977
7. Barrs DM, DeSanto LW, O'Fallon WM: Squamous cell carcinoma of the tonsil and tongue: Base region. Arch Otolaryngol 105:479, 1979
8. Barton JH, Osborne BM, Butler JJ, et al: Non-Hodgkin's lymphoma of the tonsil: A clinicopathologic study of 65 cases. Cancer 53:86, 1984
9. Bataini JP, Asselain B, Jaulerry C, et al: A multivariate primary tumour control analysis in 465 patients treated by radical radiotherapy for cancer of the tonsillar region: Clinical and treatment parameters as prognostic factors. Radiother Oncol 14:265, 1989
10. Batsakis JG: Tumors of the Head and Neck, 2nd ed, pp 144–176. Baltimore, Williams & Wilkins, 1979
11. Beahrs OH, Henson DE, Hutter RVP, Myers MH (eds): Manual for Staging of Cancer, 3rd ed, pp 34–35. Philadelphia, JB Lippincott, 1988
12. Bedwinek JM, Shukovsky LJ, Fletcher GH, Daley TE: Osteonecrosis in patients treated with definitive radiotherapy for squamous cell carcinomas of the oral cavity and naso- and oropharynx. Radiology 119:665, 1976
13. Beiler DD: Interstitial radiation in the treatment of carcinoma of the tonsillar region. AJR 128:1031, 1977
14. Bloedorn FG, Cuccia CA, Mercado R Jr: Place of interstitial gamma-ray emitters in radiation therapy: Indications, technique, examples. AJR 96:407, 1966
15. Byers RM, Anderson B, Schwarz EA, et al: Treatment of squamous carcinoma of the retromolar trigone. Am J Clin Oncol 7:647, 1984
16. Cardinale F, Fischer JJ: Radiation therapy of carcinoma of the tonsil. Cancer 39:604, 1977
17. Cheng VST, Shetty KS, Deutsch M: Carcinomas of the anterior tonsillar pillar and the soft palate-uvula: Treatment by radiation therapy. Radiology 134:497, 1980
18. Cheng VST, Wang CC: Osteoradionecrosis of the mandible resulting from external megavoltage radiation therapy. Radiology 112:685, 1974
19. Chung TS, Stefani S: Distant metastases of carcinoma of tonsillar region: A study of 475 patients. J Surg Oncol 14:5, 1980
20. Conley J, Pack GT: Melanoma of the mucous membranes of the head and neck. Arch Otolaryngol 99:315, 1974
21. Coutard H: Roentgen therapy of epitheliomas of the tonsillar region, hypopharynx and larynx from 1920 to 1926. AJR 28:313, 1932
22. Dubois JB, Broquerie JL, Delard R, Pourquier H: Analysis of the results of irradiation in the treatment of tonsillar region carcinomas. Int J Radiat Oncol Biol Phys 9:1195, 1983
23. Ensley JF, Jacobs JR, Weaver A, et al: Correlation between response to cisplatinum-combination chemotherapy and subsequent radiotherapy in previously untreated patients with advanced squamous cell cancers of the head and neck. Cancer 54:811, 1984
24. Ervin TJ, Clark JR, Weichselbaum RR, et al: An analysis of induction and adjuvant chemotherapy in the multidisciplinary treatment of squamous-cell carcinoma of the head and neck. J Clin Oncol 5:10, 1987

25. Fayos JV, Lampe I: Radiation therapy of carcinoma of the tonsillar region. AJR 111:85, 1971
26. Fletcher GH: Textbook of Radiotherapy, 3rd ed, pp 286–329. Philadelphia, Lea & Febiger, 1980
27. Fletcher GH, Lindberg RD: Squamous cell carcinomas of the tonsillar area and palatine arch. AJR 96:574, 1966
28. Fletcher GH, MacComb WH, Shalek RJ: Radiation Therapy of the Oral Cavity and Oropharynx. Springfield, IL, Charles C Thomas, 1962
29. Gall AM, Sessions DG, Ogura JH: Complications following surgery for cancer of the larynx and hypopharynx. Cancer 39:614, 1977
30. Garrett PG, Beale FA, Cummings BJ, et al: Carcinoma of the tonsil: The effect of dose-time-volume factors on local control. Int J Radiat Oncol Biol Phys 11:703, 1985
31. Gelinas M, Fletcher GH: Incidence and cause of local failure of irradiation in squamous cell carcinoma of faucial arch, tonsillar fossa and base of tongue. Radiology 108:383, 1973
32. Givens CD Jr, Johns ME, Cantrell RW: Carcinoma of the tonsil: Analysis of 162 cases. Arch Otolaryngol 107:730, 1981
33. Grant BP, Fletcher GH: Analysis of complications following megavoltage therapy for squamous cell carcinomas of the tonsillar area. AJR 96:27, 1966
34. Griffin TW, Davis R, Hendrickson FR, et al: Fast neutron radiation therapy for unresectable squamous cell carcinomas of the head and neck: The results of a randomized RTOG study. Int J Radiat Oncol Biol Phys 10:2217, 1984
35. Hussey DH, Maor MH, Fletcher GH: A detailed analysis of the MDAH-TAMVEC neutron therapy trials for head and neck cancer. In 13th International Cancer Congress, Part D, Research and Treatment, pp 267–277. New York, Alan R Liss, 1983
36. Jesse RH Jr, Fletcher GH: Metastases in cervical lymph nodes from oropharyngeal carcinoma: Treatment and results. AJR 90:990, 1963
37. Johnston WD, Byers RM: Squamous cell carcinoma of the tonsil in young adults. Cancer 39:633, 1977
38. Keus RB, Pontvert D, Brunin F, et al: Results of irradiation in squamous cell carcinoma of the soft palate and uvula. Radiother Oncol 11:311, 1988
39. Koss L, Shapiro R, Jahdu S: Small cell (oat cell) carcinoma of minor salivary gland origin. Cancer 30:737, 1972
40. Kramer S, Gelber RD, Snow JB, et al: Combined radiation therapy and surgery in the management of advanced head and neck cancer: Final report of study 73-03 of the Radiation Therapy Oncology group. Head Neck Surg 10:19, 1987
41. Larson DL, Lindberg RD, Lane E, Goepfert H: Major complications of radiotherapy in cancer of the oral cavity and oropharynx: A 10-year retrospective study. Am J Surg 146:531, 1983
42. Leborgne JH, Leborgne F, Barlocci LA, Ortega B: The place of brachytherapy in the treatment of carcinoma of the tonsil with lingual extension. Int J Radiat Oncol Biol Phys 12:1787, 1986
43. Lindberg RD: Distribution of cervical lymph node metastasis from squamous cell carcinoma of the upper respiratory and digestive tracts. Cancer 29:1446, 1972
44. Lindberg RD: Sites of first failure in head and neck cancer. Cancer Treat Symp 2:21, 1983
45. Lo K, Fletcher GH, Byers RM, et al: Results of irradiation in the squamous cell carcinomas of the anterior faucial pillar-retromolar trigone. Int J Radiat Oncol Biol Phys 13:969, 1987
46. Lusinchi A, Wibault P, Marandas P, et al: Exclusive radiation therapy: The treatment of early tonsillar tumors. Int J Radiat Oncol Biol Phys 17:273, 1989
47. MacComb WS, Fletcher GH: Cancer of the Head and Neck, pp 179–212. Baltimore, Williams & Wilkins Company, 1967
48. Maltz R, Shymrick DA, Aron BS, Weichert KA: Carcinoma of the tonsil: Results of combined therapy. Laryngoscope 81:2172, 1974
49. Mantravadi RVP, Liebner EJ, Ginde JV: An analysis of factors in the successful management of cancer of the tonsillar region. Cancer 41:1054, 1978
50. Marcial VA, Amato DA, Pajak TF: Patterns of failure after treatment for cancer of upper respiratory digestive tracts: A Radiation Therapy Oncology Group report. Cancer Treat Symp 1:33, 1983
51. Marks JE, Davis C, Gottsman V, et al: The effects of radiation on parotid salivary function. Int J Radiat Oncol Biol Phys 7:1013, 1981
52. Mazeron J-J, Langlois D, Glaubiger D, et al: Salvage irradiation of oropharyngeal cancers using iridium 192 wire implant: 5-year results of 70 cases. Int J Radiat Oncol Biol Phys 13:957, 1987
53. Mazeron JJ, Lusinchi A, Marinello G, et al: Interstitial radiation therapy for squamous cell carcinoma of the tonsillar region: The Creteil experience (1971–1981). Int J Radiat Oncol Biol Phys 12:895, 1986
54. Mendenhall WM, Parsons JT, Cassisi NJ, Million RR: Squamous cell carcinoma of the tonsillar area treated with radical irradiation. Radiother Oncol 10:23, 1987
55. Merino OR, Lindberg RD, Fletcher GH: An analysis of distant metastases from squamous cell carcinoma of the upper respiratory and digestive tract. Cancer 40:145, 1977
56. Million RR, Cassisi NJ: Oropharynx. In Million RR, Cassisi NJ (eds): Management of Head and Neck Cancer: A Multidisciplinary Approach, pp 299–314. Philadelphia. JB Lippincott, 1984
57. Mizono GS, Diaz RF, Fu KK, Doles R: Carcinoma of the tonsillar region. Laryngoscope 96:240, 1986
58. Murthy AK, Hendrickson FR: Is contralateral neck treatment necessary in early carcinoma of the tonsil? Int J Radiat Oncol Biol Phys 6:91, 1980
59. Nussbaum H, Kagan AR, Chan P, et al: Carcinoma of the tonsillar area treated with external radiotherapy alone. Am J Clin Oncol 6:639, 1983
60. Ogrady M, Doyle PJ, Flores AD: Cancer of the tonsil. J Otolaryngol 14:221, 1985
61. Oreggia F, Stefani EDE, Deneo-Pelligrini H, Olivera L: Carcinoma of the tonsil: A retrospective analysis of prognostic factors. Arch Otolaryngol 109:305, 1983
62. Perez CA, Ackerman LV, Mill WB, et al: Malignant tumors of the tonsil. AJR 114:43, 1972
63. Perez CA, Carmichael T, Devineni VR, et al: Carcinoma of the tonsillar fossa: A nonrandomized comparison of irradiation alone or combined with surgery: Long-term results. Head Neck (in press)
64. Perez CA, Emami BN, Straube W, et al: Irradiation and external hyperthermia in treatment of head and neck cancer. In Sugahara T, Saito M (eds): Hyperthermic Oncology 1988, vol 2, pp 446–449. London, Taylor & Francis, 1989
65. Perez CA, Lee FA, Ackerman LV, et al: Carcinoma of the tonsillar fossa: Significance of dose of irradiation and volume treated in the control of the primary tumor and metastatic neck nodes. Int J Radiat Oncol Biol Phys 1:817, 1976
66. Perez CA, Lee FA, Ackerman LV, et al: Non-randomized comparison of preoperative irradiation and surgery versus irradiation alone in the management of carcinoma of the tonsil. AJR 126:248, 1976
67. Puthawala AA, Syed AMN, Eads DL, et al: Limited external irradiation and interstitial 192 iridium implant in the treatment of squamous cell carcinoma of the tonsillar region. Int J Radiat Oncol Biol Phys 11:1595, 1985
68. Quenelle DJ, Crissman JD, Shumrick DA: Tonsil carcinoma: Treatment results. Laryngoscope 89:1842, 1979
69. Radiation Therapy Oncology Group Protocol No. 79-13: Hyperfractionated photon radiation therapy in the treatment of advanced squamous cell carcinoma of the oral cavity, pharynx, larynx, and sinuses, using radiation therapy as the only planned treatment modality. Philadelphia, RTOG, 1979
70. Remmler D, Medina J, Byers RM, et al: Treatment of choice for squamous carcinoma of the tonsillar fossa. Head Neck Surg 7:206, 1985
71. Rider WD: Epithelial cancer of the tonsillar area. Radiology 78:760, 1962
72. Rubin P: Clinical Oncology: A Multidisciplinary Approach, 6th ed. New York, American Cancer Society, 1983
73. Scanlon PW, Devine KD, Wooner LB, McBean JB: Cancer of the tonsil: 131 patients treated in the 11 year period 1950 through 1960. AJR 100:894, 1967

74. Seydel HG, Scholl H: Carcinoma of the soft palate and uvula. Am J Roentgenol Radium Ther Nucl Med 120:603, 1974
75. Seydel HG, Scholl H: Permanent implants in the management of head and neck cancer by radiotherapy. AJR 117:565, 1973
76. Shukovsky LJ, Baeza MR, Fletcher GH: Results of irradiation in squamous cell carcinomas of the glossopalatine sulcus. Radiology 120:405, 1976
77. Shukovsky LJ, Fletcher GH: Time-dose and tumor volume relationships in the irradiation of squamous cell carcinoma of the tonsillar fossa. Radiology 107:621, 1973
78. Spiro RH, Koss LG, Hajdu SI, Strong EW: Tumors of minor salivary origin. Cancer 31:117, 1973
79. Strong EW: Sites of treatment failure in head and neck cancer. Cancer Treat Symp 2:5, 1983
80. Tapley N, Evans RA, Kligermann MM, Jacox HW: Carcinoma of the tonsillar area: Factors influencing the results of treatment. AJR 82:626, 1959
81. Tarpley JL, Chretien PB, Alexander JC, et al: High dose methotrexate as a preoperative adjuvant in the treatment of epidermoid carcinoma of the head and neck. Am J Surg 130:481, 1975
82. Terz JJ, Farr HW: Carcinoma of tonsillar fossa. Surg Gynecol Obstet 125:621, 1973
83. Tuyns AT, Esteve J, Raymond L, et al: Cancer of the larynx/hypopharynx, tobacco and alcohol: IARC International case-control study of Turin and Varese (Italy), Zaragosa and Navarra (Spain), Geneva (Switzerland) and Calvados (France). Int J Cancer 41:483, 1988
84. United States Department of Health and Human Services, SEER Program: Cancer Incidence and Mortality in United States 1973. Bethesda, MD, National Cancer Institute, 1984
85. Vallis MP, Cleeland J, Bradley PJ, Morgan AL: Radiation therapy of squamous carcinoma of the tonsil: An analysis of prognostic factors and of treatment failures. Br J Radiol 59:251, 1986
86. Wang CC: Local control of oropharyngeal carcinoma after two accelerated hyperfractionation radiation therapy schemes. Int J Radiat Oncol Biol Phys 14:1143, 1988
87. Wang CC: Improved local control for advanced oropharyngeal carcinoma following twice daily radiation therapy. Am J Clin Oncol 8:512, 1985
88. Wang CC: Management and prognosis of squamous cell carcinoma of the tonsillar region. Radiology 104:667, 1972
89. Wasserman TH, Stetz J, Phillips TL: Radiation Therapy Oncology Group clinical trials with misonidazole. Cancer 47:2382, 1981
90. Whicker JH, DeSanto LW, Devine KD: Surgical treatment of squamous cell carcinoma of tonsil. Laryngoscope 84:90, 1974
91. Wong CS, Ang KK, Fletcher GH, et al: Definitive radiotherapy for squamous cell carcinoma of the tonsillar fossa. Int J Radiat Oncol Biol Phys 16:657, 1989

33

○ ○ ○ • • •

Base of Tongue

Joseph R. Simpson
James E. Marks

ANATOMY

The posterior third of the tongue, known as the base of tongue, lies in the oropharynx, posterior and inferior to the palatoglossal arch (anterior tonsillar pillar). It is bounded anteriorly by the circumvallate papillae, laterally by the glossopharyngeal sulci and oropharyngeal walls, and inferiorly by the glossoepiglottic fossae or valleculae and the pharyngoepiglottic fold (Fig. 33-1).[52] Embryologically, its epithelium is derived from endoderm, unlike that of the oral tongue, which derives from ectoderm, and its body is formed by thick muscles continuous with those of the oral tongue. These muscles originate from the margins of the mandible and are attached to the hyoid bone. They are indispensable to the processes of articulation and deglutition. A scattered submucosal deposition of lymphoid tissue known as the lingual tonsil exists in the base of tongue and is considered the most caudal part of Waldeyer's ring, which includes the nasopharyngeal and the pharyngeal tonsils (adenoid).

EPIDEMIOLOGY

Approximately 6200 new cases of tongue cancer were diagnosed in the United States in 1991, for an incidence of 2.23 per 100,000, with about 1850 deaths or a mortality rate of 0.93 per 100,000.[7] These statistics include the oral tongue and base of the tongue and are thus in excess of the true number of patients who present with and die of cancer of the base of the tongue.

A Memorial Hospital study of tongue cancers showed that 25% to 30% arose in the base or posterior third of the organ.[23,28] These cancers more often afflict males (4 : 1) than females between 40 and 80 years of age, but they can also occur in the young. An analysis of tongue cancer cases over time has shown an increasing incidence in women, presumably because women smoke and drink more now than in the past.[11,66] Carcinogens contained in tobacco smoke are believed to be the leading cause of tongue cancer, and alcohol appears to act synergistically with tobacco.[13,48]

NATURAL HISTORY

Base of tongue cancers are usually infiltrating, with superficial ulceration. More tumor is often found on palpation than on inspection. By the time they are diagnosed, as many as three fourths of these cancers have invaded adjacent structures, including the glossopharyngeal, sulcus, pharyngeal wall, larynx, and faucial arch.[18] Tumors may infiltrate anteriorly into the oral tongue or deeply into the root because no natural anatomic barriers prevent spread. An exophytic squamous cell tumor may present as a mass; this presentation seems to be more common in the glossopharyngeal sulcus.[13,51]

The base of tongue contains a rich lymphatic plexus, the branches of which terminate for the most part in the upper anterior cervical or subdigastric lymph nodes. Bilateral and contralateral lymphatic spread is not uncommon (Fig. 33-2), and retrograde spread to retropharyngeal lymph nodes has been reported.[21,34,52] The deeply infiltrating nature of most cancers correlates with the high frequency of lymphatic metastases observed at presentation in as many as 80% of patients overall, with bilateral presentation in 30%.

Distant metastases are not uncommon in base of the tongue cancer. At Washington University, our data showed a distant metastatic rate of 20% for 101 patients who were treated with preoperative radiation therapy and surgery.[58] It may even be higher in patients with advanced nodal disease.[41]

CLINICAL PRESENTATION

Cancers of the base of the tongue, unlike those of the oral tongue, are rarely visualized by the patient and may grow to large size before detection.[23] The most common presenting symptom is local pain, often described as a sore throat aggravated by swallowing or coughing. The patient can usually point to the site of pain and the location of the tumor and sometimes complains of ipsilateral otalgia. Difficulty in swallowing because of pain is common, but dysphagia and impaired deglutition caused by massive infiltration of the tongue by tumor are un-

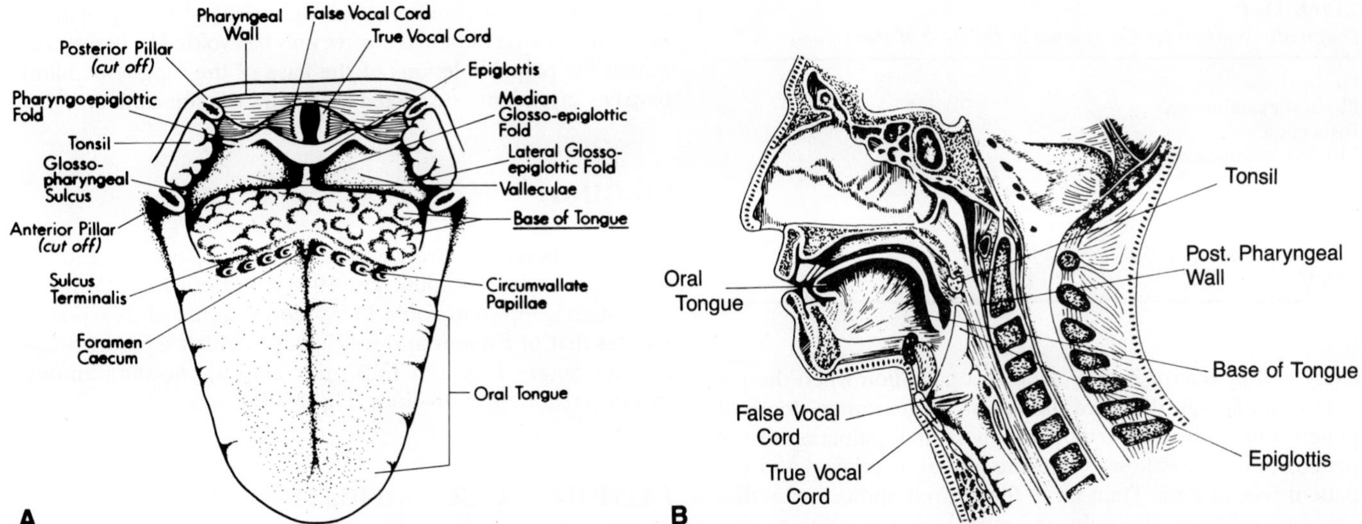

FIGURE 33–1. (**A**) Anatomy of the base of the tongue viewed from above. (**B**) Sagittal view.

usual. In advanced tumors that fix the root of the tongue, poor articulation is caused by impaired tongue mobility.

A common presentation, because of the great propensity for even small nonkeratinizing tumors of the base of the tongue to metastasize lymphatically, is a painless lump in the neck. This sign is far more likely to occur in base of the tongue, nasopharyngeal, and hypopharyngeal cancers than in cancers in other head and neck sites.

DIAGNOSTIC WORKUP

The diagnostic evaluation of patients suspected of having cancer in the base of the tongue is initially a matter of inspection and palpation (Table 33-1). Most patients present with disease limited to the oropharynx and neck that can be outlined by direct inspection, mirror examination, and palpation. Assessment of the two-dimensional tumor extent can be made rela-

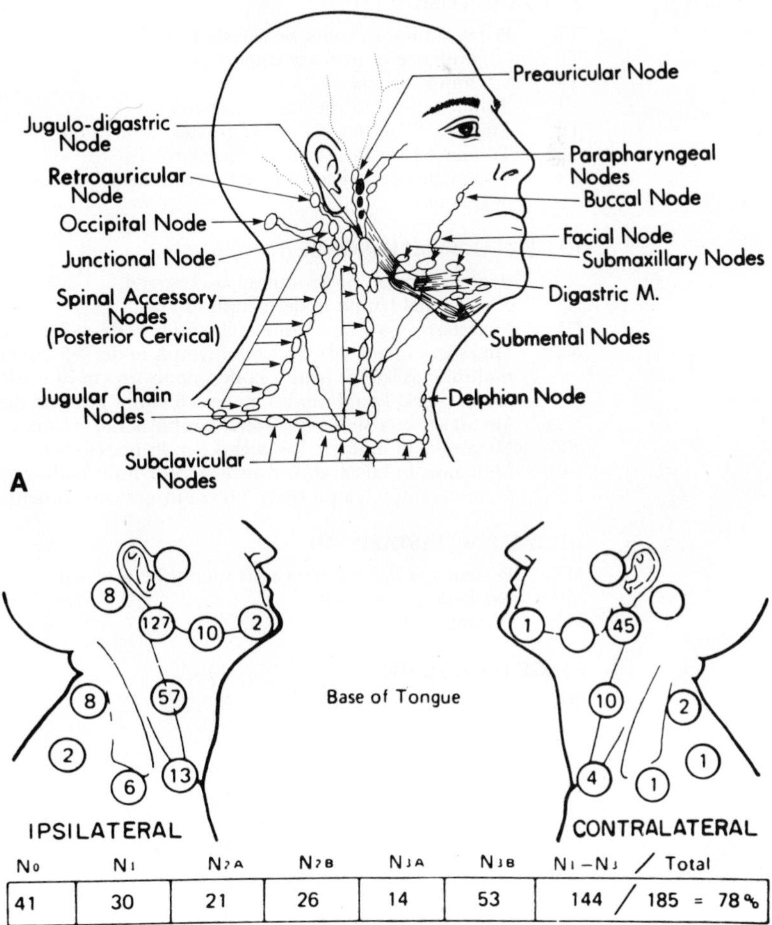

N0	N1	N2A	N2B	N3A	N3B	N1–N3 / Total
41	30	21	26	14	53	144 / 185 = 78%

FIGURE 33–2. (**A**) Lymphatics of the head and neck. Both deep (*shaded*) parapharyngeal and superficial nodes (jugulodigastric) are commonly involved. (**B**) Distribution of nodal involvement at presentation of squamous cell carcinoma of the base of the tongue. (Lindberg RD: Cancer 29:1466, 1972)

TABLE 33–1
Diagnostic Workup for Carcinoma of the Base of the Tongue

History
Physical examination
Inspection
Indirect laryngoscopy
Palpation
Direct laryngoscopy
Chest radiography
Computed tomography of head and neck
Biopsy

tively well by mirror examination and palpation when the patient is awake, but the third dimension of the tumor, depth of penetration, is best determined by bimanual palpation of the patient under anesthesia when the tongue is relaxed and the patient free of pain. Plain x-ray films rarely show disease that was not suspected clinically, and even benign conditions may simulate tumor radiographically; double contrast studies have been suggested for diagnosis of base of the tongue cancers.[1,26] Computed tomography scans may reveal retropharyngeal nodes or deep primary extension otherwise unappreciated.[38]

Biopsy is best performed in the primary site, leaving clinically apparent neck disease undisturbed before definitive therapy. Neck wound contamination by incisional biopsy of neck nodes if a primary lesion is elusive may be avoided by biopsies of nonvisible palpable lesions of the base of the tongue or blind biopsies in patients suspected of having tongue cancer.

STAGING

Staging depends on primary size, tongue fixation, and nodal size, number, and location. The 1988 American Joint Committee system is shown in Table 33-2.[3] Modifications of this system, such as that of Parsons and colleagues,[41] which separate Stage IV into Stages IVA and IVB, may help in choosing among various treatment modalities (Fig. 33-3).

PATHOLOGIC CLASSIFICATION

Squamous cell carcinomas, often poorly differentiated, account for more than 90% of cancers of the base of the tongue. Other cell types include non-Hodgkin's lymphomas (1.2%), which have a more favorable prognosis, and salivary gland tumors (*i.e.*, mucoepidermoid, adenocarcinoma or adenoid cystic type), which seem to behave more like salivary gland tumors of similar

TABLE 33–2
TNM Classification for Carcinoma of the Oropharynx

PRIMARY TUMOR (T)

TX	Primary tumor cannot be assessed
T0	No evidence of primary tumor
Tis	Carcinoma *in situ*
T1	Tumor ≤2 cm in greatest dimension
T2	Tumor >2 cm but <4 cm in greatest dimension
T3	Tumor >4 cm in greatest dimension
T4	Tumor invades adjacent structures (cortical bone, soft tissues of neck, deep [extrinsic] muscle of tongue)

REGIONAL LYMPH NODES (N)

NX	Regional lymph nodes cannot be assessed
N0	No regional lymph node metastasis
N1	Metastasis in a single ipsilateral lymph node, ≤3 cm in greatest dimension
N2	Metastasis in a single ipsilateral lymph node, >3 cm but <6 cm in greatest dimension; in multiple ipsilateral lymph nodes, none >6 cm in greatest dimension; or in bilateral or contralateral lymph nodes, none >6 cm in greatest dimension
N2a	Metastasis in a single ipsilateral lymph node, >3 cm but <6 cm in greatest dimension
N2b	Metastasis in multiple ipsilateral lymph nodes, none >6 cm in greatest dimension
N2c	Metastasis in bilateral or contralateral lymph nodes, none >6 cm in greatest dimension
N3	Metastasis in a lymph node >6 cm in greatest dimension

DISTANT METASTASIS (M)

MX	Presence of distant metastasis cannot be assessed
M0	No distant metastasis
M1	Distant metastasis

STAGE GROUPING

Stage 0	Tis	N0	M0
Stage I	T1	N0	M0
Stage II	T2	N0	M0
Stage III	T3	N0	M0
	T1	N1	M0
	T2	N1	M0
	T3	N1	M0
Stage IV	T4	N0,N1	M0
	Any T	N2,N3	M0
	Any T	Any N	M1

(Beahrs OH, Henson IE, Hutter RVF, Myers MH [eds]: Manual for Staging of Cancer, 3rd ed. Philadelphia, JB Lippincott, 1988)

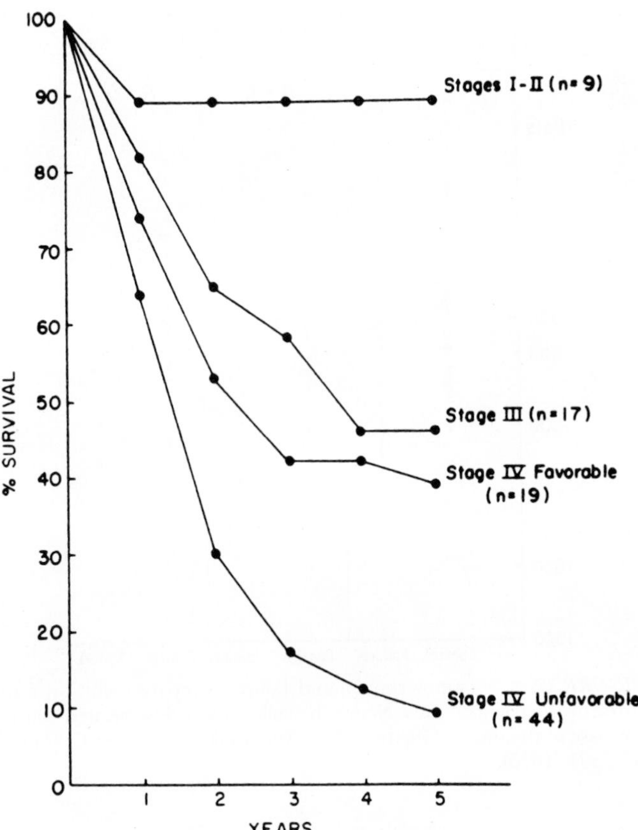

FIGURE 33–3. Survival compared with stage for base of the tongue cancer treated with radiation therapy. Notice the difference in Stage IV survival for T4N3 lesions (Stage IV, unfavorable). (Parsons JR, Million RR, Cassisi NJ: Laryngoscope 92:689, 1982)

histology in other sites than like squamous cell cancers of similar size and location.[2, 16, 23, 54, 55, 58]

PROGNOSTIC FACTORS

Treatment decisions for patients with base of the tongue cancer are best made by clinicians with a thorough understanding of the host and tumor characteristics that predict primary, nodal, or distant (TNM classification) relapse and survival. Host and tumor factors have been correlated with survival but not with primary, nodal, and distant relapses.[11, 13, 14, 20, 23] Some prognostic information has been derived from a study of oral and base of the tongue cancers and another study of cancers confined to the base of the tongue.[23, 46]

Age and sex are the *two host characteristics* that have prognostic significance. Survival declines with advancing age and is higher for females than males, presumably because of earlier detection of tumors in women.

Tumor characteristics that have prognostic significance include tumor size and extension, presence or absence of palpable lymph nodes, and location, number, and size of involved lymph nodes. Overall, base of the tongue cancers have a worse prognosis than do their oral tongue counterparts because of greater size at diagnosis, more frequent spread to adjacent structures, and higher rates of lymphatic spread. Stage for stage, they may have similar prognoses as oral tongue cancers.[31] Small tumors (*i.e.*, superficial surface lesions) have higher rates of local control by surgery or irradiation and a better prognosis than infiltrating or large tumors. Patients with tumors confined to the base of the tongue survive longer than those with tumors that extend to the faucial arch, oral cavity, or larynx and hypopharynx.[18, 21, 27, 41, 52, 58, 62] Patients with vallecular primary lesions have had a slightly poorer prognosis than those with base of the tongue primary tumors.[24] The prognosis is generally better for patients without palpable lymph nodes (N0) or better for those with small, ipsilateral, mobile lymph nodes than those with large, fixed, contralateral or bilateral nodes.[41] Treatment policies may modify these prognostic factors; our experience with preoperative irradiation and surgery showed no difference in survival for patients with N+ or those with N0 necks.[58]

GENERAL MANAGEMENT

The objectives of therapy are control of the primary tumor and regional lymph nodes, with preservation of deglutition, mandible, and phonation. Selection of tumors that can be controlled by surgery or irradiation alone is still not well understood, and the optimal combination of surgery and irradiation for control of intermediate-sized lesions with minimal complications is still debated.[8–10, 12, 21, 41] Unfortunately, many base of the tongue cancers are so large at diagnosis that total glossectomy and total laryngectomy are necessary, a choice often unpalatable to patients and surgeons alike; these patients may be irradiated for palliation.[18, 23, 27, 40, 49]

The clinical course of patients treated by surgery only or full-course irradiation requires a 2-year follow-up to detect 90% of primary and nodal recurrences, but select groups of patients treated by preoperative irradiation and surgery have required up to 4 years to manifest this fraction of recurrences.[9, 23, 46, 54, 56] Recurrence in a dissected neck is unusual, but contralateral neck failure in preoperatively irradiated patients has been the predominate type of neck failure (77%).[58, 67] Distant metastases to lung, bone, liver, and brain may occur late in follow-up, often in patients whose primary tumor and nodes have been controlled by the original treatment.[14, 58] It is likely that some who died of locoregional regrowth of tumor already harbored distant micrometastases that had not yet grown to detectable size.

Control of a base of the tongue tumor that has regrown after original treatment is difficult and uncommon. Usually the only patients salvaged by additional treatment are those who undergo neck dissection for involved lymph nodes in the contralateral neck site. Two thirds of patients die of tumor (50% local or 20% distant), and one third die of complications of treatment, chronic illness, or second primary cancers.[32, 56, 58] Second primary tumors occur in as many as 20% of the patients treated for base of the tongue cancer.[32, 41, 58]

Surgery

Surgical resection by way of a mandibular osteotomy and neck dissection has been recommended for T1 and T2 cancers. Radical neck dissection yields data for determining the need for postoperative irradiation, which is recommended in patients with disease more extensive than Stage N1. If this approach is used, almost all patients with T1 and T2 primary cancers can retain the mandible.[15] In our series from Washington University, 47% of patients treated with combined surgery and preoperative irradiation had their mandibles preserved.[58] For T3 and T4 tumors, composite resection and flap reconstruction are more often required.

Tumors of the lower base of the tongue that involve the

valleculae and extend inferiorly to the supraglottic larynx and pyriform sinus may be controlled by partial glossectomy and subtotal supraglottic laryngectomy or partial laryngopharyngectomy with preservation of voice.[46,58] Conditions required for a subtotal supraglottic laryngectomy include no gross involvement of pharyngoepiglottic fold, preservation of one lingual artery, resection of less than 80% of base of the tongue, pulmonary function suitable for supraglottic laryngectomy, and a medical condition suitable for major operation. Patients who require extensive glossectomy (*i.e.*, more than half of the base of the tongue or both lingual arteries) or those who are elderly or have poor pulmonary function require total laryngectomy to prevent subsequent chronic aspiration.[18,23,27,40,45] A surgical technique that allows base of the tongue resection with supraglottic laryngectomy and without aspiration has been described by Weisberger and Lingeman.[66] Lesions that crossed the midline were considered inoperable because they demanded sacrifice of the opposite lingual artery, both hypoglossal nerves, and the superior laryngeal nerves as well as total glossectomy.[28,40,49] Surgical resection and reconstruction may be a reasonable choice for some patients.[50]

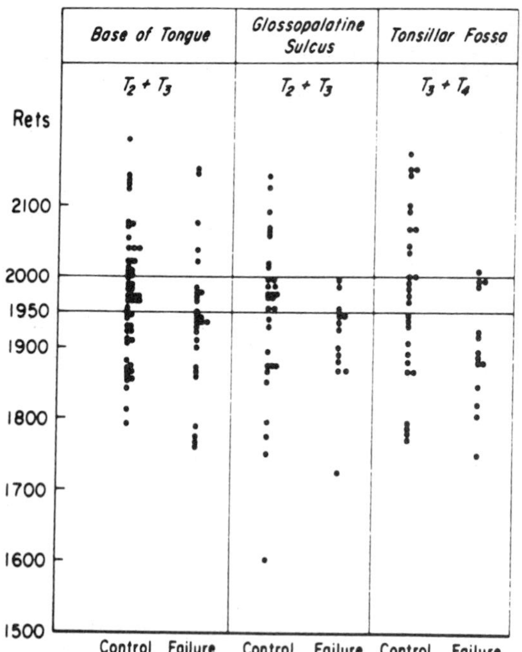

FIGURE 33–4. Tumor control and failure compared with dose for three oropharyngeal sites. Notice the lack of clear dose-related control for base of the tongue. (Spanos W Jr, Shukovsky L, Fletcher G: Cancer 37:2591, 1976)

Irradiation Alone

Irradiation alone is advocated for small tumors, surface tumors, and exophytic lesions that do not limit protrusion of the tongue, because primary and regional tumor control is quite good in these cases.[30] Base of tongue primary lesions fail more frequently and are less amenable to salvage surgery than anterior tonsillar pillar, tonsillar fossa, or soft palate primary tumors.[24]

Proper selection of patients for irradiation alone is essential to achieve good results. This requires examination of the tongue with the patient awake and asleep to accurately gauge the extent of the primary tumor.

Irradiation success is usually a function of tumor volume and morphology. Small T1 and T2 base of the tongue tumors without significant infiltration and surface or exophytic T2 and T3 lesions of the glossopharyngeal sulcus (glossopalatine sulcus) are readily controlled by high-dose radiation therapy (Fig. 33-4).[53] Size for size, surface and exophytic tumors of the glossopharyngeal sulcus regress more readily and are more easily controlled by irradiation than the usual infiltrating base of the tongue cancer. The poor response of infiltrating or endophytic base of the tongue tumors has been attributed to hypoxia.[21,53,58]

Large, unresectable base of the tongue cancers that cross the midline and infiltrate and fix the tongue are often irradiated palliatively to achieve as much tumor regression as possible. Those that prove responsive may even be controlled long term by high-dose irradiation.[41,46]

Surgery and Irradiation

Surgery combined with irradiation is best suited for intermediate or large tumors that extend beyond the base of the tongue or infiltrate and partially fix the tongue. Tumors of the upper base of the tongue confined to one side may be resected with preservation of the mandible and primary closure of the pharynx.[8,52,58,67] Bulky tumors that extend anteriorly into the oral cavity and superiorly or laterally to the faucial arch or pharyngeal wall may also be resected, but hemimandibulectomy and myocutaneous flap reconstruction are often necessary to facilitate closure.[18,57]

Adjuvant preoperative or postoperative irradiation should be routinely used for resectable T3 and T4 base of the tongue cancers to reduce the likelihood of recurrence.[42,62] Doses of 6000 cGy are necessary because of the significant primary tumor burden and the high rate of unilateral and bilateral lymphatic spread. Radiation therapy in these doses is better delivered postoperatively than preoperatively, because higher doses can be given after pharyngeal and cutaneous suture lines have healed.[17,59] Recent reviews demonstrate a trend to the more frequent use of radiation therapy after surgical resection.[6,62,63]

New Approaches

There are several new approaches in the management of base of the tongue cancers:

1. Better use of treatment planning and boost doses of irradiation with high-energy x-rays, submental electron beams, or interstitial implants to selectively increase the dose in the base of the tongue without damaging the larynx or mandible
2. Radiation sensitizers, hyperthermia, and high-linear-energy-transfer radiations in unresectable base of the tongue cancers
3. Chemotherapy in untreated patients with advanced tumors followed by surgery or radiation therapy, which should continue to be evaluated in prospective, controlled clinical trials
4. Microvascular surgery and myocutaneous flaps to improve functional results after extensive resections

RADIATION THERAPY TECHNIQUES

Definitive Irradiation

Irradiation portals for base of the tongue cancer should encompass the primary tumor and its local and regional extensions. Portals should extend superiorly to the base of skull and the floor of the sphenoid sinus to include the retropharyngeal lymphatics, anteriorly to include the faucial arch and a portion of the oral tongue, inferiorly to include the supraglottic larynx, and posteriorly to include the posterior cervical triangle. The primary tumor and both sides of the upper neck are irradiated through opposing lateral fields. Both sides of the lower neck are irradiated through a single anteroposterior field with a midline block at the junction between the upper lateral and low-neck fields to prevent spinal cord injury (Fig. 33-5).

Supine patients with bite-block immobilization receive daily treatment of all fields. The spinal cord is shielded after administration of 4000 cGy to 4500 cGy, and the posterior cervical triangles are boosted with electrons to spare the underlying spinal cord. Ellis compensators are used to ensure dose homogeneity and to prevent excessive dose to the supraglottic larynx.

After 4000 cGy to 4500 cGy with low-energy megavoltage beams, the remaining dose may be delivered with high-energy x-rays to concentrate the dose centrally and to reduce the dose to the parotids, the mandible, and the temporomandibular joints. After 6000 cGy are delivered, the field is reduced to encompass only the primary tumor, and weighted to the side involved by tumor with the high-energy beam. The boost dose after 6000 cGy may also be delivered by a submental electron beam or low-energy photon field. Doses to the primary tumor and palpable lymph nodes range from 6500 cGy to 7500 cGy delivered in 6.5 to 7.5 weeks; doses for elective irradiation of subclinical microscopic lymphatic metastases should be at least 5000 cGy. Treatment plans illustrating dose distributions are shown in Figure 33-6.

Preoperative Irradiation

Preoperative irradiation is designed to reduce the size of the primary tumor and palpable lymph nodes and to eradicate microscopic local extensions and subclinical locoregional metastases. Fields and beam direction are similar to those used for full-course irradiation. Preoperative doses of 4500 cGy to 5000 cGy are given in 4 to 5 weeks.

Interstitial Implants

Intraoral placement of radium needles into the base of the tongue is difficult, but skill in percutaneous placement of hollow steel needles and plastic afterloading tubes as described by Pierquin and associates[43] can be acquired. Employing these techniques, interstitial implantation of the base of the tongue for primary or recurrent tumors has become routine procedure in our clinic. Others have also advocated interstitial implantation as a boost for base of the tongue cancer, and a nonlooping technique has been described by several investigators.[5,25,44,60,61] Foote and associates,[22] however, reported no improvement in local control or decrease in morbidity for patients boosted with an implant compared to external irradiation for base of the tongue cancer.

Dose Response

When those few tumors treated with the lowest doses are excluded, there appears to be a slight dose-response correlation for T3 tumors, a moderate association for T1 and T2 base of the tongue cancers, and a marked dose-response relationship for T2 and T3 glossopalatine sulcus cancers (Fig. 33-7). Improved tumor control with increasing doses is a function of tumor volume and morphology; small base of the tongue cancers and exophytic cancers of the glossopalatine sulcus are more radioresponsive and controllable than large infiltrating tumors.[46] Increasing dose is strongly advocated for small, surface, and exophytic lesions but less for large, infiltrating T4 lesions, because there is less chance of improved tumor control but an increased risk of damage the mandible and larynx with higher doses. Determining optimal dose is difficult because improved tumor control and incidence of mandibular necrosis begin to increase simultaneously for doses in excess of 7000 cGy administered in 7 weeks.[4] Conservation surgery with preservation of mandible and phonatory larynx and postoperative irradiation (6000 cGy in 6 weeks) may achieve the same tumor control with

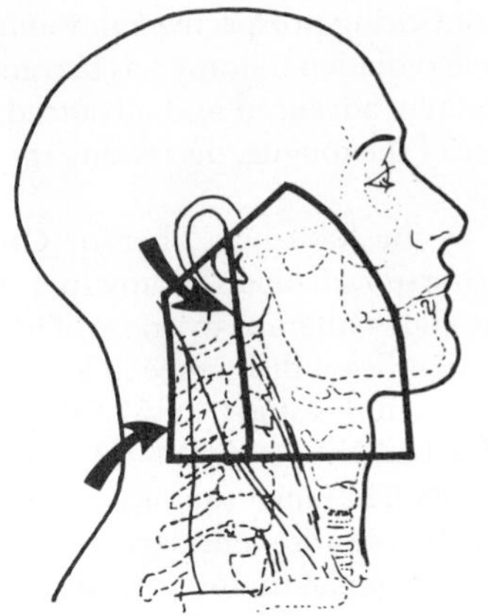

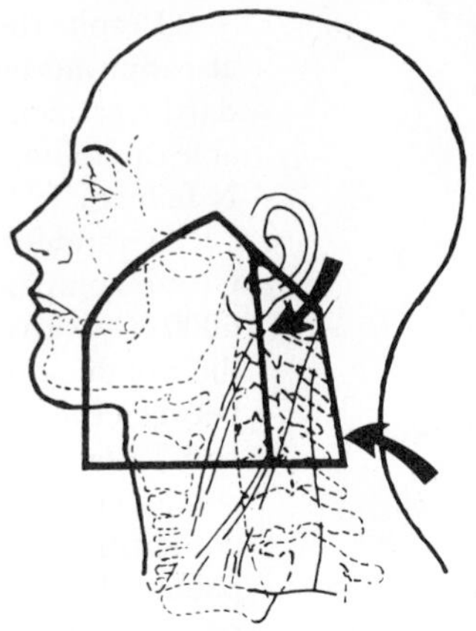

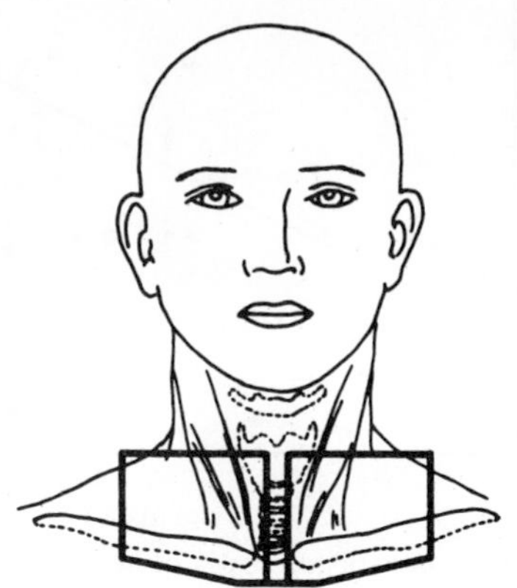

FIGURE 33–5. Portal arrangements for cancer of the base of the tongue. Field size reduction (*arrows*) after 4000 cGy to 4500 cGy protects the spinal cord.

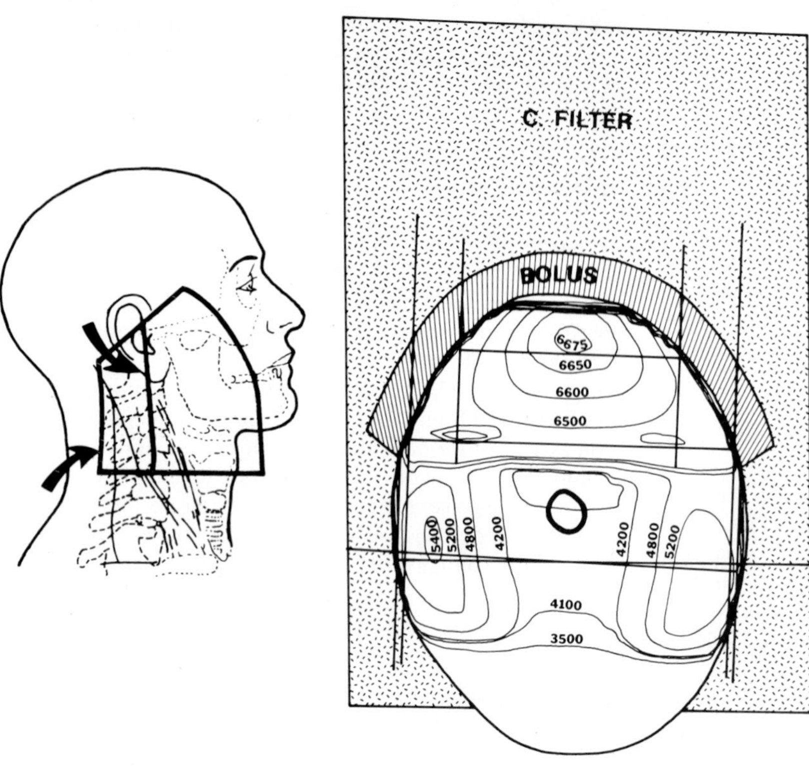

FIGURE 33–6. Isodose plan showing delivery of 6500 cGy to 6600 cGy to the primary tumor volume and 5000 cGy electively to the neck.

preservation of function and fewer complications than more radical irradiation or radical surgery.

SUMMARY OF CLINICAL TRIALS

Prospective clinical trials with combinations of irradiation and surgery for base of the tongue cancer have been few and unilluminating. Lawrence and associates[34] studied the use of 1400 cGy preoperatively in two equal fractions completed 24 hours before surgery in 69 patients with head and neck cancer, including tongue, tonsil, soft palate, and hypopharyngeal primary tumors. They compared this group with 74 patients receiving surgery alone, and found no difference in local control, morbidity, or mortality.

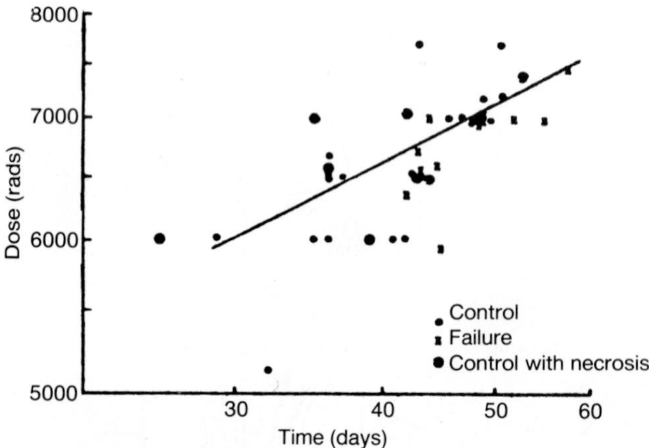

FIGURE 33–7. Dose-response curve for T2 and T3 cancers of the glossopalatine sulcus. (Spanos W Jr, Shukovsky L, Fletcher G: Cancer 37:2591, 1976)

Vandenbrouck and associates[59] attempted to deliver 5500 cGy preoperatively in 5.5 weeks, followed in 2 weeks by surgery or 5500 cGy delivered postoperatively in 6 weeks beginning less than 4 weeks after surgery to patients with hypopharyngeal primary lesions. Only 49 patients were entered before the trial was discontinued because of prohibitive morbidity and mortality (17%) in the preoperative radiation therapy group. The 5-year survival rate in the preoperative group was only 14%, significantly lower than the rate of 56% in the postoperative group, leading the authors to conclude that preoperative radiation therapy with a "curative dose" was not the best therapeutic strategy for patients with operable tumors of the hypopharynx.

Strong and colleagues[57] compared 100 patients with Stage II and III cancers of the oropharynx treated with 2000 cGy preoperatively in 5 days and surgery within 30 days or with surgery alone. There was no difference in the 5-year survival rate, which was 40% for the two groups. However, both groups had unacceptably high rates (56%) of recurrence in the neck after treatment.

Despite the lack of convincing prospective randomized trials, adjuvant postoperative radiation therapy has become standard treatment in moderately advanced and advanced, operable carcinoma of the base of the tongue, decreasing the T and N failures.[62,63]

A randomized trial by the Radiation Therapy Oncology Group comparing split-course radiation therapy to a dose of 6000 cGy with continuous-course therapy to a dose of 6600 cGy did not demonstrate any significant difference in local control between the treatment arms. In this study, 89% of the patients had T2 or T3 disease, 75% had N+, and 60% N3. All five T1 and seven of ten T2 patients had initial tumor control. When both primary and regional disease were considered, only 38% of patients became free of locoregional tumor. Five-year survival results in this group of patients were poor, with only 15% surviving. The overall locoregional failure rates were 84% in the continuous-course group and 73% in the split-course group. These results suggest that external irradiation alone to these doses is insufficient for advanced base of the tongue carcinoma.[39] Horiot and associates reported no difference in 3-year survival but a significant improvement in 3-year locoregional tumor control for bid treatment to 805 cGy versus daily irradiation to 7000 cGy.[29]

A retrospective study of accelerated fractionation showing improved local tumor control in carcinomas of the oropharynx, half of which arose in the base of the tongue, was reported by Wang.[65] At 36 months, he obtained an actuarial local control rate of 97% for T1 and T2 lesions and 77% for T3 and T4 lesions. For all stages, the local control rate was 77%. This compared with only 47% for patients treated with external irradiation using conventional rather than accelerated fractionation.

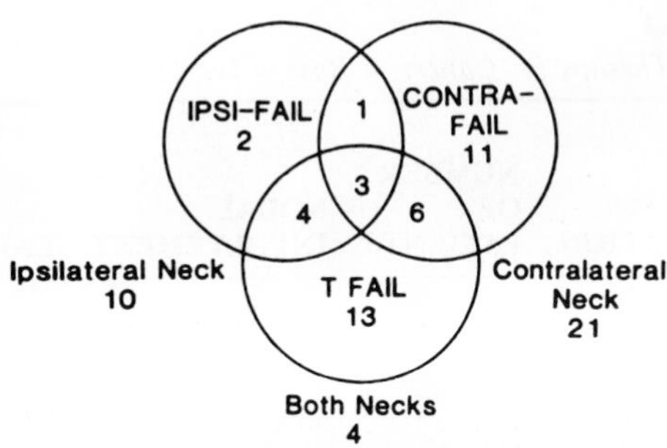

FIGURE 33–8. Venn diagram showing distribution of T and N failures in 50 patients who relapsed after preoperative (ipsilateral) radiation therapy and surgery for cancer of the base of the tongue. (Thawley SE, Simpson JR, Perez CA, et al: Ann Otol Rhinol Laryngol 92:485, 1983)

RESULTS OF THERAPY

Several authors have reported the advantages of external irradiation plus interstitial implant for treating base of the tongue lesions, particularly T1 or T2 lesions. Housset and colleagues[20] reported a local failure rate of 20% with external irradiation plus implantation but a rate of 43% with external irradiation alone.[30] Surgery plus external irradiation produced similar results, as did implantation. Because surgery was practical only for peripheral base of the tongue tumors and deemed to have rather poor functional results, external irradiation plus interstitial implant was favored for T1 and T2 lesions. Crook and coworkers[9] reported their 10-year experience with external irradiation and implant for T1 and T2 base of the tongue cancers. They had a 5-year local control rate of 85% for T1 tumors and 71% for T2 tumors. The overall disease-free survival rate at 5 years was 50%.

Puthawala and associates reported their 10-year experience with limited external-beam irradiation and interstitial implant in treating 70 patients.[44] Eighty-three percent of these were Stage T3 or T4 and had N2 or N3 neck disease. The primary site, vallecula, pharyngeal wall, glossopalatine sulcus, and tonsillar bed and pillars were routinely implanted to encompass the target volume. The neck nodes were separately implanted in these cases. Locoregional tumor control for a minimum of 2 years was obtained in 77% of all patients. The overall 5-year actuarial survival rate for the entire group was 35%. There was no difference in actuarial survival between patients with N0 and N1 neck disease, but patients with N2 or N3 disease had inferior survival rates.

Overall treatment results for base of the tongue cancer appear to be best for combinations of surgery and irradiation, intermediate for radiation therapy alone, and worst for surgery alone.[11,28,41,46,47,56,58,63,67]

There are two series that speak to the results of surgical therapy alone for base of the tongue cancer. Of 252 patients from the Memorial Sloan-Kettering Cancer Center, 56% patients subsequently failed in after resection bed or neck.[28] The 5-year survival rate was also low (21%), and there was little opportunity for salvage after primary treatment failure. The results obtained by Whicker and colleagues[68] at the Mayo Clinic are considerably better, but they reflect a different patient population. Of 102 patients, 42% survived 5 years after surgical treatment but only 55% of patients initially had neck node involvement, a low figure compared with most series. In addition, some of their patients had recurrences after primary radiation therapy for early lesions. Thirty-seven percent of patients experienced local or regional disease relapse. These results have not been duplicated in other surgical series.

Because even moderately advanced lesions of the base of the tongue have a significant propensity for bilateral neck disease, the surgical approach may be incomplete if bilateral neck exploration is not done. This limitation is not encountered in radiation therapy of base of the tongue cancers because bilateral neck treatment is routine even in the N0 cases. Ipsilateral neck treatment alone with preoperative radiation therapy yields an unacceptably high rate of contralateral neck recurrences (Fig. 33-8).[58] Control of the primary tumor and lymph nodes, along with prognosis, progressively declines with advancing T and N stages.[34,41,45,47,49,52] Table 33-3 compares the results of various therapeutic approaches.

SEQUELAE OF TREATMENT

High-dose irradiation for base of the tongue cancer causes acute side effects, such as severe mucositis, difficulty in swallowing, loss of taste, dry mouth, and weight loss. Patients must be observed carefully, and nasogastric intubation may become necessary to ensure adequate hydration and caloric intake. Late complications of high doses of irradiation occur in a fourth of the patients (Table 33-4) and cause significant morbidity. Necrosis of bone and cartilage with associated pain is a difficult management problem and can necessitate removal of the mandible. Doses of irradiation greater than 7000 cGy in 7 weeks can be avoided by using compensating filters to ensure dose homogeneity and high-energy x-rays to spare the mandible, temporomandibular joints, and subcutaneous tissues. Moderate doses of adjuvant irradiation of 5000 cGy to 6000 cGy delivered in 5 to 6 weeks in combination with conservation surgery significantly reduces the incidence of late radiation complications without compromising tumor control.

Surgery for base of the tongue cancer is associated with an operative mortality that ranges from 4% to 7%, which may be justified in view of the improved tumor control and reduction in late radiation-induced sequelae. Because of the proximity of pharyngeal and cutaneous suture lines to the carotid artery, formation of pharyngocutaneous fistulas with carotid artery rupture is an ever present danger.

MANAGEMENT OF RECURRENT TUMORS

Treatment options for recurrent tumors include surgical resection, radiation implants, external-beam irradiation, cryotherapy, laser therapy, chemotherapy, and hyperthermia. Patients with recurrences in the neck can sometimes be salvaged by

TABLE 33–3
Results of Therapy for Cancer of Base of the Tongue

INVESTIGATION	NUMBER OF PATIENTS	NODAL INVOLVEMENT	LARYNGECTOMY	MANDIBLE PRESERVED	OPERATIVE MORTALITY	5-YR SURVIVAL RATE, DETERMINATE	LOCAL FAILURE (T AND N)
SURGERY							
Harold[28]	204	70%	42%	42%	78%	21%	56%
Whicker[68]	102 (56+R)	55%	23% total (16%) partial (7%)		4%	42%	37%
(80% = T1 T3)							
RADIATION THERAPY							
Wang[64]	190	73%				34% 3-yr 39% salvage	
Parsons[41]	89	83%					
Spanos[53]	174	76%					26 (T only)
Riley[45]	97	76%				26%	53%
SURGERY AND RADIATION THERAPY							
Thawley[58]	101	74%	2% total 33% partial	41%		45%	40%
Riley[45]	28					25%	22%

radical neck dissection alone, and small primary recurrences may respond well to surgery or radiation implants. Interstitial irradiation combined with interstitial hyperthermia was believed to be superior to irradiation alone in the patient with recurrences.[19] Langois and co-workers,[33] however, reported a 67% probability of local control in 123 patients with recurrent base of the tongue cancer treated with ^{192}Ir or with second primary lesions arising in previously irradiated areas.

CHEMOTHERAPY

The role of chemotherapy has been limited. There are few agents that produce significant regression of the primary and regional tumors.[14,20,35] In view of their limited efficacy and substantial toxicity, particularly in the aged and nutritionally deprived patient, it is difficult to justify the adjuvant use of drugs in this group without a carefully designed protocol study or better predictors for therapeutic response. Because the rate of distant metastasis is significant, particularly in patients with advanced nodal involvement, there is a rationale for developing a successful systemic treatment. Newer drug combinations, usually containing cisplatin, have shown high complete response rates in nonkeratinizing head and neck cancers, and they should be tested further in prospective clinical trials.[20]

TABLE 33–4
Complications of Radiation Treatment for Cancer of the Base of the Tongue

COMPLICATION	NUMBER OF PATIENTS (%)*
Osteonecrosis of mandible	6 (6%)
Severe neck fibrosis	8 (8%)
Severe mucositis or edema	4 (4%)
C5–6 osteomyelitis	1 (1%)
Cerebral vascular accident	1 (1%)
Dehydration after irradiation	1 (1%)
Epiglottic ulcer, tracheitis, hemorrhage	1 (1%)
Bilateral hypoglossal nerve paralysis	1 (1%)
Laryngeal chondritis tracheostomy	1 (1%)
Necrosis of cricoid cartilage	1 (1%)
Patients with one or more complications	24 (23%)

** Total number of patients treated was 104.*
(Weller SA, Goffinet DR, Goode RL, et al: AJR 126:236, 1976 © by American Roentgen Ray Society, 1976)

REFERENCES

1. Apter AJ, Levine MS, Glick SN: Carcinomas of the base of the tongue: Diagnosis using double-contrast radiography of the pharynx. Radiology 15:123, 1984
2. Batsakis JG. (ed): Tumors of the Head and Neck: Clinical and Pathological Considerations, 2nd ed, pp 144–176. Baltimore, Williams & Wilkins, 1979
3. Beahrs OH, Henson DE, Hutter RVF, Myers MH (eds): Manual for Staging of Cancer, 3rd ed, pp 34–35. Philadelphia, JB Lippincott, 1988
4. Bedwinek JM, Shukovsky LJ, Fletcher GH, et al: Osteonecrosis in patients with definitive radiotherapy for squamous cell carcinomas of the oral cavity and naso- and oropharynx. Radiology 119:665, 1976
5. Blumberg A, Fu K, Phillips T: Results of treatment of carcinoma of the base of the tongue, the UCSF experience, 1957–1976. Int J Radiat Oncol Biol Phys 5:1971, 1979
6. Callery CD, Spiro RH, Strong EW: Changing trends in the management of squamous carcinoma of the tongue. Am J Surg 148:449, 1984
7. CA 41(1):28, 1991
8. Crews Q, Fletcher G: Comparative evaluation of the sequential use of irradiation and surgery in primary tumors of the oral cavity, oropharynx, larynx, and hypopharynx. AJR 111:73, 1971
9. Crook J, Mazeron J-J, Marinello G, et al: Combined external irradiation and interstitial implantation for T1 and T2 epidermoid carcinomas of base of the tongue: The Creteil experience (1971–1981). Int J Radiat Oncol Biol Phys 15:105, 1988

10. Cummings C, Goepfert H, Myers E: Squamous cell carcinoma of the base of the tongue. Arch Otolaryngol Head Neck Surg 9:56, 1986
11. Dalley V: The place of radiotherapy in the treatment of tumors of the base of the tongue. AJR 93:20, 1965
12. Davidson TM: Letter to the Editor. Arch Otolaryngol Head Neck Surg 9:312, 1987
13. del Regato JA, Spjut HJ, Cox JD (eds): Cancer: Diagnosis, Treatment, and Prognosis, 6th ed, p 336. St. Louis, CV Mosby, 1985
14. Dennington ML, Carter DR, Meyers AD: Distant metastases in head and neck epidermoid carcinoma. Laryngoscope 90:196, 1980
15. DeSanto LW, Thawley SE: Treatment of tumors of the oropharynx. In Thawley SE, Panje W, Batsakis J (eds): Comprehensive Management of Head and Neck Tumors. Philadelphia, WB Saunders, 1986
16. DeVries EJ, Johnson JT, Myers EN, et al: Base of tongue salivary gland tumors. Arch Otolaryngol Head Neck Surg 9:329, 1987
17. Donald PJ: Complications of combined therapy in head and neck carcinomas. Arch Otolaryngol Head Neck Surg 104:329, 1978
18. Dupont A, Guillamondegui O. Jesse R: Surgical treatment of advanced carcinomas of the base of the tongue. Am J Surg 114:501, 1978
19. Emami B, Marks JE, Perez CA, et al: Interstitial thermoradiotherapy in the treatment of recurrent/residual malignant tumors. Am J Clin Oncol 7:699, 1984
20. Ervin TJ, Clark JR, Weichselbaum RR: Multidisciplinary treatment of advanced squamous carcinoma of the head and neck. Semin Oncol 12:71, 1985
21. Fletcher G (ed): Textbook of Radiotherapy, 3rd ed, p 322. Philadelphia, Lea & Febiger, 1980
22. Foote RL, Parsons JT, Mendenhall WM, et al: Is interstitial implantation essential for successful radiotherapeutic treatment of base of the tongue carcinoma? Proc Am Radium Soc April 1989
23. Frazell E, Lucas J Jr: Cancer of the tongue. Cancer 15:218, 1967
24. Gelinas M, Fletcher G: Incidence and causes of local failure of irradiation in squamous cell carcinoma of the faucial arch, tonsillar fossa and base of the tongue. Radiology 108:383, 1973
25. Goffinet DR, Fee WE, Wells J, et al: ^{192}Ir pharyngoepiglottic fold interstitial implants: The key to successful treatment of base tongue carcinoma by radiation therapy. Cancer 55:941, 1985
26. Gromet M, Homer MJ, Carter BL: Lymphoid hyperplasia at the base of the tongue. Radiology 144:825, 1982
27. Hamberger AD, Fletcher GH, Guillamondegui OM, et al: Advanced squamous cell carcinoma of the oral cavity and oropharynx treated with irradiation and surgery. Radiology 119:433, 1976
28. Harrold C: Surgical treatment of cancer of the base of the tongue. Am J Surg 114:247, 1967
29. Horiot JC, LeFur R, Nguyen T, et al: Two fractions per day versus a single fraction per day in the radiotherapy of oropharynx carcinoma: Results of an EORTC randomized trial. Proceedings of the 30th Annual ASTRO meeting. Int J Radiat Oncol Biol Phys 15(Suppl 1): 179, 1988
30. Housset M, Baillet F, Dessard-Diana B, et al: A retrospective study of three treatment techniques for T1–T2 base of the tongue lesions: Surgery plus postoperative radiation, external radiation plus interstitial implantation and external radiation alone. Int J Radiat Oncol Biol Phys 13:511, 1987
31. Ildstad ST, Bigelow ME, Remensnyder JP: Squamous cell carcinoma of the tongue: A comparison of the anterior two thirds of the tongue with its base. Am J Surg 146:456, 1983
32. Jesse R, Sugarbaker E: Squamous cell carcinoma of the oropharynx: Why we fail. Am J Surg 132:435, 1976
33. Langlois D, Hoffstetter S, Malissard L, et al: Salvage irradiation of oropharynx and mobile tongue about 192 iridium brachytherapy in Centre Alexis Vautrin. Int J Radiat Oncol Biol Phys 14:849, 1988
34. Lawrence W, Terz JJ, Rogers C, et al: Preoperative irradiation for head and neck cancer: A prospective study. Cancer 33:318, 1975
35. Lester EP, Kinnealey AM, Matz GJ: Sequential combination chemotherapy for advanced squamous cell carcinoma of the head and neck. Laryngoscope 89:1921, 1979
36. Lindbergh RD: Distribution of cervical lymph node metastases from squamous cell carcinoma of the upper respiratory and digestive tracts. Cancer 29:1466, 1972
37. Lusinchi A, Eskandari J, Son Y, et al: External irradiation plus curietherapy boost in 108 base of the tongue carcinomas. Int J Radiat Oncol Biol Phys 17:1191, 1989
38. Mancuso AA, Hanafee WN (eds): Nasopharynx, oropharynx, parapharyngeal space, and floor of mouth: Normal anatomy and methodology. In Computed Tomography of the Head and Neck, p 112. Baltimore, Williams & Wilkins, 1982
39. Marcial VA, Hanley JA, Hendrickson F, et al: Split-course radiation therapy of carcinoma of the base of the tongue: Results of a prospective national collaborative clinical trial conducted by the Radiation Therapy Oncology Group. Int J Radiat Oncol Biol Phys 9:437, 1983.
40. Novak A: Treatment of carcinoma of the base of the tongue and the larynx. Laryngoscope 89:1332, 1975
41. Parsons JT, Million RR, Cassisi NJ: Carcinoma of the base of the tongue: Results of radical irradiation with surgery reserved for irradiation failure. Laryngoscope 92:689, 1982
42. Perez C, Marks J, Powers W: Preoperative irradiation in head and neck cancer. Semin Oncol 4:387, 1977
43. Pierquin B, Chassagne DJ, Chahbazian CM, et al: Brachytherapy, p 113. St. Louis, Warren G Green, 1978
44. Puthawala AA, Nisay Syed AM, Eads DL, et al: Limited external beam and interstitial ^{192}Ir irradiation in the treatment of carcinoma of the base of the tongue: A ten-year experience. Int J Radiat Oncol Biol Phys 14:839, 1988
45. Riley RW, Lee WE, Goffinet D, et al: Squamous cell carcinoma of the base of the tongue. Arch Otolaryngol Head Neck Surg 91:143, 1983
46. Rollo J, Rosenbom C, Thawley S, et al: Squamous carcinoma of the base of the tongue. Cancer 47:333, 1981
47. Scanlon PW, Soule EH, Devine KD, et al: Cancer of the base of the tongue. Radiology 1054:26, 1969
48. Schottenfeld D: Alcohol as a co-factor in the etiology of cancer. Cancer 43:1962, 1979
49. Sessions DG, Stallings JO, Brownson RJ, et al: Total glossectomy for advanced carcinoma of the base of the tongue. Laryngoscope 81:39, 1971
50. Sessions DG: Surgical resection and reconstruction for cancer of the base of the tongue. Otolaryngol Clin North Am 16:309, 1983
51. Shukovsky L, Baeza M, Fletcher G: Results of irradiation in squamous cell carcinomas of the glossopalatine sulcus. Radiology 120:405, 1976
52. Shumrick DA, Gluckman JL: Cancer of the oropharynx. In Suen JY, Myers EN (eds): Cancer of the Head and Neck. New York, Churchill-Livingstone, 1981
53. Spanos W Jr, Shukovsky L, FLetcher G: Time, dose, and tumor volume relationships in irradiation of squamous cell carcinomas of the base of the tongue. Cancer 37:2591, 1976
54. Spiro RH, Koss LG, Hajdu SI, et al: Tumors of minor salivary gland origin. Cancer 31:117, 1973
55. Spiro RH, Huvos AG, Strong EW: Adenoid cystic carcinoma of salivary origin. Am J Surg 128:512, 1974
56. Spiro RH, Strong EW: Surgical treatment of cancer of the tongue. Surg Clin North Am 54:233, 1974
57. Strong MS, Vaughan CW, Kayne HL, et al: A randomized trial of preoperative radiotherapy in cancer of the oropharynx and hypopharynx. Am J Surg 136:494, 1978
58. Thawley SE, Simpson JR, Perez CA, et al: Preoperative irradiation and surgery for carcinoma of the base of the tongue. Ann Otol Rhinol Laryngol 92:485, 1983
59. Vandenbrouck C, Sancho H, Le Fur R, et al: Results of a randomized clinical trial of preoperative irradiation versus postoperative in treatment of tumors of the hypopharynx. Cancer 39:1445, 1977

60. Vikram B, Hilaris BS: A non-looping afterloading technique for interstitial implants of the base of the tongue. Int J Radiat Oncol Biol Phys 7:419, 1981
61. Vikram B, Strong EW, Shah J, et al: A non-looping afterloading technique for base of the tongue implants: Results in the first 20 patients. Int J Radiat Oncol Biol Phys 11:1853, 1985
62. Vikram B, Strong EW, Shah JP, et al: Failure at the primary site following multimodality treatment in advanced head and neck cancer. Arch Otolaryngol Head Neck Surg 6:720, 1984
63. Vikram B, Strong EW, Shah JP, et al: Failure in the neck following multimodality treatment for advanced head and neck cancer. Arch Otolaryngol Head Neck Surg 6:724, 1984
64. Wang CC: Radiation Therapy for Head and Neck Neoplasms, p 146. Boston, John Wright, 1983
65. Wang CC: Local control of oropharyngeal carcinoma after two accelerated hyperfractionation radiation therapy schemes. Int J Radiat Oncol Biol Phys 14:1143, 1988
66. Weisberger EC, Lingeman RE: Modified supraglottic laryngectomy and resection of lesions of the base of the tongue. Laryngoscope 93:20,1983
67. Weller SA, Goffinet DR, Goode RL, et al: Carcinoma of the oropharynx: Results of megavoltage radiation therapy in 305 patients. AJR 126:236, 1976
68. Whicker JH, DeSanto LW, Devine KD: Surgical treatment of squamous cell carcinoma of the base of the tongue. Laryngoscope 82:1853, 1972

34

○ ○ ○ ● ● ●

Hypopharynx

James E. Marks
J. Gershon Spector

ANATOMY

The hypopharynx is divided into the pyriform sinus, pharyngeal wall, and postcricoid regions (Fig. 34-1). The hypopharynx communicates above with the oropharynx at the level of the pharyngoepiglottic folds and below with the cervical esophagus at the inferior margin of the cricoid cartilage. In order of decreasing frequency, hypopharyngeal cancers involve the pyriform sinus, the pharyngeal wall, and the postcricoid region.[31,39,41]

The pyriform sinus or the laryngopharyngeal sulcus is an inferior extension of the glossopharyngeal sulcus in the oropharynx, is bounded by three walls and an ill-defined apex at its inferior extent, and is open posteriorly. The medial wall is formed by the marginal structures of the larynx, including the free border of epiglottis, aryepiglottic fold, and arytenoid. The anterior wall is composed of soft tissue; the lateral wall is formed by thyroid cartilage.

The lateral wall of the pyriform sinus extends posteriorly to become the pharyngeal wall, which is formed by the superior, middle, and inferior pharyngeal constrictor muscles and lies in direct contact with prevertebral fascia and cervical vertebra.

The postcricoid region is a large mucosal surface covering the posterior surface of the cricoid cartilage, the partition between larynx and hypopharynx. It lies immediately below the interarytenoid notch, just medial and inferior to the apex of the pyriform sinus, and it forms the anterior wall of the lowest portion of the hypopharynx.

EPIDEMIOLOGY

The number of new pharyngeal cancers in the United States in 1990 was approximately 9000, and the number of deaths was 4000.[56] Because the reported incidence and mortality statistics for pharyngeal cancers may include cancers of the nasopharynx, oropharynx, and hypopharynx, the true incidence and mortality for hypopharyngeal cancers are probably less than reported.

The mean age for patients with pyriform sinus and pharyngeal wall cancers ranges from 60 to 65 years, depending on the series studied. Men are affected more often than women, with a ratio of 7 to 1 for pyriform sinus cancer and 4 to 1 for pharyngeal wall cancer.[42,43] In the United States, postcricoid cancer is rare. In Great Britain and Scandinavia, this type of cancer is more common and occurs with greater frequency in women.[1,16,24,68] In 70% of patients with postcricoid cancers originally reported by Ahlbom,[1] there was an associated triad of dysphagia, hypochromic anemia, and atrophic mucosal changes, known as Plummer-Vinson syndrome in Scandinavia and Paterson-Brown-Kelly syndrome in Great Britain.[26] The dysphagia, hypochromic anemia, and mucosal changes disappeared with adequate dietary intake of iron. The syndrome and postcricoid cancer became less frequent in Sweden after a law was passed in 1940 requiring iron fortification of flour.[1,24,68]

In the United States, almost all patients who develop hypopharyngeal cancer give a history of heavy tobacco use with or without alcohol consumption. The epidemiologic concept that tobacco is the primary etiologic agent for cancers of the larynx and hypopharynx and that alcohol in addition to tobacco merely enhances the risk of cancer has recently been challenged.[71] Tuyns and co-workers report that the carcinogenic effect of alcohol is present at the lowest levels of tobacco consumption and that alcohol influences the development of epilaryngeal and hypopharyngeal cancers more than the development of endolaryngeal cancer.[63] Presumably, alcohol bathes the mucosa of the epilarynx and hypopharynx but does not have access to the mucosa of the endolarynx. Second primary cancers of other aerodigestive sites occur in approximately one fifth of patients with hypopharyngeal cancer, indicating the multicentric nature of tobacco- and alcohol-induced neoplasia of aerodigestive epithelium exposed to common carcinogens.[28,41,65]

NATURAL HISTORY

The natural history of untreated cancers of the hypopharynx is unknown, but their clinical course after treatment is well documented. Irradiated tumors of the pyriform sinus, pharyngeal wall, and postcricoid region that recur usually do so in the primary site and neck within 1 year, as do pharyngeal wall cancers treated by preoperative irradiation and surgical excision.[37,39,41,42] Among pyriform sinus cancers treated by preoperative irradiation and surgical resection, most recurrences appear locoregionally within 2 years and spread to distant sites in lung, bone, brain, and liver a short time later. Because distant metastases appear later than primary or neck recurrences, the patient may die of locoregional disease before micrometastases

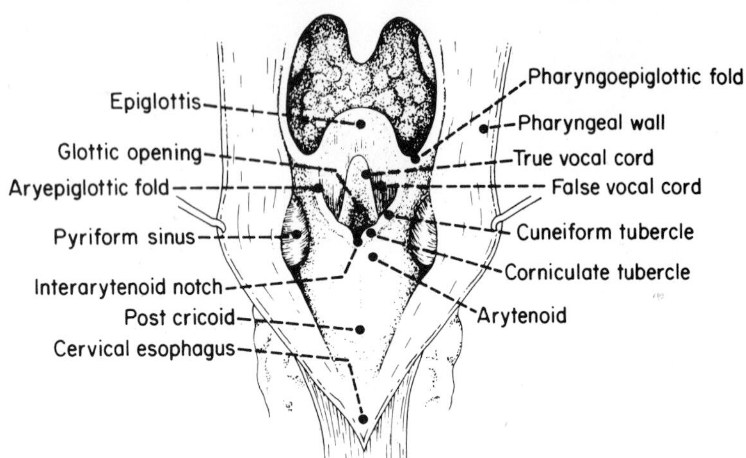

FIGURE 34–1. Posterior view of the hypopharynx, showing the topography of the pyriform sinus, pharyngeal wall, and postcricoid region. (Redrawn from Figge FHJ [ed]: Sobotta/Figge Atlas of Human Anatomy, ed 9, vol 2. Munich, Urban and Schwarzenberg, 1977)

in distant sites have enlarged to clinically perceptible size. Therefore, the incidence of distant metastases in patient populations whose locoregional disease is controlled is usually greater than the rate in populations who have locoregional recurrence.[42]

Retreatment of locally recurrent pyriform sinus or pharyngeal wall cancer is rewarded by few salvages and is usually successful only in patients who have completion laryngectomy for recurrent disease in the laryngeal remnant or in those who have neck dissection for a mobile lymph node in the opposite side of the neck.[42,65] The interval between relapse and death from hypopharyngeal cancers is short; most patients die within 1 year of treatment. The rates of relapse and death from tumor are most precipitous for pharyngeal wall cancers and large unresectable pyriform sinus and postcricoid cancers irradiated for palliation. For patients whose primary tumor and regional lymph nodes have been controlled, there exists a significant risk of developing a second epithelial cancer of the aerodigestive tract.

CLINICAL PRESENTATION

The cardinal presenting symptoms for carcinomas of the pyriform sinus, pharyngeal wall, and postcricoid region are sore throat, dysphagia, and hoarseness. This triad of symptoms also occurs with carcinomas of the supraglottic larynx, but with hypopharyngeal tumors, it is more often associated with a neck mass, otalgia, and weight loss. Emergency tracheostomy for airway obstruction is necessary in 5% to 10% of the patients with carcinomas of the pyriform sinus and pharyngeal wall.[39]

Patterns of Local Spread

Hypopharyngeal cancers, unlike laryngeal cancers, are not constrained by submucosal lymphatic compartments or barriers, and patterns of local invasion are usually more extensive.[22]

Pyriform Sinus Cancers

Cancers located on the medial wall of the pyriform sinus commonly invade the larynx and involve the aryepiglottic fold and arytenoid (Fig. 34-2).[50] They spread within the paraglottic space like transglottic cancers (Fig. 34-3) to involve the thyroarytenoid and other intrinsic muscles of the larynx.[30,50,52] They may involve the cricoarytenoid joints and the recurrent laryngeal nerves, structures intimately associated with the pyriform sinus mucosa (Fig. 34-1).[30,52] In one serial section study, three of 19 patients had invasion of the cricoarytenoid joints, and four of 19 had perineural invasion.[52]

Cancers of the lateral wall and apex of the pyriform sinus commonly invade thyroid cartilage and occasionally invade cricoid cartilage because the lateral wall and apex of the pyriform sinus are adjacent to the laryngeal skeleton (Figs. 34-2 and 34-3).[30,50,52] After penetrating the cartilaginous framework, they may also invade the thyroid gland.[50,52] They occasionally spread posteriorly around the thyroid ala to involve the external perichondrium without destroying cartilage.[50] Among 40 cases of pyriform sinus cancer involving the lateral wall studied by serial section, 20 invaded the thyroid cartilage and two invaded the cricoid ring.[30] The apex of the pyriform sinus was involved in all 22 cases, indicating that apical involvement usually is associated with invasion of the thyroid cartilage.

Pyriform sinus cancers develop ample submucosal microscopic extensions beyond the visible margins of the tumor, an average of 10 mm in one serial section study.[22,30,52]

Pharyngeal Wall Cancers

Only a few pharyngeal wall cancers have been studied by serial section technique. These showed widespread invasion of mucosa, submucosa, and muscle with tumor involving the margins of the specimen.[22] Because pharyngeal wall cancer is close to prevertebral fascia and spine, surgical excision with adequate deep margins is seldom possible.

Postcricoid Region Cancers

Postcricoid cancer commonly invades cricoid cartilage and interarytenoid and posterior cricothyroid muscles, producing hoarseness (Fig. 34-4).[52] Most lesions extend to adjacent anatomic regions, such as pyriform sinus, pharyngeal wall, and cervical esophagus. Because of this pattern of spread, Lederman[36] has suggested that the term epiesophageal should be used instead of postcricoid. One serial section study showed an average submucosal extension of 5 mm for postcricoid cancers.[22]

Patterns of Lymphatic Spread

The lymphatics in the hypopharynx are abundant, accounting for the relatively high rate of metastases to regional lymph

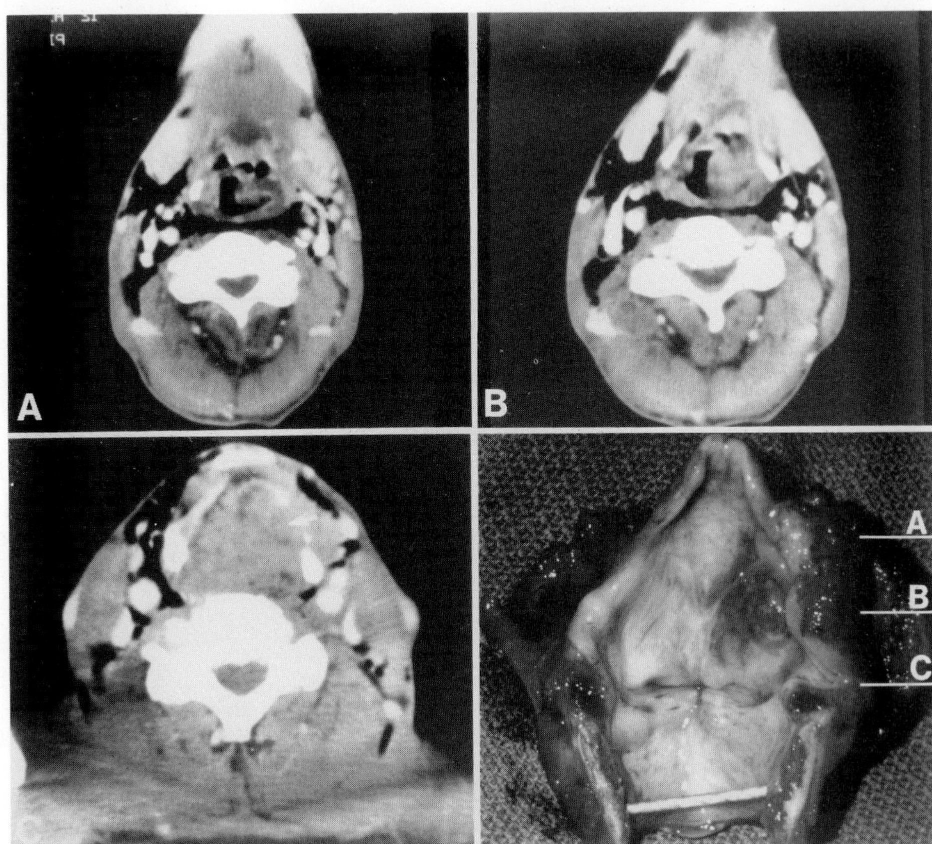

FIGURE 34–2. Computed tomography scans of the (A) upper, (B) middle, and (C) inferior pyriform sinus showing a large cancer invading the larynx, partly occluding the airway, destroying thyroid cartilage, and invading soft tissue.

nodes.[12,13,16,42,43,48,65,67] The midcervical lymph nodes are most commonly involved and the incidence of lymphatic metastasis varies according to the site of origin within the hypopharynx; the incidence of palpable lymph nodes is greatest for carcinoma of the pyriform sinus and intermediate for carcinomas of the pharyngeal wall and postcricoid region (Fig. 34-5). Although the incidence of nodal metastases progressively

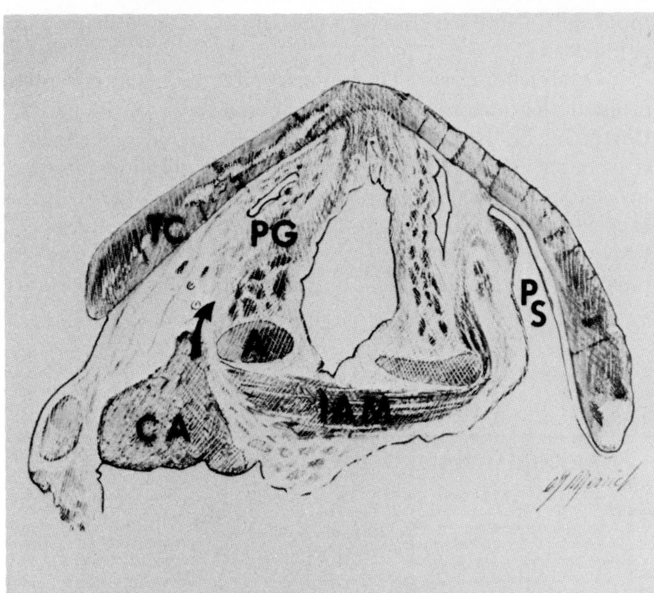

FIGURE 34–3. Horizontal cross-section of the larynx and hypopharynx, showing cancer of the pyriform sinus infiltrating the laryngeal paraglottic space. A, arytenoid cartilage; CA, cancer; IAM, interarytenoid muscle; PG, paraglottic space; TC, thyroid cartilage. (Kirchner JA: Ann Otol Rhinol Laryngol 84:793, 1975)

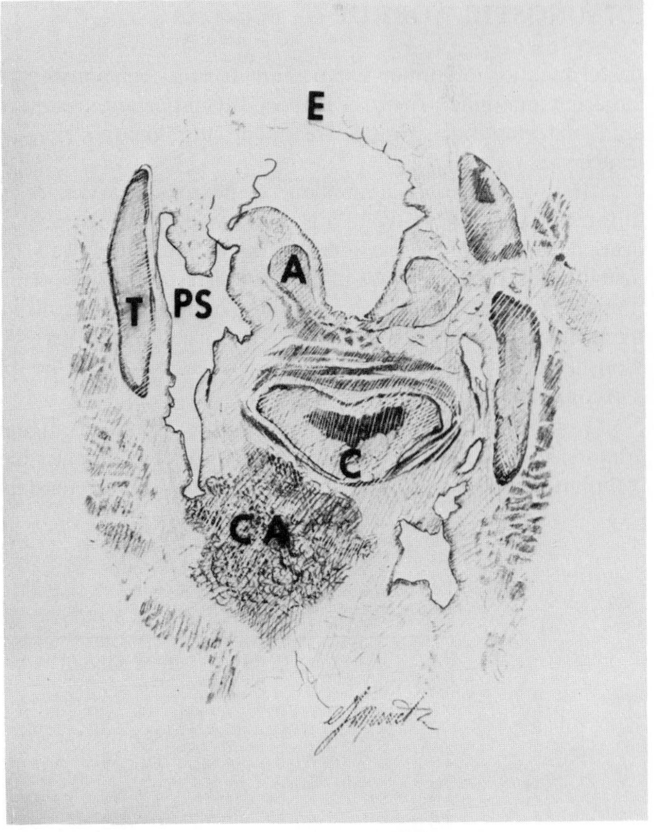

FIGURE 34–4. Coronal section of the hypopharynx, showing a postcricoid carcinoma. A, arytenoid cartilage; C, cricoid cartilage; CA, cancer; E, epiglottis; PS, pyriform sinus; T, thyroid cartilage. (Olofsson J, van Nostrand AWP: Acta Laryngol [Suppl] 308: 1, 1973)

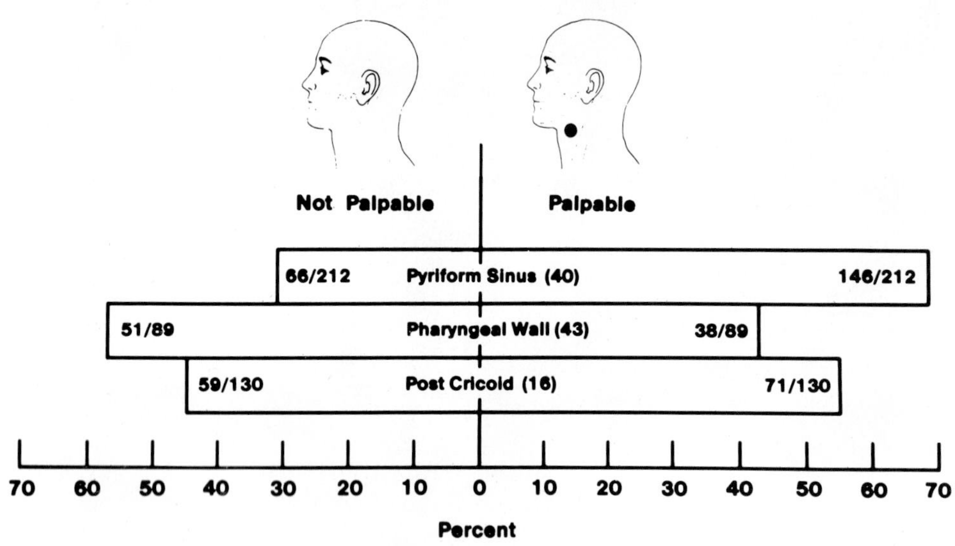

FIGURE 34–5. Bar graph showing the incidence of palpable lymph nodes for carcinomas of the pyriform sinus, pharyngeal wall, and postcricoid region.

increases with increasing tumor size for postcricoid cancers, there is only a weak association between tumor size and incidence of nodal metastases for pharyngeal wall cancer and none for carcinoma of the pyriform sinus (Table 34-1). The reasons for these differences are unclear, but they may be due to the difficulty in estimating tumor size, greater lymphatic density, or a greater proportion of nonkeratinizing tumors in the pyriform sinus than in the other two sites.

DIAGNOSTIC WORKUP

Determination of tumor extent and its exact relationship to adjacent anatomic structures is especially important in staging and determining surgical treatment for hypopharyngeal cancers.

Indirect mirror examination of the hypopharynx is an informative clinical study because it allows direct tumor visualization. Tumors of the pyriform sinus and pharyngeal wall can usually be seen, but lesions of the postcricoid region are often missed. Adequate visualization of these tumors requires direct pharyngoscopy and laryngoscopy. Tumor extent and its relationship to hypopharyngeal-laryngeal anatomy should be diagrammed carefully.

Examination of the neck is important for hypopharyngeal tumors, because these patients commonly present with palpable lymph nodes. Location, size, consistency, mobility, and tenderness are recorded for all lymph nodes. Occasionally a large, fixed mass in the neck is the result of a direct extension of pyriform sinus cancer through or posterior to the thyroid cartilage that involves the soft tissues of the neck. Tenderness usually indicates thyroid cartilage invasion, and loss of crepitation, evidenced by side-to-side movement of the larynx, indicates postcricoid tumor, with edema between the larynx, inferior hypopharynx, and spine.

Digital palpation of the tongue is necessary to detect induration caused by superior spread of tumor into the vallecula and base of the tongue.

Biopsy is performed at the time of video indirect pharyngoscopy or in the operating room during direct pharyngoscopy. Biopsy may be done using local or general anesthetic.

Radiographic studies are important in delineating tumor extent and planning treatment. Cartilage destruction may be shown by x-ray films of the larynx, xeroradiography, polytomography, computed tomography, or magnetic resonance imaging scans.

Other laboratory data are nonspecific, but it is important to evaluate the hematologic and nutritional status of the patient. Correcting low hemoglobin levels and nutritional abnormalities is essential to diminish postoperative complications and improve tolerance to radiation. Evaluation of pulmonary status is especially important because many of these patients have been heavy smokers and may tolerate anesthesia poorly. Patients who have relatively severe chronic obstructive pulmonary disease are

TABLE 34–1
Percentage of Nodal Metastases as a Function of Location and Tumor Size

SIZE OF TUMOR	PYRIFORM SINUS				PHARYNGEAL WALL			POSTCRICOID
	(12)*	(13)	(42)	(65)	(43)	(48)	(67)	(16)
T1	84	91	38	74	33	45	70	6
T2	83	82	67	83	31	36	79	17
T3	80	76	69	74	47	58	85	38
T4	98	69	63	60	70	82		50

* *The numbers in parentheses refer to studies in the reference list.*

unsuitable candidates for conservation surgery because of the risk of aspiration pneumonia. Evaluation of the liver is also important because many have been heavy drinkers.

STAGING

The American Joint Committee staging for tumors of the hypopharynx fails to describe anatomic sites within the hypopharynx involved by tumor and does not require an estimate of tumor size, both of which are prognostic and useful in selecting patients for conservation surgery or full-course radiation therapy.[2] The Ogura system for staging the primary tumor defines the anatomic sites involved and is particularly useful in selecting patients for conservation surgery.[41,42,51]

In pyriform sinus cancer, small lesions of the medial wall that secondarily involve the marginal structures of the larynx or those lesions confined to the upper two thirds of the pyriform sinus are amenable to conservation surgery, with sparing of the phonatory larynx. These same lesions are amenable to full-course irradiation. Invasion of the larynx with partial or complete fixation of vocal cord and involvement of the lateral wall or apex of the pyriform sinus (Fig. 34-2) contraindicate conservation surgery.[30,51,52] Fixation of the vocal cord by a pyriform sinus cancer that has invaded the larynx predicts poor outcome after irradiation.[4,60] In pharyngeal wall cancer, tumor size as determined at direct pharyngoscopy is important in predicting tumor control and prognosis after radiation treatment.[48,53] Tumor control and prognosis are also related to the length of tumor and invasion of the larynx by postcricoid cancers.[16,69] The American Joint Committee system for staging lymph nodes is shown in Table 34-2.

PATHOLOGIC CLASSIFICATION

Most tumors of the hypopharynx are squamous cell carcinomas. Uncommon lesions are adenocarcinomas, lymphomas, and sarcomas of various types, including liposarcomas, fibrosarcomas, and malignant fibrous histiocytomas.

In a study of 108 carcinomas of the pyriform sinus, two thirds were keratinizing and one third were nonkeratinizing.[45] The nonkeratinizing tumors were more often poorly differentiated than were the keratinizing tumors. The margins of the cancer were infiltrating in 80% and pushing in 20% of the specimens studied. Keratinization, degree of differentiation, and pattern of tumor-stromal interface had no significant association with cervical lymph node metastases.

PROGNOSTIC FACTORS

In hypopharyngeal cancers, the risk of complications after surgical treatment is significant, and knowledge of prognostic fac-

TABLE 34–2
T and N Staging for Cancers of the Hypopharynx

ANATOMIC SITE	STAGE	CHARACTERISTICS
Hypopharynx[2]	TX	Primary tumor cannot be assessed
	T0	No evidence of primary tumor
	Tis	Carcinoma *in situ*
	T1	Tumor limited to one subsite of hypopharynx
	T2	Tumor invades more than one subsite of hypopharynx or an adjacent site, without fixation of hemilarynx
	T3	Tumor invades more than one subsite of hypopharynx or an adjacent site, with fixation of hemilarynx
	T4	Tumor invades adjacent structures
Pyriform sinus[42,51]	T1	Tumor limited to one site only
	T2	Two sites involved
	T3	Three sites involved
	T4	Tumor outside inferior hypopharynx
Pharyngeal wall[41,43,48]	T1	Lesions ≤2 cm in size
	T2	Lesions >2 cm
	T3	Invasion beyond region
	T4	Invasion of bone (massive)
All sites[2]	NX	Regional lymph nodes cannot be assessed
	N0	No regional lymph node metastasis
	N1	Metastasis in a single ipsilateral lymph node, ≤3 cm in greatest dimension
	N2	Metastasis in a single ipsilateral lymph node, >3 cm but <6 cm in greatest dimension; in multiple ipsilateral lymph nodes, none >6 cm in greatest dimension; or in bilateral or contralateral lymph nodes, none >6 cm in greatest dimension
	N2a	Metastasis in a single ipsilateral lymph node, >3 cm but <6 cm in greatest dimension
	N2b	Metastasis in multiple ipsilateral lymph nodes, none >6 cm in greatest dimension
	N2c	Metastasis in bilateral or contralateral lymph nodes, none >6 cm in greatest dimension
	N3	Metastasis in a lymph node >6 cm in greatest dimension

tors helps in determining optimal treatment for each patient.[19,20,41,43] Unfortunately, studies of the prognostic factors for hypopharyngeal cancers are lacking. The information that follows is derived from study of pyriform sinus cancers and does not relate to pharyngeal wall or postcricoid cancers.[45]

Age and sex are the two host characteristics that have the most prognostic significance for carcinoma of the pyriform sinus. Survival progressively declines with advancing age, and female patients survive significantly longer than male patients, probably because they present with earlier stage cancers.[39]

Tumor characteristics that predict local failure, distant metastases, and survival are described by the clinical examiner and the surgical pathologist. Anatomic location, size of hypopharyngeal tumor, and presence or absence of palpable lymph nodes are the three factors determined by clinical examination that best correlate with relapse and prognosis.[41,42] Because they are surgically resectable and often smaller than are pharyngeal wall and postcricoid cancers, pyriform sinus cancers have the lowest rate of local failure and the best prognosis (Fig. 34-6).[14,41,42] Small tumors of any hypopharyngeal site have higher rates of local control by surgery and irradiation and better prognosis than larger tumors.

Keratinizing tumors and those with infiltrating margins are more often associated with primary and regional failure than are those without these characteristics; nonkeratinizing tumors are more frequently associated with distant metastases than keratinizing tumors (Fig. 34-7).[45]

The most favorable prognostic factors for pyriform sinus cancer are negative surgical margins, no extranodal extension of tumor, absence of cancer in lymph nodes, and granulomatous response at the primary site (Fig. 34-7).[45] In every instance, except granulomatous response, favorable prognosis is explained by lower rates of relapse. Granulomatous response was presumed to be a host-related phenomenon because it could not be shown that tumors were any more or less aggressive in patients with or without such a response.[45]

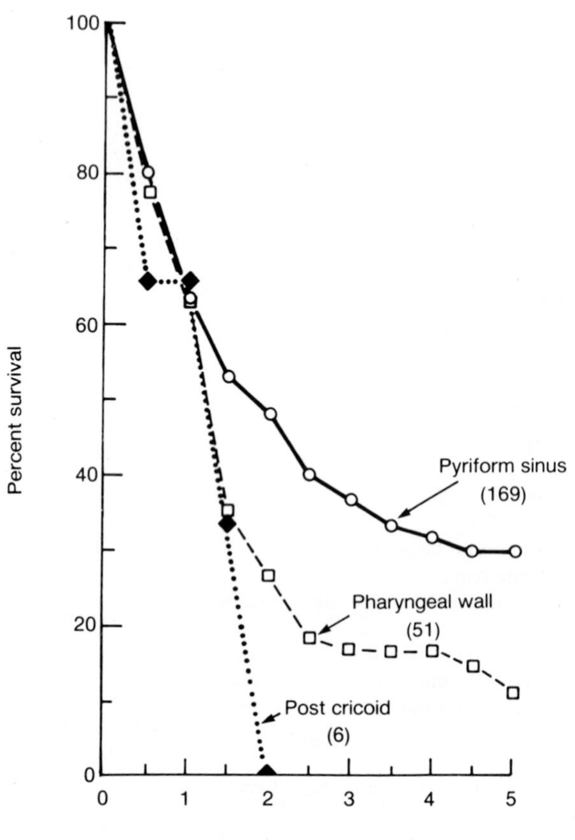

FIGURE 34–6. Survival of patients with cancer originating from different sites in the hypopharynx.[14,41,42] Number of patients is in parentheses.

GENERAL MANAGEMENT

The best treatment for hypopharyngeal carcinoma is that which most often controls the primary tumor and lymph nodes and preserves voice with the least risk to the host. Irradiation alone, surgery alone, and surgical resection with adjuvant preoperative or postoperative irradiation are the methods used to accomplish these goals.[1,3–6,8,9,12,13,15,16,18,23–25,28,31–33,35,41,42,46,47,49,54,55,62,64–68,70] Table 34-3 outlines the management of hypopharyngeal tumors.

The efficacy of chemotherapy remains unproven, but it has significant potential in the treatment of hypopharyngeal tumors because rates of locoregional failure and distant metastases are relatively high. Keane and associates[29] conducted a pilot study using mitomycin C and 5-fluorouracil infusion with split-course irradiation for advanced cancers of the larynx and hypopharynx. Of 57 patients studied, 90% completed irradiation and 70% completed chemotherapy.[29] Immunotherapy using BC6 has proven ineffective.[7]

Pyriform Sinus Cancers

Selection of Treatment

The treatment method selected for carcinoma of the pyriform sinus depends on the size and location of the primary tumor, fixation or mobility of regional lymph nodes, and the medical condition of the patient.

One fifth of the patients who present with pyriform sinus cancer receive palliative radiation therapy or chemotherapy because the primary tumor or neck nodes are unresectable or because the patient's medical condition or age prohibits more aggressive treatment; very few have proven distant metastases at initial diagnosis.[5,28,42]

For the remaining patients who have resectable tumors and are able to tolerate surgery, the choice of treatment is generally based on the size of the primary tumor, fixation of lymph nodes, and medical condition of the host. Combined surgery and irradiation more often control the primary tumor and lymph nodes than either modality alone.

Irradiation Alone

Radiation alone controls a substantial proportion of small surface lesions in the pyriform sinus.[4,47,49] Mendenhall[47] reported that 16 (64%) of 25 T1 and T2 lesions of the pyriform sinus were controlled with full-course irradiation. If irradiation alone is to be used, it is important that the radiation oncologist be present at direct pharyngoscopy or review the video pharyngoscopy findings. The best results will be obtained by selecting lesions that are confined to one or two walls of the pyriform sinus, lack bulk, and do not infiltrate the larynx or destroy thyroid cartilage.

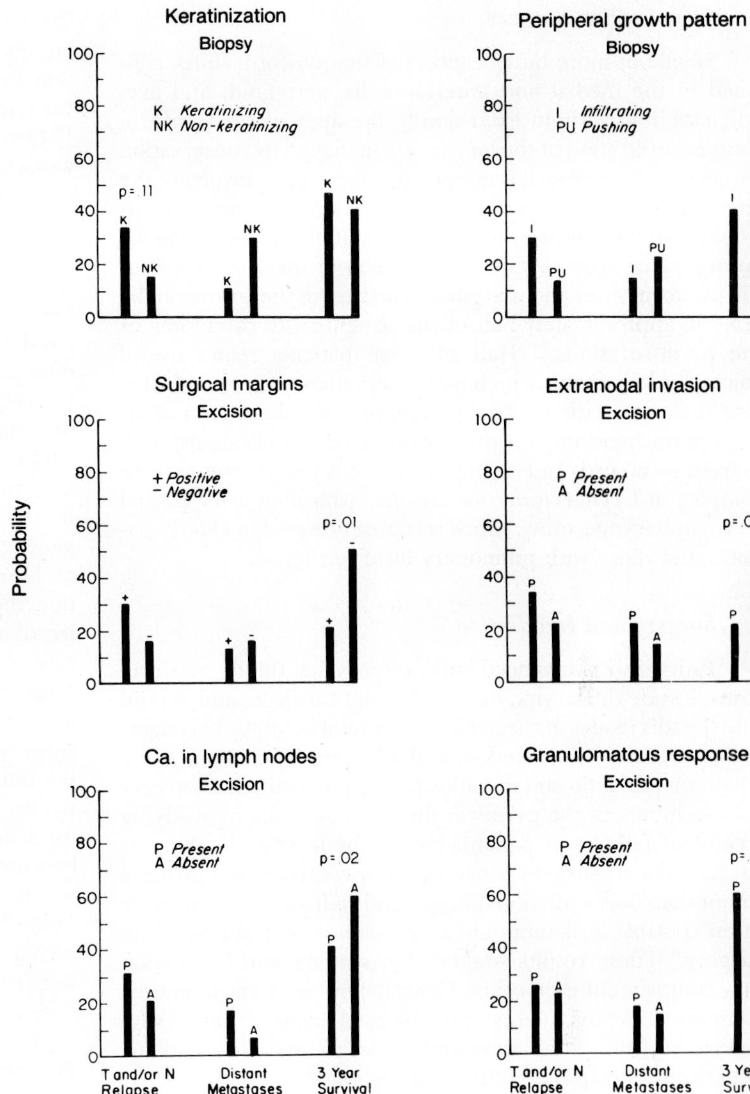

FIGURE 34–7. Histograms of tumor characteristics that predict TNM relapse and survival for pyriform sinus cancer. (Martin SA, Marks JE, Bauer W, et al: Cancer 46:1974, 1980)

TABLE 34–3
Management of Hypopharyngeal Cancer

TUMOR SITE	TREATMENT
PYRIFORM SINUS	
T1 and T2 lesions	Irradiation alone or partial laryngopharyngectomy, ipsilateral neck dissection, and postoperative irradiation (6000 cGy in 6 wk)
T3 and T4 lesions, resectable	Total laryngopharyngectomy, ipsilateral neck dissection, and postoperative irradiation (6600 cGy in 6.5 wk)
Unresectable or medically inoperable lesions	Irradiation alone and/or chemotherapy
With fixed lymph nodes	Preoperative irradiation
PHARYNGEAL WALL	
T1 lesions	Irradiation alone
T2, T3, and T4 lesions	Resection followed by adjuvant irradiation
POSTCRICOID REGIONS	Optimal treatment undefined. Surgery and postoperative radiation therapy if resectable; and radiation therapy alone if unresectable

Conservation Surgery

Small but more bulky cancers of the pyriform sinus, confined to the medial and anterior walls, arytenoid, and aryepiglottic fold without extension to the apex of the pyriform sinus or infiltration of the larynx, are managed by conservation surgery. This approach is not possible for tumors involving the lateral wall or the apex of the pyriform sinus because the cut would traverse cancer in the thyroid ala in most cases.[30] Partial laryngopharyngectomy or local excision of the medial wall of the pyriform sinus and marginal structures of the larynx can be done in approximately half of the patients with carcinoma of the pyriform sinus.[19] Half of these patients retain useful voices.[19] The patients who have conservation surgery and later lose their voice die of locally recurrent or distant tumor or require tracheostomy for therapy-induced complications, such as fixed vocal cords and laryngeal edema. A few patients require completion laryngectomy for chronic aspiration after partial laryngopharyngectomy, which is contraindicated in elderly patients and those with pulmonary insufficiency.

Surgery and Irradiation

Patients with advanced bulky tumors that fill the pyriform sinus, invade the larynx, destroy thyroid cartilage, and extend into the soft tissues of the neck require total laryngopharyngectomy, radical neck dissection, and adjuvant irradiation.

A case for adjuvant radiation therapy in addition to surgery for carcinoma of the pyriform sinus can be made by studying treatment failures of patients treated by irradiation alone or surgery alone.[8] Surgery provides better control of the primary tumor than does radiation therapy, and radiation therapy more often controls ipsilateral and contralateral neck disease than surgery.[8] These results suggest that surgery and irradiation may complement each other. Contralateral neck recurrence is common (25%) in patients with advanced primary tumors who receive adjuvant irradiation and undergo total laryngopharyngectomy and ipsilateral neck dissection.[42]

Higher doses of adjuvant radiation are better delivered postoperatively than preoperatively, because preoperative irradiation retards healing of pharyngeal and cutaneous suture lines and may cause more complications than postoperative irradiation.[6,10,64] Preoperative irradiation need not increase postsurgical complications, provided sufficient time is allowed between radiation therapy and surgery for fibroblasts to repopulate the irradiated field.[38] Preoperative irradiation is advised for patients with fixed lymph nodes because neck dissection is later possible in some of these patients.[42]

Treatment of Recurrence

Retreatment of recurrent pyriform sinus cancer in the primary site or the neck is rewarded by few salvages, because these patients have fixed lymph nodes, recurrence in the dissected neck, or diffusely recurrent cancer in the pharynx, producing an excessive complication rate.[42,65] The only patients salvaged are those who have a small recurrence in the laryngeal remnant, for which completion laryngectomy is possible, or a mobile lymph node in the opposite side of the neck that may be removed by neck dissection.

Pharyngeal Wall Cancers

External-beam irradiation of pharyngeal wall cancer yields rates of tumor control that range from 21% to 50%.[43,47,48,53,66] Tumor control is better for small than for large tumors and is enhanced by interstitial implantation with ^{192}Ir and ^{125}I.[47,59] Son and Kacinski[59] controlled 12 of 14 pharyngeal wall cancers for 6 to 88 months after external irradiation and implant with ^{192}Ir or ^{125}I. They described the implantation technique and reported necrosis of the primary tumor and reepithelialization of the pharyngeal wall. Ulceration and fibrosis of the pharynx were not mentioned.

Our thinking about the optimal treatment for pharyngeal wall cancers evolved as we analyzed the outcome of treatment by low-dose preoperative irradiation and surgery and treatment by irradiation alone.[41,43] Our first analysis of patients treated predominantly by low doses of preoperative irradiation and partial pharyngectomy showed a mortality rate of 14%, a mediocre rate of tumor control (43%), and a prohibitive rate of major postsurgical complications (>50%).[41] Others had reported reasonable rates of tumor control by irradiation alone without the mortality and high rate of complications associated with surgery.[48,66] We therefore discontinued irradiation and surgery, and in 1978, began to treat pharyngeal wall cancer with radiation therapy alone. Follow-up analysis of patients treated by irradiation alone between 1978 and 1982 showed a very poor rate of primary tumor control (25%).[43] Tumor size and nodal stage for the cohort treated by irradiation alone were comparable to the group treated by preoperative radiation therapy and surgery, but it was clear that the primary tumor regrew most of the time after doses of 6500 cGy to 7000 cGy given in 6.5 to 7 weeks. Therefore, we believed that surgery should again be used in the treatment of pharyngeal wall cancer, especially because methods of reconstructing the pharynx with myocutaneous flaps had improved during the same period (1978–1982).[21] We now resect the primary tumor, close the pharynx with a thin myocutaneous flap, and administer 6000 cGy in 6 weeks after healing of pharyngeal and cutaneous suture lines.[57]

Postcricoid Cancers

Most postcricoid cancers in Great Britain managed by radiation therapy show rather dismal results.[16,27,36,69] In one large series of 200 patients, 25% were not treated, 25% were irradiated with palliative intent, and the remaining 50% received irradiation with curative intent.[16] All untreated patients were dead within 9 months, and only 20% of those radically irradiated survived 5 years. There was an incremental decrease in survival with increasing tumor length and fixation of the vocal cord.[16,69] Larger and more extensive tumors are poorly controlled by radiation alone. Surgical resection is probably desirable for primary tumor control, especially now that improved methods of reconstructing the pharynx are available.

RADIATION THERAPY TECHNIQUES

Preoperative Irradiation

Preoperative irradiation for hypopharyngeal tumors is delivered to the larynx, pharynx, and neck, because the incidence of lymphatic metastases is high. Fields extend from the inferior margin of the mandible and mastoid to the clavicles and encompass the anterior and posterior cervical triangles. In the case of pyriform sinus cancer that extends superiorly into the oropharynx, fields are designed to encompass retropharyngeal nodes up to the base of the skull. Preoperative doses range from 4000 cGy to 4500 cGy given in 4 to 4.5 weeks.

Postoperative Irradiation

Postoperative irradiation for hypopharyngeal tumors is designed to prevent recurrence in the laryngeal remnant, pharynx, neck, tracheostoma, and superior mediastinum. A dose of 6000 cGy is routinely prescribed after successful extirpation of the tumor. If the pathologist demonstrates tumor in the margins of excision, a dose of 6600 cGy is prescribed. The radiation therapy technique most commonly used consists of three fields: two opposed upper lateral fields encompassing the primary tumor and an anterior low-neck field to irradiate the tracheostoma and lower cervical lymph nodes. The spinal cord is shielded from the lateral direction just posterior to the pharynx (Fig. 34-8). An anterior shield at the junction of the upper lateral and low neck fields is not used to avoid shielding of the pharynx, paratracheal lymph nodes, and parastomal tissues. A beam splitter is routinely used for the low-neck field to prevent upward divergence of the radiation beam and possible overlap at the junction of the three radiation fields (Fig. 34-9).

Compensating filters are routinely used for low-energy megavoltage beams to eliminate the variations in dose that result from variations in thickness of the neck. The spinal cord is shielded after 4000 cGy to 4400 cGy, and that part of the neck underlying the shield is routinely irradiated with a 9-MeV electron beam to complete the dose of 5000 cGy. The use of multiple spliced fields and electron-beam irradiation to spare the centrally located spinal cord is safe but dosimetrically imperfect. Tissues at the junction of spliced fields are generally underdosed by as much as 20% (Fig. 34-10).[44]

A technique is needed that homogeneously irradiates the tissues of the neck anterior and lateral to the spinal cord to doses that exceed the tolerance of the spinal cord. One technique that does this relatively well is the minimantle technique devised by Doppke and colleagues.[11] This technique uses opposed 10-MV beams with a posterior cervical shield to reduce dose to the spinal cord. It is less suitable for lower-energy megavoltage beams because dose to the posterior cervical lymph nodes is reduced. An isocentric, triangular, three-field technique using two anterolateral fields with compensating filters and a third posterior field with a cervical shield has been devised for lower-energy megavoltage beams.[17] This technique does not deliver doses exceeding 4500 cGy to the spinal cord and allows delivery of 5500 cGy to the target tissues anterior and lateral to the spinal cord.

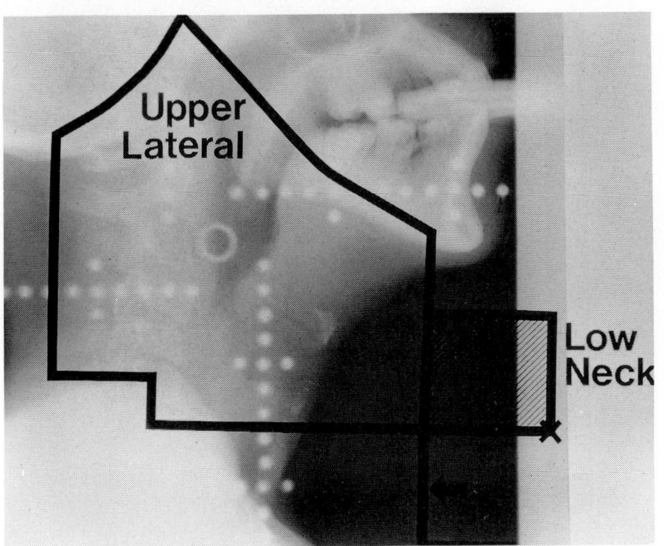

FIGURE 34–8. Upper lateral field for postoperative irradiation of a patient with cancer of the pyriform sinus. Spinal cord is shielded laterally, posterior to the pharynx and tracheostoma. Beam splitter is used superiorly on the low-neck field to prevent upward divergence of the beam.

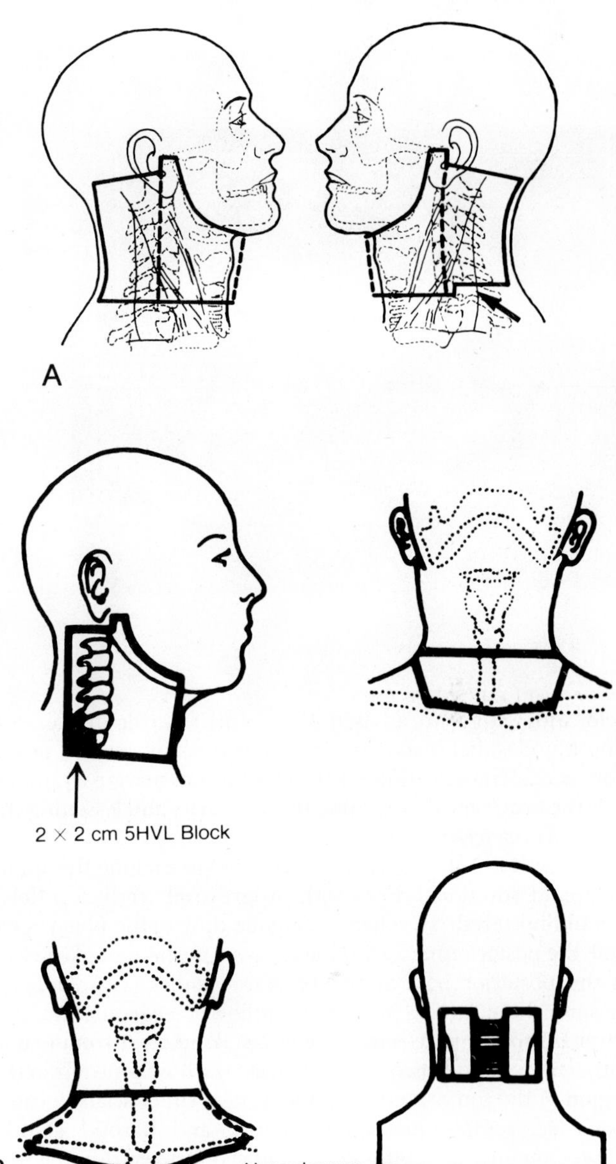

FIGURE 34–9. Diagram of portals, at the initiation of therapy, used for treatment of patients with hypopharyngeal lesions who have palpable lymphadenopathy. The posterior cervical lymph nodes are included in the photon-irradiated volume for doses up to 4400 cGy. Additional doses to the posterior neck are delivered with electron beam (usually 9 MeV). A block to avoid overlap of lateral and anteroposterior portals is shown.

Full-Course Irradiation

Full-course irradiation for pharyngeal wall cancer should encompass the nasopharynx, oropharynx, hypopharynx, and upper cervical esophagus because of the propensity of this cancer to spread submucosally.[22] The lateral beam direction encompasses the tumor with adequate superior and inferior margins, if the patient pulls on a strap looped around the feet to depress the shoulders. If the lateral beam direction inadequately encompasses the tumor, then anteroposterior or anterior oblique

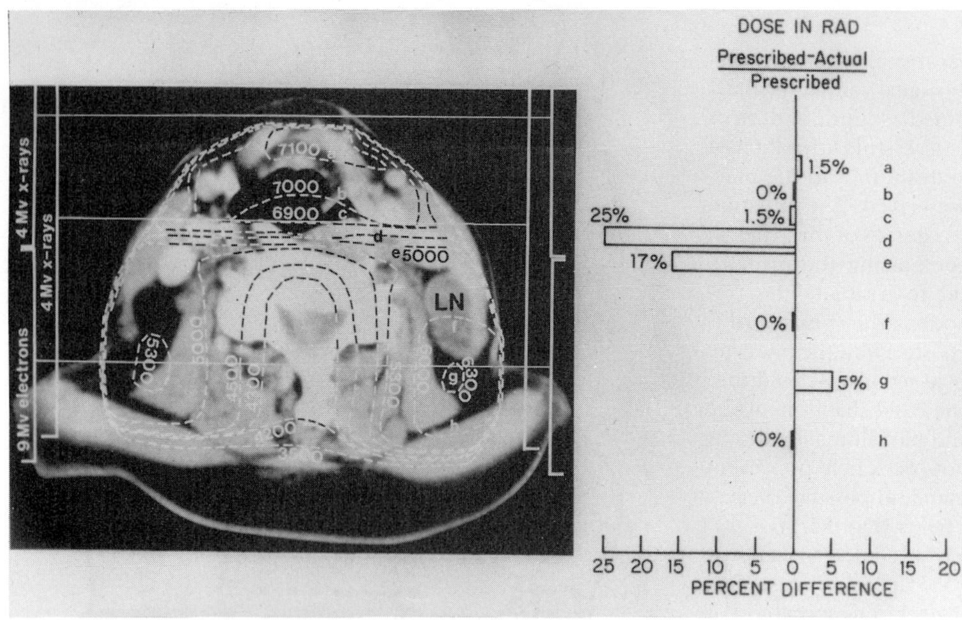

FIGURE 34–10. Dose distribution superimposed on a computed tomographic scan of a patient with cancer of the pyriform sinus and a large lymph node (LN) in the right side of the neck. The prescribed dose was 7000 cGy to the larynx and pharynx, 6000 cGy to the posterior cervical area of the right side of the neck, and 5000 cGy to the posterior cervical area of the left side of the neck. The percent difference between the prescribed and actual dose for isodose lines A through H is shown on the histogram to the right. (Marks JE, Silverman CL, Devineni VR, Simpson JR: Head Neck Surg 8:77, 1986)

fields with wedges are advised. If there are any palpable cervical lymph nodes, fields should encompass the anterior and posterior cervical triangles (Fig. 34-9). The anterior margin irradiates only the oropharynx, shielding the oral cavity and lessening the mucosal area irradiated.

After 4400 cGy, portals are reduced to exclude the spinal cord, and additional doses with progressively reducing fields are administered. To achieve adequate dose to the pharyngeal wall, the posterior margin of the off-cord portal should be close to the posterior part of the vertebral bodies (Fig. 34-11).[47] Because these tumors are often midline or near midline, it is advisable to use high-energy photons alone or in conjunction with lower energy x-rays to concentrate the dose centrally in the region of the tumor, reducing the dose to superficially located mandible, temporomandibular joints, and parotid glands. Doses range from 6500 cGy to 7000 cGy delivered in 6.5 to 7 weeks.

Dose Response

Pyriform Sinus Cancers

Improved tumor and nodal control with increasing doses has been documented for primary T1 and T2 cancers of the pyriform sinus and involved lymph nodes, regardless of size (Fig. 34-12). The dose-response curve for small tumors plateaus after 7000 cGy and is flat for larger T3 tumors within the therapeutic range of doses used. There seems to be a moderate advantage to increasing the dose for small tumors and lymph nodes, but there is no advantage in delivering doses greater than 6000 cGy for T3 cancers of the pyriform sinus.

Pharyngeal Wall Cancers

Improved tumor control with increasing doses of irradiation has been reported for T1 and T2 pharyngeal wall cancers, but the dose-response curve for advanced T3 and T4 lesions is relatively flat within the range of doses reported (Fig. 34-13). Exophytic pharyngeal wall cancers are probably more radioresponsive and easier to control than endophytic ulcerating tumors, so that tumor morphology as well as size should determine the dose selected for a given tumor. Doses of 6500 cGy to 7000 cGy administered in 6.5 to 7 weeks are recommended for T1 and T2 lesions to achieve maximal tumor control without excessive complications. Doses in excess of 6500 cGy to 7000 cGy delivered in 6.5 to 7 weeks are not advantageous for advanced ulcerated tumors because control of more-advanced tumors is unlikely and radiation-induced complications are more likely.

Data on tumor control and radiation dose have not been published for postcricoid cancers.

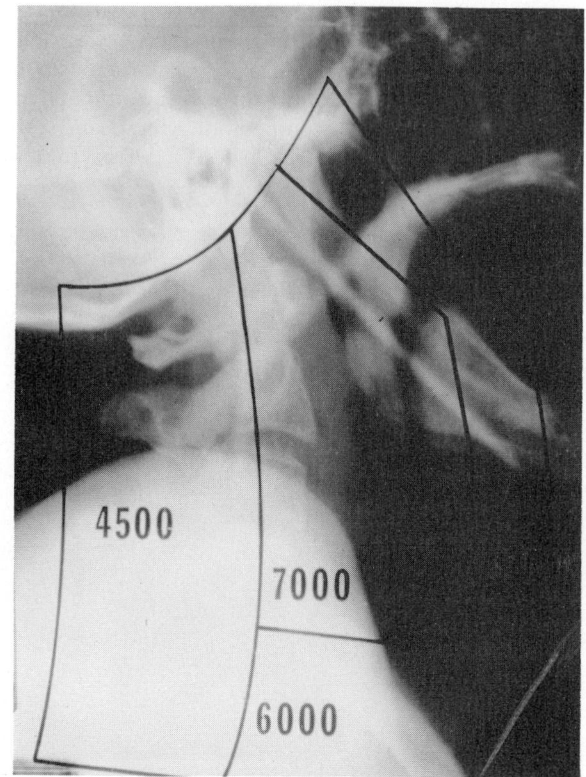

FIGURE 34–11. Shrinking fields and dose (cGy) to each field for a carcinoma of the posterior oropharyngeal wall. Notice that the posterior margin of the off-cord portal borders the posterior margin of the vertebral bodies.

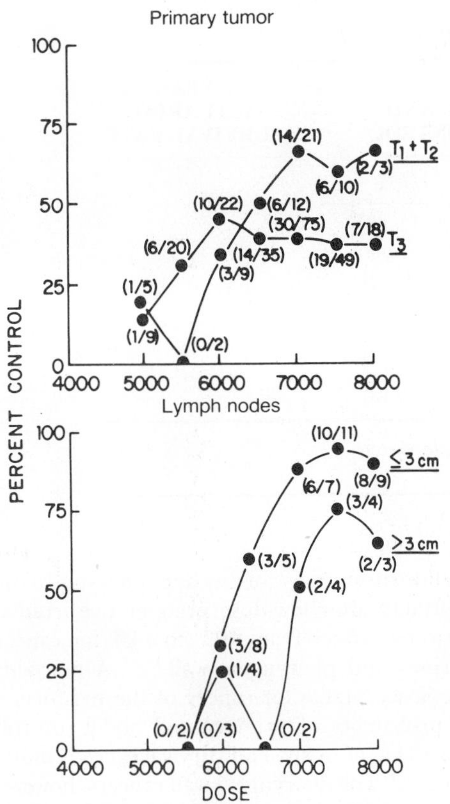

FIGURE 34–12. Dose-response curves for primary tumor and nodal control as a function of size for cancers of the pyriform sinus. (Bataini P, Brugere J, Bernier J, et al: Int J Radiat Oncol Biol Phys 8:1277, 1982)

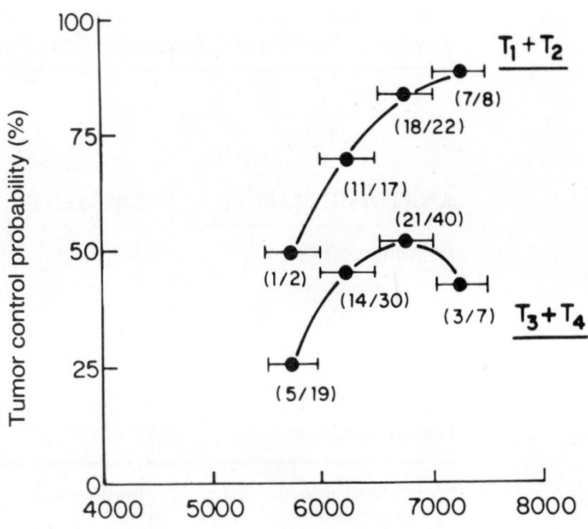

FIGURE 34–13. Dose-response curves for T1 to T2 and T3 to T4 pharyngeal wall cancers treated by irradiation alone. (Meoz-Mendez RT, Fletcher GH, Guillamondeque OM: Int J Radiat Oncol Biol Phys 4:579, 1978)

RESULTS OF THERAPY

Treatment results are summarized in Tables 34-4 and 34-5. The ability to control the primary tumor and lymph nodes progressively diminishes for carcinomas of the pyriform sinus, pharyngeal wall, and postcricoid region, an observation explained by tumor resectability and size (Fig. 34-6).[14,41,42] Pyriform sinus cancer, because of its anterior and superior location in the hypopharynx, is more easily resected and controlled than are the posteriorly and inferiorly located cancers of the pharyn-

TABLE 34–4
Primary and Nodal Control and Survival by Treatment Method for Carcinoma of the Pyriform Sinus

		PRIMARY AND NODAL CONTROL		THREE-YEAR SURVIVAL RATE
INVESTIGATOR	**TREATMENT**	PATIENTS	%	%
Kirchner and Owen[31]	Surgery alone	15/28	54	32
Jesse and Lindberg[25]	Surgery alone	47/67	70	
Carpenter et al[8]	Surgery alone	51/81	63	
Carpenter et al[8]	Irradiation alone	23/39	59	
Kirchner and Owen[31]	Irradiation alone	27/55	49	4
Lederman[36]	Irradiation alone			19
Keane et al[28]	Irradiation alone	40/98	41	24
Bataini et al[4]	Irradiation alone	205/434	47	26
Million and Cassisi[49]	Irradiation alone	24/37	65	
Dubois et al[12]	Irradiation alone	52/209	25	5*
Vandenbrouck[65]	Irradiation alone	69/152	45	25
Marks et al[42]	Irradiation and surgery	99/137	72	43
Kirchner and Owens[31]	Irradiation and surgery	27/33	82	36
Jesse and Lindberg[25]	Surgery and irradiation	42/49	86	
Carpenter et al[8]	Surgery and irradiation	13/22	59	
El Badawi et al[13]	Surgery and irradiation	111/125	89	47
Dubois et al[12]	Surgery and irradiation	55/154	35	33*
Vandenbrouck[65]	Surgery and irradiation	159/198	80	48

* *Five-year survival rate.*

TABLE 34–5
Treatment Results for Carcinomas of the Pharyngeal Wall and Postcricoid Region

ANATOMIC SITE	TREATMENT*	PRIMARY AND NODAL CONTROL PATIENTS	PRIMARY AND NODAL CONTROL %	3-YEAR ACTUARIAL SURVIVAL RATE %
Pharyngeal Wall	R+S[41]	14/29	48	17
	RA[43]	6/25	25	12
	RA[48]	98/164	60†	
	RA[53]	26/122	21	3
	RA[47]	29/62	47†	
	RA[48]	19/42	45†	
Postcricoid Region	RA[16]	30/156	19†	20

**R+S, irradiation plus surgery; RA, irradiation alone. Superscript numbers indicate references.*
† Primary control only.

geal wall and postcricoid region. Because of their relatively inaccessible locations, pharyngeal wall and postcricoid tumors are usually irradiated.[16,69] Unfortunately, they are often advanced and poorly controlled by irradiation. Control of pharyngeal wall cancers by radiation therapy progressively declines with advancing T stage or tumor size (Fig. 34-13); postcricoid or epiesophageal tumors are often larger and more difficult to control than pharyngeal wall cancer.[36,48]

SEQUELAE OF TREATMENT

Because of the aggressive nature of hypopharyngeal tumors, radiation therapy and surgery frequently have been used together, and complications have been significant (Tables 34-6 and 34-7).[20] It is apparent from both retrospective and prospective studies that the incidence of major complications, including carotid rupture, is usually greater for preoperative than for postoperative irradiation.[6,10,64] The incidence of pharyngocutaneous fistulas after pharyngectomy is the same whether the pharynx has been irradiated before or not, but the time required to heal a preoperatively irradiated fistula is significantly greater than for the unirradiated fistula.[6,64]

Balancing risk with benefit is essential in determining the optimal treatment strategy for any hypopharyngeal tumor. Operative mortality after low-dose preoperative irradiation and pharyngectomy ranges from 10% to 14% for cancers of the pyriform sinus and pharyngeal wall.[19,41] A mortality of this magnitude is acceptable for cancer of the pyriform sinus because the probability of primary and nodal control exceeds mortality by a factor of six, and survival exceeds mortality by a factor of three.[42] For pharyngeal wall cancers, however, a mortality of this magnitude is unacceptable because it is roughly equivalent to survival, and irradiation alone gives the same rate of primary and nodal control as surgery without the associated mortality.[41]

SUMMARY OF CLINICAL TRIALS

An important trial by Strong from Memorial Sloan-Kettering demonstrated the value of low-dose preoperative irradiation (2000 cGy in 1 week) in a variety of tumors that required radical neck dissection as part of treatment. Preoperative radiation decreased the recurrence rate in the neck from 34% for the surgery-alone group to 22% for the irradiated group; this approach was particularly valuable for patients with advanced nodal disease involving multiple levels in the neck.[61]

TABLE 34–6
Complications for Carcinoma of the Pyriform Sinus Treated by Preoperative Irradiation and Surgery*

COMPLICATION	PARTIAL LARYNGO-PHARYNGECTOMY (N = 85) PATIENTS	%	TOTAL LARYNGO-PHARYNGECTOMY (N = 57) PATIENTS	%	TOTAL (N = 142) PATIENTS	%
Operative mortality	10	12	4	7	14	10
Pharyngocutaneous fistula	5	6	8	14	13	9
Aspiration pneumonia	5	6	0		5	4
Esophageal stricture	1	1	4	7	5	4
Carotid rupture	1	1	1	2	2	1
Miscellaneous†	5	6	2	4	7	5

**72% of patients received 3000 cGy in 3 weeks.*
† Vocal cord paralysis, hemorrhage, wound infection, chyle fistula, Horner's syndrome.
(Modified from Freeman RB, Marks JE, Ogura JH: Laryngoscope 89:1855, 1979)

TABLE 34–7
Complications for Pharyngeal Wall Cancer by Treatment Method

COMPLICATION	PREOPERATIVE IRRADIATION AND SURGERY PATIENTS	%	IRRADIATION ALONE PATIENTS	%
MAJOR				
Pharyngocutaneous fistula	11/38	29	0	
Carotid rupture (3 deaths)	4/38	11	0	
Airway obstruction	3/38	8	7/34	21
Pharyngeal exsanguination (1 death)	1/38	3	0	
MINOR				
Pneumonia or aspiration	9/38	24	5/34	15
Wound infection	7/38	18	0	
Wound dehiscence	4/38	11	0	
Painful ulcer	3/38	8	7/34	21
Gastrointestinal bleeding	1/38	3	2/34	6
Pharyngeal stricture or dysphagia	3/38	8	4/34	12
Nonunion mandibulotomy	1/38	3	0	
Trismus	0		1/34	3
Dental caries	0		1/34	3
Neck fibrosis	0		1/34	3

(Modified from Marks JE, Smith PG, Sessions PG: Arch Otolaryngol, 111:79, 1985)

A randomized clinical trial at Gustave-Roussy Institute compared preoperative and postoperative irradiation (5500 cGy in 5.5 weeks) administered in conjunction with laryngopharyngectomy and neck dissection for carcinoma of the pyriform sinus.[6,64] The trial was terminated after it became apparent that surgical complications after high-dose preoperative irradiation were excessive. Postoperative irradiation was associated with a lesser risk and produced a significantly greater survival rate (56%) than preoperative irradiation (36%), even after exclusion of those preoperatively irradiated patients who died postoperatively of complications.

A randomized trial by Strong and associates compared surgery alone with low-dose preoperative irradiation (2000 cGy in 1 week) and surgery for oropharyngeal and hypopharyngeal tumors.[62] Tumor control and survival did not differ significantly for the two groups; complications were not analyzed.

A trial, conducted by the Radiation Therapy Oncology Group compared preoperative and postoperative irradiation plus surgery for cancers of the oral cavity, oropharynx, supraglottic larynx, maxillary sinus, and hypopharynx.[33,58] Patients received 5000 cGy in 5 weeks preoperatively and 6000 cGy in 6 weeks postoperatively. Those who received more dose postoperatively had better 4-year locoregional control (61% vs. 50%) and disease-free survival (28% vs. 18%), but improvements in tumor and nodal control and survival were not significant ($P = 0.10$). Surgical and radiation complications were comparable in both groups, and the postsurgical complications in the preoperatively irradiated patients were significantly lower than those reported in the Gustave-Roussy trial. This lower incidence of postsurgical complications is best explained by prolongation of the interval between the end of irradiation and surgery, which was 4 weeks in the Radiation Therapy Oncology Group study and 2 weeks in the Gustave-Roussy study.[33,38,58,64]

Of four trials that compared surgery alone to preoperative irradiation and surgery, only one showed an advantage to the use of preoperative irradiation.[34,61,62,64] The only trial comparing surgery alone to surgery plus postoperative irradiation demonstrated an insignificant improvement or trend in favor of the postoperatively irradiated patients, but it failed to accession an adequate number of patients.[32]

REFERENCES

1. Ahlbom HE: The results of radiotherapy of hypopharyngeal cancer at the Radiumhemmet, Stockholm 1930 to 1939. Acta Radiol 22:155, 1941
2. American Joint Committee for Cancer Staging and End Results Reporting: Manual for Staging of Cancer, pp 34–35. Philadelphia, JB Lippincott, 1988
3. Baclesse F: Roentgen therapy in cancer of the hypopharynx. JAMA 140:525, 1949
4. Bataini P, Brugere J, Bernier J, et al: Results of radical radiotherapeutic treatment of carcinoma of the pyriform sinus. Int J Radiat Oncol Biol Phys 8:1277, 1982
5. Briant TDR, Lord I: Carcinoma of the hypoppharynx. Can J Otolaryngol 2:4, 1973
6. Cachin Y, Eschwege F: Combination of radiotherapy and surgery in the treatment of head and neck cancers. Cancer Treat Rev 2:177, 1975
7. Cachin Y, Vandenbrouck C, Amiel JL, Eschwege F, Sancho-Garnier H: Preliminary results of a randomized trial with BCG immunotherapy in laryngeal and hypopharyngeal carcinoma. Int Head Neck Oncol Res Conf Abstracts 9:12, 1980
8. Carpenter RJ, Desanto LW, Devine KD, et al: Cancer of the hypopharynx: Analysis of treatment and results in 162 patients. Arch Otolaryngol 102:716, 1976
9. Cunningham MP, Catlin D: Cancer of the pharyngeal wall. Cancer 27:1859, 1967
10. Donald PJ: Complications of combined therapy in head and neck carcinomas. Arch Otolaryngol 104:329, 1979
11. Doppke K, Norack D, Wang C: Physical considerations in the treatment of advanced carcinomas of the larynx and pyriform

sinus using 10-MV x-rays. Int J Radiat Oncol Biol Phys 6:1251, 1980

12. Dubois JB, Guerrier B, Di Ruggiero JM, Pourquier H: Cancer of the pyriform sinus: Treatment by radiation therapy alone and with surgery. Radiology 160:831, 1986
13. El Badawi, Goepfert H, Fletcher GH, et al: Squamous cell carcinoma of the pyriform sinus. Laryngoscope 92:357, 1982
14. Ellis W, Marks JE: Unpublished data, 1978
15. Ennuyer A, Bataini P, Daudel R, et al: A propos de la radiotherapie des adenopathies cervicales secondaires aux epitheliomas du pharynx. Bull Cancer (Paris) 60:1, 1973
16. Farrington WT, Weighall JS, Jones PH: Postcricoid carcinoma (a ten-year retrospective study). J Laryngol Otol 100:79, 1986
17. Fields JN, Marks JE: A technique for treatment of advanced carcinomas of the larynx and hypopharynx using low-megavoltage x-rays. Radiother Oncol 7:281, 1986
18. Fletcher GH, Jesse RH: The place of irradiation in the management of the primary lesion in head and neck cancers. Cancer 39:862, 1977
19. Freeman RB, Marks JE, Ogura JH: Voice preservation in treatment of carcinoma of the pyriform sinus. Laryngoscope 89:1855, 1979
20. Gall AM, Sessions DB, Ogura JH: Complications following surgery for cancer of the larynx and hypopharynx. Cancer 29:624, 1977
21. Guillamondegui OM, Meoz R, Jesse RH: Surgical treatment of squamous cell carcinoma of the pharyngeal walls. Am J Surg 136:474, 1978
22. Harrison DFN: Pathology of hypopharyngeal cancer in relation to surgical management. J Laryngol Otol 84:349, 1970
23. Inoue T, Shigeinatsu Y, Sato T: Treatment of carcinoma of the hypopharynx. Cancer 31:649, 1973
24. Jacobsson F: Carcinoma of the hypopharynx. A clinical study of 322 cases treated at the Radium Hemmet from 1939 to 1947. Acta Radiol 35:1, 1951
25. Jesse RH, Lindberg RD: The efficacy of combining radiation therapy with a surgical procedure in patients with cervical metastases from squamous cancer of the oropharynx and hypopharynx. Cancer 35:1153, 1975
26. Jones RFM: The Paterson-Brown-Kelly syndrome, its relationship to iron deficiency and postcricoid carcinoma. Parts I and II. J Laryngol Otol 75:529, 1961
27. Kalvathi N: Factors influencing cure in the radiotherapy of postcricoid carcinoma. Clin Radiol 21:248, 1970
28. Keane TJ, Hawkins NV, Beale FA, et al: Carcinoma of hypopharynx: Results of primary radical radiation therapy. Int J Radiat Oncol Biol Phys 9:659, 1983
29. Keane TJ, Hawkins NV, Beale FA, et al: A pilot study of mitomycin C/5-fluorouracil infusion combined with split-course radiation therapy for carcinomas of the larynx and hyppharynx. J Otolaryngol 15:286, 1986
30. Kirchner JA: Pyriform sinus cancer: A clinical and laboratory study. Ann Otolaryngol Rhinol Laryngol 84:793, 1975
31. Kircher JA, Owen JR: Five hundred cancers of the larynx and pyriform sinus: Results of treatment by radiation and surgery. Laryngoscope 87:1288, 1977
32. Kokal WA, Nesfeld JP, Eisert D, et al: Postoperative radiation as adjuvant treatment for carcinoma of the oral cavity, larynx, and pharynx: Preliminary report of a prospective randomized trial. J Surg Oncol 38:71, 1988
33. Kramer, S, Gelber RD, Snow JB, et al: Combined radiation therapy and surgery in the management of advanced head and neck cancer: Final report of study 73-03 of the Radiation Therapy Oncology Group. Head and Neck Surgery 10:19, 1987
34. Lawrence WL, Terz JJ, Rogers C, King RE, Wolf JS, King ER: Preoperative irradiation for head and neck cancer: A prospective study. Cancer 33:318, 1974
35. Lederman M: Cancer of the pharyngolaryngeal groove with special reference to the sinus pyriformis. J Laryngol Otol 67:641, 1953
36. Lederman M: Carcinoma of the laryngopharynx: Results of radiotherapy. J Laryngol Otol 76:317, 1962
37. Lord IJ, Brian TDR, Rider WD, et al: A comparison of preoperative and primary radiotherapy in the treatment of carcinoma of the hypopharynx. Br J Radiol 46:175, 1973
38. Marcial VA, Gelbert R, Kramer S, Snow JB, et al: Does preoperative irradiation increase the rate of surgical complications in carcinomas of the head and neck? Cancer 49:1297, 1982
39. Marks JE: Unpublished data, 1978
40. Marks JE, Breaux S, Smith PG, et al: The need for elective irradiation of occult from cancers of the larynx and pharynx. Head Neck Surg 8:3, 1985
41. Marks JE, Freeman RB, Lee F, et al: Pharyngeal wall cancer: An analysis of treatment results, complications and patterns of failure. Int J Radiat Oncol Biol Phys 4:587, 1978
42. Marks JE, Kurnik B, Powers WE: Carcinoma of the pyriform sinus: An analysis of treatment results and patters of failure. Cancer 41:1008, 1978
43. Marks JE, Smith PG, Sessions DG: Pharyngeal wall cancer: A reappraisal after comparison of treatment methods. Arch Otolaryngol 111:79, 1985
44. Marks JE, Silverman CL, Devineni VR, Simpson JR: Success of elective irradiation of occult lymphatic metastases from cancers of the larynx and pyriform sinus. Head Neck Surg 8:77, 1986
45. Martin SA, Marks JE, Bauer W et al: Carcinoma of the pyriform sinus: Predictors of TNM relapse and survival. Cancer 46:1974, 1980
46. McGavran MH, Bauer WC, Spjut HJ, et al: Carcinoma of the pyriform sinus. Arch Otolaryngol 78:826, 1963
47. Mendenhall, WM, Parsons JT, Mancuso AA, et al: Squamous cell carcinoma of the pharyngeal wall treated with irradiation. Radiother Oncol 11:205, 1988
48. Meoz-Mendez RT, Fletcher GH, Guillamondeque OM: Analysis of the results of irradiation in the treatment of squamous cell carcinoma of the pharyngeal walls. Int J Radiat Oncol Biol Phys 4:579, 1978
49. Million RR, Cassisi NJ: Radical irradiation for carcinoma of the pyriform sinus. Laryngoscope 91:439, 1981
50. Ogura JH: Surgical pathology of cancer of the larynx. Laryngoscope 65:867, 1955
51. Ogura JH, Geeneman H: Conservative surgery of the larynx and hypopharynx: Selection of patients and results. Can J Otolaryngol 2:11, 1973
52. Olofsson J, van Nostrand AWP: Growth and spread of laryngeal and hypopharyngeal carcinoma with reflections on the effect of preoperative irradiation. Acta Otolaryngol Suppl (Stochk) 308:1, 1973
53. Pene F, Avedian V, Eschwege F, Barrett A, Schwaab G, Marandas P, Vandenbrouck C: A retrospective study of 131 cases of carcinoma of the posterior pharyngeal wall. Cancer 42:2490, 1978
54. Raven RW: Carcinoma of the hypopharynx. Am J Roentgenol Radium Ther Nucl Med 120:173, 1974
55. Shah JP, Shaha R, Spiro RH, et al: Carcinoma of the hypopharynx. Am J Surg 132:439, 1976
56. Silverberg E: Cancer statistics 1989 from NCI Surveillance, Epidemiology and End Results (SEER) Program (1983–1985). Cancer 39:12, 1989
57. Smith PG, Collins SL: Repair of head and neck defects with thin and double-lined pectoralis flaps. Arch Otolaryngol 110:468, 1984
58. Snow JB, Gelber R, Kramer S, Davis LW, Marcial VA, Lowry LD: Comparison of preoperative and postoperative radiation therapy for patients with carcinoma of the head and neck. Acta Otolaryngol (Stockh) 91:611, 1981
59. Son YH, Kacinski BM: Therapeutic concepts of brachytherapy/megavoltage in sequence for pharyngeal wall cancers. Cancer 59:1268, 1987
60. Spaulding CA, Gillenwater A, Constable WC, Hahn SS, Kersh CR: Prognostic value of vocal cord fixation with respect to treatment in cancers of the supraglottis and pyriform sinus. Layngoscope 97:1450, 1987
61. Strong EW: Preoperative radiation and radical neck dissection. Surg Clin North Am 49:271, 1969
62. Strong MS, Vaughan CW, Kayne HL, et al: A randomized trial of preoperative radiotherapy in cancer of the oropharynx and hypopharynx. Am J Surg 136:494, 1978
63. Tuyns AT, Esteve J, Raymond L, et al: Cancer of the larynx/hypopharynx, tobacco and alcohol: IARC International case-control study of Turin and Varese (Italy), Zaragosa and Na-

varra (Spain), Geneva (Switzerland) and Calvados (France). Int J Cancer 41:483, 1988

64. Vandenbrouck C, Sancho H, Lefur R, et al: Results of a randomized clinical trial to preoperative irradiation versus postoperative irradiation in the treatment of tumors of the hypopharynx. Cancer 39:1445, 1977
65. Vandenbrouck C, Eschwege F, De la Rochefordiere A, et al: Squamous cell carcinoma of the pyriform sinus: Retrospective study of 351 cases treated at the Institut Gustave-Roussy. Head Neck Surg 10:4, 1987
66. Wang CC: Radiotherapeutic management of carcinoma of the posterior pharyngeal wall. Cancer 27:894, 1971
67. Wang CC, Schulz MD, Miller D: Combined radiation therapy and surgery for carcinoma of the supraglottis and pyriform sinus. Am J Surg 124:551, 1972
68. Werner G, Baryd I: Telegamma therapy in carcinoma of the hypopharynx with special reference to histologically verified metastases in the neck. Acta Radiol 9:129, 1970
69. Willatt DJ, Jackson SR, McCormick MS, et al: Vocal cord paralysis and tumor length in staging postcricoid cancer. J Surg Oncol 13:131, 1987
70. Wookey H: The surgical treatment of carcinoma of the hypopharynx and esophagus. Br J Surg 35:249,1948
71. Wynder EL, Mushinski MH, Spivok JG: Tobacco and alcohol consumption in relation to the development of multiple primary cancers. Cancer 40:1872, 1977

35

○ ○ ○ • • •

Larynx

William M. Mendenhall
James T. Parsons
Anthony A. Mancuso
Nicholas J. Cassisi
Scott P. Stringer
Rodney R. Million

ANATOMY

The larynx is divided into the supraglottic, glottic, and subglottic regions. The supraglottic larynx consists of the epiglottis, the false vocal cords, the ventricles, and the aryepiglottic folds, including the arytenoids. The glottis includes the true vocal cords and the anterior commissure. The subglottis is located below the vocal cords (Figs. 35-1 and 35-2).[12]

The lateral line of demarcation between the glottis and the supraglottic larynx is considered clinically as the apex of the ventricle. The demarcation between the glottis and subglottis is ill-defined, but the subglottis is considered to begin 5 mm below the free margin of the vocal cord and to end at the inferior border of the cricoid cartilage and the beginning of the trachea.

The vocal cords, thicker in their midportion, are 3 mm to 5 mm thick. Technically, the vocal cords terminate posteriorly with their attachment to the vocal process. The mucosa between the arytenoids is called the posterior commissure.

The outside shell of the larynx is formed by the hyoid bone, thyroid cartilage, and cricoid cartilage; the cricoid cartilage is the only complete ring. The more mobile interior framework is composed of the heart-shaped epiglottis and the arytenoid, corniculate, and cuneiform cartilages. The corniculate and cuneiform cartilages produce small, rounded bulges at the posterior end of the aryepiglottic folds.

The thyroid and the cricoid cartilages and a portion of the arytenoid cartilage are hyaline cartilage and may partially ossify with age, particularly in men. The epiglottis is elastic cartilage; ossification does not occur, and even focal calcification is rare.[33]

The external laryngeal framework is linked together by the thyrohyoid, the cricothyroid, and the cricotracheal ligaments or membranes (Figs. 35-3 and 35-4).[12]

The epiglottis is joined superiorly to the hyoid bone by the hyoepiglottic ligament. The epiglottis is joined to the thyroid cartilage by the thyroepiglottic ligament at a point just below the thyroid notch and above the anterior commissure. The arrangement of the ligaments that connect the cricoid and arytenoid cartilages and form the vocal ligaments, which are part of the true vocal cords, is shown in Figure 35-2*B*. The conus elasticus (cricovocal ligament) is the lower portion of the elastic membrane that connects the inferior framework. It connects the upper surface of the cricoid, the vocal process of the arytenoid, and the lower thyroid cartilage; its free border is thickened into the vocal ligament.

The vocal ligaments and muscles attach to the vocal process of the arytenoid posteriorly and the thyroid cartilage anteriorly. The arrangement of the intrinsic muscles of the larynx, which primarily control the movement of the cords, is presented in Figures 35-2 and 35-3. The extrinsic muscles are concerned primarily with swallowing, except for the cricothyroid muscle, which produces tension and elongation of the vocal cords and is innervated by the superior laryngeal nerve (Fig. 35-4).

The preepiglottic and paraglottic fat spaces are one continuous space lying between the external framework of the thyroid cartilage and hyoid bone and the inner framework of the epiglottis and intrinsic muscles. This space is traversed by blood and lymphatic vessels and nerves. Because there are few capillary lymphatics arising in this area, invasion of the fat space should only indirectly be associated with lymph node metastases. The fat space is limited by the conus elasticus inferiorly; the thyroid ala, thyrohyoid membrane, and hyoid bone anterolaterally; the hyoepiglottic ligament superiorly; and the fascia of the intrinsic muscles on the medial side. Posteriorly, it is adjacent to the anterior wall of the pyriform sinus.

The laryngeal surface of the epiglottis and the free margin of the vocal cords are squamous epithelium, and the remainder is usually pseudostratified ciliated columnar epithelium. Beneath the epithelium of the free edge of the vocal cord is the lamina propria, which can be divided into three layers. There is no true submucosal layer along the free margin of the vocal fold.[27]

The laryngeal arteries are branches of the superior and inferior thyroid arteries.

The intrinsic muscles of the larynx are innervated by the

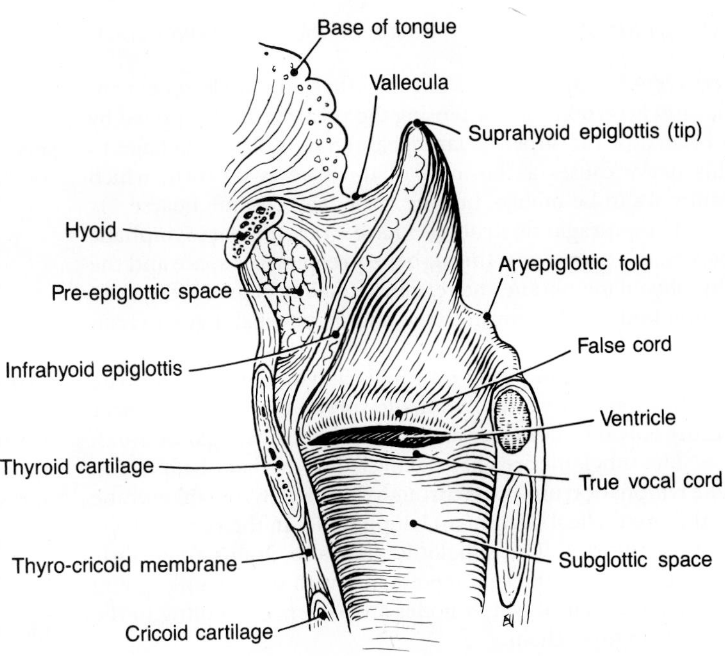

FIGURE 35–1. Diagrammatic sagittal section of the larynx. (Redrawn from Sabotta J: In Clemente CD [ed]: Anatomy: A Regional Atlas of the Human Body. Philadelphia, Lea & Febiger, 1975. Copyright © Munich, Urban & Schwarzenberg, 1975)

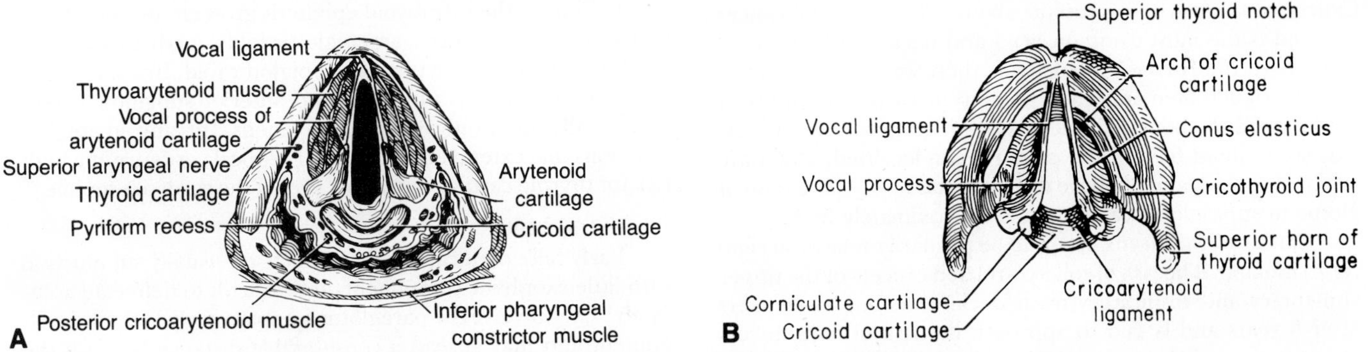

FIGURE 35–2. (**A**) Cross-section of larynx at the level of the vocal cords. (**B**) Framework of the larynx. (Redrawn from Sabotta J: In Clemente CD [ed]: Anatomy: A Regional Atlas of the Human Body. Philadelphia, Lea & Febiger, 1975. Copyright © Munich, Urban & Schwarzenberg, 1975)

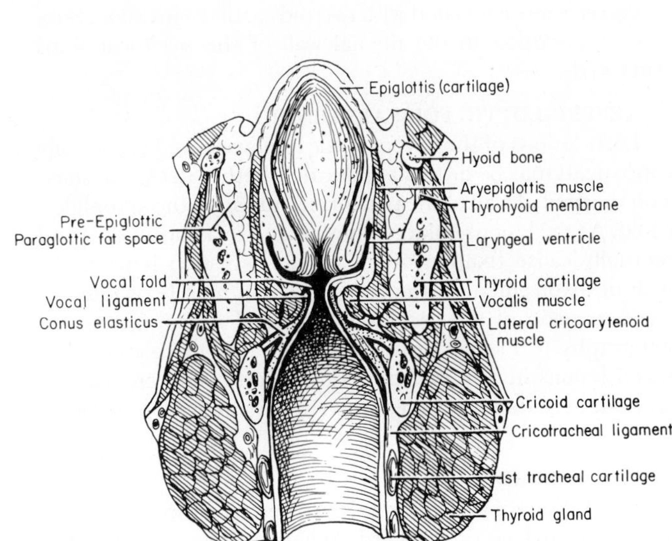

FIGURE 35–3. Diagram of the coronal view of the larynx. (Redrawn from Sabotta J: In Clemente CD [ed]: Anatomy: A Regional Atlas of the Human Body. Philadelphia, Lea & Febiger, 1975. Copyright © Munich, Urban & Schwarzenberg, 1975)

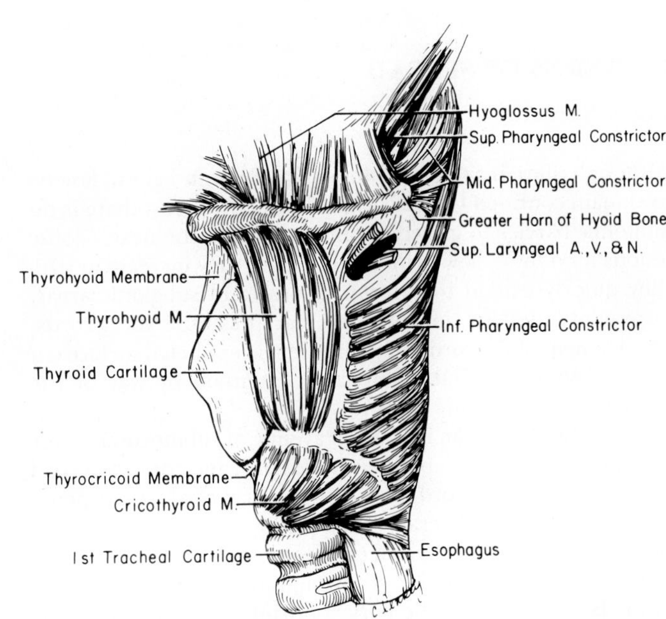

FIGURE 35–4. External view of the larynx. (Sabotta J: In Clemente CE [ed]: Anatomy: A Regional Atlas of the Human Body. Philadelphia, Lea & Febiger, 1975. Copyright © Munich, Urban & Schwarzenberg, 1975)

recurrent laryngeal nerve. The cricothyroid muscle, an extrinsic muscle responsible for tensing the vocal cords, is supplied by a branch of the superior laryngeal nerve; isolated damage to this nerve causes a "bowing" of the true vocal cord, which continues to be mobile, but the voice may become hoarse.

The supraglottic structures have a rich capillary lymphatic plexus; the trunks pass through the preepiglottic space and the thyrohyoid membrane and terminate mainly in the subdigastric lymph nodes; a few drain to the middle internal jugular chain lymph nodes.

There are essentially no capillary lymphatics of the true vocal cords; as a result, lymphatic spread from glottic cancer occurs only if tumor extends to supraglottic or subglottic areas.

The subglottic area has relatively few capillary lymphatics. The lymphatic trunks pass through the cricothyroid membrane to the pretracheal (Delphian) lymph nodes in the region of the thyroid isthmus. The subglottic area also drains posteriorly through the cricotracheal membrane, with some trunks going to the paratracheal lymph nodes and others continuing to the inferior jugular chain.

EPIDEMIOLOGY AND RISK FACTORS

Cancer of the larynx represents about 2% of the total cancer risk and is the most common head and neck cancer (skin excluded). In 1990 in the United States, there were approximately 12,300 (10,000 men and 2300 women) new cases of cancer of the larynx and about 3750 deaths from laryngeal cancer.[67] At diagnosis, about 62% of the cases remain localized, 26% have regional spread, and 8% have distant metastases.[66] The ratio of glottic to supraglottic carcinoma is approximately 3 : 1.

Cancer of the larynx seems to be primarily related to cigarette smoking. The risk of tobacco-related cancers of the upper alimentary and respiratory tracts declines among ex-smokers after 5 years and is said to approach the risk of nonsmokers after 10 years of abstention.[79] The role of alcohol in provoking laryngeal cancer remains unclear.[74] There is some evidence that heavy marijuana smoking may be associated with laryngeal cancer in young patients.

PATTERNS OF SPREAD

Local Spread

Although there is a tendency for supraglottic and glottic lesions to remain confined to their original compartments, there is no anatomic barrier to growth from one area to the next. Glottic lesions tend to be slow-growing, but after they increase in size, they quickly extend to the supraglottic and subglottic areas. Supraglottic lesions do not often start near the vocal cords. Involvement of the cords on their external epithelial surface is a late phenomenon, but submucosal extension by way of the paraglottic area occurs earlier.

The fat space is an important avenue of submucosal tumor spread for infrahyoid epiglottis, false cord, and true vocal cord lesions. As the false cord and the true vocal cord lesions penetrate anteriorly and laterally, they quickly encounter the tough perichondrium of the thyroid cartilage and then grow along the paraglottic fat space and even through the cricothyroid membrane before invading the perichondrium and cartilage. Thyroid cartilage invasion usually occurs in the ossified section of the cartilage, commonly in the region of the anterior commissure tendon or the junction of the anterior one fourth and the posterior three fourths of the thyroid lamina.[4]

Fixation of the vocal cord from laryngeal cancer is usually caused by invasion or destruction of the vocal cord muscle, invasion of the cricoarytenoid muscle or joint, or rarely, invasion of the recurrent laryngeal nerve.

Perineural spread is uncommon in laryngeal malignancies.

Supraglottic Larynx

SUPRAHYOID EPIGLOTTIS

A lesion of the suprahyoid epiglottis may produce a huge exophytic mass with little tendency to destroy cartilage or spread to adjacent structures. Other lesions may infiltrate the tip and destroy cartilage. The destructive lesions tend to invade the vallecula and preepiglottic space, the lateral pharyngeal walls, and the remainder of the supraglottic larynx.

INFRAHYOID EPIGLOTTIS

Lesions of the infrahyoid epiglottis tend to produce irregular tumor nodules and simultaneously invade the porous epiglottic cartilage and thyroepiglottic ligament into the preepiglottic fat space and extend toward the vallecula and base of the tongue. The thick hyoepiglottic ligament is an effective tumor barrier. However, the tumor may present in the vallecula and base of tongue without involving the suprahyoid epiglottis.

Lesions of the infrahyoid epiglottis grow circumferentially to involve the false cords, aryepiglottic folds, medial wall of the pyriform sinus, and the pharyngoepiglottic fold. Invasion of the anterior commissure and cords and anterior subglottic extension usually occur only in advanced lesions. Infrahyoid epiglottic lesions that extend onto or below the vocal cords are at a high risk for thyroid cartilage invasion, even if the cords are mobile.[60]

FALSE CORD

Early false cord carcinomas, which are usually submucosal with little exophytic component, are difficult to delineate accurately. They involve the paraglottic fat space early in their development and may spread a considerable distance beneath the mucosa without producing physical signs. These carcinomas extend to the perichondrium of the thyroid cartilage quite early, but cartilage invasion is a late phenomenon. Extension to the lower portion of the infrahyoid epiglottis and invasion of the preepiglottic space are common. Submucosal extension involves the true vocal cord, which may appear normal. Vocal cord invasion is often associated with thyroid cartilage invasion. Submucosal extension to the medial wall of the pyriform sinus occurs early.

ARYEPIGLOTTIC FOLD/ARYTENOID

Early lesions of the aryepiglottic fold/arytenoid are usually exophytic. It may be difficult to decide whether the lesion started on the medial wall of the pyriform sinus or on the aryepiglottic fold. As the lesions enlarge, they extend to adjacent sites and eventually cause fixation of the larynx. Fixation is usually a result of involvement of the cricoarytenoid muscle or joint or, rarely, invasion of the recurrent laryngeal nerve. Computed tomography (CT) may distinguish the cause of fixation. Advanced lesions invade the thyroid, epiglottic, and cricoid cartilages and eventually invade the pyriform sinus and postcricoid area.

VOCAL CORD

Most lesions of the true vocal cord begin on the free margin and upper surface of the cord. When diagnosed, about two thirds are confined to the cords, usually one cord. The anterior portion of the cord is the most common site. Anterior commissure involvement, which is common, is said to occur when no tumor-free cord can be seen anteriorly; if the lesion crosses to the opposite cord, anterior commissure invasion is certain. Small lesions isolated to the anterior commissure account for only 1% to 2% of all cases. Extension to the posterior commissure area is uncommon, occurring only in advanced lesions.

Tumors at the anterior commissure may extend anteriorly the short distance along the anterior commissure tendon (Broyles' ligament), which inserts directly into the thyroid cartilage and allows tumor access to the cartilage without penetrating a muscle or the perichondrium.[10] Early subglottic extension is also associated with involvement of the anterior commissure, and tumor may grow through the cricothyroid membrane.

Lesions that arise on the posterior half of the vocal cord tend to extend along the submucosa toward the medial side of the vocal process and invade the cricoarytenoid joint and posterior commissure, which is difficult to appreciate by clinical examination.

Subglottic extension may occur by simple mucosal surface growth, but it more commonly occurs by submucosal penetration through the conus elasticus. One centimeter of subglottic extension anteriorly or 4 mm to 5 mm of subglottic extension posteriorly brings the border of the tumor to the upper margin of the cricoid, the limits of performing a conventional hemilaryngectomy. Lesions may spread beneath the epithelium along the length of the vocal cord within Reinke's space.[51]

As vocal cord lesions enlarge, they extend to the false cord, vocal process of the arytenoid, and subglottic region. Infiltrative lesions invade the vocal ligament and muscle and eventually reach the paraglottic space and the perichondrium of the thyroid cartilage. The conus elasticus provides a temporary barrier to subglottic penetration. The conus elasticus may direct tumor growth toward the cricothyroid membrane. Advanced glottic lesions eventually penetrate through the thyroid cartilage or cricothyroid membrane to enter the neck, where they may invade the thyroid gland. Lesions involving the anterior commissure often extend through the cricothyroid membrane after they extend subglottically.[51]

A fixed cord with less than 1 cm of subglottic extension and no false cord involvement does not ordinarily indicate invasion of the thyroid cartilage.[29] If the false cord is also involved, cartilage invasion is likely.

Subglottic Larynx

Subglottic cancers are rare. Most involve the inferior surface of the vocal cords by the time they are diagnosed, so it is difficult to know whether the tumor started on the undersurface of the vocal cord or in the true subglottic larynx. Because early diagnosis is uncommon, most lesions are bilateral or circumferential at discovery. They involve the cricoid cartilage early, because there is no intervening muscle layer. Partial or complete fixation of one or both cords is the rule.

Lymphatic Spread

The location and stage of neck nodes detected on admission for previously untreated patients with squamous cell carcinoma of the supraglottic larynx are given in Figure 35-5.[32] The disease spreads mainly to the subdigastric area. The submandibular area is rarely involved, and there is only a small risk of spinal accessory lymph node involvement. The incidence of clinically positive nodes is 55% at the time of diagnosis; 16% are bilateral.[32] Elective neck dissection reveals pathologically positive nodes in 16% of the cases; observation of initially node-negative necks eventually identifies the appearance of positive nodes in 33% of the cases.[15,47] Spread to the pyriform sinus, vallecula, and base of the tongue increases the risk of node metastases. The risk of late-appearing contralateral lymph node metastasis is 37% if the ipsilateral neck is pathologically positive, but the risk is unrelated to whether the nodes in the ipsilateral neck were palpable before neck dissection.

In carcinoma of the vocal cord, the incidence of clinically positive lymph nodes at diagnosis approaches zero for T1 lesions and is 1.7% for T2 lesions.[40] The incidence of neck metastases increases to 20% to 30% for T3 and T4 lesions. Supraglottic spread is associated with metastasis to the jugulodigastric nodes. Anterior commissure and anterior subglottic invasion are associated with involvement of the midline pretracheal lymph node (Delphian node).

Lederman[30] reported a 10% incidence of positive lymph nodes in 73 patients with subglottic carcinoma.

CLINICAL PRESENTATION

Carcinoma arising on the true vocal cords produces hoarseness at a very early stage. Sore throat, ear pain, pain localized to the thyroid cartilage, and airway obstruction are features of advanced lesions.

Hoarseness is not a prominent symptom of cancer of the supraglottic larynx until the lesion becomes quite extensive. Pain on swallowing, usually mild, is the most frequent initial symptom, often described as a sore throat. Some patients report a sensation of a "lump in the throat." Pain is referred to the ear

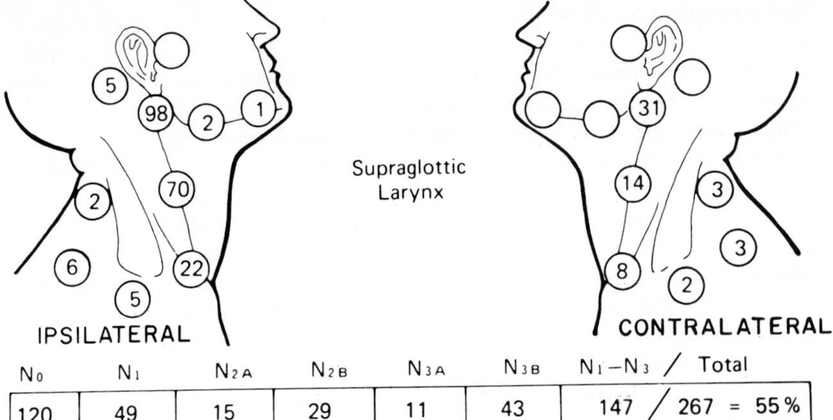

N_0	N_1	N_{2A}	N_{2B}	N_{3A}	N_{3B}	$N_1 - N_3$ / Total
120	49	15	29	11	43	147 / 267 = 55%

FIGURE 35–5. Nodal distribution on admission, M. D. Anderson Cancer Center, 1948–1965. (Lindberg RD: Cancer 29:1446, 1972)

by way of the vagus nerve and auricular nerve of Arnold. A mass in the neck may be the first sign of a supraglottic cancer. Late symptoms include weight loss, foul breath, dysphagia, and aspiration.

DIAGNOSTIC WORKUP

Physical Examination

Rigid and flexible fiberoptic illuminated endoscopes are now used routinely as a complement to the laryngeal mirror examination. The Hopkins rod with a right-angled lens gives excellent visualization of the infrahyoid epiglottis and anterior commissure, areas that may be difficult or impossible to see with a laryngeal mirror. The mirror gives a larger image of the larynx or hypopharynx than that obtained by direct laryngoscopy or by fiberoptic endoscopy. The flexible fiberoptic laryngoscope is inserted through the nose and is useful in the more difficult cases. The occasional patient who does not tolerate the mirror or flexible fiberoptic laryngoscopic examination may be successfully examined if diazepam is administered intramuscularly or intravenously before the procedure.

Determination of the mobility of the vocal cords frequently requires multiple examinations, because the subtle distinctions between mobile, partially fixed, and fixed cords are often challenging, apparently changing from examination to examination. A cord that appeared mobile to the surgeon before direct laryngoscopy may exhibit sluggish motion or even fixation after biopsy.

Ulceration of the infrahyoid epiglottis or fullness of the vallecula is an indirect sign of preepiglottic space invasion. Palpation of diffuse, firm fullness above the thyroid notch with widening of the space between the hyoid and the thyroid cartilages signifies invasion of the preepiglottic space. Lateral soft tissue roentgenograms of the neck may show irregular air cavities inferior to the vallecula in patients with lesions of the suprahyoid epiglottis invading into the preepiglottic space by way of the vallecula. The preepiglottic fat space is a low-density area on the CT scan, and changes resulting from tumor invasion are easily seen.

Postcricoid extension may be suspected when the laryngeal click disappears on physical examination. Postcricoid tumor may cause the thyroid cartilage to protrude anteriorly, producing a fullness of the neck.

Invasion of the thyroid cartilage remains a difficult clinical diagnosis. Localized pain or tenderness to palpation or a small bulge over one ala of the thyroid cartilage is suggestive.

Radiographic Studies

CT scan with contrast enhancement is the method of choice for studying the larynx (Fig. 35-6). The CT scan should be done before biopsy. CT is preferred to magnetic resonance imaging (MRI) because the longer scanning time for MRI produces motion artifact.[43] CT slices 3 mm thick are obtained at 3-mm intervals through the larynx and at 5-mm intervals for the remainder of the study. The gantry is angled so that the scan slices are parallel to the plane of the true vocal cords. It is also necessary to obtain a CT scan of the entire neck to detect positive, nonpalpable lymph nodes.

Contrast enhancement helps to outline the blood vessels and thyroid gland. Tumor is often enhanced, probably because of reactive inflammatory changes. In addition to CT, MRI may be obtained to define subtle exolaryngeal spread or early cartilage destruction. The value of MRI for detecting early cartilage destruction is open to speculation. Sagittal MRI may be useful in detecting early invasion of the base of the tongue.

Vocal Cord Carcinoma

The CT scan does not show minimal mucosal lesions and is generally not indicated for well-defined, easily visualized T1 or early T2 vocal cord carcinomas. CT is excellent for determining subglottic extension and is often used in selected T1 or T2 lesions for this reason alone. CT scanning is useful in the diagnosis of moderately advanced and advanced lesions; it is excellent for demonstrating extension outside the larynx into the soft tissues of the neck and has potential for determining thyroid or cricoid cartilage invasion, which tends to occur at the edges of the cartilage rather than on the faces. Early cartilage involvement is difficult to detect with axial scans, but it may be demonstrated by coronal or sagittal scanning techniques. If the low-density plane of the paraglottic space is intact, cartilage is probably not invaded by metastatic disease.

Archer and associates[5] of St. Louis University correlated CT findings with the incidence of cartilage or bone invasion on whole organ sections. For 12 of 14 patients with pathologic evidence of cartilage invasion, the average diameter of the tumor in two dimensions was more than 16 mm and the lesion was located below the top of the arytenoid. Lesions in which the maximum diameter lay above the top of the arytenoid had a low incidence of cartilage invasion.[5,42]

Supraglottic Carcinoma

The CT scan provides an excellent means for viewing the preepiglottic and paraglottic fat spaces. Soft tissue extension into the neck or base of the tongue can also be seen. The CT scan is also useful for determining extension to the subglottic areas.[33]

Diagnostic procedures for laryngeal cancer at the University of Florida are summarized in Table 35-1. A CT scan is not usually done for T1 or early T2 vocal cord cancers, but it is almost always done for the remainder of laryngeal lesions. Direct laryngoscopy and biopsy with frozen section are usually performed with the patient under general anesthesia. The ventricles, subglottic area, apex of the pyriform sinus, and postcricoid area must be carefully examined, because these areas are not consistently seen by indirect examinations. Fiberoptic telescopes (0 and 30 degrees) are introduced through the laryngoscope for inspection of these areas. A generous biopsy specimen is taken from the obvious lesion; additional biopsy specimens may be obtained from suspicious areas and from areas grossly involved. The mucosa of the margin of the cord may be stripped to provide adequate tissue if the lesion is distributed superficially along the cord and is not obviously a carcinoma.

STAGING

The 1988 American Joint Committee on Cancer staging system for laryngeal primary cancer is listed in Table 35-2.[2] For lesions arising in the supraglottis, the sites of origin include false cords, aryepiglottic folds, suprahyoid epiglottis, infrahyoid epiglottis, and arytenoids. Only in the early T stages can one identify the specific site of origin with certainty. As the lesion enlarges, the site of origin is an educated guess based on the location of the greatest bulk of tumor.

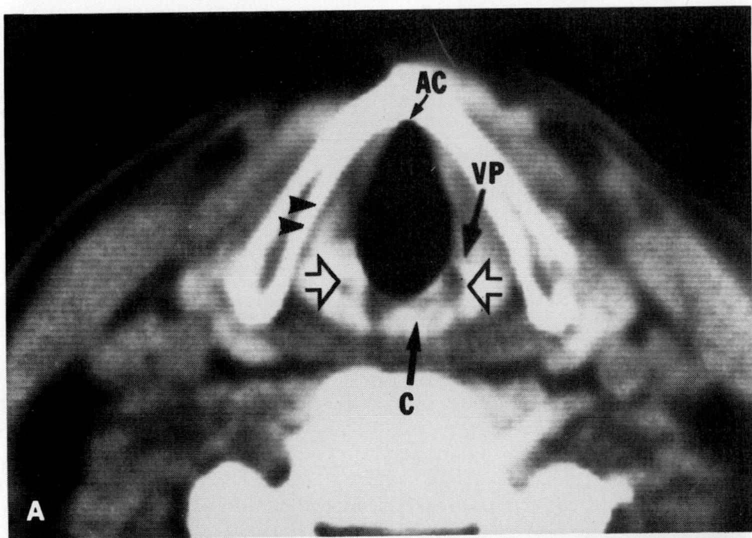

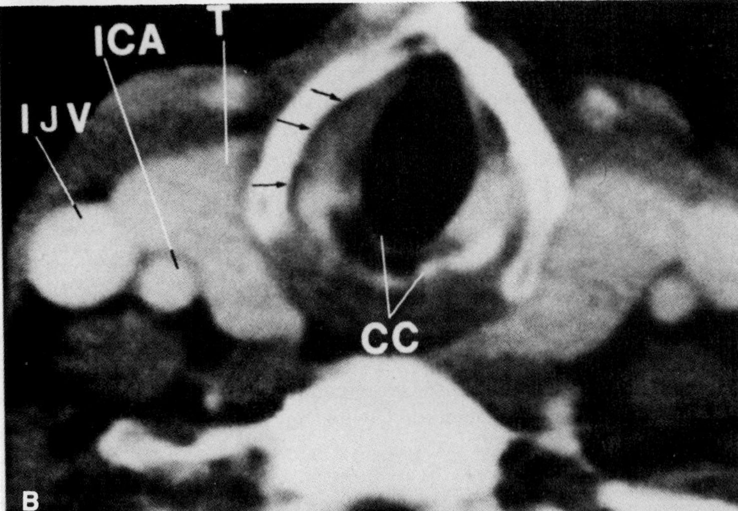

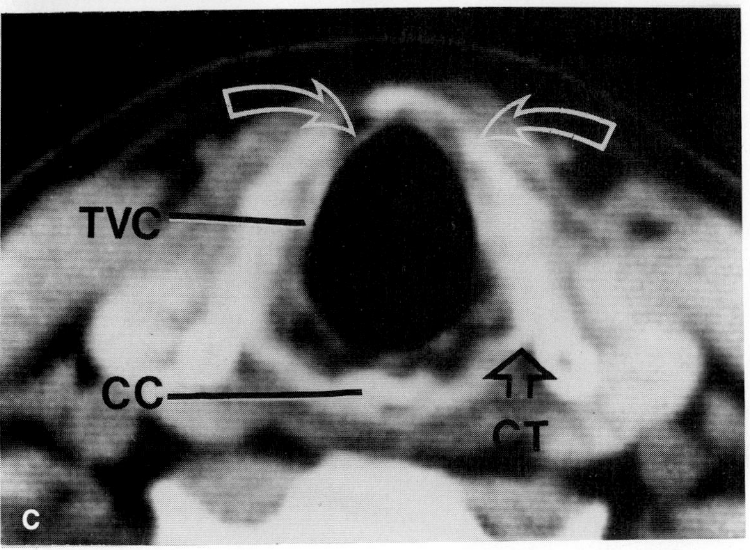

FIGURE 35–6. (**A**) Normal CT anatomy of the midplane of the true vocal cords. Open arrows indiate arytenoid cartilages. The top of the cricoid cartilage (C) is partially visualized at this level. The vocal process (VP) of the left arytenoid cartilage is demonstrated. A narrow, low-density plane is seen between the right true vocal cord and the thyroid lamina (*arrowheads*); this is the inferior part of the paraglottic fat space. Notice the complete lack of tissue at the anterior commissure (AC). Any tissue density here should be considered abnormal. (**B**) Normal CT anatomy just below the midplane of the vocal cords. Arrows indicate low-density lower paraglottic fat space. The fibrofatty tissue in this space facilitates separation of the vocal cord and the adjacent thyroid lamina. If this clear space is maintained in the face of the thyroid lamina irregularity adjacent to the tumor, the lamina abormality can be attributed to uneven calcification rather than tumor destruction. The posterior portion (lamina) of the cricoid cartilage (CC) is seen. The outer and inner cortex of the cartilage is calcified; there is an intervening marrow space that has lower density. The vertical height of the lamina is 2 cm to 3 cm. There is incomplete calcification of the thyroid cartilage anteriorly. IJV, internal jugular vein; ICA, internal carotid artery; T, thyroid gland. (**C**) Normal CT anatomy 5 mm below the free margin of the true vocal cord (TVC). The vocal cord appears thin due to abduction during scanning. There is incomplete bilateral paramedian calcification and thinning of the thyroid lamina (*arrows*). Notice the normal lack of tissue density between the airway and the anterior arch of the thyroid cartilage. CC, cricoid cartilage; CT, cricothyroid joint. (Million RR, Cassisi NJ: Larynx. In Million RR, Cassisi NJ [eds]: Management of Head and Neck Cancer: A Multidisciplinary Approach, pp 315–364. Philadelphia, JB Lippincott, 1984)

PATHOLOGIC CLASSIFICATION

Nearly all malignant tumors of the larynx arise from the surface epithelium and therefore are squamous cell carcinoma or one of its variants.

Carcinoma *in situ* occurs frequently on the vocal cords. Differentiating among dysplasia, carcinoma *in situ*, squamous cell carcinoma with microinvasion, and true invasive carcinoma is a problem that the pathologist and the clinician frequently confront. Stripping the entire cord in patients with minimal lesions serves as the biopsy of the mucosa.

Most vocal cord carcinomas are well differentiated or moderately well differentiated. In a few cases, an apparent carcinoma and sarcoma occur together, but most of these are

TABLE 35–1
Diagnostic Workup for Carcinoma of the Larynx

GENERAL

History
Physical examination, including both necks
Indirect laryngoscopy (with photography)
Direct laryngoscopy
Biopsies
Videolaryngoscopy (optional)

RADIOGRAPHIC STUDIES

Chest x-ray films
Computed tomography with contrast enhancement (before biopsy)
Magnetic resonance imaging (selected cases)

LABORATORY TESTS

Complete blood count
Blood chemistry
Urinalysis

actually a spindle-cell carcinoma (*i.e.*, squamous cell carcinoma with a spindle-cell stromal reaction). Carcinosarcoma, a rare tumor, may present in the larynx and trachea as a polypoid or pedunculated tumor with a string-like umbilical cord.

Verrucous carcinoma occurs in 1% to 2% of patients with carcinoma of the vocal cord. The histologic diagnosis is difficult and must correlate with the gross appearance of the lesion.

Small cell carcinoma ("oat cell") is rarely diagnosed in the supraglottic larynx, but it should be recognized because of its biologic potential for rapid growth, early dissemination, and responsiveness to chemotherapy.

Minor salivary gland tumors arise from the mucous glands in the supraglottic and subglottic larynx, but they are rare.[20]

TABLE 35–2
Staging of Laryngeal Cancer

TUMOR STAGE	CHARACTERISTICS
SUPRAGLOTTIS	
Tis	Carcinoma *in situ*
T1	Tumor confined to region of origin with normal vocal cord mobility
T2	Tumor involving adjacent supraglottic site(s) or glottis without vocal cord fixation
T3	Tumor limited to the larynx with vocal cord fixation and/or extension to involve the postcricoid area, medial wall of pyriform sinus, or preepiglottic space
T4	Tumor invading through the thyroid cartilage and/or extending beyond the larynx to involve the oropharynx or soft tissues of the neck
GLOTTIS	
Tis	Carcinoma *in situ*
T1	Tumor confined to vocal cord(s) with normal mobility (may involve anterior or posterior commissures)
T2	Supraglottic and/or subglottic extension of tumor and/or impaired vocal cord mobility
T3	Tumor confined to the larynx with vocal cord fixation
T4	Tumor invading through the thyroid cartilage and/or extending beyond the larynx to involve the oropharynx or soft tissues of the neck

Even rarer are chemodectoma, carcinoid, soft tissue sarcoma, malignant lymphoma, or plasmacytoma. Benign chondromas and osteochondromas are reported, but their malignant counterparts are rare.

TREATMENT

Vocal Cord Carcinoma

Selection of Treatment Modality

In treating vocal cord carcinoma, the goal is cure with the best functional result and the least risk of a serious complication. Patients may be considered to be in an early or a late group. The early group may be treated initially by irradiation or, in selected cases, by partial laryngectomy. The late group may be treated with irradiation, with laryngectomy reserved for failure, or with total laryngectomy with or without radiation therapy.

CARCINOMA *IN SITU*

Lesions diagnosed as carcinoma *in situ* may sometimes be controlled by stripping the cord. However, it is difficult to exclude the possibility of microinvasion on these specimens. Recurrence is frequent, and the cord may become thickened and the voice hoarse with repeated stripping.

We now recommend early irradiation for carcinoma *in situ*, realizing that most cases eventually receive this treatment and that earlier use of irradiation means a better chance of preserving a good voice.

Many of the cases treated as carcinoma *in situ* have obvious lesions that probably contain invasive carcinoma. We have often proceeded with radiation therapy rather than put the patient through a repeated biopsy procedure.

EARLY VOCAL CORD CARCINOMA

Early vocal cord cancer is defined as the subset that can be cured with larynx preservation. In most centers, irradiation is the initial treatment prescribed for T1 and T2 lesions, with operation reserved for salvage of irradiation failures. Although hemilaryngectomy or cordectomy produce comparable cure rates for selected T1 or T2 vocal cord lesions, irradiation is generally preferred. There is limited information available about the efficacy of laser excision.[22,52,64] The major advantages of irradiation compared with hemilaryngectomy or cordectomy are that the quality of the voice is better and that a major operation is avoided. Hemilaryngectomy finds its major use as a salvage operation in suitable cases after irradiation failure. Even if the patient has a local recurrence after a salvage hemilaryngectomy, there is a third chance with total laryngectomy, which may still be successful.[7]

Verrucous lesions have the reputation of being unresponsive to irradiation and, in some instances, converting into invasive, often anaplastic, metastasizing lesions after unsuccessful irradiation. Hemilaryngectomy is recommended for early verrucous carcinoma of the glottis, but radiation therapy is recommended if the alternative is total laryngectomy. We have observed typical verrucous lesions that have disappeared with radiation therapy and not recurred. Burns and co-workers[11] have also made this observation.

Fixed-cord lesions (T3) may be subdivided into relatively favorable or unfavorable lesions. Patients with unfavorable lesions usually have extensive bilateral disease with a compromised airway. Patients considered to have favorable lesions have disease confined mostly to one side of the larynx, have a good airway, are relatively easy to examine, and are reliable for follow-up. Some degree of supraglottic extension usually exists but does not, by itself, predict success or failure. Subglottic extension occurs frequently. Subglottic extension of 1 cm or less does not affect local control if twice-a-day fractionation is used; extension >1 cm to 2 cm reduces the chances of local control, but in two patients, this level of disease was controlled with radiation therapy alone. Women have a better chance of cure and should be seriously considered for conservative treatment, regardless of tumor extent.

The patient with a favorable lesion is advised of the alternatives of radiation therapy with surgical salvage or immediate total laryngectomy.[57] The patient must be willing to return for follow-up examinations every 1 to 2 months for the first 2 years. He must understand that total laryngectomy may be recommended purely on clinical grounds without biopsy-proven recurrence and that the risk of laryngeal osteochondronecrosis is about 5%.

Evaluation of cord mobility after 5040 cGy has not been helpful in predicting local control. Mobility evaluated 4 to 6 weeks after treatment has better predicted the local control rate. Some patients in whom the vocal cord remained fixed have had local control of the disease for 2 years or longer after irradiation.

The major difficulty in using irradiation for the more advanced lesions is differentiating radiation edema and local recurrence during follow-up examinations. Progressive laryngeal edema, persistent throat pain, or fixation of a previously mobile vocal cord frequently signify recurrent disease in the larynx, although a few patients with these findings remain disease-free with long-term follow-up.

Extended hemilaryngectomy has been used by a few surgeons in the treatment of well-lateralized fixed-cord lesions. A permanent tracheostomy is usually required because a portion of the cricoid is resected, but a useful voice may be retained.[58]

ADVANCED VOCAL CORD CARCINOMA

Advanced lesions usually show extensive subglottic and supraglottic extension, bilateral glottic involvement, and invasion of the thyroid, cricoid, or arytenoid cartilage, or frequently all three.[4,5] The airway is compromised, and there is often extension to the pyriform sinus or postcricoid area. Clinically positive lymph nodes are found in about 30% of the patients. Approximately 30% require a tracheotomy at the time of direct laryngoscopy and biopsy.

The mainstay of treatment is total laryngectomy, with or without preoperative or postoperative irradiation. The most frequent sites of local failure after total laryngectomy are around the tracheal stoma, in the base of tongue, and in the neck lymph nodes or soft tissues of the neck. If the neck is clinically negative before the operation and if postoperative irradiation is planned, neck dissection may not be done and irradiation may be used to treat both sides of the neck. However, in practice, some surgeons perform an elective neck dissection in conjunction with a total laryngectomy for T3N0 or T4N0 laryngeal cancer, even if postoperative irradiation is planned. If the lymph nodes are clinically positive, a neck dissection is done.

Postoperative irradiation may be used to control subclinical disease in the opposite neck site and to help prevent recurrence in other areas. The indications for postoperative irradiation include close or positive margins, subglottic extension, cartilage invasion, perineural invasion, extension of the primary tumor into the soft tissues of the neck, multiple positive neck nodes, and extension of tumor through the capsule of the lymph node(s).[1] Preoperative irradiation is indicated for patients who have fixed neck nodes, have had an emergency tracheotomy through tumor, or have direct extension of tumor involving the skin.

Radical irradiation is prescribed for the patient who refuses total laryngectomy or is medically unsuitable for a major operation.

Surgical Treatment

Thyrotomy with cordectomy is an excision of the vocal cord. Its use is usually confined to small lesions of the middle third of the cord. Cordectomy is generally reserved for the uncommon, postirradiation recurrence limited to the middle third of the cord with normal mobility. After cordectomy, a pseudocord is formed, and the patient has a useful, if somewhat harsh voice. A portion of the adjacent thyroid cartilage may be removed with the cord.

Hemilaryngectomy is a partial, "vertical" laryngectomy that allows removal of limited cord lesions with preservation of voice. One entire cord and as much as a third of the opposite cord is the maximum cordal involvement suitable for the operation in men; women have a smaller larynx, and usually only one vocal cord may be removed without compromising the airway. Partial fixation of one cord is not a contraindication to hemilaryngectomy, but only a few surgeons have attempted hemilaryngectomy for selected fixed-cord lesions. The maximum subglottic extension suitable for hemilaryngectomy is 8 mm to 9 mm anteriorly and 5 mm posteriorly; this limit is necessary to preserve the integrity of the cricoid. Tumor extension to the epiglottis, false cord, or both arytenoids is a contraindication to hemilaryngectomy. In properly selected cases, fewer than 5% of hemilaryngectomies are converted to total laryngectomies.

Total laryngectomy with or without neck dissection is the operation of choice for advanced lesions and as a salvage procedure for irradiation failures in lesions that are not suited for conservative operations. The entire larynx is removed, and the pharynx is reconstituted. A permanent tracheostomy is required. Speech may be reconstituted with a prosthesis, such as the Singer-Blom prosthesis or the Panje button, or with an electrolarynx.

Irradiation Technique

Irradiation for T1 or T2 vocal cord cancer is delivered by small portals covering only the primary lesion. The cervical lymph node chain is not electively treated. Radiation portals extend from the thyroid notch superiorly to the inferior border of the cricoid and fall off anteriorly. The posterior border depends on posterior extension of the tumor.[43] The field size ranges from 4 cm × 4 cm to 5 cm × 5 cm and is occasionally 6 cm × 6 cm for a large T2 lesion. Portals larger than this increase the risk of edema without increasing the cure rate. Because the portals are small and the skin of the neck is mobile, it is our practice to have the physician check the portal on the treatment table each day by palpation of the anatomic landmarks.

A commonly used dose-fractionation schedule at many institutions is 6600 cGy for T1 lesions and 7000 cGy for T2 cancers given in 200-cGy fractions. Evidence suggests that increasing the dose per fraction may improve the likelihood of local control.[3,16,25,26,78] Patients with T1 or T2 vocal cord cancer treated with once-a-day fractionation at the University of Florida are irradiated with 225-cGy fractions; the dose fractionation schemes employed are shown in Table 35-3.[44,53] Since December 1986, twice-a-day irradiation employing 120-cGy fractions

TABLE 35–3
Radiation Treatment Plan for Glottic Carcinoma at the University of Florida

TUMOR STAGE	DESCRIPTION	EXTERNAL BEAM IRRADIATION (cGy TUMOR DOSE)
T1	Early, no visible tumor	5625/25 fractions/5 weeks
T1	Moderate size	6300/28 fractions/5.5 weeks
T2	Early, normal motion	6300/28 fractions/5.5 weeks
T2	Moderate size, reduced motion	6525/29 fractions/6 weeks

(Million RR, Cassisi NJ, Clark JR: Cancer of the head and neck. In DeVita VT Jr, Hellman S, Rosenberg SA (eds): Cancer: Principles and Practice of Oncology, *3rd ed, pp 488–580. Philadelphia, J.B. Lippincott, 1989)*

to deliver a total dose of 7440 cGy has been used to treat most T2 glottic cancers.

At the University of Florida, the patients are treated in the lateral decubitus ("chicken-wing") position with the arm flexed at the elbow and tucked under the thorax (Fig. 35-7).[39] The field is set up by the physician at the treatment machine each day according to palpable anatomic landmarks, and new lines are drawn on the patient each day. This allows the treatment volume to be kept at a minimum and reduces the risk of geographic miss. The lateral decubitus position is chosen because we believe identification of the posterior border of the thyroid cartilage is easier than when the patient is supine, and the maximum lateral thickness of the patient is reduced. The technique requires no simulation, and portal films are unnecessary.[55] Freehand "stacked blocks" are used for secondary beam collimation; patients receiving an anterior boost dose are supine (Fig. 35-7).[39] A three-field technique, using ^{60}Co or 4-MV x-rays, is used to deliver approximately 95% of the dose through opposed lateral wedged fields weighted to the side of the lesion; the remaining dose is delivered by an anterior field shifted 0.5 cm toward the side of the lesion (Fig. 35-8).[43] The tumor dose is usually specified at the 95% normalized isodose line.

At other institutions, patients are treated in the supine position with parallel opposed lateral portals, usually 5 cm × 5 cm or 6 cm × 6 cm, depending on the size of the lesion, using the same reference points and doses described previously.

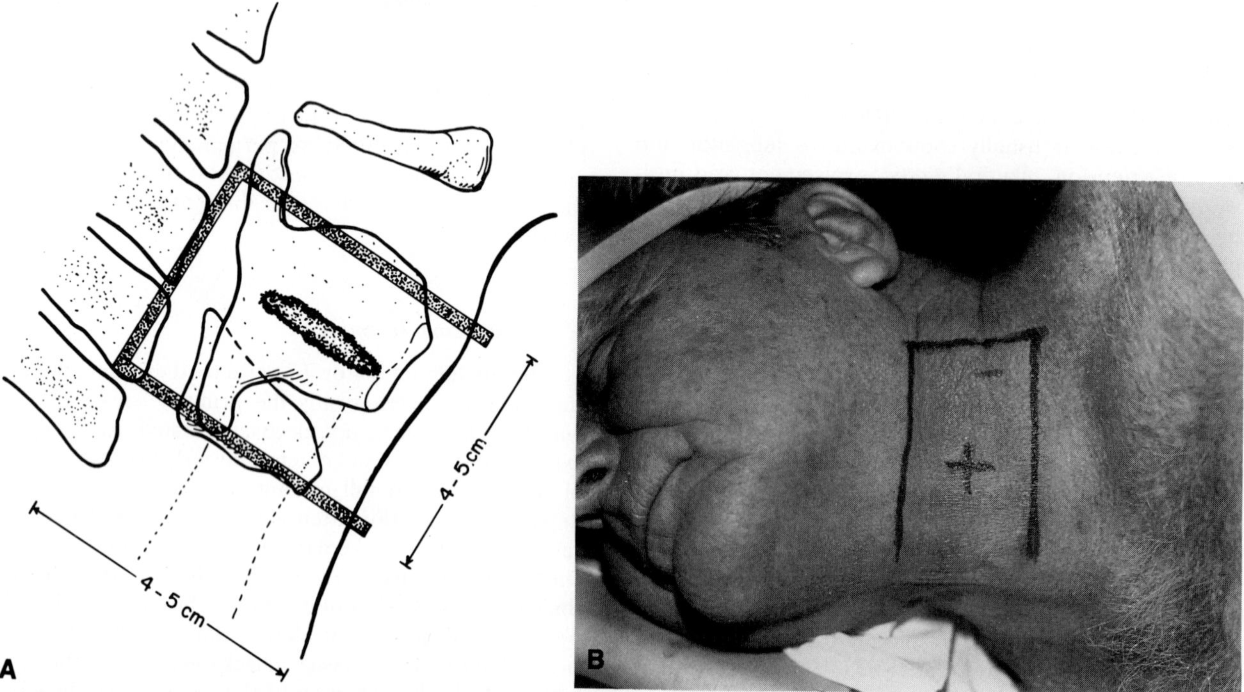

FIGURE 35–7. (**A**) Treatment portal for early glottic carcinoma. The top border is adjusted according to the lesion. The bottom of the thyroid notch is the landmark for very early lesions and the top of the notch is the marker for larger lesions or those with minimal supraglottic extension. The posterior border is the back edge of the thyroid cartilage if the lesion is confined to the anterior two thirds of the vocal cord; if the posterior one third of the vocal cord is involved, the posterior border is placed 1.0 cm to 1.5 cm behind the cartilage. The inferior border is placed at the bottom of the cricoid cartilage if there is no subglottic extension. (Million RR, Cassisi NJ: Larynx. In Million RR, Cassisi NJ [eds]: Management of Head and Neck Cancer: A Multidisciplinary Approach, pp 315–364. Philadelphia, JB Lippincott, 1984) (**B**) Patient in the lateral "chicken-wing" position for treatment of a T1N0 squamous cell carcinoma confined to the anterior two thirds of the vocal cord. (Mendenhall WM, Parsons JT, Million RR, Fletcher GH: Int J Radiat Oncol Biol Phys 15:1267, 1988)

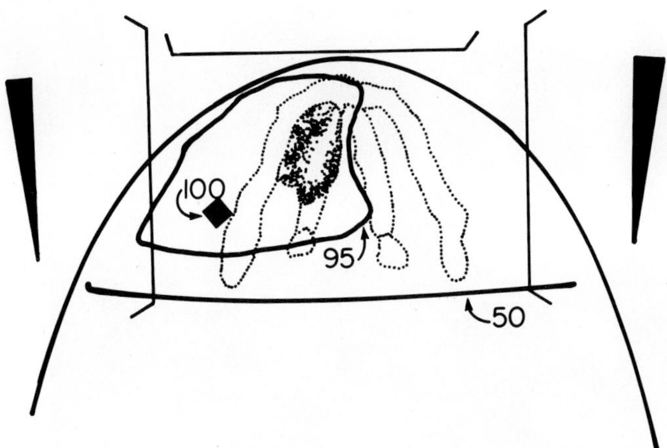

FIGURE 35–8. Normalized isodose distribution for three-field technique for treatment of a tumor involving the anterior two thirds of one true vocal cord. The dose is specified at the 95% isodose line.

Open fields and wedges are used to obtain a more homogeneous dose (Fig. 35-9).

Irradiation of T3 and T4 lesions requires larger portals, which include the jugulodigastric and middle jugular lymph nodes (Fig. 35-10).[36] The inferior jugular lymph nodes are included in a separate low-neck portal. The portals are reduced after 4600 cGy (200 cGy/fraction). The reduced portals cover only the primary lesion, and the dose per fraction is increased to 225 cGy. The final dose is 6850 cGy to 7075 cGy administered in 33 to 34 fractions.

If the patient has a short neck and there is 2 cm or more of subglottic extension, it may be difficult to adequately treat the inferior extent of the primary tumor with parallel opposed fields. In this case, the lateral fields may be angled 5 degrees to 10 degrees inferiorly, or a four-field box technique, similar to that used for lesions of the cervical esophagus, may be used.[34]

Since 1978, we have used twice-a-day fractionation (120-cGy fractions) to administer a total dose of 7440 cGy to 7680 cGy in 6.5 weeks for T3 or T4 vocal cord cancers.[56,57]

The treatment technique used for postoperative irradiation after total laryngectomy is depicted in Figure 35-11.[1] The treatment technique for preoperative irradiation is essentially the same as that employed for irradiation alone.

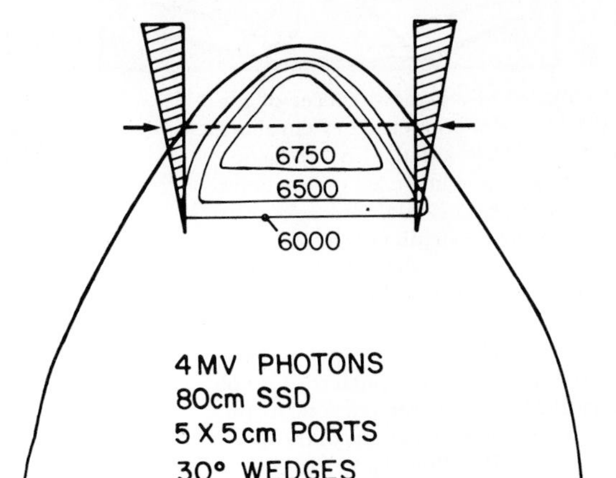

FIGURE 35–9. Composite isodose curves for irradiation of glottic tumors with parallel opposed portals, administering 50% of the dose with open fields and 50% with 30-degree wedges.

Management of Recurrence

Most recurrences appear within 18 months, but late recurrences may appear after 5 years.[19] The risk of metastatic disease in lymph nodes increases with local recurrence.[37]

RECURRENCE AFTER RADIATION THERAPY

With careful follow-up, recurrence is sometimes detected before the patient notices a return of hoarseness. There is often minimal lymphedema for 1 to 2 months after radiation therapy, which usually subsides or stabilizes. An increase in edema, particularly if associated with hoarseness or pain, suggests recurrence, even if there is no obvious tumor. Fixation of a previously mobile vocal cord usually implies local recurrence, but we have observed five patients who have developed a fixed cord with an otherwise normal-appearing larynx and who have not shown evidence of recurrence. A paralyzed left vocal cord also suggests the possibility of lung cancer.

It may be difficult to diagnose recurrence if the tumor is submucosal. Generous, deep biopsies are required. If recurrence is strongly suspected, laryngectomy may rarely be advised without biopsy-confirmed evidence of recurrence.

Irradiation failures may be salvaged by cordectomy, hemilaryngectomy, or total laryngectomy. Biller and co-workers[7] reported a 78% salvage rate by hemilaryngectomy for 18 selected patients in whom irradiation failed. Total laryngectomy was eventually required in two patients. Only two patients died of cancer. These investigators offered guidelines for using hemilaryngectomy: contralateral vocal cord is normal, arytenoid is not involved, subglottic extension does not exceed 5 mm, and vocal cord is not fixed. In our experience, 6 to 10 patients irradiated for T1 or T2 vocal cord cancers were successfully salvaged by surgery after irradiation failed.[40]

RECURRENCE AFTER SURGERY

The rate of salvage by radiation therapy for recurrences or new tumors that appear after initial treatment by hemilaryngectomy is about 50%. Lee and co-workers reported seven successes among 12 patients; one lesion was subsequently controlled by total laryngectomy.[31] Total laryngectomy can be used successfully to treat hemilaryngectomy failures not suitable for radiation therapy. Radiation therapy rarely cures a patient with recurrence in the neck or stoma after total laryngectomy.

Supraglottic Larynx Carcinoma

Selection of Treatment Modality

Patients with supraglottic larynx carcinoma may be considered to be in an early or favorable group suitable for radiation therapy or supraglottic laryngectomy or an unfavorable group often requiring total laryngectomy. Neck nodes are commonly involved and influence the overall treatment plan.

EARLY AND MODERATELY ADVANCED SUPRAGLOTTIC LESIONS

Treatment of the primary lesion for the early group is by external-beam irradiation or supraglottic laryngectomy, with or without adjuvant irradiation. Total laryngectomy is rarely indicated as the initial treatment for this group of patients and is reserved for treatment failures.[50]

Irradiation and supraglottic laryngectomy are highly successful modes of therapy for the early lesions. Approximately 50% of supraglottic laryngectomies performed at the University of Florida have been followed by postoperative radiation therapy because of positive margins or because of neck disease.

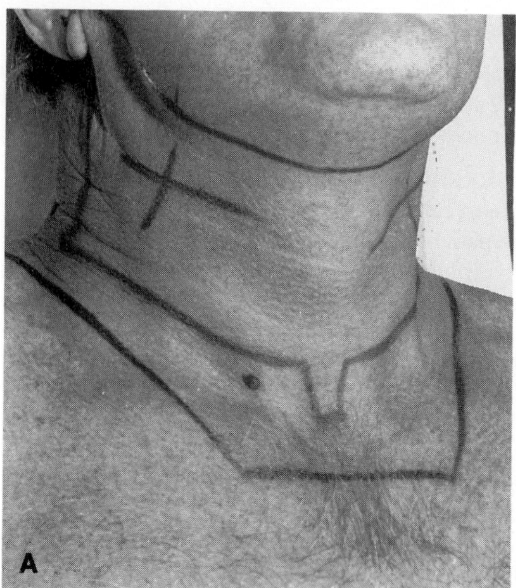

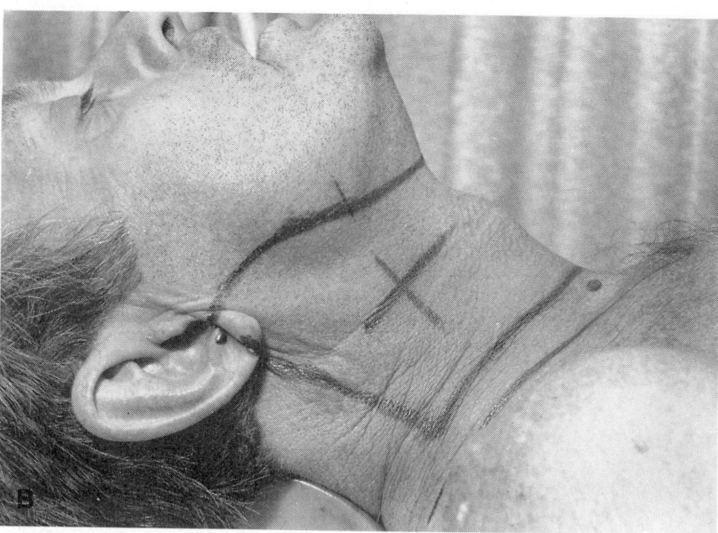

FIGURE 35–10. Radiation treatment of stage T3 glottic carcinoma by means of parallel opposed fields and anterior low-neck field with a tracheal block. (**A**) Lateral view. (**B**) Anterior view. (Mendenhall WM, Million RR, Sharkey DE, Cassisi NJ: Int J Radiat Oncol Biol Phys 10:357, 1984)

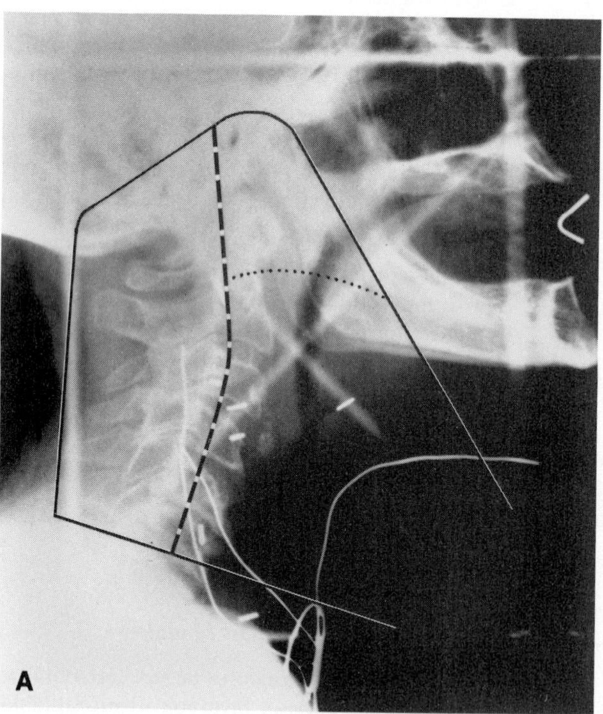

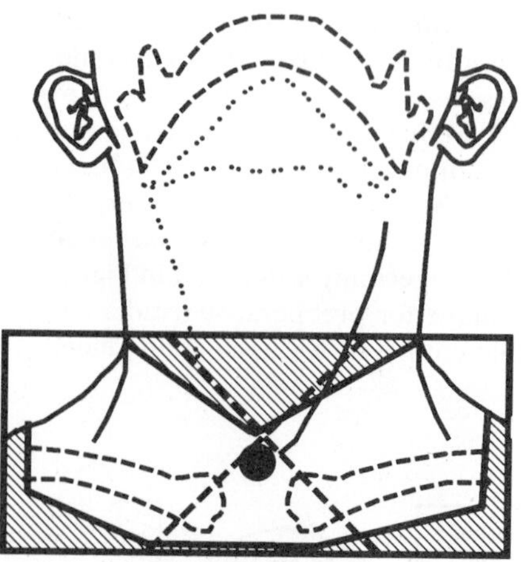

FIGURE 35–11. (**A**) Typical simulation film for postoperative treatment of advanced cancer of the laryngopharynx. If the neck is pathologically negative, the superior field border is lowered to 2 cm above the angle of the mandible. The initial "off-cord" reduction (5000 cGy) (*broken line*) and the final reduction (*dotted line*) are indicated. Wires mark the surgical scars and stoma. The slanting line used on the lower border reduces the length of spinal cord treated by the primary field, allows better caudal coverage of the mucosal surfaces while simultaneously bypassing the shoulders, and facilitates matching of the low-neck field. (**B**) Schematic diagram of low-neck field. The rectangle (*solid line*) represents the light field. The shaded areas represent the blocked portions of the field (stacked lead blocks). The superior border of the neck field is the inferior border of the primary field. The actual line is treated only in the primary field. The upper border of the low-neck field assumes a V shape. In the midline of the patient, the apex of the V generally is at or close to the central axis (*broken lines*), so that the portal that treats the spinal cord is not divergent in its upper portion and diverges away from the primary fields in its lower portion. At the junction of the three fields, a short (2–3 cm) segment of spinal cord remains untreated by any of the three fields. (Amdur RJ, Parsons JT, Mendenhall WM, et al: Int J Radiat Oncol Biol Phys 16:25, 1989)

We follow certain guidelines for selecting supraglottic laryngectomy or radiation therapy. The patient and family are sometimes instrumental in making the decision, based on their previous experience with surgery or radiation therapy. Overall, about 80% of patients are treated initially by radiation therapy. Approximately half of the patients seen in our clinic whose lesions are technically suitable for a supraglottic laryngectomy are not suitable for medical reasons (*e.g.*, inadequate pulmonary status or other major medical problems). These patients are treated by radiation therapy. Elderly or poorly motivated patients are not good candidates for supraglottic laryngectomy.

Analysis of local control by anatomic site within the supraglottic larynx shows no obvious differences in local control by radiation therapy for similarly stage lesions. Transglottic lesions are not suitable for supraglottic laryngectomy, but they may be managed by radiation therapy in favorable cases. Invasion of the preepiglottic space is not a contraindication to supraglottic laryngectomy or radiation therapy. A large, bulky infiltrative lesion, especially one with extensive preepiglottic-space invasion, is a common reason to select supraglottic laryngectomy.

The status of the neck often determines the selection of treatment of the primary lesion. Patients with clinically negative neck nodes and a high risk for occult bilateral neck disease (*e.g.*, poorly differentiated carcinoma of the suprahyoid epiglottis with midline base of the tongue involvement) may be treated by radiation therapy because of the ease of bilateral elective neck irradiation. Alternatively, supraglottic laryngectomy and bilateral conservation neck dissections may be done.

If a patient has an early-stage primary lesion but advanced neck disease (N2b or N3), combined treatment is frequently necessary to control of the neck disease. In these cases, the primary lesion is usually treated by irradiation alone, with surgery added to the treatment of the involved neck site(s). If the same patient were treated with supraglottic laryngectomy, neck dissection, and postoperative irradiation, the radiation therapy portals would unnecessarily cover the primary site and the neck. If the patient has early, resectable neck disease (N1 or N2a) and surgery is elected for the primary site, postoperative irradiation is added only because of unexpected findings (*e.g.*, positive margins, multiple positive nodes, or extracapsular extension). We prefer to avoid routine high-dose preoperative or postoperative irradiation in conjunction with a supraglottic laryngectomy because the lymphedema of the remaining larynx may be considerable, although it eventually subsides. However, Robbins and co-workers[61] from M. D. Anderson Cancer Center reported good results with combined supraglottic laryngectomy and postoperative irradiation for moderately advanced lesions.

ADVANCED SUPRAGLOTTIC LESIONS

The surgical alternative for these lesions is total laryngectomy. Selected advanced lesions, especially those that are mainly exophytic, may be treated by irradiation, and total laryngectomy is reserved for irradiation failures. Borderline lesions are given a trial of irradiation to 4500 cGy to 5000 cGy, and if the response is good, irradiation is continued for cure. If the response is unsatisfactory, irradiation is stopped and total laryngectomy is done 4 to 6 weeks later.

Lesions unsuitable for irradiation are managed by total laryngectomy. If the neck disease is resectable, surgery is the initial treatment, and postoperative irradiation is added if needed. If the neck disease is unresectable, preoperative irradiation is used (see Chap. 37). The indications for preoperative and postoperative irradiation have been previously outlined in this chapter.

Surgical Treatment

SUPRAGLOTTIC LARYNGECTOMY

Supraglottic laryngectomy is a voice-sparing operation that can be used successfully for selected lesions involving the epiglottis, a single arytenoid, the aryepiglottic fold, or the false vocal cord. Extension of the tumor to the true vocal cord, the anterior commissure, or both arytenoids; fixation of the vocal cord; or thyroid or cricoid cartilage invasion preclude supraglottic laryngectomy. The supraglottic laryngectomy may be extended to include the base of the tongue if one lingual artery is preserved. To extend the procedure for involvement of the base of the tongue, the tongue extension must be lateralized to one side and should not extend beyond the circumvallate papillae. A neck dissection on one or both sides may be added as part of the supraglottic laryngectomy; 30% to 35% of patients have histologically positive nodes even if their necks are clinically negative.

All patients have difficulty swallowing with a tendency to aspirate in the immediate postoperative period, but almost all learn to swallow again in a short time; motivation and the amount of tissue removed are key factors in learning to swallow again. Preoperatively, adequate pulmonary reserve is evaluated by blood gas determinations, pulmonary function tests, chest roentgenography, and a work test involving walking the patient up two flights of stairs to determine tolerance to pulmonary stress. The voice quality is generally normal after supraglottic laryngectomy.

Routine use of preoperative irradiation is not indicated in carefully selected cases, because the cure rate with surgery alone is quite high, and radiation therapy increases the surgical complications and promotes lymphedema without substantially affecting the cure rate. Postoperative radiation therapy may be advised for close or positive margins or if the risk of neck failure is substantial.

WIDE-FIELD TOTAL LARYNGECTOMY

The entire larynx and preepiglottic space are resected en bloc, and a permanent tracheostomy is fashioned. The strap muscles, the hyoid bone, and a portion of the thyroid gland are included with the specimen. The pharynx is reconstituted in most cases without a flap. Neck dissection is added on one or both sides, depending on the presence and extent of neck disease and whether or not adjuvant irradiation is planned.

Irradiation Technique

The primary lesion and both sides of the neck are treated with opposed lateral portals; wedges are used to compensate for the contour of the neck. The anterior midline skin is shielded, if possible (Fig. 35-12).[35] The dose for T1 lesions is 6000 cGy to 6500 cGy, and the dose for T2 or T3 lesions is 7000 cGy or, occasionally, 7500 cGy. The early lesions that are encompassed by a small treatment volume receive 200 cGy per fraction. The lesions requiring a large treatment volume are treated with 180-cGy fractions for the first 4500 cGy to 5000 cGy and 180-cGy or 200-cGy fractions for the remainder. For patients treated with twice-a-day fractionation at 120 cGy per fraction, the total dose ranges from 7440 cGy to 7680 cGy. All patients are treated with the continuous-course technique.[54] The lower neck nodes are irradiated through a separate anterior portal (Fig. 37-13).[35] An anterior submental boost portal with photons or electrons may be used for the last 500 cGy to 1000 cGy for suprahyoid epiglottis lesions that invade the vallecula (Fig. 35-14).[35]

In the case of clinically positive nodes, an electron-beam

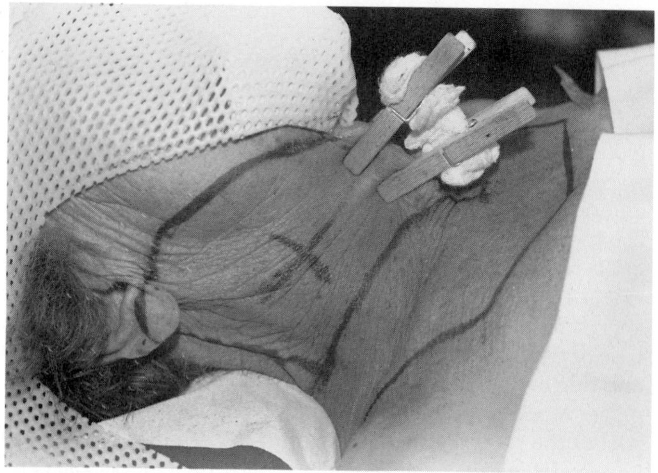

FIGURE 35–12. Radiation treatment of supraglottic larynx carcinoma. Patient in the treatment position using a nonfilled low-temperature thermal plastic (polycaprolactone) face mask to immobilize the head. Clothespins are used to increase the amount of tissue spared anteriorly. (Mendenhall WM, Million RR, Cassisi NJ: Int J Radiat Oncol Biol Phys 10:2223, 1984)

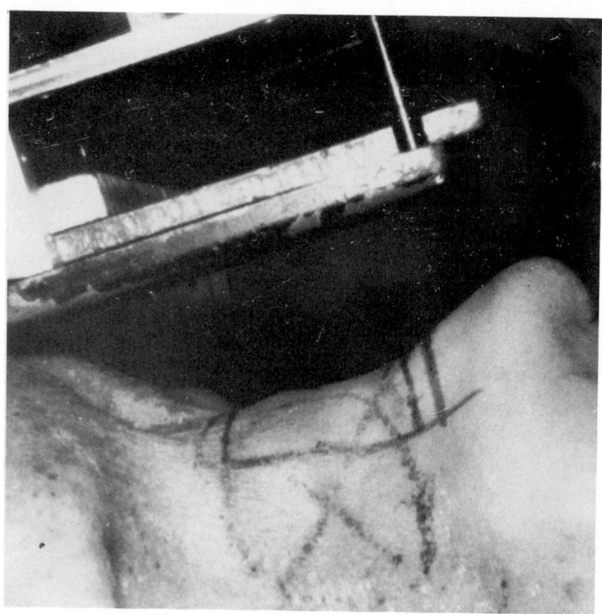

FIGURE 35–14. Radiation treatment of supraglottic larynx carcinoma: Submental boost using electron beam. (Mendenhall WM, Million RR, Cassisi NJ: Int J Radiat Oncol Biol Phys 10:2223, 1984)

portal may be used to increase the dose to the posterior cervical nodes after reducing the fields to avoid the spinal cord at 4500 cGy.[35] The addition of a neck dissection usually increases the risk of temporary lymphedema; however, neck dissection is preferable in terms of tumor control and complications to the higher doses of radiation therapy required to control large neck nodes.

Patients develop a sore throat, loss of taste, and moderate dryness during irradiation. Edema of the arytenoids may occur and give a sensation of lump in the throat. Tracheostomy is seldom necessary, even for bulky lesions.

Edema of the larynx may persist for several months to a year. Neck dissection increases the degree of lymphedema on the side of the operation. The lymphedema of the larynx and submental space resolves together. Patients who continue to smoke heighten the side-effects of dryness, dysphagia, and hoarseness.

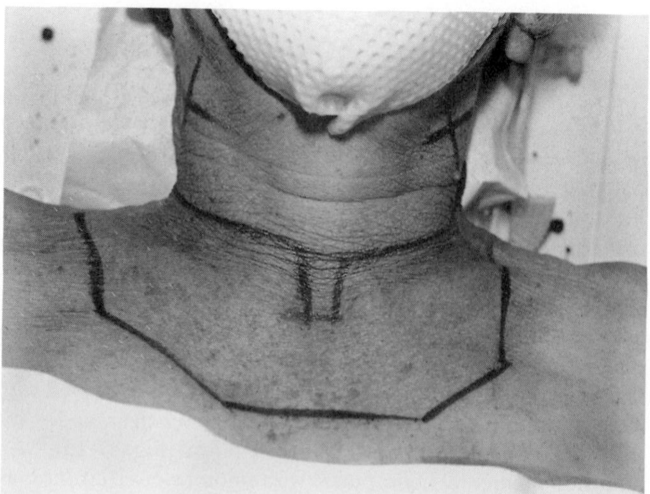

FIGURE 35–13. Radiation treatment of supraglottic larynx carcinoma: Low-neck field with midline block. (Mendenhall WM, Million RR, Cassisi NJ: Int J Radiat Oncol Biol Phys 10:2223, 1984)

Preoperative and Postoperative Treatment Technique

If total laryngectomy is required and the lesion is resectable, postoperative irradiation is preferred, because there is no evidence that preoperative irradiation produces any better locoregional control or survival rates than surgery and postoperative irradiation. Radiation therapy is added for close or positive margins, invasion of soft tissues of the neck, subglottic extension, cartilage invasion, and N2b or N3 neck disease. The high-risk areas are usually the base of the tongue and the neck. The stomal area is at risk mainly if there is subglottic extension; otherwise, it may be shielded.

The dose for postoperative irradiation as a function of known residual disease is as follows: negative margins, 6000 cGy in 30 fractions; microscopically positive margins, 6600 cGy in 33 fractions; and gross residual disease, 7000 cGy in 35 fractions. All patients are treated with continuous-course irradiation employing one fraction per day for 5 days per week. If the daily dose is lowered to 180 cGy, 500 cGy is added to the total dose in each category. The lower neck is treated with doses to 5000 cGy in 25 fractions at D_{max}. If there is subglottic extension, the dose to the stoma is boosted with electrons (usually 10–14 MeV) for an additional 1000 cGy in five fractions. The treatment technique is outlined in Figure 35-11. If postoperative irradiation is added after a supraglottic laryngectomy, the dose is lowered to 5500 cGy given in 180-cGy fractions. This dose produces acceptable rates of local control and laryngeal edema.[61]

The treatment technique employed for preoperative irradiation is essentially the same as that used for patients managed with irradiation alone, using doses of 4500 cGy to 5000 cGy.

Management of Recurrence

Failures after supraglottic laryngectomy or irradiation can frequently be controlled by further treatment; therefore, recognition of recurrence should be vigorously pursued. Salvage of patients with recurrence after combined total laryngectomy and radiation therapy is uncommon. Stomal recurrences are occasionally controlled by radiation therapy or surgery.

RESULTS OF TREATMENT

Vocal Cord Cancer

Surgical Results

Neel and co-workers[46] reported the results for 182 patients with early vocal cord carcinoma who were suitable for cordectomy; 177 had lesions that were confined to one cord. The lesions were 2 mm to 25 mm long. The follow-up was less than 3 years in 18% of the cases. Four patients developed laryngeal recurrence, and three developed neck recurrence. Only three (2%) patients died of vocal cord cancer.

Ogura and associates[49] reported a 3-year disease-free survival rate of 91% for 281 patients treated by hemilaryngectomy. The local recurrence rate was 4%, and the neck recurrence rate was 1.5%; 74% of the treatment failures were controlled by salvage therapy.

A review of 61 patients with involvement of the anterior commissure treated by hemilaryngectomy revealed an absolute survival rate of 74%.[63] There were three (9%) local recurrences and three (9%) neck recurrences.

Hemilaryngectomy including the ipsilateral arytenoid was performed for 130 cases of vocal cord carcinoma extending posteriorly to the vocal process and face of the arytenoid.[70] The cure rate for 104 patients with a T2 lesion was 74%, and for 26 patients with a T3 lesion, it was 58%.

Bauer and co-workers[6] analyzed the significance of the surgical margins in 111 hemilaryngectomy specimens. Thirty-nine (35%) patients were found to have involved margins (usually the anterior margin). The local recurrence rate was 10% with 5-year minimum follow-up. Only seven (18%) of the 39 patients with an involved margin developed a recurrence, compared with 6% with uninvolved margins. Another 5% had recurrence evident in the cervical lymph nodes. Four patients eventually died of cancer.

Ogura and co-workers[49] found that the 3-year cause-specific disease-free survival rate for patients treated by total laryngectomy with or without radical neck dissection was 80%. The local and regional recurrence rate was 21%; approximately 46% of treatment failures were successfully managed by surgery or radiation therapy, alone or combined.

The results of treatment of T4 vocal cord carcinoma from four surgical series and two irradiation series are summarized in Table 35-4.[24] The University of Florida results for total laryngectomy in T3 lesions are presented in the following section.

Radiation Therapy Results

Pene and Fletcher[59] described the results for 79 patients with carcinoma *in situ* and seven patients with dysplasia. The local failure rate was 11% for lesions with a T1 anatomic distribution and 26% for lesions with a T2 anatomic distribution. Elman and co-workers[14] reported similar results. Twelve patients with carcinoma *in situ* were treated at the University of Florida, and the disease was locally controlled in 11 (92%), with follow-up ranging from 2 to 16 years.[38]

The current local control rates reported from several institutions for invasive squamous cell carcinoma are in the range of 90% for T1, 70% for T2, and 50% to 60% for T3 or T4 disease. The surgical salvage rate is 90% to 95% for patients with T1 or T2 lesions that recur after irradiation (Tables 35-5 and 35-6).[24,39,57]

The local control rates for 304 patients with squamous cell carcinoma of the vocal cord, according to stage and surgical procedure, that we treated by irradiation at the University of Florida are given in Table 35-7.[40] Patients were excluded from analysis of local control if they died within 2 years of treatment with the primary site continuously disease-free. The overall rate of voice preservation for the entire series of 304 patients is presented in Table 35-8.[40] Extension to the anterior commissure did not affect success with irradiation. Seven patients with T2 glottic carcinomas were treated with twice-a-day fractionation employing 120-cGy fractions to a total dose of 7440 cGy, and all have remained free from local recurrence for 2 years or longer.

Local control was analyzed in the various subsets as a function of total dose and dose per fraction. In three of seven subsets, there was no dose-fractionation relationship observed; in one subset, there were no local recurrences, and in another, there were only two local recurrences. The correlation between total dose and dose per fraction in the four appropriate subsets is given in Table 35-9.[39] In general, there is a direct relationship between the rate of local control and dose per fraction, with poor results obtained particularly in the T2 lesions at 180 cGy to 190 cGy per fraction at similar or higher total doses. This is consistent with data presented in Table 35-6. At M. D. Anderson, the University of Maryland, and Princess Margaret Hospital, patients were usually treated at ≥210 cGy per fraction, compared with the University of California at San Francisco, where most patients were treated with 180-cGy fractions. Schwaibold and co-workers[62] reported a series of 56 evaluable patients who were treated with irradiation for T1N0 glottic

TABLE 35–4
Treatment of Stage T4 Glottic Carcinoma

INVESTIGATOR	TUMOR STAGE	NO. OF PATIENTS	METHOD OF TREATMENT	RESULTS (NED)*
Jesse[28]	T4 N0 – N+	48	Laryngectomy	54% at 4 yr
Ogura et al[49]	T4 N0	11	Laryngectomy	45% at 3 yr
Skolnick et al[68]	T4 N0	7	Laryngectomy	30% at 5 yr
Vermund[73]	T4 N0	31	Laryngectomy	35% at 5 yr
Stewart and Jackson[72]	T4 N0	13	Irradiation with surgery for salvage	38% at 5 yr
Harwood et al[24]	T4 N0	56	Irradiation with surgery for salvage	49% at 5 yr*

**NED, no evidence of disease.*
† Life-table method; uncorrected for deaths from intercurrent disease.
(Modified with permission from Harwood AR, Beale FA, Cummings BJ, Keane TJ, Payne D, Rider WD: Int J Radiat Oncol Biol Phys 7:1507, 1981. Copyright © 1981, Pergamon Press)

TABLE 35–5
Stage T1 or T2 Glottic Carcinoma Treated with Irradiation

INVESTIGATION	NO. OF PATIENTS		LOCAL CONTROL* (%)		ULTIMATE LOCAL CONTROL* (%)	
	T1	T2	T1	T2	T1	T2
Princess Margaret Hospital[25,26]	333	244	86	69		
M. D. Anderson Cancer Center[16]	332	175	89	74	98	94
U. of Maryland[3]	86	34	92	88	99	94
U. of California at San Francisco[78]	183	42	80	52	97	90
U. of Florida[39]	184	120	93	75	97	94

**No exclusions.*
(Mendenhall WM, Parsons JT, Million RR, Fletcher GH: Int J Radiat Oncol Biol Phys 15:1267, 1988)

TABLE 35–6
Stage T3 Glottic Carcinoma Treated with Irradiation

INVESTIGATOR	INSTITUTION	NO. OF PATIENTS	MINIMUM FOLLOW-UP (YR)	LOCAL CONTROL	ULTIMATE CONTROL AFTER SALVAGE SURGERY
Harwood et al[23]	Princess Margaret	112	3	51%	77%
Wang et al[76]	Mass. General	70	4	36%	57%
Fletcher et al[18]	M.D. Anderson	17	2	77%	
Skolyszewski and Reinfuss[69]	15 European centers	91	3	50%	
Stewart et al[71]	Manchester	67	10	57%	67%
Mills[45]	Capetown, S.A.	18	2	44%	78%
Mendenhall et al[36]	U. Florida	13*	2	54%	77%
Parsons et al[57]	U. Florida	21†	2	67%	83%

**Continuous-course, once-a-day treatment.*
† Continuous-course, twice-a-day irradiation.
(Parsons JT, Mendenhall WM, Mancuso AA, Cassisi NJ, Stringer SP, Million RR: Head Neck 11:123, 1989)

TABLE 35–7
Local Control of Stage T1 or T2 Glottic Carcinoma

TUMOR STAGE	SUB-GROUP*	SIZE	EXCLUDED†	LOCAL CONTROL‡	NO. SALVAGED/NO. ATTEMPTED: HEMI-LARYNGECTOMY	NO. SALVAGED/NO. ATTEMPTED: TOTAL LARYNGECTOMY	ULTIMATE LOCAL CONTROL
T1a	C	<5 mm	1	12/12 (100%)			12/12 (100%)
		5–15 mm	8	73/78 (94%)	3/4	0/1	76/78 (97%)
		>15 mm	2	45/50 (90%)		4/5	49/50 (98%)
T1b	HL	All	0	14/15 (93%)		0/1	14/15 (93%)
	TL	All	2	15/16 (94%)	0/1		15/16 (94%)
T2a	HL	All	5	23/27 (85%)		4/4	27/27 (100%)
	TL	All	2	27/38 (71%)	2/3	7/8	36/38 (95%)
T2b	HL	All	3	13/18 (72%)	1/2	2/3	16/18 (89%)
	TL	All	2	18/25 (72%)		4/6	22/25 (88%)

**C: suitable for cordectomy; HL: suitable for hemilaryngectomy; TL: suitable for total laryngectomy.*
† Died within 2 years of treatment with primary site continuously disease-free.
‡ Local control (no. controlled/no. treated) for 304 patients, 279 of whom were evaluable.
(Mendenhall WM, Parsons JT, Stringer SP, Cassisi NJ, Million RR: Head Neck Surg 10:373, 1988)

TABLE 35–8
Voice Preservation in 304 Patients with Stage T1–T2 Glottic Carcinoma

TUMOR STAGE	SUBGROUP*	SIZE	PROPORTION WITH VOICE PRESERVATION
T1a	C	<5 mm	13/13 (100%)
		5–15 mm	83/86 (97%)
		>15 mm	47/52 (90%)
T1b	HL	All	14/15 (93%)
	TL	All	17/18 (94%)
T2a	HL	All	28/32 (88%)
	TL	All	31/40 (78%)
T2b	HL	All	17/21 (81%)
	TL	All	20/27 (74%)

** C: suitable for cordectomy; HL: suitable for hemilaryngectomy; TL: suitable for total laryngectomy.*
(Mendenhall WM, Parsons JT, Stringer SP, Cassisi NJ, Million RR: Head Neck Surg 10:373, 1988)

carcinoma. Twenty-eight patients were treated at 180 cGy per fraction with a local control rate of 75%, which was compared with 100% local control for 28 patients treated at ≥200 cGy per fraction.

There was a correlation between the rate of disease control in the neck for 268 patients with T1N0 or T2N0 vocal cord carcinoma treated with irradiation to the primary lesion alone and primary tumor control; if the primary lesion was controlled, 0% to 3% of patients developed recurrent disease in the neck, but 20% to 22% of the patients developed recurrent neck disease if their primary lesions recurred.

The absolute and cause-specific (excluding patients who died of intercurrent disease within 5 years of treatment) survival rates for T1N0 or T2N0 vocal cord cancers treated at the University of Florida are shown in Table 35-10.[40]

The survival and control rates of patients with T3 fixed-cord lesions treated at the University of Florida are presented in Table 35-11.[36] Eleven patients in the radiation treatment group had preservation of their larynxes. Two additional patients retained their larynxes but died of other causes before 2 years of follow-up. The vocal quality varied from fair to nearly normal.

TABLE 35–9
Local Control of Stage T1 or T2 Glottic Carcinoma

TUMOR STAGE*	TOTAL DOSE (cGy)	DOSE PER FRACTION (cGy)	LOCAL CONTROL† (NO. CONTROLLED/ NO. TREATED)
T1a, C (5–15 mm)	6100–6500	225	32/32 (100%)
	6100–6700	200–220	22/25 (88%)
	5600–5700	225–230	16/18 (89%)
T2a, HL	6100–6500	225	15/16 (94%)
	6100–6500	215–220	5/6
	6500–7000	180–200	2/4
T2a, TL	6100–6500	225	17/18 (94%)
	6100–6500	215–220	2/5
	6500–7000	180–190	2/6
T2b	6100–6800	220–225	19/25 (76%)
	6100–7000	205–215	5/8
	6100–7000	180–200	6/9

** C: suitable for cordectomy; HL: suitable for hemilaryngectomy; TL: suitable for total laryngectomy.*
† Only the data for the specified ranges of total dose and dose per fraction are included in this table. Thus, the numbers of patients in a certain stage subset may not be the same as in other tables.
(Mendenhall WM, Parsons JT, Million RR, Fletcher GH: Int J Radiat Oncol Biol Phys 15:1267, 1988)

TABLE 35–10
Five-Year Survival Rates for Stage T1 or T2 N0 Glottic Carcinoma

TUMOR STAGE	SUBGROUP*	ABSOLUTE SURVIVAL†	CAUSE-SPECIFIC SURVIVAL
T1a N0	C	107/122 (88%)	107/110 (97%)
T1b N0	HL	12/13 (92%)	12/12 (100%)
	TL	11/16 (69%)	11/12 (92%)
T2a N0	HL	16/23 (70%)	16/18 (89%)
	TL	27/34 (79%)	27/28 (96%)
T2b N0	HL	11/16 (69%)	11/13 (85%)
	TL	18/22 (82%)	18/20 (90%)

** C: suitable for cordectomy; HL: suitable for hemilaryngectomy; TL: suitable for total laryngectomy.*
† Results exclude three patients with synchronous primary head and neck cancers and one patient with clinically positive neck nodes at presentation.
(Mendenhall WM, Parsons JT, Stringer SP, Cassisi NJ, Million RR: Head Neck Surg 10:373, 1988)

TABLE 35–11
Treatment of Stage T3 Glottic Carcinoma, 1965–1981

PARAMETER	IRRADIATION ALONE	SURGERY ± ADJUVANT IRRADIATION
Local control after initial treatment	11/18 (61%)	31/37 (84%)
Ultimate local control	15/18 (83%)	33/37 (89%)
Control above clavicles after initial treatment	11/19 (58%)	31/39 (79%)
Ultimate control above the clavicles	15/19 (79%)	34/39 (87%)
5-year absolute survival	8/15 (53%)	19/38 (50%)
5-year cause-specific survival	8/12 (67%)	19/28 (68%)

(Mendenhall WM, Million RR, Sharkey DE, Cassisi NJ: Int J Radiat Oncol Biol Phys 10:357, 1984)

Parsons and co-workers updated the University of Florida experience with the use of twice-a-day irradiation alone for patients with T3 vocal cord cancer.[57] With a minimum of 2 years of follow-up, local control was obtained in 12 (67%) of 18 evaluable patients. None of the patients whose disease was locally controlled developed regional or distant metastases. All six patients who developed local recurrence underwent a salvage laryngectomy. Three remain alive with no evidence of disease; one patient developed recurrence above the clavicles, a stomal failure after salvage surgery; and two died of distant metastases.

Six patients with T4 lesions of the glottic larynx have been irradiated with twice-a-day fractionation at the University of Florida, and two have had no local recurrence with 2 years or more follow-up.

Supraglottic Larynx Cancer

Surgical Results

The 3-year cause-specific survival rate for 176 patients with supraglottic carcinoma managed by supraglottic laryngectomy is shown in Table 35-12; 109 patients received preoperative radiation therapy.[50] Only 11 (6%) patients developed local recurrences; in five, salvage by total laryngectomy or radiation therapy proved successful. Seventeen had treatment failures in the neck, and salvage was achieved in nine. For patients with advanced lesions treated with preoperative radiation therapy followed by total laryngectomy and radical neck dissection, the 3- and 5-year survival rates were 70% and 67%, respectively.

TABLE 35–12
Three-Year Cause-Specific Survival Among 176 Patients After Supraglottic Laryngectomy

TUMOR STAGE	NO. SURVIVING/NO. AT RISK	
	NECK STAGE N0 (134 PATIENTS)	NECK STAGES N1–N3 (42 PATIENTS)
T1	64/78 (82%)	8/14 (57%)
T2	23/34 (68%)	8/12 (67%)
T3	7/10	2/3
T4	9/12 (75%)	8/13 (62%)

(Ogura JH, Sessions DG, Spector GJ: Laryngoscope 85:1808, 1975)

Ogura and co-workers[48] reported 59 patients with supraglottic carcinoma with extension to one arytenoid treated by supraglottic laryngectomy; 56 had preoperative radiation therapy. Five patients developed local recurrences, and six developed neck recurrences. Salvage by total laryngectomy or radiation therapy was obtained in four.

Bocca[9] reported 250 cases of T1 and T2 supraglottic carcinoma managed by supraglottic laryngectomy and bilateral elective or therapeutic neck dissection. The local recurrence rate was 11%, and the neck recurrence rate was 5%; in nine patients, salvage was achieved by further therapy. The 5-year survival rate was 80%.

Radiation Therapy Results

A recent analysis of the results of treatment by radiation therapy alone at the University of Florida is outlined in Tables 35-13 and 35-14.[41] There is no difference in local control rates as a function of site within the supraglottic larynx. There is a modest improvement in the local control rate for T2, T3, and T4 lesions irradiated twice a day. There is a high local control rate with doses of 6000 cGy to 6500 cGy for T1 lesions and 7000 cGy for T2 or T3 lesions treated with once-a-day irradiation.[17,65]

Combined Therapy Results

In patients with resectable Stage IV supraglottic carcinomas, Fletcher and Goepfert[16] reported a 5-year survival rate of 24% (19 of 78 patients) with surgery alone and a rate of 42% (16 of 38) with combined surgery and irradiation. In a similar group of patients, Goepfert and associates[21] found a rate for failure above the clavicle of 24% (28 of 116 patients) with surgery alone and a rate of 13% (seven of 53) with surgery and postoperative irradiation. The data clearly support the use of combined-modality treatment in these patients.

Comparison of Surgery and Radiation Therapy

Weems and co-workers[77] analyzed the University of Florida series of 195 patients treated with curative intent by irradiation, surgery or both. Patients treated with surgery alone were grouped with those treated with preoperative or postoperative irradiation.[26,28,35] The rates of initial and ultimate local control, local control with voice preservation, and initial and ultimate control above the clavicles are shown in Table 35-15 and 35-16. Irradiation or surgery with selected use of adjuvant irradiation offers similar results (90% to 100% 5-year cause-specific survival) for early-stage lesions but surgery offers better results than irradiation for Stage IV disease (27% and 50%, respectively).

FOLLOW-UP POLICY

Follow-up of patients with early lesions is planned for every 4 to 6 weeks for 2 years, every 3 months for the third year, and then every 6 months for life. Photographs are helpful for noticing subtle changes. Follow-up by multiple examiners should be encouraged.

Follow-up of patients with vocal cord or supraglottic larynx lesions treated by irradiation or conservative surgery is almost

TABLE 35–13
Local Control of Supraglottic Carcinoma

TUMOR STAGE*	ONCE-A-DAY IRRADIATION	TWICE-A-DAY IRRADIATION	TOTAL LOCAL CONTROL†	NO. SALVAGED/ NO. ATTEMPTED‡	ULTIMATE LOCAL CONTROL
T1	11/11	2/2	13/13 (100%)		13/13 (100%)
T2	23/29 (79%)	11/13 (85%)	34/42 (81%)	3/7	37/42 (88%)
T3	4/9 (41%)	21/32 (66%)	25/41 (61%)	9/13	34/41 (83%)
T4	2/8	1/1	3/9	3/3	6/9

** Tumor stage on system of the American Joint Committee on Cancer.*
† Control data given for 129 patients with 131 lesions. It excludes 26 patients dead <2 years from treatment with primary site continuously disease free.
‡ Surgical salvage implies continuous local control ≥12 months after salvage procedure.
(Mendenhall WM, Parsons JT, Stringer SP, Cassisi NJ, Million RR: Head Neck 12:204–209, 1990)

more important than the treatment itself, because early detection of recurrence usually results in salvage that may include cure with voice preservation.

If recurrence is suspected but the biopsy is negative, patients are reexamined at 2-week intervals until the matter is settled. The value of follow-up CT scans for detecting early local recurrence is investigational.

Wagenfield and co-workers[75] studied 740 cases of glottic larynx cancer treated from 1965 to 1974 to determine the incidence of second respiratory tract malignancies. There was a minimum follow-up of 5 years. There were 48 second respiratory tract malignancies, although only 14 were expected. Twenty-five were in the lung, and 23 were scattered among other head and neck sites. Only seven of the 23 second head and neck primary lesions resulted in death; these second lesions were frequently diagnosed in an early stage during routine follow-up for the glottic lesion.

Because the risk of a lethal lung primary lesion is nearly as great as that of dying of an early glottic carcinoma, it makes sense to obtain chest roentgenograms every 6 to 12 months.

SEQUELAE OF TREATMENT

Surgical Treatment

Neel and associates[46] reported a 26% incidence of nonfatal complications for cordectomy. Immediate postoperative complications included atelectasis and pneumonia, severe subcutaneous emphysema in the neck, bleeding from the tracheotomy site or larynx, wound complications, and airway obstruction requiring tracheotomy. Late complications included granulation tissue that had to be removed by direct laryngoscopy to exclude recurrences, extrusion of cartilage, laryngeal stenosis, and obstructing laryngeal web.

The postoperative complications and sequelae of hemilaryngectomy include chondritis, wound slough, inadequate glottic closure, and anterior commissure webs.[19] The complications associated with supraglottic laryngectomy and total laryngectomy for supraglottic carcinomas include fistula (8%) carotid artery exposure or blowout (3% to 5%), infection or wound sloughing (3% to 7%), and fatal complications (3%).[19] The risk of complication increased if tumor margins were involved by tumor; there was no change in risk associated with age, sex, race, laryngeal site, stage of primary tumor, size of primary tumor, use of low-dose preoperative irradiation, or status of the positive nodes.

The risk of severe complications for a series of 195 patients with squamous cell carcinomas of the supraglottic larynx treated at the University of Florida is shown in Table 35-17.[77] A severe complication was defined as one that necessitated surgical intervention or resulted in death. Five percent of patients treated with irradiation with or without neck dissection experienced a severe complication, compared with 17% to 23% of those treated with an operation, alone or combined with adjuvant irradiation.

TABLE 35–14
Five-Year Survival Rates for 84 Patients with Supraglottic Carcinoma

STAGE	ABSOLUTE SURVIVAL*	CAUSE-SPECIFIC SURVIVAL
I	2/6	2/2
II	10/20 (50%)	10/12 (83%)
III	9/20 (45%)	9/13 (69%)
IVA	4/9	4/6
IVB	7/29 (24%)	7/22 (32%)

** All patients had continuous-course irradiation employing once-a-day or twice-a-day fractionation. One patient with synchronous primary lesions was staged according to the more advanced lesion.*
(Mendenhall WM, Parsons JT, Stringer SP, Cassisi NJ, Million RR: Head Neck 12:204–209, 1990)

Radiation Therapy

Acute Reactions

The acute reactions from the treatment of early vocal cord cancer using a tumor dose of 225 cGy per day to administer a total dose of 5625 cGy to 6300 cGy of ^{60}Co in 5 fractions per week are relatively mild. During the first 2 to 3 weeks, the voice may improve as the tumor regresses. The voice generally becomes hoarse again because of radiation-induced changes, even though the tumor continues to regress.

A mild sore throat develops beginning at the end of the second week, but medication is usually not required.

The voice begins to improve approximately 3 weeks after completion of treatment, usually reaching a plateau in 2 to 3 months.

Patients with extensive lesions often recover a normal voice, although not as frequently as those with small tumors.

TABLE 35–15
Local Control of Supraglottic Carcinoma in 195 Patients, 1964–1984

	LOCAL TUMOR CONTROL AS A FUNCTION OF T STAGE		ULTIMATE LOCAL CONTROL AFTER SALVAGE THERAPY	
TUMOR STAGE*	RADIATION THERAPY ALONE†	SURGERY ± ADJUVANT RADIATION THERAPY†	RADIATION THERAPY ALONE†	SURGERY ± ADJUVANT RADIATION THERAPY†
T1	12/13 (92%)	9/9 (100%)	13/13 (100%)	9/9 (100%)
T2	29/36 (81%)	20/25 (80%)	32/36 (89%)	21/25 (84%)
T3	12/20 (60%)	17/18 (94%)	15/20 (75%)	18/18 (100%)
T4	4/13 (31%)	15/18 (83%)	7/13 (54%)	15/18 (83%)

** All data excludes 43 patients who died within 2 years of treatment with the primary site continuously disease-free.*
† Patients treated with continuous- or split-course irradiation. Results are given as number controlled/number treated.
(Weems DH, Mendenhall WM, Parson JT, Cassisi NJ, Million RR: Int J Radiat Oncol Biol Phys 13:1483, 1987)

TABLE 35–16
Ultimate Local Control of Supraglottic Carcinoma with Voice Preservation in 195 Patients

TUMOR STAGE	RADIATION THERAPY ALONE*	SURGERY ± ADJUVANT RADIATION THERAPY*	SIGNIFICANCE LEVEL
T1	15/16 (94%)	8/9	0.600
T2	38/45 (84%)†	12/31 (39%)	<0.001
T3	17/25 (68%)	6/26 (23%)	0.002
T4	14/21 (67%)	3/23 (13%)	<0.001

** All results presented for number controlled with voice preservation/number treated.*
† One patient had two T2 primary lesions and was counted twice.
(Weems DH, Mendenhall WM, Parsons JT, Cassisi NJ, Million RR: Int J Radiat Oncol Biol Phys 13:1483, 1987)

TABLE 35–17
Incidence of Severe Complications Among 195 Patients with Supraglottic Carcinoma

INITIAL TREATMENT	NO. OF PATIENTS WITH SEVERE COMPLICATIONS OF INITIAL TREATMENT/ NO. INITIALLY TREATED	NO. OF PATIENTS WITH SEVERE COMPLICATIONS/ NO. OF ATTEMPTED SALVAGE PROCEDURES
Radiation therapy alone	5/106 (5%)	2/20 (10%)
Surgery alone	6/26 (23%)	1/4
Preoperative radiation therapy + surgery	6/28 (21%)	0/1
Surgery + postoperative radiation therapy	6/35 (17%)	1/4

(Weems DH, Mendenhall WM, Parsons JT, Cassisi NJ, Million RR: Int J Radiat Oncol Biol Phys 13:1483, 1987)

TABLE 35–18
Incidence of Moderately Severe and Severe Complications Among 303 Patients with Stage T1 or T2 Glottic Carcinoma Correlated With Irradiation Doses

	T1 TREATMENTS, DOSE PER FRACTION*		T2 TREATMENT, DOSE PER FRACTION*	
TOTAL DOSE (cGy)	225–255 cGy†	185–224 cGy	225–245 cGy†	175–224 cGy
>7000				0/3
6700–7000		0/2	2/7	0/12
6000–6600	0/86	1/58 (2%)	1/61 (2%)	1/34 (3%)
5400–5700	0/36	0/2		0/2

** All patients were treated with once-a-day fractionation. Results given as number of complications/number of patients treated.*
† Only one patient was treated at >235 cGy per fraction.
(Mendenhall WM, Parsons JT, Million RR, Fletcher GH: Int J Radiat Oncol Biol Phys 15:1267, 1988)

Late Complications

Edema of the larynx is the most common sequela after irradiation for glottic or supraglottic lesions. The rate of clearance of the edema is related to the dose of radiation, volume of tissue irradiated, addition of a neck dissection, continued use of alcohol and tobacco, and size and extent of the original lesion. Edema may be accentuated by a radical neck dissection and may require 6 to 12 months to subside.

Soft tissue necrosis leading to chondritis occurs in fewer than 1% of the patients, usually in those who continue to smoke. Soft tissue and cartilage necroses mimic recurrence, with hoarseness, pain, and edema; a laryngectomy may be recommended as a last resort for fear of recurrent cancer, even though biopsy specimens show only necrosis.

Corticosteriods such as dexamethasone (Decadron) have been used to reduce radiation-induced edema after recurrence has been ruled out by biopsy. If ulceration and pain occur, administration of an antibiotic like tetracycline may help.

Of 304 patients with T1 or T2 vocal cord cancer treated at the University of Florida, five experienced significant complications; these included subcutaneous fat necrosis, one case of osteochondronecrosis (which healed with conservative management), and three cases of severe laryngeal edema, necessitating tracheostomy. One of the patients with edema was thought to have recurrent cancer, underwent a laryngectomy, and was found to have no tumor in the specimen. The incidence of significant complications as a function of T stage, total dose, and dose per fraction is shown in Table 35-18.[39]

In patients irradiated for supraglottic carcinoma, sore throat persists until 3 to 4 weeks after completion of treatment. There is an associated dry mouth from irradiation of the salivary and parotid glands, a loss of taste, and a sensation of a lump in the throat if the entire glottic area is included.

It is unusual for the patients to require a tracheotomy before irradiation unless they develop severe lymphedema at the time of direct laryngoscopy and biopsy. However, in patients who have recovered from the direct laryngoscopy and biopsy without obstruction, a tracheotomy has been required only once during a fractionated course of radiation therapy.

Patients treated twice a day with 120-cGy fractions (continuous-course technique) to total doses of 7400 cGy to 7680 cGy usually have more brisk acute reactions than those treated once a day with 200-cGy fractions. Approximately 10% treated with twice-a-day irradiation require nasogastric feeding tubes because they have difficulty in swallowing.

Examples of acute chondritis requiring discontinuation of treatment have not been seen, although most epiglottis lesions exhibit cartilage invasion.

The epiglottis, both suprahyoid and infrahyoid portions, remains thicker than normal for long periods of time, but this is not often associated with difficulty in swallowing, respiratory obstruction, or aspiration. The patient is cautioned to eat and drink slowly until the edema resolves. The false cords and arytenoids may develop some edema.

Lesions of the suprahyoid epiglottis frequently destroy the tip of the epiglottis, and it may require some time for the exposed cartilage to heal. Successful irradiation of infrahyoid epiglottis tumors is not associated with a high rate of necrosis, even though most of these lesions penetrate the porous epiglottic cartilage.

Shukovsky[65] analyzed the risk of severe complications for 114 patients with squamous cell carcinoma of the supraglottic larynx. There were five patients who developed necrosis and seven patients who developed severe edema. All but one of these complications appeared with doses in excess of 7000 cGy delivered in 7 weeks or with larger treatment volumes.

REFERENCES

1. Amdur RJ, Parsons JT, Mendenhall WM, Million RR, Stringer SP, Cassisi NJ: Postoperative irradiation for squamous cell carcinoma of the head and neck: An analysis of treatment results and complications. Int J Radiat Oncol Biol Phys 16:25, 1989
2. American Joint Committee on Cancer: Manual for Staging of Cancer, 3rd ed, pp 39–44. Philadelphia, JB Lippincott, 1988
3. Amornmarn R, Prempree T, Viravathana T, Donavanik V, Wizenberg MJ: A therapeutic approach to early vocal cord carcinoma. Acta Radiol Oncol 24:321, 1985
4. Archer CR, Yeager VL, Herbold DR: Computed tomography vs. histology of laryngeal cancer: Their value in predicting laryngeal cartilage invasion. Laryngoscope 93:140, 1983
5. Archer CR, Yeager VL, Herbold DR: Improved diagnostic accuracy in laryngeal cancer using a new classification based on computed tomography. Cancer 53:44, 1984
6. Bauer WC, Lesinski SG, Ogura JH: The significance of positive margins in hemilaryngectomy specimens. Laryngoscope 85:1, 1975
7. Biller HF, Barnhill FR Jr, Ogura JH, Perez CA: Hemilaryngectomy following radiation failure for carcinoma of the vocal cords. Laryngoscope 80:249, 1970
8. Biller HF, Ogura JH, Pratt LL: Hemilaryngectomy for T2 glottic cancers. Arch Otolaryngol 93:238, 1971
9. Bocca E: Supraglottic cancer. Laryngoscope 85:1318, 1975
10. Broyles EN: The anterior commissure tendon. Ann Otol Rhinol Laryngol 52:342, 1943.
11. Burns HP, van Nostrand AWP, Bryce DP: Verrucous carcinoma of the larynx: Management by radiotherapy and surgery. Ann Otol Rhinol Laryngol 85:538, 1976
12. Clemente CD: Anatomy: A Regional Atlas of the Human Body. Philadelphia, Lea & Febiger, 1975
13. Devesa SS, Silverman DT: Cancer incidence and mortality trends in the United States: 1935–1974. JNCI 60:545, 1978
14. Elman AJ, Goodman M, Wang CC, Pilch B, Busse J: *In situ* carcinoma of the vocal cords. Cancer 43:2422, 1979
15. Fletcher GH: Elective irradiation of subclinical disease in cancers of the head and neck. Cancer 29:1450, 1972
16. Fletcher GH, Goepfert H: Larynx and pyriform sinus. In Fletcher GH (ed): Textbook of Radiotherapy, 3rd ed, pp 330–363. Philadelphia, Lea & Febiger, 1980
17. Fletcher GH, Lindberg RD, Hamberger A, Horiot J-C: Reasons for irradiation failure in squamous cell carcinoma of the larynx. Laryngoscope 85:987, 1975
18. Fletcher GH, Lindberg RD, Jesse RH: Radiation therapy for cancer of the larynx and pyriform sinus. Eye Ear Nose Throat Digest 31:58, 1969
19. Gall AM, Sessions DG, Ogura JH: Complications following surgery for cancer of the larynx and hypopharynx. Cancer 39:624, 1977
20. Gindhart TD, Johnston WH, Chism SE, Dedo HH: Carcinoma of the larynx in childhood. Cancer 46:1683, 1980
21. Goepfert H, Jesse RH, Fletcher GH, Hamberger A: Optimal treatment for the technically resectable squamous cell carcinoma of the supraglottic larynx. Laryngoscope 85:14, 1975
22. Haraf DJ, Weichselbaum RR: Treatment selection in T1 and T2 vocal cord carcinoma. Oncology 2:41, 1988
23. Harwood AR, Beale FA, Cummings BJ, Hawkins NV, Keane TJ, Rider WD: T3 glottic cancer: An analysis of dose-time volume factors. Int J Radiat Oncol Biol Phys 6:675, 1980
24. Harwood AR, Beale FA, Cummings BJ, Keane TJ, Payne D, Rider WD: T4N0M0 glottic cancer: An analysis of dose-time volume factors. Int J Radiat Oncol Biol Phys 7:1507, 1981
25. Harwood AR, Beale FA, Cummings BJ, Keane TJ, Rider WD: T2 glottic cancer: An analysis of dose-time volume factors. Int J Radiat Oncol Biol Phys 7:1501, 1981
26. Harwood AR, Hawkins NV, Rider WD, Bryce DP: Radiotherapy of early glottic cancer—I. Int J Radiat Oncol Biol Phys 5:473, 1979

27. Hirano M: Structure and vibratory behavior of the vocal folds. In Sawashima M, Cooper FS (eds): Dynamic Aspects of Speech Production: Current Results, Emerging Problems, & New Instrumentation, pp 13–27. Tokyo, University of Tokyo Press, 1977
28. Jesse RH: The evaluation of treatment of patients with extensive squamous cancer of the vocal cords. Laryngoscope 85:1424, 1975
29. Kirchner JA: Staging as seen in serial sections. Laryngoscope 85:1816, 1975
30. Lederman M: Place de la radiotherapie dans le traitment due cancer du larynx (The place of radiotherapy in the treatment of cancer of the larynx). Ann Radiol (Paris) 4:433, 1961
31. Lee F, Perlmutter S, Ogura JH: Laryngeal radiation after hemilaryngectomy. Laryngoscope 90:1534, 1980
32. Lindberg R: Distribution of cervical lymph node metastases from squamous cell carcinoma of the upper respiratory and digestive tracts. Cancer 29:1446, 1972
33. Mancuso AA, Hanafee WN: Computed Tomography and Magnetic Resonance Imaging of the Head and Neck, 2nd ed, pp 241–341. Baltimore, Williams & Wilkins, 1985
34. Mendenhall WM, Million RR, Bova FJ: Carcinoma of the cervical esophagus treated with radiation therapy using a four-field box technique. Int J Radiat Oncol Biol Phys 8:1435, 1982
35. Mendenhall WM, Million RR, Cassisi NJ: Squamous cell carcinoma of the supraglottic larynx treated with radical irradiation: Analysis of treatment parameters and results. Int J Radiat Oncol Biol Phys 10:2223, 1984
36. Mendenhall WM, Million RR, Sharkey DE, Cassisi NJ: Stage T3 squamous cell carcinoma of the glottic larynx treated with surgery and/or radiation therapy. Int J Radiat Oncol Biol Phys 10:357, 1984
37. Mendenhall WM, Parsons JT, Brant TA, Stringer SP, Cassisi NJ, Million RR: Is elective neck treatment indicated for T2N0 squamous cell carcinoma of the glottic larynx? Radiother Oncol 14:199, 1989
38. Mendenhall WM, Parsons JT, Million RR, Cassisi NJ: Commentary on Urban ML, Biller HF: Management of early vocal cord cancer. Oncology 2:59, 1988
39. Mendenhall WM, Parsons JT, Million RR, Fletcher GH: T1–T2 squamous cell carcinoma of the glottic larynx treated with radiation therapy: Relationship of dose-fractionation factors to local control and complications. Int J Radiat Oncol Biol Phys 15:1267, 1988
40. Mendenhall WM, Parsons JT, Stringer SP, Cassisi NJ, Million RR: T1–T2 vocal cord carcinoma: A basis for comparing the results of radiotherapy and surgery. Head Neck Surg 10:373, 1988
41. Mendenhall WM, Parsons JT, Stringer SP, Cassisi NJ, Million RR: Carcinoma of the supraglottic larynx: A basis for comparing the results of radiotherapy and surgery. Head Neck 12:204–209, 1990
42. Million RR: The myth regarding bone or cartilage involvement by cancer and the likelihood of cure by radiotherapy. Head Neck Surg 11:30, 1989
43. Million RR, Cassisi NJ: Larynx. In Million RR, Cassisi NJ (eds): Management of Head and Neck Cancer: A Multidisciplinary Approach, pp 315–364. Philadelphia, JB Lippincott, 1984
44. Million RR, Cassisi NJ, Clark JR: Cancer of the head and neck. In DeVita VT Jr, Hellman S, Rosenberg SA (eds): Cancer: Principles and Practice of Oncology, 3rd ed, pp 488–590. Philadelphia, JB Lippincott, 1989
45. Mills EED: Early glottic carcinoma: Factors affecting radiation failures, results of treatment, and sequelae. Int J Radiat Oncol Biol Phys 5:811, 1979
46. Neel H III, Devine KD, Desanto LW: Laryngofissure and cordectomy for early cordal carcinoma: Outcome in 182 patients. Otolaryngol Head Neck Surg 88:79, 1980
47. Ogura JH, Biller HF, Wette R: Elective neck dissection for pharyngeal and laryngeal cancers: An evaluation. Ann Otol Rhinol Laryngol 80:646, 1971
48. Ogura JH, Sessions DG, Ciralsky RH: Supraglottic carcinoma with extension to the arytenoid. Laryngoscope 85:1327, 1975
49. Ogura JH, Sessions DG, Spector GJ: Analysis of surgical therapy for epidermoid carcinoma of the laryngeal glottis. Laryngoscope 85:1522, 1975
50. Ogura JH, Sessions DG, Spector GJ: Conservation surgery for epidermoid carcinoma of the supraglottic larynx. Laryngoscope 85:1808, 1975
51. Olofsson J, van Nostrand AWP: Growth and spread of laryngeal and hypopharyngeal carcinoma with reflections on the effect of preoperative irradiation: 139 cases studied by whole organ serial sectioning. Acta Otolaryngol Suppl (Stockh) 308:1, 1973
52. Ossoff RH, Duncavage JA, Fried MP: Laser laryngoscopy. In Fried MP (ed): The Larynx: A Multidisciplinary Approach, pp 359–370. Boston, Little Brown, 1988
53. Parsons JT: Time-dose-volume relationships in radiation therapy. In Million RR, Cassisi NJ (eds): Management of Head and Neck Cancer: A Multidisciplinary Approach, pp 137–172. Philadelphia, JB Lippincott, 1984
54. Parsons JT, Bova FJ, Million RR: A re-evaluation of the split-course technique for squamous cell carcinoma of the head and neck. Int J Radiat Oncol Biol Phys 6:1645, 1980
55. Parsons JT, Mendenhall WM, Bova FJ, Million RR: Irradiation technique for head and neck cancer. In Levitt SH (ed): Technological Basis of Radiation Therapy: Practical Clinical Applications. Philadelphia, Lea & Febiger (in press)
56. Parsons JT, Mendenhall WM, Cassisi NJ, Isaacs JH, Million RR: Hyperfractionation for head and neck cancer. Int J Radiat Oncol Biol Phys 14:649, 1988
57. Parsons JT, Mendenhall WM, Mancuso AA, Cassisi NJ, Stringer SP, Million RR: Twice-a-day radiotherapy for T3 squamous cell carcinoma of the glottic larynx. Head Neck 11:123, 1989
58. Pearson BW, Woods RD, Hartman DE: Extended hemilaryngectomy for T3 glottic carcinoma with preservation of speech and swallowing. Laryngoscope 90:1950, 1980
59. Pene F, Fletcher GH: Results in irradiation of the *in situ* carcinomas of the vocal cords. Cancer 37:2586, 1976
60. Pillsbury HRC, Kirchner JA: Clinical vs histopathologic staging in laryngeal cancer. Arch Otolaryngol 105:157, 1979
61. Robbins KT, Davidson W, Peters LJ, Goepfert H: Conservation surgery for T2 and T3 carcinomas of the supraglottic larynx. Arch Otolaryngol Head Neck Surg 114:421, 1988
62. Schwaibold F, Scariato A, Nunno M, Wallner PE, Lustig RA, Rouby E, Gorshein D, Wenger J: The effect of fraction size on control of early glottic cancer. Int J Radiat Oncol Biol Phys 14:451, 1988
63. Sessions DG, Ogura JH, Fried MP: The anterior commissure in glottic carcinoma. Laryngoscope 85:1624, 1975
64. Shapshay SM: Application of the Nd:YAG laser in the larynx and the trachea. In Fried MP (ed): The Larynx: A Multidisciplinary Approach. Boston, Little Brown, 1988
65. Shukovsky LJ: Dose, time, volume relationships in squamous cell carcinoma of the supraglottic larynx. Am J Roentgenol Radium Ther Nucl Med 108:27, 1970
66. Silverberg E: Cancer statistics, 1982. CA 32:15, 1982
67. Silverberg E, Boring CC, Squires TS: Cancer statistics, 1990. CA 40(1):18, 1990
68. Skolnik EM, Yee KF, Wheatley MA, Martin LO: Carcinoma of the laryngeal glottis: Therapy and results. Laryngoscope 85:1453, 1975
69. Skolyszewski J, Reinfuss M: The results of radiotherapy of cancer of the larynx in six European countries. Radiobiol Radiother 22:32, 1981
70. Som ML: Cordal cancer with extension to vocal process. Laryngoscope 85:1298, 1975
71. Stewart JG, Brown JR, Palmer MK, Cooper A: The management of glottic carcinoma by primary irradiation with surgery in reserve. Laryngoscope 85:1477, 1975
72. Stewart JG, Jackson AW: The steepness of the dose response curve both for tumor cure and normal tissue injury. Laryngoscope 85:1107, 1975
73. Vermund H: Role of radiotherapy in cancer of the larynx as related to the TNM system of staging. Cancer 25:485, 1970
74. Vincent RG, Marchetta F: The relationship of the use of to-

bacco and alcohol to cancer of the oral cavity, pharynx or larynx. Am J Surg 105:501, 1963
75. Wagenfeld DJH, Harwood AR, Bryce DP, van Nostrand AWP, DeBoer G: Second primary respiratory tract malignancies in glottic carcinoma. Cancer 46:1883, 1980
76. Wang CC: Radiation therapy of laryngeal tumors: Curative radiation therapy. In Thawley SE, Panje WR (eds): Comprehensive Management of Head and Neck Tumors, pp 906–919. Philadelphia, WB Saunders, 1987
77. Weems DH, Mendenhall WM, Parsons JT, Cassisi NJ, Million RR: Squamous cell carcinoma of the supraglottic larynx treated with surgery and/or radiation therapy. Int J Radiat Oncol Biol Phys 13:1483, 1987
78. Woodhouse RJ, Quivey JM, Fu KK, Sien PS, Dedo HH, Phillips TL: Treatment of carcinoma of the vocal cord: A review of 20 years experience. Laryngoscope 91:1155, 1981
79. Wynder EL: The epidemiology of cancer of the upper alimentary and upper respiratory tracts. Laryngoscope 88(suppl 8):50, 1978

36

Unusual Nonepithelial Tumors of the Head and Neck

Carlos A. Perez
Beatriz E. Amendola
Robert Lindberg
Victor A. Marcial-Vega

GLOMUS TUMORS

Anatomy

Glomus bodies are found in the jugular bulb and along the tympanic (Jacobson) and auricular (Arnold) branch of the tenth nerve in the middle ear or in other anatomic sites (Fig. 36-1). Depending on the location, glomus tumors (chemodectoma or paraganglioma) can be classified as tympanic (middle ear), jugulare or carotid vagal, or designated as originating from other locations, such as the larynx, adventitia of thoracic aorta, abdominal aorta, or surface of the lungs.[52] These tissues are responsive to changes in oxygen and carbon dioxide tensions and pH.

Glomus tumors consist of large epithelioid (smooth muscle) cells with fine granular cytoplasm embedded in a rich capillary network and fibrous stroma with reticulin fibers. Although histologically benign, they may extend along the lumen of the vein to regional lymph nodes, but rarely to distant sites. Metastases occur in 2% to 5% of these cases.[140]

Epidemiology

The mean age at diagnosis of carotid body tumors reported by Parry and co-workers[202] is 44.7 years, and for glomus tympanicum 52 years as reported by Larson and associates.[148] Most patients are 40 years or older at diagnosis. These tumors are three or four times more frequent in women than in men, suggesting a possible estrogen influence.[25,140,148,180] Glomus tumors may be familial, and they occur in multiple sites in 10% to 20% of the patients.[234]

Bilateral carotid glomus tumors were reported in six (38%) of 16 patients with a positive family history for these lesions but in 17 (8%) of 206 patients without such a history.[202]

Clinical Presentation

Glomus tumors may arise along the nerve roots, causing clinical signs and symptoms that are a function of the site of origin.[103] Glomus tumors of the middle ear may initially cause earache or discomfort. As they expand, they produce pulsatile tinnitus and hearing loss, and in later stages, they produce cranial nerve paralysis resulting from invasion of the base of skull in 10% to 15% of the patients. Patients endure ear symptoms for 3 to 5 years before seeking medical attention.

If the tumor invades the middle cranial fossa, symptoms may include temporoparietal headache, retroorbital pain, proptosis, and paresis of cranial nerves V and VI. If the posterior fossa is involved, symptoms may include occipital headache, ataxia, and paresis of cranial nerves V, VI, VII, IX, and XII; invasion of the jugular foramen causes paralysis of nerves IX, X, and XI.

Chemodectoma of the carotid body usually presents as a painless, slowly growing mass in the upper neck. The mass may be pulsatile and may have an associated thrill or bruit. As it enlarges, the mass may extend into the parapharyngeal space and be visible on examination of the oropharynx.[78]

Diagnostic Workup

Diagnostic evaluation for glomus tumors of the ear and the base of skull is outlined in Table 36-1. For most of the glomus tympanicum tumors, physical examination demonstrates a red, vascular middle ear mass, although it may be tinged blue or white, with the latter resembling a cholesteatoma.[148] Audiography may demonstrate conductive hearing loss in the ear involved by tumor, as reported in 33 of 49 patients evaluated by Larson and associates.[148] Six of these patients had bilateral sensorineural

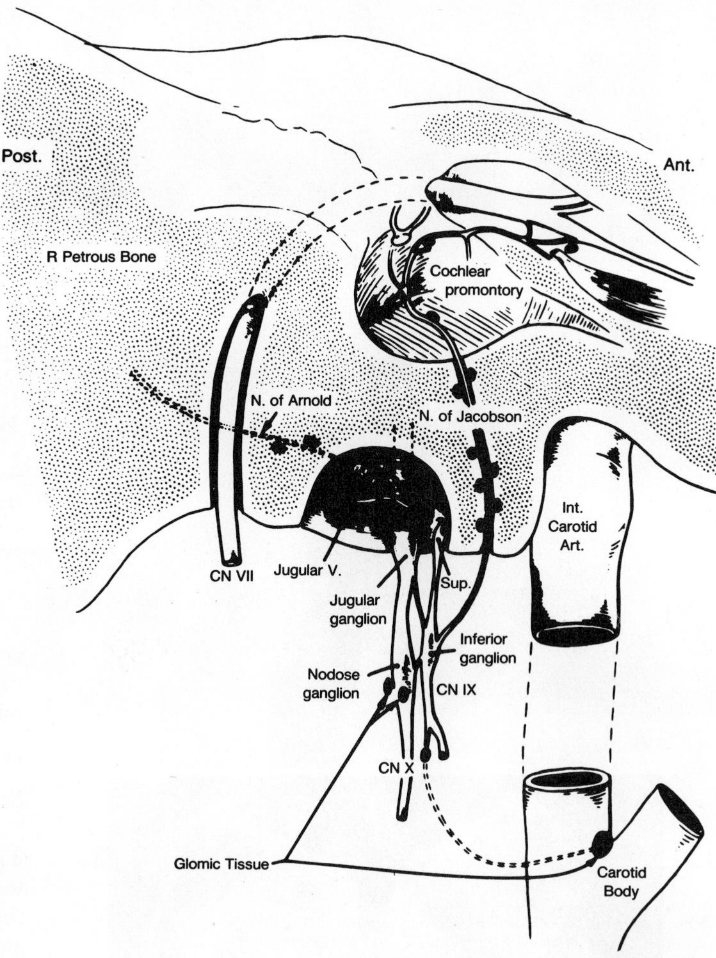

FIGURE 36–1. Anatomy of the region of the glomus jugulare. (Hatfield PM, James AE, Schulz MN: Cancer 30:1165, 1972)

hearing loss. Four of the 33 patients with conductive deficits also exhibited tympanic pulsations. Examination of the neck may rarely reveal regional lymph node metastases or a mass in the neck that may be pulsatile or have a bruit.

Radiographic studies are invaluable in the diagnosis of these tumors. High-resolution computed tomography (CT) with contrast has the highest degree of sensitivity and specificity for diagnosing this tumor if it is located in the middle ear or jugular bulb. Masses as small as 3 mm were demonstrated in the middle ear.[148] Tumor enhancement is similar to that of the temporalis muscle (Fig. 36-2).[148] In 46 patients with glomus tympanicum chemodectomas, there were no instances of local bony erosion; instead the tumors engulfed the ossicular chain, bulged or protruded through the tympanic membrane, filled the middle ear, or extended into the eustachian tube orifice or aditus and antrum. Cholesteatomas, however, typically destroy adjacent bony landmarks, including the ossicles and progressively erode the petrous bones as they enlarge.[148]

Magnification angiography is an invasive but sensitive and specific means of detecting glomus tympanicum tumors. This procedure should be performed after contrast-enhanced, high-resolution, thin-section CT scanning only if there is a question regarding the nature of the lesion or the location of the carotid canal. Biopsy of an aberrant internal carotid artery can produce major neurologic sequelae or death.[5,226]

Findings include a hypervascular middle ear mass that first appears in the middle to late arterial phase, persists through the capillary phase, and quickly disappears in the venous phase without demonstrable early draining veins. On the lateral projection, overlying dense petrous bone tends to obscure the enhanced glomus tumor positioned at the medial end of the external auditory canal.[166] Plain mastoid radiographs do not show the soft tissue mass in the middle ear, although they frequently demonstrate clouding of the mastoid air cells suggesting mastoiditis.[65,159] The role of magnetic resonance imaging (MRI) in the evaluation of these tumors is being investigated.

TABLE 36–1
Diagnostic Workup for Glomus Tumors of the Ear and Base of Skull, Hemangiopericytoma, Esthesioneuroblastoma of the Head and Neck, and Extramedullary Plasmacytoma

GENERAL

History
Physical examination

SPECIAL TESTS

Audiograms (to establish baseline hearing loss)
Histologic staining to determine presence of catecholamines

RADIOGRAPHIC STUDIES

Plain radiographs (including temporal bone views)
Polytomography of temporal bone
CT or MRI scans to define extension
Arteriography to determine bilateral involvement and collateral cerebral blood flow
Jugular phleborography (optional)

LABORATORY STUDIES

Complete blood counts on admission
Blood chemistries
Urinalysis

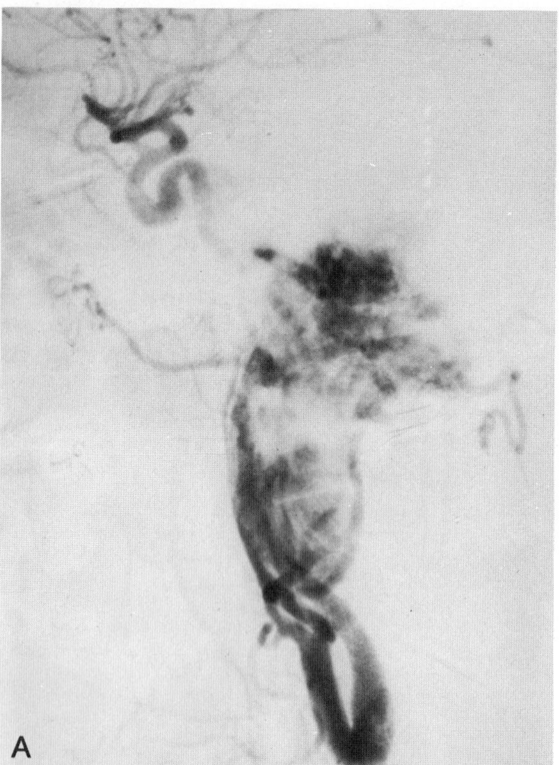

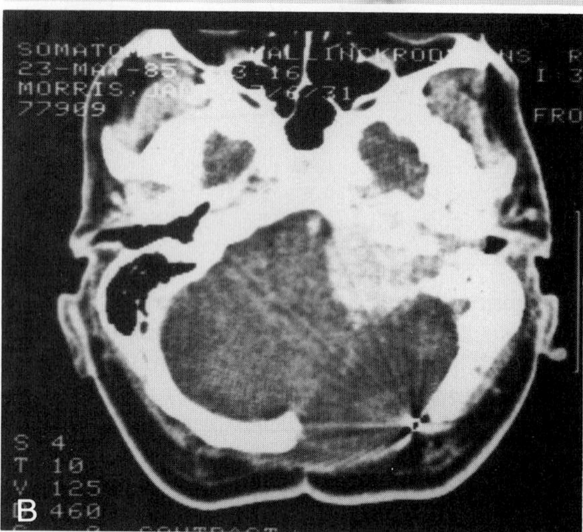

FIGURE 36–2. (**A**) Late-phase arteriogram illustrates large glomus jugulare tumor with extension into the neck. (**B**) CT scan with contrast enhancement shows intracranial component of the lesion.

In 30 patients with neck masses, scanning with a bolus injection of ^{99m}Tc-gluconate (20 mCi injected into the basilic vein) immediately followed by rapid injection of saline and scanning of the head and neck was a useful procedure for demonstrating glomus jugulare or carotid body tumors in seven patients, including two tumors unsuspected clinically.[145] The procedure was particularly useful in differentiating chemodectomas, which show marked vascularity on the scans, from other head and neck lesions, such as thyroid tumor, parathyroid tumors, cystic hygroma, bronchogenic cysts, neural tumors, sarcomas, and lymph nodes.

Cytochemical techniques have demonstrated increased levels of serotonin, epinephrine, and norepinephrine in normal glomus tissue of the carotid body.[150] Histologic staining techniques, including the chromaffin and the argentaffin reactions, identify patients with hormonally active tumors. This is important because the glomus tumor may coexist with a pheochromocytoma, which requires special preoperative preparation of the patient.

TABLE 36–2
Glasscock-Jackson Classification of Glomus Tumors

GLOMUS TYMPANICUM	
I	Small mass limited to promontory
II	Tumor completely filling middle ear space
III	Tumor filling middle ear and extending into the mastoid
IV	Tumor filling middle ear, extending into the mastoid or through tympanic membrane to fill the external auditory canal; may extend anterior to carotid
GLOMUS JUGULARE	
I	Small tumor involving jugular bulb, middle ear, and mastoid
II	Tumor extending under internal auditory canal; may have intracranial canal extension (ICE)
III	Tumor extending into petrous apex; may have ICE
IV	Tumor extending beyond petrous apex into clivus or infratemporal fossa; may have ICE

(Jackson CG, Glasscock ME III, Harris PF: Arch Otolaryngol Head Neck Surg 108:401, 1982)

Staging

The prognosis of glomus tumors is closely related to the anatomic location and the volume of the lesion, which is reflected in the Glasscock-Jackson classification shown in Table 36-2. An alternative classification proposed by McCabe and Fletcher[173] is illustrated in Table 36-3.

TABLE 36–3
Modification of McCabe and Fletcher Classification of Chemodectomas

TUMOR GROUP	CHARACTERISTICS
Group I Tympanic tumors	Absence of bone destruction on x-rays of the mastoid bone and jugular fossa; absence of facial nerve weakness; intact eighth nerve with a conductive deafness only; intact jugular foramen nerves (cranial nerves IX, X, and XI)
Group II Tympanomastoid tumors	X-ray evidence of bone destruction confined to the mastoid bone and not involving the petrous bone; a normal or paretic seventh nerve; intact jugular foramen nerves; and no evidence of involvement of the superior bulb of the jugular vein on retrograde venogram
Group III Petrosal and extrapetrosal tumors	Destruction of the petrous bone, jugular fossa, or occipital bone on x-ray films; positive findings on retrograde jugulography; evidence of destruction of the petrous or occipital bones on carotid arteriogram; jugular foramen syndrome (paresis of cranial nerves IX, X, or XI), or the presence of metastasis

(Wang M-L, Hussey DH, Doornbos JF, Vigliotti AP, Wen B-C: Int J Radiat Oncol Biol Phys 14:643, 1987)

General Management

Surgery

Surgery is generally selected for treatment of small tumors that can be completely excised. Glomus tympanicum tumors are particularly well managed with excision by a tympanotomy or mastoidectomy. Percutaneous embolization of a low-viscosity silicone polymer has been used, frequently as preoperative preparation of the tumor; embolization of feeding vessels allows meticulous microsurgery with virtually complete hemostasis.[28, 194, 224]

Surgical treatment of a glomus tumor arising in the jugular bulb, however, often consists of piece-by-piece removal, accompanied by significant bleeding with damage to adjacent neurovascular structures, and requires more complex surgical approaches involving the base of the skull.[127] Tumors that destroy the petrous bone, jugular fossa, or occipital bone or patients with jugular foramen syndrome are more reliably managed with irradiation. The local tumor control rate reported with surgery alone is only about 60%, and there is significant morbidity, particularly cranial nerve injury and bleeding.[101, 117, 139, 162, 188, 208, 212, 236, 249]

Radiation Therapy

Irradiation is frequently used in the treatment of glomus tumors, particularly in the tympanicum and jugulare bulb location.[139, 140, 180, 220] Some surgeons, such as Glasscock and associates[95] and Spector and Sobol,[237] have questioned the effectiveness of radiation therapy in the treatment of chemodectomas, because it is possible to find chromophilic cells remaining in the tumor on histologic sections obtained even many years after irradiation. However, there is also evidence of fibrosis and decreased vascularity.[237] Suit and Gallager[244] demonstrated in a murine mammary carcinoma model that morphologically intact cells may have lost their reproductive ability after irradiation, which is the ultimate end point of cell destruction. A glomus tumor rarely regrows after irradiation.

Some reports describe successful combinations of surgery with preoperative or postoperative irradiation. A postoperative approach is used if obvious tumor could not be resected, and a preoperative approach is employed to make an unresectable tumor operable.[90, 91, 235]

Radiation Therapy Techniques

Radiation therapy techniques are determined by the location and extent of the tumor, which must be defined before treatment. Limited portals should be used for relatively localized glomus tumors, whether or not the treatment is combined with surgery (Fig. 36-3). Figure 36-4 shows superior-inferior 60-degree and 45-degree wedged filtered fields. Dickens and associates[58] used a three-field arrangement with a superior-inferior wedged and lateral open field, with a weighting of 1 : 1 : 0.33. The use of electrons (15–18 MeV) with a lateral portal or combined with ^{60}Co-4-MV photons (20% to 25% of total tumor dose) renders a good dose distribution (Fig. 36-5). In patients in whom tumor has spread into the posterior fossa, it may be necessary to use parallel opposed portals. Treatment is given at the rate of 180 cGy to 200 cGy tumor dose per day with five treatments per week, for a total tumor dose of 4500 cGy to 5000 cGy in 5 weeks. Table 36-4 summarizes the doses of irradiation recommended by several investigators and the probability of tumor control. Figure 36-6 illustrates the tumor control for 14 lesions treated with various dose fractionation schedules.

Results of Therapy

The postirradiation change in tumor size is slow, with an increase in proliferative fibrosis and perivascular fibrosis and minimal alterations in the chief epithelial cells.[212, 235] Histologic evaluation of tumor cell viability is not reliable.[244] Despite the persistence of tumor clinically and angiographically, amelioration of symptoms, absence of disease progression, and occasional return of cranial nerve function have been reported.[170]

A group of 17 patients were treated for glomus tympanicum tumors at Washington University and followed up for a minimum of 5 years. In five patients, initial treatment consisted of irradiation alone, and all were tumor-free at last follow-up or at death. Seven of eight patients irradiated for surgical recurrence were free of disease from 4.5 to 19 years after irradiation.

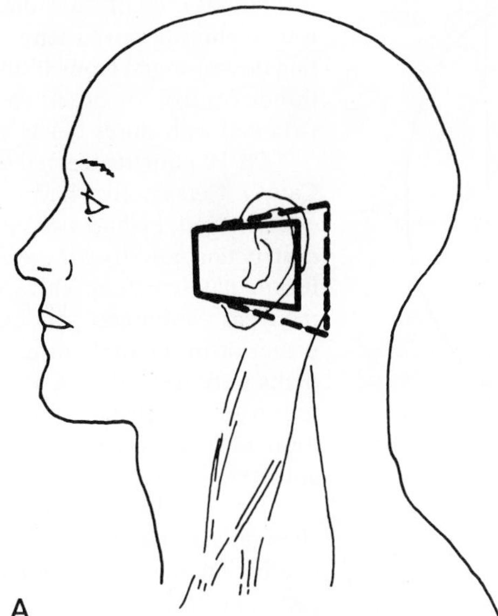

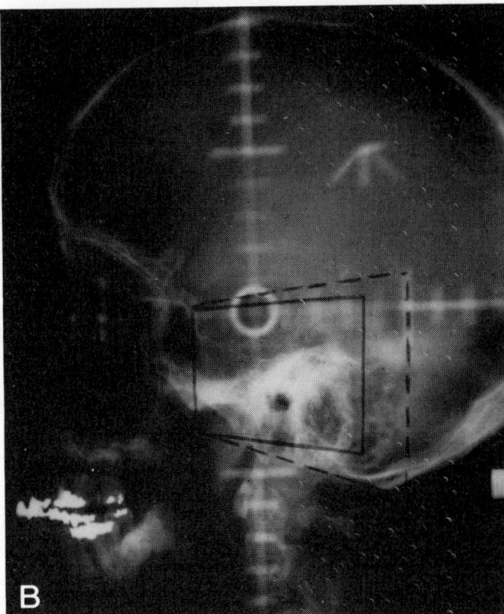

FIGURE 36–3. (**A**) Portal used for relatively localized glomus tumor. (**B**) Simulation film of patient with glomus tumor.

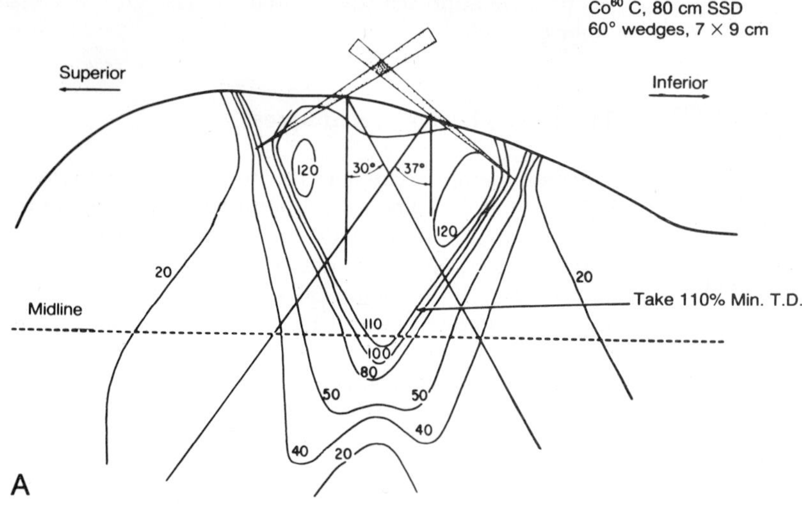

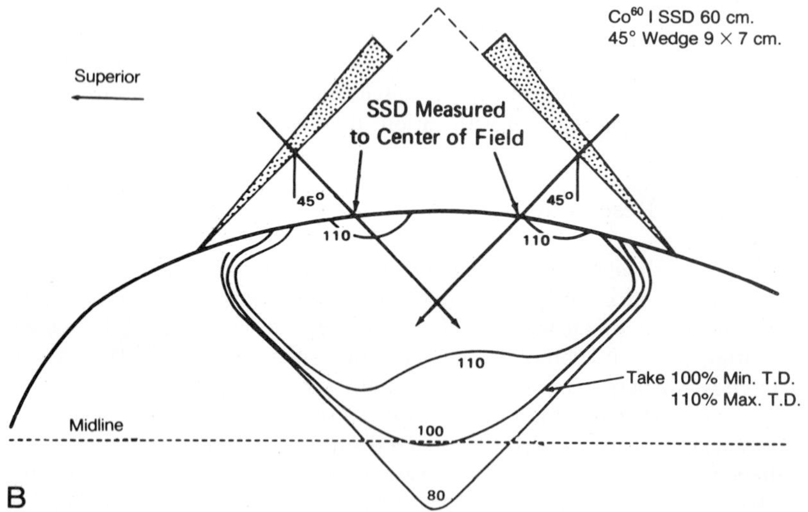

FIGURE 36–4. (**A, B**) Isodose distributions using superior-inferior pairs of 60-degree and 45-degree converging wedge-filtered ^{60}Co fields, demonstrating limited volume of irradiation. (Tidwell TJ, Montague ED: Radiology 116:147, 1975)

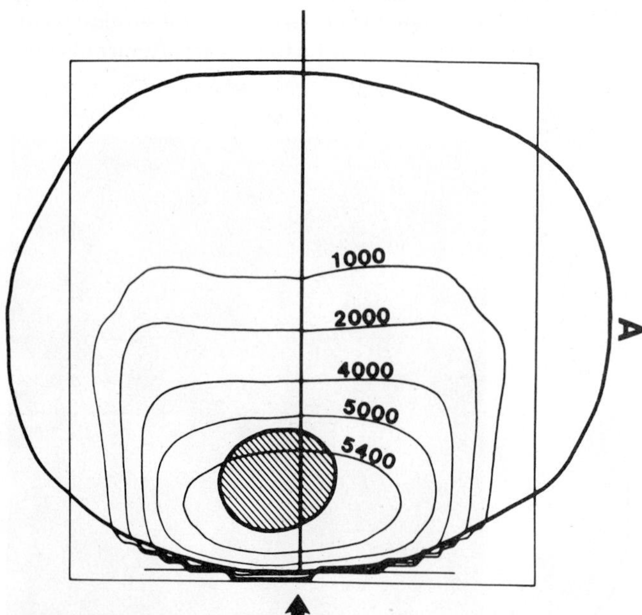

FIGURE 36–5. Isodose distribution of a mixed-beam unilateral port for glomus tympanicum lesion (80% 16-MeV electrons, 20% 4-MV photons). (Konefal JB, Pilepich MV, Spector GJ, Perez CA: Laryngoscope 97:1331, 1987)

The remaining four patients were treated preoperatively or postoperatively; only one had a recurrence, was salvaged surgically, and was tumor-free 10 years later. Of six patients with glomus jugulare lesions treated with irradiation, two with extensive lesions died of their disease, and disease was controlled in four, including two patients with intracranial extension. Irradiation doses ranged from 4600 cGy to 5200 cGy with 86% to 100% tumor control for doses over 4600 cGy and 50% (two of four patients) with doses below 4600 cGy.

Of 19 patients treated with irradiation at M. D. Anderson Cancer Center, five had only a biopsy without any surgical excision and 14 had partial excisions. Ten patients had bony destruction, and five of these had petrous pyramid and jugular foramen destruction, with accompanying multiple cranial nerve paralysis. Seventeen patients were treated with ^{60}Co anterior-posterior or superior-inferior wedged-filtered fields. Two patients were treated with a mixture (3 : 1) of electrons and photons with a single lateral field. Of 18 patients surviving a minimum of 5 years (13 survived more than 10 years), all are alive and free of disease or have subsequently died of other causes.

Wang and associates[262] reported 32 patients with tympanic chemodectomas; 13 were treated with surgery alone, 15 with irradiation alone, and four with a combination of both modalities. The initial tumor control rate was 46% with surgery alone, although ultimately 84% of the patients were tumor free after

TABLE 36–4
Local Control with Radiation Therapy for Chemodectoma of the Temporal Bone

INVESTIGATION	LOCAL CONTROL (PATIENTS)	NOMINAL DOSAGE SCHEDULE
M.D. Anderson Cancer Center[250]	16/17	4500–5000 cGy/4.5–5 wks
University of Florida[58]	14/14	3760–5640 cGy/4–6.5 wks
Princess Margaret Hospital[47]	42/45*	3500 cGy/3 wks
Geisinger Medical Center[38]	20/24	4000–5000 cGy†
Mount Sinai Hospital, New York[222]	6/6	4000–5000 cGy/4–5 wks
Royal Victoria Infirmary, Newcastle Upon Tyne[257]	11/13	5000–5500 cGy/5–5.5 wks
Queen Elizabeth Hospital, Birmingham[10]	19/20‡	4500–5000 cGy/4–5 wks
University of Washington[223]	10/13	2800–6500 cGy/4–7 wks
Arhus Municipal Hospital, Denmark[249]	13/15	5000–6000 cGy/5–6 wks
University Hospital of Wales, Cardiff[94]	12/14	4250–5000 cGy/15 fractions
Rotterdamsch Radio-Therapeutisch Instituut, Netherlands[160]	19/19	4000–6000 cGy/4–6 wks
University of Minnesota[170]	13/14	3000–6000 cGy/3.5–7.5 wks
University of Virginia[139]	26/30	4000–5000 cGy/4–5 wks
Total	221/244 (91%)	

** Two patients listed as failures were salvaged with further treatments.*
† Fractionation schedule not specified.
‡ The one patient listed as a failure was salvaged with further radiation therapy.
(Wang M-L, Hussey DH, Doornbos JF, Wen B-C: Int J Radiat Oncol Biol Phys 14:643, 1987)

salvage with additional surgery. Seventy-eight percent survived 10 years; however, 31% developed complications. Of the patients treated with irradiation, 84% had initial local tumor control, 77% survived 10 years, and only 11% developed complications. The doses of irradiation used were slightly higher (mean 5832 cGy) than those reported by others. Complications were reported in two or three patients receiving 6600 cGy. However, no improvement in tumor control occurred with higher doses.

In a compilation of many studies, Kim and colleagues[139] reported a 25% local failure rate in 83 patients receiving less than 4000 cGy and 1.4% local failure rate in 142 patients receiving more than 4000 cGy. Arthur[10] reported no recurrences in 24 patients treated with doses ranging from 4500 cGy to 5000 cGy; only one failure occurred in a patient receiving 3000 cGy in 15 fractions in 21 days. Reddy and colleagues[208] described 10 recurrences in 13 patients with glomus jugulare tumors initially treated with surgery alone, in contrast to no failures in four patients receiving postoperative radiation therapy or in seven patients treated with this modality for postsurgical recurrences. Most of the lesions were treated with 4000 cGy to 5600 cGy. Greater local control is not achieved with doses higher than 5000 cGy. If the tolerance of the brain and brain stem to irradiation is considered, doses of 4500 cGy to 5000 cGy given in 180-cGy to 200-cGy fractions are optimal for the treatment of these lesions.

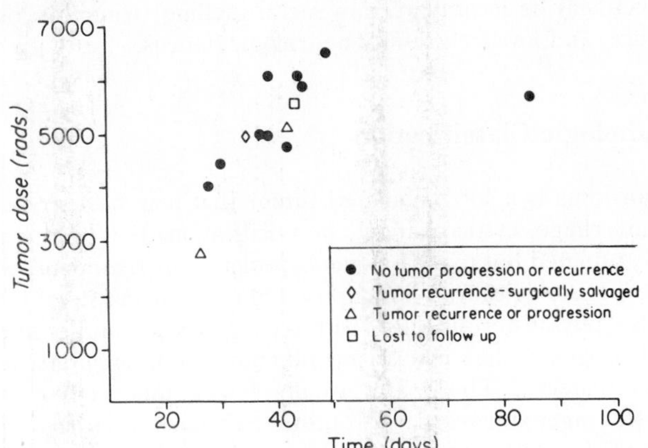

FIGURE 36–6. Time-dose relationships in 14 glomus tumors treated with various dose or fractionation schedules. (Simko TG, Griffin GW, Gendes AJ, et al: Cancer 42:104, 1978)

Mendenhall and colleagues[180] reported six chemodectomas of the carotid body and ganglion nodosum in four patients treated with radiation therapy. Doses of 4080 cGy to 4850 cGy were delivered with ^{60}Co, 8-MV x-rays, or combination of 8-MV and 17-MV x-rays. Lesions have remained stable in four of the patients for 2 to 4.5 years after irradiation. Treatment results in a few patients with this type of tumor are summarized in Table 36-5.

CHORDOMAS

Anatomy

Chordomas are rare neoplasms of the axial skeleton that arise from the remnant of the primitive notochord (chorda dorsalis). About 50% arise in the sacrococcygeal area, 35% arise intracranially, where they typically involve the clivus, and the remaining 15% occur in the midline along the path of the notochord, primarily involving the cervical vertebrae. (Fig. 36-7).[245]

TABLE 36–5
Chemodectomas of the Carotid Body and Ganglion Nodosum

INVESTIGATION	NO. OF PATIENTS	NO. OF LESIONS	DOSE (cGy)	RESULTS†
Mitchell and Clyne[184]	6	6	3750–5500	5/6 controlled at 1.5–8 years
Lybeert et al[160]	9	11	4000–6000*	9/9 controlled at 1.5–18 years
Krupski et al[143]	1	1		Controlled at 8 years
Wilson[267]	1	1		Controlled at 10 years
Endicott and Maniglia[71]	1	1	4500	Controlled at 1 year
Mendenhall et al[180]	4	6	4080–4850	4/4 controlled at 2–4.5 years

**200 cGy per fraction.*
† Control is defined as regression or stabilization of local disease; no evidence of lymph node metastases.
(Mendenhall WM, Million RR, Parsons JT, et al: Int J Radiat Oncol Biol Phys 12:2175, 1986)

Epidemiology

Chordomas are more common in patients in their fifties and sixties but can occur in all age groups. In children and young adults, the prognosis and long-term survival rate appear to be better than in older patients.[271] No risk factors have been identified. These tumors occur two or three times more often in males than in females.[122]

Natural History

Although they are slowly growing lesions, chordomas are locally invasive, destroying bone and infiltrating soft tissues. The basisphenoidal chordomas tend to cause symptoms earlier and may be difficult to differentiate histologically from chondromas and chondrosarcomas and radiographically from craniopharyngiomas, pineal tumors, and hypophyseal and pontine gliomas. However, chordomas usually present with a longer clinical history. Sacrococcygeal chordomas progress insidiously, and symptoms do not appear until after the tumor has grown for many years. The lethality of these tumors rests on their critical location, aggressive local behavior, and an extremely high local recurrence rate.

The incidence of metastases is higher than previously believed.[119,213] Metastases occur in as many as 25% of the patients, and the high rate may be related to the long clinical history. The most common sites of distant metastases are the lungs, followed by liver and bone.[261] Lymphatic spread is uncommon.

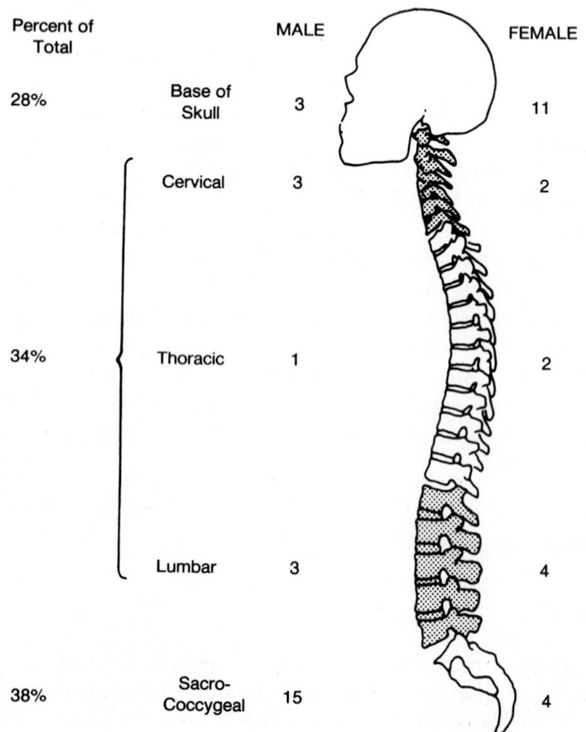

FIGURE 36–7. Sex and site distributions of patients with chordoma. (Rich TA, Schiller A, Suit HD, et al: Cancer 56:182, 1985)

Clinical Presentation

Clinical symptoms vary with the location and extent of the tumor. In the head, extension may be intracranial or extracranial, into the sphenoid sinus, nasopharynx, clivus, and sellar and parasellar areas, with a resultant mass effect. In chordomas of the sphenooccipital region, the most common presenting symptom is headache.[119,122,215] Other presentations include symptoms of pituitary insufficiency, nasal stuffiness, bitemporal hemianopsia, diplopia, and other cranial nerve deficits. Fuller and Bloom[87] recently reported on 13 patients with clivus chordoma, all of whom presented with multiple cranial nerve palsies. There was facial pain in 11 of the 13 patients.

In sacrococcygeal chordomas, the major complaint is pain, which may be accompanied by sacral swelling, urinary incontinence, and lower extremity neurologic deficits.

Pathologic Classification

Chordoma is a soft, lobulated tumor that may have areas of hemorrhage, cystic changes, or calcification. It is frequently encapsulated but may be nonencapsulated or pseudoencapsulated. Histologically, it is composed of cords or masses of large cells ("physalisferous cells") with typical vacuoles and granules of gylcogen in their cytoplasm and abundant intercellular mucoid material. There are usually few mitotic cells.[76,86,124] Heffelfinger and associates[119] postulated that a chondroid variant of chordoma may exist and be prevalent in the sphenooccipital area. Patients with this type of histologic variant have an improved chance for survival.

Prognostic Factors

In addition to the histologic features, the prognostic factors that most influence the choice of treatment are location and local extent of tumor. Surgical extirpation is unusual.[215,248,261]

Diagnostic Workup

The diagnostic workup varies with the primary location of disease. Most patients have significant bony destruction, and some may have calcifications in the tumor. Plain films and CT scans are highly useful (Table 36-6). In most cases, the soft tissue component is much more extensive than initially appreciated, and a CT scan with contrast enhancement is required to reveal it (Fig. 36-8). CT and MRI are equivalent for demonstrating the presence and site of the tumors. MRI is inferior to CT in its ability to demonstrate bony destruction and intratumoral calcification (Fig. 36-9).[197,245] However, MRI is superior to CT for delineating the extent of the tumor, which allows better treatment planning. However, given its greater availability and lower cost, CT appears to be the technique of choice for routine follow-up of previously treated patients.[44]

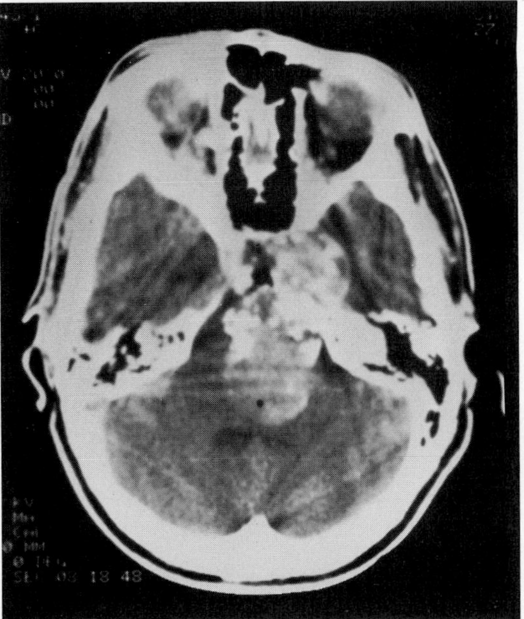

FIGURE 36–8. Contrast-enhanced axial CT scan demonstrates a large chordoma with extension into the posterior fossa and left parasellar region.

General Management

The general management of the patient is dictated by the anatomic site of the tumor and the direction and extent of spread. A surgical approach is preferred. Intracranial spread usually requires steroid coverage and therapy directed to correction of neurologic deficits. Because of the high incidence of local recurrence, combined surgical excision and irradiation is frequently used. No meaningful chemotherapeutic agent or combination of drugs has been identified.

Radiation Therapy Techniques

Radiation therapy techniques vary considerably, depending on the location of the tumor along the craniospinal axis. Basisphenoidal tumors usually are treated by a combination of parallel opposed lateral fields, anterior wedges, and combinations of photon and electron beams, depending on the extent of the neoplasm (Fig. 36-10). Precision radiation therapy planning, preferably using CT and MRI, is required because high doses of external-beam radiation therapy are required. Sacrococcygeal and spinal chordomas are treated by a combination of posterior oblique wedged fields with or without an additional boost (Fig. 36-11).

Because of the slow proliferative nature of these tumors, high linear energy transfer (LET) units may prove useful in chordoma management.[269] Proton beam boosts also have been recommended. Rich and colleagues[210] reported the results for 48 patients with chordomas: 14 of these patients were treated with surgery, 17 with a combination of partial surgical resection

TABLE 36–6
Diagnostic Workup for Chordoma

GENERAL

History
Physical examination

RADIOLOGIC STUDIES

Plain radiographs
Computed tomography scan
Magnetic resonance imaging

LABORATORY STUDIES

Complete blood counts on admission
Chemistry
Urinalysis

SPECIAL STUDIES

Endocrinologic profile (clivus)
Visual evaluations (clivus)

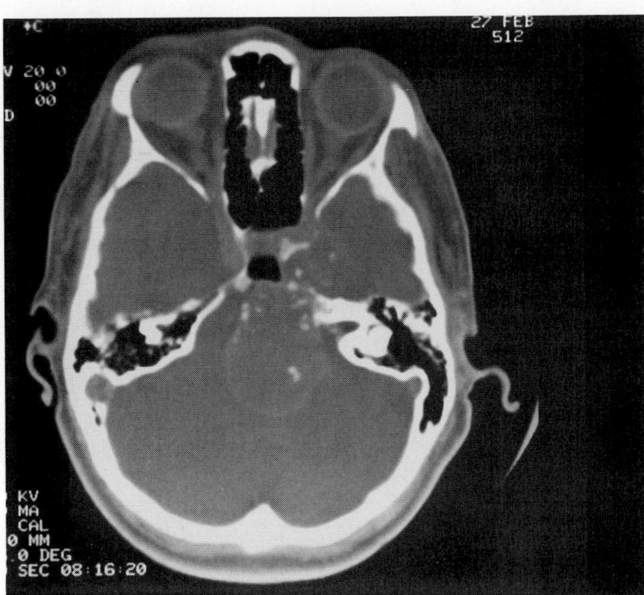

FIGURE 36–9. CT scan photographed at bone windows shows the bony destruction and intratumoral calcifications.

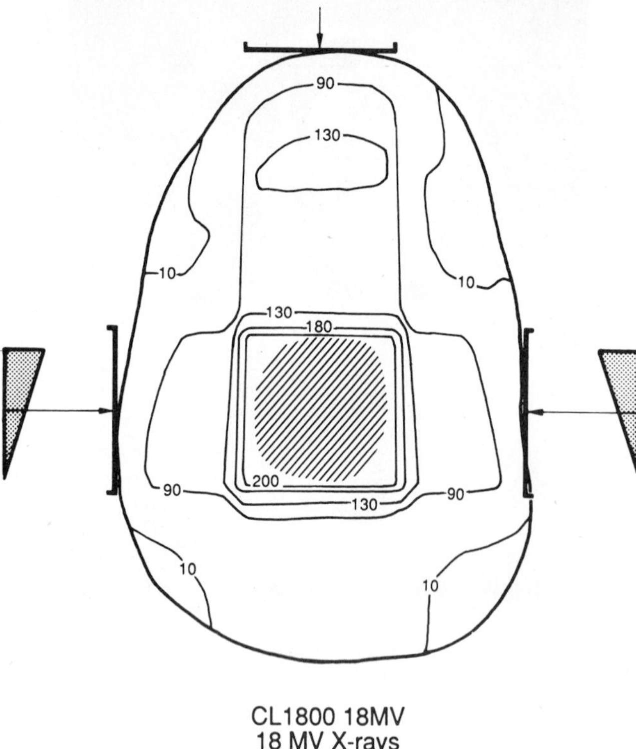

FIGURE 36–10. Treatment planning field arrangement for clivus chordoma.

and irradiation, and 15 with irradiation alone after biopsy (Table 37-7). Various techniques were employed to deliver doses of 4500 cGy to 8040 cGy with photons alone or combined with 160-MeV protons, usually 200 cGy daily. Brachytherapy for recurrent tumors of the base of skull or adjacent to the spine can be used if a more aggressive surgical exposure is offered. Three of five chordomas were rendered stable after treatment with ^{125}I implants by Gutin and others,[105] performed with CT sterotactic technique. Kumar and colleagues[144] reported the use of ^{125}I intraoperative interstitial implantation in two patients with recurrent chordomas. Disease was effectively controlled in both.

Results of Therapy

Although survival in some patients with chordoma may be long term, the salient feature of this unusual neoplasm is local recurrence with eventual death from the disease. The course may be indolent, with multiple treatments for recurrences, but the overall 5-year disease-free survival rate is less than 10% to 20%. In the series of Higinbotham and colleagues[122] of 46 patients with chordoma, only three were alive with no evidence of disease at 5, 13, and 26 years, respectively. At M. D. Anderson, of 19 patients treated definitively, three were alive and free of disease at 3, 6, and 7.5 years, respectively.[215] Dahlin and colleagues,[49] in a series of 59 cases, also showed disappointing local control. Fuller and Bloom[87] treated 25 patients with external-beam radiation therapy and produced a 96% stabilization or reduction of pain; the overall actuarial survival rates were 44% and 17% for 5 and 10 years, respectively. These results parallel our own experience with 21 patients with chordomas (11 arising from the clivus) treated with surgery followed by radiation therapy with doses ranging from 5000 cGy to 6600 cGy in 5 to 6.5 weeks.[4] Although irradiation achieved significant tumor control with remission of symptoms for 1 to 6 years, the 5-year actuarial survival rate was 50%, and the 10-year survival rate was only 20%.[4]

The best results in the treatment of chordomas have been obtained with radical surgical procedures followed by high-dose irradiation. Berson and associates[22] described their experience with 45 patients with chordoma or chondrosarcomas at the base of the skull or cervical spine who were treated by subtotal resection and postoperative irradiation. Twenty-three of these patients were treated definitively by charged particles, 13 patients with photons and particles, and nine were treated for recurrent disease. Doses ranged from 3600 cGy to 8000 cGy equivalent. There appears to be significant benefit for patients with smaller tumor volumes, who had an 80% actuarial survival

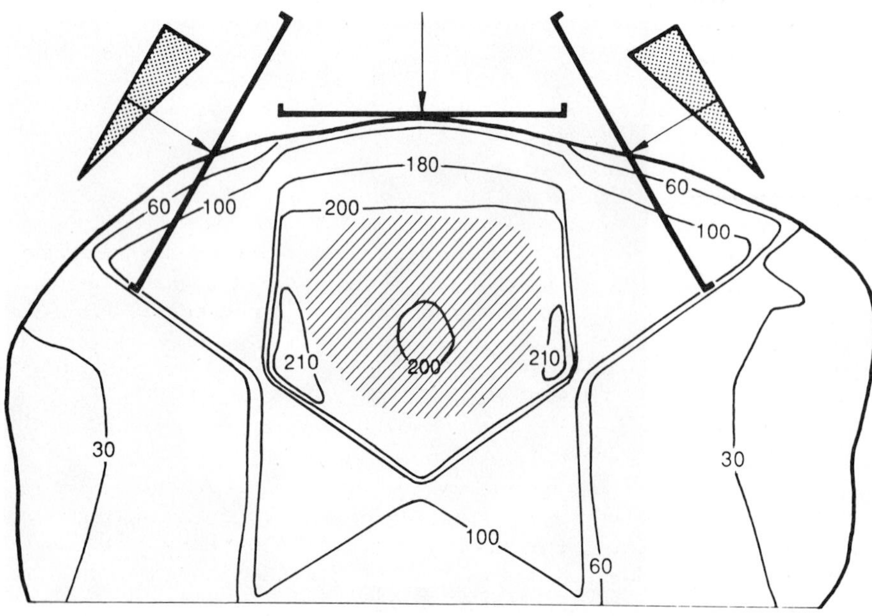

FIGURE 36–11. Field arrangement for treating sacral chordoma.

TABLE 36–7
Patient Status According to Treatment of Chordoma and Radiation Dose Level

TREATMENT					CAUSE OF FAILURE				
SURGERY	IRRADIATION	NO. OF PATIENTS	NED*	AWD	LOCAL	LOCAL + DM	DM	ID	LOST
Radical excision	None	8	4	0	2	0	0	1	1
Palliative excision	None	6	0	0	4	1	0	1	0
Partial excision	>6000 cGy	5	4	0	0	1	0	0	0
	<6000 cGy	12	0	3	6	2	0	0	1
Biopsy	>6000 cGy	9	5	2	0	1	0	1	0
	<6000 cGy	6	0	0	1	4	0	0	1
Total excision	Preop (5000 cGy)	2	1	1	0	0	0	0	0
Total		48	14	6	13	9	0	3	3

NED: no evidence of disease; AWD: alive with disease; DM: distant metastasis; ID: intercurrent death; Preop: preoperative.
(Rich TA, Schiller A, Suit HD, et al: Cancer 56:182, 1985)

rate at 5 years; the rate was only 33% for patients with large tumors. Patients treated for primary disease had a 78% actuarial local control rate at 2 years, but the rate for patients with recurrent disease was 33%.[22] Because of disappointing long-term survival rates with conventional treatment, innovative approaches, especially particle therapy, are being actively explored.

Sequelae of Treatment

In patients irradiated with high doses and with charged particles, there is an increasing probability of sequelae, including brain damage, spinal cord injury, bone or soft tissue necrosis, and xerostomia. In the report of Berson and colleagues,[22] there were three patients with unilateral visual loss, and four patients had radiation-induced injury of the brain stem. The endocrine function of patients receiving high-dose proton therapy for clivus tumors was studied by Slater and colleagues.[228] The actuarial incidence of endocrine abnormalities was 26% at 3 years and 37% at 5 years; hypothyroidism was the most frequent abnormality. The dose to the pituitary in patients with abnormalities ranged from 6310 cGy to 6770 cGy (equivalent).

HEMANGIOPERICYTOMA

Hemangiopericytoma is an unusual vascular tumor, first described as a distinct clinical entity by Stout and Murray in 1942.[243] It represents approximately 1% of all vascular neoplasms.[275] Hemangiopericytoma occurs in both sexes with equal frequency and is primarily a tumor of adults. Hemangiopericytomas are believed to originate from the pericytes of Zimmerman, a cell morphologically resembling smooth muscle that is found around the capillaries.[277] They are believed to arise from the primitive mesenchymal cells.[209] Pericytes are believed to provide mechanical support for capillaries with contractile power.

Hemangiopericytomas are composed of a proliferation of tightly packed pericytes around thin-walled endothelial-lined vascular channels ranging from capillary-sized vessels to large gaping sinusoidal spaces.[74] Hemangiopericytomas have a tendency to grow relatively slowly and invade locally into adjacent structures. Although they are always well circumscribed and partially or completely surrounded by a pseudocapsule, benign tumors may be difficult to differentiate from malignant ones.[192] However, prominent mitosis (> four per high-power field), foci of necrosis, and increased cellularity suggest malignancy.[75] The one definitive sign of malignancy is recurrence or development of metastases, which most frequently populate lungs, skeleton, and liver. Late metastases occurring after 10 years of diagnosis are not uncommon. The metastasizing rate, which depends on the site of origin, can be as high as 50% to 80%.[118] In general, tumors in the central nervous system (CNS), lower extremity, or mediastinum tend to be more malignant, with local recurrences in as many as 50% of these patients.[74]

Clinical Presentation

Although hemangiopericytomas may occur anywhere in the body, the head and neck is the third most common location after the lower extremities and the retroperitoneum.[75] Most hemangiopericytomas arise from the soft tissues of the body, and only 45 cases of primary hemangiopericytomas of bone have been described in the world literature.[51,247] Soft tissue hemangiopericytomas present as firm, painless, slowly expanding masses that are often nodular and well localized. The skin overlying the mass does not have any discoloration or redness to indicate its vascular origin because the capillaries are emptied of the blood by compression of massive numbers of pericytes surrounding them.[102]

In the head and neck, the tumor may constitute a polypoid, soft gray or reddish mass that grows slowly and may cause nasal obstruction. Epistaxis is a common symptom. The hemangiopericytoma-like tumors of the nasal passages and paranasal sinuses differ slightly from those occurring elsewhere and probably represent a related but separate entity, because they rarely recur or metastasize, regardless of the type of therapy.[39]

Orbital hemangiopericytomas account for 3% of orbital malignancies and most frequently present with painless proptosis.[44,218]

Hemangiopericytoma may occur intracranially. When it arises in the brain, it is a solid mass attached to the meninges and grossly resembles a meningioma.[126] These intracranial hemangiopericytomas carry a high risk of local failures (80%) and higher potential for dissemination. The mean time for local recurrence is 75 months.[126]

Hemangiopericytoma appears on plain radiographs as a soft tissue mass in the nasal cavity or other portions of the head and neck. A defect caused by pressure erosion of the surrounding bones may occur, and because calcifications are rare, the plain radiographic pattern does not help in diagnosing these tumors. On arteriography, according to Yaghmai,[275] hemangiopericytoma is the only vascular tumor that presents some characteristic angiographic features regardless of its location, site of origin, or clinical behavior. These features consist of radially arranged or spider-like branching vessels around and inside the tumor and a long-standing, well-demarcated tumor stain. Intracranial tumors typically have arterial blood supply from meningeal and cerebral connections, with one to three main feeders supplying many small corkscrew-like vessels.[168] The most distinctive and constant feature of this tumor is its hypervascularity, which explains the profuse bleeding that commonly occurs during surgical manipulation. This tissue characteristic may also be demonstrated with contrast-enhanced CT.[3,97] Intracranially, the diffusely enhancing tumor may resemble a meningioma on CT. However, some CT signs may suggest hemangiopericytoma rather than meningioma: lack of calcification, scarce surrounding edema, and ring-like enhancement.[198] CT and MRI scans are especially valuable in delineating the full extent of the soft tissue tumor.

General Management

Although hemangiopericytoma is rare and experience in its management is limited, it appears that surgical resection combined with preoperative embolization of the tumor is the treatment of choice.[260] More extensive surgery is required for tumors that show features of malignancy. For incompletely resected tumors, postoperative radiation therapy is used. The role of chemotherapy in this tumor is not yet determined. A few reports have described partial tumor regression in some lesions treated with cytotoxic agents. Doxorubicin (Adriamycin), alone or in combination-drug regimens, is the most effective agent for metastatic hemangiopericytomas, producing complete and partial remissions in 50% of the cases.[272] Other drugs prescribed are cyclophosphamide, dacarbazine, vincristine, and actinomycin D.[118]

Radiation Therapy Techniques

The role of radiation therapy alone in the management of hemangiopericytoma is controversial. The tumor has been considered relatively radioresistant, and Friedman and Egan[84] concluded that an effective dose for hemangiopericytoma lies in the range of 7500 cGy to 9000 cGy administered in 30 to 60 days. There have been several reports indicating a place for radiation therapy in unresectable tumors or in patients with residual disease.[131,183] Orbital hemangiopericytoma has been cured by surgery and postoperative radiation therapy in doses to 6500 cGy.[218]

The main role of irradiation is as adjuvant therapy after complete excision of the lesion or postoperatively for minimal residual disease. Tumor doses of 5500 cGy to 6500 cGy in 6 to 7 weeks are required to produce local control in the postoperative cases.[126] There appears to be a definite role for postoperative irradiation to the brain for primary hemangiopericytomas if radical surgery is performed, because these tumors tend to recur after seemingly complete removal. Jha and associates[131] reported local control in all patients treated postoperatively with adjuvant external-beam radiation therapy. Radiation therapy has also been used as a salvage procedure to treat a local recurrence after initial surgery with or without chemotherapy.

The fields of irradiation should be wide enough to encompass the tumor bed with safe margin of at least 5 cm to avoid marginal recurrence. Portal arrangement and beam selection are similar to those used in the treatment of soft tissue sarcomas.

LETHAL MIDLINE GRANULOMA

Natural History and Pathology

Lethal midline granuloma (midline malignant polymorphic reticulosis) is a clinical entity characterized by progressive, unrelenting ulceration and necrosis of the midline facial tissues. There has been considerable controversy about various disorders characterized by a necrotizing and granulomatous inflammation of the tissues of the upper respiratory tract and oral cavity. If infections and other known agents, such as cocaine use, sarcoidosis, environmental toxins, and various neoplasms, can be excluded, three clinicopathologic entities remain: Wegener's granulomatosis, lethal midline granuloma, and polymorphic reticulosis.[14] Characteristics of the three different diseases are outlined in Table 36-8.

Wegener's granulomatosis is an epithelioid necrotizing granulomatosis with vasculitis of small vessels. Systemic involvement of the kidneys and lungs is common.

Polymorphic reticulosis is an unusual disorder with distinctive clinical and pathologic features.[175] Histologically, polymorphic reticulosis is characterized by an atypical mixed lymphoid infiltration of the submucosa, with extensive areas of necrosis extending sometimes to bone or cartilage. The lesion consists of zones of small lymphocytes with scattered immunoblastic forms, abundant plasma cells with occasional eosinophilia and histiocytosis.[229] Since its first description by Eichel and colleagues[68] in 1966, it was considered a lymphoproliferative disorder. Recent investigations have shown that most or all cases of polymorphic reticulosis are peripheral T-cell lymphomas.[155,265] Several authorities believe that polymorphic reticulosis and systemic lymphomatoid granulomatosis are the same disease, with the latter predominantly involving the lungs.[92,155]

Idiopathic lethal midline granuloma describes a localized disorder not characterized by visceral lesions but by destruction of the midfacial areas that, if left untreated, is uniformly fatal. The histopathologic findings are nonspecific, with a relatively nondescript acute and chronic inflammation and necrosis. Despite specific clinicopathologic features, the distinction between lethal midline granuloma and polymorphic reticulosis is often difficult; they may even represent two phases of the same disease, with lethal midline granuloma remaining histologically benign or evolving into polymorphic reticulosis.

Lethal midline granuloma occurs more frequently in males.[81] Ages of patients range from 21 to 64 years; almost half of the patients are in their fifties at presentation. Most patients have involvement of the nasal cavity (including destruction of the septum) and the paranasal sinuses (particularly maxillary antrum). The primary lesion may extend into the orbits, the palate or gingiva of the oral cavity, and the pharynx. Destruction or ulceration of the nose may occur.

Clinical Features and Diagnostic Workup

Clinical manifestations include progressive nasal discharge, obstruction, foul odor emanating from the nose, and in later stages, pain in the nasal cavity, paranasal areas, and orbits.

TABLE 36–8
Differential Features of Three Clinicopathologic Entities

CHARACTERISTIC	WEGENER'S GRANULOMATOSIS	IDIOPATHIC MIDLINE GRANULOMA	POLYMORPHIC RETICULOSIS
Disease features	Diffuse, inflammatory disease of upper airway, predominantly sinuses and nose	Destructive extension to the palate and facial soft tissues	Destructive lesion with destruction of bone and extension through soft tissues
Systemic involvement	Lungs, kidneys, small-vessel vasculitis may not have airway involvement	No	No
Associated with lymphoma	No	May remain benign or progress to lymphoma	Usually evolves to lymphoma
Histologic features	Necrotizing vasculitis with epithelioid granulomas, giant cells, and fibrinoid necrosis	Inflammatory reaction, nonspecific; granulomas and giant cells are infrequent	Characteristic atypical and polymorphic lymphoreticular cellular infiltrate; angiocentric growth patterns may simulate vasculitis, but fibrinoid necrosis is absent in vessel walls
Treatment	Chemotherapy	Radiation therapy	Chemotherapy Radiation therapy and chemotherapy

(Modified from Bataskis JG: Head Neck Surg 1:213, 1979)

Examination discloses destructive ulceration and necrosis in the nasal cavity, perforation or destruction of nasal septum and turbinates, and ulceration of the nose. There may be edema of the face and eyelids, and the bridge of the nose may be sunken. Radiographic studies initially show soft tissue swelling, mucosal thickening, and findings consistent with chronic sinusitis. CT is invaluable in demonstrating the full extent of the tumor, including bone or cartilage destruction.

General Management and Radiation Therapy Techniques

When treatment of these patients is planned, it is extremely important to exclude the diagnosis of Wegener's granulomatosis, a benign process that is commonly treated with steroids and systemic chemotherapy.[57,186] Lethal midline granuloma does not respond to steroids. The treatment of choice is radiation therapy.[60] Target volume should encompass all areas of involvement including adjacent areas at risk (*e.g.*, for a lesion of the maxillary antrum, the volume includes the antrum and the paranasal sinuses).[107] Because marginal failures are a significant problem, wide margins are necessary for treatment of these patients.[229]

Techniques of irradiation are similar to those described for tumors of the paranasal sinuses, nasal cavity, or nasopharynx. Because of the rarity of this tumor, experience is limited. Complete responses have occurred with doses between 1000 cGy and 5000 cGy, with most patients treated with 3500 cGy to 4000 cGy in 3 to 4 weeks (Table 36-9).[60,79,82] We recommend 4500 cGy to 5000 cGy in 4.5 to 5 weeks in daily fractions of 180 cGy to 200 cGy.

TABLE 36–9
Radiation Therapy for Polymorphic Reticulosis or Lymphomatoid Granulomatosis

YEAR	INVESTIGATOR	NO. OF CASES	LOCATION	DOSE (cGy)*	RESULTS
1966	Eichel et al[68]	9	Nose	NS	9/9 NED at 5 years
1966	Liebow et al[154]	1	Neck nodes Brain	NS	Improvement in adenopathy and CNS symptoms; alive at 8 years
1976	McDonald et al[175]	20	Upper airway	4000–4200	13 NED >1-year follow-up
1978	McRemee et al[57]				2 NED <1-year follow-up One lost to follow-up Four dead, intercurrent disease
1978	Fuller et al[88]	1	Thigh Lung Liver	3000 4000 3000	Mass resolved Obstruction resolved Dead, hepatic failure
1978	Shank et al[219]	2	Brain Lung Orbital mass	4000 3000 2800	Improvement in CNS symptoms and CT Chest radiograph improved Mass regression

**NS: not specified; NED: no evidence of disease.*
(From Halperin EC, Dosoretz MD, Goodman M, et al: Br J Radiol 55:645, 1982)

Results of Therapy

Fauci and colleagues[80] reported ten patients with extensive midline granuloma who were treated with irradiation. Three received 1000 cGy, and all failed within 2 years (retreated with 4000 cGy to 4600 cGy). The remaining seven patients received between 4000 cGy and 5000 cGy. The rate of local control of disease was 77%; two patients had local recurrences, one outside the initially irradiated volume.

In a report by Eichel and co-workers,[68] of 33 patients believed to have nasal lymphoma, nine patients were found to have polymorphic reticulosis and survived for a prolonged period after radiation therapy. The Mayo Clinic has most extensive experience in treating polymorphic reticulosis and lethal midline granuloma with irradiation (4000–4200 cGy).[57,175] Of 20 patients irradiated for localized upper airway polymorphic reticulosis, 13 were alive and well for an average of 9.5 years; two were alive and well with less than 1 year of follow-up; four were dead of other disease; and one was lost to follow-up.

In a study of 34 patients with polymorphic reticulosis treated with primary radiation therapy except for one patient, Smalley and colleagues[229] found that a minimum dose of 4200 cGy or a time-dose factor of 70 was necessary to achieve long-term local control. The most frequent failure site was within the original radiation field. They believe that this problem will diminish with implementation of proper time-dose-fractionation schemes. Systemic failure occurred in 25% of their patients initially presenting with limited disease. The salvage of this subset of patients requires effective systemic chemotherapy.

Fauci and co-workers[79] published a prospective study of 15 patients with systemic lymphomatoid granulomatosis. Of 13 patients treated with cyclophosphamide and prednisone, seven sustained a complete remission (mean duration of remission, 5.2 ± 0.6 years). Two patients receiving only prednisone and six receiving cyclophosphamide and prednisone died. Six of these deaths were caused by biopsy-proven lymphoma; one was caused by a lymphoma-like illness unproven by biopsy. The eighth death was caused by adenocarcinoma in a patient with lymphoma in remission. None of these patients received radiation therapy.

CHLOROMA

Natural History and Clinical Presentation

Chloromas (granulocytic sarcomas, myeloblastomas) are solid extramedullary tumors composed of early myeloid precursors usually associated with acute myelocytic leukemia.[35] Chloromas are most commonly found in association with bone and nervous tissue, and the most common sites of presentation are in the orbit and other craniofacial bones.[264] The name "chloroma" (from the Greek "chloros," meaning green) describes the color of affected tissues caused by the presence of myeloperoxidase.[31] Because not all deposits exhibit the characteristic green tint, the term granulocytic sarcoma seems more appropriate.[207] Granulocytic sarcomas have been identified in 3% of 478 patients with acute chronic granulocytic leukemia. They are associated with other myeloproliferative disorders, including polycythemia vera, hypereosinophilia, and myeloid metaplasia.[185–187] In the absence of acute leukemia, granulocytic sarcoma is usually an ominous sign, suggesting imminent conversion to acute myelocytic leukemia or blast crisis.[187] As survival rates for myelogenous leukemias improve, the number of patients who relapse with chloromas is increasing.[185]

Children are affected more often than adults. Of 33 patients with orbital chloromas reported by Zimmerman and Font,[278] 75% were in their first decade of life. Chloromas are more frequent in children with the M4 and M5 acute myeloid leukemia subtypes of the French-American-British Cooperative Group Classification and are also associated with the 8:21 chromosomal translocation.[161] Chloromas may appear during bone marrow remission, before an increase in blasts is detected in the bone marrow, and they may herald relapse.

Intraorbital (retrobulbar) chloroma causes insidiously progressive exophthalmos or temporal swelling. Central nervous system involvement causes local pressure phenomena and generalized elevation of intracranial pressure with consequent headaches, nausea, and vomiting.

Intracerebral chloromas may manifest as the rare CNS involvement of acute nonlymphocytic leukemia.[99] Woo and colleagues[273] believe that intracerebral chloromas represent reactivation of sanctuary deposits of leukemic cells in the CNS originated from an initial hematogenous spread. ANLL in the developing world appears to have different clinical features. There is a higher incidence of gingival hypertrophy, hepatosplenomegaly, and chloromas in blacks than in whites among South African children.[161] Spontaneous regression of ANLL complicated with chloroma has been reported.[246]

Diagnostic Workup

All patients require complete hematologic and neurologic testing, as for any patient with suspected leukemia. Open biopsy remains the best diagnostic tool. Plain radiographic findings consist mainly of localized bone destruction with predominantly lytic lesions and associated soft tissue masses. CT scans show the soft tissue masses in orbital and periorbital chloromas. Intracranial chloromas may exhibit intermediate or high attenuation in unenhanced CT scans, with intense, uniform enhancement after intravenous administration of contrast material. Confusion with meningioma, hematoma, solitary metastasis, and lymphoma may occur on CT scans.[203,231]

Gallium 67 scintigraphy should be used to detect unsuspected lesions, because it demonstrates increased uptake even in small leukemic infiltrates.[157] ^{67}Ga is also useful as a marker for follow-up and for measuring response to therapy.[157]

Radiation Therapy Techniques

Chloromas are extremely radiosensitive; however, an optimal dose of radiation therapy has not yet been established. Response rates of leukemic infiltrates have been reported with doses as low as 400 cGy. However, the need for doses up to 3000 cGy in certain locations of extramedullary leukemic infiltrates is recognized. Mair[164] recommends anywhere from 600 cGy in a single dose to 1500 cGy in ten fractions to a maximum of 3000 cGy. Although there is not much information about the maximum dose needed for treatment of chloromas, it appears that 3000 cGy is the maximum required for local control. In our limited experience, there appears to be a relationship between the size of the chloroma and the total dose of external-beam radiation therapy required for control. The target volume is the tumor mass and an adequate margin (2–3 cm).

Techniques of irradiation depend on the location of the infiltrate. For superficial lesions, electron beam is recommended. Orbital chloroma may constitute a radiation therapy emergency, because visual loss is possible if the patient is not treated promptly.

ESTHESIONEUROBLASTOMA

Anatomy

Esthesioneuroblastomas are rare tumors thought to arise in the olfactory receptors in the nasal mucosa of the cribriform plate of the ethmoid bone. The olfactory nerves perforate grooves in the ethmoid bone in the cribriform plate and continue into the subarachnoid spaces, accounting for the high incidence of intracranial extension.[18,20,21,69]

Epidemiology

Hamilton and colleagues[108] and Herrold[121] induced olfactory neuroblastoma in the nasal cavity of hamsters by injection of dimethylnitrosamine and other nitroso derivatives. What role these agents may play in humans is unknown. No other risk factors have been identified. There appears to be a slight male predominance. The incidence has a bimodal distribution, with peaks at 11 to 20 years and 40 to 60 years, with the highest incidence from 51 to 60 years.[69]

Natural History

In 1924, Berger and Luc[21] first described a tumor arising in the nasal fossa, which they called olfactory esthesioneuroepithelioma. Two years later, Berger and Coutard[20] described a similar tumor. Berger and others[20] thought that esthesioneuroblastoma had an endodermal origin, arising from the olfactory placode, but others proposed an ectodermal origin. Most observers believe the tumor to be of neuroectodermal origin in the olfactory epithelium.[93,108,160,174,189] In Obert's review, most tumors were found to occur high in the vault of the nasal cavity or in the lateral wall adjacent to the ethmoids.[190]

The tumors may originate in the interior, middle, or posterior group of ethmoid cells, but the site has no clinical significance. The tumor may spread to the opposite ethmoid bone, superiorly to the frontal sinus and anterior cranial fossa, posteriorly to the sphenoid sinus, nasopharynx, and base of skull, laterally to the orbits, forward to the frontonasal angle, or inferiorly to the nasal cavity and antrum (Fig. 36-12).

Lymphatic spread may be to the subdiagastric, posterior cervical, submaxillary, or preauricular nodes and to the nodes of Rouviere. The exact incidence of distant metastases is uncertain; it has been reported to be as high as 50%, but this rate is influenced by the use of chemotherapy in high-risk patients.

Clinical Presentation

These tumors tend to be friable and bleed easily. The most common clinical symptoms are epistaxis and nasal blockage. Patients also may present with local pain or headache, visual disturbances, rhinorrhea, tearing, proptosis, or swelling in the cheek.[61,134,153,196] The symptoms may be associated with a mass in the neck.

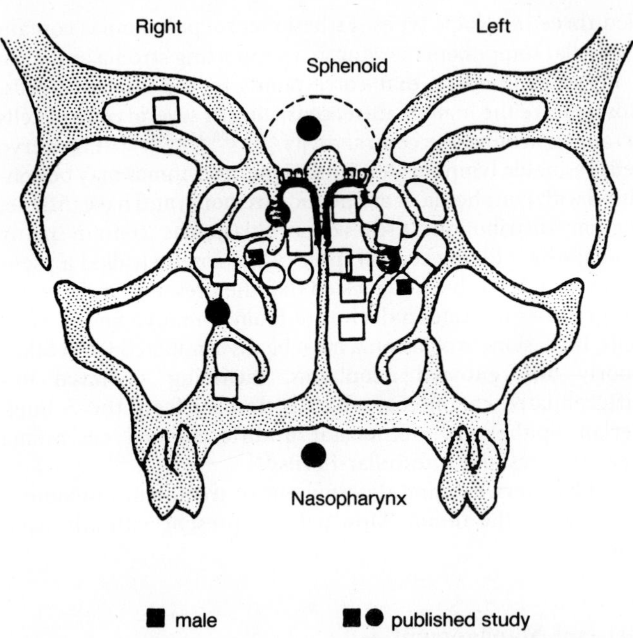

FIGURE 36–12. Demographic distribution of olfactory neuroblastomas. (Appelblatt NH, McClatchey KD: Head Neck Surg 5:108, 1982. Reprinted by permission of John Wiley & Sons)

Diagnosis Workup and Staging

Physical examination may reveal the inferior aspect of a polypoid, friable mass in the nasal cavity. Ocular changes or a mass in the nasopharynx may be present. With early lesions, radiographs or CT may show only nonspecific opacification, soft tissue swelling, or bone destruction. Table 36-1 outlines the suggested diagnostic workup.[165,193,225] MRI, especially with gadolinium contrast, may be used as a supplement or alternative to CT scanning.[152,158,216] Although dopamine β-hydroxylase and catecholamines have been produced by these tumors, their measurements or vanillylmandelic acid excretion levels have not proved clinically useful.[61,93,225] A staging system has been proposed by Kadish and others (Table 36-10).[134]

Pathologic Classification and Prognostic Implications

Esthesioneuroblastomas are polypoid, frequently red, soft, and quite vascular tumors with neuroblasts and neurocytes. Gerard-Marchant and Micheau[93] and McCormack and Harris[174] classi-

TABLE 36–10
Staging of Esthesioneuroblastoma

STAGE	CHARACTERISTIC
A	Disease confined to the nasal cavity
B	Disease confined to the nasal cavity and one or more paranasal sinuses
C	Disease extending beyond the nasal cavity or paranasal sinuses; includes involvement of the orbit, base of skull or intracranial cavity, cervical lymph nodes, or distant metastatic sites

(Kadish S, Goodman M, Wang CC: Cancer 37:1571, 1976)

fied three histologic types. Esthesioneuroepitheliomas contain epithelial components serving as a supporting stroma and have a nerve component that corresponds to the olfactory cells. Rosettes are the main feature, consisting of several rows of cells arranged around the central cavity.[20, 21, 93, 153, 162, 189] The nerve cells resemble lymphocytes. Esthesioneurocytomas may be confused with lymphoma or anaplastic carcinoma and have diffuse, regular distribution. Esthesioneuroblastomas contain many fibrils, which fill the central space of the rosette (called a pseudorosette). It has been suggested that the presence of chromaffin granules indicates a derivative from primitive neural crest cells. Esthesioneuroblastoma must be discriminated from other poorly differentiated neoplasms, including sinonasal undifferentiated carcinoma, which is derived from the Schneiderian epithelium.[85] Sinonasal undifferentiated carcinoma lacks rosettes and intercellar fibrils.[241]

The overwhelming determinant of treatment outcome is the stage of the tumor. Most patients present with advanced disease.

General Management

Rarely, early lesions involving the ethmoids with little or no bony destruction or nerve invasion can be treated adequately by complete surgical removal or by high-energy (photon or electron) radiation therapy with good cosmetic and functional results.[18, 61, 64, 69, 153, 190] Those with limited disease benefit from surgery and judicious delivery of adjuvant radiation therapy, although some clinicians argued against combined surgery and radiation therapy because of complications.[12, 18, 61, 69, 153, 190, 196, 242]

An ethmoidomaxillary resection with or without orbital sparing is usually necessary. This procedure is combined with preoperative or postoperative radiation therapy.[64, 174, 196, 227, 253] Although irradiation can control extensive lesions, the treatment of choice is combined surgery and irradiation. For advanced lesions, in which disseminated disease is likely, chemotherapy may decrease the incidence of distant metastases. The doses required for control are in the range of 5000 cGy to 6000 cGy when combined with surgery. For patients with inoperable tumor, doses of approximately 6500 cGy are necessary.

Patients with extensive disease at higher risk of intracranial extension or distant metastases benefit from the addition of chemotherapy. Extensive lesions have been treated with preoperative chemotherapy and radiation therapy. Thiotepa, cyclophosphamide (Cytoxan), doxorubicin, vincristine, nitrogen mustard, and actinomycin D have been used. Weiden and others[266] reported complete tumor regression and 2.7-year survival in a patient with extensive olfactory esthesioneuroblastoma treated with a combination of wide local excision, cyclic cisplatin, 5-fluorouracil, and irradiation (5580 cGy).

Radiation Therapy Techniques

A combination of photons and electrons with anterior fields provides good coverage for limited disease if the tumor is anterior in location. If there is intracranial or posterior extension or there is spread into the maxillary sinus, paired perpendicular (anteroposterior and lateral) portals with wedges or lateral wedge fields in combination with open anterior photon fields give excellent and uniform coverage of the treatment volume. The orbits can be spared or treated as the degree of extension dictates. Occasionally, an anterior electron-beam field may be used for boosting or supplementing low-dose areas.

For extensive disease, a combination of lateral weighted wedges with an open weighted field gives the best uniform coverage, and this basic arrangement can be modified to treat the orbit or maxillary sinus, as determined by treatment volume. A bolus may be needed for a patient treated postoperatively because there may be a significant surgical defect. Techniques of treatment are similar to those described for treatment of paranasal sinuses (see Chap. 29). A minimal tumor volume is selected, and doses of 6000 cGy to 7000 cGy are delivered, with the dose increased at the higher-risk areas. Treatment planning with CT for tumor extension determination is important.[13, 18] When the electron beam is used over the air cavities, some problems of dosimetry result. Eye blocks must be positioned precisely to avoid undesirable side effects.

Because of the low incidence (≤10%) of cervical lymph nodes, elective irradiation of the neck or a dissection is not indicated.[69, 72] Clinically palpable lymph nodes may be managed by irradiation, radical neck dissection, or a combination of these.[69]

Results of Therapy

Djalilian and co-workers[61] at the Mayo Clinic described 19 cases of esthesioneuroblastoma, 18 of which were followed. Four patients with advanced disease received radiation therapy exclusively; three soon died of disease, and one patient died 5 years later, presumably of coronary occlusion. Combination radiation therapy and rhinotomy failed in five other patients, but three were salvaged surgically. Three of nine patients treated with surgery only were free of disease at 3 to 14 years. Five of six failures were salvaged by means of irradiation and surgery.

Ahmad and Fayos[1] showed primary control in six of nine patients with surgical excision and postoperative irradiation, although three of the six developed distant metastases. The other three patients died with local recurrence and distant metastases. Appelblatt and McClatchey[8] reported 21 cases of olfactory neuroblastoma treated with various methods, including initial surgery or irradiation or combination of both for the treatment of recurrences. Local recurrence was reported in 61% of the patients and metastasis in 28%.

At M. D. Anderson, 11 patients were treated definitively with combined surgery and irradiation in most instances. Four patients are alive and disease free at 2.5, 5, 8, and 12 years, respectively. Two died of disease 4 and 5 years after treatment. One patient was lost to follow-up at 9 months with extensive disease and is presumed dead. Two patients died of intercurrent disease at 4.5 and 15 years, respectively. Two patients died of complications but were free of disease.

Elkon and co-workers[69] compiled the results reported in the literature for 97 patients treated with different modalities. The survival and tumor control in 78 of the patients, staged according to the Kadish and associates system, are summarized in Table 36-11[134]

In 1988, Spaulding and colleagues[233] compared results in 30 patients treated in two time periods, 1969 to 1975 and 1976 to 1985. With the introduction of craniofacial resection, complex field megavoltage irradiation, and chemotherapy for Stage C disease in 1976, the overall 2-year survival rate increased from 70% to 87%. For Stage C disease, the survival rate increased from 50% to 88%.

O'Connor and co-workers[191] used surgery and postoperative radiation therapy for treating seven patients, including four with Stage C disease. All patients are living free of disease at least 2 years after therapy ended.

TABLE 36–11
Treatment of Esthesioneuroblastoma by Modality and Stage

	STAGE A			STAGE B			STAGE C		
MODALITY*	INITIAL TREAT-MENT	FOR RECUR-RENCE	TOTAL CONTROL RATE (%)	INITIAL TREAT-MENT	FOR RECUR-RENCE	TOTAL CONTROL RATE (%)	INITIAL TREAT-MENT	FOR RECUR-RENCE	TOTAL CONTROL RATE (%)
Radiation therapy alone	2/5	5/5	70	4/7	3/4	64	1/5	1/1	33
Surgery alone	5/9	4/4	69	3/6	1/2	50	1/1		
Radiation therapy and surgery	7/10		70	12/30	0/1	57	7/15		47

** All results reflect treatment of 78 patients, who were followed up for 6 months to 32 years.*
(Elkon D, Hightower SI, Lim ML, et al: Cancer 44:1087, 1979)

Chemotherapy

Wade and associates[259] reported the response to chemotherapy (cyclophosphamide and vincristine) in five patients and compiled their experience with eight additional cases reported in the literature. They found that eight (63%) of 13 patients had an objective response to cytotoxic agents. In Stage B, about 30% of the patients, and in Stage C, 48% of the patients developed distant metastases, with or without local recurrence. It may be worthwhile to consider the use of adjuvant chemotherapy in the patients with more advanced stages of the disease.

Sequelae of Treatment

In a few patients, depending on the dose of irradiation, long-term sequelae include bone necrosis, blindness, or painful eye reactions requiring enucleation.[12,153,196,221]

EXTRAMEDULLARY PLASMACYTOMAS

Solitary plasmacytomas are rare tumors. Multiple myeloma occurs 40 times more often than solitary plasmacytoma.[79] The annual incidence of extramedullary plasmacytoma is 0.04 cases per 100,000 population.[200] There are four times more male patients than female patients, and 75% present between the ages of 40 and 60 years.[13,41]

Approximately 80% of all extramedullary plasmacytomas occur in the head and neck area.[62] They form only 0.5% of all upper respiratory tract malignancies. The most common sites in the head and neck are the nasopharynx, nasal cavity, paranasal sinuses, and tonsils.[13]

The usual criteria for solitary plasmacytoma, medullary or extramedullary, include a biopsy-proven plasma cell tumor with one or two solitary foci, the absence of Bence-Jones protein in the urine, bone marrow taken some distance away from the primary site not involved by the tumor (*i.e.*, <10% of plasma cells), hemoglobin of 13 g/100 ml or more, and a normal serum protein level or serum electrophoresis at the time of the diagnosis. The diagnosis of solitary plasmacytoma is made by eliminating the possibility of multiple myeloma.[41]

Extramedullary plasmacytoma of the head and neck area should be considered a separate entity because of its clinical behavior. The most common symptoms are nasal obstruction, local pain and swelling, and epistaxis. The diagnostic workup for extramedullary plasmacytoma arising in the head and neck region is shown in Table 36-1.

Grossly, plasmacytomas tend to be sessile in the nasal cavity and paranasal sinuses and pedunculated in the nasopharynx and larynx. The masses are soft, pliable, and pale gray. The clinical course is unpredictable. The lesion may remain localized or may infiltrate and destroy the surrounding soft tissue and bone. Bone destruction is not a particularly bad prognostic sign, although some physicians report that it adversely affects the prognosis.[1,69] Bony invasion is common in the more malignant types.[13] Cervical lymph node metastasis from extramedullary plasmacytoma varies with the site of the primary lesion and follows the same pattern of spread as squamous cell carcinoma arising in a similar site. The incidence of lymph node metastasis ranges from 12% to 26%.[33,73]

The association between solitary extramedullary plasmacytoma and multiple myeloma is unclear. However, approximately one third of the patients with plasmacytoma develop multiple myeloma.[251]

Pedunculated extramedullary plasmacytoma lesions may be treated by surgical excision because the chance of local recurrence is slight. The treatment of choice for all other lesions is radiation therapy.

Radiation Therapy Techniques

The radiation therapy technique varies with the location of the primary tumor. The techniques are similar to those used for primary tumors in comparable locations (*i.e.*, nasopharynx, tonsil, paranasal sinuses). Solitary plasmacytomas respond well to moderate doses of radiation therapy. Most of the recommended doses are between 4000 cGy and 5000 cGy delivered at 1000 cGy per week. The local control rate by radiation therapy alone is 84.9% (101 of 119 patients). The reported incidence of subsequent development of multiple myeloma is 22.1% (23 of 104 patients).

Harwood and colleagues[115] summarized the literature but could not draw a dose-response curve from the data because of the lack of cases receiving low-dose radiation therapy. Meyer and Schulz[181] stated that there is a high risk of local recurrence with tumor doses below 3000 cGy and a negligible risk for those treated at or above a 4000-cGy tumor dose. Table 36-12 summarizes the doses of irradiation and probability of tumor control reported by various authors. Our experience confirms the efficacy of tumor doses of 4000 cGy to 5000 cGy for local control.

TABLE 36–12
Extramedullary Plasmacytoma of Head and Neck Treated by Radiation Therapy

INVESTIGATION	NO. OF PATIENTS	NO. MALES/ NO. FEMALES	PATIENTS <50 YR	LOCAL CONTROL	NO. WITH MULTIPLE MYELOMA	RECOMMENDED TUMOR DOSE (cGy)*
Todd[251]	15	13/2	12	14/15	5	3450–3800 for 3 wk
Kotner and Wang[142]	16	10/6	12	12/16	4	4000–5000
Wiltshaw[268]	14	10/4	10	11/14	N/A	
Woodruff et al[274]	15	8/7	11	14/15	1	4000–5000
Bush et al[32]	10	5/5	5	8/10	2	5000–5500
Harwood et al[115]	22	18/4	16	18/22	4	3500 for 3 wk
Kapadia et al[136]	12	9/3	10	11/12	3	
M.D. Anderson Cancer Center†	15	12/3	12	13/15	4	5000
Total	119	85/34 (2.5:1)	88 (73.9%)	101/119 (84.9%)	23 (19.3%)	4000–5000

** 1000 cGy/week unless otherwise stated.*
† Updated data of Corwin J: Unpublished data.

Some of our patients had extensive disease, and a higher dose (5000–6000 cGy) was used, as recommended by several investigators.[41, 142, 269]

NASOPHARYNGEAL ANGIOFIBROMA

Juvenile nasopharyngeal angiofibroma, the most common benign disease in this area, is found more frequently in young pubertal boys.[270] It comprises less than 0.05% of head and neck tumors.[163] Patient age at presentation has ranged from 9 to 30 years, with a median of 15 years.[48, 241, 270] Females comprise fewer than 4% of the total cases.[45] Some researchers have suggested chromosomal studies of affected women, because this is mainly a male disease.[34] The tumor is believed to originate from the broad area of the posterolateral wall of the nasal cavity, where the sphenoidal process of the palatine bone meets the horizontal ala of the vomer and the roof of the pterygoid process, because it is always involved.[7, 34] Involution of tumor after irradiation usually occurs in this direction.[217]

It is hypothesized that this tumor represents residual erectile tissue arrested in the nasopharynx during embryologic development. This theory is strongly supported by the clinical picture of tumor growth beginning at puberty, the presence of dihydrotestosterone receptors, and its histologic similarity to erectile tissue.[7, 77, 151, 172]

Clinical Presentation

Nasopharyngeal angiofibroma may initially extend into the nasal fossae and maxillary antrum, push the soft palate downward and through the pterygopalatine fossa, and extend superoanteriorly through the inferior orbital fissure or laterally through the pterygomaxillary fissure to the cheek and temporal regions.[55]

Symptoms usually occur for 2 to 48 months before diagnosis.[46, 239] Most common complaints are nasal obstruction or epistaxis, followed by nasal voice or discharge, cheek swelling, proptosis, diplopia, hearing loss, and headaches.[46, 241] In a series by Witt and associates[270] from Memorial Hospital, 7 of 31 patients presented with anomalous sexual development.

Differential diagnosis includes fibrosarcoma, rhabdomyosarcoma, chronic sinusitis, arteriovenous malformation, lymphangioma, neurofibroma, pleomorphic adenoma, lymphoma, pyogenic granuloma, polyps, and hemangioma.[66, 133]

Diagnostic Workup

The diagnosis is usually made by the clinical picture: a pubertal male with epistaxis or nasal obstruction. After the history taking and physical examination, CT scans with and without contrast should be obtained. The pattern of enhancement in this highly vascular tumor is diagnostic, and many researchers believe carotid angiograms are unnecessary after CT diagnosis of the lesion unless embolization, which is controversial, is contemplated.[27] If there is intracranial extension and radiation therapy is contemplated, no further studies are indicated. If the lesion is extracranial and surgery is indicated, bilateral carotid angiograms can identify the feeding vessels and delineate the boundaries of the tumor (Fig. 36-13).

Biopsies are not indicated in all patients because of the potential for severe hemorrhage. It is important to perform a biopsy of the lesion if the clinical picture (*i.e.*, sex and age of patient, location and behavior of the lesion) is not consistent with juvenile nasopharyngeal angiofibroma, because some lesions have turned out to be sarcomas or chronic sinusitis.[34, 238] Two cases of fibrosarcoma have been reported in patients in their forties.[63, 276] This highly vascular tumor looks nodular and is dark red or gray.[163] Histologically, it has a spindle-shaped fibroblast background with interspersed dilated vascular channels. The vessels lack an elastic membrane, which explains the propensity of these lesions to bleed.[240]

Staging

Two staging systems have been proposed. One from Chandler and colleagues[34] is shown in Table 36-13. The second staging is a radiographic one by Sessions and associates.[217] Stage Ia is limited to the nasopharynx and posterior nares: Stage Ib extends to the paranasal sinuses; Stages IIa, IIb, and IIc extend to other extracranial locations, and Stage III is intracranial.

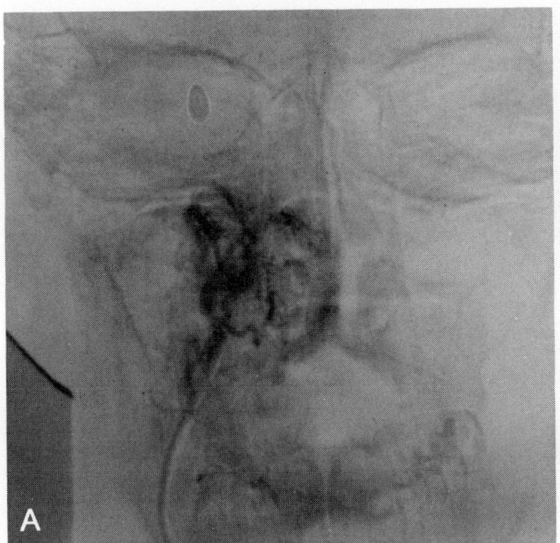

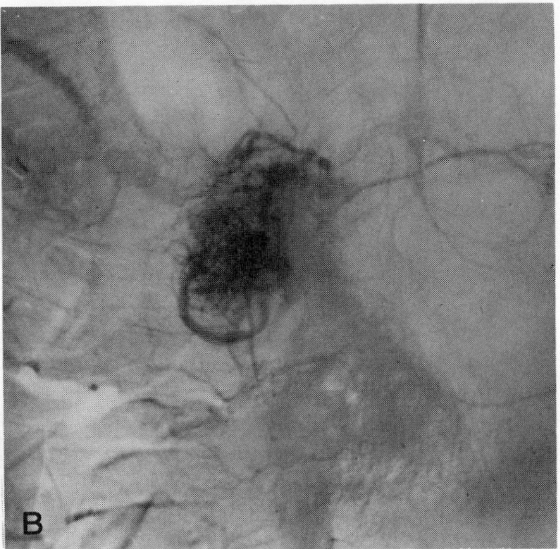

FIGURE 36–13. (**A**) Anteroposterior and (**B**) lateral arteriograms illustrate the extent of the lesion and rich vascular supply of the nasopharyngeal angiofibroma.

Management

The decision of whether surgery or radiation therapy should be employed depends in part on the initial extent of the disease. In patients with extracranial tumors, surgery is the treatment of choice and yields near-zero mortality or long-term morbidity.[270] If there is intracranial tumor extension, the risk of surgically related death is increased.[130, 270] In a literature review by Jones and co-workers,[132] the rate was found to be 14% to 84%. These patients are best managed with irradiation. Although radiation therapy is equally effective in extracranial tumors, the low but extant risk of secondary malignancies should limit its use to the most advanced tumors only.[14, 146, 232]

Some authors recommend preoperative intraarterial tumor vessel embolization at the time of diagnostic bilateral carotid angiography, claiming a decrease in operative bleeding.[2, 146, 149]

Salvage with embolizations of polyvinyl alcohol have been described.[129] There has also been anecdotal evidence of partial regression with the use of estrogens, believed to be caused by feedback inhibition of the pituitary's production of gonadotropin-releasing hormone.[70]

Radiation Therapy Techniques

Megavoltage photon irradiation should be used, and fields must be individualized to cover the tumor completely. Treatment portals are similar to those used in carcinoma of the nasopharynx (without irradiating the cervical lymph nodes) or carcinoma of the paranasal sinuses if there is involvement of those structures or the nasal cavity (Fig. 36-14). Opposing lateral portals are suitable in most patients, with larger fields and compensators used for tumors extending into the nose. More extensive disease requires three-field or wedge-pair arrangements (Fig. 36-15). In all cases, the eyes are protected. The recommended tumor dose ranges from 3000 cGy in 15 fractions in 3 weeks to 4800 cGy in 24 to 28 fractions in 5 weeks. A typical setup at Washington University uses 6-MV to 18-MV photons to treat with parallel opposed fields (Fig. 36-16).

TABLE 36–13
Staging of Nasopharyngeal Angiofibromas

STAGE	CHARACTERISTICS
I	Confined to the nasopharynx
II	Extension to nasal cavity or sphenoid sinus
III	Extension to one or more: antrum, ethmoid, pterygomaxillary and infratemporal fossae, orbit and/or cheek
IV	Intracranial extension

(Chandler JR, Goulding R, Moskowitz L, et al: Ann Otol Rhinol Laryngol 93:322, 1984)

Results of Therapy

Jones and associates[132] reported the results of 40 patients with juvenile nasopharyngeal angiofibroma treated with surgery alone. With a mean follow-up of 17 months (6–36 months), the control rates according to the Sessions staging system were: 100% (Stages I and IIa), 83% (Stage IIb), 80% (Stage IIc), and 50% (Stage III). All failures were controlled with irradiation, embolization, and surgical resection, and the other four were only observed, demonstrating the extremely high salvage rate in this disease.[8, 18, 132] This is consistent with other series reporting an initial surgical control of 86% and an ultimate control rate with surgery of 96%.[270]

Cummings and colleagues[48] treated 42 patients primarily with irradiation and 13 postsurgical failures. All but six had a biopsy. Nine had Stage IV disease according to Chandler's staging system. The dose delivered was 3000 cGy to 3500 cGy in 14 to 16 fractions over a 3-week period. Follow-up ranged from 3 to 26 years. The control rate was 80% and was equivalent for all dose ranges. The local control was 89% and 74% for three fields and two fields, respectively. The control rate was 83% if the field size was more than 6 cm x 6 cm and 55% for smaller portals, indicating the importance of accurately determining the target volume, including any potential tumor extension. The minimum craniocaudad field dimension in most successfully treated patients was 8 cm. Of the 11 patients with recurrences, eight were controlled by a second course of irradiation and three by surgery.

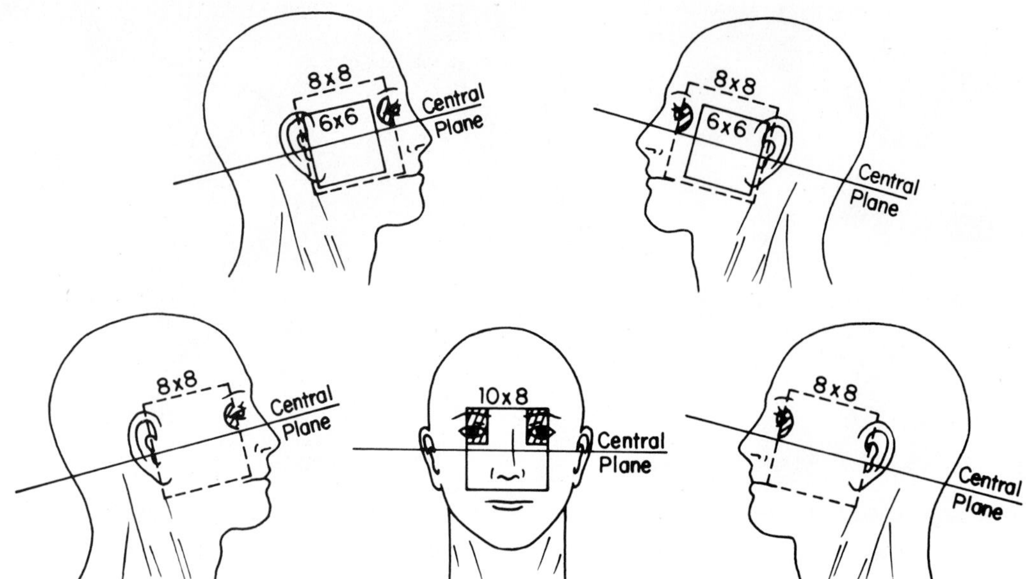

FIGURE 36–14. Diagrams of the most commonly used field arrangements: Lateral opposed field pair and three-field technique. (Cummings BJ, Blend R, Keane T: Laryngoscope 94:1601, 1984)

These tumors regress slowly, with 50% of the tumors still present at 12 months. At 24 months, 23% of the tumors were still present, and half of those recurred. Of the complete responders, only one of 33 recurred. Robinson and colleagues[211] also found that objective responses after irradiation occurred within 6 months in 60% of the patients and within 6 to 20 months in the other 40%. Symptoms, however, resolved in all patients within 6 months of treatment.

At the Mallinckrodt Institute of Radiology, Fields[83] reviewed our experience with 13 patients. Eleven were surgical failures, and two were treated primarily with irradiation. Intracranial extension was reported in 38% of the patients. Follow-up ranged from 40 to 173 months. Doses ranged from 3600 cGy to 5200 cGy, with a median of 4800 cGy given in 180-cGy to 200-cGy fractions 5 days per week. The control rate was 85%; patients failing irradiation were salvaged with embolizations. Chronic morbidity manifested mostly as xerostomia and dental decay.

Goepfert and associates[96] used chemotherapy to treat five patients with aggressive nasopharyngeal angiofibromas that recurred after extracranial resection and irradiation. One regimen of doxorubicin (60 mg/m^2 by I.V. push for 1 day) and dacarbazine (250 mg/m^2 by I.V. drip for 5 days) was given, with the courses repeated every 3 to 4 weeks. In the second regimen, vincristine, dactinomycin, and cyclophosphamide were administered at usual doses. Tumors regressed in all patients. All five patients are free of disease at 2, 3, 6, 10, and 10 years, respectively.

Tumor regression usually occurs at a slow rate after surgery, irradiation, or chemotherapy; therefore the presence of tumor up to 2 years after treatment is not an invariable sign of failure unless it is symptomatic or progressing.[48,96,167,239]

Sequelae of Therapy

The most common side effects of radiation therapy include delayed growth because of hypopituitarism and decreased bone maturation.[34] There are only four well-documented cases of radiation-induced sarcomas in the patients who received doses ranging from 6600 cGy to more than 9000 cGy.[15,232] Spagnolo and associates[232] reported on four patients who were treated with irradiation and subsequently developed sarcomas. Chen and Bauer[36] also reported a sarcoma in a patient receiving 6600 cGy and followed up for 18 years. Because this patient was 48 years old, the original diagnosis of juvenile nasopharyngeal angiofibroma does not coincide clinically with the typical profile of the disease. Cummings and co-workers[48] reported two subsequent neoplasms developing 13 and 14 years after irradiation. One was a basal cell carcinoma and one metastatic thyroid carcinoma. Both patients are alive without disease.[46] Two patients developed cataracts. Most physicians agree that surgical mortality increases if intracranial extension of the tumor is encountered.[238]

NONLENTIGINOUS MELANOMA

Malignant melanoma accounts for 11% of the primary head and neck malignancies.[11] Of all malignant melanoma cases, 20% to 35% are located in the head and neck area.[114]

Cutaneous Melanomas

In a review of the literature, Batsakis and associates[16] found that 64% to 78% of all head and neck malignant melanomas were cutaneous, 6% to 8% were mucosal, and 14% to 30% were ocular. The superficial spreading and nodular types of malignant melanoma have a metastatic potential of 10% to 30% and 50%, respectively.[114] The difference is believed to result from the predominantly horizontal growth phase of the former and the vertical growth for the latter, increasing the chances of hematogenous spread in the nodular type. Neurotropic melanoma is an uncommon variant of cutaneous melanoma, with a higher propensity to invade peripheral nerves. A thorough evaluation with CT scans should determine whether there is intracranial or base of the skull involvement.[176] Beenken and

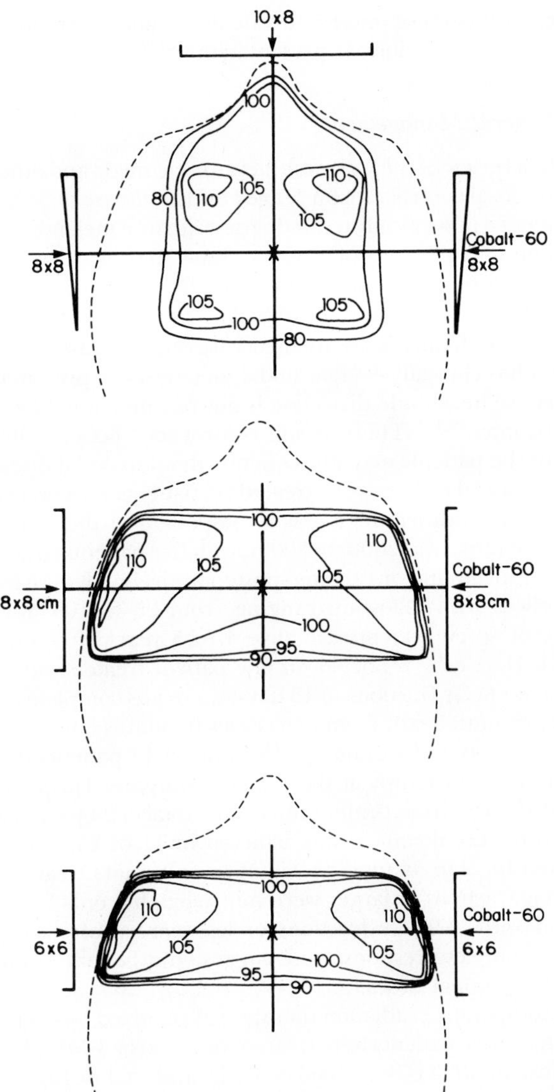

FIGURE 36–15. Dose distribution of radiation in the central plane for different field arrangements. All fields are ^{60}Co, and all dimensions are in centimeters. The radiation dose of 3000 cGy or 3500 cGy is delivered to the volume marked 100%. The three-field technique allows the greatest volume to be included. The possible effects of eye shields, for example, which would alter these distributions, are not shown. (Cummings BJ, Blend R, Keane T, et al: Larngoscope 94:1602, 1984)

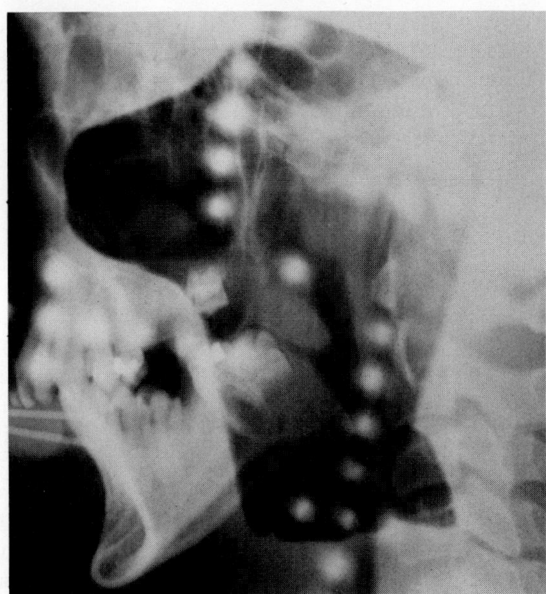

FIGURE 36–16. Example of a lateral portal used at the Mallinckrodt Institute of Radiology for a nasopharyngeal angiofibroma.

colleagues[19] reported 13 such cases, two of which failed perineurally.

The treatment of cutaneous melanomas has typically been a wide excision of the lesion with a minimum 3-cm margin.[258] Margins of at least 2 cm have been used recently in the head and neck area for Stage I melanomas with comparable success as verified by their local failure rate of 3% to 6%.[147,256] Local failures of 45% have been reported by McNeer and Cantin[178] in a review of 793 patients with Stage II disease (*i.e.,* lymphatic node metastases). Five-year survival rates of 55% have been reported for cutaneous melanomas of the head and neck.[104]

Dickson,[59] from the Princess Margaret Hospital, treated 16 patients with nodular melanomas with local excision and postoperative radiation therapy with 5000 cGy delivered in ten fractions over a 2-week period. Fourteen were locally controlled, and six of the patients are alive and well 2 to 14 years after treatment. The results at his institution were comparable to those with wide local excision alone, but with less morbidity and cosmetic alterations.[59] Later, at the same institution, Harwood[111] treated five patients with definitive radiation therapy for superficial spreading melanoma of the head and neck area. All five were locally controlled; one had a lymph node metastasis that was subsequently controlled, and one died of distant metastases.[111] He recommends treating these patients with regimens of 4500 cGy in ten fractions over 2 weeks to 5000 cGy in 15 fractions over 3 weeks.[112,113]

Harwood[111] also reported treating 74 patients with three 800-cGy fractions given on days 0, 7, and 21 with shielding of the spinal cord, brain, and eye. Thirty patients were treated postoperatively after neck dissections if they had extracapsular extension, multiple nodal involvement, >3-cm node metastasis, or residual disease. Control in the neck was achieved in 26 of 30 patients who were followed up for 1 to 4 years. In four patients who had microscopic residual disease at the primary site, this postoperative regimen controlled three of four lesions, with follow-up ranging from 1 to 3.5 years. The other 40 patients were treated for gross (13 patients) or recurrent (27 patients) cutaneous melanoma. There were complete responses in 15 of 40 lesions and partial responses in 12 of 40. In an update of his data,[113] he reported a neck control rate of 94% in 41 adjuvantly treated patients, compared with 57% in 48 patients with gross residual or recurrent tumors. He concluded that irradiation alone should be considered in superficial spreading melanomas for which surgery would be contraindicated and in all cases of nodular melanoma after a simple excision if wide excision was contraindicated because of age, location, or medical condition. For nodal disease, patients should receive postoperative radiation therapy for poor prognostic pathologic factors. Recurrent or unresectable tumors should also be irradiated.

Harwood recommended the use of high dose fractions because his local control rate was 71% if the dose per fraction was 400 cGy but 25% with lower fractions.[116] A new approach to the treatment of recurrent or unresectable cutaneous melanomas is combined hyperthermia and high-fraction radiation therapy as reported by Emami and associates[70] and Overgaard.[199] The data also support the use of high dose fractions for melanoma because Overgaard's complete response rate was 59% if fractions of more than 400 cGy were used but 33% for lower fraction sizes.

Mucosal Melanomas

Primary mucosal melanomas of the head and neck area comprise 2% to 8% of the cases seen yearly in the United States.[16] They are more commonly seen in countries such as Japan where mucosal melanoma accounts for 22% to 32% of the patients with malignant melanoma.[254] Most are seen in the fifth to seventh decades of life and are extremely rare (0.6%) in the first two decades of life.[89, 109, 169, 252, 255] Males and females are equally affected.[252] A review by Batsakis and associates[16] of 204 mucosal melanomas showed 56.4% to be from the upper respiratory tract and 44% from the oral cavity and pharynx. Nasal cavity and paranasal tumors comprise less than 1% of malignant melanomas and 2% to 9% of all head and neck melanomas.[89, 123] Pigmentation may precede the lesion for more than a year in as many as 28% of the patients.[30] In the oral cavity, as many as 80% of the melanomas arise in the hard palate, followed in order of decreasing frequency by the upper gingiva and lower gingiva.[178] In a review of the literature, Kim and colleagues[138] found only 27 cases of laryngeal melanoma.

The differential diagnosis of a pigmented lesion, especially in the oral cavity, includes amalgam tattoo from dental procedures, melanotic macule, pigmented nevus, blue nevus, junctional nevus, intramural nevus, compound nevus, chronic intestinal disorders, Peutz-Jeghers syndrome, Addison's disease, and metastatic melanoma.[67, 98, 182]

Diagnostic Workup

Mucosal melanomas may arise from the incomplete migration of melanoblasts from the neural crest to the skin along the nerve pathways.[43] This theory is supported by the finding of melanin production in some nerve endings.[135] An excisional biopsy should be performed because possible local or metastatic spread has been associated by some physicians with punch or incisional biopsy, although this has not been reported for cutaneous melanomas.[100, 205] Batsakis and associates[16] found that two thirds of the lesions produced melanin in large amounts and one third were amelanotic or produced smaller amounts that had to be detected by Fontana and other stains. Hoki and colleagues[123] reported that 25% of melanomas were amelanotic.

Metastatic disease to the mucosa of the head and neck area is less common.[214] It can be differentiated from primary tumors by the presence of normal tissue between subepidermal tumor and the basal layer of melanocytes.[128] In a review of the literature, Henderson and co-workers[120] found that the most common locations for metastases were the larynx, tongue, and tonsil.

Prognostic Factors

Batsakis and associates[16] found lesions of more than 0.5 mm to have a poor prognostic factor. Trapp and colleagues[252] offered a poor prognosis only for patients with more than 7-mm invasion. Lymph node involvement is not a prognostic factor. Mucosal melanomas fare worse than their cutaneous counterparts.[137] Possible explanations are a lack of a lymphocytic infiltrate around the mucosal tumors, suggesting a lack of immunologic competence, increased vascularity and ulceration, and more advanced lesions at presentation.[16, 137, 138, 206]

General Management

In a review of the Japanese literature, Umeda and others[255] found a local control rate for Stage I and II disease of 58% (7 of 12 patients) in surgically treated series with oral melanomas and a minimum follow-up of 3 years. Snow and associates[230] reported failure rates of 40% to 60% in different series, even with radical en bloc excisions (20% to 42%).[23] Because the main cause of treatment failure is distant metastases and because almost no patient has clinically evident nodal metastases at presentation, an elective neck node dissection is not recommended by some investigators.[24, 111] There is still controversy, because 30% to 60% of the patients may subsequently develop nodal disease.[23]

Ohya and colleagues[195] treated six patients with oral cavity melanomas with irradiation as a component of their therapy. The dose range was 2000r to 8900r, with five patients irradiated preoperatively and one treated postoperatively. All were locally controlled, with follow-up ranging from 25 to 109 months. Three of seven patients are alive 4 to 5 years after therapy ended. Harries[110] reported on one patient treated with 2400 cGy, in 800-cGy fractions in 15 days; there was complete tumor clearance until death from metastases 6 months later.

Harwood and Cummings[114] reported 12 patients treated with radiation therapy at the Princess Margaret Hospital and added 12 cases from the literature, for a total of 24 patients and 25 lesions. Local control was achieved in 11 of 24, who were followed for 9 to 54 months. Six of seven tumors treated with 400-cGy fractions or larger were controlled, but only five of 18 treated with 399-cGy fractions or less were controlled. The higher complete response rate suggested a benefit from the higher fractional doses.

Postoperative radiation therapy was reported by Panje and Moran.[201] Five patients were treated with ^{60}Co or 4-MV photons to a dose of 5000 cGy to 6000 cGy administered in 150-cGy to 200-cGy fractions over a period of 5 to 6 weeks. Only one patient showed local control, and the remainder failed 6 to 12 months after irradiation. In another case reported by McRae and colleagues,[179] 6000 cGy given in 6 weeks controlled the disease until the disease recurred locally 3 years later.

At Washington University, Marcial-Vega[169] reviewed our experience with eight patients with mucosal melanoma. Two patients treated with surgery alone developed local failures at 6 and 12 months and died of metastases at 6 and 67 months, respectively. Two patients received preoperative radiation therapy of 2000 cGy to 2600 cGy administered in 200-cGy fractions for five fractions per week. One recurred locally at 36 months; the other patient had local tumor control and died of metastases at 129 months. Of four patients treated with irradiation alone (4000–7000 cGy, 200–300-cGy per fraction, five fractions a week or 3400 cGy, 425-cGy fractions twice a week), only one was locally controlled until death from metastases at 21 months. This patient received 425 cGy fractions. The other three patients died of distant metastases. These data support the use of high fractional doses for mucosal melanomas.

Survival

Patients with nasal cavity or paranasal tumors have a median survival of 24 months.[171] Five-year disease-free survival rates of 25% have been reported.[252] Patients with laryngeal melanoma have a 13% 5-year disease-free survival rate.[138] Because of the poor results obtained and because 37% of the patients have associated adjacent pigmentation, some authors recommend prophylactic excision of all melanocytic nevi.[29,40,206] Because the results of irradiation are comparable to surgical series and because of the poor survival of these patients as a result of distant metastases, irradiation alone, with surgery saved for salvage, should be considered the primary treatment for mucosal melanomas of the head and neck.

LENTIGO MALIGNA MELANOMA

Natural History

Lentigo maligna (Hutchinson's melanotic freckle or circumscribed precancerous melanosis of Dubreuilh) and its invasive counterpart, lentigo maligna melanoma, are well-recognized clinicopathologic entities.[6,37,125] Lentigo maligna melanoma comprises about 10% of all melanomas in the head and neck region, occurs predominantly on the face and ears of elderly persons, and usually has a very long natural history, frequently reaching a large size before diagnosis.[50] Approximately one third of the lentigo maligna lesions, if left untreated, eventually transform into invasive disease.[6]

These lesions first appear circumscribed and later as more diffuse areas of hyperpigmentation of the skin. They may develop some superficial nodularity and eventual ulceration as they become more invasive. In 10% of the latter patients regional and distant metastases eventually develop.[263] The 10% metastatic spread in lentigo maligna melanoma contrasts with the 25% metastatic tendency in nodular melanomas arising in superficial spreading melanomas and a 50% chance of metastatic spread in nodular melanomas arising *de novo*.[177]

The average age of patients with lentigo maligna melanoma is 73 years, with a range from 58 to 92 years.[116]

Diagnostic Workup

The diagnostic workup of these patients is similar to that of patients suspected of having malignant melanoma. Biopsies of the lesion are required to obtain histopathologic confirmation of the diagnosis. Careful physical examination must rule out any areas of extension or regional or distant spread. Dancuart and associates[50] stated that pathologic assessment of the invasiveness of the lesion was not made in most patients. Only one third of pathologically proven lentigo maligna melanomas showed clinical evidence of nodular formation.[263]

General Management

The usual treatment of lentigo maligna and lentigo maligna melanoma has been surgery, with approximately 1-cm margin of normal skin.[17,42,53] Because of the low incidence of regional lymph node metastases, elective lymph node dissection is not indicated.[54] For larger lesions, wider surgical excision with skin grafting has given poor cosmetic results. As an alternative, electrodesiccation and curettage or topical 5-fluorouracil has been advised.[156] However, in three patients with large lentigo maligna of the head and neck treated with 5-fluorouracil, recurrences requiring further therapy developed in all patients.[156]

Radiation therapy with various techniques has been frequently used in the treatment of these patients, particularly those with larger lesions, because of minimum morbidity and generally excellent cosmetic results (Fig. 36-17).

Radiation Therapy Techniques

Portals should be carefully designed to include the entire tumor with margins of 1 cm for lesions less than 2 cm and 2 cm for

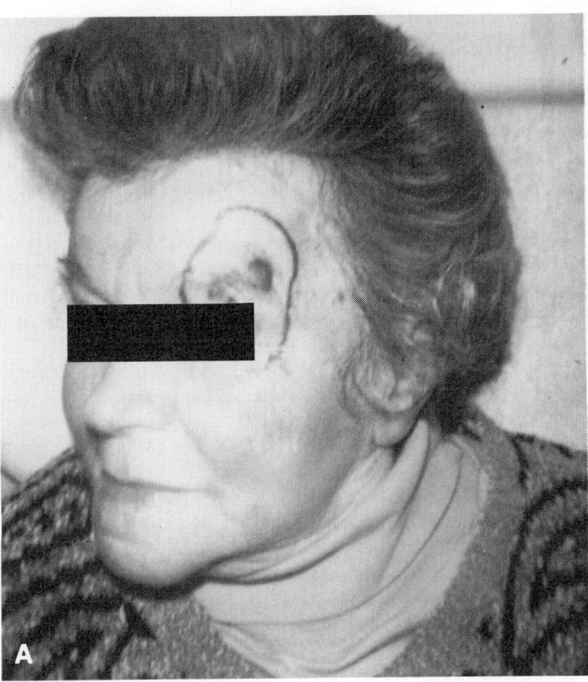

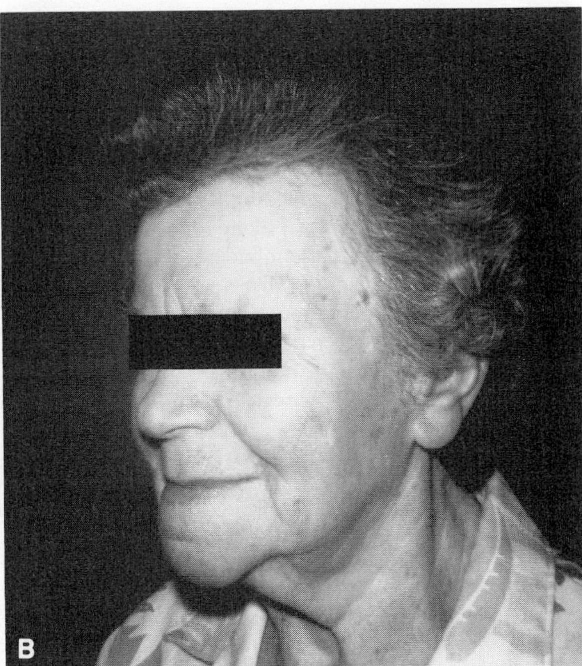

FIGURE 36–17. Lentigo maligna melanoma of the face (**A**) before and (**B**) 3 years after 5000 cGy in 25 fractions delivered with 9-MeV electrons and bolus.

larger tumors. Because Miescher's irradiation technique uses very superficial x-rays, with 50% depth dose being at approximately 1 mm, there is the possibility of local recurrence if dermal extension is unrecognized. Therefore, Dancuart and associates[50] and Harwood and Larson[116] recommend using minimum x-ray energies of 100 keVp and preferably 140 to 175 keVp. Superficial x-rays (100–200 keVp) with adequate filtration or electrons (6–9 MeV) with appropriate thickness of bolus (1.5 cm) can treat most of these patients. Doses of 4500 cGy to 5000 cGy given in 15 to 25 fractions delivered over 3 to 5 weeks adequately control the disease in most patients.

Although it has been suggested that higher fractions are more effective in the treatment of melanoma, including the lesions under discussion, a recent randomized study by Radiation Therapy Oncology Group comparing four fractions of 800 cGy given on days 0, 7, 14, and 21 and 20 fractions of 250 cGy in five weekly fractions shows no significant difference in tumor response (24.2% and 23.4% complete response, respectively, and 35% partial response).[106,204] We recommend delivering 300 cGy to 350 cGy, three times weekly, every other day, to a total of 4500 cGy to 5000 cGy, depending on the size and thickness of the lesion. Elective irradiation of the regional lymphatics is not necessary.

Dancuart and associates[50] point out that, after irradiation, the lesion-associated hyperpigmentation may take up to 18 to 24 months to completely disappear. Careful follow-up with clinical examinations and photographs of the lesion is essential to ascertain the continuing regression of the tumor.

For patients who had surgical excisions, postoperative irradiation is recommended if positive margins were found.[50] Doses are similar to those stated earlier.

Results of Therapy

Soft x-rays (≤50 KV) have been used to administer doses of 10,000 cGy in four or five treatments, with recurrences developing in only 2% of the patients.[50] However, Kopf and associates[141] reported six recurrences among 16 patients treated by this method.

Dancuart and associates[50] and Harwood and Larson[116] (updated report) described 13 patients with lentigo maligna treated with radiation therapy: 11 had local tumor control, one had an edge recurrence salvaged by irradiation, and one had residual tumor (alive and well 11 years after treatment for the recurrence). One patient alive at 2 years refused further treatment. Of 19 patients irradiated for lentigo maligna melanoma, 17 had tumor control with radiation therapy alone for periods ranging from 6 months to 6 years. One patient had a central recurrence that was salvaged by surgery and is alive and well 5 years after treatment of recurrence. One patient died of intercurrent disease less than 3 months after irradiation. No patients have developed lymph node or distant metastases in either group.

REFERENCES

1. Ahmad H, Fayos JV: Role of radiation therapy in the treatment of olfactory neuroblastoma. Int J Radiat Oncol Biol Phys 6:349, 1980
2. Allison DJ: Therapeutic embolization and venous sampling. In Taylor S (ed): Recent Advances in Surgery, vol 10, p 27. Edinburgh, Churchill-Livingstone, 1980
3. Alpern MB, Thorsen MK, Kellman GM: CT appearance of hemangiopericytoma. J Comput Assist Tomogr 10:264, 1986
4. Amendola BE, Amendola MA, Oliver E, et al: Chordoma: Role of radiation therapy. Radiology 158:839, 1986
5. Anderson JM, Stevens JC, Sundt TM Jr, et al: Ectopic internal carotid artery seen initially as middle ear tumor. JAMA 249:2228, 1983
6. Andrade R: Circumscribed precancerous melanosis (dubreuilh). In Andrade R, Gumport SL, Popkin GL, Rees TD (eds): Cancer of the Skin: Biology, Diagnosis, Management, vol 1, pp 679–702. Philadelphia, WB Saunders, 1976
7. Antonelli AR, Cappiello J, Lorenzo DD, et al: Diagnosis, staging, and treatment of juvenile nasopharyngeal angiofibroma (JNA). Laryngoscope 97:1319, 1987
8. Appelblatt NH, McClatchey KD: Olfactory neuroblastoma: A retrospective clinicopathologic study. Head Neck Surg 5:108, 1982
9. Arma-Szlachicic M, Ott F, Sotrk H: Zur Strahlen therapie der melanotischen pracancerosen (Studie anhand von 88 nach Kortrollierten Fallen). Hautarzt 21:505, 1970
10. Arthur K: Radiotherapy in chemodectoma of the glomus jugalare. Clin Radiol 28:415, 1977
11. Balch CM, Milton GW, Shaw HM, et al: Clinical management and treatment: Results worldwide. In Balch CM, Milton GW (eds): Cutaneous Melanoma, p 225. Philadelphia, JB Lippincott, 1985
12. Baron SH: Brain radiation necrosis following treatment of an esthesioneuroblastoma (olfatory neurocytoma). Laryngoscope 89:214, 1979
13. Bataskis JG: Tumors of the Head and Neck, 2nd ed, pp 474–475. Baltimore, Williams & Wilkins, 1979
14. Batsakis JG: Wegener's granulomatosis and midline (non peeling) "granuloma." Head Neck Surg 1:213, 1979
15. Batsakis JG, Klopp CT, Newman W: Fibrosarcoma arising in a "juvenile" nasopharyngeal angiofibroma following extensive radiation therapy. Am Surg 21:786, 1955
16. Batsakis JG, Regezi JA, Solomon AR, et al: The pathology of head and neck tumors: Mucosal melanomas. XIII. Head Neck Surg 4:404, 1982
17. Becker FF: Lentigo maligna and lentigo maligna melanoma: Recognition and treatment. Arch Otolaryngol Head Neck Surg 104:352, 1978
18. Becker LE, Hinton D: Primitive neuroectodermal tumors of the central nervous system. Hum Pathol 14:538, 1983
19. Beenken S, Byers R, Smith JL, et al: Desmoplastic melanoma. Arch Otolaryngol Head Neck Surg 115:374, 1989
20. Berger L, Coutard H: L'esthesioneurocytome olfactid. Bull Assoc Fr Etude Cancer 15:404, 1926.
21. Berger L, Luc R: L'esthesioneuropitheliome olfacif. Bull Cancer (Paris) 13:410, 1924
22. Berson AM, Castro JR, Petti P, et al: Charged particle irradiation of chordoma and chondrosarcoma of the base of skull and cervical spine: The Lawrence Berkeley Laboratory experience. Int J Radiat Oncol Biol Phys 15:559, 1988
23. Berthelsen A, Andersen AP, Jensen TS, et al: Melanomas of the mucosa in the oral cavity and the upper respiratory passages. Cancer 54:907, 1984
24. Blatchford SJ, Koopmann CF, Coulthard SW: Mucosal melanoma of the head and neck. Laryngoscope 96:929, 1986
25. Bratt GW, Bess FH, Miller GW, et al: Glomus tumor of the middle ear: Origin, symptomatology and treatment. J Speech Hear Disord 44:121, 1979
26. Braun-Falco O, Lukacs S, Schoenfinuis HH: Urberhandlung der melanosis circumscripta praecancerousa Dubreuilh. Hautarzt 26:207, 1975
27. Bremer JW, Neel HB III, DeSanto LW, et al: Angiofibroma: Treatment trends in 150 patients during 40 years. Laryngoscope 96:1321, 1986
28. Brismar J, Crongvist S: Therapeutic embolization in the external carotid artery region. Acta Radiol 19:5, 1978
29. Buchner A, Hansen LS: Pigmented nevi of the oral mucosa: A clinicopathologic study of 32 new cases and review of 75 cases from the literature. Oral Surg 49:55, 1980
30. Buchner A, Hansen LS: Pigmented nevi of the oral mucosa: A clinicopathologic study of 36 new cases and review of 155 cases from the literature. II. Analysis of 191 cases. Oral Surg 63:676, 1987

31. Burns A: Observation on the surgical anatomy of the head and neck. Baltimore, 386, 1823.
32. Bush SE, Goffinet DR, Bagshaw MA: Extramedullary plasmacytoma of the head and neck. Radiology 140:801, 1981
33. Carson CP, Ackerman LV, Maltby JD: Plasma cell myeloma: A clinical, pathological, and roentgenologic review of 90 cases. Am J Clin Pathol 25:849, 1955
34. Chandler JR, Goulding R, Moskowitz L, et al: Nasopharyngeal angiofibromas: Staging and management. Ann Otol Rhinol Laryngol 93:322, 1984
35. Chapman P, Johnson SAN: Mastoid chloroma relapse in acute myeloid leukemia. J Laryngol Otol 94:1423, 1980
36. Chen KTK, Bauer FW: Sarcomatous transformation of nasopharyngeal angiofibroma. Cancer 49:369, 1982
37. Clark WH, Mihm MC: Lentigo maligna and lentigo maligna melanoma. Am J Pathol 55:39, 1969
38. Cole JM: Glomus jugulare tumor. Laryngoscope 87:1244, 1977
39. Compagno J: Hemangiopericytoma-like tumors of the nasal cavity: A comparison with hemangiopericytoma of the soft tissues. Laryngoscope 88:460, 1972
40. Conley J, Pack GT: Melanoma of the mucous membranes of the head and neck. Arch Otolaryngol Head Neck Surg 99:315, 1974
41. Corwin J, Lindberg RD: Solitary plasmacytoma of bone versus extramedullary plasmacytoma and their relationship to multiple myeloma. Cancer 43:1007, 1979
42. Costello MJ, Fisher SB, Defeo CP: Melanotic freckle. Arch Dermatol 80:153, 1959
43. Cramer SF: The histogenesis of acquired melanocytic nevus. Am J Dermatol 6(Suppl 1):229, 1984
44. Croxatto J, Font RL: Hemangiopericytoma of the orbit: A clinicopathologic study of 30 cases. Hum Pathol 13:199, 1982
45. Cummings BJ: Relative risk factors in the treatment of juvenile nasopharyngeal angiofibroma. Head Neck Surg 3:21, 1980
46. Cummings BJ: The treatment of juvenile nasopharyngeal angiofibroma: The case for radiation therapy. J Laryngol Otol 8(Suppl 1):101, 1983
47. Cummings BJ, Beale FA, Garrett PG, et al: The treatment of glomus tumors in the temporal bone by megavoltage radiation. Cancer 53:2635, 1984
48. Cummings BJ, Blend R, Keane T, et al: Primary radiation therapy for juvenile nasopharyngeal angiofibroma. Laryngoscope 94:1599, 1984
49. Dahlin DC, MacCarty CS: Chordoma. A study of 59 cases. Cancer 5:1170, 1952
50. Dancuart F, Harwood AR, Fitzpatrick PJ: The radiotherapy of lentigo maligna and lentigo maligna melanoma of the head and neck. Cancer 45:2279, 1980
51. Daugaard S, Hultberg BM, Hou-Jenson K, Mouridsen HT: Clinical features of malignant haemangiopericytomas and haemangioendotheliosarcomas. Acta Oncol 27:209, 1988
52. Davidson J, Gullane P: Glomus vagale tumors. Otolaryngol Head Neck Surg 99:66, 1988
53. Davis J, Pack GT, Higgins GK: Melanotic freckle of Hutchinson. Am J Surg 113:457, 1967
54. Davis NC, McLeod GR, Beardmore GL, et al: A report from the Queensland melanoma project. CA 26:81, 1976
55. De SK, Das S, Dey D: Multiple extra-nasopharyngeal extensions of juvenile nasopharyngeal angiofibroma. J Laryngol Otol 101:1083, 1987
56. De Groot WP: Provisional results of treatment of the melanose precancereuse circonscrite Dubreuih by Bucky-rays. Dermatologica 136:429, 1968
57. DeRemee RA, Weitland LH, McDonald TJ: Polymorphic reticulosis-lymphomatoid granulomatosis: Two diseases or one? Mayo Clin Proc 53:634, 1978
58. Dickens WJ, Million RR, Cassisi NJ, et al: Chemodectomas arising in temporal bone structures. Laryngoscope 92:188, 1982
59. Dickson RJ: Malignant melanoma: A combined surgical and radiotherapeutic approach. AJR 79:1063, 1958
60. Dickson RJ: Radiotherapy of lethal midline granuloma. J Chronic Dis 12:417, 1960
61. Djalilian M, Zujko RD, Weiland LH, et al: Olfactory neuroblastoma. Surg Clin North Am 57:751, 1977
62. Dolin S, Dewar JP: Extramedullary plasmacytoma. Am J Pathol 32:83, 1956
63. Donald PJ: Sarcomatous degeneration in a nasopharyngeal angiofibroma. Otolaryngol Head Neck Surg 87:42, 1979
64. Doyle PJ, Paxton HD: Combined surgical approach to esthesioneuroepithelioma. Trans Am Acad Ophthalmol Otolaryngol 75:526, 1971
65. Duggan CA, Hoffman JC, Brylski JR: The efficacy of angiography in the evaluation of glomus tympanicum tumors. Radiology 97:45, 1970
66. Duvall AJ III, Moreano AE: Juvenile nasopharyngeal angiofibroma: Diagnosis and treatment. Otolaryngol Head Neck Surg 97:534, 1987
67. Eckardt A: Primary malignant melanoma of the oral mucosa: Report of a case. J Oral Maxillofac Surg 45:1065, 1987
68. Eichel BS, Harrison EG Jr, Devine KD, et al: Primary lymphoma of the nose including relationship to lethal midline granuloma. Am J Surg 112:597, 1966
69. Elkon D, Hightower SI, Lim ML, et al: Esthesioneuroblastoma. Cancer 44:1087, 1979
70. Emami B, Perez CA, Konefal J, et al: Thermoradiotherapy of malignant melanoma. Int J Hyperthermia 4:373, 1988
71. Endicott JN, Maniglia AJ: Glomus vagale. Laryngoscope 90:1604, 1980
72. Eneroth CM, Fluur E, Soderberg G, Anggard A: Nasal hemangiopericytoma. Laryngoscope 80:17, 1970
73. Ennuyer A, Bataini P, Chavanne G, Halevy J: Les plasmacytomaes des voies aero-digestives superieures. A propos de 248 cas dont 19 trasts a la Fondation Curi. Ann Radiol (Paris) 6:742, 1963
74. Enzinger FM, Smith BH: Hemangiopericytoma: An analysis of 106 cases. Hum Pathol 7:61, 1976
75. Enzinger FM, Weiss SW: Hemangiopericytoma. In Enzinger FM, Weiss SW (eds): Soft Tissue Tumors, 2nd ed. St. Louis, CV Mosby, 1988
76. Erlandson RA, Tandler B, Lieberman PH, et al: Ultrastructure of human chordoma. Cancer Res 28:2115, 1968
77. Farag MM, Ghanimah SE, Ragaie A, et al: Hormonal receptors in juvenile nasopharyngeal angiofibroma. Laryngoscope 97:208, 1987
78. Farr HW: Carotid body tumors: A thirty year experience at Memorial Hospital. Am J Surg 114:614, 1967
79. Fauci AS, Hayes BF, Costa J, et al: Lymphomatoid granulomatosis: Prospective clinical and therapeutic experience over 10 years. N Engl J Med 306:68, 1982
80. Fauci AS, Johnson RE, Wolff SM: Radiation therapy of midline granuloma. Ann Intern Med 84:140, 1975
81. Fechner RE, Lamppin DW: Midline malignant reticulosis: A clinicopathologic entity. Arch Otolaryngol Head Neck Surg 95:467, 1972
82. Feder BH, Shramek JH, Ikeda TS: Large-field radiotherapy in lethal midline granuloma. Radiology 81:293, 1963
83. Fields JN: Written communication, July 1989
84. Friedman M, Egan JW: Irradiation of hemangiopericytoma of Stout. Radiology 74:721, 1960
85. Frierson HF Jr, Mills SE, Fechner RE, et al: Sinonasal undifferentiated carcinoma: An aggressive neoplasm derived from Schneiderian epithelium and distinct from olfactory neuroblastoma. Am J Surg Pathol 10:771, 1986
86. Fu YS, Pritchett PS, Young TF: Tissue culture study of a sacrococcygeal chordoma with further ultrastural study. Acta Neuropathol (Berl) 23:223, 1975
87. Fuller DB, Bloom JG: Radiotherapy for chordoma. Int J Radiat Oncol Biol Phys 15:331, 1988
88. Fuller PS, Haferman DR, Byrol RB, et al: Use of irradiation in lymphomatoid granulomatosis. Chest 74:105, 1978
89. Gadeberg CC, Hjelm-Hansen M, Sogaard H, et al: Malignant tumours of the parasanal sinuses and nasal cavity: A series of 180 patients. Acta Radiol Oncol 23:181, 1984
90. Gardner G, Cocke EW, Robertson JT, et al: Glomus jugulare tumours: Combined treatment. I. J Laryngol Otol 95:437, 1981
91. Gardner G, Cocke EW, Robertson JT, et al: Glomus jugulare

tumours: Combined treatment. II. J Laryngol Otol 95:567, 1981

92. Gaulard P, Henni T, Marroleau JP, et al: Lethal midline granuloma (polymorphic reticulosis) and lymphomatoid granulomatosis. Cancer 62:705, 1988
93. Gerard-Marchant R, Micheau C: Microscopical diagnosis of olfactory esthesioneuromas: General review and report of five cases. JNCI 35:75, 1965
94. Gibbin KP, Henk JM: Glomus jugulare tumors in South Wales: A twenty-year review. Clin Radiol 29:607, 1978
95. Glasscock ME III, Jackson CG, Johnson GD, Poe DS: Radiation therapy in chemodectoma treatment (letter to the editor). Laryngoscope 98:465, 1988
96. Goepfert H, Cangir A, Lee YY: Chemotherapy for aggressive juvenile nasopharyngeal angiofibroma. Arch Otolaryngol Head Neck Surg 111:285, 1985
97. Goldman GM, Davidson AJ, Neal J: Retroperitoneal and pelvic hemangiopericytomas: Clinical, radiologic and pathologic correlation. Radiology 168:13, 1988
98. Green TL, Greenspan D, Hansen LS: Oral melanoma: Report of case. J Am Dent Assoc 113:627, 1986
99. Grier HE, Weinstein HJ: Acute non-lymphocytic leukemia. In Pizzo PA, Poplack DD (eds): Principles and Practice of Pediatric Oncology, p 367. Philadelphia, JB Lippincott, 1988
100. Griffiths RW, Briggs JC: Biopsy procedures, primary wide excisional surgery and long-term prognosis in primary clinical Stage I invasive cutaneous malignant melanoma. Ann R Coll Surg Engl 67:75, 1985
101. Grubb WV Jr, Lampe I: The role of radiation therapy in the treatment of chemodectomas of the glomus jugulare. Laryngoscope 75:1861, 1965
102. Gudrun R: Hemangiopericytoma in otolaryngology. J Laryngol Otol 93:477, 1979
103. Guild SR: The glomus jugulare: A nonchromaffin paraganglion in man. Ann Otol Rhinol Laryngol 62:1045, 1953
104. Gussak GS, Reintgen D, Cox E, et al: Cutaneous melanoma of the head and neck. Arch Otolaryngol Head Neck Surg 109:803, 1983
105. Gutin PH, Leibel A, Hosobuchi Y, et al: Brachytherapy of recurrent tumors of the skull base and spine with Iodine-125 sources. Neurosurgery 20:938, 1987
106. Habermalz HJ, Fischer JJ: Radiation therapy of malignant melanoma. Experience with high individual treatment doses. Cancer 38:2258, 1976
107. Halperin EC, Dosoretz MD, Goodman M, Wang CC: Radiotherapy of polymorphic reticulosis. Br J Radiol 55:645, 1982
108. Hamilton WJ, Boyd JD, Mossman HW: Human Embryology: Prenatal Development of Form and Function. Baltimore, Williams & Wilkins, 1945
109. Hanchard B, Salmon B: Primary malignant melanoma of the maxillary gingiva in a 4-year old girl. West Indian Med J 34:278, 1985
110. Harries MLL: Melanoma metastatic to the head and neck. J Laryngol Otol 102:842, 1988
111. Harwood AR: Melanomas of the head and neck. J Otolaryngol 12:64, 1983
112. Harwood AR: Role of radiation therapy in the treatment of melanoma. In Larson DL, Ballantyne AJ, Guillamondegui OM (eds): Cancer in the Neck: Evaluation and Treatment, p 243. New York, Macmillan, 1986
113. Harwood AR: Verbal Communication, August 8, 1989
114. Harwood AR, Cummings BJ: Radiotherapy for mucosal melanomas. Int J Radiat Oncol Biol Phys 8:1121, 1982
115. Harwood AR, Knowling MA, Bergsagel DE: Radiotherapy for extramedullary plasmacytoma of the head and neck. Clin Radiol 32:31, 1981
116. Harwood AR, Lawson VG: Radiation therapy for melanomas of the head and neck. Head Neck Surg 4:468, 1982
117. Hatfield PM, James AE, Schulz MD: Chemodectomas of the glomus jugulare. Cancer 30:1164, 1972
118. Heckmayr M, Gatzemeir U, Radenback D, et al: Pulmonary metastasizing hemangiopericytoma. Am J Clin Oncol 11:636, 1988
119. Heffelfinger MJ, Dahling DC, MacCarty CS, et al: Chordomas and cartilaginous tumors at the skull base. Cancer 32:410, 1973
120. Henderson LT, Robbins KT, Weitzner S: Upper aerodigestive tract metastases in disseminated malignant melanoma. Arch Otolaryngol Head Neck Surg 112:659, 1986
121. Herrold KM: Induction of olfactory neuroepithelial tumors in Syrian hamsters by diethylnitrosamine. Cancer 17:114, 1964
122. Higinbotham NL, Phillips RF, Farr HW, et al: Chordoma: Thirty-five year study at Memorial Hospital. Cancer 20:1841, 1967
123. Hoki K, Sambe S, Asakuru K, et al: Malignant melanoma in the maxillary sinus: A case successfully treated with radiotherapy. Auris Nasus Larynx (Tokyo) 12:81, 1985
124. Horten BC, Montague SR: *In vitro* characteristics of sacrococcygeal chordoma maintained in tissue and organ culture systems. Acta Neuropathol (Berl) 35:13, 1976
125. Hutchinson J: Notes on cancer and cancerous processes. Arch Surg 2:218, 1890
126. Jaaskelainen J, Servo A, Haltia M, et al: Intracranial hemangiopericytoma: Radiology, surgery, radiotherapy and outcome in 21 patients. Surg Neurol 23:227, 1985
127. Jackson CG, Glasscock ME, Harris PF: Glomus tumors: Diagnosis, classification, and management of large lesions. Arch Otolaryngol 108:401, 1982
128. Jackson R: Epidermotropic malignant melanoma: The distinction between metastatic and new primary lesions in the skin. Can J Surg 27:533, 1984
129. Jacobsson M, Petruson B, Svendsen P, et al: Juvenile nasopharyngeal angiofibroma: A report of eighteen cases. Acta Otolaryngol (Stockh) 105:132, 1988
130. Jafek BW, Nahum AM, Butler RM, et al: Surgical treatment of juvenile nasopharyngeal angiofibroma. Laryngoscope 83:707, 1973
131. Jha N, McNeese M, Barkley HT, et al: Does radiotherapy have a role in hemangiopericytoma management? Report of 14 new cases and review of the literature. Int J Radiat Oncol Biol Phys 13:1399, 1987
132. Jones GC, DeSanto LW, Bremer JW, et al: Juvenile angiofibromas. Arch Otolarygol Head Neck Surg 112:1191, 1986
133. Kabot TE, Goldman ME, Bergman S, et al: Juvenile nasopharyngeal angiofibroma: An unusual presentation in the oral cavity. Oral Surg 59:453, 1985
134. Kadish S, Goodman M, Wang CC: Olfactory neuroblastoma, a clinical analysis of 17 cases. Cancer 37:1571, 1976
135. Kanno J, Matsubara O, Kasuga T: Induction of melanosis in Schwann cell and peripheral epithelium by 9,10-1,2-benzathracene (DMBA) and 12-*o*-tetradecanolylphorbol-13-acetate (TPA) in BDFI mice. Acta Pathol Jpn 37:1297, 1987
136. Kapadia SB, Desai V, Cheng VS: Extramedullary plasmacytoma of the head and neck: A clinicopathologic study of 20 cases. Medicine (Baltimore) 6:317, 1982
137. Kato T, Takematsu H, Tomita Y, et al: Malignant melanoma of mucous membranes. Arch Dermatol 123:216, 1987
138. Kim H, Park CI: Primary malignant laryngeal melanoma. Yonsei Med J 23:118, 1982
139. Kim J-A, Elkon D, Lim M-L, et al: Optimum dose of radiotherapy for chemodectomas of the middle ear. Int J Radiat Oncol Biol Phys 6:815, 1980
140. Konefal JB, Pilepich MV, Spector GJH, Perez CA: Radiation therapy in the treatment of chemodectomas. Laryngoscope 97:1331, 1987
141. Kopf AW, Bart RS, Gladstein AH: Treatment of melanotic freckle with x-rays. Arch Dermatol 112:801, 1976
142. Kotner L, Wang CC: Plasmacytoma of the upper air and food passage. Cancer 30:414, 1972
143. Krupski WC, Effeney DJ, Stoney RJ, et al: Carotid body tumours. Aust NZ J Surg 53:539, 1983
144. Kumar PP, Good RR, Sulkety ME, et al: Local control of clival and sacral chordoma after interstitial irradiation with iodine-125: New techniques for treatment of recurrent or unresectable chordomas. Neurosurgery 22:479, 1988
145. Laird JD, Ferguson WR, McIlrath EM, Hamilton JRL: Radio-

nuclide angiography as the primary investigation in chemodectoma: Consise communication. J Nucl Med 24:475, 1983
146. Lang DA, McKellar NJ, Lang W: Juvenile nasopharyngeal angiofibroma: The preferred treatment. Scott Med J 28:64, 1983
147. Lang NP, Stair JM, Degges RD: Melanoma today does not require radical surgery. Am J Surg 148:723, 1984
148. Larson TC III, Reese DF, Baker HL Jr, McDonald TJ: Glomus tympanicum chemodectomas: Radiographic and clinical characteristics. Radiology 163:801, 1987
149. Lasjaunias P: Nasopharyngeal angiofibromas: Hazards of embolization. Radiology 136:119, 1980
150. LeCompte PM: Tumors of the carotid body. Am J Pathol 24:305, 1948
151. Lee DA, Rao BR, Meyer JS, et al: Hormonal receptor determination in juvenile nasopharyngeal angiofibroma. Cancer 46:547, 1980
152. Levine PA, Paling MR, Black WC, Cantrell RW: MRI versus high resolution CT scanning: Evaluation of the anterior skull base. Otolaryngol Head Neck Surg 96:260, 1987
153. Lewis JS, Hutter RV, Tollefsen HR, et al: Nasal tumors of olfactory origin. Arch Otolaryngol Head Neck Surg 81:169, 1965
154. Liebow AA, Carrington CRB, Friedman PJ: Lymphomatoid granulomatosis. Hum Pathol 3:457, 1972
155. Lippman SM, Grogan TM, Spier EM, et al: Lethal midline granulomas with a novel T-cell phenotype as found in peripheral T-cell lymphoma. Cancer 59:936, 1987
156. Litwin MS, Krementz ET, Mansell PW, Reed RJ: Topical chemotherapy of lentigo maligna and fluorouracil. Cancer 35:721, 1975
157. Luddi RE, Levy BE, Schwartz AD: ^{67}Ga scintigraphy in granulocytic sarcoma. Cancer 46:1357, 1980
158. Lund VJ, Hound DJ, Lloyd GAS, Cheesman AD: Magnetic resonance imaging of paranasal sinus tumors for craniofacial resection. Head Neck Surg 11:279, 1989
159. Lundgren N: Tympanic body tumours in the middle ear: Tumours of carotid body type. Acta Otolaryngol 37:367, 1949
160. Lybeert MLM, Van Andel JG, Eijkenboom WMH, et al: Radiotherapy of paragangliomas. Clin Otolaryngol 9:105, 1984
161. MacDougall LG, Jankowitz P, Cohn R, et al: Acute childhood Leukemia in Johannesburg. Am J Pediatr Hematol Oncol 8:43, 1986
162. Mackay B, Luna MA, Butler JJ: Adult neuroblastoma: Electron microscopic observations in nine cases. Cancer 37:1134, 1976
163. Maharaj D, Fernandes CMC: Surgical experience with juvenile nasopharyngeal angiofibroma. Ann Otol Rhinol Laryngol 98:269, 1989
164. Mair G: Hematological malignancy in the adult. In Hote-Stone HF (ed): Radiotherapy in Clinical Practice, p 258. London, Butterworths, 1986
165. Manelfe C, Bonafe A, Fabre P, et al: Computed tomography in olfactory neuroblastoma. J Comput Assist Tomogr 2:412, 1978
166. Manelfe C, Roulleau J, Julian A, et al: Glomus tympanicum tumours: Early diagnosis by arteriography. Neuroradiology 4:226, 1972
167. Mantravadi RVP: Radiation therapy for nonsquamous tumors of the head and neck. Otolaryngol Clin North Am 19:741, 1986
168. Marc JA, Takei Y, Schechter MM, Hoffman JA: Intracranial hemangiopericytomas: Angiography, pathology and differential diagnosis. AJR 125:823, 1975
169. Marcial-Vega VA: Written Communication, August 7, 1989
170. Maruyama Y: Radiotherapy of tympanojugular chemodectomas. Radiology 105:659, 1972
171. Matias C, Corde J, Soares J: Primary malignant melanoma of the nasal cavity: A clinicopathologic study of nine cases. J Surg Oncol 39:29, 1988
172. Maurice M, Milad M: Pathogenesis of juvenile nasopharyngeal fibroma (a new concept). J Laryngol Otol 95:1121, 1981
173. McCabe BF, Fletcher M: Selection of therapy of glomus jugulare tumors. Arch Otolaryngol Head Neck Surg 89:156, 1969
174. McCormack LJ, Harris HE: Neurogenic tumors of the nasal fossa. JAMA 157:318, 1955
175. McDonald TJ, DeRemee RA, Harrison EG Jr, et al: The protean clinical features of polymorphic reticulosis (lethal midline granuloma). Laryngoscope 86:936, 1976
176. McGinnis JP, Greer JL, Wolve NL: Neurotropic melanoma of the lower lip. Oral Pathol 15:445, 1986
177. McGovern VJ: Malignant Melanoma: Clinical and Histological Diagnosis, pp. 121–129. New York, John Wiley, 1976
178. McNeer G, Cantin J: Local failure in the treatment of melanoma. AJR 99:791, 1967
179. McRae RG, Bellino JP, Khasgiwala C: Control of malignant melanoma of the nasal mucous membrane: Panel discussion (continued). Laryngoscope 92:1247, 1982
180. Mendenhall WM, Million RR, Parsons JT, et al: Chemodectoma of the carotid body and ganglion nodosum treated with radiation therapy. Int J Radiat Oncol Biol Phys 12:2175, 1986
181. Meyer JE, Schulz MD: Solitary myeloma of bone. Cancer 34:438, 1974
182. Miller CS, Craig RM, Mantich NM: Blue-black macule on the maxillary palate. J Am Dent Assoc 114:503, 1987
183. Mira JH, Chu FC, Fortner JC: The role of radiotherapy in the management of malignant hemangiopericytoma: Report of 11 new cases and review of the literature. Cancer 30:1254, 1977
184. Mitchell DC, Clyne CAC: Chemodectomas of the neck: The response to radiotherapy. Br J Surg 72:903, 1985
185. Muss HB, Maloney WC: Chloroma and other myeloblastic tumors. Blood 42:721, 1973
186. Neiman RA: The peripheral cell lymphomas come of age. Mayo Clin Proc 61:504, 1986
187. Neiman RS, Barcos M, Berard C, et al: Granulocytic sarcoma: A clinicopathologic study of 61 biopsied cases. Cancer 48:1426, 1981
188. Newman H, Rowe JF Jr, Phillips TL: Radiation therapy of the glomus jugulare tumor. AJR 118:663, 1973
189. Oberman HA, Rice DH: Olfactory neuroblastomas: A clinicopathologic study. Cancer 38:2494, 1976
190. Obert GJ, Devine KD, McDonald JR: Olfactory neuroblastomas. Cancer 13:205, 1960
191. O'Connor TA, McLean P, Juillard GJF, Parker RG: Olfactory neuroblastoma. Cancer 63:2426, 1989
192. Ogilvie RF: Histopathology, 6th ed, pp 85–86. Baltimore, Williams & Wilkins, 1962
193. Ogura JH, Schneck NL: Unusual nasal tumors: Problems in diagnosis and treatment. Otolaryngol Clin North Am 6:813, 1973
194. Ogura JH, Spector GJ, Gado M: Glomus jugulare and vagal. Ann Otol Rhinol Laryngol 83:622, 1978
195. Ohya T, Kudo K, Chen C-H, et al: Primary malignant melanomas of the oral mucosa. Int J Oral Maxillofac Surg 16:496, 1987
196. Olsen KD, DeSanto LW: Olfactory neuroblastoma: Biologic and clinical behavior. Arch Otolaryngol Head Neck Surg 109:797, 1983
197. Oot RF, Melville GE, New PF, et al: The role of MR and CT in evaluating clival chordomas and chondrosarcomas. AJR 151:567, 1988
198. Osborne DR, DuBois P, Drayer B, et al: Primary intracranial meningeal and spinal hemangiopericytomas: Radiologic manifestations. AJNR 2:69, 1981
199. Overgaard J: The current and potential role of hyperthermia in radiotherapy. Int J Radiat Oncol Biol Phys 16:535, 1989
200. Pahor AL: Extramedullary plasmacytoma of the head and neck, parotid, and submandibular salivary glands. J Laryngol Otol 91:241, 1977
201. Panje WR, Moran WJ: Melanoma of the upper aerodigestive tract: A review of 21 cases. Head Neck Surg 8:309, 1986
202. Parry DM, Li FP, Strong LC, et al: Carotid body tumors in humans: Genetics and epidemiology. JNCI 68:573, 1982
203. Pomeranz SJ, Hawkins HH, Towbin R, et al: Granulocytic

sarcoma (chloroma): CT manifestations. Radiology 155:167, 1985
204. Radiation Therapy Oncology Group Protocol No 8305, 1988
205. Rampen FH: Biopsy and survival of malignant melanoma. J Am Acad Dermatol 12:385, 1985
206. Rapini RP, Golitz LE, Greer RO, et al: Primary malignant melanoma of the oral cavity: A review of 117 cases. Cancer 55:1543, 1985
207. Rappaport H: Tumors of the hematopoietic system. In Atlas of Tumor Pathology, sec 3, fasc 8, p 2410. Washington, DC, Armed Forces Institute of Pathology, 1966
208. Reddy EK, Mansfield CM, Hartman GV: Chemodectoma of glomus jugulare. Cancer 52:337, 1983
209. Rhodin JAG: Ultrastructure of mammalian venous capillaries, venules and small collecting veins. J Ultrastruct Res 25:452, 1968
210. Rich TA, Schiller A, Suit HD, Mankin HJ: Clinical and pathologic review of 48 cases of chordoma. Cancer 56:182, 1985
211. Robinson ACR, Khoury GG, Ash DV, et al: Evaluation of response following irradiation of juvenile angiofibromas. Br J Radiol 62:245, 1989
212. Rossenwasser H: Current management of glomus jugulare tumors. Ann Otol Rhinol Laryngol 76:603, 1967
213. Saunders WM, Castro JR, Chen GTY, et al: Early results of ion beam radiation therapy for sacral chordoma. J Neurosurg 64:243, 1986
214. Sawyer DR, Rennie JS: Gingival metastasis of a malignant melanoma. J Oral Med 41:35, 1986
215. Saxton JP: Chordoma. Int J Radiat Oncol Biol Phys 7:913, 1981
216. Schroth G, Gawehn J, Marquardt B, Schabet M: MR Imaging of esthesioneuroblastoma. J Comput Assist Tomogr 10:316, 1986
217. Sessions RB, Bryan RN, Naclerio RM, et al: Radiographic staging of juvenile angiofibroma. Head Neck Surg 3:279, 1981
218. Setzkorn RK, Lee DJ, Iliff NT, Green R: Hemangiopericytoma of the orbit treated with conservative surgery and radiotherapy. Arch Ophthalmol 105:1103, 1987
219. Shank BB, Kelley Cd, Nisce LZ, et al: Radiation therapy in lymphomatoid granulomatosis. Cancer 42:2572, 1978
220. Sharma PD, Johnson AP, Whitton AC: Radiotherapy for jugulo-tympanic paragangliomas (glomus jugulare tumours). J Laryngol Otol 98:621, 1984
221. Shukovsky LJ, Fletcher GH: Retinal and optic nerve complications in a high dose irradiation technique of ethmoid sinus and nasal cavity. Radiology 104:629, 1972
222. Silverstone SM: Radiation therapy of glomus jugulare tumors. Arch Otolaryngol 97:43, 1973
223. Simko TG, Griffin TW, Gerdes AJ, et al: The role of radiation therapy in the treatment of glomus jugulare tumors. Cancer 42:104, 1978
224. Simpson GT, Konrad HR, Takahashi M, et al: Immediate postembolization excision of glomus juglare tumors. Arch Otolaryngol Head Neck Surg 105:639, 1979
225. Singh W, Ramage C, Best P, et al: Nasal neuroblastoma secreting vasopressin: A case report. Cancer 56:961, 1980
226. Sinnreich AI, Parisier SC, Cohen NL, et al: Arterial malformations of the middle ear. Otolaryngol Head Neck Surg 92:194, 1984
227. Skolnik EM, Massari FS, Tenta LT: Olfactory neuroepithelioma: Review of the world literature and presentation of two cases. Arch Otolaryngol Head Neck Surg 84:644, 1966
228. Slater JD, Austin-Seymour M, Munzenrider J, et al: Endocrine function following high dose proton therapy for tumors of the upper clivus. Int J Radiat Oncol Biol Phys 15:607, 1988
229. Smalley RS, Cupps RE, Anderson JA, et al: Polymorphic reticulosis limited to the upper aerodigestive tract: Natural history and radiotherapeutic considerations. Int J Radiat Oncol Biol Phys 15:599, 1988
230. Snow GB, van der Waal I: Mucosal melanomas of the head and neck. Otolaryngol Clin North Am 19:537, 1986
231. Sowers JJ, Moody PM, Naidich TP, et al: Radiographic features of granulocytic sarcoma (chloroma). J Comput Assist Tomogr 3:226, 1979
232. Spagnolo DV, Papadimitiou JM, Archer M: Postirradiation malignant fibrous histiocytoma arising in juvenile nasopharyngeal angiofibroma and producing alpha-1-antitrypsin. Histopathology 8:339, 1984
233. Spaulding CA, Kranyak MS, Constable WC, Stewart FM: Esthesioneuroblastoma: A comparison of two treatment eras. Int J Radiat Oncol Biol Phys 15:581, 1988
234. Spector GJ, Ciralsky R, Maisel RH, et al: Multiple glomus tumors in the head and neck. Laryngoscope 85:1066, 1975
235. Spector GJ, Compagno J, Perez CA, et al: Glomus jugulare tumors: Effects of radiotherapy. Cancer 35:1316, 1975
236. Spector GJ, Fierstein J, Ogura JH: A comparison of therapeutic modalities of glomus tumors in the temporal bone. Laryngoscope 86:690, 1976
237. Spector GJ, Sobol S: Surgery for glomus tumors at the skull base. Otolaryngol Head Neck Surg 88:524, 1980
238. Standefer J, Hold GR, Brown WE Jr, et al: Combined intracranial and extracranial excision of nasopharyngeal angiofibroma. Laryngoscope 93:772, 1983
239. Stansbie JM, Phelps PD: Involution of residual juvenile nasopharyngeal angiofibroma (a case report). J Laryngol Otol 100:599, 1986
240. Stavas J: Nasopharyngeal mass in a teenage male. Neb Med J March:61, 1989
241. Stewart FM, Frierson HF, Levine PA, Spaulding CA: Esthesioneuroblastoma. In Williams CJ, Krikorian JG, Green MR, Raghavan D (eds): Textbook of Uncommon Cancer, p 63. New York, John Wiley, 1988
242. Stout AP: Hemangiopericytoma: Study of 25 new cases. Cancer 2:1027, 1949
243. Stout AP, Murray MR: Hemangiopericytoma: Vascular tumor featuring Zimmermann's pericytes. Ann Surg 116:26, 1942
244. Suit HD, Gallager HS: Intact tumor cells in irradiated tissue. Arch Pathol 78:648, 1964
245. Sze G, Jichanco LS, Brant-Zawadski MN, et al: Chordomas: MR imaging. Radiology 166:187, 1988
246. Takaue Y, Culbert SJ, Eys JV, et al: Spontaneous cure of endstage ANLL complicated with chloroma. Cancer 58:1101, 1986
247. Tang JSH, Gold RH, Mirra JM, Eckhardt J: Hemangiopericytoma of bone. Cancer 62:848, 1988
248. Tewfik HH, McGinnis WLK, Nordstrom DG, et al: Chordoma: Evaluation of clinical behavior and treatment modalities. Int J Radiat Oncol Biol Phys 2:959, 1974
249. Thomsen K, Elbrond O, Andersen AP: Glomus jugulare tumors: A series of 21 cases. J Laryngol Otol 89:1113, 1975
250. Tidwell TJ, Montague ED: Chemodectomas involving the temporal bone. Radiology 116:147, 1975
251. Todd IDH: Treatment of solitary plasmacytoma. Clin Radiol 16:395, 1965
252. Trapp TK, Fu YS, Calcaterra TC: Melanoma of the nasal and paranasal sinus mucosa. Arch Otolaryngol Head Neck Surg 113:1086, 1987
253. Tyler TC, Chandler JR, Wetli C, et al: Olfactory neuroblastoma. South Med J 67:640, 1974
254. Uehara T, Matsubara O, Kasuga T: Melanocytes in the nasal cavity and paranasal sinus. Acta Pathol Jpn 37:1105, 1987
255. Umeda M, Mishima Y, Teranobu O, et al: Heterogeneity of primary malignant melanomas in oral mucosa: An analysis of 43 cases in Japan. Pathology 20:234, 1988
256. Urist MM, Balch CM, Soong SJ, et al: Head and neck melanoma in 534 clinical stage I patients: A prognostic factors analysis and results of surgical treatment. Ann Surg 200:769, 1984
257. Van Miert PJ: The treatment of chemodectomas by radiotherapy. Proc R Soc Med 57:946, 1964
258. Veronesi U, Adamus J, Bandiero DC: Inefficacy of immediate note dissection in stage I melanoma of the limbs. N Engl J Med 297:627, 1977
259. Wade PM Jr, Smith RE, Johns ME: Response of esthesioneuroblastoma to chemotherapy: Report of five cases and review of the literature. Cancer 53:1036, 1984
260. Walike JW, Bailey BJ: Head and neck hemangiopericytoma. Arch Otolaryngol Head Neck Surg 93:345, 1971

261. Wang CC, James AE Jr: Chordoma: Brief review of the literature and report of a case with widespread metastases. Cancer 22:162, 1968
262. Wang M-L, Hussey DH, Doornbos JF, et al: Chemodectoma of the temporal bone: A comparison of surgical and radiotherapeutic results. Int J Radiat Oncol Biol Phys 14:643, 1988
263. Wayte DM, Helwig EB: Melanotic freckle of Hutchinson. Cancer 21:893, 1968
264. Weirnik PH, Serpick AA: Granulocytic sarcoma (chloroma). Blood 35:361, 1970
265. Weis JW, Winter MW, Phyliky RL, et al: Peripheral T-cell lymphomas: Histiologic, immunohistiologic and clinical classification. Mayo Clin Proc 61:411, 1986
266. Wieden PL, Yarington CT Jr, Richardson RG: Olfactory neuroblastoma: Chemotherapy and radiotherapy for extensive disease. Arch Otolaryngol Head Neck Surg 110:759, 1984
267. Wilson H: Carotid body tumors. Surgery 59:483, 1966
268. Wiltshaw E: The natural history of extramedullary plasmacytoma and its relation to solitary myeloma of bone and myelomatosis. Medicine (Baltimore) 55:217, 1976
269. Withers HR, Peters LJ: The application of RBE values to clinical trials of high-LET radiations: High-LET radiation in clinical radiotherapy. Eur J Cancer :257, 1979
270. Witt TR, Shah JP, Sternberg SS: Juvenile nasopharyngeal fibroma: A 30 year clinical review. Am J Surg 46:521, 1983
271. Wold LE, Laws ER: Cranial chordomas in children and young adults. J Neurosurg 59:1043, 1983
272. Wong PP, Yagoda A: Chemotherapy of malignant hemangiopericytoma. Cancer 41:1256, 1978
273. Woo E, Yue CP, Onann KE, et al: Intracerebral chloromas. Clin Neurol Neurosurg 88:135, 1986
274. Woodruff RK, Whittle JM, Malpas JS: Solitary plasmacytoma. I. Extramedullary soft tissue plasmacytoma. Cancer 43:2340, 1979
275. Yaghmai I: Angiographic manifestations of soft tissue and osseous hemangiopericytomas. Radiology 126:652, 1978
276. Zakzouk SM, Elgarem A, Hafiz MA: An unusual case of nasopharyngeal angiofibroma. Ear Nose Throat J 58:47, 1979
277. Zimmerman KW: Der feinere Bau der blutkapillaren. Anat Entwicklungsgesch 69:28, 1923.
278. Zimmerman LCE, Font RL: Ophthalmologic manifestations of granulocytic sarcoma: A clinicopathologic study of 33 cases. Am J Ophthalmol 75:80, 1975

37

Head and Neck: Management of the Neck

William M. Mendenhall
James T. Parsons
Anthony A. Mancuso
Scott P. Stringer
Nicholas J. Cassisi
Rodney R. Million

ANATOMY

The incidence of lymph node metastases at the time of diagnosis for each head and neck site is related to the relative density of the capillary lymphatic network (Table 37-1).[50] The nasopharynx and pyriform sinus have the most profuse capillary lymphatic networks, whereas the paranasal sinuses, middle ear, and true vocal cords have either sparse or no capillary lymphatics.[76]

The locations of the various lymph node groups in the head and neck are shown in Figure 37-1.[76] Under normal conditions, the right and left lymphatic networks do not shunt from one side to the other.[21]

The internal jugular chain (IJC) lymph nodes lie adjacent to the internal jugular vein and extend from the base of the skull to the clavicle. The most superior group of lymph nodes in this chain lies near the base of the skull in the posterior aspect of the lateral pharyngeal space and is often referred to as the parapharyngeal or junctional lymph nodes. These lymph nodes lie deep to the sternocleidomastoid muscle, the posterior belly of the digastric muscle, and the tail of the parotid gland. The remainder of the IJC lymph nodes are artificially divided into the subdigastric, middle jugular, and lower jugular groups.

The spinal accessory chain (SAC) lymph nodes (posterior cervical chain or posterior triangle lymph nodes) are distributed along the course of cranial nerve XI. The superior nodes of the SAC blend with the upper IJC nodes and are often referred to as the junctional lymph nodes.

The supraclavicular lymph nodes merge laterally with the SAC lymph nodes and medially with the lower IJC lymph nodes.

There are three to six submandibular lymph nodes. They may be either preglandular or postglandular; no lymph nodes are in the substance of the submandibular gland.

The submental lymph nodes lie in the midline between the anterior bellies of the digastric muscles, are anterior to the hyoid bone, and external to the mylohyoid muscle.

NATURAL HISTORY

The risk of lymph node metastases is influenced by the location of the primary tumor, the degree of histologic differentiation, the size of the lesion, and the availability of capillary lymphatics.[49] The estimated risk of subclinical disease in the clinically negative neck as a function of primary site and T stage is shown in Table 37-2.[48] Recurrent lesions have a higher risk of lymphatic involvement than untreated lesions.

The relative incidence of clinically positive lymph nodes in the neck is shown in Table 37-3 by anatomic site and T stage.[38] The most commonly involved lymph nodes in the head and neck are the subdigastric lymph nodes, followed by the midjugular lymph nodes. Lesions that are well lateralized almost always spread first to the ipsilateral neck nodes. Lesions on or near the midline as well as lateralized base of tongue and nasopharyngeal lesions may spread to both sides of the neck.

Theoretically, patients who have clinically positive lymph nodes on the ipsilateral side of the neck may be at risk for contralateral lymph node spread if the metastatic masses produce significant obstruction of the lymphatic trunks. In addition, patients who have undergone previous surgery on one side of the neck develop shunting of lymph across the submental region to the opposite side of the neck. When contralateral lymph node metastases occur, the subdigastric lymph nodes are most frequently involved, followed by the midjugular and lower jugular lymph node groups.

As tumor grows within a lymph node, the node becomes indurated and more rounded, and enlarges. Tumor eventually

TABLE 37–1
Incidence of Lymph Node Metastasis by Site of Primary Disease in Head and Neck Squamous Cell Carcinomas

SITE	NODES POSITIVE AT PRESENTATION (%)	NODES NEGATIVE CLINICALLY, POSITIVE PATHOLOGICALLY (%)	NODES NEGATIVE INITIALLY, BECOMING POSITIVE WITH NO NECK TREATMENT (%)
Floor of mouth	30–59 [25,27,32]	40–50 [29,77]	20–35 [4,58]
Gingiva	18–52 [14,19,25,45]	19[14]	17[4,14]
Hard palate	13–24 [17,20,45]	ND	22[4]
Buccal mucosa	9–31 [25,32]	ND	16[4]
Oral tongue	34–65 [25,27,31,32]	25–54 [10,19,26,36,78]	38–52 [26,31,58,79]
Nasopharynx	86–90 [11,40,64]	ND	19–50 [30,65]*
Anterior tonsillar pillar/ retromolar trigone	39–56 [5,33,39]	ND	10–15 [77]
Soft palate/uvula	37–56 [5,33,39]	ND	16–25 [39]
Tonsillar fossa	50–76 [11,27,33,35,40,64]	ND	22[75]†
Base of tongue	50–83 [33,64,66,70,77]	22[66]	ND
Pharyngeal walls	50–71 [33,64,66,77]	66[66]	ND
Supraglottic larynx	31–64 [27,28,77]	16–26 [66,72]	33[22,72]
Hypopharynx	52–78 [19,60,66,77]	38[66]	ND

ND: no data
** T1N0 patients only*
† Patients received preoperative irradiation.
(Mendenhall WM, Million RR, Cassisi NJ: Head Neck Surg 3:15–20, 1980)

extends through the capsule of the lymph node and invades surrounding structures. Extension to the neurovascular bundle is common and may produce a mass that is considered fixed to palpation. The incidence of tumor involvement and the likelihood of capsular penetration as a function of lymph node size are shown in Table 37-4.[74]

DIAGNOSTIC WORKUP

Physical Examination

The patient is always examined in the sitting position—the examiner behind the patient with one hand on the occiput to flex the patient's head forward and the other hand on the side of

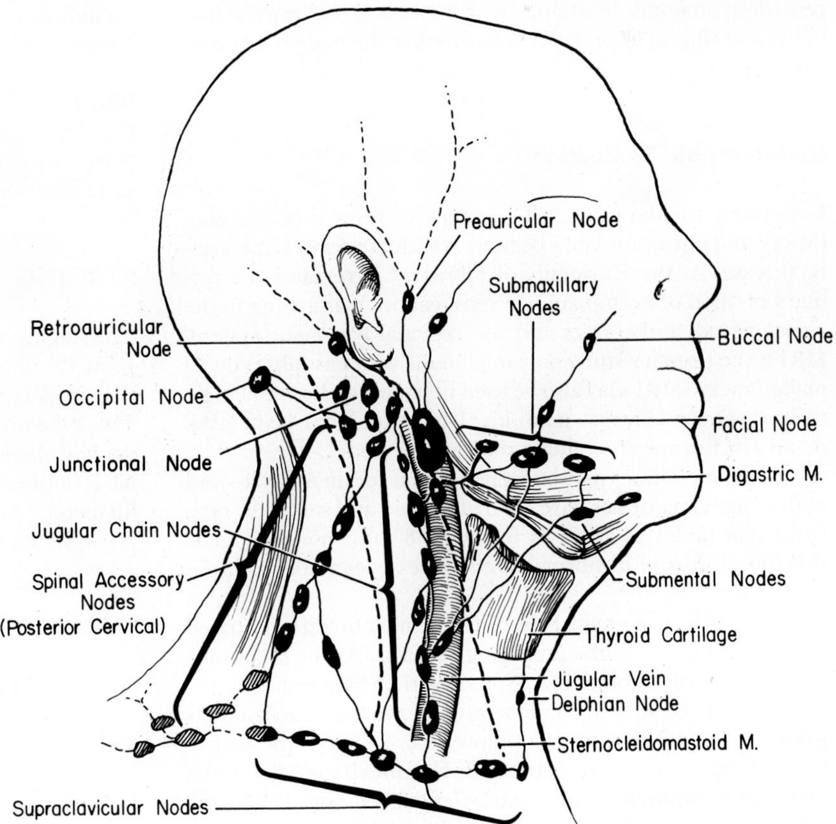

FIGURE 37–1. Arrangement of lymph nodes in the head and neck. (Redrawn from Rouviere H: Anatomy of the Human Lymphatic System, p 27. Tobias MJ [trans]: Ann Arbor. Edwards Brothers, 1938)

TABLE 37–2
Definition of Risk Groups

GROUP	ESTIMATED RISK OF SUBCLINICAL NECK DISEASE	STAGE	SITE
I Low risk	<20%	T1	Floor of mouth, oral tongue, retromolar trigone, gingiva, hard palate, buccal mucosa
II Intermediate risk	20%–30%	T1	Soft palate, pharyngeal wall, supraglottic larynx, tonsil
		T2	Floor of mouth, oral tongue, retromolar trigone, gingiva, hard palate, buccal mucosa
III High risk	>30%	T1–4	Nasopharynx, pyriform sinus, base of tongue
		T2–4	Soft palate, pharyngeal wall, supraglottic larynx, tonsil
		T3–4	Floor of mouth, oral tongue, retromolar trigone, gingiva, hard palate, buccal mucosa

(Mendenhall WM, Million RR: Int J Radiat Oncol Biol Phys 12:741–746, 1986)

the neck to be examined. To examine the IJC lymph nodes, which lie deep to the sternocleidomastoid muscle along the internal jugular vein, place the thumb and index finger around the sternocleidomastoid muscle in the form of a C and then gently proceed from the sternal notch to the angle of the mandible. Both sides of the neck should not be examined simultaneously. The submandibular and submental nodes may be evaluated by direct palpation of these areas as well as by a bimanual examination with the index finger placed in the floor of the mouth.[61,63]

The following features of metastatic lymph nodes must be recorded: anatomic location, size, consistency, tenderness, mobility, and clinical impression as to whether the node is involved with cancer.

Radiographic Evaluation

Computed tomography (CT), magnetic resonance imaging (MRI), and ultrasound may be used to evaluate cervical metastatic disease. At the University of Florida, CT remains the primary method of examination of most carcinomas arising in the upper aerodigestive tract and the regional lymphatic system. MRI is the primary study only in patients with nasopharyngeal malignancies. MRI may also be used in patients who are allergic to intravenous contrast medium. Ultrasound has been used mainly in Europe to evaluate the cervical nodes.

Small metastases may be seen as lucent foci in normal-sized nodes. Such metastases have been identified and surgically confirmed in nodes as small as 6 mm to 8 mm; however, most subclinical disease in normal-sized nodes goes undetected on CT.

Lucent foci in normal-sized nodes must be differentiated from hilar fat or volume-averaging artifacts. As the metastasis grows, the node becomes more spherical than elliptical. Areas of necrosis may be seen in 1 cm metastases and are almost always present in nodal metastases of more than 2 cm. As the metastasis enlarges, the capsule of the node becomes hyperemic and is seen radiographically as a contrast-enhanced rim. When the capsule becomes indistinct and irregular along its outer margin, it is highly suggestive of early capsular penetration. Continued growth causes obliteration of the fat planes surrounding the nodes. Finally, no clear plane of normal tissue lies between the mass and the adjacent structures, at which point the clinician usually notes fixation (Fig. 37-2). Penetration of the prevertebral fascia and fixation to the scalene muscles are uncommon in untreated patients.

If a node shows evidence of capsular penetration and envelops more than 50% of the circumference of the carotid artery, clinical evidence of fixation to the artery is likely. Ultrasound and MRI may prove useful in evaluating tumor extension to the carotid, as suggested by CT. MRI tends to be better at excluding extension to the neurovascular bundle when it is "suspected" on CT, whereas ultrasound can help show invasion of the vessel wall, thus confirming focal extension to the artery. When tumor extension to the carotid is strongly suspected on CT, MRI, or ultrasound, test-balloon occlusion of the carotid before surgery is suggested, so that the artery may be resected with a reasonable margin of safety if this becomes necessary.

STAGING

The staging system shown in Table 37-5 is that of the American Joint Committee on Cancer (AJCC).[2] Stage N3C is rare and should alert the clinician to search for another primary lesion. The 1988 update of the AJCC staging system classifies bilateral or contralateral nodes, not more than 6 cm in diameter, as N2C; N3 is defined as a metastasis in a lymph node more than 6 cm in diameter.[3] All University of Florida data presented in this chapter were analyzed using the 1983 AJCC staging system.

SURGERY

General Management

Standard radical neck dissection involves removal of the superficial and deep cervical fascia with its enclosed lymph nodes in continuity with the sternocleidomastoid muscle, omohyoid muscle, internal and external jugular veins, spinal accessory nerve, and submandibular gland. The indication for this opera-

TABLE 37–3
Clinically Detected Nodal Metastases on Admission, by T Stage

PRIMARY SITE	T STAGE	N0 (%)	N1 (%)	N2–N3 (%)
Oral tongue*	T1	86	10	4
	T2	70	19	11
	T3	52	16	31
	T4	24	10	66
Floor of mouth*	T1	89	9	2
	T2	71	18	10
	T3	56	20	24
	T4	46	10	43
Retromolar trigone/ anterior tonsillar pillar†	T1	88	2	9
	T2	62	18	20
	T3	46	21	33
	T4	32	18	50
Soft palate†	T1	92	0	8
	T2	64	12	24
	T3	35	26	39
	T4	33	11	56
Tonsillar fossa†	T1	30	41	30
	T2	32	14	54
	T3	30	18	52
	T4	10	13	76
Base of tongue†	T1	30	15	55
	T2	29	14	56
	T3	26	23	52
	T4	16	8	76
Oropharyngeal walls†	T1	75	0	25
	T2	70	10	20
	T3	33	22	44
	T4	24	24	52
Supaglottic larynx‡	T1	61	10	29
	T2	58	16	26
	T3	36	25	40
	T4	41	18	41
Hypopharynx§	T1	37	21	42
	T2	30	20	49
	T3	21	26	54
	T4	26	15	58
Nasopharynx¶	T1	8	11	82
	T2	16	12	72
	T3	12	9	80
	T4	17	6	78

(2044 patients, M. D. Anderson Hospital, 1948–1965)
** T stage defined by Lindberg*[38]
† T stage defined by Fletcher et al[23]
‡ T stage defined by Fletcher et al[24]
§ T stage defined by MacComb et al[41]
¶ T stage defined by Chen and Fletcher[16]
(Lindberg R: Cancer 29:1446–1449, 1972)

tion is clinically positive lymph nodes. Sacrifice of cranial nerve XI often, but not always, results in atrophy of the trapezius muscle, with shoulder drop and discomfort.

Radical neck dissection sparing cranial nerve XI is performed in patients with clinically positive nodes in which the metastatic masses can be removed without sacrificing the nerve, although this does not guarantee that trapezius function will remain.

Functional neck dissection (Bocca neck dissection) removes the superficial and deep cervical fascia with its enclosed lymph nodes and leaves intact the sternocleidomastoid and digastric muscles, internal jugular vein, and spinal accessory nerve. This operation is usually selected for patients in whom no clinically positive lymph nodes are present. The advantages of the functional neck dissection are less cosmetic deformity and better function.

TABLE 37–4
*Relationship Between Node Size, the Presence of Tumor in the Node, and Capsular Penetration in 519 Nodes**

	SIZE OF NODE (CM)				
	1	2	3	4	≥5
No. of nodes	177	183	84	17	58
Percent positive	33	62	81	88	100
Percent positive with capsular penetration	14	26	49	71	76

** Institut Gustav-Roussy*
(Modified from Richard JM, Sancho-Garnier H, Micheau C, et al: Laryngoscope 97:97–101, 1987)

Supraomohyoid neck dissection is a functional neck dissection that removes the lymph nodes above the omohyoid muscle and usually includes the subdigastric, midjugular, submandibular, and upper posterior cervical lymph nodes. The sternocleidomastoid muscle is preserved, and cranial nerve XI is spared. At the University of Florida, the supraomohyoid dissection has generally been replaced by complete functional neck dissection, which incurs little or no added morbidity or operating time.

Bilateral neck dissections may be done simultaneously or separately in patients with bilateral neck disease as long as one internal jugular vein can be preserved. Fewer complications occur and operative mortality is lower when the neck dissections are performed as two different procedures, allowing the patient to recover between operations.[46,73]

Complications

Complications after neck dissection include hematoma, seroma, lymphedema, wound infection, wound dehiscence, chyle fistula, damage to cranial nerves VII, X, and XII, carotid expo-

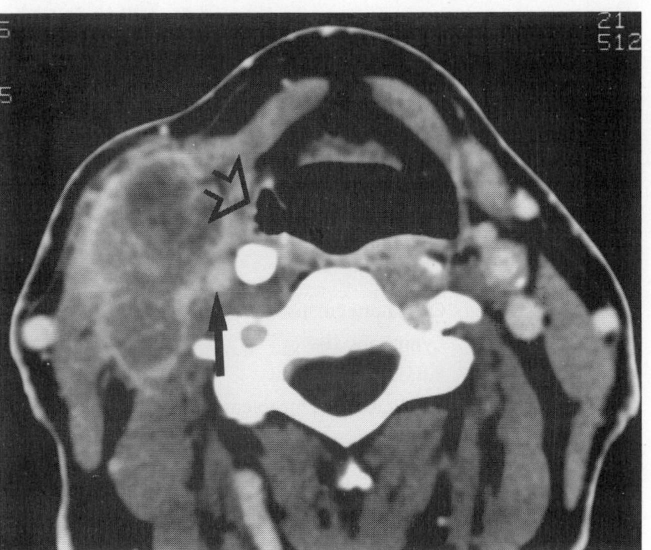

FIGURE 37–2. T1 squamous cell carcinoma of the lateral wall of the right pyriform sinus (*open arrow*) and a fixed N3A neck node that abuts but does not surround the carotid artery (*solid arrow*).

TABLE 37–5
1983 American Joint Committee on Cancer Staging for Neck Lymph Nodes

STAGE	DEFINITION
NX	Nodes cannot be assessed
N0	No clinically positive nodes
N1	Single clinically positive homolateral node 3 cm or less in diameter
N2	Single clinically positive homolateral node more than 3 cm but not more than 6 cm in diameter or multiple clinically positive homolateral nodes, none more than 6 cm in diameter
N2A	Single clinically positive homolateral node more than 3 cm but not more than 6 cm in diameter
N2B	Multiple clinically positive homolateral nodes, none more than 6 cm in diameter
N3	Massive homolateral node(s), bilateral nodes, or contralateral node(s)
N3A	Clinically positive homolateral node(s), one more than 6 cm in diameter
N3B	Bilateral clinically positive nodes (in this situation, each side of the neck should be staged separately; i.e., N3B: right, N2A; left, N1)
N3C	Contralateral clinically positive node(s) only

(American Joint Committee on Cancer: Manual for Staging of Cancer, 2nd ed, p 27. Philadelphia, JB Lippincott, 1983)

sure, and carotid rupture. The incidence of complications is higher when neck dissection is combined with resection of the primary lesion or when it follows a course of radiation therapy. The postoperative mortality rate for unilateral neck dissection following irradiation was 3% for patients treated between 1964 and 1982.[51]

Tables 37-6 and 37-7 show the incidence of postoperative complications in a series of patients treated with radiation therapy to the primary lesion and neck followed by unilateral or bilateral neck dissection(s).[51] The incidence of complications was higher for maximum subcutaneous doses over 6000 cGy and for bilateral simultaneous dissection than for bilateral staged neck dissection.[69]

RADIATION THERAPY

General Management

Radiation therapy may be used in the management of cervical lymph node metastases as elective treatment when there are no palpable lymph nodes, as the only treatment for clinically positive lymph nodes, or as preoperative or postoperative treatment in combination with neck dissection for clinically positive lymph nodes.

The regional lymph nodes are considered in the treatment planning of the primary lesion. With clinically negative neck nodes, treatment planning depends on the estimated risk of subclinical disease in the nodes. With clinically positive lymph nodes, the plan is influenced by the number of lymph nodes, their size, and their location.

Elective Irradiation of Cervical Lymph Nodes When the Primary Tumor Is Treated by Radiation Therapy

The factors that influence the decision to irradiate the neck electively are site and size of the primary lesion, histologic grade, difficulty in neck examination, relative morbidity for adding lymph node coverage, likelihood of the patient's returning for follow-up examinations, and suitability of the patient for a radical neck dissection if the tumor appears in the neck at a later date. Patients in whom the primary lesion is to be treated by radiation therapy, who have clinically negative nodes, and in whom the risk of subclinical disease is 20% or greater usually receive elective neck radiation to a minimum dose equivalent to 4500 cGy to 5000 cGy over 4.5 to 5 weeks (see Table 37-2). Patients with lesions arising in the lip, nasal vestibule, nasal cavity, or paranasal sinuses have a low risk of subclinical neck disease, and the neck is not treated electively unless the lesion is recurrent, advanced, or poorly differentiated. Similarly, the

TABLE 37–6
Postoperative Complications of Unilateral Neck Dissection Following Irradiation to the Primary Lesion and Neck (143 Patients)

COMPLICATION	NUMBER OF COMPLICATIONS	NUMBER OF SECOND OPERATIONS TO REPAIR COMPLICATION	DEATH
Salivary fistula	1	0	0
Wound breakdown	23	15	0
Bleeding	2	1	1
Pneumonia	2	0	1
Orocutaneous fistula	1	1	0
Lymphatic fistula	2	0	0
Pulmonary embolus	1	0	0
Cardiovascular problem	2	0	1
Sepsis	1	0	1
Total complications	35*	17	4†
Incidence	33/143 (23%)	17/143 (12%)	4/143 (3%)

**35 complications in 33 patients*
† Deaths occurred 6, 7, 8, and 35 days after surgery.
(Mendenhall WM, Million RR, Cassisi NJ: Int J Radiat Oncol Biol Phys 12:733–740, 1986)

TABLE 37–7
Postoperative Complications in Patients Undergoing Bilateral Neck Dissection Following Irradiation to the Primary Lesion and Neck (18 Patients)

	SIMULTANEOUS (N = 12)		STAGED (N = 6)	
COMPLICATION*	NUMBER	SECOND OPERATION	NUMBER	SECOND OPERATION
Acute laryngeal edema	2	2	0	0
Wound breakdown	4	2	2	1
Chylous fistula	1	1	0	0
Total (incidence)	7 (58%)	5 (42%)	2 (33%)	1 (17%)

** No postoperative deaths*
(Mendenhall WM, Million RR, Cassisi NJ: Int J Radiat Oncol Biol Phys 12:733–740, 1986)

risk of occult neck disease is essentially zero for T1 and 1.7% for T2 glottic carcinomas, and elective neck irradiation is not indicated.[55,57]

The lateral treatment portals used to encompass cancers in the oropharynx, supraglottic larynx, and hypopharynx include the upper jugular and often the midjugular chain lymph nodes. Radiation portals used for primary lesions of the oral cavity, nasopharynx, glottis, nasal cavity, and paranasal sinuses must be enlarged to include the lymph nodes. The treatment portals for irradiation of the cervical lymph nodes must be designed in such a way as to minimize additional mucosal irradiation.

Elective neck irradiation for early oral cavity lesions includes the submaxillary and subdigastric lymph nodes. The midjugular and low jugular lymph nodes are treated as well, using a narrow anterior field. For primary lesions located in the oropharynx, nasopharynx, supraglottic larynx, and hypopharynx, the lower neck nodes are also routinely included. The low neck is treated with a single anterior field (Figs. 37-3 and 37-4).[67–70] A tapered midline larynx/trachea shield is added to protect the spinal cord, the larynx, and the pharynx. For primary lesions lying below the thyroid notch, a small midline tracheal block is placed in the low neck field primarily to avoid field overlap at the spinal cord. A 5 mm wide midline block made of Lipowitz's metal may be used to shield the trachea, esophagus, and spinal cord below the level of the cricoid; this results in an 18 mm midline gap between the 90% isodose lines using ^{60}Co when the block is placed 15 cm to 18 cm above the patient (SSD 80). Great care must be used to ensure that this block does not shield the midjugular and low jugular lymph

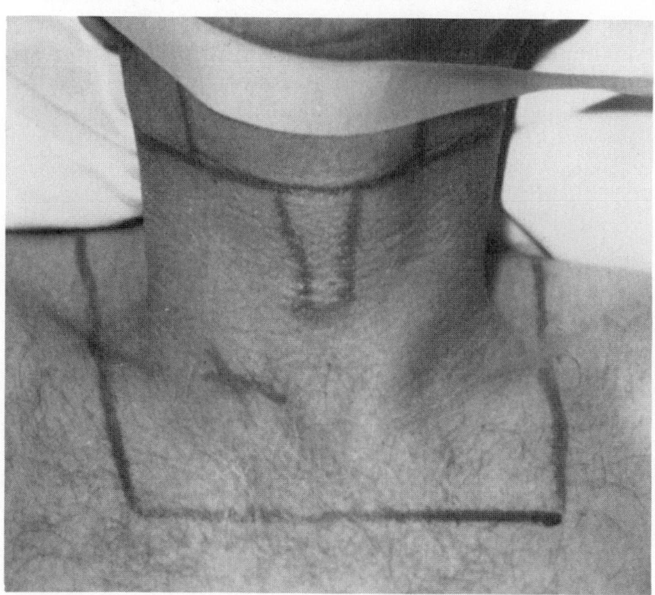

FIGURE 37–3. *En face* field for irradiation of the lower neck in conjunction with lateral base of tongue portals. The larynx and portions of the upper trachea, the cervical spinal cord, the cervical esophagus, and sometimes the thyroid isthmus may be shielded by an individually fitted, tapered midline block. More or less of the supraclavicular fossae may be irradiated, depending on the clinical stage of each side of the neck. (Parsons JT, Million RR, Cassisi NJ: Laryngoscope 92:689–696, 1982)

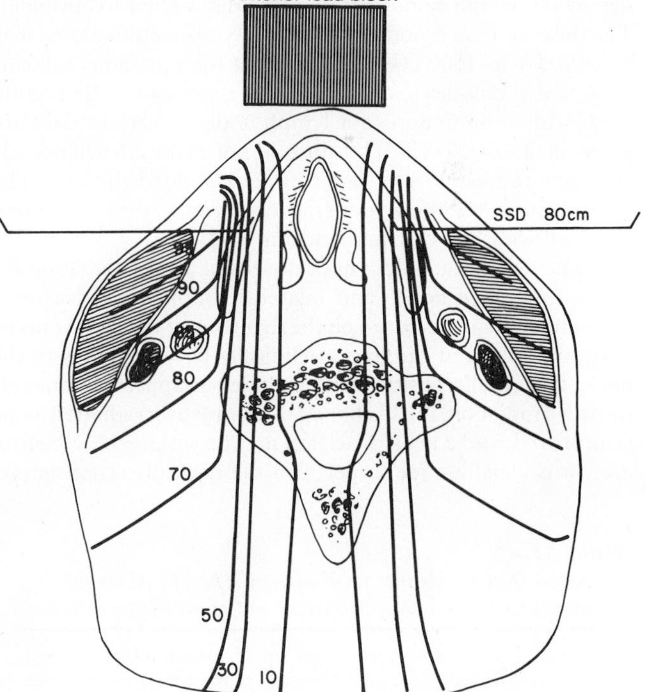

FIGURE 37–4. Dose distribution for ^{60}Co lower neck irradiation. Contour is through the level of the true vocal cords. The SSD is placed on the anterior surface of the sternocleidomastoid opposite the cricoid cartilage. The jugular chain lymph nodes receive a minimum dose that is 80% to 85% of the maximum dose. When 5000 cGy is administered to D_{max}, these nodes receive more than 4000 cGy. The larynx and spinal cord are shielded by an anterior lead block. SSD: source-skin distance. (Parsons JT: Time-dose-volume relationships in radiotherapy. In Million RR, Cassisi NJ [eds]: Management of Head and Neck Cancer: A Multidisciplinary Approach, p 141. Philadelphia, JB Lippincott, 1984)

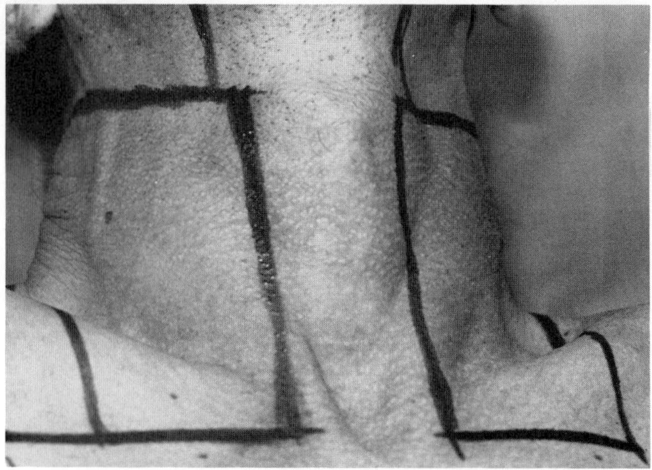

FIGURE 37–5. Improperly designed midline block. Note that the block shields the low jugular lymph nodes that lie under the sternocleidomastoid muscle in the low neck.

nodes. *Improper design of the midline larynx/trachea block is a common error* (Fig. 37-5).

Management of Clinically Positive Cervical Lymph Nodes When the Primary Lesion Is Treated by Radiation Therapy

The dose required to control clinically positive lymph nodes that are included within the radiation portals depends on the size of the lymph node and, to some degree, on its histology. The dose for lymph nodes involved by lymphoepithelioma may be 500 cGy to 1000 cGy less than that for squamous cell carcinoma if the nodes show rapid early regression. The recommended minimum doses for lymph nodes of various sizes are given in Table 37-8.[62] The dose is not reduced when early complete regression occurs during fractionated therapy. The control rates at 180 cGy per fraction are not as good as those obtained with 200 cGy per fraction.[49]

The decision to add a neck dissection after irradiation for multiple positive nodes and bilateral lymph node disease is individualized and is based on the diameter of the largest node, node fixation, and number of clinically positive nodes in the neck. If clinically positive lymph nodes disappear completely during irradiation, the likelihood of control by irradiation alone is improved, and a neck dissection may be withheld.[7–9,42] However, it is usually safer to perform the neck dissection immediately after irradiation because detection of lymph node recurrence may be difficult, due to fibrosis of subcutaneous tissues of the neck and because of poor salvage of neck recurrence.[12,51]

If a neck dissection is to follow radiation therapy in patients with clinically positive lymph nodes, the preoperative dose varies with the size and location of the lymph node, fixation, and response to irradiation. Preoperative doses of 5000 cGy are sufficient for mobile lymph nodes 3 cm to 4 cm in size, but ≥6000 cGy is recommended for 5 cm to 6 cm nodes and for fixed nodes. Lymph nodes 7 cm to 8 cm are almost always fixed to adjacent structures and often require doses of 7000 cGy to 7500 cGy for the surgeon to achieve a complete resection. If the lymph node lies behind the plane of the spinal cord, electrons may be used to boost the dose after the primary fields have been reduced off the spinal cord after 4500 cGy to 5000 cGy.[52]

Another technique commonly used for boosting the dose to the neck mass after spinal cord tolerance has been reached and the treatment to the primary lesion has been completed is opposed anterior and posterior fields with wedges. The final dose to the neck node (not to the entire neck) may be 7000 cGy to 8000 cGy without exceeding the spinal cord tolerance (Fig. 37-6). The anterior and posterior wedge-pair technique is preferable to an appositional electron boost field because high-energy electron beams increase the skin and mucosal dose.

When the cervical lymph nodes are located superficially, sometimes within 1 cm from the skin or fixed to it, treatment with high-energy photon beams (≥6 MV) may underdose these nodes. Treatment should be initiated with ^{60}Co or 4 MV x-rays for the initial 4500 cGy to 5000 cGy, after which a higher-energy photon beam can be used to continue irradiation of the primary tumor if the neck nodes are clinically negative or if a neck dissection is planned to follow radiation therapy (Fig. 37-7). Parallel opposed 6 MV x-ray beams may adequately treat the upper neck nodes included in the primary treatment fields; however, the supraclavicular nodes in the *en face* low neck field may be underdosed with a 6 MV beam. Although electrons alone may be used to treat cervical nodes, it is preferable to combine them with photons because of the high surface dose with high electron energies. Use of both 20 MeV electrons and 17 MV x-rays is compared with treatment by 20 MeV electrons alone in Figure 37-8 in a patient with a lateralized lesion of the

TABLE 37–8
Radiation Dose Guidelines for Radiation Therapy Alone for Squamous Cell Carcinoma Metastatic to Cervical Lymph Nodes

	DOSE (cGy)	
NODE SIZE (CM)	1000 cGy/wk	900 cGy/wk
≤1.0	6000	6500
1.5–2.0	6500	7000
2.5–3.0	7000	7500
3.5–6.0	7500	8000

(*Million RR, Cassisi NJ: General principles for treatment of cancers in the head and neck: Radiation therapy. In Million RR, Cassisi NJ [eds]: Management of Head and Neck Cancer: A Multidisciplinary Approach, pp 77–90. Philadelphia, JB Lippincott, 1984*)

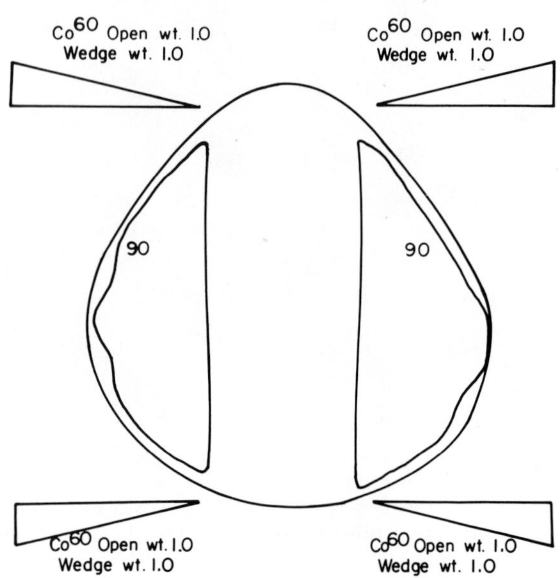

FIGURE 37–6. Dose distribution for anterior and posterior wedge ^{60}Co portals, both fields weighted 1.0.

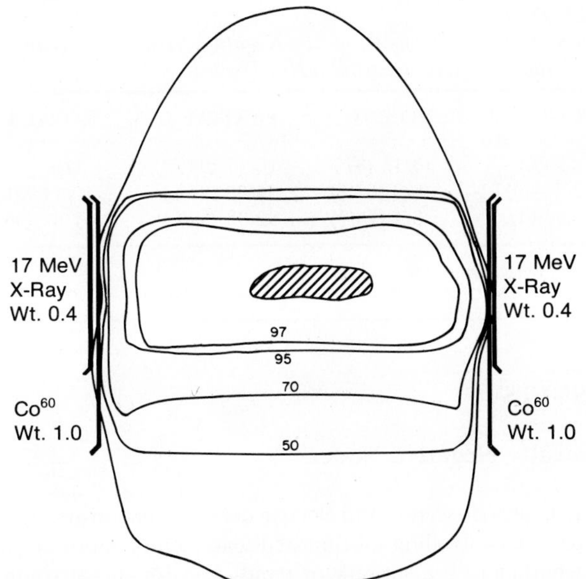

FIGURE 37–7. Dose distribution for parallel opposed ^{60}Co portals, each weighted 1.0, with reduced 17 MV x-ray portals, each weighted 0.4.

oropharynx.[13] The addition of the 17 MV x-rays to the 20 MeV electrons decreases the surface dose while still adequately irradiating the cervical nodes that are within the primary field. The addition of these x-ray beams also produces a dose distribution that is less affected by bone than that from the electron beam alone.

Large lymph nodes may not show much regression during the course of radiation therapy but often show a major regression from completion of treatment to the time that the patient returns for neck dissection, usually after 4 to 6 weeks. The mass frequently has a thick capsule that facilitates its removal at the time of neck dissection. It is preferable to add a neck dissection rather than treat with high-dose irradiation alone, because the rate of disease control is higher, neck fibrosis is less pronounced, cranial nerve XII palsy due to entrapment is less frequent, and attempted salvage of a patient with neck failure after high-dose irradiation alone is seldom successful and often morbid.

Patients with bilateral neck disease require individualized joint treatment planning by the radiation oncologist and the surgeon. If the disease is minimal on one side, then irradiation alone may be used to control the disease on that side of the neck, and a neck dissection may be used on the side with more disease. If major bilateral disease is present, bilateral neck dissection should follow radiation therapy.

The complications of neck irradiation include subcutaneous fibrosis and lymphedema of the larynx and face. The latter complication may be minimized by sparing an anterior strip of skin when designing the parallel opposed lateral portals used to include the primary lesion. Clothespins may be used to retract additional skin and subcutaneous tissues out of the radiation field and thereby further decrease the risk of edema (Fig. 37-9).[52] A 5 mm wide midline block in the *en face* low neck field may also diminish the likelihood of postirradiation edema. The probability of complications is directly related to the radiation dose with little, if any, morbidity observed with the doses used for elective irradiation of the neck.

Complications of neck treatment in patients who receive both radiation therapy and surgery to the primary site are essentially the same as those occurring after neck dissection. However, they occur with an increased incidence relevant to the radiation dose and extent of the surgery.

Management of the Neck After Incisional or Excisional Biopsy

Open biopsy of a clinically positive neck node before definitive treatment potentially spills tumor cells along tissue planes that may not be removed with a radical neck dissection. McGuirt and McCabe[47] reported that incisional/excisional biopsy of positive

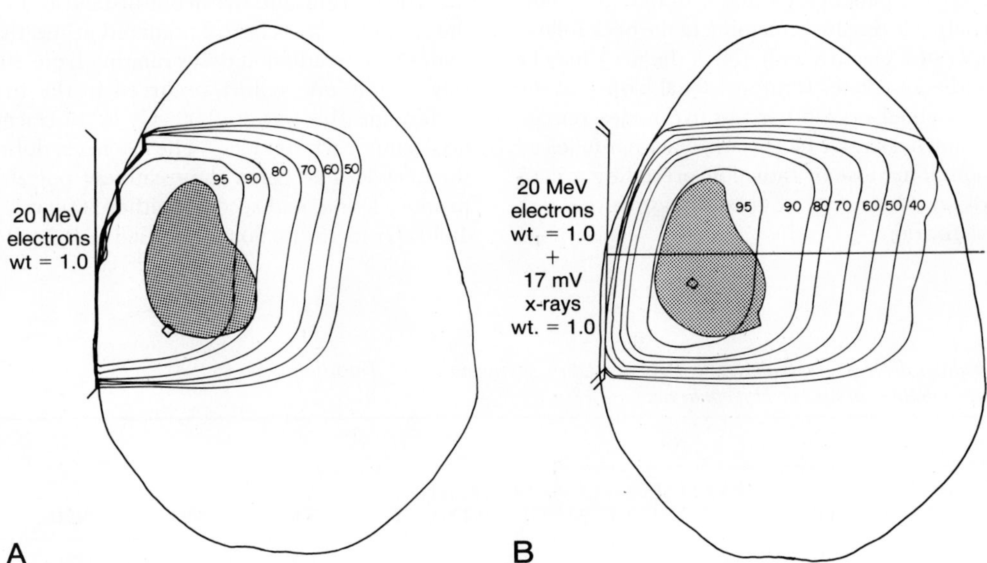

FIGURE 37–8. (**A**) Dose distribution for 20 MeV electrons, field size 8.5 cm × 8.5 cm, SSD 100 cm. (**B**) Dose distribution for 20 MeV electrons, field size 8.5 cm × 8.5 cm, and 17 MV x-rays, field size 7 cm × 7 cm. SSD 100 cm for both. The given doses are weighted 1 to 1. The addition of the 17 MV x-ray beam reduces the surface dose and gives a dose distribution that is affected less by bone. (Bova FJ: Treatment planning for irradiation. In Million RR, Cassisi NJ [eds]: Management of Head and Neck Cancer: A Multidisciplinary Approach, p 226. Philadelphia, JB Lippincott, 1984)

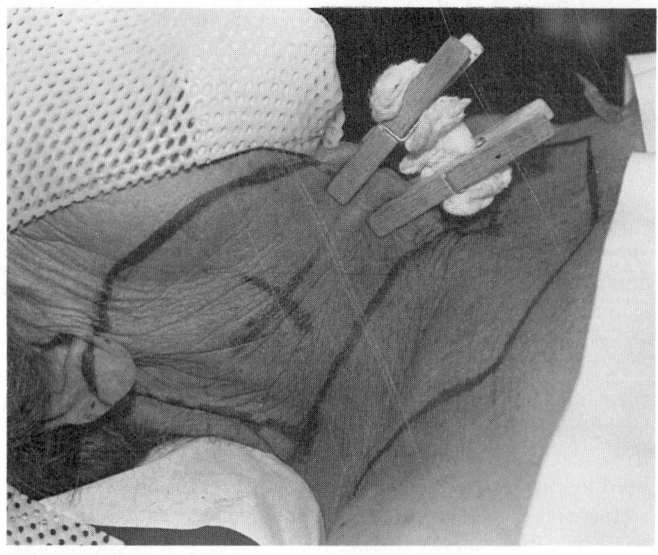

FIGURE 37–9. Parallel opposed portals with clothespins are used to increase the amount of tissue spared anteriorly. (Mendenhall WM, Million RR, Cassisi NJ: Int J Radiat Oncol Biol Phys 10:2223–2230, 1984)

neck nodes before definitive surgery increased the risk of neck failure and worsened the prognosis for patients with squamous cell carcinoma of the head and neck. Parsons and co-workers[71] reported the experience with incisional/excisional biopsy of positive neck nodes followed by irradiation as the initial step in the management of the patient. Following excisional biopsy of a single lymph node, radiation therapy alone to the primary lesion and to the neck resulted in a 96% rate of neck control. If residual disease occurred in the neck following biopsy, radiation therapy followed by neck dissection was more successful than irradiation alone for controlling neck disease (see Table 37-20).

If the primary lesion is to be treated surgically, the patient is treated with preoperative irradiation to the primary lesion and neck, followed by resection. If the primary lesion is to be managed with irradiation, the patient is treated with radiation therapy. If there is no palpable disease remaining in the neck following excisional biopsy of a positive node (NX), the neck may be managed with irradiation alone. If an incisional biopsy of the node has been performed or if other positive nodes remain following an excisional neck node biopsy, irradiation is followed by a neck dissection. The dose of radiation preceding a neck dissection depends on the amount of gross disease in the neck and the degree of fixation.[51]

TABLE 37–9
Control of Disease in the Clinically Negative Neck with Elective Neck Irradiation (No. Controlled/No. Treated)

RISK GROUP	NO ENI	PARTIAL ENI	TOTAL ENI
I (<20%)	13/15 (87%)	16/17 (94%)	1/1
II (20%–30%)	6/9 (67%)	34/38 (89%)	10/11 (91%)
III (>30%)	3/4 (75%)	32/33 (97%)	61/62 (98%)

ENI: elective neck irradiation
(Mendenhall WM, Million RR: Int J Radiat Oncol Biol Phys 12:741–746, 1986)

RESULTS

Clinically Negative Nodes

Elective neck dissection and elective neck irradiation are equally effective in controlling subclinical disease. The decision regarding whether to use surgery or irradiation for the purpose of electively treating the neck nodes depends largely on the method used to manage the primary lesion. Patients whose primary lesion is treated surgically may undergo an elective neck dissection, and those whose primary lesion is to be treated with radiation therapy should be considered for elective neck irradiation. Patients with a relatively early primary lesion and clinically negative nodes should be treated with one modality.

The results of elective neck irradiation at the University of Florida for patients with squamous cell carcinoma of the head and neck in whom the primary lesion was controlled are shown in Table 37-9.[48,50] Patients were divided into three risk categories based on the estimated risk of subclinical disease in the neck as follows: group I—low risk (<20% likelihood of occult disease); group II—moderate risk (20% to 30% risk of occult disease); and group III—high risk (>30% likelihood of occult disease). There were six neck failures (21%) in 28 patients who did not receive elective neck irradiation (ENI) and eight neck failures (5%) in 162 patients who received ENI. Of the eight failures in patients receiving ENI, two occurred within the irradiation fields, one at the field margin, and five in out-of-field areas. No correlation of the rate of tumor control occurred at the first-echelon lymph nodes with irradiation doses ranging from 4000 cGy to ≥ 5500 cGy.[48] Only one failure occurred in the first-echelon lymph nodes, and this was at 4800 cGy in 25 fractions using continuous-course irradiation.[48] The low neck, defined as that part of the neck located below the treatment portals used to treat the primary lesion, had received either 5000 cGy in 25 fractions or 4050 cGy in 15 fractions, specified at D_{max}. Both of these dose-

TABLE 37–10
Failure of Initial Ipsilateral Neck Treatment: 596 Patients with Carcinoma of the Tonsillar Fossa, Base of Tongue, Supraglottic Larynx, or Hypopharynx

	N0							
TREATMENT	NO TREATMENT	PARTIAL TREATMENT	COMPLETE TREATMENT	N1	N2A	N2B	N3A	N3B
Irradiation		15%	2%	15%	27%	27%	38%	34%
Surgery	55% (16/29)	35%	7%	11%	8%	23%	42%	41%
Combined		1/5	0/6	0	0	0	23%	25%

M.D. Anderson Hospital, 1948–1967
(Modified from Barkley HT Jr, Fletcher GH, Jesse RH, Lindberg RD: Am J Surg 124:462–467. 1972)

TABLE 37–11
*Five-Year Rate of Neck Control by 1983 AJCC Stage and Treatment (459 Patients; 593 Heminecks)**

	RT ALONE		RT + NECK DISSECTION		
STAGE	NO. OF HEMINECKS	CONTROL	NO. OF HEMINECKS	CONTROL	**SIGNIFICANCE**
N1	215	86%	38	93%	$P = 0.28$
N2A	29	79%	24	68%	$P = 0.6$
N2B	138	70%	80	91%	$P < 0.01$
N3A	29	33%	40	69%	$P < 0.01$

**Excludes 67 heminecks on which incisional or excisional biopsy was done before treatment.*
(Unpublished University of Florida data; patients treated 10/64–10/85, analysis 12/88 by Eric R. Ellis, M.D.)

fractionation protocols are equally effective in sterilizing subclinical disease in the low neck.[56]

No evidence suggests that elective irradiation to the neck is less effective for certain anatomic sites. If the primary lesion recurs, however, there is a renewed risk of lymphatic spread to the neck even after elective neck radiation has been administered because of the possibility of reseeding the neck lymphatics. In patients in whom primary failure occurs in addition to failure in the clinically negative nodes, the chances of surgical salvage are poor. In patients in whom the primary lesion is controlled and in whom failure develops in the initially negative neck, the chances of salvage with neck dissection are approximately 60%.

Clinically Positive Nodes

The incidence of treatment failure in the neck by N stage and treatment category has been reported by the M. D. Anderson Cancer Center (Table 37-10) and the University of Florida (Table 37-11).[6,51] In patients treated with combined modalities, radiation therapy precedes surgery when the primary site is to be treated with irradiation or when the node is fixed. Surgery precedes irradiation when the primary site is to be treated operatively and the nodes are resectable.

When the initial treatment is surgery, a neck dissection is sufficient treatment for patients with a single positive lymph node unless there is extracapsular spread of disease. Radiation therapy may be added for control of subclinical disease in the contralateral side of the neck (Table 37-12). The presence of multiple positive nodes in the surgical specimen is an indication for postoperative irradiation of the neck, especially when positive nodes are found at more than one level.[37,74] The postoperative dose prescribed is usually 6000 cGy in 30 fractions to 6500 cGy in 35 fractions over 6 to 7 weeks for patients with negative margins; higher doses may be prescribed when residual disease is present in the neck.[1,44,59] If radiation therapy is to be added following surgery, it is usually initiated within 4 to 6 weeks after the operation, although it has been reported that a delay to 10 weeks is not associated with an increased risk of neck failure.[1]

TABLE 37–12
Cervical Metastasis Appearing in the Contralateral N0 Neck: 596 Patients with Carcinoma of the Tonsillar Fossa, Base of Tongue, Supraglottic Larynx, or Hypopharynx

	STAGE				
TREATMENT	N0	N1	N2A	N2B	N3A
Irradiation	4%	2%	9%	7%	0%
Surgery	25%	17%	23%	43%	33%
Combined	0%	0%	0%	11%	0%

(M.D. Anderson Hospital, 1948–1967)
(Modified from Barkley HT Jr, Fletcher GH, Jesse RH, Lindberg RD: Am J Surg 124:462–467, 1972)

Table 37-13 shows the rate of control for neck nodes treated with radiation therapy alone as a function of node size, treatment scheme, and dose. Radiation therapy alone is sufficient for patients with N1 (up to 2 cm) disease as long as the fraction size (200 cGy) and the total dose are sufficient.[49] Irradiation combined with neck dissection has provided better rates of disease control than irradiation alone for patients with more advanced neck disease. The rate of neck disease control for patients treated with twice-daily radiation alone or followed by neck dissection is depicted in Figure 37-10 and shows a significant improvement in the control rates when neck dissection was added in selected cases.[68,69] At least 5000 cGy should be given preoperatively to the lymph nodes, although doses vary according to the size and degree of fixation of the lymph node. For example, large, fixed lymph nodes require 7000 cGy to 7500 cGy of preoperative radiation (Table 37-14).[52] The likelihood of disease control in each side of the neck treated with irradiation and neck dissection is decreased when the node is fixed before treatment or when residual tumor is found in the pathologic specimen (Tables 37-15 and 37-16). There is no difference in the rate of control as a function of the interval between radiation therapy and neck dissection when patients operated on within 6 weeks of completing radiation therapy are compared with those undergoing neck dissection more than 6 weeks after irradiation.[51] In the event of a subsequent local recurrence, prior combined treatment of the neck does not diminish the chance of successful surgical salvage of the patient.[53] The likelihood of disease control at the primary site was not found to be related to neck stage at diagnosis in patients treated with radiation alone or followed by neck dissection at the University of Florida.[54]

Clinically Positive Nodes with Incisional or Excisional Biopsy

Patients who present following an incisional or excisional biopsy of a metastatic lymph node prior to referral do not have an increased risk of neck failure or a decreased cure rate if radiation therapy is the next step in their treatment.[71] The likelihood of control and the cure rate are probably diminished

TABLE 37–13
Lymph Node Disease Control by Radiation Treatment Technique (No. Controlled/No. Treated)

NODE SIZE (CM)	CONTINUOUS COURSE	SPLIT COURSE	EXCLUDED*	TOTAL
<1.0	5/5	2/2	1/1	8/8
1.0	29/35 (83%)	19/23 (83%)	3/4	51/62 (82%)
1.5–2.0	43/49 (88%)	20/24 (83%)	5/9	68/82 (83%)
2.5–3.0	14/19 (74%)	10/18 (56%)	0/3	24/40 (60%)
3.5–6.0	14/20 (70%)	10/17 (59%)	0/1	24/38 (63%)
≥7.0	0/2	0/5	0/1	0/8

*<5000 cGy for nodes ≤ 1.0 cm and <5500 cGy for nodes ≥ 1.5 cm
(Mendenhall WM, Million RR, Bova FJ: Int J Radiat Oncol Biol Phys 10:639–643, 1984)

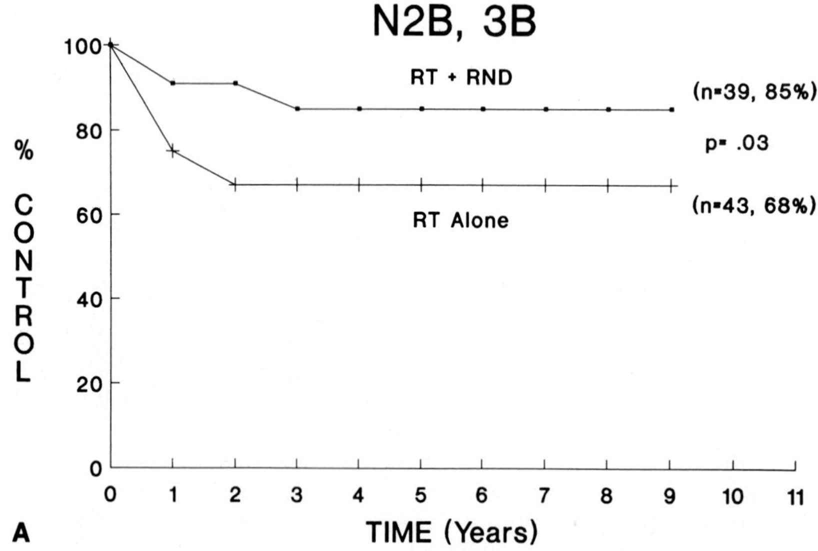

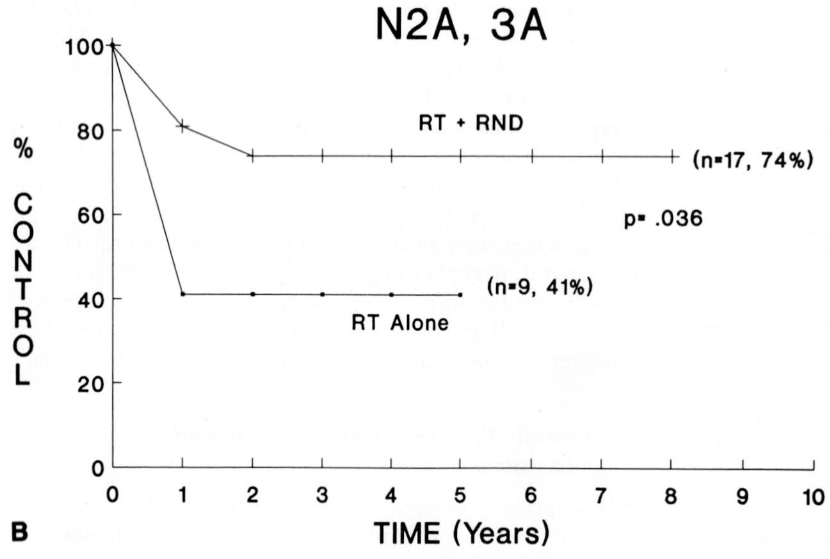

FIGURE 37–10. Rate of neck disease control (life-table method[18]) for patients treated with twice-daily irradiation alone (RT) or combined with neck dissection (RT + RND) for clinically positive neck nodes. (**A**) N2B, N3B. (**B**) N2A, N3A. (Parsons JT, Mendenhall WM, Cassisi NJ, et al: Head Neck 11:400–404, 1989)

TABLE 37–14
Cervical Lymph Node Disease Control with Radiation Therapy Followed by Neck Dissection, with Primary Lesion Managed Initially by Radiation Therapy (No. Controlled/No. Treated)

MAXIMUM NODE DIAMETER (CM)	MINIMUM NODE DOSE (cGy)			
	<5000	5000–5999	6000–6999	≥7000
<3	5/5	1/2	5/5	3/3
3–4	6/8	10/14	9/9	5/7
5–6	4/7	5/5	7/8	4/4
7–8	2/3	2/4	4/6	3/4
≥9	No data	1/1	2/4	0/1

Patients treated with once-a-day fractionation, continuous- or split-course technique; 91 patients, 100 heminecks (University of Florida, October 1964 to December 1982; analysis, December 1984 by W.M. Mendenhall, M.D.)

if an operation without prior radiation therapy follows incisional or excisional biopsy of a metastatic neck node because of the risk during the biopsy procedure of disseminating tumor cells into tissues that are not removed by a neck dissection.[47]

CERVICAL LYMPH NODE METASTASIS WITH UNKNOWN PRIMARY TUMOR

In a small percentage of patients who present with enlarged cervical lymph nodes, the primary lesion cannot be found, even after extensive evaluation. Patients who present with enlarged lymph nodes in the upper neck have a good prognosis when treated aggressively, compared with those who present with enlarged lymph nodes in the low internal jugular chain or supraclavicular fossa. The latter group is much more likely to have a primary lesion located below the clavicles, which carries with it a much worse prognosis. The majority of patients are found to have either squamous cell carcinoma or poorly differentiated carcinoma. Those with adenocarcinoma almost always have a primary lesion below the clavicles, although if the nodes are located in the upper neck, one must exclude salivary gland, thyroid, or parathyroid primary tumor. This section deals with patients presenting with squamous cell or poorly differentiated carcinoma in the upper or middle neck.

Patients should be evaluated with a thorough physical examination including careful evaluation of the head and neck. A needle biopsy, an incisional biopsy, or, if possible, an excisional biopsy of a small solitary node should be performed. Following chest roentgenography, a CT or MRI scan of the head and neck is obtained to detect an unknown primary lesion arising from the mucosa of the head and neck. Direct laryngoscopy and examination under anesthesia are performed with blind biopsies of the nasopharynx, tonsils, base of the tongue, and pyriform sinuses, and of any abnormalities noted on CT/MRI or suspicious mucosal lesions noted at laryngoscopy. However, if the primary lesion is not found on repeated physical examination by multiple examiners or is not found on the CT or MRI scan of the head and neck, it is unlikely that direct laryngoscopy with blind biopsies will locate the primary lesion. The diagnostic evaluation for the patient with cervical metastasis from an unknown head and neck primary lesion is summarized in Table 37-17.

Some patients may be cured with treatment directed only to the involved area of the neck; however, we usually irradiate the nasopharynx, oropharynx, hypopharynx, and larynx as well as both sides of the neck. It is not necessary to irradiate the oral cavity unless the patient presents with submandibular adenopathy, in which case we either do a neck dissection and observe the patient or irradiate the oral cavity and oropharynx and do not irradiate the nasopharynx, larynx, or hypopharynx. Patients are treated with parallel opposed fields at 180 cGy per fraction to a midline dose of 5500 cGy to 6000 cGy with reduction off the

TABLE 37–15
Control of Disease in the Neck as a Function of Node Mobility (109 Patients; 121 Heminecks)

SIZE (CM)	PROPORTION OF FIXED NODES	NO. HEMINECKS CONTROLLED/ NO. TREATED	
		MOBILE OR TETHERED	FIXED
<3	1/23	19/22 (86%)	1/1
3–4	4/44 (9%)	33/40 (83%)	2/4 (50%)
5–6	9/27 (33%)	17/18 (94%)	6/9 (67%)
7–8	10/21 (48%)	8/11 (73%)	5/10 (50%)
≥9	3/6 (50%)	2/3 (67%)	1/3 (33%)

(Mendenhall WM, Million RR, Cassisi NJ: Int J Radiat Oncol Biol Phys 12:733–740, 1986)

TABLE 37–16
Neck Disease Control as a Function of Pathologic Findings in Neck Dissection Specimen (108 Patients; 120 Evaluable Heminecks)*

SIZE (CM)	PROPORTION WITH POSITIVE SPECIMEN	NO. HEMINECKS CONTROLLED/NO. TREATED	
		NEGATIVE SPECIMEN	POSITIVE SPECIMEN
<3	10/23 (43%)	13/13 (100%)	7/10 (70%)
3–4	22/43 (51%)	20/21 (95%)	14/22 (64%)
5–6	10/27 (37%)	17/17 (100%)	6/10 (60%)
7–8	12/21 (57%)	8/9 (89%)	5/12 (42%)
≥9	4/6 (67%)	2/2 (100%)	1/4 (25%)

** One patient was excluded because data were unavailable.*
(Mendenhall WM, Million RR, Cassisi NJ: Int J Radiat Oncol Biol Phys 12:733–740, 1986)

TABLE 37–17
Diagnostic Workup for Cervical Lymph Node Metastases: Unknown Primary Tumor

GENERAL

History

Physical examination
- Careful examination of the neck and supraclavicular regions
- Examination of oral cavity, pharynx, and larynx (indirect laryngoscopy)

RADIOGRAPHIC STUDIES

Chest roentgenogram

Computed tomography or magnetic resonance imaging scans of head and neck (special attention to nasopharynx, paranasal sinuses, pharynx, and larynx)

Upper gastrointestinal series and barium enema (in patients with adenocarcinoma involving supraclavicular lymph nodes)

LABORATORY STUDIES

Complete blood cell count

Blood chemistry profile

Urinalysis

DIRECT LARYNGOSCOPY AND BLIND BIOPSIES

Nasopharynx, both tonsils, base of tongue, both pyriform sinuses, and any suspicious or abnormal mucosal areas

INCISIONAL/EXCISIONAL BIOPSY OF CERVICAL LYMPH NODE

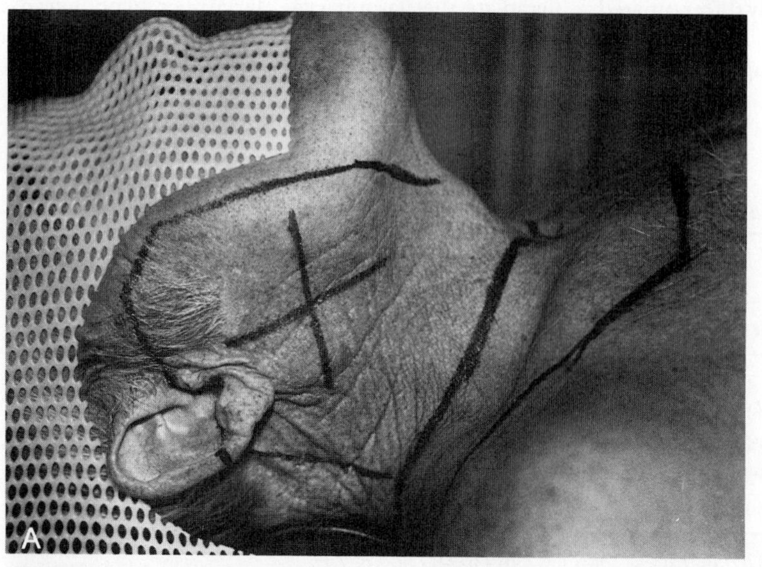

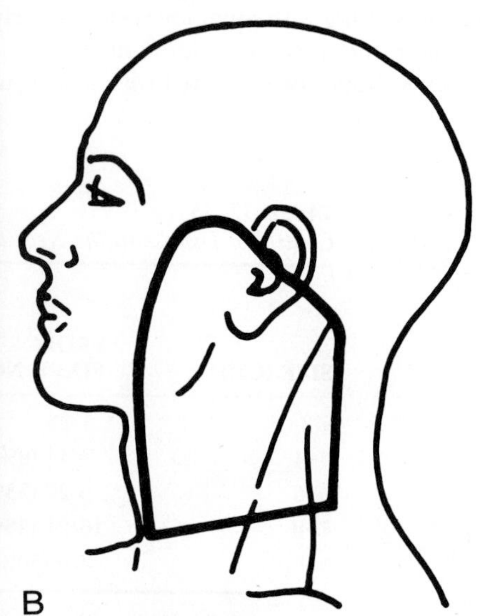

FIGURE 37–11. Parallel opposed lateral fields are used to treat an unknown head and neck primary lesion. A strip of skin is spared anteriorly over the larynx, and clothespins are used to increase the amount of unirradiated tissue in this area.

TABLE 37–18
Metastatic Cervical Lymph Nodes, Unknown Primary: Location of Primary Lesion Appearing After Treatment (184 Patients)

	TYPE OF TREATMENT		
LOCATION	SURGERY	RADIATION THERAPY	COMBINATION THERAPY
Hypopharynx	6	1	1
Tonsil or faucial arch	4	0	1
Base of tongue, valleculum	4	0	0
Oral cavity, salivary glands	2	2	0
Nasopharynx	2	0	0
Maxillary antrum	0	0	1
Aryepiglottic fold, epiglottis	1	0	1
Cervical esophagus	1	0	0
Thyroid	1	0	0
Total head and neck	21/104 (20%)*	3/52 (6%)†‡	4/28 (14%)‡
Below clavicle	5	3	1

** Primary lesion was subsequently controlled in 14/21 (8 by radiation therapy, 6 by surgery)*
† Portals covered Waldeyer's ring in 45/52
‡ Primary lesion was controlled in 2/7 (by surgery).
(Jesse RH, Perez CA, Fletcher GH: Cancer 31:854–859, 1973)

spinal cord at 4500 cGy tumor dose (Fig. 37-11). The lower neck is treated through a separate *en face* anterior field. If there is a suspected primary site of focus, an additional 500 cGy may be delivered to that site, particularly if a total dose of 5500 cGy has been selected. Management of the neck depends on the extent and location of the adenopathy.

The location of the primary lesion as a function of the type of treatment is given in Table 37-18 for a series of patients at M. D. Anderson Cancer Center.[34] It is noteworthy that in patients treated with surgery alone, a primary lesion appeared in the head and neck in only 20%. It is probable that the percentage of patients who subsequently developed a "local recurrence" would have been higher if the data had been analyzed by the actuarial method. The failure rate of the initial treatment in the treated side of the neck as a function of the treatment group is given in Table 37-19. When the primary lesion appeared, the survival rate was 50% lower than when the primary lesion did not appear after treatment of the neck. The absolute survival at 3 years is shown in Table 37-20 as a function of treatment group and disease stage.

Carlson and associates reported their experience with 120 patients with involved cervical lymph nodes, unknown primary tumor, 93 of whom were treated with curative intent.[15] Twenty patients received radiation therapy to the neck only, 26 to the nasopharynx, oropharynx, and neck, and 47 to the nasopharynx, oropharynx, and hypopharynx as well as to the neck. In 86 of 93 patients (92.5%), there was eventual control of disease above the clavicles. Fourteen patients later developed tumor at a primary site or recurrence of disease in the neck; in nine patients, the recurrent disease was located in areas not previously irradiated. Of 73 patients in whom the nasopharynx was irradiated with 5000 cGy, one primary tumor developed at this site. Of the 93 patients, 22 died of cancer and 36 died of other causes.

The main complication of radiation therapy for patients treated for an unknown head and neck primary tumor is xerostomia. The complications of treatment of the neck, which have been discussed previously, depend on whether a neck dissection is added.

TABLE 37–19
Metastatic Cervical Lymph Nodes, Unknown Primary: Failure of Initial Treatment in Treated Side of Neck (184 Patients)

	TYPE OF TREATMENT		
STAGE	SURGERY	RADIATION THERAPY	COMBINATION THERAPY
NX–N1	6/45 (13%)	2/12 (17%)	0/6
N2–N3	19/59 (32%)	9/40 (22%)	4/22 (18%)

(Jesse RH, Perez CA, Fletcher GH: Cancer 31:854–859, 1973)

TABLE 37–20
Metastatic Cervical Lymph Nodes, Unknown Primary: Three-Year Disease-Free Absolute Survival

	TYPE OF TREATMENT		
STAGE	SURGERY	RADIATION THERAPY	COMBINATION THERAPY
NX	31/39 (79%)	8/9	3/3
N1	4/6	1/3	1/3
N2	10/22 (45%)	3/4	5/9
N3	14/37 (38%)	13/36 (36%)	4/13 (31%)
Total	59/104* (57%)	25/52† (48%)	13/28† (46%)

(M.D. Anderson Hospital; 184 patients, July 1948–June 1968)
** Salvage in eight patients by radiation therapy and in six patients by surgery.*
† Salvage in one patient by surgery
(Jesse RH, Perez CA, Fletcher GH: Cancer 31:854–859, 1973)

REFERENCES

1. Amdur RJ, Parsons JT, Mendenhall WM, Million RR, Stringer SP, Cassisi NJ: Postoperative irradiation for squamous cell carcinoma of the head and neck: An analysis of treatment results and complications. Int J Radiat Oncol Biol Phys 16:25–36, 1989
2. American Joint Committee on Cancer: Manual for Staging of Cancer, 2nd ed, pp 25–54. Philadelphia, JB Lippincott, 1983
3. American Joint Committee on Cancer: Manual for Staging of Cancer, 3rd ed, p 29. Philadelphia, JB Lippincott, 1988
4. Ash CL: Oral cancer: A twenty-five year study. Am J Roentgenol Radium Ther Nucl Med 87:417–430, 1962
5. Barker JL, Fletcher GH: Time, dose and tumor volume relationships in megavoltage irradiation of squamous cell carcinomas of the retromolar trigone and anterior tonsillar pillar. Int J Radiat Oncol Biol Phys 2:407–414, 1977
6. Barkley HT Jr, Fletcher GH, Jesse RH, et al: Management of cervical lymph node metastases in squamous cell carcinoma of the tonsillar fossa, base of tongue, supraglottic larynx, and hypopharynx. Am J Surg 124:462–467, 1972
7. Bartelink H: Prognostic value of the regression rate of neck node metastases during radiotherapy. Int J Radiat Oncol Biol Phys 9:993–996, 1983
8. Bartelink H, Breur K, Hart G: Radiotherapy of lymph node metastases in patients with squamous cell carcinoma of the head and neck region. Int J Radiat Oncol Biol Phys 8:983–989, 1982
9. Bataini JP, Bernier J, Jaulerry C, Brunin F, Pontvert D, Lave C: Impact of neck node radioresponsiveness on the regional control probability in patients with oropharynx and pharyngolarynx cancers managed by definitive radiotherapy. Int J Radiat Oncol Biol Phys 13:817–824, 1987
10. Beahrs OH, Devine KD, Henson SW Jr: Treatment of carcinoma of the tongue: End-results in one hundred sixty-eight cases. AMA Arch Surg 79:399–403, 1959
11. Berger DS, Fletcher GH, Lindberg RD, et al: Elective irradiation of the neck lymphatics for squamous cell carcinomas of the nasopharynx and oropharynx. Am J Roentgenol Radium Ther Nucl Med 111:66–72, 1971
12. Bernier J, Bataini JP: Regional outcome in oropharyngeal and pharyngolaryngeal cancer treated with high dose per fraction radiotherapy: Analysis of neck disease response in 1646 cases. Radiother Oncol 6:87–103, 1986
13. Bova FJ: Treatment planning for irradiation of head and neck cancer. In Million RR, Cassisi NJ (eds): Management of Head and Neck Cancer: A Multidisciplinary Approach, pp 209–230. Philadelphia, JB Lippincott, 1984
14. Cady B, Catlin D: Epidermoid carcinoma of the gum. A 20-year survey. Cancer 23:551–569, 1969
15. Carlson LS, Fletcher GH, Oswald MJ: Guidelines for radiotherapeutic techniques for cervical metastasis from an unknown primary. Int J Radiat Oncol Biol Phys 12:2101–2110, 1986
16. Chen KY, Fletcher GH: Malignant tumors of the nasopharynx. Radiology 99:165–171, 1971
17. Chung CK, Rahman SM, Lim ML, et al: Squamous cell carcinoma of the hard palate. Int J Radiat Oncol Biol Phys 5:191–196, 1979
18. Cutler SJ, Ederer F: Maximum utilization of the life table method in analyzing survival. J Chronic Dis 8:699–712, 1958
19. Del Regato JA, Spjut HJ: Ackerman and del Regato's Cancer: Diagnosis, Treatment, and Prognosis, ed 5, pp 264, 281, 341–342, 345. St. Louis, CV Mosby, 1977
20. Eneroth CM, Hjertman L, Moberger G: Squamous cell carcinomas of the palate. Acta Otolaryngol (Stockh) 73:418–427, 1972
21. Fische U: Lymphographische untersuchungen uber das zervicale lymphsystem. Fortschritte der Hals-Nasen-Ohren Heilkunde, vol 14, pp 53–162. Basel, S Karger, 1966
22. Fletcher GH: Elective irradiation of subclinical disease in cancers of the head and neck. Cancer 29:1450–1454, 1972
23. Fletcher GH, Jesse RH, Healey JE Jr, Thoma GW Jr: Oropharynx. In MacComb WS, Fletcher GH (eds): Cancer of the Head and Neck, pp 179–212. Baltimore, Williams & Wilkins, 1967
24. Fletcher GH, Jesse RH, Lindberg RD, et al: The place of radiotherapy in the management of the squamous cell carcinoma of the supraglottic larynx. Am J Roentgenol Radium Ther Nucl Med 108:19–26, 1970
25. Fletcher GH, MacComb WS, Braun EJ: Analysis of sites and causes of treatment failures in squamous cell carcinomas of the oral cavity. Am J Roentgenol Radium Ther Nucl Med 83:405–411, 1960
26. Frazell EL, Lucas JC Jr: Cancer of the tongue: Report of the management of 1554 patients. Cancer 15:1085–1099, 1962
27. Goffinet DR, Gilbert EH, Weller SA, et al: Irradiation of clinically uninvolved cervical lymph nodes. Can J Otolaryngol 4:927–933, 1975
28. Golder SL: Carcinoma of the supraglottic larynx. 10th Annual Radiation Therapy Clinical Research Seminar, April 24–26, 1980, pp 237–247. Gainesville, FL, Division of Radiation Therapy, University of Florida, 1981
29. Hardingham M, Dalley VM, Shaw HJ: Cancer of the floor of the mouth: Clinical features and results of treatment. Clin Oncol 3:227–246, 1977
30. Ho JHC: An epidemiologic and clinical study of nasopharyngeal carcinoma. Int J Radiat Oncol Biol Phys 4:181–198, 1978
31. Horiuchi J, Adachi T: Some considerations on radiation therapy of tongue cancer. Cancer 28:335–339, 1971
32. Jesse RH, Barkley HT Jr, Lindberg RD, et al: Cancer of the oral cavity: Is elective neck dissection beneficial? Am J Surg 120:505–508, 1970
33. Jesse RH, Fletcher GH: Metastases in cervical lymph nodes from oropharyngeal carcinoma. Treatment and results. Am J Roentgenol Radium Ther Nucl Med 90:990–996, 1963
34. Jesse RH, Perez CA, Fletcher GH: Cervical lymph node metastasis: Unknown primary cancer. Cancer 31:854–859, 1973
35. Kaplan R, Million RR, Cassisi NJ: Carcinoma of the tonsil: Results of radical irradiation with surgery reserved for radiation failure. Laryngoscope 87:600–607, 1977
36. Kremen AJ: Results of surgical treatment of cancer of the tongue. Surgery 39:49–53, 1956
37. LeFebvre JL, Castelain B, De La Torre JC, et al: Lymph node invasion in hypopharynx and lateral epilarynx carcinoma: A prognostic factor. Head Neck Surg 10:14–18, 1987
38. Lindberg RD: Distribution of cervical lymph node metastases from squamous cell carcinoma of the upper respiratory and digestive tracts. Cancer 29:1446–1449, 1972
39. Lindberg RD, Barkley HT Jr, Jesse RH, et al: Evolution of the clinically negative neck in patients with squamous cell carcinoma of the faucial arch. Am J Roentgenol Radium Ther Nucl Med 111:60–65, 1971
40. Lindberg RD, Jesse RH: Treatment of cervical lymph node metastases from primary lesions of the oropharynx, supraglottic larynx, and hypopharynx. Am J Roentgenol Radium Ther Nucl Med 102:132–137, 1968
41. MacComb WS, Healey JE Jr, McGraw JP, et al: Hypopharynx and cervical esophagus. In MacComb WS, Fletcher GH (eds): Cancer of the Head and Neck, pp 213–240. Baltimore, Williams & Wilkins, 1967
42. Maciejewski B: Regression rate of metastatic neck lymph nodes after radiation treatment as a prognostic factor for local control. Radiother Oncol 8:301–308, 1987
43. Mancuso AA, Hanafee WN: Computed Tomography and Magnetic Resonance Imaging of the Head and Neck, 2nd ed. Baltimore, Williams & Wilkins, 1985
44. Marcus RB Jr, Million RR, Cassisi NJ: Postoperative irradiation for squamous cell carcinoma of the head and neck: Analysis of time-dose factors related to control above the clavicles. Int J Radiat Oncol Biol Phys 5:1943–1949, 1979
45. Martin CL, Craffey EJ: Cancer of the gums. Am J Roentgenol Radium Ther Nucl Med 67:420–427, 1952
46. McGuirt WF, McCabe BF: Significance of node biopsy before definitive treatment of cervical metastatic carcinoma. Laryngoscope 88:594–597, 1973
47. McGuirt WF, McCabe BF: Bilateral radical neck dissections. Arch Otolaryngol 106:427–429, 1980

48. Mendenhall WM, Million RR: Elective neck irradiation for squamous cell carcinoma of the head and neck: Analysis of time-dose factors and causes of failure. Int J Radiat Oncol Biol Phys 12:741–746, 1986
49. Mendenhall WM, Million RR, Bova FJ: Analysis of time-dose factors in clinically positive neck nodes treated with irradiation alone in squamous cell carcinoma of the head and neck. Int J Radiat Oncol Biol Phys 10:639–643, 1984
50. Mendenhall WM, Million RR, Cassisi NJ: Elective neck irradiation in squamous cell carcinoma of the head and neck. Head Neck Surg 3:15–20, 1980
51. Mendenhall WM, Million RR, Cassisi NJ: Squamous cell carcinoma of the supraglottic larynx treated with radical irradiation: Analysis of treatment parameters and results. Int J Radiat Oncol Biol Phys 10:2223–2230, 1984
52. Mendenhall WM, Million RR, Cassisi NJ: Squamous cell carcinoma of the head and neck treated with radiation therapy: The role of neck dissection for clinically positive neck nodes. Int J Radiat Oncol Biol Phys 12:733–740, 1989
53. Mendenhall WM, Parsons JT, Amdur RJ, Cassisi NJ, Million RR: Squamous cell carcinoma of the head and neck treated with radiotherapy: Does planned neck dissection reduce the chance for successful surgical management of subsequent local recurrence? Head Neck Surg 10:302–304, 1988
54. Mendenhall WM, Parsons JT, Amdur RJ, et al: Squamous cell carcinoma of the head and neck treated with radiation therapy: The impact of neck stage on local control. Int J Radiat Oncol Biol Phys 14:249–252, 1988
55. Mendenhall WM, Parsons JT, Brant TA, et al: Is elective neck treatment indicated for T2 NO squamous cell carcinoma of the glottic larynx? Radiother Oncol 14:199–202, 1989
56. Mendenhall WM, Parsons JT, Million RR: Elective lower neck irradiation: 5000 cGy/25 fractions versus 4050 cGy/15 fractions. Int J Radiat Oncol Biol Phys 15:439–440, 1988
57. Mendenhall WM, Parsons JT, Stringer SP, Cassisi NJ, Million RR: T1–T2 vocal cord carcinoma: A basis for comparing the results of radiotherapy and surgery. Head Neck Surg 10:373–377, 1988
58. Million RR: Elective neck irradiation for TxNO squamous carcinoma of the oral tongue and floor of mouth. Cancer 34:149–155, 1974
59. Million RR: Squamous cell carcinoma of the head and neck: Combined therapy: Surgery and postoperative irradiation. Int J Radiat Oncol Biol Phys 5:2161–2162, 1979
60. Million RR, Cassisi NJ: Radical irradiation for carcinoma of the pyriform sinus. Laryngoscope 91:439–450, 1981
61. Million RR, Cassisi NJ: General principles for the treatment of cancers in the head and neck: Selection of treatment for the primary site and for the neck. In Million RR, Cassisi NJ (eds): Management of Head and Neck Cancer: A Multidisciplinary Approach, pp 43–62. Philadelphia, JB Lippincott, 1984
62. Million RR, Cassisi NJ: General principles for treatment of cancers in the head and neck: Radiation therapy. In Million RR, Cassisi NJ (eds): Management of Head and Neck Cancer: A Multidisciplinary Approach, pp 77–90. Philadelphia, JB Lippincott, 1984
63. Million RR, Cassisi NJ, Clark JR: Cancer of the head and neck. In DeVita VT Jr, Hellman S, Rosenberg SA (eds): Cancer: Principles and Practice of Oncology, 3rd ed. pp 488–590. Philadelphia, JB Lippincott, 1989
64. Million RR, Fletcher GH, Jesse RH Jr: Evaluation of elective irradiation of the neck for squamous cell carcinoma of the nasopharynx, tonsillar fossa, and base of tongue. Radiology 80:973–988, 1963
65. Moench HC, Phillips TL: Carcinoma of the nasopharynx. Review of 146 patients with emphasis on radiation dose and time factors. Am J Surg 124:515–518, 1972
66. Ogura JH, Biller HF, Wette R: Elective neck dissection for pharyngeal and laryngeal cancers. An evaluation. Ann Otol Rhinol Laryngol 80:646–651, 1971
67. Parsons JT: Time-dose-volume relationships in radiotherapy. In Million RR, Cassisi NJ (eds): Management of Head and Neck Cancer: A Multidisciplinary Approach, pp 137–172. Philadelphia, JB Lippincott, 1984
68. Parsons JT, Mendenhall WM, Cassisi NJ, et al: Hyperfractionation for head and neck cancer. Int J Radiat Oncol Biol Phys 14:649–658, 1988
69. Parsons JT, Mendenhall WM, Cassisi NJ, et al: Neck dissection after twice-a-day radiotherapy: Morbidity and recurrence rates. Head Neck 11:400–404, 1989
70. Parsons JT, Million RR, Cassisi NJ: Carcinoma of the base of the tongue: Results of radical irradiation with surgery reserved for irradiation failure. Laryngoscope 92:689–696, 1982
71. Parsons JT, Million RR, Cassisi NJ: The influence of excisional or incisional biopsy of metastatic neck nodes on the management of head and neck cancer. Int J Radiat Oncol Biol Phys 11:1447–1454, 1985
72. Putney FJ: Elective versus delayed neck dissection in cancer of the larynx. Surg Gynecol Obstet 112:736–742, 1961
73. Razack MS, Baffi R, Sako K: Bilateral radical neck dissection. Cancer 47:197–199, 1981
74. Richard JM, Sancho-Garnier H, Micheau C, et al: Prognostic factors in cervical lymph node metastasis in upper respiratory and digestive tract carcinomas: Study of 1,713 cases during a 15-year period. Laryngoscope 97:97–101, 1987
75. Rolander TL, Everts EC, Shumrick DA: Carcinoma of the tonsil: A planned combined therapy approach. Laryngoscope 81:1199–1207, 1971
76. Rouviere H: Anatomy of the Human Lymphatic System. Trans MJ Tobias, pp 1–28, 77–78. Ann Arbor, MI, Edwards Brothers, 1938
77. Southwick HW: Elective neck dissection for intraoral cancer. JAMA 217:454–455, 1971
78. Southwick HW, Slaughter DP, Trevino ET: Elective neck dissection for intraoral cancer. AMA Arch Surg 80:905–909, 1960
79. Spiro RH, Strong EW: Discontinuous partial glossectomy and radical neck dissection in selected patients with epidermoid carcinoma of the mobile tongue. Am J Surg 126:544–546, 1973

38

○ ○ ○ • • •

Lung

Bahman Emami
Carlos A. Perez

ANATOMY

The right lung is composed of three lobes: upper, middle, and lower.[21] The lobes are separated from one another by two fissures—the oblique or major and the horizontal or minor fissure. The left lung is composed of two lobes, which are separated by a single fissure.[21] The lingular portion of the left upper lobe corresponds to the middle lobe on the right. The trachea enters the superior mediastinum and bifurcates approximately at the level of the fifth thoracic vertebra.[92] The hila of the lungs contain the bronchi, pulmonary arteries and veins, various branches from the pulmonary plexus, bronchial arteries and veins, and lymphatics.[92]

Lymphatics

The lung has a rich network of lymphatic vessels throughout its loose interstitial connective tissue, ultimately draining into the various lymph node stations, which may be divided into the following groups[5]:

I: Intrapulmonary nodes (along the secondary bronchi)
II: Bronchopulmonary nodes (hilar nodes)
III: Mediastinal nodes
IV: Supraclavicular and scalene nodes

The intrapulmonary lymph nodes may be related to segmental bronchi or lie in the bifurcation of the branches of the pulmonary artery (Fig. 38-1).

The bronchopulmonary lymph nodes, situated either alongside the lower portions of the main bronchi (hilar lymph nodes) or at the bifurcations of the main bronchi into lobar bronchi (interlobar nodes),[20] from a radiotherapeutic viewpoint comprise the hilar nodes (see Fig. 38-1).

The mediastinal lymph nodes are divided in two groups: (1) superior, located above the bifurcation of the trachea (carina), including the upper paratracheal, pretracheal, retrotracheal, lower paratracheal nodes (azygos nodes) and a group of nodes located in the aortic window, and (2) inferior, situated in the subcarinal region and inferior mediastinum (see Fig. 38-1), including the subcarinal, paraesophageal, and pulmonary ligament nodes.

Routes of Efferent Lymph Flow

The drainage for each pulmonary lobe is shown in Fig. 38-2.[175] The lymph from the right upper lobe flows to the tracheobronchial lymph nodes.

The lymph from the left upper lobe flows not only to the venous angle of the same side but to the venous angle of the opposite superior mediastinum. The right and left lower lobe lymphatics drain into the subcarinal nodes and from there to the right superior mediastinum (the left lower lobe also may drain into the left superior mediastinum) and directly into the inferior mediastinal lymph nodes.

EPIDEMIOLOGY

The incidence of lung cancer is increasing rapidly in both sexes.[246] It is estimated that lung cancer was diagnosed in 101,000 males and 60,000 females in the United States in 1991. About 90% of these patients die of the disease.[4]

Although the incidence of lung cancer ranks fourth after breast, colon, and uterus cancer in females, breast cancer and lung carcinoma are the leading causes of death in women (death rate, 18% for each).[246] The male–female ratio for patients in the United States has decreased from 6 : 1 in 1950 to 3 : 1.[240] Johnson has reported on 2580 patients diagnosed with lung cancer over a 15-year period from Duke University Medical Center.[123] During the first 5 years, the relative incidences of the various types of lung cancers were squamous cell carcinoma (43.1%), large cell undifferentiated carcinoma (22.5%), adenocarcinoma (18.6%), small cell undifferentiated carcinoma (11.6%), and bronchial alveolar carcinoma (3.5%). During the second and third 5-year periods, squamous cell carcinoma remained the most common neoplasm, but its incidence declined to 35.7%,

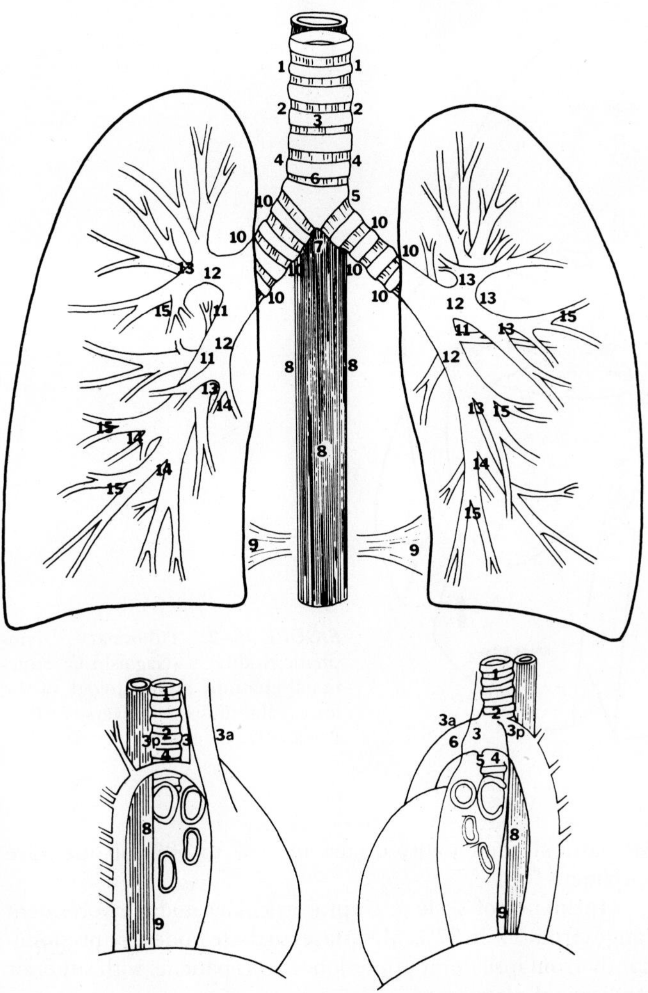

FIGURE 38–1. Lungs and mediastinum—sites of lymph nodes. N2 nodes—superior mediastinal nodes: 1: highest mediastinal; 2: upper paratracheal; 3: pre- and retrotracheal; 4: lower paratracheal (including azygous nodes). Aortic nodes—5: subaortic (aortic window); 6: paraaortic (ascending aorta or phrenic). Inferior mediastinal nodes—7: subcarinal; 8: paraesophageal (below carina); 9: pulmonary ligament. N1 nodes—10: hilar; 11: interlobar; 12: lobar; 13: segmental (proximal). N0 nodes—14, 15: segmental (distal).

whereas adenocarcinoma became the second most common lung cancer at 22%. Adenocarcinoma was the most common primary lung cancer in women.[123] Similar findings were reported by Galietti and associates,[82] who studied 3398 cases of lung cancer in Italy. The majority of cases for both sexes occurred in patients in the age range of 35 to 75 years, with a peak at age 55 to 65 years.

Since 1964, many reports have stressed the causative relation of cigarette smoking to lung cancer.[279] A survey by Doll and Hill[62] of 40,000 British doctors showed that of 36 cases of lung cancer, 25 involved smokers. The risk of lung cancer for heavy smokers was 20 times greater than that for nonsmokers. Studies by Hammond and Horn[102] on mortality rate show that lung cancer death occurred in 54.3 per 100,000 for persons who smoked ten to 20 cigarettes per day; this rate rose to 217.3 per 100,000 for persons who smoked over 40 cigarettes a day. Parallel conclusions were reported by Denoix and co-workers.[60] In addition to these epidemiologic data, other experimental studies confirm the above relationship.[7,277]

Other agents found in the industrial environment such as asbestos, coal tar fumes, nickel, chromium, arsenic, and radioactive materials have been related to the development of lung cancer. Atmospheric pollution and genetic factors are also implicated in the development of lung cancer, but their role is more difficult to pinpoint.

NATURAL HISTORY

The natural history of lung cancer begins with exposure of a susceptible host to carcinogenic agents, which leads to progressive changes from metaplasia, to atypia and dysplasia, and ultimately to carcinoma *in situ* and invasive cancer.[133]

It is often difficult to determine the site of origin of lung cancer. Garland and colleagues[84] studied 463 patients, 150 of whom had less advanced tumors that were suitable for determination of the site of origin. In their series the site of origin was the right lung in 58% and left lung in 42% of cases.

Herman and Crittenden[110] studied 600 autopsies of patients with lung cancer for determination of site of origin. In their series, the location was in the main stem of the bronchus in 32%, in the lobar or segmental bronchus in 48%, and in the peripheral bronchus in 14% of cases. In 6% of cases in their series, the site could not be determined.

Once established, the tumors are likely to grow with a constant doubling time at least during the early stages of their development.[177] The technique of measuring doubling time (DT) was developed by Collins and colleagues.[46] For various histologic types of lung cancer, the lowest DT is for adenocarcinoma and the fastest DT for small cell carcinoma.[31] More detailed information on doubling time and lung cancer can be found elsewhere.[59]

Patterns of Spread

The spread pattern of lung cancer may be divided conveniently into three different pathways: local (intrathoracic), regional (lymphatic), and distant (hematogenous). Progression of lung cancer can be by any of these pathways in no particular order.

A relationship has been described between the incidence of local, regional, and distant spread and histologic types. Undifferentiated small cell carcinoma (oat cell cancer) has a higher incidence of distant metastasis than non-small cell cancers (see Table 38-2). Of the latter group, adenocarcinoma has shown higher potential for distant metastasis (Table 38-1).

Analysis of patients in a protocol by the Radiation Therapy Oncology Group (RTOG) demonstrated that in patients with non-small cell carcinoma of the lung, the ultimate incidence of distant metastases was 75% to 80%, regardless of histologic type. This is not too different from the incidence with small cell undifferentiated carcinoma. Metastases developed more promptly in patients with adenocarcinoma or large cell undifferentiated carcinoma than in those with squamous cell carcinoma. Patients with small cell carcinoma developed metastases within 2 to 3 years.[204,219] The true incidence of cardiac metastasis from lung cancer is not known, because it is not commonly diagnosed before death. From autopsy series, cardiac metastasis can occur in 15% to 35% of patients with lung cancer.[14,151,258] Analysis of 418 autopsy cases by Strauss and associates[258] shows that pericardial metastases are more common than myocardial metastases, and the majority of patients have both.

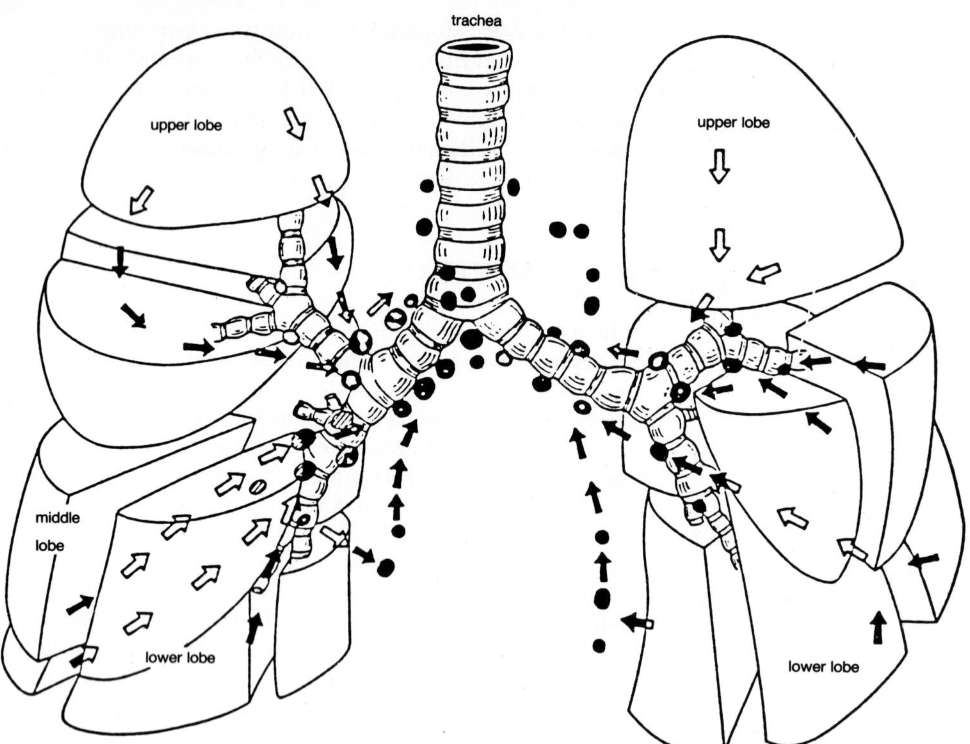

FIGURE 38–2. Pulmonary lymphatic drainage. (Nagaishi C: Functional anatomy and histology of the lung. Baltimore, University Park Press, 1972)

Lymphatic Spread

Although hematogenous spread is one pathway for dissemination of lung cancer, lymph node metastasis is another closely related phenomenon. Croxatto and Barcat[52] found lymph node metastasis in 90% of patients with distant dissemination. Overall incidence of nodal involvement in lung cancer varies in reported series, depending on patient selection. It is lowest in lobectomy series (37%) and highest in necropsy series (94%).[20, 113, 182, 183, 187, 217, 234, 249, 277, 278]

Hilar lymph node metastases from lung cancer occur in about 60% of right upper lobe and middle lobe lesions. The incidence of hilar node metastasis from lower lobes is approximately 75%.[239]

Mediastinal nodal involvement in lung cancer has also been studied both in surgical series (early cases) and in autopsy series. Mediastinal adenopathy occurs in 40% to 50% of operative specimens.[8]

Incidence of scalene (supraclavicular) nodal involvement ranges from 2% to 37%. Metastases to these nodes are predominantly from ipsilateral upper lobes or in patients with superior mediastinal metastases.

Extrathoracic Spread

Hematogenous spread with multiple organ involvement is frequently reported. Table 38-1 shows the site of metastases correlated with the histologic type of tumor in approximately 6000 autopsies.[144] Hansen and Muggia,[104] in a group of 83 patients with limited nonresectable carcinoma and 67 patients with extensive bronchogenic carcinoma, reported an incidence

TABLE 38–1
Site of Metastasis Related to Histologic Type (at Autopsy)

SITE OF METASTASES	SQUAMOUS	OAT CELL	ANAPLASTIC	ADENO-CARCINOMA
Lymph Nodes	137 (54%)	163 (85%)	135 (76%)	42 (75%)
Liver	58 (23%)	122 (64%)	67 (38%)	26 (47%)
Adrenals	54 (21%)	84 (44%)	69 (39%)	17 (30%)
Bones	59 (23%)	75 (39%)	53 (30%)	23 (41%)
Brain	26 (17%)	45 (42%)	30 (24%)	13 (39%)
Kidney	39 (15%)	28 (14.5%)	24 (13.5%)	11 (20%)
Pancreas	9 (3.5%)	46 (24%)	25 (14%)	3 (5%)
Lung	31 (12%)	13 (7%)	15 (8%)	8 (14%)
Pleura	18 (7%)	21 (11%)	9 (5%)	3 (5%)
Total	255	191	179	56

(Line DH, Deeley TJ: Br J Dis Chest 65:238–242, 1971)

of 3.6% positive bone marrow biopsy for tumor invasion in patients with epidermoid carcinoma, 12.5% for large cell carcinoma, 18.5% for adenocarcinoma, and 46.4% for small cell carcinoma. Peritoneoscopy and liver biopsies were performed on 47 patients with limited small cell undifferentiated bronchogenic carcinoma and 11 patients with extensive tumors. Only one of 47 patients with limited disease was found to have detectable hepatic metastasis, whereas three of 11 patients with extensive tumors showed hepatic metastasis. Brain metastases are also common; their incidence, correlated with histologic cell type in a group of 134 patients reported by Hansen and Muggia,[104] was comparable to the autopsy material described by Line and Deeley.[144]

Adrenal metastasis has been reported in 27.4% of patients with epidermoid carcinoma, 35% to 40% of patients with small or large cell undifferentiated carcinoma, and 42.9% of patients with adenocarcinoma.[5] The abdominal lymph nodes were reported to be involved in over 50% of patients with small cell undifferentiated carcinoma.[104]

CLINICAL PRESENTATION

Carcinoma of the lung is among the most insidious of all neoplasms.[57] Signs and symptoms may arise from local tumor growth, invasion of adjacent structures, regional growth, and distant metastatic sites (hematogenous dissemination), or from a secondary effect of the tumor (paraneoplastic syndromes).[43]

Cough is a major symptom in 75% of patients and is severe in 40%. Hemoptysis has been described in 57% of patients and was the first symptom in 4%. Other common symptoms found in approximately 15% of the patients are dyspnea and chest pain resulting from involvement of the pleura, chest wall, or mediastinal structures. Nonspecific initial symptoms such as weight loss, weakness, anorexia, and malaise may occur in 10% to 15% of the patients. Less common are febrile respiratory episodes.

Involvement of intrathoracic structures may result in specific symptomatology. Tumors located in the apex of the lungs usually grow by local extension and involve cervical and thoracic nerves, resulting in Pancoast's or superior sulcus tumor syndrome,[193, 194] characterized by shoulder pain radiating to the arm along the distribution of the ulnar nerve. Sympathetic nerve involvement results in Horner's syndrome, which consists of enophthalmos, ptosis, meiosis, and ipsilateral loss of sweating. Entrapment or involvement of the recurrent laryngeal lymph node may lead to paralysis of the nerve and hoarseness. Because of the longer intrathoracic course of the laryngeal nerve on the left side, this symptom is more common in tumors of the left lung. Involvement of the phrenic nerve can result in paralysis of the hemidiaphragm with resulting dyspnea. Dysphagia may result from a mechanical compression of the tumor on the esophagus. Primary tumors located in the right lung or metastatic tumor in the right mediastinal lymph nodes may cause superior vena cava syndrome (SVC).[248] Large tumors in the upper lobes with massive upper mediastinal lymph adenopathy may cause thoracic inlet obstruction with severe respiratory distress. Tumor involvement of the pericardium and the heart may result in pericardial tamponade and congestive heart failure.

Approximately 2% of patients with lung cancer develop manifestations of "paraneoplastic syndromes" or "remote effects" of malignancy.[101]

DIAGNOSTIC WORKUP

Radiologic Examination

Garland and colleagues[84] estimated that when a tumor of the lung is first detected on a chest x-ray film, it has already completed 75% of its natural history. Rigler[218] observed that x-ray abnormality frequently antedates the first symptoms or signs of the disease by 7 months or more.

Routine chest x-ray studies, posteroanterior and lateral, are by far the most commonly used radiologic examination in patients with lung cancer.[55, 280] Computed tomography (CT) is the most important and valuable radiologic tool in diagnostic evaluation and therapeutic planning of lung cancer (Fig. 38-3),[229, 230] because it is highly accurate in predicting the likelihood of curative surgical resection in the majority of patients

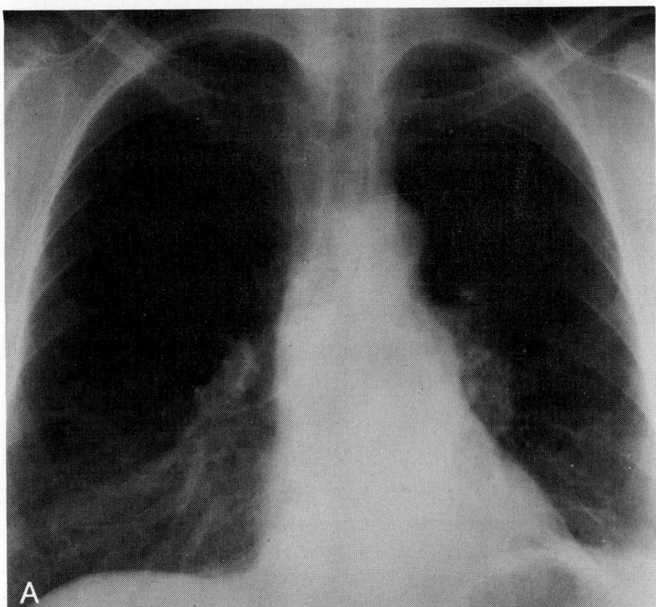

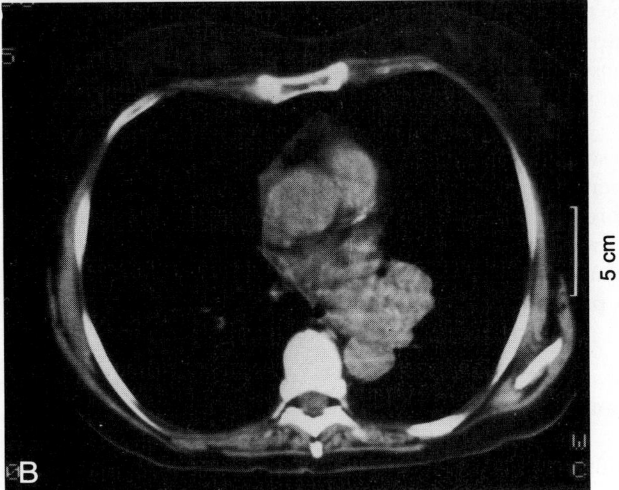

FIGURE 38–3. Sixty-six-year-old white female with undifferentiated small cell carcinoma of the left lung. (**A**) Chest x-ray was read as left hilar mass with associated volume loss in the left hemithorax. (**B**) CT scan clearly delineates the tumor with extension to the mediastinum. Enlarged pretracheal, aortopulmonary window and left hilar lymph nodes were also present.

with bronchogenic carcinoma.[10,85,215] Staging of lung cancer by CT clearly is superior to conventional radiologic techniques for the demonstration of direct extension of the primary neoplasm into the mediastinum or chest wall and the detection of enlarged mediastinal lymph nodes.[160,166,188,211] However, CT cannot differentiate inflammatory disease from neoplasia. Also, CT fails to detect microscopic metastatic disease in normal-sized lymph nodes.[98]

Recognizing the above-mentioned diagnostic criteria, Sagel[230] indicated that mediastinal nodes less than 1 cm in diameter are considered unlikely to contain metastatic disease, and nodes 1 cm to 2 cm in diameter are considered intermediate. Enlargement may be caused either by neoplasms or by granulomatous disease. Mediastinal nodes more than 2 cm in diameter in a patient with known primary bronchogenic carcinoma almost certainly result from neoplastic involvement. A new approach has been proposed by Buy and associates,[29] who considered mediastinal nodes abnormal when the short access of the largest mediastinal node in the lymphatic drainage territory of the cancer was ≥10 mm and the difference between this node and the largest node in the other territories was more than 5 mm. In 47 patients Buy and associates reported a 78% sensitivity, a 99% specificity, a 95% positive predictive value, a 94% negative predictive value, and a 94% accuracy. In general, histologic confirmation of neoplasm in the mediastinal nodes is recommended.

The staging CT examination for bronchogenic carcinoma should include scans for assessment of the adrenals. In suspicious cases, percutaneous needle biopsy of an adrenal mass under CT-directed guidance may be useful to confirm distant metastasis.

Computed tomography also has proven to be extremely useful for radiation therapy treatment planning in bronchogenic carcinoma.[70,212] In a study by Emami and coworkers,[70] use of chest CT scans in preradiation therapy evaluation of 32 patients with lung cancer resulted in a clearer delineation of the tumor extent in 75%, changes in assessment in the size of the lesion in 43%, changes of disease stage in 40%, demonstration of the inadequacy of the treatment plan in 28%, and changes in the volume of the normal tissue irradiated in 40% of the patients. Overall, CT scan was thought to be essential for treatment planning in 53% of the patients. Similar results have been reported by other investigators.[212,241] One of the most important potential uses of CT scans is in three-dimensional treatment planning in radiation therapy.[74]

Magnetic resonance imaging (MRI) has recently been used to study patients with lung cancer.[42,83,86] MRI has occasionally been useful in differentiating recurrent cancer from radiation fibrosis.[86] MRI has not shown superiority over CT scan, and the advantages and limitations are similar.[12,98] MRI is not recommended as a routine study or as a replacement for CT scanning in patients with a diagnosis of lung cancer.

Radioisotope Procedures

Multiple organ system scanning (liver-spleen, brain, and bone scan) as part of the routine workup for all histologies of lung cancer is not indicated,[53,58,60,75,159,213,223] because in the absence of signs or symptoms of the specific organ, such investigations are usually unrewarding. One probable exception is obtaining a brain CT scan in the workup of small cell carcinoma because of the high incidence of brain metastasis.

Special Diagnostic Procedures

Pulmonary Function Tests

Pulmonary function tests are also important predictors of the patient's ability to undergo surgical resection or withstand irradiation. Table 38-2 lists important tests that can be used in evaluating patients with lung cancer.

Bone Marrow Biopsy and Aspiration

Bone marrow involvement is present in 11% to 47% of patients with small cell carcinoma.[119] In recent years, as patients with less-advanced disease have entered chemotherapy trials, the incidence of marrow involvement at diagnosis has declined to about 20%.

Sputum Cytology

The rate of success of sputum cytology depends on the amount of sputum produced and the quality of technical procedures, but in many cases it is possible to determine the presence of malignancy as well as the cell type. Sputum cytology has diagnosed malignancy in 65.2%[268] to 75%[76] of patients.

Bronchoscopy

Bronchoscopic examination provides important data even in the presence of preoperative cytologic proof of cancer.[129] In patients with lung cancer, 59% to 74% of lesions were seen through the fiberoptic scope; biopsy and brushing gave a true positive diagnosis in 86% to 96% of patients.[63,216] The combination of bronchial brushings and biopsy gave an overall accuracy of 79% including 66% to 78% of peripheral lesions and 86% of central lesions.[63,216] The false-positive rate was very low (0.8%). When a flexible fiberoptic scope was used, transbronchial forceps biopsy of peripheral lung lesions under fluoroscopic control yielded diagnosis in 70% to 75% of patients.[67,129]

Thoracic Fine-Needle Aspiration Biopsy

In patients with suspicious, undiagnosed peripheral lung lesions seen on x-rays films, percutaneous biopsy can be per-

TABLE 38–2
Tests Used in Evaluating Patients with Lung Cancer and Impaired Function

PARAMETER	TEST
Ventilatory function	Forced expired volume (FEV_1), vital capacity (VC), maximum breathing capacity (MBC)
Gas exchange	PO_2, PCO_2, A-aDO_2, diffusing capacity
Circulatory studies	EKG, vascular pressures, cardiac output, scanning techniques
Integrated function	Exercise evaluation
Regional pulmonary function	Quantitative ventilation-perfusion isotope scans

(Kanarek OJ: Assessment of pulmonary function in lung cancer. In Choi NC, Grillo HC [eds]: Thoracic Onology, pp 103–113. New York, Raven Press, 1983)

formed under fluoroscopic control.[124,231,250] Analysis of the two large series[231,250] showed a correct diagnosis in 91% of patients with up to 71% having cytologic evidence of malignancy. There were 2.4% false-positive and 0.23% false-negative diagnoses. In the report by Sagel and associates,[231] one aspiration procedure provided malignant cells in 87% of patients; this figure rose to 96% after two procedures. In the two above-mentioned studies combined, pneumothorax occurred in 27% of patients, 14% of whom required chest tube; hemoptysis occurred in 2% to 5%; 4% to 11% had local bleeding around the lesion; and in only one case implantation of metastasis was observed.

Other procedures used in establishing the diagnosis of lung cancer are mediastinoscopy, scalene node biopsy, exploratory thoracotomy, and biopsy of any accessible metastatic site.

STAGING

The American Joint Committee on Cancer has adopted the TNM classification, originally proposed by Mountain and Carr,[174] primarily based on surgical findings. This staging system has recently been revised.[171–173] Table 38-3 shows the revised TNM staging system adopted by RTOG. It is critical to differentiate between those patients in whom local control by irradiation is possible and those with extremely advanced regional or metastatic disease for whom palliation is the only goal.

PATHOLOGIC CLASSIFICATION

Many histologic classifications of lung tumors have been suggested. With only minor differences reflecting individual preferences, all are variations of the WHO classification system (Table 38-4). The proposed classification is cumbersome for clinical usage and has been reduced to a smaller number of categories by various authors. We have found the classification system proposed by the Armed Forces Institute of Pathology to be simple and practical (Table 38-5).[30]

Pathologic classification has prognostic value (Table 38-6). It is generally believed that epidermoid carcinoma has the best prognosis, followed by adenocarcinoma and undifferentiated large cell carcinoma. Until recently, undifferentiated small cell carcinoma had the poorest prognosis, but because of more aggressive combined modality treatments prognosis will most likely change in the near future.

PROGNOSTIC FACTORS

Numerous reports in the literature deal with the prognostic significance of anatomic extent of disease[172,173,254] and non-anatomic factors[172,173,191] in carcinoma of the lung. The prognostic significance of the extent of disease, *staging*, was best demonstrated by Mountain.[172,173] Stanley[254] evaluated 77 prognostic factors in approximately 5000 patients with inoperable

TABLE 38–3
Staging System for Lung Cancer

PRIMARY TUMOR (T)

TX	Primary tumor cannot be assessed, or tumor proven by presence of malignant cells in sputum or bronchial washings but not visualized by imaging or bronchoscopy
T0	No evidence of primary tumor
Tis	Carcinoma *in situ*
T1	Tumor 3 cm or less in greatest dimension, surrounded by lung or visceral pleura, without bronchoscopic evidence of invasion more proximal than the lobar bronchus
T2	Tumor with *any* of the following features of size or extent: More than 3 cm in greatest dimension Involves main bronchus, 2 cm or more distal to the carina Invades the visceral pleura Associated with atelectasis or obstructive pneumonitis that extends to the hilar region but does not involve the entire lung
T3	Tumor of any size that directly invades any of the following: chest wall (including superior sulcus tumors), diaphragm, mediastinal pleura, parietal pericardium; or tumor in the main bronchus less than 2 cm distal to the carina but without involvement of the carina; or associated atelectasis or obstructive pneumonitis of the entire lung
T4	Tumor of any size that invades any of the following: mediastinum, heart, great vessels, trachea, esophagus, vertebral body, carina; or tumor with a malignant pleural effusion

LYMPH NODE (N)

NX	Regional lymph nodes cannot be assessed
N0	No regional lymph node metastasis
N1	Metastasis in ipsilateral peribronchial or ipsilateral hilar lymph nodes, including direct extension
N2	Metastasis in ipsilateral mediastinal or subcarinal lymph node(s)
N3	Metastasis in contralateral mediastinal, contralateral hilar, ipsilateral or contralateral scalene or supraclavicular lymph node(s)

DISTANT METASTASES (M)

MX	Presence of distant metastasis cannot be assessed
M0	No distant metastasis
M1	Distant metastasis

STAGE GROUPING

Occult Carcinoma	TX	N0	M0
0	Tis	N0	M0
I	T1	N0	M0
	T2	N0	M0
II	T1	N1	M0
	T2	N1	M0
IIIA	T1	N2	M0
	T2	N2	M0
	T3	N0	M0
	T3	N1	M0
	T3	N2	M0
IIIB	Any T	N3	M0
	T4	Any N	M0
IV	Any T	Any N	M1

(Mountain CF: Chest 89[Suppl]:225S–233S, 1986)

TABLE 38–4
World Health Organization (WHO) Histologic Classication of Lung Cancer

I. Epidermoid carcinoma
II. Small cell anaplastic carcinoma
  1. Fusiform cell type
  2. Polygonal cell type
  3. Lymphocyte-like (oat cell) type
III. Adenocarcinoma
  1. Bronchogenic
    a. Acinar, with or without mucin formation
    b. Papillary
  2. Bronchoalveolar
IV. Large cell carcinoma
  1. Solid tumors with mucin-like content
  2. Solid tumors without mucin-like content
  3. Giant cell carcinoma
  4. Clear cell carcinoma
V. Combined epidermoid and adenocarcinoma
VI. Carcinoid tumors
VII. Bronchial gland tumors
  1. Cylindromas
  2. Mucoepidermoid tumors
  3. Others
VIII. Papillary tumors of surface epithelium
  1. Epidermoid
  2. Epidermoid with goblet cells
  3. Others
IX. "Mixed" tumors and carcinomas
  1. Mixed tumors
  2. Carcinosarcoma of embryonal type (blastoma)
  3. Other carcinomasarcomas
X. Sarcomas
XI. Unclassified
XII. Mesotheliomas
  1. Localized
  2. Diffuse

TABLE 38–5
Pathologic Types of Bronchogenic Carcinoma

TUMOR TYPE	APPROXIMATE INCIDENCE
Squamous Cell Carcinoma	40%
Well-Differentiated	6%
Moderately Differentiated	18%
Poorly Differentiated	16%
Small Cell Carcinoma	20%
Lymphocyte-like (Oat Cell)	3%
Polygonal (Intermediate)	14%
Other and Combined	3%
Adenocarcinoma	20%
Well-Differentiated	6%
Moderately Differentiated	5%
Poorly Differentiated	6%
Bronchioalveolar	3%
Large Cell Carcinoma	20%
Large Cell Undifferentiated	19%
Giant Cell	1%
Clear Cell	0%
Combined Squamous Cell and Adenocarcinoma	1%

(Carter D, Eggleston JC: Tumors of the lower respiratory tract. In Atlas of Tumor Pathology, Fascicle 17, 2nd series. Washington, DC, Armed Forces Institute of Pathology, 1980)

carcinoma of the lung from Veterans Administration Lung Group Protocols. The three most important prognostic factors affecting survival were performance status (Karnofsky's score), extent of disease, and weight loss. Other factors, such as tumor size and histologic type, appear to be important when considered alone but not in multivariate analysis. Bonomi and colleagues,[19] in an analysis of 66 patients with Stage III non-small cell lung cancer, found that performance status and eligibility for surgery were the most important prognostic factors. Maurer and Pajak[158] also noted that the extent of disease and performance status were the major prognostic factors.

NON-OAT CELL CARCINOMA

General Management

Non-oat cell carcinoma of the lung, whenever resectable, should be treated surgically.[176] Generally accepted criteria as contraindications to curative surgery are the following[178]: spread of tumor beyond the hemithorax, including supraclavicular lymph node involvement; malignant pleural effusion; recurrent laryngeal nerve paralysis; medical inoperability; patient refusal; and presence of mediastinal lymph node metastasis. However, some surgeons do operate on patients with limited mediastinal lymph node metastasis. In the pre-CT era approximately 30% of patients would have been considered operable, and radical resection would have been carried out in 15% (resectability rate of 50%). With the current meticulous use of CT scan for patient selection for surgery, approximately 20% of patients are operated on, with a resectability rate of 92% to 94%.[221] Only about

TABLE 38–6
Overall Five-Year Survival Rates for Major Histologic Types of Lung Cancer

	5-YEAR SURVIVAL RATE (%)		
HISTOLOGIC TYPE	ALL CASES (N = 2155)	RESECTED CASES (N = 835)	RESECTABLE CASES (%)
Epidermoid carcinoma	25	37	60
Adenocarcinoma	12	27	38*
Large cell carcinoma	13	27	38*
Small cell carcinoma	1	0	11

** Combined in AJC report*
(Data from Matthews MJ, Gordon PR: Morphology of pulmonary and pleural malignancies. In Strauss MJ [ed]: Lung Cancer Clinical Diagnosis and Treatment. New York, Grune & Stratton, 1977; Mountain CF, Carr DT, Martini N, et al: Staging of Lung Cancer, 1979. American Joint Committee for Cancer Staging and End Results Reporting. Chicago, Task Force on Lung Cancer, 1980)

20% of all patients presenting with lung cancer are suitable for curative surgery.

Definitive Radiation Therapy

In patients with early stage disease (T1, T2-N0, N1) for whom surgery is not possible because of medical reasons, curative radiation therapy is a reasonable alternative.[222] Some authors[56] found no advantage in survival rate in patients treated with modest doses of radiation over the control group given a placebo. Some authors, such as Rubin,[225] Salazar,[233] Choi,[37] Mantravadi,[153] and Perez and their colleagues,[201,205] have shown improved survival times of up to 3 years after irradiation in patients receiving higher doses of radiation. Patients with advanced disease localized to the chest, with good performance status, should be treated with 6500 cGy to 7500 cGy to the primary tumor, 6000 cGy in 6 to 7 weeks to the regional nodes harboring gross disease seen on CT, and 5000 cGy to other thoracic nodal regions in an effort to sterilize both the primary tumor and the metastasis in the regional nodes.[49]

Payne[196] and Cohen[44] have questioned this aggressive approach in the light of the natural history of non-oat cell tumor, with a high incidence of distant metastases and low probability of long-term survival (5% at 5 years). Palliative effects of radiation therapy, an important objective, are also dose-dependent. Teo and associates[260] reported on 291 patients with inoperable advanced non-oat cell carcinoma of the lung: 18 were excluded from the study for defaulting treatment, and 27 of the remaining 273 were inevaluable for treatment response because of death. The patients were randomized to be treated with either 4500 cGy without correction for lung attenuation in 18 fractions over 4.5 weeks or 3120 cGy in four fractions in 4 weeks. Survival was the same in both arms, with median survival of 20 weeks. However, 71% of patients who received the higher dose achieved symptomatic palliation compared with 54% of patients treated with 3120 cGy ($P < 0.02$). Treatment complications were mild and comparable in both arms.

Patients with distant metastasis should receive palliative irradiation to the thorax consisting of 4000 cGy to 5000 cGy tumor dose in 4 to 5 weeks. Metastatic sites can be treated palliatively with doses of 3000 cGy to 4000 cGy delivered in 2 to 3 weeks.

Results

Surgery

For Stage I disease (T1N0 and T2N0), surgery has resulted in 5-year survival rates of 53% to 70%.[13] For Stage II disease (T1N1 and T2N1), results of surgery have ranged from 48% to 56%.[13] In a report from Memorial Hospital[154] of a total of 706 patients with N2 disease, complete resection was carried out in 151 patients. With the addition of postoperative radiation therapy to this group, 27% of these patients were alive and well at 5 years. Similar results were achieved by Neptune.[179] Without the addition of postoperative radiation therapy, the survival rates in patients with T3N0 and T3N1 or N2 disease were 33% and 0% at 5 years, respectively.[172] Non-small cell lung cancer invading the mediastinum (T3) has also been treated with surgery. Of 225 patients with T3 lesions who underwent surgical resection, 49 patients had complete resection, and a 5-year survival rate of 9% has been achieved. Perioperative mortality rate in this group was 2.7%, and the major complication rate was 13%.[28]

Preoperative Irradiation

Despite initial encouraging results of an institutional trial by Bloedorn and co-workers,[17] two national collaborative studies have failed to show any improvement in survival with the use of preoperative radiation therapy.[243,274] Many aspects of study design and stratification were far from optimal: all stages and histologies were included, and no appropriate stratification was carried out. Treatment planning by simulators and megavoltage equipment were not used in either study.

Sherman and associates[242] reported encouraging results with preoperative radiation therapy in a selected group of patients who were designated as "marginally resectable." Most of these patients received 3000 cGy in ten fractions over 2 weeks, and their surgery was carried out within 2 weeks of completion of radiation therapy. Resectability was increased from marginal to complete resectability in 83% of patients, and the 5-year survival rate was 18%.

Recently the results of a prospective randomized multi-institution trial of 478 patients with lung cancer was reported in which patients receiving preoperative radiation therapy (2000 cGy in five fractions) followed by surgery were compared with patients with surgery alone. There was no difference in the 5-year survival rate of patients with Stage I and Stage II disease. However, the 3-year and 5-year survival rates for Stage III patients were 49.4% and 29.2%, respectively, for the combined group compared with 28.1% and 15.8% for the surgery-alone group.[262]

Postoperative Irradiation

We recommend a course of postoperative radiation therapy in all patients with disease confined to one hemithorax who have hilar or mediastinal nodal metastasis or positive surgical margins. The recommended dose is 5000 cGy at the rate of 200 cGy per day to all hilar and mediastinal lymph nodes with an additional 1000 cGy to 1500 cGy with reduced portals to the volume of known metastatic involvement.

A great deal of controversy exists on the use of postoperative radiation therapy in lung cancer. Van Houtte and colleagues[270] reported on 224 patients, 175 of whom were randomized to be treated by surgery alone or by surgery combined with radiation therapy (6000 cGy/TD [target (tumor) dose] in 6 weeks delivered with ^{60}Co). All patients had disease confined to the hemithorax without lymph node metastasis and had complete resection of the lesion. No significant difference in survival rate was found within the two groups. Moreover, in the patients with T2 lesions, the 5-year survival rate was 43% for pneumonectomy alone compared with 16% for patients receiving postpneumonectomy irradiation. This randomized study confirms the observation of other authors that patients without hilar or mediastinal nodal metastasis do not benefit from adjuvant postoperative radiation therapy.

Postoperative radiation therapy has been used in patients with Stage II and Stage III, N1, and N2 disease.[69,134,255]

Other comparative studies[9,38,41,96,120,131,195] in a selected group of patients with metastatic regional lymph nodes in the thorax demonstrated increased survival and intrathoracic tumor control with postoperative radiation therapy (Table 38-7). Approximately a 40% 3- to 5-year survival rate was achieved in these studies (Fig. 38-4). The Lung Cancer Study Group (LCSG)[275] reported on the results of a randomized trial in patients with Stages II to III epidermoid carcinoma of the lung; after complete resection, these patients received postoperative radiation therapy or no treatment. The conclusion of

TABLE 38–7
Survival with Postoperative Irradiation in Non-Small Cell Carcinoma of the Lung

AUTHOR	SURVIVAL (YEARS)	NO. UNDERGOING SURGERY ALONE	NO. UNDERGOING RADIATION THERAPY	MEDIAN DOSE (cGy)
Bangma[9]	1	25/37 (67%)	19/36 (53%)	Not specified
Choi et al[38]	5* (Adenocarcinoma)	/21 (8%)	/40 (43%)	4500
Choi et al[38]	4* (Squamous cell)	/29 (33%)	/46 (42%)	—
Chung et al[41]	3	3/29 (10%)	15/38 (40%)	4600
Green et al[97]	5	1/30 (3%)	23/66 (35%)	5000
Israel et al[120]	3*	/126 (50%)	/104 (70%)	5000
Kirsh et al[131]	5	0/20 —	16/69 (23.1%)	5000
Paterson and Russell[192]	3	36/99 (36.4%)	33/103 (33%)	4500
Pavlov et al[195]	5	/301† (24%)	/212 (38%)	4500
VanHoutte et al[270]‡	5	/92 (45%)	/83 (20%)	6000
Weisenburger et al[275]	5	57/108 (53%)	57/102 (56%)	5000

**Actuarial NED survival*
† Patients treated with combination of surgery and chemotherapy
‡ Patients without metastatic tumor in hilar or mediastinal nodes
(Modified from Perez CA: Int J Radiat Oncol Biol Phys 8:2019–2022, 1982)

this randomized study was that postoperative radiation therapy significantly reduced the rate of local recurrence without any benefits to survival (Fig. 38-5). The following are four significant fallacies in the design and conduct of this study: only squamous cell carcinoma was included; 11% of patients had no regional lymph node metastasis and thus would not have been advised to have postoperative radiation therapy; among patients who were assigned to receive postoperative radiation therapy, only 74% received within 5% of the total dose prescribed; and no other comments were made about the adequacy of the irradiated volume. Therefore, it is critical to determine in appropriately controlled randomized studies whether postoperative radiation therapy (6000 cGy TD in 6 weeks with decreasing fields and modern techniques) will improve tumor control and survival in patients with resectable bronchogenic carcinoma who have metastatic hilar or mediastinal nodes.

Definitive Radiation Therapy

Results of radiation therapy alone in early stage, technically operable patients are shown in Table 38-8. Most clinical results available today have been obtained with doses ranging from 4000 cGy to 6500 cGy.[35,153] In 376 patients with Stages T1 to T3, N0 to N2 carcinoma of the lung tumors accessioned to an RTOG randomized study[142] to evaluate different doses of radiation, a better 3-year survival rate (15%) was observed with 6000 cGy compared with lower doses of radiation (4000 cGy or 5000 cGy; Fig. 38-6). Patients treated with 6000 cGy had an overall intrathoracic failure rate of 33% at 3 years compared with 42% for those treated with 5000 cGy, 44% for patients receiving 4000 cGy with split-course, and 52% for those treated with 4000 cGy continuous-course radiation therapy (Fig. 38-7).

Patients surviving 6 to 12 months treated with 5000 cGy to 6000 cGy radiation doses showing intrathoracic tumor control had a 3-year survival rate of 22% compared with 10% for those with thoracic failure ($P = 0.05$). In patients treated with 4000 cGy (split- or continuous-course), the respective survival rates were 25% with intrathoracic tumor control and 5% if the tumor was not controlled. In another RTOG study for patients with more advanced tumors (T4 or N3), those with local tumor control at 12 months had a 3-year survival rate of 25% compared with 5% for those with thoracic failures. Differences are statistically significant. It is concluded that higher doses of radiation yield a greater proportion of complete response, higher intrathoracic tumor control, and better survival up to 3 years in non-oat cell medically inoperable or unresectable carcinoma of the lung.

In RTOG 73-01, tumors less than 3 cm in diameter had a tumor control of 60% compared with only 40% for larger lesions.[206] These observations support the need for higher doses

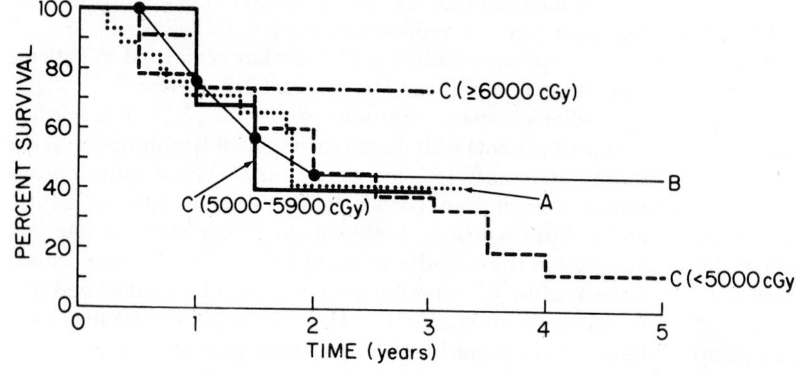

FIGURE 38–4. Results of surgery plus postoperative radiation therapy in Stages II and III of non-small cell lung cancer. (A, Data from Herskovic AM, Bauer M, Seydel HG, et al: Int J Radiat Oncol Biol Phys 14:37–42, 1988; **B,** Data from Steinfeld AD, Glicksman AS: J Surg Oncol 26:154–157, 1984; C, Data from Emami B, Kim T, Roper C, et al: Radiology 164:251–253, 1987)

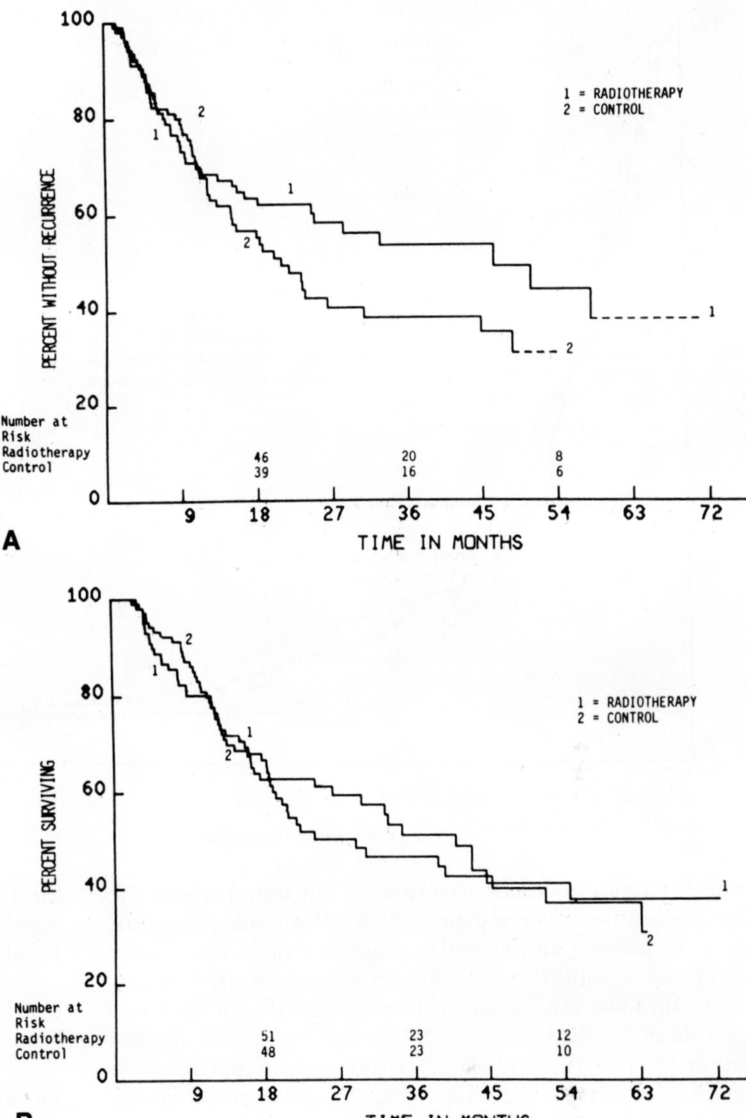

FIGURE 38–5. (**A**) Time to recurrence of epidermoid cancer (including second primary tumors) among 210 patients, according to study group. The difference between the groups was not significant ($P = 0.188$, log-rank test). (**B**) Time to death (from any cause), according to study group. The difference between the groups was not significant ($P = 0.678$ log-rank test). (Reprinted with permission of The Lung Cancer Study Group, N Engl J Med 315:1377–1381, 1986).

of radiation to control larger tumors. However, this need must be tempered by awareness of the effect of increasing doses of radiation on the surrounding normal tissues and by the possibility of inducing life-threatening or fatal complications. It may be possible to selectively increase the tumor dose to volumes with larger cell burden, without unduly increasing complica-

TABLE 38–8
Results of Radical Radiation Therapy in Early Stage, Technically Operable Non-Small Cell Lung Cancer

AUTHOR	NO. OF PATIENTS	3-YEAR SURVIVAL RATE	5-YEAR SURVIVAL RATE
Haffty et al[100]*	43	36%	21%
Zhang et al[281]	44	55%	32%
Noordijk et al[184]†	50	56%	16%

**In this study 11 patients were treated with continuous course and 32 patients with split-course irradiation. Five-year survival rates for the two subgroups were 45% and 12%, respectively.*
† Elderly patients with poor cardiopulmonary condition

tions. In RTOG 83-12, which uses CT scan, computed treatment planning, and dose optimization procedures, 7500 cGy in 28 fractions is delivered to the gross tumor volume seen on chest x-ray film or CT scan, whereas the rest of the potentially involved lymph nodes in the hila and mediastinum received 5040 cGy in 28 fractions.[73] The results of fractionation trials are summarized in Table 38-9.

Seydel and associates[240] reported on a pilot RTOG study in which ten patients received a total radiation dose of 5040 cGy, 20 patients received 6000 cGy, 79 patients received 6960 cGy, and 11 patients received 7440 cGy with a twice-daily fractionation regimen. A complete response rate of 22% to 26% was achieved, and toxicity was acceptable. Later the RTOG conducted a multi-institution prospective phase II study on the effect of hyperfractionation in tumor control and the survival of patients with non-small cell lung cancer.[48] Fractions of 120 cGy were administered twice daily (at 4- to 6-hour intervals). Patients were randomized to minimum total doses of 6000 cGy, 6480 cGy, 6960 cGy, 7440 cGy, and 7920 cGy. Among 519 patients, 248 had favorable prognostic signs (performance status 70 to 100 and weight loss of less than 5%); 271 were unfavorable (performance status 50 to 69 or weight loss over 5%). No signifi-

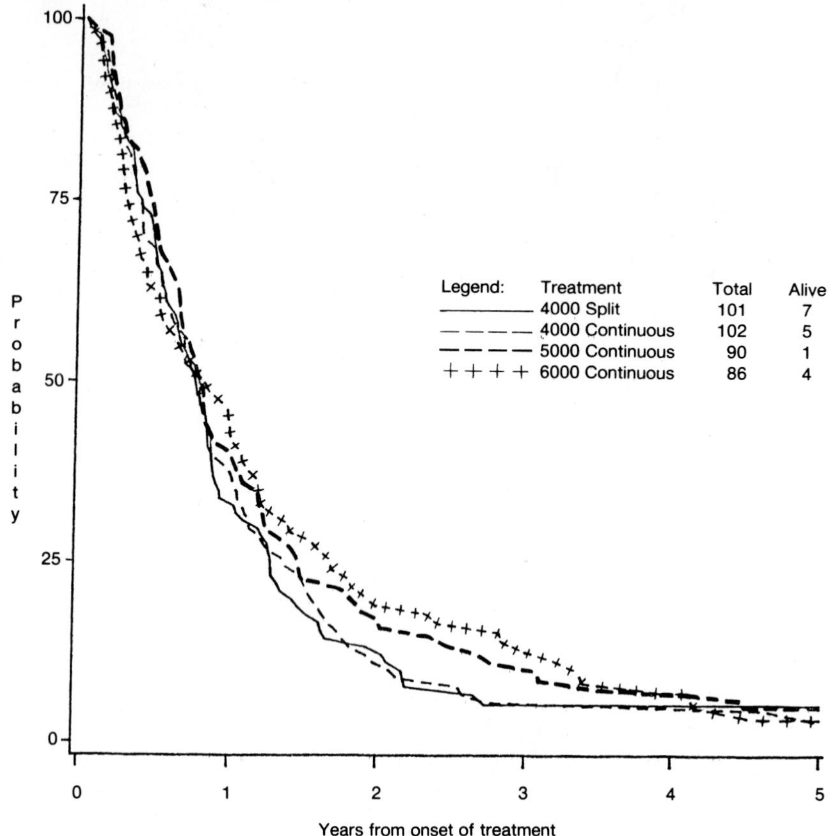

FIGURE 38–6. Correlation of doses of irradiation with survival in unresectable non-small cell carcinoma of the lung.

cant difference in disease-free survival was found among the five arms of the study in patients with unfavorable prognostic signs. In patients with favorable prognostic signs, there was a significant benefit ($P > 0.04$) in survival and disease-free survival with 6960 cGy radiation dose compared with the lower total doses (median 14.8 months survival and 2-year survival rate of 33%). No further benefit was found with hyperfractionation at 7440 cGy and 7920 cGy. No significant differences in the risks of acute or late effects in normal tissue were found among the five arms of therapy, nor was there increased risk over standard fractionation based on previous RTOG study analyses. Results of this study are shown in Table 38-10.

Patterns of Failure of Non-Small Cell Carcinoma

The locoregional or intrathoracic failure rate within the irradiated volume is dose-dependent. In a study by Perez and associ-

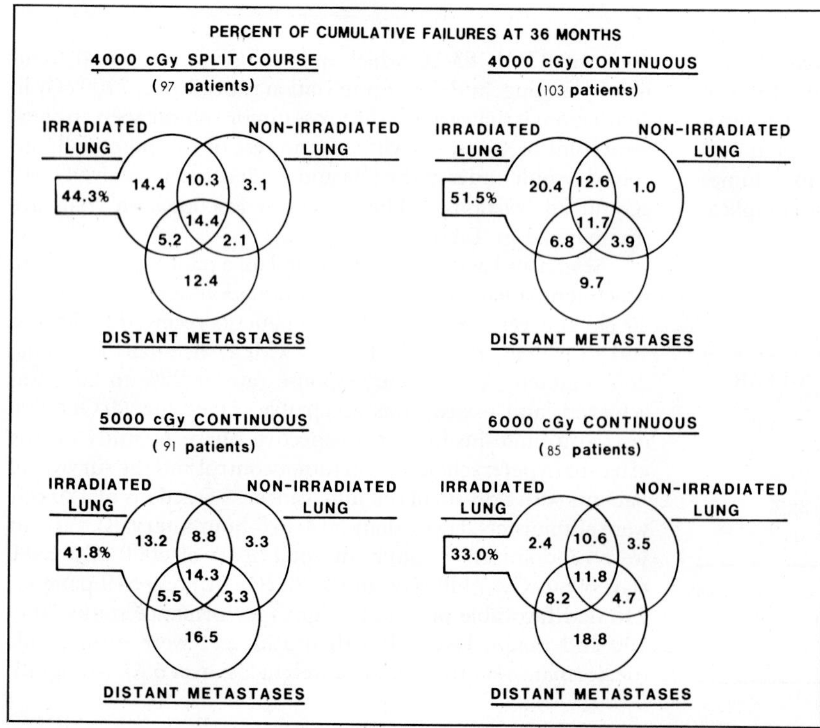

FIGURE 38–7. Patterns of failure in patients with non-small cell lung cancer treated with irradiation (RTOG studies). (Perez CA, Bauer M, Edelstein S, et al: Int J Radiat Oncol Biol Phys 12:539–547, 1986)

TABLE 38–9
Non-Small Cell Carcinoma of the Lung: Dose–Time Factors and Results of Therapy (Randomized Studies)

AUTHOR	TOTAL DOSE (cGy)	NUMBER FRACTIONS/ DOSE (cGy)	REGIMEN TYPE*	NO. OF PATIENTS	TUMOR RESPONSE % CR	TUMOR RESPONSE % CONTROL	% SURVIVAL 1 YR	% SURVIVAL 2 YR
Emami et al[71]	5000–6000	25–30/200	C	76		58.5		
Emami et al[71]	5000	10/250	S(3)	24		45.4		
Guthrie et al[99]	6000	20/300	S(4)	46			34	
Guthrie et al[99]	4000	10/400	S(4)	51			12	
Holsti[117]	5500–6200	25–30	C	90			18 NED	12
Holsti[117]	5400–6000	20/270–300	S(2)	118			23 NED	15
Holsti and Mattson[118]	5000	25/200	C	158†				27
Holsti and Mattson[118]	5500	18/300	S(2)	205†				29
Landgren et al[135]	5000–6000	25/300	C	32				19
Landgren et al[135]	6000	20/300	S(2)	34				12
Lee et al[138]	5000	25/200	S(3–4)	71	45		~40	~15
Lee et al[138]	5000	25/200	C	59	40		~40	~15
Levitt et al[140]	6000	30/200	C				7	
Levitt et al[140]	3600	6/600	S(4)				20	
Perez et al[206]	4000	20/200	C	97	19	33	40	15
Perez et al[206]	5000	25/200	C	91	22	36	48	20
Perez et al[206]	6000	30/200	C	84	24	50	48	20
Perez et al[206]	4000	10/400	S(2)	100	9	35	40	15
Scruggs et al[237]	3500–4000	17–20/200	C	93			27	15
Scruggs et al[237]	4000	10/400	S(2)	128			30	19
Simpson et al[247]	3000	10/300	C	102	17	30		
Simpson et al[247]	4000	20/200	C	105	15	32		
Simpson et al[247]	4000	10/400	S(2)	109	12	36		

**Numbers in parentheses indicate weeks of rest period.*
† Includes 24 (C) and 25 (S) patients with small cell carcinoma
CR: complete response; C: continuous; S: split course
(Perez CA: Cancer Treat Symp 2:131–142, 1985)

ates[203] of two randomized trials of lung cancer by RTOG, the tumor failure rate within the irradiated volume was 48% with 4000 cGy continuous radiation, 38% with 4000 split-course or 5000 cGy continuous regimen, and 27% for patients receiving 6000 cGy continuously. The failure rate in the nonirradiated lung ranged from 25% to 30% in various groups. The incidence of distant metastasis was 50% to 80% in various groups, most frequently in bone, brain, and liver.

Elective Brain Irradiation in Non-Small Cell Carcinoma

Brain metastases, which have been the subject of great interest in patients with small cell carcinoma of the lung, were noted as the ultimate site of failure in 16% of patients with squamous cell carcinoma and in 30% of those with adenocarcinoma or large cell undifferentiated carcinoma.[198]

TABLE 38–10
Survival for Regional Stage III Non-Small Cell Carcinoma Patients with Performance Status of 70 to 100 and Weight Loss Under 5%

ASSIGNED TREATMENT	NO. OF PATIENTS	NO. OF FAILURES	MEDIAN SURVIVAL (MONTHS)	1-YEAR SURVIVAL RATE	2-YEAR SURVIVAL RATE
Conventional RT (CALGB 84-33)	78	62	8.7	40%	13%
VBL + DDP + RT (CALGB 84-33)	78	53	13.8	55%	24%
69.6 Gy HFX RT (RTOG 83-11)	89	77	13.0	56%	29%
Standard RT 60 Gy (RTOG 83–21)	98	89	8.9	34%	10%

(Cox JD, Azarnia N, Byhardt RW, et al: Hyperfractionated radiation therapy [1.2 Gy b.i.d.] with 69.6 Gy total dose increases survival in favorable patients with stage III non-small cell carcinoma of the lung: Report of RTOG 83-11. J Clin Oncol 8:1543–1555, 1990)

The RTOG conducted a randomized trial (84-03) to assess the value of elective brain irradiation (3000 cGy in 15 fractions) in patients with non-small cell carcinoma of the lung treated with definitive radiation therapy.[28] No difference was found in the results of any of the end points analyzed.[2]

SUPERIOR SULCUS LUNG CARCINOMA

A lung cancer located at the lung apex is considered to be a superior sulcus lung cancer. When it is associated with Horner's syndrome, it is called Pancoast's tumor.[189] The majority of patients present with pain of variable intensity at front or back of the upper chest, neck, shoulder region, arm, or forearm. Vertebral involvement may be present, but large tumors rarely involve the spinal cord.

Treatment

Traditionally, these tumors have been treated by a combination of preoperative radiation therapy with doses ranging from 3000 cGy to 5000 cGy, followed by *en bloc* resection.[164, 193, 194] A summary of the literature of patients treated in this manner is shown in Table 38-11. The dose of preoperative radiation therapy influences the final outcome. A study by Hilaris and Martini[114] compared 2000 cGy preoperative radiation therapy, followed by thoracotomy 1 week later, with another group receiving 4000 cGy in 4 weeks followed by surgery in 4 to 6 weeks. The local control rates were 61% and 85% and 5-year survival rates were 6% and 25% in the two groups, respectively. Radiation therapy alone has also been used for superior sulcus tumors.

Hilaris and Nori[114] reported a 3% 5-year survival rate when irradiation was used as a palliative measure. However, with definitive doses of radiation therapy (5000–6500 cGy) and adequate portals, the results were comparable to those obtained with preoperative radiation therapy and surgery. Komacki and associates[132] reported a 23% 5-year survival rate, and Ahmad and colleagues[2] reported a 27.9% 5-year survival rate in this group of patients. The total dose of radiation therapy also influences the outcome. In the report by Ahmad and coworkers[2] only two of 22 patients receiving less than 5000 cGy were alive without disease at 5 years. However, a 5-year survival rate of 27.9% was achieved when doses over 5000 cGy were used.[269]

We recommend doses of 4500 cGy in 5 weeks given preoperatively followed by surgery in 4 to 5 weeks for those patients in whom curative surgery with an acceptable complication rate is anticipated. For unresectable, localized superior sulcus tumors, a course of definitive radiation therapy (6500 cGy in 6 to 7 weeks) is a reasonable alternative.

TABLE 38–11
Superior Sulcus Lung Tumors: Results of Preoperative Radiation Therapy Plus Surgery

AUTHOR	FIVE-YEAR SURVIVAL RATE
Paulson[193]	22%
Paulson[194]	28%
Miller et al[164]	34%
Hilaris and Nori[114]	19%
Ahmad et al[2]	15.3%

For superior sulcus tumors, the portals include the supraclavicular nodes, adjacent vertebral body, the upper lobe, and hilar nodes (Fig. 38-8). Inclusion of subcarinal nodes and, therefore, the levels of the inferior border in portals for superior sulcus tumors is controversial.

Interstitial radiation therapy has also been used for treatment of these tumors. Hilaris and Martini[115] reported a 17% 5-year survival rate with interstitial brachytherapy.

RADIATION THERAPY TECHNIQUES

Tumor Doses

When the advanced status of lung cancer patients seen in radiation therapy departments is considered, it becomes evident that modest doses of 4000 cGy to 5000 cGy are inadequate to control the tumor.[17, 108] Eisert and co-workers[66] reported local tumor control in 27% of patients receiving less than 1450 ret compared with 51% of patients treated with higher doses. Rissanen and colleagues[219] reported no carcinoma in the tumor volume of 30% of patients treated with radiation up to 6000 cGy. In contrast, seven patients whose therapy was interrupted after doses of 2000 cGy or 3000 cGy all showed evidence of malignancy at autopsy.

From basic principles advocated by Fletcher,[78] it is obvious that doses in the range of 8000 cGy to 10,000 cGy are required to sterilize the size of tumors frequently treated in bronchogenic carcinoma.

Fractionation

For biologic reasons, split-course irradiation has been proposed by some authors to be superior to continuous fractionation. However, none of the studies reported has shown superiority of split-course irradiation over continuous regimens.[199]

Numerous nonrandomized retrospective studies have been published on the results of radiation therapy with various fractionation schedules in patients with non-oat cell carcinoma, with tumor doses ranging from 4000 cGy to 6000 cGy. Most split-course fractionation schedules deliver doses of 250 cGy to 300 cGy TD in 2 to 3 weeks with a 2- to 4- week rest period between the two split courses. Continuous radiation was delivered with doses of 200 cGy daily, five weekly fractions.

Multiple daily fractions have been advocated to deliver higher doses of radiation to the tumor without increasing morbidity in the normal tissues.[46]

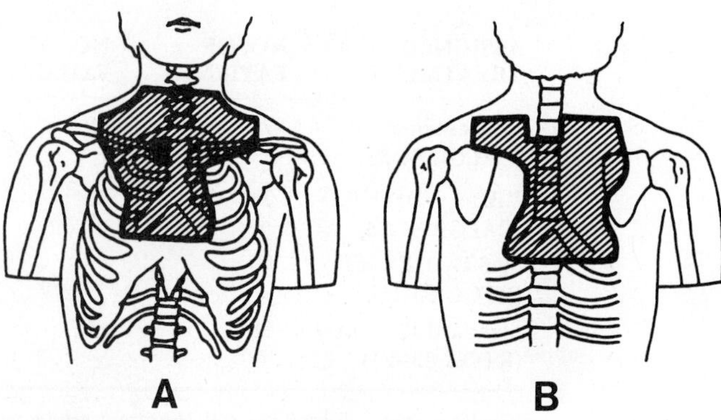

FIGURE 38–8. Examples of portal arrangements for superior sulcus tumors of the lung. (**A**) Anteroposterior. (**B**) Posteroanterior.

Volume, Portals, and Beam Arrangement

The volume to be treated and the configuration of the radiation portals are determined by size and location of the primary tumor, areas of lymphatic drainage in the hila and mediastinum, histologic type, and the equipment and beam energy available. It is common practice to design treatment portals with a 2 cm margin around any gross tumor seen on posteroanterior radiographs and approximately a 1 cm margin around electively treated regional lymph node areas. Irregularly shaped fields are preferred, which requires special secondary blocking to spare as much of the normal tissue as possible. Design of treatment portals used for various types of tumors, depending on location, stage, and histology, are illustrated in Fig. 38-9.

Often, oblique portals are required to deliver the tumor boost. Examples of oblique portal simulation films are illustrated in Figure 38-10. Lateral portals are used in some institutions to deliver supplemental doses of radiation to the primary tumor and hilar and mediastinal lymph nodes. However, at the Mallinckrodt Institute of Radiology we discourage this practice. Because of the lateral thickness of the chest, relatively significant doses of radiation can be delivered to the lung with this technique (Fig. 38-11), which may increase the risk of pneumonitis.

A technique that also should be discouraged is the use of a posterior spinal cord block (five half-value layers, 2 cm wide), because it results in substantial underdosage of the mediastinum (Fig. 38-12). Therefore, if this technique must be used, it should be used only for a small portion of the treatment.

When portals are designed to cover potential lymphatic drainage, the following general principles are recommended:

1. If the primary tumor is in an upper lobe, both supraclavicular regions should be included in the treatment portals. The inferior margin of the portal should be 5 to 6 cm below the carina.
2. If the primary tumor is located in a middle or lower lobe

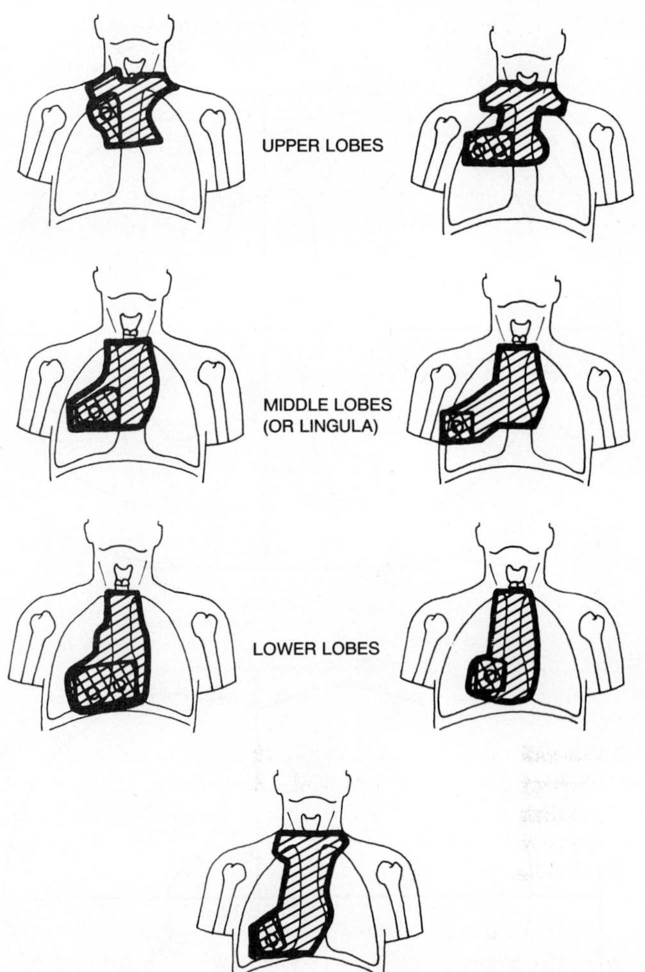

FIGURE 38–9. Examples of portals used for irradiation of non-small cell carcinoma of the lung, depending on the anatomic location of the primary. The tumor and grossly enlarged lymph nodes are treated to higher doses (cross-hatched pattern).

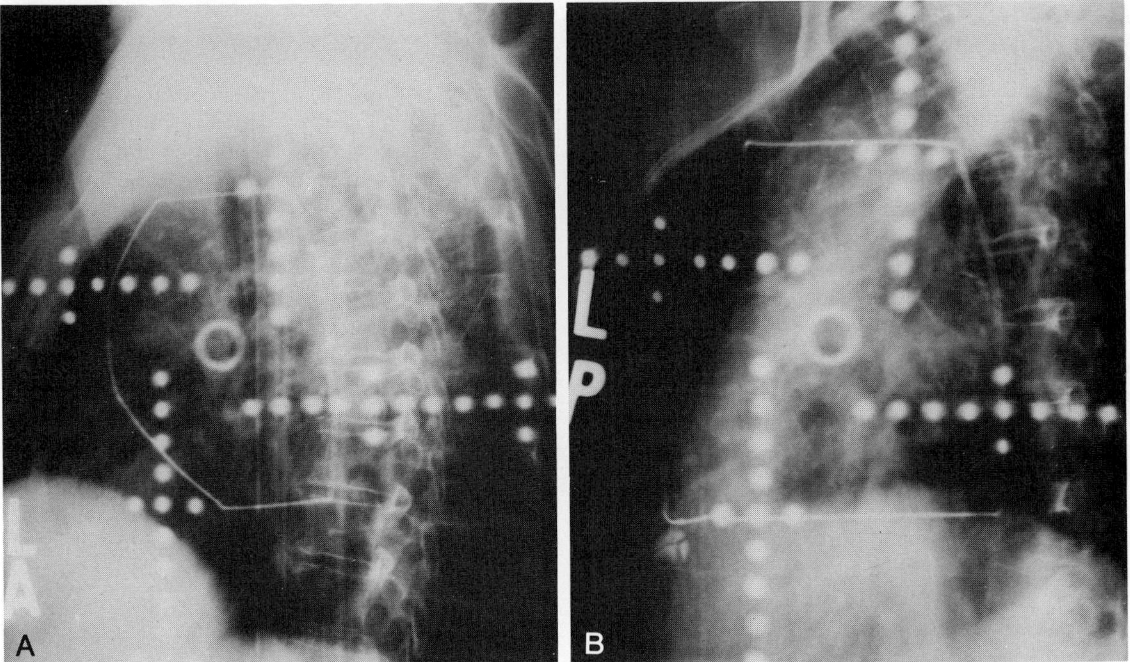

FIGURE 38–10. Examples of oblique portals. These portals are usually selected to spare spinal cord and minimize the irradiated normal lung volume.

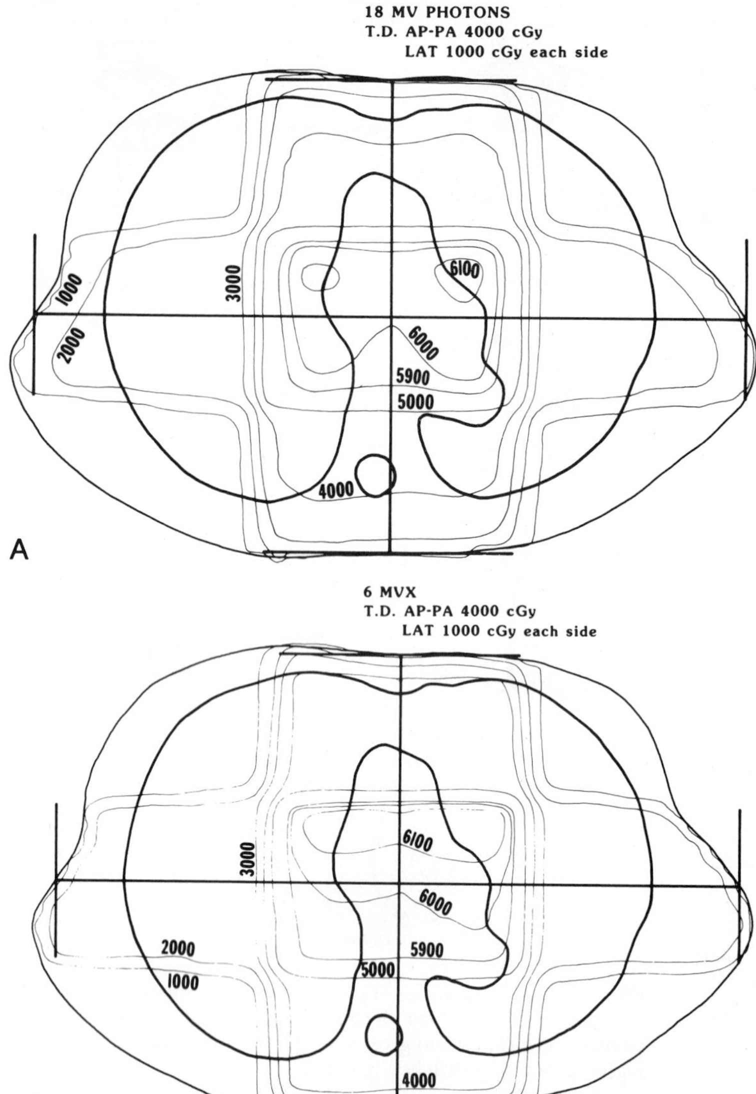

FIGURE 38–11. Irradiation treatment plan with isodose curves demonstrating excess dose to normal lung when lateral beams are used to boost the primary central tumor.

and no mediastinal lymphadenopathy is present, there is no need to treat the supraclavicular areas.

3. If there is a gross mediastinal tumor demonstrated on the CT scan or established by mediastinoscopy, inclusion of both supraclavicular areas within the treated volume is desired.
4. For a tumor located in the lower lobe, the lower border of the mediastinal portal should encompass the entire length of the mediastinum down to the diaphragm.

Figure 38-13 illustrates a CT scan of the chest and various anteroposterior (AP), oblique, and reduced AP fields as well as the isodose curves used in the definitive irradiation of a patient with a primary adenocarcinoma of the right upper lobe.

For small cell undifferentiated carcinoma, portal arrangements are a subject of controversy. Some authors[204] advocate more generous portals that include the primary lesion with generous margins as well as both hilar regions, the entire mediastinum, and both supraclavicular areas. However, others argue that only limited portals encompassing the prechemotherapy primary tumor with a 1 cm margin and high-risk, nodal-bearing areas are adequate, because with effective chemotherapy taking care of subclinical or microscopic disease, there is no need for generous portals. Moreover, judiciously tailored portals may result in a significant reduction of complications due to combined modality therapy of radiation and chemotherapy.[167]

It is extremely important not to exceed the maximum doses tolerated by sensitive and intrathoracic structures such as lung, spinal cord, and heart. Special care should be exercised to restrict the radiation dose to the normal lung (below 1800 cGy, uncorrected for inhomogeneity), whenever possible. Figure 38-14 shows examples of optimized beam arrangements used in bronchogenic carcinoma.

Brachytherapy in Carcinoma of the Lung

External radiation therapy, even in high doses, still is unable to achieve a high rate of locoregional control of locally extensive tumors. Interstitial irradiation, first reported in 1933,[89] is considered the treatment of choice by some institutions for such localized large, unresectable cancers.

Indications for use of brachytherapy are the following: a patient with limited pulmonary reserve, in whom adequate resection necessitates removal of lung tissue beyond the toler-

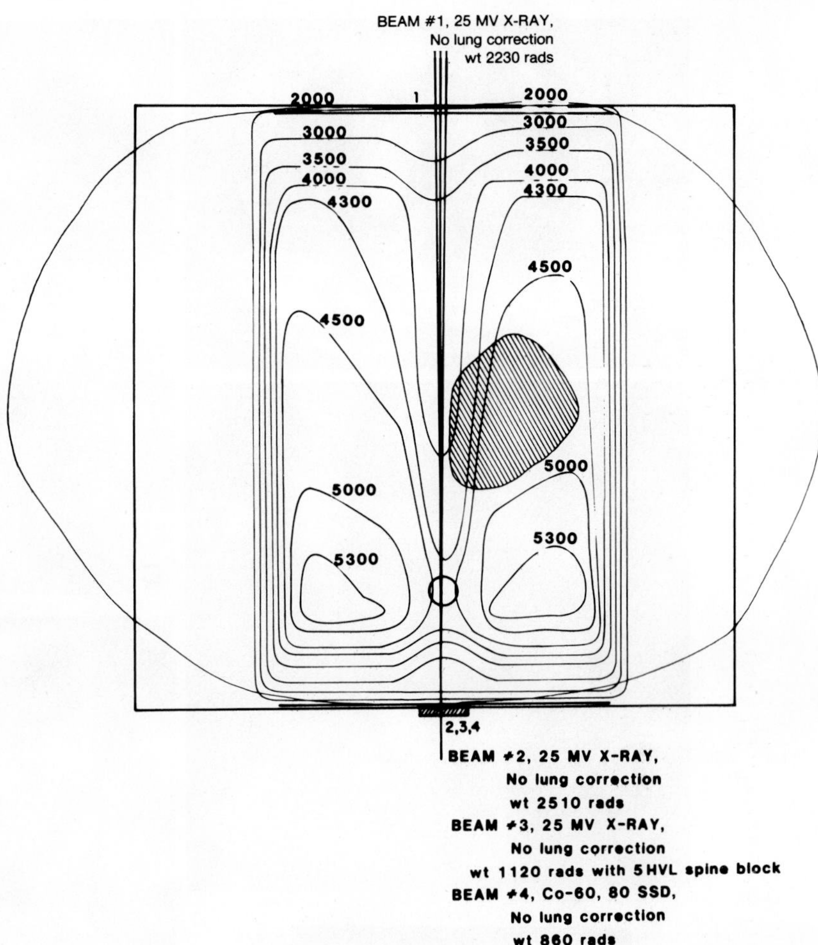

FIGURE 38–12. Isodose curves of a treatment plan with posterior spinal cord block demonstrating underdosage of the posterior part of the mediastinum.

ance of the patient; the presence of hilar tumors adherent to the major vessels with no clearance for safe dissection or division of hilar structures; the presence of tumors extending to the mediastinum and attached to the trachea, esophagus, aorta, or superior vena cava; and the presence of tumors with extensive involvement of chest wall or spine that cannot be completely excised. Brachytherapy in lung cancer may be administered by permanent ^{125}I interstitial implants performed intraoperatively, removable ^{192}Ir implants through intraoperative insertion of Teflon catheters in the tumor, and intrabronchial low- or high-dose-rate ^{192}Ir implants.

Brachytherapy has not been used in highly anaplastic tumors such as small cell cancer or in tumors with distant metastasis. Henschke reported median survival of 7.4 months with three patients living 3 to 5 years after treatment.[109] Hilaris and co-workers,[114,115] reporting on 88 patients with mediastinal nodal metastasis treated with permanent ^{125}I implant of the primary lung and a temporary ^{192}Ir implant of the mediastinum, as well as postoperative external-beam radiation therapy, observed a local control of 76%, a median survival of 26 months, and a 2-year actuarial survival rate of 51%.

Intraluminal brachytherapy has also been used in patients with lung cancer.[236] Preliminary reports with this technique in patients with compromised airway have been reported.[163,185,235] Subjective response (improvement of dyspnea, ventilatory pulmonary function, and lung perfusion scans) has been reported in 60% to 79% of patients. Significant complications such as hemorrhage and fistula have also been described.

SMALL CELL CARCINOMA

General Management

Small cell lung cancer (SCLC) accounts for 20% of all primary lung tumors. SCLC has a high growth fraction, grows rapidly, and is usually widely disseminated when the disease is diagnosed. Bronchial obstruction is associated with 30% to 40% of patients, and in 14% of cases a solitary peripheral mass is found.

The tumors are sensitive to many chemotherapeutic agents. Multiagent drug combinations are more effective than single agents.[87] Intensive initial chemotherapy has been shown to induce a complete response rate of 40% to 68% in patients with limited disease and 18% to 40% in those with extensive disease.[24,54,87]

Surgery

There has been a current interest in including surgery in the multidisciplinary management of limited small cell carcinoma.[88,122] However, prospective studies have shown that few small cell carcinoma lung cancer patients are actually candidates for thoracotomy before or after chemotherapy.[122] Occasionally the denominator of these studies has been changed from the total number of patients to the number of operable patients or to the number of resectable patients or to the number of patients completely resected in order to augment the

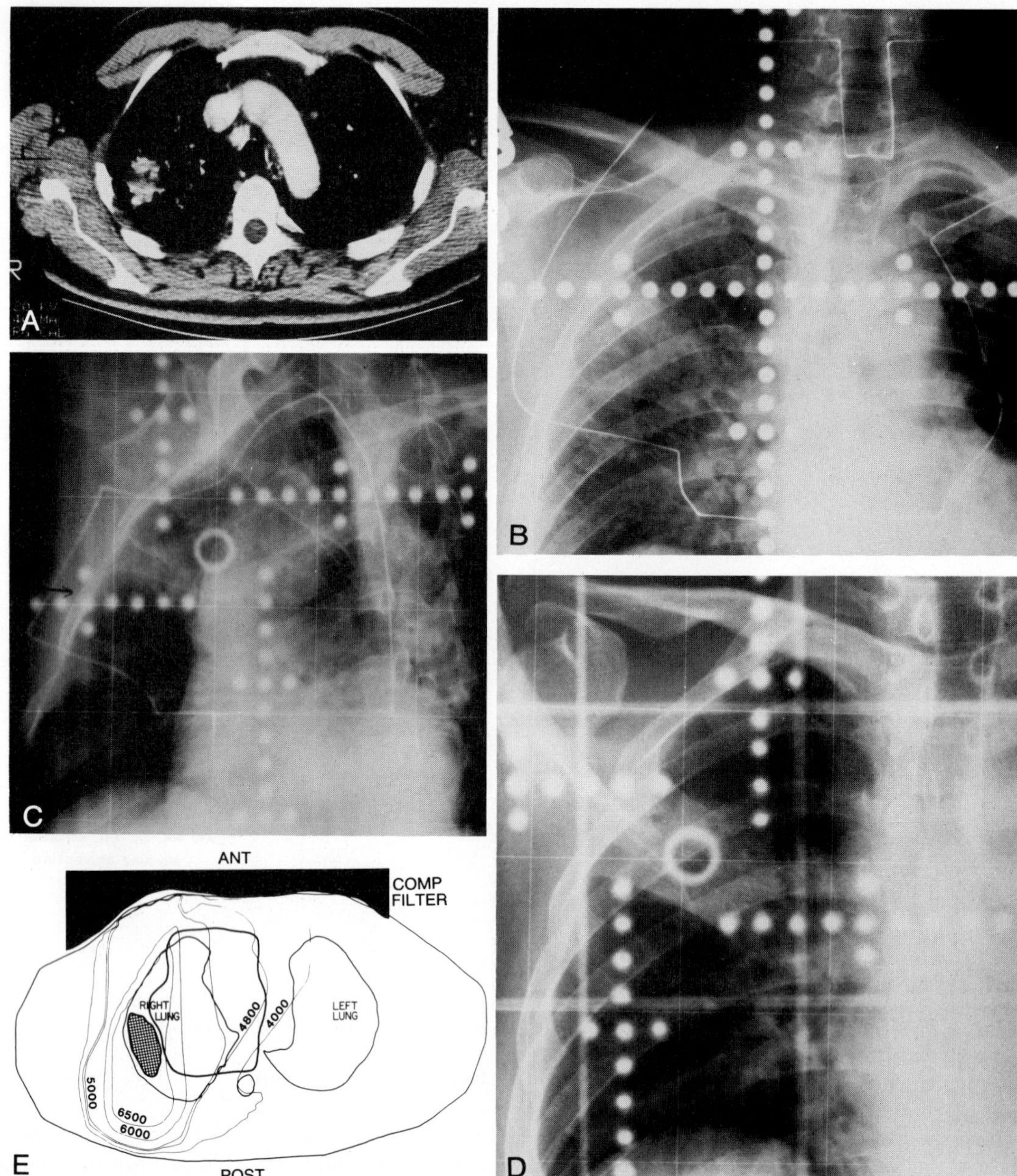

FIGURE 38–13. A 58-year-old man with a T2N2M0 adenocarcinoma in the posterior segment of the right upper lobe. Because of the presence of mediastinal lymph nodes, it was decided to treat the patient with radiation therapy. (**A**) CT scan of the chest demonstrating tumor in the posterior segment of the right upper lobe and some enlarged mediastinal lymph nodes. (**B**) Simulation film of the initial portal, used to deliver 4500 cGy. The right upper lobe, higher mediastinum, and supraclavicular lymph nodes are included. Compensating filters were used. (**C**) Oblique portal used to deliver an additional 1500 cGy to the right upper lobe and regional lymph nodes. (**D**) Reduced PA portal to deliver additional 500 cGy to the primary tumor only. (**E**) Composite isodose curve depicting total doses delivered to the primary tumor and hilar and mediastinal nodes.

success rate. Overall, approximately 10% of limited small cell carcinomas are amenable to surgery. Patients in this group have approximately 50% chance of complete response to chemotherapy alone. Thus, submitting these patients to surgery, which has a 2% to 3% mortality rate and a 10% to 20% major complication rate, does not appear to be justified.

Thoracic Irradiation Including Technical Considerations

Because of the high incidence of distant metastasis, some medical oncologists question the indication for thoracic irradiation.[45,94] Nevertheless, thoracic irradiation enhances tumor control within the irradiated volume.[16,87,168,202] Locoregional (intrathoracic) recurrences are reported in 30% to 60% of patients receiving thoracic radiation, whereas 75% to 80% of patients treated with chemotherapy alone exhibit this type of failure.[168] In a retrospective review of the literature between 1977 and 1979, Salazar and Creech[232] showed average tumor relapse in the thorax of 82% in patients receiving chemotherapy alone, 33% in patients treated with radiation alone, and 28% in patients receiving a combination of both modalities. Perez and co-workers,[202] in a randomized study involving 304 patients, reported an intrathoracic failure rate of 52% in patients receiving multiagent chemotherapy not treated with thoracic irradia-

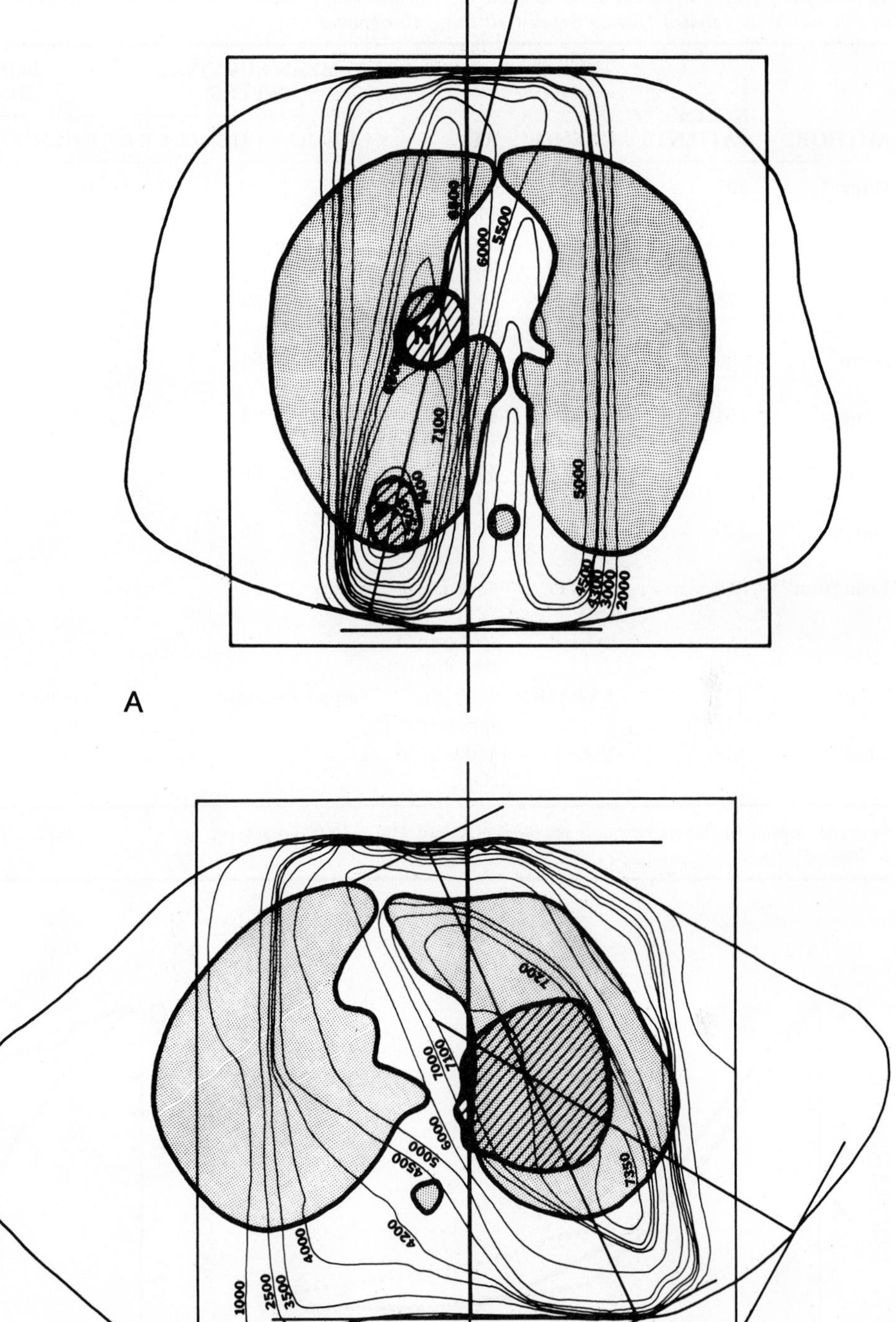

FIGURE 38–14. Examples of optimized treatment plans. (**A**) Isodose curves for treatment of a patient with a right lower lobe lesion and gross right hilar node on CT scan. Small right posterior oblique portal directed to both primary tumor and node delivers 7500 cGy to the primary tumor and 6500 cGy to the gross nodal disease. This patient was treated according to RTOG protocol 83-11 with twice-daily fractionation. Dose to spinal cord is limited to 4500 cGy and minimal volume of normal lung is irradiated to high dose. (**B**) Isodose curves of a patient with huge left upper lobe lesion. In this case two left posterior oblique ports were used, each encompassing gross tumor volume with small margin, thus limiting the volume of the normal lung in high dose area. Spinal cord dose is less than 4500 cGy.

tion and 36% rate in those receiving it. The 2-year survival rate was 23% in the group not receiving thoracic irradiation compared with 40% in those receiving thoracic irradiation. The difference between the two groups was statistically significant ($P = 0.04$). Unfortunately, these results were not maintained after 3 years.

Bunn and Ihde[24] observed a 2-year disease-free survival rate of 17% in patients treated with chemotherapy and radiation therapy in contrast to 7% in those treated with chemotherapy alone.

Perry and colleagues[207] conducted a prospective, randomized study to clarify the role of radiation in treatment of the primary tumor and the timing of chemotherapy/irradiation in limited small cell cancer of the lung. The chemotherapy consisted of cyclophosphamide, etoposide (VP16-213), and vincristine, with doxorubicin subsequently replacing etoposide in alternate cycles 7 through 18. Radiation therapy consisted of 4000 cGy in 6 weeks to the primary tumor followed by a 1000 cGy "boost" directed to the residual disease. All patients received prophylactic whole-brain irradiation. A total of 426 patients were enrolled; 399 were evaluable. There was a statistically significant difference in the number of complete responses in favor of the two radiation therapy regimens ($P = 0.0013$; Table 38-12). Relapse-free survival was also longer with these two regimens ($P < 0.001$; Fig. 38-15*A*), as was the interval before treatment failure in the chest ($P < 0.001$; Fig. 38-15*B*)

TABLE 38–12
Summary of Several Reported Series Comparing Chemotherapy Alone with Chemotherapy Plus Chest Irradiation in Patients With Limited Disease Small Cell Lung Carcinoma

AUTHOR	NO. OF PATIENTS	CHEMO	RT	MEAN SURVIVAL (WEEKS)		LONG-TERM SURVIVAL		PATIENTS WITH CHEST RELAPSE (%)	
				CHEMO	CHEMO + RT	CHEMO	CHEMO + RT	CHEMO	CHEMO + RT
Perez[202]	291	CAV	4000 cGy/ 14 fr/7 wk	49	60	19	28	52	36
Perry[207]	247	CAV/ CVPV	5000 cGy/ 5 wk	Similar response		Similar response		11	20
Fox[79]	73	CAVM	4000 cGy/ 20 fr	62	68	4	25	68	32
Bunn[25]	96*	CMC/ ProAV	4000 cGy/ 15 fr/3 wk	47 (Median)	64	12	28	67	29
Hansen[103]	134	CMV- CCNU	4000 cGy/ 10 fr/5 wk	60	48	10	4		
Looper[149]	123	CAV → CM	3500 cGy/ 10 fr/6 wk	43	60	14	29	69	26
Souhami[252]	129	AV/CM	4000 cGy/ 4 wk	56	56			32	28
Livingston[147]	333	VMVP/ CAV → CUP	4800 cGy/ 22 fr/6 wk split-course responders	67	97			(11/12)	(5/11)
Kies[130]	473	VVPAMC	4800 cGy split-course	Similar response		Similar response		72	50
Choi[34]	148	Varied	4400–5400 cGy	11	13	0	21	80	25

** Complete response for chemotherapy alone and chemo + RT was 43% and 81%, respectively.*
fr: fractions

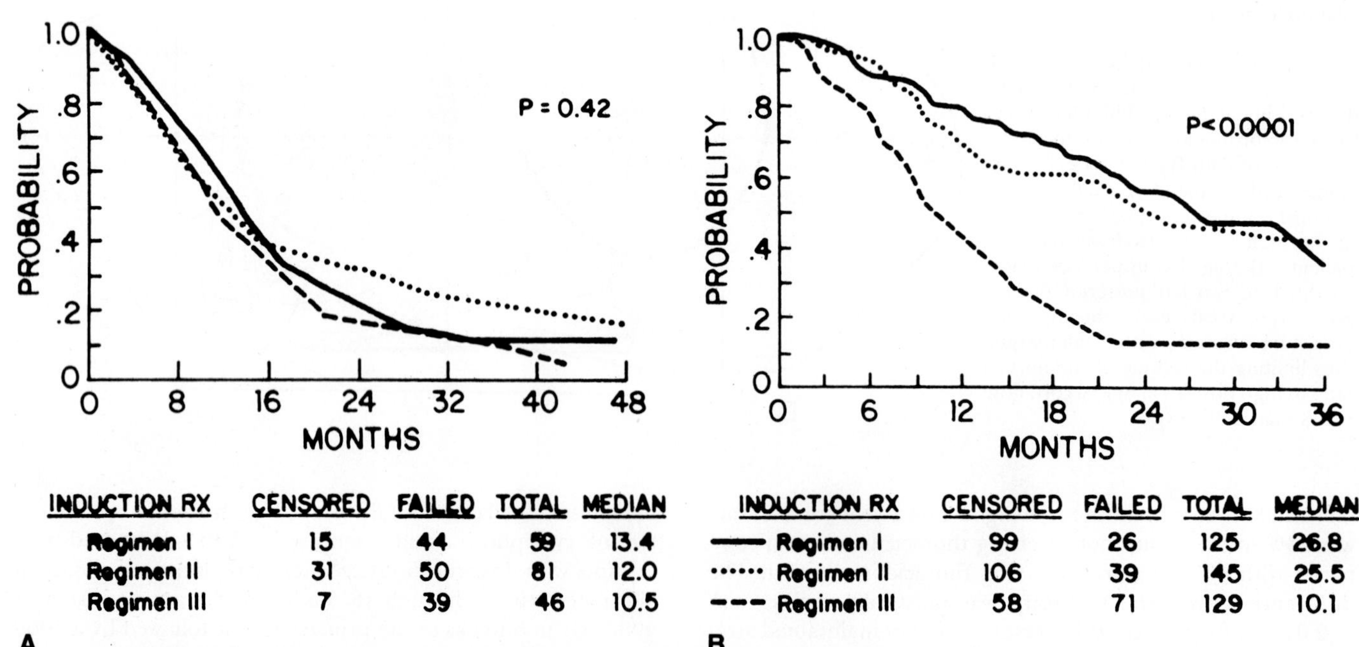

FIGURE 38–15. (**A**) Disease-free survival in patients on the three regimens. Disease-free survival (calculated from the date of complete response) was not significantly different with any regimen (P = 0.42). (**B**) The length of time from entry into the study until treatment failure in the chest. The interval was longer with the two radiation therapy regimens ($P < 0.0001$). (Perry MC, Eaton WL, Propert KJ, et al: N Engl J Med 316:912–918, 1987)

and overall survival ($P = 0.0099$). As expected, toxic effects—chiefly neutropenia—were also increased in the radiation therapy and chemotherapy arms.

To summarize, of six recent randomized trials, four demonstrated a benefit from added chest irradiation, including all three with concurrent chemoradiotherapy. In addition, the most recent Southwest Oncology Group (SWOG) trial,[87] although nonrandomized, involved a large number of patients and seemed to show a survival advantage in the concurrent use of chest and brain irradiation with cisplatin and VP16.[87] Table 38-12 shows a summary of several series reported in the literature documenting the value of thoracic irradiation in SCLC.

Doses and Fractionation of Irradiation

With the current recognition of the superior results of combined modality treatments over chemotherapy alone,[80,106,207] many radiation oncologists are asking important questions about sequencing, timing, and dose-time relationship in thoracic irradiation combined with systemic chemotherapy. Coy and coworkers[51] reported the results of a Canadian multicenter randomized trial in which patients receiving locoregional thoracic irradiation were randomized to receive either 2500 cGy in ten fractions (low dose) over 2 weeks or 3750 cGy in 15 fractions over 3 weeks (high dose). The overall response rate after combined radiation therapy and chemotherapy was 94% (complete response 67%, partial response 27%). The complete response rate for low-dose radiation was 65% and for high-dose radiation was 69%. Locoregional relapse rates, however, were very high for both arms of the trial. Lung and mediastinal recurrence rates for the lower dose arm were 53% and 27%, respectively; for the higher dose arm, 46% and 17%. These results clearly indicate that the doses of radiation used were very low. In studies using "routine" radiation doses of 4500 cGy TD, the tumor recurrence rate in the irradiated volume is about 30%, and the total intrathoracic failure rate is about 50%.[142] Thus, Choi and colleagues[33,34,36] strongly suggest that doses over 5000 cGy are necessary to achieve better tumor control (Fig. 38-16). We concur with this suggestion.

Other fractionation radiation therapy regimens have also been used in oat cell and undifferentiated small cell carcinoma of the lung. Choi and colleagues[40] reported on a phase II study of the Cancer and Leukemia Group B, which used accelerated radiation therapy followed by chemotherapy for locally recurrent small or persistent small cell carcinoma of the lung. Radiation therapy consisted of 5000 cGy in 30 fractions in 21 days to the chest. Chemotherapy was given 2 weeks after the completion of radiation therapy and was repeated every 3 weeks for 13 months. Of 29 potentially eligible patients with locally recurrent small cell lung cancer after first-line chemotherapy alone, 12 were enrolled initially in this study, including one patient who died immediately after the start of radiation therapy. Analysis of the remaining patients reveals complete remission in 72% (eight of 11) and partial remission in three patients. At the time of the report, survival ranged from 2 to 20 months, with a median survival of 6 months.

A preliminary report by Turrisi and co-workers[264] on 23 patients with small cell lung cancer treated with concurrent cisplatin and etoposide (VP16) chemotherapy and a twice-daily 150 cGy dose to a total dose of 4500 cGy in 3 weeks with modern radiation therapy treatment techniques showed that 21 patients achieved complete response (91%). Esophagitis occurred in 73% (13% severe) and hematologic toxicity in 65%. Median follow-up at the time of the report was 22 months with an actuarial projected 2-year survival rate of 56%. A recent update of this trial[265] with 30 patients shows a 93% complete response rate and a 54% actuarial survival rate of 2 years. This is an important study, currently being tested by several cooperative groups. Johnson and associates[121] from the National Cancer Institute (NCI) reported on 23 patients with limited stage small cell lung cancer treated with the same regimen as that in the Turrisi study.[264] Of 18 patients who completed the course of treatment, 16 achieved complete response (89%), and two achieved partial response (11%), with an overall response rate of 100%.

Volume

Optimal volume to be treated, optimal fractionation schedule, and the most effective combination of chemotherapeutic agents also have not been definitely established.[167] Kies and colleagues[130] reported on a randomized study (SWOG) of patients with limited small cell carcinoma of the lung treated with large fields outlined to cover the prechemotherapy tumor volume or smaller fields encompassing only the residual disease following two courses of multiagent chemotherapy. Patients

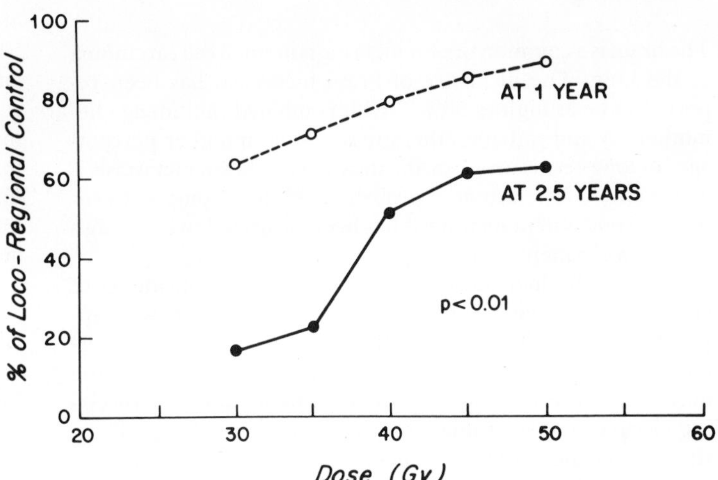

FIGURE 38–16. Locoregional control rates measured at 1 and 2.5 years for different levels of radiation doses. The actuarial method was used. (Choi NC, Carey RW: Int J Radiat Oncol Biol Phys 17:307–310, 1989)

randomized to the large field technique had slightly improved median survival (51 *versus* 46 weeks) and remission duration (31 *versus* 30 weeks), but these differences were not significant.

Sequence of Irradiation and Chemotherapy

The timing of chemotherapy and irradiation poses problems: Should chemotherapy and radiation therapy be used concomitantly or sequentially? It is important to realize that the toxicity caused by one form of treatment should not interfere with the optimal dose of the other.

Papac and co-workers[190] reported on 26 patients with limited small cell carcinoma of the lung treated with 6000 cGy to the thorax and cyclic combination chemotherapy with cyclophosphamide, VP16, and methotrexate. Of the 26 patients with limited disease, 57% achieved complete response after chemotherapy. Only one patient (3.8%) who received 6000 cGy to the thorax failed locally.

The following general guidelines for the management of patients with small cell carcinoma of the lung are suggested: All patients, after adequate workup and staging, should receive multiagent chemotherapy (four to six cycles). After this induction chemotherapy, the patient should be re-staged. Complete and partial responders should receive thoracic and elective brain irradiation. Thoracic irradiation should encompass the initial tumor volume (before chemotherapy) and adjacent hilar and mediastinal nodal-bearing areas plus or minus supraclavicular regions. The tumor dose should be biologically equivalent to 5000 cGy in 5 to 6 weeks (180–200 cGy, five weekly fractions). At Washington University, we administer 4000 cGy in 15 fractions over a 3-week period. With this regimen the spinal cord dose is limited to 3500 cGy.

An alternate approach to the "traditional" sequential treatment is concomitant chemotherapy and radiation therapy. In a study by the Southwest Oncology Group, 147 patients with limited disease received concurrent cisplatin and VP16 plus vincristine and continuous fractionated irradiation to a total dose of 4500 cGy in 5 weeks (180 cGy per fraction) as well as elective whole-brain irradiation. After three induction cycles, chemotherapy was continued with other active drugs according to an alternating schema. The most recent actuarial projection, demonstrated that 40% of all patients were alive at 2 years and showed an apparent survival plateau at 35%.[61]

Elective Cranial Irradiation in Small Cell Carcinoma of the Lung

The brain is a common site for metastasis in small cell carcinoma of the lung. The incidence of brain metastasis has been reported to be as high as 50%.[26] With combined multidrug chemotherapy and radiation therapy resulting in higher percentages of long-term survivors, the incidence of brain metastasis is increasing.[186] The actuarial probability of developing any central nervous system metastasis has been projected to be as high as 80% for patients surviving 5 years.[186]

Elective brain irradiation decreases the overall incidence of cranial brain metastasis to below 5% in comparison with approximately 30% in unirradiated patients.[50] In a review of literature by Pederson and associates,[197] among 715 patients the incidence of central nervous system relapse in those not receiving elective cranial irradiation was 22% compared with 6% in those receiving radiation. There was no survival advantage with prophylactic cranial irradiation in any of the studies. Dementia, psychomotor retardation, organic mental syndrome, optic atrophy, and hemiparesis have been reported following elective cranial irradiation combined with chemotherapy,[32,81,136,137,150,265] especially with concomitant Vinca alkaloids and nitrosoureas.[112] A review of literature reveals that almost all cases of neurotoxicity involve high doses of radiation per fraction; a review by Herskovic and Orton[112] correlated this high-dose fractionation schedule with moderate to severe neurologic problems in up to 45% of patients. However, very little toxicity has been reported with the use of conventional (180–200 cGy) fractionation. Another critical factor is the timing of prophylactic cranial irradiation. A long delay of prophylactic cranial irradiation enhances the risk of central nervous system relapse, whereas early cranial irradiation, at the peak of interaction of radiation therapy and chemotherapy, contributes to higher toxicity. In a study by Turrisi and colleagues,[266] elective cranial irradiation was initiated on week 24 in an attempt to reduce late effects. The dose was 2400 cGy in eight to 12 fractions. They reported no complications. At Washington University, elective cranial irradiation is given to patients who have achieved a complete or partial response to initial inductive chemotherapy. We deliver 3000 cGy in 15 fractions to the whole brain. No clinical neurotoxicity has been observed.

TREATMENT OF RECURRENT BRONCHOGENIC CARCINOMA

Although many patients who fail definitive treatment for lung cancer have both local and distant metastases, approximately 10% to 20% of patients develop an isolated intrathoracic recurrence after curative surgery or definitive radiation therapy.[95,97,156,244,253] Aggressive and judicious management by local or radiation therapy has resulted in both subjective and objective responses and even long-term survival.

Green and Kern[95] reported on 46 patients who had local recurrences after curative surgery and were treated by irradiation. Sixty-three percent had subjective improvement and 61% had objective improvement. Of the total group, 64% survived 6 months, 38% survived 1 year, and 10% survived 2 years. Of the patients who received 4000 cGy or more, 70% had a favorable response, compared with 33% who received less than 4000 cGy. Subjective response for dyspnea, hemoptysis, pain, and superior vena cava obstruction was noted in 50%, 75%, 73%, and 100% of the patients, respectively.

Retreatment of 29 patients with local recurrence after definitive radiation therapy was described by Green and Melbye.[97] Forty-eight percent favorable subjective responses and 74% objective responses were noted. The range of survival was 1 to 54 months, with a median survival of 5 months. It should be emphasized that in retreatment of patients with thoracic recurrences after definitive radiation therapy, careful planning is mandatory to avoid excessive radiation dose to critical structures such as the spinal cord or heart. Depending on the original dose of radiation given, subsequent treatment with doses ranging from 4000 cGy to 5000 cGy (180–200 cGy fractions), using limited treatment volumes, may be safely delivered.

CHEMOTHERAPY IN LUNG CANCER

Non-Small Cell Carcinoma

In contrast to small cell carcinoma, current results of chemotherapy in non-small cell carcinoma are not encouraging. The results of single agent chemotherapy from ten studies reported in the literature have been summarized by Hansen and Rorth.[105] Of 240 patients compiled from ten studies, there were two complete responses (0.7%) and 40 partial responses (14%). Combination chemotherapy administered to 189 patients collected from six reported series resulted in seven complete responses (3.7%) and 44 partial responses (23.3%). Median duration of response ranged from 1 to 20 months.

Rapp and associates[214] reported on a Canadian multicenter randomized trial in which patients with locally advanced non-small cell carcinoma were randomly allocated to receive cyclophosphamide (Cytoxan), doxorubicin (Adriamycin), and cisplatin (CAP) or vindesine and cisplatin (VP) or a placebo. Two-hundred fifty-one patients were entered; evaluation was done on only 172 patients. Median survival was 24.7 weeks with CAP, 32.6 weeks with VP, and 17 weeks with placebo/basic supportive care. Both chemotherapy trial arms were superior to basic supportive care ($P = 0.02$). Significant toxicity was encountered with chemotherapy.

In a randomized study,[126] patients with inoperable non-small cell carcinomas were randomized to receive 4200 cGy radiation in 15 fractions over 3 weeks *versus* chemotherapy (cisplatin and etoposide) repeated every third week to a maximum of four cycles. One-hundred-eighteen patients received radiation therapy, and 116 received chemotherapy. The median survival was 10.6 months with radiation therapy *versus* 10.5 months with chemotherapy. The objective response rate (CR + PR) was 42% with radiation and 21% with chemotherapy. This difference was statistically significant ($P = 0.009$).

Chemotherapy has also been used as an adjuvant to surgery (before or after) and to radiation therapy.[116, 139, 259] Shields and associates[245] reported no beneficial effect of adjuvant chemotherapy after surgical resection in 417 patients.

In another randomized study,[263] 360 patients were treated with surgery, and 360 patients were treated with surgery followed by chemotherapy consisting of cyclophosphamide (Cytoxan), methotrexate, and 5-FU (5-fluorouracil). One-, 3-, and 5-year survival rates were identical for both groups (34.4% and 34.2%, respectively). For patients with Stage I and Stage II disease (without nodal metastasis), surgical treatment was superior to combined therapy: 5-year survival rate for surgery was 51.3% compared with 38.7% for combined treatment. Only in Stage III patients with squamous cell histology was the combined therapy superior (33.3% 5-year survival rate compared with 23.3% for surgery alone).

In a prospective randomized study by the Lung Cancer Study Group,[134, 228, 245] patients with incompletely resected non-small cell lung cancer were treated with either postoperative radiation therapy alone or in combination with chemotherapy (cyclophosphamide, doxorubicin, and cisplatin). At 2 years, all study parameters (recurrence rate, death rate from all causes, death rate from cancer) were identical in both groups. Three-year overall survival rate, approximately 20%, was also similar in both arms of the study. The only positive point of this study was the median time to recurrence: 14 months for the chemotherapy plus irradiation arm compared with 8 months for the radiation therapy-alone arm.

The subject of so-called neoadjuvant chemotherapy treatment before surgery, especially in patients with Stage III non-small cell carcinoma, has gained much recent attention. The number of patients is extremely small, and the follow-up is very short in all the reports. The most widely acclaimed study of this type is the one by Memorial Hospital in New York.[90, 91] The median survival of 19.5 months is not significantly different from 15.8 months median survival with radiation therapy alone. Neoadjuvant chemotherapy in Stage III non-small lung cancer have been eloquently discussed by Einhorn.[65]

Encouraging results have recently been published on the use of preoperative chemotherapy plus radiation therapy in Stage III patients with non-small cell lung cancer.[64, 128, 210, 266] In a study from Rush University Medical Center in Chicago,[128] 130 patients with Stage III non-small cell lung cancer were treated with one of two protocols using simultaneous chemotherapy and radiation therapy followed by surgery when eligible. Sixty-four patients received cisplatin and infusion of 5-FU concurrently with split-course irradiation, whereas 66% of patients received the same regimen plus VP16. Of 85 patients preclassified as eligible for surgery, 62 underwent thoracotomy. Thirty patients (23%) remain alive with no evidence of disease with a median follow-up of 3.3 years. Nineteen patients (10.8%) died of concurrent medical problems, and six patients (4.6%) died of treatment-related toxicity.

In patients with inoperable non-small cell lung cancer, radiation therapy has also been compared with a combination of radiation therapy and adjuvant chemotherapy. A summary of prospective randomized trials is shown in Table 38-13. These data show that the addition of chemotherapy has not had a significant benefit over radiation therapy alone in terms of survival, except in the study by Dillman and associates (CALGB).[61]

In a review of the literature on chemotherapeutic trials in lung cancer, several points need further clarification.[65] The results reported from single institutions, which usually include smaller numbers of patients, have not been reproduced in larger trials. For example, the BACON regimen (bleomycin, doxorubicin, CCNU, vincristine, nitrogen mustard) was initially reported to have a 45% response rate in a single institution,[146] but when subjected to a cooperative group study only a 21% response rate was found.[145]

One of the most common methods of analyzing the results of treatment for a non-small cell lung cancer is to compare survival for responders with nonresponders. Using such a comparison, authors frequently find statistically significant differences in favor of the responders, depending on the selected variables. With a "significant *P* value," the authors come to the "logical" conclusion that the treatment was responsible for the difference. There are several pitfalls in this kind of analysis, as pointed out by Aisner and Hansen.[3] For example, comparison of responders and nonresponders may simply represent a selection of patients with good general condition who are likely to survive longer.

Small Cell Carcinoma

The role of chemotherapy in small cell carcinoma has been reviewed extensively.[25, 54, 105, 161, 276] Hansen and Rorth[105] reported on the effect of single agent chemotherapy in this disease. From a total of 184 cases compiled from 11 reported series in the literature, there were nine complete responses (4.9%) and 24 partial responses (13%). The duration of response in three studies was 2, 3, and 8 months. Combination chemotherapy has been shown to be substantially more effective than single agents. Hansen and Rorth[105] also reported on a total of 270 patients from eight reports in the literature who were treated with combined chemotherapy. There were 82 (30.3%) complete responses and 107 (39.6%) partial responses. Median duration of the response for all these trials ranged from 3 to 13 months. A combination of radiation therapy and multidrug chemotherapy has increased both local control and survival, as discussed previ-

TABLE 38–13
Summary of Prospective, Randomized Trials of Radiation Therapy and Radiochemotherapy in Inoperable Non-Small Cell Lung Carcinoma

AUTHOR	DOSE (cGy)	CHEMOTHERAPY	NUMBER OF PATIENTS	MEDIAN SURVIVAL (MONTHS)	% SURVIVAL (YEAR) 1	3	5
Mattson et al[157] (1988)	5500 S	—	119	10.3	41	11	—
	5500 S	CAP	119	11.0	41	7	—
Morton et al[170] (1988)	6000 C	—	53	9.6	43	—	—
	6000 C	MACC	54	10.4	47	—	—
Dillman et al[61] (1988)	6000 C	—	62	8.5	31	10	—
	6000 C	VBL + CDDP	68	16.5	55	22	—
Soresi et al[257] (1988)	5000 C	—	50	11	40*		—
	5000 C	CDDP	45	16	40		—
Robinow et al[220] (1989)	4000 S	CAP	38	14.8	61	13	3
	4000 S	V-CAP	39	16.2	67	26	18
	4000 S	T-CAP	25	14.6	56	20	16

*At 18 months
S: split course; C: continuous course; CAP: Cytoxan, Adriamycin, cisplatin; MACC: methotrexate, doxorubicin, Cytoxan, and CCNU; VBL: Vinblastine; CDDP: cisplatin; V-CAP: VP16 (etoposide) + CAP; T-CAP: Triazinate + CAP

ously. However, optimal doses of various drugs, doses of radiation, and optimal sequencing of these two modalities remain to be established.

SUPERIOR VENA CAVA SYNDROME

Superior vena cava syndrome is a medical emergency occasionally seen in patients with malignant neoplasia that requires immediate therapeutic action.[235] Currently the majority of cases (80%) of superior vena cava syndrome result from bronchogenic carcinoma.[6] Malignant lymphoma represents 10% to 18% of the cases, and benign causes, such as goiter, account for 2% to 3%.

This syndrome is produced by extrinsic compression of the superior vena cava or intracaval thrombosis, which is seen in approximately 40% to 50% of patients with this syndrome. Workup and establishment of diagnosis for patients with this syndrome depend on the severity of the symptoms. In patients with an earlier symptomatology and less severe respiratory distress, appropriate workup including chest x-ray studies, CT scan, bronchoscopy, and biopsy of tumor can be carried out. However, in patients with full-blown superior vena cava syndrome and severe respiratory distress, emergency therapy should be initiated and can be carried out without tissue diagnosis.

Although it is generally believed that these patients have an extremely poor prognosis, approximately 10% to 20% survive longer than 2 years.[6,248] Therefore, in the absence of distant metastasis, aggressive management and support are indicated.

Radiation Therapy

Radiation therapy should be initiated as soon as possible, sometimes without a definitive histologic diagnosis. Patients should initially be given high dose fractions (400 cGy tumor dose),[226] for 2 or 3 days followed by additional daily doses of 180 cGy to 200 cGy to complete the definitive course of radiation therapy. The recommended total dose for patients with localized bronchogenic carcinoma is 6000 cGy to 7000 cGy in 6 to 7 weeks, whereas patients with malignant lymphoma should receive a 4000 cGy to 4500 cGy tumor dose. In patients diagnosed with small cell carcinoma presenting with superior vena cava syndrome, the mode of initial therapy is controversial; both radiation therapy and chemotherapy are effective.

Portals of radiation therapy should encompass the mediastinal, hilar, and any adjacent pulmonary parenchymal lesions. Supraclavicular nodal areas should also be included.

Rubin and co-workers[225,227] described the effectiveness of and tolerance to high dose-fraction irradiation. Experimental animal data and results of patients treated with higher fractions (over 400 cGy) show a faster regression of symptoms and physical findings than those treated with low dose-fraction schedules.

Symptomatic Relief

Excellent symptomatic relief (disappearance of dyspnea, edema of the face, and distention of the neck and thoracic veins) has been observed in approximately 20% of patients with bronchogenic carcinoma and 75% of patients with malignant lymphoma. Good and symptomatic improvement has also been noted in an additional 50% of patients with bronchogenic carcinoma and 20% of patients with malignant lymphoma. Only 15% of patients with bronchogenic carcinoma had minimal improvement, and 15% showed no significant response.[248]

Survival Rates

In 84 patients, Armstrong and co-workers,[6] reported a 25% 1-year survival and a 10% 3-year survival. In the report by Armstrong and co-workers,[6] patients were treated with initial high-dose radiation therapy followed by conventional therapy, which provided faster and more durable symptomatic relief compared with patients treated with conventional fractionation at the initiation of the treatment (70% *versus* 56%). Patients exhibiting symptomatic relief within 30 days had a significantly better survival rate than those who did not ($P = 0.002$). Addition of chemotherapy to radiation at the initiation of treatment did not have any effect on the final outcome in the two studies.[6,141]

In general, patients with lymphoma have a better prognosis than those with small cell carcinoma, and the latter have a better prognosis than patients with non-small cell bronchogenic carcinoma.[6]

SEQUELAE OF THERAPY OF LUNG CANCER

The most frequently reported sequelae noted in the RTOG trials were pneumonitis (approximately 10% grade 2 and 4.6% grade 3), pulmonary fibrosis (approximately 20% grade 2 and 8% grade 3 or greater), esophagitis (about 12% grade 2 and 3% grade 3), and esophageal stricture (about 1%). Thoracic spinal cord myelopathy was observed in four of 1380 patients (0.3%).[198]

The grade 2 toxicity incidence appeared to correlate with the total doses of radiation (27% with less than 4000 cGy and 34% with doses greater than 5000 cGy). There was no significant correlation between the daily fraction and the incidence of grade 2 toxicity (between 27% to 35%)

The frequency of grade 3 complications as a function of total dose is shown in Table 38-14. The highest incidence of toxicity (15.5% to 17.6%) was reported with 3600 cGy in six fractions, 4000 cGy with a split course of 400 cGy fractions each, or 6000 cGy with conventional fractionation, compared with 8.6% to 11.4% in the patients treated with conventional fractionation or doses higher than 6000 cGy with twice-daily fractionation.

Acute radiation esophagitis usually begins in the third week of radiation therapy, at the dose of approximately 3000 cGy.[224] In five patients reported on by Seaman and Ackerman[238] with severe damage and four with moderate damage of the normal esophagus, the suggested dose for 5% incidence of esophageal injury was 6300 cGy in 30 fractions and for 50%, 6650 cGy in 30 fractions (without lung inhomogeneity corrections).

The combination of irradiation and chemotherapy may significantly increase the incidence of esophageal injury.[93,180] Johnson and associates[125] reported severe esophagitis in 13 and esophageal strictures in three of 21 patients receiving 3000 cGy to 4000 cGy in 3 to 4 weeks combined with intensive chemotherapy (doxorubicin, 40 mg/m^2, vincristine, 2 mg/m^2, and cyclophosphamide, 1200 to 1500 mg/m^2).

In the acute stage of esophageal injury, mucosal anesthetics such as lidocaine hydrochloride (1 tablespoon 10 to 15 minutes before food ingestion) may improve swallowing. Other analgesics decrease the odynophagia. Taking liquid analgesics or dissolving pills or capsules in water or fruit juices makes administration easier. Liquid antacids (aluminum or magnesium hydroside) every 2 hours decrease symptoms in many patients.

If symptoms do not improve and nutritional status is compromised, insertion of a nasogastric tube or even a temporary gastrostomy or intravenous hyperalimentation may be necessary. Superimposed moniliasis should be ruled out; if present, it should be treated with appropriate medication (*e.g.,* Mycostatin).

Long-term esophageal problems, such as stenosis, ulceration, and fistula formation, are very rare, although recessional stenosis has been reported.[238]

The threshold dose for radiation pneumonitis is 2000 cGy to 2500 cGy.[142,181,209] The incidence and degree of radiation pneumonitis depend on the total dose, fractionation, and volume of lung irradiated.[261] The maximum lung volume that can be included in a high-dose zone without significant clinical symptoms is 25% to 30% of the total lung volume.[152,224]

Decreased pulmonary blood flow can be demonstrated in nuclide ventilation perfusion scanning. Pulmonary function studies in patients with lung cancer receiving radiation demonstrated decreased compliance, diffusing capacity, and lung volumes.[4,17,39,56] Phillips and Margolis[209] indicated that a 50% incidence of clinical pneumonitis occurs with doses below 3000 cGy delivered with small fractions (less than 150 cGy). With dactinomycin (Actinomycin-D), they noted a 50% incidence of clinical pneumonitis with doses below 2650 cGy delivered in 20 fractions. Similar observations have also been reported with other drugs.[65,237,271]

Treatment of the acute phase of radiation pneumonitis includes absolute bed rest, use of bronchodilators, and corticosteroid therapy. In severe cases, it may be necessary to use positive pressure oxygen. There is no indication for antibiotics

TABLE 38–14
Non-Oat Cell Carcinoma of the Lung: Grade 3 or Worse Toxicity by Total Radiation Dose (RTOG Protocols)

	PERCENT WITH TOXICITY						
	3600 cGy	SPLIT 4000 cGy	4000 cGy	5000 cGy	5000–6000 cGy	6000 cGy	BID >6000 cGy*
Pneumonitis	4.6%	5.0%	0%	3.3%	4.4%	4.8%	3.3%
Pulmonary fibrosis	1.9%	8.0%	1.0%	1.1%	3.4%	4.8%	4.1%
Esophagitis	7.4%	2.0%	1.9%	1.1%	1.6%	1.2%	3.0%
Esophageal stricture	2.8%	0%	1.0%	0%	0.2%	1.2%	0.3%
Myelopathy/myelitis	1.9%	0%	0%	1.1%	0%	0%	0%
All other toxicities	4.6%	3.0%	5.7%	2.2%	2.6%	6.0%	2.3%
No. of evaluable patients	108	100	105	92	496	84	394
Total percent with toxicity	17.6%	16.0%	8.6%	8.7%	9.9%	15.5%	11.4%

* *Hyperfractionation*

TABLE 38–15
Neurologic Sequelae of Elective Cranial Irradiation and Concomitant Chemotherapy in Small Cell Carcinoma of the Lung

REPORT	NO. OF PATIENTS	CLINICAL	RADIOLOGIC	CHEMOTHERAPY	DOSE/FRACTIONS
Lee (M.D. Anderson)[137]	24	12.5%		Various; no nitrosoureas	3000 cGy/10
	14	0.0%	70%	Various; no nitrosoureas	3000 cGy/10
	10		70%	Various; no nitrosoureas; procarbazene; MTX	3000 cGy/10
	5	0.0%		Various	Not Reported
Looper	18	77%		Various	3500–3600 cGy split
(Indiana University)[149]	6	75%		Various; no nitrosoureas	
Licciardello[143]	7	42%		CAV or CV + VP16	Not Reported
Ellison[68]	10	40%		Cyclo-MTX; VCR-CCNU	Not Reported
Livingston[147]	17	6%–12%		CAV + maintenance CA-C + MTX	3000 cGy/10

until there is associated secondary infection. It should be emphasized that after control of acute symptoms, corticosteroid use should be tapered over a period of several weeks. Abrupt discontinuation of the steroids may result in activation of subclinical radiation injuries in the lung.

Radiation-induced cardiac disease following radiation therapy for lung cancer is relatively rare. Radiation pericarditis is the most common form of clinical cardiac damage caused by irradiation.[169,256] Factors involved in this complication include the volume of irradiated heart and the radiation dose. Stewart and Fajardo[257] reported on incidence of cardiac complications of 6.6% after a mean dose of 4281 cGy. Similar findings have been observed by others.[142] Certain chemotherapeutic agents, such as doxorubicin, are not only cardiotoxic by themselves but also have synergistic cardiotoxicity with radiation. Extreme caution is required when radiation is combined with such drugs.

Since its original description,[18] this complication has been the subject of numerous reviews in the literature.[1,148,208,273] Review of the literature discloses that the following factors are important in the development of permanent radiation damage to spinal cord: total radiation dose, length of the irradiated cord, and fractionation schedule. It appears that with conventional fractionation (200 cGy per day, 5 days per week) and the length of spinal cord within the radiation volume equal to or less than 10 cm, the threshold dose is about 4500 cGy. A shorter length cord may possibly tolerate a slightly higher dose, but it is advisable even in this case to limit the dose to an absolute maximum of 5000 cGy. Longer segments of cord or higher daily fractions should mandate the lowering of the total dose.[247]

Toxicity of Elective Brain Irradiation

Several authors have described clinical and radiologic findings indicative of various types and degrees of brain injury, including neurologic deficit, memory loss, and dementia.[8,13,23,24,267] This syndrome has been associated with concomitant administration of chemotherapy and moderate doses of radiation (Table 38-15). The physiopathologic lesion seems to be a diffuse degenerative encephalopathy affecting higher cortical functions (cognition, speech, mental ability), although disorders of equilibrium and gait may be seen.[8] Symptoms appear between a few months to several years after cranial irradiation. The majority of patients have a progressive course leading to death in 1 to 26 months.[8]

The most effective suggested management for these undesirable sequelae of brain irradiation is use of lower doses of radiation (2500–3000 cGy) delivered with daily fractionation of 180 cGy to 200 cGy in five weekly fractions.

REFERENCES

1. Abbatucci JS, Delozier T, Quint R, et al: Radiation myelopathy of the cervical spinal cord: Time, dose and volume factors. Int J Radiat Oncol Biol Phys 4:239–248, 1978
2. Ahmad K, Fayos JV, Kirsh MM: Apical lung carcinoma. Cancer 54:913–917, 1984
3. Aisner J, Hansen HH: Commentary: Current status of chemotherapy for non-small cell lung cancer. Cancer Treat Rep 65(11–12):979–986, 1981
4. American Cancer Society: 1991 Cancer Facts and Figures. Atlanta, American Cancer Society, 1991
5. American Joint Committee on Cancer: Lung. In Beahrs OH, Myers MH (eds): Manual for Staging of Cancer, 2nd ed, p 99. Philadelphia, JB Lippincott, 1983
6. Armstrong BA, Perez CA, Simpson JR, Hederman MA: Role of irradiation in the management of superior vena cava syndrome. Int J Radiat Oncol Biol Phys 13:531–539, 1987
7. Auerbach O, Stout AP, Hammond EC, et al: Changes in bronchial epithelium in relation to cigarette smoking and in relation to lung cancer. N Engl J Med 265:253, 1961
8. Baird JA: The pathways of lymphatic spread of carcinoma of the lung. Br J Surg 52:868–875, 1965
9. Bangma PJ: Post-operative radiotherapy. In Deeley TJ (ed): Modern Radiotherapy. Carcinoma of the Bronchus, pp 163–170. New York, Appleton-Century-Crofts, 1972
10. Baron RL, Levitt RG, Sagel SS, et al: Computer tomography in the preoperative evaluation of bronchogenic carcinoma. Radiology 145:727–732, 1982
11. Basso-Ricci, et al: Report on 42 cases of post irradiation lesions of the brachial plexus and their treatment. Tumori 66(1):117–122, 1980
12. Batra P, Brown JD, Collins CO, et al: Evaluation of intrathoracic extent of lung cancer by plain chest radiography, computed tomography, and magnetic resonance imaging. Am Rev Respir Dis 137:1456–1462, 1988
13. Beattie EJ, Raskin NM: Progress in lung cancer: Non-oat cell (non-small cell lung cancer). Jpn J Surg 17:313–322, 1987
14. Bisel HF, Wroblewski F, LaDue JS: Incidence and clinical manifestations of cardiac metastases. JAMA 153:712–715 1953
15. Bitran JD, Gololmb HM, Hoffman PC, et al: Protochemotherapy in non-small cell lung carcinoma: An attempt to increase surgical resectability and survival. A preliminary report. Cancer 57:44–53, 1986

16. Bleehan NM, Bunn PA, Cox JD, et al: Role of radiation therapy in small cell anaplastic carcinoma of the lung. Cancer Treat Rep 67:11–19, 1983
17. Bloedorn FG, Cowley RA, Cuccia CA, et al: Combined therapy: Irradiation and surgery in the treatment of bronchogenic carcinoma. AJR 85:175–181, 1961
18. Boden G: Radiation myelitis of the cervical spinal cord. Br J Radiol 21:464–469, 1948
19. Bonomi P, Gale M, Rowland K, et al: Prognostic factors in stage 3 non-small cell lung cancer (NSCLC) patients receiving combined modality treatment (Abstract). Proc Am Soc Clin Oncol 8:233, 1989
20. Borrie J: Primary carcinoma of the bronchus: Prognoses following surgical resection (Hunterian Lecture). Ann R Coll Surg Engl 10:165–186, 1952
21. Boyden EA: Segmental Anatomy of the Lungs. New York, McGraw-Hill, 1955
22. Brantigan OC, Moszkowski E: Bilateral biopsy of non-palpable cervical lymph nodes. Diagnosis and prognosis of carcinoma of the lung. Dis Chest 50:464–469, 1966
23. Bunn PA, Cohen M, Lichter A, et al: Randomized trial of chemotherapy versus chemotherapy plus radiotherapy in limited stage small cell lung cancer (Abstract). Proc Am Assoc Cancer Res 24:200, 1983
24. Bunn PA, Ihde DC: Small cell bronchogenic carcinoma: A review of therapeutic results. In Livingston RB (ed): Lung Cancer I, pp 169–208. Hague, Martinus Nijhoff, 1981
25. Bunn PA, Lichter AS, Makuch RW, et al: Chemotherapy alone or chemotherapy with chest radiation therapy in limited stage small cell lung cancer. Ann Intern Med 106:655–662, 1987
26. Bunn PA, Nugent JL, Matthews MJ: Central nervous system metastases in small cell bronchogenic carcinoma. Semin Oncol 5:314–322, 1978
27. Burkes R, Ginsberg R, Shepherd F, et al: Neo-adjuvant trial with MVP (Mitomycin-C + Vindesine + Cisplatin) chemotherapy for stage III (T1–3, N2 MO) unresectable non-small cell lung cancer (NSCLC) (Abstract). Proc Am Soc Clin Oncol 8:221, 1989
28. Burt ME, Pomerantz AH, Bains MS, et al: Results of surgical treatment of stage III lung cancer invading the mediastinum. Surg Clin North Am 67:987–1000, 1987
29. Buy JN, Ghosian MA, Poirson F, et al: Computed tomography of mediastinal lymph nodes in nonsmall cell lung cancer: A new approach based on the lymphatic pathway of tumor spread. J Comput Asst Tomogr 12:545–552, 1988
30. Carter D, Eggleston JC: Tumors of the Lower Respiratory Tract. Washington, DC, Armed Forces Institute of Pathology Publication, 1980
31. Chahinian AP, Israel L: Rates and patterns of growth of lung cancer. In Israel L, Chahinian AP (eds): Lung Cancer: Natural History, Prognosis and Therapy, pp 63–79. New York, Academic Press, 1976
32. Chak LY, Zatz LM, Wasserstein P, et al: Neurologic dysfunction in patients treated for small cell carcinoma of the lung: A clinical and radiological study. Int J Radiat Oncol Biol Phys 12:385–389, 1986
33. Choi NC: Reassessment of the role of radiation therapy relative to other treatment in small-cell carcinoma of the lung. In Choi NC, Grillo HC (eds): Thoracic Oncology, pp 233–256. New York, Raven Press, 1983
34. Choi NC, Carey RW, Kaufman D, et al: Small cell carcinoma of the lung: A progress report of 15 years' experience. Cancer 59:6–14, 1987
35. Choi NC: Curative radiation therapy for unresectable non-small cell carcinoma of the lung: Indications, techniques, results. In Choi NC, Grillo HC (eds): Thoracic Oncology, pp 163–199. New York, Raven Press, 1983
36. Choi NC, Carey RW: Importance of radiation dose in achieving improved loco-regional tumor control in limited stage small-cell lung carcinoma: An update. Int J Radiat Oncol Biol Phys 17:307–310, 1989
37. Choi NC, Doucette JA: Improved survival of patients with unresectable non-small-cell bronchogenic carcinoma by an innovated high-dose en-bloc radiotherapeutic approach. Cancer 48:101–109, 1981
38. Choi NC, Grillo HC, Gardiello M, et al: Basis for new strategies in postoperative radiotherapy of bronchogenic carcinoma. Int J Radiat Oncol Biol Phys 6:31–35, 1980
39. Choi NC, Kanarek DJ, Kazemi H: Physiological changes in pulmonary function after thoracic radiotherapy for patients with lung cancer and role of regional pulmonary function studies in predicting postradiotherapy pulmonary function before radiotherapy. Cancer Treat Symp 2:119–130, 1985
40. Choi NC, Propert K, Carey R, et al: Accelerated radiotherapy followed by chemotherapy for locally recurrent small-cell carcinoma of the lung: A phase II study of cancer and leukemia group B. Int J Radiat Oncol Biol Phys 13:263–266, 1987
41. Chung CK, Stryker JA, O'Neill M Jr, et al: Evaluation of adjuvant postoperative radiotherapy for lung cancer. Int J Radiat Oncol Biol Phys 8:1877–1880, 1982
42. Cohen AM, Creviston S, LiPuma JP, et al: NMR evaluation of hilar and mediastinal lymphadenopathy. Radiology 148:739–742, 1983
43. Cohen MH: Signs and symptoms of bronchogenic carcinoma. In Straus MJ (ed): Lung Cancer Clinical Diagnosis and Treatment, pp 85–94. New York, Grune & Stratton, 1977
44. Cohen MH: Is immediate radiation therapy indicated for patients with unresectable non-small cell lung cancer? No. Cancer Treat Rep 67:333–336, 1983
45. Cohen MH: Is thoracic radiation therapy necessary for patients with limited-stage small cell lung cancer? No. Cancer Treat Rep 67:217–221, 1983
46. Collins VP, Loeffler R, Tivey H: Observations on growth rates for human tumors. AJR 76:988, 1956
47. Cox JD, Azarnia N, Byhardt RW, et al: Hyperfractionated radiation therapy (1.2 Gy b.i.d.) with 69.6 Gy total dose increases survival in favorable patients with stage III non-small cell carcinoma of the lung. Report of RTOG 83-11. J Clin Oncol 8:1543–1555, 1990
48. Cox JD, Bauer M: Therapeutic ratio and fractionation in cancer of the lung. Front Radiat Ther Oncol 22:121–126, 1988
49. Cox JD, Komaki R, Byhardt RW: Is immediate chest radiotherapy obligatory for any or all patients with limited-stage non-small cell carcinoma of the lung? Yes. Cancer Treat Rep 67:327–331, 1983
50. Cox JD, Stanley K, Petrovich Z, et al: Cranial irradiation in cancer of the lung of all cell types. JAMA 245(5):469–472, 1981
51. Coy P, Hodson I, Payne DG, et al: The effect of dose of thoracic irradiation on recurrence in patients with limited stage small cell lung cancer initial results of a Canadian multicenter randomized trial. Int J Radiat Oncol Biol Phys 14:219–226, 1988
52. Croxatto OC, Barcat JA: Lymph node metastasis in bronchogenic carcinoma: Study on its role in dissemination. Johns Hopkins Med J 126:121–129, 1970
53. Cunningham JJ: Gray scale echography of the lung and pleural space: Current applications of oncologic interest. Cancer 41:1329–1339, 1978
54. Daniels JR, Chak LY, Sikic BI, et al: Chemotherapy of small cell carcinoma of lung: A randomized comparison of alternating and sequential combination chemotherapy protocols. J Clin Oncol 2:1193–1199, 1984
55. Davies DF: A review of detection methods for the early diagnosis of lung cancer. J Chronic Dis 19:819–895, 1966
56. Deeley TJ: A clinical trial to compare two different tumor dose levels in the treatment of advanced carcinoma of the bronchus. Clin Radiol 17:299–301, 1966
57. del Regato JA, Spjut HJ: Cancer: Diagnosis, Treatment, and Prognosis, 5th ed, p 378. St Louis, CV Mosby, 1977
58. DeLaude FH, et al: ^{67}Ga-citrate imaging in untreated primary lung cancer: Preliminary report of cooperative group. J Nucl Med 15:408, 1974
59. DeMeester TR, et al: Gallium-67 scanning for carcinoma of the lung. J Thorac Cardiovasc Surg 72:699, 1976
60. Denoix PF, Schwartz D, Anguera G: L'enquête française sur

l'étiologie du cancer bronco-pulmonaire. Analyse detaillée. Bull Assoc Fr Cancer 26:1085, 1958
61. Dillman RO, Seagren SL, Propert KJ, et al: Induction chemotherapy improves survival in regional non-small cell lung cancer: A study of Cancer and Leukemia Group B. N Engl J Med (submitted for publication)
62. Doll R, Hill AB: A study of the etiology of carcinoma of the lung. Br Med J 2:1271, 1952
63. Dvale PA, Bode FR, Kini S: Diagnostic accuracy in lung cancer: Comparison of techniques used in association with flexible fiberoptic bronchoscopy. Chest 69:752–757, 1976
64. Eagan RT, Ruud C, Lee RE, et al: Pilot study of induction therapy with cyclophosphamide, doxorubicin, and cisplatin (CAP) and chest irradiation prior to thoracotomy in initially inoperable stage III MO non-small cell lung cancer. Cancer Treat Rep 71:895–900, 1987
65. Einhorn LW: Neoadjuvant therapy of stage III non-small cell lung cancer. Ann Thorac Surg 46:362–365, 1988
66. Eisert DR, Cox JD, Komaki R: Irradiation for bronchial carcinoma: Reasons for failure. Cancer 37:2665–2670, 1976
67. Ellis JH: Transbronchial lung biopsy via the fiberoptic bronchoscopy: Experience with 107 consecutive cases and comparison with bronchial brushing. Chest 68:534–531, 1975
68. Ellison N, Bernath A, Kane R, et al: Disturbing problems of success: Clinical status of long-term survivors of small cell lung cancer (SCLC). Proc Am Soc Clin Oncol 1:C-579, 1982
69. Emami B, Kim T, Roper C, et al: Postoperative radiation therapy in the management of lung cancer. Radiology 164:251–253, 1987
70. Emami B, Melo A, Carter BL, et al: Value of computed tomography in radiotherapy of lung cancer. AJR 131:63–67, 1978
71. Emami B, Munzenrider JE, Lee DJ, et al: Radical radiation therapy of advanced lung cancer. Evaluation of prognostic factors and results of continuous and split-course treatment. Cancer 44:446–456, 1979
72. Emami B, Perez CA: Radiation therapy in the management of carcinoma of the lung and esophagus. In Levitt SH, Tapley ND (eds): Technological Basis of Radiation Therapy: Practical Clinical Applications, vol 2. Philadelphia, Lea & Febiger (in press)
73. Emami B, Perez, CA Herkovic A, Hederman MA: Phase I/II study of treatment of locally advanced (T3 T4) non-oat cell lung cancer with high dose radiotherapy (rapid fractionation): Radiation Therapy Oncology Group Study. Int J Radiat Oncol Biol Phys 15:1021–1025, 1988
74. Emami B, Purdy JA, Manolis J, et al: Three dimensional treatment planning for lung cancer. Int J Radiat Oncol Biol Phys (submitted for publication)
75. Ernst H, Kruger J, Vassal K: Lung scanning as a screening method for cancer of the lung. Cancer 23:508, 1969
76. Erozan YS, Frost JK: Cytopathological diagnosis of lung cancer. Semin Oncol 1(3):191–198, 1974
77. Feinstein AR, Gelfman NA, Yesner R: Observer variability in the histopathologic diagnosis of lung cancer. Am Rev Respir Dis 101:671–684, 1970
78. Fletcher GH: Clinical dose-response curves of human malignant epithelial tumours. Br J Radiol 46:1–12, 1973
79. Fox RM, Tattersall MHN, Woods RL: Radiation therapy as an adjuvant in small cell lung cancer treated by combination chemotherapy: A randomized study (Abstract). Proc Am Soc Clin Oncol 22:502, 1981
80. Fox RM, Woods RL, Brodie GM, et al: A randomized study: Small cell anaplastic lung cancer treated by combination chemotherapy and adjuvant radiotherapy. Int J Radiat Oncol Biol Phys 6:1083–1085, 1980
81. Grytak S, Shaw JN, O'Neill BP, et al: Leukoencephalopathy in small cell lung cancer patients receiving prophylactic cranial irradiation. Am J Clin Oncol (CCT) 12:27–33, 1989
82. Galietti F, Giorgis GE, Toffola AD, et al: Epidemiological study of 3,398 cases of lung cancer histologically ascertained in 1973–84. Panminerva Med 30:16–22, 1988
83. Gamsu B, Webb WR, Sheldon P, et al: Nuclear magnetic resonance imaging of the thorax. Radiology 147:473–480, 1983
84. Garland LH, Beier RL, Coulson W, et al: The apparent sites of origin of carcinomas of the lung. Radiology 78:1–11, 1962
85. Glazer HS, Kaiser LR, Anderson DJ, et al: Indeterminate mediastinal invasion of bronchogenic carcinoma: CT evaluation. Radiology 173:P37–42, 1989
86. Glazer HS, Levitt RG, Lee JKT, et al: Differentiation of radiation fibrosis from recurrent pulmonary neoplasm by magnetic resonance imaging. AJR 143:729–730, 1984
87. Goodman GE, Livingston RB: Small cell lung cancer. Curr Probl Cancer 13:7–55, 1989
88. Graham BL, Balducci L, Khansur T, et al: Surgery in small cell lung cancer. Ann Thorac Surg 45:687–692, 1988
89. Graham EA, Singer JJ: Successful removal of an entire lung for carcinoma of the bronchus. JAMA 101:1371–1374, 1933
90. Gralla RJ: Preoperative and adjuvant chemotherapy in nonsmall cell lung cancer. Semin Oncol 15:8–12, 1988
91. Gralla RJ, Kris MG: Chemotherapy in non-small cell lung cancer: Results of recent trials. Semin Oncol 15:2–5, 1988
92. Gray H: Anatomy of the Human Body, 29th ed. Philadelphia, Lea & Febiger, 1973
93. Greco FA, Brereton HD, Kent H, et al: Adriamycin and enhanced radiation reaction in normal esophagus and skin. Ann Intern Med 85:294–298, 1976
94. Greco FA, Perez C, Einhorn LH: Combination chemotherapy with or without concurrent thoracic radiotherapy in limitedstage small cell lung cancer. A phase III trial of the Southeastern Cancer Group (Abstract). Proc Am Soc Clin Oncol 5:178, 1986
95. Green N, Kern W: The clinical course and treatment results of patients with post resection locally recurrent lung cancer. Cancer 42:2478–2482, 1978
96. Green N, Kurohara SS, George FW III, et al: Postresection irradiation for primary lung cancer. Radiology 116:405–407, 1975
97. Green N, Melbye RW: Lung cancer: Retreatment of local recurrence after definitive irradiation. Cancer 49:31–34, 1982
98. Grenier PH, Dubray B, Carette MF, et al: Preoperative thoracic staging of lung cancer: CT and MR evaluation. Diagn Intern Radiol 1:23–28, 1989
99. Guthrie RT, Ptacek JJ, Hass AC: Comparative analysis of two regimens of split-course radiation in carcinoma of the lung. AJR 117:605–608, 1973
100. Haffty BG, Goldberg NB, Gerstley J, et al: Results of radical radiation therapy in clinical stage I, technically operable nonsmall cell lung cancer. Int J Radiat Oncol Biol Phys 15:69–73, 1988
101. Hall TC (ed): Paraneoplastic syndromes. Ann NY Acad Sci 230:1–577, 1974
102. Hammond EL, Horn D: Smoking death-rates report on forty-four months of follow-up of 187,783 men. JAMA 166:1159, 1958
103. Hansen HD, Dombernowsky P, Hansen HS, et al: Chemotherapy versus chemotherapy plus radiotherapy in regional small-cell carcinoma of the lung: A randomized trial (Abstract). Proc Am Assoc Cancer Res 20:277, 1979
104. Hansen HH, Muggia FM: Staging of inoperable patients with bronchogenic carcinoma with special reference to bone marrow examination and peritoneoscopy. Cancer 30:1395–1401, 1972
105. Hansen HH, Rorth M: Lung Cancer. In Pinedo HM, Chabner BA (eds): Cancer Chemotherapy, pp 307–325. New York, Elsevier, 1983
106. Hansen M, Hansen HH, Dombernowsky P, et al: Long term survival in small cell carcinoma of the lung. JAMA 244:247–250, 1980
107. Haratake J, Horie A, Tokudome S, et al: Inter- and intrapathologist variability in histologic diagnoses of lung cancer. Act Pathol Jpn 37:1053–1060, 1987
108. Hellman S, Kligerman MM, VonEssen CF, et al: Sequelae of radical radiotherapy of the lung. Radiology 82:1055–1081, 1964
109. Henschke UK: Interstitial implantation in the treatment of primary bronchogenic carcinoma. AJR 79:981–987, 1958

110. Herman DL, Crittenden M: Distribution of primary lung carcinomas in relation to tissue as determined by histochemical techniques. J Natl Cancer Inst (in press)
111. Herskovic AM, Bauer M, Seydel HG, et al: Postoperative thoracic irradiation with or without Levamisole in non-oat cell lung cancer: The results of a Radiation Therapy Oncology Group study. Int J Radiat Oncol Biol Phys 14:37–42, 1988
112. Herskovic AM, Orton CG: Editorial: Elective brain irradiation for small cell anaplastic lung cancer. Int J Radiat Oncol Biol Phys 12:427–429, 1986
113. Higginson JF: Block dissection in pneumonectomy for carcinoma. J Thorac Surg 25:582–592, 1953
114. Hilaris BS, Nori D: The role of external radiation and brachytherapy in unresectable non-small cell lung cancer. Surg Clin North Am 67:1061–1071, 1987
115. Hilaris BS, Martini N: The current state of intraoperative interstitial brachytherapy in lung cancer. Int J Radiat Oncol Biol Phys 15:1347–1354, 1988
116. Holmes EC: Current status of adjuvant chemotherapy in the treatment of non-small cell lung cancer. In DeVita VT, Hillman S, Rosenberg SA (eds): Important Advances in Oncology, pp 259–272. Philadelphia, JB Lippincott, 1988
117. Holsti LR: Clinical experience with split-course radiotherapy: A randomized clinical trial. Radiology 92:591–596, 1969
118. Holsti LR, Mattson K: A randomized study of split-course radiotherapy of lung cancer: Long term results. Int J Radiat Oncol Biol Phys 6:977–981, 1980
119. Ihde DC, Hansen HH: Staging procedures and prognostic factors in small cell carcinoma of the lung. In Greco FA, Oldham RK, Bunn PA (eds): Small Cell Lung Cancer, pp 261–284. New York, Grune & Stratton 1981
120. Israel L, Bonadonna G, Sylvester R: Members of the EORTC Lung Cancer Group: Controlled study with adjuvant radiotherapy, chemotherapy, immunotherapy, and chemoimmunotherapy in operable squamous carcinoma of the lung. In Rozencweig M, Muggia F (eds): Lung Cancer: Progress in Therapeutic Research, pp 443–452. New York, Raven Press, 1979
121. Johnson BE, Grayson E, Woods AF, et al: Limited (LTD) stage small cell lung cancer (SCLC) treated with concurrent etoposide/cisplatin (VP/PLAT) plus bid chest radiotherapy (RT) (Abstract). Proc Am Soc Clin Oncol 8:228, 1989
122. Johnson DH, Einhorn LH, Mandelbaum I, et al: Post-chemotherapy resection of residual tumor in limited stage small cell lung cancer. Chest 92:241–246, 1987
123. Johnson WW: Histologic and cytologic patterns of lung cancer in 2,580 men and woman over a 15-year period. Acta Cytol 32:163–168, 1988
124. Johnson WW: Fine needle aspiration biopsy versus sputum and bronchial material in the diagnosis of lung cancer: A comparative study of 168 patients. Acta Cytol 32:641–646, 1988
125. Johnson RE, Brereton HD, Kent CH: Small-cell carcinoma of the lung: Attempt to remedy causes of past therapeutic failure. Lancet 2:289–291, 1976
126. Kaasa S, Thorud E, Host H, et al: A randomized study evaluating radiotherapy versus chemotherapy in patients with inoperable non-small cell lung cancer. Radiother Oncol 11:7–13, 1988
127. Kanarek OJ: Assessment of pulmonary function in lung cancer. In Choi NC, Grillo HC (eds): Thoracic Oncology, pp 103–113. New York, Raven Press, 1983
128. Kaplan EH, Bonomi P, Faber LP, et al: Patterns of failure in patients (PTS) with stage III non-small cell lung cancer (NSCLC) treated with combined modality therapy (Abstract). Proc Am Soc Clin Oncol 8:225, 1989
129. Khan MA, Whitcomb ME, Snider GL: Flexible fiberoptic bronchoscopy. Am J Med 61:151–155, 1976
130. Kies MS, Mira JG, Crowley JJ, et al: Multimodal therapy for limited small-cell lung cancer: A randomized study of induction combination chemotherapy with or without thoracic radiation in complete responders; and with wide-field versus reduced-field radiation in partial responders. A Southwest Oncology Group Study. J Clin Oncol 5:592–600, 1987
131. Kirsh MM, Rotman H, Argenta L, et al: Carcinoma of the lung: Results of treatment over ten years. Ann Thorac Surg 21:371–377, 1976
132. Komaki R, Roh J, Cos J, et al: Superior sulcus tumors: Results of irradiation of 36 patients. Cancer 48:67–72, 1981
133. Kotin P: Carcinogenesis of the lung. In Liebow AA, Smith DE (eds): The Lung, p 203. Baltimore, Williams & Wilkins, 1968
134. Lad T, The Lung Cancer Study Group, Rubinstein L, et al: The benefit of adjuvant treatment for resected locally advanced non-small-cell lung cancer. J Clin Oncol 6:9–17, 1988
135. Landgran RC, Hussey DH, Barkley HT, et al: Split-course irradiation compared to split-course irradiation plus hydroxyurea in inoperable bronchogenic carcinoma: A randomized study of 53 patients. Cancer 34:1598–1601, 1974
136. Laukkanen E, Klonoff H, Allan E, et al: The role of prophylactic brain irradiation in limited stage small cell lung cancer: Clinical, neuropsychologic, and CT sequelae. Int J Radiat Oncol Biol Phys 14:1109–1117, 1988
137. Lee JS, Umsawasdi T, Lee YY, et al: Neurotoxicity in long-term survivors of small cell lung cancer. Int J Radiat Oncol Biol Phys 12:313–321, 1986
138. Lee RE, Carr DT, Childs DS: Comparison of split-course radiation therapy and continuous radiation therapy for unresectable bronchogenic carcinoma: Five year results. AJR 126:116–122, 1976
139. Legha SS, Muggia FM, Carter SK: Adjuvant chemotherapy in lung cancer: Review and prospects. Cancer 39:1415–1424, 1977
140. Levitt SH, Bogardus CR, Ladd G: Split-course intensive radiation therapy in the treatment of advanced lung cancer: A randomized study. Radiology 88:1159–1161, 1967
141. Levitt SH, Jones TK Jr, Kilpatrick SJ Jr, et al: Treatment of malignant superior vena caval obstruction. Cancer 24:447–451, 1969
142. Libshitz HI, Southard ME: Complications of radiation therapy: The thorax. Semin Roentgenol 9(1):41–49, 1974
143. Licciardello J, Bromer R, Karp D, et al: Delayed neurotoxicity after prophylactic cranial irradiation or mediastinal irradiation with chemotherapy for patients with small cell lung cancer. Proc Am Soc Clin Oncol 2:C-737, 1983
144. Line DH, Deeley TJ: The necropsy findings in carcinoma findings in carcinoma of the bronchus. Br J Dis Chest 65:238–242, 1971
145. Livingston RB: Combination chemotherapy of bronchogenic carcinoma. I. Non-oat cell. Cancer Treat Rev 4:153–165, 1977
146. Livingston RB, Fee WH, Einhorn LH, et al: BACON (bleomycin, Adriamycin, CCNU, Oncovin and nitrogen mustard) in squamous lung cancer. Cancer 37:1237–1242, 1976
147. Livingston RB, Mira JG, Chen TT: Combined modality treatment of extensive small cell lung cancer: A Southwest Oncology Group Study. J Clin Oncol 2(6):585–590, 1984
148. Locksmith JP, Powers WE: Permanent radiation myelopathy. AJR 102(4):916–926, 1968
149. Looper JD, Hornback NB: The role of chest irradiation in limited cell carcinoma of the lung treated with combination chemotherapy. Int J Radiat Oncol Biol Phys 10:1855–1860, 1984
150. Lucas CF, Robinson B, Hoskin PJ, et al: Morbidity of cranial relapse in small cell lung cancer and the impact of radiation therapy. Cancer Treat Rep 70:565–570, 1986
151. Luomanen RKJ, Watson WL: Autopsy findings. In Watson WL (ed): Lung Cancer: A Study of Five Thousand Memorial Hospital Cases. St Louis, CV Mosby, 1968
152. Mah K, van Dyke J, Kaene T, et al: L Acute radiation-induced pulmonary damage: A clinical study on the response to fractionated radiation therapy. Int J Radiat Oncol Biol Phys 13:179–188, 1987
153. Mantravadi RVP, Gates JO, Crawford JN, et al: Unresectable non-oat cell carcinoma of the lung: Definitive radiation therapy. Radiology 172:851–855, 1989
154. Martini N, Flehinger B: The role of surgery in N2 lung cancer. Surg Clin North Am 67:1037, 1987
155. Matthews MJ, Gordon PR: Morphology of pulmonary and pleural malignancies. In Strauss MJ (ed): Lung Cancer Clini-

cal Diagnosis and Treatment. New York, Grune & Stratton, 1977

156. Matthews MJ, Kanhouwa S, Pickren J: Frequency of residual and metastatic tumor in patients undergoing curative resection for lung cancer. Cancer Chemother Rep 4(Suppl 4):63–67, 1973
157. Mattson K, Holsti LR, Holsti P, et al: Inoperable non-small cell lung cancer: Radiation with or without chemotherapy. Eur J Cancer Clin Oncol 24:477–482, 1988
158. Maurer LH, Pajak TF: Prognostic factors in small cell carcinoma of the lung: A Cancer and Leukemia Group B study. Cancer Treat Rep 65:767–774, 1981
159. Maxfield WS, Hatch HB Jr, Nelson JR: Forecast of prognosis after radiotherapy. In Deeley TJ (ed): Carcinoma of the Bronchus. New York, Appleton-Century-Crofts, 1971
160. McCloud TC, Wittenberg J, Ferrucci JT: Computed tomography of the thorax and standard radiographic evaluation of the chest: A comparative study. J Comput Assist Tomogr 3:170–180, 1979
161. McCracken JD, Janaki LM, Taylor SA, et al: Concurrent chemoradiotherapy for limited small cell carcinoma of the lung. In Ishagami J (ed): Recent Advances in Chemotherapy: Proceedings of the 14th International Congress of Chemotherapy, pp 1138–1139. Tokyo, University of Tokyo Press, 1985
162. McDermot RS: Cobalt 60 beam therapy: Post irradiation effects in breast cancer patients. J Can Assoc Radiol 22:195, 1971
163. Macha HN, Koch K, Stadler M, et al: New technique for treating occlusive and stenosing tumours of the trachea and main bronchi: Endobronchial irradiation by high dose iridium-192 combined with laser canalisation. Thorax 42:511–515, 1987
164. Miller J, Mansour K, Hatcher C: Carcinoma of the superior pulmonary sulcus. Presented at the 25th Annual Meeting of the Southern Thoracic Surgical Association, November 2–4, 1978, Marco Island, Florida
165. Minna JD, Bunn PA: Paraneoplastic syndromes. In DeVita VT Jr, Hellman S, Rosenberg SA (eds): Cancer: Principles and Practice of Oncology, pp 1476–1517. Philadelphia, JB Lippincott, 1982
166. Mintzer RA, Malave SR, Neiman HL, et al: Computed vs. conventional tomography in the evaluation of primary and secondary pulmonary neoplasms. Radiology 132:653–659, 1979
167. Mira JG, Livingston RB: Evaluation of radiotherapy implications of chest relapse patterns in small cell lung carcinoma treated with radiotherapy-chemotherapy: Study of 34 cases and review of the literature. Cancer 46:2557–2565, 1980
168. Mira JG, Livingston RB, Moore TN, et al: Influence of chest radiotherapy in frequency and patterns of chest relapse in disseminated small cell lung (A Southwest Oncology Group Study). Cancer 50:1266–1272, 1982
169. Morton DL, Kagan AR, Roberts WC, et al: Pericardiectomy for radiation-induced pericarditis with effusion. Ann Thorac Surg 8:195–208, 1969
170. Morton RF, Jett JR, Maher L, et al: Randomized trial of thoracic radiation therapy (TRT) with or without chemotherapy for treatment of locally unresectable non-small cell lung cancer (NSCLC) (Abstract). Proc Ann Meet Am Soc Clin Oncol 7:200, 1988
171. Mountain CF: The new international staging system for lung cancer. Surg Clin North Am 67:925–935, 1987
172. Mountain CF: Prognostic implications of the international staging system for lung cancer. Semin Oncol 15:236–245, 1988
173. Mountain CF: A new international staging system for lung cancer. Chest 4S:225S–232S, 1989
174. Mountain CF, Carr DT, Anderson WAD: A system for the clinical staging of lung carcinoma. AJR 120:130, 1974
175. Nagaishi C: Functional Anatomy and Histology of the Lung. Baltimore, University Park Press, 1972
176. Nakhashi H, Yasumoto K, Ishida T, et al: Results of surgical treatment of patients with T3 non-small cell lung cancer. Ann Thorac Surg 46:178–181, 1988
177. Nathan MH, Collins VP, Adams RA: Differentiation of benign and malignant pulmonary nodules by growth rate. Radiology 79:221, 1962
178. Nealon TF: Choice of operation and technique for cancer of the lung. Proceedings of the Sixth National Cancer Conference. Philadelphia, JB Lippincott, 1970
179. Neptune WB: Primary lung cancer surgery in stage II and stage III. Arch Surg 123:583–585, 1988
180. Newburger PE, Cassady JR, Jaffe N: Esophagitis due to Adriamycin and radiation therapy for childhood malignancy. Cancer 42:417–423, 1978
181. Newton KA, Spittle MF: Analysis of 40 cases treated by total thoracic irradiation. Clin Radiol 20:19–22, 1969
182. Nohl-Oser HC: The Spread of Carcinoma of the Bronchus. Chicago, Year Book Medical Publishers, 1962
183. Nohl-Oser HC: An investigation of the anatomy of the lymphatic drainage of the lungs. Ann R Coll Surg Engl 51:157, 1972
184. Noordijk EM, v.d. Poest Clement E, Hermans J, et al: Radiotherapy as an alternative to surgery in elderly patients with resectable lung cancer. Radiother Oncol 13:83–89, 1988
185. Nori D, Hilaris BS, Martini N: Intraluminal irradiation in bronchogenic carcinoma. Surg Clin North Am 67:1093–1102, 1987
186. Nugent JL, Bunn PA, Matthews MJ, et al: CNS metastasis in small cell bronchogenic carcinoma. Cancer 44:1885–1893, 1979
187. Ochsner A, Dixon JL, DeBakey M: An analysis of 190 cases, 58 of which were successfully treated by pneumonectomy, with a review of the literature. Clinics 3:1187, 1945
188. Pagani JJ, Libshitz HI: CT manifestations of radiation-induced change in chest tissue. J Comput Assist Tomogr 6:243–248, 1982
189. Pancoast HK: Superior pulmonary sulcus tumor. JAMA 99:1391, 1932
190. Papac RJ, Son Y, Bien R, et al: Improved local control of thoracic disease in small cell lung cancer with higher dose thoracic irradiation and cyclic chemotherapy. Int J Radiat Oncol Biol Phys 13:993–998, 1987
191. Pater JL, Loeb M: Non-anatomic prognostic factors in carcinoma of the lung. Cancer 50:326–331, 1982
192. Paterson R, Russell MH: Clinical trials in malignant disease. Part IV-Lung Cancer. Value of post-operative radiotherapy. Clin Radiol 13:141–144, 1962
193. Paulson DL: The role of preoperative radiation therapy in the surgical management of carcinoma in the superior pulmonary sulcus. Front Radiat Ther Oncol 5:177–187, 1970
194. Paulson DL: Management of superior sulcus carcinomas. In Choi NC, Grillo HC (eds): Thoracic Oncology. New York, Raven Press, 1983
195. Pavlov A, Pirogov A, Trachtenberg A: Results of combination treatment of lung cancer patients: Surgery plus radiotherapy and surgery plus chemotherapy. Cancer Chemother Rep 4:133–135, 1973
196. Payne DG: Non-small-cell lung cancer: Should unresectable stage III patients routinely receive high-dose radiation therapy. J Clin Oncol 6:552–558, 1988
197. Pedersen AG, Kristjansen PEG, Hansen HH: Prophylactic cranial irradiation and small cell lung cancer. Cancer Treat Rev 15:85–103, 1988
198. Perez CA, Azarnia N, Cox JD, Shapiro SJ: Sequelae of definitive irradiation in the treatment of carcinoma of the lung. In Motta G (ed): Lung Cancer: Advanced Concepts and Present Status. Genoa, Italy, 1989
199. Perez CA: Is postoperative irradiation indicated in carcinoma of the lung? (Editorial) Int J Radiat Oncol Biol Phys 8:2019–2022, 1982
200. Perez CA: Non-small cell carcinoma of the lung: Dose-time parameters. Cancer Treat Symp 2:131–142, 1985
201. Perez CA, Bauer M, Edelstein S, et al: Impact of tumor control on survival in carcinoma of the lung treated with irradiation. Int J Radiat Oncol Biol Phys 12:539–547, 1986
202. Perez CA, Einhorn RK, Oldham FA, et al: Randomized trial of radiotherapy to the thorax in limited small cell carcinoma of the lung treated with multiagent chemotherapy and elective

brain irradiation: A preliminary report. J Clin Oncol 2(11):1200–1207, 1984
203. Perez CA, Pajak TF, Rubin P, et al: Long-term observations of the patterns of failure in patients with unresectable non-oat cell carcinoma of the lung treated with definitive radiotherapy: Report by the Radiation Therapy Oncology Group. Cancer 59:1874–1881, 1987
204. Perez CA, Purdy J, Razek A: Radiation therapy of carcinoma of the lung and esophagus. In Levitt SH, Tapley ND (eds): Technological Basis of Radiation Therapy: Practical Clinical Applications, pp 138–171. Philadelphia, Lea & Febiger, 1984
205. Perez CA, Stanley K, Grundy G, et al: Impact of irradiation technique and tumor extent in tumor control and survival of patients with unresectable non-oat cell carcinoma of the lung. Cancer 50:1091–1099, 1982
206. Perez CA, Stanley K, Rubin P, et al: A perspective randomized study of various irradiation doses and fractionation schedules in the treatment of inoperable non-oat-cell carcinoma of the lung. Cancer 45:2744–2753, 1980
207. Perry MC, Eaton WL, Propert KJ, et al: Chemotherapy with or without radiation therapy in limited small-cell carcinoma of the lung. N Engl J Med 316:912–918, 1987
208. Phillips TL, Buschke F: Radiation tolerance of the thoracic spinal cord. AJR 104:659–664, 1969
209. Phillips T, Margolis L: Radiation pathology and the clinical response of lung and esophagus. In Vaeth JM (ed): Frontiers of Radiation Therapy and Oncology, vol 6, pp 254–273. Baltimore, University Park Press, 1972
210. Pincus M, Reddy S, Lee MS, et al: Preoperative combined modality therapy for stage III MO non-small cell lung carcinoma. Int J Radiat Oncol Biol Phys 15:189–195, 1988
211. Platt JF, Glazer GM, Gross BH, et al: CT evaluation of mediastinal lymph nodes in lung cancer: Influence of the lobar site of the primary neoplasm. AJR 149:683–686, 1987
212. Prasad S, Pilepich MV, Perez CA: Contribution of CT to quantitative radiation therapy planning. AJR 136:123–128, 1981
213. Ramsdell JW, et al: Multiorgan scans for staging lung cancer. J Thorac Cardiovasc Surg 73:653–659, 1977
214. Rapp E, Pater JL, Willan A, et al: Chemotherapy can prolong survival in patients with advanced non-small-cell lung cancer: Report of a Canadian multicenter randomized trial. J Clin Oncol 6:633–641, 1988
215. Rea HH, Shevland JE, House AJS: Accuracy of computer tomographic scanning in assessment of the mediastinum in bronchial carcinoma. J Thorac Cardiovasc Surg 81:825–829, 1981
216. Richardson RH, Zavala DC, Jukerjee PK, et al: The use of fiberoptic bronchoscopy and brush biopsy in the diagnosis of suspected pulmonary malignancy. Am Rev Respir Dis 109:63–66, 1974
217. Rienhoff WF: The present status of the surgical treatment of carcinoma of the lung. Ann Surg 125:541, 1947
218. Rigler LG: The earliest roentgenographic signs of carcinoma of the lung. JAMA 195:655, 1966
219. Rissanen PM, Tikka U, Holsti LR, et al: Autopsy findings in lung cancer treated with megavoltage radiotherapy. Acta Radiol (Stockh) 7:433–442, 1968
220. Robinow JS, Shaw EG, Eagan RT, et al: Results of combination chemotherapy and thoracic radiation therapy for unresectable non-small cell carcinoma of the lung (in press)
221. Roper C: Personal communication, 1984
222. Roswit B, Higgins GA, Shields W, Keehn RJ: Preoperative radiation therapy for carcinoma of the lung: Report of a national VA controlled study. In Vaeth JM (ed): Frontiers of Radiation Therapy and Oncology, vol 5, pp 163–176. Baltimore, University Park Press, 1970
223. Rubenstein JH, Richter MP, Moldofsky PJ, et al: Prospective prediction of post-radiation therapy lung function using quantitative lung scans and pulmonary function testing. Int J Radiat Oncol Biol Phys 15:83–87, 1988
224. Rubin P, Casarett GW: Clinical Radiation Pathology. Philadelphia, WB Saunders, 1968
225. Rubin P, Ciccio S, Setisarn B: The controversial status of radiation therapy in lung cancer. Proceedings of the Sixth National Cancer Conference, pp 855–865. Philadelphia, JB Lippincott, 1970,
226. Rubin P, Ciccio S: High daily dose for rapid decompression. In Deeley TJ (ed): Modern Radiotherapy. Carcinoma of the Bronchus, pp 276–297. New York, Appleton-Century-Crofts, 1971
227. Rubin P, Green J, Holzwasser G, et al: Superior vena caval syndrome: Slow low dose versus rapid high dose schedules. Radiology 81:388–401, 1963
228. Sadeghi A, Payne D, Rubinstein L, et al: Combined modality treatment for resected advanced non-small cell lung cancer: Local control and local recurrence. Int J Radiat Oncol Biol Phys 15:89–87, 1988
229. Sagel SS: Special Procedures in Chest Radiology. Philadelphia, WB Saunders, 1976
230. Sagel SS: Lung, pleura, pericardium and chest wall. In Lee JKT, Sagel SS, Stanley RJ (eds): Computed Body Tomography. New York, Raven Press, 1983
231. Sagel SS, Ferguson TB, Forrest JV, et al: Percutaneous transthoracic aspiration needle biopsy. Ann Thorac Surg 26:399–405, 1978
232. Salazar OM, Creech RH: "The state of the art" towards defining the role of radiation therapy in the management of small cell bronchogenic carcinoma. Int J Radiat Oncol Biol Phys 6:1103–1117, 1980
233. Salazar OM, Rubin P, Brown JE, et al: The assessment of tumor response to irradiation of lung cancer: Continuous versus split-course regimes. Int J Radiat Oncol Biol Phys 1:1107–1118, 1976
234. Salzer G, Wenzl M, Jenny EH, et al: Das bronchuscarcinoma. Wien, Springer-Verlag, 1952
235. Schechter MM: The superior vena cava syndrome. Am J Med Sci 227:46–56, 1954
236. Schray MF, McDougall JC, Martinez A, et al: Management of malignant airway compromise with laser and low dose rate brachytherapy. Chest 93:264–269, 1988
237. Scruggs H, El-Mahdl A, Marks RD, et al: The results of split-course radiation therapy in cancer of the lung. Am J Roentgenol 121:754–760, 1974
238. Seaman WB, Ackerman LV: The effect of radiation on the esophagus: A clinical and histologic study on the effects produced by the betatron. Radiology 68:534–541, 1957
239. Seydel HG, Chait A, Gmelich JT: Cancer of the Lung. New York, John Wiley & Sons, 1975
240. Seydel HG, Diener-West M, Urtasun R, et al: Hyperfractionation in the radiation therapy of unresectable non-oat cell carcinoma of the lung: Preliminary report of a RTOG pilot study. Int J Radiat Oncol Biol Phys 11:1841–1847, 1985
241. Seydel HG, Kutcher GJ, Steiner RM, et al: Computed tomography in planning radiation therapy for bronchogenic carcinoma. Int J Radiat Oncol Biol Phys 6:601–606, 1980
242. Sherman DM, Neptune W, Weichselbaum RR, et al: An aggressive approach to marginally resectable lung cancer. Cancer 41:2040–2045, 1978
243. Shields TW: Pre-operative radiotherapy in the treatment of bronchial carcinoma. Cancer 30:1388–1394, 1972
244. Shields TW, Higgins GA, Keehn RJ: Factors influencing survival after resection for bronchial carcinoma. J Thorac Cardiovasc Surg 64:391–399, 1972
245. Shields TW, Humphrey EW, Eastridge CE, et al: Adjuvant cancer chemotherapy after resection of carcinoma of the lung. Cancer 40:2057–2062, 1977
246. Silverberg E, Boring CC, Squires TS: Cancer—A cancer journal for clinicians. Cancer Stat 40(1):9–26, 1990
247. Simpson JR, Francis ME, Perez-Tamayo R, et al: Palliative radiotherapy for inoperable carcinoma of the lung: Final report of a RTOG Multi-Institutional Trial. Int J Radiat Oncol Biol Phys 11:751–758, 1985
248. Simpson JR, Perez CA, Presant CA, et al: Superior vena cava syndrome. In Yarbro JW, Bornstein RS (eds): Oncologic Emergencies, pp 43–72. New York, Grune & Stratton, 1980
249. Simpson SL: Primary carcinoma of the lung. Q J Med 22:413–449, 1929
250. Skinner WN: Pulmonary neoplasms diagnosed with transthoracic needle biopsy. Cancer 43:1533–1540, 1979

251. Soresi E, Clerici M, Grilli R, et al: A randomized clinical trial comparing radiation therapy versus radiation therapy plus cis-Dichlorodiammine Platinum (II) in the treatment of locally advanced non-small cell lung cancer. Semin Oncol 15:20–25, 1988
252. Souhami RL, Geddes DM, Spiro SG, et al: Radiotherapy in small cell cancer of the lung. Br Med J 288:1643–1646, 1984
253. Spjut HJ, Mateo LE: Recurrent and metastatic carcinoma in surgically treated carcinoma of the lung. Cancer 18:1462–1466, 1965
254. Stanley KE: Prognostic factors for survival in patients with inoperable lung cancer. J Natl Cancer Inst 65:25–32, 1980
255. Steinfeld AD, Glicksman AS: Postoperative adjuvant mediastinal radiation in lung cancer. J Surg Oncol 26:154–157, 1984
256. Stewart JR, Fajardo LF: Radiation-induced heart disease: Clinical and experimental aspects. Radiol Clin North Am 9:511–531, 1971
257. Stewart JR, Fajardo LF: Dose response in human and experimental radiation-induced heart disease: Application of the nominal standard dose (NSD) concept. Radiology 99:403–408, 1971
258. Strauss BL, Matthews MJ, Cohen MH, et al: Cardiac metastasis in lung cancer. Chest 71:607–611, 1977
259. Taylor SG, Trybula M, Bonomi PD, et al: Simultaneous cisplatin fluorouracil infusion and radiation followed by surgical resection in regionally localized stage III, non-small cell lung cancer. Ann Thorac Surg 43:87–91, 1987
260. Teo P, Tai TH, Damon C, Tsui KH: A randomized study on palliative radiation therapy for inoperable non-small cell carcinoma of the lung. Int J Radiat Oncol Biol Phys 14:867–871, 1988
261. Thomas ED, Clift RA, Hersman J, et al: Marrow transplantation for acute nonlymphoblastic leukemia in first remission using fractionated or single-dose irradiation. Int J Radiat Oncol Biol Phys 8:817–821, 1982
262. Trakhtenberg AK, Kiseleva ES, Pitskhelauri VG, et al: Preoperative radiotherapy in the combined treatment of lung cancer patients. Neoplasma 35:459–465, 1988
263. Trakhtenberg AK, Zakharchenkov AV, Zhiglov MA, et al: Combined treatment including postoperative chemotherapy in lung cancer patients. Neoplasma 35:351–358, 1988
264. Turrisi AT, Glover DJ, Mason BA: A preliminary report: Concurrent twice-daily radiotherapy plus platinum-etoposide chemotherapy for limited small cell lung cancer. Int J Radiat Oncol Biol Phys 15:183–187, 1988
265. Turrisi AT, Glover DJ, Mason BA, et al: Concurrent twice-daily multi-field radiotherapy (2X/D XRT) and plantinum-etoposide chemotherapy (P/E) for limited small cell lung cancer (SCLC) (Abstract). Proc Am Soc Clin Oncol 7:211, 1988
266. Turrisi AT, Glover DJ, Mason BA, et al: Prophylactic cranial irradiation (PCI) after chemotherapy as part of a combined modality platinum (DDP)-etoposide (VP-16) and twice-daily chest radiotherapy (BID-TRT) for limited small cell lung cancer (LSCLC) (Abstract). Proc Am Soc Clin Oncol 8:245, 1989
267. Twijnstra A, Boon PJ, Lormans ACM, et al: Neurotoxicity of prophylactic cranial irradiation in patients with small cell carcinoma of the lung. Eur J Cancer Clin Oncol 23:983–986, 1987
268. Umiker WO: Relative accuracy of various procedures in the diagnosis of bronchogenic carcinoma. JAMA 195:6–7, 1966
269. Van Houtte P, MacLennan I, Poulter C, et al: External radiation in the management of superior sulcus tumor. Cancer 54:223–227, 1984
270. Van Houtte P, Rocmans P, Smets P, et al: Postoperative radiation therapy in lung cancer: A controlled trial after resection of curative design. Int J Radiat Oncol Biol Phys 6:983–986, 1980
271. Verschoore J, Lagrange JL, Boublil JL, et al: Pulmonary toxicity of a combination of low-dose doxorubicin and irradiation for inoperable lung cancer. Radiother Oncol 9:281–288, 1967
272. Wara WM, Phillips TL, Margolis LW, et al: Radiation pneumonitis: A new approach to the derivation of time-dose factors. Cancer 32:547, 1973
273. Wara WM, Phillips TL, Sheline GE, et al: Radiation tolerance of the spinal cord. Cancer 35:1558–1562, 1975
274. Warren J: Pre-operative irradiation of cancer of the lung: Final of a therapeutic trial. Cancer 36:914–925, 1975
275. Weisenburger T, The Lung Cancer Study Group, et al: Effects of postoperative mediastinal radiation on completely resected stage II and stage III epidermoid cancer of the lung. N Engl J Med 315:1377–1381, 1986
276. Weiss RB: Small cell carcinoma of the lung: Therapeutic management. Ann Intern Med 88:522–531, 1978
277. Wiklund TH: Bronchogenic carcinoma, a clinical study of 259 cases, 100 of which were resected, follow-up study of the resected cases. Acta Chir Scand 117(Suppl):162, 1951
278. Willis RA: Pathology of Tumors, 3rd ed. London, Butterworths, 1960
279. Wynder EL, Hoffmann D: Tobacco and tobacco smoke: Studies in experimental carcinogenesis. New York, Academic Press, 1967
280. Yerushalmy J: The statistical assessment of the variability in observer perception and description of roentgenographic pulmonary shadows. Radiol Clin North Am 7(3):381–392, 1969
281. Zhang HX, Yin WB, Zhang LJ, et al: Curative radiotherapy of early operable non-small cell lung cancer. Radiother Oncol 14:89–94, 1989

39

Mediastinum and Trachea

Bahman Emami

ANATOMY

The boundaries of the mediastinum are the thoracic inlet superiorly (at the level of the first thoracic vertebra and the first rib), the diaphragm inferiorly, the sternum anteriorly, the vertebral column posteriorly, and the parietal pleura laterally.[110] The mediastinum can be divided into three compartments: anterior, medial, and posterior. Some authors have suggested that the superior mediastinum is a separate compartment, whereas others have included the superior mediastinum as part of the anterior mediastinum.[21] The anatomic structures normally found in the different mediastinal compartments and the tumors arising from those structures are listed in Table 39-1 and illustrated in Figure 39-1.

In adults, a majority of thyroid tumors, thymomas, mediastinal germ cell tumors, and teratomas are located in the superior and anterior mediastinum; 80% of neurogenic tumors are located in the posterior mediastinum, and 50% of mediastinal lymphomas are in the middle mediastinum.[71] In adults the incidence of anterosuperior, middle, and posterior mediastinal tumors is about 54%, 20%, and 26%, respectively.[38] However, in children the posterior mediastinum contains 63% of the lesions, the anterior mediastinum contains 26%, and the middle mediastinum contains 11%.[67]

Primary mediastinal tumors are relatively rare. About ten to 25 cases per year are seen in the typical major medical center.[21] The relative incidence of mediastinal tumors is listed in Table 39-2. In the adult population the ratio of benign to malignant tumors is about 60 to 40 (Table 39-3). The relative incidence of malignant mediastinal tumors in children is about 50%.[55] Neurogenic tumors, lymphomas, esophageal tumors, and tumors of the heart and great vessels are discussed in other chapters of this book. In this chapter, thymomas, mediastinal germ cell tumors, and tracheal tumors are discussed.

DIAGNOSTIC WORKUP

The diagnostic workup for mediastinal tumors is outlined in Table 39-4. Computed tomography (CT) is the most valuable radiologic technique in the evaluation of the mediastinum.[96,136,138] The size, contour, tissue density, and homogeneity of a mediastinal lesion can be defined as well as its relationship to or invasion of other mediastinal structures (Fig. 39-2). CT is well suited for staging of these tumors and is helpful as a baseline for monitoring response to treatment with irradiation or chemotherapy. It is also useful for planning radiation therapy portals in patients with mediastinal tumors.[7] Magnetic resonance imaging (MRI) has not been shown to yield more information than the CT scan.[26] MRI, however, has the advantage of differentiating vascular structures, thus eliminating potential risk of using contrast medium.[26,38]

Because most mediastinal tumors are surgically removed, tissue diagnosis is most often done at thoracotomy. Mediastinoscopy and anterior mediastinotomy may yield the diagnosis, especially when enlarged lymph nodes are present.[145]

THYMOMAS

Epidemiology

Thymomas are the most common tumors of the anterior mediastinum. Most patients with thymomas are adults, with an average age of 48 years and a median age of 52 years. There is an equal overall sex incidence.[8,14,93,138]

Natural History

Embryologically, the thymus gland originates in the lower portion of the third pharyngeal pouch on each side. These cords of epithelial cells subsequently constitute the medullary areas of the lobules of the thymus.[131] Along with proliferation of epithelial cords, lymphocytes appear within the spaces of epithelial cells. The process of differentiation into mature thymocytes is under the influence of the humoral factor thymosin, which is produced by the epithelial cells. Despite its epithelial origin, the fully developed thymus is considered a lymphatic organ. The medullary areas of the lobules are largely composed of epithelial cells. Germinal centers and lymphoid follicles are usually not found in the thymus.

Clinical Presentation

About 30% of thymomas are asymptomatic, and the tumor is usually an incidental finding on chest x-ray examination. Symptoms are generally the result of impingement on surrounding mediastinal structures. Of all diagnoses of thymoma, approx-

TABLE 39–1
Classification of Mediastinal Structure and Tumors by Anatomic Location

ANTEROSUPERIOR MEDIASTINUM	MIDDLE MEDIASTINUM	POSTERIOR MEDIASTINUM
ANATOMIC STRUCTURES		
Aorta and great vessels	Heart and pericardium	Sympathetic chain vagus
Thymus gland	Trachea and major bronchi	Esophagus
Lymph nodes	Pulmonary vessels	Thoracic duct
	Lymph nodes	Descending aorta
		Lymph nodes
MEDIASTINAL TUMORS AND CYSTS		
Thymic tumors	Lymphomas	Neurogenic tumors
Lymphomas	Sarcoidosis	Lymphomas
Germinal cell tumors	Cardiac and pericardial tumors	Esophageal tumors
Endocrine	Tracheal tumors	Endocrine tumors
Thyroid tumors	Vascular tumors	Tumors of spinal column
Parathyroid tumors	Lung cancer	Lung cancer
Mesenchymal tumors	Cysts	Cysts
Lung cancer		
Cysts		

imately 50% are associated with myasthenia gravis, 5% with red cell aplasia, and 5% with hypogammaglobulinemia.[27,73,74,80,81,120,128,132]

Myasthenia gravis is an autoimmune disease. By radioimmunoassay, 87% of patients with myasthenia gravis have anti-acetylcholine receptor antibodies. Pathophysiologically, myasthenia gravis is characterized by rapid exhaustion of voluntary muscular contractions with a slow return to the normal state. The most common clinical feature is neuromuscular fatigue. Ocular muscles are involved in 90% of patients. Next in frequency of involvement are facial and pharyngeal muscles, progressing to fatigue of proximal limb girdle muscles and respiratory suppression.[40]

Of patients with myasthenia gravis, approximately 25% have a normal-sized thymus and 75% have thymic abnormalities; 15% are associated with thymoma, and the remaining 60% have thymic lymphoid hyperthermia.[132] The association of thymomas with myasthenia gravis carries a prognosis poorer than that of myasthenia gravis without thymomas.[11]

Staging

Staging of thymomas is generally based on degree of invasiveness. One of the staging systems proposed for thymomas is by Bergh and colleagues.[13]

Stage I Intact capsule or a growth within the capsule
Stage II Pericapsular growth into the mediastinal fat tissue

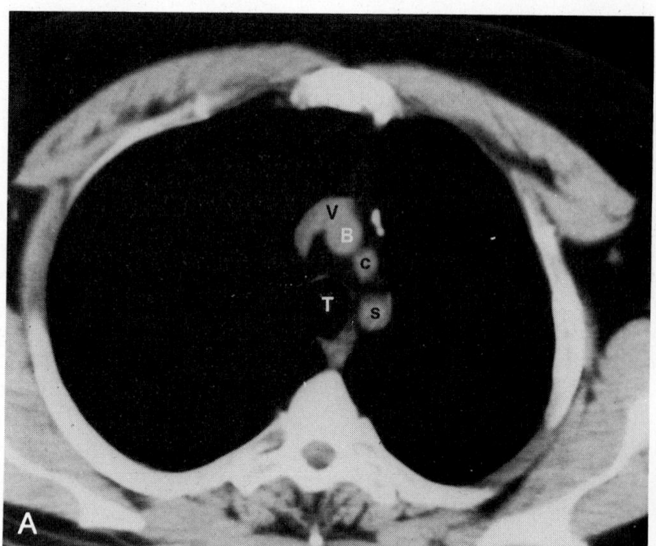

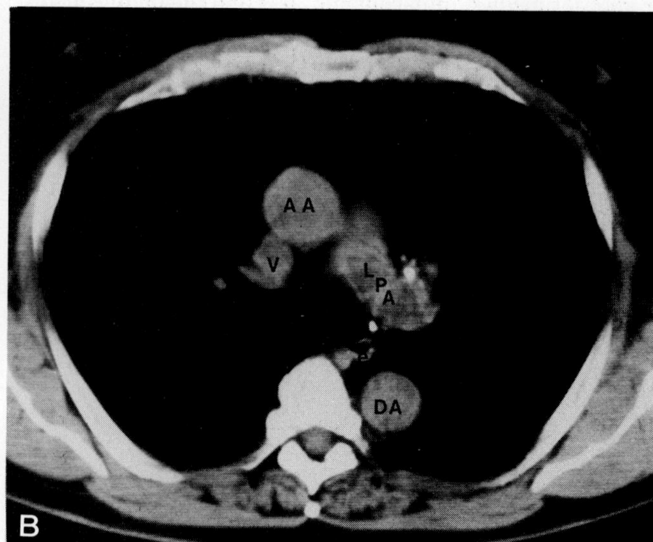

FIGURE 39–1. CT scans of two levels of mediastinum depicting various anatomic structures. (**A**) One centimeter below carina. (V: Innominate vein; B: brachiocephalic artery; C: left common carotid artery; T: trachea; S: subclavian artery) (**B**) One centimeter above aortic arc. (AA: ascending aorta; V: superior vena cava; LPA: left pulmonary artery; DA: descending aorta)

TABLE 39–2
Primary Mediastinal Tumors and Cysts in 2399 Patients

TYPE OF TUMOR	NO. OF PATIENTS	%
Neurogenic tumors	496	20.7
Thymomas	458	19.1
Lymphomas	301	12.5
Germ cell tumors	239	10.0
Primary carcinoma	111	4.6
Mesenchymal tumors	143	6.0
Endocrine tumors	154	6.4
Cysts	439	18.3
Other	58	2.4

(Modified from Davis RD, Oldham HN, Sabiston DC: Ann Thorac Surg 44:229–237, 1987)

Stage III Invasive growth into the surrounding organs or intrathoracic metastases or both

Of the reported studies, 40% of thymomas were Stage I, 19% were Stage II, and 41% were Stage III.[13] The pleura was the most common site of metastasis in the Stage III patients, occurring in about 50% of cases.

The most widely accepted classification of thymomas comprises two categories: invasive and noninvasive. The incidence of invasive compared with noninvasive thymomas from the reported literature is shown in Table 39-5.

Distant metastases with thymomas are rare. Seventeen cases of metastatic thymomas are reported.[11] In most cases (13 of 17) metastases were associated with an invasive primary tumor. The liver, lung, and bones are the most common sites of distant metastasis.

Pathologic Classification

Several classifications of thymomas have been proposed. The most widely used classification is that of Rosai and Levine.[131] Based on histopathology, they divided thymomas into three types, depending on the predominant cell type making up the tumor: lymphocytic, epithelial, and mixed (lymphoepithelial).

TABLE 39–3
Relative Incidence of Mediastinal Tumors and Cysts

TYPE OF TUMOR	BENIGN %	MALIGNANT %
Thymic tumors	10.2*	6.5
Neurogenic tumors	11.0	3.3
Lymphomas	—	15.5
Germ cell neoplasms	5.3	5.3
Carcinomas	—	8.5
Mesenchymal tumors	4.3	1.8
Endocrine tumors	2.0	1.0
Cysts	25.0	—
Total	57.8	41.9

** Includes thymic cysts and hyperplasia*
(Modified from Davis RD, Oldham HN, Sabiston DC: Ann Thorac Surg 44:229–237, 1987)

TABLE 39–4
Diagnostic Workup for Mediastinal Tumors

GENERAL

History
Physical examination—for male patients with mediastinal germ cell tumors, this should include a thorough examination of the testes.

RADIOGRAPHIC STUDIES

Standard
- Chest radiographs
- CT scan
- Tomography
- Barium swallow
- Fluoroscopy
- Arteriography

Complementary
- For male patients with mediastinal germ cell tumors and abnormal clinical examination of testes, ultrasonography and/or lymphangiography may be necessary.

LABORATORY STUDIES

Admission CBC, blood chemistry, urinalysis
Germ cell tumors: α-fetoprotein, human chorionic gonadotropin (HCG), carcinoembryonic antigen
Thymoma—radioimmunoassay for antiacetylcholine receptors

SPECIAL TESTS

All mediastinal tumors
- Mediastinoscopy and anterior mediastinotomy with biopsy
- Bronchoscopy, esophagoscopy with biopsy, if indicated
- Biopsy of palpable cervical or supraclavicular nodes

Some authors also suggested a fourth group, spindle cell type,[93] but this type is often considered a variant of the epithelial type. Distribution of various histologic subtypes from several reported series is shown in Table 39-6.

No correlation has been found between the histopathology of thymomas and their malignant potential (Fig. 39-3),[131,138] and no correlation has been shown between histopathologic subtypes of thymomas and the associated systemic syndromes. The malignant potential of thymomas correlates with their invasiveness,[138] which is most often diagnosed during surgery. About 40% of thymomas show invasive features and are considered malignant.

Prognostic Factors

The most important prognostic factor in thymomas is encapsulation of the tumor, which is the basis for benign or malignant potential. Less than 2% of encapsulated, noninvasive tumors recur after resection, whereas 20% of invasive tumors recur after surgery.[8,51]

Another significant prognostic factor in thymomas is the presence or absence of any associated syndromes, such as myasthenia gravis. Of all recurrences after surgical resection of thymomas, approximately 50% are associated with myasthenia gravis, and the presence of this syndrome has adverse effects on surgical results with noninvasive, encapsulated thymomas. Age also appears to be a prognostic factor. Thymomas in children appear to have a more malignant course than those in adults.[157] Fortunately, malignant thymomas in children are extremely rare.[30]

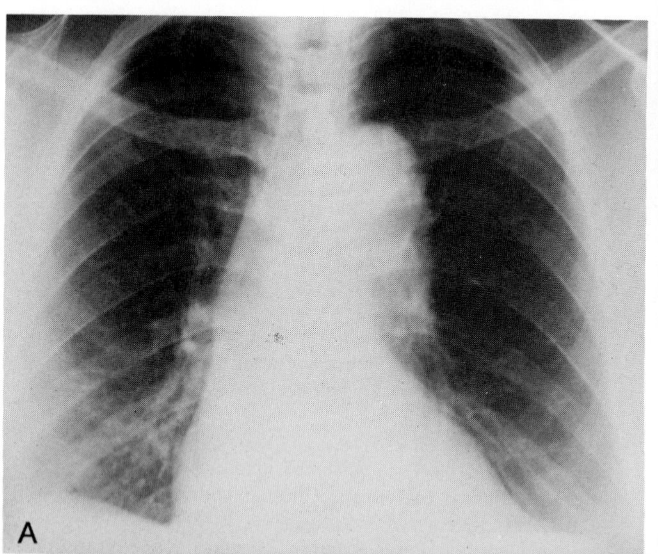

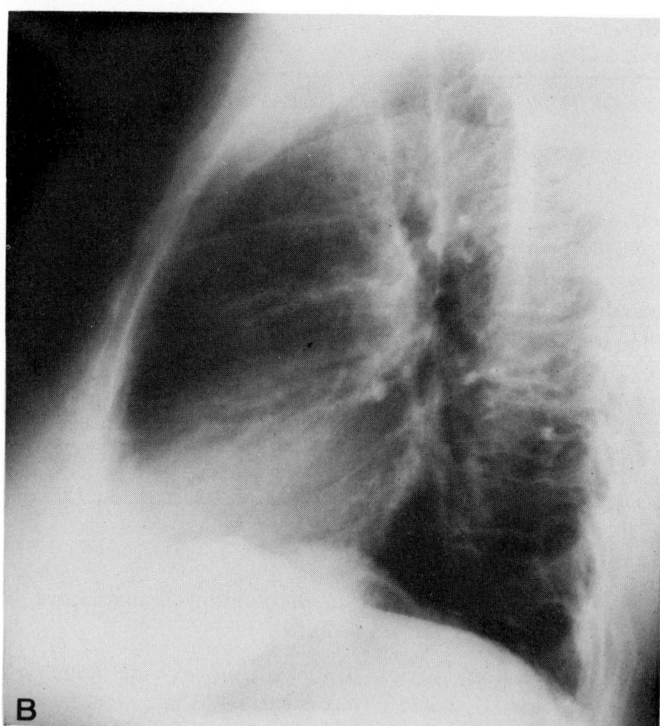

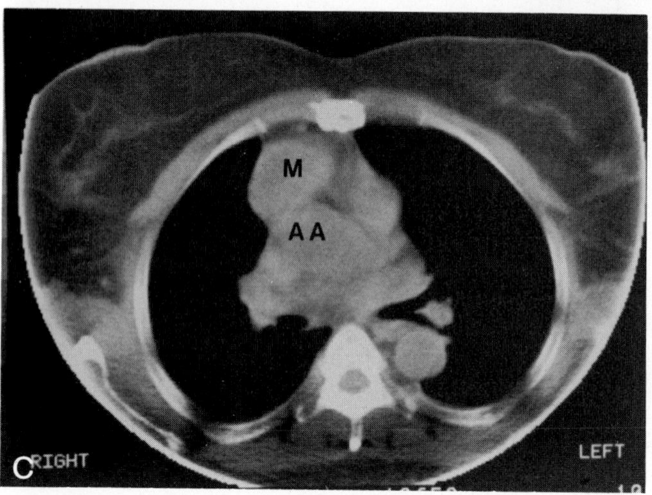

FIGURE 39–2. A 75-year-old woman with thymoma. (**A** and **B**) Posteroanterior and lateral chest x-ray examination are normal except for a tortuous aorta. No mediastinal mass is seen. (**C**) CT demonstrates a 4 cm mass (M) in the vicinity of the inferior right lobe of the thymus, anterior to the ascending aorta (AA). (Sagel SS, Aronberg DJ: Thoracic anatomy and mediastinum. In Lee JKT, Sagel SS, Stanley RJ [eds]: Computed Body Tomography, p 55, New York, Raven Press, 1983)

TABLE 39–5
Invasive and Noninvasive Thymomas

AUTHOR	STUDY YEARS	NO. OF INVASIVE CASES	NO. OF NONINVASIVE CASES
Salyer and Eggleston[138]	1931–1971	22	43
Bergh et al[13]	1954–1975	26	17
Legg[92]	1934–1961	10	36
LeGolvan and Abell[93]	1938–1972	20	26
Bernatz et al[14]	1941–1969	66	115
Batata et al[8]	1928–1972	36	18
Wilkins[160]	1939–1977	37	66
Kilman[83]	1950–1970	21	38
Fugimura et al[57]	1965–1985	35	31
Nakahara et al[111]	1957–1985	81	45
Maggi et al[100]	1956–1984	459	106
Curran et al[34]	1971–1985	57	43
Total		470 (44.6%)	584 (55.4)%

TABLE 39–6
Distribution of Histologic Subtypes of Thymomas

		NUMBER OF TUMORS			
AUTHOR	STUDY YEARS	LYMPHOCYTIC	MIXED	EPITHELIAL	SPINDLE CELL
Salyer and Eggleston[138]	1931–1971	23	12	30	—
Bergh et al[13]	1954–1975	10	15	18	—
Lattes[91]	—	42	—	20	26
Legg[92]	1934–1961	8	—	14	29
LeGolvan and Abell[93]	1938–1972	—	23	12	11
Bernatz et al[14]	1941–1969	60	43	31	47
Batata et al[8]	1928–1972	10	4	36	4
Sellors[143]	1947–1967	2	16	25	16
Nakahara et al[111]	1957–1985	36	77	26	—
Maggi et al[100]	1956–1984	20	107	36	—
Total		211	297	248	133

General Management

Complete surgical resection remains the treatment of choice for all thymomas regardless of invasiveness, except for rare cases with extrathoracic metastasis and extensive intrathoracic metastasis. When an encapsulated thymoma without associated myasthenia gravis is removed without disturbing the integrity of the capsule, the chance for recurrence is extremely rare.[8] For encapsulated, noninvasive thymomas not associated with myasthenia gravis, survival is excellent.[57, 100] The presence of associated myasthenia gravis has marked adverse effects on the surgical results for noninvasive thymomas.[100] Results of surgery for invasive thymomas, regardless of presence or absence of myasthenia gravis, are poor. In a series reported by Fugimura and associates,[57] 10-year survival rates for invasive and noninvasive thymomas were 49.4% and 74.3%, respectively. Similar results are reported by Maggi and colleagues.[100] An aggressive surgical approach to invasive tumors should be taken to remove as much of the lesion as possible at the time of surgery.

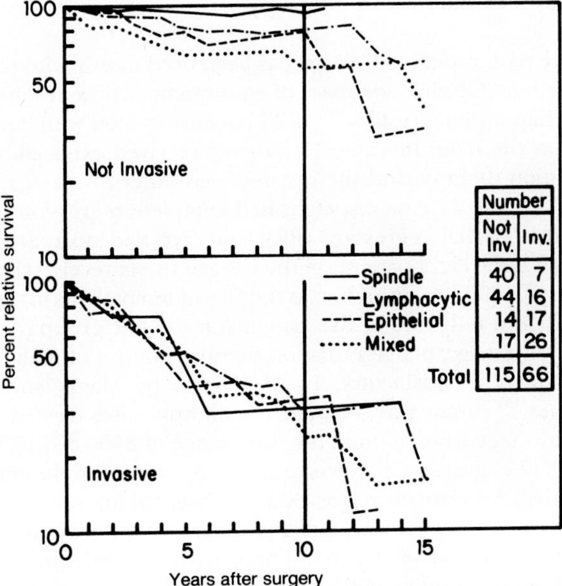

FIGURE 39–3. Survival rate for different histologic types of thymoma shown at each point on graph calculated by direct method (actual number of patients surviving for indicated time period divided by total number of patients actually available for follow-up during all that time period). (Bernatz PE, Khonsari S, Harrison EG, et al: Surg Clin North Am 3:885, 1973)

Radiation therapy is an excellent adjuvant therapy for invasive thymomas. Thymomas are generally radioresponsive. The surgeon should delineate the extent of the tumor and specify the areas of invasion with metallic clips for future radiation therapy planning.

Adjuvant (postoperative) radiation therapy to encapsulated, noninvasive thymomas is still controversial. We believe that when thymomas are well encapsulated and completely excised and integrity of the capsule is well documented at the time of pathology, no postoperative adjuvant therapy is required. These patients, however, should be followed up closely, and in case of recurrence a second resection and postoperative radiation therapy is recommended (4500 cGy to 5000 cGy in 23 to 25 fractions).

For invasive thymomas, postoperative radiation therapy is necessary, regardless of the completeness of the operation. Invasive thymomas completely resected carry a much poorer prognosis than noninvasive tumors.[11, 121] A mediastinal recurrence rate of 33% (six of 18) at 5 years was reported for surgery alone compared with a local failure rate of 0% for total resection plus radiation therapy and 21% for subtotal resection plus irradiation.[34] In cumulative series from the literature, the thoracic failure rates for total resection alone and total resection with radiation therapy were 28% and 5%, respectively. The 5-year survival rates for noninvasive and invasive tumors is 83% and 54%, respectively.[8] A Mayo Clinic study reported 10-year survival rates for noninvasive and invasive tumors of 65% and 30%, respectively.[14]

Limited experience with chemotherapy has demonstrated some effectiveness in thymomas (Table 39-7). Unsustained partial remissions have been observed with doxorubicin (Adriamycin),[18, 58, 143] maytansine,[27, 29, 77] cisplatin,[151] and corticosteroids.[62, 125, 144] Various combination therapies have also demonstrated partial remission (see Table 39-7). Complete remissions have been noted with the COPP (cyclosphamide, vincristine, prednisone, procarbazine) regimen[133] and doxorubicin plus cisplatin[27, 77, 113, 159] with radiation therapy as consolidations. The PAC (platinum, doxorubicin, cyclophosphamide) regimen, CAV (cyclophosphamide, doxorubicin, vincristine) regimen, and single agent cisplatin therapy have also induced complete remissions.[25, 113, 159]

TABLE 39–7
Responses to Different Chemotherapeutic Regimens in Treatment of Thymoma

CHEMOTHERAPEUTIC REGIMEN	NO. OF PATIENTS	NO. OF RESPONSES*	DURATION
SINGLE AGENT			
Corticosteroids[18,27,62,144]	8	3 PR	
Doxorubicin (Adriamycin)[18]	1	PR	
Nitrogen mustard[18]	2	0	
Chlorambucil[18]	4	0	
Cyclophosphamide (Cytoxan)[18]	2	0	
Vincristine[18]	2	0	
Maytansine[18,29,77]	7	5 PR	
Azacytidine[27]	1	0	
Azathioprine[27]	1	0	
L-Asparaginase[27]	2	0	
Cisaplatin[113,151]	2	1 PR, 1 CR	
COMBINATION THERAPY			
MOPP (mechlorethamine/vincristine/procarbazine/prednisone)[18]	2	2 PR	3 months, 3 weeks
COPP (cyclophosphamide/vincristine/procarbazine/prednisone)[49]	5	4 PR	12, 33, 33, 34 months
PAC (cisplatin/Adriamycin/cyclophosphamide)[25]	1	CR	
Cytoxan/vincristine/prednisone[63]	1	CR	
Adriamycin/cisplatin[27,77,159]	4	1 CR	
Bleomycin/cisplatin/Adriamycin/prednisone[27]	5	2 PR	4, 12 months
Cytoxan/methotrexate/vincristine[27]	1	0	
Nitrogen mustard/vincristine/procarbazine/vinblastine[18]	2	2 PR	
BAPP (bleomycin/Adriamycin/cisplatin/prednisone)[28]	9	1 CR	
Adriamycin/cisplatin[106]	1	1 CR	9 months
Cisplatin/Adriamycin/Cytoxan[25]	1	1 CR	12 months
Cisplatin ± etoposide[59]	5	2 PR	1, 27 months
Cisplatin/vinblastine/bleomycin + RT[41]	4	2 CR	
Cytoxan/Adriamycin/vincristine[37]	2	2 CR	4, 8 months
Cisplatin/Adriamycin/Cytoxan/vincristine[54]	11	4 CR	5, 8, 29, 29 months
CCNU/vincristine/Cytoxan/prednisone[38]	9	4 CR	31, 33, 41, 62 months
Cytoxan/Adriamycin/Oncovin/prednisone[73]	1	—	—

**CR: complete response; PR: partial response*

Invasive thymomas therefore appear to be both chemosensitive and radiosensitive. A total experience with these agents alone or in combination suggests that PAC chemotherapy may be useful in the treatment of invasive thymomas. A national collaborative investigation through an intergroup study is underway to evaluate this matter.

Radiation Therapy Techniques

The recommended radiation dose for malignant thymomas, after resection, is 4500 cGy in 23 to 25 fractions; however, doses up to 5600 cGy have been used, with excellent local control rates with all doses above 4000 cGy. After surgical removal of as much tumor as possible, a dose of 4500 cGy, 180 cGy to 200 cGy daily, 5 days a week, is sufficient for tumor control. Several local recurrences have been reported with doses less than 4000 cGy. Occasionally, major resection is impossible and surgery is limited. In these cases, an additional 500 cGy boost is justified.

The volume treated should include the entire mediastinum and part of the involved adjacent lung when there is parenchymal involvement or as delineated by CT scan or surgical clips, plus at least a 1 cm margin (Fig. 39-4). Mediastinal treatment is usually given through anteroposterior (AP) portals with various combinations of photon beams (not shown here) and anterior wedge oblique portals (isodoses shown in Fig. 39-5).

Results of Radiation Therapy

In the past, radiation therapy has been used mostly with palliative intent. Often inadequacy of equipment or dose resulted in less than optimal results.[91] Of 23 patients treated with irradiation as the main therapy, 17 patients received external-beam radiation therapy, and the rest received other forms of radiation.[8] Of the 23 patients, eight had complete regression (CR), ten had partial regression (PR), and five had no regression (NR). Of the eight patients in the CR group, six received tumor doses of 4000 cGy or higher, as did five of ten patients in the PR group and only one of five patients in the NR group.

With megavoltage radiation therapy, control of malignant thymomas is satisfactory. In the report by Marks and colleagues,[101] tumor was controlled in all nine cases treated with megavoltage irradiation in the dose range of 3500 cGy to 4800 cGy. The average follow-up was 5.5 years (minimum 30 months). Ariaratnam and associates[3] observed tumor control in eight of 11 patients with malignant thymoma for a minimum follow-up period of 2 years. Three patients died; two of the three received only 3000 cGy in 3 weeks to the mediastinum.

Postoperative radiation therapy has resulted in improved survival of patients with invasive thymomas, after both complete and incomplete resections. Recently, Nakahara and associates[111] have reported a 5-year survival rate of 91.5% for patients with Stage II and 87.8% for patients with Stage III disease who

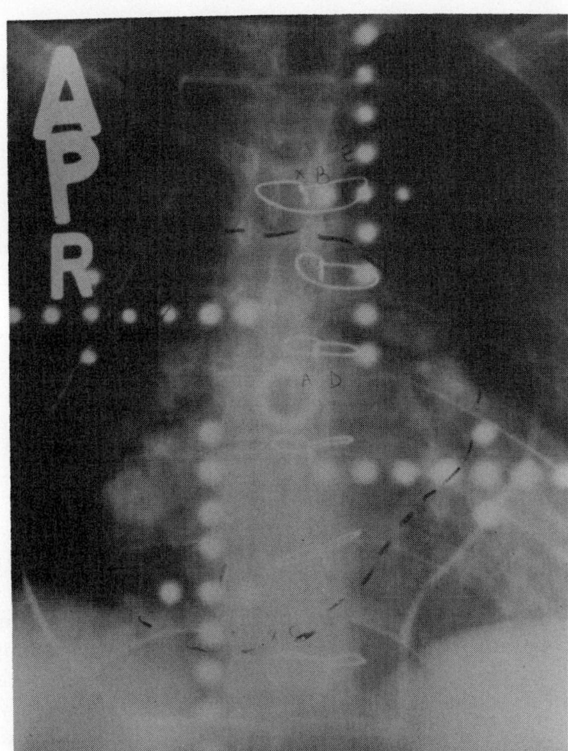

FIGURE 39–4. Treatment portal used in treatment of a 58-year-old woman with malignant thymoma. A 3:2 loading favoring the anterior port can be quite satisfactory. Various other portal arrangements with wedged beams can be used (Fig. 39-5). If a pleural metastasis is present, the entire hemithorax and lung can be irradiated by the moving-strip method using ^{60}Co or with open fields (1600 cGy to 1800 cGy in 2 weeks, ten fractions)

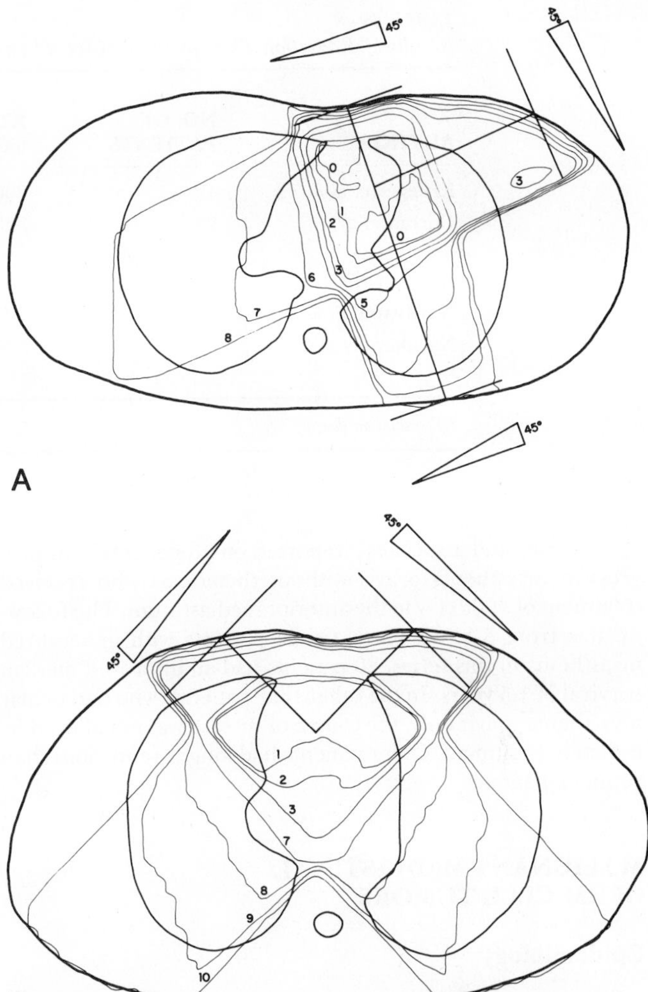

FIGURE 39–5. Isodose curves of optimized treatment plan used in treatment of mediastinal tumors. (**A**) Three-wedge portal (RAO, LAO, and LPO) arrangements. (**B**) Two anterior wedge portals (RAO and LAO). Note that in both plans the isodose curves are normalized to line 1 (100%) with subsequent lines representing a 10% reduction in total dose in decreasing order. (RAO: right anterior oblique; LAO: left anterior oblique; LPO: left posterior oblique)

were treated with postoperative radiation therapy. A summary of reported literature is shown in Table 39-8.

Sequelae of Treatment

In reported studies, the most common sequelae have been radiation pneumonitis, pericarditis, and, rarely, myelitis. In the studies reported by Marks and colleagues,[101] one patient died of myelitis; tumor dose was stated to be 4000 cGy, but because of the technique used, the spinal cord dose to a 20 cm segment was 4340 cGy. One port was treated each day. Autopsy showed no evidence of disease.

MYASTHENIA GRAVIS

Medical treatment consists mainly of administration of an anticholinesterase such as pyridostigmine bromide. In patients who have failed on anticholinesterase therapy and other modalities, adrenal corticosteroids have been suggested.[40] The surgical approach to the therapy of myasthenia gravis has been removal of the thymus. Buckingham[20] analyzed two groups of patients matched for age, sex, and severity and duration of myasthenia gravis. One group was treated medically, and the other was treated surgically. In a report by Evoli and associates,[50] thymectomy resulted in major improvement of myasthenia gravis in 30 of 75 patients (40%) with thymomas and in 100 of 161 patients (62%) without thymomas. Similar results have been reported by Jaretzki and colleagues.[78] Schulz and Schwab[142] reported a 17% improvement with no treatment or with medication alone and 65% improvement with surgery.

Braitman and colleagues[19] analyzed the results in 33 patients with thymic tumors, 17 of whom had associated myasthenia gravis. Response of myasthenia gravis to removal of the thymic tumor was good to excellent in 44% of the patients with an average follow-up of 5.5 years.

The results of thymic irradiation for myasthenia gravis have been similar to those of surgery.[123] In a report from the Massachusetts General Hospital,[141] 45 patients diagnosed with myasthenia gravis were treated with thymic irradiation only. In ten patients who had associated thymic tumors, improvement rate was 60%. In an additional 35 patients who had no thymic tumor, a 54% improvement rate was seen when the thymus was irradiated. A total of 27 patients in this series were treated by thymectomy followed by thymic irradiation; overall improvement rate was 66%. Again, no significant difference in results was found between patients harboring an associated tumor and those having no tumor. The dose of radiation to the thymic area in these studies ranged from 1500 cGy to 3000 cGy with conventional fractionation.

TABLE 39–8
Results of Radiation Therapy in Invasive Thymomas

AUTHOR	NO. OF PATIENTS	RT DOSE (cGy)	LOCAL CONTROL	5-YEAR SURVIVAL RATE
Krueger et al[87]	12	3000–5600	67%	75%
Curran et al[34]	25	3200–6000	84%	86% Stage II 69% Stage III
Kersh et al[82]	10	4600–5200	60%	57%
Nordstrom et al[115]	20	4000–5000	55%	50%
Nakahara et al[111]	4	3000–5000		91.5% Stage II 87.8% Stage III

RT: radiation therapy

Currier and associates[35] reported on 28 patients with progressive myasthenia gravis without thymomas who received treatment of 3000 cGy to the anterior mediastinum. The follow-up was from 5 to 18 years. Of 24 patients with generalized myasthenia in this series, 20 patients had an improved median survival of 1.5 years. In the other four patients, who had ocular myasthenia gravis only, the course of disease was not altered by radiation treatment. Older patients had longer remissions than younger patients.

MALIGNANT MEDIASTINAL GERM CELL TUMORS

Epidemiology

Malignant mediastinal germ cell tumors account for 5% to 13% of malignant mediastinal tumors[33,38] and about 2.5% of all mediastinal neoplasms.[162] The disease is most common in males. Of 150 patients with mediastinal germ cell tumors reported in seven series, 126 (84%) were males and 24 (16%) were females.[33,80,81,102,135,158]

Pure seminomas are most common in the third decade of life, followed by the fourth and second decades. Nonseminomatous germ cell tumors (pure or mixed histology) occur in young adults, the majority being in the 15- to 35-year age group.

Natural History

The majority of mediastinal germ cell tumors are located in the anterosuperior mediastinum.[17] In a review by Martini and colleagues,[102] the tumor was located in the anterior mediastinum in all 30 of the reported patients.

Mediastinal germ cell tumors have the same morphologic appearance as that of germinal tumors of the testes. The ratio of metastatic germ cell tumors in the chest to primary mediastinal germ cell tumors is 47 to 1.4.[102] However, these metastases were found anywhere in the chest. Primary testicular tumors that metastasize to the anterior mediastinum are very rare. If anterior mediastinal metastases are present, middle and posterior mediastinal lymph nodes as well as retroperitoneal nodes are frequently involved.[99]

Rather and associates,[128] after detailed histologic examination of patients with disseminated germ cell tumors, have described fibrotic scars in the testes. However, Luna and Tamariz[99] found evidence of a scar or occult tumor in the testes in only two of 20 cases of mediastinal germ cell tumors.

The histogenesis of these extragonadal germ cell tumors remains controversial. Two theories have gained the most popularity: the theory of somatic aberration by Schlumberger[141] and the theory of germ cell origin by Friedman.[55] The theory of somatic aberration by Schlumberger suggests that extragonadal germ cell tumors develop as a result of dislocation of germ cell layers during embryogenesis and that the mediastinal tumors derive from thymic origin, constituting an abnormality in thymic development. The location of germ cell tumors and thymomas, both commonly in the anterior mediastinum, supports this theory. However, the presence of other midline extragonadal germ cell tumors, such as primary tumors from the pineal area and retroperitoneum, argues against it.

Clinical Presentation and Diagnostic Workup

Patients with mediastinal germ cell tumors may be entirely asymptomatic, particularly when the tumor is a benign teratoma or seminoma.[102,118] A review of the literature[118] showed that in approximately 25% to 30% of patients, the first sign of disease was an abnormal "routine" chest x-ray examination. Anterior mediastinal tumors, because of their location, produce substernal pressure and pain radiating to the neck and the arms in 30% to 60% of patients.[38,135] The tumors impinge on the venous system, producing superior vena cava syndrome in 10% of patients.[33] Embryonal cell carcinoma, teratocarcinoma, and choriocarcinoma are more aggressively infiltrating neoplasms, resulting in substernal pleuritic pain, which is occasionally associated with dyspnea, cough, and hemopytysis. Approximately 40% of patients with choriocarcinoma show gynecomastia.[32,53,102,118]

As with evaluation of other mediastinal tumors, CT is the radiologic method of choice (see Table 39-3).[17,96] Direct extension of tumor to adjacent mediastinal structures can be evaluated by transverse CT sections. In the presence of abnormalities in the testes, appropriate radiologic examinations should be obtained for a testicular or retroperitoneal neoplasm (ultrasonography, CT, and possibly lymphangiography).

Germ cell tumors, in general, elaborate two proteins that are extremely useful in patient evaluation. The β-subunit of human chorionic gonadotropin (β-HCG) is found in elevated levels in the serum of 60% of patients with nonseminomatous germ cell tumors and 7% of patients with pure seminomas.[38,46,79,149] All patients with choriocarcinoma have elevated urinary and serum β-HCG levels. The α-fetoprotein (AFP), an α_1-globulin, is produced in the liver, yolk sac, and gastrointestinal tract of the fetus. Approximately 70% of the patients with nonseminomatous germ cell tumors have elevated levels of AFP, which often correlates with the presence of embryonal or yolk sac components.[22,38] Over 90% of patients with germ cell tumors have elevated levels of one or both of these markers.[79]

Serum measurements of these biomarkers are helpful in monitoring the response of the tumor to therapy and also can be used to detect recurrences[43,79]; therefore, the determination of pre- and posttreatment baseline levels is essential. The biomarkers have been studied extensively with testicular tumors; however, several reports indicate that they are of similar value with extragonadal germ cell tumors.[22,38,43]

In most cases of mediastinal tumors, a thoracotomy is necessary to establish a histopathologic diagnosis. When surgical removal of the tumor is not indicated or possible, an open biopsy can be done. A needle biopsy is usually inadequate for establishing diagnosis. Occasionally some of these tumors (*e.g.*, seminomas) are very difficult to differentiate from other anterior mediastinal tumors such as lymphomas, small cell tumors, and thymomas.

Pathologic Classification

Rosai and Levine[131] divided mediastinal germ cell tumors into germinomas (seminomas), adult teratomas, embryonal carcinomas, teratocarcinomas, choriocarcinomas, and yolk sac tumors (endodermal sinus tumors). However, a simpler system of classification is one that divides these tumors into pure seminomas or nonseminomatous carcinomas.[102]

In over 450 patients with mediastinal germ cell tumors reported in the English literature, pure seminomas comprise about 40% and nonseminomatous tumors about 60% of the cases. Therefore, the relative incidence of seminomas among germ cell tumors in the mediastinum is comparable to that in the testes (40%).

Prognostic Factors

As in the testis, the most important prognostic factor in anterior mediastinal extragonadal germinal tumors is histologic type. Seminomas are highly curable by radiation therapy and carry a substantially better prognosis than nonseminomatous germ cell tumors, which are mildly radiosensitive, often treated by surgery and combination chemotherapy, and carry a poorer prognosis.

In a review of the literature by Cox,[33] of 18 patients with nonseminomatous germ cell tumors, all died of their tumor within 1 year of the time of diagnosis, except two patients, both with mixed histology of embryonal carcinoma and seminoma. The mean survival time of all patients who died with disease correlates with the histopathologic diagnosis: seminoma, 16 months; embryonal carcinoma, 6.2 months; teratocarcinoma, 3.9 months; and choriocarcinoma, 1 month.

In a report of 24 patients with mediastinal seminomas,[85] patients under 35 years old tended to do better (ten of 17 with no evidence of disease) than those over 35 years (two of six with no evidence of disease). In this series there was complete resection in nine patients and incomplete resection or biopsy in the remaining 15. Six of nine patients in the first group and six of 15 in the second group were NED at the time of the report.

General Management

Among all seminoma cases reported in the literature, thoracotomy with radical intent has been performed in approximately 50% of patients who had surgery; in only 40% to 50% of patients undergoing radical surgery was complete tumor removal possible.[85] In the remaining patients, a diagnosis was established by mediastinoscopy, limited thoracotomy, or supraclavicular biopsy. Of 36 patients from the literature on whom surgery was performed with curative intent, only 17 had this as the only type of treatment. In the remaining 19 patients, adjuvant radiation therapy was used after complete surgical resection. The results of surgery alone and of complete removal of the tumor with postoperative radiation therapy are shown in Tables 39-9 and 39-10. Orchiectomy, in the absence of any clinical or radiographic indication of abnormality in the testes, is not recommended.[1,6,33,39,102,140]

Combination chemotherapy has been used in metastatic testicular seminomas as well as in mediastinal seminomas[56,71,92] with some success. Einhorn and Williams[47] have reported on 19 patients with disseminated seminomas treated with a combination of cisplatin, vinblastine, bleomycin, and (sometimes) doxorubicin. Of 19 patients, 12 (63%) achieved complete responses with a median duration of 18 months. Minimum follow-up was 1 year, and four patients have been in complete remission for over 2 years. In a series of 229 patients with disseminated germ cell tumors reported by Roth and co-workers[134] treated with cisplatin-based combination chemotherapy, 26 had seminomas; 14 of the 26 patients survived for a median of 26.6 months.

The role of radiation therapy in treatment of nonseminomatous germ cell tumors of the mediastinum is questionable. Neither irradiation nor surgery has been successful in the management of local or metastatic disease. In a report by Economou and colleagues,[43] only three of 17 patients (18%) with primary mediastinal nonseminomatous germ cell tumors were alive and free of disease. One patient was treated by operation alone and survived 15 years. Two other patients, treated aggressively by operation, irradiation, and combination chemotherapy, were alive and free of disease at 6 months and 3 years. In a report by Martini and associates,[102] all patients with nonseminomatous mediastinal germ cell tumors were dead of disease within 5 years after initiation of treatment, except one

TABLE 39–9
Results of Surgery Alone in Mediastinal Seminomas

AUTHOR	RESULTS OF FOLLOW-UP*
Taniguchi et al[152]	Operative death (2)
Kountz et al[86]	Alive at 6 years
Inada and Nakano[75]	Alive at 8 years
O'Gara et al[117]	Alive at 17 years
Lattes[90]	Alive at 7.5 years (1), alive at 4.5 years (1)
Schantz et al[140]	Alive at 4 years (5)
Beznyak et al[15]	Operative death
Levine[95]	Dead
Martini et al[102]	Alive at 20 years
Das and Deodhare[36]	Operative death
Hurt et al[74]	Alive at 13 years
Dosios et al[39]	Local recurrence at 3 years; then received radiation therapy (4000 cGy)

* *Single cases except as indicated in parentheses*

TABLE 39–10
Primary Seminomas of the Mediastinum: Results of Resection Followed by Irradiation

AUTHOR	DOSE OF RADIATION (cGy)	RESULTS OF FOLLOW-UP*
Woolner et al[161]	6000	Alive 3 years (metastasis after 6 months—irradiated)
O'Gara et al[117]	5500	Alive 6 years
Oberman and Liboke[116]	4000	Alive 5 years
Inada and Nakano[75]	2000 (split)	Alive 8 years
Andier et al[4]	4800	Alive 3 years
Pachter and Lattes[118]	6000 (in 5 months)	Dead in 6 months (local recurrence)
Edland et al[44]	NS	Alive 1 year
Schantz et al[140]	NS	Alive 11 years
Medini et al[105]	3500	Alive 17 years (1); alive 5 years (1)
Hurt et al[74]	3000	Alive 17 years (1); alive 5 years (1)
	3325	Alive 5 years
	3700	Died 12 years later with metastases
	2500	Alive 11 years
	4270	Dead at 11 months with metastases
Aygun et al[5]	NS	Alive 2 years (1); alive 12 years (1)
Raghavan and Barrett[127]	4500	Alive 10 years (preaortic nodal radiation therapy 2 months later)
Knapp et al[85]	1326–4900†	Alive without tumor (12), average 143 months' follow-up Alive with tumor (3), average 51 months Died with tumor (9), average 49.6 months

NS: not specified
** Single cases except as indicated in parentheses*
† 21 of 24 patients received radiation therapy.

patient with mixed histology of embryonal cell-choriocarcinoma who was alive at the time of publication of the report. The latter was treated with resection, radiation therapy, and chemotherapy.

Recently, following very encouraging results of treating testicular nonseminomatous germ cell tumors with combination chemotherapy (vinblastine, dactinomycin, bleomycin, and cisplatin),[46, 94, 134, 155] the same combination chemotherapy was applied to mediastinal germ cell tumors. A series of 203 patients with disseminated nonseminomatous germ cell tumors were treated with cisplatin-based combination chemotherapy. Of 203 patients, 133 survived for a median of 26.6 months (range 14.2 to 48.5 months). Reynolds and colleagues[129] reported an objective response of 53% (ten of 19 patients) with mediastinal germ cell tumors treated with combination chemotherapy. Two of these patients had complete remission of the disease. In a series of 32 patients with primary nonseminomatous mediastinal germ cell tumors treated with surgery and combination chemotherapy four survived with relapse, although follow-up was short.[85] Beattie[10] predicts that the 60% 5-year survival rate for Stage III germ cell tumors of the testes can be duplicated for the same tumors of the mediastinum by the use of multimodality therapy.

Radiation Therapy Techniques

Of all germ cell tumors, seminomas are the most curable with radiation therapy. The treatment technique is the same as for thymomas. Both supraclavicular areas may be irradiated as recommended by Bagshaw and associates.[6] A review of the literature indicates that doses ranging from 2000 cGy to 6000 cGy have been used. Cox[33] analyzed the dose-time relationship in the radiation therapy of germ cells tumors. Based on his data from Walter Reed and the Massachusetts General Hospital, he suggests that 3000 cGy given in 15 fractions over 3 weeks is adequate. However, Bagshaw and colleagues[6] recommend 4000 cGy to 5000 cGy in 4 to 4.5 weeks to the mediastinum and the supraclavicular lymph nodes. In an update of the Stanford experience by Bush and colleagues,[23] 13 patients were treated with definitive megavoltage radiation therapy and were available for 5-year follow-up. The actuarial 10-year survival rate was 69%, and the relapse-free survival rate was 54%. No patients receiving more than 4700 cGy to the primary lesion had local or systemic relapse. Our recommendation is 3000 cGy in 15 fractions over 3 weeks for minimal disease. For gross tumors we suggest 4000 cGy (180 cGy to 200 cGy daily, 5 days a week) to the large field encompassing mediastinum and both supraclavicular areas, followed by an additional 1000 cGy with reduced portals to the gross tumor volume (visible on CT scan).

Results of Radiation Therapy

The results of radiation therapy as the main modality of treatment for mediastinal seminomas (after biopsy or incomplete resection), summarized from the literature, are shown in Table 39-11. Of 22 patients who died of disease, two had locoregional

TABLE 39–11
Results of Radiation Therapy as Main Mode of Treatment in Mediastinal Seminomas

TOTAL DOSE (cGy)	NO. OF PATIENTS	ALIVE*	DEAD WITH DISEASE	DEAD OF INTERCURRENT DISEASE
Unspecified	7	4	3	—
<3000	15	7 (4)	8	—
≥3000	26	19 (1)	5	2
≥4000	30†	24 (3)	5	1
≥5000	9	9 (1)	—	—
≥6000	4	3	1	—
Total	91	66 (9)	22	3

**Numbers in parentheses represent patients alive with distant metastases.*
† One patient had complete resection before and one patient had surgery after radiation therapy.
Data from the following references: 5, 6, 23, 33, 45, 74–76, 81, 84, 86, 89, 102, 104, 105, 112, 114, 116–118, 124, 127, 140, 147, 148, 151, 162

recurrence (9.1% local failure rate). Of 78 patients receiving less than 5000 cGy, 54 are alive (eight with distant metastasis), and 21 died of disease. Of 13 patients who received 5000 cGy and over, 12 are alive and one died of disease. It appears that higher doses are needed to control seminomas of the mediastinum compared with testicular origin, most likely because of the larger size (tumor burden) of the mediastinal tumor compared with the testicular counterpart. Results of treatment of nonseminomatous germ cell tumors from the literature, as reviewed by Cox,[33] show that of 85 patients with teratocarcinoma, 18 with embryonal carcinoma, and 23 with choriocarcinoma, only two patients with embryonal carcinoma are known to be cured.

TRACHEAL TUMORS

Epidemiology

Primary malignant tumors of the trachea are rare. Gilbert and colleagues[60] have reported on 546 cases of primary tracheal tumors in adults (93.2%) and children (6.8%). Of 509 adult cases, 49.1% were malignant. Of the malignant tumors, 79% were carcinomas. About one tracheal carcinoma occurs for every 180 bronchogenic or 75 laryngeal carcinomas.[9] Over 800 cases of primary carcinomas of the trachea have been reported. Of these, 50% are squamous cell carcinomas, and 20% to 35% are adenoid cystic carcinomas.[137] The same etiologic relationship that exists between lung cancer and smoking and other environmental carcinogens applies to tracheal tumors (see Chap. 39). The age range and peak incidence are similar to those with laryngeal cancers (see Chap. 35). There is no sex predominance.

Natural History

Squamous cell cancer has a predilection for the distal third of the trachea, with over 60% of cases originating in the posterior or lateral wall. Approximately one third of patients have mediastinal spread or pulmonary metastases when first seen. The tumor first involves adjacent lymph nodes, and by direct extension to the mediastinal structures, metastases to distant organs (lungs, liver, bone) are common. Twenty percent of patients with tracheal tumors may present with synchronous or metachronous second carcinoma.

Adenoid cystic carcinomas and adenocarcinomas have a tendency to appear in the upper third of the trachea. These carcinomas may extend for a greater distance in the tracheal wall with only a portion of tumor presenting intratracheally. Therefore, with both surgery and radiation therapy, larger margins of clearance are needed. Extension beyond the trachea occurs three times more frequently with the adenoid cystic carcinomas (58%) than with squamous cell carcinomas.[9]

Clinical Presentation

The most common presenting signs and symptoms of tracheal tumors are upper airway obstruction, cough, hemoptysis, and recurrent pneumonia. Shortness of breath, initially on exertion and with progression of disease at rest, is common. In a Washington University series,[52] the most common symptoms were hemoptysis (60%), dyspnea (56%), hoarseness (40%), and cough (36%).[52]

Diagnostic Workup

Patients with the previously mentioned nonspecific symptoms may have a normal chest x-ray film. Bronchoscopy can be helpful for determination of resectability and relief of obstruction in occasional life-threatening situations. A rigid bronchoscope is usually used, but in recent years laser resection has been used more frequently.[88]

As with other mediastinal tumors, CT scan appears to be the radiologic study of choice for delineation of tumor extent.[156] Use of contrast material has been found to be unnecessary,[66] and careful study using air as a contrast medium gives adequate information.[107]

Prognostic Factors

Squamous cell carcinoma has a poorer prognosis than does adenoid cystic cancer.[52] In the report by Fields and associates,[52] patients with adenoid cystic carcinoma had a significantly better median survival (126 months) than those with squamous cell carcinoma (6.5 months) ($P = 0.03$). Tumor extent also has significant prognostic value.

General Management

Surgical resection with primary anastomosis or reconstruction is considered the treatment of choice for tracheal tumors.[64, 154, 163] Although endoscopic removal offers significant palliation for adenoid cystic carcinomas, it is usually associated with late local recurrences and protracted, incapacitating terminal illness. For localized lesions, sleeve resection and an end-to-end anastomosis are occasionally recommended.[103] Operative mortality of up to 16% has been reported.[122] Of 110 patients with primary malignant tumors of the trachea at Massachusetts General Hospital,[66] 54 underwent primary resection and reconstruction. Results are reported in Table 39-12. The follow-up period ranged from 1 to 20 years (median period was not mentioned). Adjuvant preoperative or postoperative radiation therapy was used in some patients.[120] Eschapasse,[48] in a collective series, and Perelman and Koroleva[122] have reported similar results.

In many patients irradiation has been used because the tumor was either recurrent after initial surgical failure or initially too extensive for surgical resection. In the report by Hajdu and colleagues,[69] four patients died without any evidence of tumor. Two of the four were treated surgically and lived 10 to 12 years; another patient received 7000 cGy in 3 weeks and lived 13 years; the last patient was treated with 5000 cGy external-beam and radon seed implant and survived 8 years. Houston and associates[72] reported that four patients with adenoid cystic carcinomas treated with radiation therapy alone lived 4, 7, 9, and 25 years.

In a report by Rostom and Morgan,[133] 13 of 44 patients received doses of less than 5000 cGy. In a study by Pearson and colleagues,[120] irradiation, usually preoperative, consisted of 3500 cGy to 4000 cGy in 21 days. In a series reported by Birt,[16] eight of 23 patients were treated with nonmegavoltage equipment, and dose range in this series was from 2000 cGy in 19 days to 6600 cGy in 65 days. In a report by Fields and colleagues,[52] local tumor control was achieved in six of seven (86%) patients who received more than 6000 cGy and in one of 11 (9%) patients treated to less than 6000 cGy ($P = 0.001$). The 5- and 10-year survival rates for their entire series were 23% and 13%, respectively.

Chemotherapy alone has not been shown to be useful,[42] but its use in conjunction with other modalities has been recommended.[148]

Radiation Therapy Techniques

CT scan and megavoltage energy are mandatory for proper treatment planning. Owing to the high incidence of mediastinal nodal involvement, almost the entire mediastinum (low border at least 6 cm below the carina) and both supraclavicular regions should be encompassed within the initial portal up to a dose of at least 4500 cGy.

A portion of the treatment can be with parallel opposed portals up to the spinal cord tolerance. In curative cases, additional boost (to a total tumor dose of 6500 cGy to 7000 cGy) can be delivered through anterior oblique portals with wedges (Fig. 39-6).

Planned preoperative radiation therapy up to 5000 cGy and surgery 4 to 6 weeks later seems to be most appropriate. Anastomotic sites should be out of the high-dose region (maximum 4500 cGy). If surgery cannot be performed, the total dose of radiation therapy should be 6500 cGy to 7000 cGy in 6 to 7 weeks. If CT scan shows massive tumor extension through the tracheal wall and if surgery is ruled out, high risk of fistula precludes a radical dose of radiation therapy. In this situation,

TABLE 39–12
Results of Therapy for Tracheal Tumors

AUTHOR	THERAPY*	TOTAL NO. OF PATIENTS	NO. ALIVE WITH TUMOR	NO. ALIVE WITHOUT TUMOR	NO. DEAD WITH TUMOR	NO. DEAD WITHOUT TUMOR
Hajdu[69]	S	6	2	1	1	2
	S + R	8	—	2	6	—
	R	22	1	1	18	2
	None	5	—	—	5	—
Houston[72]	S	21	—	7	14	—
	R	16	—	1	15	—
	None	8	—	—	8	—
Bennetts[12]	R	10	—	3	7	—
Roston and Morgan[133]	R	44	—	6	32	6
Richardson [130]	R	1	—	1	—	—
Grillo[65]	S ± R	54†	3	39‡	7	1
Pearson and Thompson[120]	R + S	16§	—	8	5	—
Cheung[31]	R	21	—	2	19	—
	S + R	2	1	—	1	—
	None	1	—	—	1	—
Fields[52]	R	18 }	—	3	20	1
	S + R	6 }				

** S: surgery; R: radiation therapy*
† Four operative deaths
‡ Some patients with short follow-up
§ Seventeen resections in six patients; four postoperative deaths.

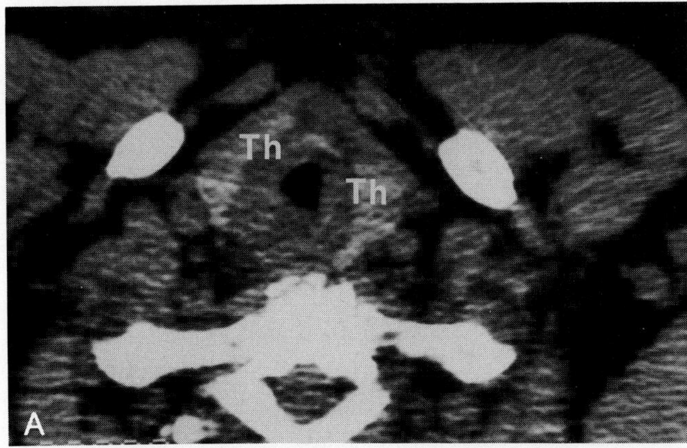

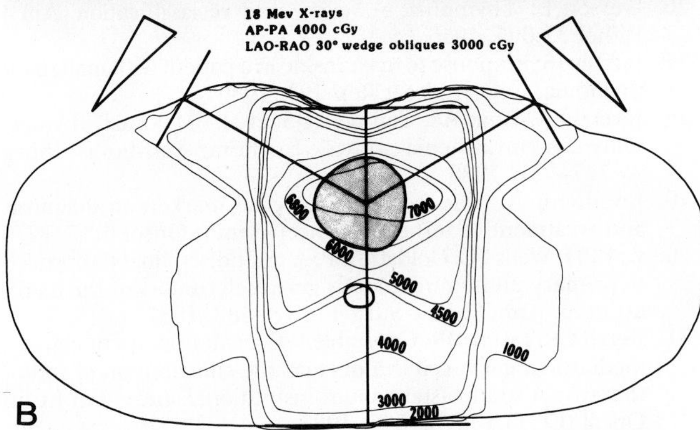

FIGURE 39–6. Treatment plan of a patient with primary tracheal carcinoma. (**A**) CT scan demonstrating a large tumor narrowing the trachea and displacing the thyroid gland (Th) laterally. (**B**) Optimized treatment plan used in radiation therapy: two PA-AP portals followed by two anterior wedge oblique portals (boost)

as well as in any condition in which the patient cannot tolerate high doses of radiation, a protracted palliative dose of 4500 cGy in 4 to 5 weeks can be used.

REFERENCES

1. Antoniades J: Uncommon malignant tumors. In DeVita VT Jr, Brady LW (eds): Cancer Management. New York, Masson, 1982
2. Applequist P, Kostianen S, Franssila K, et al: Treatment and prognosis of thymoma. Surg Oncol 20:265–268, 1982
3. Ariaratnam LS, Kalnicki S, Mincer F, et al: The management of malignant thymoma with radiation therapy. Int J Radiat Oncol Biol Phys 5:77, 1979
4. Audier M, Dor J, Picard D, et al: Thymoma "pseudo-seminoma." Presse Med 68:574, 1960
5. Aygun C, Slawson RG, Bajaj K, et al: Primary mediastinal seminoma. Urology 23:109, 1984
6. Bagshaw MA, McLaughlin WT, Earle JD: Definitive radiotherapy of primary mediastinal seminoma. AJR 105:86, 1969
7. Baron RL, Lee JKT, Sagel SS, et al: Computed tomography of the abnormal thymus. Radiology 142:127, 1982
8. Batata MA, Martini N, Nuvos AG, et al: Thymomas: Clinicopathologic features, therapy, and prognosis. Cancer 34:389, 1974
9. Batsakis JG: Tumors of the head and neck. In Batsakis JG (ed): Clinical and Pathological Considerations, 2nd ed, p 90. Baltimore, Williams & Wilkins, 1979
10. Beattie EJ Jr: Mediastinal germ cell tumors. Semin Oncol 6:109, 1979
11. Bematz P: Thymoma: Factors influencing prognosis. Surg Clin North Am 54:884, 1973
12. Bennetts FE: Tracheal tumors. Postgrad Med J 45:446, 1969
13. Bergh NP, Gatzinsky P, Larsson S, et al: Tumors of the thymus and thymic region. I. Clinicopathological studies of thymomas. Ann Thorac Surg 25:91, 1978
14. Bernatz PE, Khonsari S, Harrison EG, et al: Thymoma: Factors influencing prognosis. Surg Clin North Am 53:885, 1973
15. Besznyak I, Sebesteny M, Kuchar F: Primary mediastinal seminoma: A case report and review of the literature. J Thorac Cardiovasc Surg 65:930, 1973
16. Birt BD: The management of malignant tracheal neoplasms. J Laryngol Otol 84:723, 1970
17. Blomlie V, Lien HH, Fossa SD, et al: Computed tomography in non-seminomatous germ cell tumors of the mediastinum. Acta Radiol 29:289–292, 1988
18. Boston B: Chemotherapy of invasive thymoma. Cancer 38:49, 1976
19. Braitman H, Li Wei I, Hermann C, et al: Surgery for thymic tumors. Arch Surg 103:14, 1971
20. Buckingham J: The value of thymectomy in myasthenia gravis. Ann Surg 194:453, 1976
21. Burkell CC, Cross JM, Kent HP, et al: Mass lesions of the mediastinum. In Ravitch M (ed): Current Problems in Surgery. Chicago, Year Book Medical Publishers, 1969
22. Burt ME, Javadpour N: Germ cell tumors in patients with apparently normal testes. Cancer 47:1911, 1981
23. Bush SE, Martinez A, Bagshaw MA: Primary mediastinal seminoma. Cancer 48:1877, 1981
24. Butler WM, Diehl LF, Taylor HG, et al: Metastatic thymoma with myasthenia gravis. Cancer 50:419–422, 1982
25. Campbell MG, Pollard R, Al-Sarraf M: A complete response to metastatic malignant thymoma to cis-platinum, doxorubicin and cyclophosphamide. Cancer 48:1315, 1981
26. Casamassima F, Villari N, Fargnoli R, et al: Magnetic resonance imaging and high-resolution computed tomography in tumors of the lung and the mediastinum. Radiother Oncol 11:21–29, 1988
27. Chahinian AP, Bhardwaj S, Meyer RJ, et al: Treatment of invasive or metastatic thymoma. Cancer 47:1752, 1981
28. Chahinian AP, Holland JF, Bhardwaj S: Chemotherapy for malignant thymoma. Ann Intern Med 99:136, 1983
29. Chahinian AP, Mogrire C, Ohnuma T, et al: Phase I study of weekly maytansine given by IV bolus or 24-hour infusion. Cancer Treat Rep 63:1953, 1979
30. Chatten J, Katz SM: Thymoma in a 12 year old boy. Cancer 37:953, 1976
31. Cheung AYC: Radiotherapy for primary carcinoma of the trachea. Radiother Oncol 14:279–285, 1989
32. Cohen BA, Needle MA: Primary mediastinal choriocarcinoma in a man. Chest 67:106, 1975
33. Cox J: Primary malignant germinal tumors of the mediastinum: A study of 24 patients. Cancer 36:1162, 1975
34. Curran WJ, Kornstein MJ, Brooks JJ, et al: Invasive thymomas: The role of mediastinal irradiation following complete or incomplete surgical resection. J Clin Oncol 6:1722–1727, 1988
35. Currier RD, Routh A, Hickman CT, et al: Thymus irradiation for myasthenia gravis. Radiology 146:199, 1983
36. Das PB, Deodhare SG: Giant mediastinal seminoma (germinoma). Int Surg 61:563, 1976
37. Daugaard G, Hansen HH, Rirth M: Combination chemotherapy for malignant thymoma. Ann Intern Med 99:189–190, 1983
38. Davis RD, Oldham HN, Sabiston DC: Primary cysts and neoplasms of the mediastinum: Recent changes in clinical presentation, methods of diagnosis, management, and results. Ann Thorac Surg 44:229–237, 1987
39. Dosios T, Sbokos C, McMillan IKR, et al: Primary malignant mediastinal germ cell tumors. A study of 3 cases. J Surg Oncol 15:367, 1980
40. Drachman DB: Myasthenia gravis. N Engl J Med 298:136, 186, 1978
41. Dy C, Calvo FA, Mindan JP, et al: Undifferentiated epithelial-

rich invasive malignant thymoma: Complete response to cisplatin, vinblastine, and bleomycin therapy. J Clin Oncol 6:536–542, 1988
42. Eby LS, Johnson DS, Baker HW: Adenoid cystic carcinoma of the head and neck. Cancer 29:1160, 1972
43. Economou JS, Trump DL, Holmes EC, et al: Management of primary germ cell tumors of the mediastinum. J Thorac Cardiovasc Surg 83:643, 1982
44. Edland RW, Levine S, Serfas LS, et al: Seminoma-like tumor in the hyperplastic thymus gland: A case report and literature review. AJR 103:25, 1968
45. Effler DB, McCormack IJ: Thymic neoplasms. J Thorac Surg 31:60, 1956
46. Einhorn LH, Donohue J: Cisdiamminedichloroplatinum, vinblastine, and bleomycin combination chemotherapy in disseminated testicular cancer. Ann Intern Med 87:293, 1977
47. Einhorn LH, Williams SO: Chemotherapy of disseminated seminoma. Cancer Clin Trial 3:307, 1980
48. Eschapasse H: Les tumeurs tracheales primitives: Traitement chirurgical. Rev Fr Malad Resp 2:425, 1974
49. Evans WK, Thompson DM, Simpson WJ, et al: Combination chemotherapy in invasive thymoma. Cancer 46:1523–1527, 1980
50. Evoli A, Batocchi AP, Provenzano C, et al: Thymectomy in the treatment of myasthenia gravis: Report of 247 patients. Neurology 235:272–276, 1988
51. Fechner RE: Recurrence of noninvasive thymomas. Cancer 23:1423, 1969
52. Fields JN, Rigaud G, Emami B: Primary tumors of the trachea: Results of radiation therapy. Cancer 63:2429–2433, 1989
53. Fine G, Smith RW Jr, Puchter MR: Primary extragenital choriocarcinoma in the male subject: Case report and review of the literature. Am J Med 32:726, 1962
54. Fornasiero A, Daniele O, Sperandio P, et al: Chemotherapy of invasive or metastatic thymoma: Report of 11 cases. Cancer Treat Rep 68:1205–1210, 1984
55. Friedman NG: The comparative morphogenesis of extragenital and gonadal teratoid tumors. Cancer 6:625, 1951
56. Fuen LG, Samson MK, Stephens RL: Vinblastine (VLB), bleomycin (BLEO), cis-diamminedichloroplatinum (DDP) in disseminated extragonadal germ cell tumors. Cancer 45:2543, 1980
57. Fujimura S, Kondo T, Handa M, et al: Results of surgical treatment for thymoma based on 66 patients. J Thorac Cardiovasc Surg 93:708–714, 1987
58. Gerein AN, Srivastana SP, Burgess J: Thymoma: A ten year review. Am J Surg 136:49, 1978
59. Giaccone G, Musella R, Bertetto O, et al: Cisplatin-containing chemotherapy in the treatment of invasive thymoma: Report of five cases. Cancer Treat Rep 69:695–697, 1985
60. Gilbert JG, Mazzerella LA, Feit LJ: Primary tracheal tumors in the infant and adult. Arch Otolaryngol 58:1, 1953
61. Gravanis M: Metastasizing thymoma. Am J Clin Pathol 49:690, 1967
62. Green JD, Forman WH: Response of thymomas to steroids. Chest 65:114, 1974
63. Griffin JD, Aisenberg AC, Long JC: Lymphyocytic thymoma associated with T-cell lymphocytosis. Am J Med 64:1075, 1978
64. Grillo HC: Tracheal tumors: Surgical management. Ann Thorac Surg 26:112, 1978
65. Grillo HC: Management of tracheal tumors. Am J Surg 143:697, 1982
66. Grillo, HC: Tracheal tumors: Diagnosis and management. In Choi NC, Grillo HC (eds): Thoracic Oncology, p 271. New York, Raven Press, 1983
67. Grosfeld JL, Weinberger M, Kilman JW, et al: Primary mediastinal neoplasms in infants and children. Ann Thorac Surg 12:179, 1971
68. Gullian R: Malignant thymoma associated with myasthenia gravis, and evidence of extrathoracic metastases. Cancer 27:823, 1971
69. Hajdu SI, Huvos AG, Goodner JT, et al: Carcinoma of the trachea. Clinicopathological study of 41 cases. Cancer 25:1148, 1970
70. Hammon JW Jr, Sabiston DC Jr: The mediastinum. In Ellis HE, Goldsmith HS (eds): Thoracic Surgery. Hagerstown, MD, Harper & Row, 1985
71. Herlitzka AJ, Gale JW: Tumors and cysts of the mediastinum. Arch Surg 76:697, 1958
72. Houston HE, Payne S, Harrison EG, et al: Primary cancers of the trachea. Arch Surg 99:132, 1969
73. Hu E, Levine J: Chemotherapy of malignant thymoma: Case report and review of the literature. Cancer 57:1101–1104, 1986
74. Hurt RD, et al: Primary anterior mediastinal seminoma. Int Surg 49:1658, 1982
75. Inada K, Nakano A: Germinoma of mediastinum: Case report with special reference to histogenesis of mediastinal teratoma. Dis Chest 36:438, 1959
76. Iverson L: Thymoma: A review and reclassification. Am J Pathol 32:695, 1956
77. Jaffrey IS: Response to maytansine in a patient with malignant thymoma. Cancer Treat Rep 193, 1980
78. Jaretzki A, Penn AS, Younger DS, et al: "Maximal" thymectomy for myasthenia gravis. J Thorac Cardiovasc Surg 95:747–757, 1988
79. Javadpour N: The value of biological markers in diagnosis and treatment of testicular cancer. Semin Oncol 6:37, 1979
80. Kay PH, Wells FC, Goldstraw P: A multidisciplinary approach to primary nonseminomatous germ cell tumors of the mediastinum. Ann Thorac Surg 44:578–582, 1987
81. Kersh CR, Eisert DR, Constable WC, et al: Primary malignant mediastinal germ-cell tumors and the contribution of radiotherapy: A southeastern multi-institutional study. Am J Clin Oncol (CCT) 10:302–306, 1987
82. Kersh CR, Eisert DR, Hazra TA: Malignant thymoma: Role of radiation therapy in management. Radiology 156:207–209, 1985
83. Kilman J: Thymoma. Am J Surg 121:710, 1971
84. Kleitsch WP, Tarricco A, Haslam GJ: Primary seminoma (germinoma) of mediastinum. Ann Thorac Surg 4:249, 1967
85. Knapp RH, Hurt RD, Payne WS: Malignant germ cell tumors of the mediastinum. J Thorac Cardiovasc Surg 89:82–89, 1985
86. Kountz SI, Connolly JF, Cohn R: Seminoma-like (or seminomatous) tumors in anterior mediastinum: Report of four new cases and review of literature. J Thorac Cardiovasc Surg 45:289, 1963
87. Krueger JB, Sagerman RH, King GA: Stage III thymoma: Results of postoperative radiation therapy. Radiology 168:855–858, 1988
88. Laforet EG, Berger RI, Vaughan CW: Carcinoma obstructing the trachea. Treatment by laser resection. N Engl J Med 294:941, 1976
89. Larmi RHI, Karkola P: Mediastinal seminoma. Ann Chir Gynaecol 63:351, 1974
90. Lattes R: Thymoma and other tumors of the thymus: An analysis of 107 cases. Cancer 15:1224, 1962
91. Lattes R: Thymoma and other tumors of the thymus. Cancer 15:1224, 1964
92. Legg M: Pathology and clinical behavior of thymomas. Cancer 18:1121, 1965
93. LeGolvan DP, Abell MR: Thymomas. Cancer 39:2142, 1977
94. Levi JA, Thomson D, Sandeman T, et al: A prospective study of cisplatin-based combination chemotherapy in advanced germ cell malignancy: Role of maintenance and long-term follow-up. J Clin Oncol 6:1154–1160, 1988
95. Levine GD: Primary thymic seminoma: A neoplasm ultrastructurally similar to testicular seminoma and distinct from epithelial thymoma. Cancer 31:729, 1973
96. Levitt RG, Husland JE, Glazer HS: CT of primary germ cell tumors of the mediastinum. AJR 142:73, 1984
97. Loehrer PJ, Bonomi P, Goldman S, et al: Remission of invasive thymoma due to chemotherapy: Two patients treated with cyclophosphamide, doxorubicin, and vincristine. Chest 87:377–380, 1985

98. Lewis JE, Wick MR, Scheithauer BW, et al: Thymoma: A clinicopathological review. Cancer 60:2727–2743, 1987
99. Luna M, Tamariz JV: Germ-cell tumors of the mediastinum: Post-mortem findings. Am J Clin Pathol 65:450, 1976
100. Maggi G, Giaccone G, Donadio M, et al: Thymomas: A review of 169 cases, with particular reference to results of surgical treatment. Cancer 58:765–776, 1986
101. Marks RD Jr, Wallace KM, Pettit H S: Radiation therapy control of nine patients with malignant thymoma. Cancer 41:117, 1978
102. Martini N, Golbey RB, Hajdu SI, et al: Primary mediastinal germ cell tumors. Cancer 33:763, 1974
103. McCafferty GJ, Parker LS, Suggit SC: Primary malignant disease of the trachea. J Laryngol Otol 78:331, 1964
104. Meares EM, Briggs EM: Occult seminomas of the testis masquerading as primary extragonadal germinal neoplasms. Cancer 30:300, 1972
105. Medini E, Levitt SH, Jones TK, et al: The management of extratesticular seminoma without gonadal involvement. Cancer 44:2032, 1979
106. Mitrov PS, Bergmann L, Tuengerthal S: Induktion einer kompletten remission mit Adriamycin und cis-platin bei einem invasiv wachsenden thymoma. Dtsch Med Wochenschr 44:1667, 1982
107. Momose KR, MacMillan AS Jr: Roentgenologic investigations of the larynx and trachea. Radiol Clin North Am 16:327, 1978
108. Monden Y, Nakahara K, Iioka S, et al: Recurrence of thymoma: Clinicopathological features, therapy, and prognosis. Ann Thorac Surg 39:165–169, 1985
109. Monden Y, Uyama T, Taniki T, et al: The characteristics of thymoma with myasthenia gravis: A 28-year experience. J Surg Oncol 38:151–154, 1988
110. Nagaishi C: Functional Anatomy and Histology of the Lung. Baltimore, University Park Press, 1972
111. Nakahara K, Ohno K, Hashimoto J, et al: Thymoma: Results with complete resection and adjuvant postoperative irradiation in 141 consecutive patients. J Thorac Cardiovasc Surg 95:1041–1047, 1988
112. Nazari A, Gagnon ED: Seminoma-like tumor of the mediastinum: Case report. J Thorac Cardiovasc Surg 51:751, 1966
113. Needles B, Kemeny N, Urmacher C: Malignant thymoma: Renal metastasis responding to cis-platinum. Cancer 42:223, 1981
114. Nickls J, Franssila K: Primary seminoma of the anterior mediastinum. Acta Pathol Microbiol Scand (A) 80:260, 1972
115. Nordstrom D: Thymoma: Therapy and prognosis as related to operative staging. Int J Radiat Oncol Biol Phys 5:2059, 1979
116. Oberman HA, Liboke JH: Malignant germinal neoplasms of the mediastinum. Cancer 17:498, 1964
117. O'Gara RW, Horn RC Jr, Enterline HT: Tumors of anterior mediastinum. Cancer 11:562, 1958
118. Pachter MR, Lattes R: Germinal tumors of the mediastinum: A clinicopathologic study of adult teratomas, teratocarcinomas, choriocarcinomas, and seminomas. Dis Chest 45:301, 1964
119. Papatestas A, Genkins G, Kornfeld P, et al: Effects of thymectomy in myasthenia gravis. Ann Surg 206:79–88, 1987
120. Pearson FG, Thompson DW, Weissberg D, et al: Adenoid cystic carcinoma of the trachea. Ann Thorac Surg 18:16, 1974
121. Penn CRH, Hope-Stone HF: The role of radiotherapy in the management of malignant thymoma. Br J Surg 59:533, 1972
122. Perelman MI, Koroleva N: Surgery of the trachea. World J Surg 4:583, 1980
123. Phillips TL, Busckke F: The role of radiation therapy in myasthenia gravis. Calif Med 106:282, 1967
124. Polansky SM, Barwick KW, Ravin CE: Primary mediastinal seminoma. AJR 132:17, 1979
125. Posner J, Howleson J, Civitkovic E: "Disappearing" spinal cord compression: Oncolytic effect of glucosteroids (and other chemotherapeutic agents) on epidural metastasis. Ann Neurol 2:409, 1977
126. Rachmanioff R: Thymoma with metastasis to the brain. Am J Clin Pathol 41:61, 1964
127. Raghavan D, Barrett A: Mediastinal seminomas. Cancer 46:1187, 1980
128. Rather LJ, Gardiner WR, Fredricks JB: Regression and maturation of primary testicular tumors with progressive growth of metastasis: Report of 6 new cases and review of literature. Stanford Med Bull 12:12, 1954
129. Reynolds TF, Yagoda A, Vogrin D, et al: Chemotherapy of mediastinal germ cell tumors. Semin Oncol 6:113, 1979
130. Richardson JD, Graver F, Trinkle JK: Adenoid cystic carcinoma of the trachea. Thorac Cardiovasc Surg 66:311, 1973
131. Rosai J, Levine GD: Tumors of the thymus. In Atlas of Tumor Pathology, second series, fascicle 13. Washington, DC, Armed Forces Institute of Pathology, 1976
132. Rosenberg JC: Neoplasms of the mediastinum. In DeVita VT Jr, Hellman S, Rosenberg SA (eds): Cancer: Principles and Practice of Oncology, p 475. Philadelphia, JB Lippincott, 1982
133. Rostom AY, Morgan RL: Results of treating primary tumors of the trachea by irradiation. Thorax 33:387, 1978
134. Roth BJ, Greist A, Kubilis PS, et al: Cisplatin-based combination chemotherapy for disseminated germ cell tumors: Long-term follow-up. J Clin Oncol 6:1239–1247, 1988
135. Saabye J, Elbirk A, Andersen K: Teratomas of the mediastinum. Scand J Thorac Cardiovasc Surg 21:271–272, 1987
136. Sagel SS, Aronberg DJ: Thoracic anatomy and mediastinum. In Lee JKT, Sagel SS, Stanley RB (eds): Computed Body Tomography, p 55. New York, Raven Press, 1983
137. Salm R: Primary carcinoma of the trachea: A review. Br J Dis Chest 58:61, 1964
138. Salyer WR, Enggleston JC: Thymoma: A clinical and pathological study of 65 cases. Cancer 37:229, 1976
139. Sawyers JL, Foster JH: Surgical treatment of thymomas. Arch Surg 96:814, 1968
140. Schantz A, Sewell W, Castleman B: Mediastinal germinoma: A study of 21 cases with an excellent prognosis. Cancer 30:1189, 1972
141. Schlumberger HG: Teratoma of the anterior mediastinum in the group of military age: A study of sixteen cases and a review of theories of genesis. Arch Pathol 41:398, 1966
142. Schulz MD, Schwab RS: Results of thymic (mediastinal) radiation in patients with myasthenia gravis. Ann NY Acad Sci 183:303, 1971
143. Sellors TH, Thackray AC, Thompson AD: Tumors of the thymus. Thorax 22:193, 1967
144. Shellito J, Khandekar JD, McKeever WP, et al: Invasive thymoma responsive to oral corticosteroids. Cancer Treat Rep 62:1397, 1978
145. Shields TW: Primary tumors and cysts of the mediastinum. In Shields TW (ed): General Thoracic Surgery, p 927. Philadelphia, Lea & Febiger, 1983
146. Shields TW, Fox RT, Lees WM: Thymic tumors: Classification and treatment. Arch Surg 92:617, 1966
147. Steinmetz WH, Hays RA: Primary seminoma of the mediastinum: Report of a case with an unusual site of metastasis and review of the literature. AJR 86:669, 1961
148. Steinoff NG, Harris HS, Mari J: An analysis of cylindroma of the head and neck. J Surg Oncol 5:17, 1973
149. Stepanas AV, Samaan NA, Schultz PN, et al: Endocrine studies in testicular tumor patients with and without gynectomastia: A report of 45 cases. Cancer 41:369, 1978
150. Sterchi M, Cordell AR: Seminoma of the anterior mediastinum. Ann Thorac Surg 19:371, 1975
151. Talley RW, Gutterman JU, Brownlee RW, et al: Clinical evaluation of toxic effects of cis-diamminedichloroplatinum (NSC 119875) phase I study. Cancer Chemother Rep 57:465, 1973
152. Taniguchi H, Pai TJ, Amdkata Y: Two cases of seminomatous tumors originating from anterior mediastinum. Gann 48:639, 1957
153. Verley JM, Hollmann KH: Thymoma: A comparative study of clinical stages, histologic features, and survival in 200 cases. Cancer 55:1074–1086, 1985
154. Vieta JO, Maier HC: The treatment of adenoid cystic carcinoma (cylindroma) of the respiratory tract by surgery and radiation therapy. Dis Chest 31:493, 1957
155. Vugrin D, Whitmore WF, Bains M, et al: Role of chemo-

therapy and surgery in the treatment of thoracic metastasis from nonseminomatous germ cell testis tumor. Cancer 50:1056, 1982

156. Weber AL, Grillo HC: Tracheal tumors: A radiological clinical and pathological evaluation of 84 cases. Radiol Clin North Am 16:227, 1978
157. Welch KJ, Tapper D, Vawter GP: Surgical treatment of thymic cysts and neoplasms in children. J Pediatr Surg 14:691, 1979
158. Whelan AJ, Hughes CF. Flynn PWP, et al: Primary malignant non-seminomatous germ cell tumour of the mediastinum treated by surgery and chemotherapy. Aust NZ J Surg 58:251–254, 1988
159. Wick MR, Nichols WC, Ingle JN, et al: Malignant predominantly lymphocytic thymoma with central and peripheral nervous system metastases. Cancer 47:2036, 1981
160. Wilkins EW: Thymoma: A continuing survey at Massachusetts General Hospital. Ann Thorac Surg 28:252, 1978
161. Woolner IB, Jamplis RW, Kirklin WJ: Seminoma (germinoma) apparently primary in the anterior mediastinum. N Engl J Med 252:653, 1955
162. Wychoulis AR, Payne WS, Clagett OT, et al: Surgical treatment of mediastinal tumors: A 40 year experience. J Thorac Cardiovasc Surg 62:379, 1971
163. Zunker HO, Moore RL, Baker DC, et al: Adenoid cystic carcinoma (cylindroma) of the trachea: Case report with 9 year follow-up. Cancer 23:699, 1969

40

○ ○ ○ • • •

Esophagus

Scot A. Fisher
Luther W. Brady

TOPOGRAPHIC ANATOMY

The esophagus is a thin-walled, hollow tube with an average length of 25 cm. The normal esophagus is lined with stratified squamous epithelium similar to the buccal mucosa. There are many methods of subdividing the esophagus, all of which are arbitrary. The cervical esophagus begins at the cricopharyngeal muscle (C7) and extends to the thoracic inlet (T3). The thoracic esophagus represents the remainder of the organ, going from T3 to T10 or T11.[89]

The American Joint Committee on Cancer (AJCC) divides the esophagus into four regions: cervical, upper thoracic, midthoracic, and lower thoracic.[9] Figure 40-1 correlates the basic anatomy of the esophagus with the subdivision schemes described above.

Lymphatic Drainage

The esophagus has a dual longitudinal interconnecting system of lymphatics. As a result of this system, lymph fluid can travel the entire length of the esophagus before draining into the lymph nodes,[89] so that the entire esophagus is at risk for lymphatic metastasis. In "skip areas," up to 8 cm of normal tissue can exist between gross tumor and micrometastasis within lymph fluid traveling in the esophagus.[110] Lymphatics of the esophagus drain into nodes that usually follow arteries, including the inferior thyroid artery, the bronchial and esophageal arteries from the aorta, and the left gastric artery (celiac axis).[98] Figure 40-2 illustrates the major lymph node groups draining the esophagus.

EPIDEMIOLOGY AND RISK FACTORS

Carcinoma of the esophagus represents roughly 1% of all cancer in the United States, excluding skin and *in situ* lesions. In 1990, there were an estimated 10,600 new esophageal cancer patients (7400 men and 3200 women).[99] Patients usually present with the disease between 55 and 65 years of age.[90] In the United States, the rates for whites are 4.8 and 1.6 per 100,000 for men and women, respectively. In blacks the rates are 16.9 and 4.5 per 100,000 for men and women, respectively. Puerto Rican men have a rate similar to that of black men.[114] The estimated deaths in 1990 totaled 9500 (7000 men, 2500 women).[99]

Carcinoma of the esophagus is found in many regions and the world-wide incidence usually varies from 2.5 to 5.0 per 100,000 in men and 1.5 to 2.5 per 100,000 in women.[95] Perhaps the highest rates in the world are found in Iran and the Soviet Union around the Caspian Sea.[56,65,90] The population in those areas is largely Moslem, with generally no alcohol consumption and low tobacco use.[90] However, the climate is an important factor, with high-risk areas having an arid climate with alkaline soil.[64] In China, the prevalence of esophageal carcinoma extends to northern China with an incidence of more than 100 per 100,000 in persons over 30 years old.[113]

In North America and western Europe, alcohol and tobacco use are the major risk factors and are associated with 80% to 90% of all cases.[95] Schottenfeld postulated possible mechanisms by which alcohol contributes to cancer formation,[94] including local cytotoxicity affecting mucosal permeability, low levels of carcinogens in alcoholic beverages, alcoholic liver injury that may affect chemical detoxification, nutritional deficiencies, and decreased immune response.

Certain high-risk groups consume corn, wheat, millet, and small amounts of fruits, vegetables, and animal products.[95] Patients with Plummer-Vinson (Paterson-Kelly) syndrome, are at an increased risk for oral cavity, hypopharyngeal, and esophageal cancer. Dietary intake of nitrosamines, nitrosamides, and N-nitroso compounds induces tumors in many species. Pickled vegetables, alcoholic beverages, cured meats, and fish are common sources of these nitrates. Fungal contamination may increase the synthesis of nitrosamines.[61,72]

Other risk factors are associated with carcinoma of the esophagus. Adenocarcinoma of the esophagus occurs in 2.4% to 8.5% of patients with Barrett's esophagus.[41,77,84] Sarr and associates found a 15% incidence of adenocarcinoma in patients who had Barrett's esophagus with symptoms of gastroesophageal reflux.[93] Achalasia of long duration (25 years or more) is associated with a 5% incidence of squamous cell carcinoma of the esophagus.[112] Caustic burns, especially lye corrosion, are related to the development of esophageal cancer.[8,44] Patients who have had burns tend to be younger with a more favorable prognosis. Patients with tylosis (hyperkeratosis of the palms and soles and papilloma of the esophagus) have a 37.5% chance of developing esophageal cancer at a mean age of 45 years.[40,95]

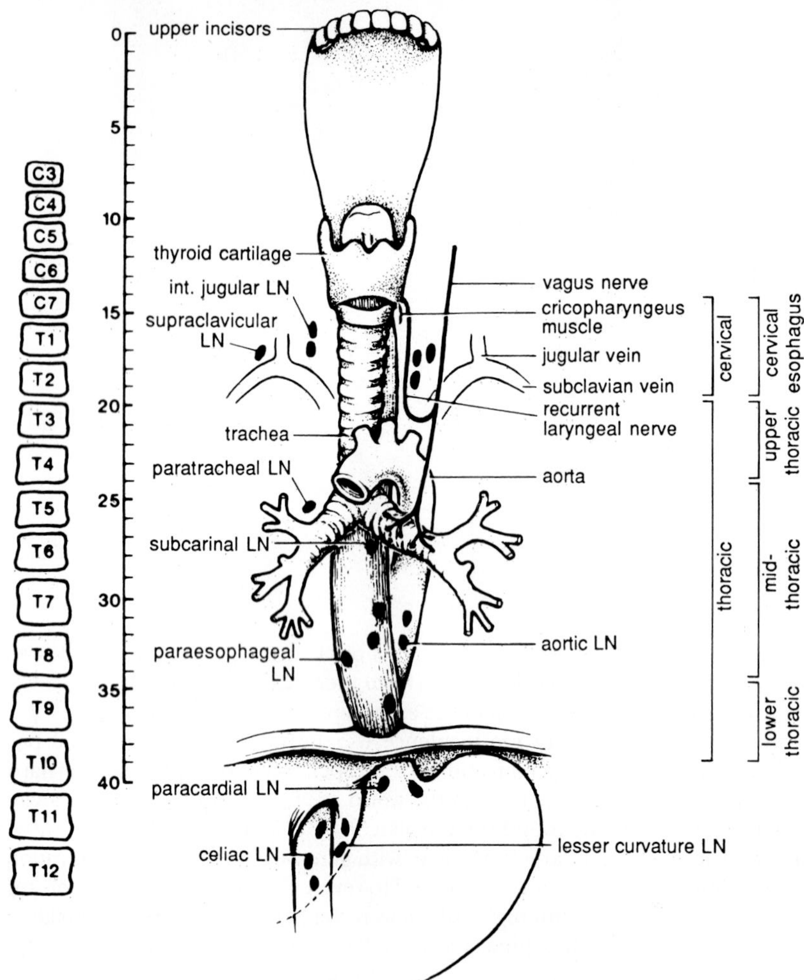

FIGURE 40–1. Basic anatomy of the esophagus. Note the lengths of the various segments of the esophagus from the upper central incisors and the two classification schemes for subdividing the esophagus. (LN: lymph node)

Finally, 2% to 4% of patients with head and neck cancer develop carcinoma of the esophagus.[14]

NATURAL HISTORY AND PATTERNS OF SPREAD

Squamous cell carcinoma is characterized by extensive local growth and lymph node metastases before it becomes widely disseminated.[38] Because the esophagus has no serosa, direct invasion of contiguous structures occurs very early.[82] Various authors have estimated the incidence of squamous cell cancer in each third of the esophagus: upper third, 10% to 25%; middle third, 40% to 50%; lower third, 25% to 50%.[45,73] If extra-esophageal extension occurs in the mediastinum, tracheo-esophageal or bronchoesophageal fistulas may occur. Mediastinitis, massive hemorrhage, and empyema are other catastrophic events that can result from direct invasion.[45]

Lymph node metastases are found in roughly 70% of patients at autopsy (see Fig. 40-2).[6,11,23]

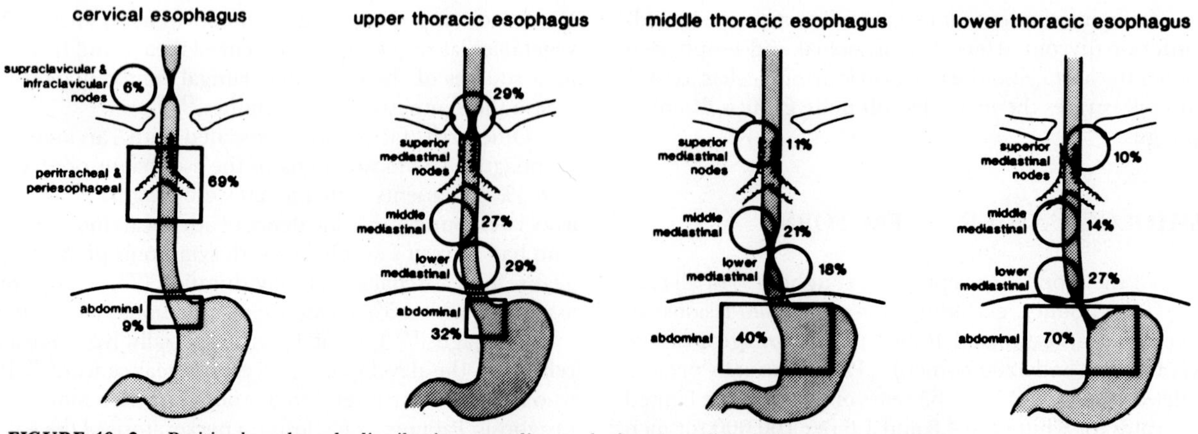

FIGURE 40–2. Positive lymph node distribution according to the location of the primary tumor. (Modified from Akiyama H, Tsurumaru M, Kawamura T, et al: Ann Surg 194:438, 1981; Dormans E: Z Krebforsch 49:86, 1939)

TABLE 40–1
Distribution of Metastases by Anatomic Site

SITE	NUMBER OF PATIENTS	PERCENT	SITE	NUMBER OF PATIENTS	PERCENT
Lymph nodes	58	73	Thyroid	5	6
Lung	41	52	Gastrointestinal serosa	5	6
Liver	37	47	Aorta	4	5
Adrenals	16	20	Peritoneum	4	5
Diaphragm	15	19	Small bowel	4	5
Bronchus	13	17	Appendix	2	3
Pleura	13	17	Brain	1	1
Stomach	12	15	Skin	1	1
Bone	11	14	Thoracic wall	1	1
Kidneys	10	13	Prostate	1	1
Trachea	10	13	Omentum	1	1
Pericardium	9	11	Large bowel	1	1
Pancreas	9	11	Bladder	1	1
Heart	7	9	Ureter	1	1
Spleen	6	8			

Anderson LL, Lad TE: Cancer 50:1587–1590, 1982

Sannohe and colleagues reported an incidence greater than 15% of positive supraclavicular nodes for thoracic esophagus lesions.[92] Metastasis can occur at almost any site (Table 40-1).

PATTERNS OF FAILURE

Aisner and colleagues[3] reviewed the patterns of failure in esophageal cancer after radical irradiation, radical surgery, and a combination of both. Table 40-2 summarizes these findings. These data suggest that a very high rate of local recurrence is found when either irradiation or surgery is used alone. Long-term survivors risk developing a second malignancy. Fogel and co-workers[32] estimated that at 5 years after surgery or irradiation, there is a 25% risk of developing a second primary tumor in the upper aerodigestive tract.

CLINICAL PRESENTATION

Symptoms of esophageal cancer usually start 3 to 4 months before diagnosis. Dysphagia and weight loss are seen in over 90% of patients. Odynophagia (pain on swallowing) is present in up to 50% of patients.[90] Infrequent initial symptoms also may be hoarseness, cough, and glossopharyngeal neuralgia.[73]

Advanced lesions can produce signs and symptoms from tumor invasion into local structures. Hematemesis, hemoptysis, and melena, and persistent cough secondary to esophagotracheal or esophagobronchial fistula may occur. Compres-

TABLE 40–2
Patterns of Failure in Esophageal Cancer

MODALITY	NO. OF PATIENTS	RECURRENCE (%) LOCAL	MARGINAL	NECK	MEDIASTINAL	DISTANT
Irradiation alone (3000–8000 cGy)	517	25–84	25	10–43		23–65
Radical surgery alone	266	21–50		44	33	17–69 33 Abdominal nodes 17 Liver 6 Lung
Combined (Primarily preoperative irradiation, 3500–5000 cGy usual dose)	2078	22–87	53*		20*	17–43 15–41 Abdominal nodes 7 Liver* 7–29 Lung† 7 Bone*

**From one study*
†From two studies
(Aisner J, Forastiere A, Aroney R: Patterns of recurrence for cancer of the lung and esophagus. In Wittes RE [ed]: Cancer Treatment Symposia: Proceedings of the Workshop on Patterns of Failure After Cancer Treatment, vol 2, p 87. Washington, DC, U.S. Department of Health and Human Services, 1983)

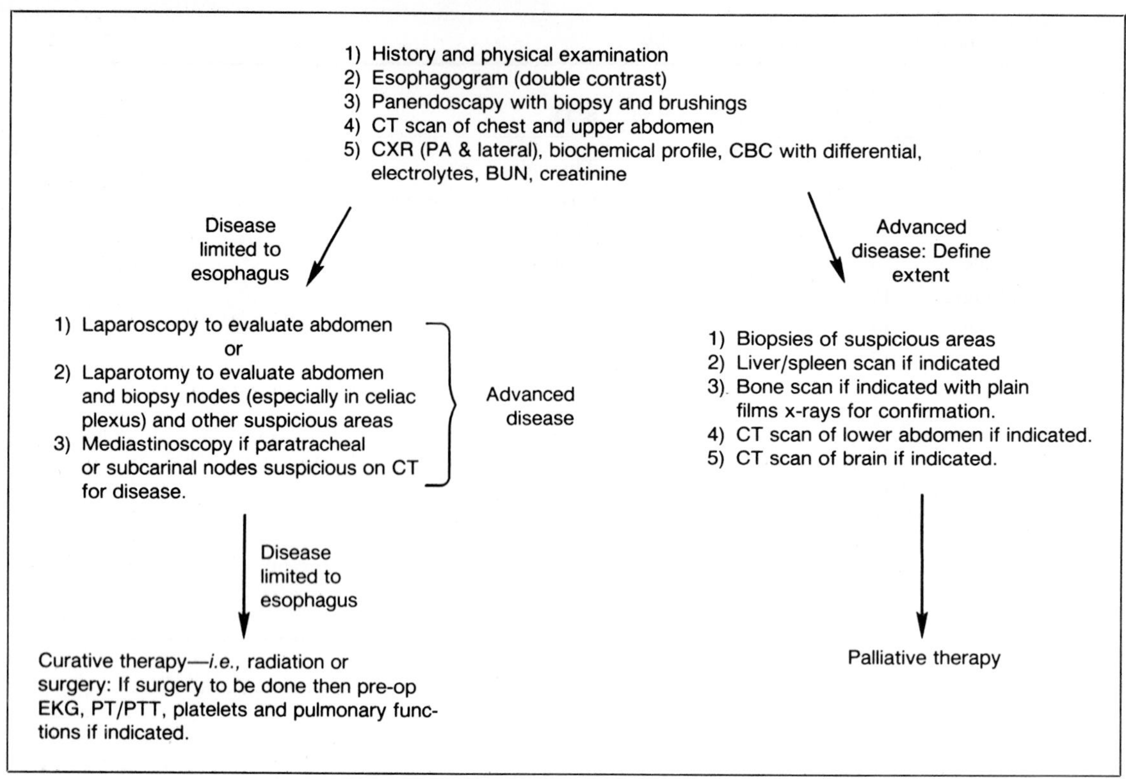

1) History and physical examination
2) Esophagogram (double contrast)
3) Panendoscopy with biopsy and brushings
4) CT scan of chest and upper abdomen
5) CXR (PA & lateral), biochemical profile, CBC with differential, electrolytes, BUN, creatinine
Disease limited to esophagus
Advanced disease: Define extent
1) Laparoscopy to evaluate abdomen
or
2) Laparotomy to evaluate abdomen and biopsy nodes (especially in celiac plexus) and other suspicious areas
3) Mediastinoscopy if paratracheal or subcarinal nodes suspicious on CT for disease.
Advanced disease
1) Biopsies of suspicious areas
2) Liver/spleen scan if indicated
3) Bone scan if indicated with plain films x-rays for confirmation.
4) CT scan of lower abdomen if indicated.
5) CT scan of brain if indicated.
Disease limited to esophagus
Curative therapy—i.e., radiation or surgery: If surgery to be done then pre-op EKG, PT/PTT, platelets and pulmonary functions if indicated.
Palliative therapy

FIGURE 40–3. Diagnostic workup for patients with esophageal cancer.

sion or invasion of the left recurrent laryngeal nerve or the phrenic nerves can cause dysphonia or paralysis of a hemidiaphragm. Superior vena cava syndrome and Horner's syndrome can also appear. Finally, pleural effusion and exsanguination resulting from aortic communication can occur.[90] Distant metastasis may be detected. However, most deaths are caused by the primary tumor.[73]

DIAGNOSTIC WORKUP

After a thorough history and physical examination, all patients with suspected esophageal cancer should have a workup similar to that outlined in Figure 40-3.

The esophagogram can characterize the lesion,[106] although this is not of prognostic significance.[74] Deformity of the esophageal axis can be seen (Fig. 40-4). Unfortunately, it is difficult to assess the true length of a tumor with routine esophagograms.[5] However, the double contrast esophagogram may be better at this and may improve detection of early lesions.[37] Computed tomography (CT) of the thorax can demonstrate extramucosal extension of disease. The CT scan of the thorax should be extended below the diaphragm to include the liver, upper abdominal nodes, and adrenals. The CT scan may not adequately assess periesophageal lymph node involvement or accurately show the true length of the primary tumor.[59,75,83] Routine CT of the brain should not be done because of the low incidence of metastasis (less than 1%) in this organ.[86] Nuclear magnetic resonance imaging (MRI) for esophageal cancer seems to have the same limitations as CT scanning.[87] Liver ultrasonongraphy is useful only for the evaluation of possible abdominal metastasis, especially in the hepatobiliary system, and is not routinely used.[106]

Esophagoscopy, using either flexible or rigid techniques, should be performed. Biopsies and brushings should be done on any areas suspected of containing metastasis. Because of the high incidence of second tumors, a thorough examination of the oral cavity, pharynx, larynx, and tracheobronchial tree should also be performed at the time of esophagoscopy.[89] Mediastinoscopy may be a useful study in the peritracheal or subcarinal nodes.[49,76]

Palpable nodes can have a direct biopsy. Biopsies can also be

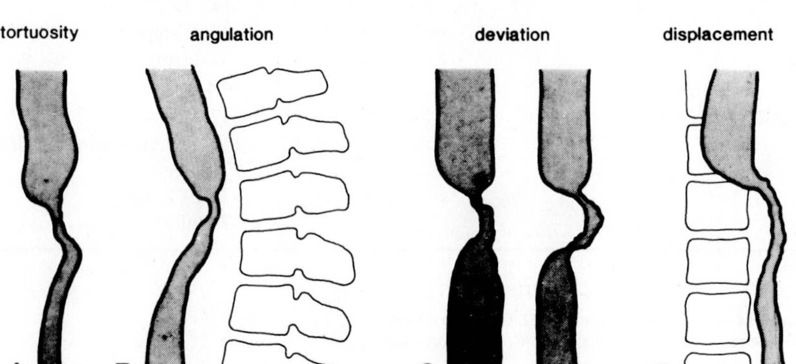

FIGURE 40–4. Abnormalities of the esophageal axis seen in esophagograms of unresectable tumors. (**A**) Tortuosity of the esophageal axis proximal to the tumor. (**B**) Angulation of the esophageal axis. (**C**) Axis deviation above and below the tumor and axis deviation of the tumor itself. (**D**) Abnormality of the distance from the spine. (Adapted and reproduced with permission from Akiyama H: Surgery for carcinoma of the esophagus. In Ravitch MM, et al [eds]: Current Problems in Surgery. Copyright © 1980 by Year Book Medical Publishers, Inc., Chicago 1980)

performed at the time of laparoscopy or laparotomy because up to 30% of superior gastric nodes can be positive even in upper thoracic lesions.[6]

Laparoscopy can be useful in evaluating malignant ascites, liver metastatis, and stomach involvement.[89] Laparotomy can be used to obtain information that would prevent a curative procedure (*e.g.*, tumor in the abdomen) or as part of an overall curative operation.

STAGING SYSTEMS

A number of staging systems have been proposed. Table 40-3 represents the AJCC clinical and pathologic staging system. The Japanese have a similar staging system,[47] which is based on operative findings. The Rotterdam group has used still another staging system. Patients are grouped as operable-curable, inoperable-curable, operable-incurable, or inoperable-incurable.[109]

PATHOLOGIC CLASSIFICATION

Table 40-4 lists the pathologic classification of esophageal tumors according to the World Health Organization.[79] Ninety percent of all esophageal tumors are squamous cell carcinomas. Some authors believe that the degree of differentiation affects survival,[115] but others think that it has no impact on survival or lymph node involvement.[89]

Pseudosarcoma is a variant of a poorly differentiated squamous cell carcinoma with spindle-shaped cells in the stroma resembling fibroblasts. Verrucous carcinoma is another variant of squamous cell carcinoma. It is well differentiated and papillary in appearance.[89] The last variant of squamous cell carcinoma is carcinoma *in situ*, which is rare in the United States[12,66,104] and should be distinguished from dysplasia.

Adenocarcinoma is an epithelial tumor of the esophagus that usually represents extension from gastric adenocarcinoma. Turnbull and co-workers reported a 2.4% incidence of adenocarcinoma in a review of 1918 cases of cancer of the esophagus.[107] Adenocarcinoma may arise from foci of ectopic gastric mucosa, intrinsic esophageal glands, or Barrett's esophagus. Submucosal spread is not as common as in squamous cell carcinoma. Spread usually occurs by transverse penetration through the full thickness of the wall.[21] Turnbull and colleagues found a 2.2% 5-year survival rate for adenocarcinoma compared with a 1.5% rate for squamous cell carcinoma. When a small focus of squamous cell metaplasia is found in an adenocarcinoma, the tumor is called an *adenoacanthoma*.[106]

Adenoid cystic carcinomas, mucoepidermoid tumors, and adenosquamous carcinomas are rare and have poor prognoses.[107] Undifferentiated carcinomas resemble small cell carcinomas and originate in the argyrophil cells in the esophagus. These carcinomas are found predominantly in the middle and lower esophagus in men.[46] They are highly malignant and may produce paraneoplastic syndromes, such as antidiuretic hormone secretion and hypercalcemia.[22] The clinical course of small cell carcinoma of the esophagus is similar to that of small cell carcinoma of the lung.[46,107]

Nonepithelial tumors of the esophagus are rare. Among these, leiomyosarcomas are the most common. Twenty-five percent of patients with this tumor have metastasis.[34,80,86] Histologically, these tumors have interlacing bundles of spindle-shaped cells. The less aggressive forms have fewer mitotic figures and less anaplasia. Turnbull and associates state that leiomyosarcoma has a prognosis more favorable than that of squamous cell carcinoma.[107]

Malignant melanoma is very rare and can occur as a primary esophageal tumor or as metastasis. Generally large and bulky, it is covered by intact squamous mucosa with focal areas of ulceration. Spread is usually submucosal, and mean survival is 7 months.[63,103]

Metastases to the esophagus occur. The most common source is the breast, but other reported sites include the phar-

TABLE 40–3
TNM Staging for Cancer of the Esophagus

Primary Tumor (T)	
TX	Primary tumor cannot be assessed
T0	No evidence of primary tumor
Tis	Carcinoma *in situ*
T1	Tumor invades lamina propria or submucosa
T2	Tumor invades muscularis propria
T3	Tumor invades adventitia
T4	Tumor invades adjacent structures
Regional Lymph Nodes (N)	
NX	Regional lymph nodes cannot be assessed
N0	No regional lymph node metastasis
N1	Regional lymph node metastasis
Distant Metastasis (M)	
MX	Presence of distant metastasis cannot be assessed
M0	No distant metastasis
M1	Distant metastasis

(Beahrs OH, Henson DE, Hutter RV, Myers MH [eds]: Manual for Staging of Cancer, 3rd ed. Philadelphia, JB Lippincott, 1988)

TABLE 40–4
Pathologic Classification of Malignant Esophageal Tumors

EPITHELIAL TUMORS

Squamous Cell Carcinoma
- Well differentiated
- Moderately differentiated
- Poorly differentiated

Variants of Squamous Cell Carcinoma
- Spindle cell carcinoma
- Pseudosarcoma and carcinosarcoma
- Verrucous carcinoma
- *In situ* carcinoma

Adenocarcinoma
- Adenoacanthoma

Adenoid cystic carcinoma (cylindroma)
Mucoepidermoid carcinoma
Adenosquamous carcinoma
Carcinoid
Undifferentiated carcinoma

NONEPITHELIAL TUMORS

Leiomyosarcoma
Malignant melanoma
Rhabdomyosarcoma
Myoblastoma
Choriocarcinoma
Lymphoma

(Rosenberg JC, Lichter AS, Leichman LP: Cancer of the esophagus. In DeVita VT, Hellman S, Rosenberg SA [eds]: Cancer: Principles and Practice of Oncology, 2nd ed, p 499. Philadelphia, JB Lippincott, 1989)

ynx, tonsil, larynx, lung, stomach, liver, kidney, prostate, testis, bone, and skin.[90]

PROGNOSTIC FACTORS

Many factors can influence the decision to seek either curative or palliative treatment for esophageal tumor. The location of the tumor is important; patients with lesions in the upper third of the esophagus do better than those with lesions in the lower two thirds.[45,81]

Tumor size is also important. Hussey and colleagues[45] found 2-year survival rates of 19.2% and 1.9% for tumors smaller than 5 cm and larger than 9 cm, respectively. The extent of a tumor is also correlated with its size. Tumors smaller than 5 cm are localized 40% of the time; tumors larger than 5 cm are unresectable for cure or have distant metastasis 75% of the time.[17,30,71]

Additional prognostic factors influence outcome. Women tend to fare better than men.[45,81] Race may be a factor; Hussey and co-workers[45] found that whites do better than blacks. Age was found to be significant, with patients older than 65 years doing worse.[81] Weight loss and low overall performance status also indicate poor prognosis.[45] Deep ulceration of the tumor, sinus tract formation, and fistula formation are other poor prognostic factors.[90]

GENERAL MANAGEMENT

Treatment for esophageal carcinoma can be broadly divided into curative and palliative. According to Pearson,[81] of every 100 patients with cancer of the esophagus, only 20 have tumor that is truly localized to the esophagus. Hence, 80 of every 100 patients have locally extensive or distant disease from the time of diagnosis and thus are not amenable to local treatment alone.

Curative Surgery

Curative surgery of the thoracic esophagus involves a subtotal or total esophagectomy. It should include a cuff of stomach and go as high up in the proximal esophagus as possible. A laparotomy can be performed before or concurrently with esophagectomy to rule out any disease below the diaphragm. Multiple reconstruction options are available after definitive surgery. Esophagogastrostomy is the most widely used. Colon interposition, preferably with the left colon, can also be used.[89]

Squamous cell carcinoma of the cervical esophagus presents a very difficult situation. If surgery is performed, it usually requires removal of portions of the pharynx, the entire larynx and thyroid gland, and the proximal esophagus. Radical neck dissections are also carried out.[90] For this reason radiation therapy to this portion of the esophagus is preferable. Survival is essentially the same as with surgery, but irradiation does not cause the major functional impairments or the high morbidity and mortality rates of surgery.[39]

Curative Radiation Therapy

Curative irradiation with external-beam therapy for esophageal cancer also requires careful patient selection. Patients with tumors up to 10 cm in length with disease limited to the locoregional nodes without evidence of tracheoesophageal fistula are good candidates for irradiation.[90] If tumors appear to infiltrate the tracheobronchial tree with impending fistula development or if the adventitia of the aorta is involved with impending rupture, the daily dose should be reduced from the conventional 180 cGy or 200 cGy per fraction to 150 cGy. This may prevent rapid tumor regression with consequent fistula formation or vessel rupture.[89]

Chemotherapy

Chemotherapy has been used in combination with irradiation and surgery for esophageal cancer. Single agents were tried initially, using bleomycin, cisplatin, mitomycin-C, doxorubicin (Adriamycin), 5-fluorouracil, methotrexate, lomustine (CCNU), methyl-GAG, vindesine, and VP-16-213 (etoposide). Response rates varied from 15% to 22%.[53]

Currently, most trials use multiagent chemotherapy, with cisplatin, 5-fluorouracil, and mitomycin C being the most frequently used drugs. Kelsen reported a response range of 15% to 80% in reviewing 256 patients from combined series using multiagent chemotherapy.[53]

Palliative Treatment

Palliative treatment is chosen only for the relief of symptoms of esophageal carcinoma, especially dysphagia.[101] The best surgical palliation involves resection and reconstruction, if possible. This removes the bulk of the disease and can potentially prevent abscess and fistula formation as well as bleeding. Substernal bypass with colon or gastric tube or with the entire stomach if necessary can also be carried out.[101]

Intraluminal intubation is good for extremely debilitated patients with tracheoesophageal fistula or invasion of vital structures. There are two types of tubes. Push-through tubes are good for segments smaller than 10 cm in the upper and middle third of the esophagus. Examples are the Mackler and Souttar tubes. Pull-through tubes are used more frequently for middle and lower third lesions and are attached to the stomach by suture. Examples are the Celestin, Mousseau-Barbin, Fell, and Haering tubes.[90]

Dilatation is another reasonable alternative. When the lumen of the esophagus is dilated to 15 mm, dysphagia is no longer experienced. Attempts should be made to get 17 mm of dilatation and maintain this with weekly or monthly dilatations.[90]

Both the Nd : YAG laser and photoradiation with an argon laser, together with presensitization of tumor with intravenous hepatoporphyrin derivative, have provided palliation with minimal risk.[29,50,69]

Palliative irradiation can be used to control the primary disease as well as distant metastasis. The resolution of symptoms, especially pain and dysphagia, can reach 80%.[89] Palliative treatment regimens range from 3000 cGy over 2 weeks[73] to 5000 cGy over 5 weeks or 6000 cGy over 6 weeks.[89] These can be continuous- or split-course regimens. Chemotherapy can also be used for palliation alone or in combination with the above options.

RADIATION THERAPY TECHNIQUES

When designing a treatment plan for esophageal tumor, the radiation oncologist should make sure that the volume treated adequately encompasses the tumor and a margin of normal tissue. This concept applies to both radical and palliative treatment because local control of the tumor is desired. A margin of 5 to 6 cm above and below the tumor is generally recommended.[90]

Frontal and lateral radiographs of the patient in the treatment position should be obtained whether or not there is a simulator, with barium in the esophagus to delineate the tumor.[45] Some authors recommend placing the patient in the prone position for treatment to move the esophagus away from the spinal cord.[102] Without a simulator, the position of the esophagus can be delineated by using a plastic tube containing lead beads passed through the tumor, if possible. After this is done, portal films are taken on the treatment machine to visualize the lead beads.[45] Contours should be obtained at the level of the tumor and at the superior and inferior margins of the treatment fields. This can be done with solder wire, plaster of Paris, or CT scans.

If CT planning is available, the scan should be done with the patient in the exact treatment position on a flat surface (Fig. 40-5). Anterior or posterior and lateral radiopaque markers should be used to define the isocenter. With the tumor volume outlined on CT, various field arrangements are tried using the CT in connection with a treatment planning computer.

Appropriate blocks (Cerrobend) to define the portals must be cut. In addition, wedges, compensators, bolus, and field weightings should be used as needed to deliver an adequate dose to the target volume minimizing radiation to surrounding normal tissues.

Because of the changing contour from the neck to the thoracic inlet, treatment of lesions of the upper third of the esophagus presents difficult technical problems. Usually, lesions in the upper cervical or postcricoid esophagus are treated from the laryngopharynx to the carina. Supraclavicular and superior mediastinal nodes are irradiated electively. This can be achieved with lateral parallel opposed or oblique portals to the primary tumor and a single anterior field for the supraclavicular and superior mediastinal nodes.[45]

Another technique devised at the University of Florida treats lesions in this region by means of a four-field box technique. A wax bolus is used to build up the lack of tissue above the shoulders, acting as a compensator. A high-energy beam (17 MV) is used because the apices of the lungs are in the treated volume, and both sides of the neck are treated prophylactically. The four-field box is taken to 4500 cGy in 5 weeks and then coned down. Lateral portals are taken to 7000 cGy to 8000 cGy.[70] Other methods of treating lesions of the thoracic inlet include 140-degree arc rotations, anterior wedged pairs, and three- or four-field techniques using posterior oblique portals combined with a single anterior portal or AP-PA fields.[45] Figure 40-6 demonstrates some of the isodose curves for these techniques for lesions in the cervical and thoracic esophagus.

Lesions in the lower two thirds of the esophagus (thoracic esophagus) are easier to treat. The Hahnemann University Hospital technique includes the entire thoracic esophagus as well as bilateral supraclavicular nodes in the initial treatment volume. The inferior margin of the initial fields always includes the esophagogastric junction and, for lower-third lesions, the celiac plexus. At least 5 cm of normal tissue is included above and below the gross disease. The initial fields are anteroposterior/posteroanterior (AP-PA) opposed portals and are taken to 3000 cGy.

At the Mallinckrodt Institute of Radiology, 4500 cGy is delivered with AP-PA portals and high-energy photons. At these dose levels two posterior oblique portals with wedges are started to spare the spinal cord. The superior and inferior margins are kept the same, and the dose is taken to 5000 cGy. The fields are reduced to boost the gross disease to 6000 cGy to 7000 cGy. Another method used to cone down on middle-third lesions is a 360-degree rotation. Figure 40-7 shows the initial simulation and portal films for a typical thoracic esophageal lesion. Oblique fields are used to spare the spinal cord after 4200 cGy to 4500 cGy is delivered with AP-PA portals (Fig. 40-8).

In patients with tumors in the distal third and even in large lesions (> 5 cm) in the middle or upper third of the thoracic esophagus, the treatment portals are modified to include the celiac axis lymph nodes, because of their frequent metastatic involvement (see Fig. 40-2). CT scans may help in determining the exact location of enlarged lymph nodes.

Doses of Radiation

Based on data from squamous cell carcinoma of the upper aerodigestive tract, 5000 cGy at 180 cGy to 200 cGy per fraction over 5 weeks should control more than 90% of subclinical disease. At least 6000 cGy to 7000 cGy is needed for gross disease in fractions of 180 cGy to 200 cGy per day, 5 days per week.[111]

In addition to external-beam therapy, intracavitary therapy can be used as part of a radical or palliative treatment plan. At Hahnemann University we use an ^{192}Ir afterloading technique. A No.16 French Levin-type nasogastric tube has three

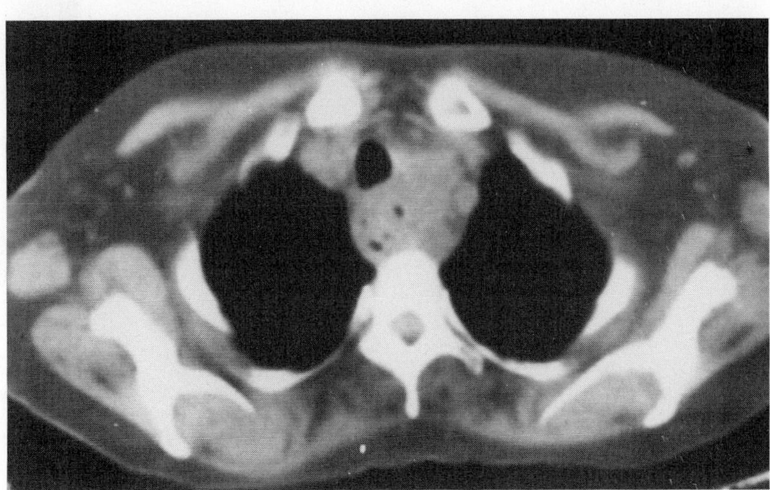

FIGURE 40–5. CT scan of the upper thorax demonstrating marked thickening of the esophageal wall, some compression of the anterior wall of the trachea with displacement to the left, and tumor infiltration of the periesophageal soft tissues.

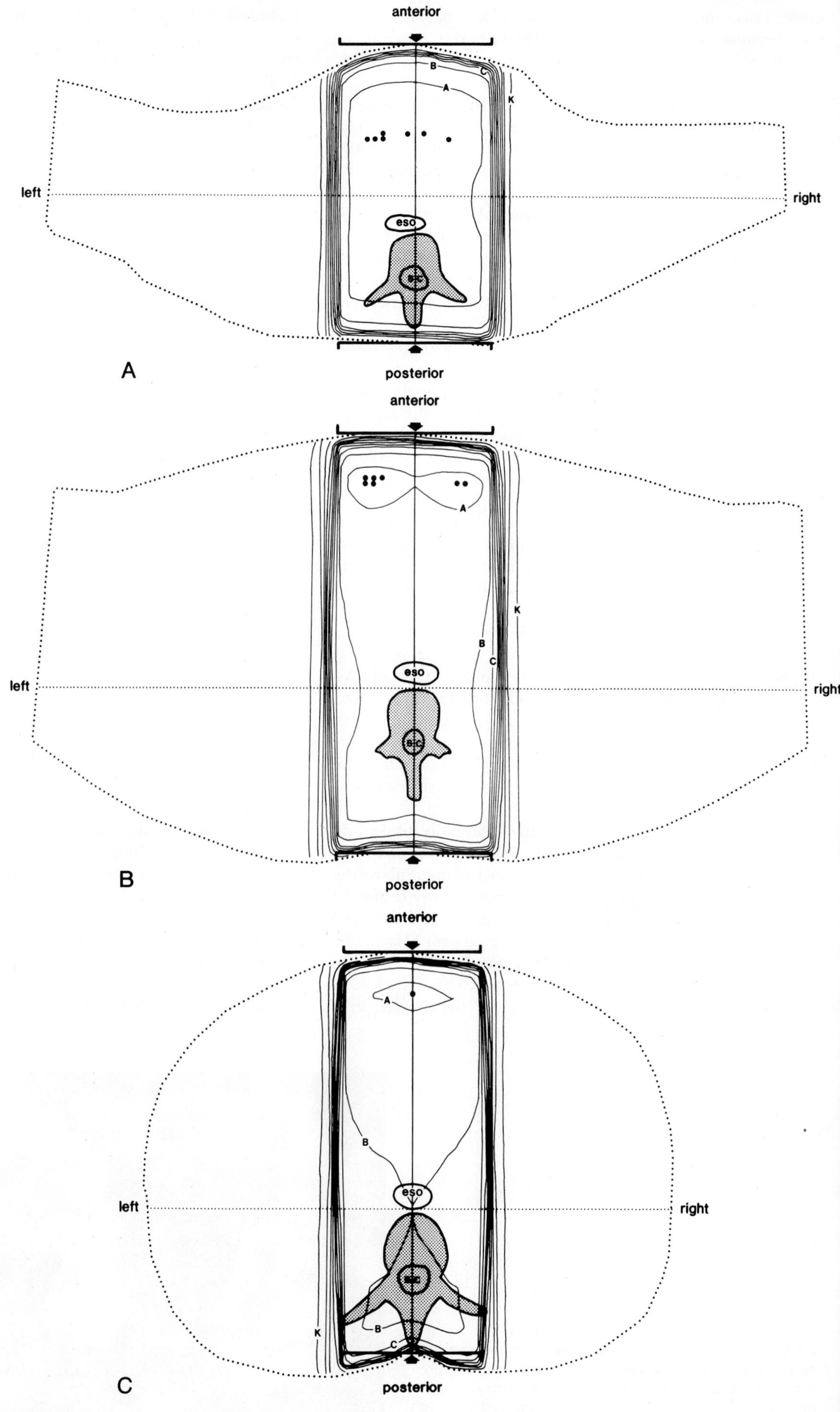

anterior
B
C
A
K
left
right
eso
posterior
A
anterior
A
K
B
C
left
eso
right
posterior
B
anterior
A
B
left
eso
right
K
B
C
posterior
C

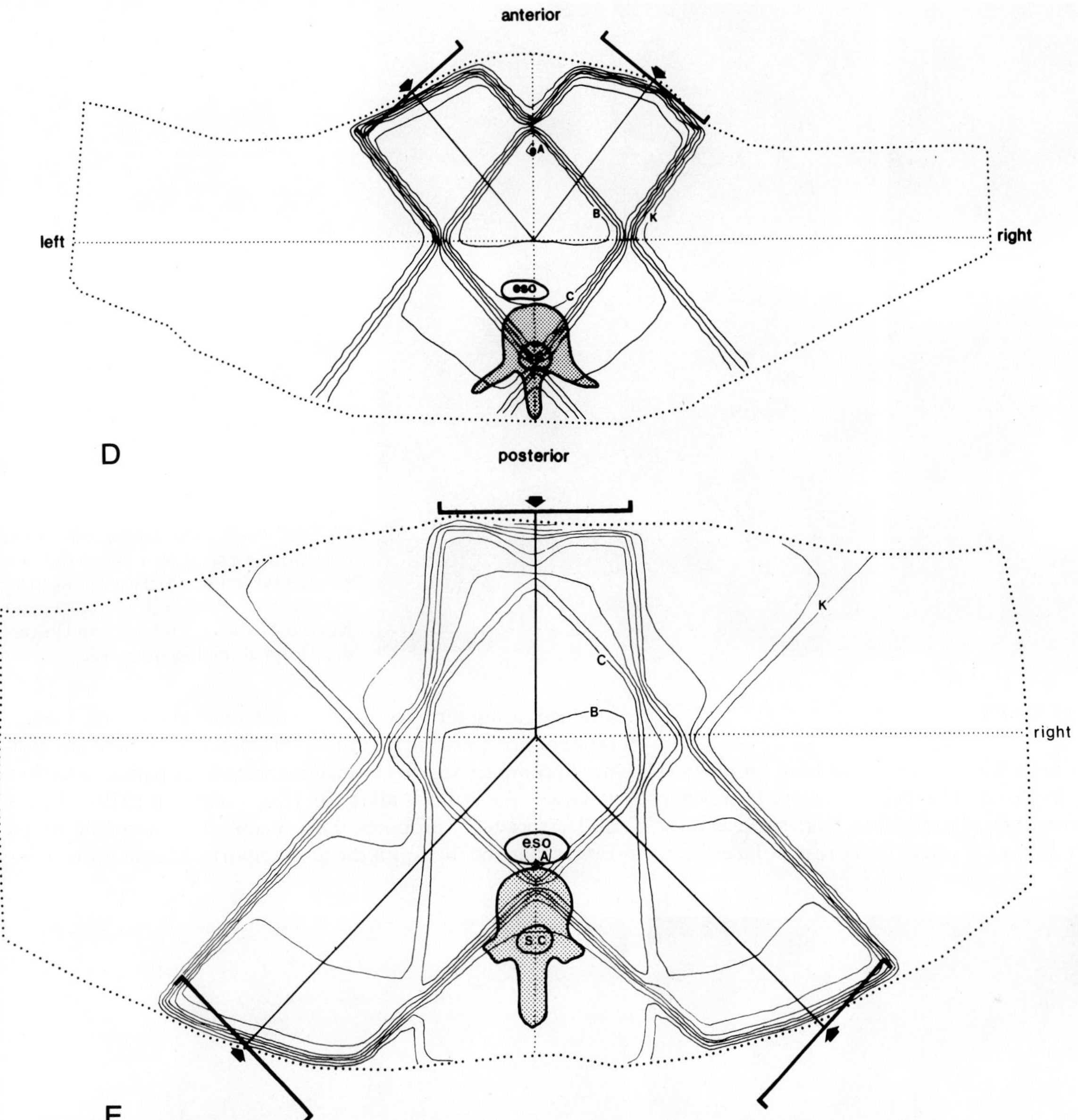

FIGURE 40–6. Radiation therapy techniques for lesions in the cervical and thoracic esophagus. The A-line is 110%. B-Line is 100%. C-line is 90%. K-line is 10%. **(A)** AP-PA opposed portals 8 cm above the central axis with equal weighting at the level of the clavicles. **(B)** AP-PA opposed portals at the central axis with equal weighting at the level of the tracheal bifurcation. **(C)** AP-PA opposed portals at 8 cm below central axis with equal weighting at the level of the diaphragm. **A, B,** and **C** are taken from 8 cm × 20 cm AP-PA parallel opposed portals at 100 cm source-skin distance. **(D)** Anterior oblique fields with equal weighting at the level of the clavicles. Each field is 6 cm × 10 cm at 100 cm source-axis distance (SAD). **(E)** Two posterior oblique portals and a single anterior field, all with equal weighting at the level of the tracheal bifurcation. Each field is 8 cm × 10 cm at 100 cm SAD. All summations are taken from an Alderson Rondo Phantom for a 10-MV linear accelerator. eso: esophagus; sc: spinal cord (Courtesy of Department of Radiation Oncology and Nuclear Medicine, Hahnemann University Hospital, Philadelphia, PA, with special thanks to Raymond Croce, dosimetrist)

afterloading tubes inserted into the lumen and fixed to the distal end. The nasogastric tube is passed into the patient, and the ^{192}Ir strands are inserted into the afterloading tubes with the patient on the simulator. A previous barium swallow is used to locate the primary tumor in relation to anatomic landmarks, which are verified with the simulator. Figure 40-9 shows dosimetry films (*A,B*), the dose distribution (*C*), and the nasogastric tube (*D*) for treatment in this fashion. We deliver 1500 cGy to 2000 cGy over 20 to 30 hours with this technique.

A radium bougie has also been used at Hahnemann University and has been described by others.[25] Dubois described an intraluminal brachytherapy technique using a modified Haering prosthesis with ^{192}Ir wires 1 to 2 months following external-beam irradiation. Recently high dose-rate remote afterloading devices have been used with ^{192}Ir sources to treat esophageal carcinoma (either palliatively or as a boost after external irradiation). Doses of 700 cGy at 1 cm are delivered two or three times at weekly intervals.[31,43]

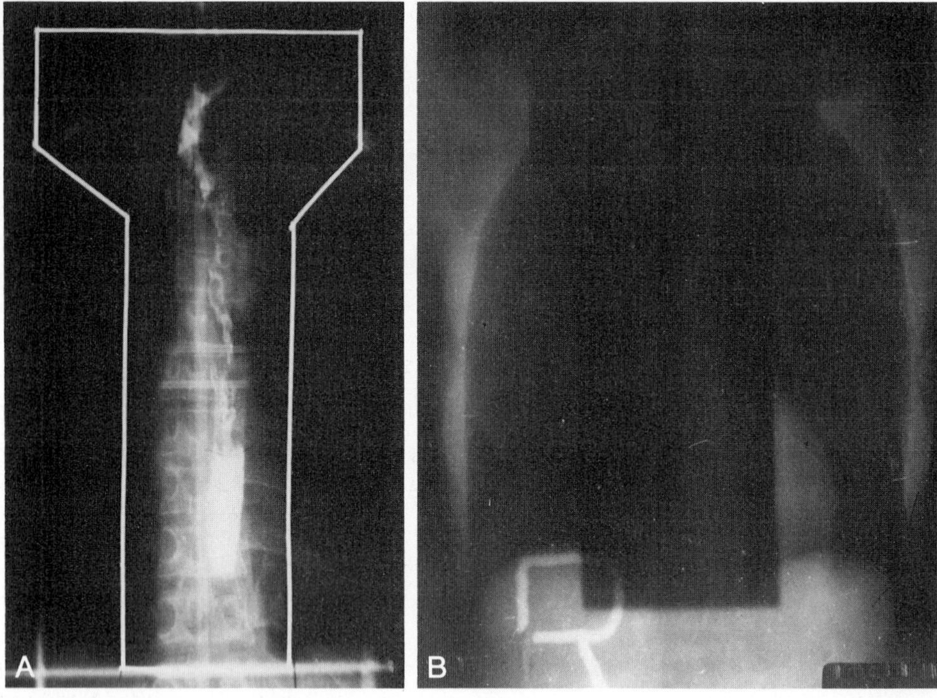

FIGURE 40–7. (**A**) Initial simulation film with portal drawn for a thoracic esophageal lesion. (**B**) Portal film. (Department of Radiation Oncology and Nuclear Medicine, Hahnemann University Hospital, Philadelphia, PA)

RESULTS OF THERAPY

The best results are seen with patients who have esophageal tumors that are truly localized and are either removed surgically or treated with curative doses of irradiation. High survival rates range from 25% to 35% at 5 years; these results have been attained using surgery alone, irradiation alone, and various types of preoperative treatment. Problems arise when attempting to compare various modalities because of patient selection. Review of the Princess Margaret Hospital data in 1979 by Beatty and associates[10] supports the concept that extent of tumor rather than the therapy is the most important factor influencing

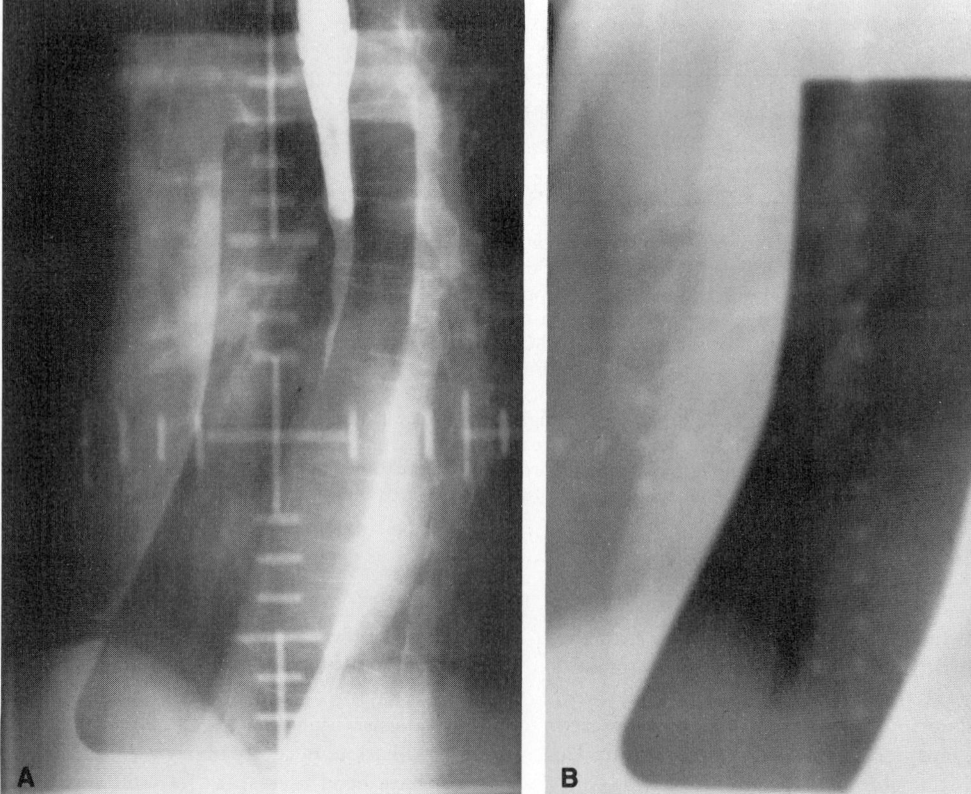

FIGURE 40–8. (**A**) Simulation film. (**B**) Portal film. Anterior oblique field used to treat tumor in the lower third of the thoracic esophagus. AP and PA portals were used to deliver 4200 cGy to the midplane of the thorax. Additional 1800 cGy was delivered with oblique fields, sparing the spinal cord. The patient was treated with 18 MV photons.

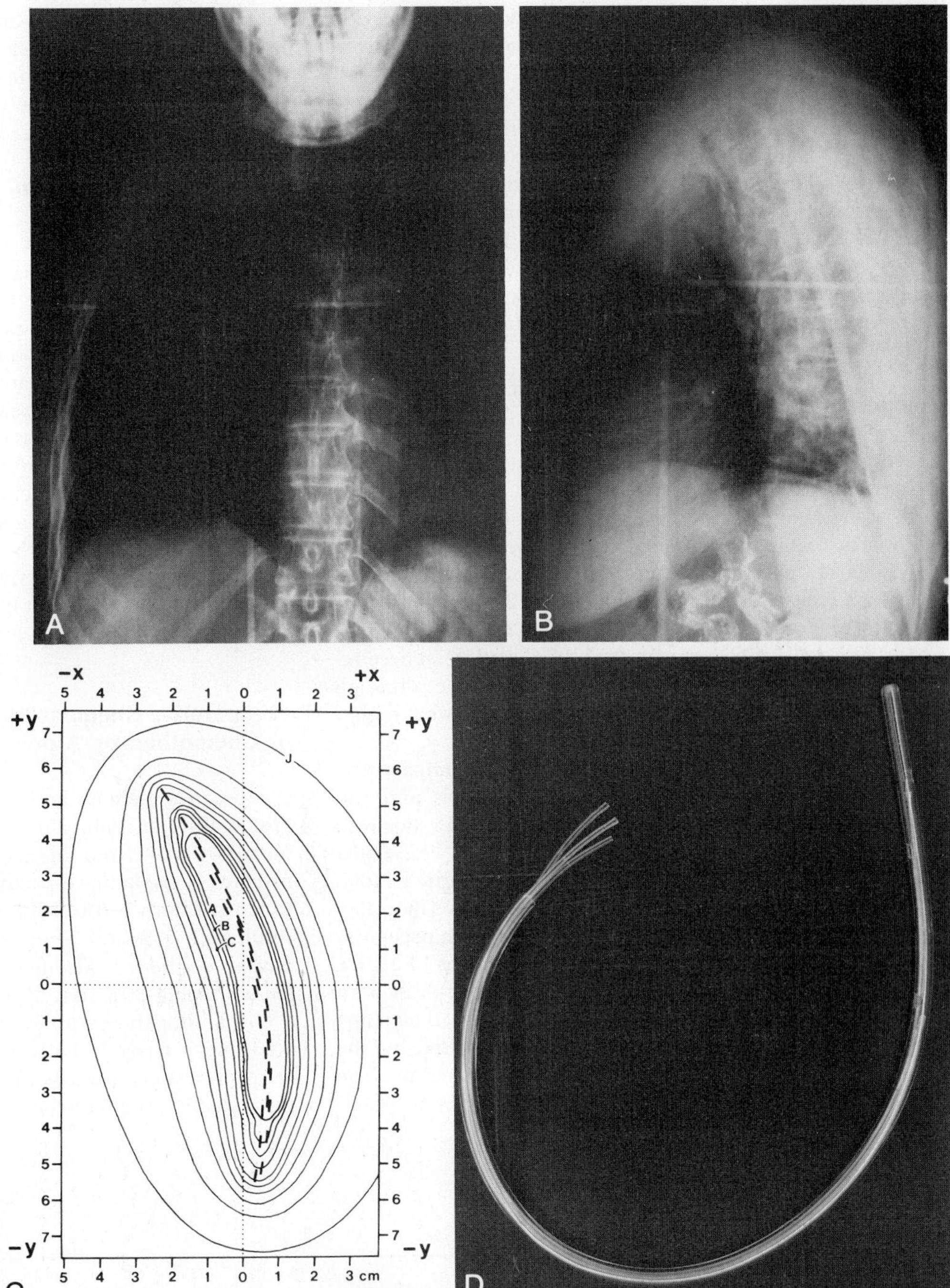

FIGURE 40–9. (**A** and **B**) PA and lateral views of ^{192}Ir implant. (**C**) ^{192}Ir isodose display for an esophageal intracavitary placement. There are 36 seeds with 0.502 mg radium equivalent activity each. (A-line, 70 cGy/hr; B-line, 60 cGy/hr; C-line, 50 cGy/hr). (Courtesy of the Department of Radiation Oncology and Nuclear Medicine, Hahnemann University Hospital, with special thanks to Bizhan Micaily, M.D., and John L. Day, Ph.D.) (**D**) Nasogastric tube with three ^{192}Ir afterloading tubes inserted into the lumen.

survival. They found a significant correlation between T stage and response to treatment. T1 lesions showed a 100% response rate, whereas T2 and T3 lesions had a 68% and 58% response rate, respectively. They also found differences in survival according to T stage, M stage, and overall stage. Almost 20% of Stage I patients were alive at 3.5 years, whereas only 11% of Stage II patients were alive after the same interval. All Stage III patients died by approximately 1.5 years after therapy.

Surgery Alone

In 1980, Earlam and Cunha-Melo reviewed 122 series involving over 83,000 patients treated primarily by surgery.[26] When palliative surgery was performed, the death rate was 10% to 43%. The overall 5-year survival rate for patients with resected tumors was 12%. Patients treated with palliative intent had a survival range of 2 to 6 months. Several recent studies are in basic agreement with the findings of Earlam and Cunha-Melo.[2,36,58,81,96,100] Operability ranged from 20% to 100%. Resectability ranged from 58% to 86%, and resection mortality rate ranged from 11% to 30%. The overall, operated, and resected 5-year survival rates ranged from 2% to 14%, 9.3% to 14%, and 5.3% to 20%, respectively.

Radiation Therapy Alone

In general, irradiation alone has been given when cases are deemed inoperable because of tumor extent or medical contraindications. Exceptions are patients with lesions in the cervical esophagus who are treated with primary radiation therapy in many institutions.

Earlam and Cunha-Melo also reviewed 49 series with over 8400 patients treated primarily with irradiation.[27] They found overall 1-, 2-, and 5-year survival rates of 18%, 8%, and 6%, respectively. They stated that in three series that were comparable to surgical series, the 1-, 2-, and 5-year survival rates ranged from 42% to 46%, 8% to 27%, and 6% to 20%, respectively. These figures are as good as those in most surgical series without the operative mortality rate. Table 40-5 outlines the results of treatment in several series using irradiation alone.

Preoperative Radiation Therapy

In general, preoperative regimens are given as a short course, such as 2000 cGy over 4 to 5 days, followed in several days by surgery, or as a long course, such as 4000 cGy to 6000 cGy over 4 to 7 weeks, followed by surgery in 4 to 8 weeks.

Table 40-6 shows the results of several preoperative series. The resectability rate ranges from 54% to 82%. The operative mortality rate ranges from 12% to 25%, and the 5-year survival rate in resected patients ranges from 9.5% to 25%. These results are similar to those reported with surgery alone, although the 5-year survival rate with resection may be somewhat higher in the preoperative series.

Two randomized studies were undertaken to compare preoperative irradiation with surgery alone. Launois and colleagues in 1981 reported using 4000 cGy over 8 to 12 days with surgery 8 days later compared with surgery alone.[58] Resection rates were similar, being 70% and 58% for preoperative irradiation and surgery alone, respectively. The operative mortality rate of 23% was the same as that found in those with preoperative irradiation. The resected 5-year survival rate was 11.5% for those with surgery alone compared with 9.5% for those with irradiation and surgery. This series has been criticized on many levels, including the unusual fractionation scheme used, but the results between the two groups are not very different. The second randomized study was the trial of the European Organization for Research on Treatment of Cancer (EORTC) started in 1976, using 3300 cGy over 12 days.[35] There was no significant difference in survival. At the present time, one cannot conclude that preoperative radiation therapy is beneficial.

Postoperative Radiation Therapy

Postoperative irradiation is usually used for esophageal cancer patients who have unresectable disease with gross tumor left behind or in whom there is microscopic residual. Generally, these patients have very poor prognoses. Drucker and co-workers in 1979 reported on 23 of 45 patients treated with 4000 cGy to 6000 cGy postoperatively compared with 22 of 45 who had no irradiation.[24] At 3 years, both groups had 20% survival rates, whereas at 5 years less than 5% survival rate was found in the postoperative group and no survival in the surgery-alone group. Kasai and co-workers, using 6000 cGy postoperatively, showed an improvement in survival rate over that of patients treated by surgery alone when no lymph node metastases were found at the time of surgery. Patients with lymph node metastases had no survival benefit but did have improved local tumor control.[51]

Preoperative Chemoradiotherapy or Chemotherapy Alone

Preoperative chemoradiotherapy has been used in several series (Table 40-7), including the Wayne State experience.[33,60] The initial two trials from this group used 5-fluorouracil and mitomycin-C or cisplatin, respectively, concomitantly with 3000 cGy in ten fractions before surgery. These preoperative regimens resulted in 25% and 33%, respectively, of resected specimens having no tumor. Mortality rates were significant in these studies, being 30% and 27%, respectively, following surgery.

Following these studies, the SWOG[85] and the RTOG[97] initiated similar trials. In both studies, 5-fluorouracil and cisplatin were given concomitantly with 3000 cGy in 15 days. Postoperative radiation therapy consisting of 2000 cGy in 2 weeks was

TABLE 40–5

Results with Radiation Therapy Alone for Esophageal Cancer

AUTHOR	YEAR	NUMBER OF PATIENTS		DOSE	2-YEAR SURVIVAL	5-YEAR SURVIVAL
Pearson[81]	1977	288		5000 cGy/4 wk (250 cGy/fr)		17% (48/288)
Beatty[10]	1979	344	176 curative*	>4000 cGy/<19fr >4500 cGy/<23fr >5000 cGy/<3 mo	21%	0%
			168 palliative	Less than the above doses	0%	0%
VanAndel[109]	1979	234	Curative operable/unresectable	6000–6600 cGy/10–10.5 wk (200 cGy/fr)	4% (2/52)	0%
			Curative/inoperable, palliative	Split course as above	4.3% (5/115)	0.8% (1/115)
				3000–4000 cGy/2–4 wk (250–300 cGy/fr)	0%	0%
Schuchmann[96]	1980	127		>4500 R		0%
				<4500 R		0%
Newaishy[78]	1982	444	All curative	5000–5500 cGy/4 wk (250–275 cGy/fr)		9%

fr: fraction
**Thirty of the 176 radically treated patients had surgery plus irradiation.*

TABLE 40–6
Results with Preoperative Irradiation for Esophageal Cancer

AUTHOR	YEAR	NO. PATIENTS WITH PREOP. IRRAD./TOTAL NO. OF PATIENTS	DOSE	OPERATION (%)	RESECTIONS (%)	OPERATIVE MORTALITY (%)	5-YEAR SURVIVAL RESECTIONS %	5-YEAR SURVIVAL OVERALL %
Akakura[4]	1970	117/346	5000–6000 cGy/30–40 days, 150–200 cGy/fr	100 (117/117)	82 (96/117)	20.8	25	
VanAndel[109]	1979	133/328	4000 cGy/4 wk, 200 cGy/fr	100 (133/133)	61 (81/133)	21 (17/81)*	21 (18/81)	6 (19/328)
Kelsen[54]	1981	76/110 { 57/110	4000–6000 cGy/4–6 wk, 200 cGy/fr	82 (47/57)	54 (41/76)	12 (8/66)		
		19/110	2000 cGy in 5 days, 400 cGy/fr	100 (19/19)				
Launois[58]	1981	124 Randomized { 67	4000 cGy/8–12 days	92 (62/67)	70 (47/67)	23 (14/62)	9.5	
		57	No irradiation	82 (47/57)	58 (33/57)	23 (11/47)	11.5	
Gignoux[35] (EORTC)	1987	208 Randomized { 102	3300 cGy/12 days, 330 cGy/fr	95 (97/102)	77.3	25.3	16.0	10
		106	No irradiation	100	82.1	19.5	10.0	9

fr: fraction
** This figure is resection mortality.*

given when there were positive nodes or margins. In the SWOG trial, 17% of the patients had complete eradication of tumor, whereas 28% had tumor progression before or at the time of surgery. Of the 18 complete responders, eight have died, four with tumor recurrence. The projected 3-year survival rate for complete response in resected patients was 45% *versus* 16% for all patients in the study. Acute toxicity reactions included leukopenia (two life-threatening), anorexia, mucositis, stomatitis, nausea, and vomiting. The RTOG study reported on 42 patients, with eight of 27 resected patients having no tumor in the specimen. The 2-year survival rate was 15% for all patients compared with 33% for resected patients without tumor in the specimen. All 3-year survivors had tumor-free specimens.

Other studies have used preoperative chemotherapy alone. Roth[91] compared preoperative and postoperative cisplatin, vindesine, and bleomycin to no chemotherapy (see Table 40-7). The chemotherapy group did slightly better with 35% compared with 21% complete response at surgery. Median survival was 9 months in both groups, but the actuarial 3-year survival rates were 25% and 5% in the chemotherapy and surgery-alone arms of the study, respectively. It is interesting to note that patients with less than 10% weight loss did better in both arms, and all patients who responded to preoperative chemotherapy were in this group.

Chemoradiotherapy

A number of studies have used concomitant or sequential chemoradiotherapy as primary management, reserving surgery for salvage (Table 40-8). Earle and associates[28] reported on patients randomized to radiation therapy alone compared with those who had radiation therapy and bleomycin. There was no difference in overall median survival, which was 6.2 months and 6.4 months for radiation therapy and chemoradiotherapy, respectively. Reusbeut and colleagues[88] reported on combined therapy using vincristine, methotrexate, and cisplatin (VMP) with split-course irradiation. In this series, 15 of 28 patients were treated with palliative intent. Even so, the 2-year survival rate for VMP responders was 16%. The median survival of VMP responders treated for cure was 15.5 months with 27% alive at 2 years. Keane[52] reported 48% 2-year survival rate in 15 patients receiving 5-fluorouracil and mitomycin-C with continuous-course radiation therapy.

Herskovic and colleagues[42] reported on a pilot series from Wayne State using concomitant chemoradiotherapy. The initial 18 patients received 5-fluorouracil, cisplatin, mitomycin-C, and bleomycin. The latter two agents were discontinued because of respiratory difficulties requiring steroids in six cases. Radiation therapy was 3000 cGy in 3 weeks to the tumor with 5 cm margins followed by 2000 cGy in 2 weeks as a boost. This regimen resulted in a 19.5-month overall median survival with six (28%) of 22 patients remaining alive with no evidence of disease at a median of 42 months. These results compare favorably with the initial Wayne State preoperative studies, which had an 18-month median survival compared with 19.5 months in this series.

Coia and associates[18] reported on using concomitant 5-fluorouracil and mitomycin-C with 5000 cGy to 6000 cGy. There were 30 patients with Stage I and Stage II disease who received 6000 cGy. Seven of 30 patients had adenocarcinoma; the remainder had squamous cell carcinomas. The median survival in this group was 24 months with 47% and 32% actuarial survival rate at 2 and 5 years, respectively. There was a 73% local relapse-free rate at 1 year, similar to the 79% local relapse-free rate reported by Keane. In the 20 patients with Stage III and Stage IV disease, a 64% sustained local palliation occurred with this regimen. Severe esophagitis developed in five patients and fatal mediastinitis in one patient.

John and co-workers[48] recently reported results with che-

TABLE 40–7
Results with Preoperative Chemotherapy with or without Radiation Therapy for Esophageal Cancer

		NO. OF PATIENTS COMPLETING PREOP. TREATMENT AND GOING TO SURGERY						MEDIAN SURVIVAL (MONTHS)				
AUTHOR	YEAR	TOTAL NO. OF PATIENTS	CHEMOTHERAPY	RADIATION THERAPY	%OPERATIVE MORTALITY	% RESECTED	% CR AT SURGERY	CR RESECTED PATIENTS	RESECTED PATIENTS	RESPONDERS	NON-RESPONDERS	OVERALL
Kelson[55]*	1983	34/71	DDP/vindesine/ bleomycin		5.8 (2/34)	82 (28/34)						16.2
Coonley[19]†	1984	34/70	DDP/bleomycin		19 (5/26)	76 (26/34)			13			11‡
Leichman[60]	1984	19/21	5-FU/DDP	3000 cGy/3 wks, 200 cGy/fr	27 (5/19)	79 (15/19)	33 (5/15)	24	24			18
Carey[15]§	1986	22/24	5-FU/DDP		5	86 (19/22)	53 (10/19)			20.4	6.7	
Poplin[85] (SWOG-8037)	1987	71/113	5-FU/DDP	3000 cGy/3 wks, 200 cGy/fr	11	77 (55/71)	25 (18/71)	32				12
Roth[91]	1988	39/39	19—DDP/vindesine/ bleomycin				35			20	6.2	9
	Randomized		20—No chemotherapy				21					9
Seydel[97]	1988	27/42	5-FU/DDP	3000 cGy/3 wks, 200 cGy/fr	3.7 (1/27)	100 (27/27)	29.6 (8/27)	15				13

DDP: cisplatin; 5-FU: fluorouracil; fr: fraction; CR: complete response
** Following surgery patients with T3 lesions or +nodes received 5500 cGy/fractions for 5.5 weeks.*
† Following surgery patients with T3 lesions or +nodes or unresected disease received 3200 cGy at 400 cGy/fraction twice weekly for 4 weeks.
‡ This is the median survival of the 34 patients who were considered potentially curable.
§ Following surgery, patients with invasion into the mediastinum, +nodes, or abnormal resection margins received 5000–6000 cGy in 5–6 weeks.

TABLE 40–8
Results of Chemoradiotherapy

AUTHOR	YEAR	NO. OF PATIENTS	CHEMOTHERAPY	RADIATION THERAPY	% CR	MEDIAN SURVIVAL OF RESPONDERS (MONTHS)	OVERALL SURVIVAL (MONTHS)	SURVIVAL
Byfield[13]	1980	6	5-FU	6000 cGy/11 wk, 250 cGy/fr	83 (5/6)	4 patients NED 4, 9, 10, 22 months		
Earle[28]	1980	40 (77 Randomized)	bleomycin	5000–6000 cGy/5–6 wk			6.4	
		37		5000–6000 cGy/5–6 wk			6.2	
Marcial[67]	1980	26	vincristine/bleomycin/ methotrexate	5000 cGy/4 wk 250 cGy/fr	60 (15/25)	11		
Abitol[1]	1983	9	5-FU/DDP/ methotrexate	6000 cGy/6 wk 250 cGy/fr	56 (5/9)	8.5	7.3	
Resbeut[88]	1985	28	vincristine/ methotrexate/DDP	3000 cGy/2 wk 300 cGy/fr, 2-wk rest, 3000 cGy/3 wk, 200 cGy/fr	32 (9/28)	13.5	11.5	
Keane[52]	1985	15	5-FU/mitomycin	4500–5000 cGy				48% at 2 yr
		20	5-FU/mitomycin	2250–2500 cGy twice (split course)			12	13% at 2 yr
Lokich[62]	1987	13	5-FU	4500–6900 cGy, 150–250 cGy/fr	92 (12/13)		16	22% at 3 yr
Coia[18]	1987	30 Stage, I, II	5-FU mitomycin	6000 cGy/ 6–7 wk 200 cGy/fr	87 (26/30)		24	47% at 2 yr 32% at 5 yr
		20 Stage III, IV	5-FU mitomycin	5000 cGy/5 wk 200 cGy/fr	82* 14/17		8	
Herskovic[42]	1988	22	5-FU/DDP/ bleomycin/ mitomycin	3000 cGy/3 wk 200 cGy/fr, 6-wk break, 2000 cGy, 200 cGy/fr			19.5	28% at 42 mo
John[48]	1989	30 Stage I, II, III	5-FU/DDP/ mitomycin/ methotrexate	4110 cGy/4.5 wk 180 cGy/fr, 3.5 wk break, 900 cGy/wk, 180 cGy/fr	77	15	11	29% at 2 yr
		35 Stage I, II, III	No chemotherapy	5600–6100 cGy/6–7 wk 180 cGy/fr	30	9	8	13% at 2 yr

**Freedom from dysphagia*
5-FU: 5-fluorouracil; DDP: cisplatin; NED: no evidence of disease; fr: fraction

moradiotherapy. They treated 30 patients with Stages I, II, and III disease with alternating cycles of 5-fluorouracil-mitomycin-C, 5-fluorouracil-cisplatin, and 5-fluorouracil-methotrexate concomitantly with irradiation. They treated small fields with 3 cm margins to 4140 cGy followed on the 8th week by a 900 cGy boost to the primary tumor site. These patients were compared with similar historical control patients treated with conventional radiation therapy alone to 5600 cGy to 6100 cGy. Locoregional control was 73% for patients who received chemoradiotherapy compared with 23% for those who received radiation therapy alone. The 29% 2-year survival rate for complete responders to chemoradiotherapy was also superior to the 13% 2-year survival rate for those with radiation therapy alone. Toxicity reactions in both groups were similar.

Combined chemoradiotherapy as primary management is a viable alternative to surgery with or without preoperative radiation therapy and chemotherapy. Survival figures are similar without the surgical mortality risk. These results should be viewed with caution because longer follow-up is needed. Furthermore, if significant long-term cure rates are to be obtained, more aggressive combinations of radiation therapy and chemotherapy will be needed with the increased risk of morbidity and mortality rates. However, primary chemoradiotherapy with surgical salvage seems to be a sensible extension of the preoperative studies done in the past and may emerge as the treatment of choice for cancer of the esophagus.

TREATMENT SEQUELAE

Surgery

Sequelae following surgery lead to a high rate of operative mortality and morbidity in patients with cancer of the esophagus. Anastomotic leaks and cardiopulmonary complications lead the list of problems.[89] Cukingnan and Carey reviewed the literature and stated that 8.6% of operative deaths were the result of anastomotic leaks and 8% were secondary to respiratory complications.[20] They noted that about 5% of patients develop chronic fistulas, which later become strictures.

Radiation Therapy

Pneumonitis is a potentially serious complication of radiation treatment. If fields are properly shaped, however, this risk can be minimized. If a patient develops persistent substernal pain, a high pulse rate, fever, and persistent hemorrhage, a perforation should be suspected. If this is confirmed with an esophagogram, treatment should be stopped.[45]

Long-term sequelae in normal structures can be limited with proper treatment planning. However, potentially serious problems within the tumor volume can develop. Perforation and hemorrhage, usually secondary to tumor destruction by irradiation, can develop during treatment, as stated above, or several months following treatment. Stenosis and stricture can lead to symptoms of obstruction, usually 4 to 6 months after treatment and possibly progressing for at least 1 year. This may require dilatation.[45]

NEW THERAPEUTIC APPROACHES

In the past few years, some groups have used high linear-energy transfer radiation to treat this malignant disease. A Radiation Therapy Oncology Group study conducted by Laramore and associates[57] used fast neutrons or mixed-beam therapy (neutrons and photons) in 39 inoperable patients. This study showed no improvement in survival or local control over standard photon therapy. There was also a high rate of fistula formation, although this may have been secondary to the advanced nature of the disease in these patients. Castro and co-workers[16] used helium ions on 22 patients. They had acceptable morbidity rate but a local failure rate of nearly 80%. They found no improvement in survival over conventional treatment.

Conformational therapy may enable higher doses of conventional photons to be delivered to the tumor volume while minimizing normal tissue dose. With this technique the standard collimator is replaced by a device with 20 to 30 separate pairs of leaves. These can be changed independently and continuously move as the gantry rotates around the patient. The result is a very tailored dose distribution around the tumor volume.[105]

Another interesting approach is combined preoperative hyperthermia-chemotherapy-radiation therapy. Matsufuji and associates[68] described this technique used in ten patients who were given 150 cGy to 200 cGy 1 hour before the tumor was heated with an intraluminal device to 42°C to 45°C for 30 minutes and given intravenous bleomycin or peplomycin chemotherapy. Most patients received a total of five to ten hyperthermia treatments and 3000 cGy to 4000 cGy over 3 to 5 weeks. The 34% 2-year survival rate compares favorably with that of their other patients who did not receive hyperthermia. Another potential area of research may be twice-daily irradiation with or without systemic therapy.[108]

REFERENCES

1. Abitbol A, Straus M, Franklin G, et al: Infusional chemotherapy and cyclic radiation therapy in inoperable esosphageal and gastric cardia carcinoma. Am J Clin Oncol 6:195, 1983
2. Adelstein DJ, Forman WB, Beavers B: Esophageal carcinoma: A 6-year review of the Cleveland Veterans Administration Hospital Experience. Cancer 54:918, 1984
3. Aisner J, Forastiere A, Aroney R: Patterns of recurrence for cancer of the lung and esophagus. In Wittes RE (ed): Cancer Treatment Symposia Proceedings of the Workshop on Patterns of Failure after Cancer Treatment, vol 2, p 87. Washington, DC, US Department of Health and Human Services, 1983
4. Akakura I, Nakamura Y, Kakewgawa T, et al: Surgery of carcinoma of the esophagus with preoperative radiation. Chest 57:47, 1970
5. Akiyama H: Surgery for carcinoma of the esophagus. Curr Probl Surg 17:56, 1980
6. Akiyama H, Tsurumaru M, Kawamura T, et al: Principles of surgical treatment for carcinoma of the esophagus. Analysis of lymph node involvement. Ann Surg 194:438, 1981
7. Anderson LL, Lad TE: Autopsy findings in squamous-cell carcinoma of the esophagus. Cancer 50:1587–1590, 1982.
8. Appleqvist P, Salmo M: Lye corrosion carcinoma of the esophagus. Cancer 45:P2655, 1980
9. Beahrs OH, Henson DE, Hutter RV, Myers MH: Manual for Staging of Cancer, 3rd ed. Philadelphia, JB Lippincott, 1988
10. Beatty JD, DeBoer G, Rider WD: Carcinoma of the esophagus: Pretreatment assessment, correlation of radiation treatment parameters with survival, and identification and management of radiation treatment failure. Cancer 43:2254, 1979
11. Bloedorn FG, Kasdorf H: Radiotherapy in squamous cell carcinoma of the esophagus. In Clark RL, Cumley RW, McCay JE, et al (eds): Oncology 1970 Proceedings of the Tenth International Cancer Congress, vol 4, p 111. Chicago, Year Book Medical Publishers, 1971
12. Burke EL, Sturm J, Williamson D: The diagnosis of microscopic carcinoma of the esophagus. Dig Dis 23:148, 1978.
13. Byfield JE, Barone R, Mendelsohn J, et al: Infusional 5-fluorouracil and x-ray therapy for non-resectable esophageal cancer. Cancer 45:703–708, 1980
14. Cahan WG, Castro EB, Rosen PB, et al: Separate primary carcinomas of the esophagus and head and neck region in the same patient. Cancer 37:85–89, 1976. J Natl Cancer Inst 28:495, 1962
15. Carey RW, Hilgenberg AD, Wilkins EW, et al: Preoperative chemotherapy followed by surgery with possible postoperative radiotherapy in squamous cell carcinoma of the esophagus: Evaluation of the chemotherapy component. J Clin Oncol 4(5):697–701, 1986
16. Castro JR, Saunders WM, Tobias CA, et al: Treatment of cancer with heavy charged particles. Int J Radiat Oncol Biol Phys 8:2191, 1982
17. Clayton ES: Carcinoma of the esophagus. Surg Gynecol Obstet 46:52, 1928
18. Coia L, Engstrom P, Paul A: Nonsurgical management of esophageal cancer: Report of a study of combined radiotherapy and chemotherapy. J Clin Oncol 5:1783–1790, 1987

19. Coonley CJ, Bains M, Hilaris B, et al: Cisplatin and bleomycin in the treatment of esophageal carcinoma. Cancer 54:2351, 1984
20. Cukingnan RA, Carey JS: Carcinoma of the esophagus. Ann Thorac Surg 26:274, 1975
21. Danoff B, Cooper J, Klein M: Primary adenocarcinoma of the upper esophagus. Clin Radiol 29:519, 1978
22. Doherty MA, McIntyre M, Arnott SJ: Oat cell carcinoma of the esophagus: A report of six British patients with a review of the literature. Int J Radiat Oncol Biol Phys 10:1477, 1984
23. Dormans E: Das oesophaguscarcinoma. Ergebnisse der unter mitarbeit von 39 pathologischen instituten Deutschlands durchgefuhrten erhebung uber das osephaguscarcinomon (1925–1933). Z Krebforsch 49:86, 1939
24. Drucker MH, Mansour KA, Hatcher Cr Jr, et al: Esophageal carcinoma: An aggressive approach. Ann Thorac Surg 28:133, 1979
25. Dubois SB, Balmes JL, Pujol H: An endoesophageal irradiation technique using iridium-192. Br J Radiol 57:351, 1984
26. Earlam R, Cunha-Melo Jr: Oesophageal squamous cell carcinoma. I.A critical review of surgery. Br J Surg 67:384, 1980
27. Earlam R, Cunha-Melo Jr: Oesophageal squamous cell carcinoma. II. A critical review of radiotherapy. Br J Surg 67:457, 1980
28. Earle J, Gelber R, Moertel C, et al: A controlled evaluation of combined radiation and bleomycin therapy for squamous cell carcinoma of the esophagus. Int J Radiat Oncol Biol Phys 6:821, 1980
29. Fleischer D, Kessler F, Haye O: Endoscopic Nd: YAG laser therapy for carcinoma of the esophagus. A new palliative approach. Am J Surg 143:280, 1982
30. Fleming JAC: Carcinoma of thoracic esophagus: Some notes on its pathology and spread in relation to treatment. Br J Radiol 16:212, 1943
31. Flores AD, Stoller JL, Nelems B, et al: Combined primary treatment of cancer of the esophagus and cardia by intracavitary and external irradiation. In Sirwir NY (ed): Diseases of the Esophagus, pp 745–753. New York, Springer-Verlag, 1987
32. Fogel TD, Harrison LB, Yung HS: Subsequent upper aerodigestive malignancies following treatment of esophageal cancer. Cancer 55:1882, 1985
33. Franklin R, Steiger Z, Vaishampayan G, et al: Combined modality therapy for esophageal squamous cell carcinoma. Cancer 51:1062–1071, 1983
34. Gaede JT, Postlethwait RW, Shelnurne JR, et al: Leiomyosarcoma of the esophagus. Report of two cases, one with associated squamous cell carcinoma. J Thorac Cardiovasc Surg 75:740, 1978
35. Gignoux, M, Roussel A, Paillot B, et al: The value of preoperative radiotherapy in esophageal cancer: Results of a study of the E.O.R.T.C World J Surg 11:426–432, 1987.
36. Giuli R, Gignoux M: Treatment of carcinoma of the esophagus. Ann Surg 192:44 1980
37. Goldstein HM, Zornoza J, Hopens T: Intrinsic diseases of the adult esophagus: Benign and malignant tumors. Semin Roentgenol 16:183, 1981
38. Halber MD, Daffner Rh, Thompson WM: CT of the esophagus. I. Normal appearance. AJ Radiol 133:1047, 1979
39. Hancock SL, Glatstein E: Radiation therapy of esophageal cancer. Semin Oncol 11:144, 1984
40. Harper PS, Harper RMJ, Howel-Evans AW: Carcinoma of the esophagus with tylosis. Q J Med 34:317–333, 1970
41. Hawe AW, Payne WS, Weiland LH: Adenocarcinoma in the columnar epithelial lined lower (Barrett) oesophagus. Thorax 28:541, 1973
42. Herskovic A, Leichman L, Lattin P, et al: Chemo/radiation with and without surgery in the thoracic esophagus: The Wayne State experience. Int J Radiat Oncol Biol Phys 15:665–662, 1988.
43. Hishikawa Y, Kamikonya N, Tanaka S, Miura T: Radiotherapy of esophageal carcinoma: Role of high-dose-rate intracavitary irradiation. Radiotherapy Oncol 9:13–20, 1987
44. Hopkins RA, Postlethwait RW: Caustic burns and carcinoma of the esophagus. Ann Surg 194:146, 1981
45. Hussey DH, Barakley T, Bloedorn F: Carcinoma of the esophagus. In Fletcher GH (ed): Textbook of Radiotherapy, 3rd ed, p 688. Philadelphia Lea & Febiger, 1980
46. Imai T, Sannohe Y, Okano H: Oat cell carcinoma (apudoma) of the esophagus. Cancer 41:358, 1978
47. Japanese Society for Diseases: Guidelines for the clinical and pathologic studies on carcinoma of the esophagus. Jpn J Surg 6:69, 1976
48. John MJ, Marshall SF, Mowry PG, et al: Radiotherapy alone and chemoradiation for nonmetastatic esophageal carcinoma. Cancer 63:2397–2403, 1989
49. Just-Viera, JO, Silva JE: Esophageal carcinoma. Ann Thorac Surg 19:688, 1975
50. Karlin DA, Fisher RS, Krevsky B: Prolonged survival and effective palliation in patients with squamous cell carcinoma of the esophagus following endoscopic laser therapy. Cancer 59(11):1969–1972, 1987.
51. Kasai M, Mori S, Watanabe T: Follow-up results after resection of thoracic resection of thoracic esophageal cancer. World J Surg 2:543, 1978
52. Keane TJ, Harwood AR, Elhakim T, et al: Radical radiation therapy with 5-fluorouracil infusion and mitomycin C for oesophageal squamous cell carcinoma. Radiother Oncol 4:205–210, 1985
53. Kelsen D: Chemotherapy of esophageal cancer. Semin Oncol 11:159, 1984
54. Kelsen DP, Ahuja R, Hopfan S, et al: Combined modality therapy of esophageal carcinoma. Cancer 48:34, 1981
55. Kelsen DP, Hilaris B, Coonley C, et al: Cisplatin, vindesine and bleomycin chemotherapy of local-regional and advanced esophageal cancer. Am J Med 75:645, 1983
56. Kmet J, Mahboubi E: Esophageal cancer in the Caspian littoral of Iran: Initial studies. Science 175:846, 1972
57. Laramore GI, Davis RB, Olson MH, et al: RTOG phase I study on fast neutron teletherapy for squamous cell carcinoma of the esophagus. Int J Radiat Oncol Biol Phys 9:465, 1983
58. Launois B, Delarue D, Campion JP, et al: Preoperative radiotherapy for carcinoma of the esophagus. Surg Gynecol Obstet 153:690, 1981
59. Lea JW, Prager RL, Bender H: The questionable role of computed tomography in preoperative staging of esophageal cancer. Ann Thorac Surg 38:479, 1984
60. Leichman I, Steiger Z, Seydel HG, et al: Preoperative chemotherapy and radiation therapy for patients with cancer of the esophagus: A potentially curative approach. J Clin Oncol 2(2):75–79, 1984.
61. Lijinsky W: Current concepts in the toxicology of nitrates, nitrites and nitrosoamines. In Mehlman MA, Shapiro RE, Blumenthal H (eds): Advances in Modern Toxicology, vol 1. New Concepts in Safety Evaluation (part 2), p 149. Washington, Hemisphere Publishing, 1979
62. Lokich J, Shea M, Chaffey J: Sequential infusional 5-fluorouracil followed by concomitant radiation for tumors of the esophagus and gastroesophageal junction. Cancer 60:275–279, 1987
63. Ludwig ME, Shaw R, Suto-nagy GD: Primary malignant melanoma of the esophagus. Cancer 48:2528, 1981
64. Mahboubi NE, Day NE, Ghadrian P: The neglible role of alcohol and tobacco in the etiology of esophageal cancer in Iran: A case-control study. In Nieburgs H (ed): Prevention and Detection of Cancer, Part II, p 1149. New York, Marcel Dekker, 1978
65. Mahboubi ME, Kmet J, Cook PJ: Esophageal cancer studies in the Caspian littoral of Iran: The Caspian cancer registry. Br J Cancer 28:196, 1973
66. Maimon HN, Dreskin RB, Coco AE: Positive esophageal cytology without detectable neoplasm. Gastrointest Endosc 20:156, 1974
67. Marcial V, Velezgarcia F, Clintron J, et al: Radiotherapy preceded by multidrug chemotherapy in carcinoma of the esophagus. Cancer Clin Trials 3:127, 1980
68. Matsufuji F, Kuwano H, Kai H, et al: Preoperative hyperthermia combined with radiotherapy and chemotherapy for patients with incompletely resected carcinoma of the esophagus. Cancer 62(5):889–894, 1988.

69. McCaughan JS, Hicks, WM, Laufman L, et al: Palliation of esophageal malignancy with photoradiation therapy. Cancer 54:2905, 1984
70. Mendenhall WM: Carcinoma of the cervical esophagus. In Million RR, Cassisi NJ (eds): Management of Head and Neck Cancer: A Multidisciplinary Approach, p 393. Philadelphia, JB Lippincott, 1984
71. Merendiono KA, Maerk VJ: An analysis of 100 cases of squamous cell carcinoma. II. With special references to its theoretical curability. Surg Gynecol Obstet 94:110, 1952
72. Miao C, Guo FC, Zhang JZ: The relationship between fungi and nitrosoamines and their precursors (2). The action of fungi isolated from grains in Linxian. Med Ref 2:46, 1978
73. Moertel CG: The esophagus. In Holland JF, Frei E III (eds): Cancer Medicine, 2nd ed, p 1753. Philadelphia, Lea & Febiger, 1982
74. Mori S, Kasai M, Watanabe T, et al: Preoperative assessment of resectability for carcinoma of the thoracic esophagus. I. Esophagograms and azygogram. Ann Surg 190:100, 1979
75. Moss A, Schnyder P, Thoeni RF, et al: Esophageal carcinoma: Pre-therapy staging by computed therapy. AJR 136:1051, 1981
76. Murray GF, Wilcox BR, Starek JK: The assessment of operability of esophageal carcinoma. Ann Thorac Surg 23:393, 1977
77. Naef AP, Savary M, Ozzello L: Columnar-lined lower esophagus: an aquired lesion with malignant predisposition. J Thorac Cardiovasc Surg 70:826, 1975
78. Newaishy GA, Read GA, Duncan W, et al: Results of radical radiotherapy of squamous cell carcinoma of the oesophagus. Clin Radiol 33:347, 1982
79. Oota K, Shin LH: Histological Typing of Gastric and Oesophageal Tumors. Geneva, World Health Organization, 1977
80. Partyka EK, Sanowsksi RA, Kozarek RA: Endoscopic diagnosis of a giant esophageal leiomyosarcoma. Am J Gastroenterol 75:135, 1981
81. Pearson JG: The present status and future potential of radiotherapy in the management of esophageal cancer. Cancer 39:882, 1977
82. Pearson JG, Leroux BT: Malignant tumors of the esophagus. In Vantaappgen G, Hellman J (eds): Diseases of the Esophagus, p 447. New York, Springer-Verlag, 1974
83. Picus D, Balfe DM, Koehler R, et al: Computed tomography in staging esophageal carcinoma. Radiology 146:433, 1983
84. Poleynard GD, Marty AT, Birnbaum WB, et al: Adenocarcinoma of the columnar-lined (Barrett) esophagus. Case Reports and review of the literature. Arch Surg 112:997, 1977
85. Poplin F, Fleming T, Leichman L, et al: Combined therapies for squamous cell carcinoma of the esophagus: Southwest Oncology Group Study (SWOG-8037). J Clin Oncol 5(4):622–628, 1987
86. Postlethwait RW, Sealy WC: Surgery of the Esophagus, p 341. New York, Appleton-Century-Crofts, 1979
87. Quint LE, Glazer L, Orringer MB: Esophageal imaging by MR and CT: Study of normal anatomy and neoplasms. Radiology 156:727, 1985
88. Resbeut M, Le Prise Fleury E, Ben Hassel M, et al: Squamous cell carcinoma of the esophagus: Treatment by combined vincristine-methotrexate plus folinic acid rescue and cisplatin before radiotherapy. Cancer 56(6):1246–1250, 1985
89. Rosenberg JC, Franklin R, Steiger Z: Squamous cell carcinoma of the thoracic esophagus: An interdisciplinary approach. Curr Probl Cancer 5:6, 1981
90. Rosenberg JC, Lichter AS, Leichman LP: Cancer of the esophagus. In DeVita VT, Hellman S, Rosenberg SA (eds): Cancer: Principles and Practice of Oncology, 3rd ed, p 725. Philadelphia, JB Lippincott, 1989
91. Roth JA, Pass HI, Flanagan MM, et al: Randomized clinical trial of preoperative and postoperative adjuvant chemotherapy with cisplatin, vindesine, and bleomycin for carcinoma of the esophagus. J Thorac Cardiovasc Surg 96(2):242–248, 1988
92. Sannohe Y, Hiratsuka R, Koki K: Lymph node metastases in cancer of the thoracic esophagus. Am J Surg 141:216, 1981
93. Sarr MG, Hamilton SR, Marrone GC, et al: Barrett's esophagus: Its prevalence and association with adenocarcinoma in patients with symptoms of gastroesophageal reflux. Am J Surg 149:187, 1985
94. Schottenfeld D: Alcohol as a co-factor in the etiology of cancer. Cancer 43:1962, 1979
95. Schottenfeld D: Epidemiology of cancer of the esophagus. Semin Oncol 11:92, 1984
96. Schuchmann GF, Heydorn WH, Hall RV, et al: Treatment of esophageal carcinoma. A retrospective review. J Thorac Cardiovasc Surg 79:67, 1980
97. Seydel HG, Wichman L, Byhhardt R, et al: Preoperative radiation and chemotherapy for localized squamous cell carcinoma of the esophagus. A RTOG study. Int J Radiat Oncol Biol Phys 14:33–35, 1988
98. Shapiro AL, Robillard GL: The esophageal arteries. Ann Surg 131:171, 1950
99. Silverberg E, Boring CC, Squires TS: Cancer statistics, 1990. CA 40(1):1, 1990
100. Skinner DB: En bloc resection for neoplasms of the esophagus and cardia. J Thorac Cardiovasc Surg 85:59, 1983
101. Skinner DB: Surgical treatment for esophageal carcinoma. Semin Oncol 11:136, 1984
102. Smoron G, O'Brien C, Sullivan C: Tumor localization and treatment technique for cancer of the esophagus. Radiology 111:735, 1974
103. Son YH: Primary mucosal malignant melanoma. Appraisal of role of radiation therapy. Acta Radiol Oncol 19:177, 1980
104. Sotus PC, Majmudar B, Symbas PN: Carcinoma *in situ* of the esophagus. JAMA 239:335, 1978
105. Tate T, Brace JA, Morgan H, Skeggs DBL: Conformation therapy: A method of improving the tumour treatment volume ratio. Clin Radiol 37:267, 1986
106. Thompson WM: Esophageal cancer. Int J Radiat Oncol Biol Phys 9:1533, 1983
107. Turnbull AD, Rosen P, Goodner JT, et al: Primary malignant tumors of the esophagus other than typical epidermoid carcinoma. Ann Thorac Surg 15:463, 1973
108. Turrisi AT III, Glover DJ, Mason BA: A preliminary report: Concurrent twice-daily radiotherapy plus platinum-etoposide chemotherapy for limited small cell lung cancer. Int J Radiat Oncol Biol Phys 15:183–187, 1988
109. van Andel JG, Dees J, Dijkhuis CM, et al: Carcinoma of the esophagus: Results of treatment. Ann Surg 190:684, 1979
110. Watson WL, Goodner JT, Miller TP, et al: Torek esophagectomy: The case against segmental resection for esophageal cancer. J Thorac Surg 32:347, 1956
111. Withers HR, Peters LJ: Basic principles of radiotherapy: Basic clinical parameters. In Fletcher GH (ed): Textbook of Radiotherapy, 3rd ed, p 180. Philadelphia, Lea & Febiger, 1980
112. Wychulis AR, Woolam GL, Anderson HA: Achalasia and carcinoma of the esophagus. JAMA 215:1638, 1971
113. Yang CS: Research on esophageal cancer in China: A review. Cancer Res 40:2633, 1980
114. Young JL Jr, Pollack ES: The incidence of cancer in the United States. In Schottenfeld D, Fraumeni JF Jr (eds): Cancer Epidemiology and Prevention, p 141. Philadelphia, WB Saunders, 1982
115. Younghusband JD, Aluwihare APR: Carcinoma of the esophagus: Factors influencing survival. Br J Surg 57:422,1970

41

Heart and Blood Vessels

Bahman Emami
John Antoniades

ANATOMY

The heart is a hollow muscular organ, which rests on the diaphragm between the lower part of the two lungs. It is located at the lower part of the middle mediastinum. In the adult, the heart measures about 12 cm in length, 8 cm to 9 cm in breadth, and 6 cm in width. It is enclosed in a special membrane, the pericardium. The wall of the heart is composed of three layers: an outer visceral pericardium, a middle myocardium, and an inner endocardium. The heart consists of four chambers: two large ventricles with thick muscular walls, which compose the bulk of the organ, and two smaller atria with thin muscular walls. The septum, which separates the ventricles, also extends between the atria.[35]

EPIDEMIOLOGY

Primary cardiac tumors are rare, with an incidence of between 0.0017% and 0.8% in reported autopsy series.[14,64] The relative incidence of primary tumors of the heart and pericardium has been reported by McAllister and Fenoglio[45]; from 533 primary cardiac tumors reviewed, 75% were benign and 25% were malignant. This relative incidence is true for adults. In infants (under 1 year), 96% of the tumors are benign and only 4% are malignant.[45] In children (1 to 15 years of age), 91% are benign and 9% are malignant.[45] The ratio of primary malignant tumors to benign tumors is greater in the pericardium (1 : 1) than in the heart (1 : 3).[29] Metastatic neoplasms of the heart are reported to occur 13 to 39 times more frequently than primary tumors.[29] Of 533 primary tumors and cysts of the heart and pericardium from the files of the Armed Forces Institute of Pathology (AFIP),[41] 444 (83.3%) were found in adults, 89 (16.7%) in children 1 to 15 years of age, and 48 (9%) in infants less than 1 year old.

Gender incidence varies, depending on the type of tumor. Pericardial tumors occur among men twice as frequently as among women. The reported male : female ratio for myxomas varies from no sex predominance to 1 : 3 male : female ratios.[23,55] Malignant tumors of the heart involve men slightly more frequently than women, with a ratio of 1.4 : 1.

NATURAL HISTORY

Pericardial Tumors

Mesothelioma, the most common malignant pericardial tumor, may be confined to the pericardial sac or may involve the myocardium or mediastinal structures. Thirty to fifty percent of cases are associated with metastasis. The most common sites of metastatic spread are regional lymph nodes and lungs; less often, the tumor metastasizes to the liver, kidneys, adrenal glands, or bones. The duration of life, from the onset of signs and symptoms, is usually less than 2 years. The most common causes of death have been cardiac tamponade, vena cava obstruction, and invasion of the myocardium.

Tumors of the Myocardium and Endocardium

Myxomas are the most common tumors of the heart in adults; 25% of all tumors and cysts and 40% of benign cardiac tumors are myxomas.[45] Approximately 95% of these tumors arise from one of the atria; the left atrium is affected three to four times as often as the right atrium,[26] most frequently in the region of the fossa ovalis. The morphology of the tumor and the extended duration of symptoms[30,66] (reported to be as long as 17 and 43 years, respectively) are indicative of slow growth and minimal invasiveness; if not removed, however, tumor will eventually cause embolization and total cardiac failure. The local recurrence rate after surgery has been reported to be 0%[40] to 5.4%.[56] Very rare cases of metastasizing atrial myxomas have also been reported.[60]

Malignant Tumors of the Myocardium

Sarcomas are the most common malignant tumors of the heart. The right side of the heart is more frequently involved than the left; a ratio of 2 : 1 was reported in one series.[29] The interval between onset of symptoms and death is short, usually less than 2 years. Of 27 rhabdomyosarcomas in one series, 24 had metastasized.[29] The most common sites of metastasis were the lung (50%), liver (30%), and lymph nodes (25%).

CLINICAL PRESENTATION

Patterns of clinical presentation of cardiac tumors are congestive heart failure, thromboembolic episodes, hemodynamic obstruction, arrhythmias, pericardial involvement (effusion), and no symptoms. In intramural tumors, congestive heart failure (CHF) and arrhythmias are the most prevailing signs. Rapidly progressive congestive heart failure of recent onset, which remains refractory to treatment, is characteristic of a cardiac tumor. If a tumor protrudes into the heart cavity, it may produce hemodynamic obstruction and thromboembolic episodes, mostly to the central nervous system. Occasionally, cardiac tumors may present with superior vena caval obstruction.

No specific electrocardiogram (ECG) changes are found in patients with cardiac tumors. The ECG commonly shows nonspecific ST-T changes, but low voltage or bundle branch block may also occur.[12] Laboratory findings may be anemia, erythrocytosis, thrombocytopenia, thrombocytosis, leukocytosis, and elevated sedimentation rate.[51]

DIAGNOSTIC WORKUP

Procedures used in the diagnosis of cardiac tumors are listed in Table 41-1.

The chest radiograph frequently reveals generalized cardiac enlargement, although irregularity of the heart borders and a distorted cardiac silhouette may be observed.[1] An abnormality, albeit inconclusive, is found in 87% of the cases.[16] Calcification in cardiac tumors, seen on plain chest x-ray films, has been reported in 2%[15] to 20% of cases.[1]

Echocardiography, M-mode and two-dimensional, is considered by some authors to be the most useful diagnostic tool in detecting cardiac tumors.[16] Abnormal findings, diagnostic of cardiac tumors in most cases, have been demonstrated in 94% of cases studied.[16] This technique is now the most commonly used diagnostic procedure for cardiac tumors.[17]

Cardiac catheterization has been performed in 50% of reported cases. Findings were abnormal in 80% and normal in 20% of cases.[16] The abnormal findings, indicative of cardiac obstruction, were in cases with tumors protruding into the cardiac lumen.

Radionuclide imaging has been occasionally used in the workup of patients suspected of having cardiac tumors. In 16 patients in which radionuclides were used, ten had myxomas, and all were diagnosed by gated cardiac blood pool scintigraphy.[16]

Angiography has been used in 64% of the reported series in the literature. Results were abnormal in 94% and normal in 6% of the cases.[16,50] Some findings in the latter group were said to be the result of technical difficulties.

Computed tomography (CT) and magnetic resonance (MR) scanning have also recently been used in the workup of patients with suspected cardiac tumors[7,12,19] and have been found to be quite informative. Further studies are needed in this area.

TABLE 41–1
Diagnostic Workup for Tumors of the Heart

ROUTINE
History
Physical examination

RADIOGRAPHIC STUDIES
X-ray examination of chest
Computed tomography scans
Echocardiography (special esophageal echocardiography)

LABORATORY STUDIES
Complete blood count
SMA-12
Urinalysis

OPTIONAL STUDIES (AS INDICATED)
Cardiac catheterization
Radionuclide imaging (scintigraphy)
Angiography
Magnetic resonance imaging

CLASSIFICATION

Cardiac tumors can be classified as primary or secondary. Primary cardiac tumors can be further classified according to their site of involvement (Table 41-2). Mesotheliomas are the most common primary tumors of pericardial origin. The majority of benign cardiac tumors in children are rhabdomyomas, whereas myxomas constitute about 50% of all adult benign tumors.

Sarcomas are by far the most prevalent malignant tumors of the myocardium. In a review of the literature between 1971 and 1977,[15] of 44 malignant cardiac tumors, there were 14 angiosarcomas, 12 rhabdomyosarcomas, five malignant mesenchymomas, and 13 other tumors including other sarcomas.

No staging system is available for cardiac tumors.

TABLE 41–2
Tumors of the Heart and Pericardium

PRIMARY TUMORS
Tumors arising from faulty embryogenic development
- Teratomas
- Thyroid nest tumors

Benign pericardial tumors
- Mesotheliomas
- Angiomas
- Fibromas

Benign heart tumors
- Rhabdomyomas
- Myxomas

Malignant heart tumors
- Mesotheliomas
- Sarcomas

Tumors arising from major vessels
- Aorta
- Pulmonary artery
- Pulmonary vein
- Superior vena cava
- Inferior vena cava

METASTATIC TUMORS OF THE HEART
- Carcinomas
- Sarcomas
- Melanomas
- Lymphomas

MANAGEMENT OF CARDIAC TUMORS

In a review of English literature between 1971 and 1977, it was found that more than 75% of 219 primary cardiac tumors were diagnosed during life. Surgery remains the treatment of choice for patients with cardiac tumors. The use of radiation therapy has been reported only in isolated case reports.

Primary Pericardial Tumors

Radical surgery is possible in localized pericardial tumors, that is, primary pericardial mesothelioma (PPM). Only palliative surgery, pericardiosynthesis, and drainage can be performed in the diffuse forms of these tumors. Primary pericardial mesotheliomas are believed to be resistant to radiation, like their pleural counterparts. Nevertheless, it is notable that two patients with a diagnosis of PPM, who were treated with biopsy and postoperative irradiation, had no evidence of disease at 7 months and 5 years, respectively (Table 41-3).[6]

For patients with localized malignant pericardial tumors not suitable for curative surgery, we recommend a course of radiation therapy either alone (after biopsy) or postoperatively. The total radiation dose is determined by the heart tolerance. A total dose of 4500 cGy in 25 fractions (180 cGy per day) appears to be appropriate. Additional doses (1000 cGy to 1500 cGy) may be delivered through small portals when indicated.

Treatment volume should include the entire pericardial content with a 1 cm to 2 cm margin. Appropriate margin, especially at the left and inferior borders, should be allowed for cardiac motion, to ensure adequate coverage. In this case, simulation of the patient under fluoroscopy is highly recommended. In mesothelioma, mediastinal nodes should also be included in the irradiated volume. Use of parallel opposed portals with differential loading, favoring the anterior portal, appears to be adequate at least for the first part of the treatment (Fig. 41-1). However, for the boost treatment, other techniques such as two anterior wedged portals are desirable to avoid excess dose to the spinal cord. Occasionally, the entire treatment can be given with the latter technique (Fig. 41-2).

Benign Endocardial and Myocardial Tumors

Myxomas and rhabdomyomas are usually treated surgically with low morbidity rate and excellent results.[58] Of 23 cardiac tumors reported by Poole and associates,[53] 17 were diagnosed antemortem. Of these 17, 14 were benign tumors (11 myxomas). Twelve of 14 patients were reported to be alive with no evidence of recurrence after a follow-up of 55 months. The other two patients died of intercurrent disease. Bogren and colleagues[16] reviewed the English literature on cardiac tumors between 1972 and 1977. Patients with myxomas have an excellent 5-year survival rate of 86%; overall those with benign cardiac tumors show a 5-year survival rate of 80%. In Bogren's series patients with benign and malignant pediatric cardiac tumors had 5-year survival rates of 57% and 33%, respectively.[16] Livi and associates[43] reported on 38 patients with cardiac myxomas treated with radical surgery. Two patients died within 1 month of the operation. The remaining 36 patients

TABLE 41–3
Summary of Literature on Radiation Therapy of Malignant Primary Cardiac Tumors

AUTHOR	TUMOR TYPE	SURGERY	IRRADIATION	SURVIVAL
Poole[53]	Fibrosarcoma	RS	4000 cGy/4 wk	Decrease in tumor size but patient died at 4 mo
Anderson[6]	PPM	PS	?	NED 7 mo
Anderson[6]	PPM	PS	?	NED 5 yr
Sytman and MacAlpin[65]	PPM	—	5125 cGy	Progression (died few months later) with local tumor
Furman[32]	PPM	PS	5100 cGy	
Hollingsworth and Sturgill[39]	Pericardial angiosarcoma	B	5400 cGy (+ chemo)	NED→ 10 mo
Allaire et al[4]	Pericardial angiosarcoma	?	?	Progression
Matloff[48]	Rhabdomyosarcoma	Recurrence after S	4950 cGy (+ chemo)	34-mo survival
Gerdes et al[33]	Metastatic rhabdomyosarcoma from lung	B	5500 cGy	24-mo survival; died with local tumor
Dong et al[25]	Fibrosarcoma	?	5392 cGy	12 mo→ died of brain metastasis
Sagerman[57]	Fibrosarcoma	PS S	6300 cGy	12 mo→ died of brain metastasis (local control)
Baldelli et al[11]	Fibrosarcoma	B	5400 cGy	1-yr survival
Goldstein and Mahoney[34]	Fibrosarcoma	Resection	7000 cGy	Died 6 mo with metastasis
Borggio[15]	Fibrosarcoma	B	?	Progression→ died 2 yr later with local tumor
Larrieu[42]	Rhabdomyosarcoma	RS	? (+ chemo)	Died <8 mo
Larrieu[42]	Skeletal angiomatosis	RS	? (+ chemo)	Died <8 mo
Larrieu[42]	Malignant melanoma	RS	? (+ chemo)	Died <8 mo

RS: radical resection; PS: partial or palliative resection; B: biopsy; S: surgery; NED: no evidence of disease; ?: radiation therapy given, dose unknown; PPM: primary pericardial mesothelioma

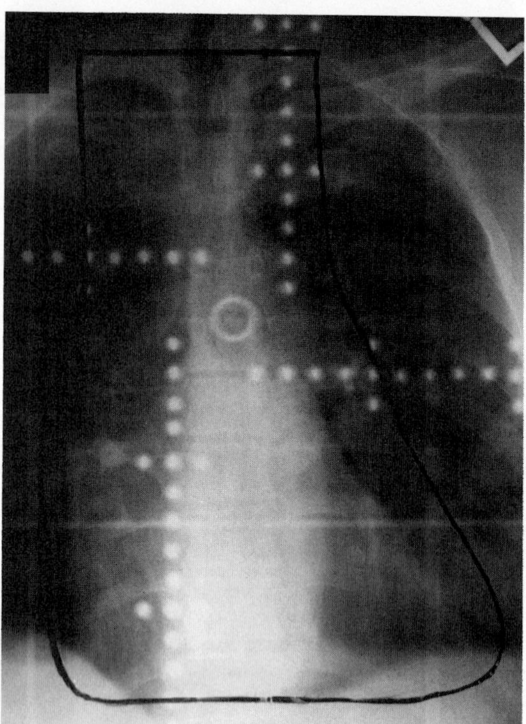

FIGURE 41–1. Radiation therapy portal in a patient with malignant pericardial mesothelioma; note the coverage of the mediastinal nodes.

were reported to be alive with no recurrence and an average follow-up of 5.2 years.

Primary Malignant Cardiac Tumors

Approximately 25% of all primary cardiac tumors are malignant, and almost all of these are sarcomas. Over 50% of these tumors show local extension to the pericardium.[13] Metastasis of cardiac sarcomas has been reported in 30% to 75% of cases.[47] Metastasis occurs most frequently to the lungs (60% to 80%), mediastinal lymph nodes (30%), and liver (30%).[49]

Surgery is the treatment of choice. However, local resection has nearly always been incomplete because of the extent and invasiveness of the tumor. Bogren and associates[16] reported a 14% 5-year survival rate for adults and a 33% rate for children with cardiac tumors. More recent reports do not show significant improvement.[49,56] In spite of the high rate of local extension, the value of radiation therapy in primary malignant cardiac tumors has not been fully evaluated, and the role of chemotherapy is even less clear.

A summary of the literature on cases with primary malignant cardiac tumors in which irradiation was part of the treatment is listed in Table 41-3. Despite some encouraging results, the data are anecdotal, and no firm conclusion can be drawn. Nevertheless, a course of radiation therapy for all primary malignant tumors is recommended, either alone (after biopsy) or postoperatively. The total dose is determined by the heart tolerance. A total dose of 5040 cGy in 28 fractions (180 cGy per day) appears to be appropriate; an additional dose of 1000 cGy may be delivered to small volumes. Treatment volume should encompass the entire content of the pericardium with a margin of 2 cm. The entire mid- and lower mediastinum should be included in the treatment volume because of the high incidence of metastasis to the mediastinal nodes. In spite of the high incidence of distant metastasis, the role of systemic therapy in

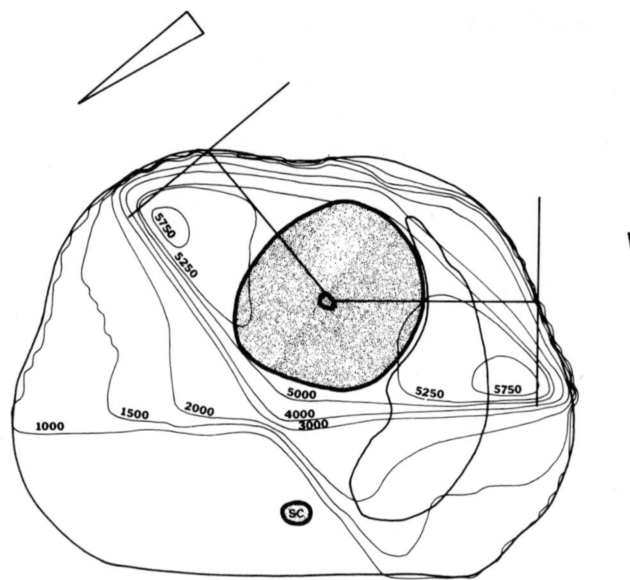

FIGURE 41–2. Two anterior oblique wedged portals used in treatment of a patient with isolated metastatic cardiac tumor from primary lung tumor. Patient is alive and well 8 months after cardiac irradiation and 26 months after primary course of radiation therapy to the lung cancer.

the treatment of these cardiac tumors is virtually unknown. Unfortunately, the major toxicity reaction of the most effective chemotherapeutic agent against sarcomas, doxorubicin (Adriamycin), is cardiac. There is evidence of increased cardiotoxicity when doxorubicin is combined with irradiation.[27]

Secondary Tumors of the Heart and Pericardium

Metastatic tumors to the heart are more prevalent than primary cardiac tumors,[55] and the incidence is increasing as antineoplastic treatment results in longer survival.[44] At autopsy of patients who die of cancer, 5% have metastases to the heart and 13% to the pericardium.[20] Table 41-4 lists the primary tumors that most frequently metastasize to the heart and pericardium. A detailed summary of an earlier autopsy series is reported by Hamfling.[36] The primary cancers that most often spread to the heart are lung and breast carcinomas and malignant melanomas.[46,52,64] Cardiac metastases from other primary sites are rare.[9,38] In children rhabdomyosarcomas are frequently primary tumors.[54] The left ventricular myocardial wall is the most common site of metastasis.[1]

TABLE 41–4
The Primary Site of Cardiac Metastasis

PRIMARY TUMOR	NUMBER OF PATIENTS
Lung	58 (32.4%)
Breast	37 (20.6%)
Lymphoma and leukemia	29 (16.2%)
Malignant melanoma	10 (5.6%)
Miscellaneous (other)	45 (25.2%)
Total	179 (100.0%)

(Data compiled from Adenle AD, Edwards JE: Chest 81:116–169, 1982; Cham WC, Frisman AH, Carstens PHB, et al: Radiology 14:701–704, 1985; Fabian JT, Rose AG: S Afr Med J 16:71–77, 1982)

Survival of patients with metastatic tumors to the heart is poor. Overall, only a 7% 5-year survival rate has been reported.[16]

Palliative surgery is most commonly used as a therapeutic measure. Radiation therapy has occasionally been used. Cham and associates[18] reported on the radiotherapeutic management of 38 patients with cardiac and pericardial metastasis. The radiation dose was 2500 cGy to 3500 cGy in 3 to 4 weeks except for cases of leukemia and lymphoma (1500 cGy to 2000 cGy in 1.5 to 2 weeks). Clinical improvement was achieved in 60% of patients, with durations of 12 to 35 months. The best palliative results were in patients with leukemia and lymphomas (six of seven), followed by those with breast (11 of 16) and lung (two of seven) cancer.

Malignant pericardiac effusion/tamponade is a life-threatening complication of malignant pericardial invasion. Emergency pericardiotomy in such cases is both diagnostic and therapeutic.[8] A median survival of 4 months has been reported in this group of patients.[8] Intrapericardial tetracycline installation to induce sclerosis has also been a useful palliative procedure. Complete control of the initial signs and symptoms of effusion and tamponade was achieved in 30 of 33 patients in one series.[22]

TUMORS OF THE MAJOR BLOOD VESSELS

The Aorta

Histologically, most tumors of the aorta can be classified as fibromyxosarcomas. On the basis of their growth pattern, they can be divided into polypoid, which appear as masses within the lumen; infiltrating, which progress by extension-forming plaques; and adventitial, which grow essentially away from the vessel.[59]

The clinical diagnosis of fibromyxosarcomas is very difficult because of the rarity of the disease and the vagueness of the symptoms. Metastases are often to the bones, liver, and kidneys.[40,59,62] There are no survivors among the 15 cases we have reviewed; radiation therapy was used in none of these cases.

The Pulmonary Artery

Microscopically, tumors of the pulmonary artery are sarcomas; most of them are leiomyosarcomas, fibrosarcomas, and undifferentiated sarcomas.[3,15,31] Obstruction to the right ventricular outflow tract causes pulmonary hypertension and eventually failure of the right heart. Thus, the patients present with congestive heart failure that does not respond to the usual therapeutic measures. Chest x-ray examinations show a prominence of the pulmonary artery component. Angiography reveals large filling defects.[24,41] Metastases to the lungs are common, occurring in over 66% of cases.

Surgery with vascular grafting has been performed in recent years. Haythorn and co-workers[38] described a case in which radiation therapy was applied to a fibromyxosarcoma of the pulmonary artery without success. Patient survival has ranged from 1 to 39 months.[37,61]

The Superior and Inferior Venae Cavae

Vena caval tumors occur more frequently in females than in males. Inferior vena caval tumors, for purposes of clinical correlation, have been subdivided into three main groups by Staley and associates[63]: those occurring in the inferior vena cava from the junction of the common iliac to the renal veins[4]; those occurring in the segment between the renal vein and the hepatic vein[5]; and those occurring at the superior segment from the hepatic vein to the right atrium. The liver forces tumors of the middle and superior segment to propagate in an intraluminal fashion. Tumors arising in the lower part may grow extraluminally.[63]

Histologically, for practical purposes all primary tumors of the venae cavae are leiomyosarcomas. Generally, they are of low grade and metastasize late.[63]

The diagnosis usually has been made by venacavography. Improved surgical techniques have made feasible the surgical resection of a good number of these lesions. Human venous grafts and synthetic grafts have been used.[10,63] Radiation therapy has been used in combination with the surgical procedure. Davis and associates[21] treated a patient with leiomyosarcoma of the superior vena cava with 5500 cGy of radiation postoperatively. Four years later, the patient had survived without signs of recurrence or distant metastases.[21] Allan and colleagues obtained pain relief in a patient with a recurrent tumor after a course of palliative radiation therapy.[5] Improved surgical techniques have resulted in increased survival and possibly in cures among patients with tumors of the superior and inferior venae cavae.[21]

REFERENCES

1. Abrams HL, Adams DF, Grant HA: The radiology of tumors of the heart. Radiol Clin North Am 9:299–326, 1971
2. Adenle AD, Edwards JE: Clinical and pathologic features of metastatic neoplasms of the pericardium. Chest 81:166–169, 1982
3. Ali MY, Lee GS: Sarcoma of the pulmonary artery. Cancer 17:1220, 1964
4. Allaire FJ, Grimm CA, Taylor LM, et al: Primary hemangioendothelioma of the heart. Rocky Mt Med J 61:34, 1964
5. Allan J, Burnett W, Lee FD: Leiomyosarcoma of the inferior vena cava. Scott Med J 9:352, 1964
6. Anderson JA, Hansen BF: Primary pericardial mesothelioma. Dan Med Bull 21(5):195–200, 1974
7. Andreou J, Leitman BS, McCauley DI, et al: The use of computed tomography in the assessment of cardiac masses. Comput Radiol 7(6):355–359, 1983
8. Appelgvist P, Maamies T, Grohn P: Emergency pericardiotomy as primary diagnostic and therapeutic procedure in malignant pericardiac tamponade: Report of three cases and review of literature. J Surg Oncol 21:18–22, 1982
9. Arvold DS: Right ventricular metastasis of endometrial carcinoma: A case report. Gynecol Oncol 29:231–233, 1988
10. Bailey RV, Stribling J, Weitzner S, et al: Leiomyosarcoma of the inferior vena cava: Report of a case and review of the literature. Ann Surg 184:169, 1976
11. Baldelli P, De Angeli D, Dolara A, et al: Primary fibrosarcoma of the heart. Chest 62:234, 1972
12. Becker RC, Hobbs RE, Ratliff NB: Cardiac rhabdomyosarcoma: Case report with review of clinical and pathologic features. Cleve Clin Q 51:83–88, 1984
13. Bemis EL, Pemberton AH, Lurie A: Rhabdomyosarcoma of the heart. Cancer 29:924–929, 1972
14. Benjamin HS: Primary fibromyxoma of the heart. Arch Pathol 27:950, 1939
15. Boggio RR: Primary fibrosarcoma of the heart. Arch Pathol Lab Med 108:533, 1984
16. Bogren HG, DeMaria AN, Mason DT: Imaging procedures in the detection of cardiac tumors with emphasis on echocardiography: A review. Cardiovasc Intervent Radiol 3:107–125, 1980
17. Cacciapuoti F, Arpino G, D'Avino M: Reliability of echocar-

diography in the detection of metastatic malignant pericardial masses. Int J Cardiol 18:109–112, 1988
18. Cham WC, Frisman AH, Carstens PHB, et al: Radiation therapy of cardiac and pericardial metastasis. Radiology 114:701–704, 1975
19. Cholankeril JV, Millman AE, Ramamurti S, et al: Computerized tomography in intracardiac tumors. Comput Radiol 7(5):311–318, 1983
20. Davies MJ: Tumors of the heart and pericardium. In Pomerance A, Davies MJ (eds): The Pathology of the Heart, pp 413–439. Philadelphia, JB Lippincott, 1975
21. Davis GL, Bergman M, O'Kane H: Leiomyosarcoma of the superior vena cava: A first case with resection. J Thorac Cardiovasc Surg 72:408, 1976
22. Davis S, Rambotti P, Grignani F: Intrapericardial tetracycline sclerosis in the treatment of malignant pericardial effusion: An analysis of thirty-three cases. J Clin Oncol 2(6):631–636, 1984
23. Differding JT, Gardner RE, Roe BB: Intracardiac myxomas with report of two unusual cases and successful removal. Circulation 23:929–941, 1961
24. DiGilio MM, Tatooles CJ, Rosen KM, et al: Myxosarcoma of the pulmonary valve. Chest 62:639, 1972
25. Dong E Jr, Hurley EJ, Shumway NE: Primary cardiac sarcoma. Am J Cardiol 10:871, 1962
26. Doohen DJ, Greer JW, Diorio N, et al: Emergency excision of a myxoma of the right ventricle which was obstructing the right ventricular outflow tract. J Thorac Cardiovasc Surg 47:342–348, 1964
27. Eltringham JR, Fajardo LF, Stewart JR: Adriamycin cardiomyopathy: Enhanced cardiac damage in rabbits with combined drug and cardiac irradiation. Radiology 115:471–472, 1975
28. Fabian JT, Rose AG: Tumors of the heart: A study of 89 cases. S Afr Med J 16:71–77, 1982
29. Fine G: Neoplasms of the pericardium and heart. In Gould SE (ed): Pathology of the Heart and Blood Vessels, pp 851–883. Springfield, IL, Charles C Thomas, 1968
30. Frankenfeld RH, Waters CH, Steiner RC: Bilateral myxomas of the heart. Ann Intern Med 53:827–838, 1960
31. Friedman HM, Smith CK: Leiomyosarcoma of the pulmonary artery. JAMA 203:809, 1968
32. Furman R, Bryant LR, Srivastava TN, et al: Right ventricular mesothelioma with pulmonary obstruction. Chest 63:642, 1973
33. Gerdes AJ, Parker RG, Berry HC: Pleomorphic rhabdomyosarcoma: Response to irradiation. Radiol Clin (Basel) 44:97, 1975
34. Goldstein S, Mahoney EB: Right ventricular fibrosarcoma causing pulmonic stenosis. Am J Cardiol 17:570, 1966
35. Gray H, Gross CM (eds): Anatomy of the Human Body, pp 527–727. Philadelphia, Lea & Febiger, 1973
36. Hamfling SM: Metastatic cancer to the heart: Review of literature and report of 127 cases. Circulation 22:474–483, 1960
37. Hayashi Y, Iwasaka T, Hachisuga T, et al: Malignant pericardial effusion in endometrial adenocarcinoma. Gynecol Oncol 29:234–239, 1988
38. Haythorn SR, Ray WB, Wolff RA: Primary fibromyxosarcomas of the heart and pulmonary artery. Am J Pathol 17:261, 1941
39. Hollingsworth JH, Sturgill BC: Treatment of primary angiosarcoma of the heart. Am Heart J 78:254, 1969
40. Kattus AA Jr, Longmire WP, Cannon JA, et al: Primary intraluminal tumor of the aorta producing malignant hypertension. N Engl J Med 262:694, 1960
41. Killebrew E, Gerbode F: Leiomyosarcoma of the pulmonary artery diagnosed preoperatively by angiocardiography. Replacement with composite graft. J Thorac Cardiovasc Surg 71:469, 1976
42. Larrieu AJ, Jamieson WRE, et al: Primary cardiac tumors: Experience with 25 cases. J Thorac Cardiovasc Surg 83:339–348, 1982
43. Livi U, Bortolotti U, Valente M, et al: Cardiac myxomas: Results of 14 years' experience. Thorac Cardiovasc Surg 32:143–147, 1984
44. Lockwood WB, Broghamer WL: The changing prevalence of secondary cardiac neoplasms as related to cancer therapy. Cancer 45:2659–2662, 1980
45. McAllister HA, Fenoglio JJ: Tumors of the cardiovascular system. In Atlas of Tumor Pathology. Washington, Armed Forces Institute of Pathology, 1978
46. McKenna RJ, Ali MK, Ewer MS, et al: Pleural and pericardial effusions in cancer patients. Curr Probl Cancer 9:1–44, 1985
47. McNalley MC, Kelble D, Pryor R, et al: Angiosarcoma of the heart: Report of a case and review of literature. Am Heart J 65:244, 1963
48. Matloff JM, Bass H, Dalen JE: Rhabdomyosarcoma of the left atrium: Physiologic responses to surgical therapy. J Thorac Cardiovasc Surg 61:451, 1971
49. Mori K, Itoh H, Kanaya H, et al: Malignant fibrous histiocytoma of the heart. Jpn Circ J 47:188–193, 1981
50. Nakamura Y, Nishiya Y, Kawada, et al: Primary hemangiopericytoma of the heart associated with pseudoaneurysm of the pulmonary artery: A case report. Angiology 38:788–792, 1987
51. Peters MN, Hall RJ, Colley DA, et al: The clinical syndrome of atrial myxoma. JAMA 230:695–701, 1974
52. Pinto MM: Malignant pericardial effusion and cardiac tamponade. Acta Cytol 30:657–661, 1986
53. Poole GV, Breyer RH, Holiday RH, et al: Tumors of the heart: Surgical considerations. J Cardiovasc Surg 25:5–11, 1984
54. Pratt CB, Dugger DL, Johnson WW, et al: Metastatic involvement of the heart in childhood rhabdomyosarcoma. Cancer 31:1492–1497, 1973
55. Prichard RW: Tumors of the heart: Review of the subject and report of 150 cases. Arch Pathol Lab Med 51:98–128, 1951
56. Reece AJ, Cooley DA, Frazier OH, et al: Cardiac tumors: Clinical spectrum and prognosis of lesions other than classical benign myxomas in 20 patients. Thorac Cardiovasc Surg 88:439–446, 1984
57. Sagerman RH, Hurley E, Bagshaw MA: Successful sterilization of a primary cardiac sarcoma by supervoltage radiation therapy. AJR 92:942, 1964
58. St. John Sutton MG, Mercier LA, Guiliani ER, et al: Atrial myxomas: A review of clinical experience in 40 patients. Mayo Clin Proc 55:371–376, 1980
59. Salm R: Primary fibrosarcoma of the aorta. Cancer 29:73, 1972
60. Seo IS, Warner TFCS, Colyer RA, et al: Metastasizing atrial myxoma. Am J Surg Pathol 4:391–399, 1980
61. Shmookler BM, Marsh HB, Roberts WC: Primary sarcoma of the pulmonary trunk and/or right or left main pulmonary artery: A rare cause of obstruction to right ventricular outflow. Report on two patients and analysis of 35 previously described patients. Am J Med 63:263, 1977
62. Sladen RA: Neoplasia of the aortic intima. J Clin Pathol 17:602, 1964
63. Staley CJ, Valaitis J, Trippel OH, et al: Leiomyosarcoma of the inferior vena cava. Am J Surg 113:211, 1967
64. Straus R, Merliss R: Primary tumor of the heart. Arch Pathol 39:74, 1945
65. Sytman AL, MacAlpin RN: Primary pericardial mesothelioma: Report of two cases and review of the literature. Am Heart J 81:760, 1971
66. Thomas GI, Edmark KW, Jones TW, et al: Myxoma of the left ventricle: A case report. J Thorac Cardiovasc Surg 46:220–226, 1963

42

Breast: Stage Tis, T1, and T2 Tumors

Carlos A. Perez
Delia M. Garcia
Robert R. Kuske
Seymour H. Levitt

ANATOMY

Breast anatomy has been described in great detail in numerous publications[89, 163] and will only be sketched here.

The breast is made up of the mammary gland, fat, blood vessels, nerves, and lymphatics (Fig. 42-1). The surface of the breast has deep attachments of fibrous septa, called *Cooper's ligament,* which runs between the superficial fascia (attached to the skin) and the deep fascia (covering the pectoralis major and other muscles of the chest wall).[89]

The mammary gland lies over the pectoralis major muscle and extends from the second to the sixth rib in the vertical plane and from the sternum to the anterior axillary line.[89] In older and obese women with pendulous breasts, the breast tissue can fall to the midaxillary line or even farther posteriorly. An additional layer of mammary tissue extends laterally into the axilla to a variable degree. This axillary projection, often called the "tail," is sometimes very prominent.

The retromammary bursa lies between the deep layer of the superficial fascia and the deep fascia; it contains loose areolar tissue that allows for mobility over the chest wall.[163] It is crossed by projections of the deep layer of the superficial fascia that join with the deep pectoral fascia to form the posterior suspensory ligaments of the breast. Deep projections of mammary parenchyma may extend between the muscle bundles of the pectoralis major muscle. The *mamma* consists of glandular tissue arranged in multiple lobes composed of lobules connected in ducts, areolar tissue, and blood vessels. The smallest lobules consist of clusters of rounded alveoli that open into the small branches of the lactiferous ducts (Fig. 42-2); these unite and form larger ducts that eventually converge into single canals in the nipple, corresponding to each lobe of the gland (15 to 20 galactophores).[218]

A network of lymphatics is formed over the entire surface of the chest, neck, and abdomen and becomes dense under the areola. Mammary gland lymphatics begin in the interlobular or prelobular spaces, follow the ducts, and end in the subareolar network of lymphatics of the skin.[89, 163] The following lymphatic pathways originate mostly in the base of the breast. The axillary or principal pathway passes from the upper and lower halves of the breast to the lateral chain of nodes situated between the second and third intercostal space; the transpectoral pathway passes through the pectoralis major muscle to the supraclavicular lymph nodes; and the internal mammary pathway passes through the midline, through the pectoralis major and intercostal muscles, usually close to the sternum, to the nodes of the internal mammary chain. The main lymphatic channels of the breast are illustrated in Figure 42-3.

EPIDEMIOLOGY

In the United States in 1991, approximately 175,900 new cases of breast cancer were diagnosed; 44,800 women died of the disease.[4] Breast and lung cancer are the foremost causes of cancer deaths in women. The breast cancer mortality rate has been stable for the last 50 years; yet recently it was strongly suggested that there is a slight overall decline in breast cancer age-adjusted mortality, in contrast to pronounced peaks in incidence.[15] Nearly all the increase (83%) is accounted for by early diagnosis of *in situ* or invasive lesions less than 2 cm in hospitals with screening mammography programs.

Although one in every ten women in the United States is projected to develop carcinoma of the breast, 80% to 92% of all breast masses are benign.[78, 256] Approximately 1% of breast cancer occurs in men.

The risk factors for breast cancer in women are well documented: age over 50 years, personal or family history of breast cancer, nulliparous, and first child delivered after age 30.[487] The increase in incidence in breast cancer over the last two decades has occurred mostly among women aged 45 to 74 years, with a further increase among black women.[210]

Breast cancer is observed more frequently in specific groups of women: whites more than nonwhites; Jewish women

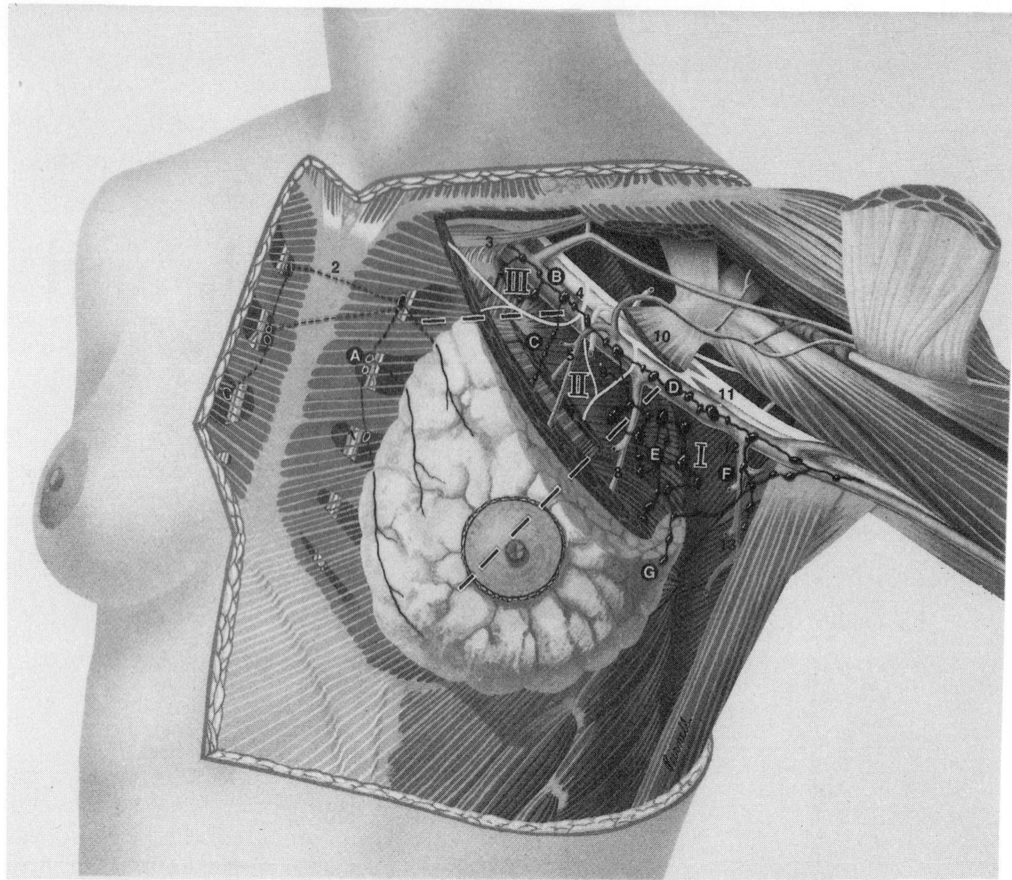

FIGURE 42–1. Anatomy of the breast and lymphatic drainage. (Osborne MP: Breast development and anatomy. In Harris JR, Hellman S, Henderson IC, Kinne DW [eds]: Breast Diseases, pp 1–14. Philadelphia, JB Lippincott 1987)

more than non-Jewish women; women from upper socioeconomic classes more than those from lower socioeconomic classes; women who have never been married more than married women; nulliparous women more than those who have had children; and those with strong family history of breast cancer (mother, aunts, and so on). Low incidence and low mortality rates for female breast cancer are found in most Asian and African countries, intermediate incidence and mortality rates in southern European and South American countries, and high incidence and mortality rates in North American and northern European countries.[210] Several explanations for this variability are possible, such as environmental factors and diet. Studies have shown that after two or three generations, the incidence of female breast cancer among descendants of Japanese immigrants to Hawaii or to the mainland of the United States approaches that of many-generation residents.[210]

Exposure to ionizing radiation during or after puberty increases the risk of developing carcinoma of the breast. Land and associates[237] reviewed reports on three populations of patients: a report by Tokunaga and colleagues[443] on survivors of the atomic bombings in Hiroshima and Nagasaki; a report by Boice and Monson[38] on women of Massachusetts who had mul-

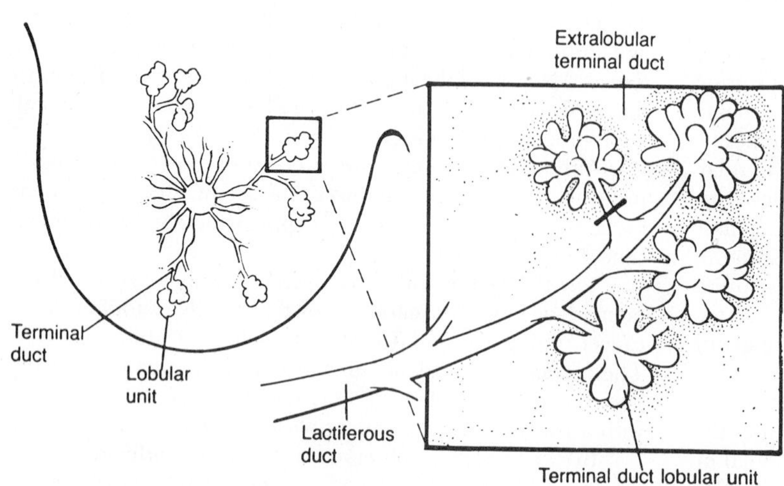

FIGURE 42–2. Microscopic structure of mammary gland. Ducts extend back from the nipple independent of one another, each defining a lobe of the breast. The major ducts arborize, culminating in the terminal lobular units. The ducts are lined by an epithelial layer in which ductal cancer is thought to arise. Most cancer is thought to arise in the extralobular terminal duct. (Kopans DB: Breast Imaging. Philadelphia, JB Lippincott, 1989)

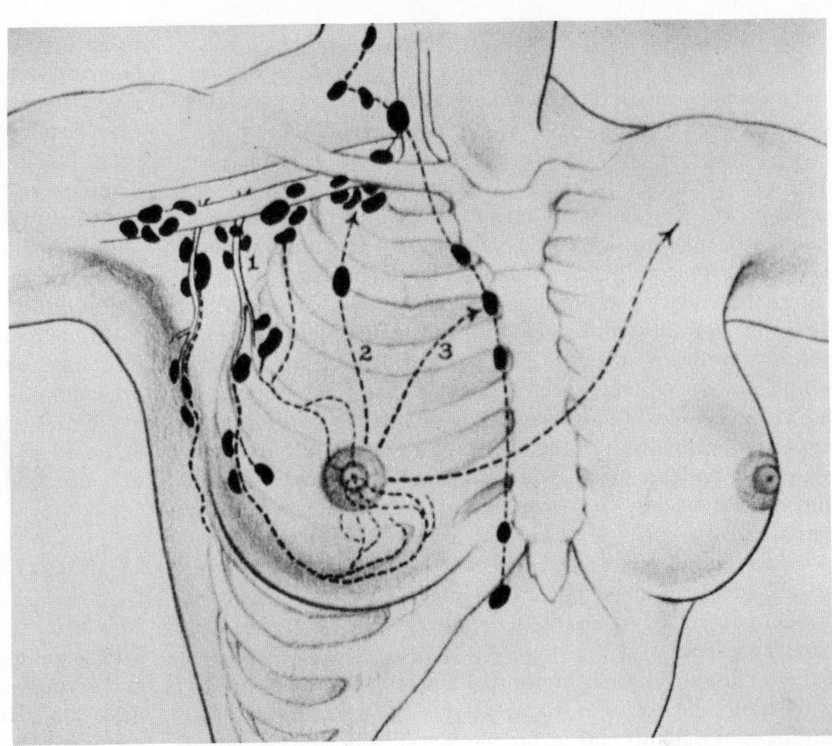

FIGURE 42–3. Anatomy of the lymphatic routes of the breast. (del Regato JA, Spjut HJ, Harlan J, Cox J: Ackerman and del Regato's Cancer: Diagnosis, Treatment, and Prognosis, 6th ed. St. Louis, CV Mosby, 1985)

tiple fluoroscopic examinations of the chest for pulmonary tuberculosis; and a study by Shore and co-workers[396] on patients with postpartum mastitis who were exposed to multiple x-ray examinations, in which nonexposed civilians were used as a control group. Conclusions were that the risk of radiation-induced cancer of the breast increased approximately linearly according to amount of doses and was heavily dependent on age at exposure. These observations were subsequently confirmed by other investigators. In a study of 31,710 women who had tuberculosis and were examined with repeated fluoroscopic studies, a substantial proportion (26.4%) received doses to the breast of 10 cGy or more.[286] The risk was greatest among women who had radiation exposure between the ages of 10 and 14 (relative risk of 4.5 per cGy and an additive risk of 6.1 per 10^4 person-years per cGy), with substantially less excess risk with increasing age at first exposure.

In a study of 1030 women with scoliosis who had multiple radiographic examinations over an average period of 8.7 years, 11 cases of breast cancer were reported, compared with six expected (1.82 risk factor).[196] Risk also increased with the number of x-ray examinations and estimated radiation dose to the breast (mean 13 cGy). Furthermore, in a cohort of 1201 women who received x-ray treatment in infancy for an enlarged thymus gland (estimated mean absorbed dose of radiation to the breast was 690 cGy), after an average of 36 years of follow-up, 22 breast cancers were diagnosed, compared with 12 in 2469 nonirradiated sisters (adjusted risk factor of 3.6).[194] The dose-response relationship was linear with a relative risk of 3.48 per 100 cGy and an additive excess risk of 5.7 per 10^4 person-years per cGy.

It should be stressed that the risk of breast cancer associated with radiation exposure decreases sharply with increasing age at exposure, and even a small benefit to women of screening mammography would outweigh any possible risk of radiation-induced breast cancer.[286]

Higher alcohol consumption has been correlated with increased risk of breast cancer.[484] Several large-scale studies have failed to demonstrate a correlation between the prolonged use of oral contraceptives and breast cancer.[206,257,328,360,413,445,467,468] A study of over 100,000 women showed no association between smoking and risk of breast cancer.[262] A study of 2201 women between the ages of 30 and 62 years showed no significant association between the degree of adiposity and the incidence of breast cancer, but suggested that increased central to peripheral body fat distribution may be a more specific marker over premalignant hormonal pattern predisposing to this disease.[19]

NATURAL HISTORY

The most common site of origin of breast cancer is the upper outer quadrant (38.5%), followed by the central area (29%), the upper inner quadrant (14.2%), the lower outer quadrant (8.8%), and the lower inner quadrant (5%).[163] These rates correlate with the amount of breast tissue in the various quadrants. Cancer is somewhat more common in the left breast than in the right; it is unusual for cancer to appear in both breasts simultaneously (1% to 2%). Metachronous bilateral carcinoma of the breast has been observed in 7% to 8% of patients.[163]

The growth rate of a tumor in the breast is thought to be constant from the date of origin.[163] Using estimates of doubling time, it would take an average of approximately 5 years for a tumor to reach palpable size, and those lesions with slower doubling time would have an even longer latent period.[163]

As the cancer grows, it travels along the ducts, eventually breaking through the basement membrane of the duct, invading adjacent lobules, ducts, fascial strands, and mammary fat, spreading through the breast lymphatics and into the peripheral lymphatics. The prognostic and therapeutic implications of tumor multicentricity and multifocality are discussed in detail later in this chapter (see Prognostic Factors). The tumor can grow through the wall of blood vessels, spread into the deep lymphatics of the dermis, and produce edema of the skin (*peau d'orange*); this usually indicates that the superficial lymphatics as well as the deeper ones are involved. Ulceration and infiltration of overlying skin may develop late in the course of the disease and is usually preceded by fixation and localized redness of the skin over the tumor.[163]

A common route taken by breast carcinoma as it metastasizes is first through the axillary lymph nodes; the incidence of metastases to these lymph nodes increases with larger tumors.[97] About 40% of newly diagnosed Stage T1 and T2 breast cancers have pathologic evidence of axillary nodal metastases. The higher the axillary level of lymph node metastases, the worse the prognosis; supraclavicular node involvement is generally evidence of advanced disease. The number of involved axillary lymph nodes definitely influences prognosis.[121] Metastasis to the axillary nodes is most frequently seen from lesions of the upper outer quadrant of the breast. Metastasis to the internal mammary nodes is most frequently seen from the medial half and central lesions; these metastases occur more frequently when axillary nodes are involved (Table 42-1). The supraclavicular lymph nodes may be the target of metastatic deposits, usually after the high axillary or internal mammary lymph nodes are involved by tumor, depending on the location of the primary lesion.

Vascular invasion by tumor and hematogenous metastases to the lungs, pleura, bone, brain, eyes, liver, ovaries, and adrenal and pituitary glands may be observed even with small tumors.

An attempt was made to determine whether the patterns of failure after mastectomy are different in patients with various stages of disease.[243] Valagussa and colleagues,[455] in their study of operable breast cancer patients treated with radical surgery, noted that node-negative patients had fewer failures than node-positive patients, but that the proportion of locoregional and distant metastases was essentially the same in both groups.

Fowble and associates[142] performed a pattern of failure analysis after mastectomy and chemotherapy for node-positive patients entered into an Eastern Cooperative Oncology Group trial. No radiation therapy was given. Isolated locoregional recurrence was found to correlate with the presence of four to seven positive lymph nodes, T3 tumors, positive surgical margins, and high nuclear grade. Patients with one to three positive nodes had a lower incidence of locoregional recurrence. Patients with more than seven positive nodes tended to fail systemically as well as locally, minimizing the incidence of isolated locoregional recurrence.

DePietro and co-workers[91] found that in 800 patients with first recurrence of carcinoma at various sites after mastectomy, visceral metastases were more common in patients under 50 years of age, whereas local recurrence was more common in patients over 50 years. The survival rate after recurrence for patients with first metastasis confined to soft tissues was higher than for those with bone or visceral metastases. A study by Hagemeister and colleagues[171] consistently found more tumor involvement than had been clinically suspected in 166 patients who died of breast cancer and had autopsy; most of these patients had received treatment that included chemotherapy. There were 325 unsuspected metastases. Areas of tumor involvement were the endocrine organs (40%), liver (30%), lungs (28%), cardiovascular system (21%), and genitourinary system (21%). Major causes of death were pulmonary insufficiency (26%), infection (24%), cardiac disease (15%), and hepatic insufficiency (14%). The primary cause of death was metastatic disease to various organs, accounting for 45% of all the deaths; infection was the second most common cause of death.

The patterns of failure in intraductal, lobular *in situ,* and Stage T1 and T2 breast cancer after breast conservation surgery are analyzed in detail in various sections of this chapter.

CLINICAL PRESENTATION

The majority of patients with T1 or T2 breast cancers present with a painless breast mass or have an abnormal screening mammogram. Occasionally, patients have mammary tenderness, skin changes, bloody nipple discharge, or change in shape and size of breast. Rarely, patients may present with axillary lymphadenopathy (occasionally painful) or even distant metastasis.

SCREENING MAMMOGRAPHY

With wider use of screening mammography, a growing percentage of patients are seen with clinically silent carcinomas. Approximately 40% of lesions reported by Austin and associates[15] were detected by mammography only. They noted an increasing proportion of carcinoma *in situ* and early stages diagnosed in San Francisco–Oakland from 1974 through 1986 as a result of greater use of screening mammography.[15] In another series approximately 50% of lesions detected by mammography only and 36% by mammography and physical examination were infiltrating carcinomas smaller than 1 cm.[18]

A pessimistic attitude toward the curability of breast cancer and a skeptical view regarding the effectiveness and high economic cost of mammography were expressed by Skrabanek.[402] However, evidence is increasing that early treatment after screening by clinical breast examination and mammography is associated with reduced breast cancer mortality for women 50 years of age and older.[307] Sixteen-year results from the Health Insurance Plan (HIP), which involved two systematically se-

TABLE 42–1
Internal Mammary (IM) Node Involvement Related to Location of Primary and Axillary Node Involvement

% IM INVOLVEMENT	UIQ	LIQ	CENTRAL	UOQ	LOQ
Total	27% 67/248	33% 20/61	32% 70/216	14% 54/382	13% 12/93
Axilla not involved	14% 20/143	6% 2/36	7% 5/76	4% 7/170	5% 2/40
Axilla involved	45% 47/105	72% 18/25	46% 65/140	22% 47/212	19% 10/53

(Handley RS: Ann R Coll Surg 57:59–66, 1975)

lected, randomly sampled groups of about 31,000 women aged 40 to 64 years, demonstrated that mortality rate was reduced by about one third in women 50 to 59 years of age.[394,395] Women in the HIP study were offered screening examinations. Sixty-five percent of those who appeared for an initial evaluation were offered three additional examinations at annual intervals unless early follow-up or biopsy was indicated. Screening consisted of a clinical examination, usually by a surgeon, mammography in which two views were taken (cephalocaudad and lateral), and an interview to obtain relevant demographic information. The control group was observed and followed. Large differences in general mortality between the study women who participated in the screening program and those who refused have been recognized. Death from breast cancer among cases detected, starting 3 to 3.5 years after screening ended became very similar for study and control groups of women.

Figure 42-4 demonstrates the complex changes that occur in cumulative case survival rate (CSR) in a screening program; the survival difference between mammography-only and clinical examination-only cases appears 7 to 10 years after diagnosis. Thus, only additional years of observation can determine whether this difference represents the start of real separation of the curves or chance variation. Although the greatest difference in mortality between screened and control groups was detected in women 50 to 59 years of age when they entered the study, the differences are in favor of the study of groups at all ages (Table 42-2). However, in the age 40 to 49 subgroup the difference is not yet statistically significant.

A Swedish study[147] reported on 40,000 women aged 40 to 64 years who were invited for screening mammography (single view) and 20,000 women who served as controls. Of 128 breast cancers detected in the first round, 37 were Stages II to IV, and in the second 21 of 95 were Stage II or greater, indicating a reduction in the number of advanced cancers detected in the screening group from the first to the second round. The cumulative number of Stage II or greater breast cancers in the

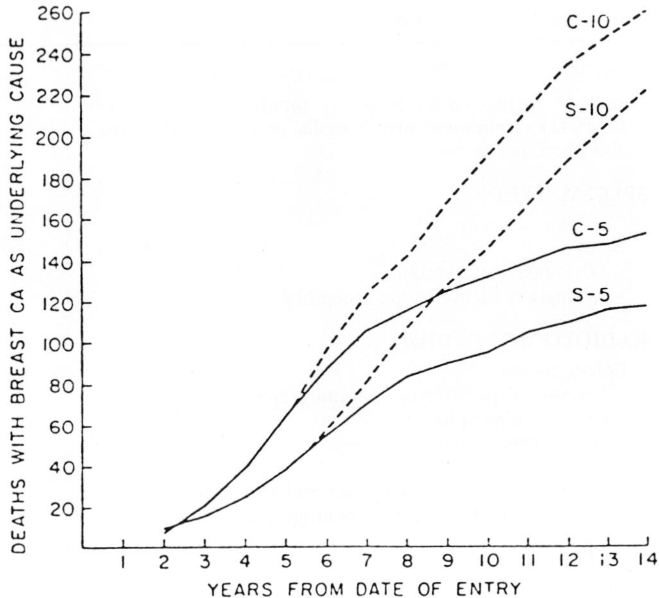

FIGURE 42–4. Cumulative breast cancer deaths by time interval from date of entry in mammography screening program. S-5 and C-5 refer to breast cancer deaths among cancers diagnosed within 5 years of entry. S-10 and C-10 refer to corresponding situation for cancers diagnosed within 10 years of entry. (S: total study; C: controls) (Shapiro S, Venet W, Strax P, et al: J Natl Cancer Inst 69:349, 1982)

TABLE 42–2
*Breast Cancer Deaths in Screening Mammography Program by Age at Entry, 5 and 14 Years from Entry**

AGE AT ENTRY (YR)	NO. OF DEATHS THROUGH FOLLOWING YEARS AFTER ENTRY			
	5		14	
	STUDY	CONTROL	STUDY	CONTROL
Total	39	63	118	153
40–49	19	20	46	61
40–44	9	11	18	26
45–49	10	9	28	35
50–59	15	33	53	68
50–54	8	23	29	36
55–59	7	10	24	32
≥60	5	10	19	24

**Included are deaths with breast cancer as an underlying cause among breast cancers diagnosed during the first 5 years after entry.*
(Shapiro S, Venet W, Strax P, et al: J Natl Cancer Inst 69[2]:349–355, 1982)

screening and control populations at various ages was comparable. After 5 years the number of tumors found in the study population exceeded the number in the control population by 45%, with a tendency toward more favorable stages in the screened women between the ages of 40 and 64 years. A breakdown by age suggests an effect in the 50- to 59-year age group but not in women 40 to 49 or 60 to 64 years old.

Several reports have shown the usefulness of cumulative incidence of Stage II or worse tumors detected during a screening trial as an early indicator of mortality outcome.[428,429] Anderson and associates[6] reported on a study conducted in Malmö with about 21,000 women invited for screening and 21,195 in the control group. A total of 588 women in the study group and 447 in the control group were found to have carcinoma of the breast, a large percentage (26%) of them being noninvasive carcinomas; cancers of Stage II or greater accounted for 33% of the cancers in the study group and 52% in the control group. The percentage of advanced cancers in women who did not attend for screening was 72% compared with 50% in the control group. Overall, women in the study group aged 55 years or older had a reduction in breast cancer mortality (35% *versus* 44%).

A large trial was conducted in the United Kingdom[451] involving 45,841 women aged 45 to 64 years who were offered annual screening by clinical examination and mammography; 63,636 were taught breast self-examination, and 127,117, for whom no extra services were provided, constituted a control population. No significant reduction in mortality from breast cancer was observed during the first 5 years among the various groups. However, thereafter there was a 14% reduction in mortality rate, which rose to 20%, in the women undergoing mammographic screening. No significant difference in mortality occurred between the groups who were taught breast self-examination and the control group.

Peeters and co-workers[319] reported on a mammographic screening program carried out in Nijmegen in 23,000 women aged 35 to 64 years in the first group, 7700 women in the second group, and 3900 younger women in the third group. At the time of the first screening examination, 21% of tumors were 10 mm or less, whereas 20% were over 20 mm. At later examination 33% of the cancers were less than 10 mm and 20% were over 20 mm. Detection rates of carcinoma were highest for elderly women at first examination (9.5 per 1000 screened). The corresponding values were 5.6 per 1000 for women aged 50 to 64 years and 2.3 per 1000 for women younger than 50 years. This was not a randomized study, and mortality reduction, which was 50% in the screened population, was evaluated by means of a case control study.

Verbeek and associates[461] reported decreased breast cancer mortality in a screened population. Likewise, high survival rates were observed in 4240 women found to have carcinoma of the breast in the Breast Cancer Diagnosis Demonstration Project (BCDDP). The relative 5- and 10-year survival rates were 88% and 79%, respectively.[391]

No randomized trial has been carried out comparing the effectiveness of different screening intervals. The American Cancer Society and the American College of Radiology recommend a baseline mammogram at the age of 35 years (30 in high-risk groups). Repeat examinations should be carried out every 2 years beginning at age 40. In women over age 50, mammograms should be performed annually. It has been suggested that screening mammography every 30 to 36 months may reduce breast cancer mortality. Risk factor information could be used to determine the optimal frequency of screening.

Hendee and Kellie[189] reviewed the economic aspects of mammographic screening. They concluded in 1984 that the net increase in cost associated with annual mammographic screening of 4.5 million women 40 to 49 years old was estimated to be approximately $400 million per year. The savings in initial treatment and subsequent terminal care charges for those dying of breast cancer would be offset by the cost of medical care in women who died of other causes. Eddy and associates[106] reviewed the value of mammography screening in women under 50 years of age and reached conclusions that did not strongly support mammographic screening for all 40- to 49-year-old women. They recommended a flexible policy for asymptomatic women who are willing to bear the cost, in consultation with their physicians.

Moskowitz[296] carried out a detailed cost/benefit analysis of breast cancer screening and concluded that the cost/benefit ratio for mammographic screening of a large population of asymptomatic women is within the range accepted for other areas in health care.

With regard to risk, some authors believe that little evidence suggests significant induction of breast cancer from x-ray exposure of periodic mammographic examinations.[115]

SCREENING BY PHYSICAL EXAMINATION

There are no controlled studies evaluating the effectiveness of screening by breast self-examination (BSE) alone, except the United Kingdom trial. Using Breast Cancer Registry data, Foster and Constanza[75,137] found fewer deaths from breast cancer (14% *versus* 26%) and improved estimated 5-year survival rates (75% *versus* 59%) among women who reported performing BSE compared with those who did not. No significant difference has been reported in tumor size in patients reporting regular BSE or not. In the Breast Cancer Detection Demonstration Project (BCDDP),[391] the estimated overall sensitivity of breast self-examination in detecting breast cancer was 26% compared with 75% for the combination of clinical breast examination and mammography.

Baines and associates[17] reviewed the potential value of breast physical examination in 89,835 women participating in the Canadian National Breast Screening Study, 50% of whom did not have mammography and had only physical examinations performed by nurses. No significant difference was noted between nurse and physician examiner findings; the authors concluded that physical examination of the breast by trained nurses was useful and cost-effective.

DIAGNOSTIC WORKUP

The workup of a patient with a breast mass is summarized in Table 42-3. The patient should be examined in several positions, including sitting up and lying down. Careful inspection of both breasts should be made, noting size, form and symmetry, changes in pigmentation, scaling or discharge from the nipple, and dilated veins or edema of the skin in a nonpregnant breast. The location, size, and mobility of the palpable tumor should be recorded. It is useful to draw and photograph the projection of any suspicious or palpable masses on the skin of the breast or nodal areas.

In addition to examination of the breast, careful evaluation of the axilla and supraclavicular areas is required. The number, consistency, mobility or fixation, and size of lymph nodes should be noted. In approximately 20% to 35% of cases (depending on tumor size), clinically node-negative patients have pathologic involvement, whereas no tumor is found in 25% to 30% of patients with clinically palpable axillary nodes. Examination of the abdomen for liver enlargement or nodules and evaluation for bony pain are also essential. Finally, a complete pelvic examination should be done.

Laboratory studies include a complete blood count and chemistry profile, with particular emphasis on alkaline phosphatase level as well as liver function tests (SGOT, SGPT, LDH, bilirubin, and others).

TABLE 42–3
Diagnostic Workup for Carcinoma of the Breast

GENERAL
- History: menstrual status, parity, family history of cancer
- Physical examination: breast, axilla, supraclavicular area, abdomen, pelvis

SPECIAL TESTS
- Needle aspiration
- Biopsy
  - Histologic examination
  - Evaluation for hormone receptors

RADIOLOGIC STUDIES
- Before biopsy
  - Mammography or xeromammography
  - Chest radiographs
- After positive biopsy
  - Bone scan
  - After bone scan positive, liver and spleen scan
  - Internal mammary lymphoscintigraphy

LABORATORY STUDIES
- CBC, blood chemistry
- Urinalysis

OPTIONAL
- Growth fraction (DNA index)
- Oncogene assays

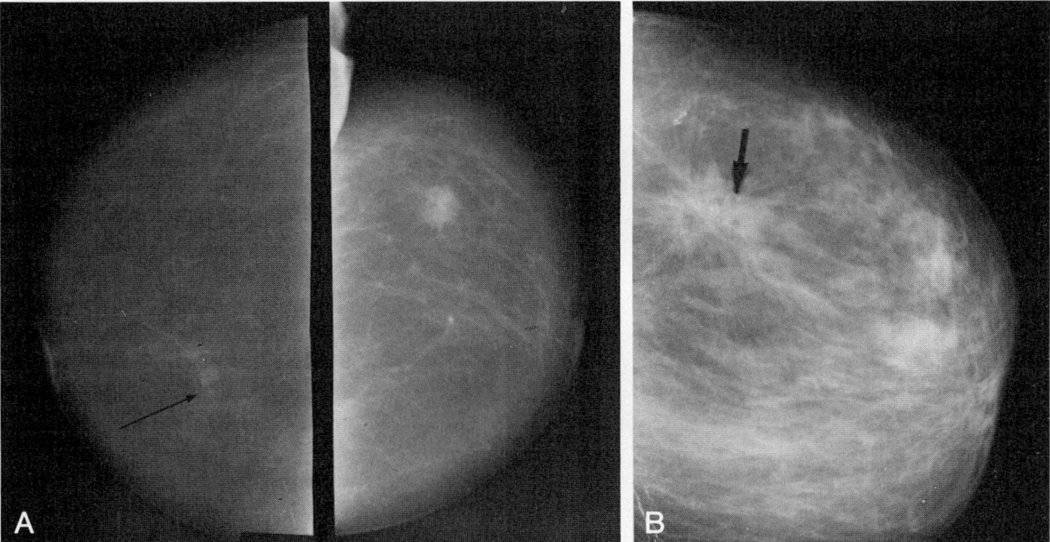

FIGURE 42–5. (**A**) This patient demonstrates the value of screening mammography. A lesion 1 cm in diameter was palpated in the left breast and is apparent on the mammogram. A second lesion, a nonpalpable invasive ductal carcinoma less than 0.5 cm in diameter, was detected on the mammogram of the contralateal breast (*arrow*). (**B**) A mammogram showing classic ductal carcinoma of the breast with a mass and a radiating pattern into the adjacent tissues and microcalcifications (*arrow*). This type of lesion usually is also detected on physical examination.

Imaging Techniques in Breast Cancer

Radiographic studies include chest x-ray examination, bilateral mammograms if they were not obtained as part of the initial screening process, and plain radiographs of symptomatic bones if clinically warranted.

Kopans and associates[219] reviewed the various diagnostic imaging techniques available for evaluation of patients with breast cancer and their advantages or disadvantages. Mammography with dedicated mammographic units and high-sensitivity screen film (or Xerox) techniques have been described.[94,427] Classically, breast carcinoma is seen as an ill-defined mass that may have spiculated margins (Fig. 42-5), although rarely cancers may also be seen with a knobby, lobulated, or even smooth contour (ultrasonography may distinguish them from cystic masses). Architectural distortion of the breast tissue may be present. The appearance of linear, radiated, or spiculated changes about a central focus should always be considered suspicious for carcinoma. The tumor may be hidden by dense parenchyma; review of previous mammograms is very important in detecting subtle interval changes in the appearance of the breast.

Calcifications can be associated with either benign or malignant conditions of the breast. However, calcifications associated with malignant tumors are typically 100 μ to 300 μ in size and are rod-like, tubular, branching, or punctate. Clusters of microcalcifications (more than five) are suggestive of intraductal disease, and in nonpalpable lesions excisional biopsy done after needle localization aids in the diagnosis (Fig. 42-6). About 30%

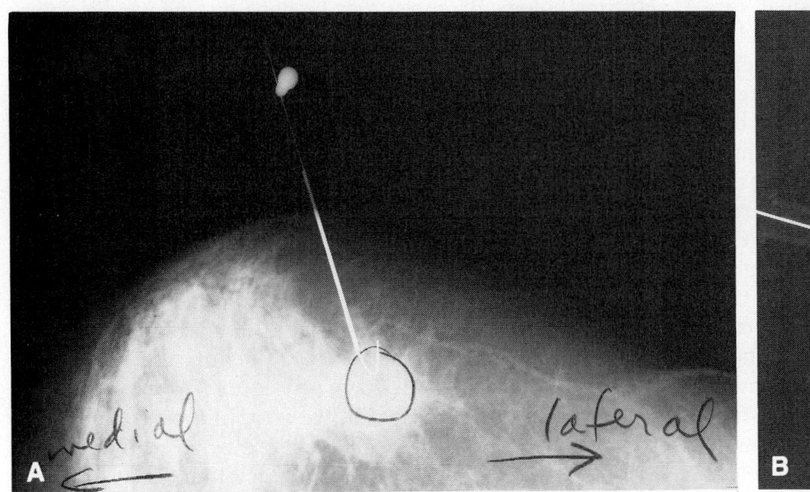

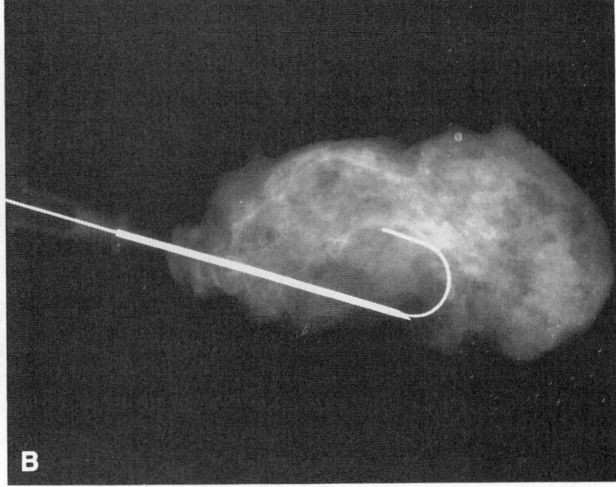

FIGURE 42–6. (**A**) Mammogram demonstrating microcalcifications in central portion of the breast with needle localization on site. (**B**) Radiograph showing microcalcifications in central portion of wide, excisional biopsy specimen. Pathologic diagnosis was intraductal carcinoma. Posttylectomy mammogram showed no residual calcifications in the breast. Patient was treated with conservation surgery and irradiation 4 years ago and remains tumor-free.

of biopsies (51 of 173) of patients with clusters of at least five microcalcifications without palpable findings showed malignancy; 56% of the lesions were noninfiltrating, and 37% were invasive ductal carcinoma. Solin and associates,[408] in a review of 1507 cases of breast cancer, noted that mammographic needle localization breast biopsy increased from 3% in 1977 to 1978 to 26% (111 of 421) in 1987 to 1988. The incidence of intraductal carcinoma referred for breast conservation therapy rose from 6% (two of 32) to 13% (53 of 421).

The average sensitivity of mammography is about 90%, and the specificity is 94% with wide ranges (sensitivity of 60% to 95% and specificity of 50% to 98%). The positive predictive value is approximately 8% to 14% for screened patients, but is significantly higher for patients with symptoms or palpable masses.[219] If microcalcifications were initially present, posttylectomy mammography is important to rule out residual disease for patients considering breast conservation therapy.

Ultrasonography has a reported sensitivity of 73% and a specificity of 95%.[404] However, to achieve this level of accuracy a high degree of expertise and dedication to the interpretation of the test are required.[404] Major disadvantages of ultrasonography are its inability to image microcalcifications and great difficulty in imaging lesions less than 1 cm in diameter. Medullary cancer, with its frequently sharp margins, may simulate a benign fibroadenoma. In addition, fatty breast tissue is poorly examined because of its high echogenicity.[487]

Transillumination, the use of infrared or near-infrared light as a possible screening test for breast disease, was evaluated. The sensitivity of the test is generally low because of inability to detect small or deep tumors. Monsees and associates[288,289] reported a 58% sensitivity, and Gisuold and coworkers[152] reported 67%, whereas others reported higher figures (85% to 88%).[99,475]

Thermography has been shown to have no significant value for either screening or diagnosis of breast disease because of its low sensitivity and specificity.[485]

Magnetic resonance imaging (MRI) is being evaluated for imaging breast diseases, and some authors suggest a sensitivity and specificity comparable to those of mammography.[86,192] However, cost and availability are major deterrents at the present time. Use of gadolinium DTPA, a paramagnetic agent, increases the contrast between normal and malignant tissues. Heywang and associates[193] were able to visualize 20 small carcinomas with MRI, three of which would have been missed by non-contrast-enhanced imaging, and two carcinomas in dense breast that were not visible on mammography. Magnetic resonance spectroscopy provides information about cellular biochemical processes by measuring the concentration of energy systems and metabolism, particularly of organic phosphorus.[265] Degani and colleagues[88] studied postoperative specimens from five benign and nine malignant breast tumors and showed that the concentrations of nucleosides, triphosphates, and phosphomonoesters are consistently higher by a factor of 3 in the carcinomas than in benign lesions. The studies have been conducted *in vitro,* and there is no foreseeable clinical application.

Computed tomography has been shown to outline tumors or lymph nodes greater than 1 cm in size. The need for iodine contrast material to differentiate benign from malignant conditions, high radiation dose, cost per study, and inability to detect small lesions preclude the use of tomography as a screening method.

Bone scan is frequently used to evaluate asymptomatic bony metastases. In patients with Stage I disease, the incidence of abnormal bone scan is about 2%, but a significantly greater incidence of abnormalities is found in Stage II (20%) and Stage III (over 30%).[48,66] Of over 20,000 women operated on for breast cancer in Denmark,[438] 7604 had a bone scan; of these about 5% had abnormal studies. The incidence of abnormal scans was greater in patients over 60 years (8%) than in the younger age group (3%), most likely because of the many benign bone disorders frequently seen in older women. Routine bone scan at the time of initial treatment of Stage I and Stage II breast cancer is of limited value and should be reserved for those patients with bone pain.[361,437]

Lymphoscintigraphy, a procedure in which ^{99m}Tc-labeled colloid is injected subcutaneously into the abdominal wall or into webbed spaces of the fingers, has been used to visualize the internal mammary or axillary lymph nodes, respectively. McLean and Ege[281] reported a sensitivity of 76% and a specificity of 67% in 62 patients with axillary lymphoscintigraphy when compared with the findings at axillary dissection. A very critical factor of this technique is that it indicates disease by the absence of normal tissue uptake rather than by demonstrating the disease itself.[365]

Internal mammary lymphoscintigraphy in patients treated with irradiation has been advocated on the basis that 15% of the patients demonstrate cross-drainage between parasternal lymphatics, and in 30% of the patients parasternal lymph nodes have been shown to lie outside typical radiation therapy portals.[107] Ege and Clark[108] reported on 524 patients with carcinoma of the breast treated with partial mastectomy and irradiation, who had internal mammary lymphoscintigraphy. The authors observed a statistically significant difference in actuarial survival rates in patients with normal and abnormal scanning of internal mammary lymph nodes. Bourgeois and associates[41] also suggested using postoperative lymphoscintigraphy of axillary lymph nodes. In 313 patients who had undergone a radical mastectomy with axillary dissection, they noted that only 36% had total absence of visualization of residual nodes. They observed that patients showing interruption of the lymphatic pathways of the arm had a greater incidence of upper extremity edema. However, in the United States this test has not gained significant popularity.

Pathologic Studies

Histopathologic diagnosis may be done by fine-needle aspirations of cystic or solid masses or biopsies of solid masses. Any fluid aspirated from the breast should be examined for malignant cells. Fine-needle aspiration of the breast is a simple, low-cost, accurate diagnostic technique that has been used for many years in Europe, particularly Sweden, for diagnosis and pretreatment evaluation of breast cancer.[495,496] This technique is gaining increasing acceptance in the United States.[31,476,487] Many centers are currrently performing fine-needle aspiration using a special stereotactically guided mammography device.

Breast biopsy of any suspicious mass is extremely important. In nonpalpable lesions needle localization and radiographic techniques are necessary to identify the tissue to be removed. Although a one-stage procedure (frozen section and mastectomy) was advocated in the past, in recent years a two-step approach has gained wide acceptance, in many instances because of patient preference. If conservation breast surgery is considered, the surgeon must have as much knowledge of the nature of the mass as possible, because if malignancy is suspected a wide local excision with adequate margins should ideally be carried out.

The surgeon should prepare the specimen accordingly, and the margins of the resected breast tissue should be inked.

The pathologist should be made aware of the nature of the lesion, for appropriate handling of the specimen. The biopsy usually can be done under local anesthesia; the patient can be informed as to the nature of the lesion to allow for her greater participation in therapeutic decisions. No evidence exists that delay in treatment of up to 2 weeks following biopsy causes any significant worsening of prognosis.[119] Radiation oncologists should be aware of the implications of the diagnostic procedures for carcinoma of the breast if they are active participants in a breast preservation therapeutic approach.

Estrogen and progesterone receptor assays are routinely done in the United States in patients with breast cancer, because these parameters not only have been correlated with prognosis but also with response to chemotherapeutic and hormonal agents.[259,277,489] Immunohistochemical techniques have been developed for qualitative (not quantitative) estrogen and progesterone receptor assessment if no fresh tissue is available.

Growth fraction cellular assays measure the S phase (growth fraction) of tumors, either by thymidine labeling index (TLI) or flow cytometry methods.[284,285] The growth fraction assay is a stage-independent prognostic variable and is also hormonal receptor-independent.

STAGING SYSTEMS

There are three widely used staging systems for breast cancer: the American Joint Committee (AJC),[28] the Union Internationale contre le Cancer (UICC),[450] and the Columbia System[163] (Tables 42-4 and 42-5). Figure 42-7 depicts the various clinical stages according to T and N characteristics.

PATHOLOGIC CLASSIFICATION

The World Health Organization (WHO)[375] classified proliferative conditions and tumors of the breast into the following categories: benign mammary dysplasias, benign or apparently benign tumors, carcinoma, sarcoma, carcinosarcoma, and unclassified tumors.

The American Joint Committee on Cancer[28] has developed an alternate system of histologic typing of breast tumors, shown in Table 42-6.

Numerous detailed reports and monographs describe the pathologic features and clinical implications of carcinoma of the breast. For a concise review the reader is referred to publications

TABLE 42–4
AJC Definition of TNM

PRIMARY TUMOR (T)

Definitions for classifying the primary tumor (T) are the same for clinical and for pathologic classification. If the measurement is made by physical examination, the examiner will use the major headings (T1, T2, or T3). If other measurements, such as mammographic or pathologic, are used, the telescoped subsets of T2 can be used.

TX		Primary tumor cannot be assessed
T0		No evidence of primary tumor
Tis*		Carcinoma *in situ*: Intraductal carcinoma, lobular carcinoma *in situ*, or Paget's disease of the nipple with no tumor
T1		Tumor 2 cm or less in greatest dimension
	T1a	0.5 cm or less in greatest dimension
	T1b	More than 0.5 cm but not more than 1 cm in greatest dimension
	T1c	More than 1 cm but not more than 2 cm in greatest dimension
T2		Tumor more than 2 cm but not more than 5 cm in greatest dimension
T3		Tumor more than 5 cm in greatest dimension
T4†		Tumor of any size with direct extension to chest wall or skin
	T4a	Extension to chest wall
	T4b	Edema (including *peau d'orange*) or ulceration of the skin of the breast or satellite skin nodules confined to the same breast
	T4c	Both (T4a and T4b)
	T4d	Inflammatory carcinoma

REGIONAL LYMPH NODES (N)

NX	Regional lymph nodes cannot be assessed (*e.g.*, previously removed)
N0	No regional lymph node metastasis
N1	Metastasis to movable ipsilateral axillary lymph node(s)
N2	Metastasis to ipsilateral axillary lymph node(s) fixed to one another or to other structures
N3	Metastasis to ipsilateral internal mammary lymph node(s)

PATHOLOGIC CLASSIFICATION (pN)

pNX			Regional lymph nodes cannot be assessed (*e.g.*, previously removed or not removed for pathologic study)
pN0			No regional lymph node metastasis
pN1			Metastasis to movable ipsilateral axillary lymph node(s)
	pN1a		Only micrometastasis (none larger than 0.2 cm)
	pN1b		Metastasis to lymph node(s), any larger than 0.2 cm
		pN1bi	Metastasis in 1 to 3 lymph nodes, any more than 0.2 cm and all less than 2 cm in greatest dimension
		pN1bii	Metastasis to 4 or more lymph nodes, any more than 0.2 cm and all less than 2 cm in greatest dimension
		pN1biii	Extension of tumor beyond the capsule of a lymph node metastasis less than 2 cm in greatest dimension
		pN1biv	Metastasis to a lymph node 2 cm or more in greatest dimension
	pN2		Metastasis to ipsilateral axillary lymph nodes that are fixed to one another or to other structures
	pN3		Metastasis to ipsilateral internal mammary lymph node(s)

DISTANT METASTASIS (M)

MX	Presence of distant metastasis cannot be assessed
M0	No distant metastasis
M1	Distant metastasis (includes metastasis to ipsilateral supraclavicular lymph node[s])

** Paget's disease associated with a tumor is classified according to the size of the tumor.*
† Chest wall includes ribs, intercostal muscles, and serratus anterior muscle but not pectoral muscle.
(Beahrs OH, Henson DE, Hutter RWP, Myers MH [eds]: Manual for Staging of Cancer, 3rd ed. Philadelphia, JB Lippincott, 1988)

TABLE 42–5
Carcinoma of the Breast: The Columbia Clinical Classification

Stage A: No skin edema, ulceration, or solid fixation of tumor to chest wall
Axillary nodes not clinically involved

Stage B: No skin edema, ulceration, or solid fixation of tumor to chest wall
Clinically involved nodes, but less than 2.5 cm in transverse diameter and not fixed to overlying skin or deeper structures of axilla

Stage C: Any one of five grave signs of advanced breast carcinoma
1. Edema of skin of limited extent (involving less than one-third of the skin over the breast)
2. Skin ulceration
3. Solid fixation of tumor to chest wall
4. Massive involvement of axillary lymph nodes (measuring 2.5 cm or more in transverse diameter)
5. Fixation of the axillary nodes to overlying skin or deeper structures of axilla

Stage D: All other patients with more advanced breast carcinoma, including
1. A combination of any two or more of the five grave signs listed under Stage C
2. Extensive edema of skin (involving more than one third of the skin over the breast)
3. Satellite skin nodules
4. The inflammatory type of carcinoma
5. Clinically involved supraclavicular lymph nodes
6. Internal mammary metastases as evidenced by a parasternal tumor
7. Edema of the arm
8. Distant metastases

(Haagensen CD: Disease of the Breast, 2nd ed. Philadelphia, WB Saunders, 1971)

by Fisher and associates[128, 129] and by Rosen.[350] The radiation oncologist should be familiar with the histologic characteristics of carcinoma of the breast, because many of them affect prognosis and may have important therapeutic implications.

Brief descriptions of several varieties of carcinoma of the breast follow:

Intraductal carcinoma (IDC) is a noninvasive lesion with a probability of recurrence or progression to invasive ductal carcinoma within 10 years in about 30% to 35% of patients if treated by biopsy alone.[114] The term "invasive intraductal carcinoma" is contradictory and should be avoided.

In describing the different histologic types of noninvasive ductal breast cancer, some disagreement is noted. For example, some investigators consider solid intraductal carcinoma to represent an earlier form of comedocarcinoma. Others note a higher incidence of high nuclear grade and microinvasion with comedocarcinoma than with the solid subtype, supporting each histology as distinct.[316] Papillary and micropapillary intraductal carcinoma are distinct entities, with the former having invaginations of a fibrovascular core within the lumen of the duct that are completely absent in the micropapillary histology. Cribriform intraductal carcinoma is histologically distinctive, with a sieve or "Swiss cheese" appearance within the lumen of the duct. Table 42-7 lists the various types of intraductal carcinomas and some important pathologic features.

General statements can be made regarding the biologic behavior of two subtypes of intraductal breast cancer: Comedo-intraductal carcinoma is more likely to have a higher nuclear grade,[233, 316] higher thymidine labeling index,[284] foci of microinvasion,[233, 316] and possibly a higher local recurrence rate after tylectomy alone [233, 400]; and micropapillary intraductal carcinoma is more likely to be multicentric or diffuse throughout a significant portion of the breast.[182]

Lobular carcinoma in situ (LCIS) is a noninvasive proliferation of abnormal epithelial cells in the lobules of the breast. The cells are large, with indistinct borders and round nuclei; mitoses are rarely seen. Because the lobules of the breast atrophy after menopause, LCIS is primarily a premenopausal incidental finding; most are nonpalpable and mammographically silent.

Infiltrating ductal carcinoma is the most common type of breast cancer, comprising more than 50% of all cases. It appears as solid cords or groups of tumor cells varying in size and cytoplasmic content.[128] Necrosis is rare, but lymphatic invasion may be present. An *in situ* component is frequently seen.

Tubular carcinoma is composed of tubular structures typically lined by a single layer of well-differentiated epithelium. The tubular cells simulate those of normal ducts or ductules.[55] These tumors have tubular elements arranged in

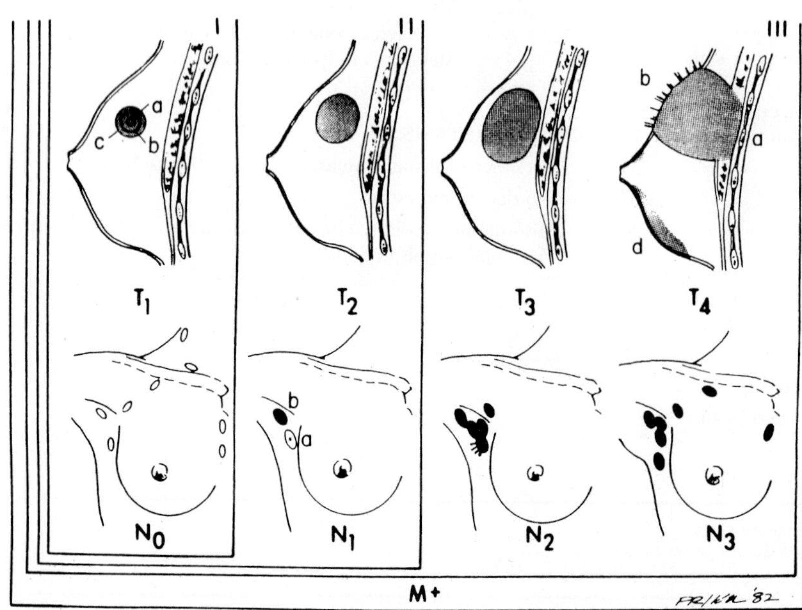

FIGURE 42–7. Clinical staging of carcinoma of the breast. Stages in part reflect curability by locoregional modes of surgery and radiation therapy. The equivalence of T and N categories prognostically are T2 = N1, T3 = N2, T4 = N3. AJC[28] and UICC[450] use similar categories and stages. (Modified from AJC, UICC, Rubin P [ed]: Clinical Oncology: A Multidisciplinary Approach, 6th ed. New York, American Cancer Society, 1983; courtesy of Philip Rubin, M.D.)

TABLE 42–6
AJC Histopathologic Classification of Breast Tumors

Cancer, NOS
Ductal
- Intraductal (*in situ*)
- Invasive with predominant intraductal component
- Invasive, NOS
- Comedo
- Inflammatory
- Medullary with lymphocytic infiltrate
- Mucinous (colloid)
- Papillary
- Scirrhous
- Tubular
- Other

Lobular
- *In situ*
- Invasive with predominant *in situ* component
- Invasive

Nipple
- Paget's disease, NOS
- Paget's disease with intraductal carcinoma
- Paget's disease with invasive ductal carcinoma

Other

NOS: not otherwise specified
(Beahrs OH, Henson DE, Hutter RWP, Myers MH [eds]: Manual for Staging of Cancer, 3rd ed. Philadelphia, JB Lippincott, 1988)

multiglandular cribriform or adenocystic configurations and are frequently associated with other *in situ* carcinomas of the breast[276]; perineural invasion may be seen. Tubular tumors have a nonaggressive growth pattern; axillary lymph node involvement is reported in about 10% of the patients.

Medullary carcinomas are composed of cords and masses of large cells with reticular pleomorphic nuclei containing prominent nucleoli. There is a scant fibrous stroma, but lymphoid infiltrate is prominent. These tumors are microscopically and grossly well circumscribed. Prognosis, in general, is better than for other tumors.

Lobular invasive carcinomas may be interspersed with lobular carcinomas *in situ*; the cells appear to be solitary or in small clusters in a targetoid or Indian file pattern. Some scirrhous carcinomas probably are invasive lobular lesions; these tumors tend to be aggressive and multicentric and are likely to develop distant metastases. du Toit and coworkers[100] reported five subtypes of lobular carcinomas in 171 cases and observed a 12-year actuarial survival rate of 100% for the tubulolobular subtype and only 47% for the solid variant. The other three subtypes had intermediate prognoses.

Mucinous carcinoma, also called mucoid or colloid carcinoma, has been observed in older women with relatively long duration of symptoms.[398] It is slow-growing with a pushing border and has a low incidence of axillary lymph node metastasis.[398] This tumor has a greater likelihood of being devoid of a cellular reaction; necrosis and lymphatic invasion are rare. Survival is appreciably better than with infiltrating ductal carcinoma.[306]

Adenocystic carcinoma is rarely found in the breast. Histologic features and clinical behavior are similar to its counterparts in the salivary gland and the upper respiratory tract.

Papillary carcinoma is a rare neoplasm, histologically characterized by frond-like projections with fibrous supporting stalks. Its delicate or nonexisting fibrovascular cord, nuclear hyperchromatism, and absence of double layer of cells and apocrine changes distinguish papillary carcinoma from intraductal papillomas.[221] These lesions have a low incidence of invasion and metastasis to the regional lymph nodes.

Paget's disease describes involvement of the nipple by tumor. Most investigators agree that it represents extensions of neoplasms from subjacent ducts in the nipple[204] or metastases from an underlying carcinoma.[61,297] The tumor seems to travel linearly down the ducts and may appear to be multicentric. There may be an associated subareolar tumor.

Carcinosarcoma is a rare tumor, characterized by nodular, circumscribed, or irregular masses without encapsulation. Squamous differentiation with carcinoma was noted in 15 of 70 tumors reported by Wargotz and Norris.[478] The sarcoma was predominantly polymorphous tumor, frequently resembling malignant fibrous histiocytoma in 40 and fibrosarcomatous neoplasias in 28. Cellularity of the sarcoma component was high (97%). Thirteen (26%) of 50 patients had axillary lymph node metastasis. Only one of 11 patients had hormonal receptors. The 5-year survival rate was 49% for those with carcinosarcoma compared with 64% for those with spindle cell carcinoma.

Cystosarcoma phyllodes was named in 1838 by James Muller who emphasized its benign nature. Within broad fibrous "leaf-like" beads, cystic clefts are lined by a single layer of cells. These tumors are large, usually encapsulated, without invasion of the adjacent breast. The lesions frequently develop from preexisting fibromas and have a long initial period of slow growth followed by sudden, rapidly increas-

TABLE 42–7
Histologic Types of Intraductal Breast Cancer: Frequency of Pathologic Features

	NUMBER (%)	HIGH NUCLEAR GRADE (%)	MICRO-INVASION (%)	MEAN NO. OF DUCTS INVOLVED	MULTI-CENTRICITY (%)
Comedo	19 (35)	17 (89)	12 (63)	78	7 (37)
Papillary	15 (27)	1 (7)	1 (7)	112	6 (40)
Micropapillary	10 (18)	2 (20)	3 (30)	198	8 (80)
Cribriform	6 (11)	0 (0)	0 (0)		
Solid	5 (9)	0 (0)	0 (0)	20	3 (27)
Total	55	20 (38)	16 (29)	98	24 (44)

(Patchefsky AS, Schwartz GF, Finkelstein SD, et al: Cancer 63:731–741, 1989)

ing size. The grade (mitotic rate) and surgical margins have prognostic importance; El-Naggar and colleagues[109] performed DNA analysis in 30 cystosarcoma phyllodes and concluded that DNA ploidy, proliferative index, number of mitoses, and tumor margin were significantly associated with prognosis. Several authors have reported a few cases in which these tumors metastasized to the other breast, axillary lymph nodes, mediastinum, and lungs. In a report by Treves and Sunderland,[446] 18 lesions in 77 patients were classified as malignant, 18 as borderline, and 41 as benign. Nine of the patients with malignant tumors developed distant metastases.

Other unusual tumors occassionally described in the breast are sarcomas, pure squamous cell carcinoma, basal cell carcinoma, and malignant lymphoma.

PROGNOSTIC FACTORS

The prognostic factors influencing local relapse and survival can be divided into intrinsic, related to the characteristics of the tumor (*e.g.*, histologic features, lymph node metastases), and extrinsic (*e.g.*, host factors, type and adequacy of treatment).

Intrinsic Prognostic Factors

Involvement of Axillary Nodes by Tumor

Haagensen[165] and Valagussa and associates[455] demonstrated a direct relation between the number of involved axillary nodes and chest wall recurrence and an inverse relation between number of lymph nodes involved and survival of patients treated with radical mastectomy or treated with modified radical mastectomy.

Valagussa and associates[455] also noted that patients who had involved internal mammary nodes had more recurrences than those who did not (10-year relapse rate in patients with negative axillary nodes, 27.9%; in patients with negative axillary nodes and involved internal mammary nodes, 60%). The Primary Therapy of Breast Cancer Study Group[329] and others[108, 124, 356, 385, 444, 493] confirm these findings. Fisher and associates[127] described diminishing survival after mastectomy with a greater number of metastatic axillary lymph nodes.[121] Lash and colleagues[238] described lower survival rates and a greater incidence of local recurrences in patients with positive axillary nodes after partial mastectomy. A study from the Institut Gustave-Roussy[373] of 356 patients treated with conservation surgery plus irradiation (BCT) noted that local recurrence developed in 26% of patients with involved nodes compared with 6.5% of patients without nodal involvement; the greater the number of nodes involved, the more likely the occurrence of local failures and the lower the survival rate.[97] Increased incidence of breast relapses was also reported by van Limbergen and colleagues[460] in patients with N1b (eight of 42, or 19%) or when three or more lymph nodes were positive or the apical axillary lymph nodes contained metastatic tumor (four of 14, or 28.6%) compared with those with N0 or N1a lymph nodes (14 of 187, or 7.5%).

Tumor Size (Stage)

In a few series of breast conservation therapy, a correlation was noted between the size of the tumor and the incidence of local recurrence, whereas this observation is not reported by other authors (Table 42-8).[85] This is probably related to the treatment techniques (completeness of tumor excision, radiation boost). In general, patients with Stage T1 tumors have better disease-free and overall survival than patients with Stage T2 tumors.

Diffuse, infiltrating tumors have a higher incidence of local recurrence than localized tumors. In patients treated with mastectomy, analysis of skin changes (edema, erythema, and ulceration of the breast) showed that only edema was statistically significant for increased local recurrence.[97]

Presence of Multiple Primary Tumors (Multicentricity)

In 657 mastectomy specimens, Gump and associates[161] noted multifocal disease in 19% of patients with invasive ductal carcinoma, compared with 81% of 42 patients with intraductal carcinoma and 50% of 92 patients with invasive lobular carcinoma. Although in invasive ductal carcinoma, tumor multicentricity was related to size (12% in lesions <2 cm and 23% in tumors >2 cm), this was not observed in invasive lobular carcinoma, in which the corresponding multicentricity values were 54% and 45%.

Leopold and associates[239] reported on four of ten patients with failure of two or more separate breast cancers after conservation surgery and irradiation compared with 11% failures in 707 patients with single lesions ($P = 0.02$). Six of eight patients in this group had extensive intraductal component compared with 33% incidence in patients with solitary lesions. Therefore the use of conservation therapy in patients with more than one primary lesion should be considered with caution.

Histologic Features and Tumor Grade

Incidence of local recurrence was greater and survival decreased with undifferentiation and necrosis of the tumor, higher nuclear grade, vascular invasion, and inflammatory infiltrate.[97, 111]

TABLE 42–8
Conservation Surgery and Irradiation in Breast Cancer: Local Recurrence According to Initial Tumor Stage

	LOCAL RECURRENCE	
AUTHOR	STAGE T1 or I	STAGE T2 or II
Amalric[2]	21% (62)*	20% (60)
Barr[22]	12% (101)	12% (255)
Bartelink[23]	2% (360)	2% (197)
Calle[51]	7% (190)	11% (113)
Clarke[72]	6% (305)	3% (95)
Delouche[90]	6% (220)	14% (190)
Dubois[101]	10.8% (231)	16.1% (161)
Fisher, NSABP[126]	7% (298)	10% (256)
Kuske[230]	4.7% (235)	7% (159)
Leung[240]	7.4% (158)	12.8% (335)
Montague[291]	7% (94)	5% (78)
Solin[409]	5% (217)	8% (166)
Stotter[420]	10% (249)	12% (241)
van Limbergen[460]	5% (57)	11.5% (104)
Veronesi[466]	4% (701)	—

* *Total number of patients in study in parentheses*

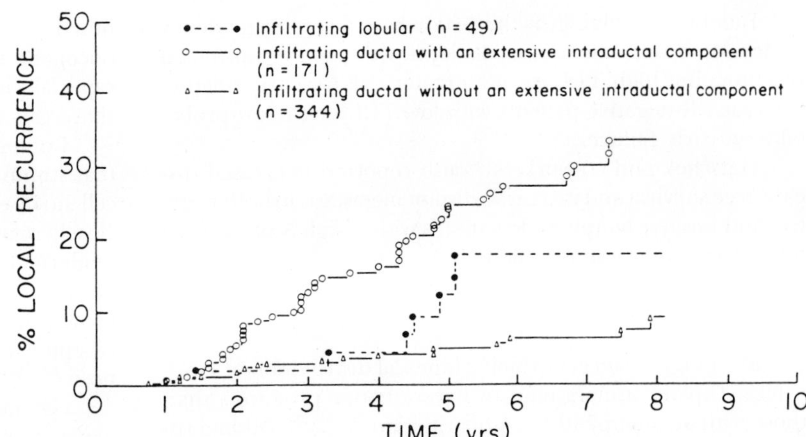

FIGURE 42–8. Actuarial local recurrence curves for patients with infiltrating lobular carcinoma, infiltrating ductal carcinoma with extensive intraductal component, and infiltrating ductal carcinoma without extensive intraductal component. (Schnitt SJ, Connally JL, Recht A, et al: Cancer 64:448, 1989)

Schnitt and associates[383] compared the results of tumor excision and irradiation in 49 patients with infiltrating lobular Stage I and Stage II carcinoma and 561 patients with similar stages of infiltrating ductal carcinoma. The 5-year actuarial risk of local recurrence was similar for both groups (12% *versus* 11%). The 12% local recurrence rate for infiltrating lobular carcinoma was between that for infiltrating ductal carcinoma with or without an extensive intraductal component (23% and 5%, respectively; Fig. 42-8). The patterns of recurrence in the breast were similar in the infiltrating lobular and ductal carcinoma patients; 80% occurred in the vicinity of the primary tumor. The conclusion was that the combination of conservation surgery and irradiation is a reasonable treatment option for patients with infiltrating lobular carcinoma, contrary to previous reports that emphasized the multicentric nature of lobular carcinoma.[130,340]

Extensive Intraductal Carcinoma

Extensive intraductal carcinoma (EIC) involving the primary tumor and adjacent tissues has been reported by some groups, particularly Harvard University[178,384] and Marseilles,[226] to be associated with a high incidence of breast recurrences.

In contrast to the above-mentioned experience, Clarke and associates,[72] Fisher and colleagues,[132] and van Limbergen and co-workers[460] found no significant impact on local tumor control with extensive intraductal extension. This may be related to the pathologic criteria used in the definition of extensive intraductal carcinoma and the adequacy of tumor excision. According to the Harvard definition of EIC, 25% or more of the primary tumor mass is intraductal carcinoma and intraductal carcinoma is seen outside (adjacent to) the infiltrating border.

Fourquet and associates[139] reported a 20% incidence of extensive intraductal component in 185 women under 45 years of age compared with 10.4% in 279 older women. As suggested by Kurtz and colleagues,[225] these two prognostic parameters may be interdependent.

Recently Holland and associates[198] stated that an extensive intraductal component is highly associated with subsequent breast recurrence because of the presence of residual intraductal carcinoma in these patients. In a series of 214 women who underwent mastectomy, 71% of those with extensive intraductal component had residual intraductal carcinoma compared with 28% of those without that pathologic feature (Fig. 42-9). In particular, 44% of EIC-positive patients had prominent residual tumor compared with 3% of those with EIC negative ($P < 0.00001$). Carefully assessed negative surgical margins and adequate irradiation may decrease or eliminate the significance of EIC for local failure.

Thymidine Labeling Index

Meyer and co-workers[284] demonstrated a significant correlation of thymidine labeling index (TLI) with survival in 278 primary breast cancer patients. TLIs below the median of 4.55% carried a 20% probability of relapse at 4 years, in contrast to 52% with TLI above the median. The probability of relapse significantly correlated with the TLI, independent of tumor stage, axillary lymph node status alone, estrogen receptor (ER) content, or menopausal status. In another study[449] it was reported that the higher the TLI, the shorter the intervals from initial treatment to first relapse or from first relapse to death. Also, the proportion of relapses was smaller in patients with a low TLI. These findings were confirmed by Tubiana and co-workers[448] in 128 patients with breast cancer followed up for more than 15 years; significantly improved disease-free survival and overall survival was observed in patients with TLI index less than 0.25, compared with those with higher values.

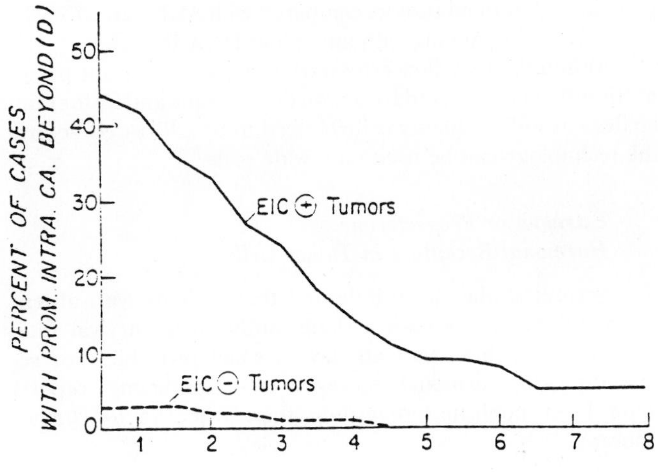

FIGURE 42–9. Percentage of mastectomy cases with prominent (≥ 6 LPF) intraductal carcinoma at or beyond certain distances (D) from edge of primary tumor (at 0.5 cm intervals). Wilcoxon test of amount of intraductal carcinoma in EIC+ cases *versus* EIC− cases at or beyond 2 cm from edge of tumor, $P = 1 \times 10^{-8}$; at or beyond 4 cm, $P = 5 \times 10^{-8}$. EIC: extensive intraductal carcinoma (Holland R, Connally JL, Gelman R, et al: J Clin Oncol 8:113–118, 1990)

Patients with high growth fraction have a greater tendency to develop distant metastases. Patients with positive hormonal receptors but high TLI are at a greater risk for early relapse, whereas ER-negative patients with low TLI have a low probability of early failure.

Hatschek and co-workers[183] also reported decreased disease-free survival and increased distant metastasis in both negative and positive lymph node patients with a high S-phase fraction on cytofluorometric studies.

DNA Ploidy Index

Most breast cancers exhibit a bimodal distribution of DNA values. Diploid tumors tend to have a better prognosis than those with an aneuploid DNA distribution.[12,110,208] Diploid tumors also tend to be estrogen receptor-positive, whereas aneuploid tumors are frequently estrogen receptor-negative.[14] Older patients are more likely to have hyperdiploid tumors.[433] DNA ploidy as measured by flow cytometry correlates with nuclear grade; low-grade tumors are diploid and high-grade tumors are aneuploid.[317] Premenopausal patients with aneuploid tumors have been found to have more axillary metastases and an inferior disease-free survival than those with diploid tumors.[186]

In a study of 1331 breast tumors reported by Clark and colleagues,[67] 57% were aneuploid. The median S-phase fraction was 10.3% for aneuploid tumors compared with 2.6% for diploid lesions. Ewers and co-workers[112] assessed DNA content in over 500 primary breast cancers; 60% had aneuploid tumors. In patients with Stage I or Stage II tumors the recurrence rate for aneuploidy was twice that for the diploid group.

Toikkanen and co-workers,[442] in 351 tumors of patients followed up for a minimum of 22 years, observed a 28% 25-year survival rate for patients with nondiploid tumors in contrast to 48% for those with diploid DNA pattern.

In a report by Fallenius and associates[113] of patients with negative lymph nodes, the disease-free survival rate was 60% for aneuploid tumors compared with 90% for those with diploid DNA index. On the other hand, Keyhani-Rofagha and associates,[212] in 165 node-negative adenocarcinomas of the breast, described 5- and 10-year survival rates of 87.8% and 73.4% in patients with diploid tumors compared with 84.1% and 75.5%, respectively, in patients with aneuploid DNA index.

Although DNA flow cytometry provides important prognostic information, standardization of technique and histogram analysis as well as quality control need to be addressed before the technology can be used on a wide scale.[309]

Estrogen or Progesterone Hormonal Receptors in Tumor Cells

Several studies have indicated that patients with absent hormonal receptors have a significantly lower survival rate. Furthermore, these patients have a small probability of responding to hormonal therapy.[277,489] Conflicting reports have been published regarding their response to chemotherapy.[214,259]

Oncogenes

Abnormal DNA content may be a gross indicator of a tumor genome characterized by rearranged, amplified, or deleted genetic sequences.[309] Several oncogenes, including HER-2 (also called c-erb B-2 or neu), probably code for a surface membrane receptor that interacts with an unidentified growth factor. Amplification or overexpression of this gene has been noted in breast cancer tissue. Several studies suggest that this oncogene is an important prognostic factor in breast cancer, especially in patients with positive nodes, whereas others do not share this view.[403,458]

Epidermal growth factor (EGF) is a polypeptide hormone that stimulates cell proliferation through specific binding to a cell surface receptor. Many oncogenes have been found to be closely related to known growth factors or their receptors, and epidermal growth factor receptor is homologous to a known oncogene (c-erb B-1). The epidermal growth factor receptor content in breast cancer tissue is inversely related to estrogen receptor content and may be a predictor of poor prognosis.[320,367]

Garcia and associates[148] reported amplification of the c-myc gene in 18% of 125 primary breast cancers and reported a significant association of this gene's amplification with inflammatory carcinoma. The c-erb B-2 gene was amplified in 22% of the tumors, and this alteration was significantly linked to histologic grade 3 tumors and absence of estrogen and progesterone receptors. Heintz and colleagues[187] reported amplification of the c-erb B-2 oncogene in 17 of 50 patients (34%) with infiltrating ductal carcinoma. However, the gene amplification was not significantly correlated with the presence of estrogen and progesterone receptors, survival, recurrence, and metastasis rates.

In contrast, Thor and associates,[439] in a study of a c-erb B-2 oncogene expression in 313 patients treated for carcinoma of the breast, described a significant correlation between the amplification of the oncogene and status of estrogen receptors, lymph node status, and survival. In patients with strongly reactive tumors the 6-year survival rate was 0% compared with 55% in those with negative to weakly reactive tumors.

Cathepsin D Assay

Cathepsin D is an estrogen-induced lysosomal protease that is secreted in excess by breast cancer cells and is under the influence of estrogen regulation. Although the cathepsin D level has been found to be very low or negligible in normal breast tissue, it is elevated in both benign and malignant ductal proliferative diseases of the breast. Thorpe and associates[440] found cathepsin D levels to be an independent prognostic factor for disease-free survival with about the same importance as lymph node status for both menopausal groups; patients with elevated cathepsin D levels had a shorter disease-free survival and a trend toward shorter overall survival. Tanon and colleagues[431] found in a multivariate analysis that the presence of high levels of cathepsin D was the most important independent prognostic factor in node-negative breast cancer. Spyratos and co-workers[416] also found that the predictive value of cathepsin D was greater in axillary lymph node-negative patients than in node-positive patients. These studies, however, used an ELISA or Western blot technique, which in association with the tumor included inflammatory cells that also contain cathepsin D. Later, Henry and associates[190] studied cathepsin D using an immunohistochemical staining technique, which may be more specific to tumor cells. The authors found an opposite prognostic impact, with a significant trend toward increase in overall disease-free and absolute survival when cathespin D values were elevated in node-positive but not node-negative patients.

Extrinsic Prognostic Factors

Although the most important parameters in determining prognosis and patterns of failure are the intrinsic factors, extrinsic (host) factors and adequacy of treatment are also relevant.

TABLE 42–9
Young Age as Risk Factor for Breast Recurrence

	LOCAL RECURRENCES	
SOURCE	YOUNGER THAN 40 YEARS	40 YEARS OR OLDER
Curie[471]	11/79 (14%)	7/235 (3%)
Charlebourg[90]	14/71 (19.7%)	26/239 (7.9%)
Villejuif[72]*	3/29 (10.3%)	21/403 (5.2%)
Harvard[335]*	47 (26%)†	560 (10%)†
van Limbergen[460]	— (21.3)†	— (5% to 10%)†
Marseille[227]	41/210 (19.5%)	106/1172 (9%)
Solin[411]	8/88 (9%)	65/808 (8%)

** Threshold at 35 years*
† 5-year actuarial calculation
(Kurtz JM, Spitalier JM, Amalric R, et al: Int J Radiat Oncol Biol Phys 15:271, 1988)

Age

Young age may be a risk factor for breast recurrence in conservation surgery and irradiation. Different investigators have used various age cutoffs such as 50, 40, 35, and 30 years. Vilcoq and co-workers[471] found a locoregional recurrence rate of 35% and 4% in women under and over 30 years, respectively.

Kurtz and associates[227] reported 19% incidence of local recurrence in 210 women under 40 years old compared with 9% in 1172 older women. This observation correlated with the presence of EIC, high tumor grade, and a major mononuclear cell reaction. The Harvard University Joint Center's inferior results in younger women also correlated with the presence of EIC.[336] These findings have been reported by other authors (Table 42-9).[72,90,460,471]

Pregnancy

Although in the past it was thought that pregnancy after the diagnosis of breast cancer was associated with a worse prognosis, recent evidence suggests the contrary.[202] Some physicians recommend that patients not consider pregnancy for the first 3 years following treatment, because this is the period of the highest probability of recurrence.

Multivariate Analysis of Prognostic Factors

Zafrani and associates,[494] in 434 patients with infiltrating ductal carcinoma treated with limited surgery and irradiation, found that incomplete surgical excision, lymphatic invasion, and the presence of an extensive *in situ* component were pathologic predictors of local breast recurrence. The corresponding predictors of survival were the three features just mentioned in addition to size of the primary tumor and histologic high grade of the tumor. Tables 42-10 and 42-11 summarize the differences in breast local tumor control and survival for the various predictive parameters.

Locker and associates,[261] in an analysis of 263 patients treated with local excision and irradiation, reported that patient age, axillary nodal status, tumor size, definite vascular invasion, adjacent intraductal carcinoma, and histologic grade were independent predictors of local recurrence.

Toikkanen and co-workers,[442] in 351 patients with breast cancer, reported independent prognostic factors for survival to be axillary lymph node status, tumor size, histologic tumor grade, extent of tumor necrosis, histologic type, and type of tumor margin (defined or diffuse).

Kurtz and co-workers,[225] in 496 patients with Stages I or II infiltrating ductal carcinoma treated with breast conservation therapy (BCT), identified extensive intraductal component, tumor histologic grade, and mononuclear cell reaction as significant prognostic factors in Cox multivariate analysis.

Analysis by Epstein and associates[111] of 438 patients with infiltrating ductal carcinoma treated with conservation surgery and irradiation showed that the predictors of distant relapse were comparable to those reported in patients treated with radical mastectomy.

Survival in Untreated Breast Cancer

A classic paper by Bloom and associates[36] outlined the natural history of breast cancer in 356 patients seen between 1805 and 1933, not treated by surgery or irradiation, 250 of whom had pathologic diagnosis of cancer. No patients had Stage I disease, 2.4% had Stage II disease, 23% had Stage III disease, and 74% had Stage IV disease (Manchester system).[318] The survival of the untreated group was compared with that of a later group of patients treated with radical or modified radical mastectomy

TABLE 42–10
Pathologic Factors Influencing Local Breast Tumor Control

	NO. OF PATIENTS*	NO. OF BR	10-YEAR LCB RATE†	*P* VALUE‡
Adequacy of Surgical Excision				
Incomplete	59	15	76%	<0.0001
Complete	374	31	91%	
Lymphatic Invasion				
Present	25	6	74%	<0.02
Absent	401	39	90%	
DCIS Component				
Extensive	63	12	77%	= 0.03
Nonextensive	361	33	95%	

BR: breast recurrence; LCB: local control in the breast
** Because this study was retrospective, complete pathologic analysis could not be performed for all patients.*
† Kaplan-Meier estimates
‡ Log-rank test
(Zafrani B, Vielh P, Fourquet A, et al: Eur J Cancer Clin Oncol 25:1645, 1989)

TABLE 42–11
Pathologic Factors in Breast Cancer Influencing Survival

	NO. OF PATIENTS*	NO. OF DEATHS	10-YEAR SURVIVAL RATE†	*P* VALUE‡
Adequacy of Surgical Excision				
Incomplete	59	16	75%	<0.007
Complete	374	43	88%	
Lymphatic Invasion				
Present	25	12	60%	< 0.0001
Absent	401	45	89%	
Intraductal Cancer Component				
Absent	166	31	79%	< 0.008
Present	258	27	90%	
Tumor Size				
>1 cm	193	26	83%	<0.03
≤1 cm	121	7	95%	
Histologic grade				
I	104	4	98%	
II	250	39	84%	<0.005
III	33	6	79%	

** Because this study was retrospective, complete pathologic analysis could not be performed for all patients.*
† Kaplan-Meier estimates
‡ Log-rank test
(Zafrani B, Vielh P, Fourquet A, et al: Eur J Cancer Clin Oncol 25:1645, 1989)

with or without irradiation. Bloom and co-workers reported an overall 10-year survival rate of 34% in the treated patients and 3.6% in the untreated group; survival in both groups was dependent on the histologic grade of the tumor.

GENERAL MANAGEMENT

Since the beginning of this century, based on Halsted's hypothesis of tumor spread, the predominant surgical treatment of carcinoma of the breast was a radical mastectomy (with several modifications).[119]

Halsted[173] proposed that breast cancer spreads by direct extension, rather than tumor cell embolization. Based on this premise, the wider the surgical extirpation, the greater the chance for cure. McWhirter[282,283] popularized a lesser surgical procedure (total mastectomy) in combination with radiation to the chest wall and regional lymphatics, a technique that was shown to yield results comparable to those of radical mastectomy.[120,207]

Another treatment for breast cancer that was initially described by Keynes in 1929 and 1937[213] combines conservation surgery (ranging from biopsy to wide local tumor excision to segmental mastectomy or quadrantectomy) and definitive irradiation.[3,50,179,180,241,300,321,331,471] This approach, popular in Europe since 1950, has progressively gained acceptance in the United States in the past 20 years.

Management of Intraductal Carcinoma and Lobular Carcinoma *in Situ*

Because of greater use of screening mammography, an increasing number of patients are being referred for treatment of noninvasive lesions called intraductal carcinoma or lobular carcinoma *in situ*. Several authors have reported subsequent development of invasive carcinoma of the breast in about 30% of patients who have had not had definitive treatment after initial diagnosis of intraductal carcinoma. Those with lobular carcinoma *in situ* also have a tendency to develop invasive lesions (35% to 45% in 10 to 20 years).[34,114,131,235,314,352]

Treatment for Intraductal Carcinoma

Two recent series have shown an incidence of intraductal carcinoma (IDC) of 15% to 20% in women undergoing mammography for screening.[18,461] The reported incidence of multicentricity in women with IDC is approximately 35% but depends on the sampling techniques of the pathologist. Some of the studies in the literature showed an incidence of 33% by Brown,[45] 38% by von Rueden,[473] 40% by Tinnemans,[441] 41% by Schwartz,[388] and 34% by Holland.[199]

The incidence of residual intraductal carcinoma after biopsy is high, an important consideration if local excision alone is advocated for treatment. Rosen and associates[357] observed a 57% incidence of residual DCIS after biopsy in 53 women treated with mastectomy. In reports by Wanebo[477] and Carter[56] and their colleagues, residual DCIS after biopsy were seen in 60% and 66% of mastectomy specimens, respectively. However, it is uncertain whether the surgeons attempted to obtain negative margins at the time of biopsy.

Fisher and associates[131] reported multicentricity in 27 (39.7%) of 68 patients with intraductal carcinoma treated with a total mastectomy on whom multiple random sections of all quadrants of the breast were analyzed. This material was part of a randomized study comparing segmental mastectomy alone or combined with irradiation or a total mastectomy in invasive carcinoma of the breast less than 4 cm in diameter. The majority of the patients were followed up for a minimum of 2 years; median follow-up was 5 years. Of 22 patients treated with segmental mastectomy only, five (23%) developed recurrence in contrast to two of 29 (7%) patients receiving radiation therapy after tumor excision.

Unlike lobular carcinoma *in situ*, intraductal lesions involve

TABLE 42–12
Breast Recurrence Following Wide Excision Alone for Intraductal Carcinoma

AUTHOR	PERIOD OF TREATMENT	NUMBER OF PATIENTS	DETECTION	HISTOLOGIC PATTERN	TUMOR SIZE	BREAST RECURRENCE* (% NONINVASIVE)	INTERVAL TO RECURRENCE (YEARS)	DEAD OF DISEASE
Lewis and Geschickter[253]	1918–1936	8	Mass	Comedo	50% >5 <9 cm	75% (NS)	1–4 +	0
Kraus and Neubecker[221]	Before 1961	4	Mass	Papillary	NS	50% (NS)	10 & 12	NS
Rosen et al[351]	1940–50	15	Incidental	Micropapillary	Microscopic	67% (13)	9.7	30%
Farrow[114]	1949–67	25	NS	NS	NS	20% (NS)	1–8	NS
Millis and Thynne[287]	1948–68	8	Mass	All	1–5 cm	25% (NS)	.5 & 7	0
Page et al[314]	1952–68	28	Incidental	Cribriform, micropapillary	Microscopic	25% (0)	3–10	43%
Fisher et al[131]	1976–84	22	Mass	All	2.2 cm ± 1.3 cm	23% (9)	.3–1.5	0
Lagios et al[235]	1972–80	20	Mass 20% Mammogr 65% Incidental 10%	All	8 mm median	15% (NS)	.75, 1.3†	0
Lagios et al[232]	1972–87	79	Mass 6% Mammogr 92% Incidental 1%	All	5 mm median	10% (5)	.75–7.2	0

NS: not stated
**Total breast recurrence includes invasive and noninvasive recurrence. Parentheses indicate % of all patients with noninvasive recurrence.*
† One patient recurred at .75 year, one patient at 1 year, and one at 3 years.
(Fowble B: Oncology 3:51–58, 1989)

a low risk of contralateral carcinoma of the breast. Webber and co-workers[479] showed a 3.4% risk of contralateral breast cancer with an average follow-up of 9 years (four of 116 patients). On the other hand, Kinne and associates[216] reported on 25 patients with bilateral *in situ* carcinoma of the breast. Eight of the patients developed metachronous invasive carcinoma, two with positive axillary lymph nodes, probably the result of undetected invasive carcinoma.

The ideal treatment of patients with intraductal carcinoma must be based on the natural history of the disease, extent of the tumor, and histologic features. Several reports are found in the literature of patients treated with biopsy only, with recurrences ranging from 10% in selected patients[232,235] to 75%.[221,253] Various reports are summarized in Table 42-12. In our opinion, excision alone should be offered only on protocol (NSABP B1-7, randomizing excision with negative margins alone *versus* excision plus irradiation). More effective treatment options for intraductal carcinoma are total mastectomy and, more recently, wide tumor excision followed by breast irradiation. Silverstein and associates[400] reported a 4% recurrence rate with mastectomy compared with 11% with conservation surgery and irradiation in patients with comedocarcinoma. Nonpalpable micropapillary and papillary lesions should also have treatment to the whole breast (mastectomy or BCT), whereas small cribriform or solid IDC may be treated with wide local excision and careful observation.

Intraductal cancers rarely metastasize to axillary lymph nodes. In six series totaling over 400 patients[9,56,131,216,337,399] the incidence of positive axillary lymph nodes was less than 1% (Table 42-13). Thus, only the breast needs to be addressed when considering treatment, whether mastectomy or irradiation. A possible exception would be the large or extensive intraductal cancer (*e.g.*, ≥4 cm), which is known to have a small but finite incidence of axillary spread, probably the result of pathologic sampling error (undetected invasive carcinoma). Results described with mastectomy are shown in Table 41-14.

Several reports have described satisfactory results in women treated with local excision and irradiation for intraductal cancers. At M. D. Anderson Cancer Center, of 34 consecutive patients treated with 5000 cGy radiation to the breast and 1000 cGy boost, only one recurrence was noted in the untreated ipsilateral axilla of a patient (3 to 17 years' follow-up).[291] Recht and colleagues[337] reported on 40 women with intraductal carcinoma treated with excisional biopsy and irradiation (4600 cGy

TABLE 42–13
Incidence of Axillary Lymph Node Involvement in Intraductal Carcinoma

AUTHOR	POSITIVE NODES (%)
Ashikari[9]	1/109 (1)
Carter[56]	1/31 (3)
Kinne[216]	1/128 (0.8)
NSABP[131]	0/78 (0)
Recht[337]	0/13 (0)
Silverstein[399]	0/100 (0)
Total	3/459 (0.6)

TABLE 42–14
Intraductal Carcinoma: Local Recurrence After Mastectomy

AUTHOR	NO. OF PATIENTS	% LOCAL RECURRENCES	% CANCER DEATHS (DOD)	FOLLOW-UP (YEARS)
Ashikari, 1971[9]	111	2	1	1–10
Brown, 1976[45]	40	0	0	5
Carter, 1977[56]	38	8	8	—
Farrow, 1970[114]	147	4	2	—
Fentiman, 1986[116]	82	1	1	4.7 median
Fisher, 1986[131]	28	4	3	3.2 mean
Kinne, 1989[216]	80	1	1	11.5 median
Lagios, 1982[235]	53	6	2	—
Millis, 1975[287]	20	0	0	<5 to >15
Ozzello, 1983[313]	22	5		
Rosner, 1980[359]	182	10	2	5
Schuh, 1986[386]	51	0	2	5.5 mean
Silverstein, 1987[399]	49	2	0	2.3 median
Sunshine, 1985[423]	70	4	4	>10
Temple, 1986[434]	116	0	0	7.5 mean
VonRueden, 1984[473]	47	2	0	—
Westbrook, 1975[482]	64	2	0	—

to 5000 cGy); 26 of the patients also received a boost of 1000 cGy to 2000 cGy at the primary excision site. With a follow-up ranging from 1 to 8 years, four patients had recurrences (10%). Three recurrences were subareolar and may possibly be related to incomplete excision of the tumor. They were successfully retreated with a mastectomy. All patients are well without metastases from 0 to 15 months after treatment of the recurrence.

Zafrani and associates[494] reported on 54 patients treated with local excision and irradiation with an average follow-up of 55 months; 6% had recurrences in the breast, and one patient later died of recurrent tumor.

Stotter and colleagues[421] reported a 10-year locoregional tumor control rate of 91% and a disease-specific survival rate of 96% in 44 breasts treated for intraductal carcinoma with limited surgery and irradiation. At Washington University, of 70 patients treated with BCT including irradiation, three (4.3%) developed a breast relapse in contrast to three of seven treated with wide local excision alone.[230]

Although the reported results of treating intraductal cancers with conservation surgery and breast irradiation represent limited numbers of patients and short follow-up, the incidence of local recurrence (Table 42-15) is not significantly different from that seen after mastectomy. More important, survival is comparable, and patients who have recurrences after lumpectomy and irradiation can be salvaged with a mastectomy.

Treatment for Lobular Carcinoma in Situ

Of 211 cases of lobular carcinoma *in situ* (LCIS), it was noted that 90% were in premenopausal women.[166] This lesion is almost always nonpalpable and is usually discovered incidentally after biopsy of a clinically palpable benign lesion.[426] Lobular carcinoma *in situ* has a high incidence of multicentricity ranging from 48% to 80%[32,357,387] and bilaterality ranging from 18% to 67%.[56,114,423] In Farrow's study[144] of 270 women with lobular carcinoma *in situ,* 33 women had simultaneous bilateral

TABLE 42–15
Results of Conservation Surgery and Irradiation in Intraductal Carcinoma of the Breast

	NO. OF PATIENTS	MEDIAN FOLLOW-UP (YEARS)	% LOCAL RECURRENCE	CANCER DEATHS
Fisher[131]	29	3.2*	7	0
Fowble[143]	46	2.9	4	0
Kurtz[226]	47	5	4	2
Kuske[230]	70	3.8	4	1
Montague[291]	34	5.5	3	0
Recht[337]	40	3.6	10	0
Silverstein[399]	97	2.1	8	0
Stotter[421]	42	7.6	9	4
Zafrani[493]	54	4.5	6	2

* *Mean follow-up*

LCIS, and 16 developed subsequent contralateral LCIS (bilateral disease in 18%); 70 (26%) had previous, simultaneous, or subsequent cancer.

One important issue is whether patients with LCIS subsequently develop invasive carcinoma that would warrant therapeutic intervention at initial diagnosis. Overall, 25% to 35% of women with LCIS develop invasive cancer with the risk in either breast being fairly equal, although the frequency varies in several series.[5,166,355,483] In the series from Haagensen and associates[166] of 211 untreated cases of LCIS with a mean follow-up of 14 years, overall probability of developing invasive cancer in the ipsilateral breast was 10% and in the contralateral breast, 9%. In patients followed up for 16 to 25 years, the risk of invasive cancer increased to 22% in the ipsilateral breast compared with 15% in the contralateral breast. Haagensen and associates recommended close follow-up because of the equal risk of cancer in both breasts and the long interval to the development of invasive cancer.

Confirming these findings, Rosen and colleagues[355] reported on 84 patients with LCIS with an average follow-up of 24 years after biopsy only. The incidence of subsequent invasive carcinoma in the ipsilateral breast was 14%, whereas the risk in the contralateral breast was 14%, and 8% for bilateral cancers. Overall, 36% of the patients subsequently developed invasive cancer. In contrast, in a study of 149 patients with carcinoma of the breast in whom a diagnosis of carcinoma *in situ* was confirmed, in those treated by local excision, ipsilateral cancers were subsequently seen in 12% of patients with ductal carcinoma *in situ* and in 13% of the patients with lobular carcinoma *in situ*.[435] Contralateral metachronous invasive cancers were seen in 6% of the ductal carcinoma *in situ* patients and 3% of the lobular carcinoma *in situ* patients. No lymph node involvement was seen in any of these patients, either with prophylactic dissection or in follow-up. Seventeen of 109 patients with intraductal lesions treated with local excision had a local recurrence (12%), whereas in seven of 40 patients with lobular carcinoma *in situ* lesions treated by local excision, two had recurrences and one additional patient developed invasive tubular carcinoma in the ipsilateral breast. The authors concluded that both *in situ* lesions had similar clinical courses; treatment (ranging from local excision to modified or radical mastectomy) did not appear to affect prognosis and lymph node dissection was not necessary.

Treatment options for LCIS are complete local excision of the lesion and close follow-up, ipsilateral total mastectomy with or without contralateral "mirror" biopsies, bilateral mastectomies, and hormonal manipulation in investigational protocols.[425] However, since 20% to 30% of women with LCIS subsequently develop invasive carcinoma in either breast, often after a great number of years, excisional biopsy with close follow-up appears to be the most reasonable approach. Currently, no information is available regarding the use of breast irradiation in the LCIS type of tumor. Physicians are encouraged to register their LCIS patients on NSABP protocol B-17.

Treatment for Invasive Tumors

The management of invasive breast cancer varies considerably among institutions and physicians. However, it should be based on the clinical extent and pathologic characteristics of the tumor, in addition to the age of the patient (menopausal status), some biologic prognostic factors, and the desires and psychologic profile of the patient.

A radical or modified radical mastectomy was considered for many years the standard therapy for operable patients.[119,164,165,167,453,454] Total mastectomy combined with irradiation of the chest wall and regional lymphatics has been used with comparable results.[125,207,282,283] Alternatively, for over 40 years Stage I and Stage II tumors (T2, T2, N0, or N1) have been treated with complete local excision of the breast tumor and radiation therapy.

Tannock[432] noted that in a questionnaire mailed to 2405 oncologists of all three oncologic disciplines and 60 oncology nurses in the United States, over 60% felt that either modified radical mastectomy or conservation surgery and irradiation were equal options for patients with Stage T1 and Stage T2 carcinoma of the breast. In addition, 31% of surgical oncologists favored the former, whereas 35% of radiation oncologists favored the latter approach. Medical oncologists were almost equally divided between the two procedures, 14% and 18%, respectively. Thus, patients with lesions less than 5 cm in diameter and with some specific characteristics to be discussed later should be offered both options, with each modality thoroughly discussed. In some states legislation has been enacted requiring treating physicians to comply with the practice of offering all options.

However, a modified radical mastectomy should be recommended, even in small tumors, in patients with any of the following characteristics: belief that cosmesis is not important or desire to avoid 5 to 7 weeks of irradiation; larger tumors in small breasts in which a lumpectomy would remove so much tissue that the cosmetic outcome would be severely compromised; tumors larger than 5 cm; tumors with high probability of local recurrence (*e.g.*, extensive intraductal component where negative margins have not been attained); presence of skin or connective tissue diseases that could be complicated by irradiation; and unreliable follow-up.

Occasionally, following radical or modified radical mastectomy, postoperative irradiation of the chest wall and peripheral lymphatics is indicated in selected patients with high-risk characteristics, regardless of the initial clinical stage or the administration of adjuvant chemotherapy.[142,267] Although claims have been made that postoperative irradiation is harmful,[197,418] several analyses demonstrate that no evidence has been found of a deleterious effect of postoperative radiation therapy.[248,249] A recent study in which adequate doses and fields of radiation were used demonstrated a longer disease-free survival in patients treated with preradical or postradical mastectomy irradiation compared with those treated with mastectomy alone.[422] Postoperative irradiation is discussed in detail in Chapter 43.

Premenopausal patients who have poor prognosis following a mastectomy or breast conservation therapy also are treated with adjuvant chemotherapy. Levitt and associates[244–246,250,251] noted problems with interpretation of data in some of the major clinical studies of adjuvant chemotherapy. Essentially, they concluded that only premenopausal patients with fewer than three positive nodes show a benefit from this treatment. Present evidence does not demonstrate a definite advantage to the treatment of postmenopausal patients with adjuvant chemotherapy.[244]

Hormonal therapy has been extremely useful in many patients, particularly those with positive estrogen/progesterone receptors.[211,258] The procedures included oophorectomy and adrenalectomy. At one time either bilateral salpingo-oophorectomy or radiation ablation was the initial treatment of choice for premenopausal patients with metastatic breast cancer. Estrogens have been used in premenopausal and postmenopausal patients as well. In women who are 4 years or more postmenopausal, estrogen administration was successful in approximately 35%, with remissions lasting from several months to many years. Adrenal hormones, corticosteroids, progestins, and antiestrogens such as tamoxifen have been found to be beneficial.[258]

Treatment for Bilateral Carcinoma of the Breast

Two pathologic studies have demonstrated unsuspected contralateral breast carcinoma in a relatively high proportion of patients, although the clinical significance of these findings is uncertain. In a series by Nielsen and co-workers,[304] 68% of 84 patients with a clinical diagnosis of invasive breast carcinoma were found to have contralateral breast cancer on autopsy. Of the contralateral lesions, 49% were invasive and 51% were *in situ*. Ringberg and colleagues[341] reported a 40% incidence of unsuspected bilateral carcinoma and 44% in patients with an initial carcinoma *in situ* in a group of 73 women with known unilateral breast carcinoma on whom contralateral subcutaneous mastectomy was performed as part of reconstructive surgery. Among factors that have been reported as associated with increased risk of bilateral breast carcinoma are younger age,[1,37,60,195,254] family history of breast cancer,[37,59,195,304,390] lobular carcinoma,[195,201,254] multicentric disease,[304] histologic differentiation of primary tumor,[344] parity status,[285] and positive progesterone receptor assay.[201]

Patients with bilateral carcinoma have been treated with total or modified radical mastectomy.[216] Definitive irradiation combined with tumor excision is an acceptable alternative therapy for appropriately selected women with bilateral carcinoma of the breast. Solin and associates[410] reported on 30 women receiving radiation therapy after breast conservation surgery (11 with concurrent and 19 with bilateral carcinoma). A dose of 4500 cGy to 5000 cGy was delivered to both breasts with tangential fields in addition to a boost of 1000 cGy to 1500 cGy delivered with either iridium implant or electrons of varying energies. Adjuvant chemotherapy was given to ten patients. The tangential fields were matched in the midline in 17 patients and overlapped by up to 3 cm in ten patients. The 5-year actuarial disease-free survival rate following treatment of the first breast cancer was 79%, and the 5-year actuarial overall disease-free survival rate was 72%. For the 60 treated breasts the 5-year actuarial local failure rate was 6%. In 25 treated breasts with a minimum of 2 years' follow-up, 68% had excellent and 24% had good cosmetic results. The incidence of arm edema was 6%, similar to that reported in patients with unilateral disease.

Treatment for Cystosarcoma Phyllodes

Treatment for cystosarcoma phyllodes is either mastectomy or generous wide local excision, depending on the degree of malignancy or size of the lesion. Histologic grade appears to be the most important factor. Only about 10% of benign tumors recur. Size of tumor has not been shown to be a significant prognostic factor but may influence surgical margins. However, the presence of underlying or clearly malignant changes is associated with a higher recurrence rate and evidence of distant metastases.[446,474] In a series of 17 patients from the Radium Center, Copenhagen,[446] 12 tumors were classified histologically as benign and five as malignant. In three of five patients treated by local excision only, there was evidence of recurrence, in contrast to three of seven patients treated with simple mastectomy. Of the five patients in the malignant group, one failed after a local excision. The other four patients were treated with simple mastectomy; two patients had local recurrence, one with distant metastases also, and a third patient had distant metastases only. The authors stated that poor correlation was found between the biologic behavior and the histologic appearance of the tumor.

Although no data support the use of radiation therapy in patients with malignant cystosarcoma phyllodes,[474] from our experience with other histologic types of breast tumors, it appears that adjuvant radiation therapy may decrease the incidence of chest wall recurrences but may not have a significant impact on survival. Patients with malignant cystosarcomas and positive or close surgical margins and those who have a local recurrence should be offered radiation therapy to the chest wall (5000 cGy) followed by a boost (1000 cGy to 1500 cGy), depending on the presence of residual microscopic or gross disease. Because of the low incidence of axillary lymph node metastases, we do not advocate irradiation of the regional lymphatics.

Treatment for Paget's Disease of the Breast

This is a rare form of breast cancer, accounting for 1% to 4% of all breast tumors.[10,138] In 40% of patients no evidence of a breast mass is found on clinical or radiographic examination. The role of limited surgery in the management of these patients has not been established; Lagios and associates[236] noted one recurrence in five selected patients treated with limited surgery only, and Paone and Baker[315] observed no recurrences in five patients treated with nipple excision and wedge resection of the underlying breast. Many of these patients have been treated with mastectomy with favorable results.[264,303]

A few reports have been published on conservation surgery and irradiation; Rissanen and associates[343] described results in 12 patients with Paget's disease of the breast without palpable mass and a minimum follow-up of 5 years. Nine patients had conservative treatment, eight of whom had limited surgery and radiation therapy. Tumor recurred in three patients, and one died of breast cancer. In those eight patients, radiation therapy was delivered with 200 kV x-rays, and doses were lower than actual standards. Fourquet and colleagues[138] reported on 20 patients treated conservatively with radiation therapy alone (17 patients) or limited surgery and irradiation (three patients). The 7-year actuarial disease-free survival rate was 81%, and the overall actuarial survival rate was 93%. Three patients had recurrence in the treated breast (nipple or areola) at 21, 27, and 49 months after diagnosis. One of these patients was treated with a modified radical mastectomy and the other two patients with simple mastectomy. All three patients were surviving with disease at 28, 77, and 98 months after salvage surgery. No axillary failures have been observed. Most of the patients received 5000 cGy to 5500 cGy to the breast and axillary lymph nodes and 4000 cGy to 4500 cGy to the external mammary and supraclavicular lymph nodes. Cosmetic results were satisfactory in approximately 70% of the patients. Although Fourquet and associates irradiated the axilla, at the present time this is not recommended, because of the low incidence of axillary lymph nodes.[303]

Treatment for Angiosarcoma of the Breast

Angiosarcoma is a rare tumor accounting for 3% to 9% of all breast sarcomas; it accounts for about 1% of all breast primary malignancies.[52] These tumors tend to be large, soft, and ill-defined, frequently with focal areas of hemorrhagic necrosis; they are somewhat difficult to diagnose histologically because of the normal appearance of some of the blood vessels.[62] The tumors are anaplastic, composed of unevenly dilated vascular channels lined by flat endothelial cells. Proliferation of endothelial cells projected into the vascular lumina is observed, along with highly cellular nodules of varying sizes with hemorrhagic centers. Because of the innocuous appearance of some of the blood vessels, in a series reported by Chen and co-workers,[62] 37% were misinterpreted as benign tumors at initial biopsy. Some authors have correlated survival with the degree of histologic tumor differentiation.

Simple excision of the tumor is frequently followed by local recurrence[62]; therefore a simple mastectomy or generous wide local excision and radiation therapy are the recommended methods of treatment. More radical procedures may be required for larger tumors, particularly those invading adjacent structures. Lymph node metastases are very uncommon, and according to Bundred and associates,[46] axillary node sampling or dissection appears unnecessary because the main mode of tumor spread is hematogenous. Sellke and associates[393] stated that, of 164 cases that had been reported in the literature, 21 patients survived longer than 5 years and 8 longer than 10 years without evidence of disease.

Radiation therapy has been occasionally used in the treatment of angiosarcoma patients, but no specific reports are available. If a patient requires irradiation for angiosarcoma, we recommend doses and techniques similar to those outlined for the treatment of breast carcinoma. Several authors, including Donnell and associates[98] and Rosner,[358] have reported better survival with adjuvant chemotherapy. Antman and colleagues[7] described the treatment of five patients with angiosarcoma who were treated with combination of surgery, postoperative irradiation, and adjuvant chemotherapy (doxorubicin alone or combined cyclophosphamide with dacarbazine), some of whom survived 20 to 38 months following therapy. Bundred and associates[46] believe that adjuvant chemotherapy cannot be justified even in women with poorly differentiated angiosarcoma of the breast, because the behavior of the tumor is so unpredictable.

Treatment for Adenocarcinoma in Axillary Lymphadenopathy Without Detectable Breast Primary Cancer (Stage T0N1b)

The radiation oncologist is sometimes presented with a puzzling clinical presentation, isolated axillary lymphadenopathy with adenocarcinoma, with no clinical or radiologic evidence of a primary tumor in the breast or any other anatomic site.[217,469,470] Patients with this presentation should have the same workup as any other patient suspected of having a breast malignancy. In addition to a careful physical examination including breast examination, bilateral mammograms and chest radiographs should be obtained. An exhaustive radiographic workup including CT scan of the chest, upper gastrointestinal tract, barium enema, and intravenous pyelogram is not warranted.[53] Often, after careful examination of mastectomy specimens, the primary tumor in the breast cannot be demonstrated (Table 42-16). Patients with this condition have a relatively good prognosis, with survival rates of 50% to 80% at 5 and 10 years.[117,312,481]

Whereas some authors advise mastectomy and axillary dissection in Stage T0N1b patients,[11] an alternative is irradiation of the breast and regional lymphatics. Even though a primary tumor many times is not identified on mammograms and boost doses cannot be delivered to the breast in general, the breast is treated with doses of 5000 cGy and 5000 cGy to the axillary/supraclavicular lymph nodes, with a boost of 1000 cGy to 1500 cGy to the axillary fossa where the initial lymph nodes were palpated. Because of the excellent prognosis of these patients and the rarity of distant metastases, adjuvant chemotherapy may not be warranted.[469]

TABLE 42–16
Patients with Isolated Axillary Adenopathy and Histologically Negative Mastectomy Specimens

AUTHOR	NO. OF MASTECTOMY SPECIMENS EXAMINED	NO. (%) OF NEGATIVE SPECIMENS
Owen et al[312]	25	10 (40)
Feuerman et al[117]	10	3 (30)
Westbrook and Gallager[481]	12	3 (25)
Total	47	16 (34)

(Vilcoq JR, Calle R, Fem F, et al: Arch Surg 117:1136–1138, 1982)

Campana and associates[53] reported on 31 patients, some of whom were previously included in publications by Vilcoq and colleagues.[469,470] Initial treatment consisted of resection of the involved lymph nodes followed by irradiation in 14 patients, axillary dissection followed by radiation therapy in eight patients, radiation therapy followed by axillary dissection in six patients, combination of irradiation and modified radical mastectomy in one patient, and irradiation alone in two patients. The radiation therapy techniques included breast irradiation in 30 patients using standard techniques.[470] Dose delivered to the midpoint of the breast was 6200 cGy. All 31 patients received radiation therapy to the regional lymphatics (axillary, supraclavicular, and internal mammary chains) to doses of 6000 cGy or higher. Ten patients received adjuvant chemotherapy.

All 31 cases have been followed, with a median follow-up of 9 years. Eight locoregional recurrences have been detected; all were histologically proven infiltrating ductal carcinomas. Four of the eight patients had isolated breast recurrences that appeared at 63, 90, 136, and 162 months following treatment. Three of these four patients were salvaged by modified radical mastectomy, and one of four was given further irradiation for a recurrence in an initially underdosed region. Three of the eight patients had breast recurrences associated with axillary relapse at 7, 19, and 46 months, and one developed isolated low cervical lymph node recurrence. Two contralateral breast tumors occurred 1 and 9 years after treatment of the ipsilateral lesion. The overall 5- and 10-year actuarial survival rates were 76% and 71%, respectively. The risk of locoregional recurrence at 5 and 10 years was 14% and 25%, respectively. The risks of developing distant metastases were 23.5% and 29% at 5 and 10 years, respectively. Cosmetic results were evaluable in 24 of the 31 patients. Of the 24 women who retained their breasts, cosmesis was reported to be good in 19 (75%) and fair in five. Therapy was in general well tolerated; six patients had limitation of shoulder movement, two had arm edema, and two had asymptomatic focal pulmonary fibrosis.

Baron and co-workers[21] reported on 35 patients with axillary metastasis without evidence of breast cancer, even with mammographic evaluation. Twenty-eight patients were treated with mastectomy, whereas seven were managed by limited resection or axillary dissection and irradiation. Twenty-two of the 33 breast specimens (67%) contained carcinoma (invasive carcinoma in 18, *in situ* carcinoma in four). The actuarial 5-year survival rate was 77% after mastectomy and 65% after breast-preserving surgery and irradiation. A total of five patients had contralateral breast cancer treated either before or after therapy for the axillary carcinoma with occult breast tumors. The 5-year survival was comparable for patients receiving or not receiving adjuvant chemotherapy (79% and 77%, respectively).

RADIATION THERAPY IN CARCINOMA OF THE BREAST

Irradiation as the primary treatment for breast cancer is indicated in several situations, alone or usually combined with various surgical procedures (Table 42-17).

Combination of Irradiation With Wide Local Excision (Tylectomy) for Stage I and Stage II Primary Tumors

In addition to tumor control and survival, conservation of the breast with optimal cosmetic results is a crucial goal of irradiation with wide local excision for Stage I and Stage II primary tumors, which is associated with improved psychoemotional adjustment of the patient to the diagnosis and treatment of carcinoma of the breast. It also enhances the acceptance by women of mammographic screening for early detection of this disease.[24,487]

Patient and Tumor Selection

It is extremely important to select the appropriate patients and tumors for the above-mentioned therapy, with the surgeon and the radiation oncologist in close consultation and after thorough discussion of therapeutic alternatives with the patient and her significant others.

The following are guidelines for the selection of these patients:

The patient must be psychologically prepared for a conservation procedure and place emphasis on cosmetic appearance. Occasionally, a patient feels better when a mastectomy is performed.

In general, lesions less than 4 cm in diameter can be adequately treated with conservation surgery and irradiation, although tumors up to 5 cm have been treated in this fashion.[126]

Some authors have suggested that patients at a higher risk of developing a local recurrence should not be treated with conservation surgery. High-risk patients are those with extensive intraductal carcinoma, multiple breast microcalcifications, or subareolar location of the tumor.

With increasing experience it is apparent that many of these patients can be effectively treated with irradiation and tylectomy. It is appropriate to note that even though the failure rate in this subset of patients is high (25% to 30%), over 70% of these breasts can be preserved, and the breast failures are effectively treated with total or modified radical mastectomy.[83,223,225] Perhaps more important, refinements such as careful pathologic margin assessment, adequate irradiation, and the integration of chemotherapy may eliminate these poor prognostic subsets.

Danoff and Goodman,[83] in 674 patients with Stage I and Stage II breast cancer treated with conservation surgery and irradiation, isolated 48 patients for whom modified radical mastectomy was recommended because of the presence of gross multicentric disease (24 patients), diffuse microcalcifications (16 patients), or subareolar primary tumor (eight patients). According to the authors, these findings suggested that more than one quadrant of the breast was involved, and a high percentage of positive axillary nodes was noted (16 of 40).

Harris and colleagues,[177,178] in a retrospective review of 221 women with infiltrating ductal carcinoma treated with wide local tumor resection and irradiation, identified 53 cases in which the excision specimen showed (1) prominent intraductal carcinoma component in the tumor, (2) intraductal carcinoma in the adjacent tissue, and (3) poorly differentiated nuclei. In patients with all three pathologic features, the actuarial risk of local recurrence was 37% compared with 11% for 79 patients with two features, 9% for 62 patients with one feature, and 0% for 32 patients with none of the three features. Pathologic assessment of surgical margins was not done. It is noteworthy that additional dose of radiation (boost) to the primary site did not reduce the risk of local recurrence (34%) significantly in patients with all three features, compared with those patients not receiving supplemental radiation (49% recurrence). At 6 years the survival rate was 69% for the high-risk group and 90% for the other patients.

Schnitt and associates[384] updated this report with observations on 356 patients with Stage I and Stage II infiltrating ductal carcinoma. Again, they noted that patients with extensive intraductal component had a 24% risk of local recurrence at 5 years compared with only 2% in the other patients. The risk of distant failure at 5 years was similar for patients with or without extensive intraductal involvement (20% and 21%).

Surgical Techniques of Tumor Excision

There are several types of breast-preserving surgery: wide local excision (tylectomy, tumorectomy, lumpectomy), segmental or partial mastectomy, or quadrantectomy. Because cosmesis is a critical goal for performing tumor excision and irradiation instead of mastectomy, wide local excision with microscopically negative margins is preferable to segmental mastectomy or quadrantectomy. The latter procedures without a radiation boost are inferior cosmetically to a tylectomy with an electron beam or implant boost dose to the tumor bed.

Surgeons should familiarize themselves with the principles of breast conservation surgery. The National Surgical Adjuvant Breast Project (NSABP) has recommended specific types of incisions, depending on the location of the tumor (Fig. 42-10). The radiation oncologist may play an advisory role, because

TABLE 42–17
Role of Irradiation in Primary Management of Breast Cancer

Combined with wide local excision or segmental mastectomy (T1, T2 tumors)
After modified radical mastectomy
a. T3, any N, T4, N2
b. T2 primary with fascia involvement, lymphatic permeation, or more than 4 positive axillary nodes
Combined with total mastectomy (McWhirter's technique)
Preoperative irradiation combined with chemotherapy in unresectable breast primary or lymph nodes
Alone (or combined with chemotherapy) in inoperable tumors, inflammatory carcinoma

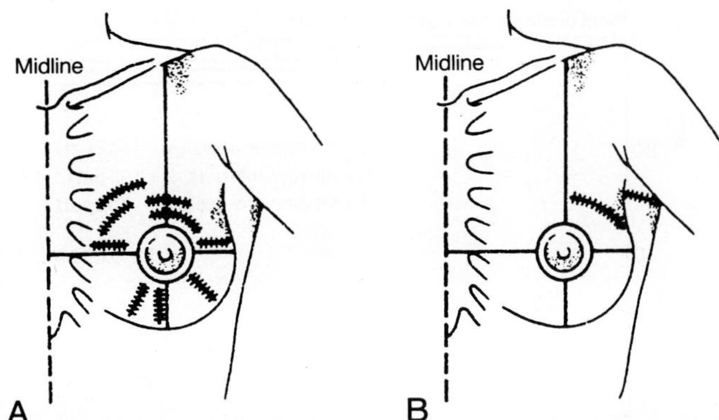

FIGURE 42–10. (**A**) NSABP recommendation for the direction of incisions used for tumorectomy. (**B**) NSABP recommendation for the incision used for axillary node dissection. (Courtesy of Bernard Fisher, M.D. Chairman, National Surgical Adjuvant Breast Project. Bedwinek JM: Int J Radiat Oncol Biol Phys 7:1553, 1981)

ideally all patients should be evaluated by both the surgeon and the radiation oncologist before any operation.

In 131 selected mastectomy specimens (tumor less than 3 cm) Muller and co-workers[302] simulated segmental resections with a 2 cm wide margin of normal tissue surrounding the primary lesion. Following these resections, residual primary tumor was found in 19% of the cases and multicentric tumor foci in 24% of the remaining breasts. The volume of residual tumor was significantly larger than the volume of the multicentric foci. These findings were confirmed by Holland and associates,[200] who reported on the incidence of multifocal carcinoma in breast tumors 2 cm or smaller in diameter, as a function of the distance from the edge of the primary tumor; 17% had additional tumor within 1 cm, 28% had carcinoma *in situ,* and 14% had invasive carcinoma within 2 cm from the edge of the tumor (Fig. 42-11). These findings provide a strong rationale for the irradiation of the entire breast and the use of boost dose at the primary site after wide local excision. Muller and co-workers noted that irradiation could be omitted only under exceptional circumstances in controlled studies.[302]

Reports on the impact of type of excision on tumor control are not consistent. van Limbergen and associates[460] noted poorer local tumor control in 20 patients treated with subtotal resection compared with those treated with tumorectomy or segmentectomy (Fig. 42-12*A*). On the other hand, Bartelink and associates[23] observed no significant impact on tumor control rate with the degree of completeness of the excision (Fig. 42-12*B*). This may be related to the treatment technique, which included 5000 cGy to the breast in 5 weeks and ^{192}Ir volume implant to the tumor excision site (2500 cGy).

Kantorowitz and associates[209] observed a local recurrence rate of 26% in 99 women treated with segmental mastectomy without irradiation in contrast to 7.6% for 146 women treated with segmental mastectomy and irradiation. In the women treated with segmental mastectomy alone, very little advantage was found in enlarging the extent of resection, failure rates being observed in 15.5% and 12.5% of the patients, respectively. By contrast, only 2.8% of women treated with quadrantectomy and irradiation and 22.2% of patients treated with quadrantectomy only failed.

In another report, three patients treated with bilateral subcutaneous mastectomy and cosmetic implants for fibrocystic disease or carcinoma *in situ* subsequently developed invasive breast carcinoma, which strongly suggests that this procedure is inappropriate for the patient likely to harbor occult invasive breast carcinoma.[157]

Tumor Reexcision

The percentage of patients with residual tumor at the time of reexcision varies widely, depending on the criteria used for returning a patient to the operating room for more breast surgery. The overall incidence of positive reexcisions ranges from 32% to 62%.[273,291,382,406] When the initial margins of resection are positive, 55% to 69% of reexcision specimens will contain cancer cells,[273,382] compared with 49% of specimens with unknown margins[406] and 33% of specimens with negative margins.[382]

Surgical removal of additional breast tissue surrounding the original excision site is indicated when it is highly probable that the tumor cell burden exceeds that which can be controlled by the typical doses of radiation (5000 cGy to the breast and 1000 cGy boost). Solin and colleagues[406] reported on 253 patients with clinical Stage I or Stage II tumors who underwent a reexcisional biopsy before definitive radiation therapy. Of 127 Stage T1 tumors, 57 (47%) and 37 of 60 (62%) T2 lesions showed residual tumor in reexcision specimens. Of the excised positive specimens, 134 (85%) had an invasive component of tumor and 24 (15%) had noninvasive disease. In 66 patients in whom the initial biopsy was described as incisional, 64 (97%)

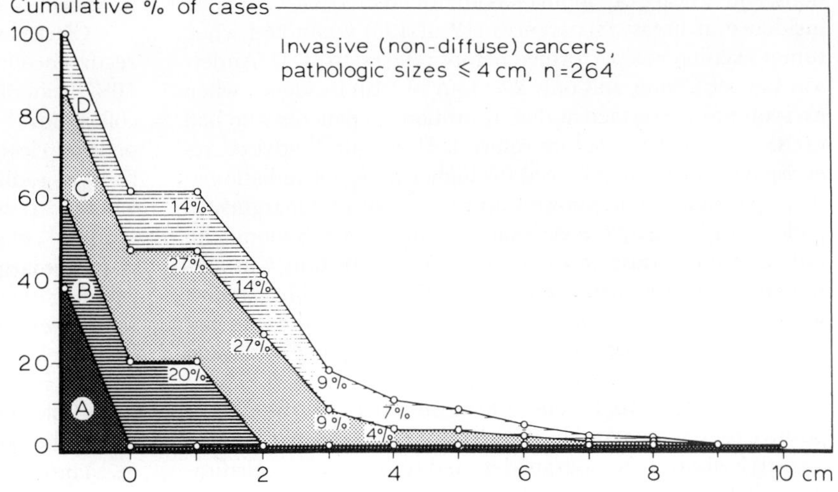

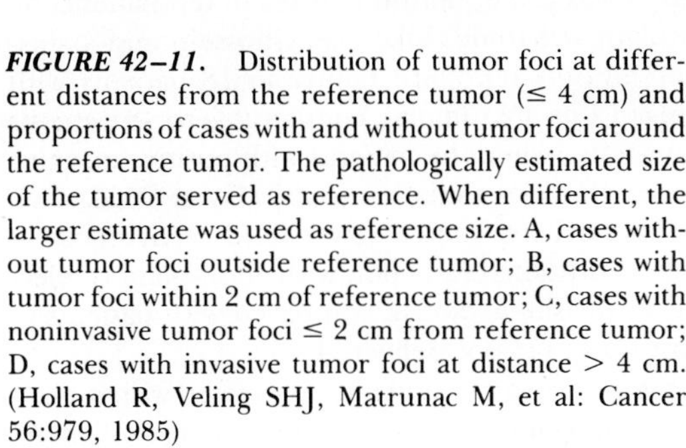

FIGURE 42–11. Distribution of tumor foci at different distances from the reference tumor (≤ 4 cm) and proportions of cases with and without tumor foci around the reference tumor. The pathologically estimated size of the tumor served as reference. When different, the larger estimate was used as reference size. A, cases without tumor foci outside reference tumor; B, cases with tumor foci within 2 cm of reference tumor; C, cases with noninvasive tumor foci ≤ 2 cm from reference tumor; D, cases with invasive tumor foci at distance > 4 cm. (Holland R, Veling SHJ, Matrunac M, et al: Cancer 56:979, 1985)

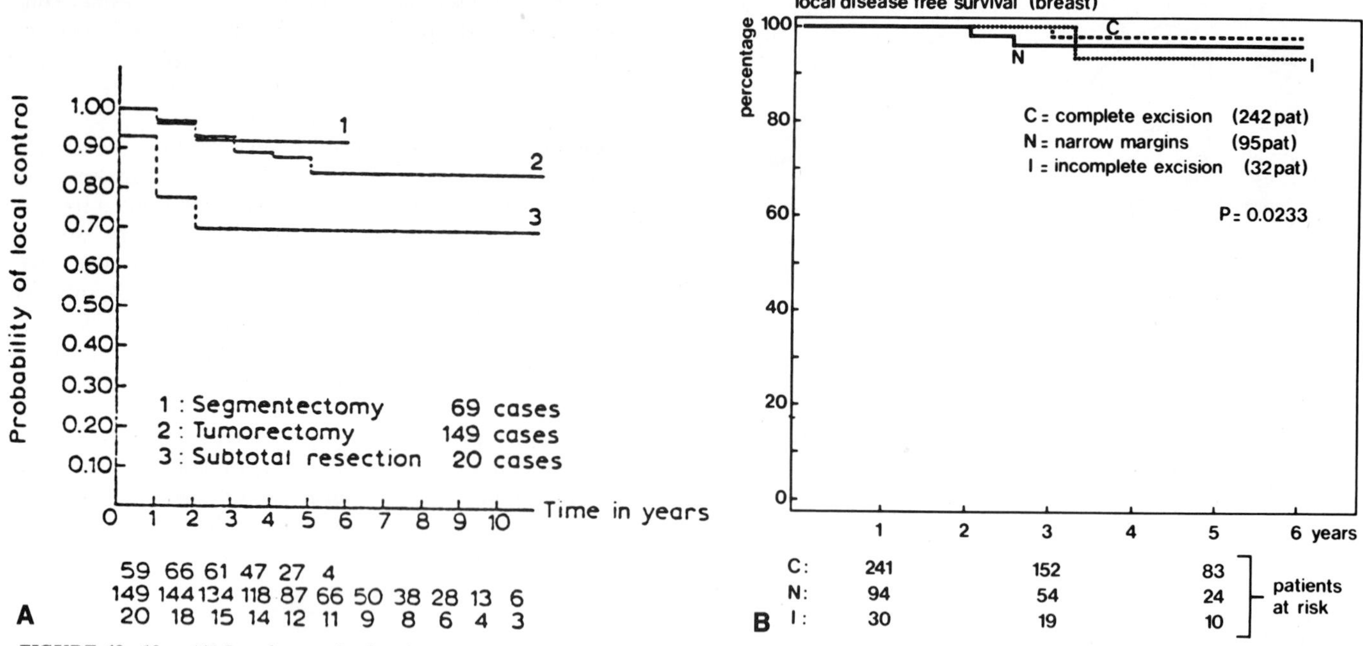

FIGURE 42–12. (**A**) Local control related to extent of conservation surgery. (van Limbergen E, van den Bogaert W, van der Schueren E, et al: Radiother Oncol 8:1, 1987) (**B**) Local disease-free survival in the breast in patients with a microscopically complete excision. C: margin > 0.5 cm; N: narrow margins, 0 to 0.5 cm; I: incomplete excision. (Bartelink H, Borger JH, van Dogen JA, et al: Radiother Oncol 11:297, 1988)

had residual tumor in contrast to 94 (50%) of 187 patients who had an initial excisional biopsy. When the pathologic margin of the initial excisional biopsy specimen was described as positive, 15 (60%) of 25 had residual tumor. Of 160 patients for whom the pathologic margin of the specimen was unknown, 79 (49%) had residual tumor in the reexcision specimen.

Furthermore, Brenner and co-workers[43] reported on 180 patients with Stage I and Stage II carcinoma of the breast who underwent reexcision after an initial excisional procedure of the primary tumor. Reexcision was performed for close or positive margins and/or extensive intraductal component. Residual disease was identified in the reexcision specimen in 128 patients (71%).

Some authors have published policies for reexcising the primary site when the biopsy was performed at an outside hospital with unknown resection margins. Of 210 patients having surgery at M. D. Anderson Cancer Center, 67 underwent a reexcision after biopsies had been performed at other institutions, and invasive carcinoma was identified in 57%.[291] An 8.2% incidence of breast recurrences (12 of 135) was noted when tumor excision was performed before referral to M. D. Anderson Cancer Center and only 2% (four of 210) incidence when excision was performed at that institution. In patients who had excisions performed before referral, Montague[291] advised reexcision to eliminate the need for higher doses for radiation in those patients with unknown status of the surgical margins. In patients with negative reexcision specimens for carcinoma, no radiation boost dose was delivered. At the Institut Gustave-Roussy,[72] breast recurrence rate of 10% was noted in patients who had outside excisions, compared with 5% in those who had tumor excision at the Institut. Patients undergoing reexcision experienced only a 3% breast failure rate.

Two other factors seem to have an impact on the rate of positive reexcisions. At the University of Pennsylvania[406], when a posttylectomy mammogram detected residual microcalcifications, 86% of the reexcisions contained tumor. At Harvard University,[382] when extensive intraductal carcinoma (EIC—defined as intraductal carcinoma in ≥25% of the primary tumor mass plus extension beyond infiltrating margin) was detected on the initial biopsy, 88% of the reexcisions were positive compared with 48% when EIC was absent.

Tumor size is usually not considered an indication for reexcision in the absence of other factors. The Harvard University data revealed no difference between the positive reexcision rate of T1 and T2 tumors,[382] but the University of Pennsylvania found a rate of 62% for T2 compared with 45% for T1 tumors.[406]

The presence of residual tumor in the reexcision specimen or the status of the margins has not consistently been correlated with prognosis if adequate doses of radiation are administered. Kantorowitz and associates[209] reported that after conservation surgery and irradiation, patients with negative margins had a 3% locoregional failure rate (one of 31), in contrast to 12.6% (14 of 111) in patients when the specimen had close, positive, or unknown margins.

Clarke and associates[72] described a 4.6% incidence of local recurrence in patients with negative margins (12 of 262) and 10% incidence with positive margins (eight of 80). Harris and colleagues[176] reported a 38% local failure rate in eight patients on whom less than excisional biopsy was done and no additional boost of radiation was given, but no failures in ten patients on whom ^{192}Ir implant was done. Likewise, Ghossein and associates[150, 151] observed only one local failure in 18 patients with positive margins (T1 or T2 tumors), comparable to 18 patients with negative margins, when the patients with positive margins were given higher doses of radiation (6500 cGy to 7000 cGy). Bedwinek and co-workers[30] noted fewer local recurrences in patients receiving additional radiation with an implant or electrons following an incisional biopsy, compared with patients to whom the boost dose was not delivered.

The decrement in cosmetic outcome associated with reexcision must be weighed against possible improved local control. At

Washington University, 85% of 153 patients without reexcision had good-to-excellent cosmetic results compared with 60% of 70 reexcised patients ($P < 0.001$). Based on these findings, we recommend reexcision at the primary tumor site when an initial incisional biopsy is done; when pathologic margins on the initial excisional biopsy are not adequately assessed or are shown to be involved by tumor; when excision specimen shows extensive intraductal component and no clearly negative margins; or when residual microcalcifications are seen on posttylectomy mammogram.

Surgical Evaluation of the Axillary Lymph Nodes

In patients with carcinoma of the breast with clinically negative lymph nodes, approximately 35% to 40% have pathologic evidence of lymph node metastases.[82, 125, 166] Yet in patients with Stage I and Stage II breast cancer with clinically negative axillary lymph nodes, failure to perform axillary dissection results in about a 21% incidence of axillary recurrence.[125] The axillary contents are divided into three levels: level I represents tissue between the axillary vein and the latissimus dorsi muscle and the lateral border of the pectoralis minor muscle; level II is located between the lateral and medial borders of the pectoralis minor muscle; and level III is between the medial border of the pectoralis minor and Halsted's ligament (apex of the axilla).[82] The 3-year survival rate was 87% for patients with level I positive nodes, 75% for those with level II, and 36% for those with level III.[33] Axillary recurrences after complete dissection range from 1% to 2%.[125] Twenty percent to 30% of patients with a clinically positive axilla have no histologic evidence of nodal metastatic disease.[82, 125, 163, 166]

In most patients treated with conservation surgery, an axillary node dissection is carried out in addition to excision of the tumor. This is most important for premenopausal women because the axillary nodal status will determine whether to use adjuvant chemotherapy or which drug combination should be given. If the results of surgical axillary staging are not going to offset systemic therapies, we occasionally treat the axilla with irradiation alone, provided that the axilla is clinically negative. Haffty and associates[168] reported a 97% actuarial 5-year nodal control rate and a 96% nodal control rate at 10 years for 244 patients receiving radiation alone without axillary dissection and 167 treated with radiation to the supraclavicular and internal mammary lymph nodes after axillary dissection.

NSABP (protocol 06) advises an incision for the axillary surgery different from that used for the excision of the breast tumor. The exception in our experience is when only a small (less than 3 cm) segment of breast will remain between the two incisions, because of the possibility of necrosis in the remaining breast tissue between the excised sites.

The extent of axillary dissection in patients treated with conservation surgery and irradiation has been the subject of intense debate, because dissection of level III carries greater morbidity (arm edema).

Pigott and associates[327] reported on 146 patients treated with radical mastectomy (either modified or Halsted) for invasive ductal or lobular carcinoma of the breast. Eighty (55%) patients had histologically proven axillary lymph node metastases. If only the low (level I) axillary lymph nodes had been removed, 18 patients (25%) would have had metastases confined to levels II and III that would have gone undetected. Medial quadrant lesions exhibited this tendency more than lateral quadrant lesions (50% *versus* 20%). However, only 1.4% of patients showed positive level III lymph nodes when level I and II nodes were negative.

Danforth and colleagues[82] reviewed the pathologic findings in 71 patients treated with a modified radical mastectomy and 65 patients treated with conservation surgery of the breast and irradiation for clinical Stage I and Stage II breast carcinoma. Thirty-nine percent of the lymph nodes removed were contained in level I, 41% in level II, and 20% in level III. In patients with clinically negative nodes 23% of those with T1 tumors (ten of 43) and 47% of those with Stage T2 lesions (31 of 66) had pathologically positive lymph nodes. Although the authors emphasized that 29% of the node-positive patients had metastases to level II or III without level I involvement, only two of 65 patients (3.1%) had isolated level III metastases. Table 42-18 depicts the location of metastatic axillary node metastases reported by several authors.[82] Thus thorough dissection of level I and II lymph nodes is the minimum procedure to be performed on these patients. Complete axillary dissection, including level III, would be performed only in patients with clinically positive lymph nodes. However, a higher incidence of breast and arm edema has been noted with a level III axillary node dissection,[333] and the benefit of dissecting the level III lymph nodes has not been demonstrated. Axillary sampling is to be strongly discouraged.

Axillary dissection, when properly carried out, is well toler-

TABLE 42–18
Anatomic Location of Axillary Breast Cancer Metastases: Summary of Series Evaluating Complete Axillary Lymph Node Dissection

AXILLARY LEVEL	PIGOTT ET AL[327]	SMITH ET AL[405]	BOOVA ET AL[40]	ROSEN ET AL[354]	DANFORTH ET AL[82]
N*	72	304	80	281	65
I	18.0	29.6	48.8	48.4	30.8
II	19.4	10.5	6.3	1.4	21.5
III	1.4	9.9	1.3	0	3.1
I, II	21.0	15.1	23.8	22.1	20.0
I, III	2.7	7.6	5.0	1.1	1.5
II, III	4.2	6.6	1.3	1.1	4.6
I, II, III	33.3	20.7	13.8	26.0	18.5

**N represents the number of lymph node-positive patients in the respective series. All figures represent the percentage of lymph node-positive patients with metastases to the corresponding axillary level(s).*
(Danforth DN, Findlay PA, McDonald HD, et al: J Clin Oncol 4[5]:655–662, 1986)

ated in most patients. Rose and associates[347] reported five transient nonsurgical complications and one case of cellulitis resulting in a frozen shoulder requiring corrective surgery in 176 patients on whom low axillary dissection was performed. The authors emphasized the importance of carrying the axillary dissection up to but without dissecting the axillary vein to decrease morbidity.

Irradiation of Regional Lymph Nodes in Patients Without Clinical or Pathologic Evidence of Axillary Metastatic Lymph Nodes

Considerable controversy exists regarding the subject of whether to irradiate regional lymph nodes with no of evidence of metastasis, although most authors today agree that it is not necessary if an adequate axillary dissection was performed.[492] This view is supported by a report by Sarrazin and colleagues,[373] who carried out a randomized study comparing 88 patients treated with tumorectomy and irradiation with 91 patients treated with mastectomy. A second randomization was done in this study, in which patients with positive axillary lymph nodes in the first randomization were randomized to be treated with nodal irradiation or not. No significant difference in overall survival occurred between the two groups (Fig. 42-13).

Clark and associates[70] reported similar survival and breast recurrence rates (9% and 12%) whether the axillary lymph nodes were irradiated or not. Likewise, the axillary relapse rates were comparable with or without axillary irradiation (6.8% *versus* 9.6%), when the breast was irradiated. If no radiation was given, the axillary relapse rate was 19%.

Dewar and associates[93] reported on 558 patients with T1 and small T2 tumors treated with conservation therapy, including a lower axillary dissection in 374 patients (67%) and axillary clearance in 184 patients (33%). Axillary lymph node metastases were evident in 36% of the patients. In patients with metastatic lymph nodes in the lower axilla, a complete axillary dissection was performed, usually in combination with irradiation. Only five patients relapsed in the axilla (probability of relapse at 5 years = 1.2%). No axillary recurrences were found in node-positive patients who had axillary clearance, whether or not radiation was delivered.

Gerard and associates[149] reported a 1.2% probability of axillary recurrence after axillary dissection without irradiation in 195 patients with Stage T1 and Stage T2 tumors treated with a conservation approach and breast irradiation.

Yarnold[492] pointed out the advisability of withholding lymphatic irradiation in patients treated with conservation therapy on whom an adequate axillary dissection had been performed and whose lymph nodes were found to be negative.

Irradiation of Lymphatics in Patients With Positive Axillary Lymph Nodes Receiving Adjuvant Chemotherapy

The question of whether to irradiate lymphatics in patients with positive axillary nodes who are receiving chemotherapy is an extremely controversial issue that may give rise to heated discussions among both radiation and medical oncologists. Whereas in current practice some radiation oncologists still favor irradiation of the regional lymphatics in addition to the breast, several cooperative groups are not following this policy and are irradiating only the breast. Yarnold[492] advised elective irradiation of the axilla and the supraclavicular fossa in selected patients, such as those with four or more metastatic axillary lymph nodes, involvement of the apex of the axilla, and extracapsular extension, even if these patients are to receive adjuvant chemotherapy. Careful follow-up determines whether adjuvant chemotherapy alone effectively prevents regional nodal recurrences and improves survival in this subpopulation of patients.

Follow-Up of Patients Treated With Conservation Surgery and Irradiation

It is extremely important to follow up closely patients treated with conservation surgery and irradiation, because early detection of a local recurrence may allow for even another wide local excision or a total mastectomy, without significantly compromising the overall survival of the patient.[144,181,223]

Frequent physical examinations (every 3 months for the first 2 years, every 4 months in the third year, and every 6 months thereafter) should be emphasized. A posttreatment mammogram should be obtained within 6 months after completion of irradiation as a baseline for comparison with subsequent studies. Diagnostic mammograms of the treated breast should be repeated every 6 to 12 months for the first 2 years, and thereafter on a yearly basis.

At times, these patients are difficult to evaluate. Posttreatment hematomas, fat necrosis, seromas, cysts, and scar tissue pose frequent dilemmas. Consultation with an experienced mammographer is essential. When in doubt, repeat biopsies may be indicated. Recht and Harris[338] reported on 1233 patients with clinical Stage I or Stage II carcinoma of the breast treated with excisional biopsy and irradiation who were followed up periodically. Thirty-eight had pathologically negative post-

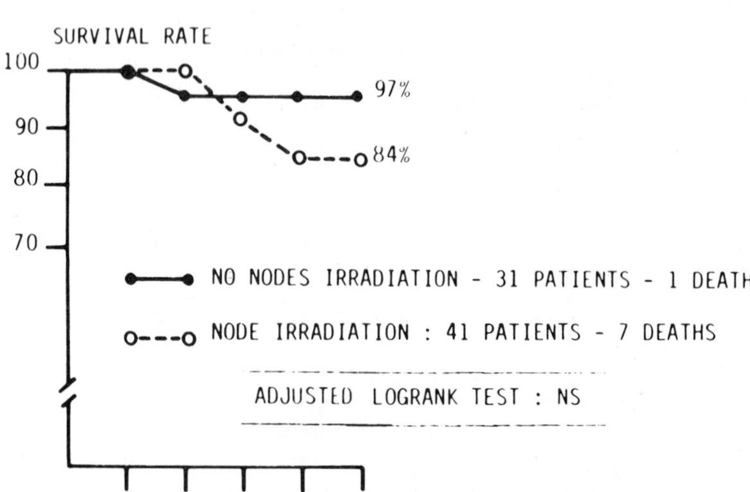

FIGURE 42–13. Survival curves by lymph node irradiation in patients treated with breast conservation therapy. (Sarrazin D, Le M, Rouesse J, et al: Cancer 53:1209, 1984)

treatment ipsilateral breast biopsies at different times (from 5 to 59 months; median 26 months). The most common findings just before the first biopsy were palpable mass with or without induration in 15 patients (39%) and thickening of the breast or fullness without a mass in 20 patients (53%). Only 21 patients had mammograms within 4 months prior to the biopsy. Three of these patients showed a mass only (14%); four had breast findings without a mass (19%), and one had both findings. Eleven of the 21 patients (52%) had no suspicious findings. Two of the patients undergoing biopsies (5%) subsequently developed breast failures.

Stomper and colleagues[419] reported on 50 of more than 1600 patients with Stage I and Stage II invasive breast cancer treated with conservation surgery and irradiation on whom biopsies were performed within 4 months of a mammogram for suspected recurrence in the irradiated breast. The most common radiographic findings were calcifications, with or without a mass, or a mass. Histologic evidence of recurrent cancer was found in 23 of 45 biopsy specimens (51%). Sixty-five percent of the patients had recurrences at the primary site and 22% in other sites; 13% of recurrences were multifocal. In these patients the tumor was suspected on mammogram in only eight (35%), on physical examination in nine (39%), and on both in six patients (26%). The authors believed that whenever there is evidence of suspicious microcalcifications, masses, or architectural distortions of the breast after conservation surgery and irradiation, a biopsy should be obtained to rule out a recurrence. In ten (7%) of 152 patients who underwent reexcision of breast tissue because of suspicious microcalcifications after excisional biopsy and irradiation, six had benign and four had malignant calcifications on mammography.[334]

Radiation Therapy to the Chest Wall and Lymph Node-bearing Areas Combined With Total Mastectomy

Irradiation of the chest wall and node-bearing areas in addition to total mastectomy (McWhirter's technique) was used in selected Stage I and Stage II (high-risk groups) and resectable Stage III tumors. The regional lymph nodes are treated even when no palpable axillary lymph nodes are found because of the probability of subsequent appearance of lymphadenopathy (18% of patients) if irradiation is not given.[125] The techniques of irradiation are described in detail in Chapter 43.

RADIATION THERAPY TECHNIQUES FOR THE INTACT BREAST

Following wide local excision, segmental mastectomy, or quadrantectomy, the breast is irradiated with lateral and medial tangential portals.

Treatment Volume

The entire breast and underlying chest wall with a small portion of lung should be included in the irradiated volume. Radiopaque surgical clips placed at the margin of the tumor bed may assist in defining the tumor volume.[407] In general, when combined with a supraclavicular portal, the upper margin of the portal is placed at the first or second intercostal space (latter at Louis' angle). If the regional lymph nodes are not to be irradiated (such as in patients with intraductal disease or negative axillary lymph nodes or in those with positive axillary lymph nodes who are receiving adjuvant chemotherapy), the upper margin of the portals should be placed at the head of the clavicle to include the entire breast (Fig. 42-14). The medial margin, if no internal mammary portal is used, should be at the midline or 1 cm over. If an internal mammary field is used, the medial tangential portal is located at the lateral margin of the internal mammary field (Fig. 42-15). The lateral/posterior margin should be placed 2 cm beyond all palpable breast tissue, which is usually near the midaxillary line. The inferior margin is drawn 1 cm to 2 cm below the inframammary fold.

Usually 2 cm to 3 cm of underlying lung is included in the tangential portals. The amount of lung included in the irradiated volume is greatly influenced by the portals used. Roberson and colleagues,[345] using computed tomography data, demonstrated the impact of tangential breast fields (medial border

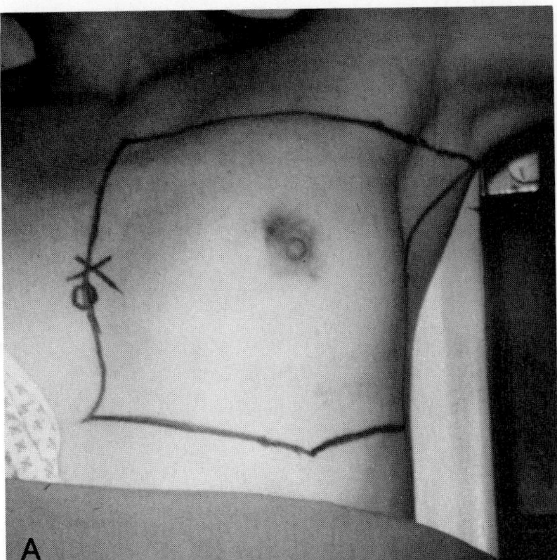

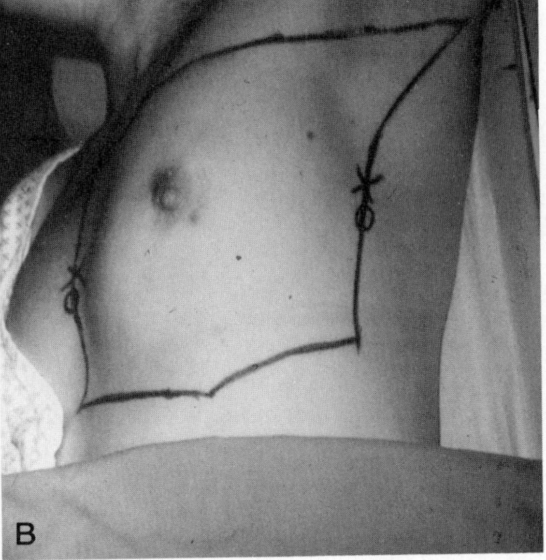

FIGURE 42–14. (**A**) AP photograph of patient with intraductal carcinoma of the breast illustrating the treatment portal for the breast only, without fields for irradiation of peripheral lymphatics. (**B**) Tangential photograph of the same patient. In premenopausal patients with axillary node involvement who receive adjuvant chemotherapy, similar portals are sometimes used for invasive tumors to treat the breast only. This policy is still controversial.

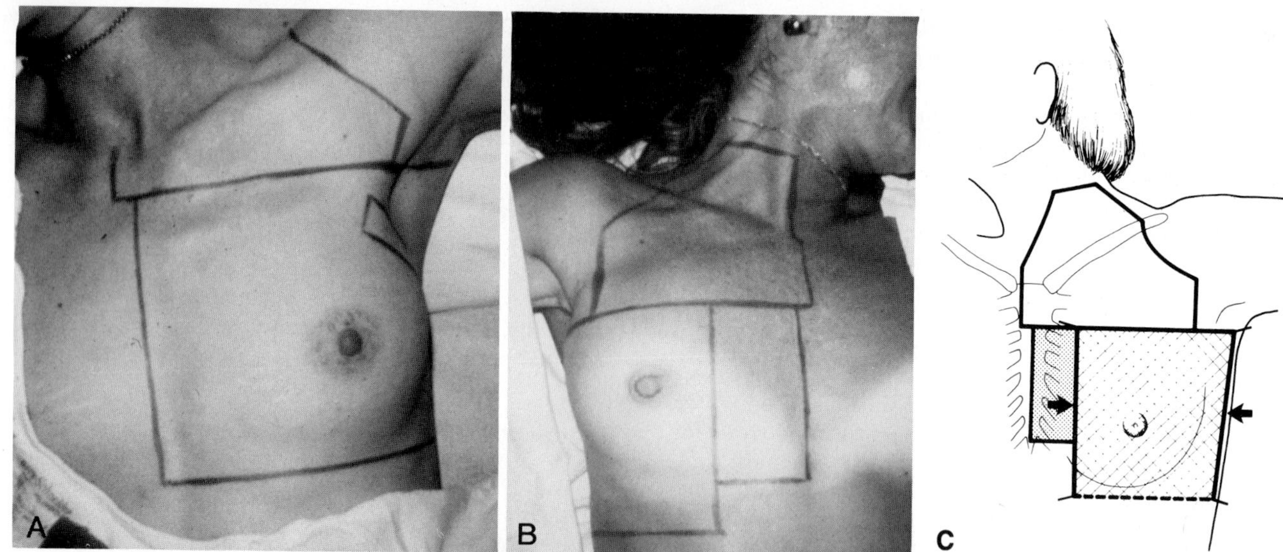

FIGURE 42–15. (**A**) Example of portals for definitive radiation therapy in a patient with T1N0M0 ductal carcinoma of the left breast treated with wide local excision of tumor and irradiation. Because the bridge separation was 18 cm and the primary tumor was located in the lateral quadrant, a separate internal mammary portal was not used. Treatment was given in 1974, at which time axillary dissection was not carried out. Because of this the regional lymph nodes were irradiated. (**B**) Example of portals for irradiation of the breast and regional lymphatics in a patient with a periareolar T2N0M0 tumor of the right breast. See text for a description of portal design. (**C**) Diagrammatic representation of volume treated in patients with lesions eligible for conservation surgery and irradiation when treatment of the peripheral lymphatics is indicated (in the axilla, volume dissected is excluded except when there is extranodal tumor extension).

1 cm or 3 cm to 4 cm beyond midline) and internal mammary portal on percentage of lung volume irradiated using photons or electrons (Fig. 42-16). Careful individualized planning and use of appropriate energy electrons for all or a major portion of the internal mammary node irradiation are necessary to minimize dose to the underlying lung.

The standard portals must be modified to accommodate topographic features of the patient or location of the tumor excision site to avoid junction of fields at the scar (Fig. 42-17). In some patients the breast falls superiorly toward the supraclavicular area in the supine position. An inclined board placed on the treatment table can correct this problem.

A modified lateral decubitus position with an immobilization device has been suggested for women with large breasts (Fig. 42-18*A*). The dose distribution with a "mock wedge" is satisfactory (Fig. 42-18*B*).

Alignment of the Tangential Beam With the Chest Wall Contour

The anterior chest wall in most women slopes downward from the midchest to the neck. To make the posterior edge of the tangential beam follow this downward sloping contour, the collimator of the tangential beam is usually rotated. An alternative technique is used at the Mallinckrodt Institute of Radiology; the posterior edge of the tangential beam is made to follow the chest wall contour by means of a rotating beam splitter mounted on a tray (Fig. 42-19) without rotating the collimator. In this way the superior edge of the tangential beam remains in the true vertical and matches perfectly the vertical inferior edge of the supraclavicular field. Examples of localization films for tangential portals are shown in Figure 42-20.

Doses and Beams

Minimal tumor doses of 4500 cGy to 5000 cGy are delivered to the entire breast in 5 to 6 weeks (180 cGy to 200 cGy dose [TD] daily, five weekly fractions). Doses of 4500 cGy (180 cGy daily fraction) are preferred for patients with large, pendulous breasts or when radiation is combined with chemotherapy.[181]

^{60}Co or x-ray energies of 4 MV to 6 MV should be used to treat the breast. Photon energies greater than 6 MV may underdose superficial tissues just beneath the skin surface, but 6 MV to 10 MV photons may be helpful in large breasts to decrease the integral breast dose. Chin and associates[63] in a breast phantom study with various energy photons demonstrated that the areas of high dose (hot spots) noted along the periphery of the breast were less with high-energy photons (6 MV and 8 MV). At the same time a decreased dose was delivered to the skin and superficial portions of the breast (Fig. 42-21). Inhomogeneity in the dose distribution (as much as 25% from central axis dose) is enhanced at the inferior portion of the breast, where the entrance-exit distance of the two tangential beams is significantly shorter than at the central plane. This is not easily appreciated on a two-dimensional treatment plan; fortunately no significant fibrosis is observed in this area.

Wedges or compensating filters must be used for a portion of the treatment to achieve a uniform dose distribution within the breast (10% or less dose variance from the base to the apex; Fig. 42-22).

It is unnecessary to apply a bolus to the entire breast or to the excision site because the skin is usually not at risk for recurrence following complete excision of a T1 or T2 lesion as is the skin of the chest wall following a mastectomy. The use of bolus can result in impaired cosmetic results.

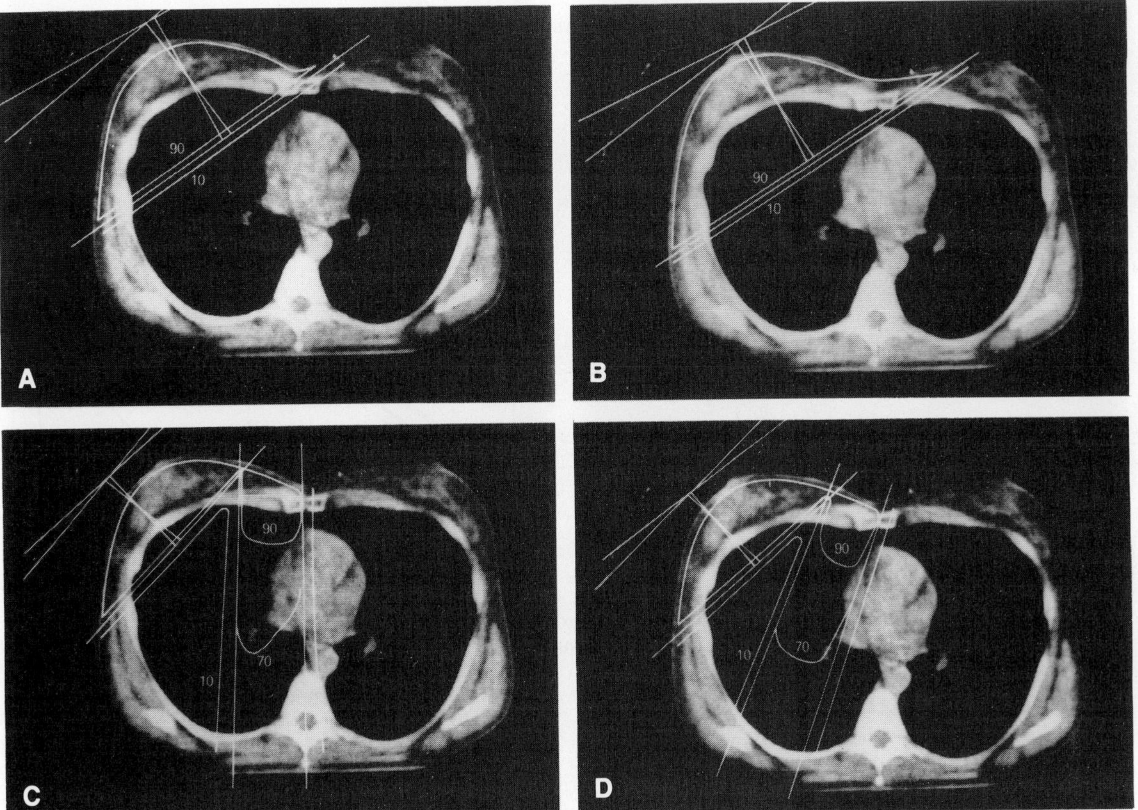

FIGURE 42–16. Irradiation of the breast. Field configurations and isodose lines for 6 MV photons. (**A**) "Standard tangents" technique. (**B**) Deep tangents technique. (**C**) *En face* IMF technique. (**D**) Twenty-degree IMF technique. (Roberson PL, Lichter AS, Bodner A, et al: Int J Radiat Oncol Biol Phys 9:97, 1982.)

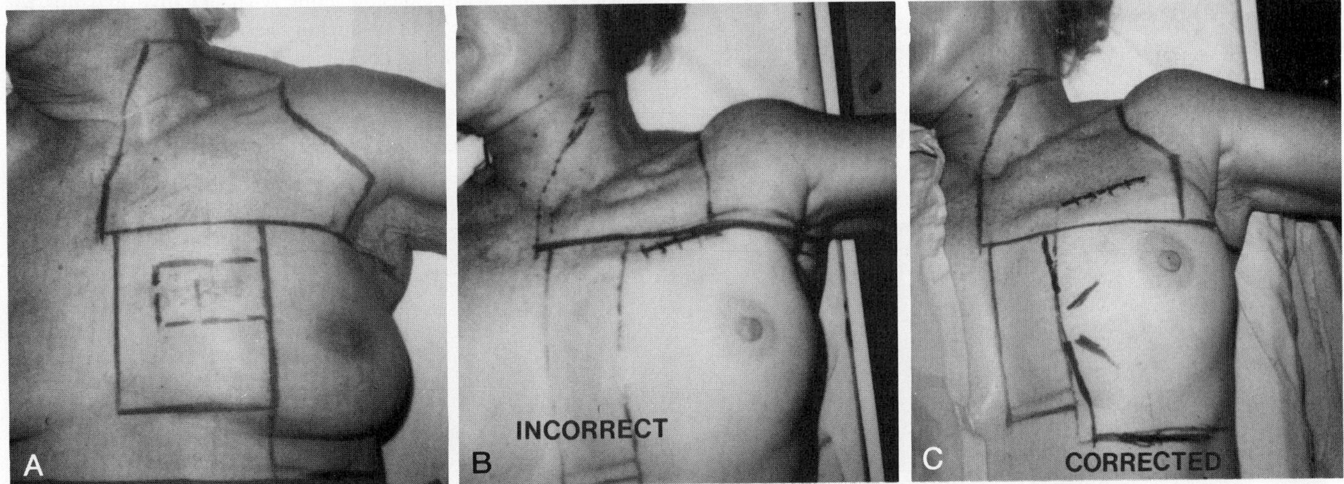

FIGURE 42–17. Modification of treatment portals to adjust to topography of tumor. (**A**) A 70-year-old woman had a 3 cm ductal carcinoma of the upper inner quadrant and no palpable axillary lymph nodes. Axillary dissection was not carried out because of her age. The internal mammary field was drawn wider to accommodate the entire excision site as an alternative to having the junction of the internal and tangential fields "cutting" the excision scar. Boost volume is outlined. (**B** and **C**) Patient with T2N0M0 ductal carcinoma of the left breast treated with wide local excision, axillary dissection, and definitive irradiation. The excision site (**B**) in an unusually high location would have been at the junction of the tangential and supraclavicular fields, which is undesirable. Modification of the portal (**C**) increases the height of the supraclavicular portal. Note that the low and midaxillary lymph nodes are not included in the supraclavicular field.

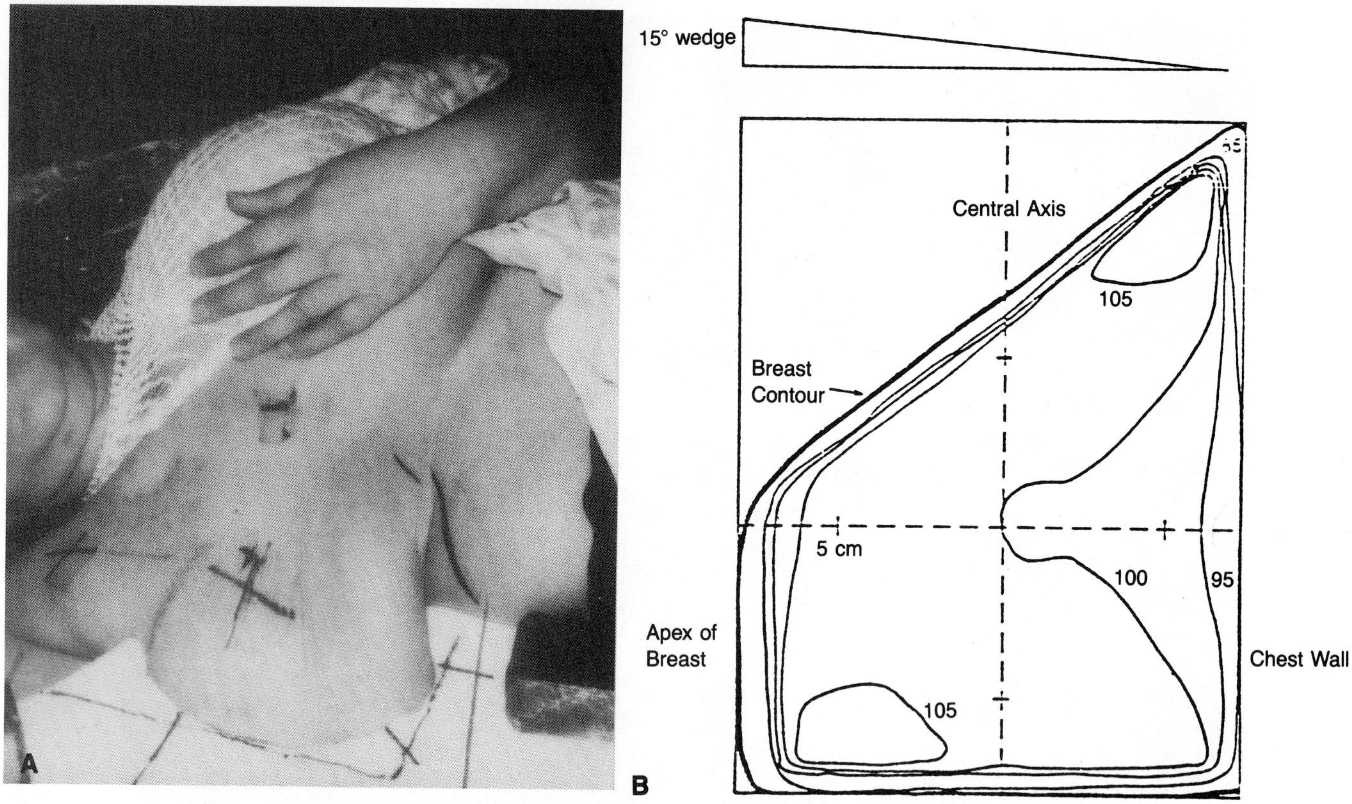

FIGURE 42–18. (**A**)Patient with large pendulous breast in lateral decubitus treatment position. (**B**) Lateral decubitus isodose distribution with 15-degree wedge. (Cross M, Elson HR, Aron BS: Int J Radiat Oncol Biol Phys 17:199, 1989)

Boost to Tumor Site

In recent years, careful pathologic examination of mastectomy specimens[199, 200, 302] in patients who were candidates for breast conservation therapy (with margins of 1 cm to 2 cm) demonstrated that residual microscopic tumor can be detected in 20% to 40% of patients within 2 cm of the primary tumor. Therefore a significant residual tumor burden may be present after an excisional biopsy with negative pathologic margins, a finding that correlates well with the NSABP B-06 12% breast recurrence rate following excision alone with negative margins for invasive carcinoma.[126] Most authors report that 65% to 80% of breast recurrences after conservation surgery and irradiation occur around the primary tumor site.[51, 132, 144, 182, 225, 340] These data provide a strong rationale for a tumor bed boost, although the issue has not been elucidated and the role of the boost in

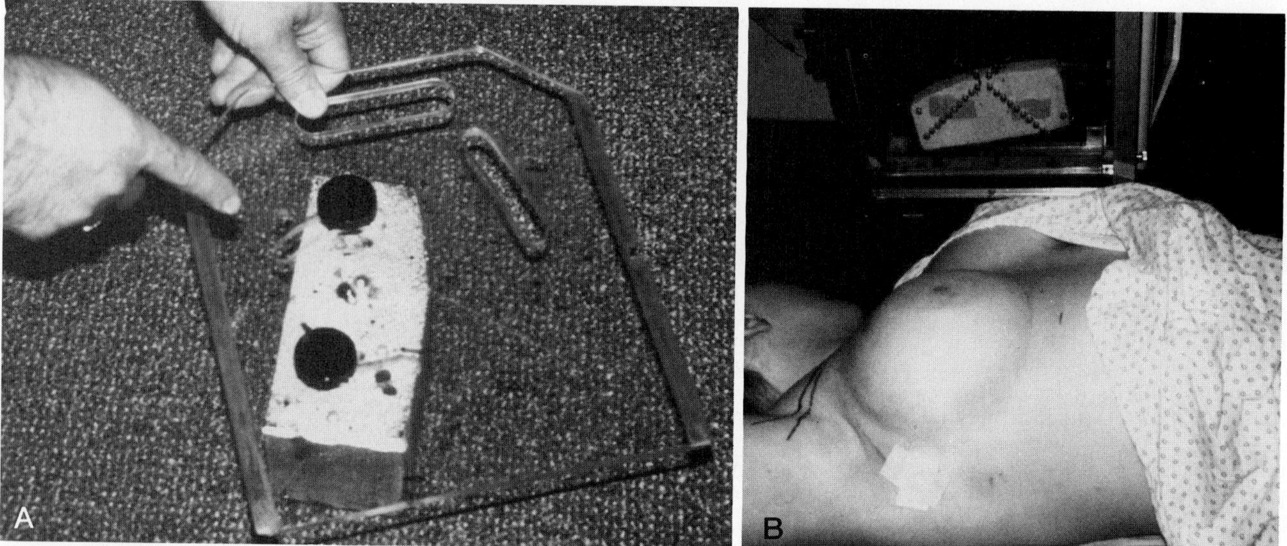

FIGURE 42–19. (**A**) Beam splitter used for tangential beams for irradiation of the breast (or chest wall). Block is made of Cerrobend, and several configurations can be designed to match the sloping anterior contour of the chest wall. (**B**) Patient and tangential beam splitting block in the treatment position.

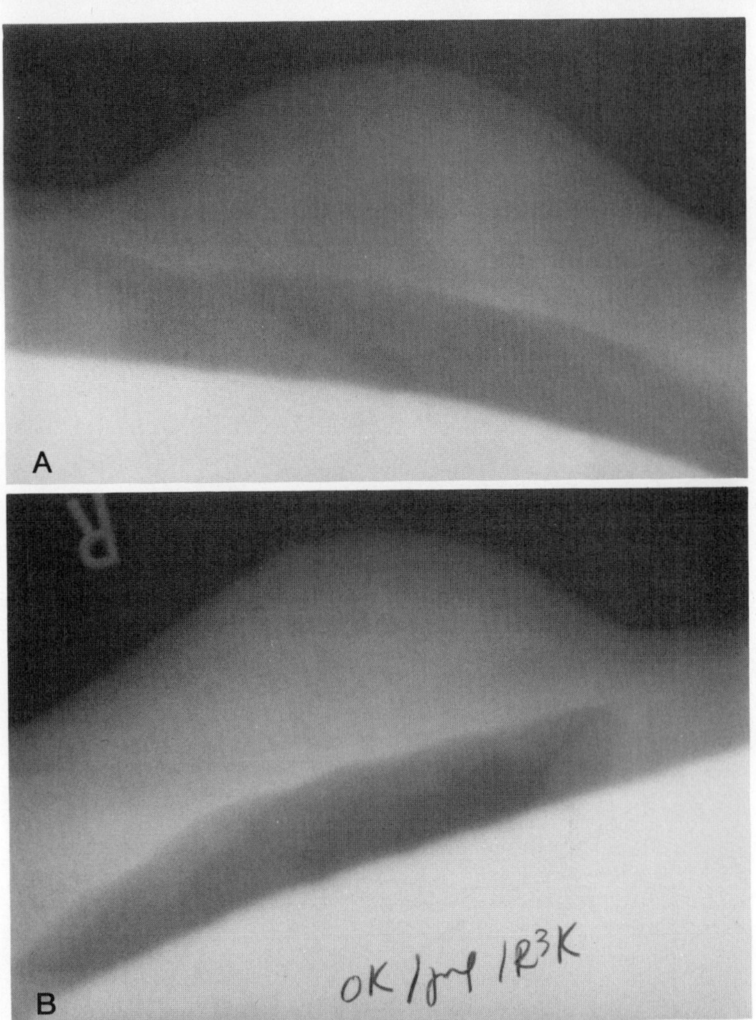

FIGURE 42–20. Examples of localization films of tangential breast portals demonstrating the amount of lung to be included in the field.

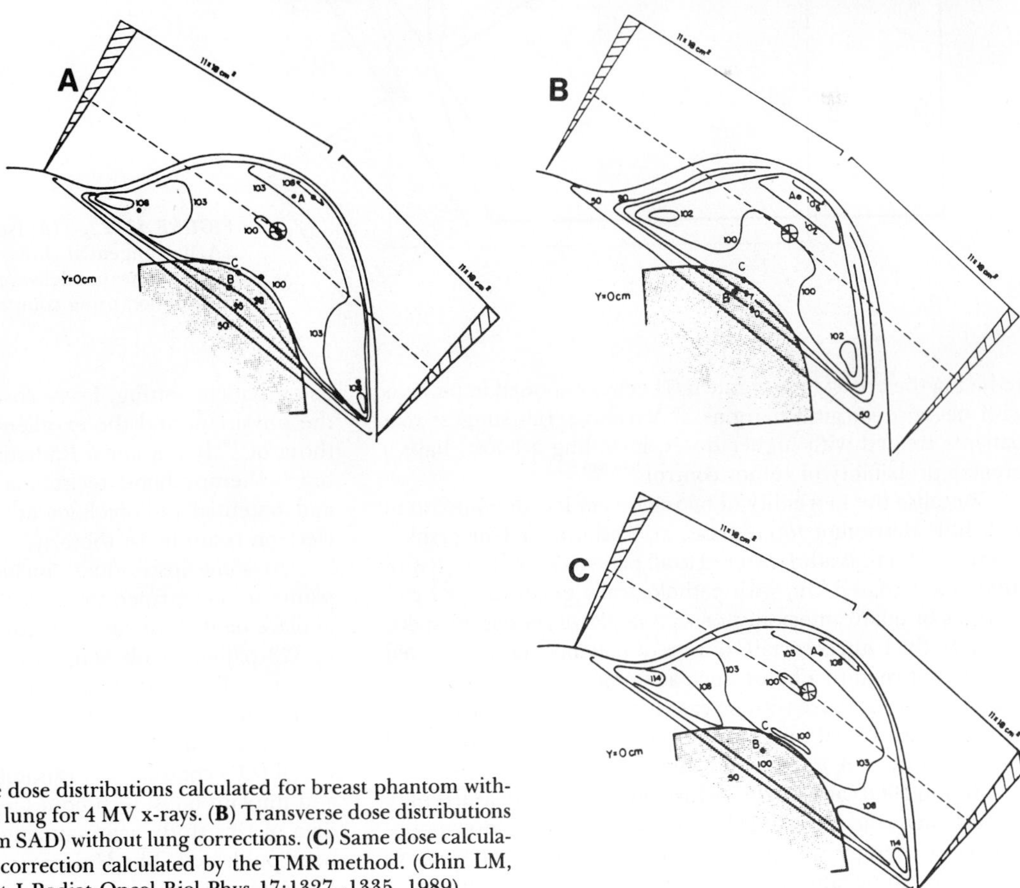

FIGURE 42–21. (**A**) Transverse dose distributions calculated for breast phantom without correction for presence of the lung for 4 MV x-rays. (**B**) Transverse dose distributions calculated for 8 MV x-rays (100 cm SAD) without lung corrections. (**C**) Same dose calculations for 4 MV x-rays with lung correction calculated by the TMR method. (Chin LM, Cheng CW, Siddon RL, et al: Int J Radiat Oncol Biol Phys 17:1327–1335, 1989)

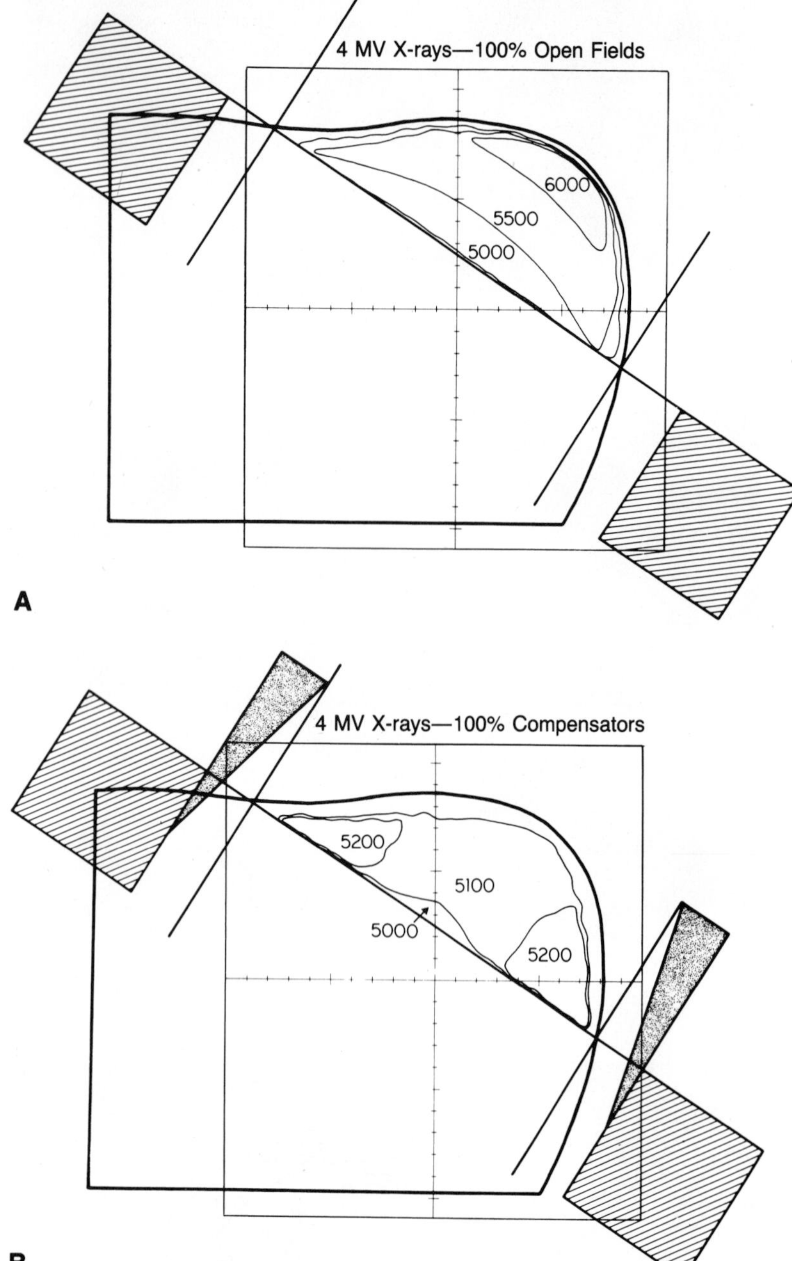

FIGURE 42–22. (**A**) Isodose curves for 4 MV x-rays (80 cm SAD), tangential breast portals without compensators. Higher doses are delivered to the apex of the breast. (**B**) Dose distribution using compensators for all treatments.

reducing the breast failure rate has been questioned in patients with negative surgical margins.[126] Various series suggest that patients treated with higher doses, including a boost, have a greater probability of tumor control.[339,340]

Because the morbidity of boosts is very low to nonexistent with little detriment to cosmesis, at Washington University a tumor bed boost is administered to all patients except those with tumors less than 1 cm, with pathologically generous (>2 cm) margins or quadrantectomy, or with negative reexcision specimens. In the future, certain subsets of patients may be defined who do not require a boost, such as women over age 40, those with T1 tumors, those with no extensive intraductal carcinoma or mononuclear-cell infiltrate, negative surgical margins, and those with neither necrosis nor high-grade tumors.

In the 1960s and 1970s, before the widespread availability of electron beam, interstitial brachytherapy or cone-down photon boost therapy was popular. Many institutions have preferred electron-beam boost because of its relative ease in setup, its outpatient setting, lower cost, decreased time demands on the physician, and the excellent results when compared with those of ^{192}Ir implants. Radiation oncologists who prefer the brachytherapy boost technique point to decreased skin dose and potential radiobiologic advantages when compared with electron-beam boost therapy.

At some institutions (including ours) intraoperative implants are performed to reduce cost and enhance the accuracy of placement of the catheters for the radioisotope. Mansfield,[266] in 323 patients with Stage T1-2N0-1 tumors reported 6-year actuarial disease-free survival rates of 96% and 98%, a local tumor control rate of 97%, and good to excellent cosmesis in 95% of the patients.

RTOG conducted a randomized trial comparing electron and implant boost techniques in T1-2N0-1 breast cancer. The data of this study are maturing, and the results have not yet been published. The University of Cincinnati and Washington University analyzed their combined results in 417 breast can-

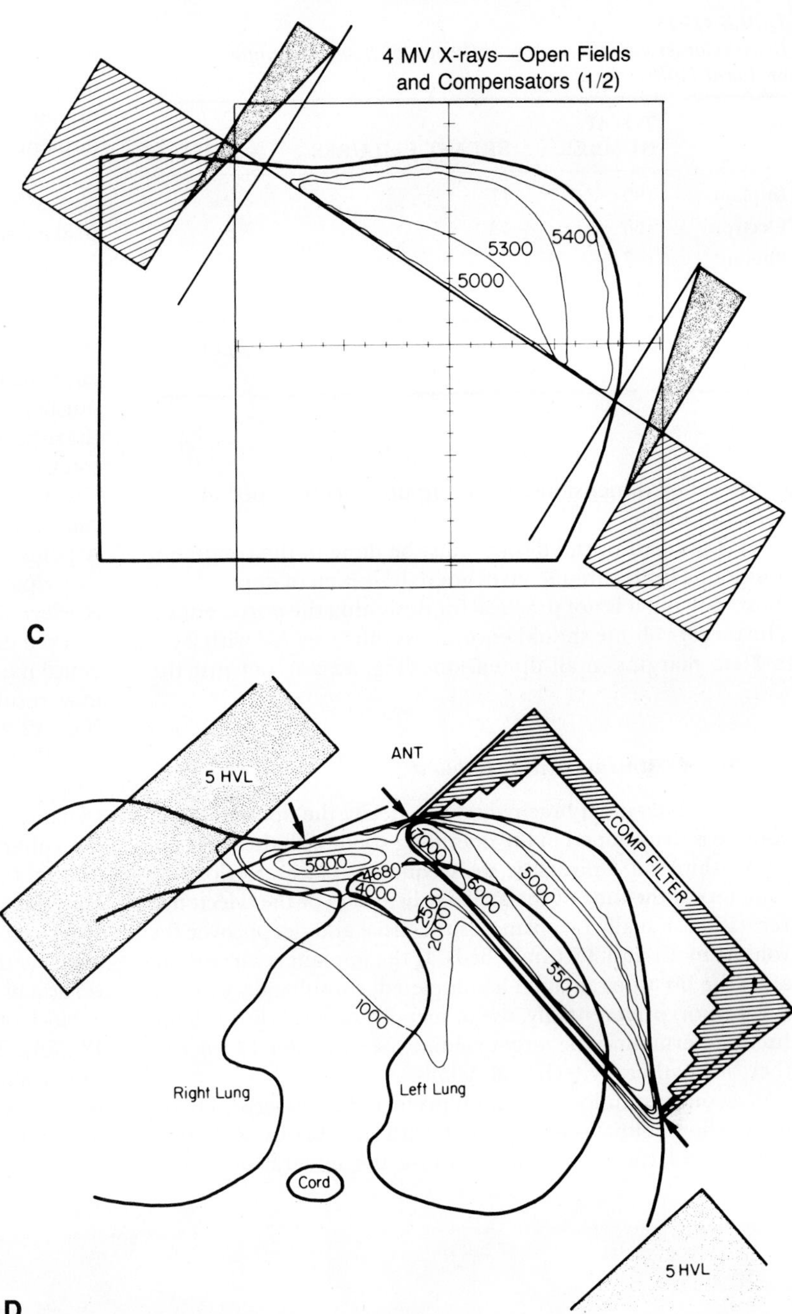

FIGURE 42–22. (*Continued*) (**C**) Isodose curves using open fields for half of the treatment and compensators for the other half. (**D**) Composite isodose curves for customized 2-dimensional compensating filters, beam splitter for tangential fields, and internal mammary portal treated with 4 MV photons (1600 cGy) and 12 MeV electrons (3000 cGy).

cers with a minimum follow-up period of 5 years.[231] Treatment philosophies were similar at the two institutions, with the exception that implant boosts were preferred at Cincinnati, whereas electron boosts were more frequently used at Washington University. No difference in tumor control could be detected between the two boost techniques (Table 42-19). In addition, a previous analysis showed no difference in cosmetic outcome as a function of boost technique.[232] Other investigators have observed better cosmetic results with electrons than with implants.[332,447]

Boost With Electron Beam

The clinical setup for electron boosts involves marking the projection of the postoperative induration on the skin and adding 2 cm to 3 cm in all directions. Ideally the skin markings should be placed and photographed at the time of initial simulation, not after 5 weeks of tangential whole-breast irradiation. The patient is positioned with the arm above the head to flatten the breast contour and then rolled so that the tylectomy scar is parallel with the table and the simulator (accelerator) head can point straight down onto the target volume. An electron energy is selected that covers the target volume depth (9 MeV, 12 MeV to 16 MeV). The 90% prescription isodose line is limited to the pectoral fascia to avoid substantial dose into the lung.

Accurate target volume definition is critical with any boost technique. Methods may vary from the simple and unsophisticated (as described in the previous paragraph) to the complex and expensive, such as surgical clips, ultrasonography, and CT definition of the target volume.

The surgical clip method requires the cooperation of the surgical team. Despite the fact that it would theoretically take an infinite number of clips to define every extension of a typical tylectomy cavity, in practice six clips suffice (superficial, deep, medial, lateral, cephalad, and caudal).[407] Ultrasonography can provide the depth of the biopsy cavity, as well

TABLE 42–19
Breast Conservation Therapy: Influence of Boost Technique on Local Failure

	TOTAL NUMBER	BREAST FAILURES	% FAILURE
Implant	199	17	8.5
Electron	166	13	7.8
Photon	7	1	14.3
No boost	45	4	8.9

(*Kuske RR, Compaan P, Cross M, et al: Int J Radiat Oncol Biol Phys 17[1]:235–236, 1989*)

as the other dimensions, for designing electron portal borders and energy.

CT-guided portal design must be done in the treatment position. This technique gives good definition of depth of the chest wall, but it is not practical for designing the portal edges. The target volume should encompass the *tumor bed* with 2 cm to 3 cm margins in all dimensions (Fig. 42-23), not just the scar.

Boost With Interstitial Implant

With interstitial brachytherapy, ideally the optimal target volume is determined in the operating room with the surgeon. At Washington University, we frequently place afterloading catheters at the time of the axillary dissection or the tylectomy/reexcision. Usually two planes (superficial and deep) cover the volume in T1 and T2 tumor beds. If the implant is carried out after the breast irradiation is completed, consultation with the surgeon or, preferentially, use of metallic surgical clips is helpful in determining the target volume. See Chapter 13 for further brachytherapy technical details.

At our institution, implant is preferred over electron boost in two clinical situations: in patients with large breasts with deep tumors (≥4 cm below skin), because the integral dose with electrons is high and there can be exit dose into the lung, and in patients with microscopically positive or unknown margins with no reexcision or other poor pathologic features, because a higher dose can more easily be delivered at depth with the implant (2000 cGy to 2500 cGy).

Matching the Tangential Fields With the Supraclavicular Field

A hot spot caused by divergence of the tangential beams into the supraclavicular field and of the supraclavicular beam into the tangential fields can exist just beneath the skin surface at the junction of the inferior border of the supraclavicular field and the superior border of the tangential fields.[29] The M. D. Anderson Cancer Center experience with the penumbra characteristics of ^{60}Co is such that this matchline is probably not enough to cause significant late problems. Yet, approximately 60% of their patients developed matchline fibrosis, which was detected only by palpation. On the other hand, the sharp beam of a linear accelerator and the "horns" at the edge of this beam produce a marked increase in dose beneath the matchline when the divergence mentioned above is not corrected. This increase in dose may result in severe matchline fibrosis or even rib fracture (Fig. 42-24).

The divergence of the tangential fields can be eliminated by angling the foot of the treatment couch away from the radiation source to direct the tangential beams inferiorly so that the superior edge of these beams lines up perfectly with the inferior border of the supraclavicular field (Fig. 42-25). In addition, the collimator must be rotated to geometrically eliminate overlap at this junction, or the "hanging block" technique developed at the Harvard Joint Center may be used, in which a vertical block is affixed to the superior portion of the collimator to block off the nonvertical portion of the tangential beam (Fig. 42-26*A*). The inferior divergence of the supraclavicular beam can be eliminated by blocking off the inferior half of this beam with a "beam splitter" so that the central nondiverging portion of the beam becomes the inferior border of this field (Fig. 42-26*B*).

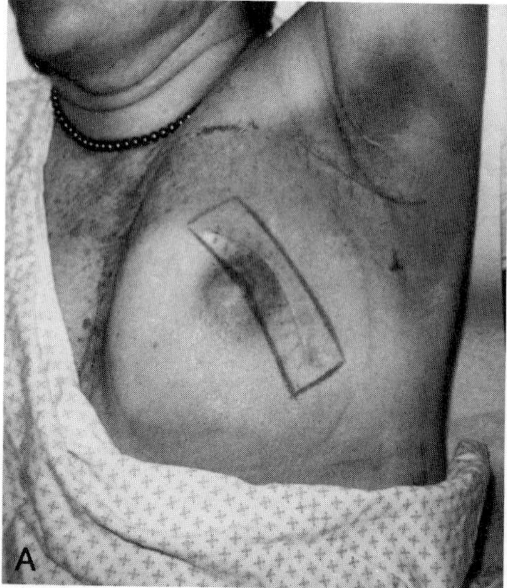

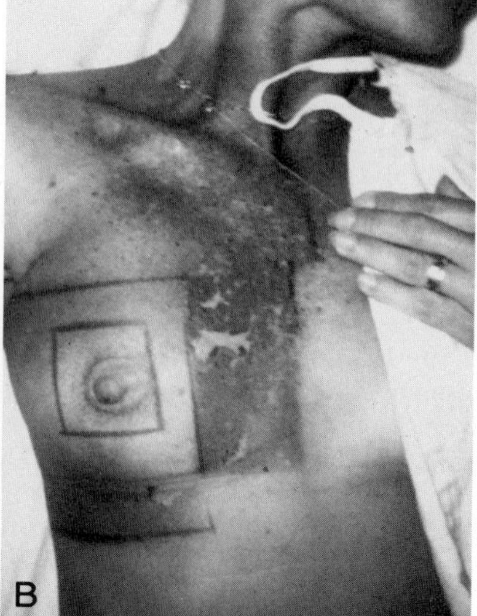

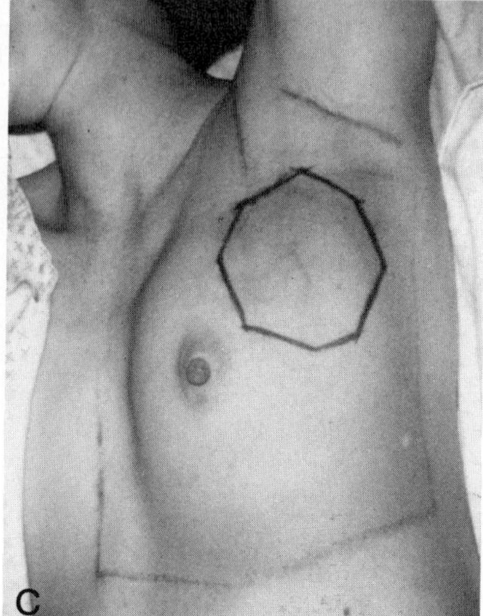

FIGURE 42–23. Examples of reduced portals used to deliver a "boost dose" to the excision site following breast irradiation. Margins in general are 2 cm from the scar, depending on size of lesion and adequacy of surgical margins.

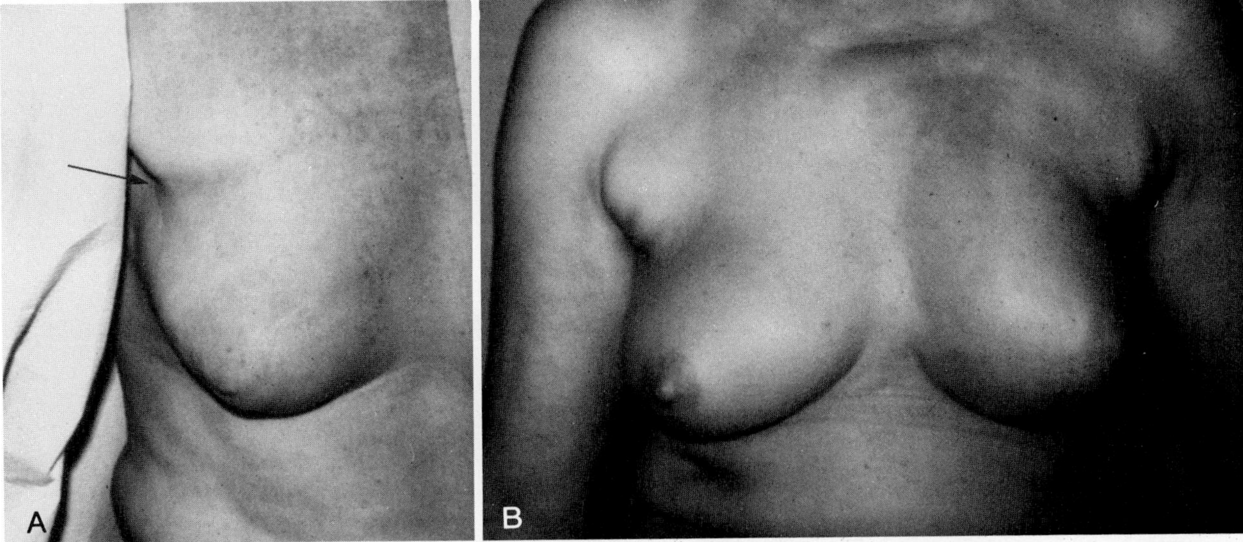

FIGURE 42–24. (**A**) Photograph of a patient 5 years after irradiation and tumor excision for carcinoma of the breast. A line of subcutaneous fibrosis is noted at the junction of the supraclavicular and tangential portals (*arrow*). (**B**) Photograph of another patient 10 years after treatment with tumor excision and radiation therapy to breast and regional lymph nodes. Some fibrosis at the junction of the supraclavicular and tangential portals and minimal atrophy and fibrosis of the breast are present.

Matching the Tangential Fields With the Internal Mammary Field

The match between the medial tangential field and the internal mammary field can be a problem when a significant amount of breast tissue lies beneath this matchline. In this situation a cold spot can exist (Fig. 42-27*A*), which may be negligible when the breast tissue beneath this matchline is thin (Fig. 42-27*B*); or it can be avoided by not using a separate internal mammary field (Fig. 43-27*C*). When this is done, it is necessary to be certain that the internal mammary nodes are included in the tangential beams (CT scan, radionuclide scintigraphy). Usually this can be achieved by moving the medial border 3 cm to 5 cm across the midline. The portal films should be inspected to ensure that an excessive amount of lung or heart is not being irradiated. There is no good solution to this matchline problem in large-chested women who also have a significant amount of breast tissue beneath the tangential-internal mammary matchline. To solve this problem Woudstra and van der Werf[491] described a technique using an oblique incidence of the internal mammary portal matching the orientation of the adjacent medial tangential portal (Fig. 42-28*A*), which results in a more homogeneous dose distribution at the junction of the two fields (Fig. 42-28*B*).

Irradiation Dose to the Contralateral Breast

Fraass and colleagues[145] measured dose to the contralateral breast in 16 women treated to the intact breast with tangential fields and performed phantom measurements. The contralateral breast received 50 cGy to 200 cGy for a typical treatment of 5000 cGy. The use of tangential fields merely resulted in more dose delivered to the surface area of the opposite breast, whereas the use of internal mammary field in addition to the tangential portals gave more dose deeper in the breast (ranges 1% to 4% from the lateral to the medial portions of the opposite breast). The volume of breast irradiated has minimal effect, but the use of portals for the regional lymph nodes increases dose to the contralateral breast.

The authors pointed out that the use of a 2.5 cm thick lead shield over the contralateral breast when treated with a medial tangential field reduces the dose to 35% of its original value. Similar shields used on the lateral tangent have essentially no protective effect. They also recommend that, whenever possible, wedges be used on the lateral tangential fields rather than on the medial fields to decrease the dose of contralateral breast.

Tercilla and associates,[436] measuring the dose with thermoluminescent dosimetry in 15 patients treated with tangential fields of ^{60}Co to the breast, demonstrated that the contralateral breast receives 6% to 13% of the prescribed dose with the source-skin distance (SSD) technique compared with 4% to 9% with the isocentric source-axis distance (SAD) technique. The doses ranged from 325 cGy to 650 cGy for the SSD method and from 200 cGy to 450 cGy for the SAD technique. They concluded that the increase in doses could be attributed mainly to transmission of radiation through the Cerrobend block. The highest doses were measured within 2 cm from the beam edge, a region containing the penumbra. A greater contribution of the dose is given from the medial tangential than from the lateral tangential beam. The doses described with the SAD technique by these authors are higher than those measured by Fraass and associates,[145, 146] who believe the discrepancy could be attributed to the difference in treatment wedges used.

It follows that attention should be focused on the medial beam in attempting to reduce the contralateral breast dose, which could be accomplished by treating without a wedge on the medial beam. However, this compromises the dose distribution. Increasing the thickness of the beam splitter on the medial field could lower the contralateral breast dose, but the greater weight makes the handling of the block by the technologist more difficult. The clinical significance of this inadvertent radiation dose to the opposite breast is uncertain; various investigators have failed to show an increased risk of contralateral breast malignancy following treatment of the original breast by radiation therapy.

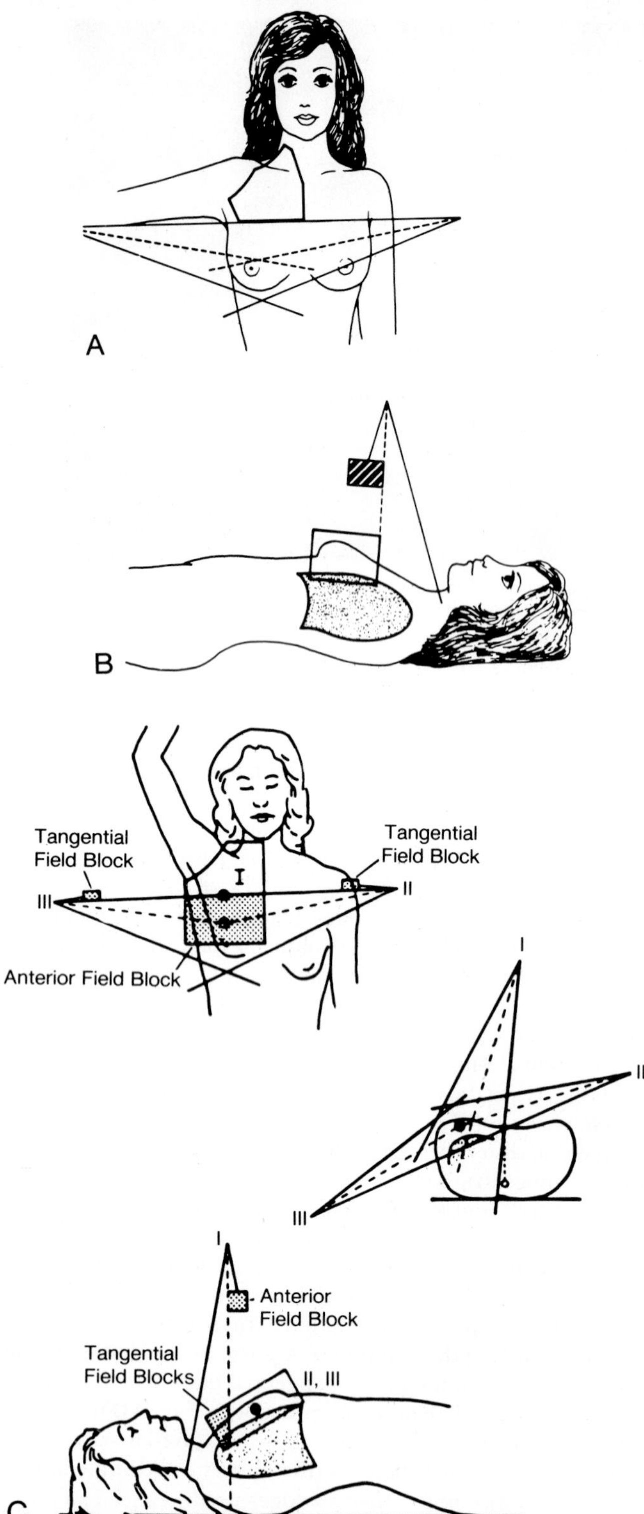

FIGURE 42–25. (**A**) Inferior angulation of the tangential beams eliminates their divergence into the supraclavicular field. (**B**) Splitting the supraclavicular beam eliminates its divergence into the tangential field. (Bedwinek JM: Int J Radiat Oncol Biol Phys 7:1553, 1981) (**C**) Three-field treatment beam geometry in irradiation of the intact breast and supraclavicular fields illustrated in coronal, cross-sectional, and sagittal projections. The supraclavicular and tangential field blocks are shaded. (Svensson GK, Chin LM, Siddon RL, et al. Breast treatment techniques at the Joint Center for Radiation Therapy. In Harris JR, Hellman S, Silen W [eds.]: Conservative Management of Breast Cancer: New Surgical and Radiotherapeutic Techniques. Philadelphia, JB Lippincott, 1983)

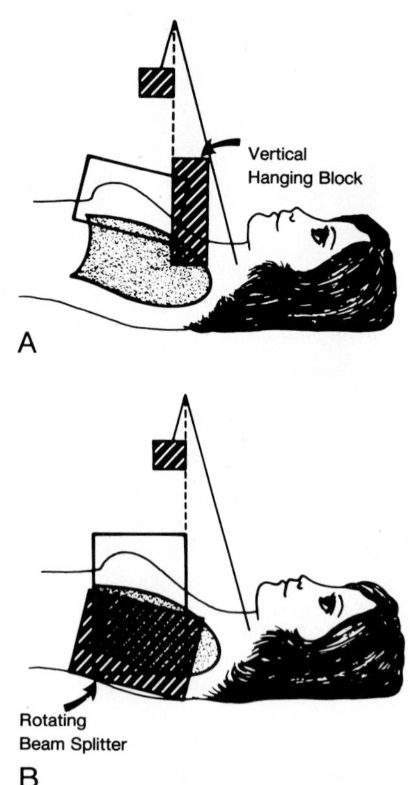

FIGURE 42–26. (**A**) The superior edge of the tangential beams can be made perfectly vertical by means of the "hanging block" technique or (**B**) by avoiding collimator rotation with the use of a rotating beam splitter. (Bedwinek JM: Int J Radiat Oncol Biol Phys 7:1553, 1981)

Irradiation of Regional Lymphatics

Internal Mammary Lymph Nodes

The medial border of the internal mammary field is the midline; the lateral border is 5 cm to 6 cm lateral to the midline; the superior border abuts the inferior border of the supraclavicular field; and the inferior border is at the xiphoid. If only the internal mammary nodes are to be treated, the superior border of the field is at the superior surface of the head of the clavicle. The field is set as described, with an oblique incidence to match the medial tangential portal (Fig. 42-29). The dose to the internal mammary field (4500 cGy to 5000 cGy at 180 cGy to 200 cGy/day) is calculated at a point 4 cm beneath the skin surface. To spare underlying lung, mediastinum, and spinal cord, electrons in the range of 13 MeV for a portion of the treatment are preferred. The usual proportion is 1440 cGy delivered with 4 MV to 6 MV photons and 3060 cGy with electrons (180 cGy daily).

Supraclavicular Lymph Nodes

If the apex of the axilla alone is treated (after modified radical mastectomy or axillary dissection), the inferior border of the supraclavicular field is the first or second intercostal space. The medial border is 1 cm across the midline, extending upward, following the medial border of the sternocleidomastoid muscle to the thyrocricoid groove. The lateral border is a vertical line at the level of the anterior axillary fold. The humeral head is blocked as much as possible without compromising coverage of the high axillary lymph nodes.

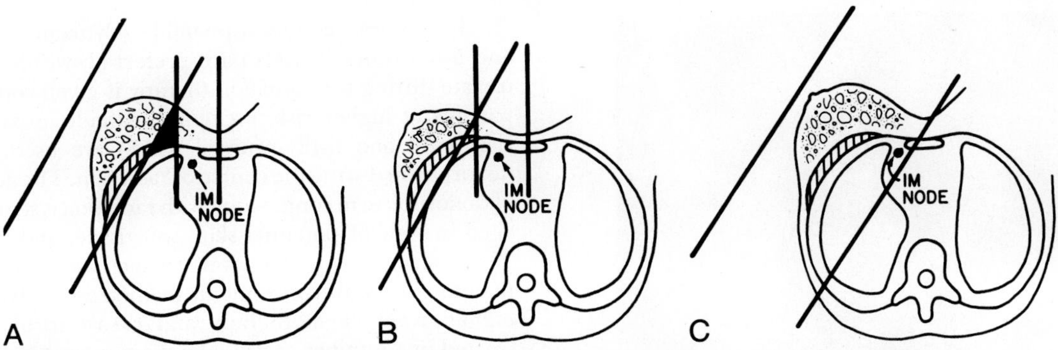

FIGURE 42–27. Diagrams showing several relationships between internal mammary and tangential fields. (**A**) A significant cold region exists when the internal mammary (IM)-tangential matchline overlies a large amount of breast tissue. (**B**) The cold area may be negligible when the breast tissue beneath the matchline is thin. (**C**) The lack of a separate IM field can result in the irradiation of an excessive volume of lung, particularly in large-chested patients. (Bedwinek JM: Int J Radiat Oncol Biol Phys 7:1553, 1981)

This field is angled about 15 degrees laterally to spare the spinal cord (Fig. 42-30).

The low axilla is treated only when the tumor breaks through the capsule of the lymph nodes or when axillary dissection is not performed. Here, the supraclavicular field is modified: The inferior border comes down to split the second rib (Louis' angle), and the lateral border is drawn to just block fall-off across the skin of the anterior axillary fold.

The total dose delivered to the supraclavicular field is 4600 cGy at 200 cGy/day in five weekly fractions to a point 3.0 cm beneath the skin surface. An alternative time-dose schedule is 5040 cGy at 180 cGy/day.

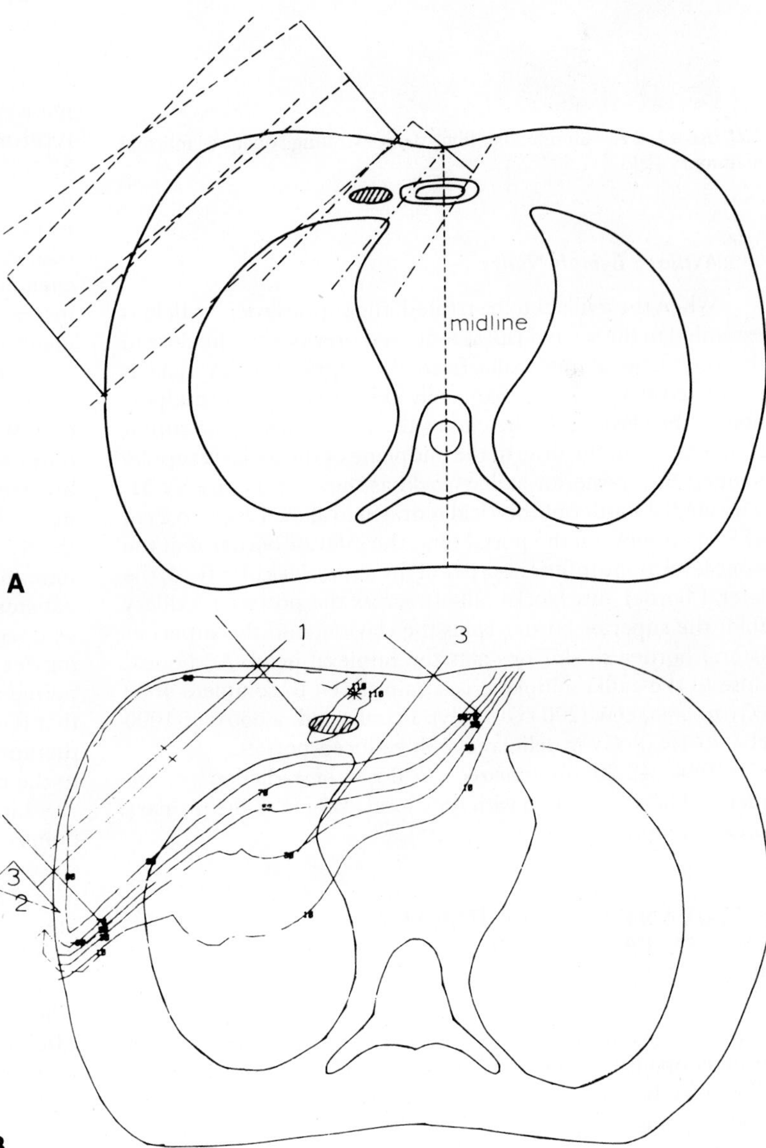

FIGURE 42–28. (**A**) An obliquely incident electron beam matched to the usual tangential beams. (**B**) Isodose presentation of optimal matching of an oblique incident electron beam to the tangential beams. The target volume is enclosed by the 90-isodose line (= 4050 cGy). Electron beam: 16 MeV; photon beam: 6 MV. (Woudstra E, van der Werf H: Radiother Oncol 10:209, 1987)

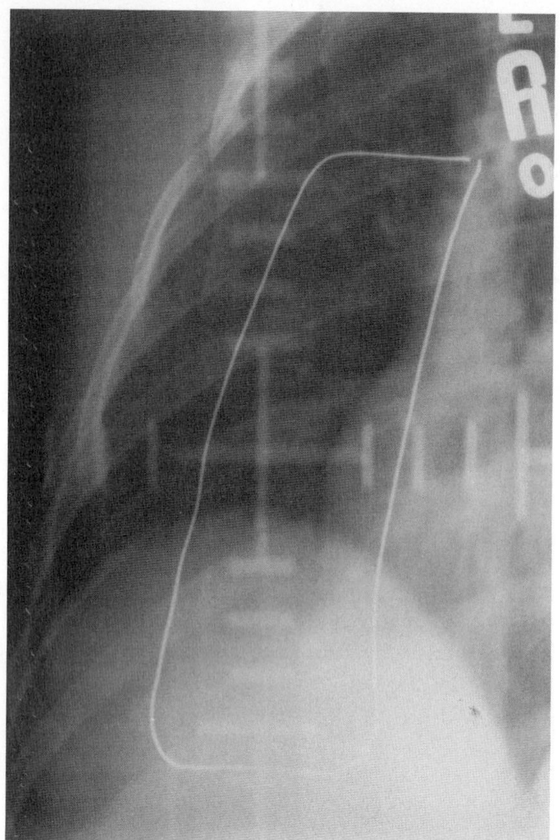

FIGURE 42–29. Simulation film demonstrating oblique internal mammary field.

Axillary Lymph Nodes

When the axilla is to be treated, the supraclavicular field is extended to the second rib, as indicated previously. The dose to the midplane of the axilla from the supraclavicular field is calculated at a point approximately 2 cm inferior to the midportion of the clavicle. At the end of the treatments to the supraclavicular field, the dose to the midplane of the axilla is supplemented by a posterior axillary field as shown in Figure 42-31. The medial border of this field is drawn to allow 1.5 cm to 2 cm of lung to show on the portal film; the inferior border is at the same level as the inferior border of the supraclavicular field; the lateral border just blocks fall-off across the posterior axillary fold; the superior border splits the clavicle; and the superior-lateral border shields or splits the humeral head. Additional dose to the axilla midplane is administered to complete 4600 cGy to 5000 cGy (200 cGy daily). If indicated, a boost of 1000 cGy to 1500 cGy is delivered with reduced portals.

Table 42-20 summarizes the doses of radiation recommended in combination with wide local excision of the primary breast tumor.

ADJUVANT CHEMOTHERAPY IN THE TREATMENT OF T1-2N0-1 BREAST CANCER

Adjuvant chemotherapy has been shown to improve survival of premenopausal women with positive axillary lymph nodes at diagnosis. It is being used increasingly for women with negative nodes. Thus, with the rising numbers of women opting for breast conservation therapy for early breast cancer, coordination of chemotherapy and irradiation is a pressing issue.

In general, cyclophosphamide (Cytoxan), methotrexate, and 5-fluorouracil (CMF) are preferred, withholding methotrexate during the radiation therapy if given concurrently. In patients at higher risk, cyclophosphamide, doxorubicin (Adriamycin), and 5-fluorouracil (CAF) are used, withholding doxorubicin during the course of radiation. The administration of doxorubicin in conjunction with radiation is strongly discouraged in view of potential skin, soft tissue, and heart toxicity. There is some concern about an increased risk of radiation pneumonitis with concomitant methotrexate. Women requiring adjuvant chemotherapy and breast irradiation can be treated in a number of ways: by the two treatments given concomitantly, with the above adjustments; by a sequential approach, with radiation given first; or by use of a sandwich technique with the radiation interposed between courses of chemotherapy. No approach has proven to be superior in terms of the ability to control tumor locally or distantly. However, because of increasing normal tissue reactions with either drug combination plus radiation, it is common practice to initiate chemotherapy after completion of irradiation.

Patients opting for breast conservation therapy who also receive adjuvant chemotherapy may have less favorable cosmetic results when compared with those of women not receiving chemotherapy.[333] Not only are the long-term cosmetic results in women treated with both modalities less satisfactory, also an increase in early skin reaction occurs in patients receiving combined therapy.[27,333]

Rose and colleagues[349] recently updated the Harvard cosmesis data.[27] They reported that at 3 years, 68% of women not receiving chemotherapy had an excellent result compared with 37% of women who received chemotherapy. These figures were maintained at 5 years. Conversely, of the patients who did not receive chemotherapy, 9% were judged to have fair or poor cosmetic results compared with 24% of those who received chemotherapy. These differences were mostly the result of an increase in breast retraction and, to a lesser extent, the development of telangiectasia.

Concern has been voiced regarding the potential difficulty in administering adequate doses of chemotherapy after irradiation. Weiss and associates[480] analyzed the ability to deliver full doses of adjuvant chemotherapy in 764 women treated with breast conservation therapy compared with women treated with mastectomy. Although more leukopenia was noted in the group treated with breast conservation therapy and a slightly longer time to deliver all the therapy was required compared with patients treated with mastectomy, the percentage of women who received more than 85% doses was high, no life-threatening degree of leukopenia was observed, and skin reactions and pulmonary fibrosis were rarely severe. Thus, this study showed that it is possible to administer high doses of adjuvant chemotherapy to patients treated concurrently with radiation therapy to the breast.

Lippman and co-workers[260] reported on a prospective randomized trial comparing modified radical mastectomy to breast conservation therapy and evaluated whether irradiation negatively affected the ability to administer adjuvant cyclophosphamide and doxorubicin in women with positive axillary lymph nodes. All women were treated identically, with a third cycle of chemotherapy given during radiation therapy. No significant differences were found in the amount of chemotherapy administered to either treatment group, and no differences were found in the recurrence rates as a function of the quantity of drug received.

In the 8-year results of the NSABP (B-06),[126] it was found that women with positive axillary lymph nodes who were treated with lumpectomy, breast irradiation, and adjuvant che-

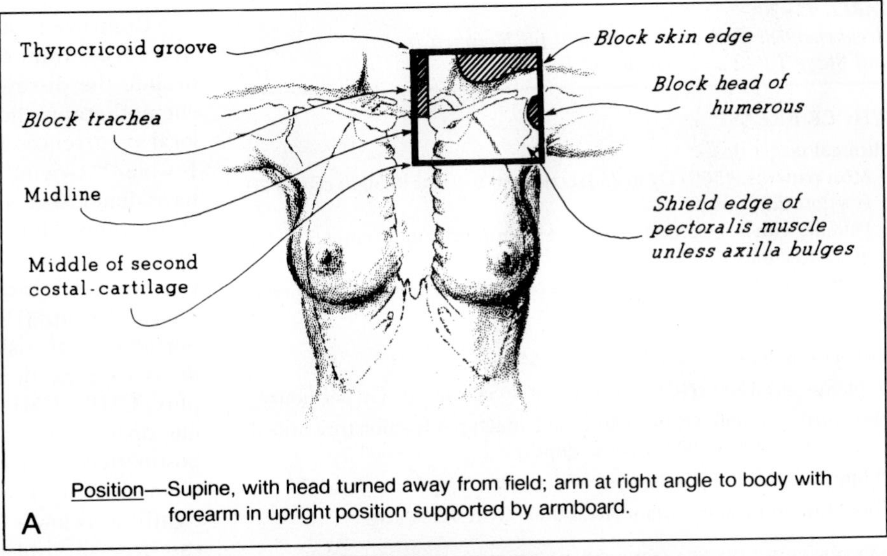

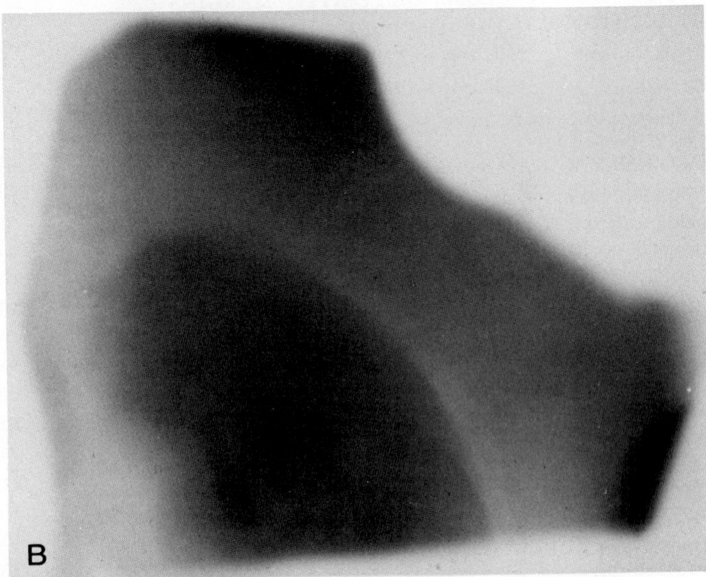

FIGURE 42–30. (**A**) Diagram illustrating the supraclavicular portal. When a 15-degree lateral angulation is used to avoid the spinal cord, the medial margin is 1 cm across the midline up to the sternal notch. The humeral head is at least partially blocked. (**B**) Localization film of the supraclavicular portal.

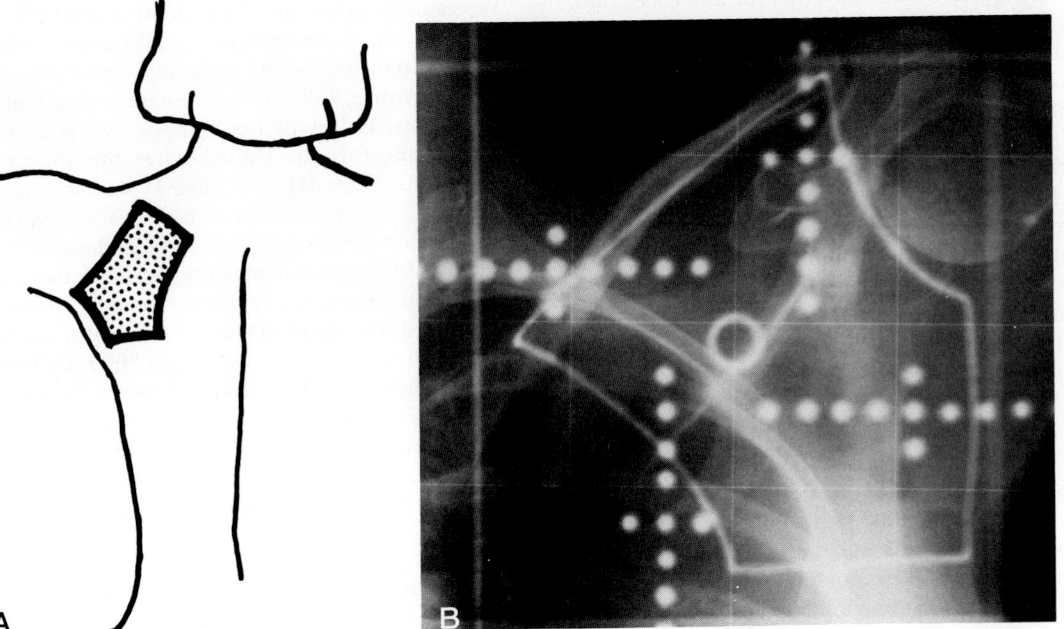

FIGURE 42–31. (**A**) Posterior left axillary field used to supplement the dose at midplane of the axilla. (**B**) Simulation film of a posterior right axillary field. Notice the small amount of lung included and shielding of the humeral head (whenever possible).

TABLE 42–20
Recommended Policies of Treatment for Noninvasive and Stage T1–T2 Carcinoma of Breast

WHOLE BREAST

Minimal target doses:

Most patients: 4500 cGy in 25 fractions in 5 weeks to 5040 cGy in 28 fractions in 6 weeks

Patients with large breasts or bridge separation over 22 cm: 4500 cGy in 25 fractions in 5 weeks

Patients in whom chemotherapy has been administered or is planned: 4500 cGy in 25 fractions in 5 weeks

BREAST BOOST

Implant: 1500 cGy to 2000 cGy at 40 cGy to 50 cGy per hour

Electrons: 1000 cGy to 1600 cGy at 200 cGy per fraction (prescribed at the 90% isodose depth)

Photons: 1000 cGy to 1600 cGy at 200 cGy per fraction

Total dose to primary tumor site: 6000 cGy to 6500 cGy

PATIENTS WITH "CLOSE" OR POSITIVE MARGINS IN EXCISION SPECIMEN(S)

Boost implant: 1800 cGy to 2500 cGy

Electrons: 1500 cGy to 2000 cGy

Total dose to primary tumor site: 6500 cGy to 7000 cGy

INTERNAL MAMMARY NODES

If treated, the internal mammary nodes should be included in tangent fields with the entire breast (lower nodes) or in the *en face* supraclavicular/axillary field. Use electrons (3000 cGy) combined with photons (1600 cGy) to decrease lung irradiation.

AXILLARY LYMPH NODES

If treated, the axillary lymph nodes should receive 4500 cGy to 4600 cGy in 23 to 25 fractions over a period of 4.6 to 5 weeks. When extracapsular disease is present, axillary nodes should be boosted to a total dose of 5000 cGy to 5400 cGy. For gross residual disease, a boost to a total dose not exceeding 6000 cGy should be used.

motherapy had a lower breast tumor recurrence rate (6%) than women with negative axillary lymph nodes treated with surgery and breast irradiation only (12%).

These findings were confirmed by Rose and colleagues,[348] who reported an actuarial risk of breast failure of 5% in 74 patients with positive nodes treated with adjuvant chemotherapy in addition to conservation surgery and irradiation of the breast, in contrast to 17% local failure in 192 patients who received no adjuvant chemotherapy. These findings suggest that chemotherapy and irradiation may have an additive or synergistic effect. However, adjuvant chemotherapy alone was unable to prevent breast cancer recurrences. Of women treated with segmental mastectomy without breast irradiation in NSABP (B-06), who also received chemotherapy because of involved axillary lymph nodes, 43% developed recurrent tumor in the breast.[126]

For many years there has been controversy concerning the benefit of adjuvant chemotherapy (ACT) in the treatment of T1 and T2 breast cancer with positive axillary nodes.[39, 57, 95, 154, 156, 252, 330] A recent review evaluated a large number of studies using the process of meta-analysis, and a consensus was developed that premenopausal patients with T1,T2,N1 disease or patients with one to three positive nodes benefited from adjuvant chemotherapy (CMF, CMFVP, and others). No such positive finding for the use of adjuvant chemotherapy was found in postmenopausal patients with positive nodes. These patients demonstrated a positive survival benefit from the use of tamoxifen.[103]

Controversy still exists regarding the overall survival benefit from adjuvant radiation therapy.[133, 255] It is noteworthy that, despite the disease-free survival improvement with adjuvant chemotherapy, the role of adjuvant irradiation in preventing local recurrences still exists. A number of authors including Fowble,[142] Griem,[160] Marcial,[268] Levitt,[244] and their colleagues have demonstrated that there is a definite rationale for postmastectomy adjuvant radiation therapy in addition to chemotherapy or hormonal therapy in patients with four or more positive nodes. In a study from the Danish Breast Cancer Cooperative Group (DBCCG), Overgaard and co-workers[294] reported on high-risk breast cancer patients. Premenopausal patients were randomized to receive postmastectomy radiation plus CMF, CMF alone, or CMF plus tamoxifen. Postmenopausal patients were randomized to receive tamoxifen, postmastectomy irradiation plus tamoxifen alone, or CMF plus tamoxifen. At 4 years, the locoregional recurrence rate was significantly lower in the irradiated patients. Furthermore, disease-free survival was improved in both premenopausal and postmenopausal irradiated patients compared with those who had systemic treatment only. At the time of the report, significant survival differences existed in the treatment groups.

Rutqvist and colleagues[366] reported on a trial comparing postoperative irradiation (4600 cGy in 4.5 weeks to chest wall and regional lymph nodes) or 12 courses of CMF (cyclophosphamide, 100 mg/m^2 by mouth on days 1 to 14; methotrexate, 40 mg/m^2 intravenously on days 1 and 8; and 5-FU, 600 mg/m^2 intravenously on days 1 and 8). During the first 18 months of the study, cyclophosphamide was replaced by chlorambucil (10 mg to 15 mg by mouth). Eighty-five percent of the patients were treated with CMF. Analysis of the study of 706 evaluable women, which is still open, shows that the actuarial 7-year disease-free survival rate is about 10% higher for patients receiving postoperative radiation therapy ; however, the difference is not statistically significant. The greatest difference in disease-free survival rate was noted in postmenopausal patients treated with irradiation (57%) compared with those receiving chemotherapy (36%; $P = 0.01$). No significant difference was noted in the premenopausal patients. The overall survival is comparable in the various groups (Fig. 42-32). In the entire group of patients, locoregional recurrences were noted in 12% of patients receiving postoperative irradiation and in 22% of those receiving adjuvant chemotherapy only. Distant metastases were noted in 33% and 36% of the patients, respectively.

In France, 250 patients were treated with neoadjuvant chemotherapy and irradiation without surgery for various stages of breast cancer. In the United States, this approach is limited to those with Stage III and Stage IV tumors. Jacquillat and colleagues[205] reported 5-year disease-free survival rates of 100% in 19 patients with Stage I, 82% in 86 in those with Stage IIA, and 61% in 51 Stage IIB patients receiving three to six cycles of vinblastine, thiotepa, methotrexate, and 5-fluorouracil with or without doxorubicin in combination with ^{60}Co radiation (4500 cGy to the breast and 2000 cGy to 3000 cGy boost to the initial tumor site with ^{192}Ir implant). About 30% complete responses and 41% to 75% partial responses, depending on initial tumor size, were observed after initial chemotherapy. The actuarial locoregional recurrence rate was zero in T1 and 13% in T2 tumors. Breast preservation at 5 years was 94%.

Adjuvant Chemotherapy in Node-Negative Patients

Radiation oncologists are well aware of the controversy inspired by what was believed by some to be a premature clinical alert disseminated by the National Cancer Institute (NCI) on the use

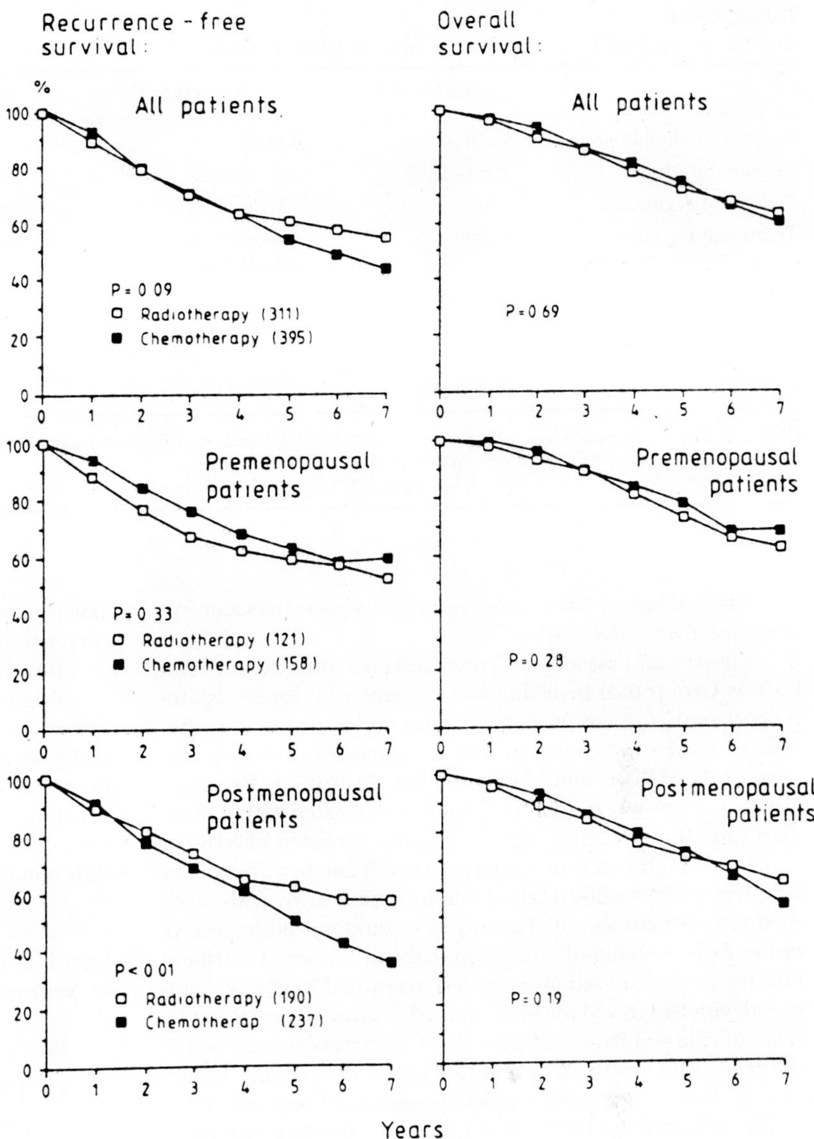

FIGURE 42–32. Trial of postoperative radiation therapy *versus* adjuvant chemotherapy: recurrence-free and overall survival by menopausal status. (Rutqvist LR, Cedermark B, Glas U, et al: Int J Radiat Oncol Biol Phys 16:629, 1989)

of adjuvant chemotherapy in node-negative (N0) breast cancer patients, based on what was considered to be inadequate statistically valid data. This was shortly followed by the publication of several clinical trials in the *New England Journal of Medicine*.[122, 123, 263, 267] Wolmark[490] analyzed the merits and possible negative repercussions of the publicized NCI clinical alert. The characteristics of the patients in the four trials are shown in Table 42-21, which unfortunately failed to include data showing no significant overall survival benefits for patients treated with adjuvant chemotherapy in any of the trials. Thus, the benefit of the demonstrated prolongation of disease-free survival must be weighed against the toxicity and cost of adjuvant therapy in these patients.

Very critical to the issue of adjuvant chemotherapy in node-negative patients is the identification of high-risk subgroups to whom it is justifiable to administer cytotoxic agents. This category may include patients with a high growth fraction (greater than 5.2% S phase), high aneuploid DNA index, expression of epidermal growth factor receptor, oncogene analysis, tumors larger than 3 cm, negative hormonal receptors, lymphatic or vascular permeation, or high nuclear grade indicating poor tumor differentiation. From several studies[76, 298, 397] patients with negative axillary lymph nodes have been classified into low or high risk, depending on several parameters (Table 42-22).

Many medical oncologists do not believe that T1 lesions that are less than or equal to 1 cm in diameter or that are estrogen receptor-positive require adjuvant chemotherapy. In addition, other oncologists of equal prominence disagree with the conclusion of the NCI suggestions and note the cost and toxicity involved in this program in which there is not so far an increase in overall survival, but merely an increase in recurrence-free interval of approximately 4% to 5%. Obviously, this subject remains controversial. The reader is advised to read the literature carefully and peruse the editorial by McGuire that appeared in the same journal as the reported studies.[92, 122, 123, 155, 267, 278, 279]

ADJUVANT HORMONAL THERAPY

Tamoxifen, an antiestrogen, has been frequently used as an adjuvant, particularly in postmenopausal patients. A recent review of 28 randomized trials involving over 16,000 women demonstrated reductions in mortality in women receiving tamoxifen compared with those not receiving the hormone, particularly in women 50 years or older.[103] Furthermore, in NSABP (B14), patients randomized to receive tamoxifen (10 mg twice daily) showed a significant reduction in incidence of

TABLE 42–21
Accrual and Patient Eligibility Criteria in Four Clinical Trials Assessing Adjuvant Chemotherapy in Node-Negative Breast Cancer Patients

	LUDWIG V[263]	INTERGROUP[267]	NSABP 13[123]	NSABP 14[122]
Number of eligible patients	1275	406	679	2644
Accrual duration	1981–1985	1981–1988	1981–1988	1982–1987
Treatment regimen	CMF	CMFP	M→F	Tamoxifen
Treatment duration	9 days	6 months All ER Neg, Er Pos ≥ 3 cm	13 months ER Neg ONLY	5 to 10 years ER Pos ONLY
Operation	Mastectomy	Mastectomy	Mastectomy or lumpectomy	Mastectomy or lumpectomy
Disease-free survival benefit (p)	$P = 0.04$ at 4 years	$P = 0.0001$ at 3 years	$P = 0.003$ at 4 years	$P < 0.00001$ at 4 years
Overall survival	Not reported	Not reported	87% *versus* 86% ($P = 0.8$)	92% *versus* 93% ($P = 0.3$)

CMF: cyclophosphamide, methotrexate, 5-fluorouracil; CMFP: cyclophosphamide, methotrexate, 5-fluorouracil, prednisone; ER Neg: estrogen-receptor negative; ER Pos: estrogen-receptor positive
(Modified from Wolmark N: PPO Updates 3[12]:1–10, 1989)

contralateral breast cancer, underscoring its potential value in a hormone preventive setting.[490]

Rutqvist and associates[366] reported on a Stockholm Breast Cancer Group trial involving 891 patients with lower risk tumors (less than 3 cm in diameter and no lymph node metastasis), 146 of whom were treated with breast-conserving surgery, axillary dissection, and radiation therapy to the breast (5000 cGy in 5 weeks); the remainder was treated with a modified radical mastectomy. Another group consisted of 516 patients with high-risk tumors (larger than 3 cm or with axillary lymph node metastases), all of whom were treated with modified radical mastectomy. Patients were randomized to receive or not receive 40 mg of tamoxifen daily for 2 years. Treatment failures in the tamoxifen group occurred in 173 (24%), compared with 214 (31%) in the untreated control group ($P < 0.1$). A significant reduction in locoregional recurrences occurred in the tamoxifen group (.61 event rate ratio), whereas the reduction in distant metastasis was less pronounced and not statistically significant (.84 event rate ratio). The 6-year recurrence-free survival rate was superior in the tamoxifen-treated groups (86% *versus* 77% in the lower-risk and 59% *versus* 51% in the high-risk patients). There was no significant correlation in the results between tumor stage and the high- or low-risk patient groups.

RESULTS OF THERAPY IN PRIMARY BREAST CANCER

Radical Surgery

No single operative procedure can be used for all primary breast cancers. Among the best results reported for patients treated with radical mastectomy alone are those of Haagensen.[165] The 10-year survival rates in 1001 patients were 70.5% in Stage A and 44% in Stage B. The Stage A and B cases with proven subclavicular or internal mammary metastases (triple biopsy) were treated by irradiation only in this series; their 10-year survival rate was 21%. The radiation technique used in this study differed markedly from modern radiation therapy techniques. Numerous reports with results of radical or modified radical mastectomy have been published and are not further reviewed here. Ten-year survival rates vary from 75% to 80% for patients with small tumors and negative lymph nodes to 30% to 40% with more advanced lesions and four or more axillary metastatic lymph nodes. Likewise, the incidence of recurrences in the chest wall ranges from 10% to 45%, depending on tumor stage and status of the regional lymph nodes.[96]

Patients who were good operative risks and who had a high risk of early metastatic spread to the internal mammary lymph nodes were treated at some institutions with extended radical mastectomy. The 10-year survival rate was 56% when only internal mammary node metastases were present and 29% when both axillary and internal mammary nodes were involved with metastatic cancer.[453]

Local Tumor Excision (Tylectomy, Lumpectomy) or Segmental Mastectomy and Breast Irradiation

Early Reports

In 1937 Keynes[213] stated that "widespread operations based upon the permeation theory on lymphatics and fascial planes have no real justification and the idea of conservative treatment of cancer of the breast may become less repugnant to us [surgeons]." He treated 325 patients with local removal of breast tumor and radium implantation at the site of local incision as well as in the axilla. In 250 evaluable patients the 5-year survival rate was 71% for group 1 (disease confined to the breast), 29% for group 2 (disease apparently confined to breast and axilla), and 23.6% for group 3 (advanced disease or inoperable). At the time, the results were comparable to those of a radical mastectomy. Rissanen[342] in 1969 reported on 415 pa-

TABLE 42–22
Factors Affecting Risk of Recurrence in Node-Negative Breast Cancer

PROGNOSTIC FACTOR	LOW	HIGH
Nuclear grade	I	III
Estrogen receptor	Positive	Negative
Tumor size	<1 cm	>2 cm
Ploidy	Diploid	Aneuploid
S phase cell cycle	Low*	High

** The cut-off value should be determined for each laboratory; some laboratories use the median value.*
(Osborne MP: PPO Updates 4[3]:1, 1990)

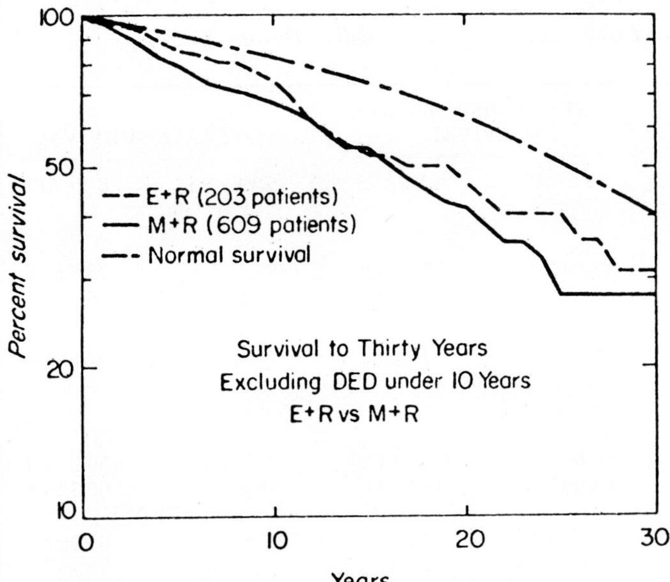

FIGURE 42–33. Comparison of long-term survival for carcinoma of the breast with local excision and irradiation (E + R) or radical mastectomy and irradiation (M + R). DED: death from extraneous disease. (Peters MV: Int J Radiat Oncol Biol Phys 2:1151, 1977)

tients with Stage T1, T2, N0M0 mammary carcinoma treated with local tumor excision and irradiation (2500 cGy to 3500 cGy in 2 weeks) to the breast and regional lymph nodes. The 5-year survival rate was 79% and the 10-year rate 71%, compared with 82% and 71.5%, respectively, in 593 patients treated during the same period with radical mastectomy and irradiation. Local recurrences were noted in 23.6% of the patients with T1 tumors and in 27.6% of those with T2 lesions. Morbidity was lower than in the mastectomy patients.

Mustakallio[301] updated two previous reports[299, 300] and described results in 702 patients with Stage I carcinoma of the breast treated with local resection of the tumor and breast irradiation. The 10-year disease-free survival rate was 72% (257 of 418), and the local recurrence rate was 24%. In these patients the axillary lymph nodes were not dissected, and approximately 25% developed regional recurrences after an average of 4 years.

Skepticism regarding the long-term effectiveness of conservation surgery and irradiation to match the results of radical mastectomy should be dispelled by the reports of long-term results, such as those reported at 30 years by Peters[321] (Fig. 43-33). The results of these trials are summarized in Table 42-23.

Randomized Studies

The earliest prospective randomized trial comparing breast conservation and radical mastectomy was conducted at Guy's Hospital in London, England.[13] Between 1961 and 1971, 370 women with Stage I and Stage II breast cancer were randomized to a standard radical mastectomy or a wide local excision and irradiation. Although survival or distant metastasis was not significantly different according to treatment for Stage I disease, the recurrence rates in the breast and axilla were higher in the group treated with local excision and irradiation. In Stage II disease, not only were the breast and axillary recurrence rates higher in patients treated with wide excision and irradiation, but the survival rates were significantly lower because of a higher distant metastatic rate. Major weaknesses of this study are the low doses of radiation used: 3500 cGy to 3800 cGy to the breast and 2500 cGy to 2700 cGy to the axilla and probably patient selection as well as surgical techniques.

Veronesi and associates[462, 464] reported on 701 patients with tumors less than 2 cm in diameter without palpable axillary nodes randomized to be treated with either a quadrantectomy and axillary dissection plus irradiation (5000 cGy in 5 weeks to the breast and 1000 cGy boost) or a radical (Halsted) mastectomy. All women with positive axillary lymph nodes also received 12 cycles of adjuvant chemotherapy with CMF. The actuarial overall and disease-free survival rates are comparable in both groups (83% and 85%, and 77% and 80% at 8 years). The incidence of local failure is comparable.

Fisher and colleagues[126] updated a previous report published in 1985 conducted by the National Surgical Adjuvant Breast Project (Protocol B-06) on 1843 women with Stage I and Stage II carcinoma of the breast less than 4 cm in diameter. Patients were randomized to be treated with total mastectomy or lumpectomy (segmental mastectomy) with or without irradiation. The margins of the lumpectomy specimens were required to be tumor-free. Patients with margin involvement underwent total mastectomy. Posttreatment occurrence of tumor in the same breast after lumpectomy was not designated as an end point event in determining disease-free survival; those patients underwent a total mastectomy. Irradiated patients received 5000 cGy to the breast through tangential fields. Supplemental radiation boost to the operative site was not given.

The 5- and 8-year survival rates were comparable in the three treatment groups and were analyzed according to the status of the axillary lymph nodes (Table 42-24; Fig. 42-34). Disease-free survival was superior in the patients treated with lumpectomy and irradiation (Fig. 42-35). A significant difference was found in the overall probability of tumor control in patients with lumpectomy and irradiation (90%) compared with

TABLE 42–23
Early Reports on Conservation Surgery and Irradiation in Breast Cancer

AUTHOR	NO. OF PATIENTS	STAGE	IRRADIATION (cGy)	LOCAL TUMOR CONTROL	DISEASE-FREE SURVIVAL	YEARS AFTER TREATMENT
Keynes[213]	75	I	? (radium implant)	—	71%*	5
	66	II	? (radium implant)	—	29%*	5
Mustakallio[300]	702	I		76%	72%	10
Crile et al[79]	173	I		88%	76%	10
Rissanen[342]	415	T1, 2N0	2500–3500	T1 76% T2 72%	71%	10
Peters[321]	203	T1, 2N0	4500–6000	92%	40%*	20

**Results comparable to patients treated with mastectomy*

TABLE 42–24
*NSABP Protocol 06: Comparison of Total Mastectomy with Lumpectomy and with Lumpectomy and Radiation Therapy According to Nodal Status**

NODAL STATUS AND TREATMENT GROUP	NO.	DISEASE-FREE SURVIVAL 5 YEARS	DISEASE-FREE SURVIVAL 8 YEARS	DISTANT DISEASE-FREE SURVIVAL 5 YEARS	DISTANT DISEASE-FREE SURVIVAL 8 YEARS	OVERALL SURVIVAL 5 YEARS	OVERALL SURVIVAL 8 YEARS
NEGATIVE NODES							
Total mastectomy	366	75.1±2.3	65.5±3.3	81.5±2.1	73.8±3.2	87.7±1.8	78.7±3.2
Lumpectomy	392	67.6±2.4	60.7±2.8	74.5±2.2	69.6±2.6	87.1±1.8	76.6±2.8
Overall *P* value		0.05		0.03†		0.5	
Lumpectomy and irradiation	399	77.3±2.2	65.6±3.3	80.9±2.0	70.7±3.2	88.3±1.7	82.9±2.3
Overall *P* value		0.7		0.6		0.8	
POSITIVE NODES‡							
Total mastectomy	224	53.5±3.4	44.5±4.0	60.8±3.3	50.7±4.2	77.2±3.1	59.9±4.1
Lumpectomy	244	55.4±3.3	41.6±4.1	63.9±3.2	49.1±4.6	75.6±2.9	60.3±4.5
Overall *P* value		0.6		0.4		0.7	
Lumpectomy and irradiation	230	59.0±3.3	46.6±4.1	62.8±3.3	53.1±3.9	77.2±2.9	68.3±3.9
Overall *P* value		0.2		0.6		0.3	

**The values are life-table estimates of the results 5 and 8 years after surgery and are expressed as mean (±SE) percentages. The P values are for comparisons with the total mastectomy group.*
†In our first paper[132] the P value for this comparison was incorrectly published as 0.2 instead of the correct value of 0.02.
‡The values have been adjusted for the number of positive nodes (1 to 3, 4 to 9, or ≥10).
(Fisher B, Redmond C, Paisson R, et al: N Engl J Med 320[13]:822–828, 1989)

those who received no radiation after lumpectomy (61%; Fig. 42-36). The benefit of irradiation was more noticeable in patients with positive nodes (94% tumor control) in comparison with those treated with segmental mastectomy alone (57% tumor control) despite the fact that these patients received adjuvant chemotherapy ($P < 0.001$). In patients with negative axillary lymph nodes, the probability of tumor control was 88% with irradiation and 63% without it.

The Institut Gustave-Roussy conducted a prospective randomized trial[373] comparing mastectomy with local excision plus irradiation for women with cancers measuring 2 cm or less.[372] Eighty-eight patients were treated with conservation surgery and irradiation (4500 cGy in 18 fractions, 250 cGy daily, four fractions per week) and a boost of 1500 cGy in six fractions, and 91 were treated with a modified radical mastectomy without excision of the pectoral muscle. All patients had a low axillary dissection with immediate histologic examination; those with positive axillary lymph nodes had a complete axillary dissection immediately. The 5-year disease-free survival rate was 85% for the tumorectomy group compared with 74% for the mastectomy group, and 10-year rates were 65% and 55%, respectively. The overall survival rates were 95% and 91%, respectively. The 5-year local recurrence rate was 5% in the conservation surgery and irradiation group compared with 12% in the mastectomy group. Distant metastases were noted in 12% of the former and 18% of the latter group. Table 42-25 summarizes the main characteristics of several randomized trials comparing these treatment modalities.

The EORTC Breast Cancer Cooperative Group[459] conducted a randomized trial of 903 patients, 745 with Stage II cancer, the remainder with Stage I, comparing modified radical mastectomy with breast conservation therapy (BCT). Survival and disease-free survival were comparable in both arms of the trial. The actuarial 8-year local tumor control was 91% in the

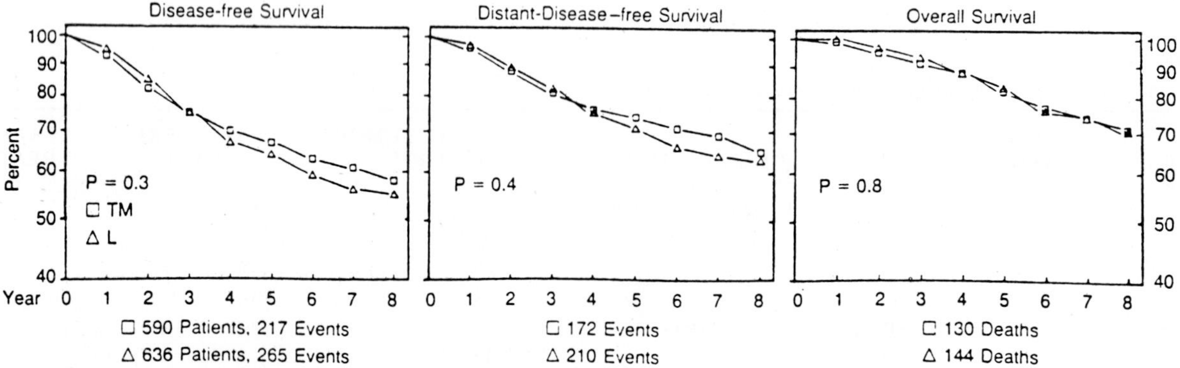

FIGURE 42–34. Life-table analysis showing rates of disease-free survival, distant disease-free survival, and overall survival of patients treated with total mastectomy (TM) or lumpectomy (L), with or without irradiation. The results have been adjusted for the number of positive nodes. (Fisher B, Redmond C, Poisson R, et al: N Engl J Med 320:822, 1989)

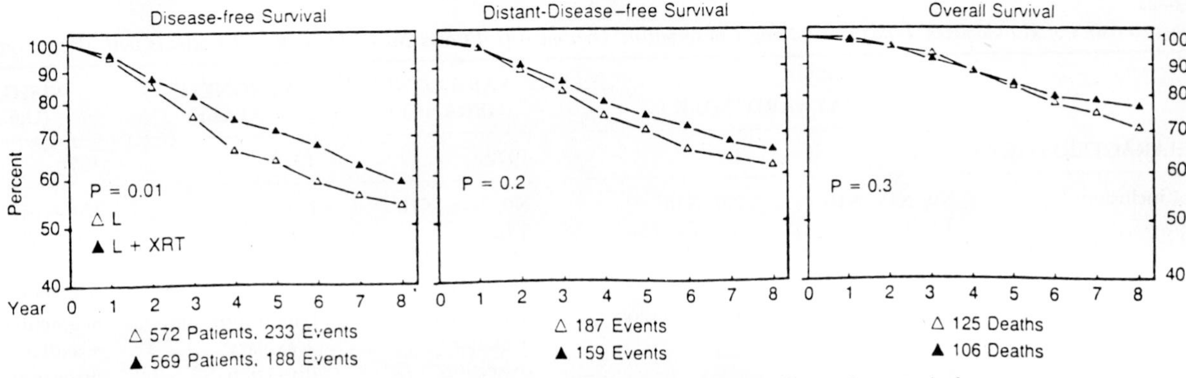

FIGURE 42–35. Life-table analysis showing rates of disease-free survival, distant disease-free survival, and overall survival of patients treated with lumpectomy (L) or with lumpectomy and irradiation (L + XRT) who had tumor-free specimen margins. The results have been adjusted for the number of positive nodes. (Fisher B, Redmond C, Poisson R, et al: N Engl J Med 320:822, 1989)

mastectomy and 87% in the BCT groups (differences not statistically significant). One axillary recurrence was seen in the mastectomy and three in the BCT patients.

A Danish Cooperative Study[35] carried out a similar randomized trial in 405 women (another 248 patients were treated with mastectomy or BCT without randomization, according to preference). In high-risk patients (tumor >5 cm, invasion to skin or deep fascia, metastatic axillary lymph nodes) treated with BCT the regional lymph nodes were irradiated. Also, in high-risk patients treated with mastectomy the same target volume was irradiated as in BCT patients. All high-risk patients received adjuvant CMF. At 6 years the recurrence-free survival rate in 430 BCT patients was 70% and in 429 patients in the mastectomy arm, 66%. Overall survival rates were 79% and 82%, respectively. Twelve breast relapses occurred in the BCT patients (3%) and 19 chest wall recurrences (4%) in the mastectomy group. In the BCT group 31% of patients had excellent and 41% had satisfactory cosmesis.

The US National Cancer Institute[153] recently updated results of a randomized study in which 122 patients with T1–2N0M0 were treated with a modified radical mastectomy and 125 with breast conservation therapy (4500 cGy to 5000 cGy to breast plus 1500 cGy to 2000 cGy boost). With a median follow-up of 6.5 years the actuarial 8-year disease-free survival rates were 76% in the mastectomy and 66% in the lumpectomy/radiation therapy arms; overall survival was 79% and 85%, respectively. The 8-year risk of locoregional failure was 6% for the mastectomy and 19% for the BCT groups. Cosmesis was excellent in 40% and good in 29% of the BCT patients.

Recently the Uppsala-Orebro Breast Cancer Study Group[452] reported on a trial in which 187 women with histopathologic Stage I invasive breast carcinoma were treated with sector resection and axillary dissection plus postoperative irradiation (5400 cGy to the breast), and 194 women were randomized to be treated with the same surgical procedures alone. The actuarial local recurrence rate after 3 years was 2.9% in the irradiated group and 7.6% with surgery only. The 3-year disease-free survival rates were 96% and 90%, respectively, and the 5-year survival rates 86.5% and 85%.

In these trials local tumor excision (tylectomy, lumpectomy), segmental mastectomy, or quadrantectomy combined with radiation to the breast has been shown to yield survival rates and tumor control similar to those with modified or classic radical mastectomy (Table 42-26).[30,73,188,332,464]

Nonrandomized Reports

Of the numerous reports on the subject only a few of the earlier studies will be commented on. Crile and associates initially in 1965[77] and later in 1980[79] reported the results in patients treated with partial mastectomy with or without irradiation, with irradiation being administered only to about 25% of the patients. The local control rate was 88% and in the axilla was 92%. The actuarial 5-year survival rates were 76% and 44% at

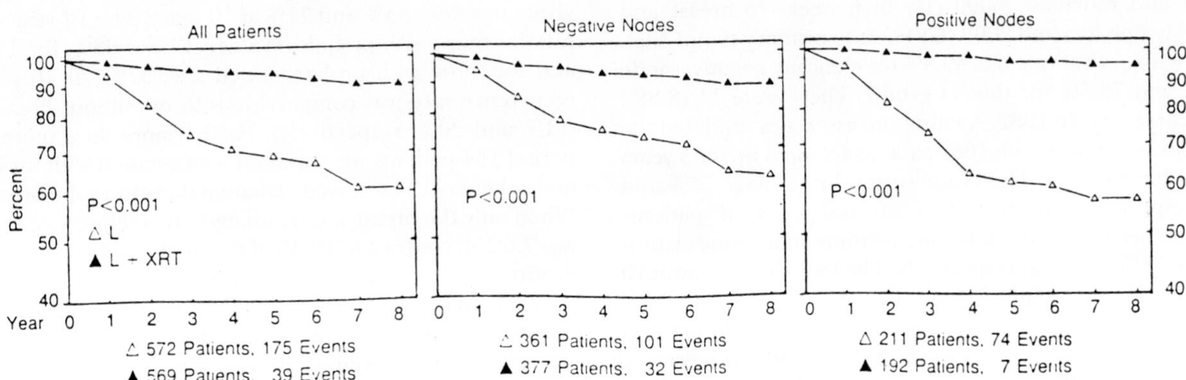

FIGURE 42–36. Life-table analysis showing the percentage of patients who remained free of breast tumor after lumpectomy (L) or after lumpectomy and breast irradiation (L + XRT). The results for all patients and for patients with positive nodes have been adjusted for the number of positive nodes. (Fisher B, Redmond C, Poisson R, et al: N Engl J Med 320:822, 1989)

TABLE 42–25
Main Characteristics of Randomized Trials Comparing Conservative Treatment (CT) and Mastectomy in M0 Patients with Breast Cancer

	HAYWARD[185] (U.K.)		SARRAZIN[372] (FRANCE)	VERONESI[464] (ITALY)	FISHER[120] (U.S.A.)
MAIN CHARACTERISTICS	1961	1971	1972	1973	1976
Criteria of inclusion	N0, N1a, N1b T1, T2, T3a age > 50	N0, N1a T1, T2, T3a	N0, N1a, N1b T1a Macroscopic diameter ≤20 mm	N0 T1	N0, N1a, N1b T1, (T2)[a] Clinical size ≤40 mm
Surgical technique CT group	Wide excision	Wide excision	Tumorectomy + axillary dissection	Quadrantectomy + axillary dissection	Segmentectomy + axillary dissection
Control group	Halsted	Halsted	Radical modified mastectomy	Halsted	Halsted
Breast RT (CT group)	Systematic RT 38 Gy linear accelerator	Systematic RT 38 Gy linear accelerator	Systematic RT 45 Gy tumor bed 60 Gy (^{60}Co)	Systematic RT Maximum 50 Gy tumor bed 60 Gy (^{60}Co)	RT randomly allocated Maximum 50 Gy linear accelerator
Adjuvant therapy for N+patients	Systematic nodal RT 3000 cGy (300 kV)	Systematic nodal RT 30 Gy (300 kV)	Nodal RT randomly allocated 45 Gy (^{60}Co)	Systematic nodal RT (or CMF) 45 Gy (^{60}Co)	Systematic chemotherapy
Five-year rates					
Survival (stage)†	(I) (II)	(I)	(I + II)	(I)	(I + II)
Mastectomy	69% 68%	88%	92%	90%	75%
CT + breast RT	73% 46%§	76%§	92%	92%	84%‡
CT without breast RT	—	—	—	—	85%‡
Relapse-free survival					
Mastectomy	—	—	77%	85%	67%
CT + breast RT	—	—	83%	88%	70%§
CT without breast RT					63%

**A part of T_2*
† Stage I: patients with N_0, or $N_0 - N_{1a}$; Stage II: patients with N_{1b}
‡ Comparison between mastectomy and CT: $P < 0.05$
§ Comparison between mastectomy and CT: $0.05 < P < 0.10$
(Sarrazin D, Le MG, Arriagada R, et al: Radiother Oncol 14:177–184, 1989)

10 years; 63 of the patients were followed up for that period of time.

Montague[391] noted a locoregional recurrence rate of 4.9% in 345 patients treated with conservation surgery compared with 5.6% in patients treated with radical or modified radical mastectomy. No significant difference was found in 10-year disease-free survival between the two groups (78% *versus* 80% for Stage I and 73% *versus* 65% for Stage II, respectively).

Spitalier and associates[414] in 1977 reported on 160 patients with T1, T2, and a few with T3 breast cancer treated with local excision and radiation (6000 cGy in 6 weeks to breast and regional lymphatics and 2000 cGy boost to primary tumor site). The 5-year survival rate was 89.8% for clinically negative-node patients and 78.6% for the N1 group. There were 11 (8.8%) local recurrences. In 1982, Amalric and associates[2] updated the Marseilles experience with 1083 patients followed up for 5 years and 234 for 10 years. The crude survival rates were 73% and 68%, respectively. Comparative survival rates in patients treated before 1960 with radical mastectomy at the same institution were 78% and 68%, respectively. The local failure rate at 10 years was 20% in T1 and 21% in T2 tumors.

Calle and colleagues[49] described the results in 514 patients with T1,T2,T3N0–N1 breast cancer treated with lumpectomy and radiation (5000 cGy to breast and regional lymphatics, 1500 cGy to lumpectomy site, and 1000 cGy to lower axilla). The absolute 5-year disease-free survival rate was 85% (102 of 120 patients) and 94% with the breast being preserved. The 10-year disease-free survival rate was 75% (50 of 68), with 88% of the patients having breast preservation. Local recurrences developed in 13% (16 of 120) of the patients within 5 years. Eight of 14 patients (57%) retreated surgically survived 5 years without tumor. Cosmesis was excellent to good in 60% and good to fair in 37.5% of the patients.

Clark and colleagues[69] reported on 680 patients with Stage I and Stage II disease followed up over a period of 21 years after treatment with local excision of the primary tumor and irradiation of the breast and peripheral lymphatics. The 5-year survival rates were 83% and 71% at 10 years. The 10-year survival rate for those with pathologic Stage T1 was 63%, for T2, 62%, and for those with undetermined size, 57%. At 10 years the recurrence rate was comparable with or without breast boost (21% and 20%, respectively). Furthermore, in a more recent period 154 patients were treated with excision without irradiation, whereas 195 received radiation therapy to the breast only. When only the breast was irradiated, the relapse rate at 5 years was 7.6% in contrast to 12.3% if the breast and any lymph node group were irradiated. The relapse rate was 24.4% when no radiation to the breast was delivered (despite the fact that these patients had the more favorable tumors).

Clarke and associates[72] described the results in 436 patients with Stage T1 and T2 tumors treated with tumor excision and irradiation. The actuarial probability of tumor control was 93% at 5 years and 90% at 10 years. Prognostic factors of significance for prediction of breast recurrences included Bloom (histologic)

TABLE 42–26
Conservation Surgery and Irradiation in Stage I and II Carcinoma of the Breast: Results of Randomized Comparisons With Radical or Modified Mastectomy

			CONSERVATION SURGERY + RADIATION THERAPY		MASTECTOMY	
TRIAL	**NO. OF PATIENTS***	**TUMOR SIZE (cm)**	TUMOR CONTROL (%)	DISEASE-FREE SURVIVAL (%)	TUMOR CONTROL (%)	DISEASE-FREE SURVIVAL (%)
Guy's[13]	182/188	<4	T1 80 T2 30	80 25	T1 90 T2 80	80 60
Milan[465]	352/349	≤2		77†		76†
NSABP[126]	624/590	≤4	90	59‡	92	54‡
NCI[153]	125/122	≤5	80	66‡	88	76‡
EORTC[459]	452/422	≤5	87		91	
DBCG[35]	430/429	≤5	97	70	96	66
G. Roussy[371]	88/91	≤2	95	85†	88	74†

** Conservation surgery plus radiation therapy/mastectomy*
† Ten years
‡ Eight years actuarial

grade and tumor doses to the excision site greater or lower than 1840 cGy (NSD 2.3% *versus* 7%, respectively).

Danoff and associates[85] reported 82% survival rate at 4 years for 85 patients with pathologic Stage I and 70% for patients with Stage II carcinoma of the breast treated with conservation surgery and irradiation. The cumulative failure rate was 5%. Cosmesis was good or excellent in 90% of the patients. Results described by multiple authors are summarized in Table 42-27. Nonrandomized comparison of survival with radical mastectomy breast conservation therapy at various institutions in Europe and North America is illustrated in Table 42-28.

CHRONOLOGIC RATE AND LOCATION OF BREAST CANCER RELAPSES

The majority of breast cancer relapses (65% to 86%) after BCT occur around the primary tumor site and may be seen many years after therapy. Recht and associates,[339] in an analysis of 607 patients with clinical Stage I or Stage II invasive carcinoma, described a 5-year cumulative actuarial probability of failure of 10% and a 10-year probability of 16%. The hazard rate in the first 5 years was approximately 2% per year until about 5 years after treatment and decreased to 0.5% per year at 8 years.

Fourquet and associates[139] reported on 518 patients treated with conservation surgery and irradiation (5700 cGy to 6500 cGy to the breast and 900 cGy to 1200 cGy boost to tumor site). An increasing incidence of breast recurrences was noted with time, reaching over 20% at 20 to 25 years; 46% (26 of 56) of those recurrences were located in the same quadrant as the primary tumor.

Haffty and colleagues[169] reported 67% local recurrences at or near the primary site. Fisher and co-workers[132] reported that 95% of recurrences in 1108 patients involved the mammary parenchyma, and the rest involved the skin or nipple only, or both. Eighty-six percent of recurrences were localized masses within or close to the quadrant of the initial primary tumor. In 14% the recurrence involved the initial quadrant and extended to remote areas.

Kurtz and co-workers[223] in 1593 patients with clinical Stage I and Stage II disease treated with conservation surgery and irradiation noted a yearly actuarial risk of breast recurrence of 1.5% during both of the first two 5-year periods. After 10 years following therapy, the yearly risk decreased to 1.1%. During the first 10 years, about 80% of the recurrences were located in the vicinity of the primary tumor. With the increasing interval from primary treatment, only 45% of the breast carcinoma recurrences were near the primary tumor.

Kurtz and associates[224] analyzed the fate of 300 of these patients who were disease-free 10 years following initial treatment. Sixteen patients (5.3%) developed recurrent carcinoma in the treated breast beyond the tenth year.

Factors Influencing Breast Tumor Control

There are several important considerations in the analysis of results of combined segmental mastectomy or tumor excision and irradiation.

Tumor Excision

Complete resection of gross tumor eliminates the need for higher doses of radiation and improves tumor control and cosmetic results. Amalric and colleagues[2] reported results in 1440 women treated for infiltrating breast carcinoma with irradiation alone or combined with conservation surgery who had more than 5 years of follow-up. At 10 years the failure rate in patients treated with tumor excision and irradiation was 20% (25 of 122) compared with 38% in patients irradiated without prior tumor excision (43 of 112). Calle and associates[49] described a 10-year disease-free survival rate of 40% (32 of 82) in patients with Stages T2, T3, N0N1 treated with irradiation alone compared with 75% (50 of 68) when treatment was combined with tumor excision. Fifty-five percent of patients required surgery for either persistent or recurrent disease.

Irradiation of the Breast

Some authors question the need for irradiation, even though breast recurrences have been reported, ranging from 15% after quadrantectomy alone,[159] 20% with segmental mastectomy,[234] to 37% to 43% following wide local excision alone.[126,430] Clark and associates[70] reported a 14% breast re-

TABLE 42–27
Conservation Surgery and Irradiation in Stage I and II Breast Cancer: Results of Selected Nonrandomized Recently Reported Studies

AUTHOR	NO. OF PATIENTS	STAGE	IRRADIATION DOSE (cGy)		LOCAL TUMOR CONTROL (%)	EXCELLENT/ GOOD COSMESIS (%)	10-YEAR DISEASE-FREE SURVIVAL (%)
			BREAST	BOOST			
Amalric[3]	1440	I, II	6000	1500–2000	80	90	74
Baeza[16]	171	T1, T2	5000	1400	96.5	79	77
Barr[22]	411	I, II, III	4840	2000	88	—	—
Bartelink[23]	585	T1, T2	5000	2500	98	—	T1 92*
							T2 85
Calle[50]	411	I, II	5000	1000	89	88	78
Cedermark[58]	262	I	5000		97	92	
Clark[70]	1504	T1,2N0	4000/3 wk	500–1500	86	—	70
Clarke[72]	436	T1, T2	4500	1500	90	—	
Danoff[85]	189	T1, T2	4500–5000	1500–2000	95	93	75†
Delouche[90]	410	T1, T2	5000–6000	Yes	94 (T1)	{93	62.5
					86 (T2)		
Dubois[101]	231	I	4500	1000–1500	91 (I)	90	I 84
	161	II			84 (II)		II 75
Durand[102]	265	T1, T2	5500	1000	92	75	84
Fourquet[139]	518	T1, T2	5700–6200	500–1200	90	—	—
Gerard[149]	195	T1, T2	5000	2000	96	70	81‡
Haffty[169, 170]	278	I, II	4600	1000–2000	91	—	81
	281	I			81	—	75
		II	<4600	1000–2000	79		57
Hallahan[172]	207	I, II	4600	1400–1600	92	93	80‡
Harris and Hellman[180]	225	I, II	5000	1000–2000	97 (I)		93
					87 (II)		84
Kantorowitz[209]	146	I, II	5000	1000–2500	90	—	89‡
Kurtz[223]	1593	I, II	5000–6000	2000	89		86
Kuske[231]	417	I, II	5000	1000–2000	91	81	I 80
							II 52
Montague[291]	134	I	5000	1500–2000	94	—	78
	157	II	5000	1000–2000	95	—	73
Osborne[310]	263	T1, T2	4500	1000	85 (I)	—	54
					81 (II)	—	29
Pierquin[326]	177	I, II	5000	1000–2000	95	82	80‡
Prosnitz[331]	293	I, II	5000	1000–2000	92		64
Recht[340]	366	I, II	5000	1000	96 (I)	—	
					90 (II)		
Sarrazin[373]	179	T1smT2	4500	1500	95	92	85‡
Schmidt-Ullrich[380]	108(115)	I, II	5000	1000–2000	100	66	I 95‡
						for all	II 80‡
Solin[409]	217	T1	4500–5000	1000–1500	95	90	T1 80‡
	166	T2	4500–5000	1000–1500	92	90	T2 69‡
Steeves[417]	124	Tis, 1, 2, 3	5000	1600	95	82	82‡
van Limbergen[460]							T1 75.4
	235	T1, T2(3)	4000–6500	800–2000	90		T2 61.9
Vilcoq[471]	314	T1, T2	5000–5500	1000–2000	90		84‡

** Six-year disease-free survival*
† Four-year disease-free survival
‡ Five-year disease-free survival

lapse rate in 1108 patients with conservation surgery and irradiation, in contrast to 29% in 374 patients who received no irradiation (at 10 years). Thus it is obvious that tumor excision or chemotherapy alone does not reduce the probability of breast recurrences, whereas irradiation combined with local excision, alone or with chemotherapy, enhances tumor control. Table 42-29 compares the breast relapse rate in patients with or without irradiation after local tumor excision.

Technique and Dose of Radiation

The techniques and doses of radiation play a crucial role in the success of conservation treatment of breast cancer. Atkins and associates[13] and Hayward[184] reported a 37% local relapse rate at 10 years in patients with clinical Stage I disease treated with doses of radiation of 3500 cGy. van Limbergen[460] reported a correlation between the dose of radiation and the probability

TABLE 42–28
Survival Comparisons According to Treatment for Stage I–II Breast Carcinoma in Nonrandomized Studies

		CONSERVATION SURGERY AND RADIATION THERAPY		RADICAL AND MODIFIED MASTECTOMY	
AUTHOR	**CLINICAL STAGE**	NO. OF PATIENTS	5-YEAR SURVIVAL NED	NO. OF PATIENTS	5-YEAR SURVIVAL NED
Amalric[2]	I–II	1099	72%	121	78%
Montague[291]	I–II	134	85%	224	88%
		157	78%	370	77%
Peters[321]	I–II	203	86%	609	82%
Rissanen[342]	I–II	415	79%	593	82%

NED: no evidence of disease

of local tumor control (67% for doses less than 1600 ret, 83.9% for 1600 ret to 1800 ret, and 96% to 100% for higher doses). The dose effect was more noticeable in T2 lesions with doses greater than 2000 ret (Fig. 42-37). Unfortunately, but predictably, the higher doses were associated with poorer cosmetic results. Recht and co-workers[340] found that patients receiving 6000 cGy or more had a 6% recurrence rate of the primary tumor at 6 years compared with 12% for those receiving lower doses ($P = 0.37$). Fourquet and associates[139] noted no improvement in recurrence rate with higher doses of radiation, possibly because patients with inadequate surgical margins were selected to receive the higher doses.

Additional Dose to Primary Tumor Site (Boost)

Fisher and associates[120] raised the question of the need for a radiation dose boost at the excision site. However, the delivery of a boost dose to the site of tumor excision increases the probability of tumor control, as reported by Bedwinek and associates,[30] Hellman and co-workers,[188] Harris and colleagues,[176] Clark and associates,[70] and others (Table 42-30). Clark and coworkers[70] in 1504 patients reported a greater incidence of failures at 10 years in patients to whom no boost was delivered (17%) compared with other patients receiving doses from 500 cGy to 1500 cGy at the primary excision site (11%; $P = 0.03$). Other series with unknown surgical margins have noted lower breast failure rate (6% to 11%) with boost compared with no boost (9% to 20%).[64, 340]

Kuske and associates,[231] in 417 patients with T1 or T2, N0 or N1 carcinoma of the breast treated with conservation surgery and irradiation including a boost, noted a locoregional failure rate of 3.7% for T1 and 4.9% for T2. A higher incidence of breast recurrences (18%) was noted in patients with inner quadrant primary tumors. Breast tumor control and cosmesis were comparable in 217 patients treated with ^{192}Ir implant and 154 patients given electron-beam boost.

No evidence exists that either an iridium implant or an electron-beam boost of radiation may be superior to the other. Results with either method are comparable (Table 42-31).

Status of Surgical Margins at Primary Tumor Site

The presence of positive margins with less than complete tumor excision increases the incidence of breast relapses when radiation therapy is not given in sufficiently high doses.[2, 30, 176] Ghossein and colleagues[151] reported on a group of 201 patients, 53 (26%) of whom had positive margins after limited surgery for carcinoma of the breast without reexision. In these patients,

TABLE 42–29
Tumor Recurrence Rate After Tumor Excision Alone or Combined with Irradiation in Stage I and II Carcinoma of Breast

			TUMOR RECURRENCE	
AUTHOR	**TUMOR SIZE**	**SURGERY**	TUMOR EXCISION ONLY	TUMOR EXCISION AND IRRADIATION
Cedermark[58]	≤2 cm	Partial mastectomy	9/58(15.5%)	6/204(2.9%)
Clark et al[70]	≤5 cm	Local excision	396(29%)	1108(14%)*
Fisher[126]†	≤4 cm	−Axillary Nodes	13/361(37%)	45/377(12%)
		+Axillary Nodes	9/211(43%)	11/192(6%)
Kantorowitz[209]	≤5 cm	Local excision	22/77(18.6%)	15/106(14.2%)
		Quadrantectomy	4/18(22.2%)	1/36(2.8%)
Uppsala-Orebro[452]	≤2 cm‡		2/194(10.2%)	5/187(2.9%)

** Ten-year actuarial relapse*
† Eight-year actuarial relapse
‡ Five-year actuarial relapse

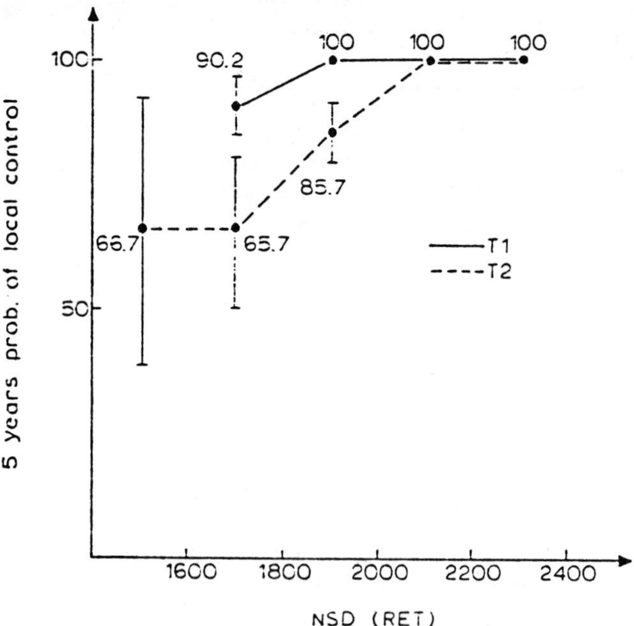

FIGURE 42–37. Breast conservation therapy: local control related to radiation dose to the breast. (van Limbergen E, van den Bogaert W, van der Schueren E, et al: Radiother Oncol 8:1, 1987)

treated with 5000 cGy to the breast and 2000 cGy boost to the tumor excision site, the breast tumor recurrence rate at 5 years was 14%, which was less than half the incidence reported with limited surgery alone (15% to 37%).

Schmidt-Ullrich and associates[380] reported results in 115 breasts treated in 108 women with conservation surgery and irradiation (5000 cGy, and boost dose with interstitial ^{192}Ir implants delivered to doses of 1000 cGy, 1500 cGy, or 2000 cGy, depending on the status of the surgical specimen). No local failures were noted, and only two patients developed regional lymph node recurrences in unirradiated areas.

In 366 patients with clinical Stage I or Stage II disease treated with local excision and radiation therapy, Recht and associates[336] noted a 4% probability of a marginal miss at 5 years, which was not related to the dose or the volume of the boost used. The probability of local recurrence was significantly higher if less than a complete excisional biopsy had been performed (Fig. 42-38).

Pezner and co-workers[322] treated 54 breasts in 53 patients on whom the inked specimen margins showed no evidence of tumor with 5000 cGy to the breast without a boost and noted a local tumor control of 100% with a mean follow-up of 38 months. In contrast, in 28 treated breasts in 27 patients on whom the tumor excision specimen was not evaluated for margins, followed by radiation to the breast and additional boost by either interstitial ^{192}Ir implant or electron beam, the actuarial local control rate at 48 months was 87%. Among patients with clear surgical margins who received a local boost, one of nine developed a local recurrence. Among those with tumor in specimen margins who received a local boost, one of eight developed a local recurrence. Local recurrences were more frequently seen in poorly differentiated tumors (two of 11) than in those with other invasive carcinomas (three of 91).

Surgical Techniques

The impact of the type of surgical excision on control rates is controversial, especially in view of the known adverse effect of larger resection on cosmetic results. This issue is the subject of a present trial in Milan, randomizing quadrantectomy *versus* tylectomy. The breast failure rate in the initial Milan trial with quadrantectomy was no different from that of the WHO trial with tylectomy.

TABLE 42–30
Correlation of Incidence of Recurrence in the Breast Following Conservation Surgery and Irradiation

AUTHOR	STAGE (T)	NO. OF PATIENTS	DOSE (cGy) BREAST	BOOST	RECURRENCES AT 5 YEARS
Atkins[13]	1, 2	70	3600	—	48
Rissanen[342]	1, 2	415	2500–3500	—	25
Osborne et al[310]	1, 2	263	4000	1000	15–19
Clark et al[70]	1, 2	1504	4000	No	13 (17)*
			5000	Yes	7 (11)*
Fisher et al[120]	1, 2	625	5000	—	10
Peters[321]	1, 2	66	4500	—	10
Calle et al[49]	1, 2	120	5000	1000	10
Wise and Ackerman[488]	1, 2	96	6100	—	9
Bataini[26]	1, 2	39	5500	1000–2000	9
Harris et al[176]	1, 2	176	5000	1500–2500	7
Hellman[188]	1, 2	184	5000	1000–2000	6
Montague[291]	1, 2	345	5000	1000–2000	5
Danoff et al[85]	1, 2	189	4600–5000	1500–2000	5
Kuske[229]	1, 2	215	5000	1000–2000	3.3
Veronesi et al[466]	1	352	5000	1000	2(4)†

* *Recurrence rate at 10 years*
† *Recurrence rate at 12 years*

TABLE 42–31
Conservation Surgery and Irradiation in Cancer of the Breast: Impact of Method of Boost on Outcome

	TUMOR CONTROL (%)		EXCELLENT—GOOD COSMESIS (%)	
AUTHOR	ELECTRONS/ PHOTONS	^{192}Ir IMPLANT	ELECTRONS/ PHOTONS	^{192}Ir IMPLANT
Clark[70]	93			
Fowble[140]	98	96	96	88
Gerard[149]	90	96	70	70
Hery[191]	94		98	
Hunig[203]	94		80	
Kuske[231]	92	91	82	80
Mate[271]	92		—	
Nobler[305]	91.5	92	80	
Pezner[322]	93	86	—	—
Ray[332]	99		91	52
Sarrazin[371]	95		92	
Triedman[447]	92	91	96	88
van Limbergen[460]	90			
Veronesi[463]	96		67	

Histologic Features

Fisher and co-workers[132] described the pathologic findings in 110 local breast recurrences observed in 1108 patients in NSABP 06. Histologically, high nuclear grade and intralymphatic extension were associated with higher probability of recurrence. This trend was not observed for tubular or scar cancers. Kurtz and associates[225] recently correlated an inflammatory cellular infiltrate within the tumor with a higher incidence of breast failure, as did tumor necrosis in a study by Epstein and associates.[111] Recht and colleagues[340] noted in 607 patients with Stage I and Stage II cancer a probability of failure substantially higher in the presence of extensive intraductal carcinoma (EIC; 33% at 10 years) compared with patients without EIC (8%). The greater probability of failure in patients with an extensive intraductal component is confirmed in an updated report by the same group.[311] Furthermore, a greater recurrence rate was noted (27% at 5 years and 71% at 8 years) in patients with *macroscopic* pattern EIC compared with 18% at 5 and 8 years with those with *microscopic* EIC pattern.

Survival was not affected by the histologic pattern or the higher local recurrence rate of EIC, suggesting that this event is not related to systemic tumor dissemination. The higher failure rate in patients with EIC is believed to be related to the high incidence of significant posttylectomy tumor burden and doses of radiation given. Residual carcinoma was found in more reexcision specimens (88%) compared with 48% in patients who had questionable margins but not histologic evidence of EIC.[382] Table 42-32 summarizes reports on breast relapse incidence correlated with the presence of extensive intraductal carcinoma.

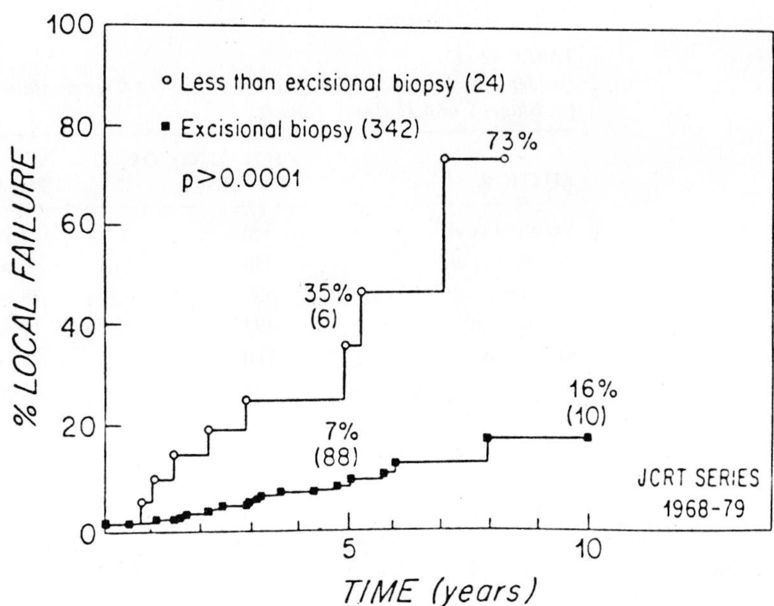

FIGURE 42–38. Breast conversation therapy: actuarial probability of local recurrence by type of biopsy. (Recht A, Silver B, Schmitt S, et al: Int J Radiat Oncol Biol Phys 11:1271–1276, 1985)

TABLE 42–32
Incidence of Tumor Relapse Correlated With Extensive Intraductal Carcinoma (EIC) Component in Primary Breast Tumor or Adjacent Breast

	% TUMOR RECURRENCE AT 5 YEARS*	
AUTHOR	EIC PRESENT	EIC ABSENT
Bartelink[23]	9 (79)	2 (208)
Eberlein[104]	27 (166)	7 (418)
Koper[220]	10 (283)	13 (283)
Kurtz[225]	18 (106)	8 (390)
Recht[337]	23 (143)	5 (302)
Schnitt[381]	15 (113)	1 (98)
Zafrani[494]	11 (63)	6 (361)

**Number of patients in parentheses*

Stage of Primary Tumor and Lymph Nodes

The size of the tumor (stage) may influence local recurrence rate and prognosis, although results are not consistent. Osborne and colleagues[310] noted in 263 patients a 10-year locoregional relapse rate of 22% with T1 or T2N0N1a tumors and 52% in patients with T1T2N1b lesions. The overall relapse rate in the breast was 12% at 10 years for T1 tumors with an additional 3% by 20 years compared with 16% at 10 years for the T2 tumors, with a 3% subsequent relapse. The 5-year disease-free survival rate for Stage I tumors was 70% and for Stage II, 37%; at 10 years the rates were 54% and 29%, respectively. Kuske and co-workers[231] noted a locoregional failure rate of 6.5% (16 of 246) in T1 tumors compared with 11% (17 of 151) in T2 tumors. Harris and colleagues[176] reported 6.3% failure in 80 patients with T1 and 5.8% local failure in 86 patients with T2 tumors treated in a similar fashion. Bartelink and co-workers[23] reported a comparable local recurrence rate in 585 patients with Stage I and Stage II tumors.

Danoff and co-workers[85] noted a 4-year actuarial disease-free survival rate of 82% in 109 patients with pathologic T1 tumors and 70% in 80 patients with T2 lesions treated with conservation surgery and irradiation (4500 cGy to 5000 cGy to breast and regional lymph nodes plus 1500 cGy to 2000 cGy boost to primary site with ^{192}Ir implant or electrons). The local failure rate was 5% in both T1 and T2 tumors, and the regional failure rate was 8%. Results reported by various authors are summarized in Table 42-8.

The presence of lymph node involvement worsens the prognosis and local tumor control probability in the absence of chemotherapy. Unpublished data by Spitalier indicate that in 143 patients with T1-2N0 tumors, 13 (9%) developed a breast recurrence as opposed to 11 of 47 (23%) with T1-T2N1 tumors.

Harris and associates[176] reported a higher incidence of failures in patients with pathologically positive axillary lymph nodes (13%) in contrast to 5% for negative nodes. However, Recht and colleagues[339] found no significant difference in breast tumor control between these two groups (12% and 10% at 5 years, respectively). The impact of chemotherapy on local control in more recent years at Harvard University may explain these differences.

Regional Lymph Node Recurrence

Fowble and colleagues[144] reported a 3% isolated regional node recurrence rate (without simultaneous distant metastases) in 990 patients with clinical Stage I and Stage II breast cancer treated with conservation surgery and irradiation; 914 patients had limited axillary dissection. The most common site of regional failure was the axilla (17 patients), followed by the supraclavicular lymph nodes (13 patients). Salvage therapy was effective in ten of 14 patients with axillary failure with or without breast failure. Noteworthy is that only one patient developed an internal mammary node tumor recurrence associated with simultaneous distant metastases. Treatment of patients with regional recurrences in addition to a surgical resection, when feasible, included combination of chemotherapy or hormonal therapy. All eight patients with concurrent axillary and breast failures treated with mastectomy and axillary dissection followed by CMF, chemotherapy (five patients), or tamoxifen (two patients) have experienced subsequent local or regional relapse. Only the number of axillary lymph nodes removed at the time of initial axillary dissection was shown to be a significant prognostic factor for axillary recurrences. Age of patient (under 35 years) was correlated with the risk of supraclavicular recurrence. Table 42-33 summarizes reports on the incidence of regional lymph node relapse following conservation surgery and irradiation in Stage I and Stage II breast cancer.

TABLE 42–33
Incidence of Regional Node Relapse Following Conservation Surgery and Radiation Therapy for Stages I and II Breast Cancer

AUTHOR	TOTAL NO. OF PATIENTS	FOLLOW-UP	% REGIONAL NODE RELAPSE
Veronesi et al[465]	352	8 years median	2.3
Pierquin et al[325]	3353	>5 years median	3
Sarrazin et al[370]	592	78 months median	2
Leung et al[240]	493	10 years mean	1.2
Mate et al[271]	180	5 years actuarial	5
van Limbergen et al[460]	235	80 months median	3
Fisher et al[120]	625	38.9 months mean	2.2
Delouche et al[90]	410	11 years median	1.2
Calle et al[51]	324	5 years minimum	2.1
Fowble et al[144]	990	5 years actuarial	3

(Fowble B, Solin LJ, Schultz DJ, et al: Int J Radiat Oncol Biol Phys 17:703–710, 1989)

COSMESIS

Surgical, radiotherapeutic, chemotherapeutic, and host factors may influence cosmetic outcome. Some surgical factors to be considered are the extent of surgical resection, reexcision, the orientation and length of the scar, closure or no closure of the tylectomy cavity, separate or continuous axilla tylectomy scars, the extent of the axillary dissection, and whether or not an ellipse of skin over the tumor was removed. Some radiotherapeutic factors to be considered are the prescribed doses to the whole-breast tangential portals, the gradient of dose through the breast tissues (use of wedge or compensating filters), bolus, fractionation, overall duration of therapy including breaks, type and dose of the boost machine energy, volume treated, and peripheral lymphatic irradiation. Chemotherapy issues include the cytotoxic agents used, timing and sequence relative to radiation therapy, and doses and combinations of drugs. Host factors are the size and shape of the breast, age, race, compliance with regard to care and hygiene, concurrent medical illnesses (hypertension, diabetes, collagen vascular disease), and intrinsic sensitivity to radiation.

Different methods have been used to evaluate breast cosmesis after BCT. Some of these methods are flawed because they do not establish strict guidelines or criteria for objectively judging cosmetic outcome. Pezner and co-workers[323] used scales and standard procedures for obtaining color slides to assess the cosmetic results of breast conservation therapy. Other scales designed by various investigators were given to patients for comparison. The study demonstrated that observer-based consensus of cosmetic results is difficult to obtain with two commonly used scales, but by changing the scale gradations from four to two (0 to 1 *versus* 2 to 3 = satisfactory results), consensus exceeding 85% of observers can be obtained.

van Limbergen and associates[460] proposed a quantitative scoring system consisting of multiple measurements obtained with the plotting device of the treatment planning system of the position of the nipple and the inferior and lateral borders of the breast contour on photographs taken under standard conditions projecting on a bidimensional screen system. In 142 patients with Stage I and Stage II breast cancer treated with tumor excision and external irradiation, this system disclosed 46% satisfactory, 26.8% moderate, and 22.5% poor cosmetic results.

At Washington University, specific guidelines have been established for each cosmetic end point. Questionnaires were completed by 224 patients and their radiation oncologists at regular 6-month intervals after treatment. Significant radiotherapeutic factors adversely affecting cosmesis were use of bolus, lack of tissue compensation, whole-breast dose higher than 5000 cGy, and peripheral lymphatic irradiation. Boost type or dose did not have an impact on the cosmetic results. Table 42-34 summarizes our results. Figure 42-39 illustrates examples of cosmetic results obtained in some of our patients.

With regard to impact of boost technique, Ray and Fish[332] reported excellent cosmetic results in 91% of 107 patients given the boost dose with electrons compared with 52% in 12 of 23 patients treated with an interstitial iridium implant. Olivotto and the Harvard Group,[308] in 593 patients treated with conservation surgery and irradiation, reported excellent or good cosmetic results of 90% at 5 years and 78% at 10 years. In 497 patients receiving a boost with interstitial implant, the 3-year excellent cosmesis score was 58%, compared with 85% for those given a boost with photons or electrons and 85% when no boost dose was administered ($P = 0.03$). This may be related to the volume implanted and dose delivered because in patients with implants containing fewer than 70 ^{192}Ir seeds, only 15% had poor or fair cosmesis compared with 38% with implants containing 100 or more seeds ($P < 0.01$). Rose and co-workers[349] reviewed additional aspects of cosmetic results in these patients. Adjuvant chemotherapy affected cosmesis negatively (40% excellent compared with 71% without chemotherapy) as did tumor size (73% of patients with T1 and 55% of patients with T2 tumors had excellent cosmesis). Cosmetic results were stable at 3 to 5 years, with only 5% deteriorating from good or excellent to fair results. These results are similar to those reported by Spitalier and colleagues.[415]

Hallahan and associates[172] observed only 61% (of 207 patients) excellent or good cosmetic results in patients with scar length more than 8 cm and 68% satisfactory cosmesis in patients with large volumes of breast tissue resected with segmental mastectomy. The boost technique did not have a significant impact on cosmetic results (95% excellent to good results in 40 patients with ^{192}Ir implant and 94% in 151 patients receiving boost with electrons or photons). Chemotherapy did not have an impact on cosmesis; 90% of 34 patients receiving adjuvant chemotherapy (CMF or CAF) and 93% of 166 patients given no adjuvant chemotherapy or only tamoxifen had excellent/good cosmetic results.

It should be emphasized that surgical procedures have a profound effect on the cosmetic results of breast conservation therapy, such as amount of tissue removed, size and location of incision, and so on (Fig. 42-40).

Adjuvant chemotherapy may have a significant deleterious influence on cosmetic results (Table 42-35). In several studies, the main effect is a switch from the "excellent" to the "good" category. Gore and colleagues[158] also demonstrated that the sequencing of chemotherapy and radiation therapy was important in cosmetic outcome.

At Washington University, no significant difference was found between the percentage of good to excellent results with the use of chemotherapy. This is probably a result of our policy to rarely administer concurrent chemoradiotherapy in favor of sequencing chemotherapy after irradiation. Overall, 70% to 90% of patients treated with breast conservation therapy can be expected to have a good or excellent cosmetic outcome.

Management of Local Recurrences After Breast Conservation Therapy

Unlike local failures on the chest wall after radical mastectomy, the prognosis for patients who fail within the breast after conservation therapy is more favorable. As high as 80% of women who develop chest wall tumor recurrences after mastectomy will manifest distant metastases,[65] whereas 50% or less of the women who develop isolated breast failure after conservation therapy develop distant disease.[223] A significant percentage of women who have recurrences locally following breast conservation therapy can be salvaged with additional surgery, resulting in a 5-year survival fairly comparable to the 5-year survival of women initially treated by a mastectomy (Table 42-36).[13]

The majority of the recurrences during the first 10 years after wide local excision and irradiation occur in the vicinity of the original primary tumor site.[49, 134, 136] Kurtz and colleagues[224, 225] suggest that the treatment of localized recurrences after wide local excision and irradiation may be effectively accomplished in selected patients with resection of the recurrent tumor without resorting to mastectomy (Fig. 42-41). Kurtz and colleagues[225] reported on 178 patients (11% of original group) with Stage I and Stage II breast cancer surgically

TABLE 42–34
*Factors Influencing Cosmetic Results with BCT**

	% GOOD–EXCELLENT RESULTS		P VALUE	
	PATIENTS	PHYSICIANS	PATIENTS	PHYSICIANS
SURGICAL FACTORS				
Quadratectomy *vs*	72	54	0.0000	0.0000
limited surgical excision	92	86		
Re-excision *vs*	82	68	0.0043	0.0000
single tylectomy	93	87		
Continuous tylectomy-axilla scar *vs*	79	59	0.012	0.0024
separate scars	92	82		
Scar orientation non-NSABP *vs*	83	67	0.0085	0.0000
per NSABP	93	87		
No nodes removed *vs*	86	84	0.20	0.52
fewer than 11 nodes removed *vs*	85	77		
11 or more nodes removed	92	80		
Surgeon (breast specialist) *vs*	98	96	0.032	0.0054
all other referring surgeons	88	78		
RADIATION THERAPY FACTORS				
Whole breast dose ≥ 5000 cGy *vs*	78	71	0.0005	0.0095
<5000 cGy	93	84		
Bolus applied to skin *vs*	79	75	0.0011	0.13
no bolus	92	83		
No compensation *vs*	60	52	0.0000	0.0002
compensating filters	91	83		
Peripheral lymphatic RT *vs*	79	70	0.0001	0.0002
breast only RT	95	87		
Implant boost *vs*	86	80	0.28	0.80
electron boost *vs*	91	82		
no boost	83	77		
Total dose to tumor bed				
≥6000 cGy	89	78	0.97	0.19
<6000 cGy	89	84		
CHEMOTHERAPY FACTORS				
Chemotherapy	85	78	0.31	0.55
No chemotherapy	90	81		
HOST FACTORS				
Large size				
(bridge separation ≥20 cm) *vs*	90	81	0.90	0.89
small size (<20 cm)	89	80		
Menopausal status				
Premenopausal *vs*	94	85	0.12	0.23
perimenopausal *vs*	86	86		
postmenopausal	87	78		
Age				
≤45 years	92	81	0.37	0.82
>45 years	88	80		
Race				
White	89	82	0.85	0.15
Black	90	72		
Tumor size				
T1 (≤2 cm)	89	79	0.47	0.52
T2 (2–5 cm)	86	75		

**Cosmetic results were obtained from questionnaire completed at the most recent follow-up visit.*
RT: radiation therapy

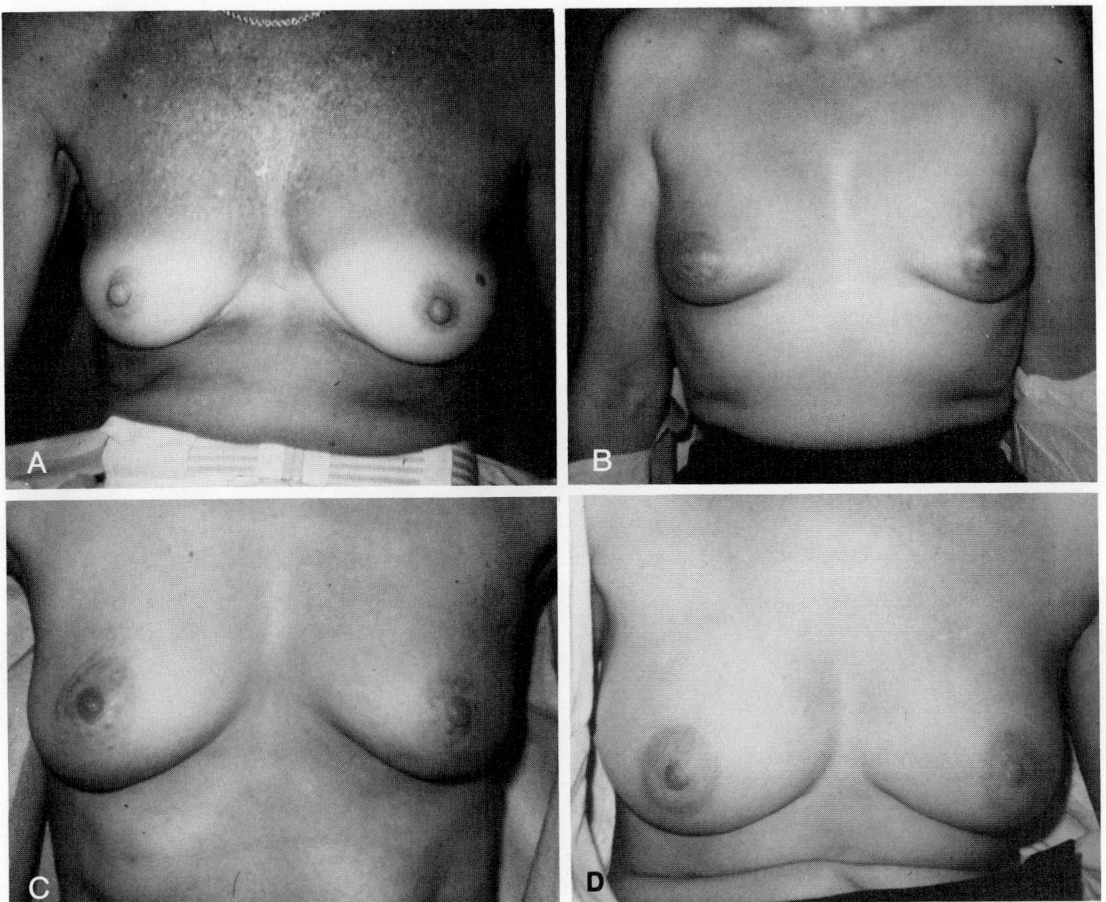

FIGURE 42–39. Photographs of patients showing excellent cosmetic results obtained with conservation surgery and irradiation for patients with T1 and T2 carcinomas of the breast. The patient in **C** has minimal telangiectasis in the area treated with a boost (upper quadrant of left breast).

treated for isolated mammary recurrences after conservation surgery and irradiation. In 66 patients, a mutilating operation was performed (simple mastectomy in eight patients, modified radical mastectomy in 39 patients, and radical mastectomy in 19 patients). Additional wide local excision was carried out in 34 patients and wide local excision with axillary dissection in 18 patients. Follow-up from time of salvage surgery ranged from 12 months to 20 years with a median of 7 years. At the time of the report, 34 (29%) of the women had developed distant metastases, and 38% had died. Actuarial survival rate from time of salvage surgery was 72% at 5 years and 58% at 10 and 15 years. Haffty and colleagues[169] noted a greater incidence of subsequent breast relapses after treatment of a diffuse local recurrence (four of nine, or 44%) and distant metastases (five of nine, or 55%) than in patients with localized breast failures (no local relapse and three of 22, or 14% distant failures).

Calle and associates[49] published their 10-year experience with 120 patients treated with lumpectomy and irradiation; 16 developed locoregional recurrences: three in the axilla, one in the supraclavicular fossa, and 12 in the breast. Of these 16 patients, 10 had mastectomy and four had limited resection. Eight of the 14 patients (57%) survived 5 years without disease.

Clark and associates[69] reported on 680 women treated with local excision and irradiation. The 10-year breast relapse rates for T1 tumors were 20% and for T2 tumors 23%. The 5-year survival rate after the time of first relapse for the women who relapsed locally was 55% in contrast to only 7% for 550 women treated with mastectomy who had recurrences in the chest wall. Women who relapsed in the breast only had the same survival as those who never relapsed at any site.

Delouche and colleagues[90] reported on 410 patients treated with tumor excision and irradiation and followed up for a minimum of 5 years. Thirty-five women (8.5%) had recurrences within the breast; 30 of them had additional surgery (25 were treated by mastectomy), with 14 patients remaining free of tumor. Thus of the approximately 10% of patients who failed locally, 75% had operable disease and only 2% went on to manifest uncontrolled local disease.

In a report on 276 patients by Kurtz and associates,[226] 63% of the breast tumor recurrences after local excision and irradiation occurred within 5 years, with a few recurrences taking place after 10 years. The proportion of failures occurring late was greater for T1 than for T2 tumors (53% *versus* 25%). Seventy-four percent of early recurrences were operable compared with all the recurrences taking place after 5 years. The early recurrences had an adverse impact on the 10-year survival rate (41%) in contrast to the good prognosis in the few patients with late breast local failures (94% 10-year survival), similar to patients who did not develop recurrences. Prognosis was similar to that of 20 patients who developed contralateral breast carcinoma. These observations were confirmed by Fourquet and associates,[139] who reported a 73% 5-year survival rate following recurrence in 56 patients of 518 initially treated patients failing after conservation surgery and irradiation. The survival rate was 44% for those patients having recurrences in the first 3 years, in contrast to 87% for those with late recurrences.

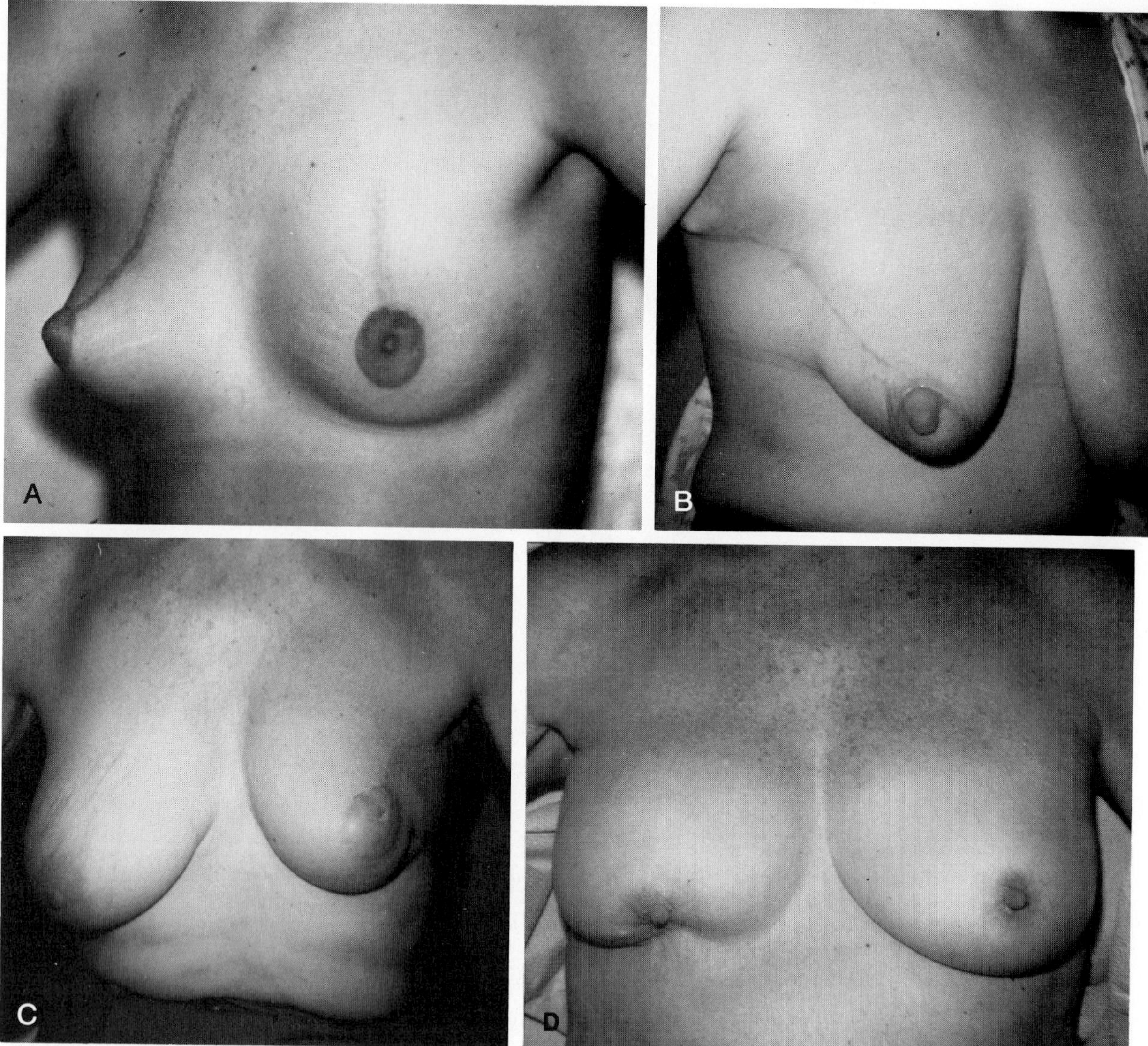

FIGURE 42–40. Photographs of patients illustrating poor cosmetic results with technically poor surgical procedures. The direction of the incision, the amount of tissue removed, and the continuity of the incision used to remove the primary tissue in the upper outer quadrant of the breast with axillary dissection are contributing factors.

Results With Total Mastectomy and Radiation Therapy

Following the report by McWhirter,[283] in which he reported survival rates in total mastectomy and irradiation patients that were comparable to those obtained with radical mastectomy, other randomized studies have confirmed his observations. Kaae and Johansen,[207] in the latest update of their randomized series for Stage I and Stage II carcinoma of the breast, showed the same survival and recurrence rates in the treated areas of Stage I and Stage II carcinoma treated with total mastectomy and irradiation or an extended radical mastectomy (with internal mammary lymph node dissection). The results are summarized in Figure 42-42 and Table 42-37.

TABLE 42–35
Impact of Adjuvant Chemotherapy on Cosmesis in Breast Conservation Therapy

	% GOOD–EXCELLENT COSMESIS	
INSTITUTION	RADIATION THERAPY WITHOUT CHEMOTHERAPY	RADIATION THERAPY WITH CHEMOTHERAPY
Harvard University[27]	92	67
Palo Alto[332]	88	73
NCI[118]	80	70
University of Pennsylvania[183]	89	81
Washington University[232]	81	78

TABLE 42–36
Survival Following Salvage Surgery for Isolated Breast Recurrence

AUTHOR	NO. OF PATIENTS	5-YEAR SURVIVAL RATE
Calle[49]	19	74%
Amalric[3]	62	72%
Kurtz[222]	159	69%
Clark[70]	87	55%
Montague[291]	16	67%
Clarke[72]	11	81%
Osborne[310]	12	50%
Recht[340]	65	63%
Fowble[139]	52	81%
Haffty[169]	25	48%
Dubois[101]	30	70%

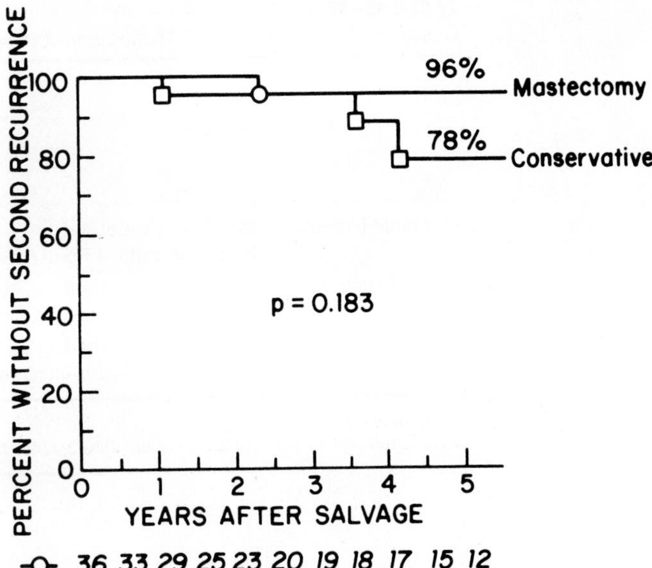

FIGURE 42–41. Actuarial locoregional recurrence-free survival rate after treatment of operable late recurrence in the breast, comparing salvage mastectomy with conservative salvage surgery. No events were observed after 5 years. The numbers under the time axis represent the patients at risk for the particular interval. (Kurtz JM, Spitalier JM, Amalric R, et al: Int J Radiat Oncol Biol Phys 18(1):87, 1990)

Brinkley and Haybittle[41] reported no significant differences in results in 204 patients with Stage II breast cancer treated with a radical or simple mastectomy followed by x-ray therapy (50% and 57% 5-year disease-free survival rates, respectively). In the Cancer Research Campaign trial,[54] with 2243 evaluable patients with clinical Stage I and Stage II breast cancer randomized to be treated with simple mastectomy alone (watch group) or combined with irradiation, no difference in overall 5-year survival rate was noted (69% and 72%, respectively). However, a threefold greater incidence of local recurrences was noted in the watch group (345 patients) compared with the irradiated group (122 patients). Local recurrence-free 5-year survival rates were 70% and 89%, respectively.

The 5-year survival rates reported with total mastectomy and radiation therapy for Stages I, II, and III breast cancer are similar to those obtained with more radical operations. The local failure rate is 5% to 10%, depending on the stage of tumor and the dose of radiation given.[207]

Fisher and the NSABP[124] described the latest results in protocol 04, which compared patients with total mastectomy alone (and delayed axillary dissection) with or without irradiation with those with radical mastectomy. Patients with comparable lesions and clinically negative axillary lymph nodes had about a 60% 5-year disease-free survival rate and a 47% rate at 10 years, which was observed in patients treated with total mastectomy alone or combined with irradiation or with a radical mastectomy (Fig. 42-43*A*). The overall survival was 57% at 10 years (Fig. 42-43*B*). Patients treated with total mastectomy alone had an 18% incidence of axillary lymph node failures, which were subsequently treated with a dissection. The incidence of first chest wall and regional lymph node recurrences is lower in patients treated with total mastectomy and irradiation (less than 4%) compared with those treated with radical mastectomy (6.6%) or total mastectomy alone (9.3%).

Patients with clinically palpable axillary lymph nodes treated with total mastectomy and irradiation have the same disease-free survival rate as those treated with a standard radical mastectomy (about 40% to 45% at 5 years and 25% to 29% at 10 years). The overall survival rate was 60% at 5 years and 38%

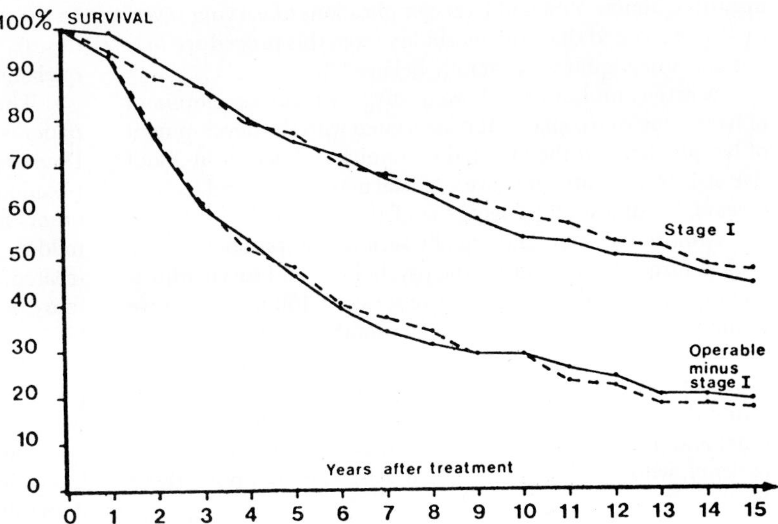

FIGURE 42–42. Crude survival rates for clinical Stage I and operable minus Stage I with McWhirter's method (*solid line*) and extended radical mastectomy (*broken line*). (Kaae S, Johansen H: Int J Radiat Oncol Biol Phys 2:1163, 1977)

TABLE 42–37
Comparison of McWhirter's Method and Extended Radical Mastectomy*

		NO. OF PATIENTS	CRUDE SURVIVAL RATE (%) 5 YEARS	10 YEARS	15 YEARS
Operable patients	McWhirter's method	219	66	46	36
	Extended radical mastectomy	206	67	50	37
Clinical Stage I	McWhirter's method	149	75	54	44
	Extended radical mastectomy	141	77	59	47
Operable minus clinical Stage I	McWhirter's method	70	46	29	19
	Extended radical mastectomy	65	48	29	17

**Reference 283*
Kaae S, Johansen H: Int J Radiat Oncol Biol Phys 2:1164, 1977

at 10 years. A lower incidence of chest wall recurrences was noted in the total mastectomy and irradiation patients (about 4%) compared with 10.5% in the radical mastectomy group, but a 10% incidence of axillary lymph node failures was seen in the former patients compared with 2% of those treated with radical mastectomy.

SEQUELAE OF THERAPY

Radical Surgery

A review of the literature and current textbooks yields little information about the complications of radical surgery for breast cancer. One of the most comprehensive articles is that from the Ellis Fischel State Cancer Hospital,[374] which detailed the incidence of complications following radical mastectomy in 1531 patients with carcinoma of the breast treated between 1940 and 1965. Complications in the radical mastectomy alone group (1198 patients) included death (1.2%), skin flap necrosis (36%), hematoma under the flap (4%), serum collection under the flap (40%), wound dehiscence (3%), chest wound infection (14%), loss of skin graft (32%), and arm edema (31%). Additional surgical complications of radical mastectomy were pneumothorax (6%) and infection of the donor site (8%).

A second article observed that among 211 patients treated with radical mastectomy at 36 university centers and cancer institutes, almost 50% had local complications of varying severity.[74] It was noted that "the morbidity from this procedure may not be as negligible as generally believed."

A rare complication following surgery is the development of lymphangiosarcoma.[270] It is associated with the development of lymphedema in the affected extremity and occurs in about five of 1000 patients who have a radical mastectomy and survive 5 years.[102] Almost all patients die of the disease.

A more common and equally serious complication of the radical surgical procedure is the psychologic and social adjustment to mastectomy. A consecutive series of 160 postoperative women was assessed at 3, 12, and 24 months for marital adjustment, sexual adjustment, interpersonal relationships, work adjustment, depression, and personality characteristics.[295] It was found that more than 25% of patients had failed to adjust by 2 years and also that the course of recovery was not smooth for patients who did recover.[295] Other studies support these findings.[369]

Conservation Surgery and Irradiation

Complications most frequently associated with conservation surgery plus irradiation are arm or breast edema, breast fibrosis, painful mastitis or myositis, pneumonitis, and rib fracture. Although apical pulmonary fibrosis is frequently noted when the regional lymph nodes are irradiated, in a report of 151 patients only 12% had symptomatic pneumonitis and 9% had some degree of arm edema.[292] An increase in incidence of symptomatic radiation pneumonitis has been described with larger volume of lung irradiated.[363, 364]

Danoff and colleagues[85] reported arm edema in 7% of 189 patients, symptomatic pneumonitis in 1%, rib fractures in 1%, pericarditis in 1%, and pleural effusion in 1%. Kantorowitz[209] reported moderate sequelae of therapy in 6.8% of 146 patients treated with segmental mastectomy and irradiation, consisting mostly of breast and arm edema, shoulder, arm, and chest wall myositis, and breast pain. Subcutaneous fibrosis has been reported in about 10% of patients.[290]

Schmidt-Ullrich and associates[380] treated 115 breasts in 108 women with conservation surgery and irradiation. Moderate breast edema, fibrosis, and discomfort were noted in about 9% of patients, and severe sequelae were recorded in about 2% of patients.

At the Foundation Curie in Paris,[49] of patients treated with lumpectomy plus irradiation, 27% were found to have moderate radiation changes and none had severe radiation sequelae. In the group of patients treated with radiation alone (to higher doses), 20% had minimal sequelae, 33% had moderate sequelae, and 1% had severe sequelae.

The Radiation Therapy Oncology Group evaluated 234 patients treated with primary irradiation for Stage I and Stage II adenocarcinoma of the breast.[30] Six patients had severe complications (2.6%), all of which were breast fibrosis. Fourteen others had complications, approximately 5% of which were of mild or moderate severity. In a report comparing 21 patients treated with BCT and 27 treated with modified radical mastectomy, it was shown that the BCT patients had a significantly better range of shoulder (arm) motion in the immediate postoperative period. After 3 months no difference was seen after physical therapy in the flexion and abduction of the arm in the two groups.[162]

The incidence of breast edema after conservation therapy has varied, with most authors reporting between 20% and 40%, depending on posttreatment time. This may be related to the

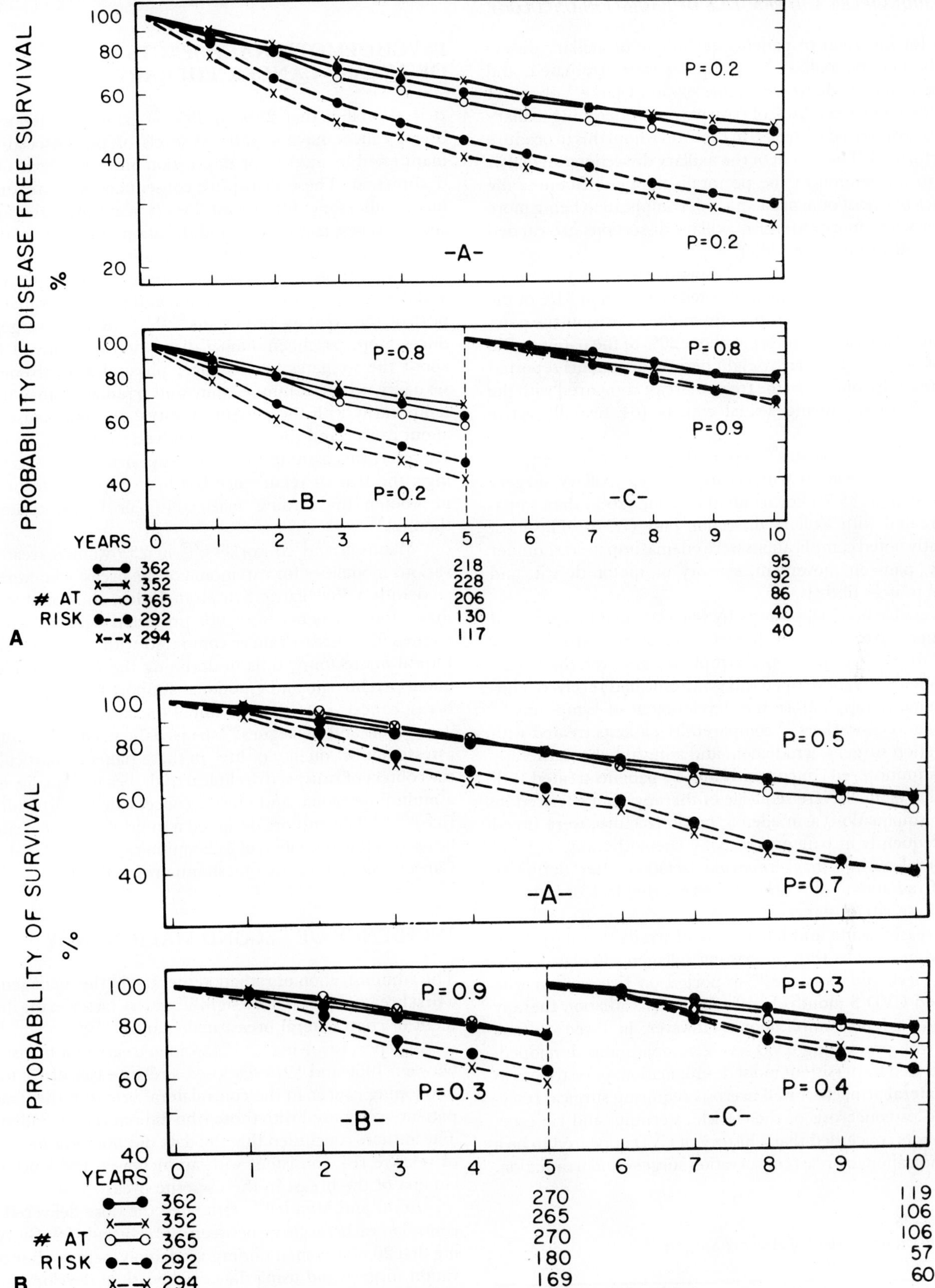

FIGURE 42–43. (**A**) Disease-free survival through 10 years (part A), during the first 5 years (part B), and during the second 5 years (part C) for patients free of disease at the end of the fifth year in NSABP protocol 04. Patients were treated by radical mastectomy (*solid circle*), total mastectomy plus irradiation (X), or total mastectomy alone (*open circle*). There were no significant differences among the three groups of patients with clinically negative nodes (*solid line*) or between the two groups with clinically positive nodes (*broken line*). (**B**) Survival through 10 years (part A), during the first 5 years (part B), and during the second five years (part C) for patients alive at the end of the fifth year. Patients were treated by radical mastectomy (*solid circle*), total mastectomy, and irradiation (X), or total mastectomy alone (*open circle*). No significant differences were found among the three groups of patients with clinically negative nodes (*solid line*) or between the two groups with positive nodes (*broken line*). (Fisher B, Redmond C, Fisher C, et al: N Engl J Med 312:674, 1985)

criteria for inclusion of patients, technique of axillary dissection, whether the axillary lymph nodes were irradiated, and doses of radiation delivered (Table 42-38). Clarke[71] observed breast edema in about 20% of patients not undergoing axillary dissection compared with 80% in those on whom this procedure was performed. The extent of the axillary dissection (medial or lateral to the tendon of the pectoralis minor) influences the incidence of breast or arm edema, this complication being more frequent when more extensive axillary dissections are carried out (beyond group 2—middle).[333]

McCormick and associates[273] showed in a survey that breast swelling was the most frequently noted symptom in 31% of the patients, followed by muscle pain (in motion), incision-site pain, and general breast discomfort in about 20% of the patients. Rib pain was noted by 13%. Forty-eight percent of patients reported more breast discomfort in the treated breast compared with the untreated breast during sexual activity (64 sexually active patients).

Dewar and associates[93] reported a greater incidence of upper limb sequelae in patients undergoing axillary surgery and irradiation (33.7%) or irradiation alone (26%) than in patients treated with axillary dissection only (7.2%). The most frequently noted complications were edema, impaired shoulder mobility, pain on movement, sensory or motor deficit, and pectoral muscle fibrosis.

Reversible brachial plexopathy was evaluated in a group of 565 patients treated at the Joint Center at Harvard.[368] Only 1.4% of the patients developed symptoms; however, the majority of patients who developed this syndrome had received adjuvant chemotherapy before the development of symptoms.[368]

Ray and co-workers[333] compared 51 patients treated with conservation surgery, irradiation, and adjuvant chemotherapy (CMF) administered concurrently and 83 patients treated with irradiation alone. Severe sequelae of therapy, characterized by moist desquamation, arm edema, or rib fracture, were noted more frequently in patients receiving chemotherapy.

Several authors have reported lactation after definitive doses of radiation.[87,346] Others have reported lack of lactation under these circumstances.[47,362]

Increased acute and late effects of irradiation have been reported in patients with preexisting collagen vascular disease (CVD). Fleck and associates[133] reported on five women who developed CVD 3 months to 10 years after radiation therapy and who had no complications. However, in three of four women with preexisting CVD severe complications developed, characterized by persistent moist desquamation, paresthesias in the ipsilateral arm, chest wall necrosis requiring surgical resection, and osteonecrosis of the clavicle, sternum, and rib cage. The authors concluded that a history of CVD appeared to be a contraindication to breast conservation surgery and irradiation.

TABLE 42–38
Breast Edema and Extent of Axillary Surgery in Conservation Therapy

AUTHOR	DISSECTION	
	FULL	LIMITED
Clarke (1982)[71]	26/33 (79%)	5/43 (12%)
Montague (1983)[293]	9/9 (100%)	10/77 (13%)
Ray (1983)[332]	50/90 (56%)	6/40 (15%)
Pezner (1985)[324]	14/36 (39%)	2/11 (18%)
Beadle (1983)[27]	44/109 (40%)	24/96 (25%)
Kuske (1990)[231]	7/46 (15%)	10/121 (8%)

PSYCHOEMOTIONAL ASPECTS OF BREAST CANCER THERAPY

It is estimated that 25% to 35% of patients diagnosed with breast cancer have significant levels of psychosocial distress manifested by anxiety or depression and some level of sexual dysfunction. These disruptive consequences of treatment remain bothersome for at least 2 years after initial therapy. The specific types, magnitude, and duration of emotional dysfunction of women undergoing conservation breast therapy compared with those treated with mastectomy are highly variable, and they also require the attention and psychotherapeutic support of the treating physicians.[24,264,376] Radical surgery produces more psychoemotional disruption in terms of feelings about the woman's body image, physical attractiveness, and sexuality, whereas lumpectomy and irradiation may interfere temporarily with the patient's lifestyle and may cause worries about cancer and the perceived adverse effects of irradiation. However, this assumption is not supported by research findings; the fear of recurrence has been reported to be similar in women undergoing mastectomy or breast conservation therapy.[377]

Maunsell and co-workers,[272] in 235 women treated with various modalities for carcinoma of the breast who were evaluated with a Psychiatric Symptom Index, showed that partial mastectomy patients were not protected against psychologic distress after breast cancer compared with a group treated by radical mastectomy, thus underlining the importance of adequate psychologic and emotional support for all patients with breast cancer, regardless of initial therapy.

Levine and colleagues[242] stressed the need to quantitate the assessment of "quality of life" in these patients, particularly in the context of prospective clinical trials, because quality of life is a multidimensional and elusive concept that is difficult to define.[379,457] The authors designed a multiple-question survey to be used in the evaluation of a chemotherapy clinical trial (Breast Cancer Chemotherapy Questionnaire = BCQ).

INCIDENCE OF SECOND MALIGNANCY

The administration of radiation therapy in the management of a first breast cancer is not a significant risk factor in the development of contralateral breast malignancy.[20,25,201,274,275,378]

A report involving 27,175 women treated for breast cancer between 1960 and 1975 disclosed a relative risk of 1.2 to 1.4 of developing cancer in the contralateral breast in the irradiated patients, compared with those who did not receive radiation.[175] The authors concluded that the data did not indicate a pattern of relative risk consistent with an increased incidence of carcinoma of the breast in the opposite breast.

Levitt and Mandell[247] estimated the dose delivered to the contralateral breast to be between 100 cGy and 400 cGy. Assuming that 20,000 women undergo radiation therapy after conservation surgery and using data on the risk of developing breast cancer after various doses of ionizing radiation, the authors concluded that fewer than one additional case of breast cancer would occur after 10 years.

Montague[291] reported six second breast primary tumors in 316 patients (1.9% incidence) treated with conservation surgery and irradiation in contrast to 30 of 576 (5.2%) after radical or modified radical mastectomy alone.

Contralateral breast cancer developed during the second decade in five of 300 patients reported on by Kurtz and associates,[224] with a cumulative risk of 6.5% at 20 years. Clark and

TABLE 42–39
Incidence of Contralateral Breast Cancer in Carcinoma of Breast Treated with Conservation Surgery and Irradiation or Mastectomy

STUDY	CONSERVATION TREATMENT	MASTECTOMY
Clark and colleagues[70]	45/1504 (3%)	
Kurtz and colleagues[224]	6/300 (6.5%)*	—
Montague[291]	6/316 (1.9%)†	30/576 (5.2%)
Recht and colleagues[340]	366 (9%)‡	—
Sarrazin and associates[371]	5/88 (9%)§	6/91 (9%)
Veronesi[463]	18/349 (5%)¶	16/352 (5%)¶

** Actuarial risk at 20 years*
† Excludes simultaneous bilateral cancer
‡ Actuarial risk at 5 years
§ Actuarial relapse at 10 years
¶ Actuarial risk at 12 years

colleagues[70] reported only 3% incidence of contralateral breast primary tumors in 1504 patients and Recht[340] in 9% of 357 patients treated with conservation surgery and irradiation (Table 42-39).

Rosen and associates[353] reported on 644 patients with T1 breast carcinoma treated primarily with mastectomy; 76 received adjuvant radiation therapy to the internal mammary and supraclavicular lymph nodes; 47 received radiation to the regional nodes, and five had irradiation of the chest wall. Subsequent contralateral breast carcinoma was found in 10.9% of patients receiving adjuvant irradiation compared with 9.4% of those who did not receive postoperative irradiation. Curtis and colleagues,[81] in an analysis of the Surveillance, Epidemiology and End Results (SEER) Program of 59,115 women with breast cancer diagnosed between 1973 and 1980, reported no cases of leukemia in a group of 1988 women who received radiation therapy. In contrast, six cases of leukemia were observed (compared with 1.58 expected) in 6040 patients receiving chemotherapy in their first course of therapy. Five of the six cases occurred in the third to seventh year after therapy. Parenthetically, the risk of developing leukemia in patients treated with surgery alone did not differ significantly from that of the general population.

Rarely sarcomas have been reported after mastectomy and postoperative irradiation of the chest wall. Souba and coworkers[412] described ten patients with carcinoma of the breast in a group of 16 patients with radiation-induced chest wall sarcoma. Of the ten tumors, six were malignant fibrohistiocytomas, two were osteosarcomas (one of the rib and one of the sternum), one was a fibrosarcoma, and one was a supraclavicular mesenchymoma. The latency period between irradiation and diagnosis of chest wall sarcoma ranged from 5 to 28 years, with a mean of 13 years and a median of 10 years. Prognosis for these patients is extremely poor, with only one surviving past 2 years (died at 48 months after treatment for sarcoma). The mean survival time is about 13 months. Most patients are treated surgically, if the tumor is resectable. Chemotherapy has shown minimal efficacy.

REFERENCES

1. Adami H, Bergstrom R, Hansen J: Age at first primary as a determinant of the incidence of bilateral breast cancer: Cumulative and relative risks in a population-based case-control study. Cancer 55:643–647, 1985
2. Amalric R, Santamaria F, Robert F, et al: Radiation therapy with or without primary limited surgery for operable breast cancer. Cancer 49:30–34, 1982
3. Amalric R, Santamaria F, Robert F, et al: Conservation therapy of operable breast cancer: Results of 5, 10 and 15 years in 2216 consecutive cases. In Harris HR, Hellman S, Silen W (eds): Conservative Management of Breast Cancer: New Surgical and Radiotherapeutic Techniques, pp 15–21. Philadelphia, JB Lippincott, 1983
4. American Cancer Society. Cancer Facts and Figures. Atlanta, ACS, 1991
5. Andersen J: Lobular carcinoma *in situ:* An approach to rational treatment. Cancer 39:2597–2602, 1977
6. Anderson I, Aspegren K, Janzon L, et al: Mammographic screening and mortality from breast cancer: The Malmö mammographic screening trial. Br Med J 297:943–948, 1988
7. Antman KH, Corson J, Greengerger J, et al: Multimodality therapy in the management of angiosarcoma of the breast. Cancer 50:2000–2003, 1982
8. Arriagada R, Le MG, Mouriesse H, et al: Long-term effect of internal mammary chain treatment: Results of a multivariate analysis of 1195 patients with operable breast cancer and positive axillary nodes. Radiother Onncol 11:213–222, 1988
9. Ashikari R, Hajdu SI, Robbins GF: Intraductal carcinoma of the breast. Cancer 28:1182–1187, 1971
10. Ashikari R, Park K, Huvos AG, et al: Paget's disease of the breast. Cancer 26:680–685, 1970
11. Ashikari R, Rosen PP, Urban JA, et al: Breast cancer presenting as an axillary mass. Ann Surg 183:415–417, 1976
12. Atkin NB, Kay R: Prognostic significance of modal DNA value and other factors in malignant tumors, based on 1465 cases. Br J Cancer 40:210, 1979
13. Atkins H, Hayward JL, Klugman DJ, et al: Treatment of early breast cancer: A report after 10 years of a clinical trial. Br Med J (Clin Res) 2:423–429, 1972
14. Auer GU, Caspersson TO, Gustafsson SA, et al: Relationship between nuclear DNA distribution and estrogen receptors in human mammary carcinomas. Anal Quant Cytol Histol 2:280, 1980
15. Austin DF, Reynolds P, Boyd PT, et al: Progress in the war against cancer (Letter). N Engl J Med 321(17):1197–1198, 1989
16. Baeza MR, Sole J, Leon A, et al: Conservative treatment of early breast cancer. Int J Radiat Oncol Biol Phys 14:669–676, 1988
17. Baines CJ, Miller AB, Bassett AA: Physical examination: Its role as a single screening modality in the Canadian National Breast Screening Study. Cancer 63:1816–1822, 1989
18. Baker LH: Breast cancer detection demonstration project: Five year summary report. CA 32:194–225, 1982
19. Ballard-Barbash R, Schatzkin A, Carter CL, et al: Body fat distribution and breast cancer in the Framingham Study. J Natl Cancer Inst 82(4):286–290, 1990
20. Baral E, Larsson L, Mattisson B: Breast cancer following irradiation of the breast. Cancer 40:2905–2910, 1977
21. Baron PL, Moore MP, Kinne DW, et al: Occult breast cancer presenting with axillary metastases. Arch Surg 125:210–215, 1990
22. Barr LC, Brunt AM, Goodman AG, et al: Uncontrolled local recurrence after treatment of breast cancer with breast conservation. Cancer 64:1203–1207, 1989
23. Bartelink H, Borger JH, van Dogen JA, et al: The impact of tumor size and histology on local control after breast-conserving therapy. Radiother Oncol 11:297–303, 1988
24. Bartelink H, Van Dam F, Van Dongen J: Psychological effects of breast conserving therapy in comparison with radical mastectomy. Int J Radiat Oncol Biol Phys 11:381–385, 1985
25. Basco VE, Coldman AJ, Elwood JM, et al: Radiation dose and second breast cancer. Br J Cancer 52:319–325, 1985
26. Bataini JP, Picco C, Martin M, et al: Relation between time-dose and local control of operable breast cancer treated by tumorectomy and radiotherapy or by radical radiotherapy alone. Cancer 42:2059–2065, 1978
27. Beadle GF, Come S, Henderson C, et al: The effect of adjuvant chemotherapy on the cosmetic results after primary radi-

ation treatment for early stage breast cancer. Int J Radiat Oncol Biol Phys 10:2131–2137, 1984

28. Beahrs OH, Henson DE, Hutter RWP, Myers MH (eds): Manual for Staging of Cancer, 3rd ed. Philadelphia, JB Lippincott, 1988
29. Bedwinek J: Treatment of stage I and II adenocarcinoma of the breast by tumor excision and irradiation. Int J Radiat Oncol Biol Phys 7:1553, 1981
30. Bedwinek J, Perez C, Kramer S, et al: Irradiation as the primary management of Stage I and II adenocarcinoma of the breast. Cancer Clin Trials 3:11, 1980
31. Bell DA, Hajdu SI, Urban JA, et al: Role of aspiration cytology in the diagnosis and management of mammary lesions in office practice. Cancer 51:1182–1189, 1983
32. Benfield JR, Jacobson M, Warner NE: *In situ* lobular carcinoma of the breast. Arch Surg 91:130–135, 1965
33. Berg JW: The significance of axillary node levels in the study of breast carcinoma. Cancer 8:776–778, 1955
34. Betsill WL Jr, Rosen PP, Lieberman PH, et al: Intraductal carcinoma. Long-term follow-up after treatment of biopsy alone. JAMA 239:1863–1867, 1978
35. Blichert-Toft M: A Danish randomized trial comparing breast conservation with mastectomy in mammary carcinoma. NIH Consensus Development Conference, pp 28–31. June 18–21, 1990
36. Bloom HJG, Richardson WW, Harries EJ: Natural history of untreated breast cancer (1805–1933). Br Med J 2:213–221, 1962
37. Bodian C, Haagensen CD: Bilateral carcinoma of the breast. In Haagensen CD (ed): Diseases of the Breast, 3rd ed, pp 440–461. Philadelphia, WB Saunders, 1986
38. Boice JD Jr, Monson RR: Breast cancer in women after repeated fluoroscopic examinations of the chest. J Natl Cancer Inst 59:823–832, 1977
39. Bonadonna G, Valagussa P: Current status of adjuvant chemotherapy for breast cancer. Semin Oncol 14(1):8–22, 1987
40. Boona RS, Bonanni R, Rosato FE: Patterns of axillary nodal involvement in breast cancer: Predictability of level one dissection. Ann Surg 196:642–644, 1982
41. Bourgeois P, Fruhling J, Henry J: Postoperative axillary lymphoscintigraphy in the management of breast cancer. Int J Radiat Oncol Biol Phys 9:29, 1983
42. Boyages J, Recht A, Connolly, et al: Factors associated with local recurrence as a first site of failure following conservative treatment of early breast cancer. Rec Results Cancer Res 115:92–102, 1989
43. Brenner MJ, Schnitt SJ, Connolly JL, et al: The use of re-excision in primary radiation therapy for stage I and II breast carcinoma (Abstract). Int J Radiat Oncol Biol Phys 11(1):186, 1985
44. Brinkley D, Haybrittle JL: Treatment of stage II carcinoma of the female breast. Lancet 2:292–295, 1966
45. Brown PW, Silverman J, Owens E, et al: Intraductal "non-infiltrating" carcinoma of the breast. Arch Surg 111:1063–1067, 1976
46. Bundred NJ, O'Reilly K, Smart JG: Long term survival following bilateral breast angiosarcoma. Eur J Surg Oncol 15:263–264, 1989
47. Burns PE: Absence of lactation in a previously radiated breast. Int J Radiat Oncol Biol Phys 13:1603–1604, 1987
48. Butzelaar RMJM, VanDongen JA, Van der Schoot JB, et al: Evaluation of routine preoperative bone scintigraphy in patients with breast cancer. Eur J Cancer 13:19–21, 1977
49. Calle R, Pilleron J, Schlienger P, et al: Conservative management of operable breast cancer: Ten years' experience at the Foundation Curie. Cancer 42:2045–2053, 1978
50. Calle R, Pilleron JP, Vilcoq JR, et al: Breast carcinoma: Experience of Curie Institute. In Ames FC, Blumenschein GR, Montague ED (eds): The Proceedings of 1982 Clinical Conference: Current Controversies in Breast Cancer, pp 121–128. Austin, University of Texas Press, 1983
51. Calle R, Vilcoq JR, Zafrani B, et al: Local control and survival of breast cancer treated by limited surgery followed by irradiation. Int J Radiat Oncol Biol Phys 12:873–878, 1986
52. Callery DCH, Rosen PR, Kinne WD: Sarcoma of the breast: A study of 32 patients with reappraisal of classification and therapy. Ann Surg 201:527–532, 1985
53. Campana F, Fourquet A, Ashby MA, et al: Presentation of axillary lymphadenopathy without detectable breast primary (TON1b breast cancer): Experience at Institut Curie. Radiother Oncol 15:321–325, 1989
54. Cancer Research Campaign Working Party: Cancer Research Campaign (King's/Cambridge) Trial for Early Breast Cancer: A detailed update at the tenth year. Lancet 2:55–60, 1980
55. Carstens PHB, Huvos AG, Foote FW Jr, et al: Tubular carcinoma of the breast: A clinicopathologic study of 35 cases. Am J Clin Pathol 58:231–238, 1972
56. Carter D, Smith RRL: Carcinoma *in situ* of the breast. Cancer 40:1189–1193, 1977
57. Cascinelli N, Greco M, Leo E: Comments on primary and adjuvant treatments of breast cancer. Eur J Cancer Clin Oncol 24(3):487–491, 1989
58. Cedermark B, Askergren J Alveryd A, et al: Breast-conserving treatment for breast cancer in Stockholm, Sweden, 1977 to 1981. Cancer 53:1253–1255, 1984
59. Chaudary MA, Millis RR, Bulbrook RD, Hayward JL: Family history and bilateral primary breast cancer. Breast Cancer Res Treat 5:201–205, 1985
60. Chaudary MA, Millis RE, Hoskins EOL, et al: Bilateral primary breast cancer: A prospective study of disease incidence. Br J Surg 71:711–714, 1984
61. Cheatle GL, Cutler M: Paget's disease of the nipple. Arch Pathol 12:435–466, 1931
62. Chen, KTK, Kirkegaard, DD, Bocian JJ: Angiosarcoma of the breast. Cancer 46:368–371, 1980
63. Chin LM, Cheng SW, Siddon RL, et al: Three-dimensional photon dose distributions with and without lung corrections for tangential breast intact treatments. Int J Radiat Oncol Biol Phys 17:1327–1335, 1989
64. Chu AM, Cope O, Russo R, et al: Treatment of early stage breast cancer by limited surgery and radical irradiation. Int J Radiat Oncol Biol Phys 6:25–30, 1980
65. Chu FC, Lin FJ, Kim JH, et al: Locally recurrent carcinoma of the breast. Cancer 37:2677–2681, 1986
66. Citrin DL, Tormey Dc, Carbone PP: Implications of the ^{99m}Tc diphosphonate bone scan on treatment of primary breast cancer. Cancer Treat Rep 61:1249–1252, 1977
67. Clark GM, Dressler LG, Owens MA: Prediction of relapse or survival in patients with node-negative breast cancer by DNA flow cytometry. N Engl J Med 320:627–633, 1989
68. Clark RM: Alternatives to mastectomy: The Princess Margaret Hospital experience. In Harris JR, Hellman S, Silen W (eds): Conservative Management of Breast Cancer, pp 35–46. New York, JB Lippincott, 1983
69. Clark RM, Wilkinson RH, Mahoney LJ, et al: Breast cancer: A 21 year experience with conservative surgery and radiation. Int J Radiat Oncol Biol Phys 8:967–975, 1982
70. Clark RM, Wilkinson RH, Miceli PN, et al: Breast cancer: Experience with conservation therapy. Am J Clin Oncol (CCT) 10(6):461–468, 1987
71. Clarke DR: Breast edema following staging axillary node dissection in patients with breast carcinoma treated by radical radiotherapy. Cancer 49:2295, 1982
72. Clarke DR, Le MG, Sarrazin D, et al: Analysis of local-regional relapses in patients with early breast cancers treated by excision and radiotherapy: Experience of the Institut Gustave-Roussy. Int J Radiat Oncol Biol Phys 11:137–145, 1985
73. Clarke D, Martinez A, Cox RS: Analysis of cosmetic results and complications in patients with stage I and II breast cancer treated by biopsy and irradiation. Int J Radiat Oncol Biol Phys 9:1807–1813, 1983
74. Cohn I, Slack NYH, Fisher B: Complications and toxic manifestations of surgical adjuvant chemotherapy for breast cancer. Surg Gynecol Obstet 127:1201–1209, 1968
75. Costanza MC, Foster RSP: Relationship between breast self-examination and death from breast cancer by age groups. Cancer Detect Prev 7:103–108, 1984
76. Courdi A, Hery M, Dahan E, et al: Factors affecting relapse in

node-negative breast cancer: A multivariate analysis including the labeling index. Eur J Cancer Clin Oncol 25(2):351–356, 1989

77. Crile G Jr: Study of metastasis from involved lymph nodes after removal of primary tumors with special reference to cancers of breast. Trans South Surg Assoc 76:131, 1965
78. Crile G Jr: The relationship of surgeons and pathologists. Am J Clin Pathol 75:457–459, 1981
79. Crile G Jr, Cooperman A, Esselstyn CB: Results of partial mastectomy in 173 patients followed for from 5 to 10 years. Surg Gynecol Obstet 150:563–566, 1980
80. Cross MA, Elson HR, Aron BS: Breast conservation radiation therapy technique for women with large breasts. Int J Radiat Oncol Biol Phys 17:199–203, 1989
81. Curtis RE, Hankey BF, Myers MH, Young JL Jr: Risk of leukemia associated with the first course of cancer treatment: An analysis of the Surveillance, Epidemiology and End Results section. J Natl Cancer Inst 72:531–544, 1984
82. Danforth DN, Findlay PA, McDonald HD, et al: Complete axillary lymph node dissection for stage I–II carcinoma of the breast. J Clin Oncol 4(5):655–662, 1986
83. Danoff B, Goodman RL: Identification of subset of patients with early breast cancer in whom conservative surgery and radiation is contraindicated. Int J Radiat Oncol Biol Phys 11:104, 1985
84. Danoff BF, Goodman RL, Glick JH, et al: The effects of adjuvant chemotherapy on cosmesis and complications in patients with breast cancer treated by definitive irradiation. Int J Radiat Oncol Biol Phys 9:1625–1630, 1983
85. Danoff BF, Pajak TF, Solin LJ, et al: Excisional biopsy, axillary node dissection and definitive radiotherapy for stages I and II breast cancer. Int J Radiat Oncol Biol Phys 11:479–483, 1985
86. Dash N, Lupetin AR, Daffner RH, et al: Magnetic resonance imaging in the diagnosis of breast disease. AJR 146:119–125, 1986
87. David FC: Lactation following primary radiation therapy for carcinoma of the breast. Int J Radiat Oncol Biol Phys 11:1425, 1985
88. Degani H, Harowtiz A, Itzchak Y: Breast tumours: Evaluation with P31 MR spectroscopy. Radiology 161:53–55, 1986
89. del Regato JA, Spjut HJ, Harlan J, Cox JD (eds): Ackerman and del Regato's Cancer: Diagnosis, Treatment, and Prognosis, 6th ed. St. Louis, CV Mosby, 1985
90. Delouche G, Bachelot F, Premont M, et al: Conservation treatment of early breast cancer: Long term results and complications. Int J Radiat Oncol Biol Phys 13:29–34, 1987
91. dePietro S, Bertario L, Cantu G, et al: An analysis of 800 breast cancer patients relapsed after radical mastectomy. Tumori 62:99–112, 1976
92. DeVita VT: Breast cancer therapy: Exercising all our options. N Engl J Med 320(8):527–529, 1989
93. Dewar JA, Sarrazin D, Benhamou E, et al: Management of the axilla in conservatively treated breast cancer: 592 patients treated at Institut Gustave-Roussy. Int J Radiat Oncol Biol Phys 13:475–481, 1987
94. Dodd GD: Radiation detection and diagnosis of breast cancer. Cancer 47:1766–1769, 1981
95. Dombernowsky P, Brincker H, Hansen M, et al: Adjuvant therapy of premenopausal and menopausal high-risk breast cancer patients. Acta Oncol 27(6a):691–697, 1988,
96. Donegan W, Spratt JS Jr: Cancer of the Breast. Philadelphia, WB Saunders, 1967
97. Donegan WL, Perez-Mesa CM, Watson FR: A biostatistical study of locally recurrent breast carcinoma. Surg Gynecol Obstet 122:529–540, 1966
98. Donnell RM, Rosen PP, Lieberman PH.: Angiosarcoma and other vascular tumors of the breast: Pathologic analysis as a guide to prognosis. Am J Surg Pathol 5:629–642, 1981
99. Dowle CS, Caseldine J, Tew J, et al: An evaluation of transmission spectroscopy (light scanning) in the diagnosis of symptomatic breast lesions. Clin Radiol 38:375–377, 1987
100. du Toit RS, Locker AP, Ellis IO, et al: Invasive lobular carcinomas of the breast: The prognosis of histopathological subtypes. Br J Cancer 60:605–609, 1989
101. Dubois JB, Gary-Bobo J, Pourquier H, et al: Tumorectomy and radiotherapy in early breast cancer: A report on 392 patients. Int J Radiat Oncol Biol Phys 15:1275–1282, 1988
102. Durand JC, Poljicak M, Lefranc JP, et al: Wide excision of the tumor, axillary dissection, and postoperative radiotherapy as treatment of small breast cancers. Cancer 53:2439–2443, 1984
103. Early Breast Cancer Trialists' Collaborative Group: Effects of adjuvant tamoxifen and of cytotoxic therapy on mortality in early breast cancer. N Engl J Med 319(26):1681–1692, 1988
104. Eberlein TJ, Connolly JL, Schnitt SJ, et al: Predictors of local recurrence following conservative breast surgery and radiation therapy. Arch Surg 125:771–777, 1990
105. Eby C, Brennen M, Fine G: Lymphangiosarcoma: A lethal complication of chronic lymphedema. Arch Surg 94:223–230, 1977
106. Eddy DM, Hasselblad V, McGivney W, et al: The value of mammography screening in women under age 50 years. JAMA 259:1512–1519, 1988
107. Ege GN: Internal mammary lymphoscintigraphy—the rationale, technique, interpretation and clinical application: A review based on 848 cases. Radiology 118:101–107, 1976
108. Ege GN, Clark RM: Internal mammary lymphoscintigraphy in the conservative management of breast carcinoma: An update and recommendations for a new TNM staging. Clin Radiol 36:469–472, 1985
109. El-Naggar AK, Ro JY, McLemore D, et al: DNA content and proliferative activity of cystosarcoma phyllodes of the breast. Am J Clin Pathol 93:480–485, 1990
110. Ellis CN, Frey ES, Burnette JJ, et al: The content of tumor DNA as an indicator of prognosis in patients with T1N0M0 and T2N0M0 carcinoma of the breast. Surgery 106:133–138, 1989
111. Epstein AH, Connolly JL, Gelman R, et al: The predictors of distant relapse following conservative surgery and radiotherapy for early breast cancer are similar to those following mastectomy. Int J Radiat Oncol Biol Phys 17:755–760, 1989
112. Ewers SB, Langstrom E, Baldetrop B, et al: Flow-cytometric DNA analysis in primary breast carcinomas and clinicopathological correlations. Cytometry 5:408, 1984
113. Fallenius AG, Franzen SA, Auer GU: Predictive value of nuclear DNA content in breast cancer in relation to clinical and morphological factors. Cancer 62:521, 1988
114. Farrow JH: The James Ewing Lecture: Current concepts in the detection and treatment of the earliest of the early breast cancers. Cancer 25:468–477, 1970
115. Feig S: Radiation risk from mammography: Is it clinically significant? AJR 143:469–475, 1984
116. Fentiman JS, Fagg M, Millis RR, et al: *In situ* ductal carcinoma of the breast: Implications of disease pattern and treatment. Eur J Surg Oncol 12:261–266, 1986
117. Feuerman L, Attie JN, Rosenberg B: Carcinoma in axillary lymph nodes as an indicator of breast cancer. Surg Gynecol Obstet 114:5–8, 1962
118. Findlay P, Goodman R: Radiation therapy for treatment of intraductal carcinoma of the breast. Am J Clin Oncol (CCT) 6:281–285, 1983
119. Fisher B: Some thoughts concerning the primary therapy of breast cancer. In St. Arneautl G, Band P, Israel L (eds): Recent Results in Cancer Research. Breast Cancer: A Multidisciplinary Approach, pp 150–163. Berlin, Springer-Verlag, 1976
120. Fisher B, Bauer M, Margolese R, et al: Five year results of a randomized clinical trial comparing total mastectomy and segmental mastectomy with or without radiation in the treatment of breast cancer. N Engl J Med 312:665–673, 1985
121. Fisher B, Bauer M, Wickerham L, et al: Relation of number of positive axillary nodes to the prognosis of patients with primary breast cancer: An NSABP update. Cancer 52:1551, 1983
122. Fisher B, Constantino J, Redmond C, et al: A randomized clinical trial evaluating tamoxifen in the treatment of patients with node-negative breast cancer who have estrogen-receptor-positive tumors. N Engl J Med 320(8):479–484, 1989
123. Fisher B, Redmond C, Dimitrov NV, et al: A randomized

clinical trial evaluating sequential methotrexate and fluorouracil in the treatment of patients with node-negative breast cancer who have estrogen-receptor-negative tumors. N Engl J Med 320:473–478, 1989

124. Fisher B, Redmond C, Fisher E, et al: The contribution of recent NSABP clinical trials of primary breast cancer therapy to an understanding of tumor biology: An overview of findings. Cancer 46:1009–1025, 1980
125. Fisher B, Redmond C, Fisher E, et al: Ten-year results of a randomized clinical trial comparing radical mastectomy and total mastectomy with or without radiation. N Engl J Med 312:674–681, 1985
126. Fisher B, Redmond C, Poisson R, et al: Eight-year results of a randomized clinical trial comparing total mastectomy and lumpectomy with or without irradiation in the treatment of breast cancer. N Engl J Med 320(13):822–828, 1989
127. Fisher B, Wolmark N, Bauer M, et al: The accuracy of clinical nodal staging and of limited axillary dissection as a determinant of histological nodal status in carcinoma of the breast. Surg Gynecol Obstet 152:765–772, 1981
128. Fisher ER: Pathology of breast cancer. In McGuire WL (ed): Breast Cancer: Advances in Research and Treatment, vol 1, Current Approaches to Therapy, pp 43–123. New York, Plenum Press, 1977
129. Fisher ER, Gregorio FM, Fisher G, et al: The pathology of invasive breast cancer: A syllabus derived from findings of the National Surgical Adjuvant Breast Project (Protocol No. 4). Cancer 6:1–85, 1975
130. Fisher ER, Gregorio R, Redmond C, et al: Pathologic findings from the National Surgical Adjuvant Breast Project (Protocol 4). I. Observations concerning the multicentricity of mammary cancer. Cancer 35:247–254, 1975
131. Fisher ER, Sass R, Fisher B, et al: Pathologic findings from the National Surgical Adjuvant Breast Project (Protocol 6). I. Intraductal carcinoma (DCIS). Cancer 57:197–208, 1986
132. Fisher ER, Sass R, Fisher B, et al: Pathologic findings from the National Surgical Adjuvant Breast Project (Protocol 6). II. Relation of local breast recurrence to multicentricity. Cancer 57:1717–1724, 1986
133. Fleck R, McNeese MD, Ellerbroek NA, et al: Consequences of breast irradiation in patients with preexisting collagen vascular diseases. Int J Radiat Oncol Biol Phys 17:829–833, 1989
134. Fletcher GH: Clinical dose-and-response curves of human malignant epithelial tumors. Br J Radiol 46:1–12, 1973
135. Fletcher GH, McNeese MD, Osward MJ: Long-range results for breast cancer patients treated by radical mastectomy and postoperative radiation without adjuvant chemotherapy: An update. Int J Radiat Oncol Biol Phys 17:11–14, 1989
136. Fletcher GH, Shukovsky LJ: The interplay of radiocurability and tolerance in the irradiation of human cancers. J Radio Electro 56:383–400, 1975
137. Foster RS, Costanza MC: Breast self-examination and breast cancer survival. Cancer 53:999–1005, 1984
138. Fourquet A, Campana F, Vielh P, et al: Paget's disease of the nipple without detectable breast tumor: Conservative management with radiation therapy. Int J Radiat Oncol Biol Phys 13:1463–1465, 1987
139. Fourquet A, Campana F, Zafrani B, et al: Prognostic factors of breast recurrence in the conservative management of early breast cancer: A 25-year follow-up. Int J Radiat Oncol Biol Phys 17:719–725, 1989
140. Fowble B: Conservative surgery and radiation in the treatment of stage I and II breast cancer. Refresher Course No. 207, 31st Annual ASTRO Meeting, San Francisco, October 1–6, 1989
141. Fowble B: Intraductal noninvasive breast cancer: A comparison of three local treatments. Oncology 3:51–58, 1989
142. Fowble B, Gray R, Gilchrist K, et al: Identification of a subgroup of patients with breast cancer and histologically positive axillary nodes receiving adjuvant chemotherapy who may benefit from postoperative radiotherapy. J Clin Oncol 6(7):1107–1117, 1988
143. Fowble BL, Solin SJ, Goodman RL: Results of conservative surgery and radiation for intraductal noninvasive breast cancer (Abstract). Am J Clin Oncol (CCT) 10:110–111, 1987
144. Fowble B, Solin LJ, Schultz DJ, et al: Frequency, sites of relapse, and outcome of regional node failures following conservative surgery and radiation for early breast cancer. Int J Radiat Oncol Biol Phys 17:703–710, 1989
145. Fraass BA, Roberson PL, Lichter AS: Dose to the contralateral breast due to primary breast irradiation. Int J Radiat Oncol Biol Phys 11:485–497, 1985
146. Fraass BA, van de Geijn J: Peripheral dose from megavoltage beams. Med Phys 10:809–818, 1983
147. Frisell J, Eklund G, Hellstrom L, et al: The Stockholm Breast Cancer Screening Trial: Five year results and stage at discovery. Breast Cancer Res Treat 13:79–87, 1989
148. Garcia I, Dietrich P-Y, Aapro M, et al: Genetic alterations of c-myc, c-erb B-2, and c-Ha-ras protooncogenes and clinical associations in human breast carcinomas. Cancer Res 49:6675–6679, 1989
149. Gerard JP, Montbarbon JF, Chassard JL, et al: Conservative treatment of early carcinoma of the breast: Significance of axillary dissection and iridium implant. Radiother Oncol 3:17–22, 1985
150. Ghossein NA, Stacey P, Alpert S, et al: Local control of breast cancer with tumorectomy plus radiotherapy or radiotherapy alone. Radiology 121:455–459, 1976
151. Ghossein NA, Vilcoq J, Stacey P, et al: Is it necessary to irradiate the breast after conservative surgery for local cancer. Arch Surg 122:913–917, 1987
152. Gisuold JJ, Brown LR, Swee RG, et al: Comparison of mammography and transillumination light scanning in the detection of breast lesions. AJR 147:191–194, 1986
153. Glatstein E, Straus K, Lichter A, et al: Results of the NCI Early Breast Cancer Trial. NIH Consensus Development Conference, pp 32–33. June 18–21, 1990
154. Glick JH: Meeting highlights: Adjuvant therapy for breast cancer. J Natl Cancer Inst 80(7):471–475, 1988
155. Goldhirsch A, et al: Prolonged disease-free survival after one course of perioperative adjuvant chemotherapy for node-negative breast cancer. N Engl J Med 310(8):491–496, 1989
156. Goldie JH: Scientific basis for adjuvant and primary (neoadjuvant) chemotherapy. Semin Oncol 14(1):1–7, 1987
157. Goodnight JE Jr, Quagliana JM, Morton DL: Failure of subcutaneous mastectomy to prevent the development of breast cancer. J Surg Oncol 26:198–201, 1984
158. Gore SM, Come SE, Griem K, et al: Influence of the sequencing of chemotherapy and radiation therapy in node-negative breast cancer patients treated by conservative surgery and radiation therapy. In Salmon SE (ed): Adjuvant Therapy of Cancer. V. Orlando, FL, Grune & Stratton, 1987
159. Greening WP, Montgomery ACU, Gowing NFC: Report of pilot study on treatment of breast cancer by quadrantic excision with axillary dissection and no other therapy. J R Soc Med 71:261–264, 1978
160. Griem KL, Henderson IC, Gelman R, et al: Post-operative radiotherapy after adjuvant chemotherapy in breast cancer patients: Results of a randomized trial. J Clin Oncol 5:1546–1555, 1987
161. Gump FE, Shikora S, Habif DV, et al: The extent and distribution of cancer in breasts with palpable primary tumors. Ann Surg 204(4):385–390, 1986
162. Gutman, H, Kersz T, Barzilai T, et al: Achievements of physical therapy in patients after modified radical mastectomy compared with quadrantectomy, axillary dissection, and radiation for carcinoma of the breast. Arch Surg 125:389–391, 1990
163. Haagensen CD: Diseases of the Breast, 2nd ed. Philadelphia, WB Saunders, 1971
164. Haagensen CD: The choice of treatment of operable carcinoma of the breast. Surgery 76:685–714, 1974
165. Haagensen CD: Treatment of curable carcinoma of the breast. Int J Radiat Oncol Biol Phys 2:975–980, 1977
166. Haagensen CD, Lane N, Lattes R, et al: Lobular neoplasia (so-called lobular carcinoma *in situ*) of the breast. Cancer 42:737–769, 1978
167. Haagensen CD, Stout AP: Carcinoma of the breast. I. Results of treatment. Ann Surg 116:801, 1942
168. Haffty BG, Fischer DB, Fischer JJ: Regional nodal irradiation

in the conservative treatment of breast cancer (Abstract). Int J Radiat Oncol Biol Phys 17(Suppl 1):178, 1989
169. Haffty BG, Goldberg NB, Fischer D, et al: Conservative surgery and radiation therapy in breast carcinoma: Local recurrence and prognostic implications. Int J Radiat Oncol Biol Phys 17:727–732, 1989
170. Haffty BG, Goldberg NB, Rose M, et al: Conservative surgery with radiation therapy in clinical stage I and II breast cancer: Results of a 20-year experience. Arch Surg 124:1266–1270, 1989
171. Hagemeister FB, Buzdar AU, Luna MA, et al: Causes of death in breast cancer: Clinicopathologic study. Cancer 46:161–167, 1980
172. Hallahan DE, Michel AG, Halpern HJ, et al: Breast conserving surgery and definitive irradiation for early stage breast cancer. Int J Radiat Oncol Biol Phys 17:1211–1216, 1989
173. Halsted WS: The results of operations for the cure of cancer of the breast performed at the Johns Hopkins Hospital from June, 1889 to January, 1894. Johns Hopkins Hosp Bull 4:297, 1894–1895
174. Handley RS: Carcinoma of the breast. Ann R Coll Surg 57:59–66, 1975
175. Hankey BF, Curtis RE, Naughton MD, et al: A retrospective cohort analysis of second breast cancer risk for primary breast cancer patients with an assessment of the effect of radiation therapy. J Natl Cancer Inst 70:797–804, 1983
176. Harris JR, Botnick L, Bloomer WD, et al: Primary radiation therapy for early breast cancer: The experience at the Joint Center for Radiation Therapy. Int J Radiat Oncol Biol Phys 7:1549–1552, 1981
177. Harris JR, Connolly JL, Schnitt SJ, et al: Clinical-pathologic study of early breast cancer treated by primary radiation therapy. J Clin Oncol 1:184–189, 1983
178. Harris JR, Connolly JL, Schnitt SJ, et al: The use of pathologic features in selecting the extent of surgical resection necessary for breast cancer patients treated by primary radiation therapy. Ann Surg 201:164–169, 1985
179. Harris JR, Hellman S: Primary radiation for early breast cancer. Cancer 51(Suppl 12):2547–2552, 1983
180. Harris JR, Hellman S: The treatment philosophy, technique and results of primary radiation for early breast cancer at the Joint Center for Radiation Therapy. In Ames FR, Blumenschein GR, Montague ED (eds): Current Controversies in Breast Cancer. Austin, University of Texas Press, 1983
181. Harris JR, Hellman S: Conservative surgery and radiotherapy. In Harris JR, Hellman S, Henderson IC, Kinne DW (eds): Breast Diseases, pp 299–323. Philadelphia, JB Lippincott, 1987
182. Harris JR, Recht A, Amalric R, et al: Time course and prognosis of local recurrence following primary radiation therapy for early breast cancer. J Clin Oncol 2:37–41, 1984
183. Hatschek T, Fagerberg G, Stal O, et al: Cytometric characterization and clinical course of breast cancer diagnosed in a population-based screening program. Cancer 64:1074–1081, 1989
184. Hayward J: The surgeon's role in primary breast cancer. Breast Cancer Res Treat 1:27–32, 1981
185. Hayward JL: The Guy's Hospital trials on breast conservation. In Harris JR, Hellman, Silen W (eds): Conservative Management of Breast Cancer, pp 78–90. Philadelphia, JB Lippincott, 1983
186. Hedley DW, Friedlander ML, Taylor IW, et al: Method for analysis of cellular DNA content of paraffin-embedded pathological material using flow cytometry. J Histochem Cytochem 31:1333, 1983
187. Heintz NH, Leslie KO, Rogers LA, et al: Amplification of the c-erb B-2 oncogene and prognosis of breast adenocarcinoma. Arch Pathol Lab Med 114:160–163, 1990
188. Hellman S, Harris JR, Levene MB: Radiation therapy of early carcinoma of the breast without mastectomy. Cancer 46:988–994, 1980
189. Hendee WR, Kellie SR: Mammographic screening in women 40–49 years old. AJR 141:683–684, 1988
190. Henry JA, McCarthy AL, Angus B, et al: Prognostic significance of the estrogen-regulated protein, cathepsin D, in breast cancer: An immunohistochemical study. Cancer 65:265–271, 1990
191. Hery M, Namer M, Verschoore J, et al: Conservative treatment of breast cancer: A report of 108 patients. Int J Radiat Oncol Biol Phys 10:2185–2190, 1984
192. Heywang SH, Fenzl G, Hahn D, et al: MR imaging of the breast comparison with mammography and ultrasound. J Comput Assist Tomogr 10:615–620, 1986
193. Heywang SH, Hahn D, Schmidt H, et al: MR imaging of the breast using gadolinium DTPA. J Comput Assist Tomogr 10:199–204, 1986
194. Hildreth NG, Shore RE, Dvoretsky PM: The risk of breast cancer after irradiation of the thymus in infancy. N Engl J Med 321:1281–1284, 1989
195. Hislop TG, Elwood JM, Coldman AJ, et al: Second primary cancers of the breast: Incidence and risk factors. Br J Cancer 49:79–85, 1984
196. Hoffman DA, Lonstein JE, Morin MM, et al: Breast cancer in women with scoliosis exposed to multiple diagnostic x-rays. J Natl Cancer Inst 81:1307–1312, 1989
197. Holland JF: Major advance in breast cancer therapy (Editorial). N Engl J Med 294:440–441, 1976
198. Holland R, Connolly JL, Gelman R, et al: The presence of an extensive intraductal component following a limited excision correlates with prominent residual disease in the remainder of the breast. J Clin Oncol 8:113–118, 1990
199. Holland R, Hendriks J, Verbeek A, et al: Extent, distribution, and mammographic/histological correlations of breast ductal carcinoma *in situ*. Lancet 335:519–522, 1990
200. Holland R, Veling SHJ, Matrunac M, et al: Histologic multifocality of Tis, T1–2 breast carcinomas: Implications for clinical trials on breast conserving therapy. Cancer 56:979–991, 1985
201. Horn PL, Thompson WD: Risk of contralateral breast cancer: Associations with histologic, clinical, and therapeutic factors. Cancer 62:412–424, 1988
202. Hornstein E, Skornick Y, Rozin R: The management of breast carcinoma in pregnancy and lactation. J Surg Oncol 21:179–182, 1982
203. Hunig R, Walther E, Harder F, et al: The Basel lumpectomy protocol: 5 year experience with a prospective study for conservative treatment of breast cancer. In Harris JR, Hellman S, Silen W (eds): Conservative Management of Breast Cancer, pp 23–35. Philadelphia, JB Lippincott, 1983
204. Inglis K: Paget's disease of the nipple with special reference to the changes in ducts. Am J Pathol 22:1–33, 1946
205. Jacquillat C, Weil M, Baillet F, et al: Results of neoadjuvant chemotherapy and radiation therapy in the breast-conserving treatment of 250 patients with all stages of infiltrative breast cancer. Cancer 66:119–129, 1990
206. Jick H, Walker AM, Watkins RN: Oral contraceptives and breast cancer. Am J Epidemiol 112:577–585, 1980
207. Kaae S, Johansen H: Does simple mastectomy followed by irradiation offer survival comparable to radical procedures? Int J Radiat Oncol Biol Phys 2:1163–1166, 1977
208. Kallioniemi OP, Blanco G, Alavaikko M, et al: Tumour DNA ploidy as an independent prognostic factor in breast cancer. Br J Cancer 56:637, 1987
209. Kantorowitz DA, Poulter CA, Rubin P, et al: Treatment of breast cancer with segmental mastectomy alone or segmental mastectomy plus radiation. Radiother Oncol 15:141–150, 1989
210. Kelsey JL: A review of the epidemiology of human breast cancer. Epidemiol Rev 1:74–109, 1979
211. Kennedy BJ: New role of endocrine therapy in breast cancer. Int J Radiat Oncol Biol Phys 4:469–472, 1978
212. Keyhani-Rofagha S, O'Toole RV, Farrar WB, et al: Is DNA ploidy an independent prognostic indicator in infiltrative node-negative breast adenocarcinoma? Cancer 65:1577–1582, 1990
213. Keynes G: Conservative treatment of cancer of the breast. Br Med J 2:643–649, 1937
214. Kiang DT, Frenning DH, Goldman AI, et al: Estrogen receptors and responses to chemotherapy and hormonal therapy in advanced breast cancer. N Engl J Med 299:1330–1334, 1978

215. Kinne DW, Kopans DB: Physical examination and mammography in the diagnosis of breast disease. In Harris JR, Hellman S, Henderson IC, Kinne DW (eds): Breast Diseases, pp 55–86. Philadelphia, JB Lippincott, 1987
216. Kinne DW, Petrek JA, Osborne MP, et al: Breast carcinoma *in situ.* Arch Surg 124:33–35, 1989
217. Klopp CT: Metastatic cancer of axillary lymph node without a demonstrable primary lesion. Ann Surg 131:437–439, 1950
218. Kopans DB: Breast Imaging. Philadelphia, JB Lippincott, 1989
219. Kopans DB, Meyer JE, Sadowsky N: Breast imaging. N Engl J Med 310:960–967, 1984
220. Koper PCM, van Putten WLJ, Wÿnmaalen AJ, et al: Breast conserving surgery and radiotherapy in early stage breast cancer. Int J Radiat Oncol Biol Phys (in press)
221. Kraus FT, Neubecker RD: The differential diagnosis of papillary tumors of the breast. Cancer 15:444–455, 1962
222. Kurtz JM, Amalric R, Brandone H, et al: Results of salvage surgery for mammary recurrence following breast-conserving therapy. Ann Surg 207:347–351, 1988
223. Kurtz JM, Amalric R, Brandone H, et al: Local recurrence after breast-conserving surgery and radiotherapy: Frequency, time course, and prognosis. Cancer 63:1912–1917, 1989
224. Kurtz JM, Amalric R, Delouche G, et al: The second ten years: Long-term risks of breast conservation in early breast cancer. Int J Radiat Oncol Biol Phys 13:1327–1332, 1987
225. Kurtz JM, Jacquemier J, Amalric, et al: Risk factors for breast recurrence in premenopausal and postmenopausal patients with ductal cancers treated by conservation therapy. Cancer 65:1867–1878, 1990
226. Kurtz JM, Spitalier JM, Amalric R: Late breast recurrence after lumpectomy and irradiation. Int J Radiat Oncol Biol Phys 9:1191–1194, 1983
227. Kurtz JM, Spitalier JM, Amalric R, et al: Mammary recurrences in women younger than forty. Int J Radiat Oncol Biol Phys 15:271–276, 1988
228. Kurtz JM, Spitalier JM, Amalric R, et al: The prognostic significance of late local recurrences after breast conserving therapy. Int J Radiat Oncol 18:87–93, 1990
229. Kuske RR, Compaan PJ, Aron BS: Breast conservation therapy for breast cancer: A report on 215 patients. Int J Radiat Oncol Biol Phys 11(S1):184, 1985
230. Kuske RR, Bean JM, Garcia D, et al: Breast conservation therapy for ductal carcinoma *in situ.* (unpublished data)
231. Kuske R, Compaan P, Cross M, et al: Breast conservation therapy: 417 breast cancers with a minimum follow-up period of five years. Int J Radiat Oncol Biol Phys 17(1):235–236, 1989
232. Kuske RR, Garcia DM, Perez CA, et al: Cosmesis after breast conservation therapy. Int J Radiat Oncol Biol Phys 15(Suppl 1):239, 1988
233. Lagios MD, Margolin FR, Westdahl PR, et al: Mammographically detected duct carcinoma *in situ.* Frequency of local recurrence following tylectomy and prognostic effect of nuclear grade on local recurrence. Cancer 63:618–624, 1989
234. Lagios MD, Richards VE, Rose MR: Segmental mastectomy without radiotherapy: Short-term follow-up. Cancer 52:2173–2179, 1983
235. Lagios MD, Westdahl PR, Margolin FR, et al: Duct carcinoma *in situ*: Relationship of extent of noninvasive disease to frequency of occult invasion, multicentricity, lymph node metastases and short term treatment failures. Cancer 50:1309–1314, 1982
236. Lagios MD, Westdahl PR, Rose MR, et al: Paget's disease of the nipple: Alternative management in cases without or with minimal extent of underlying breast carcinoma. Cancer 54:545–551, 1984
237. Land CE, Boice JD Jr, Shore RE, et al: Breast cancer risk from low-dose exposure to ionizing radiation. J Natl Cancer Inst 65:353–376, 1980
238. Lash RH, Bauer TW, Medendorp SV: Prognostic significance of the proportion of intraductal and infiltrating ductal carcinoma in women treated by partial mastectomy. Surg Pathol 3:47–57, 1990
239. Leopold KA, Recht A, Schnitt S, et al: Results of conservative surgery and radiation therapy for multiple synchronous cancers of the breast. Int J Radiat Oncol Biol Phys 16:11–16, 1989
240. Leung S, Otmezguine Y, Calitchi E, et al: Local regional recurrences following radical external beam irradiation and interstitial implantation for operable breast cancer: A 23 year experience. Radiother Oncol 5:1–10, 1986
241. Levene MB: Interstitial therapy of breast cancer. Int J Radiat Oncol Biol Phys 2:1157–1161, 1977
242. Levine MN, Guyatt GH, Gent M, et al: Quality of life in stage II breast cancer: An instrument for clinical trials. J Clin Oncol 6(12):1798–1810, 1988
243. Levitt SH: Patterns of failure in breast cancer. Cancer Treat Symp 2:123–129, 1983
244. Levitt SH: The role of adjuvant CMF chemotherapy in breast cancer: What is it? Proceedings of the 1983 R.A.T.I.0.3 International Workshop on Radiodiagnostic and Integrated Oncotherapy, Rome, Italy, 1983
245. Levitt SH: Controversies in the treatment of breast cancer: A need for return to the three Rs in clinical research. Am J Clin Oncol 7:583–591, 1984
246. Levitt SH, Khan FM, Boen JR, et al: Multimodal therapy in the treatment of breast cancer. Am J Clin Oncol (CCT) 6:387–391, 1983
247. Levitt SH, Mandell J: Benefits versus risks in conservation surgery with irradiation for breast cancer. Am J Med 77:93–100, 1984
248. Levitt SH, McHugh RB: Radiotherapy in the postoperative treatment of operable cancer of the breast. I. Critique of the clinical and biometric aspects of the trials. Cancer 39:924–932, 1977
249. Levitt SH, McHugh RB, Song CW: Radiotherapy in the postoperative treatment of operable cancer of the breast. Cancer 39:933–940, 1977
250. Levitt SH, Potish RA: The role of radiation therapy in the treatment of breast cancer: The use and abuse of clinical trials, statistics and unproven hypotheses. Int J Radiat Oncol Biol Phys 6:791–798, 1980
251. Levitt SH, Potish RA: The case for adjuvant CMF chemotherapy in breast cancer: Has it been made? Cancer Clin Trials 4:363–369, 1981
252. Levitt SH, Potish RA, Aeppli D, Lindgren B: The consensus statement on adjuvant chemotherapy in breast cancer. Am J Clin Oncol 11(1):73–76, 1988
253. Lewis D, Geshickter CF: Comedo carcinoma of the breast. Arch Surg 36:225–234, 1938
254. Lewis TR, Casey J, Buerk CA, et al: Incidence of lobular carcinoma in bilateral breast cancer. Am J Surg 144:635–638, 1982
255. Lichter AS: Is radiation therapy in conjunction with mastectomy indicated for the treatment of operable breast cancer? Cancer Invest 5(3):243–261, 1987
256. Linsk JA, Franzen S: Clinical Aspiration Cytology, pp 105–137. London, JB Lippincott, 1983
257. Lipnick RJ, Buring JE, Hennekens CH, et al: Oral contraceptives and breast cancer: A prospective cohort study. JAMA 255:58–61, 1986
258. Lippman ME, Allegra JC: Receptors in breast cancer. N Engl J Med 299:930–933, 1978
259. Lippman ME, Allegra JC, Thompson EB, et al: The relation between estrogen receptors and response rate to cytotoxic chemotherapy in metastatic breast cancer. N Engl J Med 298:1223–1228, 1978
260. Lippman ME, Edwards BK, Findlay P, et al: Influence of definitive radiation therapy for primary breast cancer on ability to deliver adjuvant chemotherapy. NCI Monogr 1:99–104, 1986
261. Locker AP, Ellis IO, Morgan DAL, et al: Factors influencing local recurrence after excision and radiotherapy for primary breast cancer. Br J Surg 76:890–894, 1989
262. London SJ, Colditz GA, Stampfer MJ, et al: Prospective study of smoking and the risk of breast cancer. J Natl Cancer Inst 81:1625-1631, 1989
263. Ludwig Breast Cancer Study Group: Prolonged disease-free

survival after one course of perioperative adjuvant chemotherapy for node-negative breast cancer. N Engl J Med 320:491–496, 1989

264. Maier WP, Rosemond GP, Harasym Jr EL, et al: Paget's disease in the female breast. Surg Gynecol Obstet 128:1253–1263, 1969

265. Maisey MN: Imaging techniques in breast cancer. What is new? What is useful? A review. Eur J Cancer Clin Oncol 24(1):61–68, 1988

266. Mansfield CM: Intraoperative Ir-192 implantation for early breast cancer. Cancer 66:1–5, 1990

267. Mansour EG, Gray R, Shatila AH, et al: Efficacy of adjuvant chemotherapy in high-risk node-negative breast cancer. N Engl J Med 320:485–490, 1989

268. Marcial VA, Velez-Garcia E, Bartolucci A, et al: Comparison of adjuvant chemotherapy versus loco-regional radiotherapy followed by adjuvant chemotherapy in breast cancer patients with 4 or more positive axillary nodes: A Southeastern Cancer Study Group Study (Abstract). Int J Radiat Oncol Biol Phys 17(S1):180, 1989

269. Margolis GJ, Goodman RL: Psychological factors in women choosing radiation therapy for breast cancer. Psychosomatics 25:464–469, 1984

270. Martin MB, Kon ND, Kawamoto EH, et al: Postmastectomy angiosarcoma. Am Surg 50:541–545, 1984

271. Mate TP, Carter D, Fischer DB, et al: A clinical and histopathologic analysis of the results of conservation surgery and radiation therapy in stage I and II breast carcinoma. Cancer 58:1995–2002, 1986

272. Maunsell E, Brisson J, Deschenes L: Psychological distress after initial treatment for breast cancer: A comparison of partial and total mastectomy. J Clin Epidemiol 42(8):765–771, 1989

273. McCormick B, Yahalom J, Cox L, et al: The patient's perception of her breast following radiation and limited surgery. Int J Radiat Oncol Biol Phys 17:1299–1302, 1989

274. McCredie JA, Inch WR: Prophylactic postoperative radiotherapy and consecutive primary cancers. Arch Surg 105: 297–301, 1972

275. McCredie JA, Inch WR, Alderson M: Consecutive primary carcinomas of the breast. Cancer 35:1472–1477, 1975

276. McDivitt RW, Stone KR, Craig B, et al.: A proposed classification of breast cancer based on kinetic information derived from a comparison of risk factors in 168 primary operable breast cancers. Cancer 57:269–276, 1986

277. McGuire WL: Physiological principles underlying endocrine therapy of breast cancer. In McGuire WL (ed): Breast Cancer: Advances in Research and Treatment, vol 1, Current Approaches to Therapy, pp 217–262. New York, Plenum Press, 1977

278. McGuire WL: Adjuvant therapy of node-negative breast cancer. N Engl J Med 320(8):525–527, 1989

279. McGuire WL, Abeloff MD, Fisher B, et al: Adjuvant therapy in node-negative breast cancer. Breast Cancer Res Treat 13:97–115, 1989

280. McGuire WL, Tandom AK, Allred GC, et al: How to use prognostic factors in axillary node-negative breast cancer patients. J Natl Cancer Inst 82(12):1006–1015, 1990

281. McLean RC, Ege GN: Prognostic value of axillary lymphoscintigraphy in breast carcinoma patients. J Nucl Med 27:1116–1124, 1986

282. McWhirter R: The value of simple mastectomy and radiotherapy in the treatment of cancer of the breast. Br J Radiol 21:599–610, 1948

283. McWhirter R: Simple mastectomy and radiotherapy in treatment of breast cancer. Br J Radiol 28:128–139, 1955

284. Meyer JS, Friedman MS, McCrate MM, et al: Prediction of early course of breast carcinoma by thymidine labeling. Cancer 51:1819–1886, 1983

285. Michowitz M, Noy S, Lazebnik N, et al: Bilateral breast cancer. J Surg Oncol 30:109–112, 1985

286. Miller AB, Howe GR, Sherman GJ, et al: Mortality from breast cancer after irradiation during fluoroscopic examinations in patients being treated for tuberculosis. N Engl J Med 321:1285–1289, 1989

287. Millis RR, Thynne GSJ: *In-situ* intraduct carcinoma of the breast: A long term follow-up study. Br J Surg 62:957–962, 1975

288. Monsees B, Destouet JM, Gersell D: Light scan evaluation of non palpable breast lesions. Radiology 163:467–470, 1987

289. Monsees B, Destouet JM, Totty WG: Light scanning versus mammography in breast cancer detection. Radiology 163:463–465, 1987

290. Montague ED: Radiation management of advanced breast cancer. Int J Radiat Oncol Biol Phys 4:305–307, 1978

291. Montague ED: Conservation surgery and radiation therapy in the treatment of operable breast cancer. Cancer 53:700–704, 1984

292. Montague ED, Gutierrez AE, Barke JL, et al: Conservation surgery and irradiation for the treatment of favorable breast cancer. Cancer 43:1058–1061, 1979

293. Montague ED, Pauleis DD, Schell SR, et al: Selection and followup of patients for conservation surgery and irradiation. Front Radiat Ther Oncol 17:124–130, 1983

294. Monyak D, Levitt S: The changing role of radiation therapy in the treatment of primary breast cancer. Invest Radiol 24(6):483–494, 1989

295. Morris T: Psychological adjustment to mastectomy. Cancer Treat Rev 6:41–61, 1979

296. Moskowitz M: Cost of screening for breast cancer. Radiol Clin North Am 25(5):1031–1037, 1987

297. Muir R: Further observations on Paget's disease of the nipple. J Pathol Bacteriol 49:299–312, 1939

298. Muss HB, Kute TE, Case LD, et al: The relation of flow cytometry to clinical and biologic characteristics in women with node negative primary breast cancer. Cancer 64:1894–1900, 1989

299. Mustakallio S: Uber die Moglichkeiten der Rontgentherapie bei der Behandlung des Bruskrebses. Acta Radiol 26:503–511, 1945

300. Mustakallio S: Treatment of breast cancer by tumor extirpation and roentgen therapy instead of radical operation. J Faculty Radiol 6:23–26, 1954

301. Mustakallio S: Conservative treatment of breast carcinoma: Review of 25 years follow up. Clin Radiol 23:110–116, 1972

302. Müller A, von Fournier D, Kaufmann M, et al: Whole breast irradiation and boost irradiation in breast-conserving therapy based on morphologic findings. Breast Dis 2:121–130, 1989

303. Nance FC, DeLoach DH, Welsh RA, et al: Paget's disease of the breast. Ann Surg 171:864–872, 1970

304. Nielsen M, Christensen L, Andersen J: Contralateral cancerous breast lesions in women with clinical invasive breast cancer. Cancer 57:897–903, 1986

305. Nobler MP, Venet L: Twelve years experience with irradiation as the primary treatment for breast cancer. Int J Radiat Oncol Biol Phys 7:33–42, 1981

306. Norris HJ, Taylor HB: Prognosis of mucinous (gelatinous) carcinoma of the breast. Cancer 18:879–885, 1965

307. O'Malley MS, Fletcher SW: Screening for breast cancer with breast self-examination. JAMA 257(16):2197–2203, 1987

308. Olivotto IA, Rose MA, Osteen RT, et al: Late cosmetic outcome after conservative surgery and radiotherapy: Analysis of causes of cosmetic failure. Int J Radiat Oncol Biol Phys 17:747–753, 1989

309. Osborne CK: Prognostic factors in breast cancer. PPO Updates 4(3):1, 1990

310. Osborne MP, Ormiston N, Harmer CL, et al: Breast conservation in the treatment of early breast cancer: A 20-year followup. Cancer 53:349–355, 1984

311. Osteen RT, Connolly JL, Recht A, et al: Identification of patients at high risk for local recurrence after conservative surgery and radiation therapy for stage I or II breast cancer. Arch Surg 122:1248–1252, 1987

312. Owen HW, Dockerty MB, Gray HK: Occult carcinoma of breast. Surg Gynecol Obstet 98:302–309, 1954

313. Ozzello L: Intraepithelial carcinomas of the breast. In Hollman KH, Verley JM (eds): New Frontiers in Mammary Pathology, vol 2, pp 147–164. New York, Plenum Press, 1983

314. Page DI, DuPont WD, Rogers LW, et al: Intraductal car-

cinoma of the breast: Followup after biopsy only. Cancer 49:751–758, 1982
315. Paone JF, Baker R: Pathogenesis and treatment of Paget's disease of the breast. Cancer 48:825–829, 1981
316. Patchefsky AS, Schwartz GF, Finkelstein SD, et al: Heterogeneity of intraductal carcinoma of the breast. Cancer 63:731–741, 1989
317. Patek E, Johannisson E, Krauer F, et al.: Microfluorometric grading of mammary tumors. Anal Quant Cytol 2:264, 1980
318. Paterson R: Treatment of Malignant Disease by Radium and X-rays, p 309. London, Edward Arnold & Co, 1948
319. Peeters PHM, Verbeek ALM, Hendricks JHCL, et al: Screening for breast cancer in Nijmegen: Report of six screening rounds, 1975–1986. Int J Cancer 43:226–230, 1989
320. Perez R, Pascual M, Macias A, et al: Epidermal growth factor receptors in human breast cancer. Breast Cancer Res Treat 4:189, 1984
321. Peters MV: Wedge resection with or without radiation in early breast cancer. Int J Radiat Oncol Biol Phys 2:1151–1156, 1977
322. Pezner RD, Lipsett JA, Desai K, et al: To boost or not to boost: Decreasing radiation therapy in conservative breast treatment when "inked" tumor resection margins are pathologically free of cancer. Int J Radiat Oncol Biol Phys 14:873–877, 1988
323. Pezner RD, Lipsett JA, Vora NL, et al: Limited usefulness of observer-based cosmesis scales employed to evaluate patients treated conservatively for breast cancer. Int J Radiat Oncol Biol Phys 11:1117–1119, 1985
324. Pezner RO, Patterson MP, Hill LR, et al: Breast edema in patients treated conservatively for stage I and II breast cancer. Int J Radiat Oncol Biol Phys 11:1765–1768, 1985
325. Pierquin B, Marin L: The past and future of conservative treatment of breast cancer. Am J Clin Oncol 9:476–480, 1986
326. Pierquin B, Owen R, Maylin C, et al: Radical radiation therapy of breast cancer. Int J Radiat Oncol Biol Phys 6:17–24, 1980
327. Pigott J, Nichols R, Maddox WA, et al: Metastases to the upper levels of the axillary nodes in carcinoma of the breast and its implications for nodal sampling procedures. Surg Gynecol Obstet 158:255–259, 1984
328. Pike MC, Henderson BE, Casagrande JT, et al: Oral contraceptive use and early abortion as risk factors for breast cancer in young women. Br J Cancer 43:72–76, 1981
329. Primary Therapy of Breast Cancer Study Group: Identification of breast cancer patients with high risk of early recurrence after radical mastectomy. II. Clinical and pathological correlations. Cancer 42:2809–2826, 1978
330. Pritchard KI: Current status of adjuvant endocrine therapy for resectable breast cancer. Semin Oncol 14(1):23–33, 1987
331. Prosnitz LR, Goldenberg IS, Harris JR, et al: Radiotherapy for carcinoma of the breast instead of mastectomy: An update. Front Radiat Ther Oncol 17:69–75, 1983
332. Ray GR, Fish VJ: Biopsy and definitive radiation therapy in stage I and II adenocarcinoma of the female breast: Analysis of cosmesis and the role of electron beam supplementation. Int J Radiat Oncol Biol Phys 9:813–818, 1983
333. Ray GR, Fish VJ, Marmor JB, et al: Impact of adjuvant chemotherapy on cosmesis and complications in stages I and II carcinoma of the breast treated by biopsy and radiation therapy. Int J Radiat Oncol Biol Phys 10:837–841, 1984
334. Rebner M, Pennes DR, Adler DD, et al: Breast microcalcifications after lumpectomy and radiation therapy. Radiology 170:691–693, 1989
335. Recht A, Connolly J, Schnitt S, et al: Conservative surgery and radiotherapy for early breast cancer: The effect of age on breast recurrence (Abstract). Int J Radiat Oncol Biol Phys 12(Suppl):93, 1986
336. Recht A, Connolly JL, Schnitt SJ, et al: The effect of young age on tumor recurrence in the treated breast after conservative surgery and radiotherapy. Int J Radiat Oncol Biol Phys 14:3–10, 1988
337. Recht A, Danoff B, Solin LJ, et al: Intraductal carcinoma of the breast: Results of treatment with excisional biopsy and irradiation. J Clin Oncol 3:1339–1343, 1985
338. Recht A, Harris JR: Negative breast biopsies after primary radiation therapy: Safety and accuracy (Abstract). Int J Radiat Oncol Biol Phys 11(1):131, 1985
339. Recht A, Silen W, Schnitt SJ, et al: Time-course of local recurrence following conservative surgery and radiotherapy for early stage breast cancer. Int J Radiat Oncol Biol Phys 15:255–261, 1988
340. Recht A, Silver B, Schnitt S, et al: Breast relapse following primary radiation therapy for early breast cancer. I. Classification, frequency and salvage. Int J Radiat Oncol Biol Phys 11:1271–1276, 1985
341. Ringberg A, Palmer B, Linell F: The contralateral breast at reconstructive surgery after breast cancer operation: A histopathological study. Breast Cancer Res Treat 2:151–161, 1982
342. Rissanen PM: A comparison of conservative and radical surgery combined with radiotherapy in the treatment of stage I carcinoma of the breast. Br J Radiol 42:423–426, 1969
343. Rissanen PM, Holsti P: Paget's disease of the breast. Oncology 23:209–216, 1969
344. Robbins GF, Berg JW: Bilateral primary breast cancers: A prospective clinicopathological study. Cancer 17:1501–1527, 1964
345. Roberson PL, Lichter AS, Bodner A, et al: Dose to lung in primary breast irradiation. Int J Radiat Oncol Biol Phys 9:97–102, 1982
346. Rodger A, Corbett PJ, Chetty U: Lactation after conserving therapy, including radiation therapy, for early breast cancer. Radiother Oncol 15:243–244, 1989
347. Rose CM, Botnick LE, Weinstein M, et al: Axillary sampling in the definitive treatment of breast cancer by radiation therapy and lumpectomy. Int J Radiat Oncol Biol Phys 9:339–344, 1983
348. Rose MA, Henderson C, Gelman R, et al: Premenopausal breast cancer patients treated with conservative surgery, radiotherapy and adjuvant chemotherapy have a low risk of local failure. Int J Radiat Oncol Biol Phys 17:711–717, 1989
349. Rose MA, Olivotto I, Cady B, et al: Conservative surgery and radiation therapy for early breast cancer: Long-term cosmetic results. Arch Surg 124:153–157, 1989
350. Rosen PP: The pathology of breast carcinoma. In Harris JR, Hellman S, Henderson IC, Kinne DW (eds): Breast Diseases, pp 147–209. Philadelphia, JB Lippincott, 1987
351. Rosen PP, Braun DW, Kinne DW: The clinical significance of pre-invasive breast carcinoma. Cancer 46:919–925, 1980
352. Rosen PP, Braun DW, Lyngholm B, et al: Lobular carcinoma *in situ* of the breast: Preliminary results of treatment by ipsilateral mastectomy and contralateral breast biopsy. Cancer 47:813–819, 1981
353. Rosen PP, Groshen S, Kinne DW, et al: Contralateral breast carcinoma: An assessment of risk and prognosis in stage I (T1NOMO) and stage II (T1N1MO) patients with 20-year follow-up. Surgery 106:904–910, 1989
354. Rosen PP, Lesser ML, Kinne DW, et al: Discontinuous or "skip" metastases in breast carcinoma. Ann Surg 197:276–283, 1983
355. Rosen PP, Lieberman PH, Braun DW, et al: Lobular carcinoma *in situ* of the breast: Detailed analysis of 99 patients with average follow-up of 24 years. Am J Surg Pathol 2:225–251, 1978
356. Rosen PP, Saigo PE, Braun SE, et al: Predictors of recurrence in stage I (T1NOMO) breast carcinoma. Ann Surg 193:15–25, 1981
357. Rosen PP, Senie R, Schottenfeld D, et al: Noninvasive breast carcinoma: Frequency of unsuspected invasion and implications for treatment. Ann Surg 189:377–382, 1979
358. Rosner D: Angiosarcoma of the breast: Long-term survival following adjuvant chemotherapy. J Surg Oncol 39:90–95, 1988
359. Rosner D, Bedwani RN, Vana J, et al: Noninvasive breast carcinoma: Results of a national survey of the American College of Surgeons. Ann Surg 192:139–147, 1980
360. Rosner D, Lane WW: Oral contraceptive use has no adverse effect on prognosis of breast cancer. Cancer 57:591–596, 1986
361. Rossing N, Munck O, Nielsen SP, et al: What do early bone

scans tell about breast cancer patients? Eur J Cancer Clin Oncol 18:629–636, 1982

362. Rostom AY, O'Cathail S: Failure of lactation following radiotherapy for breast cancer. Lancet 18:163, 1986
363. Rothwell RI, Kelly SA, Joslin CAF: Radiation pneumonitis in patients treated for breast cancer. Radiother Oncol 4:9–14, 1985
364. Rotstein S, Lax I, Svane G: Influence of radiation therapy on the lung-tissue in breast cancer patients: CT-assessed density changes and associated symptoms. Int J Radiat Oncol Biol Phys 18:173–180, 1990
365. Rubin P (ed): Clinical Oncology: A Multidisciplinary Approach. Atlanta, American Cancer Society, 1983
366. Rutqvist LE, Cedermark B, Glas U, et al: Radiotherapy, chemotherapy, and tamoxifen as adjuncts to surgery in early breast cancer: A summary of three randomized trials. Int J Radiat Oncol Biol Phys 16:629–639, 1989
367. Sainsbury JRC, Nicholson S, Angus B, et al: Epidermal growth factor receptor status of histological sub-types of breast cancer. Br J Cancer 58:458, 1988
368. Salner A, Botwick L, Herzog A, et al: Reversible brachial plexopathy following primary radiation therapy for breast cancer. Cancer Treat Rep 65:797–802, 1981
369. Sanger C, Rasnikoff M: A comparison of the psychological effects of breast-saving procedures with the modified radical mastectomy. Cancer 48:2341–2346, 1981
370. Sarrazin D, Dewar JA, Arriagada R, et al: Conservative management of breast cancer. Br J Surg 73:604–606, 1986
371. Sarrazin D, Le MG, Arriagada R, et al: Ten-year results of a randomized trial comparing a conservative treatment to mastectomy in early breast cancer. Radiother Oncol 14:177–184, 1989
372. Sarrazin D, Le M, Fontaine F, Arriagada R: Conservative treatment versus mastectomy in T1 or small T2 breast cancer: A randomized clinical trial. In Harris JR, Hellman S, Silen W (eds): Conservative Management of Breast Cancer, pp 101–111. Philadelphia, JB Lippincott, 1983
373. Sarrazin D, Le M, Rouesse J, et al: Conservative treatment versus mastectomy in breast cancer tumors with macroscopic diameter of 20 millimeters or less: The experience of the Institut Gustave-Roussy. Cancer 53:1209–1213, 1984
374. Say C, Donegan W: A biostatistical evaluation of complications from mastectomy. Surg Gynecol Obstet 138:370–376, 1974
375. Scarff RW, Torloni H, et al: Histological Typing of Breast Tumors. Geneva, World Health Organization, 1968
376. Schain WS: Psychosocial factors affecting treatment recommendations for primary breast cancer. NIH Consensus Development Conference, pp 38–39. June 18–21, 1990
377. Schain E, Edwards BK, Gorrell CR, et al: Psychosocial and physical outcomes of stage I primary breast cancer therapy: Mastectomy vs excisional biopsy and irradiation. Breast Cancer Res Treat 3:377–382, 1983
378. Schell SR, Montague ED, Spanos WJ, et al: Bilateral breast cancer in patients with initial stage I and II disease. Cancer 50:1191–1194, 1982
379. Schipper H, Levitt M: Measuring quality of life: Risks and benefits. Cancer Treat Rep 69:1115–1123, 1985
380. Schmidt-Ullrich R, Wazer DE, Tercilla O, et al: Tumor margin assessment as a guide to optimal conservation surgery and irradiation in early stage breast carcinoma. Int J Radiat Oncol Biol Phys 17:733–738, 1989
381. Schnitt SJ, Connolly JL, Harris JR, et al: Pathologic predictors of early local recurrence in stage I and II breast cancer treated by primary radiation therapy. Cancer 53:1049–1057, 1984
382. Schnitt SJ, Connolly JL, Khetty U, et al: Pathologic findings on reexcision of the primary site in breast cancer patients considered for treatment by primary radiation therapy. Cancer 59:675–681, 1987
383. Schnitt SJ, Connolly JL, Recht A, et al: Influence of infiltrating lobular histology on local tumor control in breast cancer patients treated with conservative surgery and radiotherapy. Cancer 64:448–454, 1989
384. Schnitt SJ, Connolly JL, Recht A, et al: Breast relapse following primary radiation therapy for early breast cancer. II. Detection of pathologic features and prognostic significance. Int J Radiat Oncol Biol Phys 11:1277–1284, 1985
385. Schottenfield D, Nasly A, Robbins G, et al: Ten year results of the treatment of primary operable breast cancer. Cancer 38:1001–1007, 1976
386. Schuh ME, Nemoto T, Penetrante RB, et al: Intraductal carcinoma: Analysis of presentation, pathologic findings and outcome of disease. Arch Surg 121:1303–1307, 1986
387. Schwartz GF: Clinically occult breast cancer: Multicentricity and implication for treatment. Ann Surg 191:8–12, 1980
388. Schwartz GF, Feig SA, Patchefsky AS: Significance and staging of nonpalpable carcinomas of the breast. Surg Gynecol Obstet 166:6–10, 1988
389. Schwartz GF, Patchefsky AS, Finkelstein SD, et al: Non-palpable *in situ* ductal carcinoma of the breast. Arch Surg 124:29–32, 1989
390. Sears HF, Janus C, McDermott A, et al: Bilateral breast carcinoma: Prospective evaluation of factors assisting diagnosis. J Surg Oncol 32:203–207, 1986
391. Seidman H, Gelb SK, Silverberg E, et al: Survival experience in the breast cancer detection demonstration project. CA 37:258–290, 1987
392. Selby P, Buick RN, Tannock I: A critical appraisal of "human tumor stem-cell assay." N Engl J Med 308:129–134, 1983
393. Sellke FW, Loughry CW, Kashkari S: Angiosarcoma of the breast: Report of two long-term survivals. Int Surg 73:193–195, 1988
394. Shapiro S, Venet W, Strax P, et al: Ten to 14 year effect of screening on breast cancer mortality. J Natl Cancer Inst 69(2):345–355, 1982
395. Shapiro S, Venet W, Strax P, et al: Selection, follow-up, and analysis in the Health Insurance Plan (HIP) Study. In Selection, Follow-up and Analysis in Prospective Studies: A Workshop, Monograph 67, pp 65–74. Bethesda, MD, National Cancer Institute, 1985
396. Shore RE, Hempelmann LH, Kowaluk E, et al: Breast neoplasms in women treated with x-rays for acute postpartum mastitis. J Natl Cancer Inst 59:813–822, 1977
397. Sigurdsson H, Baldeterp B, Borg A, et al: Indicators of prognosis in node-negative breast cancer. N Engl J Med 322:1045–1053, 1990
398. Silverberg SG, Kay S, Chitale AR, et al: Colloid carcinoma of the breast. Am J Clin Pathol 55:355–363, 1971
399. Silverstein MJ, Rosser RJ, Gierson ED, et al: Axillary lymph node dissection for intraductal breast carcinoma: Is it indicated? Cancer 59:1819–1824, 1987
400. Silverstein MJ, Waisman JR, Gamagami P, et al: Intraductal carcinoma of the breast (208 cases): Clinical factors influencing treatment choice. Cancer 66:102–108, 1990
401. Simard C: La maladie de Paget du mamelon: Cancer epidermotrope. Bull Cancer (Paris) 19:50–81, 1930
402. Skrabanek P: Screen for disease: False premises and false promises of breast cancer screening. Lancet 316–319, 1985
403. Slamon DJ, Clark GM, Wong SG, et al: Human breast cancer: Correlation of relapse and survival with amplification of the HER-2/neu oncogene. Science 235:177, 1987
404. Smallwood J, Guyer P, Dewbury K, et al: The accuracy of ultrasound in the diagnosis of breast disease. Ann R Coll Surg Engl 68:19–22, 1986
405. Smith JA, Gamez-Araujo JJ, Gallagher HS, et al: Carcinoma of the breast: Analysis of total lymph node involvement versus level of metastasis. Cancer 39:527–532, 1977
406. Solin LJ, Danoff BF, Martz, R, et al: Results of re-excisional biopsy of the primary tumor in preparation for definitive irradiation of patients with early stage breast cancer. Int J Radiat Oncol Biol Phys 12:721–725, 1986
407. Solin LJ, Danoff BF, Schwartz GF: A practical technique for the localization of the tumor volume in definitive irradiation of the breast. Int J Radiat Oncol Biol Phys 11:1215–1220, 1985
408. Solin LJ, Fowble BL, Delray J, et al: The impact of mammography on the patterns of patients referred for definitive breast irradiation. Cancer 65:1085–1089, 1990
409. Solin LJ, Fowble B, Martz KL, Goodman RL: Definitive irra-

diation for early stage breast cancer: The University of Pennsylvania experience. Int J Radiat Oncol Biol Phys 14:235–242, 1988

410. Solin LJ, Fowble BL, Schultz DJ, et al: Bilateral breast carcinoma treated with definitive irradiation. Int J Radiat Oncol Biol Phys 17:263–271, 1989
411. Solin LJ, Fowble B, Schultz DJ, et al: Age as a prognostic factor for patients treated with definitive irradiation for early stage breast cancer. Int J Radiat Oncol Biol Phys 16:373–381, 1989
412. Souba WW, McKenna RJ, Meis J, et al: Radiation induced sarcomas of the chest wall. Cancer 57:610–615, 1986
413. Spitalier JM, Amalric R: Treatment of operable mammary carcinoma with conservation of the breast at the Cancer Institute of Marseille. In Marchant DJ, Myirjesy I (eds): Breast Disease, pp 222–251. New York, Grune & Stratton, 1979
414. Spitalier JM, Brandone H, Ayme Y, et al: Cesium therapy of breast cancer: A five-year report on 400 consecutive patients. Int J Radiat Oncol Biol Phys 2:231–235, 1977
415. Spitalier JM, Gambarelli J, Brandone H, et al: Breast conserving surgery with radiation therapy for operable mammary carcinoma: A 25 year experience. World J Surg 10:1014–1020, 1986
416. Spyratos F, Brouillet J, Defrenne A, et al: Cathepsin D: An independent prognostic factor for metastasis of breast cancer. Lancet 2:1115–1118, November 11, 1989
417. Steeves RA, Phromratanapongse P, Wolberg WH, et al: Cosmesis and local control after irradiation in women treated conservatively for breast cancer. Arch Surg 149:1369–1373, 1989
418. Stjernsward J: Decreased survival related to irradiation postoperatively in early operable breast cancer. Lancet 2:1285–1286, 1974
419. Stomper PC, Recht A, Berenberg AL, et al: Mammographic detection of recurrent cancer in the irradiated breast. AJR 148:39–43, 1987
420. Stotter AT, McNeese MD, Ames FC, et al: Predicting the rate and extent of locoregional failure after breast conservation therapy for early breast cancer. Cancer 64:2217–2225, 1989
421. Stotter AT, McNeese M, Oswald MJ, et al: The role of limited surgery with irradiation in primary treatment of ductal *in situ* breast cancer. Int J Radiat Oncol Biol Phys 18:283–287, 1990
422. Strender L-E, Wallgren A, Arndt J, et al: Adjuvant radiotherapy in operable breast cancer: Correlation between dose in internal mammary nodes and prognosis. Int J Radiat Oncol Biol Phys 7:1319–1325, 1981
423. Sunshine JA, Moseley HS, Fletcher WS, et al: Breast carcinoma *in situ*: A retrospective review of 112 cases with a minimum of 10-years' follow-up. Am J Surg 150:44–51, 1985
424. Svensson GK, Chin LM, Siddon RL, et al: Breast treatment techniques at the Joint Center for Radiation Therapy. In Harris JR, Hellman S, Silen W (eds): Conservative Management of Breast Cancer: New Surgical and Radiotherapeutic Techniques, pp 239–255. Philadelphia, JB Lippincott, 1983
425. Swain M: Lobular carcinoma *in situ*: Incidence, presentation, guidelines to treatment. Oncology 3:35–40, 1989
426. Swain SM, Lippman ME: Intraepithelial carcinoma of the breast: Molecular carcinoma *in situ* and ductal carcinoma *in situ*. In Lippman ME, Lichter AS, Danforth DN (eds): The Diagnosis and Management of Breast Cancer, pp 296–325. Philadelphia, WB Saunders, 1988
427. Tabar L, Dean PB: Screen/film mammography: Quality control. In Feig SA, McLelland R (eds): Breast Carcinoma: Current Diagnosis and Treatment, pp 161–168. New York, Masson, 1983
428. Tabar L, Dean PB: The control of breast cancer through mammography screening. What is the evidence? Radiol Clin North Am 25:993–1005, 1987
429. Tabar L, Fagerberg CJG, Day NE: The results of periodic one-view mammographic screening in a randomized controlled trial in Sweden. II. Evaluation of the results. Manuscript presented at the UICC Workshop on Screening for Breast Cancer, Helsinki, Finland, 1986
430. Tagart REB: Partial mastectomy for breast cancer. Br Med J 2:178:1978
431. Tandon AK, Clark GM, Chamness GC, et al: Cathepsin D and prognosis in breast cancer. N Engl J Med 322(5):297–302, 1990
432. Tannock IF: Use of a physician-directed questionnaire to define a consensus about management of breast cancer: Implications for assessing the costs and benefits of treatment. NIH Consensus Development Conference, pp 74–77. June 18–21, 1990
433. Taylor IW, MuSgrove EA, Friedlander ML, et al: The influence of age on the DNA ploidy levels of breast tumors. Eur J Cancer 19:623, 1983
434. Temple WJ, Jenkins M, Alexander F, et al: *In situ* breast cancer in Alberta 1951–1984 (Abstract). Am J Clin Oncol 9:109–110, 1986
435. Temple WJ, Jenkins M, Alexander F, et al: Natural history of *in situ* breast cancer in a defined population. Ann Surg 210(5):653–657, 1989
436. Tercilla O, Krasin F, Lawn-Tsao L: Comparison of contralateral breast doses from 1/2 beam block and isocentric treatment techniques for patients treated with primary breast irradiation with ^{60}Co. Int J Radiat Oncol Biol Phys 17:205–210, 1989
437. Thomsen HS, Lund JO, Munck O, et al: The value of prescheduled bone scintigraphies in breast cancer. Acta Oncol 27:617–619, 1988
438. Thomsen HS, Lund JO, Munck O, et al: Experience with 7,604 bone scintigraphies at time of operation for breast cancer 1977–1987. Dan Med Bull 36:481–483, 1989
439. Thor AD, Schwartz LH, Koerner FC, et al: Analysis of c-erB-2 expression in breast carcinomas with clinical follow-up. Cancer Res 49:7147–7152, 1989
440. Thorpe SM, Rochefort H, Garcia M, et al: Association between high concentrations of M_r 52,000 cathepsin D and poor prognosis in primary human breast cancer. Cancer Res 49: 6008–6014, 1989
441. Tinnemans JGM, Wobbes T, van der Sluis RF, et al: Multicentricity in nonpalpable breast carcinoma and its implications for treatment. Am J Surg 151:334–338, 1986
442. Toikkanen S, Joensuu H, Klemi P: The prognostic significance of nuclear DNA content in invasive breast cancer: A study with long-term follow-up. Br J Cancer 60:693–700, 1989
443. Tokunaga M, Norman JE Jr, Asano M, et al: Malignant breast tumors among atomic bomb survivors, Hiroshima and Nagasaki, 1950–1974. J Natl Cancer Inst 62:1347–1359, 1979
444. Tough ICK: The significance of recurrence in breast cancer. Br J Surg 53:897–900, 1966
445. Trapido EJ: A prospective cohort study of oral contraceptives and breast cancer. J Natl Cancer Inst 67:1011–1015, 1981
446. Treves N, Sunderland DA: Cystosarcoma phyllodes of the breast: A malignant and benign tumor. Cancer 4:1286–1332, 1951
447. Triedman S, Boyages J, Silver B, et al: A comparison of local control and cosmetic outcome in patients boosted with electrons or implant in the conservative management of early breast cancer (Abstract), p 48. Proceedings 17th International Congress of Radiation Oncology. Paris, July 1989
448. Tubiana M, Pejovic MH, Koscielny S, et al: Growth rate, kinetics of tumor cell proliferation and long-term outcome in human breast cancer. Int J Cancer 44:17–22, 1989
449. Tubiana M, Pejovic MF, Renaud A, et al: Kinetic parameters and the course of the disease in breast cancer. Cancer 47:937–943, 1981
450. Union Internationale Contre le Cancer: TNM-Atlas: Illustrated Guide to the Classification of Malignant Tumours. Berlin, Springer-Verlag, 1982
451. United Kingdom Trial of Early Detection of Breast Cancer Group: First results on mortality reduction in the UK trial of early detection of breast cancer. Lancet 2:411–416, 1988
452. Uppsala-Orebro Breast Cancer Study Group: Sector resection with or without postoperative radiotherapy for stage I breast cancer: A randomized trial. J Natl Cancer Inst 82:277–282, 1990
453. Urban JA: Is there a rationale for an extended radical procedure? Int J Radiat Oncol Biol Phys 2:985–988, 1977

454. Urban JA: Management of operable breast cancer: The surgeon's view. Cancer 42:2066–2077, 1978
455. Valagussa P, Bonadonna G, Veronesi U: Patterns of relapse and survival following radical mastectomy: Analysis of 716 consecutive patients. Cancer 41:1170–1178, 1978
456. Valeriote FA, Edelstein MB: The role of cell kinetics in cancer chemotherapy. Semin Oncol 4:217–226, 1977
457. Van Dam FASM, Linssen CA, Couzijn AL: Evaluating quality of life in cancer clinical trials. In Buyse ME, Staquet MJ, Sylvester RJ (eds): Cancer Clinical Trials: Methods and Practice, pp 26–43. Oxford, Oxford University Press, 1984
458. van de Vijver M, Peterse JL, Mooi WJ, et al: Neu-protein overexpression in breast cancer. N Engl J Med 319:1239, 1988
459. van Dongen JA: Randomized clinical trial to assess the value of breast conserving therapy in stage I and stage II breast cancer: EORTC Trial 10801. NIH Consensus Development Conference, pp 25–27. June 18–21, 1990
460. van Limbergen E, van den Bogaert W, van der Schueren E, et al: Tumor excision and radiotherapy as primary treatment of breast cancer: Analysis of patient and treatment parameters and local control. Radiother Oncol 8:1–9, 1987
461. Verbeek ALM, Holland R, Sturmans F, et al: Reduction of breast cancer mortality through mass screening with modern mammography: First results of the Nijmegen project, 1975–1981. Lancet 1:1222–1224, 1984
462. Veronesi U: Conservative treatment in breast cancer of limited size. In Feig SF (ed): Breast Carcinoma: Current Diagnosis and Treatment, pp 433–438. New York, Masson, 1983
463. Veronesi U, Banfi A, DelVecchio M, et al: Comparison of Halsted mastectomy with quandrantectomy, axillary dissection and radiotherapy in early breast cancer: Long-term results. Eur J Cancer Clin Oncol 22:1085–1089, 1986
464. Veronesi U, Saccozzi R, DelVecchio M, et al: Comparing radical mastectomy with quadrantectomy, axillary dissection, and radiotherapy in patients with small cancers of the breast. N Engl J Med 305:6–11, 1981
465. Veronesi U, Zucali R, DelVecchio M: Conservative treatment of breast cancer with the QUART technique. World J Surg 9:676–681, 1985
466. Veronesi U, Zucali R, Luini A: Local control and survival in early breast cancer: The Milan trial. Int J Radiat Oncol Biol Phys 12:717–720, 1986
467. Vessey M, Baron J, Doll R, et al: Oral contraceptives and breast cancer: Final report of an epidemiologic study. Br J Cancer 47:455–462, 1983
468. Vessey MP, McPherson K, Yeates D, et al: Oral contraceptive use and abortion before first term pregnancy in relation to breast cancer risk. Br J Cancer 45:327–331, 1982
469. Vilcoq JR, Calle R, Fem F, et al: Conservative treatment of axillary adenopathy due to probable subclinical breast cancer. Arch Surg 117:1136–1138, 1982
470. Vilcoq JR, Calle R, Schlienger P: Irradiation techniques for conservative treatment of localized breast cancer. In Harris JR, Hellman S, Silen W (eds): Conservative Management of Breast Cancer, pp 213–224. Philadelphia, JB Lippincott, 1983
471. Vilcoq JR, Calle R, Stacey P, et al: The outcome of treatment by tumorectomy and radiotherapy of patients with operable breast cancer. Int J Radiat Oncol Biol Phys 8:1327–1332, 1981
472. Von Hoff DD: "Send this patient's tumor for culture and sensitivity." N Engl J Med 308:154–155, 1983
473. von Rueden DG, Wilson RE: Intraductal carcinoma of the breast. Surg Gynecol Obstet 158:105–111, 1984
474. Vorherr H, Vorherr UF, Kutvirt DM, et al: Cystosarcoma phyllodes: Epidemiology, pathohistology, pathobiology, diagnosis, therapy, and survival. Arch Gynecol 236:173–181, 1985
475. Wallberg H, Alveryd A, Sundelin P, et al: The value of diaphonography as an adjunct to tomography in breast diagnostics. Acta Chir Scand 530 (Suppl):83–87, 1986
476. Wanebo HJ, Feldman PS, Wilhelm MC, et al: Fine needle aspiration cytology in lieu of open biopsy in management of primary breast cancer. Ann Surg 199:569–579, 1984
477. Wanebo HJ, Huvos AG, Urban JA: Treatment of minimal breast cancer. Cancer 33:349–357, 1974
478. Wargotz ES, Norris JH: Metaplastic carcinomas of the breast. III. Carcinoma. Cancer 64:1490–1499, 1989
479. Webber BL, Heise H, Neifeld JP, et al: Risk of subsequent contralateral breast carcinoma in a population of patients with *in situ* breast carcinoma. Cancer 47:2928, 1981
480. Weiss RB, Valagussa P, Moliterni A, et al: Adjuvant chemotherapy after conservative surgery plus irradiation versus modified radical mastectomy. Am J Med 83:455–463, 1987
481. Westbrook KC, Gallager HS: Breast carcinoma presenting as an axillary mass. Am J Surg 122:607–611, 1971
482. Westbrook KC, Gallagher HS: Intraductal carcinoma of the breast. Am J Surg 130:667–670, 1975
483. Wheeler JE, Enterline HT, Roseman JM, et al: Lobular carcinoma *in situ* of the breast: Long-term follow-up. Cancer 34:554–563, 1974
484. Willet WC, Stampfer MJ, Calditz GA, et al: Moderate alcohol consumption and risk of breast cancer. N Engl J Med 315:1174–1180, 1987
485. Williams KL, Phillips BH, Jones PA, et al: Thermography in screening for breast cancer. J Epidemiol Commun Health 44:112–113, 1990
486. Williams PL, Warwick R, Depon M, Bannister LW (eds): Gray's Anatomy, 37th ed. New York, C. Livingston, 1989
487. Winchester DP, Bernstein JR, Paige ML, et al: The Early Detection and Diagnosis of Breast Cancer, pp 1–20. Atlanta, American Cancer Society, 1988
488. Wise L, Mason AY, Ackerman LV: Local excision and irradiation: An alternative method for the treatment of early mammary cancer. Ann Surg 174:392, 1971
489. Witliff J: Steroid-hormone receptors in breast cancer. Cancer 53(Suppl):630–643, 1984
490. Wolmark N: 1989: The year of adjuvant therapy in node-negative breast cancer. PPO Updates 3(12):1–10, 1989
491. Woudstra E, van der Werf H: Obliquely incident electron beams for irradiation of the internal mammary lymph nodes. Radiother Oncol 10:209–215, 1987
492. Yarnold JR: Selective avoidance of lymphatic irradiation in the conservative management of breast cancer. Radiother Oncol 2:79–92, 1984
493. Zafrani B, Fourquet A, Vilcoq JR, et al: Conservative management of intraductal breast carcinoma with tumorectomy and radiation therapy (Abstract). Int J Radiat Oncol Biol Phys 10(Suppl 2):140, 1984
494. Zafrani B, Fourquet A, Vilcoq JR, et al: Conservative management of intraductal breast carcinoma with tumorectomy and radiation therapy. Cancer 57:1299–1301, 1986
495. Zajdela A, Ghossein NA, Pillerson JP, et al: The value of aspiration cytology in the diagnosis of breast cancer: Experience at the Foundation Curie. Cancer 35:499–506, 1975
496. Zajicek J, Caspersson T, Jakobsson P, et al: Cytologic diagnosis of mammary tumors from aspiration biopsy smears: Comparison of cytologic and histologic findings in 2111 lesions and diagnostic use of cytophotometry. Acta Cytol 14:370–376, 1970

43

Breast: Locally Advanced (T3 and T4) and Recurrent Tumors

David Monyak
Seymour H. Levitt

NATURAL HISTORY

The local spread of advanced breast cancer results in infiltration of the deep lymphatics of the dermis causing edema of the skin. More pronounced edema (*peau d'orange*) usually indicates that the superficial lymphatics as well as the deeper ones are involved. Later in the course of the disease, fixation of the skin over the tumor and localized redness occur, followed by ulceration and infiltration of the overlying skin. Skin retraction may be caused by tumor invasion of Cooper's ligament. Further indications of extensive involvement are the appearance of satellite nodules and carcinoma *en cuirasse,* in which the skin becomes plaque-like and yellowish red-gray.[90]

Lymphatic spread to the axillary, internal mammary, and supraclavicular nodes may occur. The supraclavicular lymph nodes are usually involved after the high axillary or internal mammary lymph nodes are first involved by tumor. However, if the skin of the upper half of the breast is involved, direct spread may progress to the supraclavicular nodes.

The most common initial sites of hematogenous spread are bone, lung, and pleura—in that order.[49] Initial involvement of the liver and brain can occur but is less common.[26,204]

Local recurrence occurs in the breast or the chest wall. The most common manifestation is nodules on the skin flaps on the chest wall after mastectomy, which probably results from implantation of carcinoma cells by instruments or sponges during the operation or may represent unrecognized microscopic foci of carcinoma left on the flaps by the surgeon.

CLINICAL PRESENTATION

Patients with advanced breast cancer may present with pain or a lump in the breast, nipple soreness, bleeding, discharge, or retraction, axillary lump, ulceration or edema of the skin, or enlargement of the breast.

Inflammatory breast cancer is characterized by erythema, warmth, skin induration, and diffuse enlargement of the breast. These inflammatory changes may appear rapidly in a previously normal-appearing breast and can be mistaken for acute mastitis.

DIAGNOSTIC WORKUP

Physical examination must give special attention to documenting the locoregional extent of disease as well as carefully checking potential sites of hematogenous spread. Areas of erythema, edema, subtle subcutaneous infiltration, and small subcutaneous nodules are easily missed and could lead to marginal failures if not taken into account when radiation fields are planned. Fixation to the pectoralis muscle or fascia can be determined by assessing the mobility of the mass with the pectoralis muscle relaxed and contracted.

Laboratory studies should include a complete blood count, liver function studies, and alkaline phosphatase and calcium levels.

Radiographic studies should include chest x-ray, bone scan, and plain radiographs of symptomatic bones or suspicious areas of increased uptake on bone scan. Bone scans should be obtained in patients with Stage III and Stage IV disease even when the alkaline phosphatase level is normal.[71] About 35% of patients with apparent Stage III cancer have an abnormal bone scan.[11,31,42] If the patient has abnormal liver function values, a liver computed tomography (CT) scan should be obtained. CT scan is probably a more sensitive study for detection of liver metastases than radionuclide scan.[25,110] If the patient has any neurologic symptoms suggestive of cerebral metastases, a contrast-enhanced CT scan of the brain should be obtained. CT scans are superior to radionuclide scans for the detection of brain metastases.[29,152]

PROGNOSTIC FACTORS

Prognostic factors can be intrinsic (related to the initial inherent condition of the tumor itself, such as lymph node involvement and histology) or extrinsic (related to type and adequacy of treatment).

Donegan and colleagues[61] noted that the following intrinsic factors were most frequently related to local recurrence:

Involvement of axillary nodes by tumor. Local recurrence developed in 26% of patients with involved axillary nodes compared with 6.5% of patients without nodal involvement; the greater the number of nodes involved, the more likely the local recurrence. Fisher and associates[74] also reported diminishing survival rate with a greater number of metastatic axillary lymph nodes.

Gross characteristics of the primary tumor. Larger tumors, more diffuse tumors, and the presence of edema are associated with increased local recurrence.[61]

Histologic tumor grade. Incidence of local recurrence increased with degree of nondifferentiation of the tumor.

Meyer and co-workers[136] showed a significant correlation of the thymidine labeling index (TLI; an indication of growth fraction) with survival rate. TLIs below the median of 4.55% carried a probability of relapse of 20% at 4 years, in contrast to a 52% probability of failure with TLI above the median.

The presence or absence of estrogen or progesterone hormonal receptors in tumor cells is an important intrinsic prognostic factor for patients with breast cancer. Patients without hormonal receptors have a significantly lower survival rate and are not likely to respond to hormonal therapy.[132,205] Conflicting reports have been published on the correlation between the presence or absence of hormonal receptors and chemotherapy response.[108,122]

Fisher and colleagues[75] found that the most significant pathologic features related to estrogen receptor (ER) and progesterone receptor (PR) positivity and concordance (ER + PR +, ER − PR −) were a well-differentiated nuclear and histologic grade, slight or absent tumor lymphoid infiltration, slight or absent necrosis, and moderate or marked elastica. All these factors were directly or indirectly related to tumor differentiation. Disease-free survival decreased from concordant ER + PR + to discordant ERPR (ER + PR − or ER − PR +) with the worst prognosis in concordant ER − PR −. Chevallier and associates[39] reported that ER and PR have their own prognostic weight and should be considered among other classic prognostic factors.

McGuire and colleagues[43,133] reported on a series of patients on whom ER and PR readings, thymidine labeling index (TLI), and DNA flow cytometry were performed. In Stage II breast cancer, PR seemed to be more reliable than ER in predicting disease-free survival and was as important as ER in predicting overall survival. McGuire noted a strong correlation between tumor receptor content, the percent S phase, and aneuploidy and suggested that these measurements in concert might identify a subset of patients at increased risk for recurrence.

Nuclear DNA distribution pattern was evaluated by von Rosen and co-workers,[200] who found DNA of prognostic value in node-negative patients, but not of prognostic value in node-positive patients. Fallenius and associates[69] also noted that tumors with normal DNA content (diploid or euploid) had a better prognosis. The median S-phase fraction (SPF) is lower in diploid than in euploid tumors. Dressler and colleagues[63] noted that both an aneuploidy and a high SPF were related to absence of steroid receptors.

Epidermoid growth factor receptor (EGFr)-positive patients have a worse prognosis.[166] An excellent overview of growth factors and their mechanism of action has been published recently by McGuire and associates.[134]

Slamon and co-workers[177] reported that the HER-2/neu oncogene amplification was a significant predictor of overall survival and time to relapse. Other intrinsic prognostic factors are the detection of the circulating antigen CA 15.3 by monoclonal antibody techniques.

GENERAL MANAGEMENT AND RESULTS OF TREATMENT

Mastectomy and Adjuvant Irradiation Alone

One of the first adjuvants in the treatment of breast cancer was irradiation. The controversy over the value of adjuvant irradiation has existed since the inception of its use. Analyses of nonrandomized and randomized studies have fueled diverse and contradictory opinions. The problems with many nonrandomized studies are that they were not done in a disciplined manner, the details of radiation therapy vary, and patient follow-up is not adequate.

The most recent analysis of prechemotherapy adjuvant irradiation clinical trials is presented by Cuzick and coworkers.[50,51] They found no advantage to the treatment of patients with adjuvant irradiation. At 10 years they claimed a statistically significant increased incidence in mortality in patients who had received adjuvant radiation therapy.

In reviews and analyses by Levitt and colleagues,[118–120] numerous statistical and irradiation technique flaws were found in a majority of the studies, which led to bias and inevaluability of a number of the trials.

Unfortunately, in all the studies some variation of treatment has occurred. Probably the best two studies are the Oslo II and the Stockholm studies. In the Oslo II study,[100,101] there was an overdosage to the internal mammary node so that an increased cardiac mortality occurred in Stage I patients. All patients were castrated in addition to receiving irradiation; the added effect is not known. Overall no significant improvement in survival was noted in these patients.

In the Stockholm studies[165,184,201,202] before the use of chemotherapy, both a preoperative and a postoperative arm were compared with that of surgery alone. In the most recent analysis of the Stockholm trials,[165] a statistically significant improvement in recurrence-free survival rate has occurred in patients treated with preoperative or postoperative irradiation or both, compared with those treated with modified radical mastectomy alone. In the postoperative group, where axillary nodal status is available, the improvement has been significant for both node-positive and node-negative patients. In the node-positive patients, postoperative irradiation significantly reduced the incidence of both local and distant metastases. No significant difference in overall survival rate was found, but the trend favors the irradiation arm (Table 43-1, Fig. 43-1).

Levitt[118] noted that the Stockholm study and the Oslo trials

TABLE 43–1
Overall and Locoregional Recurrences, Distant Metastases, and Deaths by Nodal Status for Patients in the First Stockholm Trial

	POSTOP. IRRADIATION*		SURGERY ALONE†			
HISTOLOGIC NODE STATUS, TYPE OF EVENT	NO. OF PTS.	NO. OF EVENTS (%)	NO. OF PTS.	NO. OF EVENTS (%)	RATE RATIO‡ (95% CONFIDENCE INTERVAL)	P (LOG RANK)
pN0	203		197			
Treatment failure§		65 (32)		86 (44)	0.67 (0.49–0.92)	0.01
Locoregional recurrence		9 (4)		45 (23)	0.23 (0.14–0.39)	<0.001
Distant metastases		48 (24)		44 (22)	1.06 (0.70–1.59)	0.79
Death		60 (30)		60 (30)	0.97 (0.68–1.39)	0.87
pN+	118		120			
Treatment failure		72 (61)		93 (78)	0.62 (0.45–0.84)	<0.01
Locoregional recurrence		20 (17)		59 (49)	0.31 (0.20–0.48)	<0.001
Distant metastases		57 (48)		82 (68)	0.64 (0.46–0.89)	<0.01
Death		68 (58)		80 (67)	0.81 (0.59–1.12)	0.21

Note: Only patients randomized to postoperative radiation therapy or mastectomy alone are included because preoperative irradiation obscures the node status.
** Two cases excluded because data on node status were unavailable*
† Four cases excluded because data on node status were unavailable
‡ Radiation therapy versus *surgery alone*
§ End point in calculations of recurrence-free survival
(Rutqvist LE, Cedemark B, Glaz U, et al: Int J Radiat Oncol Biol Phys 16:629–639, 1989)

did not contain a sufficient number of patients to prove a statistically significant improvement in survival rate for adjuvant irradiation, even if the difference observed was clinically significant. Each trial suggested improved survival rate for the radiation therapy arm, but the number of patients required to provide a reasonable chance of proving statistical significance for these differences was greater than the actual number entered.

In one particular subset of patients—those with medial lesions—several studies have shown a consistent long-term benefit in survival from internal mammary nodal treatment.[8, 100, 101, 111, 112, 195, 202] Arriagada and colleagues[8] reported on a multivariate analysis of 1195 patients treated at the Institut Gustave-Roussy that showed a significant improvement in both survival rates (Fig. 43-2) and a risk of distant metastases in patients with medial lesions who received either surgery or postoperative irradiation to the internal mammary region.

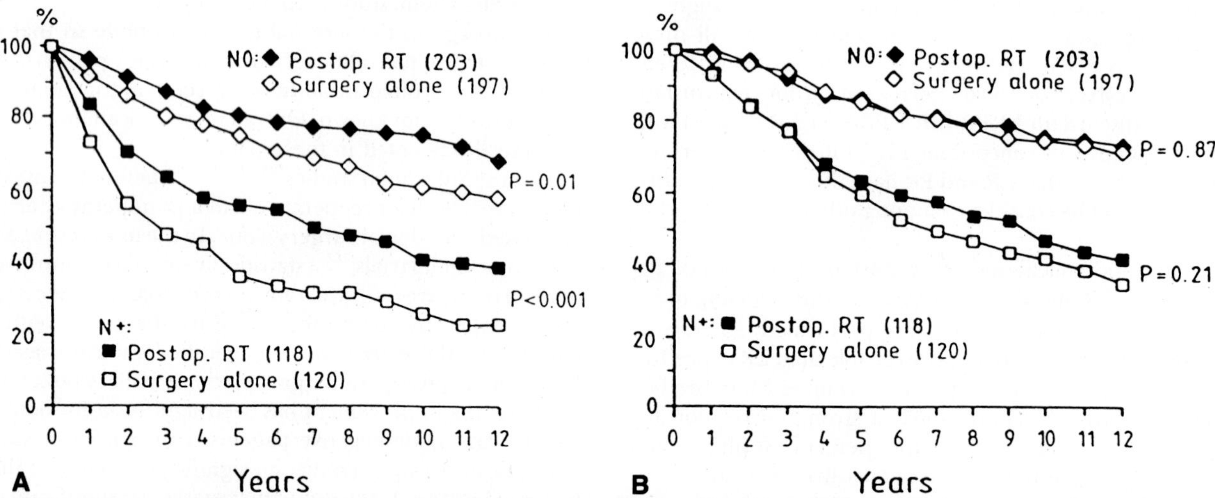

FIGURE 43–1. (**A**) Actuarial curves for recurrence-free survival rates by nodal status from the first Stockholm trial randomizing patients to mastectomy and postoperative irradiation or mastectomy alone. (**B**) Actuarial curves for overall survival rates by nodal status from the first Stockholm trial randomizing patients to mastectomy and postoperative irradiation or mastectomy alone. (Rutqvist LE, Cedemark B, Glaz U, et al: Int J Radiat Oncol Biol Phys 16:629–639, 1989)

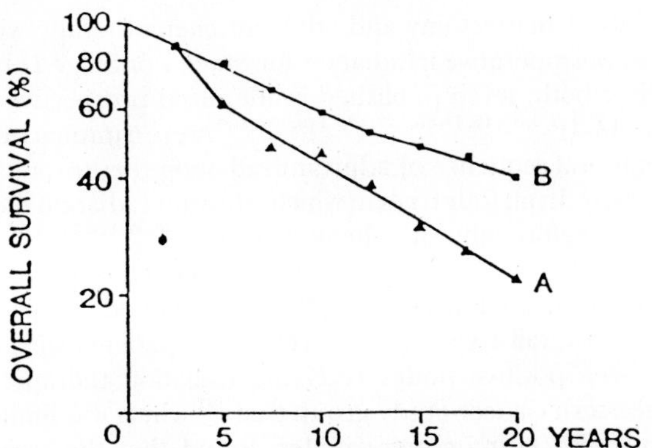

FIGURE 43–2. Actuarial survival rates for patients with medial breast tumors treated at the Institut Gustave-Roussy. Curve A indicates patients without treatment to the internal mammary nodes; curve B indicates patients with treatment (surgery, radiation therapy, or both) to the internal mammary chain (P = 0.01). (Arriagada R, Le MG, Mouriesse H, et al: Radiother Oncol 11:213–222, 1988)

Mastectomy and Adjuvant Chemotherapy or Hormonal Therapy *Versus* Irradiation

Chemotherapy has become the standard adjuvant treatment following mastectomy, and it is no longer possible to carry out a radiation therapy adjuvant trial that does not include chemotherapy.[77,116–120,188] However, three published randomized prospective trials are available comparing a radiation therapy-alone arm with a chemotherapy or hormonal therapy-alone arm.

The Royal Infirmary of Glasgow trial[179] compared CMF (cyclophosphamide, methotrexate, 5-fluorouracil) chemotherapy alone, postoperative irradiation alone, and combined postoperative irradiation and CMF. No difference in survival rate or disease-free survival rate was found between patients receiving CMF alone and those receiving postoperative radiation alone. Patients with more than three positive nodes who received CMF and irradiation had a statistically improved disease-free survival rate over those who had CMF alone or irradiation alone.

The second series of the Stockholm trials[165] compared postoperative irradiation alone with CMF chemotherapy alone in both premenopausal and postmenopausal high-risk (primary lesion >3 cm, or positive axillary nodes) patients. No significant difference in recurrence-free survival rate was found between the two groups. The subgroup of postmenopausal patients receiving postoperative radiation therapy alone had a statistically improved recurrence-free survival rate, with both decreased locoregional recurrence and distant metastases (Table 43-2).

In a third series of the Stockholm trials,[165] postmenopausal patients receiving adjuvant chemotherapy or irradiation were

TABLE 43–2
Overall and Locoregional Recurrences, Distant Metastases, and Deaths by Menopausal Status for Patients in the Second Stockholm Trial

	POSTOP. IRRADIATION		ADJUVANT CHEMOTHERAPY			
MENOPAUSAL STATUS, TYPE OF EVENT	**NO. OF PTS.**	**NO. OF EVENTS (%)**	**NO. OF PTS.**	**NO. OF EVENTS (%)**	**RATE RATIO* (95% CONFIDENCE INTERVAL)**	***P* (LOG RANK)**
Premenopausal	121		158			
Treatment failure†		53 (44)		60 (38)	1.20 (0.83–1.75)	0.33
Locoregional recurrence		14 (12)		29 (18)	0.63 (0.34–1.14)	0.13
Distant metastases		47 (39)		47 (30)	1.44 (0.95–2.18)	0.08
Death		40 (33)		39 (25)	1.28 (0.82–1.99)	0.28
Postmenopausal	190		237			
Treatment failure		74 (39)		124 (52)	0.65 (0.49–0.87)	<0.01
Locoregional recurrence		24 (13)		59 (25)	0.48 (0.31–0.74)	<0.001
Distant metastases		56 (29)		94 (40)	0.69 (0.50–0.95)	0.02
Death		63 (33)		88 (37)	0.81 (0.58–1.11)	0.19
All patients	311		395			
Treatment failure		127 (41)		184 (47)	0.82 (0.66–1.03)	0.09
Locoregional recurrence		38 (12)		88 (22)	0.53 (0.37–0.75)	<0.001
Distant metastases		103 (33)		141 (36)	0.92 (0.71–1.18)	0.49
Death		103 (33)		127 (32)	0.95 (0.73–1.23)	0.69

Note: Patients were randomized to mastectomy and postoperative irradiation versus *mastectomy and adjuvant chemotherapy.*
* *Radiation* versus *chemotherapy*
† *End point in calculations of recurrence-free survival*
(Rutqvist LE, Cedemark B, Glaz U, et al: Int J Radiat Oncol Biol Phys 16:629–639, 1989)

randomized to 2 years of tamoxifen therapy *versus* no adjuvant endocrine treatment. Tamoxifen improved the recurrence-free survival rate in the high-risk patients who also received adjuvant chemotherapy. This improvement raised recurrence-free survival rates to the levels achieved with radiation therapy alone. The addition of tamoxifen to irradiation added nothing to the recurrence-free survival rate achieved with radiation therapy alone.

In addition to these three randomized trials, a major nonrandomized series carried out at an institution in which precise performance of radiation therapy and accurate, adequate follow-up of patients are available is the subject of a report on more than 900 patients by Fletcher and colleagues from M. D. Anderson Cancer Center.[77,188] They found that patients treated with adjuvant irradiation and without chemotherapy had a 10-year recurrence-free interval and overall survival similar to those of patients with chemotherapy at Milan.

Mastectomy and Adjuvant Chemotherapy and Irradiation

In a study of 627 women entered into the Eastern Cooperative Oncology Group (ECOG) cooperative group adjuvant chemotherapy protocols, Fowble and associates[80] identified a subgroup of patients undergoing mastectomy and adjuvant chemotherapy who might benefit from the addition of radiation therapy. Premenopausal patients were randomized to CMF, CMFP, or CMFPT (cyclophosphamide, methotrexate, 5-fluorouracil, CMF with prednisone, CMF with prednisone and tamoxifen). Postmenopausal patients were randomized to observation, CMFP, or CMFPT. In a multivariate analysis, the risk factors for locoregional recurrence without distant metastases were identified.

Patients with four to seven positive nodes or tumor size over 5 cm had a high risk of developing an isolated locoregional recurrence despite adjuvant chemotherapy (Table 43-3).

Fowble and associates[80] concluded that there was a need for adjuvant locoregional treatment in patients with four or more positive nodes and tumor size over 5 cm and that such treatment could potentially improve not only locoregional control, but also overall survival.

In a separate series from the University of Pennsylvania, Fowble and co-workers[79] demonstrated the efficacy of postoperative irradiation as adjuvant locoregional treatment in a series of 63 patients at high risk for recurrence following mastectomy and adjuvant chemotherapy.

In Monyak and Levitt's[138] review of randomized prospective trials of mastectomy and adjuvant chemotherapy with or without postoperative irradiation for Stage I or Stage II breast cancer or both, seven published randomized prospective trials (Table 43-4)[2,5,33,46,47,86,127,130,140,179,199] were summarized by the temporal sequence of adjuvant radiation therapy and chemotherapy. In all four trials in which adjuvant radiation therapy was given before adjuvant chemotherapy,[33,46,47,127,130,140,179,199] locoregional control was improved in the patient groups receiving irradiation. The Glasgow study[130,179] also showed a statistically improved overall freedom from relapse in patients with more than three positive nodes receiving radiation therapy. The Southeastern Cancer Study group trial,[127] which was limited to patients with four or more nodes, found that the radiation therapy-treated patients had an improved freedom from local recurrence, a decreased overall recurrence rate, and a rate of distant metastases compared with patients receiving CMF alone.

Two studies reported on patients who were given concurrent adjuvant chemotherapy and postoperative irradiation. In the Mayo study[2] a significant improvement in locoregional recurrence rate occurred in the irradiation-plus-chemotherapy group, but no difference in overall freedom from relapse. The Arizona study[5] failed to show an improvement in locoregional recurrence rate but was marred by the inclusion of nonrandomized patients in the analysis.

In a study at the Dana Farber Cancer Institute,[86] postoperative radiation therapy was given after adjuvant chemotherapy. Significant improvement occurred in the local recurrence rate for patients with more than three nodes who received the adjuvant chemotherapy plus radiation therapy.

Overall, six of the seven trials showed some degree of reduction in locoregional recurrence rate with the addition of irradiation. Results for differences in freedom from any relapse were inconclusive.[138]

A generally accepted policy for postoperative irradiation is to recommend it for patients treated with a radical mastectomy with lesions larger than 5 cm in diameter, with any skin involvement, or with more than four positive axillary lymph nodes. It appears that such postoperative radiation may be effectively given before, concurrent with, or after the use of adjuvant chemotherapy.

LOCALLY ADVANCED BREAST CANCER

The term "locally advanced breast cancer" comprises a heterogeneous group of breast cancers that includes large primary (T3, T4) tumors, tumors with fixed ipsilateral axillary nodes

TABLE 43–3
Effect of Primary Tumor Size and Nodal Status on Isolated Locoregional Recurrence

	NO. OF PATIENTS*	% ISOLATED LR (*P* VALUES)	% DISTANT	% RECURRENCE ISOLATED LR (*P* VALUES)
1-3N+, TS <5 cm	256	6 (.23)	16	28 (.56)
1-3N+, TS ≥5 cm	51	12	22	35
4-7N+, TS <5 cm	133	10 (.001)	22	31 (.02)
4-7N+, TS ≥5 cm	47	31	19	62
>7N+, TS <5 cm	94	15 (1.00)	48	24 (1.00)
>7N+, TS ≥5 cm	41	15	44	25

N+: positive nodes; TS: tumor size
** 627 patients treated on Eastern Cooperative Oncology Group Trials of Mastectomy and Adjuvant Chemotherapy (Fowble B, Gray R, Gilchrist K, et al: J Clin Oncol 6:1107–1117, 1988)*

TABLE 43–4
*Summary of Randomized Prospective Trials of Mastectomy and Adjuvant Chemotherapy With or Without Postoperative Irradiation in Stage I and/or II Breast Cancer**

POSTOPERATIVE RADIATION THERAPY GIVEN BEFORE ADJUVANT CHEMOTHERAPY

Bowman-Gray University

Number	159 patients
Eligibility	Stage II disease
Randomization	(1) L-PAM chemotherapy alone (2) RT + L-PAM (3) CMF chemotherapy alone (4) RT + CMF
Locoregional recurrence	"Local recurrence more common in patients treated with chemotherapy alone"; percentages not given
Overall freedom from recurrence	Percent relapse-free survival was similar at 5 years for all four treatments; treatment failures at last follow-up for 1 to 3 nodes: 35% L-PAM; 35% L-PAM + RT; 21% CMF; 55% CMF + RT; for ≥ 4 nodes: 70% L-PAM; 50% L-PAM + RT; 70% CMF; 53% CMF + RT

Southeastern Cancer Study Group

Number	276 patients
Eligibility	Operable breast cancer with ≥ 4 positive axillary nodes
Randomization	(1) CMF chemotherapy × 6 mos alone (2) CMF × 12 mos (3) RT + CMF × 6 mos
Locoregional recurrence	20% CMF 6 mos; 19% CMF 12 mos; 10% RT + CMF; differences not significant
Overall freedom from relapse	50% CMF 6 mos; 44% CMF 12 mos; 62% RT + CMF; differences not significant

Royal Infirmary Glasgow

Number	322 patients
Eligibility	Operable breast cancer with positive axillary nodes
Randomization	(1) CMF chemotherapy alone (2) RT + CMF chemotherapy (3) RT alone
Locoregional recurrence	31% CMF alone; 12% RT + CMF; 16.5% RT alone
Overall freedom from relapse	Statistically improved for patients with >3 positive nodes who received radiation

M.D. Anderson Hospital and Tumor Institute

Number	238 patients
Eligibility	Operable breast cancer with positive axillary nodes
Randomization	(1) FAC chemotherapy ± BCG immunotherapy alone (2) RT + FAC chemotherapy ± BCG immunotherapy alone
Locoregional recurrence	Chest wall and nodes as site of first recurrence: 4% FAC ± BCG alone; 2% RT + FAC ± BCG
Overall freedom from relapse	No difference

POSTOPERATIVE RADIATION THERAPY GIVEN CONCURRENTLY WITH ADJUVANT CHEMOTHERAPY

Mayo Clinic

Number	293 patients
Eligibility	Operable breast cancer with positive axillary nodes and/or skin, muscle, fascia, or nipple invasion
Randomization	(1) L-PAM chemotherapy alone (2) CFP chemotherapy alone (3) RT + CFP chemotherapy
Locoregional recurrences	35% L-PAM alone; 54% CFP alone; 12% RT + CFP; difference CFP ± RT statistically significant
Overall freedom from relapse	No statistical difference

University of Arizona

Number	159 patients
Eligibility	Stage II breast cancer
Randomization	(1) AC chemotherapy alone (2) AC chemotherapy + RT
Locoregional recurrence	11% in both arms; for 1–3 positive nodes, 11% in AC alone, 0% AC + RT; for 4 or greater nodes, 12% in AC alone, 18% in AC + RT arm
Overall freedom from relapse	No statistical difference except in subgroup with 1–3 positive nodes, where AC + RT group was significantly better than AC alone group

POSTOPERATIVE RADIATION THERAPY GIVEN AFTER ADJUVANT CHEMOTHERAPY

Dana Farber Cancer Institute

Number	206 patients
Eligibility	Operable breast cancer T1–T3 with positive axillary nodes, and/or >5 cm primary
Randomization	(≥ 4 positive nodes or 1 positive apical node) (1) CA chemotherapy (2) CA chemotherapy + RT
Randomization	(1–3 positive nodes, or negative nodes and T3 primary) (1) CMF/MF chemotherapy (2) CMF/MF chemotherapy + RT
Locoregional recurrence	5% CMF/MF chemotherapy + RT; 20% CA alone; 6% CA + RT; difference in CA arm significant
Overall freedom from relapse	No significant difference for RT in either CA or CMF/MF groups

L-PAM: melphalan; RT: radiation therapy; CMF: cyclophosphamide, methotrexate, and 5-fluorouracil; FAC: 5-fluorouracil, Adriamycin, cyclophosphamide; BCG: Bacillus Calmette-Guérin; CFP: cyclophosphamide, 5-fluorouracil, Prednisone; AC: Adriamycin and cyclophosphamide; CA: cyclophosphamide, Adriamycin; MF: methotrexate, 5-fluorouracil
**Data from references 2, 5, 33, 46, 47, 86, 127, 130, 140, 179, 199*
(Monyak D, Levitt S: Invest Radiol 24:483–494, 1989)

(N2), tumors with ipsilateral supraclavicular or infraclavicular nodes, or tumors producing arm edema (N3).

In general, life expectancy is primarily determined by the high probability (about 80%) that these patients will develop blood-borne metastases.[17,154] Because of the compelling need for systemic therapy, chemotherapy has assumed a primary role in most treatment trials of patients with locally advanced breast cancer. Radiation or surgery in turn has assumed a secondary but not insignificant role of locally supplementing the chemotherapy to spare patients from the prospect of an uncontrolled, painful mass in the breast or chest wall.

For discussion here, the patients are divided into two basic treatment groups: those with technically resectable lesions and those with borderline resectable or unresectable tumors, including inflammatory carcinoma. Special mention should be made of patients with T3 primary lesions and negative axillary nodes. These patients in the past have been assigned to Stage III advanced breast cancer. However, such patients have been found to have a relatively good prognosis,[81,82] in recognition of which the 1988 revision of the American Joint Committee and Union Internationale contre le Cancer staging systems have reassigned them to Stage II.[7]

Technically Resectable Locally Advanced Breast Cancer

There is a consensus that all patients with technically resectable locally advanced breast cancer should have surgery: Controversy has centered on which adjuvant treatment is appropriate. Three published randomized prospective trials[88,109,145,180] specifically studied the efficacy of postmastectomy irradiation in these high-risk patients. Spangenberg and associates[180] randomized 131 technically resectable Stage III breast cancer patients to radiation therapy and single agent chemotherapy (cyclophosphamide) *versus* multiagent chemotherapy alone (CMF and vinblastine). The 5-year relapse-free rate was 40.4% for patients receiving irradiation and chemotherapy compared with 26.8% for patients receiving chemotherapy alone. This difference, although favoring the irradiation arm, was not significant.

Papaioannou and co-workers[145] treated patients with induction chemotherapy (cyclophosphamide, Adriamycin, vincristine, methotrexate, 5-fluorouracil [CAVMF] with tamoxifen or oophorectomy) followed by surgery; 205 patients were then randomized to irradiation or no irradiation. Both groups received postoperative chemotherapy (cyclophosphamide, Adriamycin, vincristine, methotrexate, 5-fluorouracil [CAVMF] and tamoxifen). The relapse-free rate was 79% in the irradiation group compared with 73% in the nonirradiation group. This difference, although again favoring the irradiation arm, was not statistically significant. The trial was flawed by 78 exclusions from the analysis.

In the Helsinki University Stage III trial,[88,109] 120 patients with operable Stage III breast cancer were randomized between postmastectomy irradiation, postmastectomy chemotherapy, and both postmastectomy chemotherapy and radiation therapy. The first 60 patients randomized to each arm also received levamisole. Patients receiving chemotherapy had a 25% (chemotherapy-alone arm) and 28% (chemotherapy-plus-radiation therapy arm) incidence of distant metastases compared with a 70% incidence in the radiation therapy-alone arm. Patients receiving radiation therapy had a 20% incidence (radiation-alone arm) and 8% incidence (radiation therapy-plus-chemotherapy arm) of local failure compared with a 57.5% incidence in the chemotherapy-alone arm. The reduction of both distant metastases and local failures in the arm receiving both adjuvant chemotherapy and irradiation led to a statistically significant improvement in overall freedom from relapse and in survival rate (Fig. 43-3). This important study strongly suggests that in patients at high risk for locoregional failure, postoperative irradiation added to mastectomy and adjuvant chemotherapy can make a significant impact on survival as well as on locoregional control.

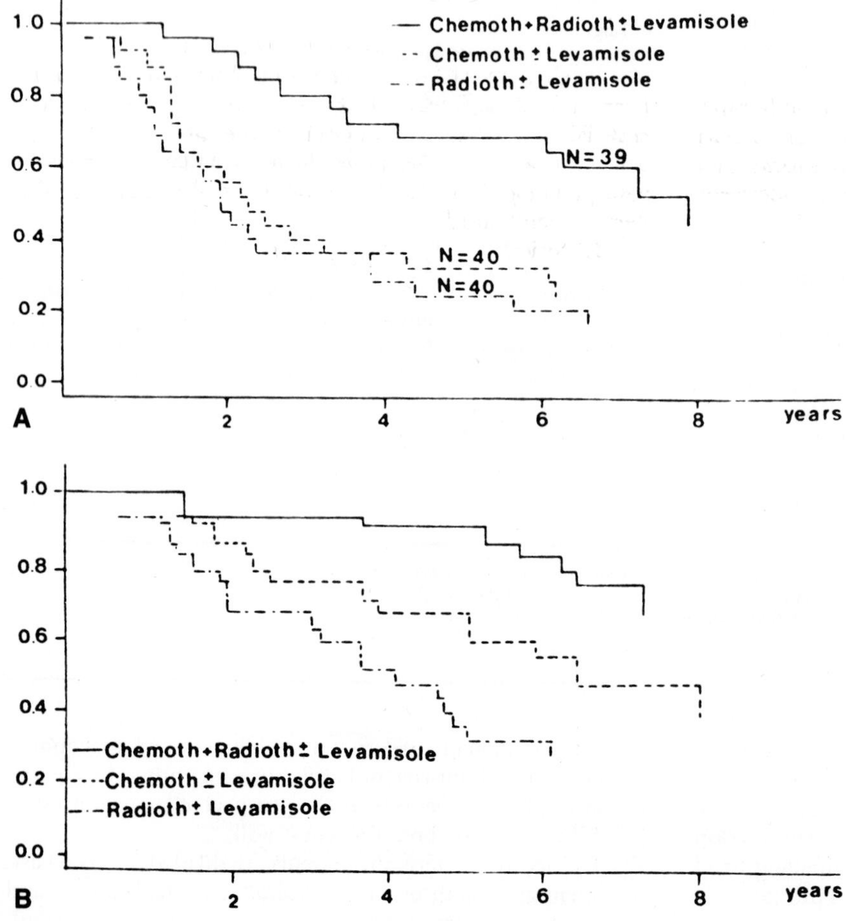

FIGURE 43–3. (**A**) Disease-free survival of patients in the Helsinki trial. (**B**) Overall survival of patients in the Helsinki trial. (Klefstrom P, Grohn P, et al: Cancer 60:936–942, 1987)

Borderline Resectable or Unresectable Locally Advanced Breast Cancer

Radiation Therapy Alone

Historically, borderline resectable or unresectable locally advanced breast cancers have been treated by radiation therapy alone. Five-year survival rates range from 10% to 25%.[17,27,40,78,87,162,194] With moderate doses of radiation, local control rates of 35% to 65% can be expected.[10,17,27,83,87] Radical doses of radiation (7000 cGy to 10,000 cGy) can yield local control rates of 70% to 100% (Table 43-5),[4,78,141,187] but carry with them a significant risk of soft tissue and lung injury.[181]

Radiation Therapy Alone Versus *Irradiation Followed by Chemotherapy*

The high rates of distant failure[17,154] in patients with borderline resectable or unresectable breast cancer highlight the need for adequate systemic therapy in these patients. Several published studies have suggested an improved freedom from relapse in patients treated with chemotherapy and irradiation compared with the historical results in patients with irradiation alone.[22,34,55,56,70,148,161,164]

Two published randomized trials compare radiation therapy alone *versus* combined chemotherapy and irradiation. Between 1977 and 1980, 118 patients were randomized at the Netherlands Cancer Institute to irradiation alone, irradiation followed by 12 cycles of CMF, or radiation therapy followed by alternating cycles of AV (Adriamycin and vincristine) and CMF. Both chemotherapy arms also received tamoxifen. The 5-year survival rate was 37% in all arms of the study. No statistically significant difference in overall freedom from relapse or locoregional recurrence rate occurred among any of the arms.[171]

Between 1978 and 1985, 231 patients with locally advanced noninflammatory carcinoma of the breast were randomized at the University of Witwatersrand and Johannesburg Hospitals to radiation therapy *versus* irradiation plus CMF chemotherapy. The chemotherapy randomization included allocation to both low-dose CMF and higher-dose CMF. It should be noted that 120 patients had technically resectable lesions and underwent mastectomy before randomization. For the combined group of technically operable and technically inoperable patients, a significant improvement in freedom from relapse was seen in premenopausal patients receiving chemotherapy; no difference occurred in overall survival. For postmenopausal women, no difference occurred in either freedom from relapse or overall survival.[57]

Chemotherapy Followed by Irradiation Versus *Chemotherapy Followed by Surgery*

In about 80% of cases, borderline inoperable or inoperable tumors treated with chemotherapy regress sufficiently to become operable.[99,150] Chemotherapy may also sensitize the tumor to local radiation. There are two published prospective trials in which patients made resectable with initial chemotherapy were randomized to mastectomy or breast irradiation: one from the National Cancer Institute of Milan[55,196] and the other from the Cancer and Leukemia Group B Study Group.[150] Neither trial showed any statistically significant difference in freedom from relapse or in survival rate between the surgery arms and the irradiation arms of the studies.

Chemotherapy, Surgery, and Radiation Therapy

Extrapolating from the superiority of the triple modality arm of surgery, radiation therapy, and chemotherapy in the Helsinki trial for operable Stage III breast cancer,[88,109] it may be persuasively argued that such triple modality treatment is most likely to yield the best treatment results in marginally unresectable or unresectable advanced breast cancer. Several single-arm protocols also suggest that this may be the case.[12,28,145,173] As yet, no randomized prospective trial has compared such triple modality treatment with lesser treatment.

INFLAMMATORY BREAST CANCER

Inflammatory carcinoma is a subset of "what was considered technically inoperable locally advanced breast cancer" that has been variously defined on the basis of both clinical or pathologic criteria. The clinical definition is the presence of color, erythema, and *peau d'orange* in the involved breast. The alternate pathologic criterion is the presence of tumor emboli in dermal lymphatics.[67,123]

Historically, inflammatory breast cancer has been charac-

TABLE 43–5
Results of Radiation Therapy for Locally Advanced T3–T4 Breast Cancer

AUTHOR	NO. OF PATIENTS	TUMOR DOSE (cGy)	LOCAL CONTROL (%)	5-YEAR SURVIVAL (%)
Rubens et al[162]	184	3600–4000	19	13
Griscom and Wang[87]	97	4000–6000	35	22
Bedwinek et al[17]	54	4000–7000	39	18
Bruckman et al[27]	116	4000–8500	64	25
Baclesse[10]	79	6000–6800	58	
Ghossein et al[83]	22	6000–8000	46	
Treurniet-Donker et al[194]	129	≤7000	78	12
Nobler and Venet[41]	36	7000	89	
Fletcher[76]	144	9000	70	10
Syed et al[186]	53	9000–10,000	89	
Alderman[4]	18	10,000	100	

(Danoff BF: The role of radiotherapy in the management of locally advanced nonmetastatic breast cancer. In Levitt S [ed]: Syllabus. A Categorical Course in Breast Cancer. Radiological Society of North America Proceedings, 1984)

terized by a high rate of locoregional recurrence after mastectomy and the rapid development of metastatic disease. This led to the widely expressed feeling that surgery was contraindicated in inflammatory breast cancer. Current increasing retrospective data suggest that chemotherapy can delay the development of metastatic disease and extend the patient's survival. This increase in survival has in turn led to a reexamination of the role of surgery as an adjunct to irradiation in locoregional control.

The largest series of inflammatory breast cancer patients is from the Institut Gustave-Roussy.[161] This series retrospectively compared the results of treatment with irradiation and hormonal manipulation (group C: 60 patients treated from 1973 to 1975), induction Adriamycin, vincristine, and methotrexate (AVM), radiation therapy, and maintenance vincristine, cyclophosphamide, 5-fluorouracil (VCF) (group A: 91 patients treated from 1976 to 1980), and induction Adriamycin, vincristine, cyclophosphamide, methotrexate, 5-fluorouracil (AVCMF), radiation therapy, and maintenance VCF (group B: 79 patients treated from 1980 to 1982). The 4-year disease-free survival rates were 15% for group C, 32% for group A, and 54% for the most intense chemotherapy regimen, group B. The corresponding survival rates at 4 years were 42%, 53%, and 74%. They concluded that a combination of intensive induction chemotherapy and maintenance chemotherapy can improve both freedom from relapse as well as survival over that achieved with irradiation alone.

At Washington University in St. Louis, between 1958 and 1985, 107 patients received radiation therapy as part of the treatment of nonmetastatic inflammatory breast cancer.[72,73] Radiation therapy alone was given to 31 patients, irradiation and mastectomy to 16, irradiation and chemotherapy to 23, and irradiation, chemotherapy, and surgery to 37. Patients who underwent surgery showed improved locoregional (LR) control as well as survival rates over those who did not; 83% (42 of 52) LR control compared with 30% (16 of 53) 5-year survival rates were 37% and 7%, respectively. Patients who received chemotherapy had improved 5-year freedom-from-relapse rates (20% *versus* 5%) and 5-year survival rates (23% *versus* 3%) over those who did not. Although they noted the limitations of their analysis because of possible selection effects, the authors were encouraged by the improved locoregional control they were able to achieve with combined irradiation and surgery.[70]

A study from M. D. Anderson Cancer Center[190] has also reported on a large retrospective series of inflammatory breast cancer patients. Patients were treated with various regimens: once-daily irradiation alone; accelerated fractionation irradiation alone; initial multiagent chemotherapy followed by accelerated fractionation irradiation; initial chemotherapy, surgery, if possible, daily or accelerated irradiation, and maintenance chemotherapy.

After 1972, no difference in the crude locoregional recurrence rate occurred among any of the treatment regimens. Researchers at M. D. Anderson Cancer Center found that a policy of performing surgery whenever possible did not result in an overall improvement in locoregional control. They did believe, however, that mastectomy in such patients could be justified because it reduced the need for high doses of radiation and subsequent problems of breast fibrosis and necrosis.

LOCOREGIONAL RECURRENCE AFTER MASTECTOMY

Locoregional recurrences in carcinoma of the breast after radical or modified radical mastectomy have been reported in 10% to 20% of patients,[61] although in Stage III and local Stage IV disease the incidence is as high as 40% to 45%.[91] Recurrence rates of 10% to 18% have been reported following administration of adjuvant chemotherapy after radical surgery.[19–21]

Untreated, locoregional tumors may cause painful, foul-smelling ulcerations of the chest wall. Arm edema, weakness, pain, and paresthesias may occur from supraclavicular or axillary nodal recurrences. An internal mammary nodal recurrence can produce pain and a parasternal mass (Fig. 43-4).

Although radiation therapy can provide significant palliation for many of these patients, the best complete remission rate obtained at any time during the patient's treatment course is only about 66%[174]; the overall local failure rate ranges from 31% to 69%.[1,16,38,41,58,94,103,125,146,159,183,192] The 5-year survival rate for patients who have an isolated locoregional recurrence without distant metastases is 22% to 40%[16,58,146,183,192]; the relapse-free rate is only about 15%.[15,41,58]

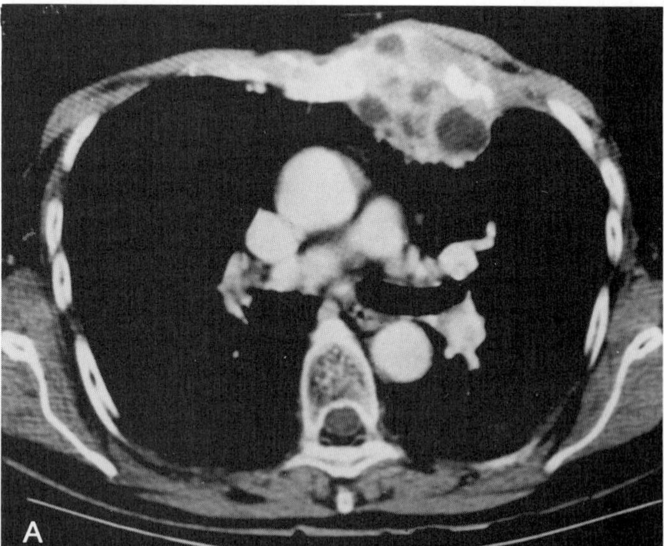

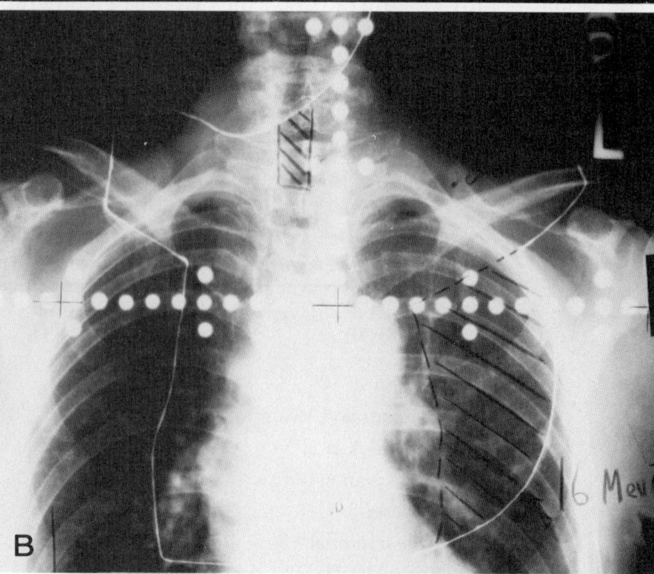

FIGURE 43–4. (**A**) A CT scan of the chest illustrating a large internal mammary recurrence. The patient also had some enlarged metastatic lymph nodes. (**B**) Example of portals used in the treatment of the same patient. First, 2000 cGy was delivered with the large field (*white contour*). Following this, an additional 2000 cGy was given to the mediastinum with AP/PA portals and 2000 cGy to the shaded area with 16 MeV electrons. A reduced AP portal was instituted at that point to deliver an additional 1000 cGy with 16 MeV electrons to the residual mass in the left chest wall. (AP: anteroposterior; PA: posteroanterior)

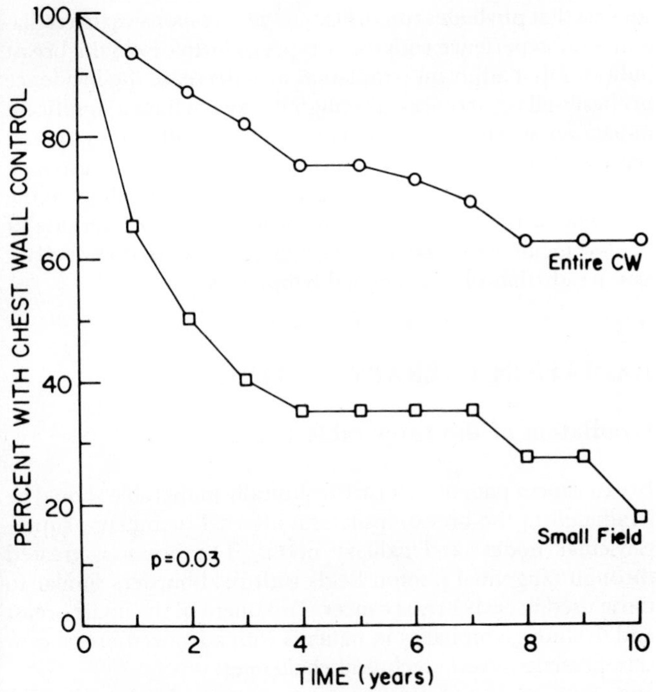

FIGURE 43–5. Actuarial risk of re-recurrence in the chest wall by treatment with small *versus* large fields. (CW: chest wall) (Halverson KJ, Perez CA, Kuske RR, et al: Int J Radiat Oncol Biol Phys 19:851–858, 1990)

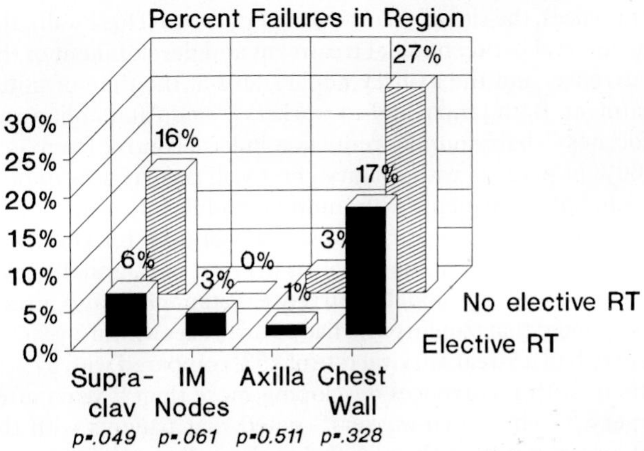

FIGURE 43–6. Regional treatment failure related to elective radiation therapy (RT) and no elective radiation therapy. Results are from Washington University (Adapted from Halverson KJ, Perez CA, Kuske RR, et al: Int J Radiat Oncol Biol Phys 19:851–858, 1990)

In the treatment of chest wall recurrences, results from Washington University[15,94] have indicated the importance of treating the entire chest wall and not merely a small local field (Fig. 43-5).[94] Others series have confirmed this observation.[58,183]

A second issue in the treatment of isolated locoregional recurrences is elective radiation treatment of the chest wall and regional lymphatic sites to prevent second recurrences in those sites. Chen and associates[138] found that 27% of their patients treated with involved field irradiation failed only in an uninvolved locoregional site. More than 50% of these recurrences occurred in the chest wall, leading them to recommend elective chest wall irradiation. At Washington University, elective treatment of the chest wall reduced second recurrences in that site from 27% to 17%, but the difference is not significant in the latest analysis (Fig. 43-6).[94] Chen and associates, however, continue to recommend elective chest wall irradiation. Other authors have also advocated elective chest wall treatment.[53,156,192]

Several authors have advocated elective radiation treatment of the supraclavicular area.[15,53,94,156,192] The series from Washington University found that elective supraclavicular irradiation reduced the second recurrence rate in that region from 16% to 5.6% (see Fig. 43-6). This difference was statistically significant.

A few authors have also advocated elective radiation treatment of the internal mammary nodal area or the axilla or both.[156,191,192] Toonkel and co-workers,[191] for example, observed a 71% probability of local tumor control at 5 years when the chest wall and comprehensive lymphatic drainage regions were treated compared with only 50% in patients treated to the chest wall or regional lymphatics only. The corresponding 5-year survival rates were 37% compared with 8%. In the Washington University experience,[15,94] recurrences in the axilla and internal mammary nodal regions were unusual, and no benefit to elective treatment could be demonstrated.

Adequate doses are also important in achieving optimal results; radiation doses of 5000 cGy should be given to the electively treated areas and to recurrent tumors that have been completely excised. For lesions less than 3 cm, doses in the range of 6000 cGy should be given. Larger masses require doses of 6500 cGy to 7000 cGy.[15,94] Several series have demonstrated a dose response for achieving local control (Table 43-6).[15,41,94,146] Haverson and colleagues[94] recommend that complete surgical excision should be considered when it can be accomplished with minimal morbidity.

Other identified factors affecting treatment outcome for locoregional recurrences after mastectomy are the number of

TABLE 43–6
Tumor Response and Radiation Dose in Patients With Chest Wall Recurrences

	COMPLETE CONTROL		PARTIAL OR NO CONTROL	
NSD	NO. OF PATIENTS	%	NO. OF PATIENTS	%
<1060 rets (3600 cGy/3.5 wk)	12/25	48	13/25	52
1060–1470 rets (3600–5000 cGy/3.5 wk)	68/98	69	30/98	31
>1470 rets	47/61	77	14/61	23

NSD: nominal standard dose
(Chu FCH, Lin F-J, Kim JH, et al: Cancer 37:2677–2681, 1976)

recurrences, the site of recurrence (nodal *versus* chest wall), the time interval between initial treatment and development of the recurrence, and the axillary nodal status at the time of initial treatment. Both Janjan and co-workers[103] and Patanaphan and associates[146] have found a reduction in local control from 50% to 60% in patients with solitary chest wall recurrences to only 20% to 25% in patients with multiple nodules. Halverson and colleagues[94] found 5-year survival rates of 50% for chest wall recurrence only, 36% for nodal recurrence only, and 19% for both chest wall and nodal recurrence. Patanaphan and associates[146] noted that patients who had recurrences within 2 years of surgery had a 5-year survival rate of 25% compared with 57% in patients with recurrences developing more than 2 years after surgery. Chen and co-workers[38] noted that patients with the best prognosis were those with histologically negative lymph nodes at the time of mastectomy and a single chest wall recurrence (78% probability of tumor control and 48% 5-year recurrence-free).

Several reports now suggest that results of irradiation alone for locoregional recurrence of breast cancer can be improved by the addition of hyperthermia to irradiation.[62, 85, 149, 174, 197] Perez and co-workers[149] reported a complete response rate of 80% for lesions 1 cm to 3 cm in diameter and 65% for lesions greater than 3 cm. Dragovic and colleagues[62] reported a complete response rate of 81% for lesions less than 5 cm and 29% for lesions more than 5 cm. Gonzalez and associates[85] divided lesions into those without skin ulceration that could easily be encompassed in a hyperthermia field with reliable thermometry (Stage I and Stage II) and those with ulceration not easily encompassed in a hyperthermia field (Stage III and Stage IV). They achieved a complete response rate of 84% (21 of 27) in their Stage I and Stage II lesions compared with only 30% (six of 20) in Stage III and Stage IV.

CYSTOSARCOMA PHYLLODES

The treatment of choice for cystosarcoma phyllodes is surgery. In general, mastectomy has been the recommended treatment,[65, 92, 106, 126, 131, 142, 203] but currently some authors have advocated more conservative resections,[89, 160, 168]

In the series from the National Cancer Institute of Milan,[168] a correlation was found between the local recurrence rate after limited surgery and tumor grade. In 24 women with benign phyllodes tumors, one of 15 (6.7%) treated with limited surgery suffered a local recurrence compared with none of nine treated with mastectomy. In women with borderline tumors, ten of 22 (45%) treated with limited surgery suffered local recurrence compared with none of four treated with mastectomy. In women with malignant tumors, three of eight (37.5%) treated with limited surgery had recurrences locally compared with none of 13 treated with mastectomy. No correlation was found between tumor size and local recurrence rate. Distant metastases occurred in 0%, 3.7%, and 4.7% of patients with benign, borderline, and malignant tumors, respectively. Other series, however, have failed to find a relationship between local recurrence rate after limited surgery and tumor grade. Haagensen,[89] for example, reported local recurrence in 17 of 37 (46%) benign tumors; Pietruszka and Barnes[151] reported local recurrence in four of 18 (22%) benign tumors. Hajdu and co-workers[93] found an 18% recurrence rate in benign tumors and an 8% recurrence rate in malignant tumors.

Axillary nodal disease is generally thought to be rare,[142] and an axillary nodal dissection is not usually recommended.

In the more recent literature, anecdotal data[6, 30, 98, 105, 189] suggest that phyllodes tumors can be very responsive to irradiation. Our experience with other types of histology in the breast indicates that adjuvant irradiation may decrease the incidence of chest wall recurrences, although it may not have a significant impact on survival. If patients are to be treated, they should receive at least a 5000 cGy radiation dose to the chest wall, followed by a boost (1000 cGy to 1500 cGy), depending on the presence of residual microscopic or gross disease. Because of the low incidence of axillary node metastases, we do not advocate irradiation of the regional lymphatics.

RADIATION THERAPY TECHNIQUES

Irradiation of the Inoperable Breast

Breast cancer patients who are technically inoperable should be irradiated to the breast, ipsilateral internal mammary, supraclavicular nodes, and axillary nodes. The breast is treated through tangential photon fields with field borders similar to those used in early breast cancer. Treatment of the intact breast and draining lymphatics in patients with advanced breast cancers presents several technical challenges:

1. Homogeneous irradiation of the breast tissue despite its half-oblate geometric shape
2. Adequate skin and dermal dose. Unlike in early breast cancer in which there is no clinical need to treat the skin and immediate dermis, in advanced breast cancer the frequent presence of gross or subclinical skin or dermal involvement must be treated.
3. Precise matching between the plane of the inferior border of the supraclavicular field with the plane of the superior border of the medial and lateral breast tangential fields. With the sharp beam edges of the modern linear accelerator, inadequate matching may result in a thin "cold plane" of tissue that may harbor a nidus for recurrence or else a thin plane of "matchline fibrosis."
4. Minimal beam divergence into the lung from the medial and lateral breast tangential fields as well as the dose to the opposite breast from the lateral breast tangential
5. Adequate coverage of the internal mammary nodes. Inclusion of the internal mammary nodes in the breast tangential fields often results in the inclusion of too much lung. On the other hand, use of a separate single anterior internal mammary field that matches the medial border of the medial breast tangential field produces a "cold wedge" of breast tissue that is often unacceptable; this cold wedge may harbor gross or subclinical deposits of cancer cells.

Adequate Skin and Dermal Dose

Adequate skin and dermal dose is of particular importance in treating advanced breast cancer. It is technically easily achieved by adding bolus over the entire area of concern. A box-shaped bolus may be used over the entire breast to provide an adequate skin and dermal dose as well as homogeneous irradiation of the breast tissue.

The more difficult clinical issue is how many bolus treatments are necessary, given the limits of normal skin tolerance. Empirical clinical experience has been to use bolus in 40% to 60% of treatments, either consecutively or every other day. When using a separate interval mammary field, it is very important to ensure adequate coverage of the skin at the junction with the medial tangential portal.

Doses

A total dose of 5000 cGy to 6000 cGy at 180 cGy to 200 cGy daily fractions should be given to the entire breast. The residual gross disease should then be excised. If this is not possible, the breast should be boosted an additional 1500 cGy to 2500 cGy with external irradiation (electrons or photons) using shrinking fields or with an ^{192}Ir implant.

Internal mammary nodes, supraclavicular fossa, and the axillary nodal areas should receive 4500 cGy to 5000 cGy over 5 to 6 weeks. Any gross nodal disease should then be boosted with an additional 1000 cGy to 1500 cGy. An appositional electron-beam field may be used.

Irradiation of the Chest Wall

Irradiation of the chest wall after mastectomy can be accomplished through use of tangential photon fields as used in the treatment of the intact breast or by using electron beams. If tangential photon fields are used, the technical challenges are similar to those encountered in the treatment of the intact breast. Adequate skin and dermal dose is achieved in the case of elective treatment of the chest wall after mastectomy by adding bolus over the entire field for one third of the treatments and adding bolus to the the scar alone for an additional third of the treatments. In treatment of chest wall recurrences, a bolus to the entire field should be used for about one third of the treatments and a bolus within a generous margin around the recurrence for most if not all of the remaining treatments.

Several electron techniques can be used as an alternative to tangential photon treatment. The simplest technique is the use of a single appositional electron field using a 9 MeV to 12 MeV beam. Bolus may be used for part of the treatment to minimize the lung dose and to increase the skin surface dose beyond the 80% to 90% typically given with these beams.

The difficulty with a single appositional electron field is poor lateral coverage (Fig. 43-7). If the lateral coverage is just marginally inadequate, a single, medially angled electron field may be added to boost the depth coverage in the lateral region. Otherwise, use of more sophisticated electron arc[113, 114, 135, 147] or pseudoarc techniques[23] may be required. Electron arc therapy is a technically demanding and time-consuming treatment. Field shaping requires the use of custom lead strips or a Cerrobend cast placed on the patient's skin. It is often unappreciated that the surface dose in the electron arc technique is much lower than that for the same single electron beam of the same energy, and the effective depth coverage is less. Use of bolus to bring up the surface dose becomes mandatory.

Field Borders

Guidelines for the anatomic landmarks defining the field borders for treatment of breast/chest wall tangentials, supraclavicular nodes, internal mammary nodes, and axilla are similar to those used in the treatment of early breast cancer.

Examples of various field arrangements for irradiation of the chest wall and regional lymphatics are shown in Figure 43-8. Table 43-7 describes the advantages and disadvantages of the four techniques.The dose distribution for two tangential fields to the chest wall and internal mammary portal are illustrated in Figure 43-9.

CHEMOTHERAPY AND HORMONAL THERAPY

Adjuvant Chemotherapy for Resectable Breast Cancer

Adjuvant chemotherapy is designed to improve the cure rate or the disease-free interval following mastectomy, based on the concept that when the rate of tumor growth is high, chemotherapy is more effective in eliminating micrometastases[172, 176]

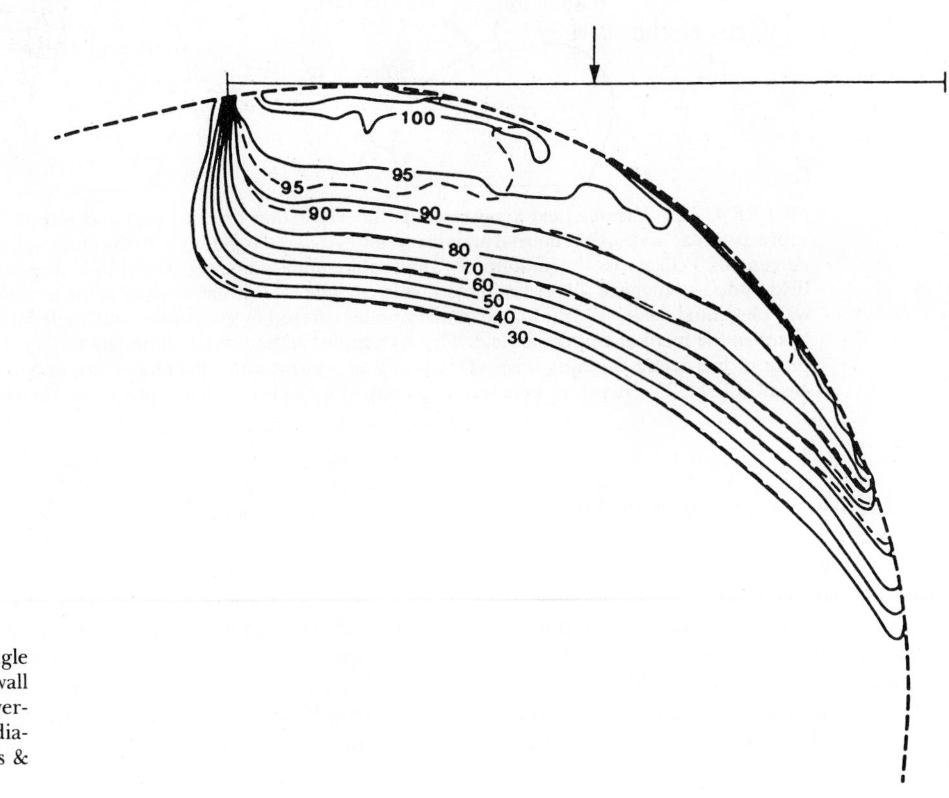

FIGURE 43–7. Isodose curves for a single appositional electron field to the chest wall shows the potentially inadequate depth coverage laterally. (Khan FK: The Physics of Radiation Therapy, p. 326. Baltimore, Williams & Wilkins, 1984)

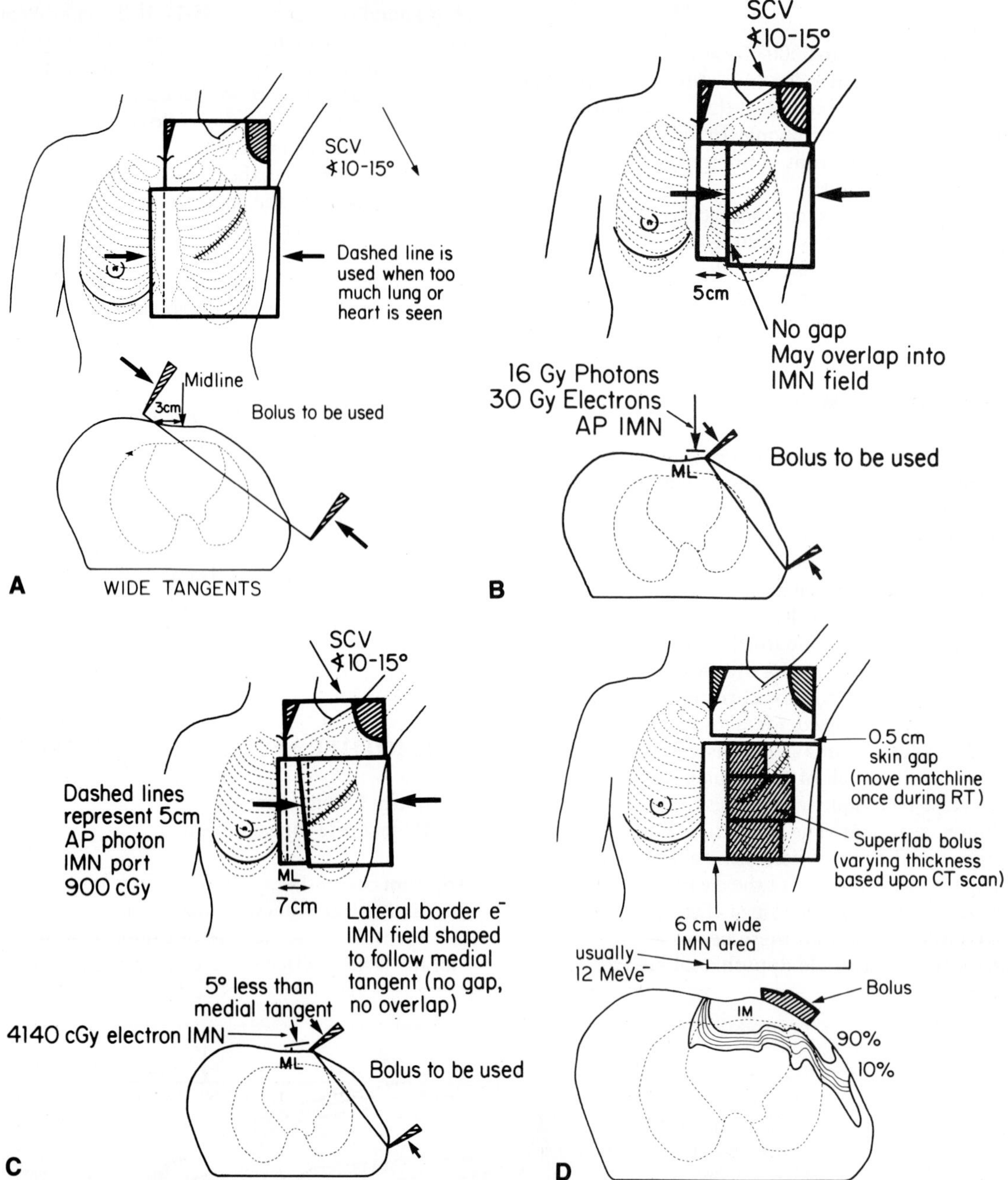

FIGURE 43–8. Various field arrangements for irradiation of chest wall and internal mammary and supraclavicular nodes. (**A**) Internal mammary nodes covered together with the chest wall by extending the tangentials 3 cm across the midline. (**B**) Internal mammary nodes covered by a separate 5 cm wide AP field. A disadvantage of this technique is a "cold triangle" of untreated tissue at the junction with the chest wall tangential fields. (**C**) Internal mammary nodes covered by a separate field angled laterally 5 degrees less than the medical tangential field. This technique can be used to eliminate the "cold triangle" at the price of increasing the lung dose. (**D**) Chest wall and internal; mammary nodes covered by anterior electron field. The depth of penetration is shaped by a custom bolus placed on the chest wall.

The 7-year follow-up results for cyclophosphamide, methotrexate, and 5-fluorouracil (CMF) adjuvant therapy in the Milan study (Table 43-8) showed an improvement in the relapse-free survival rate in premenopausal patients with involvement of one to three axillary lymph nodes. The initial analysis suggested that no benefit occurred from adjuvant therapy in the postmenopausal group, although in retrospect this absence of benefit may have resulted from reduced doses of the drug.[18] When 85% of the drug dosages were used, there was evidence of benefit in this group; the results could reflect patient selection. Carter[36] reviewed published results of several clinical trials and concluded that no evidence suggested that adjuvant chemotherapy improved disease-free survival, overall survival, or patterns of failure in postmenopausal patients (Table 43-9). Furthermore, some reports[48, 129] have described significant psychosocial and emotional repercussions with adjuvant chemotherapy in addition to the known somatic toxicity. Bonadonna[18] has shown that adjuvant chemotherapy with six cycles of CMF

TABLE 43–7
Comprehensive Chest Wall and Nodal Irradiation for Breast Cancer

TECHNIQUE A	TECHNIQUE B	TECHNIQUE C	TECHNIQUE D
ADVANTAGES			
1. Simplicity 2. No junctions, gaps, or overlaps for dose inhomogeneity 3. Possibly better control over skin tolerance	1. Assured of coverage of IM nodal region 2. Relative simplicity 3. Can reduce amount of lung or heart seen in tangential chest wall ports 4. Allows for more generous margins medially and laterally 5. IM skin surface dose lower than (C) and (D)	1. Assured of coverage of IM nodal region 2. Can minimize the amount of lung or heart within 3000 cGy isodose curve 3. More homogeneous dose distribution at the junction of the IM and tangents than (B) 4. Lowering IM skin surface dose with 1 week of AP photons	1. With good CT treatment planning, assured of coverage of IM nodal region 2. Can minimize the amount of lung and/or heart within 3000 cGy isodose curve 3. No junction at interface of IM and chest wall regions
DISADVANTAGES			
1. Uncertainty about coverage of IM nodal region 2. Large volume (3–5 cm) of lung and/or heart treated over 4500 cGy 3. Sometimes tight coverage of the chest wall laterally	1. Since medial border of chest wall tangents is rarely a straight line, matching with lateral IM border problematic, leading to gaps and/or overlaps 2. "Cold" wedge of tissue at junction of IM and chest wall tangents 3. Pericardium and paramediastinal lung can receive substantial dose 4. Moist desquamation in IM port skin possible, especially with chemotherapy	1. Complexity 2. Treatment planning CT required; good physics and dosimetry support 3. Potential for lung overdosage if IM electron energy chosen is too high 4. Moist desquamation of IM port skin possible, especially with chemotherapy 5. Small volume (~1 cm × 2 cm × 15 cm) ~10% to 15% hot spot on tangent side of IM junction (in soft tissue and ribs) 6. More dose to contralateral breast	1. Complexity 2. Treatment planning CT required; good physics and dosimetry support 3. Potential for lung overdosage if chest wall electron energy chosen is too high 4. Moist desquamation under bolus 5. Necessity of junction with SCV portal to be gapped and moved once 6. Relative underdosage of extreme lateral chest wall 7. Small volume (1 cm × 2 cm × 15 cm) hot spot underneath edge of bolus due to sidescatter away from the edge of the bolus 10% to 15%

IM: internal mammary; AP: anteroposterior; SCV: supraclavicular

has yielded results comparable to those found with 12 cycles of CMF.

Most randomized adjuvant studies have demonstrated that results of combined chemotherapy, such as cyclophosphamide, 5-fluorouracil, prednisone (CFP) or cyclophosphamide, methotrexate, 5-fluorouracil, vincristine, prednisone (CMFVP), are superior to that of melphalan alone[3,84] and that CMFVP is better than CFP.[193] These studies appear to support the notion that the more intensive the adjuvant therapy, the better the results. In studies involving an intensive regimen, the benefit of adjuvant chemotherapy was also seen in the postmenopausal group, especially in patients with a larger number of involved lymph nodes.[193] It must be borne in mind, however, that the duration of follow-up in these studies is relatively short.

Doxorubicin (Adriamycin) has been incorporated into the adjuvant program,[32,182] but because these are not randomized studies, it is difficult to assess whether a doxorubicin-containing regimen is superior to CMF or CMFVP.

Chemotherapy for Advanced Breast Cancer

Single agent cytotoxic regimens have yielded a complete plus partial remission rate of 20% to 35%.[96] Because most randomized studies have shown that multiagent chemotherapy yields a significantly higher response rate and longer survival,[196,163,178] single agents are no longer used as first-line therapy.

In general, doxorubicin, 5-fluorouracil, methotrexate, and vincristine are more cytotoxic to proliferating than to nonproliferating cells. On the other hand, mitomycin-C and nitrosoureas are equally effective against proliferative and nonproliferative cells.[64]

The first generation of combination chemotherapy was cyclophosphamide and 5-fluorouracil (CF) or CMF (CF plus methotrexate). The second generation was CFP or CMFVP, adding prednisone (P) or vincristine (V). After the introduction of doxorubicin—the most effective single agent so far—most combination therapy has included doxorubicin (Adriamycin = A). In some studies it was shown that AV is as effective as CMF,[24,54] and a two-drug combination of cyclophosphamide and vincristine can achieve a remission rate equivalent to a five-drug combination.[104]

A current effective combination yields a response rate of around 50% to 70% and a duration of response of 8 to 10 months. Following are three major areas of concern in combination chemotherapy: the plateau of response rates reached in the last half-decade[35] and the persistently low (less than 15%) com-

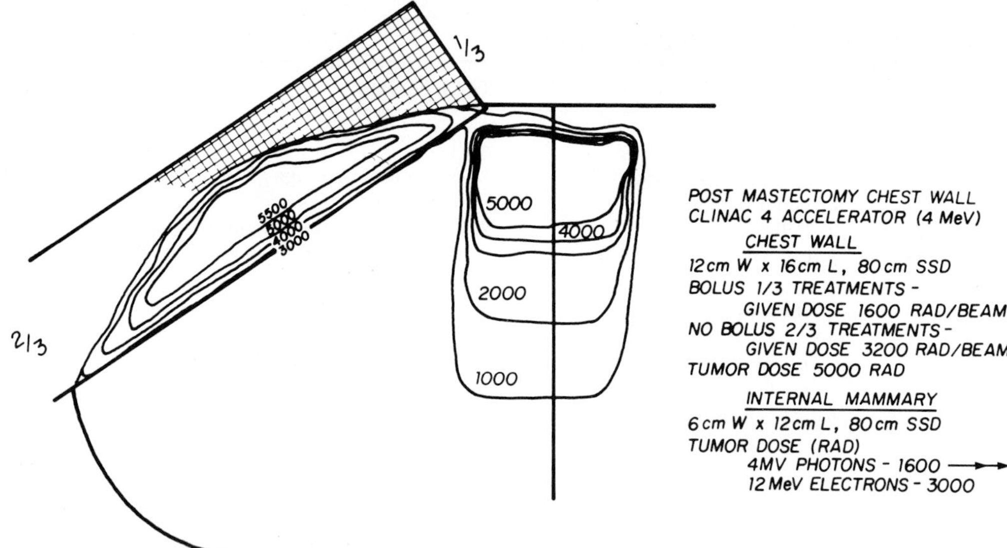

FIGURE 43–9. Isodose distribution of chest wall tangential and internal mammary fields.

plete remission rate; the lack of effective second-line chemotherapy; and the untoward side effects of chemotherapy.

Drugs frequently used for second-line chemotherapy are mitomycin-C, thiotepa, vinblastine, and dibromodulcitol.

Endocrine Therapy for Breast Cancer

Because of space limitations, this chapter cannot do justice to the literature on endocrine therapy; however, the reader should use the reference list to better appreciate the importance of adjuvant endocrine therapy in the treatment of breast cancer.

Harmsen and Porsius[95] noted four endocrine approaches in the treatment of breast cancer: additive therapy (progesterones, androgens, glucocorticoids, and high doses of estrogens), competitive therapy (antiestrogens), synthesis inhibition (aromatase inhibitors, LH-RH agonists, danazol, bromocriptine), and ablative therapy (oophorectomy, ovarian irradiation, adrenalectomy, and hypophysectomy).

Additive Agents

It has been known for some time that certain cancers are partly under the control of hormones. The cells of the normal mammary gland contain receptors for estrogen, progesterone, androgens, glucocorticoids, and prolactin.[95] The stimulating effect of estradiol (E_2) on well-differentiated breast cancers is well established and endocrine therapy is directed against this hormone. Medroxyprogesterone exerts the endometrium-transforming antiestrogenic, antiandrogenic, and antigonadotropic effects and glucocorticoid-like effects. Testosterone exerts endometrium-transforming estrogenic, antiestrogenic, androgenic, and antigonadotropic effects.[95]

For the most part, hormones have been used in advanced cancer therapy. However, with the use of estrogen and progesterone receptors, it is recommended that hormonal therapy be considered in patients at high risk of recurrence after local control of early stage cancer.

TABLE 43–8
Breast Cancer Total Relapse-free Survival Rates From CMF Adjuvant Chemotherapy

SUBGROUP	CONTROL (%)	CMF (%)	P
NUMBER OF NODES (+)			
1–3	38.5	53.6	0.001
>3	14.1	23.3	0.02
MENOPAUSAL STATUS			
Premenopausal	31.9	52.9	0.0001
Postmenopausal	31.1	34.9	0.24
Total	31.3	48.8	0.0003

CMF: cyclophosphamide, methotrexate, and 5-fluorouracil
(Bonadonna G, Valagussa P: Int J Radiat Oncol Biol Phys 3:279, 1983)

Antiestrogens

Tamoxifen is the most frequently used antiestrogen agent. Antiestrogens act as antagonists or partial agonists of circulating estrogens. The precise mechanism of action of tamoxifen is unknown. It has been hypothesized that it competes with estradiol for the cytoplasmic and nuclear estrogen receptor (ER). It is possible that there are other effects because some ER-negative tumors have been affected by tamoxifen.

The most significant side effect of tamoxifen is the possibility of developing hypercalcemia, which becomes evident a few days after treatment. Tamoxifen has been reported to be a risk factor for development of the carcinoma of corpus uteri in a Swedish report.

The Scottish Cancer Trials[13] office reported that 1312 patients under 80 years old received adjuvant tamoxifen or tamoxifen for the treatment of first relapse. They reported a highly significant delay in relapse in the adjuvant arm of the trial. This benefit superseded that from tamoxifen given as treatment for recurrent disease in control arm patients so that the benefit from tamoxifen was maintained in the overall survival rate comparisons. The improvement was independent of nodal and menopausal status. The greatest benefit in disease-free survival rate was in patients with levels of 100 fmol/mg per protein or more.

Medroxyprogesterone acetate is a progestin that requires

TABLE 43–9
Randomized Adjuvant Chemotherapy Trials in Postmenopausal Women with a Surgery-only Control Group

GROUP	STUDY OPTIONS	PREMENOPAUSAL WOMEN ALSO INCLUDED	NODE-NEGATIVE WOMEN ALLOWED	FOLLOW-UP TIME	OVERALL SURVIVAL RESULTS
NSABP	1. No Rx 2. L-PAM	Yes	No	>5 years	No difference
Milan	1. No Rx 2. CMF × 12	Yes	No	>5 years	No difference
Guys-Manchester	1. No Rx 2. L-PAM	Yes	No	Results projected to 5 years	No difference
Guys-Manchester	1. No Rx 2. CMF × 12	Yes	No	Results projected to 5 years	No difference
OSAKO	1. No Rx 2. LMF × 6 + BCG	Yes	Yes	>5 years	No difference
ECOG	1. No Rx 2. CMFP 3. CMFP + T	No	No	Results projected to 4 years	No difference
Ludwig Breast Cancer Group	1. No Rx 2. CMFP + T 3. P + T	No	No	Results projected to 5 years	No difference

L-PAM: L-phenylalanine mustard, melphalan; CMF: cyclophosphamide, methotrexate, 5-fluorouracil; P: prednisone; T: tamoxifen; L: Leukeran, chlorambucil
(Carter SK: Adjuvant chemotherapy for postmenopausal breast cancer—a disappointing clinical experiment. Proceedings of the 16th International Congress of Radiology, 1985)

estrogen priming. Drugs such as these work by producing differentiating effects in undifferentiated tissues.

Synthesis Inhibition

Aminoglutethimide is reported to perform medical adrenalectomy. It prevents conversion of cholesterol to pregnenolone in the adrenal gland and blocks the aromatase system, thereby inhibiting the extraglandular conversion of androstenedione to estrone, the chief source of estrogen production in postmenopausal women.

LH-RH agonists act to reduce steroid synthesis and decrease gonadotropin release.

Ablative Procedures

Pritchard[153] has identified Schinzinger as the first proponent of oophorectomy in 1889 for the treatment of breast cancer, which he recommended to be done at the time of the mastectomy. Oophorectomy or ovarian irradiation has an objective response rate of 53% in ER-positive tumors and 10% or less in ER-negative tumors.

Ovarian castration by irradiation has been used in conjunction with or without adjuvant radiation therapy to the breast in a number of centers in a number of trials.[116] One of the few surgical castration trials was conducted by Ravdin and associates.[155] Unfortunately it was a poorly designed and performed trial. As Levitt[116] pointed out, almost 700 patients were randomized for treatment; only 357 were judged eligible to participate. Use of castration in premenopausal women has not been adequately tested at this point and may never be.

Adrenalectomy (bilateral) has been found to be no more effective than aminoglutethimide therapy in conjunction with hydrocortisone. Hypophysectomy is no more effective than use of tamoxifen.

BREAST CARCINOMA IN THE MALE

Carcinoma of the breast accounts for only 0.2% of all cancers in men, with an annual sex-specific incidence of 0.58 cases per 100,000 males.[60] A study by Mabuchi and colleagues[124] of 52 histologically diagnosed cases with 52 controls conducted in five metropolitan United States areas found significantly more disease in Jewish than in non-Jewish controls. A significant association was found with mumps infection at the age of 20 years or older and in persons who have worked in blast furnaces, steel works, and rolling mills. It is commonly considered that Klinefelter's syndrome is a predisposing factor for male breast cancer and that gynecomastia is not. This view is supported in a recent report by van-Geel and associates.[198] Casagrande and coworkers[37] noted a relationship with obesity at age 30 and thought it was related to an increased exposure to available estrogen. Olsson and colleagues[143] noted a relationship between head trauma and prolactin-elevating drugs.

The pathologic types of breast cancer in men are essentially the same as those in women, including chromosome pattern, except that lobular carcinoma *in situ* is not found in men.[68]

The median age for breast carcinoma in men is the sixth decade; the most common presenting symptoms are a lump in the breast, nipple retraction, and local pain. The most common location of the tumor is central, perhaps due to the small size of the gland in the man. In a series conducted by Ribeiro,[157] 38% of 301 men presented with Stage I disease, 21% with Stage II disease, 26% with Stage III disease, and 15% with Stage IV disease. Estrogen and progesterone receptors were measured in 22 patients with male breast primary carcinoma and six skin metastases. Thirteen of the 16 primary tumors (81%) showed positive receptor activity (nine for both estrogen and progesterone receptors, three for estrogen receptor only, and one for progesterone receptor only). Three of the six metastatic tumors were positive for estrogen and three were positive for progesterone receptors.[157]

Treatment

As in women, the standard treatment for operable breast cancer in men has been a radical or modified radical mastectomy with or without postoperative radiation therapy.[97] Lumpectomy was performed in six of 89 patients reported on by Erlichman and associates[68]; 17 had a simple mastectomy; 46 had a modified radical mastectomy; and 16 had a radical mastectomy. Fifty-seven of the patients treated with surgery also had postoperative radiation therapy.

Patients with Stage III tumors are primarily treated with radiation therapy combined with chemotherapy or endocrine therapy. The benefit of adjuvant therapy in patients with positive axillary lymph nodes has not been documented. However, extrapolating from the experience in women, it is reasonable to expect some beneficial effect. Hormonal therapy with tamoxifen has been administered in patients with advanced tumors. An objective regression rate was noted in 37.5% of 24 patients (five complete and four partial responses).[158] Recent reports have noted a response of advanced male breast cancer to the LH-RH analogue Buserelin alone or in combination with the antiandrogen flutamide.[59]

Results

As in women, men have decreased survival with advanced clinical stage of breast cancer.[97,144] Ribeiro[157] reported a 10-year survival rate of 70% for Stage I disease, 45% for Stage II disease, and 10% for Stage III disease. As in women, the local relapse-free survival rate for patients treated with postoperative irradiation is superior to that of patients treated with surgery alone (Fig. 43-10). However, overall survival is not significantly influenced by adjuvant postoperative radiation therapy. Erlichman and associates[68] reported a 5-year survival rate of 78% in patients with negative lymph nodes compared with less than 40% in patients with positive axillary lymph nodes.

The incidence of local recurrence of breast cancer is approximately 20% in all patients and is correlated with the initial stage of the tumor. As in women, common metastatic sites are bone, lung, pleura, and brain. Erlichman and associates[68] reported no liver metastases in 46 of 89 patients who developed recurrences of their primary disease.

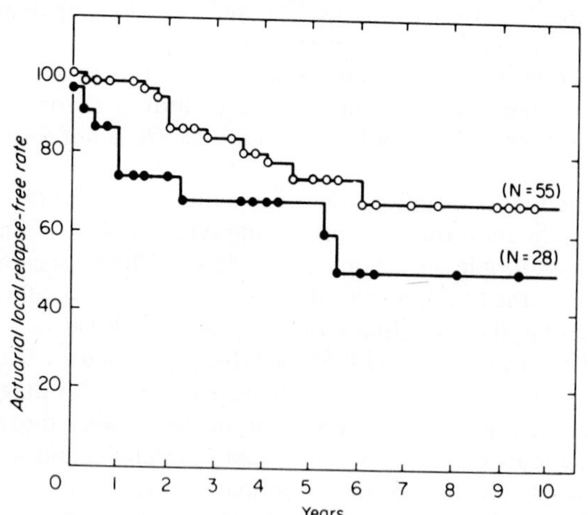

FIGURE 43–10. Survival of male patients with carcinoma of the breast, showing the efficacy of postoperative (open circles) irradiation in decreasing local recurrence. (Erlichman C, Murphy KC, Elhakim T: J Clin Oncol 2:903, 1984)

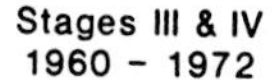

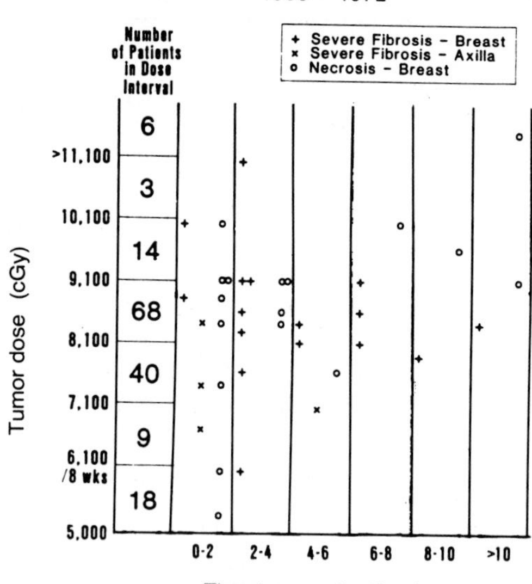

FIGURE 43–11. Time to complication versus dose in patients with locally advanced carcinoma of the breast treated with definitive irradiation alone. (Spanos WJ, Montague ED, Fletcher GH: Int J Radiat Oncol Biol Phys 6:1437–1476, 1980)

COMPLICATIONS OF RADIATION THERAPY

After definitive irradiation for advanced carcinoma of the breast at M. D. Anderson Cancer Center, 20% of patients developed severe subcutaneous fibrosis. Five to ten percent had rib fractures and symptomatic pneumonitis; a lower percentage had soft tissue and skin necrosis and ulceration.[137]

The incidence of fibrosis increases with dose[131] and may be noted even 5 and 10 years after the initial radiation therapy (Fig. 43-11). Patients treated with three weekly fractions had a higher incidence of late complications than those who received five weekly fractions.[181]

At the Joint Center at Harvard University, 1.4% of 565 patients developed symptomatic brachial plexopathy.[167] Most patients with this syndrome had received adjuvant chemotherapy before onset of symptoms.

REFERENCES

1. Aberizk WJ, Silver B, Henderson IC, et al: The use of radiotherapy for treatment of isolated localregional recurrence of breast cancer after mastectomy. Cancer 58:1214–1218, 1986
2. Ahmann D, O'Fallon S, Scanlon P, et al: A preliminary assessment of factors associated with recurrent disease in a surgical adjuvant clinical trial for patients with breast cancer with special emphasis on the aggressiveness of the therapy. Am J Clin Oncol 5:371–381, 1982
3. Ahmann DL, Scanlon PW, Bisel HF, et al: Repeated adjuvant chemotherapy with phenylalanine mustard or 5-fluorouracil, cyclophosphamide, and prednisone with or without radiation, after mastectomy for breast cancer. Lancet 1:893, 1978
4. Alderman S: Combination teletherapy and iridium implanta-

tion in the treatment of locally advanced breast cancer. Cancer 38:1936–1938, 1976

5. Allen H, Brooks R, Jones SE, et al: Adjuvant treatment for stage II (node positive) breast cancer with Adriamycin-cyclophosphamide (AC) ± radiotherapy (XRT). In Salmon SE, Jones SE (eds): Adjuvant Therapy of Cancer III, pp 453–462. New York, Grune & Stratton, 1981
6. Allen R, Nixon D, York M, Coleman J: Successful chemotherapy for cystosarcoma phyllodes in a young women. Arch Intern Med 145:1127–1128, 1985
7. American Joint Committee: Manual for Staging of Cancer, 3rd ed, pp 145–150. Philadelphia, JB Lippincott, 1988
8. Arriagada R, Le MG, Mouriesse H, et al: Long-term effect of internal mammary chain treatment: Results of a multivariate analysis of 1195 patients with operable breast cancer and positive axillary nodes. Radiother Oncol 11:213–222, 1988
9. Azzopardi JG: Problems in breast pathology. In Bennington JL (ed): Major Problems in Pathology. 11:355–359, 1979
10. Baclesse F: Roentgen therapy as the sole method of treatment of cancer of the breast. Am J Roentgenol 62:311–319, 1949
11. Baker RR, Holmes ER 3d, Alderson PO, et al: An evaluation of bone scans as screening procedures for occult metastases in primary breast cancer. Ann Surg 186:363–368, 1977
12. Balawajder I, Antich PP, Boland J: An analysis of the role of radiotherapy alone and in combination with chemotherapy in the management of advanced breast carcinoma. Cancer 51:574–580, 1983
13. Bartlett K, Eremin O, Hutcheon A, et al: Adjuvant tamoxifen in the management of operable breast cancer: The Scottish trial. Lancet 2(8552):171–175, 1987
14. Bedwinek JM: Treatment of stage I and II adenocarcinoma of the breast by tumor excision and irradiation. Int J Radiat Oncol Biol Phys 7:1553, 1981
15. Bedwinek JM, Fineberg B, Lee J, et al: Analysis of failures following local treatment of isolated local-regional recurrence of breast cancer. Int J Radiat Oncol Biol Phys 7:581, 1981
16. Bedwinek JM, Lee J, Fineberg B, Ocwieza M: Prognostic indicators in patients with isolated local-regional recurrence of breast cancer. Cancer 47:2232–2235, 1981
17. Bedwinek J, Rao DV, Perez C, et al: Stage III and localized stage IV breast cancer: Irradiation alone vs irradiation plus surgery. Int J Radiat Oncol Biol Phys 8:31–36, 1982
18. Bonadonna G, Valagussa P: Dose-response effect of adjuvant chemotherapy in breast cancer. N Engl J Med 304:11, 1981
19. Bonadonna G, Valagussa P: Chemotherapy of breast cancer: Current views and results. Int J Radiat Oncol Biol Phys 3:279, 1983
20. Bonadonna G, Valagussa, Rossi A, et al: Multimodal therapy with CMF in resectable breast cancer with positive axillary nodes: The Milan Institute experience. Recent results. Cancer Res 80: 149, 1982
21. Bonadonna G, Valagussa P, Rossi A, et al: Ten-year experience with CMF-based adjuvant chemotherapy in resectable breast cancer. Breast Cancer Res Treat 5:95, 1985
22. Boyages J, Langlands AO: The efficacy of combined chemotherapy and radiotherapy in advanced non-metastatic breast cancer. Int J Radiat Oncol Biol Phys 14:71–78, 1988
23. Boyer AL, Fullerton GD, Mira JG: An electron beam pseudoarc technique for irradiation of large areas of chest wall and other curved surfaces. Int J Radiat Oncol Biol Phys 8:1969–1974, 1982
24. Brambilla C, DeLena M, Rossi A, et al: Response and survival in advanced breast cancer after two non-cross resistant combinations. Br Med J 1:801, 1976
25. Brendel AJ, Leccia F, Drouillard J: Single photon emission computed tomography (SPECT), planar scintigraphy, and transmission computed tomography: A comparison of accuracy in diagnosing focal hepatic disease. Radiology 153:527–532, 1982
26. Bruce J, Carter DC, Fraser J: Patterns of recurrent disease in breast cancer. Lancet 1:433–435, 1970
27. Bruckman JE, Harris JR, Levene MB, et al: Results of treating stage III carcinoma of the breast by primary radiation therapy. Cancer 43:985–993, 1979
28. Brun B, Otmezguine Y, Feuilhade F, et al: Treatment of inflammatory breast cancer with combination chemotherapy and mastectomy versus breast conservation. Cancer 61:1096–1103, 1988
29. Buell U, Niendorf HP, Kazner E, et al: Computerized transaxial tomography and cerebral serial scintigraphy in intracranial tumors—rates of detection and tumor-type identification: Concise communication. J Nucl Med 19:476–479, 1978
30. Burton GV, Hart LL, Leight GS, et al: Cystosarcoma phyllodes. Effective therapy with cisplatin and etoposide chemotherapy. Cancer 63:2088–2092, 1989
31. Butzelaar RMJM, Van Dongen JA, Van der Schoot JB, Van Ulden BJG: Evaluation of routine preoperative bone scintigraphy in patients with breast cancer. Eur J Cancer 13:19, 1977
32. Budzar A, Smith T, Blumenschein G, et al: Adjuvant chemotherapy with fluorouracil, doxorubicin, and cyclophosphamide (FAC) for stage II or III breast cancer: 5-year results. In Salmon SE, Jones SE (eds): Adjuvant Therapy of Cancer, p 419. New York, Grune & Stratton, 1981
33. Buzdar AU, Blumenschein GR, Smith TL, et al: Adjuvant chemotherapy with fluorouracil, doxorubicin, and cyclophosphmide, with or without BCG and with or without irradiaton in operable breast Ca. A prospective randomized trial. Cancer 53:384–389, 1984
34. Buzdar AU, Montague ED, Barker JL, et al: Management of inflammatory carcinoma of breast with combined modality approach—an update. Cancer 47:2537–2542, 1981
35. Carbonne PP, Bauer M, Band P, et al: Chemotherapy of disseminated breast cancer. Cancer 39:2916, 1977
36. Carter SK: Adjuvant chemotherapy for postmenopausal breast cancer: A disappointing clinical experiment. Proceedings of the 16th International Congress of Radiology, 1985
37. Casagrande JT, Hanisch R, Pike MC, et al: A case-control study of the male breast cancer. Cancer Res 48:1326–1330, 1988
38. Chen KK-Y, Montague ED, Oswald MJ: Results of irradiation in the treatment of locoregional breast cancer recurrence. Cancer 56:1269, 1985
39. Chevallier B, Heintzmann F, Mosseri V, et al: Prognostic value of estrogen and progesterone receptors in operable breast cancer. Cancer 62:2517–2524, 1988
40. Chu AM, Cope O, Doucette J, Curran B: Non-metastatic locally advanced cancer of the breast treated with radiation. Int J Radiat Oncol Biol Phys 10:2299–2304, 1984
41. Chu FCH, Lin F-J, Kim JH, et al: Locally recurrent carcinoma of the breast: Results of radiation therapy. Cancer 37:2677–2681, 1976
42. Citrin DL, Tormey DC, Carbone PP: Implications of the ^{99}mTc diphosphonate bone scan on treatment of primary breast cancer. Cancer Treat Rep 61:1249, 1977
43. Clark GM, McGuire WL: Steroid receptors and other prognostic factors in primary breast cancer. Semin Oncol 15(Suppl 1):20–25, 1988
44. Cohn I, Slack NYH, Fisher B: Complications and toxic manifestations of surgical adjuvant chemotherapy for breast cancer. Surg Gynecol Obstet 127:1201, 1968
45. Conte G, Nascimben O, Turcato G, et al: Three-field isocentric technique for breast irradiation using individualized shielding blocks. Int J Radiat Oncol Biol Phys 14:1299–1305, 1988
46. Cooper MR, Muss H, Ferree C, et al: A six and one half year follow-up of a randomized adjuvant study of chemotherapy with or without radiation therapy for stage II breast cancer (Abstract). Breast Cancer Res Treat 6:169, 1985
47. Cooper MR, Rhyne AL, Muss HB, et al: A randomized comparative trial of chemotherapy and irradiation therapy for stage II breast cancer. Cancer 47:2833–2839, 1981
48. Curtis RE, Hankey BF, Myers MH, et al: Risk of leukemia associated with the first course of cancer treatment: An analysis of the surveillance, epidemiology and end results section. J Natl Cancer Inst 72:531, 1984
49. Cutler SJ, Asire AJ, Taylor SG: Classification of patients with disseminated cancer of the breast. Cancer 24:861–869, 1969
50. Cuzick J, Steward H, Peto R, et al: Overview of randomized trials comparing radical mastectomy without radiotherapy

against simple mastectomy with radiotherapy in breast cancer. Cancer Treat Rep 71:7–14, 1987

51. Cuzick J, Stewart H, Peto R, et al: Overview of randomized trials of postoperative adjuvant radiotherapy in breast cancer. Cancer Treat Rep 71:15–25, 1987
52. Danoff BF: The role of radiotherapy in the management of locally advanced nonmetastatic breast cancer. In Levitt S (ed): Syllabus. A Categorical Course in Breast Cancer. Radiological Society of North America Proceedings, Radiological Society of North America, Oak Brook, Illinois, 1984
53. Danoff-Fowble B: The role of radiotherapy in the treatment and prevention of local-regional recurrence following mastectomy for operable breast cancer. Int J Radiat Oncol Biol Phys 12:2209–2210, 1986
54. De Lena M, Brambilla C, Morabito A, et al: Adriamycin plus vincristine compared to and combined with cyclophosphamide, methrotrexate, and 5-flourouracil for advanced breast cancer. Cancer 35:1108, 1975
55. De Lena M, Varini M, Zucali R, et al: Multimodal treatment for locally advanced breast cancer: Results of chemotherapy-radiotherapy versus chemotherapy-surgery. Cancer Clin Trials 4:229–236, 1981
56. De Lena M, Zucali R, Viganotti C, et al: Combined chemotherapy-radiotherapy in locally advanced (T3b-T4) breast cancer. Cancer Chemother Pharmacol 1:53–59, 1978
57. Derman DP, Browde S, Kessel IL, et al: Adjuvant chemotherapy (CMF) for stage III breast cancer: A randomized trial. Int J Radiat Oncol Biol Phys 17:257–261, 1989
58. Deutsch M, Parsons JA, Mittal BB: Radiation therapy for local-regional recurrent breast carcinoma. Int J Radiat Oncol Biol Phys 12:2061–2065, 1986
59. Doberauer C, Niederle N, Schmidt CG: Advanced male breast cancer treatment with the LH-RH analogue Buserelin alone or in combination with the antiandrogen flutamide. Cancer 62:474–478, 1988
60. Donegan WL, Perez-Mesa CM: Carcinoma of the male breast. Arch Surg 106:273, 1973
61. Donegan WL, Perez-Mesa CM, Watson FR: A biostatistical study of locally recurrent breast carcinoma. Surg Gynecol Obstet 122:529, 1966
62. Dragovic J, Seydel HG, Sandhu T, Kdosvary A, Blough J: Local superficial hyperthermia in combination with low-dose radiation therapy for palliation of locally recurrent breast carcinoma. J Clin Oncol 7:30–35, 1989
63. Dressler LG, Seamer LC, Owens MA, et al: DNA flow cytometry and prognostic factors in 1331 frozen breast cancer specimens. Cancer 61:420–427, 1988
64. Drewinko B, Patchen M, Yang LY, et al: Differential killing efficacy of 20 antitumor drugs or proliferating and nonproliferating human tumor cells. Cancer Res 41:2328, 1981
65. Dyer NH, Bridges EI, Taylor RS: Cystosarcoma phyllodes. Br J Surg 53:450–455, 1966
66. Eby C, Brennen M, Fine G: Lymphangiogiosarcoma: A lethal complication of chronic lymphedema. Arch Surg 94:223, 1977
67. Ellis DL, Teitelbaum SL: Inflammatory carcinoma of the breast: A pathologic definition. Cancer 33:1045–1047, 1974
68. Erlichman C, Murphy KC, Elhakim T: Male breast cancer: A 13-year review of 89 patients. J Clin Oncol 2:903, 1984
69. Fallenius AG, Auer GU, Carstensen JM: Prognostic significance of DNA measurements in 409 consecutive breast cancer patients. Cancer 62:331–341, 1988
70. Fastenberg NA, Martin RG, Buzdar AU, et al: Management of inflammatory carcinoma of the breast: A combined modality approach. Am J Clin Oncol 8:134–141, 1985
71. Feig SA: The role of new imaging modalities in staging and follow-up of breast cancer. Semin Oncol 13:402–414, 1986
72. Fields JN, Kuske RR, Perez CA, et al: Prognostic factors in inflammatory breast cancer: Univariate and multivariate analysis. Cancer 63:1225–1232, 1989
73. Fields JN, Perez CA, Kuske RR, et al: Inflammatory carcinoma of the breast: Treatment results on 107 patients. Int J Radiat Oncol Biol Phys 17:249–255, 1989
74. Fisher B, Wolmark N, Bauer M, et al: The accuracy of clinical nodal staging and of limited axillary dissection as a determinant of histological nodal status in carcinoma of the breast. Surg Gynecol Obstet 152:765, 1981
75. Fisher ER, Sass R, Fisher B: Pathologic Findings from the National Surgical Adjuvant Breast Project. Cancer 59:1554–1559, 1987
76. Fletcher GH: Clinical dose-response curves of human malignant epithelial tumors. Br J Radiol 46:1, 1973
77. Fletcher GH, McNeese MD, Osward MJ: Long-range results for breast cancer patients treated by radical mastectomy and postoperative radiation without adjuvant chemotherapy: An update. Int J Radiat Oncol Biol Phys 17:11–14, 1989
78. Fletcher GH, Montague ED: Does adequate irradiation of the internal mammary chain and supraclavicular nodes improve survival rates? Int J Radiat Oncol Biol Phys 4:481–492, 1979
79. Fowble B, Glick J, Goodman R: Radiotherapy for the prevention of local-regional recurrence in high risk patients post mastectomy receiving adjuvant chemotherapy. Int J Radiat Oncol Biol Phys 15:627–631, 1988
80. Fowble B, Gray R, Gilchrist K, et al: Identification of a subgroup of patiens with breast cancer and histologically positive axillary nodes receiving adjuvant chemotherapy who may benefit from postoperative radiotherapy. J Clin Oncol 6:1107–1117, 1988
81. Fracchia AA, Evans TF, Eisenbert BL: Stage III carcinoma of the breast: A detailed analysis. Ann Surg 192:705–710, 1980
82. Garewal HS, Takasugi B, Jones SE, et al: Is T3N0M0 breast cancer with pathologically negative nodes truely stage III? (Letter). J Clin Oncol 2:242–243, 1984
83. Ghossein NA, Stacey P, Alpert S, et al: Local control of breast cancer with tumorectomy plus radiotherapy or radiotherapy alone. Radiology 121:455–459, 1976
84. Glucksberg H, Rivkin SE, Rasmussen S, et al: Combination chemotherapy (CMFVP) versus L-phenylalanine mustard (L-pAM) for operable breast cancer with positive axillary nodes: A Southwest Oncology Group Study. Cancer 50:423, 1982
85. Gonzalez DG, van Dijk JDP, Blank LECM: Chest wall recurrences of breast cancer: Results of combined treatment with radiation and hyperthermia. Radiother Oncol 12:95–103, 1988
86. Griem KL, Henderson IC, Gelman R, et al: The 5-year results of a randomized trial of adjuvant radiation therapy after chemotherapy in breast cancer patients treated with mastectomy. J Clin Oncol 5:1546–1555, 1987
87. Griscom NT, Wang CC: Radiation therapy of inoperable breast carcinoma. Radiology 79:18–23, 1962
88. Grohn P, Heinonen E, Klefstrom P, Tarkkanen J: Adjuvant postoperative radiotherapy, chemotherapy, and immunotherapy in stage III breast cancer. Cancer 54:670–674, 1984
89. Haagensen CD: Cystosarcoma phyllodes. In Haagensen CD (ed): Diseases of the Breast, 3rd ed, pp 284–312. Philadelphia, WB Saunders, 1986
90. Haagensen CD: Diseases of the Breast, 2nd ed. Philadelphia, WB Saunders, 1971
91. Haagensen CD, Stout AP: Carcinoma of the breast. I. Results of treatment. Ann Surg 116:801, 1942
92. Hafner CD, Mezger E, Wylil JH: Cystosarcoma phyllodes of the breast. Surg Gynecol Obstet 115:29–34, 1962
93. Hajdu SI, Espinosa MH, Robbins GF: Recurrent cystosarcoma phyllodes: A clinicopathologic study of 32 cases. Cancer 38:1402–1406, 1976
94. Halverson KJ, Perez CA, Kuske RR, et al: Isolated local-regional recurrence of breast cancer following mastectomy: Radiotherapeutic management. Int J Radiat Oncol Biol Phys 0:00-00, 1990
95. Harmsen HJ, Porsius AJ: Endocrine therapy of breast cancer. Eur J Cancer Clin Oncol 24:1099–1116, 1988
96. Henderson IC, Canellos GP: Cancer of the breast: The past decade. N Engl J Med 302:78, 1980
97. Hodson G, Urdaneta L, Alijurf A, et al: Male breast carcinoma. Am Surg 51:47, 1985
98. Hoover HC, Trestioreanu A, Ketcham AS: Metastatic cystosarcoma phyllodes in an adolescent girl: An unusual malignant tumor. Ann Surg 181:279–282, 1975

99. Hortobagyi GN, Blumenschein GR, Spanos W, et al: Multimodal treatment of locoregionally advanced breast cancer. Cancer 51:763–768, 1983
100. Host H, Brennhovd IO: The effect of postoperative radiotherapy in breast cancer. Int J Radiat Oncol Biol Phys 2:1061–1067, 1977
101. Host H, Brennhovd IO, Loeb M: Postoperative radiotherapy in breast cancer: Long-term results from the Oslo Study. Int J Radiat Oncol Biol Phys 12:727–732, 1986
102. Hunt MA, Kutcher GJ, Martel KM: Matchline dosimetry of a three field technique for breast treatment using cobalt or 6 MV x-rays. Int J Radiat Oncol Biol Phys 13:1099–1106, 1987
103. Janjan NA, McNeese MD, Buzdar AU, et al: Management of locoregional recurrent breast cancer. Cancer 58:1552–1556, 1986
104. Jones SE, Durie BGM, Salmon SE: Combination chemotherapy with Adriamycin and cyclophosphamide for advanced breast cancer. Cancer 36:90, 1975
105. Kenda JFN: Fatal metastatic cystosarcoma phyllodes in a young woman. Arch Surg 118:871–872, 1983
106. Kessinger A, Foley JF, Lemon HM, Miller DM: Metastatic cystosarcoma phyllodes: A case report and review of the literature. J Surg Oncol 4:131–147, 1972
107. Khan FK: The Physics of Radiation Therapy, p 326. Baltimore, Williams & Wilkins, 1984
108. Kiang DT, Frenning DH, Goldman AI, et al: Estrogen receptors and responses to chemotherapy and hormonal therapy in advanced breast cancer. N Engl J Med 299:1330, 1978
109. Klefstrom P, Grohn P, Heinonen E, Holsti L, Holsti P: Adjuvant postoperative radiotherapy, chemotherapy, and immunotherapy in stage III breast cancer. II. 5-year results and influence of levamisole. Cancer 60:936–942, 1987
110. Knopf DR, Torres WE, Fajman WJ, et al: Liver lesions: Comparative accuracy of scintigraphy and computed tomography. AJR 138:623–627, 1982
111. Lacour J, Bucalossi P, Caceres E, et al: Radical mastectomy versus radical mastectomy plus internal mammary dissection: Five year results of an international cooperative study. Cancer 37:206–214, 1976
112. Lacour J, Le MG, Hill C, et al: Is it useful to remove the internal mammary nodes for operable breast cancer patients? Eur J Surg Oncol 13:309–314, 1987
113. Leavitt DD, Peacock LM, Gibbs FA Jr, Stewart JR: Electron arc therapy: Physical measurement and treatment planning techniques. Int J Radiat Oncol Biol Phys 11:987–999, 1985
114. Leavitt DD, Stewart JR: Optimization of electron arc therapy doses by multi-vane collimator control. Int J Radiat Oncol Biol Phys 16:489–496, 1989
115. Lebesque JV: Field matching in breast irradiation: An exact solution to a geometric problem. Radiother Oncol 5:47–57, 1986
116. Levitt SH: Controversies in the treatment of breast cancer: A need for return to the three R's in clinical research. Am J Clin Oncol 7:583–591, 1984
117. Levitt SH: The role of radiation therapy as an adjuvant in the treatment of breast cancer. Int J Radiat Oncol Biol Phys 12:843–844, 1986
118. Levitt SH: Is there a role for post-operative adjuvant radiation in breast cancer? Beautiful hypothesis versus ugly facts: 1987 Gilbert H. Fletcher Lecture. Int J Radiat Oncol Biol Phys 14:787–796, 1988
119. Levitt SH, McHugh RB: Radiotherapy in the postoperative treatment of operable cancer of the breast. I. Critique of the clinical and biometric aspects of the trials. Cancer 39:924–932, 1977
120. Levitt SH, McHugh RB, Song CW: Radiotherapy in the postoperative treatment of operable cancer of the breast. II. A reexamination of Stjernsward's application of the Mantel-Haenszel statistical method. Evaluation of the effect of the radiation on immune response and suggestions for postoperative radiotherapy. Cancer 39:933–940, 1977
121. Lichter AS, Fraass BA, Van de Geijn J, Padikal TN: A technique for field matching in primary breast irradiation. Int J Radiat Oncol Biol Phys 9:263–270, 1983
122. Lippman ME, Allegra JC, Thompson EB, et al: The relation between estrogen receptors and response rate to cytotoxic chemotherapy in metastatic breast cancer. N Engl J Med 298:1223, 1978
123. Lucas FV, Perez-Mesa C: Inflammatory carcinoma of the breast. Cancer 41:1595–1605, 1978
124. Mabuchi K, Bross D, Kessler I: Risk factors for male breast cancer. J Natl Cancer Inst 74:371, 1985
125. Magno L, Bignardi M, Micheletti E, et al: Analysis of prognostic factors in patients with isolated chest wall recurrence of breast cancer. Cancer 60:240–244, 1987
126. Maier WP, Rosemont GP, Wittemberg P, Tassoni EM: Cystosarcoma phyllodes mammae. Oncology 22:145–157, 1968
127. Marcial VA, Velez-Garcia E, Moore M, et al: Radiotherapy related adjuvant chemotherapy initiation delay in breast cancer with positive nodes: Does it affect prognosis? A Southeastern Cancer Study Group report (Abstract). Int J Radiat Oncol Biol Phys 11:150, 1985
128. Martin MB, Kon ND, Kawamoto EH, et al: Postmastectomy angiosarcoma. Am Surg 50:541, 1984
129. McArdle CS, Calman KC, Cooper AF, et al: The social, emotional and financial implications of adjuvant chemotherapy in breast cancer. Br J Surg 68:261, 1981
130. McArdle CS, Crawford D, Dykes EH, et al: Adjuvant radiotherapy and chemotherapy in breast cancer. Br J Surg 73:264–266, 1986
131. McDivitt RW, Urban JA, Farrow JH: Cystosarcoma phyllodes. John Hopkins Med J 120:33–45, 1987
132. McGuire WL: Physiological principles underlying endocrine therapy of breast cancer. In McGuire WL (ed): Breast Cancer: Advances in Research and Treatment, vol 1, Current Approaches to Therapy, p 217. New York, Plenum Press, 1977
133. McGuire WL, Clark GM, Dressler LG, Owens MA: Role of steroid hormone receptors as prognostic factors in primary breast cancer. NCI Monogr 1:19–23, 1986
134. McGuire WL, Dickson RB, Osborne CK, Salomon D: The role of growth factors in breast cancer. Breast Cancer Res Treat 12:159–166, 1988
135. McNeely LK, Jacobson GM, Leavitt DD, Stewart JR: Electron arc therapy: Chest wall irradiation of breast cancer patients. Int J Radiat Oncol Biol Phys 14:1287–1294, 1988
136. Meyer JS, Friedman MS, McCrate MM, et al: Prediction of early course of breast carcinoma by thymidine labeling. Cancer 51:1819, 1983
137. Montague ED: Experience with altered fractionation in radiation therapy of breast cancer. Radiology 90:962, 1968
138. Monyak D, Levitt S: The changing role of radiation therapy in the treatment of primary breast cancer. Invest Radiol 24:483–494, 1989
139. Morris T: Psychological adjustment to mastectomy. Cancer Treat Rev 6:41, 1979
140. Muss H, Cooper R, Ferree C, et al: Long-term follow-up of L-PAM and CMF with and without radiation therapy as adjuvant treatment for stage II breast carcinoma (Abstract). Proc Am Soc Clin Oncol 3:117, 1984
141. Nobler MP, Venet L: Twelve years' experience with irradiation as the primary treatment for breast cancer. Int J Radiat Oncol Biol Phys 7:33–42, 1981
142. Norris HY, Taylor H: Relationship of histologic features to behavior of cystosarcoma phyllodes: Analysis of ninety-four cases. Cancer 20:2090–2099, 1967
143. Olsson H, Ranstam J: Head trauma and exposure to prolectin-elevating drugs as risk factors for male breast cancer. J Natl Cancer Inst 683, 1988
144. Ouriel K, Lotze M, Hinshaw J: Prognostic factors of carcinoma of the male breast. Surg Gynecol Obstet 159:373, 1984
145. Papaioannou A, Lissaios B, Vasilaros S, et al: Pre- and postoperative chemoendocrine treatment with or without postoperative radiotherapy for locally advanced breast cancer. Cancer 51:1284–1290, 1983
146. Patanaphan V, Salazar OM, Poussin-Rosillo H: Prognosticators in recurrent breast cancer: A 15-year experience with irradiation. Cancer 54:228–234, 1984
147. Peacock LM, Leavitt DD, Gibbs FA Jr, Stewart JR: Electron are

therapy: Clinical experience with chest wall irradiation. Int J Radiat Oncol Biol Phys 10:2149–2153, 1984
148. Perez C, Presant C, Philpott G, Ratkin G: Phase I–II study of concurrent irradiation and multi-drug chemotherapy in advanced carcinoma of the breast: A pilot study of the Southeastern Cancer Study Group. Int J Radiat Oncol Biol Phys 5:1329–1333, 1979
149. Perez CA, Kuske RR, Emami B, et al: Irradiation alone vs combined with hyperthermia in the treatment of recurrent carcinoma of the breast in the chest wall. Int J Hypertherm 2:179, 1986
150. Perloff M, Lesnick GJ, Korzun A, et al: Combination chemotherapy with mastectomy or radiotherapy for stage III breast carcinoma: A Cancer and Leukemia Group B Study. J Clin Oncol 6:261–269, 1988
151. Pietruszka M, Barnes L: Cystosarcoma phyllodes: A clinicopathologic analysis of 42 cases. Cancer 41:1974–1983, 1974
152. Potts DG, Abbott GF, von Sneidern JV: National Cancer Institute study: Evaluation of computed tomography in the diagnosis of intracranial neoplasms. Radiology 136:657–664, 1980
153. Pritchard KI: Current status of adjuvant endocrine therapy for resectable breast cancer. Semin Oncol 14:23–33, 1987
154. Rao DV, Bedwinek J, Perez C, et al: Prognostic indicators in stage III and localized stage IV breast cancer. Cancer 50:2037–2043, 1982
155. Ravdin RG, Lewison EF, Slack NH, et al: Results of a clinical trial concerning the worth of prophylactic oophorectomy for breast carcinoma. Surg Gynecol Obstet 131:1055–1064, 1970
156. Recht A, Hayes DF: Local recurrence. In Harris J, Hellman F, Henderson IC, Kinne DW (eds): Breast Diseases, pp 508–524. Philadelphia, JB Lipppincott, 1987
157. Ribeiro G: Male breast carcinoma: A review of 301 cases from the Christie Hospital and Holt Radium Institute, Manchester. Clin Radiol 51:115, 1985
158. Ribeiro GG: Tamoxifen in the treatment of male breast carcinoma. Clin Radiol 34:625, 1983
159. Rodger A, Stewart HJ, White GK: The efficacy of delayed radiotherapy for locoregionally recurrent postmastectomy breast cancer. Int J Radiat Oncol Biol Phys 14:665–667, 1988
160. Rosenfeld JC, De Laurentis DA, Lerner H: Cystosarcoma phyllodes: Diagnosis and management. Cancer Clin Trials 4:187–193, 1981
161. Rouesse J, Friedman S, Sarrazin D, et al: Primary chemotherapy in the treatment of inflammatory breast carcinoma: A study of 230 cases from the Institut Gustave-Roussy. J Clin Oncol 4:1765–1771, 1986
162. Rubens RD, Armitage P, Winter PJ, et al: Prognosis in inoperable stage III carcinoma of the breast. Eur J Cancer 13:805–811, 1977
163. Rubens RD, Knight RK, Hayward JL: Chemotherapy of advanced breast cancer: A controlled randomized trial of cyclophosphamide versus a four-drug combination. Br J Cancer 32:730, 1975
164. Rubens RD, Sexton S, Tong D, et al: Combined chemotherapy and radiotherapy for locally advanced breast cancer. Eur J Cancer 46:351–356, 1980
165. Rutqvist LE, Cedemark B, Glas U, et al: Radiotherapy, chemotherapy, and tamoxifen as adjuncts to surgery in early breast cancer: A summary of three randomized trials. Int J Radiat Oncol Biol Phys 16:629–639, 1989
166. Sainsbury JRC, Farndon JR, Needham GK, et al: Epidermal growth factor receptor status as predictor of early recurrence of and death from breast cancer. Lancet 1:1398–1402, 1987
167. Salner A, Botwick L, Herzog A, et al: Reversible brachial plexopathy following primary radiation therapy for breast cancer. Cancer Treat Rep 65:797, 1981
168. Salvadori B, Cusumano F, Del Bo R, et al: Surgical treatment of phyllodes tumors of the breast. Cancer 63:2532–2536, 1989
169. Sanger C, Rasnikoff M: A comparison of the psychological effects of breast-saving procedures with the modified radical mastectomy. Cancer 48:2341, 1981
170. Say C, Donegan W: A biostatistical evaluation of complications from mastectomy. Surg Gynecol Obstet 138:370, 1974
171. Schaake-Koning C, van der Linden EH, Hart G, Engelsman E: Adjuvant chemo- and hormonal therapy in locally advanced breast cancer: A randomized clinical study. Int J Radiat Oncol Biol Phys 11:1759–1763, 1985
172. Schabel FM: Concepts for systemic treatment of micrometastases. Cancer 35:15, 1976
173. Schafer P, Alberto P, Forni M, et al: Surgery as part of a combined modality approach for inflammatory breast carcinoma. Cancer 59:1063–1067, 1987
174. Scott RS, Johnson RJR, Story KV, et al: Local hyperthermia in combination with definitive radiotherapy: Increased tumor clearance, reduced recurrence rate in extended follow-up. Int J Radiat Oncol Biol Phys 10:2119–2123, 1984
175. Siddon RL, Buck BA, Harris JR, Svensson GK: Three-field technique for breast irradiation using tangential field corner blocks. Int J Radiat Oncol Biol Phys 9:583–588, 1983
176. Skipper HE: Kinetics of mammary tumor cell growth and implications for therapy. Cancer 28:1479, 1971
177. Slamon DJ, Clark GM, Wong SG, et al: Human breast cancer: Correlation of relapse and survival with amplification of the HER-2/neu oncogene. Science 235:177–182, 1987
178. Smalley RV, Murphy S, Huguley CM, et al: Combination versus sequential five-drug chemotherapy in metastatic carcinoma of the breast. Cancer Res 36:3911, 1976
179. Smith DC, Crawford D, Dykes EH, et al: Adjuvant radiotherapy and chemotherapy in breast cancer. In Jones SE, Salmon SE (eds): Adjuvant Therapy of Cancer IV, pp 283–289. New York, Grune & Stratton, 1984
180. Spangenberg JP, Nel CJC, Anderson JD, Doman MJ: A prospective study of the treatment of stage III breast cancer. S Afr J Surg 24:57–60, 1986
181. Spanos WJ, Montague ED, Fletcher GH: Late complications of radiation only for advanced breast cancer. Int J Radiat Oncol Biol Phys 6:1473–1476, 1980
182. Spitalier JM, Amalric R: Treatment of operable mammary carcinoma with conservation of the breast at the Cancer Institute of Marseille. In Marchant DJ, Myierjesy I (eds): Breast Disease, p 222. New York, Grune & Stratton, 1979
183. Stadler B, Kogelnik HD: Local control and outcome of patients irradiated for isolated chest wall recurrences of breast cancer. Radiother Oncol 8:105–111, 1987
184. Strender L-E, Wallgren A, Arndt J, et al: Adjuvant radiotherapy in operable breast cancer: Correlation between dose in internal mammary nodes and prognosis. Int J Radiat Oncol Biol Phys 7:1319–1325, 1981
185. Svensson GK, Chin LM, Siddon RL, et al: Breast treatment techniques at the Joint Center for Radiation Therapy. In Harris JR, Hellman S, Silen W (eds): Conservative Management of Breast Cancer: New Surgical and Radiotherapeutic Techniques, p 239. Philadelphia, JB Lippincott, 1983
186. Syed AMN, Puthawala A, Fleming P, et al: Combination of external and interstitial irradiation in the primary management of breast carcinoma. Cancer 46:1360, 1980
187. Syed AMN, Puthawala AA, Orr LE, et al: Primary irradiation in the management of early and locally advanced carcinoma of the breast. Br J Radiol 57:317–321, 1984
188. Tapley ND, Spanos WJ Jr, Fletcher GH, et al: Results in patients with breast cancer treated by radical mastectomy and postoperative irradiation with no adjuvant chemotherapy. Cancer 49:1316–1319, 1982
189. Thomas AMK, Ashworth BM, Blake P: Regression of recurrent cystosarcoma phyllodes after neutron therapy with development of benign calcification. Br J Radiol 57:926–929, 1984
190. Thoms WW Jr, McNeese MD, Fletcher GH, et al: Multimodal treatment for inflammatory breast cancer. Int J Radiat Oncol Biol Phys 17:739–745, 1989
191. Toonkel LM, Fix I, Jacobson LH, et al: Postoperative radiation therapy for carcinoma of the breast: Improved results with elective irradiation of the chest wall. Int J Radiat Oncol Biol Phys 8:977, 1982
192. Toonkel LM, Fix I, Jacobson LH, et al: The significance of

local recurrence of carcinoma of the breast. Int J Radiat Oncol Biol Phys 9:33–39, 1983

193. Tormey DC, Weinberg VE, Holland JF, et al: A randomized trial of five- and three-drug chemotherapy in women with operable node positive breast cancer. J Clin Oncol 1:138, 1983
194. Treurniet-Donker AD, Hop WCJ, Den Hoed-Sijtsema S: Radiation treatment of stage III mammary carcinoma: A review of 129 patients. Int J Radiat Oncol Biol Phys 6:1477–1482, 1980
195. Tubiana M, Arriagada R, Sarrazin D: Human cancer natural history, radiation induced immunodepression and post-operative radiation therapy. Int J Radiat Oncol Biol Phys 12:477–485, 1986
196. Valagussa P, Zambetti M, Pignami P, et al: T3b-T4 breast cancers: Factors affecting results in combined modality treatments. Clin Exp Metastasis 1:191–202, 1983
197. Van der Zee J, Treurniet-Donker AD, The SK, et al: Low dose reirradiation in combination with hyperthermia: A palliative treatment for patients with breast cancer recurring in previously irradiated areas. Int J Radiat Oncol Biol Phys 15:1407–1413, 1988
198. van-Geel A, van-Slooten E, Mavrunac M, et al: A retrospective study of male breast cancer in Holland. Br J Surg 72:724, 1985
199. Velez-Garcia E, Moore M, Vogel CL, et al: Post-mastectomy adjuvant chemotherapy with or without radiation therapy in women with operable breast cancer and positive axillary nodes: The Southeastern Cancer Study Group experience. Breast Cancer Res Treat 3:49–60, 1983
200. von Rosen A, Rutqvist LE, Carstensen J, et al: Prognostic value of nuclear DNA content in breast cancer in relation to tumor size, nodal status, and estrogen receptor content. Breast Cancer Res Treat 13:23–32, 1989
201. Wallgren A, Arner O, Bergstrom J, et al: The value of preoperative radiotherapy in operable breast cancer. Int J Radiat Oncol Biol Phys 6:287–290, 1980
202. Wallgren A, Arner O, Bergström J, et al: Radiation therapy in operable breast cancer: Results from the Stockholm trial on adjuvant radiotherapy. Int J Radiat Oncol Biol Phys 12:533–537, 1986
203. West TL, Weiland LH, Claget OT: Cystosarcoma phyllodes. Ann Surg 173:520–528, 1971
204. Winchester DP, Sener SF, Khandekar JD, et al: Symptomatology as an indicator of recurrent or metastatic breast cancer. Cancer 43:956–960, 1979
205. Witliff J: Steroid-hormone receptors in breast cancer. Cancer 53:630, 1984
206. World Health Organization: Histologic typing of breast tumors. Tumor 68:181–198, 1982
207. Woudstra E, Van der Werf H: Obliquely incident electron beams for irradiation of the internal mammary lymph nodes. Radiother Oncol 10:209–215, 1987

44

○ ○ ○ • • •

Stomach

Stephen R. Smalley
Leonard L. Gunderson

ANATOMY

The stomach begins at the gastroesophageal junction and ends at the pylorus. The stomach is usually apportioned into three parts. The cranial portion is the fundus. A plane passing through the incisura angularis on the lesser curvature divides the remainder of the stomach into the body and the pyloric portion. The anterior surface of the stomach is covered with peritoneum of the greater sac. At the left and cranially, it abuts the diaphragm. The right portion of the anterior surface is adjacent to the left of the liver and the anterior abdominal wall. Posteriorly, the stomach is covered with peritoneum of the lesser sac or omental bursa. The stomach contacts many important visceral structures; from superior to inferior, it is adjacent to the spleen, left adrenal gland, superior portion of the left kidney, ventral portion of the pancreas, and transverse colon. The hepatogastric ligament or lesser omentum is attached to the lesser curvature and contains the left gastric artery and right gastric branch of the hepatic artery.

The vascular supply of the stomach is derived from the celiac axis. The celiac artery usually has three branches: the left gastric artery, which supplies the upper right portion of the stomach; the common hepatic artery, which gives rise to the right gastric artery supplying the lower right portion of the stomach and right gastroepiploic branch, which supplies the lower portion of the greater curvature; and the splenic artery, which gives rise to the left gastroepiploic, which supplies the upper portion of the greater curvature, and the short gastric arteries, which supply the fundus. Variations in this normal vascular supply are common.

The lymphatic drainage of the stomach follows arterial supply. Although most lymphatics drain ultimately to the celiac nodal area, lymph drainage sites can include the splenic hilum, suprapancreatic nodal groups, porta hepatis, and gastroduodenal areas.

EPIDEMIOLOGY

In the United States, gastric cancer affected approximately 23,200 people in 1990 and resulted in about 13,700 deaths.[28] Age-adjusted gastric cancer death rates from 1930 to 1985 have decreased from approximately 28 to 5 in 100,000 females and 38 to 7 in 100,000 males. The causes of this decline, present in other industrialized countries as well, are unknown.[76]

Risk factors implicated include smoked and salted foods, low intake of fruit and vegetables, low socioeconomic status, and decreased use of refrigeration.[28,76] Pernicious anemia is associated with gastric cancer, with 5% to 10% of those with pernicious anemia developing malignancies. Prior subtotal gastrectomy for benign lesions also carries a 2% to 5% risk of subsequent malignancies, with latency periods of 15 to 40 years.[123] Villous adenomas are clearly premalignant; hyperplastic or hamartomatous polyps occur more frequently and are apparently benign. Finally, gastric ulcer may carry a small increased risk of malignancy.

DIAGNOSIS AND PATTERNS OF SPREAD

Cancer of the stomach may extend into the omenta, pancreas, diaphragm, transverse colon or mesocolon, and duodenum.

Peritoneal contamination is possible after a lesion extends beyond the gastric wall to a free peritoneal (serosal) surface.[115]

Microscopic or subclinical spread beyond the visible gross lesion occurs frequently because of the abundant lymphatic channels within the submucosal and subserosal layers of the gastric wall. The submucosal plexus is prominent in the esophagus and the subserosal plexus in the duodenum, allowing proximal and distal spread.

It is difficult to do a complete node dissection because of the numerous pathways of lymphatic drainage from the stomach (Fig. 44-1A). Initial drainage is to lymph nodes along the lesser and greater curvatures (*i.e.*, gastric and gastroepiploic nodes), but includes the celiac axis (*i.e.*, porta hepatis, splenic suprapancreatic, and pancreaticoduodenal nodes), adjacent paraaortics, and distal paraesophageal system.

Gastric venous drainage is primarily to the liver by the portal system. Liver involvement is found in as many as 30% of the patients at initial exploration, and it can occur as a result of direct extension (Fig. 44-1B).

CLINICAL PRESENTATION

The most common presenting symptoms are loss of appetite, abdominal discomfort, weight loss, weakness from anemia, nausea and vomiting, and tarry stools. Duration of symptoms is less than 3 months in almost 40% of the patients and longer than 1 year in 20%. Physical examination can reveal advanced disease,

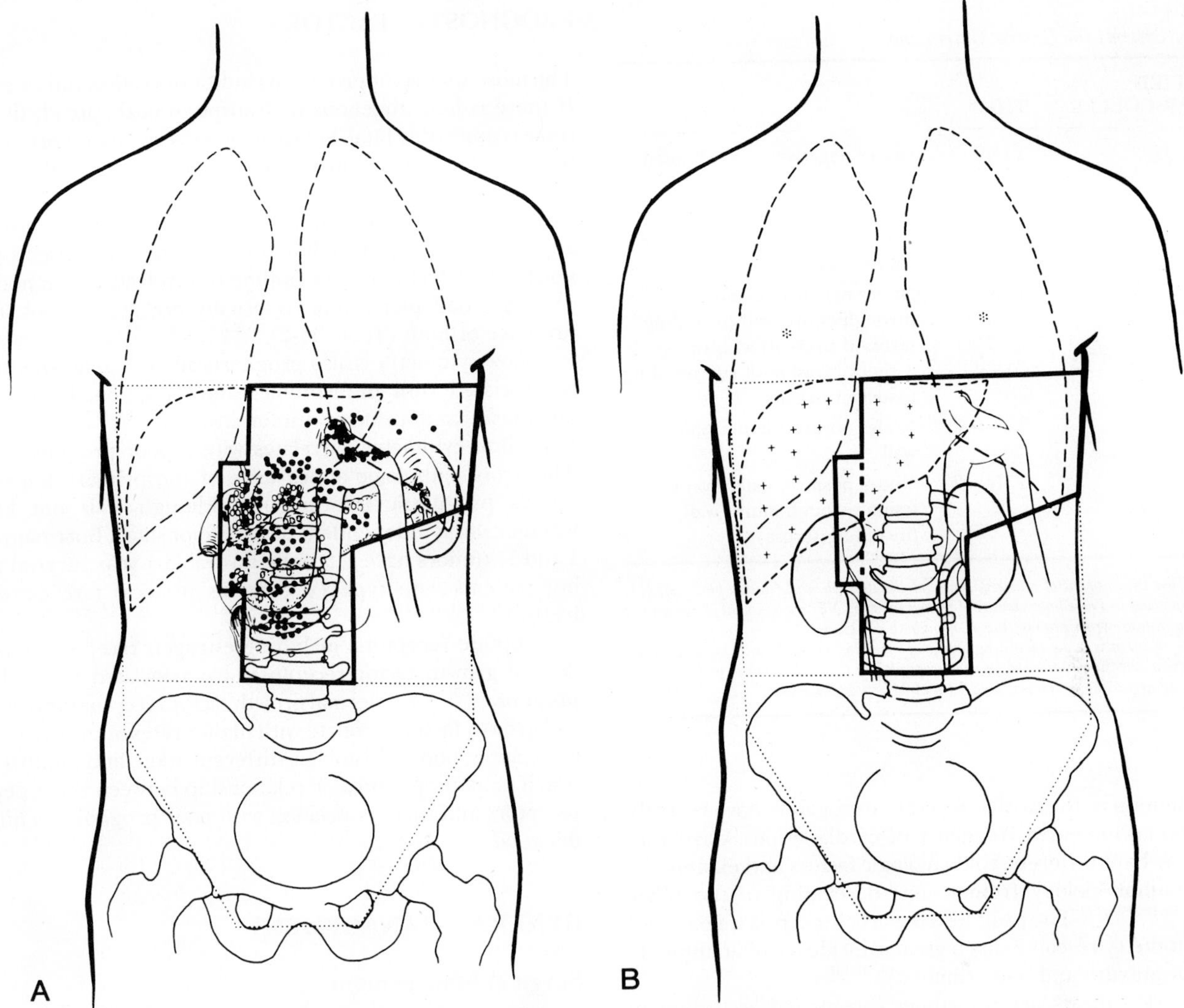

FIGURE 44–1. Patterns of failure in 82 evaluable patients in the University of Minnesota Reoperation series. (**A**) ● indicates local failures in surrounding organs or tissues; ○ indicates lymph node failures. (**B**) * indicates lung metastasis; + indicates liver metastasis. Superimposed radiation portals encompass postsurgical gastric remnant, anastomoses, duodenal stump, gastric bed structures, and primary and secondary areas of lymph node drainage; broken lines represent upper and total abdomen fields. (Modified from Gunderson LL, Sosin H: Int J Radiat Oncol Bio Phys 8:1, 1982)

which may present as an abdominal mass (epigastric mass or liver), palpable left supraclavicular nodes, or a rectal shelf (peritoneal seeding).

DIAGNOSTIC WORKUP

Diagnosis usually is confirmed by upper gastrointestinal radiography and endoscopy. Double-contrast x-rays may reveal small lesions limited to the inner layers of the gastric wall. Endoscopy with direct vision, cytology, and biopsy yields the diagnosis in 90% or more of exophytic lesions, but infiltrative (linnitus plastica), small (< 3 cm), or cardia lesions are more difficult to diagnose endoscopically.

Abdominal computed tomography (CT) studies are useful in determining the abdominal extent of disease and may help determine which lesions extend to surgically unresectable structures, but they are of little value in ruling out peritoneal spread. Distant metastases should be ruled out with chest films, liver function studies, and CT scans (which we prefer) with or without a liver scan or ultrasonography. CT scans provide valuable tumor localization information if irradiation becomes necessary.

STAGING

The TNM system presented by Kennedy and associates[81] is compared in Table 44-1 with a modification of the Astler-Coller rectal system, suitable for all alimentary tract carcinomas. The Astler-Coller system better describes the degree of extension beyond the wall (*e.g.*, T3 includes any degree of extension beyond the serosa), but the TNM system better describes nodal involvement. The original M1 designation (modified Astler-Coller B3 or C3) was occasionally used for involvement of the pancreas by direct extension.

PATHOLOGY

Adenocarcinomas account for 90% to 95% of all gastric malignancies. Lymphomas, usually with unfavorable histology, are the second most common malignancies. Rarely, leiomyosarcomas (2%), carcinoid (1%), adenoacanthoma (1%), and squamous cell carcinomas (1%) occur.

Tumors usually develop in the antrum, are less common in the body of the stomach (lesser > greater curvature), and are

TABLE 44–1
Staging Systems for Gastric Carcinoma

MODIFIED ASTLER-COLLER	TNM*	
A	T1N0	Nodes negative; lesion limited to mucosa
B1	T2N0	Nodes negative; extension of lesion through mucosa but still within gastric wall
B2†	T3N0	Nodes negative; extension through entire wall (including serosa if present) with or without invasion of surrounding tissues or organs
C1	T2N1–2	Nodes positive; lesion limited to wall
C2†	T3N1–2	Nodes positive; extension of lesion through entire wall (including serosa)

** T4: diffuse involvement of entire thickness of the stomach wall (linitus plastica); N1: perigastric nodes in immediate vicinity of primary tumor; N2: involvement of perigastric nodes at a distance from primary tumor or on both curvatures.*
† Separate notation is made regarding degree of extension through wall; m: microscopic only; g: gross extension confirmed by microscopy; B3 + C3: adherence to or invasion of surrounding organs or structures; both T3 and M1 in TNM system.

least common in the cardia. Several investigators have recently reported an increased frequency of cardia lesions. Cardia lesions may have different epidemiologic factors and exhibit different tumor biology from lesions developing in the other sites.[70,79,96,104,171] The prognosis is worse for cardia lesions, and flow cytometry reveals a much greater incidence of aneuploidy than for antrum and body tumors.[49,70,116]

Gastric cancers are sometimes categorized according to Borrmann's[13] five types: Type I tumors are polypoid or fungating; II are ulcerating lesions surrounded by elevated borders; III have ulceration with invasion of the gastric wall; IV are diffusely infiltrating (linnitus plastica); and V are unclassifiable.

PROGNOSTIC FACTORS

The most important prognostic indicators reflect tumor extent. If there is hematogenous or transperitoneal spread, the outcome is uniformly fatal. Survival rates decrease with progressive tumor extension within or beyond the gastric wall.[36,65,70,81] Lymph node involvement is not as important as the number and location of nodes affected.[38,70,81,114] Minimal node involvement adjacent to the primary lesion only moderately affects prognosis.[38,101,114] The solitary finding of involved lymph nodes or complete wall penetration is usually not as ominous as the presence of both (Table 44-2).[36,65,81,114]

Flow cytometry is also prognostically valuable; aneuploidy is associated with unfavorable tumor location, lymph node metastasis, and primary tumor invasion.[8,87,116] Unfavorable DNA flow cytometry correlates with a poor prognosis.[8,87,116] The gross pathologic appearance of the primary lesion also reveals prognostic information, although it is not known whether this is independent of the tumor stage. Borrmann type I and II tumors have relatively favorable 5-year survival rates, but patients with type IV (linnitus plastica) fare extremely badly.[6,7,33,81,101,164]

Peptide receptors, including estrogen receptors and epidermal growth factor receptors, are associated with adverse prognoses.[69,155] Epidermal growth factor receptors and epidermal growth factor correlate with higher rates of primary tumor infiltration, poorer histologic differentiation, and linnitus plastica. The pathophysiologic relationship between these peptide receptors and their association with poor prognoses is not understood.

GENERAL MANAGEMENT

Surgical Management

Operative attempts are highly successful if disease is limited to the mucosa, but the incidence of such early lesions at diagnosis is less than 5% in most U.S. series. In Japan, the incidence of lesions initially confined to the mucosa or submucosa was only

TABLE 44–2
Extent of Initial Disease Compared With Survival Rates for Cancer of the Stomach

EXTENT OF DISEASE	5-YEAR SURVIVAL RATE: DOCKERTY[36]*	5-YEAR SURVIVAL RATE: KENNEDY[81]	≥ 5-YEAR DISEASE-FREE SURVIVAL RATE: UNIVERSITY OF MINNESOTA RE-OPERATION SERIES[65]
NEGATIVE LYMPH NODES			
Mucosa only	100%	85%	
Beyond mucosa but within wall	61%	52%	
Through wall	44%	47%	
POSITIVE LYMPH NODES			
Nodal extent	15%		19%
Regional only		17%	
Nonregional		5%	
Extent of primary			
Within wall			14%
Through wall			12%

** Percentages are of those patients who left the hospital.*

TABLE 44–3
Patterns of Failure After "Curative" Resection of Gastric Cancer

PATTERN OF FAILURE	INCIDENCE IN TOTAL PATIENT GROUP (%) CLINICAL[89,90]	UNIVERSITY OF MINNESOTA REOPERATION[65]*	AUTOPSY[74,103,153,162]
Locoregional†	38	67	80–93
Peritoneal seeding	23	41	30–43
Localized		19	
Diffuse		22	
Distant metastases	52	22	49

** 107 patients at risk.*
† Local or regional failure on basis of direct extension of tumor, lymphatic spread, or operative wound implant; distant metastasis(es) on hematologic basis; abdominal involvement on basis of peritoneal seeding or peritoneal lymphatics.

3.8% in 1955 and 1956, but by 1966, due to screening procedures, this figure had increased to 34.5%, with corresponding survival rates of 90.9%.[131]

Surgical resection, curative or palliative, is possible for 50% to 60% of the patients at the time of initial disease presentation. Unfortunately, only 25% to 40% are eligible for potentially curative resection.

There are no prospectively randomized trials that definitively establish optimal surgical therapy. The preferred treatment for gastric carcinoma, especially for lesions arising in the body and antrum, is a radical subtotal resection. This operation removes approximately 80% of the stomach with the node-bearing tissue, the gastrohepatic and gastrocolic omenta, and the first portion of the duodenum. Larger or more proximal lesions require total gastrectomy. There appears to be no advantage to performing total gastrectomy if subtotal gastrectomy produces satisfactory (5 cm) margins.[42,132,144] Patients treated with total gastrectomy characteristically have 5-year survival rates of 10% to 15%, and those undergoing radical subtotal gastrectomy have 5-year survival rates of 25% to 45%.[42,132,144] The inferior survivorship of patients undergoing total gastrectomy is probably a result of the larger tumors and unfavorable proximal lesions that prompt such a procedure.

The propensity for gastric carcinoma to spread by means of submucosal lymphatics dictates the need for a 5-cm margin of normal stomach tissue as part of the resection. It may be necessary to extend the dissection to include a portion of the esophagus or duodenum to achieve adequate margins. Frozen-section pathologic evaluation of the surgical margins has been advocated to confirm the adequacy of margins.[41] The value of splenectomy has not been addressed in prospective randomized trials, but retrospective Japanese data do not support the survival benefits of this procedure.[154,158]

The extent of lymph node dissection is controversial. The Japanese advocate complete lymph node removal to improve the rates of local control and survival. Several nonrandomized clinical trials have suggested that extended lymphadenectomies may improve survival.[31,41,82,85,124] However, Gunderson and Sossin[65] and others[82] reported that increasingly radical lymphadenectomies failed to improve survival statistics or patterns of failure. Nevertheless, there is a small subset of patients with nodal metastasis in the celiac axis, superior pancreatic, superior mesenteric artery or paraaortic area who are salvaged by extended lymph node dissection.[38]

Endoscopic laser surgery has been applied successfully to patients with very early gastric cancer who are inoperable because of complicating medical illness. Small lesions that are pedunculated, noninvasive, and well differentiated have lymph node metastasis in less than 5% of cases and can be completely removed endoscopically in 75% of the cases.[57] Radiation therapy with chemotherapy may be considered as adjuvant therapy.

Noncurative gastrectomies may be indicated for lesions not resectable for "cure." Some unresectable disease may be successfully debulked, with sites of minimal residual disease marked judiciously with clips. This allows accurate delivery of postoperative radiation therapy and assessment of chemotherapy for residual disease.

Failure Patterns After Surgical Resection

Local regrowth or failures in the tumor bed and regional lymph nodes or distant failures by hematogenous or peritoneal routes are common mechanisms of failure after "curative resection" in clinical, reoperative, and autopsy series (Tables 44-3 and 44-4).[65,74,89,90,103,125,153,162]

For lesions of the esophagogastric junction, the liver and lungs are common sites of distant metastases. With gastric lesions that do not extend to the esophagus, the initial site of distant metastasis is usually the liver, and many failures could be prevented if an effective abdominal treatment could be combined with treatment to the tumor-node region. In Landry's series, 50 (57%) of 88 failing patients had disease progression within the abdomen only. Abdominal treatment could also ad-

TABLE 44–4
Patterns of Locoregional Failure After Resection of Gastric Cancer

FAILURE AREA	INCIDENCE (%) CLINICAL*	REOPERATION†	AUTOPSY‡
Gastric bed	21	54	52–68
Anastomosis or stumps	25	26	54–60
Abdminal or stab wound		5	
Lymph node(s)	8	42	52

** 130 patients at risk.[90]*
† 107 patients at risk.[65]
‡ 92 patients at risk[103] and 28 patients at risk.[162]

dress peritoneal seeding, which occurs in 23% to 43% of postgastrectomy patients.[63,74,89,103,153,162]

Locoregional failures occur commonly in organs and structures of the gastric bed and in lymph nodes (Table 44-4). Failures in anastomoses, gastric remnant, or duodenal stump also are frequent, but they were less common in clinical series or at reoperation than at autopsy (Table 44-4). Progressive extension of the operative procedure to include routine splenectomy, omentectomy, and radical lymph node dissection neither improved survival nor decreased the incidence of locoregional failures in the University of Minnesota series.[59,65] Subsequent failure in areas of initial node dissection occurred in a high percentage of patients, even with radical node dissections, indicating the difficulty of performing a complete lymph node dissection.[65]

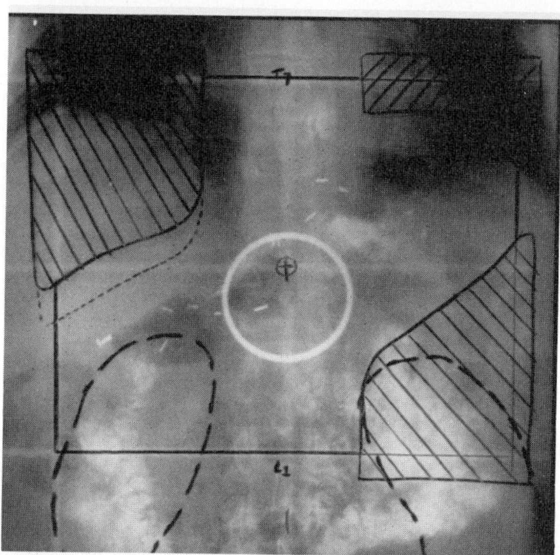

FIGURE 44–3. Inclusion of right kidney in the treatment of a distal gastric lesion. The extent of an unresectable carcinoma of the stomach was marked with clips at exploration. Because the radiation portal included almost 50% of the right kidney (*broken line*), Cerrobend blocking was used to exclude the left kidney. Other blocks (*crosshatched areas*) were used to exclude portions of the liver and heart. Additional liver blocking was added after 3500 cGy (*interrupted line*). (Macdonald B, Cohn I, Gunderson LL: Carcinoma of the stomach. In DeVita V, Hellman S, Rosenberg SA [eds]: Principles and Practice of Oncology. Philadelphia, JB Lippincott, 1985)

RADIATION THERAPY TECHNIQUES

The radiation field should include the tumor or tumor bed and major nodal chains: lesser and greater curvature; celiac axis including pancreatoduodenal, splenic, suprapancreatic, and porta hepatis; paraaortic to level of mid-L3 or mid-L4; paraesophageal with proximal lesions. The idealized portals generated from reoperative patterns of failure need to be modified on the basis of initial extent of disease.[65]

Parallel opposed anteroposterior (AP/PA) fields are the most practical arrangement for the major portion of tumor nodal irradiation, but multifield techniques should be used if they can improve long-term tolerance of normal tissue. In view of the posterior extent of the gastric fundus, it is often impractical to use lateral portals for 1000 cGy to 2000 cGy to spare spinal cord or kidney, as can be done with lesions in the head of the pancreas. Tightly contoured AP/PA fields are used to spare as much normal tissue as possible (Figs. 44-2 and 44-3).

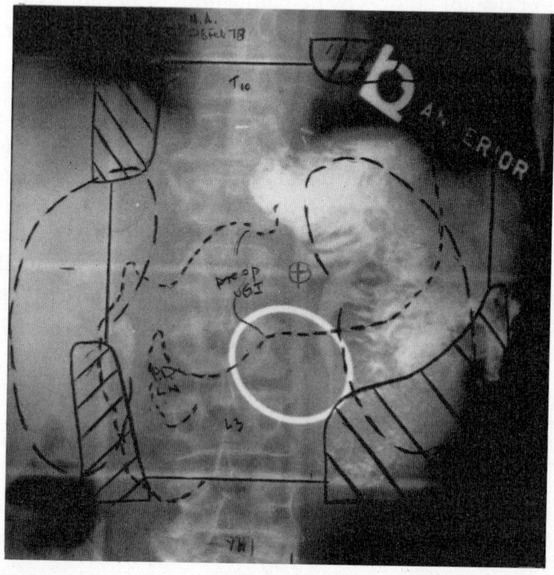

FIGURE 44–2. After subtotal gastrectomy for an adenocarcinoma of the stomach, the contrast within the residual gastric pouch and the position of the stomach on preoperative barium swallow is indicated by a broken line. Portals are within solid lines and crosshatched areas are blocks. The radiation portal included 70% of the left kidney (contrast in hilum, *interrupted lines* are renal outline). No more than 25% of the right kidney was treated. (Macdonald JS, Cohn I, Gunderson LL: Carcinoma of the stomach. In DeVita V, Hellman S, Rosenberg SA [eds]: Principles and Practice of Oncology. Philadelphia, JB Lippincott, 1985)

In the Massachusetts General Hospital and Mayo Clinic pilot series, the average radiation field measured 15 cm × 15 cm. With single daily fraction schemata, the usual dose is 4500 cGy to 5200 cGy delivered in 180-cGy to 200-cGy fractions over 5 to 5.5 weeks, with a field reduction after 4500 cGy. Tightly contoured boost fields to small areas of residual disease can sometimes be cautiously carried to doses of 5500 cGy to 6000 cGy. The authors of this chapter rarely exceed 5500 cGy in their clinical practice unless the stomach can be excluded.

In most patients, a portion of both kidneys is within the treatment field, but at least two thirds to three fourths of one kidney should be excluded. For proximal gastric lesions, 50% or more of the left kidney is commonly within the irradiation portal, and the right kidney must be appropriately spared (Fig. 44-2). For distal lesions with narrow or positive duodenal margins, a similar amount of right kidney is often included; every effort must be taken to spare enough left kidney to maintain function (Fig. 44-3). Chronic renal problems have not been encountered with these techniques.[63]

With proximal gastric lesions or lesions at the esophagogastric junction, a 3-cm to 5-cm margin of distal esophagus should be included; if the lesion extends through the entire gastric wall, a major portion of the left hemidiaphragm should be included (Fig. 44-4). In these circumstances, blocking can decrease the volume of irradiated heart. For unresectable lesions with moderate periesophageal extension, one may be unable to exclude an adequate amount of heart with AP/PA fields, and the use of lateral fields for a portion of treatment may be indicated.

During therapy, patient tolerance, weight, and blood counts are checked at least weekly. If chemotherapy is used with irradiation, blood counts are obtained twice weekly.

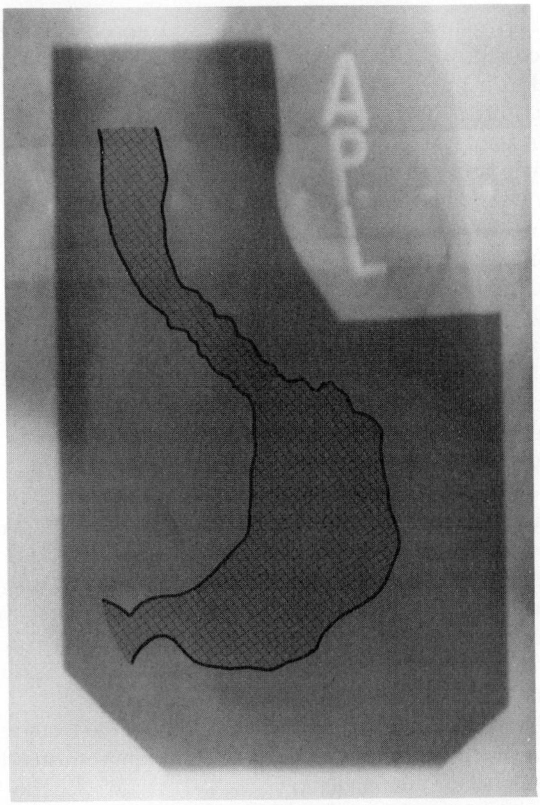

FIGURE 44–4. Localization film of anteroposterior portal used to irradiate a patient with adenocarcinoma of the esophagogastric junction and fundus of the stomach. The inclusion of the distal esophagus is illustrated.

RESULTS OF THERAPY

Preoperative Radiation Therapy

Several investigators have published experiences with preoperative radiation therapy.[62,75,80,105,152] Preoperative irradiation can produce tumor regression that appears to increase as a function of the radiation dose.[75,80] Although survival rates and toxicity with preoperative irradiation are acceptable, there are no prospectively randomized trials that provide conclusive evidence that it alters survival.[62,152] Patients with gastric carcinoma who have lesions resectable for cure should not have surgery delayed by preoperative radiation therapy. Patients with borderline resectable lesions may receive preoperative chemotherapy or radiation therapy with or without chemotherapy before surgery, or patients who present with clearly locally unresectable lesions may have their resectability status reassessed after radiation doses of 4500 cGy to 5500 cGy.

Adjuvant Radiation Therapy

Radiation therapy has no proven benefit after gross complete resections. Nevertheless, there is some rationale for considering irradiation for future gastric surgical adjuvant trials. The pattern of failure data consistently document a substantial locoregional failure problem after potentially curative surgery. Clinical, reoperative, and autopsy series reveal that more than 60% of the patients with positive lymph nodes or extension of the tumor through the serosa subsequently fail in the tumor bed, regional nodes, stump, or anastamosis.[65,89,90,103,162] Approximately 20% of all patients undergoing gastrectomy fail only in these sites.

Combination radiation therapy and chemotherapy is clearly capable of sterilizing known residual disease. Moreover, radiation therapy appears most efficacious if tumor burden is minimized.[2,6,7,23,26,139,161] It follows, then, that irradiation of the locoregional area could sterilize subclinical disease in most of the patients with involved nodes or T3 or T4 primary lesions. If radiation therapy provided substantially improved local control, especially for those destined to fail only locoregionally, the survival rates could improve.

Several phase II trials and three flawed, but prospectively randomized phase III studies using irradiation with or without chemotherapy as surgical adjuvant therapy suggest that more definitive trials are warranted.[3,33,109,157] Gunderson and associates[63] reported 43% overall disease-free survival in a small series of patients with B2, C1, C2, or C3 tumors treated with postoperative irradiation (4500–5200 cGy, 180 cGy/day), usually with chemotherapy. Robinson and Cohen[133] reported 94 consecutive Stage B and C patients treated with irradiation (3000–4000 cGy, 200 cGy/day) and 5-fluorouracil (5-FU). Those receiving adjuvant therapy had substantially improved survival if compared with historic controls, but the lack of a concurrent control group makes this trial inconclusive.

Takahashi and Abe[157] conducted a large trial in which patients were randomized on the basis of their day of hospital admission to receive surgery only or surgery plus intraoperative radiation therapy (IORT) of 2800 cGy to 3500 cGy. Results are shown in Table 44-5. Stage I outcome was not improved in the IORT group. However, 5-year survival rates were improved approximately 15% to 25% with IORT in Stages II–IV. The survival advantage seems to correlate with the 20% of patients who fail only locoregionally. Although this trial is intriguing, it is flawed because the randomization was susceptible to bias affecting treatment selection, and it failed to stratify for important prognostic factors.

Moertel and colleagues[109] performed a prospectively randomized trial among 62 patients with poor prognoses who had completely resected lesions. A nonstratified prerandomization scheme was used. Patients were randomized to surgery only or to surgery followed by irradiation (3750 cGy in 4–5 weeks) with concomitant 5-FU (15 mg/kg/day × 3 by I.V. bolus). In patients randomized to treatment, informed consent was requested. Of

TABLE 44–5
Survival of Resected Gastric Cancer Patients Randomized to Surgery Alone or Surgery Plus Intraoperative Radiation Therapy

STAGE	TREATMENT*	NO. OF PATIENTS	5-YEAR SURVIVAL RATE
I	Surgery + IORT	24	87%
	Surgery	43	93%
II	Surgery + IORT	20	84%
	Surgery	11	62%
III	Surgery + IORT	30	62%
	Surgery	38	37%
IV	Surgery + IORT	27	15%
	Surgery	18	0

**IORT: intraoperative radiation therapy.*
(Modified from Takahashi M, Abe M: Eur J Surg Oncol 12:247, 1986)

the 62 entered on the study, 39 were randomized to treatment and 23 randomized to observation. Ten of the 39 randomized to irradiation plus 5-FU refused therapy and were therefore only observed. If analyzed by initial randomized assignment, the 39 randomized to radiation therapy plus 5-FU (regardless of treatment actually received) had a statistically significant improvement in relapse-free and overall survival. Unexpectedly, however, the ten randomized to therapy but refusing it had a 5-year recurrence-free survival rate of 20%, slightly better than the rate of 17% for the 29 randomized to and receiving therapy and far superior than the rate of 4% for those randomized to observation. Locoregional recurrence was decreased (39% in the 29 randomized and treated patients versus 54% in the 33 untreated either because they were randomized to observation or refused therapy) by radiation therapy plus 5-FU. The surprisingly good outcome of those randomized to but refusing therapy complicates interpretation.

The British Stomach Cancer Group (BSCG) has recently completed a prospectively randomized trial of surgery only versus FAM chemotherapy (*e.g.*, 5-FU, doxorubicin, and mitomycin C) versus with irradiation (4500 cGy in 25 fractions ± 500-cGy boost).[3] Stratified by age, symptom duration, and stage, 436 patients were randomized and followed for a minimum of 12 months. Interpretation is complicated by the inclusion of 128 (29%) patients with resectable but residual disease (BSCG Stage IV Ai) and 78 (18%) patients with positive resection margins. These patients would not be candidates for many gastric surgical adjuvant trials. Furthermore, of 153 randomized to radiation therapy, only 104 (68%) received a dose of 4050 cGy or more, and formal evaluation of the irradiation field design was not reported. Analysis of overall survival and cause of death of all patients randomized revealed no significant differences among the three groups. Analysis of only those patients treated in compliance with protocol was not performed. Locoregional failure, as a component of initial failure, was documented in only 15 (10%) of 153 of the irradiation cohort, 39 (27%) of 145 in the surgery only arm, and 26 (19%) of 138 in the FAM group.

The methodologic flaws in both the Japanese IORT and Mayo external-beam trials and the negative results of the BSCG trial preclude definitive judgments about the value of postoperative radiation therapy. Nevertheless, it is reasonably well tolerated and clearly decreases locoregional failure.[3,33,63,109,133,157] Currently, a large U.S. intergroup protocol is nearing activation to evaluate postoperative irradiation plus chemotherapy.

Locally Unresectable or Postoperative Residual Disease

Radiation therapy has the potential of salvaging a small but reproducible percentage of patients presenting with locally advanced disease. Table 44-6 summarizes the results of treatment for locally unresectable or postoperative residual gastric cancer. These data show a 5-year survival rate ranging from zero to 20%.[2,84,108,139,140] Realistically, 5% to 10% can probably be cured with currently available therapy.[6,7,67,68,72,108,168]

Several general treatment principles emerge from reviewing these reports. Concomitant 5-FU therapy consistently improves survival and palliation.[47,72,108,118,119,133,138] The Mayo Clinic documented the value of concomitant 5-FU in a phase III trial in 48 patients histologically confirmed to have locally unresectable gastric adenocarcinoma.[27,108] Patients received 3500 cGy to 4000 cGy and were randomized in a double-blind fashion to receive 5-FU (15 mg/kg/ I.V. on days 1–3) or saline placebo on the same schedule. Overall survival was markedly improved

TABLE 44–6
Radiation Therapy With or Without Chemotherapy for Locally Advanced Gastric Cancer

INVESTIGATOR	NO. OF PATIENTS	REGIMEN†	SURVIVAL 1 YEAR	2 YEARS	3 YEARS	5 YEARS
GTSG[139]	45	(2500 cGy + 5-FU) × 2, break, 5-FU + meCCNU	(44%)	(25%)	(20%)	(20%)
Nordman[118]	19	3000–5000 cGy (37% with concomitant 5-FU)	10/19 (53%)	5/19 (26%)	3/19 (16%)	
Asakawa[7]	43	≥ 6000 cGy with concomitant 5-FU	21/43 (49%)			2/43 (5%)
Caudry[26]	30	FAM, 4000–5000 cGy, FAM × 6 cycles			6/30 (20%)	
Haas[67,68]	11	(FAM + 1500 cGy) × 3, break, FAM × 4	9/11 (82%)	1/11 (9%)	1/11 (9%)	1/11 (9%)
Thirlwell[161]	15	4600 cGy + 5-FU 500 mg/m² I.V., q wk, 5-FU + MeCCNU	7/15 (50%)	5/15 (33%)		
Klaasen[84]	26	4000 cGy + 5-FU, then 5-FU weekly	(37%)	0/26		
Asakawa[6]*	96	≥ 5000 cGy with concomitant 5-FU	55/96 (57%)	25/96 (26%)	17/96 (18%)	11/96 (11%)
MAOP[140]	30	FAM, (2250 cGy + 5-FU) × 2, FAM × 6	(70%)‡	(15%)‡		
Mayo Clinic[72,109]	25	3500–4000 cGy + 5-FU 15 mg/kg on d 1–3	(36%)‡			3/25 (12%)§
	23	3500–4000 cGy + saline	(18%)‡	0/23		0/23 (0%)§
Abe[2]	14	IORT 2000–4000 cGy	11/14 (79%)	5/14 (36%)	5/14 (36%)	3/14 (21%)
Wieland[168]	106	6000 cGy			9/106 (8%)	5/106 (5%)

* *Includes some patients from Asakawa.*[7]
† *5-FU: 5-Fluorouracil, FAM: combination chemotherapy consisting of 5-FU, doxorubicin (Adriamycin), and Mitomycin C.*
‡ *Estimated from actuarial curves.*
§ *Randomized trial.*

in the 5-FU group, with a mean survival of 6 months with placebo and 13 months with 5-FU, and 12% of the 5-FU group survived 5 years while none in the placebo group survived that long. These differences were highly statistically significant ($P<0.01$).

Patients treated with irradiation for residual disease after surgical debulking consistently survive better than those irradiated for unresectable disease and may tolerate therapy better.[7,26,63,139,161] It is not clear whether this improved survival is a result of surgical debulking or more favorable tumor biology and host resistance, which is associated with the ability to perform a debulking operation.

It is not surprising that several incompletely characterized tumor and patient variables predict prognosis in radiation therapy series. Analysis of outcome by Borrmann classification reveals improved tumor response, survival, and palliation with Borrmann types I and II.[6,7,33,164] Borrmann type III and especially type IV (linnitus plastica) patients fare especially poorly. Lower-stage tumors have superior survival to those with higher stage.[2,6,33] Females may survive better than males.[26] Patients with substantial pretreatment weight loss fare poorly, as would be expected.[84] Undoubtedly, many of these factors are interrelated, but they all underscore the influences of tumor biology and host resistance on outcome.

Palliative Radiation Therapy

Radiation therapy is capable of providing substantial palliation of local gastric cancer symptoms.[18,48,53,63,84,102,113] Table 44-7 summarizes results from several series that attempted to quantitate the benefit of palliative irradiation. It appears that 50% to 75% of patients can expect improvement of symptoms such as obstruction, pain from local tumor extension, or bleeding. The likelihood of benefit may increase with concomitant 5-FU administration, with less tumor bulk, and if the patient's performance score is better before therapy.[47,48,71,119] The median duration of palliation varies from 4 to 18 months in reports addressing this issue.[47,48,100,119]

SEQUELAE OF THERAPY

Acutely, anorexia, nausea, and fatigue are nearly universal complaints during gastric radiation therapy. Paradoxically, our understanding of these problems is quite limited.[14,35,50,149,166] Although visceral afferents may play some role in the acute emetogenic effects of radiation, other unknown factors, possibly chemical in nature and mediated by the chemoreceptor trigger zone (CTZ), appear more important. Other compounding factors may include the altered gastric motility and prolonged gastric emptying time observed in animal experiments as a response to irradiation.[14,35,50,149] Nutritional complications of treatment and myelosuppression, if chemotherapy is used, can carry substantial morbidity and even occasional mortality from therapy. The Gastrointestinal Tumor Study Group reported a minimum 13% treatment-related mortality from nutritional problems or septic events.[139] Almost 20% of Caudry's[26] patients were unable to complete therapy because of nutritional problems. However, others reported no severe or life-threatening nutritional compromise with aggressive radiation therapy.[63,140,161] The toxic gastrointestinal effects are usually managed with careful nutritional support and antiemetic therapy.

Myelosuppression, causing serious or, rarely, lethal toxicity, is also reported in many of the combined-modality trials.[63,67,84,140,161] If blood counts are monitored twice weekly during combined modality therapy, serious problems with sepsis or bleeding should be uncommon.[63,67,161]

Chronically moderate doses of 1600 cGy to 3600 cGy reduce secretion of pepsin and hydrochloric acid.[22,60,138,149] For this reason, radiation therapy was once a common and successful therapy for peptic ulcer disease. Most of the gastric ulcers healed, but they recurred in approximately 40% of the patients.[22,60,149] Gastric acid secretion decreased in almost all cases, with achlorhydria in 25% to 40%.[22,60] The gastric acid decrease usually persisted from 1 to 6 months, but 25% showed persistent decrease in acid production for 1 to 5 years or more.

Gastric late effects were categorized by the Walter Reed Group as dyspepsia, radiation gastritis, uncomplicated gastric ulcer, or gastric ulcer with perforation or obstruction.[4,15,54] The

TABLE 44–7
Radiotherapeutic Palliation of Gastric Cancer

INVESTIGATOR	NO. OF PATIENTS	REGIMEN*	PALLIATED (%)	MEDIAN DURATION OF PALLIATION (MO)
Falkson[47]	12	4500 to 6000 cGy	0	
	18	5-FU 15 mg/kg/d × 5	16	
	17	"Low-dose" irradiation + chemotherapy	18	
	139†	(300 cGy × 5 + 5-FU 12 mg/kg/d q 6 wks) × 5–6	55	6
Mantell[100]	17	3000 cGy/10 fractions	76	4
Henderson[71]	9	4000–5500 cGy	66	
Guttman[66]	5	4000–4500 cGy	80	
Nordmann[119]	32	3000–5000 cGy +/− 5-FU	22	18
Tsukiyama[164]	75	4000–7000 cGy +/− chemotherapy	70	
Falkson[48]‡	28	2000 cGy, break, 1200 cGy courses × 4–5 with 5-FU, DTIC, VCR, BCNU	36	15
Falkson[48]‡	31	2000 cGy, break, 1200 cGy courses × 4–5 with 5-FU	55	5

** 5-FU: 5-fluorouracil; VCR: vincristine; DTIC: 5-imidazole-4-carboxamide*
† 39 received larger initial irradiation dose during first cycle; 18 received additional cytostatics.
‡ Randomized trial.

TABLE 44–8
Radiation Dose Compared With Late Effects in the Walter Reed Experience

		RADIATION LATE EFFECTS (%)*			
DOSE (cGy)	NO. OF PATIENTS†	DYSPEPSIA	GASTRITIS	ULCER	COMPLICATED ULCER‡
<4000	111	5	2	3	0
4000–4499	23	0	22	0	0
4500–4999	27	4	19	11	11
5000–5499	34	0	24	18	12
5500–5999	14	0	50	14	7
>6000	8	0	0	13	38

* *Results reported as number of patients with injury/total number of patients treated with this dose.*
† *Total number of patients treated at this dose.*
‡ *Ulcers complicated by obstruction or perforation.*
(Modified from Friedman M: Proc Second Natl Cancer Conf 1:390, 1952)

associations between dose and these late effects are described in Table 44-8. These data suggest a 20% to 30% incidence of ulceration with doses of 4500 cGy to 5900 cGy, with complications of these ulcers in 30% to 50% of the treated patients. Some caution is necessary in the interpretation of this experience because the Walter Reed cohort was treated with 200-keV photons or 1-MeV photons using a 70-cm target-skin distance, usually employing only one field each day with daily fraction sizes of 300 cGy to midline, which sometimes produced daily given doses of 400 cGy to 600 cGy per day.[15,126]

Table 44-9 summarizes recent reports of late gastric and small bowel complications from paraaortic irradiation using fraction sizes of 150 cGy to 200 cGy.[9,10,16,46,51,52,61,77,78,91,117,126–129,135,137,159,167] These data suggest that gastric late effects are rare with doses of 4000 cGy to 5200 cGy using conventional fractionation. However, doses in the range of 5000 cGy to 5500 cGy may produce variable gastric late effects, which in one series reached 9%.[61] Doses of 6000 cGy carried a 5% to 15% risk of gastric late effects.[6,7,26,117] The relatively low risk of gastric late effects with doses less than 5000 cGy is corroborated by many series using radiation therapy with or without chemotherapy for locally advanced gastric cancer.[26,67,84,108,139,140,161]

The ability of H_2-blockers and sucralfate to prevent the later development of radition-induced gastric ulcerations is unproven. It may be reasonable to administer H_2-blockers prophylactically to patients receiving 4500 cGy or more to any significant volume of their stomachs or proximal duodenums.

TABLE 44–9
Late Complications of Paraaortic Irradiation

			SITE		DOSE (cGy)	
INVESTIGATOR	DIAGNOSIS*	NO. OF PATIENTS	GASTRIC	SMALL BOWEL	TOTAL/FRACTION	COMMENTS†
Piver[126]	Cx	21	3 (14%)	7 (33%)	6000/200	2, A, ii, 4
Nelson[117]	Cx	23	1 (4%)	2 (9%)	6000/200	1, A, i, 3
Tewfik[159]	Cx	23	0	8 (35%)	5000–5500/180	1, A, i, 3
Fletcher[51,52]	Cx	54		11 (20%)	4500–5500/170–200	1, A, i, 3, 5
Goldstein[61]	Cx	121	11 (9%)		4500–5500/170–200	1, A, i, 3, 5
Rubin[16,137]	Cx	16	0	3 (19%)	4000–5000/170–200	1, A, i, 4
Piver[126]	Cx	10	0	1 (10%)	4400–5000/200	1, A, i, 4
Welander[167]	Cx	26	0	6	4400/180–200	1, 2, A, i
Hughes[77]	Cx	41	0	2 (5%)	3600–5100/170	1, A, i, 3, 4
Berman[10]	Cx	11	0	1	4000–5200/—	1, A (4pts, 1 SBO), B (7 pts)
Potish[127,129]	Cx	104	0	2	4500–5000/180–200	1, 3, B (21 pts), C (83 pts), 4, 5, i
LaPolla[91]	Cx	16	0	1	4000–5000/180–200	1, A (8 pts), B (8 pts), i
Ballon[9]	Cx	18	0	0	4300–5100/—	1, B, 3, 4, i
Jolles[78]	Cx	11	0	0	4500–5000/180	1, C, 5
Emami[46]	Cx	36	0	2	4500–5000/175	1, C, i
Rotman[135]	Cx	42	0	1	4500/180	2, C, 3, i
Potish[128]	Endo	48	0	0	4500–5100/150–170	1, A (30 pts), C (18 pts), 4, 5, i
Goldstein[61]	Testes	52	1		4000–5000/—	

* *Cx: cervix; Endo: endometrium.*
† *1: AP/PA only; 2: AP/PA with rotational or lateral fields; 3: ^{60}Co; 4: 2–6 MeV; 5: >6 MeV; A: intraperitoneal staging; B: extraperitoneal staging; C: radiographic staging; i: continuous-course therapy; ii: split-course therapy.*

CHEMOTHERAPY

Disseminated Disease

Chemotherapy for disseminated gastric cancer produces response rates greater than in other gastrointestinal adenocarcinomas. However, it is clear that there is room for continued improvement, because response rates and durations of response are still far from adequate, and survival remains entirely unsatisfactory. Single agents with response rates of 20% or greater include: doxorubicin, cisplatin, 5-FU, and mitomycin C.[29,58,107,110,141] Unfortunately, complete remissions are rare; remission duration is usually 3 to 5 months, and survival is usually only 4 to 6 months for patients with measurable disease. Combination chemotherapy regimens, almost universally using a fluorinated pyrimidine, reliably obtain responses of 25% to 50%, but their practical benefit to the patient is not clear. Combination chemotherapy regimens that have produced response rates of 30% to 45% include 5-FU, doxorubicin, and mitomycin C (FAM regimen); 5-FU plus BCNU; 5-FU plus methyl-CCNU; 5-FU plus mitomycin C; 5-FU, doxorubicin (Adriamycin), and methyl-CCNU; 5-FU, doxorubicin, and BCNU; 5-FU, doxorubicin, and cisplatin.[11,12,37,58,88,92,97,110,111,113,136,160,170]

Although response rates are somewhat greater for combined-modality therapy, this does not translate into improved survival. Most of the multiagent trials report median survivals of approximately 5 to 7 months, which is similar to the survival of patients receiving single-agent chemotherapy. The North Central Cancer Treatment Group (NCCTG) reported a prospective randomized phase III trial comparing 5-FU, 5-FU plus doxorubicin, and FAM. Overall responses were similar, and there were no differences in survival.[32] After the apparent success in treating colorectal carcinoma, there were several trials using pharmacologic manipulation of 5-FU with leucovorin rescue in treating gastric carcinoma.[5,98,99] Responses varied between 11% to 50%, but despite this wide range of response rates, median survival rates were almost identical at 5.5 months. Many of these combination chemotherapy regimens have been subjected to confirmatory trials, which often failed to reproduce the initially high response rates.

Aggressive combination regimens are costly; toxicity is sometimes formidable, and remissions are rare or short. Although the occasional patient responding to therapy with substantial treatment-related morbidity may benefit from chemotherapy, patients with disseminated disease should be considered for clinical trials.

Preoperative and Postoperative Chemotherapy

Preusser and colleagues[130] generated some interest administering chemotherapy before gastric resection. They reported results of combination chemotherapy using the etoposide VP-16, doxorubicin, and cisplatin (EAP regimen) for locally advanced gastric cancer. They found a 22% complete remission rate and an overall response rate of 70%. Furthermore, a total of 15 of the 27 patients initially reported were without evidence of disease after this neoadjuvant chemotherapy with or without surgery and with or without consolidation. Their results with neoadjuvant therapy corresponded with a similar complete remission rate of 21% and an overall response rate of 73% with this same chemotherapy for advanced disease.[169] Verschueren and associates,[165] using neoadjuvant therapy consisting of 5-FU and methotrexate, were able to resect 7 of 15 patients who were inoperable at the time of initial laparotomy. Unfortunately, 5 of the 7 patients had locoregional recurrences. Neoadjuvant chemotherapy remains investigational, and the EAP regimen is quite toxic.

Adjuvant chemotherapy postoperatively has been the subject of many clinical trials but there is no conclusive evidence that any chemotherapy confers survival benefit at this time.

PROBLEMS AND FUTURE DIRECTIONS

Local Control

Local failure remains a substantial problem in radiation therapy series of locally advanced, nonmetastatic gastric cancer. Asakawa,[6,7] despite the use of high doses (≥ 6000 cGy) with concomitant 5-FU, reported all failing patients manifested a component of local failure. Klaasen and colleagues[84] reported a 29% local failure rate, Haas and co-workers[67,68] reported a 42% local failure rate, and Gunderson and associates[63] reported a 44% local failure rate. All of these series used doses of 4000 cGy or more with chemotherapy given sequentially or concomitantly. Adjuvant trials show persistently high rates of locoregional failure. The British Stomach Cancer Group observed locoregional failure as the site of first recurrence in 15 of 153 patients who were randomized to the radiation therapy arm.[3] In the Mayo Clinic randomized trial, 39% of the 29 patients actually receiving adjuvant radiation therapy plus 5-FU manifested locoregional failure as the first clinical recurrence.[109] Gunderson and associates[63] reported a 14% rate of locoregional failure after aggressive radiation therapy and chemotherapy for high-risk gastric cancer after surgical resection.

Alternative methods of improving local control must be explored, because conventional external-beam therapy is approaching normal gastric tolerance. There is interest in optimizing the interaction of radiation and chemotherapy. The mechanism by which 5-FU augments radiation effects may be additive or synergistic.[20,21,150] Several clinical trials are currently using 5-FU administered by constant intravenous infusion with concomitant radiation therapy, based on several radiobiologic experiments suggesting that constant infusion of 5-FU is more effective in producing radiosensitization than conventional bolus administration.[20,21] Two prospective randomized trials studying advanced diseases in other gastrointestinal sites show greater response rates with continuous infusion 5-FU than with conventional bolus scheduling.[94,143]

Altered dose-fractionation schemes and specialized boost techniques also warrant additional investigation. Hyperfractionated radiation therapy has been used in pilot studies for gastric cancer as well as for other upper gastrointestinal sites.[121,142,145] The Mayo Clinic pilot study of hyperfractionated radiation therapy for locally unresectable gastric cancer using 150-cGy fractions twice a day to a total dose of 4500 cGy achieved good local control but was poorly tolerated if combined with 5-FU infusions. Other hyperfractionated treatments of the upper abdomen have used fraction sizes of 100 cGy to 120 cGy to a total dose of 5040 cGy to 7000 cGy, as single-modality therapy or with combination chemotherapy.[142,145] Tolerance of hyperfractionated radiation therapy using these lower fraction doses was somewhat better.

Sindelar and Kinsella[147,148] reported a prospectively randomized trial comparing conventional external-beam radiation therapy (5000 cGy) to IORT (2000 cGy, 11-MeV electrons) after complete or subtotal resection. Actuarial survival (*i.e.*, 20.8

months with IORT and 10.2 months with external beam) and median disease-free interval (*i.e.*, 14.2 months with IORT and 6.9 months with external beam) were improved for the IORT patients, although these differences were not statistically significant. Local disease control, however, was significantly prolonged in the IORT patients; the median time to local failure was 20.8 months for IORT patients and 8 months for patients receiving external-beam therapy. IORT has been used with acceptable toxicity and provocative results as adjuvant therapy and for locally advanced disease.[1,100,147,148,163] However, there is no current evidence to suggest the IORT offers a substantial advantage over conventional external-beam therapy.

Particle therapy should be further explored to improve local control. Neutron therapy has been most thoroughly investigated.[25,43,44,83] Eichhorn and co-workers[43,44] suggested that neutron boosts produced improved rates of histologically confirmed complete responses; there were no complete responses in ten patients treated with photons only, but 34% of the 29 patients receiving neutron boost had complete responses. Catterall and associates[25,83] have substantial experience with neutron therapy, and they have observed considerable palliation and histologic tumor regression. However, complete tumor regression and cure were rare. Gastric motility was lost, and a constant progressive reduction in stomach capacity occurred with neutron therapy.

These observations underscore the complexities of predicting neutron-induced toxicities on the gut from other than empirical experience and the extreme caution necessary with clinical investigations of neutron therapy in gastrointestinal tumors.[45,149]

The Berkeley group reported results with helium charged particle therapy, which has the potential advantage of improving dose distribution but has relative biologic effectiveness values similar to that of supravoltage photon therapy.[24] The 18 patients treated had acceptable toxic effects with 33% 1-year, 15% 2-year, and 6% 5-year survival rates. Local control was achieved in 22% of the patients.

Hepatic, Peritoneal, and Distant Relapse

Most failures after curative surgery and definitive radiation therapy are intraabdominal, chiefly in the liver and peritoneum.[63,65,89] This observation spawned several pilot studies designed to address the issue of failure in the liver or peritoneum, including trials underway with whole-abdomen or hepatic irradiation in addition to irradiation of tumor-nodal fields and concomitant chemotherapy.

Peritoneal infusion of chemotherapy with locoregional radiation therapy is being explored. Several encouraging preliminary reports by Japanese groups with intraperitoneal hyperthermia with or without mitomycin C have appeared.[55,56,86] Fujimoto and associates documented clinically and histologically determined complete responses among patients with peritoneal recurrence in gastric cancer.[55,56] Koga and colleagues[86] report improved survival with intraperitoneal hyperthermic perfusions of mitomycin C after curative resection.

Supportive Care

Nutritional problems are consistently observed in many gastric radiation therapy trials.[26,139] Patients receiving radiation therapy need careful nutritional support. Routine calorie supplementation and liberal use of intravenous or enteral hyperalimentation are mandatory. Several groups routinely place jejunostomy feeding tubes before radiation therapy to obviate nutritional concerns.

Improvements in psychosocial supportive therapy deserve attention, because most of those persons in whom gastric cancer develops die of their disease, and therapies carry substantial potential morbidity, even if successful.[17,19,23,73] This subject is discussed in detail in Chapter 77.

REFERENCES

1. Abe M, Takahashi M: Intraoperative radiotherapy: The Japanese experience. Int J Radiat Oncol Biol Phys 5:863, 1981
2. Abe M, Takahashi M, Yabumoto E, et al: Clinical experiences with intraoperative radiotherapy of locally cancers. Cancer 45:40, 1980
3. Allum WH, Hallissey MT, Ward LC, Hockey MS: A controlled, prospective, randomised trial of adjuvant chemotherapy or radiotherapy in resectable gastric cancer: Interim report. Br J Cancer (in press)
4. Amory H, Brick I: Irradiation damage of the intestines following 1,000-KV roentgen therapy: Evaluation of tolerance dose. Radiology 56:49, 1951
5. Arbuck SG, Douglass HO, Trave F, et al: A phase II trial of 5-fluorouracil and high-dose intravenous leucovorin in gastric carcinoma. J Clin Oncol 5:1150, 1987
6. Asakawa H, Otawa H, Yamada S, Matsumoto K: Combination therapy of gastric carcinoma with radiation and chemotherapy. Tohoku J Exp Med 137:445, 1982
7. Asakawa H, Takeda T: High energy x-ray therapy of gastric carcinoma. J Jpn Soc Cancer Ther 8:362, 1973
8. Baba H, Korenaga D, Okamura T, et al: Prognostic significance of DNA content with special reference to age in gastric cancer. Cancer 63:1768, 1989
9. Ballon S, Berman M, Lagasse L, et al: Survival after extraperitoneal pelvic and paraaortic lymphadenectomy and radiation therapy in cervical carcinoma. Obstet Gynecol 57:90, 1981
10. Berman M, Lagasse L, Watring W, et al: The operative evaluation of patients with cervical carcinoma by an extraperitoneal approach. Obstet Gynecol 50:658, 1977
11. Benetta G, Fraschini P, Labianca R, Luporini G: The value of FAM polychemotherapy in advanced gastric cancer. Proc Am Soc Clin Oncol 1:103, 1982
12. Bitran JD, Desser RK, Kozloff MF, et al: Treatment of metastatic pancreatic and gastric adenocarcinomas with 5-fluorouracil, Adriamycin, and mitomycin C (FAM). Cancer Treat Rep 63:2049, 1979
13. Borrmann R: Geschwulste des Magens und Duodenums. In Henke F, Lanbarsch O (eds): Handbuch der Speziellen Pathologischen Anatomie and Histologie, vol 4. Berlin, Julius Springer, 1926
14. Brecher G, Cronkite E, Conard R, Smith W: Gastric lesions in experimental animals following single exposures to ionizing radiations. Am J Pathol 34:105, 1958
15. Brick I: Effects of million volt irradiation on the gastrointestinal tract. Arch Intern Med 96:26, 1955
16. Brookland R, Rubin S, Danoff B: Extended field irradiation in the treatment of patients with cervical carcinoma involving biopsy proven para-aortic nodes. Int J Radiat Oncol Biol Phys 10:1875, 1984
17. Brown JH, Paraskevas F: Cancer and depression: Cancer presenting with depressive illness: An autoimmune disease? Br J Psychiatry 141:227, 1982
18. Buffet C, Turner K: Letter to the Editor. Br J Surg 70:131, 1983
19. Bukberg J, Penman D, Holland JC: Depression in hospitalized cancer patients. Psychosom Med 46:199, 1984
20. Byfield J: Theoretical basis and clinical applications of 5-fluorouracil as a radiosensitizer. In Rosenthal C, Rotman M (eds):

Clinical Applications of Continuous Infusion Chemotherapy and Concomitant Radiation Therapy, p 113. New York, Plenum Press, 1985
21. Byfield J, Calabro-Jones P, Klisak I, Kulhanian F: Pharmacologic requirements for obtaining sensitization of human tumor cells *in vitro* to combine 5-fluorouracil or ftorafur and x-rays. Int J Radiat Oncol Biol Phys 8:1923, 1982
22. Carpender J, Levin E, Clayman C, Miller R: Radiation in the therapy of peptic ulcer. AJR 75:374, 1956
23. Cassileth BR, Lusk EJ, Hutter R, et al: Concordance of depression and anxiety in patients with cancer. Psychol Rep 54:588, 1984
24. Castro JR, Chen GTY, Pitluck S, et al: Helium charged-particle radiotherapy of locally advanced carcinoma of the esophagus, stomach, and biliary tract. Am J Clin Oncol 6;629, 1983
25. Catterall M: The treatment of advanced cancer by fast neutrons from the Medical Research Council's cyclotron at Hammersmith Hospital, London. Eur J Cancer 10:343, 1974
26. Caudry M, Escarmant P, Maire JP, et al: Radiotherapy of gastric cancer with a three field combination: Feasibility, tolerance and survival. Int J Radiat Oncol Biol Phys 13:1821, 1987
27. Childs DS, Moertel C, Holbrook MA, et al: Treatment of unresectable adenocarcinomas of the stomach with a combination of 5-fluorouracil and radiation. AJR 102:541, 1968
28. Coggon D, Barker DJP, Cole RB, Nelson M: Stomach cancer and food storage. JNCI 81:1178, 1989
29. Comis RL, Carter SK: Integration of chemotherapy into combined modality treatment of solid tumors. III. Gastric cancer. Cancer Treat Rev 1:221, 1974
30. Copeland EM, Souchon EA, MacFayen BV Jr, et al: Intravenous hyperalimentation as an adjunct to radiation therapy. Cancer 39:609, 1977
31. Csendes A: Invited commentary. World J Surg 12:398, 1988
32. Cullinan S, Moertel C, Fleming T, et al: A randomized comparison of 5-FU alone (F), 5-FU + Adriamycin (FA) and 5-FU + Adriamycin + mitomycin C (FAM) in gastric and pancreatic cancer. Proc Am Soc Clin Oncol 3:137, 1984
33. Dent DM, Werner ID, Novis B, et al: Prospective randomized trial of combined oncological therapy for gastric carcinoma. Cancer 44:385, 1979
34. DeWys WD, Walters K: Abnormalities of taste sensation in cancer patients. Cancer 36:1888, 1975
35. Dickson H: Effect of x-irradiation on glucose absorption. Am J Physiol 182:477, 1955
36. Dockerty MB: Pathologic aspects of primary malignant neoplasms of the stomach. In ReMine WH, Priestley JT, Berkson J (eds): Cancer of the Stomach, p 173. Philadelphia, WB Saunders, 1964
37. Douglass H, Lavin PT, Goudsmit A, Klaassen DJ: Phase I–II evaluation of combinations of methyl-CCNU, mitomycin C, Adriamycin and 5-fluorouracil in advanced measurable gastric cancer (Est-2277). Proceedings of the American Society of Clinical Oncology 2:121, 1983
38. Douglass HO, Clark JL, Barcewicz P, et al: Importance of the R_2 lymph node dissection in the surgical treatment of gastric cancer. Proceedings of the American Society of Clinical Oncology 8:101, 1989
39. Douglass HO, Lavin PT, Goudsmit A, et al: Phase II–III evaluation of combination of methyl CCNU, mitomycin C, Adriamycin and 5-fluorouracil in advanced measurable gastric cancer (EST 2277). Proc ASCO p 91, 1983
40. Douglass HO, Milliron S, Nava H, et al: Elemental diet as an adjuvant for patients with locally advanced gastrointestinal cancer receiving radiation therapy: A prospectively randomized study. J Parenter Enteral Nutr 2:682, 1978
41. Douglass HO, Nava HR: Gastric adenocarcinoma: Management of the primary disease. Semin Oncol 12:32, 1985
42. Dupont JB Jr, Lee JR, Burton GR, et al: Adenocarcinoma of the stomach: Review of 1497 cases. Cancer 41:941, 1978
43. Eichhorn HJ: Results of a pilot study on neutron therapy with 600 patients. Int J Radiat Oncol Biol Phys 8:1561, 1982
44. Eichhorn HJ, Lessel A, Matschke S: Comparison between neutron therapy and ^{60}Co gamma ray therapy of bronchial, gastric and oesophagus carcinomata. Eur J Cancer 10:361, 1974
45. Ellis F, Weatherburn H: RBE and clinical response in radiotherapy with neutron beams. Br J Radiol 57:817, 1984
46. Emami B, Watring W, Tak W, et al: Para-aortic lymph node radiation in advanced cervical cancer. Int J Radiat Oncol Biol Phys 6:1237, 1980
47. Falkson G: Halogenated pyrimidines as radiopotentiators in the treatment of stomach cancer. Prog Biochem Pharmacol 1:695, 1965
48. Falkson G, Van Eden EB, Sandison AG: A controlled clinical trial of fluorouracil plus imidazole carboxamide dimethyl triazeno plus vincristine plus bis-chloroethyl nitrosourea plus radiotherapy in stomach cancer. Med Pediatr Oncol 2:111, 1976
49. Fein R, Kelsen DP, Geller N, et al: Adenocarcinoma of the esophagus and gastroesophageal junction: Prognostic factors and results of therapy. Cancer 56:2512, 1985
50. Fenton P, Dickson H: Changes in some gastrointestinal functions following x-irradiation. Am J Physiol 177:528, 1954
51. Fletcher G, Lindberg R, Caderao J, Wharton J: Hyperbaric oxygen as a radiotherapeutic adjuvant in advanced cancer of the uterine cervix. Cancer 39:617, 1977
52. Fletcher G, Rutledge F: Extended field technique in the management of cancers of the uterine cervix. AJR 114:116, 1972
53. Freid JR, Goldberg H, Tenzel W, et al: Cobalt 60 beam therapy: Three year's experience at Montefiore Hospital (New York). Radiology 67:200, 1956
54. Friedman M: Calculated risks of radiation injury of normal tissue in the treatment of cancer of the testis. Proceedings of the Second National Cancer Conference 1:390, 1952
55. Fujimoto S, Shrestha RD, Kokubun M, et al: Clinical trial with surgery and intraperitoneal hyperthermic perfusion for peritoneal recurrence of gastrointestinal cancer. Cancer 64:154, 1989
56. Fujimoto S, Shrestha RD, Kokubun M, et al: Intraperitoneal hyperthermic perfusion combined with surgery effective for gastric cancer patients with peritoneal seeding. Ann Surg 208:36, 1988
57. Fukutomi H, Nakahara A: Endoscopic therapy of gastrointestinal cancer and its curability. Gan To Kagaku Ryoho 4:1132, 1988
58. Gastrointestinal Tumor Study Group: Phase II–III chemotherapy studies in advanced gastric cancer. Cancer Treat Rep 63:1871, 1979
59. Gilbertson VA: Results of treatment of stomach cancer: An appraisal of efforts for more extensive surgery and a report of 1938 cases. Cancer 23:1305, 1969
60. Goldgraber M, Rubin C, Palmer W, et al: The early gastric response to irradiation: A serial biopsy study. Gastroenterology 27:1, 1954
61. Goldstein HM, Rogers LF, Fletcher GH, et al: Radiological manifestations of radiation induced injury to the normal upper gastrointestinal tract. Radiology 117:135, 1975
62. Groves LK, Rodriguez-Antunez A: Treatment of carcinoma of the esophagus and gastric cardia with concentrated preoperative irradiation followed by early operation. Ann Thorac Surg 15:333, 1973
63. Gunderson LL, Hoskins B, Cohen AM, et al: Combined modality treatment of gastric cancer. Int J Radiat Oncol Biol Phys 9:965, 1983
64. Gunderson LL, Meyer JE, Sheedy P, et al: Radiation oncology. In Margolis AR, Bruhenne HJ (eds): Alimentary Tract Radiology, 3rd ed, p 2409. St. Louis, CV Mosby, 1983
65. Gunderson LL, Sosin H: Adenocarcinoma of the stomach: Areas of failure in a reoperation series (second or symptomatic looks): Clinicopathologic correlation and implications for adjuvant therapy. Int J Radiat Oncol Biol Phys 8:1, 1982
66. Guttmann RJ: Effect of 2 million volt roentgen therapy on various malignant lesions of the upper abdomen. AJR 74:204, 1955
67. Haas CD, Mansfield CM, Leichman LP, et al: Combined nonsimultaneous radiation therapy and chemotherapy with 5-FU, doxorubicin, and mitomycin for residual localized gastric adenocarcinoma: A Southwest Oncology Group pilot study. Cancer Treat Rep 67:421, 1983
68. Haas L, Vaitkevicius V, Bukowski R, et al: Southwest Oncology

Group (SWOG) pilot study of radiotherapy (R) + 5 fluorouracil (F) + Adriamycin (A) + mitomycin C (M) in patients with minimal residual gastric cancer. Proceedings of the American Society of Clinical Oncology: 342, 1980

69. Harrison JD, Morris DL, Ellis IO, et al: The effect of tamoxifen and estrogen receptor status on survival in gastric carcinoma. Cancer 64:1007, 1989
70. Hartley LC, Evans E, Windsor CJ: Factors influencing prognosis in gastric cancer. Aust NZ J Surg 57:5, 1987
71. Henderson IWD, Lipowska B, Lougheed MN: Clinical evaluation of combined radiation and chemotherapy in gastrointestinal malignancis. Am J Roentgenol Radium Ther Nucl Med 102:545, 1968
72. Holbrook MA: Radiation therapy. Current concepts in cancer. Gastric cancer: Treatment principles. JAMA 228:1289, 1974
73. Holland JC, Korzun AH, Tross S, et al: Comparative psychological disturbance in patients with pancreatic and gastric cancer. Am J Psychiatry 143:982, 1986
74. Horn RC: Carcinoma of the stomach: Autopsy findings in untreated cases. Gastroenterology 29:515, 1955
75. Hoshi H: Histologic study on the effect of preoperative irradiation of gastric cancer. Tohoku J Exp Med 96:293, 1968
76. Howson CP, Hiyama T, Wynder EL: The decline in gastric cancer: Epidemiology of an unplanned triumph. Epidemiol Rev 8:1, 1986
77. Hughes R, Brewington K, Hanjani P, et al: Extended field irradiation for cervical cancer based on surgical staging. Gynecol Oncol 9:153, 1980.
78. Jolles C, Freedman R, Hamberger A, Horbelt D: Complications of extended-field therapy for cervical carcinoma without prior surgery. Int J Radiat Oncol Biol Phys 12:179, 1986
79. Kalish RJ, Clancy PE, Orringer MB, Appelman HD: Clinical epidemiologic and morphologic comparison between adenocarcinomas arising in Barrett's esophageal mucosa and in the gastric cardia. Gastroenterology 86:461, 1984
80. Kamimura S, Mikuriya S, Hara O, et al: Preoperative radiotherapy of carcinoma of the stomach and breast. (Abstract) Gan To Kagaku Ryoho 14:1558, 1987
81. Kennedy BJ: TNM classification for stomach cancer. Cancer 26:971, 1970
82. Kern KA: Gastric cancer: A neoplastic enigma. J Surg Oncol Suppl 1:34, 1989
83. Kingsley D, Gad A, Catterall M: Adenocarcinoma of the stomach: Radiological and pathological correlation of effects of treatment with fast neutrons. Gut 17:624, 1976
84. Klaassen DJ, MacIntyre JM, Catton GE, et al: Treatment of locally unresectable cancer of the stomach and pancreas: A randomized comparison of 5-fluorouracil alone with radiation plus concurrent and maintenance 5-fluorouracil: An Eastern Cooperative Oncology Group study. J Clin Oncol 3:373, 1985
85. Kodama Y, Sugimachi K, Soejima K, et al: Evaluation of extensive lymph node dissection for carcinoma of the stomach. World J Surg 5:241, 1981
86. Koga S, Hamzoe R, Maeta M, et al: Prophylactic therapy for peritoneal recurrence of gastric cancer by continuous hyperthermic peritoneal perfusion with mitomycin C. Cancer 61:232, 1988
87. Korenaga D, Okamura T, Saito A, et al: DNA ploidy is closely linked to tumor invasion, lymph node metastasis, and prognosis in clinical gastric cancer. Cancer 62:309, 1988
88. Kovach JS, Moertel CG, Schutt AJ: A controlled study of combined 1,3-bis-2-chloroethyl-nitrosourea and 5-fluorouracil therapy for advanced gastric and pancreatic cancer. Cancer 33:563, 1974
89. Landry J, Tepper JE, Wood WC, et al: Patterns of failure following curative resection of gastric carcinoma. Presented at the ASTRO meeting, San Francisco, CA, October 1986
90. Landry J, Tepper J, Wood W, Moulton E: Analysis of survival and local control following surgery for gastric cancer. (Abstract). Int J Radiat Oncol Biol Phys 12:119, 1986
91. LaPolla J, Schlaerth J, Gaddis O, Morrow C: The influence of surgical staging on the evaluation and treatment of patients with cervical carcinoma. Gynecol Oncol 24:194, 1986
92. Levi JA, Dalley DN, Aroney RS: Improved combination chemotherapy in advanced gastric cancer. Br Med J 2:1471, 1979
93. Lingos T, Tepper JE, Gunderson LL, et al: Adjuvant FAM-RAD-FAM after resection of high risk gastric carcinoma. Int J Radiat Oncol Biol Phys 11:116, 1985
94. Lokich J, Ahlgren J, Gullo J, et al: A prospective randomized comparison of continuous infusion fluorouracil with a conventional bolus schedule in metastatic colorectal carcinoma: A Mid-Atlantic Oncology Program study. J Clin Oncol 7:425, 1989
95. MacDonald JS, Cohn I, Gunderson LL: Carcinoma of the stomach. In DeVita V, Hellman S, Rosenberg SA (eds): Principles and Practices of Oncology. Philadelphia, JB Lippincott, 1985
96. MacDonald WC, MacDonald JB: Adenocarcinoma of the esophagus and/or gastric cardia. Cancer 60:1094, 1987
97. Macdonald JS, Schein PS, Woolley PV, et al: 5-Fluorouracil, mitomycin C, and Adriamycin (FAM): A new combination chemotherapy program for advanced gastric carcinoma. Ann Intern Med 93:533, 1980
98. Machover D, Goldschmidt, Chollet P, et al: Treatment of advanced colorectal and gastric adenocarcinomas with 5-fluorouracil and high-dose folinic acid. J Clin Oncol 4:685, 1986
99. Machover D, Schwarzenberg L, Goldschmidt E, et al: Treatment of advanced colorectal and gastric adenocarcinomas with 5-FU combined with high-dose folinic acid: A pilot study. Cancer Treat Rep 66:1803, 1982
100. Mantell BS: Radiotherapy for dysphagia due to gastric carcinoma. Br J Surg 69:69, 1982
101. Maruta K, Shida H: Some factors which influence prognosis after surgery for advanced gastric cancer. Ann Surg 167:313, 1968
102. Maus JH, McCormick NA: Three years' clinical experience with rotation therapy with the theratron. AJR 79:382, 1958
103. McNeer G, Vandenberg H, Donn FY, et al: A critical evaluation of subtotal gastrectomy for the cure of cancer of the stomach. Ann Surg 134:2, 1957
104. Meyers WC, Damiano RJ, Postlethwait RW, Rotolo FS: Adenocarcinoma of the stomach: Changing patterns over the last 4 decades. Ann Surg 205:1, 1987
105. Mikuriya S, Oh'ami H: Radiotherapy and cellular infiltration of tumor nests. Radiat Med 1:248, 1983
106. Moertel CG: Alimentary tract cancer. In Holland J, Frei E (eds): Cancer Medicine. Philadelphia, Lea & Febiger, 1982
107. Moertel CG: Chemotherapy of gastrointestinal cancer. Clin Gastroenterol 5:777, 1976
108. Moertel CG, Childs DS Jr, Reitemeier RJ, et al: Combined 5-fluorouracil and supervoltage radiation therapy of locally unresectable gastrointestinal cancer. Lancet 2:865, 1969
109. Moertel CG, Childs DS, O'Fallon JR, et al: Combined 5-fluorouracil and radiation therapy as a surgical adjuvant for poor prognosis gastric carcinoma. J Clin Oncol 2:1249, 1984
110. Moertel CG, Lavin PT: Phase II–III chemotherapy studies in advanced gastric cancer. Cancer Treat Rep 63:1863, 1979
111. Moertel CG, Mittleman JA, Bakermeier RF, et al: Sequential and combination chemotherapy of advanced gastric cancer. Cancer 38:678, 1976
112. Moertel CG, Reitemeier RJ, Childs DS, et al: Combined 5-fluorouracil and supervoltage radiation therapy in the palliative management of advanced gastrointestinal cancer: A pilot study. Mayo Clin Proc 39:767, 1964
113. Moertel CG, Rubin J, O'Connell MJ, et al: A phase II study of combined 5-fluorouracil, doxorubicin, and cisplatin in the treatment of advanced upper gastrointestinal adenocarcinomas. J Clin Oncol 4:1053, 1986
114. Nagatomo T, Murakami E, Kondo K: Histologic criteria of serosal rupture and prognosis in gastric carcinoma. Cancer 29:180, 1969
115. Nakajima T, Harashima S, Hirata M, et al: Prognostic and therapeutic values of peritoneal cytology in gastric cancer. Acta Cytol 22:225, 1978

116. Nanus DM, Kelsen DP, Niedzwiecki D, et al: Flow cytometry as a predictive indicator in patients with operable gastric cancer. J Clin Oncol 7:1105, 1989
117. Nelson J, Boyce J, Macasaet M, et al: Incidence, significance, and follow-up of para-aortic lymph node metastases in late invasive carcinoma of the cervix. Am J Obstet Gynecol 128:336, 1977
118. Nordman E: Value of megavolt therapy in gastric carcinoma. Bull Cancer 63:217, 1976
119. Nordman E, Kauppinen C: The value of megavolt therapy in carcinoma of the stomach. Strahlentherapie 144:635, 1972
120. O'Connell MJ: Current status of chemotherapy for advanced pancreatic and gastric cancer. J Clin Oncol 3:1032, 1985
121. O'Connell MJ, Gunderson LL, Moertel CG, et al: A pilot study to determine clinical tolerability of intensive combined modality therapy for locally unresectable gastric cancer. Int J Radiat Oncol Biol Phys 11:1827, 1985
122. O'Connell MJ, Stablein DM: Randomized study of combination chemotherapy in unresectable gastric cancer. Cancer 53:13, 1984
123. Offerhaus GJA, Stadt J, Huibregtse K, et al: The mucosa of the gastric remnant harboring malignancy. Cancer 64:698, 1989
124. Okajima K: Surgical treatment of gastric cancer with specific reference to lymph node removal. Acta Med Okayama 31:369, 1977
125. Papachristou DN, Fortner JG: Local recurrence of gastric adenocarcinomas after gastrectomy. J Surg Oncol 18:47, 1981
126. Piver S, Barlow J, Krishnamsetty R: Five-year survival (with no evidence of disease) in patients with biopsy-confirmed aortic node metastasis from cervical carcinoma. Am J Obstet Gynecol 139:575, 1981
127. Potish R, Adcock L, Jones T, et al: The morbidity and utility of periaortic radiotherapy in cervical carcinoma. Gynecol Oncol 15:1, 1983
128. Potish R, Twiggs L, Adcock L, et al: Para-aortic lymph node radiotherapy in cancer of the uterine corpus. Obstet Gynecol 65:251, 1985
129. Potish R, Twiggs L, Prem K, et al: The impact of extraperitoneal surgical staging on morbidity and tumor recurrence following radiotherapy for cervical carcinoma. Am J Clin Oncol 7:245, 1984
130. Preusser P, Wilke H, Achterrath W, et al: Advanced gastric carcinoma: A phase II study with etoposide, Adriamycin and split course of cis-platin. Proc Am Soc Clin Oncol 6:75, 1987
131. Prolla J, Kobayashi S, Kirsner J: Gastric cancer: Some recent improvements in diagnosis based upon the Japanese experience. Arch Intern Med 124:238, 1969
132. ReMine WH, Priestley JT, Berkson J: Cancer of the Stomach. Philadelphia, WB Saunders, 1964
133. Robinson E, Cohen Y: The combination of surgery, radiotherapy, and chemotherapy in the treatment of gastric cancer. Recent Results Cancer Res 32:177, 1977
134. Roswit B, Malsky SJ, Reid CB: Radiation tolerance of the gastrointestinal tract. In Vaeth J (ed): Frontiers of Radiation Therapy Oncology, p 160. Baltimore, University Park Press, 1972
135. Rotman M, Moon S, John M, et al: Extended field para-aortic radiation in cervical carcinoma: The case for prophylactic treatment. Int J Radiat Oncol Biol Phys 4:795, 1978
136. Rougier P, Droz JP, Theodore C, et al: Phase II trial of combined 5-fluorouracil plus doxorubicin plus cisplatin (FAP regimen) in advanced gastric carcinoma. Cancer Treat Rep 71:1301, 1987
137. Rubin S, Brookland R, Mikuta J, et al: Para-aortic nodal metastases in early cervical carcinoma: Long-term survival following extended-field radiotherapy. Gynecol Oncol 18:213, 1983
138. Rubin P, Casarett G: Clinical Radiation Pathology, pp 153–292. Philadelphia, WB Saunders, 1968
139. Schein PS, Novak J: A comparison of combination chemotherapy and combined modality therapy for locally advanced gastric carcinoma. Cancer 49:1771, 1982
140. Schein PS, Smith FP, Dritschillo A, et al: Phase I–II trial of combined modality FAM plus split-course radiation (FAM-RT-FAM) for locally advanced gastric and pancreatic cancer: A Mid-Atlantic Oncology Program study. American Society of Clinical Oncology Abstracts, p 126, 1983
141. Schein PS, Smith FP, Woolley PV, Ahlgren JD: Current management of advanced and locally unresectable gastric carcinoma. Cancer 50:2590, 1982
142. Schuster-Uitterhoeve ALJ, Gonzalez DG, Blank LECM: Radiotherapy with multiple fractions per day in pancreatic and bile duct cancer. Radiother Oncol 7:205, 1986
143. Seifert P, Baker L, Reed M, et al: Comparison of continuous infusion 5-fluorouracil with bolus injection in treatment of patients with colorectal adenocarcinoma. Cancer 365:123, 1975
144. Serlin O, Keehn RJ, Higgins GA, et al: Factors related to survival following resection for gastric carcinoma. Cancer 40:1318, 1977
145. Seydel HG, Stablein D, Leichman L, Kinzie J: Hyperfractionated radiation therapy and chemotherapy in definitive management of unresectable localized adenocarcinoma of the pancreas. Int J Radiat Oncol Biol Phys 11:195, 1985
146. Silverberg E, Boring CC, Squires TS: Cancer statistics, 1990. CA 40(1):9, 1990
147. Sindelar WF: Intraoperative radiotherapy in carcinoma of the stomach and pancreas. Cancer 110:226, 1988
148. Sindelar WF, Kinsella TJ: Randomized trial of resection and intraoperative radiotherapy in locally advanced gastric cancer. Proceedings of the American Society of Clinical Oncology 6:91, 1987
149. Smalley SR, Evans RG: Radiation morbidity to the gastrointestinal tract and liver. In Plowman P, McElwain TJ, Meadows AT (eds): The Complications of Cancer Management. London, Butterworth, 1989
150. Smalley SR, Kimler BF, Evans RG: 5-fluorouracil modulation of radiosensitivity in cultured human carcinoma cells. Int J Radiat Oncol Biol Phys 20:207–211, 1990
151. Souba WW, Klimberg VS, Dolson DD, et al: Prophylactic glutamine protects the intestinal mucosa from radiation injury. (Abstract) Proceedings of the 71st Annual Meeting of the American Radium Society: 8, 1989
152. Stoliarov VI, Volkov ON, Kanaev SV, et al: Comparative evaluation of surgical and combined treatment of cancer of the proximal region of the stomach. Vopr Onkol 30:31, 1984
153. Stout AP: Pathology of carcinoma of the stomach. Arch Surg 46:807, 1943
154. Sugimachi K, Kodama Y, Kumashiro R, et al: Critical evaluation of prophylactic splenectomy in total gastrectomy for stomach cancer. Gan 71:704, 1980
155. Sugiyama K, Yonemura Y, Miyazaki I: Immunohistochemical study of epidermal growth factor and epidermal growth factor receptor in gastric carcinoma. Cancer 63:1557, 1989
156. Takahashi T: Studies on preoperative and postoperative telecobalt therapy in gastric cancer. Nippon Acta Radiol 24:129, 1964
157. Takahashi M, Abe M: Intra-operative radiotherapy for carcinoma of the stomach. Eur J Surg Oncol 12:247, 1986
158. Takahashi T, Sogabe K, Ichikawa J, et al: Examination of combined resection of the tail of the pancreas and spleen in advanced cancer of upper and mid stomach. Proceedings of the 35th meeting Japanese Research Society on Gastric Cancer, 1980
159. Tewfik H, Buchsbaum H, Latourette H, et al: Para-aortic lymph node irradiation in carcinoma of the cervix after exploratory laparotomy and biopsy-proven positive aortic nodes. Int J Radiat Oncol Biol Phys 8:13, 1982
160. The Gastrointestinal Tumor Study Group: A comparative clinical assessment of combination of chemotherapy in the management of advanced gastric carcinoma. Cancer 49:1362, 1982
161. Thirlwell MP, Keable HE, Kost K, et al: Combination of 5-flu-

orouracil (5-FU) plus semustine (MECCNU) with and without radiotherapy (RT) in advanced gastric and pancreatic carcinoma. Proceedings of the American Society of Clinical Oncology 22:449, 1981

162. Thomson FB, Robins RE: Local recurrence following subtotal resection for gastric carcinoma. Surg Gynecol Obstet 95:341, 1952
163. Tobe T, Hikasa Y, Matsuda S, et al: Treatment of gastric cancer with combined surgery and intraoperative radiotherapy. World J Surg 3:715, 1979
164. Tsukiyama I, Akine Y, Kajiura Y, Ogino T, Yamashita K, Egawa S: Radiation therapy for advanced gastric cancer. Int J Radiat Oncol Biol Phys 15:123, 1988
165. Verschueren R, Willemse P, Sleijfer D, et al: Combined chemotherapeutic-surgical approach of locally advanced gastric cancer. Proc Am Soc Clin Oncol 7:93, 1988
166. Wang S, Renzi A, Chinn H: Mechanism of emesis following x-irradiation. Am J Physiol 193:335, 1958
167. Welander C, Pierce V, Nori D, et al: Pretreatment laparotomy in carcinoma of the cervix. Gynecol Oncol 12:336, 1981
168. Wieland C, Hymmen U: Megavoltage therapy for malignant gastric tumors. Strahlentherapie 40:20, 1972
169. Wilke H, Preusser P, Fink U, et al: Neo-adjuvant chemotherapy with etoposide/Adriamycin/cisplatin in locally advanced gastric cancer. Proc Am Soc Clin Oncol 7:100, 1988
170. Woolley PV, Smith F, Estevez R: A phase II trial of 5-FU, Adriamycin, and cisplatin (FAP) in advanced gastric carcinoma. Proc Am Soc Clin Oncol 22:455, 1981
171. Yamada Y, Kato Y: Greater tendency for submucosal invasion in fundic area gastric carcinomas than those arising in the pyloric area. Cancer 63:1757, 1989

45

○ ○ ○ • • •

Pancreas and Hepatobiliary Tract

Leonard L. Gunderson
Christopher G. Willett

Most patients with pancreatic cancer present with lesions in the head of the pancreas that have spread beyond the local area by hematogenous or peritoneal routes or are technically unresectable because of the local extent of disease. For the latter group, the main surgical options are palliative biliary bypass alone or in combination with elective gastroenterostomy. Carcinomas of the biliary tract (gallbladder or bile duct) are uncommon compared with other gastrointestinal malignancies and reflect a wide spectrum of natural histories. Until recently, surgery was the only therapy considered for most patients, although most lesions were unresectable and only palliative procedures could be performed.

PANCREAS

Anatomy and Pathways of Tumor Spread

The pancreas lies in the retroperitoneal space of the upper abdomen at about the level of the first two lumbar vertebrae. It has intimate contact with surrounding organs, including the stomach, duodenum, jejunum, kidneys, spleen, and vessels that can be involved by direct tumor extension (Fig. 45-1). Tumors in the head of the pancreas commonly invade or compress the common bile duct, causing jaundice and dilatation of the bile ducts and gallbladder.

The abundant pancreatic lymphatics have many connections with those of the duodenum. Primary drainage is to superior and inferior pancreaticoduodenal, porta hepatis, and suprapancreatic nodes. With posterior tumor extension, paraaortic nodes are at risk. The main venous channels drain by the portal system to the liver. The lungs and pleura are also frequently involved because of posterior extension into tissues with venous drainage by the vena cava or its tributaries. Generalized peritoneal involvement is more common with carcinoma of the body and tail than with carcinoma of the head.

Epidemiology and Risk Factors

Pancreatic cancer is currently the fourth leading cause of cancer deaths in the United States, and the incidence is increasing. Approximately 28,100 new cases and 25,000 deaths occurred in the United States in 1990.[31]

Clinical Presentation

Cancer of the pancreas rarely presents at a resectable stage, because many of the symptoms are nonspecific and are not investigated early, or they result from local or systemic spread of disease. The most common presenting symptoms are jaundice, pain, anorexia, and weight loss. Positive physical findings, if any, are indicative of late-stage disease. These may include a palpable abdominal mass (*i.e.*, pancreas, liver, gallbladder resulting from biliary obstruction), supraclavicular nodes, or rectal shelf (*i.e.*, peritoneal seeding).

Diagnostic Workup

For diagnostic purposes and radiation treatment planning, a computed tomography (CT) scan is better than ultrasound or arteriograms in defining extent of disease, although they may provide complementary information. The biliary tract component of disease can be evaluated by transhepatic cholangiography and endoscopic retrograde cholangiopancreatography. Among patients with evidence of localized pancreatic cancer but without metastases demonstrated by CT, magnetic resonance imaging (MRI), or angiography, more than 40% are found to have small metastases in the liver or omentum or on parietal peritoneal surfaces that can usually be seen and sampled by laparoscopy.[37] These nodules are usually 1 mm to 2 mm in diameter and are undetectable by any other means. Table 45-1

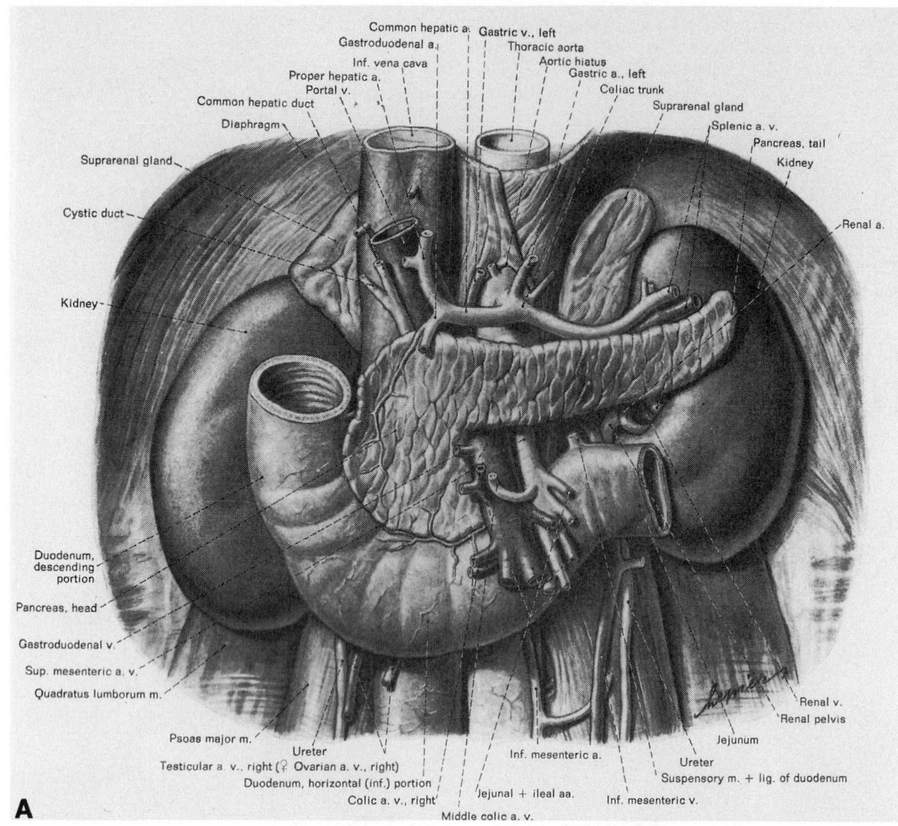

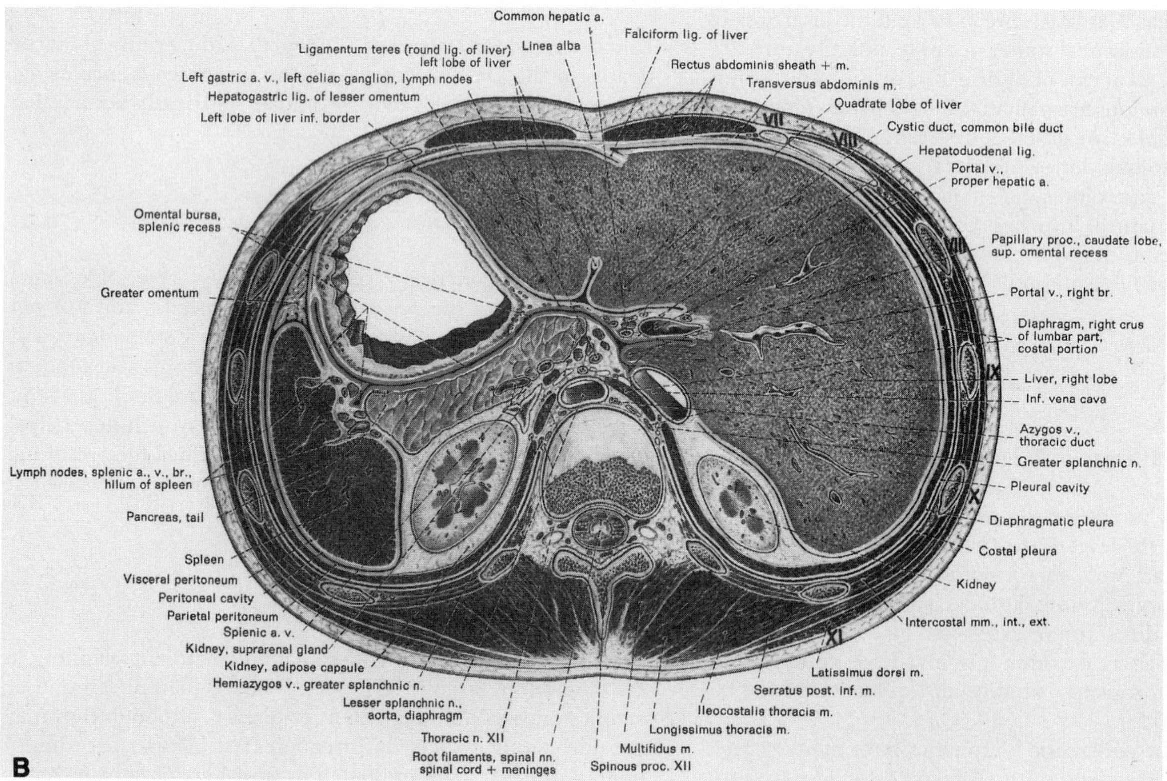

FIGURE 45–1. (**A**) Coronal view illustrating anatomy of the pancreas. (**B**) Transverse section of the upper abdomen illustrating the anatomic relationships of the pancreas to the surrounding viscera. (Figge FHJ [ed]: Sobotta-Figge Atlas of Human Anatomy, ed 9, vol 2. Munich, Urban & Schwarzenberg, 1977)

TABLE 45–1
Diagnostic Workup for Carcinoma of the Pancreas and Biliary Tree

GENERAL
- History
- Physical examination

RADIOGRAPHIC STUDIES
- Standard
  - Upper GI series
  - CT scan
  - Ultrasonography
  - Oral or I.V. cholecystography (cholangiography) if bilirubin plasma levels allow it
  - Transhepatic cholangiography
  - Endoscopic retrograde cholangiopancreatography
- Optional
  - MRI scan
  - Arteriography
  - Intravenous pyelography

LAPAROSCOPY (IF NO PRIOR ABDOMINAL SURGERY)

LABORATORY STUDIES
- Complete blood counts
- Blood chemistry profile
- Urinalysis
- Liver function studies

summarizes the diagnostic procedures used in the evaluation of patients with pancreatic cancer.

Staging

Staging has rarely been used in most published series, and tumors are instead usually classified as unresectable or resectable. The current TNM staging system is described in Table 45-2.[4]

Pathologic Classification

Most pancreatic cancers are adenocarcinomas (approximately 90%), and at least two thirds are in the head of the pancreas. Other cell types include islet cell tumors, cystadenomas, and cystadenocarcinomas; all have a much slower natural history than adenocarcinomas and are not be considered in the section on treatment.

General Management

Operative Considerations

Operability with curative intent varies from 10% to 25% in different series, but operative mortality rates of 10% to 30% are not uncommon.[23] In some of the larger series, however, operative mortality has been greatly reduced; Howard[20] reported 41 and Warren and associates[36] reported 56 consecutive procedures without a death.

Although 5-year survival rates are poor, even with resection (5% to 15%), a significant difference in survival rates exists between patients undergoing definitive resection and those receiving palliative bypass or exploration with biopsy alone.[23]

Areas of Failure and Cause of Death

Little has been done to systematically analyze areas of failure in patients with pancreatic cancer, because most lesions are

TABLE 45–2
AJC TNM Classification for Pancreatic Cancer

PRIMARY TUMOR (T)

TX	Primary tumor cannot be assessed
T0	No evidence of primary tumor
T1	Tumor limited to the pancreas
T1a	Tumor ≤ 2 cm in greatest dimension
T1b	Tumor > 2 cm in greatest dimension
T2	Tumor extends directly to the duodenum, bile duct, or peripancreatic tissues
T3	Tumor extends directly to the stomach, spleen, colon, or adjacent large vessels

REGIONAL LYMPH NODES (N)

NX	Regional lymph nodes cannot be assessed
N0	No regional lymph node metastasis
N1	Regional lymph node metastasis

DISTANT METASTASIS (M)

MX	Presence of distant metastasis cannot be assessed
M0	No distant metastasis
M1	Distant metastasis

STAGE GROUPING

Stage I	T1	N0	M0
	T2	N0	M0
Stage II	T3	N0	M0
Stage III	Any T	N1	M0
Stage IV	Any T	Any N	M1

(Beahrs OH, Henson DE, Hutter RVP, Myers MH [eds.]: Manual for Staging of Cancer, 3rd ed. Philadelphia, JB Lippincott, 1988)

initially unresectable for cure. Death most often results from hepatic failure caused by biliary obstruction by the local tumor or hepatic replacement by metastases. Peritoneal seeding occurs, but the exact frequency is not well documented.

Failure after curative resection was analyzed in a series of 31 patients from Massachusetts General Hospital in which survival was equivalent to that in other surgical series.[34] Of the 26 postoperative survivors, 22 died of disease, and reoperative or autopsy information was available for 13. The incidence of regional failure in the pancreatic bed was 50% (13 of 26 patients), and liver metastases were also common. A recent analysis from the University of Kansas indicated similar local failure rates (50%) after resection and high incidences of liver metastases (44%) and peritoneal seeding (31%) (Table 45-3).[14]

Chemotherapy

Single chemotherapeutic agents with reported response rates of at least 20% include 5-fluorouracil (5-FU), mitomycin C, and streptozotocin.[26] When these drugs are combined (*i.e.*, SMF regimen) or used with other single agents, including doxorubicin (Adriamycin) in the FAM regimen or cisplatin in the FAP regimen, objective response rates of at least 40% have been reported. However, only 5% are complete responses, and less than 10% last more than 1 year. Current data do not suggest increased survival with the addition of chemotherapy except if it is given in combination with radiation therapy.

Radiation Therapy Techniques

Dose-Limiting Tissues

The dose-limiting organs for irradiating upper abdominal cancers are the small intestine, stomach, liver, kidneys, and spinal cord. Split-course regimens or precision multifield stan-

TABLE 45–3
Patterns of Failure in Pancreatic Cancer After Surgery With or Without Irradiation

FAILURE	NO. OF FAILURE/NO. AT RISK	COMPONENTS OF FAILURE											
		LOCAL*			LIVER*			PERITONEAL*			DISTANT†		
		NO.	%	(%)	NO.	%	(%)	NO.	%	(%)	NO.	%	(%)
Initial	26/36	18	70	(50)	13	50	(36)	8	31	(22)	6	23	(17)
Total		19	62	(44)	11	42	(31)	11	42	(31)	7	27	(20)

Open percentages refer to the proportion of the failure group affected, and those in parentheses represent the percentage of postoperative survivors affected.
** Abdominal—initial and eventual failure in 26 patients (100% of failure group, 72% of patients at risk)*
† Extraabdominal failures.
(Griffin JF, Smalley SR, Jewell W, et al: Cancer 66:56, 1990)

dard fraction techniques allow delivery of higher external-beam irradiation doses than were previously accepted as tolerable (*e.g.*, split-course regimen of 6000 cGy over 10 weeks and precision irradiation techniques using 6000 cGy to 7000 cGy over 7 to 9 weeks).[6, 19, 38, 39] Although precision techniques can spare the liver, kidney, and spinal cord, portions of the stomach and small bowel remain within the field. Because the long-term survival rate is small, the actual number of patients at long-term risk for small bowel or gastric complications is also small. It is probably wrong to assume that these dose levels are as well tolerated for extended periods as they are immediately after therapy, although that possibility exists because a much smaller volume of small bowel and stomach is included within the high-dose field.

Treatment Volumes and Doses

For patients undergoing surgery, clips should be placed to mark the extent of the lesion for later external irradiation. Used sparingly (*e.g.*, a single small vascular clip placed in each location to mark superior, inferior, lateral, and medial margins), small clips produce only minimal interference on CT scans.

The patient should be supine during simulation and treatment. An initial set of anteroposterior (AP) and cross-table lateral films is obtained after injection of renal contrast to identify operative clips and renal position relative to the field center. Additional films can be obtained with contrast in the stomach and duodenal loop.

The intent of treatment is to use multifield, fractionated, external-beam techniques with high-energy photons to deliver 4500 cGy to 5000 cGy in 180-cGy fractions to unresected or residual tumor, as defined by CT and clips, and nodal areas at risk. With head of pancreas lesions, major node groups include the pancreaticoduodenal, porta hepatis, celiac, and suprapancreatic. The suprapancreatic node group is included with the body of the pancreas for a 3-cm to 5-cm margin beyond gross disease, but more than two thirds of the left kidney is excluded from the AP/PA field, because at least 50% of the right kidney is often in the field because of duodenal inclusion. The entire duodenal loop with margin is included because pancreatic head lesions may invade the medial wall of the duodenum and place the entire circumference at risk (Fig. 45-2).

With pancreatic body or tail lesions, at least 50% of the left kidney may need to be included to achieve adequate margins and include node groups at risk (*i.e.*, lateral suprapancreatic and splenic hilum). Because inclusion of the entire duodenal loop is not indicated with body or tail lesions, at least two thirds of the right kidney can be preserved, but with tailored blocks, it is usually possible to cover pancreatiocoduodenal and porta hepatis nodes adequately (Fig. 45-3).

For head of pancreas lesions, the superior field extent is at the middle or upper portion of the T11 vertebral body for adequate margins on the celiac vessels (T12, L1). The upper field extent is occasionally more superior with body lesions in order to obtain adequate margin on the primary lesion. With the lateral fields, the anterior field margin is 1.5 cm to 2.0 cm beyond gross disease. The posterior margin is at least 1.5 cm behind the anterior portion of the vertebral body to allow adequate margins on paraaortic nodes, which are at risk with posterior tumor extension in head or body lesions. The lateral contribution is usually limited to 1800 cGy to 2000 cGy because a moderate volume of kidney or liver may be in the field.

Radiation Therapy Results

Resectable Tumors

For the few patients who have resectable lesions, there is justification for adjuvant treatment on the basis of patterns of failure after resection and the results of a prospective randomized trial from the Gastrointestinal Tumor Study Group.[21] In this study, patients were randomized to receive no further treatment (*i.e.*, 22 patients in the surgery-only control arm) or irradiation plus 5-FU (*i.e.*, 23 patients received 4000 cGy in a 6-week split-course schedule with 500 mg/m^2 of 5-fluorouracil given days 1 to 3 of each sequence). A survival advantage was seen with the combined treatment, which had a 2-year survival rate of 42% and a 5-year rate of 14%, over the control arm, which had a 2-year survival rate of 15% and a 5-year survival rate of 5% ($P<0.05$). The Gastrointestinal Tumor Study Group registered 30 additional patients in the treatment group and replicated and confirmed the improved survival (Table 45-4).[10]

It is difficult to interpret the significance of the incidence of local failure in the Gastrointestinal Tumor Study Group series. Because the resection alone group had a median survival of only 10.9 months, many patients were not at risk long enough to develop symptoms of local recurrence. The incidence of local recurrence is excessive with the low doses of irradiation used in this trial (*i.e.*, 4000 cGy in 6 weeks plus 5-FU). With the use of multiple, shaped fields, the Massachusetts General Hospital and Mayo Clinic have delivered 4500 cGy to 5000 cGy in 25 to 28 fractions over 5 to 5.5 weeks in combination with 5-FU as adjuvant therapy with acceptable tolerance.

Investigators at the National Cancer Institute carried out a

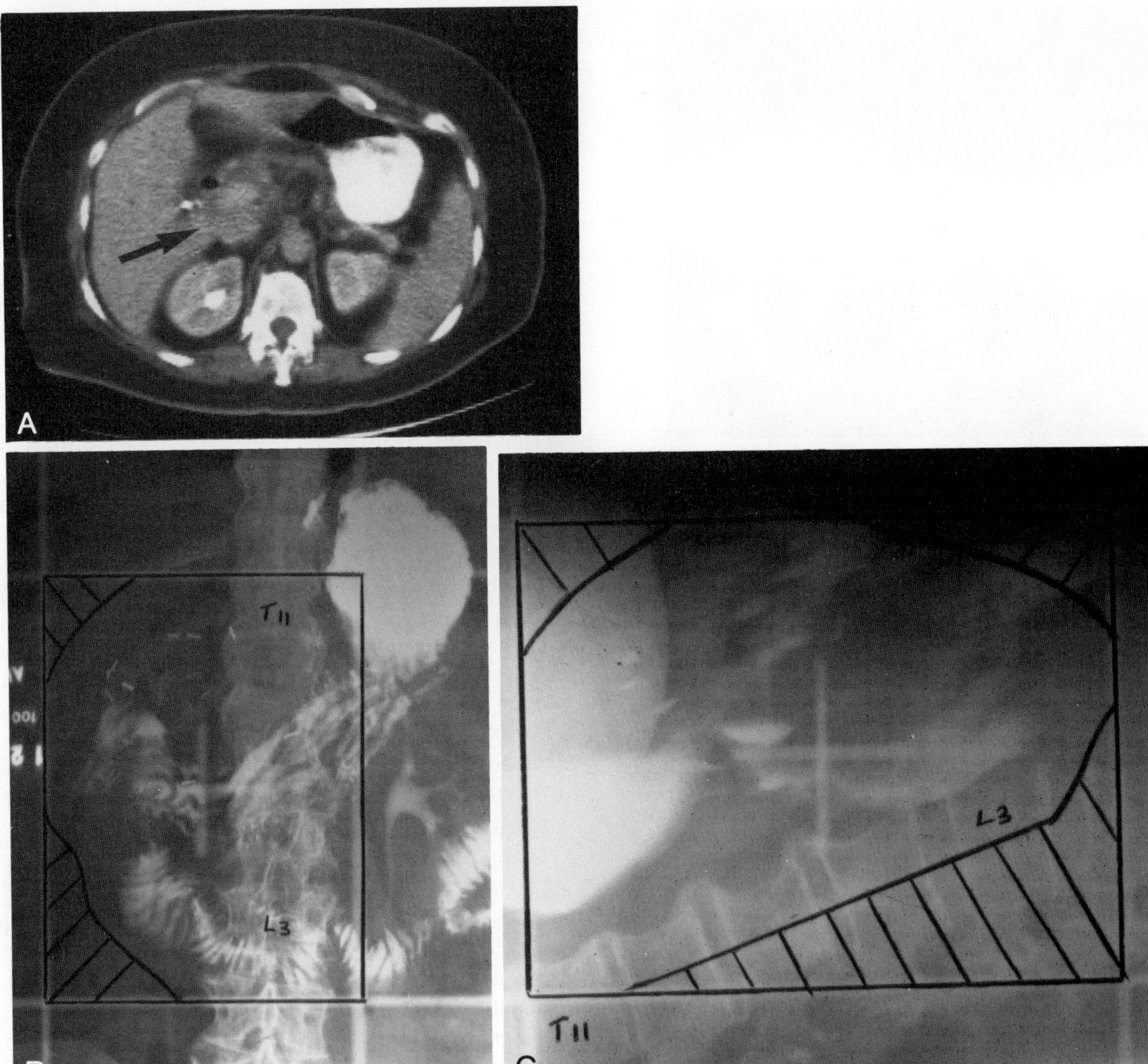

FIGURE 45–2. External-beam four-field technique for treating a pancreatic head lesion. (**A**) The lesion on CT scan. Notice dilated pancreatic duct and relation of pancreas to duodenal loop and stomach. (**B**) The AP/PA field, which includes tumor with approximately a 3-cm margin of the pancreas (body), the duodenal loop (plus approximately 50% of the right kidney), and nodal area at risk. Most of the left kidney is shielded. (**C**) The lateral field includes an anterior margin 1.5 to 2.0 cm beyond gross disease and a posterior margin at least 1.5 cm behind the front edge of vertebral body.

controlled prospective trial of adjuvant radiation therapy after curative resection.[32] Patients were randomized to receive 2000 cGy intraoperative radiation therapy (IORT) immediately after resection, followed by 5000 cGy of postoperative external-beam irradiation or 5000 cGy of postoperative external-beam irradiation only. Although overall survival time was the same for the two groups, local control and median survival were improved in patients receiving IORT.

Unresectable for Cure

EXTERNAL-BEAM IRRADIATION WITH OR WITHOUT CHEMOTHERAPY

For unresectable lesions, palliation can be obtained using external-beam irradiation techniques.[23] The duration of palliation appears to increase as the dose of radiation is increased from 4000 cGy given in 4.5 to 6 weeks to 6000 cGy to 6500 cGy given in 7 to 10 weeks, using a split-course technique with the longer time period. To deliver doses in excess of 4500 cGy to 5000 cGy with safety, the amount of normal tissue in the irradiated field must be minimized.

Survival rates for combined irradiation and chemotherapy for locally unresectable tumors are better than for radiation therapy alone or chemotherapy alone (Table 45-4). With the exception of the Eastern Cooperative Oncology Study, these results have been demonstrated in randomized studies from the Mayo Clinic and the Gastrointestinal Tumor Study Group and nonrandomized series from Duke and Thomas Jefferson Universities.[6–11,18,22,24,37,38] However, even in the high-dose series from Jefferson, local failure was documented in at least two thirds of the patients.

Pilepich and Miller[27] reported a series using preoperative irradiation in 17 patient with unresectable or borderline resectable lesions; 16 of 17 were explored, and the main cause of unresectability was vascular adherence or invasion. Irradiation was delivered in 200-cGy fractions to a total dose of 4000 cGy to

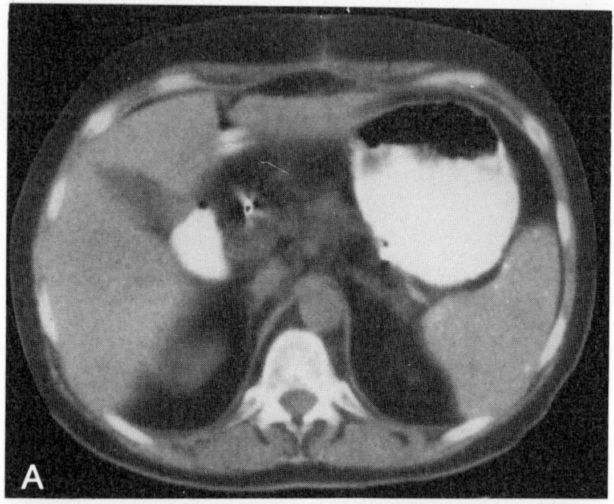

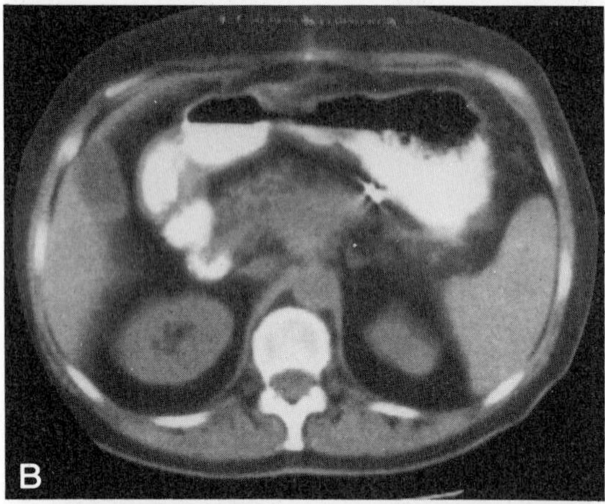

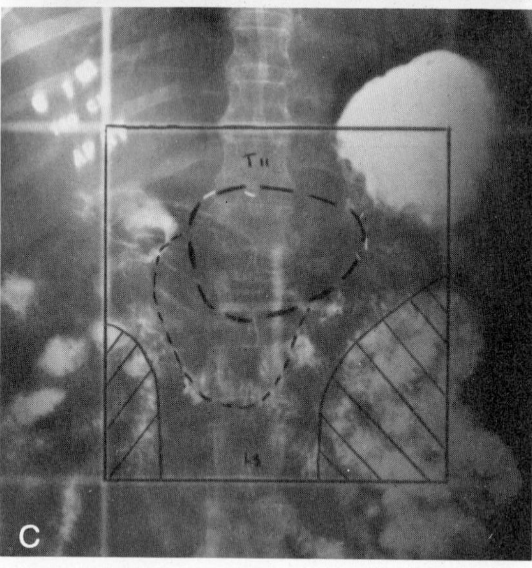

FIGURE 45–3. External-beam four-field technique for treating a body of the pancreas lesion. (**A, B**) The lesion shown on CT scan. (**A**) Right and (**B**) left tumor extent are marked with clips. (**B**) The lesion extends posteriorly; notice the proximity of the tumor to the posterior wall of the stomach anteriorly. The normal glandular appearance of the head of the pancreas and its relationship to the duodenum can be seen. (**C**) The AP/PA field with the lesion reconstructed from CT and clips (*broken line*); the head of the pancreas (*dotted line*). The field is extended to the left to get a 3-cm to 5-cm margin of uninvolved pancreas and additional nodal coverage (suprapancreatic with or without splenic); although the pancreaticoduodenal and porta hepatis nodes are included, the entire duodenal loop does not need to be treated, and at least two thirds of the right kidney can be shielded. (Gunderson LL, Meyer JE, Sheedy P, et al: Radiation oncology. In Margulis AR, Burnhenne HJ (eds): Alimentary Tract Radiology, ed 3. St. Louis, CV Mosby, 1983.)

5000 cGy in 4 to 6 weeks, with reexploration performed, usually in 6 weeks. Eleven of the 17 patients were reexplored. Radical surgery was done in six patients, all with lesions in the pancreatic head. One of the six died postoperatively. Two of the remaining five patients were alive and free of disease at 5 years, and two had recurrences.

INTRAOPERATIVE IRRADIATION

Specialized radiation therapy techniques that increase the irradiation dose to the tumor volume have been used to improve local tumor control without increasing normal tissue morbidity. These techniques include intraoperative electrons as the sole radiation modality or ^{125}I implants or intraoperative electrons for a boost dose in combination with external-beam irradiation.[1,2,12,13,15–18,25,28,29,30,35] Compared with conventional external-beam irradiation, combination techniques have produced a lower incidence of local failure in most series and improved median survival in some series, but it is uncertain whether this is the result of superior treatment or case selection (Table 45-5).

The high incidence of distant failure reported in several series prevent significant improvement in long-term survival. In the Massachusetts General Hospital and Mayo Clinic studies combining external-beam and intraoperative irradiation, local tumor control has been improved, but median survival is only approximately 12 months, and the 2-year survival rate varies from 12% to 55%. Most patients with disease progression have liver metastases, peritoneal seeding, or both.

SPECIALIZED BEAM IRRADIATION

Phase I and II pilot trials using neutrons or helium ions alone or in combination with photon irradiation have been reported. In the preliminary experience with neutrons only in the Mid-Atlantic Neutron Therapy Association study, no improvement was seen in median survival when compared with fractionated photon irradiation plus 5-FU, and toxicity was greater.[33] In TAMVEC trials, the results of treating 13 patients with neutrons plus photons were compared with the results of treating 31 patients with photons only.[3] Mean survival times were 14.5 (range, 5–42 months) and 10.4 months (range, 2–79 months), respectively. The mixed-beam approach produced good palliation and local control with minimal complications and morbidity. In the Berkeley experience with helium ions, there were no major improvements in the results.[5]

BILIARY TRACT

Topographic Anatomy

Anatomic variations of the common bile duct, hepatic artery, and portal vein, the structures comprising the portal triad, are common. Venous drainage of the gallbladder and bile ducts is into the portal vein.

The bile ducts originate within the liver with the left and right hepatic ducts joining to form the common hepatic duct. At the origin of the cystic duct, it becomes the common bile duct. The cystic duct drains bile from the gallbladder into the common duct. The gallbladder lies adjacent to the undersurface of the liver.

The primary lymphatic drainage of the biliary tract is to nodes within the porta hepatis and pancreaticoduodenal groups. A rich lymphatic network exists in the submucosa of bile ducts.

TABLE 45–4
Prospective Randomized Studies of Radiation Therapy and Chemotherapy for Pancreatic Cancer

INVESTIGATION*	NO. OF PATIENTS	MEDIAN SURVIVAL (MO)	LOCAL FAILURE IN EVALUABLE PATIENTS	2-YEAR SURVIVAL RATE
RESECTABLE				
GITSG[10,21]				
Resection only	21	10.9	7/21 (33%)	18%
Resection/EBRT (4000 cGy/6 wk)/5-FU (randomized)	19	21.0	7/15 (47%)†	46%
Resection/EBRT (4000 cGy/6 wk)/5-FU (registered)	30	18.0	11/20 (55%)†	43%
NCI[32]				
Resection + EBRT	16	12	100%	
Resection/IORT + EBRT	16	12	20%	
UNRESECTABLE				
Mayo[24]				
EBRT (3500–3750 cGy/4 wk) only	32	6.3		
EBRT (3500–3750 cGy/4 wk)/5-FU	32	10.4		
GITSG[8]				
EBRT (6000 cGy/10 wk) only	25	5.2	24%	5%
EBRT (4000 cGy/6 wk)/5-FU	83	9.6	26%	10%
EBRT (6000 cGy/10 wk)/5-FU	86	9.2	27%	10%
GITSG[9]				
EBRT (6000 cGy/10 wk)/5-FU	73	8.4	58%	12%
EBRT (6000 cGy/10 wk)/doxorubicin	70	7.5	51%	6%
GITSG[11]				
EBRT (5400 cGy/6 wk)/5-FU/SMF	31	6.5	38%	41% (1 yr)
SMF only	26	5.1	29%	19% (1 yr)
ECOG[22]				
EBRT (4000 cGy/4 wk)/5-FU	47	5.1	32%	6%
5-FU only	144	6.5	32%	13%

** GITSG: Gastrointestinal Tumor Study Group; EBRT: external-beam radiation therapy; NCI: National Cancer Institute; IORT: intraoperative radiation therapy; 5-FU: 5-fluorouracil; SMF streptozotocin, mitomycin C, and 5-FU.*
† Only 15 of 19 randomized and 20 of 30 registered to adjuvant treatment were evaluable for failure patterns.

TABLE 45–5
External-Beam and Intraoperative Radiation Therapy for Unresectable Carcinoma of the Pancreas

INVESTIGATION*	NO. OF PATIENTS	MEDIAN SURVIVAL (MO)	2-YR ACTUARIAL LOCAL FAILURE RATE (%)	2-YR ACTUARIAL SURVIVAL RATE (%)	LIVER OR PERITONEAL FAILURE (DETERMINATE) RATE (%)
Massachusetts General Hospital[28,34]					
^{125}I + EBRT (4000–4500 cGy/5 wk) ± CT	12	12	33	20	
EBRT (4500–5000 cGy/6 wk)/IORT (1500–2000 cGy) ± CT	22	16.5	69	33	
EBRT (4500–5000 cGy/6 wk)/IORT (2000 cGy)/ misonidazole ± CT	41	12.0	55	20	
Mayo Clinic[27]					
EBRT (4000–6000 cGy/6 wk) ± CT	122	12.6	80	16	56
EBRT (4500–5500 cGy/6 wk)/ IORT (2000 cGy) ± CT	37	13.4	34	12	54
Thomas Jefferson[24]					
EBRT (6300–6700 cGy/7–9 wk) ± CT	46	7.3	78 (determinate)		
EBRT (500 cGy, preimplant/^{125}I/CT (5000 cGy, postimplant)	54	12.5	12 (determinate)	18	

** EBRT: external-beam radiation therapy; IORT: intraoperative radiation therapy; CT: chemotherapy.*

Epidemiology and Risk Factors

Gallbladder carcinomas are approximately three times as common as bile duct carcinomas. The male-to-female ratio is 1 : 2.5. About two thirds of patients have associated calculi. Although implantation of foreign bodies into the gallbladder of experimental animals led to carcinoma, this effect was greatly enhanced by concomitant oral ingestion of the carcinogen dimethylnitrosamine.[81]

Bile duct carcinomas show a very slight male predominance, and approximately one third of patients have gallstones.[46] These lesions are associated with ulcerative colitis, liver-fluke infections, and congenital biliary tract cysts.[45, 84]

Pathways of Tumor Spread

Gallbladder

Both direct invasion of the liver and extension involving and obstructing the cystic and common ducts are common. Lymphatic drainage is initially to cystic and common bile duct nodes and then to the pancreaticoduodenal system, with later potential spread to the rest of the celiac axis or the superior mesenteric or aortic nodes. In combined series, regional lymph nodes were involved in 42% and 52% of patients at exploration and autopsy, respectively, and retroperitoneal lymph nodes were involved in 23% and 26% of the patients.[90]

Because of venous drainage into the hepatic division of the portal vein, liver metastasis is not uncommon. The next most frequent sites of distant involvement are peritoneal and pulmonary, with less frequent spread to ovaries, spleen, bones, and other distant organs. Peritoneal seeding at initial disease presentation has been reported for 19% of 1611 explored cases and 20% of 400 autopsy cases.[90]

Bile Duct

Biliary tumors most commonly spread by direct extension within the abundant lymphatic network in the submucosa, with extraductal involvement of surrounding organs or by metastasis to lymph nodes in the porta hepatis and celiac axis. The pancreaticoduodenal nodes are involved more frequently than with gallbladder primary tumors.

Intraabdominal spread involving peritoneal surfaces or ovaries is uncommon, with death usually occurring from local obstruction. Only seven (9%) of 77 patients explored at Lahey Clinic had any peritoneal spread.[93]

Clinical Presentation

Patients present with painless obstructive jaundice, weight loss, or a Courvoisier gallbladder. Positive physical findings are usually indicative of late-stage disease. They may include a palpable right upper quadrant mass (liver or gallbladder), periumbilical or other abdominal mass, rectal shelf (peritoneal seeding), or involved supraclavicular nodes.

Diagnostic Workup

In patients with jaundice, ultrasonography or CT can differentiate between obstructive and nonobstructive disease; obstruction causes dilated intrahepatic ducts. With extrahepatic lesions, transhepatic or endoscopic retrograde cholangiography usually reveals irregular narrowing of the ducts with dilatation proximal to the point of obstruction. Ampullary lesions may cause a filling defect in the duodenum. CT body scans and ultrasound have been used in gallbladder lesions to delineate tumor extent, liver invasion, liver metastases, and retroperitoneal adenopathy, but they are of little value in delineating lesion extent of bile duct primary tumors. A liver scan may show a solitary filling defect associated with gallbladder or common hepatic ductal lesions.

If a bile duct primary lesion is surgically violated to obtain tissue-confirmed diagnosis, the incidence of peritoneal seeding or wound implant may increase to 33% or more.[48] Thin-needle percutaneous biopsy with a transhepatic catheter in position is successful in achieving a tissue diagnosis in approximately 90% of patients and is the preferred method.

Staging

Although two pathologically oriented staging systems have been proposed, there is no commonly used clinical or TNM staging system for biliary tract lesions.

Pathologic Classification

Most lesions are adenocarcinomas, although squamous cell carcinomas have been described. Some reports state that papillary adenocarcinomas of the gallbladder and polypoid tumors of the main hepatic duct have a better prognosis than other lesions in similar locations.

Prognostic Factors

Tumors of the extrahepatic biliary tree are usually grouped by various natural histories: tumors of the distal common bile duct plus ampulla of Vater are the most resectable and have the best prognosis; gallbladder plus mid-ductal lesions (*i.e.*, cystic duct, proximal common bile duct) are prone to early regional spread and have poor prognoses; and "Klatskin" tumors (*i.e.*, common hepatic ductal region lesions) have the lowest resectability rate but can be slow growing. The relative incidence of Klatskin tumors has increased from 33% to 86% on the basis of consecutive reports from Lahey Clinic.[92–94]

In a biliary tract series with curative resection, reported by Kopelson and associates,[71] there was a high incidence of locoregional failure, regardless of tumor grade, lymph nodal status, or perineural-lymphatic-venous invasion. Nodal status and degree of local extension are the main prognostic factors.

General Management

Percutaneous or Bypass Biliary Decompression

There is no consensus for the best method of decompression if bile ducts are obstructed by a malignancy. Usual options include surgical bypass, U-tubes, or nonoperative decompression with percutaneous transhepatic catheters or a retrograde endoscopic prosthesis.[44, 74, 80, 87] Percutaneous transhepatic catheters with drainage require frequent catheter change (*i.e.*, at least every 6 months, often every 1 to 3 months in the first year) and have a substantial risk of sepsis. With proximal bile duct lesions, surgical bypass is not feasible unless the surgeon is capable of and willing to perform a hepaticojejunostomy. Devereaux and Greco[52] compared the incidence of septic deaths and time out of the hospital for 16 patients with percutaneous transhepatic catheters and 17 with surgical bypasses. The mean time from initial hospital discharge to the first major complication was 217 ± 56 days with surgical bypass and 32 ± 22 days with percutaneous transhepatic catheters; in 14 of 16 patients with catheters, the complication was sepsis. Sepsis was a component of death in one of the 17 patients receiving surgical bypasses and in seven of the 16 patients with percutaneous transhepatic catheters. Although problems with sepsis are a known risk from transhepatic catheters, the incidence of septic deaths in this series seems high compared with other reports.[74,80]

Operative Considerations

Because of anatomic location and operative limitations, many patients with gallbladder and extrahepatic biliary duct lesions have technically unresectable lesions or have gross or microscopic residual disease after attempts at resection.[72,73,75,92,93] In a Mayo series, only 5% of 78 patients with Klatskin tumors had curative resection, and there were no long-term survivors.[41] Lesions in the periampullary region or distal common duct carry a somewhat less grim prognosis; resection with a Whipple procedure may yield long-term survival in 30% to 40% of these patients.[42,83,91,94]

Patterns of Failure After Operative Treatment

Even after "curative" resection, local recurrences in the tumor bed or regional nodes (locoregional failure) are common for both gallbladder and extrahepatic biliary duct lesions.[72,73,94] In bile duct cancer, proximal and distal margins are often narrow, as are circumferential margins if lesions extend through the entire duct wall. With ductal lesions, locoregional failure is the usual cause of death. In combined series with "curative" simple cholecystectomy for gallbladder cancer, 95 (86%) of 110 patients with early relapse died with or because of local recurrences, and 11 (48%) of 25 patients alive at 5 years had local recurrences.[73] Twelve (75%) of 16 patients with radical "curative" cholecystectomy died with or because of local recurrences.[73] Hepatic metastases can occur with gallbladder and ductal tumors, but with gallbladder primary lesions, it may be difficult to differentiate liver metastasis from direct extension. Peritoneal involvement is more common with gallbladder cancer than with ductal primary tumors.

Kopelson and co-workers[71] analyzed overall patterns of failure after curative resection in a series of 28 patients with gallbladder and ductal lesions resected at Massachusetts General Hospital (Table 45-6). Of the 25 postoperative survivors, distant metastases occurred in nine (36%). Locoregional recurrence was the major mode of failure, occurring in 13 (52%). Initial spread through the wall of the organ seemed to be the best predictor of locoregional recurrence; locoregional failure occurred in four (36%) of 11 patients with lesions confined to the wall and in nine (64%) of 14 with lesions extending beyond the wall.

Chemotherapy

Single agents capable of invoking tumor response include 5-FU and mitomycin C. In single-agent trials, duration of response has been short, on the order of weeks. When both drugs were administered directly into the hepatic arteries of 13 patients with gallbladder cancer metastatic to the liver, nine (69%) patients responded.[77] Response rates of 29% to 43% have been obtained in small series with three-drug combinations of the FAM regimen or ftorafur, doxorubicin (Adriamycin), and bleomycin (FAB regimen) for metastatic biliary tract cancers.[60,62]

Irradiation Techniques

Dose-Limiting Structures

A major deterrent to improved results with external-beam irradiation is the limited tolerance of the liver, duodenum, stomach, and spinal cord and the lack of clear definition of the lesion's location relative to these dose-limiting structures. Although the superior and inferior extent of disease can often be outlined by a percutaneous cholangiogram or endoscopic retrograde cholangiopancreatography, the amount of extraductal disease is poorly defined by any noninvasive procedure. Clip placement at the time of surgical exploration or resection can be useful in outlining the extrahepatic portion of ductal lesions and in defining the bed of the gallbladder.[59] Shaped, multiple fields

TABLE 45–6
Failure After Curative Surgery for Biliary Tract at the Massachusetts General Hospital

			POSTOPERATIVE SURVIVORS: FAILURE RATE AND SITE						
				LOCOREGIONAL FAILURE*†			DISTANT FAILURE*		
SITE	NO. OF PATIENTS	CURATIVE OPERATION	TOTAL FAILURE	NUMBER	%	(%)	NUMBER	%	(%)
Klatskin	6	1	1/1 (100%)	1			0		
Gallbladder	39	12	7/11 (64%)	7	100	(64)	4	57	(36)
Common duct	15	3	1/3 (33%)	1			1		
Ampulla	15	12	7/10 (70%)	4	57	(40)	4	57	(40)
Diffuse	7	0							
Total	82	28	16/25 (64%)	13	81	(52)	9	56	(36)

* *Open percentages refer to the proportion of the failure group affected, and those in parentheses represent the percentage of postoperative survivors affected.*
† *Tumor bed, lymph nodes.*
(Modified from Kopelson G, et al: Int J Radiat Oncol Biol Phys 7:413, 1981)

and shrinking-field techniques are used to spare as much normal tissue as possible.[47,48,59,63]

Treatment Volume and Dose

Areas at risk for recurrence include the tumor bed, unresected tumor, and nodes along the porta hepatis, pancreaticoduodenal system, and celiac axis. An intravenous pyelogram should be done at the start of treatment to confirm left renal function, because one half to two thirds of the right kidney is usually included in the field of treatment. An initial set of AP and cross-table lateral simulation films can identify surgical clips and renal position relative to the field center. Contrast agent is injected into the transhepatic catheter to define the extent of ductal tumor, and the location of pancreaticoduodenal nodes is determined with contrast agent in the stomach and duodenum (nodes lie adjacent to medial wall).

The initial large-field treatment volume can be included to 4000 cGy to 4500 cGy in 170-cGy to 180-cGy fractions given 5 days a week by a three- or four-field plan (AP and laterals or AP/PA and laterals) using blocks if possible to exclude normal stomach, small intestine, kidney, and liver (Fig. 45-4).[47,48,59,63] Use of lateral fields for part of the treatment allows decreased dose to the spinal cord, right kidney, and portions of the liver. Wedge pair or arc techniques can be used in large or boost fields to alter dose distribution (Fig. 45-4*B*,*C*). Liver intolerance to irradiation may necessitate an initial field reduction after 3000 cGy to 3500 cGy and a second reduction after 4500 cGy to 5000 cGy if gross disease exists. For primary bile duct lesions, the preferred intrahepatic field margin beyond gross ductal disease is 5 cm because of the tendency for submucosal spread within lymphatics; these margins may be reduced to 2 cm to 3 cm after 3000 cGy to 3500 cGy. The upper dose level within the second boost is 5500 cGy to 6000+ cGy delivered over 6.5 to 7 weeks with external beam alone; the latter dose is used only if the boost volume is carefully defined.

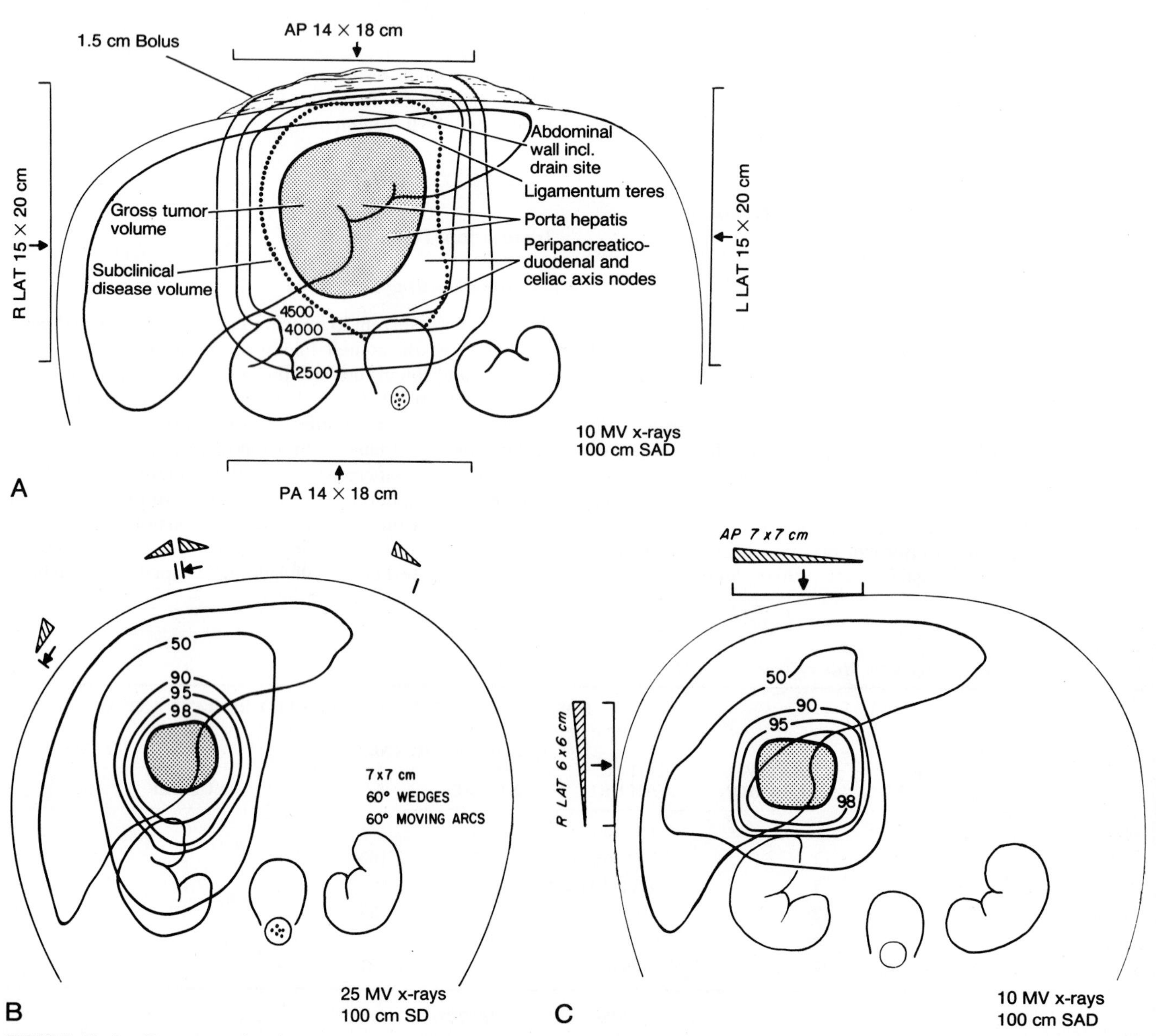

FIGURE 45–4. Treatment planning alternatives for biliary duct cancer. (**A**) Four-field technique for tumor and nodes. (**B**) Moving arcs for boost plan. (**C**) Wedge pair boost plan.

Results of Treatment

Adjuvant Irradiation

Vaittinem[90] reported 31 patients treated with curative surgery, most with simple cholecystectomy, for localized gallbladder cancer. Median survival for the 24 treated with operation alone was 29 months and 63 months for the seven who received postoperative irradiation. Two patients with ampullary cancer were alive and disease-free at more than 1 and 8 years, respectively.[70]

Primary Irradiation With or Without Chemotherapy

Until the 1980s, most authors asserted that biliary tract lesions were radioresistant without providing adequate evidence to support their pessimism.

Significant palliation and occasional long-term survival can be obtained with external-beam irradiation of unresectable or recurrent ductal lesions to doses of 4000 cGy to 6000 cGy given in 4.5 to 7 weeks, but permanent local control is uncommon (Table 45-7).[48,54,56–58,61,73,78,82,86] The higher irradiation doses can be administered with acceptable morbidity only if the tumor extent is carefully clipped at the time of surgical exploration to allow exclusion of as much of the liver as possible.

For unresectable lesions, a combination of irradiation and chemotherapy should be evaluated more extensively, because these combinations have been useful in treating other adenocarcinomas in the gastrointestinal tract.

Specialized Irradiation Modalities

The usual tumor-related cause of death after external irradiation, with or without chemotherapy, is persistent local disease. Because of the proximity of dose-limiting normal tissues, improvements in local control are not likely to occur as a result of alteration in external-beam techniques or doses. Gains will probably be achieved with specialized boost techniques, with or without irradiation dose modifiers.

Intraoperative electrons and transcatheter brachytherapy

TABLE 45–7
Irradiation for Locally Advanced Primary Bile Duct Tumors

INVESTIGATION	NO. OF PATIENTS	MEDIAN (MO)	SURVIVAL 12 MO NO. (%)	SURVIVAL 18 MO NO. (%)	COMMENTS
EXTERNAL IRRADIATION ± CHEMOTHERAPY					
Irradiation alone[73,78,82]	16	6.2	4 (25)	2 (13)	1 septic death
Irradiation/chemotherapy[73,78]	7	12.5	4 (57)	2 (29)	
Irradiation ± chemotherapy					
Hanna and Rider[61]	14	12.3			
Buskirk et al[48]	11	12.0	1 (9)	0	
Fields and Emami[54]	9	7.0	1 (11)	1 (11)	Concomitant 5-FU for 1
TRANSCATHETER ALONE					
Fletcher et al[55]	8	11+	4 (50)	3 (38)	
Karani et al[69]	30		21 (70)		
TRANSCATHETER + EXTERNAL					
Herskovic et al[64]	12		5 (42)		Septic death 3 of 16 (4 pts, no external)
Johnson et al[68]	7	12.5	4 (57)	2 (29)	1 septic death
Fields and Emami[54]	8	15	5 (63)		2 septic deaths
Buskirk et al[48]	10	12.0	8 (80)	3 (30)	
Hayes et al[63]	8	13.4	4 (50)	2 (25)	1 septic death
INTRAOPERATIVE IRRADIATION					
Todoroki et al[89]	5	8.0	2 (40)	1 (20)	
Iwasaki et al[67]*	12	15.0	7 (58)		
INTRAOPERATIVE + EXTERNAL					
Iwasaki et al[67]*	7	7.0	1 (14)		
Deziel et al[53]	5	9.0	2 (40)	2 (40)	
Bussee et al[49]	12	14.0			8 unresected
Mayo Clinic (personal communication)	12	18.7	9 (75)	6 (50)	All unresected

** Thirteen of 19 had noncurative resections before IORT; six were unresected.*

have been used as the sole treatment modality for unresectable lesions, but locoregional recurrence rates are excessive. The preferred treatment method is to deliver 4500 cGy to 5000 cGy in 25 to 28 fractions over 5 to 5.5 weeks to the primary lesion and nodal areas with external-beam multifield techniques and to use intraoperative electrons or transcatheter sources as boosts: 1500 cGy to 2000 cGy with intraoperative electrons; 2000 cGy to 3000 cGy at radii of 0.7 cm to 1.0 cm with transcatheter sources.[47] For institutions that have both options, an intraoperative electron boost may have a physical advantage over the transcatheter method because the stomach and duodenum can be displaced out of the boost field.

TRANSCATHETER BRACHYTHERAPY PLUS EXTERNAL IRRADIATION

There have been many reports of transcatheter irradiation alone or in combination with external irradiation.[47,48,50,51,54,55,57,63–66,68,69,76,79,95] There is a suggestion of improved median survival among patients treated with both external-beam irradiation and brachytherapy over treatment with either alone (Table 45-7). Deaths from sepsis are reported more commonly than in external beam only series, which is a reflection of the inherent risks of transhepatic catheters.

Because of the short follow-up and low incidence of survival beyond 1 year, the exact incidence of locoregional failure is difficult to discern. In the Mayo series, ten patients received external irradiation to doses of 4500 cGy to 5040 cGy, which was followed in 2 to 4 weeks by a transcatheter boost of 2000 cGy to 2500 cGy, calculated at a 1.0-cm radius in nine of ten patients and at 0.7 cm in one. Local failure was documented in three patients (≥30% risk).

INTRAOPERATIVE PLUS EXTERNAL IRRADIATION

In treating 11 patients for biliary tract cancer with 2500 cGy to 3000 cGy of IORT alone, Todoroki and co-workers[89] documented local persistence or progression in nine (82%), which was documented at autopsy in eight (Table 45-7).

In a recent update from that institution, 81 patients were treated for bile duct cancer between 1976 and 1986.[67] Fifty patients had curative or noncurative resection (*i.e.*, no further treatment in 33; intraoperative electron boost in 14; external irradiation in 3), and 31 had no tumor resection (*i.e.*, biliary drainage alone in 21; intraoperative electrons in 6; external irradiation in 4). There is a suggestion of an impact on the survival interval at 18 and 24 months with the addition of IORT. With biliary drainage alone, survival at 6 months was approximately 20%, with a 1-year survival rate of less than 5% and no 18-month survivors. Only one patient with noncurative resection alone was alive at 18 and 24 months, but 38% and 17% of the patients who had IORT plus noncurative resection were alive at 18 and 24 months, respectively, and 42% and 21% who had biliary drainage plus IORT were alive at these intervals. Only one (17%) of six patients without any resection survived beyond 15 months, but five (38%) of 13 patients with subtotal resections survived this interval.

Most patients in U.S. series have received both external-beam and intraoperative irradiation. In the Rush Presbyterian series, two of five patients survived 18 months or longer.[53] The single disease-free survivor at 40 months was the only patient to receive chemotherapy (5-FU plus mitomycin C) during external irradiation. Median survival in a Mayo series of 12 patients with unresectable tumors was 18.7 months, and eight (75%) of 12 survived 15 months or longer (personal communication).[48] Local tumor persistence was diagnosed in six of 12 patients, but in three who died (15, 21.5, and 37 months) of noncancer causes, tumor was documented at autopsy. Only one of 12 patients received 5-FU during external irradiation. In the Joint Center analysis, median survival was 14.0 months, and local progression or persistence was documented in 50% of the evaluable patients.[49]

A group of 39 patients were treated with curative intent for locally advanced bile duct cancer at Mayo Clinic. All received a minimum dose of 4500 cGy delivered in 25 fractions. Surgical exploration was performed in 35 of the 39, and seven had total or subtotal resections before irradiation; six had external irradiation alone, and one had external irradiation plus ^{192}Ir implant. The only survivors at 18 months or longer were two of the six patients who had total or subtotal resections before external irradiation or those who had specialized boosts (*i.e.*, three of ten with ^{192}Ir, six of 12 with IORT electrons). In patients at risk at 1 year or longer, the incidence of local progression as determined clinically on serial cholangiograms was four (67%) of six who received external irradiation with or without 5-FU, two (67%) of three who had subtotal resection plus external irradiation, two (25%) of eight who received external irradiation plus ^{192}Ir, and three (33%) of nine patients who received external irradiation plus IORT. However, it can be difficult to differentiate fibrosis from recurrent tumor on the basis of cholangiograms or other noninvasive studies. Clinical estimates of tumor control are usually falsely low, as was found in the Mayo IORT analysis, in which three additional patients with tumor persistence were discovered at autopsy.

Sequelae of Treatment

Gastric and Duodenal Tolerance

A good analysis of gastric and duodenal irradiation tolerance exists in the biliary duct analysis from Buskirk and associates.[48] For locally unresectable or residual biliary cancer, three aggressive treatment regimens were used: external irradiation alone or combined with 5-FU; 4500 cGy in 25 fractions in 5 weeks to a tumor and nodal field, with a reduced field boost for 1000 cGy to 2000 cGy in 200-cGy fractions; or similar external-beam irradiation to a tumor and nodal field combined with a boost by intraoperative electrons or brachytherapy. The distal stomach and duodenal C-loop were usually included to a dose of 4500 cGy. With brachytherapy, patients received doses of 1500 cGy to 2500 cGy, which was usually calculated at a 1-cm radius from the transcatheter iridium. With IORT, it was usually possibly to exclude duodenum and stomach.

An analysis comparing dose with complications was performed for patients who received external irradiation alone or external irradiation combined with IORT electrons. With external doses of 5500 cGy or less to the duodenum or stomach, the risk of severe gastrointestinal complications varied from 5% to 10%, depending on which parameter was evaluated. At doses greater than 5500 cGy, one third of the patients developed severe problems. In patients who received external irradiation plus iridium, the dose to the external field was limited to 5040 cGy, but most received additional irradiation to duodenum or stomach from the iridium boost (higher doses with distal lesions). There was a 30% to 40% incidence of severe complications in the duodenums or stomachs of this group of patients.

Biliary Duct Tolerance

Biliary duct tolerance to external irradiation with or without transcatheter or intraoperative boost has been evaluated in animal models as well as in clinical pilot studies. Todoroki[88] studied the effects of large single doses of irradiation to the liver hilum in rabbits and found hepatic parenchymal atrophy, significant biliary fibrosis, and necrosis at doses greater than 3000 cGy. Sindelar and co-workers[85] investigated the effects of intraoperative irradiation of the extrahepatic bile ducts in dogs and noticed dose-related fibrosis and duct stenosis at all doses over 2000 cGy. Stenosis produced secondary hepatic changes of biliary cirrhosis, which developed with time.

At the radiation dose levels used in our aggressive treatment combinations (*i.e.*, external irradiation plus transcatheter or intraoperative electron boost), temporary fibrosis and duct stenosis have occurred.[47] Transhepatic catheters or U-tubes are left in place in these patients until the degree of stenosis has stabilized or lessened on serial cholangiograms, which usually occurs within 12 to 18 months of treatment.

Hepatic Artery Tolerance

In the series reported by Iwasaki and colleagues,[67] the IORT dose for bile duct malignancies had been reduced to a maximum of 2000 cGy after curative or noncurative resection because of an excess incidence of severe complications. When IORT doses of 2000 cGy to 3500 cGy were used, four of seven patients with IORT after surgical manipulation of the hepatic artery developed stenosis, obstruction, or aneurysm. In five patients treated subsequently with IORT doses of 2000 cGy or less after resection, no severe vascular complications occurred.

LIVER

Surgery and Chemotherapy

Resection remains the treatment of choice for primary liver tumors and solitary metastatic lesions if removal is technically feasible. Infusion chemotherapy with implantable pumps can achieve significant palliation, and its potential value in treating metastatic lesions has been compared with systemic chemotherapy in randomized trials. Although response rates are higher with direct infusion, no significant difference in survival has been observed.

Irradiation Results and Tolerance

Irradiation has a significant role in treating unresectable symptomatic hemangiomas.[75, 99, 103] Long disease-free survival has been obtained with doses as low as 1300 cGy in 15 days to doses of 2000 cGy to 3000 cGy given in 3 to 4 weeks. Irradiation also has a palliative role in managing metastatic disease (*i.e.*, 50% to 75% good-to-excellent response in series with irradiation alone or in combination with infusion or systemic chemotherapy) and a possible palliative role in primary unresectable liver tumors if administered alone or in combination with chemotherapy.[75, 97, 105]

The potential impact of hyperfractionated irradiation for hepatocellular cancers was evaluated in a sequential nonrandomized Radiation Therapy Oncology Group trial involving 135 patients.[106] The standard arm consisted of daily fractions of 300 cGy to 2100 cGy plus doxorubicin and 5-FU on days 1, 3, 5, and 7, and the experimental arm used the same chemotherapy regimen with hyperfractionated irradiation of 120-cGy fractions given twice daily with 4-hour intervals between fractions, 5 days per week, to a dose of 2400 cGy. Although no benefit was observed with the hyperfractionated regimen over the standard arm (*i.e.*, response rates of 18% and 22%, respectively), toxicity in the experimental arm was greater than for the standard arm: esophagitis in 19% and 1%, respectively ($P = 0.0001$); grade 1 to 4 thrombocytopenia in 68 and 49%, respectively ($P = 0.03$).

The major factor restricting irradiation to a palliative role is the inability of the liver to tolerate more than a dose of 2500 cGy to 3000 cGy in 3 to 4 weeks. Data from Memorial Hospital and Stanford indicate that most cases of irradiation-induced hepatitis occur at or above a dose of 3500 cGy to the entire liver (≥1000 cGy/week) and that none of the cases of persistent or fatal hepatitis occurred at a dose less than 3850 cGy.[98, 100, 104] Small portions of the liver can be irradiated to doses of 5000 cGy to 6000 cGy without significant long-term morbidity. Dritshilo and associates[96] piloted the use of interstitial irradiation for metastatic lesions using ultrasound guidance. No clinically significant toxicity was reported in a group of five patients with follow-up between 2 and 6 months.

Investigators at Johns Hopkins[101, 102] explored the potential of radioimmunotherapy in combination with external-beam irradiation with or without chemotherapy. Some dramatic short-term and long-term tumor regressions were reported.

REFERENCES

Pancreas

1. Abe M, Takahashi M: Intraoperative radiotherapy: The Japanese experience. Int J Radiat Oncol Biol Phys 7:863, 1981
2. Abe M, Takahashi M, Yabumoto E, et al: Clinical experiences with intraoperative radiotherapy of locally advanced cancers. Cancer 45:40, 1980
3. Alabdula ASM, Hussey DH, Olson MH, et al: Experience with fast neutron therapy for unresectable carcinoma of the pancreas. Int J Radiat Oncol Biol Phys 7:165, 1981
4. Beahrs OH, Henson DE, Hutter RVP, Myers MH (eds): Manual For Staging Cancer, 3rd ed. Philadelphia, JB Lippincott, 1988
5. Castro JR, Quivey J, Lyman JT, et al: Current status of clinical particle radiotherapy at Lawrence Berkeley Laboratory. Cancer 46:633, 1980
6. Dobelbower RR: The radiotherapy of pancreatic cancer. Semin Oncol 6:378, 1979
7. Gastrointestinal Tumor Study Group: Comparative therapeutic trial of radiation with or without chemotherapy in pancreatic carcinoma. Int J Radiat Oncol Biol Phys 5:1643, 1979
8. Gastrointestinal Tumor Study Group: Therapy of locally unresectable pancreatic carcinoma: A randomized comparison of high dose (6000 rads) radiation alone, moderate dose radiation (4000 rads + 5-fluorouracil), and high dose radiation + 5-fluorouracil. Cancer 48:1705, 1981
9. Gastrointestinal Tumor Study Group: Radiation therapy combined with Adriamycin or 5-fluorouracil for the treatment of locally unresectable pancreatic carcinoma. Cancer 56:2563, 1985
10. Gastrointestinal Tumor Study Group: Further evidence of effective adjuvant combined radiation and chemotherapy following curative resection of pancreatic cancer. Cancer 59:2006, 1987
11. Gastrointestinal Tumor Study Group: Treatment of locally unresectable carcinoma of the pancreas: Comparison of combined-modality therapy (chemotherapy plus radiotherapy) to chemotherapy alone. JNCI 80:751, 1988
12. Goldson AL: Past, present, and future prospects of intraoperative radiotherapy (IOR). Semin Oncol 8:59, 1981
13. Goldson AL, Ashaveri E, Espinoza MC, et al: Single-dose intraoperative electrons for advanced stage pancreatic can-

cer: Phase I pilot study. Int J Radiat Oncol Biol Phys 7:869, 1981
14. Griffin JF, Smalley SR, Jewell W, et al: Patterns of failure following curative resection of pancreatic carcinoma. Cancer 66:56, 1990
15. Gunderson LL, Martin JK, Earle JB, et al: Intraoperative and external beam irradiation ± resection: Mayo pilot experience. Mayo Clin Proc 59:691, 1984
16. Gunderson LL, Martin JK, Kvols LK, et al: Intraoperative and external beam irradiation ± 5-FU for locally advanced pancreatic cancer. Int J Radiat Oncol Biol Phys 13:319, 1986
17. Gunderson LL, Shipley WU, Suit HD, et al: Intraoperative irradiation: A pilot study combining external-beam photons with "boost" dose intraoperative electrons. Cancer 49:2259, 1981
18. Gunderson LL, Tepper JE, Biggs PJ, et al: Intraoperative ± external beam irradiation. Curr Probl Cancer 7:1, 1983
19. Haslam JB, Cavanaugh PJ, Stroup SL: Radiation therapy in the treatment of unresectable adenocarcinoma of the pancreas. Cancer 32:1341, 1973
20. Howard JM: Pancreatoduodenectomy: Forty-one consecutive whipple resections without an operative mortality. Ann Surg 168:629, 1968
21. Kalser MH, Ellenberg SS, for Gastrointestinal Tumor Study Group: Pancreatic cancer: Adjuvant combined radiation and chemotherapy following curative resection. Arch Surg 120:899, 1985
22. Klaassen DJ, MacIntyre JM, Catton GE, et al: Treatment of locally unresectable cancer of the stomach and pancreas: A randomized comparison of 5-fluorouracil alone with radiation plus concurrent and maintenance 5-fluorouracil: An Eastern Cooperative Oncology Group study. J Clin Oncol 3:373, 1985
23. MacDonald JS, Gunderson LL, Cohen I: Cancer of the pancreas. In DeVita VT, Hellman S, Rosenberg SA (eds): Principles and Practice of Oncology, 2nd ed, p 563. Philadelphia, JB Lippincott, 1982
24. Moertel CT, Childs DS Jr, Reitemeir RJ, et al: Combined 5-fluorouracil and supervoltage radiation therapy of locally unresectable gastrointestinal cancer. Lancet 2:865, 1969
25. Mohiuddin M, Cantor RJ, Biermann W, et al: Combined modality treatment of localized unresectable adenocarcinoma of the pancreas. Int J Radiat Oncol Biol Phys 14:79, 1987
26. O'Connell MJ: Current status of chemotherapy for advanced pancreatic and gastric cancer. J Clin Oncol 3:1032, 1985
27. Pilepich MV, Miller HH: Preoperative irradiation in carcinoma of the pancreas. Cancer 46:1945, 1980
28. Roldan GE, Gunderson LL, Nagorney DM, et al: External beam versus intraoperative and external beam irradiation for locally advanced pancreatic cancer. Cancer 61:1110, 1988
29. Shipley WU, Nardi GL, Cohen AM: Iodine-125 implant and external beam irradiation in patients with localized pancreatic carcinoma: A comparative study to surgical resection. Cancer 45:709, 1980
30. Shipley WU, Wood WC, Tepper JE, et al: Intraoperative electron beam irradiation for patients with unresectable pancreatic carcinoma. Ann Surg 200: 289, 1984
31. Silverberg E, Boring CC, Squires TS: Cancer statistics. CA 4: 9, 1990.
32. Sindelar WF, Kinsella TJ: Randomized trial of intraoperative radiotherapy in resected carcinoma of the pancreas. Int J Radiat Oncol Biol Phys 12:148, 1986
33. Smith FP, Schein PS, MaDonald JS, et al: Fast neutron irradiation for locally advanced pancreatic cancer. Int J Radiat Oncol Biol Phys 7:1527, 1981
34. Tepper JE, Nardi GL, Suit HD: Carcinoma of the pancreas: Review of MGH experience from 1963 to 1973: Analysis of surgical failure and implications for radiation therapy. Cancer 37:1519, 1976
35. Tepper JE, Shipley WU, Warshaw AL, et al: The role of misonidazole combined with intraoperative radiation therapy in the treatment of pancreatic carcinoma. J Clin Oncol 5:579, 1987
36. Warren KW, Braasch JW, Thum CW: Carcinoma of the pancreas. Surg Clin North Am 48:601, 1968
37. Warshaw AL, Swanson RS: What's new in general surgery: Pancreatic cancer in 1988. Possibilities and probabilities. Ann Surg 208:541, 1988
38. Whittington R, Dobelbower RR, Mohiuddin M, et al: Radiotherapy of unresectable pancreatic carcinoma: A six-year experience with 104 patients. Int J Radiat Oncol Biol Phys 7:1639, 1981
39. Whittington R, Solin L, Mohiuddin M, et al: Multimodality therapy of localized unresectable pancreatic adenocarcinoma. Cancer 54:1991, 1984
40. Wood W, Shipley WU, Gunderson LL, et al: Intraoperative irradiation for unresectable pancreatic carcinoma. Cancer 49:1272, 1982

Gallbladder and Bile Duct

41. Adson MA, Farnell MD: Hepatobiliary cancer: Surgery considerations. Mayo Clin Proc 56:686, 1981
42. Akwari OE, Van Heerden J, Adson MA, et al: Radical pancreaticoduodenectomy for cancer of the papilla of Vater. Arch Surg 112:451, 1977
43. Ashayeri E, Halyard M, Goldson AL, et al: The first simultaneous intraoperative hyperthermia and radiotherapy procedure: Dog experiment and technique. J Natl Med Assoc 79:619, 1987
44. Berquist TH, May GR, Johnson CM, et al: Percutaneous biliary decompression: Internal and external drainage in 50 patients. AJR 136:901, 1981
45. Bismuth H, Malt RA: Current concepts in cancer: Carcinoma of the biliary tree. N Engl J Med 301:704, 1979
46. Braasch JW: Malignant neoplasms of the bile ducts. Surg Clin North Am 47:627, 1967
47. Buskirk S, Gunderson LL, Adson MA, et al: Analysis of failure following curative irradiation of gallbladder and extrahepatic bile duct carcinoma. Int J Radiat Oncol Biol Phys 10:2013, 1984
48. Buskirk SJ, Gunderson LL, Martenson JA, et al: Analysis of failure following curative irradiation of extrahepatic bile duct carcinoma. [ASTRO abstracts] Int J Radiat Oncol Biol Phys (Suppl) 12:120, 1986
49. Busse PM, Stone MD, Sheldon TA, et al: Intraoperative radiation therapy for biliary tract carcinoma: Results of a five year experience. Surgery 105:724, 1989
50. Chitwood WR Jr, Meyers WC, Heaston DK, et al: Diagnosis and treatment of primary extrahepatic bile duct tumors. Am J Surg 143:99, 1982
51. Conroy RM, Shahbazian AA, Edwards KC, et al: A new method for treating carcinomatous biliary obstruction with intracatheter radium. Cancer 49:1321, 1982
52. Devereaux DF, Greco RS: Biliary enteric bypass for malignant obstruction. Cancer 58:981, 1986
53. Deziel DJ, Kiel KD, Kramer TS, et al: Intraoperative radiation therapy in biliary tract cancer. Am J Surg 54:402, 1988
54. Fields JN, Emami B: Carcinoma of the extrahepatic biliary system: Results of primary and adjuvant radiotherapy. Int J Radiat Oncol Biol Phys 13:331, 1987
55. Fletcher MS, Dawson JL, Wheeler PG, et al: Treatment of high bile duct carcinoma by internal radiotherapy with iridium-192 wire. Lancet 2:172, 1981
56. Fogel TD, Weissberg JB: The role of radiation therapy in carcinoma of the extrahepatic bile ducts. Int J Radiat Oncol Biol Phys 10:2251, 1984
57. Goebel RH: Techniques for localized radiation of the biliary tree. [ASTRO proceedings] Int J Radiat Oncol Biol Phys 5:80, 1979
58. Green N, Mikkelsen WP, Kernen JA: Cancer of the common hepatic bile ducts: Palliative radiotherapy. Radiology 109:687, 1975
59: Gunderson LL, Meyer JE, Sheedy P, Munzenrider JE: Radiation oncology. In Margolis AR, Burhenne HJ (eds): Alimentary Tract Radiology, 3rd ed, p 2409. St. Louis, CV Mosby, 1982
60. Hall SH, Benjamin RS, Murphy WK, et al: Adriamycin,

BCNU, ftorafur chemotherapy of pancreatic and bile duct cancer. Cancer 44:2008, 1974
61. Hanna SS, Rider WD: Carcinoma of the gallbladder or extrahepatic bile ducts: The role of radiotherapy. Can Med Assoc J 118:59, 1978
62. Harvey JH, Smith FP, Schein PS: 5-Fluorouracil, mitomycin and doxorubicin (FAM) in carcinoma of the biliary tract. J Clin Oncol 2(suppl 11):1245, 1984
63. Hayes JK, Sapozink MD, Miller FJ: Definitive radiation therapy in bile duct carcinoma. Int J Radiat Oncol Biol Phys 15:735, 1988
64. Herskovic AM, Engler MJ, Noell KT: Radical radiotherapy for bile duct carcinoma. Endocurie Ther Hyper Oncol 1:119, 1985
65. Herskovic A, Heaston D, Engler MJ, et al: Irradiation of biliary carcinomas. Radiology 139:219, 1981
66. Ikeda H, Kiroda C, Uchida H: Intraluminal irradiation with Iridium-192 wires for extrahepatic bile duct carcinoma. Nippon Igaku 39:1356, 1979
67. Iwasaki Y, Todoroki T, Fukao K, et al: The role of intraoperative radiation therapy in the treatment of bile duct cancer. World J Surg 12:91, 1988
68. Johnson DW, Safai C, Goffinet DR: Malignant obstructive jaundice: Treatment with external beam and intracavitary radiotherapy. Int J Radiat Oncol Biol Phys 11:411, 1985
69. Karani J, Fletcher M, Brinkley D, et al: Internal biliary drainage and local radiotherapy with ^{192}Ir wire in the treatment of hilar cholangiocarcinoma. Clin Radiol 36:603, 1985
70. Kopelson G: Curative surgery for adenocarcinoma of the pancrease/ampulla of vater: The role of adjuvant pre- or postoperative radiation therapy. Int J Radiat Oncol Biol Phys 9:911, 1983
71. Kopelson G, Galdabini J, Warshaw A, et al: Patterns of failure after curative surgery for extrahepatic biliary tract carcinoma. Int J Radiat Oncol Biol Phys 7:413, 1981
72. Kopelson GK, Gunderson LL: Primary and adjuvant radiation therapy in gallbladder and extrahepatic biliary tract carcinoma. J Clin Gastroenterol 5:43, 1983
73. Kopelson G, Harisiadis L, Tretter P, et al: The role of radiation therapy in cancer of the extrahepatic biliary system: An analysis of thirteen patients and a review of the literature of the effectiveness of surgery, chemotherapy, and radiotherapy. Int J Radiat Oncol Biol Phys 2:883, 1977
74. Lokich JJ, Kane RA, Harrison DA, McDermott WF: Biliary tract obstruction secondary to cancer: Management guidelines and selected literature review. J Clin Oncol 5:969, 1987
75. MacDonald JS, Gunderson LL, Adson M: Hepatobiliary cancer. In DeVita VT, Hellman S, Rosenberg SA (eds): Principles and Practice of Oncology, 2nd ed, p 590. Philadelphia, JB Lippincott, 1982
76. Meyers WC, Jones RS: Internal radiation for bile duct cancer. World J Surg 12:99, 1988
77. Mirsa NC, Jaiswal MSD, Singh RV, et al: Intrahepatic arterial infusion of combination of mitomycin C and 5-fluorouracil in treatment of primary and metastatic liver cancer. Cancer 39:1425, 1977
78. Mittal B, Duetsch M, Iwatsuki S: Primary cancers of extrahepatic biliary passages. Int J Radiat Oncol Biol Phys 11:849, 1985
79. Molt P, Hopfan S, Watson RC, et al: Intraluminal radiation therapy in the management of malignant biliary obstruction. Cancer 57:536, 1986
80. Mueller PR, Ferrucci JT: Percutaneous biliary drainage: Current techniques. Appl Radiol :53, 1983
81. Piehler JM, Crichlow RW: Primary carcinoma of the gallbladder. Surg Gynecol Obstet 147:933, 1978
82. Pilepich MV, Lambert PM: Radiotherapy for carcinoma of the extrahepatic biliary system. Radiology 127:767, 1978
83. Piorkowski RJ: Pancreatic and periampullary carcinoma. Am J Surg 143:189, 1982
84. Ross AP: Carcinoma of the proximal bile ducts. Surg Gynecol Obstet 136:923, 1973
85. Sindelar WF, Tepper J, Travis EL: Tolerance of bile duct to intra-operative irradiation. Surgery 92:533, 1982
86. Smoron GL: Radiation therapy of carcinoma of the gallbladder and biliary tract. Cancer 40:1422, 1977
87. Terblanche J: Is carcinoma of the main hepatic junction an indication for liver transplantation or palliative surgery? A plea for the U-tube palliative procedure. Surgery 79:127, 1976
88. Todoroki T: The late effects of single massive irradiation with electrons of the liver hilum of rabbits. Jpn J Gastroenterol Surg 11:169, 1978
89. Todoroki T, Iwasaki Y, Okamura T, et al: Intraoperative radiotherapy for advanced carcinoma of the biliary system. Cancer 46:2179, 1980
90. Vaittenim E: Carcinoma of the gallbladdler. Ann Chir Gynaecol 168:1, 1970
91. Walsh DB: Adenocarcinoma of the ampulla of vater. Ann Surg 195:152, 1982
92. Warren KW: Malignant tumors of the bile ducts. Br J Surg 59:501, 1972
93. Warren KW: Primary neoplasia of the gallbladder. Surg Gynecol Obstet 126:1036, 1968
94. Warren KW: Results of radical resection for periampullary cancer. Ann Surg 181:534, 1975
95. Wong JYC, Vora NL, Chen CK, et al: Intracatheter hyperthermia and iridium-192 radiotherapy in the treatment of bile duct carcinoma. Int J Radiat Oncol Biol Phys 14:353, 1988

Liver

96. Dritshilo A, Grant EG, Harter KW, et al: Interstitial radiation therapy for hepatic metastases: Sonographic guidance for applicator placement. AJR 146:275, 1986
97. Friedman MA, Volberding PA, Cassidy MJ: Therapy for hepatocellular cancer with intrahepatic arterial Adriamycin and 5-fluorouracil combined with whole liver radiation: An NCOG study. Cancer Treat Rep 63:1885, 1979
98. Ingold JA, Reed GB, Kaplan HS, et al: Radiation hepatis. Am J Roentgenol Radium Ther Nucl Med 93:200, 1965
99. Issa P: Cancerous hemangioma of the liver: The role of radiotherapy. Br J Radiol 41:26, 1968
100. Kaplan HS, Bagshaw MA: Radiation hepatitis: Possible prevention by combined isotopic and external radiation therapy. Radiology 91:1214, 1968
101. Order SE, Leibel S, Llein JL: A phase I–II study of radiolabeled antibody integrated in multi-modal treatment of primary hepatic malignancies. [ASTRO proceedings] Int J Radiat Oncol Biol Phys 5:120, 1979
102. Order SE, Stillwagon GB, Lein J, et al: Iodine 131 antiferrin, a new treatment modality in hepatoma: A Radiation Therapy Oncology Group study. J Clin Oncol 3:1573, 1985
103. Park WC, Phillips R: The role of radiation therapy in the management of hemangiomas of the liver. JAMA 212:1496, 1970
104. Phillips R, Karnofsky DA, Hamilton LD, Nickson JJ: Roentgen therapy of hepatic metastases. Am J Roentgenol Radium Ther Nucl Med 71:826, 1954
105. Phillips R, Murikami K: Primary neoplasms of the liver: Results of radiation therapy. Cancer 13:714, 1960
106. Stillwagon GB, Order SE, Guse C, et al: 194 Hepatocellular tumors treated by radiation and chemotherapy combinations: Toxicity and response: A Radiation Therapy Oncology Group study. Int J Radiat Oncol Biol Phys 17:1223, 1989

46

○ ○ ○ • • •

Colon and Rectum

James A. Martenson, Jr.
Leonard L. Gunderson

ANATOMY

Rectum

The rectum, a continuation of the sigmoid colon, begins in front of the third sacral vertebra. At the junction of the sigmoid colon and rectum, the large bowel loses its mesentery. Peritoneum covers the upper portion of the rectum laterally and anteriorly near its junction with the sigmoid colon and only anteriorly near the peritoneal reflection. The peritoneum is reflected anteriorly onto the seminal vesicles and bladder in the male and onto the upper vagina and uterus in the female, leaving the lower half of the rectum entirely without a peritoneal covering. The location of the peritoneal reflection can have important implications in patients undergoing sphincter-preservation procedures. For example, electrocoagulation of anterior tumors above the peritoneal reflection is considered unsafe because of the risk of perforation.[23] However, location above the peritoneal reflection does not contraindicate management of selected tumors by endocavitary radiation therapy.[90]

The three transverse folds of the rectum, two on the left and one on the right, apportion it into thirds. The middle transverse fold lies approximately 11 cm from the anal verge and provides a landmark for the peritoneal reflection. The portion of the rectum below the middle valve is called the rectal ampulla; if the ampulla is resected, stool frequency often is markedly increased. This morbidity is an important factor to consider in choosing between a "radical" sphincter-sparing procedure, such as coloanal anastomosis, and a "conservative" sphincter-sparing procedure, such as endocavitary irradiation.

The principal route of lymphatic drainage for carcinomas of the rectum follows the superior rectal vessels, which empty into the inferior mesenteric nodes. Lymphatic drainage of the middle and lower rectum also occurs along the middle rectal vessels, terminating in internal iliac nodes. The lowest part of the rectum and the upper part of the anal canal share a plexus that drains to lymphatics that accompany the inferior rectal and internal pudendal blood vessels and ultimately drain to internal iliac nodes. Carcinomas of the lower rectum or those that extend into the anal canal occasionally may metastasize to superficial inguinal nodes by connections to efferent lymphatics draining the lower anus (Fig. 46-1).

Colon

The ascending and descending colon and the splenic and hepatic flexures lack a mesentery and are immobile, because of their retroperitoneal location. Cancers that extend through the bowel wall on the posterior aspect may have compromised surgical margins.

The transverse and sigmoid colon have a complete mesentery and are freely mobile. Tumors that extend through the bowel wall in these mobile segments generally can be removed surgically with satisfactory circumferential margins.

The cecum lacks a true mesentery but may have some mobility due to short folds of peritoneum that are variably present. Surgical margins may be narrow if the lesions extend posteriorly.

The lymphatic drainage of the colon follows the inferior mesenteric vessels for the left colon and the superior mesenteric vessels for the right colon. Additional lymph node groups can be at risk if adjacent organs or structures are involved by cancer. If tumors involve adjacent organs in the true or false pelvis, the iliac nodes may be at risk. Periaortic lymph nodes may be at risk when cancer invades the posterior wall. If the lower abdominal wall is involved, inguinal nodes may be at risk.

EPIDEMIOLOGY

Adenocarcinoma of the large bowel occurred in an estimated 155,000 persons in the United States in 1990 and caused approximately 61,000 deaths.[115] The incidences of large bowel cancer in males and females are approximately equal.[115] The risk of large bowel cancer is markedly increased in patients with inflammatory bowel disease and is 100% in patients with untreated familial polyposis or Gardner's syndrome.

In the past 30 to 50 years, the site of colon and rectal cancer has shifted toward the right colon.[5,17,102] Increased early detection of distal precancerous lesions has been suggested as a contributing factor.[17]

Environmental influences may have a role in the cause of large bowel cancer. For example, immigrant Japanese populations acquire higher large bowel cancer mortality rates within one generation; these rates approach those of the U.S. white

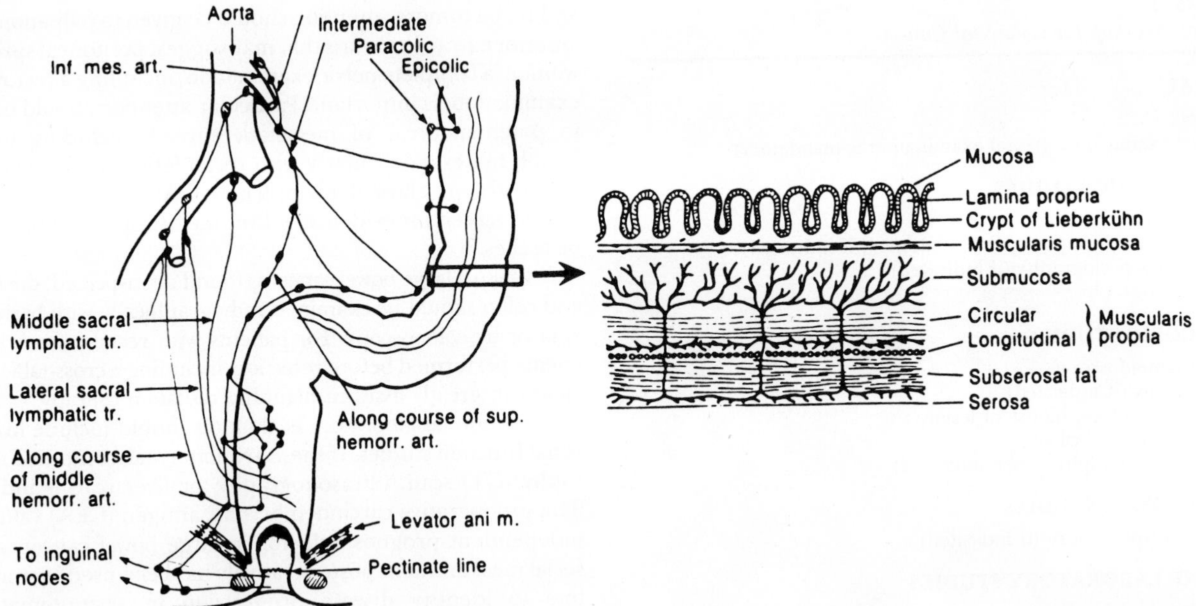

FIGURE 46–1. Lymphatic drainage of the large bowel, including the colon wall. (Modified from Villemin F, Huard P, Montague M: Rev Chir 63:39, 1925 and from Cole PP: Br Med J 1:431, 1913)

population.[54] Seventh Day Adventists and Mormons follow dietary practices that increase their fiber consumption and decrease their meat consumption. Among Seventh Day Adventists, mortality rates from colon cancer are approximately 60% to 70% of those of the general population, and the incidence of colon and rectal cancer in the Utah Mormon population is approximately 60% of that in the non-Mormon population.[75,93]

Epidemiologic evidence suggests a possible preventive role for dietary fiber in large bowel cancer. Burkitt[16] called attention to the low incidence of large bowel cancer in developing nations in which high-fiber diets are common.[128] Other studies have lent support to a protective role for dietary fiber by showing an inverse correlation between fiber intake and risk of large bowel cancer.[25,63,76,77,80]

Not all studies support a simple relationship between dietary fiber and large bowel cancer risk, however. Liu and colleagues[74] found no significant correlation between dietary fiber and mortality from colon cancer. The epidemiologic literature on the relationship between large bowel cancer and fiber has been summarized in a National Cancer Institute analysis of 40 studies.[43] Most studies found an inverse relationship between dietary fiber intake and colon cancer.

Fecal bile acids have been shown to promote carcinogenesis in an animal model, and fecal excretion of bile acids has been shown to be high in colon cancer patients.[98,99] Cholecystectomy, which results in an increase in the amount of secondary bile acids that reach the colon, might result in an increased incidence of colon cancer if secondary bile acids have a role in colon carcinogenesis in humans. Although some studies lend support to the hypothesis that cholecystectomy increases the risk of colon cancer, others do not.[11,73,124,125] A study of fecal bile acid physiology in a low-risk high-fiber-intake population in Finland suggests a possible link between promotion of colon cancer by secondary bile acids and prevention of colon cancer by high-fiber intake.[97]

Several studies indicate a positive association between fat intake and colon carcinogenesis.[3,25,27,61,74] Armstrong and Doll[3] found a strong association between mortality rates for colon cancer and total fat consumption.

A possible carcinogenic effect of dietary cholesterol was suggested by Liu and co-workers.[74] Dietary cholesterol has been hypothesized to be the fat-related substance with cocarcinogenic properties in humans.[24]

Selenium appears to inhibit carcinogenesis in laboratory animals.[44,86] Areas of the United States with high bioavailability of selenium have lower death rates from cancer in general and from cancer of the intestines and rectum in particular.[62,113]

PATTERNS OF SPREAD AND NATURAL HISTORY

Discontinuous spread of colon and rectal cancer can occur by four mechanisms: peritoneal seeding, lymphatic spread, hematogenous spread, and surgical implantation. Peritoneal spread is rare in patients with rectal cancer because most of the rectum is below the peritoneal reflection.

Extension within the bowel usually occurs only for short distances. Black and Waugh[10] found that only four of 103 patients had microscopic intramural spread greater than 0.5 cm from the gross lesion. Further evidence of the limited tendency for intramural spread was found in a study by Pollett and associates[95] in which anastomotic recurrence, local control, and survival were nearly identical in patients with less than or with greater than 2-cm longitudinal margins.

Because primary venous and lymphatic channels originate in submucosal layers of the bowel, cancers limited to the mucosa are at little risk for dissemination. Lymph node involvement is found in approximately 50% of these patients and usually is orderly and predictable. Skip metastasis or retrograde spread occurs in only 1% to 3% of node-positive patients and is generally thought to be due to lymphatic blockage.[45]

CLINICAL PRESENTATION

The most common presenting feature in patients with rectal and lower sigmoid cancer is melena. Abdominal pain is the most common presenting feature in patients with colon cancer.[96]

TABLE 46–1
Diagnostic Workup for Colorectal Cancer

GENERAL
- History
- Physical examination (rectal examination is mandatory)

RADIOGRAPHIC STUDIES
- Barium enema
- Computed tomography (pelvis, abdomen, if indicated)
- Intravenous pyelography (if indicated)
- Chest radiography

ENDOSCOPIC STUDIES
- Proctosigmoidoscopy
- Colonoscopy (if indicated)
- Excision of polyps; biopsy of lesion
- Cystoscopy (if indicated)
- Excretory urography (when indicated)

RADIOISOTOPE STUDIES
- Liver scan/spleen scan (if indicated)

ROUTINE LABORATORY STUDIES
- Complete blood count
- Urinalysis
- Blood chemistry profile

Other presenting features of large bowel cancer include a change in bowel habit, nausea, vomiting, weakness, and abdominal mass. Patients found incidentally to have microcytic anemia should be considered to have large bowel cancer until proven otherwise.

DIAGNOSTIC WORKUP

Diagnostic procedures for the evaluation of colon and rectal cancer are outlined in Table 46-1. Physical examination should produce a detailed description of the primary tumor and screen for potential sites of metastatic disease. In patients with rectal cancer, a digital rectal examination and endoscopy should provide information regarding the location of the lesion (*i.e.*, distance above the anal verge and which rectal walls are involved), whether it is exophytic or ulcerative, its size and mobility, and whether any palpable perirectal nodes are present. For colon and rectal tumors, attention should be given to palpation of any anterior extrarectal mass that may suggest peritoneal spread. In women, a complete pelvic examination, including a rectovaginal examination, is important. Particular attention should be given to potential areas of metastatic spread, including inguinal lymph nodes (particularly with rectal lesions near the dentate line) and supraclavicular lymph nodes. Abdominal examination should screen for evidence of liver metastasis, abdominal mass, or ascites.

When a large bowel cancer is found or suspected, the rectum and colon should be examined radiographically with barium enema or by colonoscopy. For patients with rectal cancer, barium enema performed before resection, including a cross-table lateral view, can greatly assist in planning radiation therapy.

Additional laboratory evaluation should include liver and renal function studies. If these are abnormal, computed tomography (CT) scan, ultrasonography, or liver scan is indicated. The preoperative carcinoembryonic antigen (CEA) value is an independent prognostic factor in large bowel cancer, and its serial measurement postoperatively has been used in some centers to identify disease progression in asymptomatic patients.[78,130] A National Institutes of Health Consensus Development Panel determined that serial CEA measurement remains the most sensitive laboratory indicator of recurrent disease.[42] However, most patients with recurrence have symptoms before the CEA value increases.[7] CEA increases in only 25% of patients with recurrent disease.[84] Moreover, patients found to have recurrent disease by this test are unlikely to be cured.[78,91]

STAGING SYSTEMS

Dukes[28] described a staging system based on the extent of disease penetration through the bowel wall and the presence or absence of nodal metastasis (Table 46-2). Dukes' staging has the disadvantage of not specifying the degree of tumor penetration through the wall of the bowel in node-positive patients. The Astler-Coller staging system allows specification of tumor penetration and nodal involvement, and its subsequent modification also permits the specification of tumor adherence to surrounding organ structures.[4,52] The Dukes, Astler-Coller, and modified Astler-Coller systems all are postoperative pathologic staging systems and cannot be used preoperatively. The TNM system of the American Joint Committee on Cancer can be used as a clinical (preoperative) or a postoperative staging system.[6]

TABLE 46–2
Staging Systems for Large Bowel Cancer

STAGING SYSTEM				
DUKES[28]	ASTLER-COLLER[4]	MODIFIED ASTLER-COLLER	TNM	DESCRIPTION
A	A	A	T1N0	Nodes negative; limited to mucosa
	B1	B1	T2N0	Nodes negative; penetration into submucosa but not through muscularis propria
B	B2	B2	T3N0	Nodes negative; penetration through muscularis propria
		B3	T4N0	Nodes negative; penetration through muscularis propria with adherence to or invasion of surrounding organs or structures
C	C1	C1	T1–2N1	Nodes positive; limited to bowel wall
	C2	C2	T3N1	Nodes positive; penetration through muscularis propria
		C3	T4N1	Nodes positive; penetration through muscularis propria and adherence to or invasion of surrounding organs or structures

TABLE 46–3
Failure Patterns in Rectal Cancer Classified by the Modified Astler-Coller System

INVESTIGATOR	MAC STAGE*	NO. OF PATIENTS AT RISK	FAILURES: LOCAL ONLY (PATIENTS)	(%)	TOTAL OR LOCAL (PATIENTS)	(%)
Rich et al[103]	A, B1	39	2	5	3	8
	B2	44	5	11	10	23
	B3	15	6	40	8	53
	C1	4	1	25	1	25
	C2	34	6	18	10	29
	C3	6	4	67	4	67
Gilbert[41]	A	1			0	0
	B1	42			6	14
	B2, B3	37			13	35
	C1	5			1	20
	C2, C3	37			24	65
Walz et al[129]	A	12	0	0	2	17
	B1	21	0	0	0	0
	B2	38	3	8	6	16
	B3	5	1	20	1	20
	C1	7	0	0	2	29
	C2	38	4	11	14	37
	C3	2	0	0	1	50

**MAC: modified Astler-Coller system.*

PATHOLOGIC FEATURES

Most malignant tumors of the large bowel are adenocarcinomas, and most are moderately well differentiated histologically. Among patients who undergo operation for cure, approximately one third have lymph node metastasis (Tables 46-3 and 46-4). Retrograde lymph node involvement and skip metastasis are unusual, and both are associated with poor prognoses.[45]

PROGNOSTIC FACTORS

From the radiation oncologist's perspective, the most useful prognostic factors are tumor penetration of the bowel wall and lymph node involvement. Both factors confer an increased risk of local recurrence (Tables 46-3 and 46-4) and, accordingly, are helpful in selecting candidates for adjuvant radiation therapy. The absolute number and the proportion of lymph nodes involved are important predictors of outcome.[22,110] The presence of both lymph node involvement and extension of disease beyond the bowel wall is more ominous than the presence of either alone.[103,110] In patients with low rectal cancer who are being considered for sphincter-sparing treatment, clinical mobility of the lesion, size of the lesion, and morphology of the lesion are predictors of prognosis.[90]

TABLE 46–4
Patterns of Failure in Colon Cancer by Stage

MAC*	NO. OF PATIENTS AT RISK	FAILURES (%): LOCAL ONLY†	LOCAL ± DISTANT
A	29	0	3
B1	89	1	2
B2	163	4	11
B3	83	11	30
C1	20	0	0
C2	100	10	32
C3	49	12	49
Total	533	6	19

**MAC: modified Astler-Coller system.*
† Defined as recurrence within the tumor bed, in adjacent organs by direct extension, or in regional node groups.
(Data from the Massachusetts General Hospital series adapted from Willett CG, Tepper JE, Cohen AM, et al: Ann Surg 200:685, 1984)

GENERAL MANAGEMENT

Operative Considerations

Surgical resection is the initial treatment of choice for most patients. The objective is removal of the tumor and primary nodal drainage with as wide a margin around both as feasible. Anterior resections are technically feasible in patients with cancers at least 6 cm to 8 cm above the anal verge, producing survival rates similar to those for abdominoperineal resection.[118]

Surgical and pathologic reports commonly refer to the longitudinal bowel margin. Nodal and circumferential (radial) margins actually may be more important, however. If a tumor spreads beyond the bowel wall in anatomically immobile segments of the large bowel, the narrowest margin of resection typically is situated laterally, anteriorly, or posteriorly rather than along the length of the bowel. A study of whole-mount sections found that 40% of the patients who underwent resection of a rectal carcinoma had a radial margin of 3 mm or less.[19]

In patients in whom postoperative irradiation may play a role, several surgical procedures assist in planning treatment and minimizing toxicity. Pelvic floor reconstruction and reperitonealization help to minimize the volume of small bowel in the pelvis. For patients in whom high-dose treatment to the pelvis is anticipated, complete exclusion of all small bowel from the pelvis can be achieved by using an absorbable mesh sling.[2,31,64] Primary closure of the perineal wound after abdominoperineal resection ensures more rapid healing and prevents delays in instituting postoperative radiation therapy. A full description of the extent of the tumor and placement of clips demarcating the tumor bed and residual disease can assist in the design of radiation therapy fields.

Preoperative irradiation in the range of 4500 cGy to 5000 cGy does not preclude the safe use of anterior resection and primary anastomosis.[106,120] An unirradiated loop of large bowel should be used for the proximal limb of the anastomosis.

Patterns of Failure After Curative Resection

Detailed information regarding anatomic sites of failure after operation for rectal cancer is available from the University of Minnesota reoperation series (Fig. 46-2).[52] Seventy-four patients thought to be at high risk for local recurrence underwent elective or symptomatic second-look operations. Of these, 52 (70%) had metastatic or locally recurrent cancer. Locoregional recurrence in the pelvis or para-aortic nodes was the sole failure in 24 (46%) of these 52 patients and occurred as a component of failure in 48 (92%) of the 52.

Table 46-3 provides information about failure in an unselected patient population. Patients with disease extension beyond the bowel wall or with nodal involvement, or both, in general have local recurrence rates of 20% to 70%. The presence of both disease extension beyond the rectal wall and nodal involvement generally is associated with a high risk of local recurrence, particularly if the tumor adheres to surrounding structures. Distant metastasis occurs in approximately 30% of

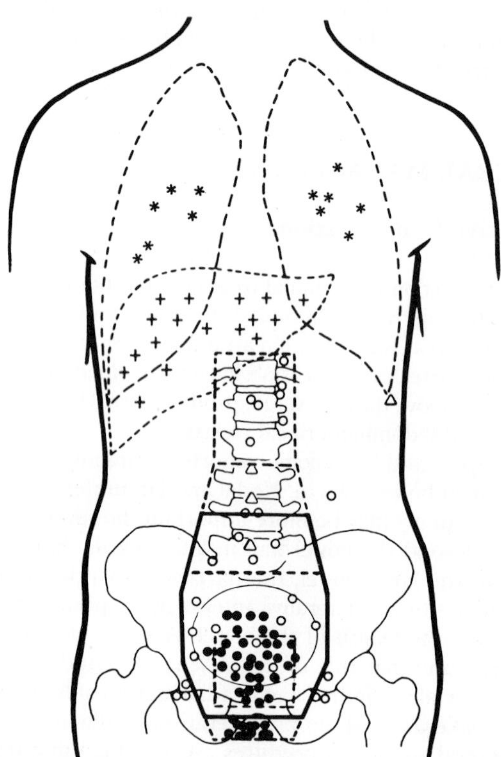

FIGURE 46–2. Sites of failure in the Minnesota reoperative series. (Gunderson LL, Sosin H: Cancer 34:1278, 1974; by permission of the American Cancer Society.)

all patients who undergo curative resection of rectal cancer, and the most common sites of involvement are liver, lung, and peritoneum.[103,134]

Patterns of failure in colon cancer have been analyzed in autopsy, clinical, and reoperation series.[53,79,107,108,133,135] Data from these series suggest that local failure is a significant problem after resection of colon cancer. Local failure is highest among patients with tumors adhering to surrounding structures and among patients with tumor extension beyond the bowel wall and with metastatically involved lymph nodes.[135]

Approximately 20% of the patients who undergo curative resection of colon cancer develop distant metastases.[79] The most common sites of distant metastases are liver, lung, and peritoneum.[107,134]

RADIATION THERAPY TECHNIQUES

A shrinking-field technique should be used, with initial radiation therapy fields designed to treat the primary tumor volume and regional lymph nodes. Smaller fields then can be used to treat the primary tumor bed to higher doses, as clinically indicated.

The width of AP/PA ports (Fig. 46-3) should cover the pelvic inlet with a 2-cm margin. The superior margin is usually 1.5 cm above the level of the sacral promontory. In patients who have had an anterior resection, the usual inferior margin is below the obturator foramina.

If the pelvis is treated, lateral fields should be used for a portion of treatment to avoid as much small bowel as possible. Bladder distention and prone position are useful techniques for displacing the small bowel out of the pelvis. The posterior field margin for lateral fields is critical because the rectum and perirectal tissues lie just anterior to the sacrum and coccyx. Accordingly, the posterior field margin should be at least 1.5 cm to 2 cm behind the anterior bony sacral margin (Figs. 46-3 and 46-4). The entire sacral canal with a 1.5-cm margin should be included in patients with locally advanced disease to avoid sacral recurrence from tumor spread along nerve roots (Fig. 46-5). The anterior margin sometimes can be shaped to decrease the amount of radiation to the femoral head and bladder inferiorly and small bowel superiorly (Fig. 46-3*C*).

The incidence of small bowel obstruction requiring reoperation after postoperative radiation therapy for rectal cancer appears to vary with treatment technique. When parallel opposed techniques, with the superior border of the field at L2, were used in the M. D. Anderson series, the incidence of small bowel obstruction was 17.5%, compared with a rate of 5% for surgery alone.[137] When the superior extent of the field was moved down to L5, the incidence of small bowel obstruction requiring operative intervention decreased to 10% to 12%. At Massachusetts General Hospital, multifield techniques and bladder distention were used.[59] The incidence of small bowel obstruction requiring surgery was 6% among patients who received postoperative irradiation and 5% in the group undergoing surgery alone.

In patients with rectal cancer, internal iliac and presacral nodes are at risk for metastatic involvement. These lymph node chains are not a standard part of the dissection for rectal cancer.[94] Accordingly, they should be included in the initial radiation therapy volume treated to 4500 cGy to 5000 cGy. External iliac nodes are not a primary lymph node drainage site and are not included unless pelvic organs with external iliac drainage (*i.e.*, prostate, upper vagina, bladder, uterus) are involved by direct extension.

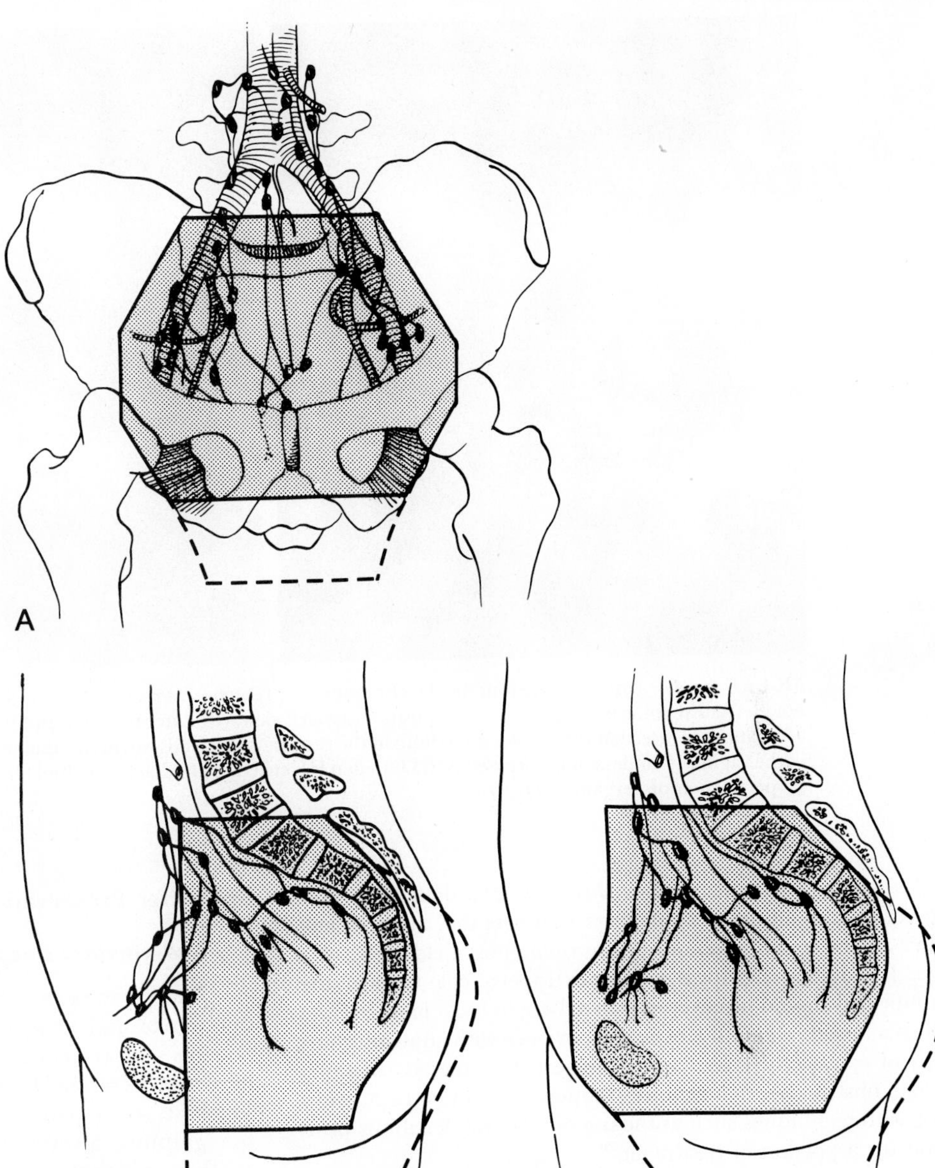

FIGURE 46–3. Radiation treatment fields before or after anterior resection or combined abdominoperineal resection (CAPR). (**A**) The AP/PA field. Notice the inferior extension (*broken line*) of the field to cover perineal tissue and scar after CAPR. (**B**) Idealized lateral field, showing inclusion of the internal iliac and presacral nodes; the posterior portion of this field is altered (*broken line*) after CAPR. (**C**) Idealized lateral field with anterior modification to include external iliac nodes. (Modified from Gunderson LL, Russell AH, Llewellyn HJ, et al: Int J Radiat Oncol Biol Phys 11:1379, 1985)

Inclusion of the entire perineum within the radiation therapy field after abdominoperineal resection is controversial.[46,123] In surgical series, the risk of perineal recurrence after abdominoperineal resection ranges from 8% to 30%.[20,85,103] Temporary, acute, moderate, or moderately severe perineal discomfort occurs in all patients whose perineums are included within radiation fields. In males, this can be partially mitigated by shifting the penis and scrotum cephalad, anterior to the symphysis pubis, during treatment. The incidence of chronic complications has not increased as a result of perineal inclusion.[59]

In one series, perineal recurrence developed in only 1.7% of 60 patients treated with the perineum within the adjuvant radiation field.[59] At the Mayo Clinic, the perineal failure rate was 2% at 5 years for patients undergoing postoperative adjuvant radiation therapy for whom the perineum was included within the radiation therapy field for the initial 4000 cGy. In contrast, if the entire perineum was not treated, the perineal failure rate was 23% at 5 years ($P=0.01$).[110] Although these results were not drawn from a randomized trial, multivariate analysis showed perineal treatment by radiation to be the only significant factor associated with perineal failure. On balance, most data suggest that inclusion of the perineum within postoperative radiation therapy fields after abdominoperineal resection decreases the risk of perineal failure from approximately 20% to 2%.

Radiopaque markers can be used to outline the extent of the perineal scar at the time of simulation for AP/PA and lateral fields (Fig. 46-6). Anteriorly, the lower third of the rectum abuts the posterior vaginal wall or prostate, and these structures should be included in patients with distal lesions. In female patients, this can be verified by placing a contrast-soaked tampon in the vagina during radiation therapy simulation. Bolus applied to the perineal scar during the PA treatment will prevent underdosage to this site.

The dose to the large fields, which include the tumor bed and regional lymph nodes, should be 4500 cGy to 5000 cGy given in 5 to 6 weeks. After this, consideration should be given to the use of a boost field to the primary tumor bed and immediately adjacent lymph nodes. If careful attention is given to technique and normal tissue tolerance, total doses of 5000 cGy to 5500 cGy delivered in 6 to 6.5 weeks are well tolerated. Boost fields are defined by methods such as barium enema studies,

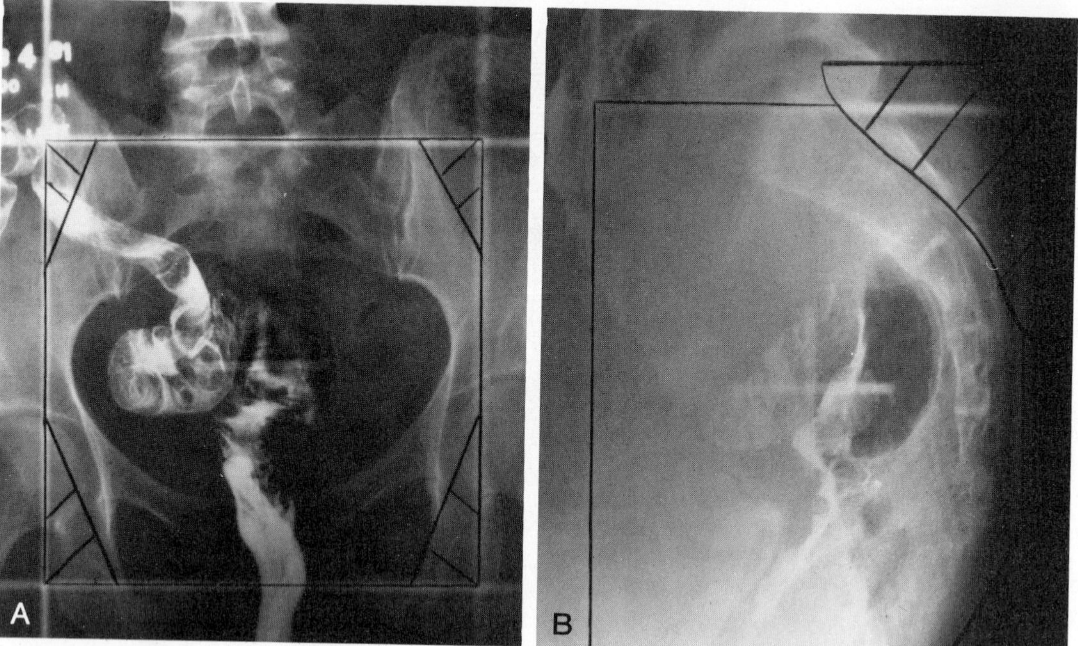

FIGURE 46–4. Postoperative four-field techniques after resection of rectal cancer and reanastomosis of bowel. (**A**) Patient is in prone treatment position, PA/AP view. (**B**) Lateral tumor and lymph node fields after anterior resection with contrast medium in the rectum, small lead shot in the anal verge, and tampon in the vagina. (Gunderson LL, Russell AH, Llewellyn HJ, et al: Int J Radiat Oncol Biol Phys 11:1379, 1985; by permission of Pergamon Press)

CT scan, and clip placement. Doses greater than 5000 cGy generally should not be administered unless there is complete shift of the small bowel out of the final boost field.

If radiation therapy is used for extrapelvic colon cancer, the tumor bed should be covered with a 3-cm to 5-cm margin. The Massachusetts General Hospital experience with adjuvant therapy of extrapelvic colon cancer suggests that the risk of small bowel obstruction that requires reoperation can be kept below 5% with techniques such as the use of a lateral decubitus position for a portion of treatment.[29]

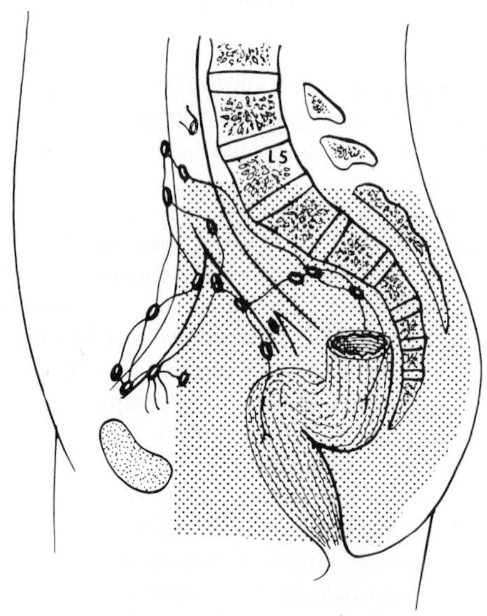

FIGURE 46–5. In a patient with locally advanced rectal cancer, the lateral field must include the entire sacral canal with a 1.5-cm margin. (Gunderson LL, Russell AH, Llewellyn HJ, et al: Int J Radiat Oncol Biol Phys 11:1379, 1985; by permission of Pergamon Press)

Sphincter Preservation

Endocavitary Radiation Therapy

Endocavitary radiation therapy produces high rates of local control and long-term survival in appropriately selected patients with rectal cancer. The indications for this technique have been described by Papillon[90] (Table 46-5). In assessing the suitability of a patient for this technique, intrarectal ultrasonography is a very accurate method for determining tumor confinement to the rectal wall.[8,58,109,132]

The treatment is performed on an outpatient basis. Local anesthesia in the anal canal occasionally is required for introducing the 3-cm-diameter applicator into the rectum. The radiation oncologist verifies the position of the applicator and coverage of the lesion. A lead apron and gloves are worn by the radiation oncologist, who holds the applicator firmly in place during the x-ray exposure.

The treatment regimen usually consists of four 3000-cGy treatments separated by intervals of approximately 2 weeks. A short-focal-distance (contact) x-ray unit is used at 50 kVp with 0.5 mm to 1.0 mm of aluminum filtration at a dose rate of approximately 1000 cGy per minute. If the size of the tumor exceeds the diameter of the applicator, several overlapping fields must be used.

For 207 patients treated by Papillon[90] with 5-year follow-up, the locoregional failure rate was 11%. Overall, 11% of the patients died of cancer, and 13% died of intercurrent disease. Distant metastases were found in only 3% of all patients. In the largest experience in the United States, similar, excellent results were obtained.[117]

At the Cleveland Clinic, 62 patients were treated between 1973 and 1984; the median follow-up was 30 months.[72] Local recurrence developed in 11 (18%) patients. In three of the 11, local recurrence was associated with distant metastasis. The remaining eight patients were rendered disease free by other

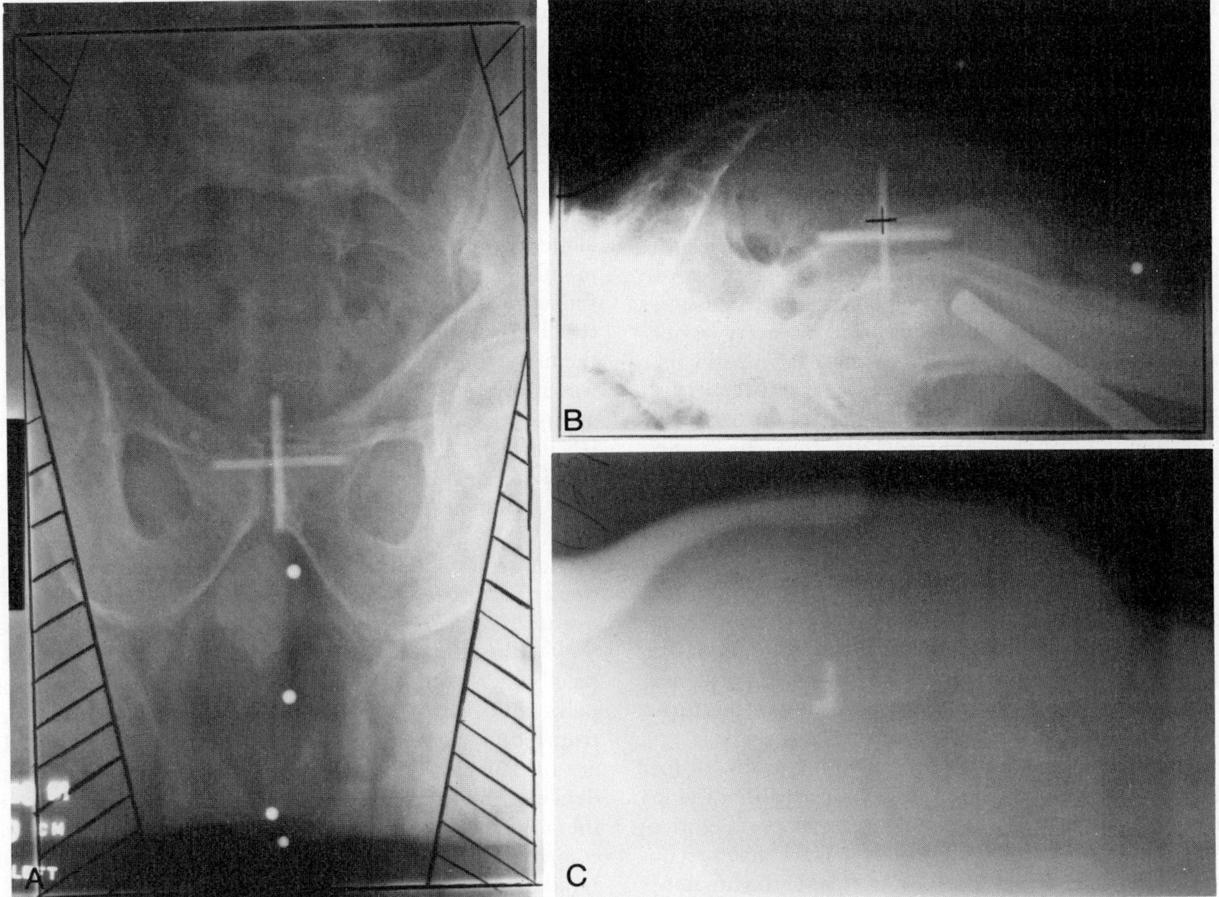

FIGURE 46–6. Postoperative four-field radiation therapy techniques after combined abdominoperineal resection; small lead shot marks the entire perineal scar. (**A**) PA/AP fields in a male patient. (**B**) Lateral fields and portal films in a female patient. The posterior extent of the scar is often more posterior than the sacrum, and (**C**) posterior fall-off of the field may be necessary on port film. (Gunderson LL, Russell AH, Llewellyn HJ, et al: Int J Radiat Oncol Biol Phys 11:1379, 1985; by permission of Pergamon Press)

treatments at a median of 20 months after recurrence. Only three patients in the entire series died of cancer.

Surgery With or Without Postoperative Radiation Therapy

In 1961, Jackman[60] reported results in 211 patients with rectal cancer treated by sphincter-sparing procedures. With follow-up ranging from 8 to 18 years, eight (4%) patients experienced local recurrence. A subsequent report described 234 patients treated mostly by local excision.[9] Forty-nine (21%) subsequently had local recurrences. The 5-year probability of local recurrence was approximately 11% for patients with *in situ* disease and 27% for patients with invasive disease.

Hager[55] described results of local excision of cancer of the rectum in 95 patients. Fifty-nine "low-risk" patients, who had a wide margin of healthy tissue at the time of local excision, were divided into those with invasion of tumor into the submucosa (group 1) and those with invasion into the muscularis propria (group 2). Local recurrence was observed in 3 (8%) of 39 patients in group 1 and 3 (15%) of 20 in group 2. The 5-year survival rate was 90% in group 1 and 58% in group 2. Thirty-six percent of patients were considered "high risk," as defined by incomplete removal of tumor. At a median follow-up of 45 months, 24% had experienced local progression, and 39% had died of cancer.

It is clear that there is a wide range in incidence of local recurrence after limited surgical procedures for rectal cancer. Interpreting the data is made difficult by the variation in selection criteria.

To minimize local recurrence, postoperative radiation therapy has been used at some institutions. Rich and colleagues[104] described results of treating 17 patients by limited surgery and postoperative radiation therapy. With a median follow-up of 26 months for surviving patients, one (6%) had local failure. Further follow-up and, ultimately, a randomized trial will be necessary to determine the benefit of radiation therapy after limited surgery.

TABLE 46–5
Selection Factors for Endocavitary Radiation Therapy for Rectal Cancer

Required characteristics
Lesion accessible by treatment proctoscope (≤10 cm from anal verge)
No evidence of disease extension beyond the bowel wall on digital rectal examination
Maximum tumor size 3 cm × 5 cm
No significant extension to anal canal
Preferred characteristics
Well or moderately well differentiated histologically
Exophytic morphology

RESULTS OF THERAPY

Rectal Cancer

Preoperative Irradiation

A theoretic advantage of preoperative irradiation is its potential to damage malignant cells that may spread locally or distantly at operation. Other potential advantages include the potential for decreased complications and increased tumor response when an undisturbed tumor is surgically treated.

Low-dose preoperative irradiation using 500 cGy in one fraction to 2500 cGy in five to ten fractions has been compared with surgery alone in four randomized prospective trials.[56, 105, 112, 121] None of these studies showed improved survival with preoperative radiation therapy (Fig. 46-7). Retrospective subgroup analysis did suggest a possible effect of preoperative treatment in two of these trials. In the Princess Margaret trial, patients with rectal cancer were randomized to surgery alone or to preoperative radiation therapy of 500 cGy given in one fraction. Although survival for all patients in the trial was virtually identical (Fig. 46-7), retrospective subgroup analysis of patients with Dukes' Stage C cancer suggested a survival advantage for preoperatively irradiated patients. Based on this observation, it was recommended that "this form of preoperative irradiation become routine."[105]

This conclusion is not justified for several reasons. If, for the entire group of patients, survival was virtually identical in the two groups, an apparent positive impact of preoperative irradiation on survival in some subgroups must be matched by an apparent negative impact in other groups. Unfortunately, analysis of subgroups complementary to the Dukes' Stage C patients was not presented. Moreover, no reliable technique is currently available to identify Dukes' Stage C patients preoperatively. Although useful for hypothesis generation, retrospective subgroup analysis is an invalid statistical technique for reaching conclusions about treatment efficacy.[37, 116] The Veterans Administration study group found better survival among the preoperatively irradiated patients (2000–2500 cGy) who underwent abdominoperineal resection.[56] The hazard of retrospective subgroup analysis was illustrated by a later Veterans Administration trial, which strongly suggested that the original evaluation favoring the preoperatively irradiated patients resulted from an imbalance in prognostic factors rather than from any effect of treatment.[57]

Interim analysis of a trial conducted by the Stockholm Rectal Cancer Study Group provides the only suggestion of a clinically measurable effect of low-dose preoperative radiation therapy.[121] In this trial, the patients were randomized to receive 2500 cGy in five fractions preoperatively or to receive surgery alone. Survival rates through 4 years of follow-up were virtually identical. Postoperative mortality was 7% in the preoperative radiation therapy group and only 2% in the surgery group ($P<0.01$). Among the patients operated on "for cure" (545 of the 694 patients), the incidence of pelvic recurrence at 4 years was approximately 17% in the preoperative radiation therapy group and approximately 31% in the surgery only group ($P<0.01$).

Retrospective studies suggest that higher doses of preoperative radiation therapy may be associated with improved survival[34, 65, 66, 100, 119] and decreased pelvic recurrence.[33, 100, 119, 120] Moderate doses (3000–4000 cGy) of preoperative radiation therapy have been formally tested in four randomized prospective trials.

At the Rotterdamsch Radio-Therapeutisch, patients with rectal cancer were randomized to 3450 cGy in 15 fractions to a pelvic and para-aortic field or to operation alone.[13] Freedom from local recurrence and survival were not significantly different in patients with T2 lesions. For patients with clinical evidence of T3 or T4 disease, 97% in the preoperative radiation therapy group subsequently had potentially curative resections, compared with only 68% in the operation-only group ($P<0.05$). Irradiated patients with T3 or T4 tumors also had better 5-year survival ($P<0.005$) and freedom from local recurrence ($P=0.08$).

A larger randomized trial, using the same preoperative dose-fractionation scheme and field design, was conducted by the European Organization for Research on Treatment of Cancer (EORTC).[39] Although local recurrence was significantly lower among patients given preoperative radiation therapy (Fig. 46-8*A*), survival was not affected (Fig. 46-8*B*).

In the second randomized trial of neoadjuvant radiation therapy conducted by the Veterans Administration Surgical Oncology Group, a preoperative dose of 3150 cGy in 18 frac-

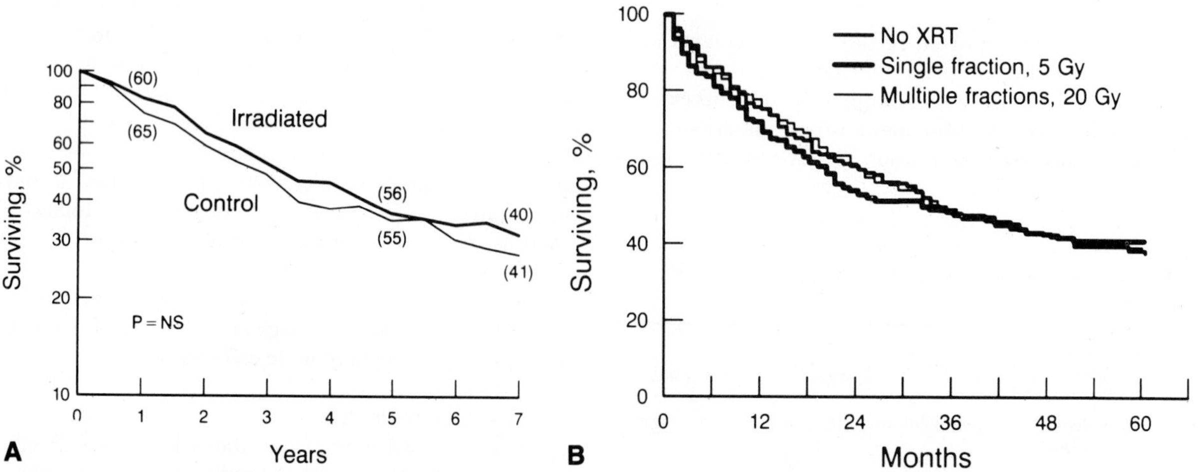

FIGURE 46–7. Survival with or without preoperative irradiation. (**A**) Results in Princess Margaret trial with 500 cGy vs. control. (Modified from Rider WD, Palmer JA, Mahoney LJ, et al: Can J Surg 20:335, 1977) (**B**) Medical Research Council study. Patients were randomized to surgery alone or to preoperative doses of 500 cGy in one fraction or 2000 cGy in ten fractions. (Modified from Second Report of an MRC Working Party: Br J Surg 71:21, 1984)

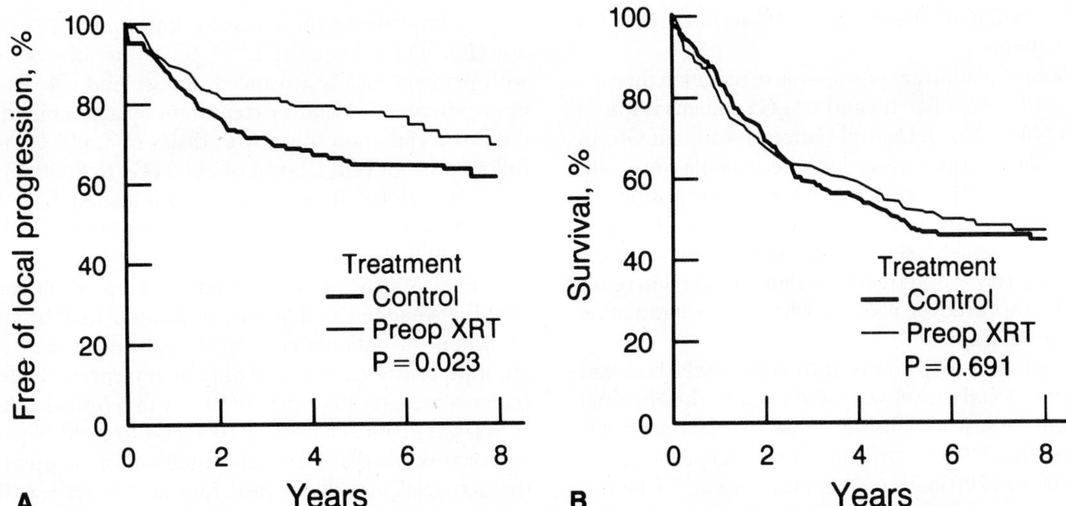

FIGURE 46–8. (**A**) Local control and (**B**) survival in the randomized European Organization for Research on Treatment of Cancer trial comparing 3450 cGy given preoperatively with surgery alone. (Modified from Gérard A, Buyse M, Nordlinger B, et al: Ann Surg 208:606, 1988)

tions to a pelvic and para-aortic field was compared with surgery alone in patients with rectal cancer.[57] Five-year survival was 50% in both arms of the study. Overall recurrence (distant and local) was also virtually identical, although a detailed analysis of patterns of failure was not reported.

Reis Neto and associates[101] reported a small clinical trial of 68 patients who were randomized to 4000 cGy in 4 weeks preoperatively or surgery alone. Five-year survival was 71% in the preoperatively treated patients and 29% in the control group. The incidence of local recurrence, with or without distant metastasis, was 15% and 47% in preoperatively irradiated and control groups, respectively.

Combined-modality preoperative therapy of radiation and 5-fluorouracil was compared with preoperative radiation therapy alone by the EORTC in a randomized clinical trial. All patients were treated with 3450 cGy in 15 fractions to pelvic and para-aortic fields, as in prior EORTC trials.[12] The addition of 5-fluorouracil had a negative effect on survival.

No benefit from low-dose preoperative radiation therapy has been observed in randomized prospective studies. Most randomized studies with higher doses of preoperative radiation suggest improved local control but not improved survival.

Postoperative Irradiation

The advantage of a postoperative approach to adjuvant therapy of rectal cancer is that it allows consideration of pathologic factors in the selection of patients for this treatment. In trials of preoperative radiation therapy, 22% to 37% of the patients randomized to surgery alone had tumors that were limited to the bowel wall and therefore were at low risk for recurrence.[18,105,112] An additional 8% to 14% were found to have distant metastases at surgery.[18,38,105,112] A postoperative approach to adjuvant therapy allows the physician to use pathologic information to exclude 30% to 50% of patients who are unlikely to benefit from adjuvant therapy.

A retrospective comparison of adjuvant postoperative irradiation with surgery alone in patients at high risk for local recurrence was performed at Massachusetts General Hospital.[59] For patients with gross extension of tumor beyond the rectal wall or with metastatically involved lymph nodes, or both, the incidence of local failure was lower after postoperative adjuvant radiation therapy. Most studies suggest that local failure can be decreased by as much as 20% if postoperative radiation therapy is used after resection of modified Astler-Coller (MAC) B2–B3 and C1–C3 tumors.[15,40,59,110,126,138] Although no prospectively acquired data are available regarding radiation dose, one retrospective analysis showed a pelvic relapse rate of 10% after more than 4500 cGy was used, but a rate of 50% if a dose of less than 4500 cGy was used.[15]

Two randomized prospective clinical trials have confirmed improved survival and local tumor control after adjuvant postoperative radiation therapy and chemotherapy in patients with MAC B2–B3 and C1–C3 tumors. The Gastrointestinal Tumor Study Group randomized patients postoperatively to four groups: no further therapy; methyl-CCNU and 5-fluorouracil; pelvic radiation therapy, 4000 cGy to 4800 cGy; or pelvic radiation therapy, 4000 cGy to 4400 cGy, and methyl-CCNU and 5-fluorouracil.[35] Overall survival was significantly better among patients treated with chemotherapy plus radiation than among patients who had no adjuvant therapy (Fig. 46-9).[36] Local recurrence rates were 24% in control patients, 27% in chemotherapy

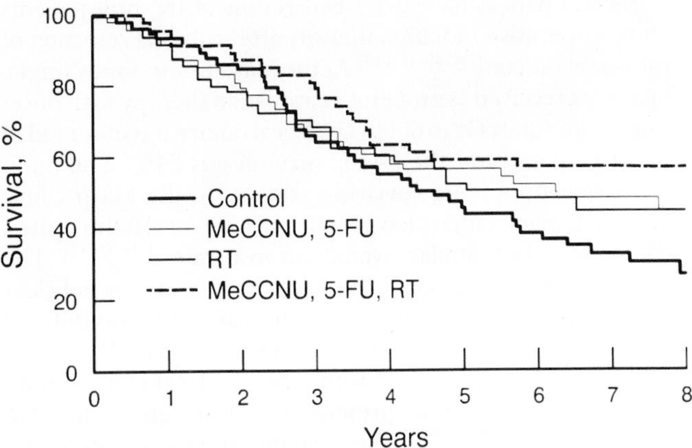

FIGURE 46–9. Survival in the Gastrointestinal Tumor Study Group trial of surgery alone (control), methyl-CCNU plus 5-fluorouracil alone, pelvic radiation therapy alone (RT), or pelvic radiation therapy plus chemotherapy (MeCCNU and 5-FU). (Modified from Gastrointestinal Tumor Study Group: N Engl J Med 315:1294, 1986)

patients, 20% in irradiated patients, and 11% in radiation plus chemotherapy patients.

Further support for adjuvant postoperative radiation therapy and chemotherapy in MAC B2–B3 and C1–C3 patients is found in a randomized Mayo–North Central Cancer Treatment Group study. After complete surgical resection, the patients were randomized to postoperative pelvic radiation therapy or postoperative pelvic radiation therapy and chemotherapy (methyl-CCNU and 5-fluorouracil). Disease-free survival, overall survival, freedom from local recurrence, and freedom from distant recurrence were significantly improved in patients who received radiation therapy and chemotherapy.[49,69,88]

A randomized trial in patients with completely resected Dukes' Stage B or C rectal cancer was conducted by the National Surgical Adjuvant Breast and Bowel Project to compare: (1) 5-fluorouracil, methyl-CCNU, and vincristine; (2) pelvic radiation therapy, 4600 to 4700 cGy; and (3) observation.[32] Chemotherapy improved survival; radiation therapy had no influence on survival. The locoregional failure rate was 16% in patients who received radiation therapy, 21% in those who received chemotherapy, and 25% in control patients ($P = 0.06$ for radiation therapy *versus* control). This study supports the value of chemotherapy in prolonging survival and also provides further evidence that radiation therapy is effective in decreasing locoregional failure.

Several randomized studies support the use of combined adjuvant postoperative radiation therapy plus chemotherapy in patients with MAC B2–B3 and C1–C3 rectal cancer. Postoperative adjuvant treatment is preferable to preoperative radiation therapy, based on evidence from randomized prospective studies supporting a survival benefit for this approach and because a postoperative adjuvant therapy allows exclusion of patients who would achieve little benefit from such treatment.

Locally Advanced Rectal Cancer

External radiation therapy alone or in combination with chemotherapy provides palliation and prolongation of life but has only minimal curative potential in patients with locally advanced rectal cancer. At the Mayo Clinic, 65 patients with locally unresectable carcinoma of the large bowel were treated with radiation therapy (3500–4000 cGy) with or without 5-fluorouracil in a randomized prospective study.[82] Survival free of progression, median duration of symptomatic control, and survival were better in patients who received 5-fluorouracil.

Several papers have described results of treating patients with postoperative radiation therapy after subtotal resection of large bowel cancer.[1,15,40,111,131] At the Mayo Clinic, for example, 17 patients received postoperative radiation therapy with doses in the range 4000 cGy to 6000 cGy. Local failure was observed in 76% of patients, and the 5-year survival was 24%. The minimum follow-up among surviving patients in the Mayo Clinic series was 5 years. Others have reported lower local failure rates, 15% to 32%, but similar overall survival rates.[1,15,40,131] The reason for the wide range of results for local control is not clear but may relate to the manner in which local failure was defined and the short duration of follow-up in some series.[111]

Preoperative irradiation with doses of 4500 cGy or more has been used in patients presenting with unresectable colon and rectal cancer.[26,30,89,119] Resectability rates after preoperative radiation therapy vary widely, ranging from approximately 50% to 75%. After resection, subsequent local failure occurs in approximately 36% to 45% of the patients, so long-term local control is achieved only in approximately 25% to 35% of these patients.

To improve on these results, intraoperative radiation therapy (IORT) has been used.[48,50,122] At the Mayo Clinic, patients with primary locally advanced disease had a 4-year survival of approximately 55% after treatment by a combination of external-beam radiation therapy to doses of 4500 cGy to 5500 cGy, followed by an IORT boost of 1000 cGy to 2000 cGy. Results in patients with locally recurrent rectal disease have been worse, with a 5-year survival rate of approximately 25%.[50] Local failure after IORT was 17%.

The Massachusetts General Hospital experience with IORT also suggests that this technique may be useful in the treatment of patients with locally advanced disease.[122] Before attempted surgical removal of primary unresectable cancer, the patients were treated with 5040 cGy in 5.5 weeks. At operation, IORT was given at a dose of 1000 cGy to 2000 cGy to the tumor bed or residual disease. With a median follow-up of 43 months, the actuarial overall survival rate at 3 years was 60% for the entire group, 70% for the patients who had undergone complete surgical resection, and 30% in those with residual tumor after local resection. Actuarial local control rate at 3 years was 87%, and the rate was highest among patients in whom complete surgical resection had been performed. As in the Mayo Clinic experience, the results at the Massachusetts General Hospital have been poorer among patients with locally recurrent disease than among patients with primary locally advanced disease.[48]

Results with external irradiation and IORT appear to be superior to those previously achieved with external irradiation alone. A randomized clinical trial has been developed by the Radiation Therapy Oncology Group to rigorously test the value of IORT.

Colon Cancer

No randomized prospective trials have examined the value of postoperative adjuvant radiation therapy for large bowel cancer above the rectum. However, several retrospective studies suggest that this would be a fruitful avenue of research.[14,29,67,68,114,136] For example, a series from the Massachusetts General Hospital showed a consistent decrease in local failure with the addition of postoperative irradiation (Table 46-6).[136] Randomized studies are needed to confirm these results. In view of recent positive results with adjuvant systemic therapy in high-risk colon cancer patients, a reasonable two-arm trial would be comparison of radiation therapy, 5-fluorouracil, and levamisole with 5-fluorouracil and levamisole alone after resection in high-risk colon cancer patients.[71,83]

Chemotherapy

Most studies using chemotherapy for advanced disease or adjuvant therapy have given disappointing results.[47,81] Several recent clinical trials, however, have produced some promising data. A Mayo–North Central Cancer Treatment Group study demonstrated improvement in Dukes Stage C patients in overall and disease-free survival with adjuvant levamisole therapy with or without 5-fluorouracil.[71] A subsequent intergroup confirmatory trial verified the value of 5-fluorouracil and levamisole for node-positive patients.[83] For patients with metastatic colorectal cancer, recent trials of 5-fluorouracil and leucovorin appear promising.[70,87,92] In a small study at the Roswell Memorial Park Institute, 74 patients with metastatic disease were randomized to receive 5-fluorouracil alone, methotrexate plus 5-fluo-

TABLE 46–6
Five-Year Actuarial Local Control Rates for Colon Cancer After Surgery Alone and After Surgery Plus Irradiation

	SURGERY ALONE		SURGERY PLUS POSTOPERATIVE IRRADIATION	
STAGE	NO. OF PATIENTS	LOCAL CONTROL RATE (%)	NO. OF PATIENTS	LOCAL CONTROL RATE (%)
B2	163	90	21	90
B3	83	69	37	92
C2	100	64	47	79
C3	49	47	28	69
Total	395	74	133	82

(Data from the Massachusetts General Hospital series adapted from Willett CG, Tepper JE, Cohen AM, et al: Ann Surg 200:685, 1984)

rouracil, or leucovorin plus 5-fluorouracil.[92] Response rates were 48% with leucovorin plus 5-fluorouracil, 11% with 5-fluorouracil alone, and 5% with 5-fluorouracil plus methotrexate. Survival was not significantly altered. A larger Mayo–North Central Cancer Treatment Group study, however, has shown improved survival for patients receiving 5-fluorouracil plus leucovorin-containing regimens.[87]

SEQUELAE

When adjuvant radiation therapy for large bowel cancer is performed carefully, long-term complications are rare. Hoskins and associates[59] found that the small bowel complication rate was not increased in patients undergoing postoperative radiation therapy for rectal cancer above that expected in patients undergoing surgery alone. In patients with extrapelvic colon cancer, surgical small bowel obstruction is uncommon if careful attention is given to radiation therapy techniques.[29]

Intracavitary radiation therapy for rectal cancer is well tolerated. Approximately 35% of patients will have minor rectal bleeding after treatment. Rectal urgency occurs in approximately 20% of the patients. These symptoms usually resolve. Approximately 75% of the patients develop ulcers after intracavitary radiation therapy, but this condition is asymptomatic and resolves in most patients.[72]

Severe sequelae of radiation therapy can occur in patients with locally advanced disease who undergo IORT. The most common sequelae of IORT are neurotoxicity, seen in approximately 32% of patients, and hydronephrosis, seen in approximately 65% of patients who have their ureter included within the field. Neurotoxicity appears to depend on the site irradiated. If the pelvic sidewall is included within the field, the incidence of neuropathy approaches 50%, but if the field is limited to the presacrum, the incidence of neuropathy is less than 10% (Edward Shaw, personal communication).

REFERENCES

1. Allee PE, Gunderson LL, Munzenrider JE: Postoperative radiation therapy for residual colorectal carcinoma. [Abstract] Int J Radiat Oncol Biol Phys 7:1208, 1981
2. Allen PIM, Fielding JWL, Middleton MD, et al: Rectal carcinoma: A new technique to allow safer postoperative irradiation of the pelvis. Eur J Surg Oncol 13:21, 1987
3. Armstrong B, Doll R: Environmental factors and cancer incidence and mortality in different countries, with special reference to dietary practices. Int J Cancer 15:617, 1975
4. Astler VB, Coller FA: The prognostic significance of direct extension of carcinoma of the colon and rectum. Ann Surg 139:846, 1954.
5. Axtell LM, Chiazze L Jr: Changing relative frequency of cancers of the colon and rectum in the United States. Cancer 19:750, 1966
6. Beahrs OH, Henson DE, Hutter RVP, et al (eds): Manual for Staging of Cancer, 3rd ed, p 75. Philadelphia, JB Lippincott, 1988
7. Beart RW Jr, O'Connell MJ: Postoperative follow-up of patients with carcinoma of the colon. Mayo Clin Proc 58:361, 1983
8. Beynon J, Roe A, Foy DM, et al: The staging of rectal cancer using endoluminal ultrasound. [Abstract] Dig Dis Sci 31(suppl 10):123S, 1986
9. Biggers OR, Beart RW Jr, Ilstrup DM: Local excision of rectal cancer. Dis Colon Rectum 29:374, 1986
10. Black WA, Waugh JM: The intramural extension of carcinoma of the descending colon, sigmoid, and rectosigmoid: A pathologic study. Surg Gynecol Obstet 87:457, 1948
11. Blanco D, Ross RK, Paganini-Hill A, et al: Cholecystectomy and colonic cancer. Dis Colon Rectum 27:290, 1984
12. Boulis-Wassif S, Gerard A, Loygue J, et al: Final results of a randomized trial on the treatment of rectal cancer with preoperative radiotherapy alone or in combination with 5-fluorouracil, followed by radical surgery: Trials of the European Organization on Research and Treatment of Cancer, Gastrointestinal Tract Cancer Cooperative Group. Cancer 53:1811, 1984
13. Boulis-Wassif S, Langenhorst BL, Hop WCJ: The contribution of preoperative radiotherapy in the management of borderline operability rectal cancer. In Jones SE, Salmon SE (eds): Adjuvant Therapy of Cancer II, p 613. New York, Grune & Stratton, 1979
14. Brenner HJ, Bibi C, Chaitchik S: Adjuvant therapy for Dukes C adenocarcinoma of colon. Int J Radiat Oncol Biol Phys 9:1789, 1983
15. Brizel HE, Tepperman BS. Postoperative adjuvant irradiation for adenocarcinoma of the rectum and sigmoid. Am J Clin Oncol 7:679, 1984
16. Burkitt DP: Epidemiology of cancer of the colon and rectum. Cancer 28:3, 1971
17. Cady B, Persson AV, Monson DO, et al: Changing patterns of colorectal carcinoma. Cancer 33:422, 1974
18. Cedermark B, Theve NO, Rieger A, et al: Preoperative short-term radiotherapy in rectal carcinoma: A preliminary report of a prospective randomized study. Cancer 55:1182, 1985
19. Chan KW, Boey J, Wong SKC: A method of reporting radial invasion and surgical clearance of rectal carcinoma. Histopathology 9:1319, 1985

20. Ciatto S, Pacini P: Radiation therapy of recurrences of carcinoma of the rectum and sigmoid after surgery. Acta Radiol Oncol 21:105, 1982
21. Cole PP: The intramural spread of rectal carcinoma. Br Med J 1:431, 1913.
22. Copeland EM, Miller LD, Jones RS: Prognostic factors in carcinoma of the colon and rectum. Am J Surg 116:875, 1968
23. Crile G Jr, Turnbull RB Jr: The role of electrocoagulation in the treatment of carcinoma of the rectum. Surg Gynecol Obstet 135:391, 1972
24. Cruse P, Lewin M, Clark CG: Dietary cholesterol is co-carcinogenic for human colon cancer. Lancet 1:752, 1979
25. Dales LG, Friedman GD, Ury HK, et al: Original contributions: A case-control study of relationships of diet and other traits to colorectal cancer in American blacks. Am J Epidemiol 109:132, 1979
26. Dosoretz DE, Gunderson LL, Hedberg S, et al: Preoperative irradiation for unresectable rectal and rectosigmoid carcinomas. Cancer 52:814, 1983
27. Drasar BS, Irving D. Environmental factors and cancer of the colon and breast. Br J Cancer 27:167, 1973
28. Dukes CE: The classification of cancer of the rectum. J Pathol Bacteriol 35:323, 1932
29. Duttenhaver JR, Hoskins RB, Gunderson LL, et al: Adjuvant postoperative radiation therapy in the management of adenocarcinoma of the colon. Cancer 57:955, 1986
30. Emami B, Pilepich M, Willett C, et al: Effect of preoperative irradiation on resectability of colorectal carcinomas. Int J Radiat Oncol Biol Phys 8:1295, 1982
31. Feldman MI, Kavanah MT, Devereux DF, et al: New surgical method to prevent pelvic radiation enteropathy. Am J Clin Oncol 11:25, 1988
32. Fisher B, Wolmark N, Rockette H, et al: Postoperative adjuvant chemotherapy or radiation therapy for rectal cancer: Results from NSABP protocol R-01. JNCI 80:21, 1988
33. Fortier GA, Krochak RJ, Kim JA, et al: Dose response to preoperative irradiation in rectal cancer: Implications for local control and complications associated with sphincter sparing surgery and abdominoperineal resection. Int J Radiat Oncol Biol Phys 12:1559, 1986
34. Friedmann P, Garb JL, Park WC, et al: Survival following moderate-dose preoperative radiation therapy for carcinoma of the rectum. Cancer 55:967, 1985
35. Gastrointestinal Tumor Study Group: Prolongation of the disease-free interval in surgically treated rectal carcinoma. N Engl J Med 312:1465, 1985
36. The Gastrointestinal Tumor Study Group: Survival after postoperative combination treatment of rectal cancer. [Letter to editor] N Engl J Med 315:1294, 1986
37. Gelber RD, Zelen M: Methodology of clinical trials. In Perez CA, Brady LW (eds): Principles and Practices of Radiation Oncology, p 122. Philadelphia, JB Lippincott, 1987
38. Gerard A, Berrod J-L, Pene F, et al: Interim analysis of a phase III study on preoperative radiation therapy in resectable rectal carcinoma: Trials of the Gastrointestinal Tract Cancer Cooperative Group of the European Organization for Research on Treatment of Cancer (EORTC). Cancer 55:2373, 1985
39. Gérard A, Buyse M, Nordlinger B, et al: Preoperative radiotherapy as adjuvant treatment in rectal cancer: Final results of a randomized study of the European Organization for Research and Treatment of Cancer (EORTC). Ann Surg 208:606, 1988
40. Ghossein NA, Samala EC, Alpert S, et al: Elective postoperative radiotherapy after incomplete resection of colorectal cancer. Dis Colon Rectum 24:252, 1981
41. Gilbert SG: Symptomatic local tumor failure following abdomino-perineal resection. Int J Radiat Oncol Biol Phys 4:801, 1978
42. Goldenberg DM, Neville AM, Carter AC, et al: CEA (carcinoembryonic antigen): Its role as a marker in the management of cancer. J Cancer Res Clin Oncol 101:239, 1981
43. Greenwald P, Lanza E, Eddy GA: Dietary fiber in the reduction of colon cancer risk. J Am Diet Assoc 87:1178, 1987
44. Griffin AC: Role of selenium in the chemoprevention of cancer. Adv Cancer Res 29:419, 1979
45. Grinnell RS: Lymphatic block with atypical and retrograde lymphatic metastasis and spread in carcinoma of the colon and rectum. Ann Surg 163:272, 1966
46. Gunderson LL: Perineal irradiation for rectal cancer. Int J Radiat Oncol Biol Phys 12:283, 1986
47. Gunderson LL, Beart RW, O'Connell MJ: Current issues in the treatment of colorectal cancer. Crit Rev Oncol Hematol 6:223, 1986
48. Gunderson LL, Cohen AC, Dosoretz DD, et al: Residual, unresectable, or recurrent colorectal cancer: External beam irradiation and intraoperative electron beam boost ± resection. Int J Radiat Oncol Biol Phys 9:1597, 1983
49. Gunderson LL, Collins R, Earle JD, et al: Adjuvant treatment of rectal cancer: Randomized prospective study of irradiation ± chemotherapy—a NCCTG, Mayo Clinic study. [Abstract] Int J Radiat Oncol Biol Phys 12:169, 1986
50. Gunderson LL, Martin JK, Beart RW, et al: Intraoperative and external beam irradiation for locally advanced colorectal cancer. Ann Surg 207:52, 1988
51. Gunderson LL, Russell AH, Llewellyn HJ, et al: Treatment planning for colorectal cancer: Radiation and surgical techniques and value of small-bowel films. Int J Radiat Oncol Biol Phys 11:1379, 1985
52. Gunderson LL, Sosin H: Areas of failure found at reoperation (second or symptomatic look) following "curative surgery" for adenocarcinoma of the rectum: Clinicopathologic correlation and implications for adjuvant therapy. Cancer 34:1278, 1974
53. Gunderson LL, Sosin H, Levitt S: Extrapelvic colon—areas of failure in a reoperation series: Implications for adjuvant therapy. Int J Radiat Oncol Biol Phys 11:731, 1985
54. Haenszel W, Kurihara M: Studies of Japanese migrants: I. Mortality from cancer and other diseases among Japanese in the United States. JNCI 40:43, 1968
55. Hager Th, Gall FP, Hermanek P: Local excision of cancer of the rectum. Dis Colon Rectum 26:149, 1983
56. Higgins GA Jr, Conn JH, Jordan PH Jr, et al: Preoperative radiotherapy for colorectal cancer. Ann Surg 181:624, 1975
57. Higgins GA, Humphrey EW, Dwight RW, et al: Preoperative radiation and surgery for cancer of the rectum: Veterans Administration Surgical Oncology Group Trial II. Cancer 58:352, 1986
58. Hildebrandt U, Feifel G: Preoperative staging of rectal cancer by intrarectal ultrasound. Dis Colon Rectum 28:42, 1985
59. Hoskins RB, Gunderson LL, Dosoretz DE, et al: Adjuvant postoperative radiotherapy in carcinoma of the rectum and rectosigmoid. Cancer 55:61, 1985
60. Jackman RJ: Conservative management of selected patients with carcinoma of the rectum. Dis Colon Rectum 4:429, 1961
61. Jain M, Cook GM, Davis FG, et al: A case-control study of diet and colo-rectal cancer. Int J Cancer 26:757, 1980
62. Jansson B, Jacobs MM, Griffin AC: Gastrointestinal cancer: Epidemiology and experimental studies. In Schrauzer GN (ed): Inorganic and Nutritional Aspects of Cancer, p 305. New York, Plenum Press, 1978
63. Jensen OM, Maclennan R: Dietary factors and colorectal cancer in Scandinavia. Isr J Med Sci 15:329, 1979
64. Kavanah MT, Feldman MI, Devereux DF, et al: New surgical approach to minimize radiation-associated small bowel injury in patients with pelvic malignancies requiring surgery and high-dose irradiation: A preliminary report. Cancer 56:1300, 1985
65. Kligerman MM: Preoperative radiation therapy in rectal cancer. Cancer 36:691, 1975
66. Kligerman MM: Radiotherapy and rectal cancer. Cancer 39:896, 1977
67. Kopelson G: Adjuvant postoperative radiation therapy for colorectal carcinoma above the peritoneal reflection. I. Sigmoid colon. Cancer 51:1593, 1983
68. Kopelson G: Adjuvant postoperative radiation therapy for colorectal carcinoma above the peritoneal reflection. II. Antimesenteric wall ascending and descending colon and cecum. Cancer 52:633, 1983

69. Krook J, Moertel CG, Wieand H, et al: Radiation versus sequential chemotherapy-radiation-chemotherapy. [Abstract] Proceedings of the American Society of Clinical Oncology 5:82, 1986
70. Laufman LR, Krzeczowski KA, Roach R, et al: Leucovorin plus 5-fluorouracil: An effective treatment for metastatic colon cancer. J Clin Oncol 5:1394, 1987
71. Laurie JA, Moertel CG, Fleming TR, et al: Surgical adjuvant therapy of large-bowel carcinoma: An evaluation of levamisole and the combination of levamisole and fluorouracil. J Clin Oncol 7:1447, 1989
72. Lavery IC, Jones IT, Weakley FL, et al: Definitive management of rectal cancer by contact (endocavitary) irradiation. Dis Colon Rectum 30:835, 1987
73. Linos DA, O'Fallon WM, Beart RW Jr, et al: Cholecystectomy and carcinoma of the colon. Lancet 2:379, 1981
74. Liu K, Moss D, Persky V: Dietary cholesterol, fat, and fibre, and colon-cancer mortality. Lancet 2:782, 1979
75. Lyon JL, Gardner JW, West DW: Cancer incidence in Mormons and non-Mormons in Utah during 1967–75. JNCI 65:1055, 1980
76. MacLennan R, Jensen OM, Mosbech J, et al: Diet, transit time, stool weight, and colon cancer in two Scandinavian populations. Am J Clin Nutr 31:S239, 1978
77. Malhotra SL: Dietary factors in a study of cancer colon from cancer registry, with special reference to the role of saliva, milk and fermented milk products and vegetable fibre. Med Hypotheses 3:122, 1977
78. Martin EW Jr, James KK, Hurtubise PE, et al: The use of CEA as an early indicator for gastrointestinal tumor recurrence and second-look procedures. Cancer 39:440, 1977
79. Minsky BD, Mies C, Rich TA, et al: Potentially curative surgery of colon cancer: Patterns of failure and survival. J Clin Oncol 6:106, 1988
80. Modan B, Barell V, Lubin F, et al: Low-fiber intake as an etiologic factor in cancer of the colon. JNCI 55:15, 1975
81. Moertel CG: Alimentary tract cancer. In Holland JF, Frei E III (eds): Cancer Medicine, p 1753. Philadelphia, Lea & Febiger, 1982
82. Moertel CG, Childs DS Jr, Reitemeier RJ, et al: Combined 5-fluorouracil and supervoltage radiation therapy of locally unresectable gastrointestinal cancer. Lancet 2:865, 1969
83. Moertel CG, Fleming TR, Macdonald JS, et al: Levamisole and fluorouracil for adjuvant therapy of resected colon carcinoma. N Engl J Med 322:352, 1990
84. Moertel CG, Schutt AJ, Go VLW: Carcinoembryonic antigen test for recurrent colorectal carcinoma: Inadequacy for early detection. JAMA 239:1065, 1978
85. Moossa AR, Ree PC, Marks JE, et al: Factors influencing local recurrence after abdominoperineal resection for cancer of the rectum and rectosigmoid. Br J Surg 62:727, 1975
86. Murphy SA, Driskell JA, Elgert KD, et al: Effects of selenium and vitamin B-6 on growth of transplanted tumors in BALB/c inbred mice. [Abstract] FASEB J 2:A859, 1988
87. O'Connell MJ: A phase III trial of 5-fluorouracil and leucovorin in the treatment of advanced colorectal cancer: A Mayo Clinic/North Central Cancer Treatment Group study. Cancer 63:1026, 1989
88. O'Connell MJ: Paper read at the 25th annual meeting of the American Society of Clinical Oncology, San Francisco, California, May 21–23, 1989
89. Påhlman L, Glimelius B, Ginman C, et al: Preoperative irradiation of primarily non-resectable adenocarcinoma of the rectum and rectosigmoid. Acta Radiol Oncol 24:35, 1985
90. Papillon J: Rectal and Anal Cancers: Conservative Treatment by Irradiation—An Alternative to Radical Surgery. Berlin, Springer-Verlag, 1982
91. Patterson DJ, Alpert E: Tumour markers of the gastrointestinal tract. In Hodgson HJF, Bloom SR (eds): Gastrointestinal and Hepatobiliary Cancer, p 189. Boston, Butterworth, 1983
92. Petrelli N, Herrera L, Rustum Y, et al: A prospective randomized trial of 5-fluorouracil versus 5-fluorouracil and high-dose leucovorin versus 5-fluorouracil and methotrexate in previously untreated patients with advanced colorectal carcinoma. J Clin Oncol 5:1559, 1987
93. Phillips RL: Role of life-style and dietary habits in risk of cancer among Seventh-Day Adventists. Cancer Res 35:3513, 1975
94. Polk HC Jr, Ahmad W, Knutson CO: Carcinoma of the colon and rectum. Curr Probl Surg 1, 1973
95. Pollett WG, Nicholls RJ: The relationship between the extent of distal clearance and survival and local recurrence rates after curative anterior resection for carcinoma of the rectum. Ann Surg 198:159, 1983
96. Postlethwait RW: Malignant tumors of the colon and rectum. Ann Surg 129:34, 1949
97. Reddy BS, Hedges AR, Laakso K, et al: Metabolic epidemiology of large bowel cancer: Fecal bulk and constituents of high-risk North American and low-risk Finnish population. Cancer 42:2832, 1978
98. Reddy BS, Narasawa T, Weisburger JH, et al: Brief communication: Promoting effect of sodium deoxycholate on colon adenocarcinomas in germfree rats. JNCI 56:441, 1976
99. Reddy BS, Wynder EL: Metabolic epidemiology of colon cancer: Fecal bile acids and neutral sterols in colon cancer patients and patients with adenomatous polyps. Cancer 39:2533, 1977
100. Reed WP, Garb JL, Park WC, et al: Long-term results and complications of preoperative radiation in the treatment of rectal cancer. Surgery 103:161, 1988
101. Reis Neto JA, Quilici FA, Reis JA Jr: A comparison of nonoperative vs. preoperative radiotherapy in rectal carcinoma: A 10-year randomized trial. Dis Colon Rectum 32:702, 1989
102. Rhodes JB, Holmes FF, Clark GM: Changing distribution of primary cancers in the large bowel. JAMA 238;1641, 1977
103. Rich T, Gunderson LL, Lew R, et al: Patterns of recurrence of rectal cancer after potentially curative surgery. Cancer 52:1317, 1983
104. Rich TA, Weiss DR, Mies C, et al: Sphincter preservation in patients with low rectal cancer treated with radiation therapy with or without local excision or fulguration. Radiology 156:527, 1985
105. Rider WD, Palmer JA, Mahoney LJ, et al: Preoperative irradiation in operable cancer of the rectum: Report of the Toronto trial. Can J Surg 20:335, 1977
106. Roberson SH, Heron HC, Kerman HD, et al: Is anterior resection of the rectosigmoid safe after preoperative radiation? Dis Colon Rectum 28:254, 1985
107. Russell AH, Pelton J, Reheis CE, et al: Adenocarcinoma of the colon: An autopsy study with implications for new therapeutic strategies. Cancer 56:1446, 1985
108. Russell AH, Tong D, Dawson LE, et al: Adenocarcinoma of the proximal colon: Sites of initial dissemination and patterns of recurrence following surgery alone. Cancer 53:360, 1984
109. Saitoh N, Okui K, Sarashina H, et al: Evaluation of echographic diagnosis of rectal cancer using intrarectal ultrasonic examination. Dis Colon Rectum 29:234, 1986
110. Schild SE, Martenson JA Jr, Gunderson LL, et al: Long-term survival and patterns of failure after postoperative radiation therapy for subtotally resected rectal adenocarcinoma. Int J Radiat Oncol Biol Phys 16:459, 1989
111. Schild SE, Martenson JA Jr, Gunderson LL, et al: Postoperative adjuvant therapy of rectal cancer: An analysis of disease control, survival, and prognostic factors. Int J Radiat Oncol Biol Phys 17:55, 1989
112. Second Report of an MRC Working Party: The evaluation of low dose pre-operative x-ray therapy in the management of operable rectal cancer: Results of a randomly controlled trial. Br J Surg 71:21, 1984
113. Shamberger RJ, Tytko SA, Willis CE: Antioxidants and cancer: Part VI. Selenium and age-adjusted human cancer mortality. Arch Environ Health 31:231, 1976
114. Shehata WM, Meyer RL, Jazy FK, et al: Regional adjuvant irradiation for adenocarcinoma of the cecum. Int J Radiat Oncol Biol Phys 13:843, 1987
115. Silverberg E, Boring CC, Squires TS: Cancer Statistics, 1990. CA 40(1):9, 1990
116. Simon R: Patient subsets and variation in therapeutic efficacy. Br J Clin Pharmacol 14:473, 1982
117. Sischy B, Hinson EJ, Wilkinson DR: Definitive radiation therapy for selected cancers of the rectum. Br J Surg 75:901, 1988

118. Slanetz CA, Herter FP, Grinnell RS: Anterior resection versus abdominoperineal resection for cancer of the rectum and rectosigmoid. Am J Surg 123:110, 1972
119. Stevens KR Jr, Allen CV, Fletcher WS: Preoperative radiotherapy for adenocarcinoma of the rectosigmoid. Cancer 37:2866, 1976
120. Stevens KR Jr, Fletcher WS, Allen CV: Anterior resection and primary anastomosis following high dose preoperative irradiation for adenocarcinoma of the recto-sigmoid. Cancer 41:2065, 1978
121. Stockholm Rectal Cancer Study Group: Short-term preoperative radiotherapy for adenocarcinoma of the rectum: An interim analysis of a randomized multicenter trial. Am J Clin Oncol 10:369, 1987
122. Tepper JE, Cohen AM, Wood WC, et al: Intraoperative electron beam radiotherapy in the treatment of unresectable rectal cancer. Arch Surg 121:421, 1986
123. Thomas PRM, Stablein DM, Kinzie JJ, et al: Perineal effects of postoperative treatment for adenocarcinoma of the rectum. Int J Radiat Oncol Biol Phys 12:167, 1986
124. Vernick LJ, Kuller LH: Cholecystectomy and right-sided colon cancer: An epidemiological study. Lancet 2:381, 1981
125. Vernick LJ, Kuller LH, Lohsoonthorn P, et al: Relationship between cholecystectomy and ascending colon cancer. Cancer 45:392, 1980
126. Vigliotti A, Rich TA, Romsdahl MM, et al: Postoperative adjuvant radiotherapy for adenocarcinoma of the rectum and rectosigmoid. Int J Radiat Oncol Biol Phys 13:999, 1987
127. Villemin F, Huard P, Montague M: Recherches anatomiques sur les lymphatiques du rectum et de l'anus: Leurs applications dans le traitement chirurgical du cancer. Rev Chir 63:39, 1925
128. Walker ARP, Burkitt DP: Colon cancer: Epidemiology. Semin Oncol 3:341, 1976
129. Walz BJ, Green MR, Lindstrom ER, et al: Anatomical prognostic factors after abdominal perineal resection. Int J Radiat Oncol Biol Phys 7:477, 1981
130. Wanebo HJ, Rao B, Pinsky CM, et al: Preoperative carcinoembryonic antigen level as a prognostic indicator in colorectal cancer. N Engl J Med 299:448, 1978
131. Wang CC, Schulz MD: The role of radiation therapy in the management of carcinoma of the sigmoid, rectosigmoid, and rectum. Radiology 79:1, 1962
132. Wang KY, Kimmey MB, Nyberg DA, et al: Colorectal neoplasms: Accuracy of US in demonstrating the depth of invasion. Radiology 165:827, 1987
133. Welch JP, Donaldson GA: Detection and treatment of recurrent cancer of the colon and rectum. Am J Surg 135:505, 1978
134. Welch JP, Donaldson GA: The clinical correlation of an autopsy study of recurrent colorectal cancer. Ann Surg 189:496, 1979
135. Willett CG, Tepper JE, Cohen AM, et al: Failure patterns following curative resection of colonic carcinoma. Ann Surg 200:685, 1984
136. Willett CG, Tepper JE, Skates SJ, et al: Adjuvant postoperative radiation therapy for colonic carcinoma. Ann Surg 206:694, 1987
137. Withers HR, Cuasay L, Mason KA, et al: Elective radiation therapy in the curative treatment of cancer of the rectum and rectosigmoid colon. In Stroehlein JR, Romsdahl MM (eds): Gastrointestinal Cancer, p 351. New York, Raven Press, 1981
138. Zucali R, Gardani G, Lattuada A: Adjuvant irradiation after radical surgery of cancer of the rectum and rectosigmoid. Radiother Oncol 8:19, 1987

47

Anal Canal

Bernard J. Cummings

ANATOMY

The anal canal is about 3 cm to 4 cm long and extends from the level of the pelvic floor to the anal verge. The superior margin is determined clinically by the palpable upper border of the anal sphincter and puborectalis muscle of the anorectal ring. The distal end of the canal at the anal verge can be defined as the level where the walls of the canal come into contact in their normal resting state and approximates to the palpable groove between the lower edge of the internal sphincter and the subcutaneous part of the external sphincter.[14] The American Joint Committee on Clinical Staging and the Union Internationale Contre le Cancer (UICC)[45] now recommend this definition of the anal canal, rather than a convention used by some centers under which carcinomas that arise above or exactly astride the dentate line are classified as anal canal tumors and those lying mainly or entirely below that line are called anal margin tumors.[11,21,22,30,43,47] Perianal carcinomas are arbitrarily considered to be cancers arising from the skin within a 5-cm to 6-cm radius of the anal verge (Fig. 47-1).

Four different types of epithelium are found within the anal region.[14] The perianal skin is similar to hair-bearing skin elsewhere and contains many apocrine glands. At the anal verge, the skin blends with a zone lined by modified squamous epithelium, which lacks hair or glandular structures. This squamous zone merges just below the dentate line (also called the pectinate line), which marks the line of the anal valves, with a transitional epithelium that incorporates features of rectal, urothelial, and squamous epithelia. The transitional zone extends proximally for about 20 mm until rectal mucosa becomes dominant.

The major lymphatic pathways pass to three lymph node systems. The perianal skin, the anal verge, and the canal distal to the dentate line drain predominantly to the superficial inguinal nodes and to the external iliac system. Lymphatics from the area about and above the dentate line flow with those from the distal rectum to the internal pudendal, hypogastric, and obturator nodes of the internal iliac system. The proximal canal drains to the perirectal and superior hemorrhoidal lymphatics of the inferior mesenteric system. There are many lymphatic connections between the various levels of the anal canal, and an intramural system connects the lymphatics of the anal canal to those of the rectum.

EPIDEMIOLOGY AND RISK FACTORS

Anal cancers are more common in women than in men, and in the United States from 1973 to 1977, the annual age-adjusted incidence rate was 0.7 per 100,000 women and about 0.5 for men.[48] Carcinomas in women arise more commonly above the dentate line, but tumors of the distal canal are more common in men. The risk of anal cancer increases with age, and the median age at diagnosis is about 60 years.[2,7,21,48]

Epidemiologic case-control studies have shown that a history of receptive anal intercourse is a risk factor for anal cancer in men, but is apparently less so in women.[10] A history of genital warts, certain genital infections, and cigarette smoking have also been associated with the risk of anal cancer.[10] The suggestion that one or more sexually transmissible agents may have an etiologic role in squamous cell cancers arising in a number of sites in the anogenital region has been strengthened by studies of human papillomaviruses (HPV). In particular, HPV-16 and, to a lesser extent, HPV-18 have been associated with anal squamous cell carcinomas.[33,38] Immunosuppression may increase the risk of anal cancer.[36]

PATHOLOGIC CLASSIFICATION

The pathologic classification used most commonly is that developed by the World Health Organization (WHO).[30] About 80% of all primary anal canal carcinomas are epidermoid, and under the WHO classification these may be further classified as squamous cell (70% to 80%), basaloid (20% to 30%), and mucoepidermoid (1% to 5%) cancers. The remaining 20% of anal carcinomas include adenocarcinomas from anal glands or fistulae or from rectal-type mucosa, melanomas, and undifferentiated carcinomas.

Most epidermoid cancers that arise above the dentate line are relatively poorly differentiated and contain little or no keratin, but those from the lower canal are usually well differentiated and produce keratin.[2,21,22] Basaloid carcinomas (also called cloacogenic or transitional carcinomas) are a variant of squamous cell carcinomas that arise from the transitional zone epithelium. Basaloid and squamous cell carcinomas generally have a similar pattern of behavior, and in most reports, they are considered simply as epidermoid carcinomas. However, the

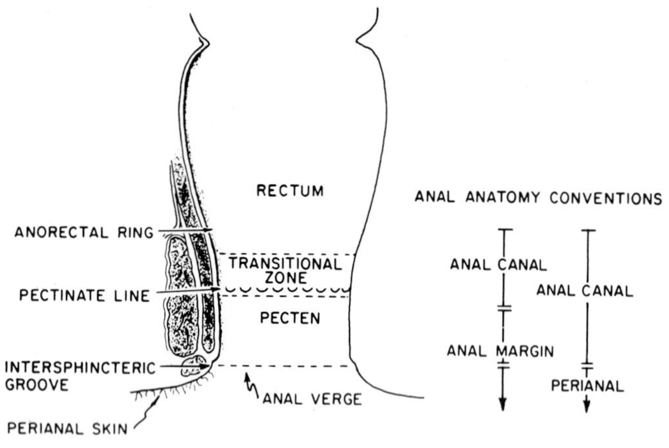

rare small cell cancers metastasize widely and rapidly and have a poor prognosis.[2]

NATURAL HISTORY

Epidermoid carcinomas of the anal canal spread most commonly by direct extension and by lymphatic pathways; hematogenous metastases are less common. Direct extension from the anal mucosa into the sphincter muscles and the perianal connective tissue spaces occurs early, and cancers were confined to the mucosa in only 12% of the patients in one large series.[2] In about half the cases, these cancers extend into the rectal wall and perianal skin.[7] Invasion of the vaginal septum and mucosa is more common than invasion of the prostate gland, and extensive tumors may infiltrate the sacrum and coccyx or the pelvic side walls.

Pelvic lymph node metastases are found in about 30% of patients treated by abdominoperineal resection, and Papillon[34] detected metastatic perirectal nodes by digital examination in 36 (30%) of 121 patients.[2,18] Inguinal metastases are present in approximately 20% of the patients at the time of initial diagnosis and are usually unilateral.[18,41,43] Stearns and associates[43] found metastases in the superior hemorrhoidal nodes in 25% (15 of 61), in the external iliac, obturator, or hypogastric nodes in 30% (eight of 27), and in the inguinal nodes in 16% (12 of 74) of patients with epidermoid carcinomas of the anal canal or anal margin. Although many investigators report mesenteric nodal metastases from fewer than 10% of carcinomas that arise below the dentate line, others have found rates of up to 40%.[11,21] Lymphatic invasion occurs relatively early, and Frost and colleagues[16] observed nodal metastases from 30% of superficial tumors and from 63% of deeply infiltrating or poorly differentiated tumors.

Extrapelvic visceral metastases are identified at the time of first presentation in about 10% of patients and are found most frequently in the liver and lungs.

Relapse after initial treatment is more common in the area of the primary tumor and the regional lymph nodes than in extrapelvic organs. The overall recurrence rate after surgical management in the Mayo Clinic series was 37% (49 of 133 patients), and this figure is typical.[2] In 73% of patients in that series, the recurrence was in the pelvis, and in a further 12%, pelvic failures occurred together with extrapelvic metastases. In a series of 51 patients treated by primary radiation, 68% (17 of 25) of the failures were at the primary sites or in the regional nodes, and all eight patients with distant metastases also had recurrences in their primary sites or nodes.[8] The risk of pelvic recurrence rises markedly if the primary tumor penetrates deeply into the sphincter muscles and if there are lymph node metastases. Late extrapelvic metastases occur in 10% to 15% of patients.[2,7,31]

PROGNOSTIC FACTORS

Prognosis is adversely affected principally by increasing size of the primary cancer[20] and the presence of lymph node metastases,[2,18] and to a lesser extent by poor histopathologic differentiation.[20] In some series, the prognosis has been reported to be better for women and better if the tumor arises in the distal rather than proximal canal.[20,21,29]

CLINICAL PRESENTATION

Bleeding and anal discomfort are the most common symptoms and are reported by about half the patients.[47] Less common complaints include awareness of an anal mass, pruritus, and anal discharge. In patients with proximal anal canal tumors, there may be an alteration in bowel habits, but this symptom is unusual with distal carcinomas.[47] The duration of symptoms does not appear to affect the prognosis. Occasionally, asymptomatic tumors are found during physical examination or in the course of investigation of an inguinal node mass.

Small carcinomas are often nodular or plaque-like, but larger tumors are more typically ulcerated. Anal sphincter tone is usually preserved and may be increased by painful spasm. Gross fecal incontinence resulting from sphincter destruction occurs in fewer than 5% of patients, although some fecal soiling is common. Synchronous inguinal node metastases are found in 10% to 30% of patients. Rarely, extrapelvic metastases may be the only symptomatic feature or finding.

DIAGNOSTIC WORKUP

The history and physical examination should stress features that delineate the extent of the primary tumor, including anal sphincter competence and possible extension to adjacent organs (Table 47-1). A biopsy of the primary tumor is necessary to establish the diagnosis and the histologic type, and general anesthesia may be needed to permit detailed pelvic and anorectal examination, which should include proctoscopy and sigmoidoscopy. Only the inguinal and low perirectal lymph nodes are accessible to clinical examination. Because lymph node enlargement may be caused by reactive hyperplasia in as many as half of those with palpable inguinal nodes, clinically suspicious nodes should be assessed by needle biopsy or simple excision.[47]

Transanorectal ultrasonography may help to identify the depth of tumor penetration into the anal wall and, in this regard, may be more accurate than digital assessment.[19] Bipedal lymphangiography gives information on the status of the external and common iliac node systems, but metastases in the internal iliac and superior hemorrhoidal node chains cannot be identified reliably by lymphangiography, computed tomography (CT), or pelvic lymphoscintigraphy. A chest film is sufficient screening for pulmonary metastases, and skeletal studies are not indicated if there are no focal symptoms. Abnormal biochemical liver function profiles should be supplemented by CT or radionuclide scans.

TABLE 47–1
Diagnostic Workup for Carcinoma of the Anal Canal

ESSENTIAL

History
Physical examination
  Regional lymph nodes and pelvic sidewalls
  Anogenital areas for concurrent malignancies
Proctoscopy
Biopsy
Chest x-ray film
Liver and renal chemistry
Urinalysis
Complete blood count

USEFUL

Colonoscopy or air contrast barium enema (to exclude other sources of lower GI tract bleeding)
Bipedal lymphangiography
Computed tomography or magnetic resonance imaging (if liver or renal biochemistry abnormal)
Transanorectal ultrasonography

TABLE 47–2
*Classification and Staging of Carcinoma of the Anal Canal**

PRIMARY TUMOR (T)

TX	Primary tumor cannot be assessed
T0	No evidence of primary tumor
Tis	Carcinoma *in situ*
T1	Tumor ≤ 2 cm in greatest dimension
T2	Tumor >2 cm but <5 cm in greatest dimension
T3	Tumor >5 cm in greatest dimension
T4	Tumor of any size invades adjacent organ(s), which should be specified (*e.g.*, vagina, urethra, bladder); involvement of the sphincter muscle(s) alone is not classified as T4

REGIONAL LYMPH NODES (N)

NX	Regional lymph nodes cannot be assessed
N0	No regional lymph node metastasis
N1	Metastasis in perirectal lymph node(s)
N2	Metastasis in unilateral internal iliac or inguinal lymph node(s)
N3	Metastasis in perirectal and inguinal lymph nodes, bilateral internal iliac, or inguinal lymph nodes

DISTANT METASTASIS (M)

MX	Presence of distant metastasis cannot be assessed
M0	No distant metastasis
M1	Distant metastasis

STAGE GROUPING

Stage 0	Tis	N0	M0
Stage I	T1	N0	M0
Stage II	T2	N0	M0
	T3	N0	M0
Stage IIIA	T4	N0	M0
	T1	N1	M0
	T2	N1	M0
	T3	N1	M0
Stage IIIB	T4	N1	M0
	Any T	N2, N3	M0
Stage IV	Any T	Any N	M1

* *The TNM classification is for the staging of cancers that arise in the anal canal only. Cancers that arise in the anal margin are staged according to cancers of the skin. (Beahrs OH, Henson DE, Hutter RVP, Myers MH [eds]: Manual for Staging of Cancer, ed 3. Philadelphia, Lippincott, 1988)*

STAGING

Several staging systems based on clinical or surgicopathologic parameters have been advocated, but none has found general acceptance. With the increasing emphasis on the preservation of anal function, clinical staging systems have become more useful than those based on histopathologic criteria. The UICC[45] and the American Joint Committee for Cancer Staging have recently proposed that the anal canal be defined as the area between the anorectal ring and the anal verge, and that carcinomas be classified according to whether they are 2 cm or smaller (T1), more than 2 cm to 5 cm (T2), more than 5 cm in diameter (T3), or invade adjacent organs such as the vagina or urethra (T4) and according to the status of the perirectal and inguinal lymph nodes (Table 47-2).

MANAGEMENT

Until the 1980s, the treatment recommended in North America for epidermoid anal cancer was usually radical resection; in Europe, radiation therapy was favored. Both treatments have been compared informally with combined-modality programs, which include chemotherapy, radiation therapy, and conservative resection. Combined-modality therapy is now favored in many centers because most patients treated by these programs retain anorectal function, with a relatively low risk of serious morbidity and with survival rates similar to those reported after radical surgery or radiation therapy.

Surgical Resection

The surgical procedure used most commonly for anal canal cancer is abdominoperineal resection with wide perineal resection and excision of the posterior vaginal wall if the cancer involves the anterior anal canal. Local excisions have limited applicability in tumors that arise above the dentate line but are favored in some centers for cancers of the distal canal.

In collected series, abdominoperineal resection yields 5-year survival rates ranging from 27% to 71%, with an average of about 50% (Table 47-3).[18,21,34] Case selection and the method of reporting contribute to this range, as they do for other treatment approaches. Abdominoperineal resection is effective but is associated with a small risk of perioperative mortality, and with the frequent psychologic and social problems of a permanent colostomy. There is also the possibility of damage to the pelvic sympathetic nerves, producing genitourinary dysfunction.

One of the objectives of radical surgery is to remove the regional lymph nodes, but only the pararectal and superior hemorrhoidal nodes are usually excised. Extending the resection to include the obturator and hypogastric nodes does not improve the survival rate, and any potential benefits from elective inguinal lymphadenectomy are outweighed by the low incidence of subclinical nodal metastases and the morbidity of the procedure.[43] If inguinal node metastases are found at the time of diagnosis, they may be managed by lymphadenectomy, although 5-year survival rates are usually only 10% to 20%, compared with 20% to 50% if the superior hemorrhoidal system is the only site of nodal metastases.[2,18,21,43] Metachronous inguinal node metastases occur in as many as 25% of patients, and if these are the only sites of failure and are resectable, 5-year survival rates of up to 60% have been obtained by lymphadenectomy, although there is a wide range of results.[2,18]

TABLE 47–3
Abdominoperineal Resection for Anal Canal Cancer

INVESTIGATOR	NO. OF PATIENTS	OPERATIVE MORTALITY (%)	5-YEAR SURVIVAL (%)	LOCOREGIONAL RECURRENCE (%)
Hardcastle[22] *	83	—	48	27‡
Dillard[11] *	40	8	45	—
Greenall[21] *	103	6	55	35‡
Boman[2] †	125	2.5	66	28‡

**Anal canal defined as anorectal junction to dentate line.*
† Anal canal defined as anorectal junction to anal verge.
‡ Sites of failure in about 5% more patients in each series are not known.

In two large series, local excision was considered an appropriate alternative to abdominoperineal resection for about 70% of cancers of the distal canal, but for only 10% of tumors arising at or above the dentate line (Table 47-4).[21,22] Even with careful selection, recurrence in the area of the canal or regional nodes was common, although secondary treatment was sometimes successful. In the upper canal, usually only small tumors that have not invaded the sphincter muscles are treated by local excision. Studies such as that by Boman and colleagues[2] of tissues removed at abdominoperineal resection have demonstrated lymph node metastases from fewer than 5% of low-grade squamous cell carcinomas less than 2 cm in diameter, but 30% to 40% of larger squamous cell carcinomas and basaloid carcinomas of any size are associated with nodal metastases. The risk of nodal metastases also increases as cancers infiltrate the sphincters. Because many believe the likelihood of nodal metastases is lower from more distally situated, well-differentiated squamous cell carcinomas, extensive local resections are sometimes performed for large tumors in the lower anal canal, with removal of up to half the circumference of the distal part of the sphincters allowing retention of anal function.[1]

The salvage rate after pelvic recurrence after abdominoperineal resection is very low, although irradiation and chemotherapy have some palliative value.[5] Greenall and associates[21] reported a median survival of 9 months after pelvic recurrence and 8 months if there were visceral metastases.

Radiation Therapy

Concern about the risk of painful anal stenosis or necrosis and doubts about the ability of orthovoltage or interstitial radiation techniques to control regional lymph node metastases contributed to the preference for radical surgery over radiation therapy in many centers.[5] However, several reports indicate that megavoltage external-beam irradiation or a combination of external-beam and interstitial irradiation can produce 5-year survival rates numerically similar to those achieved with radical surgery, with serious toxicity (*i.e.*, requiring surgical management) rates of less than 10% and no apparent increase in mortality that might be attributed to failure to control lymph node metastases (Table 47-5). A variety of different dose regimens and techniques have been successful. Minor changes in the perineum (*e.g.*, dryness, fibrosis, telangiectasia) occur in about half of the patients treated but cause few symptoms. The proportion of patients who require a colostomy as part of the management of necrosis or residual cancer is 15% to 25%. In several large series, 15% to 40% of patients treated by irradiation, often including those who presented initially with massive unresectable tumors, had residual or recurrent cancer at the primary site, but the salvage rate by abdominoperineal resection was approximately 30% to 50%.[5,9,34]

The pararectal, lower superior hemorrhoidal, and internal iliac nodes are encompassed by most external-beam techniques,

TABLE 47–4
Local Excision for Anal Canal Cancer

INVESTIGATOR	NO. TREATED BY LOCAL EXCISION/ TOTAL CASES RESECTED FOR CURE	LOCAL EXCISION CASES	
		5-YEAR SURVIVAL	LOCOREGIONAL RECURRENCE
ANAL CANAL*			
Hardcastle[22]	8/91	6/8	2/8
Greenall[21]	11/114	5/11	7/11‡
Total	19/205 (9%)	11/19 (58%)	9/19 (47%)
ANAL MARGIN†			
Hardcastle[22]	30/45	18/30	11/30‡
Greenall[21]	31/42	21/31	13/31
Total	61/87 (70%)	39/61 (64%)	24/61 (39%)

**Anal canal defined as anorectal junction to dentate line.*
† Anal margin defined as tumor mainly below dentate line to anal verge.
‡ Estimated from data in investigation report.

TABLE 47–5
Results of Radiation Therapy for Anal Canal Cancer

INVESTIGATOR	TECHNIQUE*	NO. OF PATIENTS	5-YEAR SURVIVAL (%)	RESIDUAL OR RECURRENT PRIMARY AFTER IRRADIATION (%)	COMPLICATIONS REQUIRING SURGERY (%)	PROPORTION WITH FUNCTIONAL ANUS (%)
Papillon[34]	Interstitial	88	68	14	5	88
	Combined	66	67	27	5	82
Cummings[8]	External Interstitial Combined	51	59	43	6	76
Salmon[41]	External	158	59†	33	4	73†
Eschwege[13]	External	64	46	19	14†	74
Doggett[12]	External	35	92	23	6	80

** Combined is external plus interstitial irradiation.*
† Percentage estimated from data in investigation report.

but elective irradiation of clinically normal inguinal nodes is not recommended by all radiation oncologists. Although the risk of regional recurrence is low, not all nodal metastases can be controlled if they are allowed to become clinically evident, and there is little morbidity from elective inguinal irradiation. The results shown in Table 47-6 suggest that elective inguinal irradiation is beneficial. Radiation therapy alone has had limited success in controlling unresectable inguinal node metastases.[5] Many recommend combined surgery and irradiation for established inguinal metastases, and Papillon[34] reported control at 2 years in eight of 11 patients managed in this fashion.

Combined-Modality Therapy

Because adjuvant irradiation has been given infrequently, its role has never been clearly established.[5,16,35,41] Interest in surgical adjuvant therapy increased after the report in 1974 by Nigro, Vaitkevicius, and Considine[32] of complete tumor regression in three patients who had been treated by a combination of irradiation, 5-fluorouracil (5-FU), and porfiromycin or mitomycin C before abdominoperineal resection. The protocol has been modified by many investigators, but most have reported local control rates of about 85% (Table 47-7). This treatment is no longer considered solely as an adjuvant to abdominoperineal resection, and radical resections are now usually reserved for patients who have histologically proven residual carcinoma, although even for them, local excision or further chemotherapy and radiation therapy may be an alternative.[7,15,42]

In most series, short, intensive intravenous infusions of 5-FU and bolus injections of mitomycin C have been combined with radiation. Other approaches evaluated include short-course 5-FU and split-course irradiation,[6] cyclic short-course 5-FU and irradiation, prolonged continuous-infusion 5-FU and irradiation, and daily intramuscular bleomycin and irradiation.[3,17,23] There is no evidence yet to suggest that these regimens are preferable to combinations of irradiation, 5-FU, and mitomycin C.

TABLE 47–6
Results of Elective Inguinal Node Irradiation for Anal Canal Cancer

	NO ELECTIVE NODE IRRADIATION		ELECTIVE NODE IRRADIATION	
INVESTIGATOR	RADIATION THERAPY DOSE	INGUINAL NODE ± PRIMARY FAILURE (%)	RADIATION THERAPY DOSE	INGUINAL NODE ± PRIMARY FAILURE (%)
RADIATION SERIES				
Papillon[34]	0	14/107 (13)	4500 cGy/4.5 wks	0/47 (0)
Cummings (unpublished data)	0	5/23 (22)	2400–5000 cGy/ 2.5 to 10 wks*	2/76 (3)
Rousseau[40]			6000 cGy/6 wks	3/61 (5)
Eschwege[13]	0	5/58 (7)		
SURGICAL SERIES				
Stearns[43]	0	13/53 (24)		
Boman[2]	0	15/114 (13)†		

** Radiation combined with chemotherapy in some cases.*
† Failure sites in eight other patients not known.

TABLE 47–7
Selected Combined Chemotherapy and Radiation Therapy Protocols

INVESTIGATOR	CHEMOTHERAPY*	RADIATION (cGy/FRACTIONS)	PRIMARY TUMOR COMPLETE REGRESSION		SURGERY FOR COMPLICATIONS	TUMOR SIZE
			CLINICAL	HISTOLOGIC		
Nigro[31]	A. 5-FU 1000 mg/m^2/24 hr IVI d1–4 MMC 15 mg/m^2 IVB d1 B. 5-FU 1000 mg/m^2/24 hr IVI d29–32	A. 3000/15 d1–20	97/104 (93%)	83/93 (89%)		>4 cm, 35 (34%)
Michaelson[28]	A. 5-FU 750 mg/m^2/24 hr IVI d1–5 MMC 15 mg/m^2 IVB d1	A. 3000/15 d6–25	13/27 (48%)	16/30 (53%)	None	>2 cm, 21 (70%)
Sischy[42]	A. 5-FU 1000 mg/m^2/24 hr IVI d2–5 MMC 10 mg/m^2 IVB d2 B. 5-FU 1000 mg/m^2/24 hr IVI d28–31	A. 4500/25 d1–35 1000/10 approx d36–45 B. ±1000 implant approx d73	30/33 (91%)	4/4 (100%)	None	"most large"
Flam[15]	A. 5-FU 1000 mg/m^2/24 hr IVI d1–4 MMC 15 mg/m^2 IVB d1 B. 5-FU 1000 mg/m^2/24 hr IVI d30–34 MMC 15 mg/m^2 IVB d30	A. 4000–4500/25 d1–35	27/30 (90%)	22/26 (85%)	None	Beyond canal or fixed, 15 (50%)
Papillon[35]	A. 5-FU 600 mg/m^2/24 hr IVI d1–5 MMC 12 mg/m^2 IVB d1	A. 4200/10 d1–16 B. 2000 implant approx d77	57/70 (81%)	NEB†		>4 cm, 70 (100%)
Cummings[7]	A. 5-FU 1000 mg/m^2/24 hr IVI d1–4 MMC 10 mg/m^2 IVB d1	A. 5000/20 d1–28	15/16 (94%)	NEB	3/15	>4 cm, 13 (81%)
Cummings[7]	A. 5-FU 1000 mg/m^2/24 hr IVI d1–4 MMC 10 mg/m^2 IVB d1 B. 5-FU 1000 mg/m^2/24 hr IVI d43–46 MMC 10 mg/m^2 IVB d43	A. 2500/10 d1–12 B. 2500/10 d43–54	13/14 (93%)	NEB	3/13	>4 cm, 8 (57%)
Cummings[6]	A. 5-FU 1000 mg/m^2/24 hr IVI d1–4 MMC 10 mg/m^2 IVB d1 B. 5-FU 1000 mg/m^2/24 hr IVI d43–46 MMC 10 mg/m^2 IVB d43	A. 2400/12 d1–16 B. 2400/12 d43–58	22/28 (85%)	NEB	None	>4 cm, 16 (62%)
Cummings[6]	A. 5-FU 1000 mg/m^2/24 hr IVI d1–4 B. 5-FU 1000 mg/m^2/24 hr IVI d43–46	A. 2400/12 d1–16 B. 2400/12 d43–58	16/28 (57%)	NEB	None	>4 cm, 17 (61%)
Byfield[3]	A. 5-FU 25 mg/kg/24 hr IVI d1–5 Cycle repeated approx d15, d29, etc. × 3–5	A. 1000/4 d1–4	10/10 (100%)	9/10 (90%)	None	
Hughes[23]	A. 5-FU 300 mg/m^2/24 hr IVI d1–35	A. 4500/25 d1–35 ± 1000 boost	18/24 (75%)		None	>4 cm or fixed, 10 (42%)

**5-FU: 5-fluorouracil; MMC: mitomycin C; IVI: continuous intravenous infusion; IVB: intravenious bolus injection.*
†NEB: no elective biopsy (biopsies of clinical residual cancer only).

There appear to be few contraindications to attempting to preserve anal function, other than in patients who present with massive destruction of the anal sphincters and incontinence or with vaginal fistulae. Metastatic inguinal nodes also respond well to chemotherapy and irradiation and may be managed by the same principles as the primary carcinoma.[7,31]

After chemoradiation, random biopsies from the site of the primary carcinoma are recommended by some physicians but are not necessary.[15,28,31] The correlation between clinical assessment of regression of the primary tumor and histopathologic examination of resected tissues is excellent (Table 47-7).[15,28,31] Random biopsies may miss residual carcinoma and do not preclude the need for careful follow-up. In a series of patients from several centers, on whom information was collected by questionnaire, residual carcinoma was found in the biopsy specimen taken shortly after treatment in only one of 62 patients who had

TABLE 47–8
*Influence of Size of Primary Tumor on Local Control With Preservation of Anal Function**

INVESTIGATOR	TREATMENT	PRIMARY TUMOR (≤4 CM)	PRIMARY TUMOR (>4 CM)
Papillon[34,35]	4200 cGy/2.5 wk + implant 2000 cGy	35/39 (90%)	51/77 (66%)†
Papillon[35]	4200 cGy/2.5 wk + implant 2000 cGy + 5-FU + mitomycin C		57/70 (81%)†
Cummings[6]	4500–5000 cGy/4 wk	8/11 (73%)	8/18 (44%)
Cummings[6]	4800–5000 cGy/4–10 wk + 5-FU + mitomycin C	18/19 (95%)	32/37 (86%)‡

* *Primary tumor controlled for a minimum of 12 months. Late failure was rare in all series.*
† *Mobile cancers, suitable for conservative treatment.*
‡ *Includes cancers considered fixed and unresectable at presentation.*

clinically complete regression, but 11% (seven of 61) developed local recurrences within a year after the negative biopsy findings.[31]

A biopsy specimen should be taken from any area suspected of containing cancer. Serum levels of squamous cell carcinoma-associated antigen have been studied in patients with anal epidermoid cancers, but the role of this test is not yet established.[37]

Because of the different selection criteria used, it is difficult to make comparisons of series using irradiation alone and those using chemotherapy and irradiation, but the results shown in Table 47-8 suggest that, at least for primary tumors greater than 4 cm in diameter, chemoradiation with or without conservative local surgery more frequently both controls the primary tumor and preserves anal function than does irradiation alone.

The European Organization for the Research and Treatment of Cancer and the U.K. Coordinating Committee for Cancer Research are currently conducting randomized trials in which radiation therapy alone is compared with radiation therapy combined with 5-FU and mitomycin C.

Actuarial 5-year survival rates of about 65% (cause-specific rates about 75%) were observed in the Toronto series after irradiation or irradiation plus chemotherapy, and Memorial Hospital in New York reported a 5-year survival rate of 55% for 103 patients treated by abdominoperineal resection and 78% for 18 patients treated by combined-modality therapy.[7,21] The results in other series appear to be at least equal to those achieved by surgery or by radiation therapy alone.[15,25,42]

The acute toxicity of these regimens varies with the doses of drugs and radiation used. In programs that combined irradiation, 5-FU, and mitomycin C, moderate leukopenia, thrombocytopenia, proctitis, and perineal dermatitis were recorded in about 30% of patients after doses of 2500 cGy to 3000 cGy in 2.5 to 3 weeks, and more profound marrow depression and enteroproctitis occurred in 50% after receiving 5000 cGy in 4 weeks plus chemotherapy.[7,31] Late toxicity has not been reported after doses of 3000 cGy in 3 weeks to 4500 cGy in 5 weeks, but radiation-induced enteritis or anal ulceration occurred in six (20%) of 30 patients who received 5000 cGy in 20 fractions by continuous or split-course irradiation.[6,7,15,25,28] The appearance of the perineum of a patient treated with combined high-dose irradiation and chemotherapy is shown in Figure 47-2, and

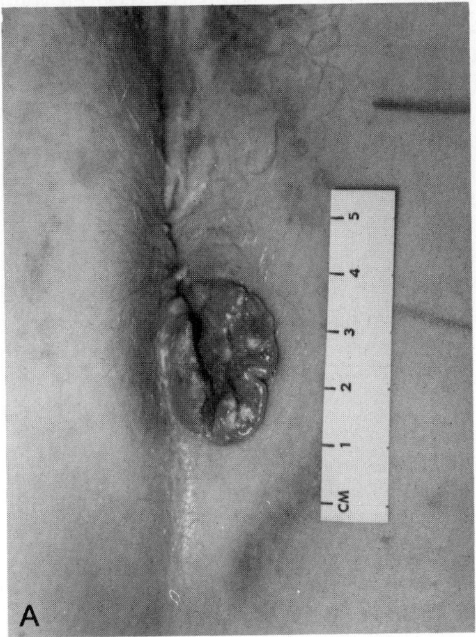

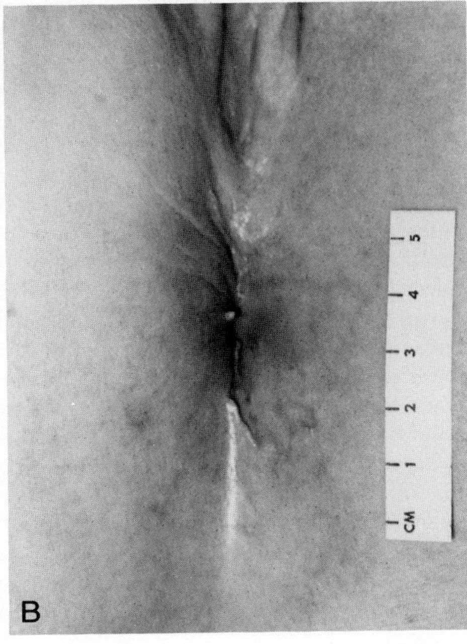

FIGURE 47–2. (**A**) A 3-cm diameter perianal extension of squamous cell carcinoma that also involved the distal 3 cm of the anal canal. (Cummings BJ, Harwood AR, Keane TJ, et al: Dis Colon Rectum 23:389, 1980) (**B**) Appearance 6 years after combined irradiation (5000 cGy in 20 fractions in 4 weeks) and chemotherapy. The patient has normal anal function. The telangiectasia is typical of that seen in about 20% of patients.

it is similar to that seen after treatment with radical radiation therapy alone.

It is not known whether chemotherapy and radiation act additively or synergistically in these programs.[44] Some laboratory studies of 5-FU and irradiation have shown only additive effects,[46] but Byfield and associates[4] concluded from *in vitro* studies of HeLa and HT29 cells that there was enhanced cell kill from combined 5-FU and x-rays that required postradiation incubation of cells in cytocidal levels of 5-FU for 48 hours. Centers that have used sequential chemotherapy and irradiation rather than concurrent treatments have observed lower tumor clearance rates, although this could be a result of the lower doses of 5-FU used and the shorter interval between radiation therapy and assessment.[28] Mitomycin C probably does not have any true sensitizing role in the doses used, but it may be of value for its relatively greater cytotoxicity for hypoxic cells.[27,39] The Radiation Therapy Oncology Group has undertaken a randomized trial to evaluate the role of mitomycin C in multimodality treatment.

Deaths resulting from distant metastases have assumed increased importance as pelvic control rates have improved. In the collected series of Nigro and colleagues[31] of 104 patients, eight of the 13 patients who died had distant metastases only, and five had both local and distant recurrence. Although Michaelson and associates reported temporary responses in 59% of patients with advanced anal cancer treated by 5-FU and mitomycin C without irradiation, there was no apparent benefit when this combination was given as adjuvant therapy for up to a year, and the drugs produced significant morbidity from myelosuppression, azotemia, and microangiopathic hemolytic anemia.[28] Other drugs that have produced responses in patients with extensive anal carcinomas when used as single agents or in combination, and those that should be considered for systemic therapy or for combination with radiation therapy include bleomycin, methyl-CCNU, vincristine, vinblastine, doxorubicin, cisplatin, and methotrexate.[5,26]

RADIATION THERAPY TECHNIQUES

Both external-beam and interstitial irradiation may be used in the treatment of anal cancers. For well-differentiated, superficial, squamous cell carcinomas involving the distal canal that are less than 3 cm in diameter and are considered to be at low risk of having regional node metastases, a direct perineal beam is sufficient. A tumor dose equivalent to 6000 cGy in 6 weeks is recommended.

For all other epidermoid carcinomas, treatment of the primary tumor and the regional nodes is recommended. The simplest field arrangement that encompasses this volume is an anterior and posterior opposed pair of fields. If the patient is prone, the anus can be readily visualized and bolus placed selectively over any perianal tumor extension. The upper border of the field may be located at the lumbosacral junction to encompass the common iliac and hypogastric nodes or at the lower border of the sacroiliac joint to include only the external iliac, lower internal iliac, and pararectal nodes.[7,12,24,28,42] The lower border is set 3 cm distal to the lower-most extension of the primary tumor, which should be indicated with a radiopaque marker during simulation. The lateral borders should cover the external iliac nodes; a lymphogram is useful for localizing this boundary. If the inguinal nodes are to be treated, this may be done by extending the anterior and posterior fields or the anterior field only, or it may be achieved by adding discontinuous anterior fields. Alternative field arrangements have been described elsewhere.[13,17,24,34,40]

All external-beam therapy is given by megavoltage apparatus. When external-beam irradiation without chemotherapy is used, a dosage of 6000 cGy to 6500 cGy delivered in 6 to 7 weeks to the primary tumor is recommended. The primary tumor and regional nodes are encompassed in the fields to yield a midplane dose of 4500 cGy administered in 4.5 to 5 weeks, after which the volume is reduced to spare the pelvic small bowel and rectosigmoid. The reduced volume includes the primary tumor and any local tumor extension, and it may be treated by interstitial therapy, by external-beam therapy with a perineal field, or by multifield techniques.[7,34,42] During simulation of the reduced fields, a thin catheter filled with barium is placed in the anal canal with a marker to indicate the anal verge. Urethral or vaginal markers may also be useful. A tumor dose of 1500 cGy to 2000 cGy in 2 weeks is given to the reduced volume. If interstitial irradiation techniques are used, a dose of 2000 cGy at 0.5 cm from the plane of the implant given in 24 hours has been recommended.[34] A template ensures regular spacing of the needles, which are usually arranged in a single plane, and the risk of stenosis or necrosis is reduced if the whole anal circumference is not implanted.[5,34,42] Proven metastases in the inguinal nodes may be given additional treatment through anterior electron-beam fields to raise the total dosage to the nodal area to between 6000 cGy and 6500 cGy in 6.5 weeks.

If irradiation and concurrent 5-FU and mitomycin C are used, some modification of these dosage guidelines is necessary, although field arrangements are the same. Midpelvic doses of 3000 cGy in 3 weeks to 4500 cGy in 5 weeks have been given without undue toxic reactions of the bowel or bladder, and split-course techniques were introduced to avoid the acute enteroproctitis and perineal reactions seen with doses at 5000 cGy in 4 weeks.[7,24,31,42] The most effective primary tumor radiation dose in these combined-modality programs has not yet been determined, and the doses used range from 3000 cGy in 3 weeks to 5500 cGy in 5 to 7 weeks (Table 47-7).

The Princess Margaret Hospital technique (Fig. 47-3) delivers half of the dose to large anterior and posterior pelvic fields with concurrent chemotherapy. Four weeks later, after any acute reaction has subsided, the second phase of the treatment is given to a reduced volume by a four-field technique, which is combined with chemotherapy. If the inguinal nodes are involved or if pelvic node metastases are demonstrated clinically or on the lymphangiogram, the fields are not reduced for the second phase of the treatment. Several dose schedules have been evaluated, and an effective and well-tolerated schedule includes the delivery of two courses of radiation, each of a total dose of 2400 cGy in 12 fractions given in 2.5 weeks to the volumes described earlier. Concomitant 5-FU (1000 mg/m^2/24 hours) is administered by continuous intravenous infusion over 96 hours, starting on the first day of each course of irradiation, and a bolus intravenous injection of mitomycin C (10 mg/m^2) is given on the first day of each course.

Although concepts of perineal tolerance have undergone some revision during the past decade, the perineum still reacts quickly and uncomfortably during treatment, and severe late reactions may require surgical management. The results obtained in several series suggest that perianal tolerance is determined by the total and the fractional radiation doses and by the amount of bolus used, by the area of the perineum irradiated, and by whether radiation beams are tangential to or directly incident on the skin surface.[7,34,42] Photon irradiation is prefer-

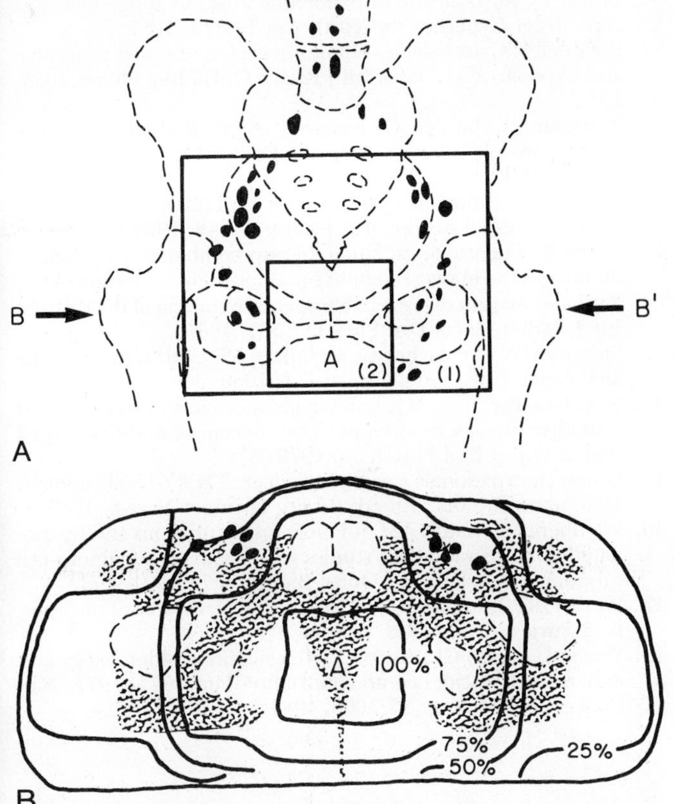

FIGURE 47–3. (**A**) Boundaries of radiation fields used in the Princess Margaret Hospital technique. Half of the tumor dose is given to the larger volume (1) by anterior and posterior opposed fields with ^{60}Co or 6-MV photons. The reduced volume (2) is treated by a four-field technique with 18-MV photons; A, anal verge marker. (**B**) Composite isodose distribution through plane B - B′ in (**A**).

red by some for perineal fields because electron-beam irradiation may cause severe late perineal reactions.[34]

Although he also obtained successful results in patients treated by interstitial therapy only, Papillon[34] now advises against such management because of the risk of necrosis and the high rates of local and lymph node failures reported.

PROSPECTIVE ISSUES

There are many unresolved issues in the management of epidermoid anal canal cancer, although substantial progress has been made in gaining acceptance of techniques that preserve anal function. Resolution of the most basic questions would require formal comparisons of radical surgery, radiation therapy alone, and combined-modality therapy. However, patients are unlikely to participate in studies in which one arm would offer a chance to avoid a colostomy and another would require it. Other questions being addressed include identification of optimal radiation techniques; detailed exploration of the mechanisms, efficacy, and toxicity of drug and radiation combinations; and identification of effective systemic chemotherapy for the management of extrapelvic metastases.

Even without formal clinical trials, however, the results reported support the use of radiation therapy alone or combined-modality therapy as the initial treatment for epidermoid anal canal carcinoma, preserving anal function whenever possible and reserving radical surgery for the patient with residual carcinoma.

REFERENCES

1. Al-Jurf AS, Turnbull RB, Fazio VW: Local treatment of carcinomas of the anus. Surg Gynecol Obstet 148:576, 1979
2. Boman BM, Moertel CG, O'Connel MJ, et al: Carcinoma of the anal canal: A clinical and pathologic study of 188 cases. Cancer 54:114, 1984
3. Byfield JE, Barone RM, Sharp TR, et al: Conservative management without alkylating agents of squamous cell anal cancer using cyclical 5-FU alone and x-ray therapy. Cancer Treat Rep 67:709, 1983
4. Byfield JE, Calabro-Jones P, Klisak I, et al: Pharmacologic requirements for obtaining sensitization of human tumor cells *in vitro* to combined 5-fluorouracil or ftorafur and x-rays. Int J Radiat Oncol Biol Phys 8:1923, 1982
5. Cummings BJ: The place of radiation therapy in the treatment of carcinoma of the anal canal. Cancer Treat Rev 9:125, 1982
6. Cummings BJ: unpublished data
7. Cummings BJ, Keane TJ, Thomas GM, et al: Results and toxicity of the treatment of anal canal carcinoma by radiation therapy or radiation therapy and chemotherapy. Cancer 54:2062, 1984
8. Cummings BJ, Thomas GM, Keane TJ, et al: Primary radiation therapy in the treatment of anal canal carcinoma. Dis Colon Rectum 25:778, 1982
9. Dalby JE, Pointon RS: The treatment of anal carcinoma by interstitial irradiation. AJR 85:515, 1961
10. Daling JR, Weiss NS, Hislop TG, et al: Sexual practices, sexually transmitted diseases, and the incidence of anal cancer. N Engl J Med 317:973, 1987
11. Dillard BM, Spratt JS, Ackerman LV, et al: Epidermoid cancer of anal margin and canal. Arch Surg 86:772, 1963
12. Doggett SW, Green JP, Cantril ST: Efficacy of radiation therapy alone for limited squamous cell carcinoma of the anal canal. Int J Radiat Oncol Biol Phys 15:1069, 1988
13. Eschwege P, Lasser P, Chary A, et al: Squamous cell carcinoma of the anal canal: Treatment by external beam irradiation. Radiother Oncol 3:145, 1985
14. Fenger C: Histology of the anal canal. Am J Surg Pathol 12:41, 1988
15. Flam MS, John MJ, Mowry PA, et al: Definitive combined modality therapy of carcinoma of the anus. Dis Colon Rectum 30:495, 1987
16. Frost DB, Richards PC, Montague ED, et al: Epidermoid cancer of the anorectum. Cancer 53:1285, 1984
17. Glimelius B, Pahlman L: Radiation therapy of anal epidermoid carcinoma. Int J Radiat Oncol Biol Phys 13:305, 1987
18. Golden GT, Horsley JS: Surgical management of epidermoid carcinoma of the anus. Am J Surg 131:275, 1976
19. Goldman S, Glimelius B, Norming U, et al: Transanorectal ultrasonography in anal carcinoma. A prospective study of 21 patients. Acta Radiol 29:337, 1988
20. Goldman S, Glimelius B, Pahlman L, et al: Anal epidermoid carcinoma: A population-based clinico-pathological study of 164 patients. Int J Colorect Dis 3:109, 1988
21. Greenall MJ, Quan HQ, Decosse JJ: Epidermoid cancer of the anus. Br J Surg 72 (Suppl):S97, 1985
22. Hardcastle JD, Bussey HJR: Results of surgical treatment of squamous cell carcinoma of the anal canal and anal margin seen at St. Mark's Hospital 1928–1966. Proc R Soc Med 61:629, 1968
23. Hughes L, Rich TA, Delclos L, et al: Radiotherapy for anal cancer: Experience at MD Anderson Hospital 1979–1987. Proceedings of the 30th annual ASTRO meeting. Int J Radiat Oncol Biol Phys 15:115, 1988
24. John MJ, Flam M, Lovalvol, et al: Feasibility of non-surgical definitive management of anal canal carcinoma. Int J Radiat Oncol Biol Phys 13:299, 1987
25. Leichman L, Nigro N, Vaitkevicius VK, et al: Cancer of the anal canal: Model for preoperative adjuvant combined modality therapy. Am J Med 78:211, 1985
26. Magill GB, Quan SHQ: Salvage chemotherapy of anal epidermoid carcinoma with cisplatin-based protocols. Proc Am Soc Clin Oncol 8:117, 1989

27. Marshall RS, Rauth AM: Oxygen and exposure kinetics as factors influencing the cytotoxicity of porfiromycin, a mitomycin C analogue, in Chinese hamster ovary cells. Cancer Res 48:5655, 1988
28. Michaelson RA, Magill GB, Quan SHQ, et al: Preoperative chemotheraphy and radiation therapy in the management of anal epidermoid carcinoma. Cancer 51:390, 1983
29. Morson BC: The pathology and results of treatment of squamous cell carcinoma of the anal canal and anal margin. Proc R Soc Med 53:416, 1960
30. Morson BC, Sobin JH: Histological typing of intestinal tumors. In International Histological Classification of Tumors, No. 25. Geneva, World Health Organization, 1976
31. Nigro ND: An evaluation of combined therapy for squamous cell cancer of the anal canal. Dis Colon Rectum 27:763, 1984
32. Nigro ND, Vaitkevicius, VK, Considine B: Combined therapy for cancer of the anal canal: A preliminary report. Dis Colon Rectum 17:354, 1974
33. Palmer JG, Shepherd NA, Jass JR, et al: Human papillomavirus type 16 DNA in anal squamous cell carcinoma. Lancet 2:42, 1987
34. Papillon J: Rectal and Anal Cancers. Conservative Treatment by Irradiation—An Alternative to Radical Surgery. Berlin, Springer-Verlag, 1982
35. Papillon J, Montbarbon JF: Epidermoid carcinoma of the anal canal. A series of 276 cases. Dis Colon Rectum 30:324, 1987
36. Penn I: Cancer is a complication of severe immunosuppression. Surg Gynecol Obstet 162:603, 1986
37. Petrelli NJ, Shawn N, Bhargava A, et al: Squamous cell carcinoma antigen as a marker for squamous cell carcinoma of the anal canal. J Clin Oncol 6:782, 1988
38. Pfister H: Relationship of papillomaviruses to anogenital cancer. Obstet Gynecol Clin North Am 14:349, 1987
39. Rockwell S: Cytotoxicities of mitomycin C and x-rays to aerobic and hypoxic cells *in vitro.* Int J Radiat Oncol Biol Phys 8:1035, 1982
40. Rousseau J, Mathieu G, Fenton J, et al: Radiotherapie des cancers malpighiens de l'anus. J Radiol Electrol Med Nucl 54:622, 1973
41. Salmon RJ, Fenton J, Asselani B, et al: Treatment of epidermoid anal canal cancer. Am J Surg 147:43, 1984
42. Sischy B: The use of radiation therapy combined with chemotherapy in the management of squamous cell carcinoma of the anus and marginally resectable adenocarcinoma of the rectum. Int J Radiat Oncol Biol Phys 11:1587, 1985
43. Stearns MW, Urmacher C, Sternberg SS, et al: Cancer of the anal canal. Curr Probl Cancer 4:1, 1980
44. Steel GG, Peckham MJ: Exploitable mechanisms in combined radiotherapy–chemotherapy: The concept of additivity. Int J Radiat Oncol Biol Phys 5:85, 1979
45. Union Internationale Contre le Cancer: TNM Classification of Malignant Tumors, 4th ed. Berlin, Springer-Verlag, 1987
46. Weinberg MJ, Rauth AM: 5-Fluorouracil infusions and fractionated doses of radiation: studies with a murine squamous cell carcinoma. Int J Radiat Oncol Biol Phys 13:1691, 1987
47. Wolfe HRI, Bussey HJR: Squamous cell carcinoma of the anus. Br J Surg 55:195, 1968
48. Young JL, Percy CL, Asire AJ: Surveillance, epidemiology and end results: Incidence and mortality data 1973–1977. Natl Cancer Inst Monogr 57:1066, 1981

48

Kidney, Renal Pelvis, and Ureter

Peter P. Lai

ANATOMY

The kidneys are located at a level between the eleventh rib and the transverse process of the third lumbar vertebra in the retroperitoneal space. The renal axis is parallel to the lateral margin of the psoas muscle. Each kidney is roughly 11 cm to 12 cm long, and the right one is usually 1 cm to 2 cm lower than the left one. The kidney in its fibrous capsule and the perinephric fat are enveloped by Gerota's fascia.

The caliceal collecting system lies on the anteromedial surface of the kidney. The ureters course posteriorly, paralleling the lateral border of the psoas muscle until they curve anteriorly to join the base of the bladder.

The lymphatics of the kidney and renal pelvis drain along the vessels in the renal hilum to the para-aortic and paracaval nodes. The lymphatic drainage of the ureter is segmented and diffuse and may involve any of the renal hilar, abdominal para-aortic, paracaval, common iliac, internal iliac, or external iliac nodes.

EPIDEMIOLOGY AND RISK FACTORS

The lesions discussed in this chapter are limited to adult renal cell carcinoma (*e.g.*, hypernephroma, Grawitz's tumor) and transitional cell carcinoma of the collecting system and ureter. Wilms' tumors, primary retroperitoneal sarcomas, and lymphomas are discussed in other chapters.

Renal Cell Carcinoma

The estimated number of new cases of kidney and other urinary cancers in the United States for 1990 was 24,000, resulting in more than 10,000 deaths.[41] These figures represent approximately 2% of all new cancers and cancer-related deaths. The average age at diagnosis is 55 to 60 years, and the tumors affect twice as many males as females.

A number of environmental (*e.g.*, exposure to cadmium, thorium dioxide, petroleum products, phenacetin-containing analgesics abuse, tobacco use), occupational (*e.g.*, leather tanners, shoe workers, asbestos workers), hormonal (*e.g.*, diethylstilbestrol), cellular, and genetic factors have been associated with the development of renal cell carcinoma.[23]

Acquired cystic kidney disease has been reported among chronic hemodialysis patients, and a small percentage of these patients develop renal cell carcinoma. Prolonged administration of diethylstilbestrol (DES) to male Syrian golden hamsters led to the development of renal tumors, which were inhibited by estrogen antagonist.[6] Renal cell cancer has been reported after DES therapy given for prostate cancer.[5] The role of hormonal therapy in the management of patients with metastatic renal cell carcinoma has been described elsewhere.[6]

The association of renal cell cancer and Hippel-Lindau disease has long been established.[11] Chromosomal analysis of tumor cells from a patient with Hippel-Lindau disease revealed a proximal deletion in the short arm of chromosome 3 in the 3p14 region.[20]

Various tumor-produced growth factors, such as parathyroid hormone-like, transforming growth factor-like, or epidermal growth factors have been described in the initiation or progression of renal cell carcinoma.[23]

Renal Pelvis and Ureter Cancer

Transitional cell carcinoma of the upper urinary tract comprises 7% of all renal neoplasms and less than 1% of all genitourinary tumors.[34] The incidence of bilateral upper urinary tract tumors is 1.5% to 2% for synchronous and 6% to 8% for asynchronous presentations.[18] Renal pelvis tumor is found two to three times more frequently in men than in women, and the peak incidence is in the fifth and sixth decades of life.[18] Upper urinary tract carcinoma is a multifocal process; patients with cancer at one site in the upper urinary tract are at greater risk of developing tumors elsewhere. About one third of patients with upper urinary tract tumor develop bladder carcinoma.[18]

Because the mucosal surfaces of the renal pelvis, ureter, and bladder have the same embryologic origin (hence the term urothelium), many of the etiologic factors for renal pelvis and ureter tumors also apply to tumors of the urinary bladder. Urban residency, tobacco use, aminophenol exposure (*e.g.*, benzidine, β-naphthylamine), renal stones, and analgesics (*i.e.*, chronic phenacetin abuse) have been associated with an increased risk of developing upper urinary tract tumors.

Balkan nephropathy, an endemic familial disease prevalent in Yugoslavia, Rumania, Bulgaria, and Greece, is a chronic tubulointerstitial nephropathy. It is associated with a high frequency of multifocal, slowly growing, superficial, papillary transitional cell carcinoma of the renal pelvis and ureter.[30]

NATURAL HISTORY

Renal Cell Carcinoma

The natural history of renal cell carcinoma is not always predictable. Riche[36] reported a series of 443 untreated patients with an overall survival rate of 4.4% at 3 years and 1.7% at 5 years. None of these patients were considered to be surgical candidates because of advanced presentation or multiple medical problems.

Tumor may spread by local infiltration through the renal capsule to involve the perinephric fat and Gerota's fascia; by direct propagation within the venous channels to the renal vein or to the inferior vena cava; by retrograde venous drainage to the ovary or testis; by lymphatic drainage to renal hilar, para-aortic, and paracaval nodes and eventually to every viscera in the body. The incidence of lymph node metastasis was 12% to 23% in the surgical series reported by Bassil and associates[2] and Robson and co-workers.[37]

Seven percent of renal cell carcinomas are diagnosed incidentally. Approximately 45% of patients with renal cell carcinoma have localized disease; 25% have advanced disease, and about 30% have radiographic evidence of metastasis at the time of diagnosis.[23] Of those with metastases, about 1% to 3% have solitary metastasis.[43] About half of the patients with renal cell carcinoma eventually develop metastatic disease.[26]

Among patients presenting with metastatic renal cell carcinoma, the sites of distribution reported by Maldazys and deKernion[24] include lung (75%), soft tissue (36%), bone (20%), liver (18%), cutaneous sites (8%), and central nervous system (8%). Pulmonary metastasis occurring 24 years after nephrectomy has been documented.[12]

Spontaneous or idiopathic regression of metastatic renal cell carcinoma after nephrectomy has been reported, but it is extremely rare: four (0.8%) of 474 patients in the series by Montie and associates[26] and three (0.3%) of 1139 in Bloom's report.[6] Based on a review of the literature and his own observations, Bloom[6] reported a total of 40 cases of spontaneous regression for untreated renal cell carcinoma and 11 cases of hormone-induced regression. Most of the spontaneous regression of renal cell carcinoma involved pulmonary metastases, and most were in males; hormonal-induced regression included other sites of metastases. However, regression is not synonymous with cure, and host endocrine or immunologic factors may influence the natural history of renal cell carcinoma.

Renal Pelvis and Ureter Carcinoma

Upper urinary tract carcinoma is a multifocal process, and patients with cancer at one site in the upper urinary tract are at greater risk of developing tumors elsewhere. The probability of multifocal occurrence is greater in patients with large lesions and in those with carcinoma *in situ*. Ureteral tumors have a tendency to occur in the distal third of the ureter.

Transitional cell carcinoma of the upper urothelial tract may spread both by direct extension and by way of blood and lymphatics. Implantation of tumor cells in the bladder has been demonstrated, especially in previously traumatized areas.[35] The incidence of lymph node metastasis ranged from 37% to 82% in patients with renal pelvis tumor and 22% to 41% in patients with ureteral tumor.[40] Almost any organ may acquire metastatic transitional cell tumors from the upper urinary tract.

CLINICAL PRESENTATION

Renal Cell Carcinoma

Renal cell carcinoma may present as an occult primary tumor or with signs and symptoms attributable to a local mass or systemic paraneoplastic syndromes. The classic triad of gross hematuria, palpable abdominal mass, and pain occurred in only 9% of patients. Thirty-six percent of patients presented with two of the three components of the triad. Gross or microscopic hematuria occurred in 59% of patients, and 7% had asymptomatic, incidental findings.[31]

A wide range of paraneoplastic syndromes or systemic symptoms of renal cell carcinoma has been described.[23,31] As a unified theory, it has been proposed that cells secreting abnormal peptide may be of primitive neural crest origin. Parathyroid-like hormones, erythropoietin, renin, gonadotropins, placental lactogen, prolactin, enteroglucagon, insulin-like hormones, ACTH, and prostaglandins have been identified in various patients with renal cell carcinoma.

Renal Pelvis and Ureter Carcinoma

Gross or microscopic hematuria occurs in 70% to 95% of patients with renal pelvic or ureteral tumor.[34] The other, less common symptoms include pain (8% to 40%), bladder irritation (5% to 10%), and other constitutional symptoms (5%).

About 10% to 20% of patients present with a flank mass secondary to tumor or associated hydronephrosis, but physical findings are otherwise unremarkable.

DIAGNOSTIC WORKUP

Renal Cell Carcinoma

Most renal masses are benign. If neoplasm is suspected, the imaging algorithm is illustrated in Figure 48-1.[25]

The diagnostic and staging workup for renal cell carcinoma is listed in Table 48-1. The diagnosis of renal cell carcinoma is established clinically and radiographically in most cases. Once a radiographic diagnosis is made, a thorough staging workup should be carried out to determine resectability. A metastatic workup, including bone scan, chest x-ray film, and computed tomography (CT) scan or magnetic resonance imaging (MRI) of the abdomen and pelvis, should be performed before surgery. If metastatic lesions are detected, histologic confirmation of the most easily accessible lesion should then be obtained.

Renal Pelvis and Ureter Carcinoma

The diagnostic workup for renal pelvis and ureter carcinoma is listed in Table 48-2. Excretory urography is frequently used to

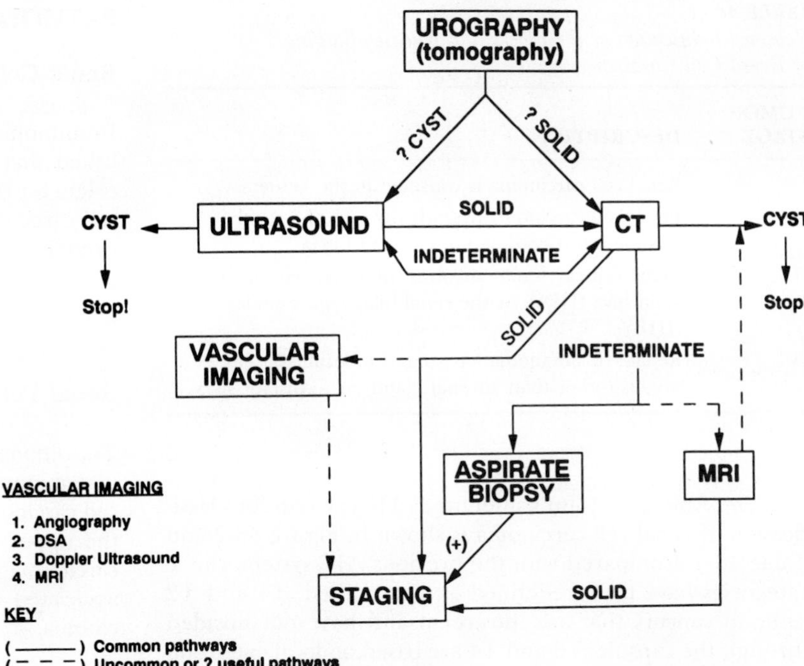

FIGURE 48–1. Imaging algorithm for renal mass. (McClennan BL, Rubin DN: Kidney. In Lee JKT, Sagel SS, Stanley RJ [eds]: Computed Body Tomography with MRI Correlation, 2nd ed. New York, Raven Press, 1988)

evaluate patients with renal pelvis carcinoma. The most common finding is a filling defect in the renal pelvis or the collecting system. Retrograde pyelography accurately delineates upper tract filling defects and defines the lower margin of the ureteral lesion. CT or MRI of the abdomen and pelvis before and after contrast administration gives useful information regarding extension of the tumor outside the collecting system. Brush cytology or biopsy from endoscopic and retrograde procedures carries a diagnostic accuracy of 80% to 90%, and urine cytology (*i.e.*, endoscopically obtained barbotage specimen) is accurate in about 80% of cases.[23]

TABLE 48–1
Diagnostic Workup for Renal Cell Carcinoma

GENERAL

History
Physical examination

RADIOGRAPHIC STUDIES

Standard
- Chest radiograph
- Intravenous pyelogram
- Ultrasonic echorenograph
- Renal arteriograph ± epinephrine
- CT or MRI scan of abdomen and pelvis
- Bone scan

Complementary
- CT and digital subtraction angiogram
- Inferior venacavogram
- CT of chest, brain, or other suspected organs

SPECIAL TESTS

Cyst puncture with fluid cytology
(if no echinococcosis is suspected)

LABORATORY STUDIES

Complete blood count
Blood chemistry
Urinalysis

STAGING

Renal Cell Carcinoma

The staging system currently used by most physicians in the United States is the Robson modification of the system proposed by Flocks and Kadesky (Table 48-3).[14] The drawback of this staging system is the subgrouping of Stage III patients with vastly different prognoses. Involvement of the renal vein or inferior vena cava (Stage IIIA) does not adversely affect survival, which is similar to Stage I or Stage II, while renal hilar, para-aortic, or paracaval adenopathy is associated with a worse prognosis.

TABLE 48–2
Diagnostic Workup for Renal Pelvis and Ureter Carcinoma

GENERAL

History
Physical examination

RADIOGRAPHIC STUDIES

Standard
- Chest radiograph
- Excretory urogram
- Retrograde pyelogram
- CT or MRI scan of abdomen and pelvis

Complementary
- Endoscopic ureteroscopy
- Percutaneous nephroscopy

SPECIAL TESTS

Urine cytology (endoscopically obtained)
Retrograde brush cytology or biopsy

LABORATORY STUDIES

Complete blood count
Blood chemistry
Urinalysis

TABLE 48–3
Robson Modification of the Flocks and Kadesky Staging of Renal Cell Carcinoma

TUMOR STAGE	DESCRIPTION
I	Renal cell carcinoma is confined to the kidneys
II	Renal cell carcinoma extends through the renal capsule but is confined to Gerota's fascia
III	Renal cell carcinoma involves the renal vein or inferior vena cava (IIIA), or the renal hilar lymph nodes (IIIB)
IV	Renal cell carcinoma has spread to local adjacent organs (other than adrenal gland) or to distant sites

The American Joint Committee (AJC) system for classification of renal cell carcinoma is shown in Figure 48-2 and Table 48-4. Compared with the previous AJC system, the T categories have been redefined and simplified. T1 and T2 refer to cancers that are intrarenal and have not invaded through the capsule. T3 and T4 are based on local extension of the primary tumor. The N classification has also been redefined and depends on the size and number of involved lymph nodes and not on laterality.

Renal Pelvis and Ureter Carcinoma

Grabstald and associates,[16] after studying 70 patients with renal pelvis tumor, proposed a classification based on tumor extension and grade. Various modifications of this staging classification have been proposed. Ureteral tumors have been given a similar staging system.

The 1988 AJC staging classification for renal pelvis and ureter carcinoma is shown in Table 48-5. The grouping of the T categories depends on the tumor extent (*i.e.*, depth of penetration of the lesion).

PATHOLOGIC CLASSIFICATION

Renal Cell Carcinoma

Immunohistologic and ultrastructural analyses have established that the proximal tubular epithelium is the tissue of origin for renal cell carcinoma. The histologic subtypes of renal cell carcinoma include clear cell carcinoma, which is the most predominate type; granular cell carcinoma; and the spindle cell (or sarcomatoid) variant. Few tumors are purely clear cell or granular cell type; most are mixtures of both.

Renal Pelvis and Ureter Carcinoma

Transitional cell carcinoma accounts for more than 90% of the malignant tumors of the renal pelvis and ureter.[23] Squamous cell carcinoma accounts for 7% to 8%, and adenocarcinoma of the upper urothelial tract is rarely reported. Squamous cell carcinoma of the renal pelvis is often deeply invasive and is associated with a worse prognosis than transitional cell carcinoma.

PROGNOSTIC FACTORS

Renal Cell Carcinoma

The major prognostic factors for survival of patients with renal cell carcinoma are stage and histologic grade of the tumor. The survival statistics for patients with different stages of renal cell carcinoma have remained essentially the same for 20 years. The 5-year survival rates reported by Robson and co-workers[37] in 1969, using the Robson modification of the Flocks and Kadesky staging classification, were 66% for Stage I, 64% for Stage II, 42% for Stage III, and 11% for Stage IV. A 1986 report by Golimbu and associates[15] reported similar 5-year survival statistics: 88% for Stage I, 67% for Stage II, 40% for Stage III, and 2% for Stage IV.

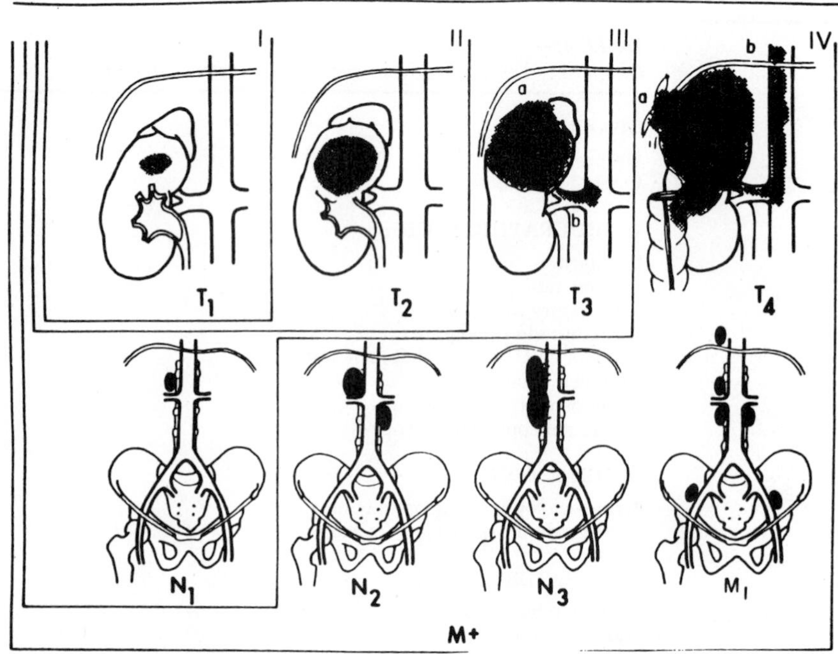

FIGURE 48–2. Staging classification for renal cell carcinoma according to the 1988 AJC system. See Table 48-5 for details. (Modified from AJC, UICC, Rubin P (ed): Clinical Oncology: A Multidisciplinary Approach, 6th ed. American Cancer Society, 1983; courtesy of Philip Rubin, M.D.)

TABLE 48–4
1988 American Joint Committee Staging Classification for Kidney Tumors

PRIMARY TUMOR (T)

TX	Primary tumor cannot be assessed
T0	No evidence of primary tumor
T1	Tumor ≤ 2.5 cm in greatest dimension limited to the kidney
T2	Tumor > 2.5 cm in greatest dimension limited to the kidney
T3	Tumor extends into major veins or invades adrenal gland or perinephric tissues but not beyond Gerota's fascia
T3a	Tumor invades adrenal gland or perinephric tissues but not beyond Gerota's fascia
T3b	Tumor grossly extends into renal vein(s) or vena cava
T4	Tumor invades beyond Gerota's fascia

REGIONAL LYMPH NODES (N)

NX	Regional lymph nodes cannot be assessed
N0	No regional lymph node metastasis
N1	Metastasis in a single lymph node, ≤ 2 cm in greatest dimension
N2	Metastasis in a single lymph node, > 2 cm but < 5 cm in greatest dimension, or multiple lymph nodes, ≤ 5 cm in greatest dimension
N3	Metastasis in a lymph node > 5 cm in greatest dimension

DISTANT METASTASIS (M)

MX	Presence of distant metastasis cannot be assessed
M0	No distant metastasis
M1	Distant metastasis

STAGE GROUPING

Stage I	T1	N0	M0
Stage II	T2	N0	M0
Stage III	T1	N1	M0
	T2	N1	M0
	T3a	N0, N1	M0
	T3b	N0, N1	M0
Stage IV	T4	Any N	M0
	Any T	N2, N3	M0
	Any T	Any N	M1

HISTOPATHOLOGIC GRADE

GX	Grade cannot be assessed
G1	Well differentiated
G2	Moderately well differentiated
G3–4	Poorly differentiated or undifferentiated

(Beahrs OH, Henson DE, Hutter RVP, Myers MH [eds]: Manual for Staging of Cancer, 3rd ed, p 199. Philadelphia, JB Lippincott, 1988)

Renal vein or vena cava involvement without corresponding regional lymph node metastasis is not a poor prognostic sign.[31] Patients with renal vein or vena cava involvement have almost the same 5- and 10-year survival rates as those of Stage I patients, provided the entire thrombus is removed (Table 48-6).

The mean survival rate for patients with metastasis at the time of diagnosis is approximately 4 months, and only about 10% of patients survive 1 year.[31]

High nuclear grade of renal cell carcinoma correlates with increased incidence of regional lymph node involvement and a decreased 5-year survival rate.[31] The sarcomatoid variant of renal cell carcinoma carries a significantly poorer prognosis than the clear cell or granular cell subtypes.[39] Forty-eight percent of the patients with sarcomatoid renal cell carcinoma were found to have bony metastases at presentation and have a median survival of 6.6 months; median survival was 19 months for other histologic types.[39]

The chance of survival improves if there is a long disease-free interval between initial nephrectomy and the appearance of metastases, if only pulmonary metastases are present, if there is a good performance status, and if the primary tumor has been removed.[23]

TABLE 48–5
1988 American Joint Committee Staging Classification for Renal Pelvis and Ureter Tumors

PRIMARY TUMOR (T)

TX	Primary tumor cannot be assessed
T0	No evidence of tumor
Tis	Carcinoma *in situ*
Ta	Papillary noninvasive carcinoma
T1	Tumor invades subepithelial connective tissue
T2	Tumor invades muscularis
T3	Tumor invades beyond muscularis into periureteric or peripelvic fat or renal parenchyma
T4	Tumor invades adjacent organs or through the kidney into perinephric fat

REGIONAL LYMPH NODES (N)

NX	Regional lymph nodes cannot be assessed
N0	No regional lymph node metastasis
N1	Metastasis in a single lymph node, ≤ 2 cm in greatest dimension
N2	Metastasis in a single lymph node, > 2 cm but < 5 cm in greatest dimension, or multiple lymph nodes, none > 5 cm in greatest dimension
N3	Metastasis in a lymph node > 5 cm in greatest dimension

DISTANT METASTASIS (M)

MX	Presence of distant metastasis cannot be assessed
M0	No distant metastasis
M1	Distant metastasis

STAGE GROUPING

Stage 0	Tis	N0	M0
	Ta	N0	M0
Stage I	T1	N0	M0
Stage II	T2	N0	M0
Stage III	T3	N0	M0
Stage IV	T4	N0	M0
	Any T	N1, N2, N3	M0
	Any T	Any N	M1

HISTOPATHOLOGIC GRADE

GX	Grade cannot be assessed
G1	Well differentiated
G2	Moderately well differentiated
G3–4	Poorly differentiated or undifferentiated

(Beahrs OH, Henson DE, Hutter RVP, Myers MH [eds]: Manual for Staging of Cancer, 3rd ed, p 205. Philadelphia, JB Lippincott, 1988)

Renal Pelvis and Ureter Carcinoma

Both stage and grade are important prognostic factors in carcinoma of the renal pelvis and ureter. Using the unified staging classification adopted by AJC and Union Interantionale Contre le Cancer (UICC), Huben and associates[18] reported that 54 patients with transitional cell carcinoma of the renal pelvis and ureter had a median survival of 91.1 months for low-stage tumors and 12.9 months for high-stage tumors. After patients

TABLE 48–6
Extent of Renal Cell Carcinoma and Survival

INVOLVEMENT	PATHOLOGIC EXTENT OF TUMOR	SURVIVAL RATE	
		5 YEARS (%)	10 YEARS (%)
Stage I—kidney only	Confined	65	56
Renal vein	Alone	66	49
	+ Vena cava	55	43
	+ Perinephric fat	50	33
	+ Regional nodes	0	0
Perinephric fat	Alone	47	20
Regional nodes	Alone	33	17
Direct extension to contiguous visceral structure		0	0

(Pritchett TR, Lieskovsky G, Skinner DG: Clinical manifestations and treatment of renal parenchymal tumors. In Skinner DG, Lieskovsky G [eds]: Diagnosis and Management of Genitourinary Tumors, pp 337–361. Philadelphia, WB Saunders, 1988)

were stratified according to tumor grade, the corresponding median survival was 66.8 months for low-grade tumors and 14.1 months for high-grade tumors. For patients who underwent conservative resection, 12 (50%) of 24 with multifocal tumors had recurrences in the remaining urothelium, but one (3%) of 34 patients with solitary lesions had a recurrence.[27]

GENERAL MANAGEMENT

Renal Cell Carcinoma

The standard treatment for patients with T1 and T2 renal cell carcinoma is radical nephrectomy, which consists of complete removal of the intact Gerota's fascia and its contents, including the kidney, adrenal, and perinephric fat. Regional lymphadenectomy is often performed at the time of radical nephrectomy, although its role in enhancing survival has yet to be demonstrated in a randomized study. Aggressive surgical approach is indicated for patients with venous extension and no evidence of distant metastasis, because their prognosis is similar to that of patients with early-stage disease. For patients with pathologic T1 and T2 disease without lymph node metastasis, radical nephrectomy is a curative procedure with a greater than 80% 5- and 10-year survival rate in some series.[40]

The role of preoperative radiation therapy before nephrectomy has yet to be defined. Based on radiobiologic principles, several theoretic advantages were enumerated by Rubin and co-workers.[38]

Tumor shrinkage and increased resectability have been reported in patients who received preoperative radiation therapy, but no survival benefit was found. Many patients had T1 or T2 tumors. Because this group of patients is least likely to benefit from preoperative radiation therapy, it is not surprising that no survival benefit was reported.

The potential benefit of postnephrectomy irradiation has not been demonstrated. Brady[7] suggested that postoperative irradiation should be considered in one or more of the following circumstances:

1. Residual tumor in the renal fossa
2. Tumor extension into the perinephric fat
3. Regional lymph node involvement that can be encompassed by a treatment portal of modest size
4. Renal vein tumor extension
5. Transection of tumor during the operative procedure
6. Spillage of tumor into the renal fossa during resection

Patients with primary renal cell carcinoma with pathologic evidence of invasion of Gerota's fascia or adjacent organs or with regional lymph nodes who have no known metastatic disease (*i.e.*, T3a, T3b, T4, or N1–3 disease) are candidates for adjuvant postoperative radiation therapy.

With the use of adjuvant irradiation, improved local control and increased resectability have been reported, but most investigators have used survival as the end point (Tables 48-7 and 48-8).[32,33,45] Moreover, the reported complication rate was unacceptably high.

The role of preoperative or postoperative irradiation is not yet defined and is best carried out under a protocol study. Definitive radiation treatment is indicated if the patient is not a candidate for surgical resection. The limitation for definitive radiation therapy for renal cell carcinoma is the inability to deliver high doses of radiation to the upper abdomen, in which most surrounding structures are dose limiting.

Chemotherapy for renal cell carcinoma, as adjuvant therapy with radical nephrectomy or as treatment for unresectable or metastatic disease, has not been shown to increase the survival rate over other treatment protocols.

For patients with metastatic renal cell carcinoma, adjuvant or palliative nephrectomy is performed to relieve pain, hemorrhage, hypercalcemia, or hypertension. It is not recommended for induction of spontaneous regression. The regression rate of metastatic foci of renal cell carcinoma after nephrectomy has been reported to be less than 1%.

Patients with a solitary bony metastasis are at risk of developing multiple metastases, but they also have a 30% to 40% chance of surviving 5 years.[21] In that regard, palliative high-dose radiation therapy should be delivered to metastatic bony lesions to ensure a long disease-free survival for these patients.

Hormonal therapy of metastatic renal cell carcinoma has resulted in an overall objective response of 6% to 33%; most responses were partial and short-lived and primarily affected pulmonary metastases.[6] There are some exciting developments in biologic therapy at the National Cancer Institute, such as adoptive cellular therapy with lymphokine-activated cells plus interleukin-2 in the management of patients with metastatic renal cell carcinoma.

TABLE 48–7
Five-Year Survival After Nephrectomy or Nephrectomy and Postoperative Irradiation for Renal Cell Carcinoma

INVESTIGATOR	STAGE	NO. OF PATIENTS	RADIATION DOSE/FRACTION SIZE (cGy)	TREATMENT*	5-YEAR SURVIVAL RATE	LOCAL RECURRENCE	COMMENTS
Peeling and associates[29] (1969)		96		N	52% (50/96)		1
		68		N + RT	25% (17/68)		
Rafla[32] (1970)	All	96		N	37% (35/94)	(25%)	2
		94		N + RT	57% (46/81)	(7%)	
	Renal vein ± others	36		N	30% (11/36)		
		40		N + RT	40% (14/35)		
	Renal pelvis ± others	50		N	32% (16/49)		
		60		N + RT	60% (30/50)		
	Renal capsule ± others	52		N	28% (15/52)		
		69		N + RT	57% (34/59)		
Rafla and Parikh[33] (1984)		135		N	18% (24/135)		3
		105	4500	N + RT	38% (40/105)		
Finney[13] (1973)		48		N	47% (17/35)	7	4
		52	5500/204	N + RT	36% (14/39)	7	
Kjaer and associates[22] (1987)	II, III	33		N	63%†	1	5
		32	5000/250	N + RT	38%†	0	

**N: nephrectomy; RT: postoperative radiation therapy.*
† Interpolated from graph; number at risk not known.
1. This is a retrospective study with incomplete staging information and no description of radiation dose or technique. Five-year survival was the endpoint, with no mention of the incidence of local recurrence.
2. This is the only report that described the beneficial effect of RT with survival and local recurrence as endpoints. There was no description of radiation dose or technique. The study was carried out before CT; therefore, local recurrence is underestimated. Subgroup analysis (involvement of renal vein, renal pelvis, renal capsule ± others) indicated an impact of RT on survival.
3. The authors also showed some data attesting to the beneficial effect of RT in patients with renal capsular, renal vein, and regional lymphatic involvement.
4. It is a randomized study, but with no staging information. The incidences of local recurrence and distant metastasis are similar. However, there were four fatal cases of liver complications among the patients who rceived RT.
5. In this randomized study, 27 of 32 patients assigned to the RT arm completed the treatment; 12 (44%) of 27 reported significant complications, with five fatal complications related to irradiation.

Renal Pelvis and Ureter Carcinoma

The management of renal pelvis or ureter carcinoma is nephroureterectomy with excision of a cuff of bladder and bladder mucosa. Less aggressive surgery, such as nephrectomy and partial ureterectomy, is accompanied by a 30% recurrence rate in the ureter stump. More conservative surgical excision has been advocated for patients with low-stage, low-grade, and solitary lesions.[27]

There are very few data on the role of adjuvant irradiation in the management of carcinoma of the renal pelvis and ureter. A retrospective review by Brookland and Richter[10] revealed decreased local failure after postoperative irradiation. Reports by Brady and associates[8] and Babaian and colleagues[1] suggested the beneficial effect of postoperative irradiation, although prospective trials are needed to demonstrate it.

Combination chemotherapy consisting of methotrexate, vinblastine, doxorubicin (Adriamycin), and cisplatin (MVAC) produced an objective response in more than 70% of patients with metastatic transitional cell carcinoma of bladder, ureter, and renal pelvis.[42] For a patient with a high-stage and high-grade tumor with periureteral, peripelvic, or perirenal extension or a patient with regional lymph node metastasis, MVAC combination chemotherapy and adjuvant irradiation offer the best chance of disease control. However, data for combined chemotherapy and radiation therapy in the primary management of cancer of the renal pelvis and ureter are not available. Less than 30% of patients with poor prognostic factors are cured by surgery alone, and about 45% of these patients develop distant metastases; it appears that combined postoperative chemotherapy and radiation therapy may offer the best chance for cure but should be carried out only under a protocol setting.

RADIATION THERAPY TECHNIQUES

Renal Cell Carcinoma

Radiation therapy has been employed in the management of primary renal cell carcinoma preoperatively, postoperatively, as definitive treatment for patients who are not surgical candidates, and for palliation of symptoms if the tumor is unresectable. Except for the total dose, the radiation therapy technique and the fractionation schedule are similar in most situations. The usual treatment volume includes the entire kidney (if the renal cell carcinoma is left in place), the renal fossa, and the para-aortic and paracaval lymph nodes. The kidneys are located in juxtaposition to the liver, small bowel, stomach, pancreas, and spinal cord, which are dose-limiting structures. For preoperative irradiation, a CT scan should be used to delineate tumor extent and for treatment planning. Before postoperative radiation therapy begins, a baseline CT scan should be obtained for later comparison.

The preoperative radiation doses reported in the literature range from 3000 cGy to 4800 cGy.[23,28] Postoperative radiation doses range from 4500 cGy to 6000 cGy.

The usual recommended dose that can be safely given to

TABLE 48–8
Five-Year Survival After Nephrectomy or Preoperative Irradiation and Nephrectomy for Renal Cell Carcinoma

INVESTIGATOR	STAGE	NO. OF PATIENTS	RADIATION DOSE/FRACTION SIZE (cGy)	TREATMENT*	5-YEAR SURVIVAL RATE	LOCAL RECURRENCE	COMMENTS
van der Werf-Messing[45] (1973)	I	21		N	88%	0	1
		22	3000/200	RT + N	85%	0	
	II	19		N	64%	1	
		12	3000/200	RT + N	62%	0	
	III	22		N	29%	3	
		30	3000/200	RT + N	27%	3	
van der Werf-Messing and associates[46] (1978)		85		N	No difference		2
		89	3000–4000/200	RT + N			
Juusela and associates[19] (1977)		50		N	63%		3
		38	3300/220	RT + N	47%		
Rubin and colleagues[38] (1975)	II			N	52%		4
			4500–4800/200	RT + N	68%		
	I			N	No difference		
			4500–4800/200	RT + N			

**N: nephrectomy; RT: preoperative radiation therapy.*
1. Five-year actuarial survival rates were interpolated from a graph. Higher survival during the first 18 months was noted for clinical Stage III patients who received RT. Seventy-three percent (22 of 30) complete resectability was reported for clinical Stage III patients who received RT, and a 50% rate (11 of 22) was found for those without RT. Thirty-four percent (43 of 126) had clinical Stage I tumors and probably would not have benefitted from RT.
2. The 126 patients reported in 1973 were apparently included in this study. The radiation dose had apparently been changed to 4000 cGy for patients treated after 1973. Five-year survival was about 50%, and "preoperative RT had no bearing on survival." There was no mention of the incidence of local recurrences.
3. Subgroup analysis by histologic grade and pathologic stage indicated no survival advantage for patients who received RT; however, there was no mention of local control or resectability.
4. Two-year survival rates were obtained by interpolation from a graph. One hundred fifty-five patients were randomized to receive RT; the number of nephrectomy patients was not specified. For only 101 of 155 patients were details of RT techniques provided; however, only 21 patients were adequately treated to the regional lymph nodes (>4000 cGy). Better survival (15% to 20% in the first 2 years) occurred among Stage II patients who received RT. No difference in survival was detected in Stage I patients. The exact number in each subgroup was not specified.

the upper abdomen with an acceptable complication rate is 5040 cGy in 180-cGy fractions over a period of 5 to 6 weeks. A boost of 540 cGy in three fractions to a smaller volume may be added to bring the total tumor dose to 5580 cGy. The remaining kidney should not receive doses above 1500 cGy. For a right-sided tumor, there may be a need for a field reduction at 3600 cGy to 4000 cGy to ensure that no more than 30% of the liver parenchyma is irradiated to a high dose. The nominal dose for the spinal cord should be limited to 4000 cGy. There is no attempt to include the entire surgical incision in the treatment field for patients who receive postnephrectomy radiation therapy unless there is specific knowledge of significant wound contamination by tumor spillage.

The patient is usually treated by a combination of parallel opposed anteroposterior/posteroanterior (AP/PA) plus oblique fields with 180-cGy fractions (Figs. 48-3 and 48-4). Rubin and colleagues[38] described several treatment plans, including a single posterior oblique field, equal-weighting parallel opposed AP/PA field, bias loading (*i.e.,* 3 : 1 or 2 : 1 posterior loading), and other rotating or wedge pair techniques. A shrinking-field technique should be employed to reduce exposure to dose-limiting adjacent structures. High-energy photons (10-MV photons or above) from linear accelerators should be used.

Renal Pelvis and Ureter Carcinoma

Postoperative radiation therapy has been used to treat renal pelvis and ureter carcinoma. The treatment portal usually includes the entire renal fossa, the entire ureteral bed, and the ipsilateral trigone. The extent of the portal is dictated by clinical information obtained at the time of surgery and from pathologic analysis of the resected specimen (Fig. 48-5). Because of the high incidence of lymph node involvement, the treatment portal should also include the para-aortic and paracaval areas. As in renal cell carcinoma of the kidney, the postoperative radiation dose is limited by the tolerance of the normal tissue in the treatment field; the dose is usually 5040 cGy given in 180-cGy fractions with a boost of an additional 540 cGy in three fractions to a total of 5580 cGy. Preoperative radiation doses of 2000 cGy in five fractions have been given.[44] Like those with renal cell carcinoma, patients should be treated with an isocentric setup with opposing AP/PA portals and 180-cGy fractions. High-energy photons from a linear accelerator should be used.

RESULTS OF THERAPY

Renal Cell Carcinoma

The role of adjuvant irradiation in conjunction with nephrectomy in the management of renal cell carcinoma is not yet defined. The most recent study comparing nephrectomy with nephrectomy and irradiation showed no benefit for patients who received postoperative radiation therapy.[22] The most comprehensive treatise on the role of adjuvant radiation therapy in the management of renal cell carcinoma has been compiled by Rafla and Parikh.[33] A summary of the selected recent series of

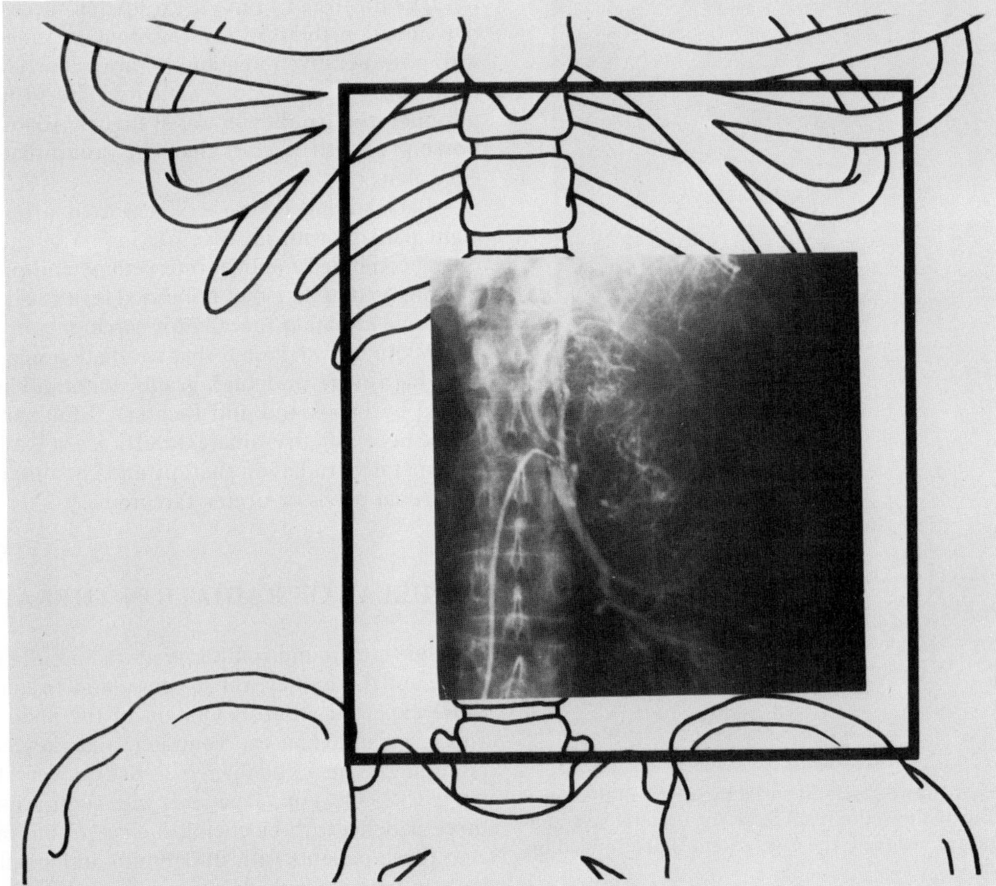

FIGURE 48–3. Radiation portal for large, left-sided renal cancer. The primary tumor and bilateral lymph nodes are included.

renal cell carcinoma patients who received postoperative radiation therapy is listed in Table 48-7.

The only study that reported a beneficial effect for postnephrectomy radiation therapy is that by Rafla.[32] However, it is not a randomized study, and the radiation doses and techniques were not specified. In a later publication, he mentioned a postoperative radiation dose of 4500 cGy.[33] Morbidity or complications from radiation therapy were not described. Two randomized studies, one by Finney[13] and the other by Kjaer and associates,[22] reported no beneficial effect of radiation therapy after radical nephrectomy. Both studies were plagued with high complication rates, possibly related to the radiation dose and the technique. There were four fatal liver complications in the Finney series[13] and five fatal complications in Kjaer's report.[22] The study by Peeling and colleagues[29] reported worse survival rates for patients who received postoperative irradiation.

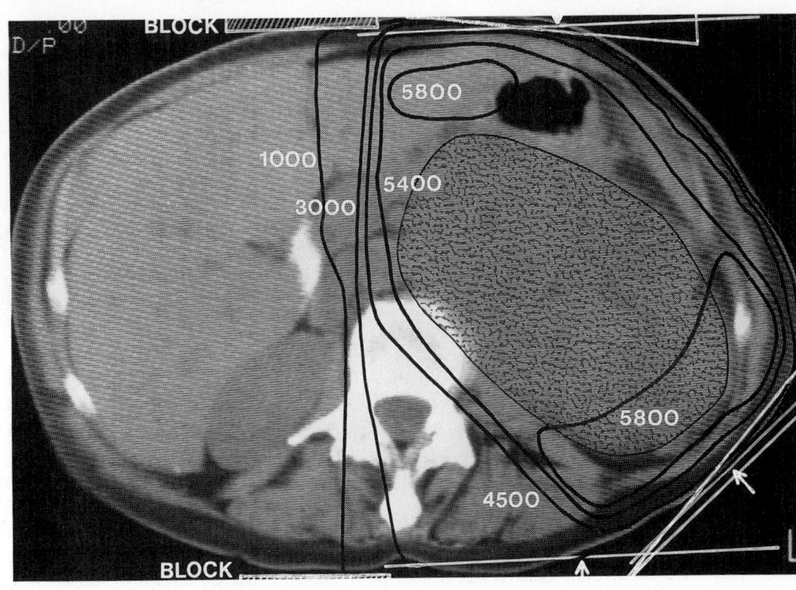

FIGURE 48–4. Radiation dose distribution corresponding to the treatment portal in Figure 48–3. Notice that a combination of AP/PA plus oblique portals with wedges is used to encompass the entire lesion with an isodose curve of 5400 cGy. Spinal cord dose is less than 4150 cGy.

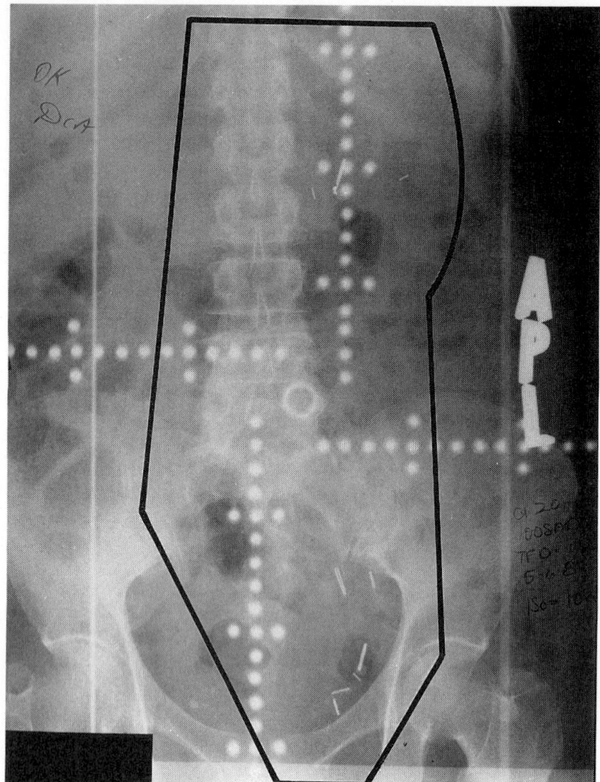

FIGURE 48–5. Postoperative radiation portal for cancer of the renal pelvis and ureter. Usually the entire renal fossa, the ureteral bed, and the ipsilateral trigone are included; the exact extent is determined by pathologic information.

The results of three randomized studies of preoperative radiation therapy before nephrectomy are summarized in Table 48-8. In the report by van der Werf-Messing,[45] there was increased resectability and better survival in the first 2 years for clinical Stage III patients who received preoperative irradiation. The report by Juusela and co-workers[19] reported no survival advantage for patients treated with preoperative radiation therapy. The study by Rubin and colleagues[38] demonstrated better 2-year survival for patients with Stage II renal cell carcinoma who received preoperative irradiation. No 5-year data were available.

Future studies should select those patients who could potentially benefit from adjuvant radiation therapy, especially those with advanced-stage, high-grade renal cell carcinoma. Patients with renal cell carcinoma tumors confined to the renal parenchyma do well with nephrectomy alone and should not be included in randomized studies.

Renal Pelvis and Ureter Carcinoma

Brookland and Richter[10] reported the retrospective analysis of patients with transitional cell carcinoma of the renal pelvis and ureter treated with surgery and postoperative radiation therapy. Eleven patients received postoperative radiation therapy (4000–6000 cGy, mean of 5000 cGy in 200-cGy fractions), all with poor prognostic factors: those with histologic grade of II or above; depth of invasion B or above (*i.e.*, parenchyma invasion); periureteral, peripelvic, or perirenal extension; or nodal or regional metastasis. The incidence of local recurrence was lower in the patients who received postoperative irradiation. One of nine patients had local failure as a component of failure; this was true for five of 11 in the group that received no postoperative radiation therapy. Overall, four of nine patients treated with postoperative radiation therapy recurred, compared with eight of 11 surgery-only patients. The group that received postoperative irradiation was at higher risk of recurrence with worse prognostic factors than the group that underwent surgery alone.

Babaian and co-workers[1] reported promising results for eight patients with invasive carcinoma of the ureter who received combined nephroureterectomy and postoperative irradiation. A compilation of published results of surgery and postoperative radiation therapy for carcinoma of ureter by Brady and Manning[9] suggested that irradiation may benefit patients with high-stage and high-grade tumors. Therefore, as suggested by Brookland and Richter,[10] multiinstitutional studies will be necessary to evaluate the efficacy of local preoperative or postoperative radiation therapy and chemotherapy in patients with renal pelvis or ureter carcinoma.

SEQUELAE OF RADIATION THERAPY

The side effects and complications from radiation treatment of cancer of the kidney, renal pelvis, and ureters are similar to those expected from irradiation of the abdomen and pelvis, which include nausea, vomiting, diarrhea, and abdominal cramping. The Copenhagen Renal Cancer Study Group reported 12 (44%) of 27 patients with significant complications: three patients with biochemical changes indicating liver damage; three patients with duodenum and small bowel stenosis, and six patients with duodenum and small bowel bleeding.[22] Surgery was performed on four of nine patients with bowel complications. Five patients died of treatment-related complications. The total radiation dose was 5000 cGy given in 250-cGy fractions, which may account for the high complication rates. Finney[13] also reported four cases of "liver failure" among the 52 patients who received postoperative radiation therapy.

The complication rate is related to the total dose and the fraction size, as well as the technique of irradiation. The complication rates reported by Kjaer[22] and Finney[13] should not be considered as the prevailing rates.

REFERENCES

1. Babaian RJ, Johnson DE, Chan RC: Combination nephroureterectomy and postoperative radiotherapy for infiltrative ureteral carcinoma. Int J Radiat Oncol Biol Phys 6:1229, 1980
2. Bassil B, Dosoretz DE, Prout GR Jr: Validation of the tumor, nodes and metastasis classification of renal cell carcinoma. J Urol 134:450, 1985
3. Beahrs OH, Henson JE, Hutter RVP, Myers MH (eds): Manual for Staging of Cancer, 3rd ed, p 199. Philadelphia, JB Lippincott, 1988
4. Beahrs OH, Henson JE, Hutter RVP, Myers MH (eds): Manual for Staging of Cancer, 3rd ed, p. 205. Philadelphia, JB Lippincott, 1988
5. Bellet RE, Squitieri AP: Estrogen-induced hypernephroma. J Urol 112:160, 1974
6. Bloom HJG: Hormone-induced and spontaneous regression of metastatic renal cancer. Cancer 32:1066, 1973
7. Brady LW: Carcinoma of the kidney: The role for radiation therapy. Semin Oncol 10:417, 1983
8. Brady LW, Gislason GJ, Faust DS, et al: Radiation therapy: A valuable adjunct in the management of carcinoma of the ureter. JAMA 206:2871, 1968
9. Brady LW, Manning DM: The role of radiation therapy in

primary carcinoma of the ureter. In Bergman H (ed): The Ureter, 2nd ed, p 417. New York, Springer-Verlag, 1981
10. Brookland RK, Richter MP: The postoperative irradiation of transitional cell carcinoma of the renal pelvis and ureter. J Urol 133:952, 1985
11. Christoferson LA, Gustafson MB, Petersen AG: Von Hippel-Lindau's disease. JAMA 178:126, 1961
12. Donaldson J, Slease R, DuFour R, et al: Metastatic renal cell carcinoma 24 years after nephrectomy. JAMA 236:950, 1976
13. Finney R: An evaluation of postoperative radiotherapy in hypernephroma treatment: A clinical trial. Cancer 32:1332, 1973
14. Flocks RH, Kadesky MC: Malignant neoplasms of the kidney: An analysis of 353 patients followed five years or more. J Urol 79:196, 1958
15. Golimbu M, Joshi P, Sperber A, et al: Renal cell carcinoma: Survival and prognostic factors. Urology 27:291, 1986
16. Grabstald H, Whitmore WF, Melamed MR: Renal pelvic tumors. JAMA 218:845, 1971
17. Harris DT: Hormonal therapy and chemotherapy of renal-cell carcinoma. Semin Oncol 10:422, 1983
18. Huben RP, Mounszer AM, Murphy GP: Tumor grade and stage as prognostic variables in upper tract urothelial tumors. Cancer 62:2016, 1988
19. Juusela H, Malmio K, Alfthan O, et al: Preoperative irradiation in the treatment of renal adenocarcinoma. Scand J Urol Nephrol 11:277, 1977
20. King CR, Schimke RN, Arthur T, et al: Proximal 3p deletion in renal cell carcinoma cells from a patient with von Hippel-Lindau disease. Cancer Genet Cytogenet 7:345, 1987
21. Kjaer M: The treatment and prognosis of patients with renal adenocarcinoma with solitary metastasis 10 year survival results. Int J Radiat Oncol Biol Phys 13:619, 1987
22. Kjaer M, Frederiksen PL, Engelholm SA: Postoperative radiotherapy in stage II and III renal adenocarcinoma. A randomized trial by the Copenhagen Renal Cancer Study Group. Int J Radiat Oncol Biol Phys 13:665, 1987
23. Linehan WM, Shipley WU, Longo DL: Cancer of the kidney and ureter. In DeVita VT, Hellman S, Rosenberg SA (eds): Cancer: Principles and Practice of Oncology, 3rd ed, p 979. Philadelphia, JB Lippincott, 1989
24. Maldazys JD, deKernion JB: Prognostic factors in metastatic renal carcinoma. J Urol 136:376, 1986
25. Mcclennan BL, Rabin, DN: Kidney. In Lee JKT, Sagel SS, Stanley RJ (eds): Computed Body Tomography with MRI Correlation, 2nd ed. New York, Raven Press, 1988
26. Montie JE, Stewart BH, Stroffon RA, et al: The role of adjunctive nephrectomy in patients with metastatic renal cell carcinoma. J Urol 117:272, 1977
27. Mufti GR, Gove JRW, Badenoch DF, et al: Transitional cell carcinoma of the renal pelvis and ureter. Br J Urol 63:135, 1989
28. Pearse HD: The kidney. In Moss WT, Cox JD (eds): Radiation Oncology: Rationale, Technique, Results, p 416. St. Louis, CV Mosby, 1989
29. Peeling WB, Mantell BS, Shepheard BGF: Postoperative irradiation in the treatment of renal cell carcinoma. Br J Urol 41:23, 1969
30. Petkovic SD: Epidemiology and treatment of renal pelvic and ureteral tumors. J Urol 114:858, 1975
31. Pritchett TR, Lieskovsky G, Skinner DG: Clinical manifestations and treatment of renal parenchymal tumors. In Skinner DG, Lieskovsky G (eds): Diagnosis and Management of Genitourinary Tumors, pp 337–361. Philadelphia, WB Saunders, 1988
32. Rafla S: Renal cell carcinoma. Cancer 25:26, 1970
33. Rafla S, Parikh K: The role of adjuvant radiotherapy in management of renal cell carcinoma. In Javadpour N (ed): Cancer of the Kidney, p 93. New York, Thieme-Stratton, 1984
34. Reitelman C, Sawczuk IS, Olsson CA, et al: Prognostic variables in patients with transitional cell carcinoma of the renal pelvis and proximal ureter. J Urol 138:1144, 1987
35. Richie JP: Carcinoma of the renal pelvis and ureter. In Skinner DG, Lieskovsky G (eds): Diagnosis and Management of Genitourinary Tumors, p 323. Philadelphia, WB Saunders, 1988
36. Riches EW: The natural history of renal tumors. In Tumors of the Kidney and Ureter, p 124. Edinburgh, Livingstone, 1964
37. Robson CJ, Churchill BM, Anderson W: The results of radical nephrectomy for renal cell carcinoma. J Urol 101:297, 1969
38. Rubin P, Keller BO, Cox C, et al: Preoperative irradiation in renal carcinoma: Evaluation of radiation treatment plans. Cancer 123:114, 1975
39. Sella A, Logothetis CJ, Ro JY, et al: Sarcomatoid renal cell carcinoma. Cancer 60:1313, 1987
40. Shipley WU: Genitourinary cancer. In Wang CC (ed): Clinical Radiation Oncology: Indications, Techniques, and Results, p 262. Littleton, MA, PSG, 1988
41. Silverberg E, Boring CC, Squires TS: Cancer statistics 1990. CA 40:9, 1990
42. Sternberg CN, Yagoda A, Scher HI, et al: Preliminary results of M-VAC (methotrexate, vinblastine, doxorubicin and cisplatin) for transitional cell carcinoma of the urothelium. J Urol 133:403, 1985
43. Tolia BM, Whitmore WF: Solitary metastasis from renal cell carcinoma. J Urol 114:836, 1975
44. Walz BJ: Carcinoma of the kidney, renal pelvis, and ureter. In Perez, CA, Brady LW (eds): Principles and Practice of Radiation Oncology, p 838. Philadelphia, JB Lippincott, 1987
45. Werf-Messing B van der: Carcinoma of the kidney. Cancer 32:1056, 1973
46. Werf-Messing B van der, Heul RO van der, Ledeboer RCH: Renal cell carcinoma trial. Cancer Clin Trials 1:13, 1978

49

○ ○ ○ • • •

Bladder

James T. Parsons
Rodney R. Million

In many centers in the United States, the role of radiation therapy for bladder cancer has diminished over the past decade. This chapter, in addition to providing an overview of bladder cancer and its treatment, outlines the situations in which radiation therapy may benefit these patients. In particular, the roles of radiation therapy in bladder preservation or as an adjunct to surgery are discussed.

TOPOGRAPHIC ANATOMY

The urinary bladder is a hollow, thick-walled, muscular organ that, if empty, lies entirely within the true pelvis. The empty bladder is roughly tetrahedral; each of its four surfaces is shaped like an equilateral triangle, with each side approximately 3 inches long.

The triangular superior surface, the only surface covered with peritoneum, has its base behind and apex in front. The apex of the bladder is directed toward the upper part of the pubic symphysis and is joined to the umbilicus by the median umbilical ligament, the urachal remnant. The sigmoid colon and coils of the small intestine rest on the superior surface; in the female, the body of the uterus overhangs this surface.

The paired inferolateral surfaces are separated from the pelvic side walls by loose areolar tissue (*i.e.*, the retropubic space) anteriorly and by the internal obturator muscles posteriorly.

The posterior surface, called the base of the bladder, faces downward and backward. In the female, the bladder base is closely related to the anterior wall of the vagina. In the male, the upper part of the bladder base is separated from the rectum by the rectovesical pouch; the lower part of the base is separated from the rectum by the seminal vesicles and the deferent duct. In the interval between the ducts, only the rectovesical fascia intervenes between the two organs.

As the bladder fills, its corners become rounded and its shape ovoid. The parietal peritoneum of the suprapubic region of the abdominal wall is displaced so that the bladder lies directly against the anterior abdominal wall without any intervening peritoneum. Therefore, the full bladder may be surgically approached through the anterior abdominal wall without traversing the peritoneum.

The ureters pierce the wall of the bladder base obliquely. The orifices of the ureters are posterolateral to the internal urethral orifice and, with the urethral orifice, define a triangle (the trigone), the sides of which are approximately 2.5 cm long in the contracted state and up to 5.0 cm in the distended state. Between the slit-like ureteral orifices is a slightly curved ridge, the interureteric crest, which appears on cystoscopic examination as a pale band and is an important landmark for locating the orifices. The internal urethral orifice pierces the bladder neck, the lowest and most fixed part of the bladder. In the male, the bladder neck rests on the prostate; in the female, it is related to the pelvic fascia surrounding the upper urethra. The internal urethral sphincter controls the neck of the bladder in males and females and is not under voluntary control.

The mucous membrane of the bladder is pale pink. It is continuous with the mucosal linings of the ureters above and the urethra below. The epithelium ("urothelium") is a transitional variety. With the bladder collapsed, the epithelium is five to seven cell layers thick; in the distended state, it is two to three layers thick. The mucous membrane is only loosely attached to the subjacent (detrusor) muscle layer by a delicate vascular submucosa (lamina propria), except over the trigone, where the mucosa is firmly attached.

EPIDEMIOLOGY AND RISK FACTORS

There are approximately 50,000 new cases of bladder carcinoma and approximately 10,000 deaths in the United States each year. The incidence peaks in the seventh decade; less than 1% of bladder cancer occurs in patients younger than 40 years old. The male-to-female ratio in most Western countries is approximately 2 : 1 or 3 : 1. In men, it is the fourth most prevalent malignant disease.[182]

Bladder cancer has a higher incidence in industrialized nations than in underdeveloped countries and is more prevalent in urban than in rural areas.[35] Although a number of occupations, including the dye, rubber, leather, paint, organic chemical, textile, printing, and electrical cable industries, have been linked to the development of bladder cancer, occupational exposure probably accounts for a relatively small portion of the total cases.[92] The usual latent interval is 15 to 25 years.

Case-control studies have consistently demonstrated a twofold to threefold increase in bladder cancer among cigarette smokers compared with nonsmokers.[35,92]

Patients whose bladders are chronically irritated by long-term catheter drainage (such as paraplegics)[100] or bladder calculi are at risk of developing squamous cell carcinoma. Chronic infection with *Schistosoma haematobium* may produce epithelial hyperplasia, dysplasia, squamous metaplasia, and eventually squamous cell carcinoma. Adenocarcinoma may occur in patients with exstrophy of the bladder.

Attempts to associate consumption of coffee and nonnutritive sweeteners with bladder cancer have been unsuccessful.[164] The consumption of large amounts of phenacetin-containing analgesics has been associated with the development of transitional-cell carcinoma of the renal pelvis and bladder, with a latency period of approximately 15 to 20 years.[62, 159] The antineoplastic agents chlornaphazin[164] and cyclophosphamide[144] may also lead to bladder cancer.

TABLE 49–1
Incidence of Histologically Positive Lymph Nodes According to Pathologic Stage

PATHOLOGIC STAGE	NUMBER OF PATIENTS	PERCENTAGE OF PATIENTS WITH POSITIVE LYMPH NODES
pT1	41	5
pT2	20	30
pT3a	13	31
pT3b	28	64
pT4	8	50

(Modified from Skinner DG, Tift JP, Kaufman JJ: J Urol 127:671, 1982)

NATURAL HISTORY

Approximately 75% to 85% of new bladder cancers are superficial (Tis, Ta, or T1). Lutzeyer and co-workers[109] reported that 75% of patients with newly diagnosed Ta and T1 lesions had single tumors, and 25% had multifocal disease at the time of presentation. Fitzpatrick and colleagues[61] found that 84% of newly diagnosed Ta (grade 1 or 2) lesions were solitary at initial diagnosis. Three hundred thirty-five (73%) of 457 patients with newly diagnosed Ta or T1 bladder cancers in the British Medical Research Council study on mitomycin C were solitary at the time of first presentation.[212] In the Medical Research Council study of thiotepa, 214 (70%) of 305 patients with Ta or T1 disease had solitary lesions at diagnosis (MKB Parmar, written communication, 1990). Heney and associates[75] found that 36 (62%) of 58 patients presenting for the first time with Ta or T1 bladder cancers at the Massachusetts General Hospital between 1973 and 1977 had single tumors.

Approximately 15% to 25% of new bladder cancers have evidence of muscle invasion at the time of diagnosis. In addition, a number of other patients with superficial disease develop muscle invasion if their tumors recur after conservative therapy. Considering all patients with muscle-invasive bladder cancer, approximately 60% had evidence of muscle invasion at the time of initial diagnosis, and the remaining 40% initially presented with more superficial disease that later progressed.[41]

The most common sites of disease are the trigone, the lateral and posterior walls, and the bladder neck. Bladder cancer spreads by direct extension into or through the wall of the bladder. In a few cases, the tumor spreads submucosally under an intact, normal-appearing mucosa.[131] Papillary tumors tend to remain superficial, but solid lesions are usually deeply invasive. Perineural invasion and lymphatic or blood vessel invasion are common after tumor has invaded muscle. Carcinoma *in situ* is commonly seen in adjacent mucosa. Noncontiguous areas of carcinoma *in situ* or superficial disease are also frequent.[114, 197] If there is multifocal or diffuse carcinoma *in situ,* intraepithelial involvement of the distal ureters, prostatic urethra, and periurethral prostatic ducts is also common.[114] The multifocality of bladder cancer probably accounts for many recurrences after transurethral resection.

Lymphatic drainage is by the external and internal iliac and the presacral lymph nodes. Skinner and co-workers[188] compared the incidence of pelvic lymph node metastases to depth of tumor invasion in the bladder wall (Table 49-1).

The most common sites of distant metastases are lung, bone, and liver.

CLINICAL PRESENTATION

Between 75% and 80% of the patients with bladder cancer have gross, painless, total (throughout urination) hematuria. Clot retention may occur. Approximately 25% of all patients have symptoms of vesical irritability. Twenty percent have no specific symptoms; their cancers are detected by microscopic hematuria, pyuria, or other means.[92] Hematuria is sometimes intermittent, occurring for a day or two, and then subsiding for a period of weeks or months. The degree of hematuria bears no relationship to the size and invasiveness of the tumor.

At least 90% of patients with carcinoma *in situ* have frequency, urgency, dysuria, and hematuria, suggesting irritative bladder disease. Because of similarities in symptoms and cystoscopic appearance, interstitial cystitis may be diagnosed. In a review of 486 patients treated for interstitial cystitis at the Mayo Clinic, carcinoma *in situ* was ultimately identified in 23% of the men and 1% of the women.[215] The most accurate test for diagnosis is exfoliative urinary cytology. On cystoscopic examination, carcinoma *in situ* usually appears as a slightly raised, cobblestone lesion that has no discrete boundaries; if the bladder is too greatly distended during cystoscopy, the lesion may be missed.

Simultaneous presentations of carcinoma of the bladder and adenocarcinoma of the prostate are not rare. These cases call for highly individualized treatment because a variety of combinations of clinical stages and presentations are possible.

DIAGNOSTIC WORKUP

Each patient should have a chest roentgenogram, urinalysis, a complete blood cell count, liver function tests, a complete cystoscopic evaluation, and bimanual examination under anesthesia both before and after endoscopic surgery (*i.e.,* biopsy or transurethral resection). An intravenous urogram should be obtained before cystoscopy so that the upper tracts may be evaluated by retrograde pyelogram, cytology, brush biopsy, or ureteroscopy at the time of cystoscopy, if indicated. Second lesions in the upper tracts are not uncommon. The number, size, and configuration of all tumors should be recorded and diagrammed. Biopsy of the mucosa of selected clinically uninvolved sites in patients with superficial disease may reveal atypia or carcinoma *in situ,* the presence of which portends an increased rate of recurrence.[190] Biopsies of the prostatic urethral mucosa and submucosa should be performed if these areas look suspicious or if diffuse carcinoma *in situ* is found.

TABLE 49–2
Comparison of Marshall and AJCC Staging Systems for Bladder Cancer

TUMOR EXTENT	MARSHALL MODIFICATION OF JEWETT-STRONG CLASSIFICATION[115]	AJCC CLASSIFICATION[12]
Confined to mucosa	O	
Nonpapillary, noninvasive		Tis
Papillary, noninvasive		Ta
Not beyond lamina propria (no mass palpable after complete TUR)	A	T1
Invasion of superficial muscle (no induration after complete TUR)	B1	T2
Invasion of deep muscle (induration after complete TUR)	B2	T3a
Invasion into perivesical fat (mobile mass after TUR)	C	T3b
Invasion of neighboring structures; muscle invasion present		
Substance of prostate, vagina, uterus	D1*	T4a
Pelvic sidewall fixation or invading abdominal wall	D1*	T4b

**In the Marshall modification of the Jewett-Strong staging system, D1 disease may involve lymph nodes below the sacral promontary (bifurcation of the common iliac artery). D2 implies distant metastases or more extensive lymph node metastases.*

Cystograms provide little precise information. Computed tomography (CT) is widely used to help detect bladder-wall thickening, extravesical extension, and lymph node metastases. We find it useful in initial evaluation and follow-up. After transurethral resection (TUR) of the bladder tumor, CT findings that suggest extravesical extension may be caused by hemorrhage and edema; therefore the results must be interpreted with caution. Bone scans are obtained for patients with T3 or T4 disease and those with bone pain. Magnetic resonance imaging (MRI) allows images to be obtained in coronal or sagittal projections, which are sometimes useful in defining tumor extent.

STAGING SYSTEMS

Two clinical staging systems, the Marshall modification of the Jewett-Strong system and the TNM system of the American Joint Committee on Cancer (AJCC), are widely used in the United States and abroad (Table 49-2).[12,115] Both systems combine histologic findings from TUR specimens and clinical findings from bimanual examination under anesthesia.

Pathologic staging is based on the histologic findings from cystectomy specimens; in the AJCC system, the stages are preceded by the prefix p (*e.g.,* pT3).

The TNM system has a separate staging system for nodal and distant metastases (Table 49-3). A shortcoming of the Marshall system is its failure to divide stage 0 into papillary and nonpapillary morphologies, because the two disease processes have strikingly different natural histories and clinical courses.

It is generally not possible for the pathologist examining TUR specimens to determine if tumor is confined to superficial muscle layers or has invaded the deep muscle.[231] Muscle invasion merely implies that the lesion is Stage B1, B2, C, D1, or D2 (T2–T4b). Although bimanual examination under anesthesia and radiography are helpful in further separating the various stages, understaging remains a common problem. Approximately 40% to 50% of patients with clinical Stage B2 or C disease are found to have Stage D cancer when cystectomy is undertaken, and 25% of patients with pathologic Stage B2 or C disease determined by the cystectomy specimen had clinical Stage B1 or lower.[141] The problem of overstaging is infrequently encountered.

Additional clues that suggest the possibility of an advanced-stage cancer are poor differentiation, because high grade is strongly correlated with high stage; a solid, sessile pattern of growth; and ureteral obstruction, which usually indicates at least T3 disease.[19]

All reports of treatment results should clearly state whether patients were staged by clinical (*i.e.,* pretreatment TUR, examination under anesthesia, radiography) or pathologic (*i.e.,* post-cystectomy) criteria.[87] The latter should be designated pTNM.

Mucosal extension to the prostatic urethra or periurethral

TABLE 49–3
AJCC Staging System for Nodal Involvement and Distant Metastases in Bladder Cancer

NODAL INVOLVEMENT (N)

NX	Minimum requirements to assess the regional nodes cannot be met
N0	No involvement of regional lymph nodes
N1	Involvement of a single homolateral regional lymph node
N2	Involvement of contralateral, bilateral, or multiple regional lymph nodes
N3	A fixed mass on the pelvic wall with a free space between it and the tumor

DISTANT METASTASIS (M)

MX	Minimum requirements to assess the presence of distant metastasis cannot be met
M0	No known distant metastasis
M1	Distant metastasis present

(Beahrs OH, Myers MH [eds]: American Joint Committee on Cancer: Manual for Staging of Cancer, 2nd ed. Philadelphia, JB Lippincott, 1983)

ducts is common in superficial bladder tumors. These tumors should be staged according to the tumor in the bladder, rather than as T4a. The T4a designation should be reserved for tumors that invade the substance of adjacent organs (*e.g.*, prostatic stroma invasion).

In many reports of treatment results, bladder cancers are categorized into two broad groupings. Carcinoma *in situ*, Ta, and T1 lesions are often referred to as "superficial" cancers, but those that invade the muscle or beyond (T2–T4) are regarded as "invasive" or "muscle-invasive" disease.

PATHOLOGIC CLASSIFICATION

Approximately 98% of bladder cancers are epithelial in origin. In the Western hemisphere, approximately 92% of epithelial tumors are transitional cell carcinomas, 6% to 7% are squamous cell carcinomas, and 1% to 2% are adenocarcinomas. Squamous or glandular differentiation can be seen in as many as 20% to 30% of transitional cell carcinomas; from a practical standpoint, the biologic behavior of these tumors does not differ significantly from that of pure transitional tumors.[92] Sarcomas, pheochromocytomas, lymphomas, and carcinoid tumors account for most of the remaining 2%; because of their rarity, they are not discussed here.

Morphologically, bladder cancers can be separated into four categories: papillary; papillary infiltrating; solid infiltrating; and nonpapillary, noninfiltrating, or carcinoma *in situ*.[132] At diagnosis, 70% are papillary; 25% show papillary or solid infiltration, and 3% to 5% are carcinoma *in situ*. Papillary cancers are usually low grade, have "pushing" borders, do not generally invade muscle, and have a relatively favorable prognosis.[197] Infiltrating lesions tend to be higher grade and are sessile, nodular, and bulky. Frequently, they invade into and beyond muscle in strands, nests, and individual cells infiltrating between normal structures. They invade blood and lymphatic spaces and generally have a worse prognosis. Carcinoma *in situ* may occur in association with invasive cancer, or it may occur *de novo*. When focally present, carcinoma *in situ* is most often seen in the area of the trigone and the ureteral orifices. More often, carcinoma *in situ* is a diffuse process, involving half or more of the bladder mucosa.[132]

When the degree of anaplasia is evaluated, a three-grade system is preferred (*i.e.*, grades 1, 2, and 3). There is a strong correlation between grade and depth of invasion.

Nonbilharzial squamous cell carcinomas are typically bulky, with ulceration and necrosis; all grades are seen. Men and women develop squamous cell carcinomas with almost equal frequency.[36,58,96] Most cancers are solitary, and almost all show evidence of muscle invasion at diagnosis.[96,166] Bladder cancers in areas where bilharziasis is endemic are usually squamous (70%) and generally well differentiated. Although they are usually locally advanced, they have a relatively low incidence of metastasis.[31]

Most primary vesical adenocarcinomas arise in the trigone or the posterior wall and are usually sessile, solid-appearing masses.[94,132] Adenocarcinomas that arise from urachal remnants are confined to the dome and anterior wall, are principally intramural with secondary involvement of mucosa, and often extend into the anterior abdominal wall. They frequently contain calcification that is visible on CT.[26,134] "Signet-ring cell" carcinoma of the bladder is a rare variant of mucus-producing adenocarcinoma that usually behaves aggressively.[23,42,84] Direct secondary invasion of the bladder by colorectal or cervical carcinoma also is possible.[230]

Small cell invasive carcinoma of the bladder is a rare, recently described variant that resembles oat cell carcinoma of the lung. Most patients are elderly men.[123] The clinical course is usually aggressive.[39,86,207] Many of the lesions have associated carcinoma *in situ*, invasive transitional cell carcinoma, adenocarcinoma, or squamous cell carcinoma.[123]

PROGNOSTIC FACTORS

Factors of prognostic importance include depth of tumor invasion (stage) and grade. The presence of blood vessel or lymphatic vessel invasion is significant, even in the absence of positive lymph nodes and even if the tumor is still confined to the lamina propria.[13,76,91,120,145] Other indicators of a poor prognosis include carcinoma *in situ*, solid tumor morphology, large tumor size, multiplicity of tumors, the presence of histologically positive lymph nodes, and obstructive uropathy.[180,235]

GENERAL MANAGEMENT

Transurethral Resection and Fulguration

Ta and T1 tumors are usually treated by transurethral resection and fulguration, with or without intravesical chemotherapy or Calmette-Guérin bacillus (BCG). Patients with diffuse grade 3, T1 disease or involvement of the prostatic urethra or ducts are difficult to treat by local means and are sometimes treated by cystectomy at the outset.[194] Transurethral resection may be done under general or spinal anesthesia. The tumor or tumors are first described (size, location, configuration) by means of cystoscopy, and a "bladder map" is made to help ensure that all tumors have been removed at the completion of the procedure, when the ability to visualize tumors is diminished. Biopsies are performed of the tumor, the adjacent mucosa, any suspicious-appearing mucosa (especially red velvety areas that may represent carcinoma *in situ*), and several areas of normal-appearing mucosa; rigid cup biopsy forceps are used. The cystoscope is removed, and the resectoscope is inserted. After the tumor has been resected to apparently uninvolved muscle fibers, all of the tumor fragments are evacuated from the bladder and are sent as the surgical specimen for pathologic evaluation. The base of the tumor and its margins are then fulgurated.

Intravesical chemotherapy is often administered after TUR for Ta (grade 2 or 3) lesions, T1 lesions, or lesions associated with carcinoma *in situ*. Most physicians withhold intravesical treatment for patients with grade 1, Ta tumors.[194] Intravesical therapy decreases the likelihood of bladder tumor recurrence and may eradicate residual disease after incomplete resection; by itself, however, it has no role in managing prostatic urethral or periurethral ductal disease.[195] Some of the most commonly used agents are thiotepa, mitomycin, doxorubicin, and BCG. The patients receive close follow-up by cystoscopy, cytology, and resection, as indicated. Failure to completely eradicate high-grade disease, progression to muscle invasion, or involvement of the prostatic urethra or prostatic periurethral ducts usually signals the need for radical cystectomy.

For carcinoma *in situ*, prompt radical cystectomy is usually curative;[215] however, most patients and urologists prefer initial attempts at more conservative management. For lesions that are smaller than 5 cm, reasonably well delineated, and without involvement of the bladder neck, prostatic urethra, or ureters, treatment consists of fulguration followed by intravesical chemotherapy or BCG; TUR alone is not advised.[148] If disease is multifocal or diffuse, intravesical BCG is usually administered, because it is considered more effective than other intravesical agents.[71] If treatment fails or if the prostatic urethra, prostatic ducts, or ureters are involved, radical cystectomy, urethrectomy, and resection of the distal 6 cm to 8 cm of the ureters are usually performed.

Bretton and colleagues[25] reported 23 patients with carcinoma *in situ* involving the prostatic urethra (19) or ducts (four) whose treatment consisted of TUR of all visible tumor and intravesical BCG; 13 remained free of recurrence at 6 to 105 months (median, 44 months). More patients, with longer follow-up periods, should be observed before this approach can be recommended with confidence, especially for patients with ductal involvement.

Definitive treatment by TUR is not applicable to most patients with muscle-invasive disease,[92] but it has been used in some carefully selected patients with small, papillary, well-differentiated T2 lesions.[244]

Partial Cystectomy

Carefully chosen patients with muscle-invasive disease or superficial disease not suitable for TUR may be treated by segmental resection (partial cystectomy). The procedure is done by an extraperitoneal approach. A cystotomy is made away from the area of the tumor, to avoid cutting across cancer, and the tumor is excised with a full thickness of the bladder wall and at least a 2-cm margin around the tumor.[16]

Eligible patients should have solitary, well-defined lesions with no prior history of vesical malignancy and no evidence of *in situ* disease or atypia elsewhere in the bladder on random cold-cup biopsies. The lesion should allow a wide excision, should be located in a mobile portion of the bladder (*i.e.*, walls or dome rather than trigone, neck, or base), and should be situated so that ureteral reimplantation is not necessary; after resection, functional bladder capacity should remain. Some physicians also consider low-grade tumors more suitable than high-grade lesions.[208]

The strict criteria limit the applicability of the procedure to 3% to 7% of patients, usually those with clinical B1 lesions.[16,21,136,138,214] Patients with cancers arising in vesical diverticula and those with urachal adenocarcinomas are particularly well suited.[245] Failure to observe the narrow indications for the procedure leads to local recurrence in 50% to 75% of B1 lesions and higher rates in B2 and C disease.[40,56,59,117,136,161,173,216] A large proportion of the recurrences are both higher stage (49%) and higher grade (40%) than the original lesion.[59] Many of the patients who are disease-free 5 years after partial cystectomy owe their survival to salvage treatment with total cystectomy, irradiation, or transurethral resection; in the Stanford series, radical cystectomy was the most successful salvage treatment.[59]

Circumferential submucosal tumor extensions in the muscle planes and lymphatic vessels within the muscularis deep to adjacent normal mucosa (as described in whole-organ sections 35 years ago)[7] and the fact that most recurrences develop at the margins of resection justify the use of preoperative irradiation or an interstitial implant adjacent to the bladder suture line at the time of segmental resection.[7,119,138,186,244] Bladder capacity is not adversely affected by preoperative irradiation.[138,185]

Radical Cystectomy

Radical cystectomy with or without preoperative irradiation differs from simple cystectomy in that the plane of dissection is the muscular pelvic wall rather than the bladder wall. The radical operation removes the bladder, the distal 1 cm to 2 cm of ureter, the perivesical fat, and the peritoneum covering the bladder. In men, the prostate, seminal vesicles, proximal vas deferens, and 1 cm to 2 cm of proximal urethra are removed; many urologists electively perform a total urethrectomy if the bladder tumor is multifocal, if it involves the bladder neck or prostatic urethra, or if there is diffuse carcinoma *in situ* because the risk or subsequent urethral involvement in this group exceeds 10%.[57,169] In women, the uterus, fallopian tubes, ovaries, anterior vaginal wall, and urethra are included.

Radical cystectomy may or may not include a formal pelvic lymphadenectomy. In patients who have undergone preoperative irradiation with 4500 cGy to 5000 cGy, lymphadenopathy is usually not performed. If no preoperative irradiation or only low-dose (*e.g.*, 2000 cGy) preoperative irradiation has been given, lymphadenectomy is generally performed for patients with muscle-invasive disease.

Until recently, cystectomy implied incontinent cutaneous diversion, usually by an ileal conduit with an external appliance and no reservoir capacity, for most patients. Two classes of continent diversions that require no external appliance have come into use. In the first type, the patient has an abdominal stoma, but unlike the ileal conduit, the stoma is "continent," requiring self-catheterization every 4 to 6 hours (continent cutaneous diversion). The most popular of the continent stomal reservoirs is the Kock pouch.[104] There are two valves, one for continence and one to prevent reflux. A small pad is worn over the stoma to prevent soiling from mucus. Reoperation, usually because of efferent valve malfunction, is necessary in 20% to 25% of patients.[104] In the second procedure, the reservoir is anastomosed directly to the male urethra (urethral continent diversion or functional diversion); the patient voids every 4 to 6 hours and rarely requires catheterization. There is only one valve, which prevents reflux. The continence mechanism is the external urinary sphincter, and voiding is accomplished by abdominal straining.[103] When the external sphincter relaxes during sleep, enuresis may occur, but patients who are carefully chosen usually achieve daytime and nighttime continence.[103]

The ileoanal reservoir, in which the Kock pouch is anastomosed to the sigmoid colon, is an alternative to urethral diversion in women, because the urethra is removed.[102] Most of the surgical techniques modify the bowel, often by opening it longitudinally and then folding and suturing it back on itself, to counteract the effects of directional peristalsis, which can produce high-pressure waves that can overcome the resistance of the external sphincter.[104,187] Because villous atrophy occurs in the reservoir, metabolic disturbances caused by shifts of solutes and water are rare.

Ahlering and associates[2] have shown that the Kock pouch urinary diversion can be safely performed at the time of salvage cystectomy after failure of high-dose (≥6000 cGy) irradiation. When previously irradiated patients were compared with a control group of patients, the operating time, estimated blood loss, length of hospitalization, and percentage of patients with urinary leaks did not differ significantly. The incidence of diarrhea was significantly greater in the irradiated patients but required medication for only 1 to 3 months in the typical patient.[2] Although specific information has not been published, it seems logical that if the Kock pouch is feasible after high-dose irradiation, it should be feasible after planned preoperative irradiation to lesser doses.

In 1982, Walsh and Donker[229] demonstrated that impotence after radical prostatectomy or radical cystectomy arises from injury to the pelvic plexus, which provides autonomic innervation to the corpora cavernosa. Because the bulk of the pelvic plexus and its branches are located lateral and posterior to the seminal vesicles, the vesicles may be used as a landmark to avoid injury to the cavernous branches. Schlagel and Walsh[172] noted that potency was preserved in 67% of patients who underwent this type of dissection; the rate of potency preservation was not adversely affected by 4000 cGy administered preoperatively. How the procedure may apply to patients with perivesical extension remains to be defined, because it leaves behind tissues that may be involved by cancer.[147]

Radical cystectomy (without preoperative irradiation) is recommended for superficial disease (Tis, Ta, T1) in which all attempts at conservative management have proven unsuccessful. This includes patients whose recurrences after each successive TUR or intravesical chemotherapy are increasing in frequency or grade or have progressed to muscle invasion. Cystectomy is also indicated for patients with recurrent tumors in whom bladder capacity has been so reduced by repeated TURs and intravesical chemotherapy that successful eradication of the tumor by the conservative means of repeat fulguration or irradiation would produce unsatisfactory functional results.

For clinical Stage T2 disease, radical cystectomy with or without preoperative irradiation is commonly used. Preoperative irradiation is recommended for large (≥4 cm) tumors or high-grade lesions, because the risk of serious understaging in these situations is high, as shown by Marshall[115] 40 years ago and repeatedly by many others. In the University of Iowa series, patients with Stage B cancers measuring more than 3 cm experienced a 50% 5-year survival rate after being treated by preoperative irradiation and cystectomy, but only 16% of patients treated by radical cystectomy alone were alive at 5 years.[77]

For T3 and resectable T4a disease, there are clear indications for the use of preoperative irradiation before radical cystectomy.[141]

Full-Dose External-Beam Irradiation

External-beam irradiation (with cystectomy reserved for salvage) is a common treatment scheme in Canada and Great Britain.[51,69,83] In the United States, initial surgery is more commonly used; irradiation is usually administered "by default" if the patient is medically unfit, refuses cystectomy, or has disease that is too advanced for surgery. Patients treated by radical irradiation ideally should have adequate bladder capacity without substantial voiding symptoms or incontinence; patients whose bladders are already contracted are poor candidates.

The largest, most comprehensively analyzed series and the only one for which long-term actuarial data on tumor control are available is the Edinburgh series.[50–52,149–155] This series is unique in that selection bias was minimal, because irradiation was the institutional policy. The rate of complete response at first follow-up cystoscopy after 5500 cGy to 5750 cGy given in 20 fractions over 4 weeks was approximately 45% for all T stages (T1–T4).[51] Roughly half of the patients who achieved complete remission later developed local recurrences, yielding 5-year local control rates of approximately 25% each for T1, T2, and T3 lesions. Five- and 10-year local control rates for T4 cancers were 16%.[153] The rate of complete response was inversely related to lesion size ($P<0.05$). For T2, T3, and T4 disease, complete response was associated with significantly improved survival rates, an observation confirmed by other investigators.[1,15,83]

Reports of the influence of gross tumor morphology (*i.e.*, papillary, solid, mixed) on local control after external-beam treatment are confusing. In the Edinburgh series of 917 patients with T1 through T4 disease, Duncan and Quilty[51] found significantly higher rates of complete response for solid tumors than for papillary or mixed tumors; when analyzed by stage, the same observation was made.[150,152] At Massachusetts General Hospital, Shipley and associates[180] found the opposite; in their analysis of 37 patients with T2 or T3 disease, the only significant and independent factor that favorably influenced local control and survival rates was papillary morphology. Because papillary tumors are generally smaller, better differentiated, and less infiltrating than solid tumors, and because it was the institutional policy at Massachusetts General Hospital to perform a "complete" TUR if possible, it is likely that the papillary tumors reported by Shipley and co-workers were mostly T2 and more often completely resected than solid tumors, which are more often T3 and not completely resectable. Data to support the idea that T2 lesions, but not T3, are completely resectable come from Jacobsen and co-workers,[89] who treated 124 patients with T2 or T3 bladder cancer with definitive radiation. Of 16 patients whose tumors could be completely resected, all had T2 cancer (AB Jacobsen, written communication, 1990). Both lower stage and smaller tumor volume after TUR would improve the results for patients with papillary tumors. Taken together, the data from the two institutions support the recommendation made by Shipley and colleagues to attempt complete resection of papillary tumors before irradiation. If stage is ignored, patients with papillary disease, which is most often grade 1 or 2 and Stage T1 or T2, have significantly higher rates of survival and lower rates of metastasis than patients with solid tumors, which are usually high grade and high stage. However, within each T stage, 5-year survival rates for patients with papillary, solid, or mixed tumors have not been shown to differ significantly after external-beam irradiation alone.[150,152]

In the Edinburgh series, the best predictor of both local control and survival within each T stage was grade.[51,150,152] The complete response and lasting local control rates were significantly higher in high-grade lesions, but paradoxically (with the exception of T1), the survival rate was significantly worse because these patients more frequently developed distant metastases.

In addition to grade and tumor morphology, other factors believed to influence local control rates include radiation dose,[82,121,130,143,150,154] tumor size,[51] hemoglobin level,[149,150] and ureteral obstruction.[180]

In addition to grade, stage, and morphology, survival rates are significantly influenced by tumor size,[15,51,60] ureteral obstruction,[32,70 180] hemoglobin level,[149] response at first follow-up cystoscopy,[14,82] radiation dose,[55,60 82] urea level,[155] and performance status.[63]

Although other factors may significantly influence prognosis, the literature is inconclusive. These factors include age,[82,122;,155,180] sex,[15,122,150,180] prior treatment,[122,180] vascular invasion, and carcinoma *in situ* elsewhere in the bladder.[180,240] Shipley and associates[180] found that completeness of TUR before radiation therapy significantly influenced local control. However, Timmer and co-workers[210] observed no such correlation; 11 of 21 patients with T2 cancer in their series who had undergone "complete" TUR developed local recurrence.

Timmer and co-workers[210] discovered that response at 4000 cGy did not predict outcome; 55% of patients whose tumors were seen at cystoscopy to have responded favorably after 4000 cGy later developed local recurrence. Veneema and colleagues[225] found that only 15 (33%) of 45 patients with T1 through T4 disease who were selected for high-dose irradiation on the basis of favorable response after 3000 cGy to 4000 cGy remained alive and without evidence of bladder recurrence at 5 years; eight others were alive, three with local persistence and five after salvage cystectomy. These results are not clearly superior to other studies in which no attempt was made to select patients on the basis of response.

Salvage Treatment After Unsuccessful Irradiation

After irradiation, patients undergo cystoscopy every 3 months for 2 years and every 6 months thereafter. Some persistent or recurrent lesions, particularly low-grade tumors, that were downstaged by radiation therapy have been successfully managed by endoscopic resection; if local tumor persists at 3 months after resection, cystectomy is indicated.[153]

Five-year survival rates after salvage cystectomy are 40% to 45%; the rates for superficial disease (Tis, T1, T2) are approximately 60% compared with 25% for more deeply invasive cancers.[64,193,206] These rates overestimate the impact of salvage cystectomy, because most patients whose tumors recur are not candidates for salvage surgery because of advanced disease, old age, poor medical condition, or refusal. Based on data from several large series, only 264 (19%) of 1377 patients with persistent local disease or recurrences underwent cystectomy.[51,64,83,121,242] The overall impact is small: 40% survival rate × 20% of the patients eligible = an 8% 5-year survival rate among patients who developed local recurrences.

"Sandwich" Radiation Therapy

There have been at least two studies of "sandwich" irradiation, in which patients with clinical B2, C, or D disease received sequentially 500 cGy (single fraction) preoperatively, radical cystectomy, and 4500 cGy postoperatively.[126,198] We think this approach has several drawbacks compared with conventional preoperative irradiation. First, after extensive surgery, many patients decline or are physically unable to withstand postoperative irradiation. Fourteen (42%) of the 33 patients treated at the University of Pennsylvania and 20 (29%) of the 68 patients in the Radiation Therapy Oncology Group(RTOG)/ Thomas Jefferson study who had pathologic indications (B2, C, or D1) to mandate postoperative irradiation never received the intended treatment.[125,126] The 5-year disease-free survival rate for these patients was only 20%.[198]

Second, irradiation administered by the sandwich technique is basically postoperative irradiation, for which few data show efficacy. Reported rates of tumor recurrence in pelvic and abdominal surgical wounds are higher after postoperative than preoperative irradiation, despite seemingly adequate postoperative doses.[122,178] It is impossible to treat the entire surgical incision and operative bed without significantly increasing the irradiated volume. Furthermore, removal of the bladder and prostate or uterus, fallopian tubes, and ovaries leaves a void into which the small bowel falls and becomes fixed. Although not statistically significant, the highest rate (18%) of small bowel obstruction in the Pennsylvania series occurred in the group that received the complete sandwich therapy.[198] The incidence of small bowel obstruction or peritonitis in the RTOG/Thomas Jefferson experience was 15% (seven of 48 patients).[126]

Concomitant Chemotherapy Plus Irradiation

In the 1960s, Woodruff and colleagues[241] and Stein and Kaufman,[201] using concomitant fluorouracil and irradiation, reported "significant benefit" compared with irradiation alone. However, two randomized trials of concomitant fluorouracil and irradiation for T3 and T4a tumors revealed no difference in 5-year survival rates compared with irradiation alone.[54,63] In a study by Rotman and associates,[163] there were eight late bowel or bladder complications in nine survivors who received concurrent fluorouracil and irradiation.

Attention has recently focused on concomitant cisplatin and irradiation.[53] Jakse and co-workers[90] and Shipley and associates[179] reported high complete response rates for T2, T3, and T4 cancers after 6000 cGy to 6500 cGy plus cisplatin. Although the 4-year survival rate (64%) for 22 cT2 patients was as high as that after cystectomy (with or without irradiation), the 4-year survival rate for cT3 and cT4 tumors combined was only 24%.[179] Sauer and co-workers[168] concluded that concomitant cisplatin and irradiation is "highly effective" for control of local disease and preservation of the bladder, but none of their patients had been observed for more than 2 years. Longer follow-up and data from randomized trials are necessary before these conclusions can be accepted.

Interstitial Implantation

In the past, permanent gold or radon seed implants were performed in the United States and abroad.[9,29,47] Interstitial therapy for bladder cancer has been largely discontinued in the United States; institutions that still perform implants use removable sources (radium, cesium, iridium, or tantalum).

Interstitial treatment may be used alone, in combination with low-dose or moderate-dose external-beam irradiation, or to treat the suture line in patients undergoing partial cystectomy. In carefully chosen patients, the technique has provided excellent long-term tumor control and bladder function. Suitable patients are those with solitary T1, T2, or T3 lesions measuring less than 5 cm whose general medical condition permits suprapubic cystotomy. The finding of carcinoma *in situ* immediately adjacent to or 2 cm from the primary lesion made no difference in the rate of local control of these lesions.[213,238]

Although the technique is infrequently used in the United States today, the excellent results obtained at an increasing number of institutions abroad should prompt trials of the technique in this country. Preliminary results of two small trials have been reported.[204,232]

Intracavitary Irradiation

Intracavitary irradiation with a central radium or cesium source inside a Foley catheter balloon was popularized by Friedman in the 1940s. The technique, often referred to as the Walter Reed technique, is still used in a few U.S. clinics for patients with superficial cancer in whom all other transurethral and intravesical chemotherapeutic treatment options have been exhausted and whose only alternative is cystectomy.[65,80,167] Patients must have adequate bladder capacity.

Solutions of radioactive gold, sodium, cobalt, or bromine in balloons are no longer used because of poor depth-dose characteristics with overtreatment of mucosal surfaces.

Intraoperative Electron-Beam Therapy

Matsumoto and associates[118] reported 116 patients with small, superficial (Ta, T1, or T2) lesions. Most patients had a solitary lesion, but a few had multiple tumors in close enough proximity to fit within the 4-cm to 6-cm diameter of an electron collimating cone. A single intraoperative dose of radiation (2500–3000 cGy, 4–6 MeV electrons) was delivered through the cone directly onto the tumor, which was exposed by cystotomy without tumor resection or fulguration. This procedure was followed 3 to 4 weeks later by external-beam irradiation of 3000 cGy to 4000 cGy over 3 to 4 weeks. Most patients retained normal bladder function, and a high rate of local control was achieved. Complications consisted of transient ureterovesical junction obstruction in three patients and a contracted bladder with bilateral hydronephrosis in one patient. No patients developed proctitis or abdominal wound recurrence.

Intraarterial Chemotherapy

Several investigators have chosen the intraarterial route of drug administration in an attempt to increase drug concentration to the bladder tumor while achieving a systemic dose comparable to that after intravenous administration.

Maatman and co-workers[110] treated 18 T3 tumors with intraarterial cisplatin (four patients), intraarterial cisplatin and doxorubicin plus intravenous cyclophosphamide (CISCA) (12 patients), or CISCA plus preoperative irradiation (two patients) before radical cystectomy. Complete pathologic response was attained in only one (6%) of 16 patients who received chemotherapy alone; both patients who received CISCA plus preoperative irradiation were staged pT0 at cystectomy, indicating perhaps that the irradiation was the more effective agent.

Recently Eapen and co-workers[53] reported 25 patients (16 T3, 9 T4), 20 of whom received either intraarterial cisplatin and concurrent irradiation to 6000 cGy and five of whom received 4000 cGy over 4 weeks with concurrent intraarterial cisplatin followed by cystectomy. A 96% complete response rate was observed. Follow-up was short (minimum 6 months, median 18 months); the authors projected a 90% 2-year survival rate. This figure will no doubt erode significantly with further follow-up, because cisplatin alone would not be expected to prevent distant metastasis in most patients with advanced cancer. There was a 46% rate of sacral neuropathy, which in some patients produced unrelenting, painful, burning pedal dysesthesias, unrelieved by medication. This report and that of Kanoh and associates,[98] who observed perineal and gluteal skin erosions and necroses after intraarterial doxorubicin, demonstrate the need for extreme caution in applying these techniques.

Neoadjuvant Chemotherapy and Adjuvant Chemotherapy

Single-agent neoadjuvant methotrexate failed to improve the rates of response, local recurrence, metastasis, or survival if given before conventional radiation therapy or preoperative irradiation plus cystectomy in 376 randomized patients with T3 bladder cancers in a Cooperative Urological Cancer Group trial.[174] Neoadjuvant cisplatin did not improve survival compared with irradiation alone in a trial conducted in Australia and England.[157,158] There are no published randomized data that compare neoadjuvant multiagent chemotherapy plus conventional therapy with conventional therapy alone. After treatment with methotrexate and cisplatin; CISCA; methotrexate, vinblastine, doxorubicin, and cisplatin (MVAC); or cisplatin, methotrexate, and vinblastine (CMV) chemotherapy regimens, the incidence of pathologically negative cystectomy specimens ranges from 15% to 25%.[27,43,170,199,239] Although several studies report higher rates of clinical complete response after multiagent chemotherapy, at least half of those patients had residual cancer in the cystectomy specimen.[27,78,239]

Because of toxicity and lack of proven benefit, neoadjuvant MVAC and CMV should now be used only in the context of clinical trials. Several randomized trials of adjuvant chemotherapy using fluorouracil, doxorubicin-fluorouracil, or cisplatin after conventional therapy have not demonstrated increased survival rates (WU Shipley, oral communication, 1986).[162,184,189]

Management of Metastatic or Unresectable Locoregional Disease

Excellent palliation of bleeding, dysuria, pain, and frequency is obtained by treatment with 3000 cGy administered in ten fractions over 2 weeks or with 1000 cGy given as a single dose and repeated in 3 to 4 weeks.

In the past 10 years, several chemotherapy regimens have been shown to be reasonably effective in the management of metastatic bladder cancer. Although CISCA, MVAC, and CMV are the most popular regimens in the United States, these are by no means the only regimens that have achieved some success, and it is still unclear which is the most effective.[28,85,226] Four randomized trials have failed to show a benefit to multiagent chemotherapy (*i.e.*, cisplatin plus methotrexate or cisplatin plus cyclophosphamide with or without doxorubicin) over cisplatin alone.[81,101,196,213] The multiagent regimens have greater toxicity.

Sternberg and co-workers[202] reported the results of MVAC in 71 patients with unresectable locoregional or distant metastatic bladder cancer. Median survival was 12 months. Complete clinical or pathologic remission was observed in 14 (20%) patients. Nine of 14 complete responders relapsed within 21 months; the other five (7% of the total) remained continuously disease-free 2 to 4 years after beginning chemotherapy. A few additional patients have remained disease-free after surgical resection of tumors that had partially responded; the significance of this observation is unclear, because occasional cures of metastatic bladder cancer have been reported after resection alone, without chemotherapy.[37] Sternberg and associates[202] reported a "major" (complete plus partial) response rate of almost 70%. There was, however, no survival difference between the partial-response group and the groups who achieved no response or whose tumors progressed; the lack of survival benefit for partial responders is confirmed by others.[3,73,85,203] Previously irradiated patients had the same response rates as those who had not been irradiated. Squamous cell carcinoma, adenocarcinoma, and carcinoma *in situ* do not respond well to MVAC.[171,202] Tannock and co-workers[209] reported the experience with MVAC at the Princess Margaret Hospital. Complete responses occurred in four (13%) of 30 patients with measurable disease, two (7%) of whom remained disease-free at 34 and 52 months after treatment of small-volume lymph node metastases.

Harker and associates[73] reported complete responses in 14 (26%) of 54 patients who received CMV. Median survival was 8 months. Two patients remained continuously free of disease at 18 and 35 months, and 4 others were free of disease 6 to 11 months after beginning chemotherapy.

Logothetis and co-workers[107] reported complete response in 35 (36%) of 97 patients with locoregional advanced (62 patients) or distant metastatic (35 patients) cancer treated with CISCA; 13 patients remained free of disease for more than 2 years. Some failures were not observed until 3 to 5 years after treatment. The 6-year actuarial disease-free survival rate for the entire population was 9%, and the median survival was 10 months. Prior irradiation did not influence the rate of complete response.

Many patients are unable to receive aggressive combination chemotherapy because of coexisting medical problems. Other means of palliation must be sought. Montie and associates[128] reported that one half of patients with unresectable bladder cancer had improvement in urinary symptoms after diversion. The survival rate was not improved by the procedure, and operative mortality, usually from myocardial infarction or embolism, was high (14%). We prefer to administer palliative irradiation and use surgery if irradiation is unsuccessful.

Follow-up Policy

Patients are observed for recurrence in the bladder, the upper urinary tracts, and the urethra. Cystoscopy, usually with cytologic examination, is performed every 3 months for 2 years and then every 6 months thereafter. Two percent to 3% of patients with bladder cancer develop upper tract disease after treatment of their bladder tumor.[139, 243] The incidence is at least 10% for patients with multifocal carcinoma *in situ* of the bladder.[243] Herr and Whitmore[79] reported that 19 (29%) of 66 patients whose bladder remained free of disease for more than 1 year after intravesical BCG treatment of multifocal carcinoma *in situ* developed distal ureteral carcinoma *in situ*. Ureteral recurrence is sometimes delayed 5 years or longer after the bladder cancer is diagnosed.[176, 243]

Bloody discharge from the penis after radical cystectomy suggests recurrent tumor in the urethra.[169] A penile or perineal mass or involved inguinal lymph nodes may exist. In patients with deeply invasive urethral recurrence, elective treatment with irradiation or surgery of the clinically negative inguinal lymph nodes should be considered.[74]

In patients with T3 or T4 disease who were irradiated, CT is usually employed in follow-up. Chest roentgenograms are obtained every 6 months for 2 years and annually thereafter.

Treatment by Histologic Tumor Types

Squamous Cell Carcinoma

In terms of radioresponsiveness (42% complete response rate at the first follow-up cystoscopy), lasting local control (34%), and 5-year survival (14% to 19%), the treatment results after full-dose irradiation do not differ significantly from those reported for transitional cell carcinoma.[96, 151] This was shown in a multivariate analysis including histology, T stage, tumor size, and hemoglobin level.[151]

Two randomized trials comparing preoperative irradiation and cystectomy with cystectomy alone have shown a statistically significant benefit for preoperative irradiation for T3 and T4 or high-grade bilharzial tumors. In both trials, the 2- and 5-year disease-free and absolute survival rates in these subgroups of patients were more than doubled if preoperative irradiation was administered (45% to 53% *versus* 19% to 20%).[5, 66]

Swanson and co-workers[205] reported a 50% 5-year actuarial survival rate among 25 patients with T2 or T3 squamous cell carcinoma of the bladder after 5000 cGy in 25 fractions over 5 weeks, followed by radical cystectomy. Downstaging (pT<cT) was reported for ten patients (40%); six patients (24%) had no residual tumor (pT0). The authors concluded that, because pelvic failure is still the predominant cause of death and current chemotherapy regimens are not effective in treating squamous cell carcinoma of the bladder, preoperative irradiation is indicated.

Adenocarcinoma

Although Johnson and associates[94] concluded that nonurachal adenocarcinomas are less radiosensitive than transitional cell carcinomas, in their own series the three patients (Stages B2, D1, and D1) who were long-term disease-free survivors (5–14 years) were treated by high-dose irradiation alone. Mostofi and associates[133] also reported local control at 14 years for one patient treated by irradiation alone. Others generally have used irradiation only for far-advanced, inoperable cancers in which little benefit would be anticipated.[88]

In the series reported from Massachusetts General Hospital, two of three patients with T2 or T3 tumors who received preoperative irradiation plus partial cystectomy were alive without cancer at 3 years, compared with two of seven treated by partial or radical cystectomy alone.[135]

We recommend the use of preoperative irradiation if partial or radical cystectomy is indicated because of several factors. Almost all patients with adenocarcinoma have muscle-invasive disease, and the 5-year survival rate after surgery alone in several large series is 5% or less.[88, 94, 97, 105] The local recurrence rate in the pelvis, bladder, and abdominal wall or wound is approximately 50% after surgery alone for urachal tumors, while the risk of distant metastasis as first site of failure is low.[93, 175] Irradiation had been efficacious in some small series, and irradiation is clearly effective in adenocarcinomas that arise in other sites (*e.g.*, breast, cervix, uterus, prostate, parotid, rectum).[94, 133] Moreover, the newer chemotherapy regimens are not effective for adenocarcinoma of the bladder.

IRRADIATION TECHNIQUES

A four-field box technique with the patient supine is used at the University of Florida (Fig. 49-1). Although other techniques of irradiation are possible (*e.g.*, anterior and posterior, rotational, or three-field portal arrangements), we favor the four-field box because of the ease of interpreting imaging films, the ease of making portal size reductions, and the satisfactory dose distribution that can be achieved. Occasionally, it is necessary to use wedges in the lateral portals to ensure homogeneity of dose throughout the volume. For simulation, the bladder is drained of urine and filled with 30 ml of contrast medium (*i.e.*, Cysto-Conray II) and 10 cc of air, and dilute barium is inserted into the rectum.

Treatment is usually with high-energy photons (6–20 MV). The cephalad margin is usually at the middle of the sacroiliac joint or sometimes between L5 and S1, depending on disease extent. The caudal margin is usually at the bottom of the obturator foramen unless there is diffuse involvement of the bladder neck or prostatic urethra with carcinoma *in situ*, in which case the portals are extended to the bottom of the ischial tuberosities so that there is a generous margin on the prostate. The regional lymph nodes are treated by including the bony pelvic side walls with approximately a 1.5-cm margin in the anterior and posterior portals. On the lateral portals, the posterior margin is set at least 3 cm behind the most posterior extent of tumor as determined by palpation or CT. It is usually possible to

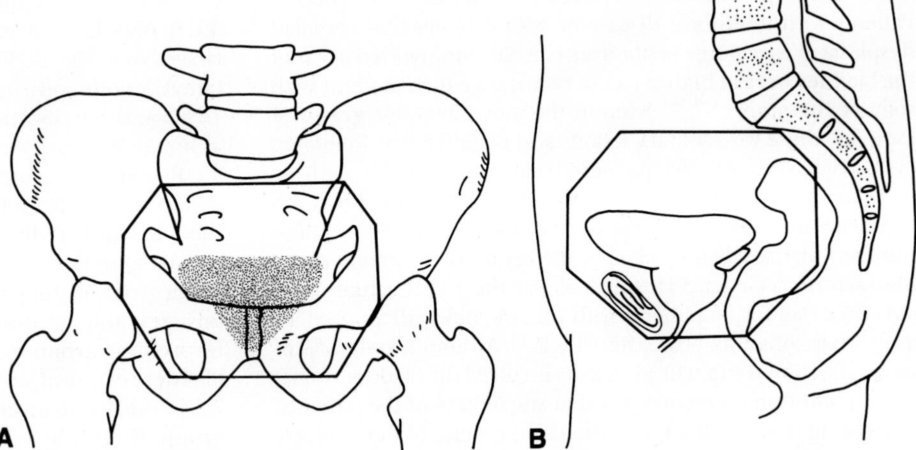

FIGURE 49–1. Radiation treatment portals for bladder cancer. (**A**) Anterior and posterior portals. (**B**) Lateral portals. (Modified from Shipley WU: Radiation therapy for patients with bladder carcinoma: Rationale, results, techniques, and possible innovations. In Bonney WW, Prout GR Jr [eds]: AUA Monographs: Bladder Cancer, vol 1, pp 243–259. Baltimore, Williams & Wilkins, 1982)

exclude the posterior half of the rectum. The anterior margin of the lateral portal is placed just in front of the bladder, and the field is shaped with Lipowitz's metal blocks to prevent fall-off over the anterior skin surface.

Because of varying degrees of bladder distention, the bladder cancer can be a "moving target." Depending on what one wishes to accomplish, the bladder may be treated empty or full. In most patients the initial treatment volume (which generally encompasses the entire bladder) is kept as small as possible by having the patient void before treatment. For patients whose tumor is confined to the bladder base or bladder neck region, the reduced portals (which often include only the involved portion of the bladder) are sometimes treated with the bladder full to displace small bowel from the pelvis.

The size of the portals is reduced after 4500 cGy to 5040 cGy (180-cGy fractions). The total dose is 6480 cGy to 6840 cGy in patients treated by irradiation alone. In most patients, the reduced portals exclude at least a portion of the uninvolved bladder (Fig. 49-2). For the past 4 years, when preoperative irradiation has been used, we have delivered a dose of 3000 cGy in ten fractions over 2 weeks followed by cystectomy in 2 to 3 weeks.

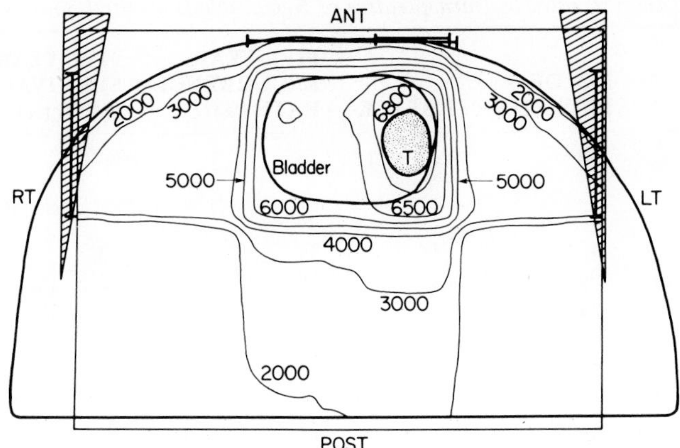

FIGURE 49–2. Isodose curves for anteroposterior (AP) and two lateral portals with wedges, using 18-MV photons to deliver 6000 cGy to the bladder and reduced AP portal for a 500-cGy boost to the tumor.

RESULTS OF TREATMENT

In reviewing results of treatment for bladder carcinoma, it is important to differentiate between clinical staging, based on TUR specimens, cystoscopic findings, and examination under anesthesia, and pathologic staging, based on cystectomy specimen findings.

Carcinoma *in Situ*

Transurethral Resection and Fulguration

After treatment of carcinoma *in situ* by transurethral electroresection (TUR) and fulguration at the Mayo Clinic, 73% of patients developed invasive cancer, and 57% died of their disease within 5 years.[215] Prout and associates[148] reported 52 patients treated by TUR alone (12 patients) or TUR plus intravesical thiotepa (40 patients). Twenty-six patients had a prior history of clinical Ta or T1 disease, without carcinoma *in situ*, and 26 others had carcinoma *in situ* at the time of initial diagnosis; ten had carcinoma *in situ* alone, and 16 had concomitant Ta or T1 disease. Only seven (13%) patients remained continuously free of disease 1 to 5 years after treatment; all seven patients had a prior history of Ta or T1 disease. Thirty-one (61%) patients required cystectomy (29 patients) for muscle invasion, prostatic invasion, or a contracted bladder and/or died (11 patients) as a result of bladder cancer.

Intracavitary Irradiation

Seven of 14 patients at the Cleveland Clinic[80] who were treated by intracavitary irradiation 1 to 3 months after diagnostic TUR remained free of disease (*i.e.*, negative cystoscopy and cytology) at 1 to 8 years (mean, 3 years).

Stage Ta or T1 Tumors

Transurethral Resection and Fulguration

Sixty percent to 80% of patients with newly diagnosed Ta or T1 disease developed recurrences at the same site or elsewhere within the bladder within 5 years after transurethral management.[41,61,190,220] Patients with T1 disease were more likely to have a recurrence than those with Ta disease. High grade and large size also correlated with risk of recurrence.[140] Patients with multifocal disease or with biopsies that revealed dysplasia or carcinoma *in situ* from clinically uninvolved areas of the bladder were at higher risk of recurrence than patients with solitary tumors.[109,190,194] Even in the most favorable group of patients, those with solitary lesions and negative first follow-up cystoscopy, 52% of 183 patients treated with TUR, with or without thiotepa instillation, in the British Medical Research Council Study, developed recurrent disease by 5 years.[140] These numbers are closely mimicked by the results of treatment at the Massachusetts General Hospital, where the 5-year actuarial recurrence rate for 36 patients with solitary, newly diagnosed Ta and T1 lesions was 60% after TUR.[75] Although only 5% of newly diagnosed superficial cancers involved the bladder dome, subsequent tumors recurred at that site in 29% of the patients, suggesting tumor cell implantation as the cause of new cancers at that site.[75]

Within 2 years of diagnosis, 3% of Ta lesions and 25% to 30% of T1 lesions developed muscle invasion. Forty percent of grade 3, T1 lesions developed muscle invasion within 2 years.[41,220]

Interstitial Irradiation

Bladder relapse rates of 15% to 20% and survival rates of approximately 75% were seen after interstitial irradiation or intraoperative electron irradiation of almost 500 newly diagnosed patients with Ta or T1 bladder cancer (Table 49-4).[11,18,118,119,220,238] The differences between these results and those for TUR with or without intravesical chemotherapy for newly diagnosed Ta or T1 disease are striking: the 5-year actuarial rates are at least four to five times higher in the TUR-alone group.[41,61,220] An additional series of 48 T1 patients demonstrated 77% tumor-free survival at 2 to 9 years after treatment with radon or gold seed implantation.[29]

In Rotterdam from 1950 to 1968, it was the institutional policy to add an interstitial implant after TUR of T1 lesions. In 1968, taking the lead from urologists in other parts of the world, the interstitial treatment was deleted if all tumor was thought to have been removed transurethrally. A retrospective comparison of results after TUR alone and TUR plus radium for T1 bladder carcinoma was reported in 1981.[220] The series was biased in favor of the group treated with TUR alone. In the TUR plus radium group, the incidence of solid tumors was twice that in the TUR group (38% *versus* 19%); poorly differentiated lesions were more than twice as common (29% *versus* 12%), and the resection was not always considered "complete," although it always was in the TUR group. The group receiving TUR alone was treated in the more modern era (1968 to 1980), with presumably more modern techniques than were used for the TUR plus radium group (1950 to 1968).

Despite the biases, the rates of bladder relapse, survival, death from bladder cancer, distant metastasis, cystectomy (for salvage), and progression to muscle invasion all significantly favored the group treated with TUR plus radium. The risk of bladder relapse at sites other than that of the original lesion was 7% in the group given radium, but it was 28% in the TUR only group. For grade 3 disease, recurrence after TUR occurred in 88% of the patients but in only 16% of those receiving TUR and radium. Most of those who relapsed after TUR underwent multiple (≥2) repeat TURs, and 65% eventually required radical cystectomy or radical irradiation. The survival and distant metastasis curves did not differ markedly until after 5 years, confirming that it often takes some time for progression to occur.

After implantation, half of the bladder relapses occurred at the same site and half occurred elsewhere in the bladder. The 7% to 11% rate of appearance of new disease elsewhere in the bladder is substantially lower than that reported after TUR alone.[11,119,220] Unfortunately, this approach to therapy has not been given a trial in the United States because most urologists simply "do not believe the results."

Intraoperative Electron-Beam Irradiation

Matsumoto and associates[118] reported 66 patients with clinical Ta or T1 lesions who were treated with intraoperative electron-beam irradiation. The 5-year recurrence rate was 9%, and the 5-year survival rate was 96%.

Radical Cystectomy

The 5-year survival rates after radical cystectomy with or without irradiation for clinical Ta or T1 disease are 70% to 80%

TABLE 49–4
Five-Year Bladder-Relapse Rates for Newly Diagnosed Ta or T1 Bladder Cancer Treated by Intraoperative or Removable Interstitial Sources

INVESTIGATOR	TREATMENT	NO. OF PATIENTS	T STAGE	FIVE-YEAR RECURRENCE RATE (%)*	FIVE-YEAR SURVIVAL RATE (%)
Matsumoto et al[118]	Intraoperative electrons (2500–3000 cGy) plus external beam (3000–4000 cGy)	66	Ta or T1	9	96
Williams et al[238]	^{182}Ta	47	T1	34	69
Van der Werf-Messing and Hop[220]	Radium ± external beam (350 cGy × 3)	196	T1	18	82
Battermann and Tierie[11]	External beam (1050–3000 cGy) plus radium	34	T1	15	72
Mazeron et al[119]	External beam (850 cGy) plus partial cystectomy plus ^{192}Ir	43	T1	23	72
Boiteux et al[18]	External beam (1050 cGy) plus partial cystectomy plus ^{192}Ir	98	T1	15†	77

** Relapse rates are for recurrences in the original site or elsewhere in the bladder.*
† Mean follow-up of 51 months.

according to Smith and associates[191] and Bracken and co-workers.[20] Neither series showed any survival benefit from the addition of preoperative irradiation. The pelvic recurrence rate is low after cystectomy alone.

External-Beam Irradiation

There is no reported role for external-beam irradiation in patients with Ta bladder cancer. Quilty and Duncan[152] employed radical irradiation (5000 cGy in 20 fractions over 4 weeks) to treat 190 patients with T1 tumors. Seventy-five patients had solitary lesions, and the rest were divided between multiple lesions and diffuse involvement of the entire bladder. The overall complete response rate was 48%; complete response did not correlate with the number of tumors or diffuseness of disease in the bladder but did significantly correlate with grade: grade 1, 37%; grade 2, 58%; grade 3, 68% ($P<0.01$). Overall, the 5-year relapse-free rate was 28% (56% at 5 and 10 years for grade 3, and 16% at 5 years and 8% at 10 years for grade 1). The results for grade 2 tumors were only slightly better than those for grade 1. Yu and associates[242] reported a similar 5-year relapse-free rate (31%) for 58 patients with T1 disease treated with irradiation to a dose of 6000 cGy to 6600 cGy in 6 to 7 weeks. Many of the failures represented new occurrences in the bladder.[165]

The 5-year survival rate in the Edinburgh and other series was 60% to 70%, a reflection of the usually indolent nature of the disease and the fact that many patients owed their survival to salvage cystectomy after irradiation failure.[227,237] There was no significant difference in survival by grade or by gross tumor morphology (most were papillary). By 10 years, the actuarial rate of distant metastasis was 37%.

Quilty and Duncan[152] concluded that external-beam irradiation for grade 1 and 2 disease contributes little, but for the small subset (19% of their patients) with grade 3 disease, external-beam irradiation should be considered early in the course of disease. At the University of Florida, the success rate after external-beam irradiation in patients who have undergone multiple TURs, fulgurations, and intravesical instillations of chemotherapy has been low; external-beam irradiation in this subset may cause severe bladder contracture, because function in many of these patients is already moderately or severely compromised.

Intracavitary Irradiation

Friedman and Lewis[65] reported 5-year disease control in seven of nine patients with T1 cancers treated by the Walter Reed technique. In the Cleveland Clinic experience, 14 (34%) of 41 patients with recurrence after transurethral attempts to control T1 lesions remained free of disease at 1 to 9 years (mean, 3.5 years) after intracavitary irradiation.[80] Russell and associates[167] observed relapse-free survival in 11 (73%) of 15 patients who received 3500 cGy to 5000 cGy by external-beam irradiation followed 3 weeks later by 2000 cGy to 3000 cGy administered by intracavitary cesium.

Summary

Either interstitial or intraoperative electron irradiation is an attractive treatment alternative for solitary, small lesions. Because 65% to 85% of newly diagnosed Ta and T1 lesions are solitary, most patients are candidates for this approach at presentation.[61,75,109,212] Survival results compare favorably with results achieved by TUR and fulguration, with or without intravesical chemotherapy. Reported rates of tumor control strongly favor the interstitial or intraoperative irradiation approach. The occurrence of new tumors elsewhere in the bladder is also markedly lower than after TUR, with or without intravesical chemotherapy. Although we have advised more widespread application of these techniques, U.S. urologists have been reluctant to explore the approach.

Stage T2 Tumors

Transurethral Resection

Barnes and associates[8] reported 5-year survival in 16 (28%) of 68 Stage B patients with grade 2, 3, or 4 lesions, 80% of which measured less than 3 cm. Approximately half of the patients suffered local recurrences. Henry and co-workers[77] reported a 35% 5-year survival rate for 43 patients with Stage B disease with similar characteristics (*i.e.*, 72% had tumors <3 cm) after treatment by TUR; ten eventually required radical cystectomy.

Herr and Whitmore[79] used repeat TUR alone to treat 45 patients, who were selected from 217 patients with muscle-invasive disease who had restaging cystoscopy at Memorial Hospital after diagnostic TUR elsewhere. This treatment was usually possible only for papillary lesions. Of the 45 patients, 37 had B1 disease, seven had B2 disease, and one had D1 disease. With 3 to 7 years of follow-up, nine patients (20%) remained continuously disease-free after the TUR performed at Memorial Hospital. Twenty-one others were free of disease and retained their bladders as of the time of the report, but had undergone multiple repeat TURs and intravesical treatment for recurrent cancer. Eleven other patients had undergone cystectomy.

Partial Cystectomy

We are aware of no data for clinical Stage B1 disease. The 5-year survival rate for patients with pathologic Stage B1 cancer is usually reported as 50% to 60%.[21,108,136,161,216] High local recurrence rates and lower survival rates are reported for patients with tumors in the fixed portion of the bladder and for patients whose tumors require ureteral reimplantation.[40,216]

Magri[113] found that combined irradiation and partial cystectomy produced a significantly higher survival rate than partial cystectomy alone. Because partial-cystectomy series report intravesical recurrence rates of 50% or more, it is notable that Mazeron and associates[119] reported only a 7% recurrence rate at the same site or elsewhere in the bladder among 30 patients with clinical Stage T2 disease (6% for 31 pT2 patients) who underwent partial cystectomy plus an ^{192}Ir implant. Boiteux and co-workers[18] likewise reported intravesical recurrence in only 18% of 66 patients with T2 lesions treated at eight institutions by partial cystectomy plus iridium.

Radical Cystectomy

Whitmore and colleagues[234] reported 5-year survival rates for clinical Stage B1 cancer of 45% to 50% after radical cystectomy alone or with 2000 cGy to 4000 cGy administered preoperatively. Few other data exist for clinical Stage B1 disease because the results are usually combined with those for Stages 0 and A or are reported only according to pathologic stage. Whitmore and co-workers[234] and other investigators have reported 5-year survival rates for pathologic Stage B (pT2) cancer of approximately 60% after radical cystectomy alone.

TABLE 49–5
Treatment of T2 Bladder Carcinoma with External-Beam Radiation Therapy Alone

INSTITUTION	NO. OF PATIENTS	5-YEAR SURVIVAL RATE (%)
Edmonton[46]	16	69
Rotterdam[217]	25	44
M.D. Anderson[122]	43	26
Stanford[68]	68	42
Michigan[60]	29	43
Bern[70]	62	35
London Hospital[82]	132	30
Radiumhemmet[55]	27*	37
	28†	33
Edinburgh[51]	298	40

**Patients treated three times a day to a total dose of 8400 cGy.*
† Patients treated with one treatment a day to a total dose of 6400 cGy.

External-Beam Irradiation

The 5-year survival rate in most series is approximately 40% (Table 49-5).[46, 51, 55, 60, 68, 70, 82, 122, 217] Failure to control the primary lesion accounts for approximately 90% of recurrences; distant metastasis alone accounts for only 10% to 15% of all recurrences.[82, 210, 242]

Intraoperative Electron-Beam Irradiation

Matsumoto and associates[118] reported a 5-year recurrence rate of 18% and a 5-year survival rate of 62% in 28 patients with T2 cancer (Table 49-6).

Interstitial Irradiation

The 5-year bladder-relapse rate in 700 patients with T2 disease treated by interstitial or intraoperative therapy was 20% to 25%. The 5-year survival rate was 55% to 60% (Table 49-6).[11, 18, 118, 119, 222, 223, 238] Two thirds of the relapses in one series were at the site of initial disease.[222] The recurrence rate elsewhere in the bladder was 7%.[119, 222]

Summary

For patients with T2 disease who are to undergo partial cystectomy, there is justification to recommend preoperative irradiation (4500 cGy in 5 weeks) or an interstitial implant at the time of cystectomy. Large or high-grade lesions for which radical cystectomy is indicated should receive preoperative irradiation.

Interstitial irradiation and intraoperative electron-beam irradiation have been highly successful means of curing T2 bladder cancer with preservation of function; neither approach is popular in the United States.

External-beam irradiation, with or without systemic chemotherapy (with cystectomy reserved for salvage), is the usual treatment offered at our institution to patients who wish to preserve their bladders. Patients receive three cycles of CMV chemotherapy, followed by concurrent external-beam irradiation and weekly low-dose cisplatin. Approximately 5% to 10% of our referral population receives irradiation alone because of medical problems that preclude chemotherapy or cystectomy.

Stage T3 Tumors

Radical Cystectomy

Forty percent to 50% of patients with clinical Stage B2 or C bladder cancer who proceed directly to cystectomy are found to have pathologic Stage D disease at operation.[141] Also, 25% of the patients with pathologic Stage B2 or C disease have tumors that were clinically Stage A or B1.[141] In comparing the results of treating pathologic Stage B2 or C disease by cystectomy alone with treating clinical Stage B2 or C disease with preoperative irradiation and cystectomy, the results are markedly biased in favor of the surgery-alone group because this group includes early-stage (clinical A or B1) cancers and excludes advanced-stage (pathologic D) cancers.

After 4000 cGy to 5000 cGy of preoperative irradiation, 50% to 75% of tumors are downstaged (*i.e.*, the pathologic stage is less than the clinical stage), and no tumor is found in 30% to

TABLE 49–6
Five-Year Bladder-Relapse Rates and Survival Rates After Treatment of T2 Bladder Carcinoma with Intraoperative or Removable Interstitial Sources

INVESTIGATOR	TREATMENT	NO. OF PATIENTS	5-YEAR BLADDER-RELAPSE RATE (%)*	5-YEAR SURVIVAL RATE (%)
Matsumoto et al[118]	Intraoperative electrons (2500–3000 cGy) plus EB† (3000–4000 cGy)	28	18	62
Williams et al[238]	^{182}Ta	76	30	41
Van der Werf-Messing et al[222]	EB (1050 cGy) plus radium	328	23	56
Battermann and Tierie[11]	EB (1050–3000 cGy) plus radium	89	26	55
Mazeron et al[119]	EB (850 cGy) plus partial cystectomy plus ^{192}Ir	30	7	55
Boiteux et al[18]	EB (1050 cGy) plus partial cystectomy plus ^{192}Ir	66	18‡	63
Van der Werf-Messing and Putten[223]	EB (4000 cGy) plus radium (within 1 wk)	48	12	73

**Relapse rates are for recurrences in the original site or elsewhere in the bladder.*
† EB: external-beam radiation therapy.
‡ Mean follow-up of 15 months.

TABLE 49–7
Five-Year Survival Results for Clinical Stage T3 Bladder Cancer After Total or Radical Cystectomy Alone

INVESTIGATOR	DATES PATIENTS ENTERED STUDY	CLINICAL STAGES	NO. OF PATIENTS	5-YEAR SURVIVAL RATE (%)
Jewett et al[91]	Not reported	B2–C	55	13
Poole-Wilson and Barnard[146]	1950–1969	T1–T3 (previously untreated)	21	24
Stadie and Kuhne[200]	1945–1965	B2–C	33	18
Brannan et al[22]	1942–1968	B2–C	22*	18†
Varkarakis et al[224]	1961–1971	B2–C–D	26‡	20
Slack et al[189]	1964–1970	T2–T4	129§	32
Marshall and McCarron[116]	1960–1971	B2–C	163	26
Whitmore et al[234]	1949–1958	B2–C	64	16
Vinnecombe and Abercrombie[228]	1966–1977	T3	17‖	35
Morabito et al[129]	1961–1978	B–C	29	24
Drago and Rohner[48]	1971–1981	"Muscle invasive"	13¶	31
Montie et al[127]	1960–1975	T3a, b; T4a	24#	40

* *Some patients received radiation therapy.*
† *Five-year survival rate was 25% for the ileal conduit group.*
‡ *Includes 21 Stage B2–C and 5 Stage D patients, of whom 18 B2–C and 4 D patients died of bladder cancer.*
§ *Fifteen percent had partial cystectomy.*
‖ *Seventeen patients had* 5-year minimum follow-up; 4000 cGy preoperative irradiation was used in an unspecified number of these patients.
¶ *Excludes seven patients treated by partial cystectomy.*
\# *Some patients received postoperative radiation therapy.*
(Parsons JT, Million RR: Int J Radiat Oncol Biol Phys 14:797, 1988)

40% of cystectomy specimens (pT0). The incidence of histologically positive pelvic lymph nodes is approximately half the incidence found in surgery-alone series.[141] Preoperative irradiation produces downstaging in papillary and solid tumors in roughly the same proportions.[17,219,233]

There has been a trend toward improved survival rates after radical cystectomy alone in recent years (Table 49-7).[22,48,91,116,127,129,146,189,200,224,228,234] The highest reported survival rate at 5 years was 40% for 24 patients, some of whom received postoperative irradiation.[127]

Tables 49-8, 49-9, and 49-10 show 5-year survival rates after 2000 cGy, 4000 cGy, and 4500 to 5000 cGy, respectively.[10,15,30,44,72,189,210,211,219] The only group for which the survival rate was consistently higher than 50% at 5 years was the high-dose (4500–5000 cGy) group. The data shown from the National Surgical Adjuvant Bladder Project exclude patients who received chemotherapy.

There have been five reported randomized trials comparing cystectomy alone with cystectomy preceded by preoperative irradiation in patients with T3 bladder cancer.[4,5,66,112,189] Four show an advantage for preoperative irradiation. The fifth study was a Veterans Administration trial that randomized only 35 patients seen over a 5-year period to either radical cystectomy or preoperative irradiation plus cystectomy. A recently reported Southwest Oncology Group trial showed no difference between cystectomy alone and preoperative irradiation plus cystectomy, but the trial included patients with Tis, Ta, T1 (high grade), T2, T3, and presumably some T4a cancers.[192] Because the trial included several subgroups (*i.e.*, Tis, Ta, and T1) for which preoperative irradiation has been shown to be of no value, and because the total dose was only 2000 cGy, the lack of an overall survival difference is not surprising.

Some investigators argue that improved survival rates in preoperatively irradiated patients are attributable to better surgical techniques than were available in the era when surgery-alone was popular.[156,183] Figure 49-3 compares "modern" cystectomy-alone series (*i.e.*, patients treated after 1960) with preoperative irradiation plus cystectomy series for all reported series with available 5-year survival results.[142] There is no evidence that contemporaneously treated cystectomy-alone patients fared as well as the preoperative irradiation group. With a single exception, the 5-year results of all preoperative irradiation series were as high as or higher than the best 5-year result (40%) reported after cystectomy alone.

TABLE 49–8
Five-Year Survival for Clinical Stage T3 Bladder Carcinoma After 2000 cGy Preoperative Irradiation Plus Cystectomy

INVESTIGATOR	DATES PATIENTS ENTERED STUDY	CLINICAL STAGE*	NO. OF PATIENTS	TREATMENT	5-YEAR SURVIVAL RATE (%)
Batata et al[10]	1966–1974	T3	106	2000 cGy/1 wk; immediate cystectomy; lymph node dissection	40

* *McGill results[160] are reported by pathologic stage and are therefore not included in the table.*
(Parsons JT, Million RR: Int J Radiat Oncol Biol Phys 14:797, 1988)

TABLE 49–9
Five-Year Survival for Clinical Stage T3 Bladder Carcinoma After 4000 cGy Preoperative Irradiation Plus Cystectomy

INVESTIGATOR	DATES PATIENTS ENTERED STUDY	CLINICAL STAGE	NO. OF PATIENTS	TREATMENT	5-YEAR SURVIVAL RATE (%)
Bloom et al[15]	1966–1975	T3	77	4000 cGy/4 wk; cystectomy and lymph node dissection 4 wk later	44*
Batata et al[10]	1959–1965†	T3	50	4000 cGy/4 wk; radical cystectomy and lymph node dissection 4–12 wk later	34
Van der Werf-Messing et al[219]	1966–1978	T3 (>5 cm)	183	4000 cGy/4 wk; simple cystectomy as soon as possible	52
Timmer et al [210]	1975+1980	T3	14‡	4000 cGy/4 wk; cystectomy 4 wk later	56

* *Cause-specific survival.*
† *Dates found in Whitmore et al.[234]*
‡ *Four of the 14 patients underwent cystoscopic reevaluation after 4000 cGy and were found to have an unfavorable tumor response.*
(Parsons JT, Million RR: Int J Radiat Oncol Biol Phys 14:797, 1988)

External-Beam Irradiation

The complete-response rate at first follow-up cystoscopy was approximately 45% in several series.[1, 15, 83, 150, 240] Complete-response rates correlated with 5-year survival rates: 50% to 70% 5-year survival for complete responders and 10% to 20% for those whose tumors persisted.[1, 15, 83, 150] The overall 5-year survival rate in most series was approximately 20% (Table 49-11).[6, 15, 46, 55, 60, 68, 70, 82, 122, 137, 150, 217] Ninety percent of treatment failures occur in the pelvis; distant metastasis alone accounts for only 10% of the failures.[82, 210, 242]

Interstitial Treatment

Bladder-relapse and survival rates after interstitial implantation of T3 bladder tumors are shown in Table 49-12.[18, 119, 221–223, 238] In the largest series, 28% of the patients developed recurrences at the site of the original lesion and 5% had recurrences elsewhere in the bladder.[222]

Summary

Some patients with T3a lesions are suitable for interstitial irradiation, usually preceded by external-beam treatment to shrink the tumor and improve the geometry of the implant. There is little experience with this approach in the United States.

If radical cystectomy is indicated, there are clear indications for administering preoperative irradiation. If neoadjuvant chemotherapy (*e.g.*, CMV or MVAC) is administered, the chemotherapy is given first, followed by irradiation, and then by cystectomy. There are no data to justify abandoning preoperative irradiation and its replacement with preoperative chemotherapy.

The indications for preoperative or interstitial irradiation in patients undergoing partial cystectomy were discussed under T2 lesions, as were the indications for external-beam irradiation with or without chemotherapy.

Stage T4 Tumors

Radical Cystectomy

Laplante and Brice[106] and Whitmore and Marshall[236] reported 49 patients with tumor invasion into their prostates and 17 with invasion into other organs (*e.g.*, cervix, uterine corpus, vagina, colon); none survived 5 years after radical cystectomy.

TABLE 49–10
Five-Year Survival for Clinical Stage T3 Bladder Carcinoma After 4500 cGy to 5000 cGy Preoperative Irradiation Plus Cystectomy

INVESTIGATOR	DATES PATIENTS ENTERED STUDY	CLINICAL STAGE	NO. OF PATIENTS	TREATMENT	5-YEAR SURVIVAL RATE (%)
Slack et al[189]	1964–1970	T2–T4	70*	4500 cGy/4–4.5 wk; cystectomy 4–8 wk later	54
DeWeerd and Colby[44]	1963–1966	T2–T4	45	4800 cGy; cystectomy; lymph node dissection	51
Chan and Johnson[30]	1969–1975	T3	89	5000 cGy/5 wk; cystectomy 6 wk later	55
Tjabbes[211]	1968–1978	T3	48	4500 cGy; immediate cystectomy	45
Hall and Heath[72]	1964–1978	T3	102	4000–4500 cGy/4–4.5 wk; cystectomy 1–6 wk later	50†

* *Received radiation therapy, cystectomy, and "no drug" or "placebo"; 5-fluorouracil patients excluded.*
† *Overall 5-year survival figure was not given in the paper, but it was calculated from available data. Survival in the 74% of patients whose tumors were downstaged was 60% and 30% in the 26% of patients whose tumors were not downstaged, giving a 5-year overall survival rate of 50.4%.*
(Parsons JT, Million RR: Int J Radiat Oncol Biol Phys 14:797, 1988)

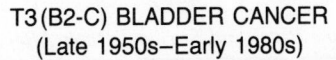

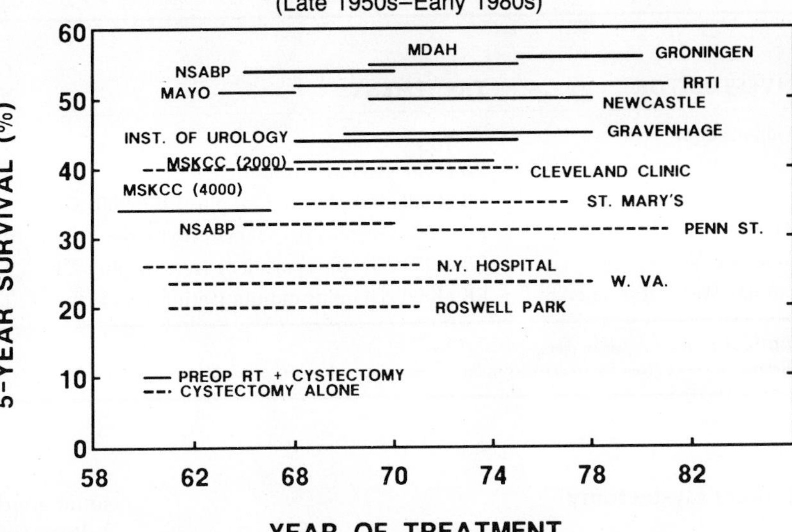

FIGURE 49–3. The 5-year survival rates (%) after total or radical cystectomy alone for seven series of patients with clinical Stage B2-C (T3) bladder cancer are depicted according to the year patients were treated (*dashed lines*). All patients were treated between 1960 and 1981. Five-year survival rates for patients treated during this period range from 20% to 40% (median, 32%). The 5-year survival rates for preoperative irradiation plus total or radical cystectomy for ten series of patients with clinical Stage B2-C (T3) bladder cancer are given according to the year patients were treated (*solid lines*). All patients were treated between 1959 and 1981. Five-year survival rates for patients treated during this period range from 34% to 55% (median, 50%). (Parsons JT, Million RR: Semin Surg Oncol 5:255, 1989)

None of the 46 pT4 patients treated by Giuliani and coworkers[67] or the 18 patients treated by Minervini and associates[124] survived 5 years after cystectomy alone. Braedel and coworkers[24] and Clark[34] each cured a single pT4 patient.

In 1977, Whitmore and associates[234] reported no 5-year survivors among 26 clinical Stage T4 patients treated by cystectomy with or without preoperative irradiation; however, there was a 13% cure rate among 116 patients with pathologic T4 disease treated by cystectomy alone and a 24% cure rate for 21 patients with pT4 disease treated by preoperative irradiation plus cystectomy, suggesting that preoperative irradiation has a role in this pathologic stage of disease.

External-Beam Irradiation

The reported 5-year survival rate in most series is approximately 10% (Table 49-13).[51, 55, 60, 63, 68, 70, 82, 122, 180, 217] Patients with T4a disease are more likely to survive than patients with T4b cancer.[63] Ninety percent of failures are due to failure to control the primary lesion; distant metastasis alone accounts for 10% of all failures.[82, 242]

TABLE 49–11
Treatment of T3 Bladder Carcinoma with External-Beam Radiation Therapy Alone

INSTITUTION	NO. OF PATIENTS	5-YEAR SURVIVAL RATE (%)
Rotterdam[217]	108	17
Coventry[16]	124	19
Edmonton[46]	23	9
M.D. Anderson Cancer Center[122]	109	20
Stanford[68]	218	28
Michigan[60]	42	19
Bern[70]	133	17
London Hospital[82]	220	38
Royal Marsden[15]	85	31
Radiumhemmet[55]	36*	37
	40†	16
Edinburgh[150]	333	26
Dublin[137]	109	20

* *Patients received three treatments per day.*
† *Patients received one treatment per day.*

Summary

For resectable T4a disease, we recommend preoperative irradiation and radical cystectomy with or without neoadjuvant chemotherapy. For patients who wish to attempt bladder preservation, external-beam irradiation with or without chemotherapy may be used.

Few patients with T4b disease are cured by any approach. We recommend treatment with CMV for three cycles and reassessment, based on response and general condition, to decide on curative treatment with irradiation plus cisplatin or low-dose palliative irradiation.

Positive Pelvic Lymph Nodes

Although some series report lower[76, 145] or higher[188] 5-year survival rates, the usual reported rates for patients with positive pelvic lymph nodes after radical cystectomy, with or without preoperative irradiation, are 15% to 25%.[15, 34, 49, 106, 160, 236]

SEQUELAE

Transurethral Resection and Intravesical Chemotherapy

Mortality rates after transurethral resection in two large series (2143 and 834 procedures) ranged from 0.6% to 1.3%.[33, 45] Severe permanent bladder contracture sometimes develops as a result of intramural fibrosis after extensive repeated TURs, with or without intravesical chemotherapy. Tiny bladder perforations, with extraperitoneal extravasation of urine, that are caused by cold-cup biopsy are probably rather common but are of no clinical significance.[181] Intraperitoneal perforations occur more rarely, but because they may cause more serious problems, they require laparotomy.[45, 245]

TABLE 49–12
Five-Year Bladder-Relapse Rates and Survival Rates After Treatment of T3 Bladder Carcinoma with Removable Interstitial Sources

INVESTIGATOR	TREATMENT*	CLINICAL STAGE	NO. OF PATIENTS	BLADDER-RELAPSE RATE† (%)	SURVIVAL RATE (%)
Williams et al[238]	^{182}Ta	T3	24	29	21
Van der Werf-Messing et al[222]	EB (1050 cGy) plus radium	T3	63	33	39
Van der Werf-Messing et al[221]	EB (1050 cGy) plus radium plus EB (3000 cGy)	T3	41		57
Mazeron et al[119]	EB (850 cGy) plus partial cystectomy plus ^{192}Ir	T3	5	0	25
Boiteux et al[18]	EB (1050 cGy) plus partial cystectomy plus ^{192}Ir	T3a	26	15	47
Van der Werf-Messing et al[223]	EB (4000 cGy) plus radium (within 1 wk)	T3	42	14	54

**EB: external-beam radiation therapy.*
† Relapse rates are given for recurrences in the original site or elsewhere in the bladder.

Radical Cystectomy

Operative mortality has declined from 15% to 20% in the 1960s to 0% to 3% in many recent cystectomy series. In several preoperative irradiation series, operative mortality was also in the 0% to 3% range, and the operative morbidity did not increase compared with cystectomy alone.[44,95,121,177,219,234]

Sequelae of Irradiation

Acute side-effects generally consist of symptoms of cystitis and diarrhea and are managed with Pyridium and Lomotil or Imodium, respectively. Patients are encouraged to drink plenty of fluids. If cystitis symptoms are severe, a urinary tract infection should be suspected; urine culture and sensitivity testing should be carried out, and antibiotic therapy initiated.

In the postirradiation period, some therapists advise their patients to delay micturation until they feel slight discomfort in an effort to "stretch" their bladders and avoid contracture that may result from fibrosis. We have no way of knowing if this is helpful, but it seems reasonable to try because no harm and some good may result. If symptoms of cystitis persist, a urine culture should be performed.

The morbidity of radical irradiation is mainly associated with complications of the bladder (8% to 10%), rectum (3% to 4%), and small bowel (1% to 2%).[51,121] The mortality rate attributable to late irradiation complications is 1%.[51]

Interstitial Irradiation

Complications in 391 patients after treatment with three 350-cGy fractions followed by an interstitial radium implant included symptomatic necrosis in four (1%) patients, stone formation in 29 (7%), severe bladder contracture in one (0.2%), and fatal complications in five (1%).[222]

Intraoperative Irradiation

Transient ureterovesical obstruction occurred in three (3%) of 116 patients treated intraoperatively with a single electron treatment of 2500 cGy to 3000 cGy followed by external-beam irradiation of 3000 cGy to 4000 cGy given over 3 to 4 weeks. Only one patient developed a contracted bladder, and no proctitis occurred.[118]

Intracavitary Irradiation

Radiation cystitis develops in 10% to 15% of patients receiving intracavitary irradiation, and in approximately 1% of those patients, it produces contracted bladders.[80,111,167]

TABLE 49–13
Treatment of T4 Bladder Carcinoma with External-Beam Radiation Therapy Alone

INVESTIGATION	NO. OF PATIENTS	5-YEAR SURVIVAL RATE (%)
Rotterdam[217]	121	12
M.D. Anderson Hospital[122]	121	9
Stanford[68]	65	8
Michigan[60]	40	11
Bern[70]	30	10
London Hospital[82]	262	9
Norwegian Radium Hospital[63]	159	16
Massachusetts General Hospital[180]	18	9
Radiumhemmet[55]	20*	22
	17†	15
Edinburgh[51]	101	12

** Patients treated three times per day.*
† Patients treated once a day.

Chemotherapy

The toxicity of MVAC is significant; Sternberg and associates[202] reported a 20% incidence of nadir sepsis and a 4% mortality. Tannock and colleagues[209] reported septic neutropenia in 18 of 41 patients and one drug-related death. The toxicity of CMV is similar, with 4% mortality and a rate of 26% for nadir sepsis.[73]

EXPERIMENTAL RADIATION THERAPY PROTOCOLS

Hyperfractionated irradiation shows some promise in the treatment of bladder cancer. In the randomized trial conducted at the Radiumhemmet from 1971 to 1978,[55] 168 patients with T2,

T3, or T4 bladder cancer were randomized to one of two treatment arms: 8400 cGy given in 100-cGy fractions three times a day (t.i.d.; 4-hour interfraction intervals) or 6400 cGy in 200-cGy fractions once a day (q.d.). In both treatment arms, there was a 2-week split after half of the total dose was administered. All patients were observed for 5 to 9 years. The 5-year survival rate of 37% for the T3 patients in the t.i.d. treatment arm was significantly better than the rate of 16% for the q.d. arm. The improvement seen in T2 patients (37% in the t.i.d. arm and 33% in the q.d. arm) and T4 patients (22% in the t.i.d. arm and 15% in the q.d. arm) was not significant. When T2, T3, and T4 patients were grouped together, the 5-year survival rates were 34% for the t.i.d. arms and 22% for the q.d. arm ($P=0.01$). There were no significant differences between the two treatment groups in the rate of severe bowel complications.

Phase I and II RTOG protocol 83-08 studied three dose levels: 6000 cGy, 6480 cGy, and 6960 cGy administered at 120 cGy twice a day.[38] Acceptable late complication rates were observed at all three dose levels.

Over the past 3 years at the University of Florida, 51 patients with muscle-invasive cancer (*i.e.*, ten with cT2; 28 with cT3; 13 with cT4) have been treated with two cycles of CMV chemotherapy followed by 6480 cGy of external-beam irradiation and concomitant cisplatin (10 mg/m^2/week) in an attempt at bladder preservation. Complete clinical response (*i.e.*, negative cystoscopy, negative cytology) was observed in 23 (45%) patients after CMV alone and in 34 (67%) patients after completion of irradiation and cisplatin. Toxic reactions were appreciable; although 90% of the patients completed two courses of chemotherapy, almost two thirds of them had dose modifications or treatment delays. There was one chemotherapy-related death. Longer follow-up is required to determine the durability of responses. These results are closely matched by those from Massachusetts General Hospital, where 50 patients had a 48% complete-response rate after two courses of CMV and a 67% complete-response rate after the addition of 4000 cGy of radiation therapy.[99] RTOG protocol 88-02 is a current phase I–II study of the use of neoadjuvant chemotherapy plus irradiation and cisplatin.

REFERENCES

1. Abratt RP, Tucker RD, Barnes DR: Radical irradiation of T2 grade III and T3 bladder cancer: Tumor response and prognosis. Int J Radiat Oncol Biol Phys 9:1213, 1983
2. Ahlering TE, Kanellos A, Boyd SD, et al: A comparative study of perioperative complications with Kock pouch urinary diversion in highly irradiated versus nonirradiated patients. J Urol 139:1202,1988
3. Akaza H: Progress and controversies in chemotherapy of advanced unresectable and/or metastatic carcinoma of the bladder. In Schröder FH, Kurth KH, Splinter TAW, et al (eds): EORTC Genitourinary Group Monograph 5: Progress and Controversies in Oncological Urology II, pp 539–548. New York, Alan R Liss, 1988
4. Anderström C, Johansson S, Nilsson S, et al: A prospective randomized study of preoperative irradiation with cystectomy or cystectomy alone for invasive bladder carcinoma. Eur Urol 9:142, 1983
5. Awwad H, Abd El-Baki HA, El-Bolkainy N, et al: Pre-operative irradiation of T3 carcinoma in bilharzial bladder: A comparison between hyperfractionation and conventional fractionation. Int J Radiat Oncol Biol Phys 5:787, 1979
6. Backhouse TW: A rotation technique for irradiation of the bladder and the results obtained. Clin Radiol 30:259, 1979
7. Baker R: Correlation of circumferential lymphatic spread of vesical cancer with dept of infiltration. Relation to present methods of treatment. J Urol 73:681, 1955
8. Barnes RW, Dick AL, Hadley HL, et al: Survival following transurethral resection of bladder carcinoma. Cancer Res 37:2895, 1977
9. Barringer BS: Radium therapy of bladder cancer: Retrospect and prospect. J Urol 68:280, 1952
10. Batata MA, Chu FCH, Hilaris BS, et al: Preoperative whole pelvis versus true pelvis irradiation and/or cystectomy for bladder cancer. Int J Radiat Oncol Biol Phys 7:1349, 1981
11. Battermann JJ, Tierie AH: Results of implantation for T1 and T2 bladder tumours. Radiother Oncol 5:85, 1986
12. Beahrs OH, Myers MH (eds): American Joint Committee on Cancer: Manual for Staging of Cancer, 2nd ed. Philadelphia, JB Lippincott, 1983
13. Bell JT, Burney SW, Friedell GH: Blood vessel invasion in human bladder cancer. J Urol 105:675, 1971
14. Bloom HJG: Pre-operative intermediate-dose radiotherapy and cystectomy for deeply invasive carcinoma of the bladder: Rationale and results. In Oliver RTD, Hendry WF, Bloom HJG (eds): Bladder Cancer: Principles of Combination Therapy, pp 151–174. London, Butterworths, 1981
15. Bloom HJG, Hendry WF, Wallace DM, et al: Treatment of T3 bladder cancer: Controlled trial of pre-operative radiotherapy and radical cystectomy versus radical radiotherapy: Second report and review (for the Clinical Trials Group, Institute of Urology). Br J Urol 54:136, 1982
16. Boileau MA: Segmental or partial cystectomy. In Johnson DE, Boileau MA (eds): Genitourinary Tumors: Fundamental Principles and Surgical Techniques, pp 457–465. New York, Grune & Stratton, 1982
17. Boileau MA, Johnson DE, Chan RC, et al: Bladder carcinoma: Results with preoperative radiation therapy and radical cystectomy. Urology 16:569, 1980
18. Boiteux J-P, Rozan R, Giraud B, et al: Interstitial iridium-192 therapy for bladder cancer. A multicentric survey (Abstract 75). J Urol 139:181A, 1988
19. Boswell WD Jr: Diagnostic imaging in genitourinary cancer. In Skinner DG, Lieskovsky G (eds): Diagnosis and Management of Genitourinary Cancer, pp 237–263. Philadelphia, WB Saunders, 1988
20. Bracken RB, McDonald MW, Johnson DE: Cystectomy for superficial bladder cancer. Urology 18:459, 1981
21. Brannan W, Ochsner MG, Fuselier HA Jr, et al: Partial cystectomy in the treatment of transitional cell carcinoma of the bladder. J Urol 119:213, 1978
22. Brannan W, Ochsner MG, Whitehead CM Jr, et al: Cystectomy and segmental resection for primary carcinoma of the bladder: Experience at Ochsner Clinic 1942–1968. South Med J 66:241, 1973
23. Braun EV, Ali M, Fayemi AO, et al: Primary signet-ring cell carcinoma of the urinary bladder: Review of the literature and report of a case. Cancer 47:1430, 1981
24. Bredael JJ, Croker BP, Glenn JF: The curability of invasive bladder cancer treated by radical cystectomy. Eur Urol 6:206, 1980
25. Bretton PR, Herr HW, Whitmore WF Jr, et al: Intravesical bacillus Calmette-Guerin therapy for *in situ* transitional cell carcinoma involving the prostatic urethra. J Urol 141:853, 1989
26. Brick SH, Friedman AC, Pollack HM, et al: Urachal carcinoma: CT findings. Radiology 169:377, 1988
27. Bukowski RM, Montie JE, Pontes EJ: Neoadjuvant chemotherapy of locally advanced transitional cell carcinoma of the bladder: Results of a phase II trial and followup (Abstract 424). Proc Annu Meet Am Soc Clin Oncol 6:108, 1987
28. Carmichael J, Cornbleet MA, MacDougall RH, et al: Cisplatin and methotrexate in the treatment of transitional cell carcinoma of the urinary tract. Br J Urol 57:299, 1985
29. Carver JH: Interstitial radiation in the treatment of selected cases of cancer of the bladder. Br J Urol 31:313, 1959
30. Chan RC, Johnson DE: Integrated therapy for invasive bladder carcinoma: Experience with 108 patients. Urology 12:549, 1978

31. Chevlen EM, Awwad HK, Ziegler JL, et al: Cancer of the bilharzial bladder. Int J Radiat Oncol Biol Phys 5:921, 1979
32. Chougule P, Young J Jr, Aygun C, et al: Radiation therapy for transitional cell bladder carcinoma: A ten-year experience. Urology 32:91, 1988
33. Cifuentes Delatte L, Garcia de la Peña E, Vela Navarrete R: Survival rates of patients with bladder tumours: An experience of 1744 cases (1950–1978). Br J Urol 54:267, 1982
34. Clark PB: Radical cystectomy for carcinoma of the bladder. Br J Urol 50:492, 1978
35. Clayson DB: Recent research into occupational bladder cancer. In Connelly JG (ed): Carcinoma of the Bladder, pp 13–24. New York, Raven Press, 1981
36. Costello AJ, Tiptaft RC, England HR, et al: Squamous cell carcinoma of bladder. Urology 23:234, 1984
37. Cowles RS, Johnson DE, McMurtrey MJ: Long-term results following thoracotomy for metastatic bladder cancer. Urology 20:390, 1982
38. Cox JD, Guse C, Asbell S, et al: Tolerance of pelvic normal tissues to hyperfractionated radiation therapy: Results of protocol 83-08 of the Radiation Therapy Oncology Group. Int J Radiat Oncol Biol Phys 15:1331, 1988
39. Cramer SF, Aikawa M, Cebelin M: Neurosecretory granules in small cell invasive carcinoma of the urinary bladder. Cancer 47:724, 1981
40. Cummings KB, Mason JT, Correa RJ Jr, et al: Segmental resection in the management of bladder carcinoma. J Urol 119:56, 1978
41. Cutler SJ, Heney NM, Friedell GH: Longitudinal study of patients with bladder cancer: Factors associated with disease recurrence and progression. In Bonney WW, Prout GR Jr (eds): Bladder Cancer, pp 35–46. Baltimore, Williams & Wilkins, 1982
42. DeFillipo N, Blute R, Klein LA: Signet-ring cell carcinoma of bladder: Evaluation of three cases with review of literature. Urology 29:479, 1987
43. Denis L, Hendrickx G: Preoperative chemotherapy in T3/T4-NX-M0 bladder cancer (Abstract 475). J Urol 135:222A, 1986
44. DeWeerd JH, Colby MY Jr: Bladder carcinoma treated by irradiation and surgery: Interval report. J Urol 109:409, 1973
45. Dick A, Barnes R, Hadley H, et al: Complications of transurethral resection of bladder tumors: Prevention, recognition and treatment. J Urol 124:810, 1980
46. Dick DAL: Carcinoma of the bladder treated by external irradiation. Br J Urol 34:340, 1962
47. Dix VW, Shanks W, Tresidder GC, et al: Carcinoma of the bladder: Treatment by diathermy snare excision and interstitial irradiation. Br J Urol 42:213, 1970
48. Drago JR, Rohner TJ Jr: Bladder cancer: Results of radical cystectomy for invasive and recurrent superficial tumors. J Urol 130:460, 1983
49. Dretler SP, Ragsdale BD, Leadbetter WF: The value of pelvic lymphadenectomy in the surgical treatment of bladder cancer. J Urol 109:414, 1973
50. Duncan W, Arnott SJ, Jack WJL, et al: A report of a randomized trial of d(15) + Be neutrons compared with megavoltage x-ray therapy of bladder cancer. Int J Radiat Oncol Biol Phys 11:2043, 1985
51. Duncan W, Quilty PM: The results of a series of 963 patients with transitional cell carcinoma of the urinary bladder primarily treated by radical megavoltage x-ray therapy. Radiother Oncol 7:299, 1986
52. Duncan W, Williams JR, Kerr GR, et al: An analysis of the radiation related morbidity observed in a randomized trial of neutron therapy for bladder cancer. Int J Radiat Oncol Biol Phys 12:2085, 1986
53. Eapen L, Stewart D, Danjoux C, et al: Intraarterial cisplatin and concurrent radiation for locally advanced bladder cancer. J Clin Oncol 7:230, 1989
54. Edland RW, Wear JB Jr, Ansfield FJ: Advanced cancer of the urinary bladder: An analysis of the results of radiotherapy alone *vs.* radiotherapy and concomitant 5-fluorouracil: A prospective randomized study of 36 cases. Am J Roentgenol Radium Ther Nucl Med 108:124, 1970
55. Edsmyr F, Andersson L, Esposti PL, et al: Irradiation therapy with multiple small fractions per day in urinary bladder cancer. Radiother Oncol 4:197, 1985
56. Evans RA, Texter JH Jr: Partial cystectomy in the treatment of bladder cancer. J Urol 114:391, 1975
57. Faysal MH: Urethrectomy in men with transitional cell carcinoma of bladder. Urology 16:23, 1980
58. Faysal MH: Squamous cell carcinoma of the bladder. J Urol 126:598, 1981
59. Faysal MH, Freiha FS: Evaluation of partial cystectomy for carcinoma of bladder. Urology 14:352, 1979
60. Fish JC, Fayos JV: Carcinoma of the urinary bladder: Influence of dose and volume irradiated on survival. Radiology 118:179, 1976
61. Fitzpatrick JM, West AB, Butler MR, et al: Superficial bladder tumors (stage pTa, grades 1 and 2): The importance of recurrence pattern following initial resection. J Urol 135:920, 1986
62. Fokkens W: Phenacetin abuse related to bladder cancer. Environ Res 20:192, 1979
63. Fosså SD, Kaalhus O, Sauer T, et al: Radiotherapy of T4 bladder carcinoma. Radiother Oncol 1:291, 1984
64. Freiha FS, Faysal MH: Salvage cystectomy. Urology 22:496, 1983
65. Friedman M, Lewis LG: Irradiation of carcinoma of the bladder by a central intracavitary radium or cobalt 60 source (the Walter Reed technique). Am J Roentgenol Radium Ther Nucl Med 79:6, 1958
66. Ghoneim MA, Ashamallah AK, Awaad HK, et al: Randomized trial of cystectomy with or without preoperative radiotherapy for carcinoma of the bilharzial bladder. J Urol 134:266, 1985
67. Giuliani L, Giberti C, Martorana G, et al: Results of radical cystectomy for primary bladder cancer: Retrospective study of more than 200 cases. Urology 26:243, 1985
68. Goffinet DR, Schneider MJ, Glatstein EJ, et al: Bladder cancer: Results of radiation therapy in 384 patients. Radiology 117:149, 1975
69. Goodman GB, Hislop TG, Elwood JM, et al: Conservation of bladder function in patients with invasive bladder cancer treated by definitive irradiation and selective cystectomy. Int J Radiat Oncol Biol Phys 7:569, 1981
70. Greiner R, Skaleric C, Veraguth P: The prognostic significance of ureteral obstruction in carcinoma of the bladder. Int J Radiat Oncol Biol Phys 2:1095, 1977
71. Guinan P, Crispen R, Rubenstein M: BCG in management of superficial bladder cancer. Urology 30:515, 1987
72. Hall RR, Heath AB: Radiotherapy and cystectomy for T3 bladder carcinoma. Br J Urol 53:598, 1981
73. Harker WG, Meyers FJ, Freiha FS, et al: Cisplatin, methotrexate, and vinblastine (CMV): An effective chemotherapy regimen for metastatic transitional cell carcinoma of the urinary tract. A Northern California Oncology Group study. J Clin Oncol 3:1463, 1985
74. Henderson RH, Parsons JT, Morgan L, et al: Elective ilioinguinal lymph node irradiation. Int J Radiat Oncol Biol Phys 10:811, 1984
75. Heney NM, Nocks BN, Daly JJ, et al: Ta and T1 bladder cancer: Location, recurrence and progression. Br J Urol 54:152, 1982
76. Heney NM, Proppe K, Prout GR Jr, et al: Invasive bladder cancer: Tumor configuration, lymphatic invasion and survival. J Urol 130:895, 1983
77. Henry K, Miller J, Mori M, et al: Comparison of transurethral resection to radical therapies for stage B bladder tumors. J Urol 140:964, 1988
78. Hermansen DK, Reuter VE, Whitmore WF Jr, et al: Flow cytometry and cytology as response indicators to M-VAC (methotrexate, vinblastine, doxorubicin and cisplatin). J Urol 140:1394, 1988
79. Herr HW, Whitmore WF Jr: Ureteral carcinoma *in situ* after successful intravesical therapy for superficial bladder tumors: Incidence, possible pathogenesis and management. J Urol 138:292, 1987
80. Hewitt CB, Babiszewski JF, Antunez AR: Update on intracavitary radiation in the treatment of bladder tumors. J Urol 126:323, 1981

81. Hillcoat BL, Raghavan D: A randomized comparison of cisplatinum (C) versus cisplatinum and methotrexate (C + M) in advanced bladder cancer (Abstract 426). Proc Annu Meet Am Soc Clin Oncol 5:110, 1986
82. Hope-Stone HF, Blandy JP, Oliver RTD, et al: Radical radiotherapy and salvage cystectomy in the treatment of invasive carcinoma of the bladder. In Oliver RTD, Hendry WF, Bloom HJG (eds): Bladder Cancer: Principles of Combination Therapy, pp 127–138. London, Butterworths, 1981
83. Hope-Stone HF, Oliver RTD, England HR, et al: T3 bladder cancer: Salvage rather than elective cystectomy after radiotherapy. Urology 24:315, 1984
84. Horne DW, Fauver HE: Primary signet-ring cell carcinoma of bladder. Urology 30:574, 1987
85. Hrushesky WJM, Roemeling RV, Wood PA, et al: High-dose intensity systemic therapy of metastatic bladder cancer. J Clin Oncol 5:450, 1987
86. Ibrahim NBN, Briggs JC, Corbishley CM: Extrapulmonary oat cell carcinoma. Cancer 54:1645, 1984
87. Jacobi GH, Engelmann U, Hohenfellner R: Classification of bladder tumours. In Zingg EJ, Wallace DMA (eds): Bladder Cancer, pp 117–139. Berlin, Springer-Verlag, 1985
88. Jacobo E, Loening S, Schmidt JD, et al: Primary adenocarcinoma of the bladder: A retrospective study of 20 patients. J Urol 117:54, 1977
89. Jacobsen A-B, Lunde S, Ous S, et al: T2/T3 bladder carcinomas treated with definitive radiotherapy with emphasis on flow cytometric DNA ploidy values. Int J Radiat Oncol Biol Phys 17:923, 1989
90. Jakse G, Frommhold H, Nedden DZ: Combined radiation and chemotherapy for locally advanced transitional cell carcinoma of the urinary bladder. Cancer 55:1659, 1985
91. Jewett HJ, King LR, Shelley WM: A study of 365 cases of infiltrating bladder cancer: Relation of certain pathological characteristics to prognosis after extirpation. J Urol 92:668, 1964
92. Johnson DE, Boileau MA: Bladder cancer: Overview. In Johnson DE, Boileau MA (eds): Genitourinary Tumors: Fundamental Principles and Surgical Techniques, pp 399–447. New York, Grune & Stratton, 1982
93. Johnson DE, Hodge GB, Abdul-Karim FW, et al: Urachal carcinoma. Urology 26:218, 1985
94. Johnson DE, Hogan JM, Ayala AG: Primary adenocarcinoma of the urinary bladder. South Med J 65:527, 1972
95. Johnson DE, Lamy SM: Complications of a single stage radical cystectomy and ileal conduit diversion: Review of 214 cases. J Urol 117:171, 1977
96. Johnson DE, Schoenwald MB, Ayala AG, et al: Squamous cell carcinoma of the bladder. J Urol 115:542, 1976
97. Jones WA, Gibbons RP, Correa RJ Jr, et al: Primary adenocarcinoma of the bladder. Urology 15:119, 1980
98. Kanoh S, Umeyama T, Nemoto S, et al: Long-term intra-arterial infusion chemotherapy with Adriamycin for advanced bladder cancer. Cancer Chemother Pharmacol 11 (Suppl):51, 1983
99. Kaufman DS, Prout GR Jr, Shipley WU, et al: Upfront MCV chemotherapy plus cisplatin and radiotherapy: Its efficacy in successful bladder preservation in 50 patients with invasive cancer (Abstract 500). Proc Annu Meet Am Soc Clin Oncol 8:129, 1989
100. Kaufman JM, Fam B, Jacobs SC, et al: Bladder cancer and squamous metaplasia in spinal cord injury patients. J Urol 118:967, 1977
101. Khandekar JD, Elson PJ, DeWys WD, et al: Comparative activity and toxicity of *cis*-diamminedichloroplatinum (DDP) and a combination of doxorubicin, cyclophosphamide, and DDP in disseminated transitional cell carcinomas of the urinary tract. J Clin Oncol 3:539, 1985
102. Kock NG, Ghoneim MA, Lycke KG, et al: Urinary diversion to the augmented and valved rectum: Preliminary results with a novel surgical procedure. J Urol 140:1375, 1988
103. Kock NG, Ghoneim MA, Lycke KG, et al: Replacement of the bladder by the urethral Kock pouch: Functional results, urodynamics, and radiological features. J Urol 141:1111, 1989
104. Kock NG, Nilson AE, Nilsson LO, et al: Urinary diversion via a continent ileal reservoir: Clinical results in 12 patients. J Urol 128:469, 1982
105. Kramer SA, Bredael J, Croker BP, et al: Primary non-urachal adenocarcinoma of the bladder. J Urol 121:278, 1979
106. Laplante M, Brice M II: The upper limits of hopeful application of radical cystectomy for vesical carcinoma: Does nodal metastasis always indicate incurability? J Urol 109:261, 1973
107. Logothetis CJ, Dexeus FH, Chong C, et al: Cisplatin, cyclophosphamide and doxorubicin chemotherapy for unresectable urothelial tumors: The M.D. Anderson experience. J Urol 141:33, 1989
108. Long RTL, Grummon RA, Spratt JS, et al: Carcinoma of the urinary bladder (comparison with radical, simple, and partial cystectomy and intravesical formalin). Cancer 29:98, 1972
109. Lutzeyer W, Rübben H, Dahm H: Prognostic parameters in superficial bladder cancer: An analysis of 315 cases. J Urol 127:250, 1982
110. Maatman TJ, Montie JE, Bukowski RM, et al: Intra-arterial chemotherapy as an adjuvant to surgery in transitional cell carcinoma of the bladder. J Urol 135:256, 1986
111. Maatman TJ, Novick AC, Montague DK, et al: Radiation-induced cystitis following intracavitary irradiation for superficial bladder cancer. J Urol 130:338, 1983
112. Madsen PO, Hoyme UB, Byar DP, et al: No differences reported in 10-year survival rates in three bladder cancer groups. (Paper presented to the North Central Section of the AUA.) Urol Times April:20, 1980
113. Magri J: Partial cystectomy: A review of 104 cases. Br J Urol 34:74, 1962
114. Mahadevia PS, Koss LG, Tar IJ: Prostatic involvement in bladder cancer: Prostate mapping in 20 cystoprostatectomy specimens. Cancer 58:2096, 1986
115. Marshall VF, The relation of preoperative estimate to the pathologic demonstration of the extent of vesical neoplasms. J Urol 68:714, 1952
116. Marshall VF, McCarron JP Jr: The curability of vesical cancer: Greater now or then? Cancer Res 37:2753, 1977
117. Masina F: Segmental resection for tumours of the urinary bladder: Ten-year follow-up. Br J Surg 52:279, 1965
118. Matsumoto K, Kakizoe T, Mikuriya S, et al: Clinical evaluation of intraoperative radiotherapy for carcinoma of the urinary bladder. Cancer 47:509, 1981
119. Mazeron J-J, Crook J, Chopin D, et al: Conservative treatment of bladder carcinoma by partial cystectomy and interstitial iridium 192. Int J Radiat Oncol Biol Phys 15:1323, 1988
120. McDonald JR, Thompson GJ: Carcinoma of the urinary bladder: A pathologic study with special reference to invasiveness and vascular invasion. J Urol 60:435, 1948
121. Miller LS: Bladder cancer: Superiority of preoperative irradiation and cystectomy in clinical stages B2 and C. Cancer 39:973, 1977
122. Miller LS, Johnson DE: Megavoltage irradiation for bladder cancer: Alone, postoperative, or preoperative? Genitourinary Cancer 10:771, 1973
123. Mills SE, Wolfe JT III, Weiss MA, et al: Small cell undifferentiated carcinoma of the urinary bladder: A light-microscopic, immunocytochemical, and ultrastructural study of 12 cases. Am J Surg Pathol 11:606, 1987
124. Minervini R, Carlino F, Fiorentini L: Total cystectomy and ureterosygmoidostomy for carcinoma of the bladder. Eur Urol 9:80, 1983
125. Mohiuddin M, Kramer S, Newall J, et al: Combined pre- and postoperative adjuvant radiotherapy for bladder cancer: Results of RTOG/Jefferson study. Cancer 47:2840, 1981
126. Mohiuddin M, Kramer S, Newall J, et al: Combined preoperative and postoperative radiation for bladder cancer: Results of RTOG/Jefferson study. Cancer 55:963, 1985
127. Montie JE, Straffon RA, Stewart BH: Radical cystectomy without radiation therapy for carcinoma of the bladder. J Urol 131:477, 1984
128. Montie JE, Whitmore WF Jr, Grabstald HM, et al: Unresectable carcinoma of the bladder. Cancer 51:2351, 1983
129. Morabito RA, Kandzari SJ, Milam DF: Invasive bladder car-

cinoma treated by radical cystectomy: Survival of patients. Urology 14:478, 1979

130. Morrison R: The results of treatment of cancer of the bladder: A clinical contribution to radiobiology. Clin Radiol 26:67, 1975
131. Mostofi FK: Pathological aspects and spread of carcinoma of the bladder. JAMA 206:1764, 1968
132. Mostofi FK, Davis CJ Jr, Sesterhenn IA: Pathology of tumors of the urinary tract. In Skinner DG, Lieskovsky G (eds): Diagnosis and Management of Genitourinary Cancer, pp 83–117. Philadelphia, WB Saunders, 1988
133. Mostofi FK, Thomson RV, Dean AL Jr: Mucous adenocarcinoma of the urinary bladder. Cancer 8:741, 1955
134. Narumi Y, Sato T, Kuriyama K, et al: Vesical dome tumors: Significance of extravesical extension on CT. Radiology 169:383, 1988
135. Nocks BN, Heney NM, Daly JJ: Primary adenocarcinoma of urinary bladder. Urology 21:26, 1983
136. Novick AC, Stewart BH: Partial cystectomy in the treatment of primary and secondary carcinoma of the bladder. J Urol 116:570, 1976
137. O'Flynn JD, Smith JM, Hanson JS: Transurethral resection for the assessment and treatment of vesical neoplasms: A review of 840 consecutive cases. Eur J Urol 1:38, 1975
138. Ojeda L, Johnson DE: Partial cystectomy: Can it be incorporated into integrated therapy program? Urology 22:115, 1983
139. Oldbring J, Glifberg I, Mikulowski P, et al: Carcinoma of the renal pelvis and ureter following bladder carcinoma: Frequency, risk factors and clinicopathological findings. J Urol 141:1311, 1989
140. Parmar MKB, Freedman LS, Hargreave TB, et al: Prognostic factors for recurrence and follow-up policies in the treatment of superficial bladder cancer with a report from the British Medical Research Council Subgroup on Superficial Bladder Cancer (Urologic Cancer Working Party). J Urol 142:284, 1989
141. Parsons JT, Million RR: Planned preoperative irradiation in the management of clinical stage B2-C (T3) bladder carcinoma. Int J Radiat Oncol Biol Phys 14:797, 1988
142. Parsons JT, Million RR: Role of planned preoperative irradiation in the management of clinical stage B2-C(T3) bladder carcinoma in the 1980s. Semin Surg Oncol 5:255, 1989
143. Parsons JT, Thar TL, Bova FJ, et al: An evaluation of split-course irradiation for pelvic malignancies. Int J Radiat Oncol Biol Phys 6:175, 1980
144. Pearson RM, Soloway MS: Does cyclophosphamide induce bladder cancer? Urology 11:437, 1978
145. Pomerance A: Pathology and prognosis following total cystectomy for carcinoma of bladder. Br J Urol 44:451, 1972
146. Poole-Wilson DS, Barnard RJ: Total cystectomy for bladder tumours. Br J Urol 43:16, 1971
147. Pritchett TR, Schiff WM, Klatt E, et al: The potency-sparing radical cystectomy: Does it compromise the completeness of the cancer resection? J Urol 140:1400, 1988
148. Prout GR Jr, Griffin PP, Daly JJ: The outcome of conservative treatment of carcinoma *in situ* of the bladder. J Urol 138:766, 1987
149. Quilty PM, Duncan W: The influence of hemoglobin level on the regression and long term local control of transitional cell carcinoma of the bladder following photon irradiation. Int J Radiat Oncol Biol Phys 12:1735, 1986
150. Quilty PM, Duncan W: Primary radical radiotherapy for T3 transitional cell cancer of the bladder: An analysis of survival and control. Int J Radiat Oncol Biol Phys 12:853, 1986
151. Quilty PM, Duncan W: Radiotherapy for squamous carcinoma of the urinary bladder. Int J Radiat Oncol Biol Phys 12:861, 1986
152. Quilty PM, Duncan W: Treatment of superficial (T1) tumours of the bladder by radical radiotherapy. Br J Urol 58:147, 1986
153. Quilty PM, Duncan W, Chisholm GD, et al: Results of surgery following radical radiotherapy for invasive bladder cancer. Br J Urol 58:396, 1986
154. Quilty PM, Duncan W, Kerr GR: Results of a randomized study to evaluate influence of dose on morbidity in radiotherapy for bladder cancer. Clin Radiol 36:615, 1985
155. Quilty PM, Kerr GR, Duncan W: Prognostic indices for bladder cancer: An analysis of patients with transitional cell carcinoma of the bladder primarily treated by radical megavoltage x-ray therapy. Radiother Oncol 7:311, 1986
156. Radwin HM: Radiotherapy and bladder cancer: A critical review. J Urol 124:43, 1980
157. Raghavan D, Pearson B, Duval P, et al: Initial intravenous cisplatinum therapy: Improved management for invasive high risk bladder cancer? J Urol 133:399, 1985
158. Raghavan D, Wallace DMA, Sandeman T, et al: First randomized trials of pre-emptive (neoadjuvant) intravenous (IV) cisplatin (CDDP) for invasive transitional cell carcinoma of bladder (TCCB) (Abstract 516). Proc Annu Meet Am Soc Clin Oncol 8:133, 1989
159. Rathert P, Melchior H, Lutzeyer W: Phenacetin: A carcinogen for the urinary tract? J Urol 113:653, 1975
160. Reid EC, Oliver JA, Fishman IJ: Preoperative irradiation and cystectomy in 135 cases of bladder cancer. Urology 8:247, 1976
161. Resnick MI, O'Conor VJ: Segmental resection for carcinoma of the bladder: Review of 102 patients. J Urol 109:1007, 1973
162. Richards B, Bastable JRG, Freedman L, et al: Adjuvant chemotherapy with doxorubicin (Adriamycin) and 5-fluorouracil in T3, NX, M0 bladder cancer treated with radiotherapy. Br J Urol 55:386, 1983
163. Rotman M, Macchia R, Silverstein M, et al: Treatment of advanced bladder carcinoma with irradiation and concomitant 5-fluorouracil infusion. Cancer 59:710, 1987
164. Rübben H, Lutzeyer W, Wallace DMA: The epidemiology and aetiology of bladder cancer. In Zingg EJ, Wallace DMA (eds): Bladder Cancer, pp 1–21. Berlin, Springer-Verlag, 1985
165. Rubin P: The impact of supervoltage irradiation on the treatment of bladder carcinoma. J Urol 86:82, 1961
166. Rundle JSH, Hart AJL, McGeorge A, et al: Squamous cell carcinoma of bladder: A review of 114 patients. Br J Urol 54:522, 1982
167. Russell KJ, Koh W-J, Russell AH, et al: Combined intracavitary and external beam irradiation for superficial transitional cell carcinoma of the bladder: An alternative to cystectomy for patients with recurrence after intravesical chemotherapy. J Urol 141:30, 1989
168. Sauer R, Schrott KM, Dunst J, et al: Preliminary results of treatment of invasive bladder carcinoma with radiotherapy and cisplatin. Int J Radiat Oncol Biol Phys 15:871, 1988
169. Schellhammer PF, Whitmore WF Jr: Transitional cell carcinoma of the urethra in men having cystectomy for bladder cancer. J Urol 115:56, 1976
170. Scher H, Reuter V, Sternberg C, et al: Pathologic response to M-VAC (methotrexate, vinblastine, Adriamycin and cisplatin) in urothelial tract tumors (Abstract 410). Proc Annu Meet Am Soc Clin Oncol 6:105, 1987
171. Scher HI, Yagoda A, Herr Hw, et al: Neoadjuvant M-VAC (methotrexate, vinblastine, doxorubicin and cisplatin) effect on the primary bladder lesion. J Urol 139:470, 1988
172. Schlagel PN, Walsh PC: Neuroanatomical approach to radical cystoprostatectomy with preservation of sexual function. J Urol 138:1402, 1987
173. Schoborg TW, Sapolsky JL, Lewis CW Jr: Carcinoma of the bladder treated by segmental resection. J Urol 122:473, 1979
174. Shearer RJ, Chilvers CED, Bloom HJG, et al: Adjuvant chemotherapy in T3 carcinoma of the bladder. A prospective trial: Preliminary report. Br J Urol 62:558, 1988
175. Sheldon CA, Clayman RV, Gonzalez R, et al: Malignant urachal lesions. J Urol 131:1, 1984
176. Sherwood T: Upper urinary tract tumours following on bladder carcinoma: Natural history of urothelial neoplastic disease. Br J Radiol 44:137, 1971
177. Shipley WU: Radiation therapy for patients with bladder carcinoma: Rationale, results, techniques, and possible innovations. In Bonney WW, Prout GR Jr (eds): AUA Monographs:

Bladder Cancer, 1:243–259. Baltimore, Williams & Wilkins, 1982

178. Shipley WU: Radiation therapy of bladder carcinoma. ASTRO refresher course, Los Angeles, CA 1983
179. Shipley WU, Prout GR Jr, Einstein AB, et al: Treatment of invasive bladder cancer by cisplatin and radiation in patients unsuited for surgery. JAMA 258:931, 1987
180. Shipley WU, Rose MA, Perrone TL, et al: Full-dose irradiation for patients with invasive bladder carcinoma: Clinical and histological factors prognostic of improved survival. J Urol 134:679, 1985
181. Sigler LJ, Addonizio JC, Fernandez R, et al: Incidence and treatment of bladder perforation following bladder biopsy. Urology 26:10, 1985
182. Silverberg E, Lubera JA: Cancer statistics, 1989. CA 39:3, 1989
183. Skinner DG: Current perspectives in the management of high-grade invasive bladder cancer. Cancer 45:1866, 1980
184. Skinner DG, Daniels JR, Lieskovsky G: Current status of adjuvant chemotherapy after radical cystectomy for deeply invasive bladder cancer. Urology 24:46, 1984
185. Skinner DG, Kaufman JJ: Management of invasive and high grade bladder cancer. In Skinner DG, deKernion JB (eds): Genitourinary Cancer, pp 269–283. Philadelphia, WB Saunders, 1978
186. Skinner DG, Lieskovsky G: Management of invasive and high-grade bladder cancer. In Skinner DG, Lieskovsky G (eds): Diagnosis and Management of Genitourinary Cancer, pp 295–312. Philadelphia, WB Saunders, 1988
187. Skinner DG, Lieskovsky G, Boyd S: Continent urinary diversion. J Urol 141:1323, 1989
188. Skinner DG, Tift JP, Kaufman JJ: High dose, short course preoperative radiation therapy and immediate single stage radical cystectomy with pelvic node dissection in the management of bladder cancer. J Urol 127:671, 1982
189. Slack NH, Bross IDJ, Prout GR Jr: Five-year follow-up results of a collaborative study of therapies for carcinoma of the bladder. J Surg Oncol 9:393, 1977
190. Smith G, Elton RA, Beynon LL, et al: Prognostic significance of biopsy results of normal-looking mucosa in cases of superficial bladder cancer. Br J Urol 55:665, 1983
191. Smith JA Jr, Batata M, Grabstald H, et al: Preoperative irradiation and cystectomy for bladder cancer. Cancer 49:869, 1982
192. Smith JA Jr, Crawford ED, Blumenstein B, et al: A randomized prospective trial of pre-operative irradiation plus radical cystectomy versus surgery alone for transitional cell carcinoma of the bladder: A Southwest Onclogy Group study (Abstract 416). J Urol 139:266A, 1988
193. Smith JA Jr, Whitmore WF Jr: Salvage cystectomy for bladder cancer after failure of definitive irradiation. J Urol 125:643, 1981
194. Soloway MS: Introduction and overview of intravesical therapy for superficial bladder cancer. Urology 31(suppl 3):5, 1988
195. Soloway MS: Diagnosis and management of superficial bladder cancer. Semin Surg Oncol 5:247, 1989
196. Soloway MS, Einstein A, Corder MP, et al: A comparison of cisplatin and the combination of cisplatin and cyclophosphamide in advanced urothelial cancer: A National Bladder Cancer Collaborative Group A study. Cancer 52:767, 1983
197. Soto EA, Friedell GH, Tiltman AJ: Bladder cancer as seen in giant histologic sections. Cancer 39:447, 1977
198. Spera JA, Whittington R, Littman P, et al: A comparison of preoperative radiotherapy regimens for bladder carcinoma: The University of Pennsylvania experience. Cancer 61:255, 1988
199. Splinter TAW, Schröder FH, Denis L, et al: A Phase-II study of neoadjuvant chemotherapy in T3-4N0-XM0 Transitional cell carcinoma of the bladder: A preliminary analysis. Eur Urol 14(suppl 1):24, 1988
200. Stadie G, Kuhne U: Late results of cystectomy in carcinoma of the urinary bladder. Int Urol Nephrol 3:379, 1971
201. Stein JJ, Kaufman JJ: The treatment of carcinoma of the bladder with special reference to the use of preoperative radiation therapy combined with 5-fluorouracil. Am J Roentgenol Radium Ther Nucl Med 102:519, 1968
202. Sternberg CN, Yagoda A, Scher HI, et al: M-VAC (methotrexate, vinblastine, doxorubicin and cisplatin) for advanced transitional cell carcinoma of the urotherlium. J Urol 139:461, 1988
203. Stoter G, Splinter TAW, Child JA, et al: Combination chemotherapy with cisplatin and methotrexate in advanced transitional cell cancer of the bladder. J Urol 137:663, 1987
204. Straus KL, Littman P, Wein AJ, et al: Interstitial iridium-192 treatment for invasive bladder carcinoma (Abstract 189). Int J Radiat Oncol Biol Phys 11(suppl 1):188, 1985
205. Swanson DA, Liles A, Zagars GK: Preoperative irradiation and radical cystectomy for stages T2 and T3 squamous cell carcinoma of the bladder. J Urol 143:37, 1990
206. Swanson DA, von Eschenbach AC, Bracken RB, et al: Salvage cystectomy for bladder carcinoma. Cancer 47:2275, 1981
207. Swanson PE, Brooks R, Pearse H, et al: Small cell carcinoma of urinary bladder. Urology 32:558, 1988
208. Tannenbaum M, Romas NA: The pathobiology of early urothelial cancers. In Skinner DG, deKernion JB (eds): Genitourinary Cancer, pp 232–255. Philadelphia, WB Saunders, 1978
209. Tannock I, Gospodarowicz M, Connolly J, et al: M-VAC (methotrexate, vinblastine, doxorubicin and cisplatin) chemotherapy for transitional cell carcinoma: The Princess Margaret Hospital experience. J Urol 142:289, 1989
210. Timmer PR, Hartlief HA, Hooijkaas JAP: Bladder cancer: Pattern of recurrence in 142 patients. Int J Radiat Oncol Biol Phys 11:899, 1985
211. Tjabbes D: Surgical treatment of 81 deep infiltrating bladder tumours after preoperative irradiation. In Pavone-Macaluso M, Smith PH, Edsmyr F (eds): Bladder Tumors and Other Topics in Urological Oncology, vol 1, pp 283–285. New York, Plenum Press, 1980
212. Tolley DA, Hargreave TB, Smith PH, et al: Effect of intravesical mitomycin C on recurrence of newly diagnosed superficial bladder cancer: Interim report from the Medical Research Council Subgroup on Superficial Bladder Cancer (Urological Cancer Working Party). Br Med J 296:1759, 1988
213. Troner M, Birch R, Omura GA, et al: Phase III comparison of cisplatin alone versus cisplatin, doxorubicin and cyclophosphamide in the treatment of bladder (urothelial) cancer: A Southeastern Cancer Study Group trial. J Urol 137:660, 1987
214. Utz DC, DeWeerd JH: The management of low grade, low stage carcinoma of the bladder. In Skinner DG, deKernion JB (eds): Genitourinary Cancer, pp 256–268. Philadelphia, WB Saunders, 1978
215. Utz DC, Farrow GM, Rife CC, et al: Carcinoma *in situ* of the bladder. Cancer 45:1842, 1980
216. Utz DC, Schmitz SE, Fugelso PD, et al: A clinicopathologic evaluation of partial cystectomy for carcinoma of the urinary bladder. Cancer 32:1075, 1973
217. Van der Werf-Messing BHP: Carcinoma of the bladder treated by suprapubic radium implants: The value of additional external irradiation. Eur J Cancer 5:277, 1969
218. Van der Werf-Messing BHP: Cancer of the urinary bladder treated by interstitial radium implant. Int J Radiat Oncol Biol Phys 4:373, 1978
219. Van der Werf-Messing BHP, Friedell GH, Menon RS, et al: Carcinoma of the urinary bladder T3NXM0 treated by preoperative irradiation followed by simple cystectomy. Int J Radiat Oncol Biol Phys 8:1849, 1982
220. Van der Werf-Messing BHP, Hop WCJ: Carcinoma of the urinary bladder (category T1NXM0) treated either by radium implant or by transurethral resection only. Int J Radiat Oncol Biol Phys 7:299, 1981
221. Van der Werf-Messing BHP, Menon RS, Hop WCJ: Carcinoma of the urinary bladder category T3NXM0 treated by the combination of radium implant and external irradiation: Second report. Int J Radiat Oncol Biol Phys 9:177, 1983

222. Van der Werf-Messing BHP, Menon RS, Hop WCJ: Cancer of the urinary bladder category T2, T3, (NXM0) treated by interstitial radium implant: Second report. Int J Radiat Oncol Biol Phys 9:481, 1983
223. Van Der Werf-Messing BHP, van Putten WLJ: Carcinoma of the urinary bladder category T2,3 NXM0 treated by 40 Gy external irradiation followed by cesium[137] implant at reduced dose (50%). Int J Radiat Oncol Biol Phys 16:369, 1989
224. Varkarakis MJ, Gaeta J, Moore RH, et al: Prognosis of bladder carcinoma in patients treated with cystectomy. Int Urol Nephrol 7:38, 1975
225. Veenema RJ, Harisiadis L, Chang C, et al: Preliminary external radiotherapy used as a means for selecting complete treatment. In Connolly JG (ed): Carcinoma of the Bladder, pp 183–191. New York, Raven Press, 1981
226. Veronesi A, Galligioni E, Lo Re G, et al: Combination chemotherapy with fluorouracil, Adriamycin, *cis*-platinum and VM-26 in advanced transitional cell carcinoma of the urinary tract. Eur J Cancer Clin Oncol 22:1457, 1986
227. Villar A, Munoz J, Aguiló F, et al: External beam irradiation for T1, T2-3 and T4 transitional cell carcinoma of the urinary bladder. Radiother Oncol 9:209, 1987
228. Vinnicombe J, Abercrombie GF: Total cystectomy: A review. Br J Urol 50:488, 1978
229. Walsh PC, Donker PJ: Impotence following radical prostatectomy: Insight into etiology and prevention. J Urol 128:492, 1982
230. Washecka R, Geisler E, Johanson K-E: Case profile: Colonic carcinoma involving the bladder. Urology 26:511, 1985
231. Webb JN: The histopathology of bladder cancer. In Zingg EJ, Wallace DMA (eds): Bladder Cancer, pp 23–51. Berlin, Springer-Verlag, 1985
232. Weiss J, Parsons J, Klimberg IW, et al: Treatment of muscle invasive transitional cell carcinoma of the bladder with external beam and interstitial radiotherapy (Abstract 73). J Urol 139:181A, 1988
233. Whitmore WF: Integrated irradiation and cystectomy for bladder cancer. Br J Urol 52:1, 1980
234. Whitmore WF Jr, Batata MA, Ghoneim MA, et al: Radical cystectomy with or without prior irradiation in the treatment of bladder cancer. J Urol 118:184, 1977
235. Whitmore WF Jr, Batata MA, Hilaris BS, et al: A comparative study of two preoperative radiation regimens with cystectomy for bladder cancer. Cancer 40:1077, 1977
236. Whitmore WF Jr, Marshall VF: Radical total cystectomy for cancer of the bladder: 230 consecutive cases five years later. J Urol 87:853, 1962
237. Whitmore WF III, Prout GR Jr: Discouraging results for high dose external beam radiation therapy in low stage (0 and A) bladder cancer. J Urol 127:902, 1982
238. Williams GB, Trott PA, Bloom HJG: Carcinoma of the bladder treated by interstitial irradiation. Br J Urol 53:221, 1981
239. Williams RD: Cystectomy following CMV chemotherapy for extensive TCC of the bladder (Abstract 426). J Urol 139:269A, 1988
240. Wolf H, Olsen PR, Højgaard K: Urothelial dysplasia concomitant with bladder tumours. A determinant for future new occurrences in patients treated by full-course radiotherapy. Lancet 1:1005, 1985
241. Woodruff MW, Murphy WT, Hodson JM: Further observations on the use of combination 5-fluorouracil and supervoltage irradiation therapy in the treatment of advanced carcinoma of the bladder. J Urol 90:747, 1963
242. Yu WS, Sagerman RH, Chung CT, et al: Bladder carcinoma: Experience with radical and preoperative radiotherapy in 421 patients. Cancer 56:1293, 1985
243. Zincke H, Garbeff PJ, Beahrs JR: Upper urinary tract transitional cell cancer after radical cystectomy for bladder cancer. J Urol 131:50, 1984
244. Zingg EJ, Plowman PN, Wallace DMA, et al: Treatment of muscle invasive bladder cancer. In Zingg EJ, Wallace DMA (eds): Bladder Cancer, pp 189–234. Berlin, Springer-Verlag, 1985
245. Zingg EJ, Wallace DMA: The treatment of superficial bladder tumours. In Zingg EJ, Wallace DMA (eds): Bladder Cancer, pp 161–187. Berlin, Springer-Verlag, 1985

50

Female Urethra

Perry W. Grigsby

ANATOMY

The female urethra is approximately 4.0 cm long and extends from the urinary bladder through the urogenital diaphragm to the vestibule, where it forms the urethral meatus. Because of the proximity of the symphysis pubis, a small curve is formed with an anterior concavity. The dorsal urethral boundary abuts the anterior vaginal wall.

The wall of the urethra consists of three layers. The muscular layer is continuous with that of the bladder. At the vesicle end of the urethra, this muscular wall forms the internal sphincter. The voluntary urethral sphincter is at the plane of the urogenital diaphragm. A thin layer of erectile tissue consisting of a plexus of veins and muscle fibers forms the middle layer of the wall. The mucous membrane is continuous with the bladder proximally and the vulva distally. This membrane consists of transitional epithelium near the bladder but distally changes to nonkeratinizing stratified squamous epithelium and pseudostratified columnar epithelium. The distal urethra also contains small mucous recesses and periurethral or Skene's glands, most of which are in the region of the meatus.

The lymphatic drainage of the urethral meatus parallels that of the vulva to the superficial and deep inguinal and external iliac lymph nodes. The primary drainage of the entire urethra is mainly to the obturator and internal and external iliac nodes.

EPIDEMIOLOGY

Carcinoma of the urethra in women is rare. Only a few cases are seen annually at major cancer centers.[11,15,21,22] About 1500 cases have been reported in the literature. Carcinoma of the female urethra makes up 0.02% of all cancers in women and accounts for about 0.1% of all gynecologic cancers. The average patient age at the time of diagnosis is 60 years, with most patients between 50 and 80 years old.[9,19,24]

NATURAL HISTORY

A tumor of the urethral meatus at an early stage may resemble a urethral caruncle or a prolapse of the mucosa through the urethral orifice.[3] As the lesion progresses, it enlarges and eventually ulcerates.[18]

During the later stages, cancers of the middle or posterior urethra tend to extend upward into the urinary bladder, downward to invade the remainder of the urethra, and posteriorly into the vaginal mucosa. Lesions involving the anterior urethra account for approximately 30% of all cases.[2,9,23]

Regional lymph node involvement is uncommon in early tumors (Stage 0) of the urethral meatus.[2] Advanced tumors (Stages II, III) of the urethra have been associated with a 35% to 50% incidence of inguinal or pelvic lymph node involvement.[2,6,8,14,19,25] Bilateral nodal involvement occurs in about one third of patients with positive nodes. Grabstald and associates[9] confirmed nodal involvement in 24 of 25 patients with clinically palpable nodes. In their series of patients with advanced disease, 26 underwent pelvic lymph node sampling, and 13 (50%) were found to have nodal involvement.

Distant metastases are found in approximately 10% of patients at presentation, and about 30% to 50% ultimately die of distant disease. The most common sites of metastasis are lung, liver, bone, and brain.[9,18]

CLINICAL PRESENTATION

Bleeding is the prevailing presenting sign.[1] About 30% of patients experience pain, difficulty in urinating, and frequent micturition. Urinary retention and overflow incontinence may occur in advanced cases. Less frequently cited signs and symptoms are a mass in the introitus (10% to 20% of patients), dyspareunia, perineal pain, and inguinal lymphadenopathy.[7,8,18] Urethrovaginal and vesicovaginal fistulae may develop in advanced, neglected cases.[3]

Small tumors involving the urethral meatus are often mistakenly diagnosed as urethral caruncle, a benign, inflammatory lesion.[3] However, larger lesions of the distal urethra are readily identified on inspection. Tumors occupying the proximal urethra produce a fusiform enlargement, which can be palpated during pelvic examination.

DIAGNOSTIC WORKUP

An outline for the diagnostic workup for carcinoma of the female urethra is presented in Table 50-1. A routine history and general physical examination should be performed for all pa-

TABLE 50–1
Diagnostic Workup for Carcinoma of the Female Urethra

GENERAL
- History
- Physical examination, including detailed pelvic examination under anesthesia

SPECIAL PROCEDURES
- Urine cytology
- Punch biopsy
- Urethroscopy
- Cystoscopy
- Rectosigmoidoscopy (advanced stages or if symptomatic)

RADIOGRAPHIC EVALUATION
- Standard
  - Chest radiographs
  - Intravenous urography
  - Computed tomography scan (abdomen and pelvis)
  - Barium enema (advanced stages or if symptomatic)
- Complementary
  - Urethrography
  - Lymphangiography

LABORATORY EVALUATION
- Complete blood count
- Chemistry profile
- Urinalysis

tients. A detailed pelvic examination under anesthesia is necessary to fully evaluate the clinical extent of the disease. This examination can be performed at the time of urethroscopy and cystoscopy.

Urine cytologic analyses have a high false-negative rate. The definitive diagnosis is made by punch or incisional biopsy.

Routine radiographic evaluation should include chest radiographs, an intravenous urogram, and a computed tomography scan of the abdomen and pelvis. Complementary studies include a barium enema for patients with symptoms or advanced disease, urethrography, and lymphangiography.

STAGING SYSTEMS

Many attempts have been made to formulate a staging system for carcinoma of the urethra. Urethral tumors can be classified in two groups: those involving the distal half of the urethra and those located in the proximal or entire urethra. Most authors have found that this classification correctly depicts the feasibility of treatment and the prognosis. A staging system based on location has been proposed by Prempree, Amornmarn, and Patanaphan (Table 50-2).[20] The TNM staging system of the American Joint Committee on Cancer is shown in Table 50-3.

PATHOLOGIC CLASSIFICATION

Squamous cell carcinoma is the most prevalent histologic category in cancer of the female urethra, representing almost 70% of all cases. Other histologic types include transitional cell carcinoma (15% to 20%) and adenocarcinoma (10% to 15%).[17,21] The remainder includes melanoma, anaplastic tumors, lymphomas, and metastatic lesions.[4,21]

TABLE 50–2
Proposed Clinical Staging System for Carcinoma of the Female Urethra

TUMOR STAGE	CHARACTERISTICS
Stage I	Disease limited to distal one half of urethra
Stage II	Disease involving entire urethra, with extension to periurethral tissues, but not involving vulva or bladder neck
Stage III	
A	Disease involving urethra and vulva
B	Disease invading vaginal mucosa
C	Disease involving urethra and bladder neck
Stage IV	
A	Disease invading parametrium or paracolpium
B	Metastasis
1	Inguinal lymph nodes
2	Pelvic lymph nodes
3	Paraaortic
4	Distant

(Prempree T, Amornmarn R, Patanaphan V: Cancer 54:729, 1984)

PROGNOSTIC FACTORS

The most important factors in determining prognosis and survival are the tumor size and location. Grigsby and associates[10] demonstrated a worsening prognosis with increased tumor size (Fig. 50-1). Eighty-one percent of patients with lesions less than 2 cm had 5-year progression-free survival, compared with 37% of those with lesions 2 cm to 4 cm and 7% of patients with lesions more than 4 cm ($P = 0.0001$). For lesions confined to the proxi-

TABLE 50–3
TNM Classification of Carcinoma of the Urethra

PRIMARY TUMOR (T)

TX	Primary tumor cannot be assessed
T0	No evidence of primary tumor
Tis	Carcinoma *in situ*
Ta	Noninvasive papillary, polypoid, or verrucous carcinoma
T1	Tumor invades subepithelial connective tissue
T2	Tumor invades corpus spongiosum or prostate or periurethral muscle
T3	Tumor invades corpus cavernosum or beyond the prostatic capsule or the anterior vagina or the bladder neck
T4	Tumor invades other adjacent organs

REGIONAL LYMPH NODES (N)

NX	Regional lymph nodes cannot be assessed
N0	No regional lymph node metastasis
N1	Metastasis in a single lymph node, ≤ 2 cm in greatest dimension
N2	Metastasis in a single lymph node, > 2 cm but < 5 cm in greatest dimension, or multiple lymph nodes, none > 5 cm in greatest dimension
N3	Metastasis in a lymph node > 5 cm in greatest dimension

DISTANT METASTASIS (M)

MX	Presence of distant metastasis cannot be assessed
M0	No distant metastasis
M1	Distant metastasis

(Beahrs OH, Henson DE, Hutter RVP, Myers MH [eds]: American Joint Committee on Cancer, Manual for Staging of Cancer, 3rd ed. Philadelphia, JB Lippincott, 1988)

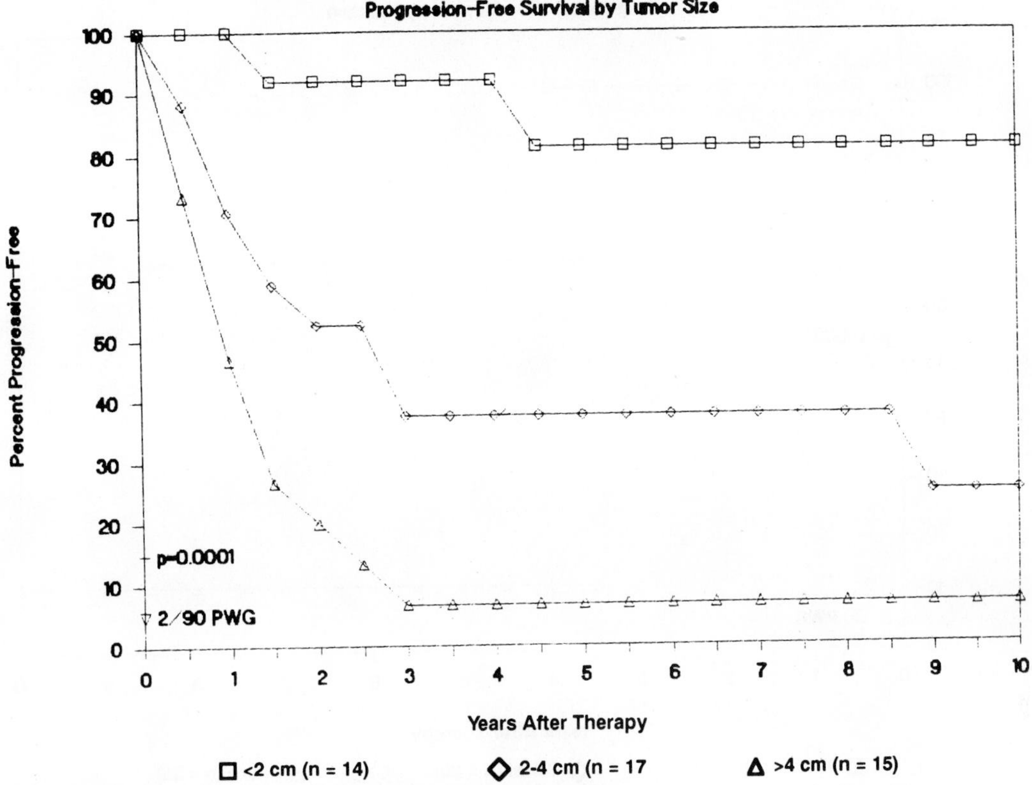

FIGURE 50–1. Progression-free survival by tumor size.

mal urethra, there was local control in all four patients. However, the patients with tumors involving the distal urethra had a 5-year progression-free survival rate of 69%, and there was a 12% survival rate for those with involvement of the entire urethra ($P=0.0001$) (Fig. 50-2). Patients with meatal tumors, if diagnosed early and treated appropriately, can achieve an 80% to 90% survival rate.[3] Bladder neck involvement, parametrial extension, and inguinal lymph node involvement have been identified as poor prognostic factors.

Patients with adenocarcinoma have been reported to have a good prognosis, but most studies have shown no difference in survival among patients with adenocarcinoma, squamous cell carcinoma, and transitional cell carcinoma.[2,5,9,19,23] Primary melanoma of the urethra, although rare, has a very poor prognosis.[24]

GENERAL MANAGEMENT

Several therapeutic approaches are employed in the management of carcinoma of the female urethra. The variety of treatments reflect the dimensions and locations of disease and the approaches of the treating physicians.

Anterior Urethral Cancer

Open excision, electroexcision, fulguration, or loser coagulation are possible for tumors at the meatus or with *in situ* involvement of the distal urethra (Stage 0). For larger and more invasive lesions (Stage I), interstitial irradiation or a combination of interstitial and external-beam irradiation are alternatives to surgical resection of the distal third of the urethra. Anterior urethral lesions treated by local excision or radiation therapy that recur may require anterior exenteration and urinary diversion.

If inguinal nodes are involved, ipsilateral node dissection or irradiation is indicated, because cure is still achievable with limited regional nodal metastases. If no inguinal adenopathy exists, node dissection is not recommended, but prophylactic groin irradiation is recommended for patients with invasive lesions.

Posterior Urethral Cancer

Cancers of the posterior or entire urethra (Stages II, III, and IV), are usually associated with invasion of the bladder and a high incidence of inguinal and pelvic lymph node metastases. The best results have been achieved with preoperative irradiation with exenterative surgery and urinary diversion. In selected patients, it is possible to remove part of the pubic symphysis and the inferior pubic rami to maximize the surgical margin. Perineal closure and vaginal reconstruction can be accomplished with the use of myocutaneous flaps.

Recurrent Urethral Cancer

Locally recurrent urethral cancer after radiation therapy should be treated by surgical excision. Locally recurrent urethral cancer after surgery alone should be considered for combination radiation therapy and wider surgical resection. Metastatic urethral cancer should be considered for investigational chemotherapy.

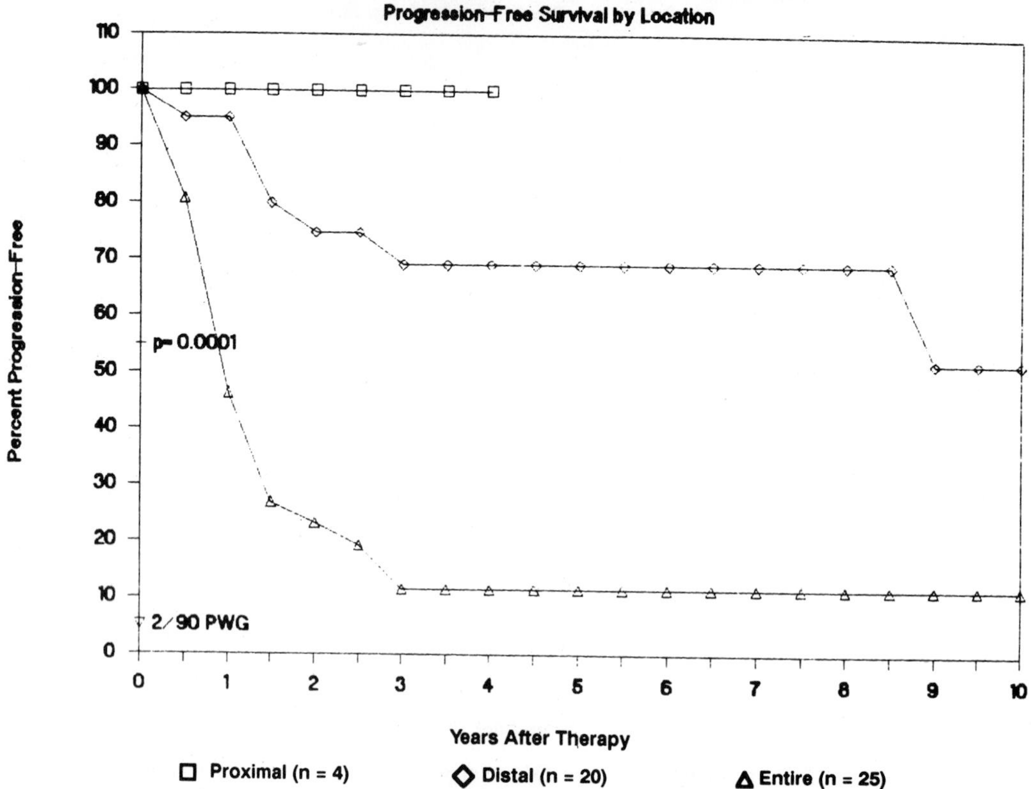

FIGURE 50–2. Progression-free survival by tumor location.

RADIATION THERAPY TECHNIQUES

Interstitial implant has been the usual method for treating meatal carcinomas. Radium needles, forming a double-plane or a volume implant, have been employed (Fig. 50-3). Afterloading implants using ^{192}Ir have replaced radium.[12] For localized disease, a volume implant composed of 8 to 12 needles arranged in an arc around the urethral orifice is used (Fig. 50-4). It is often difficult to use additional needles for crossing purposes. Increasing the active length of the needles can eliminate the need for crossed ends in most cases. After radiographs are used to verify needle placement (Fig. 50-5), a dose of 6000 cGy to 7000 cGy can be given in 6 to 7 days (40 cGy/hour to the target volume) when an implant alone is employed.

Large tumors extending into the labia, vagina, entire urethra, or base of the bladder cannot be treated with an implant alone. For these patients a combination of external-beam irradiation and implant is recommended. The external-beam portal should flash the perineum in order to cover the entire urethra. The portal should be wide enough to cover the inguinal nodes and extend cephalad to the L4–L5 interspace to include the pelvic nodes (Fig. 50-6). A bolus, appropriate for the photon energy employed, should be added to the groins when inguinal nodes are positive. The whole pelvis is treated to a dose of 2000 cGy. A midline block is added, and an additional 3000 cGy is delivered to the inguinal and pelvic nodes. A boost of 1000 cGy to 1500 cGy is delivered to positive nodes through reduced anteroposterior fields. At some institutions, the dose to the whole pelvis is 4000 cGy, with an additional dose of 1000 cGy given to the parametria with midline shielding.

In patients with advanced disease, the primary tumor is treated with a vaginal cylinder to bring the dose to the entire urethra to approximately 6000 cGy. An interstitial implant is administered to raise the total tumor dose to 7000 cGy to 8000 cGy. Intracavitary irradiation with the vaginal cylinder and an interstitial implant are almost never employed simultaneously, because of the resultant high dose rate at the vaginal mucosa interface of the intracavitary and interstitial implant. A vaginal cylinder with partial shielding posteriorly can be used in selected patients.

A limiting factor in the use of external-beam irradiation is the tolerance of the perineal skin (*i.e.*, confluent moist desquamation). Extensive disease combined with advanced age can be formidable obstacles to completing the irradiation course. Diligent personal hygiene and individualized care are necessary if patients are to complete the course of treatment.

RESULTS OF THERAPY

Surgery

Five of seven patients with early meatal tumors were cured of disease in the series reported by Grabstald and co-workers[9] after partial urethrectomy. In the remaining two patients, both local recurrences and distant metastases developed. Bracken and associates[5] reported local control in only one of four patients treated with local excision only for distal urethral lesions. Peterson and colleagues[18] reported two patients in whom squamous cell carcinomas were excised successfully. In the same

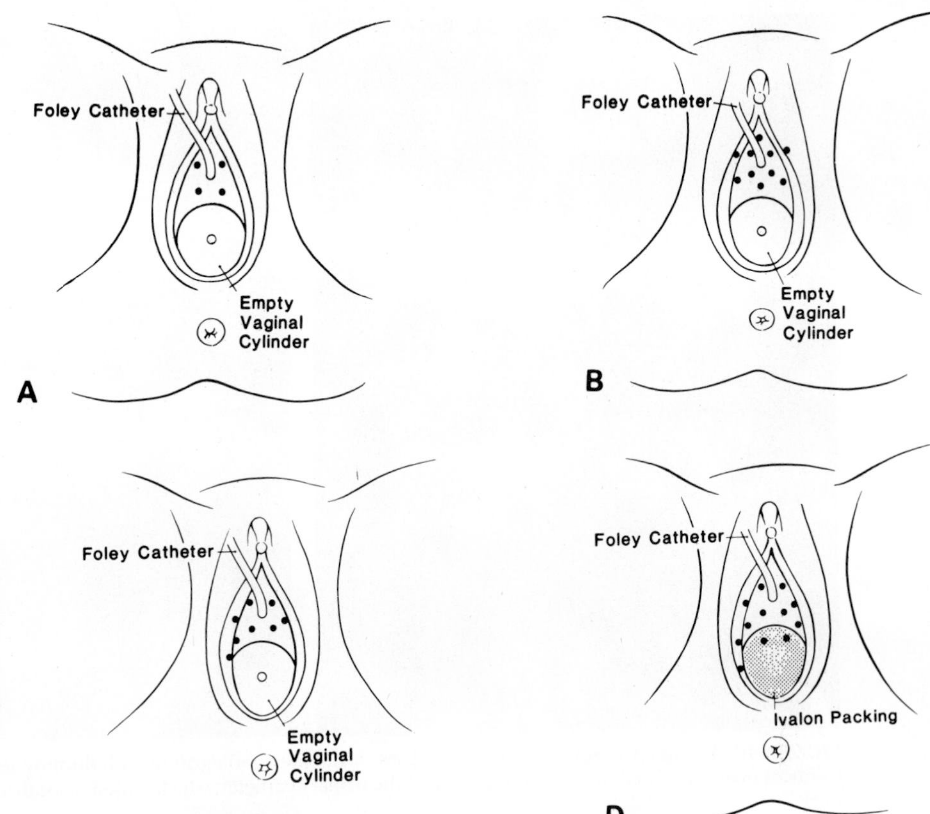

FIGURE 50–3. Diagrams of implants. (**A**) Tumor limited to the urethra. (**B**) Tumor extending to the periurethral tissues or originating in the periurethral glands. (**C**) Tumor extending into the vagina or labia minora. (**D**) Tumor involving the suburethral area. (Delclos L: Carcinoma of the female urethra. In Johnson DE, Boileau MA [eds]: Genitourinary Tumors, pp 275–286. New York, Grune & Stratton, 1982)

series, a patient with adenocarcinoma treated with local excision developed a local recurrence and left inguinal adenopathy 4 years later.

Grabstald and co-workers[9] performed radical surgery on 15 patients with advanced disease; there were only three survivors at 5 years. Peterson and others[18] performed radical surgery on seven patients, with three alive at 5 years. Primary radical cystectomy with anterior vaginectomy and total urethrectomy was performed on eight patients by Mayer and associates.[16] Only three of these patients were free of disease at 1, 4, and 11 years.

Radiation Therapy

Control of tumors of the urethral meatus or the distal urethra with irradiation alone is satisfactory. A literature review indicates that early meatal tumors have cure rates of 70% to 90%.[20]

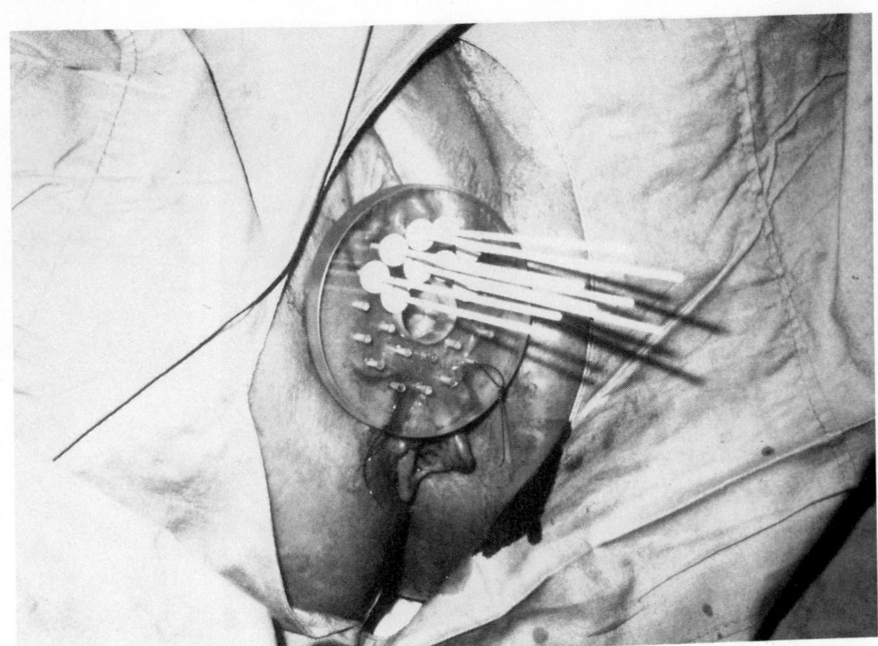

FIGURE 50–4. A template is used for a curved, double-plane implant that surrounds the urethra, The closed-end flexible catheters inserted in the periurethral or vaginal tissues are glued to the template, which is sutured to the skin. The catheters are afterloaded with ^{192}Ir.

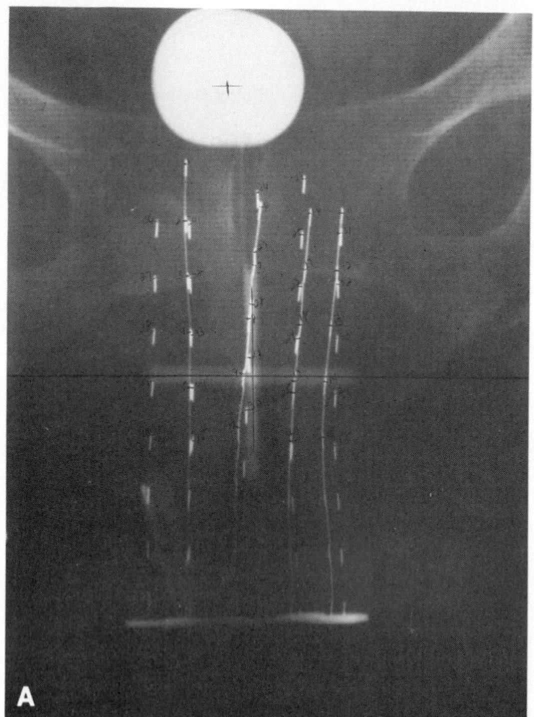
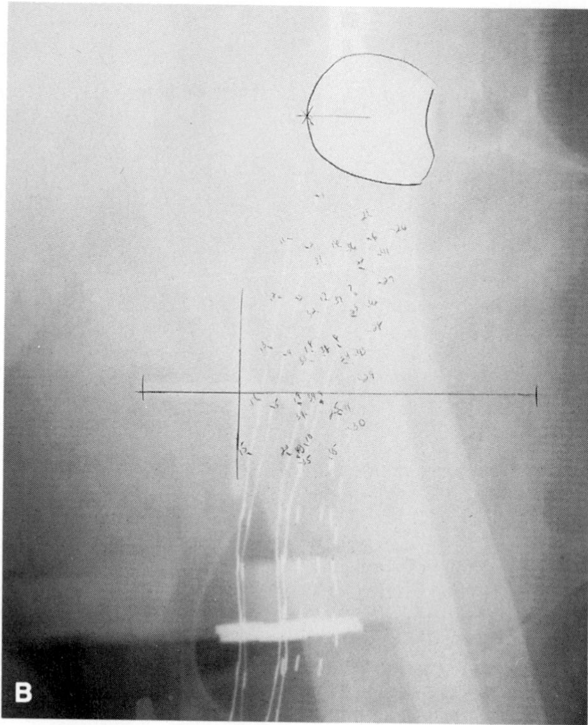

FIGURE 50–5. (**A**) Anteroposterior and (**B**) lateral simulator radiographs with dummy seeds in place. Contrast material is used to inflate the balloon of the urinary catheter, which is used to localize the bladder neck.

Chu[6] reported 5-year progression-free survival rate of 64% for 11 patients with tumor involvement of the anterior urethra treated with irradiation alone. Prempree and associates[20] treated three patients with Stage I disease with interstitial irradiation alone (5000–6500 cGy) and achieved local control in all three. In the same series, two of four patients with Stage II disease had local control and were alive 5 years after treatment. Weghaupt and co-workers[25] reported a 5-year survival rate of 71.4% for 42 patients with cancer of the anterior urethra. Their doses ranged from 5500 cGy to 7000 cGy from intracavitary and external irradiation.

Tumors of the proximal urethra or involving the entire

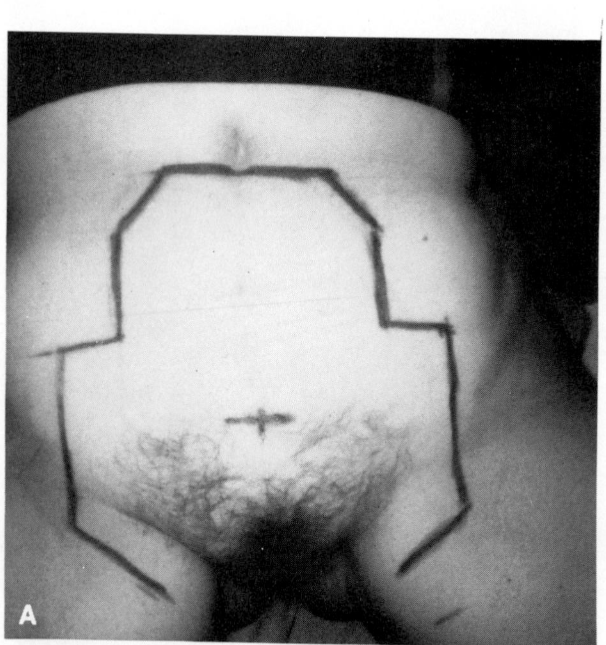
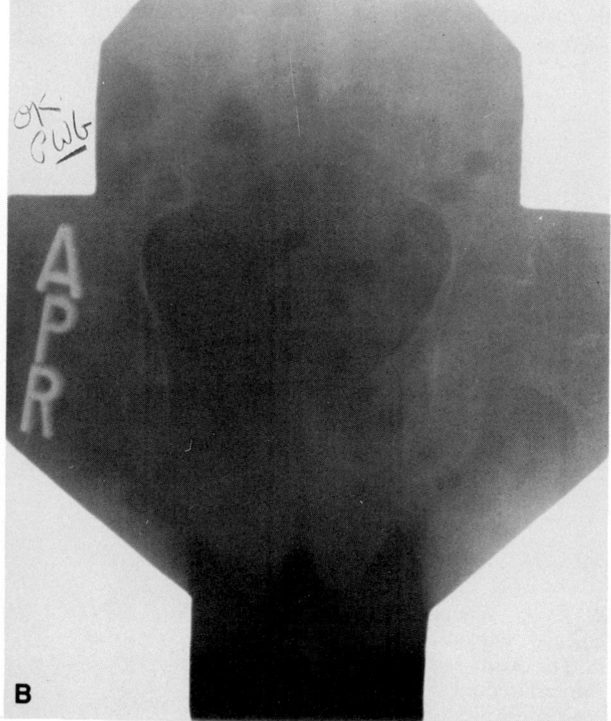

FIGURE 50–6. (**A**) External marking and (**B**) anteroposterior simulation film of a pelvic portal. Notice the lateral extension of the portal to cover the inguinal lymph nodes.

TABLE 50–4
Summary of Treatment Results

INVESTIGATOR	NO. OF PATIENTS	STAGE*	TREATMENT†	PELVIC CONTROL	5-YEAR DISEASE-FREE SURVIVAL
DeSai[7]	10	I			4/10 (40%)
	6	III			1/06 (17%)
Taggart[23]	11	I	RT	7/11	7/11 (64%)‡
Antoniades[2]	9	I	RT	8/09	8/09 (89%)
	7	III	RT	1/07	2/07 (29%)
	4	IV	RT	1/04	2/04 (50%)
	3	I	S + R	3/03	2/03 (67%)
Bracken[5]	30	I–II	RT(19), R + S(8), S(3)		(45%–50%)§
	44	III–IV	RT(35), R + S(1), S(8)		(20%–25%)§
Pointon[19]	26	I	RT		20/26 (77%)‖
	52	II–IV	RT		22/52 (42%)‖
Grabstald[8]	13	I	RT		3/13 (23%)
	10	I	S		8/10 (80%)
	3	I	R + S		2/03 (67%)
	14	III	RT		1/14 (7%)
	17	III	S		3/17 (18%)
	17	III	R + S		5/17 (29%)
Weghaupt[25]	42	I	RT		30/42 (71%)
	20	III	RT		10/20 (50%)
Peterson[18]	25	I	RT(5), R + S(6), S(14)		13/25 (52%)
	24	III	RT(15), R + S(4), S(5)		5/24 (21%)
Chu[6]	11	I	RT		7/11 (64%)
		III	RT		0/11 (0%)
Turner[24]	13	I	RT(8), S(5)		(80%)§
	7	II	RT		(20%)‡
	13	III	RT(12), S(1)		(60%)§
	6	IV	RT(5), S(1)		(20%)§
Prempree[20]	3	I	RT	3/3	3/03 (100%)
	4	II	RT	2/4	2/04 (50%)
	6	III	RT(5), R + S(1)	5/6	4/05 (80%)

** Clinical stage determined by review of the investigator's description of the tumor.*
† RT, radiation therapy; S, surgery; S + R, surgery plus radiation therapy.
‡ Disease-free survival at 2 years.
§ Estimated from survival curves.
‖ Crude 3-year survival rate.

urethra are more difficult to treat. The overall local control rate is 20% to 30%. Bracken and others[5] treated 81 patients, and the 5-year survival rate was about 25% for Stage III and 20% for Stage IV patients. Weghaupt and associates[24] reported 20 patients with tumor involvement of the posterior urethra who received irradiation alone or preoperative irradiation and surgery. The 5-year survival rate for these patients was 50%. Preoperative irradiation combined with radical surgery is an approach employed by Klein and colleagues.[14] They treated five women in this manner and achieved a 5-year survival rate of 40%. Table 50-4 summarizes treatment results.

SEQUELAE OF THERAPY

Complications as a result of surgery, irradiation, or combined modality therapy can be significant. Urethral strictures develop in some patients, necessitating dilatation or urinary diversion. Others may develop incontinence, cystitis, and vaginal stenosis. Severe complications are fistula formation, bowel obstruction, and occasionally operative mortality. In the case of advanced neoplasms, fistula formation may be unavoidable because of tumor erosion of the organ and subsequent tumor necrosis. The complication rates reported vary greatly, from 0% to 42%, because of different tumor stages, the extent of surgery, and various irradiation doses.[2,5,6,12,19,20]

CLINICAL TRIALS

A nonrandomized phase II multicenter study employing trimetrexate is available for patients with locally advanced and metastatic disease of the urothelial tract (*i.e.*, transitional cell carcinoma, adenocarcinoma, or squamous cell carcinoma). Phase II studies are also ongoing for patients with advanced or recurrent disease and transitional cell histology at Memorial Sloan-Kettering Cancer Center. One study consist of high-dose methotrexate, vinblastine, doxorubicin, and cisplatin with leucovorin rescue. A second study evaluates the use of gallium nitrate in this patient population.

REFERENCES

1. Ali MM, Klein FA, Hazra TA: Primary female urethral carcinoma: A retrospective comparison of different treatment techniques. Cancer 62:54, 1988

2. Antoniades J: Radiation therapy in carcinoma of the female urethra. Cancer 24:70, 1969
3. Antoniades J, Pilepich M: Carcinoma of the female urethra. In Perez CA, Brady LH (eds): Principles and Practice of Radiation Oncology, p 863. Philadelphia, JB Lippincott, 1987
4. Barbagli G, Natali A, Urso C, et al: Primary malignant melanoma of the female urethra: A case report with immunohistochemical findings. Urol Int 43:110, 1988
5. Bracken RB, Johnson DE, Miller JS, et al: Primary carcinoma of the female urethra. J Urol 116:188, 1976
6. Chu AM: Female urethral carcinoma. Radiology 107:627, 1973
7. Desai S, Libertino JA, Zinman L: Primary carcinoma of the female urethra. J Urol 110:693, 1973
8. Grabstald H: Tumors of the urethra in men and women. Cancer 32:1236, 1973
9. Grabstald H, Hilaris B, Henschke U, et al.: Cancer of the female urethra. JAMA 197:835, 1966
10. Grigsby PW, Corn B: Localized urethral tumors in women: Indications for conservative versus exenterative therapies. J Clin Oncol (in press)
11. Hopkins SC, Grabstald H: Benign and malignant tumors of the male and female urethra. In Walsh PC, Gittes RF, Perlmutter AD, Stamey TA (eds): Campbell's Urology, 5th ed, p 1441. Philadelphia, WB Saunders, 1986
12. Johnson DE, O'Connell JR: Primary carcinoma of the female urethra. Urology 21:42, 1983
13. Klein FA, Ali MM, Kersh R: Carcinoma of the female urethra: Combined iridium 192 interstitial and external beam radiotheraphy. South Med J 80:1129, 1987
14. Klein FA, Whitmore WF, Herr HW, et al: Inferior pubic rami resection with en bloc radical excision for invasive proximal urethral carcinoma. Cancer 51:1238, 1983
15. Levine RL: Urethral cancer. Cancer 45:1965, 1980
16. Mayer R, Fowler JE Jr, Clayton M: Localized urethral cancer in women. Cancer 60:1548, 1987
17. Meis JM, Ayala AG, Johnson DE: Adenocarcinoma of the urethra in women: A clinicopathologic study. Cancer 60:1038, 1987
18. Peterson DT, Dockerty MB, Utz DC, et al: The peril of primary carcinoma of the urethra in women. J Urol 110:72, 1973
19. Pointon RCS, Poole-Wilson DS: Primary carcinoma of the urethra. Br J Urol 40:682, 1968
20. Prempree T, Amornmarn R, Patanaphan V: Radiation therapy in primary carcinoma of the female urethra. II. An update on results. Cancer 54:729, 1984
21. Sailer SL, Shipley WU, Wang CC: Carcinoma of the female urethra: A review of results with radiation therapy. J Urol 140:1, 1988
22. Srinivas V, Khan SA: Female urethral cancer: An overview. Int Urol Nephrol 19:423, 1987
23. Taggart CG, Castro JR, Rutledge FN: Carcinoma of the female urethra. AJR 114:145, 1972
24. Turner AG, Hendry WF: Primary carcinoma of the female urethra. Br J Urol 52:549, 1980
25. Weghaupt K, Gerstner GJ, Kucera H: Radiation therapy for primary carcinoma of the female urethra: A survey over 25 years. Gynecol Oncol 17:58, 1984

51

○ ○ ○ • • •

Prostate

Carlos A. Perez

ANATOMY

The prostate gland surrounds the male urethra between the base of the bladder and the urogenital diaphragm. It is a walnut-shaped, solid organ, weighing about 20 g and consisting of fibrous, glandular, and muscular elements. The normal consistency is similar to the tip of the nose, with carcinomatous tissue having a firmer consistency.[77] The prostate is attached anteriorly to the public symphysis by the puboprostatic ligament. It is separated from the rectum posteriorly by Denovilliers' fascia (retrovesical septum), which attaches above to the peritoneum and below to the urogenital diaphragm. It is this portion of the prostatic fascia that restricts posterior extension of prostatic carcinoma into the rectum. The seminal vesicles and the vas deferens pierce the posterosuperior aspect of the gland and enter the urethra at the verumontanum (Fig. 51-1). The lateral margins of the prostate are delineated usually against the levator ani muscles forming the lateral prostatic sulci. Often there is a midline furrow that demarcates the left and right lobes of the prostate.

The prostate is divided into five histologically distinct lobes: anterior, posterior, median, and two lateral lobes. It is the posterior lobe, extending across the entire posterior surface of the gland, that is felt on rectal examination.

McNeal[249] defined four morphologic areas of the prostate:

1. The peripheral zone, constituting 70% of the glandular prostate, is the site of over 95% of carcinomas of the prostate.
2. The central zone, constituting 25% of the glandular prostate, has marked histologic differences from the peripheral zone.
3. The periprostatic region is the urethral segment proximal to the verumontanum and is the site of benign prostatic hyperplasia.
4. The anterior fibromuscular stroma forms the anterior surface of the prostate.

EPIDEMIOLOGY

Adenocarcinoma of the prostate is one of the most common tumors in men; in 1991 in the United States, an estimated 122,000 new cases were clinically diagnosed and 32,000 patients died of the disease.[4]

The incidence in the United States is higher in black than in white males (95 and 58 per 100,000, respectively). Blacks in the United States have one of the highest incidences of prostatic cancer in the world, 40 times the incidence among residents of Japan.[100] Five-year survival rates are also higher in white (63%) than in black (55%) males for those diagnosed between 1970 and 1973. Survival rates are increasing for both.[320]

Environmental factors may account for the reported differences; immigrants from low-risk countries to the United States have rates of clinical disease intermediate between those of their country of origin and that prevailing in the United States.[54,166,354]

Some studies have reported that patients had more sexual partners and higher rates of venereal disease than controls, suggesting a possible relationship between prostate cancer and viral-venereal diseases.[211,334,355] However, increased sexual activity may also be associated with greater circulating androgens.[394]

A study of the role of circumcision has also shown no correlation with development of the disease.[321,401] Japanese men exposed to atomic bomb explosions in Hiroshima and Nagasaki have not had significantly higher incidences of prostatic cancer.[36] Several authors have reported a familial tendency to develop the disease.[211,321,398]

Hormones may have some role in causing prostatic cancer, but the evidence is not firm. It is known that eunuchs do not develop these tumors, and the incidence of latent carcinoma is lower than expected in cirrhotic patients with higher than normal levels of endogenous estrogens.[144,315]

The higher incidence of carcinoma of the prostate in black males perhaps could be associated with a higher testosterone level. Ross and associates[319] reported a mean testosterone level in blacks that was 15% higher than in whites (normal subjects). Ghanadian and colleagues[138] showed that patients with carcinoma of the prostate had higher levels of serum testosterone compared with healthy controls: seven of 33 cases with cancer and only one of 42 controls had levels greater than 30 nMol/dl. Drafta and colleagues[102] also found significantly higher circulating testosterone levels in 23 patients with prostatic carcinoma compared with 63 normal controls. On the other hand, Wright and co-workers[400] found no difference in the testosterone levels in 23 urologic patients without carcinoma of the prostate and 26 patients with well-differentiated carcinoma of the gland.

No association has been found between smoking and prostatic cancer.[168]

Several studies have suggested that patients with cancer of the prostate may consume more dietary fat than control sub-

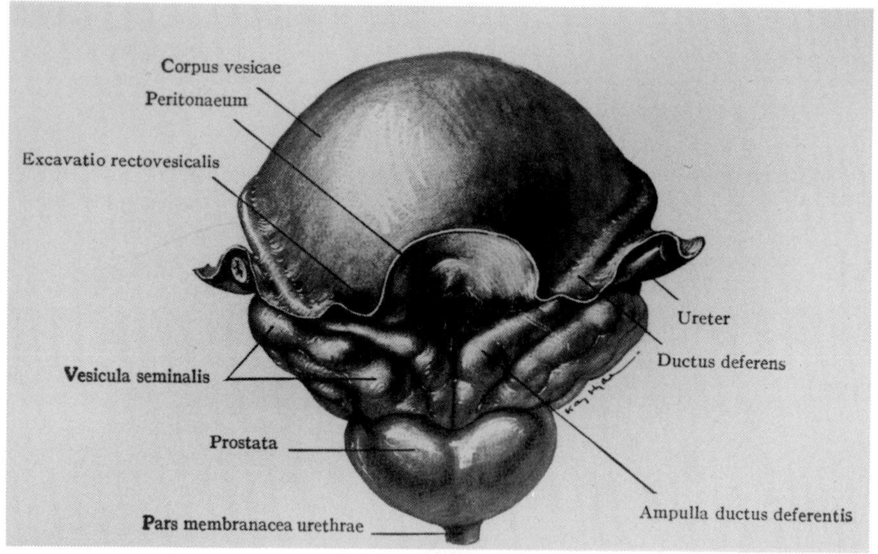

FIGURE 51–1. View of posterior urinary bladder, illustrating positions of prostate and seminal vesicles. (Anson BJ, McVay CB: Surgical Anatomy, vol 2, 5th ed, p 771. Philadelphia, WB Saunders, 1971)

jects.[155] Armenian and associates,[13] in a study of 296 benign prostatic hyperplasia cases diagnosed either histologically or clinically and 299 age-matched controls followed from 7 to 27 years, found the incidence of prostatic cancer to be 3.7 times higher in the benign prostatic hyperplasia group than in the controls. This association was not observed by Greenwald and co-workers.[161]

NATURAL HISTORY

Local Growth Patterns

Although there is an increasing incidence of cancer of the prostate in older men, the clinical incidence of Stage A tumors is about 50% of that expected on the basis of autopsy studies.[166, 167, 169, 389]

The studies of prostate morphology conducted by McNeal[251] showed that almost all prostatic carcinomas develop in the peripheral glands of the prostate, but benign prostatic hyperplasia arises from the central (periurethral) portions. McNeal believed the development of carcinoma in the gland follows predictable patterns, including early involvement of the capsule and perineural spaces.[251]

Breslow and associates[54] found that 64% of 350 carcinomas were present in a slice taken 5 mm from the distal end of the prostate. Therefore the urethra must be transected distal to the prostate to avoid leaving prostatic cancer behind. The practice of leaving a "button" of distal prostate to facilitate the urethrovesical anastomosis is a dangerous one.[47, 126, 250, 251]

There may be one nodule or many, involving any number of the lobes. Jewett[195] reported that multiple foci of disease were found throughout the prostate in 77% of prostatectomy specimens.

As it grows, the tumor may extend into and through the capsule of the gland, invade periprostatic tissues and seminal vesicles, and later involve the bladder neck or the rectum. Tumor may invade the perineural spaces, the lymphatics, and the blood vessels, producing lymphatic or distant metastases.

Regional Lymph Node Involvement

Tumor size and degree of differentiation affect the tendency of prostatic carcinoma to metastasize to regional lymphatics.[119, 124] Flocks and associates[119] in a study of 411 patients were among the first to correlate the size of the gland and the probability of lymphatic metastases. The correlations of clinical stage, histologic differentiation, and pelvic nodal metastases are shown in Table 51-1. McLaughin and co-workers[248] point out that multi-

TABLE 51–1
Incidence of Pelvic Lymph Node Metastasis Correlated with Clinical Stage and Histologic Grade

	GRADE							
	WELL DIFFERENTIATED		MODERATELY DIFFERENTIATED		POORLY DIFFERENTIATED		TOTAL	
STAGE	NO./TOTAL	PERCENT	NO./TOTAL	PERCENT	NO./TOTAL	PERCENT	NO./TOTAL	PERCENT
A1	0/28		0/12		0/1		0/41	
A2	0/7		5/19	26	3/7	43	8/33	24
B1	2/53	4	13/94	14	3/9	33	18/156	12
B2	5/27	18	29/106	27	9/21	43	43/154	28
C	5/10	50	18/44	41	13/14	93	36/68	53
Total	12/125	10	65/275	24	28/52	54	105/452	23

(Middleton RG: NCI Monogr 7:41, 1988)

ple lymph nodes are frequently found in patients with well-differentiated tumors as well as those with poorly differentiated lesions.

Periprostatic and obturator nodes are involved first, followed by external iliac, hypogastric, common iliac, and periaortic nodes (Table 51-2).[302] Approximately 7% of patients have involvement of the presacral and presciatic lymph nodes (including promontorial and middle hemorrhoidal group) without evidence of metastases in the external iliac or hypogastric lymph nodes.[302]

Prout and associates[304] described 92 patients with various stages of prostatic carcinoma undergoing pelvic lymphadenectomy. Solitary lymph node metastasis was noted in 11 of 32 patients with positive nodes. Bilateral pelvic lymph node involvement occurred in 14 (58%) of 24 patients having more than one involved lymph node. Prognosis is closely related to regional lymph node metastases; however, a single nodal metastasis is not an unfavorable prognostic sign. Prout and associates[304] reported that only two (18%) of 11 patients with a single metastasis had tumor progression, compared with 15 (76%) of 21 with multiple lymph node involvement.

Distant Metastases

Prostatic carcinoma metastasizes to the skeleton, liver, lungs, and occasionally to the brain or other sites. Batson[34] proposed the generally accepted theory that prostatic carcinoma metastasizes preferentially to the bones of the pelvis and the spine by the vertebral veins. Dodds and associates[99] disputed this, having found that the distribution of skeletal metastases from prostatic cancer is comparable with that from other primary tumors. The preponderance of metastases to the axial skeleton and proximate long bones may be a function of regional arterial blood flow and not of any specific venous drainage.

CLINICAL PRESENTATION

Because patients with localized prostatic carcinoma are frequently asymptomatic, the diagnosis is often made during a routine rectal examination. Stage A or B disease may be asymptomatic or may be diagnosed at transurethral resection for symptoms of bladder outlet obstruction caused by benign prostatic hyperplasia. Patients with larger tumors may have urethral obstruction with resulting increased frequency, nocturia, hesitancy, and narrow stream. Severe irritative bladder symptoms occasionally occur without clinical evidence of infection. Isolated hematuria or hematospermia is rare. Most patients with advanced disease present with pain or stiffness caused by bony metastases.[283]

SCREENING AND DIAGNOSTIC WORKUP

Screening

Mass screening for prostate cancer is not widely carried out because rectal examination still remains the most effective means of detecting early carcinoma of the prostate; other screening tests are not particularly sensitive or highly specific for this malignancy. Galen and Gambino[133] critically assessed the requirements for screening and Watson and Tang[388] addressed problems related to screening for prostatic cancer. Catalona[77] pointed out that efficiency of a screening test is a function of three factors: sensitivity of the test (*i.e.*, the proportion of patients with prostate cancer who have a positive test); specificity of the test (*i.e.*, proportion of men not having prostate cancer when a negative test is obtained); and the prevalence of prostatic carcinoma in the population being screened.

Digital rectal examination has about 80% sensitivity and 50% specificity. Radioimmunoassays for prostatic acid phosphatase have a sensitivity of only 10% and a specificity of 90% for malignant tumors.[77]

Prostatic-specific antigen (PSA) plasma levels are routinely obtained. This antigen, initially identified and purified by Wang and associates[386] in 1979 from prostatic tissue, is a protein with a molecular weight of 33,000 and is about 7% carbohydrate. PSA is detected in prostatic tissue (*i.e.*, normal, benign hyperplasia, malignant tumors), seminal fluid, and the sera of patients with prostatic cancer. PSA is localized within the cytoplasm of ductal epithelial cells and in secretorial materials in ductal lamina.[271] Seamonds and co-workers[339] reported a specificity of 95% in 40 newly diagnosed carcinomas of the prostate and 97.1% in 35 patients with recurrent tumors. This was superior to the positivity of prostatic acid phosphatase (60% and 55.7% in the same patients, respectively). The specificities of PSA and prostatic acid phosphatase were comparable in their experience (96.8% and 98.9%, respectively). The normal value of PSA at our institution is 0.4 to 4 ng/ml. Elevated titers at diagnosis have been associated with a greater probability of lymph node metastases or distant dissemination.

Stamey and associates[353] compared PSA and prostatic acid phosphatase as measured by radioimmunoassay of 2200 serum

TABLE 51–2
Lymph Node Involvement in Adenocarcinoma of the Prostate in 93 Patients

LYMPH NODE GROUP	PATIENTS UNDERGOING BIOPSY	PATIENTS WITH TUMOR	PERCENT OPACIFIED*
Para-aortic	74	13 (18%)	93
Common iliac	76	13 (17%)	95
External iliac	74	16 (22%)	94
Internal iliac	63	16 (24%)	87
Obturator	51	16 (31%)	94

**Refers to histologic evidence of retained contrast material within the lymph node specimen.*
(Pistenma DA, Bagshaw MA, Feiha FS: Extended-field radiation therapy for prostatic adenocarcinoma: status report of a limited prospective trial. In Johnson DE, Samuels ML [eds]: Cancer of the Genitourinary Tract. New York, Raven Press, 1979)

samples from 699 patients, 378 known to have prostatic carcinoma. The PSA level was elevated in 122 of 127 patients with newly diagnosed and treated prostatic carcinoma; the levels increased with advancing clinical stage (Fig. 51-2). On the other hand, the prostatic acid phosphatase concentration was elevated in only 57 of the patients with cancer and correlated less closely with tumor volume. However, PSA was increased in 86% and prostatic acid phosphatase was increased in 14% of the patients with benign prostatic hyperplasia. After radical prostatectomy for cancer, PSA levels routinely fell to undetectable ranges with a half-life of 2.2 days. Prostatic acid phosphatase, if initially elevated, fell to normal levels within 24 hours but always remained detectable. Several investigators concluded that PSA was more sensitive than prostatic acid phosphatase in detecting prostatic carcinoma and more useful in monitoring response and recurrence after therapy.[188,339,353]

A caveat is that both PSA and prostatic acid phosphatase may be elevated in benign prostatic hyperplasia. However, Hudson and others[188] reported only 3% of 168 men with benign prostatic hyperplasia with PSA levels greater than 10 ng/ml, compared with 44% in 231 patients with prostatic carcinoma. After radical prostatectomy, the PSA values decreased to undetectable levels (below 0.6 ng/ml) in 89% of the patients with tumor confined to the prostate gland and 87% of those with microscopically positive margins only. Levels were undetectable in only 34% with seminal vesicle or lymph node involvement. Only three (17%) of 18 patients treated with definitive radiation therapy, who appeared to be clinically free of disease, had postirradiation PSA values less than 0.6 ng/ml. The PSA values remained above 4 ng/ml in 39% of the patients during a mean follow-up period of 17.4 months (range, 9 to 59 months). None of these patients has had a clinical recurrence of tumor.

PSA may be of great value in the follow-up of irradiated patients. Stamey and associates[353] reported on 124 of 183 patients who were treated with external irradiation or ^{125}I implant for whom serial PSA determinations were performed.[20,163] Thirty-six percent of the patients had elevated PSA levels between 2.5 and 20 ng/ml, and 28% had higher levels. A total of 44 patients had multiple PSA determinations during year 1, 21 in year 2, and 59 thereafter. During the first year after completing radiation therapy, the PSA level decreased in 82% (36 of 44) of the patients, with a mean decrease rate of 9.7 ng/ml per month.

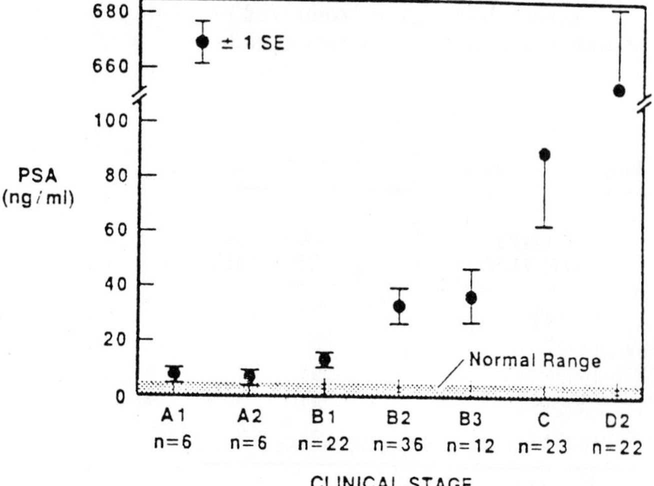

FIGURE 51–2. Relation of PSA plasma levels to the clinical stage of prostate cancer. (Stamey TA, Yang N, Hay AR, et al: N Engl J Med 317:909, 1987)

These researchers also found minimal correlation between PSA and total serum acid phosphatase values.

Landman and Juning[221] observed elevated PSA values in 46 (65%) of 71 patients treated with definitive irradiation. With serial testing and median follow-up of 18 months, PSA values returned to normal in 34 (74%) patients 6 months after therapy and in 36 (78%) 1 year after irradiation. The authors concluded that patients whose PSA values fail to normalize 6 months after irradiation carry a high risk of tumor recurrence.

Diagnosis

A complete general physical examination is mandatory. Rectal examination of the prostate is critical. The examination is best performed with a well-lubricated glove and the patient in a standing position, bent over at the waist with his elbows resting comfortably on a firm surface. The examiner should verify the size of the gland, its overall consistency, and the presence of any firm areas. A typical neoplastic nodule of prostatic carcinoma is extremely firm, often not elevated above the surface of the gland, but surrounded by compressible prostatic tissue. The examiner should determine whether the lateral sulcus is involved by the tumor and also the degree of spread superiorly. In most patients, the seminal vesicles cannot be palpated as discrete structures, and the finding of a firm area extending above the prostate suggests that the seminal vesicles are involved by malignancy. Not all areas of induration felt on prostatic examination represent carcinoma. Other causes of induration are prostatic calculi, infections, granulomatous prostatitis, prostatic infarction, and firm nodules of benign prostatic hyperplasia. Approximately 50% of prostatic nodules found on rectal examination are confirmed to be malignant on biopsy.[110,197]

In an excellent study by Guinan and associates,[163] digital rectal examination had the highest overall efficiency (sensitivity, 69%; specificity, 89%) of ten screening tests for prostatic cancer.

Although rectal examination remains the keystone for early detection, the actual diagnosis of carcinoma of the prostate can be obtained only through histologic or cytologic evaluation. The needle biopsy by the perineal or transrectal route is still the standard method employed to diagnose this tumor in the United States.

There is little current enthusiasm for the routine use of transurethral biopsy of the prostate, which should be performed only in patients with outflow obstruction. Although it allows diagnosing Stage A cancer of the prostate, it is of no value in determining the nature of a solitary nodule felt on rectal examination and may miss tumors that have not extended to the periurethral area.

In Europe and especially in Scandinavia, aspiration biopsy has been used for many years with impressive results. The most commonly used instrument is the needle described by Franzen and colleagues,[127] which is guided by the rectal examining finger to the nodule; an aspirate is obtained directly from the suspected area. No anesthesia is required. With adequate skills, unsatisfactory cell samples resulting from faulty biopsy technique are found in fewer than 1% of all specimens.[5,393] False-negative diagnoses range from less than 5% to 30%. False-positive diagnoses are relatively rare, but granulomatous prostatitis or aspiration of cells from the seminal vesicle can confuse the cytopathologist.

Esposti[113] found a significant correlation between the cytologic grade of the specimen on fine needle aspiration biopsy and clinical staging. The results with this technique were recently reviewed by Benson,[39] who concluded that this procedure has been shown to have a sensitivity and specificity equal to the standard core biopsy and that it should be used more frequently in the evaluation of patients with suspected prostatic carcinoma.

Standard Workup

The standard tests required in the evaluation of patients with prostatic carcinoma are listed in Table 51-3.

The value of serum acid phosphatase in the detection or staging of prostatic cancer is limited.[114, 122, 402] Neither radioimmunoassay nor conventional enzymatic methods are accurate enough to use as routine screening tests for carcinoma of the prostate.[114, 402] There is little evidence to warrant the routine use of bone marrow acid phosphatase in staging carcinoma of the prostate.[37] The potential value of plasma levels of PSA in determining tumor cell burden and prognosis was discussed earlier.

Brawer and associates[52] reported no significant impact of rectal examination on the plasma levels of PSA or acid phosphatase in 26 patients with various prostatic abnormalities from whom blood samples were collected before, immediately after, and 30 minutes after rectal examination of the prostate.

Lund and co-workers[237] and Merrick and colleagues[254] have stressed the value of bone scanning in the staging of patients with clinically localized carcinoma of the prostate for whom radiation therapy or a surgical procedure is planned. Abnormalities in the bone scan coupled with elevation of the plasma acid phosphatase or PSA levels are strongly suggestive of clinically unapparent metastatic disease. In a study by the Uro-oncology Research Group (UROG)[280] of 509 men with newly diagnosed prostatic adenocarcinoma, ^{99m}Tc bone scanning demonstrated bony metastases in approximately 25% of all patients judged free of disease by a routine bone survey, with incidence related to the stage of the disease. Merrick and associates[254] anticipated that repeated follow-up bone scans may help in detecting posttreatment metastases, because patients with normal bone scans live longer than those with abnormal studies. However, from a clinical standpoint, this procedure in follow-up is of questionable value, because it may not be justifiable to treat asymptomatic bone metastases. Bone scans are of substantial diagnostic help in managing patients with bone pain and normal radiographs. X-ray films may sometimes be necessary to better evaluate areas of increased uptake on the radioisotope bone scan, but routine radiographic bone surveys are of little value and add unnecessary expense to the evaluation of the patient, although occasionally a lesion seen on radiographs may not show in the bone scan.[263]

TABLE 51–3
Diagnostic Workup for Carcinoma of the Prostate

ROUTINE

Clinical history and physical examination
Rectal examination

LABORATORY

Complete blood count
Blood chemistry
Serum prostatic specific antigen (PSA)
Plasma acid phosphatases (prostatic/total)

RADIOGRAPHIC IMAGING

CT or MRI scan of pelvis and abdomen
Intravenous pyelography
Chest x-ray film
Radioisotope bone scan
Transrectal ultrasonography

CYSTOURETHROSCOPY

Needle biopsy of prostate (transrectal, transperineal)
Transurethral resection, if indicated

The lymphangiogram has shown an overall accuracy of 75% in several studies.[76, 182, 302] Pistenma and co-workers[302] described a true-negative rate of 88% (52 of 59 patients), and a true-positive rate of only 50% (15 of 30). The lymphangiogram cannot outline microscopic metastases or lymph nodes that are totally replaced by metastatic tumor. The bipedal lymphangiogram does not opacify the internal iliac and obturator nodes, which are frequently involved in early nodal tumor extension. This accounts for the relatively high incidence (22% to 40%) of false-negative results with routine lymphangiography.[182, 280, 312, 359] Asbell and co-workers[15] analyzed the results of therapy in Radiation Therapy Oncology Group (RTOG) protocol 77-06 according to the method used to evaluate lymph node status (*i.e.*, staging lymphadenectomy in 117 patients or lymphangiogram in 328 patients). The staging lymphadenectomy group showed better overall 5-year survival (87% *versus* 76%, $P = 0.02$) and 5-year disease-free survival (76% *versus* 63%, $P = 0.008$). Local tumor control was comparable in both groups (88%). Distant metastases were less frequent in the surgically staged patients (12%) than in the lymphangiogram group (18%) at 5 years. These observations reflect the shortcomings of lymphangiography in accurately detecting lymph node metastases.

Computed tomographic (CT) scanning and magnetic resonance imaging (MRI) are increasingly used in the evaluation of the primary tumor extension and regional nodes in patients with prostatic carcinoma.[186, 395] Tumor extension beyond the capsule of the gland, particularly into the seminal vesicles, can be frequently identified on CT scans (Fig. 51-3). However, the tumor itself cannot be outlined in the prostate gland. MRI may provide a more sensitive means of assessing interglandular and extracapsular tumors (Fig. 51-4). Biondetti and colleagues[44] evaluated MRI in 29 patients with clinical Stage B carcinoma and correlated the findings with surgical observations in 18 patients. The periprostatic fat signal had a sensitivity of 29%, a specificity of 100%, and an accuracy of 85% in detecting extracapsular tumor extension, but the periprostatic venous plexus had corresponding values of 57%, 86%, and 80% for detecting seminal vesicle involvement. The overall accuracy in differentiating Stage B from Stage C or D1 (positive lymph nodes) was 89% (16 of 18 patients); these findings indicate a promising role for MRI in staging prostatic carcinoma, although greater clinical experience is necessary.[59]

A CT scan cannot accurately delineate intranodal metastasis unless the nodes are enlarged more than 2 cm.[154] Large lymph nodes in a patient with prostatic cancer do not necessarily indicate metastatic tumor in the nodes, because they may be enlarged for other reasons (*e.g.*, hyperplasia). In a study by Golimbu and associates,[152] the accuracy of CT scanning was only 70% in assessing lymph node status and 47% in determining tumor extent.

CT of the pelvis and abdomen as a routine procedure in the follow-up of patients with prostatic carcinoma without clinical or laboratory evidence of tumor progression does not seem warranted. George,[136] in a study of 120 patients with asymptomatic carcinoma of the prostate managed with observation only (no anticancer therapy), abandoned routine CT studies of patients with clinically undetectable lymph nodes after 20 examinations showed no evidence of disease progression.

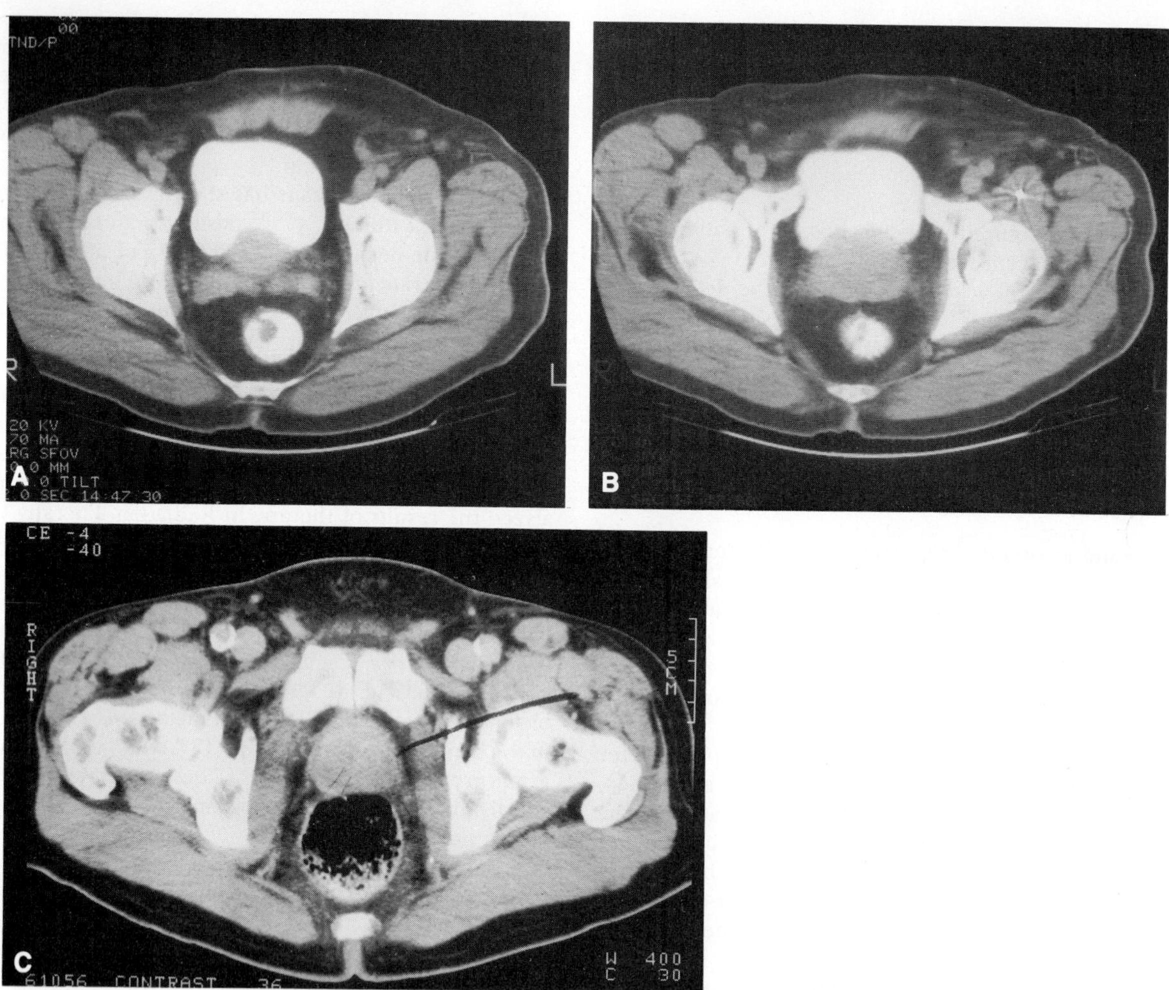

FIGURE 51–3. (**A**) CT scan of the pelvis illustrating the prostate, bladder, and seminal vesicles. (**B**) Impingement of the bladder by an enlarged median lobe of the prostate. (**C**) Close position of the prostate to the pubic symphysis, to which it is attached by the puboprostatic ligament.

Several reports have been published describing the technique of transrectal ultrasound and the anatomy of the prostate and preliminary findings in benign hyperplasia or carcinoma of the prostate.[228,313] Rifkin[313] found 130 pathologically proven cancers and 313 cases of benign prostatic disease in 443 men undergoing transrectal endosonography of the prostate. Cancers were hyperechoic in 69% of the patients and had poorly defined margins, but benign lesions were hyperechoic in only 46% of the cases and tended to be more accurately measured because of their sharper borders (Fig. 51-5). However, he concluded that there are no specific characteristics of transrectal sonograms that differentiate between many cases of benign prostatic disease and malignancy. Therefore, biopsy is always required, and a needle inserted through the perineum or the rectum can be guided to the suspicious nodule by ultrasound.

The sensitivity and specificity of ultrasound in detecting early localized carcinoma of the prostate are somewhat controversial. Carter and associates,[75] after performing preoperative transrectal ultrasound examinations for 59 patients with palpable prostate tumors clinically confined to one lobe, reported that this test detected 13 of 25 unsuspected cancers, yielding a sensitivity of 52%. Of 34 patients with no palpable contralateral lobe lesions, transrectal ultrasound was correct in 23, generating a specificity of 68%. The positive and negative predicted values of transrectal ultrasound in these patients were 54% and 66%, respectively. Chodak and others,[82] in a prospective randomized study of transrectal sonography in 216 men, reported a sensitivity of 86% but a specificity of only 41%; tumors less than 1 cm were the most difficult to detect. In the experience at Memorial Sloan-Kettering Cancer Center, only 5% of patients with a positive transrectal ultrasonogram had carcinoma confirmed on subsequent biopsy.[356]

Hricak and associates[187] compared the accuracy of ultrasonography and MRI in determining prostatic volume in 15 patients with surgical evaluation of the size of the gland. They concluded that transabdominal ultrasound was effective in determining prostatic size in patients with small to moderately enlarged glands. Combined with transrectal ultrasound, its accuracy was improved from an average difference of 14% to 8%. MRI had an accuracy of 6% average difference, but its cost does not justify its routine use. Both tests lack specificity in differentiating benign from malignant prostatic disease.

Transrectal ultrasonography has been used to monitor the response of carcinoma of the prostate after irradiation. Fujino and Scardino[131] found that the two most sensitive parameters for monitoring tumor regression were the calculated volume of the prostate and the integrity of the prostatic capsule. Another study demonstrated no correlation between the rate of tumor regression and progression of disease.[73] Fujino and Scardino[131] suggested that if the percent of change in volume per month of follow-up had been determined, as in their series, a significant difference might have become apparent.

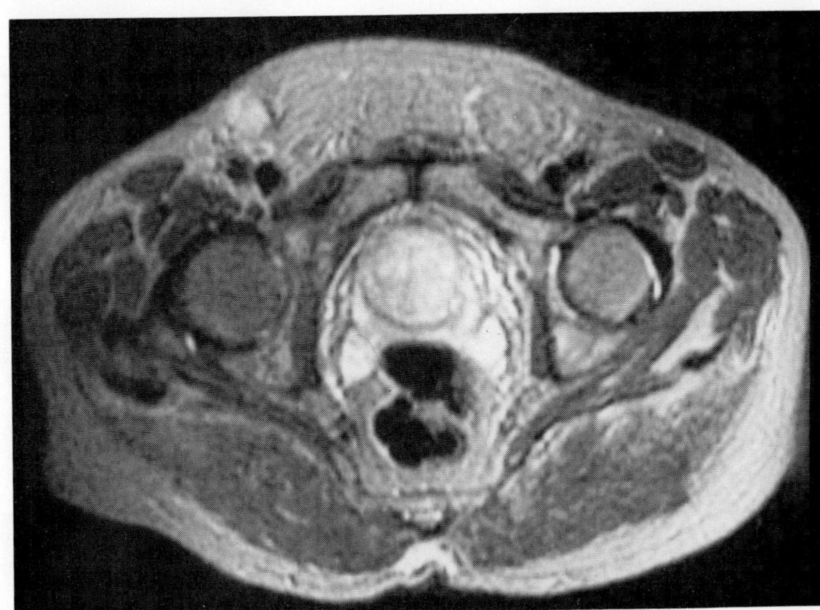

FIGURE 51–4. Transverse MRI of the pelvis demonstrating the prostate and seminal vesicles. Loss of anatomic detail and disruption of prostate capsule on left side indicate extracapsular extension.

Kabalin and colleagues[203] reported 27 patients on whom transrectal ultrasound-guided needle biopsies of the prostate were performed more than 18 months after irradiation. Sixty-seven percent of the hypoechoic areas were positive for cancer. Seminal vesicle biopsies were positive in seven (26%) patients. Ten (83%) of 12 patients with serum PSA levels below 10 ng/ml had positive biopsy results, as did all 15 with higher levels. Since the time the biopsies were performed, distant metastases have been documented in two patients.

In patients for whom multiple biopsies were performed at different times, Kiesling and associates[208] found that about one third had varying biopsy results, with most changing from negative to positive. The sampling error inherent in needle biopsies and the possibility that residual microscopic viable tumor in the prostate may be undetected could explain the failures that are sometimes seen after negative biopsies (*e.g.*, 12% in Freiha and Bagshaw's experience).[128] None of the studies compared the ultrasound findings with rectal examination or correlated the findings with outcome. This should be done before indiscriminate adoption of ultrasound in the routine follow-up of patients with prostatic carcinoma.

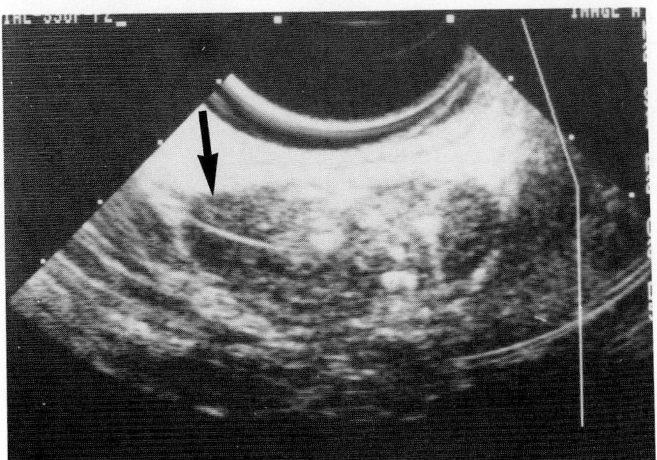

FIGURE 51–5. Ultrasound of prostate demonstrating several hyperechoic areas and a hypoechoic larger lesion in the right lobe (*arrow*).

STAGING

The American Joint Committee (AJC) and the American Urological Association schemata for staging carcinoma of prostate are shown in Table 51-4 and Figure 51-6.[36,324] Even experienced digital evaluation of the prostate yields relatively inaccurate staging information about tumor volume. Byar and Mostofi[68] reported that 855 of the nodules in 208 patients treated with radical prostatectomy were multifocal or extensive and that 17% of the patients with clinical Stage A2 and B tumors had extracapsular tumor extension in the specimen. Jewett[197] reported that after radical prostatectomy 25% of his patients with Stage A and B disease had involvement of the seminal vesicles.

Walsh[379] found capsular penetration in 6% of patients with Stage A disease, in 17% with Stage A2, in 35% with Stage B1, and in 71% with Stage B2 disease in specimens from radical prostatectomy, although the frequency of extracapsular extension was not stated. Frequency of seminal vesicle involvement ranged from 3% in Stage B1N to 10% to 15% in Stages A2 or B1 and 31% in Stage B2.

Stage A1 or T1a lesions are well-differentiated adenocarcinomas, not clinically apparent; they are incidentally found during a transurethral resection or needle biopsy of the prostate.[341] Stage A2 or T1b tumors are also subclinical, but they are more diffuse or have a larger volume, frequently with multifocal involvement of the prostate.[151]

Stage B or T2 tumors are palpable and are confined within the capsule of the prostate gland. Stage B1 or T2a tumors involve a single lobe and are less than 1.5 cm in diameter; Stage B2 or T2b represents a more extensive intraglandular palpable tumor.

Stage C or T3a–b lesions have extracapsular extensions and are subclassified as C1 or T3a if they involve the periprostatic tissues or one seminal vesicle. Tumors that involve both seminal vesicles or are larger than 6 cm are subclassified as Stage C2 or T3b. Neglia and associates[266] also place in the C2 subgroup tumors that extend into the bladder neck, rectum, or pelvic wall.

Stage D or T4 tumors are subclassified as D1 if there is metastatic disease to the regional lymph nodes or if, as used by Perez and associates,[288] there is clinically determined extensive

TABLE 51–4
Staging Systems for Carcinoma of the Prostate

AMERICAN UROLOGICAL ASSOCIATION	AMERICAN JOINT COMMITTEE	
	PRIMARY TUMOR (T)	
	TX	Minimum requirement to assess the primary tumor cannot be met.
	T0	No tumor present
A1	T1a	No palpable tumor; on histologic sections no more than three high-power fields of carcinoma found
A2	T1b	No palpable tumor; histologic sections revealing more than three high-power fields of prostatic carcinoma
B1	T2a	Palpable nodule <1.5 cm in diameter with compressible, normal-feeling tissue on at least three sides
B2	T2b	Palpable nodule >1.5 cm in diameter or nodule or induration in both lobes
C	T3	Palpable tumor extending into or beyond the prostatic capsule
C1	T3a	Palpable tumor extending into the periprostatic tissues, or involving one seminal vesicle
C2	T3b	Palpable tumor extending into the periprostatic tissues, involving one or both seminal vesicles; tumor size >6 cm in diameter
D1*	T4	Tumor fixed or involving neighboring structures
	NODAL INVOLVEMENT (N)	
	The regional nodes are those within the true pelvis; all others are distant nodes. Histologic examination is required for stages N0 through N3, except for subset "c."	
	NX	Minimum requirements to assess the regional nodes cannot be met.
	N0	No involvement of regional lymph nodes
D1†	N1	Involvement of a single homolateral regional lymph node
	N2	Involvement of contralateral, bilateral, or multiple regional lymph nodes
	N3	A fixed mass present on the pelvic wall with a free space between this and the tumor
	DISTANT METASTASIS (M)	
	MX	Minimum requirements to assess the presence of distant metastasis cannot be met
	M0	No (known) distant metastasis
D2	M1	Distant metastasis present Specify ______________
	Specify sites according to the following notations: Distant lymph nodes LYM; Pulmonary PUL; Osseous OSS; Hepatic HEP; Brain BRA; Pleura PLE; Skin SKI; Eye EYE; Other OTH	

* *Modification used at the Mallinckrodt Institute of Radiology.*
† *Surgical staging.*
(Beahrs OH, Henson DE, Hutter RVP, Myers MH [eds]: Manual for Staging of Cancer, American Joint Committee on Cancer, 3rd ed. Philadelphia, JB Lippincott, 1988)

involvement of the bladder, rectum, or pelvic tissues extending to the pelvic wall. D2 represents clinically evident metastatic carcinoma at the time of initial presentation, as determined by abnormal findings on radionuclide bone scans, liver and spleen scans, and skeletal radiographs or by surgically proven extra-pelvic soft tissue or lymph node metastases.

In general, 10% of the newly diagnosed cases of prostatic adenocarcinoma are Stage A, 15% to 20% are Stage B, 40% are Stage C, and the remainder are Stage D. The proportion of patients with Stage D2 disease has decreased from about 40% 20 years ago to 25% in recent years, a reflection of professional and public education, which has increased the awareness of the disease.[263]

Staging Lymphadenectomy

A limited pelvic lymph node dissection is begun at the bifurcation of the common iliac vessels, extends down the medial inferior margin of the external iliac artery to the pelvic floor, and is

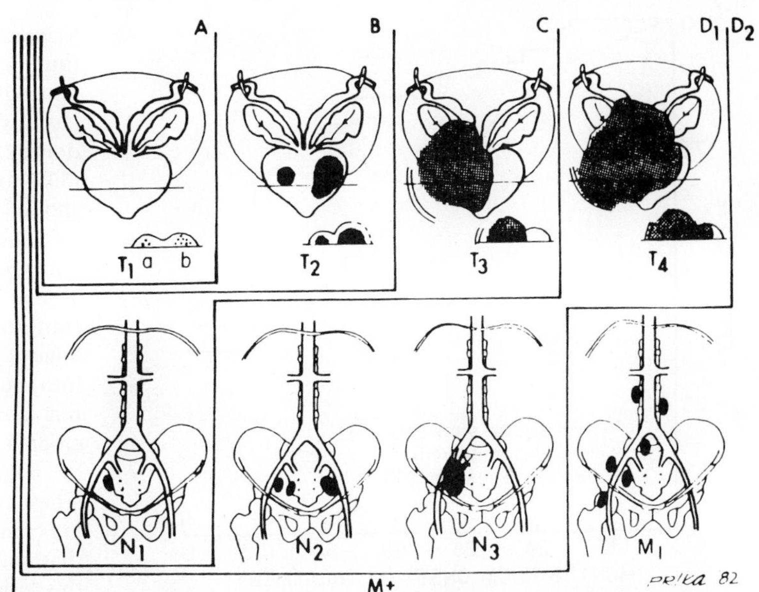

FIGURE 51–6. Anatomic staging of carcinoma of the prostate incorporating the American Urological Staging System or the TNM system used in the AJC and the UICC classifications. (Modified from AJC, UICC, Rubin P: Clinical Oncology: A Multidisciplinary Approach, 6th ed. American Cancer Society, 1983; courtesy of Philip Rubin, M.D.)

carried medially across the pelvic floor to the inferior border of the prostate and then superiorly along the hypogastric vessels back to the bifurcation of the common iliac vessels. Tissue surrounding the obturator nerve is incorporated in the specimen; the obturator artery and vein may be sacrificed, if necessary.[280] Fowler and Whitmore[124] showed that obturator lymph nodes were involved in only 60% of the patients with positive pelvic nodes, indicating that a limited lymphadenectomy cannot accurately detect all nodes involved by tumor. The UROG found no cases of positive periaortic node involvement among 54 patients with negative pelvic nodes,[280] confirming similar observations made by Flocks and associates[119] and Arduino and Glucksman.[10] However, a more extensive dissection beyond the bifurcation of the common iliac artery superiorly to the genitofemoral nerve laterally and the obturator fossa medially produces in higher morbidity and is discouraged by many surgeons.[153,277]

A staging pelvic lymphadenectomy had definite value as a predictor of prognosis. Whitmore and associates[390] reported that 40% of patients who had lymph node involvement after a pelvic lymph node dissection and insertion of an ^{125}I implant in the prostate failed within 2 years; over 75% of the patients with pelvic node involvement had evidence of distant metastases within 5 years of treatment. Hilaris and associates[182] found that patients with Stage T1 or T2 disease and no evidence of pelvic node involvement had few distant metastases; of those with T3 or T4 disease and no evidence of pelvic node involvement, about 50% had distant metastases after 5 years. Patients with positive lymph nodes, any T stage, have a 75% to 80% incidence of distant metastases during the same 5-year period. Cline and co-workers[83] in a series of patients treated with pelvic lymph node dissection and radical perineal prostatectomy found that 50% of patients with lymph node involvement failed within 2 years of treatment.

In the UROG study, almost 50% of patients with Stages IB, II, or III disease were shifted to a more advanced disease category as a result of isotope bone scans and staging lymphadenectomy.

The curative value of pelvic lymph node dissection is debatable. Barzell and colleagues[30] reported some therapeutic benefit for patients treated with interstitial irradiation and pelvic node dissection if the total tumor volume in the lymph nodes was less than 3 cc. However, a more recent study at the same institution[162] and one by Kramer and associates[212] provide evidence that in most patients staging lymphadenectomy is not a curative procedure. Kramer and associates[212] reported that, of 11 patients with Stage D1 carcinoma of the prostate who were treated with radical perineal prostatectomy plus pelvic lymph node dissection, 50% failed within 18.3 months.

If the nodes are negative, the irradiation portals should be confined to the prostate and periprostatic tissues, but for positive nodes, irradiation may be extended to pelvic or periaortic lymph nodes, although this approach is debatable. Freiha and associates[128] questioned whether radiation therapy can sterilize metastatic pelvic lymph nodes. Recently, Paulson and co-workers[278] studied 90 patients with surgical Stage D1 carcinoma; the mean time to failure was 23 months in a group receiving extended field radiation therapy (*i.e.,* inverted T field extending from the diaphragm to the prostate with lateral extension to the pelvic side walls, with a total dose of 7000 cGy delivered to the prostate and 5000 cGy to the periaortic and pelvic nodes) and 12 months in patients receiving delayed hormonal treatment ($P = 0.02$). Although radiation therapy delayed the onset of recurrent disease, it had little impact on prolonging overall survival in these patients.

PATHOLOGIC CLASSIFICATION

Adenocarcinoma, arising from peripheral acinar glands, is the most common tumor in the prostate. It is graded as well-, moderately, or poorly differentiated according to cellular characteristics, such as nuclear content, number of nuclei, pleomorphism, invasion of the stroma, and gland formation.[260]

Gleason and associates[146–148] initially proposed a prognostic classification system based on the clinical stage and the degree of differentiation of primary and secondary patterns of the tumor. Subsequently, only pathologic features were scored (up to 10). Patients with tumors with a Gleason score of less than 4 have well-differentiated lesions, with excellent prognosis; scores 5 through 7 correspond to tumors with moderate differentiation and intermediate prognosis; and scores of 8 or higher are anaplastic lesions with a poor prognosis (Fig. 51-7).

Gaeta and co-workers[132] proposed a different grading system based on glandular pattern and cellular anaplasia cate-

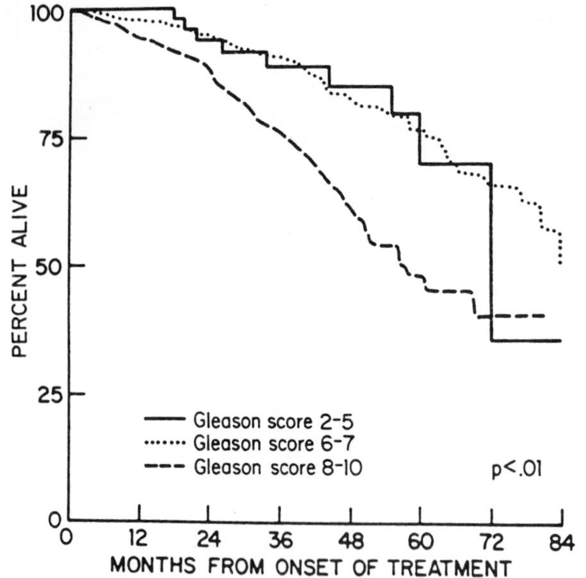

FIGURE 51–7. Incidence of locoregional recurrence by Gleason score in 539 patients with Stage A2, B, and C disease treated with external irradiation. (Pilepich MV, Krall JM, Sause WT, et al: Int J Radiat Oncol Biol Phys 13:339, 1987)

gorizing the tumors into four grades. The tumor is graded according to the worst component present in at least one third of the specimen. Washington University uses a simplified tumor grading based on histologic differentiation that correlates well with prognosis (Fig. 51-8).

One of the problems in accurately determining the histologic subtype or degree of differentiation of the tumor resides in the vagaries of needle biopsies and the amount of tissue that is submitted for analysis.

Catalona and associates,[80] comparing the histologic appearance in the needle biopsy and prostatectomy specimens from 66 patients with Stage B disease, found that the tumor was undergraded in the needle biopsies in 22 (33%) patients, overgraded in five (8%) patients, and correctly classified in 39 (60%). They reported a good correlation between the grading in prostatic needle biopsies and the incidence of lymph node metastases.

Further, the tumor histologic characteristics change with time. Brawn[53] reported 54 patients with prostatic carcinoma who each had two transurethral resections of the prostate separated by 3 to 11 years. He observed significant dedifferentiation of the tumors, evolving into higher grades, in 19 (73%) of 26 lesions that were initially grade 1, nine (75%) of 12 grade 2 tumors, and seven (88%) of 8 grade 3 tumors. A direct correlation existed between dedifferentiation and development of metastases: no grade 1 lesions in the second analysis showed evidence of metastases, but four (19%) of 21 grade 2 lesions, ten (55%) of 18 grade 3 lesions, and 28 (80%) of 35 grade 4 lesions showed distant dissemination.

Periurethral duct carcinoma is a separate clinicopathologic entity, consisting of a transitional cell type of carcinoma usually seen in histologic sections, although a mixture of glandular and transitional cells is also observed.[2,33,103,160,199,210] Large anaplastic tumor cells cluster in the periurethral ducts and spread into the stroma. Frequent mitoses are seen.[361] This tumor does not invade the perineural spaces as commonly as adenocarcinoma of the prostate.

Ductal adenocarcinoma rarely arises from the major ducts. These tumors are usually papillary and on microscopic sections are composed of tall columnar cells with eosinophilic cytoplasm that may resemble endometrial carcinoma.[72,362,407] Originally, this lesion was thought to originate in the prostatic utricle, a müllerian remnant.[252] However, most total adenocarcinomas are not derived from müllerian remnants and behave as acinar adenocarcinoma.[159]

Some investigators believe ductal adenocarcinomas are relatively benign,[33] yet most reports point to aggressive behavior, with invasion of the prostatic stroma and the bladder neck and metastases to the lymph nodes, bone, and lung. Most patients die of their tumors within 4 years.[160,199] The treatment of choice is a radical cystoprostatectomy.[397] This tumor is not hormonally responsive but is moderately sensitive to radiation therapy. Kopelson and associates[210] report a good prognosis in early stages; however, the 5-year survival rate was only 34.5% among patients with Stage C disease. They reported local tumor control rate of 78% and 5-year survival rate of 58% for patients treated with irradiation, in contrast to 14% local tumor control and 24% 5-year survival rate in patients not receiving this treatment.

Mucinous carcinoma, not arising in major ducts or in the urethra, has been detected with positive histochemical stains for prostatic acid phosphatases.[111]

Sarcomas (*i.e.*, leiomyosarcoma, rhabdomyosarcoma, or fibrosarcoma) constitute 0.1% of all primary neoplasms of the prostate.[361] Leiomyosarcoma is more common in middle-aged or older men, and rhabdomyosarcoma is found more frequently in younger patients. Several cases of malignant schwannoma have been described.[335] These tumors tend to invade lymphatics and blood vessels, causing widespread regional lymphatic and distant metastases.

Carcinosarcoma of the prostate constitutes 0.1% of prostat-

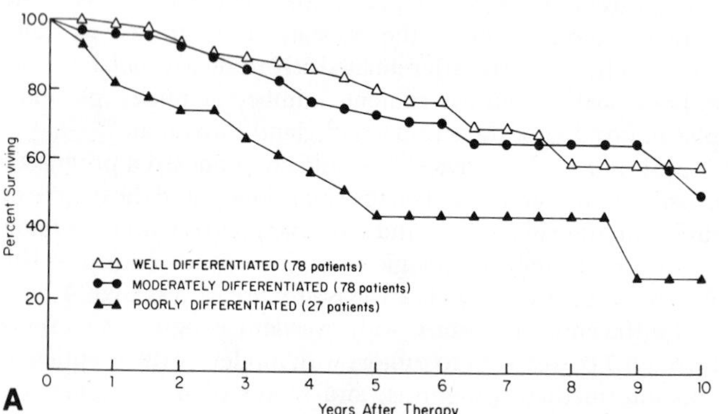

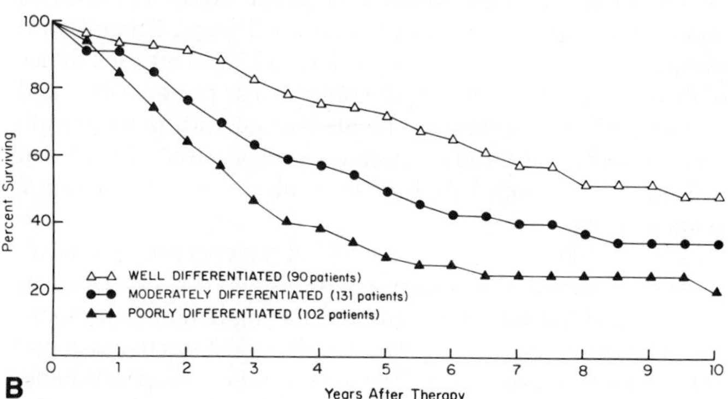

FIGURE 51–8. Disease-free actuarial survival of patients with (**A**) Stage B carcinoma or (**B**) Stage C carcinoma of the prostate according to histologic grade treated at the Mallinckrodt Institute of Radiology (1967–1983). (Perez CA, Garcia D, Simpson JR, et al: Radiother Oncol 16:1, 1989)

ic neoplasms. A mixture of adenocarcinoma invading the stroma and sarcomatous elements is seen histologically; smooth or striated muscle, fibroblasts, or other mesenchymal malignant cells may be identified.

Endometroid tumors occasionally arise from the verumontanum. Endometrial glands and cells with numerous mitotic figures may be seen. These tumors may have an exophytic configuration in the prostatic urethra or infiltrate the adjacent tissues.

Adenoid cystic carcinoma is a rare tumor in the prostate, representing less than 0.1% of all tumors of this gland. The histologic appearance is similar to that of the salivary gland counterpart.

Other epithelial tumors, such as carcinoid or small cell carcinoma, have been reported in the prostate.[3, 19, 137] The experience with these lesions is very limited, and in most of the patients, behavior is highly aggressive and fatal.[333] Squamous cell carcinoma originating primarily in the prostate is extremely rare.[156] Metastatic malignant tumors from other locations to the prostate are occasionally reported.[198]

Primary malignant lymphomas of the prostate are rare. They may be of the lymphocytic, histiocytic, or mixed type.[261] They behave similarly to extranodal malignant lymphomas in other sites and should be treated accordingly.

PROGNOSTIC FACTORS

Tumor Stage and Histologic Differentiation

As reported by multiple authors, the strongest prognostic indicators in carcinoma of the prostate are clinical stage and pathologic grade of tumor differentiation.[61, 147, 172, 229, 296] This is a consequence of the more aggressive behavior and greater incidence of lymphatic and distant metastases in the larger and less-differentiated tumors. McNeal[251] reported that 80% of the tumors less than 10 mm were focal, but 78% of those larger than 10 mm were diffuse, and 84% of the larger, diffuse lesions had penetrated and spread outside the capsule. These findings were confirmed by Scott and associates.[337] Byar and Mostofi[68] showed that the depth of penetration of the tumor in the capsule before there is periprostatic involvement has prognostic implications.

As Gleason[148] pointed out, the degree of histologic differentiation of prostatic adenocarcinoma is the simplest, strongest, and most readily available measure of the biologic malignancy of this tumor. Paulson and the UROG[280] and Kramer and associates[213] concluded that the Gleason grade of prostatic carcinoma determined by needle biopsy specimens is an accurate predictor of pelvic lymph node metastases. Others not using the Gleason grading system routinely have not shown a particularly strong correlation of these parameters.[304]

Zagars and co-workers[405] observed a worse survival rate in Stage A2 patients (74% at 5 years) than in Stage B patients (95% at 5 years) ($P = 0.02$). Multivariate analysis revealed prior endocrine therapy as the only adverse prognostic factor in disease-free survival and no prognostic factors in overall survival for Stages A2 and B. Pilepich and associates[296] reported 566 patients with Stages A2 or B disease with positive pelvic nodes or Stage C disease treated in a prospective randomized study evaluating definitive radiation therapy to the pelvic nodes and prostate, with or without elective periaortic lymph node irradiation. Multivariate analysis identified histologic grade of differentiation as the most powerful prognostic indicator for survival, relapse-free survival, and incidence of regional or distant failures.

At Washington University the histologic differentiation of the tumor was strongly correlated with incidence of distant metastases and survival, but not with locoregional failures.[286] In contrast, Pilepich and co-workers[296] observed strong correlation between Gleason score or tumor grade and incidence of locoregional recurrences. In their study, clinical stage was not a reliable prognosticator, but this is probably because only patients with Stage A2 or B disease with metastatic pelvic lymph nodes (a strong prognostic factor) were eligible for the protocol. In Pilepich's[296] analysis, tumor size correlated well with the existence of distant metastases, as did elevation of the serum acid phosphatases, but neither factor correlated with survival.

Age

The prognostic significance of age has been controversial.[67, 84, 200, 318] Decreased survival in patients younger than 50 years of age has been reported.[200] Leibel and associates[229] and Pilepich and co-workers[296] found that patients younger than 60 years had a higher locoregional failure rate than older patients; however, there was no significant difference in survival between the two groups. In the patients with Stage B disease treated at Mallinckrodt Institute of Radiology there was no difference in survival for the various age groups; however, in patients with Stage C lesions, those younger than 60 had a lower survival rate than those older than 60.[285]

Race

Several authors have observed lower survival rates for a given stage of disease in black men than in white patients.[18, 60, 92, 232, 296] Although this observation was not confirmed by us among patients with Stage A2 and B disease, it was for the patients with Stage C lesions.[18, 263, 285] This difference may be related to a lower immune competence, more biologically aggressive tumors, testosterone levels, environmental or socioeconomic conditions, and genetic or other factors.[18, 93, 255, 396] In 117 patients reported by Aziz and associates[18] with various clinical stages of disease, a greater percentage of black patients presented with high Gleason scores than white patients (43% and 27%, respectively). In Pilepich's[296] analysis, race correlated with disease-free survival if univariate analysis was used, but the prognostic significance disappeared when Cox regression analysis was applied.

Plasma Acid Phosphatases

Plasma acid phosphatase levels correlate closely with tumor dissemination and prognosis, with elevations over 25% of maximum normal values carrying poorer prognoses.[270, 402] Leibel and associates[229] found elevated plasma acid phosphatase levels to be associated with a greater incidence of recurrences (52.6%) *versus* 33.2% in patients with normal levels, but no data on survival were presented. Pilepich and co-workers[296] also found that elevated plasma acid phosphatase correlated well with the incidence of distant metastases and disease-free survival but was not a useful predictor of survival. However, Perez and associates[285] did not find this assay to be a reliable predictor of survival or patterns of failure.

Prostatic Specific Antigen

Recently Stamey and co-workers[353] concluded that PSA is more sensitive than acid phosphatases in the detection of prostatic carcinoma and more useful in monitoring response and recurrence after therapy. Several reports strongly suggest that elevated levels of PSA at time of diagnosis or during posttreatment follow-up correlate with a greater incidence of failures and poorer prognosis.[221,352] However, Lange and colleagues,[222] after evaluating PSA values in 100 consecutive patients undergoing radical prostatectomy, believed that the PSA levels did not adequately predict extracapsular tumor extension and that the test was therefore not particularly useful for staging. Nevertheless, high levels of PSA, at the time of or following prostatectomy, were associated with a higher incidence of recurrence. Persistently elevated PSA values 3 to 6 months after radical prostatectomy or definitive irradiation are sensitive indicators of persistent disease. With broader use, PSA is rapidly replacing plasma acid phosphatase in assessing prognosis after therapy.

Lymph Node Status

The evaluation of the pelvic lymph nodes and impact of lymphatic metastases on prognosis is a complex issue. The frequency and location of lymph node metastases have great prognostic significance.[182] Bagshaw and colleagues[24] reported that the disease-free survival in patients with negative lymph node involvement was 86%. If pelvic lymph nodes were involved, the survival rate was 71%, and if periaortic lymph nodes were involved, the rate was only 30%. However, Pilepich and colleagues[295] reported 448 patients treated in a randomized study to evaluate the effectiveness of elective irradiation of the lymph nodes in Stage C carcinoma of the prostate, and they observed no significant difference in survival in patients with positive or negative lymph nodes as evaluated by lymphangiogram or lymphadenectomy, suggesting that irradiation may have a beneficial effect on node-positive patients. Perez and co-workers[285] found that patients with Stage B tumors showed no significant difference in survival whether the lymph nodes were positive or negative as determined by staging lymphadenectomy or lymphangiogram, but in Stage C disease, there was a 7-year survival rate of over 80% for the patients with negative nodes and 20% for 15 patients with positive lymph nodes. These results are similar to those reported by Zincke and associates[409] in patients with Stage C tumors treated with radical prostatectomy and bilateral pelvic lymphadenectomy. Prout and colleagues[304] observed better survival of patients with negative nodes or with positive nodes if the volume of metastatic tumor was small (*i.e.*, a single node or just a few nodes involved by tumor).

At Washington University, pelvic lymph nodes are routinely treated in patients with Stage B or C tumors, although the benefit of this approach for Stage B lesions has not been demonstrated.[14,266,302,405] Bagshaw and associates[22] reported a trend toward improved survival in patients with small Stage B tumors and negative-stage lymphadenectomy after lymph nodes were irradiated; the results were superior to those observed in positive-node patients (Fig. 51-9*A*). McGowan and co-workers[246] described better survival and fewer pelvic failures in patients with Stage B2 or C tumors who were treated with larger fields encompassing the pelvic lymph nodes than for patients with similar stages treated with portals encompassing only the prostate and periprostatic tissues (Fig. 51-9*B*). On the other hand, Asbell and associates[14] reported no difference in survival or patterns of failure in a randomized study of 445 evaluable patients with Stages A2-B tumors who were treated to the pelvic nodes (4500 cGy) and the prostate (additional 2000 cGy) or to the prostate only (6500 cGy) (Fig. 51-10*A*). Elective irradiation of the periaortic lymph nodes was not found to improve survival or tumor control in patients with Stage C lesions in a prospective randomized study conducted by RTOG (Fig. 51-10*B*).[295]

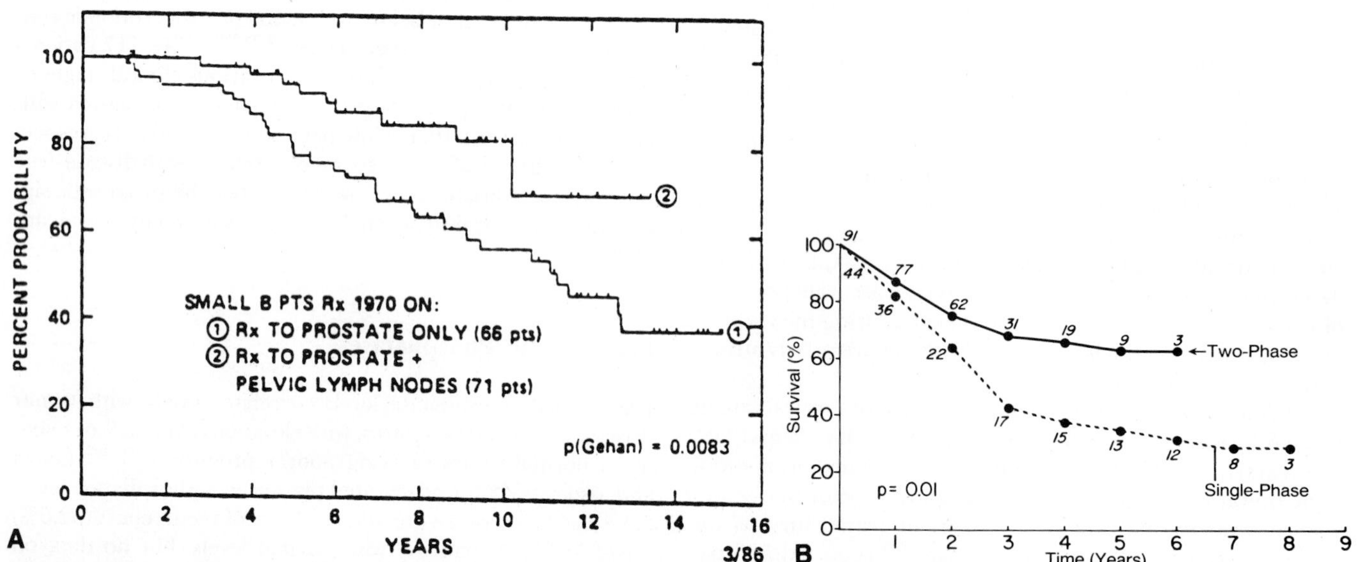

FIGURE 51–9. (**A**) Curves illustrating increase in survival for patients with small prostatic tumors on whom treatment volume included the first-echelon pelvic lymphatics compared with irradiation to prostate only. (Bagshaw MA: Int J Radiat Oncol Biol Phys 12:1721, 1986) (**B**) Comparison of disease-free survival for single-phase (small field) and two-phase (portals encompassing all of the pelvic lymph nodes in addition to prostate boost) techniques in late Stage B2 and C adenocarcinoma of the prostate. (McGowan DG: Int J Radiat Oncol Biol Phys 7:1333, 1981)

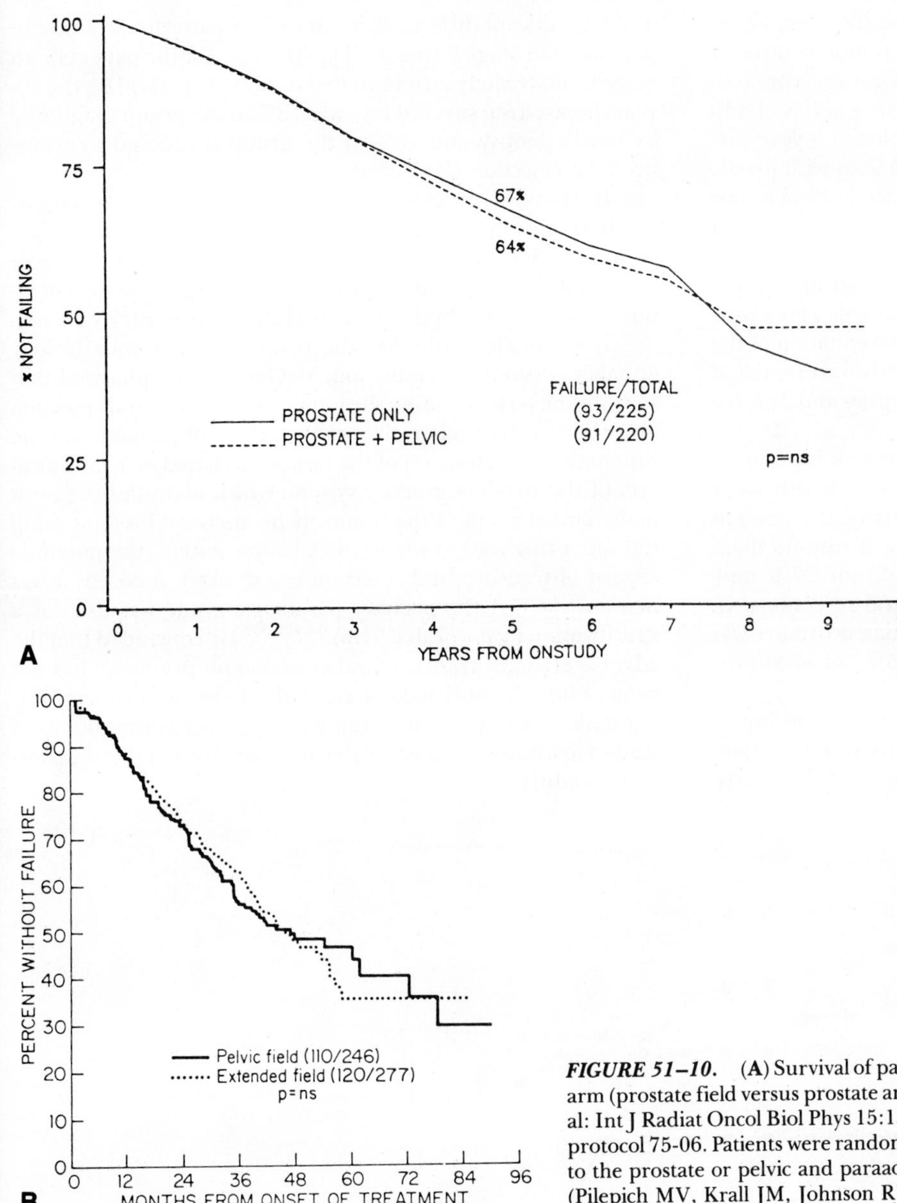

FIGURE 51–10. (**A**) Survival of patients treated on RTOG protocol 77-06 by treatment arm (prostate field versus prostate and pelvic field). (Asbell SA, Krall JM, Pilepich MV, et al: Int J Radiat Oncol Biol Phys 15:1307, 1988) (**B**) Survival of patients treated on RTOG protocol 75-06. Patients were randomized to receive pelvic irradiation followed by a boost to the prostate or pelvic and paraaortic irradiation followed by a boost to the prostate. (Pilepich MV, Krall JM, Johnson RJ, et al: Int J Radiat Oncol Biol Phys 12:345, 1986)

DNA Content

Quantitative cytologic analysis of prostatic carcinoma specimen by flow cytometry has been correlated with prognosis. Aneuploidy has usually been associated with more aggressive tumors than diploid lesions.[40,164] A technique combining flow cytometry and 5α-reductase activity in 20 prostate cancer specimens correlated favorably with the histologic grade of the tumor and course of the disease.[164] If flow cytometry was used, the disappearance of aneuploidy correlated with response to chemotherapy in small groups of patients, and reappearance of this pattern was evidence of therapeutic escape even without clinical evidence of disease progression.[50,230]

Transurethral Resection

Another controversial area is the impact of transurethral prostatic resection on survival. McGowan and colleagues[208] described lower survival in patients undergoing this procedure than for those diagnosed by needle biopsy, and this correlated with a higher incidence of distant metastases. However, the histologic degree of differentiation was not incorporated in the stratification of the patients. An updated multivariate analysis of 702 patients revealed a difference in survival in the needle biopsy and transurethral resection groups in Stages B and C combined (65% and 59% at 5 years and 50% and 43% at 10 years, respectively).[247] Yet in 255 patients with Stages B1 or B2 tumors, no difference in disease-free survival was found between the needle biopsy or the transurethral resection groups ($P=0.75$); for the more advanced Stage B2 and C tumors, better disease-free survival was found in the patients diagnosed by needle biopsy ($P=0.021$).

Pilepich and associates[293] compared the outcome in 299 patients undergoing transurethral resection with 292 patients diagnosed by needle biopsy in a protocol involving elective periarotic lymph node and pelvic irradiation for Stage C carcinoma of the prostate. Patients with T3 or T4 moderately or poorly differentiated tumors diagnosed by transurethral resections had a greater frequency of distant metastases and decreased survival than patients who had needle biopsies. There were lower survival rates and locoregional tumor control in patients with poorly differentiated tumors (Gleason score 6 to 10) regardless of the method of diagnosis. For a series of 240 patients, Forman and co-workers[120] showed lower 5-year survival rates with transurethral resection (42%) than with needle biopsy (55%); however, there was no difference in local tumor control. Kuban and co-workers[218] reported a higher, but not statistically significant, incidence of distant metastases in 162 patients undergoing transurethral resection than in 125 patients diagnosed by needle biopsy. After the patients were classified according to the stage and degree of differentiation of the tumor, the 5-year survival rate for Stage C poorly differentiated tumors was 68% for those who had needle biopsies and 38% for patients who had transurethral resections.

Patients who require transurethral resection have more bulky, usually poorly differentiated lesions, which bear poorer prognoses.[293] At Washington University, the percent of patients with poorly differentiated Stage B tumors diagnosed with needle biopsies was 13% (20 of 152) and 27% (nine of 33) for the patients who had transurethral resections. In Stage C, the proportion of poorly differentiated tumors was 29% (73 of 248) for needle biopsy and 42.5% (34 of 80) for transurethral resection.

Further analysis by Perez and associates[285] according to method of diagnosis (needle biopsy or transurethral resection) and degree of histologic tumor differentiation showed no statistically significant difference in survival or patterns of failure in patients with Stage B tumors (Fig. 51-11*A*). For the patients with Stage C moderately differentiated tumors (Fig. 51-11*B*), the 10-year disease-free survival rate was 48% in the group diagnosed by needle biopsy and 15% in the group diagnosed by transurethral resection ($P = 0.06$).

In Hanks'[176] analysis of the Patterns of Care Study, a statistically significant better survival rate occurred among 52 patients with Stage C, grade 2 and 3 tumors diagnosed by needle biopsy (50% 10-year survival rate) than among 87 patients diagnosed by transurethral resection (12% 10-year survival rate).

It is not clear whether the procedure or tumor biology enhances distant dissemination. McGowan[247] emphasized that some of the series refuting the impact of transurethral resection on prognosis had relatively small numbers of patients and the histologic differentiation of the tumor was based on a modification of the Broders grading system, which identifies the most malignant element in the tumor. If he analyzed his data using the worst (highest) grade in the Gleason system, the potential hazard of transurethral resection was masked; however, it was demonstrated if the primary pathologic grade was used as a stratification factor (Table 51-5).[94, 123, 336] He concluded that the adverse effect of transurethral resection on prognosis has not been definitely confirmed or refuted. In view of these conflicting data, it is important to carry out prospective randomized studies to assess the potential detrimental effect of this diagnostic procedure.

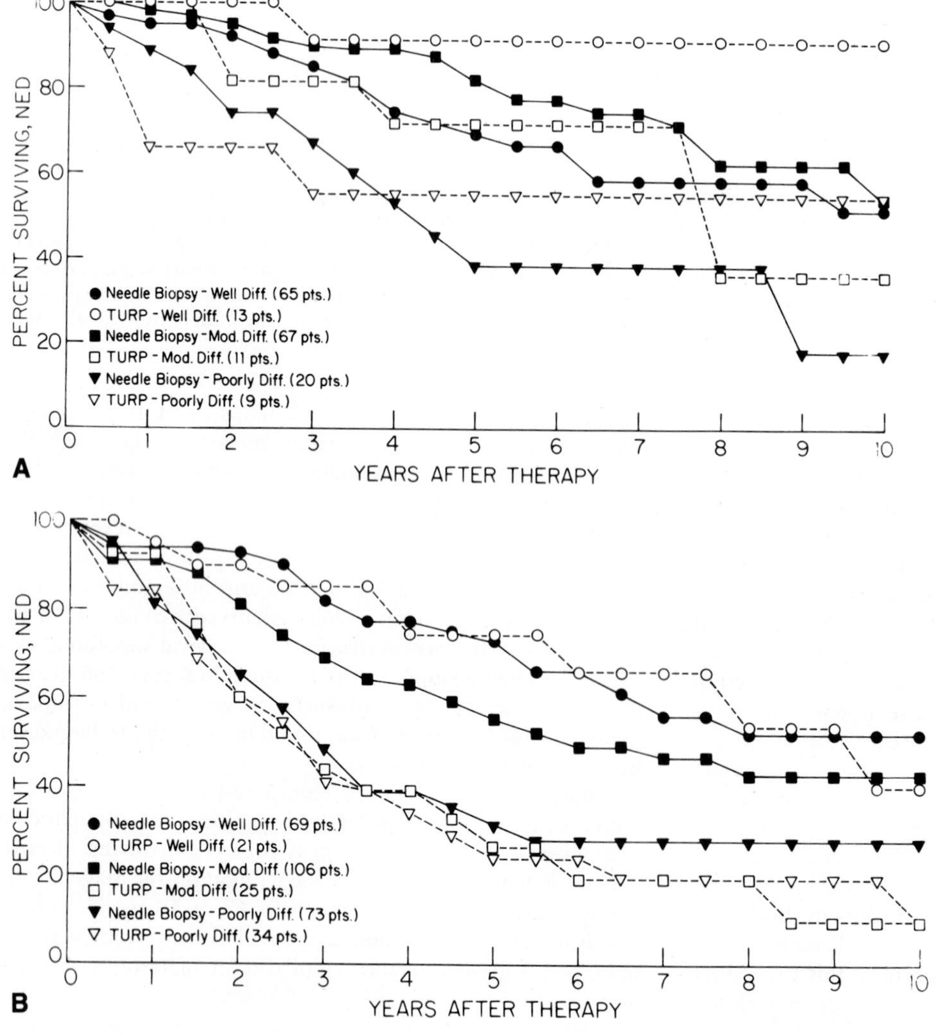

FIGURE 51–11. **(A)** Tumor-free survival according to the method of diagnosis and histologic grade for patients with Stage B carcinoma of prostate (1967–1983). **(B)** Stage C disease. (Perez CA, Garcia D, Simpson JR, et al: Radiother Oncol 16:1, 1989)

TABLE 51–5
Comparison of Observed and Expected Relapses for Needle and Transurethral Resection of Prostate (TURP) Stratified Within Worst Histologic Grade and Other Strata

WORST		OBSERVED (O)	EXPECTED (E)	O/E RATIO	SIGNIFICANCE
Early	Needle	51	48.64	1.05	Chi-square = 0.25
	TURP	38	40.36	0.94	$P = 0.62$
Late	Needle	66	68.59	0.96	Chi-square = 0.17
	TURP	96	93.41	1.03	$P = 0.68$
All	Needle	117	117.23	1.00	Chi-square = 0.0001
	TURP	134	133.77	1.00	$P = 0.98$

(McGowan DG: Int J Radiat Ocol Biol Phys 15:1057, 1988)

Adjuvant Hormonal Therapy

The experience at Washington University indicates survival and incidence of locoregional or distant metastases have not been significantly affected by the concomitant administration of hormonal therapy and initial irradiation, findings in agreement with those described by Neglia and associates[266] and van der Werf-Messing and colleagues.[372,285] On the contrary, in the multiinstitutional nonrandomized study described by Pilepich and co-workers[296] a lower incidence of distant metastases was noted in patients who received concomitant hormonal management, even though they had a higher proportion of high-grade tumors. The potential efficacy of hormonal manipulation immediately before and during radiation therapy has been discussed by Green and co-workers[158] and Pilepich and associates[296] and is the subject of a randomized trial by the RTOG.

GENERAL MANAGEMENT

There are several areas of controversy in the management of patients with prostatic carcinoma. The natural history of this tumor is variable and is influenced by multiple prognostic factors. Diverse forms of therapy can affect the quality of life and sexual function in different degrees. Proceedings of a Consensus Conference, sponsored by the National Cancer Institute, are highly recommended reading.[265] Properly designed prospective clinical trials that would resolve some of these issues are lacking and should be given high priority in the near future.

Stage A1 (T1a) disease found incidentally on a transurethral resection requires no treatment according to many urologists; it may take many years of natural evolution before it becomes a clinical problem.[351] Byar and associates[69] reported that only 6.8% of 148 patients with Stage A focal carcinoma, treated conservatively or not at all, had progression of disease; a literature review demonstrated a death rate of only 1.9% in 262 patients with Stage A1 carcinoma. Barnes and Ninan[28] reported comparable survival rates for patients with Stage A and B disease treated with radical prostatectomy or endocrine therapy.

Walsh and colleagues[379] in a report of 21 patients with Stage A1 tumors treated with nerve-sparing radical prostatectomy advocated more aggressive therapy for selected patients with these lesions. Untreated patients were not available for comparison.

Hanks and associates[174] reported 313 patients with T1N0 tumors who were treated with external irradiation. The 5-year survival rate for this group was comparable to that of a matched-age normal male group (77% and 81%, respectively), but the 10-year survival rate was below the normal life expectancy (51% and 62%, respectively). This was due to the development of distant metastases as a first recurrence in 18% of the patients. Overall, 72% of the patients were free of any recurrence, and 88% were without in-field failures at 5 years. The development of metastatic disease was related to the grade of differentiation of the tumor: a 5-year disease-free survival rate of 87% for grade 1, 79% for grade 2, and 69% for grade 3 tumors. This is in keeping with observations by Heaney and associates,[180] who reported a significantly lower survival rate for patients with poorly differentiated tumors in a group of 100 patients with Stage A1 adenocarcinoma of the prostate not definitively treated, usually with hormonal therapy only (Fig. 51-12).

Irradiation is recommended for Stage A1 moderately or poorly differentiated lesions, using small fields (7 cm × 9 cm or 8 cm × 10 cm), 120-degree bilateral arcs to a dose of 6000 cGy to 6500 cGy in 200-cGy fractions.

Patients with Stage A2 (T1b) or B (T2) tumors may be

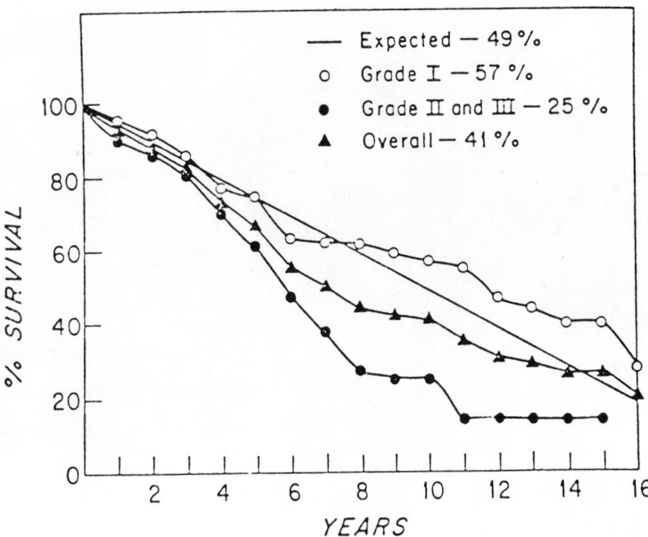

FIGURE 51–12. Survival in patients with Stage A carcinoma of the prostate receiving no initial definitive treatment according to tumor differentiation. Notice the significant difference in survival at 10 years between grade I and grades II and III ($P < 0.01$). (Heaney JA, Chang HC, Daly JJ, Prout GR Jr: J Urol 118:283, 1977)

treated with a radical prostatectomy, with an interstitial ^{125}I or ^{192}Ir implant combined with a staging pelvic lymphadenectomy, or with external irradiation.

Stage C tumors may be treated with definitive external irradiation or, in some instances, with hormonal manipulation. Stage D2 patients should be treated initially with hormonal therapy or chemotherapy; irradiation may be useful in controlling local or metastatic tumor growth.

Radical Prostatectomy

Radical prostatectomy, which was initially described by Young[404] in 1905 and popularized by Jewett,[195] is a therapeutic option only if the tumor is confined to the prostate; it has no role in the management of extracapsular disease or lymph node metastases.

Freiha and associates,[129] after reviewing 300 cases evaluated at autopsy or by specimens of radical prostatectomy, concluded that the largest optimal volume amenable to cure by radical prostatectomy is 4 cc (1.4-cm nodule), if capsular penetration is considered a proven prognostic sign.

Two approaches for radical prostatovesiculectomy are used: retropubic or perineal.[192,378] The procedure consists of complete removal of the prostate, its surrounding capsule together, the seminal vesicles, the ampulla, and the vas deferens. The prostate should be removed completely by excision of the urethra at the prostatomembranous junction, leaving no residual "button" of prostatic tissue at the apex. The fascia extending between the bladder and seminal vesicles should be removed despite the risk of damage to the posterior bladder wall and ureters.

The retropubic approach is preferred by many urologic surgeons, because they are more familiar with the pelvic anatomy than with the perineal approach. The former procedure allows the simultaneous performance of a bilateral pelvic lymph node dissection.

Radical Prostatectomy with Preservation of Sexual Function

Walsh and Donker[381] described the anatomic basis for sexual impotence after radical prostatectomy. Through detailed anatomic studies, they demonstrated that the branches of the pelvic autonomic plexus that innervate the corpora cavernosa are located between the rectum and the urethra, along the lateral aspect of the prostate, and penetrate the urogenital diaphragm near or in the midmuscular wall of the urethra (Fig. 51-13). Later they described the technique for radical retropubic prostatectomy with preservation of the neurovascular pedicle (nerve-sparing prostatectomy).[383] They reported preservation of sexual function in 73% of 250 patients treated with this operation; the incidence of sexual impotence is related to the age of the patient (Table 51-6).[379]

Catalona and Dresner,[79] reporting the results for 52 patients who had the same surgical procedure for clinical Stage A or B carcinoma of the prostate, observed that for 22 (52%) of the 42 patients who were sexually potent after surgery, there was return of erection sufficient for vaginal penetration. The erection returned in 57% of the patients younger than 60 years of age and in 43% of those older than 60. A potential problem with this surgery is the incidence of positive margins, which was reported by Catalona and Dresner[79] to be 18% (four of 22) in patients with Stage A or B1 disease and 57% (17 of 30) in patients with Stage B2 tumors. These findings were similar to

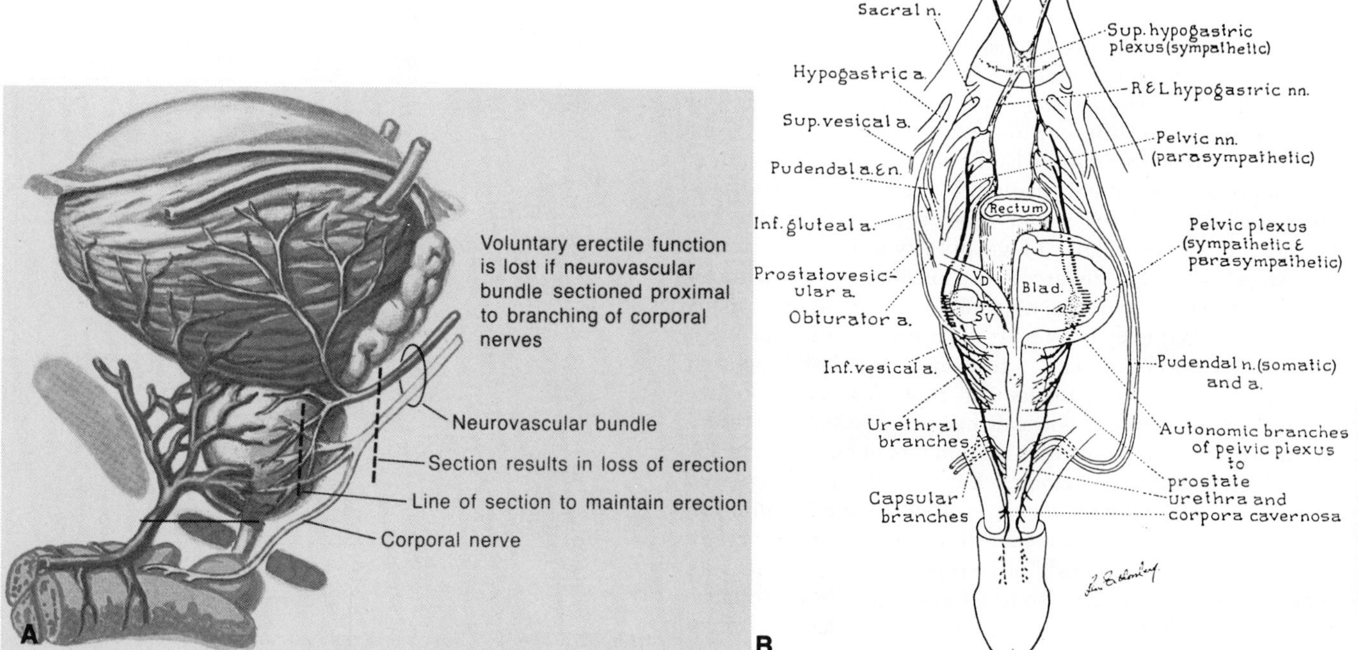

FIGURE 51–13. (**A**) Diagrammatic representation of neurovascular bundle to be spared in radical prostatectomy. (Paulson D: Clin Symp 41:2, 1989) (**B**) Detailed schematic diagram of arterial blood supply to the prostate (*left*) and the relationship of these vessels to the pelvic plexus and its branches to the corpora cavernosa (*right*). (Walsh PC, Lepor H, Eggleston JE: Prostate 4:473, 1983)

TABLE 51–6
Influence of Age and Clinical Stage of Carcinoma of the Prostate on Postoperative Potency in 250 Men Followed Up for at Least 1 Year

	AGE (YEARS)				
STAGE	30–39	40–49	50–59	60–69	70–79
A1–A2			83.3% (10/12)	77.8% (7/9)	0% (0/1)
B1–B2	100% (1/1)*	81.3% (13/16)	83.5% (71/85)	58.7% (44/75)	40% (2/5)
D0				50% (1/2)	
Total	100% (1/1)	81.3% (13/16)	83.5 (81/97)	60.5% (52/86)	33.3% (2/6)

**Numbers in parentheses represent the number of potent patients.*
(Modified from Walsh PC: NCI Monogr 7:133, 1988)

those observed with standard radical retropubic prostatectomy (Table 51-7).

RADIATION THERAPY TECHNIQUES

Interstitial Irradiation

Paschkis and Tittinger[272] first used a radium source inserted through a cytoscope to treat prostatic carcinoma. In 1911, Pasteau[273] introduced a radium source in a catheter placed in the urethra to treat some patients. Needles have been implanted by a perineal route, and special applicators have been inserted through the rectum or the prostatic urethra.[96,403] Bumpus[58] and Nitch[268] used rectal, urethral, or external applicators or interstitial implantation into the prostate gland through a suprapubic cystostomy. Barringer[29] and Smith and Pierson[346] combined brachytherapy with external x-ray therapy. Flocks[118] used interstitial injection of radioactive colloidal gold into the prostate gland, producing a local control rate of over 50% and few complications.

Iodine 125 Permanent Implants

Whitmore and associates[392] and Hilaris and colleagues[182] popularized the retropubic implantation of ^{125}I for clinical Stages A2, B, and selected C. The Memorial Sloan-Kettering group concluded that interstitial irradiation was probably unsuitable for patients with locally advanced tumors, those with grossly involved regional lymph nodes, and those with poorly differentiated tumors.[32] A limited staging lymphadenectomy is initially performed; frozen sections of obturator or suspicious external iliac or hypogastric nodes are performed. Patients with no involved nodes and selected patients with fewer than three involved lymph nodes are implanted with the radioactive sources. For technical details, the reader is referred to Chapter 13.

Iridium 192 Implants

Two groups described a perineal approach with afterloading techniques for implanting removable ^{192}Ir implants.[81,360] Syed and associates[360] performed temporary ^{192}Ir implants (3000–3500 cGy) combined with external irradiation (4000 cGy) for the treatment of patients with Stage A2, B, or C carcinoma of the prostate. Of 40 patients treated, 38 (94%) had local tumor control at the time of the report. The experience of this group was updated by Puthawala and colleagues,[305] who reported a biopsy-proven local tumor control rate of 89% and a rate of severe complications of 14% in 100 patients. Garcia and associates[134] described a modification of the technique, inserting small Teflon guides through a perineal route under ultrasound control and using ^{192}Ir to deliver 3000 cGy in combination with external irradiation of approximately 4000 cGy.

Gold 198 Permanent Implants

^{198}Au grains have been combined with external irradiation by Carlton and associates.[71] After staging pelvic lymphadenectomy is performed, gold grains are implanted into the prostate gland through a suprapubic incision to deliver 3000 cGy to 3500

TABLE 51–7
Incidence of Positive Margins With Nerve-sparing and Standard Radical Retropubic Prostatectomy

CLINICAL STAGE	NO. OF NERVE-SPARING POSITIVE MARGINS	NO. OF STANDARD POSITIVE MARGINS	SIGNIFICANCE
A1 and B1	4/22 (18%)	2/11 (18%)	$P = 1.00$
B2	17/30 (57%)	7/14 (50%)	$P = 0.68$
Total	21/52 (40%)	9/25 (36%)	$P = 0.71$*

**By chi-square analysis.*
(Catalona WJ, Dresner SM: J Urol 134:1149, 1985)

cGy, followed by external irradiation to the pelvis of approximately 4000 cGy.

External Irradiation

With the advent of megavoltage equipment, an increase in the use of external irradiation has emerged for the treatment of patients with carcinoma of the prostate.[87,95] A variety of techniques have been used, ranging from parallel anteroposterior portals with a perineal appositional field to lateral portals (box technique) or rotational fields to supplement the dose to the prostate.[23,95,246,286]

In patients on whom a transurethral resection has been carried out for relief of obstructive lower urinary tract symptoms, 4 weeks should elapse before radiation therapy is begun to decrease sequelae, including urinary incontinence and urethral strictures.

Volume Treated

If the pelvic lymph nodes are treated, as is frequently done at Washington University, the field size for Stage A2 or B lesions is 15 cm × 15 cm at the patient surface (16.5 cm at isocenter). For Stage C or D1 tumors, the field size is increased to 15 × 18 cm at the skin surface (16.5 cm × 20.5 cm at isocenter) to cover the common iliac lymph nodes. The inferior margin of the field should be at the junction of the prostatic and membranous urethra, usually at the bottom of the ischial tuberosities. The lateral margins should be about 2 cm from the lateral bony pelvis (Fig. 51-14*A*).

If lateral ports are used for the box technique (including the lymph nodes) or to irradiate the prostate with rotational techniques, it is important to delineate anatomic structures of the pelvis and the location of the prostate in relation to the bladder, rectum, and bony structures with CT or MRI.

The initial lateral field encompasses a volume similar to that treated with AP/PA portals, including the pelvic and presacral lymph nodes above the S3 segment, which permits partial sparing of the posterior rectal wall distal to this level. The anterior margins should be 0.5 cm to 1 cm posterior to the projection of the anterior cortex of the pubic symphysis (Fig. 51-14*B*). Some of the small bowel may be spared anteriorly keeping in mind the anatomic location of the external iliac lymph nodes.

The reduced field for treatment of the prostatic volume can be about 8 cm × 10 cm for Stages A2 or B to 10 cm × 12 cm or 12 cm × 14 cm for Stages C or D1 (Fig. 51-14*C*). Pilepich and associates[299] published practical guidelines on the size of the gland as determined by CT in 100 patients, and they recommended specific landmarks to determine field sizes (Fig. 51-15). However, in most institutions CT or MRI scanning is being used to determine the exact size and location of the prostate and to establish tumor extent. Low and colleagues[236] analyzed the impact of CT and three-dimensional treatment planning on defining the optimal volume to be treated in 12 patients. Their analysis showed that the guidelines provided by Pilepich and associates[299] would not have covered adequately the entire lesion in one third of the patients if treatment was given with fields encompassing the prostate with a 2 cm margin.

The seminal vesicles are located high in the pelvis and posterior to the bladder (Fig. 51-16), which is particularly critical in designing the reduced fields in patients with clinical or surgical Stage C2 (T3b) tumors. Perez and associates[284] demon-

CARCINOMA OF PROSTATE - PORTALS

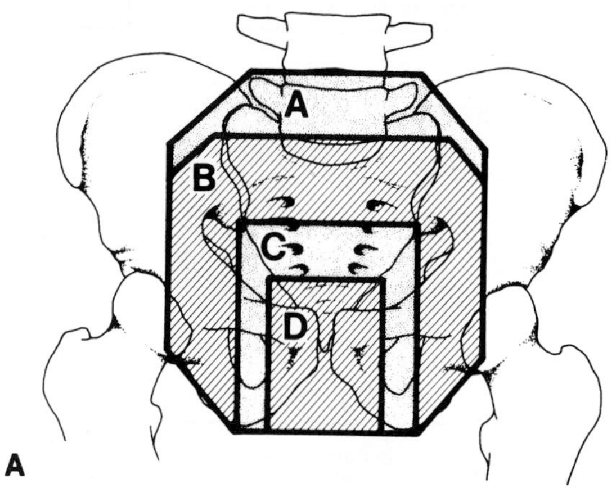

A

PROSTATE
LATERAL PELVIC FIELDS

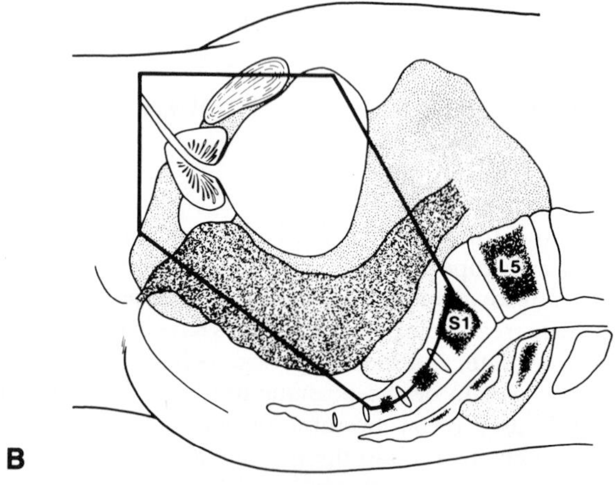

B

PROSTATE
LATERAL TUMOR BOOST FIELDS

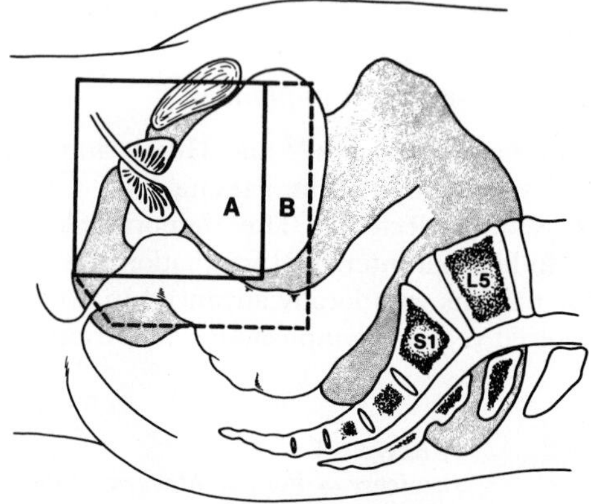

C

FIGURE 51–14. (**A**) Diagrams of the pelvis showing volume used to irradiate the prostate and pelvic lymph nodes. Lower margin is at or even 1 cm below the ischial tuberosities. At the Mallinckrodt Institute of Radiology, 15-cm × 15-cm portals at source-to-skin distance are used for Stages A2 and B disease and for selected postoperative patients, but for patients with Stage C or D1 disease, 18-cm × 15-cm portals are used to cover all of the common iliac lymph nodes up to the bifurcation of the common iliac lymph nodes. (**B**) Lateral portal used in box technique to irradiate pelvic tissues and prostate. The anterior margin is 0.5 to 1 cm posterior to projected cortex of pubic symphysis. Presacral lymph nodes are included down to S3; inferiorly posterior wall of rectum is spared. (**C**) Boost fields, lateral projection, used to irradiate the prostate.

strated a correlation between size of the reduced portal and probability of pelvic tumor control.

To simulate these portals, a small plastic rod with radiopaque markers 1 cm apart is inserted in the rectum of the supine patient to localize the posterior surface of the prostate. After thorough cleansing of the penis and surrounding areas with Betadine, using sterile technique, 40% iodinated contrast material is injected in the urethra until the patient complains of mild discomfort. This procedure documents the junction of the prostatic and bulbous urethra, accurately localizing the apex of the prostate, which is difficult to identify on CT or MRI scans. Anteroposterior and lateral radiographs are taken after the position of the small portals is determined under fluoroscopic examination.

Figure 51-17 shows simulation films outlining the anteroposterior and lateral portals used for the box technique. For the boost, the upper margin is 3 cm to 5 cm above the acetabulum, depending on extent of disease and volume to be covered (*i.e.*, seminal vesicles). The anterior margin is 1 cm posterior to the anterior cortex of the pubic bone; the inferior margin is at the ischial tuberosity, and the posterior margin is 2 cm behind the marker rod in the rectum. Figure 51-18 illustrates the reduced volume for the prostate boost.

The different boost portal sizes should be individually determined for each patient, depending on clinical and radiographic assessment of tumor extent. Policies of treatment and average field sizes are recommended in Table 51-8.

After the appropriate portals have been determined, the corners of the reduced portals and the isocenters for both portals are tattooed with India ink (Fig. 51-19).

The periaortic lymph nodes can be treated through a single portal that includes both the pelvic and periaortic lymph nodes (Fig. 51-20*A*) if large-field linear accelerator beams are available. Otherwise, a separate periaortic portal is placed above the pelvic fields, in which case calculations for an appropriate gap (≈ 3 cm) should be carried out (Fig. 51-20*B*). To cover all the periaortic lymph nodes, the portal's superior margin should be at the T12–L1 vertebral interspace. The width, which usually is about 10 cm, can be determined with the aid of a lymphangiogram or CT. If these studies are not available, the intravenous pyelogram indicates the trajectory of the ureters, which may be used as landmarks, although not 100% accurately. The dose to the distal spinal cord should be limited to 4500 cGy with a small posterior 5 half-value layer block above the L2–L3 interspace.

Beam Energy and Dose Distribution

Ideally, high-energy photons (> 10 MV) should be used to treat these patients, which simplifies techniques and decreases morbidity. Up to 4500 cGy total dose can be delivered with anteroposterior and posteroanterior portals in patients less than 20 cm in AP diameter. The additional dose is administered with lateral portals.

With photon energies below 18 MV, lateral portals are always necessary to deliver part of the dose in addition to the AP/PA portals (box technique). With photon energies above 18 MV, the lateral portals are not strictly necessary, except in patients with an anteroposterior diameter greater than 20 cm, because the improvement in the dose distribution is marginal. In our experience, the main advantage of using the box technique is a decrease in erythema and skin desquamation in the intergluteal fold, which occurs with the AP/PA portals.

For the reduced volume, a good dose distribution is obtained with bilateral 120-degree arc rotation, skipping the midline anteriorly and posteriorly (60-degree vectors). Figure 51-21 illustrates the dose distribution for 8-cm × 10-cm bilateral 120-degree arcs. The composite isodose of AP/PA portals without (Fig. 51-22*A*) and with (Fig. 51-22*B*) lateral portals can be used

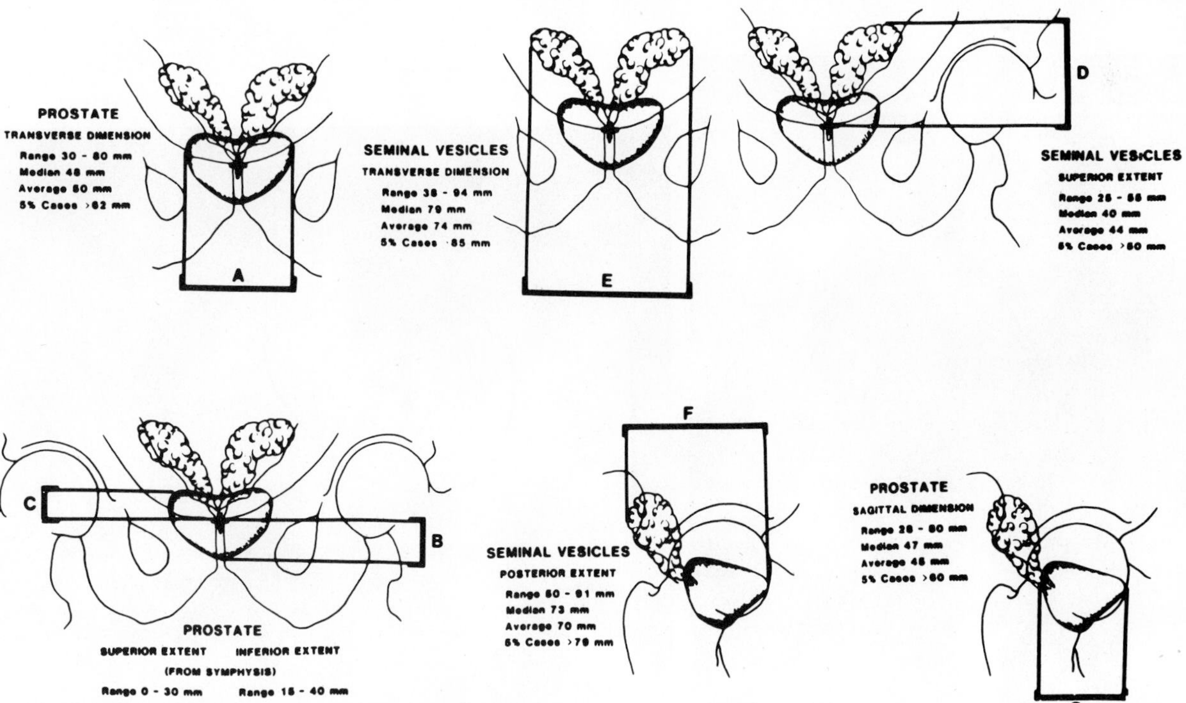

FIGURE 51–15. Diagrammatic representation of volume to be treated in various extents of carcinoma of the prostate, as derived from analysis of 100 CT scans. Dimensions would encompass 95% of the cases outlined. (Pilepich MV, Prasad SC, Perez CA: Int J Radiat Oncol Biol Phys 8:235, 1982)

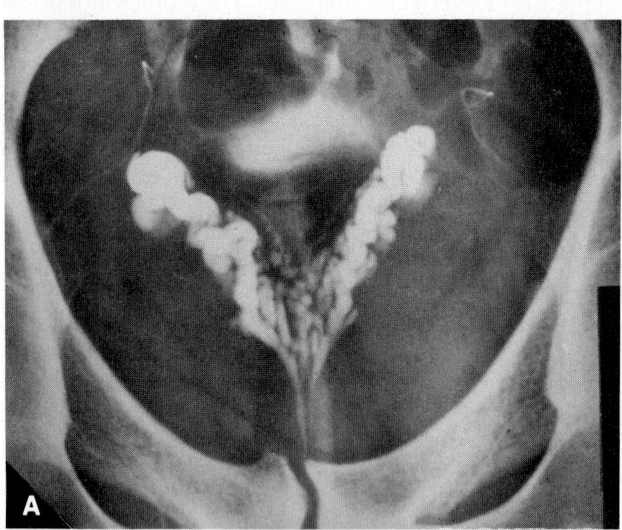

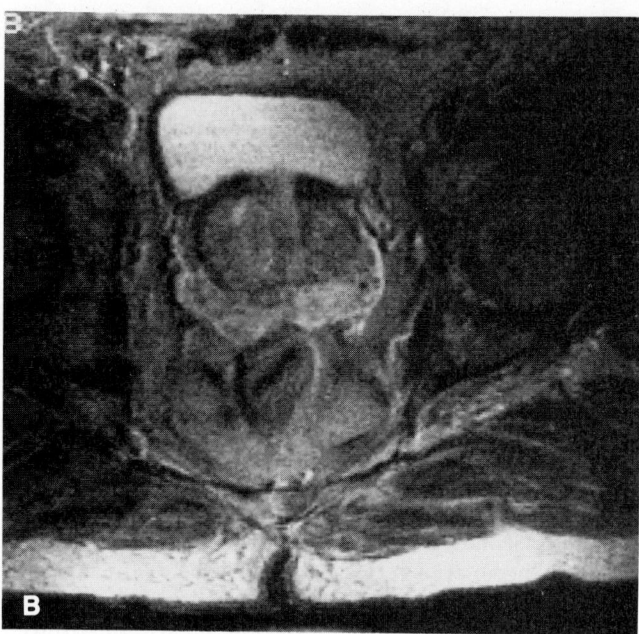

FIGURE 51–16. (**A**) Anteroposterior radiograph of seminal vesicles with contrast material showing their high location. (**B**) Cross-section of MRI scan of the pelvis illustrating position of enlarged seminal vessel. This anatomic location is important in treating patients with seminal vesicle extension, in whom the portals must be enlarged accordingly.

to plan delivery of 4500 cGy to the pelvis with the addition of a boost (2000–2500 cGy) to the prostate and surrounding tissues with bilateral 120-degree lateral arcs. Anterior and posterior oblique fields are occasionally used to irradiate the prostate. More sophisticated volume-shaping techniques using three-dimensional treatment planning have been described, but their practical advantages are yet to be documented.[236]

Doses

The usual radiation dose is 4500 cGy for the pelvic and periaortic lymph nodes, with a boost to the prostate or enlarged periaortic lymph nodes. The minimal tumor dose to the prostate for Stage A or B tumors is 6500 cGy and approximately 7000 cGy for Stage C disease. For Stage D1 lesions, treatment is

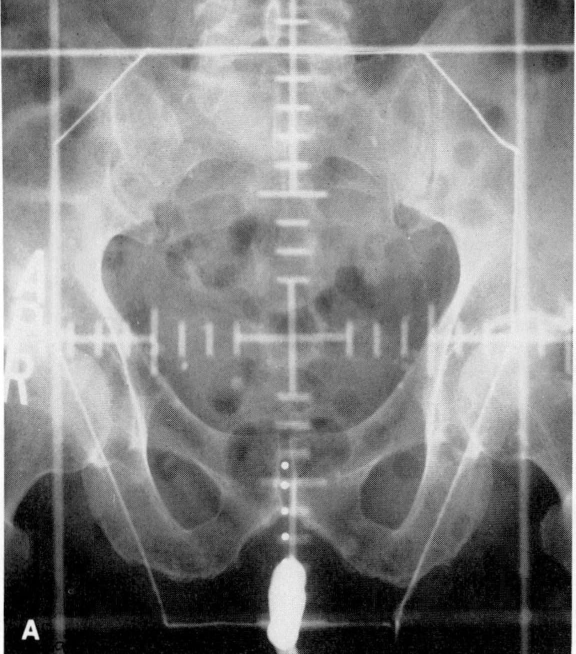

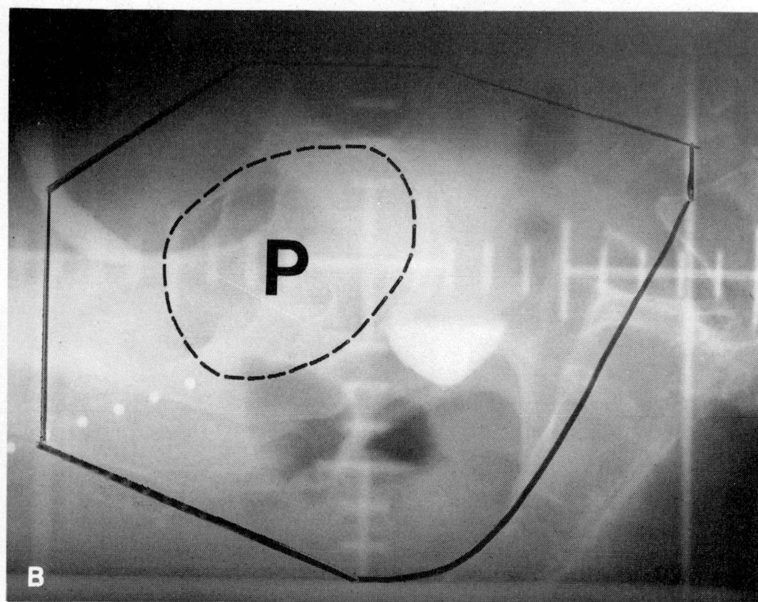

FIGURE 51–17. (**A**) Anteroposterior and (**B**) lateral portals for carcinoma of the prostate as shown on simulation films. The junction of the prostatic and bulbous urethra (distal margin of prostate) is identified by uretherogram. Notice the relationship of the portals to the roof of the acetabulum, the pubic symphysis anteriorly, and the ischial tuberosities posteriorly.

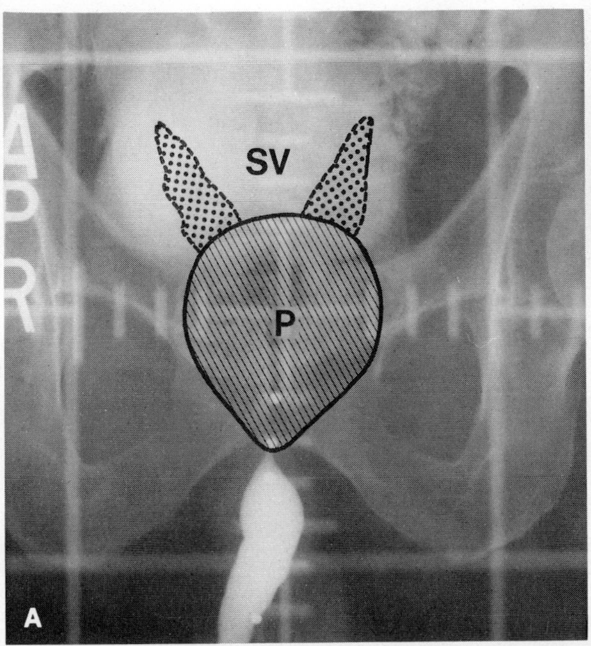

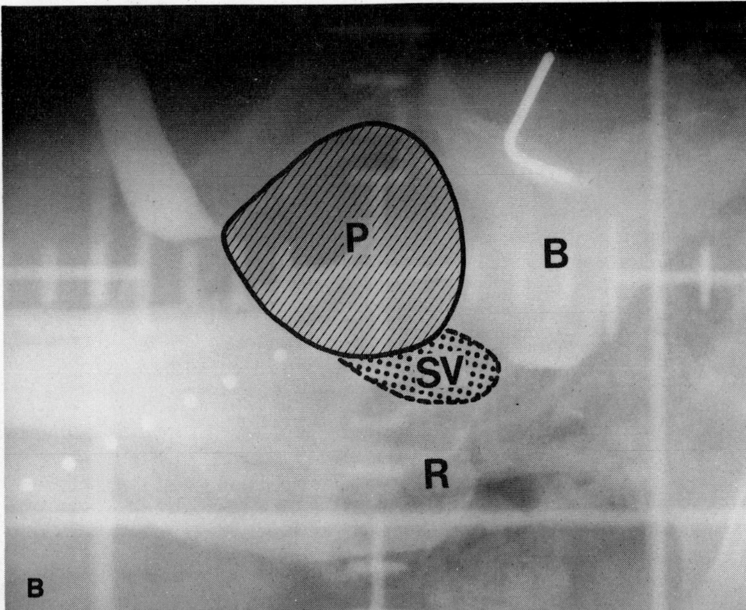

FIGURE 51–18. **(A, B)** Example of reduced volume portals for prostate boost in patient with seminal vesicle involvement.

usually palliative, and the minimal tumor dose can be held at 6000 cGy to 6500 cGy to decrease morbidity. Most institutions treat with daily fractions of 180 to 200 cGy, five fractions per week.[281,365] Lai and associates[220] found no significant correlation of pelvic tumor control or frequency of complications with various dose-time schedules. Occasionally, four weekly fractions of 225 cGy have been used.[24] At least two portals should be treated daily to improve tolerance to irradiation.

Biggs and Russell[43] described an average dose decrease of approximately 2% for patients with metallic hip prostheses who are treated with lateral portals, and an average increase of 2% for 10-MV x-rays and 5% for ^{60}Co.

TABLE 51–8
Treatment Policies for Adenocarcinoma of Prostate Using High-Energy Photons at Mallinckrodt Institute of Radiology

	PORTAL SIZE (CM AT ISOCENTER)		TECHNIQUE		TUMOR DOSES*	
STAGE	PELVIC	PROSTATE	PELVIC	PROSTATE	PELVIC LYMPH NODES (cGy)	PROSTATE BOOST (cGy)
A1 (less than well diff.)		8 × 10		120° bilateral arcs		6400/6.5 wk
A2, B (staging lymphadenectomy, negative pelvic lymph nodes)		8 × 10 or 10 × 12	None	120° bilateral arcs	0	6600/7 wk
A2, B1 (well diff.), no staging		10 × 12		120° bilateral arcs	0	6600/7 wk
A2, B (no lymphadenectomy)	16.5 × 16.5	8 × 10	AP/PA	120° bilateral arcs	4500/5 wk	2000/2 wk
A2, B (any histology, older than 70 yr)		8 × 10 or 10 × 12	None	120° bilateral arcs	0	6600/7 wk
A2, B (positive common iliac nodes, plus 4500 cGy to periaortic nodes)†	16.5 × 21	8 × 10	AP/PA	120° bilateral arcs	4500/5 wk	2000/2 wk
C (negative lymphadenectomy)	16.5 × 16.5	12 × 12 or 12 × 14	AP/PA	120° bilateral arcs	4500/5 wk	2500/2.5 wk
C (positive external iliac or hypogastric nodes by any evaluation)	16.5 × 21	10 × 12 or 12 × 14	AP/PA	120° bilateral arcs	4500/5 wk	2500/2.5 wk
C (no lymphadenectomy)	16.5 × 21	10 × 12 or 12 × 12	AP/PA	120° bilateral arcs	4500/5 wk	2500/2.5 wk
C (positive common iliac or periaortic nodes plus 4500 cGy to PA nodes)†	16.5 × 21	8 × 10 or 10 × 12	AP/PA	120° bilateral arcs	4500/5 wk	2500/2.5 wk
D1	16.5 × 21	10 × 12 or 12 × 14	AP/PA	120° bilateral arcs	4500/5 wk	2000/2 wk

* *Daily dose: Large pelvis fields, 180 cGy; prostate boosts portals, 200 cGy.*
† *In case of "grossly positive" periaortic nodes, add 500 to 1000 cGy with reduced portals. In stage C, if seminal vesicles are involved (C2), boost port may be 12 × 14 cm.*

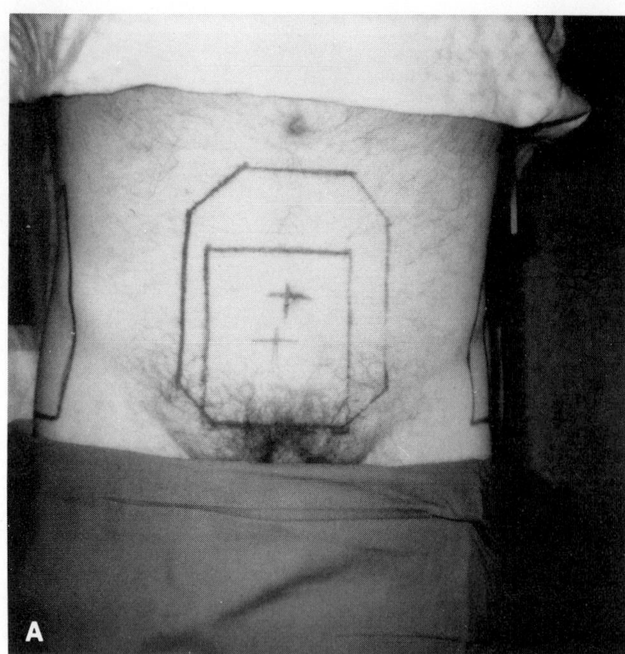

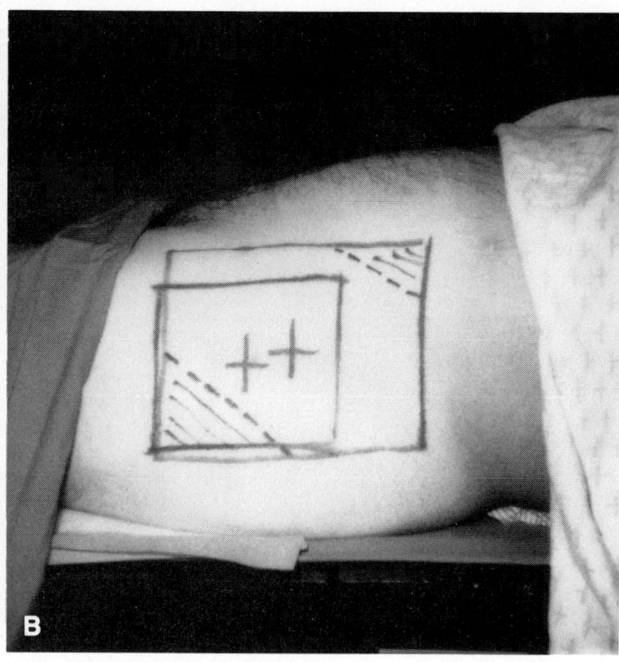

FIGURE 51–19. (**A**) Frontal and (**B**) lateral photographs of patient with Stage C prostatic adenocarcinoma showing skin markings outlining treatment portals.

Prostate Biopsies After Definitive Irradiation

Microscopic disappearance of tumor, fibrosis, obliteration of glandular structure, and calcifications in the prostate have been reported after definitive radiation therapy.[88,204,208,227] The number of positive biopsy specimens decreases with time; only those that show persistent tumor more than 18 months after radiation therapy may have some clinical significance.[88,330] Freiha and co-workers[128] reported biopsies performed in 64 of 146 patients 2 or more years after completion of irradiation; only 29% of the normal-feeling prostates contained cancer, in contrast to 85% of those that appeared abnormal on rectal examination. It is important, therefore, to determine whether biopsies were routinely done regardless of clinical findings or were specifically indicated because of clinical suspicion of tumor progression.

Cox and Kline[88] reported 46 consecutive patients, many of whom underwent serial transperineal needle biopsies of the prostate after definitive radiation therapy of 7000 cGy in 30 to 37 fractions; a decreased incidence of positive specimens was found over time, with 19% of the patients having persistent tumor after 24 months and 15% after 42 months. Perez and associates[281] recorded the time at which complete tumor regression took place after definitive radiation therapy in patients with Stage B or C carcinoma of the prostate. Figure 51-23*A* shows the superimposition of their clinical findings with the pathologic observations of Cox and Kline[88]; the clinical and histologic tumor regressions are similar, with about 20% of the tumors showing persistent tumor after using either method. Therefore, careful periodic digital examination can adequately evaluate local control in carcinoma of the prostate after irradiation. Biopsies are needed for patients who show persistent induration

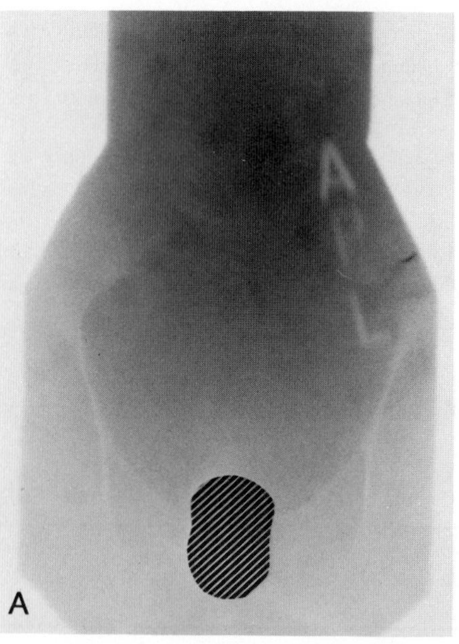

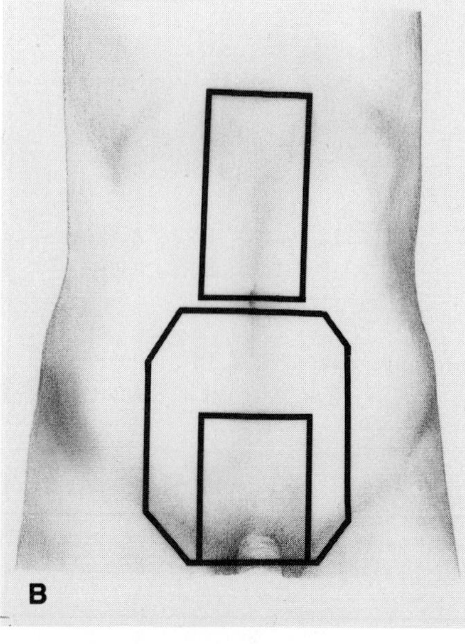

FIGURE 51–20. (**A**) Localization film showing an extended portal for irradiation of the periaortic and pelvic lymph nodes in carcinoma of the prostate. (**B**) Separate portals used for irradiation of the periaortic lymph nodes when large fields are not available. Gap separation must be calculated for each patient.

AP
BLADDER
PROSTATE
RECTUM
RT
LT
2000
3000
4000
5000
6000
6200
6400
6500
PA

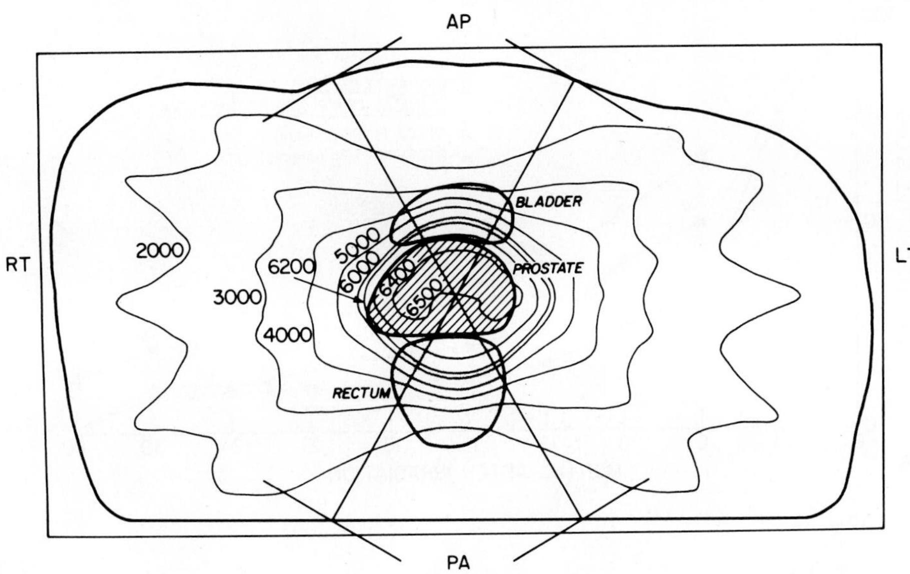

FIGURE 51–21. Isodose curves of plan delivering 6500 cGy to the prostate with 18-MV photons, bilateral 120-degree arc, skipping 60-degree anterior and posterior vectors.

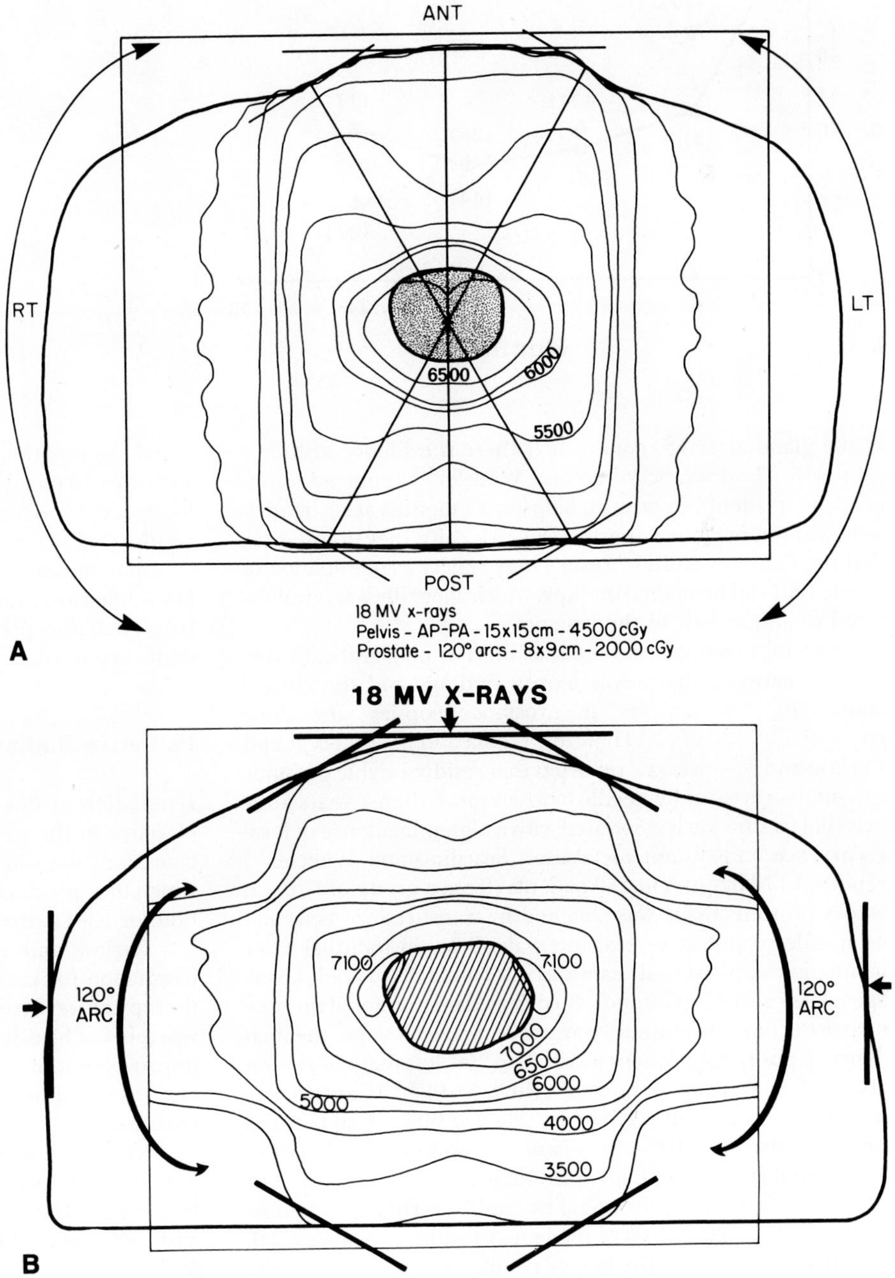

ANT
RT
LT
6500
6000
5500
POST
18 MV x-rays
Pelvis - AP-PA - 15x15cm - 4500cGy
Prostate - 120° arcs - 8x9cm - 2000 cGy
A
18 MV X-RAYS
120° ARC
120° ARC
7100
7100
7000
6500
6000
5000
4000
3500
B

FIGURE 51–22. Isodose curves for irradiation of pelvic lymph nodes and prostatic volume. (**A**) Pelvis receives 4500 cGy with AP/PA fields and prostate additional 2000 cGy with reduced portals, with bilateral 120-degree rotation arcs. (**B**) AP/PA and lateral fields are used to deliver 4500 cGy to the pelvis and 2000 cGy to prostate with reduced fields, with bilateral 120-degree arcs.

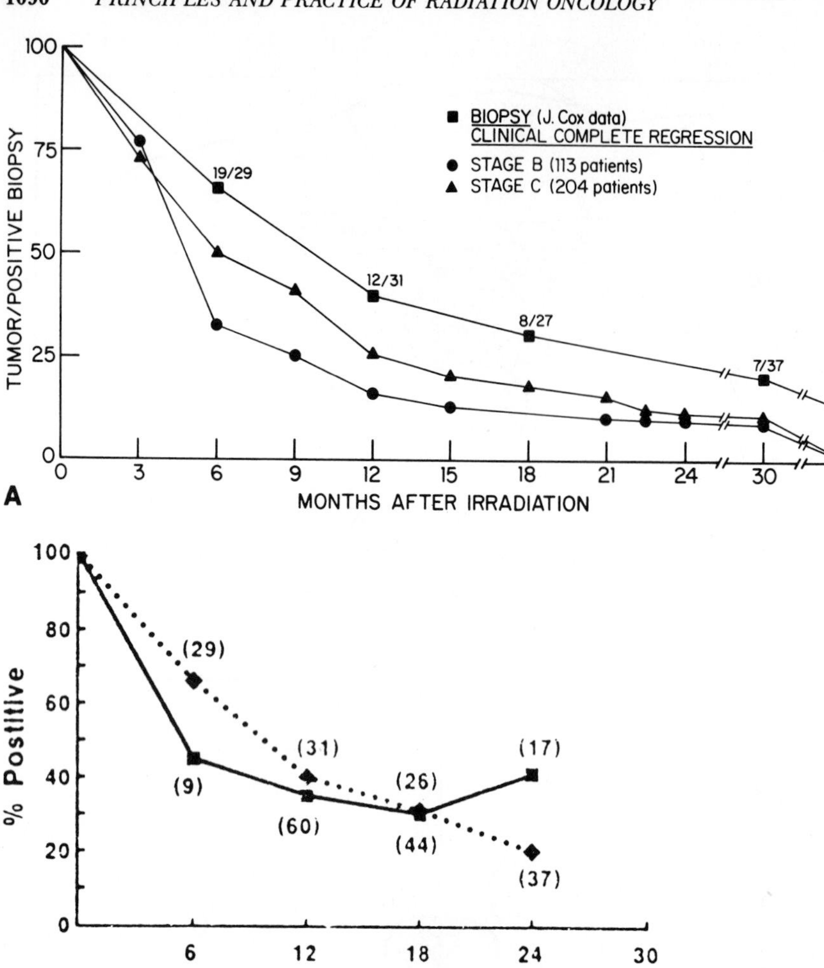

FIGURE 51–23. (**A**) Graph illustrating time to complete regression of tumor in patients with Stage B or C carcinoma of the prostate as evaluated by rectal examination (1967–1983). Comparison is made with time at which normal findings from the biopsy of the prostate were observed in another group of patients.[88] (**B**) Incidence of positive postirradiation biopsy results as a function of time after radiation therapy, reaching a minimum at 12 months in a series in which no hormonal therapy was given (*solid squares*) and 24 months in a series[89] in which hormonal therapy was widely used (*solid diamonds*). Values in parentheses are numbers of patients who had biopsies at each interval. (Scardino PT, Wheeler TM: NCI Monogr 7:95, 1988)

of the gland after 18 months or if there is evidence of tumor regrowth. However, Scardino and Wheeler[329] reported an increasing incidence of positive biopsies 18 months after irradiation, without hormonal therapy (Fig. 51-23*B*); they pointed out that the Cox and Stoffel[89] results may reflect a combination of irradiation and hormonal therapy, which allegedly was administered to almost half of the patients.

Several investigators state that there is no significant correlation between the needle biopsy findings and the clinical course of the patients if prostatic biopsies are done routinely.[88, 204, 208, 227, 281] However, Freiha and associates[128] and Carlton and co-workers[70] reported that residual viable prostatic carcinoma revealed by needle biopsies more than 2 years after external irradiation is associated with a higher incidence of local recurrence and distant metastases. Scardino and Wheeler[329] reported 170 biopsies in 140 patients (from a group of 510) on whom prostatic tissue was obtained by transurethral resection or needle biopsy at several intervals (6 to 36 months) after irradiation with external beam and interstitial ^{198}Au seeds (average total dose 6927 cGy) and who received no hormonal therapy before documented tumor recurrence. Stage by stage, the incidence of positive specimens was 20% to 25% less than those seen after external irradiation alone (Table 51-9).[329] If any biopsy was positive, the local recurrence rate was 60%; if all biopsies were negative, only 19% of the patients developed local failure. The digital rectal examination findings correlated closely with the biopsy findings: if the rectal examination results were normal, only 20% (20 of 101) of the biopsy results were abnormal, but 64% (25 of 39) of the biopsy results were abnormal if the rectal examination results were abnormal. Even in the patients with normal rectal examination and abnormal biopsy, the risk of local recurrence was greater than in patients with normal biopsy results (Fig. 51-24).

The best management for a patient with abnormal biopsy but otherwise clinically normal prostate after irradiation is controversial, and prospective clinical trials for this group of patients are needed.

Palliative Radiation Therapy for Prostatic Carcinoma

Irradiation at doses of 5000 cGy to 6000 cGy may be quite effective in the treatment of massive pelvic extensions of carcinoma of the prostate or extensive lymph node involvement, which may produce pelvic pain or hematuria, urethral obstruction, or leg edema because of lymphatic obstruction.

Carlton and associates[70] reported the results of palliative irradiation for patients who had failed to respond to estrogen therapy or were treated with hormones after irradiation. There was relief of bladder neck obstruction in 20 (50%) of 40 patients, improvement of hydronephrosis in eight (73%) of 11 patients, and disappearance of intractable hematuria in seven (100%) patients.

Kraus and associates[214] described satisfactory palliation in patients with locally advanced prostatic cancer with doses between 2250 cGy and 6600 cGy, most often between 4000 cGy and 5000 cGy. Marked improvement of rectal symptoms, including pain, constipation, and tenesmus, occurred in five

TABLE 51–9
Postirradiation Biopsy Results

	GOLD SEEDS PLUS EXTERNAL-BEAM RADIATION THERAPY		EXTERNAL-BEAM RADIATION THERAPY ALONE*	
CLINICAL STAGE	NO. OF PATIENTS	PERCENT WITH POSITIVE BIOPSY	NO. OF PATIENTS	PERCENT WITH POSITIVE BIOPSY
A2	23	35	1	0
BIN	9	11	2	0
B1	48	21	8	38
B2	27	33	22	59
C	40	55	31	74
Total	147	34	64	61

**(Data from Freiha FS, Bagshaw MA: Prostate 5:19, 1984)*
(Scardino PT, Wheeler TM: NCI Monogr 7:95, 1988)

patients (100%), and severe rectal bleeding caused by tumor invasion was controlled in one patient. Gross hematuria disappeared in 13 patients (100%), and there was definitive decrease in the size and induration of the gland in 19 (82%) of 23 patients. Symptoms of lower urinary tract obstruction improved after irradiation in 14 patients; four of five patients treated for urethral obstruction had a favorable response. Severe edema of the lower extremities improved in three patients, and perineal and inguinal pain were relieved in three patients.

Swelling during the initial phase of irradiation may cause increasing urinary difficulty in patients with partial urethral obstruction. An indwelling catheter may avert a complete blockage, but ideally, it should not be used for more than 2 or 3 weeks because of irritation and the danger of superimposed infection. A transurethral resection may be required if there is no improvement of the obstruction during the initial course of irradiation; there should be an interval of 3 or 4 weeks before resuming radiation therapy.

Irradiation is also used in the treatment of distant metastases from carcinoma of the prostate. Marked symptomatic relief occurs in more than 80% of the patients treated with doses of 3000 cGy to 3500 cGy in 2 to 3 weeks. Large portals must be used to include the entire bone, such as the extremities or the pelvis. Brain metastases may be successfully treated with doses of 3000 cGy to 3500 cGy in 2 or 3 weeks to the entire cranial contents; 75% of the patients have multiple lesions. Hemibody irradiation has been used in the palliation of disseminated bony metastases.[215] For further details the reader is referred to Chapter 76.

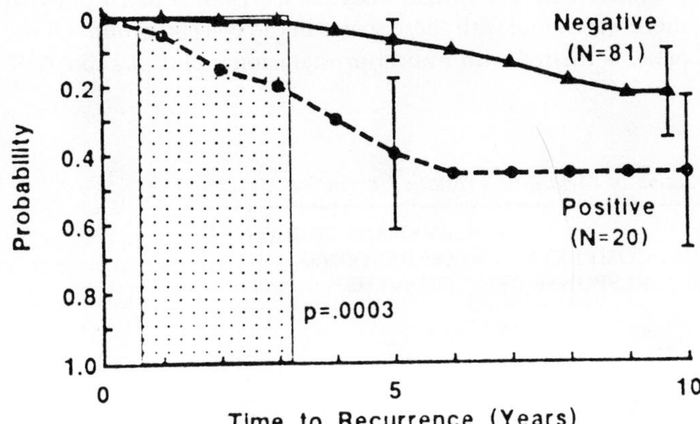

FIGURE 51–24. Development of local recurrence correlated with digital rectal examination of the prostate at the time of biopsy. An abnormal biopsy was associated with significantly greater risk of local recurrence. (Scardino PT, Wheeler TM: NCI Monogr 17:95, 1988)

Systemic ^{32}P or ^{89}Sr for Palliation of Bone Metastases

When practically all the bones of the body are involved by tumor, radioactive phosphorus (^{32}P) may be administered systemically after priming with testosterone or parathormone.[202, 205, 323, 345, 368] Testosterone cypionate (100 mg) is given intramuscularly each day for 7 to 15 days. After the first 5 or 6 days, ^{32}P is administered orally or intravenously (1.5 mCi for 6 or 7 days). Some advocate administration of a single dose of 5 mCi to 7 mCi. Edland[104] reported good to excellent relief of pain in 86% of the 42 patients treated.

Aziz and colleagues[17] reported their experience in treating 15 patients with diffuse bony metastases from carcinoma of the prostate with 10 to 12 mCi of intravenous sodium ^{32}P given in single or divided doses over a week, preceded by daily intramuscular injections of testosterone propionate (100 mg) for 5 days. Palliation of pain was achieved in 12 of the patients (80%); in seven (47%), relief was complete, and analgesics were no longer required. Maximum depression of peripheral cell counts was seen 4 to 5 weeks after therapy. The results were comparable to those reported by other investigators (Table 51-10) and similar to those described after hemibody irradiation (Table 51-11). Because of the rather delayed response to ^{32}P therapy, it has fallen out of favor.[17]

Pinck and Alexander[301] treated 32 patients with parathormone before ^{32}P administration and achieved acute pain relief in 22 (69%), with 14 of the patients maintaining pain relief for 1 year or longer. In these patients, the usual acute gastrointestinal symptoms caused by irradiation may appear, and there is some bone marrow depression.

^{89}Sr has been administered intravenously (40 μCi/kg, total dose about 3 mCi) for diffuse bone metastases, relieving pain in 80% of the patients.[46, 57, 314]

Straffon and associates[357] reported the use of ^{90}Y hypophysectomy in the palliative treatment of patients with painful, widespread bony metastases. Seven of 13 patients who had not responded to orchiectomy or estrogen therapy had good responses to this treatment.

TABLE 51–10
Relief of Bone Pain with ^{32}P Therapy in Metastatic Prostatic Carcinoma

INVESTIGATOR	NO. OF PATIENTS	TOTAL RESPONSE (%)	COMPLETE RESPONSE (%)	AVERAGE DURATION OF RESPONSE (MONTHS)
Maxfield et al[244]	21	76	47	
Vermotten et al[376]	27	75		
Joshi et al[202]	13	92	60	
Smart[345]	9	95	33	5.0
Donati et al[101]	12	91	50	6.3
Corwin et al[86]	20	70	45	3.3
Glaser et al[145]	24	58	17	5.0
Aziz et al[17]	15	80	47	6.0

(Aziz H, Choi K, Sohn C, et al: Am J Clin Oncol 9:264, 1986)

RESULTS OF THERAPY

The effectiveness of any therapy in carcinoma of the prostate is always compared with what many believe is a fairly indolent clinical course of the disease. George[136] reported 120 patients with a mean age of 74.8 years, without clinical or bone scan evidence of distant metastases, who were diagnosed as having localized prostatic carcinoma, were treated conservatively, and were followed up prospectively for a minimum of 7 years. More than 90% of the patients had been referred to the urology service for treatment of prostatic symptoms. No anticancer treatment was given other than relief of outflow tract urinary obstruction.

Increase in local tumor size was observed in 84% of the patients, and the progression was generally slow. Only a few patients developed symptoms, although most eventually had distinct T2 to T3 tumors on rectal examination. This local progression led to treatment in 23 patients (mean time to therapy, 18 months), and metastasis developed in one of the patients. Objective evidence of bony metastasis on scans emerged in 13 (11%) patients within a mean time of 35.8 months. After palliative treatment, nine patients remained well, and five (4%) patients died of prostatic cancer. Overall, 48 (40%) of the 120 patients died of other malignant tumors, cardiovascular disease, and other conditions unrelated to prostatic carcinoma. Unfortunately, follow-up compliance was inadequate, and the investigators did not correlate the initial stage or degree of differentiation of the tumor with the subsequent prognosis. They questioned the need to institute therapy in all patients with a diagnosis of asymptomatic prostatic carcinoma, without taking into consideration other parameters such as age, general condition, and associated medical problems or the fact that 23 patients required definitive treatment. They postulated that it would be difficult for any therapy to substantially improve the 80% 5-year survival rate for these elderly men treated with observation only.

However, in a study by Thompson,[367] patients treated with transurethral resection before 1940 had significantly lower survival rates compared with those receiving more aggressive therapy. Hanash and colleagues[169] reviewed 200 unstaged patients with histologically proven carcinoma of the prostate who were treated with transurethral resection only between 1934 and 1942 (probably the same population studied by Thompson). For patients with clinically latent (occult) tumors, survival was similar to that expected for a comparable normal population: the 5-year survival rate was about 50% and the 10-year survival rate for all histologic grades was 30%. However, patients with clinically apparent tumors had a 5-year survival rate of 20% for grades 1, 2, and 3 and less than 5% for grade 4. The 10-year survival rate was below 10% for all grades, significantly below the expected normal survival rate of 40%.

The Veterans Administration Cooperative Urological Research Group (VACURG) reported a randomized trial of radical prostatectomy plus placebo (37 patients) and placebo alone (29 patients) for Stage A and B tumors.[66] The results were comparable, with a median follow-up of all survivors of 7.7 years. Madsen and co-workers[239] observed that six patients in the prostatectomy group had Gleason scores of 8 to 10 but that there were none with these scores in the placebo group. Of the patients treated with radical prostatectomy plus placebo, 45%

TABLE 51–11
Relief of Bone Pain with Sequential Hemibody Irradiation of Metastatic Prostatic Carcinoma

INVESTIGATOR	NO. OF PATIENTS	TOTAL RESPONSE (%)	COMPLETE RESPONSE (%)	AVERAGE DURATION OF RESPONSE (MONTHS)
Fitzpatrick and Rider[115,116]	70	75	48	5.5
Epstein et al[112]	10	80	40	8.0
Salazar et al[327]	32	77	21	5.5
Jones et al[201]	35	86	48	5.5

(Aziz H, Choi K, Sohn C, et al: Am J Clin Oncol 9:264, 1986)

were alive at 8.5 years, and 62% of those treated with placebo alone were still alive. The differences are not statistically significant. Also, there was no significant difference in the rate of progression of Stage B prostatic carcinoma after either therapy; only two patients died with tumor.

It is practically impossible in the United States to justify delaying definitive therapy in patients with localized carcinoma of the prostate, except for selected elderly patients with well-differentiated Stage A1 (T1a) tumors.

Radical Prostatectomy

Many reports describe a 5-year survival rate of 75% to 80%, a 10-year survival rate of 60%, and a 15-year survival rate of 35% to 40% after radical prostatectomy for clinical Stage A2 and B tumors (Table 51-12).[42,91,196,197,382] The local recurrence rate ranges from 8% to 31% for patients staged pathologically and up to 43% for a group of 14 patients with clinical Stage C lesions.

A critical factor in the outcome of therapy is patient selection, because there is extracapsular extension in approximately 10% of the patients with clinical Stage A2 or B1 lesions and 50% in those with B2 tumors, significantly limiting the effectiveness of radical prostatectomy to Stage A and B1 tumors.[79,105]

In 1970, Jewett reported 111 consecutive prostatectomy patients with tumors less than 1.5 cm in size.[196] The 10-year tumor-free survival rate was 41%. The overall tumor-free survival rate was 27%. Of the 38 patients who died with disease, 17 had microscopic invasion of the seminal vesicles at the time of prostatectomy; in the remaining 21, the disease was histologically limited to the prostate. In Jewett's series of 79 patients with Stage B2 tumors, 18% survived 15 years; 50% of these patients had invasion of the seminal vesicles and only 5% lived without evidence of tumor for 15 years.

Lepor and Walsh[231] updated the results of radical perineal prostatectomy at Johns Hopkins University. Seventy patients had clinical Stage B1 disease; the 57 patients who were followed up had a 5-year survival rate of 83%, a 10-year rate of 63%, and a 15-year survival of 51%. The survival rates of these patients were virtually identical to the projected life expectancies of age-matched men in the general population. Gibbons[139] reported that 46 (84%) of 57 patients followed up for a minimum of 15 years were alive or died without evidence of tumor recurrence. These results are similar to those described by Bagshaw and associates[23] for 491 patients with clinical Stage A2 or B carcinoma of the prostate treated with radiation therapy alone, 60% of whom survived 13 years (Fig. 51-25).

Walsh and Schlegel[384] reported 320 men followed from 1 to 5 years after nerve-sparing prostatectomy. Of 259 initially sexually potent patients, 192 (74%) were potent after surgery. The authors reported a correlation of sexual potency preservation with age at the time of diagnosis (Table 51-6). In the first 100 consecutive patients, careful pathologic examination of the specimen showed that 14% had capsule penetration, but only 7% had positive surgical margins. In a review of 414 patients treated with standard radical prostatectomy, a comparable 10% had positive surgical margins. The actuarial local recurrence rate at 5 years was 10%. However, only 10 patients have been followed for 5 years, 74 for 4 years, and 142 for 3 years. Catalona and Bigg[78] reported preservation of sexual potency in 71 (63%) of 112 patients treated with bilateral nerve-sparing prostatectomy and in 13 (39%) of 33 who underwent a unilateral nerve-sparing procedure (minimum follow-up of 6 months).

Direct randomized comparison of radiation therapy or radical prostatectomy in early carcinoma of the prostate was reported by Paulson and associates[279] for 97 patients with clinical Stage A2 or B disease. Fifty-six patients received radiation therapy, and 41 were treated with radical prostatectomy. The investigators did not specify if there were any stratification criteria or satisfactorily explain why 59 patients were assigned to irradiation and 47 to radical prostatectomy in a random study. Also, seven patients in the irradiation group and nine patients in the surgical group did not receive the prescribed treatment. The actuarial disease-free survival rate was 85% for the surgical patients and 60% for the radiation therapy group. Most of the patients failed because of metastases to bone (as evidenced by an

TABLE 51–12
Results of Radical Surgery for Stages A and B Adenocarcinoma of the Prostate

	NO. OF PATIENTS			SURVIVAL (%)		
INVESTIGATOR	STAGE A	STAGE B	STAGES A & B	5-YEAR	10-YEAR	15-YEAR
Belt et al[38]		185 (c)*		78	55	31
Benson et al[41]		102 (c, No)		93 (88)†		
Boxer et al[51]			309	82	59	
		200 (p)		86	62	
Byar[63]	46			78		
Culp et al[91]		160 (cB1)			72 (27)	54 (27)
Elder et al[109]	14			100		
Gibbons et al[142]		195 (c)		95 (86)	74 (67)	55 (48)
Hodges et al[184]			119	85	53	
Jewett[195]		110 (c)		(75)	(58)	(38)
Middleton et al[257]			153 (No)	94	67	
		102 (c, No)		93 (88)		
Nichols et al[267]	28			75	60	
Veenema et al[375]			159	84	52	

**No: negative nodes by lymphadenectomy; c: clinical stage; p: pathologic stage.*
† Numbers in parentheses indicate disease-free survival.

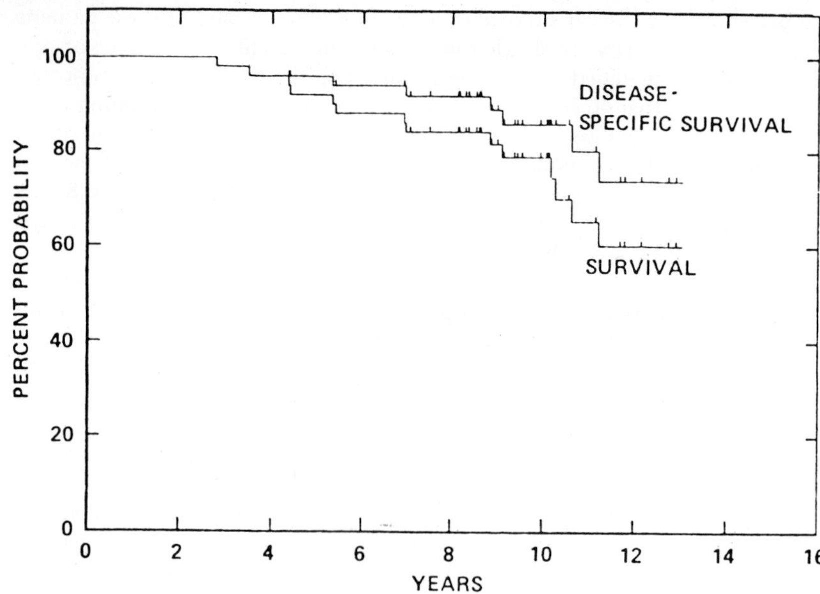

FIGURE 51–25. Long-term disease-specific and overall survival of 51 patients with Stages A2 and B prostate cancer who had no histopathologically positive lymph nodes at surgical staging (T0d, T1, T2, N0, and M0). (Bagshaw MA, Cox, RS, Ray GR: NCI Monogr 7:47, 1988)

abnormal bone scan) or other distant metastases. Paulson[275] updated the results of these patients, and again, a better actuarial tumor-free survival was found for the prostatectomy patients (76%) than for the radiation therapy group (57%) at 80 months. This difference should not have been the direct effect of the local irradiation and may be related to the initial distribution of the patients in the two study groups. There are also serious reservations regarding the statistical analysis and validity of the data.[171] The results obtained with radiation therapy in this series are inferior to those reported by other authors.[291] Figure 51-26 compares survival in patients with similar surgical tumor stages treated with radiation therapy alone at various institutions.[291] (For a more thorough discussion of the merits of this trial, the reader is referred to correspondence between Hanks and Paulson.[170, 276]) A prospective clinical trial to compare these two modalities is in progress.

Interstitial ^{125}I or ^{198}Au Irradiation

Five-year survival rates of 80% or higher have been reported for T1 and T2 tumors, and a rate of 70% for T3 was reported for tumors treated with staging lymph node dissection and ^{125}I implantation (Table 51-13).[32, 182, 183, 347] The local recurrence rate is 10% or less with doses over 15,000 cGy and 30% or higher with lower doses; overall incidence of local failures is approximately 15% in T1 and 40% to 50% for T2 or T3 tumors.[32]

Sogani and associates[347] described better tumor control with higher doses of irradiation. They also observed an overall failure rate of 5% with homogeneous distribution of the radiation dose but a failure rate of 24% with nonhomogeneous dose distribution.

Batata and colleagues[31] reported 28 patients with nodal involvement at the time of interstitial therapy and pelvic lymphadenectomy who also received irradiation to the whole pelvis alone or with the periaortic lymph nodes. These patients were compared with a group of 24 patients not given external irradiation. The determinate 5-year survival rate was 54% for both groups, and the tumor-free 5-year survival rate was 15% (two of 13) with and 21% (five of 24) without external irradiation. Similar results were described by Prout and associates,[304] who compared 16 patients given external irradiation with 16 who received no additional therapy after ^{125}I implantation of the prostate. External nodal irradiation is probably not effective because 75% to 80% of these patients develop distant metastases, and few survive over 5 years.

Morton and associates[259] compared the outcomes for 141 patients with Stage A2, B, or C disease treated with ^{125}I implants and 166 treated with external irradiation. Survival and local tumor control were similar in both groups (Table 51-14). There were significant complications in 8.5% of the patients treated with ^{125}I and 14% of those receiving external irradiation.

Shipley and associates[343] reported comparable overall survival rates (75% to 80% at 10 years) for 38 patients with Stage T2 tumors treated with ^{125}I implant and 126 similar-stage patients receiving external-beam irradiation, who had a recurrence rate of approximately 20%. Hanks[171] observed similar results in treating 65 patients with Stages A or B and negative lymph node dissection with external-beam irradiation (37 patients) or ^{125}I implant (28 patients). The overall local failure rate was 14% in both groups.

Kuban and colleagues[216] compared the results of treating 120 patients with various stages of prostatic carcinoma with ^{125}I implants and 246 patients with external irradiation alone. There were more local recurrences in patients with Stages B2 or C who were treated with interstitial ^{125}I (Table 51-15). The overall survival and disease-free survival rates were similar in both groups (Table 51-16).

Carlton and others[70, 71] treated 542 patients with ^{198}Au grains and external irradiation. Results updated by Scardino and associates[328] showed no significant difference with other techniques.

Interstitial ^{192}Ir Irradiation

Afterloading removable implants with ^{192}Ir have produced tumor control and survival comparable to other methods.[48, 55, 305, 360]

External Irradiation

The results obtained with external irradiation in treating carcinoma of the prostate have been summarized in Tables 51-17 and 51-18.

Stanford University researchers gathered information on the use of external irradiation to treat carcinoma of the prostate

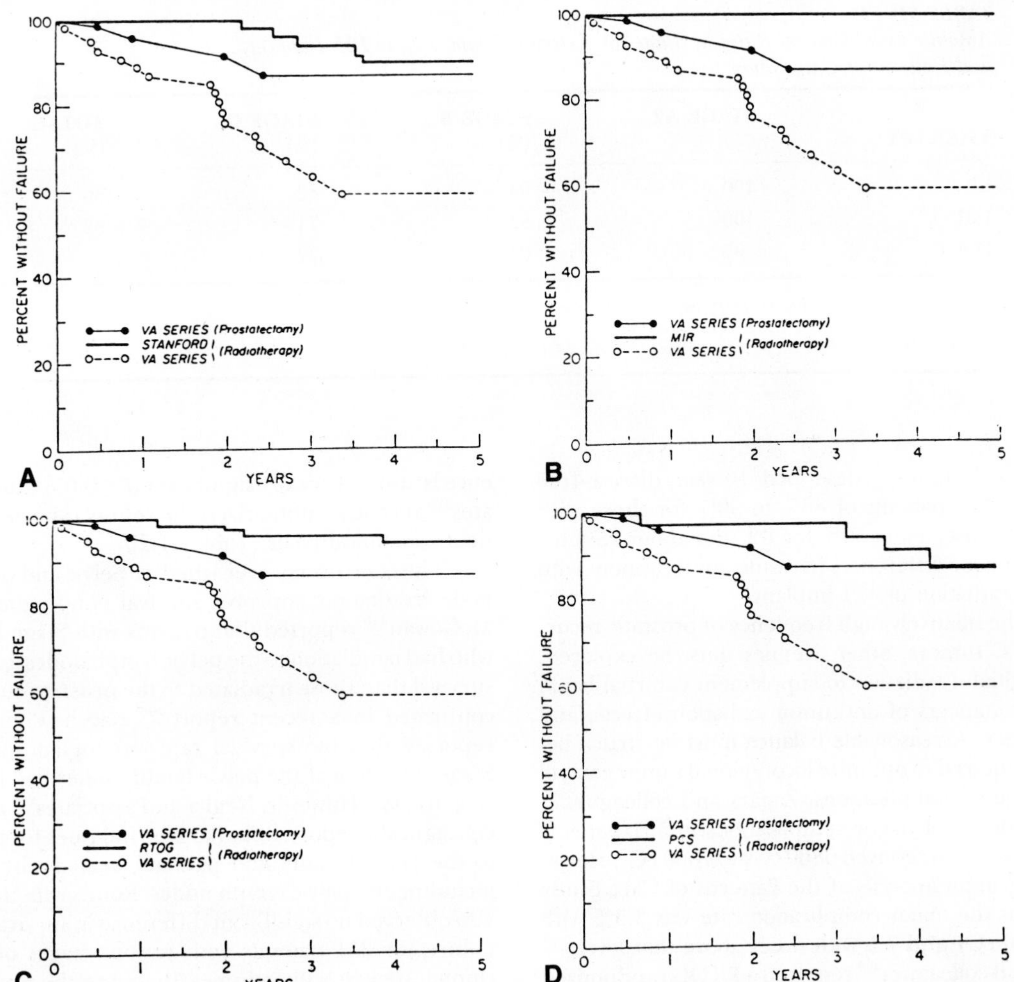

FIGURE 51–26. (**A**) Stanford University data superimposed over VA Uro-Oncology Group data. (**B**) Mallinckrodt Institute of Radiology (MIR), Washington University School of Medicine, data superimposed over VA Uro-Oncology group data. (**C**) RTOG data superimposed over VA Uro-Oncology Group data. (**D**) PCS data superimposed over VA Uro-Oncology Group data. (Pilepich MV, Bagshaw MA, Asbell SO, et al: Int J Radiat Oncol Biol Phys 13:659, 1987)

localized to the pelvis.[21–24] At 5 years, the disease-free survival rate for their patients with tumors localized to the prostate was about 75%, and at 10 years, the rate was 60%. In patients with extracapsular extension, the 5-year survival rate is 50%, and the 10-year survival rate is 30%.

Perez and colleagues[286] described results in 577 patients with carcinoma of the prostate followed up for a minimum of 3 years after radiation therapy. The actuarial disease-free 5-year survival rates were 78% for Stages A2 and B, 60% for Stage C, and 15% for Stage D1 (Fig. 51-27*A*). The overall survival was about 10% higher (Fig. 51-27*B*). Overall failure rate in patients with Stage A2 tumors was 12% (5 of 41), and it was 17% (31 of 185) in patients with Stage B tumors (Fig. 51-28); the impact of total tumor doses ranging from 6000 cGy to 7000 cGy was minimal (Fig. 51-29*A*). In Stage C patients, the failure rate was 30%, and the rate was greater for doses below 6500 cGy than with higher doses (Fig. 51-29*B*). Similar results have been reported by Hanks[175,177] in the Patterns of Care Study (Table 51-19), who also observed a difference in the incidence of in-field recurrence for patients with T2 tumors at 6000 cGy, T3 at 6500 cGy, and T4 at 7000 cGy. If a risk-time actuarial analysis is carried out, the incidence of prostatic failure is higher (Fig. 51-30). Similar observations have been made by Shipley and colleagues.[343]

Hanks and associates[175] reported the results of definitive radiation therapy (6000–7000 cGy) for 619 patients treated in the Patterns of Care Study. In Stage A, the 5-year survival rate was 75%; in Stage B, it was 85%; and in Stage C, it was 58%. At 10 years, the survival rate was 50% in Stage A2, 61% in Stage B, and 38% in Stage C. These figures are comparable to those reported at single institutions.

TABLE 51–13
Survival Rates According to Clinical Stage for ^{125}I Implants

CLINICAL STAGE	5-YEAR SURVIVAL, 1970–1976 NUMBER	(%)	OVERALL SURVIVAL, 1970–1980* NUMBER	(%)
T1	99/103	96	326/340	96
T2	39/52	76	108/123	88
T3	48/70	69	97/126	77
T4	2/15	13	4/17	24
Total	188/239	79	585/606	88

* ≥2 years.
(Batata MA, Hilaris BS, Whitmore WF: Factors affecting tumor control. In Hilaris BS, Batata MA [eds]: Brachytherapy Oncology, 1983, p 65. New York, Memorial Sloan-Kettering Cancer Center, 1983)

TABLE 51–14
Absolute Local Control Rates by Stage for External Beam, Iodine 125 Implant, and Patterns of Care Study

THERAPY*	STAGE A2 (%)	STAGE B (%)	STAGE C (%)	TOTAL (%)
EB	100	94	82	86
IMP	100	83	71	82
POC†	97	85	72	

**EB: external beam irradiation; IMP: implant; POC: Patterns of Care Study (external beam).*
† POC results are atuarial 5-year local control rates.
(Morton JD, Peschel RE: Int J Radiat Oncol Biol Phys 14:1153, 1988)

Kuban and colleagues[217] described 10-year disease-free survival rates for 414 patients of 88% to 90% for those with Stage A2 or B1 disease, about 50% for B2, and about 25% for Stage C, with no major differences in results for treatment with external-beam irradiation or ^{125}I implant.

Because of the relatively high frequency of prostatic recurrences in Stage C tumors, other avenues must be explored, including interstitial irradiation to supplement external beam doses, biologic enhancers of antitumor radiation effects, and high-LET particles. A reasonable balance must be struck between the dose required to optimize locoregional tumor control and the incidence of complications. Zagars and colleagues[406] found a 3% incidence of major complications in 551 patients with Stage C tumors who received 6800 cGy to 7000 cGy. Hanks and associates,[175] in an analysis of the Patterns of Care Study data, showed that the major complication rate was 3.5% with doses below 7000 cGy and 7% with doses above that level.

Laramore and colleagues[224] reported a RTOG randomized study of 91 patients with locally advanced adenocarcinoma of the prostate (Stages C and D1) treated with photon beam or a mixed regimen of photons and neutrons. In 78 evaluable patients (*i.e.*, no major protocol variations), the locoregional recurrence rate was 7% for the group treated with mixed beam and 22% for the group treated with photon beam. The difference is statistically significant ($P = 0.05$). For the 91 patients, the overall 5-year survival rate was 62% for the group treated with mixed beam and 35% for those receiving photons only. This difference is also statistically significant ($P < 0.05$). Russell and associates[325] recently summarized the results reported in several fast neutron clinical trials (Table 51-20).

The controversy over whether pelvic and periaortic lymph node irradiation improves survival is not completely settled. McGowan[246] reported that patients with Stage B2 or C tumors who had irradiation to the pelvic lymph nodes exhibited a better survival than those irradiated to the prostate only, observations confirmed in a recent report.[303] Bagshaw and co-workers[23] reported that the survival rate was higher for patients with Stage B2 tumor if the pelvic lymph nodes had been irradiated (Fig. 51-9*A*). However, Neglia and associates[266] and Zagars and colleagues[406] reported similar survival rates for patients treated to the prostate only and patients treated with larger portals including the pelvic lymph nodes. Rounsaville and associates[322] also observed no significant difference in survival or patterns of failure for 251 patients with various stages of prostatic carcinoma treated with volumes limited to the prostate and periprostatic tissues (90%) and for patients in other series with treated pelvic lymph nodes.

Stanford University researchers conducted a randomized study assessing the value of irradiation to the pelvic nodes in Stage B or the periaortic nodes in Stage C. Preliminary data reported by Pistenma and associates[302] suggested that survival in Stage B was similar, whether uninvolved pelvic lymph nodes are irradiated or not. However, a slightly higher survival rate was revealed for patients with nodal involvement when the

TABLE 51–15
Local Tumor Recurrence by Tumor Stage and Treatment Modality

	IODINE 125		EXTERNAL-BEAM IRRADIATION		
STAGE	NO. WITH LOCAL RECURRENCE	NO. WITH STAGE (%)	NO. WITH LOCAL RECURRENCE	NO. WITH STAGE (%)	*P* VALUE
A2	1	11 (9)	1	35 (3)	NS*
B1	1	9 (11)	2	19 (11)	NS
B2	19	68 (28)	12	85 (14)	0.028
C	14	32 (44)	28	107 (26)	0.048
Total	35	120 (29)	43	246 (17)	0.015

Recurrence rate in parentheses.
**NS, not significant.*
(Kuban D, El-Mahdi AM, Schellhammer PF: Cancer 63:2415, 1989)

TABLE 51–16
Disease-Free Survival of Carcinoma of the Prostate at 5 and 10 Years by Tumor Stage and Treatment Modality

	IODINE 125		**EXTERNAL-BEAM IRRADIATION**	
STAGE	5-YEAR DISEASE-FREE SURVIVAL (%)	10-YEAR DISEASE-FREE SURVIVAL (%)	5-YEAR DISEASE-FREE SURVIVAL (%)	10-YEAR DISEASE-FREE SURVIVAL (%)
A2	100	90	88	88
B1	88	88	81	81*
B2	77	50	72	48
C	50	14	51	35

** Results for 8 years.*
(Kuban D, El-Mahdi AM, Schellhammer PF: Cancer 63:2415, 1989)

pelvic and periaortic lymph nodes were irradiated (differences not statistically significant).[302]

RTOG conducted a randomized study of over 400 patients that assessed the value of irradiation to the pelvic nodes in Stage A2 or B tumors. Reports by Asbell and associates[14] showed similar survival and tumor control whether pelvic lymph nodes were electively irradiated or not (Fig. 51-10*A*). In another randomized trial published by Pilepich and colleagues,[295] elective irradiation of the periaortic lymph nodes (4500 cGy) in patients with clinical Stage C tumors or Stage A2 or B lesions with positive pelvic nodes also failed to improve survival (Fig. 51-10*B*).

Patients with known periaortic lymph node metastases have poor prognoses, although some survive for extended periods of time. Lawton and colleagues[226] treated 23 of these patients with 5000 cGy, in addition to irradiation to the prostate and pelvic lymph nodes. The actuarial survival rate was 80% at 5 years and 60% at 10 years, and the disease-free survival rates were 65% and 52%, respectively. No difference in survival existed between those patients shown to have periaortic lymph node metastases by biopsy or by radiographic methods without biopsy.

Perez and co-workers[286] reported an overall incidence of distant metastases of 20% in Stage B, 40% in Stage C, and 65% in Stage D1. Others have described similar results.[143, 175, 178, 191, 233, 266]

TABLE 51–17
Radiation Therapy Results for Stage A and B Adenocarcinoma of the Prostate

	NO. OF PATIENTS			**SURVIVAL (%)**		
INVESTIGATOR	STAGE A	STAGE B	STAGES A & B	5-YEAR	10-YEAR	15-YEAR
Aristizabal et al[12]	17			100		
		101		82		
Bagshaw[21]			477	81	59	
Bagshaw[20]	45			93	70	38
		461		80	58	35
Forman[121]			113	(63)†		
Hanks[172]		312		75	42 (24)	
Harisiadis et al[178]		25		90 (59)		
	13			88		
Perez et al[286]	41			(78)	(60)	
		185		(76)	(56)	
Rangala et al[307]	10			100 (56)		
		25		90 (59)		
Rosen et al[317]	25			96 (84)		
		85		77 (68)		
Rounsaville et al[322]	49			81	67	
		50		84	53	
van der Werf-Messing et al[371]		24		(61)		
Whitmore et al[391]		155*		89		
Zagars et al[405]			114	89	68	
	32			74 (94)		
		82		93 (89)	70 (85)	

** ^{125}I implant.*
† Numbers in parentheses indicate disease-free survival.

TABLE 51–18
Radiation Therapy Results in Stage C Carcinoma of the Prostate

INVESTIGATOR	NO. OF PATIENTS	SURVIVAL % 5-YEAR	10-YEAR	15-YEAR
Aristizabal et al[12]	82	60		
Bagshaw et al[23]	348	64 (46)†	35 (28)	18 (23)
	32	27 (17)	12 (7)	
Forman[121]	125	(45)		
Hanks[172]	296	58 (39)	38 (28)	
	237	65 (50)		
Harisiadis et al[178]	112	58	35	
	93	78 (69)		
Neglia[266]	97 (C1)*	72		
	53 (C2)	59		
Perez et al[286]	328	65 (58)	40 (35)	
Rangala et al[307]	93	78 (69)		
Rosen et al[317]	88	61 (53)		
Rounsaville et al[322]	140 (C1)	63	42	
	12 (C2)	32	11	
van der Werf-Messing et al[371]	247	52 (44)	32 (23)	
Zagars et al[406]	551	72 (59)	47 (46)	27 (40)

** C: clinical stage*
† Numbers in parentheses indicate disease-free survival.

Irradiation after Prostatectomy

Occasionally, patients are referred for radiation therapy after a suprapubic prostatectomy for benign hyperplasia in which tumor beyond Stage IA was found in the specimen or after a radical retropubic prostatectomy in which tumor was found at the margins of resection. In addition, some patients who initially were treated surgically for prostatic carcinoma develop isolated pelvic recurrences that require radiation therapy.

It is customary to treat smaller volumes limited to the prostate and periprostatic tissues (8-cm × 10-cm or 10-cm × 12-cm portals) in these patients. Rotational techniques with 120-degree bilateral arcs and skipping of the bladder and rectum are used at Washington University and at Stanford to deliver doses of 6000 cGy to 6500 cGy, depending on tumor extent. On rare occasions, larger volumes are irradiated to cover the seminal vesicles or pelvic lymph nodes, in which case the standard irradiation technique described previously is used.

The indications for postoperative irradiation are not accepted by all physicians. Walsh[380] in an editorial, without a statistical basis for his statements, concluded that postprostatectomy irradiation should be administered only to patients with gross residual tumor, especially at the urethra or bladder neck. He observed that there was no correlation between capsular penetration and subsequent development of local recurrence after radical prostatectomy (*i.e.*, 25% recurrences with no capsular penetration and 17% if tumor invaded periprostatic tissues or seminal vesicles). What he did not mention was that the data were based on ten autopsy cases out of an initial population of 1000 patients treated with radical prostatectomy. This editorial was refuted by Anscher and Prosnitz[8] and Randall.[306]

Most reports have documented a significant decrease in pelvic recurrences (5% to 10%) with elective adjuvant irradiation in patients with microscopic positive margins, compared with radical prostatectomy alone (25% to 40%). More difficult to document is the beneficial effect in overall survival (Table 51-21). However, some authors have observed better disease-free and overall survival rates after adjuvant irradiation.[7] Anscher and Prosnitz[7] compared the results of elective irradiation delivering 4500 cGy to 5000 cGy to the pelvis plus a boost of 1000 cGy to 1500 cGy to the prostatic bed of 46 patients, who were found to have positive surgical margins during radical prostatectomy, and the results of treating 113 similar patients with operation alone. They observed a better overall survival in the patients receiving postoperative irradiation. The 5-, 10-, and 15-year survival rates in the electively irradiated group were 96%, 90%, and 40%, respectively, in contrast to survival rates of 82%, 62%, and 21% among the patients treated with surgery only. Actuarial 15-year disease-free survival was 40% for the irradiated patients and 28% for the surgery-only group ($P = 0.34$) (Fig. 51-31). Local control was 96% in the irradiated group and 32% in the surgery-alone patients.

In a separate report, the same investigators described no difference in survival among 16 patients who received irradiation alone and 16 treated with both irradiation and hormonal therapy.[6]

Lange and colleagues[223] administered 6000 cGy to the prostatic beds of 35 patients with positive margins and to the prostates and pelvic lymph nodes of 36 patients with metastatic pelvic lymph nodes (Stage D1a). The actuarial disease-free survival rates were 75% and 72%, respectively. No local failures were reported after a mean follow-up of 62 and 48 months, respectively.

Eisbruch and associates[106] reviewed their experience with 42 patients with positive margins referred for postoperative irradiation after prostatectomy; tumors were found in nine patients at the time of suprapubic prostatectomy for benign disease and the remainder were found after radical prostatec-

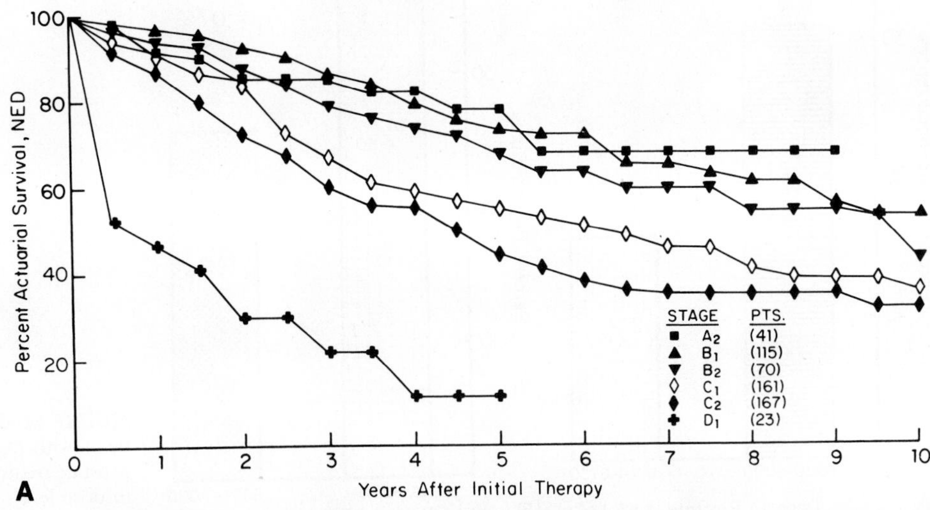

CARCINOMA OF THE PROSTATE
1967-1983
ACTUARIAL SURVIVAL BY STAGE

Stage Pts.
A2 (41)
B1 (115)
B2 (70)
C1 (161)
C2 (167)
D1 (23)
EXPECTED SURVIVAL

PERCENT ACTUARIAL SURVIVAL

YEARS AFTER THERAPY

B

FIGURE 51–27. (**A**) Disease-free survival and (**B**) actuarial 5-year survival in 577 patients with localized carcinoma of the prostate treated at Washington University. (Perez CA, Pilepich MV, Garcia D, et al: NCI Monogr 7:85, 1988)

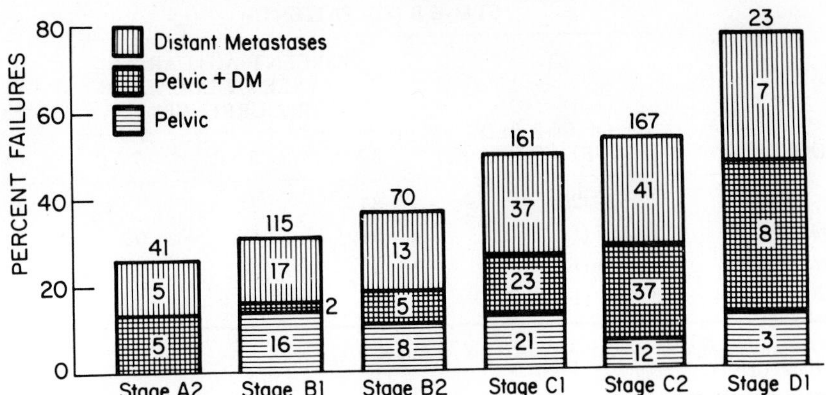

FIGURE 51–28. Anatomic sites of postirradiation failure by stage. DM, distant metastases. (Perez CA, Pilepich MV, Garcia D, et al: NCI Monogr 7:85, 1988)

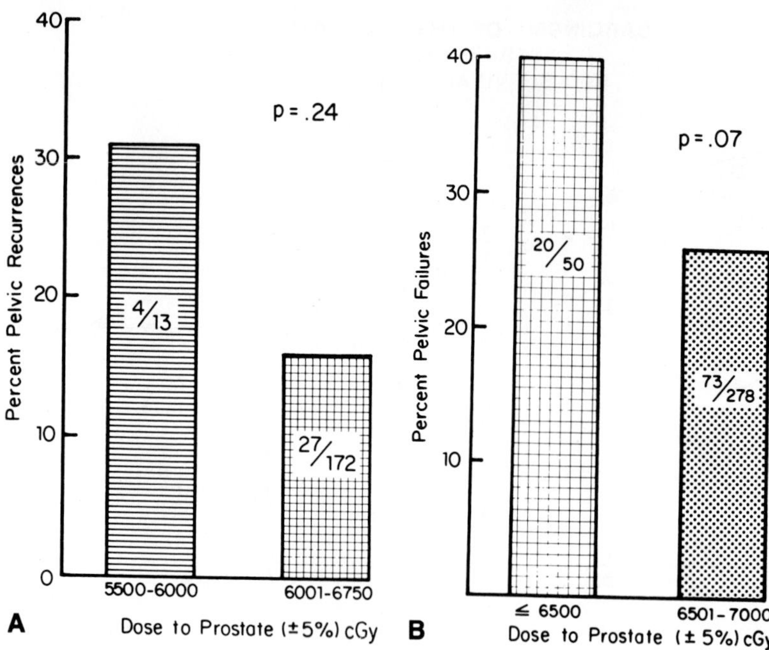

FIGURE 51–29. Incidence of pelvic recurrence in patients with (**A**) Stage B and (**B**) Stage C carcinoma of the prostate treated with definitive radiation therapy according to dose levels of irradiation (1967–1983). (Perez CA, Pilepich MV, Garcia D, et al: NCI Monogr 7:85, 1988)

tomy. The pelvic tumor control rate was 81%, and the 5-year disease-free survival rate was 66%, figures comparable to those seen in 44 patients with positive margins treated with surgery alone (Table 51-22). Complications were infrequent, consisting of urethral stricture (two patients), rectal ulcer (one), and urinary incontinence (one). There was no significant dose effect, with tumor control similar for doses of 6000 cGy or 6500 cGy (100% and 81%, respectively).

Pilepich and colleagues[300] and Ray and co-workers[309] have also reported 5-year survival rates (without evidence of tumor relapse) of 50% to 60% in small groups of patients irradiated after suprapubic prostatectomy or after radical prostatectomy when carcinoma and positive margins were found in the specimen.

Shevlin[342] reported a 10-year actuarial survival rate of 100% for 16 patients who received postoperative radiation therapy because of high-risk factors, 88% for 50 patients with tumor confined to the prostate gland treated with radical prostatectomy alone, and 72% for 57 patients who had tumor extending through the prostatic capsule, with closed or positive surgical margins or tumor extension into the seminal vesicles. The actuarial 10-year disease-free survival rates for local control were 64%, 72%, and 56%, respectively. The 10-year actuarial survival rates were 76%, 64%, and 80%, respectively.

Several other investigators have reported a significant decrease in the incidence of pelvic recurrences in surgically treated patients with carcinoma of the prostate with positive margins who received adjuvant irradiation compared with those not irradiated; improvement of overall survival is not as evident. Results obtained with prostatectomy and no elective irradiation are illustrated in Table 51-22.

It has become the policy at Washington University to irradiate patients referred for rising PSA levels without any clinical evidence of recurrent disease, employing 6000 cGy to 6400 cGy given in 6 to 6.5 weeks to fields 10 cm × 12 cm, bilateral 120-degree rotational arcs. In eight of ten patients, the PSA titers decreased shortly after irradiation. However, the follow-up period is not long enough for definitive evaluation of this therapy.[206] Similar findings have been observed by Bagshaw (Bagshaw M, Stanford University, personal communication). Irradiation can also be used in the treatment of clinically recog-

TABLE 51–19
Dose and In-Field Recurrence in Stage B and C Patients in the Patterns of Care Study

	STAGE B (724 PATIENTS)				STAGE C (624 PATIENTS)			
		PERCENT ACTUARIAL FREE OF LOCAL RECURRENCE*				PERCENT ACTUARIAL FREE OF RECURRENCE*		
DOSE cGy	NO. OF IN-FIELD FAILURES/TOTAL (%)	3 YR	5 YR	7 YR	NO. OF IN-FIELD FAILURES/TOTAL (%)	3 YR	5 YR	7 YR
<6000	22/87 (25)	85	71		17/69 (25)	72	63	
6000–6499	16/120 (13)	94	82	77	31/111 (28)	76	64	64
6500–6999	37/283 (13)	91	88	77	46/200 (23)	83	72	68
7000+	32/234 (14)	93	84	78	42/244 (17)	86	81	76

* *For unstratified linear trend,* P = *0.0021, and for Mantel,* P = *0.0203.*
(Hanks GE: NCI Monogr 7:75, 1988)

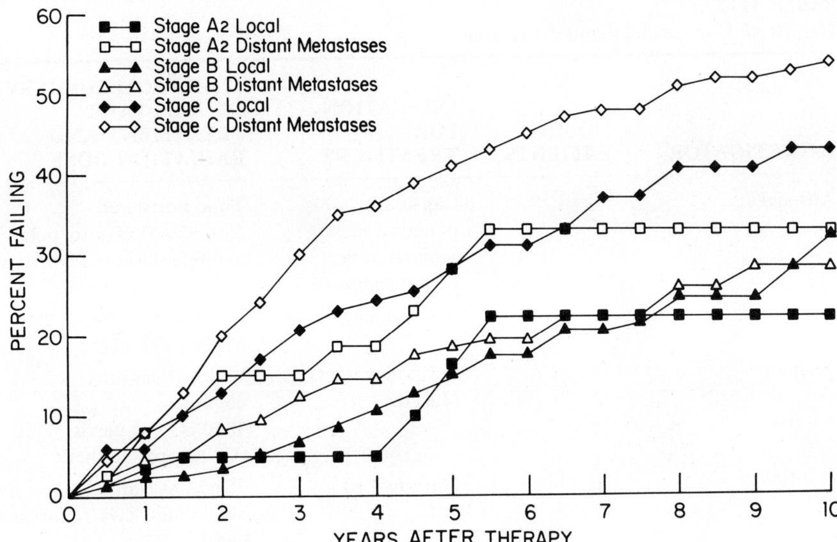

FIGURE 51–30. Actuarial probability of failures after treatment of 577 patients with carcinoma of the prostate with definitive radiation therapy at Mallinckrodt Institute of Radiology (1967–1983).

nized recurrences localized to the pelvis. Twenty-three of these patients were treated at Mallinckrodt Institute of Radiology with doses of approximately 6500 cGy in 7 weeks (180 to 200 cGy daily). The pelvic lymph nodes and prostatic bed were treated in 16 patients and the prostatic bed only in seven. The pelvic tumor control rates were 69% in the former and 57% in the latter group ($P = 0.66$), and the 5-year overall survival rates were 46% and 42%, respectively ($P = 0.54$).[106]

RECURRENT PROSTATIC CARCINOMA INITIALLY TREATED WITH IRRADIATION

In properly selected cases, overall local tumor control is achieved in 80% to 90% of the patients with Stage A2 or B disease after interstitial or external irradiation and in 65% to 70% of the patients with Stage C disease, but the radiation oncologist is sometimes faced with the need to retreat a previously irradiated patient. Selection of the appropriate method depends on the extent of the prostatic or pelvic tumor, status of metastatic dissemination, age and general condition of patient, need to preserve sexual potency, treatment modality used in initial therapy, and time span between initial therapy and retreatment.

Surgical Management

A radical prostatectomy may be attempted if technically feasible. Some urologists, including Spaulding and Whitmore[350] and Mador and others,[238] have used cystoprostatectomy or pelvic exenteration. Mador and associates[238] reported several patients who initially had been irradiated (six by external beam, one by ^{125}I implant) and who were treated surgically for recur-

TABLE 51–20
Fast Neutron Irradiation for Locally Advanced Prostate Cancer

INVESTIGATOR*	NO. OF PATIENTS	TREATMENT†	STAGE†	PERCENT SURVIVAL	YEARS
RTOG[224, 326]	55	Mixed beam	C/D1	63	8
RTOG	36	Photons	C/D1	13	8
RTOG	55	Mixed beam	C/D1	82‡	8
RTOG	36	Photons	C/D1	54‡	8
Louvain-la-neuve[312]	50	Mixed beam	A (14) C (30) D (6)	90, local control§	3
Hamburg[125]	13 (12 evaluable)	Mixed beam	T3 (7) T4 (5)	85 20	5 5
Chiba University[243]	25	Mixed beam (1) Neutrons only (15)	C (14)	77	3

** RTOG, Radiation Therapy Oncology Group.*
† Numbers in parentheses are number of patients.
‡ Adjusted to exclude intercurrent noncancer deaths.
§ Seven of ten patients observed for 3 years had no evidence of disease.
(Russell KJ, Laramore GE, Krall JM, et al: Am J Clin Oncol 12:307, 1989)

TABLE 51–21
Results of Elective Adjuvant Irradiation

INVESTIGATOR	NO. OF PATIENTS	INDICATION FOR TREATMENT	TIME FROM SURGERY TO ADJUVANT TREATMENT AND RADIATION DOSE	FOLLOW-UP (YEARS)	TUMOR CONTROL (%)	SURVIVAL (%)
Anscher[7]	46	Capsular penetration, seminal vesicle (+), margins (+)	Time not stated 4500–5000 cGy to pelvis 5500–6500 cGy to prostate	median 5	96	90*
Bahnson[25]	14	Surgical stage C	1–7 months (mean 2.4) 5000–7000 cGy	3–5	93	93
Forman[121]	28	Surgical stage C Margins (+)	Within 4 months 6500 cGy 4500 cGy to pelvis; 6500 cGy to prostate bed	median 4 range 1–8	100	90
Fried[130]	6	Margins (+)	Time not stated 5000–6500 cGy to prostate bed	median 5	100	100
Gibbons[141]	22	Surgical stage C	≤3 months 4900–7200 cGy (avg. 6300)	mean 9	95	73
Hanks[173]	11	Surgical stage C (5)	6–24 months (mean 5.4)			
		Margins (+) (6)	6000–7300 cGy	2–10; mean 7	100	100
Jacobson[194]	26	Margins (+) (3), bladder neck invasion, seminal vesicle (+), or capsular invasion (23)	1–4 months 4600–5000 cGy to pelvis 5400–7000 cGy to prostate	5	100	88
Lange[223]	35	Margins (+) Seminal vesicle (+)	1–12 months (median 3) Pelvis: 4500 cGy Prostate bed: 6000 cGy	2–10	97	86†
Perez[283]	42	Margins (+)	4500 cGy to pelvis 1500 cGy to prostate or 6000 cGy to prostate	median 5	81	65† 44*
Pilepich[300]	28	Surgical stage C (3) Margins (+) (!5) Tumor found postnucleative prostatectomy (10)	1–5 months (median 2) 4000–5000 cGy to pelvis 6500 cGy to prostate	1–10 average	96	55
Rosen[317]	16	Surgical stage C (microscopic)	Time not stated 6000–7100 cGy	median 5	94	100
Ray[308]	13	Surgical stage C (12) Margins (+) (1)	≤4 months 5400 cGy to pelvis 7000 cGy to prostate		77	

** 10-year actuarial.*
† 5-year actuarial.

rent prostatic carcinoma (three had cystoprostatectomy and urinary diversion, four underwent a radical prostatectomy). One patient died postoperatively of pulmonary edema, two had rectal lacerations (one complicated with a rectourethroperineal fistula), and two developed temporary urinary incontinence.

Carson and co-workers[74] treated 18 patients after radiation therapy with a radical prostatectomy and lymphadenectomy. Nine of the patients received additional irradiation; seven had a surgical procedure after completion of radiation therapy, and two underwent salvage prostatectomy at 16 months and 6 years after the irradiation because of local progression.

Ahlering and associates[1] treated six patients with small glands who had persistent tumor demonstrated histologically after irradiation with salvage prostatectomy. There were no postoperative complications. Three of the six patients were alive without evidence of disease 1 to 37 months at the time of the report. Three of the six patients were incontinent and needed artificial urinary sphincters. These researchers believe that salvage prostatectomy is rarely indicated and that a cystoprostatectomy may be a better procedure for these patients. They also treated nine patients with a cystoprostatectomy, one with cystoprostatectomy combined with a low anterior colon resection,

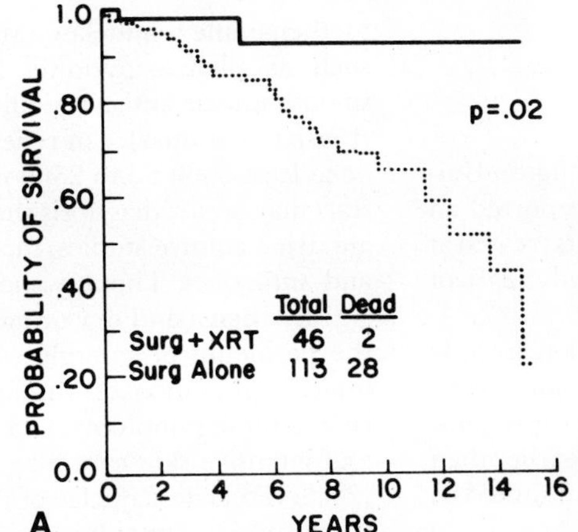

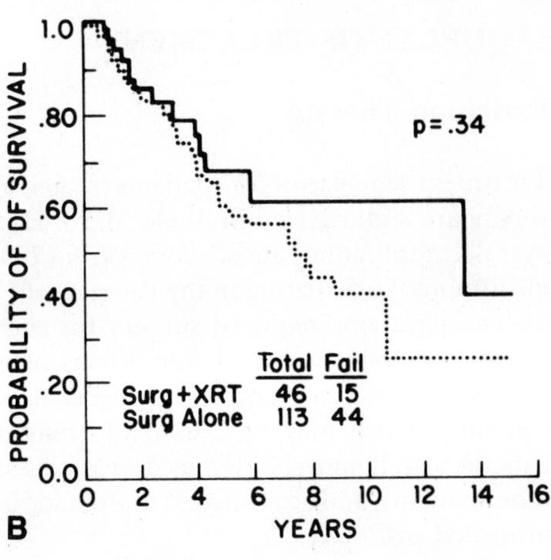

FIGURE 51–31. (**A**) Overall survival and (**B**) disease-free survival in Stage C cancer patients treated with radical prostatectomy alone (*broken line*) or with postoperative irradiation (*solid line*). (Anscher MS, Prosnitz LR: J Urol 138:1407, 1987)

and one with total pelvic exenteration.[1] Ten of the eleven patients had concurrent bilateral orchiectomy. There were no operative complications or deaths. Eight (73%) of the patients were alive without disease at 12 to 97 months, and there have been no local recurrences, although two patients developed distant metastases.

Follow-up is too short to ascertain the efficacy of these procedures. Transurethral resection may alleviate obstructive symptoms in patients with large glands or pelvic recurrences in rapidly growing tumors.

Interstitial Irradiation

Implantation with ^{125}I seeds has been carried out in patients with limited volume (<75 cc) recurrent prostatic carcinoma after external irradiation (6000–7000 cGy in 6–7 weeks).

Goffinet and colleagues[150] reported their experience with 14 of these patients who had histologically proven, locally recurrent tumor 16 to 51 months after completion of initial radiation therapy. Cystoscopy and proctosigmoidoscopy were performed to rule out bladder or rectal tumor extension. A suprapubic extraperitoneal lower abdomen approach was used for selective lymph node biopsies of suspicious nodes or for lymphadenectomy. The prostate was isolated, and the ^{125}I seeds were implanted as described in Chapter 13. The dose administered ranged from 4000 cGy to 22,500 cGy (average, 12,000 cGy).

Clinical local tumor control was observed in 11 (79%) of the 14 patients with a follow-up of 6 to 36 months after implantation, and eight (57%) of the patients were disease free at the time of the report. Complications occurred in four of the patients: two cystoproctitis, one abscess with urinary incontinence, and one vesicorectal fistula. These complications were linked to high-intensity seeds (>0.50 mCi) that were implanted in large volumes (>50 cc). Martinez and associates[242] described a technique in which a template was used to administer interstitial irradiation with afterloading ^{192}Ir to pelvic tumors. Included were six patients with recurrent prostatic tumor. Therapy was well tolerated. The authors believed that follow-up was too short to allow meaningful conclusions about tumor control.

External Irradiation

In patients initially treated with interstitial irradiation alone, it may be possible to retreat with external irradiation to the prostatic bed or the pelvis, depending on tumor extent.

A significant difficulty is the inability to protect the bladder or the anterior rectal wall without also blocking tumor. To diminish the probability of major sequelae, it is advisable to limit the total dose to 4500 cGy to 5000 cGy given in daily 180-cGy fractions five times per week. Lateral portals are preferred in an effort to decrease the dose to the bladder and the rectosigmoid.

Hormonal Therapy

Castration and exogenous hormonal manipulation, including administration of diethylstilbestrol, other synthetic estrogens, or luteinizing hormone-releasing hormone, are used in the treatment of patients with recurrent disease, particularly those with more extensive pelvic tumors or distant metastases. Palliative results are satisfactory in 75% to 80% of the patients.

TABLE 51–22
Postprostatectomy Radiation Therapy in Carcinoma of the Prostate

		5-YEAR SURVIVAL	
TUMOR EXTENT	LOCAL CONTROL	DISEASE-FREE	ACTUARIAL
Positive margins	34/42 (81%)	58%	65%
Clinical recurrence	15/23 (65.2%) [P = 0.16]	45% [P = 0.16]	44% [P = 0.25]

**Mallinckrodt Institute of Radiology data, 1966–1968.*
(Eisbruch A, Perez CA, Roessler E, et al: unpublished data)

SEQUELAE OF TREATMENT

Radiation Therapy

Treatment sequelae of 577 patients treated at Washington University are summarized in Table 51-23. Hanks[171] reported an overall complication rate of about 5% in 1293 patients treated at institutions participating in the Patterns of Care Study; 25% of the complications required surgery for correction.

Acute gastrointestinal side effects of irradiation include diarrhea, abdominal cramping, rectal discomfort, and rectal bleeding, which may be caused by transient enteroproctitis. Patients with hemorrhoids may develop discomfort earlier than other patients, and aggressive symptomatic treatment should be instituted promptly.

Diarrhea and abdominal cramping can be controlled with the administration of diphenoxylate hydrochloride with loperamide (Imodium), atropine sulphate (Lomotil), or opium preparations, such as paregoric, and emollients, such as kaolin and pectin. Proctitis and rectal discomfort can be alleviated by small enemas with hydrocortisone (Proctofoam, Cortifoam) and suppositories containing bismuth, benzyl benzoate, zinc oxide, or Peruvian balsam (Anusol, Wyanoids, Medicone). Some of the suppositories may contain cortisone. Small enemas with cod liver oil are also effective. A low-residue diet with no grease or spices usually helps to decrease gastrointestinal symptoms.

Genitourinary symptoms, secondary to cystourethritis, are dysuria, frequency, and nocturia. The urine is usually clear, although there may be microscopic or even gross hematuria.

TABLE 51–23
Complications in 577 Patients Treated with Definitive Irradiation

COMPLICATIONS	MAJOR	MODERATE
Small bowel obstruction	4	
Proctitis	1	29 (5%)
Enteritis	1*	7 (1.2%)
Rectovesical fistula	1†	
Cystitis/hematuria	2	14 (2.4%)
Bladder fistula	1	
Ureteral stricture	2	1 (.17%)
Pubic bone necrosis	1	
Rectal ulcer		1 (.17%)
Rectal stricture		1 (.17%)
Anal stricture/fissure		2 (.35%)
Urinary incontinence		
Transurethral resection (TUR)†		2 (.35%)
No TUR		4 (.69%)
Urethral stricture		
TUR‡		8/164 (4.9%)
No TUR		15/413 (3.6%)
Scrotal/penile edema		8 (1.4%)
Leg edema		
Staging laparotomy		8/83 (9.6%)
No staging laparotomy		1/494 (0.2%)
Subcutaneous fibrosis		2 (.35%)
Scrotum, skin necrosis		1 (.17%)
Bladder ulcer		1 (.17%)
Impotence		82/200 (41%)

**Acute syndrome, developed after 4020 cGy tumor dose.*
† Also recurrent pelvic tumor.
‡ 164 patients had TUR; 413 patients did not have TUR.

Methenamine mandelate (Mandelamine) and antispasmodics, such as phenazopyridine hydrochloride (Pyridium), or a smooth muscle antispasmodic, such as flavoxate hydrochloride (Urispas, Cistopaz), can relieve symptoms. Fluid intake should be at least 2000 ml to 2500 ml daily. Infections of the urinary tract may occur; diagnosis should be established with appropriate urine culture studies, including sensitivity to sulfonamides and antibiotics. Therapy should be promptly instituted.

Erythema and dry or moist desquamation may develop in the perineum or intergluteal fold. Proper skin hygiene and topical application of Vaseline, Aquaphor, or lanolin should relieve these symptoms. U.S.P. zinc oxide ointment or Desitin and intensive skin care may be needed for severe cases.

Severe, late sequelae of treatment include persistent proctitis or proctosigmoiditis. Proctitis requiring colostomy was observed in one of 577 patients treated at Washington University.[286] The incidence of grade 2 proctitis and rectal ulcers was 5%. Hazra and Giri[179] reported a 43% incidence of proctitis, with six of the patients requiring colostomy, among 32 patients with localized carcinoma of the prostate treated with 5000 cGy to the pelvic lymph nodes, 1000 cGy to the prostate and adjacent tissues with conventional fractionation, and an additional 800-cGy single-dose exposure to the pelvic girdle. The use of lateral or perineal fields to boost the prostate dose produced a 16% incidence of grade 2 diarrhea compared with a rate of 2% to 7% for other techniques.

Pilepich and colleagues,[289, 297] in a study of 453 patients randomized to treatment (6500 cGy) of the prostate only or to treatment of the prostate and the pelvic lymph nodes (the latter receiving 4500 cGy), described no significant difference in acute or late morbidity between the two techniques, except for a 20% incidence of persistent rectal bleeding (nine of 46) in patients receiving 7000 cGy to the prostate, a rate of 12% (ten of 81) with doses of 6751 cGy to 7000 cGy, and a rate of 3% to 5% with doses less than 6750 cGy. Patients treated with AP/PA fields had a somewhat higher incidence of grade 2 proctitis (seven of 81) than those treated with multiple fields (four of 139). The incidence of grade 3 proctitis was also somewhat higher with AP/PA portals (three of 81) compared with multiple fields (two of 139). The researchers did not analyze the incidence of proctitis according to beam energies.

In an analysis of 526 patients treated to the pelvis and prostate or to that volume plus the periaortic lymph nodes, Pilepich and colleagues[292] found no significant correlation between the total dose given to the regional lymphatics (4400–5100 cGy) and the incidence of bowel or bladder injuries. Except for increased diarrhea (19% incidence in 178 patients), there was no correlation between bowel or genitourinary morbidity in patients receiving 7000 cGy to the prostate compared with those receiving lower doses. Furthermore, the use of AP/PA fields or multiple portals (box technique) did not have an impact on the incidence of diarrhea or proctitis.

Schellhammer and co-workers[331] reported a somewhat higher incidence of morbidity among patients treated with ^{125}I implants than with external irradiation (14% and 5.6%, respectively).

Mameghan and associates[241] correlated a greater incidence of bowel sequelae with irradiation of larger volumes of the pelvis.

In a British study of ten men with symptomatic, chronic, radiation-induced proctitis, rectal manometry disclosed significantly lower maximum resting anal canal pressure and physiologic sphincter length than in nonirradiated sex-matched controls.[374] The squeezed pressure of the external sphincter was not significantly different. The results indicate that dysfunction of the internal anal sphincter may contribute to anal rectal discomfort after pelvic irradiation. Histologic sections in eight resected specimens showed hypertrophy of the muscularis mucosa and muscularis propria, sparse submucosal nerve plexus (Meissner's) ganglion cells, marked hypertrophy of the nerve fibers with vacuolation of the nerve sheaths in the muscular plexus of Auerbach's, and ganglion cell degeneration.[374]

Fewer than 5% of the patients develop chronic cystitis. Occasionally, with doses over 7500 cGy to the bladder, hemorrhagic cystitis may occur, requiring a cystectomy (<1%). Urethral stricture has been reported in approximately 5% of the patients, most frequently in those who had transurethral resection before or during radiation therapy.[290] A summary of the reported incidence of severe intestinal or urinary complications has been published by Dewit and associates.[97]

Sexual impotence (erectile dysfunction) has been observed in 35% to 40% of formerly potent patients treated with external irradiation, but in only 15% of those treated with interstitial ^{125}I.[23,347,286,392] Age may influence this difference, because the implants are usually performed in patients younger than those irradiated with external beam. Ziureich and colleagues[410] reported that 62% of carefully assessed patients (mean age, 67.7 years) were impotent before initiation of radiation therapy.

Banker[27] conducted a careful prospective study of 100 patients treated with external irradiation and observed preservation of sexual potency in 73% of the potent patients who admitted to more than three sexual intercourses per month; preservation was achieved in 43% of patients who had intercourse less often. Overall 54% of the 100 patients maintained potency after treatment.

Van Heeringen and associates[373] documented sexual impotence that may have been related to irradiation in three (25%) of 12 patients; in a substantial number of patients, psychogenic factors were implicated.

Sexual impotence may be a function of decreased testosterone and dihydroxytestosterone plasma levels, fibrosis or decreased external glandular secretions, pudendal or sympathetic nerve injury, vascular occlusion of penile arteries, anxiety, or depression. The potential causes of erectile impotence require a careful evaluation. Twenty (33%) of 60 patients evaluated 3 years after transurethral resection of the prostate for benign conditions noticed sexual impotence (12 complete, eight partial).[56]

Using noninvasive techniques, Mittal[258] measured the penile blood flow before and 6 to 9 months after external irradiation for prostatic carcinoma in six patients. Two of them developed impotence 2 and 4.5 months after completion of treatment; however, no significant change in penile blood flow was observed in any of the six patients.

Serial determinations of dihydroxytestosterone and testosterone plasma levels in patients treated for prostatic carcinoma with external irradiation showed no significant changes in hormonal levels after irradiation.[281]

Although extremely rare, lumbosacral plexopathy has been reported in patients treated for pelvic tumors with doses of 6000 cGy to 6750 cGy or even with doses as low as 4000 cGy in five patients treated for malignant lymphomas.[16,366,377] Characteristically these patients have motor neuron weakness of the lower legs combined with loss of deep reflexes and muscular fasciculation. Although cystometrograms demonstrated bladder atonicity in some cases, most of these men had no bladder or rectal sphincter disturbances.[16] Ashenhurst and associates[16] discovered that several of the patients previously reported as having radiation myelopathy of the lumbar spine may have suffered a lumbar and sacral nerve plexopathy, instead of or in addition to the spinal cord injury.[240] At autopsy, retroperitoneal fibrosis was seen in two cases reported by Klaua.[209] The differential diagnosis with recurrent tumors is sometimes difficult. In a comparison of 20 patients with lumbosacral plexopathy after irradiation and 30 patients with plexus damage from pelvic malignancy, Thomas and associates[366] found that indolent leg weakness occurred early in radiation-induced plexopathy, but pain was most frequently associated with tumor-induced plexopathy. Muscular weakness, numbness, and paresthesia are common in both groups. CT aided detection of pelvic masses or bone destruction caused by tumor. Electromyogram showed abnormal myokymic discharges in 57% of the patients, but this finding was very unusual in tumor-induced plexopathy.

Combined Surgery and Irradiation

There is a higher incidence of major sequelae with the combination of surgery and definitive radiation therapy.[290]

Complications of pelvic lymphadenectomy, such as prolonged serous drainage, were reported for 9% of the patients, and infection at draining sites occurred in 7%.[207,238,360,363] Pilepich and co-workers[298] described no significant edema of the lower extremities in 236 patients treated with definitive radiation therapy alone, in contrast to 15.5% (18 of 116) of the patients who had undergone limited pelvic lymph node dissection and 66% (four of six) of those treated with extended lymphadenectomy. Although symptoms related to intestinal or urinary complications improve in 80% to 90% of the patients within 2 years after therapy, leg or genital edema persists in more than 80% of the patients developing this sequela. Minimal improvement is sometimes obtained with a low-sodium diet, diuretics, postural drainage of fluid (leg raising), and elastic stockings.

Pistenma and associates[302] reported a high incidence of small bowel complications in patients who were treated with a transperitoneal periaortic lymph node dissection and 5500 cGy delivered through AP/PA portals. This incidence was significantly reduced with the use of retroperitoneal lymph node dissections and lateral portals to deliver a portion of the periaortic irradiation.

HORMONAL THERAPY

Hormonal Receptors

Seventy-five percent of patients with carcinoma of the prostate exhibit some response to hormonal therapy. Huggins and associates[189] experimentally demonstrated the correlation between prostatic tumor growth and hormonal stimulation by androgens or tumor depression by androgen deprivation or estrogen administration. In 1941, Huggins and Hodges[190] reported their historic observations on the treatment of carcinoma of the prostate with hormonal manipulation. They demonstrated prostate tumor regression and diminished serum acid phosphatase levels after orchiectomy or estrogen administration. Many types of hormonal therapy have been employed since then, all seeking to reduce androgenic stimulation of prostate carcinoma by ablation of androgen-producing tissue, suppression of pituitary gonadotropin release, inhibition of androgen synthesis, or interference with androgen action in target tissues.[253] Figure 51-32 summarizes the various mechanisms involved in hormonal therapy of prostatic carcinoma.

Some technical difficulties in the characterization of hor-

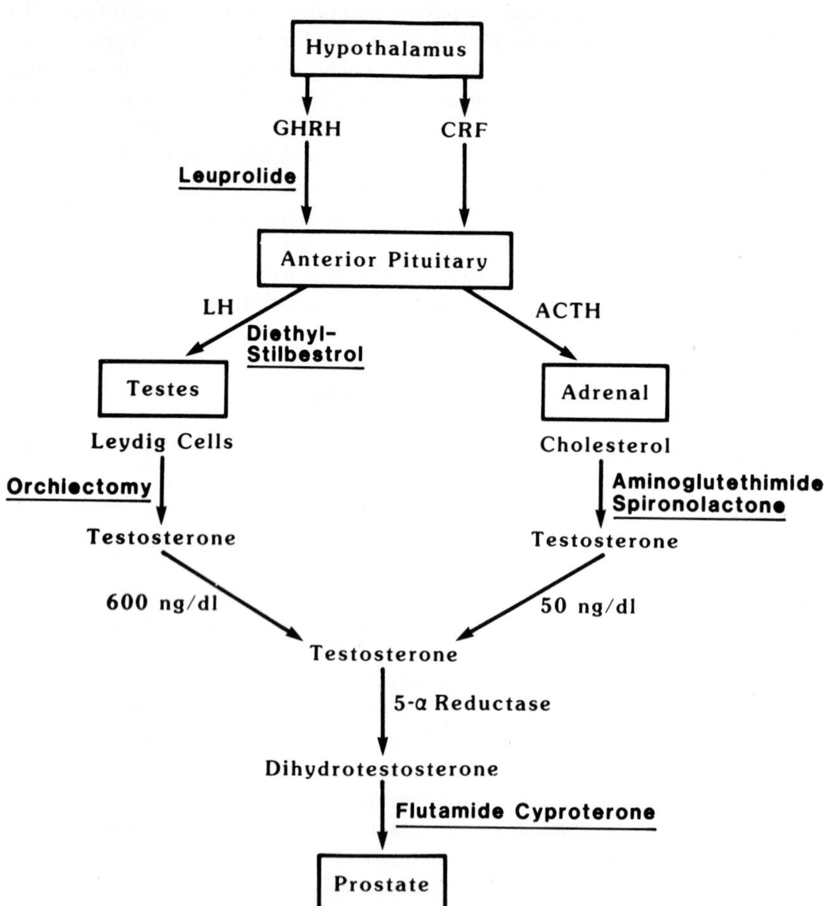

FIGURE 51–32. Flow chart illustrating anatomic sites of action of hormonal therapy agents.

monal receptors in human prostatic tissues have been identified.[108]

Nevertheless, Ekman and associates[108] in 23 patients reported a significant correlation between the presence of steroid receptors and response to hormonal therapy. Fifteen (83%) of 18 patients with "positive" receptors showed clinical tumor regression, in contrast to only one (20%) response in five patients with "negative" receptors.

Results of Hormonal Therapy

Orchiectomy removes 95% of circulating testosterone and is followed by a prompt, long-lasting decline in serum testosterone levels.[253] Estrogens appear to suppress pituitary gonadotropin, reducing stimulus for testicular testosterone synthesis, interfering with hormonal synthesis, or directly affecting the prostatic cell competing with hormonal receptors.[253] The nonsteroidal estrogen diethylstilbestrol (3 mg/day) reduces serum testosterone to castrated levels; higher doses have no additional effect.[340] Testosterone is not uniformly suppressed by 1 mg/day of diethylstilbestrol, although this dose appears to have equivalent antitumor effects. Progestational agents (Megace) suppress gonadotropin release and may also directly interfere with hormone synthesis.[135] Gonadotropin-releasing hormone agonists, such as leuprolide and Buserelin, cause an initial rise in gonadotropin levels, followed by a sharp decline within 2 to 3 weeks. Parallel changes occur in levels of circulating testosterone, interfering with androgen production in the adrenal gland.[387]

Androgen synthesis may be inhibited at several points in the synthetic pathway. Aminoglutethimide, which is administered with a glucocorticoid, inhibits the synthesis of all adrenal steroids and can further reduce serum testosterone levels in castrate patients.[399]

Progestational antiandrogens are thought to act by inhibiting formation of the dihydrotestosterone-receptor complex in prostatic nuclei, and cyproterone acetate is the most potent of these agents.[253] Flutamide is a nonsteroidal antiandrogen that does not suppress gonadotropin or testicular testosterone levels but blocks the effect of 5α-reductase, inhibiting formation of dihydrotestosterone and inhibiting androgen uptake and nuclear binding in the prostate cell; it does have estrogenic side-effects, but it infrequently produces sexual impotence.[157,348,349,364]

Tamoxifen is a nonsteroidal antiestrogen that has been studied in prostatic cancer because of preliminary evidence of the existence of estrogen receptors in neoplastic prostatic cells.[149]

Ketoconazole, an antifungal agent, impairs steroid synthesis, including testicular and adrenal androgens, and can often be administered without supplemental glucocorticoids.[364] Spironolactone, which also has some direct antiandrogenic effects, inhibits male sex hormone production further down the synthetic pathway, and estrogens and progestational agents exert these effects even more distally.[253,385]

Hormonal therapy has definite palliative value in prostatic cancer, and survival beyond 10 years occurs in 10% of patients with bony metastases responding to this treatment.[311] However, adjuvant therapy with diethylstilbestrol in patients treated with prostatic or pelvic irradiation confers no survival advantage. In a series of prospective randomized trials, VACURG found that adjuvant hormone treatment had no impact on survival for men with Stage A cancer who did not receive any locoregional therapy; diethylstilbestrol (5 mg/day) given as an adjuvant after radical prostatectomy to men with Stage A or B disease instead significantly shortened survival.[11,69]

In patients with Stage III (locally advanced) disease who were randomized to receive diethylstilbestrol (5 mg/day), orchiectomy, both treatments simultaneously, or placebo, the regimens containing estrogen shortened survival. All four treatments had similar survival effects for patients with Stage IV disease (distant metastases or elevated acid phosphatase).[45] Although fewer men given diethylstilbestrol died of cancer than those receiving only orchiectomy, the frequency of early cardiovascular deaths after treatment with diethylstilbestrol, particularly in men over 75 or with prior cardiovascular disease, obviated this therapeutic effect.[45,62]

In a subsequent VACURG study of patients with advanced disease, placebo was compared with diethylstilbestrol in doses of 5, 1, or 0.02 mg/day. Excessive cardiovascular deaths among patients with Stage III disease were again documented with 5 mg of diethylstilbestrol, but with 1 mg of diethylstilbestrol, cardiovascular deaths were not greater than with placebo.[26,64] The 1-mg and 5-mg doses of diethylstilbestrol were similar in retarding progression from Stage III and IV and in their reduction of cancer deaths overall.[64] This suggests that 1 mg of diethylstilbestrol is an effective antitumor therapy. Diethylstilbestrol (3 mg/day) has not been shown to be free of harmful cardiovascular effects.

In a third VACURG trial of Stage III and IV disease, no significant survival differences were observed among diethylstilbestrol (1 mg/day), medroxyprogesterone acetate (30 mg/day), premarin (2.5 mg/day), and the combination of diethylstilbestrol and the progestational agent.[62]

Byar and Corle,[65] reviewing the VACURG data, concluded that patients with Stages A, B, or C disease and low-grade tumors do not need hormonal therapy. However, patients with higher-grade lesions (Gleason score of 7 to 10) may benefit from hormonal therapy begun at diagnosis.

Several reports have shown similar survival, tumor control, and incidence of metastases in patients with carcinoma of the prostate localized to the pelvis after irradiation alone or with concomitant hormonal therapy.[266,286,372]

Because complete androgen blockage lacks secondary effects other than those related to hypoandrogenicity, Labrie and others[219] believe it should be initiated immediately after diagnosis of prostate cancer (for Stages C and D) to obtain remissions in more patients, to increase survival, and to minimize the appearance of clonal expansions of androgen-resistant cells. Consequently, orchiectomy, estrogens, and luteinizing hormone-releasing hormone agonists alone should not be used in this disease without the concomitant administration of a pure antiandrogen. Crawford and associates[90] reported longer progression-free survival (16.5 *versus* 13.9 months) and increased median survival (35.6 *versus* 28.3 months) for the drug-receiving portion of 303 patients with Stage D2 previously untreated carcinoma of the prostate who were randomized to receive leuprolide or a placebo.

Pilepich and colleagues[294] compared the efficacy and toxic effects of Megestrol and diethylstilbestrol as cytoreductive agents 2 months before initiation of therapy and during radiation therapy. Gynecomastia developed in 55% and fluid retention occurred in 21% of the patients receiving diethylstilbestrol, but gynecomastia occurred in only 7% and fluid retention in 6% of those treated with Megestrol. Thromboembolic phenomena were reported in 8% and 5% of the patients, respectively. Although diethylstilbestrol-treated patients showed a significantly greater median decrease in plasma testosterone levels, 3 years after initiation of therapy, 65% of all evaluable patients in both arms had evidence of local failure. The survival rate was 81% in the Megestrol group and 76% in the diethylstilbestrol-treated group.

Hormonal manipulation concurrent with irradiation has not improved survival or tumor control.[268,278,372] Therefore, it is recommended that hormonal therapy be withheld until there is evidence of tumor progression after initial therapy.

Harisiadis and co-workers[178] and Perez and associates[287] observed that patients initially treated with hormonal therapy and subsequently given radiation therapy for a nonresponsive or progressive tumor have lower survival rates than patients treated with radiation therapy at the time of diagnosis. This finding is probably a consequence of the hormone-resistant tumor being more biologically aggressive.

Irradiation of the Breast Before Hormonal Therapy

Gynecomastia is a common and unwanted side-effect of estrogen therapy, which may cause pain, discomfort, and embarrassment. Gynecomastia and related symptoms have been prevented in approximately 80% of the patients treated with superficial x-rays (1000-cGy single dose) using small appositional portals.[85,185,225,316] We employ tangential ports with ^{60}Co or 4-MV photons or appositional electron beam (9–12 MeV) portals delivering a midplane dose of 1200 cGy to each breast in three fractions. Customary field size is 8 cm × 8 cm or an 8-cm-diameter circle. The entire breast tissue must be irradiated before orchiectomy or initiation of estrogen therapy; otherwise, the glandular hyperplasia is not preventable.

CHEMOTHERAPY

Single-Agent Chemotherapy

Several drugs have been evaluated for patients who failed one or more hormonal therapies.[370] Response rates of 25% to 35% have been reported with single-agent doxorubicin (Adriamycin).[98,269,369] Cyclophosphamide was administered to 127 patients in three NPCP trials; the rate of partial response plus stable disease ranged from 26% to 41%, but only 5% of the patients had complete or partial responses.[234,332,338] 5-Fluorouracil has induced partial responses in about 10% of patients.[98,337] Hydroxyurea was administered in an NPCP study; a partial response rate of only 8% was observed.[234]

In a randomized study of patients who had failed after hormonal therapy and had not received major previous irradiation, 41% and 36% of men given cyclophosphamide or 5-fluorouracil, respectively, had no tumor progression after 12 weeks of treatment, compared with 19% receiving standard therapy.

Combination Chemotherapy

The superiority of combination chemotherapy over single drugs in metastatic prostatic cancer has not been supported by prospective randomized trials.[181,264,344] In five randomized studies comparing single-agent and combination chemotherapy, there was no or minimal difference in the percentage of patients with partial response plus stable disease in the two arms; response duration and survival were essentially the same. In the 160 patients in four studies in which NPCP response criteria were used, only 10 partial responses were reported.

Eisenberger[107] described a complete or partial response rate of less than 10% for more than 3000 patients with advanced or recurrent metastatic carcinoma of the prostate treated with various chemotherapeutic agents. A complete review of these studies is included in his publication.

Chemotherapy Combined with Hormonal Manipulation

There is no proven role for the administration of chemotherapy in combination with hormonal manipulation. The NPCP carried out a prospective randomized trial using men with newly diagnosed distant metastases who had received no prior systemic therapy; patients were treated with diethylstilbestrol or orchiectomy (standard therapy), diethylstilbestrol plus cyclophosphamide, or estramustine phosphate and cyclophosphamide. No significant differences among the treatment arms were found for complete and partial response rates, in the number of patients with progressive tumor by 12 weeks, or in time to development of disease progression.[140,262]

REFERENCES

1. Ahlering TE, Lieskovsky G, Skinner DG: Salvage options following radiotherapy failures. In Skinner DG, Lieskovsky G (eds): Diagnosis and Management of Genitourinary Cancer, pp 454–463. Philadelphia, WB Saunders, 1988
2. Albert PS, Mallouh C, Nagamatsu GR: Transitional-cell carcinoma of the prostate. Urology 2:128, 1973
3. Almagro UA: Argyrophilic prostatic carcinoma: Case report with literature review on prostatic carcinoid and "carcinoid-like" prostatic carcinoma. Cancer 55:608, 1985
4. American Cancer Society: 1991 Cancer Facts & Figures. Atlanta, American Cancer Society, 1991
5. Andersson L, Jonsson G, Brunk U: Puncture biopsy of the prostate in the diagnosis of prostatic cancer. Scand J Urol Nephrol 1:227, 1967
6. Anscher MS, Prosnitz LR: Radiotherapy vs. hormonal therapy for the management of locally recurrent prostate cancer following radical prostatectomy. Int J Radiat Oncol Biol Phys 17:953, 1989
7. Anscher MS, Prosnitz LR: Postoperative radiotherapy for patients with carcinoma of the prostate undergoing radical prostatectomy with positive margins, seminal vesicle involvement and/or penetration through the capsule. J Urol 138:1407, 1987
8. Anscher MS, Prosnitz LR: Adjuvant radiotherapy after radical prostatectomy: Is it indicated? (Letter to editor). J Urol 139:960, 1988
9. Anson BJ, McVay CB: Surgical Anatomy, vol 2, 5th ed, p 771. Philadelphia, WB Saunders, 1971
10. Arduino LJ, Glucksman MA: Lymph node metastases in early carcinoma of the prostate. J Urol 8:91, 1962
11. Arduino LJ, Bailar JC, Becker LE: Carcinoma of the prostate: Treatment comparisons. J Urol 98:516, 1967
12. Aristizabal SA, Steinbronn D, Heusinkveld RS: External beam radiotherapy in cancer of the prostate: The University of Arizona Experience. Radiother Oncol 1:309, 1984
13. Armenian HK, Lilienfeld AM, Diamond EL, et al: Relationship between benign prostatic hyperplasia and cancer of the prostate. Lancet 2:115, 1974
14. Asbell, SO, Krall, JM, Pilepich, MV, et al: Elective pelvic irradiation in stage A2, B carcinoma of the prostate: Analysis of RTOG 77-06. Int J Radiat Oncol Biol Phys 15:1307, 1988
15. Asbell SO, Martz KL, Pilepich MV, et al: Impact of surgical staging in evaluating the radiotherapeutic outcome in RTOG phase III study for A2 and B prostate carcinoma. Int J Radiat Oncol Biol Phys 17:945, 1989
16. Ashenhurst EM, Quartey GRC, Starreveld A: Lumbo-sacral radiculopathy induced by radiation. Can J Neuro Sci 4:259, 1977
17. Aziz H, Choi K, Sohn C, et al: Comparison of ^{32}P therapy and sequential hemibody irradiation (HBI) for bony metastases as methods of whole body irradiation. Am J Clin Oncol 9:264, 1986
18. Aziz H, Rotman M, Thelmo W, et al: Radiation-treated carcinoma of prostate. Comparison of survival of black and white patients by Gleason's grading system. Am J Clin Oncol 11:166, 1988
19. Azumi N, Shibuya H, Ishikura M: Primary prostatic carcinoid tumor with intracytoplasmic prostatic acid phosphatase and prostate-specific antigen. Am J Surg Pathol 8:545, 1984
20. Bagshaw MA: Current conflicts in the management of prostatic cancer. Int J Radiat Oncol Biol Phys 12:1721, 1986
21. Bagshaw MA: Potential for radiotherapy alone in prostatic cancer. Cancer 55:2079, 1985
22. Bagshaw MA: Radiotherapeutic treatment of prostatic carcinoma with pelvic node involvement. Urol Clin North Am 11:297, 1984
23. Bagshaw MA, Cox RS, Ray GR: Status of radiation therapy of prostate cancer at Stanford University. NCI Monogr 7;47, 1988
24. Bagshaw MA, Ray GR, Cox RS: Radiotherapy of prostatic carcinoma: Long-or short term efficacy (Stanford University experience). Urology 25:17, 1985
25. Bahnson RR, Garnett JE, Grayhack JT: Adjuvant radiation therapy in stages C and D1 prostatic adenocarcinoma: Preliminary results. Urology 27:403, 1986
26. Bailar JC III, Byar DP, The Veterans Administration Cooperative Urological Research Group: Estrogen treatment for cancer of the prostate: Early results with 3 doses of diethylstilbestrol and placebo. Cancer 26:257, 1970
27. Banker FL: The preservation of potency after external beam irradiation for prostatic cancer. Int J Radiat Oncol Biol Phys 15:219, 1988
28. Barnes RW, Ninan CA: Carcinoma of the prostate: Biopsy and conservative therapy. J Urol 108:987, 1972
29. Barringer BS: Radium in the treatment of prostatic carcinoma. Ann Surg 80:881, 1984
30. Barzell W, Bean MA, Hilaris BS, et al: Prostatic adenocarcinoma: Relationship of grade and local extent to pattern of metastases. J Urol 118:278, 1977
31. Batata MA, Hilaris BS, Chu FCH, et al: Radiation therapy in adenocarcinoma of the prostate with pelvic lymph node involvement on lymphadenectomy. Int J Radiat Oncol Biol Phys 6:149, 1980
32. Batata MA, Hilaris BS, Whitmore WF: Factors affecting tumor control. In Hilaris BS, Batata MA (eds): Brachytherapy Oncology, 1983 Advances in Prostate and Other Cancer, pp 65–73. New York, Memorial Sloan-Kettering Cancer Center, 1983
33. Bates HR: Transitional cell carcinoma of the prostate. J Urol 101:206, 1969
34. Batson OV: The role of the vertebral veins in metastatic processes. Ann Intern Med 16:38, 1942
35. Beahrs OH, Henson DE, Hutter RVP, Myers MH (eds): Manual for Staging of Cancer, 3rd ed, pp 177–179. Philadelphia, JB Lippincott, 1988
36. Bean MA, Yatani R, Liu PI, et al: Prostatic carcinoma at autopsy in Hiroshima and Nagasaki Japan. Cancer 32:498, 1973
37. Belleville WD, Mahan DE, Sepulveda RA, et al: Bone marrow acid phosphatase by radio-immuno assay: Three years of experience. J Urol 125:809, 1981
38. Belt E, Schroeder FH: Total perineal prostatectomy for prostate carcinoma. J Urol 107:91, 1972
39. Benson MC: Fine-needle aspiration of the prostate. NCI Monogr 7:19, 1988
40. Benson MC: Application of flow cytometry and automated image analysis to the study of prostate cancer. NCI Monogr 7:25, 1988

41. Benson RC, Tomera KM, Zincke H, et al: Bilateral pelvic lymphadenectomy and radical retropubic prostatectomy for adenocarcinoma confined to the prostate. J Urol 131:1103, 1984
42. Berlin BB, Cornwell PM, Connelly RR, Eisenberg H: Radical perineal prostatectomy for carcinoma of the prostate, survival in 143 cases treated from 1935–1958. J Urol 99:97, 1968
43. Biggs PJ, Russell MD: Effect of a femoral head prosthesis on megavoltage beam radiotherapy. Int J Radiat Oncol Biol Phys 14:581, 1988
44. Biondetti PR, Lee JKT, Ling D, Catalona WJ: Clinical stage B prostate carcinoma: Staging with MR imaging. Radiology 162:325, 1987
45. Blackard CE, Byar DP, Jordan WP: Orchiectomy for advanced prostatic carcinoma: A reevaluation. Urology 1:553, 1973
46. Blake GM, Wood JF, Wood PJ, et al: ^{89}Sr therapy: Strontium plasma clearance in disseminated prostatic carcinoma. Eur J Nucl Med 15:49, 1989
47. Blennerhassett JB, Vickery AL: Carcinoma of the prostate gland: An anatomical study of tumor location. Cancer 19:980, 1966
48. Bosch PC, Forbes KA, Prassvinichai S, et al: Preliminary observations on the results of combined temporary ^{192}Ir implantation and external beam irradiation for carcinoma of the prostate. J Urol 135:722, 1986
49. Bostwick DG, Egbert BM, Fajardo LF: Radiation injury of the normal and neoplastic prostate. Am J Surg Pathol 6:541, 1982
50. Bouffioux C: La mesure de l'adn dans le produit de cytoponction des cancers de la prostate: Interet diagnostique, prognostique et therapeutique. J Urol (Paris) 88:111, 1982
51. Boxer RJ, Kaufman JJ, Goodwin WE: Radical prostatectomy for carcinoma of the prostate; 1951–1976: A review of 329 patients. J Urol 117:208, 1977
52. Brawer MK, Schifman RB, Ahmann FR, et al: The effect of digital rectal examination on serum levels of prostatic-specific antigen. Arch Pathol Lab Med 112:1110, 1988
53. Brawn N: The dedifferentiation of prostate carcinoma. Cancer 52:246, 1983
54. Breslow N, Chan CW, Dhom G, et al: Latent carcinoma of prostate at autopsy in seven areas. Int J Cancer 20:680, 1977
55. Brindle JS, Martinez A, Schray M: Pelvic lymphadenectomy and transperineal interstitial implantation of ^{192}Ir combined with external beam radiotherapy for bulky stage C prostatic carcinoma. Int J Radiat Oncol Biol Phys 17:1063, 1989
56. Bruskewitz RC, Larsen EH, Madsen PO, Dorflinger T: 3-year follow-up of urinary symptoms after transurethral resection of the prostate. J Urol 135:613, 1986
57. Buchale K, Correns H-J, Scherer M, et al: Results of a double blind study of 89-strontium therapy of skeletal metastases of prostatic carcinoma. Eur J Nucl Med 14:349, 1988
58. Bumpus HC Jr: Radium in cancer of the prostate: Report of 217 cases. JAMA 78:1374, 1922
59. Buonocore E, Hesemann C. Pavlicek W, Montie JE: Clinical and *in vitro* magnetic resonance imaging of prostatic carcinoma. AJR 143:1267, 1984
60. Burbank F, Fraumeni JF Jr: US cancer mortality: Nonwhite predominance. JNCI 49:649, 1972
61. Byar DP: Identification of prognostic factors. In Buyse M, Staquet MJ, Silvester RJ (eds): Cancer Clinical Trials: Methods and Practice, pp 423–443. Oxford, Oxford University Press, 1984
62. Byar DP: VACURG studies on prostatic cancer and its treatment. In Tannenbaum M (ed): Urologic Pathology: The Prostate, pp 241–267. Philadelphia, Lea & Febiger, 1977
63. Byar DP: VACURG studies of post-prostatectomy survival. Scand J Urol Nephrol 55:113, 1980
64. Byar DP: The Veterans Administration Cooperative Urologic Research Group's studies of cancer of the prostate. Cancer 32:1126, 1973
65. Byar DP, Core DK: Hormone therapy for prostate cancer: Results of the Veterans Administration Cooperative Urological Research Group Studies. NCI Monogr 7:165, 1988
66. Byar DP, Corle DK: VACURG randomized trial of radical prostatectomy for stages I and II prostate cancer. Urology 17 (Suppl):7, 1981
67. Byar DP, Mostofi FK: Cancer of the prostate in men less than 50 years old: An analysis of 51 cases. J Urol 102:726, 1969
68. Byar DP, Mostofi FK, Veterans Administration Cooperative Urological Research Group: Carcinoma of the prostate: Prognostic evaluation of certain pathologic features in 208 radical prostatectomies examined by the step-section technique. Cancer 30:5, 1972
69. Byar DP, Veterans Administration Cooperative Urological Research Group: Survival of patients with incidentally found microscopic cancer of the prostate: Results of a clinical trial of conservative treatment. J Urol 108:908, 1972
70. Carlton CE Jr, Dawoud F, Hudgins P, Scott R Jr: Irradiation treatment of carcinoma of the prostate: A preliminary report based on 8 years of experience. J Urol 18:924, 1972
71. Carlton CE Jr, Hudgins PT, Guerriero WG, Scott R Jr: Radiotherapy in the management of stage C carcinoma of the prostate. Trans Am Assoc Genitourin Surg 67:70, 1975
72. Carney JA, Kelalis PP: Endometrial carcinoma of the prostatic utricle. Am J Clin Pathol 60:565, 1973
73. Carpentier PJ, Schroder FH: Transrectal ultrasonography in the follow-up of prostatic carcinoma patients: A new prognostic parameter? J Urol 131:903, 1984
74. Carson CC III, Zincke H, Utz DC, et al: Radical prostatectomy after radiotherapy for prostatic cancer. J Urol 124:237, 1980
75. Carter HB, Hamper UM, Sheth S, et al: Evaluation of transrectal ultrasound in the early detection of prostate cancer. J Urol 142:1008, 1989
76. Castellino RA: Lymphography in clinically localized prostate cancer. NCI Monogr 7:37, 1988
77. Catalona WJ: Prostate Cancer. Orlando, Grune & Stratton, 1984
78. Catalona WJ, Bigg SW: Nerve-sparing radical prostatectomy: Evaluation of results after 250 patients. J Urol 143:538, 1990
79. Catalona WJ, Dresner SM: Nerve-sparing radical prostatectomy: Extraprostatic tumor extension and preservation of erectile function. J Urol 134:1149, 1985
80. Catalona WJ, Stein AJ, Fair WR: Grading errors in prostatic needle biopsies: Relation to the accuracy of tumor grade in predicting pelvic lymph node metastases. J Urol 127:919, 1982
81. Charyulu KKN: Transperineal interstitial implantation of prostate cancer: A new method. Int J Radiat Oncol Biol Phys 6:1261, 1980
82. Chodak GW, Wald V, Parmer E, et al: Comparison of digital examination and transrectal ultrasonography for the diagnosis of prostate cancer. J Urol 135:951, 1986
83. Cline WA, Kramer SA, Farnham R: Impact of pelvic lymphadenectomy in patients with prostatic adenocarcinoma. Urology 17;129, 1981
84. Cochran JS, Kadesky MC: A private practice experience with adenocarcinoma of the prostate in men less than 50 years old. J Urol 125:220, 1981
85. Corvalan JG, Gill WM, Eggleston TA, et al: Irradiation of the male breast to prevent hormone produced gynecomastia. Am J Roentgenol Radiat Ther Nucl Med 106:839, 1969
86. Corwin SH, Maxwell M, Small M, et al: Experiences with ^{32}P in advanced carcinoma of prostate. J Urol 104:745, 1970
87. Cosgrove MD, George FW III, Terry R: The effects of treatment on the local lesion of carcinoma of the prostate. J Urol 109:861, 1973
88. Cox JD, Kline RW: Do prostate biopsies 12 months or more after external irradiation for adenocarcinoma, stage III, predict long-term survival? Int J Radiat Oncol Biol Phys 9:299, 1983
89. Cox JD, Stoffel TJ: The significance of needle biopsy after irradiation for stage C adenocarcinoma of the prostate. Cancer 40:156, 1977
90. Crawford ED, Eisenberger MA, McLeod DG, et al: A controlled trial of leuprolide with and without flutamide in prostatic carcinoma. N Engl J Med 321:419, 1989
91. Culp OS, Meyer JJ: Radical prostatectomy in the treatment of prostatic cancer. Cancer 32:1113, 1973
92. Dayal HH, Chiu C: Factors associated with racial differences

in survival for prostatic carcinoma. J Chronic Dis 35:553, 1982
93. Dayal HH, Polissar L, Dahlberg S: Race, socioeconomic status, and other prognostic factors for survival from prostate cancer. JNCI 74:1001, 1985
94. Delaney TF, Shipley WN, O'Leary MP, et al: Preoperative irradiation, lymphadenectomy, and iodine implantation for patients with localized carcinoma of the prostate. Int J Radiat Oncol Biol Phys 12:1779, 1986
95. Del Regato JA: Long term curative results of radiotherapy of patients with inoperable prostatic carcinoma. Radiology 131:291, 1979
96. Deming CL: Results of 100 cases of cancer of the prostate and seminal vesicles treated with radium. Surg Gynecol Obstet 34:99, 1922
97. Dewit L, Ang KK, Van der Schueren E: Acute side effects and late complications after radiotherapy of localized carcinoma of the prostate. Cancer Treat Rev 10:79, 1983
98. DeWys WE, Begg CB, Brodovsky H: A comparative clinical trial of Adriamycin and 5-fluorouracil in advanced prostatic cancer: Prognostic factors and response. Prostate 4:1, 1983
99. Dodds PR, Caride VJ, Lytton B: The role of vertebral veins in the dissemination of prostatic carcinoma. J Urol 126:753, 1981
100. Doll R: Geographic variation in cancer incidence: A clue to causation. World J Surg 2:595, 1978
101. Donati RM, Ellis H, Gallahar NI: Testosterone potentiated ^{32}P therapy in prostate carcinoma. Cancer 19:1088, 1966
102. Drafta D, Proca E, Zamfir Vl, et al: Plasma steroids in benign prostatic hypertrophy and carcinoma of the prostate. J Steroid Biochem 17:689, 1982
103. Dube VE, Farrow GM, Greene LF: Prostatic adenocarcinoma of ductal origin. Cancer 32:402, 1973
104. Edland RW: Testosterone potentiated radiophosporus therapy of osseous metastases in prostatic cancer. AJR 120:678, 1974
105. Eggleston JC, Walsh PC: Radical prostatectomy with preservation of sexual function: Pathologic findings in the first 100 cases. J Urol 134:1146, 1985
106. Eisbruch A, Perez CA, Rossler E, et al: Adjuvant irradiation after prostatectomy for carcinoma of prostate with positive surgical margins or treatment for clinical recurrence. J Urol (submitted for publication)
107. Eisenberger MA: Chemotherapy for prostate cancer. NCI Monogr 7:151, 1988
108. Ekman P, Snochowski M, Zetterberg A, et al: Steroid receptor content in human prostatic carcinoma and response to endocrine therapy. Cancer 44:1173, 1979
109. Elder JS, Jewett HJ, Walsh PC: Radical perineal prostatectomy for clinical stage B2 carcinoma of the prostate. J Urol 127:704, 1982
110. Emmett JL, Barber KW Jr, Jackman RJ: Transrectal biopsy to detect prostatic carcinoma: A review and report of cases. J Urol 87:460, 1962
111. Epstein JI, Lieberman PH: Mucinous adenocarcinoma of the prostate gland. Am J Surg Pathol 9:299, 1985
112. Epstein LM, Stewart HB, Antunez AR, et al: Half and total body radiation for carcinoma of the prostate. J Urol 122:3330, 1979
113. Esposti PL: Cytologic malignancy grading of prostatic carcinoma by transrectal aspiration biopsy. Scand J Urol Nephrol 5:199, 1971
114. Fair WR, Heston WDW, Kadmon D, et al: Prostatic cancer, acid phosphatase creatinine kinase-BB and race: A prospective study. J Urol 128:735, 1982
115. Fitzpatrick PJ, Rider WD: Half body radiotherapy of advanced cancer. J Can Assoc Radiol 27:75, 1976
116. Fitzpatrick PJ, Rider WD: Half body radiotherapy. Int J Radiat Oncol Biol Phys 1:197, 1976
117. Flocks RH: The treatment of stage C prostatic cancer with reference to combined surgical and radiation therapy. J Urol 109;461, 1972
118. Flocks RH: Interstitial irradiation therapy with a solution of Au198 as part of combination therapy for prostatic carcinoma. J Nucl Med 5:691, 1964
119. Flocks RH, Culp D, Porto R: Lymphatic spread from prostatic cancer. J Urol 81:194, 1959
120. Forman JD, Order SE, Zinreich ES, et al: The correlation of pretreatment transurethral resection of prostatic cancer with tumor dissemination and disease-free survival. A univariate and multivariate analysis. Cancer 58:1770, 1986
121. Forman JD, Wharam MD, Lee DJ, et al: Definitive radiotherapy following prostatectomy: Results and complications. Int J Radiat Oncol Biol Phys 12:185, 1986
122. Foti AG, Cooper JF, Herschman H, et al: Detection of prostatic cancer by solid phase radio-immunoassay of serum prostatic acid phosphatase. N Engl J Med 297:1357, 1977
123. Fowler JE Jr, Fisher HAG, Kaiser DL, Whitmore WF Jr: Relationship of pretreatment transurethral resection of the prostate to survival without distant metastases in patients treated with I-implantation for localized prostatic cancer. Cancer 53:1867, 1984
124. Fowler JE, Whitmore WF: The incidence and extent of pelvic lymph node metastases in apparently localized prostatic cancer. Cancer 47:1941, 1981
125. Franke HD, Schmidt R: Clinical results with fast neutrons (DT, 14 MeV). Radiat Med 3:151, 1985
126. Franks LM: Benign nodular hyperplasia of the prostate: A review. Ann R Coll Surg Engl 14:92, 1954
127. Franzen S, Fiertz G, Zakicek J: Cytological diagnosis of prostatic tumor by transrectal aspiration biopsy: A preliminary report. Br J Urol 32:193, 1960
128. Freiha FS, Bagshaw MA: Carcinoma of the prostate: Results of post-irradiation biopsy. Prostate 5:19, 1984
129. Freiha FS, McNeal JE, Stamey TA: Selection criteria for radical prostatectomy based on morphometric studies in prostate carcinoma. NCI Monogr 7:107, 1988
130. Fried PR, Mandell SA: Role of adjuvant radiotherapy following radical prostatectomy for microscopic residual disease. Eur Urol 15:37, 1988
131. Fujino A, Scardino PT: Transrectal ultrasonography for prostatic cancer. II. The response of the prostate to definitive radiotherapy. Cancer 57:935, 1986,
132. Gaeta JF, Asirwatham JE, Miller G, Murphy GP: Histologic grading of primary prostatic cancer: A new approach to an old problem. J Urol 123:689, 1980
133. Galen RS, Gambino SR: Beyond Normality: The Predictive Value and Efficiency of Medical Diagnosis. New York, John Wiley, 1978
134. Garcia D, Fathman A, Drzymala R, et al: Localized carcinoma of the prostate: Preliminary results of transperineal interstitial ^{192}Ir implantation and external irradiation. Unpublished data.
135. Geller J, Albert J, Yen SSC: Treatment of advanced cancer of prostate with megestrol acetate. Urology 12:537, 1978
136. George NJR: Natural history of localized prostatic cancer managed by conservative therapy alone. Lancet 1:494, 1988
137. Ghali VS, Garcia RL: Prostatic adenocarcinoma with carcinoidal features producing adrenocorticotropic syndrome: Immunohistochemical study and review of the literature. Cancer 54:1043, 1984
138. Ghanadian R. Puah CM, O'Donoghue EPN: Serum testosterone and dihydrotestosterone in carcinoma of the prostate. Br J cancer 39:696, 1979
139. Gibbons RP: Total prostatectomy for clinically localized prostate cancer: Long-term surgical results and current morbidity. NCI Monogr 7:123, 1988
140. Gibbons RP, Beckley S, Brady MF, et al: The addition of chemotherapy to hormonal therapy for treatment of patients with metastatic carcinoma of the prostate. J Surg Oncol 23:133, 1983
141. Gibbons RP, Cole BS, Richardson RG, et al: Adjuvant radiotherapy following radical prostatectomy: Results and complications. J Urol 135:65, 1986
142. Gibbons RP, Correa RJ, Brannen GE, et al: Total prostatectomy for localized prostatic cancer. J Urol 131:73, 1984
143. Gibbons RP, Mason JT, Correa RJ Jr, et al: Carcinoma of the prostate: Local control with external beam radiation therapy. J Urol 121:310, 1979

144. Glantz GM: Cirrhosis and carcinoma of the prostate gland. J Urol 91:291, 1964
145. Glaser MJ, Howard N, Waterfall N: Carcinoma of the prostate: The treatment of bone metastases by radiophosphorus. Clin Radiol 32:695, 1981
146. Gleason DF: Histologic grade, clinical state, and patient age in prostate cancer. NCI Monogr 7:15, 1988
147. Gleason DF, Mellinger GT, VACURG: Prediction of prognosis for prostatic adenocarcinoma by combined histological grading and clinical staging. J Urol 111:58, 1974
148. Gleason DF, Veterans Administration Cooperative Urological Research Group: Histologic grading and clinical staging of prostatic carcinoma. In Tannenbaum M (ed): Urologic Pathology: The Prostate, pp 171–198. Philadelphia, Lea & Febiger, 1977
149. Glick JH, Wein A, Padavic K, et al: Phase II trial of tamoxifen in metastatic carcinoma of the prostate. Cancer 49:1367, 1982
150. Goffinet DR, Martinez A, Freiha F, et al: 125 Iodine prostate implants for recurrent carcinomas after external beam irradiation: Preliminary results. Cancer 45:2717, 1980
151. Golimbu M, Morales P: Stage A2 prostatic carcinoma: Should staging system be reclassified. Urology 13:592, 1979
152. Golimbu M, Morales P, Al-Askari S, et al: CAT scanning in staging of prostatic cancer. Urology 18:305, 1981
153. Golimbu M, Morales P, Al-Askari S, Brown J: Extended pelvic lymphadenectomy for prostatic cancer. J Urol 121:617, 1979
154. Gore RM, Moss AA: Value of computed tomography in interstitial ^{125}I brachytherapy of prostatic carcinoma. Radiology 146:453, 1983
155. Graham S, Haughey B, Marshall J, et al: Diet in the epidemiology of carcinoma of the prostate gland. JNCI 70:687, 1983
156. Gray GF Jr, Marshall VF: Squamous carcinoma of the prostate. J Urol 113:736, 1975
157. Grayhack JT, Keeler TC, Kozlowski JM: Carcinoma of the prostate: Hormonal therapy. Cancer 60:589, 1987
158. Green N, Bodner H, Broth E, et al: Improved control of bulky prostate carcinoma with sequential estrogen and radiation therapy. Int J Radiat Oncol Biol Phys 10:971, 1984
159. Greene LF, Farrow GM, Ravitz JM, Tomera FM: Prostatic adenocarcinoma of ductal origin. J Urol 121:303, 1979
160. Greene LF, Mulcahy JJ, Warrant NM, Dockerty MB: Primary transitional cell carcinoma of the prostate. J Urol 110:235, 1973
161. Greenwald PKV, Polan AK, et al: Cancer of the prostate among men with benign prostatic hyperplasia. JNCI 53:335, 1974
162. Grossman HB, Batata M, Hilaris B, Whitmore WF Jr: I-125 implantation for carcinoma of prostate: Further follow-up of first 100 cases. Urology 20:591, 1982
163. Guinan P, Bush I, Ray V, et al: The accuracy of the rectal examination in the diagnosis of prostate carcinoma. N Engl J Med 303:499, 1980
164. Habib FK, Bissas A, Neill WA, et al: Flow cytometric analysis of cellular DNA in human prostate cancer: Relationship to 5α-reductase activity of the tissue. Urol Res 17:239, 1989
165. Haenszel W, Kurihara M: Studies of Japanese migrants. I. Mortality from cancer and other disease among Japanese in the United States. JNCI 40:43, 1968
166. Halpert B, Schmalhorst WR: Carcinoma of the prostate in patients 70 to 79 years old. Cancer 19:695, 1966
167. Halpert B, Sheehan EE, Schmalhorst WR, Scott R: Carcinoma of the prostate: A survey of 5000 autopsies. Cancer 16:737, 1963
168. Hammond EC: Tobacco. In Fraumeni JF (ed): Persons at High Risk of Cancer, pp 131–138. New York, Academic Press, 1975
169. Hanash KA, Utz DC, Cook EN, et al: Carcinoma of the prostate: A 15-year follow-up. J Urol 107:450, 1972
170. Hanks GE: More on the Uro-Oncology Research Group report of radical surgery *vs.* radiotherapy for adenocarcinoma of the prostate (Letter). Int J Radiat Oncol Biol Phys 14:1053, 1988
171. Hanks GE: External-beam radiation therapy for clinically localized prostate cancer: Patterns of Care Studies in the United States. NCI Monogr 7:75, 1988
172. Hanks GE: Optimizing the radiation treatment and outcome of prostate cancer. Int J Radiat Oncol Biol Phys 11:1235, 1985
173. Hanks GE, Dawson AK: The role of external beam radiation therapy after prostatectomy for prostate cancer. Cancer 58:2406, 1986
174. Hanks GE, Krall JM, Martz KL, et al: The outcome of treatment of 313 patients with T-1 (UICC) prostate cancer treated with external beam irradiation. Int J Radiat Oncol Biol Phys 14:243, 1988
175. Hanks GE, Leibel SA, Krall JM, Kramer S: Patterns of Care Studies: Dose-response of observations for local control of adenocarcinoma of the prostate. Int J Radiat Oncol Biol Phys 11:153, 1985
176. Hanks GE, Leibel S, Kramer S: The dissemination of cancer by transurethral resection of locally advanced prostate cancer. J Urol 129:309, 1983
177. Hanks GE, Martz JH, Diamond JJ: The effect of dose on local control of prostate cancer. Int J Radiat Oncol Biol Phys 15:1299, 1988
178. Harisiasdis L, Veenema RJ, Senyszyn JJ, et al: Tretter P, Romas NA, Chang CH, Lattimer JK, Tannenbaum M: Carcinoma of the prostate: Treatment with external radiotherapy. Cancer 41:2131, 1978
179. Hazra TA, Giri S: Prophylactic pelvic girdle irradiation in the treatment of prostatic carcinoma. Int J Radiat Oncol Biol Phys 7:817, 1981
180. Heaney JA, Chang HC, Daly JJ, Prout GR Jr: Prognosis of clinically undiagnosed prostatic carcinoma and the influence of endocrine therapy. J Urol 118:283, 1977
181. Herr HW: Cyclophosphamide, methotrexate, and 5-fluorouracil combination chemotherapy versus chloroethyl-cyclohexyl-nitrosourea in the treatment of metastatic prostatic cancer. J Urol 127:462, 1982
182. Hilaris BS, Whitmore WF, Batata M, Barzell W: Behavioral patterns of prostate adenocarcinoma following an 125I implant and pelvic node dissection. Int J Radiat Oncol Biol Phys 2:631, 1977
183. Hilaris BS, Whitmore WF, Batata MA, et al: ^{125}I implantation of the prostate: Dose-response considerations. Front Radiat Ther Oncol 12:82, 1978
184. Hodges CV, Pearse HD, Stille L: Radical prostatectomy for carcinoma: 30-year experience and 15-year survivals. J Urol 122:180, 1979
185. Honger B, Schwegler N: Experience with prophylactic irradiation of the breast in prostatic carcinoma patients being treated with estrogen. Helv Chir Acta 47:427, 1980
186. Hricak H: Noninvasive imaging for staging of prostate cancer: Magnetic resonance imaging, computed tomography, and ultrasound. NCI Monogr 7:31, 1988
187. Hricak H, Jeffrey RB, Dooms GC, Tanagho EA: Evaluation of prostate size: A comparison of ultrasound and magnetic resonance imaging. Urol Radiol 9:1, 1987
188. Hudson MA, Bahnson RR, Catalona WJ: Clinical use of prostate specific antigen in patients with prostate cancer. J Urol 142:1011, 1989
189. Huggins C, Hodges CV: Studies on prostatic cancer. I. The effect of castration of estrogen and of androgen injection on serum phosphatases in metastatic carcinoma of the prostate. Cancer Res 1:293, 1941
190. Huggins C, Stevens RE, Hodges CV: Studies on prostatic cancer. II. The effects of castration on advanced carcinoma of the prostate gland. Arch Surg 43:209, 1941
191. Hussey DH, Chan R, Delclos L, Howze J: Radiotherapy for carcinoma of the prostate. Cancer Bull 30:131, 1978
192. Hutch JA: A new theory of anatomy of the internal urinary sphincter and the physiology of micturition. IV. The urinary sphincteric mechanism. J Urol 97:705, 1967
193. Ihde DC, Bunn PA, Cohen MH, et al: Effective treatment of hormonally-unresponsive metastatic carcinoma of the prostate with Adriamycin and cyclophosphamide: Methods of documenting tumor response and progression. Cancer 45:1300, 1980
194. Jacobson GM, Smith JA Jr, Stewart JR: Postoperative radiation therapy for pathologic state C prostate cancer. Int J Radiat Oncol Biol Phys 13:1021, 1987

195. Jewett HJ: Radical perineal prostatectomy for palpable, clinically localized, non-obstructive cancer: Experience at the Johns Hopkins Hospital 1909–1963. J Urol 124:492, 1980
196. Jewett HJ: The case for radical perineal prostatectomy. J Urol 103:195, 1970
197. Jewett HJ: The present status of radical prostatectomy for stages A and B prostatic cancer. Urol North Am 2:105, 1975
198. Johnson DE, Chalbaud R, Ayala AG: Secondary tumors of the prostate. J Urol 112:507, 1974
199. Johnson DE, Hogan JM, Ayala AG: Transitional-cell carcinoma of the prostate. Cancer 29:287, 1972
200. Johnson DE, Lanieri JP Jr, Ayala G: Prostatic adenocarcinoma occurring in men under 50 years of age. J Surg Oncol 4:207, 1972
201. Jones PW, Bogardus CR, Anderson DW: Significance of initial "performance status" in patients receiving half body radiation. Int J Radiat Oncol Biol Phys 10:1947, 1984
202. Joshi DP, Seery WH, Goldberg LG, Goldman L: Evaluation of phosphorous32 for intractable pain secondary to prostatic carcinoma metastases. JAMA 193:621, 1965
203. Kabalin JN, Hodge KK, McNeal JE, et al: Identification of residual cancer in the prostate following radiation therapy: Role of transrectal ultrasound guided biopsy and prostate specific antigen. J Urol 142:326, 1989
204. Kagan AR, Gordon J, Cooper JF, et al: A clinical appraisal of post-irradiation biopsy in prostatic cancer. Cancer 39:637, 1977
205. Kaplan E, Fels IG, Kotlowski BR, et al: Therapy of carcinoma of the prostate metastatic to bone with P32 labeled condensed phosphate. J Nucl Med 1:1, 1960
206. Keisch ME, Perez CA, Grigsby PW, et al: Preliminary report on ten patients treated with radiotherapy after radical prostatectomy for isolated elevation of serum PSA levels. Int J Radiat Oncol Biol Phys 19:1503, 1990
207. Khan K, Crawford ED, Johnson EL: Transperineal percutaneous iridium-192 implant of the prostate. Int J Radiat Oncol Biol Phys 9:1391, 1983
208. Kiesling VJ, McAninch JW, Goebel JL, Agee RE: External beam radiotherapy for adenocarcinoma of the prostate: A clinical followup. J Urol 124:851, 1980
209. Klaua M: Radiogenic peripheral neuropathies following telecobalt radiation in abdominal cavity. Radiobiol Radiother (Berl) 15:459, 1974
210. Kopelson G, Harisiadis L, Romas NA, et al: Periurethral prostatic duct carcinoma: Clinical features and treatment results. Cancer 42:2894, 1978
211. Krain LS: Some epidemiologic variables in prostatic carcinoma in California. Prev Med 3:154, 1974
212. Kramer SA, Cline WA Jr, Farnham R, et al: Prognosis of patients with stage D-1 prostatic adenocarcinoma. J Urol 125:817, 1981
213. Kramer SA, Spahr J, Brendler CB, et al: Experience with Gleason's histopathologic grading in prostatic cancer. J Urol 124:223, 1980
214. Kraus PA, Lutton B, Weiss RM, Prosnitz LR: Radiation therapy for local palliative treatment of prostatic cancer. J Urol 108:612, 1972
215. Kuban DA, Delbridge T, El-Mahdi AM, Schellhammer PF: Half-body irradiation for treatment of widely metastatic adenocarcinoma of the prostate. J Urol 141:572, 1989
216. Kuban DA, El-Mahdi AM, Schellhammer PF: ^{192}Ir interstitial implantation for prostate cancer. What have we learned 10 years later? Cancer 63:2415, 1989
217. Kuban DA, El Mahdi AM, Schellhammer PF: Prognosis in patients with local recurrence after definitive irradiation for prostatic carcinoma. Cancer 63:2421, 1989
218. Kuban DA, El-Madhi AM, Schellhammer PF: The effect of TURP on prognosis in prostatic carcinoma. Int J Radiat Oncol Biol Phys 13:1653, 1987
219. LaBrie F, Dupont A, Gignere M, et al: Advantages of the combination therapy in previously untreated and treated patients with advanced prostate cancer. J Steroid Biochem 25:877, 1986
220. Lai PP, Perez CA, Shapiro SJ, Lockett MA: Carcinoma of the prostate stage B and C: Lack of influence of duration of radiotherapy on tumor control and treatment morbidity (Abstract). Int J Radiat Oncol Biol Phys 17(suppl 1):164, 1989
221. Landman C, Hunig R: Prostatic specific antigen as an indicator of response to radiotherapy in prostate cancer. Int J Radiat Oncol Biol Phys 17:1073, 1989
222. Lange PH, Ercole CJ, Lightner DJ, et al: The value of serum prostate specific antigen determinations before and after radical prostatectomy. J Urol 141:873, 1989
223. Lange PH, Reddy PK, Medini E, et al: Radiation therapy as adjuvant treatment after radical prostatectomy. NCI Monogr 7:141, 1988
224. Laramore GE, Krall JM, Thomas FJ, et al: Fast neutron therapy for locally advanced prostate cancer: Results of RTOG randomized study. Int J Radiat Oncol Biol Phys 11:1621, 1985
225. Larsson LG, Sundbom CM: Roentgen irradiation of the male breast. Acta Radiol Ther Phys Biol 58:253, 1962
226. Lawton CA, Glisch C, Bynhardt RW, et al: Extended-field radiation therapy for prostatic carcinoma with paraaortic lymph node metastasis. Am J Clin Oncol 9:302, 1986
227. Leach GE, Cooper JF, Kagan AR, et al: Radiotherapy for prostatic carcinoma: Postirradiation prostatic biopsy and recurrent patterns with long-term follow-up. J Urol 128:505, 1982
228. Lee F, Gray JM, McLeary RD, et al: Prostatic evaluation of transrectal sonography: Criteria for diagnosis of early carcinoma. Radiology 158:91, 1986
229. Leibel SA, Hanks GE, Kramer S: Patterns of Care Outcome Studies: Results of the national practice in adenocarcinoma of the prostate. Int J Radiat Oncol Biol Phys 10:401, 1984
230. Leistenschneider W, Nagel R: Cytological and DNA cytophotometric monitoring of the effect of therapy on conservatively treated prostatic carcinomas. Scand J Urol Nephrol [Suppl] 55:197, 1983
231. Lepor H, Walsh PC: Long-term results of radical prostatectomy in clinically localized prostate cancer: Experience at the Johns Hopkins Hospital. NCI Monogr 7:117, 1988
232. Levine RL, Wilchinsky M: Adenocarcinoma of the prostate: A comparison of the disease in blacks versus whites. J Urol 121:761, 1979
233. Lipsett JA, Cosrove MD, Green N, et al: Factors influencing prognosis the radiotherapeutic management of carcinoma of the prostate. Int J Radiat Oncol Biol Phys 1:1049, 1976
234. Loening SA, Scott WW, DeKernion J, et al: A comparison of hydroxyurea, methyl-chloroethyl-cyclohexyl-nitrosourea and cyclophosphamide in patients with advanced carcinoma of the prostate. J Urol 125:812, 1981
235. Logothetis CJ, Samuels MJ, von Eschenbach AC, et al: Doxorubicin, mitomycin-C and 5-fluorouracil (DMF) in the treatment of metastatic hormonal refractory adenocarcinoma of the prostate, with a note on the staging of metastatic prostate cancer. J Clin Oncol 1:368, 1983
236. Low NN, Vijayakumar S, Rosenberg I, et al: Beam's eye view based prostate treatment planning; Is it useful? Int J Radiat Biol Phys 19:759, 1990
237. Lund F, Smith PH, Suciu S, EORTC Urological Group: Do bone scans predict prognosis in prostatic cancer? A report of the EORTC Protocol 3762. Br J Urol 56:58, 1984
238. Mador DR, Huben RP, Wajsman Z, et al: Salvage surgery following radical radiotherapy for adenocarcinoma of the prostate. 133:58, 1985
239. Madsen PO, Corele DK, Byar DP: Radical prostatectomy for carcinoma of the prostate: Stages I and II. In Rost A, Fielder U (eds): Proceedings of the International Symposium on the Treatment of Carcinoma of the Prostate, p 46. Berlin, Berlin Urologische Klinik, Klinkium Steglitz, Freie Univ, 1980
240. Maier JG, Perry RH, Saylor W, Sulak MH: Radiation myelitis of the dorsolumbar spinal cord. Radiology 93:153, 1969
241. Mameghan H, Fisher R, Mameghan J, et al: Bowel complications after radiotherapy for carcinoma of the prostate: The volume effect. Int J Radiat Oncol Biol Phys 18:315, 1990
242. Martinez A, Edmundson GD, Cox RS, et al: Combination of external beam irradiation and multiple-site perineal applicator (MUPIT) for treatment of locally advanced or recurrent prostatic, anorectal, and gynecologic malignancies. Int J Radiat Oncol Biol Phys 11:391, 1985

243. Maruoka M, Ando K, Nozumi K, et al: Fast neutron therapy of prostatic cancer (Japanese). Nippon Hinyhokika Gakkai Zasshi 74:409, 1983
244. Maxfield JR, Maxfield JJG, Maxfield WS: The use of radioactive phosphorus and testosterone in metastatic bone lesions from breast and prostate. South Med J 51:320, 1958
245. McGowan, D.G. The effect of transurethral resection on prognosis in carcinoma of the prostate: Real or imaginary? Int J Radiat Oncol Biol Phys 15:1057, 1988
246. McGowan DG: The value of extended field radiation therapy in carcinoma of the prostate. Int J Radiat Oncol Biol Phys 7:1333, 1981
247. McGowan DG: The adverse influence of prior transurethral resection on prognosis in carcinoma of the prostate treated by radiation therapy. Int J Radiat Oncol Biol Phys 6:1121, 1980
248. McLaughlin AP, Saltzstein SL, McCullough DL, Gittes RF: Prostatic carcinoma: Incidence and location of unsuspected lymphatic metastases. J Urol 115:89, 1976
249. McNeal JE: Zonal anatomy of the prostate. Prostate 2:35, 1981
250. McNeal JE: Anatomy of the prostate: An historical survey of divergent views. Prostate 1:3, 1980
251. Meek AG, Park TL, Oberman E, Wielopolski L: A prospective study of prostate specific antigen levels in patients receiving radiotherapy for localized carcinoma of the prostate. Int J Radiat Oncol Biol Phys 19:733, 1990
252. Melicow MM, Tannenbaum M: Endometrial carcinoma of uterus masculinus (prostatic utricle). Report of 6 cases. J Urol 106:892, 1971
253. Menon M, Walsh PC: Hormonal therapy for prostatic cancer. In Murphy GP (ed): Prostatic Cancer, pp. 175–200. Littleton, MA, PSG Publishing, 1979
254. Merrick MV, Ding CL, Chisholm GD, Elton RA: Prognostic significance of alkaline and acid phosphatase and skeletal scintigraphy in carcinoma of the prostate. Br J Urol 57:715, 1985
255. Mettlin C, Natarajan N: Epidemiologic observations from the American College of Surgeons' survey on prostate cancer. Prostate 4:323, 1983
256. Middleton RG: Value of and indications for pelvic lymph node dissection in the staging of prostate cancer. NCI Monogr 7:41, 1988
257. Middleton RG, Smith JA, Melzer RB, et al: Patient survival and local recurrence rate following radical prostatectomy for prostatic carcinoma. J Urol 136:422, 1986
258. Mittal B: A study of penile circulation before and after radiation in patients with prostate cancer and its effect on impotence. Int J Radiat Oncol Biol Phys 11:1121, 1985
259. Morton JD, Peschel RE: Iodine-125 implants versus external beam therapy for stages A2, B, and C prostate cancer. Int J Radiat Oncol Biol Phys 14:1153, 1988
260. Mostofi FK: Grading of prostatic carcinoma. Cancer Chemother Rep 59:111, 1975
261. Mostofi FK, Price EB Jr: Malignant tumors of the prostate. In Tumors of the Male Genital System, Atlas of Tumor Pathology, 2nd series, fasc 8, p 253. Washington DC, Armed Forces Institute of Pathology, 1973
262. Murphy GP, Beckley S, Brady MF, et al: Treatment of newly diagnosed metastatic prostate cancer patients with chemotherapy agents in combination with hormones versus hormones alone. Cancer 51:1264, 1983
263. Murphy GP, Natarajan N, Pontes JE, et al.: The national survey of prostate cancer in the United States by the American College of Surgeons. J Urol 127:928, 1982
264. Muss HB, Howard V, Richards F, et al: Cyclophosphamide versus cyclophosphamide, methotrexate, and 5-fluorouracil in advanced prostatic cancer: A randomized trial. Cancer 47:1949, 1981
265. National Cancer Institute Monograph Number 7: Consensus Development Conference on the Management of Clinically Localized Prostate Cancer. Bethesda, National Cancer Institute, 1988
266. Neglia WJ, Hussey DH, Johnson DE: Megavoltage radiation therapy for carcinoma of the prostate. Int J Radiat Oncol Biol Phys 2:873, 1977
267. Nichols RT, Barry JM, Hodges CV: The morbidity of radical prostatectomy for multifocal stage I prostatic adenocarcinoma. J Urol 117:83, 1977
268. Nitch CAR: The conservative treatment of carcinoma of the prostate. Br J Urol 8:329, 1936
269. O'Bryan RM, Baker LH, Gottleib JE, et al: Dose response evaluation of Adriamycin in human neoplasia. Cancer 39:1940, 1977
270. Oesterling JE, Brendler CB, Epstein JI, et al: Correlation of clinical stage, serum prostatic acid phosphatase and preoperative Gleason grade with final pathological stage in 275 patients with clinically localized adenocarcinoma of the prostate. J Urol 138:92, 1987
271. Papsidero LD, Kuriyama M, Wang MC, et al: Prostate antigen: A marker for human prostate epithelial cells. JNCI 66:37, 1981
272. Paschkis R, Tittinger W: Radiumbehandlung eines prostatasarkoms. Weiner klische Wochenschrift Nr. 48, 1910
273. Pasteau O: Traitement du cancer de la prostate par le radium. Rev Mal Nutr 363, 1911
274. Paulson D: Diseases of the prostate. Clin Symp 41:2, 1989
275. Paulson DF: Randomized series of treatment with surgery versus radiation for prostate adenocarcinoma. NCI Monogr 7:127, 1988
276. Paulson DF: More on the Uro-Oncology Research Group report of radical surgery *vs.* radiotherapy for adenocarcinoma of the prostate: Rebuttal. (Letter). Int J Radiat Oncol Biol Phys 14:1053, 1988
277. Paulson DF: The prognostic role of lymphadenectomy in adenocarcinoma of the prostate. Urol Clin North Am 7:615, 1980
278. Paulson DF, Cline WA Jr, Koefott RN Jr, et al: Extended field radiation therapy versus delayed hormonal therapy in node positive prostatic adenocarcinoma. J Urol 127:935, 1982
279. Paulson DF, Lin GH, Hinshaw W, et al: Radical surgery versus radiotherapy for adenocarcinoma of the prostate. J Urol 128:502, 1982
280. Paulson DF, Uro-Oncology Research Group: The impact of current staging procedures in assessing disease extent of prostatic adenocarcinoma. J Urol 121:300, 1979
281. Perez CA: Carcinoma of the prostate: A vexing biological and clinical enigma. Int J Radiat Oncol Biol Phys 9:1427, 1983
282. Perez CA, Ackerman LV, Silber I, Royce RK: Radiation therapy in the treatment of localized carcinoma of the prostate: Preliminary report using 22-MeV photons. Cancer 34:1059, 1974
283. Perez CA, Fair WR, Ihde DC: Carcinoma of the prostate. In DeVita VT Jr, Hellman S, Rosenberg SA (eds): Cancer: Principles and Practice of Oncology, 3rd ed, pp 1023–1058. Philadelphia, JB Lippincott, 1989
284. Perez CA, Georgio A, Lockett MA: Impact of technical factors on outcome of irradiation of carcinoma of the prostate (in preparation)
285. Perez CA, Garcia D, Simpson JR, et al: Factors influencing outcome of definitive radiotherapy for localized carcinoma of the prostate. Radiother Oncol 16:1, 1989
286. Perez CA, Pilepich MV, Garcia D, et al: Definitive radiation therapy in carcinoma of the prostate localized to the pelvis: Experience at the Mallinckrodt Institute of Radiology. NCI Monogr 7:85, 1988
287. Perez CA, Pilepich MV, Zivnuska F: Tumor control in definitive irradiation of localized carcinoma of the prostate. Int J Radiat Oncol Biol Phys 12:523, 1986
288. Perez CA, Walz BJ, Zivnuska FR, et al: Irradiation of carcinoma of the prostate localized to the pelvis: Analysis of tumor response and prognosis. Int J Radiat Oncol Biol Phys 6:555, 1980
289. Pilepich MV, Asbell SO, Krall JM, et al: Correlation of radiotherapeutic parameters and treatment related morbidity: Analysis of RTOG study 77-06. Int J Radiat Oncol Biol Phys 13:1007, 1987
290. Pilepich MV, Asbell SO, Mulholland GS, Pajak T: Surgical staging in carcinoma of the prostate: The RTOG experience. Prostate 5:471, 1984
291. Pilepich MV, Bagshaw MA, Asbell SO, et al: Definitive radio-

therapy in resectable (stage A2 and B) carcinoma of the prostate: Results of a nationwide overview. Int J Radiat Oncol Biol Phys 13:659, 1987

292. Pilepich MV, Krall J, George FW, et al: Treatment-related morbidity in phase III RTOG studies of extended-field irradiation for carcinoma of the prostate. Int J Radiat Oncol Biol Phys 10:1861, 1984
293. Pilepich MV, Krall JM, Hanks GE, et al: Correlation of pretreatment transurethral resection and prognosis in patients with stage C carcinoma of the prostate treated with definitive radiotherapy: RTOG experience. Int J Radiat Oncol Biol Phys 13:195, 1987
294. Pilepich MV, Krall JM, John MJ, et al: Hormonal cytoreduction in locally advanced carcinoma of the prostate treated with definitive radiotherapy: preliminary results of RTOG 83-07. Int J Radiat Oncol Biol Phys 16:813, 1989
295. Pilepich MV, Krall JM, Johnson RJ, et al: Extended field (periaortic) irradiation in carcinoma of the prostate: Analysis of RTOG 75-06. Int J Radiat Oncol Biol Phys 12:345, 1986
296. Pilepich MV, Krall JM, Sause WT, et al: Prognostic factors in carcinoma of the prostate: Analysis of RTOG Study 75-06. Int J Radiat Oncol Biol Phys 13:339, 1987
297. Pilepich MV, Krall JM, Sause WT, et al: Correlation of radiotherapeutic parameters and treatment related morbidity in carcinoma of the prostate: Analysis of RTOG study 75-06. Int J Radiat Oncol Biol Phys 13:351, 1987
298. Pilepich MV, Pajak T, George FW, et al: Preliminary report on phase III RTOG studies on extended-field irradiation in carcinoma of the prostate. Am J Clin Oncol 6:485, 1983
299. Pilepich MV, Prasad SC, Perez CA: Computed tomography in definitive radiotherapy of prostatic carcinoma. II. Definition of target volume. Int J Radiat Oncol Biol Phys 8:235, 1982
300. Pilepich MV, Walz BJ, Baglan RJ: Postoperative irradiation in carcinoma of the prostate. Int J Radiat Oncol Biol Phys 10:1869, 1984
301. Pinck BD, Alexander S: Parathormone potentiated radiophosphorus therapy in prostatic carcinoma. Urology 1:201, 1972
302. Pistenma DA, Bagshaw MA, Freiha FS: Extended-field radiation therapy for prostatic adenocarcinoma; status report of a limited prospective trial. In Johnson DE, Samuels ML (eds): Cancer of the Genitourinary Tract, pp 229–247. New York, Raven Press, 1979
303. Ploysongsang S, Aron BS, Shehata WM, et al: Comparison of whole pelvis versus small-field radiation therapy for carcinoma of prostate. Urology 27:10, 1986
304. Prout GR Jr, Heaney JA, Griffin P, et al: Nodal involvement as a prognostic indicator in patients with prostatic carcinoma. J Urol 124:226, 1980
305. Puthawala AA, Syed AMN, Tansey LA, et al: Temporary Iridium-192 implant in the management of carcinoma of the prostate. Endocuriether Hypertherm Oncol 1:25, 1985
306. Randall HE: Adjuvant radiotherapy after radical prostatectomy: Is it indicated? (Letter to editor). J Urol 139:961, 1988
307. Rangala N, Cox JD, Byhardt RW, et al: Local control and survival after external irradiation for adenorcarcinoma of the prostate. Int J Radiat Oncol Biol Phys 8:1909, 1982
308. Ray GR, Bagshaw MA, Freiha F: External beam radiation salvage for residual or recurrent local tumor following radical prostatectomy. J Urol 132:926, 1984
309. Ray GR, Cassady JR, Bagshaw MA: External beam megavoltage radiation treatment of post-radical prostatectomy residual or recurrent tumor: Preliminary results. J Urol 114:98, 1975
310. Ray GR, Pistenma DA, Castellino RA, et al: Operative staging of apparently localized adenocarcinoma of the prostate: Results in 50 unselected patients. I. Experimental design and preliminary results. Cancer 38:73, 1976
311. Reiner WG, Scott WW, Eggleston JE, Walsh PC: Long-term survival after hormonal therapy for stage D prostatic cancer. J Urol 122:183, 1979
312. Richard F, Renard L, Wambersie A: Current results of neutron therapy at the UCL, for soft tissue sarcomas and prostatic adenocarcinomas. Bull Cancer (Paris) 73:562, 1986
313. Rifkin MD: Endorectal sonography of the prostate: Clinical implications. AJR 148:1137, 1987
314. Robinson RG, Blake GM, Preston DG, et al: Strontium-89: Treatment results and kinetics in patients with painful metastatic prostate and breast cancer in bone. Radiographics 9:271, 1989
315. Robson MC: Cirrhosis and prostatic neoplasms. Geriatrics 21:150, 1966
316. Rodriguez-Antunez A, Cook SA, Jelden GL, et al: Management of primary and metastatic carcinoma of the prostate by the radiotherapist. AJR 118:876, 1973
317. Rosen EM, Cassady JR, Connolly J, et al: Radiotherapy for localized prostate carcinoma. Int J Radiat Oncol Biol Phys 10:2201, 1984
318. Rosenberg SE: Is carcinoma of the prostate less serious in older men? J Am Geriatr Soc 13:792, 1965
319. Ross R, Bernstein L, Judd H, et al: Serum testosterone levels in healthy young black and white men. JNCI 76:45, 1986
320. Rotkin ID: Distribution and risk of prostatic cancer. In Cancer Epidemiology in the USA and USSR. NIH publication Ad-2044, pp 111–123. Washington DC, US Government Printing Office, 1980
321. Rotkin ID: Studies in the epidemiology of prostatic cancer: Expanded sampling. Cancer Treat Rep 61:173, 1977
322. Rounsaville MC, Green JP, Vaeth JM, et al: Prostatic carcinoma: Limited field irradiation. Int J Radiat Oncol Biol Phys 13:1013, 1987
323. Rubenfeld S: Treatment of bone metastases from carcinoma of the prostate with parathyroid hormone and radioactive phosphorous. Urology 1:268, 1973
324. Rubin P (ed): Clinical Oncology. New York, American Cancer Society, 1983
325. Russell KJ, Laramore GE, Griffin TW, et al: Fast neutron radiotherapy in the treatment of locally advanced adenocarcinoma of the prostate. Clinical experience and future directions. Am J Clin Oncol 12:307, 1989
326. Russell KJ, Laramore GE, Krall JM, et al: Eight years experience with neutron radiotherapy in the treatment of stages C and D prostate cancer: Updated results of the RTOG 7704 randomized clinical trial. Prostate 11:183, 1987
327. Salazar OM, Rubin P, Hendrickson FR, et al: Single-dose half body irradiation for the palliation of multiple bone metastases from solid tumors: A preliminary report. Int J Radiat Oncol Biol Phys 7:773, 1981
328. Scardino PT, Guerriero WG, Carlton CE Jr: Surgical staging and combined therapy with radioactive gold grain implantation and external irradiation. In Johnson DE, Boileau MA (eds): Genitourinary Tumors: Fundamental Principles and Surgical Techniques, pp 75–90. New York, Grune & Stratton, 1982
329. Scardino PT, Wheeler TM: Local control of prostate cancer with radiotherapy: Frequency and prognostic significance of positive results of postirradiation prostate biopsy. NCI Monogr 7:95, 1988
330. Schellhammer PF, Ladaga LE, El-Mahdi A: Histological characteristics of prostatic biospies after ^{125}I implantation. J Urol 124:700, 1980
331. Schellhammer PF, Whitmore RB III, Kuban DA, et al: Morbidity and mortality of local failure after definitive therapy for prostate cancer. J Urol 141:567, 1989
332. Schmidt JD, Scott WW, Gibbons RP, et al: Comparison of procarbaxine, imidazole-carboxmide and cyclophosphamide in relapsing patients with advanced carcinoma of the prostate. J Urol 121:185, 1979
333. Schron DS, Gipson TM, Mendelsohn G: The histogenesis of small cell carcinoma of the prostate: An immunohistochemical study. Cancer 53:2478, 1984
334. Schumman LM, Mandel J, Blackard C: Epidemiologic study of prostatic cancer: Preliminary report. Cancer Treat Rep 61:181, 1977
335. Schuppler J: Malignant neurilemmoma of prostate gland. J Urol 106:903, 1971
336. Schwemmer B, Ulm K, Potter M, et al: Does transurethral resection of prostatic carcinoma promote tumor spread? Urol Int 41:284, 1986

337. Scott WW, Gibbons RP, Johnson DE, et al: The continued evaluation of the effects of chemotherapy in patients with advanced carcinoma of the prostate. J Urol 116:211, 1976
338. Scott WW, Johnson DE, Schmidt JE, et al: Chemotherapy of advanced prostatic carcinoma with cyclophosphamide or 5-fluorouracil: Results of first national randomized study. J Urol 114:909, 1975
339. Seamonds B, Yang N, Anderson K, et al: Evaluation of prostate-specific antigen and prostatic acid phosphatase as prostate cancer markers. Urol 28:472, 1986
340. Shearer RJ, Hendry WF, Sommerville IF: Plasma testosterone: An accurate monitor of hormone treatment of prostatic cancer. Br J Urol 45:668, 1973
341. Sheldon CA, Williams RD, Fraley EE: Incidental carcinoma of the prostate: A review of the literature and critical appraisal of classification. J Urol 124:626, 1980
342. Shevlin BE, Mittal BB, Brand WN, Shetty RM: The role of adjuvant irradiation following primary prostatectomy, based on histopathologic extent of tumor. Int J Radiat Oncol Biol Phys 16:1425, 1989
343. Shipley WU, Prout GR Jr, Coachman NM, et al: Radiation therapy for localized prostate carcinoma: Experience at the Massachusetts General Hospital (1973–1981). NCI Monogr 7:67, 1988
344. Smalley RV, Bartolucci AA, Hemstreet G, Hester M: A phase II evaluation of a 3-drug combination of cyclophosphamide, doxorubicin, and 5-fluorouracil and of 5-fluorouracil in patients with advanced bladder carcinoma or stage D prostatic carcinoma. J Urol 125:191, 1981
345. Smart JG: The use of P32 in the treatment of severe pain from bone metastases of carcinoma of the prostate. Br J Urol 37:139, 1965
346. Smith GG, Pierson EL: Value of high voltage x-ray therapy in carcinoma of the prostate. J Urol 23:331, 1930
347. Sogani PC, DeCosse JJ Jr, Montie J, et al: Carcinoma of the prostate: Treatment with pelvic lymphadenectomy and ^{125}I implants. Clin Bull 9:24, 1979
348. Sogani PC, Vagalwala MR, Whitmore WF: Experience with flutamide in patients with advanced prostatic cancer without prior endocrine therapy. Cancer 54:744, 1984
349. Sogani PC, Whitmore WF: Experience with flutamide in previously untreated patients with advanced prostatic cancer. J Urol 122:640, 1979
350. Spaulding JT, Whitmore WF Jr: Extended total excision of prostatic adenocarcinoma. J Urol 120:188, 1978
351. Stamey TA: Cancer of the prostate. An analysis of some important contributions and dilemmas. Monogr Urol, 1982, pp 67–94
352. Stamey TA, Kabalin JN, Ferrari M: Prostate specific antigen in the diagnosis and treatment of adenocarcinoma of the prostate. III. Radiation treated patients. J Urol 141:1084, 1989
353. Stamey TA, Yang N, Hay AR, et al: Prostate-specific antigen as a serum marker for adenocarcinoma of the prostate. N Engl J Med 317:909, 1987
354. Staszewshi J, Haenszel W: Cancer mortality among the Polish-born in the U.S. JNCI 35:291, 1965
355. Steele R, Lees REM, Kraus AS, Rao C: Sexual factors in the epidemiology of cancer of the prostate. J Chronic Dis 24:29, 1971
356. Stone NN, Sogani PC, Rosenberg SM, et al: Screening of ambulatory patients for prostate cancer by transrectal ultrasonography. J Urol (submitted for publication)
357. Straffon RA, Kiser WS, Robitalle M, et al: Yttrium hypophysectomy in the management of metastatic carcinoma of the prostate gland in 13 patients. J Urol 99:102, 1968
358. Straus MJ, Fleit JP, Engelking C: Treatment of advanced prostate cancer with cyclophosphamide, doxorubicin and methotrexate. Cancer Treat Rep 66:1797, 1982
359. Strijk SP, Debruyne FM, Herman CJ: Lymphography in the management of urologic tumors: Radiological-pathological correlation. Radiology 146:39, 1983
360. Syed AMN, Puthwala AA, Tansey LA, et al: Management of prostate carcinoma: Combination of pelvic lymphadenectomy, temporary Ir-192 implantation and external irradiation. Radiology 149:829, 1983
361. Tannenbaum M: Histology of the prostate gland. In Tannenbaum M (ed): Urologic Pathology: The Prostate, pp 312–315. Philadelphia, Lea & Febiger, 1977
362. Tannenbaum M: Endometrial tumors and/or associated carcinomas of prostate. Urol 6:372, 1975
363. Tansey LA, Shanberg AM, Syed AMN, et al: Treatment of prostatic carcinoma by pelvic lymphadenectomy, temporary iridium-192 implant, and external irradiation. Urology 21:594, 1983
364. Tapazoglou E, Subramanian MG, Al-Sarraf M, et al: High-dose Ketoconazole therapy in patients with metastatic prostate cancer. Am J Clin Oncol 9:369, 1986
365. Taylor WJ, Richardson RG, Hafermann MD: Radiation therapy for localized prostate cancer. Cancer 43:1123, 1979
366. Thomas JE, Cascino TL, Earle JD: Differential diagnosis between radiation and tumor pelxopathy of the pelvis. Neurology 35:1, 1985
367. Thompson GJ: Transurethral resection of malignant lesions of the prostate gland. JAMA 120:1105, 1942
368. Tong ECK, Finkelstein P: The treatment of prostatic bone metastases with parathormone and radioactive phosphorous. J Urol 109:71, 1973
369. Torti FM, Astron D, Lum BL, et al: Weekly doxorubicin in endocrine-refractory carcinoma of the prostate. J Clin Oncol 1:477, 1983
370. Torti FM, Carter SK: The chemotherapy of prostatic adenocarcinoma. Ann Intern Med 92:681, 1980
371. van der Werf-Messing BHP, Menon RS, Putten van WLJ: Prostatic cancer treated by external irradiation at the Rotterdam Radiotherapy Institute. Strahlentherapie 160:293, 1984
372. van der Werf-Messing B, Sourek-Zikova V, Blonk DI: Localized advanced carcinoma of the prostate: Radiation therapy versus hormonal therapy. Int J Radiat Oncol Biol Phys 1:1043, 1976
373. Van Heeringen C, DeSchryver A, Verbeek E: Sexual function disorders after local radiotherapy for carcinoma of the prostate. Radiother Oncol 13:47, 1988
374. Varma JS, Smith AN, Busuttil A: Function of the anal sphincters after chronic radiation injury. Gut 27:528, 1986
375. Veenema RJ, Gussel EO, Lattimer JK: Radical retropubic prostatectomy for cancer: A 20-year experience. J Urol 117:330, 1977
376. Vermooten V, Maxfield JR, Maxfield JGS: The use of radioactive phosphorus in the management of advanced carcinoma of the prostate. West J Surg 67:245, 1959
377. Vibeke Schiodt A, Kristensen O: Neurologic complications after irradiation of malignant tumors of the testis. Acta Radiol Oncol 17:369, 1978
378. Vickery AL Jr, Kerr WS Jr: Carcinoma of the prostate treated by radical prostatectomy: A clinical pathological survey of 187 cases followed for five years and 148 cases followed for ten years. Cancer 16:1598, 1983
379. Walsh PC: Radical retropubic prostatectomy with reduced morbidity: An anatomic approach. NCI Monogr 7:133, 1988
380. Walsh PC: Adjuvant radiotherapy after radical prostatectomy: Is it indicated? (Editorial). J Urol 138:1427, 1987
381. Walsh PC, Donker PJ: Impotence following radical prostatectomy: Insight into etiology and prevention. J Urol 128:492, 1982
382. Walsh PC, Jewett HJ: Radical surgery for prostatic cancer. Cancer 45:1906, 1980
383. Walsh PC, Lepor H, Eggleston JC: Radical prostatectomy with preservation of sexual function: Anatomical and pathological considerations. Prostate 4:473, 1983
384. Walsh PC, Schlegel PN: Radical pelvic surgery with preservation of sexual function. Ann Surg 208:391, 1988
385. Walsh PC, Siiteri PK: Suppression of plasma androgens by spironolactone in castrated men with carcinoma of the prostate. J Urol 114:254, 1975
386. Wang MC, Valenzuela LA, Murphy GP, Chu TM: Purification of a human prostatic specific antigen. Invest Urol 17:159, 1979
387. Warren B, Worgul TJ, Drago J: Effect of very high dose D-leucine-6-gonadotropin-releasing hormone proethylamide

on the hypothalamic-pituitary testicular axis in patients with prostatic cancer. J Clin Invest 71:1842, 1983
388. Watson RA, Tang DB: The predictive value of prostatic acid phosphatase as a screening test for prostatic cancer. N Engl J Med 303:497, 1980
389. Whitmore WF Jr: The natural history of prostatic cancer. Cancer 32:1104, 1973
390. Whitmore WF Jr, Batata MA, Hilaris BS: Prostate irradiation: Iodine-125 implementation. In Johnson DE, Samuels ML (eds): Cancer of the Genitourinary Tract, pp 195–205. New York, Raven Press, 1979
391. Whitmore WF, Hilaris B, Batata M, et al: Interstitial radiation: Short-term palliation of curative therapy? Urology 25:24, 1985
392. Whitmore WF Jr, Hilaris B, Grabstald H: Retropubic implantation of Iodine 125 in the treatment of prostatic cancer. J Urol 108:918, 1972
393. Willems JS, Lowhage T: Transrectal fine needle aspiration biopsy for cytologic diagnosis in grading of prostatic carcinoma. Prostate 2:381, 1981
394. Williams RD (ed): Textbook of Endocrinology, p 323. Philadelphia, WB Saunders, 1974
395. Williams RD, Hricak H: Magnetic resonance imaging in urology. J Urol 132:641, 1984
396. Winkelstein W Jr, Ernster VL: Epidemiology and etiology. In Murphy GP (ed): Prostatic Cancer, pp 1–17. Littleton, MA, PSG Publishing, 1979
397. Wolfe JHN, Lloyd-Davis RW: The management of transitional cell carcinoma in the prosate. Br J Urol 53:253, 1981
398. Woolf CM: An investigation of the familial aspects of carcinoma of the prostate. Cancer 13:739, 1960
399. Worgul TJ, Saten RJ, Samojlik E, et al: Clinical and biochemical effect of aminoglutethimide in the treatment of advanced prostatic carcinoma. J Urol 129:51, 1983
400. Wright F, Poizat R, Bongini M, et al.: Decreased urinary (5 α-androstane-3α,17β-diol) glucuronide excretion in patients with benign prostatic hyperplasia. J Clin Endocrinol Metab 60:294, 1985
401. Wynder EL, Mabushi K, Whitmore WF Jr: Epidemiology of cancer of the prostate. Cancer 18:344, 1971
402. Yam LT: Clinical significance of the human acid phosphatase: A review. Am J Med 56:604, 1974
403. Young YH: Use of radium in cancer of the prostate and bladder. JAMA 68:1174, 1917
404. Young YH: Early diagnosis and radical cure of carcinoma of the prostate: Being a study of 40 cases and presentations of radical operation. Bull Johns Hopkins Hosp 16:315, 1905
405. Zagars GK, von Eschenback AC, Johnson DE, Oswald MJ: The role of radiation therapy in stages A2 and B adenocarcinoma of the prostate. Int J Radiat Oncol Biol Phys 14:701, 1988
406. Zagars GK, von Eschenbach AC, Johnson DE, Oswald MJ: Stage C adenocarcinoma of the prostate: An analysis of 551 patients treated with external beam radiation. Cancer 60:1489, 1987
407. Zaloudek C, Williams JW, Kempson RL: "Endometrial" adenocarcinoma of the prostate: A distinctive tumor of probably prostatic duct origin. Cancer 37:2255, 1976
408. Zincke H, Utz DC: Observations on surgical management of carcinoma of prostate with limited nodal metastases. Urology 24:137, 1984
409. Zincke HL, Utz DC, Myers RP, et al: Bilateral pelvic lymphadenectomy and radical retropubic prostatectomy for adenocarcinoma of prostate with regional lymph node involvement. Urology 19:238, 1982
410. Zinreich ES, Derogatis LR, Herpst J, et al: Pre and posttreatment evaluation of sexual function in patients with adenocarcinoma of the prostate. Int J Radiat Oncol Biol Phys 19:729, 1990

52

Testis

Gillian M. Thomas
Stephen D. Williams

ANATOMY

Knowledge of the lymphatic drainage of the testis is particularly important, because surgical and radiotherapeutic management are predicated on knowledge of the probable site of lymphatic involvement in the infradiaphragmatic and subdiaphragmatic regions.

Four to eight collecting lymphatic trunks drain from the hilum of the testis and accompany the spermatic cord up to the internal inguinal ring along the course of the testicular veins. These lymphatic trunks continue cephalad with the vessels to drain into the retroperitoneal lymph glands between the levels of T11 and L4, but they are concentrated at the level of the L1 and L3 vertebrae. These nodes lie adjacent to the aorta and vena cava with extensive intercommunicating lymphatic channels. On the right, most of the nodes lie anterior, lateral, and medial to the inferior vena cava and anterior to the aorta. On the left, most of the nodes lie lateral and anterior to the aorta. As determined by lymphogram, crossover from the right to the left side is constant, but crossover from the left to the right side is rare and occurs after the primary nodes are filled. In 15% to 20% of patients with testicular tumors, ipsilateral and contralateral nodes are involved.[45]

Previous inguinal surgery may disrupt the lymphatic drainage and redirect it through the subcutaneous lymphatics of the anterior abdominal wall into the bilateral iliac nodes. The lymphatic drainage of the skin and subcutaneous tissues of the scrotum is into the inguinal and iliac nodes. From the retroperitoneal lumbar nodes, drainage occurs through the thoracic duct to lymph nodes in the mediastinum and supraclavicular fossae and occasionally to the axillary nodes.

EPIDEMIOLOGY

Testicular cancer is rare, with an incidence of 3.8 per 100,000 males in the United States. However, it is the most common malignancy in men between 20 and 34 years old, and the incidence of testicular cancer has been increasing in the United States, United Kingdom, and Denmark.[50] There is considerable geographic variation in the incidence of testicular cancer, with the highest rates in North American whites, Scandinavians, and other Western Europeans. The lowest rates occur in Asians, Africans, Puerto Ricans, and North American blacks. The highest incidence is in Denmark at 6.7 per 100,000, over thirteen times higher than the rate of 0.5 per 100,000 males in Puerto Rico.

The origin of testicular cancer is probably related to gonadal dysgenesis. This theory is supported by data showing an increasing incidence of testicular cancer in patients with maldescended testes and by data correlating carcinoma *in situ* of the testis and the development of invasive testicular neoplasia. Approximately 10% of patients with testicular cancer have a history of testicular maldescent. Males with cryptorchidism have an increased risk of developing testicular cancer that is about 35 times that of the normal population.[39] This risk is further increased if the testis is intraabdominal. If maldescent is unilateral, there is still an increased risk of developing a tumor in the normally descended contralateral testis, compared with men with normally descended testes. In patients with a history of cryptorchidism and unilateral testicular cancer, 23% have carcinoma *in situ* in the other testis.[53]

Patients who have had one testicular tumor are at increased risk for developing a contralateral tumor. The incidence of carcinoma *in situ* of the contralateral testis in patients who have developed one testicular tumor is approximately 5%, and approximately 50% of men with carcinoma *in situ* develop invasive malignancy within 5 years.[68] Data from the Royal Marsden Hospital and Denmark show that 2.7% of patients who have had one testicular cancer develop contralateral testicular cancer.[38, 56]

Recent data have shown some chromosomal abnormalities in patients with nonseminomatous tumors.[15]

NATURAL HISTORY

Between 1976 and 1980, the Danish Testicular Cancer Study Group found that the median age at presentation of patients with seminomas was 40.5 years and 31.7 years for men with nonseminomatous tumors.[50]

Although the routes of dissemination are similar for seminomas and nonseminomatous tumors, the propensity for involvement of various sites at presentation differs. Pure seminoma has a much greater tendency to remain localized or involve only lymph nodes, but nonseminomatous germ cell tumors of the testes more frequently spread by hematogenous routes. Pure seminoma is confined to the testis (Stage I) in 84% of patients at presentation (Table 52-1). It spreads in an orderly fashion, initially to the drainage lymph nodes in the retroperitoneum. Thirteen percent of men present with Stage II

TABLE 52–1
Stage Distribution of Seminoma at Presentation and Expected Results of Current Therapy

STAGE	STAGE DISTRIBUTION (%)	EXPECTED SURVIVAL (%)	NO. OF PATIENTS CURED
I	84	99	83
IIA	9	95	9
IIB, C, D	4	75	3
III, IV	3	66	2
Total	100	97	97

disease. From the retroperitoneum, it spreads proximally to involve the next echelon of draining lymphatics in the mediastinum and supraclavicular fossae (Stage III disease). Only rarely and late does pure seminoma spread hematogenously to involve lung parenchyma, bone, liver, or brain (Stage IV). Less than 5% of patients have Stage III or IV disease at presentation.

CLINICAL PRESENTATION

A testicular tumor usually presents as a painless swelling in the scrotum, although pain, heaviness, and tenderness at presentation are not uncommon. Testicular self-examination enables earlier detection of disease. An important goal in cancer education is increasing public awareness of testicular cancer and the importance of testicular self-examination.

A history of antecedent trauma to the testis is common; it is probable that it is coincidental, rather than causative, and that it draws the patient's attention to the presence of an existing mass. Disease in the lymph nodes of the retroperitoneum may produce back pain or abdominal swelling. Widely disseminated parenchymal disease in lungs, liver, bone, or brain is rare, but if present, it may produce systemic symptoms. Occasionally patients present with metastatic germ cell malignancies that are diagnosed by biopsy or by elevated levels of serum tumor markers without evidence of a palpable mass in the testis. Occult primary disease in the testis is often detected by testicular ultrasound. If there is no evidence for a primary tumor in the testis, a diagnosis of an extratesticular germ cell tumor, usually mediastinal, retroperitoneal, or pineal, may be made.

DIAGNOSTIC WORKUP

The tests necessary to evaluate patients with testicular cancer are listed in Table 52-2. A complete history should be taken, including information about previous inguinal or scrotal surgery, maldescent, retractile testes, and orchiopexy. The physical examination should pay special attention to possible sites of lymph node metastases. Specifically, the abdomen should be examined to rule out the presence of large abdominal masses, and both supraclavicular regions should be palpated to rule out supraclavicular metastases. The contralateral testis should be examined clinically. The presence or absence of gynecomastia is an important observation.

If testicular tumor is suspected, testicular ultrasound should be performed. The appropriate surgical procedure to make the diagnosis and remove the primary tumor is a radical orchiectomy through an inguinal incision.

TABLE 52–2
Diagnostic Workup for Tumors of the Testis

GENERAL
History (document cryptorchidism and previous inguinal or scrotal surgery)
Physical examination

LABORATORY STUDIES
Complete blood count
Biochemistry profile (including lactate dehydrogenase)
Serum assays
  α-fetoprotein (AFP)
  β-human chorionic gonadotropin
  placental alkaline phosphatase

SURGERY
Radical inguinal orchiectomy

DIAGNOSTIC RADIOLOGY
Chest x-ray films, posterior/anterior and lateral views
CT scan of chest for nonseminomas
CT scan of abdomen and pelvis
Bipedal lymphangiogram (if abdomen CT normal)
Ultrasound of contralateral testis

SPECIAL STUDIES
Semen analysis

Laboratory Studies

A routine complete blood count and chemistry screen, including renal function tests, should be done. Pulmonary or renal function tests should be performed for patients who may receive bleomycin or combination chemotherapy.

Nonseminomatous germ cell tumors of the testes are uniquely associated with reliable serum tumor markers: the beta subunit of human chorionic gonadotropin (β-HCG) and α-fetoprotein. One or both of these serum markers are elevated in 80% to 85% of patients with disseminated nonseminomatous disease. The metabolic half-life of α-fetoprotein is approximately 5 days and approximately 18 to 24 hours for β-HCG. Although β-HCG may be modestly elevated in 17% of patients with pure seminomas, usually any elevation of α-fetoprotein connotes nonseminomatous disease.[25] However, recent ultrastructural studies of pure seminomas have shown cell-surface specialization that indicates carcinomatous transformation. The implication is that some tumors that appear to be pure seminoma by light microscopy may secrete α-fetoprotein.[44, 57] There is insufficient information about the clinical behavior of these tumors.

Placental alkaline phosphatase, an isoenzyme of the alkaline phosphatase group, may be a useful marker for seminoma. It appears to be elevated in 80% to 95% of men with active seminoma, although false-positive elevations may occur in patients who smoke tobacco.[22]

If a testicular cancer is suspected, serum tumor markers should be assayed both before and after orchiectomy, and interpretation of the levels of markers should take into account their metabolic half-lives. Serum tumor markers can document persistent or recurrent cancer after surgery or chemotherapy and may predict the responsiveness of nonseminomas to treatment. Thus the level of β-HCG should decrease by 90% or more every 21 days with each successful treatment cycle of chemotherapy.[30] A slow decline in β-HCG after treatment may imply suboptimal response to chemotherapy, permitting early implementation of salvage therapy before the development of overt resistance to the chemotherapy develops. The decline of α-fetoprotein is less predictable. Serum tumor markers may be elevated in other circumstances or "benign" conditions, such as laboratory error, cross-reactivity with luteinizing hormone, marijuana use, hepatitis, or the development of antibodies to the glycoproteins.

Semen analysis and banking of sperm, if the quality is adequate, should be considered for patients in whom treatment is likely to compromise fertility.

Radiographic Studies

Investigations should routinely include chest x-ray films for all patients and computed tomography (CT) of the thorax of any patient with nonseminomatous germ cell tumors of the testis. CT scans of the abdomen and pelvis should be performed to evaluate the retroperitoneal nodal areas and assess the liver. Bipedal lymphangiography should be obtained if the abdominal pelvic CT is within normal limits. The overall sensitivity of lymphangiography is 80% to 85% (*i.e.*, 15% to 20% are false-negative results).[32,54] Because it can show intranodal filling patterns, lymphangiography is more sensitive than CT for detecting abnormalities in nodes less than 2 cm in diameter. The incidence of false-positive lymphograms is approximately 5%. Intravenous pyelography is useful if it demonstrates ureteral deviation produced by large volume retroperitoneal disease, but it and inferior venacavography have been replaced by abdominal-pelvic CT scanning. Radionuclide scanning of bones is considered unnecessary unless specific symptoms in a patient with widely disseminated disease suggest bony involvement. Baseline ultrasonography of the remaining testis should be performed.

STAGING

Several staging systems have been used to describe the extent of disease at initial presentation. No one system is completely satisfactory for predicting outcome after standard treatment. Table 52-3 shows the common staging systems in use for testicular cancer. The Union Internationale Contre le Cancer (UICC)[66] and the American Joint Committee (AJC) on Cancer Staging and End-Results Reporting[33] classify patients by the features of the primary tumor (T), nodes (N), and metastases (M). Although the T stage is of important prognostic significance for nonseminomatous tumors, no such value has been shown for the T stage of pure seminomas.[12]

Three systems (Table 52-3) classify nodal disease by sizes of less than 2 cm, 2 cm to 5 cm, and greater than 5 cm in maximum dimension. Although bulk of disease is prognostically important for seminoma and nonseminoma, it is not certain that these three nodal subcategories make a difference in predicting response to standard therapies. The staging systems also are imperfect for categorizing patients with metastatic disease (M+).

Most investigators recognize that prognostic subgroups do exist for patients treated with standard chemotherapy. In several large series, patients have been assigned to risk categories that cross the definitions of the TNM systems. Patients' risks are instead defined by the bulk and site of disease and by elevations of serum tumor markers.[67]

Perhaps the most widely used system for classifying testicu-

TABLE 52–3
Staging Systems for Tumors of the Testis

ROYAL MARSDEN HOSPITAL SYSTEM

STAGE	
I	No evidence of metatases
II	Metastases confined to abdominal nodes:
A	Maximum diameter of metastases < 2 cm
B	2–5 cm
C	> 5–10 cm
D	> 10 cm
III	Involvement of supradiaphragmatic and infradiaphragmatic lymph nodes. No extralymphatic metastases. Abdominal status A,B,C,D, as Stage II.
IV	Extralymphatic metastases Abdominal status: 0,A,B,C,D as for Stage II Lung Status L1 ≤ 3 metastases L2 multiple < 2-cm diameter L3 multiple > 2 cm Liver Status H + liver involvement

UICC AND AJC SYSTEM[33, 36]

PRIMARY TUMOR (T) (PATHOLOGIC CLASSIFICATION)	
pT1	Tumor limited to testis (including rete)
pT2	Tumor invades beyond tunica albuginea or into epididymis
pT3	Tumor invades spermatic cord
pT4	Tumor invades scrotum
LYMPH NODE (N)	
N0	No regional node metastasis
N1	Metastasis in single node, ≤ 2 cm maximum diameter
N2	Metastasis in a single node 2–5 cm in maximum diameter
N3	Metastasis in a lymph node > 5 cm in maximum diameter
DISTANT METASTASIS (M)	
M0	No distant metastasis
M1	Distant metastases, specific site
STAGING GROUPINGS	
I	T1, T2, N0, M0
II	T3, T4, N0, M0
III	Any T, N1, M0
IV	Any T, N2 or N3, M0 Any T, Any N, M1

TABLE 52–4
Seminoma Staging System

STAGE	CHARACTERISTICS
I	No evidence of metastases
II	Metastases confined to nodes
A	Maximum diameter ≤ 2 cm
B	Maximum diameter > 2–5 cm
C	Maximum diameter > 5–10 cm
D	Maximum diameter > 10 cm
III	Supradiaphragmatic and infradiaphragmatic nodes; abdominal status: A, B, C, or D
IV	Extralymphatic metastases

lar seminoma is some modification of the Royal Marsden Hospital staging system, which closely resembles the Walter Reed General Hospital system. Discussion of seminoma in this chapter employs a modified Royal Marsden Hospital system, as shown in Table 52-4 and adopted at the Leeds Consensus Conference in 1989.[61]

Although the currently available staging systems for seminomatous and nonseminomatous germ cell tumors provide reasonable descriptions of extent and sites of disease, more work is necessary to define a universal staging system that may be different for seminomas and nonseminomas and that more accurately reflects the different prognoses of subgroups.

PATHOLOGIC CLASSIFICATION

The classification of testicular tumors most widely used today is that of the Armed Forces Institute of Pathology (Table 52-5).[35] Germ cell tumors account for 95% of testicular tumors. The non-germ cell tumors, including lymphomas of the testis and tumors arising from the supporting tissue (*i.e.*, Sertoli's cells and interstitial Leydig's cells), account for the remainder and are not discussed in this chapter.

Germ cell tumors may be predominantly of one histologic pattern or may be admixtures of several patterns. For the purposes of treatment, the two broad categories are pure seminomas and all others, which are lumped together under the title of nonseminomatous germ cell tumors of the testis. In the Armed Forces Institute of Pathology series, 60% of patients had tumors consisting primarily of a single cell type, and 40% had mixed tumors. In most series, 45% of the patients have pure seminomas and 55% have nonseminomas.

The testicular tumor panel of Great Britain described the other system of pathologic classification commonly used in the United Kingdom.[43]

Seminoma

There are three histologic subtypes of seminomas: classical, anaplastic, and spermatocytic. The spermatocytic type is seen very rarely, usually in older patients. There has been no convincing evidence that the pathologic subtype bears any significant prognostic value. Anaplastic seminoma has been used to describe tumors with increased mitotic activity, those with three or more mitoses per high-power field and those with more irregular and pleomorphic cells. Syncytiotrophoblastic giant cells may be present in pure seminomas, and immunocytochemical examination reveals β-HCG in about 15% of patients with tumors that, by all other criteria, are considered to be pure seminoma. In these cases, elevated serum β-HCG probably does not indicate occult nonseminomatous elements.

Ultrastructural studies generally show important differences between seminoma and carcinoma.[57] These differences lend some support to the view of Pugh[43] that seminomas and nonseminomas are separate clinicopathologic entities. The Pugh classification suggests an origin for seminoma in the germinal epithelium and an unknown origin for the teratomas. The World Health Organization and the Armed Forces Institute of Pathology classification systems recognize that both entities may arise from a common germ cell precursor, and recent ultrastructural studies suggest a close link between seminomas and nonseminomas, as does other clinical, histologic, biochemical, and xenograft data.[57] Some cases of seminoma may show cell-surface specialization that indicates early carcinomatous

TABLE 52–5
Classification of Germ Cell Tumors of the Testis

SYSTEM OF PUGH[43]	WHO SYSTEM[35]
SEMINOMA	**GERM CELL TUMORS SHOWING ONE HISTOLOGIC PATTERN**
Teratoma and teratoma differentiated (TD)	Seminoma
Malignant teratoma intermediate (MTI)	Classic
MTIA, with differentiated or organoid elements	Anaplastic
MTIB, no differentiated or organoid elements	Spermatocytic
Malignant teratoma anaplastic (MTA)	Embryonal carcinoma
Malignant teratoma trophoblastic (MTT)	Adults
Combined tumor	Polyembryoma
Seminoma and teratoma coexisting	Infantile
	Choriocarcinoma
	Teratoma
	Mature
	Immature
	GERM CELL TUMORS SHOWING MORE THAN ONE HISTOLOGIC PATTERN
	Embryonal carcinoma and teratoma (teratocarcinoma)
	Others

transformation. Subtypes of the nonseminomatous germ cell tumors also exhibit a continuum in their ultrastructural morphology.

Nonseminoma

Nonseminomatous tumors may be single-cell types or composed of multiple elements (Table 52-5). Nonseminomas are associated with a higher likelihood of nodal and distant metastases than their seminoma counterparts. They are also more radioresistant.

The most common single-cell type is embryonal carcinoma. Pure teratoma composed of elements from multiple germ layers is occasionally seen. Histologically, these tumors can appear quite benign, but they are associated with a finite risk of metastases, at least in adults, and should be treated as other nonseminomas. Yolk sac (endodermal sinus) tumors are the most common childhood testis tumor, and they pursue a relatively unaggressive course. In adults, however, this tumor has a higher propensity for dissemination and a poorer response to chemotherapy. Pure choriocarcinoma is rare and almost always is associated with widespread dissemination. These patients typically have very high levels of HCG production with resultant gynecomastia.

On careful pathologic review, most nonseminomatous tumors are composed of more than one element. The most common combination is teratocarcinoma (*i.e.*, teratoma plus embryonal carcinoma).

PROGNOSTIC FACTORS

Seminoma

Neither the histologic subtype nor elevation of serum β-HCG is of prognostic importance in seminomas. Except for stage and extent of disease in seminoma, no other prognostic factors have been identified.

In Stage I seminoma, the extent of local disease (*i.e.*, the size of primary, lesion), whether there is involvement of the tunica, rete, epididymis, or spermatic cord or involvement of lymphatic or vascular spaces is of no known prognostic importance, because cure rates with postorchidectomy irradiation are approximately 99%. It is possible that future metaanalyses of data from surveillance studies of Stage I patients treated with orchiectomy only may identify the prognostic significance of some of these factors, which are of known significance for nonseminomatous disease.

Within the Stage II category, the outcome after radiation therapy depends on the bulk of retroperitoneal disease.[1,8,34,63,72] Initially, two categories were used: patients with palpable and those with nonpalpable masses.[63] As CT scanning became more generally available, the size of retroperitoneal disease was more clearly defined. Patients with tumor masses less than 5 cm have a prognosis similar to those with microscopic retroperitoneal disease only.[63] Patients with masses greater than 10 cm in the maximum transverse diameter clearly have a much poorer prognosis after radiation therapy or chemotherapy than those with smaller tumors (Table 52-6). It is probable that patients with masses between 5 cm and 10 cm form an intermediate prognosis group for the Stage II category. The poorer prognosis associated with bulky disease occurs because of an increased propensity for forming distant metastases and a decreased chance of local control with standard radiation therapy.

Patients with Stage III or IV disease usually have worse prognoses than most patients in the Stage II category. However, a patient with Stage IID disease may have a worse prognosis than a Stage III patient who has minimal retroperitoneal disease but has involvement of a supraclavicular node. The probability of curing Stage III and IV disease has significantly improved with the successful application of cisplatin-containing combination chemotherapy.[28] The prognosis of patients with metastatic seminoma may be better defined by the newer systems of risk classification (Table 52-7) than by the current Stage III or IV categories.

Nonseminoma

Until the advent of cisplatin-containing chemotherapy for the management of testicular cancer, nonseminomatous elements conferred a significantly worse prognosis than that of pure seminoma. Cisplatin-based combination chemotherapy cures approximately 80% of patients with disseminated nonseminomatous testicular germ cell tumors. In the era before cisplatin, fewer than 10% of the patients could expect long-term survival.

Investigators have examined the prognostic significance of multiple clinical variables affecting outcome for patients with nonseminomas. It is agreed that true Stage I cancer has a significantly better prognosis than all other stages and extents of disseminated nonseminomatous disease. Virtually all patients with Stage I or II disease survive with modern management. Universal agreement has not yet been reached on which classification system best discriminates between high-risk and

TABLE 52–6
Results of Primary Radiation Therapy (With or Without Prophylactic Mediastinal Irradiation) for Stage II Seminoma by Bulk of Abdominal Disease

INVESTIGATOR	STAGE IIB (2–5 CM)	STAGE IIC (5–10 CM)	STAGE IID (>10 CM)
Zagars et al[72]	1/28*	0/10	4/8
Mason et al[34]	1/25	2/12	4/12
Evenson et al[8]	1/24	2/20	
Green et al[16]		0/3	
Smalley et al[54]		0/3	
Total	3/77 (4%)	4/48 (8%)	8/20 (40%)

* *Results are presented as number of patients relapsing/total treated.*

TABLE 52–7
Indiana University Staging System

MINIMAL EXTENT

1. Elevated markers only
2. Cervical nodes (± nonpalpable retroperitoneal nodes)
3. Unresectable nonpalpable retroperitoneal disease
4. Fewer than 5 pulmonary metastases per lung field and largest < 2 cm (± nonpalpable retroperitoneal nodes)

MODERATE EXTENT

5. Palpable (≥ 10-cm diameter) abdominal mass only (no supradiaphragmatic disease)
6. Moderate pulmonary metastases: 5–10 metastases per lung field and largest < 3 cm or solitary metastasis of any size > 2 cm (± nonpalpable retroperitoneal disease)

ADVANCED EXTENT

7. Advanced pulmonary metastases: Primary mediastinal germ cell tumor or > 10 pulmonary metastases per lung field, or multiple pulmonary metastases with largest > 3 cm (± nonpalpable retroperitoneal disease)
8. Palpable (≥ 10-cm diameter) abdominal mass plus supradiaphragmatic disease
9. Liver, bone, or central nervous system metastases

low-risk disease treated with standard cisplatin-containing chemotherapy.

Multivariate analyses have been used to evaluate the prognostic significance of cell type, volume, and number of any metastases, serum marker levels, presence of an extragonadal primary, and metastases in specific sites, such as bone, liver, or the central nervous system. It appears that the level of serum HCG is the most important factor and that the volume of metastases, serum lactate dehydrogenase, and serum α-fetoprotein are of some prognostic value. Bone, liver, nodal, or retroperitoneal metastases are not independently prognostic, but the volume of lung metastases influences most prognostic models.

With modern treatment, the influence of cell type on outcome is small. The apparent poorer outcome of patients with pure choriocarcinoma probably results from the volume of metastatic disease rather than cell type *per se*. Several prognostic formulae incorporating significant factors are available for categorizing patients with poor prognoses.[2,4,67]

GENERAL MANAGEMENT

The initial management of a suspected malignant germ cell tumor of the testis is to obtain serum α-fetoprotein and β-HCG measurements and then to perform a radical (inguinal) orchiectomy with high ligation of the spermatic cord. Although transscrotal biopsy or orchiectomy was previously condemned, data from the Princess Margaret Hospital showed that 15% of the patients had scrotal incisions, transscrotal needle biopsy, or previous inguinal surgery. None of the patients with scrotal interference or inguinal surgery developed scrotal recurrence during surveillance, and the overall relapse rate among these patients was comparable to that in the whole series.[60] Similar data from the Royal Marsden Hospital indicated that 17% of patients had scrotal interference. None of the 36 patients with scrotal interference developed scrotal recurrence during surveillance only.[24] Nevertheless, transscrotal operations are not recommended.

Further management depends on the pathologic diagnosis and the stage and extent of disease.

Seminoma

Standard treatment of patients with Stage I seminoma is postoperative irradiation of the para-aortic and ipsilateral pelvic nodes. Adjuvant irradiation of the first echelon of draining lymphatics is recommended because there is a risk that these nodes could harbor occult microscopic metastases undetected by current staging methods. With appropriate use of noninvasive staging techniques and the application of standard radiation therapy, relapse-free survival rates for Stage I seminoma are 98% to 99% (Table 52-8).[18,62]

Despite these good results, some controversy exists about the optimal management of Stage I seminoma. With improvement of staging techniques, such as CT scanning and lymphangiography, the probability of a false-negative assessment of the retroperitoneum is decreased. Even before sophisticated, noninvasive retroperitoneal staging methods were available, surgical series showed that fewer than 15% of clinical Stage I patients had disease in the retroperitoneum. With the availability of highly effective radiation therapy and chemotherapy for salvage after relapse and with a low risk of occult retroperitoneal disease in well-staged patients, several investigators are examining a policy of postorchiectomy surveillance (Table 52-9).[40,64] Based on 1 to 2 years of follow-up for available series, it appears that only 8% to 15% of carefully staged patients have relapsed after orchiectomy without radiation therapy. All those who have relapsed are alive and well after further therapy. With longer follow-up, more patients can be expected to relapse, but this indicates that only 10% to 15% of patients actually have disease beyond the testis. The maturation of these studies will determine whether postoperative surveillance produces survival rates similar to those obtained with routine postorchiectomy irradiation. Until then, a policy of surveillance is consid-

TABLE 52–8
Abdominal Relapse and Survival Rates Compared With Radiation Dose for Stage I Seminoma

INVESTIGATOR	NO. OF PATIENTS	RADIATION DOSE (cGy)	NO. OF ABDOMINAL RELAPSES	CAUSE-SPECIFIC SURVIVAL (%)
Fossa et al[9]	249	4000 (1000–5000)	1	99
	91	3600		
Hamilton et al[18]	232	3000	0	100
Lester et al[69]	33	2500	1 (1500 cGy)	93
Thomas[62]	150	2500	0	99

TABLE 52–9
Postorchiectomy Surveillance of Stage I Seminomas

INVESTIGATION	NO. OF PATIENTS	RELAPSES: ABDOMEN ONLY	RELAPSES: ANY DISTANT	RELAPSES: SECOND RELAPSE	CHEMOTHERAPY FOR RELAPSE	ALIVE WITHOUT DISEASE
Horwich et al[21]	90	9	1	3	4	90
Thomas et al[60]	119	6	1	1	2*	119
von der Maase et al[68]	140	8	2		2	140
Oliver et al[37]	53		6		6	53
Total	402	23 (6%)	33 (8%)		14 (3.5%)	402

* *Relapsed as nonseminomas.*

ered suitable only in a protocol setting because of the risk of late relapse or relapse with extensive disease.

There is a growing interest in Europe and the United Kingdom in reducing the radiation volumes used for the treatment of Stage I disease by omitting irradiation of the pelvic nodes. Probably fewer than 2% of patients have involved pelvic nodes, and it is unlikely that the reduction of the irradiated volume would cause a significant increase in relapses, but the practice of para-aortic nodal irradiation only, without ipsilateral pelvic irradiation, is currently considered nonstandard practice.

It has been a standard recommendation to modify the treatment volume to include the inguinal regions if there had been previous inguinal surgery and to include the scrotum if it had been violated. This counsel assumed a risk of dissemination of disease through the scrotal wall or altered patterns of lymphatic dissemination caused by interruption of the inguinal lymphatics. Even in modern series, 4% to 15% of patients have had previous inguinal surgery or scrotal violation. Recent data, particularly from surveillance studies, do not confirm that previous inguinal scrotal interference results in an increased risk of relapse.[24,64] Although scrotal relapse occurred in one of 33 patients in the Princess Margaret Hospital series who had scrotal interference without subsequent inguinoscrotal radiation therapy, the relapsing patient was subsequently cured with further irradiation.[60] Scrotal or inguinal relapse is extremely rare, and although inguinoscrotal irradiation can prevent those rare recurrences, the morbidity is not inconsequential. Radiation therapy delivers an unacceptable dose of radiation to the contralateral testis, which may produce infertility. Recommendations from the International Consensus Conference in Leeds in 1989 suggested that inguinoscrotal irradiation should be omitted, even if interference has occurred.[61] This is particularly important for the young man who wishes to preserve fertility.

Because of the exquisite radiosensitivity of seminoma, retroperitoneal lymphadenectomy has shown no advantage over radiation therapy alone.[31] Similarly, in Stage I seminoma, there is no role for adjuvant prophylactic mediastinal irradiation because subsequent mediastinal relapse almost never occurs.

For patients with Stage II seminoma, the recommended treatment depends on the bulk of retroperitoneal nodal disease. For patients with Stage IIA disease (<2-cm-diameter mass), irradiation of the para-aortic and ipsilateral pelvic nodes is identical to that used for Stage I disease. Similarly, for Stage IIB disease (≤5-cm-diameter mass), the para-aortic and ipsilateral pelvic nodes should be irradiated with appropriate modifications of technique and doses to encompass the larger mass.

For Stage IIA and IIB disease (nonpalpable), considerable controversy has arisen as to the necessity of prophylactic mediastinal irradiation. In the past, prophylactic mediastinal irradiation has been used in the United States. This treatment was given in the belief that the next echelon of potentially involved nodes should be irradiated to eradicate occult metastatic disease in the mediastinum. The necessity of prophylactic mediastinal irradiation in Stage II seminoma remains controversial in the United States. Compiled data from six series suggest that supradiaphragmatic relapse is extremely rare, even for relatively poorly staged patients with Stage IIA and IIB disease, if prophylactic mediastinal irradiation is withheld.[62] In the compiled series, mediastinal relapse occurred in only eight of 250 patients, and seven of the eight were salvaged with radiation therapy. Because the possible survival benefit of prophylactic mediastinal irradiation is 0.4% (one of 250), many radiation oncologists have abandoned the its use for Stage IIA and IIB disease.

Optimal therapy for patients with Stage IIC retroperitoneal disease (5–10 cm in transverse diameter) remains one of the most controversial areas in the management of testicular seminoma. Several approaches to initial management are currently being practiced:

1. Initial disease is treated with infradiaphragmatic irradiation only; subsequent relapse in the mediastinum or any other site is treated with cisplatin-containing combination chemotherapy.
2. Initial treatment is infradiaphragmatic and subdiaphragmatic irradiation; cisplatin-containing chemotherapy for subsequent relapse in any site.
3. Initial treatment is cisplatin-containing combination chemotherapy, followed by observation of residual masses, "consolidation" radiation therapy to sites of bulky disease, or surgery for residual masses.

The results of these various approaches are discussed later.

The choice of which initial modality is used should depend on the size and location of the retroperitoneal node mass. If the mass is centrally located and does not overlie most of one kidney or significantly overlap the liver, primary radiation therapy is appropriate. However, if the location of the mass is such that the radiation volume covers most of one kidney or significant volumes of the liver, then the potential morbidity of radiation therapy can be avoided by the use of primary cisplatin-containing chemotherapy.

If disease is confined to the retroperitoneum but is greater than 10 cm in transverse diameter (Stage IID), results with primary irradiation are inadequate (Table 52-6). Stage IID disease is a rare presentation, and too few patients are available to accurately assess the curative value of initial radiation therapy. Nevertheless, relapse rates in this group after radiation therapy (usually including prophylactic mediastinal irradiation) are approximately 40% (Table 52-6). Salvage chemotherapy is difficult and hazardous to deliver after infradiaphragmatic irradiation, which would necessarily include most of the whole abdomen, and prophylactic mediastinal irradiation. Therefore, these patients should be treated with primary cisplatin-containing combination chemotherapy.

For the rare patients with Stage III and IV disease (*i.e.*, supradiaphragmatic nodal disease or dissemination to parenchymal organs), the current standard therapy is four courses of cisplatin-containing combination chemotherapy. Although radiation therapy may cure as many as 35% of these patients, particularly those with nodal rather than parenchymal disease and those without bulky disease, most patients would need salvage chemotherapy, contraindicating initial radiation therapy.

There is no universally accepted approach to the use of "consolidation therapy" after chemotherapy for the original sites of bulky disease or for residual masses after chemotherapy given for Stage IID, III, and IV disease.

If primary combination cisplatin-containing chemotherapy has been used in the management of bulky abdominal or mediastinal disease, residual masses may exist in as many as 75% of patients.[41] Surgical series have shown that only 10% to 12% of residual masses have "viable" seminoma cells; most have fibrosis only. Therefore, routine irradiation of residual masses is not indicated because 82% to 85% of the patients would receive radiation therapy unnecessarily. One surgical series demonstrated that as many as 30% of the patients have seminoma cells if surgery is performed 1 month after chemotherapy for residual masses larger than 4 cm in diameter.[36] The relapse rates of 10% from other series do not support the conclusion that all of the patients with visible tumor cells 1 month after chemotherapy will relapse.[41,58] If given for residual masses, radiation therapy should be administered cautiously, because the patient's hematologic tolerance may be compromised by previous chemotherapy. If the enlarging mass is in the mediastinum and the patient has received previous bleomycin-containing chemotherapy, he may be at significant risk for pulmonary toxicity due to the combination of irradiation and bleomycin.

The 1989 Germ Cell Consensus Conference in Leeds, England, concluded from available data that patients should be observed after appropriate chemotherapy.[61] Further therapy should be given only for overt disease progression.

Seminomatous testicular tumors have similar sensitivity to the available chemotherapeutic agents as the nonseminomatous tumors; the most commonly accepted standard regimens for the management of testicular seminoma include four courses of PVB (cisplatin, vinblastine, bleomycin) or BEP (bleomycin, VP-16, cisplatin) regimens. Several investigators are exploring the use of fewer courses of cisplatin-containing combination chemotherapy and use of single-agent cisplatin, carboplatin, or ifosfamide.[20] Cure rates using any of the chemotherapeutic regimens appear to depend on the disease extent and prior therapy.[28]

Nonseminoma

Treatment is initiated by radical inguinal orchiectomy, which additionally provides histologic confirmation. Subsequent management, based on stage and tumor bulk, has evolved substantially over the last two decades. Major developments include the advent of effective cisplatin-based chemotherapy and the refinement and widespread use of modern urologic surgical techniques. Initial trials have been widely reported, and results are discussed in a later section. About 70% to 80% of patients with disseminated nonseminoma survive with contemporary treatment.[17,30]

The most important prognostic factor is tumor bulk.[2] Appropriately treated, patients with unresectable Stage II disease or limited Stage III disease usually obtain durable, complete remissions.[3,7] The patients at significant risk of treatment failure are those with liver, bone, or brain metastases or bulky disease above and below the diaphragm. With current management, only 50% of these patients survive.

One third of chemotherapy-treated patients have a radiographically apparent residual mass or masses after chemotherapy. In general, these should be excised, because approximately 40% are composed of teratoma and another 10% to 15% of carcinoma.[30] Patients in the former group have a low risk of recurrence after surgical excision, but there is presumptive evidence that unresected teratoma may give rise to later relapse or progression.[29] Patients with persistent carcinoma require additional chemotherapy but generally do well with this treatment.

Radiation therapy has no role in the management of patients with disseminated nonseminoma, with the exception of palliation or the management of brain metastases in some patients. Newly diagnosed patients with brain metastases, although rare, are still potentially curable. All need systemic chemotherapy; there is no evidence that surgery plus radiation therapy is superior to radiation therapy alone. Control of central nervous system disease is usually achieved, and the major cause of death is refractory systemic disease.[26]

After chemotherapy with or without surgery all patients should be followed monthly for 1 year and every 2 months for the second year. Recurrences later than 2 years after initiation of chemotherapy are unusual.

The development of systemic chemotherapy for advanced disease has had profound implications for the management of early-stage disease. The first area of involvement beyond the testis is usually the retroperitoneal lymphatics. Even radiographically uninvolved nodes have a 20% to 30% chance of being pathologically positive.[14] Therefore, clinical Stage I patients traditionally received additional "prophylactic" treatment of the retroperitoneal nodes. In North America, the usual approach is retroperitoneal node dissection. Radiation therapy has also had its proponents.[65] The last two decades, however, have witnessed a change in the management of clinical Stage I disease. The short- and long-term sequelae of surgery and chemotherapy are minimal. There is evidence from a randomized study from Denmark that retroperitoneal irradiation in a dose of 4000 cGy prevented retroperitoneal relapse in Stage I nonseminomas. None of 66 patients receiving radiation therapy relapsed in the retroperitoneum, compared with ten of 66 who were observed. However, an equal number (eight of 66 in each arm) relapsed at distant sites whether or not radiation therapy was employed.[48] Although irradiation can control microscopic nonseminomatous disease, it is the propensity for hematogenous dissemination and the subsequent need for chemotherapy in about 15% that led to abandoning radiation therapy in Stage I disease.

Observation after orchiectomy has been proposed as an acceptable alternative to retroperitoneal node dissection. Proponents of routine retroperitoneal node dissection cite the incidence of pathologically positive nodes and the almost 100% ultimate cure rate (Table 52-10), although about 10% of pathologic Stage I and 50% of pathologic Stage II patients have recurrences after node dissections. The morbidity of retroperitoneal node dissection is minimal, and the mortality rate is

TABLE 52–10
Retroperitoneal Node Dissection in Early-Stage Nonseminomas

	INDIANA[23]		INTERGROUP TESTIS STUDY[49]	
PATIENTS	STAGE I	STAGE II	STAGE I	STAGE II
Total	78	68	264	98
Recurred	8	31	28	48
Alive without disease	78	66	258	93

almost zero. On the other hand, selected patients observed after orchiectomy appear to have a similar rate of cure (Table 52-11). A retrospective review with long-term follow-up of patients after orchiectomy showed a 35% risk of relapse within the first 4 years. Most relapses occur during the first 2 years. At relapse, some patients required both chemotherapy and surgery to control their disease.

Both retroperitoneal node dissection and surveillance have strong proponents, and for most patients, they are probably equally acceptable. The fertility implications of both approaches are complex and do not clearly favor either approach. All patients should be followed by means of metabolic markers and chest x-ray films monthly for a year and every other month for the second year. Patients observed after orchiectomy only should have an abdominal CT scan every other visit. Lymphangiography rarely contributes to CT findings and is no longer believed to be necessary.

The initial postorchiectomy management of patients with Stage II disease varies with the treating center and the bulk of disease. In the United States, patients with radiographically involved "resectable" nodes usually undergo retroperitoneal node dissection. At Indiana University, patients with nodal masses larger than 3 cm to 4 cm are treated primarily with chemotherapy. The investigators also perform retroperitoneal node dissection for patients with persistently elevated serum markers although imaging findings are normal.

Half of the patients with pathologic Stage II disease relapse after retroperitoneal node dissection. This propensity for disease dissemination has prompted many centers in Europe to abandon retroperitoneal node dissection in favor of primary chemotherapy for all patients. Similarly, retroperitoneal irradiation, another from of "local" therapy, has been abandoned because of the high risk of disseminated disease and because of the low probability of radiation controlling even the retroperitoneal disease if disease is bulky.[65]

RADIATION THERAPY TECHNIQUES

Patients with Stage I seminoma should receive megavoltage irradiation to the para-aortic and ipsilateral pelvic nodes (Fig. 52-1). The treatment volume should include the superior plate of the T10 vertebra and should extend inferiorly to the top of the obturator foramina. It is unnecessary to include the scar in the inguinal region. The lateral borders should include the para-aortic lymph nodes as visualized by lymphogram and the ipsilateral renal hilum. The field is usually 10 cm to 12 cm wide except at the hila, where it may be wider. The ipsilateral iliac and pelvic nodes should be encompassed by a shaped field with 2-cm margins on the visualized nodes. Testicular shielding should be employed if the patient wishes to preserve fertility.[11] The irradiation technique employed is an anterior and posterior parallel opposed pair using megavoltage equipment. Both fields should be treated daily, 5 days per week, Monday to Friday. It was agreed at the 1989 Consensus Conference that the recommended dose prescription should be 2500 cGy given in 20 fractions.[61] It has been common practice in many centers to use higher doses, but all available data suggest that higher doses are unnecessary for sterilizing microscopic retroperitoneal disease (Table 52-9).

For Stage II disease, the volume irradiated and the dose employed are modified according to the bulk of the retroperitoneal disease. For Stage IIA, no modification of the volume or dose of radiation is necessary. For Stage IIB disease (2–5 cm diameter), the field width should be approximately widened to encompass the mass as visualized on CT or lymphography with a margin of 2 cm (Fig. 52-2). For masses with transverse diameters greater than 4 cm, the total radiation dose is increased to 3500 cGy. The first 2500 cGy is delivered in 20 fractions to an initial volume, and a boost of 1000 cGy in five to eight fractions is given to a reduced field that encompasses the node mass with an adequate margin if the retroperitoneal mass exceeds 4 cm in diameter. Some radiation oncologists treat the contralateral and the ipsilateral pelvic nodes. This treatment is prescribed because of the risk of retrograde spread into the contralateral nodes from a relatively large retroperitoneal mass, particularly if it is low lying. However, no data exist to estimate the risk of contralateral pelvic nodal relapse in this circumstance. If bilateral pelvic nodal irradiation is used, a central pelvic shield should be employed.

If elective mediastinal and supraclavicular irradiation is used, a dose of 2500 cGy given in 175-cGy to 200-cGy fractions is employed. The portal arrangement is that of an anterior and posterior opposed pair fields to the mediastinum, usually 10 cm

TABLE 52–11
Orchiectomy Alone in Clinical Stage I Nonseminoma

PATIENTS	ROYAL MARSDEN[23]	MEMORIAL[55]	MANCHESTER[46]
Total	126	45	45
Recurred	36 (28%)	9 (20%)	11 (24%)
Alive without disease	125	43	45

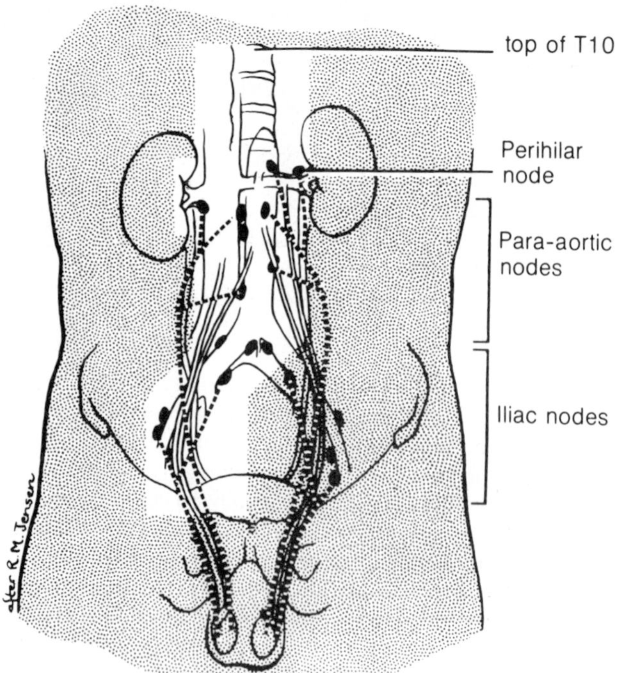

FIGURE 52–1. Lymph node drainage of the testis and radiation portals for Stage I and "small volume" Stage II disease.

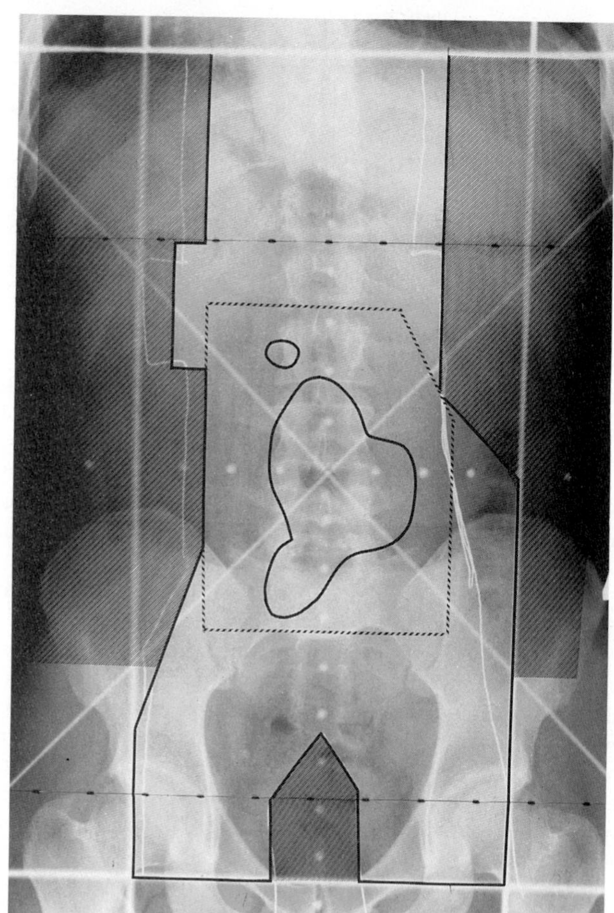

FIGURE 52–2. Example of paraaortic and pelvic irradiation portals in the treatment of Stage IIC disease. The *solid dark line* marks the initial volume treated to 2500 cGy in 20 fractions, and the *hatched line* shows the boost volume given a further 1000 cGy in seven fractions.

wide. The left supraclavicular fossa is usually adequately treated with a single anterior field. Approximately 5% to 10% of the patients have bilateral or contralateral drainage to the right supraclavicular fossa, and some radiation oncologists also treat the right-sided node-bearing area.

Stage IIC disease is treated by the same principles of radiation therapy applied to Stage IIB disease. In general, the abdominal fields are larger to encompass the known volume of disease. If a choice of primary radiation therapy has been made and the radiation field of necessity encompasses most of one kidney, the field size should be reduced as the tumor shrinks (Fig. 52-3). Initial shrinkage of large masses is often rapid, and the abdominal CT scan repeated after the first 3 weeks of radiation therapy may allow significant reduction of the treatment volume while still encompassing the tumor mass. This allows at least two thirds of the kidney to be spared total doses higher than 1800 cGy. It is probably better to use chemotherapy initially, rather than radiation therapy, if a large mass overlies one or both kidneys to an extent that the necessary radiation therapy may cause significant nephrotoxicity.

If radiation therapy is required for an enlarging mediastinal mass after treatment with chemotherapy, the mass volume should be carefully defined by CT scanning of the thorax. The radiation fields should be tightly confined to the known site of residual disease, and the radiation dose should be limited to 2500 cGy delivered in 20 fractions.

RESULTS OF THERAPY

Seminoma

Historically, the overall results for the management of patients with testicular seminoma using radiation therapy alone have been excellent. The overall survival rate of such patients was approximately 85%.[63] With the recent improvements in radiologic assessment of extensive disease, the development of serum tumor markers that largely eliminate the risk of having occult nonseminomatous disease, and the advent of platinum-based chemotherapy for treating advanced disease, overall survival rates have improved another 8% to 10% (Table 52-1).

The outcome of treatment with currently available therapies depends on the stage and extent of disease at presentation. Table 52-1 shows the stage of disease at presentation and the expected survival for each group.

For those with Stage I disease, routine irradiation of the retroperitoneum and ipsilateral pelvic nodes produces 10-year relapse-free survival rates of 96% to 98% (Table 52-9).[9,62] Approximately 1% to 4% of patients relapse after infradiaphragmatic irradiation, usually within the first 3 years of treatment. The sites of relapse are usually evenly distributed between the mediastinum and distant sites.[9,18,62] Occasional relapses occur as nonseminomatous germ cell malignancies, even after careful review of the initial tumor has shown a pure seminoma. Deaths from Stage I seminomas are extremely rare. Most relapsing patients are salvaged with subsequent treatment, usually chemotherapy.

The outcome for patients with Stage IIA disease treated with infradiaphragmatic irradiation or infradiaphragmatic plus prophylactic mediastinal irradiation is similar to Stage I, with expected survival rates of 95%.[8,62,72]

The outcome of therapy for Stage II disease depends on the bulk of disease at presentation. Radiation therapy is the treatment of choice for patients with masses less than 5 cm in diameter. The cumulative relapse rate in three series of patients

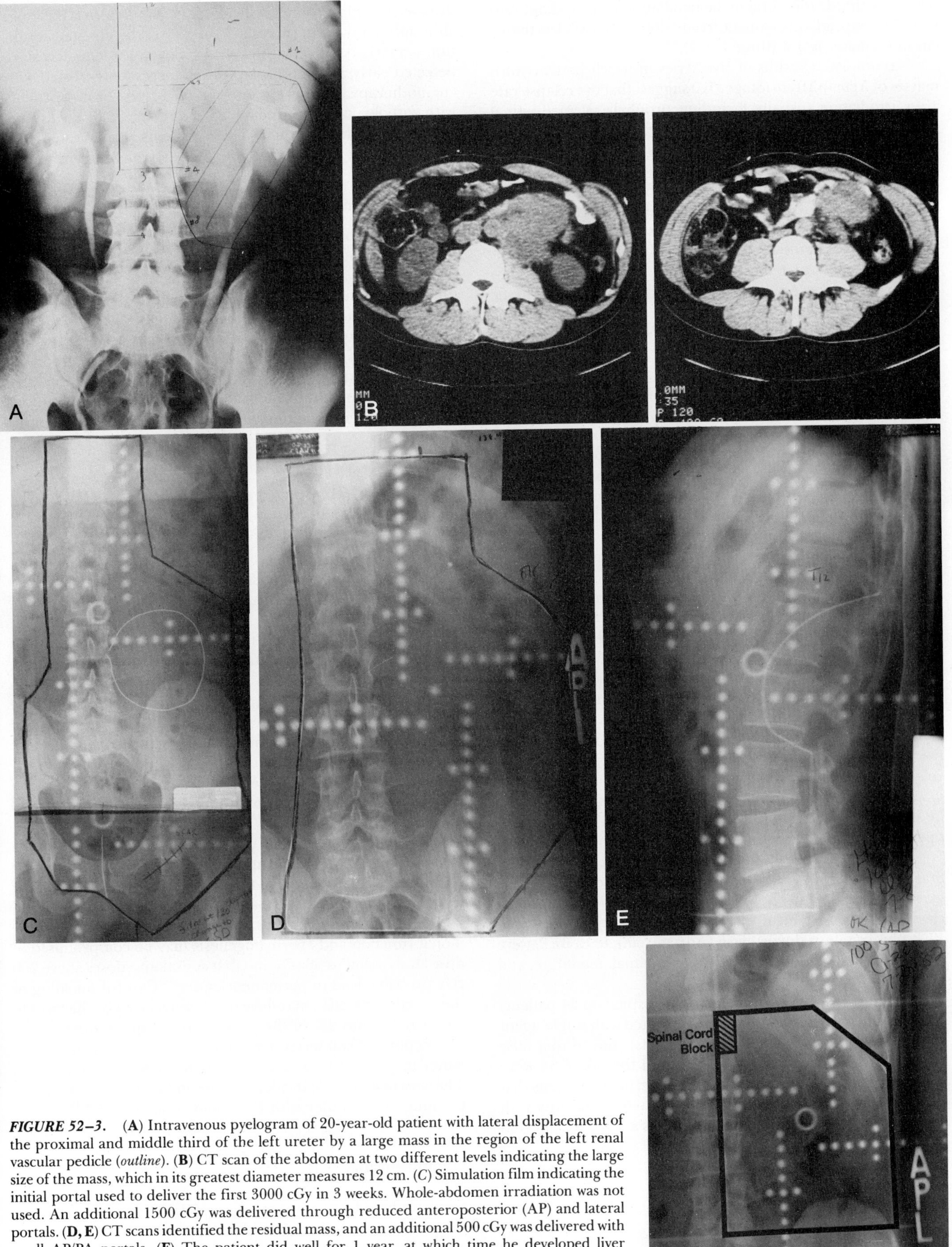

FIGURE 52–3. (**A**) Intravenous pyelogram of 20-year-old patient with lateral displacement of the proximal and middle third of the left ureter by a large mass in the region of the left renal vascular pedicle (*outline*). (**B**) CT scan of the abdomen at two different levels indicating the large size of the mass, which in its greatest diameter measures 12 cm. (*C*) Simulation film indicating the initial portal used to deliver the first 3000 cGy in 3 weeks. Whole-abdomen irradiation was not used. An additional 1500 cGy was delivered through reduced anteroposterior (AP) and lateral portals. (**D, E**) CT scans identified the residual mass, and an additional 500 cGy was delivered with small AP/PA portals. (**F**) The patient did well for 1 year, at which time he developed liver metastases. He was treated with a combination of cisplatin, vinblastine, and bleomycin. Two years after treatment of metastatic disease, he is disease free and working full time. Elective mediastinal irradiation was not given because chemotherapy might have been required later.

treated with infradiaphragmatic irradiation or infradiaphragmatic and supradiaphragmatic irradiation for masses less than 5 cm in diameter is 4% (three of 77).[8,34,72]

Accumulated results of five series in which patients with masses of 5 cm to 10 cm (Stage IIC) suggest that the relapse rate after irradiation (usually including prophylactic mediastinal irradiation) is 10% (four of 48) (Table 52-6). Although the number of patients with Stage C disease in any series is small, the overall survival rate appears to be approximately 90%. If infradiaphragmatic irradiation only is used for Stage IIC disease, the risk of subsequent relapse in the mediastinum is increased. It is estimated that 20% of patients relapse in the mediastinum or at distant sites. Chemotherapy can salvage approximately 80% of relapsing patients, producing cure rates comparable to those achieved with initial infradiaphragmatic and supradiaphragmatic irradiation.

The survival results of the three approaches to initial therapy of patients with Stage IIC disease are comparable. The potential toxicities of the three treatments must be evaluated for each patient along with other factors influencing the choice of therapy. No data from randomized trials exist to determine which initial therapy has the best therapeutic index. The Radiation Therapy Oncology Group attempted to compare initial chemotherapy with initial infradiaphragmatic irradiation, but because of the rarity of bulky Stage II disease and some physician bias, this important study closed because of lack of patient accrual.

For patients with Stage IID tumors (>10 cm in diameter), subsequent relapse occurs in approximately 50% of the patients treated with initial radiation therapy whether or not prophylactic mediastinal irradiation is given (Table 52-6). Primary chemotherapy in patients with Stage IIC or D disease has yielded a cumulative progression-free survival late of 91% (72 of 79).[10,13,51,69,72] More than half of the patients in the series, however, received later consolidation therapy, usually irradiation or surgery for initial sites of bulky disease.

The use of consolidation therapy after initial chemotherapy for bulky disease is gradually being abandoned. The role of consolidation radiation therapy has been discussed previously. Surgery to remove residual masses does not appear to be indicated and may even be contraindicated because postoperative deaths have been recorded by several investigators.[13]

The results of chemotherapy for bulky abdominal disease, Stage III and IV disease, or recurrent disease depend on the extent of disease and the previous treatment. In the Indiana classification of extent of disease, complete response rates to PVB plus or minus doxorubicin (Adriamycin), or to BEP, were 87%, 81%, and 52%, respectively, for minimal, moderate, and advanced disease.[28]

A report from the Royal Marsden Hospital on 34 patients with "advanced metastatic seminoma" treated with single-agent carboplatin (with irradiation in six patients) showed that 80% remained free of progressive disease, and that 32 of 34 were long-term survivors.[20] The high degree of efficacy suggests that single-agent chemotherapy should be tested in patients with minimal or moderate metastatic disease as a less toxic alternative to the multidrug combinations.

Nonseminoma

Early-Stage Disease

Most patients with early-stage nonseminoma survive. Patients treated with retroperitoneal node dissection who have negative nodes are observed. About 10% have recurrences of disease. The most common site of treatment failure is the lung, although many recurrences are discovered by elevated serum tumor markers only. With careful follow-up, recurrences are detected early, and most relapses are successfully treated with chemotherapy. In a recent international study of 264 patients with pathologic Stage I disease, 28 had recurrences after retroperitoneal node dissection. These patients were treated with chemotherapy, and overall, 98% (258 patients) survived.

Stage III and Bulky Stage II

Cisplatin-based treatment is now the standard of care for patients with Stage III and bulky Stage II disease. Commonly used regimens are VAB-6 (cyclophosphamide, bleomycin, dactinomycin, vinblastine) and BEP.[52] Sequential clinical trials have documented the contribution of etoposide (VP-16) and the lack of the necessity of maintenance therapy.[30,71] Overall, about 70% to 80% of patients with advanced disease are cured with appropriate chemotherapy. Most patients are in the favorable prognosis group, and over 90% survive. The poor prognosis group is smaller, but ultimately, about half of these patients die of disease.[2]

SEQUELAE OF TREATMENT

Radiation Therapy

The long-term sequelae of standard infradiaphragmatic irradiation for Stage IA and IIA disease are related to the dose of radiation employed.[1,9,18,31] There appears to be no curative advantage for doses greater than 2500 cGy. The complications associated with doses of 3000 cGy to 4000 cGy include moderate to severe dyspepsia in 5% to 6% of patients and peptic ulceration in 2% to 3%.[9,18] The Patterns of Care Study correlated the incidence of major gastrointestinal complications (*i.e.*, intestinal obstruction, peptic ulcer, or hemorrhagic gastritis) with the dose of radiation employed.[5] Below 2500 cGy, no major complications were seen, but between 2500 cGy and 3500 cGy, the incidence is 2%, and the complication rate rises to 6% for 4000 cGy to 4500 cGy.

Approximately 50% of patients with testicular seminoma have some degree of impairment in spermatogenesis at the time of presentation. Exposure of the remaining testis to therapeutic irradiation may further impair fertility, and the degree of impairment is dose dependent. Available data suggest that hormonal function and spermatogenesis may be compromised at dose levels as low as 50 cGy and that cumulative doses above 200 cGy probably lead to permanent injury.[52] Careful shielding of the remaining testis can reduce the dose received by the testis to between 1% and 2% of the patient's prescription dose.[11]

Reports of two series suggest a slight risk for second malignancy in patients receiving irradiation for Stage I seminoma. The sites of increased incidence of second malignancies include the lung and bladder with risk ratios of about 2.5.[9,19]

Chemotherapy

Cisplatin-based chemotherapy is associated with alopecia and the potential for substantial nausea and vomiting. Modern antiemetics have improved gastrointestinal reactions. Serious short-term problems are myelosuppression, bleomycin-induced pulmonary fibrosis, and rarely, cisplatin nephrotoxicity. Myelosuppression and pulmonary fibrosis are fatal in 0.5% to 4% of treated patients.

Drug-related mortality is more likely in patients with high tumor volume and previous irradiation. It is probably also related to the experience of the treating physician.

The late outcome of treatment of Indiana University patients seen between 1974 and 1979 has been reviewed.[47] The only late toxic effects occurring with any degree of frequency are distal paresthesias and cold intolerance. It has been suggested that chemotherapy is associated with myocardial infarction and stroke, but prospectively derived data demonstrate that this is unlikely. An association between chemotherapy and second malignancy has not been identified.

The fertility implications of chemotherapy are complex. These regimens cause immediate azoospermia, but with time, more than half of the patients may recover normal or nearly normal spermatogenesis.[47] In pregnancies initiated after therapy, there was no evidence of adverse fetal effects.

Surgery

Acute complications of retroperitoneal node dissection are uncommon. They include infection, pulmonary embolus, and rarely, chylous ascites and orthostatic hypotension. The operative mortality rate is less than 1%.

The major adverse effect of surgery is infertility. The autonomic nerves that control ejaculation are in close proximity to the nodes. Thus, patients who have had a classic bilateral retroperitoneal node dissection have normal potency and subjective sensation of orgasm but a dry ejaculate.

A surgical procedure has been developed that spares some of the contralateral autonomic nerves.[6,27] The operation is technically demanding but preserves ejaculation in those patients suitable for the procedure.

REFERENCES

1. Ball D, Barrett A, Peckham MJ: The management of metastatic seminoma testis. Cancer 50:2289, 1982
2. Birch R, Williams S, Cone A, et al: Prognosis factors for favorable outcome in disseminated germ cell tumors. J Clin Oncol 4:400, 1986
3. Bosl GJ, Geller NJ, Bajorin D, et al: A randomized trial of etoposide and cisplatin versus vinblastine and bleomycin and cisplatin and cyclophosphamide and dactinomycin in patients with good prognosis germ cell tumors. J Clin Oncol 6:1231, 1988
4. Bosl GJ, Geller NL, Cerrincione C, et al: Multivariate analysis of prognostic variables in patients with metastatic testicular cancer. Cancer Res 43:3403, 1983
5. Coia LR, Hanks GE: Complications from large field intermediate dose infradiaphragmatic radiation: An analysis of the Patterns of Care outcome studies for Hodgkin's disease and seminoma. Int J Radiat Oncol Biol Phys 15:29, 1988
6. Donohue JP: Preservation of ejaculation following nerve-sparing retroperitoneal lymphadenectomy (RPLND). American Urological Association annual meeting. Boston, MA, 1988
7. Einhorn LH, Williams SD, Loehrer P, et al: A Comparison of four courses of cisplatin, VP-16 and bleomycin in favourable prognosis disseminated germ cell tumors: A Southeastern Cancer Study Group protocol. J Clin Oncol 7:387, 1989
8. Evensen JF, Fossa SD, Kjellevold K, et al: Testicular seminoma: Analysis of treatment and failure for stage II disease. Radiother Oncol 4:55, 1985
9. Fossa SD, Aass N, Kaahluus: Radiotherapy for testicular seminoma stage I: Treatment results and long-term post-irradiation morbidity in 365 patients. Int J Radiat Oncol Biol Phys 16:383, 1989
10. Fossa S, Borge L, Aass N, et al: The treatment of advanced metastatic seminoma: Experience in 55 cases. J Clin Oncol 5:1071, 1987
11. Fraas BA, Kinsella TJ, Harrington FS, et al: Peripheral dose to the testes: The design and clinical use of a practical and effective gonadal shield. Int J Radiat Oncol Biol Phys 11:609, 1985
12. Freedman LS, Jones WG, Peckham MJ, et al: Histopathology in the prediction of relapse of patients with stage I testicular teratoma treated by orchiectomy alone. Lancet 1:294, 1987
13. Friedman EL, Garnick MB, Stomper PC, et al: Therapeutic guidelines and results in advanced seminoma. J Clin Oncol 3:1325, 1985
14. Fung CY, Garnick MB: Clinical Stage I carcinoma of the testis: A review. J Clin Oncol 6:734, 1988
15. Gibas Z, Prout GR, Sandberg AA: Malignant teratoma of the testis with an isochromosome No. 12, 1(12p), as the sole structural cytogenetic abnormality. J Urol 131:372, 1984
16. Green N, Broth E, George FW, et al: Radiation therapy in bulky seminoma. J Urol 5:467, 1983
17. Hainsworth JD, Greco FA: Testicular germ cell neoplasm. Am J Med 75:817, 1983
18. Hamilton C, Horwich A, Easton D, et al: Radiotherapy for stage I seminoma testis: Results of treatment and complications. Radiother Oncol 6:115, 1986
19. Hay JH, Duncan W, Kerr GR: Subsequent malignancies in patients irradiated in testicular tumours. Br J Radiol 57:597, 1984
20. Horwich A, Dearnaley DP, Duchesne GM, et al: Simple nontoxic treatment of advanced metastatic seminoma with carboplatin. J Clin Oncol 7:1150, 1989
21. Horwich A, Peckham MJ: Surveillance after orchiectomy for clinical stage I germ cell tumours of the testis: EORTC Genitourinary Group Monograph 5. Progress and Controversies in Oncological Urology II:471, 1988
22. Horwich A, Tucker DF, Peckham MJ: Placental alkaline phosphatase as a tumour marker in seminoma using the $H17E^2$ monoclonal antibody assay. Br J Cancer 51:625, 1985
23. Hoskin P, Dilly S, Eastors P, et al: Prognostic factors in stage I non-seminomatous germ cell testicular tumours managed by orchiectomy and surveillance: Implications for adjuvant therapy. J Clin Oncol 4:1031, 1986
24. Kennedy CL, Hendry WF, Peckham MJ: The significance of scrotal interference in stage I testicular cancer managed by orchiectomy and surveillance. Br J Urol 58:705, 1986
25. Lange PH, Fraley EE: Serum alpha-fetoprotein and human chorionic gonadotropin in the treatment of patients with testicular tumours. Urol Clin North Am 4:393, 1977
26. Lester SG, Morphis JG, Hornback NH, et al: Brain metastases and testicular tumours: Need for aggressive therapy. J Clin Oncol 2:1397, 1984
27. Lester SG, Morphis JG, Hornback NB: Testicular seminoma: Analysis of treatment results and failures. Int J Radiat Oncol Biol Phys 12:353, 1986
28. Loehrer PJ, Birch R Sr, Williams SD, et al: Chemotherapy of metastatic seminoma: The Southeastern Cancer Study Group experience. J Clin Oncol 5:1212, 1987
29. Loehrer PH Sr, Hui S, Clark S, et al: Teratoma following cisplatin based combination chemotherapy for non-seminomatous germ cell tumors: A clinicopathological correlation. J Urol 135:1183, 1988
30. Loehrer PJ, Williams SD, Einhorn LH: Testicular cancer: The quest continues. JNCI 80:1373, 1988
31. Maier JG, Mittenmeyer BT, Sulak MH: Treatment and prognosis in seminoma of the testis J Urol 99:72, 1968
32. Maier JG, Schamber DT: The role of lymphangiography in the diagnosis and treatment of malignant testicular tumors. Am J Roentgenol Radium Therapy Nucl Med 114:482, 1972
33. Manual for Staging of Cancer: American Joint Committee of Cancer, 3rd ed. Philadelphia, JB Lippincott, 1988
34. Mason BR, Kearsley JH: Radiotherapy for stage II testicular seminoma: The prognostic influence of tumor bulk. Clin Oncol 6:1856, 1988
35. Mostofi K, Price EB Jr: Tumors of the male genital system. In Atlas of Tumor Pathology, 2nd series, fasc 8. Washington, DC, Armed Forces Institute of Pathology, 1973
36. Motzer R, Bosl G, Heelan R, et al: Residual mass: An indication

for further therapy in patients with advanced seminoma following systemic chemotherapy. J Clin Oncol 5:1064, 1987
37. Oliver RTD: Limitations to the use of surveillance: An option in the management of stage I seminoma. J Androl 10:263, 1987
38. Osterlind A, Berthelson JG, Abeldgaard N: Incidence of bilateral testicular germ cell cancer in Denmark 1960–1984. Int J Androl 10:203, 1987
39. Peckham MJ: Testicular cancer. Rev Oncol 1:439, 1988
40. Peckham MJ, Hamilton CR, Horwich A, Hendry WF: Surveillance after orchiectomy for stage I seminoma of the testis. Br J Urol 59:343, 1987
41. Peckham MJ, Horwich A, Hendry WF: Advanced seminoma: Treatment with cisplatinum based combination chemotherapy or carboplatin (JM8). Br J Cancer 52:7, 1985
42. Pike MC, Chilver C, Peckham MJ: Effect of age at orchiopexy on risk of testicular cancer. Lancet 1:1246, 1986
43. Pugh RCG: Pathology of the Testis. Oxford, Blackwell Scientific Publications, 1976
44. Raghavan D, Sullivan AL, Peckham MJ, Neville AM: Elevated serum alpha-fetoprotein and seminoma. Cancer 50:982, 1982
45. Ray B, Hajdu SI, Whitmore WF: Distribution of retroperitoneal lymph node metastases in testicular germinal tumors. Cancer 33:340, 1974
46. Read G, Johnson RJ, Wilkinson PM, Eddleston B: Prospective study of follow-up alone on stage I teratoma of the testis. Br Med J 287:1503, 1983
47. Richie JP, Garnick MB: Limited retroperitoneal lymphadenectomy for patients with clinical stage I testicular tumour. (Abstract). Proc Am Soc Clin Oncol 4:110, 1985
48. Rorth M, von der Maase H, Nielsen ES, et al: Orchidectomy alone versus orchidectomy plus radiotherapy in stage I nonseminomatous testicular cancer: A randomized study by the Danish Testicular Carcinoma Study Group. Int J Androl 10(1): 255, 1987
49. Roth BJ, Griest A, Kublilis PS, et al: Cisplatin based combination chemotherapy for disseminated germ cell tumors: Long-term follow-up. J Clin Oncol 6:1239, 1988
50. Schultz HP, Arends J, Barlebo H, et al: Testicular carcinoma in Denmark, 1976–1980: Stage and selected clinical parameters at presentation. Acta Radiol Oncol 23:249, 1984
51. Schuette J, Niederle N, Scheulen ME, et al: Chemotherapy of metastatic seminoma. Br J Cancer 51:467, 1985
52. Shapiro E, Kinsella TJ, Makuch RW, et al: Effects of fractionated irradiation on endocrine aspects to testicular function. J Clin Oncol 3:1232, 1985
53. Skakkebaek NE: Carcinoma *in situ* of the testis: Frequency and relationship of invasive germ cell tumors in infertile men. Histopathology 2:157, 1972
54. Smalley SR, Evans RG, Richardson RL, et al: Radiotherapy as initial treatment for bulky stage II testicular seminomas. J Clin Oncol 3:1333, 1985
55. Sogani PC, Whitmore WF, Herr HW, et al: Orchiectomy alone in the treatment of clinical stage I non-seminomatous germ cell tumor of the testis. J Clin Oncol 267, 1984
56. Sokol M, Peckham MJ, Hendry WF: Bilateral germ cell tumours of the testis. Br J Urol 52:258, 1987
57. Srigley JR, MacKay B, Toth P, Ayala A: The ultrastructure and histogenesis of male germ neoplasia with emphasis on seminoma with early carcinomatous features. Ultrastruct Pathol 12:67, 1988
58. Stomper PC, Jochelson MS, Friedman EL, et al: CT evaluation of advanced seminoma treated with chemotherapy. AJR 146:746, 1986
59. Storm PB, Kern A, Loerning SA, et al: Evaluation of pedal lymphangiography in staging non-seminomatous testicular carcinoma. J Urol 118:1000, 1977
60. Thomas GM: (unpublished data)
61. Thomas GM: Consensus statement on the investigation and management of testicular seminoma. EORTC Genito-Urinary Group Monograph 7. In Newling DW, Jones WG (eds). Prostate Cancer and Testicular Cancer. Wiley-Liss, 1990
62. Thomas GM: Controversies in the management of testicular seminoma. Cancer 55:2296, 1985
63. Thomas GM, Rider WD, Dembo AJ, et al: Seminoma of the testis: Results of treatment and patterns of failure after radiation therapy. Int J Radiat Oncol Biol Phys 8:165, 1982
64. Thomas GM, Sturgeon JF, Alison R, et al: A study of post-orchiectomy surveillance in stage I testicular seminoma. J Urol 142:313, 1989
65. Tyrrell CJ, Peckham MJ: The response of lymph node metastases of testicular teratoma to radiation therapy. Br J Urol 48:363, 1976
66. UICC (International Union Against Cancer): TNM Classification of Malignant Tumours. Berlin, Springer Verlag, 1987
67. Vogelzang NJ: Prognostic factors in metastatic testicular cancer. Int J Androl 10:225, 1987
68. Von der Maase H, Giwercman A, Miller J, et al: Management of carcinoma *in situ* of the testis. Int J Androl 10:209, 1987
69. Williams SD, Birch R, Einhorn LH, et al: Disseminated germ cell tumors: Chemotherapy with cisplatin plus bleomycin plus either vinblastine or etoposide. A trial of the Southern Cancer Study Group. N Engl J Med 316:1435, 1987
70. Williams SD, Einhorn LH: Clinical stage I testis tumors: The medical oncologist's view. Cancer Treat Rep 66:15, 1982
71. Williams SD, Stablein DM, Einhorn LH, et al: Immediate adjuvant chemotherapy versus observation with treatment at relapse in pathological stage II testicular cancer. N Engl J Med 317:1433, 1987
72. Zagars GK, Babaian J: The role of radiation in stage II testicular seminoma. Int J Radiat Oncol Biol Phys 13:163, 1987

53

Penis and Male Urethra

Carlos A. Perez
Miljenko V. Pilepich

ANATOMY

The basic structural components of the penis include two corpora cavernosa and the corpus spongiosum (Fig. 53-1*A*). These are encased in a dense fascia (Buck's fascia), which is separated from the skin by a layer of loose connective tissue. Distally, the corpus spongiosum expands into the glans penis, which is covered by a skin fold known as the prepuce. The skin extends over and is firmly attached to the glans.

The male urethra is composed of a mucous membrane and the submucosa. It extends from the bladder neck to the external urethral meatus (Fig. 53-1*B*). The posterior urethra is subdivided into the membranous urethra, which passes through the urogenital diaphragm, and the prostatic urethra, which passes through the prostate. The anterior urethra passes through the corpus spongiosum and is apportioned into the fossa navicularis (a widening within the glans), the penile urethra, which passes through the pendulous part of the penis, and the bulbous urethra, the dilated proximal portion of the anterior urethra. The prostatic urethra is covered by transitional epithelium only. The distal portion of the anterior urethra is covered by stratified squamous epithelium, which changes proximally to pseudostratified columnar epithelium. The columnar epithelium gradually changes into transitional epithelium in the membranous urethra.

The lymphatic channels of the prepuce and the skin of the shaft drain into the superficial inguinal nodes located above the fascia lata. The rich anastomotic network of the lymphatics within the penis and at the base of the penis means that lymphatic drainage may be considered bilateral. There is some disagreement about whether the glans and the deep penile structures drain into the superficial or deep inguinal lymph nodes (those under the fascia lata). The so-called sentinel nodes located above and medial to the junction of the epigastric and saphenous veins have been identified as the primary drainage sites in carcinoma of the penis (Fig. 53-2).[11] A selective biopsy of this group of nodes is important in assessing tumor extent; if they are not involved by tumor, a complete nodal dissection may not be necessary. The reliability of this procedure has not been supported by some investigators.[68,69] Catalona[13] found that biopsy of the sentinel nodes showed false-negative results in 10% of Cabanas' patients who died of carcinoma.[11]

The lymphatics of the fossa navicularis and the penile urethra follow the lymphatics of the penis to the superficial and deep inguinal lymph nodes. The lymphatics of the bulbomembranous and prostatic urethra may follow three routes. Some pass under the pubic symphysis to the external iliac nodes, some go to the obturator and internal iliac nodes, and others end in the presacral lymph nodes. The pelvic (iliac) lymph nodes are rarely involved without inguinal lymph node involvement.[14]

EPIDEMIOLOGY

Carcinoma of the penis is relatively rare in the United States; the annual incidence is estimated to be one in 100,000 males, accounting for 0.03% to 1% of all cancers in men.[14] This tumor is extremely rare in circumcised Jewish men; circumcision performed early in life protects against carcinoma of the penis, but this is not true if the operation is done in adult life.[14,78] The higher incidence in some areas of South America, Africa, and Asia seems to be related to the absence of the practice of neonatal circumcision. It has been shown that male circumcision is highly effective in preventing the development of penile carcinoma in Nigeria and Uganda.[63,65] The high incidence of carcinoma of the penis in American blacks has similarly been attributed to the lower percentage of blacks undergoing neonatal circumcision. Phimosis is common in men suffering from penile carcinoma. Smegma is carcinogenic in animals, but the component of the smegma responsible for its carcinogenic effect has not been identified.[14]

Boon and associates[9] observed an increased incidence of cervical carcinoma and penile carcinoma in Bali in a Hindu population in whom circumcision is rare and phimosis in adult males is high. They suggested that human papillomavirus (HPV) infection, estimated to exist in more than 75% of the Balinese patients with genital carcinoma, may be a cofactor with impeded postcoital hygiene in genital carcinogenesis. In the Netherlands, where males are usually circumcised, the male is exclusively a vector of HPV but not a victim as in Bali. Martinez[53] in Puerto Rico and Graham and co-workers[32] in New York also reported a significantly higher incidence of carcinoma of the cervix in the wives of males with penile carcinoma. Other etiologic factors, such as viruses (herpes simplex) and venereal disease (syphilis) have been implicated, but the evidence remains inconclusive.[14,21,80]

Carcinoma of the male urethra is also rare. There are no recognized racial or geographic predisposing factors. Although the cause remains unknown, there seems to be some correlation

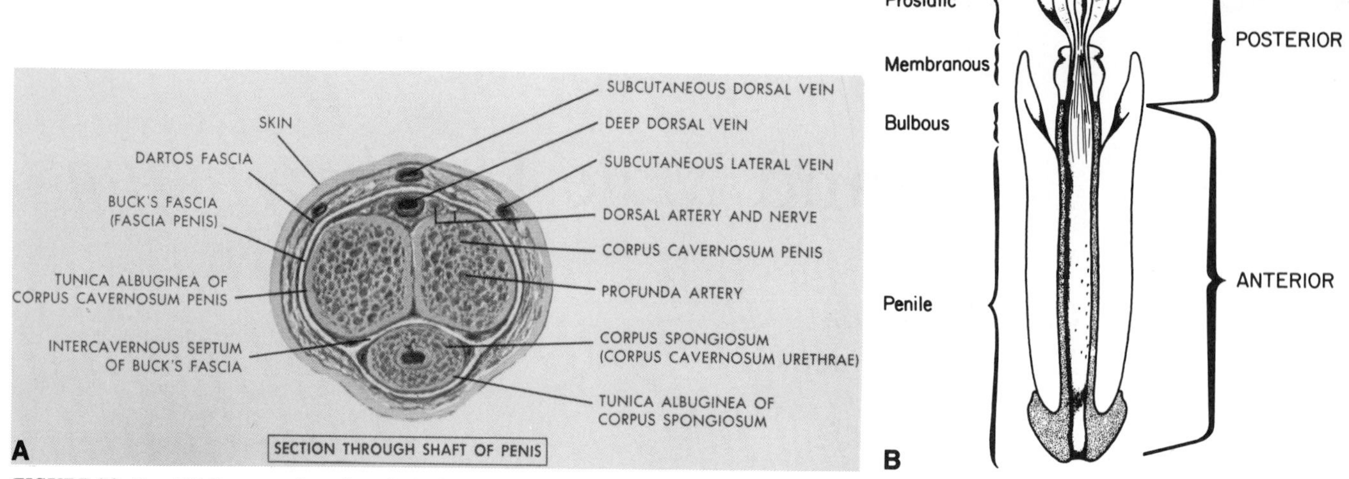

FIGURE 53–1. (**A**) Cross-section of penis shaft. (Reprinted with permission from Netter FH: The CIBA Collection of Medical Illustration, vol 2. Reproductive System. Summit, NJ, CIBA Pharmaceutical, 1972) (**B**) Anatomic subdivisions of the male urethra.

between the incidence of carcinoma of the urethra and chronic irritation produced by infection, venereal disease, and strictures. The part of the urethra covered by the transitional epithelium (prostatic and membranous urethra) may be susceptible to the same carcinogenic factors that affect the bladder and the upper urinary tract. The average age of the patients at presentation of these tumors is 58 to 60 years, although 10% occur in men younger than 40 years.[14]

NATURAL HISTORY

Most carcinomas of the penis start within the preputial area, arising in the glans, coronal sulcus, or the prepuce itself. Lesions arising in the skin of the shaft are rare. In most patients, carcinoma of the penis is characterized by slow, locoregional progression. Extensive primary lesions may involve the corpora cavernosa or even the abdominal wall. The inguinal lymph nodes are the most common site of metastatic spread. In patients with clinically nonpalpable inguinal nodes, about 20% are found to have micrometastases. Pathologic evidence of nodal metastases is reported in about 35% of all patients and in approximately 50% of those with palpable lymph nodes (Table 53-1).[11,18,21] Distant metastases are uncommon (about 10%), even in patients with advanced locoregional disease, and they usually occur in patients with inguinal lymph node involvement.[37] These patients often die of septic complications, erosion of large vessels in the groin, or a combination of the two.

The natural history of carcinoma of the anterior urethra in the male is similar to that of carcinoma of the penis. Most tumors are low grade and progress slowly at primary and regional sites rather than spread to distal areas. Tumors of the penile urethra spread to the inguinal lymph nodes first, but those of the bulbomembranous and prostatic urethra metastasize first to the pelvic lymph nodes.

CLINICAL PRESENTATION

Carcinoma of the penis may present as an infiltrative-ulcerative or an exophytic papillary lesion. Assessment of the primary lesion may be obscured by phimosis. Secondary infection and an associated foul smell are quite common. Urethral obstruction is an unusual symptom of carcinoma of the penis. Inguinal lymph nodes are palpable on presentation in 30% to 45% of the patients.[11,18,21,34,36,79] However, only half of these contain tumor; enlargement of the lymph nodes is often related to inflammatory (infectious) processes.[18] Administration of antibiotics over several weeks results in regression of inguinal lymph nodes in most patients, and many authorities have advocated this prac-

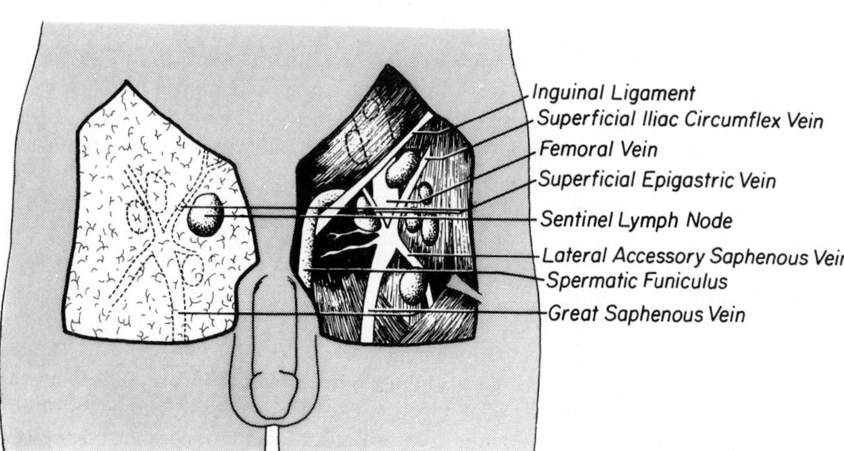

FIGURE 53–2. Anatomic landmarks for inguinal lymph node dissection. (*Left*) Skin and immediately surrounding adipose tissue are removed to expose sentinel lymph node. Deep fatty stratum remains. Other lymph nodes and great saphenous vein and tributaries are indicated (*dashed lines*). (*Right*) Sentinel lymph node and superficial and deep fascia are removed to expose other superficial and deep lymph nodes. (Cabanas RM: Cancer 39:456, 1977)

TABLE 53–1
Pathologic Incidence of Metastatic Lymph Nodes in Penile Carcinoma

INVESTIGATION	PERCENT OF CLINICALLY POSITIVE NODES	PERCENT TOTAL PATIENTS
Ekstrom[21]	51	31
Jackson[37]	27	26
Barney[4]		50
Barringer[5]		37
Lenowitz[49]		35
Bassett[6]		33
Straubitz[80]		47
Jorstad[40]		37
Dean[16]		33
Fegen[23]	20	
deKernion[18]	62	
Gentil[27]	50	
Oota[64]	28	
Paymaster[67]	50	

tice before the status of the regional lymph nodes is definitively assessed. Conversely, 20% of patients with clinically normal inguinal lymph nodes have occult metastases.[13,19,28]

Patients with urethral carcinoma may present with obstructive symptoms, tenderness, dysuria, urethral discharge, or initial hematuria. These symptoms are often attributed to urethritis or urethral stricture, which may precede the development of urethral carcinoma and may also delay diagnosis. Lesions of the distal urethra are often associated with palpable inguinal lymph nodes at presentation.

DIAGNOSTIC WORKUP

Diagnostic studies required in the evaluation of patients with suspected or confirmed carcinoma of the penis and urethra are outlined in Table 53-2.

Careful examination of the banalopreputial area may demonstrate small lesions. Urethroscopy and cystoscopy are essential. Inguinal lymph nodes should be thoroughly evaluated. A chest x-ray film and intravenous pyelogram are routinely obtained.

Assessment of the regional lymphatics by lymphangiogram in carcinoma of the penis is of questionable value. The extensive inflammatory changes that are often present in the lymph nodes make interpretation difficult. Computed tomography (CT) is useful in the identification of enlarged pelvic and periaortic lymph nodes in patients with involved inguinal lymph nodes.

In urethral carcinoma the inflammatory changes in the lymph nodes are less of a problem, and lymphangiogram results are relatively reliable. CT scans of the pelvis and abdomen are useful in evaluating the pelvic and retroperitoneal lymphatics.

STAGING

Among several staging systems proposed for classification of carcinoma of the penis, the one proposed by Jackson[37] is the most commonly used (Table 53-3). The most commonly used

TABLE 53–2
Diagnostic Workup for Carcinoma of the Penis and Male Urethra

GENERAL

History
Physical examination

SPECIAL PROCEDURES

Endoscopic examination of urethra
Cystoscopy

RADIOGRAPHIC STUDIES

Standard
- Chest radiographs
- Intravenous pyelogram
- CT scan
- Lymphangiogram (urethral tumors only)
- Bone scan
- Liver scan

Complementary
- Urethrogram

LABORATORY STUDIES

Complete blood count
Blood chemistry profile
Urinalysis

staging system for carcinoma of the male urethra has been proposed by Ray and associates (Table 53-4).[74] The American Joint Committee Staging Systems are shown in Tables 53-5 and 53-6.[7]

PATHOLOGIC CLASSIFICATION

Most malignant penile tumors are well-differentiated squamous cell carcinomas.[3] Although an apparent adverse prognostic effect of anaplasia has been reported in some series, no others have correlated histologic grade and survival.[21,36,80]

Bowen's disease is squamous cell carcinoma *in situ* that may involve the shaft of the penis and the hairy skin of the inguinal and suprapubic area. Clinically, the lesion is a solitary, dull red plaque with areas of crusting and oozing. Approximately 25% to 50% of patients with this disease have a concomitant visceral malignancy.[14]

Erythroplasia of Queyrat is an epidermoid carcinoma *in situ* that involves the mucosal or mucocutaneous areas of the prepuce or glans.[31] It appears as a reddened, elevated, or ulcerated lesion. In two reports, five of 15 patients and ten of 100 patients presenting with erythroplasia of Queyrat had invasive squamous cell carcinoma at diagnosis.[31,56] Erythroplasia of

TABLE 53–3
Staging System for Carcinoma of the Penis Proposed by Jackson

STAGE	CHARACTERISTICS
I	Tumor confined to glans or prepuce.
II	Tumor extending onto shaft of penis.
III	Tumor with malignant, but operable, inguinal lymph nodes.
IV	Inoperable primary tumor extending off the shaft of the penis or inoperable groin nodes or distant metastases.

(Jackson SM: Br J Surg 53:33, 1966)

TABLE 53–4
Staging System for Male Urethral Carcinoma Proposed by Ray and Associates

STAGE	CHARACTERISTICS
0	Tumor confined to mucosa only
A	Tumor extension into but not beyond lamina propria
B	Tumor extension into but not beyond substance of corpus spongiosum or into but not beyond prostate
C	Direct extension into tissues beyond corpus spongiosum (corpora cavernosa, muscle, fat, fascia, skin, direct skeletal involvement) or beyond prostatic capsule
D1	Regional metastasis including inguinal or pelvic lymph nodes
D2	Distant metastasis

(Ray B, Canto AR, Whitmore WF: J Urol 117:591, 1977)

Queyrat is not as frequently associated with internal malignancies as Bowen's disease.[62]

Basal cell carcinoma is infrequently reported, accounting for only 1% to 2% of all cases of penile tumors.[33,81]

Extramammary Paget's disease is a rare intraepithelial apocrine carcinoma. The most common sites are the scrotum, inguinal folds, and perineal region.[56] The lesion has a propensity to metastasize, necessitating frequent assessment of regional nodes. Radiation therapy has been recommended as palliative treatment.[56]

Soft tissue tumors are uncommon. Approximately half of the tumors are benign and may include angiomatous, neurogenous, myogenous, fibrous, and lymphoreticular tumors.[17,50] Most soft tissue tumors occur on the shaft and are malignant.

Primary lymphoma of the penis was reported in one patient with Peyronie's disease, without other evidence of lymphomatous involvement. Five cases of secondary involvement of the penis by lymphoma were reported in the literature.[86]

TABLE 53–5
AJC Staging System for Carcinoma of the Penis

PRIMARY TUMOR (T)

TX	Primary tumor cannot be assessed
T0	No evidence of primary tumor
Tis	Carcinoma *in situ*
Ta	Noninvasive verrucous carcinoma
T1	Tumor invades subepithelial connective tissue
T2	Tumor invades corpus spongiosum or cavernosum
T3	Tumor invades urethra or prostate
T4	Tumor invades other adjacent structures

REGIONAL LYMPH NODES (N)

NX	Regional lymph nodes cannot be assessed
N0	No regional lymph node metastasis
N1	Metastasis in a single superficial, inguinal lymph node
N2	Metastasis in multiple or bilateral superficial inguinal lymph nodes
N3	Metastasis in deep inguinal or pelvic lymph node(s), unilateral or bilateral

DISTANT METASTASIS (M)

MX	Presence of distant metastasis cannot be assessed
M0	No distant metastasis
M1	Distant metastasis

(Beahrs OH, Henson DE, Hutter RVP, Myers MH [eds]: Manual for Staging of Cancer, 3rd ed, p 190. Philadelphia, JB Lippincott, 1988)

Cancers metastatic to the penis are rare and usually represent late, advanced carcinomatosis. The most common neoplasms metastasizing to the penis are from the genitourinary organs, followed by the gastrointestinal and respiratory systems. The predominant cell type is carcinoma, occurring in 202 of 219 cases reported (Table 53-7). Sarcomas and tumors of unknown histologic type are rare.[72] A palpable mass, swelling, nodule, or skin change frequently occurs. Priapism as an initial presenting feature or subsequent development occurs in 40% of patients.[72]

TABLE 53–6
AJC Staging System for Carcinoma of the Urethra

PRIMARY TUMOR (T) (MALE AND FEMALE)

TX	Primary tumor cannot be assessed
T0	No evidence of primary tumor
Tis	Carcinoma *in situ*
Ta	Noninvasive papillary, polypoid, or verrucous carcinoma
T1	Tumor invades subepithelial connective tissue
T2	Tumor invades corpus spongiosum or prostate or periurethral muscle
T3	Tumor invades corpus cavernosum or beyond prostatic capsule or the anterior vagina or bladder neck
T4	Tumor invades other adjacent organs

REGIONAL LYMPH NODES (N)

NX	Regional lymph nodes cannot be assessed
N0	No regional lymph node metastasis
N1	Metastasis in a single lymph node, ≤ 2 cm in greatest dimension
N2	Metastasis in a single lymph node, > 2 cm but < 5 cm in greatest dimension, or multiple lymph nodes, none > 5 cm in greatest dimension
N3	Metastasis in a lymph node > 5 cm in greatest dimension

DISTANT METASTASIS (M)

MX	Presence of distant metastasis cannot be assessed
M0	No distant metastasis
M1	Distant metastasis

(Beahrs OH, Henson DE, Hutter RVP, Myers MH [eds]: Manual for Staging of Cancer, 3rd ed, p 210. Philadelphia, JB Lippincott, 1988)

TABLE 53–7
Primary Malignancies Associated with Secondary Cancers of the Penis in 219 Patients

SITE OF PRIMARY MALIGNANCY	NO. OF PATIENTS
Genitourinary tract	
Bladder	65
Prostate	65
Kidney	23
Testis	10
Ureter	1
Gastrointestinal tract	
Rectum/sigmoid	34
Colon	1
Anus	1
Liver	1
Pancreas	1
Respiratory tract	
Lungs	8
Nasopharynx	1
Other	
Lymphosarcoma/reticulum cell sarcoma	4
Bone	2
Burkitt's lymphoma	1
Skin (malignant melanoma)	1

(Powell BL, Craig JB, Muss HB: J Clin Oncol 3:110, 1985)

About 80% of urethral carcinomas in males can be classified as squamous cell carcinomas, which are usually well or moderately differentiated.[59] Transitional cell carcinomas, adenocarcinomas, and undifferentiated or mixed carcinomas comprise approximately 15%, 5%, and 1%, respectively. The frequency of histologic type varies with site. Over 90% of carcinomas of the prostatic urethra are of transitional cell type. Adenocarcinomas occur only in the bulbomembranous urethra.

PROGNOSTIC FACTORS

The principal prognostic factors in carcinoma of the penis are extent of the primary lesion and status of the lymph nodes. The incidence of nodal involvement is related to the extent and location of the primary lesion. Invasion of deep-seated structures (*e.g.*, corpora cavernosa) carries a high risk of deep inguinal node involvement.

Tumor-free regional nodes imply an excellent (85% to 90%) long-term survival or cure.[18,79] Patients with involvement of the inguinal nodes fare considerably worse, and only 40% to 50% survive long term.[18,79] Pelvic lymph node involvement implies a still worse prognosis; less than 20% of these patients survive.[11,18,36]

Tumor differentiation was believed to be an important prognostic factor by Fraley and associates.[24] None of nine patients with carcinoma *in situ*, one of 20 with well-differentiated, five of 13 with moderately differentiated, and three of four with poorly differentiated lesions died of their tumors. Similar observations were reported by Salaverria and colleagues.[77]

Carcinoma of the penis has been reported to have greater propensity to metastasize and poorer prognosis in patients younger than 50 years, although Marcial and colleagues[52] observed no difference in survival based on age.[24]

Overall prognosis in carcinoma of the urethra in males varies considerably with location of the primary lesions.[29,43,45,47,51,57] Distal lesions generally have a prognosis similar to that of carcinoma of the penis. Lesions of the bulbomembranous urethra are usually extensive and associated with a dismal prognosis. Tumors of the prostatic urethra have prognostic features similar to those in bladder carcinoma. Superficial lesions have a good prognosis and may be managed with transurethral resection.[47] Deeply invasive tumors have a greater tendency to develop inguinal or pelvic lymph node and distant metastases.

GENERAL MANAGEMENT

Carcinoma of the Penis

Because metastases to the regional nodes in carcinoma of the penis occur by embolization rather than through permeation of the regional lymphatics, therapeutic interventions are generally performed in two phases: initial management of the primary tumor and later treatment of the regional lymphatics.[14]

Surgical intervention at the primary site may range from local excision, or chemosurgery in a small group of highly selected cases with small lesions of the prepuce, to partial or total penectomy.[75] In patients undergoing penectomy, a margin of approximately 2 cm distal to the detectable tumor is considered adequate. Local (stump) recurrence is quite rare.[14] Although surgical resection is a highly effective and expedient treatment modality in most cases, it may not be acceptable to sexually active patients.

Bowen's disease and erythroplasia of Queyrat can be treated topically with a 5% cream of 5-fluorouracil, local excision, or superficial x-rays for a total dose of 4500 cGy to 5000 cGy given in 4 to 5 weeks.

Involved and resectable regional lymph nodes are usually managed by radical lymphadenectomy. However, the procedure is associated with a risk of wound necrosis, wound dehiscence, infection, injuries of major vessels, chronic lymphedema, and pulmonary embolism.[14]

Catalona[13] described a modified inguinal lymphadenectomy, which in his experience with six patients was shown to have significantly less morbidity than the classical groin dissection designed by Daseler and associates.[15]

The relatively low incidence (10% to 20%) of metastatic disease in patients with clinically normal lymph nodes, the morbidity associated with lymphadenectomy, and 1% to 3% mortality rates have led to management by observation, with intervention delayed until signs of nodal involvement appear, rather than by elective nodal dissection; observational management has yielded high survival rates.[77] However, Johnson and Lo[39] reported that only one of eight patients undergoing late inguinal node dissection survived 5 years. Moreover, McDougal and associates[55] found an 88% survival and 66% disease-free survival rate in patients with Stage II and III carcinoma of the penis if lymphadenectomy was performed "shortly" after treatment of the primary tumor, compared with 38% and 0%, respectively, if the primary lesion was treated locally and no lymphadenectomy was done.

As demonstrated in other tumor sites, such as the head and neck, uterine cervix, and vagina, patients with clinically negative lymph nodes who are at risk for microscopic nodal metastases (*i.e.*, primary tumor beyond Stage I or less than well-differentiated histology) can receive elective irradiation to the inguinal lymph nodes (5000 cGy at 3 cm in 5 weeks) with a high probability of tumor control and low morbidity.

Patients with metastatic inguinal lymphadenopathy can be treated with irradiation in combination with lymphadenectomy or with a radical inguinal and, if necessary, pelvic lymph node dissection.[83] Extension of the nodal dissection into the pelvis to cover the iliac lymph nodes is justified in patients with evidence of inguinal involvement (*i.e.*, positive biopsy of Cloquet's node). Approximately 20% of the patients with pelvic lymph node involvement can be salvaged by radical pelvic lymphadenectomy.[11]

The principal advantage of radiotherapeutic management of the primary lesion in carcinoma of the penis is preservation of the organ. Historically, many variations of techniques, doses, and fractionation schemes have been employed.[2,21,22,37,58,61,71] In 1924, Barringer and Dean[5] recommended only partial amputation of the penis, 1.5 cm proximal to the lesion, followed by radiation therapy to the groin. In 1931, Young[85] reported his results with partial penectomy and unilateral groin dissection for management of squamous cell carcinoma of the penis, a technique he had initiated in 1907.

Interstitial implants, molds, and contact, orthovoltage, and megavoltage irradiation have been used, often delivering total doses that would be too low by modern standards. In the past, the treatment frequently resulted in underdosage or overdosage and a high incidence of injury to normal tissues. The improvement in tumor control rate in some of the modern series employing adequate total doses and small daily doses is noteworthy, as is the decrease in the incidence of treatment-related sequelae. Most patients who do experience local failure after radiation therapy can be salvaged surgically.[22]

Irradiation of the involved regional lymph nodes in patients with carcinoma of the penis results in permanent control and cure in a substantial number of patients. In the classic series of Staubitz and associates,[80] there were 13 patients with proven involvement of regional lymph nodes who received radiation therapy to these nodes. Five (38%) of the 13 survived 5 years. Narayana and associates[59] reported that two (12%) of 16 patients with histologically proven lymph node metastases were cured with radiation therapy. No data on radiation therapy were given for either of these series, precluding an assessment of the doses and fields.

The potential value of elective regional node irradiation remains an unresolved issue. Routine regional lymphatic irradiation in patients with clinically normal groins appears ill-advised, because only a few patients harbor microscopic disease. There is a suggestion of benefit from elective irradiation in the series of Ekstrom and Edsmyr[21] and Engelstad;[22] in both series, 5-year survival rates exceeded those for patients not electively irradiated.

Carcinoma of the Male Urethra

Because of the rarity of this disease, policies of treatment in carcinoma of the male urethra are difficult to evaluate. Noninvasive carcinoma of the proximal urethra can be treated with transurethral resection. In lesions of the distal urethra, results of penectomy or radiation therapy resemble those for carcinoma of the penis, and the 5-year survival rates (50% to 60%) are comparable.[73] Involved regional lymph nodes are treated with lymphadenectomy.

Most patients, however, present with advanced, invasive lesions, which are difficult to manage with radical surgery or radiation therapy. The major problem is the high rate of local recurrence. In an attempt to improve the locoregional control rate, extended resections encompassing the inferior pubic rami, prostate, bladder, and perineum have been performed after preoperative radiation therapy. After a dose of 2000 cGy to 6000 cGy, Klein and associates[45] performed an extended resection in seven patients with proximal urethral lesions. Locoregional failure occurred in two (29%) patients.

RADIATION THERAPY TECHNIQUES

Carcinoma of the Penis

If indicated, circumcision must be performed before radiation therapy is initiated. The purpose of this procedure is to minimize the radiation therapy-associated morbidity: swelling, irritation of the skin, moist desquamation, and secondary infection.

Although external-beam therapy has become prevalent in the treatment of primary carcinoma of the penis, plastic molds or interstitial implants are still used.

Brachytherapy

A mold is usually built in the form of a box or cylinder with a central opening and channels for placement of radioactive sources (needles or wires) in the periphery of the device. The cylinder and sources should be long enough to prevent underdosage at the tip of the penis. A dose of 6000 cGy to 6500 cGy at the surface and approximately 5000 cGy at the center of the organ is delivered over 6 to 7 days. The mold can be applied continuously, in which case an indwelling catheter should be in place, or intermittently. Intermittent application requires precise time records. Alternatively, single-plane or double-plane implants can be used to deliver 6000 cGy to 7000 cGy in 5 to 7 days.[70] Salaverria and colleagues[77] point out that molds should be reserved for Stage I and II tumors. We believe the same is true for interstitial implants; for technical details, see Chapter 13. In more extensive lesions involving the shaft of the penis, it is technically difficult to obtain an adequate margin with brachytherapy procedures, similar to the problem in performing a partial penectomy.

External Irradiation

External-beam therapy requires specially designed accessories (including bolus) to achieve homogeneous dose distribution to the entire organ involved. The device usually consists of a plastic box with a central circular opening that can be fitted over the penis. The space between the skin and the box must be filled with tissue-equivalent material (Fig. 53-3). This box can then be treated with parallel opposed megavoltage beams. An ingenious alternative to the box technique is the use of a water-filled container to envelop the penis while the patient is in a prone position.[76]

Another, more complex device consists of a Perspex tube attached to a base plate resting on the skin.[25] This is placed as close as possible to the base of the penis, and a flexible tube is connected to a vacuum pump. The suction effect keeps the penis in a fixed position during treatment. Appropriate bolus is placed outside the tube. The patient can also be treated in the prone position, with the penis hanging through a small hole placed in the Perspex's cylinder.

Fraction size in most of the reported series has been 250 cGy to 350 cGy, given to a total dose of 5000 cGy to 5500 cGy, although a smaller daily fraction size of 180 cGy to 200 cGy and a higher total dose are preferable. There is a well-established association between large fraction size and late tissue damage

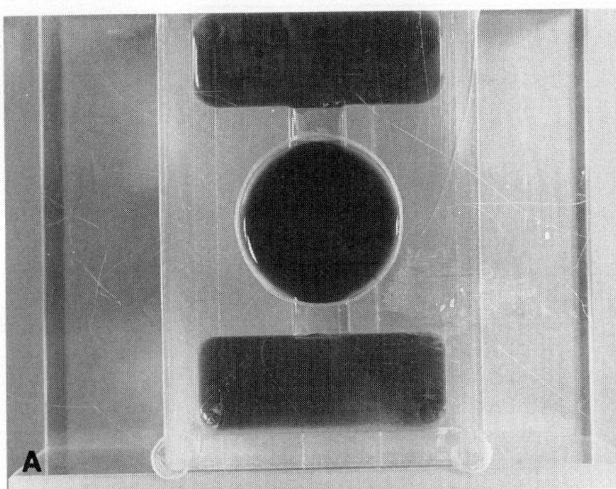

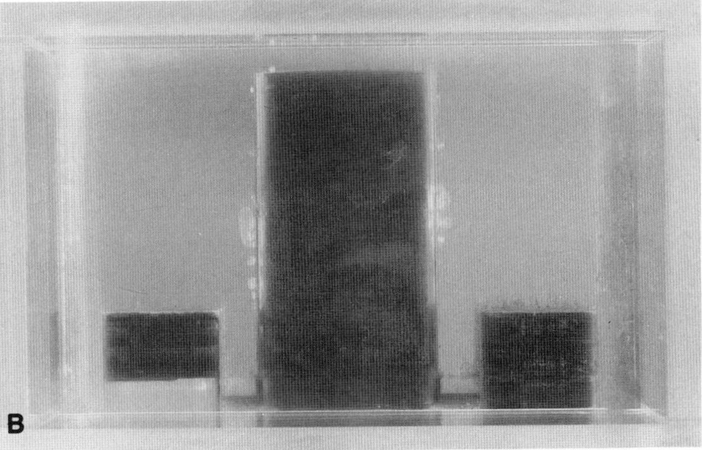

FIGURE 53–3. (**A**) View from above of plastic box with central cylinder for external irradiation of the penis. Patient is treated in the prone position. The penis is placed in the central cylinder, and water fills the surrounding volume in the box. Depth dose is calculated at the central point of box. (**B**) Lateral view.

(see Chap. 1). A total of 6500 cGy to 7000 cGy, with the last 500 cGy to 1000 cGy delivered to a reduced portal, should reduce the incidence of late fibrosis.

Regional lymphatics may be treated with external-beam megavoltage irradiation. Both groins should be irradiated. The fields should include inguinal and pelvic (external iliac and hypogastric) lymph nodes (Fig. 53-4). The posterior pelvis may be partially spared by anterior loading of the beams (see Chap. 59). Depending on the extent of the nodal disease and the proximity of detectable tumor to the skin surface or the degree of skin invasion, application of a bolus to the inguinal area should be considered. If clinical and radiographic evaluations show no gross enlargement of the pelvic lymph nodes, the dose to these nodes may be limited to 5000 cGy. In patients with palpable lymph nodes, doses on the order of 7000 cGy over 7 to 8 weeks (180–200 cGy/day) with reducing fields are advised.

Carcinoma of the Male Urethra

Radiotherapeutic treatment of patients with carcinoma of the distal urethra is quite similar to that of carcinoma of the penis; lesions of the bulbomembranous urethra can be treated with a set of parallel opposed fields covering the groins and the pelvis, followed by a perineal and inguinal boost. Lesions of the prostatic urethra can be treated with techniques similar to those used for carcinoma of the prostate.

RESULTS

Carcinoma of the Penis

Because cancer of the penis is an uncommon disease in the western world, reports of treatment results are scarce. A significant proportion of the patients have been treated surgically, with 5-year tumor control ranging from 25% to 80%, depending on the stage of the primary tumor and extent of inguinal lymph node involvement.

The use of wide local excision and lasers has been recently advocated for treating superficial tumors as an alternative to partial or total penectomy. Boon[8] reported tumor control in 13 (81%) of 16 patients with carcinoma *in situ,* T1 lesions, or T2 tumors treated in this fashion.

Radiation therapy has yielded comparable results in several institutions. A summary of tumor control rates achieved with irradiation is presented in Table 53-8. Engelstad,[22] Cade,[12] Paterson and colleagues,[66] Lederman,[48] and Thurgar[82] reported 5-year survival rates ranging from 45% to 68% in groups of patients who were between 41 and 57 years old and treated with various irradiation techniques (*e.g.,* mold, interstitial, external x-rays). The ability of irradiation to control the tumor is closely associated with the stage of the disease. Jackson[37] reported a 66% 5-year survival rate and 86% tumor control rate among 58 patients with Stage I carcinoma of the penis treated with irradiation, which compared favorably with a 70% 5-year survival rate and 81% tumor control rate for 27 surgically treated patients. In Stage II, six of 11 patients survived 5 years, and seven exhibited tumor control after irradiation; six survived 5 years

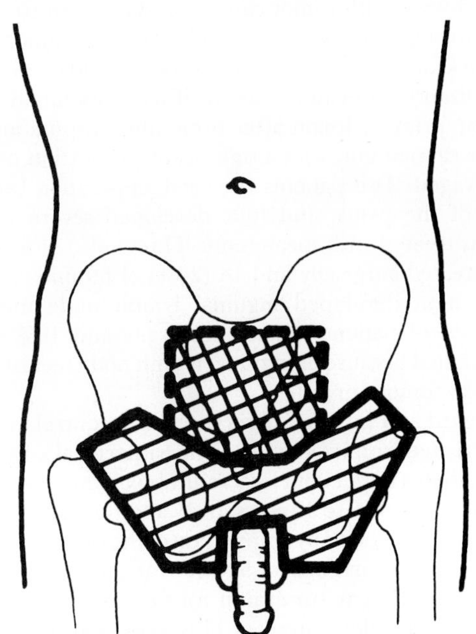

FIGURE 53–4. Portals encompassing inguinal and pelvic lymph nodes.

TABLE 53–8
Overall Control of Primary Carcinoma of the Penis with Radiation Therapy

INVESTIGATION	NO. OF PATIENTS	TREATMENT METHOD	DOSE*	LOCAL CONTROL (%)
Almgard and Edsmyr[2]	16	Radium implant External beam		87.5
Engelstad[22]	72	Mold Teleradium	3500–3700 R (500–700 R/day)	50
Jackson[37]	39	Mold (most cases) External beam (some cases)		49
Marcial et al[52]	25	External beam Interstitial Mold	4000 R in 2 weeks 5000 R in 4 weeks 5000 to 6000 R in 5–6 days	64
Murrell and Williams[58]	108	External beam	3000–6700 cGy (200 cGy/day)	52
Kelley et al[30,44]	10	External beam (electrons)	5100–5400 cGy (300 cGy/day)	100
Knudson and Brennhovd[46]	145	Mold	3500–3700 cGy in 3–5 days	32
Haile and Delclos[35]	20	Mold Implant External beam	 6000 cGy	90
Mazeron et al[54]	23	^{192}Ir implant	6000–7000 cGy	78
Pointon[71]	32	External beam	5250–5500 cGy (16 Fx in 22 days)	84.4
Sagerman et al[76]	15	External beam	4500 cGy (15 Fx in 3 weeks) to 6400 cGy (32 Fx in 6.5 weeks)	60
Salaverria et al[77]	41	Iridium mold	6000 cGy over several days	84.3

**Fx: fractions.*

and eight had tumor control in a group of 12 who were surgically treated. In Stage III, four of seven irradiated patients survived 5-years with tumor control, and of seven treated surgically, two survived for 5 years and three had tumor control.

In Jackson's[37] report, radium or cobalt molds produced the best sterilization of primary tumor; if irradiation had not controlled the primary lesion after 6 months, amputation of the penis was carried out, with a significant proportion of the patients salvaged. Two patients required amputation because of necrosis of the penis, and four developed severe phimosis, which was treated with meatotomy. Three (8%) of 37 patients initially treated surgically and 14 (20%) of 69 initially treated with radiation developed inguinal lymph node metastases. Overall, 8% of patients treated surgically and 10% of those irradiated died because of inguinal lymph node metastases and subsequent tumor spread.

Almgard and Edsmyr[2] observed tumor control in 12 of 17 patients treated with irradiation alone (superficial x-rays). Four of these patients underwent local radical excision for recurrence and survived from 10 to 30 years. In 17 additional patients, local irradiation was followed by amputation of the penis, and 16 have been free from recurrence for 5 to 32 years. Marcial and associates[52] observed 5-year survival in four of six patients who received irradiation alone, in six of 11 who were given irradiation for frank persistence after limited surgery to the penis, and in six of eight to whom irradiation was administered postoperatively. Sixteen (64%) of the 25 patients survived 5 years.

In a series of 145 patients reported by Knudsen and Brennhovd,[46] 99 (68%) had recurrences, as did five (36%) of 14 patients treated by Johnson and colleagues[38] and 24 (38%) of 63 patients reported by Murrell and Williams.[58] Haile and Delclos[35] reported tumor control and conservation of the penis in 16 (80%) of 20 patients treated with conservative radiation therapy methods. Although irradiation alone or combined with a lymph node dissection controlled lymph node metastases smaller than 2 cm in four patients, radiation therapy was successful in controlling lymph node metastases in only one of seven patients with N2 or N3 lymph nodes.

Sagerman and co-workers[76] reported tumor control in six of nine patients with Stage I, two of three with Stage II, and one of three with Stage IV disease treated with irradiation alone. Two of the patients with Stage I disease and one with Stage II disease were surgically salvaged. Doses administered ranged from 4500 cGy (15 fractions in 3 weeks) to 6400 cGy (32 fractions in 6.5 weeks) with orthovoltage x-rays or ^{60}Co and appropriate bolus. Good palliation was achieved in four of nine patients treated for inguinal lymph node metastases with doses ranging from 2000 cGy (five fractions in 1 week) to 6400 cGy. None of these patients survived more than 18 months.

Mazeron and associates[54] described tumor control in eight

of nine patients with Stage T1, 21 of 27 patients with T2, and 10 of 14 patients with T3 tumors treated with ^{192}Ir, using the Paris dosimetry system to deliver doses of 6000 cGy to 7000 cGy to the 85% minimal tumor isodose. The tumor-free 5-year actuarial survival rate was 63%. The penis was conserved in 75% of the patients followed for 8 years. Thirty-seven patients received no prophylatic treatment to the inguinal nodes, and only two (one with a T2 and the other with a T3 lesion) later developed inguinal lymph node metastases treated by inguinal node dissection and postoperative irradiation. One of the patients is alive with no evidence of disease at 10 years. Five patients with metastases to the lymph nodes at the time of diagnosis were treated with therapeutic nodal dissection and postoperative irradiation. Four of the patients had uncontrolled lymph node metastases, and all five died with distant disease.

Duncan and Jackson[20] discussed the superiority of external-beam irradiation over mold therapy, with 3-year tumor control rates of 90% and 47%, respectively. Salaverria and associates[77] reported a 5-year survival rate of 92% for 13 patients with Stage I or II tumors treated with ^{226}Ra or ^{192}Ir molds. This compared with ten (77%) of 13 patients surviving after partial penectomy. Four of six patients with Stage II disease survived 5 years after ^{192}Ir mold treatment. Ten patients with Stage III disease were treated with radical amputation, and eight survived 5 years.

Table 53-9 correlates the results of therapy with tumor stage, preservation of the organ, and morbidity.

Kearsley and associates[43] described a patient with locally advanced penile carcinoma and metastatic inguinal lymph nodes who was cured with irradiation alone, a remarkable achievement because most patients with Stage IV carcinoma die with locoregional and disseminated disease.

Carcinoma of the Male Urethra

Most patients with male urethral carcinoma are treated surgically. Bracken and associates[10] described 11 patients with tumors at or anterior to the penoscrotal junction: eight were epidermoid carcinoma, two were transitional cell carcinoma, and one was melanoma. Three of four patients treated with total penectomy and perineal urethrostomy had tumor control. Partial penectomy controlled the local tumor in two patients. The patient with melanoma had a local recurrence after surgery. Two patients were treated with radiation therapy and a third with a combination of preoperative irradiation (4500 cGy) and total penectomy. In all of these patients, tumors recurred locally. In four patients with inguinal lymph node metastases, the regional disease was controlled by bilateral lymphadenectomy. All six patients in whom local and regional tumor was controlled remain alive and disease-free 1 to 20 years later. In 16 patients, the urethral tumors arose posterior to the penoscrotal junction: 13 of the lesions were squamous cell carcinoma, two were transitional cell, and one was adenocarcinoma. Penectomy was performed in five patients, all of whom had tumor control and no evidence of recurrence 5 to 29 months after therapy. Two patients treated with local excision died of disease 14 and 18 months after surgery. Irradiation was used in three patients unsuccessfully, and all died of cancer 13 to 31 months after therapy ended.

Kaplan and colleagues[41] reported 29 patients treated at Northwestern University and reviewed 232 cases from the literature. In the analysis, lesions of the distal urethra carried the best prognosis, and those in the bulbomembranous urethra had the worst outcomes. The results of 186 cases compiled by these authors are shown in Table 53-10. Five-year survival was achieved by 16 (23%) of 71 patients with tumors in the distal urethra, ten (10%) of 99 patients with bulbomembranous urethra lesions, and four (25%) of 16 patients with prostatic urethra tumors. Radiation therapy was infrequently used to treat these patients.

CHEMOTHERAPY

Experience with chemotherapy in treating carcinoma of the penis is even more limited than for other modalities. Occasional tumor regression has been described with some antineoplastic agents, such as bleomycin, 5-fluorouracil, or methotrexate, although chemotherapy has been combined with irradiation or surgery in some instances, making assessment of the response more difficult.[84] Response to cisplatin has been reported in a few patients; Ahmed and associates[1] treated 12 patients with penile cancer with intravenous cisplatin every 3 weeks (70–120 mg/m^2) and reported three responses with durations of 2 to 8 months. Gagliano and colleagues[26] observed no complete response and only four partial responses (15.4%) among 26 patients with Stage III or IV epidermal carcinoma of the penis who received 50 mg/m^2 cisplatin intravenously on day 1 and then every 28 days. Response durations were 1 to 3 months.

TABLE 53–9
Results of Radiation Therapy for Carcinoma of the Penis

		TUMOR CONTROL			
INVESTIGATION	TREATMENT METHOD	STAGES I–II	STAGES III–IV	COMPLICATIONS	PENIS PRESERVATION
Duncan and Jackson[20]	Teletherapy	16/20 (80%)		2/20 (10%)	16/20 (80%)
Jackson[37]	Mold	20/45 (44%)		2/45 (4%)	20/45 (44%)
Haile and Delclos[35]	External beam	6/6 (100%)	2/2 (100%)		16/20 (80%)
	Brachytherapy	12/12 (100%)			
Kaushal and Sharma[42]	^{60}Co	14/16 (88%)		2/16 (12%)	13/14 (93%)
Kelley et al[44]	Electrons	10/10 (100%)			10/10 (100%)
Pierquin et al[70]	^{192}Ir	14/14 (100%)	12/31 (39%)	3/45 (6.7%)	
Sagerman et al[76]	External beam	9/12 (75%)	1/3 (33%)		2/15 (13%)
Salaverria et al[77]	Mold	12/13 (92%)			10/13 (77%)

TABLE 53–10
Treatment Results for 186 Collected Cases of Urethral Carcinoma

	DISTAL URETHRA				BULBOMEMBRANOUS URETHRA				PROSTATIC URETHRA			
TREATMENT*	SUR-VIVED >5 YEARS	DIED	FOL-LOWED <5 YEARS	LOCAL RECURR.	SUR-VIVED >5 YEARS	DIED	FOL-LOWED <5 YEARS	LOCAL RECURR.	SUR-VIVED >5 YEARS	DIED	FOL-LOWED <5 YEARS	LOCAL RECURR.
PRIMARY MODES OF TREATMENT												
Radical penile amputation	2	4	16	3	0	4	3	1				
Partial penile amputation	6	3	17	0								
Local cautery	1	0	3	1	0	0	1	0	0	1	0	0
Excision with reanastomosis of urethra	5	1	1	1	3	12	7	6				
Transurethral resection	0	1	0	0					3	4	6	1
Radical prostatectomy									1	0	0	0
Total emasculation	0	0	2	1	1	3	2	2				
Total urethrectomy					0	1	1	1				
Radical excision of perineum, urethra and prostatovesculectomy					6	16	3	3				
Radium without surgery	1	0	1	1	0	4	3	1	0	0	1	0
X-ray without surgery	1	6	0	1	0	28	1	3				
ADJUVANT MODES OF TREATMENT												
Radium	1	0	2		0	2	1		1	0	1	
Estrogen	0	1	0		0	1	0					
X-ray	1	1	2		1	7	4		2	1	2	
Inguinal node dissection	0	1	5		3	2	2					
Methotrexate					0	0	1					
^{198}Au					0	1	0		1	0	0	

** Patients are counted only once in primary modes of treatment. They may be counted more than once in adjuvant modes of treatment.*
(Kaplan GW, Bulkley GJ, Grayhack JT: J Urol 98:365, 1967)

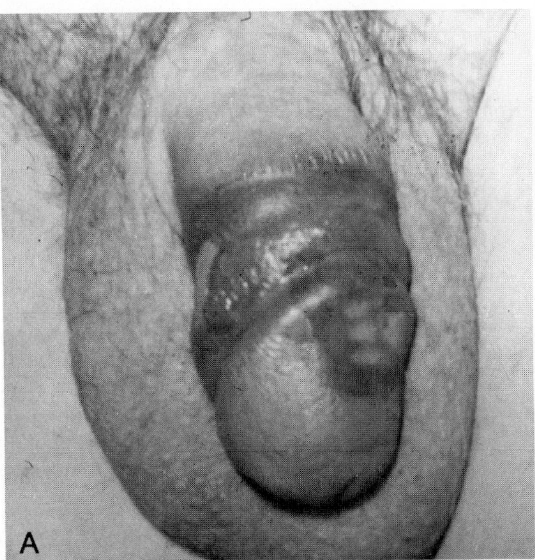

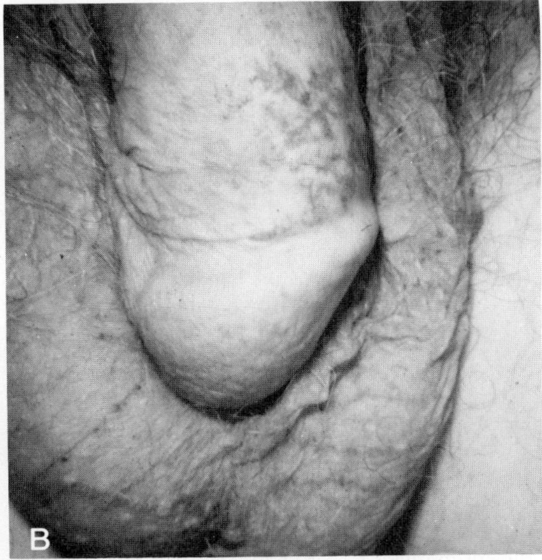

FIGURE 53–5. (**A**) Squamous cell carcinoma of the balanopreputial region with extension into the glands (Stage I). Patient was treated with 120 kVp x-rays, 0.3-mm Cu half-value layer, receiving a skin dose of 6000 cGy in 5 weeks. (**B**) Same patient 4 years later with no evidence of disease. Telangiectasis is evident.

Properly implemented phase I–II trials are needed to identify cytotoxic agents that may be effective in the treatment of patients with advanced or recurrent carcinoma of the penis.

SEQUELAE OF TREATMENT

Irradiation of the penis produces a brisk erythema, dry or moist desquamation, and swelling of the subcutaneous tissue of the shaft in virtually all patients. Although quite uncomfortable, these are reversible reactions that subside after conservative treatment within a few weeks. Telangiectasia is a common late consequence of radiation therapy and is usually asymptomatic (Fig. 53-5).

In the reported series, meatal-urethral strictures occurred with a frequency of 0% to 40%.[21,35,44,51,61] This incidence compares favorably with the incidence of urethral stricture after penectomy. Most of the strictures after radiation therapy are at the meatus.

Ulceration, necrosis of the glans, or necrosis of the skin of the shaft are rare complications. Lymphedema of the legs has been reported after inguinal and pelvic radiation therapy, but the role of irradiation in the development of this complication remains controversial. Many patients with this symptom have active tumor in the lymphatics that may be responsible for lymphatic blockage.

REFERENCES

1. Ahmed T, Sklaroff R, Yagoda A: Sequential trials of methotrexate, cisplatin and bleomycin for penile cancer. J Urol 131:465, 1984
2. Almgard LE, Edsmyr F: Radiotherapy in treatment of patients with carcinoma of the penis. Scand J Urol Nephrol 7:1, 1973
3. Barnes RD, Sarembock LA, Abratt RP, Pontin AR: Carcinoma of the penis: The Groote Schuur Hospital experience. J R Coll Surg Edinb 34:44, 1989
4. Barney JD: Epithelioma of the penis. An analysis of 100 cases. Ann Surg 46:890, 1907
5. Barringer BS, Dean AL Jr: Epithelioma of the penis. J Urol 11:497, 1924
6. Bassett JW: Carcinoma of the penis. Cancer 5:530, 1952
7. Beahrs OH, Henson DE, Hutter RVP, Myers MH (eds): Manual for Staging of Cancer, 3rd ed. Philadelphia, JB Lippincott, 1988
8. Boon IA: Sapphire probe laser surgery for localized carcinoma of the penis. Eur J Surg Oncol 14:193, 1988
9. Boon ME, Susanti I, Tasche MJA, Kok LP: Human papillomavirus (HPV)-associated male and female genital carcinomas in a Hindu population: The male as vector and victum. Cancer 64:559, 1989
10. Bracken RB, Henry R, Ordonez N: Primary carcinoma of the male urethra. South Med J 73:1003, 1980
11. Cabanas RM: An approach for the treatment of penile carcinoma. Cancer 39:456, 1977
12. Cade S: Malignant Disease and Its Treatment by Radium, p 981. Bristol, John Wright & Sons, 1940
13. Catalona WJ: Modified inguinal lymphadenectomy for carcinoma of the penis with preservation of saphenous veins: Technique and preliminary results. J Urol 140:306, 1988
14. Crawford ED, Dawkins CA: Cancer of the penis. In Skinner DG, Lieskovsky G (eds): Diagnosis and Management of Genitourinary Cancer, pp 549–563. Philadelphia, WB Saunders, 1988
15. Daseler EH, Anson BH, Reimann AF: Radical excision of the inguinal and iliac lymph glands: A study based upon 450 anatomical dissections and upon supportive clinical observations. Surg Gynecol Obstet 87:679, 1948
16. Dean AL Jr: Epithelioma of the penis. J Urol 33:252, 1935
17. Dehner LP, Smith BH: Soft tissue tumors of the penis: A clinicopathologic study of 46 cases. Cancer 25:1431, 1970
18. deKernion JB, Tynberg P, Persky L, et al: Carcinoma of the penis. Cancer 32:1256, 1973
19. Derrick FC Jr, Lynch KM Jr, Kretkowski RC, Yarbrough WJ: Epidermoid carcinoma of the penis: Computer analysis of 87 cases. J Urol 110:303, 1973
20. Duncan W, Jackson SM: The treatment of early cancer of the penis with megavoltage x-rays. Clin Radiol 23:246, 1972
21. Ekstrom T, Edsmyr F: Cancer of the penis: A clinical study of 229 cases. Acta Chir Scand 115:25, 1958
22. Engelstad RB: Treatment of cancer of the penis at the Norwegian Radium Hospital. Radiology 60:801, 1948
23. Fegen P, Persky L: Squamous cell carcinoma of the penis: Its treatment, with special reference to radical node dissection. Arch Surg 99:117, 1969
24. Fraley EE, Zhang G, Sazama R, Lange PH: Cancer of the penis. Prognosis and treatment plans. Cancer 55:1618, 1985
25. Franzen L, Henriksson R, Karlsson N-O, et al: A technical

device for irradiation in carcinoma of the penis (Letter). Acta Oncol 26:77, 1987
26. Gagliano RG, Blumenstein BA, Crawford ED, et al: Cis-diamminedichloroplatinum in the treatment of advanced epidermoid carcinoma of the penis: A Southwest Oncology Group study. J Urol 141:66, 1989
27. Gentil F, Cavalcanti S: Total managements of cancer of the penis. Rev Inst Nac Cancer (Mexico) 15:321, 1964
28. Grabstald H: Tumors of the urethra in men and women. Cancer 32:1236, 1973
29. Grabstald H: Controversies concerning lymph node dissection for cancer of the penis. Urol Clin North Am 7:793, 1980
30. Grabstald H, Kelley CD: Radiation therapy of penile cancer: Six- to ten-year follow-up. Urology 15:575, 1980
31. Graham JH, Helwig EB: Erythroplasia of Queyrat: A clinicopathologic and histochemical study. Cancer 32:1396, 1973
32. Graham S, Priore R, Graham M, et al: Genital cancer in wives of penile cancer patients. Cancer 44:1870, 1979
33. Greenbaum SS, Krull EA, Simmons EB: Basal cell carcinoma at the base of the penis: Case report. Genitourin Med 64:128, 1989
34. Gursel EO, Georgountzos C, Uson AC, et al: Penile cancer: Clinicopathologic study of 64 cases. Urology 1:569, 1973
35. Haile K, Delclos L: The place of radiation therapy in the treatment of carcinoma of the distal end of the penis. Cancer 45:1980, 1980
36. Hardner GJ, Bhanalaph T, Murphy GP, et al: Carcinoma of the penis: An analysis of therapy in 100 consecutive cases. J Urol 108:428, 1972
37. Jackson SM: The treatment of carcinoma of the penis. Br J Surg 53:33, 1966
38. Johnson DE, Fuerst DE, Ayala AG: Carcinoma of the penis: Experience with 153 cases. Urology 1:404, 1973
39. Johnson DE, Lo RK: Management of regional lymph nodes in penile carcinoma. Urology 24:308, 1984
40. Jorstad LH: Carcinoma of the penis. Am J Roentgenol 46:232, 1941
41. Kaplan GW, Bulkley GJ, Grayhack JT: Carcinoma of the male urethra. J Urol 98:365, 1967
42. Kaushal V, Sharma SC: Carcinoma of the penis. Acta Oncol 26:413, 1987
43. Kearsley JH, Roberts SJ, Bynaston B: Curative radiotherapy for stage IV carcinoma of the penis. Med J Austral 145:474, 1986
44. Kelley CD, Arthur K, Rogoff E, et al: Radiation therapy of penile cancer. Urology 4:571, 1974
45. Klein FA, Whitmore WF, Herr HW, et al: Inferior pubic rami resection with en bloc radical excision for invasive proximal urethral carcinoma. Cancer 51:1238, 1983
46. Knudsen OA, Brennhovd IO: Radiotherapy in the treatment of the primary tumour in penile cancer. Acta Chir Scand 113:69, 1967
47. Konnak JW: Conservative management of low grade neoplasms of the male urethra: A preliminary report. J Urol 123:175, 1980
48. Lederman M: Radiotherapy of cancer of the penis. Br J Urol 25:224, 1953
49. Lenowitz H, Graham AP: Carcinoma of the penis. J Urol 56:458, 1946
50. Malcaluso JN Jr, Sullivan JW, Tomberlin S: Glomus tumor of glans penis. Urology 25:409, 1985
51. Mandler JI, Pool TL: Primary carcinoma of the male urethra. J Urol 96:67, 1966
52. Marcial VA, Figueroa-Colon J, Marcial-Rojas RA, Colon JE: Carcinoma of the penis. Radiology 79:209, 1962
53. Martinez I: Relationship of squamous cell carcinoma of the cervix uteri to squamous cell carcinoma of the penis. Cancer 24:777, 1969
54. Mazeron JJ, Langlois D, Lobo PA, et al: Interstitial radiation therapy for carcinoma of the penis using iridium 192 wires: The Henri Mondor experience (1970–1979). Int J Radiat Oncol Biol Phys 10:1891, 1984
55. McDougal WS, Kirchner FK Jr, Edwards RH, Killion LT: Treatment of carcinoma of the penis: The case for primary lymphadenectomy. J Urol 136:38, 1986
56. Mikhail GR: Cancers, precancers, and pseudocancer on the male genitalia: A review of clinical appearances, histopathology, and management. J Dermatol Surg Oncol 6:1027, 1980
57. Mullin EM, Anderson EE, Paulson DF: Carcinoma of the male urethra. J Urol 112:610, 1974
58. Murrell DS, Williams JL: Radiotherapy in the treatment of carcinoma of the penis. Br J Urol 37:211, 1965
59. Narayana AS, Olney LE, Loening SA, et al: Carcinoma of the penis: Analysis of 219 cases. Cancer 49:2185, 1982
60. Netter FH: The CIBA Collection of Medical Illustrations, vol 2: Reproductive System. Summit, NJ, CIBA Pharmaceutical, 1972
61. Newaishy GA, Deeley TJ: Radiotherapy in the treatment of carcinoma of the penis. Br J Radiol 41:519, 1968
62. Nichols P: Pathology of cancer of penis. In Skinner DG, Lieskovsky G (eds): Diagnosis and Management of Genitourinary Cancer, pp 207–214. Philadelphia, WB Saunders, 1988
63. Onuigbo WI: Carcinoma of skin of penis. Br J Urol 57:465, 1985
64. Oota K: Symposium de cancer del pene. Cancer of the penis in Japan. Rev Inst Nac Cancer (Mexico) 15:289, 1964
65. Owor R: Carcinoma of the penis in Uganda. IARC Sci Publ 63:493, 1984
66. Paterson R, Tod MC, Russell MH: The Results of Radium and X-ray Therapy in Malignant Disease, p 146. Edinburgh, Livingstone, 1950
67. Paymaster JC, Gangadharan P: Carcinoma of the penis in India. J Urol 97:110, 1967
68. Perinetti E, Crane DB, Catalona WJ: Unreliability of sentinel lymph node biopsy for staging penile carcinoma. J Urol 124:734, 1980
69. Persky L: Commentary: Problems and management of squamous cell carcinoma of the penis. In Whitehead ED, Leiter E (eds): Current Operative Urology, 2nd ed, pp 1180–1183. Philadelphia, Harper & Row, 1984
70. Pierquin B, Chassagne D, Chahbazian C, Wilson J: Brachytherapy, pp 193–196. St. Louis, Warren H Green, 1978
71. Pointon RCS: External beam therapy. Proc R Soc Med 68:779, 1975
72. Powell BL, Craig JB, Muss HB: Secondary malignancies of the penis and epididymis: A case report and review of the literature. J Clin Oncol 3:110, 1985
73. Raghavaiah NV: Radiotherapy in the treatment of carcinoma of the male urethra. Cancer 41:1313, 1978
74. Ray B, Canto AR, Whitmore WF: Experience with primary carcinoma of the male urethra. J Urol 117:591, 1977
75. Rosenberg SK: Carbon dioxide laser treatment of external genital lesions. Urology 24:555, 1985
76. Sagerman RH, Yu WS, Chung CT, Puranik A: External-beam irradiation of carcinoma of the penis. Radiology 152:183, 1984
77. Salaverria JC, Hope-Stone HF, Paris AMI, et al: Conservative treatment of carcinoma of the penis. Br J Urol 51:32, 1979
78. Schrek R, Lenowitz H: Etiologic facts in carcinoma of the penis. Cancer Res 7:180, 1947
79. Skinner DG, Leadbetter WF, Kelley SB: The surgical management of squamous cell carcinoma of the penis. J Urol 107:273, 1972
80. Staubitz WJ, Lent MH, Oberkircher OJ: Carcinoma of the penis. Cancer 8:371, 1955
81. Sulaiman MZ, Polazarz SV, Partington PE: Basal cell carcinoma of the penis: Case report. Genitourin Med 64:128, 1989
82. Thurgar CJL: British Practice in Radiotherapy, p 194. London, Butterworths, 1955
83. Vaeth JM, Green JP, Lowy RO: Radiation therapy of carcinoma of the penis. AJR 108:130, 1970
84. Yagoda A, Mukherji B, Young C, et al: Bleomycin, an antitumor antibiotic: Clinical experience in 274 patients. Ann Intern Med 77:861, 1972
85. Young HH: A radical operation for the cure of cancer of the penis. J Urol 26:285, 1931
86. Yu GSM, Nseyo UO, Carson JW: Primary penile lymphoma in a patient with Peyronie's disease. J Urol 142:1076, 1989

54

○ ○ ○ • • •

Uterine Cervix

Carlos A. Perez

ANATOMY

The uterus is a muscular hollow organ located in the midplane of the true pelvis, behind the bladder and in front of the rectum (Fig. 54-1). The organ usually is in an anteverted position, but this may change with expansion of the bladder or the rectum. It is partially covered by peritoneum in its fundal portion and posteriorly; its anterior and lateral surfaces are in contact with extraperitoneal connective tissue and are related to the bladder and the broad ligaments, respectively.

The three regions of the uterus are the fundus, the corpus, and the cervix. The cervix is separated from the corpus by a subtle constriction (isthmus) and is divided into two regions: an upper or supravaginal portion above the ring containing the endocervical canal and the vaginal portion, which projects into the vault.

The uterus is attached to the surrounding structures in the pelvis by two pairs of ligaments, the broad and the round ligaments (see Fig. 54-1*A*). The broad ligament is a double layer of peritoneum extending from the lateral margin of the uterus to the lateral wall of the pelvis. It contains the fallopian tubes. An extension beyond the tube constitutes the suspensory ligament for the ovary. The two layers of peritoneum forming the broad ligament enclose the extraperitoneal connective tissue, termed the *parametrium,* as it reaches the uterus. Inferiorly, the broad ligament follows the plane of the pelvic floor and ends medially in the upper portion of the vagina.[13]

The round ligament is a true band of smooth muscle and connective tissue and contains small vessels and nerves. It extends forward horizontally from its attachment in the anterolateral portion of the uterus to the lateral pelvic wall. The cord ascending from the lateral wall of the true pelvis crosses the pelvic brim and extends laterally to reach the abdominoinguinal ring through which it leaves the abdomen to traverse the inguinal canal and terminate in the superficial fascia.

The uterosacral ligaments are paired supports for the lower uterus consisting of fibrous tissue with smooth muscle; they extend from the uterus to the sacrum and run along the recto-uterine-peritoneal fields.[13]

The uterus has a rich lymphatic network that drains principally into the paracervical lymph nodes, where they go to the external iliac (of which the obturator nodes are the innermost component) and the hypogastric lymph nodes. The pelvic lymphatics drain into the common iliac and periaortic lymph nodes. Lymphatics from the fundus pass laterally across the broad ligament continuous with those of the ovary, ascending along the ovarian vessels into the periaortic lymph nodes. Some of the fundal lymphatics also drain into the external and internal common iliac lymph nodes (Fig. 54-2).

The main artery supplying the uterus is the uterine artery, which originates from the anterior division of the hypogastric artery. The uterine artery lies first on the inner wall of the true pelvis, passing medially and slightly forward on the fascia that covers the upper surface of the elevator ani muscle in the lower margin of the broad ligament. In the parametrial tissue, enclosed by the peritoneal layers of the ligament, it arches over the ureter about 2 cm from the uterus. The uterine artery ascends as far as the fundus, supplying many branches to the anterior and posterior surfaces of the uterus, and continues laterally to divide into branches that supply the ovary and fallopian tubes.

EPIDEMIOLOGY

Carcinoma of the uterine cervix is the fourth most common malignant neoplasm in women, after carcinoma of the breast, colorectum, and endometrium. The American Cancer Society estimated in 1991 that there were 13,500 new cases of invasive carcinoma of the cervix in the United States and 6000 deaths from the disease[9] in addition to over 50,000 cases of carcinoma *in situ.* Cervical cancer is more common in Latin America and less common in Jewish and European women and Fiji Islanders.[143] Although some researchers have attributed the low incidence of cervical carcinoma in Jewish women to the circumcision of Jewish men,[381] this low incidence has not been demonstrated in sexual partners of non-Jewish circumcised men.[364] Ackerman and del Regato[4] postulated that Jewish women have a genetic resistance to tumors of the cervix. It has been shown that male circumcision provides only partial protection for cervical carcinogenesis in tropical Africa.[348]

The incidence of cervical carcinoma is substantially higher among women in low socioeconomic classes. Sexual activity and parity also appear to affect incidence. Carcinoma of the uterine cervix is more common in women who had first intercourse at an early age, who have a history of sexual promiscuity, or who have had a large number of pregnancies.[61,174,330] In contrast, carcinoma of the cervix is uncommon in nulliparous women and in those without active sexual lives such as nuns.[331,380]

Despite many theories, at the present time the causative

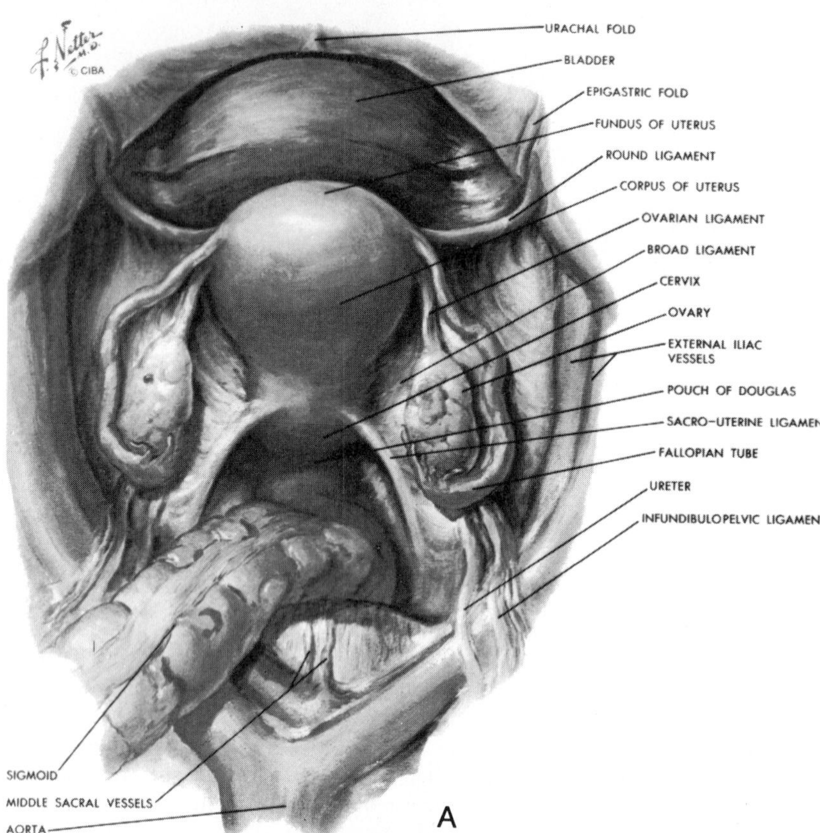

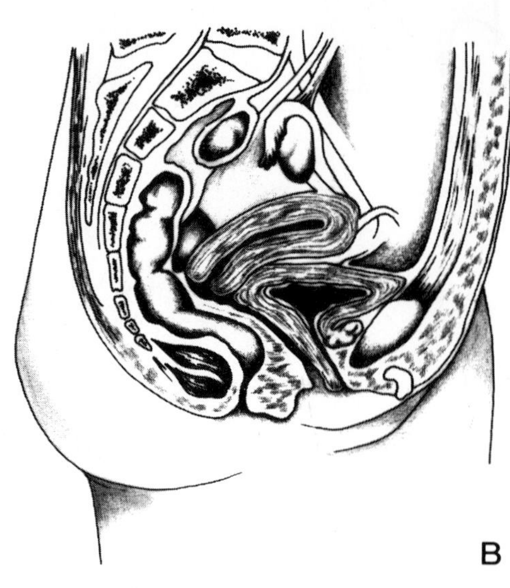

FIGURE 54–1. (**A**) Anatomy of the pelvis observed from above and (**B**) on a sagittal view, demonstrating the close relationship of the uterus to the bladder and the rectosigmoid. (A, Copyright 1954, CIBA-GEIGY Corporation. Reproduced with permission from *The CIBA Collection of Medical Illustrations* by Frank Netter, M.D. All rights reserved)

agents of cervical carcinoma are not known, although predisposing and associated factors have been reported.[255] Carcinoma of the uterine cervix can be induced in experimental animals by application of hormonal or other chemical carcinogens.[168] The association of prenatal exposure to diethylstilbestrol and development of clear cell adenocarcinoma of the cervix or vagina in young women has been reported.[130,138,140] The overall incidence is thought to be small (0.14 to 1.4 per 1000 DES-exposed women).[138] Age at time of tumor presentation ranges from slightly over 10 years up to 30 years (average age 19 years). The majority of the patients (about 90%) present with Stage I and Stage II tumors.

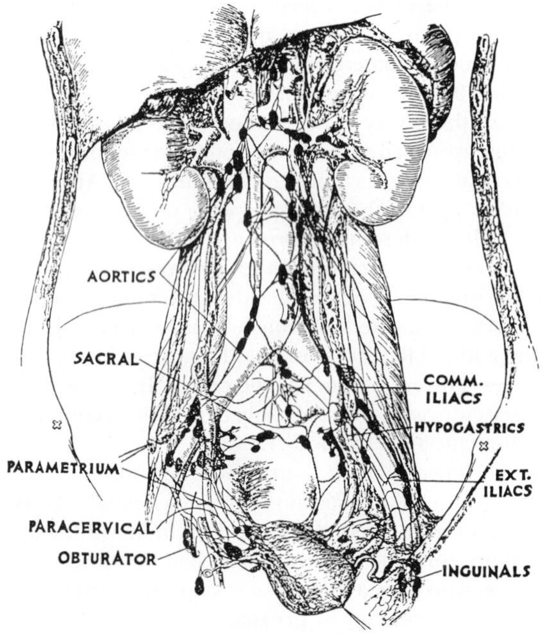

FIGURE 54–2. Lymph vessels and lymph nodes of the cervix and the body of the uterus. (Henrikson E: Am J Obstet Gynecol 58:924–942, 1949)

No definite evidence exists linking the use of oral contraceptives with carcinoma of the uterine cervix.[89,235]

The identification of herpesvirus type II and the presence of high antibody titers against this virus have been reported more often in patients with cervical carcinoma than in controls.[5,106,178,322] However, a direct etiologic role has not been established.

Boon and associates[38] suggested that human papillomavirus (HPV), estimated to be present in over 75% of the Balinese Hindu population with genital carcinomas, may be a co-factor in genital carcinogenesis along with poor postcoital hygiene. In contrast, in the Netherlands where males are usually circumcised, the male is exclusively a vector of the HPV but not a victim as in Bali. Martinez[228] in Puerto Rico and Graham and coworkers[117] in New York also noted a significantly higher incidence of carcinoma of the cervix in wives of men with penile carcinoma. Furthermore, Boon and associates[38] pointed out that even when the spouse does not have penile carcinoma, he may have contributed to the development of cervical carcinoma by being a vector of the HPV. Indeed, Kessler[179] in a study of 4178 women with cervical carcinoma in Baltimore identified 14 marital clusters instead of the expected four. At the time of their report, the associated viral agent was thought to be herpesvirus type II.

Current studies suggest that almost 50% of intraepithelial neoplasias show evidence of HPV infection,[70,325] and viral particles have been demonstrated in invasive cervical cancer.[70]

NATURAL HISTORY

Squamous cell carcinoma of the uterine cervix usually originates at the squamous columnar junction of the endocervical canal and the portio of the cervix.[324] The lesion is frequently associated with chronic cervicitis, severe dysplasia, and carcinoma *in situ*,[324,327] usually showing a progression that may take from 10 to 20 years.[23,172]

It is generally accepted that carcinoma *in situ* precedes invasive carcinoma of the cervix in the majority of cases.[63,193,197,290] The malignant process breaks through the basement membrane of the epithelium and invades the cervical stroma.[60] Formerly, if the invasion was less than 3 mm, the lesion was classified as microinvasive or superficially invasive (Stage IA1)[408]; the probability of lymph node metastasis is about 1%.[37] Invasion may progress and, according to a recent modification of the International Federation of Gynecology and Obstetrics (FIGO) staging schema,[158] when a tumor is not grossly visible but has a depth of penetration of less than 5 mm, it is classified as Stage IA2 invasive carcinoma; the incidence of metastatic pelvic lymph nodes is related to the depth of invasion, with an overall incidence of 5% to 8%.[336]

Growth of the cervical lesion may eventually be manifested by superficial ulceration, exophytic tumor in the exocervix, or extensive infiltration of the endocervix. The lesion may spread to the adjacent vaginal fornices or to the paracervical and parametrial tissues, with eventual direct invasion of the bladder, the rectum, or both (if untreated).

Carcinoma of the uterine cervix has been found to extend into the lower uterine segment and endometrial cavity in 10% to 30% of patients.[241,280] In an analysis of 473 patients, Perez and colleagues[280] noted decreased survival and greater incidence of distant metastases in patients with stromal endometrial invasion or replacement of normal endometrium by cervical carcinoma, confirming observations reported by Mitani and associates.[241]

Regional lymphatic or hematogenous spread occurs, depending on the stage of the tumor, but dissemination does not always follow an orderly sequence, and occasionally a small carcinoma may be seen infiltrating the pelvic lymph nodes, invading the bladder or rectum, or producing distant metastasis. The cervix has a rich lymphatic network that is more abundant in the muscular layers. After the tumor has invaded these structures, there is a higher probability of dissemination to the regional lymphatics. Carcinoma of the cervix may spread to the paracervical and parametrial lymphatics, metastasizing to the obturator lymph nodes (considered a medial group of the external iliac nodes), to other external iliac nodes, and to the hypogastric lymph nodes (Table 54-1). From these, there may be tumor metastases to the common iliac or periaortic lymph nodes.[31,137] The incidence of metastasis to pelvic or periaortic lymph nodes in various stages of the disease is listed in Tables 54-2 and 54-3.

In addition to the frequently described pelvic nodes, lymph nodes are distributed throughout the parametrium. Girardi and associates[109] carefully studied 359 specimens of radical hysterectomies (132 Stage IB, eight Stage IIA, and 219 Stage IIB). They found parametrial nodes in 280 patients (78%), 63 (22.5%) of whom had metastatically involved lymph nodes. The incidence of positive nodes was 11.4% in Stage IB and 21.5% in Stage IIB. Metastatic lymph nodes were found in the medial parametrium (44.4%), in the lateral parametrium (38%), or in both areas (17.5%) (Fig. 54-3). There was a close correlation between involvement of the parametrial lymph nodes and the iliac lymph nodes; with negative parametrial nodes, only 26% of patients had positive iliac lymph nodes, whereas 81% of patients with positive parametrial lymph nodes also had metastatic pelvic nodes. These data are important because they underscore the need to irradiate the parametrial tissues or carry out a complete bilateral pelvic lymphadenectomy in patients with invasive cervical carcinoma.

Hematogenous dissemination through the venous plexus and the paracervical veins occurs less frequently but is relatively high with more advanced stages. The most common metastatic sites are the lungs, mediastinal and supraclavicular lymph nodes, bones, and liver (Table 54-4).[19,54]

CLINICAL PRESENTATION

Intraepithelial or early invasive carcinoma of the cervix can be detected before it becomes symptomatic by periodic examination of cytologic smears. In patients with intraepithelial carcinoma *in situ*, no gross abnormality of the cervix may be noted, or a small central superficial ulceration may be the only finding.

Frequently the first manifestation of abnormality is postcoital spotting, which later may increase to limited metrorrhagia

TABLE 54–1
Lymph Node Group Involvement and Location in Carcinoma of the Uterine Cervix

SITE	RIGHT	LEFT	TOTAL	PERCENT		
Paracervical	3	3	3	2		69
Obturator	34	31	65	20		69
External iliac medial	50	53	103	31	47	69
External iliac anterior	15	17	32	10	47	69
External iliac lateral	10	9	19	6	47	69
Hypogastric	15	9	24	7		
Common iliac	28	18	46	14		
Periaortic	14	17	31	10		
Total number of involved node groups	169	157	323			
Total number of cases			91			
Average number of node groups per case			3.5			

(Graham JB, Sotto LSJ, Paoloucek FP: Carcinoma of the Cervix, p 192. Philadelphia, WB Saunders, 1962)

TABLE 54–2
Incidence (%) of Pelvic Node Metastases in Carcinoma of the Uterine Cervix

SITE	STAGE I	STAGE II	STAGE III
No Irradiation			
Morton et al[251]	16	32	47
Guttman[127]	11	35	
Meigs[234]	18	45	
Brunschwig et al[46]	13	30	
Christensen et al[58]	16	44	
Graham et al[116] (collected series)	15	27	66
Postirradiation Lymphadenectomy			
Morton et al[251]	9	21	17
Guttman[127]	0	4	
Rutledge et al[340]	3	14	13
Perez et al[281]	7	0	

(Perez CA, DiSaia PJ, Knapp RC, Young RC: Gynecologic tumors. In DeVita VT Jr, Hellman S, Rosenberg SA [eds]: Cancer: Principles and Practice of Oncology, 2nd ed. Philadelphia, JB Lippincott, 1985)

(intermenstrual bleeding). More prominent menstrual bleeding (menorrhagia) may occur.

Serosanguineous or yellowish foul-smelling vaginal discharge may be noted in patients with invasive carcinoma, particularly with more advanced necrotic lesions. If chronic bleeding occurs, the patient may complain of fatigue or other symptoms related to anemia.

Pain, usually in the pelvis or hypogastrium, may be noted and could be caused by tumor necrosis or associated pelvic inflammatory disease. Some patients complain of pain in the lumbosacral area, and in these cases the possibility of periaortic lymph node involvement with extension into the lumbosacral roots or hydronephrosis should be considered. Occasionally epigastric pain may be caused by metastasis to high periaortic lymph nodes.

Urinary and rectal symptoms (hematuria, rectal bleeding) may appear in advanced stages as a consequence of invasion of the bladder or rectum by the neoplasia.

DIAGNOSTIC WORKUP

Every patient with carcinoma of the cervix should be jointly evaluated by the radiation and the gynecologic oncologist. The techniques for history taking and the physical pelvic examination have been described in standard textbooks.[265] After a general physical examination with special attention to the supraclavicular (nodal) areas, abdomen, and liver, a careful pelvic examination should be carried out with as little discomfort to the patient as possible, without compromising the thoroughness of the evaluation. Pelvic examination should include inspection of external genitalia, vagina, and uterine cervix, bimanual palpation of the pelvis, and rectal examination. Cystoscopy or rectosigmoidoscopy should be performed on all patients with Stage IIB, III, and IVA disease or those with earlier stages who have a history of urinary or lower gastrointestinal tract disturbances. An outline of the diagnostic procedures for carcinoma of the cervix is presented in Table 54-5.

Cytology

Ideally, carcinoma of the cervix should be diagnosed while still a severe dysplasia or carcinoma *in situ*. The detection of carcinoma *in situ* by screening cytology and ensuing proper treatment have resulted in a decreased prevalence of invasive carcinoma and a lower mortality from these tumors.[43, 100, 128]

The American Cancer Society has recommended that asymptomatic women 20 years of age and older and those under 20 who are sexually active have a Papanicolaou smear annually

TABLE 54–3
Metastases to Paraaortic Lymph Nodes in Carcinoma of the Uterine Cervix

STUDY	STAGE IB	(%)	STAGE IIA	(%)	STAGE IIB	(%)	STAGE IIIA	(%)	STAGE IIIB	(%)	STAGE IV	(%)
Sudarsanam et al[371]	11/155	(7)	3/21	(14)	4/22	(18)	0/3	(0)	3/16	(19)	0/3	(0)
Nelson et al[259]					5/31	(16)			13/28	(46)		
Piver et al[295]					6/46	(13)			18/49	(36)	4/7	(57)
Wharton et al[416]	0/21	(0)	0/10	(0)	10/47	(21)			14/42	(33)		
Lagasse et al[206]	8/143	(5)	4/22	(18)	19/58	(33)	0/3	(0)	19/61	(31)	1/4	(25)
Buchsbaum[47]	0/23	(0)	1/12	(7)					7/20	(35)	1/2	(50)
Averette et al[18]	3/40	(8)	2/9	(22)	2/9	(22)			2/20	(10)	1/2	(50)
Welander et al[413]					8/41	(20)	2/6	(33)	8/32	(25)	4/12	(33)
Berman et al[29]	8/158	(5)	3/25	(12)	40/240	(17)	1/3	(33)	44/177	(25)	3/17	(18)
Total	30/540	(6)	13/99	(13)	94/494	(19)	3/15	(20)	128/445	(29)	14/47	(30)

(Modified from Hoskins WJ, Perez CA, Young RC: Gynecologic tumors. In DeVita VT Jr, Hellman S, Rosenberg SA [eds]: Cancer: Principles and Practice of Oncology, 3rd ed. Philadelphia, JB Lippincott, 1989)

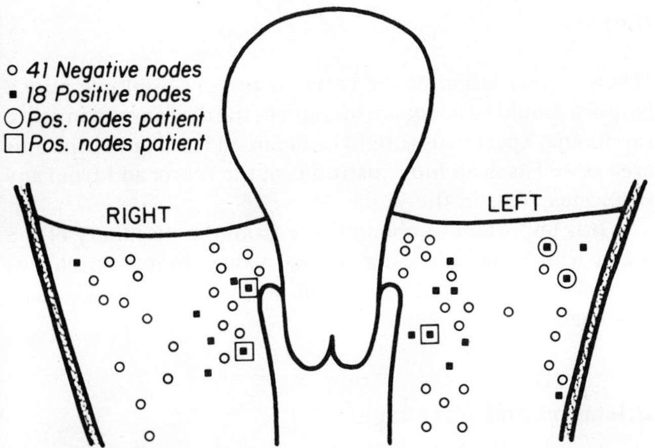

FIGURE 54–3. Location of positive and negative parametrial nodes in 12 patients with negative pelvic lymph nodes. (Girardi F, Lichtenegger W, Tamussion K, et al: Gynecol Oncol 34:206, 1989)

for 2 consecutive years and at least one every 3 years until the age of 65.[9] The American College of Obstetricians and Gynecologists[10] has strongly recommended that the practice of obtaining Papanicolaou smears be continued on an annual basis. Women who are at high risk of developing cervical carcinoma because of early age at first intercourse, multiple sexual partners, and multiparity should have a yearly smear. A complete gynecologic examination should be performed when the vaginal smear is obtained.[9]

The correlation between the cytologic diagnosis and subsequent histologic examination is over 90%.[177] Vaginal smears have been classified as follows: I (normal), II (atypical), III (dysplasia), IV (carcinoma *in situ*), and V (invasive carcinoma). However, some pathologists prefer to avoid the "class" system and describe the morphologic diagnosis on the cytologic examination.

The technique for obtaining the Papanicolaou smear has been described in standard textbooks.[265] Special attention should be directed to avoid using a lubricating agent (warm water on the speculum will suffice), to obtaining good "scrapings" from the cervix and vaginal posterior fornix (without blood), and to using a small swab to obtain an endocervical sample. If the cytologic smear shows atypia or mild dysplasia (class II), the smear should be repeated no sooner than 2 weeks, to allow representative cellular exfoliation. The patient should be instructed not to cleanse with a douche before the examination, and specimens should be obtained for studies of *Trichomonas*. If the findings persist, the patient should be followed up closely and smears repeated every 6 months.

If the cytologic smear shows dysplasia or malignant cells, directed biopsies at colposcopy should be carried out immediately. Endocervical curettage must always be performed except in pregnant women. If the biopsy results are negative, the procedure should be repeated and, if necessary, a conization should be performed.[257]

Papanicolaou smears can be useful in evaluating patients after radiation therapy. It must be remembered that dysplasia and bizarre epithelial changes following radiation therapy may be seen,[413] which makes the interpretation of cytologic smears difficult. Marcial and colleagues[225] reported on 342 patients with cervical carcinoma treated by irradiation who had a Papanicolaou smear within 4 months of therapy; approximately 90% had normal cytologic findings. A normal cytologic smear 4 to 12 months after irradiation is associated with a good prognosis with Stage I and Stage II disease, but not with Stage III and Stage IV disease. Marcial and colleagues concluded that the presence of tumor cells in the smear in the first 4 months after completion of irradiation is of no prognostic significance. However, Koss[196] reported that the presence of tumor cells 4 weeks or more following the completion of irradiation carried an ominous prognosis. The presence of tumor cells in the cytologic smear should be of concern if found 3 months after irradiation; if tumor cells are found, cervical biopsies, dilatation and curettage (D & C), and careful examination under anesthesia should be performed.

TABLE 54–4
Sites of Distant Metastases in 2220 Patients With Squamous Cell Carcinoma of the Cervix Treated Between September 1948 and December 1963

SITE	PATIENTS WITH SINGLE ORGAN METASTASIS	PATIENTS WITH MULTIPLE ORGAN METASTASES
Nodes	33 (30%)	157 (67.9%)
Supraclavicular	9	57
Paraaortic	12	54
Inguinal	8	43
Mediastinal	1	37
Iliac	1	28
Cervical	1	16
Axillary	0	12
Other	1	38
Lung	40 (36.3%)	86 (37.2%)
Bone	18 (16.3%)	67 (28%)
Abdomen	8 (7.2%)	97 (41.9%)
Generalized	0	37
Peritoneum	2	11
Liver	6	42
Gastrointestinal tract	0	24
Other	0	54
Miscellaneous	11	101

(Carlson V, Delclos L, Fletcher GH: Radiology 88:961–966, 1967)

TABLE 54–5
Diagnostic Workup for Carcinoma of the Uterine Cervix

General
- History
- Physical examination, including bimanual pelvic and rectal examinations

Diagnostic Procedures
- Cytologic smears (Papanicolaou) if not bleeding
- Colposcopy
- Conization (subclinical tumor)
- Punch biopsies (edge of gross tumor, four quadrants)
- Dilatation and curettage
- Cytoscopy, rectosigmoidoscopy (Stages IIB, III, IVA)

Radiographic Studies
- Standard
  - Chest radiography
  - Intravenous pyelography
  - Barium enema (Stage III, IVA, and earlier stages if symptoms are referable to colon or rectum)
- Complementary
  - Lymphangiography
  - Computed tomography or magnetic resonance

Laboratory Studies
- Complete blood count
- Blood chemistry
- Urinalysis

Colposcopy

Colposcopy may adequately evaluate the exocervix and a portion of the endocervix adjacent to the transition of the squamous and columnar epithelium (T zone). This examination, performed with a colposcope, provides a 10- to 15-fold magnification view of the cervix. A colposcope is essentially an instrument with a light source and a magnifying optical system; the focal length is 20 cm to 25 cm with a visual field of not less than 25 mm. To visualize the vascular system, a green filter is attached. Color photographs or television views can be obtained. Combined with cytologic examination and biopsy of grossly abnormal sites, colposcopy may be extremely useful in detecting the majority of early cervical lesions.[87,266]

Conization

Conization must be performed in specific situations such as when no gross lesion of the cervix is noted and an endocervical tumor is suspected; when the entire lesion cannot be seen with the colposcope; when diagnosis of microinvasive carcinoma is made on biopsy; when discrepancies are found between the cytologic and the histologic appearances of the lesion; and when the patient is not reliable for continuous follow-up.[257]

Conization involves a conical removal of a large portion of the exocervix and endocervix. Cold biopsy specimens should always be obtained with a scalpel or other appropriate instrument. At least 50% of the endocervical canal should be removed without compromising the internal sphincter. A curettage of the remaining endocervical canal should be carried out.

Hot conization (fulguration) should never be performed because it distorts the tissues and prevents pathologic examination.

Biopsy

When a gross lesion of the cervix is present, multiple punch biopsies should be adequate to confirm the diagnosis of invasive carcinoma. Specimens should be obtained from any suspicious area as well as in all four quadrants of the cervix and from any suspicious areas in the vagina.

It is important to obtain tissue from the periphery of the lesion with some adjoining normal tissue. Biopsy specimens from central ulcerated or necrotic areas may not be adequate for diagnosis.

Dilatation and Curettage

Because of the possibility of upper extension of the tumor that may modify the plan of therapy, fractional curettage of the endocervical canal and the endometrium is recommended at the time of initial evaluation or during the first intracavitary radioisotope insertion if the patient is treated with radiation therapy.

Laboratory Studies

For invasive carcinoma, patients should have the following laboratory studies: complete peripheral blood evaluation, including hemogram, white blood cell count, differential, and platelet count; SMA-12, with particular attention to blood urea nitrogen, creatinine, uric acid, and liver function values; and urinalysis.

Radiographic Studies

Chest radiographs and intravenous pyelograms should be obtained in all patients. A barium enema study should be performed on patients with Stage IIB, III, or IVA disease as well as on patients with earlier stages who have symptoms referable to the colon and rectum.

Lymphangiograms may provide useful information concerning lymph node involvement in the pelvis or periaortic nodes. Unfortunately, not all the lymph nodes to which carcinoma of the cervix may metastasize (such as the obturator or hypogastric nodes) are opacified by a pedal lymphangiogram. Small metastatic lesions do not produce enough modification of the architecture of the lymph node to be apparent in the lymphangiogram, and at times the metastatic tumor completely obliterates the lymph node or obstructs lymphatics, preventing visualization of the involved lymph nodes.

Piver and associates[303] reported on 102 patients on whom lymphangiograms were correlated with operative findings. Of 41 abnormal lymphangiograms, 40 were subsequently confirmed by biopsy and laparotomy (98% accuracy). In contrast, in 12 of 61 cases in which lymphangiograms were interpreted as normal, the patients had metastases in the lymph nodes at laparotomy (~20% false-negative rate). The initial enthusiasm for the use of the lymphangiogram has been replaced with a more realistic expectation.

DeMuylder and co-workers[79] reported on 100 patients with Stage IB carcinoma of the uterine cervix on whom lymphangiography was done before a radical hysterectomy with lymphadenectomy. The lymphangiograms of five patients were

TABLE 54–6
CT Scan in the Evaluation of Paraaortic Nodes

AUTHOR	NUMBER OF CASES	FIGO STAGE	SENSITIVITY (%)	SPECIFICITY (%)	ACCURACY (%)
Kilcheski et al[184]	36	I–IV, rec			80
Brenner et al[41,42]	42	I–IV, rec	77	86	83
Bandy et al[20]	44	I–IV, rec	75	91	86
DMC (1986)[52]	10	IIB–IV	67	100	90
	61	I–IV	67	100	98
Camilien et al[52]	51	IB–IIA	67	100	100
Camilien et al[52]	10	IIB–IV	67	100	90

(Modified from Camilien L, Gordon D, Fruchter RG, et al: Gynecol Oncol 30:209–215, 1988)

classified as abnormal, 15 as suspicious, and 80 as normal. Surgical/pathologic findings demonstrated pelvic lymph node metastasis in 18 patients (five with abnormal, three with suspicious, and ten with normal findings on the lymphangiogram). Thus the specificity of this test was 100%, but the sensitivity to detect metastases was low (28%). The lymphangiogram definitely is of value in outlining abnormal lymph nodes that can be included in the irradiated fields or, in the case of surgical management, those that should be removed by the surgeon for pathologic examination. Furthermore, Hammond and coworkers[133] found a correlation between lymphangiographic findings and prognosis in 215 patients with Stage IB through Stage IIIB treated with definitive irradiation.

Computed tomography (CT) is used more frequently, and at some institutions attempts are being made to replace lymphangiography with this procedure.[406] CT scan diagnostic accuracy is under evaluation. Camilien[52] reported observations in 61 patients with carcinoma of the uterine cervix who had both preoperative CT scans and exploratory laparotomy. The radiographic and surgical/pathologic findings were correlated, showing that 75% of the enlarged pelvic lymph nodes on CT scan contained metastases and 97% of the patients with negative nodes on CT scan were pathologically negative (specificity 97%). However, histologically positive pelvic nodes were often missed on CT scan (sensitivity 25%). The CT scan has been found to be more valuable in the evaluation of the paraaortic lymph nodes (specificity 100%; sensitivity 67%) by various authors (Table 54-6).

Magnetic resonance imaging is being used more frequently for assessment of extracervical extension.[152,390] Parametrial tumor was easily identified on T2-weighted images from the low-intensity cervix and uterine ligaments.[390,420] Ebner and associates[94] reported that in comparing MRI findings in 12 women with recurrent pelvic tumors and in ten with fibrotic mass (confirmed by laparotomy or biopsy in 21 patients), they were able to differentiate the two processes accurately in most instances. However, at the present time no reliable evaluation of the accuracy of this procedure is available. It is highly desirable to confirm abnormal or suspicious lymph node radiographic findings with CT-guided fine-needle aspiration biopsies.[423]

It has been emphasized by Griffin and colleagues[122] that in many instances staging procedures may have a low yield of positive findings (Table 54-7). However, these examinations must be selectively carried out, depending on the stage of the tumor. Even when normal, they have value as a baseline for evaluation of the patient following therapy.[71,273]

Surgical Staging Procedures

Some gynecologists have advocated the use of pretherapy laparotomy, particularly to evaluate the presence of periaortic lymph nodes.[206] However, it has not been demonstrated that this procedure increases the probability of survival in these patients.[169,295] In addition, a higher incidence of complications has been described when laparotomy and extensive periaortic lymph node dissection are carried out on patients who are later treated with definitive radiation therapy.[211]

TABLE 54–7
Tumor-Related Abnormalities Found in Patients with Carcinoma of the Uterine Cervix

		POSITIVE FINDINGS				
CLINICAL STAGE	NO. OF PATIENTS	CYTOSCOPY	PROCTOSCOPY	BARIUM ENEMA	INTRAVENOUS PYELOGRAM	CHEST X-RAY
I	111	0	0	0	0	0
IIA	123	0	0	0	0	0
IIB	44	0	0	0	2	1
IIIA	8	0	0	0	2	0
IIIB	37	2	5	3	24	1
IV	4	2	4	4	3	0
Total	327	4	9	7	31	2

(Griffin TW, Parker RG, Taylor WJ: Am J Roentgenol Radium Ther Nucl Med 127:825–827, 1976)

Wharton and associates[416] reported on 120 patients with squamous cell carcinoma of the uterine cervix who had a preirradiation celiotomy. Sixty-four patients had metastatic carcinoma in the lymph nodes (33% in the pelvis and 20% in the common iliac or periaortic lymph nodes or both). Sixteen had fatal complications and 32 had major intestinal complications, particularly small bowel obstruction and perforation. The majority of the patients with positive lymph nodes died with distant metastasis. Because of this negative experience, preirradiation laparotomy was discontinued at M. D. Anderson Cancer Center, and the status of the lymph nodes is investigated with lymphangiography and verified when possible with percutaneous transabdominal needle biopsy.[423]

Averette and associates[17] have reported a substantial lack of correlation between the clinical stage of patients with carcinoma of the cervix and the surgical findings (26% in Stage IB, 45% in Stage IIA, 60% in Stage IIB, 66% in Stage IIIA, and 95% in Stage IIIB). However, in other series these differences are considerably less, and the discrepancy may reflect the thoroughness of the presurgical evaluation or the search for metastatic sites (including lymph nodes) at the time of laparotomy. In a group of 48 patients with clinical Stage IB and 16 patients with Stage IIA treated with low-dose preoperative irradiation and radical hysterectomy at Washington University, only three were found to have a more advanced stage of disease at the time of the operation.[281]

Ketcham and colleagues[181] reported positive results of scalene fat pad biopsies in seven of 36 patients with Stage II, Stage III, and Stage IV carcinoma of the cervix and in four of 22 patients with postirradiation recurrences. Twenty-three patients with positive periaortic nodes described by Buchsbaum[47] had left scalene node biopsy, and eight (34.8%) had positive nodes. Buchsbaum recommends a scalene node excision prior to any treatment plan when positive aortic lymph nodes are found. However, this procedure is not routinely carried out at most institutions because of the low yield of positive specimens. For instance, Perez-Mesa and Spratt[288] noted that in 73 consecutive patients with various stages of cervical carcinoma, the scalene lymph node biopsy failed to demonstrate metastatic tumor in a single instance. Manetta and associates[222] found no scalene node metastasis in 24 patients with recurrent carcinoma of the cervix evaluated for exploration and possible pelvic exenteration.

STAGING

It is imperative that the gynecologic oncologist and the radiation oncologist jointly stage the tumor in every patient, with bimanual pelvic and rectal examination under general anesthesia. Ideally, staging should be done before institution of therapy. However, occasionally after an initial evaluation, the final staging is postponed because of logistic and economic reasons until the time of a surgical procedure or the first intracavitary radioisotope insertion, which should be done within 2 weeks from initiation of the external-beam irradiation, if the patient is treated with this modality. In surgically treated patients, the clinical staging can be done immediately before the radical hysterectomy is performed.

The initial staging system proposed in 1929 by a subcommittee of the League of Nations was later revised in 1937 and 1950. These functions were taken over by FIGO in collaboration with the World Health Organization and the International Union Against Cancer. The staging recommendations were last revised in 1987. The current criteria for the various stages are defined in Table 54-8.[158] A parallel TNM staging system has been proposed by the American Joint Committee.[24] The clinical staging groups are summarized in Figure 54-4. All histologic types should be included. When a disagreement occurs regarding the staging, the earlier stage should be selected for statistical purposes. It is noteworthy that the latest revision categorizes minimal microscopic stromal invasion as Stage IA1 and invasion of 5 mm or less in depth or 7 mm or less in horizontal spread as Stage IA2. Stage IB includes all invasive tumors larger than those in Stage IA2 limited to the cervix. Stage IB occult is no longer used. Kolstad[194] reviewed the results of therapy in 643 patients with microinvasive carcinoma reclassified as Stage IA1 or Stage IA2. Three (1.3%) of the 232 patients with Stage IA1 disease and 12 (2.9%) of 411 Stage IA2 patients had local recurrence in addition to four pelvic recurrences, confirming the validity of the staging modification. Similar conclusions were reached by Tsukamoto and co-workers.[391]

The FIGO staging system is based on clinical evaluation

TABLE 54–8
Staging of Carcinoma of the Uterine Cervix

AJC	FIGO	
PRIMARY TUMOR (T)		
TX		Primary tumor cannot be assessed
T0		No evidence of primary tumor
Tis	0	Carcinoma *in situ*
T1	I	Cervical carcinoma confined to uterus (extension to corpus should be disregarded)
T1a	Ia	Preclinical invasive carcinoma, diagnosed by microscopy only
T1a1	Iaa1	Minimal microscopic stromal invasion
T1a2	Ia2	Tumor with invasive component 5 mm or less in depth taken from the base of the epithelium and 7 mm or less in horizontal spread
T1b	Ib	Tumor larger than T1a2
T2	II	Cervical carcinoma invades beyond uterus but not to pelvic wall or to the lower third of vagina
T2a	IIa	Without parametrial invasion
T2b	IIb	With parametrial invasion
T3	III	Cervical carcinoma extends to the pelvic wall or involves lower third of vagina or causes hydronephrosis or nonfunctioning kidney
T3a	IIIa	Tumor involves lower third of the vagina, no extension to pelvic wall
T3b	IIIb	Tumor extends to pelvic wall or causes hydronephrosis or nonfunctioning kidney
T4*	IVa	Tumor invades mucosa of bladder or rectum or extends beyond true pelvis
REGIONAL LYMPH NODES (N)		
Regional lymph nodes include paracervical, parametrial, hypogastric (obturator), common, internal and external iliac, presacral and sacral.		
NX		Regional lymph nodes cannot be assessed
N0		No regional lymph node metastasis
N1		Regional lymph node metastasis
DISTANT METASTASIS (M)		
MX		Presence of distant metastasis cannot be assessed
M0		No distant metastasis
M1	IVb	Distant metastasis

**Note: Presence of bullous edema is not sufficient evidence to classify a tumor as T4. (Beahrs OH, Henson DE, Hutter RVP, Myers MH [eds]: Manual for Staging of Cancer, 3rd ed, pp 151–153. Philadelphia, JB Lippincott, 1988)*

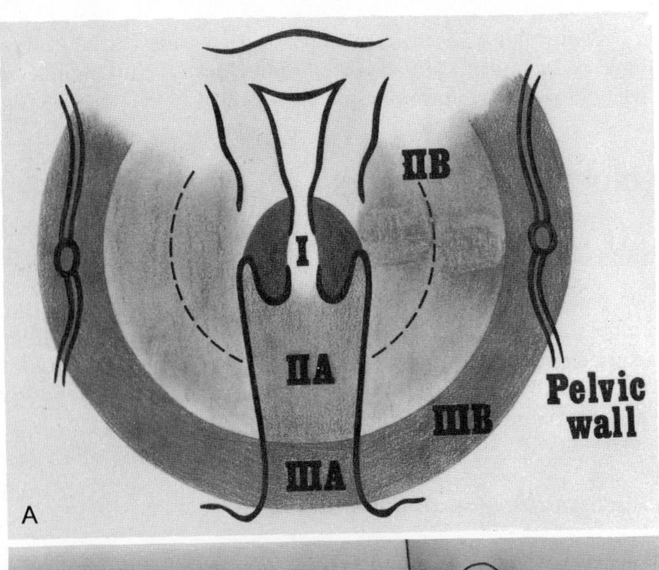

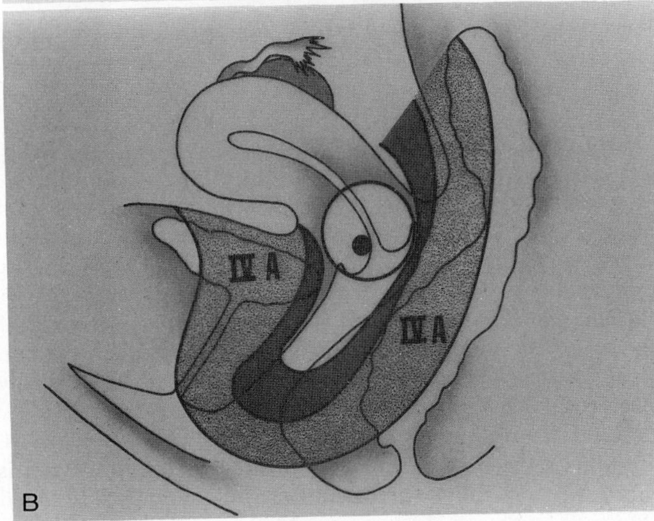

FIGURE 54–4. (**A** and **B**) Diagrammatic representation of various anatomic stages of carcinoma of the uterine cervix, according to the FIGO classification.

(inspection, palpation, colposcopy), roentgenographic examination of the chest, kidneys, and skeleton, and endocervical curettage and biopsies. Lymphangiograms, arteriograms, computed tomography findings, and laparoscopy or laparotomy findings should not be used for clinical staging.

Suspected invasion of the bladder or rectum should be confirmed by biopsy. Bullous edema of the bladder and swelling of the mucosa of the rectum are not accepted as definitive criteria for staging.

For a lesion to be classified as Stage IIIB, the tumor should definitely extend to the lateral pelvic wall, although fixation is not required.

Patients with hydronephrosis or nonfunction of the kidney ascribed to extension of the tumor are classified as Stage IIIB, regardless of the pelvic findings. The currently used staging systems could be modified to accommodate some prognostic factors that have been reported, such as the significance of endometrial extension of cervical carcinoma, stromal invasion, and tumor volume in Stage I and Stage IIA carcinoma (barrel-shaped in the cervical or bulky tumor presentations), lymphatic/vascular permeation, and involvement of the lateral parametrium in Stage IIB as opposed to the medial parametrium.[300, 332, 400]

PATHOLOGIC CLASSIFICATION

Over 90% of tumors are of the squamous cell type. Approximately 7% to 10% are classified as adenocarcinoma, and 1% to 2% are clear cell, mesonephric type.

Squamous cell or *epidermoid carcinoma* is composed of cores and nests of epithelial cells arranged in random fashion and forming multiple arborescences of different-sized configurations. The keratinizing cells show foci of keratinization with cornified pearls. The nonkeratinizing cells have well-demarcated tumor-stromal borders but no evidence of keratinization. The small cells have a spindle or small, round appearance and poorly defined tumor-stromal borders. The connective tissue stroma may be infiltrated by tumor and show edema of the collagen fibers, infiltration by leukocytes, and neovessel formation. The tumor may destroy the basement membrane and grow in large cores throughout the stroma. Electron microscopy may show desmosomes and tonofilaments. Wentz and Reagan[413] have divided squamous cell carcinoma into three types: keratinizing, nonkeratinizing, and small cell type.

Adenocarcinoma arises from the cylindrical mucosa of the endocervix or the mucus-secreting endocervical glands.[1] The endocervical adenocarcinoma may form mucosal glands lined by high columnar cells and produce tubular folds oriented in many directions. The stroma surrounds the epithelial formations. As the tumor becomes less differentiated, the cells become more bizzare, contain more mitoses, and do not have a glandular appearance. Sometimes it is difficult to differentiate a primary endocervical adenocarcinoma from an endometrial tumor. Drescher and associates[88] described a higher incidence of involvement of the uterine corpus and the regional lymph nodes in 21 patients with adenocarcinoma compared with a similar number of patients with squamous cell carcinoma. A well-differentiated cervical adenocarcinoma has been improperly designated as "adenoma malignum" when it is truly a malignant tumor that invades adjacent tissues and may produce distant metastasis.[357]

Adenosquamous carcinoma is relatively rare (2% to 5% of all cervical carcinomas) and consists of intermingled epithelial cell cores and glandular structures. The squamous component is frequently nonkeratinizing.[344] If the squamous component is benign metaplasia, the tumor is called *adenoacanthoma.* Saigo and associates[344] reported a 39% 5-year survival rate for patients with adenosquamous carcinoma compared with 51% for adenocarcinoma and 64% for clear cell carcinoma.

Glassy cell carcinoma is considered a poorly differentiated adenosquamous tumor with a distinctive histologic appearance. Survival is poor after surgery or irradiation. Ulbright and Gersell,[393] in five cases of glassy cell carcinoma evaluated by light and electron microscopy, described both glandular and squamous differentiation, with the tumor probably originating from the subcylindric reserve cells. Only two patients were alive with no evidence of disease at 15 and 24 months after therapy. Littman and associates[215] reported only four of 13 patients, the majority with Stage II disease, surviving 5 years (six had extrapelvic failures).

A small group of adenocarcinomas are *clear cell carcinomas* (mesonephric) and may grow in a tubular, glandular, papillary, or solid pattern. These tumors are composed of clear and "hobnail" cells. The clear cell is characterized by a voluminous cytoplasm filled with glycogen and the hobnail cell by single cell apical projections into the neoplastic lumina.[132, 135, 264]

In 1903, Meyer described a *mesonephric adenocarcinoma,* reports of which have occasionally appeared in the literature.[135, 155] Clear cell adenocarcinoma not related to DES exposure[139] accounts for approximately 2% of primary cervical adenocarcinomas and is thought to arise in mesonephric remnants. These tumors may appear at any time, with one third occurring in women under 30 years old.[170] Patients with mesonephric adenocarcinoma are treated with radical surgery or definitive radiation therapy. Kaminsky and Maier[170] reported on 12 of 21 women with follow-up of 4 to 23 years surviving after initial therapy. The survival rate for Stage I and Stage II patients was 77%.

Adenocystic carcinoma or *cylindroma* is an uncommon type of adenocarcinoma (less than 1%) with an appearance similar to that of its counterparts in the salivary gland or the bronchial tree.[115,321]

Some investigators believe that *small cell carcinoma* of the cervix arises from endocervical argyrophil cells or precursors, multipotential neuroendocrine cells,[276] but many small cell tumors do not contain morphologic evidence of neuroendocrine origin. Lymphatic and vascular invasion are significantly more common in small cell carcinoma (noted in 58% of patients with Stage IB; 40% of these patients had lymph node metastases at the time of radical surgery). The 5-year survival rate was 66%, which was comparable to other subtypes.[101] In contrast, Wentz and Reagan[413] reported only 17% survival 5 years after therapy.

Van Nagell and associates,[401] in an analysis of 25 patients, noted a high incidence of pelvic recurrences and distant metastases, with a 5-year survival rate of 54% for all stages compared with 68% for matched large cell nonkeratinizing squamous cell carcinomas and 74% for patients with keratinizing squamous cell carcinomas.

Gersell and associates[108] reported only three of 15 patients with small cell carcinoma alive at 5, 11, and 78 months after initial diagnosis and treatment. In the majority of the patients the cervical stroma was extensively infiltrated by single, small round cells. Invasion of vascular spaces was a prominent feature in seven tumors. Thirteen tumors showed evidence of cytokeratin on immunohistochemical studies, and at least one neuroendocrine marker was found in all 13 tumors (neuron-specific enolase, Leu-7, chromogranin, and synaptophysin).

Basaloid carcinoma, an extremely uncommon tumor, is characterized by nests or cords of small basaloid cells, prominent peripheral palisading of cells in the tumor nests, no significant stromal reaction, and an infiltrating growth pattern. It also has been called adenoid-basal carcinoma. Some authors have suggested a slow growth pattern with limited local invasiveness and low probability of lymph node metastases.[72]

Primary *sarcomas* of the cervix have been occasionally described (*e.g.*, leiomyosarcoma, rhabdomyosarcoma, stromal sarcoma, carcinosarcoma).[36,347]

Malignant lymphomas, primary or secondary in the cervix, have been sporadically reported. They behave and should be treated as other lymphomas.[326,367]

PROGNOSTIC FACTORS

Age

According to some reports, carcinoma of the cervix has the same prognosis in younger as in older patients.[28,205] Other authors have noted decreased survival rate in women under 35[315] or 40 years,[73] who have a greater frequency of poorly differentiated tumors.

Race and Socioeconomic Status

Several authors have noted a correlation between race or socioeconomic characteristics of patients and outcome of therapy.

Tumor Volume

Nahhas and colleagues,[254] in 88 patients with Stage IB and Stage IIA of the cervix, described a greater incidence of metastatic lymph nodes in the presence of deep stromal invasion or lymphatic permeation. Furthermore, these patients had a lower 2-year relapse-free survival rate and a greater incidence of recurrences. Similar observations were reported by Rotman and associates[334] and Alvarez and colleagues[8] in surgically treated patients.

Piver and Chung[298] and Van Nagell and co-workers[400] have shown a greater incidence of lymphatic and distant metastasis and lower survival rate in patients with bulky and barrel-shaped Stage IB and Stage IIA tumors treated by radical hysterectomy (Table 54-9). Similar findings were reported by Fletcher[104] and Perez and associates[281] (Fig. 54-5) in patients treated with irradiation.

Several retrospective studies have demonstrated decreased survival and a greater incidence of distant metastases in patients with endometrial extension of a primary cervical carcinoma (endometrial stroma invasion or replacement of the endometrium by tumor only).[241,281] Grimard and associates,[125] on the other hand, confirmed these findings only in patients with Stage IB tumors but not in more advanced stages.

Similar findings have been reported by Noguchi and associates[262] in 301 patients treated with radical hysterectomy (uter-

TABLE 54–9
Size of Cervical Lesion and Lymph Node Metastasis in Stages IB and IIA Cervical Carcinoma

	STAGE IB				STAGE IIA			
SIZE (cm)	NO. OF PATIENTS	NO. WITH METASTASES	PERCENT		NO. OF PATIENTS	NO. WITH METASTASES	PERCENT	
≤1	22	4	18.1	21.1	11	3	27.2	21.0
2–3	72	16	22.1		27	5	18.5	
4–5	45	16	35.5	35.2	44	19	43.1	42.1
≥6	6	3	50.0		13	5	38.4	
Total	145	39	26.8		95	32	33.6	

(Piver MS, Chung WS: Obstet Gynecol 46:507, 1975)

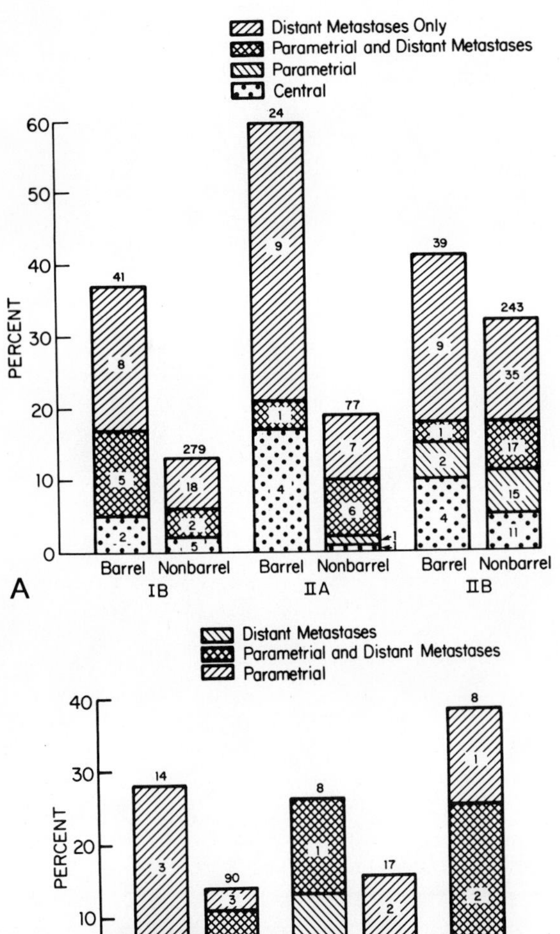

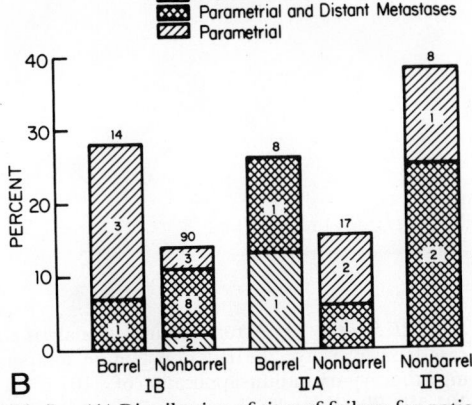

FIGURE 54–5. (**A**) Distribution of sites of failure for patients treated with irradiation alone. There is a significantly greater incidence of distant metastases for the patients with barrel-shaped cervix in Stages IB and IIA ($P < 0.01$). (**B**) Distribution of sites of failure for patients treated with irradiation and surgery. A greater incidence of distant metastases was seen in the patients with barrel-shaped cervix than in those with non-barrel-shaped cervix in all stages. (Perez CA, Kao MS: Int J Radiat Oncol Biol Phys 11:1903–1909, 1985)

ine body invasion in 7.8% of Stage IB, 25.5% of Stage IIA, and 38.2% of Stage IIB patients). Most of the patients with invasion of the uterine body had extension to other surrounding tissues (vaginal wall in 58.5%, parametrial infiltration in 87%, and pelvic lymph node metastases in 52.3%). Extension of cervical cancer in the uterine body was associated with a higher incidence of peritoneal carcinomatosis and distant metastases. Patients without uterine body invasion had a 5-year survival rate of 92.4% compared with 53.8% in patients with invasion.

Histology

Most reports have shown no significant correlation between survival or tumor behavior with the degree of differentiation of squamous cell carcinoma or adenocarcinoma of the cervix. Whereas Reagan and Fu,[323] Wentz and Reagan,[414] and Swan and Roddick[373] demonstrated prognostic value of histologic differentiation in patients treated with irradiation, others such as Goellner,[111] Gunderson,[126] and Crissman and associates[69] have failed to observe a correlation between histologic parameters and patient survival.

General Host Factors

In addition to stage and tumor volume, histologic type of lesion, and vascular or lymphatic invasion,[31] other host factors affect the prognosis of patients with cervical carcinoma. Evans and Bergsjo,[97] Bush and co-workers,[50] and Vigario and associates[403] have reported a greater incidence of pelvic recurrences and lower survival in patients with anemia (hemoglobin below 10 to 11 g/dl) (Table 54-10). The use of blood transfusions improved the response of the tumor to radiation therapy, decreasing the occurrence of pelvic failures and enhancing survival.[51] Hirst,[142] in a review of experimental and clinical physiopathologic data, emphasized that both duration and severity of hypoxia may be important in determining cell survival. Blood transfusion is generally beneficial to the anemic cancer patient, but it must be given as soon as possible before the first irradiation dose to maximize its effects.

Jenkin and Stryker[162] observed a higher incidence of pelvic recurrences and complications in patients with arterial hypertension (diastolic pressure above 110 mm Hg).

Decreased survival rate in 260 patients with oral temperatures higher than 100°F was reported by Van Herik[399] in a study of 666 patients. In 21.2% of the patients pelvic inflammatory disease was noted, and in 6.9% local infection was found. However, in 57.3% of the patients, no specific etiologic factor could be determined. The prognosis was worse with a longer duration of fever (more than 7 days). More recently, Kapp and Lawrence[171] reported similar observations in 398 patients; patients with temperatures over 101°F had a higher incidence of distant metastases (Fig. 54-6) and lower survival.

Flow Cytometry Studies on DNA and Growth Fraction

In recent years, attempts have been made to correlate the distribution of peridiploid and aneuploid tumors by flow cytometry with prognosis. Some authors have noted no significant difference in recurrence rates between patients with diploid or aneuploid tumors,[93,366] whereas others, such as Rutgers and associates,[339] observed a less favorable prognosis in tumors with a diploid or tetraploid DNA content in comparison with the non-

TABLE 54–10
The Log-Rank Adjusted Local Relapse Rate, Distant Relapse Rate, and Total Relapse for 1055 Patients With Stage IIB or III Cancer of the Cervix According to the Average Hb Level During Radiation Therapy

Hb (g/dl)	NO. OF PATIENTS	LRR	DRR	RR
<10	19	0.46	0.18	0.49
10 to 11.9	319	0.29	0.24	0.47
12 to 13.9	578	0.20	0.16	0.33
≥14	129	0.20	0.18	0.33
P value		0.002	0.1	0.0007

Hb: hemoglobin; LRR: local relapse rate; DDR: distant relapse rate; RR: total relapse rate (Bush RS: Int J Radiat Oncol Biol Phys 12:2047–2050, 1986)

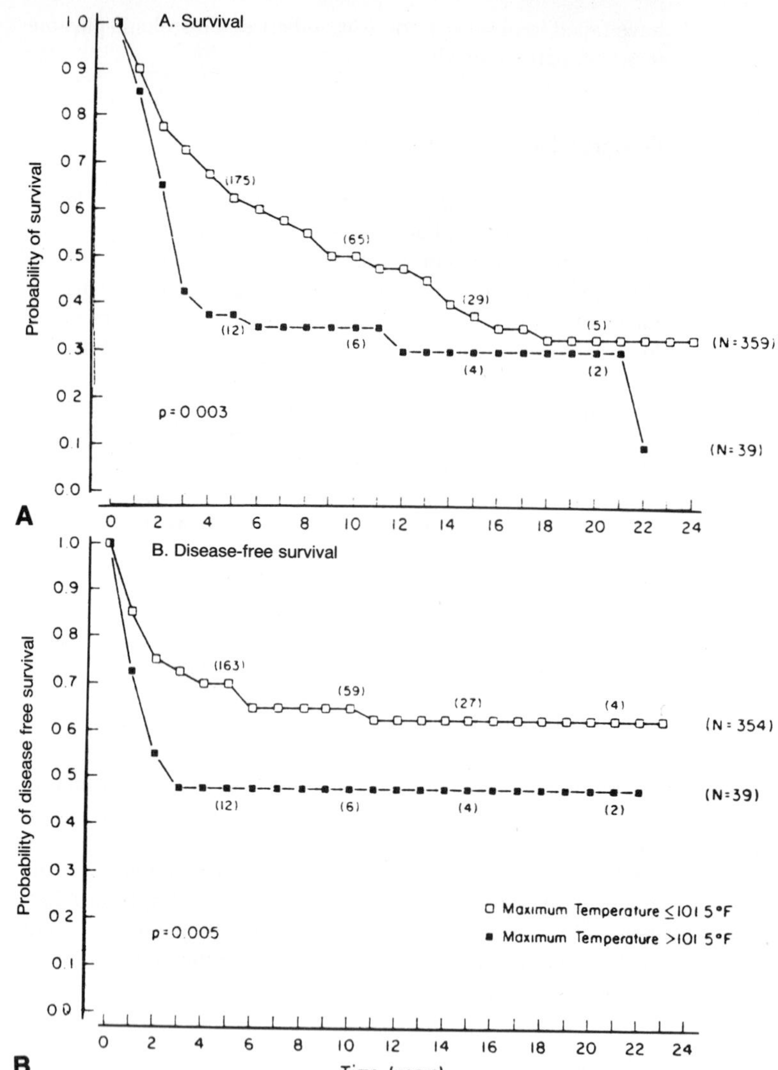

FIGURE 54–6. (**A**) Actuarial survival analysis and (**B**) disease-free survival on the basis of maximum temperature during intracavitary radium application of ≤101.5°F (□) *versus* > 101.5°F (■). (Kapp DS, Lawrence R: Int J Radiat Oncol Biol Phys 10:2281–2292, 1984)

diploid/nontetraploid tumors when the parameters were combined with age (under 51 years) and degree of differentiation of the tumor. However, the difference was not statistically significant.

Strang and associates[366] noted more relapses in tumors with S-phase rate of 20% or greater. Kelland and Steel,[175] analyzing the response to irradiation of five established carcinomas of cervix cell lines exposed to various dose rates (1.6 cGy, 3.2 cGy, or 150 cGy per minute), noted a significant difference in radiosensitivity for various cell lines, and the data were well fitted by the incomplete repair model.[383] The authors suggested that this predictive testing of intrinsic cellular radiosensitivity may be of clinical value in the treatment of these patients.

GENERAL MANAGEMENT

Controversy has existed between those who advocate either radical surgery or radiation therapy for the treatment of carcinoma of the uterine cervix. Patients should be treated with close collaboration between the gynecologic oncologist and the radiation oncologist, and an integrated team approach should be vigorously pursued.

It is critical that the results of surgical series be reported, based on the initial clinical staging, which include all patients evaluated for that therapeutic modality.

Carcinoma *In Situ*

Patients with carcinoma *in situ,* which may include those with severe dysplasia, are best treated with a total abdominal hysterectomy with or without a small vaginal cuff.[67] The decision to remove the ovaries depends on the age of the patient and the status of the ovaries.

Occasionally, when the patient wishes to have more children, carcinoma *in situ* may be treated conservatively with a therapeutic conization.[34] This procedure should be judiciously selected when the extent of tumor allows it and the patient is reliable for continued follow-up.[59]

The use of therapeutic conization is controversial due to reports of persistent or recurrent carcinoma *in situ.*[349,356] Kolstad and Klem[195] reported that, in 795 patients with carcinoma *in situ* who were treated with therapeutic conization, 19 (2.3%) developed recurrent carcinoma *in situ* and seven (0.9%) had disease that evolved to invasive carcinoma. A nonrandomized comparable group of 238 patients were treated with hysterectomy; three patients (1.2%) developed recurrent carcinoma *in situ* and five (2.1%) developed invasive carcinoma.

Although some surgeons use frozen sections of the conization specimen to decide whether hysterectomy should be performed, pathologists prefer permanent sections because a more thorough examination of the specimen can be carried out.[173] A therapeutic hysterectomy can be performed 6 weeks after the conization.

Colposcopy for periodic evaluation plays a major role in the conservation management of patients with carcinoma *in situ* of the cervix.

Irradiation may be useful for the treatment of *in situ* carcinoma, particularly in patients with strong medical contraindications for surgery or when there is extension of the lesion to the vaginal wall or multifocal carcinoma *in situ* both in the cervix and the vagina.[67,78,195]

In a group of 26 patients with carcinoma *in situ* treated at Washington University with intracavitary irradiation alone (approximately 5000 mgh—4500 cGy to point A) with tandem and ovoids, no recurrences were recorded.[277]

Stage IA

The definition of microinvasive (Stage IA) carcinoma of the cervix lacks uniformity of diagnostic criteria; the volume of tumor in the stroma may be a more reliable criterion than depth of invasion to arrive at a definition of Stage IA.[49] Depth of invasion and tumor confluence have been identified as prognostic factors that should be taken into consideration in the planning of therapy.[26,136] According to Kolstad,[194] lesions less than 1 mm in depth can be treated with conization, provided that all margins are tumor-free and that continued careful follow-up is instituted. Early invasive carcinoma of the cervix (Stage IA2) is usually treated with a total abdominal or modified radical hysterectomy, but it can be treated with intracavitary radioactive sources alone (6500 mgh to 8000 mgh [6000 cGy to 7500 cGy to point A] in one or two insertions, respectively). When the depth of penetration of the stroma by tumor is less than 3 mm, the incidence of lymph node metastasis is 1% or less, and a lymph node dissection or pelvic external-beam irradiation is not warranted.[99,257,351] With more extensive lesions a Wertheim radical hysterectomy with pelvic lymphadenectomy is the preferred treatment. Tumor control with all treatment methods is close to 100%, with patients eventually dying of intercurrent disease.[336]

Stages IB and IIA

The choice of definitive irradiation or radical surgery for Stage IB and Stage IIA carcinoma of the cervix remains highly controversial, and the preference of one procedure over the other depends on the institution, the gynecologic oncologist or radiation oncologist involved, the general condition of the patient, and the characteristics of the lesion. An operation has been preferred by some clinicians in young women because of the desire to preserve the ovaries[409] and the possibility of a more pliable vagina following surgery. According to some gynecologists, treatment with radical pelvic surgery may alter sexual function to a lesser degree than radiation therapy.[2,355] Another important alleged advantage of surgery is the opportunity to do a thorough pelvic and abdominal evaluation because a disparity exists between the clinical and surgical-pathologic stages. However, surgical staging has not been shown to improve overall patient survival.[259,416] It should be noted that exploratory laparotomy eliminates from the surgical group those patients with more advanced disease.[149]

Despite a slower regression after irradiation, which reflects cellular kinetics and a slow growth, no difference in tumor control or survival rates has been observed in adenocarcinomas when compared with those of epidermoid carcinoma.[124,342] Because of the predilection for endocervical involvement in adenocarcinoma, a combination of irradiation and conservative hysterectomy has been advocated by some authors.[341,342]

Bulky endocervical tumors and the so-called barrel-shaped cervix have a higher incidence of central recurrence, pelvic and periaortic lymph node metastasis, and distant dissemination.[104,219] Because of the inability of the intracavitary sources to encompass all of the tumor in a high-dose volume, larger doses of external radiation to the whole pelvis or extrafascial hysterectomy or both have been advocated to improve therapeutic results.[230,269] Durrance and co-workers[93] and Nelson and colleagues[256] recommended an extrafascial conservative hysterectomy 6 weeks after completion of high-dose preoperative irradiation (2000 cGy to the whole pelvis, additional 3000 cGy to the parametria with midline shielding, and one intracavitary insertion for 6000 mgh, delivering about 5500 cGy to point A).

Stages IIB, III, and IVA

Patients with Stage IIB and Stage III tumors are treated with irradiation alone. Patients with Stage IVA disease (bladder or rectal invasion) can be treated either with high doses of external-beam irradiation to the whole pelvis, intracavitary insertions, and additional parametrial irradiation or with pelvic exenteration.[21,22,76,103,189]

No known chemotherapeutic agents have proven effective in the adjuvant treatment of patients with advanced disease, which has a higher incidence of distant metastasis. However, several reports have been published on the concomitant use of irradiation and cytotoxic agents (cisplatin, 5-FU, in a few trials combined with mytomycin-C) administered to obtain a radiosensitizing effect.[82,123,165,203,386]

Management of Small Cell Carcinoma of the Cervix

Small cell carcinoma of the cervix, like its counterparts in the lung and other anatomic locations, has a high proliferation rate and marked propensity to regional lymph node and distant metastases. Therefore patients with this disease need to be evaluated in conjunction with a medical oncologist in the same manner as patients with primary tumors of the lung. The workup should include bone marrow aspiration biopsy of the iliac crest and other tests to rule out metastatic spread. Furthermore, the basic therapy should include a combination of cytotoxic agents with pelvic external-beam and intracavitary irradiation. As in carcinoma of the lung, it is probably more efficacious to administer two or three cycles of chemotherapy before the initiation of radiation therapy if there is no acute bleeding. When bleeding is present, prompt institution of radiation therapy is necessary.

At Washington University, patients with small cell cervical carcinoma are treated with the same irradiation techniques as outlined for other histologic varieties of cervical carcinoma in combination with multiagent chemotherapy. The most frequently prescribed drugs are cyclophosphamide (1000 mg/m^2), doxorubicin ([Adriamycin] 50 mg/m^2), and vincristine (1 mg/

m^2) given every 3 or 4 weeks. Etoposide (VP16) is being incorporated more frequently into some of the regimens. Depending on the patient's age and tolerance to therapy, the doses of irradiation may be decreased by approximately 10%.

Combination of Irradiation and Surgery

At some institutions the combination of preoperative irradiation and a radical hysterectomy has been used in the treatment of patients with Stage IB and Stage IIA disease.[58,251,317,320] Sometimes an intracavitary insertion alone before surgery has been used (5000 mgh to 6000 mgh). The rationale for the use of an operation has been the alleged inability of irradiation to completely eradicate the metastatic tumor in the pelvic lymph nodes.[213,251,379]

Postoperative Radiation Therapy Following Radical Hysterectomy

Patients who have undergone radical hysterectomy with no preoperative radiation therapy at Washington University are considered for postoperative radiation therapy if they have positive pelvic lymph nodes, microscopic positive margins of resection in the cervix, deep stromal invasion, or vascular/lymphatic permeation.

In patients receiving postoperative irradiation, extreme care should be exercised in designing treatment techniques, including intracavitary insertions. Because of the surgical extirpation of the uterus, the bladder and the rectosigmoid may be closer to the radioactive sources than in the patient with an intact uterus (Fig. 54-7). Furthermore, vascular supply may be affected by the surgical procedure, and adhesions can prevent mobilization of the small bowel loops that occasionally may be fixed in the pelvis.

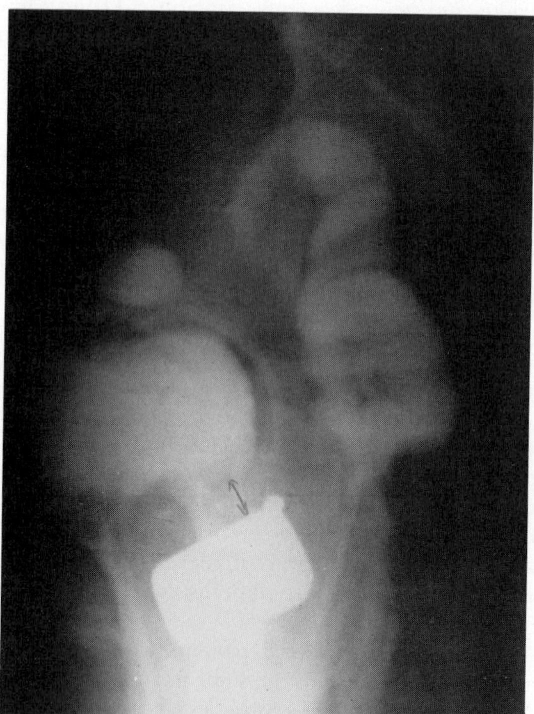

FIGURE 54–7. Lateral radiograph of the pelvis in a patient treated with an intracavitary insertion (vaginal colpostats only) following a radical hysterectomy. Close proximity of the bladder and the rectum to the applicator is evident.

When metastatic pelvic lymph nodes are present, treatment consists of 5000 cGy to the whole pelvis. Patients with positive common iliac or periaortic node metastases should receive 5000 cGy to the periaortic region as well.

In patients not irradiated preoperatively, for whom postoperative irradiation is indicated for deep stromal invasion in the cervix or close/positive surgical margins, external-beam irradiation is administered (2000 cGy to the whole pelvis and 3000 cGy to the parametria with a small midline block) in combination with an intracavitary insertion for 6500 cGy to the vaginal mucosa (about 1800 mgh) with two colpostats. The localization films and isodose curves seen with this therapy are shown in Figure 54-8. Alternatively, in some institutions external-beam irradiation alone (5000 cGy to the midplane of the pelvis) has been used.

No controlled studies are available showing improved survival with postoperative pelvic irradiation following radical surgery in the presence of positive pelvic nodes. Guttman[127] reported on 50 patients receiving postoperative pelvic irradiation (4000 cGy to 5000 cGy) in 4 to 5 weeks following radical hysterectomy. Two patients received paraaortic irradiation (4000 cGy). Eleven of 14 patients with Stage I, 24 of 31 with Stage II, and four of five with Stage III tumors survived 5 years. The overall 5-year survival rate in the entire group was 76%, and at 10 years it was 50%. Complications were uncommon.

Fuller and co-workers[107] found 71 of 431 patients with Stage IB and Stage IIA carcinoma of the uterine cervix treated with radical hysterectomy to have pelvic lymph node metastases. Postoperative radiation therapy (4000 cGy in 4 weeks) was given. In 32 patients with one to two positive nodes the 5-year survival rate in the irradiated group was slightly higher than in the nonirradiated group (about 60% *versus* 40%, respectively). Lower survival rate was observed in seven patients with three or more involved nodes who received postoperative irradiation. Nahhas and co-workers[254] noted two recurrences in nine patients treated with postoperative irradiation compared with two recurrences in four patients after a radical hysterectomy and lymphadenectomy alone.

Gonzalez and associates[112] reported that in 89 patients with Stage IB and Stage IIA with positive lymph nodes receiving postoperative irradiation, the 5- and 10-year survival rates were 60% and 51%, respectively. By comparison, 43 patients with negative lymph nodes had a survival rate of 85%. Multifactorial analysis showed that in the patients with lymph node metastasis microscopic infiltration in the parametrium, invasion of the vascular space by tumor, and histologic type of lesion were important prognostic factors. In the 89 patients with metastatic lymph nodes, 37 (41.5%) developed a recurrence, 21 (23.6%) of them in the pelvis, alone or combined with distant metastasis. In the 43 patients with negative lymph nodes, only three (7%) had a pelvic failure, two of which were combined with distant metastasis. In the surviving patients there were four gastrointestinal and seven genitourinary severe complications requiring surgical correction. In four patients asymptomatic stenosis of the uterus was detected by intravenous pyelogram performed routinely every year.

Kim and associates[186] reported on 38 patients (selected from 240 with Stage IB disease) receiving postoperative pelvic irradiation after radical hysterectomy because of close surgical margins or metastatic pelvic lymph nodes. Patients with close surgical margins were treated with intracavitary vaginal ovoid insertions (5000 cGy at 1 cm above and between the two ovoids). Patients with both positive margins and pelvic lymph nodes received external whole-pelvis irradiation only (5000 cGy to 6000 cGy in 6 weeks delivered through AP/PA portals). The

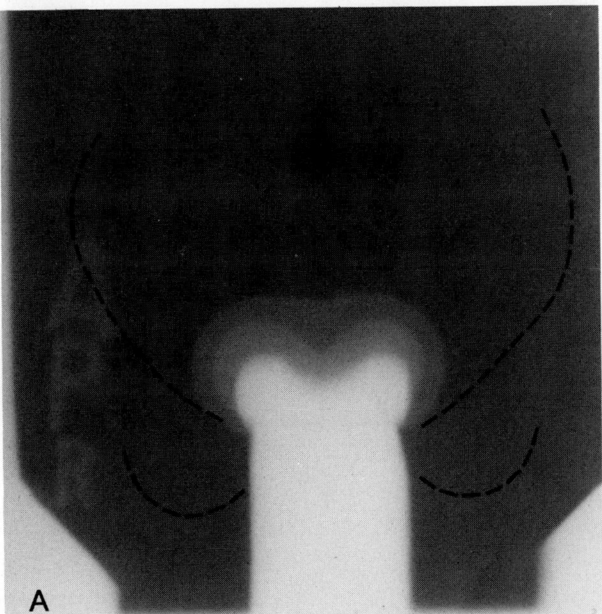

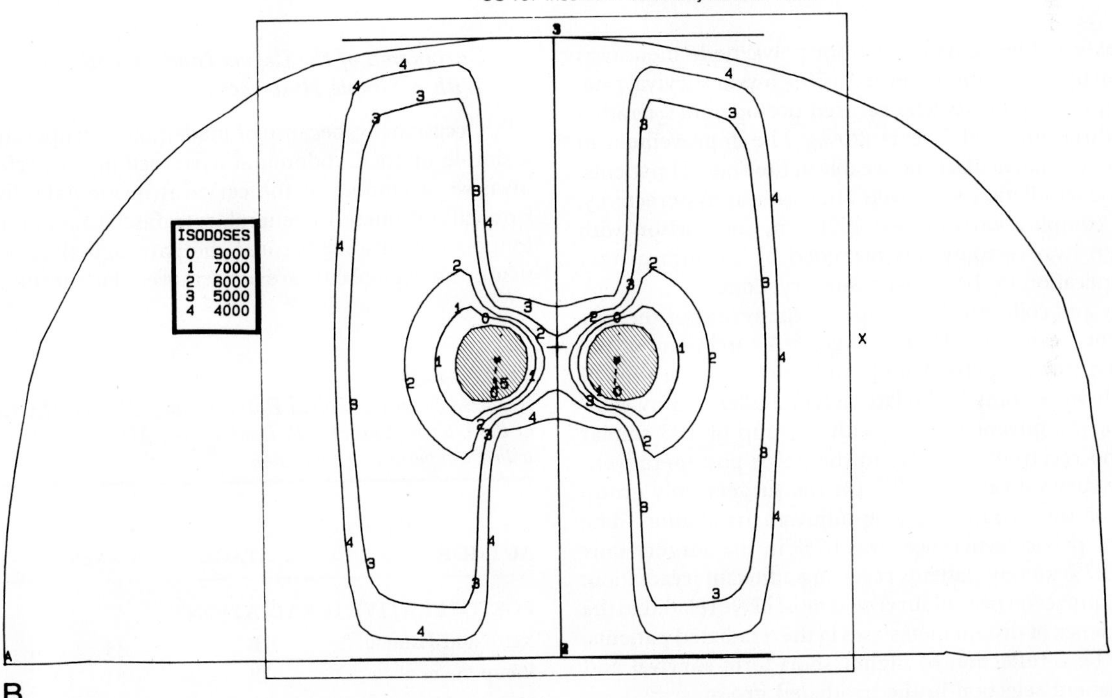

FIGURE 54–8. (**A**) Anteroposterior localization film of the pelvis with a small midline wedge in a patient receiving postoperative irradiation following a radical hysterectomy. The wedge is designed to cover only the volume irradiated with two ovoids inserted in the vaginal vault. (**B**) Composite isodose curve through the midplane of the ovoids for patient receiving postoperative irradiation (2000 cGy to the whole pelvis and 3000 cGy to the parametrium with small midline block and 6000 cGy to the vaginal mucosa with brachytherapy insertion).

overall recurrence rate was 45% (17 of 38). In patients with metastatic pelvic lymph nodes, nine (39%) of 23 had recurrences, as did five of seven with positive margins only. In the total group nine recurrences were in the pelvis (four associated with distant metastasis). Five (15%) of 33 patients treated with whole-pelvis irradiation with or without vaginal intracavitary therapy had major bowel complications requiring surgical intervention (four small bowel obstructions and one enterovesicle fistula). Five patients treated with intravaginal ovoids only had no major complications. Because of the disruption of the anatomy due to the parametrial and vaginal cuff resection, which would place potential foci of parametrial tumor at a distance from the intracavitary ovaries (Fig. 54-9), the authors recommended vaginal intracavitary irradiation alone only for those patients with carcinoma *in situ* (or with minimal invasive carcinoma, in our opinion) at the vaginal margin of resection.

The therapeutic benefit of postradical hysterectomy irradiation is controversial. Bianchi and colleagues,[32] in 60 patients

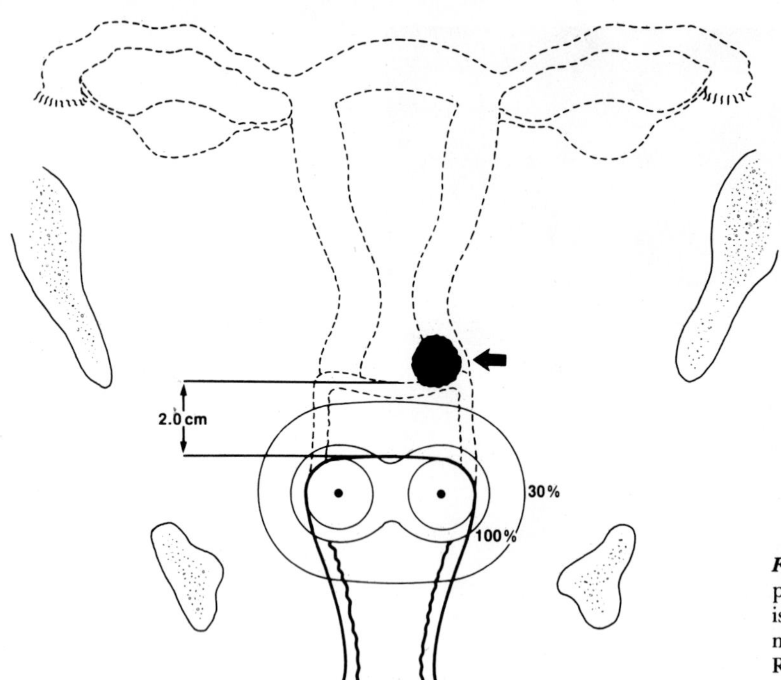

FIGURE 54–9. Isodose line of vaginal ovoid irradiation in patient with radical hysterectomy. Note that shortened vagina is away from parametrial tissue (see arrow at close paracervical margin, which is getting less than 30% of the tumor dose). (Kim RY, Slater MM, Shingleton HM: Int J Radiat Oncol Biol Phys 14:445–449, 1988)

receiving external-beam irradiation for pelvic node metastasis after radical hysterectomy, observed a 65% 5-year survival rate. In contrast, in 15 patients who refused postoperative irradiation, only three survived 5 years (20%). The improvement in survival rate was particularly noticeable in the Stage II patients. When pelvic irradiation was given after radical hysterectomy, the major complication rate was 21.1% in comparison with 19.8% when hysterectomy was preceded by an intracavitary radium application or 10.5% with surgery alone.

Kinney and colleagues[188] compared the results of therapy in 82 patients with Stage IB and Stage IIA carcinoma of the cervix found to have pelvic lymph node metastases at time of Wertheim hysterectomy and bilateral lymphadenectomy without additional adjuvant therapy with a group of 103 similar patients who received 5000 cGy to the pelvis postoperatively. The 5-year survival rate was 72% for the surgery-only group and 64% for the group receiving adjuvant irradiation. The incidence of pelvic recurrences was 67% in the surgery-only group and 27% among patients receiving adjuvant irradiation. The lack of impact on overall survival is most likely related to the higher incidence of distant metastases in the irradiated patients, which may be a reflection of higher short-term survival and high-risk patient selection in the irradiated group.

It appears that a modest gain in survival may be observed in patients with pelvic lymph node metastasis from carcinoma of the uterine cervix receiving postoperative irradiation after various types of operation (Tables 54-11 and 54-12).

However, a panel report[250] summarizing the anecdotal experience at several institutions in the United States and a review of available literature showed (1) a lack of controlled studies to evaluate postradical hysterectomy irradiation in patients with early carcinoma of the cervix having metastatic pelvic lymph nodes, (2) no difference in survival rates in irradiated and nonirradiated patients (50% to 83% 5- to 7-year survival rates), and (3) higher incidence of pelvic failures in the nonirradiated patients (84% in 57 recurrent cases) compared with those irradiated (50% in 18 recurrent patients). Prospective clinical trials, some of which are in progress, are needed to elucidate this controversy.[332]

Carcinoma of the Cervix Inadvertently Treated With a Simple Hysterectomy

Occasionally, because of inadequate preoperative workup, a simple or total abdominal hysterectomy is performed, and invasive carcinoma of the cervix is incidentally found in the surgical specimen. In general, extrafascial abdominal hysterectomy is not curative because the paravaginal/paracervical soft tissue and vaginal cuff are not removed. Furthermore, it may be

TABLE 54–11
Reported 5-Year Survival Rates in Stage IB and IIA Cancer of the Uterine Cervix with Lymph Node Metastases Treated with Postoperative Irradiation

AUTHOR	STAGE	NO. OF CASES	5-YEAR SURVIVAL RATE (%)
POSTOPERATIVE IRRADIATION			
Kelso and Funnell[176]	IB	14	57
Rampone et al[320]	IB	81	63
Masubuchi et al[232]	IB	14	57
Guttmann[127]	IB–IIA	18	61
Morrow[250]	IB	49	60
Fuller et al[107]	IB–IIA	32	43
Kjorstad et al[191]	IB	138	56
Gonzales et al[112]	IB–IIA	89	59
NO POSTOPERATIVE IRRADIATION			
Burch and Chalfant[48]	IB	23	56
Hsu et al[153]	IB	37	40
Piver and Chung[298]	IB	39	55
Morrow[250]	IB	144	59
Fuller et al[107]	IB	39	55

(Gonzalez DG, Ketting BW, van Bunningen B, vanDijk JDP: Int J Radiat Oncol Biol Phys 16:389–395, 1989)

TABLE 54–12
*Results of Elective Postoperative External Irradiation After Radical Hysterectomy in Early-Stage Carcinoma of the Cervix from Literature Review**

AUTHOR	NO. OF PATIENTS	LOCAL CONTROL (%)	SURVIVAL (%)	SURVIVAL MONTHS	SEVERE COMPLICATION† (%)
Kellso et al[176]	224	82	82	60	—
Matsuyama et al[233]	147‡	—	73	60	10
Inoue et al[156]	115	—	72	60	—
Martinbeau et al[226]	120	73	53	60	—
Tanaka et al[378]	195§	—	82	60	—
Guttman[127]	50§	—	78	60	4
Morrow et al[250]	49	63	63	24	12
Papavasiliou et al[271]	41	90	73	60	5
Sall et al[346]	40	63	63	60	3
Russell et al[338]	37‡	73	—		5
Jobson et al[164]	30	70	52	60	7
Powell et al[310]	30	—	73	24 or >?	—
Hogan et al[144]	21‡	48	48	24	24
Hoskins et al[149]	21	—	71	6–60	—
Cosbie[65]	17‡	—	47	36–120	12
Figge et al[102]	16	50	—		—
Rosseau et al[329]	14	—	50	60	—
Chung et al[62]	12‡	92	92	24	8
Benedet et al[25]	9	22	22	60 or >	—
Hsu et al[153]	7	—	14	60 or >	—
Lerner et al[212]	6	—	50	60	—
Underwood et al[396]	4	75	75		—
Ampil et al[11]	13‡	62	46	60	8

** Patients with postsurgery gross residual/recurrent disease before irradiation were excluded from the total number of cited cases.*
† Remedial surgery was performed because of bowel or bladder damage in some patients in some series.
‡ All or some of the patients had additoinal vaginal cuff irradiation.
§ Included some Stage III and IV patients.
(Ampil F, Datta R, Datta S: Cancer 60:280–288, 1987)

technically difficult to perform an adequate radical operation after previous simple hysterectomy.[11] If only microinvasive carcinoma is found when an extrafascial hysterectomy with wide cuff is performed, no additional therapy is necessary. If a less comprehensive dissection was carried out, it is critical that these patients receive radiation therapy immediately when their postoperative status allows, because the prognosis is worse when postoperative irradiation is not administered. Durrance[91] and Andras and associates[12] have reported survival rates similar to those of the intact uterus when these patients are treated appropriately.

When the cervical margins are tumor-free in the total hysterectomy specimen and invasive carcinoma is found, an intracavitary insertion with vaginal colpostats to deliver a 6000 cGy mucosal dose to the vault is sufficient. In patients with microscopic residual tumor, therapy consists of 2000 cGy to the whole pelvis and 3000 cGy to the parametria combined with an intracavitary insertion to the vaginal vault for 6000 cGy mucosal dose. If gross tumor is present in the vaginal vault, the dose to the whole pelvis should be 4000 cGy and the parametrial dose an additional 2000 cGy. An intracavitary insertion (as outlined previously) should be performed (6000 cGy mucosal dose). If residual tumor is present, an interstitial implant should be carried out to increase the dose to this volume. The specific treatment recommendations for the various categories of patients are summarized in Table 54-13.

Durrance[91] pointed out that patients with tumor at the margin of resection or gross residual tumor have a less favorable prognosis than those without residual tumor. Andras and associates[12] reported on 148 patients, 90 of whom were available for 10-year evaluation, dividing them in five groups according to tumor extent when therapy was instituted. The majority of the patients were treated with 5000 cGy whole-pelvis irradiation (with 1000 cGy parametrial boost through reduced fields), at times combined with vaginal vault intracavitary irradiation. Table 54-14 summarizes the 5-year survival rates in the various groups. Eight major complications were noted in the 148 patients. Ampil and co-workers[11] described the results in 44 patients receiving postoperative irradiation after hysterectomy for Stage IB and Stage IIA carcinoma of the uterine cervix (15 patients were treated with radical hysterectomy). Their results were similar with external-beam irradiation alone or combined with intracavitary therapy (88% and 83% local tumor control and 69% and 67% 5-year survival rates, respectively). In three patients treated with intracavitary vaginal cuff irradiation only, two had tumor control and one survived without tumor. Results reported by various authors are summarized in Table 54-15.

Green and Morris[119] reported nine of 30 patients (30%) surviving 5 years after definitive radiation therapy for the treatment of invasive cervical carcinoma after inadvertent simple hysterectomy. The same authors noted that 14 of 32 patients retreated with another surgical procedure, usually a Wertheim

TABLE 54–13
Treatment Policies for Invasive Epidermoid Carcinoma of Cervix Incidentally Found at Simple (Total) Hysterectomy

GROUP	TUMOR EXTENT	EXTERNAL IRRADIATION (cGy) WHOLE PELVIS	SPLIT FIELDS	INTRACAVITARY OVOIDS SURFACE DOSE (cGy)
I	Microinvasion (≤3 mm invasion), margins clear	0	0	6500–7000
II	Fully invasive (>3 mm), margins clear	2000	3000	6500
III	Microscopic residual (+ margins) or lymphatic permeation in groups I–II	3000	2000	7500–8000
IV	Gross residual "cut across tumor"	4000	1000–2000	7500
V	Recurrent tumor	4000	1000–2000	8000 + (interstitial radiation)

TABLE 54–14
Invasive Cervical Carcinoma Inadvertently Found at Simple Hysterectomy: Status at 5 Years After Postoperative Irradiation

GROUP	NO. OF CASES	NED NO.	NED %	DEAD OF DISEASE	ALIVE WITH TUMOR	RECURRENCE SALVAGED BY SURGERY
I	27	26	96			
II	38	32	84	3	1	
III	15	13	87		2	
IV	38	18	47	18	2	
V	30	11	37	16		2

NED: no evidence of disease
(Andras EJ, Fletcher GH, Rutledge F: Am J Obstet Gynecol 115:647–655, 1973)

TABLE 54–15
*Results of Postoperative External Irradiation After Conservative Hysterectomy in Early-Stage Carcinoma of the Cervix**

AUTHOR	NO. OF PATIENTS	LOCAL CONTROL (%)	SURVIVAL (%)	SURVIVAL MONTHS	SEVERE COMPLICATION† (%)
Cosbie[65]	119‡	—	46	60	—
Andras et al[12]	80‡	89	89	60	4
Davy et al[74]	74‡	74	61	60	3
Durrance[91]	42‡	90	90	60 or >	5
Papavasiliou et al[271]	36	89	89	60	5
Perkins et al[289]	36‡	78	67	36–120	14
Tunca et al[392]	19‡	—	53	12–60	—
Nolan[263]	16‡	31	31	19–123	—
Moore[247]	9‡	56	56	60–120	—
Ampil et al[11]	27‡	89	70	60	4

* *Patients with postsurgery gross residual/recurrent disease before irradiation were excluded from the total number of cited cases.*
† *Remedial surgery was performed because of bowel or bladder damage in some patients in some series.*
‡ *All or some of the patients had additional vaginal cuff irradiation.*
(Ampil F, Datta R, Datta S: Cancer 60:280–288, 1987)

hysterectomy, died within 5 years. Eight of nine patients with negative nodes survived, and one died of postoperative complications. The same authors pointed out that the 5-year cure rate was 30% in the patients treated within 1 year after the hysterectomy, in contrast to 16% for those treated after 1 year. Thus the time at which the patient is treated and the volume of tumor are important prognostic factors.

SURGICAL TECHNIQUES

Several types of hysterectomy are used in the management of carcinoma of the uterine cervix (Table 54-16).[301]

Total (extrafascial) abdominal hysterectomy consists of removal of the cervix and adjacent tissues as well as the upper vagina in a plane outside the pubocervical fascia. There is minimal disturbance of the ureters and the trigone of the bladder, which decreases the risk of urinary complications. When desired, a small vaginal cuff can be removed (1 cm to 2 cm).

In *modified radical hysterectomy,* the cervix and upper vagina are removed, including paracervical tissues, and the ureters are dissected in the paracervical tunnel to their point of entry into the bladder. Because the ureters are unsheathed, parametrial and paracervical tissue can be safely removed medial to the ureter.

Radical abdominal hysterectomy with bilateral pelvic lymphadenectomy consists of a wider resection of the parametrial tissues, with dissection of the ureters and mobilization of the bladder neck as well as the rectum to allow for more extensive removal of tissues. Also, a vaginal cuff of at least 2 cm to 3 cm is always included in the procedure. A bilateral pelvic lymphadenectomy is carried out.

Pelvic exenteration has been used for *en masse* removal of the pelvic viscera for presenting Stage IVA and recurrent carcinoma of the cervix. This operation, which is not done as a palliative procedure, consists of radical hysterectomy, pelvic lymph node dissection, removal of the bladder (anterior exenteration), removal of the rectosigmoid colon (posterior exenteration), or both (total exenteration). The ileum or sigmoid has been been the usual means of achieving urinary diversion. Because some patients have a pelvic recurrence following radiation therapy, the transverse colon is used for the urinary conduit. Proof that there is no fixation to the pelvic wall and no extension of disease beyond the pelvis is mandatory. Metastases outside the pelvis, including those to periaortic lymph nodes or any viscera, are absolute contraindications to the procedure. Bilateral ureteral obstruction secondary to tumor is also a relative contraindication.[44,398] In former years, pelvic exenteration was used in Stage IVA carcinoma of the cervix with extension to the bladder.[44] Modern radiation therapy makes the latter indication rarely necessary, as noted in the report of Million and coworkers[240] of 18 (34%) of 53 patients with bladder involvement who survived without disease after definitive irradiation—results comparable to those obtained with exenteration. Upadhyay and associates[397] noted 43% tumor local control and 18% 5-year survival in 44 patients with Stage IVA carcinoma of the cervix treated with definitive radiation therapy.

Pretreatment Laparotomy

Exploratory laparotomy has been performed to evaluate the presence of metastases to the pelvic or periaortic nodes without significant impact on survival (Table 54-17). In 128 patients undergoing extraperitoneal and in 156 patients undergoing transperitoneal selective paraaortic lymphadenectomy no significant difference in the sensitivity to detect nodal metastases or incidence of surgical complications was noted between the two techniques. However, if the patients had periaortic irradiation, a 11.5% incidence of major complications was noted in the transperitoneal lymphadenectomy compared with 3.9% in the extraperitoneal group (P = 0.03).[412] After retroperitoneal lymph node dissections, the use of high-energy photon beams and limitation of the tumor dose to extended volumes in the periaortic region to 5000 cGy decreases the probability of complications.

RADIATION THERAPY TECHNIQUES

Currently the two main modalities of irradiation are external photon beam and brachytherapy. External-beam irradiation is used to treat the whole pelvis and the parametria including the

TABLE 54–16
Types of Abdominal Hysterectomy

	INTRAFASCIAL	EXTRAFASCIAL TYPE I	MODIFIED RADICAL TYPE II	RADICAL TYPE III*
Cervical fascia	Partially removed	Completely removed ⟶		⟶
Vaginal cuff removal	None	Small rim removed	Proximal 1–2 cm removed	Upper third to half removed
Bladder	Partially mobilized ⟶			⟶ Mobilized
Rectum	Not mobilized	R-V septum partially mobilized ⟶		⟶ Mobilized
Ureters	Not mobilized ⟶		⟶ Unroofed in ureteral tunnel	Completely dissected to bladder level
Cardinal ligaments	Resected medial to ureters ⟶		⟶ Resected at level of ureter	Resected at pelvic sidewall
Uterosacral ligaments	Resected at level of cervix ⟶		⟶ Partially resected	Resected at postpelvic insertion
Uterus	Removed ⟶			⟶
Cervix	Partialy removed	Completely removed ⟶		⟶

* *Type IV, extended radical hysterectomy (partial removal of bladder or ureter or both), in addition to Type III*

TABLE 54–17
Carcinoma of the Uterine Cervix: Survival After Staging Laparotomy

	EXPLORED		NOT EXPLORED	
STAGE	NO. OF PATIENTS	PERCENT SURVIVING	NO. OF PATIENTS	PERCENT SURVIVING
IIB	31	64.5	14	92.8
IIIA–IIIB	28	57.1	10	60

(Nelson JH, et al: Am J Obstet Gynecol 118:749–756, 1974)

common iliac periaortic lymph nodes, whereas the central disease (cervix, vagina, and medial parametria) is primarily irradiated with intracavitary sources.

The use of radium therapy was first presented in the treatment of carcinoma of the cervix in 1913 at the Congress at Halle. The techniques described apply, with some individualization, to most patients with cervical carcinoma.

The policies for irradiation of carcinoma of the uterine cervix at the Mallinckrodt Institute of Radiology are summarized in Table 54-18.

External-Beam Irradiation

External pelvic irradiation is delivered before intracavitary insertions in patients with bulky cervical lesions to improve the geometry of the intracavitary application; with exophytic, easily bleeding tumors; with tumors with necrosis or infection; and with parametrial involvement.

Volume Treated

In the treatment of invasive carcinoma of the uterine cervix, it is important to deliver adequate doses of radiation to the pelvic lymph nodes. For Stage IB disease, 15-cm × 15-cm portals at the surface (about 16.5 cm at isococenter) are sufficient. For patients with Stages IIA, IIB, III, and IVA carcinoma, somewhat larger portals (18 cm × 15 cm at surface, 20.5 cm × 16.5 cm at isocenter) are required to cover all the common iliac nodes in addition to the cephalad half of the vagina (Fig. 54-10). A 2-cm margin lateral to the bony pelvis is adequate. If no vaginal extension is present, the lower margin of the portal is at the inferior border of the obturator foramen. When the vagina is involved, the entire length of this organ should be treated down to the introitus (Fig. 54-11). It is very important to identify the distal extension of the tumor at the time of simulation by placing a radiopaque clip or bead on the vaginal wall or inserting a small rod with a radiopaque marker in the vagina (Fig. 54-12). In these patients the portals should be modified to cover

TABLE 54–18
Carcinoma of the Uterine Cervix: MIR Policies of Treatment with Irradiation

		EXTERNAL IRRADIATION (cGy)*		BRACHYTHERAPY		
TUMOR STAGE	TUMOR EXTENT	WHOLE PELVIS	ADDITIONAL PARAMETRIAL DOSE (MIDLINE SHIELD)	TWO INSERTIONS (mg h RaEq)†	DOSE TO POINT A	TOTAL DOSE TO POINT A (cGy)
IA		0	0	6500–8000	7000	6000–7500
IB (small)	Superficial ulceration; less than 2 cm in diameter or involving fewer than two quadrants	0	4500	8000	7000	6500–7000
IB (2 to 4 cm)	Four quadrant involvement; no endocervical component or significant expansion	1000	4000	7000	6500–7500	7500–8500
IIA, IIB	Non-barrel-shaped type	2000	3000	8000	7000	8500
IB–IIA (bulky)‡, IIB, IIIA	Barrel-shaped cervix; parametrial extension	2000	3000	8000	7000	8500–9000
IIIB	Parametrial involvement	2000	4000	8000	7000	8500–9500
IIB, IIIB, IV	Poor pelvic anatomy; patients not readily treated with intracavitary insertions (barrel-shaped cervix not regressing; inability to locate external os)	4000	2000	6500	6000	8500–9500

** 180 cGy/day, five weekly fractions, using 15 or higher MV photon beams, two portals treated daily*
† 60–80 cGy/hr at point A. In patients over 65 years or with history of previous pelvic inflammatory disease or pelvic surgery, reduce doses by 10%.
‡ In Stage IB and IIA, if complete regression is not obtained, perform extrafascial conservative hysterectomy (reduce brachytherapy dose to 6000 mgh).

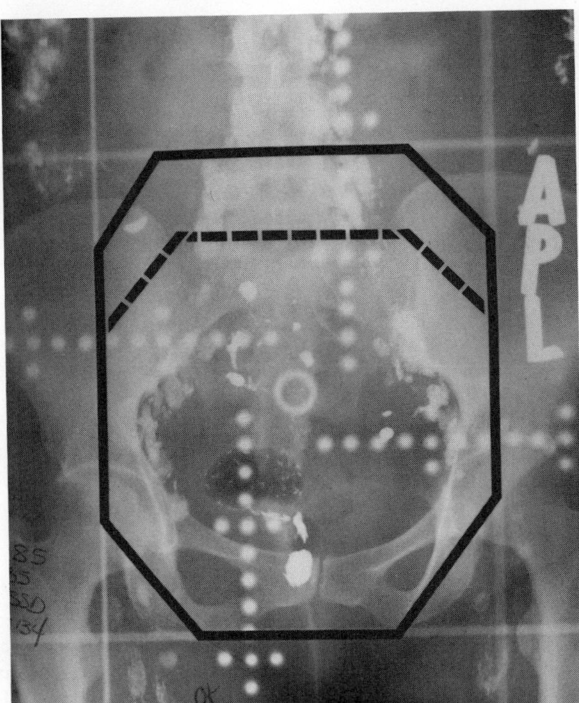

FIGURE 54–10. Anteroposterior simulation film of the pelvis illustrating portals used for external irradiation. The 15-cm × 15-cm portals at SSD are used for Stage IB (*broken line*), and 18-cm × 15-cm portals are used for more advanced disease (*solid line*). This allows better coverage of the common iliac lymph nodes. The distal margin is usually placed at the bottom of the obturator foramen. (SSD: source-skin distance)

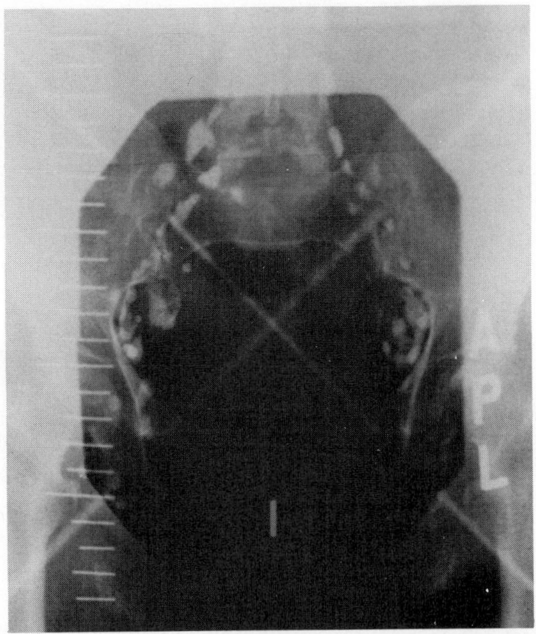

FIGURE 54–12. Anteroposterior simulation film of the pelvis showing a marker to indicate vaginal extension of tumor. The lymph nodes are opacified with contrast material.

the inguinal lymph nodes because of the increased probability of metastases (Fig. 54-13).

When parametrial tumor persists after 5000 cGy to 6000 cGy is delivered to the parametria, an additional 1000 cGy in five or six fractions may be delivered with reduced portals (8-cm × 12-cm portals for unilateral and 12-cm × 12-cm portals for bilateral parametrial coverage) (Fig. 54-14). The midline shield should be in place to protect the bladder and rectosigmoid.

If periaortic node metastases are present or suspected, the patients are treated with 5000 cGy to the periaortic area plus a 500 cGy to 1000 cGy boost dose to enlarged lymph nodes through reduced lateral or rotational portals. The retroperitoneal tissues need to be irradiated either through a separate portal or with an extended field that includes both the periaortic nodes and the pelvis (Fig. 54-15). The upper margin of the field is at the T12–L1 interspace. The width of the portals (in general 9 cm to 10 cm) can be determined by CT scans, lymphangiogram, or intravenous pyelogram outlining the ureters. The spinal cord dose (T12 to L2) should be kept below 4500 cGy by interposing a 2 cm wide 5 HVL (half-value layer) shield on the posterior portal (usually after 3800 cGy to 4000 cGy tumor dose). An effort should be made to minimize the

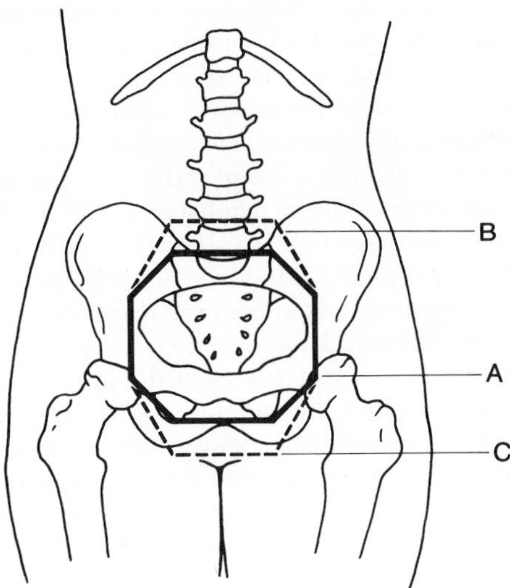

FIGURE 54–11. (**A**) Diagram of pelvic portals used in external irradiation of carcinoma of the uterine cervix. Standard portal for Stage IB tumors is outlined by solid line. (**B**) When the common iliac nodes are to be covered, the upper margin is extended to the L4–5 space. (**C**) If there is vaginal tumor extension, the lower margin of the field is drawn at the introitus.

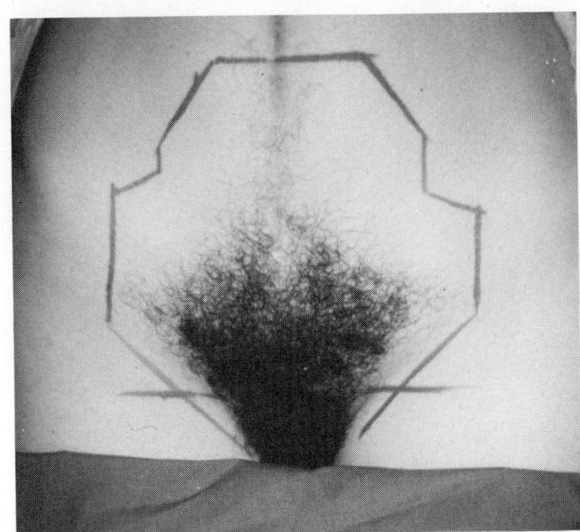

FIGURE 54–13. Lateral extension of pelvic portal to cover inguinal lymph nodes in a patient with tumor extension beyond the middle third of the vagina.

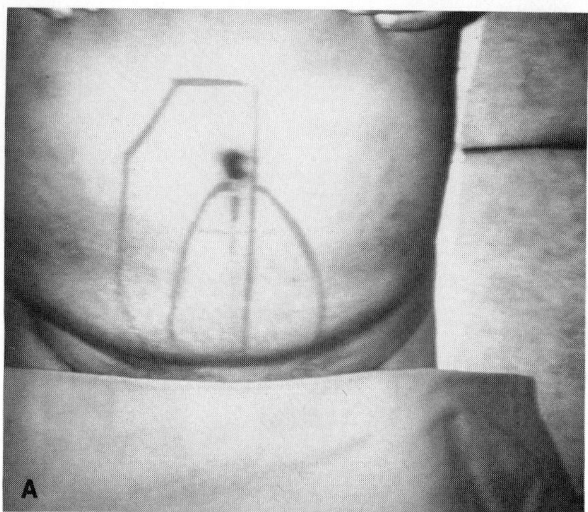

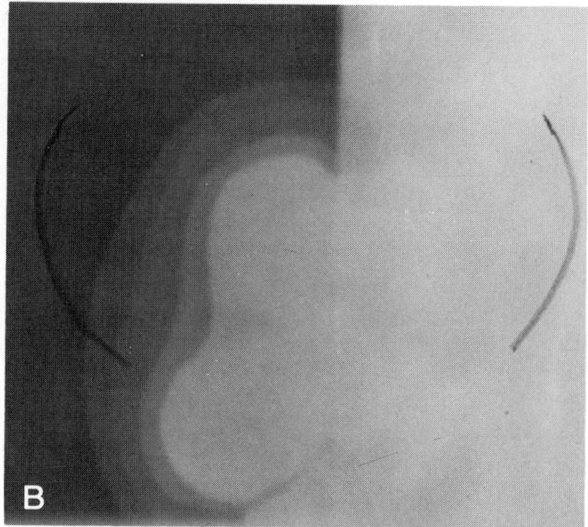

FIGURE 54–14. (**A**) Patient with reduced unilateral parametrial portal. (**B**) Localization film of a right parametrial boost portal showing the position of the midline wedge.

relatively high incidence of complications noted after extended field irradiation and laparotomy[56,258] and particularly following transperitoneal lymphadenectomy.

Beam Energies

Because of the thickness of the pelvis, high-energy photon beams are specially suited for this treatment. They decrease the dose of radiation delivered to the peripheral normal tissues (particularly bladder and rectum) and provide a more homogeneous dose distribution in the central pelvis. With lower-energy photons (^{60}Co or 4 to 6 MV x-rays), higher maximum doses must be given, and more complicated field arrangements should be used to achieve the same midplane tumor dose (three fields or four-field pelvic box or rotational techniques) while minimizing the dose to the bladder and rectum and to avoid subcutaneous fibrosis (Fig. 54-16). Biggs and Russell[33] warned that the presence of a metallic prosthesis when using lateral fields or a box pelvic irradiation technique may result in a decrease of approximately 2% for 25 MV x-rays and average increases of 2% for 10 MV x-rays and 5% for ^{60}Co.

Allt[7] and Johns,[166] in an update of the same randomized study, reported better pelvic tumor control and survival and fewer complications in a group of 65 patients with Stage IIB and Stage III cervical carcinoma treated with 23 MV photons in comparison with 61 patients treated with external-beam irradiation with ^{60}Co, in addition to intracavitary brachytherapy in both groups (Fig. 54-17).

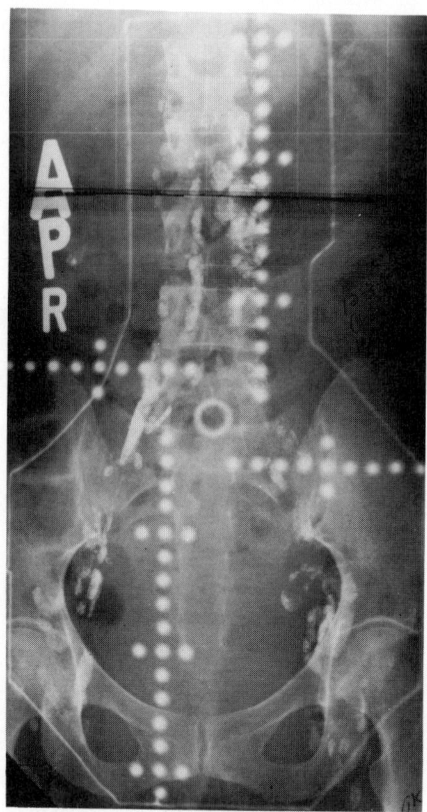

FIGURE 54–15. Simulation film of extended field for external irradiation of pelvic and periaortic lymph nodes.

Doses of Radiation

Stage IA (microinvasive) tumors are treated with intracavitary therapy only (6000 cGy in one insertion or 7500 cGy to 8000 cGy in two insertions to point A).

The optimal dose for invasive carcinoma of the cervix is delivered with a combination of whole pelvis, intracavitary, and at times interstitial therapy. Some institutions use lower doses of whole pelvis, external-beam irradiation (1000 cGy for Stage IB and 2000 cGy for Stage IIA, IIB, and III) in addition to parametrial doses to complete 5000 cGy in Stage IB and Stage IIA or 6000 cGy to the involved parametrial tissues for more advanced stages. At Washington University step wedges designed in accordance with the isodose curves of the intracavitary applications are used to block the midline (Fig. 54-18). The intracavitary insertions, usually two, deliver 7000 mgh to 7500 mgh (6500 cGy to 7000 cGy to point A) in Stage IB tumors and 7500 mgh to 8000 mgh (7000 cGy to 7500 cGy to point A) for Stages IIA, IIB, and III tumors. This technique affords a high central dose to the cervix, paracervical tissues, and parametria as well as a moderate homogeneous dose to the external iliac lymph nodes without exceeding the bladder and rectal tolerance doses (Fig. 54-19).

Other institutions prefer higher doses of whole-pelvic external-beam irradiation (usually 4000 cGy) with an additional parametrial dose (with midline 5 HVL rectangular block) to

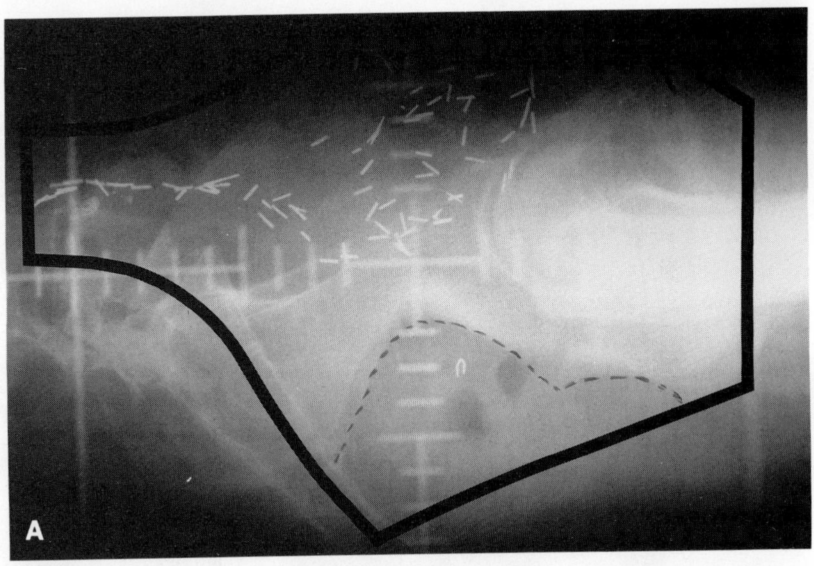

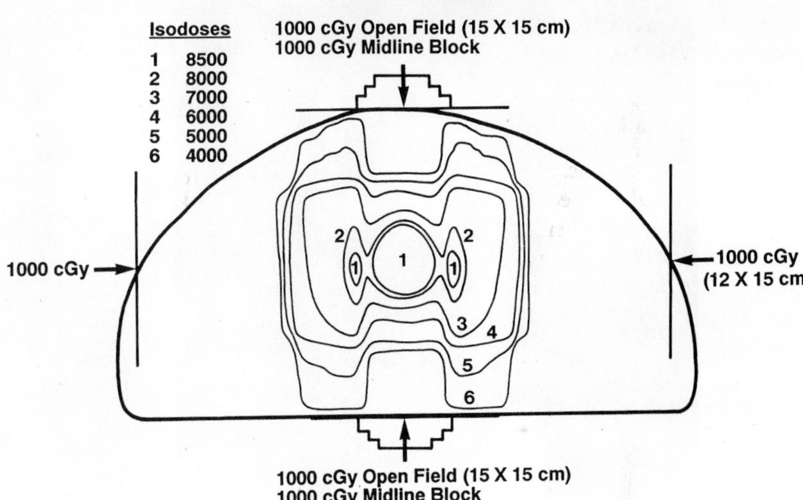

FIGURE 54–16. Examples of (**A**) lateral portal and (**B**) isodose curves for "box" irradiation of the pelvis with low-energy photons. (Perez CA, DiSaia PJ, Knapp RC, et al: Gynecologic tumors. In DeVita V, Hellman S, Rosenberg SA [eds]: Cancer: Principles and Practice of Oncology, 2nd ed. Philadelphia, JB Lippincott, 1985)

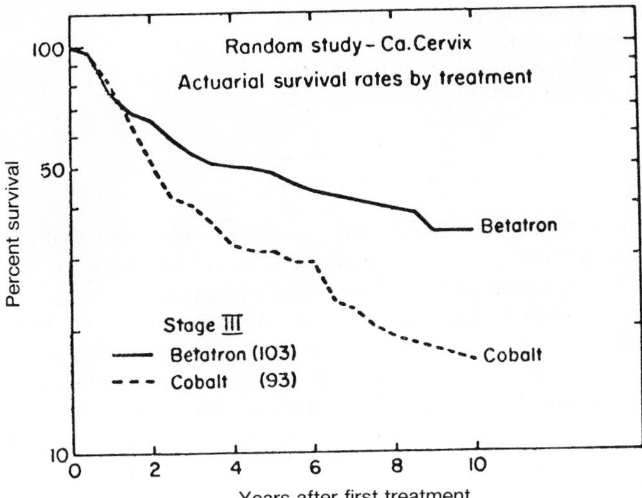

FIGURE 54–17. Survival curves for patients with Stage III carcinoma of the uterine cervix randomized to receive comparable doses of external irradiation with either betatron or ^{60}Co. (Johns HE: Optimization of energy and equipment. In Kramer S, Sunthralingam N, Zinninger GF [eds]: High-Energy Photons and Electrons, p 336. New York, John Wiley & Sons, 1976)

complete 5000 cGy in patients with Stage IB and Stage IIA tumors and 5500 cGy to 6000 cGy for patients with Stage IIB, III, or IVA tumors. This is usually combined with one or two intracavitary insertions for approximately 4500 mgh to 5500 mgh (4000 cGy to 5000 cGy to point A).

A comparison of dose profiles in the coronal and sagittal planes using the above techniques is shown in Figure 54-20. The use of different techniques may have no significant impact on outcome as long as the doses delivered are similar.

Hunter and associates[157] compared two radiation therapy techniques: (1) small field delivering 1500 cGy to point A and 3250 cGy to point B in 16 fractions in 21 days plus 6000 cGy to point A in two insertions or (2) 4000 cGy to points A and B external-beam irradiation, with large fields encompassing the whole pelvis and common iliac nodes in 20 fractions plus 3750 cGy to point A in a single intracavitary insertion using 4 MV x-rays and radium. A total of 148 patients were randomly allocated to each treatment group. The 5-year survival rates were 38.6% and 40.3%, with corrected survivals of 44.5% and 45%, respectively. Incidence of pelvic recurrences and major morbidity were comparable in both groups. It should be noted that in this trial the doses of radiation delivered were somewhat lower than those administered in the United States.

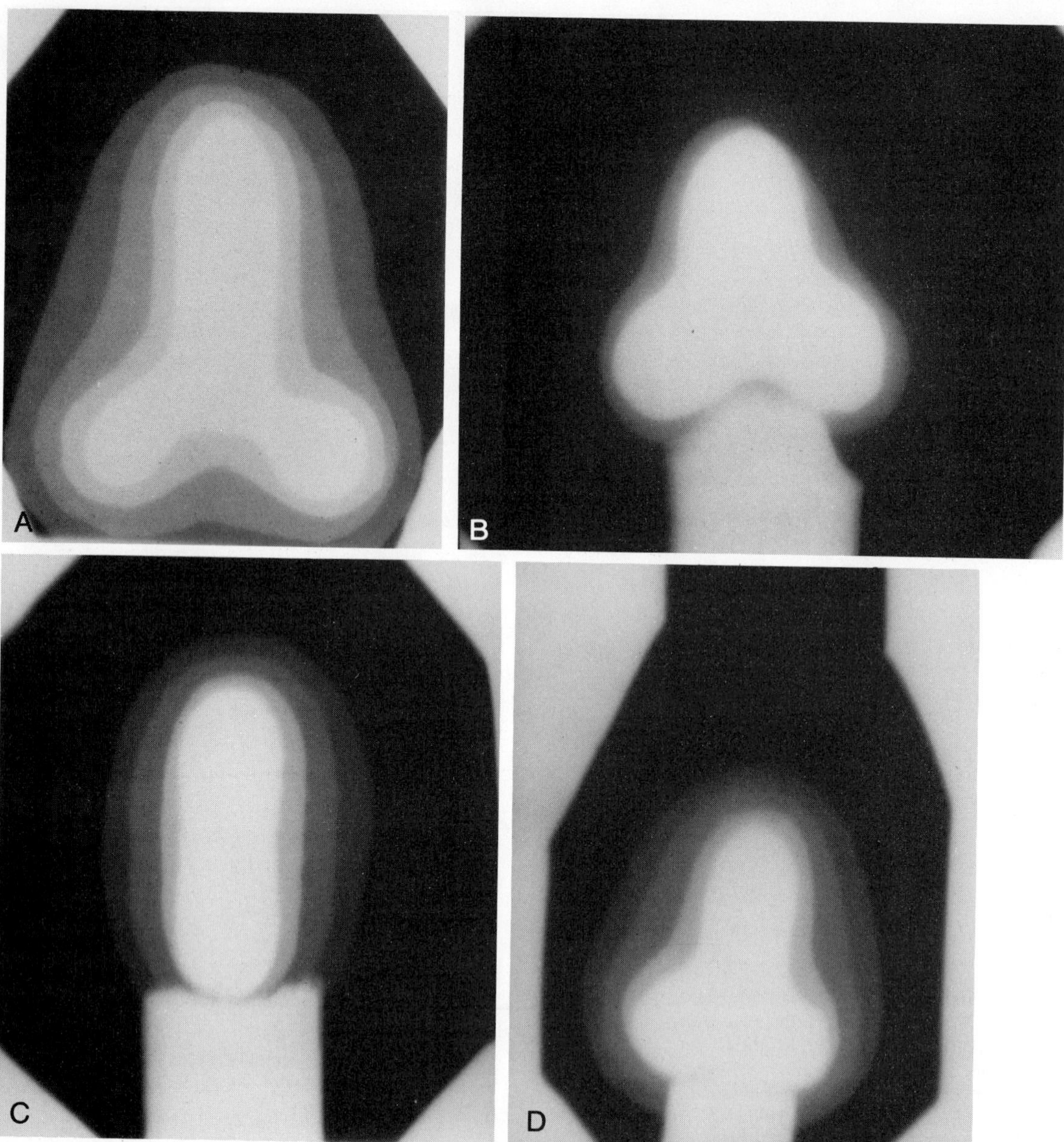

FIGURE 54–18. (**A** to **C**) Examples of different step wedges used to shield the midline during external irradiation for carcinoma of the uterine cervix. Wedges are designed according to the dose distribution obtained with brachytherapy sources. (**D**) Localization film illustrating the use of the midline wedge with a patient irradiated through extended fields. (**A** and **B**, Perez CA, DiSaia PJ, Knapp RC, et al: Gynecologic tumors. In DeVita V, Hellman S, Rosenberg SA [eds]: Cancer: Principles and Practice of Oncology, 2nd ed. Philadelphia, JB Lippincott, 1985)

Brachytherapy

Several isotopes are available, although at the present time ^{137}Cs (cesium-137) is the most popular. Brachytherapy can be delivered with intracavitary techniques using a variety of applicators consisting of an intrauterine tandem and vaginal colpostats or, when necessary, vaginal cylinders, the majority being afterloading. Radiographs are always obtained using dummy sources, and the active sources can be inserted after the films have been reviewed and the position of the applicators is judged to be satisfactory. The vaginal packing is soaked in 40% iodinated contrast material to identify it on radiographs (Fig. 54-21).

In prescribing the doses it is noteworthy that in 91 radium applications with Fletcher-Suit applicators, using linear least-square regression, Potish and associates[307] observed that although there was a moderately good correlation between the milligram hours and the doses, the dose to point A was markedly affected by the position of the colpostats and the tandem, making it difficult to formulate a simple conversion factor between the two systems. Therefore, computer-generated isodose curves provide the best means of determining the doses to point A, point B, bladder, and rectum. ICRU Report No. 38[157] defines the dose and volume specifications for reporting intracavitary therapy in gynecologic procedures.

Basic principles of clinical application of brachytherapy and the use of remote afterloading devices (low or high dose rate) are discussed in Chapter 13. In general, an intrauterine tandem with three or four sources (15 or 20-10-10-10 mCi Ra eq) is inserted in the uterus and two colpostats (2 cm in diameter, loaded with 20

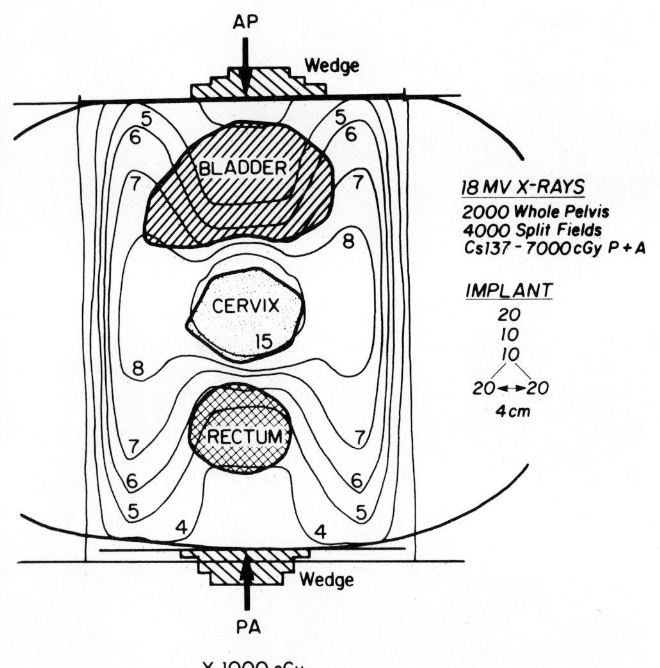

FIGURE 54–19. Composite isodose curves through point A for patient with Stage IIB carcinoma of the uterine cervix treated with external irradiation and two intracavitary insertions. Doses and source arrangement are shown. High doses can be delivered to cervix and parametrial tissues with relative sparing of the bladder and rectum.

mCi Ra eq sources) are placed in the vaginal vault and packed with iodoformed gauze.

If the vaginal vault is narrow, it may be impossible to insert regular-sized colpostats, in which case miniovoids should be used (usually loaded with 10 mCi Ra eq sources) (Fig. 54-22). When even miniovoids cannot be inserted, it is better to use a protruding source in the vaginal vault, which is inserted in the afterloading tandem (usually 20 mCi to 30 mCi Ra eq) with an overlying plastic sleeve (3 cm in diameter) (Fig. 54-23). Examples of some technical problems in achieving satisfactory intracavitary insertions are illustrated in Figures 54-24 and 54-25. Special attention should be paid to obtain as symmetric and homogeneous dose distribution as technically allowed by the geometry of the cervix/vagina and the configuration of the tumor.

Interstitial implants with ^{226}Ra, ^{137}Cs needles, or ^{192}Ir afterloading plastic catheters to limited tumor volumes are helpful in specific clinical situations (localized residual tumor, parametrial extension, and others) (Fig. 54-26).

In general, the first intracavitary insertion is scheduled after 1000 cGy to 2000 cGy of external-beam irradiation if an adequate geometry exists in the pelvis. Otherwise, 3000 cGy to 4000 cGy is delivered before the first application to decrease the size of the lesion and improve the relationship of the applicators to the cervix and vagina. The second application is performed 1 or 2 weeks later; in the meantime daily external pelvic therapy is continued.

The intracavitary therapy, with its rapid dose fall-off as a function of distance, yields a high dose to the uterus and paracervical tissues but is inadequate to treat the pelvic lymph nodes, and external-beam irradiation is necessary to supplement the dose. Therefore the parametrial dose is primarily delivered with external irradiation (Fig. 54-27).

RESULTS OF THERAPY

In the evaluation of therapeutic results in invasive carcinoma of the cervix, a direct comparison of surgically treated or irradiated patients is frought with many uncertainties, including patient selection, reporting of surgical cases using staging determined by laparotomy findings, and different treatment techniques. Zola and associates[422] reviewed 152 papers published in the United States and Europe before or during 1980 on results of treatment of Stages IA, IB, IIA, and IIB cervical carcinoma with surgery, irradiation, or combination therapy. More than half of these papers (54%) reported observations on single series without any comparison with historic or concurrently treated control patients. Two treatment arms were compared in only 56 papers (37%), and only 14 (9%) compared three treatment groups. However, in none of the reports were patients allocated at random to various therapies, and a prospectively established research protocol could not be ascertained in most studies. Identification of prognostic factors and information on imbalances on the distribution of patients between treatment groups were adequately presented in 46% of the papers. Only 13% of the papers reported frequency and severity of sequelae of therapy.

Zola and associates[422] concluded that the existing literature is of limited help in deciding the best treatment for patients with cervical carcinoma and that properly designed prospectively randomized studies with careful consideration of relevant end points are necessary to elucidate existing areas of controversy.

Patients with Stage IA cervical carcinoma are effectively treated with intracavitary ^{137}Cs insertions only. In 47 patients with microinvasive carcinoma treated at Washington University—20 with intracavitary therapy only—no local or regional failures were noted; the 5-year disease-free survival rate (corrected for intercurrent disease) was 100%. In 27 patients treated with combined external-beam irradiation and intracavitary brachytherapy, only one patient (diagnosed by conization) developed a pelvic recurrence and distant metastases; the 5-year disease-free survival rate was 96%.

Hamberger and colleagues[130] reported on 151 patients with Stage IA or Stage IB lesions less than 1 cm in diameter treated with intracavitary therapy alone to relatively high doses (9340 mgh, 13,680 mgh, and 8640 mgh, respectively). No failures were noted in 41 patients with Stage IA disease, and only four (4%) in 93 occurred in patients with Stage IB small volume disease. However, three (18%) of 17 patients with more extensive Stage IB lesions, treated with intracavitary therapy only, had regional failures. Only three (0.2%) of 151 patients developed grade 3 complications.

Volterrani and Lombardi[404] reported a 5-year survival rate of 82.6% in 23 patients with occult Stage IB carcinoma of the cervix treated with intracavitary ^{226}Ra only (using a derivation from the Paris method to deliver 7500 mgh). However, the 5-year survival rates were only 64.8% in Stage IB, 50% in Stage II, and 29.8% in Stage III disease. Unfortunately, the authors did not report the exact location of the failures. The results are substantially inferior to those obtained with a combination of intracavitary and external-beam irradiation. It is obvious that intracavitary therapy alone is grossly inadequate to irradiate the larger primary tumors, including the barrel-shaped lesions as well as any parametrial extension.

With combined external-beam irradiation and brachytherapy the typical 5-year survival rate for Stage IB cervical cancer is 86% to 92%, and for Stage IIA about 75%. The overall pelvic failure rate in Stage IB is approximately 5% to 8%, and in

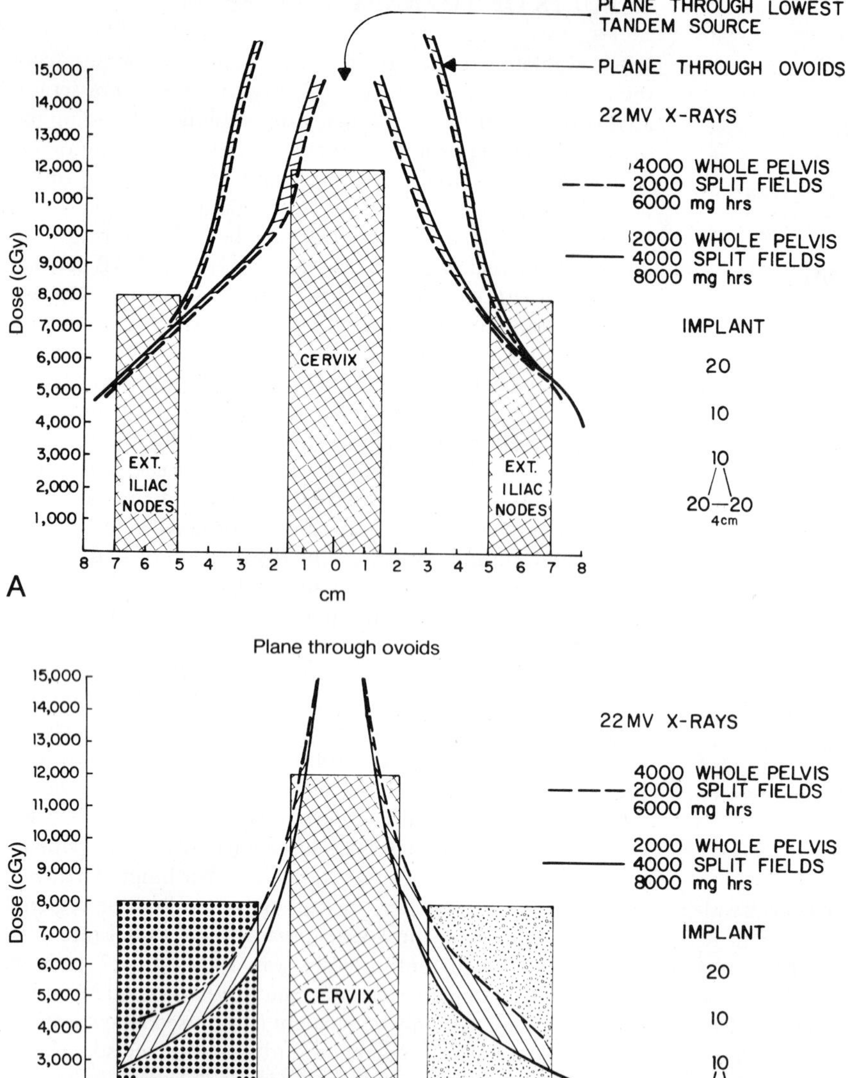

FIGURE 54–20. Dose profiles in the (**A**) coronal and (**B**) sagittal planes for patient with carcinoma of the uterine cervix treated with 2000 cGy to the whole pelvis and 8000 mgh or 4000 cGy to the whole pelvis and 6000 mgh. Additional dose to the parametria is delivered to complete 6000 cGy. The dose distributions are comparable in the coronal plane. However, on the lateral projection the technique using 2000 cGy to the whole pelvis and 8000 mgh (7200 cGy to point A) delivers about 2000 cGy less to the bladder and rectum, which should result in better tolerance for comparable tumor doses.

Stage IIA it is 15% to 20% (in 50% of the patients combined with distant metastases). Either surgery or adequate irradiation is equally effective in the treatment of Stage IB and Stage IIA carcinoma of the cervix; numerous noncontrolled studies support the merits of either modality with no significant difference in survival or pelvic tumor control[45, 272, 274, 294, 372, 406] (Tables 54-19 and 54-20; Fig. 54-28).

Newton[261] and Roddick and Greenlaw[328] reported, in prospectively randomized studies, comparable survival and pelvic recurrence rates in patients with Stage IB and Stage IIA carcinoma of the uterine cervix treated with radical hysterectomy or irradiation alone.

Kielbinska and co-workers,[183] in a long-term follow-up of 792 women treated with irradiation and 789 women treated with hysterectomy and irradiation for Stage I cervical carcinoma, found no difference in survival, general health, incidence of recurrent carcinoma, or appearance of second primary malignancies.

Piver and colleagues[300] treated 103 women with Stage IB cervical carcinoma with either radical hysterectomy and bilateral pelvic lymphadenectomy (for tumor 3 cm or less in greatest diameter) or irradiation (for tumor larger than 3 cm or medically inoperable). The 5-year estimated disease-free survival rate was 92.3% for the surgical group and 91.1% for the irradiation therapy group. Similar overall 5-year survival rates were noted in the patients treated with surgery or irradiation (Table 54-21). In the surgical group 16.4% of the patients had lymph node metastases, and 7.3% developed a recurrence after therapy. In the radiation group lesions larger than 1 cm in diameter had a 14.5% incidence of recurrence. The authors concluded that tumors less than 3 cm in diameter may be equally treated by radical hysterectomy and pelvic lymphadenectomy or radiation therapy alone; it is possible that radiation therapy could lead to even better results in a comparable younger and healthier population. The main advantage of surgical treatment is the preservation of ovarian function in women younger than 40 years of age.

Van Nagell and co-workers[402] found that the recurrence

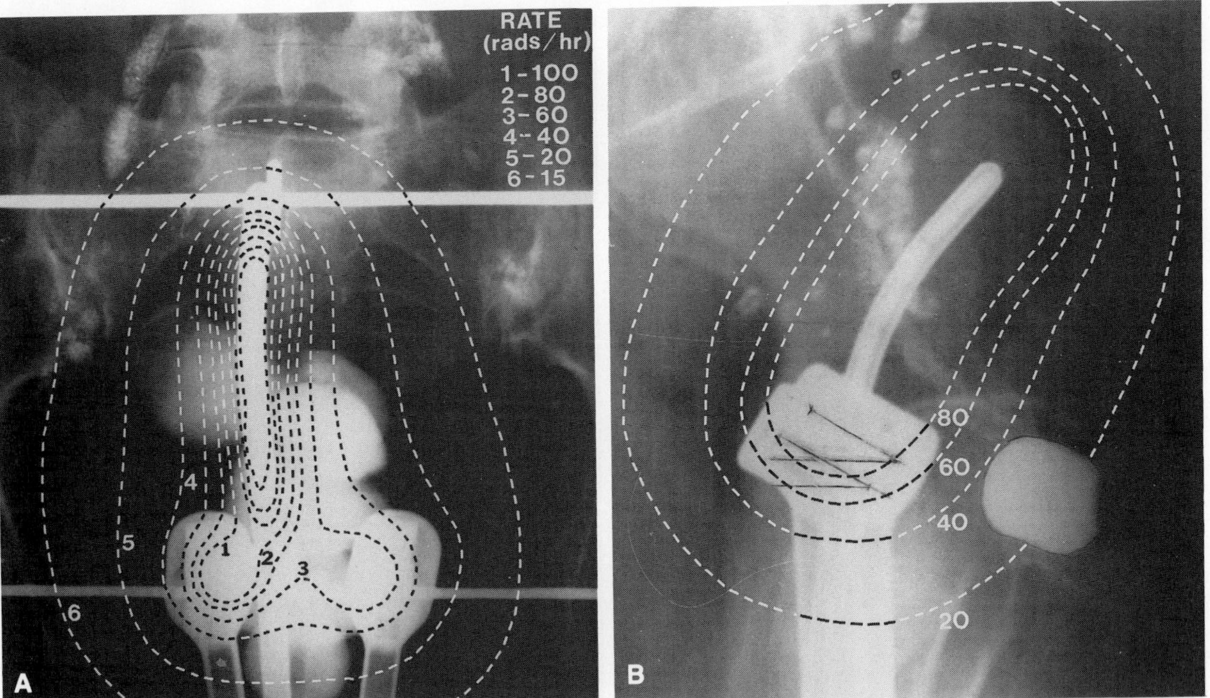

FIGURE 54–21. (**A**) Anteroposterior and (**B**) lateral radiographs of standard intracavitary insertion with afterloading Fletcher-Suit tandem and ovoids. Slight deviation of the tandem to the left is apparent. However, there is good symmetry between the tandem and the ovoids. On the lateral projection, the tandem is crossing the ovoids near the center of the long axis. Radiopaque marker is placed on the anterior lip of the cervix. A Foley balloon with Hypaque outlines the bladder neck.

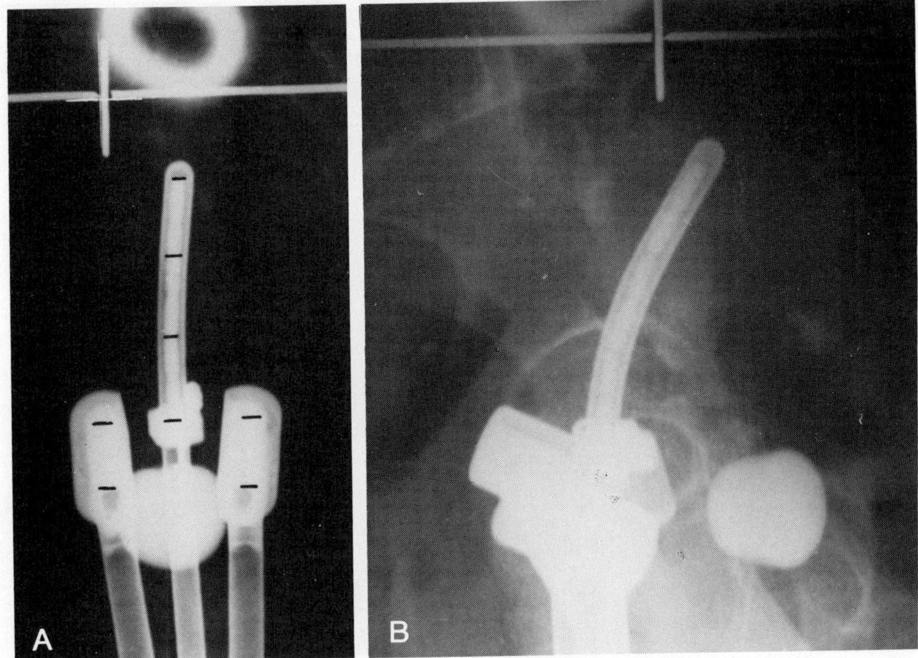

FIGURE 54–22. (**A**) Anteroposterior and (**B**) lateral radiographs of the pelvis illustrating satisfactory placement of afterloading tandem and miniovoids.

rate after radical hysterectomy or irradiation for Stage IB disease was 5% for tumors less than 2 cm in diameter treated with either modality; they recommend radical surgery for these patients. However, in lesions 2 cm to 5 cm in diameter, the failure rate was 24% with surgery but only 11% with irradiation, which should make the latter modality the preferred therapy.

Homesley and associates,[145] in 45 patients with Stage IB carcinoma treated with radiation therapy alone, reported a 5-year actuarial survival rate of 95% in 22 patients with tumors less than 4 cm in diameter and 67% in 23 patients with lesions 4 cm or greater in diameter ($P = 0.05$).

(*text continues on page 1172*)

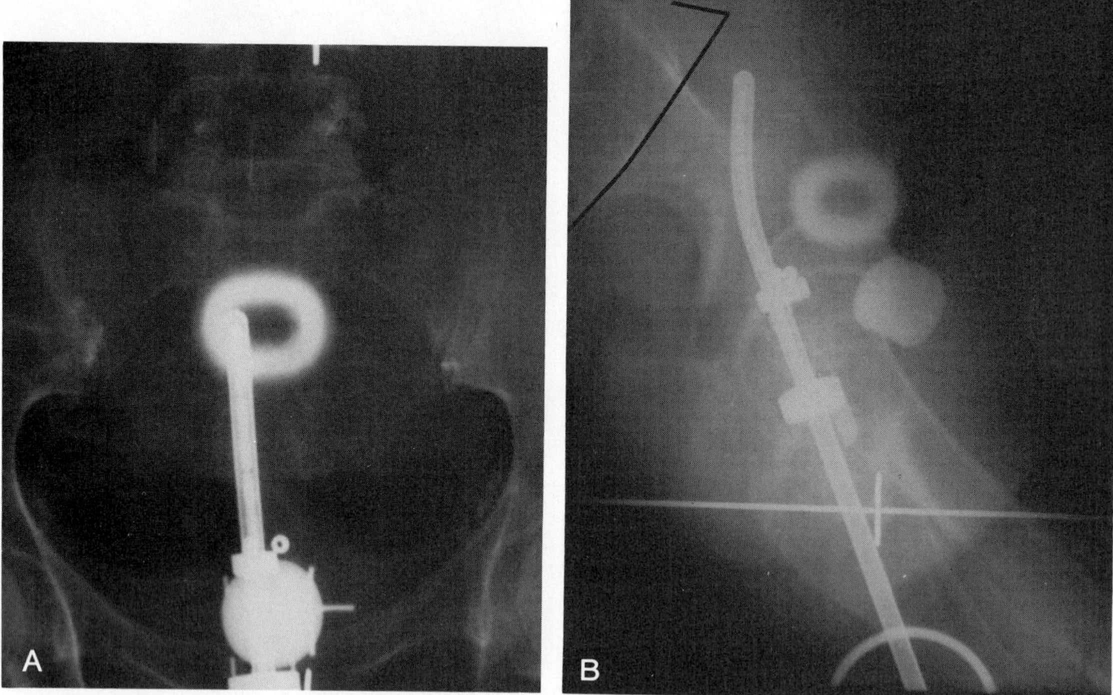

FIGURE 54–23. (**A**) Anteroposterior and (**B**) lateral radiographs of the pelvis showing insertion with afterloading Fletcher-Suit tandem without ovoids. A protruding source, usually 20 mg or 30 mg Ra eq, is placed in the upper vagina. The superior and inferior stoppers are placed above and below a plastic jacket of varying diameters, depending on the capacity of the vaginal vault.

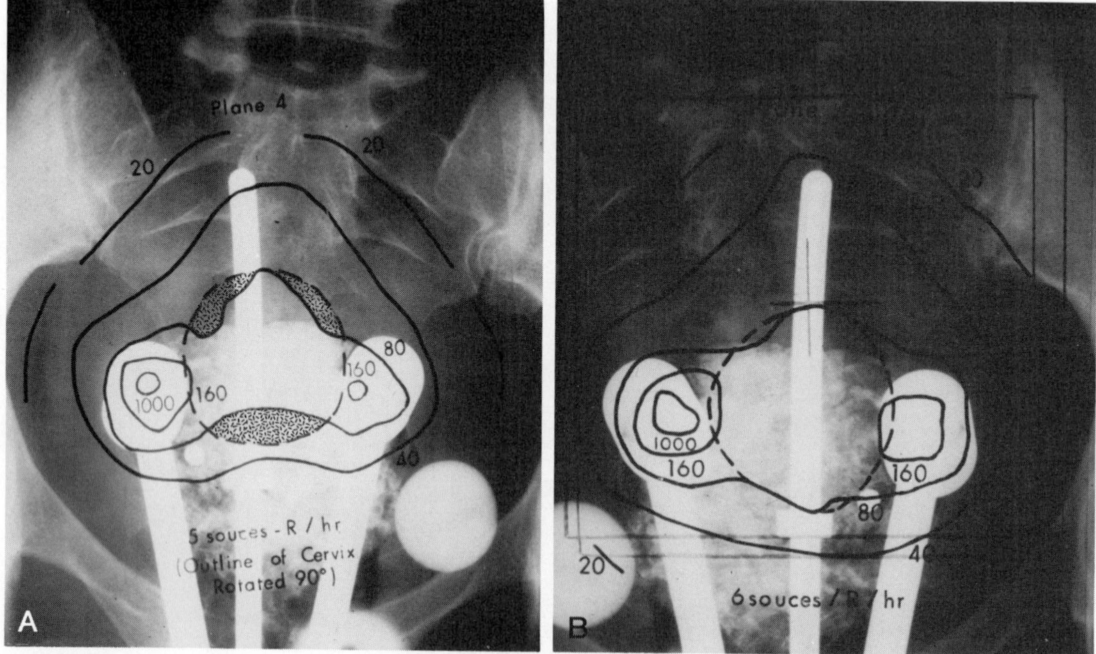

FIGURE 54–24. Radiographs of the pelvis showing intracavitary insertion in a patient with an expanded cervix. (**A**) Poor dose distribution is noted with standard 20, 10, 10 source loading in the tandem due to the dose fall-off caused by the exaggerated separation of the ovoids. (**B**) This can be corrected when a protruding 10 mg source is placed between the ovoids.

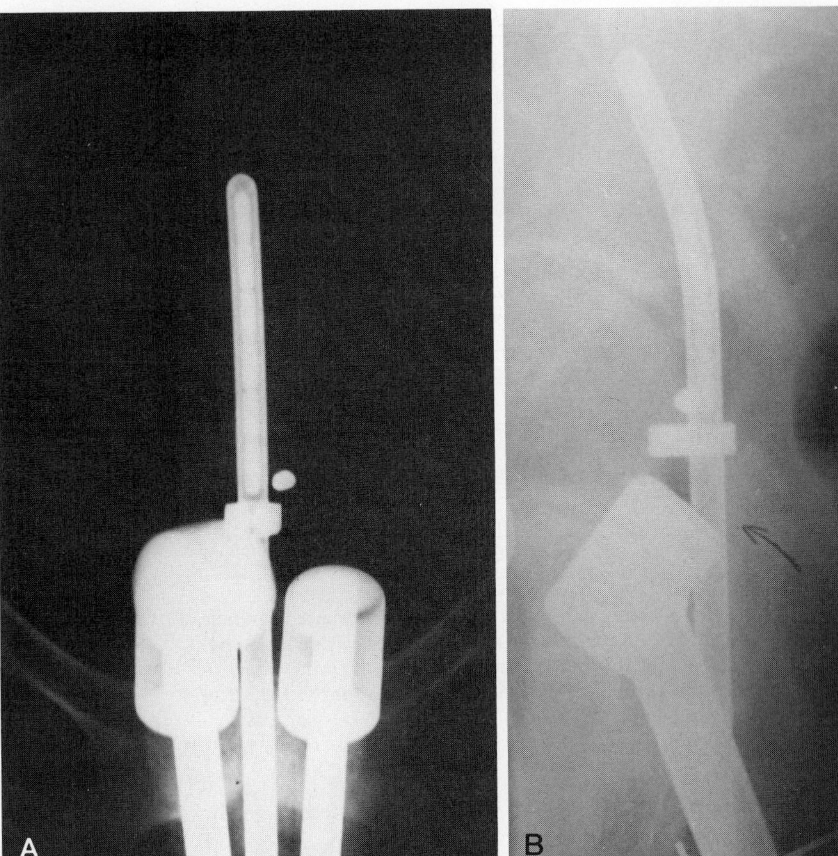

FIGURE 54–25. (**A**) Anteroposterior and (**B**) lateral radiographs of intracavitary application illustrating the importance of the lateral film. On the anteroposterior projection it is suggested that the ovoids may be placed low in the vagina. However, on the lateral projection it is evident that not only are the ovoids low, but there is an undesirable anterior location of the ovoids and posterior placement of the tandem, which will result in a substandard dose distribution.

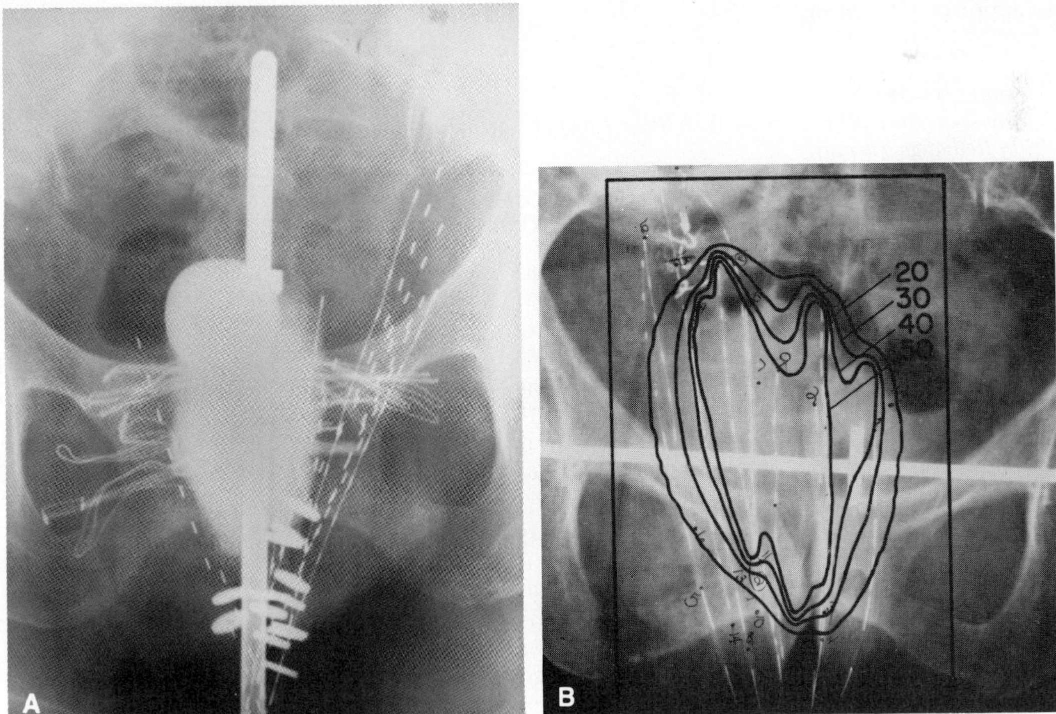

FIGURE 54–26. (**A**) Example of left parametrial implant used to boost the dose in a patient on whom only an afterloading tandem was placed in combination with whole pelvis and parametrial irradiation for treatment of Stage IIB carcinoma. (**B**) Example of afterloading iridium interstitial implant used to boost the dose in the right paravaginal and parametrial tissues in patient with Stage IIIB carcinoma of the cervix.

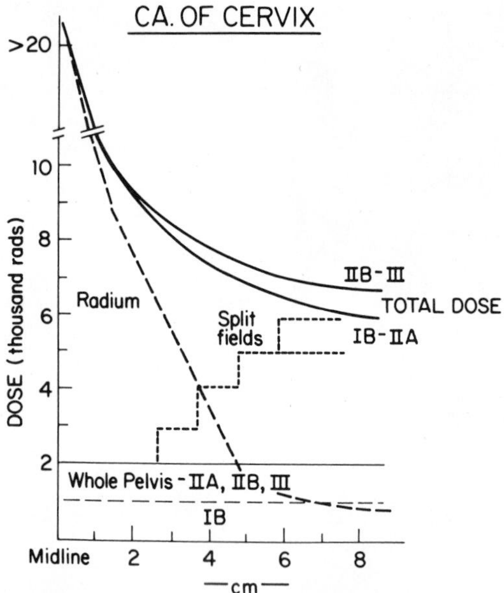

FIGURE 54–27. Dose profile in a hemipelvis, as contributed by whole pelvis, intracavitary, and parametrial doses with step-wedge block. Because of the decreasing thickness of the wedge, the increasing external-beam transmission in the lateral pelvis compensates for the fall-off of the brachytherapy dose.

In an analysis of 128 patients with barrel-shaped Stage IB, Stage IIA, and Stage IIB carcinoma of the cervix, Perez and colleagues[284] reported similar results with the combined approach or using higher intracavitary doses (7500 cGy to point A) in addition to external-beam irradiation (2000 cGy to whole pelvis and 3000 cGy to parametria with midline block) (Table 54-22). The major cause of treatment failure was distant metastases with either approach (Fig. 54-6).

Weems and associates[411] in patients with Stage IB-IIA-B carcinoma of the cervix, 6 cm or greater in diameter treated with irradiation alone or combined with a hysterectomy, also noted no significant difference in pelvic tumor control or survival with either treatment modality. These results were updated by Mendenhall and colleagues,[236] with 75 patients in each treatment group. Local control was 74% and 76%, and absolute survival 54% and 52%. The authors currently reserve combining irradiation with an extrafascial hysterectomy for those patients who have less than 25% tumor regression at the time of the first intracavitary application, who are medically operable, and in whom it is thought adequate surgical margins may be obtained.

Thoms and co-workers[389] reported on 363 patients with bulky endocervical carcinomas treated with curative intent (246 with irradiation alone and in 117 combined with surgery). Patients treated with radiation therapy alone had a 10-year survival rate of 45% compared with 64% for those with radiation therapy and surgery, but this was related to more bulky lesions being treated with radiation therapy alone. In a subset of 48 patients treated with radiation therapy alone and 45 with radiation therapy and surgery, the 10-year survival rate was comparable and pelvic tumor control was 90% and 87%, respectively.

In Stage IB and Stage IIA disease after a hysterectomy and lymphadenectomy (even combined with irradiation), patients with metastatic lymph nodes have survival rates that are approximately 50% of those for patients with negative nodes.[248, 293]

Rampone and co-workers[320] reported a 15% incidence of metastatic lymph nodes in a group of 537 patients with Stage IB carcinoma treated with two preoperative intracavitary insertions (total of 6000 mgh) that delivered 1500 cGy to the pelvic lymph nodes. All patients with positive nodes in the operative specimen had postoperative external-beam irradiation to the pelvis. The 5-year survival rate was 92.9% for 456 patients with

TABLE 54–19
Five-Year Survival of Patients With Stage I and II Carcinoma of the Uterine Cervix Treated by Radiation Therapy

STUDY	STAGE	NO. OF PATIENTS	SURVIVORS*	PERCENT SURVIVAL
Blaikley et al[35]	I	183	123	67.2
	I and II	551	296	53.7
Dickson[83]	IB	348	249	71.6
	IB and IIA	983	589	60.0
Fletcher[103]	IB	549	Actuarial	91.5
	IB and IIA	973		83.5
Kline et al[192]	IB	45	37	81.4
	IB and IIA	64	47	70.5
Kottmeier[199]	IB	611	547	89.5
	IB and IIA	1576	1244	78.9
Muirhead and Green[253]	I	194	152	78.0
	I and II	306	208	68.0
Perez et al[282]	IB	312	Actuarial	87.0
	IIA	98	NED	73.0
Wall et al[405]	I	101	87	86.4
	I and II	208	153	73.5
Average	I			83.5
	I and II			75.6

NED: no evidence of disease
** Patients dead of intercurrent disease included with survivors when data available*
(Modified from Hoskins WJ, Ford JH Jr, Lutz MH, Averette HE: Gynecol Oncol 4:278–290, 1976)

TABLE 54–20
Survival Rates for Stage I and II Carcinoma of the Uterine Cervix Treated by Radical Hysterectomy and Pelvic Lymphadenectomy

STUDY	STAGE	NO. OF PATIENTS	SURVIVORS*	PERCENT SURVIVAL
Blaikley et al[35]	IB	98	64	65.5
	IB and IIA	161	96	50.8
Brunschwig and Barber[46]	IB (A)†	173	141	81.5
	IB and IIA (B)†	308	231	76.0
Christensen et al[58]	IB	168	137	82.7
	IB and IIA	219	168	77.0
Ketcham et al[180]	IB	28	Actuarial	86.0
	IB and IIA	42		87.0
Liu and Meigs[216]	IB	116	91	78.4
	IB and IIA	165	119	72.1
Masterson[231]	IB	120	105	87.5
	IB and IIA	150	124	82.5
Park et al[272]	IB	126	Actuarial	91.0
Average	IB			81.9
	IB and IIA			74.2

** Patients dead of intercurrent disease were included with survivors when data were available*
† Surgical and pathologic classification
(Modified from Hoskins WJ, Ford JH Jr, Lutz MH, Averette HE: Gynecol Oncol 4:278–290, 1976)

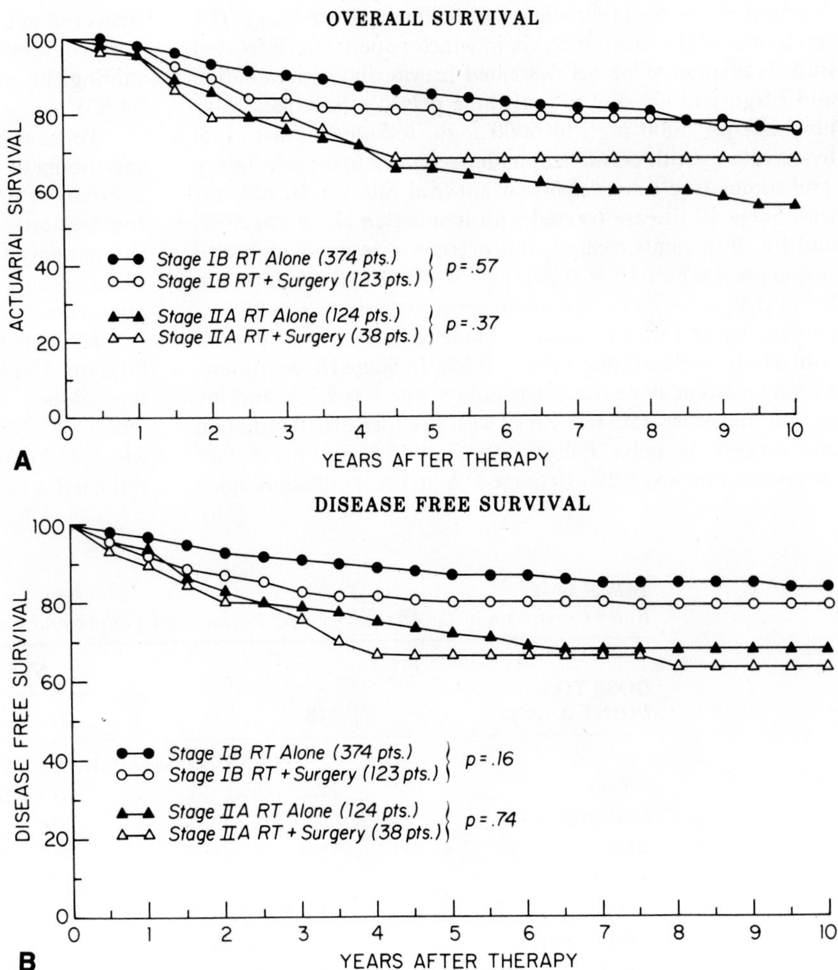

FIGURE 54–28. (**A**) Overall survival and (**B**) disease-free survival of patients with Stage IB and Stage II carcinoma of the uterine cervix treated with irradiation alone or combined with surgery (Mallinckrodt Institute of Radiology, 1959–1986).

TABLE 54–21
Stage IB Cervical Carcinoma: 5-Year Estimated Disease-Free Survival Correlated with Treatment Regimen

	RADICAL HYSTERECTOMY AND PELVIC LYMPHADENECTOMY			EXTERNAL PELVIC PLUS INTRACAVITARY IRRADIATION		
LESION SIZE (cm)	NO. OF PATIENTS	RECURRENCE	5-YEAR ESTIMATED DISEASE-FREE SURVIVAL	NO. OF PATIENTS	RECURRENCE	5-YEAR ESTIMATED DISEASE-FREE SURVIVAL
≤1	18	0	100%	14	1 (7.1%)	92.3%
1–3	34	4 (11.8%)	87.5%	20	3 (15%)	94.4%
≥3	3	0	100%	14	2 (14.3%)	84.6%
Total	55	4 (7.3%)	92.3%	48	6 (12.5%)	91.1%

(Modified from Piver MS, Marchetti DL, Patton T, et al: Am J Clin Oncol 11:21–24, 1988)

negative nodes in contrast to 52% in 81 patients with positive nodes.

Einhorn and associates,[96] in a nonrandomized study, observed 100% 5-year survival rate in 49 patients with Stage IB disease receiving combined therapy, compared with 81% in 64 patients treated with irradiation alone. No difference was observed in 25 patients with Stage IIA tumor treated with combined therapy and 40 patients treated with irradiation alone (5-year survival rate of about 75%).

Perez and colleagues[281] reported on a prospectively randomized study of 118 patients with Stage IB or Stage IIA carcinoma of the uterine cervix in which patients were treated with irradiation alone (as described previously) or irradiation and surgery (2000 cGy to the whole pelvis; one intracavitary insertion for 5000 mgh to 6000 mgh, followed by a radical hysterectomy with pelvic lymphadenectomy 2 to 6 weeks later). The tumor-free actuarial 5-year survival rate for 40 patients with Stage IB disease treated with irradiation alone was 80%, and for 48 patients treated with preoperative irradiation and surgery it was 82% (P = 0.23) (Fig. 54-29). In 16 patients with Stage IIA disease, actuarial tumor-free survival rate was 56% in patients treated with irradiation alone and 79% in 14 treated with irradiation and surgery (P = 0.13). In Stage IB carcinoma, with irradiation alone the pelvic failure rate was 2.5%, and the distant metastasis rate was 7.5%; with preoperative irradiation and surgery the pelvic failure rate was 12.5%, and the distant metastasis rate was 4.2%. In Stage IIA, in the irradiation-alone group the pelvic failure rate was 6.3%; the combined pelvic recurrence with distant metastases rate was 18.8%, and distant metastases alone rate was 12.5%. The incidence of grade 2 or 3 complications in the patients who received radiation therapy alone was 13.8% (two had vesicovaginal fistulas, one had rectovaginal fistula, and one had rectal stricture). In the patients treated with preoperative irradiation and surgery, it was 11% (one rectal stricture, one severe proctitis, one small bowel obstruction, and three ureteral strictures).

When combined therapy is used, the dose of radiation delivered to the lymph nodes, the time of the operation, and the pathologic examination of the specimens all are critical in determining the presence of postirradiation residual tumor (Table 54-23).

Perez and colleagues[280] noted that in patients with primary carcinoma of the uterine cervix who had endometrial stromal invasion or tumor only in the curettings, the addition of a hysterectomy did not improve the survival rate because most of the patients failed owing to distant dissemination. Pelvic and distant recurrences were approximately the same whether radiation therapy was used alone or in combination with surgery.

In patients with Stage IIB disease the 5-year survival rate is 60% to 65%, and practically all patients are treated with radiation alone. The pelvic failure rate ranges from 18% to 39%.[103,224,279] In an analysis of the Patterns of Care Study in which 157 patients had Stage IIB disease, Coia and associates[64] reported a better 4-year survival rate (67% and 54%) and in-

TABLE 54–22
Bulky Carcinoma of the Uterine Cervix: Parametrial Failure and Correlation With Dose to Point A

DOSE TO POINT A (cGy)	STAGE IB	STAGE IIA	STAGE IIB
	BARREL-SHAPED		
<6000	2/20 (10%)	1/5 (20%)	1/8 (12.5%)
6001 to 8000	3/13 (23.1%)	0/14	1/18 (5.6%)
>8000	0/8	0/5	1/13 (7.7%)
	NON-BARREL-SHAPED		
<6000	5/103 (4.9%)	2/28 (7.1%)	9/37 (24.3%)
6001 to 8000	5/134 (3.7%)	3/32 (9.4%)	13/123 (10.6%)
>8000	2/40 (5%)	2/17 (11.8%)	10/82 (12.2%)

(Perez CA, et al: Int J Radiat Oncol Biol Phys 11:1903, 1985)

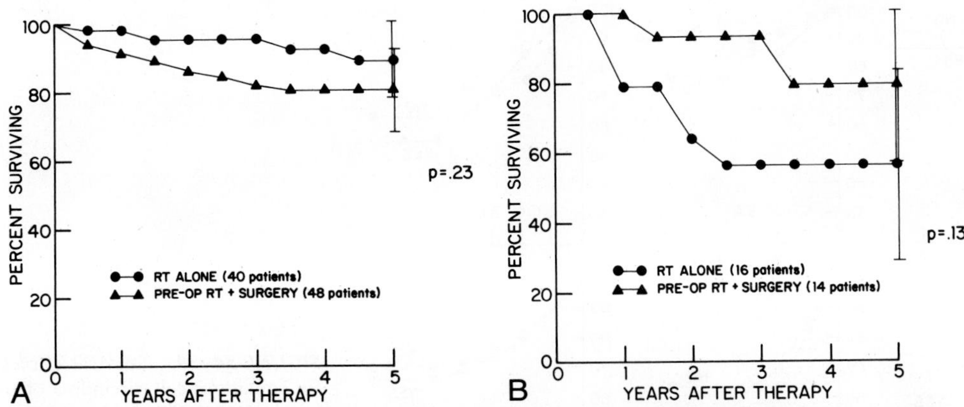

FIGURE 54–29. NED actuarial survival rates in patients with **(A)** Stage IB or **(B)** Stage IIA carcinoma of the uterine cervix treated with either irradiation alone (*circles*) or a combination of low-dose preoperative irradiation and surgery (*triangles*). Difference in survival rates is not statistically significant. (NED: no evidence of disease) (Perez CA, Camel HM, Kao MS, Askin F: Gynecol Oncol 27:129–140, 1987)

field tumor control (78% and 68%) in patients with unilateral parametrial involvement than in patients with bilateral parametrial involvement, respectively. Occasionally a conservative hysterectomy is performed 4 to 6 weeks after completion of high-dose preoperative irradiation in patients with barrel-shaped cervix and limited medial parametrial infiltration that regresses completely. Before 1965, a pelvic lymphadenectomy was carried out at M. D. Anderson Cancer Center after a full course of radiation therapy, but this procedure did not improve survival over treatment with irradiation alone (Fig. 54-30), and the complication rate was somewhat higher.[340]

In Stage IIIB carcinoma the 5-year survival rates range from 25% to 48%.[103,204,245,279] Hanks and associates,[134] reporting on the Patterns of Care Study, noted 28% probability of 5-year survival in patients with Stage III carcinoma of the cervix treated in a large number of facilities in the United States compared with 60% survival rate in selected large centers (extended survey) (Fig. 54-31). This range may be related to the socioeconomic status of the patients, extent of the disease, techniques of irradiation, and doses delivered.

The pelvic failure rate in patients with Stage IIIB disease is about 40%; in Stage IV it is 75%. In patients with Stage IVA the 5-year survival rate ranges from 18%[201] to 34%[240] after definitive irradiation.

Kramer and associates[201] reported on 48 patients with Stage IVA carcinoma of the cervix treated with definitive radiation therapy (3000 cGy to 4500 cGy to the whole pelvis with additional parametrial doses to complete 4000 cGy to 6000 cGy combined with one or two intracavitary insertions for approximately 3000 mgh to 5000 mgh) delivering 7000 cGy to 8000 cGy or more to point A. Fifteen patients also received periaortic irradiation (4000 cGy to 4500 cGy). Nine patients survived without recurrence, and the 5-year actuarial survival rate was 18%. The serious complication rate was 22%, consisting mostly of vesicovaginal fistulas in five patients and severe radiation enteritis in one patient. The degree of parametrial involvement had a significant impact on prognosis. (Patients with minimal disease had a 5-year survival rate of 46% compared with only 5% for those with extensive parametrial tumor.)

Horiot and associates[147] reported the results of a French

TABLE 54–23
Stage IB and IIA Carcinoma of the Uterine Cervix: Incidence of Metastatic Pelvic Lymph Nodes and Dose of Irradiation Delivered to Lymph Nodes

	STAGE IB		STAGE IIA		
AUTHOR	SURGERY ALONE	PREOPERATIVE RADIATION THERAPY	SURGERY ALONE	PREOPERATIVE RADIATION THERAPY	**ESTIMATED DOSE (cGy) TO NODES**
Christensen[58]	29/167 (17.4%)	—	27/104 (26%)	—	0
Morley[248]	18/143 (12.6%)	—	—	—	0
Morton[251]	9/38 (23.7%)	4/32 (12.5%)	—	—	1800
Sweeney and Douglas[374]	—	5/39 (13%)	—	9/54 (17%)	3500
Rampone[320]	—	81/537 (15%)	—	—	2000
Decker[75]	—	5/38 (13.2%)	—	11/45 (24.4%)	4000
Quigley[317]	—	13/136 (9.6%)	—	—	1800
Parker[274]	15/95 (16%)	6/73 (8%)	7/16 (44%)	20/71 (28%)	Not stated
Gray[118]	5/44 (11.4%)	3/58 (5.2%)	6/17 (35.3%)	Inc. with I	4500
Perez[281]	—	2/43 (4.6%)	—	2/24 (8.3%)	3000–4000
Perez[281]	—	0/32 (0%)	—	—	4001–5000
Rutledge[340]	—	1/30 (3.3%)	—	4/39 (10.3%)	5000

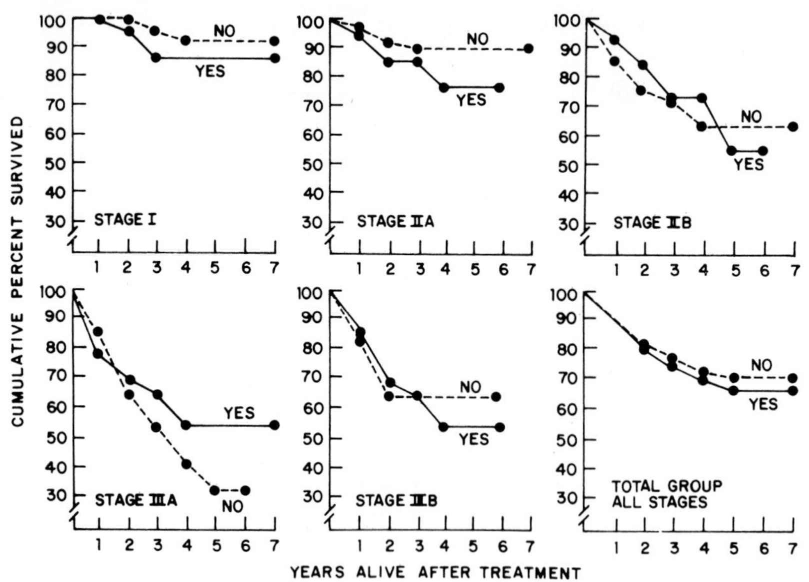

FIGURE 54–30. Survival curves of patients treated for squamous cell carcinoma of the cervix. Curves for Stages I, IIA, IIB, IIIA, and IIIB and all stages combined are shown. Patients who had lymphadenectomy added to their treatment are represented by solid line curves. The broken line curves are for patients who had irradiation only. (Rutledge FN, Fletcher GH, MacDonald EJ: Am J Roentgenol Radium Ther Nucl Med 93:607–614, 1965)

cooperative study of 1383 patients with various stages of invasive carcinoma of the intact uterus treated with irradiation alone following the M. D. Anderson Cancer Center treatment guidelines. Survival rates and locoregional tumor control rates were similar in both groups, except in those with Stage III disease, in which the pelvic and central failure rates were lower in the French patients, probably because of different amounts of tumor volume or socioeconomic factors. Major urinary complications were noted in 2% of the patients and grade 3 bowel complications in 3% of the patients with Stage I and Stage IIA disease and 7% of patients with Stage IIB and Stage III disease.

The overall survival and disease-free survival rates observed with irradiation alone at the Mallinckrodt Institute of Radiology are depicted in Figure 54-32.

Marcial and colleagues[224] described results of a prospective randomized trial of 301 patients with Stages IIB, III, and IVA carcinoma of the uterine cervix treated with split-course irradiation (ten fractions of 250 cGy, five weekly doses up to 2500 cGy, followed by a rest period of 2 weeks, and an additional 2500 cGy delivered in the same manner) or continuous irradiation consisting of 30 fractions of 170 cGy daily, five times per week (total dose 5100 cGy). In both groups, external-beam irradiation was combined with intracavitary brachytherapy for 3000 cGy to point A. There was no significant difference in tumor control, acute or late complications, or survival in the two groups, although a tendency toward better pelvic tumor control was found in the more advanced stages treated with the split-course technique. The most frequently seen severe late complication was proctitis, which occurred in 2% of the patients in the continuous-dose group and in 5% of those in the split-dose group. Cystitis and soft tissue necrosis were noted in 2% of patients in both groups.

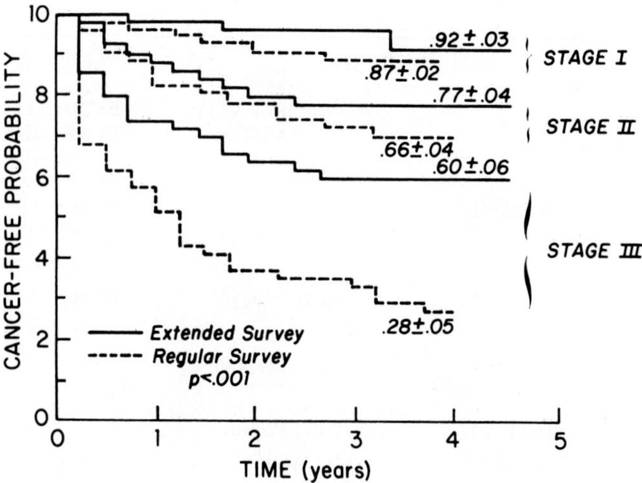

FIGURE 54–31. Patterns of Care Study analysis of disease-free survival for carcinoma of the uterine cervix treated at selected large facilities (*solid lines*) and a large number of facilities (*broken lines*). (Hanks GE, Herring DF, Kramer S: Cancer 51:959–967, 1983)

Results With Interstitial Implants

Interstitial parametrial implants have been used to supplement standard external and intracavitary techniques. Because of the inability to insert an intracavitary tandem in three patients with Stage IB and seven patients with Stage IIA disease, interstitial needle implants were used at Washington University to supplement the external radiation doses. In 30 patients with Stage IIB and in 37 with Stage III carcinoma, interstitial irradiation in the parametrium was used to supplement the dose delivered by external-beam and intracavitary brachytherapy. Despite the fact that the patients treated with interstitial implant were in a high-risk group, local control was comparable to that of patients treated with standard techniques.[286]

Pierquin and associates[291] described locoregional recurrences in 6% of 53 patients with T1, 11% of 47 patients with T2, and 42% of 19 patients with T3 primary tumors of the uterine cervix treated with a combination of external-beam irradiation and the Creteil method for interstitial implantation of ^{192}Ir sources in a plastic cervical-vaginal *moulage* and a uterine tandem.

Prempree and colleagues[312] reported a 96% local tumor control rate and 61% 5-year disease-free survival rate in 23 patients with intact uterus for Stage IIIB carcinoma of the cervix treated with a combination of external-beam irradiation and intracavitary and interstitial implant to the parametrium. They also described a 23% local failure rate and a 69% 5-year

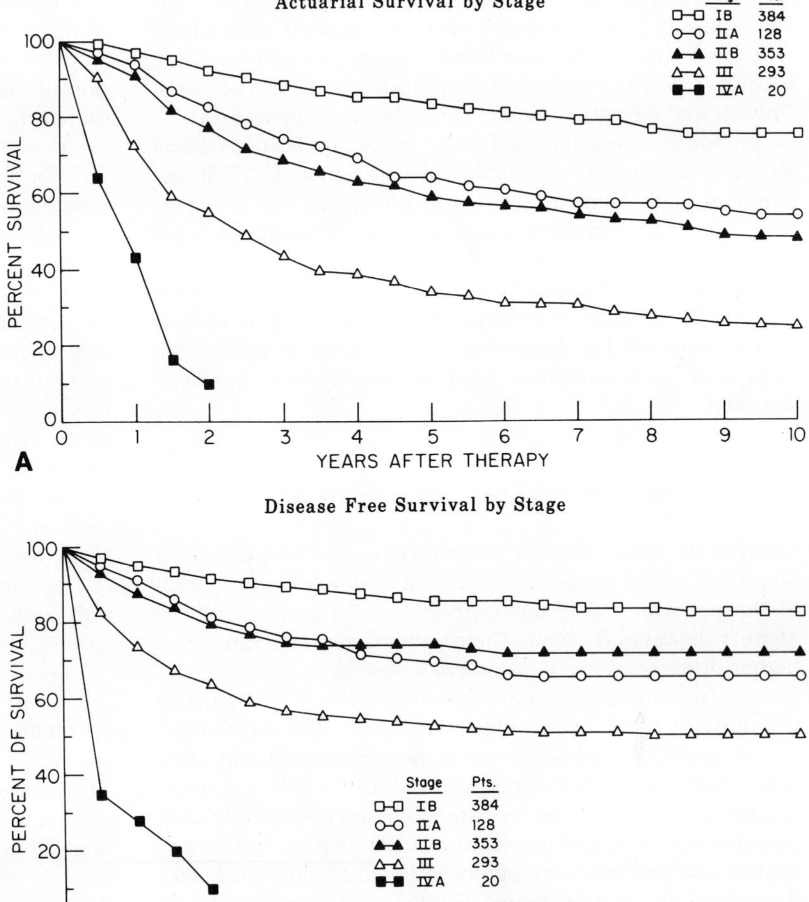

FIGURE 54–32. Overall survival (**A**) and disease-free survival rates (**B**) for 1101 patients with carcinoma of the cervix treated with irradiation alone at the Mallinckrodt Institute of Radiology (1959–1986).

survival rate in 26 patients with similar stage carcinoma of the cervix treated in the same manner but in whom the uterine cavity could not be probed or was absent. Overall, major complications were noted in 8% of the 49 patients.

Aristizabal and associates[14] treated 21 patients with locally advanced invasive carcinoma of the uterine cervix with transperineal interstitial implants using a plastic template with predrilled holes in a concentric pattern for insertion of plastic or steel guides. A central opening in the template can be used to insert the plastic vaginal cylinder. With a mean follow-up of 26 months, local tumor control was noted in 18 of the patients (85%). Seven patients (33%) developed grade 2 or 3 complications, which included one vesicovaginal fistula, one rectovaginal fistula, and one patient with both fistulas. Three patients developed severe radiation proctitis or cystitis or both (one each). The loading of the obturator needles or the use of the central cylinder sources probably contributed to the relatively high incidence of complications. The authors have discontinued the use of the obturator surface needles, except when gross residual tumor is found in the central area.

Martinez and co-workers,[227] using an applicator consisting of two acrylic cylinders, a template with an array of holes that serve as guides to localize the trocars, and a cover plate, treated 37 patients with advanced or recurrent carcinoma of the cervix and 26 with vaginal-urethral tumors. Doses in the range of 3500 cGy were given, in addition to external-beam irradiation (3600 cGy to the whole pelvis and 1400 cGy to pelvic side wall). They reported six local failures in the patients with cervical lesions and five in the group with vaginal-urethral tumors. The overall complication rate was 5.1%.

Results With Californium-252 or Neutrons

Maruyama and Muir[229] have used Californium-252(^{252}Cf)-neutron brachytherapy in conjunction with fractionated external-beam irradiation to treat carcinoma of the uterine cervix. They reported on 41 patients with Stage IB disease treated with 4000 cGy to 5000 cGy to the whole pelvis followed by a 500 cGy to 1500 cGy boost to the lateral pelvic wall. The ^{252}Cf-neutron therapy was usually delivered in a single intracavitary insertion in approximately 8 hours. A relative biologic effectiveness of 6 was assumed for the ^{252}Cf relative to the ^{137}Cs. The dose was calculated taking into consideration the contribution from the neutrons as well as from the photons of the ^{252}Cf. Nearly total tumor clearance was achieved in over 90% of the patients by the completion of therapy. Tumor regression was more rapid in the ^{252}Cf group than in similar patients treated with ^{137}Cs and the same dose of external-beam irradiation.

Maor and colleagues[223] reported results in 156 patients with locally advanced cervical carcinoma (Stages IIB, III, and IVA) treated at five institutions and randomized to receive external photons only to the pelvis (5000 cGy in 25 fractions in 5 weeks) or mixed-beam external irradiation (three fractions per week of photons) to a total relative biologic effectiveness adjusted dose of 5000 cGy over 5 weeks. All patients were scheduled to receive intracavitary brachytherapy. Of 146 evaluable patients, 80 were treated with mixed-beam and 66 with photons. Only 50% of the patients in the mixed-beam group and 75% in the photon group underwent brachytherapy applications. Local control at 2 years was 45% in the mixed-beam and 52% in the photon groups. Median survival was 1.9 and 2.3 years, respectively. Severe complications occurred in 19% of the mixed-beam and 11% of the photon-beam patients ($P < 0.13$). It was thought that the inferior outcome with neutrons may have resulted from the use of horizontal beams of varying energy and penetration. A new randomized trial using high-energy hospital-based cyclotrons with gantry-mounted beam-delivery systems has been activated.

Results With External-Beam Irradiation Alone

Occasionally brachytherapy procedures cannot be performed because of medical reasons or unusual anatomic configuration of the pelvis or the tumor (extensive lesion and inability to identify the cervical canal). These patients may be treated with higher doses of external-beam irradiation alone.

Castro and co-workers[55] reported results in 118 patients with invasive cervical carcinoma treated with 5000 cGy to 6000 cGy to the whole pelvis (four-field box technique) and additional doses to residual tumor with reduced AP-PA portals to complete the 7000 cGy tumor dose. With doses below 5000 cGy, no pelvic tumor control was obtained in 32 patients, but disease control and survival were significantly enhanced with higher doses. Complications increased with higher doses; for instance, severe sigmoiditis was not noted in 32 patients treated with 5000 cGy, but it was seen in one of 28 receiving 6000 cGy and in four of 44 in the 7000 cGy group.

Coia and co-workers,[65] in an analysis of 565 patients with various stages of cervical carcinoma treated in the Patterns of Care Study, reported better survival (67%) and pelvic tumor control (78%) rates in patients receiving brachytherapy compared with those who had no intracavitary applications (36% 4-year survival rate and 47% in-field failure). Patients treated with two intracavitary applications had a higher 4-year survival rate (73%) and in field-tumor control rate (83%) than those receiving only one application (60% 4-year survival rate and 71% in-field tumor control).

Hanks and associates[134] and Montana[245] reported a higher incidence of central pelvic recurrences in patients with Stage III cervical carcinoma treated with external-beam irradiation alone than in patients receiving brachytherapy in addition to external-beam irradiation (Table 54-24). The incidence of major complications was similar in both groups of patients.

Ulmer and Frischbier[394] treated 150 patients with external-beam irradiation alone (8000 cGy to central pelvis and 6000 cGy to pelvic wall in 6 weeks with rotational techniques) and reported tumor control in 120 of the patients (80%), depending on how the follow-up data are interpreted. The 5-year survival rates were 75% for patients with Stage II, 30% for Stage III, and 13% for Stage IV disease. Six patients developed grade 2 and six developed grade 3 complications.

Akine and associates[6] treated 104 of 2701 patients with carcinoma of the uterine cervix with external-beam irradiation alone (AP/PA or four-field box techniques) because of inability to perform intracavitary brachytherapy. The total average doses delivered were 5000 cGy to the whole pelvis followed by additional doses with reduced portals to deliver a total of 6080 cGy in 6 weeks, 7230 cGy in 7.5 weeks, and 8050 cGy in 8 weeks with a daily dose of 190 cGy or 200 cGy. The local tumor control rate was 27% for patients with Stage II, 19% for Stage III, and 15% for Stage IVA disease. The 5-year survival rates were 36%, 17%, and 5%, respectively. Four patients had major complications (usually proctitis) that required surgical treatment, and one patient died of rectal bleeding. Eight of 23 patients treated with conformation therapy had control of the tumor and survived 5 years without major complications.

Patterns of Failure

The incidence of failure at various sites in carcinoma of the uterine cervix after irradiation are closely correlated with the stage of the tumor (Table 54-25). Cervical or vaginal vault (central) recurrences should always be confirmed by biopsy. When possible, parametrial recurrences should be documented by needle biopsy. Lopez and associates[217] performed transvaginal parametrium needle biopsy in 76 patients clinically suspected of having postirradiation recurrent carcinoma of the cervix without mucosal lesions suitable for biopsy under direct vision. Needle biopsies indicated cancer in 41 patients; 20 were surgically explored, and 11 underwent total pelvic exteneration. Three patients survived longer than 5 years. In 35 patients whose parametrial biopsies were normal, eight were later shown to have progression of local and systemic disease. Twenty-seven other patients in whom biopsies were normal were cured by radiation therapy. The morbidity rate of this procedure is minimal (2.6%). However, a clinical diagnosis can nearly always be made in the presence of a "triad" consisting of sciatic pain, leg edema, and hydronephrosis. Computed tomography or lymphangiography is useful in outlining the tumor in the regional lymph nodes. Extrapelvic metastases are documented by clinical examination, radiographic or radionuclide studies, and biopsy when indicated.

Jampolis and associates,[160] analyzing postirradiation recur-

TABLE 54–24
Carcinoma of the Uterine Cervix: Incidence of Central/Pelvic Recurrences According to Method of Therapy

		INCIDENCE OF PELVIC FAILURES		
AUTHOR	**STAGE**	EXTERNAL BEAM ONLY	EXTERNAL BEAM AND INTRACAVITARY	***P* VALUE**
Hanks et al[134]	III	33/38 (86%)	55/109 (50%)	0.0002
Montana et al[245]	III	14/35 (40%)	12/37 (32%)	0.6725
Coia et al[64]	I, II, III	(53%)	(22%)	<0.01

TABLE 54–25
Carcinoma of the Uterine Cervix: Site of Failure and Stage (MIR 1959–1986)

STAGE	NO. OF PATIENTS	SITE OF FAILURE		
		PELVIC	PELVIC + DISTANT METASTASIS	DISTANT METASTASIS ONLY
IB	374	6 (1.6%)	28 (7.5%)	33 (8.8%)
IIA	124	4 (3.2%)	17 (13.7%)	23 (18.5%)
IIB	314	36 (11.5%)	35 (11.1%)	47 (15%)
III	271	48 (17.7%)	73 (26.9%)	54 (19.9%)
IVA	18	2 (11.1%)	11 (61.1%)	4 (22.2%)

rences in 916 patients with squamous cell carcinoma of the intact uterus, pointed out that central recurrences were extremely rare (2%) in Stage IB and Stage IIA disease and that in most instances they could be attributed to improper placement of the vaginal colpostats, which could produce low doses of radiation in the cervix. Parametrial recurrences in Stages I, IIA, and IIB carcinoma were correlated with lateral deviation of the radium system without compensation from the external-beam irradiation in about 75% of the patients. The overwhelming cause of failure in patients with Stage IIIB disease was massive parametrial infiltration that could not be controlled with doses of 7000 cGy.

In a review of 849 patients treated with irradiation alone (external and intracavitary), Perez and co-workers[279] illustrated a correlation of doses delivered to the medial parametrium and pelvic recurrences and disclosed no significant improvement in tumor control with increasing doses of radiation in Stage IB disease. Montana and associates[244] also failed to demonstrate significant correlation between doses to point A and probability of local/pelvic tumor control in 197 patients with Stage IB disease treated with irradiation alone (7000 cGy to 8000 cGy to point A). However, in Stage IIA, IIB, and III disease, Perez and associates[286] reported improved tumor control with total doses over 8000 cGy to 9000 cGy to point A. Moreover, higher doses delivered to the lateral parametrium in general were correlated with greater tumor control in Stage IIB and Stage III tumors. Coia and associates,[65] who reviewed the results in 565 patients treated in the Patterns of Care Study, reported a 68% 4-year survival rate in patients receiving central doses higher than 6500 cGy compared with 42% for patients treated with lower doses ($P < 0.01$). Likewise, the tumor control rate was 78% with paracentral doses higher than 6500 cGy and 59% with lower doses ($P < 0.01$).

Results in Patients With Metastatic Paraaortic Lymph Nodes

Paraaortic lymph node metastases are frequently combined with distant dissemination but are clinically apparent only in 10% to 20% of patients who have recurrences.

Nelson and associates[258] reported on 104 patients with Stage II and Stage III cervical carcinoma who had exploratory laparotomy and paraaortic lymph node biopsies; 12.5% of the patients with Stage IIA disease, 14.9% with Stage IIB, and 38.4% with Stage III disease had metastatic paraaortic lymph nodes. These patients were later treated with 6000 cGy to the paraaortic region. Within 4 years, 50% of these patients had distant metastases. Only one of 13 patients with positive paraaortic nodes was alive at the end of 4 years. Thirty-nine percent of the patients treated with paraaortic lymph node irradiation had grade 2 or 3 complications compared with 32% of the patients receiving radiation therapy to the pelvis only. No significant increase in intraperitoneal complications was found in the patients receiving paraaortic irradiation. Nelson and associates did not recommend that 6000 cGy be given to the paraaortic area. They also concluded that the main goal of exploratory laparotomy and paraaortic lymph node biopsy is to define the extent of the disease. Extended lymphadenectomies, either pelvic or paraaortic, are not therapeutic, are not substitutes for radiation therapy as a primary method of treatment, and do not enhance the success of radiation therapy.

Lovecchio and associates[218] reported a 50% 5-year survival rate in 36 patients with Stage IB and Stage IIA cervical carcinoma identified at pretherapy surgical staging laparotomy to have histologically confirmed paraaortic lymph node metastases. The patients were treated with radiation therapy, including 4500 cGy to the paraaortic lymph nodes. Fourteen of 31 evaluable patients developed pelvic recurrence (12 combined with distant metastases). Unfortunately, the authors did not specify how many patients had periaortic recurrences, although they reported four abdominal failures. Podczaski and associates[305] reported five of 35 patients with surgically documented paraaortic metastasis treated with extended field and pelvic irradiation (in seven with concurrent chemotherapy). Actuarial survival rates at 2 and 5 years were 32% and 29%, respectively. Twenty-three patients died of cervical cancer, and four patients died of intercurrent disease.

Goodman and associates[113] compiled survival statistics on patients with paraaortic lymph node metastasis and found an average 5-year survival rate of about 40% (Table 54-26).

Results of Elective Paraaortic Lymph Node Irradiation

Rotman and the Radiation Therapy Oncology Group[333] reported on a randomized study of 335 patients with Stage IIB carcinoma of the uterine cervix with no clinical or radiographic evidence of periaortic lymphadenopathy who in addition to standard pelvic irradiation were randomized to electively receive 4500 cGy to the paraaortic region. There was no significant difference in the groups ($P = 0.21$). The 5-year survival rate was 66% for patients receiving elective paraaortic irradiation and 55% for those treated to the pelvis ($P = 0.043$). Although not statistically significant, the tumor control rate was also better in the patients electively irradiated to the paraaortic area (75% *versus* 66% for the pelvic irradiated group; Fig. 54-33). Fourteen (8%) severe and six (4%) life-threatening complications occurred in the patients treated with pelvic irradia-

TABLE 54–26
Results of Extended-Field Irradiation for Paraaortic Lymph Node Metastases

AUTHOR	NO. OF PATIENTS	PARAAORTIC DOSE (cGy)	NED* SURVIVAL 2 YEARS	NED* SURVIVAL 5 YEARS	INCIDENCE OF SEVERE COMPLICATIONS (%)
Lepanto[211]	36	5000–5500	11/26 (42%)	4/8 (50%)	19.5
Delgado[77]	13	4500	38%†		46.0
Berman[30]	7	4320–5120	57%‡		—
Piver[296]	21	6000		9.6%	61.9
(two cohorts)	10	4400–5000		43.0%	10.0
Rubin[335]	14	4000–5000			36.0
Tewfik[382]	23	5000–5500	22.6§		35.0
Potish[306]	81	4350–5075		40.0%	2.4
Lovecchio[218]	36	4500	70%	50%	—
Podczaski[305]	35	4250–5100	38%	29%	9

**NED: no evidence of disease*
†Follow-up = 13 to 36 months
‡Follow-up = 4 to 25 months
§Follow-up = 45 months
(Modified from Goodman HM, Bowling MC, Nelson JH Jr: Cervical malignancies. In Knapp RC, Berkowitz RS [eds]: Gynecologic Oncology, pp 225–273. New York, Macmillan, 1986)

tion only, whereas 13 (8%) severe and 11 (7%) life-threatening complications occurred in patients irradiated to the paraaortic lymph nodes.

A similar randomized study was reported by Haie and EORTC[129] on 441 patients with cervical carcinoma who had an increased risk of lymph node metastasis and no clinical, radiographic, or surgical evidence of paraaortic lymph node involvement. In the study group the paraaortic area received 4500 cGy with external-beam irradiation. No statistically significant difference was found between the two treatment arms with regard to local control, distant metastases, and survival. However, the incidence of paraaortic and distant metastases without pelvic failure was significantly higher in patients receiving pelvic irradiation alone. The incidence of small bowel injury was 0.9% in the pelvic irradiation and 2.3% in the pelvic and paraaortic irradiation groups. A severe complication rate of 9% was observed in patients receiving paraaortic irradiation compared with 4.8% in those treated to the pelvis only.

Pelvic Tumor Control and Prognosis

Perez and colleagues,[285] in an analysis of 1054 patients, showed that control of the tumor in the pelvis was crucial to the survival of patients in all stages. One of three patients with Stage IB disease who had a pelvic failure only survived for more than 5 years after extensive surgery for treatment of the recurrence. Furthermore, patients exhibiting complete tumor regression within 30 days after completion of radiation therapy had not only a substantially lower number of pelvic recurrences but also fewer distant metastases (Table 54-27). The analysis emphasizes the need to deliver biologically effective doses of irradiation to ensure the highest probability of controlling the tumor in the pelvis, because the salvage rate in patients who failed with isolated pelvic recurrence is not optimal, even after pelvic exenteration.

In 171 patients with Stage IB tumors treated by irradiation compared with 200 patients treated with radical abdominal

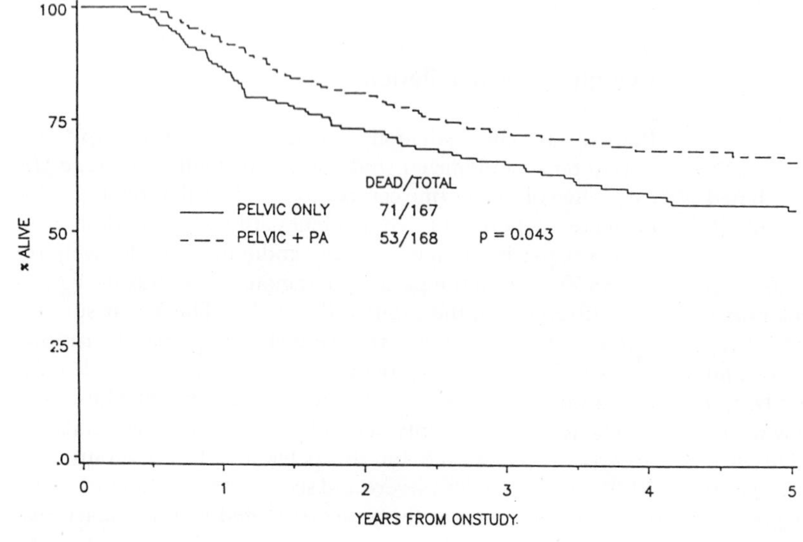

FIGURE 54–33. Survival by assigned treatment (Kaplan-Meier) for patients treated on Radiation Therapy Oncology Group protocol 79-20. Pelvic + PA: patients receiving elective periaortic irradiation. (Rotman M, Choi K, Guse C, et al: Int J Radiat Oncol Biol Phys 19:513–521, 1990)

TABLE 54–27
*Carcinoma of the Uterine Cervix: Incidence of Pelvic Recurrences and Short-Term Tumor Regression**

	TOTAL PELVIC FAILURES			TOTAL DISTANT METASTASES		
STAGE	CR†	SUSP†	PERS†	CR†	SUSP†	PERS†
IB	16/294 (5.4%)	1/3 (33.3%)	6/16 (37.5%)	35/294 (11.9%)	1/3 (33.3%)	6/16 (37.5%)
IIA	10/86 (11.6%)	2/3 (66.7%)	5/10 (50%)	24/86 (27.9%)	1/3 (33.3%)	7/10 (70%)
IIB	30/220 (13.6%)	6/11 (54.5%)	18/29 (62.1%)	40/220 (18.2%)	8/11 (72.7%)	15/29 (51.7%)
III	30/134 (22.4%)	7/19 (36.8%)	44/53 (83%)	45/134 (33.6%)	6/19 (31.6%)	37/53 (69.8%)

* *Within 30 days from completion of irradiation; MIR 1959–1982*
† *Degrees of tumor regression: CR: complete tumor regression; Susp: equivocal findings; Pers: Clinically persistent tumor*
(Perez CA, Kuske RR, Camel HM, et al: Int J Radiat Oncol Biol Phys 14:613–621, 1988)

hysterectomy and pelvic lymph node dissection, less than 20% 5-year survival rate was reported in 67 patients who developed a pelvic recurrence after primary treatment.[354]

It is important to stress the high incidence of distant metastasis in patients with Stage III and Stage IV carcinoma of the cervix that makes imperative the development of adequate adjuvant therapy to improve the prognosis of these patients. The most common metastatic sites are the lungs, mediastinal lymph nodes, liver, and bones.[54]

Results With Adenocarcinoma of the Cervix

Several authors have reported similar survival for comparable stages of adenocarcinoma or squamous cell carcinoma; the clinical stage, volume of disease,[124,185] and dose of irradiation[124] were the most important prognostic factors.

Hopkins and associates[146] reported no significant difference in survival rate among the various subtypes in 203 patients with primary adenocarcinoma of the cervix. The histologic grade of malignancy, however, played a major prognostic role, with poorly differentiated tumors having the worst prognosis.

Some authors have suggested that a combination of irradiation and surgery may be more effective than irradiation alone for patients with adenocarcinoma.[27,243] In contrast, Kilgore and associates,[185] reporting on 162 patients (67 treated with radical hysterectomy alone, 65 with irradiation alone, and the remainder with a combination of both modalities), and Grigsby and associates,[124] reporting on 79 patients treated with irradiation alone, found no significant difference in tumor control or survival in patients with squamous cell carcinoma treated in a similar manner.

Grigsby and colleagues[124] noted a 5-year disease-free survival rate (all stages combined) of 68% for 925 patients with epidermoid carcinoma compared with 64.9% for 79 patients with adenocarcinoma treated with irradiation alone ($P = 0.34$). No significant difference in the survival rate was observed when epidermoid carcinoma and adenocarcinoma were compared after stratification by clinical stage and treatment modality (Table 54-28). Prognostic variables that were significant for the development of recurrent disease in the pelvis were size of primary lesion and dose of radiation to point A. Significant factors for the development of distant metastatic disease were size of primary lesion and metastatic lymph nodes at the time of diagnosis.

Similar observations were reported by Eifel and colleagues[95] in 334 patients with adenocarcinoma of the cervix in an update of previous report by Rutledge and associates.[341] The 5-year relapse-free survival and locoregional control rates were 88% and 94%, respectively, in 91 patients with normal-sized cervix; 64% and 82%, respectively, in 102 patients with lesions 3 cm to 5.9 cm in diameter; and only 45% and 77%, respectively, in 22 patients with tumors greater than 6 cm in diameter. Decreased relapse-free survival was also strongly correlated with abnormal lymphangiograms and poorly differentiated tumors. If initial primary tumor size is taken into account, no difference was found in the previously mentioned parameters between the patients receiving irradiation alone and those treated with irradiation and extrafascial hysterectomy. The 5-year survival rates were 73% for Stage I patients, 32% for Stage II, and 31% for Stage III/IV. The incidence of distant metastasis increased with the stage and size of the tumor (Table 54-29).

Kilgore and associates,[185] in a study of 162 patients with adenocarcinoma compared with matched patients with squamous cell carcinoma, found that clinical stage and lesion size

TABLE 54–28
Carcinoma of the Uterine Cervix: 5-Year NED Survival Rates (MIR 1959–1982)

	IRRADIATION ONLY					IRRADIATION + SURGERY				
STAGE	EPIDERMOID	(%)	ADENO-CARCINOMA	(%)	*P* VALUE	EPIDERMOID	(%)	ADENO-CARCINOMA	(%)	*P* VALUE
IA	29/29	100	2/2	100	—	8/8	100	2/2	100	—
IB	265/302	87.7	32/38	84.2	0.57	81/102	79.4	14/16	87.5	0.80
IIA	73/103	70.9	5/9	55.6	0.39	22/32	68.8	1/3	33.3	0.26
IIB	165/249	66.3	10/18	55.6	0.43	32/47	68.1	—	—	—
III	83/226	36.7	3/12	25.0	0.007	13/22	59.1	—	—	—

(Modified from Grigsby PW, Perez CA, Kuske RR, et al: Radiother Oncol 12:289–296, 1988)

TABLE 54–29
Adenocarcinoma of the Cervix: Sites of Failure in Patients Treated With Curative Intent

STAGE	NO. OF PATIENTS	5-YEAR RFS	P ONLY	P + DM	DM ONLY	TOTAL P	TOTAL DM
IB <3 cm	91	88%	2 (2%)*	4 (4%)	5 (5%)	6 (6%)	9 (9%)
3–4 cm	65	65%	7 (11%)*	7 (11%)	9 (14%)	14 (22%)	16 (25%)
4.1–5.9 cm	37	62%	2 (5%)	3 (8%)	7 (19%)†	5 (14%)	10 (27%)
≥6 cm	22	45%	4 (18%)	1 (5%)	7 (32%)	5 (23%)	8 (36%)
IIA	22	38%	4 (18%)	3 (14%)	4 (18%)	7 (32%)	7 (32%)
IIB	38	28%	6 (16%)	7 (18%)	13 (34%)	14 (34%)	20 (53%)
III	46		11 (24%)	7 (15%)	11 (24%)	18 (39%)	18 (39%)

RFS: relapse-free survival; P: pelvic recurrence; DM: distant metastasis
** Six of nine patients who had pelvic recurrence of Stage I tumors ≤4 cm had been treated with radiation therapy.*
† Site of failure unknown in one Stage I, three Stage II, and two Stage III patients
(Eifel PJ, Morris M, Oswald MJ, et al: Cancer 65:2507–2514, 1990)

were the most important prognostic factors and that metastatic lymph nodes were also important prognostically (Fig. 54-34). In patients with Stage I tumors, no significant difference in survival occurred when they were treated with radical surgery, irradiation alone, or irradiation combined with hysterectomy.

Kjorstad[190] reported a worse 5-year survival rate in 102 patients with adenocarcinoma (51%) compared with that of 1900 patients with squamous cell or other differentiated carcinomas (68%). Otherwise the survival rates were comparable in 70 patients with Stages I, III, and IV disease compared with those with the other histologies. Stage I and Stage IIA patients were primarily treated by a preoperative radium implant (6000 cGy to point A) and a radical hysterectomy with bilateral lymphadenectomy. More advanced tumors were treated with external-beam irradiation and intracavitary brachytherapy.

Similarly, Berek and colleagues[27] noted comparable 5-year survival rates in patients with Stage I adenocarcinoma treated with irradiation alone or combined with surgery (81.5%); however, in Stage II disease the 5-year survival rate with irradiation alone was 39.7% (18 patients) compared with 68.2% (14 patients) with combined therapy. Moberg and colleagues[243] observed better survival in in 251 patients with Stage IB and Stage IIA disease treated with combination irradiation and surgery compared with those treated with radiation therapy alone. In their series no difference was found in 5-year survival rates between patients with adenocarcinoma and those with other cervical malignant tumors. Hopkins and associates,[146] in a review of 172 patients, noted somewhat better results with combination therapy compared with irradiation alone, although the responses were not statistically significant. Several authors have reported no difference in survival rates between patients with adenocarcinoma and those with other varieties of this histologic type.[185,243] In Stage II disease there is a greater tendency for patients to have metastatic pelvic lymph nodes,[190] which significantly affects the prognosis. In some series, patients were treated with a radical hysterectomy, followed by irradiation.[146,185] The 5-year survival rate was significantly lower in these patients (50% to 60%). We assume irradiation was delivered because of the presence of metastatic pelvic lymph nodes. Table 54-30 summarizes results of therapy with irradiation alone and with radical hysterectomy.

SEQUELAE OF TREATMENT

Irradiation Alone

The incidence of major complications of radiation therapy for Stage I and Stage IIA carcinoma of the cervix ranges from 3% to 5%, and for Stage IIB and Stage III between 10% and 15%.

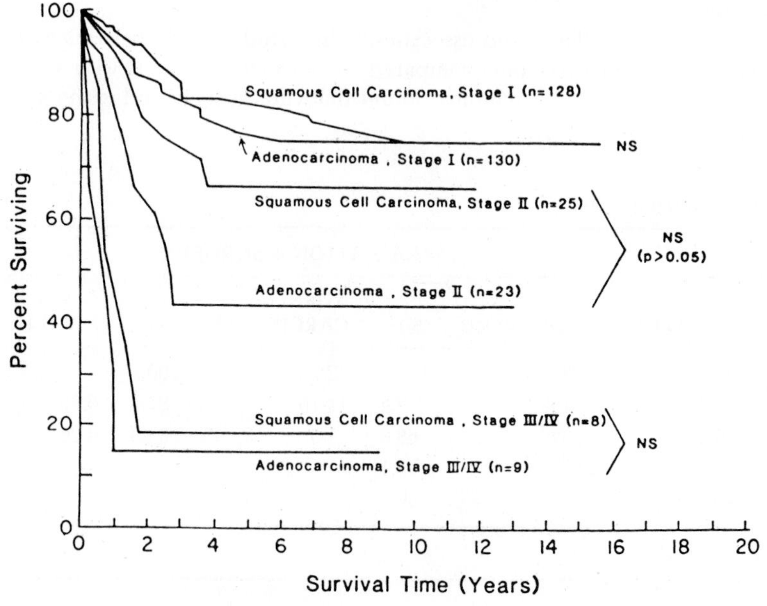

FIGURE 54–34. Survival and clinical stage in adenocarcinoma compared with squamous cell carcinoma. (NS: not significant) (Kilgore LC, Soong S-J, Gore H, et al: Gynecol Oncol 31:137–148, 1988)

TABLE 54–30
Adenocarcinoma of the Uterine Cervix: Five-Year Survival Correlated With Method of Therapy

	STAGE I		STAGE IIA	
AUTHOR	RADIATION THERAPY ALONE	RADIATION THERAPY + SURGERY	RADIATION THERAPY ALONE	RADIATION THERAPY + SURGERY
Berek[27]	16 (67.3%)	14 (83.4%)	18 (39.7%)	14 (68.2%)
Grigsby[124]	40 (85%)	18 (88.9%)	9 (5.5%)	3 (33.3%)
Hopkins[146]	15 (62%)	23 (62%)	—	—
Kilgore[185]	39 (75%)	10 (77%)	—	—
Moberg[243]	57 (79%)	25 (92%)	41 (46%)	15 (67%)
Prempree[313]	16 (81%)	15 (73%)	30 (54%)	14 (86%)
Rutledge[341]	25 (85.2%)	36 (83.8%)	13 (41.9%)	18 (53.7%)

The most common major complications for the various stages are listed in Tables 54-31 and 54-32. Injury to the gastrointestinal tract usually appears within the first 2 years after radiation therapy, whereas complications of the urinary tract are more frequently seen 3 to 4 years after treatment.[198]

Perez and colleagues,[278] Montana and associates,[245] Kottmeier,[198] and Pourquier and co-workers[309] have noted a greater incidence of complications with higher doses of irradiation. Perez and colleagues[278] and Pourquier and co-workers[309] have demonstrated that with doses below 7500 cGy to 8000 cGy delivered to limited volumes, grade 2 and 3 complications in the urinary tract and rectosigmoid were approximately 5%. How-

TABLE 54–31
Carcinoma of the Uterine Cervix: Grade 2 Sequelae (MIR 1959–1986)

	STAGE				
	IB	IIA	IIB	III	IVA
Total no. of patients treated	374	124	314	271	18
No. of complications	46 (12.3%)	16 (12.9%)	40 (12.7%)	25 (9.2%)	1 (5.6%)
INTESTINAL					
Proctitis	6	1	10	4	
Rectal ulcer	1			2	
Sigmoid stricture		2	1	1	
Diverticulitis			1		
Small bowel obstruction	2		2	3	
Small bowel perforation				1	
Malabsorption	3		1	1	
URINARY					
Chronic cystitis	2	2	6	3	
Bladder ulcer	2	1	1		
Ureteral stricture		1			
Incontinence			1		
Urethral stricture			1		
Extensive cystocele	1				
OTHER					
Pelvic abscess				1	
Pulmonary embolus			1		
Subcutaneous fibrosis	1				
Vault necrosis	6	3	1	3	
Leg edema			1		
Hemorrhage			1		
Vaginal stenosis	21	4	6	6	1
Thrombophlebitis		1	2		
Arteriosclerosis	1		3		
Thrombosis of pelvic blood vessels		1			
Neuropathy			1		

TABLE 54–32
Carcinoma of the Uterine Cervix: Grade 3 Sequelae (MIR 1959–1986)

	STAGE				
	IB	IIA	IIB	III	IVA
Total no. of patients treated	374	124	314	271	18
No. of complications	23 (6.1%)	18 (14.5%)	38 (12.1%)	29 (10.7%)	2 (11.1%)
INTESTINAL					
Rectovaginal fistula	2	1	6	7	
Rectouterine fistula	1				
Proctitis	2	1	5	2	
Sigmoid perforation			3		
Sigmoid stricture	3	4	3	2	
Small bowel perforation			3		
Enterocolic fistula	1				
Enterocutaneous fistula		1		1	
Small bowel obstruction	2	5	8	7	
Enteritis				1	
URINARY					
Vesicovaginal fistula	3		3	6	1
Cystitis	2				
Pyelonephritis					1
OTHER					
Pulmonary embolus				1	
Hemorrhage			1		
Pelvic infection	1		1		
Neuritis		1			

ever, the incidence increased to over 10% with higher doses of radiation to these organs (Fig. 54-35). Doses over 6000 cGy were also correlated with a greater incidence of small bowel injury (Fig. 54-36). The same analysis showed that patients who developed sequelae of therapy had a slightly better survival rate than patients without any complications. This was related to improved tumor control with higher doses of irradiation.[278]

Yudelev and colleagues[421] reported similar observations, with a significant increase in the incidence of rectal complications with maximum rectal doses of 7000 cGy to 8000 cGy (116–133 time-dose-factor [TDF]).

Montana and associates,[244] in 197 patients with Stage IB epidermoid carcinoma of the cervix treated with external and intracavitary irradiation (7000 cGy to 8000 cGy to point A and 5000 cGy to 5500 cGy to pelvic lymph nodes), reported increasing incidence of grade 2 and 3 complications in patients receiving mean doses of 6335 cGy to the bladder and 6810 cGy to the rectum. Eight patients (4%) developed grade 2 and seven patients (4%) developed grade 3 complications.

Strockbine and colleagues,[369] Hamberger and associates,[131] Quilty,[318] and Unal and co-workers[395] noted a greater incidence

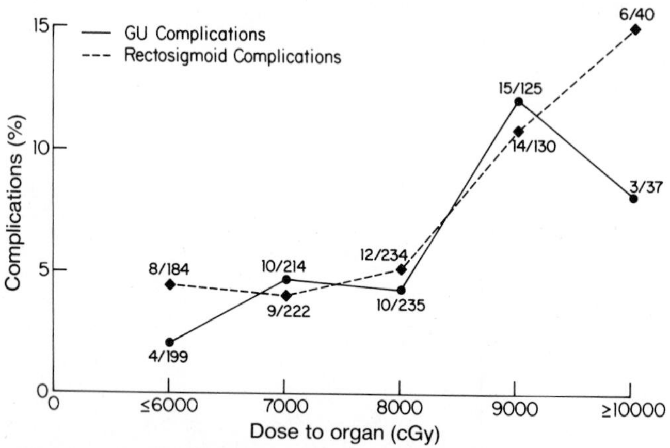

FIGURE 54–35. Incidence of grade 2 and 3 genitourinary (GU) or rectosigmoid complications in patients with carcinoma of the uterine cervix (all stages) treated with irradiation alone (external and brachytherapy). A greater incidence of complications is noted with maximum doses over 7500 cGy to 8000 cGy to the bladder or rectum. (Perez CA, Breaux S, Bedwinek J, et al: Cancer 54:235–246, 1984)

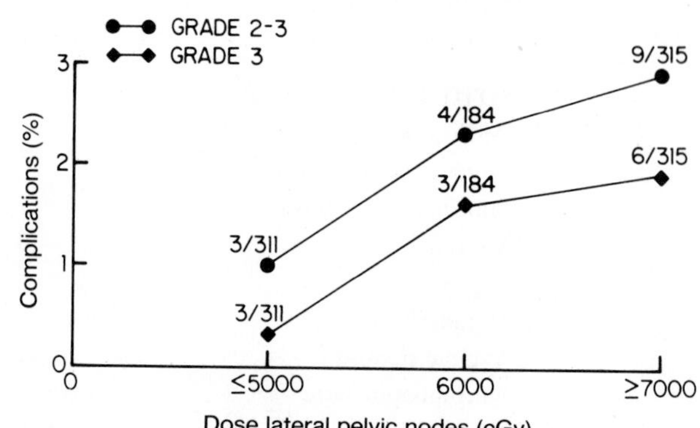

FIGURE 54–36. Incidence of grade 2 or 3 complications in the small intestine correlated with doses of irradiation. (Perez CA, Breaux S, Bedwinek J, et al: Cancer 54:235–246, 1984)

of pelvic complications in patients treated with higher doses to the whole pelvis (4000 cGy to 5000 cGy). The authors commented that the intracavitary radium dose was not correlated with severe complications. Similar observations were made by Stryker and associates[370] in 132 patients, who developed a 9% incidence of fistulas and a 14% incidence of grade 2 and 3 complications after delivery of 5000 cGy or higher to the whole pelvis combined with intracavitary insertion (180 cGy daily dose). They recommended that the whole-pelvis radiation dose should not exceed 4000 cGy to 4500 cGy when doses of approximately 4000 cGy are delivered to point A with intracavitary insertions. The authors used 10 MV photons and AP/PA portals, although a four-field box technique was used for obese patients; all fields were treated each day. It is possible that with use of higher-energy photons and the box technique, the intracavitary dose may be increased to 4500 cGy to 5000 cGy without increasing the probability of complications (total dose to point A, 8500 cGy).

Sherrah-Davies[353] reported higher morbidity when patients were treated with higher daily fractions of external-beam irradiation (4000 cGy in 16 fractions over 3 weeks).

Kuske and associates,[204] comparing the results of therapy in 99 patients with carcinoma of the cervix on whom minicolpostats were used, noted a 15% higher incidence of grade 2 and 3 complications, which was higher than the 8% rate noted in a similar group of patients treated with regular colpostats during the same period ($P = 0.08$). Perez and colleagues[278] reported that the incidence and type of complications with interstitial therapy at Washington University was approximately the same as in patients treated with intracavitary technique only.

Irradiation of the paraaortic lymph nodes has been reported to cause increased complications, particularly when it is done after staging paraaortic lymphadenectomy with a transperitoneal approach. In a randomized study reported by Rotman[333] in which 50% of the patients were given 4500 cGy to the paraaortic area in addition to the standard pelvic irradiation, a somewhat higher incidence of grade 2 and 3 complications was reported in 168 patients (31 complications in 20 patients), compared with 21 complications in 167 patients treated by pelvic irradiation only. In a similar randomized study by Haie and the EORTC,[129] the incidence of grade 3 small bowel injury was 2.3% in the paraaortic irradiation group and 0.9% in the pelvic irradiation only group. A severe complication rate of 9% was observed in patients receiving paraaortic irradiation compared with 4.8% in those treated to the pelvis only.

Less severe, but still clinically significant, sequelae have been described. Parkin and associates[275] reported a 26% incidence of severe urinary symptoms (urgency, incontinence, and frequency) in patients treated with irradiation alone for cervical carcinoma. The authors carried out urodynamic studies in 40 women, all of whom were free from disease 5 to 11 years after radiation therapy. Cystometrograms and urethral profiles of the 40 women were performed and compared with those of 28 women having urodynamic evaluations before treatment. No difference was found in the mean maximum flow rate or mean *residual* value in the two groups. However, mean volume of full bladder sensation was significantly lower in the postirradiation group than in the pretreatment group, as was the mean maximum cystometric capacity. It should be noted that this dysfunction may be noted in about 10% of the general female population[53] and that it increases in older women.[3] Although cystometrograms have demonstrated bladder atonicity in some cases, several authors have failed to observe bladder or rectal sphincter disturbances.

Although extremely rare, lumbosacral plexopathy has been occasionally reported in patients treated for pelvic tumors with doses of 6000 cGy to 6750 cGy.[16] At Mallinckrodt Institute of Radiology this syndrome has been observed twice, once in a patient with cervical carcinoma receiving 4500 cGy to the paraaortic lymph nodes (without spinal cord shielding) and once in a woman with Stage IIB carcinoma of the cervix treated with external pelvic irradiation (6000 cGy to the parametria) and brachytherapy. Characteristically, these patients have lower motor neuron weakness of the legs combined with loss of deep reflexes and muscular fasciculation.

The differential diagnosis with recurrent tumors is sometimes difficult.[220] In a comparison of 20 patients with lumbosacral plexopathy after irradiation and 30 patients with plexus damage from pelvic malignancy, Thomas and associates[388] noted that indolent leg weakness occurred early in radiation-induced plexopathy (pain occurred initially in 10% of the patients, although ultimately it was present in 50%), whereas pain is most frequently associated with tumor plexopathy. Muscular weakness, numbness, and paresthesia were common in both groups. Computed tomography is extremely helpful in the detection of pelvic masses or bone destruction caused by tumor. The authors also reported extensive retroperitoneal fibrosis of the lumbosacral plexus in two patients and femoral nerve fibrosis with plexopathy in one patient. Electromyogram (EMG) showed abnormal myokymic discharges in 57% of the patients, whereas this finding was very unusual in tumor-induced plexopathy. Unfortunately, as in radiation myelopathy, the neurologic deficit is irreversible and no effective therapy other than supportive care has been found.

Combined Irradiation and Surgery

When preoperative irradiation is combined with surgery, the complication rate tends to be higher (5% to 10%), particularly because of injury to the ureter or the bladder (ureteral stricture of ureterovaginal or vesicovaginal fistula). The dose of radiation, technique, and type of surgical procedure performed are important in determining the morbidity of combined therapy. Nelson and associates[256] reported a 17.5% incidence of severe complications in a group of 80 patients treated with irradiation and radical hysterectomy in contrast to 7.4% in a group of 95 patients treated with high-dose preoperative irradiation and a conservative extrafascial hysterectomy. Jacobs and coworkers,[159] in 102 patients with invasive cervical carcinoma treated at Washington University with low-dose preoperative irradiation and a radical hysterectomy with lymphadenectomy or high-dose preoperative irradiation and a conservative extrafascial hysterectomy, noted a major complication rate of 5%. Survival was comparable in patients with or without complications.

A significant number of complications are associated with the pretherapy staging laparotomy, particularly if irradiation (over 5000 cGy to 5500 cGy) is given when metastatic periaortic lymph nodes are found. Operative complications are pneumonia, thrombophlebitis, cardiovascular accident, hepatitis, and evisceration. Late complications include those of combined surgery and irradiation in the abdomen and pelvis. The incidence of complications has been between 5% and 20%, depending on the extent of the paraaortic lymph node dissection, the transperitoneal or retroperitoneal approach for the operation, and the dose of radiation given.[211,302,416] Coia and associates[65] reported a 23% incidence of major complications 4 years after therapy in patients on whom exploratory laparotomy was performed, compared with 11% in those without laparotomy ($P < 0.01$).

With improved anesthesia, surgical techniques, and antibiotic therapy, the mortality rate for radical hysterectomy with pelvic lymphadenectomy has decreased to 1% or less.[149] Other complications are ureterovaginal fistula (incidence has decreased to less than 3%), hemorrhage, infection, bowel obstruction, stricture and fibrosis of the intestine or rectosigmoid colon, and bladder and rectovaginal fistulas. Postsurgical complications are generally more amenable to correction than are late complications following irradiation.[377]

After pelvic irradiation or bilateral salpingo-oophorectomy, usually carried out with a radical hysterectomy in patients treated for carcinoma of the uterine cervix, symptoms of menopause may occur. These symptoms can be treated with replacement hormones, although some gynecologists have expressed reservations. Sadan and associates[343] believe hormone therapy is a safe practice, as does Ploch.[304] Usually 0.625 mg to 1.25 mg of Premarin (conjugated estrogens) daily is sufficient.

PALLIATIVE IRRADIATION

Fairly frequently the radiation oncologist is faced with the challenge of treating a patient with Stage IVB or recurrent carcinoma that requires palliation of pelvic pain or bleeding. If vaginal bleeding is the main concern, a single intracavitary insertion with tandem and colpostats for about 6000 mgh (5500 cGy to point A) suffices. If irradiation was delivered previously, lower intracavitary doses should be prescribed (4000 mgh to 5000 mgh).

Several high-dose fractionation schedules with external beam have been used. Meoz and co-workers[237] described satisfactory palliation with single doses of 1000 cGy combined with misonidasole, delivered every 3 to 6 weeks for a total of 3000 cGy. Complications in the long-term survivors were relatively high (15%).

Spanos and associates[360] reported on a phase II study of daily multifraction split-course irradiation in 142 patients (50% with recurrent or metastatic disease in the pelvis only and 50% with associated extrapelvic metastases). Irradiation consisted of 370 cGy per fraction given twice daily for two consecutive days, repeated at 3- to 6-week intervals for a total of three courses, aiming to a total tumor dose of 4440 cGy. The dose was based on linear quadratic equation considerations of acute and late effects assuming an α/β ratio of 10 for acute and 4 for late effects. Occasionally this regimen was combined with an intracavitary insertion (4500 mgh), blocking the midline for the last 1440 cGy external dose. Eighty-three (59%) of the 142 evaluable patients received three courses of radiation; 29 (20%) received two courses, and an additional 29 (20%) received only one course.

Complete response was noted in 15 of the treated patients (10.5%) and partial response in 32 (22.5%). For patients completing three courses of radiation, the complete response plus partial response rate was 45%. Twenty-seven patients survived more than 1 year. Only two cases of grade 3 toxicity (lower GI) were recorded. This is a significant decrease over the incidence reported with single doses of 1000 cGy for a total of 3000 cGy[39] and an 11% incidence of grade 3 and 19% incidence of grade 4 complications (mostly intestinal) previously reported by Spanos and associates[361] in 46 patients treated with 1000 cGy fractions given every 4 weeks for a total of 3000 cGy combined with misonidazole (4 g/m^2 administered 4 to 6 hours before irradiation). The RTOG multiple daily fractionation study has been expanded to a phase III protocol randomizing between a short (2-week) or a longer (4-week) rest period between the split courses of irradiation.[319]

TREATMENT FOR RECURRENT CARCINOMA OF THE CERVIX

After Definitive Irradiation

Reirradiation of previously irradiated patients must be undertaken with extreme caution. It is very important to analyze the techniques used in the initial treatment (beam energy, volume, doses delivered with external or intracavitary irradiation). Also, the period of time between the two treatments must be taken into consideration because it is postulated that some repair of the initial damage may take place in the interval. However, it is foolhardy to assume that previously irradiated tissues will have the same tumor as newly irradiated tissues. In general, external-beam irradiation is given to limited volumes (4000 cGy to 4500 cGy, 180 cGy tumor dose per fraction, preferentially using lateral portals). Occasionally, intracavitary or interstitial irradiation can be used to treat relatively circumscribed recurrences. In some patients this has been combined with weekly sessions of regional hyperthermia.[29]

Sommers and colleagues[359] described the results of retreatment in 376 patients with recurrent carcinoma of the uterine cervix. Table 54-33 shows the distribution of patients according to the initial stage of the tumor and the therapy administered for the recurrence. Ninety-one patients received irradiation, mostly external (86.8%), occasionally combined with brachytherapy (7.7%) to control bleeding of central recurrences; brachytherapy alone was administered in 5.5% of the patients. The mean dose of pelvic irradiation and the probability of tumor control and complications are shown in Table 54-34. The typical dose for paraaortic lymph node metastases was 4500 cGy to 5000 cGy in 5 weeks. Other metastatic sites were treated with about 3500 cGy to 4000 cGy in 3 to 4 weeks. Pelvic exenteration was attempted in 23 patients, only ten of whom were deemed to be operable (43.5%), but completed in only seven. Chemotherapy was administered to 22 patients, frequently alone, occasionally combined with surgery or irradiation. Multiple cytotoxic agent combinations were used, mostly cisplatin (50 to 75 mg/m^2) or 5-FU (750 to 1000 mg/m^2) in continuous infusion over a 4-day period. The probability of 5-year survival after treatment for recurrence was 30% for patients treated with combined surgery and external-beam irradiation, 12% for the patients treated with surgery, and 4% for patients receiving external-beam irradiation. The 5-year survival rate for the ten patients who underwent pelvic exenteration was 16%. Patients failing only in the pelvis who were reirradiated with a secondary curative aim had a 40% (two of five) 5-year survival rate. Only 1% of the untreated patients survived 5 years (Fig. 54-37). Six (4.3%) of 140 patients experienced grade 2 or 3 complications. Four of these complications were thought to be related to irradiation (one instance each of cystitis, urethral stricture, malabsorption, and leg edema) and two to surgery (pulmonary embolism, small bowel perforation).

Thomas and colleagues[387] reported a median survival of only 7 months in 242 patients with recurrent carcinoma of the uterine cervix of all stages, primarily treated with irradiation. All but one patient, who was salvaged by a hysterectomy for a central failure, died within 24 months of the treatment of the recurrence.

Puthawala and associates[316] used interstitial implants to

TABLE 54–33
Recurrent Carcinoma of the Uterine Cervix: Site of Failure and Type of Therapy (MIR 1959–1982)

SITE OF FAILURE	TYPE OF THERAPY FOR RECURRENCE				
	SURGERY*	RADIATION THERAPY	RADIATION THERAPY + SURGERY	CHEMOTHERAPY	NO TREATMENT
Stage IB					
Pelvic	2	0	0	0	1
Pelvic + DM	4	10	0	1	11
DM	2	11	2	1	12
Stage IIA					
Pelvic	0	0	0	0	2
Pelvic + DM	3	5	1	1	7
DM	1	4	0	3	12
Stage IIB					
Pelvic	3	7	2	1	19
Pelvic + DM	3	5	1	3	22
DM	4	16	0	4	22
Stage III					
Pelvic	2	3	0	0	35
Pelvic + DM	4	13	0	5	40
DM	2	7	0	3	37
Stage IV					
Pelvic	0	0	0	0	3
Pelvic + DM	0	0	0	0	11
DM	0	1	0	0	2

DM: distant metastasis
** Of the patients treated with surgery, ten had pelvic exenteration, two had modified radical hysterectomy, one had radical vulvectomy, four had diverting colostomy, three had small bowel resection, two had colon resection, and eight had exploratory laparotomy.*
(Sommers GM, Grigsby PW, Perez CA, et al: Gynecol Oncol 35:150–155, 1989)

treat 14 patients who had carcinoma of the uterine cervix recurring in the pelvis after definitive radiation therapy. Seven (50%) exhibited tumor control. Palliation of symptoms after reirradiation was obtained in about 80% of the patients. In several patients the radioactive material was implanted intraoperatively at the time of exploratory laparotomy. The technique was described in a previous publication.[375] The authors reported no postoperative mortality. Thirty percent of the patients experienced mild to moderate symptoms of proctitis and cystitis shortly after the interstitial implant. Severe complications occurred in 15% of the patients (soft tissue necrosis and one instance each of rectovaginal fistula, vesicovaginal fistula, enterovaginal fistula, and rectal stricture).

Prasasvinichai and co-workers[311] noted a 17.6% 5-year survival rate in 51 patients with recurrent tumors limited to the pelvis treated with irradiation alone, pelvic exenteration (ten patients), or a combination of exploratory laparotomy, debulking, and irradiation (ten patients). Prempree and colleagues[314] treated eight patients with advanced cervical carcinoma that recurred after primary irradiation. Three survived tumor-free for more than 5 years after retreatment.

Selected patients with limited pelvic recurrences not fixed to the pelvic wall and without evidence of extrapelvic metastases can be potentially salvaged by pelvic exenteration. In 65 patients on whom pelvic exenteration was carried out at Memorial Sloan-Kettering Cancer Center the 5-year survival rate was 23%. The operative mortality rate was 9.2%.[208] Lawhead and co-workers pointed out that the significant mortality and morbidity associated with this procedure preclude its use as palliative therapy.

Urinary diversion, either by nephrostomy or ileal bladder,

TABLE 54–34
Recurrent Carcinoma of the Uterine Cervix: Dose, Local Control, and Complications for Pelvic Reirradiation (MIR 1959–1982)

TYPE OF REIRRADIATION TO THE PELVIS	PREVIOUS POINT A DOSE (cGy)*	AVERAGE DOSE (cGy)	LOCAL CONTROL	SEVERE COMPLICATIONS
External	7684	4130	14/15	0/15
Brachytherapy	7186	3406	6/6	0/6
External and	7304	3214	3/4	1/4
brachytherapy		2529		

** Average dose to point A from the initial treatment*
(Sommers GM, Grigsby PW, Perez CA, et al: Gynecol Oncol 35:150–155, 1989)

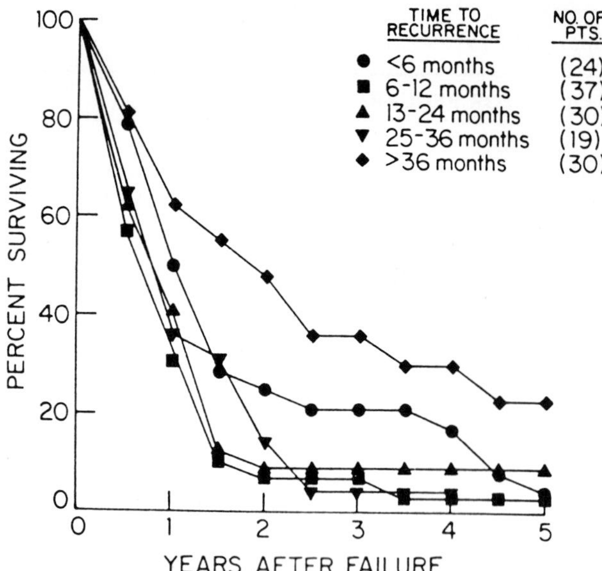

FIGURE 54-37. Actuarial survival rates after initial failure in patients treated for recurrence. (Sommers GM, Grigsby PW, Perez CA, et al: Gynecol Oncol 35:150–155, 1989)

may be of palliative value in patients with either recurrent carcinoma in the pelvis or complications.[161] It must be kept in mind that diversion may prolong life but runs the risk of denying a terminally ill cancer patient in her final days the oblivion and insensibility of uremia.[161]

A recent review by Thigpen and co-workers,[385] who evaluated the efficacy of chemotherapy for patients with recurrent cervical cancer, described a 10% to 20% response rate for single agent chemotherapy.

After Previous Surgery

It is substantially easier to treat surgical recurrences with irradiation, which can salvage about 50% of patients with localized pelvic recurrences after surgery alone.[81,107] A combination of external-beam irradiation (2000 cGy to 4000 cGy), depending on the volume of tumor, and additional parametrial dose with midline shielding for a total of 5000 cGy to 6000 cGy is needed. In addition, one or two intracavitary insertions that may cover the vaginal vault or the entire vagina, depending on tumor volume, should be delivered. The total mucosal dose to the upper vagina from the external and intracavitary therapy can approach 14,000 cGy and to the distal vagina 9500 cGy without a high risk.[141] It is extremely useful to combine these techniques with interstitial irradiation to boost the dose to the vaginal vault or the parametrium or paravaginal tissues. Doses of 2000 cGy to 3000 cGy are administered with single, double plane, or volume implants, depending on the extent of the tumor.

Jobsen and associates[163] described 16 complete responses in 18 patients (88%) with postsurgical locoregional recurrence treated with 5000 cGy to 6000 cGy to the pelvis. Five (31%) of 16 patients developed a second pelvic failure. The 5-year survival rate for the 18 patients was 44%. Evans and colleagues[98] reported on 114 patients found to have unresectable recurrent carcinoma of the cervix after primary irradiation or surgical treatment. Seventy patients were treated with irradiation (external, interstitial, or combination). Ten percent of these patients lived 15 months or longer, and 5% survived 5 or more years.

Friedman and Pearlman[106] observed a 42% tumor-free survival rate in 38 patients treated with irradiation after primary surgical therapy. Seven were irradiated electively for close or positive margins, lymphatic permeation, or pelvic lymph node involvement. Six of the seven patients were tumor-free for 2 to 5 years. Of 14 patients with limited central recurrence, eight were tumor-free from 3.5 to 9 years. The worst results were noted with persistent or recurrent peripheral pelvic tumor (three of 11 patients survived tumor-free more than 5 years) or with massive pelvic recurrences (in six patients only palliation was achieved).

Krebs and associates,[202] in 312 patients with carcinoma of the cervix treated surgically, reported 40 recurrences (13%), 11 of which were limited to the central pelvis. The 5-year salvage rate for the patients with recurrence was 13%. Webb and colleagues[410] analyzed 104 recurrences following initial surgical treatment predominantly for Stage IB tumors and found only a 5.7% 5-year survival rate after treatment for the recurrence.

Larson and associates[207] reported 27 recurrences (11%) in 249 patients treated with radical hysterectomy and pelvic lymphadenectomy for Stage IB of the cervix. Seventeen patients (63%) had tumor recurrence in the pelvis or vulva; the other ten patients developed recurrences outside the pelvis. Eight (53%) of 15 patients treated with irradiation for an isolated recurrence in the pelvis or vulva were tumor-free between 10 and 126 months after treatment of the recurrence (median 48 months).

CHEMOTHERAPY

Chemotherapy has not been extensively evaluated in cervical cancer, primarily because of effective initial therapy with other modalities and because cytotoxic agents used in patients with recurrent cervical carcinoma have shown less than optimal efficacy.[358] Other factors that complicate the effective use of chemotherapy in cervical carcinoma include decreased pelvic vascular perfusion, limited bone marrow reserve, and at times poor renal function related to ureteral obstruction from tumor or fibrosis.

Nevertheless, chemotherapy may eventually play an important role in the management of several groups of patients, including those with advanced (Stage III and IV) tumors; pelvic or paraaortic nodal metastasis with a low potential for cure with current local treatment modalities; and recurrent disease after surgery and radiation therapy.[283]

Significant activity in well-designed studies with adequate patient numbers has been documented only for 5-FU[221] and cisplatin.[384] Combination chemotherapy studies in which reasonable numbers of evaluable patients have been studied and the response rates appear to surpass those of single agents are listed in Table 54-35. However, the majority of studies have not compared combination chemotherapy regimens with standard single agent therapy, and the toxicity of these combinations is greater.

Intraarterial infusion of chemotherapeutic agents in cervical carcinoma has held considerable interest for some years, based on the distinct arterial supply to the tumor-bearing area. Unfortunately, the responses have been uncommon and of short duration, and the toxicity and complication rates have been significant.[242,249,267,268] Randomized comparisons are required to establish the benefits, if any, of intraarterial chemotherapy infusion.

Several published reports have described the use of chemotherapy as a radiosensitizer to enhance the effect of radiation

TABLE 54–35
Combination Chemotherapy in Cervical Carcinoma

REGIMEN	EVALUABLE PATIENTS	NO. OF RESPONSES	COMPLETE RESPONSES
Bleomycin and methotrexate	20	12 (60%)	0 (0%)
Bleomycin, methotrexate, and cyclophosphamide	70	22 (31%)	4 (6%)
Doxorubicin (Adriamycin) and methotrexate	59	39 (66%)	13 (22%)
	24	7 (28%)	0 (0%)
Doxorubicin and methyl-CCNU	31	14 (45%)	9 (29%)
Doxorubicin and cisplatin	19	6 (31%)	2 (10%)
Bleomycin and mitomycin-C	33	12 (36%)	5 (15%)
Mitomycin-C, vincristine, and bleomycin	91	46 (55%)	14 (15%)
Mitomycin-C, vincristine, bleomycin, and cisplatin	14	6 (43%)	4 (29%)
Methotrexate, bleomycin, and cisplatin	9	8	—

(Perez CA, DiSaia PJ, Knapp RC, Young RC: Gynecologic tumors. In DeVita V, Hellman S, Rosenberg SA [eds]: Cancer: Principles and Practice of Oncology, 2nd ed. Philadelphia, JB Lippincott, 1985)

therapy for cervical carcinoma. The two most provocative studies have used hydroxyurea, a drug with limited single-agent activity.[151,297] Piver and co-workers[297] reported that in clinical Stage IIB patients a significant improvement in 2-year survival rate was achieved for the group receiving irradiation and hydroxyurea (74%) compared with that of the control group treated with radiation therapy and a placebo (43.5%). Hreshchyshyn and associates[151] reported that among patients with Stage IIIB and Stage IV disease, the complete response rate was 68.1% for the hydroxyurea-treated group and 48.8% for the placebo group ($P = 0.5$). Duration of progression-free intervals and survival were also significantly better in patients receiving hydroxyurea. However, hematologic toxicity was more common and more severe in those patients receiving hydroxyurea. Results from both studies must be qualified because the patients were not all surgically staged and substantial numbers of randomized patients were not evaluable.

Stehman and the Gynecology Oncology Group[363] reported on 296 evaluable patients with Stage IIB, Stage III, or Stage IVA carcinoma of the uterine cervix randomized to be treated with radiation therapy and either hydroxyurea (139 patients) or misonidazole (157 patients). The median progression-free survival for all patients receiving hydroxyurea was 42.9 months and for those receiving misonidazole, 40.4 months. Failure limited to the pelvis occurred in 18% of the patients in the hydroxyurea group and in 23.6% of the misonidazole group. Mortality rates were not statistically different between the regimens, with 33.8% deaths in the hydroxyurea and 38.9% deaths in the misonidazole groups ($P = 0.25$). With effective radiation therapy alone, Fletcher[103] and Perez and colleagues[279] have noted survival and tumor control rates similar to those observed with the addition of hydroxyurea in the three series described.

Kuske and associates[203] reported preliminary results for 23 patients with advanced or recurrent gynecologic malignancy treated with definitive irradiation and synchronous sensitizing chemotherapy consisting of cisplatin (50 mg/m^2 IV rapid infusion) and a 5-day continuous infusion of 5-FU (750 mg/m^2/day). Drugs were administered every 3 to 4 weeks for a total of three cycles. Radiation therapy for implantable tumors consisted of 2000 cGy whole pelvis, 3000 cGy to 4000 cGy split field, and two intracavitary or interstitial insertions, resulting in a total dose of 7500 cGy to 8000 cGy to point A. Three courses of chemotherapy were delivered simultaneously with irradiation (during the first week of whole-pelvis irradiation and with each of the two brachytherapy procedures). Nonimplantable tumors were treated with protracted external-beam radiation therapy (5500 cGy tumor dose) and three courses of chemotherapy during weeks 1, 4, and 7 of irradiation. Twenty-one of 23 patients completed irradiation, and 18 of 23 patients completed chemotherapy as planned, but 50% had delays in either modality. Grade 2 or 3 late sequelae developed in 18% and 22% of the patients, respectively, consisting of leg edema (one), proctosigmoiditis (one), bowel obstruction (one), vesicovaginal fistula (one), and pulmonary embolus (two—one fatal). With 1 to 3 years of follow-up evaluation, 12 of 23 (52%) patients are free of disease, and nine of 22 evaluable patients (41%) have failed within the pelvis.

Grigsby and associates[123] recently updated the data in an analysis of 52 patients with advanced or recurrent gynegologic tumors who received somewhat higher doses of chemotherapeutic agents when possible (75 mg/m^2 cisplatin and 1000 mg/m^2 5-FU, continuous infusion in 4 days). The incidence of moderate and severe toxicity was 35% (eight of 23). The more significant sequelae were pulmonary embolus (two), severe proctitis (one), vesicovaginal fistula (one), and bowel obstruction (one).

Monyak and associates[246] reported on 49 patients with advanced carcinoma of the uterine cervix treated with definitive irradiation (8000 cGy to 8500 cGy to point A with external-beam irradiation and intracavitary therapy) and cisplatin (usually 20 mg/m^2 given intravenously once weekly 2 hours before irradiation). The survival rate for the entire group was 52% at 2 years and 66% for 38 patients with clinical Stages I, II, and III. Late toxicity consisted of three cases of bowel obstruction requiring surgery, one rectovaginal fistula, and one vesicovaginal fistula.

Runowicz and associates[337] noted 29 complete responses in 32 patients with various stages of cervical carcinoma (29 with Stage IIB or higher) who were treated with definitive irradiation and concomitant cisplatin (20 mg/m^2 for 5 days every 21 days). Toxicity was acceptable in most patients, although three developed rectovaginal fistulas (two associated with progression of disease) and two had radiation proctitis. Of 16 evaluable patients with Stage IIIB or Stage IVA tumors, 13 (81%) had no evidence of disease at the time of the report, with a median follow-up of 12 months.

Wong and associates[419] reported on a randomized study in which 25 patients were treated with irradiation alone, 22 patients with irradiation and weekly cisplatin, and 17 with twice-weekly cisplatin and irradiation for Stages IIB and III carcinoma of the uterine cervix. Palliative irradiation consisted of 4000 cGy in daily fractions of 250 cGy, four fractions per week, and two intracavitary applications of approximately 6000 cGy to 6500 cGy. The cisplatin was administered within 30 minutes before irradiation in bolus injections of 25 mg/m^2 on the first day and repeated weekly or twice per week (first and third days of each treatment week). Complete response after therapy was noted in 20, 14, and 15 patients in the three respective groups. Survival was similar in the three groups (Fig. 54-38). The most common side effects were nausea, vomiting, and bone marrow depression. There were no drug-related deaths. A few patients developed radiation proctitis and cystitis, and a vesicovaginal fistula was seen in one patient.

In several collected series of patients with Stages IIB and III carcinoma of the uterine cervix treated with concomitant irradiation and chemotherapy, the reported survival rate is about 60% and the pelvic tumor control rate is 75% to 80% (Table 54-36). Properly designed prospective randomized clinical trials are necessary to assess the potential value of chemotherapy in the management of patients with advanced carcinoma of the cervix as well as in other gynecologic malignancies.

HYPERBARIC OXYGEN, HYPOXIC SENSITIZERS, AND HYPERTHERMIA COMBINED WITH IRRADIATION

Several reports have been published evaluating the efficacy of hyperbaric oxygen[84] combined with irradiation in the treatment of a variety of human tumors, including carcinoma of the uterine cervix.[105,407]

Watson and associates,[407] in a randomized clinical trial involving 320 patients (Stages III and IVA) treated at four institutions, reported a 5-year survival rate of 33% in the oxygen-treated group in contrast to 27% in the control group treated in air ($P = 0.08$). The local recurrence rate was 33% in the 161 patients treated with oxygen and 53% in 159 patients treated in air ($P < 0.001$). Morbidity in the patients treated with oxygen was greater (20 severe and 13 moderate complications) than in those treated in air (six severe and eight moderate). The difference was particularly striking in the bowel (13 *versus* two severe complications, respectively). Several other reports have shown increased morbidity with hyperbaric oxygen.[105,110,407]

Dische and collaborators[86] reviewed the data in a randomized study of patients with advanced carcinoma of the cervix treated with radiation therapy and hyperbaric oxygen or air and noted that the patients treated with oxygen had improved survival at Mount Vernon and Glasgow but not at Cape Town. Data from the three centers were merged, and analysis showed that local tumor control was significantly worse in patients treated in air who had a prior blood transfusion, but in the oxygen group this effect was reversed. The same interaction was noted in the survival results ($P = 0.042$).

On the other hand, an extensive trial of carcinoma of the cervix reported by Fletcher and colleagues[105] in 233 patients with Stages IIB, III, and IV disease randomized to be treated with conventional irradiation in air or with hyperbaric oxygen demonstrated no significant benefit in survival or tumor control (20 of 109 patients treated with oxygen failed in the pelvis in contrast to 29 of 124 treated in air). Furthermore, morbidity was greater (26 complications) in patients treated with hyperbaric oxygen compared with the control group (15 complications). A smaller series of patients reported by Glassburn and associates[110] showed no benefit in survival but increased morbidity with hyperbaric oxygen.

No definite conclusions can be drawn concerning the use of hyperbaric oxygen in carcinoma of the cervix. It is possible that hyperbaric oxygen administered with fewer high-dose fractions may be more efficacious than when combined with conventional dose and fractionation schemes.[84] The trials reported have not shown an increased incidence of distant metastasis, which has been observed in a clinical study and in some animal experiments.[167]

Thomas and co-workers[397] described a phase I study of metronidazole carried out on 80 patients with various stages of carcinoma of the uterine cervix. The authors noted that a daily dose of 1.3 g/m^2 was well tolerated, but no tumor response data were reported, and phase III clinical trials were recommended. Dische[85] described preliminary observations on the use of mis-

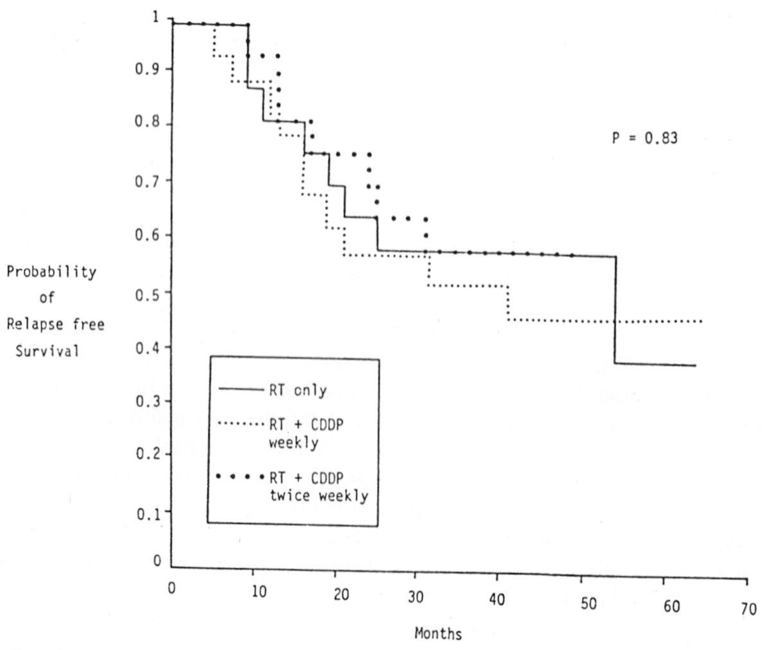

FIGURE 54–38. Disease-free and survival durations of responders in three treatment groups of patients with advanced cervix carcinoma. (Wong LC, Chao YC, Choy D, et al: Gynecol Oncol 35:159–163, 1989)

TABLE 54–36
Concomitant Chemotherapy and Irradiation in Advanced Carcinoma of the Cervix (Primary Lesion)

AUTHOR	NO. OF EVALUABLE PATIENTS	DRUGS	RADIATION THERAPY DOSE (cGy)	COMPLETE RESPONSE	SEVERE TOXICITY
Hreschyshyn et al[151] (randomized study)	51	Hydroxyurea	7000	32 (68%)	10% Thrombocytopenia Leukopenia
Piver et al[299]	60	Hydroxyurea	6000 Pelvis	—	78% Leukopenia 17% Thrombocytopenia
Potish et al[308]	29	Cisplatin	8500 Point A 4900 Periaortic	—	10% Fistula 1 Intestinal obstruction
Thomas et al[386] (26 primary, 8 recurrent)	26 8	Mit-C, 5FU	8000 Point A 3600 Periaortic	20 (74%) 3 (38%)	11% Sigmoid stricture 2 Sigmoid perforation
John et al[165]	11	Mit-C, cisplatin, 5FU	3600	10 (90%)	1 Rectal ulcer
Lipsztein et al[214]	10	Cisplatin, Mit-C, VCR, Bleo	3960 + 4000–5000 mgh	9 (90%)	None
Choo et al[57]	20	Cisplatin	4000 + 6500 mgh	55%	None
Monyak et al[246]	49	Cisplatin	8000–8500 Point A 6000 Point B	43%	3 Intestinal obstruction 2 Fistulas
Kuske et al[203]	23	Cisplatin, 5FU	Ext RT ± 1–2 ICI 8000 Point A	13/15 (86%)	1 Vaginal fistula 2 Bowel complications 2 Pulmonary emboli 14% Lympho/thrombocytopenia
Runowicz et al[337]	32	Cisplatin	180–200 in 5 fractions in 4–5 weeks Ext RT ± 1–2 ICI; 8000 Gy Point A	29 (91%)	3 Rectovaginal fistula 2 Radiation proctitis

Mit-C: mitomycin-C; 5FU: 5-fluorouracil; VCR: vincristine; Bleo: bleomycin; ICI: intracavitory cesium insertions; Ext RT: external radiation therapy
(Modified from Kuske RR, Perez CA, Grigsby PW, et al: Am J Clin Oncol 12:467–473, 1989)

onidazole in the treatment of advanced carcinoma of the cervix in ten patients. The morbidity was comparable to that observed with irradiation alone, except for some misonidazole neurotoxicity. All ten patients had over 50% tumor regression, results believed to be very promising.

Leibel and the Radiation Therapy Oncology Group[210] reported on a randomized study of 119 patients with FIGO Stage IIIB or IVA squamous cell carcinoma of the cervix to receive radiation therapy alone with or without misonidazole (400 mg/m^2 daily 2 to 4 hours before radiation therapy). With a median follow-up of 33 months 64% of the patients treated with radiation therapy alone and 54% receiving irradiation plus misonidazole were alive at 18 months. The median survival was 1.9 years and 1.6, respectively. Grade 3 and 4 toxicity was noted in five patients receiving radiation therapy alone and in three patients in the irradiation plus misonidazole group.

These findings are similar to those reported by Overgaard and associates,[270] who in a randomized study of 331 patients with Stages IIB, III, and IVA carcinoma of the uterine cervix treated with either misonidazole or a placebo and irradiation found no significant differences in local tumor control (50% *versus* 54%), disease-free survival (47% *versus* 46%), and crude survival (39% *versus* 45%) rates. Noteworthy is the fact that patients with hemoglobin levels below 7 mmol/l had significantly lower local tumor control (24% *versus* 47%).

Because of technologic limitations to the delivery of adequate heat to large parts of the body such as the pelvis, the evaluation of hyperthermia in the treatment of carcinoma of the uterine cervix has been sparse. Hornback and associates[148] described a nonrandomized study in which the combination of microwave hyperthermia and irradiation (433 MHz) resulted in improved pelvic tumor control (72%) in a group of 79 patients with Stage IIIB carcinoma compared with previously irradiated historic controls (53%). However, 5-year survival rates were comparable in both groups (22% to 30%).

Sharma and associates[352] reported a 70% disease-free survival rate at 18 months in 20 patients with Stage IIB or III carcinoma of the uterine cervix treated with a combination of irradiation and hyperthermia (13.5 MHz, 42°C to 43°C, 30 minutes before irradiation), compared with a 50% disease-free survival rate in 22 patients treated with irradiation alone. The grade 3 complication rate (8%) was similar in both groups.

CARCINOMA OF THE CERVIX IN PREGNANCY

The concurrent presence of carcinoma *in situ* or invasive carcinoma of the uterine cervix and pregnancy, although rare, poses a therapeutic dilemma to gynecologic and radiation oncologists. Boutselis[40] reported 134 intraepithelial tumors (0.14%) and 71 invasive tumors of the cervix (0.07%) in 95,000 deliveries. Because of the epithelial changes associated with pregnancy, the diagnosis of intraepithelial carcinoma may sometimes be difficult. However, Greene and Peckham[120] stressed the validity of the diagnosis of preinvasive carcinoma and the need to treat these patients adequately. If the pregnancy is to be allowed to reach full term, confirmation of the diagnosis by colposcopy and conservative management of carcinoma *in situ* with monthly Papanicolaou smears constitutes the best management.[80] Conization has frequently been performed[18]; however, Boutselis[40] reported a 20% incidence of complications, the most common being abnormal bleeding. Mikuta and co-workers[238] noted four abortions in 20 patients on whom conization was performed, and in four others premature deliveries were induced.

Punch biopsies can be obtained, but the diagnostic accuracy

is less reliable. As many as 50% of patients have residual carcinoma *in situ* after delivery. In patients with *invasive carcinoma* the lesion is usually clinically apparent. Multiple punch biopsies are adequate to confirm the diagnosis.

Greer and associates,[121] in a review of 600 infants without congenital abnormalities, pointed out that when Stage IB cervical carcinoma is diagnosed during pregnancy and fetal survival is desired, the neonatal mortality rate decreased from 30% when the fetus was delivered at 26 to 27 weeks to 2.7% when it was allowed to mature to 34 to 35 weeks.

Because there is a greater need to institute therapy for cervical carcinoma as soon as possible, the accepted method of treatment in patients in the first 6 months of pregnancy is to carry out definitive surgery or radiation therapy, as indicated by the stage of the disease.[90,389] In the third trimester of pregnancy when the fetus may be salvaged, a cesarean section, combined with a radical hysterectomy and lymphadenectomy or followed by definitive treatment postpartum, is preferred by some gynecologic oncologists.[40,120,240] However, several authors report that vaginal delivery does not affect the prognosis deleteriously.[68]

If a radical hysterectomy is performed and positive pelvic lymph nodes are found, the usual postoperative irradiation including external beam with or without intracavitary insertion should be carried out. If it is decided to terminate the pregnancy, the patient is initially treated with external-beam irradiation to the whole pelvis (4000 cGy in 4 weeks). Usually an abortion occurs, and there is some involution of the uterus. After this dose of irradiation, careful evacuation of the uterus and an intracavitary insertion may be performed under general anesthesia. If surgery is to be carried out, approximately 4000 mgh is given. If not, two intracavitary insertions for a total of 6000 mgh (5500 cGy to point A) and an additional 1000 cGy or 2000 cGy are delivered to the parametria with a midline block. The typical surgical procedure is a radical hysterectomy with lymphadenectomy except in the case of microinvasive carcinoma, for which the lymphadenectomy is not performed.

Kinch,[187] Symmonds,[376] and Creasman and co-workers[68] have reported similar 5- to 7-year survival rates in pregnant and nonpregnant patients, with the stage of the disease at the time of diagnosis being the only determining prognostic factor (Fig. 54-39). Survival is the same regardless of the trimester of the pregnancy in which definitive treatment is instituted.[66,376] Creasman and co-workers[68] reported on 98 patients: 48 treated by irradiation, 45 by irradiation followed by surgery, and five by radical hysterectomy alone. The survival rate was comparable to that of nonpregnant patients for similar stages. The survival rate for patients with Stage I disease was comparable whether vaginal delivery was allowed or a cesarean section was performed (about 85% in those with Stage I and 50% to 64% in those with Stage II disease). Also, the percentage of infants surviving (over 80%) was the same in both groups.

Senekjian and associates[350] reported no significant difference in survival or patterns of failure in 24 women who were pregnant at the time of diagnosis of clear cell adenocarcinoma of the cervix and vagina, compared with those of 408 who had never been pregnant. The 5-year and 10-year actuarial survival rates were 86% and 68% for the pregnant patients and 87% and 79%, respectively, for patients who had not been pregnant.

The practice popularized 30 years ago of administering a "restraining dose of radium" and deferring definitive radiation therapy until delivery is carried out should be strongly condemned. Strauss[368] reported two of 11 infants being born with microcephaly in addition to other complications such as alopecia, facial deformity, eye damage, and chromosomal abnormalities after this procedure.

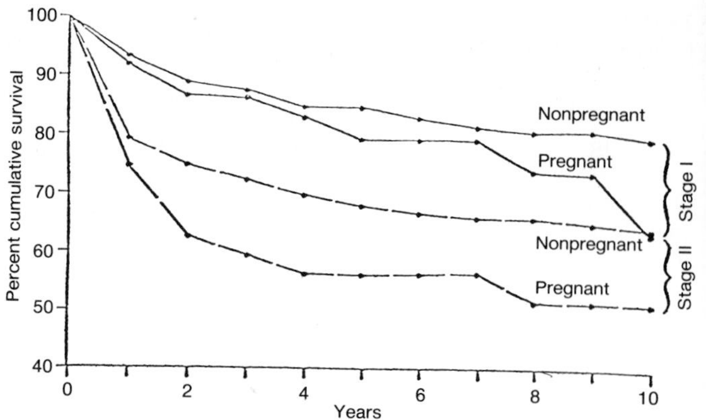

FIGURE 54–39. Actuarial survival rates for pregnant and nonpregnant women with carcinoma of the cervix. (Reprinted with permission from the American College of Obstetricians and Gynecologists. Creasman WT, Rutledge FN, Fletcher GH: Obstet Gynecol 36:495–501, 1970)

CARCINOMA OF THE CERVICAL STUMP

Subtotal hysterectomy, a relatively popular procedure for benign conditions of the uterus in past years, is rarely performed today. These patients are, of course, at risk to develop carcinoma of the uterine cervix.

It is important to divide patients with carcinoma of the cervical stump into *true,* when the first symptom occurs 3 or more years after subtotal hysterectomy, or *coincidental,* when the symptoms are noticed before the third postoperative year.[345] Moss and associates[252] recommend 2 elapsed years after hysterectomy as the time for the classification of these lesions. This separation is important because the prognosis for carcinoma of the true stump is significantly better than for coincidental lesions, in which carcinoma was probably present at the time the hysterectomy was performed.

The natural history and patterns of spread of carcinoma of the cervical stump are similar to those of the cervix in the intact uterus. The diagnostic workup, clinical staging, and basic principles of therapy are the same.

Surgery performed for Stage I tumors is somewhat more difficult because of the previous surgical procedures and the presence of adhesions in the pelvis.

When radiation is administered, the lack of a uterine cavity into which to insert a tandem containing two or three sources makes intracavitary therapy more difficult. Whenever possible, as many sources as technically feasible should be inserted in the remaining cervical canal. Occasionally, transvaginal irradiation may be used to boost the dose delivered to central disease in the stump. It is important to deliver higher whole-pelvis irradiation. In general, patients with Stage I disease are treated with a combination of 2000 cGy to the whole pelvis and 3000 cGy to the parametria with midline shielding combined with two intracavitary insertions. The dose of intracavitary therapy depends on the number of sources that can be placed in the cervical canal (1000 mgh to 3000 mgh for one to three sources).

More advanced stages of cervical carcinoma should be treated with 4000 cGy to the whole pelvis and 2000 cGy to the parametria with midline shielding, combined with the same intracavitary doses. When there is no opportunity to insert any sources in the cervical canal, the whole pelvis dose must be increased to 6000 cGy. Total dose (external and intracavitary) to the upper vaginal mucosa should not exceed 15,000 cGy.

If bulky disease is present in the cervix, parametrium, or vagina, additional interstitial therapy is advisable, if technically feasible.

When intravaginal cones are used, 3000 cGy to 4000 cGy air dose is delivered in 2 to 3 weeks, in three to five weekly fractions. Moss and associates[252] advised limiting the dose to the vaginal vault with transvaginal irradiation to 3000 cGy in 10 days.

The 5-year survival rate for carcinoma of the cervical stump treated with irradiation is similar to that reported for patients with carcinoma of the intact uterus.[182,345,417,418] The anatomic sites of failure and the incidence of recurrences are similar to those seen in patients in whom the uterus is intact. Distant metastasis also follows the same distribution.

Because of the close proximity of the bladder, rectum, and small intestine to the intracavitary sources and because of the often higher doses of external-beam irradiation given to the whole pelvis, complications are somewhat more frequent than in carcinoma of the cervix with intact uterus. Wimbush and Fletcher[417] reported five fistulas, six cases of severe proctosigmoiditis, and 12 cases of vault necrosis in 238 patients treated with definitive radiation therapy.

In 253 patients with carcinoma of the cervical stump treated at M. D. Anderson Cancer Center, median survival was 203, 140, and 32 months for Stages I, II, and III, respectively.[239] Goodman and co-workers[114] described pelvic recurrences in four of seven patients with Stage I adenocarcinoma of the cervical stump treated with external-beam irradiation (4500 cGy to 5000 cGy) to the whole pelvis and intracavitary insertions. Only one patient was alive tumor-free, and two died of intercurrent disease at 28 and 63 months. Six (66%) of nine patients with Stage IIA to IIIB tumors developed pelvic failures, and only one patient survived 5 years. It is noteworthy that three patients with adenoacanthoma survived, and none of the five with adenosquamous carcinoma survived.

Kovalic and colleagues[200] reported on 70 patients with carcinoma of the surgical stump treated with various irradiation techniques; 16 of the patients also underwent a surgical procedure. The 10-year disease-free survival rates were 100% for Stage IA, 79% for Stage IB, 66% for Stage IIB, and 39% for Stage IIIB disease. The pelvic failure rates were 10% in Stage IB (two of 19), 9% in Stage II (two of 12), and 50% in Stage IIIB (three of six). Major gastrointestinal complications were noted in 9% of the patients and urinary complications in 3.8%. The results are comparable to those seen in patients treated for invasive carcinoma of the cervix in intact uterus.

Creadick[66] reported results in 83 patients, 25 of whom were treated with radical trachelectomy and pelvic lymphadenectomy. The survival rate was 85.7% for those with squamous cell carcinoma and 50% for those with adenocarcinoma (patients with Stage I and Stage II disease).

SECOND MALIGNANCY

The possible induction of second primary cancers by pelvic irradiation is controversial. Lee and associates[209] and others[15,362] observed no significant increase in the incidence of second malignancies in patients irradiated for carcinoma of the cervix compared with the Connecticut Tumor Registry's prevailing rates. Storm[365] carried out a comprehensive analysis of the Danish Cancer Registry data on 24,970 women with invasive cervical cancer and 19,470 with carcinoma *in situ* of the cervix treated between 1943 and 1982. There was a small overall excess of second primary cancers in the lung, stomach, pancreas, rectum, and bladder, and of acute connective tissue sarcomas, although a decreased incidence of breast cancer was observed in the irradiated patients compared with that in nonirradiated patients. The significant decreased incidence of breast cancer may be attributable to the effect of ovarian ablation by radiation therapy.

In the patients irradiated for invasive carcinoma, more than 64 cases of tumors per 10,000 women per year were found in organs close to or at intermediate distance from the cervix, reaching the maximum after 30 or more years of follow-up (Table 54-37). A high risk for development of acute nonlym-

TABLE 54–37
Observed and Expected Second Primary Cancers Among Selected Patients With Carcinoma In Situ *of the Cervix Uteri Followed Up for 10 or More Years According to Treatment With or Without Radiation*

SECOND PRIMARY CANCER (ICD 7 CODE NO.)	IRRADIATED			NOT IRRADIATED		
	O	E	O/E	O	E	O/E
Stomach (151)	0	0.6	0.0	6	4.2	1.4
Colon (153)	3	1.5	2.0	10	12.4	0.8
Rectum (154)	1	0.8	1.3	4	6.7	0.6
Pancreas (157)	2	0.5	3.9	7	4.2	1.7
Lung (162)	2	1.1	1.8	29	12.4	2.3†
Breast (170)	2	4.1	0.5	50	50.7	1.0
Corpus uteri (172)	2	1.3	1.6	3	13.9	0.2‡
Ovary (175)	0	1.1	0.0	9	11.8	0.8
Other genital (176)	2	0.2	11.8*	8	1.6	4.9†
Bladder (181)	2	0.5	4.7	6	4.3	1.4
Melanoma (190)	0	0.4	0.0	4	5.5	0.7
Brain (194)	0	0.5	0.0	3	5.4	0.6
Connective tissue (197)	0	0.2	0.0	0	2.1	0.06

O: observed; E: expected; O/E: observed to expected ratio
**P <0.05*
†P <0.001
‡P <0.01
(Storm HH: Cancer 61:679–688, 1988)

phatic leukemia was observed in irradiated patients with carcinoma *in situ*, but not in those with invasive lesions. This could be explained by the lower doses of radiation delivered to the bone marrow in the *in situ* tumors treated with brachytherapy alone. Lower doses of radiation, with greater induction of mutations and less cell kill may be responsible for the leukemogenic effect.

Decreased risk was also noted for tumors of the brain, myeloma of the skin, and tumors of the colon other than rectal. Storm[365] recommended follow-up for life of irradiated patients to evaluate the long-term carcinogenic effects of irradiation.

REFERENCES

1. Abell MR, Gosling JRG: Gland cell carcinoma (adenocarcinoma) of the uterus cervix. Am J Obstet Gynecol 83:729–755, 1962
2. Abitbol NM, Davenport JH: Sexual dysfunction after therapy for cervical carcinoma. Am J Obstet Gynecol 119:181–189, 1974
3. Abrams P, Feneley RCL, Torrens M: Urodynamics. (Clinical Practice in Urology), p 160. Berlin, Springer-Verlag, 1983
4. Ackerman LV, delRegato JA (eds): Cancer: Diagnosis, Treatment, and Prognosis, pp 717–819. St. Louis, CV Mosby, 1977
5. Adam E, Rawls WE, Melnick JL: The association of herpes virus type-2 infection and cervical cancer. Prev Med 3:122–141, 1974
6. Akine Y, Hashida I, Kajiura Y, et al: Carcinoma of the uterine cervix treated with external irradiation alone. Int J Radiat Oncol Biol Phys 12:1611–1616, 1986
7. Allt WEC: Supervoltage radiation treatment in advanced cancer of the uterine cervix. Can Med Assoc J 100:792–797, 1969
8. Alvarez RD, Soong SJ, Kinney WK, et al: Identification of prognostic factors and risk groups in patients found to have nodal metastasis at the time of radical hysterectomy for early stage squamous carcinoma of the cervix. Gynecol Oncol 35:130–135, 1989
9. American Cancer Society: 1990 Facts & Figures, p 8. New York, American Cancer Society, 1990
10. American College of Obstetricians and Gynecologists Statement of Policy: Periodic Cancer Screening for Women. American College of Obstetricians and Gynecologists, June 1980
11. Ampil F, Datta R, Datta S: Elective postoperative external radiotherapy after hysterectomy in early-stage carcinoma of the cervix: Is additional vaginal cuff irradiation necessary: Cancer 60:280–288, 1987
12. Andras EJ, Fletcher GH, Rutledge F: Radiotherapy of carcinoma of the cervix following simple hysterectomy. Am J Obstet Gynecol 115:647–655, 1973
13. Anson BJ, McVay CB: Surgical Anatomy, vol 2, 5th ed, pp 800–835. Philadelphia, WB Saunders, 1971
14. Aristizabal SA, Surwit EA, Hevezi JM, Heusinkveld RS: Treatment of advanced cancer of the cervix with transperineal interstitial irradiation. Int J Radiat Oncol Biol Phys 9:1013–1017, 1983
15. Arneson AN, Schellhas HF: Multiple primary cancers in patients treated for carcinoma of the cervix. Am J Obstet Gynecol 106:1155–1170, 1970
16. Ashenhurst EM, Quartey GRC, Starreveld A: Lumbo-sacral radiculopathy induced by radiation. Can J Neurol Sci 4:259–263, 1977
17. Averette HE, Ford JH Jr, Dudan RC, et al: Staging of cervical cancer. Clin Obstet Gynecol 18:215–232, 1975
18. Averette HE, Nasser N, Yankow SL, Little WA: Cervical conization in pregnancy: Analysis of 180 operations. Am J Obstet Gynecol 106:543–549, 1970
19. Badib AO, Kurohara SS, Webster JH, Pickren JW: Metastasis to organs in carcinoma of the uterine cervix: Influence of treatment on incidence and distribution. Cancer 21:434–439, 1968
20. Bandy LC, Creasman W: Computed tomography in evaluation of extrapelvic lymphadenopathy in carcinoma of the cervix. Obstet Gynecol 65:73–76, 1985
21. Barber HRK: Relative prognostic significance of preoperative and operative findings in pelvic exenteration. Surg Clin North Am 49:431–447, 1969
22. Barber HRK, Graber EA: Treatment of advanced cancer of the cervix by pelvic exenteration. Bull NY Acad Med 49:870–886, 1973
23. Barron BA, Richart RM: Statistical model of the natural history of cervical carcinoma. II. Estimates of the transition time from dysplasia to carcinoma in situ. J Natl Cancer Inst 45:1025–1030, 1970
24. Beahrs OH, Henson DE, Hutter RVP, Myers MH (eds): Manual for Staging of Cancer, 3rd ed, pp 151–153. Philadelphia, JB Lippincott, 1988
25. Benedet JL, Turko M, Boyes DA, et al: Radiation hysterectomy in the treatment of cervical cancer. Am J Obstet Gynecol 137:254–262, 1980
26. Benson WL, Norris HJ: A critical review of the frequency of lymph node metastasis and death from microinvasive carcinoma of the cervix. Obstet Gynecol 49:632–638, 1977
27. Berek JS, Castaldo TW, Hacker NF, et al: Adenocarcinoma of the uterine cervix. Cancer 48:2734–2741, 1981
28. Berkowitz RS, Ehrmann RL, Lavizzo-Mourey R, Knapp RC: Invasive cervical carcinoma in young women. Gynecol Oncol 8:311–316, 1979
29. Berman ML, Keys H, Creasman W, et al: Survival and patterns of recurrence in cervical cancer metastatic to periaortic lymph nodes: A Gynecologic Group Study. Gynecol Oncol 19:8, 1984
30. Berman ML, Lagasse LD, Ballon SC, Watring WG, Tesler A: Modification of radiation therapy following operative evaluation of patients with cervical carcinoma. Gynecol Oncol 6:328–331, 1978
31. Beyer FD Jr, Murphy A: Patterns of spread of invasive cancer of the human cervix. Cancer 18:34–40, 1965
32. Bianchi UA, Sartori E, Pecorelli S, et al: Treatment of primary invasive cervical cancer: Considerations on 997 consecutive cases. Eur J Gynecol Oncol 9:47–53, 1988
33. Biggs PJ, Russell MD: Effect of a femoral head prosthesis on megavoltage beam radiotherapy. Int J Radiat Oncol Biol Phys 14:581–586, 1988
34. Bjerre B, Eliasson G, Linell F, et al: Conization as only treatment of carcinoma *in situ* of the uterine cervix. Am J Obstet Gynecol 125:143–152, 1976
35. Blaikley JB, Lederman M, Pollard W: Carcinoma of the cervix at Chelsea Hospital for Women, 1935–1965. Five-year and 1-year results of treatment. J Obstet Gynaecol Br Comm 76:729–740, 1969
36. Blaustein A, Immerman B: Leiomyosarcoma of the cervix. Obstet Gynecol 22:224–227, 1963
37. Bohm JW, Krupp PJ, Lee FYL, Batson HWK: Lymph node metastases in microinvasive epidermoid cancer of the cervix. Obstet Gynecol 48:65–67, 1976
38. Boon ME, Susanti I, Tasche MJA, Kok KP: Human papillomavirus (HPV)-associated male and female genital carcinomas in a Hindu population: The male as vector and victim. Cancer 64:559–565, 1989
39. Boulware RJ, Caderao JB, Delclos L, et al: Whole pelvis megavoltage irradiation with single doses of 1,000 rad to palliate advanced gynecologic cancers. Int J Radiat Oncol Biol Phys 5:333–338, 1979
40. Boutselis JG: Intraepithelial carcinoma of the cervix associated with pregnancy. Obstet Gynecol 40:657–666, 1972
41. Brenner DE, Whitley NO: Computed tomography in invasive carcinoma of the cervix: An appraisal. Obstet Gynecol 62:218–224, 1983
42. Brenner DE, Whitley NO, Umberto V: An evaluation of the computed tomographic scanner for staging of carcinoma of the cervix. Cancer 50:2323–2328, 1982
43. Breslow L: Cytology and the decline in uterine cervix mortality in California. In Clark RL, Cumley RW, McCay JE, Copeland MM (eds): Oncology 1970 (Proceedings of the Tenth International Cancer Congress), vol IV. Diagnosis and Man-

agement of Cancer: Specific Sites. Chicago, Year Book Medical Publishers, 1971
44. Brunschwig A: Complete excision of the pelvic viscera for advanced carcinoma. Cancer 1:177–183, 1948
45. Brunschwig A: The surgical treatment of cancer of the cervix stage I and II. Am J Roentgenol 102:147–151, 1968
46. Brunschwig A, Barber HRK: Surgical treatment of carcinoma of the cervix. Obstet Gynecol 27:21–29, 1966
47. Buchsbaum HJ: Extrapelvic lymph node metastases in cervical carcinoma. Am J Obstet Gynecol 133:814–824, 1979
48. Burch JC, Chalfant RL: Preoperative radium irradiation and radical hysterectomy in the treatment of cancer of the cervix. Am J Obstet Gynecol 106:1054–1064, 1970
49. Burghardt E, Holzer E: Diagnosis and treatment of microinvasive carcinoma of the cervix uteri. Obstet Gynecol 49:641–653, 1977
50. Bush RS: The significance of anemia in clinical radiation therapy. Int J Radiat Oncol Biol Phys 12:2047–2050, 1986
51. Bush RS, Jenkin RDT, Allt WEC, et al: Definitive evidence for hypoxic cells influencing cure in cancer therapy. Br J Cancer 37:302–306, 1978
52. Camilien L, Fordon D, Fruchter RG, et al: Predictive value of computerized tomography in the presurgical evaluation of primary carcinoma of the cervix. Gynecol Oncol 30:209–215, 1988
53. Cardozo LD: Detrusor instability. In Santon SL (ed): Clinical Gynecologic Urology, pp 193–203. St. Louis, CV Mosby, 1984
54. Carlson V, Delclos L, Fletcher GH: Distant metastases in squamous-cell carcinoma of the uterine cervix. Radiology 88:961–966, 1967
55. Castro JR, Issa P, Fletcher GH: Carcinoma of the cervix treated by external irradiation alone. Radiology 95:163–166, 1970
56. Chism SE, Park RC, Keys HM: Prospects for para-aortic irradiation in treatment of cancer of the cervix. Cancer 35:1505–1509, 1975
57. Choo YC, Chou TK, Wong LC, Ma HK: Potentiation of radiotherapy by cis-dichlorodiammine platinum (II) in advanced cervical carcinoma. Gynecol Oncol 23:94–100, 1986
58. Christensen A, Lange P, Neilsen E: Surgery and radiotherapy for invasive cancer of the cervix: Surgical treatment. Acta Obstet Gynecol 43:59–87, 1964
59. Christopherson WM, Gray LA, Parker JE: Microinvasive carcinoma of the uterine cervix. Cancer 38:629–632, 1976
60. Christopherson WM, Parker JE: Microinvasive carcinoma of the uterine cervix. A clinical-pathological study. Cancer 17:1123–1131, 1964
61. Christopherson WM, Parker JE: Relation of cervical cancer to early marriage and childbearing. N Engl J Med 273:235–239, 1965
62. Chung CK, Nahhas WA, Stryker JA, et al: Analysis of factors contributing to treatment failures in stages IB and IIA carcinoma of the cervix. Am J Obstet Gynecol 138:550–556, 1980
63. Clemmesen J, Poulsen H: Report of the Ministry of the Interior, Document 3, Copenhagen, 1971
64. Cosbie WG: Radiotherapy following hysterectomy performed for or in the presence of cancer of the cervix. Am J Obstet Gynecol 85:332–336, 1963
65. Coia L, Won M, Lanciano R, et al: The Patterns of Care Outcome Study for cancer of the uterine cervix. Results of the 2nd National Practice Survey. Int J Radiat Oncol Biol Phys, in press
66. Creadick RN: Carcinoma of the cervical stump. Am J Obstet Gynecol 75:565–574, 1958
67. Creasman WT, Rutledge FN: Carcinoma *in situ* of the cervix. Obstet Gynecol 3:373–380, 1972
68. Creasman WT, Rutledge FN, Fletcher GH: Carcinoma of the cervix associated with pregnancy. Obstet Gynecol 36:495–501, 1970
69. Crissman JD, Budhraja M, Aron BS, Cummings G: Histopathologic prognostic factors in stage II and III squamous cell carcinoma of the uterine cervix. Int J Gynecol Pathol 6:97–103, 1987
70. Crum CP, Levine RU: Human papillomavirus infection and cervical neoplasia: New perspectives. Int J Gynecol Pathol 3:376, 1984
71. Cunningham JJ, Fuks ZY, Castellino RA: Radiographic manifestations of carcinoma of the cervix and complications of its treatment. Radiol Clin North Am 12:93–108, 1974
72. Daroca PJ Jr, Dhurandhar HN: Basaloid carcinoma of uterine cervix. Am J Surg Pathol 4:235–239, 1980
73. Dattoli MJ, Gretz HF III, Beller U, et al: Analysis of multiple prognostic factors in patients with stage IB cervical cancer: Age as a major determinant. Int J Radiat Oncol Biol Phys 17:41–47, 1989
74. Davy M, Bentzen H, Jahren R: Simple hysterectomy in the presence of invasive cervical cancer. Acta Obstet Gynecol Scand 56:105–108, 1977
75. Decker DG, Aaro LA, Hunt AB, et al: Sequential radiation and operation in carcinoma of the uterine cervix. Am J Obstet Gynecol 92:35–42, 1965
76. Deckers PJ, Ketcham AS, Sugarbaker EV, Thomas LB: Pelvic exenteration for primary carcinoma of the uterine cervix. Obstet Gynecol 37:647–659, 1971
77. Delgado G, Coglar H, Walker P: Survival and complications in cervical cancer treated by pelvic and extended field radiation after para-aortic lymphadenectomy. Am J Roentgenol 130: 141–143, 1978
78. Del Regato JA, Cox JD: Transvaginal roentgentherapy in the conservative management of carcinoma *in situ* of the uterine cervix. Radiology 84:1090–1095, 1965
79. deMuylder X, Belanger R, Vauclair R, et al: Value of lymphography in stage IB cancer of the uterine cervix. Obstet Gynecol 148:610–613, 1984
80. DePetrillo AD, Towsend DE, Morrow CP, et al: Colposcopic evaluation of the abnormal Papanicolaou test in pregnancy. Am J Obstet Gynecol 121:441–445, 1975
81. Deutsch M, Parsons JA: Radiotherapy for carcinoma of the cervix recurrent after surgery. Cancer 34:2051–2055, 1974
82. Dewit L: Combined treatment of radiation and cis-diamoninedchloroplatinum, II. A review of experimental and clinical data. Int J Radiat Oncol Biol Phys 13:403–426, 1987
83. Dickson RJ: Late results of radium treatment of carcinoma of the cervix. Clin Radiol 23:528–535, 1972
84. Dische S: Hyperbaric oxygen: The Medical Research Council Trials and their clinical significance. Br J Radiol 51:888–894, 1979
85. Dische S: Misonidazole in the clinic at Mount Vernon. Cancer Clin Trials 3:175–178, 1980
86. Dische S, Sealy R, Watson ER: Carcinoma of the cervix: Anaemia, radiotherapy and hyperbaric oxygen. Br J Radiol 56:251–255, 1983
87. Dolan TE, Boyce J, Rosen Y, Lu T: Cytology, colposcopy, and directed biopsy: What are the limitations? Gynecol Oncol 3:314–324, 1975
88. Drescher CW, Hopkins MP, Roberts JA: Comparison of the pattern of metastatic spread of squamous cell cancer and adenocarcinoma of the uterine cervix. Gynecol Oncol 33:340–343, 1989
89. Drill VA: Oral contraceptives: Relation to mammary cancer, benign breast lesions and cervical cancer. Am Rev Pharmacol 15:367–385, 1975
90. Dudan RC, Yon JL Jr, Ford JH Jr, Averette HE: Carcinoma of the cervix and pregnancy. Gynecol Oncol 1:283–289, 1973
91. Durrance FY: Radiotherapy following simple hysterectomy in patients with stage I and II carcinoma of the cervix. Am J Roentgenol Radium Ther Nucl Med 102:165–169, 1968
92. Durrance FY, Fletcher GH, Rutledge FN: Analysis of central recurrent disease in stages I and II squamous cell carcinomas of the cervix on intact uterus. AJR 106:831, 1969
93. Dyson JED, Joslin CAF, Rothwell RI, et al: Flow cytofluorometric evidence for the differential radioresponsiveness of aneuploid and diploid cervix tumours. Radiother Oncol 8:263–272, 1987
94. Ebner F, Kressel HY, Mintz MC, et al: Tumor recurrence versus fibrosis in the female pelvis: Differentiation with MR imaging at 1.5T. Radiology 166:333–340, 1980

95. Eifel PJ, Morris M, Oswald MJ, et al: Adenocarcinoma of the uterine cervix: Prognosis and patterns of failure in 367 cases treated at the M.D. Anderson Cancer Center between 1965 and 1985. Cancer 65:2507–2514, 1990
96. Einhorn N, Bygdeman M, Sjoberg B: Combined radiation and surgical treatment for carcinoma of the uterine cervix. Cancer 45:720–723, 1980
97. Evans JC, Bergsjo P: The influence of anemia on the results of radiotherapy in carcinoma of the cervix. Radiology 81:709–716, 1965
98. Evans SR Jr, Hilaris BS, Barber HRK: External vs. interstitial irradiation in unresectable recurrent cancer of the cervix. Cancer 28:1284–1288, 1971
99. Fennell RH: Microinvasive carcinoma of the uterine cervix. Obstet Gynecol Surv 33:406–411, 1978
100. Fidler HK, Boyes DA, Worth AJ: Cervical cancer detection in British Columbia. J Obstet Gynaecol Br Comm 75:392–404, 1968
101. Field CA, Dockerty M, Symmonds RE: Small cell cancer of the cervix. Am J Obstet Gynecol 88:447–451, 1964
102. Figge DC, Tamimi HK: Patterns of recurrence of carcinoma following radical hysterectomy. Am J Obstet Gynecol 140:213–220, 1981
103. Fletcher GH: Cancer of the uterine cervix: Janeway Lecture. Am J Roentgenol Radium Ther Nucl Med 111:225–242, 1971
104. Fletcher GH (ed): Textbook of Radiotherapy, 3rd ed, pp 720–773; pp 812–828. Philadelphia, Lea & Febiger, 1980
105. Fletcher GH, Lindberg RD, Caderao JB, Wharton TJ: Hyperbaric oxygen as a radiotherapeutic adjuvant in advanced carcinoma of the uterine cervix. Preliminary results of a randomized trial. Cancer 39:617–623, 1977
106. Friedman M, Pearlman AW: Carcinoma of the cervix: Radiation salvage of surgical failures. Radiology 84:801–811, 1965
107. Fuller AF Jr, Elliott N, Kosloff C, Lewis JL: Lymph node metastases from carcinoma of the cervix, stages IB and IIA: Implications for prognosis and treatment. Gynecol Oncol 13:165–174, 1982
108. Gersell DJ, Mazoujian G, Mutch DG, Rudloff MA: Small-cell undifferentiated carcinoma of the cervix: A clinicopathologic, ultrastructural, and immunocytochemical study of 15 cases. Am J Surg Pathol 12:684–698, 1988
109. Girardi F, Lichtenegger W, Tamussino K, Haas J: The importance of parametrial lymph nodes in the treatment of cervical cancer. Gynecol Oncol 34:206–211, 1989
110. Glassburn JR, Damsker JI, Brady LW, et al: Hyperbaric oxygen and radiation in the treatment of advanced cervical carcinoma. In Fifth International Hyperbaric Congress Proceedings, II, p 813–819 (Simon Fraser University). 1974
111. Goellner JR: Carcinoma of the cervix: Clinicopathologic correlation of 196 cases. Am J Clin Pathol 66:775–785, 1976
112. Gonzalez Gonzalez D, Ketting BW, van Bunningen B, van Dijk JDP: Carcinoma of the uterine cervix stage IB and IIA: Results of postoperative irradiation in patients with microscopic infiltration in the parametrium and/or lymph node metastasis. Int J Radiat Oncol Biol Phys 16:389–395, 1989
113. Goodman HM, Bowling MC, Nelson JH: Cervical malignancies. In Knapp RC, Berkowitz RS (eds): Gynecologic Oncology, pp 225–273. New York, Macmillan, 1986
114. Goodman HM, Niloff JM, Buttlar CA, et al: Adenocarcinoma of the cervical stump. Gynecol Oncol 35:188–192, 1989
115. Gordon HW: Adenoid cystic (cylindromatous) carcinoma of the uterine cervix: Report of two cases. Am J Clin Pathol 58:51–57, 1972
116. Graham JB, Sotto LSJ, Paoloucek FP: Carcinoma of the Cervix. Philadelphia, WB Saunders, 1962
117. Graham S, Priore R, Graham M, et al: Genital cancer in wives of penile cancer patients. Cancer 44:1870–1874, 1979
118. Gray MJ, Gusberg SB, Guttman R: Pelvic lymph node dissection following radiotherapy. Am J Obstet Gynecol 76:629–633, 1958
119. Green TH, Morse WJ: Management of invasive cervical cancer following inadvertent simple hysterectomy. Obstet Gynecol 33:763–769, 1969
120. Greene RR, Peckman BM: Preinvasive cancer of the cervix and pregnancy. Am J Obstet Gynecol 75:551–564, 1958
121. Greer BE, Easterling TR, McLennan DA, et al: Fetal and maternal considerations in the management of stage IB cervical cancer during pregnancy. Gynecol Oncol 34:61–65, 1989
122. Griffin TW, Parker RG, Taylor WJ: An evaluation of procedures used in staging carcinoma of the cervix. Am J Roentgenol Radium Ther Nucl Med 127:825–827, 1976
123. Grigsby PW, Perez CA: Efficacy of 5-FU by continuous infusion and other cytotoxic agents as radiopotentiators for gynecologic malignancies. In Rotman M, Rosenthal CJ (eds): Medical Radiology: Diagnostic Imaging and Radiation Oncology. Concomitant Continuous Infusion Chemotherapy and Radiation. New York, Springer-Verlag, in press
124. Grigsby PW, Perez CA, Kuske RR, et al: Adenocarcinoma of the uterine cervix: Lack of evidence for a poor prognosis. Radiother Oncol 12:289–296, 1988
125. Grimard L, Genest P, Girard A, et al: Prognostic significance of endometrial extension in carcinoma of the cervix. Gynecol Oncol 31:301–309, 1988
126. Gunderson LL, Weems WS, Hebertson RM, Plenk HP: Correlation of histopathology with clinical results following radiation therapy for carcinoma of the cervix. Am J Roentgenol Radium Ther Nucl Med 120:74–87, 1974
127. Guttman R: Significance of postoperative irradiation in carcinoma of the cervix: A ten-year study. Am J Roentgenol Radium Ther Nucl Med 108:102–108, 1970
128. Guznick DS: Efficacy of screening for cervical cancer: A review. Am J Public Health 68:125–134, 1978
129. Haie C, Pejovic MH, Gerbaulet A, et al: Is prophylactic paraaortic irradiation worthwhile in the treatment of advanced cervical carcinoma? Results of a controlled clinical trial of the EORTC radiotherapy group. Radiother Oncol 11:101–112, 1988
130. Hamberger AD, Fletcher GH, Wharton JT: Results of treatment of early stage I carcinoma of the uterine cervix with intracavitary radium alone. Cancer 41:980–985, 1978
131. Hamberger AD, Unal A, Gershenson DM, Fletcher GH: Analysis of the severe complications of irradiation of carcinoma of the cervix: Whole pelvis irradiation and intracavitary radium. Int J Radiat Oncol Biol Phys 9:367–371, 1983
132. Hameed K: Clear cell carcinoma of the uterine cervix. Am J Obstet Gynecol 101:954–958, 1968
133. Hammond JA, Herson J, Freedman RS, et al: The impact of lymph node status on survival in cervical carcinoma. Int J Radiat Oncol Biol Phys 7:1713–1718, 1981
134. Hanks GE, Herring DF, Kramer S: Patterns of Care Outcome Studies: Results of the National Practice in Cancer of the Cervix. Cancer 51:959–967, 1983
135. Hart WR, Norris HJ: Mesonephric adenocarcinomas of the cervix. Cancer 29:106–113, 1972
136. Hasumi K, Sakamoto A, Sugano H: Microinvasive carcinoma of the uterine cervix. Cancer 45:928–931, 1980
137. Henriksen E: The lymphatic spread of carcinoma of the cervix and of the body of the uterus: A study of 420 necropsies. Am J Obstet Gynecol 58:924–942, 1949
138. Herbst AL, Cole P: Epidemiologic and clinical aspects of clear cell adenocarcinoma in young women: Intrauterine exposure to diethylstilbestrol in the human. Am Coll Ob/Gyn 2–7, 1978
139. Herbst AL, Cole P, Norusis MJ, et al: Epidemiologic aspects and factors related to survival in 384 registry cases of clear cell adenocarcinoma of the vagina and cervix. Am J Obstet Gynecol 135:876–886, 1979
140. Herbst AL, Ulfelder H, Postanzer UC: Adenocarcinoma of the vagina. N Engl J Med 284:878–881, 1971
141. Hintz BL, Kagan AR, Chan P, et al: Radiation tolerance of the vaginal mucosa. Int J Radiat Oncol Biol Phys 6:711–716, 1980
142. Hirst DG: Anemia: A problem or an opportunity in radiotherapy? Int J Radiat Oncol Biol Phys 12:2009–2017, 1986
143. Hochman A, Ratzkowski E, Schrieber H: Incidence of carcinoma of cervix in Jewish women in Israel. Br J Cancer 9:358–364, 1955
144. Hogan WM, Littman P, Griner L, et al: Results of radiation therapy given after radical hysterectomy. Cancer 49:1278–1285, 1982

145. Homesley HD, Raben M, Blake DD, et al: Relationship of lesion size to survival in patients with stage IB squamous cell carcinoma of the cervix uteri treated by radiation therapy. Surg Gynecol Oncol 150:529–531, 1980
146. Hopkins MP, Schmid RW, Roberts JA, Morley GW: Gland cell carcinoma (adenocarcinoma) of the cervix. Obstet Gynecol 72:789–795, 1988
147. Horiot J-C, Pigneux J, Pourquier H, et al: Radiotherapy alone in carcinoma of the intact uterine cervix according to GH Fletcher guidelines: A French Cooperative study of 1383 cases. Int J Radiat Oncol Biol Phys 14:605–611, 1988
148. Hornback NB, Shidnia H, Shupe RE, et al: Results comparing hyperthermia and radiation versus radiation alone in treatment of 79 patients with stage IIIB carcinoma of the uterine cervix (Abstract). Int J Radiat Oncol Biol Phys 6:1384, 1980
149. Hoskins WJ, Ford JH Jr, Lutz MH, Averette HE: Radical hysterectomy and pelvic lymphadenectomy for the management of early invasive cancer of the cervix. Gynecol Oncol 4:278–290, 1976
150. Hoskins WJ, Perez CA, Young RC: Gynecologic tumors. In DeVita VT Jr, Hellman S, Rosenberg SA (eds): Cancer: Principles and Practice of Oncology, 3rd ed. Philadelphia, JB Lippincott, 1989
151. Hreshchyshyn MM, Aron BS, Boronow RC, et al: Hydroxyurea or placebo combined with radiation to treat stages IIIB and IV cervical cancer confined to the pelvis. Int J Radiat Oncol Biol Phys 5:317–322, 1979
152. Hricak H, Lacey CG, Sandles LG, et al: Invasive cervical carcinoma: Comparison of MR imaging and surgical findings. Radiology 166:623–631, 1988
153. Hsu C, Cheng Y, Su S: Prognosis of uterine cervical cancer with extensive lymph node metastases: Special emphasis on the value of pelvic lymphadenectomy in the surgical treatment of uterine cervical cancer. Am J Obstet Gynecol 114:954–962, 1972
154. Hunter RD, Cowie VJ, Blair V, Cole MP: A clinical trial of two conceptually different radical radiotherapy treatments in stage III carcinoma of the cervix. Clin Radiol 37:23–27, 1986
155. Hurt WG, Silverberg SG, Frable RWJ, et al: Adenocarcinoma of the cervix: Histologic and clinical features. Am J Obstet Gynecol 129:304, 1977
156. Inoue T, Okumura M: Prognostic significance of parametrial extension in patients with cervical carcinoma, stages IB, IIA and IIB: A study of 628 cases treated by radical hysterectomy and lymphadenectomy with or without postoperative irradiation. Cancer 54:1714–1719, 1984
157. International Commission of Radiation Units and Measurements: Dose and Volume Specification for Reporting Intracavitary Therapy in Gynecology, ICRU Report 38. Bethesda, MD, 1985
158. International Federation of Gynecologists and Obstetricians (FIGO): Changes in the definitions of clinical staging for the cervix and ovary. Am J Obstet Gynecol 56:263–264, 1987
159. Jacobs AJ, Perez CA, Camel HM, Kao M-S: Complications in patients receiving both irradiation and radical hysterectomy for carcinoma of the uterine cervix. Gynecol Oncol 22:273–280, 1985
160. Jampolis S, Andras J, Fletcher GH: Analysis of sites and causes of failure of irradiation in invasive squamous cell carcinoma of the intact uterine cervix. Radiology 115:681–685, 1975
161. Janetschek G, Mack D, Hetzel H: Urinary diversion in gynecologic malignancies. Eur Urol 14:371–376, 1988
162. Jenkin RDT, Stryker JA: The influence of the blood pressure on survival in cancer of the cervix. Br J Radiol 41:913–920, 1968
163. Jobsen JJ, Lee JWH, Cleton FJ, Hermans J: Treatment of locoregional recurrence of carcinoma of the cervix by radiotherapy after primary surgery. Gynecol Oncol 33:368–371, 1989
164. Jobson VW, Girtanner RE, Averette HE: Therapy and survival of early invasive carcinoma of the cervix uteri with metastases to the pelvic nodes. Surg Gynecol Obstet 151:27–29, 1980
165. John M, Cooke K, Flam M, et al: Preliminary results of concomitant radiotherapy and chemotherapy in advanced cervical carcinoma. Gynecol Oncol 28:101–110, 1988
166. Johns HE: Optimization of energy and equipment. In Kramer S, Suntharalingam N, Zinninger GF (eds): High-Energy Photons and Electrons: Clinical Applications in Cancer Management, pp 333–345. New York, John Wiley & Sons, 1976
167. Johnson RJR, Walton RJ: Sequential study on the effect of the addition of hyperbaric oxygen on the 5 year survival rates of carcinoma of the cervix treated with conventional fractional irradiations. Am J Roentgenol Radium Ther Nucl Med 120:111–117, 1974
168. Joneja MG, Coulson DB.: Histopathology and cytogenetics of tumors induced by application of 7,12-dimethylbenz(a)anthracene (DMBA) in mouse cervix. Eur J Cancer 9:367–374, 1973
169. Kademian MT, Bosch A: Is staging laparotomy in cervical cancer justified? Int J Radiat Oncol Biol Phys 2:1235–1238, 1977
170. Kaminski PF, Maier RC: Clear cell adenocarcinoma of the cervix unrelated to diethylstilbestrol exposure. Obstet Gynecol 62:720–727, 1983
171. Kapp DS, Lawrence R: Temperature elevation during brachytherapy for carcinoma of the uterine cervix: Adverse effect on survival and enhancement of distant metastases. Int J Radiat Oncol Biol Phys 10:2281–2292, 1984
172. Kashigarian M, Dunn JE: The duration of intraepithelial and preclinical squamous cell carcinoma of the uterine cervix. Am J Epidemiol 92:221–222, 1970
173. Kaufman RH: Frozen section evaluation of cervical conization specimen. Clin Obstet Gynecol 10:838–852, 1967
174. Keighley E: Carcinoma of the cervix among prostitutes in a women's prison. Br J Vener Dis 44:254–255, 1968
175. Kelland LR, Steel GG: Differences in radiation response among human cervix carcinoma cell lines. Radiother Oncol 13:225–232, 1988
176. Kelso JW, Funnel JD: Combined surgical and radiation treatment of invasive carcinoma of the cervix. Am J Obstet Gynecol 116:205–213, 1973
177. Kern WH, Zivolich MR: The accuracy and consistency of the cytologic classification of squamous lesions of the uterine cervix. Acta Cytol 21:519–523, 1977
178. Kessler II: Perspectives on the epidemiology of cervical cancer with special reference to the herpes virus hypothesis. Cancer Res 34:1091–1109, 1974
179. Kessler II: Human cervical cancer as a venereal disease. Cancer Res 36:783–791, 1976
180. Ketcham AS, Hoye RC, Taylor PT, Deckers PJ: Radical hysterectomy and lymphadenectomy for carcinoma of the uterine cervix. Cancer 28:1272–1677, 1971
181. Ketcham AS, Sindelar WF, Felix EL, Bagley DH: Diagnostic scalene node biopsy in the preoperative evaluation of the surgical cancer patient. Cancer 38:948–952, 1976
182. Khint EK, Bokhman YV, Vel'gre RJ, Revazishvili TV: Prophylaxis and treatment of cervical stump cancer. Vopr Onkol 21:83–86, 1975
183. Kielbinska S, Ludwika T, Fraczek O: Studies of mortality and health status in women cured of cancer of the cervix uteri: Comparison of long-term results of radiotherapy and combined surgery and radiotherapy. Cancer 32:245–252, 1973
184. Kilcheski T, Arger P, Mikuta J: Role of computed tomography in the presurgical evaluation of carcinoma of the cervix. J Comput Assist Tomogr 5:378–383, 1981
185. Kilgore LC, Soong S-J, Gore H, et al: Analysis of prognostic features in adenocarcinoma of the cervix. Gynecol Oncol 31:137–148, 1988
186. Kim RY, Salter MM, Shingleton HM: Adjuvant postoperative radiation therapy following radical hysterectomy in stage IB ca of the cervix: Analysis of treatment failure. Int J Radiat Oncol Biol Phys 14:445–449, 1988
187. Kinch RAH: Factors affecting the prognosis of the cervix in pregnancy. Am J Obstet Gynecol 82:45, 1961
188. Kinney WK, Alvarez RD, Reid GC, et al: Value of adjuvant whole-pelvis irradiation after Wertheim hysterectomy for early-stage squamous carcinoma of the cervix with pelvic no-

dal metastasis: A matched-control study. Gynecol Oncol 34:258–262, 1989

189. Kiselow M, Butcher HR Jr, Bricker EM: Results of the radical surgical treatment of advanced pelvic cancer: A fifteen year study. Ann Surg 166:428–436, 1967
190. Kjorstad KE: Adenocarcinoma of the uterine cervix. Gynecol Oncol 5:219–223, 1977
191. Kjorstad KE, Martinbeau PW, Iversen T: Stage IB carcinoma of the cervix: The Norwegian Radium Hospital: Results and complications. III: Urinary and gastrointestinal complications. Gynecol Oncol 15:42–47, 1983
192. Kline J C, Schultz AE, Vermund H, Peckham BM: High dose radiotherapy for carcinoma of the cervix: Method and results. Am J Obstet Gynecol 104:479–484, 1969
193. Kolstad P: Carcinoma of the cervix: Stage 0; diagnosis and treatment. Am J Obstet Gynecol 96:1098–1111, 1966
194. Kolstad P: Follow-up study of 232 patients with stage Ia1 and 411 patients with stage Ia2 squamous cell carcinoma of the cervix (microinvasive carcinoma). Gynecol Oncol 33:265–272, 1989
195. Kolstad P, Klem V: Long-term follow-up of 1,121 cases of carcinoma *in situ*. Obstet Gynecol 48:125–129, 1976
196. Koss LG: Recurrent carcinoma and presence of radiation cell changes. Acta Cytol 3:418, 1959
197. Koss LG, Stewart FW, Foote FW, et al: Some histological aspects of behavior of epidermoid carcinoma *in situ* and related lesions of the uterine cervix. Cancer 16:1160–1211, 1963
198. Kottmeier HL: Complications following radiation therapy in carcinoma of the cervix and their treatment. Am J Obstet Gynecol 88:854–866, 1964
199. Kottmeier HL (ed): Annual Report on the Results of Treatment in Carcinoma of the Uterus, Vagina and Ovary, vol 15. Stockholm, International Federation of Gynecology and Obstetrics, 1973
200. Kovalic JJ, Grigsby PW, Perez CA, Lockett MA: Cervical stump carcinoma. Int J Radiat Oncol Biol Phys 20:933–938, 1991
201. Kramer C, Peschel RE, Goldberg N, et al: Radiation treatment of FIGO stage IVA carcinoma of the cervix. Gynecol Oncol 32:323–326, 1989
202. Krebs H-B, Helmkamp BF, Sevin B-Y, et al: Recurrent cancer of the cervix following radical hysterectomy and pelvic node dissection. Obstet Gynecol 59:422–427, 1982
203. Kuske RR, Perez CA, Grigsby PW, et al: Phase I/II study of definitive radiotherapy and chemotherapy (cisplatin and 5-fluorouracil) for advanced or recurrent gynecologic malignancies, preliminary report. Am J Clin Oncol 12:467–473, 1989
204. Kuske RR, Perez CA, Jacobs AJ, et al: Mini-colpostats in the treatment of carcinoma of the uterine cervix. Int J Radiat Oncol Biol Phys 14:899–906, 1988
205. Kyriakos M, Kempson RL, Perez CA: Carcinoma of the cervix in young women. Obstet Gynecol 38:930–944, 1971
206. Lagasse LD, Creasman WT, Shingleton HM, et al: Results and complications of operative staging in cervical cancer: Experience of the Gynecologic Oncology Group. Gynecol Oncol 9:90–98, 1980
207. Larson DM, Copeland LJ, Stringer CA, et al: Recurrent cervical carcinoma after radical hysterectomy. Gynecol Oncol 30:381–387, 1988
208. Lawhead RA Jr, Clark DGC, Smith DH, et al: Pelvic exenteration for recurrent or persistent gynecologic malignancies: A 10-year review of the Memorial Sloan-Kettering Cancer Center experience (1972–1981). Gynecol Oncol 33:279–282, 1989
209. Lee JY, Perez CA, Ettinger N, Fineberg BB: The risk of second primaries subsequent to irradiation for cervix cancer. Int J Radiat Oncol Biol Phys 8:207–211, 1982
210. Leibel S, Bauer M, Wasserman T, et al: Radiotherapy with or without misonidazole for patients with stage IIIB or stage IVA squamous cell carcinoma of the uterine cervix: Preliminary report of a Radiation Therapy Oncology Group randomized trial. Int J Radiat Oncol Biol Phys 13:541–549, 1987
211. Lepanto P, Littman P, Mikuta J, et al: Treatment of para-aortic nodes in carcinoma of the cervix. Cancer 35:1510–1513, 1975
212. Lerner HM, John HW III, Hill EC: Radical surgery for the treatment of early invasive cervical carcinoma (stage IB): Review of 15 years experience. Obstet Gynecol 56:413–418, 1980
213. Leveuf J, Godord H: L'exerese chirugicale des ganglions pelviens complement de la curtherapie des cancers du col de 'uterus. J Chir 43:177–187, 1934
214. Lipsztein R, Kredentser D, Dottino P, et al: Combined chemotherapy and radiation therapy for advanced carcinoma of the cervix. Am J Clin Oncol 10:527–530, 1987
215. Littman P, Clement PB, Henriksen B, et al: Glassy cell carcinoma of the cervix. Cancer 37:2238–2246, 1976
216. Liu W, Meigs JV: Radical hysterectomy and pelvic lymphadenectomy: A review of 473 cases including 244 for primary invasive carcinoma of the cervix. Am J Obstet Gynecol 69:1–32, 1955
217. Lopez MJ, Kraybill WG, Fuchs GJ, et al: Transvaginal parametrial needle biopsy for detection of postirradiation recurrent cancer of the cervix. Cancer 61:275–278, 1988
218. Lovecchio JL, Averette HE, Doinato D, Bell J: 5-Year survival of patients with periaortic nodal metastases in clinical stage IB and IIA cervical carcinoma. Gynecol Oncol 34:43–45, 1989
219. Lu T, Macasaet M, Nelson JH Jr: The barrel shaped cervix. Am J Obstet Gynecol 124:596–600, 1976
220. Maier JG, Perry PH, Saylor W, Sulak MH: Radiation myelitis of the dorsolumbar spinal cord. Radiology 93:153–160, 1969
221. Malkasian GD, Decker DG, Jorgensen EP: Chemotherapy of carcinoma of the cervix. Gynecol Oncol 5:109, 1976
222. Manetta A, Podczaski ES, Larson JE, et al: Scalene lymph node biopsy in the preoperative evaluation of patients with recurrent cervical cancer. Gynecol Oncol 33:332–334, 1989
223. Maor MH, Gillespie BW, Peters LJ, et al: Neutron therapy in cervical cancer: Results of a phase III RTOG study. Int J Radiat Oncol Biol Phys 14:883–891, 1988
224. Marcial VA, Amato D, Marks RD, et al: Split-course versus continuous pelvis irradiation in carcinoma of the uterine cervix: A prospective randomized clinical trial of the Radiation Therapy Oncology Group. Int J Radiat Oncol Biol Phys 9:431–436, 1983
225. Marcial VA, Blanco MS, DeLeon E: Persistent tumor cells in the vaginal smear during the first year after radiation therapy of carcinoma of the uterine cervix: Prognostic significance. Am J Roentgenol Radium Ther Nucl Med 102:170–175, 1968
226. Martinbeau PW, Kjorstad KE, Iversen T: Stage IB carcinoma of the cervix: The Norwegian Radium Hospital II results when pelvic nodes are involved. Obstet Gynecol 62:215–218, 1982
227. Martinez A, Edmundson GK, Cox RS, et al: Combination of external beam irradiation and multiple-site perineal applicator (MUPIT) for treatment of locally advanced or recurrent prostatic, anorectal, and gynecologic malignancies. Int J Radiat Oncol Biol Phys 11:391–398, 1985
228. Martinez I: Relationship of squamous cell carcinoma of the cervix uteri to squamous cell carcinoma of the penis. Cancer 24:777–780, 1969
229. Maruyama Y, Muir W: Human cervical cancer clearance after ^{252}Cf neutron brachytherapy versus conventional photon brachytherapy. Am J Clin Oncol 7:347–352, 1984
230. Maruyama Y, van Nagell JR, Yoneda J, et al: Dose-response and failure pattern for bulky or barrel-shaped stage IB cervical cancer treated by combined photon irradiation and extrafascial hysterectomy. Cancer 63:70–76, 1989
231. Masterson JG: The role of surgery in the treatment of early carcinoma of the cervix. Clin Obstet Gynecol 10:922–939, 1967
232. Masubuchi K, Tenjin Y, Kubo H, Kimura M: Five year cure rate for carcinoma of the cervix uteri with special reference to the comparison of surgical and radiation therapy. Am J Obstet Gynecol 103:566–573, 1969
233. Matsuyama T, Inoue T, Tsukamoto N, et al: Stage IB, IIA and IIB cervix cancer, postsurgical staging and prognosis. Cancer 54:3072–3077, 1984

234. Meigs JV: Radical hysterectomy with bilateral dissection of pelvic lymph nodes: Surgical treatment of cancer of the cervix. New York, Grune & Stratton, 1954
235. Melamed MR, Flehinger BJ: Early incidence rates of precancerous cervical lesions in women using contraceptives. Gynecol Oncol 1:290–298, 1973
236. Mendenhall WM, McCarty PJ, Morgan LS, Chafe WE, Million RR: Stage IB-IIA-B carcinoma of the cervix ≥6 cm diameter managed with irradiation: Is adjuvant hysterectomy beneficial? Int J Radiat Oncol Biol Phys 19(Suppl 1):127, 1990
237. Meoz RT, Spanos WJ, Doss L, et al: Misonidazole combined with large-fraction pelvic irradiation in the treatment of patients with advanced pelvic malignancies: Preliminary report of an ongoing RTOG phase I-II study. Am J Clin Oncol 6:417–422, 1983
238. Mikuta JH, Enterline HT, Braun TE Jr: Carcinoma *in situ* of the cervix associated with pregnancy. JAMA 204:763–766, 1968
239. Miller BE, Copeland LJ, Hamberger AD, et al: Carcinoma of the cervical stump. Gynecol Oncol 18:100–108, 1984
240. Million RR, Fletcher GH, Rutledge F: Stage IV carcinoma of the cervix with bladder invasion. Am J Obstet Gynecol 113:239–246, 1972
241. Mitani Y, Yukinari S, Jimi S, Iwasaki H: Carcinomatous infiltration into the uterine body in carcinoma of the uterine cervix. Am J Obstet Gynecol 89:984–989, 1964
242. Miura T, Oku T, Iwasaki M, et al: Surgical chemotherapy for advanced carcinoma of the cervix uteri. J Jpn Soc Cancer Ther 254, 1977
243. Moberg PJ, Einhorn N, Silfversward C, Soderberg G: Adenocarcinoma of the uterine cervix. Cancer 57:407–410, 1986
244. Montana GS, Fowler WC, Varia MA, et al: Analysis of results of radiation therapy for stage IB carcinoma of the cervix. Cancer 60:2195–2200, 1987
245. Montana GS, Fowler WC, Varia MA, et al: Carcinoma of the cervix, stage III: Results of radiation therapy. Cancer 57:148–154, 1986
246. Monyak DJ, Twiggs LB, Potish RA, et al: Tolerance and preliminary results of simultaneous therapy with radiation and cisplatin for advanced cervical cancer. Natl Cancer Inst Monogr 6:369–373, 1988
247. Moore DW: Unintentional removal of invasive epidermoid cervical carcinoma in total hysterectomy: A ten year survey at a private hospital. Am J Obstet Gynecol 89:320–325, 1964
248. Morley GW, Seski JC: Radical pelvic surgery versus radiation therapy for stage I carcinoma of the cervix (exclusive of microinvasion). Am J Obstet Gynecol 126:785–798, 1976
249. Morrow CP, DiSaia PJ, Mangan CF, Lagasse LD: Continuous pelvic arterial infusion with bleomycin for squamous carcinoma of the cervix recurrent after irradiation therapy. Cancer Treat Rep 61:1403–1405, 1977
250. Morrow CP: Panel Report: Is pelvic radiation beneficial in the postoperative management of stage IB squamous cell carcinoma of the cervix with pelvic node metastasis treated by radical hysterectomy and pelvic lymphadenectomy? Gynecol Oncol 10:105–110, 1980
251. Morton DG, Lagasse LD, Moore JG, et al: Pelvic lymphadenectomy following radiation in cervical carcinoma. Am J Obstet Gynecol 88:932–938, 1964
252. Moss WT: Radiation Oncology: Rationale, Technique, Results, pp 408–453. St. Louis, CV Mosby, 1973
253. Muirhead W, Green LS: Carcinoma of the cervix: Five-year results and sequelae of treatment. Am J Obstet Gynecol 101:744–749, 1968
254. Nahhas WA, Sharkey FE, Whitney CW, et al: The prognostic significance of vascular channel involvement and deep stromal penetration in early cervical carcinoma. Am J Clin Oncol 6:259–264, 1983
255. Nahmias AJ, Naib ZM, Josey WE: Epidemiological studies relating genital herpetic infection to cervical carcinoma. Cancer Res 34:1111–1117, 1974
256. Nelson AJ, Fletcher GH, Wharton T: Indications for adjunctive conservative extrafascial hysterectomy in selected cases of carcinoma of the uterine cervix. Am J Roentgenol Radium Ther Nucl Med 123:91–99, 1975
257. Nelson JH, Averette HE, Richart RM: Detection, diagnostic evaluation and treatment of dysplasia and early carcinoma of the cervix. CA 25:134–151, 1975
258. Nelson JH, Boyce J, Macasaet M, et al: Incidence, significance and follow-up of para-aortic lymph node metastases in late invasive carcinoma of the cervix. Am J Obstet Gynecol 128:336–340, 1977
259. Nelson JH, Macasaet MA, Lu T, et al: The incidence and significance of para-aortic lymph nodes metastases in late invasive carcinoma of the cervix. Am J Obstet Gynecol 118:749–756, 1974
260. Netter FH: The CIBA Collection of Medical Illustrations, vol 2, Reproductive System. Summit, NJ, Ciba Pharmaceutical, 1972
261. Newton M.: Radical hysterectomy or radiotherapy for stage I cervical cancer. Am J Obstet Gynecol 123:535–542. 1975
262. Noguchi H, Shiozawa I, Kitahara T, et al: Uterine body invasion of carcinoma of the uterine cervix as seen from surgical specimens. Gynecol Oncol 30:173–182, 1988
263. Nolan JF: Postoperative radiotherapy for carcinoma of the cervix: A study of 38 cases. Am J Obstet Gynecol 79:892–898, 1960
264. Noller KL, Decker DG, Dockerty MB, et al: Mesonephric (clear cell) carcinoma of the vagina and cervix. Obstet Gynecol 43:640–644, 1974
265. Novak ER, Jones GS, Jones HW (eds): Novak's Textbook of Gynecology. Baltimore, Williams & Wilkins, 1970
266. Nyberg R, Tornberg B, Westin B: Colposcopy and Schiller's iodine test as an aid in the diagnosis of malignant and premalignant lesions of the cervix uteri. Acta Obstet Gynecol Scand 39:540–556, 1960
267. Ohta A: Basic and clinical studies on the simultaneous combination treatment of cervical cancer (especially advanced cases) with a carcinostatic agent and radiation. J Tokyo Med Coll 36:529–1978
268. Oku T, Iwaskaki M, Tojo S: Study on surgical chemotherapy for advanced cancer of the uterine cervix—particularly on the problem of clinical effect and drug concentration. Acta Obstet Gynecol Jpn 31:1833, 1979
269. O'Quinn AG, Fletcher GH, Wharton JT: Guidelines for conservative hysterectomy after irradiation. Gynecol Oncol 9:68–79, 1980
270. Overgaard J, Bentzen SM, Kolstad P, et al: Misonidazole combined with radiotherapy in the treatment of carcinoma of the uterine cervix. Int J Radiat Oncol Biol Phys 16:1069–1072, 1989
271. Papavasilious C, Yiogarakis D, Pappas J, Keramopoulos A: Treatment of cervical carcinoma by total hysterectomy and postoperative external irradiation. Int J Radiat Oncol Biol Phys 6:871–874, 1980
272. Park RC, Patow WE, Rodgers RR, Zimmerman EA: Treatment for stage I carcinoma of the cervix. Obstet Gynecol 41:117–122, 1973
273. Parker RG, Friedman RF: A critical evaluation of the roentgenologic examination of patients with carcinoma of the cervix. Am J Roentgenol Radium Ther Nucl Med 96:100–107, 1966
274. Parker RT, Wilbanks GD, Yowell RK, Carter FB: Radical hysterectomy with and without preoperative radiotherapy for cervical cancer. Am J Obstet Gynecol 99:933–943, 1967
275. Parkin DE, Davis JA, Symonds RP: Urodynamic findings following radiotherapy for cervical carcinoma. Br J Urol 61:213–217, 1988
276. Pazdur R, Bonomi P, Slayton R, et al: Neuroendocrine carcinoma of the cervix: Implications for staging and therapy. Gynecol Oncol 12:120–128, 1981
277. Perez CA: Unpublished data, 1989
278. Perez CA, Breaux S, Bedwinek JM, et al: Radiation therapy alone in treatment of the uterine cervix. II. Analysis of complications. Cancer 54:235–246, 1984
279. Perez CA, Breaux S, Madoc-Jones H, et al: Radiation therapy alone in the treatment of carcinoma of uterine cervix. I. Analysis of tumor recurrence. Cancer 51:1393–1402, 1983
280. Perez CA, Camel HM, Askin F, Breaux S: Endometrial exten-

sion of carcinoma of the uterine cervix: A prognostic factor that may modify staging. Cancer 48:170–180, 1981

281. Perez CA, Camel HM, Kao MS, Askin F: Randomized study of preoperative radiation and surgery or irradiation alone in the treatment of stage IB and IIA carcinoma of the uterine cervix: Final Report. Gynecol Oncol 27:129–140, 1987
282. Perez CA, Camel HM, Walz BJ, et al: Radiation therapy alone in the treatment of carcinoma of the uterine cervix: A 20 year experience. Gynecol Oncol 23:127–140, 1986
283. Perez CA, DiSaia PJ, Knapp RC, Young RC: Gynecologic tumors. In DeVita VT Jr, Hellman S, Rosenberg SA (eds): Cancer: Principles and Practice of Oncology, 2nd ed, pp 1013–1081. Philadelphia, JB Lippincott, 1985
284. Perez CA, Kao MS: Radiation therapy alone or combined with surgery in barrel-shaped carcinoma of the uterine cervix (stages IB, IIA, IIB). Int J Radiat Oncol Biol Phys 11:1903–1909, 1985
285. Perez CA, Kuske RR, Camel HM, et al: Analysis of pelvic tumor control and impact on survival in carcinoma of the uterine cervix treated with radiation therapy alone. Int J Radiat Oncol Biol Phys 14:613–621, 1988
286. Perez CA, Kuske R, Glasgow GP: Brachytherapy techniques for gynecologic tumors. Endocurietherapy/Hyperthermia Oncology 1:153–175, 1985
287. Perez CA, Purdy JA, Korba A, et al: High-energy x-ray beams in the management of head and neck and pelvic cancers. In Kramer S (ed): High-Energy Photons and Electrons, pp 215–241. New York, John Wiley & Sons, 1976
288. Perez-Mesa C, Spratt JS: Scalene node biopsy in the pretreatment staging of carcinoma of the cervix uteri. Am J Obstet Gynecol 125:93–95, 1976
289. Perkins PL, Chu AM, Jose B, et al: Posthysterectomy megavoltage irradiation in the treatment of cervical carcinoma. Gynecol Oncol 17:340–348, 1984
290. Petersen O: Spontaneous course of cervical pre-cancerous conditions. Am J Obstet Gynecol 72:1063–1071, 1956
291. Pierquin B, Marinello G, Mege J-P, Crook J: Intracavitary irradiation of carcinomas of the uterus and cervix: The Creteil method. Int J Radiat Oncol Biol Phys 15:1465–1473, 1988
292. Pilepich MV, Myerson RJ, Emami BN, et al: Regional hyperthermia: A feasibility analysis. Int J Hyperthermia 3:347–351, 1987
293. Pilleron JP, Durand JC, Hamelin JP: Prognostic value of node metastasis in cancer of the uterine cervix. Am J Obstet Gynecol 119:458–462, 1974
294. Pilleron JP, Durand JC, Lenoble JC: Carcinoma of the uterine cervix, stages I and II, treated by radiation therapy and extensive surgery (1000 cases). Cancer 29:593–596, 1972
295. Piver MS, Barlow JJ: Para-aortic lymphadenectomy in staging patients with advanced local cervical cancer. Obstet Gynecol 43:544–548, 1974
296. Piver MA, Barlow MD, Krishnamsetty R: Five-year survival (with no evidence of disease) in patients with biopsy-confirmed aortic node metastasis from cervical carcinoma. Am J Obstet Gynecol 139:575–578, 1981
297. Piver, MS, Barlow JJ, Vongtama V, Webster J: Hydroxyurea and radiation therapy in advanced cervical cancer. Am J Obstet Gynecol 120:969–972, 1974
298. Piver MS, Chung WS: Prognostic significance of cervical lesion size and pelvic node metastases in cervical carcinoma. Obstet Gynecol 46:507–510, 1975
299. Piver MS, Krishnametty RM, Emrich LJ: Survival of nonsurgically staged patients with negative lymphangiograms who has stage IIB carcinoma of the cervix treated by pelvic radiation plus hydroxyurea. Am J Obstet Gynecol 151:1006–1008, 1985
300. Piver MS, Marchetti DL, Patton T, et al: Radical hysterectomy and pelvic lymphadenectomy versus radiation therapy for small (≤3 cm) stage IB cervical carcinoma. Am J Clin Oncol 11:21–24, 1988
301. Piver MS, Rutledge F, Smith JP: Five classes of extended hysterectomy for women with cervical cancer. Obstet Gynecol 44:265–272, 1974
302. Piver MS, Vongtama V, Barlow JJ: Para-aortic lymph node irradiation for carcinoma of the uterine cervix using split-course technique. Gynecol Oncol 3:168–175, 1975
303. Piver MS, Wallace S, Castro JR: The accuracy of lymphangiography in carcinoma of the uterine cervix. Am J Roentgenol Radium Ther Nucl Med 111:278–283, 1971
304. Ploch E: Hormonal replacement therapy in patients after cervical cancer treatment. Gynecol Oncol 26:169–177, 1987
305. Podczaski E, Stryker JA, Kaminski P, et al: Extended field radiation therapy for carcinoma of the cervix. Cancer 66:251–258, 1990
306. Potish R, Adcock L, Jones TK Jr, et al: The morbidity and utility of periaortic radiotherapy in cervical carcinoma. Gynecol Oncol 15:1–9, 1983
307. Potish RA, Deibel FC Jr, Khan FM: The relationship between milligram-hours and dose to point A in carcinoma of the cervix. Radiology 145:479–483, 1982
308. Potish RA, Twiggs LB, Adcock LL, et al: Effect of cisplatinum on tolerance to radiation therapy in advanced cervical cancer. Am J Clin Oncol 9:387–391, 1986
309. Pourquier H, Dubois JB, Deland R: Cancer of the uterine cervix: Dosimetric guidelines for prevention of late rectal and rectosigmoid complications as a result of radiotherapeutic treatment. Int J Radiat Oncol Biol Phys 8:1887–1895, 1982
310. Powell JL, Burrell MO, Franklin WE III: Radical hysterectomy and pelvic lymphadenectomy. South Med J 77:596–602, 1984
311. Prasasvinichai S, Glassburn JR, Brady LW: Treatment of recurrent carcinoma of the cervix. Int J Radiat Oncol Biol Phys 4:957–961, 1978
312. Prempree T: Parametrial implant in stage IIIB cancer of the cervix. III. A five-year study. Cancer 52:748–750, 1983
313. Prempree T, Amormarn R, Wizenberg MJ: A therapeutic approach to primary adenocarcinoma of the cervix. Cancer 56:1264–1268, 1985
314. Prempree T, Kwon T, VillaSanta U, et al: Management of late second or late recurrent squamous cell carcinoma of the cervix uteri after successful initial radiation treatment. Int J Radiat Oncol Biol Phys 5:2053–2057, 1979
315. Prempree T, Patanaphan V, Sewchand W, et al: The influence of patients' age and tumor grade on the prognosis of carcinoma of the cervix. Cancer 51:1764–1771, 1983
316. Puthawala AA, Syed AM, Fleming PA, Disaia PJ: Re-irradiation with interstitial implant for recurrent pelvic malignancies. Cancer 50:2810–2814, 1982
317. Quigley MM, Knab DR, McMahan ER: Carcinoma of the cervix: A third treatment. Obstet Gynecol 45:650–655, 1975
318. Quilty PM: A report of late rectosigmoid morbidity in patients with advanced cancer of the cervix, treated with a 6 week pelvic brick technique. Clin Radiol 39:297–300, 1988
319. Radiation Therapy Oncology Group Protocol 85-02: Phase II protocol for the evaluation of multiple daily fraction radiation for palliation in the treatment of patients with advanced pelvic malignancies. WP Spanos, Chairman. Revised 6-24-88
320. Rampone JF, Klem V, Kolstad P: Combined treatment of stage IB carcinoma of the cervix. Obstet Gynecol 41:163–167, 1973
321. Ramzy I, Yuzpe AA, Hendelman J: Adenoid cystic carcinoma of uterine cervix. Obstet Gynecol 45:679–683, 1975
322. Rawls WE, Gardner HL, Kaufman RL: Antibodies to genital herpes virus in patients with carcinoma of the cervix. Am J Obstet Gynecol 107:710–716, 1970
323. Reagan JW, Fu YS: Histologic types and prognosis of cancers of the uterine cervix. Int J Radiat Oncol Biol Phys 5:1015–1020, 1979
324. Reagan JW, Wentz WB: Genesis of carcinoma of the uterine cervix. Clin Obstet Gynecol 10:883–921, 1967
325. Reid R, Crum CP, Herschman BR, et al: Genital warts and cervical cancer. III. Subclinical papillomaviral infection and cervical neoplasia are linked by a spectrum of continuous morphologic and biologic change. Cancer 53:943, 1984
326. Retikas DG: Hodgkin's sarcoma of the cervix: Report of a case. Am J Obstet Gynecol 80:1104–1107, 1960
327. Richart RM: Natural history of cervical intraepithelial neoplasia. Clin Obstet Gynecol 10:748–784, 1967
328. Roddick JW Jr, Greenlaw RH: Treatment of cervical cancer. Am J Obstet Gynecol 19:754–764, 1971

329. Rosseau J, Fenton J, Debertrand P, Matthieu G: Carcinoma of the cervix: A 7 year study on 1212 cases treated at Foundation Curie, Paris. Radiology 103:413–418, 1972
330. Rotkin ID: Adolescent coitus and cervical cancer associations of related events with increased risk. Cancer Res 27:603–617, 1967
331. Rotkin ID: Sexual characteristics of a cervical cancer population. Am J Public Health 57:815–829, 1967
332. Rotman M, Aziz H, Boyce J: Postoperative irradiation in stage IB carcinoma of cervix. Int J Radiat Oncol Biol Phys 15:1045–1046, 1988
333. Rotman M, Choi K, Guse C, et al: Prophylactic irradiation of the para-aortic node chain in stage IIB and bulky stage IB carcinoma of the cervix: Initial treatment results of RTOG 7920. Int J Radiat Oncol Biol Phys 19:513–521, 1990
334. Rotman M, John M, Boyce J: Prognostic factors in cervical carcinoma: Implications in staging and management. Cancer 48:560–567, 1981
335. Rubin SC, Brookland R, Mikuta JJ, et al: Para-aortic nodal metastases in early cervical carcinoma: Long-term survival following extended-field radiotherapy. Gynecol Oncol 18:213–217, 1984
336. Ruch RM, Pitcock JA, Ruch WAJ: Microinvasive carcinoma of the cervix. Am J Obstet Gynecol 125:87–92, 1976
337. Runowicz CD, Wadler S, Rodriquez L, et al: Concomitant cisplatin and radiotherapy in locally advanced cervical carcinoma. Gynecol Oncol 34:395–401, 1989
338. Russell AH, Koh WJ, Markette K, et al: Radical re-irradiation for recurrent or second primary carcinoma of the female reproductive tract. Gynecol Oncol 27:226–232, 1987
339. Rutgers DH, van der Linden PM, van Peperzeel HA: DNA-flow cytometry of squamous cell carcinomas from the human uterine cervix: The identification of prognostically different subgroups. Radiother Oncol 7:249–258, 1986
340. Rutledge FN, Fletcher GH, MacDonald EJ: Pelvic lymphadenectomy as an adjunct to radiation therapy in treatment for cancer of the cervix. Am J Roentgenol Radium Ther Nucl Med 93:607–614, 1965
341. Rutledge FN, Galakatos AE, Wharton JT, Smith JP: Adenocarcinoma of the uterine cervix. Am J Obstet Gynecol 122:236–245, 1975
342. Rutledge FN, Gutierrez AG, Fletcher GH: Management of stage I and II adenocarcinomas of the uterine cervix on the intact uterus. Am J Roentgenol Radium Ther Nucl Med 102:161–164, 1968
343. Sadan O, Frohlich RP, Driscoll JA, et al: Is it safe to prescribe hormonal contraception and replacement therapy to patients with premalignant and malignant uterine cervices? Gynecol Oncol 34:159–163, 1989
344. Saigo PE, Cain JM, Kim WS, et al: Prognostic factors in adenocarcinoma of the uterine cervix. Cancer 57:1584–1593, 1986
345. Sala JM, deLeon AD: Treatment of carcinoma of the cervical stump. Radiology 81:300–306, 1963
346. Sall S, Pineda AA, Calanog A, et al: Surgical treatment of stages IB and IIA invasive carcinoma of the cervix by radical abdominal hysterectomy. Am J Obstet Gynecol 135:422–446, 1979
347. Schade FF: Sarcoma botryoides of the cervix uteri: Report of a case in an adult with survival. Obstet Gynecol 26:731–733, 1965
348. Schmauz R, Owor R: Epidemiological aspects of cervical cancer in tropical Africa. IARC Sci Publ 63:413–431, 1984
349. Schulman H, Cavanagh D: Intraepithelial carcinoma of the cervix: The predictability of residual carcinoma in the uterus from the microscopic study of the margins of the cone biopsy specimen. Cancer 14:795–800, 1961
350. Senekjian EK, Hubby M, Bell DA, et al: Clear cell adenocarcinoma (CCA) of the vagina and cervix in association with pregnancy. Gynecol Oncol 24:207–219, 1986
351. Seski JC, Abell MR, Morley GW: Microinvasive squamous carcinoma of the cervix: Definition, histologic analysis, late results of treatment. Obstet Gynecol 50:410–414, 1977
352. Sharma S, Patel FD, Sandhu APS, et al: A prospective randomized study of local hyperthermia as a supplement and radiosensitizer in the treatment of carcinoma of the cervix with radiotherapy. Endocurietherapy/Hyperthermia Oncol 5:151–159, 1989
353. Sherrah-Davies E: Morbidity following low dose rate Selectron therapy for cervical cancer. Clin Radiol 36:131–140, 1985
354. Shingleton HM, Gore H, Soong S-J, et al: Tumor recurrence and survival in stage IB cancer of the cervix. Am J Clin Oncol 6:265–272, 1983
355. Siebel M, Freeman MG, Graves WL: Carcinoma of the cervix and sexual function. Obstet Gynecol 55:484–487, 1979
356. Silbar EL, Woodruff JD: Evaluation of biopsy, cone and hysterectomy sequence in intraepithelial carcinoma of the cervix. Obstet Gynecol 27:89–97, 1966
357. Silverberg SG, Hurt WG: Minimal deviation adenocarcinoma ("adenoma malignum") of the cervix: A reappraisal. Am J Obstet Gynecol 121:971–975, 1975
358. Smith JP, Rutledge F, Burns BC Jr, Soffar S: Systemic chemotherapy for carcinoma of the cervix. Am J Obstet Gynecol 97:800–807, 1967
359. Sommers G, Grigsby PW, Perez CA, et al: Outcome of recurrent cervical carcinoma following definitive irradiation. Gynecol Oncol 35:150–155, 1989
360. Spanos W Jr, Guse C, Perez CA, et al: Phase II study of multiple daily fractionations in the palliation of advanced pelvic malignancies: Preliminary report of RTOG 8502. Int J Radiat Oncol Biol Phys 17:659–661, 1989
361. Spanos WJ, Wasserman T, Meoz R, et al: Palliation of advanced pelvic malignant disease with large fraction pelvic radiation and misonidazole: Final report of RTOG Phase I/II study. Int J Radiat Oncol Biol Phys 13:1479–1482, 1987
362. Spratt JS Jr, Hoag MG: Incidence of multiple primary cancers per man-year of follow up: 20 year review from the Ellis Fischel State Cancer Hospital. Mo Med 63:198–205, 1966
363. Stehman FR, Bundy RN, Keys H, et al: A randomized trial of hydroxyurea versus misonidazole adjunct to radiation therapy in carcinoma of the cervix: A preliminary report of a Gynecologic Oncology Group study. Am J Obstet Gynecol 159:87–94, 1988
364. Stern E, Dixon WJ: Cancer of the cervix: A biometric approach to etiology. Cancer 14:153–160, 1961
365. Storm HH: Second primary cancer after treatment for cervical cancer: Late effects after radiotherapy. Cancer 61:679–688, 1988
366. Strang P, Eklund G,M, Stendahl U, Frankendal B: S-phase rate as a predictor of early recurrences in carcinoma of the uterine cervix. Anticancer Res 7:807–810, 1987
367. Stransky GC, Acosta AA, Kaplan AL, Friedman JA: Reticulum cell sarcoma of the cervix. Obstet Gynecol 41:183–187, 1973
368. Strauss A: Irradiation of carcinoma of the cervix uteri in pregnancy. Am J Roentgenol Radium Ther Nucl Med 43:552–566, 1940
369. Strockbine MF, Hancock JE, Fletcher GH: Complications in 831 patients with squamous cell carcinoma of the intact uterine cervix treated with 3000 rads or more whole pelvis irradiation. Am J Roentgenol Radium Ther Nucl Med 108:293–304, 1970
370. Stryker JA, Bartholomew M, Velkley DE, et al: Bladder and rectal complications following radiotherapy for cervix cancer. Gynecol Oncol 29:1–11, 1988
371. Sudarsanam A, Charyulu K, Belinson J, et al: Influence of exploratory celiotomy on the management of carcinoma of the cervix: A preliminary report. Cancer 41:1049–1053, 1978
372. Surwit E, Fowler WC Jr, Palumbo L, et al: Radical hysterectomy with or without preoperative radium for stage IB squamous cell carcinoma of the cervix. Obstet Gynecol 48:130–133, 1976
373. Swan DS, Roddick JW: A clinical-pathological correlation of cell type classification for cervical cancer. Am J Obstet Gynecol 116:666–670, 1973
374. Sweeney WJ III, Douglas RG: Treatment of carcinoma of the cervix with combined radiation and extensive surgery. Am J Obstet Gynecol 84:981–991, 1962
375. Syed AMN, Feder BH: Techniques of after-loading interstitial implants. Radiol Clin 46:458–475, 1977

376. Symmonds RE: Carcinoma of the cervix associated with pregnancy. In Lewis (ed): Synopsis of Gyn, pp 181–192. 1966
377. Symmonds RE: Morbidity and complications of radical hysterectomy with pelvic lymph node dissection. Am J Obstet Gynecol 94:663, 1966
378. Tanaka Y, Sawada S, Murata T: Relationship between lymph node metastases and prognosis in patients irradiated postoperatively for carcinoma of the uterine cervix. Acta Radiol Oncol 23:455–459, 1984
379. Taussig FJ: Iliac lymphadenectomy with irradiation in the treatment of cancer of the cervix. Am J Obstet Gynecol 28:650–667, 1934
380. Taylor RS, Carroll BE, Lloyd JW: Mortality among women in 3 Catholic religious orders with special references to cancer. Cancer 12:1207–1223, 1959
381. Terris M, Wilson F, Nelson JH Jr: Relation of circumcision to cancer of the cervix. Am J Obstet Gynecol 117:1056–1066, 1973
382. Tewfik HH, Buchsbaum HJ, Latourette HB, et al Para-aortic lymph node irradiation in carcinoma of the cervix after exploratory laparotomy and biopsy proven positive aortic nodes. Int J Radiat Oncol Biol Phys 8:13–18, 1982
383. Thames HD: An "incomplete repair" model for survival after fractionated and continuous irradiations. Int J Radiat Biol 47:319–339, 1985
384. Thigpen T, Shingleton H, Homesley H, et al: Cisplatinum in treatment of advanced or recurrent squamous cell carcinoma of the cervix: A phase II study of the Gynecologic Oncology Group. Cancer 48:899–903, 1981
385. Thigpen T, Vance R, Lambuth B, et al: Chemotherapy for advanced or recurrent gynecologic cancer. Cancer 60:2104–2116, 1987
386. Thomas G, Dembo A, Beale F, et al: Concurrent radiation, mitomycin C and 5-fluorouracil in poor prognosis carcinoma of cervix: Preliminary results of a phase I-II study. Int J Radiat Oncol Biol Phys 10:1785–1790, 1984
387. Thomas GM, Rauth AM, Bush RS, et al: A toxicity study of daily dose metronidazole with pelvic irradiation. Cancer Clin Trials 3:223–230, 1980
388. Thomas JE, Cascino TL, Earle JD: Differential diagnosis between radiation and tumor plexopathy of the pelvis. Neurology 35:1–7, 1985
389. Thoms WW, Eifel PJ, Delclos L, Wharton JT, Oswald MJ: Bulky endocervical carcinomas of the uterine cervix: a 23 year experience at the M.D. Anderson Cancer Center. Int J Radiat Oncol Biol Phys 19 (Suppl 1):127, 1990
390. Togashi K, Nishimura K, Itoh K, et al: Uterine cervical cancer: Assessment with high-field MR imaging. Radiology 160:431–435, 1986
391. Tsukamoto N, Kaku T, Matsukuma K, et al: The problem of stage Ia (FIGO, 1985) carcinoma of the uterine cervix. Gynecol Oncol 34:1–6, 1989
392. Tunca JS, Dement OE: Simple hysterectomy is inadequate therapy for invasive cervical cancer. W Va Med J 73:255–257, 1977
393. Ulbright TM, Gersell DJ: Glassy cell carcinoma of the uterine cervix: A light and electron microscopic study of five cases. Cancer 51:2255–2263, 1983
394. Ulmer HU, Frischbier H-J: Treatment of advanced cancers of the cervix uteri with external irradiation alone. Int J Radiat Oncol Biol Phys 9:809–812, 1983
395. Unal A, Hamberger AD, Seski JC, Fletcher GH: An analysis of the severe complications of irradiation of carcinoma of the uterine cervix: Treatment with intracavitary radium and parametrial irradiation. Int J Radiat Oncol Biol Phys 7:999–1004, 1981
396. Underwood PB Jr, Wilson WC, Kreutner A, et al: Radical hysterectomy: A critical review of 22 years experience. Am J Obstet Gynecol 134:889–898, 1979
397. Upadhyay SK, Symonds RP, Haelterman M, Watson ER: The treatment of stage IV carcinoma of cervix by radical dose radiotherapy. Radiother Oncol 11:15–19, 1988
398. VanDyke AH, Van Nagell JR Jr: The prognostic significance of ureteral obstruction in patients with recurrent carcinoma of the cervix uteri. Surg Gynecol Obstet 141:371–373, 1975
399. Van Herik M: Fever as a complication of radiation therapy for carcinoma of the cervix. Am J Roentgenol Radium Ther Nucl Med 43:104–109, 1965
400. Van Nagell JR Jr, Donaldson ES, Wood EG, et al: The significance of vascular invasion and lymphocytic infiltration in invasive cervical cancer. Cancer 41:228–234, 1978
401. Van Nagell JR Jr, Powell DE, Gallion HH, et al: Small cell carcinoma of the uterine cervix. Cancer 62:1586–1593, 1988
402. Van Nagell JR Jr, Rayburn W, Donaldson ES, et al: Therapeutic implications of patterns of recurrence in cancer of the uterine cervix. Cancer 44:2354–2361, 1979
403. Vigario G, Kurohara SS, George FW III: Association of hemoglobin levels before and during radiotherapy with prognosis in uterine cervix cancer. Radiology 106:649–652, 1973
404. Volterrani F, Lombardi F: Long term results of radium therapy in cervical cancer. Int J Radiat Oncol Biol Phys 6:565–570, 1980
405. Wall JA, Collins VP, Hudgins PT, et al: Carcinoma of the cervix: Review of clinical experience during a 20-year period. Am J Obstet Gynecol 96:57–63, 1966
406. Walsh JW, Amendola MA, Konerding KF, et al: Computed tomographic detection of pelvic and inguinal lymph-node metastases from primary and recurrent pelvic malignant disease. Radiology 137:157–166, 1980
407. Watson ER, Halnan KE, Dische S, et al: Hyperbaric oxygen and radiotherapy: A Medical Research Council trial in carcinoma of the cervix. Br J Radiol 51:879–887, 1978
408. Way S: Microinvasive carcinoma of the cervix. Acta Cytol 8:14, 1964
409. Webb GA: The role of ovarian conservation in the treatment of carcinoma of the cervix with radical surgery. Am J Obstet Gynecol 122:476–484, 1975
410. Webb MJ, Symmonds RE: Site of recurrence of cervical cancer after radical hysterectomy. Am J Obstet Gynecol 138:813–817, 1980
411. Weems DH, Mendenhall WM, Vova FJ, et al: Carcinoma of the intact uterine cervix, stage IB-IIA-B, ≥6 cm in diameter: Irradiation alone vs preoperative irradiation and surgery. Int J Radiat Oncol Biol Phys 11:1911–1914, 1985
412. Weiser EB, Bundy BN, Hoskins WJ, et al: Extraperitoneal versus transperitoneal selective paraaortic lymphadenectomy in the pretreatment surgical staging of advanced cervical carcinoma (a Gynecologic Oncology Group study). Gynecol Oncol 33:283–289, 1989
413. Welander CE, Pierce VK, Nori D, et al: Pretreatment laparotomy in carcinoma of the cervix. Gynecol Oncol 12:336, 1981
414. Wentz WB, Reagan JW: Clinical significance of post-irradiation dysplasia of the human cervix. Am J Obstet Gynecol 106:812–817, 1970
415. Wentz WB, Reagan JW: Survival in cervical cancer with respect to cell type. Cancer 12:384–388, 1959
416. Wharton JT, Jones HW III, Day TG Jr, et al: Preirradiation celiotomy and extended field irradiation for invasive carcinoma of the cervix. Obstet Gynecol 49:333–338, 1977
417. Wimbush PR, Fletcher GH: Radiation therapy of carcinoma of the cervical stump. Radiology 93:655–658, 1969
418. Wolff JP, Lacour J, Chassagne D, Berend M: Cancer of the cervical stump: A study of 173 patients. Obstet Gynecol 39:10–16, 1972
419. Wong LC, Choo YC, Choy D, et al: Long-term follow-up of potentiation of radiotherapy by cis-platinum in advanced cervical cancer. Gynecol Oncol 35:159–163, 1989
420. Worthington JL, Balfe DM, Lee JKT, et al: Uterine neoplasms: MR imaging. Radiology 159:725–730, 1986
421. Yudelev M, Kuten A, Tatcher M, et al: Correlations of dose and time-dose-fractionation factors (TDF) with treatment results and side effects in cancer of the uterine cervix. Gynecol Oncol 23:310–315, 1986
422. Zola P, Volpe T, Castelli G, et al: Is the published literature a reliable guide for deciding between alternative treatments for patients with early cervical cancer? Int J Radiat Oncol Biol Phys 16:785–797, 1989
423. Zornoza J, Lukeman JM, Jing BS, et al: Percutaneous retroperitoneal lymph node biopsy in carcinoma of the cervix. Gynecol Oncol 5:43–51, 1977

55

Endometrium

John R. Glassburn
Luther W. Brady
Perry W. Grigsby

ANATOMY

The uterus is a hollow muscular organ situated in the midline of the pelvis, extending at a right angle from the vagina and lying between the bladder and rectum. It is divided into the corpus or body, which comprises the upper two thirds of the organ, and the cervix, which comprises the lower third. The superior-most portion of the corpus is called the *fundus*; the fallopian tubes enter the uterine cavity by piercing the fundus in each cornu. The uterine cavity is lined by a mucous membrane (endometrium) made up of columnar cells forming many tubular glands that extend into the stroma and muscular layers. A muscular layer (myometrium) is made up of smooth muscle fibers arranged in no definite pattern, which interlace randomly. The outer, serous coat (peritoneum) covers the uterus and forms laterally the broad ligaments. Further description of anatomy is given in Chapter 54.

EPIDEMIOLOGY

Carcinoma of the endometrium has surpassed carcinoma of the cervix as the most common malignant lesion arising from the female genital tract. The American Cancer Society has estimated that approximately 700,000 of the 48 million women in the United States who are 35 years of age or older will develop a malignant endometrial tumor during their lifetime.[20] The yearly incidence in the United States was projected to be 33,000 new cases in 1991, resulting in about 5500 deaths. Endometrial carcinoma accounts for 7.6% of all cancers in white women and 4.5% of cancers arising in black women.[31] The peak incidence occurs in the 50- to 70-year age group; 70% of all cases occur in postmenopausal patients.

In 1977, Casey[21] analyzed the Connecticut Tumor Registry data and demonstrated that the incidence of endometrial cancer was increasing for both premenopausal and postmenopausal age groups. Not all factors responsible for this increase are understood, but the common use of unopposed estrogens in postmenopausal women until the late 1970s and the decreased parity of the female population certainly have had significant impact. Ziel and Finkle compared a group of women with proven endometrial carcinoma with a match group of controls and found that the use of conjugated estrogen was significantly more common in the group with endometrial carcinoma.[169] Other reports have confirmed these findings and have demonstrated a direct relationship to the dose of estrogen administered.[97,101,147] Sequential oral contraceptives have also been implicated and were banned in the United States in 1976.[77,94]

Obesity and hypertension also predispose women to the development of endometrial cancer.[97] Wynder and associates found the risk to increase by a factor of 3 in women who are 21 to 50 pounds overweight and by a factor of 10 in those who are more than 50 pounds overweight.[167] Hypertension was found in 25% to 70% of women with endometrial cancer but is not a significant risk factor when not accompanied by obesity or other factors.

Diabetes mellitus also has a significant association with endometrial cancer; in most series it is found in 10% to 20% of women with demonstrated endometrial carcinoma. The relative risk for endometrial carcinoma associated with diabetes mellitus is 2.8.[97]

Parity of the patient with endometrial cancer is generally low; nulliparous women make up about 24% of the female population but account for almost 50% of women developing endometrial carcinoma.

Breast, ovary, and colon carcinomas occur more frequently in patients with a history of endometrial carcinoma than would be expected by chance alone.[97,158] A small but real increase in risk is also found in women with a family history of endometrial carcinoma or other malignancy.[93] Stein-Leventhal syndrome is present in a significant percentage of patients who develop endometrial malignancies before age 40.[36] Menopause after age 52 increases the risk by a factor of 2.4. A history of uterine irradiation also increases risk of endometrial cancer; most radiation-induced tumors, however, are sarcomas.[68]

Endometrial hyperplasia has been implicated as a precursor to endometrial carcinoma, and the two may coexist.[13] It is estimated that only 2% of patients with cystic hyperplasia develop invasive cancer.[13] However, the percentage of patients with adenomatous hyperplasia who develop invasive carcinoma is much greater. Chamlin and Taylor[22] reported that 14 of 97 premenopausal patients with endometrial hyperplasia progressed to invasive adenocarcinoma 1 to 14 years after initial diagnosis of hyperplasia, and the risk factor was 14%. Vuopala has reported that 20% of patients with adenomatous hyper-

TABLE 55–1
Histologic Grade and Depth of Invasion in Clinical Stage I Endometrial Carcinoma

DEPTH	G1	G2	G3	TOTAL
Endometrium only	44 (24%)	31 (11%)	11 (7%)	86 (14%)
Superficial	96 (53%)	131 (45%)	54 (35%)	281 (45%)
Middle	22 (12%)	69 (24%)	24 (16%)	115 (19%)
Deep	18 (10%)	57 (20%)	64 (42%)	139 (22%)
Total	180 (100%)	288 (100%)	153 (100%)	621 (100%)

(Creasman WT, Morrow CP, Bundy BN, et al: Cancer 60:2035, 1987)

plasia and 25% with atypical adenomatous hyperplasia progress to invasive cancer.[159]

NATURAL HISTORY

In most cases, endometrial carcinomas are confined to the uterus at initial diagnosis. Distribution by stage of 550 cases registered over a 20-year period at Hahnemann University Hospital is as follows: Stage I, 72%; Stage II, 5.2%; Stage III, 9.7%, and Stage IV, 13.1%. The preponderance of Stage I lesions correlates well with other series documenting stage distribution.[12, 64, 99, 140, 143, 156, 163]

Tumors arising from the mucosa commonly spread into contiguous areas. Extension into the muscle of the uterus, particularly when over 50% of the muscle wall is invaded, signifies a poor prognosis.[29, 75, 106, 139, 164] Table 55-1 documents the fact that deep myometrial invasion is more common with higher grade tumors. As depth of involvement increases, the incidence of nodal metastasis also increases (Table 55-2). Direct extension may also occur and involve the cervix, fornices of the vagina, parametrial tissue, or the bladder and rectum. It has been well documented that the incidence of pelvic lymph node involvement in Stage I disease is approximately 10%.[29, 88, 91, 130, 140] If the cervix has been involved with tumor, approximately 36% of patients have histologically proven lymphatic spread in surgical series. The periaortic nodes are less frequently involved, with the incidence varying markedly depending on tumor grade and depth of invasion (Table 55-4).[27, 29, 73, 141] Vaginal metastases are not common at presentation but have been found in 1% to 15% of patients with Stage I disease in whom no radiation therapy is used preoperatively or postoperatively.[35, 37, 40, 54, 55, 127, 129, 162] Recurrences in this area are uncommon in patients treated with combined radiation therapy and surgery (Table 55-3).[16, 35, 44, 55, 127, 136, 150, 160]

Peritoneal seeding is more common with endometrial cancer than with cervical carcinoma because endometrial lesions may penetrate the uterine wall or seed transtubally (Table 55-4). Hematogenous dissemination is infrequent with endometrial carcinoma (Table 55-5).[139]

Creasman and co-workers[28] reported that 26 of 167 patients (15.5%) with Stage I carcinoma of the endometrium treated surgically had malignant cells identified on cytologic examination of peritoneal washings. Recurrences developed in ten of these 26 patients (34%), compared with 14 of 141 (9.9%) with negative peritoneal cytology. Yazigi and associates evaluated the significance of cytologic findings in peritoneal specimens from 93 patients with Stage I endometrial carcinoma.[168] Samples from ten patients (11%) showed evidence of malignancy; in the remaining 83 patients (89%), no evidence of malignancy was found. One recurrence was seen among the patients with positive findings (10%) and six recurrences in the negative cytology group (7.2%). The 5-year survival rate was 87.5% for patients with positive findings and 93.9% for those with negative findings. No specific treatment was given to the patients with positive specimens.

Uterine sarcomas metastasize frequently by hematogenous routes; 50% to 80% develop metastasis to the lung at some time during their clinical course (Table 55-6).[11] The incidence of pelvic lymph node involvement is also high, with estimates ranging from 25% to 50% at time of presentation.

PATTERNS OF FAILURE

Incidence of pelvic failure was 8.8% and the rate of distant metastasis was 8% in a series of 553 patients with Stage I carcinoma of the endometrium treated with surgery alone.[120] The pelvic recurrence rate was 5%, and the rate of distant metastasis was 7% in 1021 patients with Stage I disease treated with radiation therapy and surgery.

In Stage II disease, the incidence of pelvic failure was about

TABLE 55–2
Grade, Depth of Invasion, and Metastases in Endometrial Carcinoma

	GRADE 1 (n = 180)		GRADE 2 (n = 288)		GRADE 3 (n = 153)	
DEPTH OF INVASION	AORTIC NODE	PELVIC NODE	AORTIC NODE	PELVIC NODE	AORTIC NODE	PELVIC NODE
Endometrium only (n = 86)	0 (0%)	0 (0%)	1 (3%)	1 (3%)	0 (0%)	0 (0%)
Superficial (n = 281)	1 (1%)	3 (3%)	5 (4%)	7 (5%)	2 (4%)	5 (9%)
Middle (n = 115)	1 (5%)	0 (0%)	0 (0%)	6 (9%)	0 (0%)	1 (4%)
Deep (n = 139)	1 (6%)	2 (11%)	8 (14%)	11 (19%)	15 (23%)	22 (34%)

(Creasman WT, Morrow CP, Bundy BN, et al: Cancer 60:2035, 1987)

TABLE 55–3
Vaginal Recurrence With and Without Preoperative Radiation Therapy Followed by Hysterectomy for Adenocarcinoma of the Corpus Uteri, Stage I

HYSTERECTOMY ONLY	PERCENTAGE OF VAGINAL RECURRENCE	IRRADIATION AND HYSTERECTOMY	PERCENTAGE OF VAGINAL RECURRENCE
Rickford[130]	14.4	Dobbie[35]	2.4
Way[162]	13.7	Stander[150]	1
Dobbie[35]	11	Gusberg et al[56]	1.1
Gusberg et al[56]	9.1	Sala and del Regato[136]	4
Price et al[127]	14	Price et al[127]	3.6
Wade et al[160]	9.3	Wade et al[160]	1.9
Frick et al[40]	2.0	Brady et al[16]	0
Whetham et al[166]	4.1		
Eifel et al[37]	1.7		

(Modified from Brady LW, Lewis GC, Antoniades J, et al: Gynecol Oncol 2:253, 1974)

12%, equal to the incidence of distant metastasis. In a small number of patients with Stage II disease treated with radiation therapy (usually including external and intracavitary irradiation), the pelvic failure rate was 18% to 37% and the incidence of distant metastasis was 32%.

In 35 patients with Stage III disease treated with irradiation alone (11 studied by Danoff and colleagues[32]; 24 by Landgren and associates[85]), the pelvic failure rate was 45%; 50% of the patients with pelvic failure also had distant metastasis. An additional 15 patients (42.9%) had distant metastasis alone; the overall incidence of distant metastasis was 65.7%.

Salazar and associates reported similar sites of failure in 364 patients according to clinical stage and method of treatment.[139]

CLINICAL PRESENTATION

The most common presenting symptom in patients with endometrial carcinoma is vaginal bleeding, which is reported by 70% to 80% of patients. Vaginal discharge, often foul-smelling, may be found in 30% of patients. Less frequently reported are bladder and bowel symptoms from pressure of the enlarged uterus on these organs, or from extension of disease to involve these structures. Low back pain radiating to the anterior abdomen may occur.

Physical findings are usually minimal; blood in the vagina emanating from the cervical os is the most common finding. Enlargement of the uterus or tumor extension to the cervix, vagina, or parametria may be found.

TABLE 55–4
Tumor Involvement Within Site from Surgical Pathology in Stage I and II Endometrial Cancer*

SITE	PERCENT POSITIVE	NUMBER POSITIVE/ NUMBER EXAMINED
Peritoneal washings†	10.3	49/476
Adnexal spread	5.3	29/544
Pelvic nodes	6.6	36/544
Aortic nodes‡	4.4	19/429*
Other sites	2.6	14/544

** Gynecologic Oncology Group protocol no. 33*
† 68 patients not examined
‡ 113 patients not examined; two gross positive not examined at biopsy
(Lewis GC, Bundy B: Cancer 48:568, 1981)

DIAGNOSTIC WORKUP

No completely satisfactory screening method is available for detecting endometrial carcinoma in asymptomatic patients. The Papanicolaou smear, which is so reliable in detecting carcinoma of the cervix, succeeded in detecting only 40% of tumors in a series of patients known to have endometrial carcinoma (from a sampling of the vaginal pool and a scraping of the cervix).[109]

Suction curettage devices such as the Vabra aspirator are effective in making the diagnosis of endometrial carcinoma in a high percentage of patients.

TABLE 55–5
Site of Distant Metastases and Nodal Failure in Endometrial Carcinoma, All Stages and All Treatments

METASTATIC SITE	NUMBER	PERCENTAGE
DISTANT METASTASES (48 PATIENTS)		
Lung	17	35
Liver	14	29
Omentum and peritoneum	12	25
GI tract	10	21
Bone	7	15
Kidney and adrenal	5	10
Brain	3	6
Breast	2	4
NODAL METASTASES (48 PATIENTS)		
Pelvic	15	38*
Periaortic	9	19
Common iliac	6	13
Cervical and supraclavicular	5	10
Inguinal	2	4

** Calculated on the basis of 40 pelvic failures. This value may be higher because nodal status was not documented in every failure.*
(Salazar OM, Feldstein ML, DePapp EW, et al: Int J Radiat Oncol Biol Phys 2:1101, 1977)

TABLE 55–6
Uterine Sarcoma: Analysis of 45 Distant Failures

	NO. OF FAILURES (PERCENTAGE OF TOTAL NO. OF FAILURES)		
DISTANT FAILURE SITE	OVERALL	SOLE DISTANT FAILURE	SOLE FAILURE
Upper abdomen	31 (69)	11 (25)	4 (9)*
Lung	27 (60)	11 (25)	7 (16)†
Upper abdomen and lung	16 (36)	11 (25)	5 (11)‡
Bone	11 (24)	2 (4)	2 (4)§
Brain	2 (4)	0 (0)	0 (0)

** All four patients with high-staged mixed mesodermal sarcomas (MMS)*
† Five MMS and two leiomyosarcomas (LMS)
‡ Three MMS and two LMS
§ Two MMS
(Salazar OM, Bonfiglio TA, Patten SF, et al: Cancer 42:1161, 1978)

A fractional dilatation and curettage and cervical biopsies should be performed in any patient in whom there is a high degree of suspicion of cancer. Approximately 28% of women with postmenopausal bleeding have a diagnosis of cancer established after appropriate workup; 50% of these lesions are of endometrial origin and 50% of cervical origin.[128]

Diagnostic studies routinely used in the clinical staging of patients with endometrial carcinoma vary with stage (Table 55-7). Chest radiography, urinalysis, complete blood count (CBC) and liver function studies are routinely done on all patients. The routine performance of a barium enema, intravenous pyelography, cystoscopy, and proctosigmoidoscopy have a low yield and should be reserved for patients who are suspected of having advanced disease or symptoms related to these organs. In a review of the cost-effectiveness of routine tests in gynecologic malignancies, the average cost quoted for each positive finding on barium enema examination, cystoscopy, or proctosigmoidoscopy was approximately $20,000.[4] Routine use of liver and bone scans is not indicated.[58] Selective use of these studies, however, in patients with advanced disease or with high-grade tumors in which hematogenous spread is more common is not discouraged. Lymphangiography in selected patients may be of use in detecting spread to the periaortic lymph nodes.

TABLE 55–7
Diagnostic Workup for Endometrial Tumors

General
- History
- Physical examination
- Pelvic examination

Special Tests
- Fractional dilatation curettage
- Biopsies of uterine cervix
- Cystoscopy
- Sigmoidoscopy (when indicated in Stages III and IV)

Radiographic Studies
- Standard
  - Chest radiography
  - CT scans of pelvis and abdomen *or*
  - Magnetic resonance imaging
- Complementary (recommended in tumors beyond Stage I *or* with high-grade tumors)
  - Intravenous pyelography
  - Barium enema
  - Liver scan
  - Bone scan

Laboratory Studies
- CBC, blood chemistry, urinalysis
- Liver function studies

Computed tomography (CT) is recommended in all patients with high-grade tumors or with Stage II or greater disease because nodal enlargement or extrauterine extension may be demonstrated. Hasumi and associates reported that computed tomography was useful in detecting the depth of myometrial invasion and the presence of cervical involvement.[60] Magnetic resonance imagining (MRI) is not particularly helpful in detecting nodal or peritoneal involvement but has been reported to have an accuracy of 82% in demonstrating the depth of myometrial invasion.[66]

Circulating tumor markers are actively being investigated in endometrial cancer. Ca-125 has been found to be elevated in 59% of patients with clinically advanced or recurrent endometrial cancer.[142]

STAGING

The most widely accepted staging system is that of the International Federation of Gynecology and Obstetrics (FIGO; Table 55-8).[70] This system should be based on bimanual pelvic examination of the patient under anesthesia as well as on the diagnostic procedures previously discussed. A new pathologic FIGO staging system was introduced in 1989 because the majority of patients are now surgically staged before institution of treatment (Table 55-9).[71]

PATHOLOGIC CLASSIFICATION

Well-differentiated adenocarcinomas have many glands with the cells showing nuclear atypia and mitosis. As the grade increases, the pattern of gland formation becomes more irregular and may display solid areas; the cells also become more atypical in configuration and mitotic figures become more common.

A variant of adenocarcinoma, *adenoacanthoma,* accounts for approximately 10% of tumors arising from the endometrium.

TABLE 55–8
Clinical Staging of Carcinoma of the Corpus Uteri

Stage 0	Carcinoma *in situ*
Stage I	Cancer is confined to corpus
IA	Uterine cavity sounds to 8 cm or less
IB	Uterine cavity sounds to over 8 cm
G1	Highly differentiated adenocarcinoma
G2	Differentiated adenocarcinoma with partially solid areas
G3	Predominantly solid or entirely undifferentiated carcinoma
Stage II	Carcinoma involves corpus and cervix
Stage III	Carcinoma extends outside corpus, but not true pelvis (it may not involve bladder or rectum)
Stage IV	Carcinoma involves bladder or rectum or extends outside true pelvis

(International Federation of Gynecology and Obstetrics: Int J Gynaecol Obstet 9:172, 1971)

TABLE 55–9
Pathologic FIGO Corpus Cancer Staging

Stage	Grade	Description
Stage IA	G123	Tumor limited to endometrium
IB	G123	Invasion to <1/2 myometrium
IC	G123	Invasion >1/2 myometrium
IIA	G123	Endocervical glandular involvement only
IIB	G123	Cervical stromal invasion
IIIA	G123	Tumor invades serosa or adnexae or positive peritoneal cytology
IIIB	G123	Vaginal metastases
IIIC	G123	Metastases to pelvic or periaortic lymph nodes
IVA	G123	Tumor invasion of bladder or bowel mucosa
IVB		Distant metastases including intraabdominal or inguinal lymph nodes

(International Federation of Gynecology and Obstetrics: Int J Gynecol Obstet 28:189–193, 1989)

TABLE 55–10
Classification of Uterine Sarcomas

Pure Sarcomas
- Homologous
  - Leiomyosarcoma
  - Stromal
  - Endolymphatic stromal myosis
  - Angiosarcoma
  - Fibrosarcoma
- Heterologous
  - Rhabdomyosarcoma
  - Chondrosarcoma
  - Osteosarcoma
  - Liposarcoma

Mixed Sarcoma
- Homologous
- Heterologous (with or without homologous elements)

Malignant Mixed Mullerian Tumors
- Homologous type
- Heterologous type

Sarcoma Unclassified

Malignant Lymphoma

(Kempson RI, Bari W: Hum Pathol 1:331, 1970)

It is composed of malignant adenomatous elements with coexisting squamous cell metaplasia. The squamous element in this case appears histologically benign.

Adenosquamous cell carcinomas account for about 20% of tumors arising from the uterus and are composed of adenomatous and squamous cells, both of which are histologically malignant. These tumors are usually of higher grade and of more advanced stage at presentation.

Although adenosquamous cell carcinomas were once believed to be more aggressive and less radiocurable than other endometrial lesions, Salazar and associates and Silverberg and colleagues found no differences in survival rates between histologic types when comparisons were made on the basis of grade and stage.[111,138,144]

Clear cell tumors may also arise from the endometrium, as they can from any area of the urogenital tract.[83,145] These tumors are extremely rare and are characterized by an abundant clear cytoplasm. Also rare are pure epidermoid carcinomas of the endometrium, which are postulated to develop from benign squamous cell metaplasia.[76] Both the clear cell tumors and the epidermoid lesions make up less than 1% of tumors arising from the lining of the endometrial cavity.

A highly malignant form of endometrial adenocarcinoma is designated as uterine papillary serous carcinoma. This particular variant tends to develop widespread abdominal carcinomatosis and ascites and carries an extremely poor prognosis.[37,62]

Also rare are sarcomatous lesions arising from the uterus. There is no agreement as to the best pathologic classification of these tumors and at times it is difficult to differentiate benign from malignant sarcomatous lesions. Kempson and Bari[79] have proposed a modification of the Ober classification that appears to have clinical usefulness (Table 55-10).[79] A sarcoma classified as pure contains a single sarcomatous element; a sarcoma classified as mixed contains two or more sarcomatous types. Both types are subclassified into homologous or heterologous. Homologous tumors contain elements derived from mesenchymal tissue normally present in the uterus. Heterologous tumors contain elements not normally found in the uterine wall, such as striated muscle, cartilage, or bone. Carcinomatous elements coexist but do not appear to influence the prognosis significantly. The mitotic index appears to be the most important criterion separating benign from malignant lesions.[59] Invasion into contiguous organs or vessels, as with most tumors, also indicates the degree of malignancy.[79]

Endometrial stromal sarcomas, however, may show vascular and myometrial infiltration without necessarily worsening the prognosis.[11] Uterine size has been found by Badid and colleagues[9] to correlate with length of survival.

The classification of sarcomas endorsed by the Gynecologic Oncology Group is more commonly used. It includes leiomyosarcoma, endometrial stromal sarcoma, mixed homologous müllerian sarcoma (carcinosarcoma), and mixed heterologous müllerian sarcoma (mixed mesodermal sarcoma). A fifth category (other uterine sarcomas) is provided for more unusual lesions.

PROGNOSTIC FACTORS

Many factors influence the prognosis of a patient with endometrial carcinoma and thus have a bearing on treatment. As with any tumors, clinical stage is one of the most important factors in prognosis.

The histologic grade of the tumor is as important as the stage of the tumor. The 5-year survival rate for patients with Stage I well-differentiated (grade 1) tumors in most reports is 90% or higher, compared with 65% to 70% with grade 3 disease.[152,160,164] As the grade of the tumor increases, so does the likelihood that the stage is more advanced. Also related to histologic grade of tumor are depth of myometrial invasion and incidence of lymph node involvement. Lewis and colleagues[91] reported that 5.5% of patients with Stage I well-differentiated lesions have positive lymph nodes, whereas 26% of patients with poorly differentiated tumors have nodal involvement. Cheon[24] and Gusberg and associates[56] have documented that the incidence of deep myometrial invasion is three to four times greater in patients with grade 3 disease than in patients with grade 1 disease. In 540 patients with Stage I tumors reported by Aalders and co-workers,[3] this finding was associated with a higher incidence of pelvic recurrence and distant metastasis.

The incidence of lymph node involvement tends to parallel histologic grade and stage (see Table 55-2). Uterine size is a less important factor in determining prognosis for patients with endometrial cancer, although in some series differences in survival have been described in patients with uterine enlargement compared with those with patients with normal-sized uterine cavities.[24,108,143,160]

The presence of lymph-vascular space involvement has been found to significantly increase the risk of tumor recurrence following surgery. Lymph node metastasis was found in 50% of patients with this involvement, and the majority developed extrapelvic recurrences.[57]

Age is also a factor in prognosis. The older the patient is at the time of diagnosis of endometrial carcinoma, the higher the chances of myometrial involvement, the greater the chances of advanced stage, and the poorer the 5-year survival rate.[24,74,140]

Residual Tumor After Radiation Therapy

In a study of 91 patients with early invasive endometrial carcinoma, Macasaet and associates[95] reported that approximately 50% had residual tumor after two intracavitary insertions delivering 6000 mgh to 8000 mgh. The authors noted a recurrence rate of 19% and probability rate of death from tumor of 23% in patients with residual tumor compared with 6% in those without residual tumor. Also an increased incidence of failure and death occurred in patients with vascular or myometrial invasion. The authors stress the unreliability of clinically staging endometrial carcinoma because 10% to 15% of patients with Stage I disease and 7% of those with Stage II disease had more advanced disease than initially ascertained by clinical evaluation, mostly because of the presence of metastatic disease in the lymph nodes.

Positive Peritoneal Cytology

Heath and co-workers reported on the prognostic significance of peritoneal cytology in 243 patients with endometrial carcinoma of all stages.[61] Sixteen percent of cytology studies were found to be positive. Of the 165 patients with negative cytology and Stage I disease, the disease-free survival rate at 3 years was 91%, and for the 25 patients with positive cytology, 56%. No difference, however, was seen in survival in those patients with less than one third myometrial invasion. Of the Stage I patients with positive cytology who received ^{32}P (chromic phosphate), the disease-free survival was 68% compared with 27% for those who had not received intraperitoneal ^{32}P colloid. Serious bowel complications were increased in those patients who received both ^{32}P and pelvic irradiation (44% *versus* 0%). In two other studies, however, no difference was found in survival rates for those patients with positive peritoneal cytology in Stage I disease.[81,168] Further work is necessary to define the significance and the treatment approach in patients with this pathologic finding.

GENERAL MANAGEMENT

Stage I Endometrial Carcinoma

The basic treatment program for all patients with Stage I endometrial carcinoma is a total abdominal hysterectomy and bilateral salpingo-oophorectomy (TAH/BSO). In all but grade 1 lesions, it is recommended that pelvic and periaortic lymph node sampling be performed at the time of surgical exploration. The incidence of nodal involvement in Stage I patients with grade 1 histology is too low to make routine sampling worthwhile, although gross nodes should be excised. Peritoneal washings are recommended for all patients at the time of surgery.

Radical hysterectomy with pelvic lymphadenectomy has also been evaluated as primary treatment of patients with Stage I disease. However, no improvement has been demonstrated in survival or results, and the rate of complications is higher for patients with Stage I disease treated in this fashion.[18,88,89,115,116]

It has been the policy at Pennsylvania Hospital to add postoperative external-beam pelvic irradiation to those patients with poor prognostic findings at the time of surgery. In patients with Stage I, grade 1 and grade 2 disease with inner third myometrial invasion only, we recommend no further therapy because the prognosis in this patient group is good.[37,164] In patients with Stage I, grade 3 disease, we generally recommend postoperative whole-pelvis irradiation (4500 cGy to 5000 cGy) in all patients with myometrial involvement because these lesions are more aggressive and there is a much greater chance of having nodal involvement.

At some institutions, irradiation is given preoperatively by intracavitary insertion to patients with grade 2 and grade 3 disease. Doses of approximately 6000 cGy are delivered to 1.5 cm depth from the surface of the uterus (3500 mgh to 4000 mgh) and 6000 cGy to 7000 cGy (1800 mgh to 2000 mgh, with 2 cm colpostats) to the vaginal mucosa. At some institutions, whole-pelvis irradiation with external beam alone in the range of 4500 cGy to 5000 cGy is prescribed.

The trend in the United States is to primarily operate on all patients with Stage I disease, regardless of tumor grade, to adequately assess the extent of disease and to allow the radiation therapy to be tailored to the pathologic findings. Even high-grade lesions limited to the endometrium alone have a very low rate of positive pelvic or periaortic nodal involvement.[29]

In medically inoperable patients, two brachytherapy placements for 8000 mgh and external irradiation to the pelvis for a total of 5040 cGy with a midline block at 2000 cGy are recommended.

Stage II Endometrial Carcinoma

Far fewer data are available to support a definitive statement about the most appropriate treatment program for patients with Stage II endometrial cancer compared with data available for those with Stage I disease. Incidence of lymph node involvement has been documented to vary between 25% and 50%, and any treatment program must ensure that the nodal areas in parametrial tissues are adequately treated.[89,91,92] Preoperative irradiation is favored when there is known cervical stroma involvement (intracavitary, external beam or combinations), preferably including the pelvic lymph nodes.

Other treatment approaches for Stage II disease have included Wertheim hysterectomy with node dissection and various combinations of irradiation and surgery (Table 55-11).[17,41,48,50,54,63,86,98,99,154,156,160] Survival rates with Wertheim hysterectomy and lymph node dissection are similar to those obtained by radiation therapy combined with surgery; however, morbidity is in general higher with the radical surgical approach.

Grigsby and associates,[54] at Washington University, treat patients with Stage II endometrial carcinoma who have only microscopic involvement of the endocervix with a preoperative

TABLE 55–11
Survival of Patients With Stage II Endometrial Carcinoma

AUTHOR	NO. OF PATIENTS	TREATMENT	5-YEAR SURVIVAL (%)
Greenberg et al[48]	19	RT	65.2
	15	Other	59.5
	34	Total	60.2 (actuarial)
Malkasian et al[99]	10	TAH-BSO	
	2	RT	
	7	Surgery + RT	
	5	Wertheim	100
	24	Total	75 (actuarial)
Homesley et al[63]	26	Wertheim	77
	10	RT + surgery	80 (disease-free)
	10	Radical hysterectomy	50
	17	Simple hysterectomy	59
Underwood et al[156]	31	Radium + surgery	73
Bruckman et al[17]	40	RT + surgery	83 (actuarial relapse-free)
Gagon et al[41]	29	RT + surgery	44.8 (absolute) 81.5 (adjusted)
Grigsby et al[54]	90	RT + surgery	78 (disease-free)
	26	RT	53 (disease-free)
Larson et al[86]	64	RT + surgery	68 (actuarial)

RT: radiation therapy; TAH-BSO: total abdominal hysterectomy and bilateral salpingo-oophorectomy

intracavitary insertion only followed by an extrafascial hysterectomy and bilateral salpingo-oophorectomy. In general, the dose is 3500 mgh to 4000 mgh to the body of the uterus and 6000 cGy to the vaginal vault (1800 mgh to 2000 mgh) with 2 cm colpostats. Madoc-Jones noted only one failure in 11 patients treated in this manner.[98] If gross or multiple quadrant microscopic involvement of the exocervix is present, in addition to the intracavitary insertion, the patient receives external irradiation (2000 cGy to the whole pelvis and a 3000 cGy additional dose to the parametria with a midline shield) followed by an extrafascial hysterectomy approximately 4 weeks later. At some institutions, preoperative external irradiation alone to the pelvis is used for this purpose (5000 cGy in 5 to 6 weeks).

Stage III Endometrial Carcinoma

Treatment for Stage III disease must be individualized. Three main patterns of tumor spread have been identified: downward to the vagina, lateral extension to the parametria, and ovarian involvement.[6] These patterns have now been included in the new pathologic FIGO staging system.

The majority of patients with vaginal or parametrial extension of tumor are not good candidates for initial surgery and may be treated with whole-pelvis (2000 cGy) and parametrial (3000 cGy) irradiation combined with two intracavitary insertions (about 8000 cGy) to ensure a high pelvic dose. When 5000 cGy to whole pelvis is delivered, the intracavitary dose should be reduced to about 5000 mgh to 6000 mgh in two insertions. Patients with obvious persistent disease following radiation therapy should be considered for an extrafascial hysterectomy.

Surgery may be considered as the initial form of treatment for the patient who has a well-defined parametrial mass that does not adhere to pelvic side wall because tumor bulk in this area can be surgically removed and a coexisting ovarian tumor is ruled out. Whole-pelvis postoperative irradiation, extended field irradiation, or whole abdominal irradiation is indicated for all patients postoperatively, depending on tumor extent pathologically.

Stage IV Endometrial Carcinoma

Patients with Stage IV carcinoma should be treated with irradiation alone. An occasional patient with bladder or rectal involvement without pelvic wall fixation who is in good medical condition may be considered for pelvic exenteration. A common treatment is pelvic irradiation (5000 cGy to 6000 cGy) with the addition of brachytherapy placements individualized, depending on the extent of disease and the whole-pelvis radiation dose. All Stage IV patients are candidates for systemic therapy. Selected patients may be candidates for whole abdominal or extended field irradiation, depending on tumor bulk.

In patients with advanced Stage IVB disease, radiation to the pelvis may be indicated for control of local symptoms such as bleeding, discharge, and pelvic pain to improve the quality of the patient's life. General policies of management used at Mallinckrodt Institute of Radiology are given in Table 55-12.

Hormonal Therapy

Many reports document that progestational agents are effective in selected patients with endometrial cancer. The overall response rate has varied from 18% to 40%.[42,78,118,132,161] The duration of response may vary widely, but it is most commonly reported to be about 30 months. A great advantage of progestational therapy is that it produces few side effects. Several months may be necessary to test response before the use of progestational agents may be deemed a failure.[107]

Intramuscular injections of hyroxyprogesterone or

TABLE 55–12
Carcinoma of the Endometrium (Mallinckrodt Institute of Radiology Treatment Policies)

STAGE AND GRADE	TUMOR EXTENT	PREOPERATIVE BRACHYTHERAPY	POSTOPERATIVE BRACHYTHERAPY	POSTOPERATIVE EXTERNAL (cGy)	
				WHOLE-PELVIS	SPLIT FIELD
MEDICALLY OPERABLE*					
IA GI	≥1/2 Myometrial penetration		6500 cGy RSD†	2000 or 5000	3000
IB GI	≥1/2 Myometrial penetration		6500 cGy RSD	2000	3000
IA G2, IB G2	<1/2 Myometrial penetration	3500 mgh to uterus; 6500 cGy RSD			
	>1/2 Myometrial penetration	3500 mgh to uterus; 6500 cGy RSD		2000	3000
IA G3, IB G3	No myometrial penetration	3500 mgh to uterus; 6500 cGy RSD			
	Any myometrial penetration	3500 mgh to uterus; 6500 cGy RSD		2000	3000
II	Cervix microscopically involved; no myometrial penetration	3500 mgh to uterus; 6500 cGy RSD			
	Cervix microscopically involved; myometrial penetration	3500 mgh to uterus; 6500 cGy RSD		2000	3000
	Cervix grossly involved	3500 mgh to uterus; 6500 cGy RSD		2000 (preop.)	3000 (preop.)
RADIATION ALONE					
IA, B		7500–8000 mgh (2 insertions)		2000	3000
II, III, IV		8000–8500 mgh (2 insertions)		2000	3000
INCIDENTALLY FOUND TUMOR AT SIMPLE HYSTERECTOMY					
I GI	<1/2 Myometrial penetration		6500 cGy RSD		
	>1/2 Myometrial penetration		6500 cGy RSD	2000	3000
I G2, G3	No myometrial penetration		6500 cGy RSD		
	Any myometrial penetration		6500 cGy RSD	2000	3000
II	No myometrial penetration		6500 cGy RSD		
III	Any myometrial penetration		6500 cGy RSD	2000	3000
			6500 cGy RSD	2000	3000
POSTOPERATIVE RECURRENCE					
			6500 cGy RSD, plus 1500 mgh needle implant‡	3000	2000

* *If periaortic diseae is present, this region receives 4500 cGy, pelvis and brachytherapy as outlined.*
† *RSD: rad surface dose (vaginal mucosal dose)*
‡ *If nodular or infiltrating disease is present*

medroxyprogesterone (1 g to 3 g loading dose and 400 mg to 800 mg per week) are indicated. Oral megestrol (160 mg per day) gives similar results. No benefit has been shown in controlled randomized trials for the prophylactic use of progestational agents in patients with Stage I disease.[90]

Chemotherapy

Multiple chemotherapeutic agents have been evaluated in the treatment of endometrial carcinoma. Doxorubicin (Adriamycin) is the principal chemotherapeutic agent used to treat patients with disseminated adenocarcinoma of the endometrium.[113,155] The median survival time of patients who showed a complete response to doxorubicin was 14 months, compared with the median survival time of 3.5 months for those who showed no response. Patients who showed a partial regression of tumor had a median survival time of 6.8 months.

Multidrug combinations have also been investigated. In a Gynecologic Oncology Group study, 358 patients with advanced recurrent disease were randomized to receive either melphalan and 5-fluorouracil (5-FU) or doxorubicin, 5-FU, and cyclophosphamide.[26] All patients received megestrol (Megace). The objective response rate in both groups was 36.8%.

Radioactive Phosphorous (^{32}P)

Intraperitoneal ^{32}P has been reported to be effective in decreasing recurrences in patients with subclinical intraperitoneal disease.[28] Soper and co-workers[148] reported on 65 patients with endometrial carcinoma who had malignant cells in peritoneal washings and were treated with colloidal ^{32}P. The actuarial survival rate at 5 years was 89% for 53 patients with Stage I disease. The 3-year survival rate for patients with clinical Stage II (nine patients) and Stage III (three patients) disease was 30%. Complications with ^{32}P alone were rare; however, five (29%) of 17 patients receiving ^{32}P and external pelvic irradiation (4000 cGy to 5500 cGy) had significant bowel complications requiring surgical correction. Unfavorable sequelae were also observed by Klaasen and associates[80] in ten (29%) of 35 patients with early high-risk ovarian carcinoma treated with 12 mCi to 15 mCi of ^{32}P and 4000 cGy to 4500 cGy in 4 to 5 weeks. They recommended that the two modalities not be combined because of excessive toxicity. Whole abdominal radiation has also been used and certainly should be considered in patients with other intraperitoneal evidence of disease.[49,125] The optimum treatment for patients with positive cytology remains to be defined.

Recurrent Endometrial Carcinoma

Success in the treatment for recurrent endometrial cancer depends on early diagnosis. We, therefore, recommend frequent follow-up examinations, particularly during the first 2 years following completion of therapy, when 70% of all relapses occur.[139] Treatment for recurrent disease depends on several factors: the site of recurrence, whether it is limited to or has spread beyond the confines of the true pelvis, and the type of therapy that the patient has previously received. Often concomitant medical problems and advanced stage of disease preclude radical surgery. Isolated vaginal recurrences are rare, particularly in patients who have received adequate initial radiation therapy. Vaginal recurrences usually coexist with more extensive pelvic disease. If no previous radiation therapy has been given, whole-pelvis irradiation combined with a vaginal intracavitary insertion or an interstitial implant is recommended based on the size and distribution of the tumor. Patients with isolated vaginal recurrences have a salvage rate of 33% to 48% with treatment. Patients who have more extensive pelvic recurrences and those who have been previously irradiated have a poor prognosis. Tumor size is a significant prognostic factor.[30,51,126]

Patients treated for recurrent disease in the pelvis who have not received previous irradiation should be treated with external-beam irradiation to the whole pelvis (4500 cGy to 5000 cGy in 5 to 6 weeks). An additional boost to the tumor bulk of 1000 cGy to 1500 cGy can be given with external-beam irradiation when the tumor involves the central pelvis or the pelvic sidewall. Lesions in the vagina can receive boost irradiation with intracavitary or interstitial irradiation to bring the total tumor dose to 7500 cGy to 8000 cGy.

Kuten and associates[84] reported the results of irradiation for 51 patients with recurrent endometrial carcinoma (vagina only in 17 patients, vagina with pelvic extension in 12, pelvis without vaginal involvement in seven, and simultaneous locoregional and distant failure in 15). The 5-year overall actuarial survival rate was 18% for all patients. The 5-year progression-free survival rates for those with an isolated vaginal recurrence and those with a vaginal recurrence with pelvic extension were 40% and 20%, respectively. None of the patients with pelvic tumor (without vaginal involvement) or those with simultaneous pelvic and distant disease survived beyond 3.5 years.

Barber and Brunschwig[10] achieved a 13.8% 5-year survival rate in a selected group of 36 patients with central recurrence without pelvic side wall extension who were candidates for pelvic exenteration.

The treatment for patients with disseminated tumor must be systemic. Progestational agents are the treatment of choice, either alone or combined with chemotherapy, depending on the status of estrogen and progesterone receptors. (Radiation may be indicated to control local symptoms.)

RADIATION THERAPY TECHNIQUES

Stage I Disease

Preoperative and postoperative techniques using external-beam irradiation and brachytherapy have been used with success, although the trend in the United States has been to use postoperative external-beam therapy on a selective basis based on histologic findings.

Brachytherapy may involve the use of Heyman capsules, Campbell capsules, Holter-Heyman capsules, Heyman-Simon capsules, or Fletcher-Suit applicators. The Heyman-Simon capsules and the Fletcher-Suit applicator have the advantage of being afterloading devices.[146] If a capsule-packing technique is used, the uterus is dilated and packed tightly with the radioactive sources (radium, ^{60}Co, ^{137}Cs) to ensure that the tumor and the entire uterine wall receive adequate radiation. Care must be taken to irradiate the lower uterine segment by placing sources in the endocervical canal. Alternatively, an afterloading tandem can be used to cover the lower uterine segment and the endometrial canal. The vaginal fornices should be irradiated with concomitant insertion of colpostats. To give an adequate distribution of irradiation to the uterus, at least four capsules should be used. If the uterus is not large enough to allow adequate placement of the capsules, the Fletcher-Suit applicator is recommended.

In patients who have preoperative placements for Stage I disease, we have used a calculated dose of 6000 cGy delivered to a 1.5 cm depth from the surface of the endometrial cavity (as outlined by the dummy sources on the implant films). A surface dose of 5000 cGy to 6000 cGy (1800 mgh to 2000 mgh) is also delivered to the surface of the vaginal fornices. Surgery is usually scheduled from 3 days to 1 week after implant removal to ensure that the true pathologic extent of the tumor can be adequately evaluated histologically. Although a much higher degree of tumor sterilization is encountered by delaying surgery 4 to 6 weeks after brachytherapy placement, the pathologic markers that can help to determine the necessity of further treatment are lost.[23,153]

A disadvantage of preoperative brachytherapy is that low radiation dose is delivered to the pelvic lymph nodes. External-beam therapy is recommended postoperatively when tumor extension to greater than 50% of the myometrium or when disease extension beyond the uterus is found at the time of surgery. Whole-pelvis fields are used with midline shielding at some point during the treatment course as determined by the bladder and rectal doses from the intracavitary insertion.

Doses and Volume to Be Treated With External Beam

The treatment fields should extend superiorly to cover the common iliac lymph nodes and inferiorly to encompass at least the upper half of the vagina. The lateral border of the treatment field should extend 1.5 cm to 2 cm beyond the border of the bony pelvis to include the pelvic lymph nodes. A localizer is placed in the vagina to demonstrate that an adequate length is included within the field (Fig. 55-1). At Pennsylvania Hospital, we prefer to use a four-field box technique, which provides a homogeneous radiation distribution to the whole pelvis. All four fields are treated daily with a minimum tumor dose of 180 cGy per treatment fraction, 5 days a week, for a total preoperative or postoperative, dose of 4500 cGy to 5040 cGy. At Washington University, patients are treated with AP-PA (anterior and posterior) portals only, using 18 MV to 25 MV photons. Examples of isodoses for both approaches are shown in Chapter 10.

In patients treated postoperatively following TAH-BSO, the same field arrangement and dose as discussed for preoperative therapy are used. If the patient has residual tumor in the pelvis, a boost to that area is indicated.

Radiation Therapy Alone

In medically inoperable patients with Stage I or II disease and those with Stage III or IV disease, we have used either a uterine packing or a Fletcher-Suit applicator to deliver 7500 mgh to 8000 mgh in two insertions including vaginal colpostats in place to deliver 6000 cGy to the vaginal surface. This is combined with external-beam therapy for an additional 2000 cGy to 4000 cGy to the whole pelvis and subsequent boosting of the lateral pelvic wall to a total of 5000 cGy with midline pelvic shield to protect the bladder and bowel.

Uterine Sarcomas

The role of radiation therapy in the treatment of uterine sarcomas is controversial; there is no clear evidence that its use either preoperatively or postoperatively improves survival.

Surgery is the mainstay of treatment for all sarcomas arising from the uterus. A TAH-BSO is the treatment of choice, although there are advocates of a more radical surgical approach for low-grade endometrial stromal sarcomas.[33] In general, lymph node dissections and sampling, although adding information about prognosis, have not improved survival rates. Local failures are common, and the majority of patients fail because of hematogenous dissemination of tumor. A primary surgical approach is preferred, with external-beam therapy added for those patients with Stage I and Stage II disease determined histologically, excluding leiomyosarcoma.

The treatment approach at the Mallinckrodt Institute for uterine sarcoma patients with Stage I or Stage II disease, excluding leiomyosarcomas, has been to perform an intracavity insertion with Simon-Heyman capsules and a Fletcher-Suit ap-

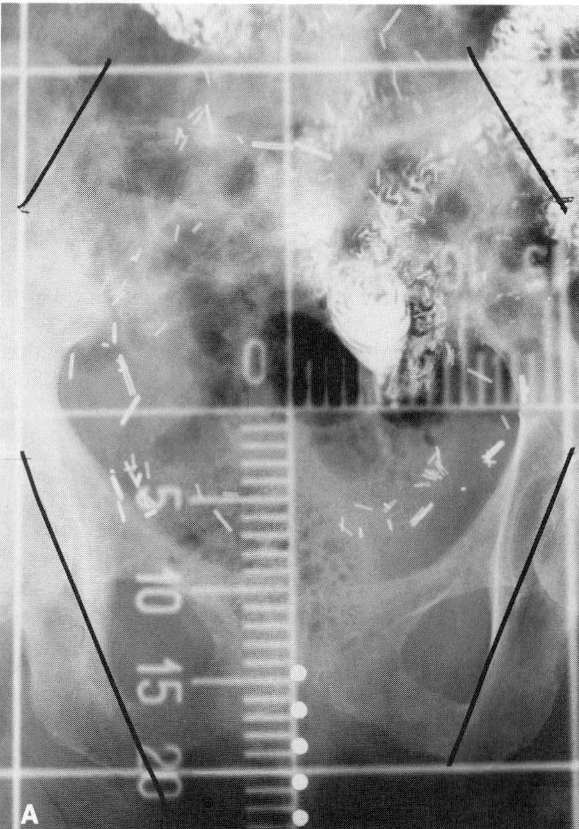

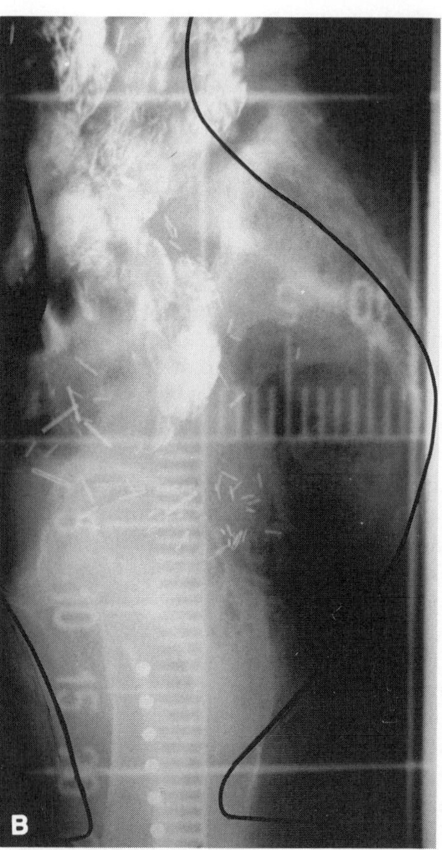

FIGURE 55–1. (**A**) Anterior and (**B**) lateral simulation films for a patient being treated postoperatively for Stage I endometrial carcinoma with areas of shielding outlined and the resulting isodose curve for the same patient on a 6 MV linear accelerator.

plicator to deliver 6000 cGy to a 1.5 cm depth from the mucosal surface of the uterus and 6000 cGy to the vaginal fornices. Patients subsequently undergo TAH-BSO. If extension is demonstrated beyond the uterus, whole-pelvis and parametrial irradiation is added with appropriate midline shielding, depending on the previous bladder and rectal dose.

In patients with Stage III or Stage IV disease who are not candidates for operation, some palliation and control of local symptoms can be achieved by use of both external-beam therapy and brachytherapy placements.

Because the major pattern of failure is disseminated tumor, either alone or in combination with local failure, effective systemic therapy must be devised for a significant improvement in survival rate to be achieved.

RESULTS OF THERAPY

Although the incidence of endometrial carcinoma has increased, the death rate has remained stable.

Stage I Endometrial Carcinoma

Several studies, both retrospective and randomized, have demonstrated that the pelvic failure rate with hysterectomy alone varies from 1.7% to 27% with an average of 12% to 15%.[37,45,53,152] With adjuvant irradiation, the incidence of vaginal recurrence can be decreased to below 3% and in the pelvis to below 5% (Table 55-13). A prospective randomized study by Graham[45] of clinical Stage I carcinoma of the endometrium described a vaginal recurrence rate of 12% with surgery alone, 3% with preoperative irradiation, and 0% (no vaginal failures) with postoperative irradiation. The 5-year survival rate was 64% (21 of 33) with surgery alone, 76% (45 of 59) with preoperative irradiation and surgery, and 81% with postoperative irradiation (25 of 31). Preoperative irradiation consisted of an intracavitary insertion for an average of 6000 mgh and in postoperative patients implant doses in the range of 2000 mgh were used.

A review of 858 patients with Stage I disease at the Mallinckrodt Institute of Radiology, of whom 538 received preoperative intracavitary therapy alone and 320 received additional

TABLE 55–13
Treatment Outcome of Stage I Disease for Carcinoma of the Endometrium

INVESTIGATOR	NO. OF PATIENTS (STAGE)	SURVIVAL (%)	NUMBER OF RECURRENCES (%)			
			VAGINA	PELVIS	PELVIS + DISTANT METASTASES	DISTANT METASTASES
Stage I—Surgery Alone						
Cheung[25]	353	87.8*		10 (1.4)	5 (1.4)	26 (7.4)
Reddy et al[129]	94	Not given		8 (8.5)		1 (1)
Salazar et al[139]	106	Not given	10 (9)	16 (15)		10 (9)
Total	553		10 (1.8)	34 (6.1)	5 (0.9)	37 (6.7)
				Pelvis 8.8%	DM 7%	
Stage I—Radiation Therapy and Surgery						
Aalders et al[3]	518	88†		31 (6)		40 (7.7)
Grigsby et al[53]	858	88.7		7 (<1%)	30 (3)	60 (7.0)
Reddy et al[129]	83 (A + B)			2 (2.4)	0	4 (4.8)
Salazar et al[139]	176			6 (3)		12 (7)
Spanos et al[149]	215 (1A) 141 (1B)			7 (3.2)‡ 8 (5.7)‡		Not reported
Total§	1635			46 (2.8)	30 (1.8)	116 (7.1)
				Pelvis 4.6%	DM 8.9%	
Stage I—Radiation Therapy Alone						
Grigsby et al[52]	69	88.1*		0	6 (8.7)	3 (4.3)
Landgren et al[85]	45 (1A) 41 (1B)	75‖ 80‖		4 (8.9) 10 (24.4)	3 (6.7) 3 (7.3)	5 (11.1) 3 (7.3)
Salazar et al[139]	25			6 (24)		8 (32)
Spanos et al[149]	30 (1A) 27 (1B)			5 (16.7)‡ 11 (40.7)‡		Not reported
Total§	180			20 (18)	12 (6.7)	19 (10.6)
				Pelvis 17.8%	DM 17.2%	

** Absolute 5-year NED (no evidence of disease)*
† 5-Years
‡ Values = combined total of recurrences in pelvis and pelvis + distant metastases in study by Spanos et al
§ Excluding Spanos et al
‖ Actuarial 5 years
(Modified from Perez CA, Bedwinek JM, Breaux SR: Cancer Treat Symp 2:226, 1983)

external-beam irradiation (usually 2000 cGy to 3000 cGy to the whole pelvis), demonstrated an overall pelvic recurrence rate of 4% for grade 1, 3% for grade 2, and 9% for grade 3.[152] Survival by grade is shown in Figure 55-2. Table 55-14 shows the 5-year survival rate for patients with Stage I disease reported in the literature.

TABLE 55–14
Stage I Endometrial Carcinoma Survival Rates

AUTHOR	NO. OF PATIENTS	5-YEAR SURVIVAL (%)
Wharam[164]	269	81 (NED)
Graham[45]	123	74 (Crude)
Malkasian[99]	409	82 (Actuarial)
Underwood[156]	220	91 (Actuarial)
Frick[40]	239	78 (Crude)
Salazar[139]	307	84 (Actuarial)
Brady[16]	99	88 (Crude)
Stokes[151]	304	87 (Actuarial)
Ritcher[131]	161	95 (Actuarial)
Nori[112]	278	85 (Actuarial—10 yr)
Grigsby[53]	858	89 (NED)

NED: no evidence of disease

Stage II Endometrial Carcinoma

Survival for patients with Stage II disease has varied widely (Table 55-15). Bruckman and colleagues[17] achieved excellent results with the use of preoperative external-beam therapy of 4000 cGy to the whole pelvis combined with a brachytherapy placement for 4000 mgh followed by a total abdominal hysterectomy and bilateral salpingo-oophorectomy. None of the 40 patients treated by this program had pelvic failures alone; three of five failures (pelvic and distant) had grade 3 disease.

Greven and Olds reported on 29 patients, 26 of whom were treated by combined surgery and irradiation—the majority postoperatively. The Kaplan-Meier 5-year survival rate estimate for all patients was 72%.[50]

Grigsby and associates[54] at the Mallinckrodt Institute of Radiology reported eight pelvic recurrences (10%) in 79 patients who received a combination of preoperative or postoperative intracavitary radiation and external irradiation for Stage II endometrial carcinoma. Eleven patients with microscopic endocervical involvement treated with a preoperative intracavitary insertion only had no pelvic or vaginal recurrences. Overall and disease-free survival rates are shown in Figure 55-3. Gross involvement of the cervix carries a worse prognosis than microscopic involvement. Grigsby and associates[53] reported a lower survival rate in patients with ectocervical tumor invasion, even if microscopic only. Patterns of failure reported by various authors in patients with Stage II endometrial carcinoma are summarized in Table 55-15.

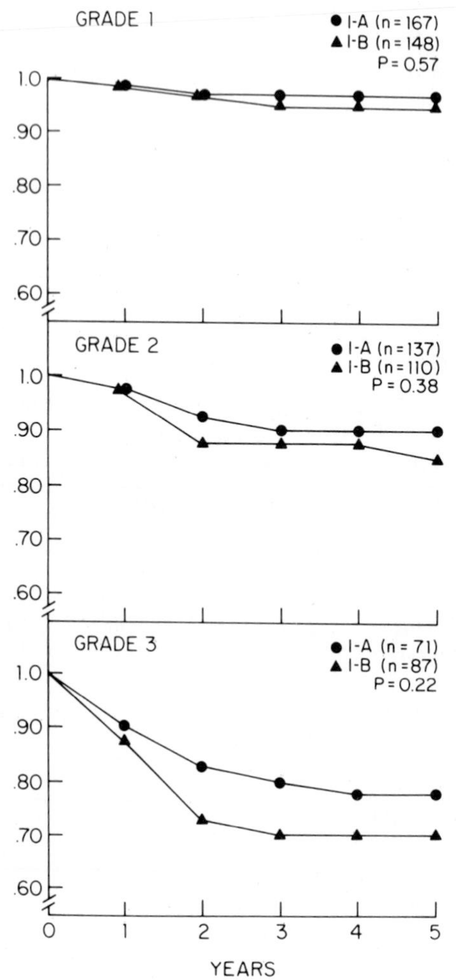

FIGURE 55–2. Disease-free survival rates for Stage IA and IB endometrial carcinoma by grade (MIR).

Stages III and IV Endometrial Carcinoma

The results of treatment for clinical Stage III endometrial carcinoma are poor. A 25% to 30% 5-year survival rate is to be expected with aggressive therapy (Table 55-16); better results (about 40% to 59% 5-year survival) were obtained in patients who had pathologic Stage III tumors.[6,32,64,82,110,134] Patients with Stage IV disease are rarely cured and most authors report a 5% 5-year survival rate.[12,140,160,163]

Recurrent Endometrial Carcinoma

The results of therapy for patients with recurrent endometrial carcinoma isolated to the vagina are shown in Table 55-17. The 5-year progression-free survival rate for this group of patients ranges from 20% to 40%. Patients with recurrent disease that extends outside the vagina and those with distant metastasis have a uniformly poor prognosis with only occasional survivors (less than 10%).

Uterine Sarcomas

Perez and co-workers[119] reported on a group of 54 patients with mixed mesodermal sarcomas of the uterus who received combined radiation therapy and surgery. In Stage I disease, a preoperative uterine packing for 6000 mgh was recommended. Treatment for patients with Stage II disease consisted of an

TABLE 55–15
Treatment Outcome of Stage II Disease for Carcinoma of the Endometrium

INVESTIGATOR	NO. OF PATIENTS	SURVIVAL (%)	NO. OF RECURRENCES (%)				
			VAGINA	PELVIS	VAGINA + PELVIS	PELVIS + DISTANT METASTASES	DISTANT METASTASES
STAGE II—RADIATION THERAPY AND SURGERY							
Gagon et al[41]	20	44.8*		1 (5)			2 (10)
Grigsby et al[54]	90	78		1 (1)		7 (8)	12 (13)
Onsrud et al[114]	44†	85			1 (2.3)		4 (9.1)
	40‡	85	2 (5)	2 (5)	3 (7.5)		4 (10)
Salazar et al[139]	20			1 (5)			3 (15)
Spanos et al[149]	61				12 (19.7)§		Not reported
Total‖	214		2 (1.6)	5 (2.3)	4 (3.2)	7 (8)	13 (10.5)
				Total pelvis 7%		Total distant metastases 9%	
STAGE II—RADIATION THERAPY ALONE							
Grigsby et al[54]	26	53		2 (8)		7 (27)	3 (12)
Landgren et al[85]	38	65¶		3 (7.9)		4 (10.5)	9 (23.7)
Salazar et al[139]	8			3 (37.5)			2 (25)
Spanos et al[149]	21				4 (19)**		Not reported
Total‖	72			8 (11.1)		11 (15.3)	14 (19.4)
				Total pelvis 26.4%		Total distant metastases 34.7%	

** 5 years*
† Radium only
‡ Radium + external
§ Value = combined total of recurrence in pelvis, vagina, vagina and pelvis, and pelvis plus distant metastases in study by Spanos et al[149]
‖ Excluding Spanos et al[149]
¶ Actuarial, 5 years
*** Value = combined total of recurrence in pelvis and pelvis plus distant metastases in study by Spanos et al*
(Perez CA, Bedwinek JM, Breaux SR: Cancer Treat Symp 2:227, 1983)

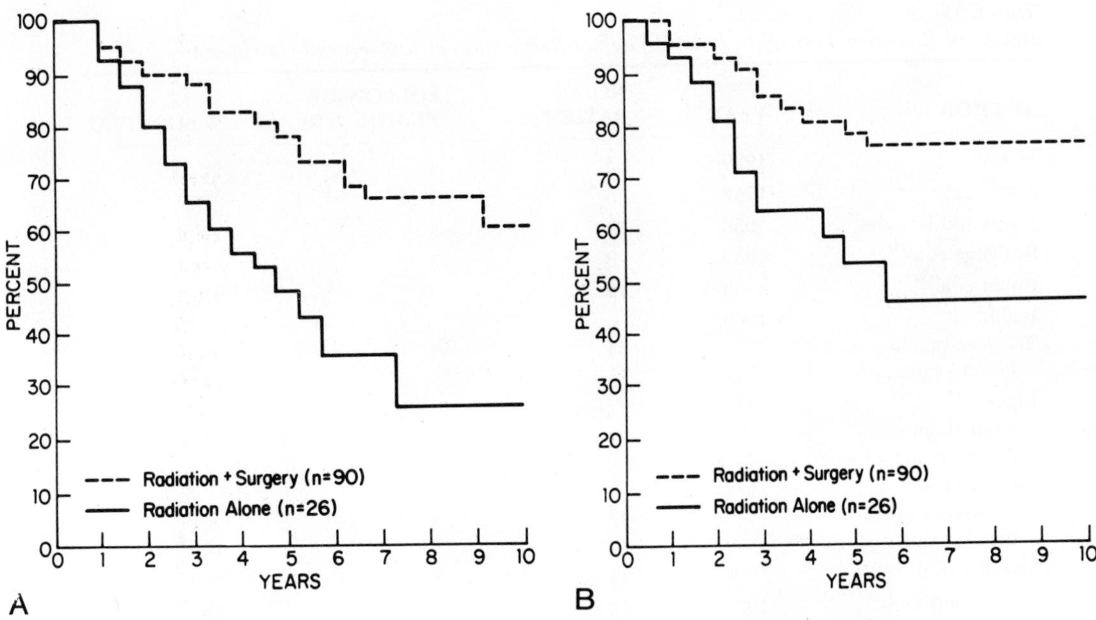

FIGURE 55–3. (**A**) Overall survival and (**B**) disease-free survival rates in 116 patients with Stage II carcinoma of the endometrium treated at Mallinckrodt Institute of Radiology (1960–1981). (Grigsby P, Perez CA, Camel HM, et al: Int J Radiat Oncol Biol Phys 11:1915, 1985)

TABLE 55–16
Five-Year Survival Rate for Stage III Endometrial Carcinoma

AUTHOR	NO. OF PATIENTS	5-YEAR SURVIVAL (%)
Antoniades et al[6]	37	25
Rutledge and Ehrlich[134]	—	21
Buchler et al[19]	32	22
Kottmeier[82]	136	30
Homesley and Lewis[64]	23	4
Boronow[14]	49	18
Geisler and Gibbs[43]	19	5.3
Ng and Reagan[110]	14	13.6
Danoff et al[32]	17	11.7
Grigsby et al[55]	27	29.7
Mackillop and Pringle[96]	62	38.5

(Modified from Danoff BF, McDay J, Louka M, et al: Int J Radiat Oncol Biol Phys 6:1491, 1980)

intracavitary insertion for 5000 mgh to 6000 mgh, combined with external-beam whole-pelvis irradiation of 2000 cGy and a 3000 cGy boost to the parametrium with a midline shield. The authors found that the incidence of local failures decreased compared with other series in which surgery alone was the treatment. This increase in local control with irradiation has been confirmed by others, and there is a tendency in the combined irradiation and surgery group toward improved survival.[33, 157, 165] However, because the numbers in most series are small and the reports are not randomized, it is difficult to make a definite statement about treatment efficacy.

Belgrad and associates[11] reviewed patients treated at four institutions and found improved 2-year survival rates in patients treated by combined irradiation and surgery for both endometrial stromal sarcomas and mixed mesodermal sarcomas. The 2-year survival rate in patients with endometrial stromal sarcomas treated by radiation therapy and surgery was 57%, whereas in those treated by surgery alone it was 37%. In the mixed mesodermal category, 35% of patients survived 2 years with combined-modality therapy and 20% with surgery only. No improvement in survival was demonstrated with the addition of irradiation for patients with leiomyosarcomas. Salazar and colleagues[137] found that local failures decreased but survival was not changed in patients who received local radiation therapy as part of their program.

In a phase III trial, the Gynecologic Oncology Group evaluated the use of doxorubicin (Adriamycin) *versus* no adjuvant therapy in Stage I and Stage II uterine sarcomas. No benefit was found for the use of chemotherapy in this patient population. Of the 149 patients, 60 received either preoperative or postoperative radiation therapy in a nonrandomized fashion. No benefit was found for radiation therapy in any group in terms of progression-free interval or absolute survival. However, in the patients with mixed mesodermal sarcoma of the uterus, pelvic recurrences were decreased from 54% to 23%.[65]

SEQUELAE OF TREATMENT

Preoperative or postoperative external-beam therapy may cause transient bowel or bladder symptoms, but chronic proctitis and cystitis are seen in less than 5% when supervoltage radiation units and judicious fractionation are used. A TAH-BSO in general has a mortality rate below 1%. However, many patients with endometrial carcinoma have concomitant medical problems such as obesity, hypertension, and heart disease, which places them in a high-risk category for complications such as infection, wound dehiscence, fistula formation, and bleeding.

Grigsby and associates[53] reported the complications in 858 patients with Stage I endometrial cancer treated with surgery and irradiation. The 5-year actuarial grade 2, 3, and 4 complication rate was 4.5% for those receiving only a postoperative vaginal cuff implant, 12.5% for those receiving postoperative external-beam whole-pelvis irradiation, 8.2% for those receiving combined postoperative implant and external beam, 3.3% for those receiving a preoperative implant and a TAH-BSO in 4 to 6 weeks, 3.7% for those receiving a preoperative implant and

TABLE 55–17
Results of Radiation Therapy in Isolated Vaginal Recurrences of Endometrial Carcinoma

AUTHOR	YEAR	NO. OF PATIENTS	FOLLOW-UP PERIOD (YR)	% SURVIVAL
Meigs[102]	1929	23	5	22
Finn[39]	1949	5	2	0
Javert and Douglas[72]	1956	40	5	20
Rutledge et al[135]	1958	9	2–5	44
Rubin et al[133]	1963	15	5	20
Badib[8]	1969			
Upper vagina		63	5	38
Lower vagina		11		27
Ingersol[69]	1971			
Vaginal apex		25		64
Anterior vaginal wall		9	5	11
Aalders et al[2]	1982			
Vaginal vault		42	3–19	26
Distal vagina		42		14
Mandell et al[100]	1985	11	5	82
Greven and Olds[51]	1987	18	3–10	33
Kuten et al[84]	1989	17	4.8	40

(Modified from Kuten A, Grigsby PW, Perez CA, et al: Int J Radiat Oncol Biol Phys 17:29–34, 1989

TABLE 55–18
Complication Rate According to Total Implant cGy (Uterus + Vagina) and Whole Pelvis External Irradiation

TOTAL cGy	NUMBER EXTERNAL	WHOLE PELVIS EXTERNAL DOSE (cGy) 3000	3000 to 4000	4000 to 5000	TOTAL
<2500	1/14		1/12	0/3	2/29 (7%)
2500 to 4500	3/46	0/10	2/8	1/2	6/66 (9%)
4500 to 6500	1/159	0/28	1/9	1/3	3/199 (2%)
≥6500	0/6	0/1	1/3		1/10 (10%)
Total	5/225 (2%)*	0/39*	5/32 (16%)*	2/8 (25)*	12/304 (4%)

* *Using trend in proportion analysis, there is a significant increase (P < 0.001) in the complication rate with increasing external whole pelvis dose. The greatest difference was at the 3000 cGy level, with a rate of 1.85 (five of 264) at 3000 cGy or less but 17.5% (seven of 40) at doses exceeding 3000 cGy (P < 0.001 by the two-tailed Fischer exact test).*
(Stokes S, Bedwinek J, Breaux S, et al: Obstet Gynecol 65:86, 1985)

preoperative external-beam irradiation and a TAH-BSO in 4 to 6 weeks, and 16.2% for those receiving a preoperative implant and postoperative external-beam irradiation. No complications occurred in 334 patients undergoing a preoperative implant followed by a TAH-BSO within 3 to 4 days after the implant. This actuarial analysis demonstrated a significant difference in complication rates by type of treatment ($P = 0.0008$).

No significant correlation was found between the incidence of complications and the number of milligram hours delivered to the uterus. There was a correlation, however, between the complication rate and the dose of external irradiation (Table 55-18) About 15% complications were observed in patients receiving over 10,000 cGy total dose to the vaginal mucosa (contribution from intracavitary and external therapy), compared with less than 7% with lower doses.

In patients with Stage II, III, or IV disease, particularly if treated by radiation therapy, a 5% to 10% incidence of proctitis or cystitis may be encountered.

SUMMARY OF CLINICAL TRIALS

Many systemic agents have been evaluated in the treatment of endometrial carcinoma. Doxorubicin appears to be as effective as doxorubicin plus cyclophosphamide (Cytoxan) in patients with advanced disease. The Gynecologic Oncology Group has two phase II trials ongoing at the present time for advanced or recurrent endometrial carcinoma. The first is with vincristine given as a weekly intravenous bolus, and the second is evaluating tumor necrosis factor (TNF). A phase III trial is comparing doxorubicin with doxorubicin plus cisplatin in patients with primary Stage III and IV or recurrent endometrial adenocarcinoma.

Ifosfamide and mesna have been found to be active in uterine sarcomas, with the highest number of responses seen in patients with mixed mesodermal tumors.

Two important trials are ongoing that deal primarily with radiation therapy. The first is aimed at evaluating surgery *versus* surgery plus adjunctive radiation therapy for patients with intermediate-risk Stage I endometrial carcinoma. The patients are randomized to receive no additional treatment or to receive 5040 cGy whole-pelvis irradiation following surgery. Hopefully this study will document the efficacy of postoperative radiation therapy in patients with intermediate or high-risk disease. The second study is aimed at evaluating total abdominal radiation therapy in patients with Stages III and IV endometrial carcinoma and all stages of papillary serous and clear cell carcinomas of the endometrium. These are extremely high-risk patients, and pilot studies with whole abdominal radiation therapy have been promising.

REFERENCES

1. Aalders JG, Abeler V, Kolstad P: Clinical (Stage III) as compared to subclinical intrapelvi extra uterine tumor spread in endometrial carcinoma: A clinical and histopathological study of 175 patients. Gynecol Oncol 17:64–74, 1984
2. Aalders JG, Abeler V, Kolstad P: Recurrent adenocarcinoma of the endometrium: A clinical and histopathological study of 369 patient. Gynecol Oncol 17:85–103, 1984
3. Aalders JG, Abeler V, Kolstad P, et al: Postoperative external irradiation and prognostic parameters in stage I endometrial carcinoma: Clinical and histopathologic study of 540 patients. Obstet Gynecol 56:419, 1980
4. Abayomi O, Dritschilo A, Emami B, et al: The value of routine tests in the staging evaluation of gynecologic malignancies: A cost effectiveness analysis. Int J Radiat Oncol Biol Phys 8:241, 1982
5. Anderson JC, Meltzer HD, Scarborough E, et al: Adenocarcinoma of the endometrium. Cancer 18:955, 1965
6. Antoniades J, Brady LW, Lewis GC: The management of stage III carcinoma of the endometrium. Cancer 38:1838, 1967
7. Austin JH, MacMahon B: Indicators of prognosis in carcinoma of the corpus uteri. Surg Gynecol Obstet 128:1247, 1969
8. Badib AO, Kurohara SS, Beitain AA, et al: Recurrent cancer of the corpus uteri: Techniques and results of treatment. Am J Roentgenol 105:596, 1969
9. Badib AO, Vontgama C, Kurohara SS, et al: Radiotherapy in the treatment of sarcomas of the corpus uteri. Cancer 24:724, 1969
10. Barber HRK, Brunschwig A: Treatment and results of recurrent cancer of the corpus uteri in patients receiving anterior and total exentration: 1947–1963. Cancer 22:949, 1968
11. Belgrad R, Elbadaw N, Rubin P: Uterine sarcoma. Radiology 114:181, 1975
12. Boronow RC: Carcinoma of the corpus. In Cancer of the Uterus and Ovary, pp 35–61. Chicago, Year Book Medical Publishers, 1969
13. Boronow RC: Endometrial cancer and endometrial hyperplasia. In Rutledge F, Boronow RC, Wharton JT (eds): Gynecologic Oncology, pp 97–116. New York, John Wiley & Sons, 1976
14. Boronow RC: Management of recurrent endometrial carcinoma. In Rutledge F, Boronow RC, Wharton JT (eds): Gynecologic Oncology, pp 117–129. New York, John Wiley & Sons, 1976
15. Boronow RC: Endometrial cancers: Staging, pretreatment evaluation, and factors in outcome. In Gray LA (ed): Endometrial Carcinoma and Its Treatment: The Role of Irradia-

tion, Extent of Surgery, and Approach to Chemotherapy, pp 38–57. Springfield, IL, Charles C Thomas, 1977
16. Brady LW, Lewis GC, Antoniades J, et al: Evolution of therapeutic techniques. Gynecol Oncol 2:253, 1974
17. Bruckman JE, Goodman RL, Murphy A, et al: Combined irradiation and surgery in the treatment of stage II carcinoma of the endometrium. Cancer 42:1146, 1978
18. Brunschwig A, Murphy A: The rationale for radical panhysterectomy and pelvic node excision in carcinoma of the corpus uteri. Am J Obstet Gynecol 68:1482, 1954
19. Buchler DA, Peckham BM, Carr WF: Treatment and results of endometrial carcinoma from 1956–1974. In Gray LA Sr (ed): Endometrial Carcinoma and Its Treatment: The Role of Irradiation, Extent of Surgery, and Approach to Chemotherapy, pp 146–150. Springfield, IL, Charles C Thomas, 1977
20. Cancer Statistics 1989: CA 37:12, 1989
21. Casey MJ: Age-specific incidence rates of endometrial cancer. JAMA 283:213, 1977
22. Chamlin DL, Taylor HB: Endometrial hyperplasia in young women. Obstet Gynecol 36:659, 1970
23. Chau PM: Technique and evaluation of preoperative radium therapy in adenocarcinoma of the uterine corpus. In Carcinoma of the Uterine Cervix, Endometrium and Ovary. Chicago, Year Book Medical Publishers, 1962
24. Cheon HK: Prognosis of endometrial cancer. Obstet Gynecol 34:680, 1969
25. Cheung AYC: Prognostic significance of negative hysterectomy specimens following intracavitary irradiation in stage I endometrial carcinoma. Br J Obstet Gynecol 88:548, 1981
26. Cohen, CJ, Bruckner HW, Deppe G, et al: Multidrug treatment of advanced and recurrent endometrial carcinoma: A Gynecologic Oncology Group Study. Obstet Gynecol 63:719, 1984
27. Creasman WT, Boronow RC, Morrow CP, et al: Adenocarcinoma of the endometrium: Its metastatic lymph node potential. Gynecol Obstet 4:239, 1976
28. Creasman WT, DiSaia PJ, Blessing J, et al: Prognostic significance of peritoneal cytology in patients with endometrial cancer and preliminary data concerning therapy with intraperitoneal radiopharmaceuticals. Am J Obstet Gynecol 141:921, 1981
29. Creasman WT, Morrow CP, Bundy, BN, et al: Surgical pathologic spread patterns of endometrial cancer. Cancer 60:2035, 1987
30. Curran WJ, Whittington R, Peters AJ, Fanning J: Vaginal recurrences of endometrial carcinoma: The prognostic value of staging by a primary vaginal carcinoma system. Int J Radiat Oncol Biol Phys 15:803, 1988
31. Cutler SJ, Young JL Jr: Third National Cancer Survey: Incidence data. Natl Cancer Inst Monogr 41:1, 1975
32. Danoff BF, McDay J, Louka M, et al: Stage III endometrial carcinoma: Analysis of patterns of failure and therapeutic implications. Int J Radiat Oncol Biol Phys 6:1491, 1980
33. DiSaia PJ, Castro JR, Rutledge FN: Mixed mesodermal sarcoma of the uterus. Am J Roentgenol Radium Ther Nucl Med 117:632, 1973
34. DiSaia PJ, Morrow CP, Boronow R, et al: Lymphatic spread pattern. Am J Obstet Gynecol 130:104, 1978
35. Dobbie BMW: Vaginal recurrences in carcinoma of the body of the uterus and their prevention by radium therapy. J Obstet Gynecol Br Emp 60:702, 1953
36. Dockerty MB, Lovelady SB, Faust ST: Carcinoma of the corpus uteri in young women. Am J Obstet Gynecol 61:966, 1951
37. Eifel P, Ross J, Hendrickson M, et al: Adenocarcinoma of the endometrium: Analysis of 256 cases with disease limited to the uterine corpus: Treatment comparisons. Cancer 52:1026, 1983
38. Fever GA, Calanog A: Endometrial Carcinoma: Treatment of positive paraaortic Nodes. Gynecol Oncol 27:104, 1987
39. Fin WF: Time, site and treatment of recurrences of endometrial carcinoma. Am J Obstet Gynecol 60:773–782, 1950
40. Frick HC, Munnell EW, Richant RM, et al: Carcinoma of the endometrium. Am J Obstet Gynecol 115:663, 1973
41. Gagnon JD, Moss WT, Gabourel LS, et al: External irradiation in the management of stage II endometrial carcinoma. Cancer 44:1247, 1979
42. Geisler HE: The use of megestrol acetate in the treatment of advanced malignant lesions of the endometrium. Gynecol Oncol 1:340, 1973
43. Geisler HE, Gibbs CP: Invasive carcinoma of the endometrium: A 5 to 16 year follow-up of 183 patients. Am J Obstet Gynecol 102:516, 1968
44. Goodman R, Hellman S: The role of postoperative irradiation in cancer of the endometrium. Gynecol Oncol 2:354, 1974
45. Graham J: The value of preoperative or postoperative treatment by radium for carcinoma of the uterine body. Surg Gynecol Obstet 132:855, 1971
46. Graham JB: Treatment of choice in cancer of the uterine corpus. N Engl J Med 254:1112, 1956
47. Gray LA: Evaluation of treatment methods of endometrial carcinoma; with particular reference to surgery alone. In Gray LA Sr (ed): Endometrial Carcinoma and Its Treatment: The Role of Irradiation, Extent of Surgery and Approach to Chemotherapy, pp 165–182. Springfield, IL, Charles C Thomas, 1977,
48. Greenberg SB, Glassburn JR, Antoniades J, et al: Management of carcinoma of the uterus stage II. Cancer Clin Trials 4:183, 1981
49. Greer BE, Hamberger AD: Treatment of intraperitoneal metastatic adenocarcinoma of the endometrium by whole abdominal moving strip technique and pelvic boost irradiation. Gynecol Oncol 16:365, 1983
50. Greven K, Olds W: Radiotherapy in the management of endometrial carcinoma with cervical involvement. Cancer 60:1737, 1987
51. Greven K, Olds W: Isolated vaginal recurrences of endometrial adenocarcinoma and their management. Cancer 60:419, 1987
52. Grigsby PW, Kuske RR, Perez CA, et al: Medically inoperable stage I adenocarcinoma of the endometrium treated with radiotherapy alone. Int J Radiat Oncol Biol Phys 13:483, 1987
53. Grigsby PW, Perez CA, Kuten A, et al: Clinical Stage I endometrial cancer: Results of adjuvant irradiation and patterns of failure. Int J Radiat Oncol Biol Phys 21:379, 1991
54. Grigsby PW, Perez CA, Camel HM, et al: Stage II carcinoma of the endometrium: Results of therapy and prognostic factors. Int J Radiat Oncol Biol Phys 11:1915, 1985
55. Grigsby PW, Perez CA, Kuske RR, et al: Results of therapy, analysis of failures, and prognostic factors for clinical and pathologic stage III adenocarcinoma of the endometrium. Gynecol Oncol 27:44, 1987
56. Gusberg SB, Yannopoulos D: Therapeutic decisions in corpus cancer. Am J Obstet Gynecol 88:157, 1964
57. Hanson MB, Van Nagell, Jr, Powell DE, et al: The prognostic significance of lymph-vascular space invasion in stage I endometrial cancer. Cancer 55:1753, 1985
58. Harbert JC, Rocha L, Smith F, Delgado G: The efficacy of radionuclide liver and bone scans in the evaluation of gynecologic cancers. Cancer 49:1040, 1982
59. Hart WR, Billman JK Jr: A reassessment of uterine neoplasia originally diagnosed as leiomyosarcomas. Cancer 41:1902, 1978
60. Hasumi K, Matsuzawa M, Chen HF, et al: Computed tomography in the evaluation and treatment of endometrial carcinoma. Cancer 50:904, 1982
61. Heath R, Rosenman J, Varia M, Walton L: Peritoneal fluid cytology in endometrial cancer: Its significance and the role of Chromic Phosphate (32P) Therapy. Int J Radiat Oncol Biol Phys 15:815, 1988
62. Hendrickson M, Ross J, Eifel P, et al: Papillary serous carcinoma: A highly malignant form of endometrial adenocarcinoma. Am J Surg Pathol 6:93, 1982
63. Homesley HD, Boronow RC, Lewis JL: Stage II endometrial adenocarcinoma—Memorial Hospital for Cancer: 1949–1965. Obstet Gynecol 49:604, 1977
64. Homesley HD, Lewis JL: Treatment of endometrial adenocarcinoma at Memorial Hospital, New York: 1884–1976. In Gray LA Sr (ed): Endometrial Carcinoma and Its Treatment: The Role of Irradiation, Extent of Surgery, and Ap-

proach to Chemotherapy, pp 99–117. Springfield, IL, Charles C Thomas, 1977

65. Hornback NB, Omura G, Major FJ: Observations on the use of adjuvant radiation therapy in patients with stage I and II uterine sarcoma. Int J Radiat Oncol Biol Phys 12:2127, 1986
66. Hricak H, Stern JL, Fisher MR: Endometrial carcinoma staging by MR imaging. Radiology 162:297, 1987
67. Hulbert M: Adjuctive pelvic irradiation in carcinoma of the endometrium. J Obstet Gynaec Br Commonw 76:624–630, 1969
68. Huynh T, Glassburn JR, Brady LW: Evaluation of treatment for sarcomas of the uterus. Cancer Clin Trials 2:145, 1979
69. Ingersol FM: Vaginal recurrences of carcinoma of the corpus: Management and prevention. Am J Surg 121:473–477, 1971
70. International Federation of Gynecology and Obstetrics classification and staging of malignant tumors in the female pelvis. Int J Gynaecol Obstet 9:172, 1971
71. International Federation of Gynecology and Obstetrics classification and staging of malignant tumors in the female pelvis. Annual Report on the Results of Treatment in Gynecological Cancer. Int J Gynecol Obstet 28:189–193, 1989
72. Javert CT, Douglas RG: Treatment of endometrial adenocarcinoma: A study of 381 cases at New York Hospital. Am J Roentgenol 75:508–515, 1956
73. Javert CT, Hofammann K: Observations on the surgical pathology, selective lymphadenectomy and classification of endometrial adenocarcinoma. Cancer 5:485, 1952
74. Jones HW: Treatment of adenocarcinoma of the endometrium. Obstet Gynecol Surv 30:147, 1975
75. Joslin CA, Vaishampayan GV, Mallik A: The treatment of early cancer of the corpus uteri. Br J Radiol 50:38, 1977
76. Kay S: Squamous cell carcinoma of the endometrium. Am J Clin Pathol 61:264, 1974
77. Kelley HW, Miles PA, Buster JE, et al: Adenocarcinoma of the endometrium in women taking sequential oral contraceptives. Obstet Gynecol 47:200, 1976
78. Kelly R, Baker W: The role of progesterone in human endometrial cancer. Cancer Res 25:1190, 1965
79. Kempson RL, Bari W: Uterine sarcomas classification, diagnosis, and prognosis. Hum Pathol 1:331, 1970
80. Klaassen D, Starreveld A, Shelly W: External beam pelvic radiotherapy plus intraperitoneal radioactive chronic phosphate in early stage ovarian cancer: A toxic combination. Int J Radiat Oncol Biol Phys 11:1801, 1985
81. Konski A, Poulter C, Beecham J, et al: The influence of positive peritoneal cytology in clinical stage I endometrial adenocarcinoma and approaches to its treatment (Abstract). Int J Radiat Oncol Biol Phys 12 (Suppl 1):128, 1986
82. Kottmeier HL: Endometrial carcinoma and its treatment: Recent experience of the Radiumhemmet, Stockholm. In Gray LA Sr (ed): Endometrial Carcinoma and Its Treatment: The Role of Irradiation, Extent of Surgery, and Approach to Chemotherapy, pp 118–126. Springfield, IL, Charles C Thomas, 1977
83. Kurman RJ, Scully RE: Clear cell carcinoma of the endometrium: An analysis of 21 cases. Cancer 37:872, 1976
84. Kuten A, Grigsby PW, Perez CA, et al: Results of radiotherapy in recurrent endometrial carcinoma: A retrospective analysis. Int J Radiat Oncol Biol Phys 17:29–34, 1989
85. Landgren RC, Fletcher GH, Delclos L, et al: Irradiation of endometrial cancer in patients with medical contraindications to surgery or with unresectable lesions. Am J Roentgenol Radium Ther Nucl Med 126:148, 1976
86. Larson DM, Copeland LJ, Gallager S, et al: Prognostic factors in stage II endometrial carcinoma. Cancer 60:1358, 1987
87. Lees D: An evaluation of treatment in carcinoma of the body of the uterus. J Obstet Gynaecol Br Commonw 76:615, 1969
88. Lefevre H: Node dissection in cancer of the endometrium. Surg Gynecol Obstet 102:649, 1956
89. Lewis GC, Bundy B: Surgery for endometrial cancer. Cancer 48:568, 1981
90. Lewis GC Jr, Slack NH, Mortel R, et al: Adjuvant progesterone therapy in the primary definitive treatment of endometrial cancer. Gynecol Oncol 2:368, 1974
91. Lewis BV, Stallworthy JA, Codwell R: Adenocarcinoma of the body of the uterus. J Obstet Gynaecol Br Commonw 77:343, 1970
92. Liu W, Meigs JV: Radical hysterectomy and pelvic lymphadenopathy. Am J Obstet Gynecol 69:1, 1955
93. Lynch HT, Kruch AJ, Larsen AL, et al: Endometrial carcinoma: Multiple primary malignancies, constitutional factors, and heredity. Am J Med Sci 252:381, 1966
94. Lyon FA: The development of adenocarcinoma of the endometrium in young women receiving long-term sequential oral contraceptive. Am J Obstet Gynecol 123:299, 1975
95. Macasaet M, Brigati D, Boyce J, et al: The significance of residual disease after radiotherapy in endometrial carcinoma: Clinicopathologic correlation. Am J Obstet Gynecol 138:557, 1980
96. Mackillop WJ, Pringle JF: Stage III endometrial carcinoma: A review of 90 cases. Cancer 56:2519, 1985
97. MacMahon B: Risk factors for endometrial cancer. Gynecol Oncol 2:122, 1974
98. Madoc-Jones H: Adenocarcinoma of the endometrium stage II: Problems in definition and management. Int J Radiat Oncol Biol Phys 6:887, 1980
99. Malkasian GD Jr, McDonald TW, Pratt JH: Carcinoma of the endometrium: Mayo Clinic Experience. Mayo Clin Proc 52:175, 1977
100. Mandell LR, Nori D, Hilaris B: Recurrent Stage I endometrial carcinoma: Results of treatment and prognostic factors. Int J Radiat Oncol Biol Phys 11:1103–1109, 1985
101. Mark TM, Pike MC, Henderson BE, et al: Estrogens and endometrial cancer in a retirement community. N Engl J Med 294:1262, 1976
102. Meigs JV: Adenocarcinoma of the fundus of the uterus. A report concerning the vaginal metastases of this tumor. N Engl J Med 201:155–160, 1929
103. Meulenaere GF: The distribution of neoplasm in patients dying after treatment of endometrial carcinoma. Br J Obstet Gynecol 83:576, 1976
104. Milton PJD, Metters JS: Endometrial carcinoma: An analysis of 355 cases treated at St. Thomas Hospital, 1945–1969, J Obstet Gynaecol Br Commonw 79: 455–464, 1972
105. Moltz A, Pomerance W, Streisfeld S: Adenocarcinoma of the endometrium. Obstet Gynecol 39:199, 1972
106. Morrow CP, DiSaia PJ, Townsend DE: Current management of endometrial carcinoma. Obstet Gynecol 42:399, 1973
107. Mortel R, Zaino R, Satyaswaroop PG: Heterogeneity and progesterone—receptor distribution in endometrial adenocarcinoma. Cancer 53:113, 1984
108. Nahhas WA, Lund CJ, Rudolph JH: Carcinoma of the corpus uteri: A 10-year review of 225 patients. Obstet Gynecol 38:437, 1970
109. Naib AM: Exfoliative Cytology. Boston, Little, Brown & Co, 1970
110. Ng ABP, Reagan JW: Incidence and prognosis of endometrial carcinoma by histologic grade and extent. Obstet Gynecol 35:437, 1970
111. Ng ABP, Reagan JW, Storaasli JP, et al: Mixed adenosquamous carcinoma of the endometrium. Am J Clin Pathol 59:765, 1973
112. Nori D, Hilaris BS, Tome M, et al: Combined surgery and radiation in endometrial carcinoma: An analysis of prognostic factors. Int J Radiat Oncol Biol Phys 13:489, 1987
113. O'Bryan RM, Luce JK, Talley RW, et al: Phase II evaluation of Adriamycin in human neoplasia. Cancer 32:1, 1973
114. Onsrud M, Aalders J, Abeler V, et al: Endometrial carcinoma with cervical involvement (stage II): Prognostic factors and value of combined radiological-surgical treatment. Gynecol Oncol 13:76, 1982
115. Park R, Patow W, Petty W, et al: Treatment of adenocarcinoma of the endometrium. Gynecol Oncol 2:60, 1974
116. Parsons L, Cesare F: Wertheim hysterectomy in the treatment of endometrial carcinoma. Surg Gynecol Obstet 108:582, 1959
117. Patanaphan V, Salazar OM, Chougule P: What can be expected when radiation therapy becomes the only curative alternative for endometrial cancer? Cancer 55:1462, 1985
118. Peck JG, Boges DA: Treatment of advanced endometrial car-

cinoma with a progestational agent. Am J Obstet Gynecol 103:90, 1969

119. Perez CA, Adkin F, Baglan RJ, et al: Effect of irradiation on mixed mullerian tumors of the uterus. Cancer 43:1274, 1979
120. Perez CA, Bedwinek JM, Breaux SR: Patterns of failure after treatment of gynecologic tumors. Cancer Treat Symp 2:217, 1983
121. Perez CA, Kuske R, Glasgow GP: Review of brachytherapy for gynecologic tumors. Endocurietherapy/Hypertherm Oncol 1:153, 1985
122. Piver SM: Progesterone therapy for malignant peritoneal cytology in surgical stage I endometrial cancer. Semin Oncol 15(Suppl1):50, 1988
123. Plentl AA, Friedman EA: Lymphatic System of the Female Genitalia. pp 85–115 Philadelphia, WB Saunders Co, 1971
124. Potish RA: Radiation therapy of periaortic node metastases in cancer of the uterine, cervix, and endometrium. Radiology 165:567, 1987
125. Potish RA, Twigg LB, Adcock LL, Ren KA: The role of whole abdominal radiation therapy in the management of endometrial cancer: Prognostic importance of factors indicating peritoneal metastases. Gynecol Oncol 21:80, 1985
126. Poulsen MG, Roberts SJ: The salvage of recurrent endometrial carcinoma in the vagina and pelvis. Int J Radiat Oncol Biol Phys 15:809, 1988
127. Price JJ, Hahn GA, Rominger CJ: Vaginal involvement in endometrial carcinoma. Am J Obstet Gynecol 91:1060, 1965
128. Procope B: An etiology of postmenopausal bleeding. Acta Obstet Gynecol Scand 50:311, 1971
129. Reddy S, Lee MS, Hendrickson FR: Pattern of recurrences in endometrial carcinoma and their management. Radiology 133:737, 1979
130. Rickford RBK: Involvement of the pelvic lymph nodes in carcinoma of the endometrium. J Obstet Gynaecol Br Commonw 75:580, 1968
131. Ritcher N, Lucas WE, Yon JL, Sanford FG: Preoperative whole pelvic external irradiation in stage I endometrial cancer. Cancer 48:58, 1981
132. Rozier J, Underwood P: Use of progestational agents in endometrial adenocarcinoma. Am J Obstet Gynecol 97:117, 1967
133. Rubin R, Gerle RD, Quick RS, et al: Significance of vaginal recurrence in endometrial carcinoma. Am J Roentgenol 89:91–100, 1963
134. Rutledge FN, Ehrlich C: Adenocarcinoma of the endometrium. In Gray LA Sr (ed): Endometrial Carcinoma and Its Treatment: The Role of Irradiation, Extent of Surgery, and Approach to Chemotherapy, pp 128–137. Springfield, IL, Charles C Thomas, 1977
135. Rutledg FN, Tan SK, Fletcher GH: Vaginal metastases from adenocarcinoma of the corpus uteri. Am J Obstet, Gynecol 75:167–174, 1958
136. Sala JM, del Regato JA: Treatment of carcinoma of the endometrium. Radiology 79:12, 1962
137. Salazar OM, Bonfiglio TA, Patten SF, et al: Uterine sarcomas: Analysis of failures with special emphasis on the use of adjuvant radiation therapy. Cancer 42:1161, 1978
138. Salazar OM, DePapp EW, Bonfiglio TA, et al: Adenosquamous carcinoma of the endometrium: An entity with an inherent poor prognosis. Cancer 40:119, 1977
139. Salazar OM, Feldstein ML, DePapp EW, et al: Endometrial carcinoma: Analysis of failures with special emphasis on the use of initial preoperative external pelvic radiation. Int J Radiat Oncol Biol Phys 2:1101, 1977
140. Sall S, Sonnenblick B, Stone ML: Factors affecting survival of patients with endometrial adenocarcinoma. Am J Obstet Gynecol 107:16, 1970
141. Schwartz AE, Brunschwig A: Radical panhysterectomy and pelvic lymph node excision for carcinoma of the corpus uteri. Surg Gynecol Obstet 105:675, 1957
142. Schwartz PE, Chambers SK, Chambers JT, et al: Circulating tumor markers in the monitoring of gynecologic malignancies. Cancer 60:353, 1987
143. Shah CA, Green TH: Evaluation of current management of endometrial carcinoma. Obstet Gynecol 39:500, 1972
144. Silverberg SG, Bolin MG, DeGiorgi LS: Adenoacanthoma and mixed adenosquamous carcinoma of the endometrium: A clinical pathologic study. Cancer 30:1307, 1972
145. Silverberg SG, DeGiorgi LS: Clear cell carcinoma of the endometrium, clinical pathologic and ultrastructural findings. Cancer 31:1127, 1973
146. Simon N, Silverstone SM: Intracavitary radiotherapy of endometrial cancer by afterloading. Gynecol Oncol 1:13, 1972
147. Smith DC, Prentice R, Thompson DJ, et al: Association of exogenous estrogen and endometrial carcinoma. N Engl J Med 293:1164, 1975
148. Soper JT, Creasman WT, Clarke-Pearson DL, et al: Intraperitoneal chromic phosphate 32P suspension therapy of malignant peritoneal cytology in endometrial carcinoma. Am J Obstet Gynecol 153:191, 1985
149. Spanos WJ, Fletcher GH, Wharton JT, et al: Patterns of pelvic recurrence in endometrial carcinoma. Gynecol Oncol 6:495, 1978
150. Stander RW: Vaginal metastases following treatment of endometrial carcinoma. Am J Obstet Gynecol 71:776, 1956
151. Stokes S, Bedwinek J, Breaux S, et al: Treatment of stage I adenocarcinoma of the endometrium by hysterectomy and irradiation: Analysis of complications. Obstet Gynecol 65:86, 1985
152. Stokes S, Bedwinek J, Kao MS, et al: Treatment of stage I adenocarcinoma of the endometrium by hysterectomy and adjuvant irradiation: A retrospective analysis of 304 patients. Int J Radiat Oncol Biol Phys 12(3):339, 1986
153. Strickland PL: Carcinoma corpus uteri: A radical intracavitary treatment. Br J Radiol 16:112, 1965
154. Surwit EA, Fowler WC, Rogoff EE, et al: Stage II carcinoma of the endometrim. Int J Radiat Oncol Biol Phys 5:323, 1979
155. Thigpen JT, Buchsbaum HG, Mangan C, et al: Phase II trial of Adriamycin in the treatment of advanced or recurrent endometrial carcinoma: A Gynecologic Oncology Group Study. Cancer Treat Rep 63:21, 1976
156. Underwood PB, Lutz MH, Kreutner A, et al: Carcinoma of the endometrium: Radiation followed immediately by operation. Am J Obstet Gynecol 128:86, 1977
157. Vongtama V, Karlen JR, Piver SM, et al: Treatment, results and prognostic factors in stage I and II sarcomas of the corpus uteri. Am J Roentgenol Rad Ther Nucl Med 126:139, 1976
158. Vongtama V, Kurohara SS, Badib AO, et al: Second primary cancers of endometrial carcinoma. Cancer 26:842, 1970
159. Vuopala S: Diagnostic accuracy and clinical application of cytological and histological methods for investigating endometrial carcinoma. Acta Scand Obstet Gynecol 56(Suppl 70):1, 1977
160. Wade MD, Kohorn EI, Morris JM: Adenocarcinoma of the endometrium. Am J Obstet Gynecol 99:867, 1967
161. Wait RB: Megestrol acetate in the management of advanced endometrial carcinoma. Obstet Gynecol 41:129, 1973
162. Way SJ: Vaginal metastases of carcinoma of the body of the uterus. J Obstet Gynaecol Br Commonw 58:558, 1951
163. Welander C, Griem JL, Newton M: Staging and treatment of endometrial carcinoma. J Reprod Med 8:41, 1972
164. Wharam MO, Phillips TL, Bagshaw MA: The role of radiation therapy in clinical stage I carcinoma of the endometrium. Int J Radiat Oncol Biol Phys 1:1081, 1976
165. Wharton JT: Sarcomas of the uterus. In Rutledge FN, Boronow RC, Wharton JT (eds): Gynecologic Oncology, pp 131–183. New York, John Wiley & Sons, 1976
166. Whetham CG, Bean JLM: Carcinoma of the endometrium. Am J Obstet Gynecol 112:339, 1972
167. Wynder EL, Escher GC, Mantel N: An epidemiological investigation of cancer of the endometrium. Cancer 19:489, 1966
168. Yazigi R, Piver MS, Blumenson L: Malignant peritoneal cytology as a prognostic indicator in stage I endometrial cancer. Obstet Gynecol 62:359, 1983
169. Ziel HK, Finkle WD: Increased risk of endometrial carcinoma among users of conjugated estrogens. N Engl J Med 293:1167, 1975

56

○ ○ ○ • • •

Ovary

Carolyn J. Horowitz
Luther W. Brady

ANATOMY

The ovary in a premenopausal woman measures 2.5 cm to 5.0 cm by 1.5 cm to 3.0 cm by 0.6 cm to 1.5 cm. Asymmetry is common; the right ovary is usually larger than the left. The anterior margin of the ovary is attached to the posterior surface of the broad ligament by the mesovarium, which contains blood vessels and nerves that enter the ovary through the hilus. The posterior surface is rounded, thick, convex, and unattached. The inferior pole is attached to the uterus by the utero-ovarian ligament. The upper pole, embraced by the fimbria of the tubes, is supported by the infundibulopelvic ligament.

The ovarian arteries arise from the aorta opposite the lower second and upper third lumbar vertebrae and pass through the infundibulopelvic ligament; they divide, the main trunk running in the folds of the broad ligament and mesovarian, anastomosing with the ascending branch of the uterine artery. The veins emerge from the hilus as two major vessels and drain in a similar fashion to the arteries. The nerve supply arises from a sympathetic plexus that is enmeshed with the ovarian vessels in the infundibulopelvic ligament. Its fibers arise from branches of the renal and aortic plexuses and from the celiac and mesenteric ganglia.

The lymphatic channels of the ovary drain almost exclusively to the periaortic lymph nodes; however, retrograde flow can lead to metastases to the uterus, vaginal fornices, and skin of the mons pubis. Retrograde flow may also account for external iliac and inguinal lymph node involvement.[99]

EPIDEMIOLOGY

In 1991, United States cancer statistics predicted 20,700 new cases of ovarian carcinoma and 12,500 deaths, making it the leading cause of gynecologic cancer death.[31] Ovarian carcinoma is the fourth most common cause of cancer death for women in the United States, exceeded only by breast, colon, and lung cancer, and the fifth most frequently diagnosed malignant solid tumor. In the United States, a 25-year trend in age-adjusted cancer deaths per 100,000 women shows approximately an 8.9% increase for ovarian carcinoma, an increase surpassed only by that for lung cancer. One woman in 80 develops ovarian carcinoma, with an expected overall cure rate of 30% for all stages.[31]

The highest incidences of ovarian carcinoma are recorded in the industrialized countries, with the exception of Japan, which has a low but increasing incidence and the lowest mortality rate worldwide of this cancer. The disease is uncommon in developing countries, perhaps because it is not often diagnosed. An association between high ovarian cancer mortality rates and high intake of total fat, particularly of animal origin, has been found. Positive correlations are present for intake of meats and milk. A negative correlation exists between mortality and vegetable/fruit intake. Obesity may also be a risk factor.[172] Carcinoma of the ovary is most frequently found in older white women, with the peak incidence being in the 50- to 70-year age group. Rarely is the disease seen before menarche; when seen, ovarian germ cell tumors predominate.

Little is known about the causes of ovarian carcinoma. Although no firm association has been documented, asbestos workers appear to have a higher than expected incidence of ovarian and peritoneal cancers.[221] Talc and asbestos-like birefringent bodies have been found in ovarian cancer specimens.[116,218] Asbestos has been a common contaminant of cosmetic talc and has been associated with condom and diaphragm use.[116] Irradiation, both diagnostic and therapeutic, has been mentioned as a potential etiologic agent of ovarian cancer, but no evidence proves this. No infectious agent has been found to be an etiologic agent; in fact, women with ovarian cancer are reported to have a lower than expected incidence of mumps and other viral infections.[221]

Higher incidences of epithelial ovarian carcinomas have been reported in women who have difficulty conceiving, nulliparous women, women with a lower mean number of pregnancies, postmenopausal women, and postmenopausal women taking stilbestrol for menopausal symptoms.[12,89,94,113] Early menarche and late menopause are also associated with increased risk.[172] On the other hand, pregnancy and oral contraceptive use seem to lower the risk.[12,174] Young age at first pregnancy may be protective.[172] One theory relates the low ovarian carcinoma rate of generations ago to the high pregnancy rates and resultant low rates of ovulation. Hormones may play a role in the observed association between breast and ovarian carcinoma. There is a threefold to fourfold increased risk of developing breast carcinoma in women diagnosed with ovarian carcinoma. Women with breast carcinoma have a twofold increase in risk of developing ovarian carcinoma.[221]

Genetic and familial associations relating to ovarian carcinoma have been reported on rare occasion. Females with Peutz-Jeghers syndrome have a 5% to 14% chance of developing ovarian tumors, which are usually benign and stromal in origin. Gonadal dysgenesis patients (46XY genotype or mosaic) tend to develop gonadoblastomas. Females with inherited basal cell nevus syndrome develop benign fibromas.[70,211] Lynch and associates[120] described three ovarian cancer-prone families, two of which contained identical twin sisters concordant for ovarian carcinoma. Vertical transmission in a pattern consonant with an autosomal dominant mode of inheritance was noted. Low serum α-L-fucosidase levels were seen in all cancer-affected patients.

An increased incidence of thecomas is reported in females receiving long-term anticonvulsant medications; this is believed to be related to variations in the ability to metabolize the drugs.[185]

McGowan[128] recently reviewed the epidemiology of ovarian cancer. Table 56-1 lists the characteristics of women at high risk for epithelial ovarian carcinoma. Black women have a proportionately greater number of gonad stromal and germ cell cancers and fewer epithelial cancers.

NATURAL HISTORY

Silent, asymptomatic growth and spread characterize ovarian carcinoma. Between 1970 and 1973, 64% of all cases presented with advanced abdominal disease compared with only 25% with localized tumor.[31] Between 65% to 75% of cases have shown intraabdominal metastasis at time of surgery.[115,154,178] Propensity to spread depends on degree of differentiation, histologic type, vascular supply, loss of cohesiveness of tumor cells, enzymatic activity, and motility of cells, as well as immunologic response of the host.[99] In addition, excrescences on the surface, fixation even though inflammatory, ascites, and extraovarian extension enhance the propensity of ovarian carcinoma to spread.

The major route of spread is transcoelomic, which occurs in 67% of cases with metastatic disease. Tumors arising in the coelomic epithelium disseminate by direct surface implantation or lymphatic spread. The tumor cells grow into nodules that eventually coat the capsules of the liver and spleen and the peritoneal surfaces of the diaphragm and bowel. The omentum often becomes heavily infiltrated with tumor, giving the appearance frequently referred to as an "omental cake." Local inflammatory response occurs, leading to adhesions, and loops of bowel may become matted, leading to mechanical obstruction. Hydronephrosis or pyelonephritis may occur secondary to obstruction and infiltration of the ureters.[99]

Particulate matter injected into the peritoneal cavity is cleared almost entirely by lymphatic capillaries lining the diaphragmatic peritoneum.[68] These capillaries form a diffuse plexus on the pleural and peritoneal surfaces of the diaphragm and are concentrated in the muscular portion of the right hemidiaphragm. From the diaphragm, drainage is primarily to the anterior mediastinal lymph nodes, which communicate with the left supraclavicular nodes.[221] This pattern of spread makes it clear that diaphragmatic metastases can be present without gross abdominal disease.[93] Ascites is related to the impairment of drainage of diaphragmatic lymphatics that are obstructed by tumor cells.

Local lymphatic invasion is seen in 20% of patients with metastatic disease. One review of the incidence of periaortic and pelvic lymph node metastasis in Stage I and Stage II disease reports approximately a 10% incidence.[160] Twenty-seven percent of 311 patients with ovarian malignancies (all stages) had either pelvic or periaortic nodal disease.[5] Autopsy findings have revealed pelvic or periaortic nodal involvement in 80% and 78% of all cases, respectively; inguinal nodes were involved in 40%, mediastinal nodes in 50%, and supraclavicular nodes in 48%.[16] At surgical staging the incidence of periaortic nodal metastases for Stage I disease has been reported to be 10.3% to 25%.[36,49,105,106,160] After the tumor cells are in the lymphatic channels, they grow by permeation, forming solid cords or tumor emboli that reach the thoracic duct and then the circulatory system, leading to wide dissemination.

The most common sites of blood-borne metastases in decreasing order of frequency are liver, lung, pleura, bone, kidney and bladder, skin, adrenal gland, and spleen (Fig. 56-1).[99]

TABLE 56–1
Characteristics of Women at High Risk for Ovarian Cancer

White
Family history of invasive disease
Having regular sexual relations, but unable to conceive
No children
No past history of hysterectomy
Menopausal hot flashes
History of difficulty getting pregnant
No severe menstrual cramps
Previous breast or colon cancer
Coexisting endometrial cancer or cervical adenocarcinoma
Peutz-Jeghers syndrome

(*McGowan L: Oncology 3:51, 1989*)

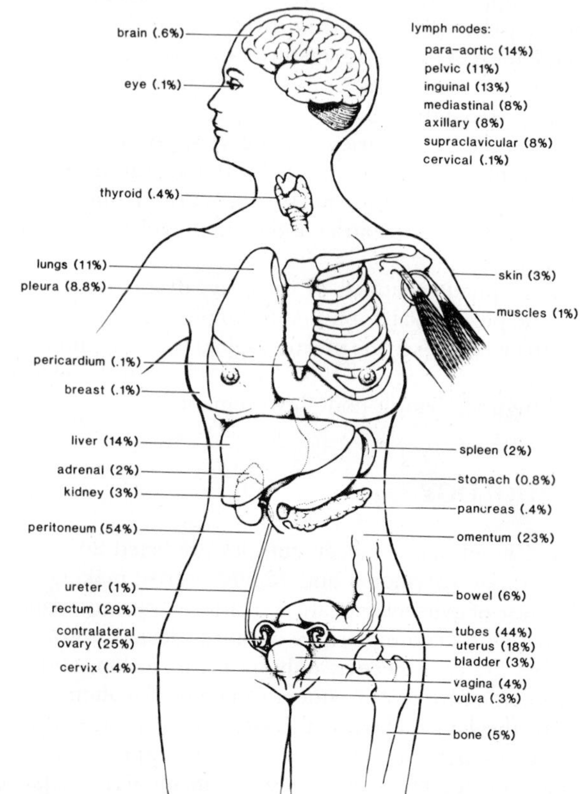

FIGURE 56–1. Distribution of mestastases from primary ovarian malignant tumors (from autopsy material). (Janovski NA, Paramanandhan TL: Ovarian tumors. In Major Problems in Obstetrics and Gynecology, vol 4. Philadelphia, WB Saunders, 1973)

Spread along epithelial-lined spaces accounts for 2% of metastatic disease, commonly seen in surface papillary tumors. Exfoliated tumor cells travel along the lumen of the tubes, the endometrial cavity, and the endocervical canal to the vagina and may implant anywhere along their path and produce metastasis. Implantation of fragments of tumor is rare (0.9%). The most common site is the surgical scar, with seeding occurring at time of surgery.

Dormant cancer may reappear suddenly, 10 to 25 years after successful removal of the primary ovarian tumor; most recurrences are intraabdominal. Possibly some immunologic derangement is responsible for this regrowth of dormant tumor cells.[99]

CLINICAL PRESENTATION

The typical presenting symptoms of ovarian carcinoma depend on the size, weight, and location of tumor and the presence of bleeding, ascites, torsion, infection, and rupture. Hormone-secreting tumors may cause symptoms, most often abnormal uterine bleeding.

Typically, women give a 2- to 6-month history of vague abdominal discomfort, dyspepsia, increasing flatulence, a sense of bloating, especially after meals, mild digestive disturbances, and pelvic unrest. Many note that their clothes no longer fit properly.

Workup of these symptoms often reveals no abnormal findings. The patient may be erroneously treated with antacids. As the tumor grows, it may invade or compress adjacent organs. Severe pain is usually associated with torsion, rupture, or invasion of nerve sheaths or organs. Occasionally an enlarged left supraclavicular lymph node may be the first presenting sign.

DIAGNOSTIC WORKUP AND STAGING

All patients should have a complete history and physical examination. Pelvic examination is essential in evaluating for possible ovarian carcinoma. The physical signs outlined in Table 56-2 may help to alert the physician to the presence of ovarian carcinoma.[10,20,83,221]

Ovarian carcinoma is staged most frequently by the International Federation of Gynecology and Obstetrics (FIGO) classification (Table 56-3); however, the American Joint Committee (AJC) on Cancer also uses TNM nomenclature (Table 56-4).[20,124] Recently FIGO changes in clinical staging have been introduced. Primarily, Stage III is better defined relative to abdominal disease.[33]

TABLE 56–3
Staging of Ovarian Carcinoma (FIGO, 1987)

Stage I	Growth limited to the ovaries.
Stage IA	Growth limited to one ovary; no ascites. No tumor on the external surface: capsule intact.
Stage IB	Growth limited to both ovaries; no ascites. No tumor on the external surfaces; capsules intact.
Stage IC	Tumor either Stage IA or IB, but with tumor on the surface of one or both ovaries; or with capsule ruptured; or with ascites present containing malignant cells or with positive peritoneal washings.
Stage II	Growth involving one or both ovaries with pelvic extension.
Stage IIA	Extension and/or metastases to the uterus and/or tubes.
Stage IIB	Extension to other pelvic tissues.
Stage IIC	Tumor either Stage IIA or IIB, but with tumor on the surface of one or both ovaries; or with capsule(s) ruptured; or with ascites present containing malignant cells or with positive peritoneal washings.
Stage III	Tumor involving one or both ovaries with peritoneal implants outside the pelvis and/or positive retroperitoneal or inguinal nodes. Superficial liver metastasis equals Stage III. Tumor is limited to the true pelvis but with histologically verified malignant extension to small bowel or omentum.
Stage IIIA	Tumor grossly limited to the true pelvis with negative nodes but with histologically confirmed microscopic seeding of abdominal peritoneal surfaces.
Stage IIIB	Tumor of one or both ovaries with histologically confirmed implants of abdominal peritoneal surfaces, none exceeding 2 cm in diameter. Nodes negative.
Stage IIIC	Abdominal implants 2 cm in diameter and/or positive retroperitoneal or inguinal nodes.
Stage IV	Growth involving one or both ovaries with distant metastasis. If pleural effusion is present there must be positive cytologic test results to allow case to Stage IV. Parenchymal liver metastasis equals Stage IV.

TABLE 56–2
Pelvic Signs of Ovarian Cancer

Mass in ovarian area
Fixation and adhesions (relative immobility)
Irregular abdominal mass
"Shotty" consistency; increased firmness
Tumors in cul-de-sac ("a handful of knuckles")
Relative insensitivity of palpable mass
Increasing mass size under observation
Bilateral pelvic findings
Nodular hepatomegaly, ascites, palpation of an omental "cake"

(Barber HRK, Hugh RK: Ovarian Carcinoma: Etiology, Diagnosis and Treatment. New York, Masson, 1978)

Ovarian carcinoma is surgically staged.[26] Surgery removes the tumor, allows identification of the primary site, determines the pattern of spread, and obtains tissue for histologic typing and grading.

In the early stages of ovarian carcinoma, no chemical, hematologic, or enzymatic abnormalities are noted; in advanced disease anemia, hypoalbuminemia, and an elevated lactate dehydrogenase level may be present.[26] Research continues on possible tumor markers, including carcinoembryonic antigen (CEA) and cancer antigen 125 (Ca-125).[23,147] The monoclonal antibody-based serum assay for Ca-125 is a reliable marker of tumor status; 80% of patients with epithelial tumors have elevated levels of Ca-125 using 35 units/ml as a normal reference value. Rising, stable, or falling levels correlate with tumor progression, stability, or regression in over 90% of patients. Monoclonal antibodies complementary to Ca-125 are also being studied. Ca 19-9 and NB/70K are examples. The use of such complementary assays may permit monitoring of the 20% of tumors not expressing Ca-125.[145] Known markers for germ cell tumors are α-fetoprotein (endodermal sinus tumors) and human chorionic gonadotropin (embryonal tumors and choriocarcinoma).[11,109]

Certain tests should be performed preoperatively (Table 56-5). Vaginal and, less frequently, cervical cytologic studies may detect abnormal cells of ovarian origin.[81,132]

Screening of 186 control patients at Roswell Park Hospital by *cul de sac* aspiration revealed only one case of ovarian neo-

TABLE 56–4
Staging of Ovarian Carcinoma

TNM	FIGO	DEFINITION
PRIMARY TUMOR (T)		
TX	FIGO	Primary tumor cannot be assessed
T0		No evidence of primary tumor
T1	I	Tumor limited to ovaries
T1a	Ia	Tumor limited to one ovary; capsule intact, no tumor on ovarian surface
T1b	Ib	Tumor limited to both ovaries; capsules intact, no tumor on ovarian surface
T1c	Ic	Tumor liminted to one or both ovaries with any of the following: capsule ruptured, tumor on ovarian surface, malignant cells in ascites, or peritoneal washing
T2	II	Tumor involves one or both ovaries with pelvic extension
T2a	IIa	Extension and/or implants on uterus and/or tube(s)
T2b	IIb	Extension to other pelvic tissues
T2c	IIc	Pelvic extension (2a or 2b) with malignant cells in ascites or peritoneal washing
T3 and/or N1	III	Tumor involves one or both ovaries with microscopically confirmed peritoneal metastasis outside the pelvis and/or regional lymph node metastasis
T3a	IIIA	Microscopic peritoneal metastasis beyond pelvis
T3b	IIIb	Macroscopic peritoneal metastasis beyond pelvis 2 cm or less in greatest dimension
T3c and/or N1	IIIc	Peritoneal metastasis beyond pelvis more than 2 cm in greatest dimension and/or regional lymph node metastasis
M1	IV	Distant metastasis (excludes peritoneal metastasis)

NOTE: Liver capsule metastasis is T3/Stage III, liver parenchymal metastasis M1/Stage IV. Pleural effusion must have positive cytology for M1/Stage IV.

REGIONAL LYMPH NODES (N)

Regional lymph nodes include hypogastric (obturator), common iliac, external iliac, internal iliac, lateral sacral, para-aortic, and inguinal.

NX	Regional lymph nodes cannot be assessed
N0	No regional lymph node metastasis
N1	Regional lymph node metastasis

TNM	FIGO	DEFINITION
DISTANT METASTASIS (M)		
MX		Presence of distant metastasis cannot be assessed
M0		No distant metastasis
M1	IV	Distant metastasis (excludes peritoneal metastasis)

NOTE: The presence of nonmalignant ascites is not classified. The presence of ascites does not affect staging unless malignant cells are present.

STAGE GROUPING

Stage IA	T1a	N0	M0
Stage IB	T1b	N0	M0
Stage IC	T1c	N0	M0
Stage IIA	T2a	N0	M0
Stage IIB	T2b	N0	M0
Stage IIC	T2c	N0	M0
Stage IIIA	T3a	N0	M0
Stage IIIB	T3b	N0	M0
Stage IIIC	T3c	N0	M0
	Any T	N1	M0
Stage IV	Any T	Any N	M1

(Beahrs OH, Henson DE, Hutter RVP, Meyers MH (eds): Cancer Manual for Staging of Cancer. 3rd ed. Philadelphia, JB Lippincott, 1988)

plasm—a teratoma.[80] A review of *cul de sac* lavage has shown only 1.2% positive cases. No cases of unsuspected ovarian carcinoma were detected.[102] Thus *cul de sac* aspiration is not recommended.

In a study by Gordon and associates, chest x-ray studies and full lung tomograms were performed on 139 and 75 patients, respectively, with ovarian carcinoma.[79] Only 17 (12.2%) abnormal and four ambiguous chest x-ray films were found. Ten (13.3%) tomograms were abnormal and two were ambiguous. It was concluded that linear tomograms are not indicated when the chest x-ray film is normal.

A barium enema is helpful in identifying primary bowel carcinoma or secondary bowel involvement by ovarian carcinoma. Abnormal findings in double-contrast barium studies to detect serosal spread were reported in nine (42.8%) of 21 new patients.[26] This study is not routinely recommended; however, it is useful to know whether there is impending obstruction.

Abnormal excreting urograms were reported in eight (11%) of 74 patients who underwent the procedure as part of the initial workup. Hydronephrosis was bilateral in one case and unilateral in seven cases. Seven of these eight patients had Stage III disease or greater.[90]

Ultrasonography is a helpful adjunct in the preoperative assessment of a pelvic mass. Generally, benign lesions are cystic without septae, whereas tumors with solid components or multiple internal echoes are considered malignant.[26] Accuracy is high, with 13 (92.8%) of 14 and 138 (87.5%) of 158 carcinomas accurately predicted in two separate studies.[45,169]

TABLE 56–5
Preoperative Studies in Ovarian Carcinoma

GENERAL
History
Physical examination

RADIOLOGIC STUDIES

STANDARD
Chest x-ray
Barium enema
Intravenous pyelography

OPTIONAL
Ultrasonography
CT scan—magnetic resonance
Upper GI series
Lymphangiography

SPECIAL PROCEDURES
Sigmoidoscopic examination
Cervical Papanicolaou smear

LABORATORY STUDIES
Admission CBC, platelets, urinalysis
Prothrombin time, partial prothrombin time
SMA-12

(Buchsbaum HJ, Lifshitz S: Semin Oncol 11:227, 1984)

Computed tomography (CT) has recently been used in assessing ovarian tumors. Although superior in detecting upper abdominal and retroperitoneal disease, its accuracy in the pelvis has not been significantly better than that of ultrasonography.[26] CT often misses serosal nodules less than 2 cm in diameter and often does not distinguish between tumor and fixed loops of bowel.[221] However, carefully performed scanning on state-of-the-art equipment may produce a higher accuracy in documenting persistent or recurrent macroscopic tumor.[130] Magnetic resonance imaging (MRI) is also being used to assess the abdomen and pelvis.

Lymphangiography (LAG) has been used to detect pelvic and periaortic lymph node metastases. In 289 consecutive patients on whom LAG was performed, Musumeci and associates[140] found evidence of nodal metastases in 88 (30%) patients. Table 56-6 presents the percentage of abnormal findings on LAG studies according to clinical stage. Pelvic nodes alone were involved in 54% of the patients; in 18%, only the periaortic chains were involved. In 28% of patients both chains were involved simultaneously. Bilateral nodal involvement was found in 63% of the cases with abnormal findings. The radiologic/histologic correlation in patients undergoing retroperitoneal node biopsies was 100% in LAG-abnormal cases. In LAG-normal cases the correlation was 81% (19% false-negative rate). Overall, the accuracy of LAG diagnosis with aortic node dissection or biopsy was 87%.

Bone scans and skeletal surveys were obtained in 104 patients with ovarian carcinoma.[133] Only four patients in the entire series had bone metastases. It was concluded that bone scan and bone survey are not indicated as a screening procedure in asymptomatic patients. Likewise, the same authors concluded that it is not necessary to do a liver/spleen scan when liver chemistries are normal.[132]

PATHOLOGIC CLASSIFICATION

The World Health Organization (WHO) and the International Federation of Gynecology and Obstetrics (FIGO) have adopted a uniform classification of the common epithelial, sex cord-stromal, and germ cell tumors (Table 56-7).[221]

Most ovarian malignancies are epithelial in origin (85% to 90%). Of these, Young and associates[221] reported that serous cystadenocarcinomas constitute 42%; mucinous cystadenocarcinomas constitute 12%; endometrial carcinomas, 15%; undifferentiated carcinomas, 17%; and clear cell carcinomas, 6%. Einhorn and co-workers[64] and Mor-Josef and colleagues[135] reported a similar distribution by histologic class. Day and associates[42] found that more anaplastic tumors were frequently assigned to the serous group because of the inability to identify mucinous or endometrioid components. Primary sex cord-stromal and germ cell tumors account for less than 10% of all ovarian malignancies.

TABLE 56–6
Results of Lymphangiography According to Clinical Stage in Ovarian Carcinoma

		POSITIVE LYMPHANGIOGRAPHY	
STAGE	**NO. OF CASES**	NO. OF CASES	PERCENT
IA	34	2	6 } 8
IB	12	2	17 }
IC	5		
IIB	7		
IIC	3		
III	90	26	29
IV	15	8	53
Recurrence	99	46	46
Restaging NED	24	4	17
Total	289	88	30

NED: no evidence of disease
(Musumeci R. Bonfi A, Bolis G, et al: Cancer 40:1444, 1977)

TABLE 56–7
World Health Organization Classification of Malignant Ovarian Tumors

COMMON EPITHELIAL TUMORS

- Malignant serous tumors
  - Adenocarcinoma, papillary adenocarcinoma, papillary cystadenocarcinoma
  - Surface papillary carcinoma
  - Malignant adenofibroma, cystadenofibroma
- Malignant mucinous tumors
  - Adenocarcinoma, cystadenocarcinoma
  - Malignant adenofibroma, cystadenofibroma
- Malignant endometrioid tumors
  - Carcinoma
    - Adenocarcinoma
    - Adenocanthoma
    - Malignant adenofibroma, cystadenofibroma
  - Endometrioid stromal sarcomas
  - Mesodermal (müllerian) mixed tumors, homologous and heterologous
- Clear cell (mesonephroid) tumors
  - Malignant
  - Malignant carcinoma and adenocarcinoma
- Brenner tumors
  - Malignant
- Mixed epithelial tumors
  - Malignant
- Undifferentiated carcinoma
- Unclassified epithelial tumors

SEX CORD—STROMAL TUMORS

- Granulosa–stromal cell tumors
  - Granulosa cell tumor
  - Tumors in the thecoma-fibroma group
  - Fibroma
  - Unclassified

SEX CORD–STROMAL TUMORS (CONTINUED)

- Androblastomas: Sertoli-Leydig cell tumors
  - Well-differentiated
    - Tubular androblastoma, Sertoli cell tumor (tubular adenoma of Pick)
    - Tubular androblastoma with lipid storage, Sertoli cell tumor with lipid storage (folliculome lipidique of Lecene)
    - Sertoli-Leydig cell tumor (tubular adenoma with Leydig cells)
    - Leydig cell tumor, hilus cell tumor
  - Of intermediate differentiation
  - Poorly differentiated (sarcomatoid)
  - With heterologous elements
- Gynandroblastoma
- Unclassified

LIPID (LIPOID) CELL AND GERM CELL TUMORS

- Dysgerminoma
- Endodermal sinus tumor
- Embryonal carcinoma
- Polyembryoma
- Choriocarcinoma
- Teratomas
  - Immature
  - Mature dermoid cyst with malignant transformation
  - Monodermal and highly specialized
    - Struma ovarii
    - Carcinoid
    - Struma ovarii and carcinoid
    - Others
- Mixed forms

GONADOBLASTOMA

- Pure
- Mixed with dysgerminoma or other form of germ cell tumor

(Serov SF, Scully RE, Solvin LH: International histological classification of tumors, No. 9. Histological Typing of Ovarian Tumors. Geneva, World Health Organization)

Mucinous and endometrioid carcinomas show higher cumulative survival rates, but this may be attributed to early detection (Fig. 56-2).[64] Similar results were reported by Dembo and Rush,[54] who ascribed the mucinous, endometrioid, and clear cell pathology subtypes to be favorable pathologies, regardless of grade. In contrast, only the well-differentiated serous tumors were favorable. In another paper, they described only the well-differentiated clear cell subtypes as favorable; however, only six patients had this histology and grade.[58] Others also reported that mucinous carcinomas have a favorable prognosis, with a 5-year survival rate of 55% to 70%.[42,139] Recently transitional cell carcinoma has been recognized as a distinct histologic type of ovarian carcinoma. Because of its favorable response to chemotherapy, improved patient survival is noted.[171]

"Tumors of borderline malignancy," which account for approximately 15% of all epithelial cancers, are often referred to as *proliferative cystadenomas.* A 10-year survival rate of approximately 95% has been reported. However, symptomatic recurrence and death may occur 20 years after therapy in a few patients.[62,221]

Sex cord-stromal tumors contain granulosa, theca, Sertoli, Leydig, and collagen-producing stromal cells or their embryonic precursors. The granulosa cell-containing tumor is seen most frequently. It generally is diagnosed at an earlier stage owing to tumor-related estrogen production and has an indo-

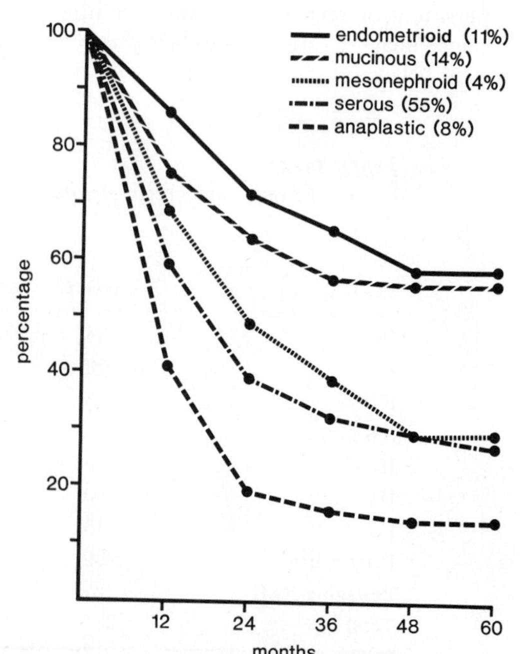

FIGURE 56–2. Carcinoma of the ovary, 1974–1979 (770 patients). Five-year cumulative survival rate for each histologic class. (Einhorn N, Milsson B, Sjovall K: Cancer 55:2019, 1985)

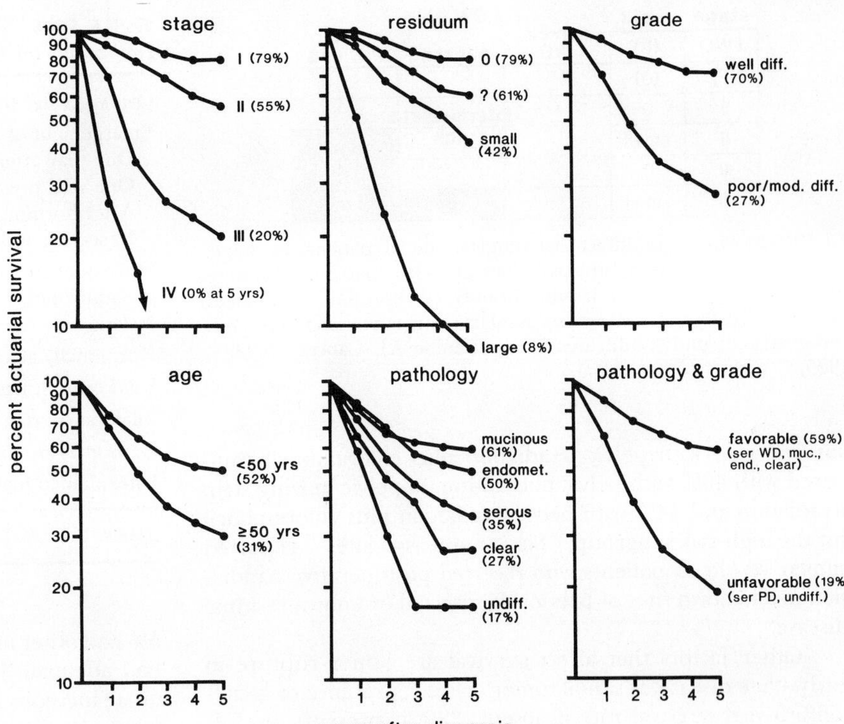

FIGURE 56–3. Univariate representation of survival by stage, residuum, grade, age, and pathology with and without grade. (Dembo AJ, Bush RS: Int J Radiat Oncol Biol Phys 8:893, 1982)

lent course. Late recurrences can sometimes be effectively managed by repeated surgery or chemotherapy.[221]

Germ cell tumors often have a mixed histology; treatment is designed to treat the most malignant component of the tumor. Malignant embyronal carcinoma, endodermal sinus tumors, and malignant teratomas have extremely poor prognoses. Aggressive surgery, irradiation, and chemotherapy are advocated.[221]

Most reports deal with epithelial carcinomas; prognosis, management, therapy techniques, and results are dealt with in the following sections. The less common sex cord-stromal and germ cell tumors are discussed where appropriate.

PROGNOSTIC FACTORS

In addition to pathologic type, stage of disease, grade of tumor, patient age, and residual bulk of disease after surgery have been extensively assessed as independent and interdependent prognostic factors (Fig. 56-3).[28,42,54,58,62,64,135,139,150,179,204] Dembo and Bush[54] made a first approximation at classifying patients into poor and good prognostic groups on the basis of stage and residuum. Many patients have been added after their original study, yielding the curve shown in Figure 56-4.[28] Patients with poor prognoses had either Stage IV disease or large residual tumor masses; very few (approximately 10%) survived 5 years. Neither irradiation nor chemotherapy (single agent or combination) has shown ability to cure in these patients; chemotherapy is the treatment of choice for palliation.[28,54]

Patients with good prognoses had Stage I, Stage II, or Stage III disease with no or uncertain residual disease and Stage II and Stage III disease with complete BSOH and small residual masses (less than 2 cm). The 5-year survival rate in this group was 61%. In an attempt to further define this group, a subgrouping was designed, incorporating pathology and grade of tumor (Fig. 56-5). The low-risk patients had Stage I well-differentiated cancer with a 5-year survival rate of approximately 95%. In the intermediate group, approximately one third of the patients were found to have relapsed, whereas in the high-risk groups patients relapsed 80% of the time (5-year survival rates of 75% and 30%, respectively). In all cases, age had a significant impact on prognosis; patients 50 years of age or older did much worse.[54] Regardless of postoperative therapy, the intermediate subgroup had a better 5-year survival rate—80% with pelvic plus abdominopelvic moving strip irradiation and 48% 5-year

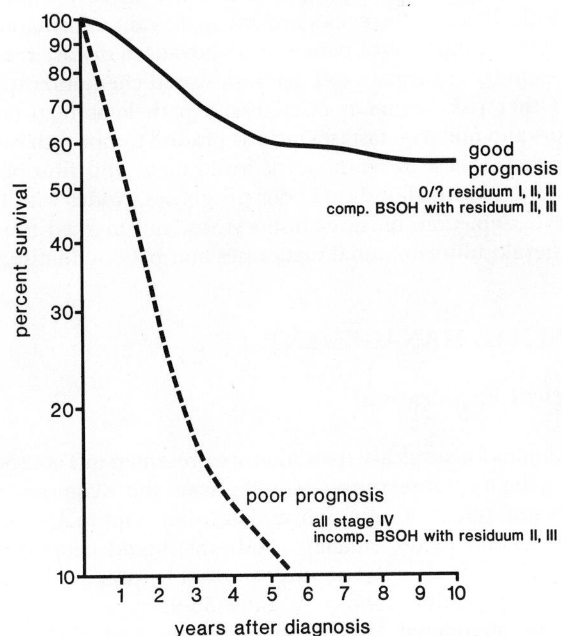

FIGURE 56–4. Actuarial survival of 810 patients seen at the Princess Margaret Hospital between April 1971 and December 1978. ? indicates uncertainty as to whether all identifiable disease has been removed (comp BSOH: complete bilateral salpingo-oophorectomy; incomp BSOH: incomplete bilateral salpingo-oophorectomy) (Bush RS: Radiology 153:17, 1984)

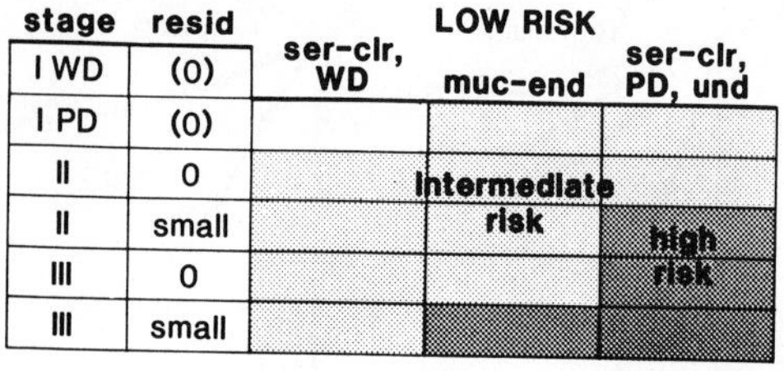

stage	resid	ser-clr, WD	LOW RISK muc-end	ser-clr, PD, und
I WD	(0)			
I PD	(0)			
II	0		Intermediate	
II	small		risk	high
III	0			risk
III	small			

FIGURE 56–5. A multifactorial subgrouping of patients by stage, postoperative residuum, and pathology/grade for patients who were treated with postoperative irradiation only. (WD: well differentiated; PD: poorly differentiated; ser: serous; clr: clear; muc: mucinous; end: endometrioid; und: undifferentiated) (Dembo AJ: Cancer 55:2285, 1985)

survival rate with pelvic irradiation plus chlorambucil compared with 40% with pelvic plus abdominopelvic moving strip irradiation and 14% with pelvic irradiation plus chlorambucil for the high-risk subgroup.[54] Schray and associates[179] reported similar results in patients who received postoperative irradiation to all known sites of previously resected or known residual disease.

Other factors that affect survival are tumor rupture in early-stage disease, residual tumor volume, presence of ascites (56% 5-year survival rate if absent; 22% if present), performance status (51% 5-year survival rate with normal activities and no symptoms; 12% with activities considerably limited by symptoms), and degree of weight loss in preceding year (45% 5-year survival rate with no weight loss; 26% with weight loss of 9 kg or more).[204] Recently, tumor ploidy as determined by flow cytometry (FCM) has emerged as a major prognostic factor in advanced ovarian carcinoma. Diploid tumors are associated with longer survival, even when a relapse has occurred. They show a better response to first-line chemotherapy, as well as to salvage therapy, than do nondiploid tumors.[177] Mitotic activity index (MAI), volume percentage epithelium (VPE), mean nuclear area (MNA), and FCM features such as cellular DNA content have also added prognostic criteria. These in combination with clinical features can provide significant information to predict the prognosis of patients with advanced disease treated with debulking surgery and platinum-based chemotherapy.[217]

Other risk factors associated with pathologic features of tumors and nodal metastases include grade 3 tumor with vascular invasion, lack of lymphocytic infiltration, and fibroblastic proliferation, which indicate poor prognoses. Nodes with lymphocyte depletion, no sinus histiocytosis, and marked fibrosis also herald ultimate nodal metastases and patient demise.[35,36]

GENERAL MANAGEMENT

Surgical Exploration

Indications for surgical exploration are presented in Table 56-8. The primary surgery not only confirms the diagnosis, but delineates tumor localization and burden. Optimal surgical cytoreduction to the smallest residuum should be performed.[6,26,50,84,87,192,216,221] The surgeon must be prepared to perform the procedures shown in Table 56-9.

The abdominal incision should be vertical, midline, or paramedian, extending from the symphysis pubis to at least halfway between the umbilicus and the xyphoid. Cephalad extension of this incision may be necessary. Piver and co-workers[162] found that 65% of the women had midline subum-

TABLE 56–8
Indications for Exploratory Surgery for Ovarian Carcinoma

Ovary greater than 7 cm in diameter
Enlargement of an "at-rest" ovary:
- One year after menopause
- One year preceding menarche
- After hormonal suppression therapy (oral contraceptives)
- In second and third trimester of pregnancy

Ovarian enlargement thought to be functional that persists after gonadotropin suppression therapy or through one or two menstrual cycles
Hormonally active ovarian neoplasm
Solid ovarian neoplasm
Bilateral ovarian neoplasms (excluding theca-lutein cysts)
Signs or symptoms suggesting torsion or rupture of an ovarian cyst
Unexplained malignant ascites

(Johnson GH: Clin Obstet Gynecol 22:903, 1979)

3% had other inadequate incisions; they believed that only 17% had adequate incisions. Young and colleagues[223] found adequate incisions in only 25% of cases referred for further treatment after initial surgery.

If ascitic fluid is present, it must be aspirated and sent for cytologic evaluation (cell block and smear). If no fluid is present, approximately 200 ml of normal saline should be instilled into the peritoneal cavity, allowed to circulate for 3 to 5 minutes, then aspirated. Each washing should be placed in a separate container so that specific sites of tumor-positive cells can be identified. Keettel and associates[102] found overall malignant cells on cytologic examination in 78.5% of 408 patients with ovarian cancer, higher than the 53.5% reported by Creasman and Rutledge.[41] Peritoneal washings were positive in 91.2% of 114 patients with Stage II or Stage III disease. The overall percentage of positive findings on cytology for Stage IA, IB, and IC tumors was 45.5%.[102] Yoshimura and co-workers[220] noted positive peritoneal cytologic findings in 46 (49%) of 94 patients with all stages. Only 18% of Stage I and Stage II tumors had positive cytology compared with 78% of higher stage tumors.

When the abdomen is entered, a biopsy must be performed on all adhesions between the parietal peritoneum and intestine or between loops of bowel; all serosal surfaces are carefully
bilical incisions, 15% had transverse Pfannenstiel incisions, and

TABLE 56–9
Primary Surgical Procedures for Ovarian Carcinoma

Vertical incision
Ascites or peritoneal washings for cytologic examination
Lysis of adhesions
Palpation, visualization, and biopsy of diaphragm
Examination of visceral and parietal peritoneum
Omentectomy
Periaortic and pelvic lymph node sampling
Total abdominal hysterectomy, bilateral salpingo-oophorectomy, and appendectomy
Cytoreductive surgery

(Buchsbaum HJ, Lifshitz S: Semin Oncol 11:227, 1984)

examined, with special attention to the undersurfaces of the diaphragm. The Gynecologic Oncology Group (GOG) is conducting protocol no. 41 to determine the patterns of spread in early ovarian carcinoma, Stage I, Stage II, and Stage III. In three (4.2%) of 72 patients thought to be clinically free from disease, tumor was found on random biopsies of the diaphragm.[26] Piver and associates[160] reviewed the incidence of diaphragmatic metastases and found an overall incidence of 15.7% (11.3% for Stage I and 23% for Stage II).

Another study[129] of 291 women with primary ovarian cancer showed that only 52% and 35%, respectively, of patients operated on by obstetricians/gynecologists and general surgeons were adequately evaluated, compared with 97% of the cases operated on by gynecologic oncologists. Piver and coworkers[162] found detailed descriptions of the diaphragm, liver, gallbladder, pancreas, kidneys, stomach, jejunum, ileum, colon, omentum, and aortic nodes in only 24% of patients reviewed, minimal description in 47%, and no description in 29%.

An infracolic omentectomy should routinely be performed. This procedure is supported by GOG data that show microscopic metastases in seven (8.9%) of 78 of cases in which the omentum was clinically negative.[26] Piver and associates,[160] however, reported only 2.7% unsuspected omental metastases for Stage I and Stage II disease. A total omentectomy should be performed for gross involvement with tumor.

Biopsy of the periaortic nodes at the level of the insertion of the ovarian arteries should be performed whether or not they are clinically suspicious. In addition, pelvic lymphadenectomy or biopsies of common, external, and internal iliac and obturator chains should be performed.[26] Pelvic nodes are reported to be involved in 8.1% of patients with Stage I disease.[160]

After appropriate staging procedures have been done, a total abdominal hysterectomy and bilateral salpingo-oophorectomy and appendectomy should be performed. Exceptions to this rule may be made in young patients who desire to retain fertility and who have borderline or well-differentiated Stage I tumor. In older patients there is a significant chance of tumor involving both ovaries simultaneously (9% to 43%).[27,139] An adenocarcinoma arising in the appendix may easily mimic ovarian cancer; for this reason an appendectomy is performed.

Cytoreductive Surgery

Cytoreductive (debulking) surgery is of major prognostic importance in ovarian carcinoma. The extent of surgery clearly depends on the spread and location of the cancer as well as the experience and judgment of the surgeon.[216]

Bowel resection in disseminated carcinoma is controversial.[32] Buchsbaum and Lifshitz[26] believe that resection of the intestines is appropriate. Hudson and Chir[97] described a radical procedure that allows intact removal of an ovarian tumor fixed in the pelvis with the whole of the peritoneum from surrounding structures still attached (including a segment of the rectum, if necessary). Blythe and Wahl[18] concluded that intestinal and bowel resection, including colostomy, did not decrease quality of life but prolonged life.

Resection of the lower urinary tract may be necessary during cytoreductive surgery. Berek and associates[14] reported on 24 patients who had either partial cystectomy, reimplantation of the ureters, or ureteral resection. Despite significant complications in 25% of the patients, the authors concluded that limited resection of the lower urinary tract may be justified to achieve optimum residuum because the patients survived longer.

Second-Look Procedures

Indications for second-look procedures are presented in Table 56-10. These operations are performed mainly to evaluate therapy results in advanced disease (Stage III and Stage IV).[15,82,167,195,196,205] When the second-look laparotomy is performed, complete exploration of the peritoneal cavity as described for the primary operation should be performed.[114] Similar recommendations are given in a recent review by Rubin.[176] If hysterectomy, bilateral salpingo-oophorectomy, and omentectomy could not be performed initially, excision of these structures should be done, if possible.[26] Stage of disease, grade of tumor, and the initial amount of residual disease have an impact on the findings at second-look laparotomy (Table 56-11). The 5-year survival rate is related to the amount of residual disease found at second-look laparotomy (Table 56-12).

Smith and Rutledge[196] reported on 103 patients who had a complete or almost complete response to chemotherapy. Sixty-five percent survived an additional 2 years, and 34% survived 5 years after second-look surgery. Overall, they concluded that patients for whom it was possible to remove all or almost all of the remaining cancer benefited by second-look surgery. Greco and co-workers[82] found that 17 (38.8%) of 45 patients who had second-look operations after combination chemotherapy had no evidence of residual tumor; nine (20%) had all known tumor resected. Sixteen of 17 patients remained in remission from 9 to 30 months. Berek and associates[15] found that optimal secondary resection (largest residual mass less than 1.5 cm) improved survival. This group had a median survival of 20 months in contrast to 5 months for the nonoptimal secondary cytoreductive surgery. When less than 1000 ml of ascites was present, median survival was 18 months compared with 5 months when more than 1000 ml was present.

Similar results were found by Tepper and co-workers[205] after combined irradiation and chemotherapy. None of the 17 patients had enough regression to allow gross total removal of tumor; all patients had microscopic disease. The 3-year survival rate was 41%. In a study conducted between 1962 and 1971, 21 (72.4%) of 29 patients able to have complete removal of residual disease at second-look surgery survived, 14 without evidence of disease.[193] Schwartz and Smith[184] reported a 27% 5-year sur-

TABLE 56–10
Indications for Second-Look Procedures

Accuracy in staging when initial operation has not clearly defined spread of disease
Cytoreductive surgery after course of radiation therapy or chemotherapy
Excision of recurrent disease
Removal of retained ovaries after complete tumor disappearance by clinical evaluations
Removal of residual tumor following reduction of tumor mass by chemotherapy or radiation therapy
Assessment of tumor status in patients who have completed initial course of treatment and demonstrate no clinical evidence of tumor by nonoperative means (it is the latter situation to which the term "second-look operation" should be applied)
Modification of subsequent treatment according to surgical findings (*i.e.*, prevent premature cessation of chemotherapy or prevent risks from needless chemotherapy)

(Smith JP, Rutledge FN: Natl Cancer Inst Monogr 42:141, 1975)

TABLE 56–11
Percent Negative at Second-Look Laparotomy

BY STAGE (1034 PATIENTS)		BY HISTOLOGIC GRADE (556 PATIENTS)		BY RESIDUAL DISEASE AT INITIAL SURGERY (753 PATIENTS)	
STAGE	PERCENT NEGATIVE	GRADE	PERCENT NEGATIVE	AMOUNT OF RESIDUAL DISEASE	PERCENT NEGATIVE
I	80	1	61	None	77
II	68	1	50	Optimal*	45
III, IV	33	3	41	Suboptimal*	25

**Definition varies in original reports.*
(Rubin SC: Oncology 1:47, 1987)

vival rate for patients who underwent total removal of residual disease at second-look surgery. They reported a 29.5% 5-year survival rate when less than 2 cm of residuum was left and a 9% 5-year survival rate when more than 2 cm remained. All patients had received prior chemotherapy. Copeland and associates[39] evaluated the prognosis of 50 of 246 patients who had microscopically positive second-look laparotomies. Analysis of recurrence, progression-free interval, and survival rates suggested that age—not more that 40 years—grade of tumor, and cytologic findings were prognostically significant. For example, patients with grade 3 disease had a 5-year survival rate of 36% compared with 79% for patients with grade 2 and 100% for patients with grade 1 disease.

Lippman and colleagues[114] found only stage and optimal disease (<2 cm residual size) after initial surgery to be significantly associated with absence of disease at second-look laparotomy. Actuarial survival after second-look laparotomy was associated with residual tumor size. Survival rate at 3 years was 80.7% ± 13.4% for no pathologic evidence of disease, 49.1% ± 13.1% for microscopic disease plus 2 cm or less of residual disease, and 29.5% ± 11.4% for gross residual disease (>2 cm). Only Raju and colleagues[167] found no statistically significant improvement in survival rate whether complete (20% 3-year survival rate) or incomplete (43% 3-year survival rate) secondary cytoreduction was performed after combination chemotherapy.

Others have examined the role of second-look laparoscopy or peritoneoscopy to evaluate the status of disease following therapy.[13, 123, 149, 163, 175, 194] Although a positive finding may spare a significant number of patients a formal laparotomy, no evidence of persistent malignancy requires second-look surgery before chemotherapy is discontinued. If the laparoscopy discloses localized residual disease, a laparotomy may be indicated because patients who have gross disease removed survive longer.[184] Overall, false-negative rates vary from 20% to 70%, and the inability to visualize the entire peritoneal cavity is high, primarily because of adhesions (6% to 24%). Berek and associates[13] noted serious sequelae (bowel perforation and hemorrhage) requiring laparotomy in 14% of their patients. Ozols and co-workers[149] reported serious sequelae in only 3% but self-limiting sequelae in 15%, for a total rate of 18%.

TABLE 56–12
Findings at Second-Look Operation Versus Survival in Patients with Ovarian Carcinoma

TUMOR VOLUME FOUND AT SECOND-LOOK OPERATION	5-YEAR SURVIVAL RATE (%)
None	80
Microscopic	50
Macroscopic	18

(Lippman SM, Alberts DS, Slymen DJ, et al: Cancer 61:2571, 1988)

Computed tomography (CT) has been tried as an alternative to second-look surgery. The false-negative rate has been high, ranging from 17.7% to 50%.[22, 200] Both studies found that CT could not be used instead of surgery. In a recent study[130] only three false negatives were seen in 19 patients; these patients were studied using newer equipment. Using older equipment, the same authors reported 11 false-negative results in 20 patients.

Adjuvant Therapy for Epithelial Ovarian Carcinoma

Radiation Therapy

The role of postoperative radiation therapy in epithelial ovarian carcinoma is controversial. Young and associates[221] point out that long-term survival data indicate that the natural history and selection of therapy depend on the amount of residual disease as well as on stage of disease. Discussion therefore is generally separated into two categories: (1) Stage I, Stage II, and Stage III with minimal residual disease and (2) advanced Stage III and Stage IV disease or any stage with bulky residual disease. Many studies, however, combine all stages.

Dembo[52] reviewed the use of radiation therapy for ovarian carcinoma and concluded that grade is the most important prognostic factor for Stage IA disease. The Princess Margaret Hospital study conducted between 1971 and 1977 showed no benefit from postoperative pelvic irradiation compared with observation alone. The nine relapses recorded in this study occurred outside the radiation field and were in the 30 patients with grade 2 or grade 3 tumors. No relapses occurred in the 24 patients with well-differentiated tumor. When treatment is indicated, therefore, the whole peritoneal cavity should be included in the fields.

Hreshchyshyn and associates[96] reported the results of a GOG study conducted between 1971 and 1978 and also found no benefit from postoperative pelvic irradiation in Stage IA grade 1 tumors. Powlis and co-workers[165] also concluded that no postoperative therapy is recommended for these tumors unless ascites or cytologic evidence of peritoneal disease is present. Webb and colleagues[212] reported that no difference was noted in survival in patients with Stage IA grade 1 tumors whether or not surgery was complete or whether or not postoperative irradiation was given. Wharton and associates[215] reviewed the use of chemotherapy and radiation therapy in the treatment of ovarian carcinoma and concluded that patients with FIGO Stage IA grade 1 carcinoma can be cured by surgical excision. They also recommend no postoperative therapy for patients with early-stage tumors of low malignant potential (borderline tumors) with minimal residual disease outside the ovary. Recently, however, 50 Stage I patients (including 20 patients with Stage IA, grade 1 carcinomas) received six to 11 courses of adjuvant melphalan (Alkeran). The actuarial survival rates of the 50 patients were 98% at 2 years and 94% at 5 years, suggesting a benefit from that therapy.[76]

It is generally agreed that patients with Stage I ovarian cancer other than Stage IA grade 1 require adjuvant therapy.[52,96,165,204] Postoperative therapy has consisted of external-beam radiation therapy, intraperitoneal instillation of radioactive colloidal gold (^{198}Au) or chromic phosphate (^{32}P), or systemic chemotherapy. Studies have shown that abdominopelvic irradiation is superior to pelvic irradiation alone.[28,55,57,155,206] Fuks and Bagshaw[73] noted that failure occurred outside the pelvis, in either the lymph nodes or in the upper abdomen (approximately 20%). Piver and associates[160] found that Stage 1 patients had 11.3% diaphragmatic and 13.3% periaortic metastases. In a review of pelvic irradiation given for Stage II ovarian carcinoma, long-term survival was not achieved in a significant number of patients (53% 5-year survival rate). Abdominopelvic irradiation or chemotherapy is recommended over pelvic irradiation.[206]

Patients with Stage II or Stage III disease with minimal or no residual disease after surgery are best managed with abdominopelvic irradiation[28,51,52,56,126,206] or chemotherapy.[194,221] These patients constitute the intermediate-risk group proposed by Dembo and Bush[54] and have either mucinous or endometrioid tumors. Included also are patients with Stage II grade 3 serous and clear cell tumors who have no residual disease after surgery. Dembo[51] reports a 5-year survival rate of approximately 70% in this group. Macbeth and associates,[121] however, report a significantly worse 57% 5-year survival rate. They found a strong correlation between histologic grade and survival. Klaassen and associates[103] report a similar result with a 62% 5-year survival rate with total abdominopelvic irradiation. Stage, grade, and histology were predictors of survival in this study. Martinez and associates[126] believe their data establish postoperative abdominopelvic irradiation (by the Martinez technique) as the standard for favorable ovarian carcinoma. Their favorable group is similar to the good prognosis group of Dembo; that is, these patients have no residual disease or single or multiple masses smaller than 2 cm in its largest dimension. This group had a 66% freedom-from-relapse rate at 5 years. As in other studies, stage, histology, and age under 40 years were indicative of statistically significant improvement in freedom from relapse.

Chromic phosphate was instilled postoperatively in patients with Stage I, II, or III completely resected tumors. A second group had the instillation after chemotherapy and second-look laparotomy yielded microscopic lesions or lesions less than 3 mm. All of the first group and 61.5% of the second group were free from relapse at 30 and 28.5 months, respectively.[168]

Smith and associates[197] compared abdominopelvic irradiation with single-agent chemotherapy (melphalan) and found equal survival rates at 5 years (approximately 71.5%). However, Dembo[52] believed that patients with more favorable disease (Stage I and Stage IIA) were in the chemotherapy arm, and information was not provided on comparisons of the treatment arms with respect to tumor grade or the presence of macroscopic tumor residuum. Dembo also believed that differing irradiation techniques between Princess Margaret Hospital and M. D. Anderson Cancer Center (mainly adequate coverage of the diaphragm) account for these results; shorter fields and the use of liver shielding with the moving strip technique may have provided a sanctuary site. Potish and colleagues[164] administered postoperative abdominopelvic radiation therapy and chemotherapy (melphalan) sequentially for Stage I and Stage II disease. They noted only possible improved survival for Stages IIB and IIC; the 5-year survival rate was 64%. Ballon and associates[9] treated patients with pelvic irradiation followed by doxorubicin (Adriamycin) and cyclophosphamide.

Klaassen and associates[103] found that abdominopelvic irradiation, melphalan, or intraperitoneal ^{32}P for treatment of early stage ovarian carcinoma yielded equal 5-year survival rates of approximately 62%. All patients were initially treated with pelvic irradiation. The ^{32}P arm was closed early because of toxicity reactions.

For patients at high risk for recurrence of ovarian carcinoma because of unfavorable histologic characteristics, high grade, and large residuum, the Princess Margaret Hospital has used a combined modality approach since 1981: six courses of combination chemotherapy (CAP = cyclophosphamide, doxorubicin [Adriamycin], cisplatin) followed by abdominopelvic radiation therapy (Fig. 56-6). Results from this approach suggest a longer disease-free survival.[51]

Patients with Stage III or Stage IV disease with macroscopic residual disease are usually treated with combined modalities. Fuks and associates[74] were the first to attempt to improve survival rates in such patients by systematically using surgery, combination chemotherapy, second-look cytoreductive surgery, and abdominopelvic radiation therapy. This aggressive therapy was tolerated with acceptable toxicity.

Hainsworth and associates[88] used abdominopelvic irradiation on 17 patients with advanced ovarian carcinoma who had minimal residual intraabdominal disease after 6 months of combination chemotherapy. Fourteen have had relapse at a median of 8 months after completion of radiation therapy. However, patients who received the entire planned dose of radiation therapy had longer disease-free survival times (median, 14 months) than did patients receiving only partial doses (median, 7 months).

The current protocol at the Princess Margaret Hospital for patients with Stage IV as well as those with large-residuum Stage II and Stage III disease is shown in Figure 56-6. It attempts to determine the relative efficacy of chemotherapy and radiation therapy after a favorable response to chemotherapy and surgery.

One report was designed to evaluate preoperative irradia-

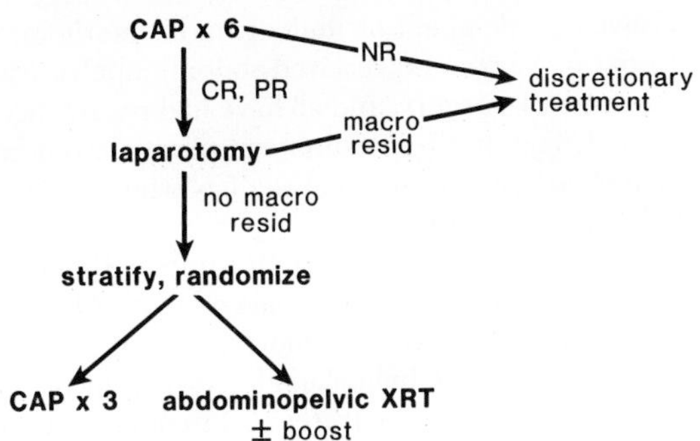

FIGURE 56–6. Combined modality protocol at the Princess Margaret Hospital. (NR: no response; PR: partial response; CR: complete response; CAP: cyclophosphamide, Adriamycin, cisplatin)

tion in large inoperable tumors fixed to surrounding tissues. Lower abdominal fields (upper margin between L3 and L4) were used in hopes of decreasing tumor volume. Some patients also received intracavitary irradiation to increase the intrapelvic dose. The 5-year survival rate among this group was 27%, with a 46% and 50% survival rate in Stages IIB and IIC, respectively, 22% in Stage III, and 0% in Stage IV. It must be kept in mind that this group as a whole belongs to an unfavorable cohort.[189]

Intraperitoneal ^{32}P was instilled as salvage therapy in 23 patients after second- or third-look laparotomy. These patients had previously received an average of ten cycles of chemotherapy. The patients were divided into those with microscopic residual disease, those with completely resected macroscopic residual disease, and those with macroscopic residual disease of less than 0.5 cm. The disease-free survival rate was 54% at 2 years and 27% at 4 years. Patients with no gross residual disease had a 27-month median survival compared with 9 months for patients with macroscopic residual disease.[198]

A later study reports the results of ^{32}P instillation after initial surgery, chemotherapy, and second-look laparotomy.[210] Of the 57 patients with no evidence of disease, 43 received 15 mCi ^{32}P immediately postoperatively. In 29 patients, microscopic or minimal residual disease (<2 cm) was found. Seven received ^{32}P, ten received ^{32}P and further chemotherapy, and 12 received chemotherapy alone. Both groups of patients who received ^{32}P had a 4-year survival rate after second-look laparotomy of 89% compared with 67% for those not receiving ^{32}P. The result was most dramatic in the minimal residual group—59% *versus* 22%. The conclusion was that ^{32}P helps survival in patients with no disease or minimal disease at second-look laparotomy. It was also concluded that patients with higher than Stage I grade 1 tumors were at high risk for failure after negative second-look laparotomy.

In a study conducted between 1970 and 1980, 50 patients were treated sequentially with six cycles of IV phenylalanine mustard (L-PAM), second-look laparotomy, and moving strip abdominopelvic irradiation. All 16 Stage I and Stage II patients survived 5 years with no evidence of disease (NED). Of the 37 Stage III patients, 26% did not respond to L-PAM, 48% were partial responders, and 26% were complete responders. Twenty-two percent of the partial responders were NED at 5 years compared with 100% of the complete responders. Factors contributing to long-term survival were residual disease at initial surgery, histology, grade, and complete response to L-PAM. It was believed that radiation therapy was relevant and may have been the factor in maintaining the complete response in patients with Stages II and III disease and in converting some partial responders into long-term survivors.[144] Hoskins and associates[95] report on eight Stage III patients with residual disease of less than 1 cm at second-look laparotomy. All but one had less than 3 cm residual disease after initial surgery, and all had received single-agent or multiagent chemotherapy (seven to 13 courses). All patients received abdominopelvic irradiation after second-look surgery, and all have had recurrences. Many patients had major gastrointestinal complications requiring surgery. These authors are some of the few who do not advocate irradiation in this setting.[95]

Rizel and associates[170] report on combined-modality therapy for 38 Stage III ovarian carcinoma patients. All patients had initial surgery with maximal tumor reduction, CHAD (cyclophosphamide, hexamethylmelamine, doxorubicin, cisplatin) combination chemotherapy (three to 14 courses), second-look laparotomy, and abdominopelvic irradiation. Of the 22 patients with large residual tumor (>2 cm) 91% responded partially or completely to chemotherapy. Twenty-eight patients had a second attempt at cytoreductive surgery. Twenty-one patients completed the radiation therapy. The actuarial survival rate for the whole group was 43% at 3 years (70% for the group with minimal residual disease after initial surgery and 41% for the group with large residual tumor after initial surgery). Combined modality was thought to be feasible and well tolerated but was of unknown curative potential in advanced disease.[170]

Steiner and associates[199] reported on 45 Stage III and Stage IV patients who received abdominopelvic irradiation in the event that microscopic or minimal disease (<2 cm) was found at second-look laparotomy. All patients initially received 11 cycles of cisplatin-doxorubicin chemotherapy. The 2-year overall survival rate was 45%. Complete responders to chemotherapy had a 2-year survival rate of 63% compared with 19% for partial responders and nonresponders. Survival was also linked to amount of residual disease left at initial surgery and grade of tumor. A similar study was conducted by Rosen and associates,[173] who treated 17 Stage III patients with multimodality therapy including initial surgery, cyclophosphamide-doxorubicin with or without cisplatin chemotherapy, second-look laparotomy, and whole abdominopelvic irradiation. Seven patients were alive with no evidence of disease 5 years after chemotherapy. No patient (of nine) with more than 0.5 cm residual disease at initial surgery survived. Seven of eight patients with no residual or 0.5 cm or less residual tumor survived. Grade of tumor also correlated with survival; four of five patients with grade 1 and 2 tumors survived compared with three of 11 patients with grade 3 tumors.

Abdominopelvic irradiation, chemotherapy, or both were evaluated in 83 ovarian carcinoma patients, 63 of whom had Stage III and Stage IV disease.[186] The patients were divided into three groups. Group 1 received primary irradiation with or without single-agent chemotherapy (chlorambucil, cyclophosphamide, 5-fluorouracil, or melphalan). Group 2 underwent irradiation after failure of chemotherapy (mainly CAP), and group 3 received CAP with subsequent or other chemotherapy for salvage. Five-year actuarial survival for group 1 was 41% and only 16% for groups 2 and 3. The authors conclude that primary irradiation with or without adjuvant single-agent chemotherapy was superior to combination chemotherapy.

Recently 28 patients with Stage III and Stage IV ovarian carcinoma were treated using four cycles of cyclophosphamide and hexamethylmelamine alternated with four cycles of concurrent cisplatin, whole abdominopelvic irradiation, and intraperitoneal misonidazole.[112] Eighteen percent of the patients had a pathologic complete response as judged by second-look laparotomy; all these survived with no evidence of disease for a median of 21.5+ months. Median survival for the whole group was 15.2 months, with Stage III patients surviving longer than Stage IV patients (24 months *versus* 12 months) and patients with less than 2 cm residual disease doing better than patients with more than 2 cm residual disease (33 months *versus* 13 months). Responders survived a median of 21 months and nonresponders a median of 8 months.[112]

Another feasibility study reported on 16 Stage IIB to Stage IV patients who completed six to 12 cycles of a cisplatin-based combination chemotherapy and who had minimal (<2 cm), microscopic, or no residual disease at second-look laparotomy. All patients received moving strip abdominopelvic irradiation; no pelvic boost was given. Of the patients with microscopic or no residual disease, only two of ten patients progressed. In patients with minimal residual disease at second-look laparotomy, the therapeutic value of sequential radiation therapy was unsatisfactory (five of six progressed). Radiation therapy was concluded to be feasible with accepted toxicity, particularly in patients pretreated with six to nine cycles of chemotherapy.[67]

Kuten and associates[110] report the results of 116 patients who received abdominopelvic irradiation following primary cytoreductive surgery and six to 11 cycles of cisplatin and doxorubicin. Patients had either Stage III or Stage IV disease (91 patients) or Stage I to Stage II grade 3 disease (25 patients). Sixty-six patients had second-look laparotomy with no clinical evidence of disease. Consolidation abdominopelvic irradiation was given to 43 patients. Because of toxicity reactions, primarily myelosuppression, irradiation was given separately to upper and lower portals. With this technique, 94% completed the planned therapy. The 5-year survival rate for all 116 patients was 28% (18% for Stage III to Stage IV patients and 67% for Stage I to Stage II patients). Irradiated patients with microscopic disease at second-look laparotomy had an actuarial 5-year survival rate of 66% in contrast to 5% (at 36 months) for patients with minimal residual disease. All five patients with no residual disease at second-look surgery survived 36 months.

A similar study of 23 patients with primarily Stage III disease was reported.[104] After initial surgery, most patients received combination cyclophosphamide and cisplatin chemotherapy for five to 11 cycles. After second-look laparotomy at which time maximum cytoreduction was achieved, the patients received abdominopelvic irradiation using a hyperfractionated split-course schedule. Two fractions each of 100 cGy were given per day with at least a 4-hour interval between fractions to a total of 1500 cGy over 1.5 weeks. After a rest period of 3 weeks, the identical course was repeated. All but one patient completed the treatment. A limited field boost (1500 cGy in 15 fractions) was given to patients with gross residual disease. Follow-up is limited (mean 16.5 months). Eight of nine patients with gross residual disease have recurrences, as have one of two with miliary peritoneal seeding, three of seven with completely resected gross disease, and two of five with microscopic disease. The highest probability of relapse was in the grade 3 tumors (ten of 14 patients).

A similar whole abdominopelvic hyperfractionation technique was described by Morgan and associates.[134] Fifteen patients were treated twice daily using 80 cGy per fraction to a total dose of 3040 cGy. All patients had Stage III disease with persistence detected at pretreatment laparotomy after cisplatin-based chemotherapy. Tumor removed at surgery was classified as microscopic (three patients), less than 1 cm (three patients), 1 cm to 3 cm (five patients), or more than 3 cm (four patients). All tumors were grade 2 (four) and grade 3 (11). Fifty-three percent of patients were alive 8 to 52 months after irradiation (mean 29 months). Overall and disease-free survival rates at 4 years were 42% and 29%, respectively. Only the absence of gross residual disease before irradiation was prognostically significant.

Schray and associates[180] used whole abdominopelvic irradiation as a curative salvage effort for 53 patients with either residual or recurrent disease after combination cisplatin-based chemotherapy. All patients had 2 cm or smaller lesions confirmed at second-look surgery. Patients received 2550 cGy to 3000 cGy to the whole abdomen with partial liver/kidney shielding and a boost to the diaphragmatic/paraaortic nodal regions to approximately 4000 cGy to 5000 cGy, respectively (Martinez technique). Actuarial overall and disease-free survival rates at 3 years were 35% and 30%, respectively. Seventy-five percent of the relapses occurred within the irradiated abdomen alone. At 3 years, 70% of the patients with well or moderately differentiated tumors were disease-free compared with 10% of those with poorly differentiated tumors. This was statistically significant as a prognosticator, as was initial residual disease before chemotherapy. Patients with high-grade tumor, residual disease of more than 2 cm after initial surgery, and macroscopic disease at second-look laparotomy did not benefit from irradiation.

The Martinez technique was also used in 38 patients treated with a protocol consisting of an initial phase induction of remission with three to 14 courses of cyclophosphamide, hexamethylmelamine, doxorubicin, and cisplatin combination chemotherapy, second-look laparotomy for resection of residual disease followed by the irradiation.[75] All patients had Stage III disease, and 76% were classified as being in pathologic complete remission after surgery. The 5-year survival and disease-free survival rates for the whole group were 27% and 17%, respectively, and for the 29 patients who received the complete sequence of prescribed protocol treatments 35% and 20%, respectively.

In a small series of ten Stage III patients, all patients had received extensive chemotherapy and had less than 2 mm residual disease after a second or third laparotomy.[30] Radiation therapy was administered to the whole abdomen (3000 cGy) area with a 1500 cGy boost to the pelvis (in selected patients discrete areas of involvement were boosted). Five recurrences were noted, and three of these patients have died. In total, five patients were alive and free from disease for 6 months to 4 years (mean 15.8 months). In a similar study, 22 Stage III patients (19 initially surgical) had persistent disease after chemotherapy; 17 patients received open whole abdominopelvic irradiation, and five patients received moving-strip technique. Eleven also received a pelvic boost. No salvages were noted in patients with macroscopic disease at second-look laparotomy. Only two of nine patients with microscopic disease at second-look were alive and disease-free at 34 and 52 months. In this study whole abdominopelvic irradiation was not an effective salvage regimen.[158]

Another study,[78] however, reports the results of a trial consisting of surgery and chemotherapy with cisplatin and melphalan with or without hexamethylmelamine (six cycles). Most of the 158 evaluable patients had Stage III and Stage IV disease. There was a significant benefit in the 3-year time to progression (TTP) in patients who received whole abdominopelvic irradiation after a pathologic complete response to chemotherapy as determined at second-look surgery (83% for those who received radiation and 49% for those who did not). Partial responders, however, gained no benefit from irradiation (3-year TTP of 21% for patients receiving no irradiation or abdominopelvic irradiation).

Overall, consolidation irradiation for advanced disease seems to be most effective in patients completely responding to chemotherapy or in those with only microscopic disease present at second-look laparotomy.

Chemotherapy

As discussed in the previous section, chemotherapy has been increasingly used to treat epithelial ovarian carcinoma. Ozols and Young[151] believe that this relates to the fact that approximately two thirds of affected women have Stage III or Stage IV disease at diagnosis, and of those whose disease is localized in the pelvis, approximately 40% eventually relapse.

Alkylating agents have been used more extensively than any other class of chemotherapeutic agent for ovarian carcinoma. Response rates of 47% to 64% were noted in a number of trials using alkylating agents alone.[66] Median survival time in trials like these is 10 to 14 months. The 5-year survival rate is approximately 7%.[151] Other classes of antitumor agents have been less extensively tested, primarily in small numbers of patients who have failed initial treatment with radiation therapy or alkylating agents. Table 56-13 presents a summary of the responses with some single agents used for advanced disease. Other single agents tried recently are ifosfamide and diaziquone (AZQ).[119,219] With ifosfamide, a 33% response rate was seen in the primary treatment group, with a median duration of remission of 13 months. AZQ was given to previously treated patients; a 6% response rate was noted. No benefit was noted compared with other agents.

Chemotherapy has been used in Stage I and Stage II disease. Ozols and Young[151] discussed these trials and pointed out that comprehensive surgical staging was not required before treatment. They cited an Ovarian Cancer Study Group study showing that careful restaging showed that 77% of the patients had Stage III disease, which explains the high relapse in the pelvic irradiation group compared with the melphalan group (30% *versus* 5%).[96] A study at the Princess Margaret Hospital showing abdominopelvic irradiation to be superior to pelvic irradiation alone or pelvic irradiation plus chlorambucil also speaks against chemotherapy for patients with Stage IB, Stage II, or asymptomatic Stage III disease.[57] A GOG study of 101 patients with Stage IA and Stage IB disease with poorly differentiated tumors and Stage IIA and Stage IIB disease with microscopic or no residual disease after surgery found that patients did equally well receiving either melphalan or radioactive ^{32}P (88% probability of 3-year survival).[151] This finding is important, considering the risk of nonlymphocytic leukemia with alkylating agents.

Good results have been reported when small-volume residual disease (Stage III and Stage IV) is treated with combination chemotherapy.[82,151,153] Parker and associates[153] reported 11 of 12 biopsy-confirmed complete responses in patients without initial palpable disease who were treated with doxorubicin and cyclophosphamide. Greco and co-workers[82] reported that 14 of 16 patients with limited residual disease had a complete response to H-CAP (hexamethylmelamine, cyclophosphamide, Adriamycin, cisplatin). Median duration of remission in these studies was 19 and 24 months, respectively.

In patients with bulky residual disease, combination chemotherapy is the initial treatment in the attempt at chemically cytoreducing the tumor and thus making optional surgical cytoreduction possible. It is hoped that the effectiveness of postoperative irradiation is enhanced. Many of the studies discussed in the previous radiation therapy section used induction combination therapy with this end in mind, but to date, no dramatic improvement in complete response rates has been noted.[148,151] In fact, there has been controversy as to the impact that combination chemotherapy has had on survival of patients with advanced disease. Several reports have failed to show a survival advantage of combination chemotherapy compared with that of single agent alkylators.[148,152] Nonetheless, most reports today describe treatment with a cisplatin-containing regimen (Table 56-14).

In the opinion of a recent editorial, cisplatin-containing regimens prolonged median survival time by 6 to 12 months over those who never received cisplatin, whether it was used as a first-line or a second-line drug. It was thought, however, that many of the reports were not mature enough to estimate a cure.[53] Louie and associates[117] treated advanced ovarian carcinoma patients with a four-drug combination (cyclophosphamide, hexamethylmelamine, 5-fluorouracil, and cisplatin [chex-UP]). Survivors of the 62 patients have been observed for a minimum of 4 years. Prolonged survival was associated with a surgically confirmed complete remission to the induction chemotherapy (12 patients). Seven of these 12 patients were randomized to six cycles of intraperitoneal (IP) 5-fluorouracil. Only 15% were alive 4 years after initiation of treatment, a rather disappointing long-term response.

In a 10-year follow-up of 56 patients receiving cisplatin, doxorubicin, and cyclophosphamide chemotherapy for advanced disease, 4-year survival was 32%, and 17% had no evidence of disease (NED).[203] Five- and 10-year survival rates were 23% and 9%, respectively, and 18% and 7% were NED in the same time frame. This study demonstrated that the rate of

TABLE 56–13
Nonalkylating Agents in Ovarian Carcinoma

AGENTS	SCHEDULE	NO. OF PATIENTS	RESPONSE RATE (%)
Antimetabolites			
5-Fluorouracil	15 mg/kg/day Then, 7.5 mg/kg every other day for 34 wk	81	32 (18–20)
	15 mg/kg IV/wk	21	33
Methotrexate	5 mg/day × 5 to 10 PO or IV 3 to 4 wk	16	25
	1 to 7.5 g/m² IV/week with leukovorin rescue	23	13
Vinca Alkaloids			
Vinblastine	0.1 to 0.15 mg/kg/day × 1 to IV	16	13
Miscellaneous			
Mexamethylmelamine	8 mg/kg/day PO or 6 mg/kg/day PO × 14 days q 4 weeks	53	41
Doxorubicin	30 mg/m²/day × 3 IV	18	28
(Adriamycin)	50 mg/m² IV q 3 weeks	33	36
Progestogens	200 to 600 mg/wk IM	50	10
Cisplatin	30 mg/m² daily IV × 3 q 28 days	34	27

IV: intravenous; IM: intramuscular; PO: by mouth
(Young RC, Knapp, RC, Perez CA: Cancer of the ovary. In DeVita VT, Hellman S, Rosenberg, SA [eds]: Cancer: Principles and Practice of Oncology. Philadelphia, JB Lippincott, 1982)

TABLE 56–14
Randomized Trials of Cisplatin + Cyclophosphamide Versus Other Drug Combinations

TRIAL DESIGN	INSTITUTION	DOSE OF CISPLATIN	RESULTS
CHAP-5 vs CP	Netherlands[143]	CHAP-5: 20 mg/m^2 day 1–5 every 5 wk CP: 75 mg/m^2 day 1 every 3 wk	Response: 80% vs 74%; complete response: 35% vs 36%; median survival: 26 mo
CP vs PAC	Cooperative Trial in N.W. Italy[38]	50 mg/m^2 day 1 every 4 wk	Complete response: 41% vs 20%; median survival: 26 mo vs 22 mo (NS)
CP vs CHAD	Mayo Clinic[63]	60 mg/m^2 day 1 every 4 wk	Overall median survival: 24.6 mo (no difference)
PAC vs CP vs P	Italian Intraregional Cooperative Trial[85]	50 mg/m^2 day 1 every 4 wk	Response: 66% vs 56% vs 49%; complete response: 26% vs 21% vs 20%; median survival: 24 mo vs 21 mo vs 19 mo (NS)
CP vs PAC	Danish Cooperative Trial[17]	50 mg/m^2 every 4 wk	No difference in long-term survival (abstract)
PAC vs CP	Gynecologic Oncology Group[146]	50 mg/m^2 every 3 wk	In optimal Stage III patients, no significant difference in response or survival (abstract)

Abbreviations: CHAP-5: cyclophosphamide, hexamethylmelamine, Adriamycin, cisplatin; P: cisplatin; NS: no significance; CP: cisplatin, cyclophosphamide; PAC: cisplatin, doxorubicin, cyclophosphamide; CHAD: cyclophosphamiude, hexamethylmelamine, doxorubicin, cisplatin
(Ozols, RF: Chemotherapy of Ovarian Cancer: Updates to Cancer—Principles and Practice of Oncology, vol 2, 2nd ed. January 1988)

relapse decreases, but does not cease, at 5 years in patients receiving cisplatin-combination therapy.

Schwartz and associates[182] reported the results of a prospective randomized trial comparing standard chemotherapy (doxorubicin, cisplatin) alone (in 51 patients) or combined with tamoxifen (in 49 patients). Both groups had an overall survival of approximately 40% to 45% at 36 months.

Intraperitoneal chemotherapy with methotrexate, 5-fluorouracil, doxorubicin, and cisplatin has been evaluated. Although the actual clinical value of the modality is not established, phase I and II trials have shown the procedure to be feasible and safe with markedly increased intraperitoneal drug level obtained.[151] Piver and associates[161] reported the results of 31 patients with Stages III and IV invasive ovarian carcinoma treated on a phase II protocol of second-line intraperitoneal cisplatin, cytarabine, and bleomycin; 26% responded. Of the 15 patients with Stage III disease, of patients with residual disease of 1 cm or less, and of patients who had responded to first-line IV cisplatin-based chemotherapy, 53% responded to second-line intraperitoneal chemotherapy. Potential uses for this therapy are listed in Table 56-15.

Other therapies for advanced ovarian carcinoma are under investigation,[151,205] including clonogenic assay-directed therapy. New platinum compounds (JM9, CHIP) are being studied.[21] Other new drugs include galactitol, prednimustine, acridinylanisidide, mitomycin, and dihydroxylbusulfan, as well as AZQ, ifosfamide, hexamethylmelamine, and Taxol (a diterpenoid plant product isolated from the western yew, *Taxus brevifolia*).[142] Whether these drugs will appear in combination chemotherapy remains to be seen.

Hormonal Therapy and Immunotherapy

The demonstration that 50% to 70% of the common epithelial tumors have estrogen receptors has led to the use of the antiestrogen tamoxifen citrate.[151, 183] Only small numbers of patients have been studied, and definite conclusions cannot be

TABLE 56–15
Potential Uses of Intraperitoneal Therapy for Ovarian Carcinoma

As a substitute for intraperitoneal radioisotopes in early ovarian cancer
After surgical debulking of advanced ovarian cancer
For remission consolidation after systemic chemotherapy or abdominal radiation therapy
As an alternate to hepatic artery infusion as a means of local chemotherapy for liver metastases
As a means of treating bulky disease with monoclonal antibodies or interferon
As a means of treating bulky disease if precautions are taken to see that therapeutic levels are also attained in the blood.

(Parker LM, Griffiths CT, Yankee RA, et al: Cancer 46:669, 1980)

drawn.[183] Progestins do not appear to have a role as single agents.[151,208]

Immunotherapy is under investigation as a treatment for ovarian carcinoma. Bacille Calmette Guérin (BCG) has augmented the activity of cyclophosphamide and doxorubicin.[1] Among other patients receiving both immunotherapy and chemotherapy, 18% had a complete response to treatment, proven on pathologic examination, whereas only 3% receiving chemotherapy alone had a similar response. The GOG is now comparing cyclophosphamide-doxorubicin-cisplatin (CAP)-BCG therapy with CAP therapy alone. The Southwest Oncology Group is completing a three-armed study comparing cyclophosphamide-doxorubicin-BCG with CAP and CAP-BCG. Others have tried intraperitoneal instillation of *C. parvum.*[11]

Recently the results of a phase I/II study of intraperitoneal ^{131}I-labeled monoclonal antibodies for ovarian cancer were presented. A total of 36 patients were studied, 33 of whom received postoperative chemotherapy (mainly with platinum-containing regimens); one patient received whole abdominal irradiation, and two received pelvic irradiation only. In 31 patients with assessable disease, no responses occurred in eight patients with gross disease (nodules >2 cm), partial response in two of 15 patients with nodules larger than 2 cm, and complete responses in three of six with microscopic disease. This type of therapy is still regarded as experimental.[201]

Management of Germ Cell and Stromal Tumors

Dysgerminoma

Dysgerminoma is the most common malignant germ cell tumor, accounting for approximately 3.5% of ovarian malignancies. Seventy-five percent occur between the ages of 10 and 30 years, but age at presentation ranges from 2 to 71 years.[60,107,111,118,137,207] Presenting symptoms most often are abdominal swelling, discomfort, pain, or abdominal mass. Less frequently the patients present with amenorrhea, nocturia, leg pain, or nonspecific illness. Approximately 5% of patients present during pregnancy, but the majority of patients are nulliparous.[60] The duration of symptoms is short, ranging generally from 0 to 3 months.[24,60,61]

Dysgerminoma is usually localized to the ovaries (Stage I), and approximately 80% are confined to one ovary. However, it is the only malignant germ cell tumor of the ovary that occurs bilaterally with any significant incidence (10% to 15%). The clinical course of this tumor is marked by early lymphatic spread to the nodes near the left kidney and to the right paraaortic nodes at the level of the third and fourth lumbar vertebrae. Hematogenous spread to the lungs, brain, or liver is rare and is almost always preceded by lymphatic metastasis. Local invasiveness and extracapsular extension are also rare, but can lead to intraabdominal spread.[60,111]

The workup of dysgerminoma should include a history and physical examination, chest x-ray studies, routine blood studies, determination of serum α-fetoprotein (AFP) and serum human chorionic gonadotrophin (HCG), intravenous pyelogram (IVP), lymphangiogram, and abdominal CT. In pure dysgerminoma, AFP is always negative, whereas HCG may be slightly elevated due to isolated gonadotropin-producing syncytiotrophoblastic giant cells.

DePalo and associates[60] reported a 35% conversion rate of clinical Stage I and II to Stage III in patients undergoing lymphangiography.

Staging is basically surgical. Slayton[191] reported that the incidence of occult metastasis to pelvic and paraaortic nodes is not known because node dissection or sampling is not routinely done. Young and co-workers[221] report a 20% incidence of metastases to regional lymph nodes.

Total abdominal hysterectomy and bilateral salpingo-oophorectomy (TAH-BSO) has been advocated for patients who have disease beyond Stage IA. It is generally agreed that patients with Stage IA well-differentiated lesions less than 10 cm, well encapsulated, which are without ascites, unruptured, without attachment to surrounding tissue, and with a normal lymphangiogram can be treated by unilateral salpingo-oophorectomy alone.[71,107,125,190,207] Wedge or sagittal biopsy of the contralateral ovary is not agreed on, but recently DePalo and associates[60] reported performing this procedure on all patients. Surgery should involve the same careful procedures outlined for epithelial tumors.

Microscopic characteristics of dysgerminomas are important. Anaplastic dysgerminomas have a poor prognosis. Asadourian and Taylor[3] found that the possibility of relapse increased from 10% to 23% when more than eight mitoses per five high-power field were found. They also report a better prognosis when a prominent lymphoid infiltrate or a granulomatous reaction is present.

Dysgerminomas are very radiosensitive. DePalo and associates[61] recommend radiation therapy for all patients with Stages I to III disease. In their Stage IA patients, the radiation is precautionary; for Stage I and Stage II patients, they recommend radiation therapy to the ipsilateral hemipelvis (with shielding of the contralateral ovary and the head of the femur), and paraaortic nodes (Fig. 56-7A) to doses of 2500 cGy to 3000 cGy. A single field incorporating these areas can be used (Fig. 56-8). In either case the upper limit of the field is at T10–T11. For Stage III retroperitoneal disease (found at surgery), the authors give curative radiation therapy in the same fashion as in Stage I and they add a precautionary field to the mediastinum and the supraclavicular nodes (Fig. 56-7C). In the presence of peritoneal involvement, the whole abdomen and pelvis, mediastinum, and supraclavicular nodes are irradiated to a dose of 2500 cGy to 3000 cGy (750 cGy to 900 cGy/week) (Figs. 56-7B, C). In curative irradiation, 3500 cGy to 4000 cGy is given; a boost (1000 cGy) is delivered to involved nodes. When irradiating above the diaphragm, DePalo and associates give 3000 cGy 3 to 6 weeks after completion of irradiation below the diaphragm. When the entire abdominal cavity is irradiated, the fields are similar to those used for epithelial tumors. The kidneys are shielded after 1800 cGy of radiation. Lawson and Adler[111] reported giving 3000 cGy (1000 cGy/week) to pelvic and paraaortic fields. Only two patients were treated to the whole abdomen—one with moving strip technique and one with open fields. The patient treated with moving strip technique received 2250 cGy to the whole abdomen and 4500 cGy to the pelvis.

Figure 56-9 illustrates portals used to treat the periaortic and left pelvic lymph nodes for Stage II disease. An example of a portal used for elective mediastinal and left supraclavicular lymph node irradiation for Stage II disease is also shown.

Others recommend a similar treatment plan. Freel and associates[71] give external pelvic irradiation for disease limited to the pelvis (2000 cGy to 3000 cGy in 2 to 3 weeks). If the paraaortic nodes are positive histologically or on lymphangiogram, the fields are extended to cover this area; in this case prophylactic radiation therapy to the mediastinum and supraclavicular nodes (2500 cGy in 2.5 to 3 weeks) is given. If extranodal spread or intraabdominal disease is found, total abdominal therapy (2500 cGy to 3000 cGy in 3 to 5 weeks) with a pelvic

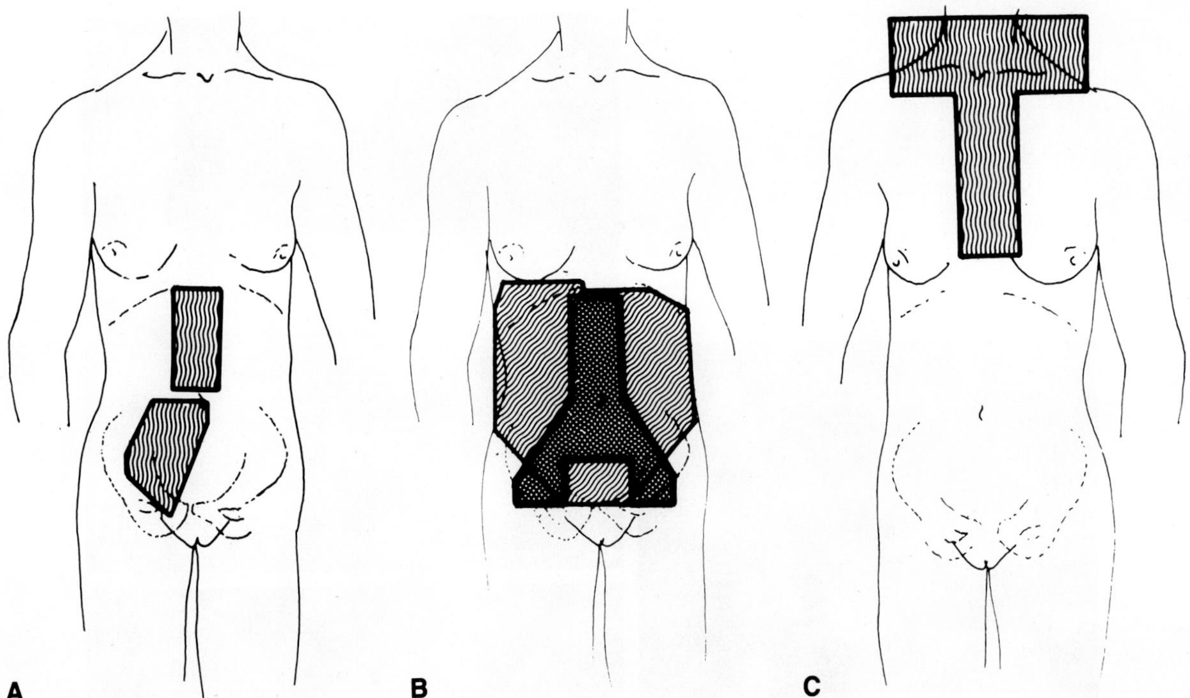

FIGURE 56–7. (**A**) Hemipelvic plus paraaortic field, precautionary in Stage I, curative in Stage III retroperitoneal. (**B**) Abdominal field plus boost on lymphatic areas, in Stage III peritoneal ± retroperitoneal. (**C**) Mediastinal and supraclavicular field, precautionary in Stage III. (DePalo G, Lattuada A, Kenda R, et al: Int J Radiat Oncol Biol Phys 13:855, 1987)

boost (1500 cGy to 2000 cGy in 1.5 to 3 weeks) and paraaortic boost (1500 cGy in 2 weeks) is recommended.[71,107,125,190]

DePalo and associates[60] reported all 13 Stage I patients (12 Stage IA and one Stage IB) alive and free from disease with a median follow-up of 77 months. The 5-year relapse-free survival rate of 12 Stage III patients was 61.4%, and the overall survival rate was 89.5%. Median follow-up was 67 months. Only one death was reported in this group. Earlier, DePalo and associates[61] reported 100% overall 5-year survival and 90% recurrence-free 5-year survival rates in 31 Stage IA, IB, and IC patients. At 4 years, an 80% overall survival rate and a 57% recurrence-free survival rate were observed in Stage III patients. Lawson and Adler[111] reported ten of 14 Stage I to Stage III patients alive with a median follow-up of 54 months. In this small series, no correlation was found between survival and either the initial stage of disease at presentation or the size of the primary tumor found at laparotomy.

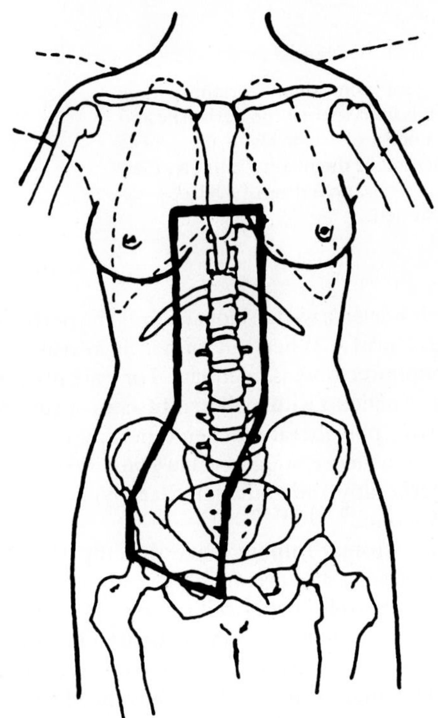

FIGURE 56–8. Ipsilateral and hemipelvic field for irradiation of dysgerminoma. (Courtesy of Carlos A. Perez, M.D., Mallinckrodt Institute of Radiology)

Recurrent disease can be surgically resected and subsequently treated with radiation therapy or chemotherapy. Eighty percent of recurrences appear within 2 years of the initial surgery and 75% within the first year. The abdomen and pelvis are the most common sites of failure, followed by the paraaortic and supraclavicular nodes.[190]

The place for chemotherapy in the treatment of dysgerminoma is uncertain. Chemotherapy is given for recurrence and advanced disease (Stages III and IV). Dactinomycin, 5-fluorouracil, and cyclophosphamide have been used in combination, as have vincristine, dactinomycin, and cyclophosphamide (VAC), and cisplatin, vinblastin, and bleomycin (PVB).[190] Lawson and Adler[111] used single-agent or combination chemotherapy (chlorambucil, thiotepa, vincristine, nitromin) in six patients and came to no clear conclusion as to its contribution. Cohen and Goldsmith[37] report a durable remission in a single case with retroperitoneal and hepatic metastases using vincristine and bleomycin for induction and methotrexate for maintenance therapy.

Other Germ Cell and Stromal Tumors

Endodermal sinus tumors are aggressive tumors of germ cell origin that reproduce the extraembryonic structures of the

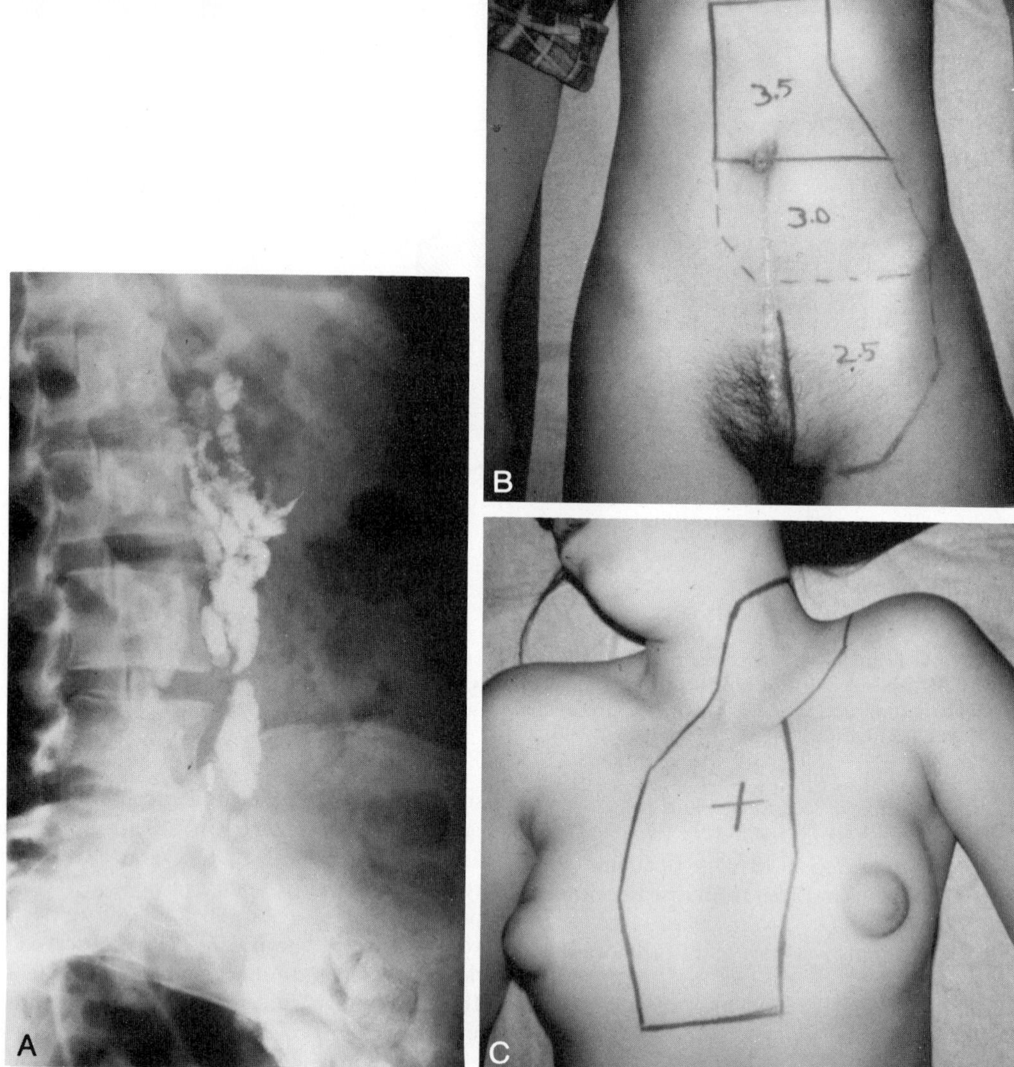

FIGURE 56–9. (**A**) Lymphangiography of a patient with ovarian dysgerminoma demonstrating a large left periaortic lymph node metastasis. (**B**) Photograph illustrating portals used to treat the periaortic and pelvic lymph nodes. The large field received 2500 cGy followed by a boost of 1000 cGy of the grossly enlarged lymph nodes. (**C**) Example of portals used for elective irradiation of the mediastinum and left supraclavicular lymph nodes in a patient with Stage II dysgerminoma of the ovary. A dose of 2000 cGy was delivered in 2 weeks. The patient is alive and well 13 years after treatment.

early embryo. They are found in girls and young women with a median age of 18 years.[190] The tumor is rarely bilateral; in a GOG series and in a study by Kurman and Norris,[108] no patient had bilateral disease.[166] For disease apparently limited to the ovary, unilateral salpingo-oophorectomy appears to be as effective as more aggressive operations.[108, 188, 190] All postoperative patients are treated with combination chemotherapy (VAC, PVB).[77, 108, 136, 190, 191] Others have used MAC (methotrexate, dactinomycin, chlorambucil).[40] Jereb and associates[100] have used postoperative radiation therapy to the whole abdomen with a boost to the periaortic nodes. Embryonal carcinoma is treated essentially the same way.[136, 190]

Choriocarcinoma is extremely rare and is best treated with chemotherapy (dactinomycin, methotrexate, and cyclophosphamide).[165]

The term *immature teratoma* has replaced older terms such as embryonal teratoma, malignant teratoma, solid teratoma, teratoblastoma, and teratocarcinoma. These tumors are usually unilateral; however, a wedge biopsy should be performed on the contralateral ovary. When no tumor is revealed, unilateral salpingo-oophorectomy is adequate. For patients with grade 2 or 3 tumor or patients with malignant ascites or ruptured tumor of any grade, postoperative chemotherapy (VAC) is recommended. No evidence suggests that combined-modality therapy (chemotherapy and radiation therapy) is superior to chemotherapy alone.[40, 122, 190, 191]

Ovarian stromal tumors make up only 1% to 3% of all ovarian neoplasms; they are mainly found to be granulosa cell, thecal cell, or Sertoli-Leydig cell tumors. If possible, a TAH-BSO is performed, but for young patients a more conservative approach is taken. Because malignant stromal cell tumors follow an indolent course, the role for adjuvant chemotherapy or radiation therapy has not been defined; postoperative radiation therapy has been advocated by some. If recurrence is found, it is generally localized to the pelvis or abdomen. Although there is no standard treatment for recurrence, generally as much tumor as possible is resected. The favorable patients receive postoperative radiation therapy; chemotherapy is reserved for bulky unresectable tumor (VAC, AcFuCy = dactinomycin, 5-fluorouracil, cyclophosphamide).[122,190,181,221]

RADIATION THERAPY TECHNIQUES

Intraperitoneal Instillation of ^{32}P

Radioactive ^{32}P or ^{198}Au has been used intraperitoneally as adjunctive therapy in Stage I, Stage II, or Stage III disease with microscopic residuum. The rationale for the procedure is to prevent seeding of cancer cells following complete resection of tumor. This modality has been combined with external-beam therapy or used alone.[4,25,44,65,92,138,159,165,202,212] The combination of intraperitoneal ^{32}P and external pelvic irradiation has been associated with a high incidence of bowel complications. Klaassen and associates[103] reported major complications in ten of 35 patients (29%) with early high-risk carcinoma who received 12 mCi to 15 mCi ^{32}P and 4000 cGy to 4500 cGy in 4 to 5 weeks. This combination therefore should be avoided or carefully planned.

The isotopes may sterilize microscopic implants but would be inadequate for large masses. Eltringham[65] pointed out that ^{32}P is more desirable than ^{198}Au because of its higher energy β-particle with greater penetration, an absence of τ-radiation (important in terms of personnel exposure and complications), ease of handling, and longer half-life, which may provide a more benign time-dose relationship resulting in fewer complications.

Generally, 15 mCi to 20 mCi of ^{32}P or 150 mCi of ^{198}Au is used. Instillation should be scheduled 1 to 3 weeks after laparotomy because postsurgical inflammatory changes will have subsided and significant adhesions, which affect uniform distribution, will not have appeared. However, some investigators recommend instillation at surgery or in the immediate postoperative period through catheters placed at surgery.

Several methods of instillation have been described; the most recent is by Sullivan and colleagues.[202] In this study fluids were administered through a peritoneal dialysis catheter placed either at surgery or by paracentesis 1 to 2 weeks later; 500 ml of normal saline with 4 mCi of ^{99m}Tc sulfur colloid was administered first to document intraperitoneal dispersion by scintillation camera scanning. Next, 15 mCi of ^{32}P suspension mixed with 500 ml of saline was given. Over the next 2 to 3 hours the patient's position was changed frequently to enhance dispersion. This method of giving the isotope (mixed with 500 ml of normal saline) was shown to be superior to that of giving the isotope as a bolus. A similar method of giving colloidal ^{198}Au (bolus followed by 600 ml of normal saline) was described by Buchsbaum and Keetel[25] and Muller.[138]

External-Beam Therapy

External-beam irradiation is given only with megavoltage equipment (^{60}Co or 4 MV to 25 MV photons). When abdominopelvic irradiation is used, the distance from target to skin should be sufficiently great (100 cm to 180 cm) to cover the volume from below the pelvic floor to above the diaphragm. During simulation, with the aid of fluoroscopy it should be ascertained that the portals include both diaphragms with 1 cm to 2 cm margins on both inspiration and expiration. Laterally, the border is beyond the peritoneal line. Two techniques have been most often described: ^{60}Co moving strip[46,59,156] and treatment by open fields (AP-PA).[47,48,209,221]

The pelvis is boosted in both techniques by an additional pelvic field afterward, by a field within a field, or by the addition of lateral fields to the pelvis (four-field). Fuks[72] calculated a nominal single dose or TDF, indicating that both techniques are essentially the same. Townsend[209] compared radiation sites, dosages, and survival rates (Table 56-16).

In the moving strip technique, lines 2.5 cm apart are marked on the front and back of the patient. On the first day, a single strip is treated on the front and an identical opposite field is irradiated from the back. Thereafter, one strip 2.5 cm in width is added daily until four strips have been irradiated both front and back. The 10 cm strip is then moved up 2.5 cm each day until the last strip is reached. The field is then reduced by one strip of 2.5 cm until on the last day a single 2.5 cm strip is irradiated.[46]

With this technique a tumor dose of 2800 cGy in the midplane of the abdomen in eight treatments is delivered in 10 to 12 elapsed days. The liver is shielded routinely on the anteroposterior-posteroanterior (AP-PA) strips and the kidneys on the AP-PA strips with 1 to 2 half-value layer (HVL) blocks. Others use blocks with 2 to 5 HVL.[47,156] The liver and kidneys receive approximately 1800 cGy (primary and scattered irradiation).[156] Figure 56-10 shows the volume, sequencing, dosimetry, and setup of this technique.

Either before or after the abdominopelvic irradiation described above, the pelvis is boosted with photon beam. Anteroposterior-posteroanterior 15-cm by 15-cm portals to a dose of approximately 3000 cGy are used.

In the open-field technique, the whole abdomen and pelvis including diaphragm are treated daily AP-PA. The inferior margin extends below the obturator foramen, and lateral borders extend beyond the peritoneum. A dose of 3000 cGy is given in 5 to 6 weeks (100 cGy to 150 cGy per fraction); the kidneys are

TABLE 56–16
Radiation Dosages, Sites, and Survival Rates in Ovarian Carcinoma

	NO. OF PATIENTS		
DOSE (cGy)	ALIVE	DEAD	TOTAL
ABDOMEN			
<2000	2	2	4
2000 to 2499	0	4	4
2500 to 2999	3	3	6
3000 to 3499	8	8	16
>3500	5	2	7
			37
PELVIS			
<2500	1	2	3
2500 to 3499	0	0	0
3500 to 4499	1	1	2
4500 to 5499	9	6	15
>5500	7	10	17
			37

(Townsend R, Glassburn JR, Brady LW, et al: Cancer Clin Trials 2:351, 1979)

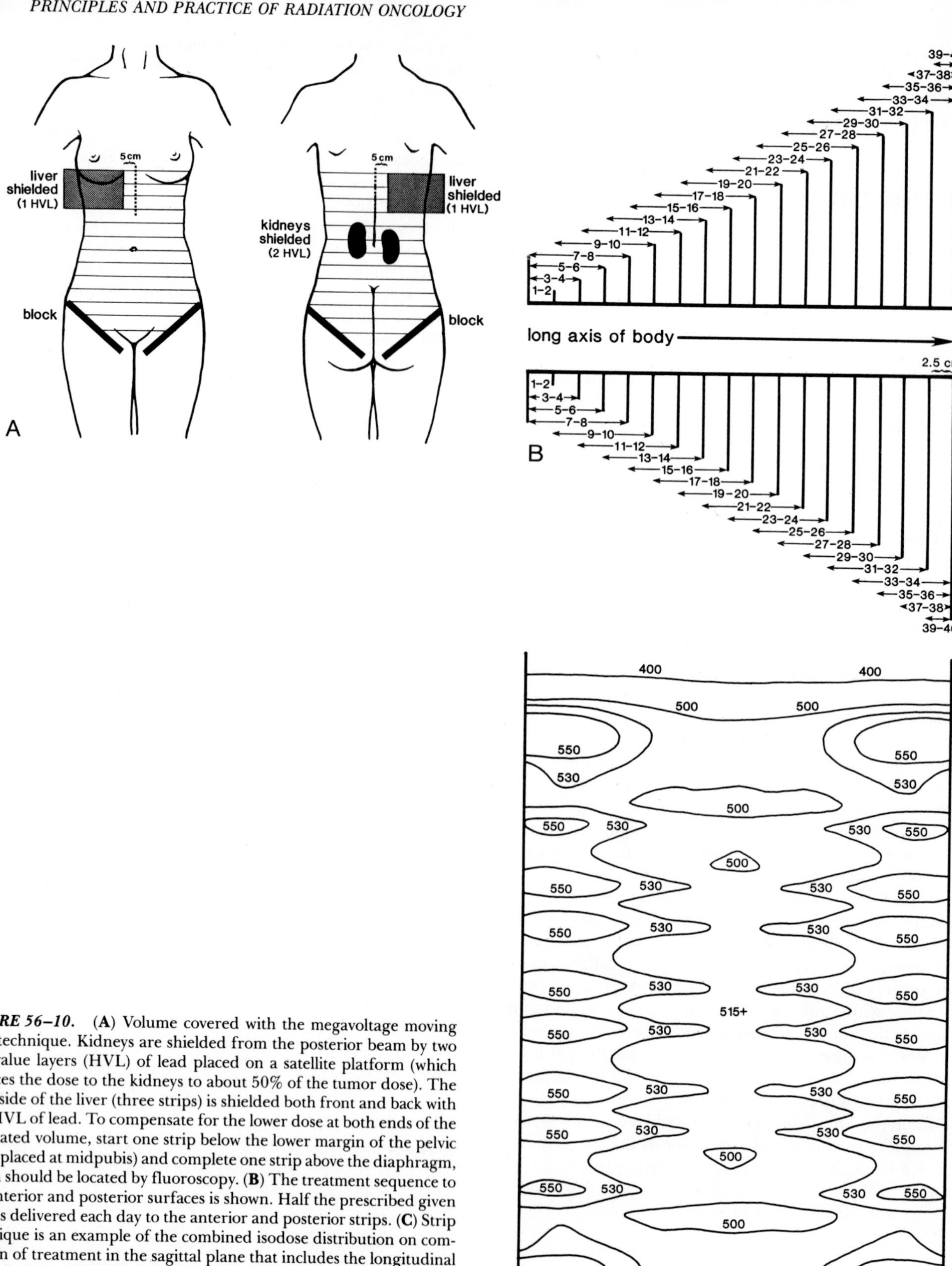

FIGURE 56–10. (**A**) Volume covered with the megavoltage moving strip technique. Kidneys are shielded from the posterior beam by two half-value layers (HVL) of lead placed on a satellite platform (which reduces the dose to the kidneys to about 50% of the tumor dose). The right side of the liver (three strips) is shielded both front and back with one HVL of lead. To compensate for the lower dose at both ends of the irradiated volume, start one strip below the lower margin of the pelvic field (placed at midpubis) and complete one strip above the diaphragm, which should be located by fluoroscopy. (**B**) The treatment sequence to the anterior and posterior surfaces is shown. Half the prescribed given dose is delivered each day to the anterior and posterior strips. (**C**) Strip technique is an example of the combined isodose distribution on completion of treatment in the sagittal plane that includes the longitudinal axis of the body. The total dose given to each strip is 100%. The distribution is computer-generated for an Eldorado 8 Cobalt Unit, source-skin distance 80 cm, trimmers at 65 cm from the source (except for a 2.5 cm field). (Delclos L, Dembo AJ: Ovaries. In Fletcher GH [ed]: Textbook of Radiotherapy. Philadelphia, Lea & Febiger, 1978)

shielded posteriorly at 1800 cGy, and the liver is shielded in the anterior portal (1 HVL).[209] Figure 56-11 shows schematically the volume covered. Figure 56-12 shows the sagittal dose distributions obtained when the abdomen and pelvis are treated AP-PA and the pelvis is boosted with an AP-PA field-within-a-field technique.

The Martinez technique[126] (Fig. 56-13) consists of three phases. The first phase treats the entire peritoneal cavity. The field extends from 1 cm above the diaphragm to the ischial tuberosity and laterally to cover the peritoneal reflections with at least a 2 cm margin. At 1000 cGy, 100% kidney blocks are introduced posteriorly only, and at 1500 cGy, 50% transmission liver blocks are placed anteriorly and posteriorly. Anterior and posterior fields are treated daily (5 days/week) to a midplane dose of 150 cGy. The upper abdomen and pelvis receive 3000 cGy each; the liver receives 2250 cGy and the kidneys receive 2000 cGy. During the second phase, the medial half of the diaphragm, the paraaortic nodes, and the true pelvis are treated by anterior and posterior fields. Eight fractions of 150 cGy are given, bringing the total dose to this area to 4200 cGy. The third and final phase treats the true pelvis anteriorly and posteriorly. A midplane dose of 180 cGy is given five times to bring the total dose to 5100 cGy. A modification of this technique is now given to patients thought to be at increased risk for late bowel injury. With the modified technique[181] the pelvis receives total radiation of 4950 cGy, the paraaortic and diaphragms 4050 cGy, and the abdomen 2550 cGy.

Kuten and associates[110] describe a split-field technique in which the lower abdomen received 3000 cGy in 3 weeks followed by the same dose to the upper abdomen. The fields were separated by a calculated gap that met at the midplane and provided approximately 157% homogenous dose. The kidneys were shielded by 3 HVL from the posterior side and the liver by 1 HVL both anteriorly and posteriorly.

Kong and associates[104] describe a split-course hyperfractionated technique. The entire peritoneal cavity was treated as previously described. Two fractions of 100 cGy each were given daily with at least a 4-hour interval between fractions. A total of 1500 cGy was given over 1.5 weeks. After a rest of 3 weeks the same course was repeated. The kidneys were protected with posterior 2 HVL lead shields from the beginning to limit the renal dose to 2000 cGy in 30 fractions. The total dose to the right lobe of the liver was limited to less than 2800 cGy by using anterior and posterior 5 HVL lead shields during the last three fractions.

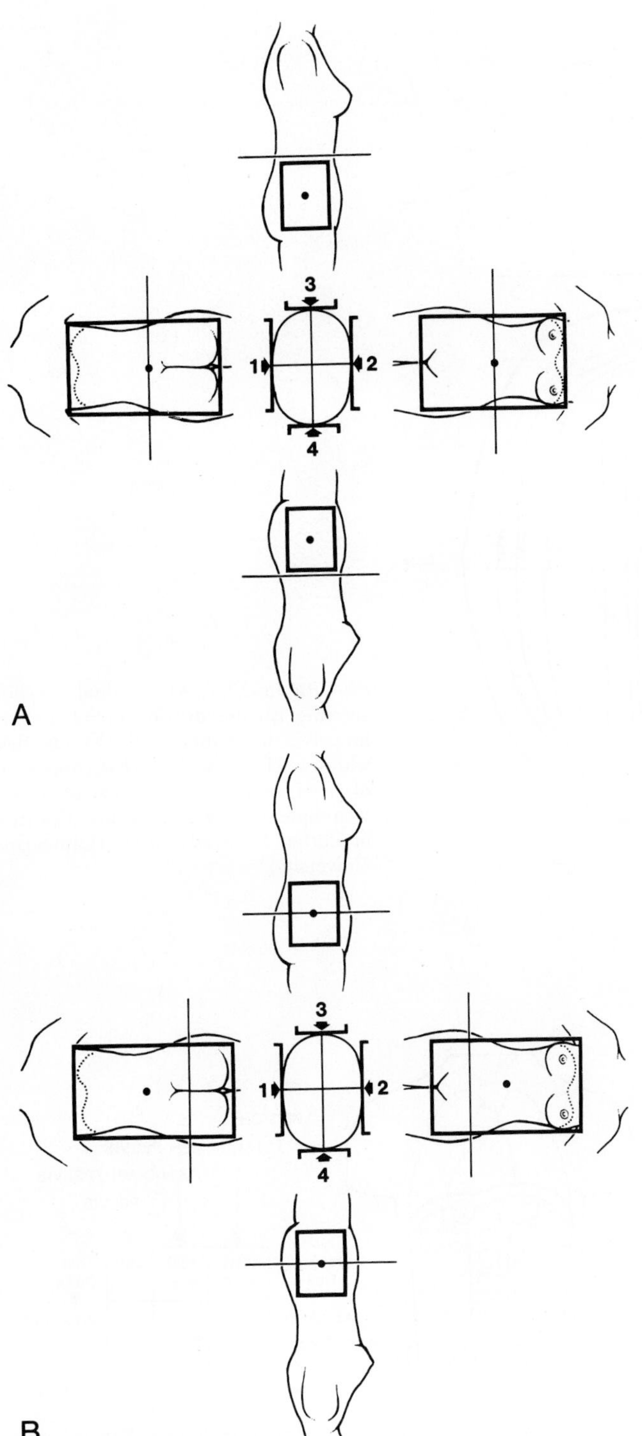

FIGURE 56–11. (**A**) Volume treated with anteroposterior abdominopelvic irradiation. The lateral pelvic fields are indicated. Line is shown through center of abdominopelvic fields. (**B**) Volume treated with lateral fields. The abdominopelvic fields are indicated. Line is shown through center of lateral fields.

RESULTS WITH STANDARD TECHNIQUES

Meaningful comparison of treatment results for ovarian carcinoma is difficult because many different modalities have been used. Perez and co-workers[157] identified other problem areas, including inaccurate surgical staging; a lack of uniformity in pathologic classification; inadequate surgical resection prior to adjuvant therapy; a lack of definite criteria for patient selection for a therapeutic modality; and, at that time, a lack of controlled, not necessarily randomized, studies to evaluate the effectiveness of the various modalities alone or in combination.

Clearly, stage, grade, and histology of tumor, and residual disease are important prognostic factors. Dembo,[51] Smith and Day,[193] Brady and associates,[19] and many others show improved survival rates under optimal conditions (*e.g.*, residuum less than 2 to 3 cm). In an earlier paper, Dembo and co-workers[57] reported improved survival when no residual disease was present. In Stage IB, Stage II, and asymptomatic Stage III patients, significantly improved survival was noted in the group without residuum who received abdominopelvic irradiation (Fig. 56-14).

Stage I disease offers the best chance for long-term survival. Smith and Day[193] reported 76% 5-year survival rate in patients treated with melphalan. Potish and associates[164] combined abdominopelvic irradiation and melphalan and reported

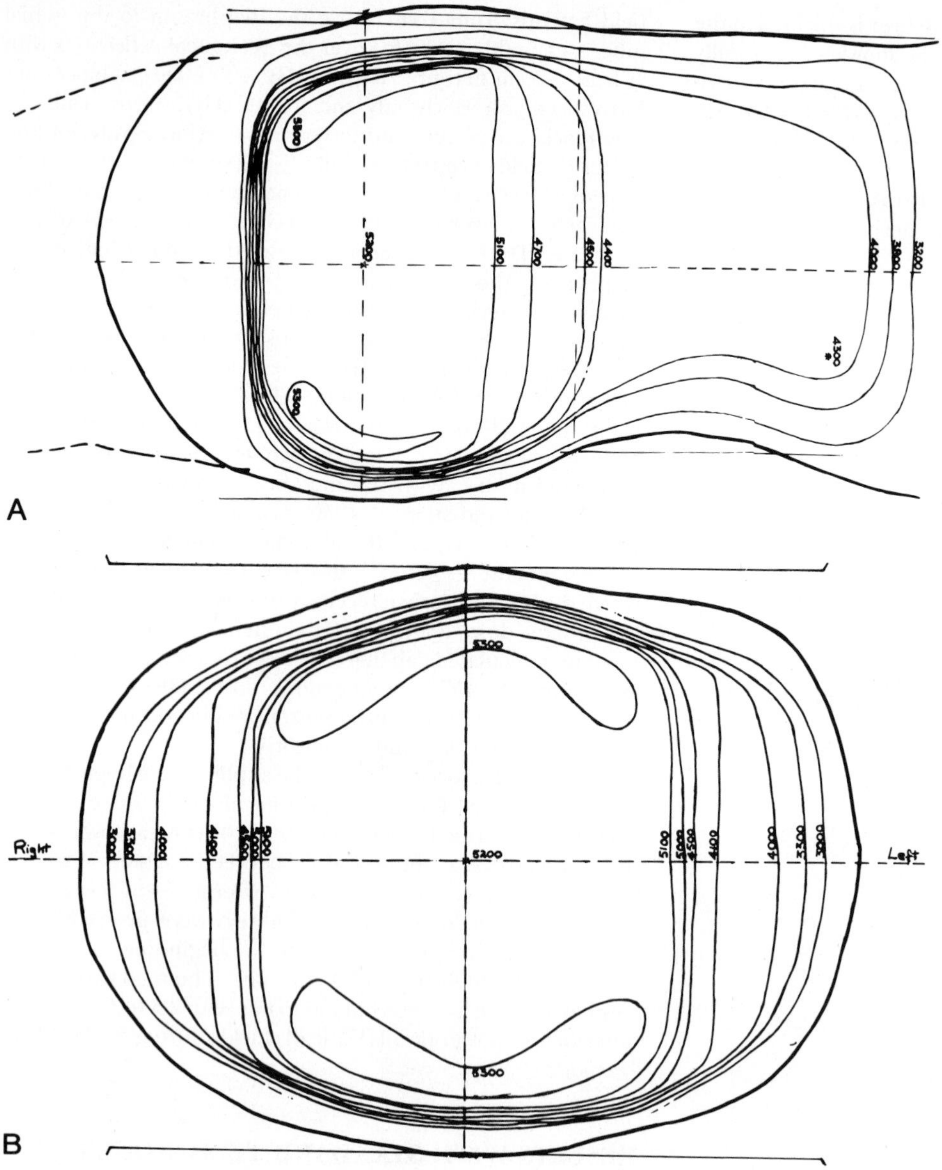

FIGURE 56–12. (**A**) Sagittal section showing isodose distribution of abdominopelvic irradiation with AP:PA field within a field pelvic boost. (**B**) Cross section of pelvis–isodose distribution of a field technique (field within a field). (Courtesy of Luther W. Brady, M.D., Hahnemann University)

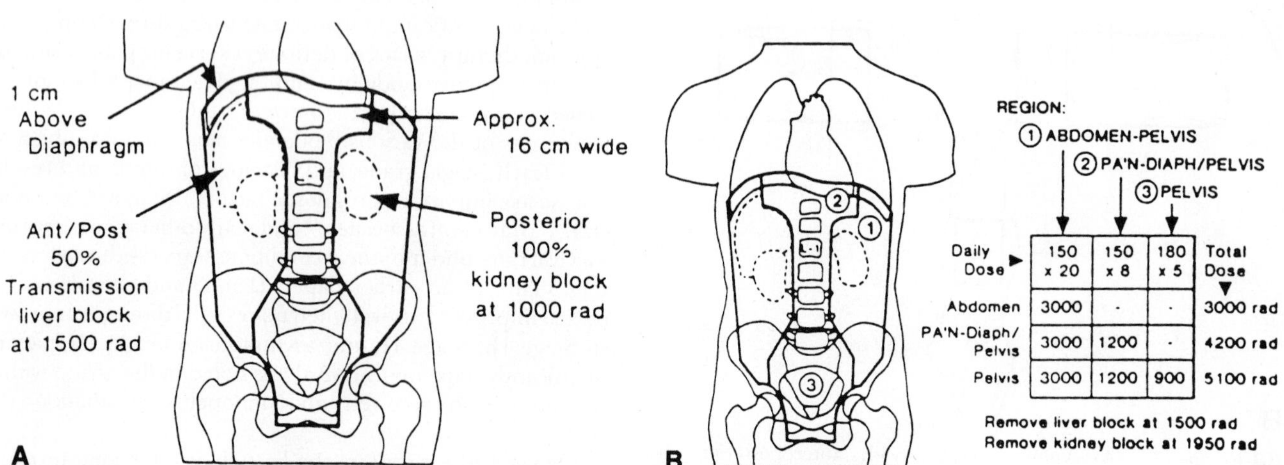

	①	②	③	
Daily Dose	150 x 20	150 x 8	180 x 5	Total Dose
Abdomen	3000	-	-	3000 rad
PA'N-Diaph/ Pelvis	3000	1200	-	4200 rad
Pelvis	3000	1200	900	5100 rad

FIGURE 56–13. (**A**) Field boundaries and blocks for treatment of gynecologic malignancies by whole-abdomen irradiation with diaphragmatic, paraaortic, and pelvic boost using the Martinez technique. (**B**) Martinez techniques and dose schedule. (PA'N: paraaortic nodes; DIAPH: diaphragm) (Martinez A, Schray MF, Howes AE, et al: J Clin Oncol 3:901, 1985)

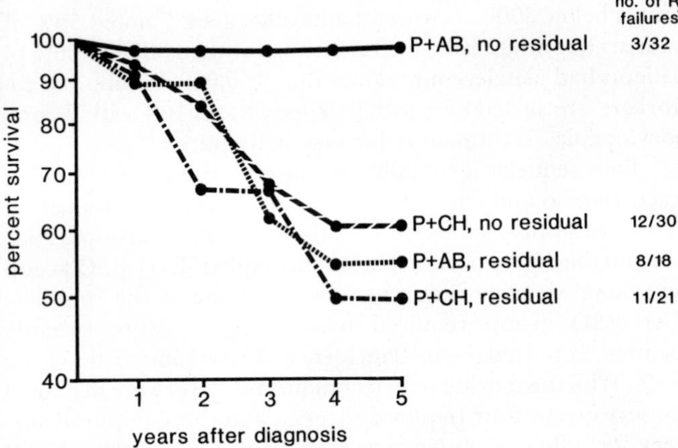

FIGURE 56–14. Actuarial survival curves by treatment and residual tumor. Proportion of patients with treatment failures is shown on the right. (P: pelvis; AB: abdomen; CH: chlorambucil) (Dembo AJ, Bush RS, Beale FA, et al: Cancer Treat Rep 63:249, 1979)

an 87% 5-year survival rate. Smith and co-workers[197] reported 90% 5-year survival rate with patients treated with melphalan. Similarly, Gallon and colleagues[76] showed 94% 5-year survival rate in patients treated with melphalan. Stage I patients treated postoperatively with abdominopelvic irradiation alone have 5-year survival rates ranging from 63.5% to 94%.[51, 86, 157, 193, 209] Grade, histology, and complete or incomplete surgery certainly affect outcome.

Stage II disease is also affected by the previously mentioned prognostic factors. Dembo[51] presented some of the best results with abdominopelvic irradiation. If the patient had no residual disease or microscopic residuum, 74% 5-year survival rate was noted. However, if the residuum was less than 2 cm, the 5-year survival rate dropped to 58%, and if the residuum was 2 cm or more, only 39% 5-year survival rate was noted. Smith and Day,[193] Haas and associates,[86] Perez,[157] Townsend and co-workers,[209] Dembo and colleagues,[57] Macbeth and associates,[121] and Martinez and co-workers[126] reported 5-year survival rates between 45% and 85%. Pelvic irradiation alone produced 5-year survival rates between 17% and 70%.[29, 56, 57, 127, 157, 211]

Most patients with Stage III and Stage IV disease are treated with combined modality. In this group also, the same prognosticators proved important. Survival overall is far less than with earlier stage disease. Patients with minimal residual disease after initial surgery had longer survival as did patients completely responding to chemotherapy or patients who could be completely resected at second-look laparotomy. Overall 5-year survival rates of approximately 30% are seen for Stage III disease.[30, 67, 75, 78, 95, 104, 110, 112, 134, 144, 158, 170, 173, 180, 186, 189, 198, 199, 210] However, Stage IV disease provides essentially no long-term survivors. Smith and Day[193] showed a 13% 5-year survival rate. Lichter and associates[112] showed 12-month median survival. Kuten and associates[110] had only an 18% survival rate for Stage III and Stage IV patients. Others have shown similar results (Table 56-17).

Recurrences are noted in the pelvis or abdomen as well as distantly. Dembo and co-workers[57] found improved control in patients receiving abdominopelvic irradiation compared with those treated to the pelvis alone and given chlorambucil. In the former group 22% failed in the pelvis; none failed in the abdomen. In the latter group 25% failed in the abdomen and 25% in the pelvis. Wallner and colleagues[211] reported that two of 24 patients treated with pelvic irradiation for Stage II failed in the pelvis, four failed in the pelvis and abdomen, and eight in the abdomen alone. Mauch and associates[127] had no relapses in the Stage II well-differentiated tumors treated with pelvic irradiation. However, nine of 18 moderately or poorly differentiated tumors failed: five in the abdomen, two in the pelvis, and two in the lungs and pleura. Haas and co-workers[86] reported six pelvic failures, ten intraabdominal failures, and 13 distant failures in 82 patients treated with abdominopelvic irradiation. Potish and colleagues,[164] Pezner and associates,[159] and Powlis and co-workers[165] also described fairly uniform distributions of failures.

When minimal residual disease is present, the data favor abdominopelvic irradiation with or without chemotherapy.[51, 57, 164] When macroscopic or bulk disease is present postoperatively, the prognosis is poor. Good data do not exist to indicate the most efficacious treatment plan. Combined modality, often with chemotherapy first, is given for advanced disease.[19, 30, 52, 67, 74, 75, 78, 88, 95, 104, 110, 112, 134, 144, 158, 164, 170, 173, 180, 186, 189, 198, 199, 210] Many studies demonstrate superior overall response, duration of response, and overall median survival with combination chemotherapy.[43, 66, 151, 221, 222] Combination chemotherapy has not been particularly successful when used after single-agent failure, and there appears to be no justification for a sequential approach of single-agent therapy followed by combinationchemotherapy at time of relapse.[151, 221, 222] Tables 56-18 and 56-19 give some of the combination regimens used and responses attained in advanced disease.

SEQUELAE OF TREATMENT

Acute complications from the moving strip or open-field technique primarily involve the gastrointestinal system. Cramps, diarrhea, nausea, and vomiting are most frequently noted. Ap-

TABLE 56–17
Disease-free Survival After Salvage Whole Abdominopelvic Irradiation Based on Residual Disease at Second-Look Surgery

	RESIDUAL DISEASE		
AUTHOR	MICROSCOPIC	MACROSCOPIC	TOTAL
Peters et al[158]	2/9	0/13	2/22
Hoskins et al[95]	0/1	0/7	0/8
Hainsworth et al[88]	3/11	0/6	3/17
Rosen et al[173]	2/3	1/9	3/12
Rizel et al[170]	4/12	—	4/12
Schray et al[180]	8/12	8/31	16/52
Total	19/57 (33%)	9/66 (14%)	28/123 (23%)

TABLE 56–18
Combination Chemotherapy Regimens in Advanced Previously Untreated Ovarian Carcinoma

REGIMEN	DOSES	RESPONSE RATE (%)
Hexa-CAF		
Hexamethylmelamine	150 mg/m² PO qd × 14	75
Cyclophosphamide	150 mg/m² PO qd × 14	
Methotrexate	40 mg/m² IV, days 1, 8	
5-Fluorouracil	600 mg/m² IV, days 1, 8	
A-C		
Cyclophosphamide	500 mg/m² IV	45
Doxorubicin (Adriamycin)	40 mg/m	
CHF		
Cyclophosphamide	100 mg/m² PO qd × 14	83
Hexamethylmelamine	150 mg/m² PO qd × 14	
5-Fluorouracil	500 mg/m² IV days 1, 8	
CHAD		
Cyclophosphamide	600 mg/m² IV day 1	90
Hexamethylmelamine	200 mg/m² PO days 8 to 22	
Adriamycin	25 mg/m² IV day 1	
Cisplatin	50 mg/m² IV day 1	
MECY		
Cyclophosphamide	250 mg/m² IV × 5 days	67
Methotrexate + CF (Citrovorum factor)	750 mg/m² IV over 4 hr followed by CF 10 mg/m² q 6 hr × 12 doses	
AP		
Adriamycin	50 mg/m² IV q 3 wk	70
Cisplatin	50 mg/m² IV q 3 wk	
PAC-1		
Cisplatin	20 mg/m² IV d × 5 q 4 wk	58
Adriamycin	50 mg/m² IV day 1 q 4 wk	
Cyclophosphamide	750 mg/m² IV day 1 q 4 wk	
CHex-UP		
Cyclophosphamide	150 mg/m² PO days 2 to 8 and days 9 to 16	74.5
Hexamethylmelamine	150 mg/m² PO days 2 to 8 and days 9 to 16	
5-Fluorouracil	600 mg/m² IV days 1 and 8	
Cisplatin	30 mg/m² IV days 1 and 8	

(Young RC, Knapp RC, Perez CA: Cancer of the ovary. In DeVita VT, Hellman S, Rosenberg SA [eds]. Cancer: Principles and Practices of Oncology, Philadelphia. JB Lippincott, 1982; and Young RC, Myers CE, Ozols RF, et al: Int J Radiat Oncol Biol Phys 8:899, 1982)

proximately 55% to 75% of the patients have one or more of these complaints, regardless of the technique used to treat the abdomen and pelvis.[56,157,209] Transient cystitis and proctitis are also noted in approximately 5% to 13% of patients.[59,209] Because of the large volume of bone marrow irradiated (50% to 60% of the adult functional marrow), leukopenia and thrombocytopenia are seen in most patients. Perez and associates[157] reported that 26.6% of patients developed white blood cell counts below 3000. Townsend and colleagues[209] noted 56% of patients had white blood cell counts lower than 3000; 43.6% of patients had platelet counts lower than 150,000. Dembo and co-workers[56] recorded 66% with leukopenia and 16% with thrombocytopenia. Treatment delay may be required.[56]

Late sequelae generally also involve the gastrointestinal tract. Dembo and co-workers[56,59] noted chronic occasional diarrhea in approximately 8% of their treatment groups. Four percent (one of 26 patients) in the incomplete TAH-BSO group had bowel damage requiring surgery; none of the complete TAH-BSO group required bowel surgery. More recently Dembo[51] reported the total incidence of bowel obstruction to be 3.1%. With the moving strip technique, two cases were managed conservatively, four required surgery, and three required surgery for adhesive obstruction with incidental radiation bowel changes. With open-field technique two obstructions were managed conservatively, two required surgery, and one (5%) required surgery for adhesive obstructions and one required diversion.

Perez and associates,[157] in 52 patients, noted one small bowel obstruction due to fibrosis and adhesions. They also had one case of rectal ulcer that was conservatively managed. Smith and associates[194] reported approximately 5% small bowel injury requiring surgery. Shelley and co-workers[187] reported 13 of 27 patients (48%) who experienced bowel obstruction after a median follow-up of 17 months. Ten (37%) required surgery. Peters and co-workers[158] noted that four of 11 patients receiving a pelvic boost had a major bowel complication, whereas none were noted in 11 patients receiving only abdominopelvic irradiation. Of the four major complications, three were bowel obstructions and one was radiation enteritis. Schray and co-workers[180] reported that 21% of their patients developed an apparently treatment-related bowel obstruction after completion of salvage irradiation. Schray and co-workers[181] analyzed toxicity of whole abdominopelvic irradiation. When it was used as primary postoperative therapy, they noted 8% severe radiation-caused bowel morbidity. Their review of the literature showed a 2% to 13% incidence of this complication. When given as salvage therapy, the above 21% morbidity was seen.

Radiation hepatitis occurred in 14 of 65 patients who received 2450 cGy to 2920 cGy to the entire liver by moving strip. The injuries to the liver were either acute (4 to 24 weeks after irradiation), subacute (8 to 28 weeks after irradiation), or chronic (24 to 39 months after irradiation). Because of this, the technique was changed to exclude part of the liver and to introduce liver shields (1 HVL).[214] Dembo[51] reported four of 226 patients with radiation hepatitis treated with moving strip (one fatal) and none with open-field technique.

Other chronic complications are basal lung fibrosis (approximately 25%) for which no therapy is required, localized varicella (4% to 9%), and raised alkaline phosphatase levels (4% to 36%).[51,59] Single cases of osteonecrosis of the pubic bone, hematuria, fever, and pulmonary embolus are also noted.[56,59,157,209] Dembo and co-workers[56,59] reported second malignancies in four patients (one ocular melanoma, one breast cancer, one thyroid lymphoma, one endometrial cancer of different histology).

When radiocolloids are used with pelvic irradiation, the incidence of bowel complications increases significantly. Pezner and associates[159] reported a 2.2% incidence of bowel complications with colloid alone and 24% with colloid and pelvic irradiation. Three of four patients in the latter group required surgery. Bakri and colleagues[8] found a major surgically confirmed complication rate of 7.4% with colloid alone compared with

TABLE 56–19
Current GOG Protocols for Ovarian Epithelial Carcinoma

GOG PROTOCOL	STAGE OF DISEASE	PROTOCOL DESIGN	PURPOSE OF PROTOCOL
52	Optimal III	CAP *versus* CP	To determine whether addition of doxorubicin to CP improves progress-free interval, frequency of negative second-look, and survival
60	III and IV	Doxorubicin cyclophosphamide, and cisplatin *versus* same drug + BCG	To see whether BCG added to chemotherapy improves remission rate, duration, or survival
67	Disease confined to abdomen (optimal) pseudomyoma peritonei	Intraperitoneal chemotherapy (doxorubicin or 5-fluorouracil)	To study response and adverse effects of intraperitoneal chemotherapy
7602A	IAii, IBii, IC, II (A, B, C)	Melphalan × 18 months *versus* ^{32}P instillation	Define natural history of patient treated on protocol Study effect of various potential prognostic factors on natural history Study patterns of relapse Study value of staging parameters
8491	III and IV suboptimal	CAP (cycle I) CAP + interferon (cycles 3–8)	To study toxicities and activity of interferon as addition to first-line therapy
95	IC, II, selected IA, IB, IAii, IBii	CP intraperitoneal ^{32}P	To compare progression-free interval and overall survival To determine patterns of relapse for each arm To define relative toxicities of each arm

CAP: cyclophosphamide, doxorubicin (Adriamycin), cisplatin; CP: cyclophosphamide, cisplatin

21% when pelvic irradiation was added. The rate rose to 42% with the addition of those diagnosed and treated by medical means only. Decker and associates[44] reported that ten of 48 patients developed small bowel obstruction when treated with ^{198}Au and external irradiation.

IMPROVING PROTOCOL DESIGN AND RESULTS IN CLINICAL TRIALS

Many studies examining the best treatment for ovarian carcinoma are in progress or under design. A joint RTOG (84-10) and NCOG (50-82-IJ) phase III protocol has been proposed to study pelvic and abdominal radiation therapy *versus* cisplatin, doxorubicin, and cyclophosphamide chemotherapy in Stage I, Stage II, and optional Stage III epithelial ovarian carcinoma. Irradiation can be given either by open field with pelvic boost or by split-field technique (Johns Hopkins University Hospital) in which the upper and lower abdomen are treated in two separate fields and a pelvic boost is given. Both techniques give 3000 cGy to the whole abdomen with an additional 1980 cGy to the pelvis. In each technique the abdominal fraction is 150 cGy and the pelvic fraction is 180 cGy.

The GOG has several ongoing protocols for epithelial carcinoma (see Table 56-19); no conclusions can yet be drawn from these studies.

Ozols and his colleagues at the National Cancer Institute are investigating mechanisms of overcoming resistance to cisplatin (Platinol) and the alkylating agents. They found that when ovarian cancer cells become resistant, they have high levels of GSH (cellular glutathione, a tripeptide involved in multiple biochemical processes). The GSH level can be lowered with a drug called BSO (buthionine sulfoximine), which has no intrinsic anticancer activity of its own. When GSH is lowered, the chemotherapy is able to become more active against the now less resistant tumor cells. Clinical studies using BSO are proposed.[91]

The challenge of the future lies in earlier diagnosis of ovarian carcinoma, which is associated with longer long-term survival. The problem lies in choosing the appropriate therapy because randomized controlled studies are few, and all modalities can be effective. No clear picture emerges indicating the best treatment, although there is a slight indication that irradiation affords better intraabdominal control, particularly in early stage ovarian cancer. Continued studies are needed to prove this.

REFERENCES

1. Alberts DS, Moon TE: Randomized trial of chemotherapy versus chemo-immunotherapy for advanced ovarian carcinoma. In National Cancer Institute Second International Conference on Immunotherapy of Cancer: Present status of trials in man, p 13. New York, 1980
2. American Cancer Society: Facts and Figures, 1983, 1984, 1985, 1989
3. Asadourian L, Taylor H: Dysgerminoma. Obstet Gynecol 33:370–378, 1969
4. Aure JC, Hoeg K, Kolstad P: Radioactive colloidal gold in the treatment of ovarian carcinoma. Acta Radiol Ther (Stockh) 10:399–407, 1971
5. Averette HE, Jaramillo BA, Sevin B: Gynecologic cancer: Possible factors in treatment failures. Cancer Treat Symp 2:211–216, 1983
6. Averette HE, Sevin B: Debulking surgery and second look operation. Int J Radiat Oncol Biol Phys 8:891–892, 1982
7. Bagley CM, Young RC, Canellos, GP, DeVita VT: Treatment of ovarian carcinoma: Possibilities for progress. N Engl J Med 287:856–862, 1972
8. Bakri YN, Given FT, Peeples WJ, Frazier AB: Complications from intraperitoneal radioactive phosphorous in ovarian malignancies. Gynecol Oncol 21:294–299, 1985
9. Ballon SC, Martinez A, Turbow MM, et al: Pelvic irradiation plus Adriamycin and cyclophosphamide in selected patients into epithelial ovarian carcinoma: A phase III study of the Northern California Oncology Group. Gynecol Oncol 19: 278–283, 1984
10. Barber, Hugh RK: Ovarian carcinoma: Etiology, diagnosis and treatment. New York, Masson, 1978
11. Bast Jr RC, Knapp RC: Immunologic approaches to the management of ovarian carcinoma. Semin Oncol 11(3):264–271, 1984
12. Beral V, Fraser P, Chilvers C: Does pregnancy protect against ovarian cancer? Lancet 1:1083–1087, 1978
13. Berek JS, Griffiths CT, Leventhal JM: Laparoscopy for second-look evaluation in ovarian cancer. Obstet Gynecol 58:192–198, 1981
14. Berek JS, Hacker NF, Lagasse LD, et al: Lower urinary tract resection as part of cytoreduction surgery for ovarian carcinoma. Gynecol Oncol 13:87–92, 1982
15. Berek JS, Hacker NF, Lagasse LD, et al: Survival of patients following secondary cytoreductive surgery in ovarian cancer. Obstet Gynecol 61:189–193, 1983
16. Bergman F: Carcinoma of the ovary: A clinicopathological study of 86 autopsied cases with special reference to mode of spread. Acta Obstet Gynecol Scand 45:211–231, 1966
17. Bertelsen K, Anderson JE, Jakobsen A, et al: A randomized study of CP versus CAP in advanced ovarian cancer: Proceedings of the European Society of Medical Oncology. Cancer Chem Ther Pharmacol 18:7, 1986
18. Blythe JG, Wahl TP: Debulking surgery: Does it increase quality of survival? Gynecol Oncol 14:396–408, 1982
19. Brady LW, Blessing JA, Slayton RE, et al: Radiotherapy (RT), chemotherapy (CT) and combined therapy in stage III epithelial ovarian cancer. Cancer Clin Trials (Summer) 111–120, 1979
20. Brady LW, Lewis GC Jr, Thigpen JT, Yaeger TE: Ovarian tumors. Oncologic Multidisciplinary Decisions in Oncology, vol 20. New York, Pergamon Press, 1984
21. Bramwell VHC, Crowther D, O'Malley S, et al: Activity of JM9 in advanced ovarian cancer: A phase I–II trial. Cancer Treat Rep 69:409–416, 1985
22. Brenner DE, Grosh WW, Jones III HW, et al: An evaluation of the accuracy of computed tomography in patients with ovarian carcinoma prior to second look laparotomy. ASCO Proc 2:149, 1983
23. Brioschi PA, Rapin C, DeRoten M, et al: Longitudinal study of CEA and CA 125 in ovarian cancer. Gynecol Oncol 21:1–6, 1985
24. Brody S: Clinical aspects of dysgerminoma of the ovary Acta Radiol (Oncol) (Stockh) 56:209–230, 1961
25. Buchsbaum HJ, Keettel WC: Radioisotopes in treatment of stage Ia ovarian cancer. Natl Cancer Inst Monogr 42:127–128, 1975
26. Buchsbaum HJ, Lifshitz S: Staging and surgical evaluation of ovarian cancer. Semin Oncol 11(3):227–237, 1984
27. Buka NJ, Macfralane KT: Malignant tumors of the ovary. Am J Obstet Gynecol 90:383–387, 1964
28. Bush RS: Ovarian cancer: Contribution of radiation therapy to patient management. Radiology 153:17–24, 1984
29. Bush RS, Allt WEC, Beale FA, et al: Treatment of epithelial carcinoma of the ovary: Operation, irradiation and chemotherapy. Am J Obstet Gynecol 127:692–704, 1977
30. Cain JM, Russell AH, Greer BE, et al: Whole abdomen radiation for minimal residual epithelial ovarian carcinoma after surgical resection and maximal first-line chemotherapy. Gynecol Oncol 29:168, 1988
31. Cancer Statistics, 1991. Ca: A Cancer Journal for Clinicians. 41(1):19, 1991
32. Castaldo TW, Petrilli ES, Ballou SC, et al: Intestinal operations on patients with ovarian cancer. Am J Obstet Gynecol 139:80–84, 1981
33. Changes in definitions of clinical staging for carcinomas of the cervix and ovary: International Federation of Gynecology and Obstetrics. Am J Obstet Gynecol 156:263–264, 1987
34. Chen SS, Lee L: Incidence of para-aortic and pelvic lymph node metastases in epithelial carcinoma of the ovary. Gynecol Oncol 16:95–100, 1983
35. Chen SS, Lee L: Prognostic significance of morphology of tumor and retroperitoneal lymph nodes in epithelial carcinoma of the ovary. I. Correlation with lymph node metastasis. Gynecol Oncol 18:87–93, 1984
36. Chen SS, Lee L: Prognostic significance of morphology of tumor and retroperitoneal lymph nodes in epithelial carcinoma of the ovary. II. Correlation with survival. Gynecol Oncol 18:94–99, 1984
37. Cohen SN, Goldsmith MA: Prolonged chemotherapeutic remission of metastatic ovarian dysgerminoma: Report of a case. Gynecol Oncol 5:299–304, 1977
38. Conte PF, Bruzzonne M, Chiara S, et al: A randomized trial comparing cisplatin plus cyclophosphamide versus cisplatin, doxorubicin and cyclophosphamide in advanced ovarian cancer. J Clin Oncol 4:965, 1986
39. Copeland LJ, Gershenson DM, Wharton JT, et al: Microscopic disease at second-look laparotomy in advanced ovarian cancer. Cancer 55:472, 1985
40. Creasman WT, Fetter BF, Hammond CB, et al: Germ cell malignancies of the ovary. Obstet Gynecol 53:226–230, 1979
41. Creasman WT, Rutledge F: The prognostic value of peritoneal cytology in gynecologic malignant disease. Am J Obstet Gynecol 110:733–781, 1971
42. Day TG, Gallager HS, Rutledge FN: Epithelial carcinoma of the ovary: Prognostic importance of histologic grade. Cancer Inst Monogr 42:15–18, 1975
43. Decker DG, Flemming TR, Malkasian GD, et al: Cyclophosphamide plus cis-platinum in combination: Treatment program for stage III or IV ovarian carcinoma. Obstet Gynecol 60:481–487, 1982
44. Decker DG, Webb MJ, Holbrook MA: Radiogold treatment of epithelial cancer of ovary: Late results. Am J Obstet Gynecol 115:751–758, 1973
45. DeLand M, Fried A, Van Nagell JR: Ultrasonography in the diagnosis of tumors of the ovary. Surg Gynecol Obstet 148:346–348, 1979
46. Delclos L, Dembo AJ: Ovaries. In Fletcher GH (ed): Textbook of Radiotherapy, pp 834–851. Philadelphia, Lea & Febiger, 1978
47. Delclos L, Quinlan EJ: Malignant tumors of the ovary managed with postoperative megavoltage irradiation. Radiology 93:659–663, 1969
48. Delclos L, Smith JP: Ovarian cancer with special regard to types of radiotherapy. Cancer Inst Monogr 42:129–135, 1975
49. Delgado G, Chun B, Caglar H, Bepko F: Para-aortic lymphadenectomy in gynecologic malignancies confined to the pelvis. Obstet Gynecol 50:418–423, 1978
50. Delgado G, Oram DH, Petrilli ES: Stage III epithelial ovarian cancer: The role of maximal surgical reduction. Gynecol Oncol 18:293–298, 1984

51. Dembo AJ: Abdominopelvic radiotherapy in ovarian cancer: A 10 year experience. Cancer 55:2285–2290, 1985
52. Dembo AJ: Radiotherapeutic management of ovarian cancer. Semin Oncol 111(3):238–250, 1984
53. Dembo AJ: Controversy over combination chemotherapy in advanced ovarian cancer: What we learn from reports of matured data. J Clin Oncol 4:1573, 1986
54. Dembo AJ, Bush RS: Choice of postoperative therapy based on prognostic factors. Int J Radiat Oncol Biol Phys 8:893–897, 1982
55. Dembo AJ, Bush RS: Radiation therapy of ovarian carcinoma. In Griffiths CT, Fuller AF (eds): Gynecologic Oncology, pp 263–298. Boston, Martinus-Nijhoff, 1983
56. Dembo AJ, Bush RS, Beale FA, et al: Ovarian carcinoma: Improved survival following abdominopelvic irradiation in patient with a completed pelvic operation. Am J Obstet Gynecol 134:793–800, 1979
57. Dembo AJ, Bush RS, Beale FA, et al: The Princess Margaret Hospital study of ovarian cancer: Stages I, II and asymptomatic III. Cancer Treat Rep 63:249–254, 1979
58. Dembo AJ, Bush RS, Brown TC: Clinicopathological correlates in ovarian cancer. Bull Cancer 69(3):292–297, 1982
59. Dembo AJ, VanDyk J, Japp B, et al: Whole abdominal irradiation by a moving strip technique for patients with ovarian cancer. Int J Radiat Oncol Biol Phys 5:1933–1942, 1979
60. DePalo G, Lattuada A, Kenda R, et al: Germ cell tumors of the ovary: The experience of the National Cancer Institute of Milan. I. Dysgerminoma. Int J Radiat Oncol Biol Phys 13:853–860, 1987
61. DePalo G, Pilotti S, Kendra R, et al: Natural history of dysgerminoma. Am J Obstet Gynecol 143:799–807, 1982
62. DiSaia PJ, Rich WM: Tumors of the Ovary. In Pilch YH (ed): Surgical Oncology, pp 807–825, New York, McGraw-Hill, 1984
63. Edmundson JH, McCormack GW, Fleming TR, et al: Comparison of cyclophosphamide and cisplatin versus hexamethylmelamine, cyclophosphamide, Adriamycin and cisplatin in combination as initial therapy for stage III and IV ovarian carcinoma. Cancer Treat Rep 69:1243, 1985
64. Einhorn N, Nilsson B, Sjovall K: Factors influencing survival in carcinoma of the ovary: Study from a well-defined Swedish population. Cancer 55:2019–2025, 1985
65. Eltringham JR: Radiation therapy for ovarian carcinoma. Clin Obstet Gynecol 22:967–992, 1979
66. Eyre HL: Chemotherapy of ovarian carcinoma: Clin Obstet Gynecol 22:957–965, 1979
67. Falcone A, Chiara S, Franzone P, et al: Moving-strip abdomino-pelvic radiotherapy after cis-platinum-based chemotherapy and second-look operation. Am J Clin Oncol 11(1):16, 1988
68. Feldman GB, Knapp RC: Lymphatic drainage of the peritoneal cavity and its significance in ovarian cancer. Am J Obstet Gynecol 119:991–994, 1974
69. Flink H, Lichter A, Rosenshein W, Order S: Maximal radiation therapy by a new treatment technique for stage III ovarian cancer. Int J Radiat Oncol Biol Phys 4:441–443, 1978
70. Fraumeni JF, Grundy GW, Greagen ET: Six families prone to ovarian cancer. Cancer 36:364–369, 1975
71. Freel JH, Cassir JF, Pierce VK, et al: Dysgerminoma of the ovary. Cancer 43:798–805, 1979
72. Fuks Z: External radiotherapy of ovarian cancer: Standard approaches and new frontiers. Semin Oncol 2:253, 1975
73. Fuks Z, Bagshaw MA: The rationale for curative radiotherapy for ovarian carcinoma. Int J Radiat Oncol Biol Phys 1:21–32, 1975
74. Fuks Z, Rizel S, Aanteby SO, Biran S: The multimodal approach to the treatment of stage III ovarian carcinoma. Int J Radiat Oncol Biol Phys 8:903–903, 1982
75. Fuks Z, Rizel S, Biran S: Chemotherapeutic and surgical induction of pathological complete remission and whole abdominal irradiation for consolidation does not enhance the cure of stage III ovarian carcinoma. J Clin Oncol 6:509, 1988
76. Gallon HH, vanNagell JR, Donaldson ES, et al: Adjuvant oral alkylating chemotherapy in patients with stage I epithelial ovarian cancer. Cancer 63:1070, 1989
77. Gershenson DM, DelJunco G, Herson J, Rutledge FN: Endodermal sinus tumor of the ovary: The M.D. Anderson experience. Obstet Gynecol 61:194–202, 1983
78. Goldhirsch A, Greiner R, Dreher E, et al: Treatment of advanced ovarian cancer with surgery, chemotherapy and consolidation at response by whole-abdominal radiotherapy. Cancer 62:40, 1988
79. Gordon RE, Mettler Jr FA, Wicks JD, Bartow SA: Chest x-ray and full lung tomograms in gynecologic malignancy. Cancer 52:559–562, 1983
80. Graham RM, Bartels JD, Graham JB: Screening for ovarian cancer by cul de sac aspiration. Acta Cytol 6:492–495, 1962
81. Graham RM, Nieerk WA: Vaginal cytology in cancer of the ovary. Acta Cytol 6:496–499, 1962
82. Greco FA, Julian CG, Richardson RL, et al: Advanced ovarian cancer: Brief intensive combination chemotherapy and second-look operation. Obstet Gynecol 58:199–205, 1981
83. Griffiths CT: The Ovary. In Kistner RW (ed.): Gynecology Principles and Practice, ed 3, pp 325–426. Chicago, Year Book Medical Publishers, 1980
84. Griffiths CT, Parker LM, Fuller AF Jr: Role of cytoreductive surgical treatment in the management of advanced ovarian cancer. Cancer Treat Rep 63:235–240, 1979
85. Gruppe Interegionale Cooperativo Oncologico Ginecologia: Randomized comparison of cisplatin with cyclophosphamide/cisplatin and with cyclophosphamide/doxorubicin/cisplatin in advanced ovarian cancer. Lancet 11:353, 1987
86. Haas JS, Mansfield CM, Hartman GV, et al: Results of radiation therapy in the treatment of epithelial carcinoma of the ovary. Cancer 46:1950–1956, 1980
87. Hacker NF, Berek JA, Lagasse LD, et al: Primary cytoreductive surgery for epithelial ovarian cancer. Obstet Gynecol 61:413–420, 1983
88. Hainsworth JD, Malcolm A, Johnson DH, et al: Advanced minimal residual ovarian carcinoma: Abdominopelvic irradiation following combination chemotherapy. Obstet Gynecol 61:619–623, 1983
89. Heintz AP, Hacker NF, Lagasse LD: Epidemiology and etiology of ovarian cancer: A review. Obstet Gynecol 66:127–135, 1985
90. Henderson JM, Mettler Jr FA, Wicks JD, et al: Urologic imaging and correlation with serum laboratory determinations in staging gynecologic malignancies. Cancer 52: 563–566, 1983
91. Highlights of a clinical conference organized by University of Southern California School of Medicine and the USC comprehensive cancer center. Oncol Comment 1(1):5–6, 1988
92. Hilaris BS, Clark DGC: The value of postoperative intraperitoneal injection of radiocolloids in early cancer of the ovary. Am J Roentgenol Radium Ther Nucl Med 112:749–754, 1971
93. Holm-Hielsen P: Pathogenesis of ascites in peritoneal carcinomatosis. Acta Pathol Microbiol Scand 33:10–21, 1953
94. Hoover R, Gray LA, Fraumeni JF: Stilbestrol and the risk of ovarian cancer. Lancet :533–534, 1977
95. Hoskins WJ, Lichter AS, Whittington R, et al: Whole abdominal and pelvic irradiation in patients with minimal disease at second-look surgical reassessment for ovarian carcinoma. Gynecol Oncol 20:271, 1985
96. Hreshchyshyn MM, Park RC, Blessing JA, et al: The role of adjuvant therapy in stage I ovarian cancer. Am J Obstet Gynecol 138:139–145, 1980
97. Hudson CN, Chir M: A radical operation for fixed ovarian tumors. J Obstet Gynaecol Br Commonw 75:1155–1160, 1968
98. Jacobs AJ, Sommers GM, Homan SM, et al: Therapy of ovarian carcinoma: The relationship of dose level and treatment intensity to survival. Gynecol Oncol 31:233, 1988
99. Janovski NA, Paramanandhan TL: Ovarian tumors. In Major Problems in Obstetrics and Gynecology, vol 4. Philadelphia, WB Saunders, 1973
100. Jereb B, Wollner N, Exelby P: Radiation in multidisciplinary treatment of children with malignant ovarian tumors. Cancer 43:1037–1042, 1979
101. Johnson GH: Pelvic mass and diagnosis of carcinoma of the ovary. Clin Obstet Gynecol 22:903–923, 1979
102. Keettel WC, Pixley EE, Buchsbaum HJ: Experience with peri-

toneal cytology in the management of gynecologic malignancies. Am J Obstet Gynecol 120:174–182, 1974

103. Klaassen D, Shelley W, Starreveld A, et al: Early stage ovarian cancer: A randomized clinical trial comparing whole abdominal radiotherapy, melphalan and intraperitoneal chromic phosphate: A National Cancer Institute of Canada Clinical Trials Group Report. J Clin Oncol 6:1254, 1988
104. Kong JJS, Peters LJ, Wharton JT, et al: Hyperfractionated split course whole abdominal radiotherapy for ovarian carcinoma: Tolerance and toxicity. Int J Radiat Biol Phys 14:737, 1988
105. Knapp RC, Friedman EA: Aortic lymph node metastases in early ovarian cancer. Am J Obstet Gynecol 119:1013–1017, 1974
106. Knipscheer RJL: Paraaortic lymph node dissection in 20 cases of primary epithelial ovary carcinoma, Stage I (FIGO): Influence of staging. Eur J Obstet Gynecol Reprod Biol 13:303–307, 1982
107. Krepart G, Smith JP, Rutledge F, Delclos L: The treatment for dysgerminoma of the ovary. Cancer 41:986–990, 1978
108. Kurman RJ, Norris HJ: Endodermal sinus tumor of the ovary: A clinical and pathological analysis of 71 cases. Cancer 38:2404–2418, 1976
109. Kurman RJ, Scardino PT, Waldmann TA, et al: Malignant germ cell tumors of the ovary and testis: An immunologic study of 69 cases. Ann Clin Lab Sci 9:462–466, 1979
110. Kuten A, Stein M, Steiner MD, et al: Whole abdominal irradiation following chemotherapy in advanced ovarian carcinoma. Int J Radiat Biol Phys 14:273, 1988
111. Lawson AP, Adler GF: Radiotherapy in the treatment of ovarian dysgerminomas. Int J Radiat Oncol Biol Phys 14:431–434, 1988
112. Lichter AS, Ozols RF, Myers CC, et al: Treatment of advanced stage ovarian carcinoma with a combination of chemotherapy, radiotherapy and radiosensitizer: Report of pilot study from the National Cancer Institute. Int J Radiat Biol Phys 13:1225, 1987
113. Lingeman CH: Etiology of cancer of the human ovary: A review. J Natl Cancer Inst 53:1603–1618, 1974
114. Lippman SM, Alberts DS, Slymen DJ, et al: Second-look laparotomy in epithelial ovarian carcinoma: Prognostic factors associated with survival duration. Cancer 61:2571, 1988
115. Llewellyn-Jones D: Fundamentals of obstetrics and gynecology. Gynecology, vol II. London, Faber & Faber, 1970
116. Longo DL, Young RC: Cosmetic talc and ovarian carcinoma. Lancet ii:349–351, 1979
117. Louie KG, Ozols RF, Myers CE, et al: Long-term results of a cisplatin-containing combination chemotherapy regimen for the treatment of advanced ovarian carcinoma. J Clin Oncol 4:1579, 1986
118. Lufcraft HH: A review of 33 cases of ovarian dysgerminoma emphasizing the role of radiotherapy. Clin Radiol 30:585–589, 1979
119. Lund B, Bramwell V, Renard J, et al: Phase II trial of diaziquone in advanced ovarian carcinoma. Cancer Treat Rep 69:339–340, 1985
120. Lynch, HT, Schuelke GS, Wells IC, et al: Hereditary ovarian carcinoma: Biomarker studies. Cancer 55:410, 1985
121. Macbeth FR, MacDonald H, Williams CJ: Total abdominal and pelvic radiotherapy in the management of early stage ovarian carcinoma. Int J Radiat Oncol Biol Phys 15:353, 1988
122. Malkasian GD, Webb MJ, Jorgensen EO: Observations on chemotherapy of granulosa cell carcinoma and malignant ovarian teratomas. Obstet Gynecol 44:885–888, 1974
123. Mangioni C, Bolis G, Molteni P, et al: Indications, advantages and limits of laparoscopy in ovarian cancer. Gynecol Oncol 7:47–55, 1979
124. Manual for Staging of Cancer, 3rd ed. American Joint Committee on Cancer. Philadelphia, JB Lippincott, 1988
125. Marks RD, Underwood PB, Othersen HB, et al: Dysgerminoma : 100% control with combined therapy in six consecutive patients with advanced disease. Int J Radiat Biol Phys 4:453–456, 1978
126. Martinez A, Schray MF, Howes AE, et al: Postoperative radiation therapy for epithelial ovarian cancer: The curative role based on a 24-year experience. J Clin Oncol 3:901, 1985
127. Mauch PM, Ehrmann RL, Griffiths CT, et al: Radiation therapy in stage III ovarian carcinoma. Cancer 45:1344–1351, 1980
128. McGowan L: Epidemiology of ovarian cancer. Oncology 3:51, 1989
129. McGowan L, Lesher LP, Norris HJ, Barnett M: Misstaging of ovarian cancer. Obstet Gynecol 65:568–572, 1985
130. Megibow AJ, Busniak MA, Ho AG, et al: Accuracy of CT in detection of persistent or recurrent ovarian carcinoma: Correlation with second-look laparotomy. Radiology 166:341, 1988
131. Menczer J, Ben-Baruch G, Modan M, et al: A comparison of postoperative radiotherapy with postoperative chemotherapy in stage II–IV ovarian cancer patients. Gynecol Oncol 17:207–212, 1984
132. Mettler FA, Christie JH, Crow NE, et al: Utility of radionuclide liver/spleen scanning and serum enzyme levels in detecting hepatic metastasis from ovarian carcinoma. Cancer 50:909–911, 1982
133. Mettler FA, Christie JH, Crow NE, et al: Radionuclide bone scan, radiographic bone survey, and alkaline phosphatase studies of limited value in asymptomatic patients with ovarian carcinoma. Cancer 50:1483–1485, 1982
134. Morgan L, Chafe W, Mendenhall W, et al: Hyperfractionation of whole-abdoman radiation therapy: Salvage treatment of persistent ovarian carcinoma following chemotherapy. Gynecol Oncol 31:122, 1988
135. Mor-Josef S, Anteby SO, Schenker JG: Trends in the incidence of ovarian cancer in a heterogenic population (1964–1976). Gynecol Oncol 21:287–293, 1985
136. Morris HHB, LaVecchia C, Draper GJ: Endodermal sinus tumor and embryonal carcinoma of the ovary in children. Gynecol Oncol 21:7–17, 1985
137. Mueller CW, Topkins P, Lapp WA: Dysgerminomas of the ovary: An analysis of 427 cases. Am J Obstet Gyncol 60:153–159, 1950
138. Muller JH: Curative aim and results of routine intraperitoneal radiocolloid administration in the treatment of ovarian cancer. Am J Roentgenol Radium Ther Nucl Med 89:533–540, 1963
139. Munnell EW: The changing prognosis and treatment in cancer of the ovary. Am J Obstet Gynecol 100:790–805, 1968
140. Musumeci R, Bonfi A, Bolis G, et al: Lymphangiography in patients with ovarian epithelial cancer: An evaluation of 289 consecutive cases. Cancer 40:1444–1450, 1977
141. Myers C: The use of intraperitoneal chemotherapy in the treatment of ovarian cancer. Semin Oncol 11:275–284, 1984
142. National Cancer Institute: Clinical Brochure: Taxol (NSC-125973), Bethesda, MD, 1983
143. Neijt JP, ten Bokkel Huinink WW, Van der Berg MEL, et al: Randomized trial comparing two combination chemotherapy regimens (CHAP 5 v. CP) in advanced ovarian carcinoma. J Clin Oncol 5:1157, 1987
144. Nevin JE, Pinzon G, Baggerly T, et al: The use of intravenous phenylalanine mustard followed by supervoltage irradiation in the treatment of carcinoma of the ovary. Cancer 51:1273, 1983
145. Niloff JM: The role of Ca-125 assay in the management of ovarian cancer. Oncology 2:67, 1988
146. Omura GA, Bundy B, Wilbanks G, et al: A randomized trial of cyclophosphamide plus cisplatin with or without Adriamycin in ovarian carcinoma. Proc Soc Clin Oncol 6:112, 1987
147. Onsrud M: Serum-mediated immunosuppression: A possible tumor marker in patients with ovarian carcinoma. Gynecol Oncol 21:94–100, 1985
148. Ozols RF: Chemotherapy of ovarian cancer. Updates to Cancer: Principles and Practice of Oncology, vol 12, 2nd ed. Philadelphia, JB Lippincott, January 1988: 1–12
149. Ozols RF, Fisher RI, Anderson T, et al: Peritoneoscopy in the management of ovarian cancer. Am J Obstet Gynecol 140:611–619, 1981
150. Ozols RF, Garvin AJ, Costa J: Advanced ovarian cancer: Correlation of histologic grade with response to therapy and survival. Cancer 45:572, 1980
151. Ozols RF, Young RC: Chemotherapy of ovarian cancer. Semin Oncol 2(3):251–262, 1984

152. Ozols RF, Young RC: Ovarian cancer. Curr Probl Cancer 11:59, 1987
153. Parker LM, Griffiths CT, Yankee RA, et al: Combination chemotherapy with Adriamycin-cyclophosphamide in advanced ovarian carcinoma. Cancer 46:669–674, 1980
154. Pearse WH, Behrman SJ: Carcinoma of the ovary. Obstet Gynecol 3:32, 1954
155. Perez CA, Bedwinek JM, Breaux SR: Patterns of failure after treatment of gynecologic tumors. Cancer Treat Symp 2:217–231, 1983
156. Perez CA, Korba A, Zivnuska F, et al: ^{60}Co moving strip technique in management of carcinoma of the ovary: Analysis of tumor control and morbidity. Int J Radiat Oncol Biol Phys 4:379–388, 1978
157. Perez CA, Walz BJ, Jacobson PL: Radiation therapy in the management of carcinoma of the ovary. Natl Cancer Inst Monogr 42:119–125, 1975
158. Peters WA, Blasko JC, Bagley CM, et al: Salvage therapy with whole-abdominal irradiation in patients with advanced carcinoma of the ovary previously treated by combination chemotherapy. Cancer 58:880, 1988
159. Pezner RD, Stevens KR, Tong D, Allen CV: Limited epithelial carcinoma of the ovary treated with curative intent by intraperitoneal instillation of radiocolloids. Cancer 42:2563–2571, 1978
160. Piver MS, Barlow JJ, Lele SB: Incidence of subclinical metastasis in stage I and II ovarian carcinoma. Obstet Gynecol 52:100–104, 1978
161. Piver MS, Lele SB, Marchetti DL, et al: Surgically documented response to intraperitoneal cisplatin, cytarabine and bleomycin after intravenous cisplatin-based chemotherapy in advanced ovarian adenocarcinoma. J Clin Oncol 6:1679, 1988
162. Piver MS, Shashikant L, Barlow JJ: Preoperative and intraoperative evaluation in ovarian malignancy. Obstet Gynecol 48:312–315, 1976
163. Piver MS, Shashikant BL, Barlow JJ: Second-look laparoscopy prior to proposed second-look laparotomy. Obstet Gynecol 55:571–573, 1980
164. Potish R, Adock L, Brooker D, et al: Sequential surgery, radiation therapy and alkeran in the management of epithelial carcinoma of the ovary. Cancer 45:2754–2758, 1980
165. Powlis WD, Mauch P, Ehrmann RL, et al: The role of postoperative local or regional irradiation in the treatment of stage I ovarian cancer. Radiology 142:747–750, 1982
166. Quinn MA, Bishop GH, Campbell JJ, et al: Laparoscopic follow-up of patients with ovarian carcinoma. Br J Obstet Gynecol 87:1132–1139, 1980
167. Raju KS, McKinna JA, Barker GH, et al: Second-look operations in the planned management of advanced ovarian carcinoma. Am J Obstet Gynecol 144:650–654, 1982
168. Reddy S, Sutton GP, Stehman FR, et al: Ovarian carcinoma: Adjuvant treatment with P-32. Radiology 165:275, 1987
169. Requard CK, Mettler FA, Wicks JD: Preoperative sonography of malignant ovarian neoplasms. Am J Roentgenol Radium Ther Nucl Med 137:79–82, 1981
170. Rizel S, Biran S, Anteby SO, et al: Combined modality treatment for stage III ovarian carcinoma. Radiother Oncol 3:237, 1985
171. Robey SS, Silver EG, Gershenson DM, et al: Transitional cell carcinoma in high-grade high-stage ovarian carcinoma: An indicator of favorable response to chemotherapy. Cancer 63:839, 1989
172. Rose DP, Boyar AP, Wynder EL: International comparisons of mortality rates for cancer of the breast, ovary, prostate, colon and per capita food consumption. Cancer 58: 2363, 1986
173. Rosen EM, Goldberg ID, Rose C, et al: Sequential multi-agent chemotherapy and whole abdominal irradiation for stage III ovarian carcinoma. Radiother Oncol 7:223, 1986
174. Rosenberg L, Shapiro A, Sloane D, et al: Epithelial ovarian cancer and combination oral contraceptives. JAMA 247:3210–3212, 1982
175. Rosenoff SH, Young RC, Chabner P, et al: Use of peritoneoscopy for initial staging and posttherapy evaluation of patients with ovarian carcinoma. Nat Cancer Inst Monogr 42:81–86, 1975
176. Rubin SC: The value of second-look laparotomy in ovarian cancer. Oncology 1:45, 1987
177. Rudenburg CJ, Cornelisse CJ, Heintz PA, et al: Tumor ploidy as a major prognostic factor in advanced ovarian cancer. Cancer 59:317, 1987
178. Schenker JG, Polishuk WZ, Steinitz P: An epidemiologic study of carcinoma of the ovary in Israel. Israel J Med Sci 4:820, 1968
179. Schray M, Martinez A, Cox R, Ballon S: Radiotherapy in epithelial ovarian cancer: Analysis of prognostic factors based on long-term experience. Obstet Gynecol 62: 373–382, 1983
180. Schray MF, Martinez A, Howes AE, et al: Advanced epithelial ovarian cancer: Salvage whole abdominal irradiation for patients with recurrent or persistent disease after combination chemotherapy. J Clin Oncol 6:1433, 1988
181. Schray MF, Martinez A, Howes AE: Toxicity of openfield whole abdominal irradiation as primary postoperative treatment in gynecologic malignancy. Int J Radiat Oncol Biol Phys 16:397, 1989
182. Schwartz PE, Chambers JT, Kohorn EI, et al: Tamoxifen in combination with cytotoxic chemotherapy in advanced epithelial ovarian cancer. Cancer 63:1074, 1989
183. Schwartz P, Kenting G, Maclusky N, et al: Tamoxifen therapy for advanced ovarian cancer. Obstet Gynecol 59:583–588, 1982
184. Schwartz PE, Smith JP: Second-look operations in ovarian cancer. Am J Obstet Gynecol 138:1124–1130, 1980
185. Schweisguth O, Gerard-Marchant R, Plainfosse B, et al: Bilateral nonfunctioning thecoma of the ovary in epileptic children under anticonvulsant therapy. Acta Paediatr Scand 60:6–10, 1971
186. Shehata WM, Meyer RL, Cormier WJ, et al: Ovarian carcinoma: Results of radiation therapy and chemotherapy in 83 patients. Radiology 163:539, 1987
187. Shelley WE, Starreveld AA, Carmichael JA, et al: Toxicity of abdominopelvic radiation in advanced ovarian carcinoma patients after cisplatin/cyclophosphamide therapy and second-look laparotomy. Obstet Gynecol 71:327, 1988
188. Simmons RI, Sciarra JJ: Treatment of late recurrent granulosa cell tumors of the ovary. Surg Gynecol Obstet 124:65–70, 1967
189. Sjovall K, Einhorn N: Preoperative therapy in advanced carcinoma of the ovary. Radiother Oncol 4:329, 1985
190. Slayton RE: Management of germ cell and stromal tumors of the ovary. Semin Oncol 11:299–313, 1984
191. Slayton RE, Hreshchyshyn MM, Silverberg SG, et al: Treatment of malignant ovarian germ cell tumors: Response to vincristine, dactinomycin and cyclophosphamide (preliminary report). Cancer 42:390–398, 1978
192. Smith WG: Surgical treatment of epithelial ovarian carcinoma. Clin Obstet Gynecol 22:939–956, 1979
193. Smith JP, Day TG: Review of ovarian cancer of the University of Texas Systems Cancer Center, M.D. Anderson Hospital and Cancer Institute. Am J Obstet Gynecol 135:984–993, 1979
194. Smith WG, Day TG Jr, Smith JP: The use of laparoscopy to determine the results of chemotherapy for ovarian cancer. J Reprod Med 18:257–260, 1977
195. Smith JP, Delgado G, Rutledge F: Second-look operation in ovarian carcinoma: Post chemotherapy. Cancer 38:1438–1442, 1976
196. Smith JP, Rutledge FN: Chemotherapy in advanced ovarian cancer. Natl Cancer Inst Monogr 42:141–143, 1975
197. Smith JP, Rutledge FN, Delclos L: Postoperative treatment of early cancer of the ovary: A random trial between postoperative irradiation and chemotherapy. Natl Cancer Inst Monogr 42:149–153, 1975
198. Soper JT, Wilkinson RH, Bandy LC, et al: Intraperitoneal chromic phosphate P32 as salvage therapy for persistent carcinoma of the ovary after surgical restaging. Am J Obstet Gynecol 156:1153, 1987
199. Steiner M, Rubinov R, Borovik R, et al: Multimodal approach (surgery, chemotherapy and radiotherapy) in the treatment of advanced ovarian carcinoma. Cancer 55:2748, 1985
200. Stern J, Buscema J, Rosenshein N, et al: Can computed to-

mography substitute for second look operations in ovarian carcinoma? Gynecol Oncol 11:82–88, 1981

201. Stewart JSW, Hird V, Snook D, et al: Intraperitoneal radioimmunotherapy for ovarian cancer: Pharmacokinetics, toxicity and efficacy of I-131 labeled monoclonal antibodies. Int J Radiat Oncol Biol Phys 16:405, 1989
202. Sullivan DC, Harris CC, Currie JL, et al: Observations on the intraperitoneal distribution of chromic phosphate (^{32}P) suspension for intraperitoneal therapy. Radiology 146:539–541, 1983
203. Sutton GP, Stehman FB, Einhorn LW, et al: Ten-year followup of patients receiving cisplatin, doxorubicin and cyclophosphamide chemotherapy for advanced epithelial ovarian carcinoma. J Clin Oncol 7:223, 1989
204. Swenerton KD, Hislop TG, Spinelli J, et al: Ovarian carcinoma: A multivariate analysis of prognostic factors. Obstet Gynecol 65:264–269, 1985
205. Tepper E, Sanfilippo LJ, Gray J, Romney SL: Second look surgery after radiation therapy for advanced stages of cancer of the ovary. Am J Roentgenol Radium Ther Nucl Med 112:755–759, 1971
206. Terada KY, Morley GW, Roberts JA: Pelvic irradiation for stage II ovarian carcinoma. Gynecol Oncol 29:26, 1988
207. Tewfik HH, Tewfik FA, Latourette HR: A clinical review of 17 patients with ovarian dysgerminoma. Int J Radiat Oncol Biol Phys 8:1705–1709, 1982
208. Thigpen JT, Vance RB, Balducci L, Khansur T: New drugs and experimental approaches in ovarian cancer treatment. Semin Oncol 11:314–323, 1984
209. Townsend R, Glassburn JR, Brady LW, Rowland J: Whole abdominal irradiation for carcinoma of the ovary. Cancer Clin Trials 2:351–358, 1979
210. Varia M, Rosenman J, Venkatraman S, et al: Intraperitoneal chromic phosphate therapy after second-look laparotomy for ovarian cancer. Cancer 61:919, 1988
211. Wallner PE, Brady LW, Lewis GC Jr, Nuss RC: Postoperative pelvic irradiation of stage II ovarian carcinoma. Int J Radiat Oncol Biol Phys 2:281–288, 1977
212. Webb MJ, Decker DG, Mussey E, Williams TJ: Factors influencing survival in stage I ovarian cancer. Am J Obstet Gynecol 116:222–228, 1973
213. Webb MJ, Snyder JA, Williams TJ, Decker DG: Second-look laparotomy in ovarian cancer. Gynecol Oncol 14:285–293, 1982
214. Wharton JT, Delclos L, Gallager S, Smith JP: Radiation hepatitis induced by abdominal irradiation with the cobalt^{60} moving strip technique. Am J Roentgenol Radium Ther Nucl Med 117:73–80, 1973
215. Wharton JT, Edwards CL, Stringer CA, et al: Chemotherapy and radiation therapy in the treatment of ovarian carcinoma of common epithelial origin. Clin Obstet Gynecol 28:806, 1985
216. Wharton JT, Herson J: Surgery for common epithelial tumors of the ovary. Cancer 48:582–589, 1981
217. Wils J, VanGeuns H, Baak J: Proposal for therapeutic approach based on prognostic factors including morphometric and flow-cytometric features in stage III–IV ovarian cancer. Cancer 61:1920, 1988
218. Woodruff J: The pathogenesis of ovarian neoplasia. Johns Hopkins Med J 144:117–120, 1979
219. Yazigi R, Wild R, Madrid J, Arraztoa J: Ifosfamide treatment of advanced ovarian cancer. Obstet Gynecol 63:163–166, 1984
220. Yoshimura S, Scully RE, Taft PD, Herrington JB: Peritoneal fluid cytology in patients with ovarian cancer. Gynecol Oncol 17:161–167, 1984
221. Young RC, Knapp RC, Perez CA, et al: Cancer of the ovary. In DeVita VT, Hellman S, Rosenberg SA (eds): Cancer: Principles and Practices of Oncology, pp 884–913. Philadelphia, JB Lippincott, 1982
222. Young RC, Myers CE, Ozols RF, Hogan WM: Chemotherapy in advanced disease. Int J Radiat Oncol Biol Phys 8:899–902, 1982
223. Young RC, Wharton JT, Decker DG, et al: Staging laparotomy in early ovarian cancer. Proc Am Assoc Cancer Res 20: 399, 1979

57

Fallopian Tube

John D. Busowski
Luther W. Brady

ANATOMY

The fallopian tubes lie between the ovaries and the uterus in the upper free border of the broad ligament, called the mesosalpinx. The tubes originate from the uterine cornua and extend to the lateral pelvic wall, opening directly into the peritoneal cavity. Each fallopian tube is 8 cm to 15 cm in length and for the purposes of description is divided into the interstitial, or intramural, portion; the isthmus; the ampulla; and the infundibulum. The interstitial portion is approximately 2 cm long and is contained within the wall of the uterus. The isthmus, the narrowest portion of the tube, lies just lateral to the uterus and extends for 2 cm to 3 cm. The ampulla is the widest and thinnest walled portion, measuring 5 cm to 8 cm long with a luminal diameter of 5 mm to 8 mm. The infundibulum is the lateral portion of the tube and terminates into approximately 25 finger-like processes known as fimbrias.[62]

The arterial blood supply has a dual origin, from the uterine artery and from the ovarian artery.[62] The end branches of the uterine and ovarian arteries anastomose in the mesosalpinx.[62]

Venous drainage of the fallopian tubes follows the arterial supply. The three plexuses become confluent in the subserosa and drain by way of tubal branches of the uterine and ovarian veins.[62]

The intrinsic lymphatics consist of three intercommunicating layers located in the mucosa, muscularis, and serosa. The efferent trunks, usually four or five in number, leave the tubal wall within the mesosalpinx.[66] From the mesosalpinx the lymphatics follow one or more of the following pathways: they pass with vessel of the uterus and anastomose with ovarian vessels to terminate in the periaortic and lumbar nodes[71]; they follow a pelvic course within the broad ligament to terminate in the internal iliac nodes[66]; occasionally, they travel a separate lymphatic channel from the ampulla to the gluteal nodes.[66]

Lymphatic drainage of the fallopian tubes is completely separate from that of the uterine lymphatics.[71]

EPIDEMIOLOGY

Carcinoma of the fallopian tube occurs most frequently in the fifth and sixth decades of life, with age at onset between 18 to 82 years.[2,6,30,39,44,75,82,86] The median age is between 52 and 58 years of age.[45,75] Approximately 50% of patients with fallopian tube carcinoma are postmenopausal. There appears to be no familial or hereditary tendency for the development of tubal carcinoma.[86] Relative infertility and nulliparity are common in patients with fallopian tube carcinoma.[3,27,30,31,75] The disease is frequently associated with chronic nonspecific salpingitis.[31,35] Little association has been found between tuberculosis and tubal carcinoma.[75]

Primary carcinoma of the fallopian tube is one of the rarest malignant tumors of the female genital tract, accounting for 0.15% to 1.8% of all primary gynecologic malignancies.[25,36,41,50] Over 1200 cases of carcinoma of the fallopian tube have been reported.[20,27,32,35,41,57,59,69,75,85]

NATURAL HISTORY

Carcinoma of the fallopian tube appears characteristically as a fusiform swelling that may involve either a portion of or the entire length of the tube.[20,27,82] Fallopian tube carcinoma may resemble a hydrosalpinx or a pyosalpinx and may be mistaken as such at the time of surgery.[36] The external surface is usually smooth but may be rough and may adhere to the pelvic side wall or visceral structures such as the bowel.[80] The fimbriated end of the tube is occluded in approximately 50% of reported cases.[27] When the tumor is encountered in an early stage, a localized swelling is usually observed at the junction of the middle and outer third of the tube.[27] The tumor may be soft initially, but later when infiltration takes place, the mass feels firm and nodular.[62]

On gross examination the tubal lumen is filled with soft-gray to pink, friable growth with areas of marked degeneration, hemorrhage, and yellow areas of necrosis.[27,82]

Bilateral tubal involvement has been reported by a number of investigators and occurs in 7.3% to 26% of cases.[24,58,74,75,79] It is unclear whether bilateral involvement is of multicentric or metastatic origin.[45,66,75,86] The absence of extratubal metastasis in the presence of bilateral tubal involvement supports the concept of independent development of bilateral tumors.[86]

Carcinoma of the fallopian tube arises from the tubal epithelium and may remain intraluminal for a long period of time. The cancer may then disseminate by direct mucosal extension or implantation into the uterus or pelvis.[3,20,32] Spread to distant sites may occur by lymphatic and hematogenous routes.[3,19,89] Sites of dissemination (in order of frequency) are the peritoneum, ovaries, uterus, intestine, vagina, and liver.[3,32,75,76] After it is seeded, the tumor may spread transcoelomically, like ovarian carcinoma.[3,13]

Lymphatic spread occurs to the inguinal, superior gluteal, internal iliac, mesenteric, and periaortic nodes.[20,27,79] Lymphatic spread may occur even when the tumor is grossly confined to the tube.[66] Blood-borne metastases to the lung and liver have been reported.[27,78,84,89,91]

Many patients have relatively early lesions at the time of diagnosis; only 15% have widespread peritoneal dissemination.[63]

An interesting finding in a number of studies is the presence of a second malignancy in patients with carcinoma of the fallopian tube.[10,67,88] Some investigators have suggested that a suppressed immune system may have a role in the development of these malignancies.

CLINICAL PRESENTATION

Carcinoma of the fallopian tube usually produces no early symptoms.[61] Diagnosis is seldom made before surgery because of the rarity of these lesions and the nonspecific nature of the physical findings. Most tubal cancers are preoperatively diagnosed as hydrosalpinx, pyosalpinx, leiomyoma, tubo-ovarian abscess, or ovarian neoplasm.[61]

The most common signs and symptoms of patients with carcinoma of the fallopian tube are intermenstrual or postmenopausal vaginal bleeding, serosanguineous or watery vaginal discharge, and crampy or intermittent lower abdominal or pelvic pain.[10,19,32,75,76,89] The triad of pain, serosanguineous vaginal discharge, and pelvic mass has been considered characteristic of carcinoma of the fallopian tube. However, in studies by Hanton and associates[30] and Yoonessi[29] only 11% and 15% of the patients, respectively, had these features.

Intermittent vaginal discharge with a diminishing adnexal mass on pelvic examination, called hydrops tubae profluens, was considered to be pathognomonic of tubal cancer.[27,49] However, the condition is more frequently associated with benign causes of tubal dilatation.[5,86]

Ascites and gastrointestinal or genitourinary complaints are infrequent findings in tubal carcinoma.[32,86]

DIAGNOSTIC WORKUP AND STAGING

Many reports suggest that evaluation of cervical cytologic specimen could lead to early diagnosis of tubal carcinoma.[4,9,22,25,26,42,73] However, many reports fail to show a correlation between cytologic findings and the presence of tubal carcinoma.[8,14,16,27,70,76] One study reported the detection of carcinoma of the fallopian tube during a vaginal hysterectomy by cytologic examination of the secretions in the space of Douglas.[48] Hysterosalpingography has been recommended by some investigators for diagnosis; others are concerned about the risk of spread of malignant cells into the peritoneum.[33,46,53,79] Also, the radiographic appearance (hysterosalpingogram) of tubal carcinoma is the same or nearly identical with that of chronic salpingitis and hydrosalpinx.[57] Laparoscopy and culdoscopy have been proposed as aids in the diagnosis of tubal cancer, but serosal involvement with tumor would be necessary for visualization and identification.[11,21,37] Therefore diagnosis of only advanced disease would be possible. The use of intravenous pyelogram (IVP) and barium enemas in the detection of fallopian tube carcinoma has been advocated by some investigators; however, these radiographic studies have identified only pelvic masses that had been palpated previously.[76] Hirai and associates reported a 60% detection rate of carcinoma of the fallopian tube using endometrial sampling.[34]

Staging of carcinoma of the fallopian tube is done at laparotomy. The presence or absence of ascitic fluid is noted. If present, the fluid is sent for cytologic evaluation and, if absent, the peritoneal cavity is washed with normal saline, which is then withdrawn for cytologic examination. The omental apron should be excised and the diaphragm and bowel should be examined for metastatic implants and direct tumor invasion.[15] Table 57-1 outlines suggested diagnostic procedures.

Several criteria have been proposed to differentiate carcinoma of the fallopian tube from metastatic disease from adjacent organs[61]:

1. The primary tubal involvement is the endosalpinx.
2. The epithelium of the endosalpinx is replaced by adenocarcinoma.
3. The neoplastic cells resemble those of normal tubal epithelium.
4. The ovaries and endometrium either are normal or they contain a small malignant lesion with histologic characteristics of tubal epithelium.
5. Transition from benign to malignant epithelium is found.
6. Tuberculosis of the tube has been excluded.[23,25]

In a few patients with extensive disease, a tumor may involve both the tube and the adjacent ovary, and it is impossible to determine the exact primary site of the tumor. Such tumors may be classified as tubo-ovarian carcinoma; however, the malignancy is probably of ovarian origin because of the higher incidence of ovarian carcinoma.[62]

There is no TNM classification of standardized staging for carcinoma of the fallopian tube. Three separate systems have been proposed (Table 57-2). Erez and colleagues proposed a staging system similar to that used for ovarian carcinoma on the premise that the two organs are closely related anatomically and the pattern of dissemination appears to be similar.[20] Dodson

TABLE 57–1
Diagnostic Workup for Carcinoma of the Fallopian Tube

General
- History
- Physical examination, including pelvic and rectal

Special Procedures
- Laparotomy
  - Cytologic examination of ascites or saline washings of peritoneal cavity
  - Removal of omental apron
  - Examination of diaphragm
  - Sampling of internal iliac and periaortic nodes
- Dilatation and curettage to exclude endometrial primary lesion

Radiographic Studies
- Standard
  - Chest x-ray
  - Intravenous pyelography
  - Ultrasonography or CT scan of abdomen and pelvis with special attention to retroperitoneal nodes
- Complementary
  - Barium enema (if large pelvic mass presents) to rule out colorectal involvement
  - Lymphangiography

Laboratory Studies
- Complete blood count
- Blood chemistry
- Urinalysis

TABLE 57–2
Staging of Primary Carcinoma of the Fallopian Tubes

EREZ AND ASSOCIATES[20]	
I	Tubal carcinoma without extension to serosa
II	Extension to serosa or adjacent pelvic viscera
III	Extension beyond pelvis but confined to peritoneal cavity
IV	Presence of extra-abdominal metastases
DODSON AND ASSOCIATES[86]*	
I	Growth limited to tube
Ia	Growth limited to one tube, no ascites
Ib	Growth limited to both tubes, no ascites
Ic	Growth in one or both tubes; ascites with malignant cells
II	Growth involving one or both tubes with pelvic extension
IIa	Extension or metastases to uterus or ovary
IIb	Extension to other pelvic tissues
III	Growth involving one or both tubes with widespread intraperitoneal metastases to abdomen (omentum, small intestine and its mesentery)
IV	Growth involving one or both tubes with distant metastases outside peritoneal cavity
SCHILLER AND SILVERBERG[74]	
0	Carcinoma *in situ* (limited to tubal mucosa)
I	Tumor extending into submucosa or muscularis but not penetrating to serosal surface of fallopian tube
II	Tumor extending to serosa of fallopian tube
III	Direct extension to ovary or endometrium
IV	Extension of tumor beyond reproductive organs (for example, to other pelvic organs, pelvic soft tissues, peritoneal implants, abdominal viscera)

* *Bilateral disease does not alter stage.*

and co-workers proposed a system based on the American College of Obstetricians and Gynecologists (ACOG) and the International Federation of Gynecology and Obstetrics staging systems for ovarian carcinoma.[16] A third staging system, proposed by Schiller and Silverberg, is similar to the Dukes system for staging colon and rectal cancer.[74] Schiller and Silverberg contend that because the fallopian tube is a hollow viscus with a muscular wall similar to that of the colon, the mechanics of tumor penetration and dissemination differ from those of ovarian malignancies and are similar to those of colon cancers.

PATHOLOGIC CLASSIFICATION

Adenocarcinoma is the most common type of malignant tumor of the fallopian tube. Other malignant tumor types are carcinosarcoma, adenoacanthoma, squamous cell carcinoma, adenosquamous carcinoma, mixed mullerian tumors, choriocarcinoma, and lymphoma.[1,29,33,43,51,52,56,60,61,75,81,83,87] As with staging, several histopathologic classifications have been suggested. The most commonly used grading classification is that devised by Hu and associates.[35]

The papillary type (grade 1) is the most common and characteristic type of fallopian tube tumor. The tumor is well-differentiated with columnar, nonciliated cells. Transition from normal epithelium to neoplastic epithelium can usually be seen. The tumor is often confined to the mucosal layer, and mitoses are few.

In the papillary-alveolar type (grade 2) of tumor, the papillary pattern persists, but gland formation and early invasion of the tubal wall are present. The tumor is less well differentiated, and the number of mitoses is increased.

In the alveolar-medullary pattern (grade 3) of fallopian tube tumor, cells are arranged in solid sheets or around gland-like spaces, and most of the papillary pattern is lost. Mitoses are common, and lymphatic invasion is present. The more anaplastic the tumor, the greater is its propensity for invasion and dissemination.

PROGNOSTIC FACTORS

The stage of the lesion is an important prognostic indicator for survival in patients with carcinoma of the fallopian tube.[3,30,31,40,45,54,82] The salvage rate of the disease is poor, primarily because of late diagnosis.[18,45,89] Early detection and adequate initial therapy are required to improve prognosis.

The overall 5-year survival rate for carcinoma of the fallopian tube varies from 5% to 44%.[8,30,35,41,79] For Stage II, Stage III, and Stage IV disease, the 5-year survival rates are 45%, 15%, and 0%, respectively.[70] Some studies associate a poorer prognosis with bilateral tubal involvement, whereas other studies show no change in prognosis.[45,62,74] Better survival rates have been reported in patients with tubal ostial closure. The assumption is that ostial closure interferes with transluminal spread and prevents dissemination of the malignancy.[89] In a study of 22 patients by Podratz and associates[67] in which peritoneal fluid or washings were obtained for cytologic analysis, the presence of malignant cells within the peritoneal cavity correlated with patient longevity. Survival at 2 and 5 years was 92% and 67% for patients with normal cytologic results and 30% and 20%, respectively, for those with positive cytologic findings ($P < 0.01$).[67]

After the tubal serosa has been involved, metastases develop regardless of the histologic grade. Hu and associates[35] and Momtazee and Kempson[57] have reported a 50% to 60% 5-year survival rate with grade 1, 40% with grade 2, and 16.7% with grade 3 lesions.

The prognostic value of histologic differentiation has been debated. Hu and associates found a relationship between grade and survival, as did Momtazee and Kempson.[35,57] In each study, poorly differentiated tumors were associated with a poorer prognosis. The results of Denham and MacLennan,[13] Hanton and colleagues,[30] Yoonessi,[89] McMurray and associates,[55] Semrad and colleagues,[76] and Young and co-workers[91] do not support this conclusion.

Peters and associates,[64] in a study of 115 women with carcinoma of the fallopian tube, reported that in 39 women with Stage I disease, only the depth of invasion within the tubal wall was a statistically significant variable. Variables tested within this group were age, grade, presence or absence of tubal occlusion, and depth of tubal invasion.

GENERAL MANAGEMENT

Because the routes of spread of tubal carcinoma are similar to those of ovarian carcinoma, it is reasonable to use the same procedures for evaluating the extent of tubal carcinoma as those used to evaluate ovarian tumor spread.[30] These procedures are peritoneal washings, inspection and biopsy of diaphragmatic surfaces, and partial omentectomy. The observation by Tamimi and Figge[79] of frequent metastasis to the pelvic and periaortic nodes suggests that lymph node dissection should be part of the initial workup in patients with disease apparently confined to the pelvis at laparotomy.

The primary treatment of carcinoma of the fallopian tube is total abdominal hysterectomy and bilateral salpingo-oophorectomy. An aggressive effort should be made to search for occult disease and to remove all gross tumor because a relationship exists between residual tumor burden and long-term survival.[33] Omentectomy should be performed because of the frequent occurrence of tumor seeding.[59] Removal of regional lymph nodes has been recommended; however, the true incidence of pelvic and periaortic nodal metastasis and the value of pelvic lymphadenectomy remain unknown. At the very least, suspicious nodes should be sampled. Some investigators recommend extensive surgery, including removal of bowel and abdominal wall and total pelvic exenteration, for locally advanced and technically resectable disease.[12] However, radical procedures add to postoperative morbidity and delay the administration of adjunctive chemotherapy or radiation therapy. If intraperitoneal colloidal chromic phosphate ^{32}P is to be used postoperatively, Silastic or polyethylene catheters should be placed in the upper right abdominal quadrant and *cul de sac.*

A unilateral salpingo-oophorectomy may be adequate surgical treatment for a small, well-differentiated tubal carcinoma confined to the mucosal layer. However, most investigators believe that a total abdominal hysterectomy is warranted even in early stage disease. Cytoreductive surgery, leaving tumor deposits no greater than 2 cm in any location, may be of value when followed by multiple agent chemotherapy or abdominopelvic irradiation.[62]

Surgery is probably sufficient treatment for well-differentiated Stage I lesions confined to the mucosa. Those patients with advanced disease require additional therapy.

Few data are available on the use of chemotherapy in the treatment of carcinoma of the fallopian tube. Yoonessi[89] and McMurray and associates[55] have shown that distant metastases are responsible for more than 50% of the failures in Stage I and Stage II disease. Semrad and colleagues reported that ten of 14 patients with recurrent disease had recurrence at sites that were extraperitoneal, and of the ten patients with extraperitoneal disease, six had metastasis above the diaphragm.[76] Consequently, adjunctive systemic therapy would be desirable.[57] Deppe and colleagues described surgically proven complete remission in two patients treated with cisplatin, doxorubicin, and progestins.[14] Eddy and co-workers reported on three additional patients treated with a variety of regimens; all demonstrated prolonged survival.[17] After second-look procedure none had evidence of disease.

In addition to progestins, tubal carcinoma has been shown to respond to thiotepa, 5-fluorouracil, melphalan, cyclophosphamide, and cisplatin.[7,14,77] Trials of combination therapy have been suggested in patients with recurrent disease and in those with large residual disease after surgery. Combinations of alkylating agents, such as 5-fluorouracil, and progestational agents with or without doxorubicin have been found to be acceptable.[13,28] The use of cyclophosphamide and cisplatin with or without doxorubicin has also be advocated. Recent studies have shown response rates of over 75% with cisplatin-containing combination chemotherapy.[38,54] The policies for suggested management for tubal carcinoma are summarized in Table 57-3.

TABLE 57–3
Suggested Management of Cancer of the Fallopian Tube

SURGICAL

Primary treatment consists of total abdominal hysterectomy and bilateral salpingo-oophorectomy, removal of all large tumor masses, omentectomy

RADIATION THERAPY

Pelvic irradiation if tumor confined to pelvic organs

Total abdominal and pelvic irradiation—small volume residual disease after cytoreductive surgery; any extrapelvic spread

Irradiation combined with systemic chemotherapy—large volume residual disease (pelvic or abdominal)

CHEMOTHERAPY

For residual, large volume, recurrent, metastatic disease—
- L-Phenylalanine mustard
- Chlorambucil
- 5-Fluorouracil
- PAC (platinum, Adriamycin, Cytoxan)

(Henderson SR, Harper RC, Salazar OM, et al: Gynecol Oncol 5:168, 1977)

RADIATION THERAPY TECHNIQUES

Postoperative radiation therapy for tubal carcinoma has been recommended by some investigators and questioned by others.[8,19,24,30,36,39,57,68,70] It is difficult to analyze the literature because of the lack of uniform staging of the disease, variability in field size, dosage, fractionation, and type of radiation used. Radiation therapy techniques include 5000 cGy to 6000 cGy whole-pelvis external-beam irradiation for the more aggressive Stage I and Stage II tumors. For Stage III disease whole-pelvis and abdominal irradiation are required. Techniques resemble those used for the treatment of ovarian cancers.[62] Instillation of radioactive colloidal gold (^{198}Au) or colloidal chromic phosphate (^{32}P) has been recommended in cases where no macroscopic disease is present in the peritoneal cavity.[3,24,31,70]

RESULTS OF THERAPY

Many studies have shown the benefits of postoperative radiation therapy for tubal carcinoma. In 1957, Engstrom[19] reported significant improvement in cases of carcinoma of the fallopian tube treated with postoperative radium and deep external-beam irradiation. Those who received postoperative radiation therapy showed a 38% 5-year survival rate compared with a 15% 5-year survival rate in those treated only with surgery. Green and Scully reported an average survival time of 2 years with postoperative irradiation and no survivors after 1 year following surgery without radiation therapy.[27] Fogh[24] demonstrated increased survival in patients treated with high-voltage radiation *versus* conventional radiation, with 2.5-year survival rates of 60% and 30%, respectively.

Boutselis and Thompson[8] reported an increased 5-year survival rate in seven of eight patients treated postoperatively with radiation therapy. Phelps and Chapman[65] described good results for patients with Stage I and Stage II disease treated with supervoltage and megavoltage irradiation. Nine patients with Stage I or Stage II disease received 2500 cGy to 5000 cGy to the pelvis or abdomen or both. Six patients also received intraperitoneal radioactive ^{198}Au or ^{32}P. Eight of the nine patients were alive at the time of publication of the study; six patients had survived for 5 years. Six patients with Stage III disease were treated with postoperative therapy; none survived.

In a series involving 12 patients reported by Henderson and associates,[32] postoperative irradiation resulted in a 50%

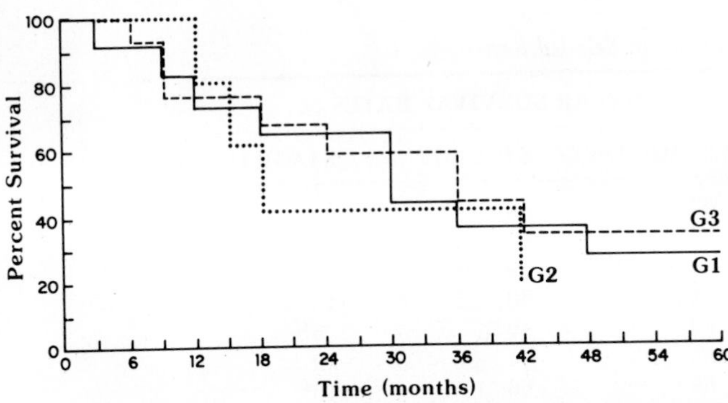

FIGURE 57–1. Survival rates in fallopian tube carcinoma according to histologic differentiation (Washington University, 1950–1981).

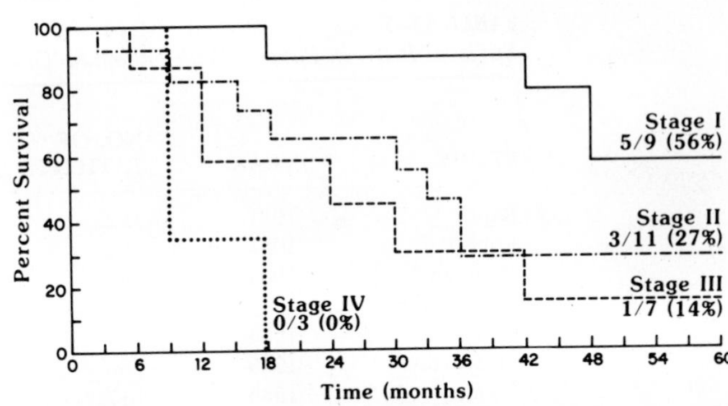

FIGURE 57–2. Survival rates in fallopian tube carcinoma according to surgical stage (Washington University, 1950–1981).

5-year survival rate compared with a 25% 5-year survival rate in those patients threated with surgery only. In a retrospective study of 34 patients at the University of Michigan Medical Center, Amendola and co-workers[2] analyzed 5-year survival rates according to the dosage of postoperative irradiation. They found that one of four patients was alive who received less than 3000 cGy, and one of four patients was alive who received between 3000 cGy and 5000 cGy. However, five of 14 patients who received more than 5000 cGy were alive and free from disease.

Brown and colleagues[10] noted that of nine patients treated with abdominopelvic or pelvic-aortic irradiation, five remained disease-free. Of the five patients who received more limited uterine or pelvic irradiation, three failures occurred, two of which were in the upper abdomen.

McMurray and co-workers[55] reported on 30 patients with adenocarcinoma of the fallopian tube treated at Washington University. Nine had Stage I disease, 11 had Stage II disease, seven had Stage III disease, and three had Stage IV disease. Histologic differentiation was grade 1 in 39%, grade 2 in 18%, and grade 3 in 43%. Primary surgical treatment consisted of total abdominal hysterectomy and bilateral salpingo-oophorectomy in 70% of the patients; 23% had more extensive surgery, and 13% had incomplete extirpation of the internal reproductive organs. Three patients with Stage I tumors were treated with surgery alone; the others received postoperative irradiation, chemotherapy, or both. Survival was unrelated to grade but was highly dependent on stage (Fig. 57-1). Disease-free survival rates at 3 years were 86% for patients with Stage I, 27% for Stage II, 29% for Stage III, and 0% for Stage IV disease (Fig. 57-2). Four of five patients treated with a combination of cisplatin, doxorubicin, and cyclophosphamide following surgery survived at least 3 years. Patterns of initial treatment failure showed 66% with a component of pelvic failure, 50% with a component of upper abdominal failure, and 44% with extraperitoneal metastases as a component of failure. Results according to method of treatment (Table 57-4) suggest that aggressive postoperative adjuvant therapy targeted at the upper abdomen and distant sites of metastasis in all lesions beyond Stage I will improve survival and tumor control.

Podratz and associates[67] assessed the results of treatment of 16 patients with disease localized to the pelvic genitalia (ten patients with Stage IA disease and six with Stage IIA disease). The patients were assessed according to whether treatment was directed to the pelvis only or beyond the true pelvis. The patients treated with surgery alone or surgery with pelvic irradiation experienced a 50% relapse rate. In contrast, among the group of six patients who received systemic or whole abdominal therapy or both, only one had a recurrence. The patient who experienced the recurrence had been treated with L-phenylalanine mustard and pelvic irradiation. Hence, this study supports the use of postoperative adjuvant radiation therapy to the entire abdomen in patients with localized disease. Table 57-5 summarizes the treatment results reported by several authors.

SEQUELAE OF TREATMENT

Complications of postoperative radiation therapy for tubal carcinoma are not often mentioned in the literature. Kinzel described a high incidence of bowel complications in patients with advanced disease.[45] Amendola and associates[2] reported mild complications in three of 22 patients, including erythematous

TABLE 57–4
Survival According to Treatment and Stage

	TREATMENT OF PATIENTS SURVIVING 3 OR MORE YEARS					
STAGE	S	S + RT	S + CT	S + PAC	S + CT + RT	TOTAL
I	3/3	1/2	3/3*	—	1/1	8/9
II	—	2/5	0/2	3/3†	0/1	5/11
III	—	—	0/3	1/2	1/2*	2/7
IV	—	—	0/1		0/2	0/3

* *Two patients received RT*
† *One patient alive with disease.*
S: surgery; RT: radiation therapy; CT: chemotherapy; PAC: cisplatin, Adriamycin (doxorubicin), and Cytoxan (cyclophosphamide)

TABLE 57–5
Survival Rates in Patients With Fallopian Tube Carcinoma in Selected Series

STUDY	YEAR	NO. OF PATIENTS	5-YEAR SURVIVAL RATES (%)		
			STAGE I	STAGE II	STAGE III
Raju[68]	1981	22	57	58	25
Roberts[70]	1981	102	77	42	6*
Denham[13]	1984	40	69	39	29
Seven series†			72	38	18
Eddy[17]	1984	71	40	40	5*
McMurray[55]	1985	30	59	44	29
Brown[10]	1985	17	60	66	16*
Podratz[67]	1986	47	64	60	18
Semrad[76]	1986	30	53	22	0*

** Stage III and Stage IV*
† Collected by Denham JW, Mallennan KA: Cancer 53:166, 1984

skin, diarrhea, and dysuria. One patient had a severe complication, a vesicovaginal fistula, after completion of 5 weeks of 5000 cGy external pelvic irradiation.

NEW APPROACHES

Early detection remains the key to increased survival of patients with carcinoma of the fallopian tube. Improved survival rates might result from earlier diagnosis, aggressive efforts to remove all gross tumor, omentectomy, postoperative radiation therapy, and adjuvant multidrug chemotherapy that includes cisplatin.

REFERENCES

1. Acosta AA, Kaplan AL, Kaufman RH: Mixed mullerian tumors of the oviduct. Obstet Gynecol 44:84, 1974
2. Amendola BE, LaRouere J, Amendola MA, et al: Adenocarcinoma of the fallopian tube. Surg Gynecol Obstet 50:223, 1983
3. Benedet JL, White GW, Fairley RN, et al: Adenocarcinoma of the fallopian tube. Obstet Gynecol 50:654, 1977
4. Benson PA: Cytologic diagnosis in primary carcinoma of the fallopian tube. Acta Cytol 18:429, 1974
5. Besserer G: Value of cytodiagnosis in detection of primary carcinoma of the fallopian tube. Geburtshilfe Frauenheilkd 13:660, 1953
6. Blaikey JB: Advanced adenocarcinoma of the fallopian tube. J Obstet Gynaecol Br Commonw 80:757, 1973
7. Bornonow RC: Chemotherapy for disseminated tubal cancer. Obstet Gynecol 42:62, 1973
8. Boutselis JG, Thompson JN: Clinical aspects of primary carcinoma of the fallopian tube. Am J Obstet Gynecol 111:98, 1971
9. Brewer JL, Guiderian AM: Diagnosis of uterine tube carcinoma by vaginal cytology. Obstet Gynecol 8:664, 1956
10. Brown MD, Kohorn EI, Kapp DS, et al: Fallopian tube carcinoma. Int J Radiat Oncol Biol Phys 11:583, 1985
11. Chalmer JA, Marshall AT: Carcinoma of the fallopian tube. Br J Obstet Gynaecol 83:580, 1976
12. Clark DGG, Brunschwig A: Total pelvic exenteration for recurrent carcinoma of the uterine tube: Report of a case. Obstet Gynecol 24:569, 1964
13. Denham JW, MacLennan KA: The management of primary carcinoma of the fallopian tube: Experience of 40 cases. Cancer 53:166, 1984
14. Deppe G, Bruckner HW, Cohen CJ: Combination chemotherapy for advanced carcinoma of the fallopian tube. Obstet Gynecol 56:530, 1980
15. DiSaia PJ, Creasman WT: Clinical Gynecologic Oncology, p 395. St. Louis, CV Mosby, 1984
16. Dodson MG, Ford JH, Averette HE: Clinical aspects of fallopian tube carcinoma. Obstet Gynecol 36:935, 1970
17. Eddy GC, Copeland, LJ, Gershenson DM, et al: Fallopian tube carcinoma. Obstet Gynecol 64:546, 1984
18. England D, Davidsohn I: Isoantigens A, B, and H in carcinoma of the fallopian tube. Arch Pathol 96:350, 1973
19. Engstrom L: Primary carcinoma of the fallopian tube. Acta Obstet Gynecol Scand 36:289, 1957
20. Erez S, Kaplan AL, Wall JA: Clinical staging of carcinoma of the uterine tube. Obstet Gynecol 30:547, 1967
21. Farber SA: Carcinoma of the fallopian tube. S Afr Med J 47:1321, 1973
22. Fidler HK, Lock DR: Carcinoma of the fallopian tube detected by cervical smear. Am J Obstet Gynecol 67:1103, 1954
23. Finn WF, Javert CT: Primary and metastatic carcinoma of the fallopian tube. Cancer 2:803, 1949
24. Fogh IB: Primary carcinoma of the fallopian tube. Cancer 23:1332, 1961
25. Frankel AN: Primary carcinoma of the fallopian tube. Am J Obstet Gynecol 72:131, 1956
26. Garret R: Extrauterine tumor cells in vaginal and cervical smears. Obstet Gynecol 14:21, 1959
27. Green TH, Scully, RE: Tumors of the fallopian tube. Clin Obstet Gynecol 5:886, 1962
28. Guthrie D, Cohen S: Carcinoma of the fallopian tube treated with a combination of surgery and cytotoxic chemotherapy. Br J Obstet Gynaecol 88:1051, 1981
29. Hanjani P, Petersen RO, Bonnell SA: Malignant mixed mullerian tumor of the fallopian tube. Gynecol Oncol 9:381, 1980
30. Hanton EM, Malkasian GD, Dahlin DC, et al: Primary carcinoma of the fallopian tube. Am J Obstet Gynecol 94:832, 1966
31. Hayden GE, Potter EL: Primary carcinoma of the fallopian tube. Am J Obstet Gynecol 79:24, 1960
32. Henderson SR, Harper RC, Salazar OM, et al: Primary carcinoma of the fallopian tube: Difficulties in diagnosis and treatment. Gynecol Oncol 5:168, 1977
33. Hershey DW, Fennell RH, Major FJ: Primary carcinoma of the fallopian tube. Obstet Gynecol 57:367, 1981
34. Hirai Y, Chen JT, Hamada T, et al: Clinical and cytologic aspects of primary carcinoma of fallopian tube carcinoma. Acta Cytol 31:834, 1987
35. Hu CY, Taymor ML, Hertig AT: Primary carcinoma of the fallopian tube. Am J Obstet Gynecol 59: 58, 1950

36. Hurlbutt FR, Nelson HB: Primary carcinoma of the uterine tube. Obstet Gynecol 21:730, 1963
37. Ingram FH, Hisley JC: Primary carcinoma of the fallopian tube. South Med J 68:1153, 1975
38. Jacobs AJ, McMurray EH, Parham J: Treatment of carcinoma of the fallopian tube using cisplatin, doxorubicin, and cyclophosphamide. Am J Clin Oncol 9:436, 1986
39. Johnson WO, Miller AJ: Primary carcinoma of the oviduct. Ann Surg 93:1208, 1931
40. Johnston, GA: Primary malignancy of the fallopian tube: A clinical review of 13 cases. J Surg Oncol 24:304, 1983
41. Jones OV: Primary carcinoma of the uterine tube. Obstet Gynecol 26:122, 1965
42. Kadziora MB, Srinivasan R: Primary carcinoma of the fallopian tube. Can J Surg 24:425, 1981
43. Kahanppa KV, Laine R, Saksela E: Malignant mixed mullerian tumor of the fallopian tube: Report of a case with 5-year survival. Gynecol Oncol 16:144, 1983
44. Kahn ME, Norris S: Primary carcinoma of the fallopian tubes. Am J Obstet Gynecol 28:393, 1934
45. Kinzel GE: Primary carcinoma of the fallopian tube. Am J Obstet Gynecol 125:816, 1976
46. Kneale BLG, Attwood HD: Primary carcinoma of the fallopian tube. Am J Obstet Gynecol 94:840, 1966
47. Krugman PI, Fisher JE: Primary carcinoma of the fallopian tube. Am J Obstet Gynecol 80:722, 1960
48. Kubler HC, Kuhn W, Rummel HH, et al: Zur diagnostik okkulter tubenkarzinome durch intraoperative peritoneal zytologis. Geburtshilfe Frauenheilkd 48:116, 1988
49. Latzko W: Linkseitiges tubenkarzinom rechtseitige karzinomatose tuboovarialcyste. Zentralbl Gynakol 40:599, 1916
50. Lofgren KA, Docketry MB: Primary carcinoma of the fallopian tubes. Surg Gynecol Obstet 82:199, 1946
51. Malinak LR, Miller GV, Armstrong JT: Primary squamous cell carcinoma of the fallopian tube. Am J Obstet Gynecol 95:1167, 1966
52. Manes JL, Taylor HB: Carcinosarcoma and mixed mullerian tumors of the fallopian tube. Cancer 38:1687, 1976
53. Martzloff HK: Primary cancer of the fallopian tube: A consideration of its incidence, clinical diagnosis, and treatment, with the report of a case diagnosed before operation. Am J Obstet Gynecol 40:804, 1940
54. Maxsom WZ, Stehman FB, Ulbright TM, et al: Primary carcinoma of the fallopian tube: Evidence for activity of cisplatin combination therapy. Gynecol Oncol 26:3053, 1987
55. McMurray EH, Jacobs AJ, Perez CA, et al: Carcinoma of the fallopian tube: Management and sites of failure. Cancer 58:2070, 1986
56. McQueeney, AJ, Carswell BL, Sheehan WJ: Malignant mixed mullerian tumor primary in uterine tube: Review of the literature and report of an additional case. Obstet Gynecol 23:338, 1964
57. Momtazee S, Kempson RL: Primary adenocarcinoma of the fallopian tube. Obstet Gynecol 32:649, 1968
58. Novak ER, Woodruff JD: Novak's Gynecologic and Obstetric Pathology, 8th ed, pp 314–318. Philadelphia, WB Saunders, 1980
59. Orthmann EG: Ueber Primares Tubencarcinom. Z Geburtshilfe Gynek 15:212, 1888
60. O'Toole RV, Tuttle SE, Shah NT: Heterologous carcinosarcoma of the fallopian tube. J Reprod Med 27:749, 1982
61. Patton GW, Goldstein DP: Gestational choriocarcinoma of the tube and ovary. Surg Gynecol Obstet 137:608, 1973
62. Pauerstein CJ: The Fallopian Tube: A Reappraisal, pp 150–185. Philadelphia, Lea & Febiger, 1974
63. Perez CA, Knapp RC, DiSaia PJ, Young RC: Gynecological tumors. In DeVita VT, Hellman S, Rosenberg SA (eds): Principles and Practice of Oncology. Philadelphia, JB Lippincott, 1985
64. Peters WA, Andersen WA, Hopkins MP, et al: Prognostic features of carcinoma of the fallopian tube. Obstet Gynecol 71:757, 1988
65. Phelps MH, Chapman EK: Role of radiotherapy in treatment of primary carcinoma of the uterine tube. Obstet Gynecol 43:669, 1974
66. Plentl AA, Friedman EA: Lymphatic System of the Female Genitalia: The Morphologic Basis of Oncologic Diagnosis and Therapy, pp 153–167. Philadelphia, WB Saunders, 1971
67. Podratz KC, Podczaski ES, Gaffey TA, et al: Primary carcinoma of the fallopian tube. Am J Obstet Gynecol 154:1319, 1986
68. Raju KS, Barker GH, Wiltshaw E: Primary carcinoma of the fallopian tube: Report of 22 cases. Br J Obstet Gynaecol 88:1124, 1981
69. Renaud F: Primary cancer of the fallopian tube. Trans Obstet Soc Lond 38:322, 1896
70. Roberts JA, Lifshitz S: Primary adenocarcinoma of the fallopian tube. Gynecol Oncol 13:301, 1982
71. Rodbard S, McMahon NJ, Denk M: Uterine structure and lymphatics. Obstet Gynecol 38:171, 1971
72. Ross WM: Primary tumours of the fallopian tube: A report of eight cases of adenocarcinoma and one case of unusual carcinoma. Can Med Assoc J 96:328, 1967
73. Scharl A, Crombach G, Krueger G, et al: Symptom harninkontinenz als hinweis auf ein tubenkarzinom. Geburtshilfe Frauenheilkd 48:113, 1988
74. Schiller HM, Silverberg SG: Staging and prognosis in primary carcinoma of the fallopian tube. Cancer 28:389, 1971
75. Sedlis A: Primary carcinoma of the fallopian tube. Obstet Gynecol Surv 16:209, 1961
76. Semrad N, Watring W, Fu YS, et al: Fallopian tube adenocarcinoma: Common extraperitoneal recurrence. Gynecol Oncol 24:230, 1986
77. Smith JP: Chemotherapy in gynecologic cancer. Clin Obstet Gynecol 18:109, 1975
78. Southland WFW: Carcinoma of the uterine tube: A review and a description of a case with unusual clinical features, presenting as an acute abdominal emergency. Br J Surg 44:487, 1956
79. Tamimi HK, Figge DC: Adenocarcinoma of the uterine tube: Potential for lymph node metastases. Am J Obstet Gynecol 141:132, 1981
80. Turunen A: Diagnosis and treatment of primary tubal carcinoma. Int J Gynaecol Obstet 7:294, 1969
81. Viniker DA, Mantell BS, Greenstein RJ: Carcinosarcoma of the fallopian tube: A case report and review of the literature. Br J Obstet Gynaecol 87:530, 1980
82. Weekes LR, Stratton EW, Elston JH: Primary carcinoma of the fallopian tube: A ten year study, 1952–1961. J Natl Med Assoc 55:268, 1963
83. Weiss PD, Mac Dougall MK, Reagan JW, et al: Primary adenosquamous carcinoma of the fallopian tube. Obstet Gynecol 55:88s, 1980
84. Willis RA: A review of 500 consecutive cancer autopsies. Med J Aust 2:258, 1941
85. Woodruff JD: Tumors of the fallopian tube and tumors and cysts of the pelvic ligaments and paraadnexal structures. In Sciarra JJ (ed): Gynecology and Obstetrics. pp 1–8. Philadelphia, Harper & Row, 1989
86. Woodruff JD, Pauerstein CJ: The Fallopian Tube: Structure, Function, Pathology and Management. p 271. Baltimore, Williams & Wilkins, 1969
87. Wu JP, Tanner WS, Fardal PM: Malignant mixed mullerian tumor of the uterine tube. Obstet Gynecol 41:707, 1973
88. Yeung HH, Bannatyne P, Russell P: Adenocarcinoma of the fallopian tubes: A clinicopathological study of eight cases. Pathology 15:279, 1983
89. Yoonessi M: Carcinoma of the fallopian tube. Obstet Gynecol Surv 34:257, 1979
90. Yoonessi M, Leberer JP, Crickard K: Primary fallopian tube carcinoma: Treatment and spread pattern. J Surg Oncol 38:97, 1988
91. Young JA, Kossman CR, Green MR: Adenocarcinoma of the fallopian tube: Report of a case with an unusual pattern of metastasis and response to combination chemotherapy. Gynecol Oncol 17:238, 1984

58

○ ○ ○ • • •

Vagina

Carlos A. Perez

ANATOMY

The vagina is a muscular, dilatable tube, approximately 7.5 cm in length, and is located posterior to the base of the bladder and urethra and anterior to the rectum. The upper fourth of the posterior wall is separated from the rectum by a reflection of peritoneum called the pouch of Douglas. At its uppermost extent the vaginal wall meets the uterine cervix, attaching at a higher point on the posterior wall than on the anterior wall, which constitutes the vaginal fornices. The vaginal wall is composed of three layers: the mucosa, the muscularis, and the adventitia. The inner mucosal layer is formed by a thick, nonkeratinizing, stratified, squamous epithelium overlying a basement membrane containing many papillae. The epithelium normally contains no glands but is lubricated by mucous secretions originating in the cervix. The muscularis layer is composed of smooth muscle fibers arranged circularly on the inner portion and longitudinally on the thicker outer portion. A vaginal sphincter is formed by skeletal muscle at the introitus. The adventitia is a thin, outer connective tissue layer that merges with that of adjacent organs.

The lymphatics in the upper portion of the vagina drain primarily through the lymphatics of the cervix, whereas those in the lowest portion of the vagina drain either cephalad to cervical lymphatics or follow drainage patterns of the vulva into femoral and inguinal nodes. The anterior vaginal wall usually drains into the deep pelvic nodes, including the interiliac and parametrial nodes (Fig. 58-1).

EPIDEMIOLOGY

Primary carcinoma of the vagina is a malignant lesion that arises in the vagina and does not involve the cervix or vulva. It is rare, representing 1% to 2% of all gynecologic malignancies.[12,23,58] A decrease in the incidence of primary vaginal tumors has been noted in recent years, possibly because of early detection with cervical cytology or more rigid diagnostic criteria that have eliminated from this category primary cancers arising from adjacent organs, such as the cervix, the vulva, and the endometrium.

Most primary vaginal cancers are squamous cell in origin. Herbst and associates[23] reviewed the literature on primary squamous cell carcinoma and noted that 47% of the patients were 60 years of age or older, with a peak incidence in the 50- to 70-year-old age group and a mean age of 60 to 65 years. They found no apparent etiology or associated factors that predisposed a patient to this malignancy.

Irradiation has been suggested as a possible cause of primary squamous cell carcinoma of the vagina.[71] In a report of 43 patients, five of whom presented with invasive carcinoma of the vagina 7 or more years after radiation therapy for invasive carcinoma of the cervix, Pride and associates[54] suggested without statistical basis that these lesions may have been induced by irradiation. However, an analysis of 1200 patients treated over a period of 20 years at Washington University failed to demonstrate an increase in the incidence of pelvic second neoplasias following radiation therapy.[34]

In the past 10 years interest has focused on an increased incidence of clear cell adenocarcinoma of the vagina in young women, which in 1971 was found to be related to the administration of diethylstilbestrol (DES) to their mothers during pregnancy.[24] The incidence of clear cell adenocarcinoma in women prenatally exposed to DES is estimated to be between 0.14 and 1.4 per 1000.[22,40] Horwitz and associates[27] noted that the incidence of DES-induced carcinoma of the vagina and cervix increased up to 1979 and decreased slightly in 1980 to 1982; therefore continued surveillance of patients exposed to DES is warranted. The median age of tumor diagnosis in these DES-exposed patients has been reported as 19 years.[24] Herbst and colleagues[24] noted a close correlation between the annual incidence of clear cell adenocarcinoma of the vagina and cervix and the estimated use of DES for pregnancy support in the United States. An association was found between the risk of developing vaginal cancer and the time of first exposure to DES; the risk was greatest for those exposed during the first 16 weeks *in utero* and declined for those whose exposure began in the 17th week or later.

NATURAL HISTORY AND PATTERNS OF FAILURE

Vaginal cancers occur most frequently on the posterior wall of the upper third of the vagina. In an extensive review of the literature, Plentl and Friedman[52] found that 51.7% of primary vaginal cancers occurred in the upper third of the vagina and 57.6% on the posterior wall.

Tumors originating in the vagina may spread along the vaginal wall to involve the cervix or vulva. However, if biopsies of the cervix or the vulva are positive at the time of initial diagnosis, the tumor cannot be considered a primary vaginal lesion.

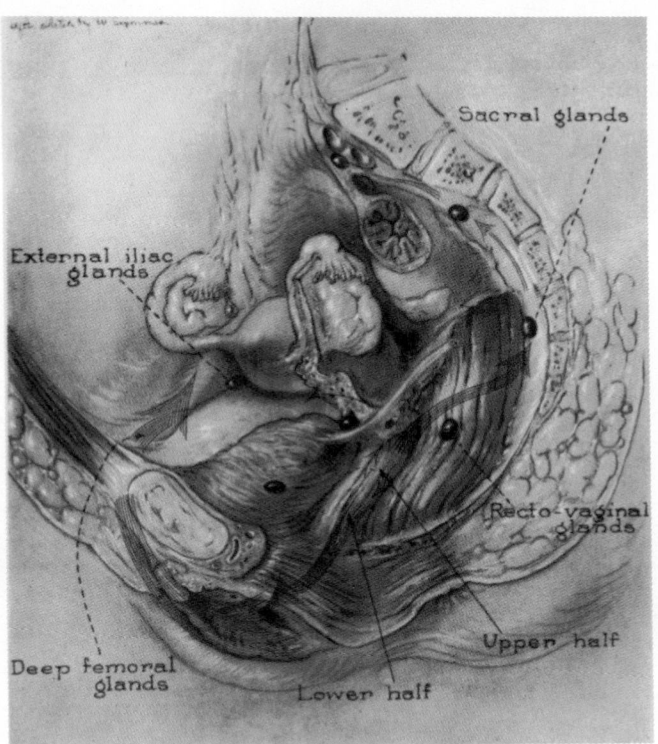

FIGURE 58–1. Lymphatic spread in carcinoma of the vagina. Lesions in the upper half drain to the same lymph node groups as carcinoma of the uterine cervix. Tumors in the lower half tend to involve the inguinal and femoral nodes preferentially and may also drain into the deep pelvic lymph nodes. (Benson RC: CA 18:2, 1968)

Because of the absence of anatomic barriers, vaginal tumors readily extend into surrounding tissues. Lesions on the anterior vaginal wall may penetrate the vesicovaginal septum; those on the posterior wall may eventually invade the rectovaginal septum. Vaginal cancer may invade the paracolpium and parametrial tissues, extending into the obturator fossa, cardinal ligaments, lateral pelvic walls, and uterosacral ligaments.

The incidence of positive pelvic nodes at diagnosis varies with the stage and location of the primary vaginal tumor. Because the lymphatic system of the vagina is so complex, any of the nodal groups may be involved regardless of the location of the lesion.[52] Involvement of inguinal nodes is most common, when the lesion is located in the lower third of the vagina. The incidence of clinically positive nodes at diagnosis is summarized in Table 58-1.

Because of the multicentricity of the disease, a few local failures (5% to 10%) are noted in patients with Stage 0 disease. Pelvic recurrences or distant metastases have not been observed. In patients with Stage I disease, the incidence of pelvic recurrence is 10% to 20%. Comparable figures are reported for distant metastases. In patients with Stage II disease, in which more paravaginal or parametrial infiltration is present, the incidence of pelvic recurrence increases to 35%, and distant metastases are more common (22%) (Table 58-2). In patients with Stage III disease, the incidence of local recurrence varies from 25% to 37%. Distant metastases have been reported in approximately 23% of patients. In patients with Stage IV disease, there is a high incidence of pelvic failure (58%) and distant metastases (approximately 30%) (Table 58-3).

In squamous cell carcinoma of the vagina, metastases to the lungs or supraclavicular nodes may occur in patients with advanced disease. However, Robboy and associates[57] reported that metastases to the lungs or supraclavicular lymph nodes represented 35% of the recurrences in young women with clear cell adenocarcinoma, a percentage much greater than that found with squamous cell carcinoma of the cervix or vagina.

TABLE 58–1
Clinically Positive Pelvic Nodes in Diagnosis of Carcinoma of the Vagina

AUTHORS	NO. OF PATIENTS	POSITIVE NODES	% POSITIVE NODES
Plentl and Friedman[52]	679	141	20.8
Whelton and Kottmeier[73]	117	8*	6.8
Brown et al[7]	76	5	6.6
Perez et al[47]	113	6	5.3

**Four had presence of tumor confirmed by biopsy.*

CLINICAL PRESENTATION

Abnormal vaginal bleeding is the presenting symptom in 50% to 75% of patients with primary vaginal tumors.[24,37,61,68] It may occur as dysfunctional bleeding or postcoital spotting. Vaginal discharge is also common. Less common presenting complaints are dysuria and pelvic pain, which occur when tumor has spread to adjacent organs.

DIAGNOSTIC WORKUP

A summary of diagnostic procedures for patients with vaginal tumors is shown in Table 58-4. In addition to a complete history and physical examination, speculum examination and palpation of the vagina are essential components of the diagnostic workup. The speculum must be rotated as it is withdrawn so that posterior wall lesions, which occur frequently, are not overlooked. Bimanual pelvic and rectal examinations are integral elements in the clinical evaluation of these patients.

Exfoliative cytology studies may detect early squamous cell lesions of the vagina, but this is not true for clear cell adenocarcinomas, which often grow in submucosal locations.[1] Schiller's test (with Lugol's solution) and colposcopy are particularly useful for directed biopsies in abnormal sites in the vagina. A metastatic evaluation including cytoscopy and proctosigmoidoscopy should be performed on patients with pathologically confirmed invasive vaginal carcinoma.

In addition to the chest radiograph, intravenous pyelogram and, when indicated, barium enema or air contrast, computed tomography, and magnetic resonance imaging (Fig. 58-2) have been increasingly used in the evaluation of patients with tumors of the vagina.[29,69] Chang and associates[8] reported the results of pelvic magnetic resonance imaging in 87 women (51 with normal vagina, two with benign cysts, and 34 with vaginal carcinoma [four of them primary, 22 metastatic, and eight recurrent]) and correlated them with surgical-pathologic findings. The positive predictive value of the test for primary and metastatic tumors was 84% and the negative predictive value, 97%. The accuracy of magnetic resonance imaging in detection of recurrent vaginal carcinoma was 82%, compared with clinical or surgical findings. The authors believed that this exam-

TABLE 58–2
Carcinoma of the Vagina: Outcome of Stage I and II Disease Treated With Radiation Therapy Alone

INVESTIGATOR	NO. OF PATIENTS (STAGE)	SURVIVAL	NO. OF RECURRENCES (%)		
			PELVIS	PELVIS + DISTANT METASTASES	DISTANT METASTASES
Stage I					
Brown et al[7]	21	85%*	1 (4.8)		1 (4.8)
Dancuart et al[11]	71	—	15 (21)	2 (2.8)	2 (2.8)
Delclos et al[13]	27	63%†		4 (14.8)‡	2 (7.4)
Marcus et al[39]	6	80%	0	0	0
Perez et al[47]	50	75%	4 (8)	3 (6)	5 (10)
Total§	175		20 (11)	5 (3)	10 (6)
Stage II					
Brown et al[7]	25	76%*	2 (8)	2‖ (8)	1‖ (4)
Dancuart et al[11]	42	—	7 (16.7)		2 (4.8)
Delclos et al[13]	47	55%†		8 (17)‡	3 (6.4)
Marcus et al[39]	10	50%†	1 (10)		2 (20)
Perez et al[47]	49 (IIA)	55%	10 (20.4)	9 (18.4)	6 (12.2)
	26 (IIB)	43%	5 (19.2)	7 (26.9)	5 (19.2)
Total§	199		25 (12.5)	18 (9)	19 (9.5)

**Determinate, 5 years*
† Absolute, 5 years, no evidence of disease
‡ Value = combined total of recurrences in pelvis and pelvis + distant metastases in study by Delclos and associates[13]
§ Excluding Delclos and associates[13]
‖ One patient had inguinal node metastasis.
(Modified from Perez CA, Bedwinek JM, Breaux SR: Cancer Treat Symp 2:217–231, 1983)

TABLE 58–3
Carcinoma of the Vagina: Outcome of Stage III and IV Disease Treated With Radiation Therapy Alone

INVESTIGATOR	NO. OF PATIENTS	SURVIVAL	NO. OF RECURRENCES (%)		
			PELVIS	PELVIS + DISTANT METASTASES	DISTANT METASTASES
Stage III					
Brown et al[7]	16	40%*	4 (25)	0	1 (6.3)
Dancuart et al[11]	42	—	10 (24)		5 (12)
Delclos et al[13]	27	37%†		10 (37)‡	0
Marcus et al[39]	3	100%†	0	0	0
Perez et al[47]	16	32%	0	6 (37.5)	4 (25)
Total§	104		14 (13.4)	6 (6)	10 (9.6)
Stage IV					
Brown et al[7]	13	0	5 (38.5)	2 (15.4)	1 (7.7)
Dancuart et al[11]	11	—	3 (27)	1 (9)	1 (9)
Delclos et al[13]	6	0		3 (50)‡	1 (16.7)
Marcus et al[39]	3	50%†	1 (33.3)	0	0
Perez et al[47]	8	10%	2 (25)	4 (50)	0
Total§	41		11 (29)	7 (17)	3 (7.3)

**Determinate, 5 years*
† Absolute, 5 years, no evidence of disease
‡ Value = combined total of recurrences in pelvis and pelvis + distant metastases in study by Delclos and associates[13]
§ Excluding Delclos and associates[13]
(Modified from Perez CA, Bedwinek JM, Breaux SR: Cancer Treat Symp 2:217–231, 1983)

TABLE 58–4
Diagnostic Workup for Vaginal Tumors

General
- History
- Physical, including careful pelvic/bimanual examination

Special studies
- Exfoliative cytology (clear cell adenocarcinomas may not be detected)
- Colposcopy and directed biopsies (including Schiller's test)
- Biopsies and examination under anesthesia to determine tumor extent
- Cytoscopy
- Proctosigmoidoscopy (as indicated)

Radiographic studies
- Standard
  - Chest radiographs
  - Intravenous pyelogram
- Complementary
  - Barium enema
  - Lymphangiogram
  - Computed tomography or magnetic resonance imaging of pelvis and abdomen

Laboratory studies
- Complete blood count
- Blood chemistry
- Urinalysis

ination could effectively differentiate between fibrotic tissue and grossly recurrent tumor, findings reported by others.[15,19] The lesions are better seen on T2 predominant images using transverse planes 5 mm thick.

STAGING

Staging is best performed jointly by the gynecologic and the radiation oncologists with the patient under general anesthesia. Multiple biopsies of the cervix are mandatory to rule out a cervical primary tumor. If a concomitant malignant lesion of the same histology is present in the cervix or if biopsies demonstrate a similar tumor, the lesion must be classified as a primary cervical carcinoma and staged accordingly.

Patients' tumors are staged according to the International Federation of Gynecology and Obstetrics (FIGO) or the American Joint Committee (AJC) staging system (Table 58-5; Fig. 58-3). It has been proposed that FIGO Stage II be subdivided into Stage IIA (subvaginal infiltration only) and Stage IIB (parametrial extension) because of the more aggressive behavior of tumors with parametrial involvement.[44]

PATHOLOGIC FEATURES

Epidermoid carcinoma accounts for more than 90% of primary vaginal tumors, most of which are nonkeratinizing and moderately differentiated.[43] Primary vaginal carcinoma *in situ* and invasive carcinoma of the vagina have been reported in a few patients who were treated for carcinoma of the uterine cervix.[30,62] It is possible that these vaginal lesions are marginal recurrences of the cervical lesions. However, Perez and coworkers[43] reported that when the vaginal tumor was detected more than 5 years after treatment of the cervical carcinoma without evidence of local recurrence in the cervix, the results after therapy were comparable to those of *de novo* primary vaginal carcinoma, and these patients should be treated with a curative aim.

Adenocarcinomas comprise approximately 5% of primary vaginal tumors. These tumors usually arise from the Bartholin or Skene submucosal glandular epithelium. Clear cell adenocarcinoma of the vagina in young patients may be found in any region of the vagina. However, Robboy and associates[58] reported that most of these tumors arise in the anterior wall, usually in the upper third. Three fourths of the tumors have a surface area of less than 12 cm^2 and most penetrate less than 3 mm into the vaginal stroma. Most are polypoid or nodular. Senekjian and associates[64] noted in 76 patients with Stage II clear cell adenocarcinoma of the vagina that the lesion involved the vesicovaginal or rectovaginal septum in 19 patients, paravaginal/parametrial tissues without extending to the pelvic wall in eight patients, and subvaginal tissue without parametrial or septal infiltration in 36 patients, and determined that the substage suggested by Perez and associates[44] showed no clinical benefit, since all subtypes showing a 5-year survival rate of 83% a 10-year rate of 62%.

Microscopic features of clear cell adenocarcinoma include cells with abundant cytoplasm filled with glycogen, and "hobnail" cells, characterized by bulbous nuclei that protrude into the lumina of tubules and cysts. Robboy and co-workers[58] noted that no squamous cell differentiation has been observed in these tumors.

Sarcomas (smooth muscle tumors) are the most common mesenchymal tumor of the vagina in adults. The clinical and pathologic features of 60 smooth muscle tumors of the vagina were reviewed by Tavassoli and Norris,[67] who concluded that a neoplasm with moderate to marked atypia and more than five mitotic figures per 10 high-power field (HPF) merits the designation of leiomyosarcoma. Five neoplasms recurred in the 60 patients, and all five primary tumors were larger than 3 cm in diameter and had more than five mitoses per 10 HPF with various degrees of atypia. Others, such as Peters and associates,[50] have included mixed mullerian tumors in this group of lesions.

Sarcoma botryoides of the vagina is a rare tumor generally found in children. It is of mesodermal origin and contains rhabdomyoblasts but rarely, if ever, cartilage or bone. The tumor may protrude from the introitus, presenting the characteristic grapelike appearance. It is locally invasive, frequently infiltrates the vesicovaginal septum, and may involve femoral, parametrial, and periaortic lymph nodes. Hematogenous metastases are common and are found predominantly in the lung, liver, and bones.

Malignant melanoma of the vagina is rare.[14,42,56] At the Armed Forces Institute of Pathology only three vaginal melanomas were listed for every 1000 cutaneous lesions.[42] In 1984, Lee and associates[36] estimated that only 106 cases had been reported previously. Average age has been reported as 55 to 60 years.[5,41] The tumor may result from malignant changes in pigment-containing remnants of the urogenital sinus. Melanoma of the vagina is a deeply pigmented ulcerative lesion that often invades adjacent organs such as the bladder, rectum, vulva, and cervix, and infiltrates the parametrium. Hematogenous and lymphatic dissemination frequently occurs, and the 5-year survival rate is less than 10%.[5]

PROGNOSTIC FACTORS

The most significant factor influencing prognosis is the clinical stage of the vaginal carcinoma, which reflects the depth of penetration into the vaginal wall or the surrounding tissues.[45]

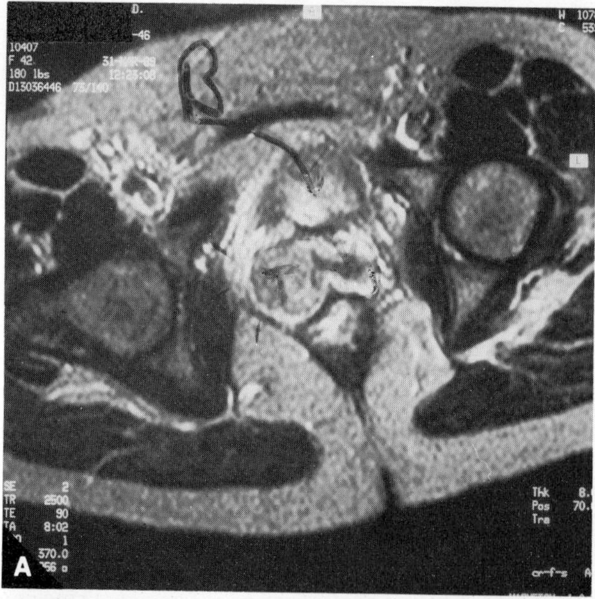

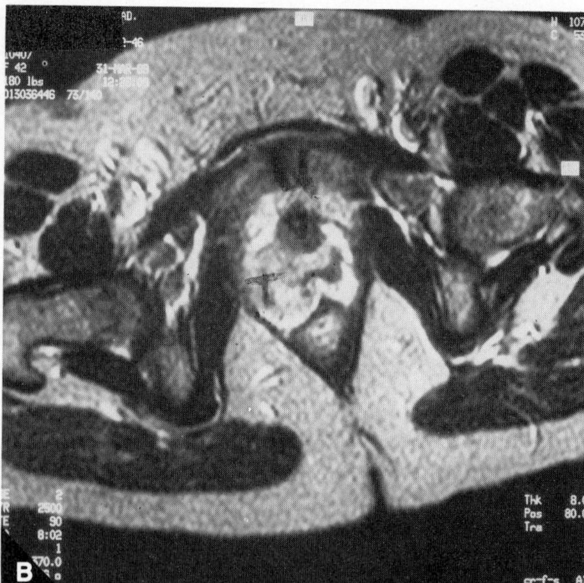

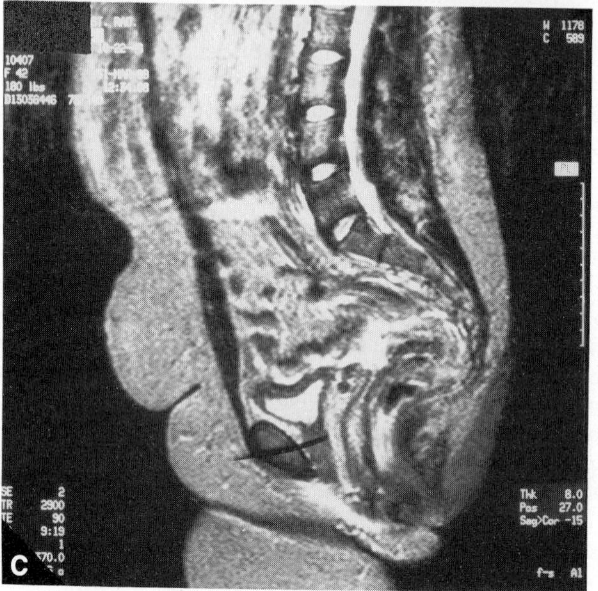

FIGURE 58–2. MRI of pelvis in patient with carcinoma of the vagina (**A**) infiltrating right paravaginal tissue and (**B**) extending into right ischiorectal fossa. (**C**) Lateral view of same patient.

TABLE 58–5
Clinical Staging of Malignant Tumors of the Vagina

AJC*	FIGO†	DESCRIPTION
Tx		Primary tumor cannot be assessed
Tis	0	Carcinoma *in situ* (intraepithelial)
INVASIVE CARCINOMA		
T1	I	Confined to vaginal mucosa
T2	II	Submucosal infiltration into parametrium, not extending out to pelvic wall
	IIA‡	Subvaginal infiltration, not into parametrium
	IIB‡	Parametrial infiltration, not extending to pelvic wall
T3	III	Tumor extending to pelvic wall
T4	IV	Tumor extension to bladder or rectum or metastasis outside true pelvis

** American Joint Committee*
† International Federation of Gynecology and Obstetrics[31]
‡ Proposed subdivision for Stage II lesions[44]

Age of the patient, extent of mucosal involvement, gross appearance of the lesion, and degree of differentiation and keratinization do not appear to be significant factors in prognosis.[43,45]

Livingstone[37] reported that patients with lesions located in the upper vagina had a better prognosis. However, other authors have found no correlation between location of the primary tumor and treatment results.[18,45,47,61,73]

Patients with nonepithelial tumors (sarcoma, melanoma) have a poor prognosis with a high incidence of local failure and distant metastasis.

GENERAL MANAGEMENT

Radiation therapy is the preferred treatment for most carcinomas of the vagina. Some authors advocate a surgical approach,[68] but operations are generally discouraged because of the excellent tumor control and good functional results obtained with adequate radiation therapy. Surgery may be reserved for the treatment of irradiation failures, for non-

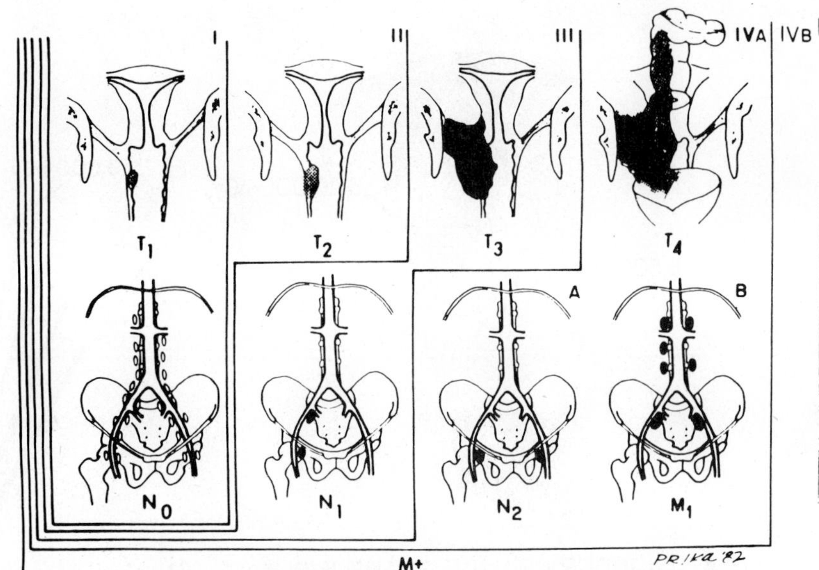

FIGURE 58–3. Clinical staging in carcinoma of vagina, FIGO system. (Modified from AJC, UICC, and Rubin P: Clinical Oncology: A Multidisciplinary Approach, 6th ed., American Cancer Society, 1983; courtesy of Philip Rubin, M.D., University of Rochester)

epithelial tumors, and for Stage I clear cell adenocarcinomas in young women.[28,72]

Several authors have discussed the complex management of patients with carcinoma of the vagina and the need for individualized radiation therapy techniques.[9] Perez and coworkers[48] reported a correlation between the doses of radiation given to patients with various stages of vaginal carcinomas and the probability of local tumor control. Paravaginal or parametrial interstitial implants or both should be considered when residual tumor is present after the planned external and intracavitary therapy is completed. Additional doses of 2000 cGy to 3000 cGy to a limited volume are usually well tolerated.[33,38,55]

A combination of irradiation and surgery has been suggested to improve therapeutic results,[6] although more complications may be seen from combined therapy.

Carcinoma *in Situ*

An intracavitary application delivering 6500 cGy to 8000 cGy to the involved vaginal mucosa is usually sufficient to control *in situ* lesions, which do not extend beyond the basement membrane of the squamous epithelium. Higher doses may cause significant vaginal fibrosis and stenosis. Because vaginal carcinoma tends to be multicentric, the entire vaginal mucosa should be treated to a dose of 5000 cGy to 6000 cGy.

Stage I

Vaginal carcinomatous lesions are invasive, are usually 0.5 cm to 1 cm thick, and may involve one or more vaginal walls. In patients with Stage I lesions, it is important to individualize radiation therapy techniques to obtain optimal functional results. Superficial tumors may be treated with only an intracavitary cylinder covering the entire vagina (6000 cGy to 7000 cGy mucosal dose) and an additional 2000 cGy to 3000 cGy mucosal dose to the tumor area.

If the lesion is thicker and localized to one wall, a single plane implant may be used with an intracavitary cylinder to increase the depth dose and limit excessive irradiation to the vaginal mucosa. A dose of 6000 cGy to 6500 cGy is delivered to the entire vaginal mucosa and an additional 1500 cGy to 2000 cGy calculated 0.5 cm beyond the plane of the implant to the gross tumor, with the involved vaginal mucosa receiving an estimated 8000 cGy to 10,000 cGy (Fig. 58-4).

Use of external-beam irradiation in Stage I disease should be reserved for aggressive lesions (more invasive, infiltrating, or poorly differentiated) to supplement intracavitary and interstitial therapy. The whole pelvis is treated with 1000 cGy or 2000 cGy; additional parametrial dose should be delivered with a midline block (5 half-value layer [HVL]) to give a total of 4500 cGy to 5000 cGy to the parametria.

Stage IIA

Patients with Stage IIA tumors have more advanced paravaginal disease without extensive parametrial infiltration. These patient should be treated with a greater external radiation dose: 2000 cGy to the whole pelvis and additional parametrial dose with a midline block (5 HVL) for a total of 4500 cGy to 5000 cGy. A combination of interstitial and intracavitary therapy may also be used to deliver a minimum of 4500 cGy to 5500 cGy 0.5 cm beyond the deep margin of the tumor (in addition to the whole-pelvis dose). Double plane implants may be necessary because of extensive tumor volume (Fig. 58-5).

Stage IIB, Stage III, and Stage IV

For advanced tumors 4000 cGy whole-pelvis and 5500 cGy to 6000 cGy total parametrial dose (with midline shielding) have been given in combination with interstitial and intracavitary insertions to deliver a total tumor dose of 7500 cGy to the vaginal tumor and 6500 cGy to parametrial and paravaginal extensions. An interstitial implant boost of 2000 cGy to 2500 cGy is sometimes given to patients with extensive parametrial infiltration (Fig. 58-6).

Boronow and associates[6] have proposed an alternative to exenterative procedures for locally advanced vulvovaginal carcinoma, using radiation therapy to treat the pelvic (internal genital) disease and a radical vulvectomy with bilateral inguinal node dissection to treat the external genital tumor. External radiation to the pelvis and inguinal nodes consisted of 4500 cGy to 5000 cGy, combined with intracavitary insertions to deliver maximum doses of 8000 cGy to 8500 cGy to the vaginal mucosa with both modalities.

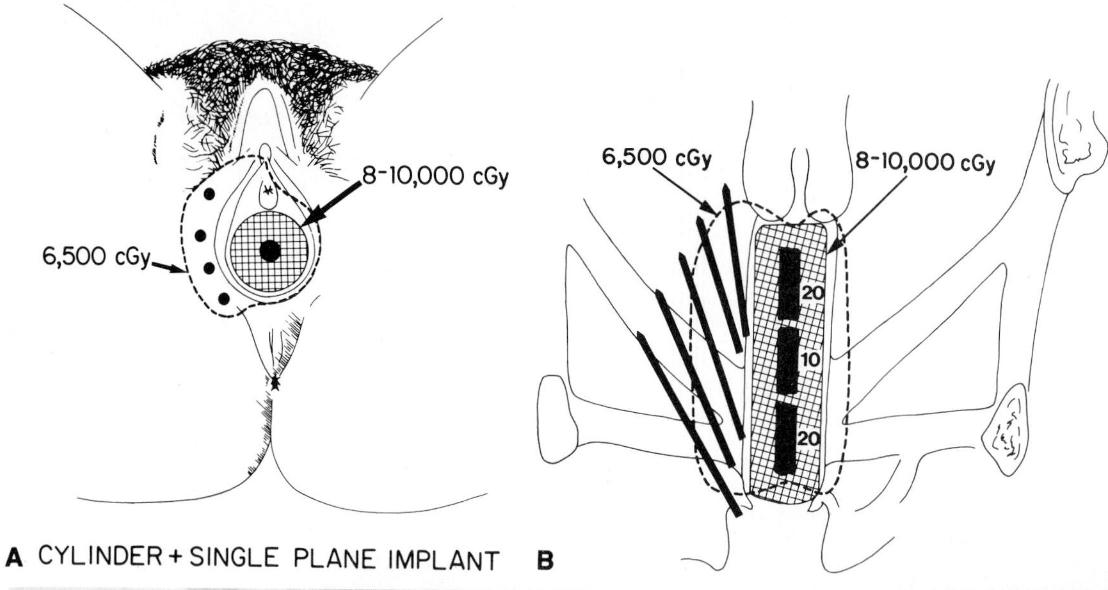

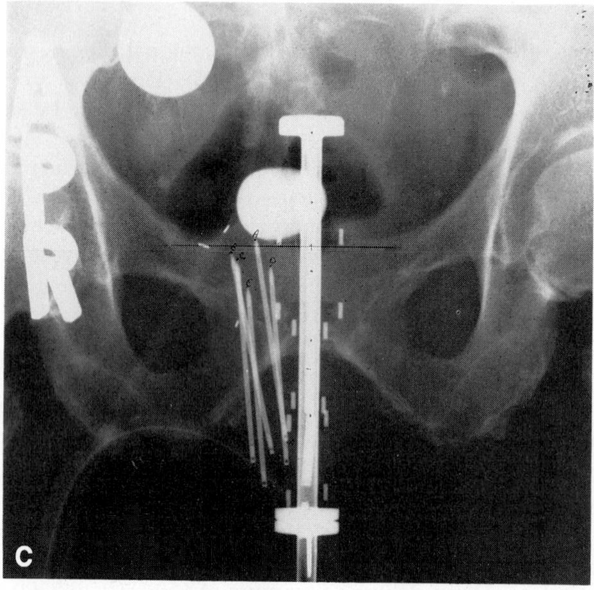

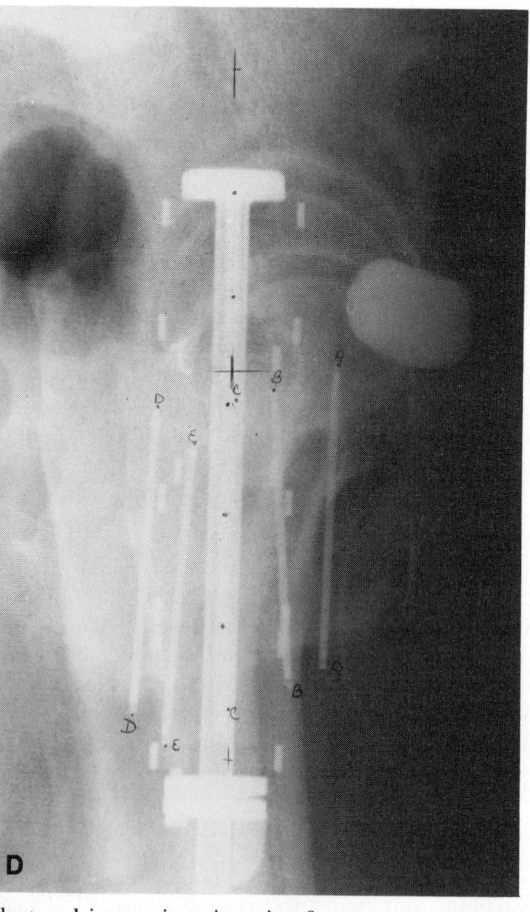

FIGURE 58–4. (**A** and **B**) Diagrams of an interstitial plane implant and intracavitary insertion for treatment of Stage I carcinoma of the vagina. (Perez CA, Korba A, Sharma S: Int J Radiat Oncol Biol Phys 2:639, 1977) Anteroposterior (**C**) and lateral (**D**) radiographs of actual single plane implant with ^{137}Cs needles and intracavitary insertion with Delclos applicator.

Treatment of Clear Cell Adenocarcinoma

Surgery for Stage I clear cell adenocarcinoma may have the advantage of ovarian preservation and better vaginal function following skin graft. Surgery for vaginal clear cell adenocarcinoma requires removal of most of the vagina and reconstructive procedures. It is important that the surgeon obtain frozen section biopsies of the distal margins of resection to determine the lower margins of the surgical resection. The vagina is dissected first before the abdominal procedure. A radical hysterectomy and lymph node dissection are necessary to encompass the area from the parametria and paracolpium to the side walls of the pelvis. Periaortic nodes should be sampled before the procedure to determine the presence of lymphatic disease beyond the pelvis. However, Fletcher[16] and Wharton and associates[72] advocate intracavitary or transvaginal irradiation for the treat-

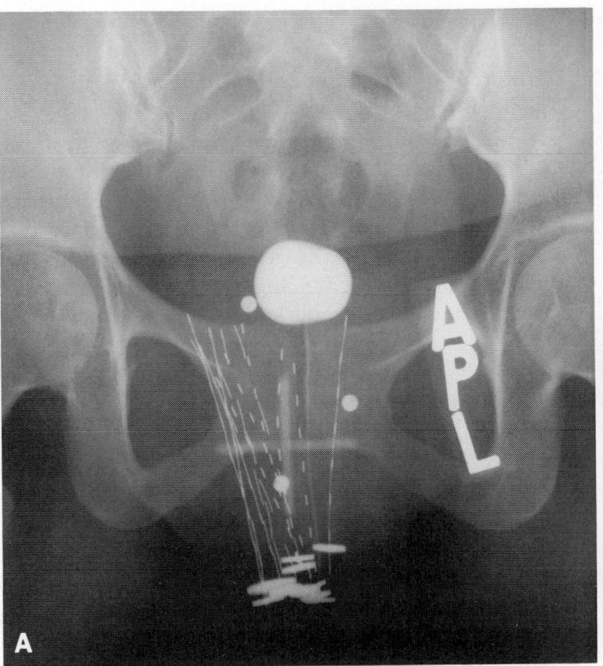

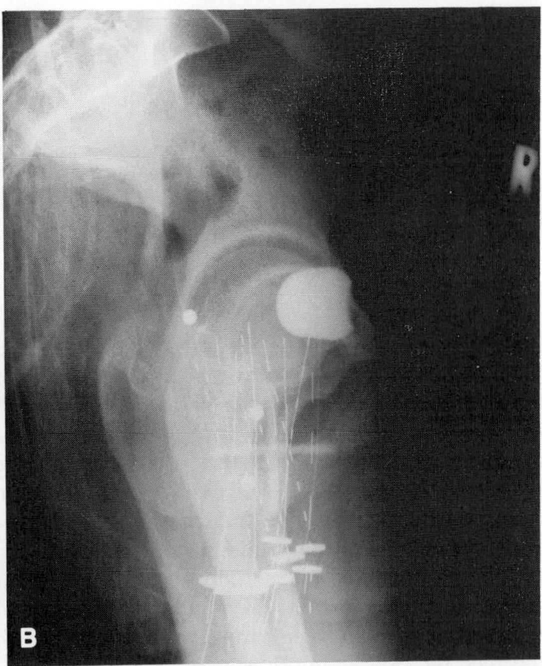

FIGURE 58–5. (**A**) Anteroposterior and (**B**) lateral radiographs of intracavitary/interstitial implant in a patient with Stage II carcinoma of the vagina.

ment of small tumors, because this may yield excellent tumor control with a functional vagina and preservation of ovarian function.

For more extensive lesions, external radiation therapy is essential. Techniques are similar to those described above.

Treatment of Vaginal Recurrences

Vaginal carcinoma can be effectively treated with surgery after postirradiation local failure. The surgical procedure may range from a wide local excision or partial vaginectomy to a posterior or total pelvic exenteration. Meticulous and regular follow-up examinations are important to detect the recurrence early.

Treatment of Nonepithelial Tumors

Rhabdomyosarcoma of the vagina is generally treated with a combination of surgical resection, irradiation, and systemic chemotherapy.[51] Melanoma and leiomyosarcoma are treated pri-

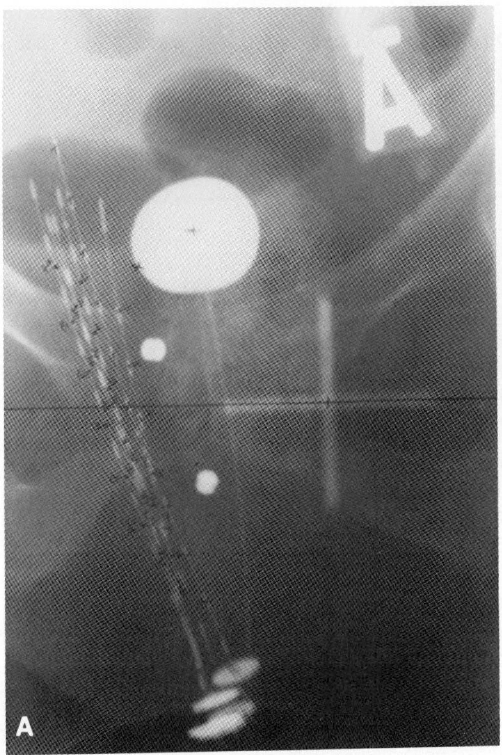

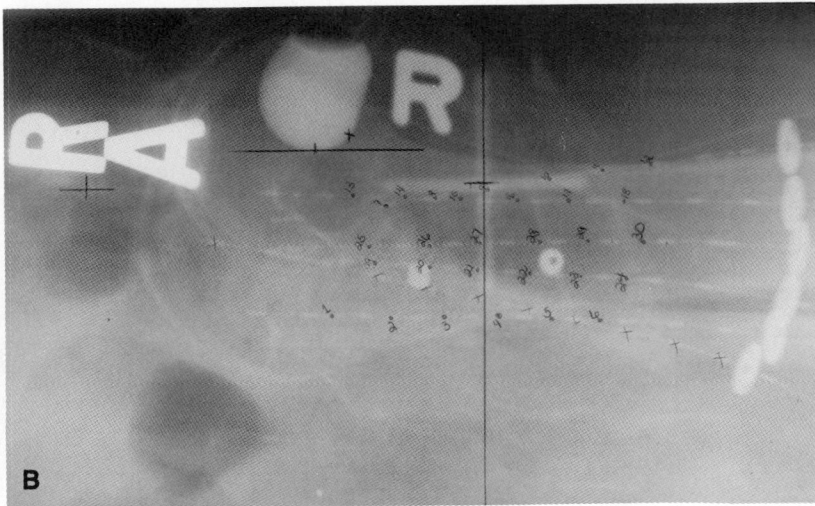

FIGURE 58–6. (**A** and **B**) Interstitial implant in paravaginal and parametrial tissues in a patient with Stage III carcinoma of the vagina.

marily with radical surgical resection (vaginectomy, hysterectomy, and pelvic lymphadenectomy).[5]

RADIATION THERAPY TECHNIQUES

Irradiation treatment policies for vaginal carcinoma are outlined in Table 58-6.

External Irradiation

The technical approach to vaginal carcinoma is similar to that for carcinoma of the uterine cervix. External irradiation should be administered using anteroposterior-posteroanterior (AP-PA) pelvic portals that encompass the entire vagina down to the introitus and the pelvic lymph nodes to the upper portion of the common iliac chain. Portals of 15 cm by 15 cm or 15 cm by 18 cm at the skin are usually adequate. The distal margin of the tumor should be identified with a radiopaque marker or bead when simulation radiographs are taken. In tumors involving the middle or lower third of the vagina, the inguinal and adjacent femoral lymph nodes should be electively treated (4500 cGy to 5000 cGy), which requires a modification of the standard portals (Fig. 58-7*A*). For patients with clinically palpable nodes, additional doses of 1500 cGy (calculated at 4 cm to 5 cm) are necessary with reducing portals (Fig. 58-7*B*). These doses can be achieved by using unequal loadings (2AP to 1PA) with 10 MV to 18 MV photons, in which case a 2 cm bolus should be used when palpable lymph nodes are present. Alternatively, equal loading with photons may be used to deliver 4500 cGy to 5000 cGy to the pelvic and inguinal nodes. If necessary, reduced AP portals are used to deliver a boost dose to the inguinal nodes with ^{60}Co or electrons (12 MeV to 16 MeV). Special attention is needed to avoid areas of overlap (Fig. 58-7*B*). A combination of 6 MV x-rays on the AP portal and 18 MV photons on the PA portal yields a higher dose to the inguinal nodes in relation to the midplane tumor dose. After a specified tumor dose is delivered to the whole pelvis (2000 cGy to 4000 cGy, depending on extent of tumor), a midline rectangular or wedge block is interposed (Fig. 58-7*C*), and additional irradiation is given to the parametrial tissues.

Brachytherapy

Intracavitary therapy is carried out using vaginal cylinders such as the Burnett, Bloedorn, Delclos, or MIRALVA applicators. The largest possible diameter should be used to improve the ratio of mucosa to tumor dose. Vaginal molds for individualized intracavitary applications have been used.[4] Interstitial therapy with ^{137}Cs, ^{226}Ra needles, or afterloading ^{192}Ir needles has been used. Depending on the extent and thickness of tumor, single plane, double plane, or volume implants should be planned (see Chap. 13, Clinical Applications of Brachytherapy).

RESULTS OF THERAPY

With adequate therapy, the survival rates of patients with carcinoma of the vagina are comparable to those reported for carcinoma of the cervix, which range from 20% to 80% at 5 years, depending on stage of the disease (Fig. 58-8).[2,7,32,48,53,60] Perez and colleagues[47] noted a somewhat higher incidence of pelvic failures in patients with carcinoma of the vagina compared with 1054 patients with invasive cervical carcinoma (Fig. 58-9), although the differences are not statistically significant.

Whelton and Kottmeier[73] reported an overall 5-year survival rate of 26.5% in 117 patients treated primarily with radiation therapy. Fifty-seven (48.8%) had persistent disease; 33 of 60 patients (55%) with no evidence of disease after treatment developed recurrent primary tumors. Rutledge[61] reported a 35% 5-year survival rate in 70 patients with invasive vaginal carcinoma (including advanced stages) treated with irradiation; some patients died of intercurrent disease.

Brown and associates,[7] Rutledge,[61] and Perez and coworkers[46] have described excellent tumor control and survival rates in patients with carcinoma *in situ* and Stage I invasive carcinoma. These authors cautioned against overly aggressive therapy in these early lesions because of the possibility of producing mucosal injury and interference with sexual function. Surgery is occasionally used for *in situ* lesions of the vagina. Lee and Symmonds[35] described 66 patients previously treated for *in situ* carcinoma of the cervix who were subsequently treated for primary carcinoma *in situ* of the vagina with wide local excision,

TABLE 58–6
Carcinoma of Vagina Treatment Policies at Mallinckrodt Institute of Radiology

	EXTERNAL RADIATION THERAPY			
FIGO STAGE	WHOLE PELVIS	PARAMETRIAL (MIDLINE BLOCK)	**BRACHYTHERAPY**	**TOTAL TUMOR DOSE (cGy)**
0	—	—	Intracavitary: 6500–8000 cGy SD to tumor 6000 cGy to entire vagina	6500–8000
I Superficial	—	—	Intracavitary: 6500–8000 cGy SD to entire vagina	6500–8000
0.5 cm thick	—	—	Intracavitary/interstitial: 6500–7000 cGy at 0.5 cm (mucosa, 10,000 cGy)	6500–7000
IIA	2000	3000	Intracavitary/interstitial: 6000–6500 cGy TD	7000–7500
IIB	2000	3000	Intracavitary/interstitial: 6500–7000 cGy TD	7500
III, IV	4000	1000*	Intracavitary: 5000–6000 cGy (interstitial: 2000–3000 cGy boost to parametrium)	8000

SD: surface dose; TD: tumor dose
** Additional 1000 cGy boost to parametrium*
NOTE: Distal vagina lesions: Inguinal lymph nodes receive 5000 cGy (at 3 cm); interstitial doses are usually calculated 0.5 cm from plane of implant.

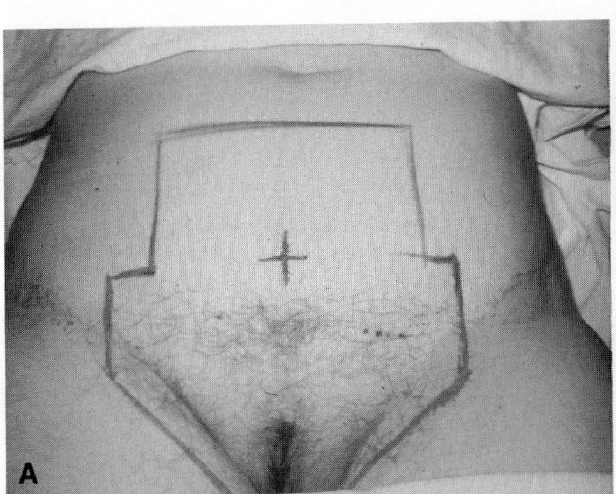

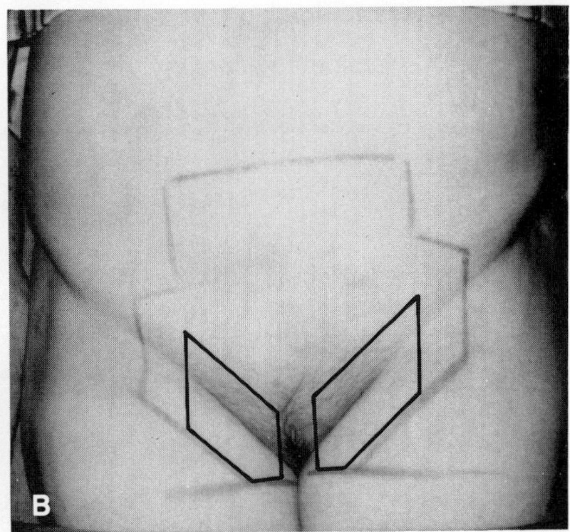

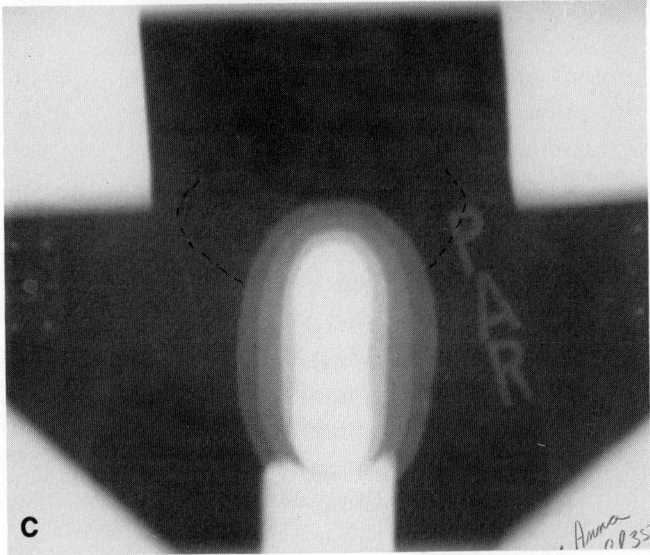

FIGURE 58–7. (**A**) Example of portal used to treat the whole pelvis and the inguinal lymph nodes in carcinoma of the vagina. (**B**) Variation of treatment portals, with small fields to boost the inguinal lymph node dose with ^{60}Co or electrons (12 MeV to 16 MeV). Overlap of this field should be carefully avoided. (**C**) A step-wedged midline block is used to shield the area treated with higher intracavitary doses (for a portion of the treatment).

partial vaginectomy, or total vaginectomy. The authors stated that 58 patients were alive and well without recurrent tumors at the time of the report; six others died of intercurrent disease without recurrent carcinoma. One patient had recurrent carcinoma of the vagina, resulting in death. These results are not superior to those reported with irradiation alone.

Perez and associates[47] noted that 15 of 16 patients (93%) with Stage 0 carcinoma of the vagina treated by various techniques had control of the tumor in the pelvis 5 years after initial irradiation. In Stage I disease, the pelvic tumor control rate was 86% (43 of 50 patients treated). In patients with more advanced tumors the pelvic control decreased significantly (40% to 50%, depending on tumor extent and techniques used; Table 58-7). Similar results were reported by Prempree and Amornmarn in 88 patients.[53]

Perez and associates[46] reported that in carcinoma *in situ* and Stage I vaginal carcinoma, tumor control in the pelvis was almost the same with or without the addition of external-beam irradiation. However, a better tumor control rate (65%) was observed in Stage II and Stage III with the addition of external irradiation compared with that seen with brachytherapy only (40%).

Prempree and Amornmarn[53] and Puthawala and coworkers[55] described tumor control rates in the pelvis ranging from 65% to 80% with a combination of external irradiation, and when appropriate, paravaginal or parametrial interstitial implant, in addition to intracavitary brachytherapy.

Dancuart and colleagues[11] reported the results in 167 patients with primary squamous cell carcinoma of the vagina treated with irradiation alone at M. D. Anderson Cancer Center. The central failure rate was 18% in 71 patients with Stage I disease, 14% in 42 patients with Stage II, 24% in 38 patients with Stage III, and 30% in 11 patients with Stage IVA disease. No significant difference was found in the failure rate when brachytherapy or external irradiation or a combination of both was used. These authors postulate that because the incidence of pelvic failures in these patients was low, there is no need to irradiate the whole pelvis. They advocate the treatment of subclinical disease in the inguinal lymph nodes with 4000 cGy or 5000 cGy radiation doses. In our experience, however, the incidence of pelvic failures in Stages IIA and IIB was relatively high, and we recommend whole-pelvis and parametrial irradiation.

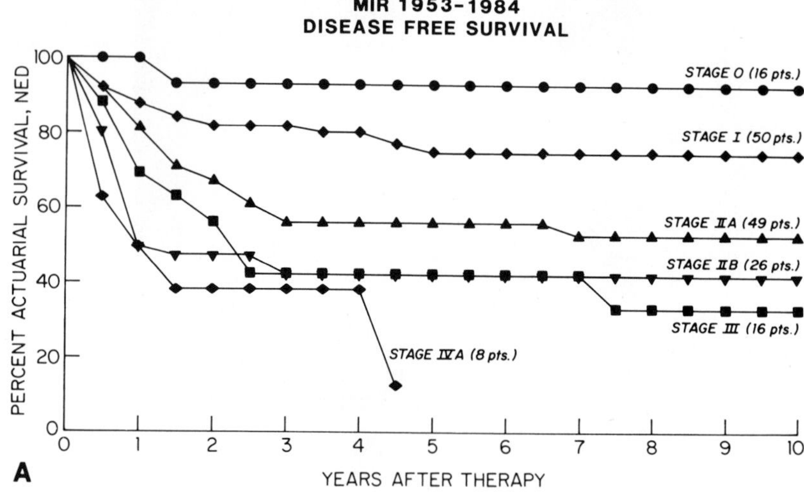

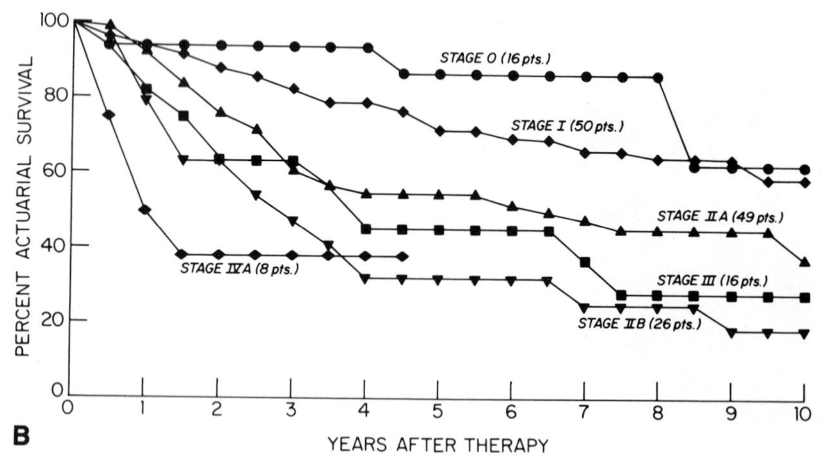

FIGURE 58–8. (**A**) Tumor-free survival for all patients with primary carcinoma of the vagina (Stages 0 through IVA). (**B**) Overall survival of patients by stage. (Perez CA, Camel HM, Galakatos AE, et al: Int J Radiat Oncol Biol Phys 15:1283–1290, 1988)

Patients With a History of Previously Treated Uterine Tumors

Perez and associates[46,47] reported that patients with carcinoma of the vagina who had a history of previously treated primary carcinoma of the cervix or the endometrium (irradiation, hysterectomy, or a combination of both) and received treatment over 5 years before the diagnosis of vaginal carcinoma had survival and tumor control rates equal to patients with *de novo* primary vaginal carcinoma (Table 58-8). The possibility of the vaginal lesion being a local recurrence or metastases was considered unlikely, because 95% of the recurrences following treatment of primary carcinoma of the cervix or the endometrium occur within 5 years after therapy. It is concluded that these lesions are most likely second primaries that should be treated with definitive radiation therapy and a curative aim.

Clear Cell Adenocarcinoma

Fletcher[16] described the results for 19 young women with clear cell adenocarcinoma treated with radiation alone (two combined with surgery), 15 of whom were followed up for more than 2 years. Eighteen patients were alive, 17 of them free from tumor. One patient with an extensive lesion had a vaginal recurrence, and one died of pulmonary embolus after removal of radium needles.

Senekjian and associates[63] reported 92% and 88% 5- and 10-year survival rates in 43 patients with Stage I clear cell vaginal carcinoma treated with local therapy (vaginectomy, local excision alone or combined with irradiation), which was comparable with the results in 126 patients treated with vaginectomy and radical hysterectomy. However, at 10 years the actuarial recurrence rate for the local excision subgroup was 45% in comparison to only 13% for the patients treated with more radical surgery. Patients who received local irradiation (with or without excision) had a recurrence rate of 27%. Recurrences were more frequently noted in patients with tumors larger than 2 cm, with invasion of 3 mm or more, and with a predominant histologic pattern other than tubulocystic. Pelvic lymph node metastases were noted at death in 12% of the patients.

Senekjian and associates also[64] reported results in 76 patients with Stage II clear cell adenocarcinomas of the vagina. Twenty-two patients were treated with surgery alone (vaginectomy with radical hysterectomy in 13 patients and vaginectomy with total or partial pelvic exenteration in nine); radiation therapy alone was used in 38 patients, and a combination of vaginec-

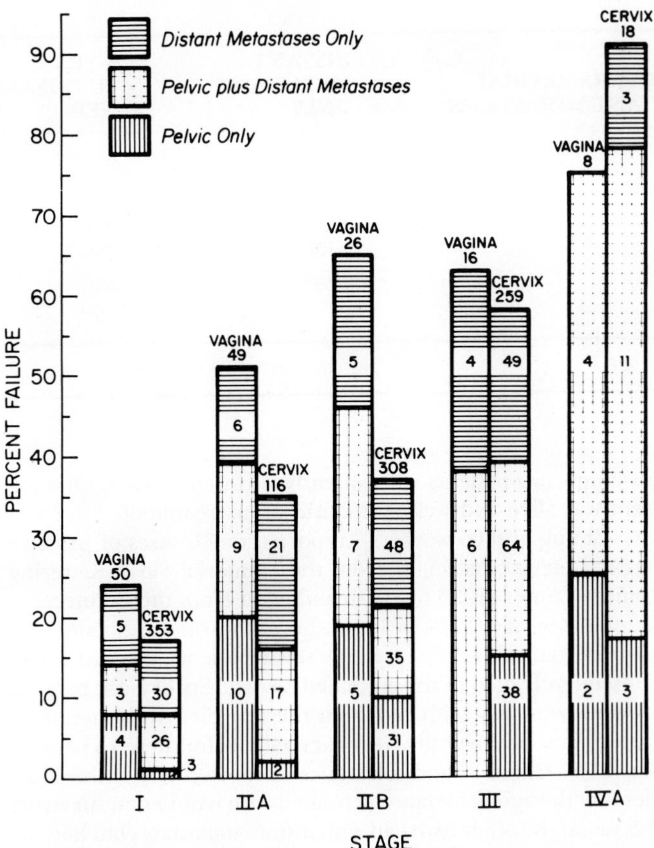

FIGURE 58–9. Comparison of anatomic sites of failure for patients with carcinoma of the vagina compared with carcinoma of the uterine cervix treated at Mallinckrodt Institute of Radiology between 1953 and 1984 illustrating the aggressive behavior of vaginal carcinoma. (Perez CA, Camel HM, Galakatos AE, et al: Int J Radiat Oncol Biol Phys 15:1283–1290, 1988)

tomy, radical hysterectomy, and external irradiation or other treatment approaches was used in 12 patients. The 5-year survival rate was approximately 80% and the 10-year survival rate 65% without significant differences among the three treatment modalities (Fig. 58-10).

Nonepithelial Tumors

Results of treatment of nonepithelial tumors have been poor. Hilgers and colleagues[25] described results in ten cases of sarcoma botryoides from the Mayo Clinic and 71 cases from the literature, most of whom were treated with surgery. Survival rates at 5 years were 20% to 30%. Peters and associates[50] reported a 36% 5-year survival rate in nine patients with leiomyosarcoma and 17% in seven patients with mixed mullerian tumors of the vagina after various forms of therapy, including pelvic irradiation. Three of four patients who underwent exenteration were tumor-free for 84 to 161 months. These results underscore the importance of local therapy, because in all 14 treatment failures the tumor first recurred within the pelvis, and in seven of 14 this was the only site of recurrence.

According to Harwood and Cummings,[21] vaginal melanomas are aggressive and less suitable for radical excision. Laufe and Bernstein[33] reviewed the literature for melanomas of the vagina in 1971 and reported that only three of 38 patients (7.9%) survived 5 years. Irradiation may have a role in the primary management of vaginal melanomas, although follow-up is short.[5,10,21,66] In a review of the literature, Morrow and DiSaia[41] found reports of one patient surviving 5 years following radiation therapy, none of ten surviving local excision, with or without irradiation, and three of 19 surviving after radical exenterative surgery. The overall 5-year survival rate was 5%, and even extended radical operations produced poor results. Harwood and Cummings[21] described a complete response in four patients with vaginal melanoma treated with irradiation,

TABLE 58–7
Carcinoma of the Vagina: Anatomic Sites of Failure (MIR 1953–1984)

STAGE	NO. OF PATIENTS	LOCAL/ PARAMETRIAL ONLY	LOCAL/PARAMETRIAL + DISTANT METASTASES	DISTANT METASTASES ONLY	DEAD OF INTERCURRENT DISEASE
0	16	1 (6.3%)	0	0	6 (37.5%)
I	50	4 (8%)	3 (6%)	5 (10%)	20 (40%)
		14%			
IIA	49	10 (20.4%)	9 (18.4%)	6 (12.2%)	15 (30.6%)
		39%			
IIB	26	5 (19.2%)	7 (26.9%)	5 (19.2%)	6 (23.1%)
		46.1%			
III	16	0	6 (36.5%)	4 (25%)	1 (6.3%)
IVA	8	2 (25%)	4 (50%)	0	1 (12.5%)
		75%			

(Perez CA, Camel HM, Galakatos AE, et al: Int J Radiat Oncol Biol Phys 15:1283–1290, 1988)

TABLE 58–8
Carcinoma of the Vagina: Sites of Failure and 5-year Survival Rates in Patients with Previous Cervix or Endometrial Primary Carcinoma (over 5 years) (MIR 1953–1984)

STAGE	NO. OF PATIENTS	LOCAL/ PARAMETRIAL ONLY	LOCAL/PARAMETRIAL + DISTANT METASTASES	DISTANT METASTASES ONLY	5-YEAR SURVIVAL, NED
0	8	1 (12.5%)	—	—	88%
I	13	2 (15.4%)	2 (15.4%)	—	72%
IIa	8	1 (12.5%)	2 (25%)	1 (12.5%)	63%
IIb	4	2 (50%)	—	1 (25%)	25%
III	3	—	1 (33.3%)	1 (33.3%)	33%
IVA	1	—	1 (100%)	—	0%

(Perez CA, Camel HM, Galakatos AE, et al: Int J Radiat Oncol Biol Phys 15:1283–1290, 1988)

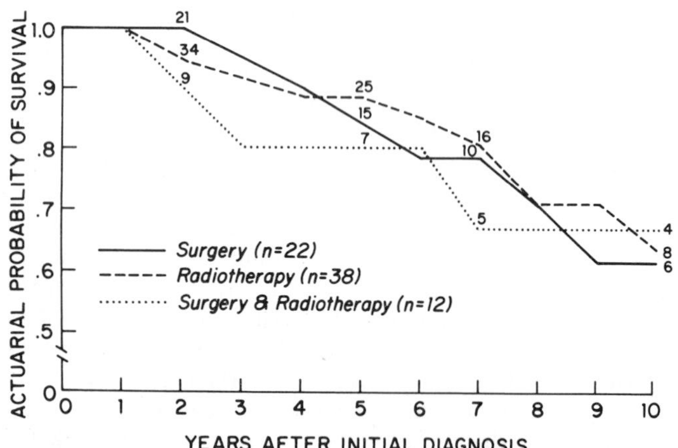

FIGURE 58–10. Survival for Stage II vaginal clear cell carcinoma by treatment modality. (Senekjian EK, Frey KW, Stone C, et al: Gynecol Oncol 31:56, 1988)

although two patients subsequently suffered relapse. One patient was alive and well 10 months after treatment.

Chung and co-workers[10] reported on 16 cases of primary vaginal melanoma: eight from the Memorial Sloan-Kettering Cancer Center (1935 to 1976) and eight from the Connecticut Tumor Registry (1934 to 1976). Local control was obtained by primary radical surgery in five of seven patients, three of whom subsequently died of disseminated disease. Six of eight patients treated primarily with radiation therapy died with metastatic melanoma. The overall 5-year survival rate for these 16 patients was 21%. Harrison and colleagues[20] reported one of three patients with vaginal melanoma treated with irradiation surviving 7.5 years; the other two died with distant metastases but had the local tumor controlled.

Bonner and associates[5] reported on ten patients with malignant melanoma, three treated with conservative surgery and six with radical surgery; no further procedures were performed on one with metastatic disease. Two patients survived over 5

TABLE 58–9
Carcinoma of the Vagina: Major Sequelae of Radiation Therapy (MIR 1953–1984)

	STAGE 0–I (66 PATIENTS)		STAGE II (75 PATIENTS)	
	BRACHYTHERAPY	BRACHYTHERAPY + EXT THERAPY	BRACHYTHERAPY	BRACHYTHERAPY + EXT THERAPY
Rectovaginal fistula				3
Vesicovaginal fistula				2
Rectal stricture		1		1
Proctitis				2*
Rectal ulcer			1	
Diverticulitis		1†		
Small bowel obstruction				1‡
Entero-cutaneous fistula				1§
Bladder neck contracture	1‖			
Urethral stricture		2		1
Cardiac arrest				1

** One patient required colostomy*
† Patient required partial colectomy
‡ Colostomy required
§ After pelvic exenteration (complication of surgery)
‖ Patient required TUR.
(Perez CA, Camel HM, Galakatos AE, et al: Int J Radiat Oncol Biol Phys 15:1283–1290, 1988)

years, one for 38 months and one for 29 months. Two patients, one treated initially with a wide local excision and the other with anterior pelvic exenteration, were alive several months after retreatment of a recurrence with high-fraction irradiation. In five of the six patients treated with radical surgery, four developed locoregional lymph node failure as the first site of recurrence (one patient had inadequate information regarding site of first relapse); all of the patients managed with local excision developed locoregional recurrent tumor.

SEQUELAE OF TREATMENT

Perez and associates[47] reported grade 2 to 3 complications in approximately 5% of patients treated for Stage 0 and Stage I and in approximately 15% of patients with Stage II lesions. No complications were reported in Stage III and Stage IV disease, probably because the patients died shortly after treatment. The most common major complications were proctitis (2), rectovesicovaginal fistulas (3), and vesicovaginal fistulas (2) (Table 58-9). The most common minor complications were fibrosis of the vagina and small areas of mucosal necrosis, which were noted in approximately 10% of patients.

Hintz and associates[26] analyzed 16 patients with cancer of the vagina locally controlled for a minimum of 18 months and indicated that doses of irradiation greater than 9800 cGy to the lower vaginal mucosa (both external and brachytherapy contributions) can result in a higher incidence of complications. The posterior wall of the vagina appears to be more sensitive to irradiation, as does the distal vaginal mucosa. In contrast, the upper vagina (vault) tolerated doses in the range of 14,000 cGy. Hintz and co-workers[26] advocated dose rates of less than 80 cGy an hour.

REFERENCES

1. Barber HRK, Sommers SC: Vaginal adenosis, dysplasia, and clear cell adenocarcinoma after diethylstilbestrol treatment in pregnancy. Obstet Gynecol 43:645–652, 1974
2. Benedet JL, Murphy, KJ, Fairey RN, Boyes DA: Primary invasive carcinoma of the vagina. Obstet Gynecol 62:715–719, 1983
3. Benson RC: Cancer of the female genital tract. CA 18:2–13, 1968
4. Bertoni F, Bertoni G, Bignardi M: Vaginal molds for intracavitary curietherapy: A new method of preparation. Int J Radiat Oncol Biol Phys 9:1579–1582, 1983
5. Bonner, JA, Perez-Tamayo C, Reid GC, et al: The management of vaginal melanoma. Cancer 62:2066–2072, 1988
6. Boronow RC, Hickman BT, Reagan MT, et al: Combined therapy as an alternative to exenteration for locally advanced vulvovaginal cancer. II. Results, complications, and dosimetric and surgical considerations. Am J Clin Oncol 10:171–181, 1987
7. Brown GR, Fletcher GH, Rutledge FN: Irradiation of "in situ" and invasive squamous cell carcinomas of the vagina. Cancer 28:1278–1283, 1971
8. Chang YCF, Hricak H, Thurnher S, Lacey CG: Vagina: Evaluation with MR imaging. II. Neoplasms. Radiology 169:175–179, 1988
9. Chau PM: Radiotherapeutic management of malignant tumors of the vagina. Am J Roentgenol 89:502–523, 1963
10. Chung AF, Casey MJ, Flannery JT, et al: Malignant melanoma of the vagina: Report of 19 cases. Obstet Gynecol 55:720–727, 1980
11. Dancuart F, Delclos L, Wharton JT, Silvo EG: Primary squamous cell carcinoma of the vagina treated by radiotherapy: A failures analysis—The M.D. Anderson Hospital experience 1955–1982. Int J Radiat Oncol Biol Phys 14:745–749, 1988
12. Daw E: Primary carcinoma of the vagina. J Obstet Gynecol Br Common 78:853, 1971
13. Delclos L: Gynecologic cancers: Pelvic examination and treatment planning. In Levitt SH, Tapley N (eds): Technological Basis of Radiation Therapy: Practical Clinical Applications, pp 193–227. Philadelphia, Lea & Febiger, 1984
14. Desai S, Cavanagh D: Malignant melanoma of the vagina. Cancer 19:632–639, 1966
15. Evner F, Kressel HY, Mintz MC, et al.: Tumor recurrence versus fibrosis in the female pelvis: Differentiation with MR at 1.5 T. Radiology 166:333–340, 1988
16. Fletcher GH (ed): Textbook of Radiotherapy, 3rd ed, pp 821–824. Philadelphia, Lea & Febiger, 1980
17. Fletcher GH: Squamous cell carcinoma of the uterine cervix. In Fletcher GH (ed): Textbook of Radiotherapy, 3rd ed, pp 720–773. Philadelphia, Lea & Febiger, 1980
18. Frick HC II, Jacox HW, Taylor HC Jr: Primary carcinoma of the vagina. Am J Obstet Gynecol 101:695–703, 1968
19. Glazer HS, Lee JKT, Levitt RG, et al.: Radiation fibrosis: Differentiation from recurrent tumor by MR imaging. Radiology 156:721–726, 1985
20. Harrison LB, Fogel TD, Peschel RE: Primary vaginal cancer and vaginal melanoma: A review of therapy with external beam radiation and a simple intracavitary brachytherapy system. Endocuriether Hypertherm Oncol 3:67–72, 1987
21. Harwood AR, Cummings BJ: Radiotherapy for mucosal melanomas. Int J Radiat Oncol Biol Phys 8:1121–1126, 1982
22. Herbst AL: The effects in the human of diethylstilbestrol (DES) use during pregnancy. In Miller RW, Takayama S, Watanabe S, et al (eds): Unusual Occurrences as Clues to Cancer Etiology, pp 67–75. Tokyo, Taylor & Francis, 1988
23. Herbst AL, Green TH Jr, Ulfelder H: Primary carcinoma of the vagina. Am J Obstet Gynecol 106:210–218, 1970
24. Herbst AL, Ulfelder H, Poskanzer DC: Adenocarcinoma of the vagina: Association of maternal stilbestrol therapy with tumor appearance in young women. N Engl J Med 284:878–881, 1971
25. Hilgers RD, Malkasian GD, Soule EH: Embryonal rhabdomyosarcoma (botryoid type) of the vagina: A clinicopathologic review. Obstet Gynecol 17:484–502, 1979
26. Hintz GL, Kagan AR, Chan P, et al: Radiation tolerance of the vaginal mucosa. Int J Radiat Oncol Biol Phys 6:711–716, 1980
27. Horwitz RI, Viscoli CM, Merino M, et al: Clear cell adenocarcinoma of the vagina and cervix: Incidence, undetected disease, and diethylstilbestrol. J Clin Epidemiol 41:593–597, 1988
28. Hoskins WJ, Perez C, Young RC: Gynecologic tumors. In DeVita VT Jr, Hellman S, Rosenberg SA (eds): Cancer: Principles and Practice of Oncology, 3rd ed, pp 1099–1161. Philadelphia, JB Lippincott, 1989
29. Hricak H, Lacey CG, Sandles LG, et al: Invasive cervical carcinoma: Comparison of MR imaging and surgical findings. Radiology 166:623–631, 1988
30. Kanbour AI, Klionsky B, Murphy AL: Carcinoma of the vagina following cervical cancer. Cancer 34:1838, 1974
31. Kottmeier HL: The classification and clinical staging of carcinoma of the uterus and vagina. J Int Fed Gynecol Obstet 1:83–93, 1963
32. Kucera H, Langer M, Smekal G, et al: Radiotherapy of primary carcinoma of the vagina: Management and results of different therapy schemes. Gynecol Oncol 21:87–93, 1985
33. Laufe LE, Bernstein ED: Primary malignant melanoma of the vagina. Obstet Gynecol 37:148–154, 1971
34. Lee JY, Perez CA, Ettinger N, et al: The risk of second primaries subsequent to irradiation for cervix cancer. Int J Radiat Oncol Biol Phys 8:207–211, 1982
35. Lee RA, Symmonds RE: Recurrent carcinoma *in situ* of the vagina in patients previously treated for *in situ* carcinoma of the cervix. Obstet Gynecol 48:61–64, 1976
36. Lee RB, Buttoni L, Dhru K, Tamimi H: Malignant melanoma of the vagina: A case report of progression from pre-existing melanosis. Gynecol Oncol 19:238–245, 1984

37. Livingstone RC: Primary Carcinoma of the Vagina. Springfield, IL, Charles C Thomas, 1950
38. MacNaught R, Symmonds RP, Hole D, Watson ER: Improved control of primary vaginal tumors by combined external beam and interstitial radiotherapy. Clin Radiol 37:29–32, 1986
39. Marcus RB, Million RR, Daly JW: Carcinoma of the vagina. Cancer 42:2507–2512, 1978
40. Melnick S, Cole P, Anderson D, Herbst A: Rates and risks of diethylstilbestrol-related clear-cell adenocarcinoma of the vagina and cervix. N Engl J Med 316:514–516, 1987
41. Morrow CP, DiSaia PJ: Malignant melanoma of the female genitalia: A clinical analysis. Obstet Gynecol Surg 31:223–271, 1976
42. Norris HJ, Taylor HB: Melanomas of the vagina. Am J Clin Pathol 46:420–426, 1966
43. Perez CA, Arneson ANA, Dehner LP, et al: Radiation therapy in carcinoma of the vagina. Obstet Gynecol 44;862–872, 1974
44. Perez CA, Arneson AN, Galakatos A, et al: Malignant tumors of the vagina. Cancer 31:36–44, 1973
45. Perez CA, Bedwinek JM, Breaux SR: Patterns of failure after treatment of gynecologic tumors. Cancer Treat Symp 2:217, 1983
46. Perez CA, Camel HM: Long-term follow-up in radiation therapy of carcinoma of the vagina. Cancer 49:1308–1315, 1982
47. Perez CA, Camel HM, Galakatos AE, et al: Definitive irradiation in carcinoma of the vagina: Long-term evaluation of results. Int J Radiat Oncol Biol Phys 15:1283–1290, 1988
48. Perez CA, Korba A, Sharma S: Dosimetric considerations in irradiation of carcinoma of the vagina. Int J Radiat Oncol Biol Phys 2:639–649, 1977
49. Perez CA, Slessinger E, Grigsby PW: Design of an afterloading vaginal applicator (MIRALVA). Int J Radiat Oncol Biol Phys 18:1503–1508, 1990
50. Peters WA III, Kumar NB, Andersen WA, Morley GW: Primary sarcoma of the adult vagina: A clinicopathologic study. Obstet Gynecol 65:699–704, 1985
51. Piver MS, Barlow JJ, Wang JJ, et al: Combined radical surgery, radiation therapy and chemotherapy in infants with vulvovaginal embryonal rhabdomyosarcoma. Obstet Gynecol 42:522–526, 1973
52. Plentl AA, Friedman EA: Lymphatic System of the Female Genitalia: The Morphologic Basis of Oncologic Diagnosis and Therapy, pp 51–74. Philadelphia, WB Saunders, 1971
53. Prempree T, Amornmarn R: Radiation treatment of primary carcinoma of the vagina: Patterns of failure after definitive therapy. Acta Radiol Oncol 24:51–56, 1985
54. Pride GL, Schultz AE, Chuprevich TW, et al: Primary invasive squamous carcinoma of the vagina. Obstet Gynecol 53: 218–225, 1979
55. Puthawala A, Syed AMN, Nalick R, et al: Integrated external and interstitial radiation therapy for primary carcinoma of the vagina. Obstet Gynecol 62:367–372, 1983
56. Ragni MV, Tobon H: Primary malignant melanoma of the vagina and vulva. Obstet Gynecol 43:658–664, 1974
57. Robboy SJ, Herbst AL, Scully RE: Clear cell adenocarcinoma of the vagina and cervix in young females: Analysis of 37 tumors that persisted or recurred after primary therapy. Cancer 34:606–614, 1974
58. Robboy SJ, Scully RE, Herbst AL: Pathology of vaginal and cervical abnormalities associated with prenatal exposure to diethylstilbesterol. J Reprod Med 15:13, 1975
59. Rubin P: Clinical Oncology: A Multidisciplinary Approach, 6th ed. American Cancer Society, 1983
60. Rubin SC, Young J, Mikuta JJ: Squamous carcinoma of the vagina: Treatment, complications, and long-term follow-up. Gynecol Oncol 20:346–353, 1985
61. Rutledge F: Cancer of the vagina. Am J Obstet Gynecol 97:635–655, 1967
62. Schiffer MA, Markles AM, Greene HJ: Carcinoma in situ of the vagina after hysterectomy. Surg Gynecol Obstet 134:652, 1972
63. Senekjian EK, Frey KW, Anderson D, Herbst AL: Local therapy in stage I clear cell adenocarcinoma of the vagina. Cancer 60:1319–1324, 1987
64. Senekjian EK, Frey KW, Stone C, Herbst AL: An evaluation of stage II vaginal clear cell adenocarcinoma according to substages. Gynecol Oncol 31:56–64, 1988
65. Sharma SC, Gerbi B, Madoc-Jhones H: Dose rates for brachytherapy applicators using ^{137}Cs sources. Int J Radiat Oncol Biol Phys 5:1893, 1979
66. Son YH: Primary mucosal malignant melanoma: Appraisal of role of radiation therapy. Acta Radiol Oncol 19(FASC 3):177, 1980
67. Tavassoli FA, Norris HJ: Smooth muscle tumors of the vagina. Obstet Gynecol 53:689–693, 1979
68. Underwood RB, Smith RT: Carcinoma of the vagina. JAMA 217:46–52, 1971
69. Togashi K, Nishimura K, Itoh K, et al: Uterine cervical cancer: Assessment with high-field MR imaging. Radiology 160: 431–435, 1986
70. Wasserman TH, Stetz J, Phillips TL: Clinical trials of misonidazole in the United States. In Brady LW (ed): Radiation Sensitizers: Their Use in the Clinical Management of Cancer, pp 387–396. New York, Masson, 1980
71. Way S: Primary carcinoma of the vagina. J Obstet Gynaecol Br Emp 55:739, 1948
72. Wharton JT, Rutledge FN, Gallagher HS, et al: Treatment of clear cell adenocarcinoma in young females. Obstet Gynecol 43:365–368, 1975
73. Whelton J, Kottmeier HL: Primary carcinoma of the vagina. Acta Obstet Gynecol Scand 41:22–40, 1962

59

Vulva

Carlos A. Perez
Perry W. Grigsby

ANATOMY

The vulva is composed of the mons veneris, the clitoris, the labia majora, and the labia minora, and blends with the urinary meatus.

Lymphatics of the labia drain into the inguinal (sometimes referred to as superficial femoral) lymph nodes, located anterior to the cribriform plate and fascia lata. The lymphatics subsequently penetrate the cribriform fascia and reach the deep femoral nodes. From these, the lymph drains into the pelvic lymphatics (external and common iliac lymph nodes). Lymphatics of the fourchette, perineum, and prepuce follow the lymphatics of the labia. The lymph from the glans clitoris, on the other hand, can drain not only to the inguinal nodes but also directly to deep femoral nodes and pelvic lymph nodes. Some of the lymphatics originating in the clitoris may enter the pelvis anterior and posterior to the symphysis and connect with the obturator and external iliac nodes, bypassing the femoral area (Fig. 59-1).

EPIDEMIOLOGY

Carcinoma of the vulva is a relatively rare malignancy, accounting for 3% to 4% of all primary genital cancer. It is a disease of the elderly, with the peak incidence for invasive tumors in the seventh and eighth decades; in the series reported by Rutledge and co-workers, 15% of patients were under age 40, and three patients were in the third decade.[89] The median age for carcinoma *in situ* is 44 years,[23,39] for microinvasive carcinoma 58 years,[65,73,81] and for invasive carcinoma 61 years.[44,85,89]

Japaze and associates[56] reported no increased incidence of vulvar cancer in any ethnic group, but Mack and Casagrande[72] noted an incidence in women of the lowest social class three times greater than in the highest social class. Medical illnesses associated with vulvar cancer are hypertension, cardiovascular disease, obesity, and diabetes.[22,36,42,72,76] A variety of sexually transmitted diseases are associated with vulvar carcinoma including lymphogranuloma venereum, syphilis, herpesvirus type II, and condyloma acuminatum.[39,58] Recent evidence suggests an association between the human papillomavirus and the herpes simplex virus and vulvar neoplasia.[8,19,29,43,59] Other associations such as leukoplakia of the vulva, genitourinary cancer, and an occupational history in the laundry and cleaning industries have been noted.[71] An increased incidence of anogenital carcinoma, especially cervical cancer, has been reported in patients with vulvar cancer.[99]

NATURAL HISTORY

Over 70% of vulvar malignancies arise in the labia majora and labia minora, 10% to 15% in the clitoris, and 4% to 5% in the area of the perineum and fourchette. The vestibule, Bartholin's glands, and the clitoral prepuce are unusual primary sites, each accounting for less than 1% of vulvar cancers.[84]

Carcinomas arising in the vulvar area ordinarily follow a predictable pattern of spread to the regional lymphatic nodes. Superficial femoral (inguinal) lymph nodes are involved first, followed by the deep femoral inguinal nodes. Although lesions arising in or involving the glans clitoris or urethra theoretically can spread to pelvic lymph nodes through the channels that bypass the inguinal areas, such metastases without inguinal node involvement occur only under exceptional circumstances.[7,37,61]

Incidence of inguinal lymph node metastasis in surgically staged patients varies between 6% and 50%, depending on tumor invasion (Table 59-1).[12,28,44,49,81,89] Plentl and Friedman[84] reported a 62% incidence of lymph node metastases in patients with clinically palpable adenopathy and 35% without clinically palpable lymph nodes. In a review of clinical staging, Franklin[35] noted that approximately 75% of patients with clinically suspicious lymph nodes proved to have nodal metastasis, and nodes that were clinically negative were found to be positive for metastasis in 11% to 43% of cases. Approximately 20% to 30% of patients with histologically proven involvement of femoral nodes show deep pelvic lymph node involvement in the event that a pelvic lymphadenectomy is performed.[7,12]

Hematogenous dissemination is unusual and is a manifestation of late disease.[99]

DIAGNOSTIC WORKUP

In addition to the vulvar/anal area and perineum, the physical examination should include the vagina and cervix, which should be thoroughly inspected. Careful bimanual pelvic examination is mandatory. In addition to careful determination of the extent of the primary lesion, an essential part of the physical examination is the assessment of the regional lymph nodes.

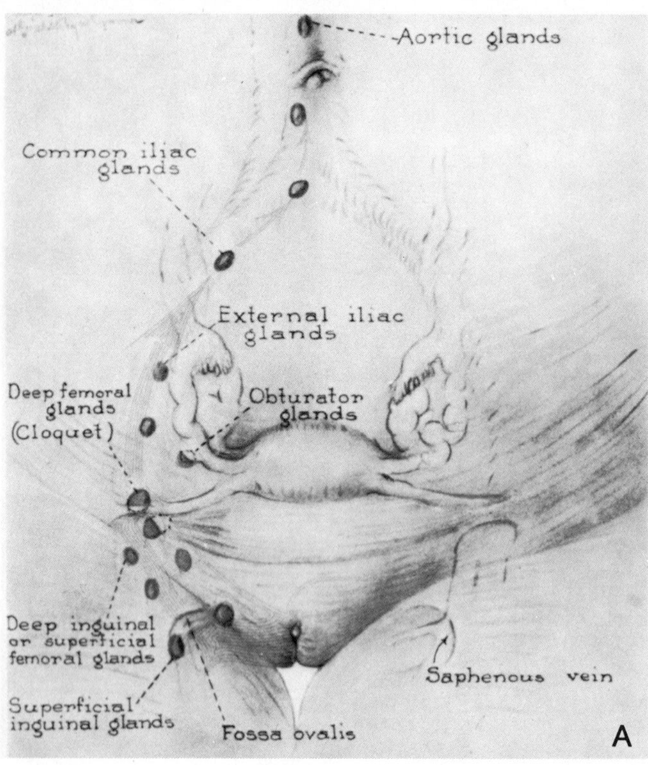

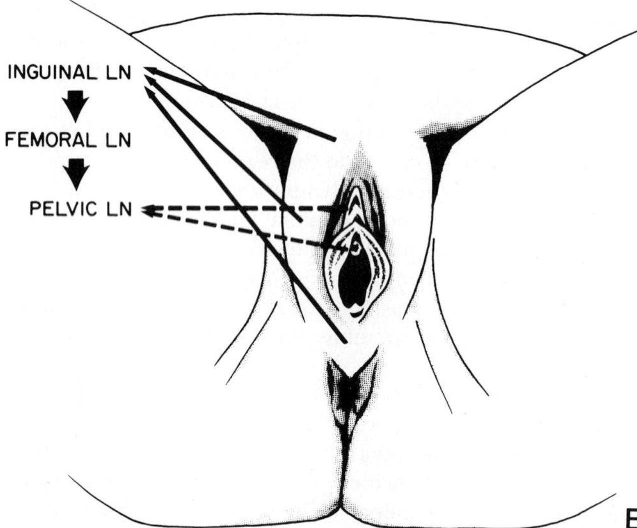

FIGURE 59–1. (**A**) Lymphatics of the groin and the pelvis (Benson RC: CA 18:4, 1968). (**B**) Schematic representation of lymphatic drainage of the vulva. (LN: lymph node)

Because of frequent inflammatory lymphadenopathy in the inguinal area, lymph node assessment in vulvar tumors is associated with a substantial rate of error. Papanicolaou smear of the cervix and vagina should be obtained.

Radiographic evaluation of regional lymphatics in carcinoma of the vulva is of limited value and is rarely used. Preoperative lymphography was evaluated at the Mallinckrodt Institute of Radiology in 32 patients with vulvar carcinoma. Correlations with the surgical specimens revealed an overall accuracy of 54.5% with a sensitivity of 15.7% and a specificity of 66.1%.[108]

Chest radiographs should be routinely obtained. Other studies include cystoscopy, proctosigmoidoscopy, barium enema, and intravenous pyelogram, when indicated. Computed tomography or magnetic resonance imaging may aid in outlining tumor extent and in evaluating the inguinal and pelvic/periaortic lymph nodes. The standard workup for these patients is described in Table 52-2.

STAGING

Clinical examination forms the basis for the currently adopted staging system (Table 59-3). The stages correlate well with treatment results. The use of 2.0 cm as the size determining the assignment of the primary lesion to T1 and T2 category has been criticized, however. Krupp and colleagues[62] and Donaldson and co-workers[28] suggest that 3.0 cm size be the determining factor for assignment of T category. The American Joint Committee (AJC) and the International Federation of Gynecology and Obstetrics (FIGO) staging systems are shown in Table 59-3.

PATHOLOGIC CLASSIFICATION

Preinvasive forms of vulvar malignancy include carcinoma *in situ* (Bowen's disease or erythroplasia of Queyrat and Paget's disease). The latter is equivalent to the same entity in the breast. Paget's disease is associated with invasive apocrine carcinoma in approximately 20% to 30% of cases.[5,48,105] Clinically these lesions may appear as flat or raised (maculopapular) or ulcerated, and they can be white (leukoplakia), red (erythroplastic), or hyperpigmented.[52,60]

Unsuspected invasion in patients with intraepithelial vulvar neoplasia was described in 13 of 69 patients (18.8%) and superficial invasion in eight patients.[20]

Basal cell carcinoma of the vulva is occasionally reported.[14,49,82]

Squamous cell carcinoma comprises over 90% of invasive lesions of the vulva. These tumors may be ulcerated and endophytic in one third of the cases; the remainder are exophytic.[38] Histologically, most of these tumors are well differentiated with keratin formation; 5% to 10% are anaplastic.[41,106] Tumors less than 2 cm in diameter and invading less than 5 mm of the basal membrane are often classified as microinvasive carcinoma.[81,109] These microinvasive carcinomas should be separated from more invasive tumors because of the excellent prognosis. Wharton and associates[109] performed lymphadenectomy in ten of 25 patients with lesions less than 2 cm in diameter and less than 5 mm of subdermal invasion and found no positive lymph nodes. Parker and colleagues,[81] using the same definition, found three patients of 37 with inguinal lymph node metastases.

Two variants of squamous cell carcinoma infrequently described are adenosquamous[67] and basaloid carcinoma. These tumors may be exophytic and well differentiated and may invade locally, but they rarely metastasize.[70]

Verrucous carcinoma of the vulva is very rare. Until 1988, the number of cases involving the female genital tract was 89.[2] Verrucous carcinoma is a slow-growing, nonaggresive tumor, with pushing margins and a rather benign histologic appearance. Incidence of lymph node metastasis is very low. The preferred treatment is wide surgical excision.

Adenoid cystic carcinoma of the Bartholin's gland constitutes approximately 10% of all carcinomas of this gland and 0.1% of all vulvar malignancies. Histologic features are similar to those found in other locations.[38] Thirty-nine cases have been described in the literature.[87] Five patients with this tumor were treated with a combination of surgery (four with wide local excision and one with hemivulvectomy) combined with post-

TABLE 59–1
Incidence of Lymph Node Involvement as a Function of Primary Tumor Size and Extent

PRIMARY TUMOR SIZE OR DEPTH OF INVASION	NO. OF PATIENTS	NUMBER OF PATIENTS WITH POSITIVE LYMPH NODES (%)
DEPTH		
≤1 mm	120	0 (0)
1.1– 2 mm	121	8 (6.6)
2.1– 3 mm	97	8 (8.2)
3.1– 4 mm	50	11 (22.0)
4.1– 5 mm	40	10 (25.0)
SIZE		
>5 mm	32	12 (37.5)
>2 cm	168	77 (45.8)
Any size primary tumor extending beyond vulva	70	38 (54.3)

(Data from Boutselis,[12] Donaldson et al,[28] Hacker,[44] Hoffman,[49] Krupp et al,[61] Parker,[81] and Rutledge et al[88].)

operative irradiation (doses ranging from 4000 cGy to 5400 cGy). Four patients are alive and well, with follow-up ranging from 2 to over 13 years. Only one patient died of disease at 5 years, 8 months.

Adenocarcinoma may also originate from the periurethral Skene's glands, but the majority arise either in Bartholin's gland or from bulboadnexal structures associated with Paget's disease.[68] Occasionally Bartholin's gland carcinoma may be a squamous cell carcinoma when it originates near the orifice of the duct, papillary when it arises from the transitional epithelium of the duct, and adenocarcinoma when it arises from the gland itself.

Melanoma represents 2% to 9% of vulvar malignancies; two varieties—nodular melanoma and superficial spreading melanoma—are described.[38] As in other locations, the depth of invasion correlates with the patterns of spread and prognosis.[4,6,13,21,52,110]

Sarcomas of the vulva are extremely rare, leiomyosarcoma being the most common. Neurofibrosarcoma, rhabdomyosarcoma, fibrosarcoma, and angiosarcoma have been reported.[5,102,105]

Metastatic carcinoma to the vulva from the uterine cervix (most common), the endometrium, or the ovary and extension or metastases from the urethra or the vagina have been described.[26]

TABLE 59–2
Diagnostic Workup for Vulva Tumors

General
- History
- Physical examination, including careful pelvic/bimanual examination

Special studies
- Exfoliative cytology of cervix and vagina
- Colposcopy and directed biopsies (including Schiller's test)
- Biopsies and examination under anesthesia to determine tumor extent
- Cytoscopy
- Proctosigmoidoscopy (as indicated)

Radiographic studies
- Standard
  - Chest radiographs
  - Intravenous pyelogram
- Complementary
  - Barium enema
  - Lymphangiogram
  - Computed tomography or magnetic resonance imaging scans of pelvis and abdomen

Laboratory studies
- Complete blood count
- Blood chemistry
- Urinalysis

TABLE 59–3
Staging of Carcinoma of the Vulva

DESIGNATION	DESCRIPTION
AJC STAGING	
Primary Tumor (T)	
Tis	Preinvasive carcinoma (carcinoma *in situ*)
T1	Tumor confined to the vulva and/or perineum, ≤2 cm in greatest dimension
T2	Tumor confined to the vulva and/or perineum, >2 cm in greatest dimension
T3	Tumor of any size with adjacent spread to the urethra and/or vagina and/or the anus
T4	Tumor of any size infiltrating the bladder mucosa and/or the rectal mucosa including the upper part of the urethral mucosa and/ or fixed to the bone
Nodal Involvement (N)	
N0	No nodes palpable
N1	Unilateral regional lymph node metastasis
N2	Bilateral regional lymph node metastasis
Distant Metastasis (M)	
M0	No clinical metastasis
M1	Distant metastasis (including pelvic lymph node metastasis)
FIGO STAGING	
Stage 0	Tis
Stage I	T1 N0 M0
Stage II	T2 N0 M0
Stage III	T3 N0 M0
	T1 N1 M0
	T2 N1 M0
	T3 N1 M0
Stage IVA	T1 N2 M0
	T2 N2 M0
	T3 N2 M0
	T4 Any N M0
Stage IVB	Any T Any N M1

(Shepherd JH: Br J Obstet Gynecol 96:889–892, 1989)

PROGNOSTIC FACTORS

The size, depth of invasion, and histologic subtype of primary tumors of the vulva, as well as degree of lymphatic and vascular invasion, correlate closely with the incidence of regional lymph node involvement and prognosis.[28,74,89,91,93] Kurzl and Messerer[66] carried out a multivariate analysis in 124 patients with various stages of vulvar carcinoma treated with simple vulvectomy and local/inguinal irradiation (4000 cGy). No inguinal lymphadenectomy was performed. They found that age, disassociated growth, lymphatic spread, tumor thickness, and ulceration were relevant prognostic factors.

Attempts have been made to identify the patients who are unlikely to develop femoral lymph node metastasis and in whom the need for inguinal dissection, with its attendant morbidity, could be obviated. Gynecologic Oncology Group protocol no. 36 was designed to assess the validity of FIGO staging relative to histopathologic prognostic factors.[51] Depth of invasion of 1 mm, 2 mm, and 3 mm corresponded to a 4.3%, 7.8%, and 17% incidence of nodal involvement. Perineural invasion was strongly associated with lymph node metastases.[88]

The incidence of lymph node involvement correlates well with the FIGO clinical staging. In the experience of Donaldson and co-workers,[28] 15% of patients in Stage I, 40% in Stage II, 80% in Stage III, and 100% of patients in Stage IV had confirmed regional lymph node involvement. Similar involvement was noted by Sedlis and colleagues,[91] who found regional node involvement in Stages I, II, III, and IV to be 8.9%, 25.3%, 31.1%, and 62.5%, respectively.

Surgical assessment of superficial femoral (inguinal) lymph nodes has become a widely accepted procedure for determination of therapeutic strategy, because survival is closely correlated with the pathologic status of the inguinal nodes (at 5 years, 80% to 85% for patients with negative nodes; 40% to 50% for those with positive nodes). Although it is generally agreed that pelvic lymph nodes do not need to be treated in patients without femoral lymph node involvement, the identification of patients with involved inguinal nodes for therapeutic management directed at the pelvis is of obvious importance. Many surgeons routinely dissect the pelvis in patients with positive inguinal areas; however, Curry and co-workers[24] suggested that the number of positive inguinal nodes serves as a predictor of deep pelvic node involvement. In their series, none of the patients with three or fewer unilaterally positive groin nodes had positive deep pelvic nodes. Similar findings have been observed by Hacker and associates.[46] Although deep pelvic node involvement is an ominous sign, one fourth to one third of patients are still salvageable, particularly when only a few nodes are involved.[12,24,37]

Extension of the primary tumor to the urethra, vagina, and anal area is associated with an increased incidence of nodal involvement and worsening of prognosis. Treatment usually involves either exenterative surgery or a combination of modalities (surgery and irradiation).

CLINICAL PRESENTATION

The most common complaint of patients with vulvar carcinoma is a mass in the vulva[76]; pruritus, bleeding, and pain are also seen. However, up to 20% of patients are asymptomatic.[16,42] A high index of suspicion and judicious use of biopsies contribute to earlier diagnosis of these tumors. Several techniques have been described to diagnose these lesions.[52]

GENERAL MANAGEMENT

The preinvasive forms of vulvar malignancies (carcinoma *in situ* and Paget's disease) can be treated in a variety of ways, including topical chemotherapy, cryocautery, and surgical resection. The preferred method of treatment is surgery, which may vary from wide local excision to partial or even total vulvectomy,[32,44,53] depending on the extent and multiplicity of intraepithelial lesions and the patient's wish to preserve the vulva. Hoskins and colleagues[52] have summarized this subject very clearly.

The accepted standard management in patients with invasive carcinoma of the vulva consists of a radical vulvectomy with inguinal lymphadenectomy.[52,55] The procedure consists of bilateral excision of the tissues in the femoral triangle and those overlying the inguinal ligament and removal of the entire vulva from the perineum to the upper margin of the mons pubis. The excision extends to the hymenal ring, pubic rami, and urogenital diaphragm. The urethral meatus is generally left *in situ*.

Whereas many surgeons have proceeded with a pelvic lymphadenectomy, current policies at some institutions reserve that procedure only for patients with clinically positive inguinofemoral lymph nodes. Attempts are being made to refine patient selection, omitting inguinal lymphadenectomy in patients with small, low-grade primary lesions and omitting pelvic lymphadenectomy in patients with three or fewer involved inguinal nodes, provided that the primary lesion does not invade the clitoris, urethra, vagina, or anal region.[27]

Because of the morbidity associated with radical vulvectomy, an attempt is being made, following biologic and therapeutic principles already validated in the head and neck, breast, and soft tissue sarcomas, to combine a wide local excision or simple vulvectomy to remove the primary tumor and, if necessary, an inguinal/femoral lymph node dissection in patients with clinically positive nodes with moderate doses of radiation therapy to the remaining vulva and regional lymph node-bearing areas (5000 cGy for subclinical disease with a boost of 1000 cGy to 1500 cGy through reduced portals for microscopically involved areas) (Fig. 59-2).

The role of radiation therapy alone in the primary management of carcinoma of the vulva remains controversial, primarily because of lack of data on the results of treatment with modern techniques and because of the traditional belief that vulvar tissues cannot tolerate high doses of radiation (over 6000 cGy). Historically, the reported control rates have been low, and the complication rate has been substantial. Radiation therapy often is used for palliation or for treatment of patients who are not amenable to surgical resection. The general principles of management for patients with various stages of carcinoma of the vulva are summarized in Table 59-4.

RADIATION THERAPY TECHNIQUES

Irradiation Alone

Vulva

In the occasional medically inoperable patient, small superficial lesions may be controlled with 6000 cGy to 6500 cGy. For larger tumors, the primary lesion needs to be irradiated to a dose of approximately 7000 cGy. It is important to use daily fractionation of 160 cGy to 180 cGy, five weekly fractions. Usually parallel opposed anterior and posterior portals are used, preferentially loaded anteriorly (or a high-energy photon single

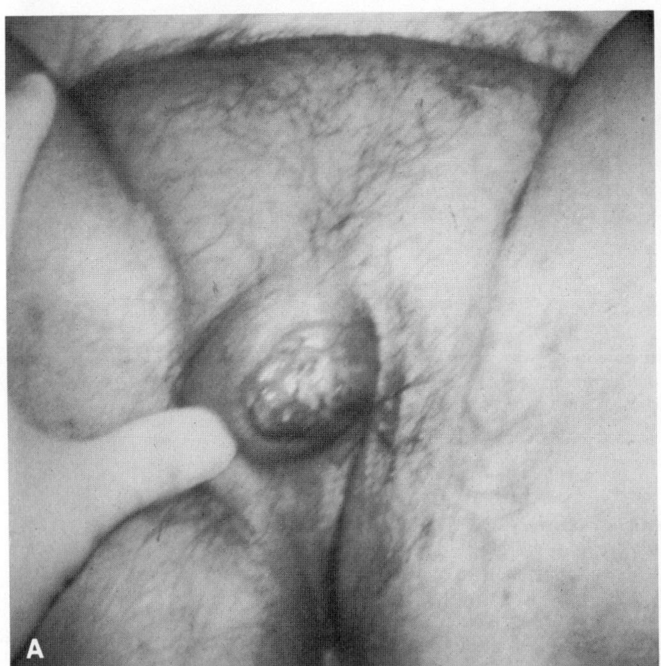

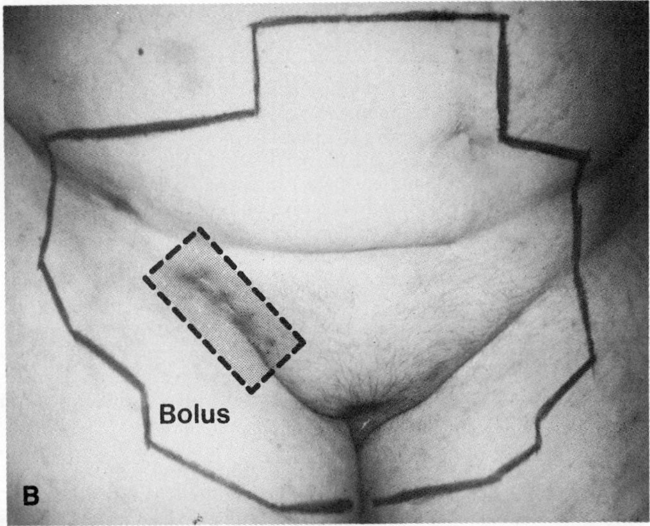

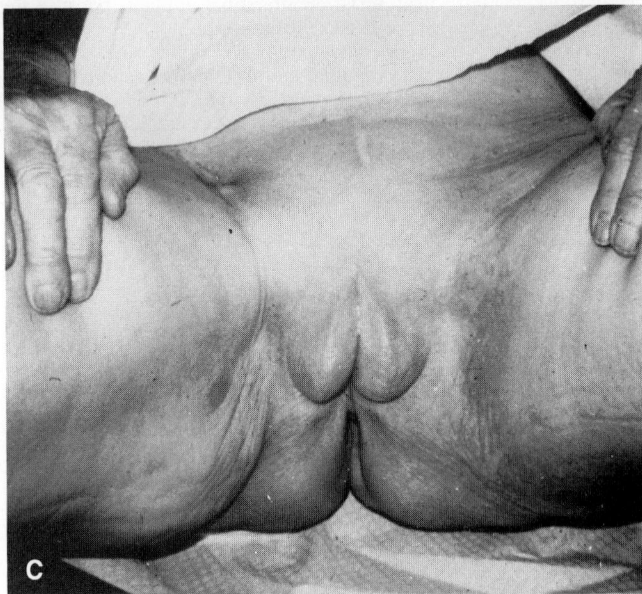

FIGURE 59–2. (**A**) Patient with a 4 cm epidermoid carcinoma in the right labia and clitoris and a 4-cm × 4-cm × 3-cm right inguinal lymph node. Wide local excision of the primary tumor and lymph nodes was carried out. (**B**) Portal used to deliver external irradiation to treat pelvic and vulvar areas to 5000 cGy. Bolus (2 cm thick) was used over right inguinal areas. Additional 1500 cGy was delivered with 12 MeV electrons to right tumor volume. (**C**) Posttreatment photograph 3 years later showing excellent cosmetic results. Patient is tumor free.

anterior beam with bolus) that covers the vulva and the regional lymphatics to deliver 4500 cGy to 5000 cGy. Appropriate bolus material over the areas of the skin (vulva) at risk for tumor involvement is essential.[80] Interruption of the radiation course is frequently necessary in the third or fourth week of treatment to prevent severe moist desquamation and maceration of the perineal skin. After a dose of 4500 cGy to 5000 cGy is delivered to the vulvar area, an electron beam (6 MeV to 9 MeV) or low-energy photon beam supplement aimed directly at the vulva is issued to deliver additional doses to gross or microscopic tumor volumes (1000 cGy to 2000 cGy). An interstitial implant may also be considered to deliver the "boost" dose to the primary tumor (Fig. 59-3).

Regional Lymphatics

In patients with primary lesions less than 2 cm in diameter, the probability of nodal involvement is low, and irradiation of the pelvic lymph nodes may be omitted when only the inguinofemoral nodes are being treated (Fig. 59-4*A*).

When an inguinal lymph node dissection is performed and only superficial node involvement is detected, postoperative irradiation is given only to the inguinofemoral lymph nodes (5000 cGy at 3 cm or 4 cm); a boost of 500 cGy to 1000 cGy may be given, depending on the number, size, or extracapsular extension of the tumor (see Fig. 59-4*A*).

Patients with metastatic deep inguinofemoral nodes found at node dissection may benefit from postoperative irradiation, including the pelvic lymphatics (5000 cGy at midplane pelvis in 5 to 6 weeks) (see Fig. 59-4*B* and *C*).

In patients with primary tumors larger than 2 cm and no clinical evidence of regional lymphatic involvement, the inguinal and pelvic lymph nodes may be treated electively to a dose of 4500 cGy to 5000 cGy (180 cGy to 200 cGy per day) in lieu of lymph node dissection (see Fig. 59-4*C*).

If palpable inguinal lymph nodes are present, doses to the inguinofemoral lymph nodes need to be in the range of 6500 cGy to 7000 cGy (with reduced fields after 5000 cGy), depending on the size of the involved nodes. When there is evidence of spread to the pelvic nodes, doses must be increased to 6000 cGy. Because some of the patients with involved pelvic lymph nodes are potentially curable, irradiation of the lower periaortic chain in the presence of pelvic lymph node involvement might be appropriate.

TABLE 59–4
Carcinoma of the Vulva: Recommended Policies of Treatment

Surgical therapy has been the standard in vulvar carcinoma.
Carcinoma *in situ* or microinvasion (≤5 mm): wide local excision
Invasive carcinoma
Stage I (Superficial, less than 2 cm in diameter); Wide local excision or simple vulvectomy
Other Stage I or Stage II: Radical vulvectomy with inguinal lymph node dissection
If clinically negative nodes, a reasonable alternative is simple vulvectomy, no lymph node dissection, elective node irradiation.
Doses of radiation therapy:
Negative lymph nodes, simple vulvectomy: 5000 cGy with 6–18 MV photons and appropriate bolus
Wide local excision, pathologically negative margins: As above. Perineal electron-beam boost to bring vulva excision site dose to 6000 cGy
Pathologically positive margins: After 6000 cGy, additional boost to positive margins or positive lymph nodes (500 cGy) with electrons or interstitial implant
Stage III: After radical vulvectomy and lymphadenectomy, indications for postoperative irradiation
a. Primary tumor ≥ 4 cm
b. Positive surgical margins
c. Three or more positive lymph nodes.
Dose: 5000 cGy to vulva and inguinal areas; boost to positive margins (1000–1500 cGy) via perineal portal or interstitial implant; boost to inguinal region via AP field (1000–1500 cGy)
Stage IV: Pelvic exenteration
Preoperative irradiation: 4500 cGy to pelvis and inguinal areas with radical vulvectomy and complete inguinal lymph node dissection.* Postoperative boost to primary (1000–1500 cGy) via interstitial and/or intracavitary and/or appositional electrons, when indicated

** In patients with palpable inguinal nodes, superficial inguinal node dissection and inguinal/pelvic irradiation may be acceptable as a less mutilating alternative.*

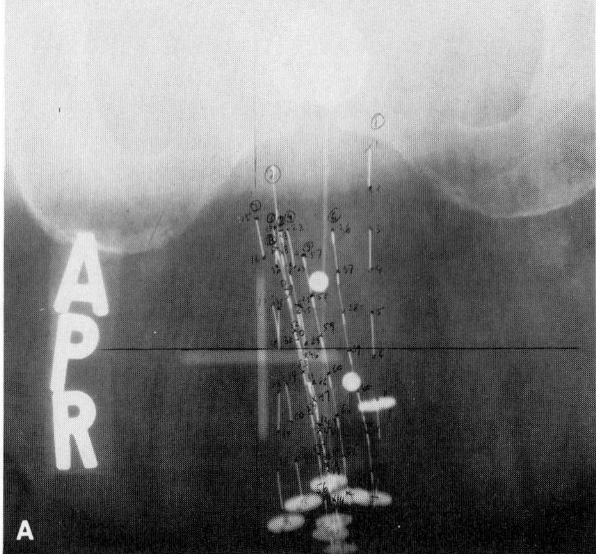

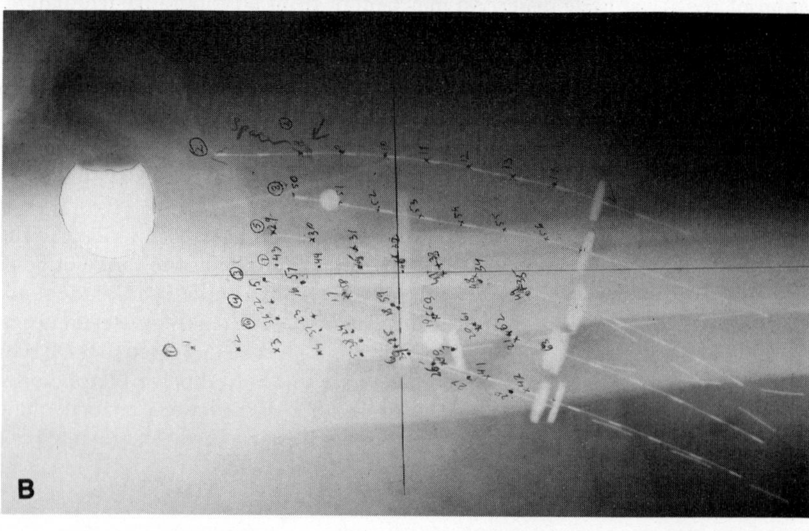

FIGURE 59–3. (**A** and **B**) Example of ^{192}Ir implant to deliver 2000 cGy to tumor excision site in combination with external irradiation in patient with T2N0M0 squamous carcinoma of the left major labium.

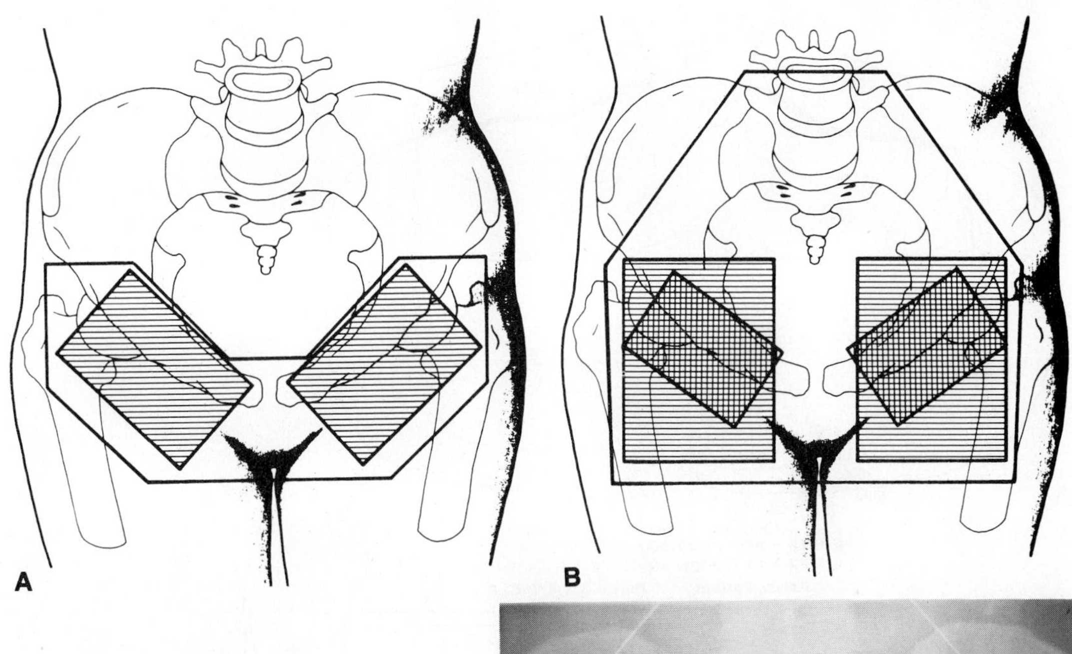

FIGURE 59–4. (**A**) Portal for elective irradiation of regional lymphatics in patients with no clinical evidence of inguinal lymph node involvement. (**B**) Portal for irradiation of pelvic and inguinofemoral lymph nodes and vulvar area. The groins are subsequently boosted to a total of 6000 cGy to 6500 cGy. A final boost of 500 cGy to 1000 cGy to the positive inguinal lymph nodes may be given with further field reduction, bringing the total dose to that area to approximately 7000 cGy. (**C**) Simulation film of portal covering pelvic and inguinofemoral lymph nodes and vulva.

In patients in whom the pelvic nodes must be treated, anterior and posterior portals covering the vulvar and regional lymphatic volumes are required.

Beams and Energies

Depending on the available equipment, either an anteroposterior beam or differentially loaded parallel opposed anteroposterior-posteroanterior (AP-PA) beams or electron beam (for part of the treatment) can be used. If only the vulva and the inguinofemoral lymph nodes are treated, ^{60}Co, 4 MV to 6 MV x-rays, or even electrons through an anterior portal may be adequate. Care should be taken to deliver adequate doses not only to the primary tumor area and superficial inguinal nodes but also to the femoral nodes and the deep pelvic nodes (Fig. 59-5). Although dry and moist desquamation are frequently observed, we still favor the use of bolus in areas potentially involved by tumor.

Higher-energy photon beams (15 MV to 18 MV) with unequal loading (AP3-PA2) and bolus on the anterior portal can be used. An alternative is to treat the anterior portal with ^{60}Co or 4 MV to 6 MV x-rays and the posterior portal with high-energy photon beam (15 MV to 18 MV; see Fig. 59-5).

Patient Positioning and Simulation

The patient is treated in the supine "frog leg" position, with the knees apart and the feet together (Fig. 59-6). A cast or alpha-cradle in the treatment position facilitates everyday repositioning.

When the patient is simulated, wires should be used to identify surgical scars or palpable/visible lesions. If the vagina or the perineum is involved, a radiopaque marker should be placed to identify these areas on radiographs. With tumors involving the urethra, a urethral catheter, if tolerated by the patient, may aid in tumor localization.

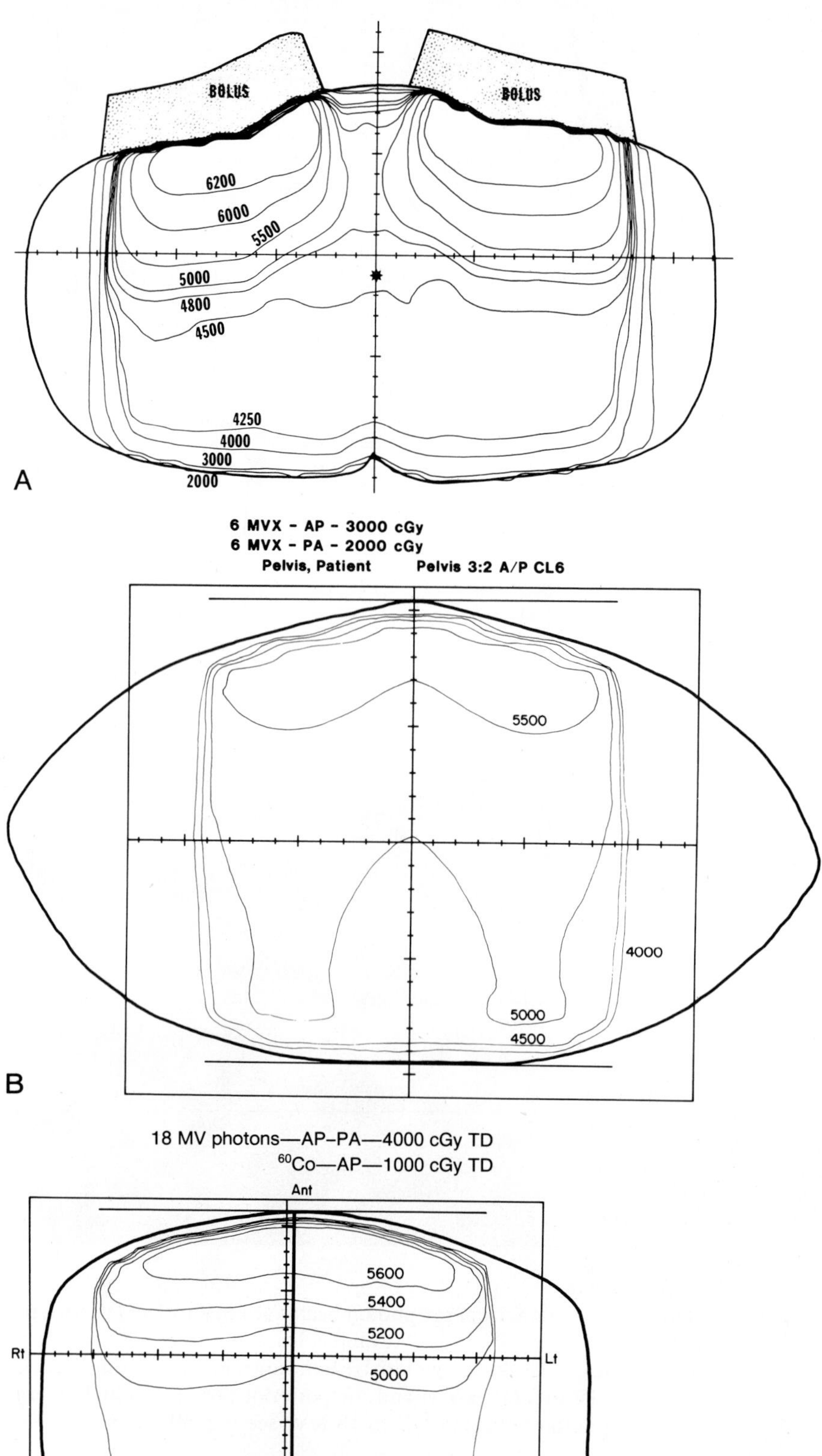

FIGURE 59–5. Representative treatment plans for irradiation of vulvar region and regional lymphatics. (**A**) Parallel opposed 18 MV photon beams, preferentially loaded anteriorly (2700 cGy anteriorly; 1800 cGy posteriorly); bolus is added over the inguinal areas to improve dose distribution in subcutaneous tissues in that area. A 1500 cGy boost using 16 MeV electrons (without bolus) is added to the groin. (**B** to **D**) Alternative setups with different beam energies and loadings.

Because of the sloping surface of the perineum, higher doses may be delivered to this area when the tumor dose is calculated at the central axis of the portal (Fig. 59-7). During simulation, consideration should be given to designing and constructing compensating filters to achieve a more homogeneous dose in the entire target volume.

Preoperative Radiation Therapy

Patients with advanced primary lesions involving surrounding structures, either of questionable resectability or clearly unresectable, should be irradiated preoperatively.[11] Moderate doses (4500 cGy to 5000 cGy in 5 to 6 weeks) may increase the resec-

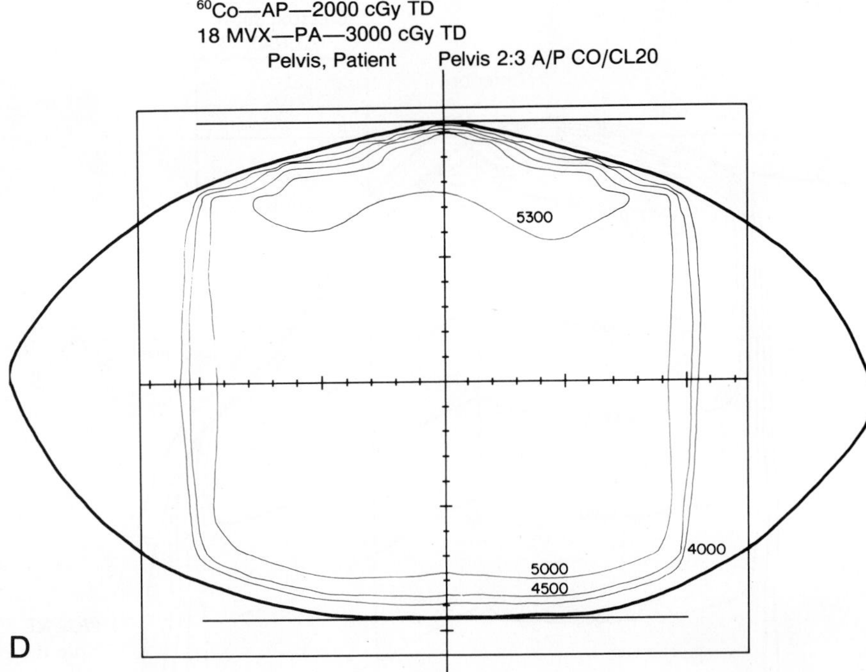

FIGURE 59–5. (*Continued*)

tability rate and also avoid mutilating procedures such as exenteration.

Postoperative Radiation Therapy

Increasingly, radiation therapy is used in combination with surgery. In patients who have undergone a radical resection of the primary lesion and the inguinofemoral lymph nodes and are considered at high risk of recurrence because of inadequate resection margins, or in patients with positive inguinal nodes (in lieu of pelvic lymph node dissection), or in patients treated with wide local tumor excision, postoperative irradiation is indicated, consisting of 5000 cGy (175 cGy to 180 cGy daily). If the resection margins are microscopically involved or if gross residual tumor exists, an additional dose (1500 cGy to 2000 cGy) needs to be administered with reduced portals or on interstitial implant.

Treatment for Recurrent Lesions

Recurrences following surgical resection remain potentially curable and need to be treated aggressively in the manner described earlier to deliver doses of 6500 cGy to 7000 cGy with reducing fields.

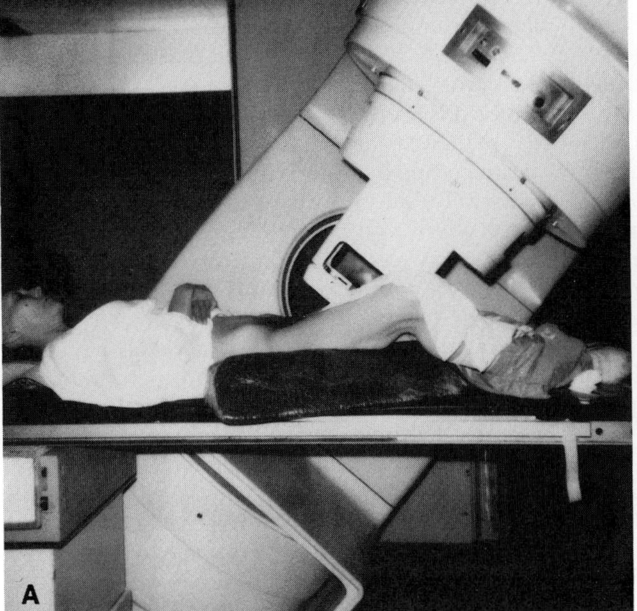

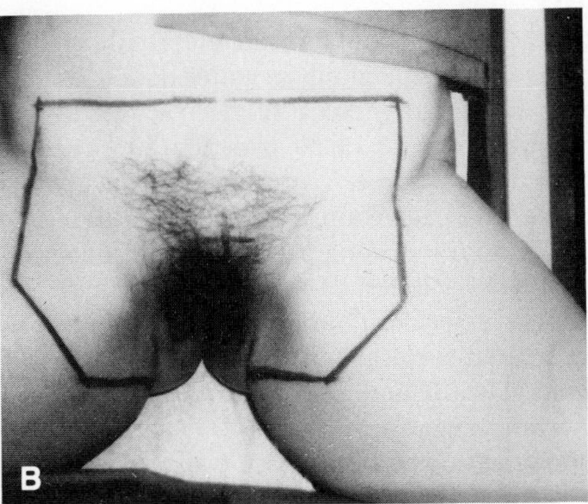

FIGURE 59–6. (**A**) Supine frog-leg position for irradiation of vulva and inguinal pelvic lymph nodes. The patient's thighs are abducted and outwardly rotated so that the inguinal folds are stretched flat. (**B**) Example of portal used for irradiation of vulva and inguinofemoral lymph nodes with patient in treatment position. (Pao WM, Perez CA, Kuske RR, et al: Int J Radiat Oncol Biol Phys 14:1123–1132, 1988)

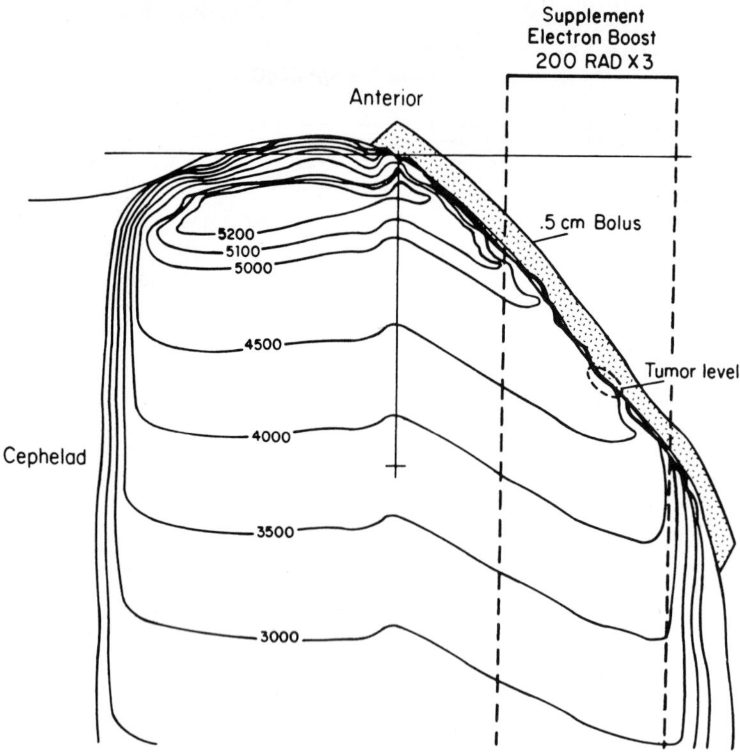

FIGURE 59–7. Sagittal isodose contours on a patient. Note the relative underdosage of the posterior vulvar region, thereby requiring a supplemental *en face* perineal electron-beam field. (Pao WM, Perez CA, Kuske RR, et al: Int J Radiat Oncol Biol Phys 14:1123–1132, 1988)

RESULTS OF THERAPY

Most reports on surgical management of carcinoma of the vulva cover a long time span, over which the philosophies of treatment, staging, and methods of reporting have varied considerably, as well as techniques of radiation therapy. Most recent reports cite an overall survival rate of approximately 50% at 5 years. Rutledge and colleagues[89] reported an actuarial survival rate of 92% for Stage I, 88% for Stage II, 70% for Stage III, and 25% for Stage IV disease. The overall actuarial survival rate at 5 years was 70%, but the absolute survival rate was only 55.7%. Boutselis[12] observed an absolute survival rate of 90% for Stage I, 63% for Stage II, 17% for Stage III, and 0% for Stage IV patients. The 5-year disease-free survival rate of 223 patients treated surgically for invasive squamous cell carcinoma of the vulva at the Mayo Clinic was 90% for patients with Stage I and 81%, 68%, and 20% for those with Stages II, III, and IV disease, respectively.[85]

Influence of nodal status on outcome is striking. In a group of 53 patients with histologically negative nodes, Rutledge and colleagues[89] did not observe a single instance of recurrent tumor; however, only 13 of 39 patients (30%) with positive nodes survived disease-free. Krupp and associates[62] noted 93% 5-year survival rate in a group of 55 patients with histologically negative groin nodes. Among patients with histologically positive inguinal lymph nodes, 24% survived 5 years.

Hacker and associates,[46] in 113 patients with invasive vulva carcinoma treated surgically, found 31 (27.4%) with positive inguinofemoral lymph nodes. The actuarial 5-year survival rate for patients with negative nodes was 96%; for those with one positive node the rate was 94%; with two positive nodes, 80%; and with three or more positive nodes, 12%. The authors pointed out that no positive pelvic nodes were found in the absence of palpable suspicious or fixed inguinal lymph nodes. The 5-year survival rate in 79 patients with clinically negative inguinal lymph nodes who did not undergo pelvic lymphadenectomy was 96%. None of six patients with metastasis to pelvic lymph nodes demonstrated at pelvic lymphadenectomy survived.

Local recurrence follows definitive surgery in 29% to 30% of patients.[22,76,94] Recurrent lesions remain potentially curable, as indicated by the report by Buechler and associates[15] (recurrences were treated by either surgical resection or irradiation).

A striking variety of techniques, doses, and fractionation schedules has been used. Following the 1930 report by Stoeckel[100] of a 12% 5-year survival rate in a group of patients treated with x-ray or radium, the results did not improve substantially until the reports by Oberhauser[79] and Frischbier and Thomsen.[40] It should be noted that patients in the report by Backstrom[3] all had T4 lesions; the 21% 5-year survival rate achieved is therefore remarkable.

Although it is difficult to critically evaluate the methods of treatment and the criteria for patient selection, an improvement in overall results has emerged with the use of adequate doses and modern equipment. The best results were reported with high-energy electrons (47.5% 5-year survival rate in 118 patients, 28% with Stage I or II and 72% with Stage III or IV disease),[40] although the advisability of a 300 cGy per day fraction in an anatomic area that is allegedly highly radiosensitive should be questioned. Twenty-four percent of the patients so treated developed ulcers, and 5% developed extensive tissue necrosis. The fractionation scheme might be responsible for the fairly high incidence of complications in that series.

Nobler[77] addressed the question of normal tissue tolerance in the vulvar area in a group of six patients treated with perineal portals to 5000 cGy to 7000 cGy in 6 to 9 weeks (200 cGy/day). No evidence of local recurrence was seen in five of the six patients for a period of 10 to 24 months. Tolerance of perineal and vulvar tissue was judged as good. The patient who developed serious complications had been treated in the past to full tumoricidal doses for carcinoma of the cervix.

Pao and associates[80] reported results in 40 patients with

primary or recurrent vulvar carcinoma treated with radiation therapy. Nineteen of the patients with primary tumors received postoperative irradiation (5000 cGy in 6 weeks). Fifteen of the 19 exhibited local tumor control. Five patients with Stage III or Stage IV disease were managed with radiation therapy alone. Four had a complete response with two currently with no evidence of disease (NED). Two patients who received preoperative irradiation with local excision were also tumor-free. The 4-year NED survival rates were 100%, 28%, 50%, 0%, and 10% for Stage I, II, III, IV, and recurrent tumors, respectively (Fig. 59-8). The poor results obtained in Stage II tumors is likely a result of selection because four of seven patients developed distant metastases. Two of the 14 patients treated for recurrent disease remain NED after local excision of their tumors before irradiation. No dose response for subclinical disease could be found for doses between 4500 cGy and 7000 cGy. Treatment morbidity was acceptable, with two patients developing severe long-term complications requiring surgical intervention.

Of 19 patients treated by Pirtoli and Rottoli[83] with definitive irradiation (200 keVp x-rays or electrons, doses of 4500 cGy to 8500 cGy to the primary tumor and 4500 cGy to 5500 cGy to inguinal lymph nodes), 17 had complete tumor regression and eight (42%) survived 5 years. Seventeen additional patients were treated for palliation, but the results were not specifically described; only one patient of five with palpable inguinal nodes showed complete tumor regression.

Table 59-5 lists some of the reported results of definitive radiation therapy.

There have been numerous attempts to combine radiation therapy and surgery to improve the therapeutic results.[1,9,10,25,34,44,63,98] Acosta and collaborators[1] found no macroscopic residual tumor in 13 patients operated on after receiving 3500 cGy to 5500 cGy. Worth mentioning is the series of Frankendal and co-workers,[34] who reported on 55 patients, 22 of whom had palpable lymph nodes considered tumorous; in 19 of these histologic confirmation of nodal involvement was observed. Primary lesions were electrocoagulated, resected, or irradiated. The regional nodes were dissected when clinically involved. Clinically negative nodes were observed unless the primary tumor was large or poorly differentiated. In such a situation, the groin was irradiated to a dose of 3000 cGy to 6000 cGy in 15 to 55 days. Of the 12 patients who were irradiated electively to the inguinal areas because of unfavorable primary lesions, none developed inguinal metastasis. In contrast, of seven patients with clinically negative nodes and early lesions who were only observed, three developed regional lymph node metastasis. Kucera and Weghaupt[63] analyzed 607 patients treated with electrocoagulation of the primary lesion and 4500 cGy (300 cGy fractions) to inguinal nodes less than 2 cm or 6000 cGy and local excision for inguinal nodes more than 2 cm. The primary excision site was not irradiated. The 5-year overall survival rates were 78%, 71%, 57%, and 12% for Stages I to IV, respectively.

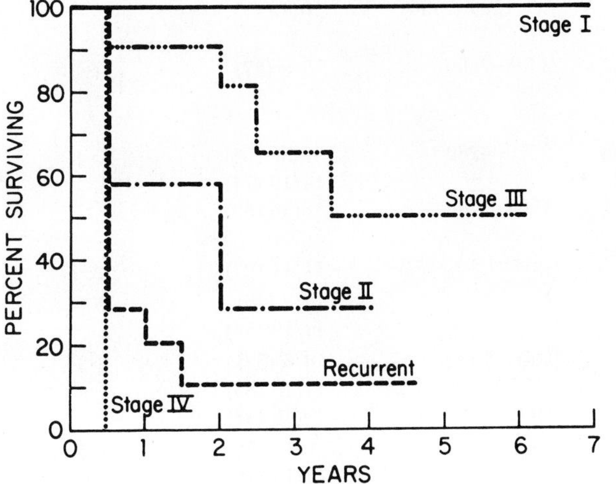

FIGURE 59–8. Actuarial no evidence of disease (NED) survival curves of 40 patients with carcinoma of the vulva by stage. (Pao WM, Perez CA, Kuske RR, et al: Int J Radiat Oncol Biol Phys 14:1123–1132, 1988)

Daly and Million[25] tested a combination of radical vulvectomy followed by elective nodal irradiation to 4500 cGy in 5 weeks. In a small series of six patients, the treatment was tolerated well with no nodal failures and no radiation complications. No delay in healing of the surgical site was recorded.

Boronow,[9] Hacker and associates,[44] and Simonsen and colleagues[98] have advocated combinations of preoperative irradiation (4400 cGy to 5400 cGy in 5 to 6 weeks) and less extensive surgery in patients with locally advanced vulvar carcinoma to decrease the size of the tumor and improve resectability. In a series of nine cases, Boronow[9] reported only one local recurrence. The incidence of operative morbidity was minimal, and five patients remained disease-free for a period of 11 months to 4.5 years. This experience was recently updated[10]; practically all of the 37 patients treated with this technique had advanced primary tumors of the vulva. The 5-year survival rate for the primary cases was 75.6%. For the patients with recurrent disease, the 5-year survival rate was 62.6%. In the majority of the patients (94.8%), the bladder and rectum were preserved. In seven of eight patients (87.5%) reported on by Hacker and associates,[44] significant regression of the tumor allowed more conservative surgical excision. Four of the eight patients had no viable tumor in the surgical specimen. Five patients (62.5%) are alive without evidence of disease at intervals ranging from 15 months to 10 years at the time of the report. One patient developed a bilateral hip necrosis and fracture.

Miyazawa and associates[75] reported results in 18 patients treated with combined irradiation and surgery and 15 patients treated with irradiation alone. In the patients treated surgically, five had a local excision or simple vulvectomy and 12 had a radical vulvectomy with or without lymph node dissection. Ten of these patients presented with local recurrence, with 60% occurring in the first 2 years after initial surgery. Seven patients were referred for irradiation because of positive lymph nodes in the surgical specimen. Of the ten patients treated for local recurrence, only two survived over 5 years. Seven patients were referred for irradiation of positive lymph nodes; only one survived 1 year. The second group consisted of 15 patients treated with irradiation alone because of associated medical problems or extensive local disease. Six had Stage III, and nine had Stage IV tumors. Thirteen of these patients were followed for up to 5 years. Four patients were alive at 1 year, two at 2 years, and one at 3 years. Severe moist desquamation, ulceration, and pain were noted in four of six patients treated with orthovoltage x-rays compared with two of 27 patients treated with megavoltage irradiation, one of whom developed an ileocutaneous fistula.

Prempree and Amormarn[86] described the results in 21

TABLE 59–5
Radiation Therapy for Vulvar Carcinoma: Literature Review

AUTHOR	TREATMENT TECHNIQUE	STAGE OF DISEASE	DOSE (cGy)	LOCOREGIONAL CONTROL (%)	FOLLOW-UP (YEARS)
Tod[104]	Radium implant only	Early Late	5500–6000	26/71 (36) 14/45 (31)	5
Ellis[30]	Radium implant + orthovoltage	I–II III–IV Recurrent	4000–6000	11/24 (46) 2/24 (08) 2/17 (12)	5
Johnson[57]	Orthovoltage inguinal treatment only with vulvar excision	NR	2100 in 3 fractions	133/175 (76)	5
Frischbier and Thomsen[40]	3–15 MeV electrons	I–II III–IV	4500–5400 300 cGy fractions	23/33 (70) 33/85 (39)	5
Backstrom et al[3]	^{60}Co	IV	5200–6900	7/19 (36)	5
Helgason et al[47]	Orthovoltage, ^{60}Co ± radium implant	I–IV Recurrent	1500–5840 3000	16/29 (55) 4/24 (17)	2–5
Frankendal et al[34]	^{60}Co inguinal treatment only with vulvar excision	I–IV	6000–6500	12/12 (100)	3
Daly and Million[24]	^{60}Co inguinal treatment only	I–III	4500–5000	6/6 (100)	0.5–3
Kuipers[64]	6–17 MeV electrons	I–II III–IV	6000–8000	3/11 (27) 12/37 (32)	5
Acosta et al[1]	^{60}Co Preoperative RT	II–III	3600–5500	13/14 (93)	.2–8
Weghaupt[107]	^{60}Co inguinal node irradiation	I–IV	6000	283/292 (97)	>5
Tafari and Magalotti[101]	^{60}Co, ^{137}Cs implants	II–IV Recurrent		7/8 (88) 2/3 (88)	1–11 1–2
Pirtoli and Rottoli[83]	Orthovoltage Electron	I–II III–IV	4500–8500	10/16 (63) 4/12 (33)	5
Iversen[54]	7, 33 MV photons ± bleomycin	IV Recurrent	1500–3000	4/9 (44) 0/4	
Boronow et al[11]	Preoperative RT	III–IV	2000 pelvis; 2000 split Implant 4500 cGy point A	24/26 (92)	1–11
Miyazawa et al[75]	Betatron, photons + electrons	III–IV Recurrent	4000–5000	2/12 (17) 2/10 (20)	2–11
Nori et al[78]	RT + Flagyl (metronidazole)	III–IV Recurrent	Implant 600 × 3 then 200 × 15	3/4 (75) 2/2 (100)	1–3
Prempree and Amornmarn[86]	^{60}Co, 15 MeV electrons + radium implant	Limited Extensive	4000–6000 + 1500–5500	8/8 (100) 0/13	>5
Hacker et al[45]	^{60}Co – 10 MV photons + ^{192}Ir implants	III–IV	4400–7800	7/8 (87)	1–10
Simonsen[97]	^{137}CS inguinal nodes only	Negative nodes Positive nodes Extranodal extension	2770–4280 4500–5400	53/56 (94) 14/19 (74) 18/36 (50)	>4
Simonsen et al[98]	RT + surgery	Recurrent		11/41 (27)	2–17
Carlino et al[18]	^{192}Ir implants only ± surgery	I–IV I–IV	NR	2/8 (25) 11/19 (58)	5
Fairey et al[31]	^{60}Co RT only RT + surgery	I–III I–III Recurrent	5000–5500 3000	4/6 (67) 11/13 (85) 19/40 (48)	>3
Pao et al[80]	Megavoltage ± implant ± surgery	I–II III–IV Recurrent	4500–7000	9/12 (75) 11/14 (79) 4/14 (29)	0.5–8

RT: radiation therapy; NR: not reported

patients with recurrent carcinoma of the vulva treated with irradiation alone (external-beam irradiation and interstitial brachytherapy); the majority of the patients received doses ranging from 5500 cGy to 8000 cGy. Patients with recurrent tumor limited to the introitus or adjacent vagina had the best prognosis, all six having tumor control and surviving over 5 years. Two of four patients with small inguinal lymph nodes were cured. None of the patients with extensive recurrences survived, although a few had transient tumor response. Buechler and colleagues[15] reported 73% tumor control rate in 18 patients presenting with postradical vulvectomy[11] or postlocal excision[7] recurrences, the majority involving only the perineum. Seven patients were treated with irradiation and 11 were treated surgically (wide local excision, radical vulvectomy, or posterior exenteration). Two patients survived for long periods (4 and 13 years).

The value of elective irradiation of the pelvic lymph nodes was demonstrated by Homesley and associates,[50] who reported on a randomized study involving 114 patients with invasive squamous cell carcinoma of the vulva and positive inguinal lymph nodes treated with radical vulvectomy and bilateral groin lymphadenectomy. The patients were randomized to receive pelvic irradiation (4500 cGy to 5000 cGy in 5 to 6 weeks) in addition to the inguinal regions or pelvic lymph node dissection. No irradiation was given to the central vulvar area. Of 59 patients randomized to irradiation, the 53 who were treated had a 68% 2-year survival rate. In contrast, the nonirradiated group had a 54% survival rate (Fig. 59-9*A*). The benefit of radiation therapy was noted only in patients with N2 or N3 lymphadenectomy (Fig. 59-9*B*). Regional lymph node recurrences were noted in seven of the 59 patients allocated to irradiation (11.9%) in contrast to 14 of 55 patients (25.4%) treated with surgery only.

Misonidazole was used as a radiosensitizer combined with high-dose radiation therapy (usually 4800 cGy to 5800 cGy) in ten patients with advanced vulvovaginal carcinoma. Nine of the patients had tumor control, and five of them were tumor-free 9 to 30 months after diagnosis. Toxicity was minimal with only one patient developing peripheral neuropathy.[78]

SEQUELAE OF TREATMENT

With a tumor at the skin or mucosal surface, which requires that the peak dose be at the surface, it is expected that literally all patients will have a significant acute (cutaneous and mucosal) reaction. Of more concern, however, is the incidence of late (chronic) sequelae, some of which can be attributed to the fractionation schemes used. Schulz and co-workers,[90] for example, reported a very high incidence of complications with 500 cGy fractions. The rate has been consistently low in patients treated with 200 cGy per day or similar fractionation schemes.[3,77] Cosmetic results with conservation surgery and irradiation may be very rewarding when appropriate surgical and irradiation techniques are applied (Fig. 59-10).

Common sequelae associated with radical surgery are those related to wound problems primarily in the form of infection and necrosis. The reported incidence of wound infection varies markedly. Iversen and co-workers[55] observed it in 5.7% of patients and Boutselis[12] in 50% of patients. The incidence of wound dehiscence and necrosis varies in most reports from 30% to 50%.[12,89] Leg edema is a serious complication of nodal dissection. Transient edema occurred in approximately 14% of patients reported on by Boutselis[12] and Rutledge and associates.[89] Chronic (persistent) edema was reported in 71% of the patients reported on by Boutselis[12] and in 20% of those reported on by Rutledge and others.[89] Operative mortality rate in most series varies from 3% to 6%.

CLINICAL TRIALS

Only a small number of clinical trials are available for the treatment of vulvar carcinoma. A phase II trial to document the rates and patterns of recurrence of early Stage I patients, all treated with ipsilateral superficial inguinal lymphadenectomy and modified radical hemivulvectomy, is in progress by the Gynecological Oncology Group (GOG-74). These patients must have pathologically negative ipsilateral superficial inguinal lymph nodes and resection margins at the dermis of more than 5 mm.

A phase III study (GOG-88) is a randomized comparison of bilateral groin irradiation with bilateral groin dissections following radical vulvectomy for Stages I, II, and III. The purpose of this protocol is to compare the therapeutic efficacy and morbidity as well as recurrence rates and survival rates in these two treatment groups.

Patients with advanced or recurrent vulvar cancer that is refractory to curative therapy or established treatments are eligible for GOG-26. This is a phase II protocol to screen new agents and drug combinations for activity in patients with advanced or recurrent pelvic malignancies.

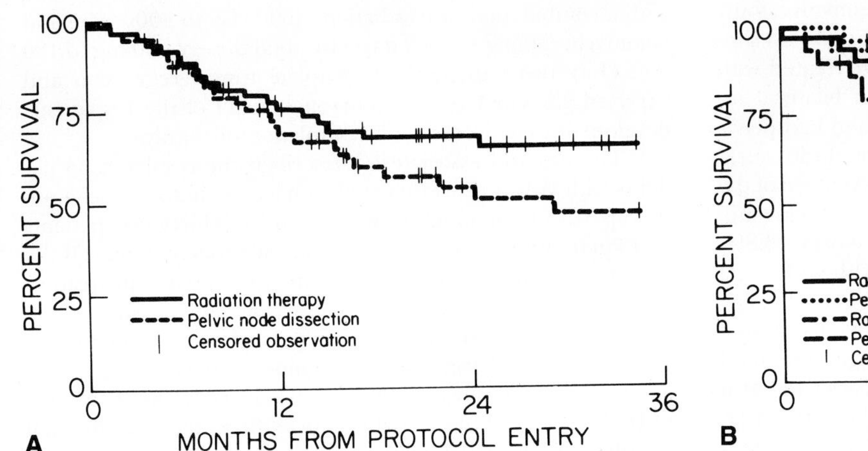

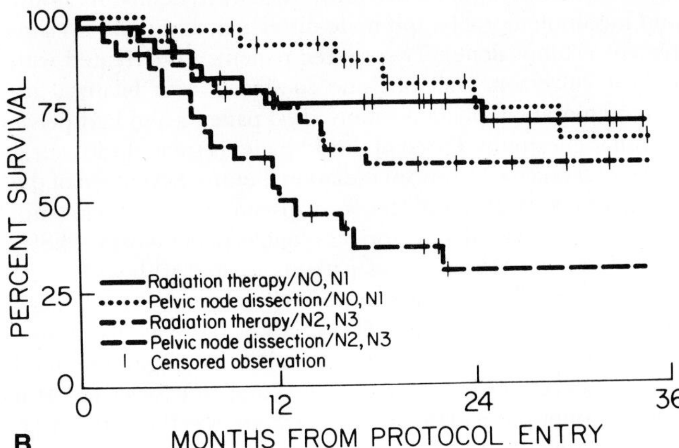

FIGURE 59–9. (**A**) Survival rate related to type of treatment. (**B**) Survival related to clinical groin node status and treatment. (Homesley HD, et al: Obstet Gynecol 68:733–740, 1986).

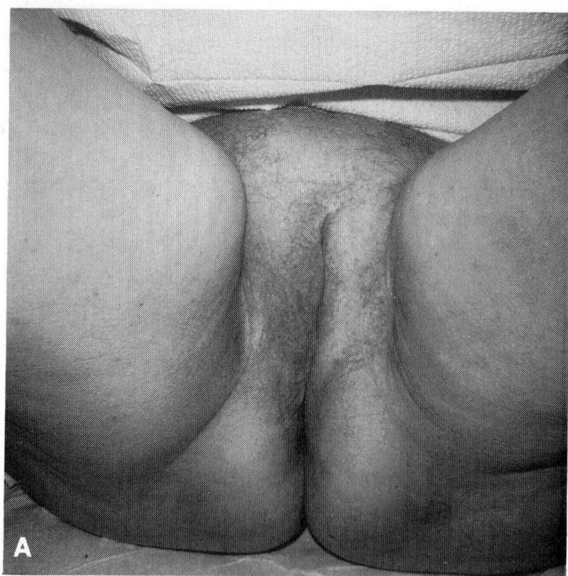

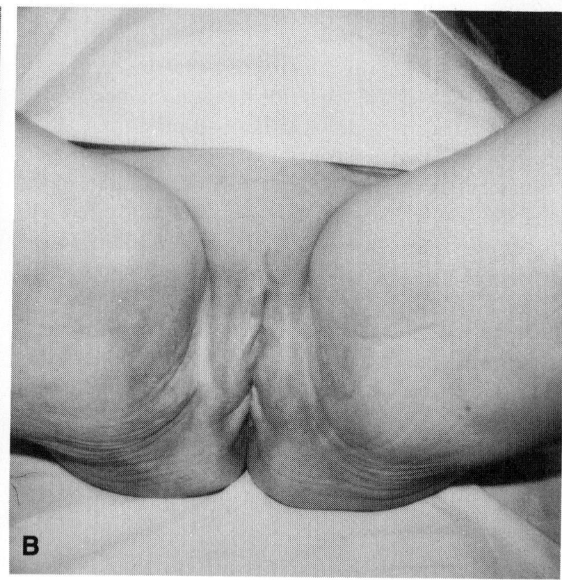

FIGURE 59–10. (**A** and **B**) Cosmetic results that can be achieved if appropriate surgical and irradiation techniques are applied.

TREATMENT FOR MALIGNANT MELANOMA

The current accepted management for vulva melanoma is radical vulvectomy and bilateral inguinal lymph node dissection for levels of invasion greater than Clark's 2. Superficial malignant melanoma of the vulva can be treated with wide local excision. Although some gynecologic oncologists recommend ipsilateral inguinal lymph node dissection, Chung and associates[21] found no lymph node metastasis in eight patients with level II malignant melanoma, and none of these patients died of the disease. The survival was closely related to depth of invasion, with only two of 25 patients with levels III through V melanoma surviving 5 years. The most common site of recurrence was the groin (nine), the perineum, vagina, and urethra (two cases in each location), and the cervix and rectum (one case in each location). All patients who died of melanoma had widespread metastases (to lungs, adrenals, brain, liver, kidneys, retroperitoneal lymph nodes).

Woolcott and associates[110] reported the results in 50 patients with primary carcinoma of the vulva, 42 of whom were treated with definitive therapy (16 with wide local excision, two with unilateral inguinofemoral and two with bilateral inguinofemoral lymphadenectomy, two with hemivulvectomy and inguinofemoral lymph node dissection, and one with simple vulvectomy alone). Twenty-tree patients were treated with radical vulvectomy, all but one combined with bilateral inguinofemoral lymphadenectomy. Two patients also had pelvic lymphadenectomy. Three of the 42 patients treated with curative intent received adjuvant radiation therapy. Seventeen of the 50 patients were alive and free from disease at the last follow-up. The 5-year survival rate for 32 eligible patients was 43.8%. Eighty percent (12 of 15) of patients treated with wide local excision were alive at 2 years, and 50% (five of ten) were alive at 5 years. Seventy-four percent (14 of 19) of the patients treated with radical vulvectomy and bilateral inguinofemoral lymphadenectomy were alive at 2 years and 50% (seven of 14) at 5 years. Depth of melanocytic penetration was the main prognostic factor. Seven of 23 patients treated with radical vulvectomy developed local recurrence; four had inguinofemoral nodal recurrences, and eight developed distant metastases. Of the 16 patients treated with wide local excision, three developed local recurrence, four had inguinofemoral recurrences, and two had distant metastases.

CHEMOTHERAPY

Topical chemotherapy has been studied for treatment of selected patients with vulvar or vaginal intraepithelial neoplasia; 5-fluorouracil (5-FU) has been the most commonly used agent.[33,95,96] Often, three 7-day courses of 5% 5-FU cream are given 2 weeks apart. A study of 25 patients treated in this manner demonstrated that although three patients required retreatment of 3, 9, and 11 months, all 25 evaluable patients were free from disease for more than 3 to 40 months after treatment.[17]

Levin and co-workers[69] have used preoperative chemotherapy (mitomycin-C and 5-FU) followed by pelvic irradiation before surgery for advanced carcinoma of the vulva. They observed marked local tumor shrinkage in six patients, which allowed more definitive surgery following the chemotherapy. Iversen[54] treated 15 patients with inoperable vulvar carcinoma with a combination of irradiation (3600 cGy to 4000 cGy) and bleomycin (30 mg every 2 days) for total doses of 90 mg to 180 mg. Only two patients had complete tumor regression and survived 2.5 and 4 years. Recurrences in 11 of the 15 patients developed a few weeks after completion of therapy.

Thomas and associates[103] described the results in 33 patients with vulvar cancer treated with a combination of chemotherapy (5-FU or mitomycin-C or both). Thirty-two patients had squamous cell carcinoma and one adenocarcinoma. Of the 18 patients with primary disease, nine were treated in an adjuvant setting (five after radical vulvectomy and inguinal node dissection, four had local excision only). Several patients had positive surgical margins. Six of the nine patients received vulva irradiation (4000 cGy to 6400 cGy) in daily fractions of 160 cGy to 180 cGy. Five of the six patients in addition received inguinal lymph node irradiation. Three of the nine patients were treated to inguinal nodes only. Six of the nine patients remain disease-free at 5 to 45 months. Two patients developed bony metastases without locoregional recurrence. One patient of the three not irradiated to the vulva had a relapse in this site. Nine other patients with primary disease received chemotherapy and irradiation as definitive management. Five of the nine patients had clinically suspicious inguinal lymph nodes. All nine patients received irradiation to the vulva, and four of the five with positive nodes also were treated to the inguinal areas. Six of the nine patients are disease-free with follow-up of 5 to 43 months. Six of the nine had an initial complete response of the vulva tumor, although three subsequently had relapses in the vulva. In the six patients with residual or recurrent vulvar carcinoma after initial chemotherapy/irradiation, five had salvage surgery (local excision in four and radical vulvectomy in one). Seven of the nine patients had vulva primary tumor control after salvage therapy. No patients developed nodal or distant metastases.

Fifteen patients were treated for recurrence after initial surgery. Ten had a previous radical vulvectomy and bilateral node dissection. Seven of these patients remain alive without disease for intervals of 5 to 45 months. Three patients treated for inguinal node recurrence never had a complete response, and all died of disease, two also having developed lung metastases. Six of the 11 patients treated for recurrence in the vulva only are alive without disease. In this group, chemotherapy and irradiation produced a complete response in eight of 15 treated patients. Four of the patients who died developed pulmonary metastases. Combined therapy was well tolerated, except for the expected oropharyngeal mucitis and hematologic toxicity of 5-FU and chemotherapy. One patient developed severe proctitis after receiving 5500 cGy in 35 fractions with electrons to the vulva. One patient developed a vascular hip necrosis following a dose of 4700 cGy in 27 fractions. These preliminary results certainly are extremely promising and suggest that patients in high-risk groups for carcinoma of the vulva may be treated effectively with combinations of surgery (ranging from wide local excision to more extensive procedures), irradiation, and systemic chemotherapy. Further assessment of long-term results is in progress.

REFERENCES

1. Acosta AA, Given FT, Frazier AB, et al: Preoperative radiation therapy in the management of squamous cell carcinoma of the vulva: Preliminary report. Am J Obstet Gynecol 132:198–205, 1978
2. Anderson ES, Sorenson IM: Verrucous carcinoma of the female genital tract: Report of a case and review of the literature. Gynecol Oncol 30:427–434, 1988
3. Backstrom A, Edsmyr F, Wicklund H: Radiotherapy of carcinoma of the vulva. Acta Obstet Gynecol Scand 51:109–115, 1972
4. Baltzer JE, Kurzl RY, Lohe KJ, Zander J: Melanoma of the vulva. J Reprod Med 31:825–827, 1986
5. Barnhill DR, Boling R, Nobles W, et al: Vulvar dermatofibrosarcoma protuberans. Gynecol Oncol 30:149–152, 1988
6. Benda JA, Platz CE, Anderson B: Malignant melanoma of the vulva: A clinical-pathologic review of 16 cases. Int J Gynecol Pathol 5:202–216, 1986
7. Benedet JL, Turko M, Fairey RN, et al: Squamous carcinoma of the vulva: Results of treatment, 1938 to 1976. Am J Obstet Gynecol 134:201, 1979
8. Bornstein J, Kaufman RH, Adam E, et al: Multicentric intraepithelial neoplasia involving the vulva: Clinical features and association with human papillomavirus and herpes simplex virus. Cancer 62:1601–1604, 1988
9. Boronow RC: Therapeutic alternative to primary exenteration for advanced vulvovaginal cancer. Gynecol Oncol 1:233, 1973
10. Boronow RC: Combined therapy as an alternative to exenteration for locally advanced vulvo-vaginal cancer: Rationale and results. Cancer 49:1085–1091, 1982
11. Boronow RC, Hickman BT, Regan MT, et al: Combined therapy as an alternative to exenteration for locally advanced vulvovaginal cancer. II Results, complications, and dosimetric and surgical consideration. Am J Clin Oncol (CCT) 10(2):171–181, 1987
12. Boutselis JG: Radical vulvectomy for invasive squamous cell carcinoma of the vulva. Obstet Gynecol 39:827, 1972
13. Brand E, Fu YS, Lagasse Ld, Berek JS: Vulvovaginal melanoma: Report of seven cases and literature review. Gynecol Oncol 33:54–60, 1989
14. Breen JL, Neubecker Rd, Greenwald E, et al: Basal cell carcinomas of the vulva. Obstet Gynecol 46:122, 1975
15. Buechler DA, Kline JC, Tynes JC, et al: Treatment of recurrent carcinoma of the vulva. Gynecol Oncol 8:180–184, 1979
16. Buscema J, Woodruff JD, Parmley TH, et al: Carcinoma *in situ* of the vulva. Obstet Gynecol 55:225, 1980
17. Calgar H, Hertzog AW, Hreschyshyn MM: Topical 5-fluorouracil treatment of vaginal intraepithelial neoplasia. Obstet Gynecol 5:580, 1981
18. Carlino G, Parisi S, Montemaggi P, et al: Interstitial radiotherapy with ^{192}Ir in vulvar cancer. Eur J Gynaecol Oncol 3:183–185, 1984
19. Carson LF, Twiggs LB, Okagaki T, et al: Human papillomavirus DNA in adenosquamous carcinoma and squamous cell carcinoma of the vulva. Obstet Gynecol 72:63–67, 1988
20. Chafe W, Richards A, Morgan L, et al: Unrecognized invasive carcinoma in vulvar intraepithelial neoplasia (VIN). Gynecol Oncol 31:154–162, 1988
21. Chung AF, Woodruff JM, Lewwis JL Jr: Malignant melanoma of the vulva. Obstet Gynecol 45:638, 1975
22. Collins CG, Lee FYL, Lopez JJ: Invasive carcinoma of the vulva with lymph node matastases. Am J Obstet Gynecol 109:446, 1971
23. Collins CG, Ramon-Lopez JJ, Lee FYL: Intraepithelial carcinoma of the vulva. Am J Obstet Gynecol 108:1187, 1987
24. Curry SL, Wharton JT, Rutledge F: Positive lymph nodes in vulvar squamous carcinoma. Gynecol Oncol 9:63, 1980
25. Daly JW, Million RR: Radical vulvectomy combined with elective node irradiation for TxN0 squamous carcinoma of the vulva. Cancer 34:161, 1974
26. Dehner LP: Metastatic and secondary tumors of the vulva. Obstet Gynecol 52:47–57, 1973
27. DiSaia PJ, Creasman WT, Rich WM: An alternative approach to early cancer of the vulva, Am J Obstet Gynecol 133:825–832, 1979
28. Donaldson ES, Powell DE, Hanson MB, et al: Prognostic parameters in invasive vulvar cancer. Gynecol Oncol 11:184–190, 1981
29. Downey GO, Okagaki T, Ostrow RS, et al: Condylomatous carcinoma of the vulva with special reference to human papillomavirus DNA. Obstet Gynecol 72:68–73, 1988
30. Ellis F: Cancer of the vulva treated by radiation. Br J Radiol 22:513, 1949
31. Fairey UN. Mackay PO, Benedet JL, et al: Radiation treatment of carcinoma of the vulva, 1950–1980. Am J Obstet Gynecol 151:591–597, 1985
32. Fiorica JV, Cavanagh D, Marsden DE, et al: Carcinoma *in situ* of the vulva: 24 years' experience in Southwest Florida. South Med J 81:589–593, 1988
33. Foster DC, Woodruff JD: The use of dinitrochlorobenzene in the treatment of vulvar carcinoma *in situ*. Gynecol Oncol 11:330, 1981
34. Frankendal B, Larsson LG, Westling P: Carcinoma of the vulva. Acta Radiol (Stockh) 12:165, 1973
35. Franklin EW: Clinical staging of carcinoma of the vulva. Obstet Gynecol 40:277, 1972
36. Franklin EW, Rutledge FD: Epidemiology of epidermoid carcinoma of the vulva. Obstet Gynecol 39:165, 1972
37. Franklin EW, Rutledge FD: Prognostic factors in epidermoid carcinoma of the vulva. Obstet Gynecol 39:892, 1971

38. Friedrich EG Jr, Wilkinson EJ: The vulva. In Blaustein A (ed): Pathology of the Female Genital Tract, pp 13–58. New York, Springer-Verlag, 1977
39. Friedrich EG Jr, Wilkinson EJ, Fu YS: Carcinoma *in situ* of the vulva: A continuing challenge. Am J Obstet Gynecol 136:880, 1980
40. Frischbier HJ, Thomsen K: Treatment of cancer of the vulva with high-energy electrons. Am J Obstet Gynecol 111:431–435, 1971
41. Gosling JRG, Abell MR, Drolette BM, et al: Infiltrative squamous cell carcinoma of the vulva. Cancer 14:330, 1961
42. Green TH: Carcinoma of the vulva: A reassessment. Obstet Gynecol 52:462, 1978
43. Gupta J, Pilotti S, Rilke F, Shah K: Association of human papillomavirus Type 16 with neoplastic lesions of the vulva and other genital sites by *in situ* hybridization. Am J Pathol 127:206–215, 1987
44. Hacker NF: Current treatment of small vulvar cancers. Oncology 4(8):21–25, 1990
45. Hacker NF, Berek JS, Juillard GJF, Lagasse LD: Preoperative radiation therapy for locally advanced vulvar cancer. Cancer 54:2056, 1984
46. Hacker NF, Berek JS, Lagasse L, et al: Management of regional lymph nodes and their prognostic influence in vulvar cancer. Obstet Gynecol 61:408–412, 1983
47. Helgason NM, Hass AC, Latourette HB: Radiation therapy in carcinoma of the vulva. Cancer 30:997, 1972
48. Helwig EB, Graham JH: Anogenital (extramammary) Paget's disease. Cancer 16:387, 1963
49. Hoffman MS, Roberts WS, Ruffolo EH: Basal cell carcinoma of the vulva with inguinal lymph node metastases. Gynecol Oncol 29:113–119, 1988
50. Homesley HD, Bundy BN, Sedlis A, Adcock L: Radiation therapy versus pelvic node resection for carcinoma of the vulva with positive groin nodes. Obstet Gynecol 68:733–740, 1986
51. Homesley HD, Sedlis A: Surgical-pathological study of women with squamous cell carcinoma of the vulva (Abstract). Soc Gynecol Oncol 17(2):259, 1984
52. Hoskins W, Perez CA: Gynecologic Tumors. In Devita VT, Hellman S, Rosenberg SA (eds): Cancer: Principles and Practice of Oncology, 3rd ed. Philadelphia, JB Lippincott, 1989
53. Husseinzadeh N, Newman NJ, Wesseler TA: Vulvar intraepithelial neoplasia: A clinicopathological study of carcinoma *in situ* of the vulva. Gynecol Oncol 33:157–163, 1989
54. Iversen T: Irradiation and bleomycin in the treatment of inoperable vulval carcinoma. Acta Obstet Gynecol Scand 61:195–197, 1982
55. Iversen T, Aalders JG, Christensen A, et al: Squamous cell carcinoma of the vulva: A review of 424 patients, 1956–1974. Gynecol Oncol 9:271, 1980
56. Japaze H, Garcia-Buneul R, Woodruff JD: Primary vulvar neoplasia. Obstet Gynecol 49:404, 1977
57. Johnson J: Radiation treatment of vulvar cancer. Geriatrics 19:447–452, 1964
58. Josey WE, Nahmais AJ, Naib ZM: Viruses and cancer of the lower genital tract. Cancer 38:526, 1976
59. Kaufman RH, Bornstein J, Adam E, et al: Human papillomavirus and herpes simplex virus in vulvar squamous cell carcinoma in situ. Am J Obstet Gynecol 158:862–869, 1988
60. Kaufman RH, Gardner HL: Intraepithelial carcinoma of the vulva. Clin Obstet Gynecol 8:1035, 1965
61. Krupp PJ, Bohm JW: Lymph gland metastases in invasive squamous cell cancer of the vulva. Am J Obstet Gynecol 130:943, 1978
62. Krupp PJ, Lee FYL, Bohm JW, et al: Prognostic parameters and clinical staging criteria in epidermoid carcinoma of the vulva. Obstet Gynecol 46:84–88, 1975
63. Kucera H, Weghaupt K: The electrosurgical operation of vulvar carcinoma with postoperative irradiation of inguinal lymph nodes. Gynecol Oncol 29:158–167, 1988
64. Kuipers T: Carcinoma of the vulva. Radiol Clin 44:475–483, 1975
65. Kunschner A, Kanbour AI, David B: Early vulvar carcinoma. Am J Obstet Gynecol 132:599, 1978
66. Kurzl R, Messerer D: Prognostic factors in squamous cell carcinoma of the vulva: A multivariate analysis. Gynecol Oncol 32:143–50, 1989
67. Lasser A, Cornorg LJT, Morris JM: Adenoid squamous carcinoma of the vulva. Cancer 33:224, 1974
68. Leuchter RS, Hacker NF, Vopet RL, et al: Primary carcinoma of the Bartholin gland: A report of 14 cases and review of the literature. Obstet Gynecol 60:361–368, 1982
69. Levin W, Rad FF, Goldberg G, et al: The use of concomitant chemotherapy and radiotherapy prior to surgery in advanced stage carcinoma of the vulva. Gynecol Oncol 25:20, 1986
70. Lucas WE, Bernischke K, Lebherz TB: Verrucous carcinoma of the female genital tract. Am J Obstet Gynecol 119:435, 1974
71. Mabuchi K, Bross DS, Kessler II: Epidemiology of cancer of the vulva. Cancer 55:1843–1848, 1985
72. Mack T, Casagrande JT: Epidemiology of gynecologic cancer. II Endometrium, ovary, vagina, vulva. In Coppleson M (ed): Gynecologic Oncology: Fundamental Principles and Clinical Practice, pp 28–30. New York, Churchill Livingstone, 1981
73. Magrina JF, Webb MJ, Gaffey TA, et al: Stage I squamous cell cancer of the vulva. Am J Obstet Gynecol 134:453, 1975
74. Malfetano JH, Piver S, Tsukada Y, Reese P: Univariate and multivariate analyses of 5-year survival recurrence, and inguinal node metastases in stage I and II vulvar carcinoma. J Surg Oncol 30:124–131, 1985
75. Miyazawa K, Nori D, Hilaris BS, Lewis JL: Role of radiation therapy in the treatment of advanced vulvar carcinoma. J Reprod Med 28:539–541, 1983
76. Morley GW: Infiltrative carcinoma of the vulva: Results of surgical treatment. Am J Obstet Gynecol 124:874, 1976
77. Nobler MP: Efficacy of a perineal teletherapy portal in the management of vulvar and vaginal cancer. Radiology 103:393, 1972
78. Nori D, Cain JM, Hilaris BS, et al: Metronidazole as a radiosensitizer and high-dose radiation in advanced vulvovaginal malignancies, a pilot study. Gynecol Oncol 16:117–128, 1983
79. Oberhauser F: Treatment of cancer of the vulva using electrons. Front Radiat Ther Oncol 2:248, 1968
80. Pao WM, Perez CA, Kuske RR, et al: Radiation therapy and conservation surgery for primary and recurrent carcinoma of the vulva: Report of 40 patients and a review of the literature. Int J Radiat Oncol Biol Phys 14:1123–1132, 1988
81. Parker RT, Duncan I, Rampone J, et al: Operative management of early invasive epidermoid carcinoma of the vulva. Am J Obstet Gynecol 123:349, 1975
82. Perrone T, Twiggs LB, Adcock LL, Dehner LP: Vulvar basal cell carcinoma: An infrequently metastasizing neoplasm. Int J Gynecol Pathol 6:152–165, 1987
83. Pirtoli L, Rottoli ML: Results of radiation therapy for vulvar carcinoma. Acta Radiol Oncol 21:45, 1982
84. Plentl AA, Friedman EA: Lymphatic System of the Female Genitalia. Philadelphia, WB Saunders, 1971
85. Podratz KC, Symmonds RE, Taylor WF, et al: Carcinoma of the vulva: Analysis of treatment and survival. Obstet Gynecol 61:63–74, 1983
86. Prempree T, Amormarn R: Radiation treatment of recurrent carcinoma of the vulva. Cancer 54:1943, 1984
87. Rosenberg P, Simonses E, Risberg D: Adenoid cystic carcinoma of Bartholin's gland: A report of five new cases treated with surgery and radiotherapy. Gynecol Oncol 34:145–147, 1989
88. Rowley KC, Gallion HH, Donaldson ES, et al: Prognostic factors in early vulvar cancer. Gynecol Oncol 31:43–49, 1988
89. Rutledge F, Smith JP, Franklin EW: Carcinoma of the vulva. Am J Obstet Gynecol 106:1117 1970
90. Schultz U, Callies R, Kruger KG: Effizienz der postoperativen electronentherapie des lekalisierten vulvarkarzinoms. Strahlentherapie 156:326, 1980
91. Sedlis A, Homesley H, Bundy BN, et al: Positive groin lymph nodes in superficial squamous cell vulvar cancer. Am J Obstet Gynecol 156:1159–1164, 1987

92. Shepherd JH: Revised FIGO staging for gynecological cancer. Br J Obstet Gynaecol 96:889–892, 1989
93. Shimm DS, Fuller AF, Orlow EL, et al: Prognostic variables in the treatment of squamous cell carcinoma of the vulva. Gynecol Oncol 24:343–358, 1986
94. Shingleton HM, Fowler WC, Palumbo L, et al: Carcinoma of the vulva. Obstet Gynecol 35:1, 1970
95. Sillman FH, Boyce JG, Macasaet MA, Nicastri AD: 5-Fluorouracil/chemosurgery for intraepithelial neoplasia of the lower genital tract. Obstet Gynecol 58:356, 1981
96. Sillman FH, Sedlis A, Boyce JG: A review of lower genital intraepithelial neoplasia and the use of topical 5-fluorouracil. Obstet Gynecol Surg 40:190, 1985
97. Simonsen E: Treatment of recurrent squamous cell carcinoma of the vulva. Acta Radiol Oncol 23:345–348, 1984
98. Simonsen E, Nordberg UB, Johnsson JE, et al: Radiation therapy and surgery in the treatment of regional lymph nodes in squamous cell carcinoma of the vulva. Acta Radiol Oncol 23:433, 1984
99. Stern BD, Kaplan L: Multicentric foci of carcinoma arising in structures of cloacal origin. Am J Obstet Gynecol 104:255, 1969
100. Stoeckel W: Zur Therapie des Vulvacarzinoms. Z Gynaekol 54:47, 1930
101. Tafari K, Magalotti M: Radiation therapy in carcinoma of the vulva. Cancer 47:686–691, 1981
102. Tavassoli FA, Norris HJ: Smooth muscle tumors of the vulva. Obstet Gynecol 53:213, 1979
103. Thomas G, Dembo A, DePetrillo A, et al: Concurrent radiation and chemotherapy in vulvar carcinoma. Gynecol Oncol 34:263–267, 1989
104. Tod MC: Radium implantation treatment of carcinoma vulva. Br J Radiol 22:508, 1949
105. Ulbright TM, Brokaw SA, Stehman FB, Roth LM: Epitheloid sarcoma of the vulva. Cancer 52:1462–1469, 1983
106. Way S: Carcinoma of the vulva. Am J Obstet Gynecol 79:692, 1960
107. Weghaupt K: Die eletrokoagulation als therapie des vulvakarzinom's methode and ergebnisse. Strahlentherapie 154:89–93, 1978
108. Weiner SA, Lee JKT, Kao MS, Moon TE: The role of lymphangiography in vulvar carcinoma. Am J Obstet Gynecol 5:1073–1075, 1986
109. Wharton JT, Gallagher S, Rutledge FN: Microinvasive carcinoma of the vulva. Am J Obstet Gynecol 118:159, 1974
110. Woolcott RJ, Henry RJW, Houghton CRS: Malignant melanoma of the vulva. J Reprod Med 33:699–702, 1988

60

○ ○ ○ • • •

Retroperitoneum

William J. Pao
Todd H. Wasserman

Primary retroperitoneal neoplasms continue to pose a major challenge to most oncologists. Data regarding these neoplasms are difficult to collect and interpret because of the tumor's diversity and uncommon occurrence. This chapter contains a discussion of tumors arising primarily from tissues in the retroperitoneal area; it does not discuss primary neoplasms arising from organs that are partially or completely retroperitoneal (*e.g.*, pancreas, kidneys, and adrenal glands).

ANATOMY

The retroperitoneum, or retroperitoneal space, is a potential space bounded anteriorly by the parietal peritoneum. Morgagni, in 1761, is credited with first describing a retroperitoneal tumor, but the term was not coined until 1829 by Lobstein. The anatomic definition has been elucidated by Donnelly,[20] Melicow,[61] and Ackerman.[02]

The retroperitoneum is that region of the trunk covered anteriorly by the parietal peritoneum. Superiorly, it is bounded by the twelfth rib and the diaphragm. The pelvic diaphragm, with the fascia of the levator ani and coccygeus muscles, forms the inferior boundary. Posteriorly, the retroperitoneum is bounded by the fascia of the muscles of the abdominal wall (Fig. 60-1). Because of the rigidity of the posterior, cephalad, and caudad boundaries, the most common route of expansion and invasion for most retroperitoneal tumors is anteriorly into the abdominal cavity.

Many vital structures are confined within the retroperitoneum, including the aorta, inferior vena cava, lumbar nerves, adrenal glands, kidneys, and ureters. The potential space itself contains loose connective tissue and is abundant in the lymphatics and paraaortic and pararenal lymph nodes. The liver, spinal cord, stomach, and intestine are in close proximity.

EPIDEMIOLOGY

Most authors attest to the rarity of primary retroperitoneal tumors. Although the incidence has been reported to be as high as 3% of all tumors,[6] this figure represents a less restrictive definition (including tumors arising from kidneys, pancreas, and other retroperitoneal organs). True primary retroperitoneal tumors represent less than 0.1% of all malignant neoplasms.[8] The incidence in two population studies was three per million.[4,8] A review of the patients reported in several large series (622 patients) shows two peak periods: one during the first decade and the other during the sixth decade.[4,6,8,18,31,34,41,60,67–69,71,91] Most infants and children develop germ cell tumors, whereas adults develop mesenchymal neoplasms such as lipomas and sarcomas in the retroperitoneal region.

NATURAL HISTORY

Most retroperitoneal tumors develop silently and tend to expand into the loose connective tissue in the potential space. The malignant tumors invade the abundant blood supply and lymphatics. The ureters are frequently involved early and with a high incidence (60% to 75%).[9,93] Most retroperitoneal tumors grow anteriorly, where there is least resistance; invasion into the posterior abdominal wall is seldom reported. The histology of the retroperitoneal tumor tends to predict the mode of invasion. Benign soft tissue and well-differentiated sarcomas (myxoid liposarcomas) tend to grow in an expansile manner. High-grade sarcomas, germ cell neoplasms, and lymphomas often invade and surround the aorta and its main tributaries and the vena cava. Small round cell tumors (neuroblastomas and rhabdomyosarcomas) can invade into the intervertebral foramina to become so-called dumbbell-shaped tumors. In several series[71,13] the incidence of adjacent organ involvement has been reported to be 60% to 70%. Hematogenous metastases at presentation are uncommon, occurring in less than 5% of patients.[70] They occur more frequently in patients with small round cell tumors, lymphomas, and high-grade sarcomas.

Because surgery has been the traditional mode of diagnosis and treatment for retroperitoneal tumors, the natural history after resection is of interest to most radiation therapists. For reasons not yet elucidated, benign-appearing tumors, especially sarcomas with low mitotic rates and no anaplasia, can recur locally and even metastasize. Azumi and associates[5] reported that 67% of 21 patients with atypical lipomatous lesions had recurrences. Shmookler and associates[82] reported that in their series of 36 leiomyosarcomas, a low mitotic rate did not predict a low recurrence rate (overall 80%). Because of the high rate of local and distant failure of retroperitoneal mesenchymal neoplasms, the clinician should scrutinize available data regarding further therapy.

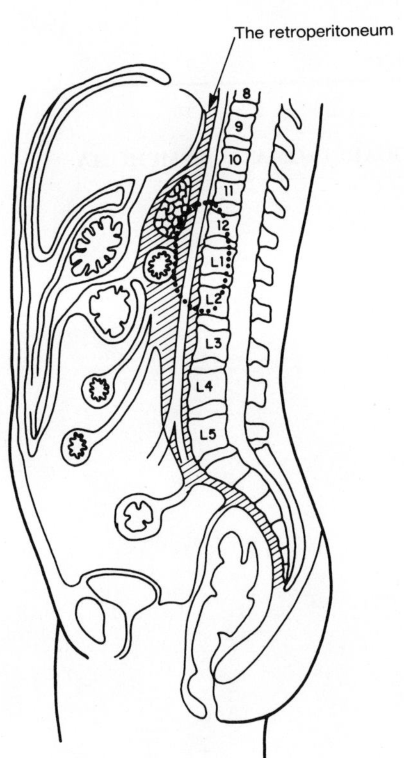

FIGURE 60–1. Sagittal view of trunk, showing the retroperitoneal space (*shaded area*). The kidney is outlined by dots.

CLINICAL PRESENTATION

Most large series of patients with retroperitoneal tumors were reported in the pre-computed tomography (CT) era. Patients presented with complaints of abdominal pain or mass in 60% to 90% of most large series. Fifty percent of patients have weight loss and loss of appetite at diagnosis.[8,9,19,39,42,70,93] The duration of symptoms ranges from 2 to 36 months; the median is usually 4 to 6 months. Patients with sarcomas tend to seek medical treatment at a later stage, whereas germ cell tumor and lymphoma patients become ill more acutely. The etiology of symptoms has been discussed by Melicow in great detail.[61] Upper retroperitoneal lesions can produce pleuritic or diaphragmatic pain radiating to the shoulder, epigastric distress, early satiety, and nausea and vomiting. With advanced disease, hematemesis and jaundice can occur. Midabdominal and high pelvic tumors can cause ureter obstruction, girdle or radicular pain, edema of the lower extremities, and hemorrhoids with constipation and dysuria. Most patients have nonspecific symptoms and usually do not recall or reveal problems unless specifically asked.

The most common clinical finding is an abdominal mass. A careful abdominal examination may reveal tenderness, approximate size, and fixation of the primary tumor. If hydronephrosis is present, the involved kidney may be enlarged. A rectal or pelvic examination can reveal tumors involving the presacral area and pelvic diaphragm; a large mass or vena caval involvement can cause hemorrhoids. Neurologic examination, including straight leg arising, can reveal any radicular nerve problems.

Several retroperitoneal tumors are associated with paraneoplastic syndromes. Germ cell tumors can cause precocious puberty in children, and neuroblastomas can produce opsoclonic myoclonus. Retroperitoneal liposarcomas or lipomas have been reported to produce intermittent hypoglycemia. Extraadrenal retroperitoneal paragangliomas, which can produce symptoms of catecholamine excess, generally invade locally and metastasize by way of the bloodstream.

DIAGNOSTIC WORKUP

The evaluation of a retroperitoneal tumor should focus on two aspects: the physiologic status of the patient and the extent of tumor involvement. In addition to a thorough history and physical examination, a complete blood count, SMA-6, liver function tests, alkaline phosphatase, serum creatinine, and creatinine clearance studies are needed to assess the baseline bone marrow, hepatic, and renal tolerance to therapy as well as any abdominal organ involvement (Table 60-1)

In the pre-CT era, intravenous pyelography (IVP) was the most commonly used test to evaluate retroperitoneal tumors. On retrospective review, 50% to 80% of patients exhibited abnormalities in their IVPs.[8,9,22,39,93] The most common finding was that of kidney or ureter displacement.[80] Plain films of the abdomen were abnormal in only 20% to 30% of patients. Selective angiography can localize tumor origins and guide operative resection of tumors.[29,55]

Computed tomography has changed the quality of detecting and staging retroperitoneal neoplasms. Unfortunately, data regarding the impact of this radiologic technique on the treatment of retroperitoneal tumors have been sparse. Few institutional clinicopathologic studies have been published that review experience from the mid-1970s onward. In a prospective survey from the Massachusetts General Hospital, the retroperitoneum was a site on which CT had a major impact. Angiography was avoided in 18 of 21 (86%) patients.[97] Delineation of tumor size and extent is a major asset of CT. Stephens and associates[88] reported on 19 patients with retroperitoneal tumors and accurately showed the extent of disease in 18 of 19 (95%) before their laparotomy. Pistolesi and co-workers[73] were able to correlate CT results with intraoperative findings; visceral organ involvement was identified in 22 of 38 (60%) patients. Organ invasion was correctly diagnosed in seven of eight (87.5%) patients with abnormal CT scan; normal CT scan, however, understates the incidence of pathologic involvement (ten of 15, or 66%). The ability of CT to predict histology has been more disappointing. Certain tumors show specific characteristics, such as lipomas and liposarcomas with their high fat content or neuroblastomas and sarcomas in which calcification is seen.[50,83] Cohan and colleagues[14] studied 33 patients with primary retroperitoneal tumors and 122 patients with lymphomas and found that CT could not distinguish the different cell types except for lipoid neoplasms. Patients who had heterogeneous masses tended to have sarcomas rather than lymphomas, which had a more homogeneous appearance.

Computed tomography is useful as a postoperative baseline study to monitor recurrence or late effects of treatment. In addition to diagnosis, CT has made it possible to obtain histologic and cytologic specimens by needle biopsy,[36,99] thus enabling the clinician to obtain a diagnosis without performing a laparotomy. The only relative contraindication to this procedure is in patients with a coagulation disorder.[30] The techniques have been described by Gothin and MacIntosh[30] and Mueller and associates[65] and are a modification of the fluoroscopy technique.

The advent of magnetic resonance imaging (MRI) provides another potential modality for the study of retroperitoneal

TABLE 60–1
Diagnostic Evaluation of Retroperitoneal Tumors by Tumor Histology

TEST	SARCOMA	GERM CELL TUMOR	ADENOCARCINOMA	LYMPHOMA
LABORATORY				
Liver function tests	++	++	++	++
Calcitonin	–	–	+	–
Prostatic acid phosphatase	–	–	+	–
β-HCG	–	++	–	–
α-Fetoprotein	–	++	–	–
CEA, Ca-125	–	–	+	–
Antigen cell surface markers	–	–	–	++
RADIOLOGY				
Chest radiograph	++	++	++	++
CT of chest, abdomen, and pelvis	++	++	++	++
Upper GI, small bowel series, barium enema	+	–	++	++
Angiogram	+	–	–	–
Lymphangiogram	–	+	–	+
IVP (if CT done)	–	–	–	–
IVP (if CT not done)	++	+	+	++
Renal scan	++	–	–	++
Testicular/pelvic ultrasonography	–	++	–	–
Bone scan	++	+	+	+

IVP: intravenous pyelography
–: Not applicable
+: Useful if clinically indicated
++: Highly suggested

tumors. A recent council report from the American Medical Association did not yet define its use in the retroperitoneum but noted that different scan sequences have been reported to distinguish histopathology in select cases[16]; in addition, the ability to construct images in any plane can aid in the evaluation of tumor extent. Earlier reports[36] stated that CT and MRI were equal in tumor delineation in soft tissue tumors. More recently, however, a study by Chang and co-workers[12] from the National Cancer Institute (NCI) showed that MRI was significantly better than CT at delineating tumor from muscle in sarcomas using T2-weighted spin echo and inversion recovery sequences in a study of 20 patients.

STAGING

Staging for retroperitoneal tumors is based on their histology. Therefore, sarcomas should be staged according to the American Joint Committee (AJC) system (1983, 1988; Chap. 67). Most pediatric neoplasms are staged by the national cooperative group systems (Intergroup Rhabdomyosarcoma Study, National Wilm's Tumor Study, and others). Germ cell tumors are staged in their urologic staging systems or AJC system. Other features that should be recorded, regardless of "stage" should be size (in two or three dimensions), location, extent, organ invasion, and lymphatic and hematogenous metastases. Although CT and MRI are currently used for staging, the role of surgery needs to be defined and reported to make various series comparable.

PATHOLOGIC CLASSIFICATION

Retroperitoneal neoplasms are extremely diverse in histopathology (Table 60-2) because of the embryologic origin of the region in which the mesoderm, urogenital ridge, and neurocrest develop.[32] Less than 25% of tumors are benign; the most common benign tumors are epithelial cysts and lipomas. As previously mentioned, many so-called benign neoplasms can recur locally if not completely excised. For example, a lipoma can recur as a liposarcoma many years later.[24,72]

Among tumors in adults, mesenchymal neoplasms predominate. Lipomas and liposarcomas are the most common histopathologic subtype. They constitute 25% to 50% of most reported studies,[33,45,59,89,91,96] most are low grade and can recur if not excised with a wide margin. Most patients who develop distant metastases have local recurrence; in the series by Kinne and associates[45] all 19 patients who had metastatic liposarcoma had local failure. Leiomyosarcomas are the next most common subtype, accounting for 10% to 50%. They behave in an aggressive manner. In the series by Hashimoto and colleagues,[34] 35 of 44 (80%) patients died of tumor; median survival was 20

TABLE 60–2
Relative Incidence of Retroperitoneal Tumors

BENIGN TUMORS (N = 198)	PERCENTAGE OF TOTAL	MALIGNANT TUMORS (N = 1080)	PERCENTAGE OF TOTAL
		Lymphoma	27.1
Lipoma	18.4	Liposarcoma	18.2
Pheochromocytoma	12.2	Fibrosarcoma	10.9
Leiomyoma	5.9	Rhabdomyosarcoma	3.7
Fibroma	3.3	Leiomyosarcoma	8.3
		Malignant fibrous histiocytoma	0.3
Hemangioma	1.3	Hemangiosarcoma	0.8
Lymphangioma	1.8	Lymphangiosarcoma	0
		Unclassified sarcoma	5.9
Myxoma	1.8	Myxosarcoma	0.7
		Mesodermal sarcoma	1.7
Neurilemoma	3.8		
Neurofibroma	4.3	Schwannoma	1.3
Ganglioneuroma	9.3	Neurofibrosarcoma	0.8
Paraganglioma	1.8	Neuroblastoma	8.2
Adenoma	1.8	Paraganglioma	0.2
		Carcinoma	2.9
Teratoma	5.8	Teratocarcinoma	1.5
		Unclassified tumor	4.4
		Metastatic tumor	2.9
Cyst	28.5		

Data from references 2, 4, 6, 8, 9, 10, 19, 20, 22, 32, 39, 42, 61, 68, 69, 70, 71, 93

months. In most histopathologic subtypes, grade is an important prognostic factor.[13,91]

In children, the most common retroperitoneal sarcoma is rhabdomyosarcoma.[17,68] Eighteen percent of patients with rhabdomyosarcoma presented with neurologic deficits from central or peripheral nervous system involvement, and 37% had distant metastases at diagnosis. Nonetheless, 40% of the patients were surviving at 3 years, attesting to the efficacy of chemotherapy and irradiation in that disease. Paragangliomas or glomus tumors rarely occur in the retroperitoneum and occasionally metastasize; they require radiation therapy if not totally excised.[48,62]

Lymphomas are the next most common tumors arising in the retroperitoneum. In children, approximately 30% have primary abdominal presentations, especially those with American Burkitt's histology.[66] Retroperitoneal presentations for lymphomas in adults are less common. The management of lymphomas is discussed elsewhere in this book.

Primary germ cell tumors of the retroperitoneum theoretically arise from the embryonic urogenital ridge. Before a definite diagnosis is reached, however, a thorough examination of the genitalia is necessary. A collection of six small series of patients shows that six of 18 (33%) patients on whom biopsy or autopsy showed malignant tumor in the testes.[7,11,56,60,63,79] The reports are probably skewed toward patients who have primary testicular tumors because routine biopsy has not been the standard of evaluation in most primary extragonadal germ cell tumor reports and because the incidence of testicular failure has been very low (less than 5%).[11,40,49,53] A physical and ultrasonographic examination is probably adequate for most patients.

Germ cell tumors are more common in children; in fact, sacrococcygeal teratoma is a common tumor of infancy. Most germ cell tumors in children are benign[23]; the malignant varieties include teratocarcinomas and endodermal sinus tumors. Germ cell tumors in adults are more often malignant than benign; with aggressive therapy, long-term cures are possible.[64]

Carcinomas that occur in the retroperitoneum are usually metastatic. The most common sites of adenocarcinomas are the endometrium, prostate, lung, pancreas, and gastrointestinal tract. Some authors[61,68] have hypothesized that urogenital ridge remnants can produce adenocarcinomas, but the survival is so poor that few patients live long enough for the primary tumor to appear. Squamous cell carcinomas can be interpreted as metastatic; the most common sites of origin are cervix, vagina, lung, and endometrium.

PROGNOSTIC FACTORS

The histology and invasiveness of retroperitoneal tumors are the major prognostic factors. In soft tissue sarcomas, the resectability and grade of tumor determine survival.[91,96] Liposarcomas, because of their better differentiation and encapsulation in a large number of tumors, tend to have a better prognosis than other sarcomas. Rhabdomyosarcomas, although invasive, are more sensitive to irradiation and chemotherapy and thus are also more curable. Size and grade have been correlated with prognosis in sarcomas.[91] In germ cell tumors, the major prognostic factors are the responsiveness to radiation therapy or chemotherapy, the size or bulk of the initial tumor, and the presence of distant metastases. Although resectability is not a major criterion, its use in removing residual tumor has been advocated.

GENERAL MANAGEMENT

In the past, surgical resection was the only means of achieving a cure in the majority of patients with retroperitoneal tumors. This is still true for the most part in soft tissue sarcomas in which resectability is a major prognostic factor. The resectability rate for these tumors has improved with refinements in anesthesia and surgery. The resectability rate has varied from 7% to 46% in the past[70]; most recently the NCI reported a resectability rate of 73% (35 of 48) in selected patients.[46] Nonresectability criteria have included involvement of the aorta, vena cava, iliac or superior mesenteric vessels, and spinal cord or nerve plexus, peritoneal seeding, and distant metastases.[13] Fortner and coworkers[25] advocated an *en bloc* technique that required removal of a portion or all the involved organ (diaphragm, abdominal wall, kidney, or major vessels). In their series from Memorial Hospital, 73% of the patients required resection of an adjacent organ to achieve complete resectability in 53% of their 60 patients. Resection of the psoas muscle and other *en bloc* techniques have been advocated[81,86] and are highly dependent on the technical skill of the surgeon. Whereas a perioperative mortality rate of 20% to 30% was the standard,[70] current studies report rates of 5% to 10%.[13,26,46]

Radiation therapy is usually required in most malignant retroperitoneal tumors. It is relatively contraindicated in tumors less than 5 cm, with a grossly wide (>2 cm) and pathologically negative margin of resection. The pathologic margin of these tumors is particularly difficult to evaluate in most patients. Because the tumors are large (usually more than 5 cm),[13,89] many have to removed in separate pieces. Inking of margins therefore becomes difficult when the specimen is not sent to the pathologist with suture or diagrams to mark the suspicious areas. Ideally, the radiation therapist should be present during the laparotomy to see where the clips for margins of resection are placed to guide treatment fields. A negative margin or a close margin in the pathology report should be reviewed. In the series of Cody and associates,[13] the local recurrence rate was 71% when residual disease was noted intraoperatively and 77% when complete excision was believed to have been achieved. On the other hand, the study by Wist and colleagues[96] showed that 30% of patients failed locally with complete excision, whereas 70% failed locally with partial excision or biopsy (Table 60-3).

CHEMOTHERAPY

The most active chemotherapeutic agent in adult sarcomas appears to be doxorubicin. The role of chemotherapy in rhabdomyosarcoma of childhood is well established; vincristine, doxorubicin, actinomycin D (dactinomycin), and cyclophosphamide are the most commonly used agents. Germ cell tumors are responsive to etoposide, cisplatin, and vincristine. In both germ cell tumors and rhabdomyosarcoma, chemotherapy is often the initial treatment, followed by surgery and irradiation. Intraarterial chemotherapy has also been used in selected patients.[95] When irradiation and chemotherapy are combined, their additive toxicities in different organ systems should be considered in radiation dose per fraction and total dose.

The use of single or multiagent chemotherapy after resection is controversial. Conflicting results are present in the literature. The most quoted results are those of Rosenberg and colleagues at the NCI.[76] One-hundred-eight patients were accrued in a prospective randomized study after removal of the primary tumor; some patients had postoperative irradiation. Among patients who were assigned to chemotherapy, survival was favorably affected in those with extremity tumors. However, patients with head and neck and truncal lesions (including retroperitoneal sarcomas) did not benefit; the 5-year survival rate was approximately 40 % in both arms. Since that time, several prospective randomized studies have not shown that truncal sarcomas benefit from adjuvant chemotherapy. Later trials conducted by the NCI in retroperitoneal sarcomas are discussed later.

RADIATION THERAPY TECHNIQUES

Irradiation should be started as soon as the patient is surgically healed after resection of retroperitoneal tumor, usually 2 to 4 weeks postoperatively. Treatment planning should be tailored to the individual. From a radiotherapeutic standpoint, retroperitoneal lesions can be divided according to right and left side in the epigastric and hypogastric areas and the pelvic region (see Fig. 60-1); often the tumors involve more than one of these regions.

Treatment planning is accomplished by two major steps: simulation and treatment planning CT scan. Ideally, surgical clips should be placed at the time of the operation to guide treatment portals; unfortunately this is not always the case because often patients are referred postoperatively. The inci-

TABLE 60–3
Retroperitoneal Sarcomas: Five-year Survival Correlated With Resection Status

	COMPLETE EXCISION		PARTIAL EXCISION OR BIOPSY	
AUTHOR	NO.	%	NO.	%
Cody[13]	19/47	40	2/62	3
McGrath[59]	12/18	60	2/29	8
Wist[95]	5/11	45	2/25	8
Karakousis[43]	18/27	66	11/41	27
Storm[89]	9/33	27	0/21	0
Solla[87]	3/7	43	0/13	0
Zhang[98]	20/42	48	0/20	0
Dalton[18]	35/63	55	12/53	22

sion, the presence of peritoneal seeding, and the closest margin of resection must be noted. In upper retroperitoneal tumors, fluoroscopy should be used to visualize the movement of the diaphragm. Intravenous pyelography is helpful to delineate the kidneys and the course of the ureters. Oral or rectal contrast studies are helpful to delineate the stomach and duodenum in upper lesions and the rectosigmoid in pelvic tumors. A treatment planning CT scan is usually required, especially when nearby critical structures are present. This can be obtained as a baseline study (in diagnostic radiology) postoperatively but with a flat insert instead of a round base to reproduce the position of the patient on the treatment couch; in this manner, a diagnostic and therapeutic planning study can be accomplished at the same time (Fig. 60-2). The role of MRI in treatment planning is not defined, although the ability to image in any plane is extremely useful in orthogonal-beam dosimetry.

Upper retroperitoneal lesions are the most difficult to plan and treat because the stomach, duodenum, and small bowel are in the field, and nausea and vomiting tend to be more severe. A more important problem is that the liver and kidneys are structures that limit the dose and volume that can be delivered. As previously mentioned, a renal scan is essential when one or both kidneys are to be treated to tolerance.[21] The contralateral kidney should be limited to 1800 cGy. The whole liver should not be treated to more than 3000 Gy, and half the liver should not be treated to above 3500 cGy. Adjustment should be made for dose according to the type and sequence of chemotherapy given. Depending on the volume at risk, an AP/PA approach can be used initially when less than two thirds of the liver is included in the high dose volume and when one kidney can be spared. However, most tumors require multiple fields or obliques to achieve an acceptable dose (Fig. 60-3). Lateral fields must be judiciously and cautiously used because a large volume of the liver and kidney can be overdosed or the portal may not include the entire target volume.

In centrally located tumors, in the epigastric or hypogastric regions, a three-way abdomen[27] or a four-field technique can be used. The patient can be treated in the supine position and the isocenter placed at the center of the tumor. High-energy photons (>10 MV) should be used to allow maximum normal tissue sparing. The initial AP (or PA) field is the tumor bed/volume, a 5 cm margin in the cranial-caudad and lateral directions, if feasible. Otherwise, 3 cm margins are used. If the tumor is anterior to the contralateral kidney, the lateral fields may be used to deliver the remaining tumor dose. The lateral field's superior and inferior borders are the same or slightly less than those of the AP/PA fields. The posterior margin, if not marked by a surgical clip, should bisect the vertebral bodies and conform to the curvature of the spine. Dose should be weighted equally to give optimal distribution to the target (Fig. 60-4).

Tumors involving the hypogastric region and pelvis can be treated by AP/PA or opposed oblique fields. Because most of the liver and the upper poles of the kidneys are absent from the initial field, the reduced and final fields can be accomplished

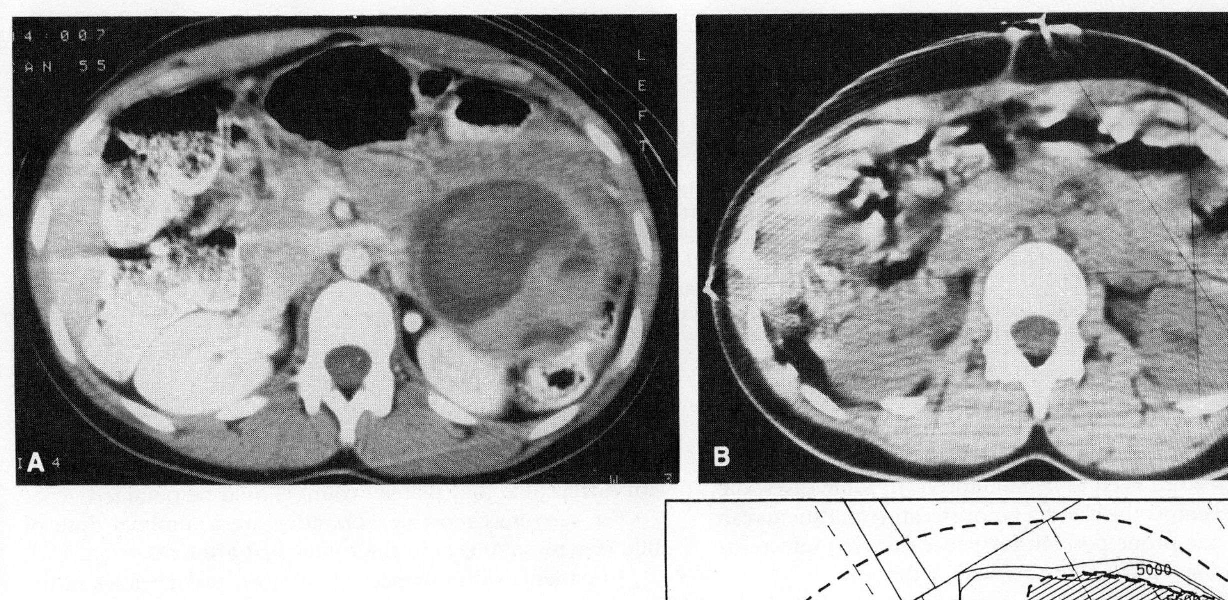

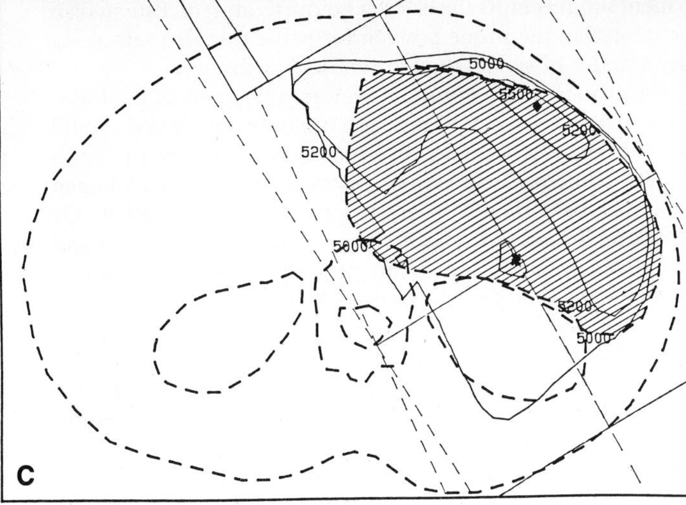

FIGURE 60–2. (**A**) A 24-year-woman with spindle cell sarcoma arising from the psoas muscle. (**B**) Postoperative treatment planning CT scan shows that displaced bowel now occupies former tumor bed. Note contrast-enhancing marks placed on the patient's skin surface denoting the cross markers for alignment lasers. (**C**) Treatment plan generated from CT scan.

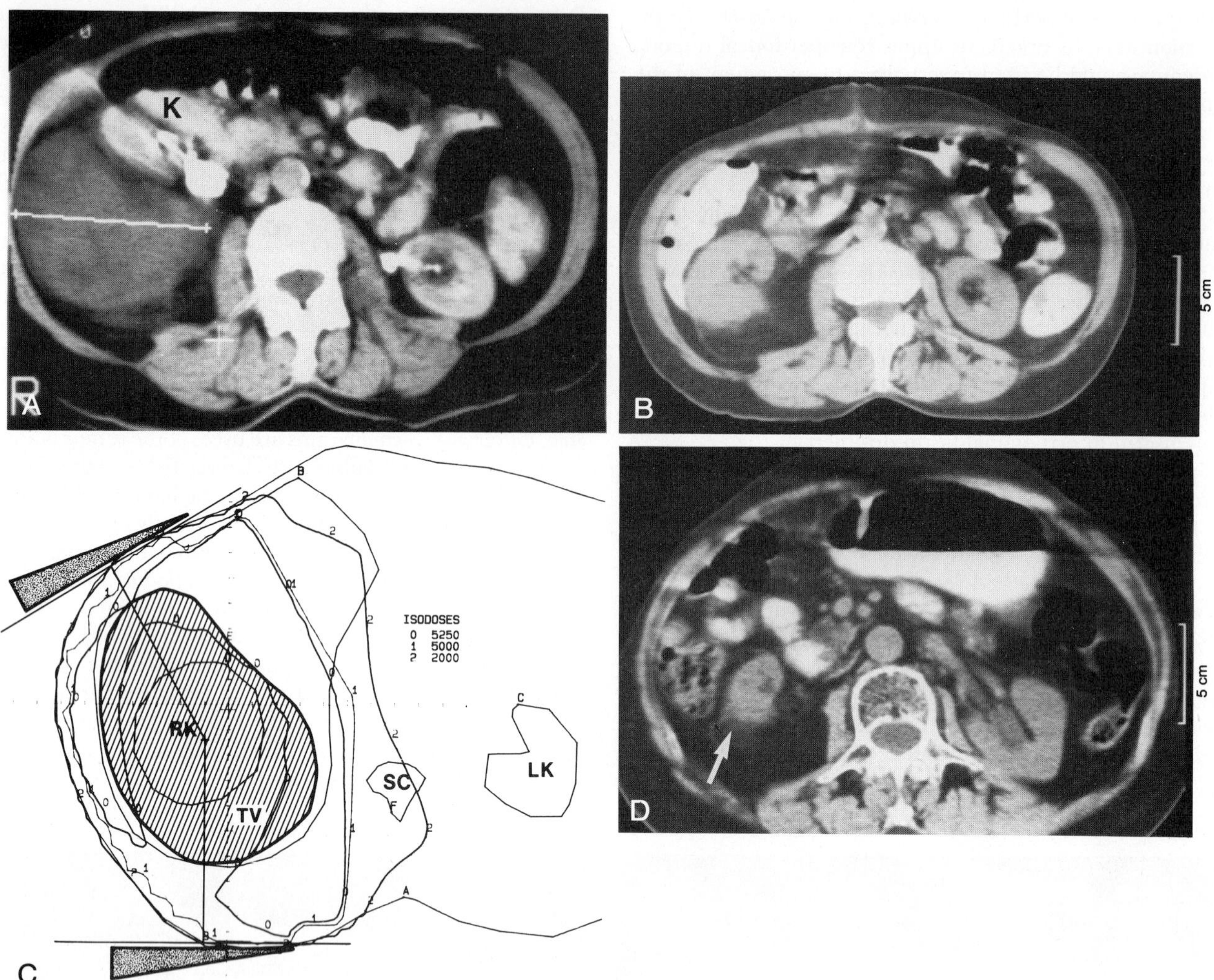

FIGURE 60–3. (**A**) A 72-year-old woman with a retroperitoneal liposarcoma displacing the right kidney (K). The tumor was grossly resected. (**B**) Postoperative CT scan shows the right kidney to be back in normal position. Renal scan showed that right kidney makes up 57% of the total renal function. (**C**) Radiation therapy using right anterior oblique and posterior fields (both with 30-degree wedges) delivered 5000 cGy to the tumor volume (TV) and included the right kidney (RK) but spared the left kidney (LK). (**D**) Follow-up CT scan obtained 27 months after completion of therapy shows no recurrence of tumor but shrinkage of right kidney (*arrow*). The patient remains disease-free.

with the same plan of therapy. The dose and volume to the bladder and rectum need to be monitored. In some cases, the patient should empty the bladder before treatment. Patients can be treated in the prone position for pelvic tumors to decrease the amount of small bowel in the field of therapy.

In patients with germ cell tumors, a large initial field with wide margins (>5 cm) around the tumor or tumor bed should be used. In cases of spillage or large (10-cm × 10-cm) tumors, a whole abdominal field may be necessary. The whole abdomen or initial field should be treated to 2500 cGy to 3000 cGy (blocking the kidneys at 1500 cGy to 1800 cGy). The tumor and lymphatic drainage, usually the paraaortics, should be treated to 4000 cGy to 4500 cGy. Gross disease should be treated to 5000 cGy with at least a 2 cm margin. The treatment of the mediastinum is somewhat controversial. If CT scan of the chest is normal, we do not recommend radiation therapy because of myelospression, which may compromise salvage chemotherapy. In general, when a large (>25-cm × 25-cm) initial field is treated, daily fractions of 180 cGy or less should be used to minimize toxicity. In addition, a weekly to twice-weekly CBC with differential and platelet count should be obtained.

For sarcomas most authors advocate a minimal dose of 5000 cGy to 5500 cGy to the tumor bed after resection.

In patients with unresectable tumors, preoperative radiation therapy may be used to decrease tumor bulk before surgery. A dose of 5000 cGy is delivered and the tumor assessed by CT scan in 4 to 6 weeks. This experience has been reproduced in other sites[51,57,90] with good results. If the lesion is unresectable after external-beam therapy, it is unlikely to be controlled by external beam alone unless the size is less than 5 cm at diagnosis.[92]

In an alternate approach used at the Massachusetts General Hospital and the NCI, intraoperative radiation therapy is used to treat grossly positive disease attached to critical structures and allow some sparing of adjacent organs.[84,85,91] Intraoperative external-beam therapy with electrons or interstitial implants has been used in a variety of intraabdominal tumors.[46,84,94] The dose of irradiation varies from 1500 cGy to

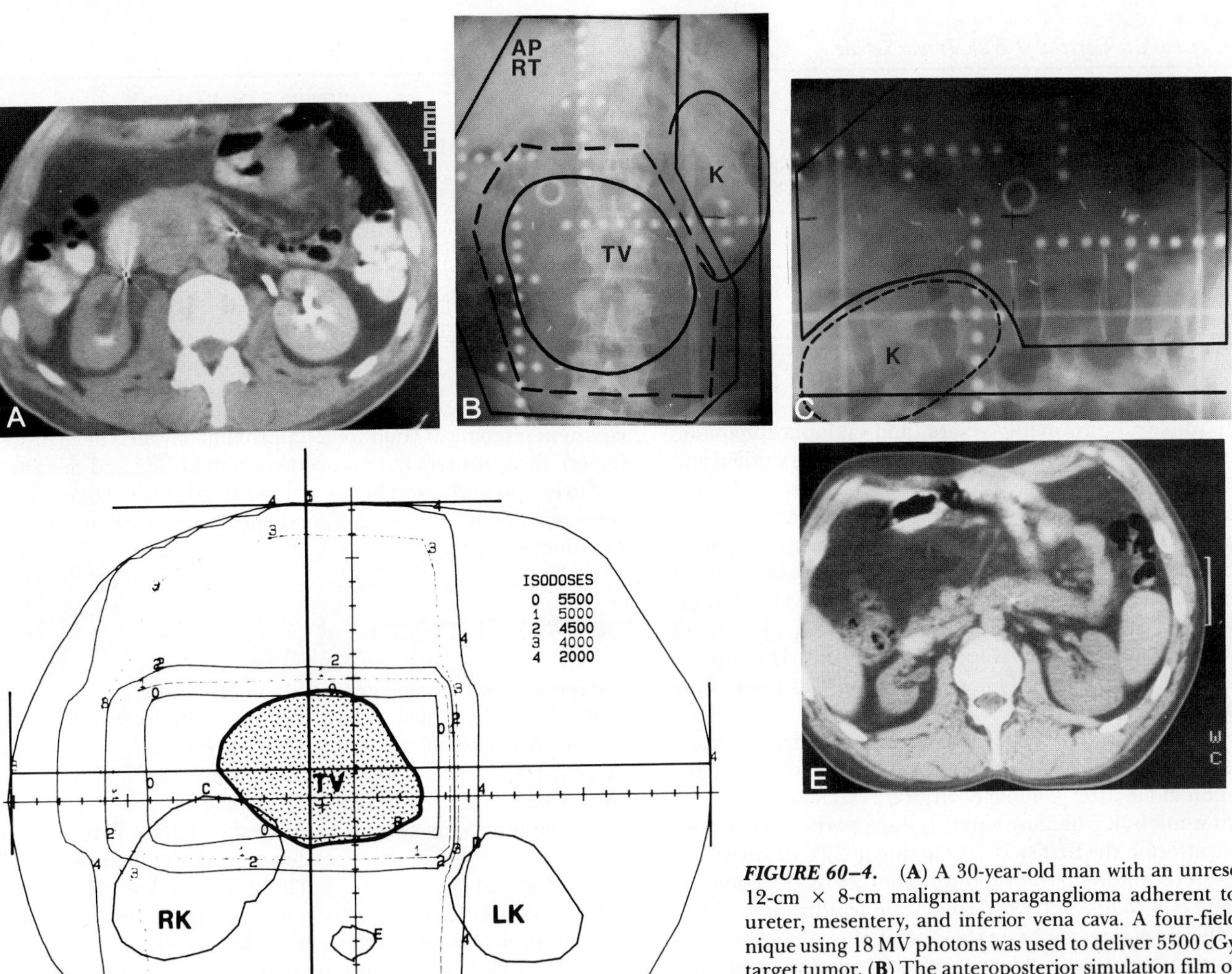

FIGURE 60–4. (**A**) A 30-year-old man with an unresectable 12-cm × 8-cm malignant paraganglioma adherent to right ureter, mesentery, and inferior vena cava. A four-field technique using 18 MV photons was used to deliver 5500 cGy to the target tumor. (**B**) The anteroposterior simulation film outlines the initial treatment area, the target volume (TV), and the boost area (*dashed lines*). Note sparing of the left kidney (K). (**C**) Lateral simulation film is shaped to avoid the kidneys. (**D**) Treatment plan indicates four-field isodoses to TV, right kidney (RK), and left kidney (LK). (**E**) CT scan of the abdomen obtained 24 months after completion of radiation therapy shows no recurrence of tumor and shrinkage of right kidney. The patient is now 5 years disease-free.

2500 cGy given in a single fraction. Multiple fields with junctures are often necessary. The major goal is to deliver a high dose to a limited volume, often as a boost or reduced field. Results of a randomized study are discussed later in this chapter.

RESULTS OF THERAPY

Soft Tissue Sarcomas

In a recent study by Zhang and associates,[98] 42 (68%) of 62 patients were able to have a complete resection with a 5-year survival rate of 48%. None of the patients who did not have complete resection survived (see Table 60-3). Local failure alone was the major cause of death in their patient population. Likewise, a recent study from Mayo Clinic by Dalton and coworkers[18] reported that 43 (68%) of 63 patients who had complete resection developed local recurrence.

The retroperitoneum is the least curable site in soft tissue sarcomas. It is probably due to the large size of the tumor when diagnosed and hence its lower rate of resectability. The major predictors of cure are resectability and grade (Table 60-4). In most series after complete gross resection, usually combined with radiation therapy, the survival rate varies from 30% to 60%. In patients with incompletely resected lesions, the survival rate varies from 0% to 25%.

Tepper and associates,[91] in 23 patients with retroperitoneal sarcomas, 17 of whom were treated with curative intent, reported a 54% 5-year actuarial survival and local tumor control rate (Table 60-5). Five of seven patients (71%) with complete resection, four of seven (57%) with incomplete removal, and one of three with no resection exhibited local tumor control. Furthermore, only two of 11 patients (18%) treated with 6000 cGy or less had tumor control in contrast to five of six (83%) receiving higher doses.

In the past decade, the NCI has launched two consecutive protocols in the treatment of retroperitoneal soft tissue sarcomas. In the first study,[26] the patients were randomized after surgery and radiation therapy (4500 cGy) to either chemo-

TABLE 60–4
Patterns of Failure Correlated With Tumor Grade

GRADE	NO. OF PATIENTS	NO. OF TOTAL RESECTIONS	NO. NED	PATTERNS OF FAILURE		
				LOCAL ONLY	LOCAL AND DISTANT	DISTANT ONLY
Low	28	10	10	9	1	8
High	25	8	7	7	4	6

(Data from Tepper JE, Suit HD, Wood HC: Int J Radiat Oncol Biol Phys 10:825–830, 1984; and Wist E, Sofheim OP, Blom P: Acta Radiol Oncol 24:305–310, 1985)

therapy (doxorubicin, methotrexate, and cyclophosphamide) or observation. From 64 patients evaluated, 37 were studied and 15 prospectively randomized. No significant differences were seen in the two groups, either studied or prospectively randomized, in disease-free or actuarial survival rates. The actuarial survival rate at 3 years was 47%, and the authors concluded that chemotherapy did not appear to affect survival. Of interest, only one of 37 patients failed in-field, although 30% of patients developed peritoneal seeding regionally. Intraoperative radiation therapy (IORT) was used in a select subset of the patients.

In the next study,[46] 35 patients were randomized to study whether an intraoperative boost was superior to conventional irradiation alone after complete surgical resection. It was decided to study IORT because enteritis was a particularly troubling side effect in the first study, occurring in 22% of survivors. Patients were randomized to receive, after gross resection, either 4500 cGy to 5000 cGy external-beam irradiation or 3500 cGy to 4000 cGy external-beam irradiation plus 2000 cGy intraoperatively. At 5 years, 40% of patients are alive, and 20% remain disease-free. No significant differences were noted in the two treatment arms, although the locoregional control rate (80%) was superior in the intraoperative arm compared with the conventional arm (35%) at 5 years. In addition, the incidence of enteritis was significantly decreased from 60% in the conventional arm to 7% in the IORT arm.

Rhabdomyosarcomas deserve special mention. The most common sarcoma of childhood (approximately 50% of all histologies), these tumors have a propensity to invade and metastasize to lymph nodes and hematogenously to lung and bone. The retroperitoneum is also the worst site in terms of survival in rhabdomyosarcoma.[17,78]

GERM CELL TUMORS

Primary retroperitoneal germ cell tumors are very rare. In the report from the British Tumor Registry, they account for only 1% of all germ cell tumors,[15] which are usually gonadal in origin. The tumor sample obtained for histologic diagnosis should be scrutinized for mixed pathology.

Seminomas (or germinomas) tend to have a better prognosis than the other subtypes because of their sensitivity to irradiation and chemotherapy. This is one subtype of tumor in which optimal surgical resection may not be necessary for improved survival. Several retrospective series show a survival rate of 60% to 70% in patients treated with irradiation with or without resection (Table 61-6). Recent reports show that the bulk of disease may influence distant failure, with a distant failure rate of up to 30% in patients with disease greater than 10 cm.[53] Because many series are retrospective and do not include optimal chemotherapy, use of chemotherapy for primary or salvage treatment should improve survival in subsequent studies.

TABLE 60–5
Results of Treatment of Retroperitoneal Sarcomas

INSTITUTION	No.	MEDIAN FOLLOW-UP (YEARS)	5-YEAR RESULTS (% OF ALL PATIENTS)		PATTERNS OF FAILURE (% OF ALL PATIENTS)		
			DFS	OS	LF	LF and DM	DM
NCI[47]	35*	1.3†	20	40	9	34	14
UCLA[89]	54	≈3	28‡	33		70‡§	12‡
NCI[26,75]	37	2.4	38	23	14	22	11
MGH[92]	23	2	NR	54¶	29¶	6¶	18¶
MSKCC[25]	78	5†	16**	31**	NR	NR	NR

NR: not reported; DFS: disease-free survival; OS: overall survival; LF: local failure; DM: distant metastasis
** Randomized trial of intraoperative irradiation plus external beam (15 patients) versus external beam alone (20 patients)*
† Minimum follow-up
‡ Based on 33 completely resected patients undergoing surgery alone
§ Includes LF and LF + DM
¶ Results from 17 patients treated with curative intent
*** Results from 32 patients completely resected treated with or without irradiation*
(Courtesy of Lawrence TS, Lichter AS, Department of Radiation Oncology, University of Michigan Medical Center, Ann Arbor, Michigan)

TABLE 60–6
Treatment Results in Retroperitoneal Seminoma

AUTHOR	NO. OF PATIENTS	NO. OF COMPLETE RESECTIONS	NUMBER NED	PATTERNS OF FAILURE* LOCAL AND DISTANT	DISTANT ONLY
Abell[1]	10	3	7	9†	1
Buskirk[11]	12	3	7	2‡	1
Green[31]	17	0	16	0	3
TOTAL	39	6	30	4	5

NED: No evidence of disease
** No "local only" failures*
† 3000 and 4000 roentgens
‡ 1800 cGy and 1900 cGy

Treatment results of teratocarcinoma, choriocarcinoma, or mixed tumors have improved in the past decade. The use of multiagent chemotherapy combined with surgical resection has made an impact on the natural history of the disease. The major prognostic factors appear to be the response to chemotherapy and subsequent surgical resection.[77] The disease-free survival rate for patients who had complete responses was 75% to 90% compared with less than 5% in patients who did not completely respond. If disease is present after retroperitoneal dissection, a radiation dose of 4000 cGy to 4500 cGy can be delivered.[38,49]

ADULT FORMS OF PEDIATRIC TUMORS

Adult Wilms' tumor is a very rare disease. In a study by Kilton and associates,[44] only 25 cases were found in reports between 1905 and 1980. In a study of 335 patients in Sweden by Jereb and Eklund, only six patients (2%) were 18 years or older.[41] The treatment is not different from that for children except perhaps that more aggressive therapy may be necessary because anaplasia (unfavorable histology) is more common in older patients.[3] In addition to vincristine, cyclophosphamide, and dactinomycin, cisplatin-based regimens may be necessary. Radiation to the tumor bed to 3000 cGy to 3500 cGy is recommended. The result of therapy is dependent on the presence of anaplasia and stage. Although the prognosis is worse in adults, long-term survival was reported in one third of patients reviewed.

Neuroblastoma in adults is also a rare neoplasm. Its natural history is similar to that of tumors that arise in children. Metastatic disease, even to lymph nodes, carries a very poor prognosis. Cases of prolonged survival are reported in the literature.[54]

SEQUELAE OF TREATMENT

The acute sequelae of treatment with irradiation are nausea and vomiting. When a large volume of the abdomen and pelvis is treated, neutropenia and thrombocytopenia are distinct possibilities. Patients need to be watched for dehydration and signs of anemia; intravenous fluid replacement or blood transfusions are occasionally necessary. The long-term major sequela of surgery and irradiation is small bowel enteropathy, which is linked to the number of laparotomies to which the patient has been subjected.[74] In the study by Wist and colleagues,[96] five of 36 patients developed enteritis, and one of the patients had life-threatening ileus. In the NCI prospective trials,[26,46] use of intraoperative radiation decreased the incidence of small bowel obstruction from 35% to 7% in long-term follow-up. A troubling problem noted by the authors was the development of radicular neuropathy in 27% of the IORT patients. The authors did not note any renal or hepatic toxicity in their long-term survivors. Nephritis can occur with high-dose irradiation (>3000 cGy), and hypertension can result.

GUIDELINES FOR FUTURE CLINICAL TRIALS

Retroperitoneal neoplasms are too uncommon for screening to be feasible. Future studies should focus on the staging and treatment of this type. The role of surgical staging needs to be defined in terms of CT and MRI; information on the efficacy of diagnostic imaging in the determination of adjacent organ involvement, resectability, and regional/distant metastases is forthcoming. Because surgical resection is still the primary therapy for sarcomas, the role of radiation (teletherapy, brachytherapy, IORT) needs to be further explored. Although chemotherapy given postoperatively has not yielded improved survival in several studies, the role of combination chemotherapy and irradiation or so-called neoadjuvant chemotherapy can be explored. To develop a clinically and statistically meaningful study, large number of patients need to be accrued.

REFERENCES

1. Abell MR, Fayos JV, Lampe I: Retroperitoneal germinomas (seminomas) without testicular involvement. Cancer 18:273, 1965
2. Ackerman LV: Tumors of the retroperitoneum, mesentery, and peritoneum. In Atlas of Tumor Pathology, Section VI, Fasc. 23–24, p 10. Washington, DC, Armed Forces Institute of Pathology, 1954
3. Adolphs HD, Knopfle G, Vogel J, et al: Wilms' tumor in the adolescent and adult. Eur Urol 9:281, 1983
4. Armstrong JR, Cohn IC: Primary malignant retroperitoneal tumors. Am J Surg 110:937, 1965
5. Azumi N, Curtis J, Kempson RL, Hendrickson MR: Atypical and malignant neoplasms showing lipomatous differentiation. Am J Surg Pathol 11:161–183, 1987
6. Bek V: Primary retroperitoneal tumors. Neoplasma 17:253, 1970
7. Böhle A, Studer UE, Sonntag RW, Scheidegger JR: Primary or secondary extragonadal germ cell tumors? J Urol 135:939–943, 1986
8. Bose B: Primary malignant retroperitoneal tumours: Analysis of 30 cases. Can J Surg 22:215, 1979

9. Braasch JW, Mon AB: Primary retroperitoneal tumors. Surg Clin North Am 47:663, 1967
10. Bryant RL, Stevenson DR, Hunton DW, et al: Primary malignant retroperitoneal tumors. Am J Surg 144:646, 1982
11. Buskirk SJ, Evans RG, Farrow GM: Primary retroperitoneal seminoma. Cancer 49:1934, 1982
12. Chang AE, Matory YL, Dwyer AJ, et al: Magnetic resonance imaging versus computed tomography in the evaluation of soft tissue tumors of the extremities. Ann Surg 205:340–348, 1987
13. Cody HS, Turnbull AD, Fortner JG: The continuing challenge of retroperitoneal sarcomas. Cancer 47:2147, 1981
14. Cohan RH, Baker ME, Cooper C, et al: Computed tomography of primary retroperitoneal malignancies. J Comput Assist Tomogr 12:804–810, 1988
15. Collins DH, Pugh RCB: Classification and frequency of testicular tumors. Br J Urol 36(Suppl):1, 1964
16. Council on Scientific Affairs: Magnetic resonance imaging of the abdomen and pelvis. JAMA 261:420–433, 1989
17. Crist WM, Raney RB, Tefft M: Soft tissue sarcomas arising in the retroperitoneal space in children. Cancer 56:2125, 1985
18. Dalton RR, Donohue, JH, Mucha P, et al: Management of retroperitoneal sarcomas. Surgery 106:725, 1989
19. Donhauser JL, Bigelow NH: Primary retroperitoneal tumors. Arch Surg 71:234, 1955
20. Donnelly BA: Primary retroperitoneal tumors. Surg Gynecol Obstet 83:705, 1946
21. Dubovsky EV, Russel ED: Quantitation of renal function with glomerular and tubular agents. Semin Nucl Med 12:308, 1982
22. Duncan RE, Evans AT: Diagnosis of primary retroperitoneal tumors. J Urol 117:19, 1977
23. Engel RM, Elkins RC, Fletcher BD: Retroperitoneal teratoma. Cancer 22:1068, 1968
24. Evans HL, Soule EH, Winkelmann RK: Atypical lipoma, atypical intramuscular lipoma, and well-differentiated retroperitoneal liposarcoma. Cancer 43:574, 1979
25. Fortner JG, Martin S, Hajdu S, et al: Primary sarcoma of the retroperitoneum. Semin Oncol 8:180, 1981
26. Glenn J, Sindelar W, Kinsella T, et al: Results of multimodality therapy of resectable soft-tissue sarcomas of the retroperitoneum. Surgery 97:316, 1985
27. Goffinett DR, Fuks Z, Glatstein E, et al: Abdominal irradiation of non-Hodgkin's lymphomas. Cancer 37:2797, 1976
28. Goldman SM, Davidson AJ, Neal J: Retroperitoneal and pelvic hemangiopericytomas: Clinical, radiologic, and pathologic correlation. Radiology 168:13–17, 1988
29. Goldman SM, Hartman DS, Weiss SW: The varied radiographic manifestations of retroperitoneal malignant fibrous histiocytoma revealed through 27 cases. J Urol 135:33–38, 1986
30. Gothin JH, MacIntosh PK: Interventional radiology in the assessment of the retroperitoneal lymph nodes. Radiol Clin North Am 17:461, 1979
31. Green N, Broth E, George FW, et al: Radiation therapy in bulky seminoma. Urology 21:467, 1983
32. Hansmann GH, Budd JW: Massive unattached retroperitoneal tumors. Am J Pathol Bacteriol 7:631, 1931
33. Harrison LB, Gutierrez E, Fischer JJ: Retroperitoneal sarcomas: The Yale experience and a review of the literature. J Surg Oncol 32:159–164, 1986
34. Hashimoto H, Tsuneyoshi J, Enjoj M: Malignant smooth muscle tumors of the retroperitoneum and mesentery: A clinicopathologic analysis of 44 cases. J Surg Oncol 28:177, 1985
35. Herdman JP: Primary retroperitoneal tumours. Br J Surg 40:331, 1953
36. Hudson TM, Hamlin DJ, Enneking WF: Magnetic resonance imaging of bone and soft tissue tumors: Early experience in 31 patients compared with computed tomography. Skeletal Radiol 13:134, 1985
37. Husband JE, Golding SJ: The role of computed tomography-guided needle biopsy on an oncology service. Clin Radiol 34:255, 1983
38. Hussey DH, Luk KH, Johnson DE: The role of radiation therapy in the management of germinal cell tumors of the testis other than pure siminomas. Radiology 123:175, 1977
39. Jacobsen S, Juul-Jorgensen S: Primary retroperitoneal tumors. Acta Chir Scand 140:498, 1974
40. Jain KK, Bosl GJ, Bains MS, et al: The treatment of extragonadal seminomas. J Clin Oncol 2:820, 1984
41. Jereb B, Eklund G: Factors influencing the cure rate in nephroblastoma Acta Radiol Oncol 12:84–106, 1973
42. Johnson Ah, Searls HH, Grimes OF: Primary retroperitoneal tumors. Am J Surg 88:155, 1954
43. Karakousis CP, Velez AF, Einrich LJ: Management of retroperitoneal sarcomas and patients survival. Am J Surg 150:376, 1985
44. Kilton L, Mathews MJ, Cohen MH: Adult Wilms' tumor: A report of prolonged survival and review of the literature. J Urol 124:1, 1980
45. Kinne DW, Chu FCH, Huvos AG: Treatment of primary and recurrent retroperitoneal liposarcoma. Cancer 31:53, 1973
46. Kinsella TJ, Sindelar WF, Lack E, et al: Preliminary results of a randomized study of adjuvant radiation therapy in resectable adult retroperitoneal soft tissue sarcomas. J Clin Oncol 6:18–25, 1988
47. Kinsella TJ, Sindelar WF, Rosenberg SA, et al: Wide excision combined with intraoperative radiotherapy and external beam therapy in retroperitoneal soft tissue tumors (Abstract). Int J Radiat Oncol Biol Phys 9(Suppl):92, 1983
48. Lack EE, Cubilla AL, Woodruff JM, Lieberman PH: Extra-adrenal paragangliomas of the retroperitoneum: A clinicopathologic study of 12 tumors. Am J Surg Pathol 4:109–120, 1980
49. Lack EE, Travis WD, Welch KJ: Retroperitoneal germ cell tumors in childhood. Cancer 56:602, 1985
50. Lane RH, Stephens DH, Reiman HM: Primary retroperitoneal neoplasms: CT findings in 90 cases with clinical and pathologic correlation. AM J Roentgenol 152:83–89, 1989
51. Leibel S: Soft tissue sarcomas: Therapeutic results and rationale for conservative surgery and radiation therapy. In Phillips TL, Pistenma DA (eds): Radiation Oncology Annual. New York, Raven Press, 1984
52. Lindberg R: Treatment of localized soft tissue sarcomas in adults in M.D. Anderson Hospital and Tumor Institute (1960–1980). Cancer Treat Symp 3:59–65, 1985
53. Logothetis CJ, Samuels ML, Selig DE, et al: Chemotherapy of extragonadal germ cell tumors. J Clin Oncol 3:316, 1985
54. Lopez R, Korakousis C, Rao U: Treatment of adult neuroblastoma. Cancer 45:840, 1980
55. Lowman RM, Grnja V, Peck DR, et al: The angiographic pattern of primary retroperitoneal tumors. Radiology 104:259, 1972
56. Malkin RB, Hotchkiss RS: Germinal carcinomas without evident testicular involvement. J Urol 101:360–365, 1969
57. Mansson E, Willems J, Aparisi P, et al: Preoperative radiation therapy of high malignancy grade soft tissue sarcoma. Acta Radiol Oncol 22:461–463, 1983
58. Mason BR, Kearsley JH: Radiotherapy for stage 2 testicular seminoma: The influence of bulk. J Clin Oncol 6:1956–1862, 1988
59. McGrath PC, Neifeld JP, Lawrence W, et al: Improved survival following complete excision of retroperitoneal sarcomas. Ann Surg 200:200, 1984
60. McLeod DG, Taylor HG, Skoog SJ, et al: Extragonadal germ cell tumors: Clinicopathologic findings and treatment experience in 12 patients. Cancer 61:1187–1191, 1988
61. Melicow MM: Primary tumors of the retroperitoneum: A clinicopathologic analysis of 162 cases. J Int Coll Surg 19:401, 1953
62. Mikhail RA, Moore JB, Reed DN Jr, Abbott RR: Malignant retroperitoneal paragangliomas. J Surg Oncol 32:32–36, 1986
63. Montague DK: Retroperitoneal germ cell tumors with no apparent testicular involvement. J Urol 113:505, 1975
64. Moss JF, Slayton RE, Economou SG: Primary retroperitoneal pure choriocarcinoma: Two long-term complete responders from a rare fatal disease. Cancer 62:1053–1054, 1988
65. Mueller PR, Wittenberg J, Ferruci JT: Fine-needle aspiration biopsy of abdominal masses. Semin Roentgenol 16:52, 1981
66. Murphy S, Hustu O: A randomized trial of combined modality therapy of non-Hodgkins lymphomas. Cancer 45:630–637, 1980

67. Neifeld JP, Walsh JW, Lawrence W, et al: Computed tomography in the management of soft tissue tumors. Surg Gynecol Obstet 155:535, 1982
68. Newman HR, Pinck BD: Primary retroperitoneal tumors: A summation of 33 cases. Arch Surg 60:879, 1950
69. North JP: Primary tumors of the retroperitoneum. Ann Surg 151:693, 1970
70. Oriana S, Bonardi P, Preda F: Primary retroperitoneal tumors. Tumori 63:397, 1977
71. Pack GT, Tabah EJ: Primary retroperitoneal tumors: A study of 120 cases. Int Abstr Surg 99:313, 1954
72. Parkinson MC, Chabrel CM: Clinicopathological features of retroperitoneal tumours. Br J Urol 56:17, 1984
73. Pistolesi GF, Procacci C, Caudanna R, et al: CT criteria of the differential diagnosis in primary retroperitoneal masses. Eur J Radiol 4:127, 1984
74. Potish RA: Importance of predisposing factors in the development of enteric damage. Am J Clin Oncol 5:189–194, 1982
75. Potter DA, Glenn J, Kinsella T, et al: Patterns of recurrence in patients with high-grade soft tissue sarcomas. J Clin Oncol 3:353, 1985
76. Rosenberg SA: Prospective randomized trials demonstrating the efficacy of adjuvant chemotherapy in adult patients with soft tissue sarcomas. Cancer Treat Rev 9:1067, 1984
77. Roth BJ, Greist A, Kublis PS, et al: Cisplatin-based combination chemotherapy for disseminated germ cell tumors: Long-term follow-up J Clin Oncol 6:1239–1247, 1988
78. Ruymann FB: Rhabdomyosarcoma in children and adolescents: A review. Hematol Oncol Clin North Am 4:621–654, 1987
79. Saltzman B, Pitts WR, Vaughan ED Jr: Extragonadal retroperitoneal germ cell tumors without apparent testicular involvement: A search for the source. Urology 27:504–507, 1986
80. Schulte TL, Emmett JL: Urography as the differential diagnosis of retroperitoneal tumors. J Urol 42:215, 1939
81. Shafir M, Holland J, Cohen B, et al: Radical retroperitoneum tumor surgery with resection of the psoas major muscle. Cancer 56:929, 1985
82. Shmookler BM, Lauer DH: Retroperitoneal leiomyosarcoma: A clinicopathologic analysis of 36 cases. Am J Surg Pathol 7:269, 1983
83. Siegel MJ, Balfe DM, McClennan BL, et al: Clinical utility of CT in pediatric retroperitoneal disease: Five years' experience. Am J Roentgenol 138:1011, 1982
84. Sindelar WF, Hoekstra HJ, Kinsella TJ: Surgical approaches and techniques in intraoperative radiotherapy for intra-abdominal, retroperitoneal, and pelvic neoplasms. Surgery 107:247–256, 1988
85. Sindelar WF, Kinsella T, Tepper J: Experimental and clinical studies with intra-operative radiotherapy. Surg Gynecol Obstet 157:205, 1983
86. Skinner DG: Technique of the thoracoabdominal approach to retroperitoneal surgery. Surg Rounds 14:12, 1980
87. Solla JA, Reed K: Primary retroperitoneal sarcomas. Am J Surg 152:496–498, 1986
88. Stephens DH, Sheedy PF, Hattery RR, et al: Diagnosis and evaluation of retroperitoneal tumors by computed tomography. Am J Roentgenol 129:395, 1977
89. Storm FK, Eilber FR, Mirra J: Retroperitoneal sarcomas. A reappraisal of treatment. J Surg Oncol 17:1, 1981
90. Suit HD, Mankin HJ, Wood MC, et al: Treatment of the patient with stage MO soft tissue sarcoma. J Clin Oncol 6:854–862, 1988
91. Tepper JE, Suit HD, Wood WC, et al: Radiation therapy of retroperitoneal soft tissue sarcomas. Int J Radiat Oncol Biol Phys 10:825, 1984
92. Tepper JE, Suit HD: Radiation therapy alone for sarcoma of soft tissue. Cancer 56:475, 1985
93. Wagenknecht LV, Schumpelick V, Winkler R: Urological aspects of primary retroperitoneal tumors. Eur Urol 2:15, 1976
94. Whittington R, Dobelbower RR, Mohiudden M, et al: Radiotherapy of unresectable pancreatic carcinoma: A six-year experience with 104 patients. Int J Radiat Oncol Biol Phys 7:1637, 1981
95. Wiley AL, Wirtanen GW, Joo P, et al: Clinical and theoretical aspects of the treatment of surgically unresectable retroperitoneal malignancy with intra-arterial actinomycin-D and radiotherapy. Cancer 36:107, 1975
96. Wist E, Sofheim OP, Blom P: Primary retroperitoneal sarcoma. Acta Radiol Oncol 24:305, 1985
97. Wittenberg J, Fineberg HV, Ferruci JT, et al: Clinical efficacy of computed body tomography. II. Am J Roentgenol 132:1111, 1980
98. Zhang G, Chen KK, Manivel C, et al: Sarcomas of the retroperitoneum and genitourinary tract. J Urol 141:1107, 1989
99. Zomoza J, Jonsson K, Wallace S, et al: Fine-needle aspiration biopsy of retroperitoneal lymph nodes and abdominal masses: An updated report. Radiology 125:87, 1977

61

○ ○ ○ • • •

Adrenal Gland

Luther W. Brady
Felipe A. Calvo

ANATOMY

The paired suprarenal (adrenal) glands are located on the upper anteromedial surface of each kidney. The right suprarenal gland relates to the diaphragm posteriorly, to the liver and inferior vena cava on its anterior surface, and to the duodenum inferiorly. The left suprarenal gland is positioned in the middle of the left crux of the diaphragm, and the omental bursa separates it from the stomach. The pancreas and splenic vessels overlap the lower surface of the suprarenal gland.[44]

The lymphatic drainage follows the superior suprarenal artery, the middle suprarenal artery, or the suprarenal vein. The superior lymphatic trunks end in lymph nodes located at the origin of the celiac artery and inferior vena cava, whereas the inferior lymphatic trunks end in lateroaortic nodes above the renal pedicle. Some trunks may pass through the diaphragm, following the splanchnic nerves, and end in a retroaortic node in the posterior mediastinum. In the right side, some lymphatic trunks may penetrate the liver.[38]

The blood supply to the adrenal gland is derived from multiple branches of the inferior phrenic artery as well as from small branches derived from the aorta and the renal arteries. A large central vein that leaves the anterior surface of the gland at the hilum provides venous drainage.

The adrenal gland is composed of the cortex and the medulla. Although in intimate contact, these two portions are essentially different organs with separate embryologic origins.

EPIDEMIOLOGY

Adrenal Cortex Tumors

Benign tumors of the adrenal cortex can appear in 20% to 25% of patients with Cushing's syndrome. Carcinomas are rare, with an incidence of about 0.2 per 100,000.[29] Calculations from the National Cancer Institute's SEER database suggests 75 to 115 new cases each year. Virilization associated with corticoadrenal tumor is often seen in patients under 12 years of age. About 130 new cases of adrenocortical carcinoma occur in the United States each year.[4]

At autopsy approximately 2% of all adults have adrenal adenomas, compared with approximately 33% of those with a family history of multiple endocrine syndromes. Of patients with hypertension, 20% have adrenal adenomas and as many as 30% of elderly, obese diabetics have this tumor.[4]

Adrenal Medulla Tumors

Ganglioneuromas are rare, benign tumors of the adrenal medulla seen in children and young adults.[32] Neuroblastomas are the most common malignant tumors of the suprarenal gland.[33] Malignant pheochromocytomas make up about 10% of all pheochromocytomas diagnosed; approximately 400 new cases are expected each year in the United States.[22,36,40] Pheochromocytoma may occur at any age,[13] but peak incidence is in the fifth decade.[13] Evidence suggests that an inherited abnormality is involved.[7,11,14,24,43] Bilateral pheochromocytomas occur in the familial syndrome. The incidence of pheochromocytoma is increased in patients with medullary carcinoma of the thyroid (Sipple's syndrome; bilateral tumors in 70%), with neurofibromatosis of von Recklinghausen (4% to 25%), and with cerebelloretinal hemangioblastomatosis of von Hippel and Lindau, as reported by Mullholland and associates.[34]

NATURAL HISTORY

The adrenal glands were described in the 16th century but were first called glands by Lancisi in 1714.[46] Cushing's syndrome caused by a confirmed adrenal tumor was described in 1913 by Turney[48] and in 1926 by Parkes-Weber.[35]

Carcinomas of the adrenal cortex usually are large tumors, 4 cm to 15 cm in diameter. The tumor may break through the capsule and invade surrounding tissues. Adrenal cortical tumors metastasize to the lungs, liver, brain, and regional lymph nodes. Malignant pheochromocytomas have a similar pattern of spread, but bones may also be involved. Ninety percent are intraabdominal. Sex distribution is equal; however, more women have the functional type of tumor. The average age at presentation is 40 to 50 years. In children, two age peaks have been suggested: an early peak at 1 to 2 years with a decline to age 7, after which there is a more even distribution through ages 9 to 16 years.

CLINICAL PRESENTATION

Patients may present with either functional or nonfunctional tumors of the adrenal cortex. Nonfunctional tumors are detected late because increasing tumor burden is often the main indicator of the problem. Detection of functional tumors frequently depends on the main hormone synthesized by the tumor cells. Hydrocortisone, corticosterone, 11-hydroxyandrostenedione, and aldosterone are among the major hormones produced by the adrenal cortex.[4, 5, 12]

Nonfunctioning carcinomas are usually found in adults with mild associated symptoms of asthenia, low-grade fever, and loin pain.[42] Functional tumors commonly present as excessive production of glucocorticoid resulting in the features of Cushing's syndrome. Because of the biochemical involvement in this disease (increased gluconeogenesis, glucose intolerance, and inhibition of amino acid uptake and protein synthesis), the signs and symptoms most frequently found are muscle wasting, striae, bruising, impaired wound healing, and osteoporosis. Excessive production of corticosteroids induces a typical clinical appearance: rounded facies, buffalo hump, striae, mild hypertension, truncal obesity, and redistribution of truncal fat.[4] Depression and psychotic behavior may occur. Virilization or feminization should arouse suspicion of an adrenal neoplasm. Conn's syndrome (primary hyperaldosteronism) manifests as sodium retention, increased total plasma volume and renal artery pressure, and inhibition of renin secretion.

Approximately 10% of all pheochromocytomas are nonfunctioning.[26] In up to 50% of cases involving pheochromocytomas, patients have intermittent episodes of hypertension with normal blood pressure otherwise. Nausea and vomiting along with chest pain or abdominal pain have also been documented.[4, 12, 40] Some pheochromocytomas produce predominantly α-adrenergic effects due to norepinephrine production: pallor, headache, and hypertension. Other pheochromocytomas produce predominantly β-adrenergic effects due to epinephrine production: flushing, sweating, palpitation, tachycardia, anxiety, and hyperglycemia. Frequently, both α- and β-adrenergic effects occur.

DIAGNOSTIC WORKUP AND STAGING

Suspected functional adrenocortical tumors are confirmed with easy laboratory tests that indicate an evening serum cortisol level of more than 15 μg/dl and a urine free cortisol level higher than 100 μg/24 hours. Table 61-1 outlines the complete diagnostic workup. These tests should be followed by the determination of morning serum cortisol (> 10 μg/dl). After 1 mg of dexamethasone at 11:00 PM urine 17-OHCS is not suppressed (< 25 μg/25 hours) by dexamethasone 0.5 mg every 5 hours for 48 hours.[4] The next step in the diagnosis of adrenocortical carcinoma is the finding of an abdominal mass. Computed tomography (CT) can recognize masses in the region of the adrenal gland; on CT scans, tumor enlargement or venous invasion may indicate the presence of malignant disease (Fig. 61-1)[4] Ultrasonography is reliable in the identification of adrenal tumors more than 3 cm in diameter.[2, 8] Arteriography is an important aid in the diagnosis of adrenal tumors.[199] Adrenal venography and adrenal venous sampling are needed to obtain serum for diagnostic biochemical determinations. Scans using ^{131}I-iodocholesterol can reveal adrenal tumors.[47]

Central necrosis on CT scan and large size are among the factors predictive of carcinoma. The most important factor is the presence of vena cava involvement in right-sided lesions. This can often be determined by CT or cavogram. The advent of quality CT and magnetic resonance imaging (MRI) scans has largely eliminated the need for vena cavography; if there is any doubt, however, this study should still be performed to allow preoperative and postoperative surgical preparation.

A staging system proposed for adrenocortical carcinoma is shown in Table 61-2.[3]

TABLE 61–1
Diagnostic Workup for Adrenal Tumors

General
- History
- Physical examination

Radiographic Studies
- Standard
  - Chest radiography
  - Computed tomography
  - Magnetic resonance imaging
  - Ultrasonography
  - Arteriography and venography
- Complementary
  - ^{131}I-iodocholesterol scan

Laboratory Studies
- Admission CBC, blood chemistry, urinalysis
- Serum and urine cortisol studies
- Serum and urine catecholamine studies

PATHOLOGIC CLASSIFICATION

An accepted classification of tumors arising in the adrenal gland is shown in Table 61-3. Benign tumors usually are small and found at autopsy. Aldosterone-functioning tumors rarely are malignant.[16]

Zones of hemorrhage and necrosis are observed macroscopically. Numerous mitotic figures and cellular undifferentiation are common findings on microscopic examination. Large adrenocortical carcinomas, invasion of surrounding tissues and veins, and many mitotic figures are poor prognostic factors.

Pheochromocytomas show malignant features in less than

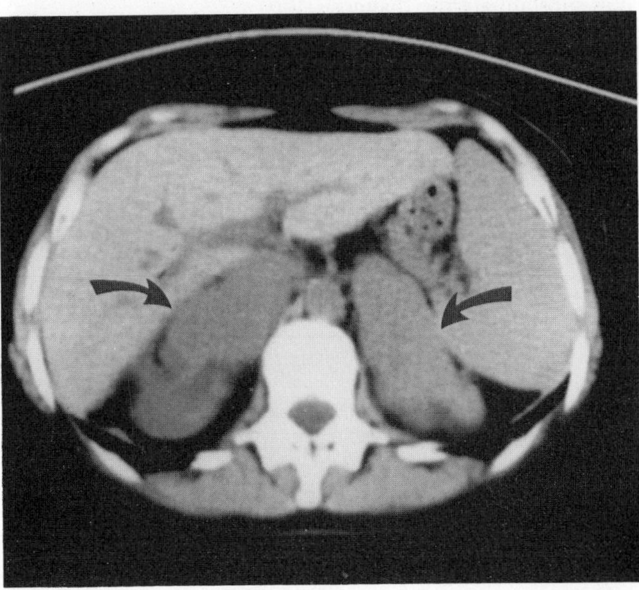

FIGURE 61–1. CT scan of abdomen illustrating large adrenal glands.

TABLE 61–2
Staging for Tumors of the Adrenal Gland

T	**EXTENT OF PRIMARY TUMOR**
1	<5 cm and confined to adrenal gland
2	>5 cm but <10 cm or adherence to kidney
3	>10 cm or invasion of surrounding structures including renal vein
M	**PRESENCE AND TYPE OF METASTASES**
0	No demonstrable metastases
1	Regional lymphatics
2	Distant metastases (*e.g.,* liver, lung, bone)
R	**TISSUE REMAINING AFTER RESECTION**
0	Tumor completely excised
1	Tumor entered at operation
2	Tumor tissue remaining after resection
D	**DEGREE OF HISTOLOGIC DIFFERENTIATION**
1	Differentiated; no capsular or vascular invasion
2	Moderately undifferentiated; either capsular or vascular invasion
3	Anaplastic; both capsular and vascular invasion

Stage I = 3 or fewer; for example, T1M0R0D1
Stage II = 4 and 5; for example, T2M0R1D2
Stage III = 6 and 7; for example, T3M1R1D2
Stage IV = 8 or more; for example, T3M2R2D3

(Bradley EL: Surg Gynecol Obstet 141:507, 1975, by permission of Surgery, Gynecology and Obstetrics)

TABLE 61–3
Classification of Adrenal Tumors

TUMORS DERIVED FROM CORTEX (EPITHELIAL)
Adenoma
 Functioning
 Nonfunctioning
Carcinoma

TUMORS DERIVED FROM MEDULLARY TISSUE (NERVOUS SYSTEM TUMORS)
Ganglioneuroma
Pheochromocytoma
Neuroblastoma
Mixed type (ganglioneuroblastoma)

TUMORS DERIVED FROM CONNECTIVE TISSUE
Myelolipomas
Lipomas
Myomas
Angiomas
Fibromas
Fibrosarcomas

10% of cases.[37,41] Size of tumor at the time of diagnosis may vary. Macroscopically, pheochromocytomas tend to be encapsulated with areas of cystic changes, hemorrhage, and necrosis. The capsule is frequently invaded, but invasion does not constitute a malignant characteristic. Histologically, cell size, nuclear size, and arrangements of cells are variable. A twisted cell cord pattern, basophilic or cytophilic staining with fine intracytoplasmic pigment granules, and PAS-stained secretory droplets aid in the diagnosis. Epinephrine-containing cytoplasmic granules can be demonstrated by ultrastructure studies. Excessive levels of plasma or urinary catecholamines or their metabolites substantiate the diagnosis.

GENERAL MANAGEMENT

Surgery is the primary treatment for adrenocortical carcinoma. Curative surgery is feasible in only a few patients because of the size of tumor at the time of diagnosis. Complete extirpation has been reported in 47% of patients initially suitable for radical surgery.[28] Surgery can be used as a palliative procedure in incurable functional tumors; partial resections are attempted to improve endocrine manifestations that cannot be controlled medically and to relieve local symptoms. Careful attention must be given to preoperative, intraoperative, and postoperative steroid replacement because the contralateral adrenal gland is often atrophied.[20,30]

Responses and good palliation have been achieved with the use of external-beam irradiation for the treatment of soft tissue and bone metastases.[6,27,36] The use of postoperative irradiation for gross or microscopic residual disease has been explored, but benefit in terms of delayed recurrence of the tumor after treatment has been minimal.[27]

Markoe and associates[31] have recently reported positive objective long-term tumor control with definitively carried out radiation therapy.

The first chemotherapeutic agent to show antitumor effect in clinical trials of carcinoma of the adrenal cortex was o,p'DDD (1, 1-dichloro-2(o-chlorophenyl)-2-(p-chlorophenyl) ethane; mitotane [Lysodren]) in 1960 by Bergenstel and associates.[1] Agent o,p'-DDD has shown an objective tumor regression rate of 10% to 61%.[14,18,19,28] There is no agreement about the impact of the agent on survival.

Doxorubicin (Adriamycin) in combination with cisplatin

TABLE 61–4
Length of Survival of Patients With Adrenal Carcinoma Treated by Three Different Methods

TREATMENT METHOD	NO. OF PATIENTS	SURVIVAL (MO) MEAN	RANGE	MEDIAN
Surgery ± radiation therapy	6	10.3 ± 8.7	1–24	8.5
Surgery + o,p'DDD	17	46.6 ± 42.7	1–120	24
Surgery + adjuvant o,p'DDD	4	74 ± 33	36–108	

(Modified from Schteingart DE, Motazedi A, Noonan RA, et al: Arch Surg 117:1142–1146, 1982)

TABLE 61–5
Survival in Adrenocortical Carcinoma

AUTHORS	YEAR	NO. OF PATIENTS	FIVE-YEAR SURVIVAL RATE (%)	COMMENTS
Henley et al[18]	1983	31	32	Curative resection
King and Lack[25]	1979	21	43	
Cohn et al[8]	1986	47	25	Median survival 1.7 years (range 2 months to 15 years)
Javadpour et al[22]	1980	58	30	Median survival 16% with disease

also has demonstrated antitumor activity.[12] Other cytotoxic drugs, including vinblastine, melphalan, 5-fluorouracil, medroxyprogesterone acetate, hydroxyurea, daunorubicin, and cyclophosphamide plus methyl-CCNU plus doxorubicin, have not been active in individual cases.[15]

RADIATION THERAPY TECHNIQUES

The occasional reports that discuss the clinical aspects of these tumors have suggested that adrenocortical carcinoma is radioresistant.[21,28] Symptomatic relief and palliation of metastatic disease to bone has been described.[6,27]

Radiation therapy is being explored more intensively in the multidisciplinary treatment of adrenocortical carcinomas. Locoregional disease control remains a major problem with this tumor; however, recent reports clearly indicate the potential for long-term regional control.[30] The clinicotherapeutic situations in which radiation therapy could be considered for combined approach in adrenocortical carcinomas are the following: preoperative irradiation in patients with large, unresectable tumors masses; postoperative irradiation in patients with residual disease or who are at high risk for locoregional relapse; and radical external-beam radiation therapy in patients with major contraindications for surgical procedures.

External-beam irradiation, intraoperative radiation therapy, and interstitial intraoperative implantation may be possible in the management of adrenocortical carcinomas. The impact of these procedures on patient survival is unknown.

Percarpio and Knowlton[36] have reported the experience at the Yale University School of Medicine in the radiation therapy treatment of 14 patients with adrenocortical carcinoma. Preoperative irradiation was used in two patients because of unresectable primary tumors, and one of them was subsequently resected without local recurrence. Four patients received postoperative radiation therapy to the flank for unresectable local disease or tumor spillage, and one of these had no local recurrence for 11 years. Twelve courses of palliative radiation therapy were given to relieve pain or obstruction; adequate palliation was achieved in all 12 patients. We recommend palliative radiation therapy for patients with painful metastases or obstructive disease to doses of 3000 cGy to 4000 cGy in 2 to 3 weeks.

RESULTS OF THERAPY

Radical surgery for adrenocortical carcinoma with complete resection of the primary tumor can achieve a 47% survival rate with an average of 7.2 years' postoperative follow-up period.[25] Results are similar for functional and nonfunctional tumors.[28] Prolonged survival can occur in patients with metastatic disease, although recent reports show an average survival period of 8 and 10 months.[23,25] The overall 5-year survival rate for patients with adrenocortical carcinoma is less than 20%[22] (Tables 61-4 and 61-5).

REFERENCES

1. Bergenstel DM, Herz R, Lipsett MB, et al: Chemotherapy of adrenocortical cancer with o,p'-DDD. Ann Intern Med 53:672, 1960
2. Bernadino ME, Goldstein HM, Green G: Gray-scale ultrasonography of adrenal neoplasms. Am J Roentgenol 130:741, 1978
3. Bradley EL: Primary and adjunctive therapy in carcinoma of the adrenal cortex. Surg Gynecol Obstet 141:507, 1975
4. Brennan MF: Cancer of the endocrine system. The adrenal gland. In DeVita VT, Hellman S, Rosenberg SA (eds): Cancer: Principles and Practice of Oncology, pp 985–1000. Philadelphia, JB Lippincott, 1982
5. Brennan MF, Dunnick NR: Localization of functional adrenal tumors. In Nayarian JS, Delaney P (eds): Breast and Endocrine Surgery. Chicago, Year Book Medical Publishers, 1981
6. Bulger AR, Correa RJK: Experience with adrenal cortical carcinoma. Urology 10:12–18, 1977
7. Carman CT, Brashear RE: Pheochromocytoma as an inherited abnormality. N Engl J Med 263:419, 1960
8. Cohn K, Gottesman L, Brennan MF: Adrenocortical carcinoma. Surgery 100:1170–1177, 1986
9. Davidson JK, Morley P, Harley GD, et al: Adrenal venography and ultrasound in the investigation of the adrenal gland: An analysis of 58 cases. Br J Radiol 48:435, 1975
10. del Regato JA, Spjut HJ: Tumors of the suprarenal gland. In Ackerman L, del Regato JA (eds): Cancer: Diagnosis, Treatment and Prognosis, ed 5, pp 697–716. St. Louis, CV Mosby, 1977
11. Farquhar JW: Phaeochromocytoma in childhood: Case report and a brief review of 56 others recorded in the literature. J R Coll Surg Edinb 3:301,1958
12. Goldsmith MA, Chahinian P, Perloff M, et al: Chemotherapy of the adrenal cortical cancer (unpublished data)
13. Graham JB: Pheochromocytoma and hypertension: An analysis of 207 cases. Int Abstr Surg 92:105, 1951; In Surg Gynecol Obstet February 1951
14. Greenberg RE, Gardner LK: Pheochromocytoma in father and son: Report of the eighth known affected kindred. J Clin Endocrinol Metab 19:351, 1959
15. Hajjar RA, Hickey RC, Samaan NA: Adrenal cortical carcinoma: A study of 32 patients. Cancer 35:549, 1975
16. Harrison JH, Mahoney EM, Bennett AH: Tumors of the adrenal cortex. Cancer 32:1227, 1973
17. Harrison TS, Bartlett JD, Seaton JF: Current evaluation and management of pheochromocytoma. Ann Surg 168:701, 1968
18. Henley DJ, van Heerden JA, Grant CS, et al: Adrenal cortical

carcinoma: A continuing challenge. Surgery 94:926–931, 1983

19. Hoevels J, Ekelund L: Angiographic findings in adrenal masses. Acta Radiol (Diagn) 20:337, 1979
20. Hoffman DL, Mattox VR: Treatment of adrenocortical carcinoma with o,p'-/DDD. Med Clin North Am 56:999, 1972
21. Hutter AM, Kayhoe DE: Adrenal cortical carcinoma: Results of treatments with o,p'-DDD in 138 patients. Am J Med 41:581, 1966
22. Javadpour N, Woltering E, Brennan MF: Adrenal neoplasms. Curr Probl Surg 17:1, 1980
23. Kelly WF, Barnes AJ, Cassar J, et al: Cushing's syndrome due to adrenocortical carcinoma. Acta Endocrinol (Copenh) 91:303, 1979
24. Kelsall AR, Ross EJ: Bilateral pheochromocytoma in two sisters. Lancet 2:273, 1955
25. King DR, Lack EE: Adrenal corticol carcinoma: A clinical and pathological study of 49 cases. Cancer 44:239, 1979
26. Levitt RG, Stanley RJ, Dehner LP: Angiography of a clinical nonfunctioning pheochromocytoma. JAMA 233:268, 1975
27. Lewinsky BS, Grigor KM, Symington T, et al: The clinical and pathologic features of "non-hormonal" adrenocortical tumors. Cancer 33:778, 1974
28. Lipsett MB, Hertz R, Ross GT: Clinical and pathophysiologic aspects of adrenocortical carcinoma. Am J Med 35:374, 1963
29. Lubitz JA, Freeman L, Okum R: Mitotane use in inoperable adrenal cortical carcinoma. JAMA 223:1109, 1973
30. Macharlane DA: Cancer of the adrenal cortex. Ann R Coll Surg Engl 23:155, 1958
31. Markoe AM, Serber W, Micaily B, Brady LW: Radiation therapy for adjunctive treatment of adrenal cortical carcinomas. Am J Clin Oncol 14:170, 1991
32. McFarland J: Ganglioneuroma of retroperitoneal origin. Arch Pathol 11:118, 1931
33. Miller RW, Fraumeni JF, Hill JA: Neuroblastoma: Epidemiologic approach to its origin. Am J Dis Child 115:253, 1968
34. Mulholland SG, Atuk NO, Walzak MP: Familial pheochromocytoma associated with cerebellar hemangioblastoma. JAMA 207:1709, 1969
35. Parkes-Weber F: Cutaneous striae, high blood pressure, amenorrhea and obesity of the type sometimes connected with cortical tumors of the adrenal glands, occurring in the absence of any such tumor: With some remarks on the morphogenetic and hormonic effects of true hypernephromata of the adrenal cortex. Br J Dermatol Physiol 38:1, 1926
36. Percarpio B, Knowlton AH: Radiation therapy of adrenal cortical carcinoma. Acta Radiol Diagn (Stockh) 15:288, 1976
37. ReMine WH, Chong GC, VanHeerden JA: Current management of pheochromocytoma. Ann Surg 179:740, 1974
38. Rouviere H: Anatomie des Lymphatiques de l'Homme. Paris, Masson et Cie, 1932
39. Schteingart DE, Motazedi A, Noonan RA, et al: Treatment of adrenal carcinomas. Arch Surg 117:1142–1146, 1982
40. Scott HW, Oates JA, Nies AS, et al: Pheochromocytoma: Present diagnosis and management. Ann Surg 183:587, 1976
41. Sherwin RP: Histopathology of pheochromocytoma. Cancer 12:861, 1959
42. Shons AR, Gamble WG: Nonfunctioning carcinoma of the adrenal cortex. Surg Gynecol Obstet 138:705, 1974
43. Smits M, Huiziaga J: Familial occurrence of phaeochromocytoma. Acta Genet (Basel) 11:137, 1961
44. Sommers SC: Adrenal glands. In Anderson WAD (ed): Pathology, vol 2, ed 6, pp 1464–1487, St. Louis, CV Mosby, 1970
45. Tang CK, Gray GF: Adrenocortical neoplasms: Prognosis and morphology. Urology 5:691, 1975
46. Thorn GW: The adrenal cortex. I. Historical aspects. Johns Hopkins Med J 123:49, 1968
47. Thrall JM, Freitas JE, Beierwaltes WH: Adrenal scintigraphy. Semin Nucl Med 8:23, 1978
48. Turney HG: Discussion of disease of the pituitary body. Proc R Soc Med 6:119, 1913
50. Van Way C, Scott HW, Page DL, et al: Pheochromocytoma. Curr Probl Surg 6:1–59, 1974

62

Hodgkin's Disease

Richard T. Hoppe
Eli Glatstein
Todd H. Wasserman

The management of Hodgkin's disease has evolved dramatically in the past three decades. Advances in staging have included improved imaging studies and the use of staging laparotomy and splenectomy to identify clinically occult disease. More refined radiation therapy techniques as well as the discovery of effective combination chemotherapy have led to a marked improvement in patient survival. With this improved outcome, the potential long-term complications of staging and treatment have become more apparent, and this has led to the development of more refined management programs, tailored to specific clinical situations.[53]

ANATOMY

Hodgkin's disease virtually always begins in lymph nodes. Isolated extralymphatic involvement in the absence of nodal disease is exceedingly rare. Although any lymph node may potentially be involved by Hodgkin's disease, there is a peculiar axial predisposition, resulting in cervical, mediastinal, or periaortic node disease in most patients. More than 80% of patients with Hodgkin's disease present with cervical lymph node involvement, and more than 50% have mediastinal disease.

EPIDEMIOLOGY AND RISK FACTORS

Hodgkin's disease accounts for only 0.75% of all cancers diagnosed in the United States each year.[126] There is a slight male predominance. Hodgkin's disease is rare in children under the age of 10 years; the median age of patients at the time of diagnosis is 26 years. The incidence of Hodgkin's disease has a bimodal peak when adjusted for age.[145] The early peak shows approximately five cases per 100,000 from ages 25 to 30. A second peak of approximately seven cases per 100,000 occurs at ages 75 to 80.

Although clusters of patients with Hodgkin's disease have been reported, no conclusive evidence supports an infectious etiology.[45] A relationship between Hodgkin's disease and prior infection with Epstein-Barr virus (EBV) has been proposed. Weiss and co-workers[140] have identified components of the EBV genome in the cellular DNA of Reed-Sternberg cells in lymph nodes involved by Hodgkin's disease. In addition, Mueller and associates[99] identified elevated levels of IgG and IgA against the EBV capsid antigen and elevated levels of antibody against the EBV nuclear antigen and early antigen D in the serum of patients with Hodgkin's disease 3 to 156 months *prior* to the diagnosis of Hodgkin's disease. Studies attempting to link occupational exposures or other etiologic factors with the development of Hodgkin's disease have been inconclusive or contradictory.[45]

NATURAL HISTORY AND CLINICAL PRESENTATION

The patient with Hodgkin's disease usually presents with painless lymphadenopathy. Some patients note systemic symptoms such as unexplained fevers, drenching night sweats, weight loss, generalized pruritus, and alcohol-induced pain in tissues involved by Hodgkin's disease. Still other patients are diagnosed after the detection of a mediastinal mass on a routine chest radiograph.

If contiguity is assumed among the supraclavicular lymph nodes and upper paraaortic nodes/celiac axis/spleen, 90% of patients present with contiguous sites of involvement.[72, 118] Furthermore, the pattern of spread among patients treated with limited irradiation also occurs in a contiguous fashion in most instances.[72] The theory of contiguity of spread and the development of treatment programs including presumptive treatment of uninvolved sites were important conceptual advances in the treatment of Hodgkin's disease.[75]

Visceral involvement may be secondary to extension from adjacent lymph node regions, for example, spread from enlarged mediastinal or bronchopulmonary (pulmonary hilar) lymph nodes directly into the pulmonary parenchyma. Disease may also extend from retroperitoneal or paravertebral lymph nodes into vertebral bodies causing blastic changes to develop in the involved bone and a characteristic "ivory vertebra" appearance on radiograph. Similar bony involvement may be noted in the pelvis, sternum, or ribs.

The mechanism of spread of disease to the spleen is unclear. However, the likelihood of disseminated disease increases as the extent of disease in the spleen increases.[73] Nearly all patients with hepatic or bone marrow involvement by Hodgkin's disease have (or have had) extensive involvement of the spleen.[58] This observation supports management programs with a systemic component when the spleen is extensively involved.

Unlike non-Hodgkin's lymphomas, Hodgkin's disease only rarely involves the gut-associated lymphoid tissues such as Waldeyer's ring and the Peyer's patches. In addition, although involvement by Hodgkin's disease occurs in the lungs, liver, bone marrow, and skeletal system, it is uncommon for it to involve other organ systems such as the upper aerodigestive tract, central nervous system, skin, and gastrointestinal tract.[72]

Although the pattern of spread of Hodgkin's disease is often predictable, the rapidity of growth and spread is not. Occasionally, a slow evolution of disease can be demonstrated on x-ray films or suspected by clinical history over a period of several years. It is unusual for disease to progress during the evaluation and staging process, which may require several weeks to complete.

One third of patients present with one of the three B symptoms: fever, night sweats, or weight loss. Patients with fever may describe a classic Pel-Ebstein pattern of waxing and waning fevers. The night sweats may be drenching, requiring a change of bedclothes. The presence of B symptoms often may be correlated with more extensive disease, and the natural history is generally worse than that of those who are asymptomatic. However, even patients with only one or two involved lymph node regions may provide a history of significant B symptoms. Recent data suggest that night sweats may be an unimportant B symptom, whereas patients who have both weight loss and fevers have a particularly poor prognosis.[26]

Patient age may have an effect on the natural history of Hodgkin's disease. Children with this disease have a particularly good prognosis compared with adults; thus, different treatment strategies have been developed for children.[33,50]

In the elderly, the presence of intercurrent illness often affects the aggressiveness of staging and treatment procedures, and is likely to have a detrimental effect on outcome.[3]

Hodgkin's disease may be diagnosed during pregnancy, and it is common for pregnancy to follow successful treatment. However, no evidence is found that pregnancy *per se* has any effect on the natural history of the disease.[66,72]

Accumulating data suggest that patients infected with the human immunodeficiency virus (HIV-1) display an unusual natural history if they develop Hodgkin's disease. Although HIV-infected patients do not appear to be at increased risk for the development of Hodgkin's disease, the disease tends to present in a more advanced stage, is more likely to be associated with systemic symptoms, and often has unusual patterns of involvement.[123] This may be secondary to an impaired host response against the disease. Treatment of these patients is challenging because they have poor tolerance for chemotherapy, and opportunistic infections are common.

TABLE 62–1
Diagnostic Workup for Hodgkin's Disease

HISTORY

Systemic B symptoms: unexplained fever, night sweats, weight loss > 10% of body weight in the last 6 months
Other symptoms: alcohol intolerance, pruritus, respiratory problems, energy loss

PHYSICAL EXAMINATION

Palpable nodes (note number, size, location, shape, consistency, mobility)
Palpable viscera

LABORATORY STUDIES

Standard
- Complete blood count
- Platelet count
- Liver and renal function tests
- Blood chemistries
- Thyroid function tests: T4, sensitive TSH

Complementary
- Erythrocyte sedimentation rate
- Serum copper

RADIOGRAPHIC STUDIES

Standard
- Chest radiograph: PA and lateral
- CT or MRI scan of thorax for disease detection and treatment planning purposes
- Bipedal lymphogram
- CT scan of abdomen and pelvis

Complementary
- Gallium scan, bone scan, if indicated

SPECIAL TESTS

Standard
- Cytologic examination of effusions, if present
- Bone marrow, needle biopsy (if subdiaphragmatic disease or B symptoms)

Complementary
- Echocardiogram (if large mediastinal mass is present)
- Percutaneous liver biopsy
- Peritoneoscopy
- Staging laparotomy with splenectomy, liver biopsy, selected lymph node biopsy, and open bone marrow biopsy

DIAGNOSTIC WORKUP

Staging procedures commonly used for Hodgkin's disease are listed in Table 62-1. Factors such as patient age and the presence of intercurrent disease should influence the selection of staging studies.

The physical examination should include a thorough lymph node examination. Routine hematologic evaluation should include a complete blood count and platelet count. Occasionally patients may display anemia, leukopenia, lymphopenia, or thrombocytosis. This is often a paraneoplastic effect, but may be indicative of bone marrow involvement. The serum alkaline phosphatase level may serve as a nonspecific marker of tumor activity or hepatic, bone marrow, or bone disease. If the alkaline phosphatase level is elevated, it is appropriate to examine other liver enzymes and to obtain a radionuclide bone scan, even in the absence of bony pain. The erythrocyte sedimentation rate and serum copper level may also be obtained because they occasionally serve as useful markers to assess response to treatment and subsequent disease activity.[41,113,131,133]

Radiographic evaluation should include a posteroanterior and lateral chest radiograph. A convenient definition of the extent of mediastinal adenopathy is to measure the maximum single width of the mediastinal mass and divide it by the maximum intrathoracic diameter (near the level of the diaphragm), as shown in Figure 62-1. When this ratio exceeds 1 : 3, the disease may be defined as bulky.[105] A computed tomography (CT) scan of the chest should also be obtained, because it provides ancillary information regarding the extent of intrathoracic disease and assists in treatment planning.[18,62]

The retroperitoneal lymph nodes are evaluated most accurately by bipedal lymphography (Fig. 62-2). The lymphogram reveals abnormalities not only in size of lymph nodes, but also in the internal architecture. The sensitivity, specificity, and overall

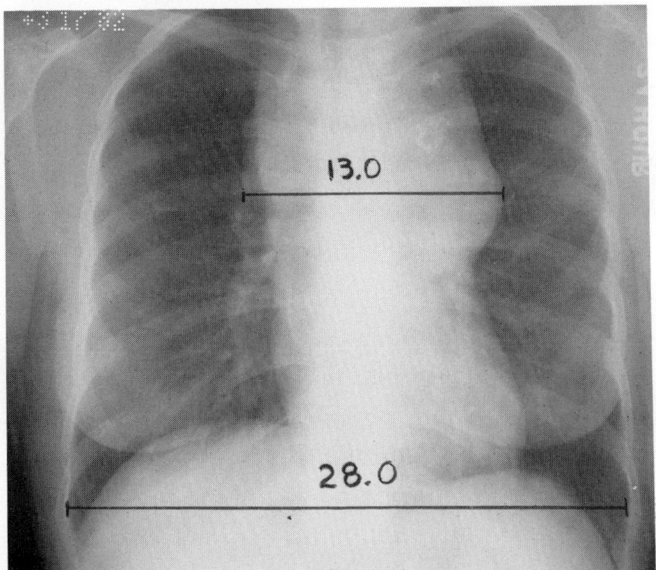

FIGURE 62–1. The mediastinal mass ratio (MMR). The ratio is defined as the maximum single horizontal mediastinal mass measurement divided by the maximum intrathoracic diameter (usually near the diaphragm). In this instance, MMR is 13.0/28.0 = 0.46.

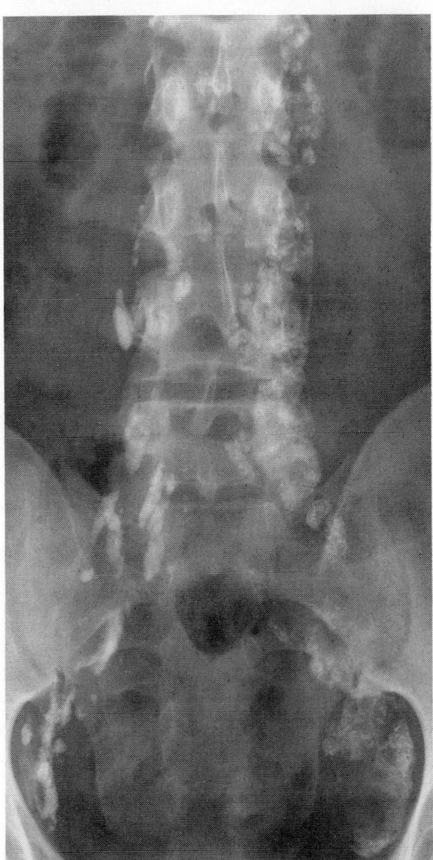

FIGURE 62–2. Example of a positive lymphogram. In this bipedal lymphogram, the nodes throughout the left side (paraaortic, common iliac, and external iliac) all are involved, demonstrating generalized enlargement and a foamy internal architectural pattern. Compare with the nodes opacified on the right (paracaval, common iliac, and external iliac), all of which appear normal.

accuracy of the lymphogram are 85%, 98%, and 95%, respectively.[20]

In the absence of adequate expertise for the performance of a lymphogram or in the presence of medical contraindication such as iodine allergy or chronic pulmonary disease, an abdominal and pelvic CT scan should be obtained. However, the CT scan is less sensitive, specific, and accurate (65%, 92%, and 87%) than the lymphogram.[20] Even in the spleen, where the risk of the presence of disease is high, the CT scan has an overall accuracy rate of only 58%. In addition, the CT scan is less useful than the lymphogram for the purposes of identification of isolated abnormal nodes for the surgeon, radiation therapy treatment planning, and subsequent follow-up evaluation.

Gallium scanning is used routinely at some centers. Its value depends on the quality of the study and the skill of the interpreter. The use of high-dose gallium provides the most valuable images. This technique may be especially helpful in evaluation of the mediastinum, including evaluation of residual disease after treatment.[2]

New modalities such as magnetic resonance imaging (MRI)[100, 142, 147] and ultrasonography[127] are being investigated to determine their usefulness. MRI scanning may prove to be especially useful in the evaluation of possible recurrent or residual disease.[100]

A posterior iliac crest, needle bone marrow biopsy may be done in selected patients. Because the yield is exceeding low in asymptomatic patients with limited clinical disease, it should be restricted to patients who have B symptoms or clinical evidence of subdiaphragmatic disease. The overall incidence of bone marrow involvement in Hodgkin's disease is only 5%.

The role of laparotomy in the staging of Hodgkin's disease remains controversial. The procedure includes a splenectomy, selected lymph node biopsies, liver biopsies, and an open bone marrow biopsy.[43] Premenopausal women also undergo a bilateral midline oophoropexy.[80] Laparotomy became a routine part of the staging evaluation at many centers in the late 1960s and early 1970s. However, as the quality of radiographic imaging has improved and our experience has provided a better ability to predict the yield of laparotomy in different clinical situations, the use of staging laparotomy has become more selective. In addition, concern has been raised regarding potential long-term toxicities of splenectomy, including overwhelming sepsis[34] and a possible increased risk of secondary leukemia among patients who later receive chemotherapy.[117, 136]

The primary role of laparotomy is the identification of patients who are candidates for treatment with irradiation alone; it need not be performed when clinical characteristics mandate the use of chemotherapy, such as in most patients with bulky mediastinal disease (if combined modality therapy is planned), patients with clinical Stage IIIB to IV disease, and all patients with a positive percutaneous needle bone marrow biopsy (pathologic Stage IV_{M+}). Other exceptions include the elderly and persons with intercurrent medical problems. In some patients, the yield of laparotomy is so small that it need not be done, as in nodular sclerosing Hodgkin's disease with clinical disease limited to intrathoracic sites or lymphocyte predominance Hodgkin's disease limited to the high cervical region.

The yield of laparotomy in 915 patients with clinical Stage I or II Hodgkin's disease treated at Stanford University was reviewed recently.[81] Table 62-2 shows the yield of laparotomy in different clinical situations. Subgroups of patients who have a very low probability of disease being identified below the diaphragm included the following: (1) patients with clinical disease limited to intrathoracic sites (yield = 0%), (2) Stage I females (yield = 6%), (3) Stage I males with lymphocyte predominance or interfollicular histology (yield = 4%), and (4) Stage II

TABLE 62–2
Yield of Laparotomy According to Major Clinical Characteristics: Results in 915 Patients Staged at Stanford

CHARACTERISTIC	NUMBER OF PATIENTS	POSITIVE LAPAROTOMY	PERCENT YIELD
Sex			
Male	519	174	36
Female	396	82	21
Symptoms			
A	841	217	26
B	174	57	33
Histology			
LPHD, NSHD	769	194	25
MCHD	128	58	45
Clinical Stage I			
Right neck	43	8	19
Left neck	61	15	25
Mediastinum	12	0	0
Axilla (right or left)	18	4	22
Clinical Stage			
I	137	27	20
II	778	229	29
Total group	915	256	28

LP: lymphocyte predominance; NS: nodular sclerosis; MC: mixed cellularity
(Modified from Leibenhaut MH, Hoppe RT, Efron B, et al: J Clin Oncol 7:81, 1989)

females with three or fewer sites of clinical involvement *and* younger than 27 years (yield = 9%). For all other clinical groups the yield of laparotomy was 20% or greater.

STAGING

The Ann Arbor staging system for Hodgkin's Disease, used since 1971, is outlined in Table 62-3.[14] The lymphoid regions defined in this system are shown in Figure 62-3. The Ann Arbor system includes designation of a clinical stage (CS), based on the results of the initial biopsy and clinical staging studies, and a pathologic stage (PS), based on the results of any subsequent biopsies. Deficiencies of the Ann Arbor system include its failure to consider bulk and the lack of a more precise definition of the E-lesion.[23]

Modifications of the Ann Arbor system have been suggested. For example, the concept of substaging in PS III has been proposed and widely adopted.[29] PS III_1 indicates involvement limited to the upper abdomen (spleen, splenic hilar, celiac, and portahepatic nodes), whereas PS III_2 includes involvement of the paraaortic, mesenteric, or pelvic lymph nodes. A description of the extent of splenic involvement may also be useful.[61] PS III_{S+} minimal indicates fewer than five nodules visible in the resected splenectomy specimen, and PS III_{S+} extensive indicates that five or more nodules were identified.

PATHOLOGIC CLASSIFICATION

The diagnostic cell of Hodgkin's disease is the Reed-Sternberg cell, which has a classic appearance in fixed sections stained with hematoxylin and eosin. It is typically binucleate, with a prominent, centrally located nucleolus in each nucleus, a well-demarcated nuclear membrane, and eosinophilic cytoplasm with a perinuclear halo. However, these cells usually account for less than 1% of the cells in a specimen involved by Hodgkin's disease. The majority of the cells are lymphoid cells, eosinophils, plasma cells, and other normal cells.

The nature of the Reed-Sternberg cell is controversial. The cell of origin has been reported to be a B cell, T cell, lymphoid precursor cell, macrophage, monocyte, and dendritic reticulum cell.[35,67] In most instances, the Reed-Sternberg cells stain positively with the antigranulocyte monoclonal antibody Leu-M1 (CD15), the macrophage marker Leu-M3, and the Ki-67 marker for actively proliferating cells; they also express the IL2

TABLE 62–3
Ann Arbor Staging Classification

Stage I	Involvement of a single lymph node region
Stage II	Involvement of two or more lymph node regions on the same side of the diaphragm (II) or localized involvement of an extralymphatic organ or site and of one or more lymph node regions on the same side of the diaphragm (IIE)
Stage III	Involvement of lymph node regions on both sides of the diaphragm (III), which may also be accompanied by involvement of the spleen (IIIS) or by localized involvement of an extralymphatic organ or site (IIIE) or both (IIISE)
Stage IV	Diffuse or disseminated involvement of one or more extralymphatic organs or tissues, with or without associated lymph node involvement

The absence or presence of fever, night sweats, and/or unexplained loss of 10% or more of body weight in the 6 months before diagnosis is denoted by the suffix letters A or B, respectively.

Patients are assigned a clinical stage (CS) based on the initial biopsy and all subsequent nonsurgical staging studies. A pathologic stage (PS) is assigned based on all clinical studies as well as subsequent surgical staging procedures such as bone marrow biopsy, staging laparotomy, and splenectomy.

(Modified from Carbone PP, Kaplan HS, Mushoff K, et al: Cancer Res 31:1860, 1971)

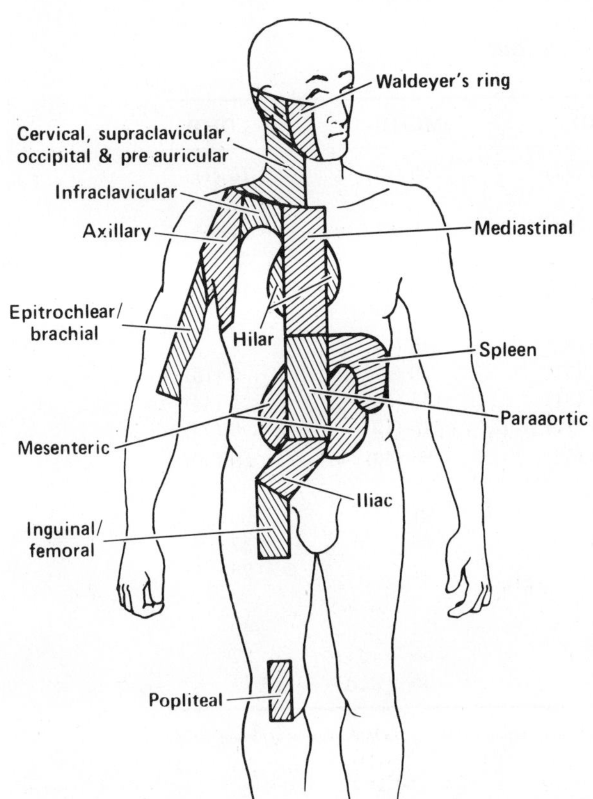

FIGURE 62–3. The lymphoid regions as defined in the Ann Arbor staging system. Note that the cervical, supraclavicular, occipital, and preauricular nodes are included in a *single* region. The mediastinum and hila make up *three* regions. (Hoppe RT: Curr Probl Cancer 11(6):379, 1987)

receptor (TAC) and HLA-DR antigens. They stain negatively with pan-B cell markers such as B-1 and the leukocyte common antigen LCA (CD45).[21,35,141]

An exception to this pattern is nodular lymphocyte predominance Hodgkin's disease, in which the Reed-Sternberg cells are strongly reactive for leukocyte common antigen and negative for Leu-M1.[104] This observation, together with reports of a different clinical behavior of the nodular form of lymphocyte predominance Hodgkin's disease, suggests that this entity may actually be a form of non-Hodgkin's lymphoma.[104,106,114]

There are four histologic subtypes of Hodgkin's disease as defined by the Rye modification of the Lukes and Butler system.[90]

Lymphocyte predominance Hodgkin's disease (LPHD) is characterized by an abundance of normal-appearing lymphocytes and a scarcity of abnormal cells. It is often diagnosed in young people. Patients frequently present with early stage disease, and systemic symptoms are uncommon (<10%). The natural history is the most favorable of the histologic subtypes. Both diffuse and nodular subtypes have been described. The diffuse form has a relapse and survival pattern similar to other forms of Hodgkin's disease, whereas the nodular form demonstrates a pattern of late relapse but good survival, similar to that of the low-grade lymphomas.[114]

Nodular sclerosis Hodgkin's disease is the most common histologic subtype of Hodgkin's disease in the United States. Involved nodes are traversed by broad bands of birefringent collagen that surround nodules of cells consisting of lymphocytes, eosinophils, plasma cells, and tissue histiocytes, intermixed with a variable proportion of atypical mononuclear cells and Reed-Sternberg cells. These cells may be in empty (lacunar) spaces, artifacts of formalin fixation. Clinically, the mediastinum is often involved. One third of patients have B symptoms. The natural history of nodular sclerosis is less favorable than that of lymphocyte predominance.

Mixed cellularity Hodgkin's disease is characterized by a diffuse effacement of lymph nodes by lymphocytes, eosinophils, plasma cells, and relatively abundant atypical mononuclear and Reed-Sternberg cells. Patients with mixed cellularity Hodgkin's disease present more commonly with advanced disease and tend to be slightly older than those with nodular sclerosing or lymphocyte predominance. The natural history of mixed cellularity Hodgkin's disease is less favorable than that of nodular sclerosing.

Lymphocyte depletion Hodgkin's disease is characterized by a paucity of normal-appearing cells and an abundance of abnormal mononuclear cells, Reed-Sternberg cells, and Reed-Sternberg variants. This subtype may occasionally be difficult to differentiate from pleomorphic large cell lymphoma. This form of Hodgkin's disease is the least common in the United States. It tends to occur in older patients and is more likely to be associated with advanced disease and B symptoms. It has the worst prognosis of all histologic subtypes of Hodgkin's disease.

Interfollicular Hodgkin's disease is an uncommon pattern of focal involvement of a lymph node in which there is reactive hyperplasia with a small focus of Hodgkin's disease in the interfollicular zone. It is easy to confuse these cases with reactive lymphoid hyperplasia.[32]

Review by a good hematopathologist is indicated in all cases of Hodgkin's disease. Other diseases, including varieties of non-Hodgkin's lymphoma, may mimic the appearance of Hodgkin's disease. Benign reactive processes associated with viral illnesses or diphenylhydantoin use also may be confused with Hodgkin's disease.

Table 62-4 summarizes the characteristics of patients treated at Stanford from 1968 to 1988, according to histologic subtype. These characteristics are similar to those reported from many other large centers in the United States and Western Europe. However, the distribution of histologic subtypes and clinical behavior reported from South America, Asia, Africa, Eastern Europe, and even some parts of the United States indicates a greater proportion of unfavorable histologies and more aggressive clinical behavior in these regions.[65]

PROGNOSTIC FACTORS AND THERAPEUTIC IMPLICATIONS

Patient-related prognostic factors are gender, age, and the presence of intercurrent disease. Disease-related prognostic factors are histology stage, bulk, presence of B symptoms, number of involved sites, serum markers of disease activity, general distribution of disease (*e.g.*, III_1 *versus* III_2), and extent of splenic involvement.

Age

The challenge of managing Hodgkin's disease in children is complicated by the potential complications of growth impairment and soft tissue deformity secondary to high-dose irradiation. Doses of more than 1500 cGy to 2500 are associated with subsequent abnormalities in height and soft tissue development. Therefore, programs incorporating high-dose irradia-

TABLE 62–4
Histologic Subtype Versus Clinical Characteristics of 1745 Patients Treated for Hodgkin's Disease at Stanford (1968–1988)

	LPHD	NSHD	MCHD	LDHD
No. (%)	87 (5)	1348 (77)	295 (17)	15 (1)
Age				
range	4–65	2–82	4–81	11–65
median	31	26	30	38
Male:female ratio	73:14	708:640	240:55	10:5
Stage				
I (%)	37 (43)	86 (6)	40 (14)	—
II (%)	33 (38)	691 (51)	79 (27)	2 (13)
III (%)	16 (18)	415 (31)	133 (45)	5 (33)
IV (%)	1 (1)	156 (12)	43 (15)	8 (53)
B Symptoms (%)	2 (2)	438 (32)	88 (30)	9 (60)
Actuarial survival (%)*				
5-year	95	88	81	65
10-year	80	79	69	37
15-year	70	72	54	25
Actuarial FFR (%)				
5-year	90	72	74	40
10-year	82	69	68	27
15-year	79	69	65	13

HD: Hodgkin's disease; LP: lymphocyte predominance; NS: nodular sclerosis; MC: mixed cellularity; LD: lymphocyte depletion; FFR: freedom from relapse
**Actuarial survival data include all causes of death.*

tion have been abandoned. Most investigators advocate the use of chemotherapy plus low-dose (1500 cGy to 2000 cGy) irradiation,[33,69] whereas others advocate the use of chemotherapy alone.[5,36]

The treatment of Hodgkin's disease in elderly patients also poses a challenge.[3] Affected persons more frequently have intercurrent disease and cannot tolerate the aggressive staging and management programs used for younger persons. These patients should be treated with slower fractionation programs and observed carefully for signs of weight loss or general deterioration.

Gender

Many large series report a slightly worse outcome for men than for women. Gender may influence the choice of treatment based on consideration of toxicities, especially reproductive complications. Although fertility may be preserved in most men who require pelvic irradiation,[103] chemotherapy programs that contain alkylating agents cause sterility in most men. In women, if pelvic lymph node irradiation is required, the ovaries cannot be protected completely, even when an oophoropexy has been performed.[80] Women over 30 are very likely to have menopausal symptoms after pelvic irradiation.[64]

Histology

The histologic subtype of Hodgkin's disease has a minor impact on therapy. Reproducibility and agreement of different pathologists are not perfect.[24] After the extent of disease has been determined, histologic subtype seems to have little additional impact on prognosis.

Ann Arbor Stage

The Ann Arbor stage is the most important prognostic factor influencing therapy. Data generated at a time when the treatment of many patients was suboptimal show a marked impact of stage on prognosis. With current management programs, this distinction has been blurred. However, although the prognostic value of stage may have been lost, it is a very important factor in determining the appropriate treatment program.

Bulk

Bulk of disease is important, especially in the mediastinum. Bulk may be defined by absolute measurements, ratios of mass to anatomic measurements, surface area on radiographs, or volumetric determinations. Most series report that the risk of relapse after treatment with single-modality therapy is greater in the presence of bulky mediastinal disease than in nonbulky disease.[8,57,93,144,146] In some instances, the special problems associated with bulky disease may be addressed by modifications of radiation therapy techniques.[55,79] At other times, it is more rational to simply use a combined modality approach.[52,84]

Disease Extent

Other measurements of disease extent that may influence treatment selection for Hodgkin's disease are the presence of B symptoms, the number of sites of involvement, the presence of disease in the lower abdomen (III_2 *versus* III_1), the presence of extensive splenic involvement, and the elevation of serum markers such as erythrocyte sedimentation rate.

GENERAL MANAGEMENT

Radiation Therapy

Irradiation is the most effective single agent for the treatment of patients with Hodgkin's disease. Optimal irradiation technique requires the use of megavoltage photon beams, large fields contoured to the patient's anatomy and tumor configuration, a tumoridical dose, opposed-field fractionated treatment, pretreatment simulation, and port film verification during therapy. Careful attention must be paid to every detail of therapy.

The use of a linear accelerator that produces 6 MV to 10 MV photons permits the treatment of large fields at an extended distance and provides a modest amount of skin sparing. Routine field simulation and port film verification provide optimal field design and documentation that the proposed treatment is executed properly. The recommendations for a tumoricidal dose of irradiation range from 3500 to 4400 cGy,[47,74] fractionated at a rate of 750 cGy to 1000 cGy per week. Evenly weighted opposed-field treatments are generally used; all fields are treated daily with fractions of 150 cGy to 200 cGy, depending on field size, patient tolerance, and other factors. A key component in curative irradiation programs is the use of prophylactic treatment to clinically uninvolved areas. The dose necessary to eradicate minimal disease in this setting is uncertain, but a minimum of 3000 cGy to 3600 cGy is usually recommended.

Chemotherapy

The effective use of combination chemotherapy in Hodgkin's disease has led to an improved prognosis for patients with advanced stage disease. The key concept of combination chemotherapy is the use of drugs that are effective as single agents but do not have overlapping toxicities. The drugs are administered intermittently, with periods of rest that permit normal tissue recovery (especially hematologic) between periods of intensive therapy. The initial drug combination that proved so successful in treating Hodgkin's disease was nitrogen mustard, vincristine, procarbazine, and prednisone (MOPP), reported by DeVita and associates from the National Cancer Institute.[30,31] The schedule of drug administration is shown in Table 62-5.

The acute toxicities of MOPP are nausea, vomiting, peripheral neuropathy, constipation, leukopenia, and thrombocytopenia. A number of MOPP-like programs that achieve comparable results with similar drugs but with less toxicity have been developed; however, MOPP remains a "gold standard."

With the advent of doxorubicin (Adriamycin), completely novel drug combinations were developed. The most successful of these is ABVD, which includes doxorubicin. bleomycin, vinblastine, and decarbazine.[7,10] Some trials suggest that ABVD is at least as good as, if not better than, MOPP in advanced Hodgkin's disease.

Different combinations of drugs have been combined in an alternating fashion, to prevent the emergence of resistant clones of cells. Most notable among these "alternating non-cross-resistant" regimens is the MOPP/ABVD combination, in which monthly cycles of MOPP are alternated with monthly cycles of ABVD.[9] A more recent innovation has been the MOPP/ABV hybrid program.[77] Table 62-5 summarizes the dosages and scheduling of these drug combinations.

Combined-Modality Therapy

Important considerations in combined-modality therapy are the selection of drugs, the sequence of therapy, the dose of radiation, the fields to be treated, and overlapping toxicities. It is logical to initiate treatment with chemotherapy. This has the advantage of treating all sites of disease at the outset (in Stage III to IV) and reducing bulky disease to facilitate subsequent irradiation (in the mediastinum). An entire course of chemotherapy may be administered before any irradiation,[110] but some combined-modality programs incorporate a split-course or alternating-treatment approach.[60] The radiation dose used

TABLE 62–5
Common Drug Combinations Used in the Treatment of Hodgkin's Disease

DRUG COMBINATION	AGENTS	DOSE (mg/m²)	ROUTE	TREATMENT DAY(S)	CYCLE DURATION (DAYS)
MOPP[31]	nitrogen mustard	6	IV	1, 8	28
	vincristine	1.4†	IV	1, 8	
	procarbazine	100	PO	1–14	
	prednisone	40	PO	1–14	
ABVD[10]	doxorubicin*	25	IV	1, 15	28
	bleomycin	10	IV	1, 15	
	vinblastine	6	IV	1, 15	
	dacarbazine	375	IV	1, 15	
MOPP/ABVD[9]	MOPP			1–14	56
	ABVD			29, 43	
MOPP/ABV[7]	MOPP			1–7	28
	doxorubicin*	35	IV	8	
	bleomycin	10	IV	8	
	vinblastine	6	IV	8	
	prednisone	40	PO	8–14	

IV: intravenous; PO: oral
** Adriamycin*
† Maximum = 2.0 mg

in combined modality studies ranges from 2500 cGy to 4000 cGy.[60,110]

RADIATION THERAPY TECHNIQUES

The use of a linear accelerator is essential in the technique of delivering optimal irradiation for patients with Hodgkin's disease. The physical characteristics of the specific machine must be known in detail by the radiation oncologist. Dose rate, depth dose characteristics, and the availability of large-field sizes at practical distances with relatively flat isodose contours all are important features of these machines. It is essential to verify the flatness of the isodose distribution for large fields at long distances; for some machines, a special beam-flattening filter may be required to eliminate very high-dose regions near the lateral edges of large fields at superficial depths.

The principal objective of the irradiation program is to treat the contiguous lymphatic chains to a dose that offers a strong probability of tumor eradication. This requires a well-collimated megavoltage beam with skin sparing and minimal penumbra. Meticulous treatment planning, simulation, and frequent verification by portal films are also crucial factors in the success of treatment.[72,76]

Several techniques for shaping large fields have been described. Kaplan first described a technique using nondivergent lead blocks placed on a table moderately close to the patient and positioned by means of a template.[72] The most common adaptation today is the use of divergent Cerrobend blocks attached to a Lucite plate and mounted to the head of the machine. Treatment at an extended distance (110 cm to 140 cm SSD [source-skin distance]) may be necessary to achieve the large field sizes required. Opposed-field treatment technique generally requires alternate prone and supine positioning of the patient; however, new extended travel distance couches may permit opposed-field treatment without changing patient position. Use of body molds made of supporting plastic foam reduces body movement and rotation and may increase patient comfort.

Large field size, treatment at an extended SSD, irregular-shaped blocks, and the presence of slanting body contours produce an inhomogeneous dose distribution. Treatment planning computers facilitate these dose calculations and should include the effects of both primary and scattered radiation to each point of calculation. The minimum dosimetry should include an irregular field point calculation for each important nodal region within the field. The dose variation determined by these calculations must be compensated for by individually designed compensators or selective area blocking.[51]

When patients require separate treatment to adjacent regions, the calculation of field separation (gap) is exceedingly important.[91] Special additional cord blocking should be used when adjacent fields overlie the spinal cord.

The Mantle

The mantle field includes all the major lymph node regions above the diaphragm. These regions are involved or are at high risk for involvement in most patients with Hodgkin's disease. The field extends from the inferior portion of the mandible nearly to the level of the insertion of the diaphragm. Individually contoured lung blocks are designed to conform to the patient's anatomy and tumor distribution.

A typical example of mantle field blocking is shown in Figure 62-4. In addition to the lung blocks, blocks can be placed over the occipital region and spinal cord posteriorly, the larynx anteriorly, and the humeral heads both anteriorly and posteriorly. Special spinal cord blocking may not be needed when the

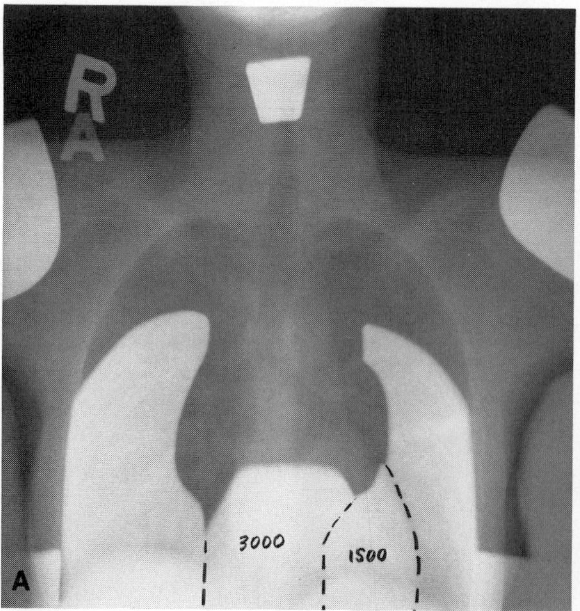

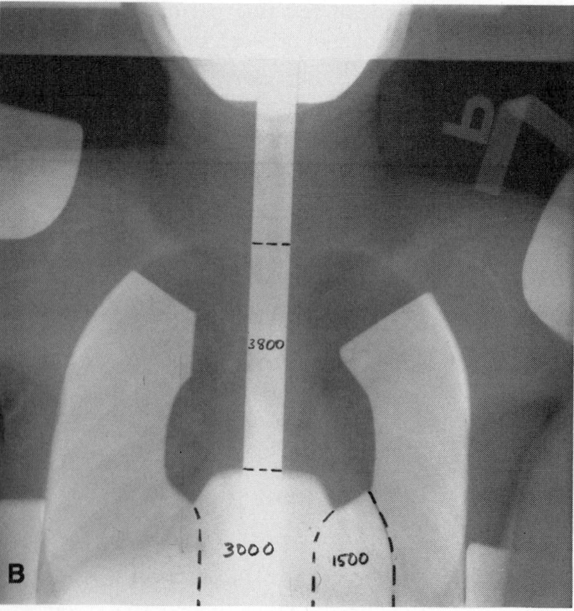

FIGURE 62–4. Anterior and posterior port films showing the configuration of blocks within the mantle field. In typical instances (mediastinum involved, but no bulky disease), the entire cardiac silhouette is treated to 1500 cGy. The apex of the heart is blocked after 1500 cGy and the subcarinal portion of the heart after 3000 cGy to 3500 cGy. (**A**) Note on the anterior field that the infraclavicular fossa is exposed. Blocks are placed over the larynx, humeral heads, and axillary skin folds. (**B**) On the posterior field, the occipital portion of the skull and cervical cord are shielded from the outset. The posterior cord block is extended over the thoracic spine at a dose calculated to limit the dose to the thoracic spinal cord to 3600 to 3800 cGy. Cord blocking should be used when the prescribed dose to the mantle field is ≥ 4000 cGy. When lower doses are prescribed, cord-blocking techniques can be modified.

prescribed tumor dose is only 3600 cGy, but it is required when the dose is 4400 cGy. At Stanford University, the mantle is treated by evenly weighted anterior-posterior opposed technique, 150 cGy to 180 cGy per fraction, five days per week, with both fields treated daily. When a dose of 4000 cGy or more is prescribed, a posterior cord block (5 half-value layers) is inserted over the cervical cord from the outset of treatment (unless contraindicated). The posterior cord block is extended over the thoracic cord at a dose calculated to limit the cord dose to 3600 cGy to 3800 cGy, depending on whether the mediastinum is involved or uninvolved and whether treatment is with irradiation alone or combined-modality therapy. A small trapezoidal block is placed anteriorly over the larynx from the outset, except in the presence of immediately adjacent lymphadenopathy. In the presence of any mediastinal disease, the entire cardiac silhouette is irradiated to 1500 cGy, with a block over the apex of the heart thereafter to shield a portion of the pericardium. After a dose of 3000 cGy to 3500 cGy has been delivered, a block is placed in the subcarinal region (approximately 5 cm below the carina), shielding even more of the pericardium and heart.[16,50,72]

Partial transmission blocks can be used to deliver low-dose irradiation to the lungs. For example, if the pulmonary hilar lypmh nodes are involved and a patient is being treated with irradiation alone, a 37% transmission lung block can be used to deliver 1500 cGy to 1650 cGy to the lung.[101] This appears to be an adequate dose for the treatment of occult microscopic disease in the pulmonary parenchyma, thus decreasing the risk of failure in that site.[16]

The mantle field may be modified during therapy. When patients with large mediastinal masses are treated, as the disease regresses, wider blocks should be cut to protect more of the lungs (shrinking-field technique). When the mediastinal mass is large, treatment may be given slowly (150 cGy per day to a total dose of 1500 cGy). Therapy is then interrupted for 7 to 14 days to permit further regression of disease and redesign of the lung blocks. An example of this shrinking-field technique is shown in Figure 62-5. In some patients, low-dose mantle irradiation

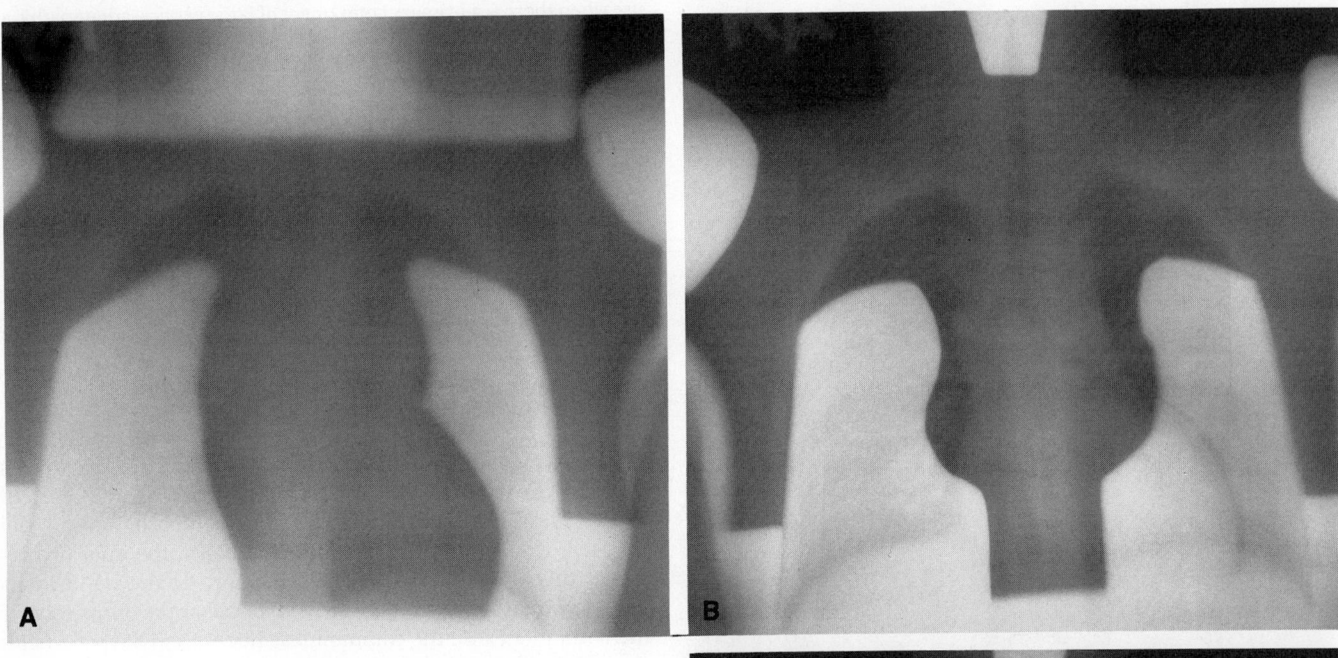

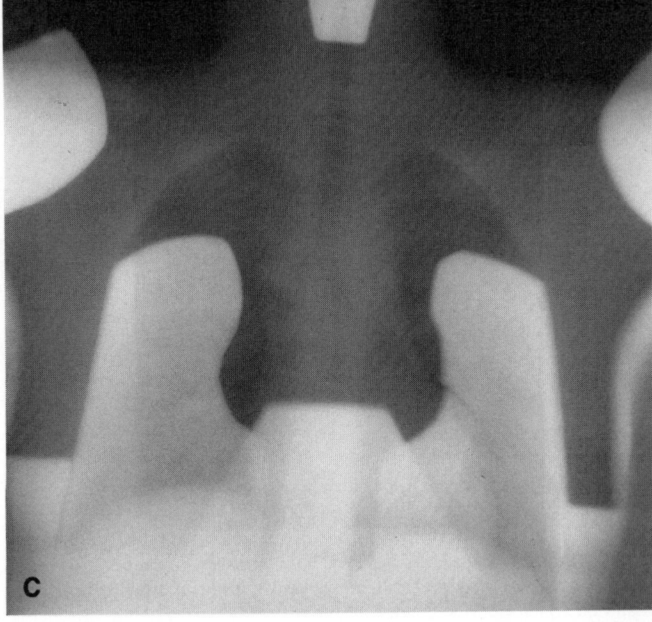

FIGURE 62–5. Example of the shrinking mantle field technique in a patient with a large mediastinal mass. (**A**) Initial anterior port film. Note that the entire cardiac silhouette is included in the field. A lower mantle field border is chosen such that the entire pericardium is included in the mantle field, minimizing the risk of recurrence in the cardiophrenic angles. (**B**) After a dose of 1500 cGy has been delivered to the mediastinum, substantial regression of mediastinal disease occurred. Wider lung blocks are cut, and a block is placed over the apical portion of the pericardium. (**C**) After a dose of 3000 cGy has been delivered to the mediastinum, a block is placed over the subcarinal portion of the heart and pericardium.

should be completed before staging laparotomy to avoid problems with intubation or anesthesia.[105]

Significant individualization of the mantle field may be indicated. For example, disease may extend anteriorly into the chest wall. If the areas of extension are otherwise within the normal boundaries of the mantle, bolus can be used on the anterior field to build up the dose in that region. However, in some instances disease may extend more laterally in the chest wall, underneath the lung blocks. In this situation normal lung blocks can be used; however, the disease that extends under the lung blocks must be boosted with electrons or tangential photon fields if irradiation alone is to be used.

Preauricular Field

The preauricular ("small Waldeyer") field is designed to encompass the preauricular lymph nodes (Fig. 62-6). This field can be treated with opposed lateral or unilateral photons or, preferably, with a unilateral 6 MeV to 9 MeV electron field to spare the contralateral parotid. This region should be treated when there is clinical involvement of the preauricular nodes. In addition, when the cervical lymph nodes are involved at a level superior to the thyroid notch, the preauricular nodes are at risk for contiguous spread, and this field may be treated prophylactically to 3600 cGy.

In some instances, the primary site of enlarged nodes may include bulky high cervical nodes, extending very near the upper border of the typical mantle field. In this setting, large opposed lateral Waldeyer fields can be used to encompass the upper cervical and adjacent nodes (Fig. 62-7). The upper border of the mantle field is then matched to the lower border of this field in the low neck.[56]

It is almost always possible to ensure that the teeth are outside the primary radiation field whether preauricular nodes are treated or not. However, if a patient has difficulty extending the neck, the superior border of the mantle field may pass through the teeth. In this case a simple midline block should be used to protect the teeth and oral cavity.

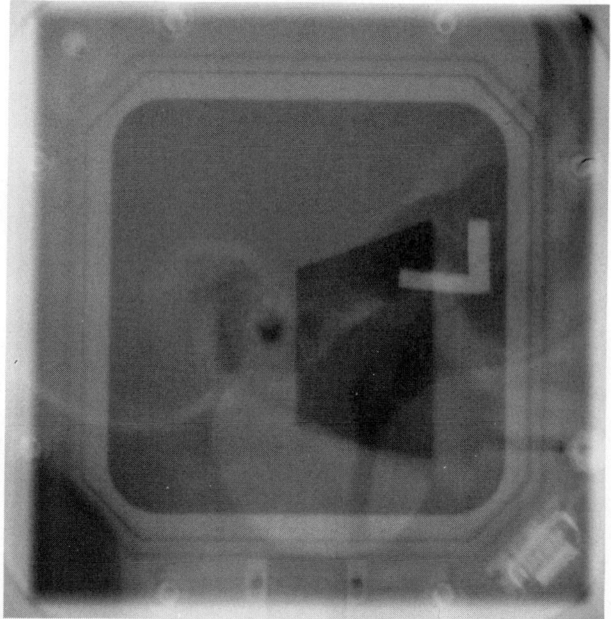

FIGURE 62–6. The small preauricular field. A unilateral preauricular field may be treated with 6 MeV to 9 MeV electrons. Note in this portal film that the posterior border of the field is just anterior to the external auditory canal; the superior border bisects the sphenoid sinus; the anterior border is posterior to the teeth; and the inferior border is matched to the mantle field.

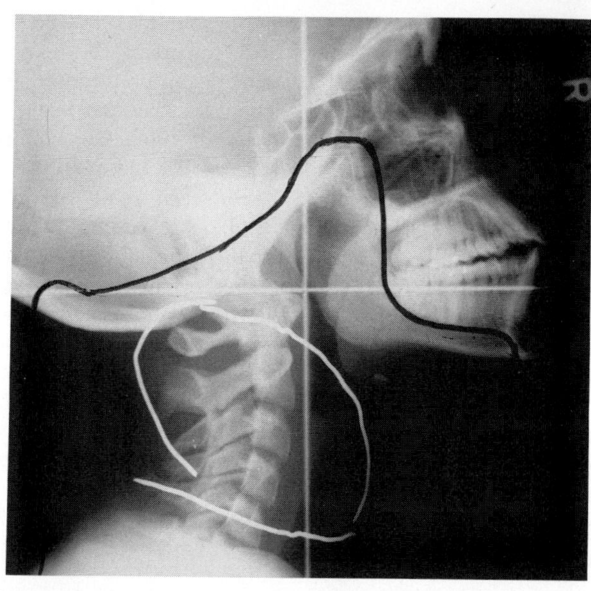

FIGURE 62–7. The large Waldeyer field. This field is appropriate to use when there is a primary component of large cervical adenopathy, as outlined by a lead wire in this setup film. This field should include the submandibular, preauricular, occipital, and high cervical nodes. The inferior border of the field is matched to the mantle low in the neck, below the cervical adenopathy. In most instances, regression of disease in the first 2500 cGy to 3000 cGy permits switching to a standard mantle with high superior border, matched to a small preauricular field.

Subdiaphragmatic Fields

The classic subdiaphragmatic irradiation field for Hodgkin's disease is the inverted Y, which includes the retroperitoneal and pelvic lymph nodes. With current treatment programs, a full inverted Y is rarely treated. More commonly, the inferior border of the subdiaphragmatic field is drawn at the L4–5 interspace (paraaortic/splenic pedicle field) or below the bifurcation of the aorta to include the common iliac nodes as well (spade field) (Fig. 62-8). If the spleen is intact, the entire spleen, not simply the splenic hilar region, is included in the field. Sequential treatment to a mantle and inverted-Y field is referred to as *total lymphoid irradiation.* When the subdiaphragmatic field does not include the pelvis, the term *subtotal lymphoid irradiation* is used.

Low-dose irradiation to the liver can be achieved with a partial transmission liver block.[124] A 50% transmission block delivers 2000 cGy to 2200 cGy to the liver during the same period of time in which the paraaortic nodes receive 4000 cGy to 4400 cGy. Hepatic irradiation can be used when there is splenic involvement, when irradiation alone is being used as primary treatment, or in combined-modality programs when the liver is involved.

Careful blocking considerations are required when the pelvic region is treated. Because the volume of marrow in the pelvis is substantial, the fields must be shaped carefully to minimize the amount of marrow treated (Fig. 62-9). If a lymphogram has been performed, more precise delineation of the pelvic field is possible and more bone marrow can be spared. Gonadal toxicity may also be an issue. In women, the ovaries normally overlie the iliac lymph nodes. To avoid irradiation-induced amenorrhea, an oophoropexy must be performed. This procedure is done by

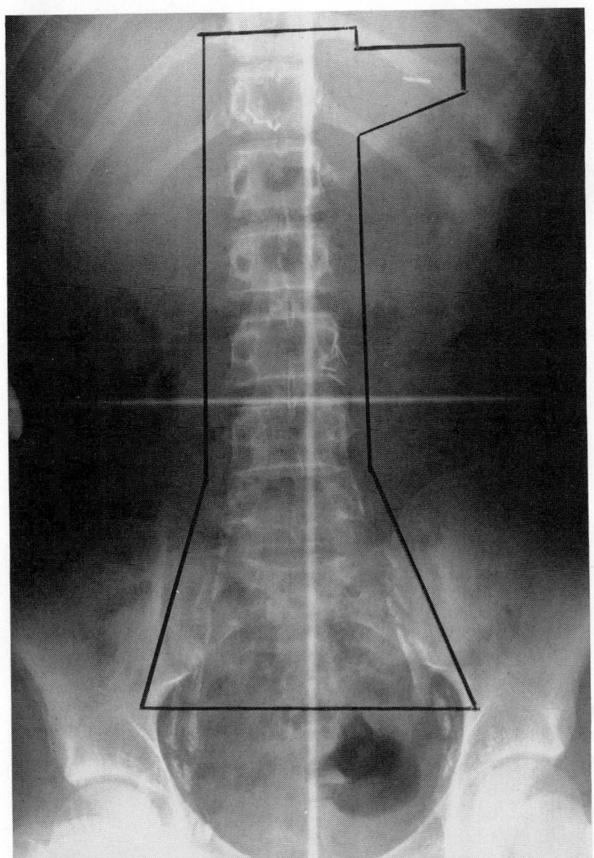

FIGURE 62–8. The spade field. In this setup film, note inclusion of the splenic pedicle region (marked by a surgical clip). The kidneys have been localized by previous CT scan and confirmed to be outside the irradiation field. The lower border of the field is chosen to include the common iliac nodes. Note how the lymphogram permits maximum tailoring of the field to minimize the amount of pelvic irradiation. In females, the inferior border of the field is drawn at a higher level if there has not been an oophoropexy or if the transposed ovaries are high up behind the uterus. A paraaortic/splenic pedicle field would have its inferior border at the L4–5 interspace.

medial transposition of the ovaries and is accomplished most readily at the time of staging laparotomy. The surgeon marks the ovaries with radiopaque sutures or clips and places them medially and as low as possible behind the uterine body. A double-thickness (10 HVL) midline block is then used; its location is guided by the position of the opacified nodes and transposed ovaries. When the ovaries are at least 2 cm from the edge of this block, the dose is limited to 8% of that delivered to the iliac nodes.[80]

In males, if no special blocking is provided for the testes, the testicular dose may be as high as 10% of the dose delivered to the inguinal-femoral nodes. Use of a double-thickness midline block and specially constructed testicular shield can reduce this dose to 0.75% to 3.0%, which is largely secondary to internal scatter. The precise dose depends on the position of the testes relative to the inferior margin of the inguinal-femoral field.

RESULTS OF THERAPY

An evaluation of efficacy of management programs involves the assessment of freedom from relapse, freedom from second relapse, survival, and risk of various complications. The results achieved at Stanford using contemporary treatment techniques are displayed in Figure 62-10.

Given the high degree of responsiveness of Hodgkin's disease to both irradiation and chemotherapy, it is not surprising that a variety of management programs have been proposed as appropriate for patients with different stages of the disease. These programs have achieved similar survival rates; however, there are important differences in freedom from relapse or potential complications of therapy. It is difficult to compare the results reported from different treatment centers because of variation in patient selection, staging evaluation, definition of response criteria, and so on. The results described in the following sections emphasize treatment programs that have been identified as "state of the art" by the Hodgkin's Disease Consensus Committee of the Patterns of Care Study (PCS) of the American College of Radiology.[51]

Supradiaphragmatic Stages I to IIA Disease

The majority of patients with Stages I to II disease can be managed effectively with irradiation alone. Ninety percent of these patients have supradiaphragmatic disease. After a staging laparotomy, appropriate treatment consists of mantle irradiation (3600 cGy to 4400 cGy) followed by a prophylactic spade or paraaortic/splenic pedicle field (3000 cGy to 4000 cGy).

Series that use this management program report a 10-year survival rate of nearly 90% and a 10-year relapse-free rate of 75% to 80% (Table 62-6). Similar results can be achieved using "extended mantle" irradiation, which includes prophylactic irradiation to the level of L4.[37]

Important management questions in this group of patients regard the necessity for treatment below the diaphragm and the efficacy of treatment without performing a staging laparotomy.

Treatment to the mantle only in laparotomy-staged patients was the standard approach at The Royal Marsden Hospital from 1970 to 1978.[138] They reported a 10-year relapse-free rate of 66%, which is slightly inferior to results reported from series in which prophylactic subdiaphragmatic treatment was used (Table 62-6). The majority of relapses in these patients were subdiaphragmatic, most commonly in paraaortic nodes. This observation supports the use of subdiaphragmatic irradiation in this group.

At centers where staging laparotomy has not been available, patients with Stages I to II disease are treated with mantle and paraaortic/spleen fields. Between 1972 and 1976, the EORTC group conducted a clinical trial in which patients were randomized to undergo laparotomy or clinical staging only.[132] All patients received prophylactic subdiaphragmatic irradiation (including the spleen, if no splenectomy had been performed). The 7-year relapse-free survival rate was 62% in the nonlaparotomy group and 69% in the surgically staged patients (Table 62-6).

At Princess Margaret Hospital in Toronto, staging laparotomy is performed only in selected circumstances. Prognostic groups that have different outcomes after treatment with irradiation alone were identified.[129] A favorable group included patients with clinical Stages IA to IIA disease with favorable histologies, patients with Stages IA to IIA with unfavorable histologies who were under 50 years old, and patients with Stages IB to IIB with favorable histologies *and* who are under 50 years old. In the favorable group treated with irradiation alone, the relapse rate was 44% after treatment with involved field irradiation, and 30% after treatment with mantle plus inverted-Y or upper abdominal field.

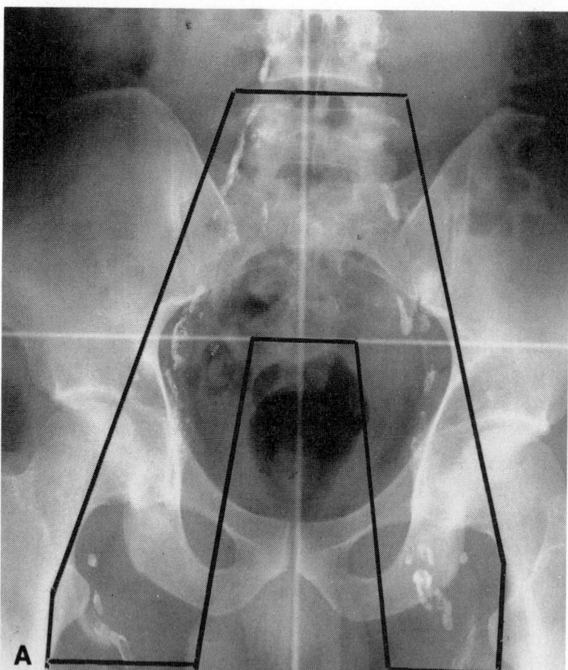

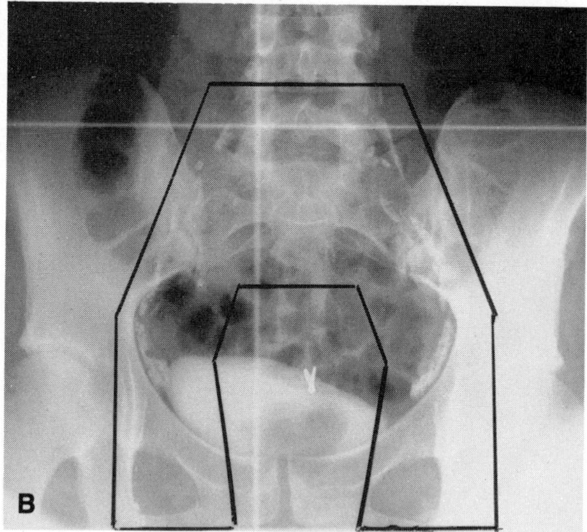

FIGURE 62–9. Typical setup films for pelvic irradiation. Note that the opacified nodes from the lymphogram permit maximum tailoring of the field to minimize the amount of bone marrow being irradiated. The field is matched superiorly to the paraaortic/splenic pedicle field, or the two fields can be treated together (inverted Y). When the pelvic nodes are involved, the midline pelvic block is deleted. (**A**) Male pelvic field. A narrow midline block protects the rectum, anus, and genitalia. A testicular shield is used during therapy. (**B**) Female pelvic field. A wide, double-thickness (10 HVL) midline block protects the rectum, anus, and ovaries. The ovaries have been transposed to the midline and are marked by wire sutures (in this case, surgical clips). Every attempt should be made to ensure that the ovaries are no closer than 2 cm from the edge of the block.

A particularly favorable presentation of Hodgkin's disease is clinical Stage IA lymphocyte predominance limited to the high neck with a negative lymphogram, in which a staging laparotomy may be avoided, and treatment may be limited to supradiaphragmatic sites.[121,129] A reasonable program includes a mantle (limiting the mediastinal dose to 3000 cGy) or minimantle (supramediastinal mantle) plus an ipsilateral preauricular field.

Another favorable presentation is nodular sclerosing Hodgkin's disease limited to intrathoracic sites. A staging laparotomy can be avoided in this group as well, but the overall treatment program typically includes subdiaphragmatic irradiation.[71]

Many trials have explored the use of combined-modality *versus* radiation therapy alone in pathologic Stage I or II disease.[1,119,134] The results of these trials demonstrate improved freedom from relapse but equivalent survival with combined-modality therapy. Given the incremental hazards of combined-modality treatment and the success of salvage therapy after initial treatment with irradiation, combined-modality therapy should not be used routinely in these patients; it should be reserved for particularly unfavorable subsets of patients, such as those with large mediastinal masses.

Supradiaphragmatic Stage I or IIB Disease

Approximately 15% to 20% of patients with Stage I or II disease have B symptoms. With comprehensive staging, which includes laparotomy, patients with pathologic Stage I or IIB can be managed effectively with radiation therapy alone. A staging laparotomy is essential, however, because any amount of subdiaphragmatic disease in this patient group (pathologic Stage IIIB) mandates the use of systemic therapy.

The largest published series of patients with pathologic Stage I to IIB Hodgkin's disease is a collaborative report from Stanford and the Joint Center[27]; 180 patients were staged with laparotomy and treated with either irradiation alone (103 patients) or combined-modality therapy (77 patients). An optimal outcome was achieved by treatment with mantle/paraaortic (or subtotal lymphoid) irradiation alone, with 10-year survival and freedom-from-relapse rates of 88% and 78%, respectively. No benefit was seen from the addition of either pelvic irradiation or chemotherapy. However, a very unfavorable subgroup of these patients was identified, who had both fevers and weight loss (with or without night sweats). Those patients had 10-year survival and relapse-free rates of only 57% and 48%, respectively, regardless of the type of therapy administered. It is possible that these patients should be managed with programs used for Stage IIIB patients.

Stage I or II Hodgkin's Disease With Bulky Mediastinal Involvement

Patients with bulky mediastinal Hodgkin's disease are difficult to categorize using the Ann Arbor staging criteria, have a poor outcome when treated with single-modality therapy, and are at special risk for development of complications related to aggressive treatment programs. For these reasons, management programs for these patients should be individualized.[52]

A staging laparotomy is not indicated in these patients if a

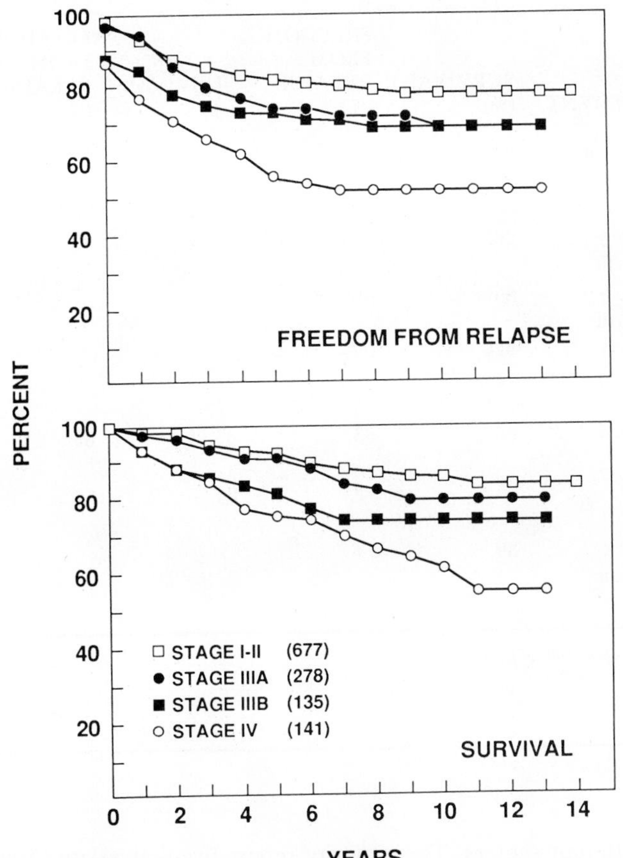

FIGURE 62–10. Actuarial freedom-from-relapse and survival rates of 1231 patients treated for Hodgkin's disease at Stanford University between 1974 and 1988. Number of patients in each stage is shown in parentheses. All causes of death are included in the survival analysis. (Hoppe RT: Radiology 169:297, 1988)

combined-modality program is planned. Indeed, it may be contraindicated because difficulty in extubation of these patients after the administration of general anesthesia has been reported.[105]

Several reports show that patients with bulky mediastinal disease are at greater risk for *relapse* after treatment with irradiation alone than after treatment with combined-modality therapy.[57,85,144] However, there may be no difference in *survival* of patients treated with either approach (Table 62-7). Despite the lack of a survival benefit, many consider it inappropriate to accept a relapse risk as high as 50% and recommend that these patients be treated with combined-modality therapy.

Chemotherapy should be administered first to decrease the mediastinal bulk and permit the use of more trim radiation therapy fields. In addition, occult microscopic disease, which is especially likely in intrathoracic sites, is treated from the outset. In some programs, only two or three cycles of chemotherapy are given,[42] but more frequently a minimum of six cycles of chemotherapy is used. In choosing the chemotherapy, the potential overlapping toxicity of doxorubicin and bleomycin with irradiation (cardiac and pulmonary effects) should be considered.

Irradiation can be administered after the completion of an entire course of chemotherapy or in a "sandwich" approach. The recommended dose of irradiation varies from 2500 cGy to 4400 cGy, but the higher range should be used when the response to chemotherapy is incomplete or the chemotherapy course is abbreviated.[52]

For some patients with bulky mediastinal Hodgkin's disease, irradiation alone may be warranted. Some mediastinal masses are technically "bulky," but their location in the superior mediastinum and lack of extension to adjacent organs permit the use of high-dose irradiation with curative intent and expectations,[55] especially with careful CT scanning to facilitate treatment planning.[54,120]

Careful identification of disease on the CT scan is essential to confirm that none of it will be inadvertently blocked. Special techniques of irradiation are warranted, including use of prophylactic whole-lung irradiation and boosts to the chest wall.[55,86] A shrinking field technique should almost always be used to minimize the volume of lung irradiated (see Fig. 62-6). The outcome of treatment in these patients may be similar to that achieved with combined-modality therapy.[4]

Subdiaphragmatic Stage I or II Disease

Approximately 10% of patients with Stage I or II Hodgkin's disease present with involvement limited to subdiaphragmatic sites.[78,82] Lymphography is an important component of their staging evaluation. Patients with inguinal-femoral presentations, especially with lymphocyte predominance histology, do not require a staging laparotomy when the lymphogram is normal in other sites. Treatment to the inverted Y and spleen may be sufficient therapy. If involvement of iliac or paraaortic nodes is detected by lymphogram, a bone marrow biopsy and staging laparotomy may be performed to define further management, because the spleen will be involved in approximately 40% of cases. If splenic involvement is absent, treatment can proceed with irradiation alone, but should include prophylactic treatment above the diaphragm (total lymphoid irradiation). When the spleen is involved, the treatment programs should be more analogous to those for Stage III disease. In general, the outcome of treatment for patients with subdiaphragmatic disease is equivalent to that for patients with supradiaphragmatic disease.[78]

Stage IIIA Disease

Stage IIIA is a heterogeneous group. The most useful practical descriptors of the extent of disease in Stage IIIA are anatomic substage and extent of splenic involvement. Only the most favorable subgroup of Stage IIIA patients, those with anatomic Substage III_1 and either an uninvolved spleen or only limited splenic involvement, should be treated with irradiation alone. This group accounts for one third of patients with Stage IIIA disease. A staging laparotomy is necessary to identify this favorable subgroup.

If a laparotomy is not performed, treatment with irradiation alone provides for a relapse-free rate of less than 40% in Stage IIIA[6,12] (Table 62-8). If a staging laparotomy is performed, but no further selection criteria are used, long-term relapse-free rates of 43% to 60% have been reported.[58,128] If patients are selected according to anatomic substage or extent of splenic involvement, relapse-free rates exceed 50% when irradiation, alone is used.[58,86,107]

Investigators at the University of Pennsylvania and the Harvard Joint Center for Radiation Therapy reported a free-

TABLE 62–6
Primary Radiation Therapy in Stage I–IIA Hodgkin's Disease

INSTITUTION	NO. OF PATIENTS	ACCRUAL YEARS	STAGING LAPAROTOMY	TREATMENT	5-YEAR SURVIVAL (%)	5-YEAR FREEDOM FROM RELAPSE (%)	10-YEAR SURVIVAL (%)	10-YEAR FREEDOM FROM RELAPSE (%)
Stanford University Hospital[57]	385	1968–1988	Yes	Subtotal or total lymphoid	94	78	87	75
Harvard, JCRT[96]	315	1969–1984	Yes	Mantle + paraaortic	96‡	86‡	90	82
EORTC[133]	202*	1972–1976	Yes (n = 94)	Mantle + paraaortic	85‡	69‡		
			No (n = 108)	Mantle + paraaortic + spleen	82‡	62‡		
University of Chicago[37]	135†	1968–1983	Yes	Extended mantle	96	83	83	83
Royal Marsden[138]	114	1970–1978	Yes	Mantle	95	72	84	66
Massachusetts General Hospital[144]	108	1975–1981	Yes	Mantle + paraaortic	89	74		

Note: These series did not exclude patients with large mediastinal masses, which likely accounted for about 10% of patients.
**Excludes patients with mixed cellularity and lymphocyte depleted histology. Data are at 7 years.*
† Includes 12 patients with B symptoms
‡ Estimated from published data.

dom from relapse of 54% in a carefully staged group of pathologic Stage III_1A patients treated with mantle and paraaortic irradiation alone.[107] The majority of initial relapses were in iliac or inguinal lymph nodes. In contrast, long-term relapse-free survival rates of 72% to 80% have been reported for programs that include irradiation of pelvic lymph nodes and low-dose hepatic irradiation in the presence of splenic involvement.[58,86] Extensive treatment of this type appears to be required to achieve results comparable with those achieved by combined modality therapy.

The majority of patients with Stage IIIA disease may be treated effectively with combined-modality therapy. The parameters of irradiation and chemotherapy vary in programs at different centers. The majority report five-year relapse-free rates of 80% to 90% (Table 62-9).

Few data exist regarding the use of chemotherapy alone in Stage IIIA Hodgkin's disease. Although patients with Stage IIIA disease are included in some series, their outcome is generally not analyzed separately from the larger group of patients with Stage IIIB or Stage IV disease. Three series from the United Kingdom have been reported recently. The drug combination most commonly used was MVPP (melphelan, vinblastine, procarbazine, and prednisone), a minimum of six cycles; the total number of patients reported was 75. The 5-year survival rates ranged from 72% to 90%, and the 5-year freedom-from-relapse rates ranged from 47% to 84%.[12,28,87]

TABLE 62–7
Outcome of Treatment in Hodgkin's Disease: Large Mediastinal Mass

INSTITUTION	NO. OF PATIENTS	10-YEAR FREEDOM FROM RELAPSE: IRRADIATION ALONE	10-YEAR FREEDOM FROM RELAPSE: COMBINED MODALITY	10-YEAR SURVIVAL: IRRADIATION ALONE	10-YEAR SURVIVAL: COMBINED MODALITY
Stanford University Hospital[57]	41	45%	81%	84% †	74% †
Harvard Joint Center[85]	54	49%	83%	83%	82%
Massachusetts General Hospital[144] *	35	45% *	100% *	96%*	100% *
Yale Hospital[109]	24	55%		90%	

Note: Large mediastinal mass is defined as a maximum mediastinal mass width that exceeds one third of the maximum intrathoracic diameter.
** Five-year data*
† All causes of death included (disease-related and non-disease-related)

TABLE 62–8
Radiation Therapy Alone in the Treatment of Stage IIIA Hodgkin's Disease

INSTITUTION	NO. OF PATIENTS	ACCRUAL YEARS	SUBGROUP	TREATMENT	SURVIVAL (%)			FREEDOM FROM RELAPSE (%)		
					5-YR	7–8-YR	10-YR	5-YR	7–8-YR	10-YR
STAGING LAPAROTOMY NOT PERFORMED ROUTINELY										
Royal Marsden[12]	59	1963–1985	all IIIA	Total nodal	86		68	49		38
CALGB 7451[6]	29	1974–1981	all IIIA					39*		
STAGING LAPAROTOMY PERFORMED ROUTINELY—ALL IIIA INCLUDED										
Stanford[58]	99	1968–1980	all IIIA	TLI (low dose liver if S+)	86	76	70	62	60	54
Collaborative[128]	85	1969–1976	all IIIA	TLI		61			43	
Yale[111]	48	1966–1975	all IIIA	TLI	80	80		35	35	
STAGING LAPAROTOMY PERFORMED ROUTINELY—RESULTS IN SELECTED SUBGROUPS										
University of Pennsylvania, JCRT[107]	63	1969–1983	III_1A	TLI MPA	88* 78	79† 78†		57* 54	51 54	
Stanford University[58]	46	1968–1980	minimal S+	TLI + low dose hepatic irradiation	93		80	82		80
University of Minnesota[86]	26	1975–1983		TLI + low dose hepatic irradiation	89	89		72	72	

TLI: total lymphoid irradiation; MPA: mantle + paraaortic/splenic pedicle irradiation
** Data estimated from published curves*
† Survival excludes death from intercurrent causes

Stage IIIB or IV Disease

The spectrum of patients included in Stage IIIB and Stage IV varies widely. Systemic chemotherapy is the mainstay of treatment for patients with advanced Hodgkin's disease. The majority of reported studies have used MOPP, MOPP-like combinations, ABVD, or alternating combinations of MOPP and ABVD.

Table 62-10 summarizes the results of selected experiences in the management of Stage IIIB and Stage IV Hodgkin's disease in which follow-up of at least 5 years has been reported. Response rates to chemotherapy are high (generally approximately 80%). Treatment with MOPP or MOPP-like combinations achieves 5-year survival rates of approximately 60% and 5-year relapse-free rates of 50% to 60%.[89] The randomized trial from the Tumor Institute in Milan[9] reports a possible improvement in outcome using alternating MOPP/ABVD compared with MOPP alone (8-year survival rate: 84% *versus* 64%; 8-year freedom-from-relapse: 65% *versus* 36%). A report from the Cancer Control Agency of British Columbia suggests an even better outcome with MOPP/ABV hybrid (with limited irradiation in some instances) (see Table 62-5); however, the follow-up is short-term.[77]

Several large series of combined-modality therapy, primarily in Stage IIIB, have been reported as well (see Table 62-10). Five-year survival rates of 60% to 80% and 5-year relapse-free rates of 60% to 75% are generally observed.

Although comparison of data from different centers suggests superiority of a combined-modality approach compared with the use of chemotherapy alone, this interpretation must be made with caution, because the patient populations vary substantially from one series to another. Unfortunately, clinical trials to compare the results of treatment with chemotherapy alone with combined-modality therapy have been designed poorly, often with a poor choice of chemotherapy or with different drug combinations in the single-modality *versus* the combined-modality arms of the study.

Pediatric Treatment

In the development of pediatric management programs, two special issues concerning staging are important. The first relates to lymphography, which may be superior to CT scans. It may be more challenging to perform a lymphogram in a child; however, a skilled person can perform this examination without difficulty even in children under 5 years. The second issue relates to laparotomy and splenectomy. Many people believe that a splenectomy should not be performed in a child younger than 5 years because before this age the spleen may still be important in the development of the normal immune system. Children older than 5 years may not be at especially high risk for complications related to splenectomy (infection and sepsis), especially when routine pneumococcal, meningococcal, and *Haemophilus* immunizations are performed before splenectomy and prophylactic antibiotics are administered afterward.[33] However, a more important issue relevant to laparotomy is the fact that the findings have only a minor impact on the overall treatment program, because most contemporary treatment programs for children include a systemic component. Therefore, most institutions have abandoned staging laparotomy and splenectomy in children and base treatment decisions on clinical stage only.

Occasionally a child may present with a solitary peripheral site of involvement, such as in the inguinal-femoral region or high neck, with lymphocyte predominance histology. In these patients, especially if they are older, it is reasonable to use modest dose (3000 cGy to 3600 cGy) involved field irradiation with close follow-up. In the majority of children, the evolution of

TABLE 62–9
Combined-Modality Therapy in the Management of Stage IIIA Hodgkin's Disease

INSTITUTION	NO. OF PATIENTS	ACCRUAL YEARS	CHEMO-THERAPY	IRRADIATION	SURVIVAL (%)			FREEDOM FROM RELAPSE (%)			COM-MENTS
					5-YR	7–8-YR	10-YR	5-YR	7–8-YR	10-YR	
Stanford[57]	183	1968–1988	MOPP × 6 (n = 102) PAVe × 6 (n = 55) Other (n = 26)	TLI or STLI (4000–4000 cGy)	93	87	82	86	86	85	
M.D. Anderson Cancer Center[48]	76	1970–1984	MOPP × 2	TLI or STLI (3000–4000 cGy)	88*	88*	86*	84	84	84	1
Tumor Institute, Milan[122]	63		MOPP × 6 (n = 30) ABVD × 6 (n = 33)	STLI or TLI (3000–3500 cGy)					65 92		2
CALGB 7451[6]	51	1974–1981	BOPP × 6	TLI				46, 84			3
Royal Marsden[12]	50	1963–1985	MOPP, MVPP or ChlVPP × 6	Mantle or TLI (3500 cGy)	84		81	70		63	4
Collaborative[128]	45		MOPP or variant × 6	TLI (3600–4000 cGy)		86			88		
Bologna[97]	38	1970–1980	MOPP × 6	TLI (3600 cGy)	73			60			
Massachusetts General Hospital[143]	38	1975–1981	MOPP × 6	STLI or TLI (4000–4500 cGy)	83			83			5
Manchester[28]	30	1975–1982	MVPP × 8	IF (3000 cGy)	80†	72†		85†	85†		
Yale, Duke[108]	24	1976–1982	MVVPP or MOPP × 6	IF (2000–2500 cGy)	91†	91†		91†	84†		6
Joint Center[92]	23	1969–1982	MOPP × 6	MPA or TLI (3600–4000 cGy)			90*			94	7

COMMENTS:
1. All patients had staging laparotomy. TLI or STLI included 3000 cGy to whole abdomen. Only patients with Substage III_1 are included.
2. One third of patients had staging laparotomy.
3. Staging laparotomy optional. Five-yr freedom from relapse FFR 46% for BOPP-TLI sequence; 84% for TLI-BOPP sequence. BOPP = BCNU, vincristine, procarbazine, and prednisone.
4. Two thirds of patients had staging laparotomy.
5. Uninvolved sites received 3600–4000 cGy.
6. Excludes patients with most favorable presentations (PS III_1A with S^- or spleen minimally involved); 50% of patients underwent staging laparotomy.
7. Data at 12 years.
** Survival excludes deaths from intercurrent causes.*
† Data are estimated from published curves.
MPA: mantle + paraaortic/splenic pedicle irradiation; STLI: subtotal lymphoid irradiation; TLI: total lymphoid irradiation

treatment programs has been toward lower doses of irradiation combined with chemotherapy. The most effective treatment programs thus far reported combine chemotherapy with MOPP, MOPP-like drugs, ABVD, or MOPP/ABVD and low-dose involved field irradiation. To limit growth effects, limitation of irradiation doses to 1500 cGy to 2500 cGy is warranted unless a particularly bulky disease has not responded to chemotherapy. Children treated with these programs, all stages combined, are reported to achieve 5-year survival rates of approximately 90% and relapse-free rates of at least 80%.[33,69]

Treatment for Relapse

Treatment for relapse must be individualized. Initial disease characteristics, initial treatment, relapse sites, and general patient status all must be considered in developing an effective secondary treatment program. In general, patients who were treated initially with irradiation alone should receive chemotherapy as the primary salvage treatment.[94,115] The efficacy of combination chemotherapy in this setting is at least as good as when chemotherapy is used in primary patient management.[31] The role of additional irradiation with salvage chemotherapy programs has not been defined, but it is advocated by some investigators.[110,115] After the completion of chemotherapy, low-dose (1500 cGy to 2500 cGy) irradiation can be delivered to previously irradiated sites, and higher doses (3500 cGy to 4400 cGy) to unirradiated regions.

Management of relapse is much more challenging when chemotherapy is included initially.[13] In the asymptomatic patient with disease limited to lymph nodes, comprehensive irradiation programs may provide durable responses.[40,95,116] However, the more common approach is to use chemotherapy with individual drugs that were not included in the primary treatment program.[13] Irradiation can also be incorporated into these salvage programs. In situations of multiple relapse or in the

TABLE 62–10
Treatment of Stage IIIB–IV Hodgkin's Disease

INSTITUTION	NO. OF PATIENTS	ACCRUAL YEARS	STAGE	TREATMENT	SURVIVAL (%) 5-YR	SURVIVAL (%) 7–8-YR	SURVIVAL (%) 10-YR	FREEDOM FROM RELAPSE (%) 5-YR	FREEDOM FROM RELAPSE (%) 7–8-YR	FREEDOM FROM RELAPSE (%) 10-YR
CHEMOTHERAPY ALONE										
NCI[89]	188†	1964–1976	95% III–IV	MOPP × 6	63*	56*	51*	58*	55*	54*
Tumor Institute, Milan[9]	88		IVA (61)	MOPP × 12 (n = 43)		64			36	
			IVB (27)	MOPP/ABVD × 6/6 (n = 45)		84			65	
Royal Marsden[12]	34	1963–1985	IIIB	MVPP, MOPP, or ChlVPP	59		43	49		41
COMBINED MODALITY THERAPY										
Stanford[57]	119	1974–1988	IIIB	MOPP (n = 71) or PAVe (n = 48) + TLI (3000–4000 cGy)	84	77	77	74	71	71
Duke, Yale[110]	102‡	1969–1982	IIIB (34) IVA (!6) IVB (52)	MVVPP, MOPP, or MOPP/ABVD + IF (2500 cGy)	74*	70*	66	66	66	66
Tumor Institute, Milan[122]	70	1974–1982	IIIB	MOPP + STLI or TLI (n = 36)					61	
				ABVD + STLI or TLI (3000–3500 cGy) (n = 34)					80	
Bologna[97]	58	1970–1980	IIIB	MOPP × 6 + TLI (3600 cGy)	66			60		
Joint Center[92] §	43	1969–1981	IIIB	MOPP × 6 + MPA or TLI (3600–4400 cGy)			76			79
Royal Marsden[12]	41	1963–1985	IIIB	MVPP, MOPP, or ChlVPP + Mantle or TLI (3500 cGy)	83		69	66		66

** Data estimated from published curves*
† Twenty-eight patients with CS IIIB disease received TLI after completion of MOPP. FFR figures are based on 84% CR rate.
‡ Survival data include 82 previously treated patients.
§ Data are at 12 years.
MPA: mantle + paraaortic/splenic pedicle irradiation; STLI: subtotal lymphoid irradiation; TLI: total lymphoid irradiation; FFR: freedom from relapse.

presence of unfavorable relapse characteristics,[98] more aggressive investigational treatment programs such as autologous bone marrow transplantation should be considered.[15,68]

FOLLOW-UP AND SEQUELAE

Patients should be followed carefully after the completion of therapy for Hodgkin's disease, although the frequency of visits can decrease as the risk of relapse diminishes. However, even 3 years after the completion of therapy, as many as 13% of patients may still be without evidence of disease who will later relapse.[49] Typical follow-up intervals include every 2 to 3 months during the first 2 years, every 4 to 6 months during the third and fourth years, and annually thereafter. Follow-up studies include an interim history and physical examination, chest and abdominal radiographs (provided that there is residual lymphographic contrast). A repeat chest CT scan should be obtained after the completion of treatment both to assess response and to provide a new "baseline" for subsequent comparison. If a pretreatment gallium scan was performed, this study should also be repeated. Hematologic evaluation at the time of each follow-up visit should include a CBC with platelet count and alkaline phosphatase level. The erythrocyte sedimentation rate or serum copper level should be obtained in selected patients in whom these markers were abnormal at the time of presentation. A serum T4 and sensitive TSH (thyroid-stimulating hormone) should be obtained annually to detect subclinical hypothyroidism.

As a general rule, the first relapse of Hodgkin's disease should be documented by biopsy. Reactive hyperplasia is especially common in unirradiated lymph nodes just outside the previous radiation portals, justifying biopsy documentation before initiating any therapy.[17]

A challenging problem in follow-up evaluation is the interpretation of residual mediastinal abnormality on chest radiograph or chest CT scan.[70,130] Comparison of pretreatment and posttreatment gallium images is helpful in some situations.[2] MRI can also provide useful information regarding the significance of residual abnormalities.[100] In the absence of other clinical suspicion, it is reasonable to follow these patients carefully for as long as the abnormality remains the same or regresses, with additional diagnostic procedures reserved for patients who appear to have a progression of disease. When patients are followed up, many prove to have no later evidence of disease[55,97]; however, patients treated initially with chemotherapy alone more often have subsequent evolution of disease associated with the residual mass.[112]

The acute side effects of radiation therapy for Hodgkin's disease are occipital hair loss, mild skin reaction, sore throat, perhaps an altered sense of taste, transient dysphagia from radiation esophagitis, dry cough, nausea, occasional vomiting, and rarely diarrhea. Most of these sequelae can be managed symptomatically without major difficulty.

Common complications that may arise in the early phase of the follow-up program are mild radiation pneumonitis, hypothyroidism, herpes zoster, Lhermitte's sign, and xerostomia.

Radiation pneumonitis usually develops within 6 to 12 weeks after completion of mantle irradiation. The likelihood of developing this complication is related to the volume of lung irradiated, total dose, and fraction size. Less than 5% of patients develop symptomatic pneumonitis, manifested by cough, fever, pleuritic chest pain, and infiltrate on chest radiograph that often conforms to the radiation fields.[16] Symptomatic management is generally adequate; however, a small proportion of patients requires treatment with corticosteroids. The initiation of corticosteroid therapy commits one to a course of at least 4 to 6 weeks with careful tapering to avoid exacerbation of symptoms.

Radiation carditis after well-executed mantle therapy is seen in less than 5% of patients. Radiation pericarditis manifests itself by an acute febrile syndrome associated with chest pain and friction rub, an asymptomatic pericardial effusion diagnosed by chest radiograph or echocardiogram, or constrictive pericarditis or tamponade. The first of these syndromes is usually managed with conservative medical treatment that includes analgesics and nonsteroidal antiinflammatory agents; it usually clears up after a few weeks. The syndrome of tamponade or constrictive pericarditis is the most serious. It is seen in approximately 1% of patients who receive treatment to the mantle and may require surgical correction. It is important to differentiate this syndrome from recurrent Hodgkin's disease. Cardiopulmonary changes that represent a latent radiation injury can occur with steroid withdrawal such as may be seen with postradiation MOPP chemotherapy.[19]

Subclinical hypothyroidism develops in approximately one third of patients with Hodgkin's disease. It can be detected by an elevation of the sensitive TSH even with a normal T4 level. Thyroid replacement therapy is recommended by using L-thyroxine, with an initial dose of 0.1 mg/day. The T4 and sensitive TSH values are monitored regularly to make adjustments in the dose. Evidence has been found that thyroid replacement therapy in this setting reduces the risk for developing benign thyroid nodules.[39]

Herpes zoster can occur during treatment for Hodgkin's disease or within the first 1 to 2 years after treatment in 15% to 20% of patients. The outbreak is generally limited to one or two contiguous dermatomes. Cutaneous dissemination is uncommon, and visceral involvement is extremely rare. If the cutaneous eruption is identified within 72 hours of its onset, treatment with acyclovir can be initiated. This may limit the duration and intensity of the infection and decrease the likelihood of cutaneous or visceral dissemination.

Lhermitte's sign develops in approximately 10% to 15% of patients after mantle therapy. This sign is marked by paresthesias extending into the arms and legs on neck flexion and may be related to transient demyelinization of the spinal cord. Its onset is usually insidious, occurring 6 weeks to 3 months after completion of the mantle; it resolves spontaneously after several weeks to a few months. This sequela is not related to the more serious problem of transverse myelitis.

Because partial xerostomia results from radiation therapy, careful dental care is required permanently, with frequent prophylaxis and use of fluoride supplements.

A potentially serious complication, which is uncommon, is overwhelming sepsis after splenectomy or splenic irradiation.[34] The most serious infections occur with gram-positive organisms including *Streptococcus pneumoniae,* meningococcus, and *Haemophilus* strains. This risk can be minimized by prior immunization against these organisms.[125] Some clinicians prescribe long-term antibiotic prophylaxis as well, but the additional benefit this treatment provides is not known.

An important concern to many patients with Hodgkin's disease is the possible effects of treatment on reproductive potential. Both irradiation and chemotherapy may have detrimental effects. In men, pelvic irradiation may be followed by azoospermia if no special precautions are taken to shield the testes. However, with appropriate testicular shielding, azoospermia is usually only transient, with subsequent recovery of sperm counts to fertile levels.[103] Chemotherapy programs such as MOPP or MOPP-like combinations that include alkylating agents cause sterility in most men. However, the ABVD regimen seems to spare male fertility.[7]

In women, treatment effects are influenced by patient age.[63] Even with a proper oophoropexy and well-planned pelvic irradiation, the scattered dose of irradiation may be sufficient to affect ovarian function and cause menopausal symptoms in women over 30 years olds, whereas younger women may not be affected. A similar observation relates to the effects of chemotherapy containing alkylating agents; normal menstrual function usually continues in women under 25 years, but is altered in women over 30. With combined chemotherapy and pelvic irradiation programs, menstrual function and fertility may even be affected in younger women. However, in contrast to MOPP, the ABVD combination appears to spare female fertility.[7]

Long-term follow-up is essential to detect late relapse and to identify potential long-term complications of treatment.[11,46,49,137] Patients should be monitored for the development of secondary cancers.[135] Leukemia may develop after treatment with chemotherapy programs that include alkylating agents (MOPP) with a latent period of 3 to 7 years. The occurrence of leukemia after treatment with irradiation alone is exceedingly rare. It remains controversial whether the risk is greater after combined-modality therapy or after chemotherapy alone. Secondary solid tumors may be related either to chemotherapy or to radiation therapy and generally have a longer latent period (at least 7 to 10 years) than leukemia. Patients who smoke should be counseled to stop because of an inordinately high risk of lung cancer when combined with irradiation. Women should undergo mammography according to the American Cancer Society guidelines. In addition, younger women should begin mammogram screening 10 years after they have completed mantle irradiation.

A group of sequelae that has received little attention until recently includes psychosocial problems. The type and incidence of problems were investigated by standardized self-administered questionnaires and interviews in a large group of patients at Stanford University.[38] Results showed that most patients had suffered a sensation of decreased energy after treatment that returned after 6 to 18 months in many; however, more than one third still had impaired energy levels. Patients with energy loss often were depressed as well. Marital difficulties included a moderately high divorce rate, concerns regarding infertility, and decreased sexual interest. Most men returned to work; fewer women did so.

Difficulties related to employment were reported by 42% of patients. These included denial of insurance and other employment benefits, lost job opportunities, and conflicts with supervisors. Identification of these problems may promote the development of rehabilitation programs to anticipate and deal with these issues early in the course of treatment programs for Hodgkin's disease.

CURRENT CLINICAL TRIALS

Provocative single-institution and cooperative group trials for Hodgkin's disease are in progress.[139] There are several lines of investigation in early stage disease. The EORTC group is examining the need for staging laparotomy in a favorable subset of patients with clinical Stage I to II disease by randomizing them to staging laparotomy *versus* no laparotomy (H6 trial). The treatment of patients who undergo laparotomy is determined by the extent of disease identified below the diaphragm, whereas those who do not undergo laparotomy received treatment to a mantle and paraaortic/spleen field.[132] The treatment of patients who undergo laparotomy and remain pathologic Stage I to II is randomized between mantle irradiation alone and mantle field plus paraaortic splenic pedicle irradiation.

Other trials in early stage Hodgkin's disease are examining the efficacy of treatment with chemotherapy alone. Investigators at both the National Cancer Institute[88] and a cooperative Italian group[22] are comparing treatment with MOPP chemotherapy to mantle plus paraaortic field irradiation in patients with pathologic Stage I to II disease. The NCI trial suggests a superiority of the MOPP treatment with respect to freedom from relapse. The Italian studies suggest a similar initial outcome of treatment for both groups but better salvage treatment for patients treated initially with irradiation. The additional observation of greater toxicity among patients treated with MOPP led this group to conclude that the irradiation approach was preferred.

A cooperative group in Argentina (GATLA) is testing CVPP chemotherapy (cyclophosphamide, voncristine, procarbazine, and prednisone) alone compared with CVPP chemotherapy plus involved field irradiation in pathologic Stage I to II disease.[102] Early results indicate a similar efficacy for both treatment approaches for patients with favorable clinical characteristics, but a superior outcome in the combined-modality group for patients with unfavorable clinical characteristics such as age over 45 years, more than two regions involved, and bulky disease.

Another novel approach in the management of patients with early stage disease is to test the efficacy of chemotherapy with less potential toxicity than is associated with MOPP or ABVD. A Stanford University study has examined the use of vinblastine, bleomycin, and methotrexate (VBM) chemotherapy as an adjuvant after involved field irradiation in pathologic Stage I to II disease.[63] Early results indicate that VBM is effective in controlling occult disease and is comparable to MOPP plus involved field irradiation in historical comparisons. A new study is testing the efficacy of VBM chemotherapy combined with regional irradiation in patients who have undergone clinical staging *only*.

For patients with bulky mediastinal disease, investigators in the EORTC and at Stanford University are comparing combined-modality programs with different chemotherapy combinations: MOPP or PAVe (procarbazine, Alkeran [L-phenylalanine mustard], and Velban [vinblastine]) plus mantle irradiation *versus* ABVD plus mantle irradiation. The efficacies of the different chemotherapy programs appear to be equivalent; however, an important component of these studies is the long-term toxicity evaluation.[59,132] Increased pulmonary toxicity may occur with ABVD compared with that of MOPP.[25]

In patients with advanced stage Hodgkin's disease at Stanford University, a program of alternating non-cross-resistant chemotherapy using MOPP/ABVD is being compared with a combined-modality program using PAVe and total lymphoid irradiation.[59] Preliminary results show no difference in outcome. The Eastern Cooperative Oncology Group (ECOG) is comparing ABVD consolidative therapy with radiation therapy consolidation after bleo-MOPP induction therapy.[44] A Southwest Oncology Group (SWOG) trial randomizes patients to involved field irradiation *versus* no further treatment after induction therapy with MOPP-BAP (bleomycin, Adriamycin [doxorubicin], and prednisone) chemotherapy.

New modalities are being tested for patients with recurrent or resistant disease. These include radiolabeled antiferritin antibodies[83] and high-dose chemotherapy with or without fractionated total-body irradiation prior to bone marrow transplantation.[15,68]

REFERENCES

1. Anderson H, Deakin DP, Wagstaff J, et al: A randomized study of adjuvant chemotherapy after mantle radiotherapy in supradiaphragmatic Hodgkin's disease PS IA-IIB: A report from the Manchester lymphoma group. Br J Cancer 49:695, 1984
2. Anderson KC, Leonard RCF, Canellos GP, et al: High-dose gallium imaging in lymphoma. Am J Med 75:327, 1983
3. Austin-Seymour MM, Hoppe RT, Cox RS, et al: Hodgkin's disease in patients over sixty years old. Ann Intern Med 100:13, 1984
4. Behar R, Hoppe RT: Radiation therapy in the management of bulky mediastinal Hodgkin's disease. Cancer 66:75, 1990
5. Behrendt H, Van Bunningen BNFM, Van Leeuwen EF: Treatment of Hodgkin's disease in children with or without radiotherapy. Cancer 59:1870, 1987
6. Bloomfield CD, Pajak TF, Glicksman AS, et al: Chemotherapy and combined modality therapy for Hodgkin's disease: A progress report on cancer and leukemia group B studies. Cancer Treat Rep 66:835, 1982
7. Bonadonna G: Chemotherapy strategies to improve the control of Hodgkin's disease. The Richard and Hinda Rosenthal Foundation Award Lecture. Cancer Res 42:4309, 1982
8. Bonadonna G, Valagussa P, Santoro A: Prognosis of bulky Hodgkin's disease treated with chemotherapy alone or combined with radiotherapy. Cancer Surv 4:440, 1985
9. Bonadonna G, Valagussa P, Santoro A: Alternating non-cross resistant combination chemotherapy or MOPP in stage IV Hodgkin's disease. Ann Intern Med 104:739, 1986
10. Bonadonna G, Zucali R, Monfardini S, et al: Combination chemotherapy of Hodgkin's disease with Adriamycin, bleomycin, vinblastine, and imidazole carboxamide versus MOPP. Cancer 36:252, 1975
11. Bookman MA, Longo DL: Concomitant illness in patients treated for Hodgkin's disease. Cancer Treat Rep 13:77, 1986
12. Brada M, Ashley S, Nicholls J, et al: Stage III Hodgkin's disease—long term results following chemotherapy, radiotherapy and combined modality therapy. Radiother Oncol 14:185, 1989
13. Buzaid AC, Lippman SM, Miller TP: Salvage therapy of advanced Hodgkin's disease. Critical appraisal of curative potential. Am J Med 83:523, 1987
14. Carbone PP, Kaplan HS, Mushoff K, et al: Report of the

committee on Hodgkin's disease staging classification. Cancer Res 31:1860, 1971

15. Carella AM, Congiu AM, Gaozza E, et al: High-dose chemotherapy with autologous bone marrow transplantation in 50 advanced resistant Hodgkin's disease patients: An Italian study group report. J Clin Oncol 6:1411, 1988
16. Carmel RJ, Kaplan HS: Mantle irradiation in Hodgkin's disease. An analysis of technique, tumor eradication, and complications. Cancer 37:2813, 1976
17. Castellino RA, Billingham M, Dorfman RF: Lymphographic accuracy in Hodgkin's disease and malignant lymphoma with a note on the "Reactive" lymph node as a cause of most false-positive lymphograms. Invest Radiol 9:155, 1984
18. Castellino RA, Blank N, Hoppe RT, et al: Hodgkin Disease. Contributions of chest CT in the initial staging evaluation. Radiology 160:603, 1986
19. Castellino RA, Glatstein E, Turbow MM, et al: Latent radiation injury of lungs or heart activated by steroid withdrawal. Ann Intern Med 80:593, 1974
20. Castellino RA, Hoppe RT, Blank N, et al: Computed tomography, lymphography and staging laparotomy: correlations in initial staging of Hodgkin's disease. Am J Radiol 143:37, 1984
21. Chittal SM, Caveriviere P, Schwarting R, et al: Monoclonal antibodies in the diagnosis of Hodgkin's disease. The search for a rational panel. Am J Surg Pathol 12:9, 1988
22. Cimino G, Biti GP, Anselmo AP, et al: MOPP chemotherapy versus extended field radiotherapy in the management of pathological stages I-IIA Hodgkin's disease. J Clin Oncol 7:732, 1989
23. Connors JM, Klimo P: Is it an E lesion or stage IV? An unsettled issue in Hodgkin's disease staging. J Clin Oncol 2:1421, 1984
24. Coppleson LW, Factor RM, Strum SB, et al: Observer disagreement in the classification and histology of Hodgkin's disease. J Natl Cancer Inst 45:731, 1970
25. Cosset JM, Henry-Amar M, Thomas J, et al: Increased pulmonary toxicity in the ABVD arm of the EORTC H6-U trial (Abstract). Proc ASCO 8:253, 1989
26. Crnkovich MJ, Hoppe RT, Rosenberg SA: Stage IIB Hodgkin's disease. The Stanford experience. J Clin Oncol 4:472, 1986
27. Crnkovich MJ, Leopold K, Hoppe RT, et al: Stage I to IIB Hodgkin's disease. The combined experience at Stanford University and the Joint Center for Radiation Therapy. J Clin Oncol 5:1041, 1987
28. Crowther D, Wagstaff J, Deakin D, et al: A randomized study comparing chemotherapy alone with chemotherapy followed by radiotherapy in patients with pathologically staged IIIA Hodgkin's disease. J Clin Oncol 2:892, 1984
29. Desser RK, Golomb HM, Ultmann JE, et al: Prognostic classification of Hodgkin's disease in pathologic stage III, based on anatomic considerations. Blood 49:883, 1977
30. DeVita VT, Hubbard SM, Longo DL: The chemotherapy of lymphomas: Looking back, moving forward—The Richard and Hinda Rosenthal Foundation Award Lecture. Cancer Res 47:4810, 1987
31. DeVita VT, Serpick AA, Carbone PP: Combination chemotherapy in the treatment of advanced Hodgkin's disease. Ann Intern Med 73:881, 1970
32. Doggett RS, Colby TV, Dorfman RF: Interfollicular Hodgkin's disease. Am J Surg Pathol 7:145, 1983
33. Donaldson SS, Link MP: Combined modality treatment with low-dose radiation and MOPP chemotherapy for children with Hodgkin's disease. J Clin Oncol 5:742, 1987
34. Donaldson SS, Moore MR, Rosenberg SA, et al: Characterization of postsplenectomy bacteremia among patients with and without lymphoma. N Engl J Med 287:69, 1972
35. Drexler HG, Leber BF: The nature of the Hodgkin cell. Blut 56:135, 1988
36. Ekert H, Waters KD, Smith PJ, et al: Treatment with MOPP or ChIVPP chemotherapy only for all stages of childhood Hodgkin's disease. J Clin Oncol 6:1845, 1988
37. Farah R, Ultmann J, Griem M, et al: Extended mantle radiation therapy for pathologic stage I and II Hodgkin's disease. J Clin Oncol 6:1047, 1988
38. Fobair P, Hoppe RT, Bloom J, et al: Psychosocial problems among survivors of Hodgkin's disease. J Clin Oncol 4:805, 1986
39. Fogelfield L, Wiviott MBT, Shore-Freedman E, et al: Recurrence of thyroid nodules after surgical removal in patients irradiated in childhood for benign conditions. N Engl J Med 320:835, 1989
40. Fox KA, Lippman SM, Cassady JR, et al: Radiation therapy salvage of Hodgkin's disease following chemotherapy failure. J Clin Oncol 5:38, 1987
41. Friedman S, Henry-Amar M, Cosset JM, et al: Evolution of erythrocyte sedimentation rate as predictor of early relapse in posttherapy early-stage Hodgkin's disease. J Clin Oncol 6:596, 1988
42. Fuller LM, Hagemeister FB, North LB, et al: The adjuvant role of two cycles of MOPP and low-dose lung irradiation in stage IA through IIB Hodgkin's disease. Preliminary results, Int J Radiat Oncol Biol Phys 14:683, 1988
43. Glatstein E, Trueblood HW, Enright LP, et al: Surgical staging of abdominal involvements in unselected patients with Hodgkin's disease. Radiology 97:425, 1970
44. Glick J, Tsiatis A, Prosnitz L, et al: Improved survival with sequential BLEO-MOPP follow by ABVD for advanced Hodgkin's disease. Proc ASCO 3:237, 1984
45. Grufferman S, Delzell E: Epidemiology of Hodgkin's disease. Epidemiol Rev 6:76, 1984
46. Hancock SL, Hoppe RT, Horning SJ, et al: Intercurrent death after Hodgkin's disease therapy in radiotherapy and adjuvant MOPP trials. Ann Intern Med 109:183, 1988
47. Hanks GE: The patterns of care study outcome survey in Hodgkin's disease. PCS Newsletter of the Patterns of Care Outcome Study, January 1983
48. Henkelmann GC, Hagemeister FB, Fuller LM: Two cycles of MOPP and radiotherapy for stage III_1A and stage III_1B Hodgkin's disease. J Clin Oncol 6:1293, 1988
49. Herman TS, Hoppe RT, Donaldson SS, et al: Late relapse among patients treated for Hodgkin's disease. Ann Intern Med 102:292, 1985
50. Hoppe RT: Radiation therapy in the management of Hodgkin's disease. Semin Oncol 17:704, 1990
51. Hoppe RT: Hodgkin's disease. Patterns of Care Study Newsletter, American College of Radiology. 1990–1991, No. 3
52. Hoppe RT: The management of bulky mediastinal Hodgkin's disease. Hematology/Oncology Clinics of North America 3:265, 1989
53. Hoppe RT: The contemporary management of Hodgkin disease. Radiology 169:297, 1988
54. Hoppe RT: Treatment planning in the radiation therapy of Hodgkin's disease. In Vaeth J, Meyer J (eds): Treatment Planning in the Radiation Therapy of Cancer, p 285, Basel, S Karger, 1987
55. Hoppe RT: The management of stage II Hodgkin's disease with a large mediastinal mass: A prospective program emphasizing irradiation. Int J Radiat Oncol Biol Phys 11:349, 1985
56. Hoppe RT, Burke JS, Glatstein E, et al: Non-Hodgkin's lymphoma: Involvement of Waldeyer's ring. Cancer 37:2797, 1978
57. Hoppe RT, Coleman CN, Cox RS, et al: The management of stage I–II Hodgkin's disease with irradiation alone or combined modality therapy: The Stanford experience. Blood 59:455, 1982
58. Hoppe RT, Cox RS, Rosenberg SA, et al: Prognostic factors in pathologic stage III Hodgkin's disease. Cancer Treat Rep 66:743, 1982
59. Hoppe RT, Horning SJ, Hancock SL, et al: Current Stanford clinical trials for Hodgkin's disease. In Diehl V, Pfreundschuh M. (eds): Recent Results in Cancer Research: New Aspects in the Diagnosis and Treatment of Cancer, p 182, Heidelberg, Springer-Verlag, 1989
60. Hoppe RT, Portlock CS, Glatstein E, et al: Alternating chemotherapy and irradiation in the treatment of advanced Hodgkin's disease. Cancer 43:472, 1979
61. Hoppe RT, Rosenberg SA, Kaplan HS, et al: Prognostic factors in Pathological stage IIIA Hodgkin's disease. Cancer 46:1240, 1980

62. Hopper KD, Diehl LF, Lesar M, et al: Hodgkin disease: Clinical utility of CT in initial staging and treatment. Radiology 169:17, 1988
63. Horning SJ, Hoppe RT, Hancock SL, et al: Vinblastine, bleomycin, and methotrexate: An effective adjuvant in favorable Hodgkin's disease. J Clin Oncol 6:1822, 1988
64. Horning SJ, Hoppe RT, Kaplan HS, et al: Female reproductive potential after treatment for Hodgkin's disease. N Engl J Med 304:1377, 1981
65. Hu E, Huffort S, Lukes R, et al: Third-world Hodgkin's disease at Los Angeles County–University of Southern California Medical Center. J Clin Oncol 6:1285, 1988
66. Jacobs C, Donaldson SS, Rosenberg SA, et al: Management of the pregnant patient with Hodgkin's disease. Ann Intern Med 95:669, 1981
67. Jaffe ES: The elusive Reed-Sternberg cell. N Engl Med 320:529, 1989
68. Jagannath S, Armitage JO, Dicke KA, et al: Prognostic factors for response and survival after high-dose cyclophosphamide, carmustine, and etoposide with autologous bone marrow transplantation for relapsed Hodgkin's disease. J Clin Oncol 7:179, 1989
69. Jenkin D, Chan H, Freedman M, et al: Hodgkin's disease in children: Treatment results with MOPP and low-dose, extended-field irradiation. Cancer Treat Rep 66:949, 1982
70. Jochelson M, Mauch P, Balikian J, et al: The significance of the residual mediastinal mass in treated Hodgkin's disease. J Clin Oncol 3:637, 1985
71. Johnson DW, Hoppe RT, Cox RS, et al: Hodgkin's disease limited to intrathoracic sites. Cancer 52:8, 1983
72. Kaplan HS: Hodgkin's disease, 2nd ed. Cambridge, Harvard University Press, 1980
73. Kaplan HS: On the natural history, treatment, and prognosis of Hodgkin's disease. Harvey Lectures, 1968–1969, pp 215, New York, Academic Press, 1970
74. Kaplan HS: Evidence for a tumoricidal dose level in the radiotherapy of Hodgkin's disease. Cancer Res 26:1221, 1966
75. Kaplan HS: The radical radiotherapy of regionally localized Hodgkin's disease. Radiology 78:553, 1962
76. Kinzie JJ, Hanks GE, Maclean CJ, et al: Patterns of care study: Hodgkin's disease relapse rates and adequacy of portals. Cancer 52:2223, 1983
77. Klimo P, Connors JM: MOPP/ABV hybrid program: Combination chemotherapy based on early introduction of seven effective drugs for advanced Hodgkin's disease. J Clin Oncol 3:1174, 1985
78. Krikorian JG, Portlock CS, Mauch PM: Hodgkin's disease presenting below the diaphragm: A review. J Clin Oncol 4:1551, 1986
79. Lee CKK, Aeppli DM, Bloomfield CD, et al: Hodgkin's disease: A reassessment of prognostic factors following modification of radiotherapy. Int J Radiat Oncol Biol Phys 13:983, 1987
80. LeFloch O, Donaldson SS, Kaplan HS: Pregnancy following oophoropexy and total nodal irradiation in women with Hodgkin's disease. Cancer 38:2263, 1976
81. Leibenhaut MH, Hoppe RT, Efron B, et al: Prognostic indicators of laparotomy findings in clinical stage I–II supradiaphragmatic Hodgkin's disease. J Clin Oncol 7:81, 1989
82. Leibenhaut MH, Hoppe RT, Varghese A, et al: Subdiaphragmatic Hodgkin's disease: Laparotomy and treatment results in 49 patients. J Clin Oncol 5:1050, 1987
83. Lenhard RE, Order SE, Spunberg JJ, et al: Isotopic immunoglobulin: A new systemic therapy for advanced Hodgkin's disease. J Clin Oncol 3:1296, 1985
84. Leopold KA, Canellos G, Rosenthal D, et al: Stage IA–IIB Hodgkin's disease: Staging and treatment of patients with large mediastinal adenopathy. J Clin Oncol 7:1059, 1989
85. Leslie NT, Mauch PM, Hellman S: Stage IA to IIB supradiaphragmatic Hodgkin's disease. Long-term survival and relapse frequency. Cancer 55:2072, 1985
86. Levitt SH, Lee CKK, Aeppli DM, et al: Radical treatment of Hodgkin disease with radiation therapy: Results of a 15-year clinical trial. Radiology 162:623, 1987
87. Lister TA, Dorreen MS, Faux M, et al: The treatment of stage IIIA Hodgkin's disease. J Clin Oncol 1:745, 1983
88. Longo D. Glatstein E, Young R, et al: Randomized trial of MOPP chemotherapy vs subtotal nodal radiation therapy in patients with laparotomy—Documented early stage Hodgkin's disease. Proc Am Soc Clin Oncol 6:A812, 1987
89. Longo DL, Young RC, Wesley M, et al: Twenty years of MOPP therapy for Hodgkin's disease. J Clin Oncol 4:1295, 1986
90. Lukes RJ, Butler JJ: The pathology nomenclature of Hodgkin's disease. Cancer Res 31:1063, 1966
91. Lutz WR, Larsen RD: Technique to match mantle and paraaortic fields. Int J Radiat Oncol Biol Phys 9:1753, 1983
92. Mauch P, Goffman T, Rosenthal DS, et al: Stage III Hodgkin's disease: Improved survival with combined modality therapy as compared with radiation therapy alone. J Clin Oncol 3:1166, 1985
93. Mauch P, Goodman R, Hellman S: The significance of mediastinal involvement in early stage Hodgkin's disease. Cancer 42:1039, 1978
94. Mauch P, Ryback ME, Rosenthal D, et al: The influence of initial pathologic stage on the survival of patients who relapse from Hodgkin's disease. Blood 56:892, 1980
95. Mauch P, Tarbell N, Skarin A, et al: Wide-field radiation therapy alone or with chemotherapy for Hodgkin's disease. J Clin Oncol 5:544, 1987
96. Mauch P, Tarbell N, Weinstein H, et al: Stage IA and IIA supradiaphragmatic Hodgkin's disease: Prognostic factors in surgically staged patients treated with mantle and paraaortic irradiation. J Clin Oncol 6:1576, 1988
97. Mazza P, Miniaci G, Lauria F, et al: Prognostic significance of lymphography in stage III_S Hodgkin's disease (HD). Eur J Cancer Clin Oncol 20:1393, 1984
98. Meakin CJ, Horning SJ, Hoppe RT: Prognostic factors in Hodgkin's disease. Impact of clinical and treatment parameters on survival of patients who relapse after treatment which includes chemotherapy. Identification of a poor prognostic group (Abstract) Int J Radiat Oncol Biol Phys 15(Suppl 1):168, 1988
99. Mueller N, Evans A, Harris NL, et al: Hodgkin's disease and Epstein-Barr virus. Altered antibody pattern before diagnosis. N Engl J Med 320:689, 1989
100. Nyman RS, Rehn SM, Glimelius BLG, et al: Residual mediastinal masses in Hodgkin disease: Prediction of size with MR imaging. Radiology 170:435, 1989
101. Palos B, Kaplan HS, Karzmark CJ: The use of thin lung shields to deliver limited whole-lung irradiation during mantle-field treatment of Hodgkin's disease. Radiology 101:441, 1971
102. Pavlovsky S, Mashio M, Santarelli MT, et al: Randomized trial of chemotherapy versus chemotherapy plus radiotherapy for stage I–II Hodgkin's disease. J Natl Cancer Inst 80:1466, 1988
103. Pedrick TJ, Hoppe RT: Recovery of spermatogenesis following pelvic irradiation for Hodgkin's disease. Int J Radiat Oncol Biol Phys 12:117, 1986
104. Pinkus GS, Said JW: Hodgkin's disease, lymphocyte predominance type, nodular—A distinct entity? Unique staining profile for L&H variants of Reed-Sternberg cells defined by monoclonal antibodies to leukocyte common antigen, granulocyte-specific antigen, and B-cell-specific antigen. Am J Pathol 118:1, 1985
105. Piro AJ, Weiss DR, Hellman S: Mediastinal Hodgkin's disease: A possible danger for intubation anesthesia. Intubation danger in Hodgkin's disease. Int J Radiat Oncol Biol Phys 1:415, 1976
106. Poppema S, Timens W, Visser L: Nodular lymphocyte predominance type of Hodgkin's disease is a B cell lymphoma. Adv Exp Med Biol 186:963, 1985
107. Powlis WD, Mauch P, Goffman T, et al: Treatment of patients with "minimal" stage IIIA Hodgkin's disease. Int J Radiat Oncol Biol Phys 13:1437, 1987
108. Prosnitz LR, Cooper D, Cox EB, et al: Treatment selection for stage IIIA Hodgkin's disease patients. Int J Radiat Oncol Biol Phys 11:1431, 1985
109. Prosnitz LR, Curtis AM, Knowlton AH, et al: Supradiaphrag-

matic Hodgkin's disease: significance of large mediastinal masses. Int J Radiat Oncol Biol Phys 6:809, 1980
110. Prosnitz LR, Farber LR, Kapp DS, et al: Combined modality therapy for advanced Hodgkin's disease: 15-year follow-up data. J Clin Oncol 6:603, 1988
111. Prosnitz LR, Montalvo RL, Fischer DB, et al: Treatment of stage IIIA Hodgkin's disease: Is radiotherapy alone adequate? Int J Radiat Oncol Biol Phys 4:781, 1978
112. Radford JA, Cowan RA, Flanagan M, et al: The significance of residual mediastinal abnormality on the chest radiograph following treatment for Hodgkin's disease. J Clin Oncol 6:940, 1988
113. Ray GR, Wolf PH, Kaplan HS: Value of laboratory indicators in Hodgkin's disease: Preliminary results. Natl Cancer Inst Monogr 36:315, 1973
114. Regula DP, Hoppe RT, Weiss LM: Nodular and diffuse types of lymphocyte predominance Hodgkin's disease. N Engl J Med 318:214, 1988
115. Roach M, Hoppe RT, Brophy N: An analysis of prognostic factors for patients relapsing following radiotherapy for early stage Hodgkin's disease. J Clin Oncol 8:623, 1990
116. Roach M, Kapp DS, Rosenberg SA, et al: Radiotherapy with curative intent: An option in selected patients relapsing after chemotherapy for advanced Hodgkin's disease. J Clin Oncol 5:550, 1987
117. Rosenberg SA: Exploratory laparotomy and splenectomy for Hodgkin's disease: A commentary. J Clin Oncol 6:574, 1988
118. Rosenberg SA, Kaplan HS: Evidence for an orderly progression in the spread of Hodgkin's disease. Cancer Res 26:1225, 1966
119. Rosenberg SA, Kaplan HS: The evolution and summary results of the Stanford randomized clinical trials of the management of Hodgkin's disease: 1962–1984. Int J Radiat Oncol Biol Phys 11:5, 1985
120. Rostock RA, Giangreco A, Wharam MD, et al: CT scan modification in the treatment of mediastinal Hodgkin's disease. Cancer 49:2267, 1982
121. Russell KJ, Hoppe RT, Colby TV, et al: Lymphocyte predominant Hodgkin's disease: Clinical presentation and results of treatment. Radiother Oncol 1:197, 1984
122. Santoro A, Bonadonna G, Valagussa P, et al: Long-term results of combined chemotherapy-radiotherapy approach in Hodgkin's disease: Superiority of ABVD plus radiotherapy versus MOPP plus radiotherapy. J Clin Oncol 5:27, 1987
123. Schoeppel SL, Hoppe RT, Dorfman RF, et al: Hodgkin's disease in homosexual men with generalized lymphadenopathy. Ann Intern Med 102:68, 1985
124. Schultz HP, Glatstein E, Kaplan HS: Management of presumptive or proven Hodgkin's disease of the liver: A new radiotherapy technique. Int J Radiat Oncol Biol Phys 1:1, 1975
125. Siber GR, Gorham C, Martin P, et al: Antibody response to pretreatment immunization and post-treatment boosting with bacterial polysaccharide vaccines in patients with Hodgkin's disease. Ann Intern Med 104:467, 1986
126. Silverberg E, Lubera JA: Cancer statistics, 1988. CA-A Cancer J Clin 38:5, 1988
127. Sommer FG, Hoppe RT, Fellingham L, et al: Spleen structure in Hodgkin disease: Ultrasonic characterization. Radiology 153:219, 1984
128. Stein RS, Golomb HM, Wiernik PH, et al: Anatomic substages of stage IIIA Hodgkin's disease: Followup of a collaborative study. Cancer Treat Rep 66:733, 1982
129. Sutcliffe SB, Gospodarowicz MK, Bergsagel DE, et al: Prognostic groups for management of localized Hodgkin's disease. J Clin Oncol 3:393, 1985
130. Thomas F, Cosset JM, Cherel P, et al: Thoracic CT-scanning follow-up of residual mediastinal masses after treatment of Hodgkin's disease. Radiother Oncol 11:119, 1988
131. Tubiana M, Henry-Amar M, Burgers MV, et al: Prognostic significance of erythrocyte sedimentation rate in clinical stages I–II of Hodgkin's disease. J Clin Oncol 2:194, 1984
132. Tubiana M, Henry-Amar M, Carde P, et al: Toward comprehensive management tailored to prognostic factors of patients with clinical stages I and II in Hodgkin's disease. The EORTC lymphoma group controlled clinical trials: 1964–1987. Blood 73:47, 1989
133. Tubiana M, Henry-Amar M, Hayat M, et al: The EORTC treatment of early stages of Hodgkin's disease: The role of radiotherapy. Int J Radiat Oncol Biol Phys 10:197, 1984
134. Tubiana M, Henry-Amar M, van der Werf-Messing B, et al: A multivariate analysis of prognostic factors in early stage Hodgkin's disease. Int J Radiat Oncol Biol Phys 11:23, 1985
135. Tucker MA, Coleman CN, Cox RS, et al: Risk of second cancers after treatment for Hodgkin's disease. N Engl J Med 318:76, 1988
136. van der Velden JW, van Putten WLJ, Guinee VF, et al: Subsequent development of acute non-lymphocytic leukemia in patients treated for Hodgkin's disease. Int J Cancer 42:252, 1988
137. van Rijswijk REN, Verbeek J, Haanen C, et al: Major complications and causes of death in patients treated for Hodgkin's disease. J Clin Oncol 5:1624, 1987
138. Verger E, Easton D, Brada M, et al: Radiotherapy results in laparotomy-staged Hodgkin's disease. Clin Radiol 39:428, 1988
139. Wasserman TH, Tubiana M: Lymphoma: Radiation therapy in lymphoma treatment. Int J Radiat Oncol Biol Phys 14: S187, 1988
140. Weiss LM, Movahed LA, Warnke RA, et al: Detection of Epstein-Barr viral genomes in Reed-Sternberg cells of Hodgkin's disease. N Engl J Med 320:502, 1989
141. Weiss LM, Strickler JG, Hu E, et al: Immunoglobulin gene rearrangements in Hodgkin's disease. Hum Pathol 17:1009, 1986
142. Weissleder R, Elizondo G, Stark DD, et al: The diagnosis of splenic lymphoma by MR imaging: Value of superparamagnetic iron oxide. AJR 152:175, 1989
143. Willett CG, Linggood RM, Meyer J, et al: Results of treatment of stage 3A Hodgkin's disease. Cancer 59:27, 1987
144. Willett CG, Linggood RM, Meyer J, et al: Results of treatment of stage IA and IIA Hodgkin's disease. Cancer 59:1107, 1987
145. Young J, Percy C, Asire A, et al: Surveillance, epidemiology, and end results: Incidence and mortality. Natl Cancer Inst Monogr 57:72, 1981
146. Young RC, Canellos GP, Chabner BA, et al: Patterns of relapse in advanced Hodgkin's disease treated with combination chemotherapy. Cancer 42:1001, 1978
147. Young SW, Ballerio C, Carrol CL: Visual fuzzy cluster analysis of MR images. AJR 152:19, 1989

63

Non-Hodgkin's Lymphomas

Todd H. Wasserman
Eli Glatstein

Non-Hodgkin's lymphomas constitute a varied and complex group of diseases that must be differentiated from Hodgkin's disease. The latter almost always begins in lymph nodes and spreads primarily in an axial fashion; non-Hodgkin's lymphomas may begin either in lymph nodes or in extranodal tissue and can spread both in an axial fashion and centrifugally.[28]

Because of changes in pathology terminology and the introduction of a classification using cell surface markers, many prognostic groups of patients with lymphomas have evolved. Therapeutic choices and prognosis are greatly influenced by variations in anatomic site and extent of disease.

EPIDEMIOLOGY

The American Cancer Society estimates that 37,200 new cases and 19,600 deaths occurred from lymphomas in 1991.[1] Malignant lymphomas of the non-Hodgkin's type tend to occur in older persons; the median age is approximately 50 years. Nodular or follicular lymphomas are rarely seen in persons under the age of 25. The male-to-female patient ratio is approximately 1.7 to 1.

The incidence of lymphomas appears to be increasing, although the cause remains unknown. A lot of speculation has been given to a viral etiology. Recent NCI SEER data show a 25% increase in incidence from 1976 to 1986. Oncogenes and chromosomal translocations have been identified in some patients.

NATURAL HISTORY

Because the principal cellular component of lymphoma is the lymphocyte, the tumor may arise in any area of lymphoid aggregation such as the bone marrow, lymph nodes, spleen, Waldeyer's ring, and gastrointestinal tract, as well as in other tissues in which lymphoid cells may be circulating. Recent improvements in surface markers and monoclonal antibodies have subclassified the lymphocyte population.

The natural history of non-Hodgkin's lymphomas is primarily related to histopathologic subtypes. Nodular or follicular disease within the lymph nodes tends to run a moderately indolent course that can be associated with prolonged survival, as originally categorized under the heading of Brill-Symmers disease. The cells of follicular lymphoma appear to be of B-cell origin within the follicle.[38] Despite the fact that many patients with non-Hodgkin's lymphoma may present with advanced disease (including bone marrow involvement), median survival is fairly long (5 to 7 years).[41]

Lymphomas in which the nodal architecture has been grossly altered to an essentially diffuse sheet of malignant lymphoid cells tend to run more virulent courses.[41] Paradoxically, many patients who have a diffuse pattern in the lymph nodes may present with relatively local or regional disease. Nonetheless, spread can be rapid and fulminant, often initially to nodes but frequently to extralymphatic sites as well.[22]

The case for lymphatic contiguity is much weaker for patients with non-Hodgkin's lymphomas than for those with Hodgkin's disease. However, at presentation most patients have disease that appears to be contiguous.[22] Despite the frequency of extranodal extension, the most common site of initial relapse in these patients, if carefully followed up, appears to be the lymphatics,[22,35] whether the patient is managed with chemotherapy or radiation therapy.[73] Nonetheless, the nodal involvement can be atypical, compared with that of patients with Hodgkin's disease. Waldeyer's ring, rarely involved in patients with Hodgkin's disease, is commonly involved in patients with non-Hodgkin's lymphomas. Epitrochlear and brachial nodes are often involved, especially in patients with follicular lymphoma or nodular lymphoma. Investigation with surgical staging of patients who have non-Hodgkin's lymphomas has demonstrated that the most striking difference between patients who have Hodgkin's disease and those who have non-Hodgkin's lymphomas is the marked increase in the incidence of bone marrow and mesenteric lymph node involvement in the latter group.[28,32] Mesenteric, epitrochlear, and Waldeyer's ring involvement necessitates some technical alteration in treatment planning for optimal radiation therapy.[34,79,90]

DIAGNOSTIC WORKUP

Diagnostic evaluation defines the extent of disease and assists in decisions on treatment. Table 63-1 and Figure 63-1 indicate diagnostic procedures for malignant lymphomas.

Because of advanced age or associated medical illnesses, many patients are not appropriate candidates for intensive radiation therapy or intensive chemotherapy. Conservative management, possibly even deferred treatment,[76] may be desirable for such patients, especially if they have asymptomatic nodular

TABLE 63–1
Diagnostic Workup for Non-Hodgkin's Lymphoma

GENERAL

History, including systemic symptoms (unexplained fever, night sweats, weight loss > 10% of body weight)
Physical examination: special attention to lymphatic sites, organomegaly
  For palpable lymph nodes: note and record number, size, location, shape, texture, and mobility.
Mirror examination of pharynx and oral cavity

SPECIAL TESTS

Standard
  Bilateral iliac crest bone marrow biopsy
  Review of slides by expert hematopathologist
  Cytologic evaluation, if any effusion present
Complementary
  Peritoneoscopy with liver biopsy
  Staging laparotomy with splenectomy, wedge liver biopsy, selected biopsies of periaortic and mesenteric nodes, and open bone marrow biopsy
    Sites of nodal biopsies and splenic pedicle should be marked with radiopaque clips

RADIOGRAPHIC STUDIES

Standard
  Posteroanterior and lateral chest films
  CT scans of abdomen and pelvis; CT scans of chest and neck if disease is present in these sites
  Isotopic bone scan
Complementary
  Gallium whole-body scan
  Upper gastrointestinal or small bowel series when clinically indicated
  CT scan of brain when clinically indicated
  Bilateral lower extremity lymphangiogram if abdominopelvic CT scan is normal

LABORATORY STUDIES

Standard
  Admission CBC (including platelet count, reticulocyte count), blood chemistries (including BUN, creatinine, uric acid levels), urinalysis
  LDH, liver function tests, including serum alkaline phosphatase
Complementary
  Erythrocyte sedimentation rate
  Serum electrophoresis
  Baseline T3, T4, TSH if neck irradiation is to be used

NON-HODGKIN'S LYMPHOMAS

NAME ______________ # ______________
PATH. DIAGNOSIS ______________ DATE ______________
AGE ______ SEX ______
HISTORY:

PATHOLOGY
ORIGINAL BX
Site
Diagnosis
Date
Date Barnes path. review
BONE MARROW
W-J BX
Aspirate
Open BX

EXAM:

LABORATORY
CBC
SMA-12
Serum copper
Fract. alk. p'tase
Thyroid studies

LAPAROTOMY FINDINGS
Lap date
Liver
Spleen
Splenic hilum
P.A. nodes
Mesenteric
Other

X-RAYS
Chest
Lung tomos
Lymphangiogram
Bone
Panorex
IVP
UGI
BE
CT scan
  Chest
  Abdomen

(SHOW SITES OF DISEASE)

FINAL DIAGNOSIS: ______________
CLINICAL STAGE: ______________ PATHOLOGICAL STAGE: ______________

TREATMENT PLAN: ______________

FIGURE 63–1. A one-page staging sheet used to easily document the initial extent of disease by clinical and pathologic workup. The original stage is never changed, even after relapse.

lymphoma. Adequate information about the extent of the initial disease is essential for proper follow-up of these patients; even the decision to withhold initial treatment implies the eventual necessity for later treatment. The need for careful follow-up is obvious in judging the tempo of disease activity.

Staging Laparotomy

Use of staging laparotomy in patients with non-Hodgkin's lymphoma remains controversial.[32] Most patients with non-Hodgkin's lymphoma present with advanced disease,[40] and the curative therapeutic options are somewhat limited. If laparotomy findings will not truly influence decisions regarding therapy, such a procedure is hard to justify, except on an investigational basis. Patients with non-Hodgkin's lymphomas tend to be older and more debilitated and to have more extensive tumor than patients with Hodgkin's disease. Consequently, laparotomy is associated with more morbidity in patients with non-Hodgkin's lymphoma.

The introduction of computed tomography (CT) scanning, particularly of the abdomen and pelvis, has enabled the identification of sites of disease that could not have been previously visualized without staging laparotomy.[52,84,94] Some gastrointestinal (GI) extranodal primary lesions, although not clearly visible on barium studies, are visible on CT scans. CT scans are best for showing mesenteric lymph node disease (Fig. 63-2*A*). The incidence of abnormal scans has decreased the need for staging laparotomy. Use of CT scans enables proper definition of tumor volume and dose-limiting normal structures (kidneys and liver) and enhances treatment planning using a simulator and therapy computer (Fig. 63-2*B*).

Some patients have a diagnostic rather than a staging laparotomy; that is, they present with abdominal disease, and the original pathology is obtained at laparotomy, with the disease often having been previously demonstrated on CT scan. It is debated as to whether more than the necessary biopsies should be done at the time of surgery. Occasionally, a bowel diversion or splenectomy may be indicated. If liver disease is not known to be present, liver biopsies should be done. The role of splenectomy in patients with non-Hodgkin's lymphomas is not clear.

Lymphangiogram

The question arises as to whether a lymphangiogram should be done when a patient is going to have a staging laparotomy or has already had a diagnostic laparotomy. If the result of a CT scan is normal, the lymphangiogram is important because it can give diagnostic information about the status of specific retro-

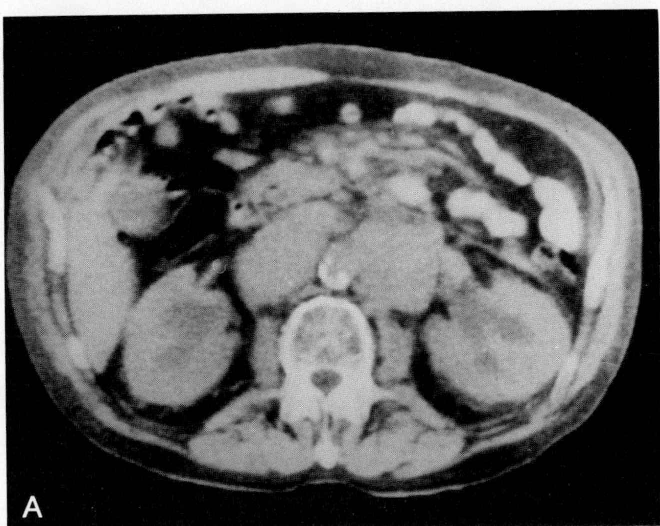

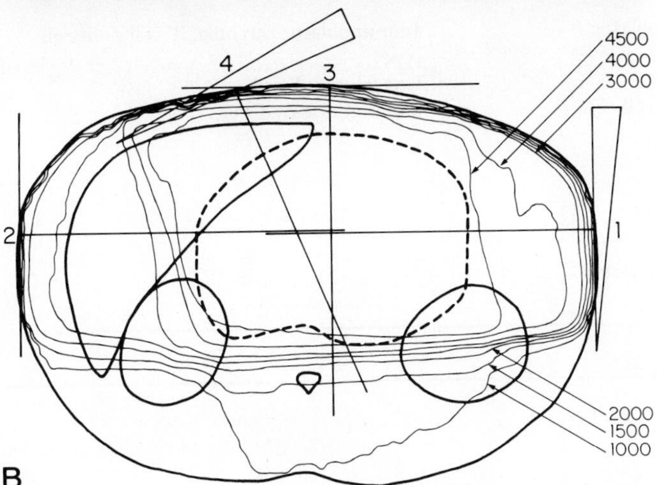

FIGURE 63–2. (**A**) CT scan showing mesenteric and retroperitoneal disease at the level of the renal hilum. (**B**) Isodose curve from a multifield radiation treatment plan to provide an idealized tumor dose of 4500 cGy to the defined target volume, with lesser dose to the liver volume (median 3000 cGy) and to the kidneys (median 2000 cGy).

peritoneal nodes and because it assesses nodal architecture instead of mere size. If radiation therapy is to be used, the lymphangiogram is valuable for localization of radiation portals. In addition, the lymphangiogram is easy to follow with a simple flat plate of the abdomen on a routine (monthly) basis.

Gallium Scan

Approximately 75% to 85% of patients with non-Hodgkin's lymphomas have uptake of gallium, depending on the histology. When tumors are found to be gallium-avid initially, repeat gallium scans can be useful after treatment to evaluate residual masses for active tumor. These studies are complementary with CT scans and MRI.[44,98]

STAGING SYSTEM

The staging classification usually used for non-Hodgkin's lymphomas is the Ann Arbor staging system for Hodgkin's disease.[13] However, this classification is not entirely satisfactory for patients with non-Hodgkin's lymphomas, because many patients have relatively advanced disease and because survival differences for patients with nodular lymphoma are marginal (except in Stage I disease) for each stage according to the different histopathologic types.[82]

The lymphoma classification system is predicated primarily on the gross distribution of nodal involvement, with subclassification based on extralymphatic spread and the presence or absence of systemic B symptoms, defined exclusively as unexplained fevers, unexplained weight loss, and night sweats. The Ann Arbor staging classification is shown in Chapter 62 (see Table 62-3). It should be noted that Stage IE disease represents disease without any lymphatic involvement. Such primary extranodal lymphomas are occasionally seen in patients with non-Hodgkin's lymphomas.

The current Ann Arbor staging system fails to account for important prognostic factors such as bulk of disease and age. The diaphragm is an insignificant barrier with the use of current clinical evaluation procedures such as CT and modern gallium scanning.

PATHOLOGIC CLASSIFICATION

The histopathologic classification of non-Hodgkin's lymphomas has been a challenge to both pathologists and clinicians for decades. The older classification of "reticulum cell sarcoma, lymphosarcoma, and giant follicular lymphoma" failed to demonstrate usefulness because these designations apparently did not represent single disease entities. The Rappaport histopathologic classification system (Table 63-2) clearly showed clinical relevance by distinguishing groups of patients who have major survival differences.[41,78] Nodular or follicular lymphoma tends to run a relatively indolent course, and patients have prolonged survival; diffuse lymphoma tends to run a relatively fulminant course, and patients have relatively poor prognosis for survival. The exception to the poor survival rates with diffuse lymphoma is found in the category of diffuse lymphocytic lymphoma, well-differentiated, which appears to run an indolent clinical course similar to that of chronic lymphatic leukemia. Even this relatively simple system, however, requires expert hematopathologic interpretation of nodal biopsies if valid comparisons are to be made from the literature.[24,39]

Some dissatisfaction has occurred with the Rappaport classification system because many of the large cell lymphomas, termed *histiocytic* on morphologic grounds, have clearly been shown by ultrastructural and immunologic techniques to be composed of large or transformed lymphocytes rather than true histiocytes.

A complication in the classification of lymphomas is the significant proportion of patients who have divergent histologies in the same or different biopsy sites. Also, histologic progression from low to high grade during the clinical course is common. Technically, a composite lymphoma is one in which two different and well-delineated types of lymphoma occur in the same anatomic site.

Several newer pathologic classifications have been proposed that are more histologically or functionally distinct than the Rappaport system (see Table 63-2). Large retrospective reviews have tested the reproducibility and prognostic value of these systems with mixed results.[18,69]

With techniques that enabled recognition of T and B cells, it became clear that disorders classified by the Rappaport system represented heterogeneous groups of disease. Malignant B-cell lymphomas represented approximately 70% of the cases,

TABLE 63–2
Pathologic Classification of Non-Hodgkin's Lymphomas

RAPPAPORT CLASSIFICATION	WORKING FORMULATION OF NON-HODGKIN'S LYMPHOMAS FOR CLINICAL USAGE	LUKES AND COLLINS CLASSIFICATION
	Low grade	
Diffuse lymphocytic, well-differentiated	ML, small lymphocytic	Small lymphocytic and plasmacytoid lymphocytic
Nodular, poorly differentiated lymphocytic	ML, follicular, predominantly small cleaved cell	Small cleaved FCC, follicular only or follicular and diffuse
Nodular, mixed lymphocytic-histiocytic	ML, follicular, mixed small cleaved and large cell	Small cleaved FCC, follicular; large cleaved FCC, follicular
	Intermediate grade	
Nodular histiocytic	ML, follicular, predominantly large cell	Large cleaved or noncleaved FCC, follicular
Diffuse lymphocytic, poorly differentiated	ML, diffuse small cleaved cell	Small cleaved FCC, diffuse
Diffuse mixed lymphocytic-histiocytic	ML, diffuse, mixed small and large cell	Small cleaved, large cleaved or large noncleaved FCC, diffuse
Diffuse histiocytic	ML, diffuse large cell	Large cleaved or noncleaved FCC, diffuse
	High grade	
Diffuse histiocytic	ML, large cell immunoblastic	Immunoblastic sarcoma, T cell or B cell type
Lymphoblastic convoluted/nonconvoluted	ML, lymphoblastic	Convoluted T cell
Undifferentiated, Burkitt's and non-Burkitt's	ML, small noncleaved cell	Small noncleaved FCC
	Miscellaneous	
	Composite	
	Mycosis fungoides	
	Histiocytic	
	Extramedullary plasmacytoma	
	Unclassifiable	

ML: malignant lymphoma; FCC: follicular center cell

and those of T-cell origin, 20% of the cases. A better prognosis was found for B-cell lymphomas compared with T-cell lymphomas. True histiocytic lymphomas were found in less than 1% of the cases.

A significant contribution of the Lukes and Collins classification is the definition of lymphoblastic (convoluted T-cell) lymphoma as a distinct pathologic and clinical entity. This lymphoma occurs predominantly in young male patients and often presents as a large mediastinal mass. Early central nervous system (CNS), bone marrow, and peripheral blood involvement are common. Before the use of modern chemotherapeutic regimens, this disease was associated with a median survival time to less than 1 year.

In 1982, *Working Formulation of the Non-Hodgkin's Lymphomas for Clinical Usage* was published.[72] This is a clinicopathologic classification that enables translation among the six major existing systems of classifying non-Hodgkin's lymphoma. The classification defines 20 distinct subtypes of lymphoma according to morphology, clinical features, and prognosis (see Table 63-2). It retains and supports the notion that a follicular (nodular) histology confers a better prognosis than does diffuse histology. It does not use techniques to characterize the surface markers of lymphoid cells but does emphasize important morphologic differences, as proposed by Lukes and Collins.[56] The classification, for example, accommodates data that have shown a better prognosis for diffuse large cell lymphoma than for immunoblastic lymphoma (both classified as diffuse histiocytic lymphoma by the Rappaport system).

Even with the Rappaport classification system, among patients who have at least two evaluable biopsy specimens of tumor at the time of presentation, the incidence of multiple histologic types is approximately 20% to 25%.[28] Thus, a significant portion of patients represent dilemmas of categorization. In addition, many patients have nodal architecture that shows both partly nodular and partly diffuse elements. In general, when a major component of the node shows a nodular pattern, the survival of such patients appears to be comparable to that of patients who have only nodular lymphomas—that is, favorable. Hence, such patients who have dual elements in the nodal architecture are usually considered under the more favorable category of nodular lymphoma.

An update of the NCI-sponsored non-Hodgkin's lymphoma pathology project[93] gives the long-term follow-up of 1153 patients treated between 1971 and 1975 with a median follow-up of 11.2 years. Ten-year survival rates were 45% for low-grade, 26% for intermediate-grade, and 23% for high-grade lymphomas.

Approximately 50% of patients with non-Hodgkin's lymphoma have a diffuse pattern and 50% have a nodular pattern.[41] Of the diffuse patterns, diffuse histiocytic lymphoma, which tends to be among the most fulminant, paradoxically appears to be curable in many patients. Most patients who fail treatment for diffuse histiocytic lymphoma do so within the first 2 years. Patients with other forms of diffuse lymphoma who fail treatment also do so within the first few years, although later relapses may be seen. Patients with diffuse mixed and diffuse lymphocytic lymphoma, poorly differentiated, have a finite cure rate with radiation therapy when disease is limited to one side of the diaphragm. Diffuse undifferentiated lymphoma, of both Burkitt's and non-Burkitt's type, is particularly difficult to treat with radiation therapy alone. Diffuse lymphocytic lymphoma, well differentiated, is a clinical variant of chronic lymphatic leukemia. Accordingly, relatively conservative treatment appears to be indicated, because the expected survival rate in this one subgroup of patients with diffuse lymphoma is generally good.

Scant evidence at the present time shows that patients with nodular lymphomas are curable. Because of the chronic nature of these lymphocytic diseases, any early judgment on the patient's curability must be deferred. Nodular lymphoma tends to present with advanced disease (Stage III or IV).[82] Patients who have localized disease appear to be curable to a finite degree with radiation therapy alone.[25] Moreover, patients with nodular lymphoma of Stage III extent may have some modest potential for curability with radiation therapy alone.[26] Evidence that Stage IV patients are curable is generally lacking; nodular lymphocytic lymphoma appears to have a continuous relapse rate for as long as patients are followed.[2,25,26,41,76,85] Patients who have nodular mixed lymphoma, by contrast, have been reported to be curable by the National Cancer Institute after intensive chemotherapy[2,85]; confirmation of these results is needed. Nodular lymphocytic lymphoma, well-differentiated, is a very rare diagnosis; it should be made only by expert hematopathologists.

Bone marrow involvement is much more common among patients who have non-Hodgkin's lymphomas than among those who have Hodgkin's disease (Table 63-3). Among patients who have nodular lymphocytic lymphoma, poorly differentiated, the probability of bone marrow involvement may be as high as 80%.[82,83] Yet circulating malignant cells (a leukemic syndrome) are infrequently reported (5% to 10%). Circulating "cleaved" cells associated with nodular lymphoma have a different prognostic significance from circulating blast cells in a true acute lymphocytic leukemia because the survival rate among patients in the former group is still comparatively good. Indeed, no conclusive evidence exists that bone marrow involvement with nodular lymphoma significantly compromises survival in patients with Stage IV involvement.[76,82] Circulating blast cells commonly occur in those with childhood lymphoma, especially with diffuse lymphoblastic lymphoma or "convoluted cell" lymphoma with mediastinal involvement at presentation.[68] Circulating blast cells in this setting herald a fulminant course.

The distinction between well-differentiated lymphocytic lymphoma and chronic lymphocytic leukemia cannot be made by lymph node biopsy alone. The circulating white blood cell count, the degree of circulating lymphocytes, and the results of a careful bone marrow examination all must be taken into account.

PROGNOSTIC FACTORS

Many factors appear to have prognostic importance in the management of patients with non-Hodgkin's lymphomas. The most important of these are age, symptoms, histology, stage, site, bulk, and tempo of disease.

Age

Non-Hodgkin's lymphoma in pediatric patients tends to be a relatively fulminant disease and is virtually always the diffuse type.[75] Many patients have mediastinal involvement and convoluted neoplastic cells of apparent T-cell origin; such patients appear to have high predilection for dissemination to bone marrow and the central nervous system. In general, for each histologic type, older patients tend to have a worse prognosis than younger ones.[41] The precise explanation for this observation is not clear; presumably the difference is a reflection of steady decline in tolerance to treatment beyond age 50. For this reason elderly patients who are not symptomatic and who appear to have relatively indolent lymphoma with a nodular histology may be appropriately managed with conservative treatment policies.

Symptoms

Systemic symptoms, seen fairly frequently in Hodgkin's disease, are comparatively uncommon with non-Hodgkin's lymphomas. Fever, night sweats, or weight loss are manifested in approximately 10% to 15% of patients at presentation.[28,41] In non-Hodgkin's lymphomas, conclusive evidence is lacking that systemic symptoms of fevers, night sweats, and weight loss indicate a particularly poor prognosis.[41]

Histology

The importance of histology in the selection of treatment must be tempered by the knowledge of the difficulty involved with reproducing histopathologic classification from pathologist to pathologist.[39] The major distinction is made between the nodular and the diffuse varieties. In general, the significance of the individual cell types is more modest.[41]

TABLE 63–3
Histology, Pathologic Stage, and Bone Marrow Involvement at the Time of Presentation for Non-Hodgkin's Lymphoma

HISTOLOGY	STAGE			POSITIVE BONE MARROW (%)
	I (%)	II (%)	III AND IV (%)	
Small lymphocytic	3	8	89	71
Follicular, small cleaved cell	8	10	82	51
Diffuse, small cleaved cell	9	19	72	32
Diffuse large cell	16	3	54	10
Large cell, immunoblastic	23	29	58	12
Lymphoblastic	7	20	74	50

Stage

It is difficult to distinguish the clinical importance of histology from that of stage in non-Hodgkin's lymphoma (see Table 63-3).

Extranodal Extension

The site of limited extranodal extension is another prognostic feature of importance in non-Hodgkin's lymphoma. A small but definite percentage of patients with Waldeyer's ring involvement have gastrointestinal (GI) disease.[22] The converse is also true; primary GI lesions have a finite probability of association with Waldeyer's ring involvement. Occasionally, patients treated for anaplastic carcinoma in the tonsillar or nasopharyngeal regions with high-dose irradiation subsequently develop subdiaphragmatic tumor that proves to be diffuse histiocytic lymphoma. The initial tumor in the Waldeyer's region was almost certainly diffuse histiocytic lymphoma that initially could not be categorized pathologically.

Shigematsu and associates[88] from Japan reviewed 142 patients with Stage I and Stage II non-Hodgkin's lymphomas of the head and neck. They found no 5-year difference in freedom from relapse between patients with Stage I and Stage II disease. In a multivariate regression analysis, they showed that primary site, use of multiagent chemotherapy, and tumor bulk were independent factors. Waldeyer's ring lymphomas did better than other nodal or extranodal lymphomas. Pathologic grade using the working formulation was also a prognostic factor.[88]

Gastrointestinal lesions usually require wide-field radiation techniques. Such lesions typically are considered to be comparatively unfavorable if they have grown to a large size.[31]

A growing problem occurring with the successful general management of lymphomas is central nervous system relapse. It has a high degree of morbidity and mortality, because the CNS is a potential sanctuary of lymphoma cells that are unresponsive to chemotherapy.

GENERAL MANAGEMENT

When any therapy for lymphoma is planned, it is first necessary to determine whether the patient is a candidate for a potentially curative approach or whether he or she should be managed palliatively.

Typically, non-Hodgkin's lymphomas confined to one side of the diaphragm, either nodular or diffuse, are usually managed by high-dose radiation therapy. This usually consists of treatment to the site(s) of involvement with additional coverage of draining nodal groups on the same side of the diaphragm. Total lymphoid irradiation for Stages I and II disease is not commonly used in the United States, although the results are reasonably encouraging.[7,25] Evidence for superiority of total lymphoid irradiation over local-field irradiation in the management of Stages I and II nodular lymphoma is lacking.[25,29] More recent experience with high-dose total lymphoid irradiation for Stages I and II diffuse lymphoma suggests some improvement over previous experience.[7,25]

Currently, for Stage I disease of nodular or diffuse histopathologic subtype, radiation therapy alone is standard management, with at least 4000 cGy being used. Extranodal lesions or large Stage I disease frequently is treated to 5000 cGy.[62] Draining regional lymphatics are usually included. It is unclear whether adjuvant chemotherapy or prophylactic radiation therapy on the opposite side of the diaphragm is more beneficial.[10,25,45,46]

Stage II disease of nodular histopathologic subtype also is usually managed with radiation therapy alone. The optimal management of Stage II disease of diffuse type is still a subject of controversy. Several investigators prefer to use total lymphoid radiation therapy[7,25] with radiation on both sides of the diaphragm, including the whole abdomen, on the basis of the high incidence of mesenteric lymph node involvement discovered by staging laparotomy.[48] Others advocate local radiation therapy for known disease plus adjuvant chemotherapy[46] or intensive chemotherapy alone.[31]

Stage III and Stage IV lymphomas are frequently grouped together for therapeutic decisions. For Stage III nodular lymphoma, it is suggested that high-dose total lymphoid irradiation may be associated with prolonged disease-free survival in a significant percentage of patients.[26] In disease as notoriously indolent as nodular lymphoma, one hesitates to say that such patients are cured; nonetheless, one third of patients with Stage III nodular lymphoma appear to be in initial remission at 10 years after high-dose total nodal irradiation. By contrast, the results of total lymphoid irradiation in Stage III diffuse lymphoma are extremely poor, with approximately only 10% of the patients alive and well, free from disease, at 10 years.[26] Consequently, for patients with Stage III diffuse lymphoma, total lymphoid irradiation alone is probably inappropriate. It remains to be seen whether radiation therapy plays a major role in Stage III disease of an unfavorable histologic type. However, systemic management is usually employed.[2,12,19,83,85] It may consist of chemotherapy alone, either single alkylating agent or combination chemotherapy. Whole-body irradiation is also used for Stage III and Stage IV nodular lymphoma as a palliative technique. Combined-modality treatment for Stage III and Stage IV nodular and diffuse lymphomas is under investigation.

For Stage III and Stage IV lymphomas of diffuse histopathologic subtype, combination chemotherapy is usually the standard of treatment.[2,85] Although there is some suggestion that irradiation to the nodes may be beneficial[25] as an adjunct to chemotherapy, this technique of combined-modality treatment remains investigational. Radiation therapy alone for the treatment of Stage III or Stage IV diffuse histopathologic subtypes is considered inadequate.

For Stage IV disease of the nodular histopathologic type, several treatment options exist. Chemotherapy is clearly a mainstay; for patients with nodular histology, even single alkylating agent chemotherapy,[76] as well as combination chemotherapy,[2,85] may be beneficial. In addition, whole-body irradiation for nodular lymphoma of advanced stage appears to be a useful therapeutic tool, although not obviously superior to chemotherapy.[12,101] It is difficult to recommend one treatment approach over another because the survival in these groups of patients appears to be comparable, regardless of the method of treatment. No conclusive evidence has been found that patients with advanced nodular lymphoma are curable, with the possible exception of patients who have nodular mixed lymphoma and are treated with intensive chemotherapy (cyclophosphamide, Oncovin [vincristine], procarbazine, and prednisone [C-MOPP]).[2,85]

If Waldeyer's ring is involved, the entire region, including draining neck nodes down to the clavicle, should be included in the treatment volume. Primary involvement of oral cavity, sinuses, or orbit clearly requires individualized treatment planning. As soon as disease has spread to regional lymphatic glands, it is important to plan to treat draining nodes as well as the primary tumor mass. Evidence is lacking to support prophylactic treatment of nodal groups when the tumor has not obviously extended to nodes. Nonetheless, regional nodes are usually included in the field because later treatment might prove difficult for optimal matching of fields.

Typically, only a biopsy or simple resection of a GI primary tumor has been performed with very few nodes sampled. In such an instance, it is difficult to know whether the patient has disease confined to the GI primary tumor. Consequently, the use of wide-field irradiation has become routine, unless many nodes were sampled at the time of a resection and all were found to be negative. Not only does such wide-field treatment minimize the probability of marginal recurrences, but it also takes into account the common finding of multiple sites of GI tract involvement and minimizes subsequent matching of portals, if later intraabdominal relapse occurs. When wide-field treatments are used, the dose rate rarely exceeds 150 cGy per day. Slow, protracted fractionation to a high cumulative dose minimizes a tendency for perforation, which is rarely seen with this technique. Patients with GI lesions should have postoperative GI contrast studies and a CT scan as a baseline before treatment.

Bony lesions, if localized after thorough staging evaluation, are usually treated with radiation therapy alone.[17] The entire involved bone is usually treated to the full dose. An appropriate amount of peripheral soft tissue must be excluded from the high-dose volume to minimize the risk of lymphedema.

Better definition of characteristics associated with a high rate of central nervous system relapse and the use of prophylactic CNS therapy, including irradiation and intrathecal chemotherapy, may reduce the risk of CNS relapse.[49,57]

RADIATION THERAPY TECHNIQUES

Dose

Dose is an important consideration in the treatment of non-Hodgkin's lymphomas. Known tumor volume carries the least probability of recurrence when radiation doses over 3500 cGy are used.[23] Typically, doses are increased to 4000 cGy and frequently 5000 cGy, especially for diffuse histiocytic lymphoma. Lower doses of 2500 cGy may be useful for palliation. Doses larger than 4000 cGy for nodular lymphoma are associated with virtually no local recurrence rate. If high doses are used for diffuse lymphomas, the local recurrence rate varies from 15% to 20% for most histologies. Diffuse histiocytic lymphoma does not have a clear dose-response curve, which is probably a reflection of the multitude of different diseases that make up diffuse histiocytic lymphoma by light microscopy.

Volume Treated

The entire lymphatic region involved must be incorporated in the radiation volume with appropriate margin. In practice, the appropriate margin as a minimum consists of contiguous lymphatic regions on the same side of the diaphragm.

Mantle Technique

For patients with mediastinal disease, the mantle technique is used; it is described in detail for Hodgkin's disease in Chapter 62. A few points should be stressed with respect to mantle irradiation for patients with non-Hodgkin's lymphomas. Extension into mediastinal nodes is a very uncommon type of failure in non-Hodgkin's lymphomas of any histology, if the patient did not present with mediastinal tumor.[22] Consequently, under certain circumstances it may be appropriate to eliminate the mediastinal component of the mantle. The supramediastinal mantle, or "minimantle," is appropriate for patients with non-Hodgkin's lymphomas under the following conditions: no obvious disease is detectable in the mediastinum by radiographs or CT scans; no supraclavicular disease is present; and no upper abdominal disease is present. Supraclavicular adenopathy may extend microscopically into upper mediastinal regions; upper abdominal disease may extend into the posterior mediastinum or retrocrural area and not be recognized by routine chest radiographs but may be seen on CT scans.

If the mediastinum is to be eliminated from the mantle field, the lower margin of the minimantle at the midline is set at the level of the inferior portion of the head of the clavicles on the anterior field; posteriorly, blocks are usually set to match the inferior surface of the shaft of the clavicles. The reason for this discrepancy is to allow infraclavicular adenopathy to be adequately treated only by the anterior field. If clinically significant infraclavicular adenopathy is noted, a small direct anterior field of electron-beam treatment may be used as a supplement to increase the dose to this area. The minimantle is centered on the suprasternal notch to facilitate any eventual matching of fields (Fig. 63-3). Omission of the mediastinum, if clinically appropriate, minimizes the risks of high-dose radiation complications and also preserves a significant portion of unirradiated bone marrow.

Preauricular Radiation

The superior margin of the mantle approaches the inferior border of the mandible; consequently preauricular nodes are excluded from a true mantle field. These nodes are frequently involved in non-Hodgkin's lymphomas and are at high risk in patients who have high cervical adenopathy, above the level of the thyroid notch. In such patients, preauricular irradiation is desirable. To encompass the preauricular area for prophylactic

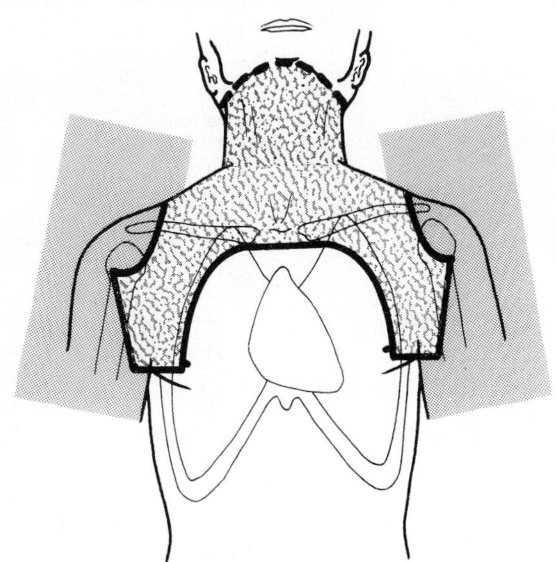

FIGURE 63–3. Example of minimantle field used to treat the cervical, supraclavicular, and, if necessary, axillary lymph nodes in patients with non-Hodgkin's lymphoma.

treatment, a repair of lateral opposing fields is set up.[36] The inferior margin of this lateral field is matched at the midplane to the superior margin of the mantle. The superior margin of the preauricular field should be above the level of the zygomatic arch and on portal films includes the floor of the sphenoid sinus. Posteriorly, the margin of the field begins at the tragus, whereas the anterior margin of the field is arranged posterior to the teeth. The morbidity with such a field, termed a "Waldeyer's ring field," is significant. Commonly, xerostomia and dental complications develop; careful dental prophylaxis, including frequent cleaning and regular administration of fluoride solution, is important. When this region is being treated on a prophylactic basis, the dosage usually is reduced to 3600 cGy midplane over approximately 4 weeks.

When Waldeyer's ring is overtly involved, a larger field is necessary, which is also appropriate for patients with high neck disease at the upper margin of the true mantle. Large lateral fields are usually initiated below the angle of the mandible (thyroid notch), and the upper margin of the mantle is reduced accordingly. In this setting, the lateral fields and mantle portal should not overlap. Because of dosimetric fall-off at the edge of large fields, it is possible to underdose known disease present at the angle of the mandible with the minimantle port. Consequently, when patients present with high neck disease, large lateral fields are appropriate for the first 2000 cGy to be certain that tumor has been fully dosed in the initial period of treatment. The large lateral fields should extend back into the occipital region, which would ordinarily be included in the diverging part of the superior portion of the anterior mantle. When such large lateral fields are being used over the preauricular and Waldeyer's region, marked reduction in tumor volume typically has occurred by 2000 cGy; a shrinking field approach can be used by reducing the lateral fields and raising the matchline to the level of the inferior mandible to deliver additional dose to the Waldeyer's ring.

Supradiaphragmatic and Subdiaphragmatic Treatment

If radiation therapy is to be delivered on both sides of the diaphragm, an appropriate gap must be calculated between the fields at the surface of the skin on the AP and PA portals to account for the normal divergence of the beam from each of the two fields. The objective of this calculation is to have the 50% isodose lines of the superior and inferior fields match exactly at the midplane.

When total lymphoid irradiation is planned, attention must be paid at the time of the initial setup to localize the appropriate level of the future matchline between supradiaphragmatic and subdiaphragmatic fields. The matchline should not knowingly be placed through a tumor mass.

Whole Abdominal Treatment

For patients with non-Hodgkin's lymphomas, mesenteric lymph node involvement is exceedingly common. Consequently, the radiation therapist must consider the high risk of such involvement in formulating the treatment strategy for this disease. One such approach is the treatment of the whole abdominal cavity based on isocentric setup (Figs. 63-4 and 63-5).[27] The upper abdominal field is set up on a four-field basis on a simulator. Initial treatment consists of simple anterior and posterior fields from the dome of the diapghragm to approximately the level of the iliac crests (assuming that the inferior margin does not cut across known tumor) (Fig. 63-6). When massive tumor occurs at this level, the entire abdominal content from diaphragm to the floor of the pelvis is treated in one large field. When possible, lead blocks are placed over the lateral portions of each ilium to attempt to protect iliac bone marrow. With large fields of this nature, the maximal dose rate should not exceed 150 cGy per day; the tumor dose goes to approximately 1500 cGy over 2 to 3 weeks to these large anterior and posterior fields. Throughout the initial portion of treatment, the right lobe of the liver is protected by a lead block to minimize the dose that the liver receives; this will be compensated in the second portion of treatment to the abdominal field.

The second portion of the abdominal treatment continues to treat the upper abdominal field but from lateral fields based on the initial isocentric setup. In the presence of massive abdominal disease, a pelvic (an iliofemoral) portion of the radiation field may continue by opposing anteroposterior techniques. The upper abdominal field receives opposing cross-table lateral fields with the patient in the supine position and with blocks to protect both kidneys. The localization of the

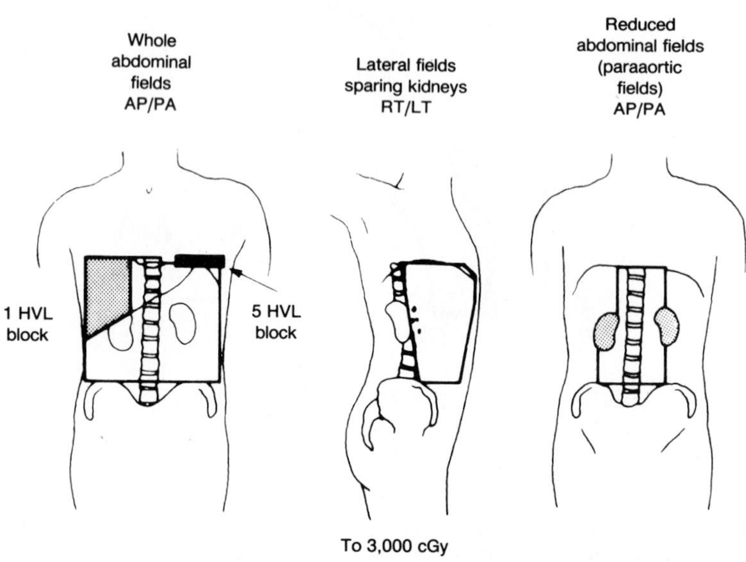

FIGURE 63–4. Schematic drawing of a multifield abdominal radiation technique. This technique uses three sets of radiation fields.

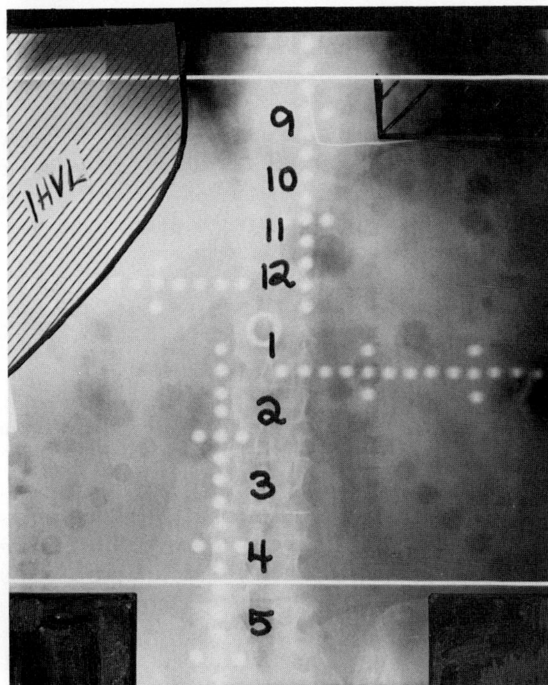

FIGURE 63–5. Simulation film showing the initial whole-abdomen field, with a 1 HVL liver block. The bottom of the field is at the top of the pelvis, and the top of the field is at the dome of the diaphragm. The lateral margins are at the abdominal wall bilaterally.

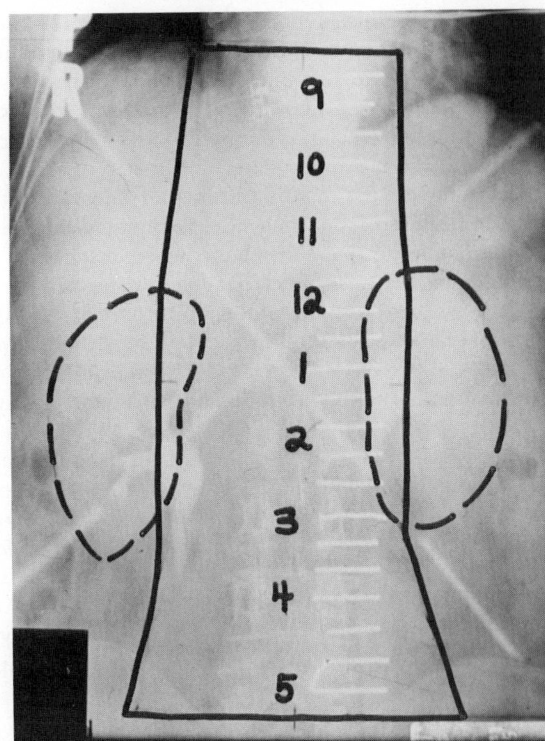

FIGURE 63–6. Simulation film of a periaortic boost field, showing the same top and bottom line but with the lateral lines wide enough to include the periaortic disease, encompassing only the medial third of the kidneys.

kidneys is obtained by CT scans or by an infusion of contrast material in the treatment position on a simulator. The posterior margin of the lateral radiation portal is placed anterior to the kidneys but posterior to opacified periaortic nodes, which are easily visualized by the lymphangiogram or CT scan. The anterior margin of the lateral portal should extend to the anterior abdominal wall. Full-thickness (5 half-value layer [HVL]) blocks are required to protect the kidneys in their posterior position while the patient is being treated from the lateral field. By use of these two opposing lateral fields, with carefully positioned kidney blocks, the upper abdomen, including the liver, receives another 1500 cGy over approximately 2 weeks, which brings the dose to periaortic nodes to approximately 3000 cGy over approximately 4 to 5 weeks.

If abdominal surgery has been performed, it may be known that retroperitoneal disease is present on the posterior abdominal wall, thus precluding kidney shielding by this technique. In addition, in some patients, the kidneys may be seen anteriorly on the lateral setup and may lie in the same plane as the periaortic nodes. This, too, may prevent adequate lateral protection of the kidneys in the attempt to treat the tumor volume. CT scans are useful in identifying these patients. When the kidney location prevents the use of the lateral field technique, anteroposterior radiation techniques are required, and the use of 5 cm thick lead kidney blocks is necessary posteriorly to keep the total renal dose under 2500 cGy.

The final portion of the upper abdominal technique is a very wide (10 cm to 12 cm) periaortic field using anterior and posterior fields. Bilateral 5 HVL thick shaped blocks are required to protect the kidneys from the anterior and posterior fields for the final 1500 cGy. The lateral width of the upper portion of this wide periaortic field extends from the lateral margin of one kidney to the lateral margin of the opposite kidney. This portal delivers the full dose to the root of the mesentery by a shrinking field technique. The right lobe of the liver is excluded throughout this portion of irradiation, after having been treated during the lateral field exposures. Thus, the total dose delivered to the central abdomen is 4500 cGy over approximately 6 to 7 weeks.

Pelvic irradiation may continue on an anterior/posterior basis throughout the period of abdominal irradiation if blood counts permit or in a separate field after completion of the upper abdominal portals. Caution should be used when blood counts are low or whenever prior chemotherapy has been used, and pelvic therapy can be deferred until the upper abdominal irradiation is completed, unless the pelvic tumor is massive or symptomatic.

It is important when one treats the pelvis of a patient with non-Hodgkin's lymphoma to maintain the height of midline pelvic blocks no higher than the symphysis pubis. Midline adenopathy can develop under higher central blocks; thus, for young female patients who have a non-Hodgkin's lymphoma, no attempt is made to preserve ovarian function when the pelvis is to be treated.

Total-Body Irradiation

In patients who have nodular lymphocytic lymphoma or nodular mixed lymphoma of advanced stage, total-body irradiation may be used for palliation.[12] This type of treatment is not well tolerated if the patient already has marrow compromise with significant leukopenia or thrombocytopenia from prior tumor treatment. Prolonged or intensive prior chemotherapy may also compromise this technique, even though peripheral hematologic parameters appear normal at the beginning of treatment because of diminished bone marrow reserve. The mechanism of action of total-body irradiation is obscure, but the rationale is based on the combination of marked radiation sensitivity of lymphocytic lymphoma and a high incidence of dissemination. Treatment is usually administered with a linear accelerator or cobalt unit at approximately a 3 meter distance. The patient is usually seated, holding his or her knees, and treatment is administered from each side. Depending on the dosimetry, compensating filters may be required to achieve a relatively homogeneous dose. Fractionation can be delivered in numerous ways, but typically a dose of approximately 150 cGy midplane over 5 weeks is administered, often at the rate of 30 cGy per week in two or three fractions per week (10 cGy to 15 cGy per fraction). Total-body irradiation is tolerated well symptomatically.

The major complication of total-body irradiation is marked thrombocytopenia or leukopenia; in particular, platelet counts should be plotted and watched carefully, with blood counts before every treatment, because a rapid decline may herald the need to discontinue treatment until platelet counts have stabilized, even though the absolute level may be greater than 100,000. The absolute nadir of thrombocytopenia may not occur for 2 to 3 weeks after treatment has been interrupted.

RESULTS OF THERAPY

Low Stage Nodular Lymphomas

For Stage I and Stage II nodular lymphoma, patients treated with radiation therapy alone have excellent survival. Indeed, for such patients with pathologic Stage I and Stage II nodular lymphomas, no clear evidence shows that treatment on the opposite side of the diaphragm is beneficial. The overall survival rate at 5 years ranges from 80% to 100%.[10,14,25] These data assume that the patient has been staged pathologically. Because surgical staging has become more difficult to justify in these patients, the incidence of unsuspected disease in the abdomen of patients with clinical Stage I and Stage II nodular lymphoma is high.[28] Consequently, if patients are to be treated with clinical staging, the highest probability of freedom from relapse can probably be seen when patients are treated with a total lymphoid approach.

Reddy and colleagues from Chicago[79,80] reviewed their experience with Stage I and Stage II non-Hodgkin's lymphomas treated for cure by radiation therapy between 1964 and 1977; 116 patients were followed up for a minimum of 8 years. Patients with Stage I tumors, both extranodal and nodal, had survival and recurrence-free survival rates of 80% and 74%, respectively. Stage II patients did significantly worse with recurrence-free survival rate of approximately 30% at 10 years. The authors were not able to analyze for bulk of disease.

The Stanford group[43] reviewed the records of 148 consecutive patients with Stage I and Stage II large cell lymphoma treated with primary irradiation with or without chemotherapy. In a multivariate analysis, the significant prognostic variables were number of sites of disease and bulk of disease less than or greater than 10 cm. In a univariate analysis of prognostic factors, stage, extralymphatic disease, constitutional symptoms, and age were prognostic factors. The number of sites of involvement were one or two in the favorable group and more than two in the unfavorable group. Patients with favorable factors can apparently be successfully treated with irradiation alone or with limited chemotherapy plus limited radiation therapy. Patients with unfavorable factors require more aggressive treatment.

In an analysis from the National Cancer Institute of Stage I and Stage II patients with favorable lymphomas, it was established that some patients could have long-term disease-free survival with irradiation alone.[47] Prognostic factors included age of patient and current overall survival; stage is a factor only in disease-free survival. Because a great percentage of failures were in sites of nodal disease, the authors believe that investigation of total lymphoid irradiation in these early stage, favorable lymphoma patients should be undertaken.

Localized Stage I and Stage II Large Cell Lymphomas

Several investigators have shown excellent results in pathologically staged patients with radiation therapy.[7,25,50,51,95,97,99] Adjuvant chemotherapy after treating only the site of involvement has been reported to be beneficial by some investigators,[37,46,60,66,71] but not by others.[25] Some groups use chemotherapy as the primary treatment with or without adjuvant irradiation with good results but questionably more morbidity.[11,55,64]

In a review from Stanford, 94 patients with Stage I and Stage II large cell lymphomas treated from 1978 to 1986 with combination chemotherapy and irradiation are presented.[77] Ninety-three percent of these patients had diffuse large cell lymphomas; 25% had Stage I or Stage IE, and 75% had Stage II or Stage IE disease; 37% of the patients had bulky disease greater than 70 cm; 45% had an elevated lactate dehydrogenase (LDH) level. The mean follow-up was 33 months, and the projected 5-year freedom from relapse is 72% of all patients, with Stage I patients doing better than Stage II patients (not statistically significant). The important prognostic factors appear to be initial LDH level, tumor bulk greater than 10 cm, and treatment sequence with chemotherapy (irradiation/chemotherapy was apparently best). This Stanford series should be contrasted with that of Kaminski and associates,[43] who reviewed the results of primary irradiation of Stage I and Stage II large cell lymphoma in which the 5-year relapse-free rates were 62% for Stage I and 38% for Stage II patients.

In a review at the Farber Cancer Center of the patterns of relapse in large cell lymphomas treated with aggressive chemotherapy using M or mBACOD chemotherapy, there was no indication that likely relapse patterns were in sites of original bulk disease exclusively. The authors question the value of adjuvant radiation therapy in this setting.[91]

The Vancouver group[16] published their early results with a short course of CHOP chemotherapy for three cycles followed by involved field radiation to the original sites of disease (3000 cGy in ten fractions) for limited stage aggressive lymphomas. This group is now treating patients with 6 weeks of ACOB chemotherapy and involved field irradiation.[15]

The Vancouver study is one of several series that suggest that chemotherapy plus radiation therapy is better than the initial treatment for patients with early stage large cell lymphomas. Some authors think that chemotherapy alone is the correct approach for these patients.[63] A subset of patients, however, could be treated with irradiation alone; patients with early stage large cell lymphomas present with supradiaphragmatic disease that is nonbulky; they do not have B symptoms with normal LDH level and are under 60 years of age. This cohort of patients may represent approximately 20% of the patients with Stage I or Stage II disease.

In a recent review from the Mallinckrodt Institute of Radiology, it was found that in 57 patients with disease presenting above the diaphragm and treated with radiation therapy alone, bulk of disease was the most important prognostic factor. Thirty patients had clinical Stage I and 27 had clinical Stage II, but this was not as important as knowing the total tumor area in square centimeters for all sites of disease. Bulky Stage I patients did worse than small volume Stage II patients. These patients all had large cell lymphomas, and none was treated with chemotherapy initially because of their presentation predominantly in the head and neck region. With a median follow-up of 9.4 years, 51% of patients had no relapse and died free from disease or were alive free from disease. The best subgroup of patients were those with disease less than or equal to 16 cm^2 who were fully staged with a relapse-free survival rate in 19 patients of 47%, and NED survival rate after salvage therapy of 95%. Thus, there is a subpopulation of patients with clinical Stage IA or IIA disease presenting above the diaphragm without bulky disease who have an excellent chance of long-term disease control treated by radiation therapy alone, with chemotherapy reserved for salvage.

In a recent series of publications[42,54,55] the controversy as to the best treatment for localized aggressive lymphomas is discussed. Jones and associates[42] published their updated series and included the Vancouver patients who received CHOP chemotherapy with or without involved field irradiation. An excellent complete response rate and an 82% NED survival rate at 5 years were observed. They continue to show that Stage II patients do less well than Stage I patients, but they fail to show any significant advantage of chemotherapy plus radiation therapy over chemotherapy alone. However, they feel that the trend is toward improvement with irradiation. In Vancouver, all patients received combined treatment. The authors also discussed the advantages of using involved field irradiation after only three cycles of chemotherapy in terms of late effects. Longo and co-workers at the NCI[54] reported on 47 patients treated with a reduced dose eight-drug combination chemotherapy regimen (proMACE-MOPP) followed by 4000 Gy involved field radiation therapy. They had a 96% complete response rate with no relapses with a median follow-up time of 42 months. This regimen was well-tolerated. There was a discussion[54] as to whether other chemotherapy regimens can be made more active than CHOP in long-term survival without increased toxicity and whether involved field radiation therapy is necessary to improve the durability of the complete remissions. It appears that there are definite subsets of patients in whom the abbreviated chemotherapy regimen and irradiation offer the best form of treatment.

High Stage Indolent Lymphomas

In the treatment of nonaggressive lymphomas, many options are available, including no treatment, single-agent adjuvant chemotherapy, combination chemotherapy, combination chemotherapy with irradiation to sites of bulky disease, low dose total-body irradiation alone or with chemotherapy, total lymphoid irradiation, total nodal irradiation and combination chemotherapy, and chemotherapy with total-body irradiation and bone marrow transplant.

For Stage III nodular lymphoma, excellent 5- and 10-year survival data can be expected with conservative management[76,81] in patients who present without symptoms and are feeling well. Such management may include deferred treatment until symptomatic manifestations of tumor require treatment. At that time, the treatment may be simply small-field, low-dose radiation therapy for relief of symptoms or even simple oral alkylating agent therapy.[76,81] Intensive combination chemotherapy for Stage III nodular lymphoma appears to be associated with a high probability of complete response but with a continuous relapse rate throughout the first 5 years of follow-up.[2,76,85] At the present time, nothing suggests that such chemotherapy is associated with cure, with the possible exception of nodular mixed lymphoma treated with the regimen of C-MOPP.[2,85]

Data from the small series reported by the NCI need confirmation from other sources. Total lymphoid radiation therapy for Stage III nodular lymphoma is associated with approximately a 30% freedom-from-relapse rate at 10 years.[26] Whole-body irradiation can also be expected to result in excellent long-term survival,[12,101] although again the rate of relapse after this form of treatment appears to be continuous. Similar results are expected in Stage IV disease, with the exception that high-dose total lymphoid radiation therapy is not considered appropriate for this stage.

In a recent report, the University of Florida group[61] updated their series of patients treated between 1972 and 1977 with whole-body irradiation. Follow-up data for 10 years or more show 5- and 10-year survival rates of 41% and 22%, respectively. Patients could be salvaged after relapse. This method is thus a form of palliative treatment. The authors' preferred technique is 100 cGy to 150 cGy at 10 cGy per fraction, five fractions per week, followed by rest for 2 or 3 weeks and an additional 170 cGy.

For Stage III and Stage IV lymphoma of diffuse histology, the mainstay of treatment is chemotherapy.[2,19,85,96] Various results have been achieved by a wide variety of different combinations. The most important results suggest that intensive combination chemotherapy, in the form of either C-MOPP or BACOP (bleomycin, Adriamycin, cyclophosphamide, Oncovin, prednisone) can be expected to achieve 40% long-term freedom-from-relapse rates in patients with advanced histiocytic lymphoma. The results in lymphomas of other histologic types appear much less impressive. Ongoing prospective studies suggest that it may be possible for boost nodal irradiation to add significantly to disease-free probabilities in patients with unfavorable histologic subtypes of Stage III and Stage IV disease.[25]

CENTRAL NERVOUS SYSTEM LYMPHOMAS

The incidence of central nervous system lymphomas is increasing, not only because of their association with patients with the acquired immunodeficiency syndrome and immunosuppressed patients who are transplant recipients, but also because of an increase in the disease in patients who do not fall into either category. The median age at diagnosis of CNS lymphoma is 55 years, and most patients present with generalized neurologic symptoms. Two thirds of patients present with cerebral disease, with only a subset having meningeal, spinal cord, or ocular disease. Pathologies are mostly of diffuse histology, predominantly B-cell tumors.

Surgery is necessary to make the diagnosis, but excision of the tumor is not necessarily therapeutic. Radiation therapy improves the median survival but only to approximately 15 months. Radiation fields are usually whole brain with an extension to the upper cervical spinal cord and occasionally to the orbit. It appears that doses above 5000 cGy may lead to longer survival.[67] In a recent Radiation Therapy Oncology Group (RTOG) study,[70] age of less than 60 years was shown to be a prognostic factor as was Karnofsky score.

In our review of the literature,[6,20,21,33,53,67,70,74] of 133 patients in whom patterns of failure could be analyzed, 100 patients failed; 92% were local failures, and 17% were distant failures. Distant failures included other areas of the central nervous system, not associated with the initial disease.

Chemotherapy has shown some responsiveness in this disease and has been integrated in the current RTOG study as initial therapy followed by radiation therapy. The schema of this study is presented in Figure 63-7. Similar studies are also being proposed by other cooperative groups. Central nervous system lymphomas are also discussed in Chapter 23.

GASTRIC LYMPHOMAS

Gastrointestinal lymphomas are the most common extranodal non-Hodgkin's lymphomas. Among the gastrointestinal lymphomas, the gastric location is the most common site.[8,30,92] Patients most frequently present with diffuse, large cell pathology. Prognostic factors are age, histology, depth of penetration, lymph node involvement, and size of initial tumor.[5] Many patients today present with a gastric symptom or sign, and diagnosis is made from an endoscopic biopsy. Endoscopic biopsies have been improved by better CT localization of the bulk of the tumor, better fiberoptic scopes, special histochemical stains for making the diagnosis of smaller volume of tissue, and flow cytometry.

With the advent of endoscopic biopsy and CT scan to stage the tumor, the question is to what extent is surgery necessary? Surgery has the advantage of prompt tumor removal and limits the low risk of perforation or hemorrhage. However, surgery delays use of chemotherapy, causes some morbidity from functional loss of the stomach in part or whole, and has a 10% mortality rate. One third of patients are found to have unresectable disease at the time of surgery. The advantage of a biopsy diagnosis is that no functional loss occurs, and adequate local control appears to be achievable by radiation therapy. Chemotherapy can be used early in the onset of the disease, and a measure of chemotherapy responsiveness can be made by the CT response of the bulk tumor. The potential morbidity of hemorrhage or perforation secondary to tumor lysis appears to be less common than originally believed.

Currently, several series have been done in which patients were treated with surgery and chemotherapy; with biopsy, chemotherapy, and irradiation; or with biopsy and irradiation. These series are summarized in Table 63-4. The M. D. Anderson series[59] and the Netherlands Cancer Institute series,[9] which had no surgery, also had no patients developing perforations or bleeding. Current clinical research trials are being proposed to treat patients with clearly resectable disease with surgery plus chemotherapy *versus* with chemotherapy plus irradiation. In patients with unresectable disease, patients will be randomized to those receiving chemotherapy alone *versus* those receiving chemotherapy plus irradiation; chemotherapy will be more intense in patients with unresectable disease. We anticipate that in the future the role of surgery in gastric lymphomas will diminish, leading to less morbidity and equal survival.

SEQUELAE OF TREATMENT

Side effects of therapy for lymphoma have been discussed in Chapter 62.

RADIATION THERAPY ONCOLOGY GROUP
RTOG #88-06

Phase I/II Protocol for the Treatment of Primary Central Nervous System Lymphoma

SCHEMA

REGISTER		TREATMENT
Performance Status	40-70 80-100	CHOD 2 cycles* CT scan brain No Progression → CHOD 1 cycle → Radiation Therapy Progression → Radiation Therapy 4140 cGy whole brain 1800 cGy boost 5940 cGy total dose
Age	<40 40-60 >60	

CHOD REGIMEN

Cyclophosphamide	750 mg/m^2 iv day 1
Doxorubicin	50 mg/m^2 iv day 1
Vincristine	1.4 mg/m^2 iv day 1 (max dose 2.0 mg)
Dexamethasone	6 mg/m^2 po days 1-5

Chemotherapy cycles repeated every 21 days

*Intrathecal (IT) Methotrexate

Only patients with cytologically positive CSF determined at time of diagnosis are to receive IT methotrexate. IT methotrexate, 12 mg per dose, via lumbar puncture or Omaya reservoir twice weekly for 3 weeks, then once per week for 3 weeks.

FIGURE 63–7. Phase I/II protocol for the treatment of primary central nervous system lymphomas.

TABLE 63–4
Gastric Lymphomas: 5-Year NED Survival Rates

GROUP	STAGE	NO.	THERAPY	5-YEAR NED SURVIVAL (% ALIVE)
Mallinckrodt Institute of Radiology (1983)[65]	All	37	Surg ± XRT ± Chemo	61
	I_E	22	Surg ± XRT ± Chemo	57
	II_E	15	Surg ± XRT ± Chemo	67
Massachusetts General Hospital (1983)[89]	I and II_E	26	Surg ± XRT	58
M.D. Anderson Cancer Center (1984)[58]	All	79	Surg ± XRT ± Chemo	54
	I_E	35		76
	II_E	44		42
Australia (1985)[87]	All	18	Surg + Chemo (CVP)	94 (3.5-yr NED)
	I_E	10		
	II_E	4		
M.D. Anderson Cancer Center (1988)[59]	All	35		69
	I_E	20	Biopsy + Chemo (CHOP-BLEO) + XRT	
	II_E	15		
Toronto (1988)[86]	All	26	Surg + Chemo (COPP or CHOP)	72 (not NED)
	I_E	12		
	II_E	14		
Netherlands (1988)[9]	I_E	24	Biopsy + XRT	83 (4-yr NED)

NED: no evidence of disease; surg: surgery; chemo: chemotherapy; XRT: radiation therapy; CVP: cyclophosphamide, vincristine, prednisone; CHOP: cyclophosphamide, doxorubicin, vincristine, prednisone; COPP: cyclophosphamide, vincristine, procarbazine, prednisone; BLEO: bleomycin

SUMMARY OF CLINICAL TRIALS

At the present time, ongoing trials have yet to show in patients with Stage I and Stage II nodular lymphoma any major advantage of radiation therapy on both sides of the diaphragm as opposed to involved field treatment only.[100] However, the natural history of nodular lymphoma is such that a prolonged time period is required before final conclusions can be made. For Stage I and Stage II lymphomas of diffuse histopathologic types, several investigators report radiation therapy on both sides of the diaphragm to be associated with major improvements compared with controls. Whether adjuvant combination chemotherapy adds to this remains controversial.

For patients with Stage III and Stage IV nodular lymphoma, the true survival benefit from any form of treatment is still controversial. Although nodular mixed lymphoma has been reported to be associated with prolonged disease-free intervals after C-MOPP, and although patients with Stage III nodular lymphoma appears to do relatively well with total lymphoid radiation therapy, the overall survival in experienced hands after conservative treatment remains comparable. Thus, for patients who have advanced stage nodular lymphoma but are asymptomatic, a major question remains whether the disease should be treated aggressively at the time of presentation or whether treatment should be deferred and the patient merely followed up carefully, with treatment to be initiated only when significant symptoms develop. Another question to be answered by prospective studies is whether irradiation of nodes after the induction of a complete remission by intensive chemotherapy affects the overall survival and duration of remission in patients with nodular lymphoma.

Various prospective studies are assessing a wide range of chemotherapeutic regimens in Stage III and Stage IV patients with disease of an unfavorable histologic type. Ongoing studies suggest that adding radiation to the nodes may be of some benefit, but the precise dose and volume to be irradiated remain controversial.

NEW APPROACHES

New approaches in the management of non-Hodgkin's lymphoma appear to center around alternating, non-cross-resistant, chemotherapeutic regimens, with boost irradiation to be considered. Whole-body radiation therapy at the present time is considered a palliative approach for advanced lymphocytic lymphoma patients without extensive prior chemotherapy.

The use of bone marrow transplantation has undergone increased activity in clinical research trials in the lymphomas. Such transplants have involved allogeneic or autologous marrow as therapy for relapse or for primary disease of aggressive cell types. The preparative regimens may involve whole-body irradiation.[3,4]

REFERENCES

1. American Cancer Society: Cancer Facts and Figures, 1991
2. Anderson T, Bender RA, Fisher RI, et al: Combination chemotherapy in non-Hodgkin's lymphoma: Results of a long-term follow-up. Cancer Treat Rep 61:1057, 1977
3. Appelbaum FR, Thomas ED: Review of the use of marrow transplantation in the treatment of non-Hodgkin's lymphoma. J Clin Oncol 1:440, 1983
4. Appelbaum FR, Thomas ED, Buckner CD, et al: Treatment of non-Hodgkin's lymphoma with chemotherapy and allogenic marrow transplantation. Hematol Oncol 1:149–157, 1983
5. Azab MB, Henry-Amar M, Rougier P, et al: Prognostic factors in primary gastrointestinal non-Hodgkin's lymphoma. Cancer 64:1208–1217, 1989

6. Berry MP, Simpson WJ: Radiation therapy in the management of primary malignant lymphoma of the brain. Int J Radiat Oncol Biol Phys 7:55–59, 1981
7. Bitran JD, Kinzle J, Sweet DL, et al: Survival of patients with localized histiocytic lymphoma. Cancer 39:342, 1977
8. Brooks JJ, Enterline HT: Primary gastric lymphomas. A clinicopathologic study of 58 cases with long-term follow-up and literature review. Cancer 51:701–711, 1983
9. Burgers JMV, Taal BG, van Heerde P, et al: Treatment results of primary stage I and II non-Hodgkin's lymphoma of the stomach. Radiother Oncol 11:319–326, 1988
10. Bush RS, Gospodarowicz M: The place of radiation therapy in the management of patients with localized non-Hodgkin's lymphoma. In Rosenberg SA, Kaplan HS (eds): Malignant Lymphomas, pp 485–502. London, London Academic Press, 1982
11. Cabanillas F: Chemotherapy as definitive treatment of stage I–II large cell and diffuse mixed lymphomas. Hematol Oncol 3:25, 1985
12. Carabell S, Chaffey JT, Rosenthal DS, et al: Results of total body irradiation in the treatment of advanced non-Hodgkin's lymphomas. Cancer 43:994, 1979
13. Carbone PP, Kaplan HS, Musshof K, et al: Report of the committee on Hodgkin's disease staging classification. Cancer Res 31:1860, 1971
14. Chen MG, Prosnitz LR, Gonzalez-Serva A, et al: Results of radiotherapy in control of stage I and II non-Hodgkin's lymphomas. Cancer 43:1245, 1979
15. Connors JM, Fairey R, Klimo P, et al: ACOB: 6 week chemotherapy and involved field radiotherapy (IFRT) for limited stage large cell lymphoma, initial results (Abstract). Proc ASCO 7:224, 1988
16. Connors JM, Klimo P, Fairey RN, Voss N: Brief chemotherapy and involved field radiation therapy for limited-stage histologically aggressive lymphoma. Ann Intern Med 107:25, 1987
17. Dosoretz DE, Murphy GF, Raymond AK, et al: Radiation therapy for primary lymphoma of bone. Cancer 51:44, 1983
18. Ersboll J, Schultz HB, Hougaard P, et al: Comparison of the working formulation of non-Hodgkin's lymphoma with the Rappaport, Kiel, and Lukes and Collins classifications. Cancer 55:2442, 1985
19. Fisher RI, Hubbard SM, DeVita VT, et al: Factors predicting long-term survival in diffuse, mixed, histiocytic or undifferentiated lymphoma. Blood 58:45, 1981
20. Formenti SC, Gill PS, Lean E, et al: Primary central nervous system lymphoma in AIDS: Results of radiation therapy. Cancer 63:1101, 1989
21. Freeman CR, Shustik C, Brisson M-L, et al: Primary malignant lymphoma of the central nervous system. Cancer 58:1106–1111, 1986
22. Fuks Z, Glatstein E, Kaplan HS: Patterns of presentation and relapse in the non-Hodgkin's lymphomata. Br J Cancer 31(Suppl II):286, 1975
23. Fuks Z, Kaplan HS: Recurrence rates following radiation therapy of nodular and diffuse lymphomas. Radiology 108:675, 1973
24. Glatstein E: Hodgkin's disease and non-Hodgkin's lymphomas: How important is histology? Front Radiat Ther Oncol 9:203, 1974
25. Glatstein E, Donaldson SS, Rosenberg SA, et al: Combined modality therapy in malignant lymphomas. Cancer Treat Rep 61:1199, 1977
26. Glatstein E, Fuks Z, Goffinet DR, et al: Non-Hodgkin's lymphoma of stage III extent: Is total lymphoid irradiation appropriate treatment? Cancer 37:2806, 1976
27. Goffinet DR, Glatstein E, Fuks Z, et al: Abdominal irradiation of non-Hodgkin's lymphomas. Cancer 37:2797, 1976
28. Goffinet DR, Warnke R, Dunnick NR, et al: Clinical and surgical (laparotomy) evaluation of patients with non-Hodgkin's lymphomas. Cancer Treat Rep 61:981, 1977
29. Gospodarowicz MK, Bush RS, Brown TC, et al: Prognostic factors in nodular lymphomas: A multivariate analysis based on the Princess Margaret Hospital experience. Int J Radiat Oncol Biol Phys 10:489, 1984
30. Gospodarowicz MK, Bush RS, Brown TC, Chua T: Curability of gastrointestinal lymphoma with combined surgery and radiation. Int J Radiat Oncol Biol Phys 9(1):3–9, 1983
31. Hande KR, Fisher RI, DeVita VT, et al: Diffuse histiocytic lymphoma involving the gastrointestinal tract. Cancer 41:1984, 1978
32. Heifetz LJ, Fuller LM, Rodgers RW, et al: Laparotomy findings in lymphangiogram-staged I and II non-Hodgkin's lymphomas. Cancer 39:843, 1977
33. Hochberg FH, Miller DC: Primary central nervous system lymphoma. J Neurosurg 68:835, 1988
34. Hoppe RT: The role of radiation therapy in the management of non-Hodgkin's lymphomas. Cancer 55:2176, 1985
35. Hoppe RT: Patterns of failure after treatment for the non-Hodgkin's lymphomas. Cancer Treat Symp 2:133, 1983
36. Hoppe RT, Burke JS, Glatstein E, et al: Non-Hodgkin's lymphoma. Involvement of Waldeyer's ring. Cancer 42:1096, 1978
37. Jacobs C, Hoppe RT: Non-Hodgkin's lymphomas of head and neck and neck extranodal sites. Int J Radiat Oncol Biol Phys 11:357, 1985
38. Jaffe ES, Shevach EM, Frank MM, et al: Nodular lymphoma: Evidence for origin from follicular B lymphocytes. N Engl J Med 290:813, 1974
39. Jones SE, Butler JJ, Byrne GE, et al: Histopathologic review of lymphoma cases from the Southwest Oncology Group. Cancer 39:1071, 1977
40. Jones SE, Fuks Z, Bull M, et al: Non-Hodgkin's lymphomas. IV. Clinicopathologic correlation in 405 cases. Cancer 31:806, 1973
41. Jones SE, Fuks Z, Kaplan HS, et al: Non-Hodgkin's lymphomas. V. Results of radiotherapy. Cancer 32:682, 1973
42. Jones SE, Miller TP, Connors JM: Long-term follow-up and analysis for prognostic factors for patients with limited-stage diffuse large-cell lymphoma treated with initial chemotherapy with or without adjuvant radiotherapy. J Clin Oncol 7(9):1186–1191, 1989
43. Kaminski MS, Coleman CN, Colby TV, et al: Factors predicting survival in adults with stage I and II large-cell lymphoma treated with primary radiation therapy. Ann Intern Med 104:747–756, 1986
44. Kaplan WD, Jochelson MS, Herman T, et al: Gallium-67 imaging: A predictor of residual tumor viability and clinical outcome in patients with diffuse large cell lymphoma. J Clin Oncol 8:1966–1970, 1990
45. Lamb DS, Hudson GV, Easterling MJ, et al: Localized grade 2 non-Hodgkin's lymphoma: Results of treatment with radiotherapy. Clin Radiol 35:253, 1984
46. Lattuada A, Bonadonna G, Milani F, et al: Adjuvant chemotherapy with CVP after radiotherapy (RT) in Stage I–II non-Hodgkin's lymphomas. In Salmon SE, Jones SE (ed): Adjuvant Therapy of Cancer, p 537. Amsterdam, Elsevier/North Holland, 1977
47. Lawrence TS, Urba WJ, Steinberg SM, et al: Retrospective analysis of stage I and II indolent lymphomas at the National Cancer Institute. Int J Radiat Oncol Biol Phys 14:417–424, 1988
48. Lester JN, Fuller LM, Conrad FG, et al: The role of staging laparotomy, chemotherapy, and radiotherapy in the management of localized diffuse large cell lymphoma: A study of 75 patients. Cancer 49:1746, 1982
49. Levitt LJ, Dawson DM, Rosenthal DS, et al: CNS involvement in the non-Hodgkin's lymphomas. Cancer 45:545, 1980
50. Levitt SH, Bloomfield CD, Frizzea G, et al: Curative radiotherapy for localized diffuse histiocytic lymphoma. Cancer Treat Rep 64:175, 1980
51. Levitt SH, Lee CKK, Bloomfield CD, et al: The role of radiation therapy in the treatment of early stage large cell lymphoma Hematol Oncol 3:33, 1985
52. Lewis E, Bernardino ME, Salvador PG, et al: Posttherapy CT detected mass in lymphoma patients: Is it viable tissue? J Comput Assist Tomogr 6:792, 1982
53. Loeffler JS, Erwin TJ, Mauch P, et al: Primary lymphomas of the central nervous system: Patterns of failure and factors that influence survival. J Clin Oncol 3:490, 1985
54. Longo DL: Editorial: Combined modality therapy for lo-

calized aggressive lymphoma: Enough or too much? J Clin Oncol 7(9):1179–1181, 1989

55. Longo DL, Glatstein E, Duffey PL, et al: Treatment of localized aggressive lymphomas with combination chemotherapy followed by involved-field radiation therapy. J Clin Oncol 7(9):1295–1302, 1989
56. Lukes RJ, Collins RD: New approaches to the classification of the lymphomata. Br J Cancer 31(Suppl II):1, 1975
57. Mackintosh FR, Colby TV, Podolsky WJ, et al: Central nervous system involvement in non-Hodgkin's lymphoma: An analysis of 105 cases. Cancer 49:586, 1982
58. Maor MH, Maddux B, Osborne BM, et al: Stages IE and IIE non-Hodgkin's lymphoma of the stomach: Comparison of treatment modalities. Cancer 54:2330–2337, 1984
59. Maor MH, Velasquez WS, Fuller LM: Stomach conservation in stages IE and IIE gastric non-Hodgkin's lymphoma (NHL). Int J Radiat Oncol Biol Phys 15(Suppl1):209, 1988
60. Mauch P, Leonard R, Sharin A, et al: Improved survival following combined radiation therapy and chemotherapy for unfavorable prognosis stage I–II non-Hodgkin's lymphomas. J Clin Oncol 3:1301, 1985
61. Mendenhall NP, Noyes WD, Million RR: Total body irradiation for stage II–IV non-Hodgkin's lymphoma: Ten-year follow-up. J Clin Oncol 7(1):67–74, 1989
62. Mill WB, Lee FA, Franssila KO: Radiation therapy treatment of stage I and II extranodal non-Hodgkin's lymphomas of the head and neck. Cancer 45:653, 1980
63. Miller TP: Therapy of localized non-Hodgkin's lymphomas. Princ Prac Oncol Updates 3:6, 1989
64. Miller TP, Jones SE: Initial chemotherapy for clinically localized lymphomas of unfavorable histology. Blood 62:413, 1983
65. Mittal B, Wasserman TH, Griffith R: Non-Hodgkin's lymphoma of the stomach. Am J Gastroenterol 78(12):781–787, 1983
66. Monfardini S, Banfi A, Bonnadonna G, et al: Improved 5-year survival after combined radiotherapy for stage I–II non Hodgkin's lymphoma. Int J Radiat Oncol Biol Phys 6:125, 1980
67. Murray K, Kun L, Cox J: Primary malignant lymphoma of the central nervous system: Results of treatment of 11 cases and review of the literature. J Neurosurg 65:600, 1986
68. Nathwoni BN, Kim H, Rappaport H: Malignant lymphoma, lymphoblastic. Cancer 38:964, 1976
69. NCI Non-Hodgkin's Classification Project Writing Committee: Classification of non-Hodgkin's lymphomas: Reproducibility of major classification systems. Cancer 55:91, 1985
70. Nelson DF, et al: Definitive radiation therapy in the treatment of primary non-Hodgkin's lymphoma of the central nervous system, non-AIDS related: Report of RTOG study 83-15. J Neurosurg (in press), 1991
71. Nissen NI, Ersboll J, Hansen HS, et al: A randomized study of radiotherapy versus radiotherapy plus chemotherapy in stage I–II non-Hodgkin's lymphoma. Cancer 52:1, 1983
72. The Non-Hodgkin's Lymphoma Pathologic Classification Project: National Cancer Institute-sponsored study of classifications of non-Hodgkin's lymphomas: Summary and description of a working formulation for clinical usage. Cancer 49:2112, 1982
73. Peterson BA, Bloomfield CD, Oliphant TH, et al: Patterns of relapse following chemotherapy in non-Hodgkin's lymphoma. Cancer Treat Symp 2:137, 1983
74. Pollack IF, Lunsford LD, Flickinger JC, Dameshek HL: Prognostic factors in the diagnosis and treatment of primary central nervous system lymphoma. Cancer 63:939–947, 1989
75. Poplack DG, Kun LE, Cassady JR, Pizzo PA: Leukemias and lymphomas of childhood. In DeVita VT Jr, Hellman S, Rosenberg SA (eds): Cancer: Principles and Practice of Radiation Oncology, 3rd ed, pp 1671–1695. Philadelphia, JB Lippincott, 1989
76. Portlock CS, Rosenberg SA: Chemotherapy of the non-Hodgkin's lymphomas: The Stanford experience. Cancer Treat Rep 61:1049, 1977
77. Prestidge BR, Horning SJ, Hoppe RT: Combined modality therapy for stage I–II large cell lymphoma. Int J Radiat Oncol Biol Phys 15:633–639, 1988
78. Rappaport H: Tumors of the Hematopoietic System. In Atlas of Tumor Pathology, Section 3, Fascicle 8. Washington, DC, Armed Forces Institute of Pathology, 1966
79. Reddy S, Pellettiere E, Saxena V, et al: Extranodal non-Hodgkin's lymphoma. Cancer 46:1925, 1980
80. Reddy S, Saxena VS, Pellettiere EV, Hendrickson FR: Stage I and II non-Hodgkin's lymphomas: Long-term results of radiation therapy. Int J Radiat Oncol Biol Phys 16:687–692, 1989
81. Rosenberg SA: The low-grade non-Hodgkin's lymphomas: Challenges and opportunities. J Clin Oncol 3:299, 1985
82. Rosenberg SA: Validity of Ann Arbor staging classification for the non-Hodgkin's lymphomas. Cancer Treat Rep 61:1023, 1977
83. Rosenberg SA: Bone marrow involvement in the non-Hodgkin's lymphomata. Br J Cancer 31(Suppl II):261, 1975
84. Schaner EG, Head GL, Doppman JL, et al: Computed tomography in the diagnosis, staging and management of abdominal lymphoma. J Comput Assist Tomogr 1:176, 1977
85. Schein PS, Chabner BA, Canelos GP, et al: Potential for prolonged disease-free survival following combination chemotherapy of non-Hodgkin's lymphoma. Blood 43:181, 1974
86. Shepherd FA, Evans WK, Kutas G, et al: Chemotherapy following surgery for stages IE and IIE non-Hodgkin's lymphoma of the gastrointestinal tract. J Clin Oncol 6:253–260, 1988
87. Sheridan WP, Medley G, Brodie GN: Non-Hodgkin's lymphoma of the stomach: A prospective pilot study of surgery plus chemotherapy in early and advanced disease. J Clin Oncol 3:495–500, 1985
88. Shigematsu N, Kondo M, Mikata A: Prognostic factors of stage I and II non-Hodgkin's lymphomas of the head and neck: The value of the working formulation and need for chemotherapy. Int J Radiat Oncol Biol Phys 15:1111–1118, 1988
89. Shimm DS, Dosoretz DE, Anderson T, et al: Primary gastric lymphoma. An analysis with emphasis on prognostic factors and radiation therapy. Cancer 52:2044–2048, 1983
90. Shimm DS, Doseretz DE, Harris NL, et al: Radiation therapy of Waldeyer's ring lymphoma. Cancer 54:426, 1984
91. Shipp MA, Klatt MM, Yeap B, et al: Patterns of relapse in large-cell lymphoma patients with bulk disease: Implications for the use of adjuvant radiation therapy. J Clin Oncol 7(5):613–618, 1989
92. Shiu MH, Nisce LZ, Pinna A, et al: Recent results of multimodal therapy of gastric lymphoma. Cancer 58:1389–1399, 1986
93. Simon R, Durrleman S, Hoppe RT, et al: The non-Hodgkin lymphoma pathologic classification project. Long-term follow-up of 1153 patients with non-Hodgkin lymphomas. Ann Intern Med 109:939–945, 1988
94. Stewart FM, Williamson BR, Innes DJ, et al: Residual mass lesions following treatment for diffuse histiocytic lymphoma: Diagnostic and therapeutic implications. Cancer 55:620, 1985
95. Sutcliffe SB, Gospodarowicz MK, Bush RS, et al: Role of radiation therapy in localized non-Hodgkin's lymphoma. Radiother Oncol 4:211–223, 1985
96. Sweet DL, Golomb HM: The treatment of histiocytic lymphoma. Semin Oncol 7:302, 1980
97. Sweet DL, Kinzie J, Gaike ME, et al: Survival of patients with localized diffuse histiocytic lymphoma. Blood 58:1218, 1981
98. Tumeh SS, Rosenthal DS, Kaplan WD, et al: Lymphoma: Evaluation with Ga-67 SPECT. Radiology 164:111–114, 1987
99. Vokes EE, Ultmann JE, Golomb HM, et al: Long-term survival of patients with localized diffuse histiocytic lymphoma. J Clin Oncol 3:1309, 1985
100. Wasserman TH, Tubiana M: Lymphoma: Radiation therapy in lymphoma treatment. Int J Radiat Oncol Biol Phys 14:S187–S201, 1988
101. Young RC, Johnson RE, Canellos GP, et al: Advanced lymphocytic lymphoma: Randomized comparisons of chemotherapy and radiotherapy, alone or in combination. Cancer Treat Rep 61:1153, 1977

APPENDIX 63-1

Glossary to Abbreviated Chemotherapy Drug Combinations

ACOB	doxorubicin, cyclophosphamide, vincristine, bleomycin
ABVD	doxorubicin, bleomycin, vinblastine, DTIC
BACOP	bleomycin, doxorubicin, cyclophosphamide, vincristine, prednisone
BLEO	bleomycin
C-MOPP	cyclophosphamide, oncovin procarbazine, prednisone
CCNU	(1-(2-chloroethyl)-3-cyclohexyl-1-nitrosourea)
CHOD	cyclophosphamide, doxorubicin, vincristine, dexamethasone
CHOP	cyclophosphamide, doxorubicin, vincristine, prednisone
CHOP-BLEO	cyclophosphamide, doxorubicin, vincristine, prednisone, bleomycin
COPP	CCNU, vincristine, procarbazine, prednisone
DTIC	5-(3,3-dimethyl-1-triazino)imidazole-4-carboxamide
mBACOD	methotrexate, bleomycin, doxorubicin, cyclophosphamide, vincristine, dexamethasone
M	methotrexate
MOPP	nitrogen mustard, vincristine, procarbazine, prednisone
proMACE	prednisone, methotrexate, doxorubicin, cyclophosphamide, etoposide (VP-16)
proMACE-MOPP	prednisone, methotrexate, doxorubicin, cyclophosphamide, etoposide (VP-16)-nitrogen mustard, vincristine, procarbazine, prednisone

64

Multiple Myeloma and Plasmacytomas

Todd H. Wasserman

EPIDEMIOLOGY

The incidence of plasma cell tumors has been gradually increasing and is now approximately the same as that of Hodgkin's disease and chronic lymphocytic leukemia (two to three per 100,000). The American Cancer Society[8] estimates that in 1991 there were 12,300 new cases (1% of all cancers) and 6200 deaths. The peak incidence is in the sixth and seventh decades, with a male : female ratio of approximately 1 : 1. The age-adjusted mortality rate for nonwhites is approximately twice that for whites.[20] The incidence of plasma cell tumors increases with age.

The specific etiology of plasma cell tumors is unknown, but possible contributing factors are chronic inflammatory conditions[46,70,72,78] and radiation. Anderson and Ishida[9] report a very marked increase in the number of deaths from multiple myeloma in Hiroshima survivors who were within 1400 m of the hypocenter (418 cases) compared with the number of deaths in those who were unexposed (104 cases). Also, in one survey the incidence of multiple myeloma in radiologists was found to be higher than expected.[60]

NATURAL HISTORY AND CLINICAL PRESENTATION

Multiple Myeloma

Plasma cell neoplasms are associated with proliferation and accumulation of immunoglobulin-secreting cells derived from B-cell lymphocytes. They are believed to be monoclonal tumors derived from a single transformed cell.

Myeloma is a low-growth fraction tumor with only a small percentage of tumor cells in cycle at any given time. The subclinical phase can take 1 to 3 years; the clinical phase can last 1 to 10 years or more.

Malignant plasma cell tumors present in several forms, comprising a spectrum from small localized lesions to diffuse dissemination. The most common presentation is that of disseminated disease (multiple myeloma) with involvement of multiple skeletal sites. Common presenting complaints are bone pain (68%), infections (12%), bleeding (7%), and easy fatigability.[55] Peripheral blood examination usually reveals anemia. Thrombocytopenia or granulocytopenia or both are present in one third of patients. Hyperglobulinemia can cause disturbances of the clotting mechanism and usually produces an elevation of the erythrocyte sedimentation rate. Hypercalcemia is present in 50% of patients. Skeletal radiographs demonstrate one of three common patterns: diffuse osteoporosis, well-demarcated lytic lesions, or localized cystic osteolytic lesions. Osteosclerosis is very uncommon in untreated myeloma[31,33,77] and is estimated to occur in 3% of cases.

Plasma cell tumors secrete a measurable "paraprotein" in 95% to 99% of cases.[18] These proteins are structurally normal immunoglobulins, or fragments thereof, but functional antibody specificity has not been demonstrated. The incidence of each type of paraprotein produced is approximately the same as that of that same immunoglobulin in normal serum. IgG is found in 50% to 60% of cases and IgA in 20% to 25%; in approximately 20% of cases only light chain or Bence Jones proteins are found.[18] These paraproteins constitute a unique tumor marker. The serum level of the paraprotein has been demonstrated to correlate with tumor cell burden.[32]

A quantitative relationship exists between the serum myeloma protein concentration and tumor weight in a mouse myeloma. Other studies using animal models have described their cellular kinetics[19] and response to various chemotherapeutic agents.[1,37,38,41]

Between 1.6% and 22% of patients either present with or later develop plasma cells in the peripheral blood.[19,56,57,86] Treatment of plasma cell leukemia has not been very effective, but new multiagent chemotherapy regimens offer some hope for improvement.[84]

Solitary Plasmacytomas

Localized lesions of bone or soft tissue (solitary plasmacytomas) account for 2% to 10% of the total plasma cell diseases.[69] Solitary plasmacytomas of bone most frequently involved the vertebral bodies or pelvic bones. After localized radiation therapy, the reported length of survival varies from a few months to 30 years.[71] Elevated serum immunoglobulin levels have been found in some cases of solitary plasmacytoma of bone. Meyer and co-workers[65] reported that out of 12 cases, two patients had a definite serum immunoglobulin elevation and one had a questionable elevation. In one of these patients the increased serum immunoglobulin disappeared after radiation therapy, and the patient was without evidence of disease for 12 years. Other investigators have reported a similar occurrence.[68,71] Most patients presenting with a solitary plasmacytoma of bone ultimately develop dissemination.[23,25,69] In spite of this, the long survival with a prolonged disease-free interval warrants aggressive primary treatment.

A second type of localized presentation occurs in soft tissue (extramedullary plasmacytoma) and arises most frequently in the upper respiratory tract (nasal cavity, nasopharynx, paranasal sinuses), the lung, lymph nodes, spleen, and gastrointestinal tract.[22,40,73,98] Wiltshaw reported a paraprotein in one of nine patients with localized extramedullary plasmacytoma.[98] Lymph node metastases occur in association with extramedullary plasmacytomas, with the reported incidence ranging from 10% to 25%.[52,74,98] Survival of patients with extramedullary plasmacytoma is much better than in patients with multiple myeloma. Wiltshaw reports a 40% survival rate at 10 years.[98] In her series of 33 patients (27 with localized disease and six with regional node involvement), local recurrence occurred in ten (30%). Local recurrence occurred in one of five patients treated with surgery alone, three of 14 treated with irradiation alone, and five of 13 treated with both irradiation and surgery. Forty-eight percent of patients ultimately developed disseminated disease.

Knowling and colleagues[50] at Princess Margaret Hospital in Toronto compared their experience with extramedullary plasmacytoma, solitary plasmacytoma of bone, and multiple myeloma. Of the 822 patients seen from 1958 to 1980, 25 had solitary plasmacytomas of bone (3%) and 25 had extramedullary plasmacytomas (3%). The median age of the first group was 50 years, compared with the median age of 61 years in multiple myeloma patients. Median survival for patients with solitary plasmacytoma of bone was 86 months; for extramedullary plasmacytoma patients, 101 months, and for multiple myeloma patients, 24 months. A distinct male predominance was found in the patients with extramedullary plasmacytoma. Of the 25 patients with extramedullary plasmacytoma, only five had progression of disease after initial radiation therapy: one as a single bony lesion, two as myeloma, and two as multiple extramedullary plasmacytoma. Seventy-one percent of patients with extramedullary plasmacytoma were progression-free at 10 years.

In contrast, of the patients with solitary plasmacytoma of bone, 13 of 29 developed disease at other sites: one had another isolated bone plasmacytoma, and 12 developed multiple myeloma. The median time to progression was 6.5 years. The authors note that regional lymph node treatment should be part of the primary irradiation when extramedullary plasmacytomas are treated. The younger age and obvious progression of disease in patients with solitary plasmacytoma of bone suggest that this is the same disease process as multiple myeloma but in an earlier phase. The predominant occurrence of extramedullary plasmacytoma in males and in the region of the upper airway passages, as well as its tendency to remain localized despite regional node involvement, suggests that it may be a different disease entity.

DIAGNOSTIC WORKUP

Recommendations for the evaluation of patients presenting with plasma cell tumors have been made by the Chronic Leukemia-Myeloma Task Force of the National Cancer Institute.[28] The diagnostic workup procedures are listed in Table 64-1.

The value of isotopic bone scans in determining the extent of disease in multiple myeloma is limited. Radioactive strontium is deposited in areas of new bone formation.[26] New bone formation is not usually seen in multiple myeloma[23,33,86] except after a fracture.[96] Hubner and associates[45] scanned 24 patients with multiple myeloma with several scanning agents, including gallium-67 (^{67}Ga) citrate, technetium-99m (^{99m}Tc) polyphosphate, and ^{99m}Tc diphosphonate. Gallium-67 imaging revealed lesions in 11 of 17 patients with bone lesions apparent on radiographs. The ^{99m}Tc compounds demonstrated lesions in seven of ten patients, but only 24 of 45 (53%) lesions seen on radiographs were confirmed on scan.

The diagnostic criteria for plasma cell tumors were defined by the Chronic Leukemia-Myeloma Task Force[28] as follows:

Patients with a paraimmunoglobulinopathy must have one or more of the following:

1. Marrow plasmacytosis of greater than 5%
2. Biopsy tissue demonstrating replacement and distortion of normal tissue by plasma cells
3. More than 500 plasma cells/mm^3 in the blood
4. Osteolytic lesions unexplained by other causes

Patients without paraimmunoglobulinopathy must have radiographic evidence of osteolytic lesions or palpable tumors plus one or more of the following:

1. Marrow plasmacytosis greater than 20% (in the absence of another disease capable of causing reactive plasmacytosis)
2. Tissue biopsy specimens demonstrating replacement and distortion of normal tissue by plasma cells

Skeletal survey is more sensitive than a bone scan with ^{99m}Tc in detecting bony lesions.[11,87,93] The false-negative rate for radionuclide scans and the underestimation of the extent of skeletal involvement have been constant problems in the radiographic evaluation of myeloma.

Recent evaluation of myeloma patients by computed tomography (CT) scanning has shown that CT scanning in selected patients can be useful to define early disease when bone pain is present and when the films are nonspecific or normal. CT scanning also often demonstrates a greater extent of disease than can be seen on radiographs. This modality is of particular

TABLE 64–1
Diagnostic Workup for Plasma Cell Tumors

Routine Studies
- General history
- Physical examination
- Bone marrow biopsy

Radiographic Studies
- Chest film
- Skeletal survey
- MRI or CT scan of painful weight-bearing areas

Laboratory Tests
- Complete blood cell count
  - Serum β_2-microglobulin
  - Plasma chemistry profile (SMA-12), including serum calcium, albumin, renal function studies, liver function studies
- Protein studies
  - Quantitative serum protein electrophoresis
  - Quantitative immunoglobulin assay
  - Antigenic typing of the light and heavy chains of the serum and/or urinary protein
  - Qualitative test for urine protein—if positive, additional tests are recommended to define quantity and type
  - Tests for cryoglobulins

Biopsies
- Any mass suspected to be either myeloma or amyeloid deposits

importance in defining the extent of extraosseous plasmacytomas that may have bone involvement by direct extension and in guiding the use of radiation therapy in treatment planning.[83]

Magnetic resonance imaging (MRI) of the spine in multiple myeloma can show more extent of disease than is evident on plain radiographs or CT scan and may be particularly useful in areas of persistent pain and in early detection of pending spinal cord compression.[61]

Beta$_2$-microglobulin is a low molecular mass protein that is a function of both myeloma cell mass and renal function, and therefore the serum level, has been useful in staging and prediction of survival.

PATHOLOGIC CLASSIFICATION

Plasma cell tumors are characterized by an increased proliferation of plasma cells of varying degrees of differentiation. Plasma cells are found primarily in the tissues and organs of the lymphoreticular system, especially in the bone marrow, lymph nodes, liver, and upper respiratory and gastrointestinal tract mucosa. It has been suggested that plasma cells may be derived from B lymphocytes, which develop from primitive reticular stem cells found scattered throughout all tissues, thus making it possible to find these tumors in nearly any tissue or organ.[94]

The classification of plasma cell tumors proposed by Azar and Potter[10] is as follows:

- multiple plasma cell myeloma (multiple myeloma)
- disseminated nonosteolytic myelomatosis
- solitary myeloma (of bone)
- extraskeletal plasmacytomas (extramedullary)
- plasma cell leukemia
- plasmacytic lymphoreticulosis (including some of the heavy-chain diseases)
- malignant lymphomas with M-component

In addition, benign reactive plasmacytosis and plasma cell granuloma must be considered in the differential diagnosis of the lesions.

PROGNOSTIC FACTORS

The Southwest Oncology Group (SWOG) reported a review of prognostic parameters in 482 patients.[4] Those over 65 years of age had a median survival of 20 months, whereas those under 55 years of age had a median survival of 26 months. Additional findings associated with a shortened survival or shortened remission duration were severe anemia, hypercalcemia, blood urea nitrogen greater than 40 mg/dl, markedly elevated M protein, hypoalbuminemia, and a high tumor cell burden. Patients presenting with advanced renal disease in addition to multiple myeloma have a poor prognosis. Also, as noted previously,[42] those patients responding rapidly had a shorter median survival and remission duration than those responding more slowly. Durie and Salmon[32] have demonstrated a correlation between survival and myeloma cell mass at time of presentation and on the basis of these factors suggested a staging system. A recent review by Bataille and associates[12,13] analyzed multiple prognostic factors in myeloma, including standard bone marrow involvement, tumor mass, renal status, chromosome ploidy, intrinsic drug sensitivity, and kinetic parameters. However, the most easily measurable and quantifiable and highly predictive parameters are the serum β_2-microglobulin level and the serum albumin level. Using these two factors, three prognostic groups can be identified, as shown in Table 64-2.

GENERAL MANAGEMENT

Chemotherapy

The mainstay of chemotherapy in myeloma for the past two decades has been melphalan, frequently in combination with prednisone. This combination improved the response time in good-risk patients from 30 months with melphalan alone to 53 months with melphalan and prednisone in one cooperative group study.[30] The reported response rates range from 45% to 70% of evaluable patients.[5–7,30,35] The median duration of response is approximately 24 months, with a median survival of 30 months.[7] Additional agents with demonstrated efficacy are cyclophosphamide,[51] BCNU,[17,59] doxorubicin,[2] and vincristine.[80]

The use of alternating combination chemotherapy has been proposed by several groups; however, it has not been substantiated that it has improved the outlook of patients. Some researchers have considered that the curability of myeloma with chemotherapy using currently available agents is small.[15]

The duration of chemotherapy is controversial. The cessation of therapy may result in relapse, and response to the retreatment may be more difficult. Continued chemotherapy may lead to refractory anemia or development of secondary acute leukemia.[44,99] Bone marrow transplantation from identical twins has yielded equivocal results. Thus, progress in the systemic treatment of multiple myeloma in the past 20 years, since the introduction of alkylating agents, has been a disappointment.[54]

Despite the lack of an advance in the curative use of chemotherapy, most patients receive chemotherapy as part of their

TABLE 64–2
Stratification of Myeloma Patients According to $S\beta_2M$ and Serum Albumin Levels

STRATIFICATION	NUMBER OF PATIENTS	% ALIVE	MEDIAN SURVIVAL (MONTHS)
Low risk: $S\beta_2M < 6$ μg/ml, and SA > 3.0 g/dl	81	78	55
Intermediate risk: $S\beta_2M \geq 6$ μg/ml, but SA > 3.0 g/dl	46	41	19
Poor risk: SA ≤ 3.0 g/dl	18	33	4

$S\beta_2M$: serum β_2-microglobulin; SA: serum albumin
(Modified from Bataille R, Durie BGM, Grenier J, et al: J Clin Oncol 4[1]:80–87, 1986)

palliative treatment.[53,55] A detailed discussion of the role of chemotherapy in the treatment of myeloma may be found elsewhere.[81]

Supportive care is extremely important and includes treatment for anemia, hypercalcemia, hyperuricemia, azotemia, and frequent infections. Fluorides have been tried in an effort to effect the resorption of calcium from the bones but have not been effective.[39]

Both chemotherapy and radiation therapy are effective in the palliation of myeloma. Curative therapy for myeloma has not been established.

Radiation Therapy

Radiation therapy plays an essential role in the management of plasma cell tumors, primarily as an adjuvant in multiple myeloma. The indications for radiation therapy are as follows:

As primary treatment in localized presentations (solitary plasmacytomas of bone and extramedullary plasmacytomas)
For palliation of pain not controlled by chemotherapy from bone lesions of disseminated disease
For prevention of pathologic fractures in weight-bearing bones
For relief of spinal cord compression or nerve root compression

TOTAL-BODY AND HEMIBODY IRRADIATION

Because myeloma is a radioresponsive disease, the possible use of systemic radiation therapy is being studied. Total-body irradiation (TBI) was used in a small number of patients with partial success.[16,27,43] Its main limitation is profound bone marrow toxicity in patients who have had extensive prior chemotherapy and local field irradiation.

A potentially promising technique is that of hemibody irradiation (HBI), which allows the delivery of a higher dose per fraction with less bone marrow toxicity. In some patients a second course of radiation to the opposite half of the body is both desirable and tolerable. The technique of HBI is clearly of value in patients who have diffusely painful sites of disease. Several reports indicate that treatment may also be appropriate in symptomatic patients who are chemotherapy-resistant as the appropriate second-line treatment. Several authors have reported on a small series of patients treated with single-dose HBI alone or with sequential double HBI treatments.[21,48,75,79,88,89] The five series report a total of 53 cases, and subjective responses of predominant pain relief were achieved in 80% to 90% of patients. Objective responses as measured by decrease in paraprotein levels or decrease in the percentage of plasma cells in follow-up bone marrow studies occurred in 32% to 45% of patients. Median survivals after this treatment are consistent with that of second-line chemotherapy in these chemotherapy-resistant patients.

The toxicity of HBI is mostly hematologic, and many patients cannot complete both courses of hemibody treatment. Gastrointestinal toxicity reactions, stomatitis, and pulmonary toxicity reactions may be related to technical factors and can be reduced with proper technique. Bone marrow toxicity may be more difficult to reduce, because these patients have decreased bone marrow reserve due to prior treatments and decreased ability to produce more bone marrow elements due to the primary disease process.

The median dose used by these five studies was 750 cGy to 850 cGy. In another study using 300 cGy to 400 cGy, the subjective response rate was only 67%, and, more important, the duration of response was significantly shorter.[66]

In a report[85] of a series of 41 patients with melphalan-resistant multiple myeloma treated with single HBI or double HBI, the authors report good palliation of widespread bony disease with 69% of patients having pain relief, most within 7 days. Patients were given 750 cGy to upper hemibody and 850 cGy to lower hemibody. No patient was treated within 6 weeks of previous chemotherapy. Twenty-four percent of the patients had greater than 50% reduction in paraprotein levels. Although the median survival of all patients was only 4.5 months, patients in more favorable prognostic groups had median survival of more than 18 months. Twenty-one of the 41 patients received double HBI treatment, and the toxicity was tolerable; only one treatment-induced death occurred from postirradiation pneumonitis.

It is likely that TBI or HBI can induce equivalent log cell kill to that induced by chemotherapy as first suggested in 1971[16]; more clinical studies are necessary.

A study by Jacobs and co-workers, from the University of Capetown, South Africa,[47] reports on 46 previously treated patients with multiple myeloma who were prospectively randomized to systemic irradiation or to chemotherapy with melphalan and prednisone. Objective response, defined as a greater than or equal to 50% reduction in plasma of the paraprotein level or disappearance of light change in urine, was achieved in 60% of the patients receiving irradiation and in 40% of the patients receiving chemotherapy. The rate of fall in paraprotein levels and the return of these toward normal levels were faster in the irradiated group. Survival rates were not significantly different in the two groups at 42 months, with 56% in the irradiated group and 64% in the chemotherapy group. The authors conclude that systemic irradiation has minimal side effects and offers a practical alternative to melphalan and prednisone chemotherapy in the management of previously untreated patients with myeloma. The systemic irradiation used was sequential HBI to a midplane dose of 600 cGy without correction for lung absorption. The lower hemibody was generally treated first. The use of systemic irradiation did not impair the secondary use of chemotherapy for those patients whose myeloma progressed after irradiation.

RADIATION THERAPY TECHNIQUES

Volume

Solitary Plasmacytomas

The radiation volume (portals) for the treatment of solitary plasmacytomas of bone should include the entire involved bone plus a 2 cm to 3 cm margin of surrounding normal tissue (Figs. 64-1 to 64-3). Plasmacytomas frequently extend into the adjacent soft tissues, requiring diligent evaluation for the true tumor extent. Computed tomography is particularly helpful in defining paravertebral extension. The treatment portals for extramedullary plasmacytomas should often include the primary draining lymph nodes.

Multiple Myeloma

The treatment of patients with symptomatic bony lesions of multiple myeloma should involve portals that encompass the entire bone if possible, such as in the extremity. In the vertebral column, at Mallinckrodt Institute of Radiology (MIR) we treat

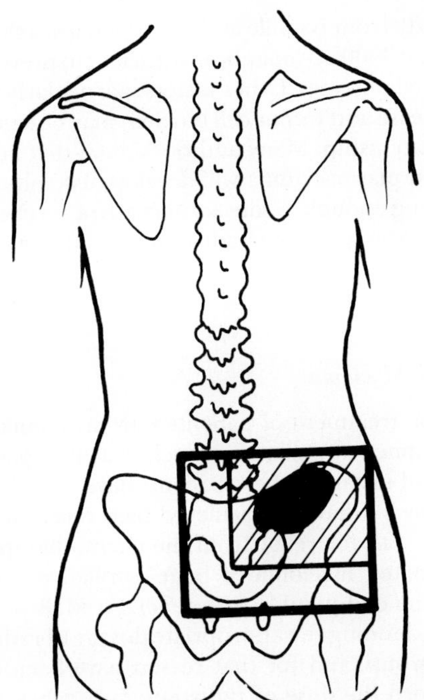

FIGURE 64–1. Portal diagram for the treatment of solitary plasmacytoma of the right ilium and sacroiliac joint region. The larger portal was given 5000 cGy. The smaller portal, delineated by cross-hatching, was given an additional 500 cGy.

the vertebrae involved and usually two vertebrae above and below the extent of the disease process (see Fig. 64-3). It is important to provide skin tattoos over the spine to assess the location of the field for future possibilities of retreatment. It is also important to assess the depth of the anterior aspect of the vertebral body either from a CT scan, which may have been available for diagnostic evaluation, or from a lateral simulation film with some appropriate depth marker. It is mandatory to keep fields in the pelvis and areas involving a lot of bone marrow activity as small as possible to save as much marrow function as possible for future chemotherapy. It is important to document the treatment of rib lesions carefully, including both rib number and geometric location. Tattoos or good diagrams are necessary.

In patients with large lytic lesions in weight-bearing bones such as the femur, orthopedic support should be used before irradiation (Fig. 64-4).

Dose

Solitary Plasmacytomas

The results of radiation delivered by various authors for solitary plasmacytoma (bone or extramedullary) and the ensuing local tumor control are summarized in Table 64-3. In all these reports, doses in the range of 4000 cGy to 5000 cGy in 4 to 5 weeks were recommended for better results. The Princess Margaret Hospital group[40] did not show a definite relationship between radiation dose and local control of extramedullary plasmacytoma. At MIR we recommend high local doses of 5000 cGy and field sizes sufficient to cover the primary mass, all its extensions, and the regional lymph nodes. Other data support this.[100]

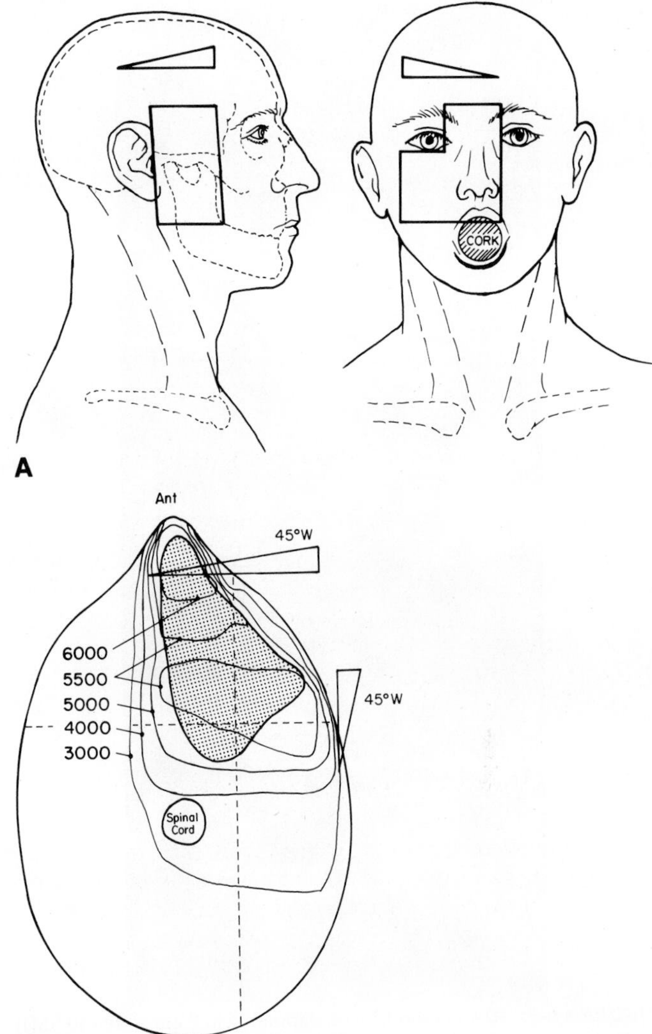

FIGURE 64–2. (**A**) Portal diagrams for the treatment of a solitary extramedullary plasmacytoma involving the right nasal fossa with clouding of the right maxillary antrum (using wedges). (**B**) Isodose distributions for the portal diagrams in (**A**).

Figure 64-5 is a scattergram of dose-response data combining ten MIR cases of solitary plasmacytoma of bone and six cases of extramedullary plasmacytoma with ten solitary plasmacytoma of bone and 17 extramedullary plasmacytoma cases from the literature.[67] The criteria for selection of the cases taken from the literature were adequate description of dose and fractionation, survival greater than 1 year in patients who did not have a local recurrence, and primary treatment with external-beam irradiation without interstitial implants. No apparent difference was found in local control of solitary plasmacytomas of bone (20 of 25) and extramedullary plasmacytomas (17 of 23), and therefore the data were combined. It is clear that these dose-response data do not define an optimal dose-time prescription that would avoid local failure.

In a study of 15 patients at the University of Florida,[63] the authors also did a retrospective review of the literature and a time-dose scattergram of all patients with solitary plasmacytoma. They suggested that a radiation dose of 4000 cGy was sufficient for control in 94% of the patients, with 6% having local failure, in the 81 patients studied. They observed no differences in local control for bony *versus* nonbony lesions.

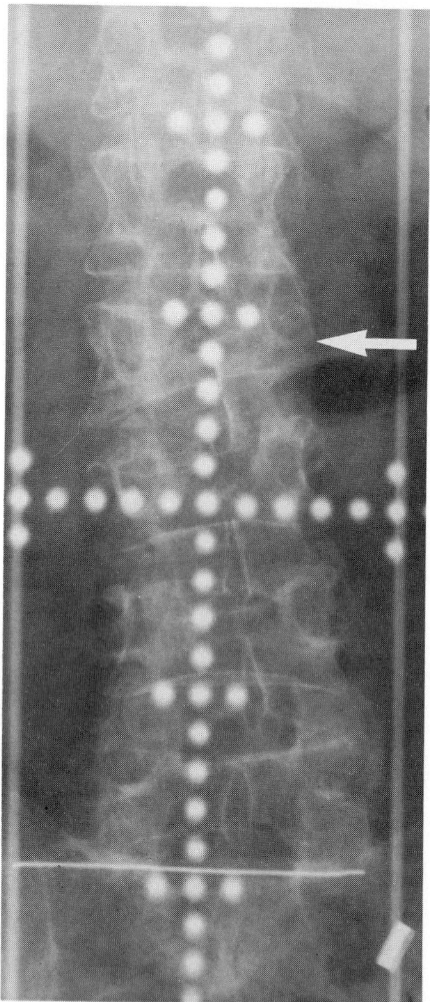

FIGURE 64–3. Simulation film of a spinal field 8 cm wide (80 SSD) with involvement at L2 (*arrow*). Top of field is at top of photo at T11–12 interspace.

The study from Bataille and Sany[13] suggests that radiation doses less than 3500 cGy may be insufficient to prevent progressive disease in bony sites. Other factors, particularly the size and extent of disease and tumor cell burden, may obscure the dose-response relationship. Many authors believe that most patients with localized plasmacytoma will develop disseminated disease if they live long enough. Some authors advocate chemotherapy after local-field high-dose irradiation, although its efficacy remains unproven.

Multiple Myeloma

Radiation treatment of patients with disseminated disease is primarily aimed at palliation, which usually is pain relief. In the majority of instances these patients have already started on chemotherapy but have not achieved pain relief, or the pain is too severe to wait for relief from the chemotherapy.

Disseminated myeloma of bone is relatively sensitive to radiation if the end point is pain relief. At MIR we have been interested in defining the appropriate dosage of radiation therapy in this group, and for that reason have been making an effort to record the dose of radiation given when the patient first reports some pain relief. This dose was recorded in 34 of 185 treatments. The distribution of the doses recorded in which pain relief was first noted is given in Figure 64-6. The median dose range was between 1001 cGy and 1500 cGy. The treatments were given with 200 cGy to 250 cGy fractions, 5 days per week.

An additional consideration is how often patients require retreatment with radiation to the same area. If the original dose of radiation was too low and the combined irradiation-chemotherapy tumor cell kill was inadequate, retreatment should be frequent. In fact, in our experience only 6.2% (17 of 276) of sites were retreated. The initial doses given in those who were retreated are shown in Figure 64-7.[67] No apparent increase in numbers of retreatments was found with low ini-

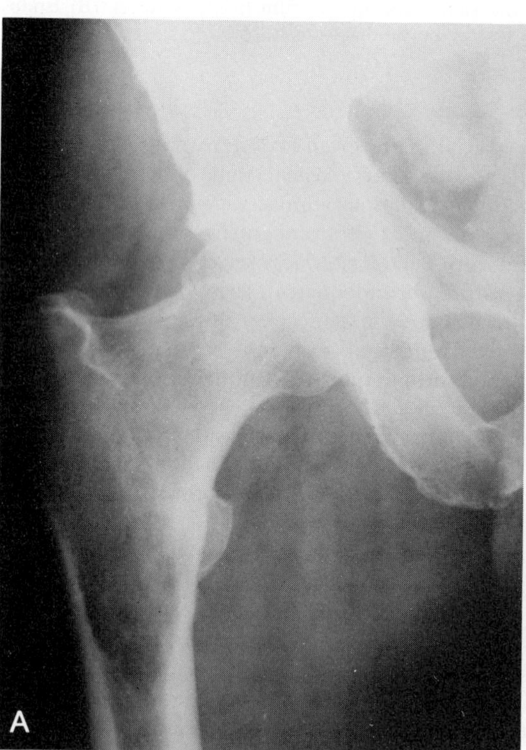

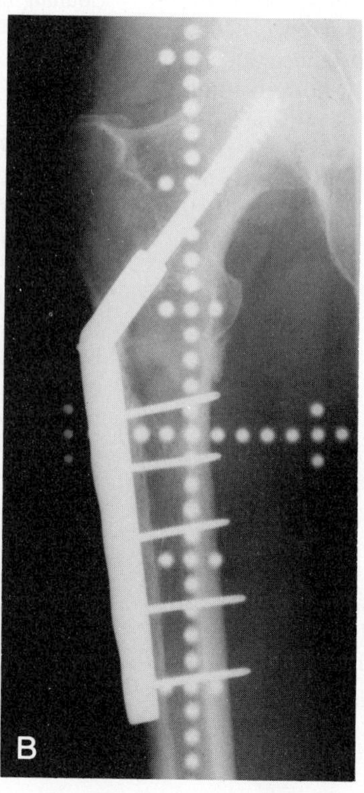

FIGURE 64–4. (**A**) Large lytic area involving the cortex in the subtrochanteric area of the femur. (**B**) Simulation film after orthopedic stabilization. Bottom of field includes the whole femur.

TABLE 64–3
Comparison of Findings of Six Studies of Solitary Plasmacytoma of Bone (SPB) and Extramedullary Plasmacytoma (EP)

	MALLINCKRODT INSTITUTE OF RADIOLOGY 1989[92]		PRINCESS MARGARET HOSPITAL 1983[50]		M.D. ANDERSON HOSPITAL 1979[29]		STANFORD 1987[24]		MAYO CLINIC 1989[34]		UNIVERSITY OF IOWA 1989[62]	
	SPB	EP	SPB	EP	SPB	EP	SPB	EP	SPB	EP	SPB	EP
Number of patients	32	14	25	25	12	12	20	NA	46	NA	17	13
Median survival (months)	50+	63+	86	101	43+	124	47	NA	96	NA	49	69
Local response	94%	93%	92%	96%	92%	83%	95%	NA	89%	NA	88%	92%
Conversion to myeloma	53%	36%	48%	8%	50%	17%	56%	NA	54%	NA	47%	23%

NA: not applicable

tial doses compared with that found with high initial doses. For these reasons, we advocate a palliative dose of 1500 cGy to 2000 cGy in disseminated myeloma, with the exact dose determined by the rapidity of pain relief and the patient's general condition. In general, patients with rapidly advancing disease receive lower doses.

Treatment of hospitalized patients two times per day with 6 hours between treatments has provided no increased complications in our experience. In patients who require retreatment, particularly over the spinal column, it is necessary to be cognizant of total dose to the cord as well as total given dose to the skin, because these patients often are recumbent and it is necessary to avoid skin ulceration from pressure.

It is unknown from our data or from the literature how often patients develop significant recalcification of bone after radiation treatment.

RESULTS OF THERAPY

Solitary Plasmacytomas

When the results of radiation treatment in solitary plasmacytoma are assessed, two distinct parameters can be measured: local control and incidence of dissemination. In our initial series of patients with solitary plasmacytomas, 13 have been followed up for a minimum of 3 years.[67] Ten of these have locally controlled disease. Dissemination has occurred in four patients. Local control in the total group of patients with plasmacytomas reviewed (our group plus those from the literature) is 77% (34 of 43). Eighty percent of the local failures occurred within 3 years.[67] Meyer and Schulz[65] report dissemination in nine of 12 patients with solitary plasmacytomas of bone; in four of these patients dissemination occurred as late as 6 to 10 years

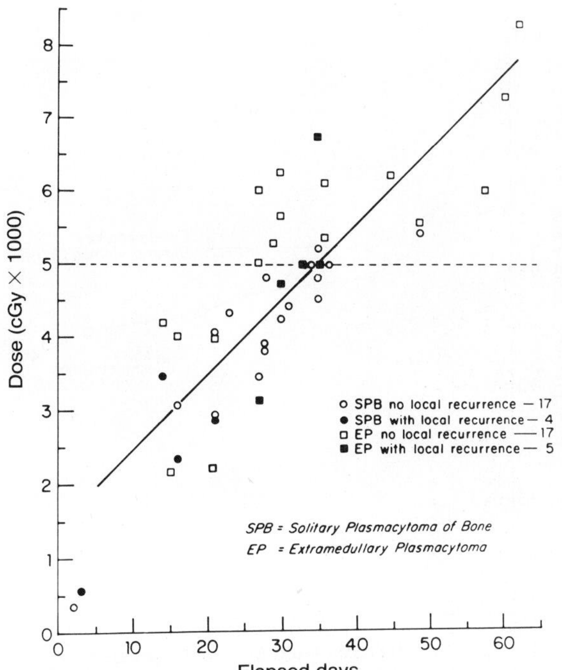

FIGURE 64–5. Dose response in 45 solitary plasmacytomas of bone and extramedullary plasmacytomas. (Mill WB, Griffith R: Cancer 45:647, 1980)

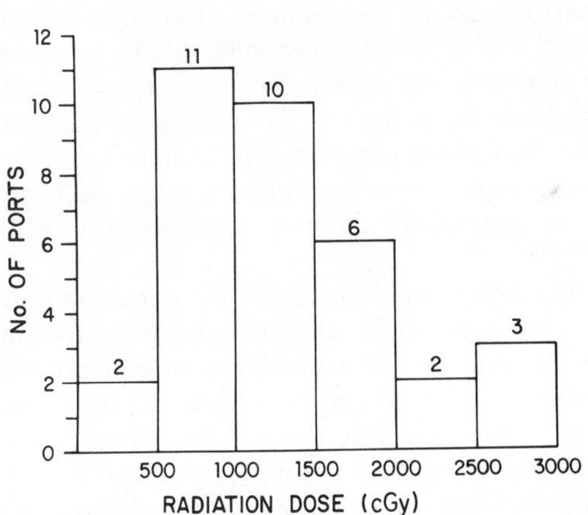

FIGURE 64–6. Distribution of minimum radiation dose producing partial subjective pain relief in 34 evaluable patients with multiple myeloma. (Mill WB, Griffith R: Cancer 45:647, 1980)

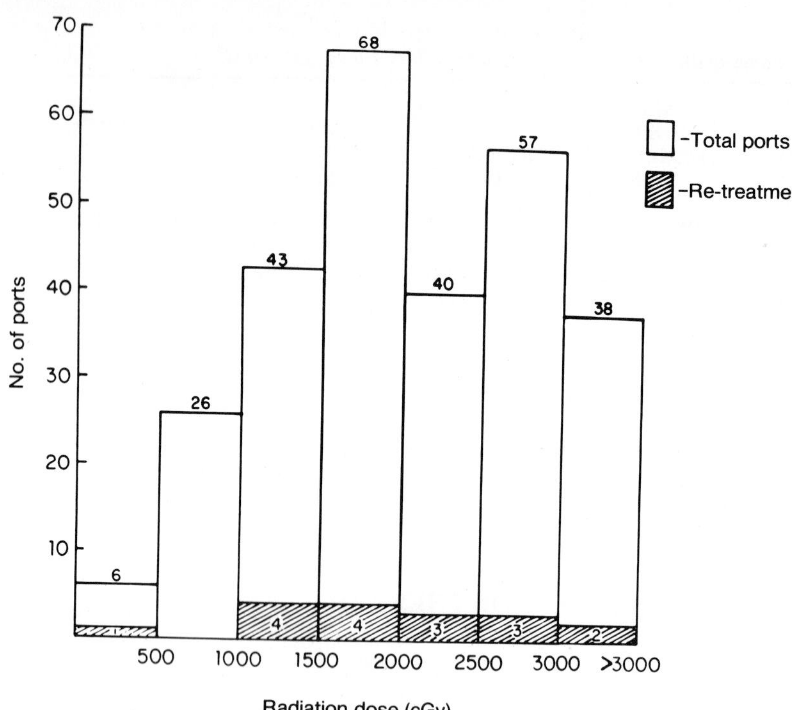

FIGURE 64–7. Radiation dose distribution of 278 portals in patients treated for multiple myeloma. Shaded area is number of portals at that dose that were later retreated to the same volume for recurrent symptoms. (Mill WB, Griffith R: Cancer 45:647, 1980)

after initial treatment. The incidence of dissemination in the total group reviewed is 37% (16 of 43).

Whitshaw[98] reviewed 272 cases of extramedullary plasmacytoma and found that 60 (22%) recurred locally and 109 (40%) recurred at other locations. This undoubtedly increases with follow-up time, but it is low enough to suggest that many of these patients may die of other causes before the disease disseminates. In 15 patients the interval from initial diagnosis to dissemination was available; 80% had disseminated disease by 6.5 years after initial treatment.[67] In 109 patients analyzed by Wiltshaw,[98] the most common sites of dissemination were bones, 41; lymph nodes; 41; subcutaneous tissues, 22; liver, 18; and lungs and pleura, ten. The reported survival rates in patients with localized plasmacytoma are 50% to 60% at 5 years and 15% to 20% at 10 years (Fig. 64-8).[13]

Most reviews of clinical experiences of solitary plasmacytoma of bone *versus* extramedullary plasmacytoma and the relationship to multiple myeloma have shown a more favorable outlook for patients with extramedullary plasmacytoma. This is because of the ability to gain local control with adequate doses of radiation and because solitary plasmacytoma of bone is a common precursor to the development of multiple myeloma (Table 64-3).[29,50,62,63,67,90] Because 20% to 50% of patients with solitary plasmacytoma of bone do not progress to multiple myeloma and because criteria are not reliable for patients at presentation who will not progress, it is recommended that all patients with apparent solitary plasmacytoma of bone receive high-dose, potentially curative local therapy with radiation.[24,91,101]

An elevated paraprotein level is not necessarily indicative of myeloma but needs to be observed after local treatment.[13,91] Because the response of abnormal protein levels in patients with localized plasmacytomas may be variable, it is important before and after local radiation therapy to obtain serial immunoglobulin determinations in patients who initially had a monoclonal gammopathy. A decrease in the level may indicate successful treatment; a level remaining abnormal or rising is a sign of progression to multiple myeloma or to the development of other localized lesions or a localized recurrence.

In a series of solitary plasmacytomas of bone from the Mayo Clinic with a review of 46 patients,[34] evidence of abnormal serum or urine protein was found in 54% of the patients, but neither disease-free survival nor overall survival was influenced by the presence of the abnormal proteins even when they persisted after radiation. As can be seen in Table 64-3, 54% of the patients developed myeloma. The mean survival from the time of development of myeloma was 39 months.

Patients with solitary plasmacytoma, either of bone or an extramedullary site, may develop solitary lesions at other sites without progressing to myeloma. These additional sites should

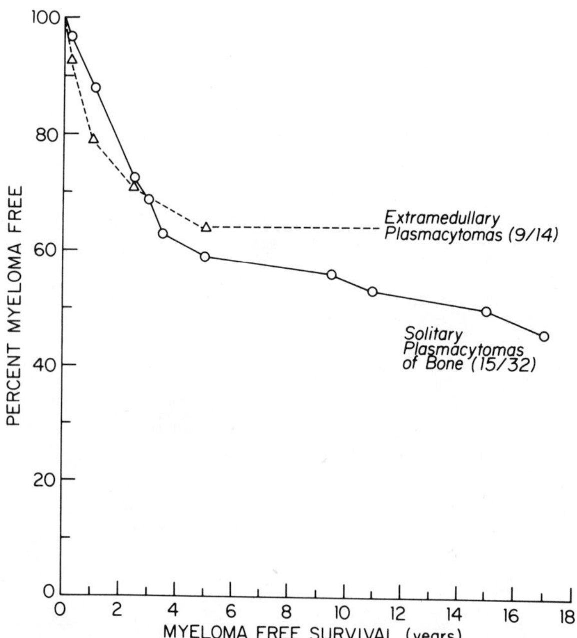

FIGURE 64–8. Myeloma-free survival for MIR patients with solitary plasmacytoma treated with irradiation alone. (Holland J, Wasserman TH, Trenkner D, et al: Prognosis of solitary plasmacytoma. Cancer, in press, 1991)

be treated aggressively, as should local recurrences, when no signs of dissemination are found after the standard workup.

At MIR we have reviewed our experience with 46 cases of solitary plasmacytoma treated with irradiation between 1961 and 1988.[92,95] Thirteen of these cases had been previously reported by Mill and Griffith.[67] Thirty-two cases were solitary plasmacytoma of bone, and 14 cases were extramedullary plasmacytoma. Both solitary plasmacytoma of bone and extramedullary plasmacytoma had a high rate of local response to radiation therapy (94% and 93%, respectively). Seventeen cases of solitary plasmacytoma of bone converted to myeloma (53%) whereas five cases of extramedullary plasmacytoma converted to myeloma (36%), suggesting separate plasma cell tumor entities. Median time of conversion to myeloma for solitary plasmacytoma of bone was 31 months (3 to 204 months). Patients with solitary plasmacytoma of bone remaining free from myeloma have had a median follow-up of over 84 months. Median time of conversion to myeloma for extramedullary plasmacytoma was 13 months. Patients with extramedullary plasmacytoma remaining free from myeloma have had a median follow-up of over 74 months (see Table 64-3). Seven cases behaved as a distinct subset of solitary plasmacytoma characterized by the development of sequential multiple solitary plasmacytomas at different sites over many years without progression to myeloma.

Prophylactic chemotherapy appears to have no established role in the prevention of conversion of solitary plasmacytoma of bone to myeloma. In our series, 64% receiving chemotherapy subsequently converted to myeloma compared with 41% not receiving chemotherapy converting to myeloma. Chemotherapy seemed to delay the time to conversion (59 months *versus* 29 months). The survival of our patients who developed myeloma after that conversion was equal to that of patients who present *de novo* with myeloma, with a median survival of 25 months.

Trends of serum protein levels, lesion size, site of involvement, and radiation dose as prognostic factors in the conversion of solitary plasmacytoma to myeloma are being reviewed.[92]

Multiple Myeloma

From 1961 to 1975, 128 patients were treated at MIR through 278 portals for disseminated multiple myeloma.[67] Eleven patients (4%) were treated for pathologic fractures of long bones. Four of these were treated with internal fixation plus irradiation. The remaining seven were treated with irradiation plus external immobilization; six of these had lesions of the upper extremities. An additional 40 lesions of long bones were treated, only one of which later fractured (immediately after radiation therapy).

In our experience, partial pain relief was achieved in 70% of patients, complete pain relief in 22%, and no pain relief in 8%. Many of the patients not obtaining relief had very advanced disease. Responses even with bulky tumors masses can often be rapid and complete.

SEQUELAE OF TREATMENT

The risk of complications is related to the dose of radiation given and the sensitivity of the normal tissues included in the treatment volume.[64] In the treatment of spinal vertebral lesions with or without extradural extension, the dose of radiation must be limited to that of spinal cord tolerance, which is usually 4000 cGy to 4500 cGy in 5 to 6 weeks, depending on the length of the segment of spinal cord included.

The development of acute nonlymphocytic leukemia is being reported with increasing frequency in myeloma.[36,49,57] Nonhematologic malignancies have also occurred in 8% to 19% of reported cases.[14,58,76,97] It is not clear whether these patients had a predisposition to a second malignancy or whether the treatment induced them.

SUMMARY OF CLINICAL TRIALS

Appropriate criteria should be developed for predicting patients at high risk for progression of localized plasmacytoma to multiple myeloma. Currently no evidence suggests that delay in the use of systemic treatments (chemotherapy) in patients with localized plasmacytoma, or even in patients with indolent multiple myeloma, affects the long-term outlook of the patients.[3] There is a need for controlled clinical trials in this group of patients and for more expansion of the data base to establish better criteria for staging at the time that the patient initially presents with localized disease. Newer methods are needed for measuring response in myeloma by quantitation of pain relief, paraprotein levels, serum β_2-microglobulin levels, and plasma cell percentage in the bone marrow.

Ongoing cooperative study group protocols are primarily testing new chemotherapy agents for activity in multiple myeloma and new combinations of chemotherapy agents. Sequential hemibody treatments allow systemic or total-body treatment, which may be useful as an adjuvant in induction therapy.[66]

An abstract of a Southwest Oncology Group randomized study of hemibody irradiation *versus* combination chemotherapy for remission consolidation in multiple myeloma was recently published.[82] The study began in 1982, and 621 patients received combination chemotherapy for remission induction with a complete response (CR) achieved in 37% and a partial response (PR) is 23%. The most important pretreatment prognostic factor for survival was serum β_2-microglobulin level. Of those achieving a CR, 183 patients were randomized to consolidation of sequential hemibody irradiation plus vincristine and prednisone or combination chemotherapy. The hemibody irradiation was given in five daily 150 cGy fractions. Upper and lower hemibody irradiation was separated by 6 weeks. For patients with CR who were randomized to the consolidation therapy, survival from the start of consolidation was better for combination chemotherapy patients (44 months) than for the hemibody patients (26 months; $P = 0.02$). Life-threatening myelosuppression was more common with hemibody irradiation.

REFERENCES

1. Abraham D, Carbone PP, Venditti HM, et al: Evaluation of chemical agents against the plasma cell tumor LPC-1 mice. Biochem Pharmacol 16:665–673, 1967
2. Alberts DS, Salmon SE: Adriamycin in the treatment of alkylator-resistant multiple myeloma. Cancer Chemother Rep 59:345–350, 1975
3. Alexanian R: Localized and indolent myeloma. Blood 56:521–525, 1981
4. Alexanian R, Balcerzak S, Bonnet JD, et al: Prognostic factors in multiple myeloma. Cancer 36:1192–1201, 1975
5. Alexanian R, Balcerzak S, Gehen E, et al: Remission mainte-

nance therapy for multiple myeloma. Arch Intern Med 135:147–152, 1975

6. Alexanian R, Bonnet J, Gehen E, et al: Combination chemotherapy for multiple myeloma. Cancer 30:382–389, 1972
7. Alexanian R, Salmon S, Bonnet J, et al: Combination therapy for multiple myeloma. Cancer 40:2765–2771, 1977
8. American Cancer Society: Cancer Facts and Figures, 1991
9. Anderson RE, Ishida K: Malignant lymphoma in survivors of the atomic bomb in Hiroshima. Ann Intern Med 61:853, 1964
10. Azar HA, Potter M: Multiple Myeloma and Related Disorders, vol I. Hagerstown, MD, Harper & Row, 1973
11. Bataille R, Chevalier J, Rossi M, Sany J: Bone scintigraphy in plasma-cell myeloma. Radiology 145:801–804, 1982
12. Bataille R, Durie BGM, Grenier J, et al: Prognostic factors and staging in multiple myeloma: A reappraisal. J Clin Oncol 4(1):80–87, 1986
13. Bataille R, Sany J: Solitary myeloma: Clinical and prognostic features of a review of 114 cases. Cancer 48:845–851, 1981
14. Bell R, Sullivan JR, Fone DJ, et al: Carcinoma of the breast: Occurrence after treatment with melphalan for multiple myeloma. JAMA 236:1609, 1976
15. Bergsagel DE: Editorial: Progress in the treatment of plasma cell myeloma? J Clin Oncol 1:510, 1983
16. Bergsagel DE: Total body irradiation for myelomatosis. Br Med J 2:325, 1971
17. Bergsagel DE: Plasma cell myeloma: An interpretive review. Cancer 30:1588–1594, 1972
18. Bergsagel DE, Griffith KM, Haut A, et al: The treatment of plasma cell myeloma. Adv Cancer Res 10:311–359, 1967
19. Bergsagel DE, Ogawa M, Librach SL: Mouse myeloma: A model for studies of cell kinetics. Arch Intern Med 135:109–113, 1975
20. Blattner WA, Blair A, Mason TJ: Multiple myeloma in the United States 1950–1975. Cancer 48:2547–2554, 1981
21. Bosch A, Frias Z: Radiotherapy in the treatment of multiple myeloma. Int J Radiat Oncol Biol Phys 15:1363–1369, 1988
22. Bush S, Goffinet DR, Bagshaw MA: Extramedullary plasmacytoma of the head and neck. Radiology 140:801, 1981
23. Carson CP, Ackerman LV, Maltby JD: Plasma cell myeloma: A clinical pathologic and roentgenologic review of 90 cases. Am J Clin Pathol 25:849–888, 1955
24. Chak LY, Cox RS, Bostwick DG, Hoppe RT: Solitary plasmacytoma of bone: Treatment, progression, and survival. J Clin Oncol 5:1811–1815, 1987
25. Charkes ND, Durant J, Barry WE: Bone pain in multiple myeloma. Arch Intern Med 130:53–58, 1972
26. Charkes ND, Young I, Sklaroff DM: The pathologic basis of strontium bone scan. JAMA 206:2482–2488, 1968
27. Coleman M, Saletan S, Wolf D, et al: Whole bone marrow irradiation for the treatment of multiple myeloma. Cancer 49:1328–1333, 1982
28. Committee of the Chronic Leukemia-Myeloma Task Force, National Cancer Institute: Proposed guidelines for protocol studies. II. Plasma cell myeloma. Cancer Chemother Rep 4:145–158, 1973
29. Corwin J, Lindberg RD: Solitary plasmacytoma of bone vs. extramedullary plasmacytoma and their relationship to multiple myeloma. Cancer 43:1007–1013, 1979
30. Costa G, Engle RL, Schilling A, et al: Melphalan and prednisone: An effective combination for the treatment of multiple myeloma. Am J Med 54:589–599, 1973
31. Courey RW: Osteoblastic lesions of unusual nature. JAMA 219:377–378, 1972
32. Durie BG, Salmon SE: A clinical staging system for multiple myeloma. Correlation of measured myeloma cell mass with presenting clinical features, response to treatment and survival. Cancer 36:842–854, 1975
33. Evison G, Evans KT: Bone sclerosis in multiple myeloma. Br J Radiol 40:81–90, 1967
34. Frassica DA, Frassica FJ, Schray MF, et al: Solitary plasmacytoma of bone: Mayo Clinic experience. Int J Radiat Oncol Biol Phys 16:43–48, 1989
35. George RP, Poth JL, Gordon D, et al: Multiple myeloma: Intermittent combination chemotherapy compared to continuous therapy. Cancer 29:1665–1670, 1972
36. Gonzalez F, Trujillo JM, Alexanian R: Acute leukemia in multiple myeloma. Ann Intern Med 86:440–443, 1977
37. Griswold DP, Schabel FM Jr, Wilcox WS, et al: Success and failure in the treatment of solid tumors. I. Effect of cyclophosphamide (NSC-26271) on primary and metastatic plasmacytoma in the hamster. Cancer Chemother Rep 52:345–387, 1968
38. Griswold DP Jr, Simpson-Herren L, Schabel FM Jr: Altered sensitivity of a hamster plasmacytoma to cytosine arabinoside (NSC-63878). Cancer Chemother Rep 54:337–346, 1970
39. Harley JB, Schilling A, Glidewell O: Ineffectiveness of fluoride therapy in multiple myeloma. N Engl J Med 24:1283–1288, 1972
40. Harwood AR, Knowling MA, Bergsagel DE: Radiotherapy of extramedullary plasmacytoma of the head and neck. Clin Radiol 32:31–36, 1981
41. Hiramoto RN, Chanta VK: Chemotherapy and rate of kill of tumor cells in a mouse plasmacytoma. Cancer Res 34:1738–1742, 1974
42. Hobbs JR: Growth rates and responses to treatment in human myelomatosis. Br J Haematol 16:607–617, 1969
43. Holder DL: Total-body irradiation in multiple myeloma. Radiology 84:83–86, 1965
44. Hoogstraten B: Multiple myeloma: A therapeutic enigma. Am J Clin Oncol 5:13, 1982
45. Hubner KF, Andrews GA, Hayes RL, et al: The use of rare-earth radionuclides and other bone-seekers in the evaluation of bone lesions in patients with multiple myeloma or solitary plasmacytoma. Radiology 125:171–176, 1977
46. Isobe T, Osserman EF: Pathologic conditions associated with plasma cell dyscrasias: A study of 806 cases. Ann NY Acad Sci 190:507, 1971
47. Jacobs P, King HS, LeRoux I: Systemic irradiation compared to chemotherapy as primary treatment for multiple myeloma (in press)
48. Jaffe JP, Bosch A, Raich PC: Sequential hemi-body radiotherapy in advanced multiple myeloma. Cancer 43:124–128, 1979
49. Karchmer RK, Amare M, Larsen WE, et al: Alkylating agents as leukemogens in multiple myeloma. Cancer 33:1103–1107, 1974
50. Knowling MA, Harwood AR, Bergsagel DE: Comparison of extramedullary plasmacytomas with solitary and multiple plasma cell tumors of bone. J Clin Oncol 1:255, 1983
51. Korst DR, Clifford GO, Fowler WM, et al: Multiple myeloma II. Analysis of cyclophosphamide therapy in 165 patients. JAMA 189:758–762, 1964
52. Kotner LM, Wang CC: Plasmacytoma of the upper air and food passages. Cancer 30:414–418, 1972
53. Kyle RA: Long-term survival in multiple myeloma. N Engl J Med 308:314, 1985
54. Kyle RA: Treatment of multiple myeloma: A small step forward? N Engl J Med 310:1382, 1984
55. Kyle RA: Subject review: Multiple myeloma: Review of 869 cases. Mayo Clin Proc 50:29, 1975
56. Kyle RA, Maldonado JE, Bayrd ED: Plasma cell leukemia: Report on 17 cases. Arch Intern Med 133:813–818, 1974
57. Kyle RA, Pierre RV, Bayrd ED: Multiple myeloma and acute myelomonocytic leukemia: Report of four cases possibly related to melphalan. N Engl J Med 21:1121–1125, 1970
58. Law IP, Blom J: Second malignancies in patients with multiple myeloma. Oncology 34:20–24, 1977
59. Lee BJ, Sahakian G, Clarkson BD, et al: Combination chemotherapy of multiple myeloma with Alkeran, Cytoxan, vincristine, prednisone and BCNU. Cancer 33:533–538, 1974
60. Lewis EB: Leukemia, multiple myeloma, and aplastic anemia in American radiologists. Science 142:1492–1494, 1963
61. Ludwig H, Fruhwald F, Tscholakoff D, et al: Magnetic resonance imaging of the spine in multiple myeloma. Lancet 2:364–366, 1987
62. Mayr NA, Wen B-C, Hussey D, et al: The role of radiation therapy in the treatment of solitary plasmacytomas. Int J Radiat Oncol Biol Phys 15(Suppl 1):209, 1988
63. Mendenhall CM, Thar TL, Million RR: Solitary plas-

macytoma of bone and soft tissue. Int J Radiat Oncol Biol Phys 6:1497–1501, 1980
64. Merriam GR, Szechter A, Focht EFL: The effect of ionizing radiation on the eye. In Vaeth JM (ed): Radiation Effects and Tolerance, Normal Tissue. Baltimore, University Park Press, 1970
65. Meyer JE, Schulz MD: "Solitary" myeloma of bone: A review of 12 cases. Cancer 34:438–440, 1974
66. Mill W, Brown G, Cohen HJ, et al: Hemi-body irradiation in multiple myeloma in patients relapsing after or resistant to chemotherapy: Report of a phase II protocol of the Southeastern Cancer Study Group. Clin Res Bull 2:3, 1985
67. Mill WB, Griffith R: The role of radiation therapy in the management of plasma cell tumors. Cancer 45:647, 1980
68. Muruyama Y, Thomson J Jr: Radiotherapeutic response of plasma cell tumors associated with monoclonal gammopathy. Cancer 26:110, 1970
69. Osserman EF: Plasma-cell myeloma II. Clinical Aspects. N Engl J Med 261:952–960, 1959
70. Osserman EF, Takatsuki K: Considerations regarding the pathogenesis of the plasmacytic dyscrasias. Scand J Haematol 4:18, 1964
71. Pankovich AM, Griem ML: Plasma-cell myeloma: A thirty-year follow-up. Radiology 104:521–522, 1972
72. Penny R, Hughes S: Repeated stimulation of the reticuloendothelial system and the development of plasma cell dyscrasias. Lancet 1:77, 1970
73. Petrovich Z, Fishkin B, Hittle RE, et al: Extramedullary plasmacytoma of the upper respiratory passages. Int J Radiat Oncol Biol Phys 2:723–730, 1977
74. Poole AG, Marchetta FC: Extramedullary plasmacytoma of the head and neck. Cancer 22:14–21, 1968
75. Qasim MM: Techniques and results of half body irradiation (HBI) in metastatic carcinomas and myelomas. Clin Oncol 5:65, 1979
76. Robins SM, Chopra D: Multiple myeloma and multiple neoplasms. JAMA 236:1609, 1976
77. Rodriguez AR, Lutcher CL, Coleman FW: Osteosclerotic myeloma. JAMA 236:1872–1874, 1976
78. Rosenblatt J, Hall CA: Plasma cell dyscrasia following prolonged stimulation of reticuloendothelial system. Lancet 1:301, 1970
79. Rostom AY, O'Cathail SM, Folkes A: Systemic irradiation in multiple myeloma: A report on nineteen cases. Br J Haematol 58:423–431, 1984
80. Salmon SE: Expansion of the growth fraction in multiple myeloma with alkylating agents. Blood 45:119–129, 1975
81. Salmon SE, Cassady JR: Plasma cell neoplasms. In DeVita VT Jr, Hellman S, Rosenberg SA (eds.): Cancer: Principles and Practice of Oncology, 3rd ed. Philadelphia, JB Lippincott, 1989
82. Salmon SE, Tesh D, Crowley J, et al: Combination chemotherapy is superior to hemibody irradiation (HXRT) for remission consolidation in multiple myeloma (MM): A Southwest Oncology Group (SWOG) study. Proc ASCO 8:250, 1989
83. Schreiman JS, McLeod RA, Kyle RA, Beabout JW: Multiple myeloma: Evaluation by CT. Radiology 154:483–486, 1985
84. Shaw MT, Twele TW, Nordquist RE: Plasma cell leukemia: Detailed studies and response to therapy. Cancer 33:619–625, 1974
85. Singer CRJ, Tobias JS, Giles F, et al: Hemibody irradiation: An effective 2nd-line therapy in drug-resistant multiple myeloma. Cancer 63:2446–2451, 1989
86. Snapper I, Turner LB, Moscovitz HL: Multiple myeloma, p 168. New York, Grune & Stratton, 1963
87. Tamir R, Gianz I, Lubin E, et al: Comparison of the sensitivity of Tc 99m-bone scan with the skeletal x-ray survey in multiple myeloma. Acta Haematol 69:236, 1983
88. Thomas RJ, Daban A, Bontoux D: Double hemibody irradiation in chemotherapy: Resistant multiple myeloma. Cancer Treat Rep 68:1173, 1984
89. Tobias JS, Richards JDM, Blackman GM, et al: Hemibody irradiation in multiple myeloma. Radiother Oncol 3:11, 1985
90. Todd IDH: Treatment of solitary plasmacytoma. Clin Radiol 16:395, 1965
91. Tong D, Griffin TW, Laramore GE, et al: Solitary plasmacytoma of bone and soft tissues. Radiology 135:195–198, 1980
92. Trenkner D, Wasserman T, Holland J, et al: Prognosis of solitary plasmacytomas Cancer (in press) 1991
93. Wahner HW, Kyle RA, Beabout JW: Scintigraphic evaluation of the skeleton in multiple myeloma. Mayo Clin Proc 55:739, 1980
94. Warner NL, Potter M, Metcalf D: Multiple myeloma and related immunoglobulin producing neoplasms. International Union Against Cancer Technical Report Series, vol 13, p 18. Geneva, IUCC, 1974
95. Wasserman TH: Diagnosis and management of plasmacytomas. Oncology 1(2):37–41, 1987
96. Weinmann JP, Sicher H: Bone and Bones: Fundamentals of Bone Biology, p 404. St. Louis, CV Mosby, 1947
97. Weitzel RA: Carcinoma coexistent with malignant disorders of plasma cells. Cancer 11:546–549, 1958
98. Wiltshaw E: The natural history of extramedullary plasmacytoma and its relation to solitary myeloma of bone and myelomatosis. Medicine 55:217–238, 1976
99. Woodruff R: Treatment of multiple myeloma. Cancer Treat Rev 8:225–270, 1981
100. Woodruff R: Solitary plasmacytoma, extramedullary soft tissue plasmacytoma. Cancer 43:2340–2343, 1979
101. Woodruff R.: Solitary plasmacytoma, solitary plasmacytoma of bone. Cancer 43:2344–2347, 1979

65

Thyroid

Larry D. Greenfield
Kenneth H. Luk

ANATOMY

The thyroid gland consists of the right and left lobes, joined by the isthmus, which crosses the trachea at the second or third cartilaginous ring. A pyramidal lobe may extend superiorly from the isthmus or one of the thyroid lobes (Fig. 65-1*A*). The thyroid gland has an average weight of 20 g. The parathyroid glands lie on the posterior surface of both thyroid lobes, and the recurrent laryngeal nerves are in a cleft between the trachea and esophagus, medial to the lateral aspect of both thyroid lobes. Readers interested in the embryologic development of the thyroid are referred to the literature.[64,175]

The four major arteries supplying the thyroid are the paired superior thyroid arteries and the paired inferior thyroid arteries. The thyroidea ima, a fifth artery, arises from the aortic arch and enters the midline of the thyroid. A venous plexus forms under the fibrous capsule and contributes to confluences forming the superior and the middle thyroid veins; these veins enter the internal jugular veins. Occasionally, arising from the inferior poles are the inferior thyroid veins, which enter the innominate vein.

Innervation of the gland is by the sympathetic and parasympathetic divisions of the autonomic nervous system.

Lymphatic drainage from the thyroid is in the superior, lateral, and inferior directions and generally follows the branches of the superior and inferior thyroid blood vessels (Fig. 65-1*B*).[66] The superior lymphatic pathways drain the anterior and posterior portions of the thyroid lobes and the medial aspect of the gland adjacent to the isthmus. The collection trunks may cross anterior and superior to the isthmus and may communicate with the prelaryngeal nodes. A pyramidal lobe, if present, is included in the prelaryngeal collecting system. The collecting pathways from the prelaryngeal region and the anterior and medial aspects of the upper poles follow the blood vessels and continue to the superior subdigastric nodes of the internal jugular chain. The posterior portion of the upper lobes empties into collecting lymphatics that usually end in the superior and anterior internal jugular nodes. The lateral pathways follow the middle thyroid veins to the inferior and lateral nodes of the internal jugular chain; they chiefly drain the lateral lower half of each thyroid lobe. The inferior pathway drains the lower portion of the isthmus, the inferior poles, and the medial and posterior lower half of each thyroid lobe; they empty into the pretracheal and paratracheal lymph nodes.

Drainage pathways may lie adjacent to the thymus, and nodes in the area of the innominate veins may show metastatic disease from the lower poles and inferior aspect of the isthmus. There appears to be free communication between the retropharyngeal and retroesophageal nodes and the recurrent laryngeal and paratracheal nodes. Anterior superior mediastinal nodes are secondary nodes to the recurrent laryngeal and pretracheal nodal groups.

EPIDEMIOLOGY

Thyroid cancer is diagnosed in 45 of every million persons in the United States annually. It comprises 1.3% of all malignancies and accounts for 0.4% of all cancer deaths.[41,67]

According to the American Cancer Society, the number of new thyroid cancer cases for 1991 was estimated to be 12,100 (3200 male and 8900 female), with an estimated 1025 deaths (375 male and 650 female) from the disease.[227]

The National Cancer Institute's Surveillance Epidemiology and End Results (SEER) program[160] found that for males and females combined the cancers with the highest 10-year relative survival rates were thyroid (90%), melanoma (68%), bladder (63%), breast (60%), and Hodgkin's disease (57%). For males, testicular cancer had a 10-year relative survival rate of 74%, second only to thyroid cancer at 88%. For females, corpus uteri cancer patients had a 10-year rate of 87%, which was exceeded only by that of thyroid cancer patients at 91%.

Radiation-Induced Thyroid Cancer

Thyroid gland exposure to ionizing radiation, particularly before puberty, is the only well-documented etiologic factor in thyroid cancer. One quarter of patients who received between 2 cGy and several hundred centigrays of external radiation to the thyroid gland develop goiters; one fourth of these or 7% of all individuals who receive external irradiation to the thyroid develop cancer, usually papillary adenocarcinoma.[82,158,171,198,206,208,235,272] Iodine-131 and x-rays are equally effective in inducing thyroid cancer at doses under 1000 cGy.[128]

The Japanese population exposed to the atomic bomb in 1945 has been studied. The Hiroshima bomb contained a significant neutron component, but the Nagasaki bomb delivered almost pure γ-rays. Of a fixed population of 20,000 heavily and lightly exposed individuals systematically examined every sec-

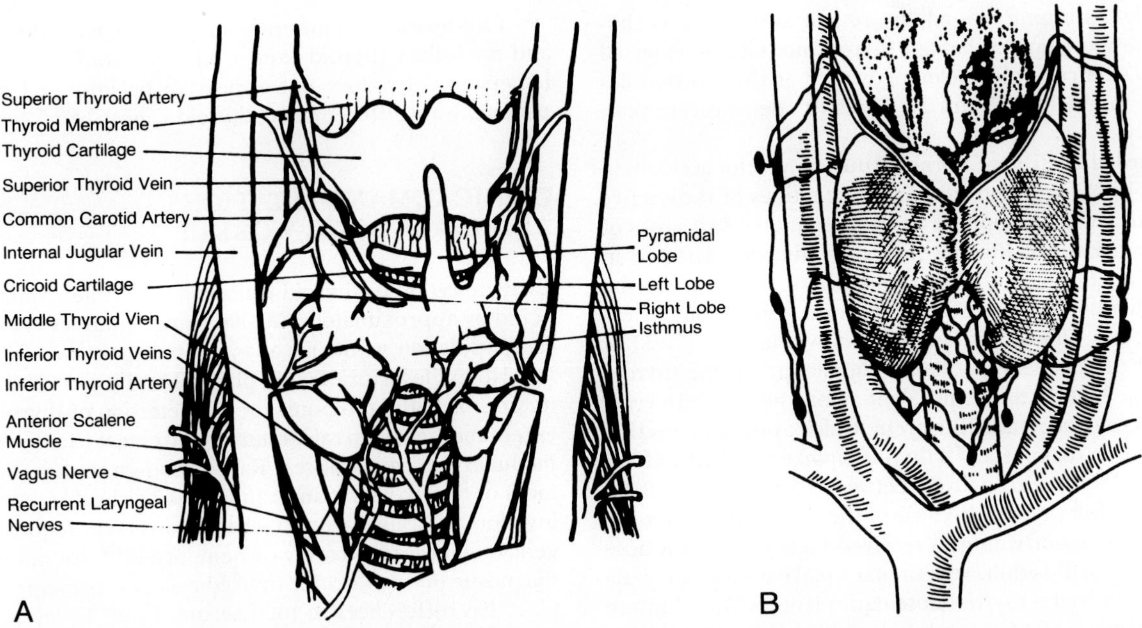

FIGURE 65–1. (**A**) Anatomy of the thyroid. (**B**) Lymphatic drainage of the thyroid. (Mahomer HR, Caylor HD, Schlottnauer CF, Pemberton J de J: Anat Rec 36:341, 1927)

ond year since 1959, approximately 0.2% have developed thyroid cancer, mostly papillary adenocarcinoma. The study found that females between 10 and 19 years old at the time of the bombings and exposed to more than 50 cGy have a risk of developing thyroid cancer 8.8 times higher than females of the same age exposed to less than 1 cGy.[97,168,182,197,221]

In 1954, Marshall Islanders were exposed to radioactive fallout from a nuclear test. Exposed persons (229) and nonexposed persons (311) from nearby uncontaminated islands have been systematically studied annually. Thyroid gland irradiation was mainly due to several short-lived internally deposited radioiodine nuclides; external γ and β irradiation also contributed. According to the 1974 survey, 34 of those exposed have developed thyroid lesions; three (1.3%) of the 34 lesions were cancers. The highest incidence of thyroid nodularity occurred in 19 persons who were irradiated before the age of 20. Their whole-body dose was estimated at 175 cGy and their thyroid dose at 1200 cGy.[97] This Polynesian population has been further reported in a 1982 publication.[248]

In the United States from the 1930s into the 1950s, there was a widespread practice of treating almost any benign disease, particularly in the very young, with x-rays or radium. These practices account for most of the large number of thyroid cancers during the past 20 years.

Among irradiated American populations, the highest incidence of thyroid cancer is in patients whose thyroid glands had been in the primary beam (*e.g.*, treatment of tonsillitis). In two Chicago studies of patients with histories of tonsillitis treated with x-rays, 6% of those in one study and 7% in the other developed thyroid cancer.[65,198] Thyroid cancer developed in 5% of a subgroup of Rochester patients with nasopharyngeal lymphoid hyperplasia; the x-ray beam had been directed at the tonsillar region.[98] Table 65-1 is a summary of the results of the Rochester study. Other studies have shown that about 30% of patients with nodular disease after irradiation develop thyroid cancer.[54,60] The incidence of carcinoma in radiation-exposed patients has been reported to be approximately 60%.[91,204] The prevalence of occult thyroid cancer found in two autopsy series of controls without radiation exposure was 0% and 2%.[91]

Modan's group[164] reported a high incidence of thyroid carcinoma in 11,000 children who received x-ray treatments to the scalp for tinea capitis. The estimated thyroid dose in these children was 6 cGy, which approximates the incidence at 6 cGy on the linear dose-response curve of the Rochester study.[104] This suggests that there is no threshold for radiation-induced thyroid cancer or, if a threshold exists, it is less than 6 cGy.

According to Maxon and associates,[149] external irradiation of the thyroid at doses greater than 2000 rem is not clearly associated with thyroid cancer induction. With less than 2000 rem of external irradiation, a linear no-threshold model suggests that children have absolute risks for thyroid cancer and for thyroid nodules of 4.2 and 12.3 cases/10^6 persons/rem/year,

TABLE 65–1
Estimated Risks of Thyroid Cancer in the Rochester Population

CHARACTERISTIC	RISK
Sex	All females have 2.3 times the risk of males; young adult females have a five-fold greater risk than males.
Age	After the 5-year latent period, the risk remains constant for 5 to 40 years after irradiation at about 28 times expectation.
Dose	Risk increases proportionately with the thyroid absorbed dose. Absolute risk: three cases per year per 10^6 persons, each with a thyroid dose of 1 cGy, or three cases per year per 10^4 persons, each with a thyroid dose of 100 cGy.
Time	Minimum latent period after irradiation in infancy was 5 years for thyroid cancer and 10 years for benign thyroid tumors.[98] Cancer occurs later in girls than in boys. There may be a 10-year minimal latent period in those irradiated as adults.[182]

(Hempelmann LH, Hall WJ, Phillips M, et al: JNCI 55:519. 1975)

respectively. Assuming that adults are half as sensitive as children to the induction of benign thyroid nodules by external irradiation, the risks of developing cancer or thyroid nodules for adults would be 4.2 and 8.2 cases/10^6 persons/rem/year, respectively.

In April of 1986, the Chernobyl nuclear reactor accident in the Soviet Union released substantial quantities of radioactive materials into the atmosphere and contaminated vast areas of Western and Eastern Europe. The radionuclides detected in the air included ^{131}I, ^{137}Cs, ^{99}Mo, and others. Iodine 131 is the easiest radionuclide to screen for in large populations of exposed persons. One study tested 58 individuals, 45 (78%) of whom had detectable quantities of radioiodine in the thyroid gland.[36] The highest dose equivalent among adults (>18 years of age) was calculated as 5180 mrem, which approximates that received from a diagnostic ^{131}I thyroid uptake test: 5 μCi of ^{131}I administered by mouth delivers between 6500 mrem to 9000 mrem to an adult thyroid. Because of the smaller thyroid mass, children (18 years or younger) received higher radiation dose equivalents than did adults with similar uptake values. A 1-year-old infant received a thyroid dose equivalent to 37,000 mrem for an uptake of 0.82 μCi; an adult thyroid gland concentrating this amount of ^{131}I would receive 471 mrem. Most of the test population, including two pregnant women, received negligible radiation dose equivalents to the thyroid.

In another study of the Chernobyl accident from Sweden, the time-activity curve for ^{131}I showed immediate uptake, with maximum uptake between 18 and 26 days after the accident.[247] No measurable levels were observed after 93 days. This may lead to a 0.1% increase in the incidence of thyroid cancer during a 25-year period.

Thyroid function abnormalities after neck irradiation for Hodgkin's disease have been reported.[12,141,167] In one study, among 50 disease-free patients 2 to 16 years after neck irradiation, 25 had abnormal thyroid studies: eight were hypothyroid; two were hypothyroid and had abnormal scans; and 15 had abnormal scans. Of 15 patients with abnormal scans, one had elevated levels of thyroid-stimulating hormone (TSH) and another developed exophthalmos. Graves' disease has also been reported to develop after radiation therapy for Hodgkin's disease.[141]

Thyroid cancer has been encountered in patients who received mantle irradiation for Hodgkin's disease.[157] The number of patients developing thyroid cancer after high-dose neck irradiation is, however, less than would be anticipated.

There have been isolated reports of thyroid cancer occurring years after ^{131}I therapy for hyperthyroidism.[154,156] Many careful studies have concluded, however, that there is no correlation between the development of thyroid cancer and ^{131}I therapy for hyperthyroidism.[106,200,213,243] One study concluded that the number of thyroid cancers found in patients previously treated with radioiodine is considerably less than would be anticipated by chance.[156] No increase has been shown in infertility, spontaneous abortions, or congenital abnormalities among patients treated for hyperthyroidism with ^{131}I.[213]

Autoimmune Aspects of Thyroid Cancer

Several investigators have reported a higher antibody titer against thyroidal components in thyroid cancer patients than in the normal population.[264] The incidence of positive antithyroglobulin and antimicrosomal antibody titers were increased in one group of patients with naturally occurring thyroid cancer, but not in those with radiation-induced tumors.[201]

Cell-mediated immunity in patients with differentiated and medullary thyroid cancer has been studied, and delayed hypersensitivity does not appear to be impaired initially in patients with differentiated thyroid cancer.[4,202,264]

CLINICAL MANIFESTATIONS AND DIAGNOSTIC WORKUP

Early detection of thyroid cancer in the United States is hampered by approximately 300,000 benign nodules in the American population with clinically apparent goiters.[67,227]

No single historic factor, physical finding, or clinical laboratory test is pathognomonic for the detection of thyroid cancer, except for the serum calcitonin measurement used for detecting medullary thyroid cancer. Rarely, benign and malignant tumors of the thyroid gland can lead to tracheal compression or invasion and cause acute tracheal obstruction requiring emergency total thyroidectomy or hemoptysis.[138] An outline of the diagnostic procedures for thyroid cancer is presented in Table 65-2. No differences in total serum T_4 or T_3 levels occur in benign and malignant disease.[220,264]

A significant increase in the incidence of HLA-DR7 has been found among nonradiation-associated thyroid cancer patients compared with normal controls. This finding was most noticeable with follicular and mixed papillary follicular cancers. The frequency of HLA-DR7 was not increased in patients with radiation-associated thyroid cancer, but the interval from the date of irradiation to the onset of thyroid cancer was shorter in HLA-DR7-positive patients than in HLA-DR7-negative patients.[245]

The thyroid gland has been reported to contain the creatine kinase isoenzymes MM and BB.[84,172,229,231]

Because medullary thyroid cancer often metastasizes to the anterior mediastinum, widening of that area on a radiograph in a patient with palpable thyroid abnormalities should result in the inclusion of medullary thyroid cancer in the differential diagnosis; however, this mediastinal finding is also seen with other types of thyroid cancers. In some patients, recognition of paraneoplastic syndromes associated with advanced medullary thyroid cancer can facilitate diagnosis.

Approximately 20% to 30% of patients with proven medullary thyroid cancer, particularly those with metastatic disease, complain of persistent diarrhea.[15,209] Prostaglandins, vasoactive intestinal polypeptide, and serotonin that may be produced by the tumor may singly or in combination be responsible for the diarrhea.[111] Indomethacin and aspirin, which block prostaglandin synthesis, may alleviate the diarrhea. Nutmeg may also be used, although its mechanism of action is speculative. A trial of steroids may be warranted if the diarrhea is the result of elevated levels of vasoactive intestinal polypeptide.[15]

Serotonin may be responsible for a carcinoid syndrome, including diarrhea. Trials of antiserotonin agents, such as cyproheptadine, may be warranted.

Cushing's syndrome may be caused by secretion of adrenocorticotropic hormone by medullary thyroid cancer. This association requires the inclusion of this thyroid lesion in the differential diagnosis of "ectopic" Cushing's syndrome.[205]

Levels of carcinoembryonic antigen (CEA) are elevated with locally advanced or metastatic medullary thyroid cancer. In general, the highest CEA levels are found in patients with the highest calcitonin levels, both markers reflecting total body tumor burden.[274]

Serum calcitonin with or without the use of calcium or pentagastrin stimulation testing is the key marker in detecting

TABLE 65–2
Diagnostic Workup for Thyroid Tumors

PROCEDURE	FINDING	SIGNIFICANCE
GENERAL		
History	External irradiation to head or neck between infancy and early adulthood	Known etiology of thyroid cancer; may also result in benign lesions[65]
	Family history of medullary thyroid cancer	Inherited in an autosomal dominant pattern
	Family or personal history of pheochromocytoma or hyperparathyroidism with or without mucosal neuromata	Suggestive of multiple endocrine neoplasia syndromes II or III with medullary thyroid cancer
	Diarrhea	Common in medullary thyroid cancer
Physical examination	Solitary thyroid nodule	Cancers more frequently found in solitary nodules
	Multiple nodules with a predominant or rapidly enlarging nodule	In multiple nodules containing cancer, neoplasm is usually in predominant nodule
	Thyroid fixation to adjacent structure	May indicate cancer
	Enlarged cervical lymph nodes in young person	May be only presenting symptom of occult thyroid cancer[276]
	Goiter with unilateral vocal cord paralysis	Unusual except for anaplastic cancer
SPECIAL TESTS		
Fine-needle aspiration and biopsy	See text	See text
Catheterization		
IMAGING STUDIES		
X-ray	Psammomatous calcifications	Suggests thyroid nodule is malignant
Ultrasound	Differentiates solid from cystic nodules	Solid nodules more often malignant
Computed tomography	Extent of primary tumor, metastases	Assists in treatment planning, assesses extent of tumor and response to therapy
Magnetic resonance imaging	See text	See text
Radionuclide procedures		
^{99m}Tc or radioiodine imaging	Cold, warm, or hot nodule; single or multiple nodule	See text
^{201}Tl		
^{123}I or ^{131}I-MIBG		
Monoclonal antibodies		
Fluorescent imaging		
LABORATORY STUDIES		
Thyroglobulin	Postoperative value elevated	Indicates residual, recurrent, or metastatic differentiated thyroid cancer and correlates well with ^{131}I imaging detection of thyroid cancer[54,264]
	Preoperative value elevated	Cannot distinguish between tumor and differentiated thyroid cancer[264]
	Normal value	Supportive but not conclusive evidence of lack of disease
Calcitonin	Preoperative value elevated (basal or stimulated)	Indicates C-cell hyperplasia or medullary thyroid cancer (spontaneous or familial)[73]
	Postoperative value (basal or stimulated)	Indicates residual, recurrent, or metastatic medullary thyroid cancer (spontaneous or familial)
	Normal level postoperatively after stimulation	Indicates lack of disease

medullary thyroid cancer and its precursor C-cell hyperplasia and in managing postoperative patients, especially those with residual disease and metastases.[14,274] A raised calcitonin level may be seen with other neoplasms, chronic renal failure, pregnancy, and use of oral contraceptives.[188]

Medullary thyroid cancer may be recognized and treated early in its well-recognized familial syndromes.[14,188,274] A thorough discussion of the multiple endocrine neoplasia (MEN) syndromes, including radiologic evaluation, diagnosis of medullary thyroid cancer in families at risk, and screening for familial medullary thyroid cancer, can be found elsewhere.[14,15,53,59,194,274]

Imaging Studies

Standard Radiographs

The most common radiographic feature associated with thyroid nodules is intraglandular calcification, four types of which have been described: vascular calcifications, amorphous calcifications (usually large with irregular edges), plaque-like linear or curvilinear calcifications, and psammomatous calcifications that are multiple, small, and discrete and suggest a malignant tumor.[186] Psammomatous calcifications are detectable radiographically in 50% of histologic specimens of papillary carcinoma, but clinical radiographs reveal them in only 10% of patients with papillary carcinoma. The radiographic evaluation of medullary thyroid cancer is thoroughly reviewed in several publications.[53,59,194]

Radionuclide Thyroid Imaging

Indications for thyroid imaging in suspected or proven thyroid cancer are:

1. Anatomic and functional evaluation of a palpable thyroid nodule
2. Detection of occult or minimal cancer in high-risk patients
3. Detection of primary tumor in a patient with known regional or distant thyroidal metastases
4. Detection of regional or distant thyroid cancer metastases
5. Assessment of therapeutic effects

The four radiopharmaceuticals most commonly employed for radionuclide imaging of the thyroid are ^{131}I, ^{125}I, ^{123}I, and ^{99m}Tc (Table 65-3).[81] The use of ^{131}I for routine thyroid imaging has diminished because it delivers a substantial radiation dose to the thyroid; ^{123}I and ^{99m}Tc provide better physical characteristics for imaging and deliver much lower radiation doses to the thyroid. Unlike ^{123}I and the other radioiodine imaging agents that are trapped and then organified by the thyroid, ^{99m}Tc is trapped by the thyroid but does not undergo organification. Iodine 131 may be used, however, when a patient is being evaluated for mediastinal thyroid tissue, and it is preferred in the postoperative management of differentiated thyroid cancer when searching for residual functioning thyroid gland tissue and functioning residual, recurrent, or metastatic thyroid tumor.

The times of thyroid imaging for ^{99m}Tc and the radioiodines differ. Thyroid imaging with ^{99m}Tc may be done 20 to 30 minutes after radionuclide administration, but imaging with radioiodines is performed 6 to 24 hours after radionuclide administration.

Pertechnetate imaging has one major disadvantage compared with radioiodine imaging: some thyroid nodules have been found to be "hot" with ^{99m}Tc, but "cold" with radioiodine. Most of these lesions have been benign (*i.e.*, colloid nodules, follicular adenomas, or thyroiditis), although 10% to 15% were cancers. Therefore, nodules that are hot with ^{99m}Tc should be restudied with ^{123}I. The theoretic basis for the discordance is that, although the trapping mechanism in these lesions is intact, organification is disrupted.[67,147,211,215] Reverse discordance (*i.e.*, cold with ^{99m}Tc, activity with ^{123}I) has been reported.

There are three categories of thyroid nodules on thyroid imaging:

1. Cold: absence of radionuclide or radionuclide concentration markedly lower than in the rest of the thyroid
2. Warm: radionuclide concentration equal to or slightly higher than in the rest of the thyroid
3. Hot: radionuclide concentration markedly higher than in the rest of the thyroid

About 15% to 25% of single cold nodules are thyroid cancers (Fig. 65-2); the other 75% to 85% are usually adenomas or colloid cysts. Other, less common diagnoses include thyroiditis, infection (*e.g.*, as abscess), hemorrhage (*e.g.*, in adenomas), lymphoma, metastases, parathyroid adenoma, large lymph nodes, and laryngeal nerve schwannoma. Oblique views of the thyroid, in addition to the usual anterior view, are often of value in disclosing hidden cold nodules.

If multiple cold nodules are found on thyroid imaging, the chance of thyroid cancer markedly decreases. Less than 5% of thyroid glands with multiple nodules contain cancer, particularly in adults. The most likely diagnosis is multinodular goiter; thyroiditis often gives the same appearance. There are two exceptions: the incidence of thyroid cancer is higher in multinodular glands exposed to external irradiation than in nonexposed glands, and the incidence of multinodular goiters is so low in children that all cold nodules, whether solitary or multiple, should be suspected of malignancy.[186,193] The incidence of thyroid cancer is low with warm nodules and rare with hot nodules.[170] Recent evidence shows that some thyroid cancers, especially follicular tumors, are hot on ^{99m}Tc thyroid imaging, but cold on radioiodine imaging.[67,147,186,211,215]

Rarely, a patient with thyroid cancer presents with a palpable cervical node that accumulates radioiodine and a thyroid gland that appears normal on imaging. These lesions are usually metastatic well-differentiated follicular carcinomas. Most metastatic differentiated thyroid tumors do not accumulate radioiodine until all normal thyroid tissue has been ablated.

A recent study proposed several indications for ^{67}Ga imaging in patients with thyroid disease: suspected anaplastic thyroid carcinoma or malignant lymphoma of the thyroid, detection of distant metastasis of anaplastic thyroid cancer and malignant lymphoma, evaluation of therapeutic effect, suspected metastasis to the thyroid gland from other malignancies, and differentiation of malignant lymphoma from chronic thyroiditis. Strengths, limitations, and potential pitfalls of ^{67}Ga imaging of the thyroid are discussed elsewhere.[99]

[^{18}F]2-fluoro-2-deoxy-D-glucose (FDG) may be used in im-

TABLE 65–3
Radionuclides Used for Thyroid Imaging

RADIONUCLIDE	DOSE	PRINCIPAL IMAGING ENERGY (keV)	PHYSICAL HALF-LIFE	RADIATION DOSE (mGy/MBq) TOTAL BODY	THYROID
^{99m}Tc	185–370 MBq, iv	140	6.02 h	0.003–0.005	0.032–0.054
^{123}I	3.7–14.8 MBq, po	159	13.2 h	0.005–0.011	2.973–5.405
^{123}I-MIBG	370 MBq, iv	159	13.2 h	0.005	0.595
^{125}I	1.85–3.7 MBq, po	28, 35	60.7 d	0.004–0.011	10.81–21.62
^{131}I	1.11–1.85 MBq, po	364	8.06 d	0.135–1.081	297.3–432.4
^{131}I-MIBG	18.5 MBq, iv	364	8.06 d	0.027	9.459
^{201}Tl	37–111 MBq, iv	68–80	73 h	0.016–0.081	0.116–0.251

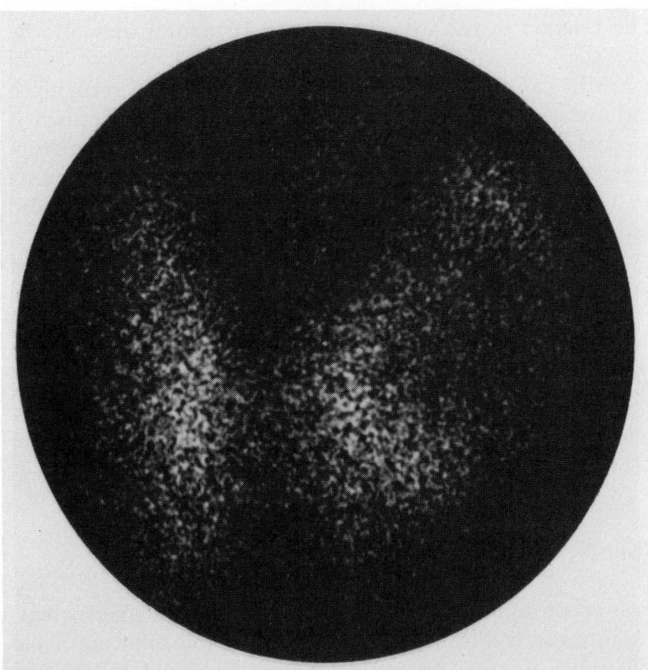

FIGURE 65–2. Iodine-123 anterior image of thyroid showing a large area of decreased uptake in the left lobe. The mass was differentiated thyroid cancer.

aging metastasis from advanced differentiated (papillary and follicular) thyroid carcinoma. FDG imaging may be useful in following patients with advanced thyroid carcinoma, because it may reveal metastases that did not accumulate ^{131}I. FDG scanning may be useful in confirming complete remission after treatment with ^{131}I.[113]

The chloride compound of ^{201}Tl has been used to evaluate cold nodules and patients with known thyroid cancer. Accumulation of thallium in a lesion that is cold on a ^{99m}Tc or radioiodine scan is a highly sensitive indicator for cancer, but it is not specific, because adenomas and thyroiditis also concentrate thallium.[67,242] Delayed thallium imaging seems to improve the specificity of this technique; most cancers retain thallium, but benign lesions tend to clear thallium quickly.[67,177]

We have developed a protocol for postoperative management of thyroid cancer. After surgery or ablative or therapeutic doses of ^{131}I, all patients with differentiated thyroid cancer are screened with a 5-mCi ^{131}I imaging procedure and with ^{201}Tl imaging.[104] When the outcome is negative, further follow-up consists of ^{201}Tl scintigraphy (yearly) and tumor marker assays (twice a year); ^{131}I scintigraphy is performed only after either test or any other clinical or radiologic information suggests metastasis to see if it is amenable to ^{131}I therapy. Another study concluded that thallium imaging alone cannot be recommended as the only modality for following patients with differentiated thyroid cancer, because its overall sensitivity in detecting tumor sites is relatively poor, even though its effectiveness is better for extraosseous lesions than ^{131}I imaging.[29] Imaging with ^{201}Tl may be helpful in localizing metastases, especially metastatic lymph nodes in patients with abnormal levels of serum thyroglobulin and those for whom results of ^{131}I scans are negative.

Technetium 99m (V)-dimercaptosuccinic acid (DMSA) has been shown to accumulate in the primary tumor in medullary thyroid cancer and its metastatic sites. These findings hold promise of a potentially useful imaging agent for the diagnosis and follow-up of this rare malignancy.[62,178,179] Medullary thyroid cancer, within the neck and at distant skeletal and extraosseous sites, has been shown to accumulate the ^{99m}Tc phosphates used for skeletal imaging; hepatic metastases may be detected with routine ^{99m}Tc-sulfur colloid liver imaging.[92,115]

[^{131}I]*m*-iodobenzylguanidine (^{131}I-MIBG) has been demonstrated to image medullary thyroid cancer, pheochromocytoma, and neuroblastoma.[63,217,240] This agent may prove to be useful in the treatment of medullary thyroid cancer.[216]

Radiolabeled monoclonal antibodies may soon be valuable in diagnosing thyroid cancer.[1,77,120,133,178,188,242] Used in association with SPECT imaging, monoclonal antibodies tagged with ^{131}I that react to CEA have been useful in gastrointestinal and medullary thyroid cancer.[189]

Fluorescent Thyroid Imaging

Fluorescent thyroid scanning compares the qualitative and quantitative distribution of stable iodine (^{127}I) that is normally present in a nodule with the thyroid gland. An iodine content ratio above 0.60 was found to be an excellent indicator of benign lesions, with a 63% sensitivity and 99% specificity.[183]

Ultrasonography

Ultrasonography is a valuable tool for evaluating thyroid nodules because it differentiates solid from cystic nodules. It is ideally performed with a high-resolution, high-frequency (7.5 MHz or 10 MHz) transducer.[46] If a cold nodule less than 4 cm in diameter on radionuclide thyroid imaging appears cystic on ultrasonography, there is a probability of less than 0.5% that the nodule is malignant. A nodule found to be solid on ultrasound scan has a 30% probability of being malignant.[219]

Often a 1-mm to 2-mm echolucent rim or "halo" is seen at the periphery of an adenoma, but this finding is occasionally seen in cases of malignant nodules with an echolucent halo.[46,192]

Thyroid cancers tend to be less echogenic than normal thyroid tissue and often show acoustic attenuation.[137] Most thyroid cancers are mixed papillary-follicular lesions and are seen as complex, predominantly solid masses on ultrasound scans.

Two recent studies have examined the use of ultrasound in the postoperative evaluation of thyroid cancer patients.[230,249] In one study, 10-MHz ultrasound was used to detect recurrent thyroid cancer in 73 patients with papillary, 16 with medullary, ten with follicular, and one with small cell cancer.[230] Of the 36 patients with normal sonograms, 35 had no other evidence of recurrence, and one had surgical proof of recurrence. Of 25 patients with abnormal ultrasound findings confirmed with surgery or ^{131}I imaging, palpation was negative in 17. Thirty-two patients with abnormal sonographic findings had no objective clinical proof of recurrence. The second study also used 10-MHz ultrasound. Ultrasound demonstrated cervical mass, lymphadenopathy, or both during postoperative follow-up of 52 patients who had undergone surgery for thyroid cancer.[249] Percutaneous biopsy with ultrasound guidance was performed in all 52 masses, 44 of which were nonpalpable. Ninety-four percent of biopsy results were assigned as either positive (56%) or negative (38%) for malignancy. Ultrasound-guided biopsy became an integral part of the evaluation for recurrent thyroid malignancy in postthyroidectomy patients.

Computed Tomography

High-resolution computed tomography (CT) provides an additional modality for thyroid cancer evaluation by defining the morphology of the thyroid gland, the anatomic extent of thyroid abnormalities in relation to the normal structures of the mediastinum and neck, and assisting in the radiologic detection of lung metastases and the assessment of therapy (Fig. 65-3).[121, 185, 228, 229, 239] As with cancers in other locations, CT is particularly valuable in radiation therapy treatment planning. The tumor volume and the isodose distribution can be accurately determined (Fig. 65-3).[112] Primary thyroid lymphoma may also be evaluated with CT.[252] Use of CT to assess MEN syndrome has been described.[53, 194]

Magnetic Resonance Imaging

Because magnetic resonance imaging (MRI) may not be able to differentiate benign from malignant tumors or determine functional status, it may have a limited role in the evaluation of patients with thyroid nodules or goiters.[174] MRI does have three indications: assessment of substernal goiters, depiction of the overall extent of the thyroid mass and involvement of muscles, and identification of sites of thyroid cancer recurrence.[10, 98]

As with CT, MRI is useful for showing the substernal extension of goiters; a coronal image provides a composite image of both the cervical and thoracic components of goiters. The relation of the mass to vascular structures may also be shown.

MRI can be used for identifying thyroid bed recurrence and involvement of regional lymph nodes. If skeletal muscle is used as a standard, thyroid bed scar produces a low-intensity signal on T2-weighted images, and recurrent cancer produces a medium- to high-intensity signal on T2 images. MRI can also define recurrence in cervical lymph nodes.

MRI has been used in the evaluation of primary thyroid lymphoma.[98]

Catheterization

Selective arterial and venous catheterization is very useful in locating sites of medullary thyroid cancer metastases.[14, 59]

Fine-Needle Aspiration Biopsy

Fine-needle aspiration biopsy, which has been receiving increasing interest, is a technique for obtaining follicular epithelial cells and minute tissue fragments for cytologic evalua-

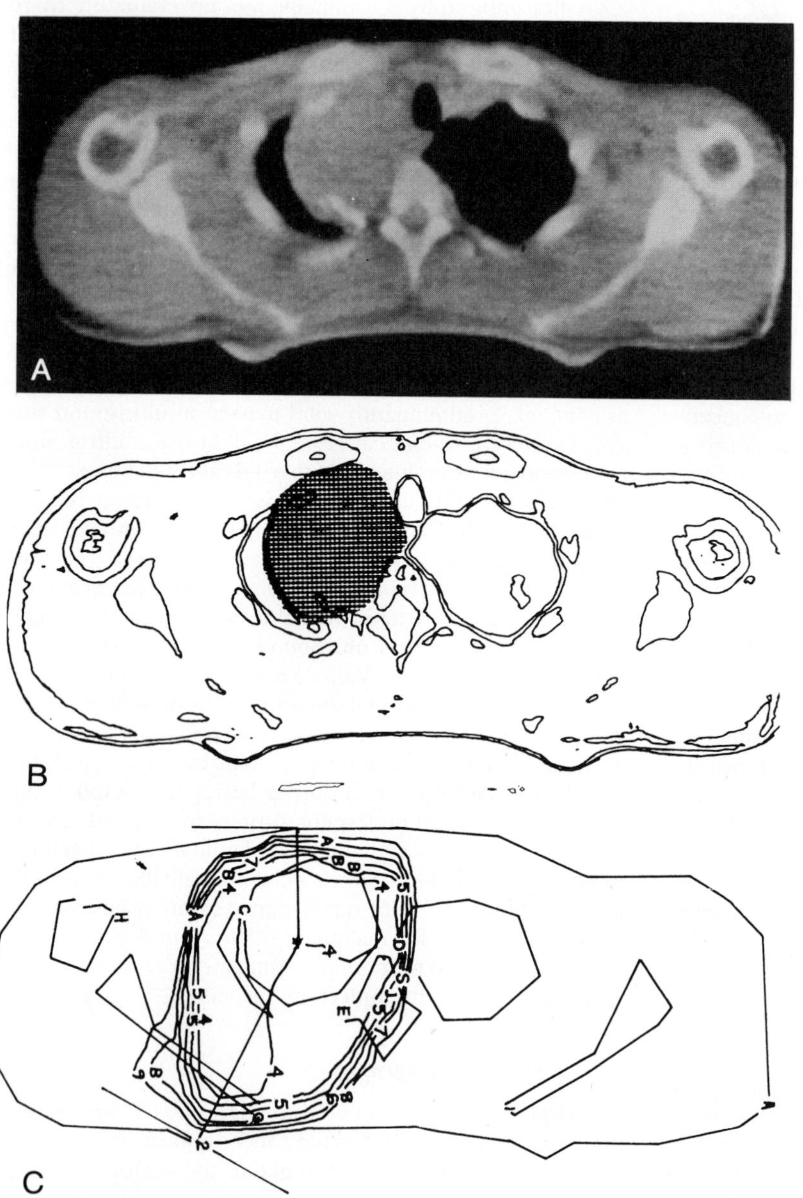

FIGURE 65–3. (**A**) Patient with superior mediastinal and left upper lobe lung metastases from thyroid cancer. (**B**) Contour plot with tumor involvement (*dotted area*). (**C**) Isodose distribution corrected for tissue inhomogeneities. (Jelden GL: CT scanning and computerized radiation therapy treatment planning. In Maruyama Y [ed]: New Methods of Tumor Localization, p 313. Lexington, University of Kentucky, 1977)

tion.[74,83,88,169,278] It is employed for thyroid nodules at least 1 cm in diameter and is occasionally used for smaller, superficially located nodules. The best results are obtained with nodules ranging in size from 1 cm to 3 cm. The technique is widely used to differentiate benign from malignant nodules and has a reported accuracy as high as 95%.[28,87,169,222,269]

This technique improved the presurgical evaluation of solitary nodules.[87] Sixty-four patients had been examined before the technique was introduced, and 147 patients were examined after its introduction. Overall management improved because the proportion of patients who underwent thyroid operation decreased from 67% to 43% and the yield of carcinoma increased from 14% to 29%; the cost of medical care per patient decreased 25%.

Cutting-needle biopsy using the Vim-Silverman or Tru-cut needles may be used to obtain larger tissue fragments for routine histologic examination. The technique should be employed cautiously, if at all, for thoracic inlet nodules because large vessels at the inlet present a risk of acute airway obstruction from bleeding. Generally, cutting-needle biopsy is applied to nodules at least 2 cm in diameter and preferably larger.

STAGING

Because the histologic diagnosis and patient age are important in determining the behavior and prognosis of thyroid cancer, these factors have to be accounted for in the staging system (Table 65-4).

Since publication of the 1983 edition of *Manual for Staging of Cancer,* the following changes have been made in the staging of thyroid cancers: 4 cm is now the dividing measurement between definitions of T2 and T3, and age division is no longer used for medullary and undifferentiated cancers, although an age split at 45 years is used for papillary and follicular cancers.

Pathologic staging of thyroid cancer tumors should be based on the World Health Organization International Classification of Diseases for Oncology[277]; this publication is identical in the morphologic classification of neoplasms with the Systematized Nomenclature of Medicine (SNOMED) published by the College of the American Pathologists in 1976.

PATHOLOGIC CLASSIFICATION

Malignant thyroid neoplasms have been designated as four main types: papillary and mixed papillary-follicular, follicular, medullary, and anaplastic.

Rare tumors, comprising fewer than 5% of malignant tumors of the thyroid, are lymphoma, plasmacytoma, squamous cell and mucin-producing carcinoma, teratoma, sarcoma, carcinosarcoma, hemangioendothelioma, metastatic carcinoma to the thyroid, and thyroid cancer at unusual sites, including median aberrant thyroid, lateral aberrant thyroid, and struma ovarii.

The pathologic characteristics, prognostic factors, and management of the four main types are discussed below and elsewhere.[67,140,152,275] For a thorough discussion of the rare

TABLE 65–4
Staging Categories for Papillary, Follicular, Medullary, and Undifferentiated Thyroid Cancer

PRIMARY TUMOR (T)

All categories may be subdivided: (a) solitary; (b) multifocal—measure the largest for classification

TX	Primary tumor cannot be assessed
T0	No evidence of primary tumor
T1	Tumor ≤1 cm in greatest dimension, limited to the thyroid
T2	Tumor >1 cm but <4 cm
T3	Tumor >4 cm in greatest dimension, limited to the thyroid
T4	Tumor of any size extending beyond the thyroid capsule

LYMPH NODES (N)

Regional nodes are the cervical and upper mediastinal lymph nodes

NX	Regional lymph nodes cannot be assessed
N0	No regional lymph node metastasis
N1	Regional lymph node metastasis
N1a	Metastasis in ipsilateral cervical lymph nodes
N1b	Metastases in bilateral, midline, or contralateral cervical or mediastinal lymph nodes

DISTANT METASTASES (M)

MX	Presence of distant metastasis cannot be assessed
M0	No distant metastasis
M1	Distant metastasis

Specify

NODAL INVOLVEMENT

Cervical unilateral ________
Cervical bilateral ________
Delphian ________
Mediastinal ________
Indicate on diagram primary tumor and regional nodes involved.

HISTOPATHOLOGIC GRADE (G)

GX	Grade cannot be assessed
G1	Well differentiated
G2	Moderately well differentiated
G3	Poorly differentiated

STAGE GROUPING

Separate stage groupings are recommended for papillary and follicular, medullary, and undifferentiated

Papillary or Follicular
(Patient under 45 years)

Stage I	Any T, Any N, M0
Stage II	Any T, Any N, M1

(45 years and over)

Stage I	T1, N0, M0
Stage II	T2, N0, M0
	T3, N0, M0
Stage III	T4, N0, M0
	Any T, N1, M0
Stage IV	Any T, Any N, M1

Medullary

Stage I	T1, N0, M0
Stage II	T2, N0, M0
	T3, N0, M0
	T4, N0, M0
Stage III	Any T, N1, M0
Stage IV	Any T, Any N, M1

Undifferentiated
All cases are Stage IV

Stage IV	Any T, Any N, Any M

(Beahrs OH, Henson DE, Hutter RVP, Myers MH [eds]: Manual for Staging of Cancer, 3rd ed. Philadelphia, JB Lippincott, 1988)

tumors including tumors metastatic to the thyroid, the reader is referred to the literature.[6,27,43,55,75,76,100,105,110,116,121,127,139,140,145,146,155,159,162,163,166,176,196,210,224,226,237,251,252,257,267]

Differentiated Thyroid Cancer

Differentiated thyroid cancer consists of papillary, mixed papillary-follicular, and follicular adenocarcinoma. These tumors arise from the thyroid follicular cells (*i.e.*, endodermal origin) and can be treated with ^{131}I and thyroid hormone suppression.

Papillary and Mixed Papillary-Follicular Cancers

Despite the differences in their histologic patterns, papillary and mixed papillary-follicular cancers are considered to represent a spectrum of neoplasms because they show biologic and clinicopathologic similarities. These neoplasms, the most common type of thyroid cancer, are usually slowly growing and indolent, with an excellent prognosis. They are multifocal in as many as 75% of patients, contain papillary structures, and may have a large follicular component, with psammoma bodies. These tumors are usually infiltrative and metastasize to regional lymph nodes through lymphatic channels; hematogenous metastases are uncommon.

Papillary cancer, including mixed papillary-follicular cancer, comprises 33% to 73% of malignant thyroid lesions. More than 90% of thyroid neoplasms found incidentally at autopsy are papillary cancers. This histologic type is the one most frequently encountered in thyroid glands previously exposed to radiation.[140,261,275] It is two to four times more common in females than in males and occurs mostly in the third to the fifth decades, although it may occur at any age. Papillary cancer accounts for 80% of thyroid cancers in the prepubertal age group.

Follicular Cancers

Follicular cancers are unifocal, have a marked tendency to invade vascular channels, and metastasize hematogenously to distant sites. Lymph node metastases are uncommon. These cancers lack papillae, psammoma bodies, and ground glass nuclei. They have the strongest propensity to concentrate ^{131}I.

Hürthle cell and primary clear cell carcinoma are classified as variants of follicular carcinoma.

Follicular cancer comprises 14% to 33% of primary thyroid cancers and affects females two to three times as frequently as men. The average age at diagnosis ranges from 50 to 58 years; it is rarely seen in children.[140,275]

Medullary Thyroid Cancer

Medullary thyroid cancer is derived from parafollicular or C cells that arise from the neuroectoderm. It comprises 5% to 10% of all thyroid cancers. Approximately 80% of cases arise spontaneously, without apparent evidence of familial disease. The other 20% occur within familial multiple endocrine neoplasia syndromes (*i.e.*, MEN IIa or MEN IIb or III).

Medullary thyroid cancer in the spontaneous or familial forms has no gender predilection. An equal gender incidence would be expected in the familial types of the disease because autosomal dominant inheritance has been proven. The spontaneous form of the tumor tends to occur more often from the fifth decade on; with the familial form, initial disease has been detected in patients younger than 10 years and in patients 80 years old.[14,15,140,274]

The characteristics of medullary thyroid cancer include nonfollicular cell derivation (APUDoma), stromal amyloid, and the tumor marker calcitonin. C-cell hyperplasia is considered to be the premalignant lesion. Medullary thyroid cancer is bilateral in all familial cases. Its clinical behavior varies from rapidly fatal to slowly growing. Regional spread usually precedes distant metastases and is seen in as many as 50% of the patients at diagnosis. Metastases, disseminated by blood and lymphatic routes, involve mainly cervical lymph nodes (58% to 70%), lung, liver, and bone. The survival rate at 5 years for medullary thyroid cancer without lymph nodes involvement is 90%, and at 10 years, it is 85%; if lymph nodes are involved, survival at 5 years is 70% and 42% at 10 years.[140,188,209]

Although medullary thyroid cancer itself does not concentrate ^{131}I, residual tumor in remaining thyroid gland tissue after surgery may be treatable with radioiodine because of iodine accumulation in follicular cells immediately adjacent to the medullary cancer cells; metastases may be treatable with ^{131}I-tagged monoclonal antibodies.[14,95,189,212]

Medullary thyroid cancer has a worse prognosis than papillary cancer, mixed papillary-follicular cancer, and possibly follicular cancer, but it carries a much better prognosis than anaplastic cancer.

Anaplastic Cancer

Anaplastic cancer originates from the follicular cells of the thyroid; the disease features three histologic types: small cell, spindle cell, giant cell. Tumors of this kind grow rapidly. Local invasion of structures, such as the trachea, is followed by or concurrent with distant metastases, and death usually occurs within 12 months of diagnosis.

Anaplastic cancer comprises about 10% of all malignant lesions of the thyroid. Patients range in age from 40 to 90 years, and women outnumber men four to one. There is a history of goiter in 80% of these patients. It has been hypothesized that there is a transformation from a benign or low-grade malignant lesion to a highly malignant one.[102,140]

Radiation-Induced Thyroid Cancer

The pathology of thyroid cancers in irradiated thyroids resembles that of spontaneous thyroid cancers; the well-differentiated papillary, follicular, and mixed papillary-follicular cancers predominate.[97] The incidence of radiation-induced and spontaneous medullary and anaplastic thyroid cancers appears to be the same.[97]

Even though radiation-induced thyroid cancers have a well-differentiated appearance and respond well to treatment, they have a tendency to invade locally and recur. Between one half and one third of patients had regional lymph node metastases when first operated on.[65,181] Distant metastases, usually to the lungs, existed in approximately 10% of patients at the time of initial surgery.[98,181]

PROGNOSTIC FACTORS

Differentiated Thyroid Cancer

The most significant prognostic factors for papillary, mixed papillary-follicular, and follicular cancers are histologic pattern, extent of local involvement, and patient age at diagnosis.

Histology and Invasiveness

There are three types of papillary cancers.[140,275] Occult sclerosing lesions, which comprise 12% to 28% of papillary cancers, are up to 1.5 cm in diameter, confined to the thyroid, usually not palpable, and discovered incidentally during thyroid exploration after presentation with cervical lymph node metastases. Intrathyroidal lesions, which comprise 34% to 78% of papillary cancers, are apparent preoperatively, are larger than occult lesions, and are confined to the thyroid. Extrathyroidal lesions, which comprise 2% to 39% of papillary lesions, extend beyond the thyroid capsule to adjacent structures.

In the Mayo Clinic series, no patient with occult cancer died of the disease during follow-up averaging 15 years and extending up to 40 years. Within the intrathyroidal group, only 2.5% of the patients died during a follow-up period averaging 11 years and extending up to 26 years. However, 38% of patients with extrathyroidal tumors died.[276] The extent of capsular involvement was found to be an important prognostic factor in pure follicular cancers.[276] Only 3% of patients with no or minimal capsular invasion died. Among the patients with moderate to marked capsular invasion, one third presented initially with metastases, and 50% were dead of the cancer after a mean survival of 6 years. Mazzaferri and associates[152] discovered similar prognostic correlations.

Young and co-workers[280] reviewed the effect of therapy in 214 patients with follicular thyroid cancer. Their study indicated that patients likely to die of this cancer have distant metastases at the time of initial presentation. If disease is confined to the neck at presentation, the overall prognosis is good, but it can be altered with the type of medical therapy. Both ^{131}I therapy and thyroid hormone therapy decreased the recurrence rate.

Among those presenting with disease confined to the neck, the recurrence rate if thyroid nodules were less than 1.5 cm was 10%, and with nodules greater than 1.5 cm, the recurrence rate was 8%. Neither lymph node involvement nor the extent of lymph node surgery affected recurrence rate. The recurrence rate was 7% if lymph nodes were involved but 11% if they were not. The duration of follow-up was not sufficient to allow conclusions about improved survival in patients with little or moderate invasion of the vasculature or thyroid nodule capsule.[280]

Age

The Mayo series showed age to be an important prognostic factor. Only 3% of patients younger than 40 years old with papillary disease (*i.e.*, occult, intrathyroidal, or extrathyroidal) died of the cancer, but 13% of older patients died of their disease. With follicular cancer, the age association was less certain, because most patients were over 40 years old at presentation.[276]

Mazzaferri and associates[152] reported that papillary cancer patients younger than 30 years of age had a higher recurrence rate than patients 30 years or older; patients 40 years of age or older had a higher mortality rate than patients younger than 40 years.

In their study of differentiated thyroid cancer, Cady and associates[34] found that the overall recurrence risk was 10% and death risk was 3% among women younger than 50 years old; among patients with recurrent disease or metastases, only 30% died of disease. For women over 50 years of age, the respective figures are 32%, 30%, and 89%.

Lymph Node Involvement

The Mayo series revealed that the extent of cervical nodal disease at the time of the initial operation had no adverse effect on survival.[276] In a Lahey Clinic series, survival was higher among patients with a greater number of involved lymph nodes in all histologically comparable groups.[35]

Medullary Thyroid Cancer

Medullary thyroid cancer has the potential for local and distant virulence in some patients but may act benignly in others. There are no firm predictive parameters.

Anaplastic Thyroid Cancer

The prognostic factors for anaplastic thyroid cancer are the consequences of the dramatic clinical characteristics of the disease, which include presentation as a large, firm, bulky mass severely distorting the normal neck contour, frequent obstruction of the larynx, trachea, and esophagus by direct tumor extension, and poor response to any treatment modality. Although cervical lymph nodes are usually involved with tumor, they may be difficult to detect because of the extent of the primary tumor. Because the size of the tumor may make tracheostomy difficult or impossible, some degree of thyroidectomy may be required to establish an airway. Anaplastic cancer and other thyroid cancers can lead to superior vena cava obstruction. Most patients may also have metastases outside the neck at the time of diagnosis.

GENERAL MANAGEMENT

The treatment of spontaneous and radiation-induced thyroid cancers is the same. The treatment modalities include surgery, thyroid hormone therapy, ^{131}I therapy, external irradiation, interstitial irradiation, and chemotherapy. The treatment of radiation-induced thyroid cancers has been thoroughly reviewed.[52,262] The management of pediatric thyroid cancer has also been described.[43,44,96,146,257]

Differentiated Thyroid Cancer

Figure 65-4 is a flow diagram that offers a guide to the postoperative management and follow-up of patients with differentiated thyroid cancer; variations may occur in different medical centers.[80]

Surgery

The recommended initial therapy for differentiated thyroid cancer is near-total or total thyroidectomy. The exceptions are occult differentiated cancers and completely excised pure papillary cancers.[80] A near-total or total thyroidectomy is necessary if additional management with ^{131}I is being considered.

Radical neck dissection has been abandoned in favor of the modified radical neck dissection for metastatic adenopathy. Limited dissections of metastatic adenopathy in the cervical, jugular, paratracheal, and upper mediastinal lymph nodes are performed with increasing frequency. Prophylactic node dissection is no longer used.

Mazzaferri and co-workers[152] showed that the extent of cervical lymph node surgery, ranging from radical neck to limited nodal dissection, did not affect recurrence or survival in patients with papillary thyroid cancer. Patients with metastatic

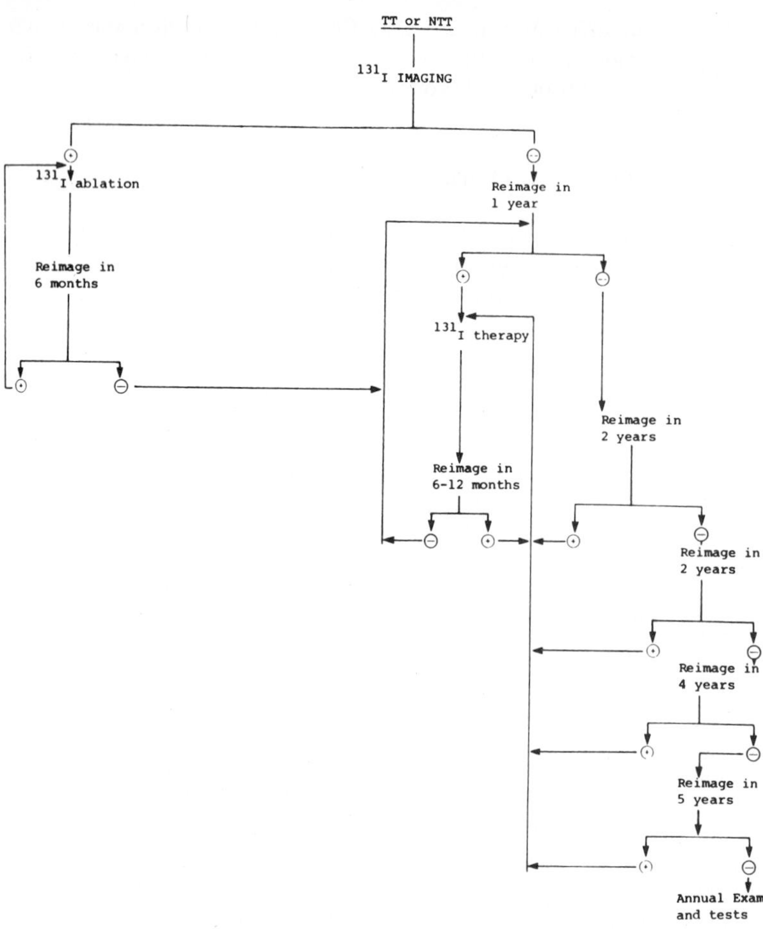

FIGURE 65–4. Flow diagram for the postoperative management and follow-up of differentiated thyroid cancer.

cervical adenopathy had the same rates of recurrence regardless of the extent of surgery.[152,280]

After total thyroidectomy for papillary cancer, the recurrence rate was 7.1%, and the death rate was 0.3%; with subtotal thyroidectomy, the recurrence and death rates were 18.4% and 1.5%, respectively. If only medical treatment (*i.e.,* ^{131}I and thyroid hormone suppression) was given after total thyroidectomy, the recurrence rate was 2.6%, and the death rate was 0%. The use of thyroid hormone only also resulted in a 0% mortality rate, but the recurrence rate was 10%. Without ^{131}I and thyroid hormone therapy, the recurrence rate was 40%, and the death rate 13.3%.[152]

Young and co-workers,[280] in a study of 214 patients with follicular thyroid carcinoma, found that the overall recurrence rate was not affected by positive cervical nodes or the extent of thyroid surgery. An increase in the recurrence rate was associated with extensive histologic invasion of the nodule capsule and thyroid. The postoperative recurrence rate was decreased by radioiodine and by thyroid hormone therapy. At 4 years, the recurrence rate was about 4% with thyroid hormone use only, 6% with ^{131}I and thyroid hormone together, and 22% without ^{131}I and thyroid hormone. But at 10 years, the recurrence rate was slightly greater than 10% with only thyroid hormone, 6% with both ^{131}I and thyroid hormone, and 33% without any medical therapy. The only deaths in their study attributable to thyroid cancer occurred in patients who presented with distant metastases.[280]

The death rates for differentiated thyroid cancer in hundreds of patients have been compared by Beierwaltes.[19] From 1935 to 1955, when less aggressive surgery was done, and there was less use of ^{131}I, the death rate was 12.5% for papillary cancer and 11.7% for follicular cancer. Between 1957 and 1972, with more adequate surgery and more routine use of ^{131}I, the death rates for papillary and follicular cancer were 2.4% and 3.1%, respectively.

Iodine 131

Radioactive iodine is used to treat some papillary, mixed papillary-follicular, and follicular cancers. Hürthle cell cancer, a variant of follicular cancer, may respond to ^{131}I therapy. (See Appendix I at the end of the chapter for procedures for administration of ^{131}I.)

The indications for ^{131}I therapy in thyroid cancer are inoperable primary tumor, thyroid capsule invasion, thyroid ablation, postoperative residual disease in the neck, recurrent disease, cervical or mediastinal nodal metastases, and distant metastases.[68]

Iodine 131 delivers a high radiation dose to normal thyroid and thyroid cancer cells. One estimate is 10 cGy per μCi of ^{131}I per gram of thyroid cancer tissue. Another estimate considering a biologic half-life for ^{131}I of 4 days and a 0.1% uptake of the ^{131}I therapy dose per gram of tumor or tissue is 15000 cGy/mCi.[19,67,109]

Thyroid tissue remaining in the thyroid bed after thyroidectomy should be ablated with ^{131}I.[67] The ablation dose, administered within 2 months after the thyroidectomy, may vary from 50 mCi to 100 mCi; more than one dose may be required. Because normal thyroid has a much greater affinity for iodine, including ^{131}I, than differentiated thyroid cancer, demonstration of metastatic disease with ^{131}I total body imaging is enhanced after ablation. With subtotal thyroidectomy and no

^{131}I ablation, metastatic disease is revealed by ^{131}I imaging in a very small percentage of patients. Other reasons for thyroid ablation include the multifocality of differentiated tumors, the high frequency of contralateral lobe disease, and the possibility of a residual site of differentiated thyroid tumor transforming to anaplastic cancer.[67,80,119]

Thyroid ablation with ^{131}I given after near-total or total thyroidectomy prepares the patient for more definitive therapy by elevating thyroid-stimulating hormone (TSH) levels enough to expose cancerous tissue to TSH, thus facilitating ^{131}I uptake into metastases for localization and therapy and removing normal thyroid tissue to eliminate extraneous thyroglobulin sources. Thyroid ablation decreases the recurrence and mortality rates of differentiated thyroid cancer.[109]

The question of appropriate doses of ^{131}I for the ablation of thyroid remnants remains controversial.[18–20,51,130,139,187,195,225,256,257,267] Some investigators advocate the use of 30 mCi or less of ^{131}I in an attempt to decrease the morbidity and hospitalization associated with large radioiodine doses.[18,51,130,195,225] Studies indicate that the higher the initial dose of ^{131}I, the more successful the ablation, and the less need for repeat administration of lower doses of ^{131}I.[20,51,195] Beierwaltes and colleagues[19,20] recommend a dose of not less than 100 mCi for residual ^{131}I uptake in the thyroid bed. They also suggest that an ablation dose of 100 mCi to 149 mCi constitutes adjuvant therapy for occult metastases not detected by ^{131}I scanning (1–5 mCi), especially when pretreatment uptake of ^{131}I is low (<4%).

Although no studies have confirmed whether low or high ablation doses are preferable, lower death and recurrence rates have been seen in patients in whom all traces of residual ^{131}I uptake are ablated.[20,67,165,270] The use of 100 to 149 mCi ^{131}I as an empiric ablation dose is attractive given its apparent success in eliminating residual ^{131}I uptake after a single dose.[20,67] Other investigators recommend that the amount of ^{131}I for adequate ablation should be determined by the individual patient's clearance of a tracer dose of radioiodine.[17,18,109,255] If necessary, another dose of 75 mCi to 100 mCi of ^{131}I may be administered 6 months later after the initial dose.

Iodine 131 may also be used to treat recurrent differentiated thyroid carcinoma, postoperative residual disease in the neck or elsewhere, nodal metastases in cervical, mediastinal, hilar, or other sites, distant metastases in lungs, liver, brain, bone, or other locations, and inoperable primary tumors (Fig. 65-5). The dose per treatment should be 150 mCi to 200 mCi of ^{131}I, depending on the clinical situation.[67,80] Individual doses less than 150 mCi are considered inadequate. The recommended maximum total dose (*i.e.*, ablation and therapy) of ^{131}I is 1000 mCi, although a few patients have received 2000 mCi to 3000 mCi.[80,114]

Iodine 131 therapy may be combined with external and interstitial radiation therapy.[80,250] The dose to metastases from ^{131}I may be calculated using SPECT imaging. The SPECT dose estimates correlate with the clinical course of disease and may provide prognostic information.[129,189,255]

In patients with unresectable or inoperable primary tumors, ^{131}I does not seem to appreciably affect the rate of tumor regression or prolong survival. A combination of ^{131}I and external radiation therapy seems to offer the best results.[257]

Beierwaltes and associates[21] established a threefold increase in survival time in patients whose metastases were eliminated by ^{131}I. Nemec and colleagues[173] showed that survival duration was significantly greater in patients treated with ^{131}I and that prognosis was adversely affected by bone metastases. In another study with ^{131}I, no patient with bone metastases was alive 10 years after treatment, and 11 (54%) of 20 patients with lung metastases were alive and free of disease 10 years after their initial therapy.[30]

The reasons for failure of ^{131}I therapy can be summarized as follows:

1. Inadequate pretherapy surgery
2. Patient off thyroid medication for insufficient time
3. Inadequate detection of ^{131}I uptake in areas to be treated immediately before therapy
4. Single therapeutic dose of ^{131}I of less than 150 mCi

Total-body imaging is done 5 to 10 days after an ^{131}I ablation or therapy dose. No additional ^{131}I is given, and no preparation of the patient is performed. This imaging is performed because an ablative or therapeutic dose of ^{131}I may reveal addi-

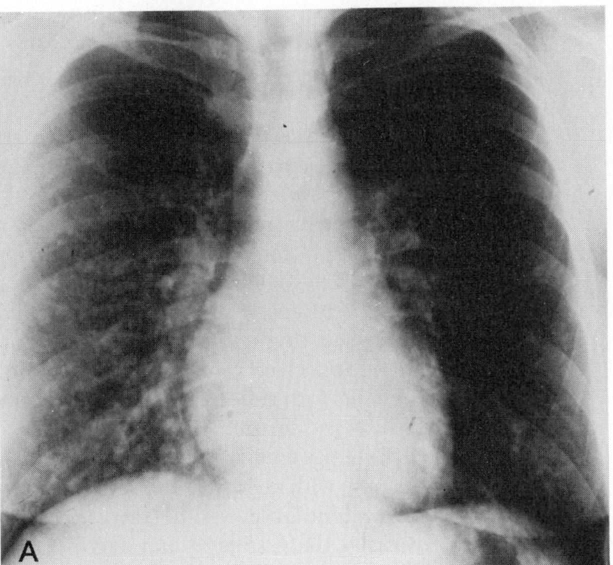

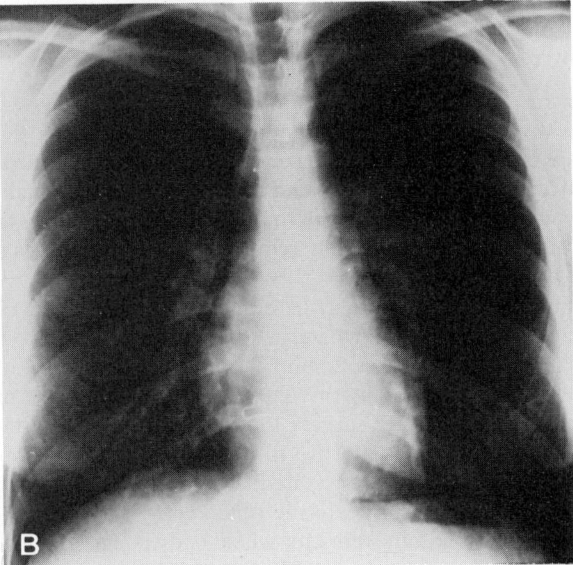

FIGURE 65–5. (**A**) Posteroanterior chest radiograph of a patient with diffuse nodular bilateral pulmonary metastases from cancer of the thyroid. (**B**) Posteroanterior radiograph of the same chest 1 year after administration of 150 mCi of ^{131}I. The pulmonary metastases have completely disappeared.

tional lesions not detected with the lower scanning dose of ^{131}I used before ablation or therapy. Studies have confirmed this rationale.[11,67,173]

Thyroid Hormone

Thyroid hormone suppression therapy is effective in the management of differentiated thyroid cancer.[67,80] All patients, regardless of the surgical procedure and between ^{131}I treatments, should be maintained on suppressive doses of long-acting thyroid medication, preferably L-thyroxine rather than desiccated thyroid, except for the patient who will not tolerate L-thyroxine.

Because differentiated thyroid cancer grows under the stimulation of TSH, the goal of suppressive thyroid medication is to achieve a TSH level that is as low as possible. Periodic thyroid hormone measurements should be obtained to assess the degree of TSH suppression to avoid inducing iatrogenic hyperthyroidism.[13,109] Currently, the thyrotropin-releasing hormone (TRH) stimulation test is considered the best means of assessing the adequacy of TSH suppression; if there is no TSH response to TRH, serum TSH levels are undetectably low.[109,241]

Suppressive thyroid medication decreases the recurrence and mortality rates associated with differentiated thyroid cancer, particularly in patients with a large tumor burden, in whom the initial ^{131}I therapy may not be totally successful in eradicating all sites of thyroid cancer metastases and who might require subsequent ^{131}I treatment or other therapy.

The effect of withdrawal of suppressive thyroid hormone therapy on serum biochemical and blood profiles was studied in athyreotic thyroid cancer patients; these patients were withdrawn from suppressive thyroid hormonal therapy of 200 μg L-thyroxine per day.[271] After 14 days off L-thyroxine therapy, nine of the ten patients studied were still clinically and biochemically euthyroid. After another 14 days without thyroid hormones, severe clinical and biochemical hypothyroidism resulted. At 28 days, certain biochemical parameters changed significantly: creatine phosphokinase activity increased (above normal in half the patients), and activities of serum glutamic-oxaloacetic transaminase, serum glutamic-pyruvic transaminase, and lactic acid dehydrogenase (means and standard deviations within the respective normal ranges).

Thyroid-Stimulating Hormone

Serum TSH has the greatest influence on ^{131}I uptake by normal thyroid cells and differentiated thyroid cancers; the latter are derived from follicular cells and have TSH receptors. The differentiated cancers respond to TSH in a fashion qualitatively similar to normal thyroid. In most, however, exposure to high concentrations of TSH is required to induce maximal uptake of ^{131}I.[109]

Although TSH levels may be elevated within 2 weeks of total or near-total thyroidectomy, it is preferable to wait 6 to 8 weeks after surgery before administering ^{131}I for ablation of residual normal functioning thyroid tissue or the treatment of thyroid cancer (*e.g.*, after surgery for recurrences or metastases). Ablation may be ineffective if attempted too soon after surgery, perhaps because of elevated levels of serum inorganic iodine or poor blood supply to the remnant.[135]

Before ^{131}I is administered for whole-body imaging, initial ablation dose (if the patient was placed on thyroid medication after surgery), repeat ablation dose, or ^{131}I therapy, thyroid hormone or L-thyroxine must be discontinued 4 to 6 weeks to allow the blood level of thyroid hormone to decrease and the TSH level to rise, enabling maximal stimulation of ^{131}I uptake. Alternatively, to shorten the period of symptomatic hypothyroidism, long-acting medications are discontinued and T_3 (*e.g.*, Cytomel) is administered for 3 weeks and then withdrawn 2 weeks before imaging or therapy. A TSH level of 50 μIU/ml or greater is preferred before ^{131}I whole-body imaging, ^{131}I ablation, or therapy is begun. Occasionally, older patients have TSH levels that rise to 30 to 50 μIU/ml, which is considered satisfactory because of their age.[84] Therapy can usually be instituted if ^{131}I uptake is adequate for imaging thyroid metastases.[67] However, if the TSH level is greater than 50 μIU/ml and there is no obvious ^{131}I uptake, radioiodine therapy may be inappropriate, because there may be insufficient uptake for destruction of malignant tissues.[67]

Twenty-four to 72 hours after an ^{131}I ablation or therapy dose has been administered, the patient is gradually administered suppressive thyroid medication. TSH and thyroid function levels are monitored and maintained as described elsewhere in this chapter.[67,80]

Low-iodine diets and diuretic therapy to waste iodine, which are advocated by some investigators, may enhance ^{131}I radioiodine uptake by normal thyroid tissue remnants and thyroid cancer metastases.[67,72,86,109,132,148,191] The increased uptake may be caused by prolonged ^{131}I retention. This prolonged retention also results in an increased whole-body and blood radiation dose; iodine depletion techniques should therefore be used with caution.

Lithium inhibits thyroid hormone release without affecting iodine transport. These characteristics might be used to increase the ^{131}I dose retained by residual thyroid tissue or differentiated thyroid cancer metastases. Prospective protocols are needed to determine if lithium has an adjuvant therapeutic role with ^{131}I in the treatment of differentiated thyroid cancer.[33,68,80,161,199]

Thyroglobulin

Thyroglobulin is produced only by the thyroid gland. Serum thyroglobulin levels are elevated in most patients with differentiated thyroid cancer before surgery, in most patients with follicular adenoma, and in some patients with other benign thyroid diseases. An elevated thyroglobulin level, therefore, cannot differentiate benign from malignant lesions preoperatively; very high levels of thyroglobulin suggest metastatic thyroid cancer.[80,109,264] Athyreotic patients should not have circulating thyroglobulin.

In patients with differentiated thyroid cancer after total thyroidectomy, the presence of serum thyroglobulin should indicate recurrent or residual thyroid neoplasm.[109,264] Many studies have compared serum thyroglobulin levels and ^{131}I whole-body imaging for detecting recurrent disease.[26,39,45,61,136,207] Thyroglobulin levels may be assessed whether the patient is receiving suppressive thyroid hormones or not. Nonsuppressed thyroglobulin values are not significantly greater than suppressed values in patients without residual disease. In patients with residual neoplasm, nonsuppressed values usually rise as the serum TSH level rises.

In 80% to 85% of patients, the thyroglobulin levels and ^{131}I imaging results agree, with abnormal ^{131}I scans seen in patients with elevated thyroglobulin levels; the reverse also holds. In 15% to 20% of cases, the results do not agree. Elevated thyroglobulin levels with normal ^{131}I scan results are believed to reflect greater sensitivity of the serum thyroglobulin for occult disease that is not detectable with imaging.[9,24,26,136,218] Normal serum thyroglobulin levels in conjunction with an abnormal ^{131}I scan occur in 1.5% of patients and probably reflect some decrease in tumor function or tumor differentiation.

Patients with bone and lung metastases tend to have the highest thyroglobulin levels, and those with lymph node metastases have the lowest.[109,218]

Serum thyroglobulin assay is useful for most patients with differentiated cancer who have had a total thyroidectomy by surgery alone or surgery with ^{131}I ablation. The value of thyroglobulin assays for patients with residual normal thyroid tissue is limited. Serial thyroglobulin levels should be obtained in all patients after total thyroidectomy to assist in their follow-up; these levels can be measured while the patient is receiving full suppressive thyroid medication. The serum thyroglobulin assay will eventually eliminate the necessity for follow-up ^{131}I whole-body imaging in some thyroid cancer patients, but the appropriate group has not yet been defined.[67]

Medullary and anaplastic cancers do not secrete thyroglobulin; therefore serum thyroglobulin levels cannot be used to follow the clinical status of these patients.[61]

Medullary Thyroid Cancer

Optimal management of medullary thyroid cancer involves early removal of the tumor, especially because localized medullary thyroid cancer has the capacity to metastasize early, whether or not the patient develops a virulent form of the disease.[14] A schema for the evaluation and management of patients with medullary thyroid cancer is presented in Figure 65-6.

The surgical management and postoperative follow-up of patients with spontaneous or familial medullary thyroid cancer are similar. The operative procedure of choice is total thyroidectomy, especially because all patients with the hereditary form of medullary thyroid cancer have bilateral involvement of the thyroid; even if tumor is seen only on microscopic examination (*i.e.,* C-cell hyperplasia or microinvasive medullary thyroid cancer), the disease is usually multifocal. Because clinically occult medullary thyroid cancer that is grossly visible on cut section of the thyroid may have regional lymph node metastases, all lymph nodes in the central zone of the neck, from the hyoid bone to the sternal notch and laterally to the jugular veins, are resected. In patients with macroscopic lymph node involvement, a modified radical neck dissection is performed. More extensive local surgery has not been shown to be more efficacious.[14,15]

Before a thyroidectomy is performed for familial or sporadic medullary thyroid cancer, the presence of a pheochromocytoma must be excluded; if an unsuspected adrenal tumor is present, general anesthesia may induce a hypertensive crisis and death. If a pheochromocytoma is detected, proper management with α-blockade is needed until the patient's symptoms and signs revert to normal. An abdominal exploration is then done, with both adrenal glands visualized because the incidence of bilateral pheochromocytomas in MEN IIa or MEN IIb ap-

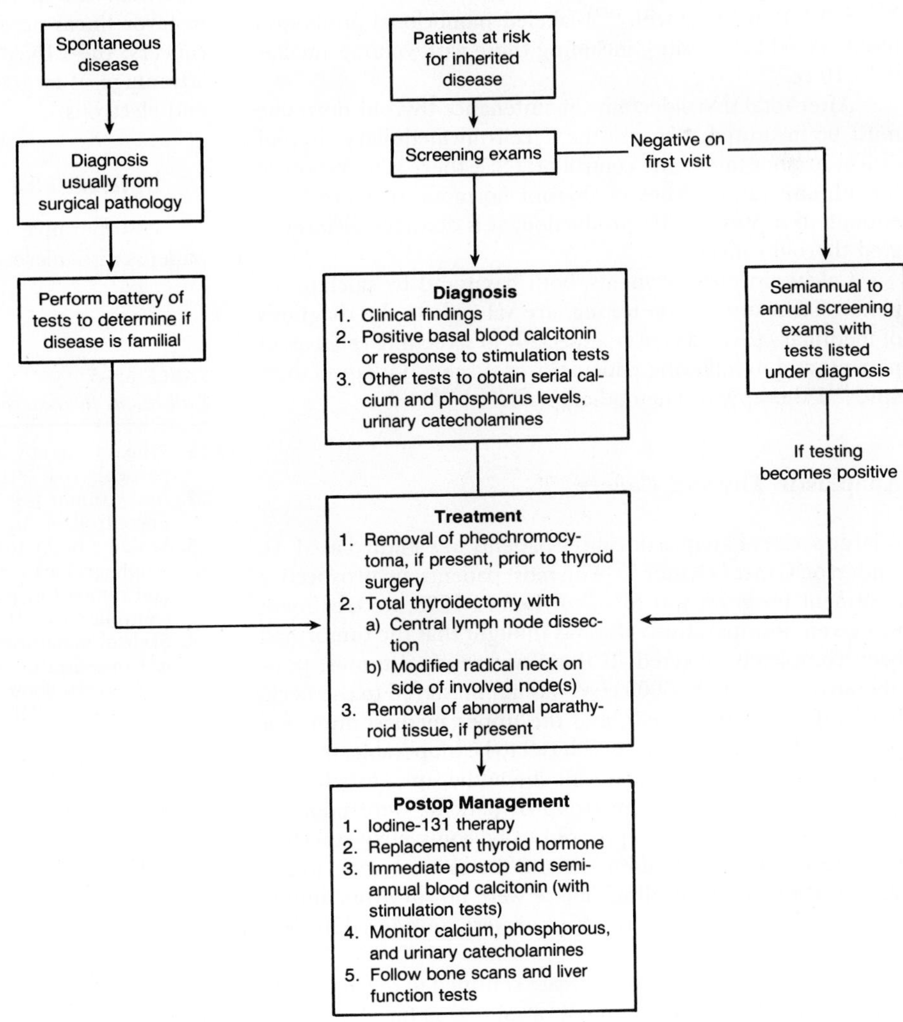

FIGURE 65–6. Schema for evaluation and management of sporadic and familial medullary thyroid cancer.

proaches 80%. The thyroidectomy is performed after the patient has recovered from the adrenalectomy.

In MEN IIa, hyperparathyroidism is common. Usually, chief cell hyperplasia is evident; the best therapy is total parathyroidectomy and autotransplantation of tissue to the forearm muscle.[14] In patients without hyperparathyroidism, every attempt is made to preserve the parathyroids *in situ.*[14]

With familial medullary thyroid cancer, early surgical intervention is important to render the patient biochemically and clinically free of apparent disease.

The C cells in medullary thyroid cancer do not concentrate iodine and are not part of the thyroid follicular apparatus. After total thyroidectomy, however, there may be remaining follicular cells whose trapping of iodine, particularly ^{131}I, is enhanced by the high levels of serum TSH.

Iodine 131 therapy may be a valuable treatment adjunct in medullary thyroid cancer patients whose disease appears limited to the thyroid at the time of surgery and in whom calcitonin is elevated postoperatively, basally, or after calcium- or pentagastrin-stimulation testing.[14] Irradiating residual medullary thyroid cancer cells with ^{131}I before local or distant spread occurs could eliminate local disease and perhaps improve survival.[50,95,212] Iodine 131 (*e.g.,* 150 mCi) has been used to treat local residual medullary thyroid cancer after total thyroidectomy.[95] The philosophy is that ^{131}I is taken up by the follicular cells and irradiates the adjacent C cells. This suggests that the C cells are radiosensitive.[50,95] Iodine 131 therapy is usually not appropriate for the treatment of metastases to lymph nodes, bone, liver, lungs, or other sites, because such metastases lack follicular cells and contain only C cells.[161,242]

SPECT imaging with ^{131}I-labeled monoclonal antibodies has detected tumor sites, including those with volume smaller than 10 cc.[189]

After total thyroidectomy, maintenance thyroid hormone must be instituted. Because the C cells in medullary thyroid cancer are not under the control of TSH, there is no rationale for administrating doses of thyroid hormone that are large enough to suppress TSH production, as is done for differentiated thyroid cancer.

Calcitonin measurements, both basal and by calcium- or pentagastrin-stimulation testing, are valuable in the diagnosis of medullary thyroid cancer, especially in screening relatives of patients and in following patients after surgery, radiation therapy, ^{131}I therapy, or chemotherapy.[14,15,73,274]

Anaplastic Thyroid Cancer

A large series of anaplastic cancer patients was studied at M. D. Anderson Cancer Center.[102] With most patients, no prospective treatment program was followed. Before 1965, no treatment was given postoperatively if it was thought that the tumor had been completely resected. If there was residual tumor, postoperative irradiation (6000 cGy) was administered to the neck, both supraclavicular areas, and the upper mediastinum. For patients whose tumor was considered to be inoperable, irradiation alone or in combination with chemotherapy was administered. Results in this latter group of patients were poor. In patients in whom tumor appeared to be completely resected, local recurrence and often distant metastases were found shortly after wound healing. There were no survivors among patients who had a partial resection or were considered inoperable.

Since 1965, patients with disease confined to the neck have been treated by surgical removal of all tumor (or as much as possible), by irradiation of the neck, both supraclavicular areas, and upper mediastinum to a dose of 6000 cGy, and by chemotherapy. Chemotherapy alone or combined with irradiation has been given to patients with distant metastases.

Patients treated with combined surgery, irradiation, and chemotherapy had the best results. Although the numbers were small, two factors seemed significant in the group of survivors. They had a limited amount of disease, and all but one were treated with a combined therapeutic approach. The treatment of anaplastic cancer is discussed further in the next section.

RADIATION THERAPY TECHNIQUES

External Irradiation

In contrast to ^{131}I, which is used for diagnosis and therapy for distant metastases of many thyroid cancers, external radiation therapy is effective for locoregional control of disease and in select metastatic sites. External radiation therapy can be used alone or in combination with ^{131}I and is well tolerated. The indications for external irradiation in thyroid cancers are listed in Table 65-5.

Definitive external radiation therapy for thyroid cancers requires careful treatment planning, because high doses are needed, and serious injuries may occur. The recommended treatments can be found in the sections dealing with the specific tumor types. In general, carcinomas require higher doses of up to 7000 cGy administered in 7.5 weeks, but lymphomas need only about 4500 cGy in 4.5 to 5 weeks. The larger penumbra and lesser skin sparing of ^{60}Co have caused radiation oncologists to favor linear accelerators for treatment of primary thyroid cancers; the LINACS produce a sharper beam and have the advantage of larger field sizes and the availability of photons and electrons.

Differentiated Thyroid Cancer

Postoperative external irradiation is rarely indicated for patients with microscopic or gross residual disease, as in the case

TABLE 65–5
Indications for External Irradiation in Thyroid Cancer

1. Primary therapy of thyroid cancer if unresectable locally, particularly if ^{131}I does not concentrate in tumor
2. Bulky tumor (*e.g.,* mediastinal disease) large enough that it is uncontrollable by ^{131}I alone
3. Residual bulky tumor in the central neck, tracheal, and/or esophageal area or cervical nodal regions after thyroid surgery and removal of malignant cervical adenopathy that may not be controlled by ^{131}I alone
4. Skeletal metastases
   a. Concentration of ^{131}I small or absent
   b. Concern about a pathologic fracture, regardless of the degree of ^{131}I concentration
5. Brain metastases
6. Hepatic metastases if symptomatic or other treatment methods have been unsuccessful
7. Relief of pressure symptoms occurring in vital areas caused by soft tissue masses
8. Superior vena cava syndrome
9. Continually recurring thyroid cancer regardless of ^{131}I accumulation
10. Recurrent or metastatic thyroid cancer occurring after maximal ^{131}I therapy
11. In sequence or conjunction with chemotherapy, particularly in anaplastic cancer
12. Preoperative therapy

of gross capsular invasion. External irradiation is indicated for patients with recurrence or extensive inoperable disease.

In follicular (including Hürthle cell tumors) or mixed papillary-follicular cancer, the tumor and its metastatic sites usually take up ^{131}I after ablation of normal thyroid tissue. Indications for external irradiation include inoperable or recurrent disease, capsular infiltration, macroscopic or microscopic residual disease, failure after ^{131}I treatment, and critical metastases.

If ^{131}I uptake is inadequate for therapeutic purposes after surgery for differentiated tumors, external irradiation is indicated if the tumor is inoperable, there is gross residual disease in the operative field, the connective tissue is invaded, or there is extensive infiltration of the cervical lymph nodes.[5,80,139]

External irradiation may be used in conjunction with ^{131}I treatment if the cancer is nonfunctional (*i.e.*, does not accumulate ^{131}I). This situation may occur in recurrent follicular cancers previously treated with ^{131}I and may indicate that the cancer is becoming less differentiated and less functional. With gross residual disease, external irradiation may be given with up to 250 mCi of ^{131}I concurrently administered. Some researchers, however, caution that external irradiation should not precede ^{131}I therapy, because it may jeopardize the success of the radioiodine treatment.[25]

The external beam field should encompass the thyroid bed and adjacent neck tissues. Electron beam therapy may be used to take advantage of the rapid fall-off of radiation dose; 9-MeV to 15-MeV electron energies may be selected, based on the depth of penetration desired. Only the rare patient with a very thick neck would require 16-MeV to 20-MeV electrons. Treatment planning with CT is very helpful in ascertaining the depth and doses to the spinal cord.

Lindberg[139] described the treatment technique used at M. D. Anderson Cancer Center. A large anterior field encompassing the neck, supraclavicular fossae, and mediastinum was treated with ^{60}Co to a dose of 5000 cGy to the supraclavicular area. Adding a posterior boost field of ^{60}Co or 25-MV photons to the mediastinum only, the tumor dose was brought to 5000 cGy and the spinal cord dose to about 4000 cGy in 5 weeks.

Sheline and associates[223] advocated external irradiation for residual microscopic infiltrating papillary carcinoma. They reported that locally persistent papillary carcinoma may remain clinically undetectable with arrested growth for more than 25 years; 11 (65%) of 17 patients survived more than 5 years after radiation therapy for incomplete surgery.

Tubiana and colleagues[258] also advocated postoperative irradiation for microscopic or macroscopic residual disease. Since 1956, they have delivered 5000 cGy in 25 fractions in 5 weeks to the neck with a boost of 500 cGy to 1000 cGy to residual disease with ^{60}Co teletherapy. The spinal cord dose was limited to 4200 cGy. They obtained a 5-year survival rate of 94% (62 of 66) for patients with complete surgery and 78% (76 of 97) for patients with incomplete surgery.

At the Princess Margaret Hospital in Toronto, the prescription for irradiation is 4000 cGy given in 15 fractions in 3 weeks for microscopic residual disease, with a boost of 1000 cGy in five fractions in 1 week directed to areas of gross tumor.[233]

Inoperable, bulky disease should be approached with curative intent. Inoperable papillary thyroid carcinoma treated with local external radiation has regressed markedly or disappeared, with patients surviving as long as 25 years.[76] The treatment field should encompass the entire thyroid tumor, neck, and superior mediastinum (Fig. 65-7). A tumor dose of 6500 cGy to 7000 cGy in 7 to 8 weeks with 180-cGy to 200-cGy fractions is recommended.

Based on the physical characteristics of the available equipment, optimal treatment plans may be generated. Judicious use of mixtures of photon and electron beams, differential weighing of doses, tissue compensators, and special spinal cord blocks all contribute to achieving satisfactory dose distribution. For example, 4500 cGy can be given to the midplane of the neck and mediastinum with AP/PA portals using ^{60}Co or 4-MV or 6-MV photons, and an additional 2000 cGy to 2500 cGy to the neck may be administered with 9-MeV to 13-MeV electrons. The boost field may also be arranged with oblique portals using a wedge. The spinal cord dose should not exceed the equivalent of 4500 cGy in 25 fractions in 5 weeks.

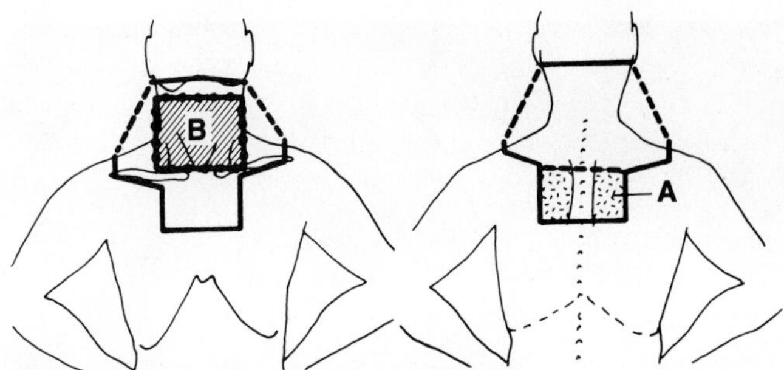

FIGURE 65–7. Diagrams of portals used in treatment of thyroid carcinoma. (*Right*) The A area represents the posterior mediastinal port used to increase the dose to these structures after the tolerance dose of the spinal cord has been reached with the large field (4500 cGy). (*Left*) Additional radiation is also delivered through an anteroposterior portal in the B area to the thyroid.

Another elaborate technique of external irradiation incorporates a rotational field with a wedge. A central blocking of the neck is used while the mediastinal field is open without blocking.[254] The resulting isodose distribution has the shape of a saddle in the neck region, with a high dose in the tumor and lower dose in the spinal cord (Fig. 65-8).

Painful osseous metastases can be palliated by external radiation therapy, and prevention of pathologic fractures is a worthwhile goal.

In long bones, a medullary rod should be placed before external irradiation is administered if pathologic fracture is imminent or has already occurred.[77,80] Brain, skeletal, hepatic, or subcutaneous metastases that press on vital structures should be treated with palliative external irradiation, ^{131}I therapy, or both. A dose of 3000 cGy in ten fractions in 2 weeks to 4500 cGy in 25 fractions in 5 weeks is adequate to achieve palliation. The patient's performance status and normal tissue tolerance must be considered in selecting the proper dose schedule.

Medullary Thyroid Cancer

The effectiveness of external irradiation for medullary cancer is still controversial, but recent data indicate that it can be used in the curative treatment of patients with microscopic residual or gross disease.[15,42,78,79,85,144,153,232,234,246,257] The radiosensitivity of medullary cancer probably falls between that of differentiated cancers and anaplastic cancers.[76] Survival rates are similar for patients who received postoperative irradiation and for those who received surgery alone, despite having more advanced local disease.[209,258] Irradiation is also used for postoperative treatment of surgically inaccessible residual disease.[76,101,103] The recommended dose is 6000 cGy administered in 6 to 7 weeks. Because of the high incidence of cervical and mediastinal nodal involvement by medullary cancer, the treatment portals must be quite large and should include the primary lesion, bilateral cervical supraclavicular lymph node areas, and the superior mediastinum. External irradiation should be

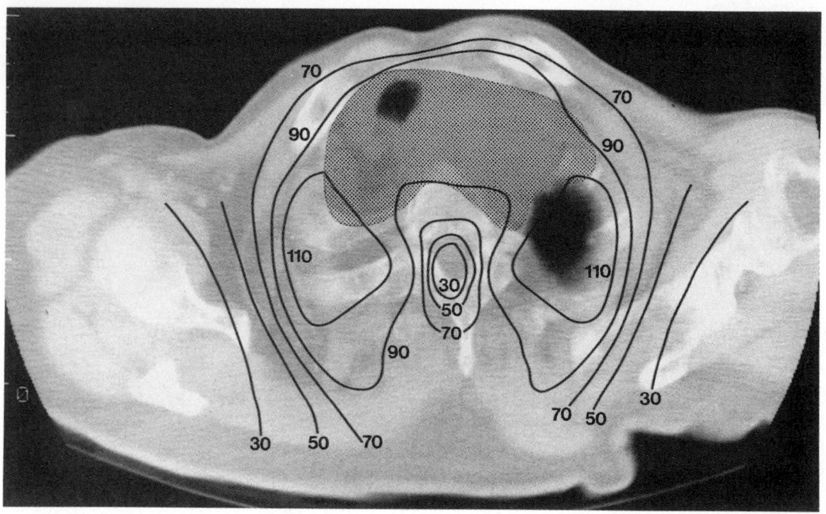

FIGURE 65–8. A "flying wedge" technique that gives a saddle-shaped dose distribution to the treatment volume with tolerable dose to the spinal cord. The treatments were given with 6-MV photon energy, a 45-degree wedge, and ± 60-degree rotation from vertical, with the beam centered on the spinal cord using a 2-cm full-thickness cord block. (Courtesy of Bruce Forell, Department of Radiation Physics, City of Hope National Medical Center)

considered for inoperable tumors; 6500 cGy to 7000 cGy is recommended, with reduced fields after 5500 cGy to 6000 cGy.[233] With bony or mediastinal lymph node metastases, external irradiation is the most effective therapy and gives prolonged palliation in 75% of the patients.[209] Tumor regression after radiation therapy is very slow, necessitating a follow-up of many years to assess the therapeutic effects.[209,257]

Anaplastic Cancer

Maximal debulking surgery should leave the least amount of tumor burden for radiation therapy. Tracheostomy may be necessary before radiation therapy to provide an adequate airway during irradiation.[203] Because of its radioresistance, higher doses tend to be delivered to anaplastic cancer; even 6000 cGy in 6 weeks cannot bring about satisfactory control or survival rates. However, a few long-term survivors have been reported.[76]

Because of very poor therapeutic response, unconventional treatments have been tried. These include large fraction sizes and hyperfractionation schemes.[234] Chemotherapy in combination with surgery and radiation therapy may be the best hope for these patients.[203]

Interstitial Irradiation

Interstitial irradiation is valuable in the treatment of primary thyroid cancer and metastatic cancer to the thyroid from other primary cancers, including head and neck neoplasms.[250] Removable (^{192}Ir) and permanent (^{125}I) interstitial implants were used in five patients with primary thyroid cancer and two patients with metastatic cancer to the thyroid with excellent local control of thyroid or metastatic neck masses. Four of the five patients with primary thyroid cancer and one of the two patients with metastases to the thyroid are alive with no evidence of disease 12 to 48 months after interstitial irradiation. Complications from the irradiation are minimal and manageable, and results are encouraging.

RESULTS OF THERAPY

In Finland, postoperative radiation therapy in the treatment of thyroid cancer has found wide use.[93] Of 231 patients with thyroid cancer, 74% received postoperative irradiation; 109 patients with primary thyroid lymphoma treated at Mayo Clinic died of their disease, 40 of them from local infiltration. In a later series of 76 patients with residual thyroid cancer after surgery, 29 received postoperative irradiation for papillary, follicular, or anaplastic thyroid cancer that was deeply infiltrating or showed neuromuscular involvement. Over 7 weeks, between 4000 cGy and 5000 cGy was administered to the thyroid bed using ^{60}Co in addition to ^{131}I.[117]

A retrospective analysis of 359 patients with differentiated medullary, anaplastic, and other types of thyroid cancer treated by external irradiation and ^{131}I was reported.[259] Doses of 5000 cGy to 6000 cGy were well tolerated, and the therapy was most effective for papillary, follicular, and medullary cancers.

Other clinical studies have described the benefits of external radiation therapy alone or with ^{131}I in controlling differentiated, medullary, or anaplastic cancers.[42,153,257]

Lymphoma of the Thyroid

Primary lymphoma of the thyroid gland is rare, comprising only 4% to 8% of all thyroid tumors and only 1.3% of all lymphomas. The predominant histologic type is diffuse histiocytic lymphoma; other types are poorly differentiated lymphocytic or mixed-cell lymphoma and Hodgkin's disease. As in other head and neck lymphomas, distant manifestation is common. Locally, the tumor may be quite bulky and may cause compression symptoms. Extension into the thoracic inlet and retrosternum is frequent.

Treatment of thyroid lymphomas may involve the different modalities of surgery, radiation therapy, and chemotherapy. After a debulking surgical procedure, postoperative radiation therapy of the neck and superior mediastinum to a minimum dose of 4000 cGy to 4500 cGy should be adequate for local control of disease for most tumors. Among 46 cases of primary lymphomas of the thyroid at the Royal Marsden Hospital treated between 1948 and 1980, the highest rates of local control and long-term survival were seen in patients who had complete surgical removal of gross tumor followed by radiation therapy ($P<0.005$). For those tumors with adverse prognostic factors, such as large bulk, fixation, extracapsular extension, or retrosternal extension, Tupchong and associates[260] recommended the addition of chemotherapy because of the high risk of distant disease and local failure (Fig. 65-9).

Blair and colleagues[27] described their experience with 38

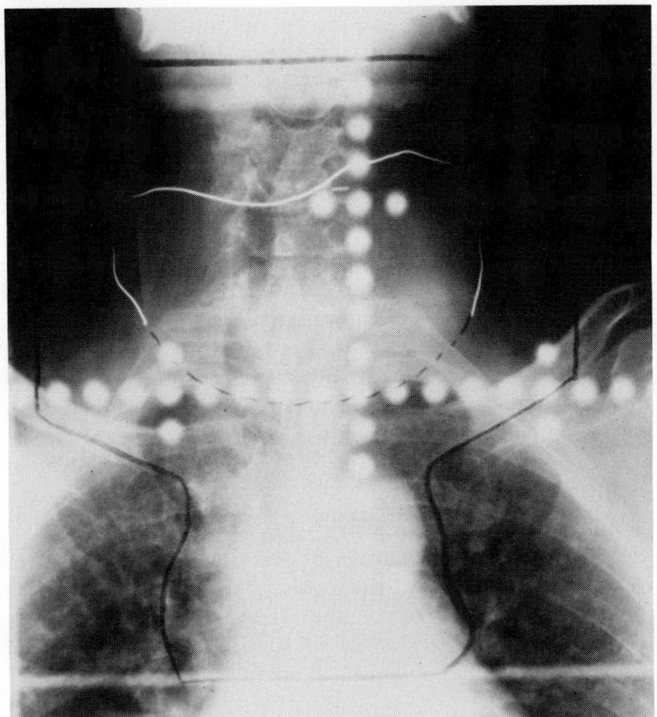

FIGURE 65–9. Anteroposterior simulation film of the initial large field, including the neck and mediastinum in a patient with a large malignant lymphoma of the thyroid.

between 1965 and 1979. All patients were irradiated to approximately 4000 cGy (range, 2400–6000 cGy) to the neck alone or to the neck and mediastinum. The 5-year disease-free survival rate was 59%. Patients with no gross residual disease at the beginning of radiation therapy had the least likelihood of recurrence. For stage IE and IIE primary thyroid lymphomas, they suggested that the radiation portal should include the neck, axillae, and mediastinum to a dose of 4000 cGy.

Vigliotti and associates[267] treated a series of patients with stage IE and IIE thyroid lymphomas at the M. D. Anderson Cancer Center. Of 38 patients, 29 received radiation therapy: 15 alone and 14 combined chemotherapy and irradiation. All patients received 4000 cGy to the neck and upper mediastinum and 3000 cGy to 3500 cGy to the lower mediastinum in 20 fractions over 4 weeks with cobalt teletherapy. The overall 5-year survival and disease-free survival rates were 72% and 64%, respectively. They concluded that radiation therapy alone was satisfactory for disease limited to the thyroid, with or without cervical adenopathy. However, they recommended combination chemotherapy for patients who had mediastinal tumor extensions.

SEQUELAE OF THERAPY WITH RADIOACTIVE IODINE

Serious complications are rare after single doses of 200 mCi or less of ^{131}I.[19,26,109] They are more common after larger single treatments or large cumulative doses. Van Nostrand and associates[265] reviewed the side-effects of ^{131}I therapy for metastatic well-differentiated thyroid cancer after a mean follow-up of 15 months.

Early Complications

Early complications occur within 3 months of treatment. Acute radiation sickness (*i.e.*, fatigue, headache, nausea, vomiting) may occur within 12 hours after ^{131}I has been administered; vomiting occurs in about 5% of patients.[109] These problems may be averted with antinausea premedication, such as prochlorperazine.[67]

Sialadenitis (*i.e.*, swelling and pain in the salivary glands) occasionally occurs shortly after ^{131}I administration or after discharge from the hospital and may last for a few days. Rarely, a dry mouth may last for months and years; a metallic taste may last for weeks. These side-effects are caused by irradiation of the salivary glands.[3,67,109,244]

To avoid cystitis, patients are asked to void hourly during the day and every other hour at night.

Edema of the neck after ^{131}I ablation of the thyroid has been reported in several patients.[71] The clinical features of early neck edema after ^{131}I ablation are similar to those of angioneurotic edema. The neck edema responded well to corticosteroids.

Transient hyperthyroidism may occur after massive thyroid tissue destruction and subsequent release into circulation of large amounts of thyroid hormone. Thyroid storm is a potential complication in patients who are hyperthyroid from functioning metastatic disease.[37,38,47,109,190,238] Pretreatment with antithyroid drugs, including β-adrenergic agents, can mediate the thyroid hormone storm after ^{131}I therapy.[37] Patients with follicular thyroid cancer may rarely have hyperthyroidism produced by secretion of large amounts of thyroid hormone by the tumor.[47]

Bone marrow suppression can be observed in almost all patients receiving ^{131}I therapy.[67] Transient anemia, leukopenia, and thrombocytopenia have been reported.[67,109] Permanent or severe marrow suppression has been reported with blood radiation doses greater than 200 cGy.[23,135]

Transient vocal cord paralysis after ^{131}I ablation of residual thyroid gland after a near-total thyroidectomy has been reported.[134]

Pain, hemorrhage, and swelling in metastases after therapy presumably results from radiation-induced swelling and is analogous to radiation-associated thyroiditis.[67,109] Sudden hemorrhage into functioning cerebral metastases and severe fatal cerebral edema in a patient with functioning cerebral metastases have been reported.[107,109] Pretreatment with corticosteroids may avert serious complications of therapy, especially with brain metastases.[109]

Long-term Complications

Long-term complications occur 3 months or longer after treatment. Radiation pneumonitis and pulmonary fibrosis have been associated with ^{131}I therapy, especially if there were diffuse functioning lung metastases. To prevent radiation pneumonitis in this circumstance, Benua and associates[23] recommend a maximum of 80 mCi ^{131}I retained in the whole body 48 hours after treatment. Pneumonitis and pulmonary fibrosis may be managed with corticosteroids.

Permanent bone marrow suppression is rare, occurring primarily in patients who received large cumulative doses of ^{131}I for bone metastases.[109]

Preleukemia, a myelodysplastic disorder, usually occurs in patients over 50 years of age. Myelodysplastic disorders may be secondary to radiation therapy and/or chemotherapy or may arise *de novo.* Preleukemia has been reported after radioiodine therapy alone and after the use of external radiation therapy in association with ^{131}I treatment.[279]

Leukemia as a complication of ^{131}I therapy is rare (<2%).[19,67,109] Patients who received the largest amount of ^{131}I (over 500 mCi total dose) in the shortest time interval appear to be the most susceptible to leukemia, especially if over 50 years of age.[109,279] Acute myelogenous leukemia is the most frequent type. Some authorities suggest waiting a year between ^{131}I therapies if the clinical situation is stable, but others suggest a 6- to 12-month interval.[14,80,135]

Some authors have suggested that treatment with ^{131}I or external irradiation may be responsible for the occasional transformation of differentiated thyroid cancer to anaplastic cancer.[67,109] However, Mazzaferri and associates[151,152] found that more than half the patients who developed anaplastic cancers did not receive prior ^{131}I therapy. This finding suggests that the anaplastic transformation may relate more to the natural history of thyroid cancer.[280]

Ovarian failure and azoospermia have been reported in patients after treatment with ^{131}I.[58,89,90] In a series of patients previously treated with ^{131}I for thyroid cancer before the age of 20, there were no differences in infertility, miscarriage rate, prematurity, or congenital abnormalities compared with the general population.[214]

We recommend that women do not become pregnant for 6 months after their last ^{131}I dose and that men do not father a child for 3 months.[109] This does not preclude nonprocreative sexual activity.

CHEMOTHERAPY

Single-Agent Chemotherapy

Of 53 patients with thyroid cancer treated with doxorubicin (Adriamycin), about one third achieved significant tumor regression and prolonged survival.[32] Pulmonary metastasis was the most commonly responsive disease, followed by bone and regional metastatic disease in the neck. Another one third of the patients manifested arrest of previously progressive metastatic disease. Patients with differentiated and medullary cancer had the most significant responses, but doxorubicin exhibited limited effectiveness in patients with anaplastic cancer.

Differentiated Thyroid Cancer

Twenty-eight patients were studied, including ten with mixed papillary-follicular cancer, nine with Hürthle cell, six with follicular, two with papillary, and one with unclassified primary thyroid tumor that was differentiated.[32] All patients had undergone total or subtotal thyroidectomy (some with neck dissection), and 24 had received prior radiation therapy with ^{131}I, external irradiation, or both. In these 28 patients, the most common sites of metastatic disease at the time of chemotherapy were the soft tissues and lymph nodes of the neck (21 patients), lungs, skeleton, and liver.[2,9,21] Ten of the 28 patients achieved a partial remission of their disease. The median duration of response and survival from the initiation of chemotherapy were 8 and 17 months, respectively. Partial remissions occurred in four patients with mixed papillary-follicular cancer, in three with Hürthle cell cancer, in two with follicular cancer, and in the one patient with unclassified tumor. Median duration of survival for 11 patients with no change in their disease was 12 months. Seven patients showed progressive disease despite doxorubicin chemotherapy; the median survival was only 6 months.

Medullary Thyroid Cancer

Seven patients (six males and one female) with medullary thyroid cancer previously treated with thyroid surgery, neck dissection, ^{131}I, or external irradiation in various combinations were given doxorubicin.[32] The median durations of disease before chemotherapy was initiated and the subsequent survival were 36 months and 19 months, respectively. Of the seven patients, three achieved a partial response of disease lasting 2, 21, and 39 months; another three patients showed no change for 4, 6, and 9 months; one patient died only 3 days after beginning chemotherapy and was considered an early death.

Anaplastic Thyroid Cancer

In 18 patients (median age, 68 years) with anaplastic cancer treated with doxorubicin, the median duration of disease from the time of diagnosis to chemotherapy was 4 months.[32] Only four of the 18 patients showed any significant response to doxorubicin; three other patients had no change in their disease for brief periods.

Median survival was 2 months; six died within 3 weeks of beginning therapy, and two survived beyond 24 months from the initiation of therapy (28 and 38 months).

Combination Chemotherapy

The Southeastern Cooperative Oncology Group had a protocol for advanced thyroid carcinoma comparing cisplatin with doxorubicin and cisplatin. The Eastern Cooperative Oncology Group had a protocol employing streptozotocin in combination with 5-fluorouracil for the treatment of APUDomas, possibly including medullary thyroid cancer. The results of various combinations of chemotherapy or single-agent (doxorubicin) chemotherapy in medullary thyroid cancer have been inconsistent.[81]

MULTIMODALITY THERAPY

A subgroup of thyroid tumors deserves consideration for chemotherapy in combination with surgery and radiation therapy. In lymphomas, the addition of chemotherapy can lead to improved local control and treatment of distant disease.

Another subgroup of thyroid tumors, anaplastic giant and spindle cell cancers, is extremely malignant and seldom controlled with radiation therapy alone. Chemotherapy has been advocated for this type of thyroid cancer.[123,124,126] Tallroth and associates[253] reported the Swedish experience with anaplastic giant cell cancer at the Radiumhemmet. Of nine patients who received a three-drug program of bleomycin, cyclophosphamide, and 5-fluorouracil and radiation therapy, only one patient (11%) survived and lived 12 years. Another group of 25 patients received three-drug chemotherapy and two-fractions-per-day radiation therapy. Three patients (12%) were free of disease, and the remaining 22 patients died of local disease and metastases. A third group of patients had preoperative and postoperative irradiation, three-drug chemotherapy, and surgery during remission, and the survival rate beyond 3 years was 12% (three of 24 patients). The most recent protocol was that of weekly doxorubicin and radiation therapy. One of five patients remained alive more than 10 months after treatment.

Kim and Leeper[126] updated a report on a prospective protocol at Memorial Sloan-Kettering Cancer Center. Since 1979, 41 patients with locally advanced thyroid cancers were treated with a combination of low-dose doxorubicin and external-beam radiation therapy. Group 1 consisted of 22 patients with well-differentiated papillary, follicular, or mixed type tumors. They received doxorubicin (10 mg/m^2) once a week before radiation therapy, which was given at a daily dose of 200 cGy, 5 days per week, to a total dose of 5600 cGy. Group 2 had 19 patients with anaplastic giant and spindle cell cancers. They were given the same dose of doxorubicin, but received their radiation twice a day, 3 days per week, at 160 cGy per fraction to a total dose of 5760 cGy in 40 days. Local control rates at 2 years were 77% and 68%, respectively. Median survival was 4 years for group 1 and 1 year for group 2.

Another multimodality study evaluated patients with anaplastic and well-differentiated tumors who received chemotherapy (melphalan, doxorubicin, bleomycin, and vincristine). Five of the patients with anaplastic cancer had received no prior therapy, and three of five responded. The responses with anaplastic cancer were encouraging.[31]

Another study described the treatment of locally advanced thyroid carcinoma with doxorubicin before radiation therapy. Local tumor control at 1 year was 85% and 77% for the differentiated and anaplastic tumor groups, respectively.[125]

The limitations of these multimodality approaches are the severe local complications, which are to be expected because of the overlapping cutaneous and mucosal toxic effects of external irradiation and various chemotherapeutic agents.

HYPERTHERMIA

Pilot clinical trials of combined hyperthermia and radiation therapy have consistently yielded local control results averaging twice as good as with radiation alone.[7,108,122,143,180] A randomized study conducted by the Radiation Therapy Oncology Group confirmed the therapeutic advantage in a subset of patients with smaller lesions.[184]

Because thyroid cancer is relatively rare and because most reported series contain small numbers of patients, hyperthermia for thyroid cancer has not been specifically mentioned. Currently, hyperthermia may be indicated in the palliative treatment of cancers that have been previously irradiated or have a low probability of control with radiation therapy alone. External hyperthermia using microwaves, ultrasound, or radiofrequencies or interstitial hyperthermia using microwaves or radiofrequency local current fields may be appropriate.[49,142]

IMMUNOTHERAPY

Immunotherapy is receiving increasing attention.[263] One study attempted to evaluate the response of a small number of patients with widespread metastatic differentiated thyroid cancer to immunotherapy, but the results were inconclusive.[4] It has been suggested that immunotherapy by specific stimulation with irradiated tumor cells or by nonspecific stimulation by *Corynebacterium,* BCG, or other vaccines should be considered in the management of undifferentiated thyroid cancer.[85] Radiolabeled monoclonal antibodies in therapy may prove valuable in the near future.[1,77,120,133,178,188,242]

Acknowledgment

The authors recognize the support and assistance of Ms. Connie Povilat and her staff, without whose patience and guidance this chapter would not have been written.

REFERENCES

1. Abdel-Nabi H, Hinkle GH, Falko JM, et al: Labeled anti-CEA antibodies uptake by Hürthle cell carcinoma. Clin Nucl Med 10:713, 1985
2. Abe Y, Ichikawa Y, Muraki T, et al: Thyrotropin (TSH) receptor and adenylate cyclase activity in human thyroid tumors: Absence of high affinity receptor and loss of TJH responsiveness in undifferentiated thyroid carcinoma. J Clin Endocrinol Metab 52:23, 1986
3. Allweiss P, Braunstein GD, Katz A, et al: Sialadenitis following I-131 therapy for thyroid carcinoma. [Concise Communication] J Nucl Med 25:755, 1984
4. Amino N, Pyscher T, Cohen EP, et al: Immunologic aspects of human thyroid cancer. Cancer 36:963, 1975
5. Ampil FL: Postoperative external irradiation in thyroid carcinoma: A clinical experience of 20 treated patients and literature radiotherapy review. J Surg Oncol 30:83, 1985
6. Antoinades J: Uncommon Malignant Tumors. New York, Masson, 1982
7. Arcangeli G, Cividalli A, Nervi C, et al: Tumor control and therapeutic gain with different schedules of combined radiotherapy and local external hyperthermia in human cancer. Int J Radiat Oncol Biol Phys 9:1125, 1983
8. Arnstein NB, Carey JE, Spaulding SA, Sisson JC: Determination of iodine 131 diagnostic dose for imaging metastatic thyroid cancer. J Nucl Med 27:1764, 1986
9. Ashcroft MW, Van Herle AJ: The comparative value of serum thyroglobulin measurements and iodine 131 total body scans in the follow-up study of patients with treated differentiated thyroid cancer. Am J Med 72:806, 1981
10. Auffermann W, Clark OH, Thurnher S, et al: Recurrent thyroid carcinoma: Characteristics on MR images. Radiology 168:753, 1988
11. Balachandran S, Sayle BA: Value of thyroid carcinoma imaging after therapeutic doses of radioiodine. Clin Nucl Med 6:162, 1981
12. Bantle JP, Lee CKK, Levitt SH: Thyroxine administration during radiation therapy to the neck does not prevent subsequent thyroid dysfunction. Int J Radiat Oncol Biol Phys 11:1999, 1985
13. Bayer MF, Kriss JP, McDougall IR: Clinical experience with sensitive thyrotropin measurements: Diagnostic and therapeutic implications. J Nucl Med 26:1248, 1985
14. Baylin SB, Wells SA Jr: Management of hereditary medullary thyroid carcinoma. Clin Endocrinol Metab 10:367, 1981
15. Baylin SB, Wells SA Jr: Management of medullary thyroid cancer. In Greenfield LD (ed): Thyroid Cancer, pp 151–163. Boca Raton, CRC Press, 1978
16. Beahrs OH, Henson DE, Hutter RVP, Myers MH (eds): Manual for Staging of Cancer, 3rd ed. Philadelphia, J.B. Lippincott, 1988
17. Becker DV, Hurley JR: Current status of radioiodine (I-131) treatment of hyperthyroidism. In Freeman LH, Weissman HS (eds): Nuclear Medicine Annual 1982, pp 265–290. New York, Raven Press, 1982
18. Becker DV, Hurley JR, Motazedi, et al: Ablation of postsurgical thyroid remnants in patients with differentiated thyroid cancer can be achieved with less whole body radiation. [Abstract] J Nucl Med 23:43, 1982
19. Beierwaltes WH: The treatment of thyroid carcinoma with radioactive iodine. Semin Nucl Med 8:79, 1978
20. Beierwaltes WH, Rabbani R, Dmuchowski et al: An analysis of "Ablation of thyroid remnants" with I-131 in 511 patients from 1947–1984: Experience at the University of Michigan. J Nucl Med 25:1287, 1984

21. Beierwaltes WH, Nishiyama RH, Thompson NW, et al: Survival time and "cure" in papillary and follicular thyroid carcinoma with distant metastases: Statistics following University of Michigan Therapy. J Nucl Med 23:561, 1982
22. Ben-Hur E, Elkind MM, Bronk BV: Thermally enhanced radioresponse of cultured Chinese hamster cells: Inhibition of repair of sublethal damage and enhancement of lethal damage. Radiat Res 58:38, 1974
23. Benua RS, Cicale NR, Sonenberg M, et al: The relation of radioiodine dosimetry to results and complications in the treatment of metastatic thyroid cancer. AJR 87:171, 1962
24. Black EG, Gimlette TMD, Maisey MN, et al: Serum Thyroglobulin in thyroid cancer. Lancet 2:443, 1981
25. Blahd W: Nuclear medicine therapy of thyroid cancer. In Thawley S, Panje W, Batsakis J, Lindberg R (eds): Comprehensive Management of Head and Neck Tumors, p 1614. Philadelphia, WB Saunders, 1987
26. Blahd WH, Drickman MV, Porter CW, et al: Serum thyroglobulin, a monitor of differentiated thyroid carcinoma in patients receiving thyroid hormone suppression therapy. [Concise Communication] J Nucl Med 25:673, 1984
27. Blair TJ, Evans RG, Buskirk GJ, et al: Radiotherapeutic management of primary thyroid lymphoma. Int J Radiat Oncol Biol Phys 11:365, 1985
28. Block MA: Needle aspiration of the thyroid gland. West J Med 142:537, 1985
29. Brendel HA, Guyot M, Jeandot R, Lefeort G, Manciet G: Thallium-201 imaging in the follow-up of differentiated carcinoma. J Nucl Med 29:1515, 1988
30. Brown AP, Greening WP, McCready VR, et al: Radioiodine treatment of metastatic thyroid carcinoma in the Royal Marsden Hospital experience. Br J Radiol 57:323, 1984
31. Bukowski RM, Brown L, Weick JK, et al: Combination chemotherapy of metastatic thyroid cancer. Am J Clin Oncol 6:579, 1983
32. Burgess MA, Hill GS Jr: Chemotherapy in the management of thyroid cancer. In Greenfield LD (ed): Thyroid Cancer, pp 233–245. Boca Raton, CRC Press, 1978
33. Burrow GN, Spaulding SW: Role of lithium in radioiodine therapy. In Spencer RP (ed): Therapy in Nuclear Medicine, pp 113–118. New York, Grune & Stratton, 1978
34. Cady B, Sedgwick CE, Meissner WA, et al: Risk factor analysis in differentiated thyroid cancer. Cancer 43:810, 1979
35. Cady B, Sedgwick CE, Meissner WA, et al: Changing clinical, pathologic, therapeutic and survival patterns in differentiated thyroid carcinoma. Ann Surg 184:541, 1976
36. Castronovo FP Jr: Iodine-131 thyroid burdens of European travelers returning to Boston after the Chernobyl accident. [Letter to the Editor] N Engl J Med 315:1679, 1986
37. Cerletty JM, Listwan WJ: Hyperthyroidism due to functioning metastatic thyroid carcinoma: Precipitation of thyroid storm with therapeutic radioactive iodine. JAMA 242:269, 1979
38. Chapman CN, Sziklas JJ, Spencer RP, et al: Hyperthyroidism with metastatic follicular thyroid carcinoma. J Nucl Med 25:466, 1984
39. Charles MA: Comparison of serum thyroglobulin with iodine scans in thyroid cancer. J Endocrinol Invest 5:267, 1982
40. Chatzkel S, Cole-Beuglet C, Breckenridge JW, et al: Ultrasound diagnosis of hypernephroma metastatic to thyroid and external jugular vein. Radiology 142:165, 1982
41. Clark DE: Association of irradiation with cancer of the thyroid in children and adolescents. JAMA 159:1007, 1955
42. Chung CT, Sagerman RH, Ryoo MC: External irradiation for malignant thyroid tumors. Radiology 136:753, 1980
43. Clayton GW: Tumors of the endocrine glands. In Sutow WW, Fernbach DJ, Vietti TJ (eds): Clinical Pediatric Oncology, pp 761–774. St. Louis, CV Mosby, 1984
44. Clayton GW, Kirkland RT: Cancer of the thyroid in children. In Greenfield LD (ed): Thyroid Cancer, pp 207–221. Boca Raton, CRC Press, 1978
45. Colacchio TA, LoGerfo P, Calacchio DA, et al: Radioiodine total body scan versus serum thryoglobulin levels in follow-up of patients with thyroid cancer. Surgery 91:42, 1982
46. Cole-Beuglet C: Superficial structures. In Goldberg BB, Wells PNT (eds): Ultrasonics in Clinical Diagnosis, 3rd ed, pp 180–202. New York, Churchill Livingstone, 1983
47. Cooper DJ, Ridgway EC, Maloof F: Unusual types of hyperthyroidism. Clin Endocrinol Metab 7:199, 1978
48. Corry PM, Robinson MS, Getz BS: Hyperthermic effects on DNA repair mechanisms. Radiology 123:475, 1977
49. Corry PM, Spanos WJ, Tilchen EJ, et al: Combined ultrasound and radiation therapy treatment of human superficial tumor. Radiology 145:165, 1982
50. Deftos IJ, Stein MF: Radioiodine as an adjunct to the surgical treatment of medullary thyroid carcinoma. J Clin Endocrinol Metab 50:967, 1980
51. DeGroot, LJ, Reilly M: Comparison of 30 and 50 mCi dose of iodine-131 for thyroid ablation. Ann Intern Med 96:51, 1982
52. DeGroot LJ, Frohman LA, Kaplan EL, et al: Radiation Associated Thyroid Carcinoma. New York, Grune and Stratton, 1977
53. Demos TC, Blonder J, Schey WL, et al: Multiple endocrine neoplasia (MEN) syndrome type IIB: Gastrointestinal manifestations. AJR 140:73, 1983
54. Denny JD, Marty R, Van Herle AJ: Serum thyroglobulin: A sensitive indicator of metastatic well differentiated thyroid carcinoma. Presented at the Society of Nuclear Medicine Western Regional Meeting, Las Vegas, 1977
55. Devine RM, Edis AJ, Banks PM: Primary lymphoma of the thyroid: A review of the Mayo Clinic experience. World J Surg 5:33, 1981
56. Dewey WC, Hopwood LE, Sapareto SA, et al: Cellular responses to combinations of hyperthermia and radiation. Radiology 123:464, 1977
57. Dewhirst MW, Sim DA, Sapareto SA, et al: Importance of minimum tumor temperature in determining early and long-term responses of spontaneous canine and feline tumors to heat and radiation. Cancer Res 44:43, 1984
58. Dobyns BM, Maloof K: The study and treatment of 199 cases of carcinoma of the thyroid with radioactive iodine. J Clin Endocrinol 11:1323, 1951
59. Dodd GD: The radiologic features of multiple endocrine neoplasia types IIA and IIB. Semin Roentgenol 20:64, 1985
60. Duffy BJ Jr, Fitzgerald PJ: Thyroid cancer in children in childhood and adolescence: A report on 28 cases. Cancer 3:1018, 1950
61. Echenique RL, Kasi L, Haynie TP, et al: Critical evaluation of serum thyroglobulin levels and I-131 scans in posttherapy patients with differentiated thyroid carcinoma. [Concise Communication] J Nucl Med 23:235, 1982
62. Endo K, Otha H, Torizuka K, et al: Technetium-99m(V)-DMSA in the imaging of medullary thyroid carcinoma. [Letter to the Editor] J Nucl Med 28:252, 1987
63. Endo K, Shiomi K, Kasagi K, et al: Imaging of medullary thyroid cancer with 131-I-MIBC. Lancet 2:233, 1984
64. Ephgrave KS, Laycock R: Thyroid hemiagenesis. Contemp Surg 27:67, 1985
65. Favus MJ, Schneider AB, Stachura ME, et al: Thyroid cancer occurring as a late consequence of head and neck irradiation: Evaluation of 1056 patients. N Engl J Med 294:1019, 1976
66. Feind CR: The head and neck. In Haagensen LD, Feind CR, Hertner FP, et al (eds): The Lymphatics in Cancer, p 59. Philadelphia, WB Saunders, 1972
67. Freitas JE, Gross MD, Ripley S, et al: Radionuclide diagnosis and therapy of thyroid cancer: Current status report. Semin Nucl Med 15:1606, 1985
68. Gershengorn MC, Izumi M, Robbins J: Use of lithium as an adjunct to radioiodine therapy of thyroid carcinoma. J Clin Endocrinol Metab 42:105, 1976
69. Gerweck LE, Dalhberg WK, Greco B: Effect of pH on single or fractionated heat treatments at 42°C–45°C. Cancer Res 43:1163, 1983
70. Gerweck LE, Gillette EL, Dewey WC: Effect of heat and radiation on synchronous Chinese hamster cells: Killing and repair. Radiat Res 64:611, 1975
71. Goolden AWG, Kam KC, Fitzpatrick ML, Munro AJ: Oedema of the neck after ablation of the thyroid with radioactive iodine. Br J Radiol 59:583, 1986
72. Goslings BM: Effect of a low iodine diet on I-131 therapy in

follicular thyroid carcinomata. [Abstract] J Endocrinol 64:30, 1975
73. Graze K, Spiler IJ, Tashjian AH Jr, et al: Natural history of familial medullary thyroid carcinoma: Effect of program for early diagnosis. N Engl J med 299:980, 1985
74. Greenebaum E, Koss LG, Elequin F, Silver CE: The diagnostic value of flow cytometric DNA measurements in follicular tumors of the thyroid gland. Cancer 56:2011, 1985
75. Greenfield LD: Management of miscellaneous thyroid malignancies. In Greenfield LD (ed): Thyroid Cancer, pp 177–187. Boca Raton, CRC Press, 1978
76. Greenfield LD: Radiation therapy in the management of thyroid cancer. In Greenfield LD (ed): Thyroid Cancer, pp 223–231. Boca Raton, CRC Press, 1978
77. Greenfield LD: Thyroid cancer: The role of radiotherapy in treatment. Int J Radiat Oncol Biol Phys 2(suppl 2):131, 1977
78. Greenfield LD, George III FW: The role of radiotherapy in the management of medullary thyroid cancer. Int J Radiat Oncol Biol Phys 5(suppl 1):81, 1979
79. Greenfield LD, Ucmakli A, George FW III, et al: The role of radiation therapy in the treatment of medullary thyroid cancer. Contemp Surg 18:59, 1981
80. Greenfield LD, Paladugu RR, Jacobs ML: Postoperative management of differentiated thyroid cancer. Contemp Surg 15:52, 1979
81. Greenfield LD, Small RC, Byfield JE: Medullary thyroid carcinoma. [Letter to the Editor] JAMA 229:1864, 1974
82. Greenspan FS: Radiation exposure and thyroid cancer. JAMA 237:2089, 1977
83. Greenspan FS: Fine-needle aspiration biopsy of thyroid. West J Med 143:89, 1985
84. Guzy PM: Creatine phosphokinase-MB (CPK-MB) and the diagnosis of myocardial infarction. West J Med 127:455, 1977
85. Halnan KF: The non-surgical treatment of thyroid cancer. Br J Surg 62:769, 1975
86. Hamburger JI: Diuretic augmentation of I-131 uptake in inoperable thyroid cancer. N Engl J Med 280:1091, 1969
87. Hamburger B, Gharib H, Melton LJ III, et al: Fine-needle aspiration biopsy of thyroid nodules. Am J Med 73:381, 1982
88. Hamburger JI, Miller JM, Kini SR (eds): Clinical-Pathological Evaluation of Thyroid Nodules Handbook and Atlas. Limited Edition, Private Publication, 1979
89. Handelsman DJ, Turtle JR: Testicular damage after radioactive iodine (I-131) therapy for thyroid cancer. Clin Endocrinol 18:465, 1983
90. Handelsman DJ, Conway AJ, Donnelly PF, et al: Azoospermia after iodine-131 treatment for thyroid carcinoma. Br Med J 281:1527, 1980
91. Hanson GA, Komorowski RA, Cerlett JM, et al: Thyroid gland morphology in young adults: Normal subjects versus those with prior low-dose neck irradiation in childhood. Surgery 94:984, 1983
92. Hartshorne MF, Karl RD Jr, Cawthon MA, et al: Multiple imaging techniques demonstrate a medullary carcinoma of the thyroid. Clin Nucl Med 8:628, 1983
93. Haynie TP, Nofal MM, Bierewaltes WA: Treatment of thyroid carcinoma with I-131. JAMA 183:303, 1963
94. Heath H, Hodgson JF, Kennedy MA: Primary hyperparathyroidsm: Incidence, morbidity and potential economic impact in a community. N Engl J Med 302:189, 1980
95. Hellman DE, Kartchner M, Van Antwerp JD, et al: Radioiodine in the treatment of medullary carcinoma of the thyroid. J Clin Endocrinol Metab 48:451, 1979
96. Herzog B: Thyroid gland diseases and tumors: Surgical aspects. Prog Pediatr Surg 16:15, 1983
97. Hempelmann LH, Furth J: Etiology of thyroid cancer. In Greenfield LD (ed): Thyroid Cancer, pp 37–49. Boca Raton, CRC Press, 1978
98. Hempelmann LH, Hall WJ, Phillips M, et al: Neoplasms in persons treated with x-rays in infancy: Fourth survey in 20 years. JNCI 55:519, 1975
99. Higashi T, Ito K, Nishikawa Y, et al: Gallium-67 imaging in the evaluation of thyroid malignancy. J Clin Nucl Med 13:792, 1988
100. Higgins CB, Auffermann W: MR imaging of thyroid and parathyroid glands: A review of current status. AJR 151:1095, 1988
101. Hill CS Jr: Medullary carcinoma of the thyroid gland. In Clarke RE, Stanley WM, Arje SL (eds): Seventh National Cancer Conference Proceedings, p 163. Philadelphia, JB Lippincott, 1972
102. Hill CS Jr, Aldinger KA: Management of anaplastic cancer of the thyroid. In Greenfield LD (ed): Thyroid Cancer, pp 165–176. Boca Raton, CRC Press, 1978
103. Hill CS Jr, Ibanez ML, Samaan NA: Medullary (solid) carcinoma of the thyroid gland: An analysis of the MD Anderson Hospital experience with patients with the tumor, its special features, and its histogenesis. Medicine (Baltimore) 52:141, 1973
104. Hoefnagel CA, Delprat CC, Marcuse HR: Role of TL-201 total body scintigraphy in follow-up of thyroid carcinoma. J Nucl Med 27:1854, 1986
105. Holm L-E, Blomgren H, Lowhagen T: Cancer risks in patients with chronic lymphocytic thyroiditis. N Engl J Med 312:601, 1985
106. Holm L-E, Dahlquist I, Israelsson A, et al: Malignant thyroid tumors after iodine-131 therapy. N Engl J Med 303:188, 1980
107. Holmquest DL, Lake P: Sudden hemorrhage in metastatic thyroid carcinoma of the brain during treatment with iodine-131. J Nucl Med 17:307, 1976
108. Hornbeck NB, Shupe RE, Shidnia H, et al: Preliminary clinical results of combined 433 megahertz microwave therapy and radiation therapy on patients with advanced cancer. Cancer 40:2854, 1977
109. Hurley RJ, Becker DV: The use of radioiodine in the management of thyroid cancer. In Freeman LM, Weissman HS (eds): Nuclear Medicine Annual 1983, pp 329–384. New York, Raven Press, 1983
110. Ivy HK: Cancer metastatic to the thyroid: A diagnostic problem. Mayo Clin Proc 59:856, 1984
111. Iwanaga T, Koyama H, Uchiyama S, et al: Production of several substances by medullary carcinoma of the thyroid. Cancer 41:1106, 1978
112. Jelden GL: CT scanning and computerized radiation therapy treatment planning. In Maruyama Y (ed): New Methods of Tumor Localization, p 313. Lexington, University of Kentucky, 1977
113. Joensuu H, Ahonen A: Imaging and metastasis of thyroid carcinoma with fluorine-18 fluorodeoxyglucose. J Nucl Med 28:910, 1987
114. Johnson D: Personal communication, 1960
115. Johnson DG, Coleman RE, McCook TA, et al: Bone and liver scans in medullary carcinoma of the thyroid. J Nucl Med 25:419, 1984
116. Johnson LA, Polga JP: Follicular adenocarcinoma arising in a thyroglossal duct remnant. Clin Nucl Med 13:378, 1988
117. Kagan AR, Nussbaum H, Chan P, et al: Thyroid carcinoma: Is postoperative external irradiation indicated? Oncology 29:40, 1974
118. Karo JJ, Maas LC, Kaine H, et al: Ultrasonography and parathyroid edema. JAMA 239:2163, 1972
119. Kasai N, Sakamoto A: Malignant transformation of thyroid cancer: Poorly differentiated cancer and anaplastic cancer transformation. Gan No Rinsho 29:A-7, 1983
120. Keenan AM, Harbert JC, Larson SM: Monoclonal antibodies in nuclear medicine. J Nucl Med 26:531, 1985
121. Kier R, Silverman PM, Korobkin M, et al: Malignant teratoma of the thyroid in an adult: CT appearance. J Comput Assist Tomogr 9:174, 1985
122. Kim JH, Hahn EW, Ahmed S: Combination hyperthermia and radiation therapy for malignant melanoma. Cancer 50:478, 1982
123. Kim JH, Leeper RD: Treatment of anaplastic giant and spindle cell carcinoma of the thyroid gland with combination Adriamycin and radiation therapy. Cancer 52:954, 1983
124. Kim JH, Leeper RD: Combination Adriamycin and radiation therapy for locally advanced carcinoma of the thyroid gland. Int J Radiat Oncol Biol Phys 9:565, 1983

125. Kim JH, Leeper R: Treatment of locally advanced thyroid carcinoma with combination Adriamycin and radiation therapy. Int J Radiat Oncol Biol Phys 11(suppl 1):90, 1985
126. Kim JH, Leeper RD: Treatment of locally advanced thyroid carcinoma with combination doxorubicin and radiation therapy. Cancer 60:2372, 1987
127. Kimler JC, Muth WF: Primary malignant teratoma of the thyroid: Case report and literature review of cervical teratoma in adults. Cancer 42:311, 1978
128. Kivel M (ed): Center findings on thyroid cancer induction confirmed by NCI. Radiol Health Bull 22: 1988
129. Koral KF, Alder RS, Carey JE, et al: Two-orthogonal-view method for quantification of rad dose to neck lesions in thyroid cancer therapy patients. Med Phys 9:497, 1982
130. Kuni CC, Klingensmith WC III: Failure of low doses of I-131 to ablate residual thyroid tissue following surgery for thyroid cancer. Radiology 137:773, 1980
131. LaFlamme L, Taillefer R, Duranceau A, et al: Medullary thyroid carcinoma: Localization of a mediastinal metastasis with I-131 MIBG. Clin Nucl Med 13:577, 1988
132. Lakshmanan M, Schaffer A, Robbins J, et al: A simplified low iodine diet in I-131 scanning and therapy of thyroid cancer. Clin Nucl Med 13:866, 1988
133. Larson SM: Radiolabeled monoclonal anti-tumor antibodies in diagnosis and therapy. J Nucl Med 26:538, 1985
134. Lee TC, Harbert JC, Dejter Sw, et al: Vocal cord paralysis following I-131 ablation of a postthyroidectomy remnant. J Nucl Med 26:49, 1985
135. Leeper RD, Simaoka K: Treatment of metastatic thyroid cancer. Clin Endocrinol Metab 9:383, 1980
136. Lemish I, Bennett F, Marten C, et al: A sensitive human thyroglobulin RIA to define clearly the presence or absence of functioning thyroid tissue. J Nucl Med 254:49, 1984
137. Leopold GR: Ultrasonography of superficially located structures. Radiol Clin North Am 18:161, 1980
138. Lim RO: Emergency thyroidectomy for tracheal obstruction. Contemp Surg 29:30, 1986
139. Lindberg RD: External beam irradiation in thyroid cancers. In Fletcher GH (ed): Textbook of Radiotherapy, 3rd ed, pp 384–388. Philadelpha, Lea & Febiger, 1980
140. LiVolsi VA: Pathology of thyroid cancer. In Greenfield LD (ed): Thyroid Cancer, pp 83–141. Boca Raton, CRC Press, 1978
141. Loeffler JS, Mauch PM, Leslie NT, et al: The development of Grave's disease following radiation therapy in Hodgkin's disease. Proceedings of the American Society for Therapeutic Radiology and Oncology, 27th Annual Meeting, vol II, suppl 1, p 156, September, 1985
142. Luk KH: Clinical indications for interstitial hyperthermia. In Steeves RA, Paliwal BR (eds): Syllabus: A Categorical Course in Radiation Therapy/Hyperthermia, pp 111–116. Oak Brook, IL, Radiological Society of North America, 1987
143. Luk KH, Francis ME, Perez CA, et al: Combined radiation and hyperthermia: Comparison of two treatment schedules based on data from a registry established by the Radiation Therapy Oncology Group (RTOG). Int J Radiat Oncol Biol Phys 10:801, 1984
144. Lynn J, Gamrros OI, Taylor S: Medullary carcinoma of the thyroid. World J Surg 5:27, 1981
145. Mailander JC, Graves VB: A thyroid nodule representing metastatic renal carcinoma. Clin Nucl Med 10:650, 1985
146. Martinez JS: Neonatal respiratory distress and thyroid teratoma. Contemp Surg 21:91, 1982
147. Massin JP, Planchon C, Perez R: Comparison of 99m Tc-pertechnetate and 131-I in scanning of thyroid nodule. Clin Nucl Med 2:324, 1977
148. Maxon HR, Thomas SR, Boehringer A, et al: Low iodine diet in I-131 ablation of thyroid remnant. Clin Nucl Med 8:123, 1983
149. Maxon HR, Thomas SR, Saenger EL, et al: Ionizing irradiation and the induction of clinically significant disease in the human thyroid gland. Am J Med 63:967, 1977
150. Mayo Clinic: Fine-needle aspiration of the thyroid. Clinical Update: Current Trends in the Practice of Medicine. [Newsletter] 3:2, 1987
151. Mazzaferri EL, Young RL: Papillary thyroid carcinoma: A 10 year follow-up report of the impact of therapy in 576 patients. Am J Med 70:511, 1981
152. Mazzaferri EL, Young RL, Oertel JE, et al: Papillary thyroid carcinoma: The impact of therapy in 576 patients. Medicine 56:171, 1977
153. McDay JB, Danoff BF: External beam radiotherapy in the management of locally invasive carcinoma of the thyroid. Int J Radiat Oncol Biol Phys 4(suppl 2):226, 1978
154. McDougall IR: Thyroid cancer after iodine-131 therapy. JAMA 227:438, 1974
155. McDougall IR, Krasne D, Handvery JW, et al: Metastatic malignant struma ovarii presenting as paraparesis from a spinal metastasis. J Nucl Med 30:407, 1989
156. McDougall IR, Nelsen TS, Kempson RL: Papillary carcinoma of the thyroid seven years after I-131 therapy for Grave's disease. Clin Nucl Med 6:368, 1981
157. McDougall IR, Saunders W, Coleman CN, et al: Thyroid cancer after high dose neck irradiation for Hodgkin's disease. Third Annual Western Regional Meeting of the Society of Nuclear Medicine, October, 1978
158. Meadows AT, Silber J: Delayed consequences of therapy for childhood cancer. CA 35:271, 1985
159. Meyer JE: Radiographic evaluations of metastatic melanoma. Cancer 42:127, 1978
160. Myers MH, Ries LAG: Cancer patient survival rates: SEER Program results for 10 years of follow-up. CA 39:21, 1989
161. Michael BE, Forouhar FA, Spencer RP: Medullary thyroid carcinoma with radioiodide transport: Effects of iodine-131 therapy and lithium administration. Clin Nucl Med 10:274, 1985
162. Mill WA, Gowing NFC, Reeves B, et al: Carcinoma of the lingual thyroid treated with radioactive iodine. Lancet 1:76, 1959
163. Mill WB, Lee FA, Franssila KO: Radiation therapy treatment of stage I and II extranodal non-Hodgkin's lymphoma of the head and neck. Cancer 45:653, 1980
164. Modan B, Ron E, Werner A: Thyroid cancer following scalp irradiation. Radiology 123:741, 1977
165. Moheshwari YK, Hill CS Jr, Haynie TP III, et al: I-131 therapy in differentiated thyroid carcinoma. Cancer 47:664, 1981
166. Moreno AJ, Sanders LR, Battafarano NJ, Doran TM, Turnbull GL: Non-Hodgkin's lymphoma. Clin Nucl Med 11:801, 1986
167. Morgan GW, Freeman AP, McLean RG, et al: Late cardiac, thyroid, and pulmonary sequelae of mantle radiotherapy for Hodgkin's disease. Int J Radiat Oncol Biol Phys 11:1925, 1985
168. Morimoto J, Yoshimoto Y, Sato K, et al: Serum TSH, thyroglobulin, and thyroidal disorders in atomic bomb survivors exposed in youth: 30-year follow-up study. J Nucl Med 28:1115, 1987
169. Muller N, Cooperberg PL, Suen KCH, et al: Needle aspiration biopsy in cystic papillary carcinoma of the thyroid. AJR 144:251, 1985
170. Nagai GR, Pitts WC, Basso L, Cisco JA, McDougall IR: Scintigraphic hot nodules in thyroid carcinomas. Clin Nucl Med 12:123, 1987
171. National Council on Radiation Protection and Measurements: Induction of thyroid cancer by ionizing radiation: Report no. 80. Bethesda, NCRP Publications, 1985
172. Nelson RM, Bucciarelli RL, Eitzman DV, et al: Serum creatine phosphokinase MB fraction in newborns with transient tricuspid insufficiency. N Engl J Med 295:146, 1978
173. Nemec J, Rohling S, Zamrazid V, et al: Comparison of the distribution of diagnostic and thyroablative I-131 in the evaluation of differentiated thyroid cancers. J Nucl Med 20:92, 1979
174. Noma S, Kanaoka M, Minami S, et al: Thyroid masses: MR imaging and pathological correlation. Radiology 168:759, 1988
175. Nunez EA, Gershon MD: Development of follicular and parafollicular cells of the mammalian thyroid gland. In Greenfield LD (ed): Thyroid Cancer, pp 1–22. Boca Raton, CRC Press, 1978
176. Ober KP, Cowan RJ, Sevier RE, Poole GJ: Thyrotoxocosis caused by functioning metastatic thyroid carcinoma. Clin Nucl Med 12:345, 1987

177. Ochi H, Sawa H, Fukuda T, et al: Thallium-201 chloride thyroid scintigraphy to evaluate benign and/or malignant nodules. Cancer 50:236, 1982
178. Ohta H, Yamamoto K, Endo K, et al: A new imaging agent for medullary carcinoma of the thyroid. J Nucl Med 25:323, 1984
179. Ohta H, Endo K, Fujita T, et al: Sipple's syndrome with liver tumors examined by iodine-131 MIBG and technetium-99m(V)-DMSA. J Nucl Med 29:1130, 1988
180. Overgaard J: Fractionated radiation and hyperthermia: Experimental and clinical studies. Cancer 48:1116, 1981
181. Paloyan E, Lawrence AM, Brooks, MH, et al: Total thyroidectomy and parathyroid autotransplantation for radiation-associated thyroid cancer. Surgery 80:70, 1976
182. Parker LN, Belsky JL, Yamamoto T, et al: Thyroid carcinoma after exposure to atomic radiation: A continuing survey of a fixed population, Hiroshima and Nagasaki, 1958–1971. Ann Intern Med 80:600, 1974
183. Patton JA, Dandler MP, Partain CL: Prediction of benignancy of the solitary "cold" thyroid nodule by fluorescent scanning. J Nucl Med 26:461, 1985
184. Perez CA, Pajak TF, Hornbeck N, et al: Randomized comparison of irradiation plus hyperthermia and radiation alone in superficial malignant tumors. Int J Radiat Oncol Biol Phys 15(suppl 1):122, 1988
185. Piekarski J-D, Schlumberger M, Leclere J, et al: Chest computed tomography (CT) in patients with micronodular lung metastases of differentiated thyroid carcinoma. Int J Radiat Oncol Biol Phys 11:1023, 1985
186. Pinsky S, Bekerman C, Hoffer P: Imaging techniques in the detection of thyroid cancer. In Greenfield LD (ed): Thyroid Cancer, pp 59–84. Boca Raton, CRC Press, 1978
187. Pochin EE: Radioiodine therapy of thryroid cancer. Semin Nucl Med 1:503, 1971
188. Ponder BAJ: Screening for familial medullary thyroid carcinoma: A review. J R Soc Med 77:585, 1984
189. Podoloff DA: SPECT of cancer patients moves into clinical arena. Diagn Imag 11:98, 1989
190. Pont A, Spratt D, Shinn JB: T3 toxicosis due to nonmetastatic follicular carcinoma for the thyroid. West J Med 136:2455, 1982
191. Powell MR, Blum AS: Maximizing radiation dose in radioiodine ablation of normal thyroid tissue and of thyroid cancer metastases. Clin Nucl Med 9(suppl 1):5, 1984
192. Propper RA, Skolnick M, Weinstein BJ, et al: The nonspecificity of the thyroid halo sign. J Clin Ultrasound 8:129, 1980
193. Puylaert JBCM, Pauwels EKJ, Goslings BM, Van Daal WAJ: Thyroid scintigraphy for the detection of radiation-induced thyroid cancer. Clin Nucl Med 10:646, 1985
194. Radin DR, Rosenstein H, Boswell WD, et al: Computed tomography of Sipple syndrome. J Comput Assist Tomogr 8:169, 1984
195. Ramacciotti C, Pretorius HT, Line BR, et al: Ablation of nonmalignant thyroid remnants with low doses of radioactive iodine. [Concise Communication] J Nucl Med 23:483, 1982
196. Ramos-Gabatin A, Pretorius HT: Radionuclide turnover studies on ectopic thyroid glands: Case report and survey of the literature. J Nucl Med 26:258, 1985
197. Razack MS, Sako K, Shimaoka K, et al: Radiation-associated thyroid carcinoma. J Surg Oncol 14:287, 1980
198. Refetoff S, Harrison J, Karanfilski BT, et al: Continuing occurrence of thyroid carcinoma after irradiation to the neck in infancy and childhood. N Engl J Med 292:171, 1975
199. Robbins J: The role of TRH and lithium in the management of thyroid cancer. In Andreoli M, Monaco F, Robbins J (eds): Advances in Thyroid Neoplasia, pp 233–244. Rome, Field Educational Italia, 1981
200. Robertson JS, Gorman CA: Gonadal radiation dose and its genetic significance in radioiodine therapy of hyperthyroidism. J Nucl Med 17:826, 1976
201. Rochman H, De Groot LJ, Rieger CHL: Carcinoembryonic antigen and humoral antibody response in patients with thyroid carcinoma. Cancer Res 35:2689, 1975
202. Rocklin RE, Gagel R, Feldman Z, et al: Cellular immune responses in familial medullary thyroid carcinoma. N Engl J Med 296:835, 1977
203. Rogers JD, Lindberg RD, Hill CS Jr, et al: Spindle giant cell carcinoma of the thyroid: A different therapeutic approach. Cancer 34:1328, 1974
204. Rojeski MT, Gharib H: Nodular thyroid disease: Evaluation and management. N Engl J Med 313:428, 1985
205. Rosenberg EM, Hahn TJ, Orth DN, et al: ACTH-secreting medullary carcinoma of the thyroid presenting as severe idiopathic osteoporosis and senile purpura: Report of a case and review of the literature. J Clin Endocrinol Metab 47:255, 1978
206. Rosenberg RD, Mettler FA Jr, Moseley RD Jr, et al: Thyroid radiation absorbed dose from diagnostic procedures in U.S. population. Radiology 156:183, 1985
207. Roti E, Robuschi G, Emanuele R, et al: The value of serum thyroglobulin measurement as a marker of cancer recurrence in the follow-up for patients previously treated for differentiated thyroid tumor. J Endocrinol Invest 5:43, 1982
208. Roudebush CP, Asteris GT, DeGroot LJ: Natural history of radiation-associated thyroid cancer. Arch Intern Med 138:1631, 1978
209. Rougier P, Parmentier C, Laplanche A, et al: Medullary thyroid carcinoma: Prognostic factors and treatment. Int J Radiat Oncol Biol Phys 9:161, 1983
210. Rudders RA, Ross ME, DeLellis RA: Primary extranodal lymphoma: Response to treatment and factors influencing prognosis. Cancer 42:406, 1978
211. Ryo UY, Vaidya P, Schneider A, et al: Histopathology of thyroid lesions that caused discrepant findings between Tc-99m and I-123 scan. [Abstract] J Nucl Med 20:678, 1979
212. Saad MF, Guido JJ, Samaan NA: Radioactive iodine in the treatment of medullary carcinoma of the thyroid. J Clin Endocrinol Metab 57:124, 1983
213. Safa AM, Schumacher OP, Rodriguez-Autenez A: Long-term follow-up results in children and adolescents treated with radioiodine (^{131}I) for hyperthyroidism. N Engl J Med 292:167, 1975
214. Sarker SD, Beierwaltes WH, Gill SP, et al: Subsequent fertility and birth histories of children and adolescents treated with I-131 for thyroid cancer. J Nucl Med 17:460, 1976
215. Shambaugh GE, Quinn JL, Oyasu R, et al: Disparate thyroid imaging: Combined studies with sodium pertechnetate Tc-99m and radioactive iodine. JAMA 228:866, 1974
216. Sandler MP: The expanding role of MIBG in clinical medicine. [Editorial] J Nucl Med 29:1457, 1988
217. Shapiro B, Copp JE, Sisson JC, et al: Iodine-131 metaiodobenzylguanidine for the locating of suspected pheochromocytoma: Experience in 400 cases. J Nucl Med 26:576, 1985
218. Schatz H, Maser E, Teuber J, et al: The significance of serum thyroglobulin determination for monitoring of patients after thyroidectomy for differentiated thyroid carcinoma. Verh Dtsch Ges Inn Med 87:587, 1981
219. Scheible W, Leopold GR, Woo VL: High resolution real-time ultrasonography of thyroid nodules. Radiology 13:413, 1979
220. Schneider AB, Favus MJ, Stachura ME, et al: Plasma thyroglobulin in detecting thyroid carcinoma after childhood head and neck irradiation. Ann Intern Med 86:29, 1977
221. Schull WJ, Kato H: Malignancies and exposure of the young to ionizing radiation. Cancer Bull 34:84, 1982
222. Schwartz AE, Nieburgs HE, Davies TF, et al: The place of fine needle biopsy in the diagnosis of nodules of the thyroid. Surg Gynecol Obstet 155:54, 1982
223. Sheline GE, Galante M, Lindsay S: Radiation therapy in the control of persistent thyroid cancer. AJR 97:923, 1966
224. Shimaoka K, Sokal JE, Pickren JW: Metastatic neoplasms in the thyroid gland: Pathological and clinical findings. Cancer 15:557, 1962
225. Siddiqui AR, Edmondson J, Wellman HN, et al: Feasibility of low doses of I-131 for thyroid ablation in postsurgical patients with thyroid carcinoma. Clin Nucl Med 6:158, 1986
226. Silver L: Squamous cell carcinoma cell of the thyroid. Clin Nucl Med 13:346, 1988
227. Silverberg E, Boring CC, Squires TS: Cancer statistics, 1990. CA 40(1):9, 1990
228. Silverman PM, Newman GE, Korobkin M, et al: Computed tomography in the evaluation of thyroid disease. AJR 141:897, 1984
229. Silverman PM, Degesys GE, Ferguson BJ, Bierre AR: Case

report: Papillary carcinoma in thyroglossal duct. CT findings. J Comput Assist Tomogr 9:806, 1985
230. Simeone JF, Daniels GH, Hall DA, et al: Sonography in a follow-up of 100 patients with thyroid carcinoma. AJR 148:45, 1987
231. Simon GE: Creatine kinase isoenzymes. West J Med 141:101, 1984
232. Simpson W, Palmer J, Rosen I, et al: Management of medullary carcinoma of the thyroid. Am J Surg 144:420, 1982
233. Simpson W, Sutcliffe S, Gospodarowicz M: The thyroid. In Moss W, Cox J (eds): Radiation Oncology: Rationale, Technique, Results, p 262. St. Louis, CV Mosby, 1989
234. Simpson WJ: Radiotherapy in thyroid cancer. Can Med Assoc J 113:115, 1975
235. Simpson CL, Hempelmann LN, Fuller LM: Neoplasia in children treated with x-rays in infancy for thymic enlargement. Radiology 64:840, 1955
236. Singer PA: Fine-needle aspiration biopsy of thyroid nodules. Current Topics in Thyroid Diseases [Newsletter] 8:1, 1986
237. Singer PA: Primary lymphoma of the thyroid. Current Topics in Thyroid Disease [Newsletter] 9:1, 1987
238. Smith R, Blum C, Benua RS, Fawwaz RA: Radioactive iodine treatment of metastatic thyroid carcinoma with clinical throtoxicosis. Clin Nucl Med 10:874, 1985
239. Som PM, Sacher M, Lanzieri CF, et al: Two benign CT presentations of thyroid-related papillary adenocarcinoma. J Comput Assist Tomogr 9:162, 1985
240. Sone T, Fukunaga M, Otsuka N, et al: Metastatic medullary thyroid cancer: Localization with iodine-131 meta-iodobenzylguanidine. J Nucl Med 26:604, 1985
241. Spencer CA, Lai-Rosenfeld AO, Guttler RB: Thyrotropin secretion in thyrotoxic and thyroxine treated patients: Assessment by a sensitive immunoenzymometric assay. J Clin Endocrinol Metab 63:349, 1986
242. Spencer RP: Medullary thyroid carcinoma: Radiotracers in therapy and evaluation of primary or metastatic sites. J Nucl Med 25:514, 1984
243. Spencer RP, Chapman CN, Rao H: Thyroid carcinoma after radioiodine therapy for hyperthyroidism: Analysis based on age, latency, and administered dose of I-131. Clin Nucl Med 8:216, 1983
244. Spiegel W, Reiners C, Borner W: Sialadenitis following iodine-131 therapy for thyroid carcinoma. [Letter to the Editor] J Nucl Med 26:816, 1985
245. Sridama V, Hara Y, Fauchet R, De Groot LJ: Association of differentiated thyroid carcinoma with HLA-DR7. Cancer 56:1086, 1985
246. Steinfeld AD: The role of radiation therapy in medullary carcinoma of the thyroid. Radiology 123:745, 1977
247. Strand S-E, Erlandsson K, Löwenhielm P: Thyroid uptake of ^{131}I and ^{133}I from Chernobyl and the population of Southern Sweden. J Nucl Med 29:1719, 1988
248. Sutow WW, Conard RA, Thompson KH: Thyroid injury and effects on growth and development in the Marshallese children accidentally exposed to radioactive fallout. Cancer Bull 34:90, 1982
249. Sutton RT, Reading CC, Charboneau JW: US-guided biopsy of neck masses and postoperative management of patients with thyroid cancer. Radiology 168:769, 1988
250. Syed AMN, Greenfield LD: The role of interstitial irradiation in the treatment of thyroid cancer. Contemp Surg 17:36, 1980
251. Sziklas JJ, Matthews J, Spencer RR, et al: Thyroid carcinoma metastatic to the pituitary. J Nucl Med 9:1097, 1985
252. Takashima S, Akezoe J, Morimoto S, et al: Primary thyroid lymphoma: Evaluation with CT. Radiology 168:765, 1988
253. Tallroth E, Wallin G, Lundell G, et al: Multimodality treatment in anaplastic giant cell thyroid carcinoma. Cancer 60:1428, 1987
254. Thambi V, Pedapatti PJ, Murthy A, et al: A radiotherapy technique for thyroid cancer. Int J Radiat Oncol Biol Phys 6:239, 1980
255. Thomas SR, Maxon HR, Kereiakes JG, et al: Quantitative external counting techniques enabling improved diagnostic and therapeutic decisions in patients with well-differentiated thyroid cancer. Radiology 122:731, 1977
256. Tubiana M: External radiotherapy and radioiodine in the treatment of thyroid cancer. World J Surg 5:75, 1981
257. Tubiana M: Thyroid cancer. In Beckers C (ed): Thyroid Diseases, pp 187–227. Paris, Pergamon, 1982
258. Tubiana M, Haddad E, Schlumberger M, et al: External radiotherapy in thyroid cancers. Cancer 55:2062, 1985
259. Tubiana M, Lacour J, Monnier JP, et al: External radiotherapy and radioiodine in the treatment of 359 thyroid cancers. Br J Radiol 48:894, 1975
260. Tupchong L, Phil D, Hughes F, et al: Primary lymphoma of the thyroid: Clinical features, prognostic factors, and results of treatment. Int J Radiat Oncol Biol Phys 12:1813, 1986
261. Turrin A, Pilotti S, Ricci SB: Characteristics of thyroid cancer following irradiation. Int J Radiat Oncol Biol Phys 11:2149, 1985
262. U.S. Dept of Health, Education and Welfare: Information for Physicians: Irradiation-Related Thyroid Cancer. Washington, DC, United States Department of Health, 1977
263. University of Texas System Cancer Center, M.D. Anderson Hospital and Tumor Institute: Immunotherapy of Human Cancer: Second Annual Clinical Conference on Cancer. New York, Raven Press, 1978
264. Van Herle AJ: Pathophysiology of thyroid cancer. In Greenfield LD (ed): Thyroid Cancer, pp 23–36. Boca Raton, CRC Press, 1978
265. Van Nostrand D, Neutze J, Atkins F: Side effects of "rational dose" iodine-131 therapy for metastatic well differentiated thyroid carcinoma. J Nucl Med 27:1519, 1986
266. Velchik MG, Alavi A, Kressel H, et al: Localization of pheochromocytoma: MIBG, CT and MRI correlation. J Nucl Med 30:328, 1989
267. Vigliotti A, Kong JS, Fuller LM, et al: Thyroid lymphomas stages IE and IIIE: Comparative results for radiotherapy only, combination chemotherapy only, and multimodality treatment. Int J Radiat Oncol Biol Phys 12:1807, 1986
268. VonNoll L, McEwan A, Shapiro B, et al: Iodine-131 MIBG scintigraphy of neuroendocrine tumors other than pheochromocytoma and neuroblastoma. J Nucl Med 28:979, 1987
269. Walts AE: Fine needle aspiration of the thyroid-review of a valuable diagnostic technique. Clin Otolaryngol 7:205, 1982
270. Waxman A, Ramanna L, Chapman N, et al: The significance of I-131 scan dose in patients with thyroid cancer: Determination of ablation. [Concise Communication] J Nucl Med 22:861, 1981
271. Weissel M, Kainz H, Höfer R: Changes in biochemical parameters during complete thyroid hormone deficiency of short duration in athyreotic patients. J Nucl Med 27:1528, 1986
272. Winship T, Rosvoll RV: Thyroid carcinoma in childhood: Final report on a 20-year study. Clin Proc Child Hosp Natl Med Center 26:327, 1970
273. Winzelberg GG, Hydovitz JD, O'Hara KR, et al: Parathyroid adenomas evaluated by Tl-201/Tc-99m pertechnetate subtraction scintigraphy and high-resolution ultrasonography. Radiology 155:231, 1985
274. Wolfe HJ, Delellis RA: Familial medullary thyroid carcinoma and C cell hyperplasia. Clin Endocrinol Metab 10:351, 1981
275. Wool MS: Management of papillary and follicular cancer. In Greenfield LD (ed): Thyroid Cancer, pp 143–150. Boca Raton, CRC Press, 1978
276. Woolner LB, Beahrs OH, Black BM, et al: Thyroid carcinoma: General considerations and follow-up data on 1181 cases. In Young S, Inman DR (eds): Thyroid Neoplasia, p 51. New York, Academic Press, 1968
277. World Health Organization: International Histological Classification of Tumors, vols 1–25. Geneva, WHO, 1957–1981
278. Yagi Y, Yagi S, Saku T: The localization of cytoskeletal proteins and thyroglobulin in thyroid microcarcinoma in comparison with clinically manifested thyroid carcinoma. Cancer 56:1967, 1985
279. Yoosufani Z, Slavin JD Jr, Hellman RM, Sethi SS, Spencer RP: Preleukemia following large dose radioiodide therapy for metastatic thyroid carcinoma. J Nucl Med 28:1348, 1987
280. Young RL, Mazzaferri EL, Rahe AJ, et al: Pure follicular thyroid carcinoma: Impact of therapy in 214 patients. J Nucl Med 21:733, 1980

APPENDIX 65-1

Procedures for Administration of ^{131}I

PLANNING

Order ^{131}I at least 48 hours in advance. Schedule patient for hospital admission.

ROOM PREPARATION

Charcoal filters in room air system and exhaust vent in hallway. Must cover with plastic bags: telephone receiver, telephone, food table, basin faucet handles, nurse call set. Disposable mats next to bed, commode, and shower. Seat liners for commode. Two radiation waste containers in room for laundry and foods/paper.

PATIENT PREPARATION

Instruct how to replace and dispose of covers and mats. Instruct to keep outside door closed and bathroom door open at all times. Obtain vital signs, blood and urine samples before ^{131}I administration.

ADMINISTRATION

Patient must wear hospital gown with a "chuck" around neck and in lap. Personnel administering ^{131}I should wear gown, gloves, and mask.

Vial containing ^{131}I should be vented in nuclear medicine hood to allow any volatile ^{131}I to escape just before administration. During administration, the patient should sit on the side of the bed in front of the ^{131}I, which is in a lead vial on a covered table. Instruct patient to open vial with T-bar, insert drinking straw, put small amount of water in vial (along straw so it doesn't splash). Patient takes ^{131}I through straw with additional water placed in lead vial to remove as much ^{131}I as possible. Swish and swallow several cups of water to rinse ^{131}I from oral cavity. Do not remove straw from vial; bend it over and carefully place lead cap on.

INITIAL SURVEY

Within 15 minutes, measure the radiation exposure rate at 1 m from the midline of patient's abdomen in both anteroposterior and lateral directions. Calculate the average. Patient may be released when same readings show less than 30 mCi of ^{131}I, which is usually about 48 to 72 hours after 100 mCi was given, but that is highly variable.

Posted on room door must be room diagram showing safety shield positions, inventory or survey form with initial activity and exposure rate, nursing instructions, and decontamination form. Do not collect urine unless lead container is available, and there is a specific reason.

SAFETY

Nursing recommendations: No pregnant nurses. Nurse should not be assigned to care for more than one radioactive patient a month. At <30 mCi ^{131}I, discharge (or exposure rate of 5 mr/hr at 1 meter).

Visiting discouraged: limit 0.5 hr/day/visitor; no children under 18 years or pregnant women. Visitors should wear gown, gloves, and mask and sit in designated chair across room. If they come close to patient, they should sit behind lead shield.

Patients should wear hospital gowns, not personal clothing (^{131}I in sweat, breath) and should leave bed only to go to bathroom or designated chair. They should drink copious amounts of water to speed release of unused radioactivity, shower frequently, flush toilet several times after each use. Males should urinate seated. There should be no personal items except those to be disposed of at discharge.

After discharge, patients should sleep alone for 3 days, and sleep alone for 1 week if wife is pregnant. Don't hold children closely for 3 days.

66

Bone

Robert J. Bertoli
Luther W. Brady

With a special section on
EWING'S SARCOMA

Patrick R.M. Thomas

Primary malignant bone neoplasms are relatively rare. The most common skeletal tumors, osteosarcoma, Ewing's sarcoma, chondrosarcoma, fibrosarcoma, malignant fibrous histiocytoma of bone, giant cell tumor, and aneurysmal bone cyst, are discussed in this chapter.

ANATOMIC CONSIDERATIONS

Approximately 50% to 60% of osteosarcomas are located in the distal femur or proximal tibia; the third most common site is the proximal humerus. In 75% of the patients, the disease occurs in tubular long bones, although in patients over 24 years of age, 41% of lesions are located in flat bones (Paget's disease association). Classic osteosarcoma is characteristically metaphyseal in origin, with only 9% developing in diaphyseal sites and 1% in epiphyseal sites.[25,26,71] Chondrosarcomas are truncal (including the shoulder girdle and proximal femur and humerus) in 75% of the patients. Chondrosarcoma most commonly involves the femur, with a striking predilection for the secondary ossification centers.[25,71,106] Chondrosarcomas arising *de novo* present most commonly in the femur; secondary chondrosarcomas are most prevalent in the ilium (31%). Most long bone chondrosarcomas are metaphyseal or diaphyseal.[51,85,106]

Primary skeletal fibrosarcomas, malignant fibrous histiocytomas, and malignant giant cell tumors arise most commonly in tubular long bones, usually the femur or tibia. Most fibrosarcomas are metaphyseal or epiphyseal in origin. Malignant fibrous histiocytomas are usually metaphyseal, and giant cell tumors are epiphyseal.[25,71,85] Aneurysmal bone cysts can present in almost any bone but have a predilection for the long tubular bones (usually lower extremity) and the vertebrae, including the sacrum.[49,106]

EPIDEMIOLOGY

Osteosarcoma is the most common primary bone tumor (excluding myeloma), comprising 20% of all primary skeletal malignancies. Peak incidence is in the second decade of life (60% of cases); 85% occur before age 35. Lichtenstein[71] reported a second, smaller peak in older patients with Paget's disease. The male-to-female ratio is 3 : 2 in patients older than 15 years, but it is equal among patients younger than 15 years.[25,71] Osteosarcomas usually arise *de novo*. An increased incidence has been reported for taller patients.[85,106] No association with previous trauma has been established.

Chondrosarcoma is approximately half as common as osteosarcoma and accounts for 10% to 20% of malignant primary bone tumors. Patient ages range from 7 to 73 years, but most tumors are diagnosed in patients between 30 and 60 years of age. Clear cell chondrosarcoma is not seen in children; the average age for mesenchymal chondrosarcoma is 26 years. Males predominate slightly in most chondrosarcoma and clear cell chondrosarcoma series, but mesenchymal chondrosarcoma occurs more frequently in women. Conditions that predispose to chondrosarcoma include Ollier's disease, Paget's disease, Maffucci's syndrome, previous intravenous Thorotrast exposure, chondromyxoid fibroma, and previous radiation therapy.[7,25,49,71]

Fibrosarcoma of bone represents 2% to 6% of primary malignant bone lesions. Most patients present between the ages of 30 and 70. Approximately one third are associated with predisposing factors such as Paget's disease, fibrous dysplasia, osteomyelitis, bone infarcts, bone cysts, benign giant cell tumors, desmoplastic fibromas, or previous radiation treatment. The tumors occur equally in males and females.[51,85,106]

Malignant fibrous histiocytoma of bone accounts for less than 1% of primary bone malignancies and has a slight male predominance. Incidence peaks occur in the third and sixth decades of life. Cases have been reported of malignant fibrous histiocytomas developing within previously irradiated fields.[52,106,110]

Giant cell tumors account for 4% to 8% of all primary bone tumors and 0.5% of all malignant primary bone lesions. Approximately 7.5% to 15% of all giant cell tumors are malignant. Most occur in the third and fourth decades. There is a slight female predominance, which is more prominent among patients younger than 20 years. Postirradiation malignant degeneration of benign giant cell tumors has been widely reported.[25,50,71,106]

Aneurysmal bone cysts account for 1% of primary bone lesions. There is a slight female predominance, and 70% occur in patients between 5 and 20 years of age. Aneurysmal bone cysts may arise secondarily from chondroblastomas, giant cell tumors, chondromyxoid fibromas, xanthomas, or fibrous dysplasias.[25,80,85]

NATURAL HISTORY

Before the advent of active chemotherapeutic agents, the 5-year survival rate was approximately 20% for patients with osteosarcomas without metastatic disease. Approximately 17% of patients have distant metastases at presentation.[25] The primary mode of metastasis for osteosarcoma is hematogenous, and metastases are usually to the lungs initially. Farrell and coworkers[37] found that approximately 80% of patients who had lung metastases developed them within 18 months of presentation. Uribe-Botero and colleagues[124] described pulmonary metastases in 98% of osteosarcoma patients at autopsy; bone metastases were present in 37%, and the pleura and heart were involved in 33% and 20%, respectively. Jeffree and associates[59] found extrapulmonary metastases in 83% of patients at autopsy and also confirmed the finding that the median time for presentation of lung metastases in patients with radiographically normal lungs at the outset was 5 to 6 months. Lymph node metastases are uncommon.

Parosteal osteosarcomas are usually low-grade malignant lesions. They are commonly localized, and pulmonary metastases are rare. Between 80% and 90% are curable with surgery alone.[74] Periosteal osteosarcomas are clinically less aggressive than classic osteosarcomas; only four of 23 patients in the Mayo Clinic series succumbed to distant metastatic disease.[121] Small cell osteosarcoma resembles Ewing's sarcoma and may behave in a similar manner clinically.[25,79] Long-term survival has been reported with combined irradiation and multiagent chemotherapy, but the reported number of cases is small.[25] Matsuno and associates[81] found that telangiectatic osteosarcoma had a worse prognosis than classical osteosarcoma, but this was not confirmed in the Memorial Sloan-Kettering experience.[53] Mandibular osteosarcomas are much less frequently associated with hematogenous dissemination and have a 3-year survival rate of 80%.[25,113] Low-grade central intramedullary osteosarcomas are usually associated with protracted histories and a lower rate of distant metastases.[25]

Chondrosarcomas are locally aggressive lesions with a high propensity for local recurrence, which usually occurs within 5 years of treatment. Head and truncal chondrosarcomas have as much as an 85% chance of recurring at the primary site.[48,71] Chondrosarcomas generally follow a more indolent course than classic osteosarcoma. The most common site of distant metastasis is the lungs; less frequent sites of involvement include bone, liver, kidney, breast, and brain.[71,106] Up to 10% of chondrosarcomas can dedifferentiate into aggressive fibrosarcomas or osteosarcomas.[25] Chondrosarcomas in the pediatric age group are clinically aggressive lesions and behave like classic osteosarcoma.[106]

Fibrosarcomas are locally aggressive lesions with a metastatic potential related to histologic grade. High-grade lesions behave like classic osteosarcomas and have a 27% 5-year survival rate.[25,56] Periosteal and low-grade fibrosarcomas are less aggressive. Five-year and 10-year survival rates for periosteal fibrosarcomas are both approximately 50%.[51]

Malignant fibrous histiocytomas of bone are also very aggressive locally with a high propensity for metastatic dissemination, most frequently to lungs; involvement of other bones, soft tissues, liver, and skin has been reported. Five-year survival rates range from 15% to 67%. Most recurrences appear within 21 months of diagnosis.[27,130]

Benign giant cell tumors have a high propensity for local recurrence. In rare instances these benign tumors may metastasize to lung without malignant transformation.[25,106] The dedifferentiated lesions are usually high-grade fibrosarcomas. The local recurrence rate ranges from 45% to 60%.[24,76] Hutter and associates[50] found that initial surgery effected a cure in 38% of their patients, and 81% of the recurrences appeared within 2 years of therapy. Sixty-nine percent of the patients were cured after a second surgery. Malignant transformation must be strongly suspected if recurrence is discovered more than 5 years after treatment. The mortality rate in patients with malignant giant cell tumor is 70%. Hutter and co-workers[50] observed that malignant degeneration after only surgical therapy tends to appear earlier, usually 1 to 2 years after surgery, and is usually of a lower histologic grade than lesions appearing after radiation therapy. Sacral giant cell tumors have a more aggressive clinical course and a worse prognosis than giant cell tumors of other sites.[86]

CLINICAL PRESENTATION

Patients with osteosarcoma usually present with nonspecific local pain and swelling in the involved area. Joint effusions and pathologic fractures are uncommon.[40,61] Parosteal osteosarcoma has a more prolonged, indolent history.[25]

Chondrosarcoma, fibrosarcoma, malignant fibrous histiocytoma, and giant cell tumor of bone have clinical presentations similar to that of osteosarcoma although duration of symptoms may be somewhat longer.[25] Pathologic fractures are more common with malignant fibrous histiocytoma and fibrosarcoma.[71,85,106] Other presenting symptoms and signs include neurologic abnormalities in vertebral lesions, decreased range of motion of the involved extremity, and muscular atrophy.[25,106]

DIAGNOSTIC WORKUP

The suggested diagnostic workup for osteosarcoma, chondrosarcoma, fibrosarcoma, malignant fibrous histiocytoma, and malignant giant cell tumor is outlined in Table 66-1.

Radiographically, classic osteosarcoma is usually a metaphyseal, ill-defined lesion with evident osteoid formation. Bone destruction with highly irregular periosteal new bone formation ("sunburst appearance") is evident. Codman's triangle is not specific for osteosarcoma or even for malignancy. An accompanying soft tissue mass immediately adjacent to the destroyed bone helps in making the diagnosis.[28] Parosteal osteosarcoma usually presents in the popliteal fossa as a dense, lobulated mass of homogeneous new bone that extends from the cortex.[25]

Computed tomography (CT) and magnetic resonance imaging (MRI) can assist in evaluating intramedullary and extraosseous soft tissue extent of disease and are useful in planning radiation therapy or surgery. CT scans (1-cm sections) of the chest are more accurate than chest radiography and conventional tomography in detecting early lung metastases. Angiography is used to delineate tumor blood supply preoperatively, for intraarterial chemotherapy, and for ra-

TABLE 66–1
Diagnostic Workup for Bone Tumors

GENERAL
History
Physical examination

SPECIAL STUDIES
Biopsy-open, avoiding incision over area not to be irradiated
Bone marrow aspiration and biopsy (for Ewing's sarcoma)

RADIOGRAPHIC STUDIES
Standard
- Plain radiography of bone and chest
- Computed tomography of affected bone, surrounding soft tissue, and lungs
- Radionuclide bone scan
- Magnetic resonance imaging of affected bone and surrounding soft tissue

Optional
- Angiography

LABORATORY STUDIES
Complete blood count on admission
Blood chemistry
Urinalysis
Erythrocyte sedimentation rate

diosensitizer infusion.[74,129] Bone scans are indicated in the initial evaluation of the patient with osteosarcoma and for routine reevaluation.[109]

Laboratory and radiologic workup for chondrosarcoma, fibrosarcoma, malignant fibrous histiocytoma, and malignant giant cell tumor is similar to that for osteosarcoma.

Classic chondrosarcoma is characterized on radiography by "fluffy" or "windblown," irregular, mottled calcifications differing in appearance from the osteosarcoma osteoid.[28] A thickened or scalloped cortex is possible with fusiform bone expansion, but significant cortical destruction is a late finding.[51] Mesenchymal chondrosarcoma more often involves the ribs and mandible and is primarily lytic; 75% of lesions have tumoral calcifications.[25]

Fibrosarcomas are lytic with no reactive sclerosis. High-grade lesions are permeative with cortical destruction and periosteal reaction (less than osteosarcomas); a soft tissue mass is not uncommon.[106] Except for the lack of osteoid production, there is little to differentiate fibrosarcomas and osteosarcomas on x-ray examination.[25]

The primary bone lesions of malignant fibrous histiocytoma are radiolucent and ill-defined; there is often cortical destruction and soft tissue extension. Periosteal reaction is rare. Pathologic fractures, however, are common. The lesion is predominantly metaphyseal and frequently shows epiphyseal extension.[28,51,110]

Typical radiographic findings with giant cell tumors of bone include thinning and expansion of the cortex by a predominantly lytic lesion in the epiphysis. Periosteal reaction is usually lacking. Soft tissue extension and pathologic fracture are possible, and extension to the articular end of the bone is common. Arteriography reveals marked tumor vascularity with arteriovenous fistula formation. It is not possible to differentiate benign from malignant giant cell tumors by radiographic examination.[25,28] After irradiation, the lesion may ossify over a few years. The Herendeen phenomenon is a rare, paradoxical enlargement of a giant cell tumor shortly after radiation therapy. The lesion may remain large for months but confers no worsening of the prognosis.[17,51]

Aneurysmal bone cysts are metaphyseal or diaphyseal expansile lesions characterized by a "blow-out" appearance with internal septae and ridges.[28] They are usually well defined and purely osteolytic. Aneurysmal bone cysts can involve the epiphysis only after closure of the growth plate.[106]

STAGING

There is no universally accepted staging system for primary bone sarcomas. The Enneking staging system classifies tumors according to grade, local extent of disease, and presence or absence of distant metastases (Table 66-2).[33]

PATHOLOGIC CLASSIFICATION

Osteosarcomas

Classic osteosarcoma is usually poorly differentiated; 85% of lesions are grade 3 or grade 4 and less than 1% are grade 1. The tumors may be predominantly osteoblastic (50%), fibroblastic (25%), or chondroblastic (25%); there is no major prognostic difference among the three groups.[25]

Osteosarcoma commonly breaches the cortex and extends to the soft tissue. There are usually varying amounts of cyst

TABLE 66–2
Enneking Staging System for Bone Sarcomas

GRADE (G)	
G1, low grade	Parosteal osteosarcoma
	Endosteal osteosarcoma
	Secondary chondrosarcoma
	Fibrosarcoma, low grade
	Atypical malignant fibrous histiocytoma
	Giant cell tumor
	Adamantinoma
G2, high grade	Classic osteosarcoma
	Radiation-induced sarcoma
	Paget's sarcoma
	Primary chondrosarcoma
	Fibrosarcoma, high grade
	Malignant fibrous histiocytoma
	Giant cell sarcoma
LOCAL EXTENT (T)	
T1, intracompartmental	Intraosseous
	Paraosseous
	Intrafascial
T2, extracompartmental	Soft tissue extension
	Extrafascial or deep fascial extension
METASTASES (M)	
M0	No distant metastases
M1	Distant metastases exist

STAGE GROUPING

Stage			
IA	G1	T1	M0
IB	G1	T2	M0
IIA	G2	T1	M0
IIB	G2	T2	M0
III	G1 or G2	T1 or T2	M1

(Enneking WF, Spanier SS, Goodman MA: Clin Orthop 153:106, 1980)

formation, hemorrhage, and necrosis, which is an important point when the radiosensitivity of these lesions is being considered. The lesion can spread extensively in the marrow cavity.[71] Enneking has stressed the importance of skip metastases. A skip metastasis is a second smaller focus of osteosarcoma in the same bone or a second bone lesion on the opposing side of a joint space with no gross or microscopic continuity or pulmonary metastases. Enneking and Kagan[31,32] found that skip metastases occurred in 25% of their series of osteosarcoma specimens. Simon and Hecht[108] reported invasion of articular cartilage by osteosarcoma in 35% of their patients and a high incidence of extension along the cruciate ligaments. Enneking and Kagan[32] also found a high proportion of transepiphyseal spread (preclosure) of tumor cells, presumably along vascular channels.

Lichtenstein,[71] Dahlin and Coventry,[23] and Schajowicz[106] found stump recurrences at the site of transmedullary amputation of the involved bone only rarely and skip metastases infrequently.[25] In fact, Springfield[111] and the Florida group found that there was no decrease in local control rate for a wide surgical margin with a functional limb remaining compared with treatment by amputation. Parosteal (juxtacortical) osteosarcoma is less aggressive and constitutes approximately 4% of these lesions.[25] Cortical disruption is unusual. Almost all juxtacortical osteosarcoma is in the femur, tibia, or humerus; the posterior distal shaft of the femur (popliteal fossa) is the most common site. Luck and associates[74] found areas of high-grade sarcoma in some parosteal osteosarcomas (usually low-grade malignancies); this finding and medullary extension worsened the prognosis.

Periosteal or peripheral osteosarcoma comprises 1% of all osteosarcomas and is slightly more aggressive histologically than parosteal osteosarcoma. The lesions are predominately cartilaginous and have a predilection for the femur and tibia, often at or near the midshaft.[25,46] Involvement is frequently limited to the cortex and periosteum. Small cell osteosarcoma resembles Ewing's sarcoma but is characterized by the production of an osteoid matrix and is rare.[80] Mandibular osteosarcoma presents in an older age group and is characterized by a significantly more differentiated histology. Telangiectatic osteosarcoma shows prominent areas of hemorrhage and only scant osteoid production. The lesions are usually metaphyseal and primarily lytic, with an increased incidence of pathologic fractures compared with other types of osteosarcoma.[36,53]

Chondrosarcomas

The chondrosarcoma lesions are graded 1 to 3 (3 is least differentiated); grade is an important prognostic indicator.[15,67] In the M. D. Anderson Cancer Center study, 43% of the chondrosarcoma lesions were grade 1, 32% were grade 2, and 25% were grade 3.[97] The number of mitoses and the degree of cellularity are important in determining grade.[25,106]

Histologic analysis reveals that chondrosarcoma may invade the adjacent joint and infiltrate beyond the x-ray "margin" of the tumor within the marrow cavity.[85] Average lesion size in the femur is 11 cm; the average pelvic tumor is 13 cm (range, 2–32 cm).[51]

Clear cell chondrosarcoma is usually low grade and may represent the malignant transformation of a chondroblastoma.[122] Mesenchymal chondrosarcoma is an undifferentiated, vascular neoplasm.[25] Juxtacortical chondrosarcoma arises from the external surface of the involved bone and is usually low grade; it seldom infiltrates the cortex.[106]

Malignant Fibrous Histiocytomas

Malignant fibrous histiocytoma of bone is a primitive, undifferentiated pleomorphic sarcoma with histiocytic and fibroblastic differentiation. The histiocyte or macrophage is the probable cell of origin. The extent of local spread on pathologic examination is almost always greater than is visible by routine radiography.[25,110,130]

Giant Cell Tumors

Giant cell tumors or osteoclastomas are characterized by a uniformly distributed increase in multinucleated giant cells. Grading is not prognostically reliable.[24,45] Malignant giant cell tumors are characterized by a massive spindle cell sarcomatous stroma.[51,71]

Aneurysmal Bone Cysts

Aneurysmal bone cysts are composed of fibro-osseous septae without endothelial coverings surrounded by nonclotted blood. There is no anaplasia. The walls may contain slivers of osteoid, woven bone, inflammatory cells, or osteoclasts.[25]

PROGNOSTIC FACTORS

The most important prognostic factor in osteosarcoma is metastasis at presentation. The Mayo Clinic cited five unfavorable prognostic factors in their case review of osteosarcoma: treatment before 1969, duration of symptoms for less than 6 months, male sex, proximal extremity primary lesion, and patient age less than 10 years.[118] Dahlin[25] reported a worse prognosis for radiation-induced osteosarcoma. Sutow and associates[116] found no significant difference in survival rates for patients treated for metastatic disease when sex, race, primary site, and site of first metastasis were compared.

Prognostic factors in chondrosarcoma include histologic grade, size, cell type, location, stage at presentation, patient age, degree of local aggressiveness, and presence or absence of pain at presentation.[51] In the M. D. Anderson series, metastases from chondrosarcoma developed in none of the grade 1 patients, in 10% of the grade 2 patients, and in 73% of the grade 3 patients; 5-year survival rates were 90%, 81%, and 43% for grade 1, grade 2, and grade 3, respectively.[109] Similar rates of metastatic spread were found in the Bristol review.[104] In the Mayo Clinic report, 10-year survival rates were 77%, 55%, and 35% for grade 1, grade 2, and grade 3, respectively.[25] Corresponding 10-year survival rates at the M. D. Anderson Cancer Center were 87%, 64%, and 29%.[97]

Mesenchymal and dedifferentiated chondrosarcomas are more virulent; clear cell and juxtacortical lesions are less aggressive than classic chondrosarcoma.[25,88,106,122] Patients with chondrosarcoma have a better median survival (27 months) than those with osteosarcoma (13.5 months). The 2-year survival rate in the chondrosarcoma group examined by Huvos[51] was 54%; the 5-year survival rate was 37%. Dahlin[25] reported 5- and 10-year survival rates of 61% and 41% for chondrosarcoma; Schajowicz[106] reported survival rates of 48.5% and 23% for 5 and 10 years, respectively.

The metastatic rate for low-grade fibrosarcoma is 5% to 15%, compared with the rate of distant metastases for high-grade fibrosarcoma, which is equal to that of osteosarcoma.[85,106] The overall survival rate is 34% at 5 years, 28% at 10 years, and 25% at 20 years. Duration of survival for patients with periosteal fibrosarcoma is about twice that for patients with medullary lesions.[51]

Malignant fibrous histiocytoma is very aggressive. Spanier and co-workers[110] reported a 2-year survival rate of less than 50%. This poor prognosis was confirmed by Schajowicz.[106] The Mayo Clinic patients fared better, with 58% and 43% 5- and 10-year survival rates, respectively.[25] Researchers at Johns Hopkins also found that these lesions were less aggressive than either fibrosarcomas or osteosarcomas.[82] Mirra[85] found a worse prognosis for malignant fibrous histiocytomas of bone than for those of soft tissue.

GENERAL MANAGEMENT

Osteosarcoma

The best treatment for osteosarcoma includes systemic chemotherapy and surgical resection. Amputation has historically been the treatment of choice for nonmetastatic classic osteosarcoma. Limb-salvage procedures have, however, become increasingly popular in treatment of osteosarcoma of the extremities. The incision must be planned to include the biopsy tract in the subsequent resection or radiation treatment field. A small incision and meticulous closure promote healing. The biopsy should be done by the surgeon who will perform the resection.[127]

Past nonrandomized trials evaluating the use of adjuvant systemic chemotherapy had been faulted for small series sizes, use of historic controls with less extensive radiologic evaluations, and inclusion of favorable histologic subsets of osteosarcoma or lesions not confirmed pathologically as osteosarcoma.[14,22,107,119] However, Link and colleagues,[73] in a large intergroup study in 1986, and Eilber and group,[29] at UCLA in 1987, reported results of randomized controlled trials demonstrating a benefit to adjuvant systemic therapy with increased disease-free and overall survival rates. Truncal lesions and parosteal, periosteal, low-grade central intramedullary, mandibular, multicentric, postirradiation, and Paget's-related osteosarcomas must be considered separately.

Marcove[76–78] has written extensively about en bloc resections and prosthetic replacement of removed bone, with pulmonary metastatectomies in some patients and adjuvant chemotherapy in all, and has judged functional results to be good with low local recurrence rates in the short term. This was confirmed in similar studies by Jaffe and associates,[58] Eilber and co-workers,[30] and Springfield and colleagues.[111] Historic controls were used in all studies. Weisenberger and colleagues[129] combined preoperative radiation (3500 cGy in ten fractions) to the primary lesion with intraarterial doxorubicin, followed by en bloc resection with metallic endoprosthetic replacement. Adjuvant postoperative chemotherapy was also employed. The 2-year disease-free survival rate was 55%, with long-term evaluation awaited.

Parosteal osteosarcoma may be treated with less radical surgery. En bloc resection with at least a 2.5-cm clear margin is required for low-grade lesions less than 5 cm in diameter without cortical disruption. In popliteal lesions, careful dissection of the neurovascular bundle and distal resection extending 0.5 cm to 1.0 cm into the articular cartilage is performed. The posterior capsule is resected. Some popliteal lesions may require more aggressive surgery, as may recurrent lesions or more histologically aggressive tumors.[74]

Adjuvant chemotherapy has proven value in nonmetastatic classic osteosarcoma. Link[73] and Eilber's[29] studies demonstrated superior disease-free 2-year survivals in the adjuvant chemotherapy arm: 55% to 66% with adjuvant therapy compared with 7% to 20% without chemotherapy. The UCLA group also observed improved overall survival at 2 years in the adjuvant therapy group (80%) compared with patients not receiving chemotherapy (48%).[29,72,73] Active agents in these and previous nonrandomized trials have included doxorubicin, bleomycin, cyclophosphamide, dactinomycin, high-dose methotrexate with citrovorum factor rescue, cisplatin, and vincristine.[5,15,21,60,110,112]

An aggressive multimodal approach is taken for patients with osteosarcoma with distant metastases. Rosen and colleagues[99,101] reported a response rate of 77% with doxorubicin, vincristine, high-dose methotrexate, and cyclophosphamide. In patients whose disease has stabilized, an aggressive surgical approach is applied to the primary tumor and pulmonary metastases. Rosen and associates[101] and Jaffe and co-workers[56,57] found that high-dose methotrexate and irradiation have additive effects in treating osteosarcoma metastases. Combined radiation therapy and chemotherapy was recommended by Memorial Sloan-Kettering for extrapulmonary metastases and for small primary lesions in patients with metastatic disease.[101]

Resection of pulmonary metastases is commonly performed, with possible improvements in patient survival.[41,77,87,99] It is contraindicated, according to Marcove and colleagues,[77] if there is tumor involvement of the bronchial tree, myocardium, or pleura. Solitary pulmonary metastases exist in approximately 3% of patients with osteosarcoma. Postoperative chemotherapy is indicated for these patients. Historic controls, consisting of patients who developed pulmonary metastases, had a 3-year survival rate of 5%. In the Memorial Sloan-Kettering metastatectomy series, the 3-year survival rate was 45%.[77]

Chondrosarcoma

The 5-year survival rate for patients with chondrosarcoma is only 6% with biopsy alone; the average survival without therapy is 1.8 years.[51] Chondrosarcoma of bone has historically been treated aggressively with surgery; this is still the treatment of choice for most lesions.

Long-term survival is possible with proper therapy for 50% to 70% of patients.[25,49,51] The standard surgical procedure is a wide total excision and, in some cases, amputation.[49,97] The biopsy tract must be excised and the tumor should not be exposed during the operative procedure.[97] The recurrence rate can vary from 15% with "adequate" surgery to 87% with inadequate procedures.[106] Because relapses can occur 10 years or more postoperatively, close follow-up is necessary.

For rib chondrosarcoma, Memorial Sloan-Kettering Cancer Center recommends excision and stripping of the involved pleura for lesions smaller than 4 cm in diameter (*i.e.*, less than the usually adequate margins) or en bloc resection if the tumor is larger than 4 cm.[76]

The 5-year survival rates for radical curative pelvic surgery are 47%, 37%, and 15% for grade 1, grade 2, and grade 3 lesions, respectively.[78]

Mesenchymal and clear cell chondrosarcoma should also be treated with aggressive surgery.[7,54] Preoperative chemotherapy, with or without radiation therapy, for mesenchymal lesions is under investigation at Memorial Sloan-Kettering Cancer Center.[54] There is evidence that the small cell component of mesenchymal chondrosarcoma is relatively radiosensitive.[7,25]

Although many authors have asserted that chondrosarcoma is radioresistant, success has been achieved with radiation treatment of inoperable lesions (*i.e.*, poor location or extensive local disease) and for palliation.[17,48,65,103,114] Chemotherapy trials are underway; no definitive results are available.

Fibrosarcoma of Bone

Nonmetastatic fibrosarcoma of bone is managed with aggressive surgical resection. Low-grade lesions may be treated with en bloc resection and prosthetic replacement.[76] Dahlin and coworkers[25] reported long-term survival of approximately one third of the patients at the Mayo Clinic. Fibrosarcoma is not highly radiosensitive, but irradiation is recommended for inoperable tumors, postoperative residual disease, and palliation. Doses of at least 6600 cGy to 7000 cGy are recommended with a shrinking-field technique if radiation therapy is necessary to attempt to control a skeletal fibrosarcoma. The Bristol experience with irradiation of primary bone fibrosarcoma revealed infrequent success in controlling disease at doses ranging from 1980 to 9176 cGy and employing a variety of therapy machines (*i.e.*, ^{60}Co, radium, cesium, superficial x-rays, orthovoltage).[34]

Malignant Fibrous Histiocytoma of Bone

The primary approach to treatment of malignant fibrous histiocytoma of bone is radical surgical resection, amputation, or disarticulation.[25] Trials with radical or limited surgical procedures combined with preoperative or postoperative chemotherapy are underway.[27,64] Responses and occasional cures have been reported with definitive radiation therapy, with and without chemotherapy, and irradiation can have palliative benefit. Responses occurred most often in patients with predominately histiocytic rather than fibrocytic histologies.[51,96,110]

Giant Cell Tumors of Bone

Surgery is the preferred therapy for giant cell tumor of bone. "Benign" giant cell tumors are treated in several ways, including curettage and bone grafting with or without cauterization, filling of the cavity with cement, application of liquid nitrogen after curettage (cryosurgery), or surgical excision if the functional result permits.[17,25,50,68,71,76,83,86] Local recurrence rates for benign giant cell tumors range from 30% or 50% after curettage; 6% to 15% recur with malignant transformation.[50]

Many cases of transformation of benign giant cell tumor into malignant giant cell tumors, fibrosarcomas, or osteosarcomas after radiation treatment have been reported, but radiation therapy for these patients frequently employed low doses, orthovoltage irradiation, and protracted fractionation schemes.[4,17,25,51] Amputations may be required to sufficiently treat some large benign lesions. Radical surgery is recommended if malignant transformation occurs; only 20% of these patients are alive at 5 years after surgery.[25,83]

Cassady[17] recommended surgery for the giant cell tumor as primary therapy, with irradiation reserved for cases in which surgery would create significant functional disability or for inoperable lesions, local recurrences despite definitive surgery, or incomplete resection.

Aneurysmal Bone Cysts

The preferred treatment of aneurysmal bone cysts is surgery with curettage and bone grafting or cryosurgery if possible.[106] Resection may be performed in noncritical locations (*e.g.*, ribs, fibula, ulna, patella). The local recurrence rate was 16.6% in the series by Clough and Price.[20] Nobler and colleagues[90] found a decrease in local recurrences from 32% to 8% with 2000 cGy to 3000 cGy delivered postoperatively. Radiation therapy is recommended for definitive treatment of vertebral lesions or for recurrent disease and for cysts in surgically inaccessible sites. Doses of 2500 cGy to 3000 cGy administered in 18 to 24 days are recommended.

RADIATION THERAPY TECHNIQUES AND RESULTS

Osteosarcoma

Definitive radiation therapy requires meticulous planning and patient immobilization. Customized lead alloy shielding and sparing of a strip of skin (1.5 to 2.0 cm if possible) on one side of an extremity are essential to limit distal extremity edema and constrictive fibrosis. Electron beam availability, tissue compensators, and the daily treatment of each field can also improve the therapeutic results. Physical therapy and braces for bone support should be instituted as early as possible in the treatment course to optimize the final functional result.[9,17,63]

Urtasun and McConnachie[125] compared osteogenic sarcoma growth before and after irradiation in tissue culture using 6000 cGy to 6500 cGy in 30 to 35 fractions in 8 weeks. They showed significantly decreased clonogenicity in the central and peripheral areas of the osteosarcomas studied. Gaitan-Yanguas[43] histologically examined osteosarcomas resected 6 months after radiation therapy. They found that a tumoricidal dose could be delivered with acceptable side-effects if elapsed treatment time was more than 45 days. Radionecrosis of normal tissues occurred in patients who received 8000 cGy in 20 days or less. Patients who received doses above 3200 cGy in 10 days to 8000 cGy to 10000 cGy in 60 to 70 days had substantial tumor necrosis.

In 1940, Ferguson[39] reviewed 400 cases in the Registry of Bone Sarcomas of the American College of Surgeons and found that patients treated with early amputation (*i.e.*, within 7 months of diagnosis) had worse 5-year survival rates than those who had radiation therapy to the primary lesion followed 6 months later by surgery. MacDonald and Budd,[75] however, found that many of the cases considered to be osteosarcomas were actually chondrosarcomas or fibrosarcomas. In their analysis, one half of the cured and noncured groups of true osteosarcomas had radiation therapy and delayed amputation.

Seeing many needless amputations in patients succumbing rapidly to their disease with early lung metastases, Cade[13] in 1955 suggested radiation therapy to the primary tumor in patients with no evidence of metastatic disease at presentation, followed by a 4- to 6-month waiting period. Reevaluation was then performed, and if no metastases were found, the patient underwent amputation. Seven patients in this series were not treated with surgery because there was control of the primary lesion with irradiation or they had a surgically unresectable lesion. Local recurrences during the 4- to 6-month waiting period were treated with amputation. The radiation therapy was delivered with a 2 MeV van de Graaff generator; 7000 cGy to 8000 cGy was delivered at 1000-cGy per week. The 5-year disease-free survival rate was 21.8%. The functional result was reported to be good in nonamputated patients.[12]

Other investigators who used the same approach found no difference, and in some cases, they found improved survival with irradiation and delayed surgery compared with immediate amputation: Allen and Stevens[1] applied 10,000 cGy in 180-cGy fractions using ^{60}Co or 2-MV photons; Lee and Mackenzie[70] applied 6000 cGy to 8000 cGy in 230-cGy fractions using 2-MV photons; Farrell and Raventos[38] administered 6000 cGy to 8000 cGy in 200-cGy fractions using orthovoltage or 2-MV photons; Sweetnam[117] (Cade's method) and Phillips and Sheline[93] administered 7000 cGy to 8000 cGy in 3 months. This approach has not been recommended for patients whose local lesions were so advanced that the functional capacity of the irradiated limb would be worse than that of a prosthesis.[6] Phillips and Sheline[93] carried the dose to as high as 11,000 cGy in patients who developed visible lung metastases during the waiting period. Amputations were avoided in most patients who developed metastatic disease within the first 6 months after presentation.[93]

Jenkin[60–62] at the Princess Margaret Hospital found radiation therapy with delayed surgery to be inadequate; many patients had relapses soon after irradiation. He recommended radiation therapy for surgically unresectable lesions and palliation only. Suit[113] found that extremities bearing large tumors usually were not reasonably functional after irradiation, but he did consider Cade's approach viable for smaller lesions. Suit also stated that upper extremity lesions smaller than 5 cm in diameter could be treated with radiation therapy alone to doses of 7000 cGy to 8000 cGy at 200 cGy or less per fraction in 8 to 10 weeks, with field size reduction from whole bone to the area of primary involvement at 4400 cGy. This was combined with chemotherapy.

Caceres and Zaharia[12] treated 34 cases of osteosarcoma preoperatively using ^{60}Co external-beam therapy to doses of 8000 cGy to 12,000 cGy at 1000 cGy to 1200 cGy per fraction and found no difference in survival between their patients and a historic group treated by amputation alone.

No benefit has been found for radiation delivered under conditions of local tissue hypoxia or combined with arterial perfusion with hydrogen peroxide or cytotoxic drugs.[69,112,126] Split-course radiation therapy also conferred no advantage.[105] Beck and co-workers[3] observed no improvement in survival and palliative benefit for only 50% of the patients treated with irradiation and delayed surgery.

Goffinet and associates[44] at Stanford University employed BUdR as a radiosensitizer in three patients. Total doses of 4200 cGy to 4800 cGy given in seven to eight fractions were delivered in conjunction with methotrexate. Local control was obtained in all three, but local subcutaneous fibrosis, muscular atrophy and fibrosis, and peroneal neuropathy were observed in each patient. Two patients developed lung metastases.

Weichselbaum and Cassady[128] recommended definitive irradiation only for older patients who refuse surgery or for patients who have surgically unresectable lesions; 4000 cGy in 200-cGy fractions with five treatments a week is given to the entire bone, with field reduction to the original tumor volume and treatment to 6600 cGy to 7000 cGy.

Suit[113] emphasized the need for supervoltage equipment, precise immobilization, shaped (Cerrobend) fields, and daily treatment of all fields. Use of electrons, if applicable, bolus over the scar site for the first 5000 cGy, and exclusion of skin areas of poor vascularity (*e.g.*, over the tibia anteriorly) were also advised.

The treatment of mandibular osteosarcomas requires special attention. Chambers and Mahoney[18] reported that these tumors cause death mainly by local recurrence and not by early metastasis. Thirty-three patients treated at Walter Reed Army Hospital first had holes drilled in the diseased area of the mandible. Radium needles were implanted to deliver 10,000 cGy to 16,000 cGy to the tumor volume. A wide surgical excision (*i.e.*, hemimandibulectomy and excision of surrounding soft tissue) was performed within 4 weeks after removal of the needles. The 5-year disease-free survival rate was 73%. Eighty-two percent of patients were treated with curative intent. Suit[113] agreed that preoperative radiation therapy for mandibular osteosarcoma was recommended. Long-term survival rates with surgery alone are 25% to 40%.

Adjuvant Pulmonary Irradiation

Because pulmonary metastases occur frequently, many trials have evaluated adjuvant pulmonary irradiation.

Newton and Barrett[89] treated the primary lesions of 14 patients with classic osteosarcoma with 6000 cGy in 6 weeks. Also, the entire thorax was irradiated to a dose of 1950 cGy (estimated 2425 cGy to lungs considering increased transmission). If no metastases were detected in 6 to 9 months, amputation was performed. The 5-year survival rate was 42.8%, with a 44-month median survival. No hematologic or pulmonary toxicity was seen.

A randomized study conducted by Rab and associates[95] showed that 1500 cGy to the lung midplane, in addition to concomitant dactinomycin, conferred no survival benefit over amputation alone. No radiation pneumonitis or fibrosis occurred.

Jenkin[61] treated six patients adjuvantly to the lungs with 1500 cGy in 14 days. Dactinomycin was given to four patients simultaneously with radiation therapy; no benefit was observed. Caceres and Zaharia[12] also found no advantage in a small series when comparing whole-lung irradiation and doxorubicin therapy with the published results of studies that used doxorubicin alone. Perez and associates[91] warned of increased risk of cardiomyopathy among patients treated with adjuvant lung irradiation who also received doxorubicin adjuvantly or may later require it.

Breur and co-workers[10] treated patients with whole-lung portals to 1750 cGy in ten fractions in 12 elapsed days (no correction for absorption in pulmonary tissue with an actual lung dose of slightly less than 2000 cGy). Eighty-six patients were randomized between amputation plus adjuvant whole-lung irradiation and amputation alone. A significant disease-free survival benefit was discovered for patients younger than 17 years of age in the adjuvant radiation therapy group, with a 3-year disease-free survival rate of 48% compared with 28% for those who had surgery alone. The European Organization for Research on Treatment of Cancer continued the investigation with a randomized trial evaluating pulmonary irradiation (2000 cGy); systemic chemotherapy with high-dose methotrexate with citrovorum factor rescue, vincristine, cyclophosphamide, and doxorubicin; and pulmonary irradiation given with a shorter, limited chemotherapy regimen.[11] All 205 patients had classic osteosarcoma of the extremity without evidence of metastatic disease. Forty-three percent overall survival and 24% disease-free survival rates were reported for the entire group, with no regimen producing a superior survival rate. Less therapy-related toxicity occurred in the group receiving pulmonary irradiation alone.

Chondrosarcoma

Several studies demonstrate a definite role for radiation therapy in the treatment of chondrosarcoma. M. D. Anderson Cancer Center reported a series of 20 chondrosarcoma patients treated with supervoltage irradiation, neutrons, or a photon-neutron combination for disease in the pelvis, sacrum, femur, and maxilla; they had an overall survival rate of 65% (13 of 20). Eleven were treated with irradiation alone; five (45%) of these were reported alive with local disease control, and six patients failed locally with one surgical salvage. Six of the remaining nine patients are alive without locally progressive disease. Two patients are alive without progressive local disease after radiation therapy failure and surgical salvage. A dose of 4000 cGy to 7000 cGy at 1000 cGy per week was employed using multiple fields. Combination photon-neutron therapy was superior to neutron therapy alone. The average length of follow-up was 38 months.[84,97]

Thirty-one patients at the Princess Margaret Hospital with unfavorable prognoses (39% mesenchymal or dedifferentiated chondrosarcoma, predominantly central lesions) were treated with definitive photon therapy and achieved a complete response rate of 50%; 25% of the patients were disease-free at 15 years. No progression of local disease occurred in any of the patients studied, and in some, tumor regression continued slowly for 2 to 3 years after therapy. A dose of 5000 cGy was delivered in 4 to 5 weeks. The entire bone was treated if there was medullary involvement.[48]

A British study using irradiation and the radiosensitizer Razoxane (ICRF 159) revealed five complete responders and two partial responders among 12 patients with chondrosarcoma after 5000 cGy to 6000 cGy; two of the complete responders were free of disease at 2.5 years.[103] Kim and co-workers[65] reported responses in seven patients treated between 1961 and 1976 with 5000 cGy to 6000 cGy, delivered with a cobalt machine in six cases and with radium needles in one.

Suit and associates[114] treated chondrosarcoma of the cervical spine and base of skull with combined photon-proton radiation therapy. Total doses ranged from 6530 to 7500 rad-equivalents, with photon doses between 2130 cGy and 3960 cGy and proton doses from 2870 to 4000 rad-equivalents. The proton field was used as the coned-down boost field. No central nervous system toxic effects were reported; survival times without evidence of disease ranged from 4 to 74 months.

Radioactive ^{35}S has been used for treatment of metastatic chondrosarcoma. At the Memorial Sloan-Kettering Cancer Center, a test dose of ^{35}S was given intravenously, and a biopsy of the chondrosarcoma lesions was done. If good relative isotope uptake occurred, 5 mCi/kg of ^{35}S was given therapeutically; this was repeated at various intervals, depending on the clinical situation. Pronounced hematologic toxic reactions with severe aplastic anemia has limited this approach to patients with end-stage disease.[71,76]

Malignant Fibrous Histiocytoma of Bone

Reagan and associates[96] treated 17 patients with malignant fibrous histiocytoma with megavoltage therapy without brachytherapy. A bolus or mixed photon-electron technique (10–12 MeV) was employed if higher skin doses were desired. Most patients were treated with doses ranging from 4594 cGy to 6642 cGy (median, 6000 cGy in 43 days). Five of 17 had irradiation alone; the remainder were treated postoperatively after excision of the gross tumor. The local control rate overall was 65%, with a postoperative control rate of 75%. Eleven of 14 patients with at least 2 cm of tumor had local tumor control; two of the three recurrences were marginal. No tumors larger than 7 cm in diameter were controlled. Distant metastases developed in 41% of the patients between 2 and 52 weeks after diagnosis.

Giant Cell Tumors of Bone

When radiation therapy is used in the treatment of giant cell tumors of bone, the recommended tumor dose is 4500 cGy to 5500 cGy in 5 to 6 weeks with megavoltage irradiation.[17,47,115] Harwood and colleagues[47] reported long-term control with no sequelae in eight of nine patients treated with 3500 cGy in 15 treatments in 21 days. Friedman and Pearlman[42] found good response and control of these tumors with doses of 4000 cGy to 4500 cGy in 35 to 42 days in adults and 3000 cGy to 5700 cGy in 25 to 60 days (split course) in children. Chen and associates[19] treated 35 patients postoperatively or with radiation therapy alone and achieved a local control rate of over 80%. Irradiation is also recommended for palliation.

SEQUELAE OF THERAPY

Chondroblasts are more radiosensitive than osteoblasts. Abnormalities in growth delay become clinically apparent after 6 months in infants and 1 year in older children. The magnitude of the effects are related directly to dose and field volume and are inversely related to age at the time of therapy. Growth delays may result in limp joint dislocation secondary to underdeveloped joint fossa and mandibular or craniofacial abnormalities and dentition delay.[35,102]

Scoliosis after vertebral irradiation is possible but is usually not progressive and frequently compensated by pelvic tilt. Including the entire width of the vertebral body in the treatment field does not appear to decrease the incidence of scoliosis.[35]

Because of radiation-induced vascular changes, irradiated bone is more sensitive to infection, fracture, and necrosis.[35,102]

Postirradiation skeletal sarcomas comprise 1.5% of all primary bone malignancies. Phillips and Sheline[92] reported that postirradiation sarcomas arose in 0.3% of all irradiated patients. Brady[8] and Cahan[14] provided criteria to categorize a skeletal malignancy as secondary to radiation treatment (Table 66-3).

Ewing's Sarcoma

Patrick R.M. Thomas

The second most common childhood neoplasm of bone, Ewing's sarcoma, is more radioresponsive than osteosarcoma, and therefore radiation therapy is frequently employed.

Epidemiology

In 1921, James Ewing[144] described as diffuse endothelioma of bone the highly malignant small cell tumor that bears his name.[138] The disease is more common in males, but is very rare

TABLE 66–3
Cahan's and Brady's Criteria for Defining Postirradiation Bone Sarcoma

CAHAN (1948)[13]	BRADY (1979)
Histologic or radiologic evidence of nonmalignant nature of initial bone problem	No histologic or radiologic evidence of abnormality in bone at time of radiation therapy
Lesion must arise in irradiated area	Significant radiation dose delivered (1100 rets)
Five-year latency period required	Relatively long symptom-free latency period (median, 11 yr)
Histologic proof of sarcoma	Microscopic evidence of sarcoma
	No exposure to other known carcinogens

in blacks.[135, 139, 149] Taller people are more likely to be affected.[146]

Natural History

Virtually any bone can be the site of the primary lesion, but the lower half of the body is much more frequently involved than the upper half. In the first Intergroup Ewing's Sarcoma Study (IESS-I) for patients with nonmetastatic disease at diagnosis, the femur was the most common site, occurring in 55 (22%) of 251 patients.[168] Other sites were innominate (pelvic) bone in 47 patients, fibula in 29, humerus in 28, tibia in 27, ribs in 16, vertebra in ten, scapula in nine, sacrum in seven, hands and feet in nine, skull and facial bones in six, clavicle in three, and other locations in five.

Although the disease can occur in any part of the bone, the diaphysis is more commonly involved than the metaphysis. Epiphyseal involvement is rare.[140] Periosteal Ewing's sarcoma has been reported, and extraosseous primary lesions are recognized but considered to be variants of rhabdomyosarcoma (see Chap. 72).[132, 174]

If untreated, the disease becomes relentless and widespread, with hematogenous metastases to almost any visceral site. Pulmonary and skeletal spread are common.[176] Lymph node spread is rare (<10%). The central nervous system was considered to be a major sanctuary site, but results from the Intergroup Ewing's Sarcoma Study and the National Cancer Institute have not confirmed this.[162, 179]

Clinical Presentation

The patient usually presents with localized pain, tenderness, and swelling in the region of the involved bone. There is frequently associated pyrexia.

Duration of symptoms before diagnosis in the IESS-I patients was longer than 3 months in 41%, 1 to 3 months in 47%, and shorter than 1 month in only 12%.[166] Metastases are often present at diagnosis.

Diagnostic Workup

Physical examination usually reveals a tender, warm, swollen area over the affected bone. If metastases exist, these signs may be multifocal, suggesting multiple bone lesions.

Ewing's sarcoma is usually suggested by its classical appearance on plain radiographs—a diaphyseal tumor with permeative involvement of the medullary cavity. There is no new bone formation, but periosteal reaction (*i.e.*, classic "onion-skin" appearance) and a soft tissue mass are frequently observed. However, there are many different manifestations of this tumor; any bone abnormality that appears malignant could be a Ewing's tumor. Furthermore, osteosarcoma or secondary involvement by other tumors, particularly neuroblastoma, can simulate a classic Ewing's tumor appearance.

The soft tissue mass may be more extensive than can be demonstrated on plain radiography. CT has made delineation of soft tissue masses more accurate, and CT of the entire affected bone and surrounding anatomic areas should be routinely performed.[133] The advent of MRI has further defined soft tissue extension and medullary involvement.[4]

Routine evaluation of a new patient with Ewing's sarcoma should also include an isotope (usually ^{99m}Tc) bone scan, because it detects asymptomatic skeletal metastases and helps to delineate the extent of medullary involvement of the tumor.[145, 156] Frequently, there is increased uptake over a greater extent of bone than is demonstrated on radiography.[145]

Routine hematologic parameters (*e.g.*, complete blood count, differential, and platelets) should be obtained before therapy, because anemia requires correction, and chemotherapy and large-field radiation therapy suppress the counts. It has also been suggested that leukocytosis or high total lymphocyte count is associated with a poor prognosis, although the opposite was true in the larger experience of IESS-I.[147, 169] The erythrocyte sedimentation rate may be elevated.

Biochemical abnormalities possibly associated with a poor prognosis include elevated levels of serum glutamic oxaloacetic transaminase and serum lactate dehydrogenase.[135, 147]

The most important investigation of the patient with suspected Ewing's sarcoma, is the biopsy, because no radiologic investigation is pathognomonic of Ewing's sarcoma. Because aspiration needle biopsy alone may not be sufficient to differentiate Ewing's sarcoma from neuroblastoma or other small round cell tumors of bone in the pediatric age group, open biopsy is preferred.[173] In certain circumstances, the biopsy may be excisional or, rarely, an amputation may first be performed.

A suitable soft tissue mass, if there is one, is the recommended site of biopsy because this avoids violating the bone cortex. Every effort must be made to avoid causing instability, which results in pathologic fracture. In addition, the incision scar should be included in the irradiation portals.

A bone marrow aspiration and biopsy should also be done to exclude diffuse metastatic involvement. Because of the rarity of central nervous system spread, routine lumbar puncture is no longer recommended.[179]

Pathologic Classification

There is no pathognomonic feature for Ewing's sarcoma. The differential diagnosis from osteosarcoma is usually easily made because of the absence of osteoblasts, but there are other small round cell tumors involving bone that must be considered, such as non-Hodgkin's lymphoma, rhabdomyosarcoma, neuroblastoma, and acute leukemia.

Microscopic evidence of cytoplasmic glycogen was originally thought to be diagnostic of Ewing's sarcoma, especially in the differential diagnosis with non-Hodgkin's lymphoma.[173] However, this is not invariably so, and 10% of neuroblastomas may contain glycogen.[159, 167, 180]

After a review of the pathology from 303 patients in IESS-I, Kissane and associates[159] recognized several microscopic patterns. The most common are a diffuse pattern, which corresponds to the classic description; lobular, in which fibrovascular septa separate the multicellular aggregates; and filagree, in which tumor tissue is found in roughly bicellular strands and is separated by filmy fibrovascular stroma.[160] The filagree pattern is relatively uncommon and carries a poorer prognosis than other patterns.[160] Immunohistochemistry to determine the B-lymphocyte marker (MB2) may be a beneficial tool.[158] N-*myc* amplification is not likely to be demonstrated in Ewing's sarcoma.[178]

Prognostic Factors

Analysis of IESS-I for prognostic factors has been reported by Gehan and colleagues.[147] Primary site was the most important factor; the pelvis was the least favorable, followed by proximal sites (*i.e.*, femur and humerus). Rib primary lesions had an intermediate outcome, with distal (*i.e.*, tibia, fibula, radius, and ulna) and other sites having relatively good prognoses. In this series females did better than males, as did patients with less than 1 month between the onset of symptoms and diagnosis. A high lymphocyte count was favorable. Those having resections had a slight advantage over those having biopsy, but this observation may have been influenced by the size and site of the primary lesion.

General Management

Controversy about the roles of surgery and radiation therapy in the local management of Ewing's sarcoma has clouded the main issue, that control of clinical and subclinical metastases is still the most important problem in increasing overall survival. In IESS-I, although the overall local primary control rate was approximately 90%, 40% of the patients developed metastases despite chemotherapy.[165, 166, 168] Management therefore includes a multimodal approach that employs aggressive chemotherapy, local irradiation, and surgery.

The arguments surrounding the use of surgery or radiation therapy for local control have been presented in review articles by Thomas and associates,[177] Neff,[164] and Pritchard.[171]

We recommend surgery as the treatment of choice for lower extremity lesions in children with unfused epiphyses or if there is an actual or impending pathologic fracture or the bones are excisable and "expendable," such as the fibula, clavicle, or certain ribs. Surgery may also be preferable treatment in the hand, especially if wide local resection is possible.[164]

Although single-agent chemotherapy has been used, combination therapy has proven to be more effective.

General supportive care of the patient is critical because irradiated volumes can be large and chemotherapy intensive. Blood transfusion, use of antibiotics, and routine skin care are very important. In addition, late effects of irradiation can be minimized by using careful techniques and by a regular program of physical therapy during and after treatment.[160] Side-effects of irradiation can be acceptable if these precautions are taken.[155]

Radiation Therapy Techniques

Strict attention to detail is necessary in pediatric patients, because growing normal tissue is more prone to radiation-associated injury. This is especially true in Ewing's sarcoma, in which adequate, yet not excessive, margins are required because of the microscopic spread around an intramedullary tumor extension. Uninvolved soft tissues, particularly lymphatics in the extremities, should be avoided or kept out of the boost field if close to the lesion.

Radiation therapy alone resulted in a local control rate of between 65% and 75%. After chemotherapy was added to adequate irradiation, this figure rose to between 90% and 95% (Table 66-4).

Data from IESS-I[38] showed that there was no radiation therapy dose response for local control. Local failure was more likely if only vincristine, dactinomycin, and cyclophosphamide were employed, rather than using these drugs plus doxorubicin (Adriamycin). If patients were irradiated with inadequate portals and received four drugs (regimen I), the local control rate was higher (87% to 90%) than it was in patients treated with three cytotoxic agents. However, these differences are not statistically significant ($P \geq 0.13$) (Table 66-5). In most instances, the recurrences were reported at the site of the initially bulky tumors.[171] The St. Jude Children's Research Hospital results, using lower doses, demonstrated that the dose of irradiation is important.[152]

In IESS-I, there was a suggestion (not statistically significant) that inadequate treatment volumes (*i.e.*, entire bone not irradiated or boost <5 cm around gross tumor) were more likely to result in lower local tumor control rates. Further analysis of IESS patients and other studies have shown that the tumor volume is clearly prognostically important.[136, 148, 150] On the basis of these data, IESS-II required doses of 4500 cGy to the whole bone with two boosts of 500 cGy each (including soft tissue mass) to tumor margins of 5 cm and 1 cm, respectively.[168] Exceptions were made when the tumor was at or near the end of a long bone. The noninvolved epiphysis was spared to reduce late effects (Fig. 66-1).

Although not proven, tailored portals (Fig. 66-2) are becoming the standard therapy given to patients not on a protocol. The initial results of the Pediatric Oncology Group study (POG-8346) showed no advantage for whole-bone irradiation compared with tailored portal irradiation.[142]

Results of Therapy

Multimodal therapy has been responsible for increasing the 2-year survival rate from 14% in patients treated by irradiation only at M. D. Anderson between 1964 and 1969 to 74% with

TABLE 66–4
Local Control of Primary Lesion In Nonmetastatic Ewing's Sarcoma

RADIATION DOSE (cGy)	CHEMOTHERAPY* DRUGS	CHEMOTHERAPY* DURATION	MINIMUM FOLLOW-UP	NO. OF PATIENTS	LOCAL CONTROL NUMBER	LOCAL CONTROL (%)	INVESTIGATION
3000–5000			5 yr	6	3	50	Roswell Park Memorial Institute
4000–5000	CY	1 yr	3 yr	6	3	50	Roswell Park Memorial Institute
2500–4400			5 yr	8	4	50	Memorial Hospital, NY
4000–6000			5 yr	25	14	56	M.D. Anderson, Houston
4000			5 yr	7	5	71	University California, San Francisco
4500			5 yr	11	8	73	University California, San Francisco
6000–7400			5 yr	15	10	67	M.D. Anderson, Houston
6000–8000			5 yr	8	5	63	Memorial Hospital, NY
4000–5000	CY + VCR ADR + AMD	1.5 h	3 yr (median)	58	49	84	IESS
5500–6000	CY + VCR + AMD + ADR		160 wk (median)	115	105	91	IESS
6000–7500	CY + VCR + AMD + ADR (×2)	2 yr	36 mo	17	14	82	Memorial Hospital, NY
4700–6300	CY + VCR	1–2 yr	4–91 mo	15	14	93	St. Jude, Memphis
6000	CY + VCR	34 wk	14–36 mo	19	18	95	M.D. Anderson, Houston
6000–7000	CY + VCR + AMD	1.5 yr	6 yr	331	282	85	IESS-I (1989)
5600	CY + VCR + ADR	1.5 yr	5.6 yr	214	195	91	IESS-II (non-pelvic)
5500	CY + ADR + VCR + AMD	1.5 yr	5.5 yr	59	51	89	IESS-II (pelvic only)
3000–3500	CY + ADR induction VCR, AMD, BCNU, CY, ADR	10 mo	2 yr	28	16	57	St. Jude (1989)

**CY: cyclophosphamide; VCR: vincristine; ADR: doxorubicin (Adriamycin); AMD: actinomycin D; BCNU: bischloroethyl nitrosourea; IESS: Intergroup Ewing's Sarcoma Study.*
(Modified from Perez CA, Tefft M, Nesbit ME, et al: JNCI 56:263, 1981)

four-drug therapy plus local treatment on the best arm of IESS-I.[141,165]

Although there appears to be better survival and local control for patients surgically treated than for those treated with radiation therapy at the Mayo Clinic and in the IESS-I study, close analysis of the latter data suggests that there may be patient selection bias, because smaller tumors, which have a better prognosis, are more likely to be excised.[136,170,171] Data from the University of Florida also have shown that patients with smaller tumors have better outcomes.[161]

Results of Clinical Trials

Since the demonstration of the effectiveness of multimodality therapy in Ewing's sarcoma, there have been many clinical trials testing a variety of agents singly or in combination with irradia-

TABLE 66–5
Local Control of Ewing's Sarcoma Achieved with Radiation Therapy and Chemotherapy

TUMOR DOSE (cGy)	ADEQUATE VOLUME REGIMEN I	ADEQUATE VOLUME REGIMENS II AND III	INADEQUATE VOLUME (MAJOR) REGIMEN I	INADEQUATE VOLUME (MAJOR) REGIMENS II AND III	INADEQUATE VOLUME (MINOR) REGIMEN I	INADEQUATE VOLUME (MINOR) REGIMENS II AND III
3000–3999	6/6*	3/3*	1/1*	1/1*	0/0*	0/0*
4000–4999	23/24	15/16	4/5	3/4	1/1	3/6
5000–5999	30/34	58/65	11/12	5/7	3/4	7/8
≥6000	21/21	35/38	2/2	1/2	3/3	6/8
Total	80/85 (94%)	111/112 (91%)	18/20 (90%)	10/14 (71.4%)	7/8 (87.5%)	16/22 (72.7%)

**Total demonstrating local control/total treated. Regimen I, VAC − ADR; Regimen II, VAC; Regimen III, VAC + pulmonary irradiation.*
(Perez CA, Tefft M; Nesbit ME, et al: JNCI 56:263, 1981)

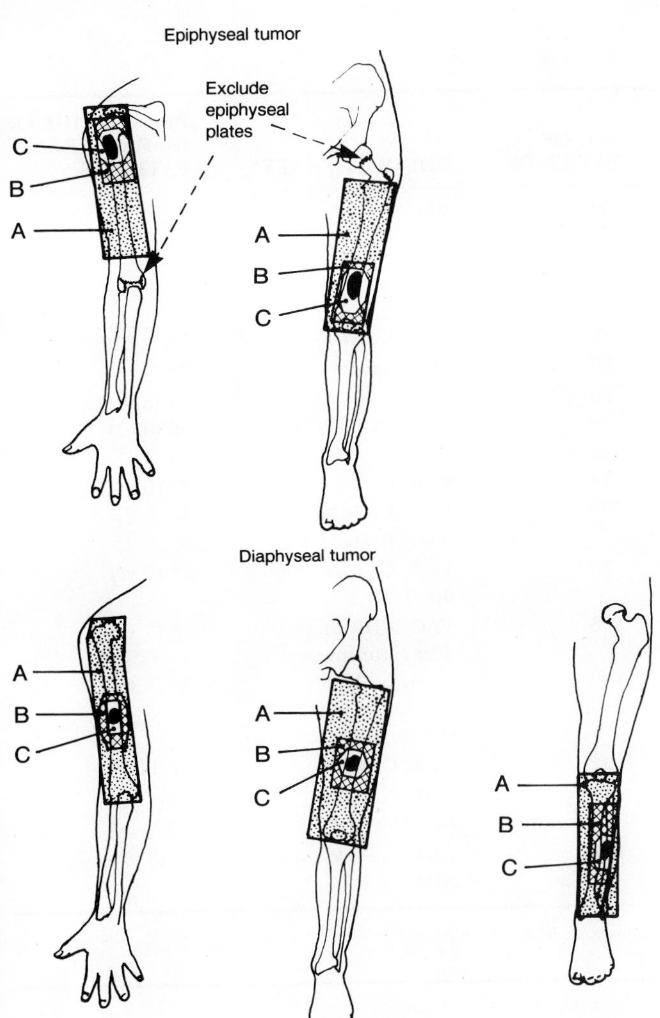

FIGURE 66–1. Examples of treatment portals used in the Second Intergroup Ewing's Sarcoma Study protocol. If the eccentric location of the tumor permits, one of the epiphyseal centers is spared to diminish growth disturbances. (*Top*) Epiphyseal tumor. (*Bottom*) Diaphyseal tumor. A, entire bone; B, tumor with 5-cm margins; C, portal used for a boost to the residual primary tumor. (Perez CA, Tefft M, Nesbit ME, et al: JNCI 56:263, 1981)

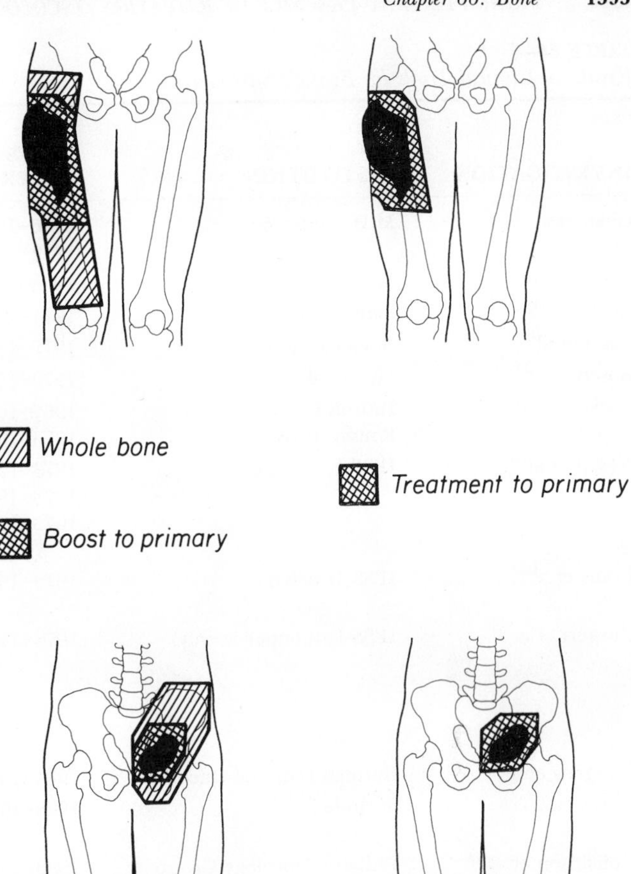

FIGURE 66–2. Examples of portals used in the Pediatric Oncology Group study.

tion or surgery for the primary tumor. Because of the paucity of patients at any one institution, these studies have been mainly single-arm designs; the major randomized studies have been done by the IESS and lately by the Pediatric Oncology Group. The results of various trials are summarized in Table 66-6.

The IESS-I studies showed that the addition of either doxorubicin or bilateral pulmonary irradiation (1500–1800 cGy at 150–200 cGy/day) to vincristine, cyclophosphamide, and dactinomycin (VAC) significantly increased disease-free status and improved the survival rate over using the three drugs alone.[166] Mature analysis showed that VAC plus doxorubicin was superior to VAC plus irradiation for relapse-free survival ($P<0.05$) and survival ($P=0.001$).[165]

The initial findings of IESS-I prompted the start of the second Intergroup Ewing's Sarcoma Study (IESS-II) in 1978. In this study, there were separate protocols for the pelvic and sacral primary tumors. This was a one-arm study that consisted of initial high-dose intermittent chemotherapy of vincristine, doxorubicin, and cyclophosphamide followed by an assessment at day 42 for resection or radiation therapy. Radiation therapy was given if resection was not performed or if there was gross or microscopic residual tumor after surgery. A dose of 4500 cGy was given to the whole bone plus original soft tissue extension, as determined by CT scan, and two boosts of 500 cGy each were administered. After radiation therapy, chemotherapy of vincristine, cyclophosphamide, and doxorubicin, alternating with dactinomycin was given. Of 59 eligible patients, seven (12%) had local recurrence, and the relapse-free survival and actuarial survival rates at 5 years were 55% and 63%, respectively.[143] Local recurrence, 5-year relapse-free survival, and survival were all significantly improved compared with the pelvic patients on IESS-I. Nonpelvic primary tumors received radiation therapy at the start (dosages as for pelvic primary tumors) with a randomization between high-dose intermittent chemotherapy (vincristine, dactinomycin, cyclophosphamide, and doxorubicin) and the same drugs on a weekly basis. The results showed a significant advantage in 5-year relapse-free survival and survival rates for high-dose intermittent chemotherapy (73% and 77%, respectively) over moderate-dose continuous-dose chemotherapy (56% and 63%, respectively) in 215 eligible patients.[137]

Metastatic Ewing's sarcoma has also been studied by the IESS. In the first study, patients were given lower-dose irradiation (4500 cGy) to the primary tumor with smaller doses to metastases and four-drug chemotherapy (vincristine, cyclophosphamide, dactinomycin, and doxorubicin).[175] Because 17 of 44 patients continued in complete remission, a second study was started using the same four drugs plus 5-fluorouracil with delayed (day 70) radiation therapy in dosages similar to those used for nonmetastatic disease.

TABLE 66–6
Results of Clinical Trials for Ewing's Sarcoma

INVESTIGATION	INSTITUTION	DATES ENTERED	NO. OF PATIENTS	CHEMOTHERAPY*	PERCENTAGE OF DISEASE-FREE PATIENTS
Chan et al[138]	M.D. Anderson	1966–1972	21	V, C	47
		1972–1975	15	V, A, C, ADR	65
Hustu et al[153]	St. Jude's	1964–1972	15	V, C	63
Jaffe et al[154]	Sidney Farber	1971–1975	14	V, A, C	78
Bacci et al[131]	Bologna, Italy	1972–1978	80	V, A, C, ADR	39
Rosen et al[172]	Memorial, NY	1970–1979	67	Many agents	79
Zucker et al[181]	Institut Gustav	1967–1972	30		23 (6 yr)
	Roussy, Paris	1973–1976	30	V, C, ADR, PCA	50 (6 yr)
Nesbit et al[166]	IESS-I	1973–1978	148	V, A, C, ADR	59
		1973–1978	74	V, A, C	22 (6 yr)
		1973–1978	109	V, A, C, + bilateral pulmonary XRT	42
Evans et al[143]	IESS-II pelvis	1978–1982	59	V, A, C, ADR (high dose)	55 (5 yr)
Burgert et al[137]	IESS-II (nonpelvic only)	1978–1982	108	VAC, ADR (high dose, intermittent)	73 (5 yr)
			106	V, A, C, ADR (moderate dose, continuous)	56 (5 yr)
Juergens et al[157]	German Pediatric Oncology	1981–1986	93	V, A, C, ADR	51 (6.5 yr)
Hayes et al[151]	St. Jude's	1978–1986	52	ADR, C → V, A, C/ BCNU→ADR, C	72 (3 yr)
Donaldson et al[142]	Pediatric Oncology Group	1983–1988	127	ADR, C → V, A, C, ADR	54 (3 yr)

* *V: vincristine; C: cyclophosphamide; A: actinomycin D; PCA: procarbazine; ADR: doxorubicin (Adriamycin); BCNU: bischloroethyl nitrosurea; XRT: external radiation therapy; IESS: Intergroup Ewing's Sarcoma Study.*

At St. Jude Children's Research Hospital, all patients with newly diagnosed metastatic and nonmetastatic Ewing's sarcoma were treated with sequential cyclophosphamide and doxorubicin in five 15-day cycles, followed by reevaluation, surgery for those in complete remission with expendable bones, or biopsy. Radiation therapy was given with limited portals to a dose of 3000 cGy to 3500 cGy, unless complete excision had been achieved (no radiation therapy) or gross disease was still present (5000 cGy). This was followed by maintenance chemotherapy. Fifty of 52 patients achieved complete or partial remission, but of 17 relapses, 14 failed locally. Additional data from St. Jude suggested that long-term survival may be possible in relapsed disease.[153]

A Pediatric Oncology Group study used similar induction therapy. Radiation therapy was randomized to standard (whole bone plus boost) volumes or tailored (original tumor with a 2-cm margin). Dosages (4000 cGy plus 1500-cGy boost) were conventional (Fig. 66-2). Results were disappointing, with a 3-year event-free survival rate of 54% and survival of 59% in patients with localized disease.[142] Metastatic disease was the predominant cause of failure.[151]

The German Pediatric Oncology Cooperative Ewing's Sarcoma Study also used vincristine, dactinomycin, cyclophosphamide, and doxorubicin with radiation therapy or definitive surgery delayed until week 18.[157] A disease-free survival rate of 51% at 6.5 years in 93 patients was recorded.

Recent results from the National Cancer Institute have shown excellent response rates (16 of 17) in recurrent Ewing's sarcoma using ifosfamide with mesna uroprotection and etoposide.[163] The Children's Cancer Study Group and Pediatric Oncology Group recently embarked on a joint clinical trial evaluating this combination. The test regimen consists of these three drugs in addition to the standard vincristine, doxorubicin, cyclophosphamide, and dactinomycin as induction therapy. This regimen is compared with one using standard drugs alone. After induction, all patients receive tailored radiation therapy to a dose of 5580 cGy given in 180-cGy fractions starting at week 19. Chemotherapy (test or standard) is given during radiation therapy and as maintenance.

The modern approach has become induction chemotherapy followed by radiation therapy and maintenance chemotherapy. The dose and volume of radiation therapy are being evaluated, although results have suggested that it is preferable to reduce volume rather than dose.

Another approach includes supralethal chemotherapy and autologous bone marrow transplantation.[160] These approaches may also be applicable to those who relapse.

Sequelae of Treatment

There are some patients for whom the late effects of irradiation are such that an amputation at diagnosis would have been preferable (*e.g.*, foot and lower extremity in a very young patient). As reported by Thomas and associates[177] and Neff,[164] patients in IESS-I experienced multiple long-term sequelae, particularly in the weight-bearing bones. Two thirds of the patients with femoral primary lesions developed shortening of 2 cm or more, and one third of the patients developed pathologic fractures. One patient in four required amputation after irradiation of a tibial primary tumor. Meticulous planning can help reduce late effects.[136,155]

Second malignant neoplasms have been a concern since a report from M. D. Anderson Cancer Center showed that 4 of 24 patients irradiated with a median dose of 6100 cGy developed a second malignancy within the portal.[175] Happily, the IESS-I patients received doses of less than or equal to 6000 cGy. The British study of 67 patients with a median dose of 5250 cGy but with a short median time on study has not reported any in-field second malignancies.[136]

REFERENCES

Bone

1. Allen CV, Stevens KR: Preoperative irradiation for osteogenic sarcoma. Cancer 31:1365, 1973
2. Baeza MR, Barkley HT, Fernandez CH: Total lung irradiation in the treatment of pulmonary metastases. Radiology 116:151, 1975
3. Beck JC, Wara WM, Bovill EG, et al: The role of radiation therapy in the treatment of osteosarcoma. Radiology 120:163, 1976
4. Bell RS, Harwood AR, Goodman SB, et al: Supervoltage radiotherapy in the treatment of difficult giant cell tumors of bone. Clin Orthop 174:208, 1983
5. Benjamin RS: Adjuvant chemotherapy for osteosarcoma. In Wiernik PH (ed): Controversies in Oncology, pp 175–188. New York, John Wiley, 1982
6. Berg NO, Hakansson CH, Lovdahl R, et al: Radiotherapy and surgery in 50 cases of osteosarcoma treated without adjuvant chemotherapy. Acta Orthop Scand 48:580, 1977
7. Bertoni F, Picci P, Bacchini P, et al: Mesenchymal chondrosarcoma of bone and soft tissue. Cancer 52:533, 1983
8. Brady LW: Radiation-induced sarcomas of bone. Skeletal Radiol 4:72, 1979
9. Brady LW, Wallner PE: Radiation therapy in skeletal disorders. In Murray RO, Jacobsen HG (eds): The Radiology of Skeletal Disorders, pp 1863–1878. New York, Churchill Livingstone, 1976
10. Breur K, Schweisguth O. Cohen P, et al: Prophylatic irradiation of the lungs to prevent development of pulmonary metastases in patients with osteosarcoma of the limbs. NCI Monogr 56:233, 1981
11. Burgers JMV, van Glabbeke M, Busson A, et al: Report of the E.O.R.T.C.–S.I.O.P. 03 trial 20781 investigating the value of adjuvant treatment with chemotherapy and/or prophylactic lung irradiation. Cancer 61:1024, 1988
12. Caceres E, Zaharia M: Massive preoperative radiation therapy in the treatment of osteogenic sarcoma. Cancer 30:634, 1972
13. Cade S: Osteogenic sarcoma: A study based on 133 patients. J Coll Surg Edinb 1:79, 1955
14. Cahan WG, Woodward HQ, Higinbotham NL, et al: Sarcoma arising in irradiated bone. Cancer 1:3, 1948
15. Companacci M: Giant-cell tumor and chondrosarcomas: Grading, treatment and results (studies of 209 and 131 cases). In Grundmann E (ed): Malignant Bone Tumors, pp 257–262. New York, Springer-Verlag, 1976
16. Carter SK: The dilemma of adjuvant chemotherapy for osteogenic sarcoma. Cancer Clin Trials 3:29, 1980
17. Cassady JR: Radiation therapy in less common primary bone tumors. In Jaffee N (ed): Solid Tumors in Childhood, pp 205–214. Boca Raton, FL, CRC, 1983
18. Chambers RG, Mahoney WD: Osteogenic sarcoma of the mandible: Current management. Am Surg 36:783, 1970
19. Chen ZX, Gu DZ, Yu ZH, et al: Radiation therapy of giant cell tumor of bone: Analysis of 35 patients. Int J Radiat Oncol Biol Phys 12:329, 1986
20. Clough JR, Price CHG: Aneurysmal bone cyst: Pathogenesis and long-term results of treatment. Clin Orthop 97:52, 1973
21. Cortes EP, Holland JF, Glidewell O: Osteogenic sarcoma studies by the cancer and leukemia group B. NCI Monogr 56:207, 1981
22. Dahlin DC: The problems of assessment of new treatment regimens of osteosarcoma. Clin Orthop 153:81, 1980
23. Dahlin DC, Coventry MB: Osteogenic sarcoma: A study of 600 cases. J Bone Joint Surg [A] 48:1, 1967
24. Dahlin DC, Cupps, RE, Johnson EW: Giant-cell tumor. A study of 195 cases. Cancer 25:1061, 1970
25. Dahlin DC, Unni KK: Bone Tumor: General Aspects and Data on 8,542 Cases. Springfield, IL, Charles C Thomas, 1986
26. Duncan W, Arnott SJ, Jack WJL: The Edinburgh experience of treating sarcomas of soft tissues and bone with neutron irradiation. Clin Radiol 37:317, 1986
27. Dunham WK, Wilborn WH: Malignant fibrous histiocytoma of bone. J Bone Joint Surg [A] 61:939, 1979
28. Edeiken J: Roentgen Diagnosis of Diseases of Bone, 3rd ed. Baltimore, Williams & Wilkins, 1981
29. Eilber F, Giuliano A, Eckardt J, et al: Adjuvant chemotherapy for osteosarcoma: A randomized prospective trial. J Clin Oncol 5:21, 1987
30. Eilber FR, Morton DL, Grant TT: En block resection and allograft replacement for osteosarcoma of the extremity. In Jaffee N (ed): Bone Tumors in Children, pp 159–68. Littleton, MA, PSG, 1979
31. Enneking WF, Kagan A: The implications of "skip" metastases in osteosarcoma. Clin Orthop 3:33, 1975
32. Enneking WF, Kagan A: Intramarrow spread of osteosarcoma. In Management of Primary Bone and Soft Tissue Tumors, pp 171–178. Chicago, Year Book Medical Publishers, 1976
33. Enneking WF, Spanier SS, Goodman MA: A system for the surgical staging of musculoskeletal sarcoma. Clin Orthop 153:106, 1980
34. Eyre-Brook AL, Price CHG: Fibrosarcoma of bone. J Bone Joint Surg [B] 51:20, 1969
35. Fajardo LF: Pathology of Radiation Injury. New York, Masson Publishing, 1982
36. Farr GH, Juvos AG, Marcove RC, et al: Telangiectatic osteogenic sarcoma: A review of 28 cases. Cancer 34:1150, 1974
37. Farrell C, Kramer S, Torpie RJ, et al: Experiences in radiation therapy for the treatment of osteosarcoma. In Symposium Ossium. London, E & S Livingston, 1970
38. Farrell C, Raventos A: Experiences in treating osteosarcoma at the Hospital of the University of Pennsylvania. Radiology 83:1080, 1964
39. Ferguson AB: Treatment of osteogenic sarcoma. J Bone Joint Surg 22:916, 1940
40. Ferguson AB: Orthopedic Surgery in Infancy and Childhood, 5th ed. Baltimore, Williams & Wilkins, 1981
41. Filler RM: Surgical treatment of pulmonary metastases from osteosarcoma. In Jaffee N (ed): Solid Tumors in Children, pp 169–182. Littleton, MA, PSG, 1979
42. Friedman M, Pearlman AW: Benign giant-cell tumor of bone. Radiation dosage for each type. Radiology 91:1151, 1968
43. Gaitan-Yanguas M: A study of the response of osteogenic sarcoma and adjacent normal tissues to radiation. Int J Radiat Oncol Biol Phys 7:593, 1981
44. Goffinet DR, Kaplan HS, Donaldson SS, et al: Combined radiosensitizer infusion and irradiation of osteogenic sarcoma. Radiology 117:211, 1975
45. Goldenburg RR, Campbell CH, Bonfiglio M: Giant-cell tumor of bone. J Bone Joint Surg [A] 52:619, 1970
46. Hall RB, Robinson LH, Malawar MM, et al: Periosteal osteosarcoma. Cancer 55:165, 1985
47. Harwood AR, Fornasier VL, Rider WD: Supervoltage irradiation in the management of giant-cell tumor of bone. Radiology 125:223, 1977
48. Harwood AR, Krajbich JI, Fornasier VL: Radiotherapy of chondrosarcoma of bone. Cancer 45:2769, 1980
49. Henderson ED, Dahlin DC: Chondrosarcoma of bone: A study of two hundred and eighty-eight cases. J Bone Joint Surg [A] 45:1450, 1963

50. Hutter RVP, Worcester JW, Francis KC, et al: Benign and malignant giant-cell tumors of bone. Cancer 15:653, 1962
51. Huvos AG: Bone Tumors: Diagnosis, Treatment and Prognosis. Philadelphia, WB Saunders, 1979
52. Huvos AG: Primary malignant fibrous histiocytoma of bone. NY State J Med 76:552, 1976
53. Huvos AG, Rosen G, Bretsky SS, et al: Telangiectatic osteogenic sarcoma: A clinicopathologic study of 124 patients. Cancer 49:1679, 1982
54. Huvos AG, Rosen G, Dabska M, et al: Mesenchymal chondrosarcoma. Cancer 51:1230, 1983
55. Jaffee N, Goorin A, Link M, et al: High-dose methotrexate in osteogenic sarcoma. Adjuvant chemotherapy and limb salvage results. Cancer Treat Rep 65:99, 1981
56. Jaffee N, Link MP, Cohen D, et al: High-dose methotrexate in osteogenic sarcoma. NCI Monogr 56:201, 1981
57. Jaffee N, Prudich J, Knapp J, et al: Treatment of primary osteosarcoma with intraarterial and intravenous high-dose methotrexate. J Clin Oncol 1:428, 1983
58. Jaffe N, Watts H, Fellows KE, et al: Resection for limb preservation. Cancer Treat Rep 62:217, 1978
59. Jeffree GM, Price DHG, Sissons HA: The metastatic patterns of osteosarcoma. Br J Cancer 32:87, 1975
60. Jenkin RDT: Radiation treatment of Ewing's sarcoma and osteogenic sarcoma. Can J Surg 20:530, 1977
61. Jenkin RDT: The treatment of osteosarcoma with radiation: Current indications. In Management of Primary Bone and Soft Tissue Tumors, pp 151–162. Chicago, Year Book Medical Publishers, 1977
62. Jenkin RDT, Allt WEC, Fitzpatrick PJ: Osteosarcoma: An assessment of management with particular reference to primary irradiation and selective delayed amputation. Cancer 30:393, 1972
63. Jentzch K, Binder H, Cramer H, et al: Leg function after radiotherapy for Ewing's sarcoma. Cancer 47:1267, 1981
64. Kahn LB, Webber B, Mills E, et al: Malignant fibrous histiocytoma (malignant fibrous xanthoma; xanthosarcoma) of bone. Cancer 42:640, 1978
65. Kim RY, Salter MM, Brascho PJ: High-energy irradiation in the management of chondrosarcoma. South Med J 76:729, 1983
66. Kinsella TJ: Limited surgery and radiation therapy for sarcomas of the hand and foot. Int J Radiat Oncol Biol Phys 12:2045, 1986
67. Kreicbergs A, Boquist L, Borsson B, et al: Prognostic factors in chondrosarcoma. Cancer 50:577, 1982
68. Larrson S-E, Lorentzon R, Boguist L: Giant-cell tumor of bone. J Bone Joint Surg [A] 57:167, 1975
69. Lee ES: Treatment of bone sarcoma. Proc Soc Med 64:1179, 1971
70. Lee ES, MacKenzie DH: Osteosarcoma: A study of the value of preoperative megavoltage radiation therapy. Br J Surg 51:252, 1964
71. Lichtenstein L: Bone Tumors, 5th ed. St. Louis, CV Mosby, 1977
72. Link MP: Adjuvant therapy in the treatment of osteosarcoma. In DeVita VT, Hellman S, Rosenberg SA (eds). Important Advances in Oncology. Philadelphia, JB Lippincott, 1986
73. Link MP, Goorin AM, Miser AW, et al: The effect of adjuvant chemotherapy on relapse-free survival in patients with osteosarcoma of the extremity. N Engl J Med 314:1600, 1986
74. Luck JV, Luck JV, Schwinn CP: Parosteal osteosarcoma: A treatment-oriented study. Clin Orthop 153:92, 1980
75. MacDonald I, Budd JW: Osteogenic sarcoma: A modified nomenclature and a review of 118 five year cures. Surg Gynecol Obstet 77:413, 1943
76. Marcove RC: The Surgery of Tumors of Bone and Cartilage. New York, Grune & Stratton, 1981
77. Marcove RC, Martini N, Rose G: The treatment of pulmonary metastases in osteogenic sarcoma. Clin Orthop 111:65, 1975
78. Marcove RC, Mike V, Hutter RVP, et al: Chondrosarcoma of the pelvis and upper end of the femur. J Bone Joint Surg [A] 54:501, 1972
79. Martin SE, Dwyer A, Kissane JM, et al: Small cell osteosarcoma. Cancer 50:990, 1982
80. Martinez A, Goffinet DR, Donaldson SS, et al: Intraarterial infusion of radiosensitizer (BUdR) combined with hypofractionated irradiation and chemotherapy for primary treatment of osteogenic sarcoma. Int J Radiat Oncol Biol Phys 11:123, 1985
81. Matsuno T, Unni KK, McLeod RA, et al: Telangiectatic osteosarcoma. Cancer 38:2538, 1976
82. McCarthy EF, Matsuno T, Dorfman HD: Malignant fibrous histiocytoma: A study of 35 cases. Hum Pathol 10:57, 1979
83. McGrath PJ: Giant cell tumor of bone. J Bone Joint Surg [B] 54:216, 1972
84. McNaney D, Lindberg RD, Ayala AG, et al: Fifteen year radiotherapy experience with chondrosarcoma of bone. Int J Radiat Oncol Biol Phys 8:187, 1982
85. Mirra JM: Bone Tumors: Diagnosis and Treatment. Philadelphia, JB Lippincott, 1980
86. Mnaymneh WA, Dudley HR, Mnaymneh LG: Giant cell tumor of bone. J Bone Joint Surg [A] 46:63, 1964
87. Mountain CF: The role of surgery in the management of pulmonary metastases. In Management of Primary Bone and Soft Tissue Tumors, pp 423–432. Chicago, Year Book Medical Publishers, 1976
88. Nakashima Y, Unni KK, Shives TC, et al: Mesenchymal chondrosarcoma of bone and soft tissue: A review of 111 cases. Cancer 57:2444, 1986
89. Newton KA, Barrett A: Prophylactic lung irradiation in the treatment of osteogenic sarcoma. Clin Radiol 29:493, 1978
90. Nobler MP, Higgihbotham NL, Phillips RF: The cure of aneurysmal bone cyst: Irradiation superior to surgery in an analysis of 33 cases. Radiology 90:1185, 1968
91. Perez C, Herson J, Kimball JC, et al: Prognosis after metastases in osteosarcoma. Am J Clin Oncol 1:315, 1978
92. Phillips TL, Sheline GE: Bone sarcoma following radiation therapy. Radiology 81:992, 1963
93. Phillips TC, Sheline GE: Radiation therapy of malignant bone tumors. Radiology 92:1537, 1969
94. Pritchard DJ: Is adjuvant chemotherapy of osteosarcoma of proved value? In Wiernik PH (ed): Controversies in Oncology, pp 195–206. New York, John Wiley, 1982
95. Rab GT, Ivins JC, Childs DS, et al: Elective whole lung irradiation in treatment of osteogenic sarcoma. Cancer 38:939, 1976
96. Reagan MT, Clowry LJ, Cox JD, et al: Radiation therapy in the treatment of malignant fibrous histiocytoma. Int J Radiat Oncol Biol Phys 7:311, 1981
97. Romsdahl MM, Evans HL, Ayala AG: Surgical treatment of chondrosarcoma. In Management of Primary Bone and Soft Tissue Tumors. Chicago, Year Book Medical Publishers, 1976
98. Rosen G, Caparros B, Huvos AG, et al: Preoperative chemotherapy for osteogenic sarcoma: Selection of postoperative adjuvant therapy based on response of primary tumor to preoperative chemotherapy. Cancer 49:1221, 1982
99. Rosen G, Marcove RC, Caparros B, et al: Primary osteogenic sarcoma: The rationale for the timing of thoracic surgery. Cancer 43:2163, 1979
100. Rosen G, Nirenberg A, Caparros B, et al: Osteogenic sarcoma: Eighty percent three-year disease-free survival with combination chemotherapy. NCI Monogr 56:213, 1981
101. Rosen G, Tefft M, Martinez A, et al: Combination chemotherapy and radiation therapy in treatment of metastatic osteogenic sarcomas. Cancer 35:622, 1975
102. Rubin P, Casaret GW: Clinical Radiation Pathology. Philadelphia, WB Saunders, 1968
103. Ryall RDH, Bates T, Newton KA, et al: Combination of radiotherapy and Razoxane (^{150}IRF) for chondrosarcoma. Cancer 44: 891, 1979
104. Sanerkin NG: The diagnosis and grading of chondrosarcoma of bone. Cancer 45:582, 1980
105. Scanlon PW: Split-course radiotherapy for radioresistant bone and soft tissue sarcoma: Ten years' experience. Am J Radiol 114:544, 1972
106. Schajowicz F: Tumors and Tumorlike Lesions of Bones and Joints. New York, Springer-Verlag, 1981
107. Sim FH, Ivins JC, Pritchard DJ: Surgical treatment of osteogenic sarcoma at the Mayo Clinic. Cancer Treat Rep 62:205, 1978

108. Simon MA, Hecht JD: Invasion of bones and joints by primary bone sarcomas in adults. Cancer 50:1649, 1982
109. Simon MA, Kirchner PT: Scintigraphic evaluation of primary bone tumors. J Bone Joint Surg [A] 62:758, 1980
110. Spanier SS, Enneking WF, Enriques P: Primary malignant fibrous histiocytoma of bone. Cancer 36:2084, 1975
111. Springfield DS, Schmidt R, Graham-Pole J, et al: Surgical treatment for osteosarcoma, J Bone Joint Surg [A] 70:1124, 1988
112. Suit HD: Radiation therapy given under conditions of local tissue hypoxia for bone and soft tissue sarcomas. In Tumors of Bone and Soft Tissue, pp 143–163. Chicago, Year book Medical Publisher, 1969
113. Suit HD: Role of therapeutic radiology in cancer of bone. Cancer 35:930, 1975
114. Suit HD, Goiten M, Munzenrider J, et al: Definitive radiation therapy for chordoma and chondrosarcoma of base of skull and cervical spine. J Neurosurg 56:377, 1982
115. Sung HW, Kuo DP, Shu WP, et al: Giant cell tumor of bone: Analysis of two hundred and eight cases in Chinese patients. J Bone Joint Surg [A] 64:755, 1982
116. Sutow WW, Herson J, Perez C: Survival after metastases in osteosarcoma. NCI Monogr 56:227, 1981
117. Sweetnam R, Knoweldon J, Sedon H: Bone sarcoma: Treatment by irradiation, amputation, or a combination of the two. Br Med J 2:363, 1971
118. Taylor WF, Ivins JC, Dahlin DC, et al: Trends and variability in survival from osteosarcoma. Mayo Clin Proc 53:695, 1983
119. Taylor WF, Ivins JC, Pritchard DJ, et al: Trends and variability in survival among patients with osteosarcoma: A 7-year update. Mayo Clin Proc 60:91, 1985
120. Tochner Z, Kinsella T, Rowland J, et al: Treatment of unresectable sarcoma (SA) with hyperfractionated irradiation (XRT) and iododeoxyuridine (IUdR). [Abstract] Proc Am Soc Clin Oncol, 24th Annual Meeting, J Clin Oncol 1988
121. Unni KK, Dahlin DC, Beabout J, et al: Periosteal osteogenic sarcoma. Cancer 37:2476, 1976
122. Unni KK, Dahlin DC, Beabout JW, et al: Chondrosarcoma: Clear cell variant. J Bone Joint Surg [A] 58:675, 1976
123. Urban C, Rosen G, Huvos AG, et al: Chemotherapy of malignant fibrous histiocytoma of bone. Cancer 51:795, 1983
124. Uribe-Botero G, Russell WO, Sutow WW, et al: Primary osteosarcoma of bone: A clinicopathologic investigation of 243 cases, with necrophic studies in 54. Am J Clin Pathol 67:427, 1977
125. Urtasun RC, McConnachie PR: Disappearance of osteogenic sarcoma after irradiation: Immunologic observations. J Can Assoc Radiol 27:80, 1976
126. van den Brenk HAS, Kerr RC, Madigan JP, et al: Results from tourniquet hypoxia and hyperbaric oxygen techniques combined with megavoltage treatment of sarcoma of bone and soft tissue. Am J Radiol 96:760, 1966
127. Watts HG: Introduction to resection of musculoskeletal sarcomas. Clin Orthop 153:31, 1980
128. Weichselbaum RR, Cassady JR: Radiation therapy in osteosarcoma. In Jaffe N (ed): Solid Tumors in Childhood, pp 183–190. Boca Raton, FL, CRC Press, 1983
129. Weisenberger TH, Eilber FR, Grant TT, et al: Multidisciplinary "limb salvage" treatment of soft tissue and skeletal sarcomas. Int J Radiat Oncol Biol Phys 7:1495, 1981
130. Weiss SH, Enzinger FM: Malignant fibrous histiocytoma. An analysis of 200 cases. Cancer 41:2250, 1978

Ewing's Sarcoma

131. Bacci GM, Picci P, Gitelis S, et al: The treatment of localized Ewing's sarcoma. Cancer 49:1561, 1982
132. Bator SM, Bauer TW, Marke KE, et al: Periosteal Ewing's sarcoma. Cancer 58:1781, 1986
133. Berger PE, Kuhn JP: Computed tomography of tumors of the musculoskeletal system in children and clinical applications. Radiology 127:171, 1978
134. Boyko OB, Cory DA, Cohen MD, et al: MR imaging of osteogenic and Ewing's sarcoma. AJR 148:317, 1987
135. Brereton HD, Simon R, Pomeroy TC: Pretreatment serum lactate dehydrogenase predicting metastatic spread of Ewing's sarcoma. Ann Intern Med 83:352, 1975
136. Brown AP, Fixsen JA, Plowman PN: Local control of Ewing's sarcoma: An analysis of 67 patients. Br J Radiol 60:261, 1987
137. Burgert EO, Nesbit ME, Garnsey LA, et al: Multimodality therapy for the management of non-pelvic localized Ewing's sarcoma of the bone: An Intergroup Study (IESS-II). J Clin Oncol 8:1514, 1990
138. Chan RC, Sutow WW, Lindberg RD, et al: Management and results of localized Ewing's sarcoma. Cancer 43:1001, 1979
139. Cutler SJ, Young JF: Third national cancer survey: Incidence data. NCI Monogr 41:412, 1975
140. Dahlin DC, Coventry M, Scanlan P: Ewing's sarcoma: A clinical analysis of 165 cases. J Bone Jont Surg [A] 43:184, 1961
141. Dahlin DC, Unni KK, Matsuno T: Malignant (fibrous) histiocytoma of bone: Fact or fancy? Cancer 39:1508, 1977
142. Donaldson SS, Shuster J, Andreozzi C: The Pediatric Oncology Group (POG) experience in Ewing's sarcoma of bone. Med Pediatr Oncol 17:283, 1989
143. Evans RG, Nesbit ME, Gehan EA, et al: Multimodal therapy for the management of localized Ewing's sarcoma of pelvic and sacral bones: A report from the Second Intergroup Ewing's Sarcoma Study (IESS-II). J Clin Oncol 9:1173, 1991
144. Ewing J: Diffuse endothelioma of bone. Proc NY Pathol Soc 21:17, 1921
145. Frankel RS, Jones AF, Cohen JA, et al: Clinical correlations of ^{67}Ga and skeletal whole body radionuclide studies with radiography in Ewing's sarcoma. Radiology 110:597, 1975
146. Fraumeni JF: Stature and malignant tumors of bone in childhood and adolescene. Cancer 20:967, 1967
147. Gehan EA, Nesbit ME, Burgert EO, et al: Prognostic factors in Ewing's sarcoma. JNCI 56:273, 1981
148. Gilula L: Personal communication, 1990
149. Glass AG, Fraumeni JF: Epidemiology of bone cancer in children. JNCI 44:187, 1970
150. Goebel V, Juergens H, Etpuler G, et al: Prognostic significance of tumor volume in localized Ewing's sarcoma of bone in children and adolescents. Cancer Res Clin Oncol 113:187, 1987
151. Hayes FA, Thompson EI, Kumar M, et al: Long-term survival in patients with Ewing's sarcoma relapsing after completing therapy. Med Pediatr Oncol 15:254, 1987
152. Hayes FA, Thompson EI, Meyer WH, et al: Therapy for localized Ewing's sarcoma of bone. J Clin Oncol 17:208, 1989
153. Hustu HO, Pinkel D, Pratt CB: The treatment of clinically localized Ewing's sarcoma with concurrent radiotherapy and chemotherapy. Cancer 30:1522, 1972
154. Jaffe N, Traggis D, Sallan S, et al: Improved outlook for Ewing's sarcoma with combination chemotherapy (vincristine, Adriamycin-D, and cyclophosphamide) and radiation therapy. Cancer 38:1925, 1976
155. Jentzsch K, Binder H, Cramer H, et al: Leg function after radiotherapy for Ewing's sarcoma. Cancer 47:1267, 1981
156. Jones GR, Miller JH, White L, et al: Improved detection of metastatic Ewing's sarcoma with the use of bone marrow scintigraphy. Med Pediatr Oncol 15:78, 1987
157. Juergens H, Bier V, Dunst J, et al: The GPO Cooperative Ewing's Sarcoma Studies CESS 81/86: Report after 6.5 years. Klin Pediatr 200:243, 1988
158. Kahn HJ, Thorner PS: Monoclonal antibody MB2: A potential marker for Ewing's sarcoma and primitive neuroectodermal tumor. Pediatr Pathol 9:153, 1989
159. Kissane JM, Askin FB, Foulkes M, et al: Ewing's sarcoma of bone: Clinicopathologic aspects of 303 cases from the Intergroup Ewing's Sarcoma Study. Hum Pathol 14:773, 1983
160. Marcus RB Jr, Graham-Pole JR, Springfield DS, et al: High-risk Ewing's sarcoma: End-Intensification using autologous bone marrow transplantation. Int J Radiat Oncol Biol Phys 15:53, 1988
161. Marcus RB, Million RR: The effect of primary tumor size in the prognosis of Ewing's sarcoma. [Abstract] Int J Radiat Oncol Biol Phys 24:88, 1984

162. Marsa GW, Johnson RE: Altered pattern of metastases following treatment of Ewing's sarcoma with radiation and adjuvant chemotherapy. Cancer 27:1051, 1971
163. Miser JS, Kinsella TJ, Triche TJ, et al: Ifosfamide with Mesna uroprotection and etoposide: An effective regimen in the treatment of recurrent sarcomas and other tumors of children and young adults. J Clin Oncol 5:1191, 1987
164. Neff JR: Nonmetastatic Ewing's sarcoma of bone: The role of surgical therapy. Clin Orthop 204:111, 1986
165. Nesbit ME, Gehan EA, Burgert EO, et al: Multimodal therapy for the management of primary nonmetastatic Ewing's sarcoma of bone: A long term follow-up of the first Intergroup Study (IESS-I). J Clin Oncol 8:1664, 1990
166. Nesbit ME, Perez CA, Tefft M, et al: Multimodal therapy for the management of primary non-metastatic Ewing's sarcoma of bone: An intergroup study. NCI Monogr 56:255, 1981
167. Nesbit ME, Robinson LL, Dehner LP: Round cell sarcoma of bone. In Sutow WW, Fernbach DJ, Vietti TJ (eds): Clinical Pediatric Oncology, pp 710–733. St. Louis, CV Mosby, 1984
168. Perez CA, Tefft M, Nesbit ME, et al: Radiation therapy in the multimodal management of Ewing's sarcoma of bone: Report of the Intergroup Ewing's Sarcoma Study. JNCI 56:263, 1981
169. Pomeroy TC, Johnson RE: Prognostic factors for survival of Ewing's sarcoma. AJR 123:598, 1975
170. Pritchard DJ: Surgical experience in the management of Ewing's sarcoma of bone. NCI Monogr 56:169, 1981
171. Pritchard DJ: Small round cell Tumors. Orthop Clin North Am 20:367, 1989
172. Rosen G, Caparros B, Huvos AG, et al: Preoperative chemotherapy for osteogenic sarcoma: Selection of postoperative adjuvant chemotherapy based on response of primary tumor to preoperative chemotherapy. Cancer 49:1221, 1982
173. Schajowicz F: Ewing's sarcoma and reticulum cell sarcoma of bone with special reference to the histochemical demonstration of glycogen as an aid to differential diagnosis. J Bone Joint Surg [A] 41:349, 1959
174. Shimada H, Newton WA, Soule EH, et al: Pathologic features of extraosseous Ewing's sarcoma: A report from the Intergroup Rhabdomyosarcoma Study. Hum Pathol 19:442, 1988
175. Strong LC, Herson J, Osborne BM et al: Risk of radiation-related subsequent malignant tumors in survivors of Ewing's sarcoma. JNCI 62:1401, 1979
176. Telles NC, Rabson AS, Pomeroy TC: Ewing's sarcoma: An autopsy study. Cancer 41:2321, 1978
177. Thomas PRM, Perez CA, Neff JR, et al: The management of Ewing's sarcoma: Role of radiotherapy in local tumor control. Cancer Treat Rep 68:703, 1984
178. Triche TJ, Cavazzana AO, Navarro S, et al: N-myc protein expression in small round cell tumors. Neuroblastoma Res 2:475, 1988
179. Trigg ME, Glaubiger D, Nesbit ME: The frequency of isolated CNS involvement in Ewing's sarcoma. Cancer 49:2404, 1981
180. Yunis EJ, Walpusk JA, Agoshini RM, et al: Glycogen in neuroblastomas: A light and electron microscopic study of 440 cases. Am J Surg Pathol 3:313, 1979
181. Zucker JM, Henry-Amar M, Sarrazin D. et al: Intensive systemic chemotherapy in localized Ewing's sarcoma in childhood. Cancer 52:415, 1983

67

Soft Tissue Sarcomas (Excluding Retroperitoneum)

Theodore S. Lawrence
Allen S. Lichter

ANATOMY

Soft tissue sarcomas constitute a relatively rare group of malignancies that occur in tissues derived from the embryologic mesenchyme. Although nerve sheath tumors actually arise from cells of ectodermal origin, they are traditionally included in the soft tissue sarcoma category. Despite the diversity of tissues and locations of origin, these tumors are grouped together because of overall similarities in natural history and treatment. The soft tissue tumors discussed in this chapter are distinct from the pediatric sarcomas, such as Ewing's sarcoma or rhabdomyosarcoma (see Chaps. 66 and 72), and from visceral sarcomas, such as uterine or bladder sarcomas, which are discussed in the chapters describing tumors of those organs.

Although soft tissue sarcomas can arise in any part of the body, some general anatomic principles on which treatment is based can be described. Although soft tissue sarcomas can occur in subcutaneous tissues, most occur within muscle groups. These tumors usually respect fascial boundaries and remain confined within the muscular compartment of origin.[41] However, subclinical disease can exist 5 cm to 10 cm from the gross tumor, representing longitudinal extension along the muscular compartment. Surgical resection changes the potential pattern of spread. After tumor cells are released through surgical manipulation, they can be carried by dissecting hematomas throughout the compartment. Both the surgical and radiotherapeutic principles of treatment are based on these anatomic patterns of presentation and spread.

EPIDEMIOLOGY AND RISK FACTORS

Approximately 5600 cases of soft tissue sarcomas occur each year, resulting in 3000 deaths. Men and women are approximately equally affected; the male-to-female ratio is 1.15 : 1.[18] These tumors can occur in any age group, with a recent large series showing that 52% of the patients were over 60 years of age at diagnosis, 28% were 40 to 60 years of age, and 20% were younger than 40 years.[65]

Although no indisputable cause can be determined for most soft tissue sarcomas, several environmental toxins have been implicated as possible etiologic agents. For instance, vinyl chloride appears to increase the risk of hepatic angiosarcomas.[29] Some, but not all, studies have suggested that pesticides containing phenoxyacetic acids increase the risk soft tissue sarcomas.[51,54,72]

Therapeutic irradiation unquestionably produces a small but detectable risk of soft tissue sarcoma. Cahan and associates[20] proposed standards for concluding that an observed sarcoma is radiation-induced. It should develop within the radiation portal, be histologically distinct from the primary lesion, and occur within a latency period consistent with biologic principles of tumor growth, which was initially suggested as 5 years, although 3 years may be more realistic.[20] These distinctions are not always obvious. For instance, it was initially concluded that therapeutic irradiation was responsible for the high incidence of osteogenic sarcoma in patients with congenital retinoblastoma until it was discovered that these second tumors occurred in patients who had never received irradiation.[2] These criteria have been met in patients reported to develop bone and soft tissue sarcomas after receiving radiation therapy for benign and malignant disease.[50,64,107] Although the rarity of radiation-induced soft tissue sarcomas makes it difficult to be precise, the overall risk of soft tissue sarcoma in patients who have survived for 5 years after the therapeutic irradiation is approximately 0.5%.

Genetic factors also appear to be involved in a small fraction of soft tissue sarcomas. Although central nervous system gliomas are the dominant tumors found in patients with von Recklinghausen's neurofibromatosis, there appears to be an increased risk of neurosarcomas as well.[94] A family cancer syndrome (Li-Fraumeni syndrome) has been identified in which patients exhibit an increased risks of breast cancer and soft tissue sarcomas.[12,70]

A history of trauma can be elicited from many patients presenting with soft tissue sarcoma, but there are no data establishing a cause-and-effect relationship. There does, however, appear to be an increase in lymphangiosarcoma in patients with breast cancer with chronic lymphedema after axillary dissection with or without axillary irradiation.[112]

NATURAL HISTORY

The chief pattern of spread of extremity soft tissue sarcomas is along the longitudinal axis of muscle compartments. At the time of surgery, lesions often appear to be encapsulated. However, this is a pseudocapsule, representing compressed normal tissue and reactive fibrosis.[41] In the less common sites of the trunk and head and neck, disease tends to invade into adjacent muscle groups. For these tumors the periosteum and fascia present partial barriers to tumor spread, and deep invasion is less common.

High-grade and, to a lesser extent, intermediate-grade lesions do have the potential to metastasize. Lymph nodes are infrequently involved, with an overall metastatic rate of approximately 4%. In a review of the pooled results from more than 5000 patients, the histopathologic subtypes that most commonly involve lymph nodes were synovial cell, epithelioid, and rhabdomyosarcomas, and only 14% to 20% of patients with these subtypes had involved lymph nodes.[8,74,108] It is for this reason that routine lymph node sampling is not performed as part of radical surgery for these patients.

Hematogenous metastasis occurs frequently in patients with high-grade lesions. These metastases typically occur within the first 2 years of diagnosis.[21,86] Approximately 50% of metastases are to the lungs.[86,104] Bone, liver, and skin metastases occurred in fewer than 5% of patients.[104] Retroperitoneal sarcomas display a somewhat different metastatic pattern. Although lung still predominates as a metastatic site, liver metastases and peritoneal carcinomatosis cause death in a substantial minority of patients.[86,95]

CLINICAL PRESENTATION

Although soft tissue sarcomas can occur in any site, over half are found in the extremities (Table 67-1). Patients usually present with a fairly long history of a slowly growing, painless mass. The median period between noticing the mass and presenting to the physician is approximately 4 months, and for some patients, years elapse between the appearance of a mass and its subsequent diagnosis as a sarcoma.[65] Patients with extremity sarcomas occasionally present with numbness, pain, or edema caused by tumor-induced neurovascular compromise. In the case of buttock or retroperitoneal tumors, masses can often attain an enormous size before coming to clinical attention.

DIAGNOSTIC WORKUP

In patients suspected of harboring a soft tissue sarcoma, the history should focus on whether the patient has a genetic predisposition, such as von Recklinghausen's neurofibromatosis, or has been exposed to therapeutic irradiation in the past. It is also important to assess the rate of tumor growth, because tumors that grow rapidly tend to be high grade. The physical examination must detail the size of the mass, because this is an important prognostic factor. In addition, evidence of neurovascular compromise and fixation to the bone should be sought, because the chance of performing a limb-sparing procedure in a patient with these findings is greatly decreased. A careful lymph node examination should always be performed.

The general staging evaluation for patients with soft tissue sarcomas is described in Table 67-2. Needle aspiration cytology rarely yields enough material to determine both the histopathologic subtype and grade, although it can be useful in diagnosing metastatic disease in patients with a history of soft tissue sarcoma.[4,63] The preferred procedure for diagnosing all but the smallest sarcomas (<3 cm) is an incisional biopsy, because an excisional biopsy may compromise the assessment of pathologic margins and the subsequent definitive procedure.

After the diagnosis has been established, a computed tomography (CT) scan of the involved site is critical in establishing tumor extent. The CT scan has decreased the need for routine tests such as the bone scan and angiography. Recent evidence suggests that magnetic resonance imaging (MRI) may have some advantages over CT scanning, because it better delineates individual muscles and compartments affected by the tumor.[3,22,31] Bone scans, however, are still useful in clarifying bone or periosteal involvement for tumors adjacent to bone.[40] Angiography remains important in determining both the vascular supply to tumors before surgery and the resectability of a lesion.

It is important to obtain a chest CT scan, especially in intermediate- or high-grade lesions. A chest roentgenogram can detect approximately two thirds of pulmonary metastases in soft tissue sarcoma.[77] However, additional lesions are found with full lung tomographs and CT scanning, and it appears that the latter is superior.[33,81]

Positron emission tomography (PET) scanning and MR spectroscopy have the potential to provide noninvasively information on tumor metabolism and grade, although the clinical role of these tests remains to be determined.[30,58]

TABLE 67–1
Occurrence of Soft Tissue Sarcomas by Site

INVESTIGATION	NO. OF PATIENTS	HEAD AND NECK (%)	TRUNK (%)	UPPER EXTREMITY (%)	LOWER EXTREMITY (%)	RETRO-PERITONEUM (%)	MEDIA-STINUM (%)
AJC Task Force[91]	1211	14.6	18.0	13.3	40.4	13.0	0.7
Christie Hospital[15]	189	5.8	17.5	13.2	45.4	15.9	2.1
M.D. Anderson[71]	300	8.7	17.7	21.0	45.7	7.0	NR†
American College of Surgeons[65] *	4550	8.9	17.9	13.1	46.4	12.5	1.3
Massachusetts General Hospital[97]	347	7.2	17.0	18.7	47.4	9.5	NR†
Total	6597	9.8	17.8	13.8	45.3	12.3	1.1

* *Patterns of Care summary.*
† *Not reported.*

TABLE 67–2
Diagnostic Workup for Patients With Soft Tissue Sarcoma

ROUTINE STUDIES
History and physical examination
Complete blood count and chemistries
Plain roentgenogram of involved area
CT scan or magnetic resonance imaging of involved site
Chest roentgenogram
CT scan of chest

COMPLEMENTARY STUDIES
Bone scan
Arteriogram
Lymphangiogram
Ultrasound

STAGING SYSTEM

The American Joint Committee staging system groups patients into distinct prognostic groups (Table 67-3). For Stages I to III, stage is virtually synonymous with grade. This is appropriate because grade is the most important prognostic factor for patients with soft tissue sarcomas. The prognostic significance of size is also recognized. The Stage IV category includes patients with regional (Stage IVA) or distant (Stage IVB) metastases.

TABLE 67–3
TNM Staging for Soft Tissue Sarcomas

PRIMARY TUMOR (T)

TX	Minimum requirements to assess primary tumor cannot be met
T0	No demonstrable tumor
T1	Tumor ≤ 5 cm in diameter
T2	Tumor > 5 cm in diameter

NODAL INVOLVEMENT (N)

NX	Minimum requirements to assess regional nodes cannot be met
N0	No histologically verified metastasis to lymph nodes
N1	Histologically verified regional lymph node metastasis

DISTANT METASTASIS (M)

MX	Minimum requirements to assess presence of distant metastasis cannot be met
M0	No known distant metastasis
M1	Distant metastasis present (specify site)

TUMOR GRADE (G)

G1	Well differentiated
G2	Moderately well differentiated; undifferentiated

STAGE GROUPING

Stage IA	G1	T1	N0	M0
Stage IB	G1	T2	N0	M0
Stage IIA	G2	T1	N0	M0
Stage IIB	G2	T2	N0	M0
Stage IIIA	G3–4	T1	N0	M0
Stage IIIB	G3–4	T2	N0	M0
Stage IVA	any G	any T	N1	M0
Stage IVB	any G	any T	any N	M1

(Beahrs OH, Henson DE, Hutter RVP, Myers MH [eds]: Manual for Staging of Cancer, 3rd ed. Philadelphia, JB Lippincott, 1988)

PATHOLOGIC CLASSIFICATION

Several pathologic classification systems employed to describe soft tissue sarcomas attempt to group lesions according to their histogenic origin.[17,42,75] One example is given in Table 67-4. However, these distinctions are difficult to reproduce among institutions and observers. One example is the diagnosis of malignant fibrous histiocytoma, which was rarely made 20 years ago and is now one of the most common subgroups described. It is more likely that this represents changing pathologic distinctions rather than a dramatic change in the tumors themselves. Another example comes from a review of Southeastern Cancer Study Group soft tissue sarcoma protocols.[87] Of the 207 evaluable cases submitted for review to a referee panel of patholo-

TABLE 67–4
Classification of Soft Tissue Sarcomas by Histogenic Origin

TISSUE		SARCOMA
I.	Fibrous	1. Fibrosarcoma
		a. Adult type
		b. Congenital and infantile
		c. Postirradiation
		d. Scar (burn, chronic infection, etc.)
II.	Muscular	1. Leiomyosarcoma
		2. Rhabdomyosarcoma
		a. Embryonal
		b. Botryoid
		c. Alveolar
		d. Pleomorphic
III.	Fat	1. Well differentiated
		a. Lipoma-like
		b. Inflammatory
		c. Sclerosing
		2. Myxoid type
		3. Pleomorphic type
		4. Round cell type
		5. Dedifferentiated
IV.	Neural	1. Malignant schwannoma
		2. Neuroblastoma
		3. Malignant paraganglioma
		4. Neuroepithelioma
		5. Clear cell sarcoma of tendon sheath
V.	Vascular	1. Hemangiosarcoma
		2. Kaposi's sarcoma
		3. Malignant hemangiopericytoma
		4. Lymphangiosarcoma
VI.	Histiocytic	1. Malignant fibrous histiocytoma
		a. Storiform-pleomorphic
		b. Myxoid
		c. Giant Cell
		d. Inflammatory
		e. Angiomatoid
		f. Post-scar (burn, chronic infection, etc.) and radiation
VII.	Synovial	1. Synovial sarcoma (mono- and biphasic)
VIII.	Osseous	1. Osteosarcoma
		2. Chondrosarcoma
		3. Mesenchymal chondrosarcoma
IX.	Multipotent	1. Malignant mesenchymoma
X.	Uncertain	1. Alveolar soft part sarcoma
		2. Epithelioid sarcoma
		3. Ewing's sarcoma
		4. Undifferentiated

(Mirra JM: Pathology of soft tissue sarcomas. In Eilber FR, Morton DL, Sondak VK [eds]: The Soft Tissue Sarcomas, p 11. Orlando, FL, Grune & Stratton, 1987)

gists, 12 (6%) were not considered to be sarcomas. In 58 (28%) of these cases, there was disagreement between the primary institution and the reviewer. In some pathologic categories, such as liposarcoma and fibrosarcoma, the panel and primary institution were in agreement less than 50% of the time. Recent advances in immunohistochemical analysis may make these assessments more reproducible.[110] For soft tissue sarcomas in adults, clinical decisions rarely depend on histopathologic subtype alone but incorporate grade as the most critical factor.

The assessment of grade is based on cellularity, nuclear pleomorphism, frequency of typical and atypical mitoses, degree of necrosis, and infiltrative pattern.[69,75] In a review of the National Cancer Institute series, the degree of necrosis was found to be the most important factor in determining outcome.[28] Grade I lesions were defined as having no necrosis, grade II as having less than 15% necrosis, and grade III as having greater than 15%. A clinically useful grading system that incorporates necrosis and histologic type is presented in Table 67-5.

It is clear that, as was the case with histopathologic subtype, the definition of grade is subjective. In the Southeastern Cancer Study Group study, there was approximately 25% disagreement on grade between the primary institution and the referee panel, with the least disagreement concerning grade 1 lesions (17%).[87] Although it is possible that the assessment of chromosomal changes or Ki-67 content (which may reflect proliferative capability) may improve pathologic subtyping, more experience is needed with these techniques before they can be used on a routine basis.[57,76,103]

PROGNOSTIC FACTORS

Despite its subjective nature, grade is the most important predictor of both overall survival and disease-free survival in patients with soft tissue sarcoma. For instance, among 565 patients presented to Memorial Sloan-Kettering Cancer Center with soft tissue sarcomas, the 5-year overall survival rate was 90% for low-grade tumors and 60% for high-grade tumors.[102] Among the 297 patients reviewed by the American Joint Committee task force, the 5-year recurrence-free survival rate decreased with increasing grade, from 68% for grade I to 50% for grade II to 25% for grade III.[52]

Another prognostic factor is tumor size, with increasing size corresponding to decreased local control and a higher risk of distant disease.[27,71,96] The presence of positive nodes, although rare, definitely decreases survival.[74] Because the American Joint Committee staging system is based on grade and nodal status, it is logical that stage has also been found to be a predictor.[91] Additional factors that influence local control are the presence of symptoms at presentation, a positive surgical margin, and the location of the tumor.[11,21,27,86]

GENERAL MANAGEMENT

Surgery

Surgical approaches to soft tissue sarcoma can be grouped into four categories.[21,41,92]

Intralesional debulking refers to partial removal of the

TABLE 67–5
Grading of Soft Tissue Sarcomas

MORPHOLOGIC CRITERIA	SPECIFIC TYPES
Grade 1 lesions	
Histologic type or subtype	Lipoma-like liposarcoma Myxoid liposarcoma Epithelial hemangioendothelioma Infantile fibrosarcoma
Histologic type and location	Deep-seated dermatofibrosarcoma protuberans Subcutaneous myxoid malignant fibrous histiocytoma
Histologic type, mitoses, and differentiation	Well-differentiated malignant hemangiopericytoma Well-differentiated malignant leiomyosarcoma Well-differentiated malignant neurofibrosarcoma Well-differentiated malignant fibrosarcoma Myxoid chondrosarcoma
Grade 2 or 3 lesions Histologic type and necrosis (N ≤ 15% G2; N > 15% G3)	Pleomorphic liposarcoma Round-cell liposarcoma Fibrosarcoma Malignant fibrous histiocytoma Malignant hemangiopericytoma Synovial sarcoma Epithelial sarcoma Neurofibrosarcoma Leiomyosarcoma Angiosarcoma Unclassified sarcoma
Grade 3 lesions Histologic type	Alveolar rhabdomyosarcoma Neuroblastoma Extraskeletal Ewing's sarcoma Mesenchymal chondrosarcoma

(Leyvraz S, Costa J: Semin Surg Oncol 4:3, 1988)

lesion. It is typically performed to accomplish an incisional biopsy or by inadvertently cutting through tumor as part of another procedure.

With a simple excisional biopsy ("shell out"), the margin is the pseudocapsule. Because the pseudocapsule represents the compressed edge of normal tissue with surrounding reactive fibrosis produced by the invading tumor, there is a high likelihood that subclinical disease is left behind. The local recurrence rate after this procedure is approximately 80%. After a more extensive excision has been performed after a simple excisional biopsy, gross residual tumor has been reported in 49% of the specimens.[46]

In wide local excision, the tumor is removed with a margin of at least several centimeters of normal tissue from within the same muscle compartment. This operation can encompass many procedures, ranging from little more than a simple excision to slightly less than a compartmental resection. The local recurrence rates from this operation reflect this variability, ranging from 30% to 60%.

Radical excision, refers to an operation that removes en bloc the tumor and the complete compartment. It can be accomplished while sparing the limb by performing a compartmental resection, in which muscles are removed from origin to insertion. Radical excision can sometimes be accomplished only by an amputation. The local control rate under these conditions is approximately 80% to 90%.

Surgery can be combined with radiation therapy to replace amputations with limb-sparing procedures for most patients without a significant sacrifice in local control.[36,71,86,96] However, the effectiveness of radiation therapy is greatly influenced by the quality of the surgical procedure. For instance, if there is doubt concerning the amount of residual tumor or the adequacy of excision, reexcision should be employed, because positive margins greatly increase the change of local recurrence, even if postoperative irradiation is given.[11,89] Surgical scars, which are at risk for subclinical disease, should be oriented longitudinally in the extremity; otherwise circumferential limb irradiation, which is hazardous to apply, might be required. It is important to use surgical clips to define the tumor bed and tumor volume to allow assessment of the unique positions often required to minimize the treatment of normal tissues.[99]

Chemotherapy

Chemotherapy has been used in the treatment of metastatic sarcoma and as adjuvant therapy. For metastatic disease, the traditional agents are cyclophosphamide, doxorubicin, and dacarbazine (DTIC). The response rate using these drugs is approximately 30%.[5,9,13,83] Ifosfamide administered with mesna to prevent hemorrhagic cystitis has recently been shown to be an active agent in treating this disease.[6]

With only modest responses seen in metastatic disease, it is not surprising that the role of adjuvant chemotherapy is controversial. The use of a control (observation) arm is particularly important, because historic controls do significantly worse than concurrent controls receiving no adjuvant treatment.[34] In six randomized studies, single-agent doxorubicin therapy did not improve overall survival and improved disease-free survival in only one study.[5,39] Combination chemotherapy appears to prolong disease-free survival but not overall survival for patients with high-grade extremity sarcomas.[23,35] However, this improvement does not extend to nonextremity sarcomas, because it has been shown that adjuvant chemotherapy is of no benefit in truncal or head and neck sarcomas and is potentially harmful in the treatment of retroperitoneal sarcomas.[47,48] Currently, adjuvant chemotherapy should be confined chiefly to clinical investigation. Many tumor biopsies express cell-surface P-glycoprotein, which has been associated with multidrug resistance and may account for the resistance to doxorubicin seen in some patients.[45]

Radiation Therapy

Radiation therapy can be used preoperatively, postoperatively, or as a "sandwich" technique, with part of the dose delivered before and some delivered after surgical resection. All three approaches have been successful when applied carefully in selected cases. Our preference is for postoperative irradiation if the tumor can be resected with clean surgical margins. If the tumor is bulky and unresectable and limb-sparing treatment is still desired, preoperative therapy is undoubtedly warranted. Radiation can also be delivered with radical or palliative intent for patients who refuse surgery or who have unresectable sarcomas.[19,93,100]

The role of radiation therapy in treating low-grade tumors has not been thoroughly studied. For lesions that have been widely excised with negative margins, we do not typically recommend postoperative treatment, because a substantial fraction of these patients are cured by this procedure. Local recurrences of low-grade lesions can often be reexcised with organ conservation, unlike the intermediate- and high-grade sarcomas, which require amputation. Radiation therapy is usually reserved for patients with positive or questionable margins in a location where local recurrence would require amputation.

Two major issues remain with regard to local control of extremity, truncal, and head and neck sarcomas. First, 10% to 30% of patients with extremity sarcomas still require amputation to achieve clear proximal margins. Clinical investigation must be directed either to treat these patients preoperatively or to deliver higher doses postoperatively so that limb sparing procedures can be performed in this group currently undergoing amputation. Second, although some patients with unresectable sarcomas can be cured with radiation therapy, the local failure rate for these patients is unacceptably high. It is possible that one of several new approaches, such as using the radiosensitizer iododeoxyuridine, intraarterial chemotherapy, hyperthermia, or neutrons, may lead to improvements in these areas.[14,25,32,60,68]

Readers requiring additional information are directed to two recent monographs on soft tissue sarcomas.[38,84]

RADIATION THERAPY TECHNIQUES

Although soft tissue sarcomas can be present in virtually any part of the body, principles of treatment can be organized according to the three major sites of soft tissue sarcomas: extremity, trunk, and retroperitoneum. Radiation therapy treatment techniques for treating sarcomas of the trunk and extremities are discussed here; retroperitoneal sarcomas are discussed in Chapter 60.

Compartmental Nature of Soft Tissue Sarcomas

Before commencing a course of irradiation as part of the limb-sparing treatment, the radiation oncologist must define the muscle and compartment of involvement, comprehend the origin and insertion of the muscle, and evaluate the anatomic extent of the compartment that contains the primary tumor. The thigh is partitioned into three compartments: an extensor group, a flexor group, and an adductor group. Knowing the anatomic location of these muscle groups allows the oncologist to position the limb appropriately for irradiation of any of the compartments.

Volume at Risk

After the involved muscle compartment is defined, the extent of the initial radiation treatment volume is determined. Some authorities recommend treating the entire compartment ("origin-to-insertion") because hematoma can theoretically track cells to the farthest reaches of a muscle compartment.[24] Others have recommended a margin of 10 cm beyond high-grade neoplasms and 5 cm beyond low-grade neoplasms.[98] Lymph node-bearing regions are rarely at risk in extremity sarcomas, except in the case of rhabdomyosarcomas or sarcomas of synovial or epithelioid histology. Therefore, it is only with these histologies that prophylactic regional lymph node irradiation should be considered.

Positioning the Extremity

After the initial volume of treatment is determined, the next step in the treatment process is to determine the optimal position of the extremity. This involves rotating the extremity to treat the affected compartment with minimal exposure of uninvolved tissues. Examples of common treatment positions for soft tissue sarcomas are illustrated in Figures 67-1 to 67-3. Muscle groups in the thigh can often be treated in the "frogleg" position. The thigh is rotated and abducted, which separates the anterior compartment from the flexor and adductor compartments. Elevating one leg above the other is often an ideal position. For treating the posterior compartment, resting the leg on the patient couch is a good position for treatment to the anterior compartment. In the arm, the "throwing" position, which separates effectively the biceps compartment from the triceps compartment, is often used.

Positioning patients can sometimes be difficult. Some patients cannot move their extremities with great ease because of the effects of tumor or surgery. If the extremity is placed at too extreme an angle, CT scanning cannot be performed in the treatment position. It is often necessary to assess multiple limb positions to discover the optimal setup; the use of a fluoroscopic simulator is invaluable in these cases.

After the patient's position has been established, the next phase of the setup process is to immobilize using a device such as a foam cradle, a plaster mold, or a thermoplastic cast (Figs. 67-4 and 67-5). An attempt should be made to immobilize the joint above and below the treatment area, because this prevents the extremity from rotating out of position.

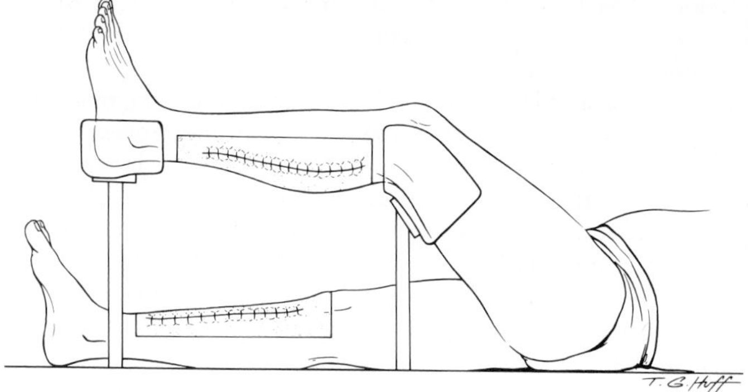

FIGURE 67–2. Elevating the leg on a support stand can facilitate treatment in the lower extremity. The elevated leg is in an excellent position for posterior compartment lesions, and the leg resting on the table is in a useful position for treatment of the anterior compartment of the leg.

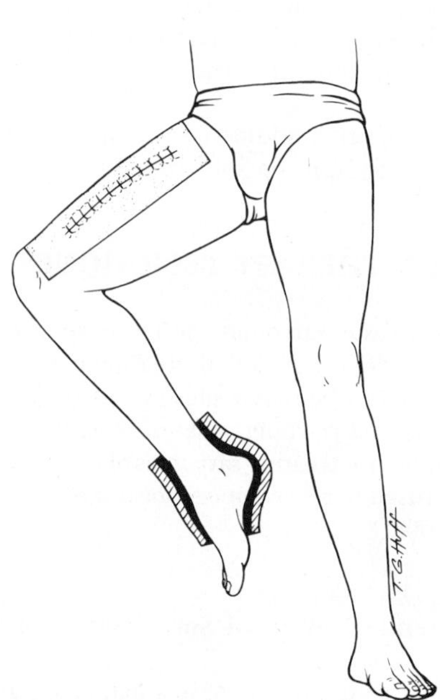

FIGURE 67–1. To treat anterior thigh musculature, the leg is often placed in the "frogleg" position. This separates the anterior thigh from the flexor and adductor compartments.

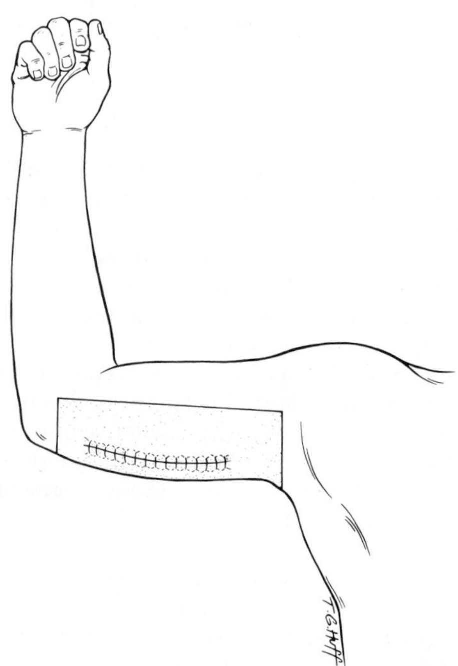

FIGURE 67–3. To treat lesions in the arm, the "throwing" position is often used. This adequately separates the biceps from the triceps compartment.

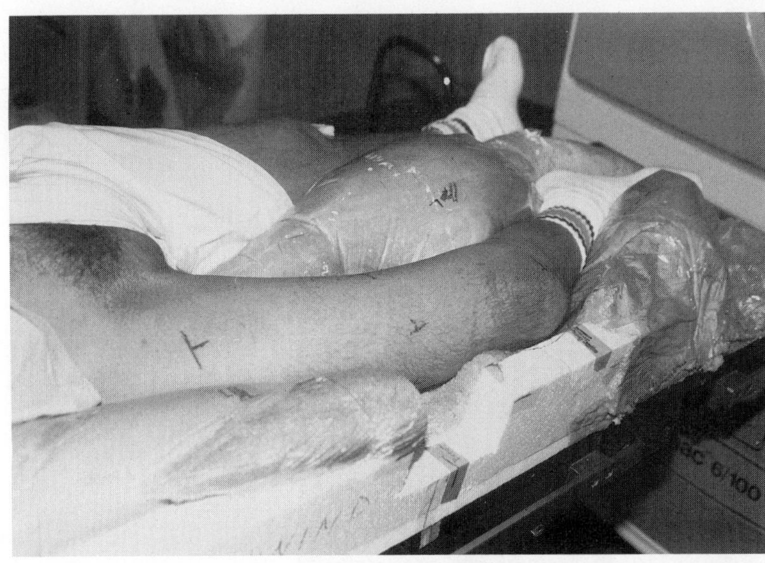

FIGURE 67–4. A custom foam cast immobilizes the right extremity for treatment of this sarcoma of the thigh.

Field Size

In most cases, three sets of treatment fields are used: the original volume, which encompasses the primary tumor with wide or complete coverage of the compartment; the secondary volume; which cones down to the tumor mass with a 5-cm to 6-cm margin; and the final tumor boost, which cones down on the clipped tumor volume with a 2-cm to 3-cm margin. In some circumstances, the original tumor is too long to be included in a single field. In such cases, fields must be gapped, and the match line between the fields is shifted each week to avoid excessive hot or cold dose areas. Full-dose irradiation should be delivered to the surgical scar. If the scar is being struck tangentially by the radiation fields, no bolus is necessary. However, if the scar is being irradiated with a direct perpendicular field, a bolus should be applied to ensure a brisk skin reaction and full dose over the scar itself. It is imperative that at least a 1-cm strip of soft tissue be spared in the treatment of an extremity to avoid subsequent edema and functional deficit in the limb.[24]

Treatment of thin regions of anatomy, such as the hand, foot, and the forearm, presents additional technical concerns. In such cases, skin-sparing by high-energy photon beams can produce underdosed regions inside the tumor volume, and bolus of the entire treatment volume may be necessary. Treatment of the involved region inside a water bath ensures uniform dosage to the affected area.[61,80]

After the fields are set up and simulation films obtained, contours are taken to allow the generation of a treatment plan. At least three contours are taken, usually at 2 cm from the inferior and superior margins of the field and at the central axis. Additional contours are often taken in regions that show significant changes in thickness, such as a surgical defect. Volumes are placed inside the contours by taking orthogonal films and plotting the location of the clips inside the contoured region (Fig. 67-6). In other cases, CT scanning in the treatment position is possible and of considerable help (Fig. 67-7). Wedge filters are usually necessary to improve the homogeneity for extremity sarcoma treatment.

Radiation Dose

Sarcomas are generally treated to high doses, even in the adjuvant setting. Low-energy photons are recommended with a maximum of approximately 6 MV, because higher energies could potentially spare too much superficial tissue. The initial volume is usually treated with 4000 cGy to 4500 cGy, the first conedown to 5400 cGy, and the final conedown to 6300 cGy, all

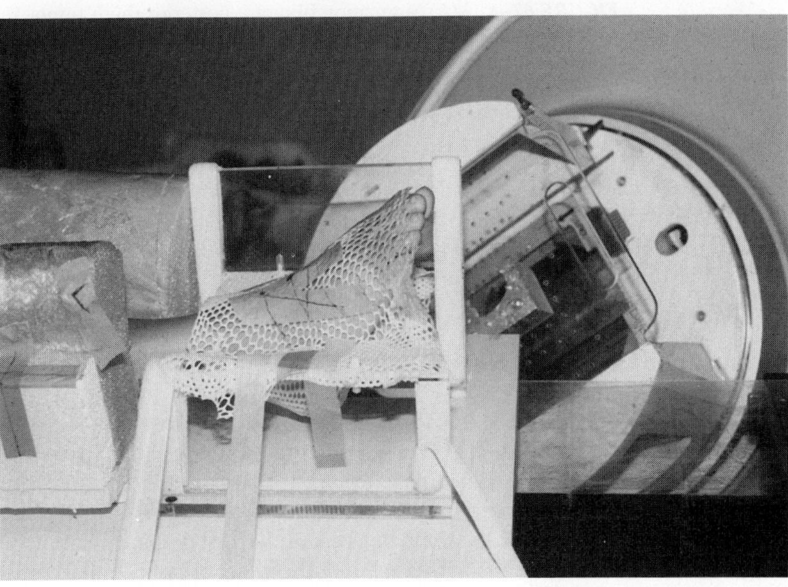

FIGURE 67–5. A thermoplastic cast immobilizes the foot for treatment of a synovial sarcoma involving the dorsum of the foot.

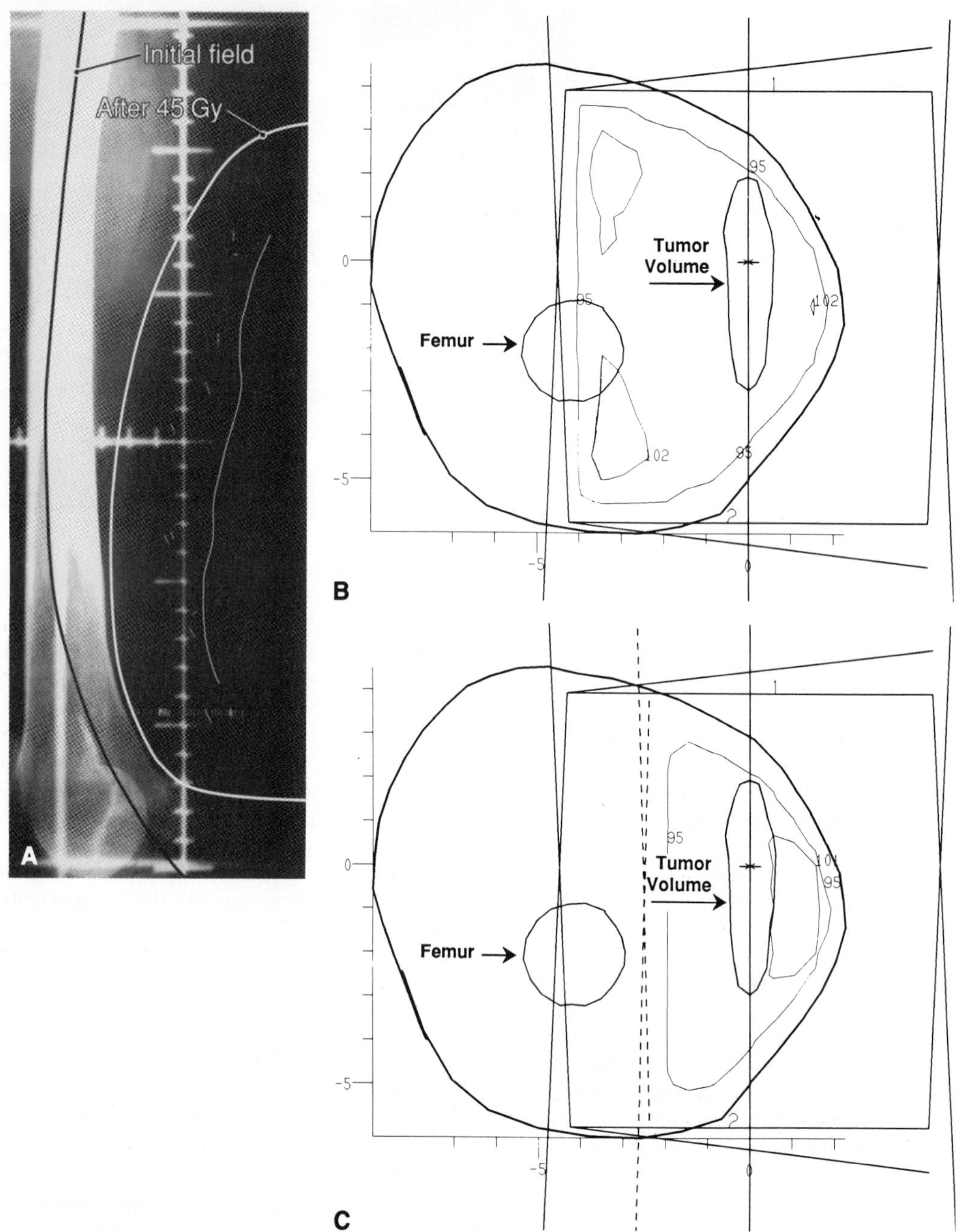

FIGURE 67–6. (**A**) Simulation film of a posterior thigh tumor for a patient with a grade 2 malignant fibrous histiocytoma. The original field treats part of the femur. The conedown field treats the tumor with a 2-cm margin around the surgical clips. (**B**) Isodose plan of the initial treatment field. Wedge filters are used to create a homogeneous dose. Ample margins are allowed around the tumor bed. (**C**) Final conedown tumor volume restricts the dose to the tumor bed plus a 2-cm margin.

with 180-cGy fractions, five fractions per week. In the case of unresectable sarcomas, doses of up to 7500 cGy are used, although the volume that receives greater than 6000 cGy is limited to the tumor plus a minimal margin.

Truncal and Head and Neck Sarcomas

Tumors arising in the trunk are generally more superficial than extremity sarcomas. As is the case for sarcomas at other sites, surgical clips are critical to outline the boundaries of the surgical bed for subsequent radiation (Fig. 67-8). Tumors on the chest wall, abdomen, and back can often be treated with oblique tangential fields analogous to the treatment of the intact breast. After 4500 cGy of photon irradiation, a boost with a direct electron field confined to the surgical bed can be used to deliver a total dose of 6300 cGy without excessive treatment of underlying critical structures, such as the bowel. High-dose electron-beam therapy can be used successfully in face and scalp angiosarcomas, which are particularly infiltrative and prone to local recurrence after surgery alone.[49,55]

Interstitial Therapy

Interstitial therapy can be used in selective cases to boost the tumor bed. In our institution, this technique is used only in selected cases, although excellent results have been reported for

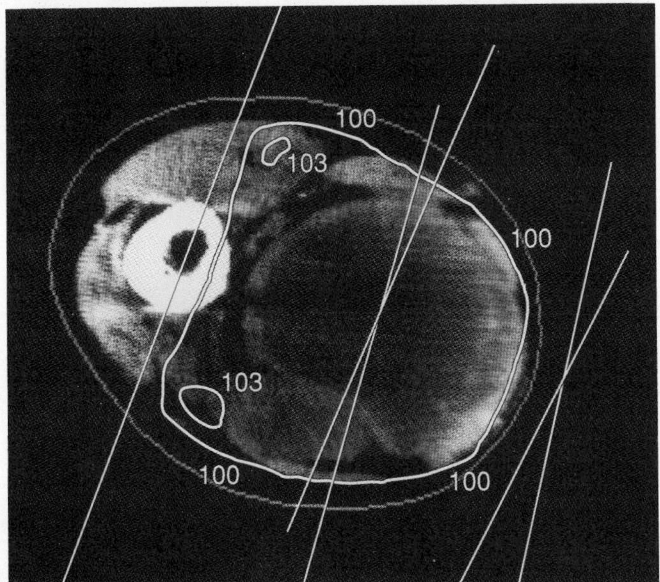

FIGURE 67–7. A treatment plan superimposed on the CT scan of a huge inoperable grade 3 neurofibrosarcoma located in the posterior right thigh. After preoperative irradiation (4500 cGy, administered as 150 cGy twice daily with the radiosensitizer 5-iodo-2′-deoxyuridine [IdUrd]), successful surgical removal was accomplished. Postoperatively, the tumor bed was boosted with an additional 3000 cGy using twice daily treatment and IdUrd.

interstitial therapy used on a routine basis to deliver all or part of the radiation.[16, 53] For interstitial therapy, afterloading catheters are placed intraoperatively at approximately 1-cm intervals to surround the target volume. Surgical clips placed at the margin of the tumor bed permit the target volume to be delineated for planning purposes. Catheters are loaded with ^{192}Ir seeds 4 to 7 days after surgery to permit adequate wound healing before irradiation. Approximately 2000 cGy to 2500 cGy delivered at 40 cGy/hour can usually be safely given in this fashion as booster treatment to the tumor bed after external-beam treatment of the operative bed (Fig. 67-9). Alternatively, 4500 cGy can be given as the total treatment without additional external-beam therapy.

RESULTS OF STANDARD TREATMENT

Extremity, Truncal, and Head and Neck Sarcomas

Many retrospective reports and a randomized trial have demonstrated conclusively that, in most patients with extremity lesions, limb-sparing surgery plus adequate irradiation produces local control and survival rates similar to those achieved with amputation.[16, 36, 71, 89, 96] The patterns of failure for patients with high-grade sarcomas who had wide local excisions and irradiation are presented in Table 67-6. These results were obtained using a variety of approaches, with irradiation delivered preoperatively or postoperatively, with and without adjuvant chemotherapy. The fact that these different techniques produce remarkably similar and excellent local control further validates the basic concept that radical treatment can be carried out with limb preservation. The somewhat higher local recurrences rate from M. D. Anderson probably resulted from the fact that many patients underwent only "shell out" of the tumor, rather than a true wide local excision.[71] Even for patients with high-grade lesions, a local control rate of approximately 90% can be achieved using limb-sparing wide local excision and meticulous radiation therapy technique.

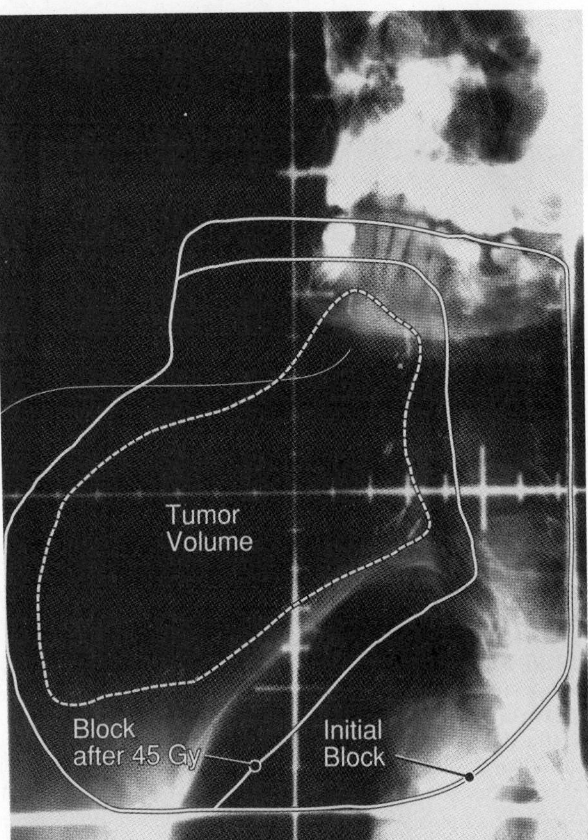

FIGURE 67–8. Simulation film of a patient with a grade 3 neurofibrosarcoma involving the brachial plexus. The proximal surgical margins were microscopically positive in the upper neck at the neural foramina. The initial volume included a small amount of the anterior oral cavity because of the patient's limited neck motion.

Despite the increased technical demands, similar local control rates with limb-sparing procedures have been described for patients with sarcomas of the distal extremities. Local recurrences can be salvaged with additional surgery (amputation) and irradiation (if the amputation removed previously irradiated tissue) with no apparent decrement in survival.[61, 80, 106, 109] Although the head and neck represents another technically challenging site, because it is difficult to obtain a wide margin without significant morbidity, local control rates have also been reported in the 75% to 90% range when irradiation was used after wide local excision.[1, 49, 78]

The overall survival and disease-free survival rates from several recent trials for patients with soft tissue sarcomas are shown in Table 67-7. Although local control rates are high, the aggressive systemic nature of intermediate- and high-grade sarcomas is evident by the fact that disease-free survival rates are consistently 20% to 30% below the local control rates. Although adjuvant chemotherapy has been shown in several trials to prolong disease-free survival, no large trial showed a statistically significant increased survival.

The local control rate for grade I (low-grade) lesions is also excellent (Table 67-8). Unlike the high- and intermediate-grade lesions, low-grade tumors have virtually no metastatic potential. Thus, local control is tantamount to cure in this group.

Unresectable Sarcomas

Some patients have unresectable soft tissue sarcomas that have remained local. Early studies by Cade[19] and McNeer and associ-

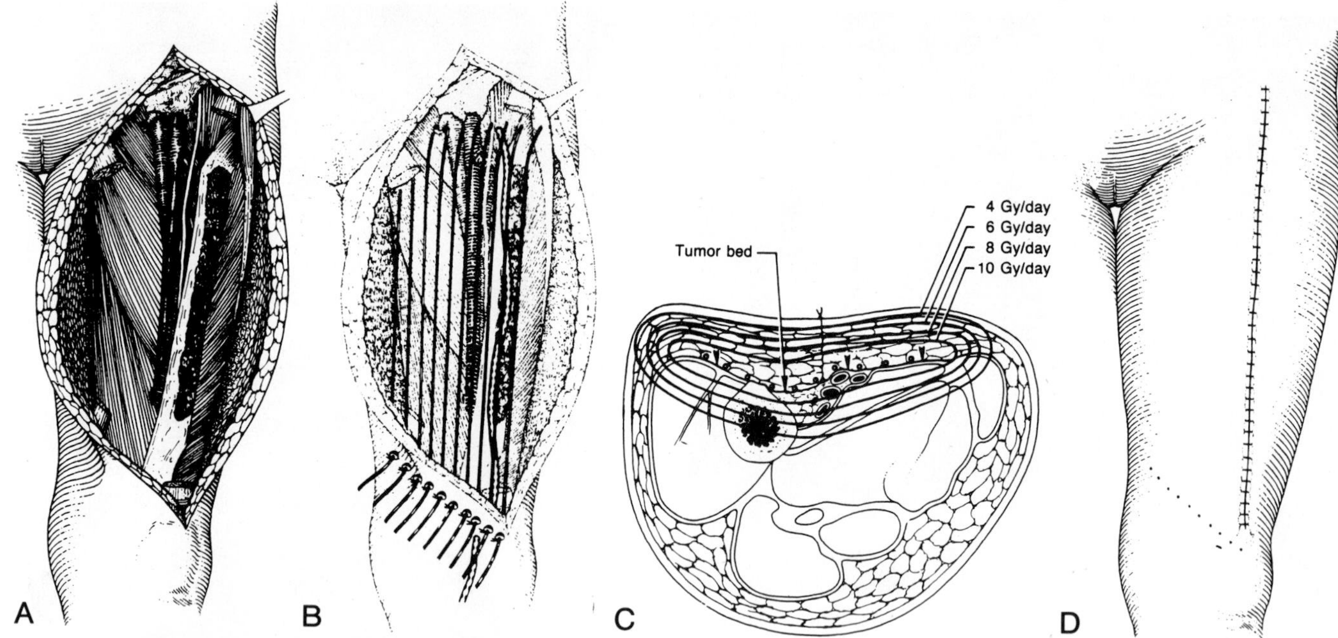

FIGURE 67–9. Endocurietherapy using ^{192}Ir afterloading removable implant after resection. (**A**) Resection has been completed and the femoral artery, vein, and nerve have been preserved. The tumor invaded the neurovascular structures. (**B**) A series of parallel catheters are inserted percutaneously and secured onto the tumor bed. (**C**) Dose distribution around the ^{192}Ir planar implant is shown in a transverse central plane. The isodose contours indicate dose in Gy/day. (**D**) The ^{192}Ir seeds and afterloading catheters are removed after completion of the prescribed treatment. The catheter exit sites require no special care. (Hilaris BS, Shiu MH, Nori D, et al: Endocuriether Hypertherm Oncol 1:17, 1985)

ates[79] demonstrated that radiation therapy alone can cure patients with unresectable soft tissue sarcomas. This has been demonstrated recently at several institutions, using both photons and neutrons (Table 67-9).[26,60,82,93,100] Although the optimal treatment of sarcomas depends on complete excision, these data show that a significant chance of cure exists for unresectable tumors if high-dose irradiation is employed.

Aggressive Fibromatosis and Dermatofibrosarcoma Protuberans

Aggressive fibromatosis (desmoid tumor) and dermatofibrosarcoma protuberans represent a special category of tumors that virtually never metastasize but are very locally invasive. Their microscopic appearance is characterized by a general lack of cellularity and the absence of mitotic figures. Although complete surgical excision alone is usually curative for these tumors, this is sometimes not possible because of their size and location.

Desmoid tumors appear to arise within the skeletal muscle or its fascial coverings. Radiation therapy has been used postoperatively in patients with positive margins and for radical treatment in patients whose tumors are unresectable. Both external-beam radiation therapy and brachytherapy have been used successfully to produce local control, even in tumors that exceed 10 cm in diameter.[59,67,5] Radical irradiation should be strongly considered for any patient who would require amputation for tumor excision, because irradiation failures can be salvaged with amputation without any decreased risk of survival. It should also be considered for patients with unresectable

TABLE 67–6
Patterns of Failure for Intermediate- and High-Grade Sarcomas

INVESTIGATION	NO. OF PATIENTS	FOLLOW-UP (YEARS)	PATTERNS OF FAILURE* (% OF ALL PATIENTS)			RADIATION THERAPY
			LF	LF AND DM	DM	
National Cancer Institute[86]	271	1–8	6	3	28	Postoperative
M.D. Anderson[71]	190	5–16	21	7	25	Postoperative
Massachusetts General Hospital[96]	180	2–16	4	7	25	Preoperative
UCLA[56]	255†	2–15	5	2	24	Preoperative + doxorubicin

** Retroperitoneal excluded. LF: Local failure; DM: distant metastasis.*
† Extremity only.

TABLE 67–7
Overall Survival and Disease-Free Survival Rates for Patients with Soft Tissue Sarcomas

			5-YEAR RESULTS* (% OF ALL PATIENTS)				
			OVERALL SURVIVAL		DISEASE-FREE SURVIVAL		
INVESTIGATION	**NO. OF PATIENTS**	**MEDIAN FOLLOW-UP (YEARS)**	(OBS)	(CHEMO)	(OBS)	(CHEMO)	**ELIGIBLE**
ECOG/MGH DFCI[111]†	75	4.1	66	68	62	74	All sites, grades 2, 3
Mayo[35]	61	5.3	77	90	50	70‡	All sites, all grades
Mayo[35]	116	>5	71		NR§		All sites, all grades
UCLA[56]	255	≈5	65		54		Extremity, grades 2, 3
NCI[23]	67	7.1	60	82	54	75‡	Extremity, grade 2, 3
NCI[23]	88	4.4		75		72	Extremity, grade 2, 3
MGH[96]	220	≈5	NR		70		Retroperitoneal excluded, all grades
M.D. Anderson[71]	300	≈5	NR		64		All sites, all grades

**All studies were limited to patients without metastatic disease at presentation who were completely resected. Randomized trials of adjuvant chemotherapy (chemo)* versus *observation (obs) are listed separately. Otherwise, reports reflect patients who underwent chiefly limb-sparing surgery with pre- or postoperative irradiation, with or without adjuvant chemotherapy. The two listings from the Mayo Clinic and NCI are independent series from the same institution.*
† ECOG, Eastern Cooperative Oncology Group; MGH, Massachusetts General Hospital; DFCI, Dana Farber Cancer Institute; NCI, National Cancer Institute.
‡ Differs from no chemotherapy ($P < 0.05$).
§ Not reported.

lesions in other sites. Some reports suggest that nonsteroidal antiinflammatory agents and tamoxifen have limited activity against desmoid tumors.[105]

Dermatofibrosarcoma protuberans appears to arise from the dermis, and has a high propensity for local recurrences. Radiation therapy has been used successfully to achieve local control in patients with positive margins after surgery or as the sole treatment.[73]

Metastatic Disease

Because of the propensity of high-grade sarcomas to metastasize to the lung as a sole site, it was hypothesized that surgical resection of isolated pulmonary metastases could potentially render a patient free from disease. Investigators at the National Cancer Institute found that thoracotomy in patients with fewer than four pulmonary nodules demonstrated on CT scan was associated with a 23-month median survival, which was far superior to those with greater than four nodules (<6 months).[88] Similar results have been reported by the group from UCLA.[56] These findings suggest that a selected subset of patients with metastatic pulmonary disease can have prolonged survival after surgical resection. However, the disease-free survival curves for these patients show a relentless downward trend over time without evidence of a plateau.

SEQUELAE

Short-term sequelae of radiation therapy are usually limited to moist desquamation in the high-dose volume if the beams are tangent to the skin, particularly if patients are receiving concurrent doxorubicin. This can be very uncomfortable in patients with proximal thigh tumors, and care should be taken to limit treatment of the perineum. Patients undergoing treatment for truncal tumors may experience nausea or thrombocytopenia. Major wound complications requiring surgical revision occur in fewer than 5% of patients, although this rate may be somewhat higher in patients treated with brachytherapy.[7,36,71]

TABLE 67–8
Patterns of Failure for Low-Grade Soft Tissue Sarcomas

			PATTERNS OF FAILURE* (% OF ALL PATIENTS)			
INVESTIGATION	**NO. OF PATIENTS**	**FOLLOW-UP (YEARS)**	LF	LF AND DM	DM	**RADIATION TREATMENT**
M.D. Anderson[71]	63	5–16	5	0	0	Postoperative
Massachusetts General Hospital[96]	40	2–16	3	3	0	Preoperative

**LF: local failure; DM: distant metastasis.*

TABLE 67–9
Treatment of Unresectable Soft Tissue Sarcomas

INVESTIGATION	NO. OF PATIENTS	MINIMUM FOLLOW-UP (YR)	RADIATION TREATMENT	5-YEAR RESULTS* (% OF ALL PATIENTS)		PATTERN OF FAILURE* (% OF ALL PATIENTS)		
				LOCAL CONTROL	OS	LF	LF AND DM	DM
Massachusetts General Hospital[100]	51	1	Photons	33	25	11‡	36‡	22‡
National Cancer Institute[60]	29	1.5†	Photons	72§	NR¶	20§	NR	20§
M.D. Anderson[93]	72	2	Photons/ neutrons‖	29	NR	33	31	17
Hammersmith[82]	50	2	Neutrons	≈20#	≈25	48**	NR	NR
Femilab[26]	26	2	Neutrons	NR	38††	50	NR	12

** OS: overall survival; LF: local failure; DM: distant metastasis.*
† Median follow-up.
‡ Results from 36 patients receiving irradiation with TDF ≥ 105.
§ Results from 15 patients presenting without metastatic disease.
¶ Not reported.
‖ 57 patients treated with photons, 3 patients with neutrons only, and 12 patients with mixed beams.
 # Disease-free survival.
*** Unspecified percentage with LF and DM.*
†† Two-year data.

Several long-term sequelae are possible. A significant decrease in mobility of the extremity, which can defeat the goal of limb preservation, can be avoided through several maneuvers. Careful sparing of a strip of normal tissue that is as wide as possible allows lymphatic drainage from the extremity and spares uninvolved muscle from the trauma of irradiation. Excluding the joint spaces after a dose of 4000 cGy to 4500 cGy avoids fibrotic constriction of joint capsules. Collaboration with a physical therapist is essential in minimizing disabilities after treatment of soft tissue sarcomas. Mobility of the extremity should be stressed, and patients should begin an exercise and range-of-motion program early in the course of therapy. Fractures can occur in as many as 10% of the patients receiving multimodality therapy, particularly when periosteal stripping is required.[37]

In the treatment of patients with truncal sarcomas, it is particularly important to use conedown fields to limit the volume of bowel that receives 5000 cGy and eliminate bowel receiving more than this dose. With attention to these details, a high local control rate can be achieved with minimum sequelae.

High-dose irradiation does not appear to compromise the viability of skin grafts used to repair defects after sarcoma surgery if adequate time is allotted for healing (at least 3 weeks).[66] Fertility can be preserved in men undergoing irradiation for lower extremity sarcomas through use of a gonadal shield to decrease testicular dose.[44]

REFERENCES

1. Abbatucci JS, Boulier N, de Ranieri J, et al: Local control and survival in soft tissue sarcomas of the limbs, trunk walls and head and neck: A study of 113 cases. Int J Radiat Oncol Biol Phys 12:579, 1986
2. Abramson DH, Ellsworth RM, Kitchin FD, et al: Second nonocular tumors in retinoblastoma survivors: Are they radiation-induced? Ophthalmology 91:1351, 1984
3. Aisen AM, Martel W, Braunstein EM, et al: MRI and CT evaluation of primary bone and soft-tissue tumors. AJR 146:749, 1986
4. Akerman M, Rydholm A, Persson BM: Aspiration cytology of soft-tissue tumors. Acta Orthop Scand 56:407, 1985
5. Antman KH, Elias AD: Chemotherapy of advanced soft-tissue sarcomas. Semin Surg Oncol 4:53, 1988
6. Antman KH, Ryan L, Elias A, et al: Response to ifosfamide and mesna: 124 previously treated patients with metastatic or unresectable sarcoma. J Clin Oncol 7:126, 1989
7. Arbeit JM, Hilaris BS, Brennan MF: Wound complications in the multimodality treatment of extremity and superficial truncal sarcomas. J Clin Oncol 5:480, 1987
8. Ariel, IM: Incidence of metastases to lymph nodes from soft-tissue sarcomas. Semin Surg Oncol 4:27, 1988
9. Baker LH, Frank J, Fine G, et al: Combination chemotherapy using Adriamycin, DTIC, cyclophosphamide, and actinomycin D for advanced soft tissue sarcomas: A randomized comparative trial. J Clin Oncol 5:851, 1987
10. Beahrs OH, Henson DE, Hutter RVP, Myers MH (eds): Manual for Staging of Cancer, 3rd ed. Philadelphia, JB Lippincott, 1988
11. Bell RS, O'Sullivan B, Liu FF, et al: The surgical margin in soft-tissue sarcoma. J Bone Joint Surg [A] 71:370, 1989
12. Birch JM, Hartley AL, Marsden HB, et al: Excess risk of breast cancer in the mothers of children with soft tissue sarcomas. Br J Cancer 49:325, 1984
13. Borden EC, Amato DA, Rosenbaum C, et al: Randomized comparison of three Adriamycin regimens for metastatic soft tissue sarcomas. J Clin Oncol 5:840, 1987
14. Bramwell VHC: Intraarterial chemotherapy of soft-tissue sarcomas. Semin Surg Oncol 4:66, 1988
15. Bramwell VHC, Crowther D, Deakin DP, et al: Combined modality management of local and disseminated adult soft tissue sarcomas: A review of 257 cases seen over 10 years at the Christie Hospital & Holt Radium Institute, Manchester. Br J Cancer 51:301, 1985
16. Brennan MF, Hilaris B, Shiu MH, et al: Local recurrence in adult soft-tissue sarcoma: A randomized trial of brachytherapy. Arch Surg 122:1289, 1987
17. Broders AC, Hargrave R, Meyerding HW: Pathological features of soft tissue fibrosarcoma. Surg Gynecol Obstet 69:267, 1939

18. Cancer Statistics. CA 39:3, 1989
19. Cade S: Soft tissue tumours: Their natural history and treatment. Proc R Soc Lond 44:19, 1950
20. Cahan WG, Woodward HQ, Higinbotham NL, et al: Sarcoma arising in irradiated bone: Report of eleven cases. Cancer 1:3, 1948
21. Cantin J, McNeer GP, Chu FC, et al: The problem of local recurrence after treatment of soft tissue sarcoma. Ann Surg 168:47, 1968
22. Chang AE, Matory YL, Dwyer AJ, et al: Magnetic resonance imaging *versus* computed tomography in the evaluation of soft tissue tumors of the extremities. Ann Surg 205:340, 1987
23. Chang AE, Kinsella T, Glatstein E, et al: Adjuvant chemotherapy for patients with high-grade soft-tissue sarcomas of the extremity. J Clin Oncol 6:1491, 1988
24. Chang AE, Rosenberg SA, Glatstein EJ, et al: Sarcomas of soft tissues. In DeVita VT, Hellman S, Rosenberg SA (eds): Cancer: Principles and Practice of Oncology, 3rd ed, p 1345. Philadelphia, J.B. Lippincott, 1989
25. Cohen L, Hendrickson FR: Neutron therapy for nonresectable radioresistant tumors. Arch Surg 124:294, 1989
26. Cohen L, Hendrickson F, Mansell J, et al: Response of sarcomas of bone and of soft tissue to neutron beam therapy. Int J Radiat Oncol Biol Phys 10:821, 1984
27. Collin CF, Friedrich C, Godbold J, et al: Prognostic factors for local recurrence and survival in patients with localized extremity soft-tissue sarcoma. Semin Surg Oncol 4:30, 1988
28. Costa J, Wesley RA, Glatstein E, et al: The grading of soft tissue sarcomas: Results of a clinicohistopathologic correlation in a series of 163 cases. Cancer 53:530, 1984
29. Creech JL, Johnson MN: Angiosarcoma of liver in the manufacture of polyvinyl chloride. J Occup Med 16:150, 1974
30. Daly PF, Cohen JS: Magnetic resonance spectroscopy of tumors and potential *in vivo* clinical applications: A review. Cancer Res 49:770, 1989
31. Demas BE, Heelan RT, Lane J, et al: Soft-tissue sarcomas of the extremities: Comparison of MR and CT in determining the extent of disease. AJR 150:615, 1988
32. Di Filippo F, Calabro AM, Cavallari A, et al: The role of hyperthermic perfusion as a first step in the treatment of soft tissue sarcoma of the extremities. World J Surg 12:332, 1988
33. Duda RB, Beatty JD, Kokal WA, et al: Radiographic evaluation for pulmonary metastases in sarcoma patients. J Surg Oncol 38:271, 1988
34. Edmonson JH: Role of adjuvant chemotherapy in the management of patients with soft tissue sarcomas. Cancer Treat Rep 68:1063, 1984
35. Edmonson JH, Fleming TR, Ivins JC, et al: Randomized study of systemic chemotherapy following complete excision of nonosseous sarcomas. J Clin Oncol 2:1390, 1984
36. Eilber FR, Eckhardt J, Morton DL: Advances in the treatment of sarcomas of the extremity. Cancer 54:2695, 1984
37. Eilber FR, Morton DL, Eckardt J, et al: Limb salvage for skeletal and soft tissue sarcomas. Cancer 53:2579, 1984
38. Eilber FR, Morton DL, Sondak VK, et al (eds): The Soft Tissue Sarcomas. Orlando, FL, Grune & Stratton, 1987
39. Elias AD, Antman KH: Adjuvant chemotherapy for soft-tissue sarcoma: A critical appraisal. Semin Surg Oncol 4:59, 1988
40. Enneking WF, Chew FS, Springfield DS, et al: The role of radionuclide bone-scanning in determining the resectability of soft-tissue sarcomas. J Bone Joint Surg [A] 63:249, 1981
41. Enneking WF, Spanier SS, Malawar MM: The effect of the anatomic setting on the results of surgical procedures for soft parts sarcoma of the thigh. Cancer 47:1005, 1981
42. Enzinger FM, Weiss SW: Soft Tissue Tumors. St. Louis, CV Mosby, 1983
43. Fortner JG, Martin S, Hajdu S, et al: Primary sarcoma of the retroperitoneum. Semin Oncol 8:180, 1981
44. Fraass BA, Kinsella TJ, Harrington FS, et al: Peripheral dose to the testes: The design and clinical use of a practical and effective gonadal shield. Int J Radiat Oncol Biol Phys 11:609, 1985
45. Gerlach JH, Bell DR, Karakousis C, et al: P-glycoprotein in human sarcoma: Evidence for multidrug resistance. J Clin Oncol 5:1452, 1987
46. Giuliano AE, Eilber FR: The rationale for planned reoperation after unplanned total excision of soft-tissue sarcomas. J Clin Oncol 3:1344, 1985
47. Glenn J, Kinsella T, Glatstein E, et al: A randomized, prospective trial of adjuvant chemotherapy in adults with soft tissue sarcomas of the head and neck, breast, and trunk. Cancer 55:1206, 1985
48. Glenn J, Sindelar WF, Kinsella T, et al: Results of multimodality therapy of resectable soft-tissue sarcomas of the retroperitoneum. Surgery 97:316, 1985
49. Greager JA, Patel MK, Briele HA, et al: Soft tissue sarcomas of the adult head and neck. Cancer 56:820, 1985
50. Halperin EC, Greenberg MS, Suit HD: Sarcoma of bone and soft tissue following treatment of Hodgkin's disease. Cancer 53:232, 1984
51. Hardell L, Eriksson M: The association between soft tissue sarcomas and exposure to phenoxyacetic acids. Cancer 62:652, 1988
52. Heise HW, Myers MH, Russell WO, et al: Recurrence-free survival time for surgically treated soft tissue sarcoma patients. Cancer 57:172, 1986
53. Hilaris BS, Shiu MH, Nori D, et al: Limb-sparing therapy for locally advanced soft-tissue sarcomas. Endocuriether Hypertherm Oncol 1:17, 1985
54. Hoar SK, Blair A, Holmes F, et al: Agricultural herbicide use and risk of lymphoma and soft-tissue sarcoma. JAMA 256:1141, 1986
55. Holden CA, Spittle MF, Jones EW: Angiosarcoma of the face and scalp: Prognosis and treatment. Cancer 59:1046, 1987
56. Huth JF, Eilber FR: Patterns of metastatic spread following resection of extremity soft-tissue sarcomas and strategies for treatment. Semin Surg Oncol 4:20, 1988
57. Karakousis CP, Dal Cin P, Turc-Carel C, et al: Chromosomal changes in soft-tissue sarcomas: A new diagnostic parameter. Arch Surg 122:1257, 1987
58. Kern KA, Brunetti A, Norton JA, et al: Metabolic imaging of human extremity musculoskeletal tumors by PET. J Nucl Med 29:181, 1988
59. Kiel KD, Suit HD: Radiation therapy in the treatment of aggressive fibromatoses (desmoid tumors). Cancer 54:2051, 1984
60. Kinsella TJ, Glatstein E: Clinical experience with intravenous radiosensitizers in unresectable sarcomas. Cancer 59:908, 1987
61. Kinsella TJ, Loeffler JS, Fraass BA, et al: Extremity preservation by combined modality therapy in sarcomas of the hand and foot: An analysis of local control, disease free survival and functional result. Int J Radiat Oncol Biol Phys 9:1115, 1983
62. Kinsella TJ, Sindelar WF, Lack E, et al: Preliminary results of a randomized study of adjuvant radiation therapy in resectable adult retroperitoneal soft tissue sarcomas. J Clin Oncol 6:18, 1988
63. Kissen MW, Fisher C, Webb AJ, et al: Value of the fine needle aspiration cytology in the diagnosis of soft tissue tumours: A preliminary study on the excised specimen. Br J Surg 74:479, 1987
64. Laskin WB, Silverman TA, Enzinger FM: Postradiation soft tissue sarcomas: An analysis of 53 cases. Cancer 62:2330, 1988
65. Lawrence W, Donegan W, Natarajan N, et al: Adult soft tissue sarcomas: A Pattern of Care Survey of the American College of Surgeons. Ann Surg 205:349, 1987
66. Lawrence WT, Zabell A, McDonald HD: The tolerance of skin grafts to postoperative radiation therapy in patients with soft-tissue sarcoma. Ann Plast Surg 16:204, 1986
67. Leibel SA, Wara WM, Hill DR, et al: Demoid tumors: Local control and patterns of relapse following radiation therapy. Int J Radiat Oncol Biol Phys 9:1167, 1983
68. Leopold KA, Harrelson J, Prosnitz L, et al: Preoperative hyperthermia and radiation for soft tissue sarcomas: Advantage of two *vs* one hyperthermia treatments per week. Int J Radiat Oncol Biol Phys 16:107, 1989
69. Leyvraz S, Costa J: Histological diagnosis and grading of soft-tissue sarcomas. Semin Surg Oncol 4:3, 1988
70. Li FP, Fraumeni JF: Prospective study of a family cancer syndrome. JAMA 247:2692, 1982

71. Lindberg RD, Martin RG, Romsdahl MM, et al: Conservative surgery and postoperative radiotherapy in 300 adults with soft-tissue sarcomas. Cancer 47:2391, 1981
72. Lynge E, Storm HH, Jensen OM: The evaluation of trends in soft tissue sarcoma according to diagnostic criteria and consumption of phenoxy herbicides. Cancer 60:1896, 1987
73. Marks LB, Suit HD, Rosenberg AE, et al: Dermatofibrosarcoma protuberans treated with radiation therapy. Int J Radiat Oncol Biol Phys 17:379, 1989
74. Mazeron JJ, Suit HD: Lymph nodes as sites of metastases from sarcomas of soft tissue. Cancer 60:1800, 1987
75. Mirra JM: Pathology of soft tissue sarcomas. In Eilber FR, Morton DL, Sondak VK (eds): The Soft Tissue Sarcomas, p 11. Orlando FL, Grune & Stratton, 1987
76. Molenaar WM, Dejong B, Buist J: Chromosomal analysis and the classification of soft tissue sarcomas. Lab Invest 60:266, 1989
77. Moody DL, Edlich RF, Gedgoudas E: The roentgenologic identification of pulmonary metastases: Evaluation of an operatively proved series. Dis Chest 51:306, 1967
78. McKenna WG, Barnes MM, Kinsella TJ, et al: Combined modality treatment of adult soft tissue sarcomas of the head and neck. Int J Radiat Oncol Biol Phys 13:1127, 1987
79. McNeer GP, Cantin J, Chu F, et al: Effectiveness of radiation therapy in the management of sarcoma of the soft somatic tissues. Cancer 22:391, 1968
80. Okunieff P, Suit HD, Proppe KH: Extremity preservation by combined modality treatment of sarcomas of the hand and wrist. Int J Radiat Oncol Biol Phys 12:1923, 1986
81. Pass HI, Dwyer A, Makuch R, et al: Detection of pulmonary metastases in patients with osteogenic and soft-tissue sarcomas: The superiority of CT scans compared with conventional linear tomograms using dynamic analysis. J Clin Oncol 3:1261, 1985
82. Pickering DG, Stewart JS, Rampling R, et al: Fast neutron therapy for soft tissue sarcoma. Int J Radiat Oncol Biol Phys 13:1489, 1987
83. Pinedo HM, Verweij J: The treatment of soft tissue sarcomas with focus on chemotherapy: A review. Radiother Oncol 5:193, 1986
84. Pinedo HM, Verweij J (eds): Treatment of Soft Tissue Sarcomas. Boston, Kluwer Academic, 1989
85. Posner MC, Shiu MH, Newsome JL, et al: The desmoid tumor—not a benign disease. Arch Surg 124:191, 1989
86. Potter DA, Glenn J, Kinsella T, et al: Patterns of recurrence in patients with high-grade soft-tissue sarcomas. J Clin Oncol 3:353, 1985
87. Presant CA, Russell WO, Alexander RW, et al: Soft-tissue and bone sarcoma histopathology peer review: The frequency of disagreement in diagnosis and the need for second pathology opinions: The Southeastern Cancer Study Group experience. J Clin Oncol 4:1658, 1986
88. Putnam JB, Roth JA, Wesley MN, et al: Analysis of prognostic factors in patients undergoing resection of pulmonary metastases from soft tissue sarcomas. J Thorac Cardiovasc Surg 87:260, 1984
89. Rosenberg SA, Kent H, Costa J, et al: Prospective randomized evaluation of the role of limb-sparing surgery, radiation therapy, and adjuvant chemotherapy in the treatment of adult soft-tissue sarcomas. Surgery 84:62, 1978
90. Rosenberg SA, Tepper J, Glatstein E, et al: The treatment of soft-tissue sarcomas of the extremities. Ann Surg 196:305, 1982
91. Russell WO, Cohen J, Enzinger F, et al: A clinical and pathological staging system for soft tissue sarcomas. Cancer 40:1562, 1977
92. Shiu MH, Castor EB: Surgical treatment of 297 soft tissue sarcomas of the extremity. Ann Surg 182:597, 1975
93. Slater JD, McNeese MD, Peters LJ: Radiation therapy for unresectable soft tissue sarcomas. Int J Radiat Oncol Biol Phys 12:1729, 1986
94. Sørensen SA, Mulvihill JJ, Nielsen A: Long-term follow-up of von Recklinghausen neurofibromatosis. N Engl J Med 314:1010, 1986
95. Storm FK, Eilber FR, Mirra J, et al: Retroperitoneal sarcomas: A reappraisal of treatment. J Surg Oncol 17:1, 1981
96. Suit HD, Mankin HJ, Wood WC, et al: Treatment of the patient with stage MO soft tissue sarcoma. J Clin Oncol 6:854, 1988
97. Suit HD, Tepper JE, Mankin HJ, et al: Sarcomas of soft tissue and bone. In Wang CC (ed): Clinical Radiation Oncology, p 331. Massachusetts, PSG Publishing, 1988
98. Tepper JE: Tumors of bone and soft tissue. In Wilson JF (ed): Syllabus: A Categorical Course in Radiation Therapy, p 65. Oak Brook, IL, Radiological Society of North America, 1988
99. Tepper JE Rosenberg SA, Glatstein E: Radiation therapy in soft tissue sarcomas of the extremity: Policies of treatment at the National Cancer Institute. Int J Radiat Oncol Biol Phys 8:263, 1982
100. Tepper JE, Suit HD: Radiation therapy alone for sarcoma of soft tissue. Cancer 56:475, 1985
101. Tepper JE, Suit HD, Wood WC, et al: Radiation therapy of retroperitoneal soft tissue sarcomas. Int J Radiat Oncol Biol Phys 10:825, 1984
102. Torosian MH, Friedrich C, Godbold J, et al: Soft-tissue sarcoma: Initial characteristics and prognostic factors in patients with and without metastatic disease. Semin Surg Oncol 4:13, 1988
103. Ueda T, Aozasa K, Tsujimoto M, et al: Prognostic significance of Ki-67 reactivity in soft tissue sarcomas. Cancer 63:1607, 1989
104. Vezeridis MP, Moore R, Karakousis CP: Metastatic patterns in soft-tissue sarcomas. Arch Surg 118:915, 1983
105. Waddell WR, Gerner RE, Reich MP: Nonsteroid antiinflammatory drugs and tamoxifen for desmoid tumors and carcinoma of the stomach. J Surg Oncol 22:197, 1983
106. Walker MJ, Wood DK, Briele HA, et al: Soft tissue sarcomas of the distal extremities. Surgery 99:392, 1986
107. Weatherby RP, Dahlin DC, Ivins JC: Postradiation sarcoma of bone: Review of 78 Mayo Clinic cases. Mayo Clin Proc 56:294, 1981
108. Weingrad DW, Rosenberg SA: Early lymphatic spread of osteogenic and soft tissue sarcomas. Surgery 84:231, 1978
109. Wexler AM, Eilber FR, Miller TA: Therapeutic and functional results of limb salvage to treat sarcomas of the forearm and hand. J Hand Surg [Am] 13:292, 1988
110. Wick MR, Swanson PE, Manivel JC: Immunohistochemical analysis of soft tissue sarcomas. Appl Pathol 6:169, 1988
111. Wilson RE, Wood WC, Lerner HL, et al: Doxorubicin chemotherapy in the treatment of soft-tissue sarcoma: Combined results of two randomized trials. Arch Surg 121:1354, 1986
112. Woodward AH, Ivins JC, Soule EM: Lymphangiosarcoma arising in chronic lymphedematous extremities. Cancer 30:562, 1972

68

Pediatric Tumors: An Overview

Giulio J. D'Angio

Childhood cancer is rare, with only about 110 new cases seen annually per million children under 16 years of age. Despite its rarity and the major therapeutic advances made in recent years, it remains the leading cause of death from disease in this age group. Its obvious importance in pediatrics becomes magnified for other reasons. First, the sick child affects the functioning of the entire family, which often is just emerging as a social and economic unit. The disruption of normal life and the prolonged and costly care impinge on the family at a crucial point in its development.[16] A second important consideration is that long-term survival in children is not measured in quinquennia or decades, but in half and three quarter centuries. The after effects of treatments used to cure the child today can produce the chronically ill adult of tomorrow.

Solutions to the social problem rest largely within Society. The quality of life for the long-term survivor, however, can be influenced by the physicians who manage children with cancer. Cure is and must remain the principal objective, but late complications caused by overapplication of rigorous, multimodal therapies commonly used in pediatric oncology can be crippling.[10] Treatment should be carefully adjusted to known risks and kept to the minimum needed to achieve the intended goal.

UNIQUE ASPECTS OF PEDIATRIC ONCOLOGY

The management of the child with a malignant tumor often differs markedly from that provided an adult. The types of neoplasms are different: tumors in adults most often affect epithelial surfaces and linings, the genitourinary apparatus, and the glandular tissues, but the supporting structures and the parenchymal and bone marrow cells are more common sites of origin in children.[27] The rapidly growing and developing tissues and structures of children are more susceptible to the antimitotic influences of radiation therapy and chemotherapy than are their counterparts in adults.[20] These basic differences impose modifications on therapy. With irradiation, adjustments may involve the daily and total doses used, portal arrangements, modality used (photons or electrons), and other technical details.

Equally important factors that affect management are related to the characteristics of the neoplastic processes of early life. Many seemingly monolithic entities now appear to be mosaics of disease with exceedingly complex natural histories.[27] Some of the neoplasms that appear to the microscopist to have identical cytohistologic patterns have very different clinical evolutions, depending on such variables as age and stage. How much irradiation to give and to which target sites depends on accurate identification of the risks imposed by the neoplasm. It is essential, therefore, that those treating children be intimately familiar with the clinical evolution of the cancers of childhood if either overtreatment or undertreatment is to be avoided. This sometimes entails abrogation of the rules that apply to the management of adults with malignant diseases.[9]

Better understanding of these differences can perhaps be gained by first considering a benign condition, such as the mixed capillary-cavernous hemangioma seen in infants. These tumors are important chiefly because they are unsightly. It is well known that most of them disappear spontaneously with time and that there is little or no residual deformity to mark the site of involvement. However, they can occasionally constitute a threat to life; for example, hemangioma of the larynx can cause asphyxia and death. Clearly, a hands-off policy in such circumstances is inappropriate. Insertion of a tracheostomy tube is an obvious solution; however, in some patients, the paralaryngeal tissues are involved with the hemangioma, making the surgical approach difficult, if not hazardous, and threatening disaster through erosion of the tracheostomy tube into an adjoining hemangiomatous pocket. It also is difficult to wean children from the tube, and underdevelopment of the larynx is not an infrequent consequence.

Under such circumstances, modest doses of radiation to the neck to speed spontaneous resolution should be considered, despite the known hazard of thyroid carcinoma. Radiation therapy can be directed to the specific area of involvement. There is no need to use high doses or to irradiate the entire lesion in those patients who might have an associated massive hemangioma of the head and neck region. The healing process, once initiated, spreads throughout the entire lesion, and resolution occurs more rapidly. One useful technique is to deliver 150 cGy to the larynx on each of 2 successive days and to observe evidence of healing during the ensuing 4 to 6 weeks. Another course of similar dosage can be administered at that time if needed.

Two concepts are illustrated in this example. First, low doses are appropriate because they are used merely to initiate spontaneous healing processes. Second, the entire implicated volume need not be included in the beam, for the same reason. Hemangioma of the liver can be approached in the same way if other means of management (steroid therapy, embolization, chemotherapy) have failed. The technique and doses are those used for Stage IV-S neuroblastoma (Fig. 68-1).[8]

Another predominantly benign condition, histiocytosis X, now termed Langerhans' cell histiocytosis, can be used to exemplify a third precept: accurate definition of the role radiation therapy plays in producing a given result.[7] Langerhans' cell histiocytosis can affect many organs and structures. The cell type is morphologically similar in involved skeletal bone, liver, and lung, which led Farber and Green[18] to suggest that eosinophilic granuloma of bone, Hand-Schüller-Christian syndrome, and Letterer-Siwe disease might be different manifestations of the same process. Perhaps this is so, but there is an enormous difference between the prognoses if only bone lesions are present contrasted with the outlook when there is extensive involvement of the soft tissues.

Management of an individual patient must be geared to the hazards posed by the disease in that patient. There are few who would advocate an aggressive, systemic chemotherapeutic regimen for a patient with a solitary Langerhans cell histiocytosis lesion in bone. It is generally agreed that local measures suffice. Yet, there has been considerable uncertainty about the radiation dose that should be delivered when radiation therapy is indicated. Doses ranging from a few hundred centigrays to 3000 cGy or more have been advocated by different authorities over the years.[25] A retrospective review by investigators at the University of Minnesota established that better results are not obtained if doses higher than approximately 600 cGy (*e.g.*, 150 cGy/day for 4 days) are used in these patients.[26] They and others have shown that the disease is self-limited and that no treatment is needed unless there are associated signs and symptoms or unless needed to prevent further collapse of the involved bone.[28]

The three concepts—low doses, partial volumes, and tailored therapy—can be applied to the management of specific malignant neoplasms of childhood.

Children with neuroblastoma provide the best examples. Their management has been improved by a better understanding of the natural histories of the disease complexes that masquerade under a common name.[17] It has now been shown conclusively that stage, age, histologic type, serum markers, and cytogenic patterns are all potent prognostic indices, especially if used together.[17,21,24,27] Infants with tumors confined to the organ or structure of origin (Stage I) have an almost 100% survival after simple surgical removal of the tumor. The addition of chemotherapy and radiation therapy does not influence that result. On the other hand, older children with widely metastatic disease in the skeleton (Stage IV) have a very poor prognosis. More than 80% of these children die. If the other prognostic factors are used, patients in the intermediate stages also can be accurately divided among those who have a better than 80% chance of survival and those with less than 20% life expectancy.[17]

There is an important subset of neuroblastoma patients. They have tumors in the usual axial or suprarenal sites that fit Stage I or II criteria and widely disseminated foci affecting the liver, skin, or bone marrow, but they have no roentgenographic or bone scan evidence of bone involvement. These children, usually infants, have been assigned to Stage IV-S.[6] Disease foci in Stage IV-S patients can disappear spontaneously, emphasizing the importance of tailoring therapy for each patient.[14] It is clear that, age for age, the outcome for Stage IV-S children is vastly different from that for Stage IV patients.

There is a wide spectrum of clinical behavior within what appears at first to be a single malignant process. Indications for treatment appropriate for one subset of neuroblastoma patients cannot be extrapolated to another. Administration of aggressive multimodal therapy thought appropriate for Stage III and IV neuroblastoma may actually worsen the outcome for the baby with Stage IV-S disease. Toxic deaths have been reported for these infants.[5,22] It is therefore important in reaching therapeutic decisions to recognize the paradoxically good survival rates for Stage IV-S patients who receive little, if any, treatment.

As with hemangiomas, however, there are individual Stage IV-S patients who require help, almost invariably because of massive hepatomegaly. The huge liver, which can completely fill the abdomen, raises the diaphragm, compresses the renal vasculature, and compromises pulmonary function, renal function, or both. The effect can be lethal, especially in the first few weeks of life. Liver failure is rarely a problem, but life can also be threatened by the associated coagulopathy that is sometimes seen in patients with massively enlarged livers. For these patients, the management principles for dose and treatment volume can be applied. The whole liver need not be treated, and only low doses are required.[9] The technique at the Children's Hospital of Philadelphia entails the use of opposing lateral fields oriented across the table, with the posterior margin placed at the anterior border of the vertebral body. The beam axis is directed 5 to 10 degrees above the horizontal to avoid the consequences of beam divergence. The kidneys and the ovaries in girls are excluded from the beam and so are the posterior recesses of the liver. Three daily doses of 150 cGy (total, 450 cGy) are given, and the effect is observed over a 10- to 12-day period. This treatment usually arrests tumor growth, but if the liver continues to enlarge, a second course of 450 cGy can be given. The objective is to initiate the anticipated spontaneous resolution of the disease process by irradiating a portion of the affected volume with a low dose (Fig. 68-1).

Some of the same considerations apply to Wilms' tumor. It is now understood that there are several kinds of childhood kidney neoplasms, some of which were previously considered variants of Wilms' tumor. The mesoblastic nephroma, a largely benign kidney tumor, was sequestered from the Wilms' tumor category years ago.[3] Several investigators began to identify cytohistologic kidney tumor patterns that could be correlated with different clinical evolutions. These have been grouped by Beckwith and Palmer[2] into two broad categories: tumors of favorable histology and those of unfavorable histology. For the patients with favorable-histology tumors, they reported 2-year survival rates of better than 90% in the First National Wilms' Tumor Study and rates of 40% for children with tumors of unfavorable histology. Moreover, unfavorable tumors with anaplastic or sarcomatous patterns have fairly specific clinical evolutions. For example, bone metastases, which are rare with true Wilms' tumors, tend to be associated with renal clear cell sarcoma, which also metastasizes to the brain. The "rhabdoid" kidney tumor is associated with separate primary and secondary brain tumors, but not with bony deposits. These observations about the clear cell and rhabdoid lesions have obvious diagnostic and therapeutic connotations.[4,12,13]

Retrospective reviews and prospective trials of the radiation therapy administered to Wilms' tumor patients have been rewarding. It is now clear that no postoperative radiation therapy is needed for Stage I or II Wilms' tumors with favorable histology. Vincristine added to dactinomycin provides better

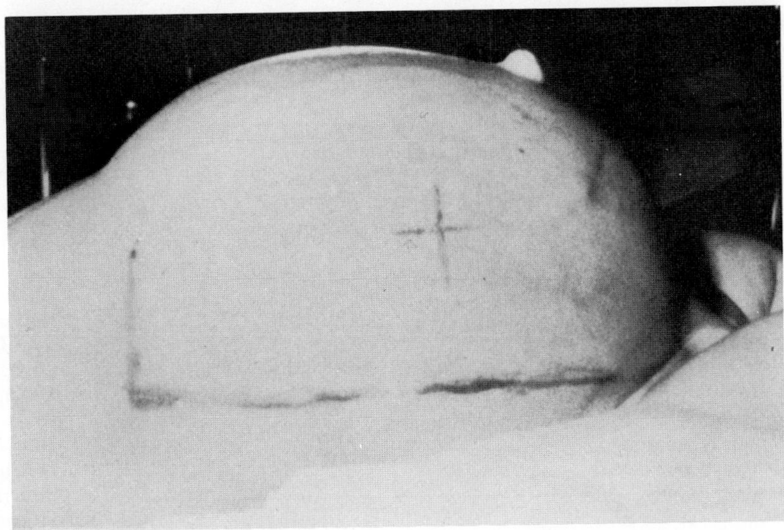

FIGURE 68–1. The skin marks indicate one of the two portals used and the central beam axis when treating massive liver enlargements in patients with neuroblastoma stage IVS disease. Across the table lateral fields are employed, tilted 5 degrees to 10 degrees above the horizontal to avoid beam divergence along the posterior margin of the opposing fields. (D'Angio GJ. In van Eys J, Sullivan MP [eds]. Status of the Curability of Childhood Cancers, pp 5–16. New York, Raven Press, 1980)

coverage of microfoci of metastatic disease and adds an element of protection at the primary tumor site. The 4-year survival rate for these unirradiated children is better than 95%.[13] Another important concept has been established: that effective chemotherapy can sometimes substitute for postoperative irradiation of the tumor bed in ablating residual microfoci of local disease. The "dose-equivalence" between the chemotherapy employed and the radiation dose depends on the tumor type and the chemotherapy employed. It is now clear that it would be wrong to give routine postoperative irradiation to all children with Wilms' tumor, as was done in the past. Similarly, the histologic type and stage of any tumor and the efficacy of the drugs employed must be assessed before valid decisions about radiation therapy can be reached.

There has been a surge of interest in pediatric brain tumors. They commonly are incorrectly grouped among the childhood cancers, although some clearly are not (*e.g.*, craniopharyngiomas).[15] Others display some of the same peculiarities of behavior that were described previously. Examples are the gliomas of the optic pathways and the pilocytic astrocytoma of the posterior fossa, lesions that can remain quiescent for long periods after partial treatment. They sometimes regress.[15] Listing these lesions among the malignant neoplasms colors thinking and hampers understanding.

CHANGES IN THERAPEUTIC PHILOSOPHY

The increasing success of therapy brings with it some unanticipated problems in the interpretation and application of past results. Prognostic criteria have become useful only in identifying the most recalcitrant subtypes among single tumor entities. The inherently more ominous nature of some neoplasms becomes obscured because their lethal potential has been suppressed by effective treatment to the same level as those that are intrinsically less aggressive. The prognostic importance of the elements used in staging and tumor grading systems does not remain static when treatment results are changing; the two evolve together.[1]

ROLE OF SYSTEMIC THERAPIES

The roles of surgery and irradiation change as better systemic therapeutic measures are discovered. For example, less radical surgical and radiation procedures can now be employed in patients with rhabdomyosarcoma, as can limb-salvaging maneuvers in the management of children with osteogenic sarcoma.

The roles of the treatment team members also have changed dramatically over the years. Not long ago, the surgeon was the sole figure. If total removal did not lead to cure, little or nothing more could be done. Radiation therapy added a new and important partner, but the real revolution occurred when effective chemotherapy came of age. Dramatic leaps in cure rates followed as each of the newer modalities was added to the therapeutic armamentarium.[19] Adjuvant chemotherapy has become an indispensable part of the management of most pediatric malignant conditions. Chemotherapy ablates micrometastases, improving relapse-free survival rates. It also makes possible centigray doses and portal size reductions, lessening delayed therapeutic adversities. The degree and frequency of these often are related to the irradiation dose and the volume treated.[10,20]

Because of continuous therapeutic advances, carefully coordinated treatment programs are essential to the care of the pediatric patient with cancer. All members of the management team must maintain a flexible attitude and be willing to explore novel treatment approaches. Reconsiderations of treatment policies must be based on experience with the vagaries of pediatric malignant diseases, their varying expressions, and the changing "rules" as treatments increase in effectiveness. It is prudent to maintain a degree of skepticism in ascribing clinical events—favorable or unfavorable—to the therapies given. Conclusions that may have both logic and validity in general oncology often do not apply to cancer in children.[9]

Delayed complications of therapy can be especially pronounced in children because of the sensitivity of pediatric anatomic structures. Many of the chemotherapeutic agents used in pediatric oncology have radiation-enhancing and radiation-reactivating properties. The reactivating characteristics have been called "flare" reactions. The consequences of the flare responses can be reduced by giving one or two courses of the radiation-enhancing and reactivating agents (*e.g.*, doxorubicin and dactinomycin) before initiating radiation therapy. This permits the reduction of field sizes in some circumstances. It also lessens the augmentation of radiation effects in normal tissues by reducing the number of potential flare reactions. Other methods include the use of split-course or double split-course and shrinking-field techniques to minimize combined treatment effects.[11,20] The local protection provided by systemic

TABLE 68–1
Late Effects of Therapy

FUNCTIONAL IMPAIRMENTS

Effects on growth and development in children
Gonadal
  Hormonal effects
  Fertility impairment
  Genetic effects
Neuropsychologic
  Neuromyeloencephalopathies
  Psychologic effects
  Intellectual impairment
Effects on other organs and structures (*e.g.*, heart, lung)

ONCOGENESIS

Benign neoplasms
Malignant neoplasms

chemotherapy has encouraged some to lower the total centigray dose for the same reason.

All these measures are designed to reduce the late deleterious consequences of successful cancer treatment, which can be divided into two broad categories: those that disturb normal function and those that are associated with the appearance of tumors (Table 68-1). Parents express particular concern about the effects of treatment, especially irradiation, on normal growth, intellectual capacity, and sexual maturation and fertility. It is for this reason that these aspects are emphasized in Table 68-1, not because dysfunctions of other critical organs are less important. All potential disturbances (except for growth) apply to adults as well as to children.

SUMMARY

The cure rate for childhood cancer has risen from less than 20% a few score years ago to at least 60%.[19,23] A new endemic entity has been created for the young adult population: the cured cancer patient. Meadows and co-workers[23] pointed out that one in every 1000 persons aged 20 is a survivor of childhood cancer. This approximates the attack rate for poliomyelitis when that disease was endemic.[10] Increasingly, more young men and women are vulnerable to the known and as yet unknown late complications of treatment. As they mature, they are no longer under the care of pediatricians, but are seen by internists and others devoted to the care of adults. Nonpediatric oncologists must become familiar with these aspects of medicine, because the problems of childhood cancer survivors are becoming theirs to recognize and solve.[10]

REFERENCES

1. Beckwith JB: Grading of pediatric tumors. In Care of the Child with Cancer, pp 39–44. New York, American Cancer Society, 1979
2. Beckwith JB, Palmer N: Histopathology and prognosis of Wilms' tumor: Results of the National Wilms' Tumor Study. Cancer 41:1937, 1978
3. Bolande RP, Brough AJ, Izant RJ Jr: Congenital mesoblastic nephroma of infancy. Pediatrics 40:272, 1967
4. Breslow N, Churchill G, Beckwith JB, et al: Prognosis for Wilms' tumor patients with nonmetastatic disease at diagnosis: Results of the Second National Wilms' Tumor Study. J Clin Oncol 3:521, 1985
5. Breslow N, McCann B: Statistical estimation of prognosis for children with neuroblastoma. Cancer Res 31:2098, 1971
6. Brodeur GM, Seeger RC, Barrett A, et al: International criteria for diagnosis, staging and response to treatment in patients with neuroblastoma. International conference on neuroblastoma staging and response criteria. J Clin Oncol 6:1874, 1988
7. Chu T, D'Angio GJ, Favara B, et al: Histiocytosis syndromes in children (By the Writing Group of the Histiocyte Society). Lancet 1:208, 1987
8. Cornelius AS, Womer RB, Jakacki R: Multiple hemangioendotheliomas of the liver. Proceedings of the Tumor Board of The Children's Hospital of Philadelphia. Med Pediatr Oncol 17:501, 1989
9. D'Angio GJ: It ain't necessarily so. In van Eys J, Sullivan MP (eds): Status of the Curability of Childhood Cancers, pp 5–16. New York, Raven Press, 1980
10. D'Angio GJ: The child cured of cancer: A problem for the internist. Semin Oncol 9:143, 1982
11. D'Angio GJ: Radiotherapy for solid tumors. In Welch K, Randolph JD, Ravitch MM, et al (eds): Pediatric Surgery, 4th ed, pp.249–256. Chicago, Year Book Medical Publishers, 1986
12. D'Angio GJ, Green DM: Primary renal tumors of childhood. In Holland JF, Frei EM III, Bast RC, Kufe DW, Morton DL, Weichselbaum RR (eds): Cancer Medicine, 3rd ed. Malvern, Lea and Febiger (in press)
13. D'Angio GJ, Breslow N, Beckwith JB, et al: The treatment of Wilms' tumor: Results of the Third National Wilms' Tumor Study. Cancer 64:349, 1989
14. D'Angio GJ, Evans AE, Koop CE: Special pattern of widespread neuroblastoma with a favorable prognosis. Lancet 1:1046, 1971
15. D'Angio GJ, Rorke LB, Packer R, et al: Key problems in the management of children with brain tumors. Int J Radiat Oncol Biol Phys 18:805, 1990
16. D'Angio GJ, Ross JW: The cured cancer patient: A new problem in attitudes and communication. In Proceedings of the American Cancer Society Third National Conference on Human Values and Cancer, pp 45–49. Washington, DC, American Cancer Society, 1981
17. Evans AE, D'Angio GJ, Propert K, et al: Prognostic factors in neuroblastoma. Cancer 59:1853, 1987
18. Green WT, Farber S: Eosinophilic or solitary granuloma of bone. J Bone Joint Surg 24:499, 1942
19. Hammond GD: Multidisciplinary clinical investigation of the cancers of children. Cancer 55:1215, 1985
20. Kun LE, Moulder JE: General principles of radiation therapy. In Pizzo PA, Poplack DG (eds): Principles and Practice of Pediatric Oncology, pp 233–262. Philadelphia, JB Lippincott, 1989
21. Marangos P: Clinical studies with neuron-specific enolase. In Evans AE, D'Angio GJ, Seeger RC (eds): Advances in Neuroblastoma Research, pp 285–294. New York, Alan R Liss, 1985
22. McWilliams NB, Hayes FA, Smith IE, et al: IV-S neuroblastoma: Chemotherapy *vs* observation. [Abstract 830] Proc Am Soc Clin Oncol 5:211, 1986
23. Meadows AT, Krejmas NL, Belasco JB: The medical cost of cure: Sequelae in survivors of childhood cancer. In van Eys, J, Sullivan MP, (eds): Status of the Curability of Childhood Cancers, pp 263–276. New York, Raven Press, 1980
24. Seeger RC, Brodeur GM, Sather H, et al: Association of multiple copies of the N-*myc* oncogene with rapid progression of neuroblastomas. N Engl J Med 313:1111, 1985
25. Slater JM, Swarm OJ: Eosinophilic granuloma of bone. Med Pediatr Oncol 8:151, 1980
26. Smith DG, Nesbit ME, D'Angio GJ, et al: Histiocytosis X: Role of radiation therapy in management with special reference to dose levels employed. Radiology 106:419, 1973
27. Triche TT, Cavazzana AO: Pathology in pediatric oncology. In Pizzo PA, Poplack DG (eds): Principles and Practice of Pediatric Oncology, pp 93–125. Philadelphia, JB Lippincott, 1989
28. Womer RB, Raney RB, D'Angio GJ: Healing rates of treated and untreated bone lesions in histiocytosis X. Pediatrics 76:286, 1985

69

Brain Tumors in Children

Larry E. Kun

ANATOMY AND DEVELOPMENT

The anatomy of the brain was described in Chapter 23. There is no significant difference in the configuration of the structures of the central nervous system in the adult and the child, except for the proportions of volume in some of the anatomic sites. Figure 69-1 identifies some important anatomic landmarks.

The central nervous system (CNS) in children reaches morphologic maturation by 12 to 18 months of age. At birth, the brain's neuronal complement and organization are essentially complete. Lacking are the myelin sheaths that cover the long nerve processes forming the connecting tracts or "white matter" of the brain and spinal cord. The process of myelinization occurs in an orderly and anatomically specific sequence early in life, beginning with the corpus callosum centrally and ending with the white matter of the peripheral hemispheres at 12 to 24 months.[23]

Although anatomically mature at 18 months, the brain develops motor and sensory coordination and intellectual capacities throughout childhood. After therapy for CNS tumors, the type and degree of neurologic and neuropsychologic alterations correlate with the age of the child during treatment.

EPIDEMIOLOGY

CNS tumors account for 20% of all neoplasms in children, and brain tumors are exceeded in frequency only by the leukemias. The incidence of 2.5 cases per 100,000 children younger than 18 years old is equivalent to approximately 1700 new cases annually in the United States.[203]

At diagnosis, 15% of the CNS tumors occur in infants between birth and 2 years of age, 30% in those 2 to 5 years old, 30% in children 5 to 10 years old, and 25% in those 11 to 18 years old. Most (55%) tumors arise in the posterior fossa. Supratentorial tumors account for 40%, which predominate in infants younger than 1 year, and 5% are spinal cord presentations.[38,53] In children between 1 and 10 years of age, infratentorial tumors account for 60% of the cases.

The frequency of specific types of brain tumors is defined largely by histology. Site-specific diagnoses are included in Table 69-1 for locations that are infrequently sampled by biopsy or for those identified in the literature by clinical diagnosis.

Children meeting the criteria for neurofibromatosis (*i.e.*, ≥6 years old, cafe au lait spots, or peripheral neurofibromas) have a high incidence of CNS tumors and represent up to 10% to 20% of cases of optic chiasmatic or hypothalamic gliomas. Low-grade cerebral tumors are associated with tuberous sclerosis, and hemangioblastomas are associated with von Hippel-Lindau disease. Other hereditary associations include Torcot's syndrome, marked by colonic polyposis and CNS tumors, and the breast cancer-sarcoma-brain tumor familial relationship known as the Li-Fraumeni syndrome, which includes brain neoplasms in childhood.[133] Associated primarily with medulloblastoma is the nevoid basal cell syndrome; the CNS component usually occurs in infancy and sometimes precedes the cutaneous signs.[147]

Familial medulloblastoma has been described.[195] An association exists between rhabdoid tumors of the kidney and CNS tumors (*i.e.*, medulloblastoma, malignant glioma, primitive embryonal tumor).[28]

There is concern about the development of secondary malignant CNS tumors in children surviving treatment for acute lymphocytic leukemia (ALL). Although the incidence of malignant gliomas has yet to be quantified, preliminary reports suggest an actuarial occurrence approaching 1% to 5% at 5 to 15 years.[150] Most cases have followed treatment that included cranial irradiation and methotrexate with or without alkylating agents.

MEDULLOBLASTOMA

Medulloblastoma is a malignant tumor of neuroectodermal origin characterized by local infiltration and dissemination within the neuraxis and systematically.[171] The tumor usually arises in the region of cerebellar vermis, extending anteriorly to fill and obstruct the fourth ventricle. The tumor grows anteriorly to invade the brain stem, laterally through foramen of Luschka to the cerebellopontine angle or prepontine cistern, superiorly toward or beyond the tentorial notch (*i.e.*, growth to and beyond the level of the pineal region), or inferiorly into the cervical spine. Local meningeal involvement is apparent in most cases at surgery, identified as "sugar coating" of the posterior fossa meninges; the prognostic implication is not clear.[199] Deutsch[49] reported disease beyond the posterior fossa in 46% of patients studied postoperatively with cranial CT (supratentorial seeding, 6%), myelography (drop metastases in the spinal canal, 28%), and cerebrospinal fluid (CSF) cytology (positive in 14%).[49]

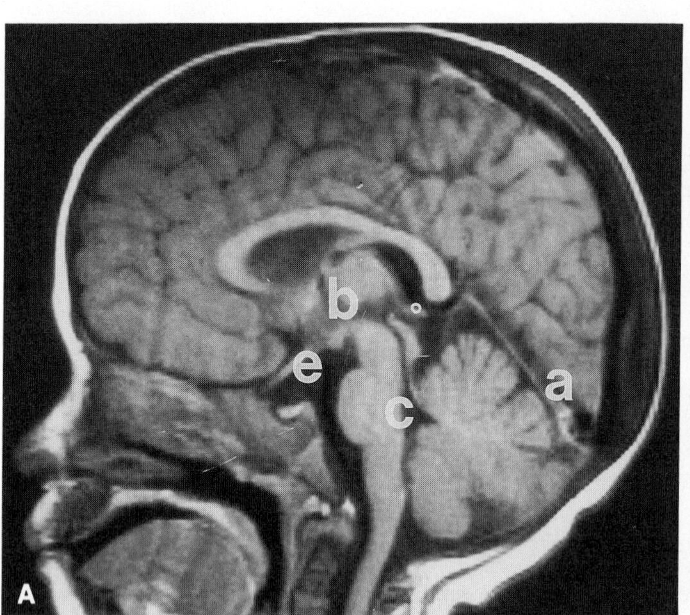

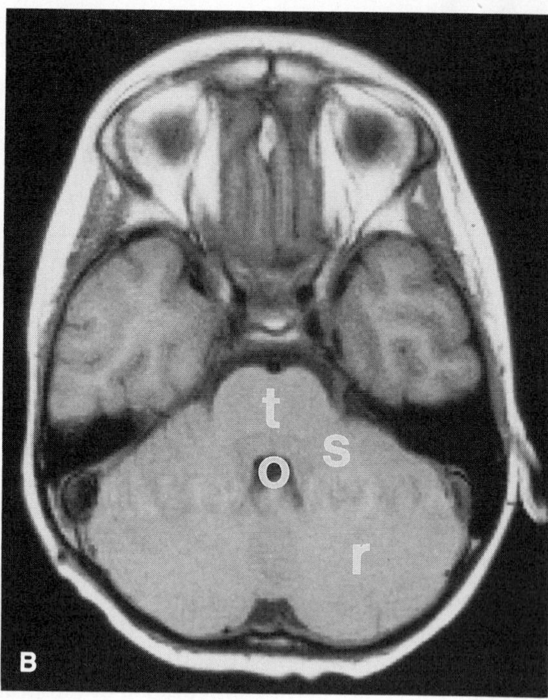

FIGURE 69–1. (**A**) Midplane sagittal MR scan of the brain. Notice the tentorium (a), separating the supratentorial compartment, above and anterior, and the posterior fossa below. The third ventricle (b) and fourth ventricle (c) are connected by the aqueduct. The suprasellar region (e) includes the hypothalamus above, the stalk, and the pituitary below. The pineal gland (o) lies below the posterior aspect of the corpus callosum. (**B**) Axial MR scan through the posterior fossa shows the cerebellum (r), fourth ventricle (o), region of the cerebellopontine peduncle (s), and brain stem (t).

The tumor is a small round cell tumor of childhood, characterized as an undifferentiated lesion that may demonstrate differentiation toward neuronal or glial cell lines.[41] Although a correlation between cellular differentiation and prognosis has been reported, there are no consistent data relating outcome to histologic factors.[32,155]

General Management

The intent of initial surgery for medulloblastoma is usually radical, seeking to resect macroscopic tumor. Contemporary series indicate complete or subtotal resection in more than 70% of the patients.[159,192] With current techniques, operative mor-

TABLE 69–1
Brain Tumors in Children

DIAGNOSIS	RELATIVE FREQUENCY	PEAK AGE GROUP (YR)
Astrocytoma*	35%	2–10
Supratentorial	22%	>6
Infratentorial	13%	2–10
Malignant glioma (anaplastic astrocytoma and glioblastoma multiforme)	8%	<1, >6
Brain stem glioma	8%	3–9
Oligodendroglioma	2%	>6
Medulloblastoma	20%	1–10
Ependymoma	8%	
Supratentorial	5%	>6
Infratentorial	3%	1–5
Craniopharyngioma	7%	8–14
Pineal region and germ cell tumors	4%	<2, >6
Choroid plexus tumors	2%	<1
Others: ganglioglioma, meningioma, neuroblastoma, primitive embryonal tumors	<2% each	

**Astrocytoma includes two primary histologic subtypes in children: pilocytic (20% of pediatric CNS tumors) and fibrillary (7%). (Data from Childhood Brain Tumor Consortium: J Neurooncol 6:9, 1988; Duffner PK, Cohen ME, Myers MH, et al: Neurology 36:597, 1986; Rubinstein LJ: Tumors of the nervous system. In Atlas of Tumor Pathology, fasc G. Washington, DC, Armed Forces Institute of Pathology, 1972)*

tality is 2% or less.[3,159] Significant postoperative morbidity, neurologically identified as the "posterior fossa syndrome," which includes respiratory and swallowing dysfunctions in addition to ataxia and lateralizing long tract signs, may follow aggressive surgery for tumors extending to the brachium pontis or floor of the fourth ventricle. Signs of bulbar and cerebellar dysfunction are reversible to a large degree.

Radiation therapy is potentially curative and is central in the management of medulloblastoma. Application of irradiation to the entire neuraxis (*i.e.*, craniospinal irradiation) was first reported soon after Cushing's description of this tumor.[43,44]

Medulloblastoma is sensitive to chemotherapy. Responses in recurrent tumors have been documented with alkylating agents (*e.g.*, cyclophosphamide), cisplatin or carboplatin, vincristine, and nitrosoureas.[63,68] Preirradiation chemotherapy has been effective in achieving partial or complete tumor regression investigationally; in young children, prolonged chemotherapy have produced a rate of approximately 40% for long-term responses, measured for intervals of 1 to 2 years before irradiation.[6,16,87,135] Prospective trials of chemotherapy by the Children's Cancer Study Group and the International Society of Pediatric Oncology showed improvement with lomustine (CCNU) and vincristine, primarily in cases categorized as high-risk medulloblastoma: children younger than 2 to 5 years, those with incompletely resected tumors, and those with overt neuraxis tumor dissemination at diagnosis.[61] A Pediatric Oncology Group study evaluating the addition of mechlorethamine, vincristine, procarbazine, and prednisone (MOPP regimen) to craniospinal irradiation showed an overall survival advantage with combined-modality therapy.[117] Preliminary reports of single-institution trials combining radiation therapy and chemotherapy have recently shown impressive control rates.[113,152] Current studies of patients with moderate- or high-risk features who are receiving chemotherapy before or after irradiation are testing the impact of chemotherapy on ultimate outcome and functional integrity.[63,113]

Radiation Therapy Techniques

Volume

Full craniospinal irradiation is mandatory for curative treatment.[95,122] Incomplete coverage of the subarachnoid space has resulted in excessive failures in the neuraxis or locally in the difficult-to-encompass subfrontal region.[99]

The volume of craniospinal irradiation includes the entire subarachnoid space. The cranial portals are indicated in Figure 69-2. The cribriform plate represents the inferior-most site subfrontally and is sometimes difficult to include because of proximity to the eyes (Fig. 69-2). Notice also the lower margin of the temporal fossa.

The preferred technique for craniospinal irradiation uses a prone position to facilitate daily setup at the junction over the cervical spine and to achieve maximal chin extension, diminishing exit through the mandible. An individually fabricated cast is a simple aid for ensuring daily reproducibility and immobilization (Fig. 69-3). Lateral craniocervical fields adjoin a posterior spinal field at the midcervical or lower cervical spine (Fig. 69-4). The spinal volume may be divided into two adjoining, appropriately gapped fields when necessary because of patient height; in such instances, it is desirable to join the fields below L2 (*i.e.*, caudal to the spinal cord).

Angles are used to correct for divergence in three dimensions. A gantry angle is optional but often desirable to avoid divergence toward the contralateral or exit eye. The collimator angle (Fig. 69-4*A*) is calculated to match the angle of divergence of the posterior spinal field, achieving a parallel "match" to avoid a more inhomogeneous junction in the lower cervical spine. With these angles alone, it is possible visually to align a junction in the midline at the back of the neck, which implies a gap of approximately 5 mm on the lateral surface of the neck. The lateral gap reflects the divergence of the craniocervical fields caudally. Further correction for this divergence can be achieved by rotating the treatment couch (Fig. 69-4*B*) through an arc of 3 to 5 degrees, which eliminates divergence in this dimension at the junction. Accomplishing a "precise match" by careful daily alignment obviates the need for any gap.

Use of a moving junction distributes the inhomogeneity at the field margins over a wider anatomic space. Increasing or decreasing the height of the craniocervical fields by 1 cm to 2 cm every five or six spinal fractions minimizes clinically significant variation in dose. In cases requiring two spinal fields, a junction change at the level of the interspinal field junction should be effected with the same frequency.

The spinal field covers the subarachnoid space inferiorly to the level of S2. A width adequate to cover the dorsal root foramina appears to be appropriate (Fig. 69-5). A cross-table lateral view on the simulator facilitates accurate calculation of depth from the posterior spinal field and allows an estimate of inhomogeneities caused by differences in depth along the length of the spinal canal.

A report detailing 15-MeV to 17-MeV electron irradiation to the spine indicates apparently adequate dose distribution within the spinal canal, at least in children younger than 4 years, whose size permits a single electron field, often at extended skin-to-source distances.[138] It is Important to abut the posterior electron field with the lateral craniocervical photon fields at the level of the cervical spine, a match requiring calculations of the electron field penumbra and cord depth.[51]

The limits of the posterior fossa field are designed to encompass the entire infratentorial compartment with some margin. An example of protocol-directed posterior fossa irradiation is depicted in Figure 69-2.

The sequence of treatment is typically craniospinal irradiation and subsequent treatment to the posterior fossa, but equivalent results are reported with the opposite sequence.[22,42,132] In treating medulloblastoma with combined modalities, it is often necessary to consider initial irradiation of the posterior fossa or interposition of posterior fossa irradiation during unscheduled interruptions in craniospinal irradiation because of hematosuppression.

Dose

Medulloblastoma is a radiosensitive tumor. A high degree of local tumor control in the posterior fossa can be achieved at dose levels within the tolerance of the nervous system. Table 69-2 indicates the reported dose-response associations for posterior fossa disease control and survival. There has been uniform agreement in recommending doses of 5000 cGy to 5500 cGy to the posterior fossa, usually reduced to 4500 cGy to 5000 cGy for young children younger than 2 to 3 years of age.[25]

There is much less information about appropriate doses for the craniospinal axis. Most recent reports documenting survival rates of 50% or more are based on cranial doses of 3500 cGy to 4000 cGy and spinal doses of 3000 cGy to 3500 cGy.[22,26,77,80,111,186] Initial reports of reduced neuraxis doses using 2500 cGy to the cranium and spine appear to support the

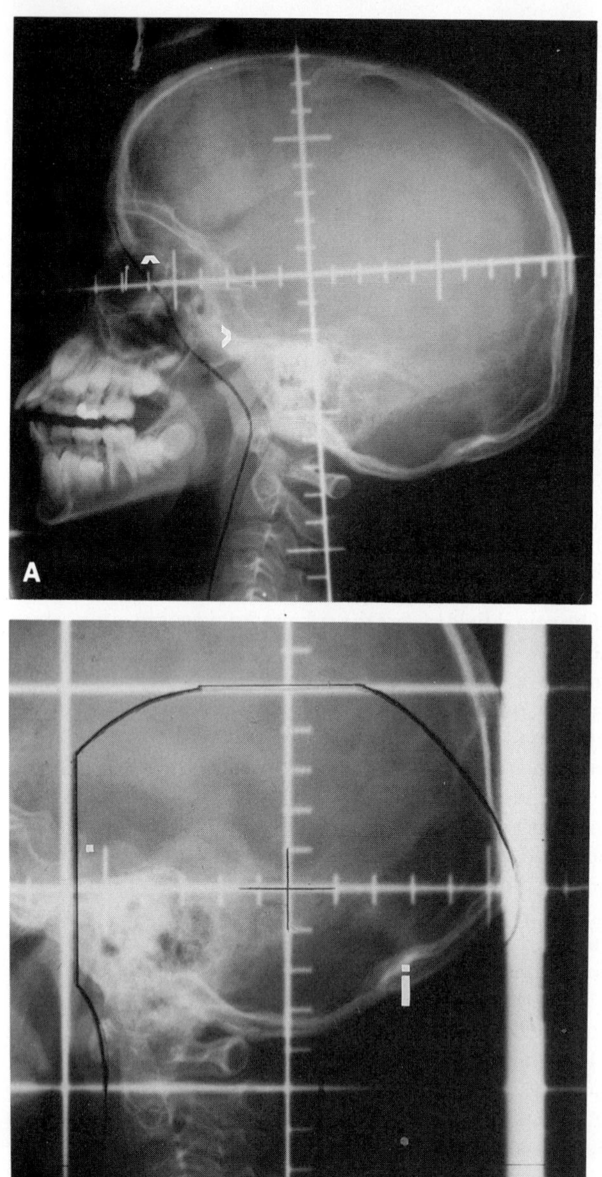

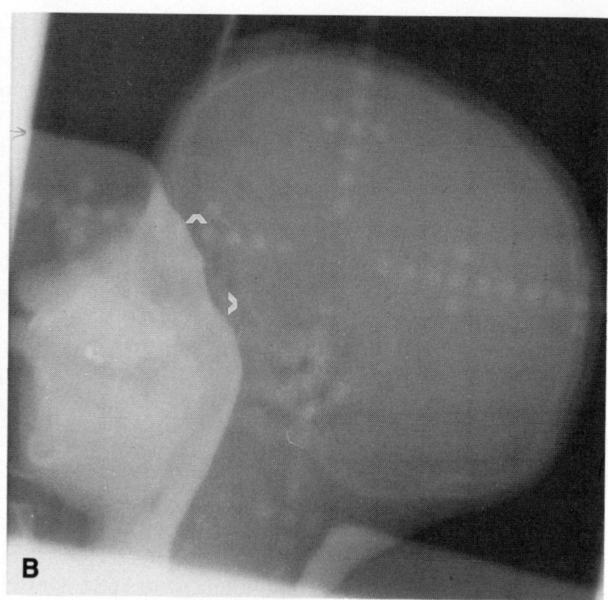

FIGURE 69–2. Treatment of medulloblastoma. (**A**) Simulation and (**B**) portal films for cranial fields, showing the cribriform plate (∧) and the lower aspect of the temporal fossa (>). (**C**) The posterior fossa field generously covers the infratentorial space from the posterior insertion of the tentorium at the inion (i) to include the posterior clinoid (□).

lower dose for medulloblastoma of limited extent after total resection.[99] A retrospective comparison of children treated with spinal doses of less than 2700 cGy (median, 2400 cGy) in conjunction with cranial doses approximating 3150 cGy showed a 5-year survival rate equivalent to that achieved with higher dose levels.[91] Combining chemotherapy (*i.e.*, procarbazine and hydroxyurea) with neuraxis doses of 2500 cGy produced 5-year survival rates equal to those achieved with reduced-dose irradiation alone.[132] An ongoing trial testing standard 3600 cGy and a reduced neuraxis dose of 2400 cGy has been conducted jointly by the Pediatric Oncology Group and Children's Cancer Study Group. Preliminary results of this study indicate an excess of failures with the lower neuraxis dose; standard dose levels (3600 cGy) are recommended.[50a]

Fraction size for neuraxis irradiation has varied between 150 and 180 cGy; treatment to the posterior fossa is most often given with 180-cGy fractions. The only available data addressing the influence of dose on survival indicate a significant decrease in 5-year survival rates for patients requiring interruption of treatment: 37% for interrupted therapy and 62% for continuous irradiation.[22]

Results of Treatment

Major series in the supervoltage era indicate 5-year survival rates approximating 55% to 60% and a 10-year survival rate of 45% (Table 69-3). The consistency of these results over the past 15 years indicates the improvement in operative and radiotherapeutic techniques compared with the "standard" in Bloom's 1969 report of a 5-year survival rate of 35% and 10-year survival rate of 26%.[25] A decrease in the survival rate of 10% to 15% between 5 and 10 years reflects the occurrence of late failures despite the fact that most disease progression occurs within the first 2 to 3 years after treatment.[49,91,128]

Treatment failures occur predominantly in the posterior fossa: 50% to 70% of all recurrent or progressive lesions have been identified in the primary site or as multisite failures that

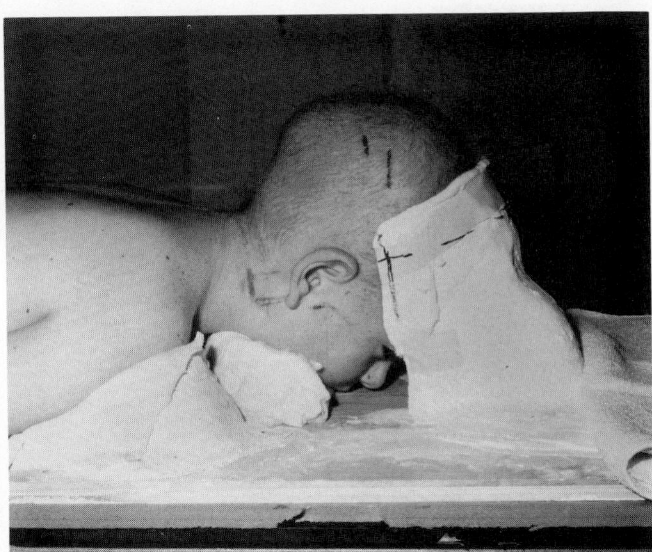

FIGURE 69–3. Immobilizing cast for prone craniospinal irradiation technique. The plaster cast is used to fix the shoulders, chin, and frontal regions. The cast allows visualization of the critical treatment setup around the eyes.

include the posterior fossa.[49,91,118] Neuraxis failures outside the posterior fossa account for 20% to 30% of recurrences, equally represented by supratentorial and spinal disease. Approximately 8% of cases fail with extraneural disease involving predominantly the bone and bone marrow.[107,118]

A staging system for medulloblastoma has been formulated by Chang and associates.[37] Table 69-4 exhibits the Chang classification and a modification to simplify disease categorization based on computed tomography (CT) and magnetic resonance imaging (MRI). A division of low-stage disease (*i.e.*, T1–T3a, M0) and high-stage disease (*i.e.*, T3b–T4, M1–M3) is now used for protocol eligibility by the Pediatric Oncology Group and the Children's Cancer Study Group.

Factors affecting outcome include:

1. Age: Children younger than 2 to 5 years old generally show decreased survival.[27,32,61,91,192]
2. Local tumor extent: Survival rates for T1 or T2 disease are 55% to 80% survival, but the rates are 25% to 50% for T3 or T4 tumors.[27,41,61,77,111,192]
3. Brain stem infiltration: Infiltration is associated with a less favorable outcome.[26,159]
4. Disease dissemination: Radiographically overt subarachnoid metastasis is associated with a decrease in survival from 60% to 70% to 0% to 50%; the impact of positive cytology alone is undefined.[49,61,77,111]
5. Surgical resection: Patients treated with biopsy or limited resection for any reason have 5-year survival rates of 30% to 40%. After total or subtotal resection, the 5-year survival rates are 50% to 70%.[61,91,159,192]

There is a group of patients with medulloblastoma with a favorable prognosis: children older than 2 to 5 years with limited disease extent (*i.e.*, T1–T3a, M0 in Chang's system, without brain stem infiltration), with total or near-total excision. Approximately 30% of children with medulloblastoma are now included within this group; long-term survival of these patients after standard irradiation approaches 65% to 70%.[123,192]

For patients with more advanced disease, data from prospective randomized trials show an apparent benefit with combined-modality treatment in cases with locally extensive or metastatic disease.[27,61,63,117] The high disease-free survival rates among patients receiving cisplatin-based chemotherapy support the use of aggressive coordinated chemotherapy and irradiation.[113,135,152,192]

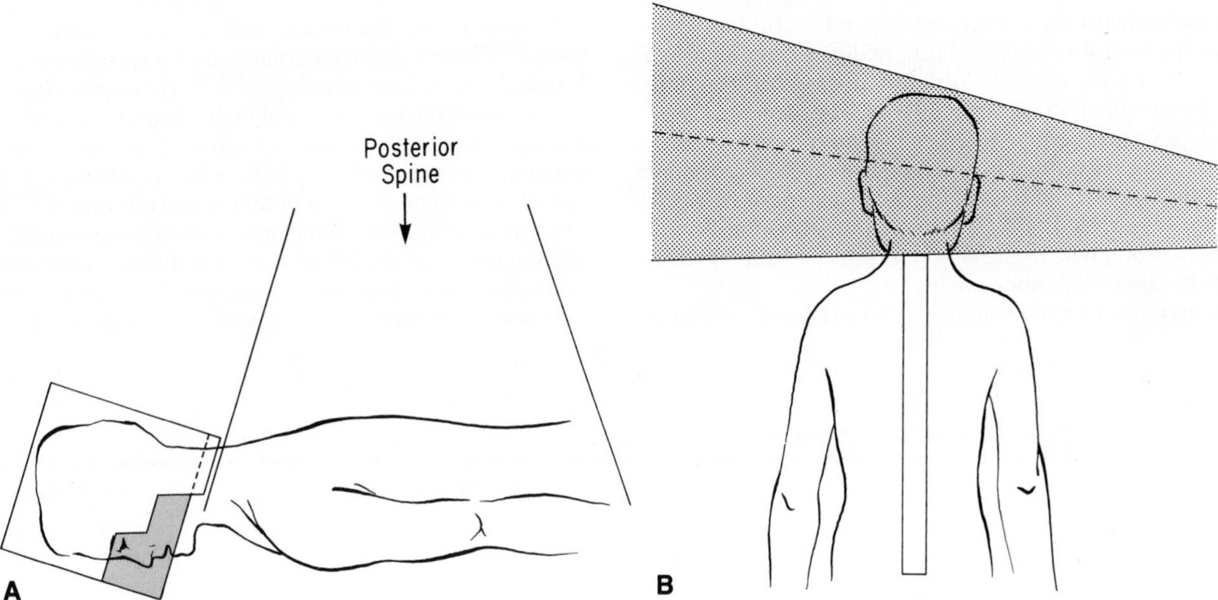

FIGURE 69–4. Schematic of craniospinal irradiation. (**A**) Lateral craniocervical field, with a collimator angle to parallel the configurations of the posterior spinal beam. (**B**) A couch angle is used for the craniocervical fields, achieving a parallel beam at the junction zone. With the three-dimensional junction incorporating both angles for the craniocervical fields, an exact match is used at the upper border of the spinal field.

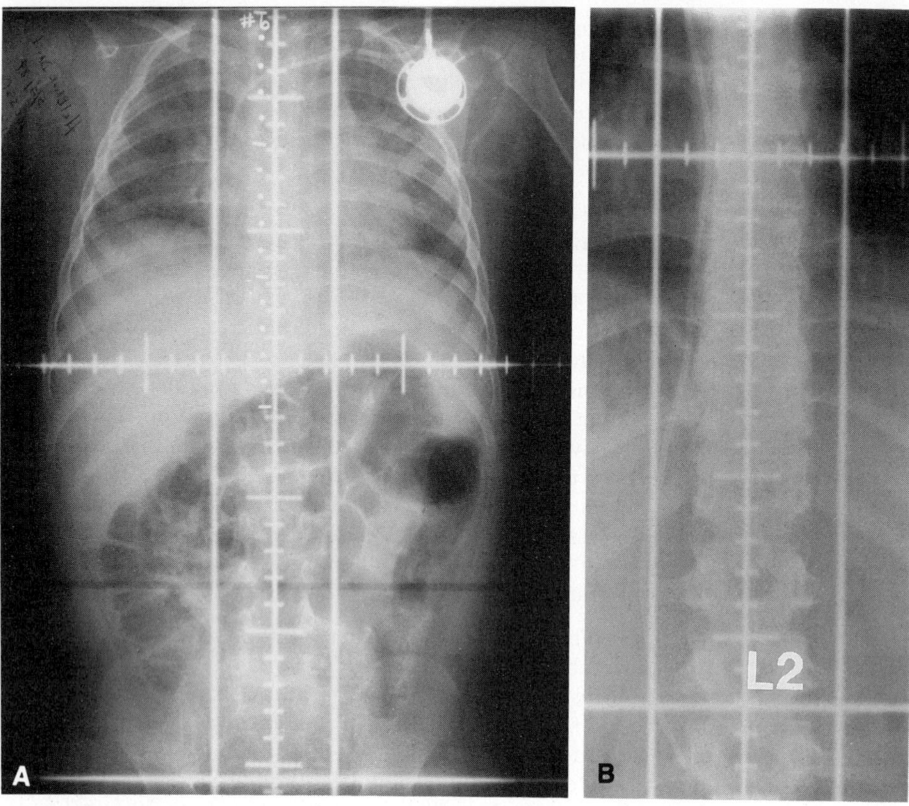

FIGURE 69–5. Spinal fields are shown for the (**A**) whole spine or (**B**) adjoining thoracic and lumbar fields, joined at L2. Notice the inferior margin below S2.

EPENDYMOMA

Ependymomas are neoplasms derived from the ependymal cells that line the ventricular system and the central spinal canal. Ependymal tumors occur throughout the CNS. In children, 90% present as intracranial lesions; 60% to 70% arise in the posterior fossa, most often within the fourth ventricle. Only 10% present as primary spinal tumors in this age group.

Tumors of the fourth ventricle typically fill the ventricle, causing obstructive hydrocephalus (Fig. 69-6). Infiltration occurs at the lateral cerebellopontine peduncles and along the floor of the fourth ventricle. Invasion into the brain stem has been documented in 25% to 50% of the patients.[92, 148, 197] Tumor grows through the foramen magnum in almost 50% of these patients, most often as a tongue-like projection of tumor extending to the C1 or C2 level; the caudal extension may reach to C3 or C5 (Fig. 69-6)[148, 194, 197] Less frequently, posterior fossa tumors may originate in the lateral medullary velum, presenting in the cerebellopontine angle.

Supratentorial ependymomas occur predominantly in the parietal and frontal lobes and present as intracerebral lesions, often contiguous with the lateral ventricles but only rarely as intraventricular neoplasms. Tumors peripheral to the ventricular system are believed to arise from cerebral hemispheric extensions of subependymal elements that migrate during embryogenesis.[92]

Ependymomas classically have ependymal rosettes (*i.e.,* discrete, rounded collections of epithelioid cells with fine cytoplasmic processes oriented toward a central lumen), fibrillary perivascular pseudorosettes, and tubular epithelial structures.[171] Clinical series generally report a correlation between histologic grade and survival.[27, 174, 182] Neuropathologists are less certain of the significance of high-grade or anaplastic ependymoma as typically defined for astrocytic tumors; three leading pediatric neuropathologists have independently reported a lack of correlation between histology and outcome.[165, 169, 170] A practical classification for the more common intracranial ependymomas categorizes 75% of tumors as differentiated and 25% as anaplastic ependymomas; the anaplastic tumors have historically been considered more aggressive with a greater potential

TABLE 69–2
Posterior Fossa Dose, Disease Control, and Survival for Medulloblastoma

INVESTIGATOR	TREATMENT INTERVAL	END-POINT	<5000 cGy RESULT	<5000 cGy NO. OF PATIENTS	≥5000 cGy RESULT	≥5000 cGy NO. OF PATIENTS
Silverman[186]	1954–1978	Survival (5 yr)	.36	29	.85	21
		PF Control	.38	29	.80	20
Berry[22]	1958–1978	Survival (5 yr)	.50	33	.63	86
Harisiadis[77]	1963–1975	Survival (5 yr)	.35	17	.46	38
Hughes[91]	1968–1984	PF Control	.33	18	.79	42

TABLE 69–3
Survival After Surgery and Radiation Therapy for Medulloblastoma

INVESTIGATOR	TREATMENT INTERVAL	NO. OF PATIENTS	SURVIVAL RATE (%)	
			5 YEAR	10 YEAR
Bloom[25]	1950–1969	90	35	26
Bloom[27]	1970–1981	53	53	46
Kopelson[111]	1962–1979	43	56	56
Harisiadis[77]	1963–1975	59	40	31
Hirsch[80]	1964–1976	44	71	
Hughes[91]	1964–1984	60	68	44
Lefkowitz[128]	1970–1983	44	54	41
Deutsch[49]	1974–1987	45	63	
Park[159]	1975–1980	50	60	

for neuraxis dissemination.[27,38,118,120] Recent clinical series question the implications of histologic grade.[148,197]

Ependymoblastoma is a rare tumor of young children, usually supratentorial and characterized by diffuse small round cells with focal areas of ependymal differentiation.[170]

General Management

Initial resection of a fourth ventricular ependymoma is technically challenging because the tumor often invades the cerebellar peduncle or ventricular floor and brain stem. Current data indicate complete resections have been possible in 30% to 50% of the patients.[148,197] For supratentorial ependymomas, resection may be difficult because of the size and location of the tumors.

Radiation therapy adds significantly to disease control and survival in ependymomas.[139,144,182,206] The occurrence in young children may compromise outcome in requiring dose reduction for those younger than 2 to 3 years of age.[139] Debate about treatment of ependymomas has focused primarily on the desirability of craniospinal irradiation for specific presentations.[27,120,130,170,174,182]

Ependymomas have proven to be relatively sensitive to chemotherapy. Significant responses have been demonstrated with alkylating agents (*e.g.*, cyclophosphamide, aziridinylbenzoquinone-AZQ), cisplatin and carboplatin, vincristine, and the nitrosoureas.[34,68,131,180] Preirradiation trials using cyclophosphamide alone or multiagent regimens including cyclophosphamide, vincristine, CDDP, and VP-16; MOPP; or "8-in-1" have produced objective and often durable responses.[6,88,160,202] Prospective trials of adjuvant chemotherapy have shown no improvement in 5-year survival rates.[26,27,63,127]

TABLE 69–4
Staging for Medullobastoma

CHANG OPERATIVE STAGING SYSTEM

T1	Tumor < 3 cm in diameter and limited to classic position in vermis, roof of fourth ventricle, and cerebellar hemisphere
T2	Tumor ≥ 3 cm in diameter and further invading one adjacent structure or partially filling fourth ventricle
T3a	Tumor further invading two adjacent structures or completely filling fourth ventricle, with extension into aqueduct or foramina of Magendie or Luschka with marked internal hydrocephalus
T3b	Tumor arising from floor of fourth ventricle or brain stem and filling fourth ventricle
T4	Tumor penetrates aqueduct to involve third ventricle or midbrain or extends to cervical cord

IMAGING MODIFICATION OF CHANG OPERATIVE STAGING

T1	Tumor < 3 cm in diameter
T2	Tumor ≥ 3 cm in diameter
T3a	Tumor with extension into the aqueduct of Sylvius or into the foramen of Luschka
T3b	Tumor with unequivocal extension into the brain stem
T4	Tumor with extension past the aqueduct of Sylvius or the foramen magnum

Surgical staging may confirm extension into the brain stem without imaging evidence.
(Langston J: Personal communication, 1989)
(Chang CH, Housepian EM, Herbert C Jr: Radiology 93:1351, 1969)

Radiation Therapy Techniques

Volume

Higher rates of failure have occurred after partial cranial irradiation (45% and 88%) than after full cranial or craniospinal irradiation (33%), although differences fail to reach statistical significance.[175,182] The high proportion of cases failing at the

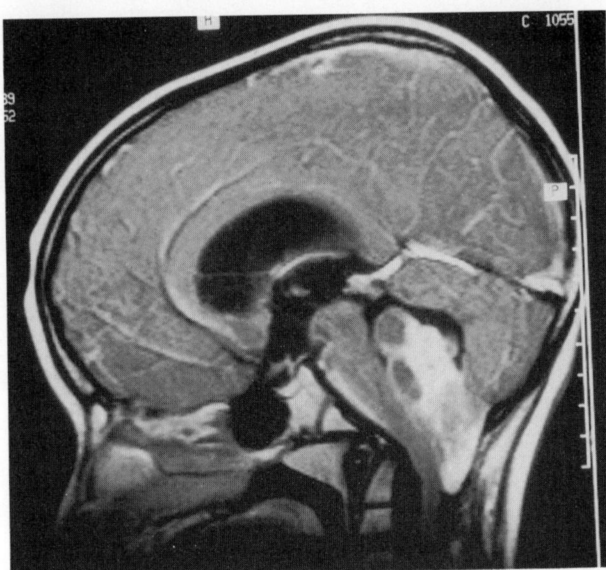

FIGURE 69–6. Fourth ventricular ependymoma, demonstrating direct extension through foramen magnum to the C1 level.

primary tumor site and more recent improvements in neuroimaging suggest that wide local fields are probably adequate.[120, 130, 139, 148, 175, 182, 197]

The major uncertainty influencing treatment volume, especially in children, is the frequency of subarachnoid dissemination. Collected series indicate an overall frequency of neuraxis seeding in 12% of intracranial lesions (*i.e.*, about 10% for supratentorial and 25% for posterior fossa).[27, 130, 162, 175] For differentiated ependymomas, most instances of spinal or remote intracranial seeding have occurred with or after recurrence at the primary site.[139, 148, 170, 182, 197] Almost 80% of patients with CNS dissemination have high-grade ependymomas of the fourth ventricle.[118, 130, 174] In more recent series addressing posterior fossa ependymomas, the number of cases demonstrating initial failure beyond the primary tumor site is small, regardless of histology.[148, 197] Results with limited fields appear to be comparable to those with full cranial or craniospinal irradiation for low-grade or differentiated tumors.[27, 148, 197]

Local treatment fields for fourth ventricular ependymomas are similar to the posterior fossa volume described for medulloblastoma, lengthening the field to include the cervical spine to at least the C2–3 interspace. In cases with documented tumor growth below the foramen magnum, the lower field margin is defined as two vertebral levels caudal to the preoperative tumor extent and administered at least to 4500 cGy, after which more narrow coverage may be adequate (Fig. 69-7). Inherent in the use of a limited volume is accurately staging the neuraxis before treatment, even with differentiated fourth ventricular tumors. Patients with positive spinal imaging or CSF cytology require craniospinal irradiation.

For fourth ventricular anaplastic ependymomas, craniospinal irradiation has been the standard. Histologic correlations with prognosis indicate the desirability of studying local fields, but treatment of the nonprotocol patient is best defined as craniospinal irradiation similar to that for medulloblastoma. With craniospinal irradiation, the boost should include the upper spine (Fig. 69-7).

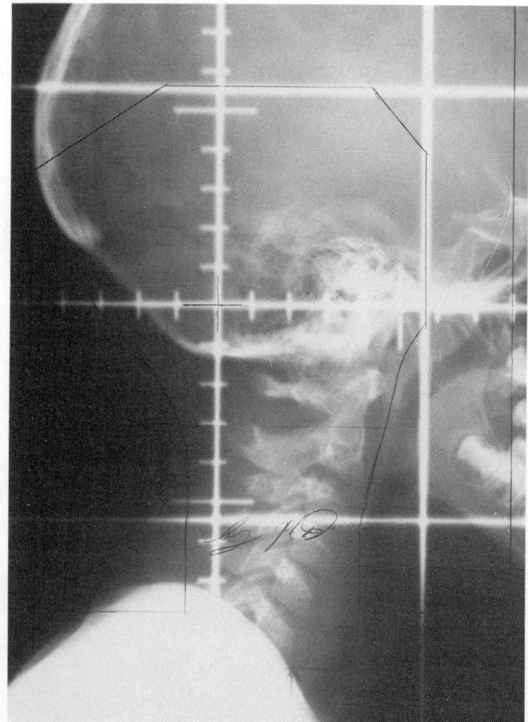

FIGURE 69–7. Simulation film of the posterior fossa volume for the fourth ventricular ependymoma. Notice the lower extension to the C3–4 interface.

In treating supratentorial ependymoma, the argument for entire cranial irradiation may be based on the inadequate imaging in older series.[130] With modern neuroimaging, it is likely that wide local fields with 2-cm to 3-cm margins around the preoperative tumor are adequate.

Dose

A dose-response association exists for fourth ventricular ependymoma; a local control rate of more than 70% and a survival rate of almost 50% have been reported after doses of 4500 cGy or more.[72, 139, 175] It has been more difficult to identify a dose relationship for supratentorial primary lesions.[139]

The relative frequency of local failure despite adequate radiation therapy and surgery has prompted recommendations for posterior fossa dose levels approaching CNS tolerance: 5400 cGy to 5500 cGy using conventional fraction sizes of approximately 180 cGy per day in children older than 2 to 3 years. Tolerance for wide-field cerebral irradiation dictates a similar dose for local fields in treating supratentorial ependymomas. A dose of 3500 cGy to 4000 cGy is recommended for supratentorial lesions requiring wide fields; in cases requiring craniospinal irradiation, spinal irradiation is also advised to a dose of 3500 cGy to 3600 cGy.

Results of Treatment

Single-institution series differ widely in reporting outcome for intracranial ependymomas. Survival rates at 5 years vary from 15% to 60%.[72, 148, 162, 175, 182, 197] Bloom and colleagues[27] reported a 50% survival rate at 5 years, falling to 30% by 15 years. Among children younger than 2 years with posterior fossa tumors, the 5-year survival rate is only 15%.[148, 197] Results appear to be better for children older than 3 to 5 years: 40% to 60%.[27, 53, 148]

Differentiation has been correlated with survival in major radiation therapy series. Shaw and associates[182] reported histologic grade as the only prognostic factor: patients with low-grade tumors had a 5-year relapse-free survival rate of 70% compared with a rate of 29% for patients with high-grade ependymomas. There have been conflicting reports from neuropathologists: Ross and Rubeinstein[170] describe long-term survival for 67% of their patients with malignant ependymoma.

Failures occur early in ependymal tumors; the median time to recurrence is 18 to 24 months.[175, 197] The predominant pattern of failure is local, emphasizing investigational approaches to increase cumulative radiation dose (*e.g.*, altered fractionation studies) and explore combinations of chemotherapy and irradiation.[120, 139, 197]

BRAIN STEM GLIOMA

Tumors of the brain stem are commonly identified as an "anatomic group" of neoplasms because of the lack of histologic information. Pontine gliomas predominate. The more generic term of brain stem glioma includes tumors of the midbrain (mesencephalon), pons, or medulla. Brain stem gliomas occur in children and adults; in children, the peak age group is 3 to 9 years.

Clinicopathologic correlations relate site of origin to histology. Intrinsic brain stem neoplasms are uniformly glial. Pontine gliomas are generally high-grade or malignant gliomas.[2,4,59] Presenting symptoms include cranial nerve and long tract deficits, often of less than 2 months' duration. Tumors of the midbrain are usually low-grade astrocytomas, frequently presenting with hydrocephalus and oculomotor signs.[2,56] Lesions of the medulla are also low-grade astrocytomas.[58]

General Management

Surgical management is controversial and evolving. Beyond providing histologic confirmation of the aggressive nature of most pontine tumors, there is little to be gained from biopsy of typical, diffusely infiltrating gliomas of the pons.[17,59]

Hoffman[83] identified a unique and relatively uncommon tumor that is exophytic.[188] This so-called dorsally exophytic benign brain stem glioma occurs in young children as a low-grade tumor that fills the fourth ventricle from the floor, demonstrating minimal if any invasion into the brain stem (Fig. 69-8). Surgery alone has achieved disease stabilization with little likelihood of tumor progression measured at 5 to 7 years.[83] Epstein's experience with surgical resection for cervicomedullary junction astrocytomas has similarly established long-term disease control without radiation therapy for an uncommon subset of brain stem gliomas.[58]

For most children presenting with brain stem gliomas, primary management is radiation therapy. Symptomatic improvement occurs in 75% of cases; long-term disease control has been described in only a small proportion of these cases.[2,57,106] The lack of histologic confirmation of most brain stem gliomas has led influential neurosurgeons to question the diagnosis in any child surviving after treatment.[140] Modern imaging techniques, frequent documentation of malignant glioma in autopsy series, and recent improvement in radiation therapy results have confirmed the role of irradiation.[2,56,67,151]

Chemotherapy has shown little effectiveness in brain stem gliomas. Despite documented response to preirradiation chemotherapy, outcome has mirrored that with radiation therapy alone.[131] A prospective trial of CCNU and vincristine demonstrated benefit in combined treatment.[97]

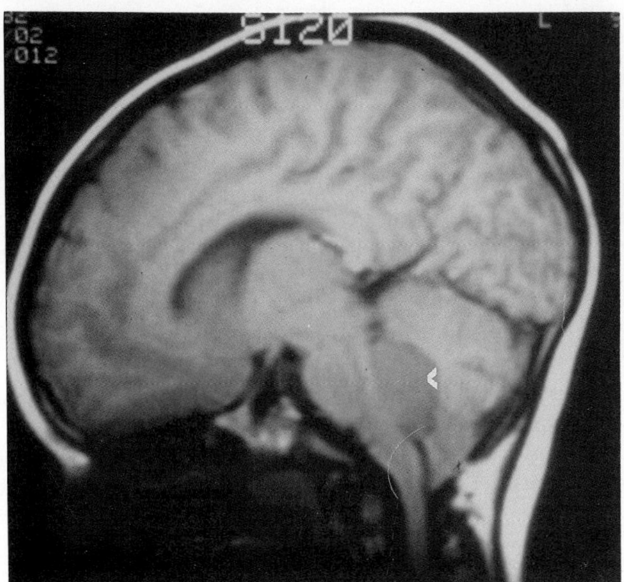

FIGURE 69–8. Dorsally exophytic brain stem astrocytoma.

Radiation Therapy Techniques

Volume

Pontine gliomas are infiltrating neoplasms that extend longitudinally to involve the midbrain and medulla and axially to involve the brachium pontis or cerebellum.[17] The treatment volume is indicated in Figure 69-9, including the brain stem from the midbrain to the cervicomedullary junction at C1. The width of the treatment volume extends from the sella anteriorly to the midcerebellum. Opposed lateral fields provide adequate coverage for the midline tumor; high-energy photons are preferable.

More focal irradiation is indicated for midbrain tumors (Fig. 69-10). Local volumes including the tumor site with 1-cm to 2-cm margins are often adequate.

Subarachnoid dissemination has been reported in as many as 15% to 20% of the children with brain stem gliomas.[57,151] The uniform pattern of disease progression at the primary site favors local irradiation techniques.[56,57,151]

Dose

Data substantiating survival in 20% to 30% of patients with brain stem gliomas has been based on dose levels of 5000 cGy to 5500 cGy with conventional fractionation for tumors in all anatomic sites.[57,106] The failure to achieve disease control in patients with typical, infiltrating pontine gliomas has led to trials of dose escalation using hyperfractionation.[208] With doses of 7200 cGy delivered in 100-cGy fractions twice daily, survival at 2 years was documented in more than 30% of the children with brain stem gliomas; among those with diffuse lesions, a median survival time of 1 year was reported.[56] A dose-response association with hyperfractionation is apparent in two series, suggesting improved survival beyond 1 year and an apparent "plateau" of survival beyond 2 years in high-risk patients with pontine gliomas treated with 7020 cGy (117 cGy twice daily) or 7200 cGy (100 cGy twice daily).[17,67,151] It is unlikely that current cooperative group trials testing 7800 cGy (100 cGy twice daily) and 7560

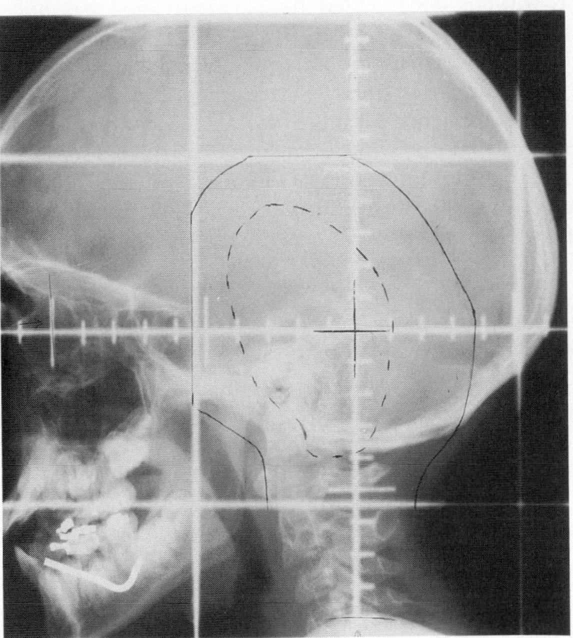

FIGURE 69–9. Treatment volume (*solid line*) and target volume (*dotted line*) for infiltrating glioma of the brain stem (pons).

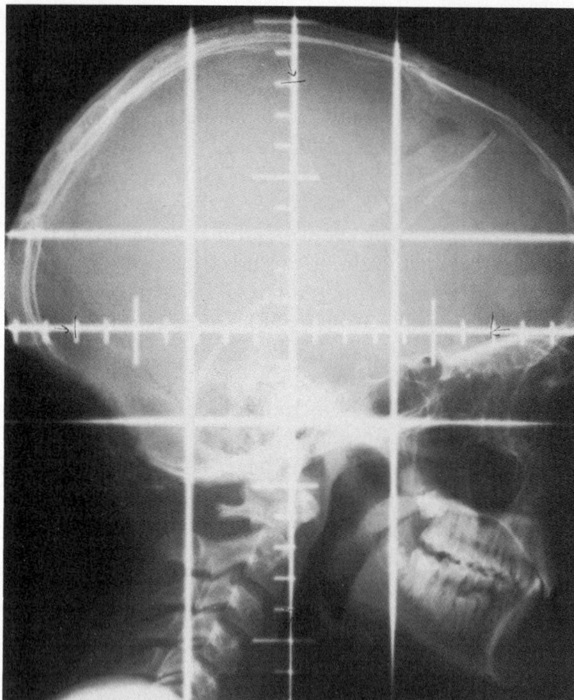

FIGURE 69–10. Lateral field used for a midbrain astrocytoma. The limited target volume and central location favor a high-energy beam using lateral or arc configurations.

TABLE 69–5
Prognostic Factors for Brain Stem Glioma

CHARACTERISTIC	2-YEAR SURVIVAL RATE (%)
Site	
Midbrain	100
Medulla	50
Pons	20
Growth	
Diffuse	23
Focal	88
Confined to one anatomic site	55
Extension beyond primary site	20
No or minimal brain stem expansion	50
Moderate or marked expansion	20
Special features	
"Benign" dorsally exophytic type	100
Cyst formation	100

(Modified from Preuss Foundation review of 87 children treated with hyperfractionated irradiation. Focal tumors are defined as lesions limited to one anatomic site (i.e., *pons or midbrain or medulla)* and *occupying less than half of the normal volume of that structure. "Brain stem expansion" refers to size based on axial MRI. The "benign" dorsally exophytic subtype is defined in the text.[83])*

cGy (126 cGy twice daily) will be followed by further dose escalation.

Hyperfractionated irradiation doses to 7000 cGy or more has been associated with instances of intralesional necrosis, hemorrhage, or cystic degeneration within 2 to 4 months after treatment. These events appear to represent a pattern of tumor response; after surgical intervention or spontaneous resolution, many of these patients have been among the long-term survivors.[67,151] Extralesional white matter changes have been documented after hyperfractionated techniques, but late brain necrosis without documented tumor progression has not been observed.[56,67,151]

The results of high-dose, hyperfractionated irradiation for focal tumors are impressive if treatment is early; use of such treatment for benign or more favorable lesions of the midbrain or medulla may be appropriate, particularly in a study.[17,56] In diffusely infiltrating pontine tumors, results at 7000 cGy to 7200 cGy in 100-cGy to 120-cGy fractions twice daily indicate a potential advantage over conventional fractionation.

Results of Therapy

Response to radiation therapy includes clinical improvement in 70% to 80% of the children.[2,56,67,106] Impressive reduction in tumor size on serial MRI has occurred after hyperfractionated irradiation in as many as one third of the patients.[67,151]

Some tumor factors influence the interpretation of clinical series (Table 69-5). Clinical parameters that correlate with better prognosis include duration of symptoms longer than 2 months and lack of cranial nerve palsies, features that often identify tumors outside the central pons.[4,56] Tumors that are focal (*i.e.*, well-demarcated lesions confined to one anatomic site and involving less than half of the structure of origin), outside the pons, and smaller (*i.e.*, degree of brain stem enlargement on axial imaging) enjoy a relatively more favorable prognosis.[17] Tumors with cyst formation are associated with more differentiated histology and improved outcome.[2,17] Studies using conventional fractionation have reported a survival rate of 50% at 2 to 5 years for focal or localized tumors.[2,118]

Survival rates in the more typical diffuse pontine lesions exceed 10% to 20% only in the more recent hyperfractionation trials.[2,51,56,67,97] Median time to progression is typically 6 to 8 months. There is a trend toward improved survival among patients with responses, as measured by CT or MRI, 6 to 8 weeks after radiation therapy.[56]

For a subset of patients treated with hyperfractionated irradiation who have stable or improved disease documented by MRI, prolonged corticosteroid therapy is necessary.[56,67] A degree of lymphopenia and the occurrence of opportunistic infection may be caused by corticosteroid use or unique treatment-related immune suppression.[56,208]

SUPRATENTORIAL GLIOMAS

Astrocytomas are the most common group of CNS tumors in children. Low-grade astrocytomas predominate, usually presenting in the cerebellum, diencephalon, or temporal lobes. Standard histopathologic classification lists the several subtypes in children[171]:

1. Fibrillary tumors occur as brain stem gliomas or as circumscribed lesions of the cerebellum or diencephalon.
2. Protoplasmic lesions present primarily as temporal lobe tumors.
3. Gemistocytic tumors are rare cerebral lesions, which often progress to glioblastoma. Fibrillary, protoplasmic, and gemistocytic tumors are often grouped as ordinary astrocytomas.
4. Pilocytic lesions are common tumors in childhood, defined by the piloid or hair-like appearance microscopically. Tumors arise in the cerebellum or diencephalon as circum-

scribed lesions; in the region of the internal capsule, corpus callosum, or optic chiasm, the tumors tend to infiltrate along the white matter tracts. Cyst formation is common.

5. Subependymal giant cell tumors are low-grade or hemartomatous tumors lining the ventricular walls in children with tuberous sclerosis.
6. Pleomorphic xanthoastrocytoma are infrequent tumors of the peripheral cerebral hemispheres with local invasion and frequent dural infiltration. The lesions look aggressive histologically, but behave in a benign fashion.[104]

Natural history and prognosis of low-grade astrocytomas vary with anatomic location and histologic grade. Tumors of the cerebellum and suprasellar region are more likely to be biologically benign than similar lesions in the cerebral hemispheres or thalamus. Oligodendrogliomas and mixed gliomas (primarily oligoastrocytoma) occur predominately in the cerebral hemispheres and behave like similar tumors in adults. Gangliogliomas, biologically indolent tumors composed of glial elements and mature ganglion cells, occur preferentially in this age group.[48,73] At the opposite end of the spectrum, malignant gliomas (anaplastic astrocytoma and glioblastoma) account for 15% to 30% of glial neoplasms in children.[27,149]

Malignant gliomas present as aggressive cerebral hemispheric thalamic or brain stem tumors. Hemispheric astrocytomas are usually well demarcated; almost 50% are cystic.[81,142] Thalamic tumors may infiltrate along white matter tracts, extending to the optic pathways, contralateral thalamic region, or longitudinally into the midbrain.

Seizures are the most frequent presenting symptoms in cerebral gliomas.[81] Headaches or focal neurologic signs predominate in malignant glioma or thalamic tumors.[21,52] Cyst formation occurs in 25% of the thalamic gliomas; histologically, 25% to 50% are malignant.[5,21] The incidence of clinically discernible leptomeningeal dissemination is high in childhood malignant glioma; 30% to 40% of children show diffuse subarachnoid or spinal metastases.[52,154,201]

General Management

The role of surgery in the management of low-grade hemispheric gliomas increased during the 1980s. Complete resection, if feasible, appears to achieve long-term disease control in a high proportion of cases.[81,142] Pilocytic astrocytomas and well-demarcated ordinary astrocytomas are most likely to be totally excised.[81,181,205] Series from the 1950s to 1980 indicate complete resections were possible in 15% to 50% of the children.[126,183,205] Recent reports suggest a potential for excision in as many as 90% of the patients.[81]

Surgical intervention for thalamic gliomas has rapidly evolved from hesitant biopsy to attempted removal in patients with apparently localized low-grade tumors.[5,21,103] Radical, if often subtotal, excision has been performed for 35% of the children; selected use of CT-directed stereotactic operative techniques has resulted in complete resections for 65% of a group of patients with limited follow-up.[21,103]

Aggressive resection has been less enthusiastically addressed in malignant gliomas. Patterns of infiltration, necrosis, and hypervascularity limit the frequency of complete resection for malignant gliomas regardless of location.[52,187]

Most controversial in the management of low-grade supratentorial gliomas is the role of radiation therapy. The efficacy of irradiation in achieving tumor reduction, symptomatic improvement, and prolongation in disease control interval has been suggested in numerous series.[5,29,57,126,129,181,183,205,213] Whether treatment results in ultimate disease control or only retards tumor progression for several years after irradiation is uncertain.[129,143,205,213] The availability of accurate neuroimaging, increasing sophistication of the general population assuring regular follow-up, and recognition of risks of surgery and irradiation allow some judgment in the timing of radiotherapeutic intervention. A national pediatric trial is ongoing for low-grade gliomas to measure disease control intervals after total or near-total resection, compare disease control intervals with and without postoperative irradiation for incompletely resected or biopsied lesions, and evaluate the impact of surgery and radiation therapy on functional integrity. Future trials must address the timing of radiation therapy and the relative merits of delayed surgery or irradiation.

Indications for radiation therapy include incompletely resected lesions in children older than 3 to 5 years, particularly if location or extent makes subsequent resection unlikely.[27,130] For children younger than 3 to 5 years lacking significant neurologic signs or changes indicative of rapid tumor growth, careful follow-up with the expectation of intervention at the time of documented tumor progression is appropriate.[21,143,193] A decision to follow an incompletely resected lesion at any age implies a commitment for regular monitoring and appropriate therapeutic intervention, often including radiation therapy, at the time of tumor progression.

The systematic role of radiation therapy in malignant hemispheric gliomas is based on documented efficacy in the adult population.[130,204] High-grade thalamic tumors similarly require irradiation.[27,57] Outcome for children that slightly exceeds that for adults indicates the importance of exploring modifications of radiation therapy delivery (*e.g.*, time-dose relationship, volume, use of interstitial implantation).[52,60]

Chemotherapy has been infrequently assessed for low-grade gliomas outside the hypothalamic-optic chiasmal site. In patients with disease progression after surgery and radiation therapy, alkylating agents (*e.g.*, cyclophosphamide, aziridinylbenzoquinone, carboplatin) have demonstrated some efficacy.[10,34,68] For malignant gliomas in children, a prospective trial has reported improvement in event-free survival and outcome using CCNU, vincristine, and prednisone.[187] The limited number of patients in this study indicate some caution in adopting the regimen as standard, but the results encourage further exploration of coordinated chemotherapy and irradiation.[187]

Radiation Therapy Techniques

Volume

Low-grade gliomas require local irradiation techniques. Hemispheric tumors may be treated with 2-cm margins, preferably based on MRI scans (Fig. 69-11). The tendency for thalamic gliomas to extend along white matter tracts indicates the need for detailed imaging studies and margins of at least 2 cm, with attention to the corpus callosum and midbrain. It is generally desirable to use multiple fields, potentially including wedged pairs or arc configurations in the coronal or axial planes to limit the high-dose volume (Fig. 69-11). Leptomeningeal spread has been reported only anecdotally for patients with low-grade tumors.[39]

For malignant gliomas, the principles of irradiation are similar to those for adults. Wide local fields are standard. Identification of clinically significant neuraxis dissemination is problematic in 25% to 40% of children.[52,201] Distant intracranial or

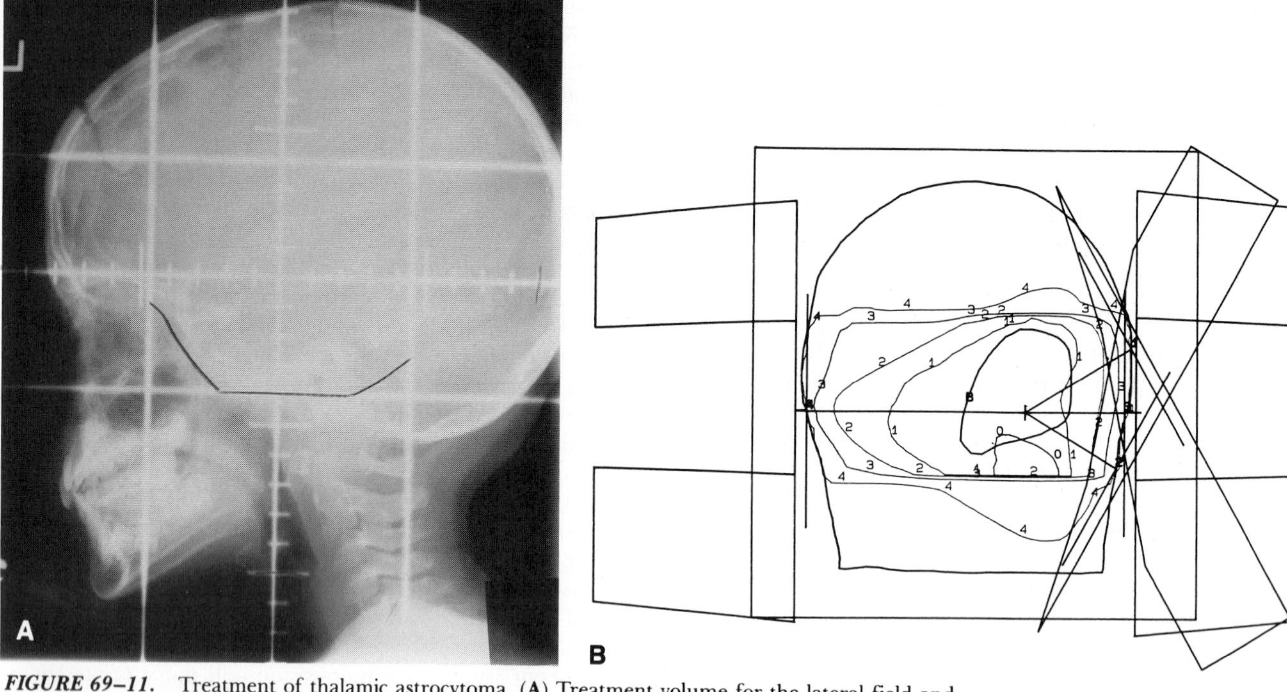

FIGURE 69–11. Treatment of thalamic astrocytoma. (**A**) Treatment volume for the lateral field and (**B**) dosimetry. Isodose curves demonstrate doses of (1) 5500 cGy, (2) 5000 cGy, (3) 4000 cGy, and (4) 2000 cGy from a composite treatment plan using unequally weighted opposed lateral and ipsilateral coronal wedged pair configurations (10-MV photons).

spinal meningeal disease may exist at diagnosis; more often, dissemination is diagnosed at the time of primary disease progression.[52] Indications for craniospinal irradiation are limited to children with overt neuraxis metastasis at diagnosis; myelography (or enhanced spinal MRI) is indicated before irradiation is begun.

Interstitial irradiation has been reported in pediatric diencephalic tumors, with 10-year follow-up suggesting treatment outcome similar or superior to that achieved with conventional irradiation.[60]

Dose

A dose-response association for astrocytomas has been reported at doses of 4500 cGy to 5300 cGy.[5,129,183] Recommendations for current management include doses of 5000 cGy to 5500 cGy given in 150-cGy to 180-cGy fractions daily. The use of smaller fraction size (*i.e.*, 150 cGy) to a maximum dose of 5000 cGy is appropriate for children 3 to 5 years old.

There are few pediatric data on the dose-response association for malignant gliomas, although dose levels of 5500 cGy to 6000 cGy are standard for adolescents. Investigations of hyperfractionated irradiation are planned at levels already established for brain stem gliomas.

Results of Treatment

Results in low-grade gliomas require long-term follow-up; treatment failures beyond 5 to 10 years are not infrequent.[27,129,205] Overall survival among patients with hemispheric astrocytoma has been reported as high as 85% at 15 years.[126,179,183,205] Hirsch and co-workers[81] reported recurrence in only three of 40 patients with completely resected lesions, with a projected 12-year relapse-free survival of 80%. For pilocytic astrocytomas, recurrence after complete resection is virtually anecdotal.[181,205] After limited surgery and irradiation, survival for ordinary hemispheric astrocytomas approximates 50% at 10 years.[27,149,183,213]

Postoperative irradiation improves 5-year survival for patients with astrocytomas, although the impact is more difficult to confirm in the pediatric age group.[130,181] Among the factors determining the indications for radiation therapy is the likelihood of malignant degeneration of tumors that recur or progress. Histologic examination of recurrent astrocytomas shows progression to more malignant or anaplastic types in as many as 50% of the patients.[126,146,171] Whether earlier irradiation can diminish or may increase the likelihood of malignant evolution is unknown.[143,146,193]

Thalamic gliomas have an intermediate prognosis, with overall survival rates in radiation therapy series of 40% at 5 years and 30% at 10 years.[27,57] Long-term survival in five of ten children with surgery only has been reported; adequate follow-up of stereotactic surgery is yet unavailable.[21,103] Results in thalamic tumors indicate survival in those with low-grade gliomas; survival of patients with malignant tumors is uncommon.[21,57]

Results of therapy for malignant glioma outside the brain stem represent a continuum of the inverse relationship between age and survival reported in adults.[130,163] Survival at 5 years approximates 25% to 30%, with median survival times of 1 to 2 years.[27,52,53] Children 4 to 12 years old have more favorable outcome.[52,149]

OPTIC CHIASMATIC AND HYPOTHALAMIC GLIOMAS

Optic pathway tumors typically involve the optic chiasm, potentially extending posteriorly to include the optic tract or radiation. Extension to the hypothalamus is common (Fig. 69-12). Arbitrarily, lesions involving the visual tracts (*i.e.*, nerve or tract) have been defined as optic pathway tumors of the chiasm rather

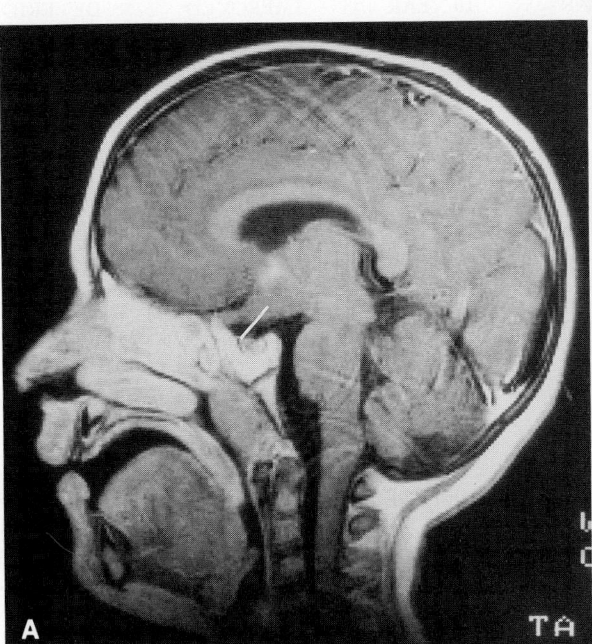

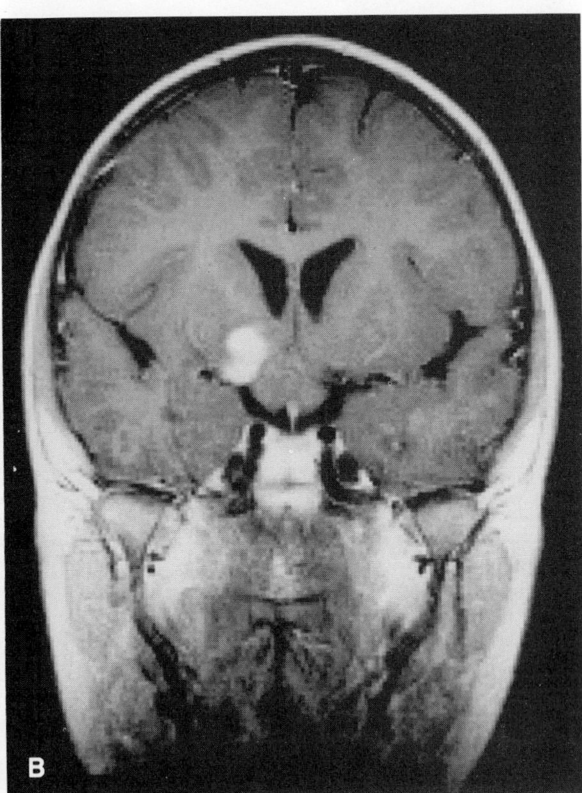

FIGURE 69–12. Optic pathway glioma. (**A**) The chiasmatic tumor (/) has extensive MR signal changes demonstrating involvement of the optic tract and (**B**) the lateral geniculate body.

than primary hypothalamic tumors, but the natural history of anterior diencephalic tumors is similar, whether defined as chiasmal or hypothalamic.[158, 179, 193]

Gliomas of the suprasellar region are most prevalent in young children; as many as 25% occur before 1 year of age.[158] Symptoms include visual disturbance and increased intracranial pressure. Precocious puberty or pituitary-hypothalamic deficiency is common at diagnosis.[167] The diencephalic syndrome, expressed in young children as cachexia and hyperactivity, is infrequent but characteristic of lesions involving the hypothalamus. Neurofibromatosis is present in 10% to 20% of children with optic pathway or hypothalamic gliomas.[161, 167, 179]

Tumors limited to the optic nerve appear to be hamartomatous, exhibiting longitudinal infiltration to the chiasm in fewer than 25% of the patients.[11] Although the natural history of chiasmatic or hypothalamic tumors varies, lesions of this region are obviously neoplastic. Histologically, chiasmatic lesions are astrocytomas (80%), mixed gliomas that include oligodendroglial elements (10% to 20%), or malignant gliomas, including anaplastic astrocytoma or malignant mixed glioma (5% to 15%).[5, 212]

General Management

Tumors confined to the optic nerve are usually treated by resection. Chiasmatic tumors exhibiting longitudinal extension beyond the region of the chiasm may be managed without histologic identification.[153] Biopsies have been obtained primarily in patients with tumors characterized as hypothalamic.[212] Visual deterioration after biopsy occurs in 10% to 15% of the patients.[167, 179] Ventriculoperitoneal shunt insertion is often required.

Tumors of the optic chiasm or hypothalamus respond well to irradiation. Significant decreases in tumor volume, including complete or almost complete tumor regression, have been described in 40% to 50% of the cases.[167, 179] Improvement in visual acuity occurs in 20% to 40% of the children (Table 69-6). Treatment-associated increased tumor size, described as a "ballooning" of the often cystic suprasellar glioma, and increased intracranial pressure with attendant visual deterioration may occur in 10% to 15% of the patients during or after radiation therapy.[45, 65, 66, 158] Improvement in the diencephalic syndrome after radiation therapy has been documented.[167]

The role of chemotherapy has recently been explored for optic pathway tumors in children younger than 5 years of age. Packer and associates[153] reported objective responses to dactinomycin and vincristine in 35% of these children. Progression-free survival is documented in 45% of the children 5 years after initiating chemotherapy.[153] Tumor progression during or after chemotherapy occurred at a median time of 3 years, suggesting the ability to delay irradiation until greater CNS maturation occurs in young children with chiasmatic or hypothalamic tumors.[158]

Radiation Therapy Techniques

Treatment of tumors infiltrating along the visual pathways generally incorporates all areas of abnormal signal defined by MRI. Large fields may be required to encompass involvement of the optic tracts (Fig. 69-13). Tumors confined to the hypothalamus may be more narrowly approached, including use of coronal arcs to limit the dose to the centrally affected area (Fig. 69-14).

Dose levels of 4500 cGy to 5000 cGy are recommended, with improvement in progression-free survival after doses of 5000 cGy.[11, 66, 189, 212] For children younger than 3 years, 4500 cGy in 150-cGy fractions has been advised.[90]

TABLE 69–6
Radiation Therapy for Optic Chiasm Gliomas

INVESTIGATOR	TIME INTERVAL	NO. OF PATIENTS	SURVIVAL RATE (%)		VISION AFTER THERAPY (%)*	
			5 YEAR	10 YEAR	IMPROVED	DETERIORATED
Danoff[45]	1958–1977	18	83	73	33	22
Packer[158]	1960–1980	18	88 (47)†	50	6	17
Horwich[90]	1951–1981	29	100	90	43	9
McLaurin[141]	1970–1985	18	93 (70)†			
Flickinger[66]	1965–1983	29	93	87	9	14
Rodriquez[167]	1977–1987	24	93	74	20	21
Pierce[161]	1971–1986	24	100	100	30	8

* *Change in vision after irradiation for patients with documented and evaluable vision deficits before irradiation.*
† *Number in parentheses indicates progression-free survival.*

Results of Treatment

Survival of patients with optic pathway or hypothalamic gliomas is excellent, exceeding most other CNS presentations. In a review of 372 cases, survival rates approached 80% and 70% at 10 and 20 years, respectively.[11] The progression-free survival rate 10 to 15 years after irradiation is 85% in several series.[66,90,179] Other institutions report progressive disease in as many as 50% to 80% of their patients by 5 to 6 years after treatment.[158,167] Criteria for patient selection and means of follow-up probably explain the differences in long-term survival after radiation therapy. Results in hypothalamic gliomas parallel those for the optic chiasmatic lesions.[141]

CEREBELLAR ASTROCYTOMA

Astrocytomas of the cerebellum are biologically benign tumors, accounting for 15% of all CNS neoplasms in children. The tumor rarely presents in infants and is most common in young children 2 to 5 years old. Findings at diagnosis include ataxia and symptoms of increased intracranial pressure resulting from obstruction of the fourth ventricle. Cysts are visible by CT or MRI in 50% of the cases; classically, the tumor includes a single large cyst and a mural tumor nodule along the cyst wall.

Histologically, 80% to 85% of the tumors are classified as pilocytic or juvenile types of astrocytoma.[74,94,171] The remaining 15% are identified as "common types" of diffuse astrocytomas. A classification of posterior fossa gliomas according to favorable prognosis (Gilles A) or more aggressive disease (Gilles B) identifies pilocytic or juvenile astrocytomas as Gilles A lesions and an eclectic group classically diagnosed as ependymomas or intermediate- or high-grade astrocytomas as Gilles B.[211]

General Management

Resection is the treatment of choice for most cerebellar astrocytomas. Current operative techniques permit gross total resection in 75% to 80% of the children.[71,93,211]

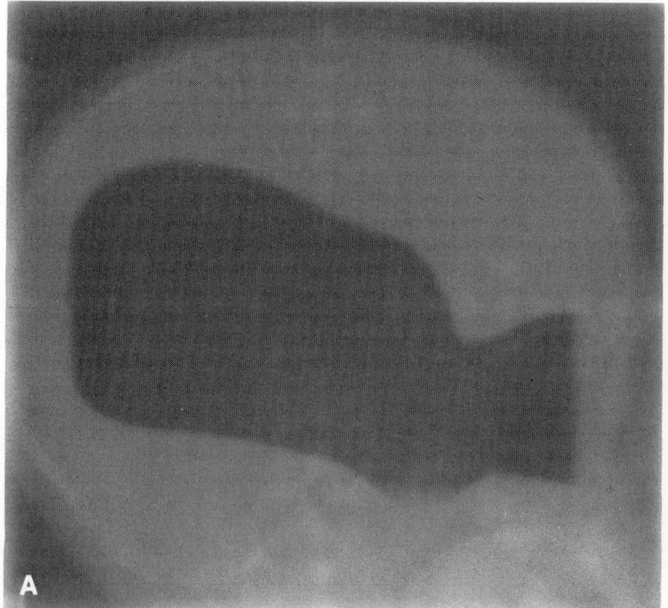

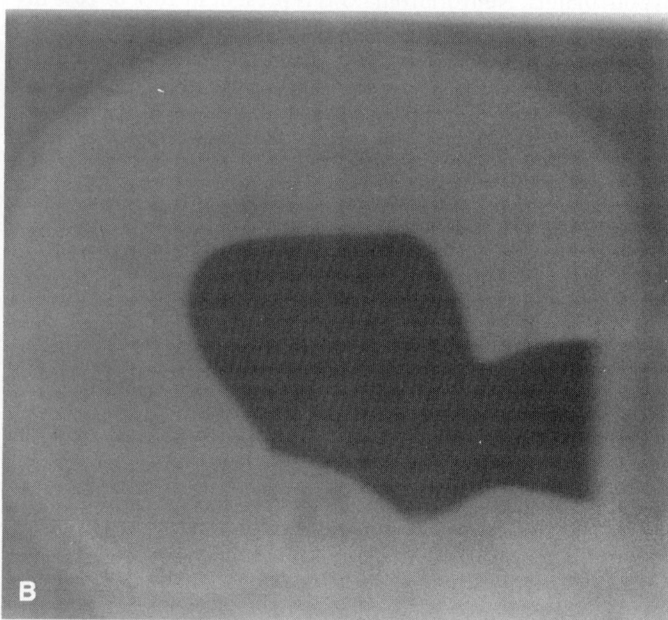

FIGURE 69–13. Portal films for optic pathway glioma in Figure 69-12. (**A**) "Full volume" treated to 4000 cGy and (**B**) "reduced volume" treated to 5000 cGy in a 3-year-old child.

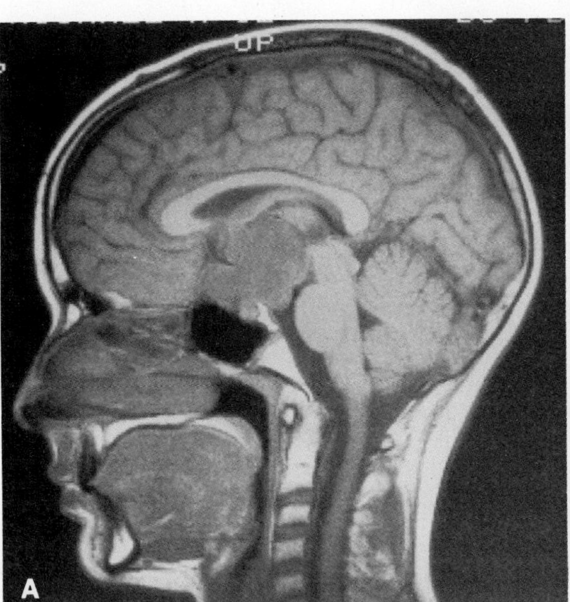

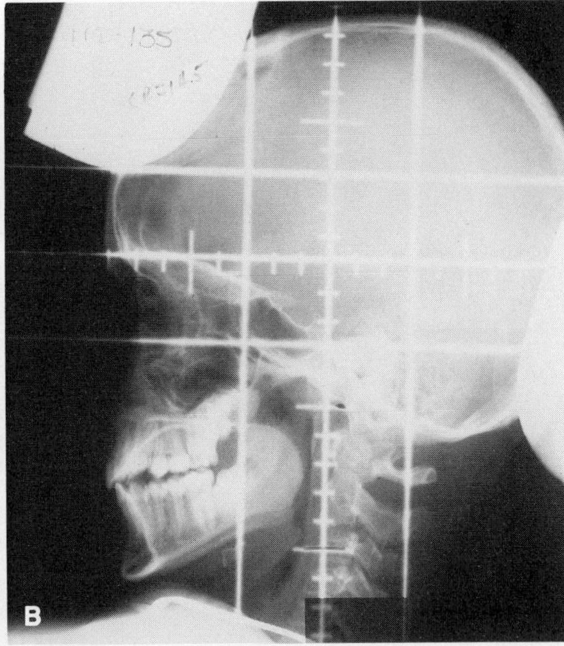

FIGURE 69–14. (**A**) Hypothalamic astrocytoma and (**B**) limited treatment volume using a coronal arc similar to that in Fig. 69–17.

The role of radiation therapy has been inadequately defined for cerebellar astrocytomas. Adjuvant irradiation is not indicated for totally resected lesions. Although several series indicate that the prognosis is excellent with radiation therapy after incomplete excision, similar survival rates are recorded after surgery alone.[15,40,70,76,94,124,129,205] Radiation therapy significantly delays tumor recurrence, but comparative data for early postoperative irradiation and for further surgical resection at the time of disease progression are unavailable.[15,70,71,93] Tumors with brain stem infiltration or those with unequivocal malignant histology require postoperative radiation therapy.[15,36]

Radiation Therapy Techniques

Treatment is limited to the posterior fossa for cases with brain stem involvement or those with clearly unresectable disease. Although controversial, the majority opinion favors craniospinal irradiation for the rare malignant or anaplastic glioma in this location.[36,102,110,173,185]

The lack of dose-response data indicates treatment toward the tolerance level: 5000 cGy to 5400 cGy using conventional 180-cGy fractions daily.

Results of Treatment

Long-term survival rates for patients with cerebellar astrocytomas are excellent: 85% to 90% at 20 to 25 years, respectively.[15,71,94,124,211] Results after total resection approach 90% to 95% survival in recent analyses.[15,70,76,93] Prolonged progression-free survival has occurred after incomplete resection; "ultimate" survival after subtotal resection exceeds 80% at 5 years and 65% to 80% at 10 to 20 years. The long-term rates demonstrate the indolent biology of cerebellar gliomas and the ability of subsequent surgery to salvage a high proportion of relapsed children.[15,71,93,124]

CRANIOPHARYNGIOMA

Craniopharyngioma is a benign tumor arising from squamous cell rests in the region of the pituitary stalk. The tumor is technically extraaxial, originating outside the brain but adhering to or invading the pituitary stalk. Intrasellar craniopharyngioma (15% of cases) may represent "epidermoid cysts" of this location; they are small cystic lesions infrequently extending into the adjacent cavernous sinus.[85,171] Prechiasmatic lesions (30%) grow between the optic nerves, pushing the chiasm posteriorly without invading the suprasellar structures. The more common retrochiasmatic tumors (55%) extend superiorly to fill the third ventricle, adhering to the hypothalamus; growth superiorly or posteriorly, even to the posterior fossa, is common.[85,171,198] Craniopharyngiomas are typically cystic and are composed of solid, often densely calcified, suprasellar tumor with solid and cystic extensions (Fig. 69-15). The cyst fluid is described as "crank case oil," a high-protein fluid with cholesterol granules.

Craniopharyngioma most frequently occurs in children 8 to 14 years old. The predominant symptoms are visual, with decrease in acuity or visual fields in 70% of the children at presentation. Increased intracranial pressure usually exists.[18,86,210] Pituitary-hypothalamic dysfunction is documented at diagnosis in 30% to 70% of these children, including deficient growth hormone or thyroid-stimulating hormone, diabetes insipidus, or gonadotropin abnormalities (*e.g.*, precocious puberty or delayed secondary sexual characteristics).[33,85,209]

General Management

Evaluation of craniopharyngioma requires CT and MRI. A ventriculoperitoneal shunt is usually required.

Surgical resection is potentially curative in a proportion of children with craniopharyngioma. The strategic location requires exquisite techniques to remove the circumscribed, if usually extensive and adherent, tumor.[85,198] In 1969, Matson[140]

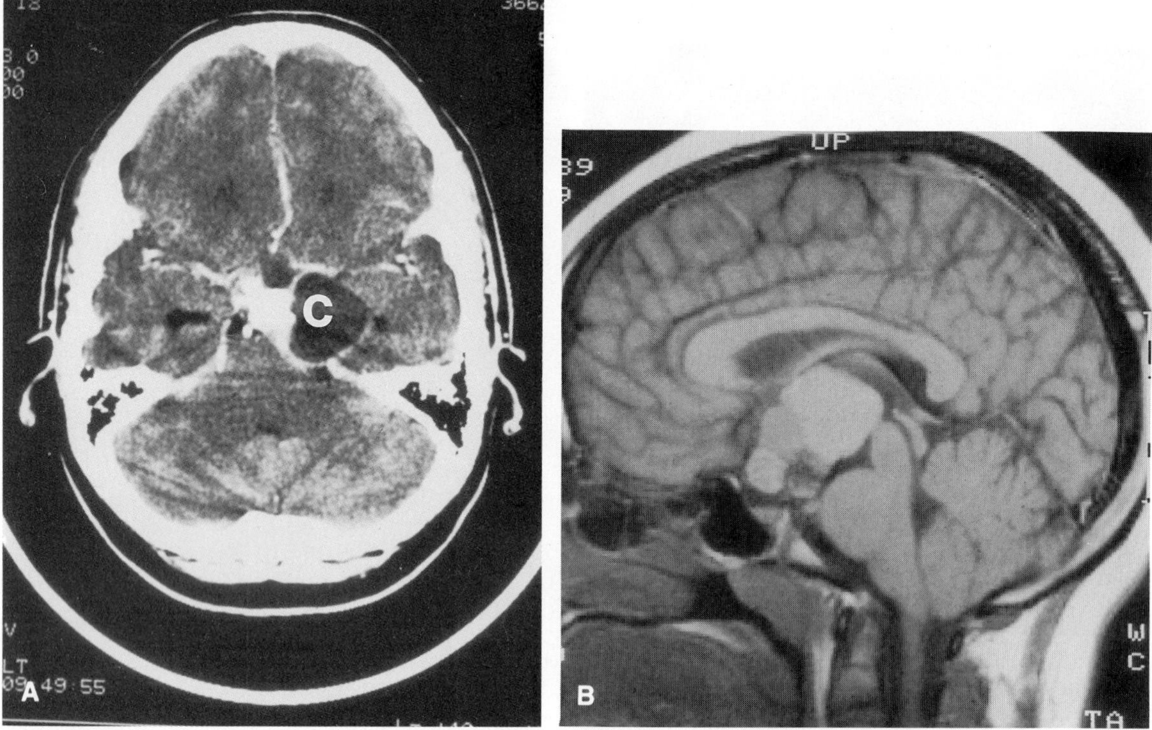

FIGURE 69–15. Craniopharyngioma. (**A**) CT demonstrates calcified suprasellar mass and adjacent cyst (c). (**B**) Tumor and cystic areas on the sagittal MR scan indicate extension to the third ventricular region.

described total resection in 34 of 40 children operated on early in the era of modern microsurgery. Institutions oriented toward primary surgery report total removal of tumor in 50% to 80% of the children.[18,33,82,85,198,209,210] Resection is more likely to be total in prechiasmatic or intrasellar lesions and in tumors less than 3 cm to 4 cm in diameter.[85,198,209] Postoperative imaging has shown residual calcification or "apparently active enhancing tumor" in as many as 50% of the "totally removed" lesions.[12,18,82,209] The correlation with subsequent tumor progression is uncertain (Table 69-7).[12,82]

Kramer and colleagues[114] first described control of craniopharyngioma using limited surgery and irradiation in 1961, later updating their experience to document progression-free survival all six of the treated children 15 years after receiving doses of 5000 cGy to 6500 cGy.[115] Numerous reports indicate excellent disease control with radiation therapy after simple cyst aspiration, limited decompressive surgery, or incomplete resection (Table 69-7).[27,31,46,190,209,210]

The merits of radical surgical extirpation compared with limited surgery and irradiation are disputed. Local recurrence after complete resection is relatively infrequent. However, the toxic effects of surgery have been considerable; despite Matson's lack of operative mortality, recent series indicate a 2% to 5% mortality and major morbidity in at least 10% of cases.[18,35,125,140,210] Data regarding intellectual deficits suggest significant and unique frontal lobe changes after surgery.[35,64] Within the population treated by conservative surgery and irradiation, functional alterations appear to be more significant in those subjected to more substantial surgery.[31,64]

The results of incomplete surgical removal without radiation therapy indicate surprisingly rapid disease progression: 70% of the patients had recurrences within 3 years.[18,31,82,190,209] The opportunity for a conservative follow-up approach and curative secondary resection is limited. There is decreased likelihood of total resection at the time of second or subsequent surgery, and morbidity and mortality rates are significantly higher for the second surgery.[198]

For tumors that recur after radiation therapy, treatment with intracystic radionuclides (*e.g.*, ^{32}P) has achieved prolonged stabilization.[108,136]

Radiation Therapy Techniques

Treatment fields for craniopharyngioma are narrowly confined to the tumor volume, including the solid tumor and cyst(s). In cases with cyst aspiration or limited resection, it is important to cover the cyst walls. It is appropriate to limit the irradiated volume to the postoperative residual tumor after removal of large cystic components, assuming confidence in the completeness of the cyst wall resection in areas not included within the target volume. High-energy (6–10-MV photons) opposed lateral fields are often reported in the literature; rotational arcs (primarily coronal) or multiple arc configurations more appropriately spare the uninvolved temporal lobes (Figs. 69-16 and 69-17).[46,64,209]

There is limited information about dose and survival. The Royal Marsden series indicates better 5- to 15-year survival with doses of 5000 cGy to 5500 cGy than with doses less than 5000 cGy.[27] Whether doses beyond 5500 cGy add to disease control is uncertain; improvement has been suggested but it lacks statistical significance.[27] Conventional fractionation of 180 cGy to 200 cGy five times daily has been standard.

Results of Treatment

Survival for children with craniopharyngioma is excellent: results after the selected use of total resection or applicable combination of limited surgery and radiation therapy indicate sur-

TABLE 69–7
Limited Surgery and Irradiation for Craniopharyngioma

INVESTIGATOR	TIME INTERVAL	AGE GROUP*	NO. OF PATIENTS	PARAMETER†	RESULTS (%) 5 YR	10 YR	15 YR
Fischer[64]	1972–1981	C	23	S	100		
				PFS	78‡		
Carmel[33]	1952–1977	C	14	S	92	78	
				PFS	78	78	
Manaka[137]	1950–1979	C	21	S	86	63	
Danoff[46]	1961–1978	C	19	S	69	66	
Wen[210]	1961–1986	C	11	PFS	91		
Bloom[27]	1950–1969	C	46	S	87	78	73
	1970–1981	C	27	S	100	96	96
Sung[190]	1950–1977	C+A	32	S	82	71	
				PFS	76	44	
Cabezudo[31]	1967–1980	C+A	16	PFS	94	94	
Baskin[18]	1969–1985	C+A	58	S	93		
Manaka[137]	1960–1969	C+A	26	S	89	77	
	1970–1979	C+A	13	S	92	92	

** C, children; C+A, children + adults in series with ≥40% pediatric cases.*
† Parameter: S, survival; PFS, progression-free survival.
‡ Includes four cases requiring cyst aspiration within 2 years of irradiation as failures despite subsequent prolonged disease control.

vival rates beyond 10 years approaching 90%.[18, 27, 31, 82, 137, 198, 209] Series comparing radical surgery to limited surgery combined with radiation therapy show no difference in the results measured up to 15 years.[18, 27, 33, 137, 190]

Surgical decompression is important in cases with visual impairment.[18, 35, 64, 125, 209] After attempted resection, diabetes insipidus or panhypopituitarism has been recorded in over three fourths of the cases.[18, 35, 64, 82, 198, 209] Growth hormone deficiency follows irradiation.[18, 46, 64] Series comparing overall functional levels suggest less long-term detriment with limited surgery and radiation therapy than with radical resection.[35, 64, 209]

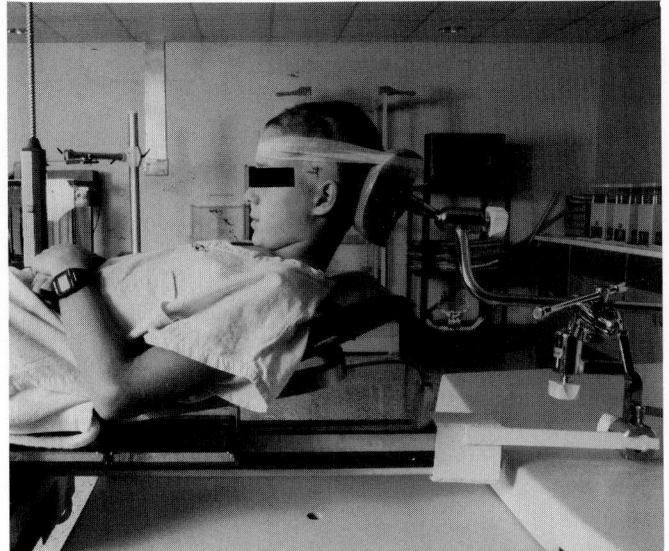

FIGURE 69–16. Immobilization device to permit coronal arc irradiation. Attachments to a standard linear accelerator treatment couch permit daily positioning.

PINEAL REGION AND INTRACRANIAL GERM CELL TUMORS

Tumors of the pineal region represent a histologically diverse group of neoplasms arising in and around the pineal gland. There is a striking male predominance for pineal germ cell tumors, especially germinomas, occurring primarily in the second decade.[24, 98, 176]

Increased intracranial pressure is common because of aqueductal compression. Tumors in the pineal and posterior third ventricular region frequently present with Parinaud's syndrome, a constellation of ocular signs including upward gaze palsy; impaired or absent pupillary response to light, with preserved constriction during accommodation, and retractory or convergence nystagmus. Subependymomal extension around the third ventricle is common in pineal germinomas, accounting for diabetes insipidus, delayed or precocious puberty, or growth deficit. As many as 25% to 35% of the pineal germ cell tumors exhibit signs of third ventricular dissemination or multiple midline tumors.[100, 166]

Pineal parenchymal tumors include the primitive pineoblastoma, often arising in young children with a marked propensity for neuraxis seeding, and the pineocytoma, which is more frequent in adults.[79, 156]

Suprasellar germ cell tumors, previously called ectopic pinealomas, are less common than primary pineal region tumors of similar histology. The suprasellar tumors occur more equally in the first and second decades, with no male dominance.[24, 98, 177] Symptoms include diabetes insipidus, pituitary deficiency, precocious puberty, or decreased visual fields or acuity. Supresellar germ cell tumors other than germinomas are rare.[98, 178]

Evaluation of pineal region tumors includes serum and CSF marker determinations. Although typically marker negative, germinomas may exhibit limited elevations of β-human chorionic gonadotropin (β-HCG).[24, 100] The α-fetoprotein level is elevated in endodermal sinus tumor or embryonal carcinoma;

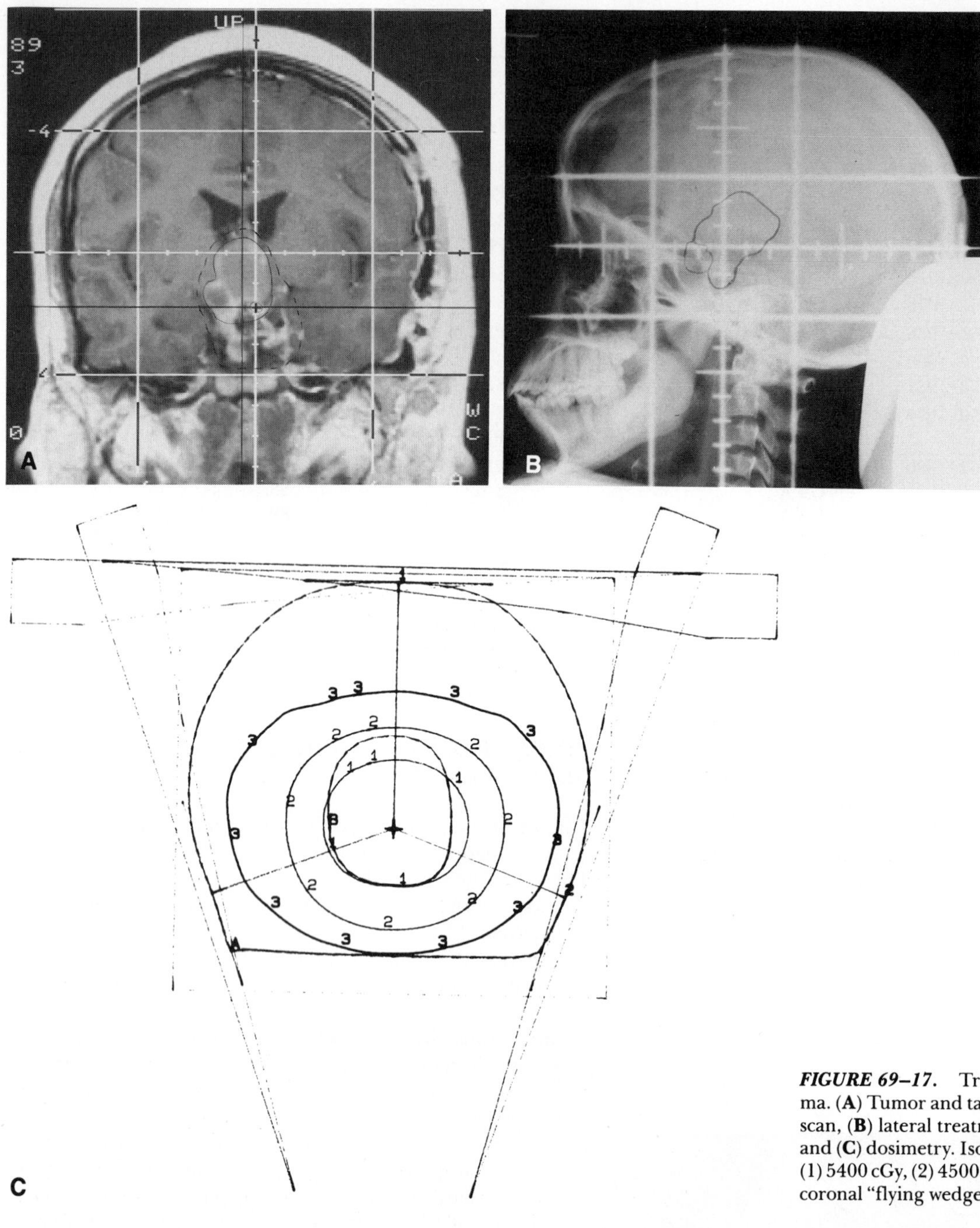

FIGURE 69–17. Treatment of craniopharyngioma. (**A**) Tumor and target volume on planning MR scan, (**B**) lateral treatment volume for coronal arc, and (**C**) dosimetry. Isodose curves indicate doses of (1) 5400 cGy, (2) 4500 cGy, and (3) 2000 cGy using a coronal "flying wedged pair" with 10-MV photons.

marked elevation of β-HCG implies choriocarcinomatous elements.[47,55]

General Management

Treatment of pineal region tumors and suprasellar germinomas has been primarily by radiation therapy. The confluence of veins surrounding the pineal region historically produced unacceptable rates of operative morbidity and mortality.[164] Recent series report operative mortality approaching zero in children undergoing open or stereotactic biopsies.[9,55,156] Postoperative neurologic deterioration is reported in as many as 25% of the cases, with long-term neurologic deficits in 10%.[55,156,164]

The relative frequency of germinomas, improved diagnostic imaging, and high rates of disease control with radiation therapy have led to a "radiodiagnostic" approach in several centers. Serial imaging after 2000 cGy has been used to test the radioresponsiveness of pineal region tumors. Lesions showing substantial early reduction are presumed to be germinomas or other highly sensitive tumor types, and radiation fields are modified, often to include cranial or craniospinal volumes, to continue primary irradiation. Lesions with minimal early response have been examined by biopsy or resected, or limited-volume irradiation has continued to higher doses because the tumor is presumed to be a glioma.[1,27,47,166]

The relative safety of biopsy procedures and the desirability of identifying the 15% to 25% of patients with pineoblastoma or germ cell tumors other than germinoma who could benefit from more aggressive radiation therapy or added chemotherapy justify histologic confirmation.[9,55,134,156,157,164,189] Elevation of α-fetoprotein or significant elevation of β-HCG provide evidence of aggressive germ cell elements without necessitating biopsy.[55,110] Biopsy does not increase the risk of neuraxis seeding.[55,164,207]

Tumors of the suprasellar region have long been approached surgically for histologic diagnosis.[9,47,178,191]

If treatment is offered without histologic examination, it is important to recognize imaging characteristics associated with tumors other than germinomas: inhomogeneous or irregular lesions on routine and enhanced CT, extensive calcifications, or cyst formation.

Chemotherapy is effective for intracranial germ cell tumors. Response to cyclophosphamide- and cisplatin-containing regimes has been impressive (Fig. 69-18).[7,109,166] Adjuvant chemotherapy has been reported for germ cell tumors other than germinoma, although controlled trials are yet unavailable.[55] Allen and co-workers[8] reported success using postoperative cyclophosphamide or a combination of cisplatin, cyclophosphamide, vinblastine, and bleomycin in conjunction with delayed, reduced-dose irradiation.[8] Long-term results are available for only a limited number of cases.[8]

Radiation Therapy Techniques

Volume

The major controversy in radiation therapy for pineal region tumors is the treatment volume.[96] Biopsy-proven gliomas or pineocytomas are adequately treated with local fields. Pineoblastomas and germ cell tumors other than germinomas require craniospinal irradiation because of the likelihood of neuraxis seeding.[79,156]

Germinomas are problematic. There is reasonable agreement that wide-field cranial irradiation should be used to deliver the initial dose of 2000 cGy to 4000 cGy to include the ventricular system or the full brain.[1,47,130,134] The rationale for a component of wide-field therapy (alone or as part of craniospinal irradiation) is tumor extension around the third ventricle in an estimated 25% to 40% of these patients.[98,134,166] The 15% to 20% incidence of intracranial failure after more limited treatment volumes is virtually eliminated with this approach.[47,130,134,189] A subsequent boost volume includes the identifiable tumor site(s) with 1-cm to 2-cm margins.

Spinal irradiation for germinomas is indicated for patients with neuraxis dissemination at diagnosis.[47,134] Positive neuraxis staging (*i.e.*, CSF cytology, imaging evidence of disease beyond the third ventricle in the cranium, spinal metastasis) has been reported in 10% to 50% of patients with pineal germinomas.[9,100,134,166,177]

Sung and colleagues[189] reported an actuarial risk of spinal failure in 40% of these patients, which was higher with suprasellar than with pineal region germinomas. Reviews by numerous authors indicate a risk of spinal seeding of zero to 25%, which is increased in suprasellar tumors and after biopsy.[30,98,130,134,177,207] Table 69-8 presents data in recent, largely pediatric series that address outcome and patterns of failure related to radiation therapy volume. Whether an estimated 5% to 10% risk of spinal failure in pineal region tumors justifies routine craniospinal irradiation is conjecture. Linstadt and others[134] reported only one of 31 spinal failures after local irradiation, including none among 13 patients with biopsied germinomas. Craniospinal irradiation is always indicated for patients with extensive intracranial disease, multifocal involvement, or operative spill; craniospinal irradiation is preferred by the author in all patients with intracranial germinomas.

Elimination of spinal failures and suggested improvement in disease-free survival (Table 69-8) after systematic craniospinal irradiation compare favorably with the low incidence of seeding and high survival rates after limited irradiation.[47,134,166,184,189,207]

Dose

Despite the radioresponsiveness of intracranial germinomas, differences of 50% to 60% local control at doses of 4000 cGy or less and local control rates of 85% to 90% using doses of 5000 cGy or more have been reported.[1,166,189] Dose to the neuraxis can be limited to 2000 cGy to 2500 cGy with negative neuraxis staging and 3000 cGy to 3500 cGy with positive cytology alone.[47,166]

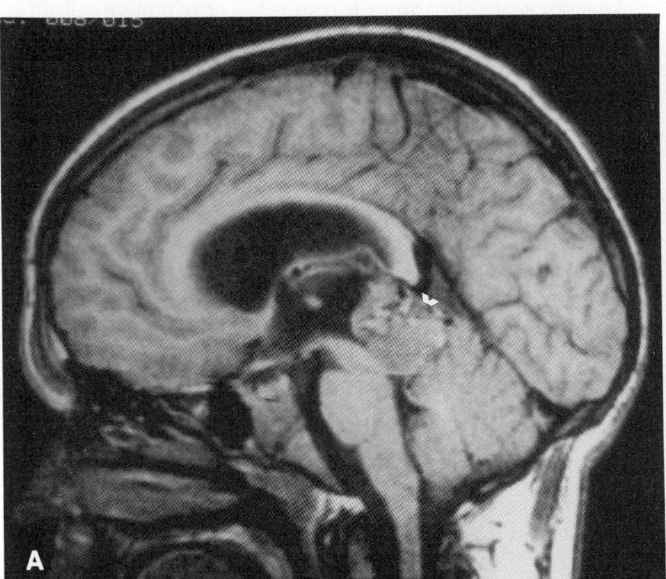

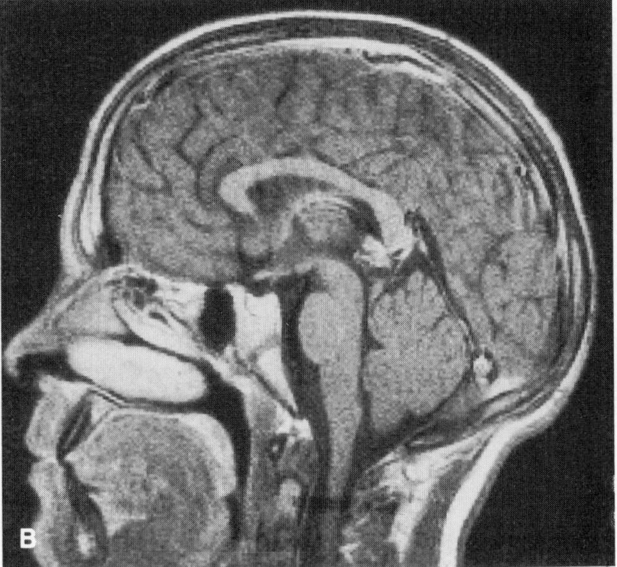

FIGURE 69–18. Malignant pineal region teratoma (>) (**A**) before chemotherapy and (**B**) after four cycles of cisplatin/VP-16. Tumor was controlled 2 years after subsequent craniospinal irradiation.

TABLE 69–8
Correlation of Biopsy, Radiation Therapy Volume, and Outcome for Localized Pineal Region Tumors and Intracranial Germinomas

INVESTIGATOR	TIME INTERVAL	HISTOLOGY	NO. OF PATIENTS	LOCAL-CRANIAL IRRADIATION*	CRANIOSPINAL IRRADIATION	5-YEAR DISEASE-FREE SURVIVAL (%)	SPINAL FAILURE†
Abay[1]	1950–1978	No biopsy	26	24	—	62 (combined)	5 (3)
				—	2		
Rich[166]	1972–1982	Germinoma	4	—	4	3	1 (1)
		No biopsy	8	—	8	8 (combined: 91)	0
Shibamoto[184]	1962–1986	Germinoma	39	19	—	82	0
				—	20	88	1
		No biopsy	27	19	—	90	0
				—	8	97	0
Glanzman[75]	1960–1985	Germinoma	4	3	—	2	1 (1)
				—	1	1 (combined: 3/4)	
		No biopsy	25	23	—	78	0
				—	2	2 (combined: 80)	1 (1)
							0
Linstadt[134]	1956–1986	Germinoma	13	12	—	100 (combined)	0
				—	1		0
		No biopsy	20	19	—	73 (combined)	1
				—	1		0
Dearnaley[47]	1962–1987	Germinoma No biopsy	9 25	32	2	87	2 (1)
Combined series		Germinoma	66	41	—	77	2 (1)
				—	25	86	2 (1)
Combined series		Pineal region	97	78	—	79	6 (4)
				—	19	99	0
Combined series		Germinoma and pineal region	163	119	—	78	8 (5)
				—	44	92	2 (1)

**Local-cranial radiation therapy includes local, ventricular, or full cranial fields, without spinal irradiation*
† Spinal failure, patients with failure at first recurrence of disease. The numbers in parentheses indicate the number of patients with concurrent intracranial failure.

Patients with germ cell tumors other than germinomas or with pineoblastomas require neuraxis therapy to doses approaching tolerance, 3600 cGy to 4000 cGy. Primary boost fields are treated to 5400 cGy. Local treatment for gliomas is recommended to doses of 5500 cGy.

Results of Treatment

The overall survival rate for pineal region tumors is 75% beyond 5 years.[75,166] Improvement in visual symptoms and pituitary-hypothalamic deficits is documented after radiation therapy for suprasellar tumors in 25% of the patients.[166]

For intracranial germinomas, 5-year survival rates of 85% to 100% have been recorded (Table 69-8).[47,134,166,184] In other types of intracranial germ cell tumors, results are not favorable, with long-term survival rates of only 5% to 35%.[47,98,166,178,207] For pineal region tumors other than those of germ cell origin, the 5-year survival rate is 65%.[47]

PRIMITIVE NEUROECTODERMAL TUMORS

Initially described in 1973 by Hart and Earle,[78] the primitive neuroectodermal tumor (PNET) is a highly malignant, undifferentiated supratentorial lesion that occurs primarily in young children.[78,112] The PNET presents as a large, often well-demarcated tumor with cystic and hemorrhagic components. Histologically, the tumor is composed of primitive cells of neuroectodermal origin with limited but divergent differentiation toward neuronal and one or more glial cell lines.[13,78] PNETs frequently seed the neuraxis and may be multicentric at diagnosis.[13,112]

There is controversy about a proposed "unifying" neuropathologic concept for embryonal tumors in children. Rorke[168] initially proposed the broader PNET term to include histologically similar tumors long recognized as medulloblastoma or pineoblastoma in addition to the supratentorial PNET as described by Hart and Earle, cerebral neuroblastoma, ependymoblastoma, and other undifferentiated lesions that share the "small round blue cell" of embryonal pediatric CNS neoplasms and a tendency for subarachnoid dissemination. In practice, the concept has been oversimplified and overused to designate embryonal or anaplastic tumors, regardless of site, as PNETs.[62,172] Although recognizing some of the common clinical and histologic features of such tumors, many investigators prefer the classical histologic designations for these entities.[62,172] A proposed international neuropathology classification will probably encompass the PNET concept but specifically define several of the classical embryonal tumors.[19]

The supratentorial PNETs of Hart and Earle require maximal surgical resection followed by craniospinal irradiation and, usually, chemotherapy.[13,112] Neuraxis techniques are identical to those described for medulloblastoma, with boost irradiation to the supratentorial tumor site(s) to cumulative dose levels of 5400 cGy to 5500 cGy. Outcome has generally been poor; survival at 1 year is reported for only 10% to 15% of these children.[69,112]

CEREBRAL NEUROBLASTOMA

Cerebral neuroblastoma is a malignant neoplasm arising predominantly in the frontal lobes in children 5 to 10 years of age.[89] The frequency of subarachnoid dissemination was reported as 40% in Horten's[89] neuropathologic review but as uncommon in Berger's[20] clinical series. Surgical resection is often possible; postoperative therapy includes craniospinal irradiation and a local boost similar to that outlined for the Hart and Earle type of PNET. Outcome may correlate with pathologic characteristics; cyst formation and differentiation are reported to be favorable prognostic factors.[20,69]

BRAIN TUMORS IN INFANTS AND YOUNG CHILDREN

Fifteen percent to 20% of pediatric brain tumors occur in infants and children younger than 2 or 3 years.[54] Several unique factors have resulted in poor outcome for this group:

1. A high proportion of young children present with histologically malignant tumors. Supratentorial lesions predominate, especially in the first year of life. Although hypothalamic and optic pathway gliomas are common and are usually low-grade tumors, there are high incidences of malignant gliomas, PNETs, and pineoblastomas.[101,200] Infratentorial tumors are almost always aggressive medulloblastomas, ependymomas, or anaplastic astrocytomas; the benign cerebellar astrocytoma is rare.
2. Many children have subarachnoid dissemination at diagnosis.[54,154]
3. Surgery is more difficult in the myelinating infant brain, with high rates of operative complications and mortality.[101,200]
4. The therapeutic index for radiation therapy is restrictive in youngsters with rapidly maturing CNS tissue. Concerns regarding neurotoxicities have led to obligatory dose reductions of 10% to 20% for infants younger than 2 years.[25] Dose-response associations presage diminished tumor control.[50,88]
5. Even with specific attention to surgical and radiotherapeutic maneuvers to minimize treatment-related toxic effects, the functional outcome of survivors has generally been unfavorable.[119,145]

Benign tumors, including a substantial number of choroid plexus tumors (usually papillomas), can be addressed by primary surgery.[21,196] Radiation therapy for astrocytomas or other low-grade neoplasms is reserved for patients with significant neurologic deficits in unresectable locations.[21] Careful observation of incompletely resected tumors, including thalamic or hypothalamic astrocytomas and dorsally exophytic brain stem tumors, may permit delayed radiation therapy until the child is older.[21,83] The therapeutic index appears to be improved with any significant gain in age. If radiotherapeutic intervention is delayed, the physician must closely monitor the child and establish a level of understanding with the family and other clinicians that permits appropriate radiation therapy when indicated.

For malignant tumors, initial chemotherapy can achieve prolonged intervals of disease control for approximately 50% of the children with medulloblastoma, malignant glioma, or ependymoma.[16,88,54] A policy of delayed but systematic radiation therapy on completion of 1 to 2 years of chemotherapy has the theoretic advantage of allowing many youngsters to mature enough that they could undergo radiation therapy with diminished neurologic and neuropsychologic sequelae.[87,135] The use of reduced neuraxis doses for children without measurable residual after surgery or chemotherapy who require craniospinal irradiation appears to be reasonable.[88,135] Doses of 2400 cGy to 2500 cGy to the neuraxis with a subsequent boost to a cumulative dose of 5000 cGy to the primary tumor site have been successful.[88] For children older than 2 or 3 years of age with residual disease at the completion of chemotherapy, full-dose irradiation that includes a neuraxis dose of 3000 cGy to 3500 cGy with a local boost to 5000 cGy to 5500 cGy (dose depends on age) is appropriate. Horowitz and co-workers[88] reported ultimate freedom from progression for over 2 years in eight of 12 infants with this approach. For all but the youngest children, it is important to intervene with radiation therapy if there is tumor progression during chemotherapy.[121]

The prolonged response to chemotherapy in this age group that was initially reported by van Eys and associates[202] has led to anecdotal strategies of primary chemotherapy, obviating irradiation except for those with disease progression.[16,116,135] Baram and colleagues[16] reported an actuarial 5-year survival rate of 75% in a group of nine children treated only with MOPP chemotherapy postoperatively; irradiation had been given to only one patient. The follow-up report of Ater and co-workers[14] indicates freedom from progression in seven of 13 children with primary chemotherapy and no radiation therapy; the ultimate 5-year survival rate, including irradiation for disease progression, was 55%. Confirmation of disease control without irradiation for medulloblastoma is extremely limited.[116,135] Chemotherapy without obligatory irradiation must be considered as highly investigational.

Acknowledgment

The author expresses appreciation to James Langston, M.D., and Douglas Coffey, M.S., for assistance and to Carole Obst and Sandra Gaither for manuscript preparation.

REFERENCES

1. Abay EO, Laws ER Jr, Grado GL, et al: Pineal tumors in children and adolescents: Treatment by CSF shunting and radiotherapy. J Neurosurg 55:889, 1981
2. Albright AL, Guthkelch AN, Packer RJ, et al: Prognostic factors in pediatric brain-stem gliomas. J Neurosurg 65:751, 1986
3. Albright AL: Surgical aspects of medulloblastoma. In Zeltzer PM, Pochedly C (eds): Medulloblastomas in Children: New Concepts in Tumor Biology, Diagnosis and Treatment, p 155. New York, Praeger, 1986
4. Albright AL, Price RA, Guthkelch AN: Brain stem gliomas of children: A clinicopathological study. Cancer 52:2313, 1983
5. Albright AL, Price RA, Guthkelch AN: Diencephalic gliomas of children: A clinicopathologic study. Cancer 55:2789, 1985
6. Allen JC, Helson L, Jereb B: Preradiation chemotherapy for newly diagnosed childhood brain tumors: A modified phase II trial. Cancer 52:2001, 1983
7. Allen JC, Bosl G, Walker R: Chemotherapy trials in recurrent primary intracranial germ cell tumors. J Neurooncol 3:147, 1985

8. Allen JC, Kim JH, Packer RJ: Neoadjuvant chemotherapy for newly diagnosed germ-cell tumors of the central nervous system. J Neurosurg 67:65, 1987
9. Allen JC: Management of primary intracranial germ cell tumors of childhood. Pediatr Neurosci 13:152, 1987
10. Allen JC, Walker R, Luks E, et al: Carboplatin and recurrent childhood brain tumors. J Clin Oncol 5:459, 1987
11. Alvord EC, Lofton S: Gliomas of the optic nerve or chiasm: Outcome by patients' age, tumor site, and treatment. J Neurosurg 68:85, 1988
12. Amacher AL: Craniopharyngioma: The controversy regarding radiotherapy. Childs Brain 6:57, 1980
13. Ashwal S, Hinshaw DB, Bedros A: CNS primitive neuroectodermal tumors of childhood. Med Pediatr Oncol 12:180, 1984
14. Ater JL, Woo SY, van Eys J: Update on MOPP chemotherapy as primary therapy for infant brain tumors. [Abstract] Pediatr Neurosci 14:153, 1988
15. Austin EJ, Alvord EC Jr: Recurrences of cerebellar astrocytomas: A violation of Collins' law. J Neurosurg 68:41, 1988
16. Baram TZ, Van Eys J, Dowell RE, et al: Survival and neurologic outcome of infants with medulloblastoma treated with surgery and MOPP chemotherapy: A preliminary report. Cancer 60:173, 1987
17. Barkovich AJ, Krischer J, Kun L, et al: MR characteristics of brain stem gliomas: Correlation with survival statistics in a three-center study. J Pediatr Neurosurgery 1991 (submitted)
18. Baskin DS, Wilson CB: Surgical management of craniopharyngiomas: A review of 74 cases. J Neurosurg 65:22, 1986
19. Becker L.: Primitive neuroectodermal tumors: Views on a working classification. In Fields WS (ed): Primary Brain Tumors: A Review of Histologic Classification. New York, Springer-Verlag, 1989
20. Berger MS, Edwards MSB, Wara WM, et al: Primary cerebral neuroblastoma: Long-term follow-up review and therapeutic guidelines. J Neurosurg 59:418, 1983
21. Bernstein M, Hoffman HJ, Halliday WC, et al: Thalamic tumors in children: Long-term follow-up and treatment guidelines. J Neurosurg 61:649, 1984
22. Berry MP, Jenkin RDT, Keen CW: Radiation treatment for medulloblastoma: A 21-year review. J Neurosurg 55:43, 1981
23. Bird CR, Hedberg M, Drayer BP, et al: MR assessment of myelination in infants and children: Usefulness of marker sites. Am J Neurol Radiol 10:731, 1989
24. Bjornsson J, Scheithauer BW, Okazaki H, et al: Intracranial germ cell tumors: Pathobiological and immunohistochemical aspects of 70 cases. J Neuropathol Exp Neurol 44:32, 1985
25. Bloom HJG, Wallace ENK, Henk JM: The treatment and prognosis of medulloblastoma in children. AJR 105:43, 1969
26. Bloom HJG: Medulloblastoma in children: Increasing survival rates and further prospects. Int J Radiat Oncol Biol Phys 8:2023, 1982
27. Bloom HJG, Glees J, Bell J: The treatment and long-term prognosis of children with intracranial tumors: A study of 610 cases, 1950–1981. Int J Radiat Oncol Biol Phys 18:723, 1990
28. Bonnin JM, Rubinstein LJ, Palmer NF, et al: The association of embryonal tumors originating in the kidney and in the brain: A report of seven cases. Cancer 54:2137, 1984
29. Bouchard J (ed): Radiation Therapy of Tumors and Diseases of the Nervous System. Philadelphia, Lea & Febiger, 1966
30. Bradfield JS, Perez CA: Pineal tumors and ectopic pinealomas: Analysis of treatment failures. Radiology 103:399, 1972
31. Cabezudo JM, Vaquero J, Areitio E, et al: Craniopharyngiomas: A critical approach to treatment. J Neurosurg 55:371, 1981
32. Caputy AJ, McCullough DC, Manz HJ, et al: A review of the factors influencing the prognosis of medulloblastoma. J Neurosurg 66:80, 1987
33. Carmel PW, Antunes JL, Chang CH: Craniopharyngiomas in children. Neurosurgery 11:382, 1982
34. Castleberry RP, Ragab AH, Steuber CP, et al: aziridinylbenzoquinone (AZQ) in the treatment of recurrent pediatric brain and other malignant solid tumors: A Pediatric Oncology Group Phase II Study. Investigational New Drugs 8:401–406, 1990
35. Cavazzuti V, Fischer EG, Welch K, et al: Neurological and psychophysiological sequelae following different treatments of craniopharyngioma in children. J Neurosurg 59:409, 1983
36. Chamberlain MC, Silver P, Levin VA: Poorly differentiated gliomas of the cerebellum: A study of 18 patients. Cancer 65:337, 1990
37. Chang CH, Housepian EM, Herbert C Jr: An operative staging system and a megavoltage radiotherapeutic technic for cerebellar medulloblastomas. Radiology 93:1351, 1969
38. Childhood Brain Tumor Consortium: A study of childhood brain tumors based on surgical biopsies from 10 North American institutions: Sample description. J Neurooncol 6:9, 1988
39. Civitello LA, Packer RJ, Rorke LB, et al: Leptomeningeal dissemination of low-grade gliomas in childhood. Neurology 38:562, 1988
40. Conway PD, Oechler HW, Kun LE, et al: Importance of histology and treatment of pediatric cerebellar astrocytoma. Cancer 67:2772–2775, 1991
41. Cruz-Sanchez FF, Rossi ML, Hughes JT, et al: Medulloblastoma: An immunohistological study of 50 cases. Acta Neuropathol 79:205, 1989
42. Cumberlin RL, et al: Medulloblastoma: Treatment results and effect on normal tissues. Cancer 43:1014, 1979
43. Cushing H: Experiences with the cerebellar medulloblastomas. Acta Pathol Microbiol Scand 7:1, 1930
44. Cutler EC, Sosman MC, Vaughan WW: The place of radiation in the treatment of cerebellar medulloblastoma. AJR 35:429, 1936
45. Danoff BF, Kramer S, Thompson N: The radiotherapeutic management of optic nerve gliomas in children. Int J Radiat Oncol Biol Phys 6:45, 1980
46. Danoff BF, Cowchock FS, Kramer S: Childhood craniopharyngioma: Survival, local control, endocrine and neurologic function following radiotherapy. Int J Radiat Oncol Biol Phys 9:171, 1983
47. Dearnaley DP, A'Hern RP, Whittaker AK, et al: Pineal and CNS germ cell tumors: Royal Marsden Hospital experience 1962–87. Int J Radiat Oncol Biol Phys 18:773, 1990
48. Demierre B, Stichnoth FA, Hori A, et al: Intracerebral ganglioglioma. J Neurosurg 65:177, 1986
49. Deutsch M: Medulloblastoma: Staging and treatment outcome. Int J Radiat Oncol Biol Phys 14:1103, 1988
50. Deutsch M: Radiotherapy for primary brain tumors in very young children. Cancer 50:2785, 1982
50A. Deutsch M, Thomas P, Boyett J, et al: Low stage medulloblastoma: A Children's Cancer Study Group (CCSG) and Pediatric Oncology Group (POG) randomized study of standard vs. reduced neuraxis irradiation (Abstr). Proc Am Soc Clin Oncol 10:124, 1991
51. Dewitt L, VanDam J, Rijnders A, et al: A modified radiotherapy technique in the treatment of medulloblastoma. Int J Radiat Oncol Biol Phys 10:231, 1984
52. Dropcho EJ, Wisoff JH, Walker RW, et al: Supratentorial malignant gliomas in childhood: A review of 50 cases. Ann Neurol 22:355, 1987
53. Duffner PK, Cohen ME, Myers MH, et al: Survival of children with brain tumors: SEER program, 1973–1980. Neurology 36:597, 1986
54. Duffner P, Cohen M, Horowitz M, et al: Postoperative chemotherapy and delayed RT in infants with intracranial ependymomas: A POG group wide protocol. [Abstract] Ann Neurol 30:1991 (in press)
55. Edwards MSB, Hudgins RJ, Wilson CB, et al: Pineal region tumors in children. J Neurosurg 68:689, 1988
56. Edwards MSB, Wara WM, Urtasun RC, et al: Hyperfractionated radiation therapy for brain-stem glioma: A phase I–II trial. J Neurosurg 70:691, 1989
57. Eifel PJ, Cassady JR, Belli JA: Radiation therapy of tumors of the brain stem and midbrain in children: Experience of the Joint Center for Radiation Therapy and Children's Hospital

Medical Center (1971–1981). Int J Radiat Oncol Biol Phys 13:847, 1987
58. Epstein F: Intraaxial tumors of the cervicomedullary junction in children. Concepts Pediatr Neurosurg 7:117, 1987
59. Epstein F, McCleary EL: Intrinsic brain-stem tumors of childhood: surgical indications. J Neurosurg 64:11, 1986
60. Etou A, Mundinger F, Mohadjer M, et al: Stereotactic interstitial irradiation of diencephalic tumors with iridium 192 and iodine 125: 10 years' follow-up and comparison with other treatments. Child Nerv Syst 5:140, 1989
61. Evans AE, Jenkin RDT, Sposto R, et al: The treatment of medulloblastoma: Results of a prospective randomized trial of radiation therapy with and without CCNU, vincristine, and prednisone. J Neurosurg 72:572, 1990
62. Fields WS (ed): Primary Brain Tumors: A Review of Histologic Classification. New York, Springer-Verlag, 1989
63. Finlay JL, Goins SC: Brain tumors in children. III. Advances in chemotherapy. Am J Pediatr Hematol Oncol 9:264, 1987
64. Fischer EG, Welch K, Belli JA, et al: Treatment of craniopharyngiomas in children: 1972–1981. J Neurosurg 62:496, 1985
65. Fletcher WA, Imes RK, Hoyt WF: Chiasmal gliomas: Appearance and long-term changes demonstrated by computerized tomography. J Neurosurg 65:154, 1986
66. Flickinger JC, Torres C, Deutsch M: Management of low-grade gliomas of the optic nerve and chiasm. Cancer 61:635, 1988
67. Freeman CR, Krischer J, Sanford RA, et al: Hyperfractionated radiotherapy in brain stem tumors: Results of treatment at the second dose level of Pediatric Oncology Group Study #8495. Cancer 1991 (in press)
68. Friedman HS, Oakes WJ: The chemotherapy of posterior fossa tumors in childhood. J Neurooncol 5:217, 1987
69. Gaffney CC, Sloane JP, Bradley NJ, et al: Primitive neuroectodermal tumours of the cerebrum: Pathology and treatment. J Neurooncol 3:23, 1985
70. Garcia DM, Latifi HR, Simpson JR, et al: Astrocytomas of the cerebellum in children. J Neurosurg 71:661, 1989
71. Garcia DM, Marks JE, Latifi HR, et al: Childhood cerebellar astrocytomas: Is there a role for postoperative irradiation? Int J Radiat Oncol Biol Phys 18:815, 1990
72. Garrett PG, Simpson WJK. Ependymomas: Results of radiation treatment. Int J Radiat Oncol Biol Phys 9:1121, 1983
73. Garrido E, Becker LF, Hoffman HJ: Gangliogliomas in children. Child Brain 4:339, 1978
74. Gjerris F, Klinken L: Long-term prognosis in children with benign cerebeller astrocytoma. J Neurosurg 49:179, 1978
75. Glanzmann CH, Seelentag W: Radiotherapy for tumours of the pineal region and suprasellar germinomas. Radiother Oncol 16:31, 1989
76. Griffin TW, Beaufait D, Blasko JC: Cystic cerebellar astrocytomas in childhood. Cancer 44:276, 1979
77. Harisiadis L, Chang CH: Medulloblastoma in children: A correlation between staging and results of treatment. Int J Radiat Oncol Biol Phys 2:833, 1977
78. Hart MN, Earle KM: Primitive neuroectodermal tumors of the brain in children. Cancer 32:890, 1973
79. Herrick MK, Rubinstein LJ: The cytological differentiating potential of pineal parenchymal neoplasms (true pinealomas): Clinicopathological study of 28 tumours. Brain 102:289, 1979
80. Hirsch JF, Renier D, Czernichow P, et al: Medulloblastoma in childhood: Survival and functional results. Acta Neurochir 48:1, 1979
81. Hirsch JF, Rose CS, Pierre-Kahn A, et al: Benign astrocytic and oligodendrocytic tumors of the cerebral hemispheres in children. J Neurosurg 70:568, 1989
82. Hoffman HJ, Chuang S, Ehrlich R, et al: The microsurgical removal of craniopharyngiomas in childhood. Concepts Pediatr Neurosurg 6:52, 1985
83. Hoffman HJ: Benign brain stem gliomas in children. Prog Exp Tumor Res 30:154, 1987
84. Hoffman HJ: Transcallosal approach to pineal tumors and the Hospital for Sick Children series of pineal region tumors. In Neuwelt EA (ed): Diagnosis and Treatment of Pineal Region Tumors, p 223. Baltimore, Williams & Wilkins, 1984
85. Hoffman HJ: Craniopharyngiomas. Prog Exp Tumor Res 30:325, 1987
86. Hoogenhout J, Otten BJ, Kazem I, et al: Surgery and radiation therapy in the management of craniopharyngiomas. Int J Radiat Oncol Biol Phys 10:2293, 1984
87. Horowitz ME, Kun LE, Mulhern RK, et al: Feasibility and efficacy of preirradiation chemotherapy for pediatric brain tumors. Neurosurgery 22:687, 1988
88. Horowitz ME, Mulhern RK, Kun LE, et al: Brain tumors in the very young child: Postoperative chemotherapy in combined-modality treatment. Cancer 61:428, 1988
89. Horten BC, Rubinstein LJ: Primary cerebral neuroblastoma: A clinicopathological study of 35 cases. Brain 99:735, 1976
90. Horwich A, Bloom HJG: Optic gliomas: Radiation therapy and prognosis. Int J Radiat Oncol Biol Phys 11:1067, 1985
91. Hughes WN, Shillito J, Sallan SE, et al: Medulloblastoma at the Joint Center for Radiation Therapy between 1968 and 1984 Cancer 61:1992, 1988
92. Ilgren EB, Stiller CA, Hughes JT, et al: Ependymomas: A clinical and pathologic study, survival features. Clin Neuropathol 3:122, 1984
93. Ilgren EB, Stiller CA: Cerebellar astrocytomas: Therapeutic management. Acta Neurochir 81:11, 1986
94. Ilgren EB, Stiller CA: Cerebellar astrocytomas: Clinical characteristics and prognostic indices. J Neurooncol 4:293, 1987
95. Jenkin RDT: Medulloblastoma in childhood: Radiation therapy. Can Med Assoc J 190:51, 1969
96. Jenkin RDT, Simpson WJK, Keen CW: Pineal and suprasellar germinomas: Results of radiation treatment. J Neurosurg 48:99, 1978
97. Jenkin RDT, Boesel C, Ertel I, et al: Brain-stem tumors in childhood: A prospective randomized trial of irradiation with and without adjuvant CCNU, VCR, and prednisone. J Neurosurg 66:227, 1987
98. Jennings MT, Gelman R, Hochberg F: Intracranial germ-cell tumors: Natural history and pathogenesis. J Neurosurg 63:155, 1985
99. Jereb B, Reid A, Ahuja RK: Patterns of failure in patients with medulloblastoma. Cancer 50:2941, 1982
100. Jooma R, Kendall BE: Diagnosis and management of pineal tumors. J Neurosurg 58:654, 1983
101. Jooma R, Hayward RD, Grant DN: Intracranial neoplasms during the first year of life: Analysis of 100 consecutive cases. Neurosurgery 14:31, 1984
102. Kandt RS, Shinnar S, D'Souza BJ, et al: Cerebrospinal metastases in malignant childhood astrocytomas. J Neurooncol 2:123, 1984
103. Kelly PJ: Stereotactic biopsy and resection of thalamic astrocytomas. Neurosurgery 25:185, 1989
104. Kepes JJ, Rubinstein LJ, Eng LF: Pleomorphic xanthoastrocytoma: A distinctive meningocerebral glioma of young subjects with relatively favorable prognosis. A study of 12 cases. Cancer 44:1839, 1979
105. Kim YH, Fayos JF: Intracranial ependymomas. Radiology 124:805, 1977
106. Kim TH, Chin HW, Pollan S, et al: Radiotherapy of primary brain stem tumors. Int J Radiat Oncol Biol Phys 6:51, 1980
107. Kleinman GM, Hochberg FH, Richardson EP: Systemic metastases from medulloblastoma: Report of two cases and review of the literature Cancer 48:2296, 1981
108. Kobayashi T, Kageyama N, Ohara K: Internal irradiation for cystic craniopharyngioma. J Neurosurg 55:896, 1981
109. Kobayashi T, Yoshida J, Ishiyama J, et al: Combination chemotherapy with cisplatin and etoposide for malignant intracranial germ-cell tumors: An experimental and clinical study. J Neurosurg 70:676, 1989
110. Kopelson G, Linggood R: Infratentorial glioblastoma: The role of neuraxis irradiation. Int J Radiat Oncol Biol Phys 8:999, 1982
111. Kopelson G, Linggood RM, Kleinman GM: Medulloblastoma: The identification of prognosis subgroups and implications for multimodality management. Cancer 51:312, 1983

112. Kosnik EJ, Boesel CP, Bay J, et al: Primitive neuroectodermal tumors of the central nervous system in children. J Neurosurg 48:741, 1978
113. Kovnar EH, Kellie SJ, Horowitz ME, et al: Preirradiation cisplatin and etoposide in the treatment of high-risk medulloblastoma and other malignant embryonal tumors of the central nervous system: A phase II study. J Clin Oncol 8:330, 1990
114. Kramer S, McKissock W, Concannon JP: Craniopharyngiomas: Treatment by combined surgery and radiation therapy. J Neurosurg 18:217, 1961
115. Kramer S, Southard M, Mansfield CM: Radiotherapy in the management of craniopharyngiomas: Further experiences and late results. AJR 103:44, 1968
116. Kretschmar CS, Tarbell NJ, Kupsky W, et al: Preirradiation chemotherapy for infants and children with medulloblastoma: A preliminary report. J Neurosurg 71:820, 1989
117. Krischer JP, Ragab AH, Kun L, et al: Evaluation of MOPP adjuvant chemotherapy in the treatment of localized medulloblastoma: A Pediatric Oncology Group study. J Neurol Surg (submitted)
118. Kun LE: Patterns of failure in tumors of the central nervous system. Cancer Treat Symp 2:285, 1983
119. Kun LE, Mulhern RK, Crisco JJ: Quality of life in children treated for brain tumors: Intellectual, emotional, and academic function. J Neurosurg 58:1, 1983
120. Kun LE, Kovnar EH, Sanford RA: Ependymomas in children. Pediatr Neurosci 14:57, 1988
121. Kun LE, Horowitz M, Douglass E, et al: Medulloblastoma in young children: Radiation therapy results following failure of primary chemotherapy. [Abstract] Pediatr Neurosci 15:9, 1990
122. Landberg TG, et al: Improvements in the radiotherapy of medulloblastoma, 1946–1975. Cancer 45:670, 1980
123. Laurent JP, Cheek WR: A staging system of primitive neuroectodermal tumor (medulloblastoma) of the posterior fossa in children. Concepts Pediatr Neurosurg 7:81, 1987
124. Laws ER, Bergstralh, Taylor WF: Cerebellar astrocytoma in children. Prog Exp Tumor Res 30:122, 1987
125. Laws ER: Craniopharyngiomas in children and young adults. Prog Exp Tumor Res 30:335, 1987
126. Laws ER Jr, Taylor WF, Clifton MB, et al: Neurosurgical management of low-grade astrocytoma of the cerebral hemispheres. J Neurosurg 61:665, 1984
127. Lefkowitz J, Evans A, Sposto R, et al: Adjuvant chemotherapy of childhood posterior fossa (PF) ependymoma: Craniospinal radiation with or without CCNU, vincristine (VCR) and prednisone (P). J Clin Oncol 8:87, 1989
128. Lefkowitz IB, Packer RJ, Ryan SG, et al: Late recurrence of primitive neuroectodermal tumor/medulloblastoma. Cancer 62:826, 1988
129. Leibel SA, Sheline GE, Wara WM, et al: The role of radiation therapy in the treatment of astrocytomas. Cancer 35:1551, 1975
130. Leibel SA, Sheline GE. Review article: Radiation therapy for neoplasms of the brain. J Neurosurg 66:1, 1987
131. Levin VA: Chemotherapy of primary brain tumors. Neurol Clin 3:855, 1985
132. Levin VA, Rodriguez LA, Edwards MSB, et al: Treatment of medulloblastoma with procarbazine, hydroxyurea, and reduced radiation doses to whole brain and spine. J Neurosurg 68:383, 1988
133. Li FP, Fraumeni JF: Rhabdomyosarcoma in children: Epidemiologic study and identification of a familial cancer syndrome. JNCI 43:1364, 1969
134. Linstadt D, Wara W, Edwards M, et al: Radiotherapy of primary intracranial germinomas: The case against routine craniospinal irradiation. Int J Radiat Oncol Biol Phys 15:291, 1988
135. Loeffler JS, Kretschmar CS, Sallan SE, et al: Preradiation chemotherapy for infants and poor prognosis children with medulloblastoma. Int J Radiat Oncol Biol Phys 15:177, 1988
136. Lunsford LD, Gumerman L, Levine G: Stereotactic intracavitary irradiation of cystic neoplasms of the brain. Appl Neurophysiol 48:146, 1985
137. Manaka S, Teramoto A, Takakura K: The efficacy of radiotherapy for craniopharyngioma. J Neurosurg 62:648, 1985
138. Maor MH, Fields RS, Hogstrom KR, et al: Improving the therapeutic ratio of craniospinal irradiation in medulloblastoma. Int J Radiat Oncol Biol Phys 11:687, 1985
139. Marks JE, Adler SJ: A comparative study of ependymomas by site or origin. Int J Radiat Oncol Biol Phys 8:37, 1982
140. Matson D: Neurosurgery of infancy and childhood, 2nd ed, pp 469–477. Springfield, IL, Charles C Thomas, 1969
141. McLaurin RL, Breneman J, Aron B: Hypothalamic gliomas: Review of 18 cases. Concepts Pediatr Neurosurg 7:19, 1987
142. Mercuri S, Russo A, Palma L: Hemispheric supratentorial astrocytomas in children: Long-term results in 29 cases. J Neurosurg 55:170, 1981
143. Morantz RA: Radiation therapy in the treatment of cerebral astrocytoma. Neurosurgery 20:975, 1987
144. Mork SJ, Loken AC: Ependymoma: A follow-up study of 101 cases. Cancer 40:907, 1977
145. Mulhern RK, Horowitz ME, Kovnar EH, et al: Neurodevelopmental status of infants and young children treated for brain tumors with preirradiation chemotherapy. J Clin Oncol 7:1660, 1989
146. Muller W, Schroder R: Supratentorial recurrences of gliomas: Morphological studies in relation to time intervals with astrocytomas. Acta Neurochir 37:75, 1977
147. Naguib MG, Sund JH, Erickson DL, et al: Central nervous system involvement in the nevoid basal cell carcinoma syndrome: Case report and review of the literature. Neurosurgery 11:52, 1982
148. Nazar GB, Hoffman HJ, Becker LE, et al: Infratentorial ependymomas in childhood: Prognostic factors and treatment. J Neurosurg 72:408, 1990
149. Nishio S, Takeshita I, Fujii K, et al: Supratentorial astrocytic tumours of childhood: A clinicopathologic study of 41 cases. Acta Neurochir 101:3, 1989
150. Ochs J, Hancock M, Kun L, et al: Risk of subsequent central nervous system tumors in children treated for acute lymphoblastic leukemia. Proc Am Assoc Cancer Res 31:196, 1990
151. Packer RJ, Allen JC, Goldwein JL, et al: Hyperfractionated radiotherapy for children with brain stem gliomas: A pilot study using 7200 cGy. Ann Neurol 27:167, 1990
152. Packer RJ, Siegel KR, Sutton LN, et al: Efficacy of adjuvant chemotherapy for patients with poor-risk medulloblastoma: A preliminary report. Ann Neurol 24:503, 1988
153. Packer RJ, Sutton LN, Bilaniuk LT, et al: Treatment of chiasmatic/hypothalamic gliomas of childhood with chemotherapy: An update. Ann Neurol 23:79, 1988
154. Packer RJ, Siegel KR, Sutton LN, et al: Leptomeningeal dissemination of primary central nervous system tumors of childhood. Ann Neurol 18:217, 1985
155. Packer RJ, Sutton LN, Rorke LB, et al: Prognostic importance of cellular differentiation in medulloblastoma of childhood. J Neurosurg 61:296, 1984
156. Packer RJ, Sutton LN, Rosenstock JG, et al: Pineal region tumors of childhood. Pediatrics 74:97, 1984
157. Packer RJ, Sutton LN, Rorke LB, et al: Intracranial embryonal cell carcinoma. Cancer 54:520, 1984
158. Packer RJ, Savino PJ, Bilaniuk LT, et al: Chiasmatic gliomas of childhood: A reappraisal of natural history and effectiveness of cranial irradiation. Child Brain 10:393, 1983
159. Park TS, Hoffman HJ, Hendrick EB, et al: Medulloblastoma: Clinical presentation and management. J Neurosurg 58:543, 1983
160. Pendergrass TW, Milstein JM, Geyer JR, et al: Eight drugs in one day chemotherapy for brain tumors: Experience in 107 children and rationale for preradiation chemotherapy. J Clin Oncol 5:1221, 1987
161. Pierce SM, Barnes PD, Loeffler JS, et al: Definitive radiation therapy in the management of symptomatic patients with optic glioma: Survival and long-term effects. Cancer 65:45, 1990
162. Pierre-Kahn A, Hirsch JF, Roux FX, et al: Intracranial epen-

dymomas in childhood-survival and functional results of 47 cases. Child Brain 10:145, 1983
163. Prados M, Levin V: Malignant supratentorial gliomas in childhood. Pediatr Neurosci 13:144, 1987
164. Raimondi AJ, Tomita T: Pineal tumors in childhood: Epidemiology, pathophysiology, and surgical approaches. Child Brain 9:239, 1982
165. Rawlings CE III, Giangaspero F, Burger PC, et al: Ependymomas: A clinicopathologic study. Surg Neurol 29:271, 1988
166. Rich TA, Cassady JR, Strand RD, et al: Radiation therapy for pineal and suprasellar germ cell tumors. Cancer 55:932, 1985
167. Rodriguez LA, Edwards MSB, Levin VA: Management of hypothalamic gliomas in children: An analysis of 33 cases. Neurosurgery 26:242, 1990
168. Rorke LB: The cerebellar medulloblastoma in its relationship to primitive neuroectodermal tumors: Presidential address. J Neuropathol Exp Neurol 42:1, 1983
169. Rorke LB: Relationship of morphology of ependymoma in children to prognosis. Prog Exp Tumor Res 30:170, 1987
170. Ross GW, Rubinstein LJ: Lack of histopathological correlation of malignant ependymomas with postoperative survival. J Neurosurg 70:31, 1989
171. Rubinstein LJ: Tumors of the central nervous system. In Atlas of Tumor Pathology, fasc G. Washington, DC, Armed Forces Institute of Pathology, 1972
172. Rubinstein LJ: Embryonal central neuroepithelial tumors and their differentiating potential. J Neurosurg 62:795, 1985
173. Salazar OM: Primary malignant cerebellar astrocytomas in children: A signal for postoperative craniospinal irradiation. Int J Radiat Oncol Biol Phys 7:1661, 1981
174. Salazar OM: A better understanding of CNS seeding and a brighter outlook for postoperatively irradiated patients with ependymomas. Int J Radiat Oncol Biol Phys 9:1231, 1983
175. Salazar OM, Castro-Vita H, VanHoutte P, et al: Improved survival in cases of intracranial ependymoma after radiation therapy: Late report and recommendations. J Neurosurg 59:652, 1983
176. Sano K: Diagnosis and treatment of tumours in the pineal region. Acta Neurochir 34:153, 1976
177. Sano K: Pinealoma in children. Child Brain 2:67, 1976
178. Sano K, Matsutani M: Pinealoma (germinoma) treated by direct surgery and postoperative irradiation: A long-term follow-up. Child Brain 8:81, 1981
179. Scott EW, Mickle JP: Pediatric diencephalic gliomas: A review of 18 cases. Pediatr Neurosci 13:225, 1987
180. Sexauer CL, Khan A, Burger PC, et al: Cisplatin in recurrent pediatric brain tumors: A POG phase II study, a Pediatric Oncology Group study. Cancer 56:1497, 1985
181. Shaw EG, Daumas-Duport C, Scheithauer BW, et al: Radiation therapy in the management of low-grade supratentorial astrocytomas. J Neurosurg 70:853, 1989
182. Shaw EG, Evans RG, Scheithauer BW, et al: Postoperative radiotherapy of intracranial ependymoma in pediatric and adult patients. Int J Radiat Oncol Biol Phys 13:1457, 1987
183. Shaw EG, Scheithauer BW, Gilbertson DT, et al: Postoperative radiotherapy of supratentorial low-grade gliomas. Int J Radiat Oncol Biol Phys 16:663, 1989
184. Shibamoto Y, Abe M, Yamashita J, et al: Treatment results of intracranial germinoma as a function of the irradiated volume. Int J Radiat Oncol Biol Phys 15:285, 1988
185. Shinoda J, Yamada H, Sakai N, et al: Malignant cerebellar astrocytic tumours in children. Acta Neurochir 98:1, 1989
186. Silverman CL, Simpson JR: Cerebellar medulloblastoma: The importance of posterior fossa dose to survival and patterns of failure. Int J Radiat Oncol Biol Phys 8:1869, 1982
187. Sposto R, Ertel IJ, Jenkin RDT, et al: The effectiveness of chemotherapy for treatment of high grade astrocytoma in children: Results of a randomized trial. A report from the Children's Cancer Study Group. J Neurooncol 7:165, 1989
188. Stroink AR, Hoffman JH, Hendrick EB, et al: Diagnosis and management of pediatric brain-stem gliomas. J Neurosurg 65:745, 1986
189. Sung DI, Harisiadis L, Chang CC: Midline pineal tumors and suprasellar germinomas: Highly curable by irradiation. Radiology 128:745, 1978
190. Sung DI, Chang CH, Harisiadis L, et al: Treatment results of craniopharyngiomas. Cancer 47:847, 1981
191. Sung DI: Suprasellar tumors in children: A review of clinical manifestations and managements. Cancer 50:1420, 1982
192. Sutton LN, Packer RJ, Siegel K, et al: Current management of medulloblastoma: A modest proposal. Concepts Pediatr Neurosurg 9:91, 1989
193. Sutton LN: Current management of low-grade astrocytomas of childhood. Pediatr Neurosci 13:98, 1987
194. Svien H, Mabon RF, Kernohan JW, et al: Ependymomas of the brain: Pathologic aspects. Neurology 3:1 1953
195. Thomas M, Adams JH: Doyle D: Neuroectodermal tumors in the cerebellum in two sisters. J Neurol Neurosurg Psychiatry 40:886, 1977
196. Tomita T, McLone G, Flannery AM: Choroid plexus papillomas of neonates, infants and children. Pediatr Neurosci 14:23, 1988
197. Tomita T, McLone DG, Das L, et al: Benign ependymomas of the posterior fossa in children. Pediatr Neurosci 14:277, 1988
198. Tomita T: Management of craniopharyngiomas in children. Pediatr Neurosci 14:204, 1988
199. Tomita T, McLone D: Medulloblastoma in childhood: Results of radical resection and low-dose neuraxis radiation therapy. J Neurosurg 64:238, 1986
200. Tomita T, McLone DG: Brain tumors during the first 24 months of life. Neurosurgery 17:913, 1985
201. Ushio Y, Arita N, Hayakawa T, et al: Leptomeningeal dissemination of primary brain tumors in children: Clinical and experimental studies. Prog Exp Tumor Res 30:194, 1987
202. Van Eys J, Cangir A, Coody D, et al: MOPP regimen as primary chemotherapy for brain tumors in infants. J Neurooncol 3:237, 1985
203. Walker AE, Robins M, Weinfeld FD: Epidemiology of brain tumors: The national survey of intracranial neoplasms. Neurology 35:219, 1985
204. Walker MD, Strike TA, Sheline GE: An analysis of dose-effect relationship in the radiotherapy of malignant gliomas. Int J Radiat Oncol Biol Phys 5:1725, 1979
205. Wallner KE, Gonzales MF, Edwards MSB: Treatment results of juvenile pilocytic astrocytoma. J Neurosurg 69:171, 1988
206. Wallner KE, Wara WM, Sheline GE, et al: Intracranial ependymomas: Results of treatment with partial or whole brain irradiation without spinal irradiation. Int J Radiat Oncol Biol Phys 12:1937, 1986
207. Wara WM, Jenkin RDT, Evans A, et al: Tumors of the pineal and suprasellar region: Children's Cancer Study Group treatment results 1960–1975. A report from Children's Cancer Study Group. Cancer 43:698, 1979
208. Wara W, Edwards MSB, Levin VA, et al: A new treatment regimen for brain-stem glioma: A pilot study of the Brain Tumor Research Center and Children's Cancer Study Group. Int J Radiat Oncol Biol Phys 12:143, 1986
209. Weiss M, Sutton L, Marcial V, et al: The role of radiation therapy in the management of childhood craniopharyngioma. Int J Radiat Oncol Biol Phys 17:1313, 1989
210. Wen B-C, Hussey DH, Staples J, et al: A comparison of the roles of surgery and radiation therapy in the management of craniopharyngiomas. Int J Radiat Oncol Biol Phys 16:17, 1989
211. Winston K, Gilles FH, Leviton A, et al: Cerebellar gliomas in children. JNCI 58:833, 1977
212. Wong JYC, Wara WM, Sheline GE: Optic gliomas: A reanalysis of the University of California, San Francisco, experience. Cancer 60:1847, 1987
213. Woo SY, Donaldson SS, Cox RS: Astrocytoma in children: 14 years' experience at Stanford University Medical Center. J Clin Oncol 6:1001, 1988

70

○ ○ ○ ● ● ●

Wilms' Tumor

Patrick R.M. Thomas

EPIDEMIOLOGY

Wilms' tumor is a highly malignant embryonal tumor of the kidney. It is the most common malignant lesion of the genitourinary tract in children and has an annual incidence of about 7.8 cases per million black and white children 1 to 14 years old.[47]

It is predominantly a disease of children under 5 years of age, and some cases are hereditary.[41] Various congenital abnormalities have been associated with Wilms' tumor, including aniridia, hemihypertrophy, and abnormalities of the genitourinary tract.[28,29,31,33] A recent review of the International Society of Pediatric Oncology (SIOP) data suggested, however, that the hereditary fraction of Wilms' tumor is small.[32] In these cases, chromosome 11 is most likely to be abnormal.[10]

NATURAL HISTORY

The disease is often localized at diagnosis, as evidenced by the fact that surgery and radiation therapy can cure almost 50% of the patients.[19] Spread throughout the peritoneal cavity also may occur, especially if there has been preoperative rupture or the disease has been spilled at surgery. However, the results of the Second National Wilms' Tumor Study (NWTS-2) demonstrated that tumor spillage at surgery, if localized to the flank, is less important prognostically than was formerly believed.[13,16] This study also showed the importance of lymph node involvement as a prognostic factor. There were 326 patients with favorable histology and negative lymph nodes. The 2-year disease-free survival rate was 88% for the patients with negative lymph nodes, and the rate was 56% for 67 patients with favorable histology and positive lymph nodes. The lungs are the most common metastatic site, followed by the liver. In NWTS-2, there were 57 (11.4%) patients with metastases at diagnosis. Forty-seven of these had pulmonary metastases only.[13]

CLINICAL PRESENTATION

The classic presentation for Wilms' tumor is that of a healthy child in whom abdominal swelling is discovered by the child's mother, pediatrician, or family practitioner during a routine physical examination. A smooth, firm, nontender mass on one side of the abdomen is felt. Gross hematuria occurs in as many as 25% of these cases.[23] The child may be hypertensive or have nonspecific symptoms, such as malaise or fever.[42] Only rarely does a patient present with symptomatic metastases.

DIAGNOSTIC WORKUP

The differential diagnosis of Wilms' tumor includes other malignant lesions of the kidney of children, neuroblastoma, and benign conditions such a hydronephrosis, polycystic disease, and splenomegaly in left-sided tumors. Plain films of the abdomen may demonstrate calcifications, which occur in 60% to 70% of neuroblastomas but in only 15% of Wilms' tumors. An intravenous pyelogram can differentiate the renal tumor from the other conditions. Cysts often appear as radiolucent areas. Ultrasonography may also be helpful because the kidney cannot be seen on intravenous pyelogram in as many as 10% of the Wilms' tumor patients. In these cases, the tumor appears solid rather than cystic.

The advent of computed tomography (CT) has reduced the popularity of invasive studies like arteriography. Abdominal CT delineates the intrarenal tumor and demonstrates gross extrarenal spread, lymph node involvement, liver metastases, and the status of the opposite kidney (Fig. 70-1). A direct comparison of CT with ultrasonography suggests that CT is a better diagnostic tool overall.[38] Clinical impression does not, however, obviate the need for inspection at laparotomy.

Plain chest radiography is also essential because asymptomatic pulmonary metastases are common. Chest CT scans may reveal some early lesions not visible on routine radiography; its role in routine preoperative investigation of Wilms' tumor has yet to be evaluated, but small lesions seen only on CT scans frequently represent metastatic tumor.[45] Of 124 patients with Wilms' tumors who had normal chest radiographs, 11 had abnormal chest CT scans.[45] Because four of these patients had relapses, it was believed that some of the lesions represented metastatic disease.

A complete blood count and a urinalysis should be performed. Wilms' tumor patients can be anemic from hematuria. Serum blood urea nitrogen and creatinine levels and liver function tests are routine. If neuroblastoma is not ruled out, a test for urinary catecholamines should be performed. Table 70-1 outlines the pretreatment investigations recommended in NWTS-4.

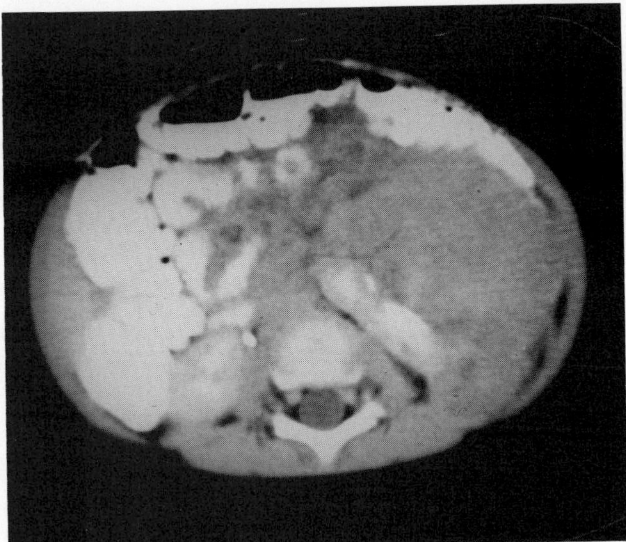

FIGURE 70–1. CT scan of a patient with large left-sided Wilms' tumor showing displacement and caliceal involvement. The intestines are mainly displaced to the right.

STAGING

Tumor staging is performed by carefully examining the operative and histopathologic findings. The most widely used staging system was devised by the National Wilms' Tumor Study (Table 70-2),[16] after analysis of the results of NWTS-1 and NWTS-2 where a grouping system had been used.

PATHOLOGIC CLASSIFICATION

It has long been recognized that there are many variants of Wilms' tumor and that these might affect prognosis.[35] Although histopathologists had attempted to relate appearance to prognosis, no generally acceptable classification was available until the report of Beckwith and Palmer[3] from the First National Wilms' Tumor Study (NWTS-1).

Wilms' tumor is usually a solitary tumor that is well demarcated from the normal kidney. It may occur in any part of either kidney; it is sometimes encapsulated and can show necrosis with cavitation and sometimes gross hemorrhage.[4]

The microscopic appearances of Wilms' tumor are varied. The tumor is derived from metanephros and from mesoderm; therefore, the appearances reflect a mixture of epithelial and stromal elements in various proportions.[1,3,4,7] Their origin from nephrogenic rests is well defined.[2]

The NWTS classifies all tumors as having favorable histology or unfavorable histology for purposes of treatment.[3,19,21,37]

The unfavorable histologic category accounts for about 12% of Wilms' tumor cases in NWTS-1 and NWTS-2.[3,19] Anaplastic tumors, strictly defined according to nuclear size, hyperchromatism, and abnormal mitotic size, are either focal or diffuse. Prognosis depends on this criterion and on stage.[3,7]

There are two monoplastic sarcomatous varieties that are no longer considered true Wilms' tumors.[1] Clear cell sarcoma consists of cells with poorly stained cytoplasm and indistinct margins. They infiltrate the parenchyma rather than form pseudocapsules and have the propensity to metastasize to bone.[39] A skeletal survey and bone scan should be part of the workup for these patients. Malignant rhabdoid tumors of the kidney are the most lethal renal neoplasms in children. They consist of sheets of polygonal cells with abundant acidophilic cytoplasm. There is no conclusive evidence of skeletal muscle origin for this tumor, but a neuroepithelial derivative has been postulated.[19] This tumor is associated with morphologically

TABLE 70–1
Pretreatment Investigations for Patients With Renal Mass Suspected of Wilm's Tumor According to NWTS-4 Recommendations

History	Record preexisting conditions, family history of cancer, or congenital anomalies
Physical examination	Blood pressure, weight, height, presence of masses, congenital anomalies, particularly genitourinary, hemihypertrophy, and aniridia
Laboratory	Hemoglobin, white cell and differential counts, platelets, urinalysis, serum BUN, creatinine, SGOT, SGPT, alkaline phosphatase
Roentgenogram	Posteroanterior and lateral chest films, excretory urogram (IVP), with specical attention to opposite kidney
Optional	Ultrasound to detect small foci in opposite kidney and tumor deposits in vena cava Skeletal survey for clear cell sarcoma Computed tomography scans of chest and abdomen (brain if rhabdoid sarcoma) Angiography to document size of tumors in both kidneys and monitor treatment in bilateral cancer

TABLE 70–2
National Wilms' Tumor Study Staging System

STAGE	DESCRIPTION
I	Tumor limited to kidney and completely excised; surface of renal capsule intact; tumor not ruptured before or during removal; no residual tumor apparent beyond margins of resection
II	Tumor extends beyond kidney but is completely excised; regional extension of tumor (*i.e.*, penetration through outer surface of renal capsule into perirenal soft tissues); vessels outside kidney substances infiltrated or contain tumor thrombus. Tumor may have been examined on biopsy, or there has been local spillage of tumor confined to flank. No residual tumor apparent at or beyond margins of excision.
III	Residual nonhematogenous tumor confined to abdomen Any of the following occur:
A	Lymph nodes on biopsy found to be involved in hilus, periaortic chains, or beyond
B	Diffuse peritoneal contamination by tumor such as spillage of tumor beyond flank before or during surgery or by tumor growth that has penetrated through peritoneal surface
C	Implants found on peritoneal surfaces
D	Tumor extends beyond surgical margins either microscopically or grossly
E	Tumor not completely excisable because of local infiltration into vital structures
IV	Hematogenous metastases; deposits beyond Stage III (*e.g.*, lung, liver, bone, brain)
V	Bilateral renal involvement at diagnosis; attempt should be made to stage each side according to the above criteria on the basis of extent of disease before biopsy

(Farewell VT, D'Angio GJ, Breslow N, et al: Cancer Clin Trials 4:167, 1981)

similar tumors in the central nervous system, particularly in the posterior fossa.

Eighty-eight percent of Wilms' tumors have favorable histologic patterns. Essentially, they are mixed tumors of the kidney that do not meet the criteria for anaplasia.

GENERAL MANAGEMENT

The diagnosis of Wilms' tumor is usually made preoperatively and confirmed at surgery. An incorrect diagnosis was made in only 30 (5%) of 606 patients registered on NWTS-1.[13] Nevertheless, preoperative therapy is not commonly practiced in the United States, although it has been examined in clinical trials. Meticulous surgical techniques for exploring the abdomen through a transperitoneal (*i.e.*, transverse, paramedian, or midline) rather than an extraperitoneal (flank) incision is essential.[22] The surgeon must excise all tumor without spillage, if possible. Thorough assessment and sampling of lymph nodes and inspection of the liver and opposite kidney should be performed.

Treatment depends on stage and histology. In general, tumors with favorable histology are responsive to radiation therapy and chemotherapy. Because of the potential long-term deleterious effects of radiation therapy, this modality plays a relatively minor role compared with that of chemotherapy. Tumors with unfavorable histology are less responsive to either modality and are generally treated with aggressive multimodality regimens.

TABLE 70–3
Recommended Radiation Therapy Doses

CHARACTERISTIC	DOSE	
STAGE		
Stage I and II FH*	No radiation therapy	
Stage III FH + II and III CCSK	1000 cGy to flank or whole abdomen plus 1000 cGy to gross residual†	
Stage IV FH + IV CCSK	No radiation therapy to abdomen (if operative abdominal Stage I or Stage II) 1000 cGy to flank or whole abdomen* plus 1000 cGy boost to gross residual (if abdominal Stage III) 1200 cGy (150-cGy fractions) to whole lungs	
Anaplastic	Sliding scale based on age at diagnosis (see below) except for Stage I where no radiation therapy is given	
	Age (months)	
	Birth–12	1200–1800 cGy
	13–18	2100 cGy
	19–30	2700 cGy
	31–40	3300 cGy
	41 or more	3800 cGy

**FH: favorable histology; CCSK: clear cell sarcoma.*
† All radiation therapy to begin within 10 days of surgery. Whole abdomen if gross residual, diffuse peritoneal implants, preoperative anterior rupture, or diffuse abdominal operative spillage.
(Based on the recommendations of the Fourth National Wilms' Tumor Study)

RADIATION THERAPY TECHNIQUES

Results of NWTS-1 and NWTS-2 show that although irradiation does not need to be given immediately after operation, as was originally suggested by Gross and Neuhauser,[18] treatment timing is important. Patients in whom irradiation was delayed for 10 days or more from surgery had a significantly higher chance of abdominal relapse, particularly those with tumors with unfavorable histology. In NWTS-1, 10% (three of 29) of children who had initiation of radiation therapy 10 or more days after surgery had relapses in operative site.[14,44] This rate was higher ($P = 0.01$) than for patients with shorter delays. In NWTS-2, eight of 99 patients with 10 or more days delay had relapses in the abdomen, but only two of 251 with shorter delays had abdominal relapses.[44] Because the pathologist cannot always rule out unfavorable histology quickly, all patients with Wilms' tumor should be scheduled to start radiation therapy within 10 days after surgery. Most patients will not be treated, but it is easier to cancel than to make arrangements to initiate irradiation for a small child on short notice.[44]

In NWTS-1, radiation dosages to the operative bed were given according to the age of the patient. In 96 patients receiving less than 100% of the protocol dosage, 27 (28%) relapses were recorded, but 45 (31%) of 144 patients receiving the protocol dose or higher doses had relapses.[14] Thus, no significant dose-response association was detected.[14,44] Because most relapses occur in patients with anaplastic tumor histology, irradiation doses for this group should remain high. However, it appears that the irradiation doses previously used for patients with favorable tumor histology are too high.[11] The recommendations for dose by stage and histology in NWTS-4 are presented in Table 70-3.

Although there did not appear to be a correlation between field size and outcome in NWTS-1, this was not so in NWTS-2.[14,44] When all factors leading to abdominal relapse were correlated with a multivariate Cox regression analysis, small field size remained a significant contributing factor ($P = 0.002$). Patients with disease confined to the operative site need only have the flank irradiated, even if there has been local spillage of tumor. Parallel opposed fields using 4-MV or 6-MV photons are preferred. The treatment portals should encompass the tumor bed and the site of the excised kidney with a 2-cm to 3-cm margin. The medial border must cross the midline to include the entire width of the vertebrae to minimize growth disturbances. A tangential abdominal wall shield can be used. An example of portals for flank irradiation is presented in Figure 70-2.[14] When whole-abdomen irradiation is administered, shaped portals must be used, and the femoral heads and acetabulum must be shielded (Fig. 70-3). This reduces the effects on epiphyseal growth or development of slipped femoral epiphysis; however, these complications did not occur at doses below 2000 cGy.[40] Whole-lung irradiation is used if there are lung metastases (Fig. 70-4). Shaped fields spare normal soft tissues. Dosages for favorable-histology bilateral Wilms' tumor should be limited to 1000 cGy to the second kidney.

RESULTS OF THERAPY

Because Wilms' tumor is rare and the major advances in its treatment have come from randomized clinical trials, there are few reports from single-institution studies. At Washington University Clouse and co-workers[9] reported 74 patients treated between 1949 and 1978 who had marked improvement in prog-

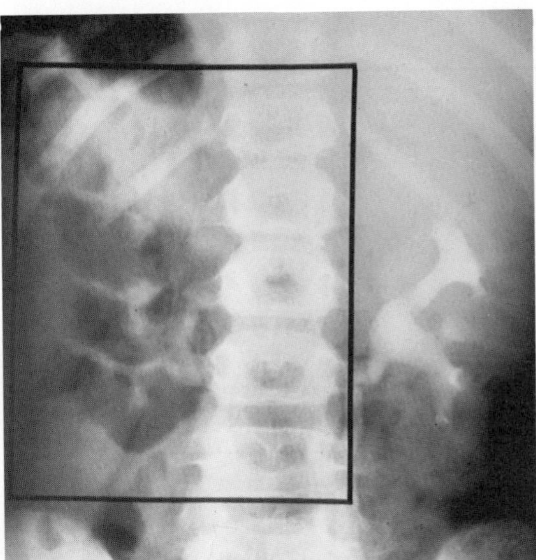

FIGURE 70–2. Simulation film of anteroposterior portal of the flank showing inclusion of the entire width of the vertebral body in the irradiated volume.

nosis for Stage II and III disease after the advent of systemic chemotherapy in 1965.

Because of the difficulty of designing studies for synchronous bilateral disease, no clinical trials defining treatment have been devised. Patients with disease of this kind, however, usually have a good prognosis and are followed but not randomized by the NWTS.[36] In a review of 30 (5.4%) NWTS-1 registrants, Bishop and associates[5] reported that bilateral Wilms' tumors were not unduly aggressive. In an analysis of NWTS-2 and NWTS-3 data, Blute and colleagues[6] found that 15 patients in whom one tumor had unfavorable histology fared much worse than 129 with two tumors with favorable histology ($P<0.001$). The investigators recommended avoiding nephrectomy and performing excisional biopsies, followed by chemotherapy appropriate for the stage of the most advanced side. Second-look laparotomy with removal of all tumor should be performed within 6 months. If it is not possible to excise all tumor, further chemotherapy and radiation should be given.

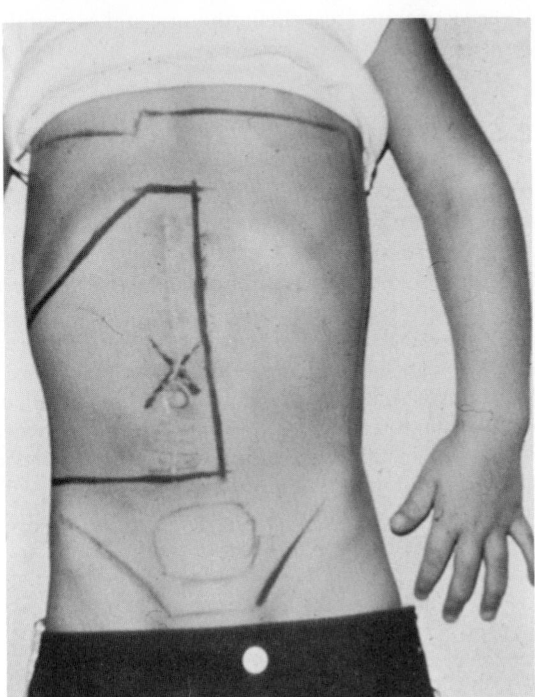

FIGURE 70–3. Anteroposterior portal for the whole-abdomen and flank portals used in irradiation of patients with stage III Wilms' tumors. The upper margin of the abdominal field must include the diaphragm. The acetabulum and femoral head should be excluded from the irradiated volume to decrease the probability of slipped femoral epiphysis. Whole-abdomen irradiation is no longer frequently used in Wilms' tumor.

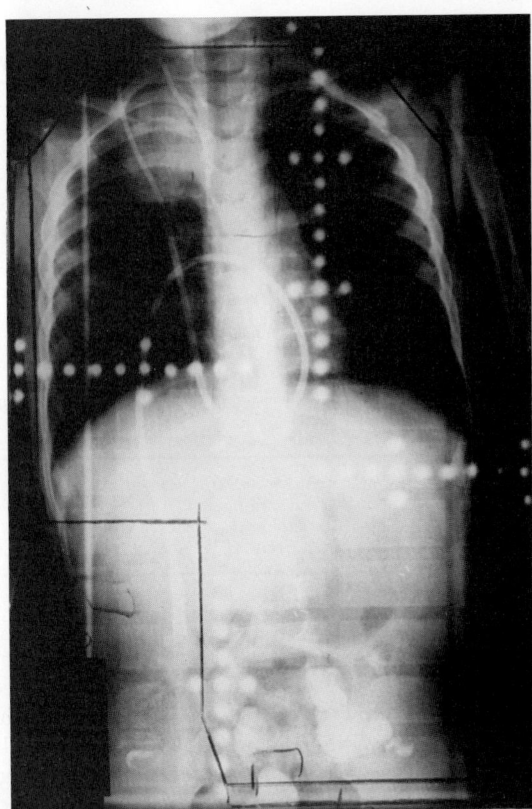

FIGURE 70–4. Patient receiving partial-abdominal plus whole-lung irradiation en bloc. Notice that the portals come below the apparent costophrenic angles and that there is a single, large, right upper lobe metastasis, an unusual finding in Wilms' tumor.

SUMMARY OF CLINICAL TRIALS

There is no tumor that has been studied by clinical trials as thoroughly and effectively as Wilms' tumor. The NWTS, under the expert guidance of Dr. Giulio J. D'Angio, has been active in North America since 1969, and there have also been successful studies run by SIOP and the Medical Research Council of the United Kingdom. In NWTS-1, it was shown that postoperative irradiation was not necessary for children under 2 years of age with group I tumors and that combined dactinomycin and vincristine for irradiated patients with groups II and III tumors was better than either agent alone (Table 70-4).[13] The addition of preoperative vincristine for group IV patients was not advantageous.

The design of NWTS-2 was based entirely on the results from NWTS-1. Because dactinomycin and vincristine achieved better results than dactinomycin alone in more advanced dis-

TABLE 70–4
Results of the First National Wilms' Study

GROUP	THERAPY	NO. OF PATIENTS	DISEASE-FREE (%)	P VALUE
Group I (<2 years old)	Radiation therapy	38	89	NS
	No radiation therapy	36	80	
Group I (>2 years old)	Radiation therapy	39	77	0.04
	No radiation therapy	41	58	
Groups II and III	AMD*	63	57	
	VCR	44	55	
	Combination	59	81	0.002
Group IV	Preoperative VCR	13	29†	
	No preoperative VCR	13	83†	0.02‡

**AMD: dactinomycin; VCR: vincristine.*
† Two-year actuarial survival.
‡ Possibly selected sample.
(D'Angio GJ, Evans AE, Breslow NE, et al: Cancer 38:633, 1976)

ease, it was postulated that vincristine could substitute for postoperative irradiation for group I patients (Table 70-4). Because the prognosis in group I was good, the question was whether 15 months of dactinomycin plus vincristine therapy could be reduced to 6 months. For irradiated patients in group II, group III, and group IV, the question was whether doxorubicin, if added to vincristine and dactinomycin, would improve the results obtained with these two agents alone. The findings showed that administering dactinomycin plus vincristine over 6 months to patients in these groups was comparable to results obtained over 15 months in group I patients.[12] Addition of doxorubicin was beneficial to patients in groups II through IV (Table 70-5).

The Medical Research Council, using schedules of chemotherapy that differed from those in NWTS, demonstrated that vincristine given weekly and then biweekly after postoperative dactinomycin therapy produced better results than continuing therapy with dactinomycin alone.[30]

NWTS-3, conducted from 1979 to 1985, studied the effects of both chemotherapy and radiation therapy. The overall object of the study was to reduce therapy for low-risk patients (Stages I to III with favorable histology) and to intensify treatment by adding a fourth drug, cyclophosphamide, for Stage IV tumors with favorable histology and all tumors with unfavorable histology. The results are presented in Table 70-6.[11] The less-intensive therapies did not result in significantly increased relapses in low-risk patients, and it appears that approximately 60% of these children need neither irradiation nor the potentially cardiotoxic doxorubicin. Detailed analysis showed a trend in favor of the addition of doxorubicin for Stage III tumors with favorable histology and that patients receiving doxorubicin or 2000 cGy had fewer abdominal relapses than those receiving 1000 cGy without doxorubicin. Although patients with Stage IV tumors with favorable histology treated with cyclophosphamide had a slightly higher relapse-free rate, it was not significant, and there was no proof that cyclophosphamide benefited patients with high-risk tumors.

The SIOP studies have mainly used preoperative therapy. The first SIOP trial found that preoperative irradiation reduced the incidence of tumor spillage but did not increase survival.[24] SIOP-5, reported in 1983, showed that preoperative vincristine was as effective as preoperative irradiation plus dactinomycin in preventing tumor rupture.[25] In SIOP-6, all patients receive preoperative chemotherapy and are randomized by operative stage.

LATE EFFECTS OF TREATMENT

The cure rate for Wilms' tumor was about 90% in NWTS-3.[11] The study of late effects is therefore of paramount importance, to prevent these survivors from becoming chronically sick adults. Although Wilms' tumor is radioresponsive, the role of radiation therapy has been reexamined because of the real and potential late effects.[20,40,43] Heaston and associates[20] reported that the skeletal effects of megavoltage irradiation were as frequent but not as severe as those of orthovoltage irradiation. A series at Washington University also confirmed a high incidence of scoliosis (14 of 26 patients) but suggested that functional disability was minimal.[43] Preliminary results of the NWTS Late Effects Study showed 66 musculoskeletal abnormalities in 86

TABLE 70–5
Two-Year Disease-Free Survival Rate in the Second National Wilms' Tumor Study

GROUP	AMD + VCR* (6 MONTHS)	AMD + VCR (15 MONTHS)	VCR + AMD + ADR (15 MONTHS)
Group I (FH + UH)*	83 (94%) of 88	83 (91%) of 91	
Groups II, III, IV (FH + UH)		106 (63%) of 159	126 (71%) of 157

P = 0.0004.
**FH, favorable histology; UH, unfavorable histology; AMD, dactinomycin; VCR, vincristine; ADR, doxorubicin.*
(D'Angio GJ, Evans AE, Breslow NE, et al: Cancer 47:2302, 1981)

TABLE 70–6
Results of the Third National Wilms' Tumor Study

STAGE	REGIMEN†	NO. OF PATIENTS	RELAPSE FREE AT 4 YEARS (%)
Stage I FH*	AMD + VCR 10 wk *vs* 6 months	607	89 *vs* 92
Stage II FH	AMD + VCR + ADR *vs* AMD + VCR	278	87 *vs* 89
Stage II FH	2000 cGy *vs* no XRT	278	89 *vs* 88
Stage III FH	AMD + VCR + ADR *vs* AMD + VCR	275	84 *vs* 74
Stage III FH	2000 cGy *vs* 1000 cGy	275	81 *vs* 77
Stage IV FH	AMD + VCR + ADR *vs* AMD + VCR + ADR + CY	120	72 *vs* 78
All UH	AMD + VCR + ADR *vs* AMD + VCR + ADR + CY	159	64 *vs* 60

**FH: favorable histology; UH: unfavorable histology.*
† ADR: doxorubicin; AMD: dactinomycin; CY: cyclophosphamide; VCR: vincristine; XRT: external radiation therapy.
(D'Angio GJ, Breslow N, Beckwith JB, et al: Cancer 64:349, 1989)

surviving irradiated group I patients and seven of 93 nonirradiated children. No increases in cardiac abnormalities were noticed in those patients receiving doxorubicin.[15]

A second malignant neoplasm also may occur in long-term survivors. At the Sidney Farber Cancer Institute, ten new cancers were identified among 487 Wilms' tumor patients treated over a 44-year period; nine of the ten were in the irradiated field.[26] The Late Effects Study Group demonstrated that 208 (68%) of 308 second malignant neoplasms in 292 patients (any primary pediatric malignancy) developed in irradiated sites; however, although Wilms' tumor was responsible for 36 of these neoplasms, approximately one third of the patients had evidence of hereditary factors.[27] The NWTS conducted a review of 2438 patients enrolled between 1969 and 1982 and found 15 second malignant neoplasms.[8] The expected number was 1.77. There was a suggestion that the rate would increase as patients were followed for more than 10 years.

FUTURE CONSIDERATIONS

Although it is difficult to improve on the overall cure rate of 90%, there are still important issues in Wilms' tumor that are yet to be resolved. The current protocol, NWTS-4, was opened in 1986, and it is summarized in Table 70-7. The objectives include testing whether pulsed intensive courses of dactinomycin are as effective as the standard 5-day course, potentially saving time and money in an era of soaring medical costs. In addition, for Stages II through IV with favorable histology and Stages I through IV clear cell sarcoma, the duration of therapy is being

TABLE 70–7
Outline of the Fourth National Wilms' Tumor Study

STAGE	TREATMENT†	
Stage I, FH* Stage I, anaplastic	Surgery, no RT	A + V 24 wk P/I A + V 18 wk
Stage II, FH	Surgery, no RT	A + V 22 wk A + V 65 wk P/I A + V 18 wk P/I A + V 60 wk
Stage III, FH Stage III, high-risk‡	Surgery, 1080 cGy Surgery, RT‡	A + V + D 26 wk A + V + D 65 wk P/I A + V + D 24 wk P/I A + V + D 54 wk
Stage II–IV, anaplastic	Surgery, RT	A + V + D 65 wk A + V + D + C 65 wk

**FH: favorable histology.*
† RT: radiation therapy; A: dactinomycin; V: vincristine; P/I: pulse intensive; D: doxorubicin; C: cyclophosphamide.
‡ High-risk patients include those with clear cell sarcoma or Stage IV FH. Flank dose is 1080 cGy for these tumors if the primary would otherwise be Stage III.

tested (6 months *versus* 15 months). For anaplastic tumors Stages II through IV, NWTS-3 data suggested that cyclophosphamide added to doxorubicin, dactinomycin, and vincristine might be beneficial, and this randomization is continued in NWTS-4. All patients with Stages III or IV tumors with favorable histology and all patients with unfavorable-histology tumors, except Stage I anaplastic, are receiving irradiation. There are no preliminary results of the randomization; however, hepatic toxic effects have been reported with the pulsed intensive regimens, resulting in a decrease of the dose of dactinomycin from 60 μg/kg to 45 μg/kg.[17]

REFERENCES

1. Beckwith JB: Wilms' tumor and other renal tumors of childhood. Hum Pathol 14:481, 1983
2. Beckwith JB, Kiviat NB, Bonadio JB: Nephrogenic rests, nephroblastomatosis, and the pathogenesis of Wilms' tumor. Pediatr Pathol 10:1, 1990
3. Beckwith JB, Palmer NJ: Histopathology and prognosis of Wilms' tumor. Cancer 41:1937, 1978
4. Belasco JB, Chatten J, D'Angio GJ: Wilms' tumor in clinical pediatric oncology. In Sutow WW, Fernbach DJ, Vietti TJ (eds): Clinical Pediatric Oncology, pp 588–621. St. Louis, CV Mosby, 1983
5. Bishop HC, Tefft M, Evans AE, et al: Bilateral Wilms' tumor: Review of 30 National Wilms' Tumor Study cases. J Pediatr Surg 12:631, 1977
6. Blute ML, Kelalis PP, Offord KP, et al: Bilateral Wilms' tumor. J Urol 138:968, 1987
7. Bonadio JF, Norkool P, Farewell VT, et al: Anaplastic Wilms' tumor: Clinical and pathologic studies. J Clin Oncol 3:513, 1985
8. Breslow NE, Norkool PA, Olshan A, et al: Second malignant neoplasms in survivors of Wilms' tumor: A report from the National Wilms' Tumor Study. JNCI 80:592, 1988
9. Clouse JW, Thomas PRM, Griffith RC, et al: The changing management of Wilms' tumor over a thirty-year period, 1949–1978. Cancer 56:1484, 1985
10. Cowell J, Pritchard J: The molecular genetics of retinoblastoma and Wilms' tumor: CRC clinical review. Oncol Hematol 7:153, 1987
11. D'Angio GJ, Breslow N, Beckwith JB, et al: The treatment of Wilms' tumor: Results of the Third National Wilms' Tumor Study. Cancer 64:349, 1989
12. D'Angio GJ, Evans AE, Breslow NE, et al: The treatment of Wilms' tumor: Results of the National Wilms' Tumor Study. Cancer 38:633, 1976
13. D'Angio GJ, Evans AE, Breslow NE, et al: The treatment of Wilms' tumor: Results of the Second National Wilms' Tumor Study. Cancer 47:2302, 1981
14. D'Angio GJ, Tefft M, Breslow NE, et al: Radiation therapy of Wilms' tumor: Results according to dose, field, postoperative timing and histology. Int J Radiat Oncol Biol Phys 4:769, 1978
15. Evans AE, Breslow N, Norkool P, et al: Complications in long-term survivors of Wilms' tumor. Proc Am Assoc Cancer Res 27:204, 1986
16. Farewell VT, D'Angio GJ, Breslow N, et al: Retrospective validation of a new staging system for Wilms' tumor. Cancer Clin Trials 4:167, 1981
17. Green DM, Finklestein J, Norkool P, et al: Severe hepatic toxicity after treatment with single-dose dactinomycin and vincristine. Cancer 62:270, 1988
18. Gross RE, Neuhauser EBD: Treatment of mixed tumors of the kidney in childhood. Pediatrics 6:843, 1950
19. Haas JE, Palmer NF, Weinberg AC, et al: Ultrastructure of malignant rhabdoid tumor of kidney. Hum Pathol 12:646, 1981
20. Heaston DK, Libshitz HJ, Chan RC: Skeletal effects of megavoltage irradiation in survivors of Wilms' tumor. AJR 133:389, 1979
21. Howell CG, Othersen HB, Kiviat NE, et al: Therapy and outcome in 51 children with mesoblastic nephroma. J Pediatr Surg 17:826, 1982.
22. Leape LL, Breslow NE, Bishop HC: The surgical treatment of Wilms' tumor. J Epidemiol Community Health 33:253, 1979
23. Ledlie EM, Mynors LS, Draper GJ, et al: Natural history and treatment of Wilms' tumour: An analysis of 335 cases occurring in England and Wales 1962–1966. Br Med J 4:195, 1970
24. Lemerle J, Voute PA, Tournade MF, et al: Preoperative versus postoperative radiotherapy, single versus multiple courses of actinomycin D in the treatment of Wilms' tumor. Cancer 38:647, 1976
25. Lemerle J, Voute PA, Tournade MF, et al: Effectiveness of preoperative chemotherapy in Wilms' tumor. Results of an International Society of Pediatric Oncology (SIOP) trial. J Clin Oncol 1:604, 1983
26. Li FP, Yan JC, Sallan S, et al: Second neoplasms after Wilms' tumor in childhood. JNCI 71:1205, 1983
27. Meadows AT, Baum E, Fossati-Bellani F, et al: Second malignant neoplasms in children: An update from the Late Effects Study Group. J Clin Oncol 3:532, 1985
28. Mesrobian H, Kelalis PP, Hrabovsky E, et al: Wilms' tumor in horseshoe kidneys: A report of the National Wilms' Tumor Study Group. J Urol 133:1002, 1985
29. Miller RW, Fraumeni JF, Manning MD: Association of Wilms' tumor with aniridia, hemihypertrophy and other congenital malformations. N Engl J Med 270:922, 1964
30. Morris-Jones PH: Medical Research Council's working party on embryonal tumors in childhood: Management of nephroblastoma in childhood. Arch Dis Child 53:112, 1979
31. Palmer NF, Evans AE: The association of aniridia and Wilms' tumor: Methods of surveillance and diagnosis. Med Pediatr Oncol 11:73, 1983
32. Pastore GD, Carli M, Lemerle J, et al: Epidemiological features of Wilms' tumor: Results of studies by the International Society of Pediatric Oncology (SIOP). Med Pediatr Oncol 16:7, 1988
33. Pendergrass TW: Congenital anomalies in children with Wilms' tumor: A new survey. Cancer 37:403, 1976
34. Penumetcha SR, Breslow NE, Koepsell T: Paternal occupation as a possible factor for Wilms' tumor. Cancer Res Bull 1:4, 1984
35. Perez CA, Kaiman HA, Keith J, et al: Treatment of Wilms' tumor and factors affecting prognosis. Cancer 32:609, 1973
36. Ragab AH, Vietti TJ, Crist W, et al: Bilateral Wilms' tumor: A review. Cancer 30:983, 1972
37. Raney RB, Palmer NF, Sutow WW, et al: Renal cell carcinoma in children. Med Pediatr Oncol 11:91, 1983
38. Reiman TAH: Siegel MJ, Shackleford GD: Wilms' tumor in children: Abdominal CT and US evaluation. Radiology 160:501, 1986
39. Sandstedt BE, Delemarre JFM, Harms D, et al: Wilms' tumour with clear cells and hyalinazation: A study of 38 tumours in children from the SIOP nephroblastoma file. Histopathology 11:273, 1987
40. Silverman CL, Thomas PRM, McAlister WH, et al: Slipped femoral capital epiphyses in irradiated children: Dose, volume and age relationships. Int J Radiat Oncol Biol Phys 7:1357, 1981
41. Strong LC: Genetic and hereditary aspects of Wilms' tumor. In Pochedly C, Miller D (eds): Wilms' Tumor, pp 65–77. New York, John Wiley & Sons, 1975
42. Suharochana K, Tolentino W, Ketsewetter WB: Wilms' tumor and hypertension. J Pediatr Surg 7:573, 1972
43. Thomas PRM, Griffith KD, Fineberg BB, et al: Late effects of treatment for Wilms' tumor. Int J Radiat Oncol Biol Phys 9:651, 1983
44. Thomas PRM, Tefft M, Farewell VT, et al: Abdominal relapses in the Second National Wilms' Tumor Study patients. J Clin Oncol 2:1098, 1984
45. Wilimas JA, Douglass EC, Magill HL, et al: Significance of pulmonary computed tomography at diagnosis in Wilms' tumor. J Clin Oncol 6:1144, 1988
46. Wilkins JR, Sinks TH: Occupational exposures among fathers of children with Wilms' tumor. J Occup Med 26:427, 1984
47. Young JL, Miller RW: Incidence of malignant tumors in US children. J Pediatr 86:254, 1975

71

Neuroblastoma

Patrick R.M. Thomas

Despite recent progress and optimism, treatment of neuroblastoma has remained problematic. Disseminated disease is often fatal, and dissemination at diagnosis is much more common in neuroblastoma (70%) than in Wilms' tumor (20%).[13] At Washington University, in a series of 119 patients treated between 1949 and 1978, only 32 (26.8%) had Stage 1 or Stage 2 disease.[49] However, recent advances in the treatment of younger patients and the identification of biologic markers have increased our understanding of the disease and currently present a more encouraging picture.

EPIDEMIOLOGY

Many neuroblastomas are clinically apparent at birth, and there may be associated congenital defects.[38] Neuroblastomas show nonrandom deletions of the short arm of chromosome 1 in approximately 70% of the patients, and in 20%, the long arm of chromosome 1 and 17 may be abnormal.[23] It may be that some neuroblastomas should be considered as anomalies of development consistent with Knudson's two-hit hypothesis.[32]

NATURAL HISTORY

Neuroblastoma, along with ganglioneuroma and ganglioneuroblastoma, may arise initially from any site along the craniospinal axis because the origin of the tumor is from the neural crest. In a composite series, approximately 33% of all neuroblastomas were found to arise from the adrenal medulla and 55% from all nonpelvic abdominal sites. The pelvis accounted for 25%, the thorax for 13%, and the head and neck for 7%.[21]

Neuroblastoma is the most common malignant tumor in early childhood and possesses unusual features. It has the highest spontaneous remission rate of any neoplasm in humans, usually by maturation to ganglioneuroma.[20] Microscopic neuroblastomas have been found in the autopsy material of the adrenal glands of young infants at more than 40 times the expected rate of occurrence. It has been suggested that most potential neuroblastomas are never clinically manifested because of spontaneous regression.[2] Despite these peculiarities, neuroblastoma is frequently a progressive, relentless disease, spreading by lymph nodes and the bloodstream.

CLINICAL PRESENTATION

Clinical manifestations may be related to the primary tumor abdominal mass, spinal cord symptoms to a dumbbell-shaped tumor, or to metastases (*e.g.*, bone pain, bony swelling, or hepatomegaly). Metastatic neuroblastoma has a predilection for bones of the skull. Orbital swelling or proptosis is a common presenting sign. Widespread neuroblastomas may produce nonspecific symptoms,such as weight loss, failure to thrive, fever, or pallor caused by anemia.

DIAGNOSTIC WORKUP

The specific workup depends on the location of the tumor. Thus, a suspected abdominal neuroblastoma requires investigations of the site of the mass, which is frequently palpable. The plain radiograph may show a calcified mass. An intravenous pyelogram usually differentiates a Wilms' tumor from an adrenal neuroblastoma (Fig. 71-1). Presacral neuroblastomas may also cause extrinsic pressure on the bladder and therefore be demonstrable on intravenous pyleogram. Computed tomography (CT) is invaluable in defining the extent of abdominal and other tumors. Magnetic resonance imaging (MRI) can accurately delineate disease before surgery.[11]

Thoracic neuroblastomas, which arise in the posterior mediastinum, may appear with symptoms and signs of spinal cord compression because of tumor extension through an intervertebral foramen (*i.e.*, dumbbell tumor). Thoracic neuroblastomas are usually well demonstrated on routine radiographs, CT, and MRI. Myelography or spinal MRI is often indicated in suspected spinal canal involvement.

Above the clavicle, the tumor most commonly involves one of the sympathetic ganglia or the olfactory bulb. A tumor of the cervical sympathetic ganglia usually presents as a neck mass, and Horner's syndrome may be present with only a small mass that might otherwise not be detectable. The site of the tumor is best delineated with a CT scan. Neuroblastoma of the olfactory bulb is known as esthesioneuroblastoma and is more common in adults.

All patients with neuroblastoma should be investigated for metastases. A complete blood count is usually normal with a localized tumor, but pancytopenia or lowering of one or more of the blood cell counts suggests metastases in the absence of other

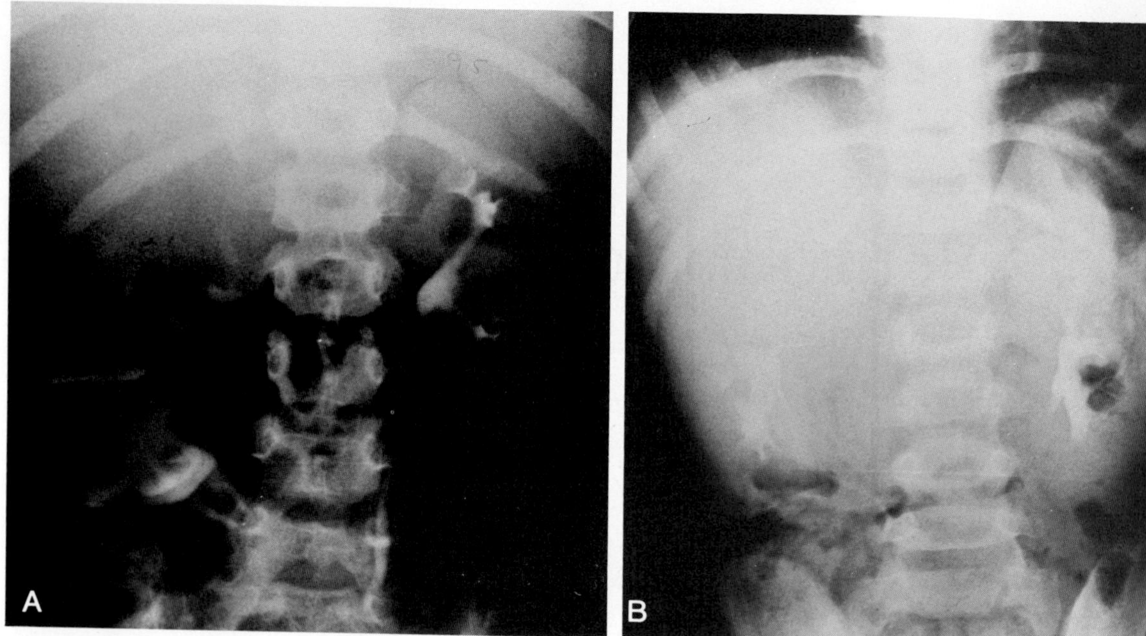

FIGURE 71–1. Intravenous pyelograms of (**A**) Wilms' tumor and (**B**) adrenal neuroblastoma. (**A**) Notice the enlargement of the right kidney, with an abnormal caliceal pattern and (**B**) the displacement of an otherwise normal right kidney, downward and laterally.

causes. Bone marrow examination is also mandatory, especially because metastases may be demonstrated in patients with normal blood counts and normal bone scans. Characteristically, the cells appear in clumps (pseudorosettes), but the absence of pseudorosettes does not eliminate the possibility of neuroblastoma. Electron microscopy may help to discriminate neuroblastoma cells from other tumors involving the marrow.[35]

Because neuroblastoma has a predilection for bony metastases, a skeletal survey and radionuclide bone scan are mandatory investigations. A bone scan may offer the only evidence of bone involvement. Other sites of metastases are lymph nodes, liver, and skin. Radioimaging of all metastatic sites can be achieved with ^{131}I-metaiodobenzylguanidine (MIBG). The overall sensitivity is about 90%.[50] Liver function tests and radionuclide liver scans should be performed routinely.

All patients with neuroblastoma should have measurements of the urinary catecholamine levels. In a pooled series, 82% of 320 patients had elevated levels of vanillylmandelic acid.[21] The standard method is the 24-hour collection, but a rapid bedside screening diagnostic test is also available.[24] The results of the two tests correlate well. A patient may present with symptoms and signs similar to those of pheochromocytoma because of catecholamine production. These include flushing, headaches, and tachycardia.

A human cellular DNA sequence related to the c-*myc* protooncogene, called n-*myc,* is selectively amplified in human neuroblastoma.[47] Monoclonal antibodies and serum neuron-specific enolase are also being investigated.[47,52]

A summary of the clinical findings and the diagnostic workup are shown in Table 71-1.

STAGING

The most frequently used staging system is that devised by Evans and colleagues (Table 71-2) based on extent of disease at diagnosis.[16] Alternative surgical systems have been devised by St. Jude's Hospital and the Pediatric Oncology Group (POG) (Table 71-3).[40,51] A recently published international staging system (Table 71-4) incorporates much of the older systems.[5]

PATHOLOGIC CLASSIFICATION

The tumors are derived from sympathetic ganglia, which originate from primitive neural crest cells and neuroblasts migrating from the mantle layer of the developing spinal cord. Three types of tumor, representing different degrees of differentiation, are recognized.

Ganglioneuroma consists of mature ganglion cells and is benign in appearance and nature. It is frequently calcified. It has been suggested that all ganglioneuromas are matured neuroblastomas.[51] Cases of maturation, spontaneously or after therapy, of proven neuroblastomas to ganglioneuromas have been reported.[20]

Ganglioneuroblastoma is the intermediate form between glangioneuroma and neuroblastoma. Both mature ganglion cells and undifferentiated neuroblasts are evident; the proportion may vary from one part of the tumor to another.

Neuroblastoma is at the undifferentiated end of the spectrum and may have no recognizable form, consisting of small round cells with darkly staining nuclei. Frequently, rosettes can be seen and characteristic neurofibrils identified. Hemorrhage can occur in the tumor, and calcification is common.

PROGNOSTIC FACTORS

Prognostic factors are crucial to the understanding and management of this disease. Stage, age at diagnosis, histology, tumor site, and biologic markers are all important prognostic variables.[7,9,40]

Multivariate analyses of groups of patients with neuroblastoma have demonstrated that stage of the cancer at diag-

TABLE 71–1
Clinical Findings and Diagnostic Workup

COMPONENT	SYMPTOMS	EXAMINATION	USEFUL INVESTIGATIONS
Primary Tumor			
Abdominal	Abdominal pain Motor or sensory changes Pain in back or legs Urinary tract or bowel dysfunction	Mass palpable Neurologic defects (spinal or peripheral nerve)	Plain x-ray films Intravenous pyelogram CT scan, MR scan Myelogram
Thoracic	Pain in back or legs Motor or sensory changes Urinary tract or bowel dysfunction	Mass palpable Neurologic defects (spinal or peripheral nerve)	Chest x-ray film CT scan, MR scan Myelogram
	Dypsnea Tightness in chest Swelling of face	Signs of tracheal or bronchial obstruction Superor vena cava syndrome	Venogram
Cervical	Mass noticeable	Palpable mass Horner's syndrome	Base-of-skull x-rays CT scan
Nasal	Nose pain Obstructed sinusitis	Tenderness Superior cranial nerve signs Mass	CT scan Sinus views
Metastases	General malaise Bone pain Enlarging abdomen Liver failure Skin of subcutaneous nodules Enlarging masses	Pallor Ecchymoses Tenderness Deformities Hepatomegaly Ascites Nodules Palpable lymph nodes	Complete blood count Bone marrow examination Bone scan Skeletal survey Liver scan Liver function tests Biopsy CT scan ^{131}I MIBG scan
Secretions of Tumor	Headaches Flushing Sweating Palpitations	Tachycardia Hypertension	Urinary catecholamines
Tumor Markers			n-*myc* amplification Monoclonal antibodies Serum neuron-specific enolase Serum ferritin

TABLE 71–2
Evans Staging of Neuroblastoma

STAGE	DESCRIPTION
I	Tumor confined to the organ or structure of origin
II	Tumors extending in continuity beyond the organ or structure of origin but not crossing the midline Regional lymph nodes on the homolateral side may be involved*
III	Tumors extending in continuity beyond the midline Regional lymph node groups may be involved bilaterally
IV	Remote disease involving skeleton, organs, soft tissues, or distant lymph node groups
IV-S	Patients who would otherwise be Stage I or II but who have remote disease confined only to one or more of the following sites: liver, skin, or bone marrow (without radiographic evidence of bone metastases on complete bone survey)

** For tumors arising in a midline structure, penetration beyond the capsule and involvement of lymph nodes on the same side shall be considered Stage II.*
(Evans AE, D'Angio GJ, Randolph J: Cancer 27:374, 1971)

TABLE 71–3
Pediatric Oncology Group Staging for Neuroblastoma

STAGE	DESCRIPTION
Stage A	Complete gross resection of primary tumor, with or without microscopic residual; intracavitary lymph nodes, not adhered to and removed with primary (nodes adhered to or within tumor resection may be positive for tumor without upstaging patient to Stage C). If primary in abdomen or pelvis, liver is histologically free of tumor.
Stage B	Grossly unresected primary tumor; nodes and liver same as Stage A
Stage C	Complete or incomplete resection of primary; intracavitary nodes not adherent to primary histologically positive for tumor; liver as in Stage A
Stage D	Any dissemination of disease beyond intracavitary nodes (*i.e.*, extracavitary nodes, liver, skin, bone marrow, bone)
Stage D (S)	Evans stage IV-S

(Nitschke R, Smith R, Shochat S, et al: J Clin Oncol 6:1271, 1988)

TABLE 71–4
International Staging System for Neuroblastoma

STAGE	DESCRIPTION
Stage 1	Localized tumor confined to the area of origin; complete gross excision, with or without microscopic residual disease; identifiable ipsilateral and contralateral lymph nodes negative microscopically
Stage 2A	Unilateral tumor with incomplete gross excision; identifiable ipsilateral and contralateral lymph nodes negative microscopically
Stage 2B	Unilateral tumor with complete or incomplete gross excision; with positive ipsilateral regional lymph nodes; identifiable contralateral lymph nodes negative microscopically
Stage 3	Tumor infiltrating across the midline with or without regional lymph node involvement; or unilateral tumor with contralateral regional lymph node involvement; or midline tumor with bilateral regional lymph node involvement
Stage 4	Dissemination of tumor to distant lymph nodes, bone, bone marrow, liver, or other organs (except as defined in Stage 4-S).
Stage 4-S	Localized primary tumor as defined for Stages 1 or 2 with dissemination limited to liver, skin, or bone marrow

(Brodeur GM, Seeger RC, Barrett A, et al: J Clin Oncol 6:1874, 1988)

nosis is the most important prognostic variable.[10,13,49] Oncogenes are also highly prognostic, as are other markers, such as serum ferritin and neuron-specific enolase.[6,12,47]

The Stage 4-S (IV-S) subgroup, as described by Evans and co-workers,[16] is important because the prognosis is usually good and the temptation to treat vigorously should be avoided. These are patients, usually younger than 1 year of age, who would otherwise be classified as having Stage 1 or Stage 2 disease but who have evidence of metastases (often massive) to the liver and sometimes to the skin and bone marrow. Patients with large primary tumors or frank bone metastases must be excluded, whatever their age. Stage 4-S tumors have an excellent chance of spontaneous maturation and may require no treatment at all, although not all patients survive with minimal or no treatment.[19,46] Most patients with Stage 4-S disease have only a single copy of n-*myc*, and those who have multiple copies may have a worse prognosis.[9] It is becoming evident that Stage 4-S, along with Stages 1 and 2, can be regarded as biologically different from the aggressive Stages 3 and 4.

Age is an independent prognostic variable.[4] In general, the younger the patient, the better the prognosis, stage for stage. However, it has been suggested that the prognosis improves if the patient is older than 6 years.[22]

Histology is an important prognostic variable, with ganglioneuroblastomas being more favorable lesions than neuroblastomas.[49] Although the site of the tumor has less independent prognostic significance than the other variables, abdominal primary tumors (particularly adrenal) fare worse than thoracic neuroblastomas. Gender does not seem to have any prognostic effect.[10,49]

At St. Jude's Hospital, the prognostic significance of involved lymph nodes that are separated from the main mass of tumor has been reported, but results from the Sidney Farber Cancer Center do not confirm this finding.[26,44]

GENERAL MANAGEMENT

The overriding problem in the general management of neuroblastoma is the treatment of metastases; the therapy of the local tumor by surgery or radiation therapy is, however, important in a small but curable minority of patients. If the tumor is apparently localized and resectable, complete excision with surgical staging should be performed, including a biopsy of local lymph nodes and inspection of neural foramina. In one series of abdominal neuroblastomas, nine (90%) of ten patients with Stage 1 disease survived for at least 2 years.[33]

Radiation therapy is not indicated if complete tumor excision is confirmed by the pathologist. It is also of doubtful value in Stage 2 tumors with or without residual disease in children younger than 1 year of age. In the surgical series, all three patients younger than 1 year of age with Stage 2 abdominal neuroblastomas were disease free with a follow-up of at least 2 years, but none of the five patients older than 2 years of age with Stage 2 disease survived, suggesting a role for postoperative irradiation.[33] However, the need for postoperative irradiation in this group of patients has been recently questioned.[17,36,37]

The management of Stage 3 neuroblastoma presents problems. The condition is relatively uncommon (*i.e.*, 10% of the Washington University series), and it appears that the combination of radiation therapy and chemotherapy may be warranted because local and distant relapses are possible.[49] The use of second-look surgery and excision of residual disease after chemotherapy also need to be evaluated.

Stage 4 neuroblastoma (exclusive of Stage 4-S) remains one of the most depressing situations in pediatric oncology, although there is now some cause for optimism. The disease has been the most common presenting form (52% of the Washington University patients), and the survival rate (6%) was grim.[49] It has been demonstrated that combination chemotherapy can produce responses in 70% or more of patients, and this should be the principal mode of therapy. Recent results from the Dana Farber Cancer Center suggest that cures can be obtained with aggressive therapy for Stage 4 patients younger than 1 year of age.[34]

The value of radiation therapy for symptomatic relief should not be underestimated, because supportive and palliative approaches are frequently necessary. The use of ^{131}I-MIBG and bone marrow transplantation for treating metastasis is under investigation.[41,45] Multiple copies of the n-*myc* oncogene probably indicates that more aggressive therapy is indicated than if a single copy is identified.[47]

RADIATION THERAPY TECHNIQUES

Because no clinical trials of radiation therapy in neuroblastomas comparing field size or dosages have been performed, it is necessary to use retrospective analysis alone to determine the optimal radiation therapy. The task is complicated by the variability of prognosis with age and the propensity for maturation of the tumor. In children, it is particularly appropriate to consider that a small gain in tumor control could be offset by a greater complication rate.

In general, it is necessary to encompass the entire tumor bed with at least a 2-cm margin. This allows for slight variation in setup and for subclinical disease. Whole-abdominal irradiation is now seldom used, because patients with Stage 3 disease usually also receive aggressive myelosuppressive chemotherapy.

Because neuroblastoma is relatively responsive to irradiation, it is the treatment of choice for painful bony metastases and orbital lesions. Portals should cover the entire lesion (or orbit) with at least a 2-cm margin.

Special situations in treating neuroblastomas are worthy of more detailed consideration.

Paraspinal neuroblastomas frequently are incompletely excised. Radiation therapy to a generous volume (at least 2-cm margin from all known tumor) is often indicated. Myelography, CT, and MRI may assist in determining the extent, especially when the surgeon has not attempted to remove the tumor. Often a single posterior photon field suffices, because the dose gradient is not great. In extensive lesions, a wedged pair of fields or a combination of photons and electrons may give a better dose distribution. At present, these patients sometimes receive a trial of chemotherapy at diagnosis.

Olfactory neuroblastomas occur in adults and arise in the upper part of the nasal cavity. The management of the patient with tumor confined to the nasal cavity can be with irradiation or surgery alone; in the advanced stages a combination of both modalities is preferred but is less likely to be successful.[27] The treatment methods described in Chapter 29 are appropriate.

Total-body irradiation has been used in many situations in neuroblastoma. Recently, it has usually been as part of a preparatory regimen for bone marrow transplantation. In one report, the autologous bone marrow was purged using an immunomagnetic procedures, and the preparatory regimen consisted of induction with cisplatin, etoposide, and cyclophosphamide, followed by surgery, vincristine, melphalan, and 1200 cGy in six fractions given twice daily.[31,41] The initial results of a 2-year survival rate of 39% for Stage IV patients were promising, but good results have also been reported with a polychemotherapy preparatory regimen without total-body irradiation.[25]

Preoperative irradiation can sometimes be applied with good effect to make unresectable lesions resectable.

The "ideal" dose for neuroblastoma is unknown; however, there is evidence that the response to dose may depend on patient age.[28] Infants may require only 1200 cGy for local control, but local failures were observed with doses up to 4500 cGy in patients 3 years of age or older. A study of postoperative irradiation from the University of Florida is in general agreement with these dose levels, as is the Washington University series.[29,49] Palliative effects can often be achieved with a single fraction of 500 cGy; however, if the patient is not immediately terminal, a course of five fractions of 300 cGy each may be preferable.

For olfactory neuroblastoma (esthesioneuroblastoma), higher doses should be used as tolerated. Advanced lesions, may recur locally with doses greater than 6000 cGy given in 6 to 7 weeks, although overall results with these doses are good.[1]

RESULTS OF THERAPY

Although there are numerous prognostic indicators other than stage, it is simpler to consider it as the principal variable in discussing results. Even stage has been made more complicated, because different reports tend to use different staging systems.

Stage 1

The results of treatment for Stage 1 disease with surgery alone are uniformly good, and it is clear that there is no role for adjuvant irradiation or chemotherapy. Koop and Schnaufer[33] from Children's Hospital of Philadelphia reported that nine of ten patients survived with surgical excision alone, and the Children's Cancer Study Group (CCSG) reported no recurrences among 27 patients, although some patients with incompletely excised lesions received irradiation.[14] POG, using their own surgical staging system (Table 71-3), reported a 2-year disease-free survival rate of 89% for 101 Stage A patients.[40]

Stage 2

The results for Stage 2 patients are very good with surgical excision and postoperative irradiation, although the value of radiation therapy is doubtful. The CCSG studied by questionnaire 156 patients with Evans Stage II neuroblastoma and found a progression-free survival rate of 90% and an overall 5-year survival rate of 96%.[36] Neither the extent of resection nor the dose of adjuvant irradiation or chemotherapy was a significant factor because 75 patients had surgery alone. These results confirm earlier studies with smaller numbers of patients.[17,37]

Stage 3

Patients with Stage 3 disease are among the most difficult to manage because they often have large, bulky primary tumors that tend to metastasize early and widely. All three modalities are often used to their fullest, with chemotherapy given after initial biopsy or surgical debulking (completed excision is seldom achieved). Second-look surgery may be attempted, followed by radiation therapy to tolerance. Results using such programs are largely anecdotal at present, but the POG study for Stage C patients 1 year or older at diagnosis currently reports that the addition of local and nodal radiation therapy to cyclophosphamide and doxorubicin is of significant benefit for response, survival, and event-free survival ($P>0.05$).[7]

Stage 4

Although cures are still rare in Stage 4 patients older than 1 year of age, aggressive therapy for infants has achieved a few cures.[34,43] Many agents are active in neuroblastoma, including vincristine, cyclophosphamide, doxorubicin, teniposide, etoposide, and cisplatin. The POG protocols 8104 and 8441 show that complete remission rates of about 35% can be expected with a combination of cyclophosphamide plus doxorubicin, platinum plus teniposide (VM-26), or all four drugs combined. Adding partial remissions, an 80% response rate was achieved with four drugs, significantly better than with either two-drug combination.[42]

Because most patients with Stage 4 neuroblastoma ultimately relapse, attempts are being made to improve survival by intensification with bone marrow transplantation or methods like ^{131}I-MIBG.[25,41,45] Although the results are preliminary, they can be regarded as encouraging.

Stage 4-S

Results of therapy for Stage 4-S disease are essentially irrelevant because of its natural history. The early experience of Bodian[3] with vitamin B_{12} was largely in children with Stage 4-S disease.

More aggressive therapy was used at Washington University with good survival; 12 (86%) of 14 lived 2 years or more.[48] However, the CCSG surveyed 35 Stage 4-S patients and found a disease-free survival rate of 97%. Seven of these patients received no treatment.[39]

SEQUELAE OF TREATMENT

Early Complications

The standard short-term complications of radiation therapy are those that could be expected for a child and for the tissues irradiated. The immediate toxic effect of the chemotherapy is that of the agent used. If irradiation and chemotherapy are employed simultaneously, great care must be taken, as exemplified in Figure 71-2.

Late Complications

The long-term effects of irradiation and chemotherapy are just beginning to be appreciated. The complications observed in the Washington University series are presented in Table 71-5.[49] Two of these patients died free of disease. The long-term complications of aggressive management of advanced disease will be manifested as survival improves.

SUMMARY OF CLINICAL TRIALS

Randomized clinical trials have only recently contributed to our knowledge of neuroblastomas. The CCSG study of adjuvant oral cyclophosphamide for Stage 1, 2, and 3 failed to show an advantage for the treated patients.[15] A later CCSG study of three-drug chemotherapy was also negative.[18] POG studies were discussed earlier.[7,42,44]

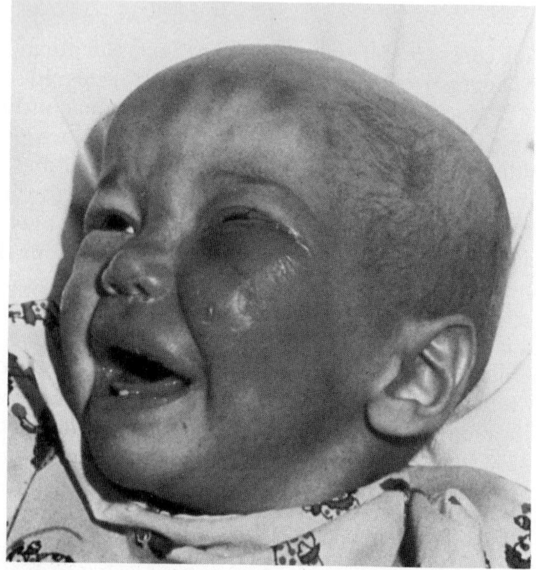

FIGURE 71–2. Fourteen-month-old child with disseminated neuroblastoma involving the left orbit and maxilla. A severe reaction occurred after irradiation with 1500 cGy and 2 days after cyclophosmamide (1500 mg/m²).

TABLE 71–5
Washington University Neuroblastoma Study of Long-Term Sequelae Related to Radiation Therapy

COMPLICATION	NO. OF PATIENTS	DOSE (cGy)
Scoliosis (mild)	6	800–3000
Scoliosis (severe)	6	1600–3700
Muscle hypoplasia	3	2800–3000
Bone hypoplasia	4	2800–3000
Breast hypoplasia	5	2800–3000
Kidney hypoplasia	2	3000–3300
Pulmonary hypoplasia	3	2800–3000
Lung fibrosis	1	4800–(possibly fatal)
Liver fibrosis	1	3950–(fatal)
Rib necrosis	1	4800
Thyroid adenocarcinoma	1	2000
Chondrosarcoma	1	2000
Cataracts	1	2000
Hypopituitarism	1	2000
Urinary tract infection	1	2000
Thyroid adenoma	1	1800
Total	38	

REFERENCES

1. Ahmad K, Fayos JV: Role of radiation therapy in the treatment of olfactory neuroblastoma. Int J Radiat Oncol Biol Phys 63:49, 1980
2. Beckwith JB, Perrin EV: In situ neuroblastomas: A contribution to the natural history of neural crest tumors. Am J Pathol 43:1089, 1963
3. Bodian M: Neuroblastoma. Pediatr Clin North Am 6:449, 1959
4. Breslow N, McCann B: Statistical estimation of prognosis for children with neuroblastoma. Can Res J 31:1098, 1971
5. Brodeur GM, Seeger RC, Barrett A, et al: International criteria for diagnosis, staging and response to treatment in patients with neuroblastoma. J Clin Oncol 6:1874, 1988
6. Brodeur GM, Seeger RC, Sather H, et al: Clinical implications of oncogene activation in human neuroblastoma. Cancer 58:541, 1986
7. Castleberry R, Kun L, Shuster J, et al: Radiotherapy improves the outlook for children older than one year with POG stage C neuroblastoma. Proc Am Soc Clin Oncol 1158:297, 1989
8. Chatten J, Voorhess ML: Familial neuroblastoma. N Engl J Med 227:1230, 1967
9. Cohn SL, Herst CV, Maurer HS, et al: N-*myc* amplification in an infant with stage IVS neuroblastoma. J Clin Oncol 5:1441, 1987
10. Coldman AJ, Fryer CJH, Elwood JM, et al: Neuroblastoma: Influence of age at diagnosis, stage, tumor site, and sex on prognosis. Cancer 46:1896, 1980
11. Dietrich RB, Kangarloo H, Lenarsky C, et al: Neuroblastoma: The role of MR imaging. Am J Radiol 148:937, 1987
12. Evans AE, D'Angio GJ, Propert K, et al: Prognostic factors in neuroblastoma. Cancer 59:1853, 1987
13. Evans AE: Staging and treatment of neuroblastoma. Cancer 45:1799, 1980
14. Evans AE, Albo V, D'Angio GJ, et al: Factors influencing survival of children with nonmetastatic neuroblastoma. Cancer 38:661, 1976
15. Evans AE, Albo V, D'Angio GJ, et al: Cyclophosphamide treatment of patients with localized and regional neuroblastoma. Cancer 38:655, 1976
16. Evans AE, D'Angio GJ, Randolph J: A proposed staging for children with neuroblastoma. Cancer 27:374, 1971
17. Evans AE, D'Angio GJ, Koop CE: The role of multimodal

therapy in patients with local and reginal neuroblastoma. J Pediatr Surg 19:77, 1984

18. Evans AE, Brand W, de Lorimier A: Results in children with local-regional neuroblastoma managed with and without vincristine, cyclophosphamide and imidazole carbxamide. Am J Clin Oncol 6:3, 1984
19. Evans AE, Chatten J, D'Angio GJ, et al: A review of 17 IV-S neuroblastoma patients at the Children's Hospital of Philadelphia. Cancer 45:833, 1980
20. Everson EC, Cole WH: Spontaneous Regression of Cancer, pp 88–163, Philadelphia, WB Saunders, 1966
21. Fernbach DJ, Williams TE, Donaldson MH: Neuroblastoma. In Sutow WW, Vietti TJ, Fernbach DJ (eds): Clinical Pediatric Oncology, 2nd ed, pp 506–537. St. Louis, CV Mosby, 1977
22. Finkelstein JZ, Klemperer MR, Evans AE, et al: Multiagent chemotherapy for children with metastatic neuroblastoma: A report from the Children's Cancer Study Group. Med Pediatr Oncol 6:179, 1979
23. Gilbert F, Feder M, Balaban G, et al: Human neuroblastomas and abnormalities of chromosomes 1 and 17. Cancer Res 44:5444, 1984
24. Gitlow SE, Bertani LM, Rausen A, et al: Diagnosis of neuroblastoma by qualitative and quantitative metabolites in urine. Cancer 25:1377, 1970
25. Hartmann O, Benhamou E, Beaujean F, et al: Repeated high-dose chemotherapy followed by purged autologous bone marrow transplantation as consolidation therapy in metastatic neuroblastoma. J Clin Oncol 5:1205, 1987
26. Hayes FA, Hustu HO, Green AA: Surgicopathologic staging of neuroblastoma: Prognostic significance of regional lymph node metastases. Pediatrics 102:59, 1982
27. Homzie MJ, Elkon D: Olfactory esthesioneuroblastoma: Variables predictive of tumor control and recurrence. Cancer 46:2509, 1980
28. Jacobson GM, Sause WT, O'Brien RT: Dose-response analysis of pediatric neuroblastoma to megavoltage irradiation. Am J Clin Oncol 7:693, 1984
29. Jacobson HM, Marcus RB, Thar TL: Pediatric neuroblastoma: Postoperative radiation therapy using less than 2000 rad. Int J Radiat Oncol Biol Phys 9:501, 1983
30. Kemshead JT, Lashford LS, Garson J, et al: Neuroblastoma: New approaches to diagnosis. Cancer Surv 6:227, 1987
31. Kemshead JT, Treleaven JG, Gibson FM, et al: Monoclonal antibodies and magnetic microspheres for the depletion of magnetic cells from bone marrow. In Dicke KA, Spitzer G, Zander AT (eds): Autologous Bone Marrow Transplantation, pp 409–414. Houston, University of Texas, 1985
32. Knudson AG: Hereditary cancer, oncogenes and antioncogenes. Cancer Res 45:1437, 1985
33. Koop CE, Schnaufer L: The management of abdominal neuroblastoma. Cancer 35:905, 1975
34. Kretschmar CS, Frantz CN, Rosen EM, et al: Improved prognosis for infants with stage IV neuroblastoma. J Clin Oncol 2:799, 1984
35. Mackay B, Masse SR, King OY, et al: Diagnosis of neuroblastoma by electron microscopy of bone marrow aspirates. Pediatrics 56:1045, 1975
36. Matthay KM, Sather HN, Seeger RC, et al: Excellent outcome of stage II neuroblastoma is independent of residual disease and radiation therapy. J Clin Oncol 7:236, 1989
37. McGuire WA, Simmons D, Grosfeld JL, et al: Stage II neuroblastoma: Does adjuvant irradiation contribute to cure? Med Pediatr Oncol 13:117, 1985
38. Miller RW, Fraumeni JF, Hill JA: Neuroblastoma: Epidemiologic approach to its origin. Am J Dis Child 115:253, 1968
39. Nickerson HJ, Nesbit ME, Grosfeld JL, et al: Comparison of stage IV and IV-S neuroblastoma in the first year of life. Med Pediatr Oncol 13:261, 1985
40. Nitschke R, Smith EI, Shochat S, et al: Localized neuroblastoma treated by surgery: A Pediatric Oncology Group Study. J Clin Oncol 6:1271, 1988
41. Philip T, Bernard JL, Zucker JM, et al: High-dose chemoradiotherapy with bone marrow transplantation as consolidation treatment in neuroblastoma: An unselected group of stage IV patients over 1 year of age. J Clin Oncol 5:266, 1987
42. POG 8104 and POG 8441. Unpublished data
43. Rosen EM, Cassady JR, Frantz CN, et al: Neuroblastoma: The Joint Center for Radiation Therapy/Dana Farber Cancer Institute/Children's Hospital experience. J Clin Oncol 2:719, 1984
44. Rosen EM, Cassady JR, Kretschmar C, et al: Influence of locoregional lymph node metastases on prognosis in neuroblastoma. Med Pediatr Oncol 12:260, 1984
45. Schwabe D, Sahm S, Gerein V, et al: ^{131}I-meta-iodobenzylguanidine therapy of neuroblastoma in childhood. Eur J Pediatr 146:246, 1987
46. Schwartz AD, Dadas-Zadeh M, Lee H, et al: Spontaneous regression of disseminated neuroblastoma. J Pediatr 85:760, 1974
47. Seeger RC, Brodeur GM, Sather H, et al: Association of multiple copies of the N-*myc* oncogene with rapid progression of neuroblastomas. N Engl J Med 31:1111, 1985
48. Stokes SH, Thomas PRM, Perez CA, et al: Stage IV-S neuroblastoma results with definitive therapy. Cancer 53:2084, 1984
49. Thomas PRM, Lee JY, Vietti TJ, et al: An analysis of neuroblastoma at a single institution. Cancer 63:3079, 1984
50. Voute PA, Hoefnagel CA, De Kraker J: ^{131}I-meta-iodobenzylguanidine in diagnosis and treatment of neuroblastoma. Bull Cancer 75:107, 1988
51. Willis RA: The Pathology of Tumors in Children, pp 7–17. Springfield, IL, Charles C Thomas, 1962
52. Zeltzer PM, Marangos PJ, Evans AE, et al: Serum neuron-specific enolase in children with neuroblastoma. Cancer 57:1230, 1986

72

○ ○ ○ • • •

Rhabdomyosarcoma

Sarah S. Donaldson

ANATOMY

Rhabdomyosarcoma is a highly malignant soft tissue sarcoma that can arise in any site in the body containing striated muscle or its mesenchymal anlage. The most frequently involved site is the head and neck (37%). Genitourinary sites account for 21% of tumors. The trunk and retroperitoneum represent 15%, and the extremities are the sites of 20%.[10]

EPIDEMIOLOGY

Soft tissue sarcomas in childhood are rare, accounting for a U.S. annual incidence of 8.4 per million whites and 3.9 per million blacks.[71] Among these, rhabdomyosarcoma is the most common, with an annual incidence of 4.4 per million whites and 1.3 per million blacks.[71]

Rhabdomyosarcoma most commonly occurs in the childhood and adolescent years, with two peak age frequencies: one between ages 2 and 6, the second in adolescence. There is a slight male predominance of 1.1 to 1.9, which does not appear to carry prognostic significance.[54]

Although the cause of rhabdomyosarcoma is unknown, it is associated with disorders in development. In an autopsy study, 75% of the children entered onto Intergroup Rhabdomyosarcoma (IRS) protocols were found to have central nervous system, genitourinary, gastrointestinal, or cardiovascular anomalies.[61] Rhabdomyosarcoma is associated with several congenital disorders, including neurofibromatosis and basal cell nevus syndrome.[2,48] Small groups of families have been described with an increased frequency of breast cancer in the relatives of children with rhabdomyosarcoma.[5,40,41] Other familial associations include a higher incidence of rhabdomyosarcoma in siblings of children with adrenocortical carcinoma, brain tumors, or other sarcomas.[40,42,52]

Genetic factors appear to play a role in rhabdomyosarcoma. Cytogenetic studies show a consistent chromosomal translocation between chromosomes 2 and 13 and chromosomes 2 and 11 in children with rhabdomyosarcoma.[10,14,63,64,70] Although investigation of the genetics of rhabdomyosarcoma is in its infancy, it is likely that cytogenetics will soon be used to confirm diagnoses, particularly for difficult-to-classify tumors.

NATURAL HISTORY

Rhabdomyosarcoma is a locally invasive tumor, often with a pseudocapsule, and has the potential for direct extension along fascial or muscle planes. The risk of lymphatic and hematogenous spread is common and varies as a function of the site of the primary lesion. The incidence of lymphatic extension has been underestimated. It is recognized that lymph node metastases are rare if tumors are confined to the orbit, but they may occur in approximately 15% of the cases with tumors at other head and neck sites, most commonly the nasopharynx. Accounting for staging inaccuracies, regional lymph node metastases occur in at least 24% of children with genitourinary tumors, in 40% of those with paratesticular primary tumors, and in 20% of patients with extremity and truncal primary tumors.[57] Routine bipedal lymphography performed for patients with tumors in subdiaphragmatic sites indicates that more than half of the lymphograms are positive, most commonly among those with lower extremity tumors of the alveolar histologic subtype.[3]

Hematogenous metastases are detected at the time of presentation in approximately 20% of patients, particularly those with extremity and truncal primary tumors.[18] The most common sites of hematogenous dissemination are the lungs, bone marrow, bone, liver, brain, distant muscle, and breast.[54]

CLINICAL PRESENTATION

Because rhabdomyosarcoma can occur in virtually any part of the body, there are a variety of clinical signs and symptoms. Rhabdomyosarcoma usually presents as an asymptomatic mass. If symptoms exist, they communicate a mass effect in involved organs and tissues. There may also be pain associated with the primary mass or metastatic disease. Rhabdomyosarcoma spreads by three routes: locally by direct soft tissue extension, by lymphatic extension, and by hematogenous dissemination. Accordingly, the appropriate workup must be dictated by the site of the primary lesion.

DIAGNOSTIC WORKUP

Determination of the extent of the primary tumor is best done with a multidisciplinary approach by a radiation oncologist, pediatric oncologist, and appropriate subspecialty surgeon. Expeditious local and systemic workup is essential, because these tumors have the potential to grow rapidly and cause distressing symptoms. Recommended baseline evaluations are shown in Table 72-1. The initial assessment by all members of the team permits accurate staging of the tumor and the formulation of a uniform treatment plan specific for the patient.

TABLE 72–1
Recommended Workup for Tumors at Various Sites

ALL PATIENTS	OPTIONAL
History	
Physical examination by several observers	Examination under anesthesia in younger children
Laboratory studies	
Complete blood count	
Liver function tests	
Renal function tests	
Urinalysis	
Radiographic studies	
Chest x-ray films	Abdomen-pelvis CT or MRI scan
Chest CT scan	Plain films of bones abnormal on scan
Bone scan	
CT or MRI of primary tumor	
Bone marrow aspirate and biopsy	
HEAD AND NECK	
MRI or CT scan of head and neck	Plain films of area Skull or paranasal sinus films Dental films
Lumbar puncture with cytologic examination of fluid in parameningeal primary tumors	MRI of spine or myelogram if CSF positive or patient is symptomatic
GENITOURINARY	
CT or MRI of abdomen-pelvis Pelvic examination under anesthesia	Ultrasound of abdomen-pelvis Lymphangiogram IVP, voiding cystourethrography, cystoscopy Barium enema Arteriogram Myelogram as indicated
EXTREMITY AND TRUNCAL LESIONS	
MRI or CT with contrast of primary lesion Plain films of primary site	Lymphangiogram IVP for retroperitoneal tumors Ultrasound Arteriogram Barium GI contrast studies

STAGING

Currently there is no universally accepted staging system for rhabdomyosarcoma. The IRS grouping system (Table 72-2) is actually a surgical-pathologic system, primarily based on whether surgical resection is accomplished, with clinical extent of disease a secondary consideration.[45] More recently, a pretreatment clinical TNM (tumor-node-metastasis) staging system, which emphasizes local invasiveness, nodal status, and metastasis, has been proposed.[11] The International Union Against Cancer (UICC) has adopted a similar TNM classification that emphasizes the size of the primary lesion.[22] In retrospective analysis, noninvasiveness, small size, and absence of metastasis have been shown to influence prognosis.[38,53] Furthermore, lymph node involvement correlates closely with invasiveness and large tumor size. Adopting the TNM approach, the IRS investigators now propose a pretreatment staging system that includes TNM, size, and site of primary lesion (Table 72-3).

The site of the primary tumor has been shown previously to affect prognosis.[38,60] In the IRS-IV study, patients are designated as Stage I if the tumor is in a favorable site (*i.e.,* orbit, paratesticular tissue, vagina, uterus, vulva, and head and neck nonparameningeal sites). Stage II tumors are smaller than 5 cm, are localized, and are in unfavorable sites of the genitourinary tract (*i.e.,* bladder and prostate), extremity, parameningeal area, and others. Stage III tumors include those in the same sites as in Stage II that are larger than 5 cm or those smaller than 5 cm with regional lymph node involvement. Stage IV is reserved for tumors that have metastasized.

TABLE 72–2
IRS Clinical Grouping Classification

Group I	Localized disease, completely resected
A	Confined to organ or muscle of origin
B	Infiltration outside organ or muscle of origin; regional nodes not involved
Group II	Compromised or regional resection
A	Grossly resected tumor with microscopic residual disease
B	Regional disease, completely resected, in which nodes may be involved or extension of tumor into adjacent organ may exist
C	Regional disease with involved nodes, grossly resected, but with evidence of microscopic residual disease
Group III	Incomplete resection or biopsy with gross residual disease
Group IV	Distant metastases at diagnosis

(Mauer HM: J Pediatr Surg 10:977, 1975)

TABLE 72–3
IRS Pretreatment Staging System

STAGE	SITE*	INVASIVENESS†	SIZE	NODAL STATUS	METASTASES
I	Favorable	T1 or T2	a or b	N0 or N1	M0
II	Unfavorable	T1 or T2	a	N0	M0
III	Unfavorable	T1 or T2	b	N0	M0
			a or b	N1	M0
IV	Any Site	T1 or T2	a or b	N0 or N1	M1

**Favorable sites: orbit, head and neck (nonparameningeal), genitourinary (non-bladder-prostate); unfavorable sites: genitourinary (bladder-prostate), extremity, parameningeal, other*
† T1: tumor confined to site or organ of origin; T2: regional extension beyond the site or organ of origin; a: 5 cm or less; b: more than 5 cm; N0: no evidence of regional node involvement; N1: evidence of regional node involvement; M0: no distant metastasis; M1: evidence of distant metastasis.

PATHOLOGIC CLASSIFICATION

The histogenesis of rhabdomyosarcoma can be traced from mesoderm to mesenchyme and ultimately to striated muscle tissue. On the basis of gross and histologic appearance, these tumors have been assigned to three histologic categories: embryonal, alveolar, and pleomorphic.[8,30] Sarcoma botryoides, considered the polypoid variant of embryonal rhabdomyosarcoma, is so called because of its gross appearance (*i.e.*, a bunch of grapes). Histologically, there is a characteristic cambium layer and a submucosal cellular layer of spindle cells, containing little cytoplasm. In other areas, the gross appearance is firm and fleshy; occasionally, it is vascular and necrotic.

If the conventional histopathologic categorization is used, the embryonal form is the most common, accounting for approximately 60% of these tumors. Embryonal tumors are by nature primitive, composed of ovoid and spindle-shaped undifferentiated cells that require differentiation from the other common small round cell tumors of childhood, such as Ewing's sarcoma, lymphoma, and neuroblastoma.[13] Approximately 15% to 20% of these tumor contain cross-striations, demonstrating their origin from striated muscle. Often they demonstrate a diastase-digestible PAS material in the cytoplasm. When differentiation is lacking, ultrastructural studies may reveal glycogen and cytoplasmic myofilaments, alternating between thick (myosin) and thin (actin) filaments. Z-band material, myofilaments, and cross-striations confirm the diagnosis of rhabdomyosarcoma.

The alveolar subtype most commonly occurs in adolescents and accounts for approximately 20% of cases. Histologically, this tumor is characterized by a pseudoalveolar pattern of connective tissue trabeculae, lined by large tumor cells (rhabdomyoblasts) and multinucleated giant cells.

The pleomorphic type is rare; many cases formerly classified as pleomorphic rhabdomyosarcoma are currently considered to be examples of malignant fibrous histiocytoma.

Fifteen percent to 20% of these tumors do not fit into a conventional classification and are categorized as mixtures.[49] One of these, extraosseous Ewing's sarcoma, is histologically identical to classic osseous Ewing's sarcoma yet responds to treatment similarly to rhabdomyosarcoma and accounts for 5% of tumors entered onto IRS protocols I and II. Despite adequate tissue, special stains, electron microscopy, and immunophenotyping, at least 15% of these sarcomas defy classification and remain either undifferentiated type indeterminate or unclassifiable tumors. Patients with the undifferentiated or unclassifiable tumors have a survival similar to those with the alveolar subtype.[10,49]

There is a clear association between histologic subtype and anatomic site of presentation.[10] Of the genitourinary tumors, 90% are either embryonal or botryoid subtypes. Among the extremity tumors, the alveolar type is seen in 50% of the cases. In the head and neck, the embryonal type is commonly seen, and in the trunk and retroperitoneum, there is a high percentage of alveolar and undifferentiated or unclassifiable tumors.

GENERAL MANAGEMENT

A multidisciplinary approach using surgery, irradiation, and chemotherapy is important in the management of rhabdomyosarcoma; however, the optimal sequence and specific application of each modality are still being investigated. Although it is agreed that the primary goal remains long-term cure, improving therapeutic results necessitates considerations of quality of life among survivors, with particular attention to maximizing functional and cosmetic results.

Surgery

Before the era of multidisciplinary therapy in rhabdomyosarcoma, surgical ablation resulted in a long-term survival rate of approximately 20% of those treated by resection, or only 8% of all patients.[33] Certain primary sites represented exceptions to these data, including the orbit, in which more than 50% with localized disease survived after orbital exenteration,[34] and 70% of patients with urinary bladder tumors were cured after total cystectomy.[67] However, with effective adjunctive treatment, preservation of function and appearance became major goals. The concept of reasonable surgery evolved: removing the bulk tumor with maximal conservation of anatomic structures, including enhanced preservation of bladder, bowel, and sexual function in patients with tumors of genitourinary origin, limb function in patients with extremity tumors, and vision, voice, deglutition, and appearance in patients with head and neck tumors.

Tumor resection from normal surrounding tissues is technically challenging and difficult to judge. Only 15% of tumors are located in sites where complete excision can be readily accomplished without an undesirable loss of function or cosmesis. An additional 25% of the patients have compromised surgical procedures, leaving microscopic residual disease. Sixty percent of patients are amenable to biopsy only or present with metastatic disease and are not candidates for primary resection.[10] Combined-modality therapy provides for local control of the primary tumor, even after subtotal excision.[12,31,32] Among patients with extremity rhabdomyosarcoma subjected to amputation for control of the primary tumor, more than 80% subsequently suffer a relapse.[27] When the IRS surgical grouping system is used, patients with tumor amenable to complete excision have been shown to fare better than those with subtotal resection or biopsy alone. However, tumors that are most accessible to surgical excision are small, noninvasive, and confined to their organ or structure of origin. Assessment using a TNM system demonstrates, that prognosis is dictated by tumor size and invasiveness rather than by the initial surgical approach.[53]

In cases of suspected rhabdomyosarcoma, the initial surgical procedure should be an incisional biopsy to allow consultation with an oncologist and radiation therapist about therapeutic options. The need for initial radical surgical extirpation is usually obviated by using primary chemotherapy and radiation therapy or by recommending a delayed second-look procedure. Amputation of an extremity, orbital exenteration, mutilating excision of the head and neck, therapeutic lymphadenectomy, and radical neck dissection are procedures reserved if initial therapy fails.[33,36] In contrast to other soft tissue sarcomas of childhood, adequate irradiation and chemotherapy can sterilize gross residual primary and nodal disease in rhabdomyosarcoma.

Chemotherapy

Chemotherapy is a necessary facet of the management of all children with rhabdomyosarcoma. Several drugs have demonstrated single-agent activity against rhabdomyosarcoma, including vincristine (59% response rate), dactinomycin (24%), cyclophosphamide (54%), doxorubicin (31%), dacarbazine (11%), mitomycin C (36%), cisplatin (15% to 21%), and etoposide (15% to 21%).[1,7,21] Agents with known activity in central nervous system tumors, such as the nitrosoureas and methotrexate, have not been shown to be useful in treating rhabdomyosarcoma.

The most extensive experience in combination chemotherapy is with the VAC regimen (vincristine, dactinomycin, cyclophosphamide) or VAC plus doxorubicin (VACA). The efficacy of 2 years of VAC therapy for patients with microscopic residual or nodal involvement has been studied, revealing that if radiation therapy is routinely given, the addition of cyclophosphamide and a 2-year course of chemotherapy results in no improvement in relapse, disease-free survival, or survival rate over 1 year of vincristine plus dactinomycin.[46]

Intensive pulse VAC has been compared with VACA, each with radiation therapy, among patients with large tumors who have gross residual or metastatic disease, with no advantages observed from the addition of doxorubicin in length of complete remission or in survival.

Some subsets of patients, such as those with tumors of unfavorable histology and those with extensive tumor burden, continue to fare poorly. Thus, more intensive therapeutic approaches are being studied using combinations of cisplatin, etoposide, dacarbazine, ifosfamide, and melphalan, in addition to the standard VAC or VACA regimens.

Initial intensive chemotherapy is now being used as a means of providing pharmacologic debulking, potentially allowing for a more conservative surgical approach or more localized radiation therapy. However, if chemotherapy alone is used for tumors in special sites, such as the head and neck or pelvis, most children require radiation therapy or a follow-up surgical procedure because of incomplete response or local recurrence.[69] Among selected children with head and neck or urogenital primary lesions treated with primary VAC chemotherapy, only 29% were alive without evidence of disease, with a median survival of 37 months.[69] Forty-two percent eventually required surgical management to achieve disease-free status, with a mean survival of 50 months. Of concern were 29% of patients with head and neck primary tumors who developed local recurrences with intracranial extension and died of uncontrolled locoregional disease. If chemotherapy is used alone, before initiation of radiation therapy, 16% of patients have been shown to develop local recurrence or direct extension to adjacent tissues.[66] Definitive local therapy, either surgery or irradiation, is necessary for cure of disease. Nevertheless, the approach of initial debulking with chemotherapy may be particularly applicable in the management of infants and very young children in whom late effects of radical surgery or high-dose, large-volume radiation are particularly severe.

RADIATION THERAPY

There is abundant evidence of the role of irradiation in the local control of microscopic or gross residual rhabdomyosarcoma. This was first demonstrated in the management of children with orbital primary tumor and subsequently in all head and neck sites.[12,16,62] Local control rates of 90% have been reported.[68]

Adequate irradiation implies careful attention to volume and dose. It is essential to evaluate the soft tissue extent of the primary lesion by computed tomographic scan, arteriography, or magnetic resonance imaging. Because rhabdomyosarcoma tends to infiltrate tissue planes widely, tumors often extend beyond a fascial compartment and beyond the obvious visible margins. Careful examination by a radiation oncologist at the time of initial diagnosis, even if the treatment plan calls for new adjuvant chemotherapy, is essential to establish the appropriate tumor volume.

Treatment portals should be designed to encompass the involved region at the time of presentation before chemotherapy, with wide margins encompassing surgical sites and biopsy tracks. When the tumor volume is adequately delineated by physical examination, surgical findings, and radiographic procedures, it is sufficient to treat the tumor volume with margin, but not necessarily the whole muscle compartment or the entire involved muscle from origin to insertion.

A biopsy should be performed on clinically suspicious lymph nodes, or they should be included in the radiation therapy portal. Prophylactic lymph node irradiation is not necessary in children with clinically negative findings who will be receiving combination chemotherapy.

Patients with tumors at parameningeal sites have developed meningeal extension of tumor when inadequate radiation portals were used.[19] However, patients with cranial nerve palsy, bone destruction adjacent to the meninges, intracranial extension, or intradural seeding, as demonstrated radiographically, or cytologic evidence of malignant cells in cerebrospinal fluid do not have a significantly decreased 5-year survival rate compared with patients with parameningeal primary lesions with no initial meningeal involvement.[4]

High-dose irradiation is necessary to ensure local control even if concomitant multiagent chemotherapy is given. Local control of gross disease requires doses of 5000 cGy to 5500 cGy, but microscopic disease can often be controlled with doses of less than 5000 cGy.[32] The IRS investigators have been unable to generate a strict dose-response curve but have observed an association with age, which suggests that lower doses, which may be given to infants and youngsters, are often associated with high relapse rates.[55] They also suggest that local control is greater for tumors less than 5 cm than for those 5 cm or greater, supporting the adult experience with soft tissue sarcoma.[68] If chemotherapy is given in addition, most radiation therapists now believe that 4140 cGy to 5040 cGy given in 4.5 to 5.5 weeks is necessary for microscopic disease, with 5040 cGy to 5580 cGy in 5.5 to 6 weeks recommended for gross residual disease.

The IRS investigators are currently studying the efficacy of a higher radiation dose, 5940 cGy, given in a hyperfractionated program for children with gross residual disease. Outside a protocol setting, radiation therapy should be given in daily fractions of 150 cGy to 180 cGy, five times a week as tolerated. In the International Society of Pediatric Oncology rhabdomyosarcoma trial, patients with bulky unresectable disease who received radiation therapy to between 4000 cGy and 4500 cGy had a high incidence of local recurrence, even if multiagent chemotherapy was administered.[9]

All children receiving external-beam radiation therapy should be simulated and treated with megavoltage units, with all fields treated daily. Special attention should be paid to the use of shrinking fields and isocentric techniques, using shaped fields to minimize toxic effects.[43] Immobilization techniques that ensure reproducible portals are essential. Often sedation or anesthesia is necessary to ensure adequacy of the treatment plan. These complex programs are best conducted in regional centers by an experienced team of physicians, including a pediatric surgeon, pediatric anesthesiologist, pediatric oncologist, and a radiation oncologist.

Interstitial radiation therapy may play an important role as primary treatment or as booster treatment after external-beam therapy for selected sites.[15,18,20,44] The advantages of precise shaping of the dose distribution, sharp fall-off of radiation dose, and shortening of overall treatment time are especially attractive in dealing with infants and youngsters. Current recommendations are for temporary implants, because the late effects data from these procedures administered to children are not yet available.

The timing of radiation therapy must be carefully coordinated with planned surgical intervention and combination chemotherapy schedule to ensure optimization of drug doses and unimpaired postoperative healing. Adherence to schedule is important, because there are toxic effects from the use of radiation with many of the active chemotherapeutic agents (*e.g.*, dactinomycin and doxorubicin). It is better to deliver radiation between courses of drugs rather than simultaneously.

Newer approaches using intraoperative radiation therapy, hyperfractionation, hyperthermia, and radiation sensitizers are considered experimental.

PROGNOSTIC FACTORS AND THERAPEUTIC CONSIDERATIONS

As rhabdomyosarcoma is protean in presentation, factors such as site, stage, extent of disease, and pathologic characteristics of the tumor influence therapeutic decisions. These prognostic factors are interrelated and are best discussed as a function of specific site. Figure 72-1 demonstrates survival differences for individual anatomic sites.

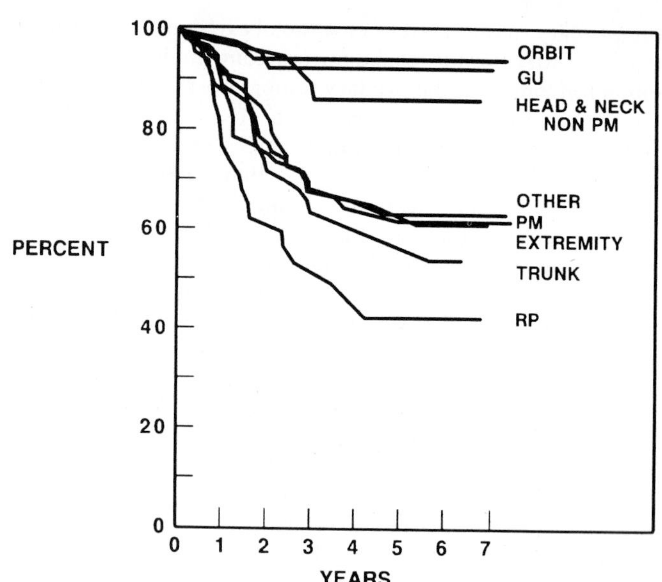

FIGURE 72–1. Survival curves for 505 children with nonmetastatic rhabdomyosarcoma entered onto Intergroup Rhabdomyosarcoma Study II are shown by the anatomic sites of the primary tumors. (Modified from Lawrence W, Gehan EA, Hays DM, et al: J Clin Oncol 5:46, 1987)

Orbit

The orbit has long been recognized as a favorable site. In addition to prompt recognition of the tumor, the paucity of lymphatics in this area means that lymphatic extension is rare. In the absence of extraorbital extension, orbital exenteration alone was curative in more than 50% of patients.[34] Radiation therapy alone has been shown to provide local control in 90% of cases treated with adequate doses and volumes, while preserving good quality vision. Although multiagent chemotherapy is commonly used and recommended, its role for patients with tumors confined to the orbit and managed by primary radiation therapy has not yet been made clear by a randomized trial. Traditionally, if irradiation alone was used, the entire orbit was considered at risk and recommended to be included in the tumor volume. However, with a combined-modality approach, the orbit can be treated to the site of tumor involvement with a margin without necessarily including the entire orbit. These techniques allow beam-shaping devices and corneal and lens protection to be employed (Figs. 72-2 and 72-3).

In individualizing the management for orbital tumors, it is generally agreed that biopsy only should be undertaken to provide the diagnosis and that primary treatment should be radiation therapy. Orbital exenteration should be reserved for salvage treatment, and enucleation for management of posttreatment ocular complications. Extension of disease beyond the orbit is associated with hematogenous metastasis, necessitating multiagent chemotherapy.

Head and Neck

Although extraorbital head and neck sites are often discussed as a group, there is much variation among these sites, which requires individualization of therapy. Tumors of the scalp, larynx, cheek, oral cavity, parotid gland, and oropharynx have a more favorable course than do those of other head and neck sites, such as the nasopharynx, nasal cavity, paranasal sinuses, middle

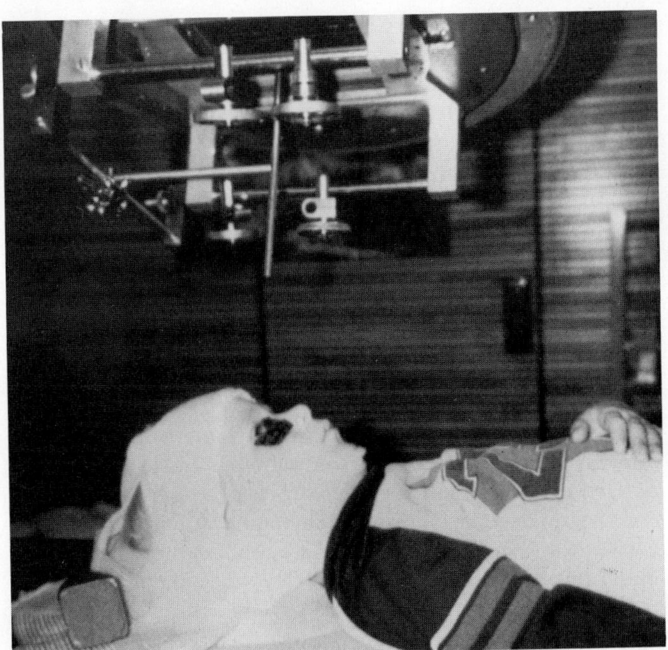

FIGURE 72–2. A 4-year-old boy with an inferior and medial right orbital tumor lying comfortably with a small cast over his forehead and chin to provide immobilization. He was instructed to look superiorly at an anteriorly placed eyebar used to shield the lens. Bolus was used along the inferior orbit to bring up the dose to the involved superficial tissues. After 8 years of follow-up, he remains disease free, with normal vision and acceptable cosmetic appearance.

ear, mastoid, pterygopalatine fossa, and infratemporal fossa. The less favorable parameningeal sites have the potential to extend intracranially, to erode the base of skull, and to cause cranial nerve palsies.

Previously, it was thought that as many as 35% of the children with tumor arising in a parameningeal site subsequently developed meningeal extension.[65] However, extension does not occur if adequate radiation portals providing coverage of the base of the skull coverage are used.[4,19] Patients with known parameningeal primary tumors,with or without base of skull erosion or cranial nerve palsy, currently receive wide local field irradiation with margin including the local meninges. Patients with known meningeal dissemination should receive craniospinal radiation therapy.[65]

Because the chemotherapeutic agents that can be administered by intrathecal route have limited efficacy in rhabdomyosarcoma, central nervous system radiation therapy should not be compromised in favor of chemotherapy for patients with a high risk of advanced disease. Adequate doses and volumes of radiation are capable of achieving local control, leading to high rates of complete remission.[17]

Because the nasopharynx has a rich lymphatic network, it is commonly associated with regional lymph node involvement. If a biopsy is not done, any suspicious regional lymph node should be considered positive and included in a radiation therapy portal.

Extremity

Tumors arising in the extremity are often alveolar or undifferentiated subtypes, are large and deeply invasive at diagnosis, and are associated with a high probability of lymphatic

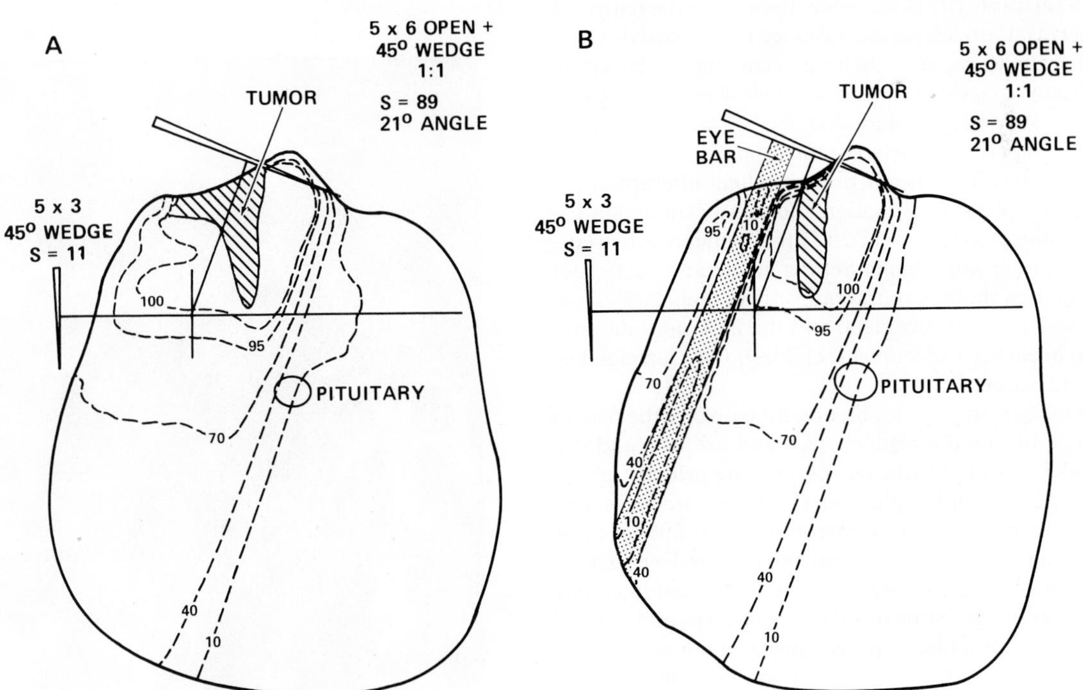

FIGURE 72–3. (**A**) Isodose distribution at the central axis of the field when an oblique open and wedged field and a direct lateral wedged field are used, showing a homogeneous distribution to the orbit for the child shown in Figure 72–2. The therapeutic unit is a 4-MV 80-SAD linear accelerator. Isodose curves are shown as percentages of the tumor dose. (**B**) A superiorly placed anterior eyebar is used to protect the lens; it lowers the dose to approximately 10% under the shadow of the eyebar. In this superior plane, the tumor is located medially and receives the full dose, but the lens dose is less than 10% of the tumor dose.

and hematogenous metastases. They have been considered to have a relatively poor prognosis.[28] However, several series show that if combined-modality treatment is given, the prognostic significance of anatomic site analysis by TNM stage is used.[53,58] Complete surgical resection is difficult to achieve, usually requires extensive dissection, and is associated with a high risk of residual disease. Children with extremity tumors subjected to amputation and chemotherapy have a relapse rate of greater than 83%.[27] Because radiation therapy and multiagent chemotherapy have been shown to provide excellent local control, it is possible to avoid disfiguring and mutilating surgical procedures with their attendant functional disabilities.

There are no data to show that lymph node dissection offers therapeutic advantage. If recommended, it is for purpose of staging, not for treatment.

Radiation therapy for extremity primary tumors requires careful immobilization techniques, sparing of nonirradiated skin for lymphatic drainage, and shrinking fields. Routine physical therapy during and after radiation therapy is important in obtaining an optimal functional result.

Pelvis

Although tumors arising in various sites of the pelvis are often grouped together, each site should be considered individually, because the natural history, spread, and sequelae of treatment are quite specific for each site.

Urinary bladder tumors are more common in males, often superficial and polypoid, and are usually the sarcoma botryoides subtype. These tumors tend to remain localized until late in the disease and spread diffusely laterally within the superficial tissues. Metastasis to regional lymph nodes and distant sites is a relatively late occurrence. Because of the nature of diffuse superficial spread, segmental resection or partial cystectomy alone leads to rapid early local recurrence.[23] However, total cystectomy is associated with a survival rate of approximately 70%.[67] Recently, emphasis has been on attempts to limit radical surgery, specifically pelvic exenteration, and to spare the bladder if possible. The use of primary chemotherapy in an attempt to avoid pelvic exenteration and pelvic irradiation has been disappointing. Only two of 29 IRS-II patients achieved a successful outcome with chemotherapy alone, and most later required radiation therapy or tumor excision. Only 52% of the survivors had functional bladders, and the 27% mortality was poorer than in earlier IRS studies if children were managed by anterior exenteration.[24,25]

Tumors arising in prostatic tissues often involve the base of the bladder, infiltrate the bladder neck and urethra, and disseminate widely through tissue planes. Prostate primary lesions are enmeshed in a rich lymphatic network and are associated with regional lymph node involvement in at least 20% of these patients.[54] Patients have poor survival and disease-free survival rates, regardless of age or stage and despite multimodality therapy. IRS protocols testing initial chemotherapy and delayed irradiation have shown biopsy-proven persistent disease in 70% of the children, suggesting that irradiation should be used earlier and routinely in all patients with prostate, bladder neck, and trigone lesions.

Because of ejaculatory impotence, lymphadenectomy is not routinely recommended for children with pelvic primary tumors. Suspicious or proven regional lymph node disease requires local irradiation to draining nodal sites with combination chemotherapy.

Paratesticular tumors arise from the ductus deferens or existing skeletal muscle in this area. As with prostatic primary tumors, the lymphatic network is rich, draining directly to the retroperitoneal nodes along the external iliac and spermatic vessels, the aorta, and vena cava. The observed incidence of para-aortic and renal hilar lymph node involvement is 40%.[39,57] Radical orchiectomy and unilateral lymph node dissection with sampling of suspicious contralateral lymph nodes have been recommended as a staging procedure, with postoperative radiation therapy to sites of nodal drainage reserved for proven nodal involvement.[57] Considering the effectiveness of multiagent chemotherapy in sterilizing micrometastasis, the necessity of lymphadenectomy after orchiectomy in a child with a normal lymphogram is now questioned.[50]

Female genital tract (*i.e.*, vaginal, uterine, vulval) primary tumors are embryonal or botryoid subtypes and are often associated with favorable prognoses.[23] Selected cases may be successfully managed with primary chemotherapy and limited surgery (*i.e.*, hysterovaginectomy and oophorectomy)[37,59] or with initial chemotherapy followed by interstitial implantation.[15,18,20,44]

Other pelvic sites include perianal, perirectal, and perineal primary sites. Regional lymph node involvement may also be high in these sites. The location of these primary tumors creates surgical and radiation challenges. Combined chemotherapy and radiation therapy programs are recommended instead of primary surgical procedures if excision demands exenteration with urinary and fecal diversion procedures (Fig. 72-4)

Increasing emphasis on use of primary chemotherapy with limited surgery or delayed irradiation has been recommended in an attempt to avoid pelvic exenteration, impotency, sterility, contracted bony pelvis, and urinary diversion.[51,59,69] These programs have resulted in several observations[47,56]:

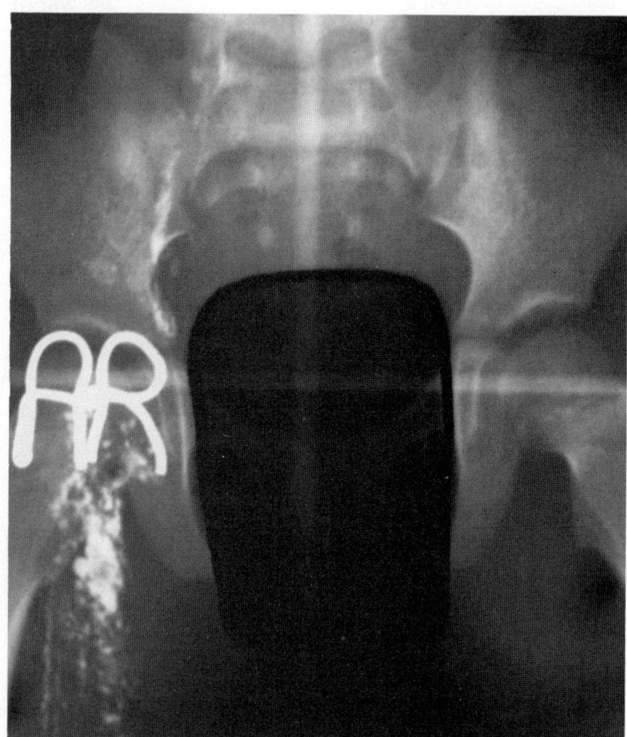

FIGURE 72–4. A shaped Cerrobend field was designed to encompass a perineal tumor with adequate margins while avoiding the bony pelvis in a 3-year-old girl. With 7 years of follow-up, she remains disease free and without detectable sequelae of therapy.

1. A dramatic response to initial pulse chemotherapy is frequently observed.
2. Approximately 20% of rhabdomyosarcomas are not sensitive to intensive pulse chemotherapy.
3. Chemotherapy alone is associated with a high local failure rate and a poor relapse-free survival rate. Only 46% of patients with bladder, prostate, or vagina tumors treated on IRS-II are relapse-free 3 years after treatment.
4. When primary chemotherapy with or without radiation therapy or limited surgery was administered to patients with prostate, bladder, or vagina primary tumors on IRS studies, survival rates were approximately 70%, but only 25% of these patients retained their bladders.
5. Although immediate cystectomy is not necessary at the time of diagnosis, if primary chemotherapy is used, radiation therapy is usually necessary for patients with prostate and bladder primary tumors, and partial vaginectomy is often needed for those with vaginal primary lesions.

RESULTS OF THERAPY

Adjuvant chemotherapy was first tested in a prospective randomized trial, showing the value of dactinomycin and vincristine among children with completely resected tumors who were receiving irradiation; 82% of these group I patients remained in remission after 2 years with adjuvant chemotherapy, compared with 47% if no chemotherapy was employed, but without survival advantages.[29]

The IRS tested the efficacy of chemotherapy and radiation therapy as a function of surgical stage. The first IRS study (IRS-I) entered 686 evaluable patients during a 6-year period. Results of that study are shown in Figure 72-5. For this study, radiation therapy was given initially for patients with IRS group I and II disease and was delayed until week 6 for those with group III and IV disease. All patients received multiagent chemotherapy for 2 years. This study made several important observations, including the following[28,46]:

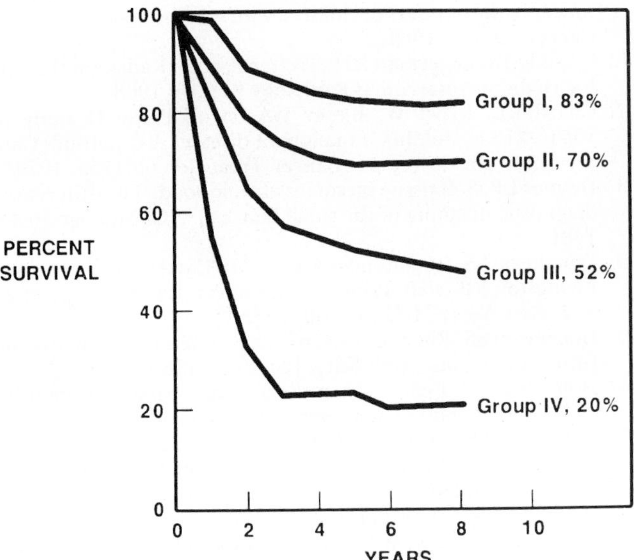

FIGURE 72–5. Survival curves of 686 children with rhabdomyosarcoma entered onto Intergroup Rhabdomyosarcoma Study I are shown by their initial groupings. (Modified from Maurer EM, Beltangady M, Gehan EA: Cancer 61:209, 1988)

1. For localized tumors amenable to complete resection (IRS group I), postoperative radiation therapy is unnecessary if the patient is given 2 years of vincristine, dactinomycin, cyclophosphamide (VAC regimen) chemotherapy. For these patients, the relapse-free survival rate at 5 years is 80%, and the 5-year survival rate is 81% to 93%.
2. Three-drug chemotherapy (VAC) fails to improve results obtained with intensive two-drug chemotherapy (vincristine, dactinomycin) for patients with group II disease if postoperative radiation therapy is given. For these patients, the relapse-free survival rate at 5 years is 65% to 72%, and the 5-year survival rate is 72%.
3. Four-drug VACA chemotherapy (vincristine, dactinomycin, cyclophosphamide, doxorubicin) provides no advantage over three-drug chemotherapy (VAC; without doxorubicin) for patients with group III disease (gross residual) or group IV disease (metastasis) if routine radiation therapy is used in addition. The complete remission rate for group III patients was 69% and 50% for group IV patients. Those who achieved a complete remission had a 60% chance of staying in remission for 5 years in group III and 30% for group IV. The survival at 5 years was 52% for group III patients and 20% for group IV patients.
4. The 5-year survival rate for the entire group was 55%.
5. Survival after relapse was poor, 32% at 1 year and 17% at 2 years.
6. The risk of distant metastasis was much greater than the risk of local recurrence.
7. Primary tumors of the orbit and genitourinary tract carried the best prognosis, and tumors of the retroperitoneum had the worst prognosis.
8. The alveolar histologic subset had a poor prognosis, especially in extremity lesions.

A second IRS study was initiated in 1978 and was built on the findings of IRS-I. Over 1000 patients were entered onto IRS-II. Following are results from this study[47]:

1. The 5-year survival rate for the IRS-II group was 62%, a 7% improvement over the IRS-I rate.
2. Patients in group I (excluding extremity alveolar patients) had better disease-free status with the VAC regimen (82%) than those receiving only vincristine and dactinomycin (68%), but they had similar survival rates (82% and 88%) at 5 years. Cyclophosphamide cannot be withdrawn safely from the standard VAC regimen if radiation therapy is omitted from patients with group I disease.
3. Intensive (cyclic-sequential) two-drug therapy of vincristine and dactinomycin is as effective as repetitive pulse VAC therapy for patients with group II disease, if all patients receive postoperative irradiation. At 5 years, 68% to 75% remain disease free, and 77% to 90% are alive, with no differences between the groups.
4. Repetitive pulse chemotherapy for 2 years increases survival in children with group III disease but not for those with group IV disease; doxorubicin and dactinomycin have comparable efficacy in the pulse regimens used. The complete remission rates are 72%. At 5 years, 70% remain in complete remission, with 64% surviving.
5. Local meningeal irradiation, with or without intrathecal chemotherapy, prevents meningeal recurrence and increases survival in patients with parameningeal primary tumors.
6. Primary repetitive pulse VAC chemotherapy for patients with special pelvic primary tumors (*i.e.*, bladder, prostate, uterus, vagina) does not reduce the frequency of total

cystectomy or produce durable bladder salvage, although survival is not compromised.

7. Survival after relapse is only 17% at 5 years.

These IRS data are reported by group (stage) without reference to site, age, tumor burden, or nodal status, which can be misleading if a physician searches for specific data relative to individual patients. Specific observations pertinent to individual sites are listed in the site-specific section on prognostic factors.

Investigators from the Institut Gustave Roussy conducted a retrospective analysis of 193 children with rhabdomyosarcoma treated with coordinated multiagent chemotherapy.[16] Using a TNM staging system, they observed a benefit from the aggressive chemotherapy program only in children with Stage II disease (invasive primary tumor) and in those patients with tumors of head and neck or genitourinary origin. They failed to show any significant improvement with aggressive chemotherapy in children with Stages I, III, or IV disease or in those with extremity primary tumors. The role of combined-modality treatment and the value of adjuvant therapy as a function of individual site, tumor bulk, and nodal status should be evaluated.

SEQUELAE OF TREATMENT

Acute side-effects from surgery are primarily postoperative complications that are reversible and not serious. The acute toxicity of combined-modality programs is primarily related to chemotherapy and includes nausea, vomiting, mucositis, alopecia, and hematopoietic suppression. Drug-induced granulocytopenia significantly increases the risk of fever and infection. With the VAC and VACA programs, these toxic effects are rarely life-threatening. The newer protocols using more aggressive therapy, including cisplatin, dacarbazine, etoposide, and other agents carry more acute side-effects, including renal and electrolyte imbalance, which demand close monitoring.

Acute radiation toxicity is related to the regions irradiated and the dose administered. It can be especially pronounced for tumors of the head and neck, abdomen, and pelvis. The additional toxic effects from drugs known to augment radiation reaction, such as dactinomycin and doxorubicin, can be severe and may require modification of treatment plans. Both dactinomycin and doxorubicin are known to accentuate a "recall" of radiation injury if given during or immediately after the course of radiation therapy. Prompt attention to skin care is important; erythema should be treated with steroid creams and moist desquamation with Domeboro soaks, or radiation therapy may be temporarily delayed.

After the orbit is treated, an acute inflammatory reaction with pain and sometimes photophobia may be seen within weeks of completion of irradiation to the cornea and conjunctiva. In the region of the eye, steroids should be administered under the direction of an ophthalmologist.

Acute otitis externa or media with hyperemia and swelling of the membranes of the eustachian tube is common during or soon after treatment of head and neck areas. Decongestants are helpful in reducing the swelling.

Erythematous mucositis leading to a patchy fibrinous exudate is seen after head and neck radiation therapy, after drug therapy, and almost universally if the two are used simultaneously. Mouthwashes with salt and soda or 1% hydrogen peroxide rinses partially alleviate the reaction. Bacterial or fungal superinfection requires specific drug management. Attention to dental care with frequent brushing, use of dental floss, and fluoride dental preparations is important.

Acute gastrointestinal sequelae, such as vomiting and diarrhea, are usually managed by supportive care. Nutritional support with hyperalimentation is often necessary to prevent protein-calorie malnutrition, including the use of indwelling central venous catheters.

Major emphasis has been given to the late effects of radiation therapy, and less attention is given to those of chemotherapy. Long-term sequelae related to specific drugs are usually site-specific, and the morbidity may be accentuated by radiation therapy. This includes cyclophosphamide-induced cystitis and doxorubicin-related cardiac injury. Radiation-related effects on bone and soft tissue growth are commonly discussed, but precise data relating to age at the time of treatment, radiation dose given, and potential outcome are lacking. Nevertheless, it is clear that radiation-related complications are most pronounced in infants and youngsters. Cataracts, hypopituitarism, altered bone growth, gonadal dysfunction, induction of a second malignant tumor, and chronic organ dysfunction should be considered.

The complications of radical surgical treatment depend on the primary tumor site and include major disfigurement and loss of function. Of greatest long-term severity are consequences of fecal and urinary diversion and ejaculatory impotence after retroperitoneal lymph node dissection.

REFERENCES

1. Baum ES, Gayvon P, Greenberg L, et al: Phase II trial of cisplatin in refractory childhood cancer: Children's Cancer Study Group report. Cancer Treat Rep 65:815, 1981
2. Beddis I, Mott M, Bullimore J: Case report: Nasopharyngeal rhabdomyosarcoma and Gorlin's naevoid basal cell carcinoma syndrome. Med Pediatr Oncol 11:178, 1983
3. Bergiron C, Markovits P, Benjaafar M, et al: Lymphography in childhood rhabdomyosarcoma. Radiology 133:627, 1979
4. Berry MD, Jenkin RP: Parameningeal rhabdomyosarcoma in the young. Cancer 48(suppl 2):281, 1981
5. Birch JM, Hartley AL, Marsden HB, et al: Excess risk of breast cancer in the mothers of children with soft tissue sarcomas. Br J Cancer 49:325, 1984
6. Cassady JR, Sagerman RH, Tretter P, et al: Radiation therapy for rhabdomyosarcoma. Radiology 91:116, 1968
7. Chard RL, Krivit W, Bleyer WA, et al: Phase II study of VP-16-213 in childhood malignant disease: A Children's Cancer Study Group report. Cancer Treat Rep 63:1755, 1979
8. Dehner LP: Soft tissue sarcomas of childhood: The differential diagnostic dilemma of the small blue cell. NCI Monogr 56:43, 1981
9. Donaldson SS: Rhabdomyosarcoma. In Carter SK, Glatstein E, Livingston RB (eds): Principles of Cancer Treatment, pp 852–862. New York, McGraw Hill, 1982
10. Donaldson SS: Rhabdomyosarcoma: Contemporary status and future directions. Arch Surg 124:1015, 1989
11. Donaldson SS, Belli JA: A rational clinical staging system for childhood rhabdomyosarcoma. J Clin Oncol 2:135, 1984
12. Donaldson SS, Castro JR, Wilbur JR, et al: Rhabdomyosarcoma of the head and neck in children: Combination treatment by surgery, irradiation and chemotherapy. Cancer 31:26, 1973
13. Donaldson SS, Hendrickson MR: Patterns of failure in childhood solid tumors: Wilms' tumor, neuroblastoma, and rhabdomyosarcoma. Cancer Treat Symp 2:267, 1983
14. Douglass EC, Valentine M, Etcubanas E, et al: A specific chromosomal abnormality in rhabdomyosarcoma. Cytogenet Cell Genet 45:148, 1987

15. Flamant F, Chassagne D, Cosset J, et al: Embryonal rhabdomyosarcoma of the vagina in children: Conservative treatment with curietherapy and chemotherapy. Eur J Cancer 15:527, 1979
16. Flamant F, Hill C: The improvement in survival in childhood rhabdomyosarcoma: A historical comparison of 345 patients in the same center. Cancer 53:2417, 1984
17. Gasparini M, Lombardi F, Gianni C, et al: Childhood rhabdomyosarcoma with meningeal extension: Results of combined therapy including central nervous system prophylaxis. Am J Clin Oncol 6:393, 1983
18. Gerbaulet A, Panis X, Flamant F, et al: Iridium afterloading curietherapy in the treatment of pediatric malignancies. The Institut Gustave Roussy experience. Cancer 56:1274, 1985
19. Gerson JM, Jaffe N, Donaldson MH, et al: Meningeal seeding from rhabdomyosarcoma of the head and neck with base of the skull invasion: Recognition of the clinical evolution and suggestions for management. Med Pediatr Oncol 5:137, 1978
20. Goffinet DR, Martinez A, Pooler D, et al: Pediatric brachytherapy. In George FW (ed): Modern Interstitial and Intracavitary Radiation Cancer Management, vol 6, pp 57–70. New York, Masson Publishing, 1981
21. Green DM, Jaffe N: Progress and controversy in the treatment of childhood rhabdomyosarcoma. Cancer Treat Rev 5:7, 1978
22. Harmor MH (ed): TNM Classification of Pediatric Tumors. Geneva, International Union Against Cancer, 1982
23. Hays DM, Raney RB, Lawrence W, et al: Rhabdomyosarcoma of the female urogenital tract. J Pediatr Surg 16:828, 1981
24. Hays DM, Raney RB, Lawrence W, et al: Bladder and prostatic tumors in the Intergroup Rhabdomyosarcoma Study (IRS-I) results of therapy. Cancer 50:1472, 1982
25. Hays DM, Raney RB, Lawrence W, et al: Primary chemotherapy in the treatment of children with bladder-prostate tumors in The Intergroup Rhabdomyosarcoma Study (IRS-II). J Pediatr Surg 17:812, 1982
26. Hays DM, Shimada H, Raney RB, et al: Clinical staging and treatment results in rhabdomyosarcoma of the female genital tract among children and adolescents. Cancer 61:1893, 1988
27. Hays DM, Soule EH, Lawrence W, et al: Extremity lesions in the Intergroup Rhabdomyosarcoma Study (IRS-I): A preliminary report. Cancer 49:1, 1982
28. Heyn R, Beltangady M, Hays D: Results of intensive therapy in children with localized alveolar extremity rhabdomyosarcoma: A report from the Intergroup Rhabdomyosarcoma Study. J Clin Oncol 7:200, 1989
29. Heyn RM, Holland R, Newton WA, et al: The role of combined chemotherapy in the treatment of rhabdomyosarcoma in children. Cancer 34:2128, 1974
30. Horn RC, Enterline HT: Rhabdomyosarcoma: A clinicopathological study and classification of 39 cases. Cancer 11:181, 1958
31. Jaffe N, Murray J, Traggis D, et al: Multidisciplinary treatment for childhood sarcoma. Am J Surg 133:405, 1977
32. Jereb B, Cham W, Lattin P, et al: Local control of embryonal rhabdomyosarcoma in children by radiation therapy when combined with concomitant chemotherapy. Int J Radiat Oncol Biol Phys 1:217, 1976
33. Johnson DG: Trends in surgery for childhood rhabdomyosarcoma. Cancer 35:916, 1975
34. Jones IS, Reese AB, Kraut J: Orbital rhabdomyosarcoma: An analysis of 62 cases. Trans Am Ophthalmol Soc 63:223, 1965
35. Kilman JW, Clatworthy HW, Newton WA, et al: Reasonable surgery for rhabdomyosarcoma: A study of 67 cases. Ann Surg 178:346, 1973
36. Kingston JE: The management of rhabdomyosarcoma. Cancer Surv 3:719, 1984
37. Kumar APM, Wrenn EL, Fleming ID, et al: Combined therapy to prevent complete pelvic exenteration for rhabdomyosarcoma of the vagina or uterus. Cancer 37:118, 1976
38. Lawrence W, Gehan EA, Hays DM, et al: Prognostic significance of staging factors of the UICC system in childhood rhabdomyosarcoma: A report from the Intergroup Rhabdomyosarcoma Study (IRS-II). J Clin Oncol 5:46, 1987
39. Lawrence W, Hays DM, Moon TE: Lymphatic metastasis with childhood rhabdomyosarcoma. Cancer 39:556, 1977
40. Li FP, Fraumeni JP: Soft tissue sarcomas, breast cancer, and other neoplasms: A familial syndrome? Ann Intern Med 71:747, 1969
41. Li FP, Fraumeni JP: Prospective study of a family cancer syndrome. JAMA 247:2692, 1982
42. Lynch HT, Katz DA, Bogard PJ, et al: The sarcoma, breast cancer, lung cancer, and adreno-cortical carcinoma syndrome revisited. Am J Dis Child 139:134, 1985
43. Martinez A, Donaldson SS, Bagshaw MA: Special setup and treatment techniques for the radiotherapy of pediatric malignancies. Int J Radiat Oncol Biol Phys 2:1007, 1977
44. Martinez A, Goffinet DR, Donaldson SS, et al: The use of interstitial therapy in pediatric malignancies. Front Radiat Ther Oncol 23:91, 1978
45. Maurer HM: The Intergroup Rhabdomyosarcoma Study: Objectives and clinical staging classification. J Pediatr Surg 10:977, 1975
46. Maurer HM, Beltangady M, Gehan EA: The Intergroup Rhabdomyosarcoma Study-I. Cancer 61:209, 1988
47. Maurer HM, Gehan EA, Beltangady M, et al: The Intergroup Rhabdomyosarcoma Study-II. Cancer, (in press).
48. McKeen EA, Bodurtha JK, Meadows AT, et al: Rhabdomyosarcoma complicating multiple neurofibromatosis. J Pediatr 93:992, 1978
49. Newton WA, Soule EH, Homoudi AB, et al: Histopathology of childhood sarcomas. Intergroup Rhabdomyosarcoma Studies I and II: Clinicopathological correlation. J Clin Oncol 6:67, 1988
50. Olive D, Flamant F, Zucker JM, et al: Paraaortic lymphadenectomy is not necessary in the treatment of localized paratesticular rhabdomyosarcoma. Cancer 54:1283, 1984
51. Ortega JA: A therapeutic approach to childhood pelvic rhabdomyosarcoma without pelvic exenteration. J Pediatr 94:205, 1979
52. Parry DM, Mulvihill JJ, Miller RW, et al: Sarcomas in a child and her father. Am J Dis Child 133:130, 1979
53. Pedrick TJ, Donaldson SS, Cox RS: Rhabdomyosarcoma: The Stanford experience utilizing a TNM staging system. J Clin Oncol 4:370, 1986
54. Pizzo PA: Rhabdomyosarcoma and the soft tissue sarcomas. In Levine AS (ed): Cancer in the Young, pp 615–632. New York, Masson, 1982
55. Ragab A, Heyn R, Tefft M, et al: Infants younger than 1 year of age with rhabdomyosarcoma. Cancer 58:2606, 1986
56. Raney RB, Gehan EA, Hays DM, et al: Primary chemotherapy with or without radiation therapy and/or surgery for children with localized sarcoma of the bladder, prostate, vagina, uterus and cervix: A comparison of the results of The Intergroup Rhabdomyosarcoma Studies I and II. Cancer 66:2071, 1990
57. Raney RB, Hays DM, Lawrence W, et al: Paratesticular rhabdomyosarcoma in childhood. Cancer 42:729, 1978
58. Ransom JL, Pratt CB, Shanks E: Childhood rhabdomyosarcoma of the extremity: Results of combined modality therapy. Cancer 40:2810, 1977
59. Rivard G, Ortega J, Hittle R, et al: Intensive chemotherapy as primary treatment for rhabdomyosarcoma of the pelvis. Cancer 36:1593, 1975
60. Rodary C, Rey A, Olive D, et al: Prognostic factors in 281 children with nonmetastatic rhabdomyosarcoma (RMS) at diagnosis. Med Pediatr Oncol 16:71, 1988
61. Ruymann FB, Maddux HR, Ragab A, et al: Congenital anomalies associated with rhabdomyosarcoma: An autopsy study of 115 cases. A report from the Intergroup Rhabdomyosarcoma Study Committee (representing the Children's Cancer Study Group and the Pediatric Intergroup Statistical Center). Med Pediatr Oncol 16:33, 1988
62. Sagerman RH, Tretter P, Ellsworth RM: The treatment of orbital rhabdomyosarcoma of children with primary radiation therapy. Am J Roentgenol 114:31, 1972
63. Scrable H, Witte D, Wang-Wuu F, et al: Molecular definition of rhabdomyosarcoma subtypes. Am J Hum Genet 39:A40, 1986

64. Seidal T, Mark J, Hagmar B, et al: Alveolar rhabdomyosarcoma: A cytogenetic and correlated cytological and histological study. Acta Path Microbiol Immunol Scand [A] 90:345, 1982
65. Tefft M, Fernandez CH, Donaldson MH, et al: Incidence of meningeal involvement by rhabdomyosarcoma of the head and neck in children: A report of The Intergroup Rhabdomyosarcoma Study (IRS). Cancer 48(suppl 2):253, 1978
66. Tefft M, Fernandez CH, Moon TE: Rhabdomyosarcoma: Response with chemotherapy prior to radiation in patients with gross residual disease. Cancer 39:665, 1977
67. Tefft M, Jaffe N: Sarcoma of the bladder and prostate in children: Rationale for the role of radiation therapy based on a review of the literature and a report of 14 additional patients. Cancer 32:1161, 1973
68. Tefft M, Lindberg RD, Gehan EA: Radiation therapy combined with systemic chemotherapy of rhabdomyosarcoma in children: Local control in patients enrolled in the Intergroup Rhabdomyosarcoma Study. NCI Monogr 56:75, 1981
69. Voute PA, Vos A, deKraker J, et al: Rhabdomyosarcoma: Chemotherapy and limited supplementary treatment program to avoid mutilation. NCI Monogr 56:121, 1981
70. Wang-Wuu S, Soukup S, Ballard E, et al: Chromosomal analysis of 16 human rhabdomyosarcomas. Cancer Res 48:983, 1988
71. Young JL, Miller RW: Incidence of malignant tumors in U.S. children. J Pediatr 86:254, 1975

73

○ ○ ○ ● ● ●

Lymphomas in Children

Patrick R.M. Thomas

The challenge in the management of lymphomas in children is no longer merely the overall increase in cure, but rather the recognition of the various disease patterns and the application of curative but potentially damaging therapy to the young patient. Hodgkin's disease is a similar process in children and adults, but pediatric non-Hodgkin's lymphomas differ from one another and from adult varieties.

HODGKIN'S DISEASE IN CHILDREN

The success of treatment for Hodgkin's disease in childhood should be comparable to that of adults. In inexperienced hands, however, a natural tendency to underinvestigate and undertreat can lead to an increased number of relapses, and overtreatment may lead to unnecessary complications.

Epidemiology

Hodgkin's disease is very rare in infants but becomes increasingly common with increasing age, reaching a peak in young adulthood.[23,44,52] The clinical presentations are essentially those of adult Hodgkin's disease (Chap. 62).[23] Little is known of etiologic factors, but viral activation has been postulated.[18] There is tentative evidence that incidence is increased in black children and children of lower socioeconomic levels.[45]

Natural History

Spread patterns of pediatric Hodgkin's disease are essentially the same as those for adults (Chap. 62).

Diagnostic Workup

The principles of investigation in adults are applicable to childhood Hodgkin's disease. Arguments pertaining to the use of computed tomography (CT) or lymphangiography are relevant in diagnosing children and adults, but lymphangiography may not be warranted in young children because of anesthesia. Abdominal CT is more accurate if there is fat around the retroperitoneal lymph nodes, which is more likely in adults.[4]

Laparotomy requires careful appraisal for the pediatric age group. Laparotomy for diagnostic and staging purposes carries a risk of morbidity and therefore should be performed only if the findings may substantially influence treatment. For instance, if the patient is already clinical Stage IV, if treatment will not be altered by staging, or if chemotherapy alone is to be used, laparotomy for diagnostic purposes only is contraindicated.[11,24,38] At institutions where the therapy depends on pathologic stage, approximately 30% of cases are either upstaged or downstaged by laparotomy and splenectomy; the procedure appears justified in these situations.[1,3,14,30] There is no accurate noninvasive diagnostic test for splenic involvement.

The possibility of an increased risk of sepsis must be carefully considered before splenectomy is used.[17] In the Intergroup Hodgkin's Disease Study, the incidence of sepsis was 2.1% (five of 234 patients) at 5 years.[19,20] However, this may be an underestimate of the final percentage. None of the cases of sepsis was fatal, and most of the patients were receiving prophylactic antibiotics (74%) and had received polyvalent pneumococcal vaccine (83%).

It seems prudent to follow the recommendation that prophylactic penicillin be given to all pediatric patients undergoing splenectomy, although the exact length of time necessary to treat is unclear.[5,8,30,44] The use of the polyvalent pneumococcal vaccine has been evaluated, but immunologic responses varied and made determination of effectiveness difficult.[9] It has been recommended that the lower age limit for splenectomy should be about 5 years in order to preserve the immature immune system.[45] Partial splenectomy has been suggested.[21,39]

The Ann Arbor staging system is generally used for Hodgkin's disease (see Table 73-2).[3]

Pathologic Classification

The Rye histologic classification is also applicable to pediatric Hodgkin's disease.[32] The influence of pathologic subtype alone, independent of stage or prognosis, has not been demonstrated.

Prognostic Factors

Treatment with high-dose, wide-field irradiation, although often indicated in an adult, may be inappropriate in children because of the arrest of bone and soft tissue growth that may follow. The results of chemotherapy alone are highly encouraging, but the very long-term effects of chemotherapy they are just emerging.[38] Six courses of MOPP (mechlorethamine, vincristine, procarbazine, and prednisone) therapy, for example, for all Stage I patients would increase early toxic effects, potentially sterilize male patients, and enhance the risk of second neoplasms.[38,50] It could also be dangerous in the long term. For this reason, other combinations including ABVD (doxorubicin [Adriamycin], bleomycin, vinblastine, dimethyltriazeno-imidazole carboxamide) or combinations of MOPP and ABVD are increasingly popular.

There is undoubtedly a higher chance of relapse in patients who are treated with local irradiation alone or extended-field irradiation alone, especially in those with mediastinal involvement, than in patients who have had both irradiation and chemotherapy even in early disease.[13,24,41] Not all patients who relapse after radiation therapy are doomed, and the overall survival rate, as opposed to the disease-free survival rate, may not be improved significantly by initial combined modality treatment for all patients.[41] The increased risk of leukemia in patients receiving a combination of radiation therapy and chemotherapy is also an important factor for consideration.

For early disease (Stages I and II), fundamental management is more controversial. Chemotherapy alone, chemotherapy plus low-dose irradiation, and irradiation alone in some situations have all been advocated and are being studied. For advanced disease (Stages III and IV), there is little argument that primary management is by chemotherapy because of the effects of standard-dose, whole-field irradiation. Questions remain about how much and which type of chemotherapy and whether results are improved by adding low-dose irradiation.

Radiation Therapy Techniques

The general principles of radiation therapy for Hodgkin's disease are outlined in Chapter 62. In children, involved field, rather than extended-field therapy, is usually employed. Protection of normal tissues is even more important than in adults. This does not, however, mean that involved-field therapy should be inadequate therapy, because coverage of lymphoid tissue at risk is vital. Examples of involved fields for several anatomic sites are shown in Figure 73-1.

Use of linear accelerators (rather than Telecobalt) sharpen the beam. In view of the superficiality of neck and inguinal nodes and the smaller size of children, treatment with low-energy (4–6 MV) accelerators is preferable to the use of the higher-energy machines. If the para-aortic nodes are to be irradiated, higher-energy photons (10–18 MV) may be used, especially in teenagers.

Custom-made blocks are also particularly indicated for children for protection of normal tissue and coverage of lymphoma tissue at risk. Specifically, shielding the teeth, the epiphyseal (especially the humeral) plates, and the uninvolved lung, heart, spinal cord, and gonads requires meticulous attention. Excessive shielding, however, may lead to local or marginal relapse.

Asymmetric growth defects are more obvious because the patient acts as his or her own control. The loss of subcutaneous adipose tissue in the neck, a very common late effect for a child or adolescent treated by irradiation only with doses of 3500 cGy to 4000 cGy given in 4 to 5 weeks is often only noticeable to the patient if it is unilateral.

Standard adult doses of radiation (*i.e.*, 3500–4000 cGy in 4–5 weeks with or without 500 cGy boost to bulky disease) should always be used if irradiation is used alone; there is no place for reduced-dose treatment in such situations. In combination with multiagent chemotherapy, lower doses to areas involved at diagnosis appear justifiable (2000–2500 cGy in 2.5–3 weeks), especially if the patient has already undergone one or more courses of chemotherapy and the tumor has responded promptly.

Results of Therapy

The results of radiation therapy alone are more difficult to assess in children than in adults because of the relative rarity of childhood disease and the variety of treatments that have been used.

Radiation therapy alone in Hodgkin's disease in children is in most centers more of historic interest. Nevertheless, there may be a role for radiation therapy alone in certain situations. Although only 69% of the Stanford series of 26 surgically staged patients treated with irradiation only were free from relapse at 10 years, this figure included eight of nine Stage I patients.[42] Jereb and colleagues[25] concluded that involved-field irradiation with chemotherapy only on relapse was suitable treatment for Stages I and IIa. Of 51 patients treated initially with involved-field radiation therapy alone, 15 had relapses, but most of these relapsing patients were salvaged by combination chemotherapy, and the 10-year survival rate was 93%. Mauch and colleagues[34] at Dana Farber Cancer Institute reported that only six of 49 patients with pathologic Stage I or IIA disease treated with irradiation alone had relapses, and only one of these subsequently died.

Management of all Stages of Hodgkin's disease in children by chemotherapy alone was originally reported from Uganda,[38] and substantial experience has been recently accumulated in

STAGE I
Unilateral Neck - Involved Fields

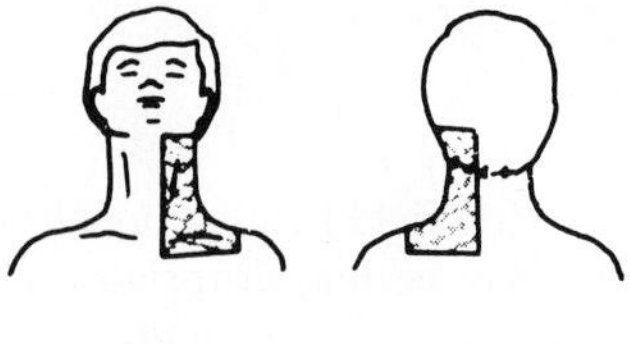

STAGE II
Unilateral Axilla and Ipsilateral Neck - Involved Fields

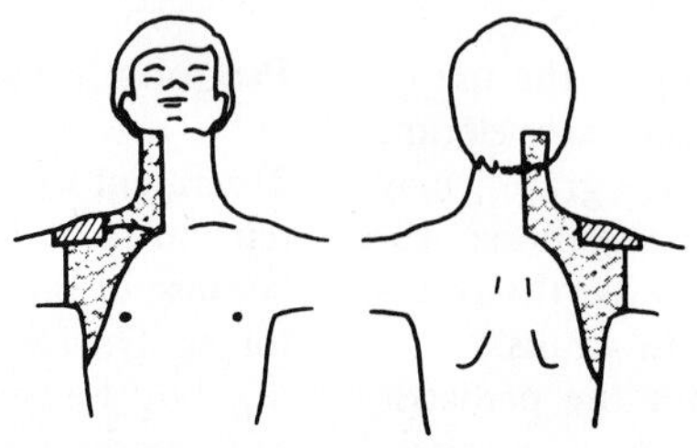

STAGE II
Mediastinum and Neck - Involved Fields

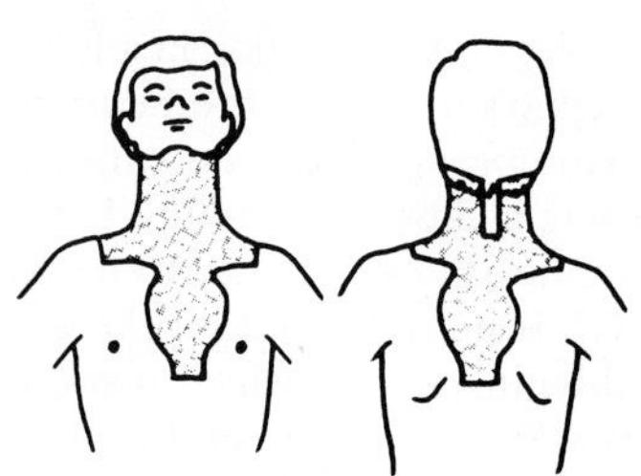

FIGURE 73–1. Examples of involved fields for several anatomic sites.

Australia.[11,12] The 4-year disease-free survival rate for 34 patients (all stages) treated with either MOPP or ABVD was 88%. However, two patients treated with MOPP died of toxic effects thought to result from cytomegalovirus in transfused blood. In the Netherlands, 21 selected children with tumors less than 4 cm in diameter were treated with six courses of MOPP only; the disease-free survival rate was 100%, with a median follow-up of 59.6 months.[2]

Much experience has been gained from the use of lower-dose irradiation (2000–2500 cGy) plus chemotherapy. The theory that less radiation is necessary with chemotherapy has been borne out in many series (Table 73-1).[7,10,24,28,51]

Sequelae

The acute complications for children are the same as those of radiation therapy for adults (Chap. 62). However, the tissues of very young children can be more acutely sensitive to radiation than those of adults. Because of the extended life expectancy of children, complications assume an added importance. Hypothyroidism, seen in approximately 48% of Hodgkin's patients younger than 10 years of age, may become more common with longer periods of follow-up.[15,36] Regular examination and, if necessary, investigation by physicians competent in the field should be performed at intervals throughout the patient's life.

In children, the special effects of radiation therapy are almost exclusively growth disturbances. If the breast bud in a prepubertal female is included in the mantle portal, hypoplasia of the breast will occur, usually leading to gross asymmetry. Irradiation of the spine can lead to reduction in the sitting height.[40] This reduction is more marked in children treated under the age of 6 and at puberty. This evidence indicates that total nodal irradiation and extended-field irradiation should be avoided if possible in childhood and early adolescence.

Pericarditis, myocardial fibrosis, and myocardial insufficiency may occur in children receiving full adult radiation doses, which could lead to premature death.[45] A survey of 12 patients who had received mantle irradiation 7 or more years earlier showed abnormal echocardiographs, pulmonary function tests, or exercise tests in nine patients, eight of whom were asymptomatic.[26] Similar abnormalities have been reported in another series.[44]

The ovaries will not function if irradiated in childhood to the dose used in the treatment of lymphoma.[43] At oophoropexy, the ovaries should be transposed laterally out of the beam or behind the uterus.[31,37]

The risk of developing second malignant neoplasms is greater in patients receiving combined radiation therapy and chemotherapy, although the evidence for this is mainly from adult patients.[6,10,33,48] Because of this risk, many investigators prefer ABVD to MOPP therapy. At Memorial Hospital, 17 second malignancies were identified in 320 patients treated between 1949 and 1983.[27] Acute nonlymphocytic leukemia, non-Hodgkin's lymphoma, and bone tumors predominated in the first 10 years after therapy ended.

Psychosocial late effects in this disease are relatively rare.[49] Of 40 patients surveyed, 95% felt that they had some good experience from having cancer. The major concerns were discrimination in employment and health insurance. Recommendations for follow-up of patients treated for childhood Hodgkin's disease have been made by Lange and Meadows.[29]

Summary of Clinical Trials

The Intergroup Hodgkin's Disease in Children Study compared the use of involved-field radiation therapy, involved-field radiation therapy and MOPP, and extended-field radiation therapy in pathologic Stages I and II Hodgkin's disease.[46] Preliminary results showed that although only eight (3%) of 279 patients died of disease, the length of initial disease control was significantly better with extended-field therapy than with involved-field radiation therapy. However, because 28% of patients were considered not evaluable for radiation therapy and because the length of follow-up was short, no therapeutic recommendations were made.

In early Hodgkin's disease, the Pediatric Oncology Group is currently investigating whether involved-field irradiation (2550 cGy) is a necessary addition to two courses of MOPP and two of ABVD. For advanced disease, four courses of MOPP and four courses of ABVD are given, and the randomization is to 2100 cGy total nodal irradiation or no additional radiation therapy for those in complete remission.

The British National Lymphoma Investigation reported an overall 5-year survival rate of 87% for 68 patients, with a variety of treatments.[33]

TABLE 73–1
Combined Modality Therapy for Pediatric Hodgkin's Disease

INVESTIGATION	STAGES*	CHEMOTHERAPY†	RADIATION THERAPY (cGy)	NO. OF PATIENTS	DISEASE-FREE SURVIVAL (%)
Toronto[18]	CS I–IV	6 × MOPP	2000–2500, extended field	27	90
Philadelphia[20]	CS IIB–IV	6 × COPP	2000, involved field	34	60
Stanford[78]	PS I–IV	6 × MOPP	1500–2500, involved field	55	89
St. Jude[79]	PS IIA–IV (large mediastinum only)	VCR, CY, 1 yr procarbazine 4×	2000	55	82
France[80]	CS I–IV	4 ABVD + 2 MOPP or 3 MOPP + ABVD	2000	157	88

**CS: clinical stage; PS: pathologic stage.*
† MOPP: mechlorethamine, vincristine, procarbazine, and prednisone; COPP: cyclophosphamide, vincristine, procarbazine, and prednisone; VCR, vincristine; CY: cyclophosphamide; ABVD: doxorubicin, bleomycin, vinblastine, and dimethyltriazene carboxamide.

NON-HODGKIN'S LYMPHOMAS IN CHILDREN

Epidemiology

Although it is established that African Burkitt's Lymphoma is linked to the Epstein-Barr virus, the cause of most types of non-Hodgkin's lymphoma in children remains obscure.[69] Immunosuppression may possibly be a factor, as is indicated by the increased risk in organ transplant patients.[82] Non-Hodgkin's lymphomas can occur in children with acquired immunodeficiency syndrome (AIDS).

The male-to-female patient ratio among children is approximately 3 : 1.[77] Non-Hodgkin's lymphoma is very rare in children younger than 3 years of age.[62,80]

Natural History

Non-Hodgkin's lymphoma in children should be considered as a disease entity separate from the adult disease. However, childhood non-Hodgkin's lymphomas share with their adult counterparts the propensity for variable patterns of spread or extranodal presentations, although the latter are even more likely to occur in children than in adults. Abdominal disease is most common (Fig. 73-2), followed by mediastinal, head and neck, and peripheral node presentations.

In the recent St. Jude Children's Research Hospital series, involved peripheral nodes outside the neck were discovered at diagnosis in only 6.5% of the patients, and bone, skin, epidural space, and thyroid were involved in 7%.[62]

The spectrum of histologies is different in children and adults. In adults, approximately half have nodular histology and half diffuse; in children, the nodular variety is very rare.[60,68] This difference explains why pediatric non-Hodgkin's lymphomas can behave very aggressively. This aggressiveness, however, parodoxically makes the pediatric disease curable in most instances.

Diagnostic Workup

Diagnostic workup must include a careful history and physical examination, a complete blood count, biochemical profiles, and a chest roentgenogram. In addition, because of the propensity of non-Hodgkin's involvement of the bone marrow and the central nervous system (CNS) and of leukemic transformation, a bone marrow aspirate and examination of the cerebrospinal fluid are mandatory. Abdominal CT should be performed routinely. Chest CT scans are obtained to assess a mediastinal mass and magnetic resonance imaging (MRI) scans should also be considered.

Laparotomy for staging purposes in Hodgkin's disease is indicated only if the treatment is likely to be altered by the findings; consequently, in childhood non-Hodgkin's lymphoma, laparotomy for staging purposes alone is practically eliminated because treatment is primarily systemic, whatever the stage.

The Ann Arbor classification was designed for Hodgkin's disease and is frequently applied to non-Hodgkin's lymphoma.[56] Although this classification may be of prognostic sig-

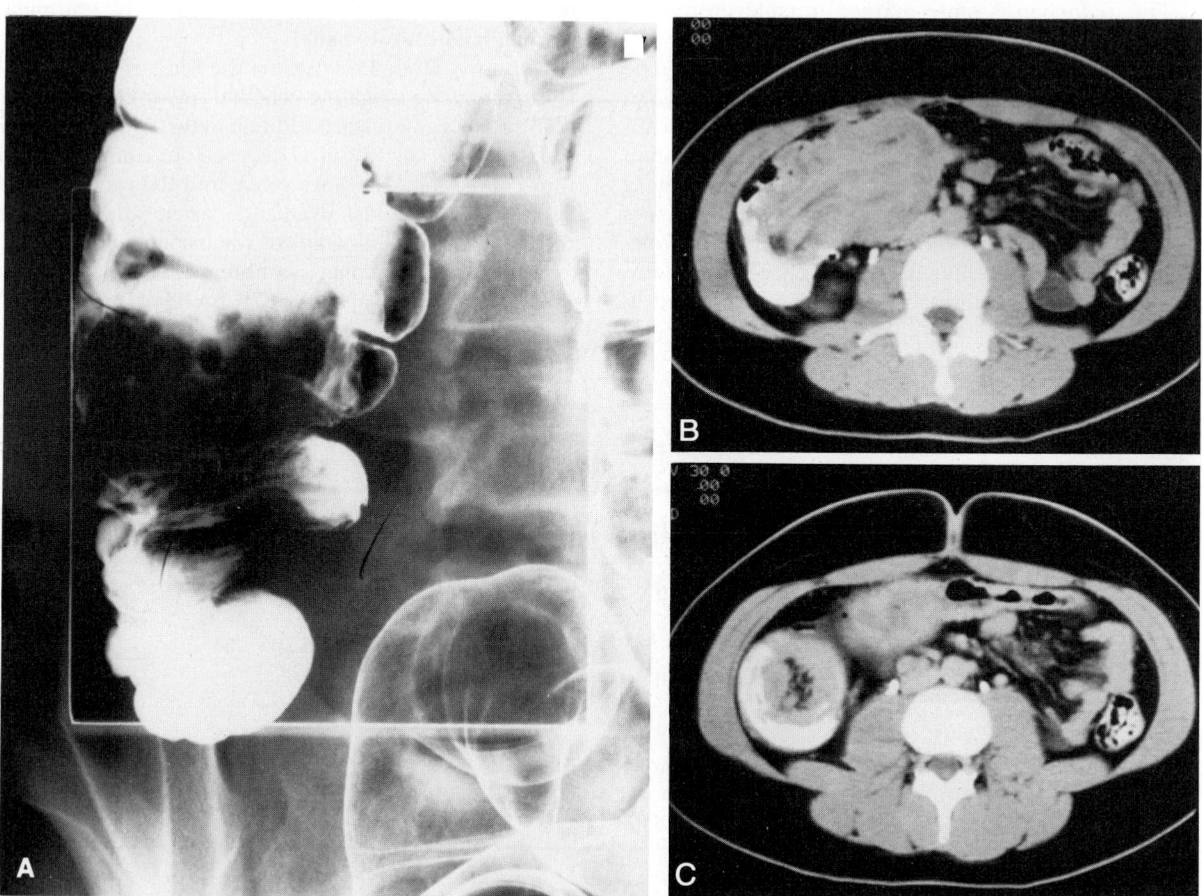

FIGURE 73–2. (**A**) Barium enema and (**B, C**) CT scans of a 12-year-old girl with ileocecal histiocytic lymphoma. Notice the (**B**) extensive involvement and (**C**) intussusception.

nificance in adults, in children it is less appropriate because of the different pace of the disease, the frequency of extranodal presentation, and the tendency for central nervous system disease and leukemic conversion.[68] Alternative classifications have been proposed by Murphy[77] and Wollner and associates[87] (Table 73-2). Because of its somewhat different features, Burkitt's lymphoma is usually staged using the system devised by Ziegler and co-workers,[90] which takes into account tumor burden.

Pathologic Classification

The Rappaport classification[84] is applicable in pediatrics, but some important reservations remain, especially in view of the paucity of nodular disease in this age group. Dehner[58] found in a cumulated review that poorly differentiated lymphocytic, lymphoblastic, and histiocytic types account for 94% of the childhood lymphomas. The classification of Lukes and Collins[71] is also applicable, and the National Cancer Institute has produced recommendations.[81]

The poorly differentiated lymphocytic and lymphoblastic tumors frequently occur in the mediastinum and often undergo leukemic transformation. The lymphoblastic variant is a disease of T lymphocytes and the undifferentiated tumors (*i.e.*, Burkitt's and non-Burkitt's) are of B cell origin.

Burkitt's lymphomas were originally described in Africa, where they often involve the head and neck (particularly the mandible), but they also occur in other countries. Gastrointestinal presentations are common. Although common in certain parts of Africa, in Dehner's[58] composite series, they accounted for only 3% of the cases. The main significance of the Burkitt's subgroup is that these lymphomas grow rapidly and may need more aggressive therapy.[77,91] The histiocytic variety only occasionally presents in the mediastinum but commonly involves the abdomen or head and neck. The reader is referred to an excellent article by Magrath[74] for a more detailed discussion on histology and immunology.

Prognostic Factors Influencing Treatment

The pathologic type of the tumor is of prognostic significance and influences the choice of treatment. The likelihood of leukemic transformation and the relatively unpredictable patterns of spread indicate systemic therapy for all patients.

Most authors regard staging as relevant in the choice of treatment; notable exceptions have been Wollner and her colleagues, who have successfully used the LSA_2-L_2 protocol for all stages.[53,57,65,78,87–89]

General Management

In view of the excellent results obtained with chemotherapy, systemic treatment for all patients is justified.[67] The goal of treatment should be eradicating the disease and curing the patient.

General principles of physiologic and psychological support apply, particularly if highly aggressive regimens are used.

Radiation Therapy Techniques

The management of pediatric non-Hodgkin's lymphoma by radiation therapy alone is of historic interest only. Radiation therapy can be used to treat bulky tumor, although the indications are few, and it may be used in certain circumstances for meningeal prophylaxis.[53,57]

Standard radiation therapy techniques are used. Specific node groups and extranodal involvement are treated as in Hodgkin's disease, except that extended-field treatment is seldom indicated. However, extensive abdominal involvement is so common that, if radiation is to be given, the whole abdomen must often be treated.

Considerable care should be employed with the timing and dosage of radiation therapy in view of both the aggressive

TABLE 73–2
Classification of Pediatric Hodgkin's and Non-Hodgkin's Lymphoma

STAGE	ANN ARBOR[56] (H AND NHL)	MURPHY[76] (NHL)	WOLLNER ET AL[86] (NHL)
I	Involvement of single lymphatic region (I) or single extralymphatic site without regional nodes (IE)	A single tumor (extranodal) or single anatomic area (nodal), with the exclusion of mediastinum or abdomen	One single site
II	Involvement of two or more lymphatic regions on the same side of the diaphragm (II), which may include the spleen (IIS), or localized extralymphatic involvement with draining regional lymph node involvement (IIE)	A single tumor (extranodal) with regional node involvement Two or more nodal areas in the same side of the diaphragm Two single (extranodal) tumors	Two or more sites on the same side of the diaphragm
III	Involvement of lymphatic regions on both sides of diaphragm (III), including spleen (IIIS), localized extralymphatic involvement (IIIE), or both (IIISE)	Two single tumors (extranodal) on opposite sides of the diaphragm Two or more nodal areas above the diaphragm All the primary intrathoracic tumors (mediastinal, pleural, thymic) All extensive primary intraabdominal disease All paraspinal or epidural tumors, regardless of other tumor site(s)	Disseminated disease without tumor or CNS involvement
IV	Disseminated extralymphatic involvement including bone marrow (IVM), liver (IVH), or pleura (IVP)	Any of the above with initial CNS or bone marrow involvement	Any of the above with bone marrow or CNS involvement

myelosuppression and the potentiation of the effects of radiation caused by chemotherapy. Radiation therapy may be better tolerated during the maintenance phase. This is particularly so if advanced (Stages III and IV) disease is to be treated. These are radiation-responsive tumors, and with intensive chemotherapy, the doses for advanced disease (Stages III and IV) should not exceed 2500 cGy in 3 weeks (2000 cGy in 3 to 4 weeks to the whole abdomen). Doses in excess of this are likely to be toxic and may limit the amount of chemotherapy given.[57,78] It seems that the standard dose of 3500 cGy given in 4 weeks with chemotherapy for early-stage (I and II) non-Hodgkin's lymphoma in children may be excessive. Current studies use lower doses.

Meningeal prophylaxis may be achieved by standard lateral cranial parallel opposed fields covering all the meninges as far as the second cervical vertebra (Fig. 73-3). Great care must be taken to avoid a geographic miss of the meninges around the orbit. The maximum dosage should be 2400 cGy administered in 2.5 weeks. Because this dosage in combination with intrathecal methotrexate may have long-term adverse effects on the brain and pituitary and because CNS prophylaxis is often satisfactorily achieved without craniospinal irradiation, radiation therapy is often not used in CNS prophylaxis for childhood lymphoma.[75,85] Cranial irradiation is almost always used if there is established CNS disease, and a spinal field may sometimes be used. In spinal irradiation, a field 6 cm to 7 cm wide is employed, treating to the bottom of the subarachnoid space (S2). If a prompt response of a mediastinal mass causing superior vena caval obstruction is not obtained with chemotherapy, irradiation in low doses (250 cGy in three fractions) provides rapid relief in most cases.

Other indications for radiation therapy are for treating primary bone lymphoma and primary lymphoma of the CNS, both of which are rare in children. Primary bone lymphoma has been successfully treated at Dana Farber Cancer Center with 4000 cGy to 4500 cGy to the whole bone plus a boost of 500 cGy to the primary lesion along with doxorubicin, prednisone, and vincristine (APO regimen).[71] Primary CNS lymphomas associated and not associated with AIDS are becoming increasingly common in adults, and there will probably be an increase in the incidence in children.

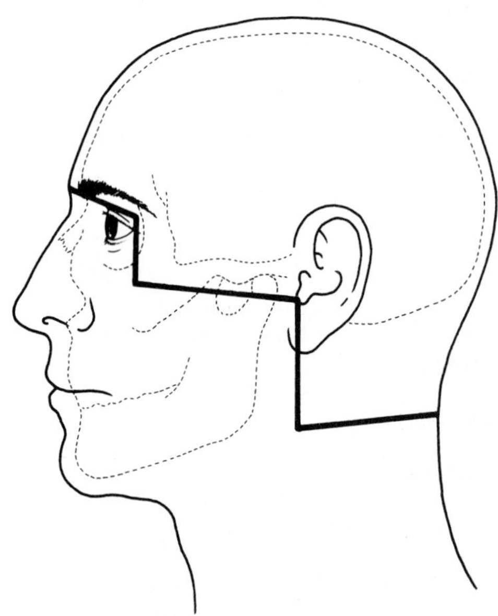

FIGURE 73–3. Standard lateral cranial parallel opposed fields covering all the meninges as far as the second cervical vertebra.

Results of Therapy

Although radiation therapy alone in one series cured approximately 55% of patients with Ann Arbor Stage I lymph node presentations, non-Hodgkin's lymphomas in children are much more curable by combined-modality therapy.[61] The 2-year disease-free survival rate can be considered the cure rate for this disease.

With radiation therapy to bulky sites (2000–3600 cGy, depending on extent) starting at the third week, combined with a relatively simple program of induction followed by maintenance chemotherapy, Brecher and colleagues[53,54] reported three of four Stage I patients (Ann Arbor classification) and nine of nine Stage II patients alive and disease-free 28 to 65 months after diagnosis. Less optimal results were obtained for patients with advanced disease.

Murphy and Hustu[78] treated 21 patients with Murphy Stages I and II disease (Table 73-2) with an induction regimen of vincristine, prednisone, and cyclophosphamide with radiation therapy (3000–3500 cGy) to bulky sites from the beginning, followed for patients with Stage II disease by randomization to CNS prophylaxis or not; all patients then received maintenance with 6-mercaptopurine and oral methotrexate. Ninety percent of patients remained disease-free.

After this experience, reduced-intensity therapy was used with involved-field (2000 cGy) irradiation in addition to induction chemotherapy (vincristine, cyclophosphamide, and prednisone), which was followed by maintenance with oral methotrexate and 6-mercaptopurine for 15 months. Of 28 patients, 24 were in complete remission at 2 years; all four failures were local in patients with tumors that had undifferentiated histologies.[79] Recently published results from St. Jude Children's Research Hospital have shown good results for patients with Stages I, II, or III disease. The 2-year event-free survival rates for 154 patients are 97% for Stage I, 86% for Stage II, 73% for Stage III, and 47% for Stage IV.[80] The results for children younger than 3 years of age from the same institution have been separately reported and showed that only six (37.5%) of 16 were long-term survivors.[62] The National Cancer Institute has also reported good results with more intensive chemotherapy over a shorter period (6 months) without irradiation.[73] Mediastinal T-cell lymphoma has been successfully treated with a six-drug leukemia regimen with cranial but no thoracic irradiation.[55]

With much more intensive therapy for all stages (Table 73-1), Wollner and associates[86,87] used the LSA_2-L_2 protocol consisting of cyclophosphamide, prednisone, vincristine, daunomycin, intrathecal methotrexate, cytosine arabinoside, thioguanine, L-asparaginase, BCNU, and hydroxyurea with local radiation therapy up to 4500 cGy in 4 weeks. Updated results have recently been published.[88] Of 60 patients with lymphoblastic lymphoma, 50 are surviving off therapy (median, 10 years). For Memorial Stages I, II, and III, the disease-free survival rate was 100%; for Stage IV it was 70%. For 114 patients with nonlymphoblastic lymphoma, the disease-free survival rate was 73%.

A highly intensive regimen was devised for children with nonlymphoblastic lymphomas consisting of induction with cyclophosphamide, doxorubicin, vincristine, and prednisone (CHOP), consolidation with triple intrathecal therapy and CHOP, alternating cytosine arabinoside and 6 thioguanine, oral methotrexate and etoposide, and CHOP. Twenty-three of 30 patients were disease-free at intervals between 21 and 65 months.[59]

The management of Burkitt's lymphoma with multimodality therapy, including aggressive surgery, has been summarized by Ziegler.[91] Approximately 50% can be cured. Conventional radiation therapy has been disappointing.[91] An actuarial survival rate of 75% was reported in one recent series with alternating doses of methotrexate and cyclophosphamide used for induction.[86] However, results from the Pediatric Oncology Group and St. Jude Children's Research Hospital showed no significant differences in any parameters, including survival for Burkitt's and non-Burkitt's, small non-cleaved cell (undifferentiated) lymphomas.[63]

The results of high-dose cytosine arabinoside therapy, total-body irradiation, and bone marrow transplantation in advanced (relapsed or never in remission) lymphoma were disappointing. There were no survivors among the four patients under 18 years of age.[83]

Sequelae of Treatment

The short-term toxicity depends on the intensity of the regimen. Thus, the LSA_2-L_2 protocol has many more toxic effects than the regimen reported by Brecher and co-workers, who reported one toxic death and otherwise only transient toxicity.[53,54,87,88] There have been deaths from measles and chickenpox, reversible renal shutdown, and profound myelosuppression with the LSA_2-L_2 protocol.[88] It has also given rise to problems with radiation therapy. For example, 4500 cGy to the nasopharynx is badly tolerated with such intense chemotherapy.

Murphy and Hustu[78] reported moderate toxicity except for one death from *Pneumocystis carinii* and one case of transverse myelitis that developed in a boy 2 months after induction with 3500 cGy given in 32 days to the mediastinum and a course of vincristine, cyclophosphamide, prednisone, and doxorubicin. After therapy for early-stage non-Hodgkin's lymphoma was reduced, the toxic effects were correspondingly less.[80]

Summary of Clinical Trials

The results of St. Jude Children's Research Hospital's earlier study for Murphy Stages III and IV showed that involved-field (3000–3500 cGy) or whole-abdominal (2000–2500 cGy) irradiation increased toxicity but provided no survival or disease-free survival benefit over chemotherapy alone.[77]

A randomized trial comparing a four-drug COMP regimen (cyclophosphamide, vincristine, methotrexate and prednisone) with a modified LSA_2-L_2 regimen was reported by the Children's Cancer Study Group.[67] All patients in both arms received maintenance intrathecal methotrexate; most received irradiation to bulk disease. Patients with lymphoblastic mediastinal presentation did better with the LSA_2-L_2 modification, but for those with diffuse undifferentiated histology, the COMP regimen was superior. Another randomized clinical trial conducted by the Children's Cancer Study Group showed that 6 months of COMP produced identical results to 18 months for patients with nonlymphoblastic (diffuse undifferentiated) histologies.[76]

The Pediatric Oncology Group has conducted several studies. For localized disease (Murphy Stages I and II), a randomized trial comparing 6 months of modest multiagent chemotherapy (vincristine, cyclophosphamide, doxorubicin, 6-mercaptopurine, and methotrexate) alone with this multiagent chemotherapy plus involved-field (2700 cGy) irradiation showed identical 4-year event-free survivals in both arms (87%) for 129 patients followed for a median of 38 months.[70]

Other Pediatric Oncology Group studies have shown the prognostic effects of histologic subclassification of diffuse undifferentiated lymphomas into large cell and small non-cleaved cell groups. Patients with the small cell disease did much better with doxorubicin, vincristine, cyclophosphamide, prednisone, methotrexate, 6-mercaptopurine, and irradiation (ACOP+).[64] Extended maintenance therapy for nonlymphoblastic (Burkitt's and non-Burkitt's) disease was found to be unnecessary in a study that compared two with six courses of maintenance high-dose methotrexate.[63]

REFERENCES

Hodgkin's Disease

1. Bell MJ, Land VJ, Ternberg JL: Staging laparotomy for Hodgkin's disease in children. Am J Surg 133:582, 1977
2. Behrendt H, Van Bunningen B, Van Leeuwen E: Treatment of Hodgkin's disease in children with or without radiotherapy. Cancer 59:1870, 1987
3. Carbone PP, Kaplan HS, Musshoff K, et al: Report of the Committee on Hodgkin's Disease Staging Classification. Cancer Res 31:1860, 1971
4. Castellino RA, Marglin SI: Imaging of abdominal and pelvic lymph nodes: Lymphography or computed tomography? Invest Radiol 17:433, 1982
5. Chilcote RR, Baehner RL, Hammond D: Septicemia and meningitis in children splenectomized for Hodgkin's disease. N Engl J Med 295:798, 1976
6. Coltman CA, Dixon DO: Second malignancies complicating Hodgkin's disease: A Southwest Oncology Group 1-year follow-up. Cancer Treat Rep 66:1023, 1982
7. Dionet C, Oberlin O, Habrand JL, et al: Initial chemotherapy and low-dose radiation in limited fields in childhood Hodgkin's disease: Results of a joint cooperative study by the French Society of Pediatric Oncology (SFOP) and Hospital Saint-Louis, Paris. Int J Radiat Oncol Biol Phys 15:341, 1988
8. Donaldson SS, Glatstein E, Vosti KL: Bacterial infections in pediatric Hodgkin's disease. Cancer 41:1949, 1978
9. Donaldson SS, Vosti K, Berberick FR, et al: A comparison of responses to pneumococcal vaccine among children with Hodgkin's disease. Proc Am Soc Clin Oncol 21:393, 1980
10. Donaldson SS, Link MP: Combined modality treatment with low-dose radiation and MOPP chemotherapy for children with Hodgkin's disease. J Clin Oncol 5:742, 1987
11. Ekert H, Waters KD, Smith PJ, et al: Treatment with MOPP or CHEVPP chemotherapy only for all stages of childhood Hodgkin's disease. J Clin Oncol 6:1845, 1988
12. Ekert H, Waters KD, Smith PJ, et al: Treatment with MOPP or CHEVPP chemotherapy only for all stages of childhood Hodgkin's disease. J Clin Oncol 6:1845, 1988
13. Fuller LM, Madoc-Jones H, Hagemeister FB, et al: Further follow-up of the 90 laparotomy negative stage I and II Hodgkin's disease patients: Significance of mediastinal and nonmediastinal presentations. Int J Radiat Oncol Biol Phys 6:799, 1980
14. Girvan D: Staging laparotomy for Hodgkin's disease in children. Can J Surg 21:409, 1978
15. Glatstein E, McHardy-Young S, Brast N, et al: Alterations in serum thyrotrophin (TSH) and thyroid function following radiotherapy in patients with malignant lymphoma. J Clin Endocrinol 32:833, 1979
16. Glicksman AS, Pajak TF, Gottlieb A, et al: Second malignant neoplasms in patients successfully treated for Hodgkin's disease. Cancer Treat Rep 66:1035, 1982
17. Green DM, Stutzman L, Blumenson LE, et al: The incidence of postsplenectomy sepsis and herpes zoster in children and adolescents with Hodgkin's disease. Med Pediatr Oncol 7:285, 1979

18. Gutensohn N, Cole P: Childhood social environment and Hodgkin's disease. N Engl J Med 304:135, 1989
19. Hays DM, Ternberg JL, Chen TT, et al: Complications relating to 234 staging laparotomies performed in the Intergroup Hodgkin's Disease Study. Surgery 96:471, 1984
20. Hays DM, Ternberg JL, Chen TT, et al: Post-splenectomy sepsis and other complications following staging laparotomy for Hodgkin's disease in childhood. J Pediatr Surg 21:628, 1986
21. Hoekstra HJ, Kamps WA: Indications for staging laparotomy and partial splenectomy. In Kamps WA, Humphrey GB, Poppema S (eds): Hodgkin's Disease in Children, pp 121–128. Boston, Kluwer Academic Publishers, 1989
22. Jenkin RDT, Berry MP: Hodgkin's disease in children. Semin Oncol 7:202, 1980
23. Jenkin RDT, Brown TC, Peters MV, et al: Hodgkin's disease in children. Cancer 35:979, 1975
24. Jenkin RDT, Freedman M, McLure P, et al: Hodgkin's disease in children: Treatment with low-dose irradiation and MOPP without staging laparotomy. Cancer 44:80, 1979
25. Jereb B, Tan CTC, Bretsy S, et al: Involved field (IF) irradiation with or without chemotherapy in the management of children with Hodgkin's disease. Med Pediatr Oncol 12:325, 1984
26. Kadota RP, Burgert EO, Driscoll DJ, et al: Cardiopulmonary function in long-term survivors of childhood Hodgkin's lymphoma: A pilot study. Mayo Clin Proc 63:362, 1988
27. Kushner BH, Zauber A, Tan CRC: Second malignancies after childhood Hodgkin's disease: The Memorial Sloan-Kettering Cancer Center experience. Cancer 62:1364, 1988
28. Lange B, Littman P: Management of Hodgkin's disease in children and adolescents. Cancer 51:1371, 1983
29. Lange BJ, Meadows AT: Late effects of Hodgkin's disease treatment in children. Cancer Treat Res 41:195, 1989
30. Lanskowsky P, Shende A, Kasayalcin G, et al: Staging laparotomy and splenectomy treatment complication of Hodgkin's disease in children. Am J Hematol 1:393, 1976
31. LeFloch O, Donaldson SS, Kaplan H: Pregnancy following oophoropexy and total nodal irradiation in women with Hodgkin's disease. Cancer 38:2263, 1976
32. Lukes RJ, Craver LF, Hall TC, et al: Report of the nomenclature committee. Cancer Res 26:1311, 1966
33. Makepeace AR, Maclennan KA, Hudson GV, et al: Hodgkin's disease in childhood: The British National Lymphoma Investigation experience (BNLI Report No. 27). Clin Radiol 38:7, 1987
34. Mauch PM, Weinstein H, Botnick LE, et al: An evaluation of long-term survival and treatment complications of children with Hodgkin's disease. Cancer 51:925, 1983
35. Mefferd JM, Donaldson SS, Link MP: Pediatric Hodgkin's disease: Pulmonary, cardiac, and thyroid function following combined modality therapy. Int J Radiat Oncol Biol Phys 16:679, 1989
36. Mill WB, Palmer Hanes LA, Purdy JA, et al: Extended field radiation therapy in Hodgkin's disease. Cancer 40:2896, 1977
37. Nahas WA, Nisce LZ, D'Angio GJ, et al: Lateral ovarian transposition: Ovarian relocation in patients with Hodgkin's disease. Obstet Gynecol 38:785, 1971
38. Olweny CLM, Katonggole M'bidde E, et al: Childhood Hodgkin's disease in Uganda. Cancer 42:787, 1978
39. Pringle KC, Hays DM: Current management and controversies: A surgeon's view in Hodgkin's disease in children. In Kamps WA, Humphrey GB, Poppema S (eds): Hodgkin's Disease in Children, pp 109–119. Boston, Kluwer Academic Publishers, 1989
40. Probert JC, Parker BR, Kaplan HS: Growth retardation in children after megavoltage irradiation of the spine. Cancer 32:634, 1973
41. Rosenberg SA, Kaplan HS, Glatstein E, et al: Combined therapy of Hodgkin's disease. Cancer 35:55, 1975
42. Russell KJ, Donaldson SS, Cox RS, et al: Childhood Hodgkin's disease: Patterns of relapse. J Clin Oncol 2:80, 1984
43. Shalet SM, Beardwell CG, Jones PHM, et al: Ovarian failure following abdominal irradiation in children. J Cancer 33:655, 1976
44. Smith IE, Peckham MJ, McElwain TJ, et al: Hodgkin's disease in children. Br J Cancer 36:120, 1977
45. Sullivan MP, Fuller LM, Butler JJ: Hodgkin's disease in children. In Sutow WW, Vietti TJ, Fernbach DJ (eds): Clinical Pediatric Oncology, 3rd ed. St. Louis, CV Mosby, 1983
46. Sullivan MP, Fuller LM, Chen T, et al: Intergroup Hodgkin's Disease in Children study of stages I and II: A preliminary report. Cancer Treat Rep 66:937, 1982
47. Tan C, D'Angio GJ, Exelby PR, et al: The changing management of Hodgkin's disease. Cancer 35:808, 1975
48. Tester WJ, Kinsella TJ, Waller B, et al: Second malignant neoplasms complicating Hodgkin's disease: The National Cancer Institute experience. J Clin Oncol 2:762, 1984
49. Wasserman AL, Thompson EI, Wilimas JA, et al: The psychological status of survivors of childhood/adolescent Hodgkin's disease. Am J Dis Child 141:626, 1987
50. Whitehead E, Shalet SM, Morris Jones PM, et al: Gonadal function after combination chemotherapy for Hodgkin's disease in childhood. Arch Dis Child 57:287, 1982
51. Wilimas JA, Thompson EI: Results of therapy for Hodgkin's disease at St. Jude's Hospital. In Kamps WA, Humphrey GB, Poppema S (eds): Hodgkin's Disease in Children. Boston, Kluwer Academic Publishers, 1989
52. Young RC, DeVita VT, Johnson RE: Hodgkin's disease in childhood. J Hematol 163, 1973

Non-Hodgkin's Lymphomas

53. Brecher ML, Sinks LF, Thomas PRM, et al: Non-Hodgkin's lymphoma in children. Cancer 41:1997, 1978
54. Brecher ML, Thomas PRM, Sinks LF, et al: Updated results on the treatment of childhood non-Hodgkin's lymphoma. Proc Am Soc Clin Oncol 20:438, 1979
55. Camitta BM, Lanes SJ, Casper JT, et al: Effectiveness of a six-drug regimen (APO) without local irradiation for treatment of mediastinal lymphoblastic lymphoma in children. Cancer 56:738, 1985
56. Carbone PP, Kaplan HS, Musshoff K, et al: Report of the Committee on Hodgkin's Disease Staging Classification. Cancer Res 31:1860, 1971
57. Cebrian Bonesena A, Schvartzman E, Roca-Garcia C, et al: Non-Hodgkin's lymphoma in children: An analysis of 122 cases from Argentina. Cancer 41:2372, 1978
58. Dehner LP: Non-Hodgkin's lymphomas and malignant histiocytosis. Semin Oncol 4:273, 1977
59. Finlay JL, Trigg ME, Link MP, et al: Poor-risk non-lymphoblastic lymphoma of childhood: Results of an intensive pilot study. Med Pediatr Oncol 17:29, 1989
60. Frizzera G, Murphy SB: Follicular lymphoma in childhood: A rare clinicopathological entity. Cancer 44:2218, 1979
61. Glatstein E, Kim H, Donaldson SS, et al: Non-Hodgkin's lymphoma. VI. Results of treatment in childhood. Cancer 34:204, 1974
62. Hutchison RE, Pui C-H, Murphy SB, et al: Non-Hodgkin's lymphoma in children younger tha n 3 years. Cancer 62:1371, 1988
63. Hutchison RE, Murphy SB, Fairclough DL, et al: Diffuse small noncleaved cell lymphoma in children, Burkitt's *versus* non-Burkitt's types. Cancer 64:23, 1989
64. Hvizdala EV, Berard CW, Callihan T, et al: Non-lymphoblastic lymphoma in children: Histology and stage related response to therapy. A Pediatric Oncology Group Study. Proc Am Soc Clin Oncol 6:192, 1987
65. Jaffe N, Buell D, Cassady JR, et al: Role of staging in childhood non-Hodgkin's lymphoma. Cancer Treat Rep 61:1001, 1977
66. Jenkin RDT: Radiation in the treatment of non-Hodgkin's lymphoma in children. Semin Oncol 4:311, 1977
67. Jenkin RDT, Anderson JP, Chilcote RR, et al: The treatment of localized non-Hodgkin's lymphoma in children: A report from the Children's Cancer Study Group. J Clin Oncol 2:88, 1973
68. Jones SE, Fuks Z, Kaplan HS, et al: Non-Hodgkin's lymphomas. V. Results of radiotherapy. Cancer 32:682, 1973

69. Klein G: The Epstein Barr virus and neoplasia. N Engl J Med 293:1353, 1975
70. Link MP, Donaldson SS, Berard CW, et al: Results of treatment of childhood localized non-Hodgkin's lymphoma with combination chemotherapy with or without radiotherapy. N Engl J Med 322:1169, 1990
71. Loeffler JS, Tarbell NJ, Kozakewich H, et al: Primary lymphoma of bone in children: Analysis of treatment results with Adriamycin, prednisone, and vincristine (APO) and local radiation therapy. J Clin Oncol 4:496, 1986
72. Lukes R, Collins RD: Immunologic characterization of human malignant lymphomas. Cancer 34:1488, 1972
73. Magrath IT, Janus C, Edwards BK, et al: An effective therapy for both undifferentiated (including Burkitt's) lymphomas and lymphoblastic lymphomas in children and young adults. Blood 63:1102, 1984
74. Magrath IT: Malignant non-Hodgkin's lymphomas in children. Hematol Oncol Clin North Am 1:577, 1987
75. Mandell LR, Wollner N, Fuks A: Is cranial irradiation necessary for CNS prophylaxis in pediatric NHL? Int J Radiat Oncol Biol Phys 13:359, 1987
76. Meadows AT, Sposto R, Jenkin RDT, et al: Similar efficacy of 6 and 18 months of therapy with four drugs (COMP) for localized non-Hodgkin's lymphoma of children: A report from the Children's Cancer Study Group. J Clin Oncol 7:92, 1989
77. Murphy SB: Classification, staging and end results of treatment of childhood non-Hodgkin's lymphoma: Dissimilarities from lymphomas in adults. Semin Oncol 7:332, 1980
78. Murphy SB, Hustu HO: A randomized trial of combined modality therapy of childhood non-Hodgkin's lymphoma. Cancer 45:630, 1980
79. Murphy SB, Hustu HO, Rivera G, et al: End results of treating children with localized non-Hodgkin's lymphoma with a combined modality approach of lessened intensity. J Clin Oncol 1:326, 1983
80. Murphy SB, Fairclough DL, Hutchison RE, et al: Non-Hodgkin's lymphomas of childhood: An analysis of the histology, staging, and response to treatment of 338 cases at a single institution. J Clin Oncol 7:186, 1989
81. National Cancer Institute sponsored study of classifications of non-Hodgkin's lymphomas. Summary and description of a working formulation for clinical usage. Cancer 49:2112, 1982
82. Penn I: Second malignant neoplasms associated with immunosuppressive medications. Cancer 37:1024, 1976
83. Petersen FB, Appelbaum CL, Bigelow CD, et al: High-dose cytosine arabinoside, total body irradiation and marrow transplantation for advanced malignant lymphoma. Bone Marrow Transplant 4:483, 1989
84. Rappaport H: Tumors of the hemopoietic system. In Atlas of Tumor Pathology, sec 3, fasc 8. Washington, DC, US Armed Forces Institute of Pathology, 1966
85. Rowland JH, Glidewell OJ, Sibley RF, et al: Effects of different forms of central nervous system prophylaxis on neuropsychobiologic function in childhood leukemia. J Clin Oncol 2:1327, 1984
86. Sullivan MP, Ramirez I: Curability of Burkitt's lymphoma with high-dose cyclophosphamide–high-dose methotrexate therapy with intrathecal chemoprophylaxis. J Clin Oncol 3:627, 1985
87. Wollner N, Burchenal JH, Exelby PR, et al: Non-Hodgkin's lymphoma in children: A comparison of two modalities of therapy. Cancer 37:123, 1976
88. Wollner N, Exelby PR, Lieberman PH: Non-Hodgkin's lymphoma in children: A progress report on the original patients treated with LSA_2-L_2 protocol. Cancer 44:1990, 1979
89. Wollner N: Non-Hodgkin's lymphoma in children diffuse lymphoblastic histology diffuse non-lymphoblastic histology LSA_2-L_2 experience. An Esp Pediatr 29(suppl 34):122, 1988
90. Ziegler JL, DeVita VT, Graw RG, et al: Combined modality treatment of American Burkitt's lymphoma. Cancer 38:2225, 1976
91. Ziegler JL: Management of Burkitt's lymphoma. An update. Cancer Treat Rep 6:95, 1979

74

Radiation Treatment of Benign Disease

William Serber
Beatriz E. Amendola

The radiation oncologist's primary concern is treatment of patients with malignant tumors. Recognizing the risks of late skin injury, carcinogenesis, leukemogenesis, and genetic damage from all ionizing radiation, radiation therapy continues to be accepted treatment for those benign diseases that do not respond to other methods of therapy and in the unusual instance of a life-threatening benign disease that cannot be surgically or medically managed.

TECHNICAL CONSIDERATIONS

The report of the Committee on Radiation Treatment of Benign Disease of the Bureau of Radiological Health recommends the following[16]:

1. Before instituting therapy, consider the quality of radiation, total dose, overall time, underlying organs at risk, and shielding factors.
2. Infants and children should be treated with ionizing radiation only in very exceptional cases and after careful evaluation of the potential risk compared with the expected benefit.
3. Direct irradiation of the skin areas overlying organs that are particularly prone to late effects (*e.g.*, thyroid, eye, gonads, bone marrow, and breast) should be avoided.
4. Meticulous radiation protection techniques, including cones and lead shields, should be used in all instances.
5. The depth of penetration of the x-ray beam should be chosen in accordance with the depth of the pathologic process.

As part of the same study, Kopicky and Order[72] analyzed the current use of radiation therapy for benign disease by radiation oncologists, using a questionnaire survey of 23 academic and 21 private practice centers. On the basis of the replies, 70 diseases mentioned in the questionnaire were divided into categories of those acceptable for treatment and those that were unacceptable by most of the centers. The data show that there are very great differences in opinion among therapists about optimal dose and fractionation for treatment of most of the diseases. Further, the benefits of irradiation may greatly outweigh the risks, which are frequently minimal.

RADIATION THERAPY TECHNIQUES

As in all radiation treatment, the choice of beam energy depends on the depth of the target volume, and every effort is made to spare normal underlying tissue in superficial lesions. Absorption data for x-ray therapy are readily obtained from standard depth-dose tables.[45]

In many facilities, medical linear accelerators with 6-MeV to 20-MeV electrons are more frequently available than low-energy x-ray equipment. These electrons are commonly used for treating superficial lesions. Generally, the effective depth of treatment is 0.3 cm/MeV, and the maximum range of the electrons is 0.5 cm/MeV. Because dose to the skin with low-energy (≤9 MeV) electrons may be less than 90% of the maximum dose, the use of a 1-cm to 1.5-cm layer of wet gauze or water-density bolus is recommended to increase the dose to the skin. Shielding of normal structures is used extensively. The thickness of lead required to absorb 95% of the radiation is shown for x-rays in Table 74-1.[45] For low-energy x-rays, including orthovoltage, 1- to 3-mm-thick lead sheets or a 1-cm to 3-cm thickness of putty containing 38% elemental lead placed directly on the skin is common.

The effect of lead on electron beams is shown in Figure 74-1. Shielding for megavoltage electron beams is best placed close to the skin to maintain a desirable distribution of dose. The thickness of lead required for shielding electrons increases with energy. Use of 0.5 mm/MeV produces a residual dose slightly in excess of 0.5%/MeV at the surface.

Internal lead shields placed in oral or nasal cavities tend to increase the dose to overlying tissue for both x-ray and electron-beam treatments. This increase is caused by backscattered electrons and may be minimized by encasing the shields in plastic.

TABLE 74–1
Lead Shielding for Transmission of 5% or Less

RADIATION	LEAD THICKNESS
120 kV or less	1 mm or 1/32 inch
200–300 kV	
HVL, 1–2-mm Cu*	1.5 mm or 1/16 inch
HVL, 2.5-mm Cu	2.5 mm or 1/8 inch
^{60}Co or 2 MV	5.0 cm or 2 inches
4 MV	6.0 cm or 2 1/4 inches

* *HVL, half-value layer.*
(Adapted from Goodwin PN, Quimby EH, Morgan RH: Physical Foundations of Radiology, 4th ed, p 195. New York, Harper & Row, 1970)

EYE

Pterygium

The treatment of pterygium is surgical, but the recurrence rate is 20% to 30% without further treatment.[17] Van den Brenk[112] reported recurrences in only 1.4% of 1300 pterygia in 1064 patients, using prophylactic postoperative β-ray treatment with an ^{90}Sr applicator. Treatment consists of 800 cGy to 1000 cGy given for each of three applications on days 0, 7, and 14 after the operation.

Cooper[27] advises long-term follow-up of patients, because late recurrences are possible and can be successfully retreated. Bahrassa and Datta[11] have also reported good treatment results administering 500 cGy weekly for five fractions; 700 cGy in four fractions also appears to be effective.[2] Recurrence rates are reduced to 6% to 8% with these techniques. Results of a prospective study in 54 patients and 54 eyes demonstrated that a 2000-cGy single dose after surgical removal is as effective as any fractionated regimen.[9]

In our experience with 48 recurrent pterygia in 42 patients, there were no recurrences if patients received 3000 cGy to 5000 cGy total dose delivered in three to five weekly fractions (1000 cGy weekly).[18] None of the patients developed cataracts or serious complications.

An alternative treatment is instillation of thiotepa solution postoperatively by various schedules, varying from 1 day to 6 weeks after treatment.[8,70]

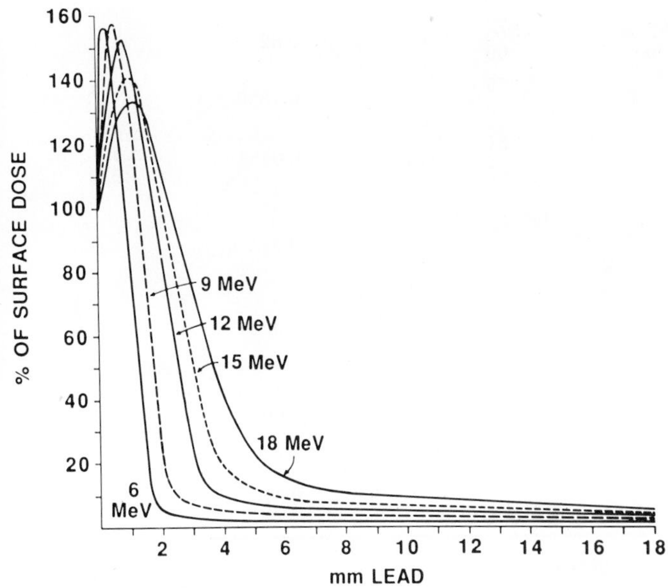

FIGURE 74-1. Shielding for electrons: surface dose compared with lead thickness.

Exophthalmos

Exophthalmos in patients with Graves' disease results from an inflammatory reaction in the periorbital tissues, particularly the extraocular muscles, with lymphocytic infiltration and edema possibly caused by a hypersensitivity reaction.[31,97] Because lymphocytes are especially radiosensitive, local radiation therapy is a logical method of treatment. Systemic corticosteroids are customarily used, but they must be given for long periods of time, increasing the risk of side-effects, and they are not always effective. Surgical orbital decompression is sometimes performed, but complications occur frequently.

In a series reported by Donaldson and co-workers,[31] 15 (65%) of 23 patients treated by orbital radiation therapy had excellent or good response occurring shortly after treatment. Severe asymmetric extraocular paresis was not relieved, and if six patients with this presenting complication are excluded, the response rate was 15 of 17 (88%). An enlarged series reported more recently presents equally good results.[32] Soft tissue changes were relieved in 78% of 29 patients treated at UCLA with 2000 cGy, and proptosis was reduced in 52%. Ophthalmoplegia was not palliated adequately in this series.[90] Thirteen of 29 patients underwent surgery for residual signs and symptoms, indicating the need for a combined approach in advanced ophthalmopathy.[99] Computed tomography (CT) is advised to rule out pseudotumor in patients without hyperthyroidism. In Ravin's series the patients with visual loss secondary to optic nerve involvement, but minimal proptosis or extraocular muscle symptoms, responded best.[97]

Megavoltage external-beam irradiation using precise planning with high-resolution CT scans and complete patient immobilization is recommended. All of these factors allow optimization of dose distribution and avoid unwanted radiation to sensitive structures, such as the lens and pituitary gland.[53]

Small bilateral orbital fields are used. Lead shielding is sometimes required to protect the lens, or a 5-degree posterior angulation may also be used. The total dose is 2000 cGy to the midplane given in ten fractions over 2 weeks. Special care should be exercised in the selection of beams and the calculation of doses to avoid excessive dose to the optic nerve and other sensitive ocular structures. Photons of 4-MV to 6-MV energies delivered with lateral fields contribute a significant dose to the contralateral eye, and this must be taken into account in calculating total tumor doses.

Orbital Pseudotumor

Idiopathic orbital inflammation can simulate Graves' exophthalmos or tumor and may be unilateral or bilateral. Extensive lymphocytic infiltration produces inflammatory signs, periorbital swelling, decreased ocular motility, and pain. There may be palpable mass or proptosis with progressive loss of vision. CT is helpful in differentiating pseudotumor from Graves' disease if the retroocular muscles are primarily involved, but biopsy is usually required, especially if the disease is unilateral. Patients are often misdiagnosed as having Graves' disease or orbital lymphoma.[33,39,71]

Radiation treatment is effective, although corticosteroids are usually administered first. A 4-MV to 6-MV beam is used with unilateral or bilateral temporal fields posterior to the lens. Donaldson[33] uses a split-beam technique for better lens protection. The dose is 2000 cGy in ten fractions over a 2-week period. Rao and co-workers[96] suggested 2000 cGy, but Fitzpatrick and Macko[39] have used doses as high as 3500 cGy. The principal cause of failure has been progression to widely metastatic lymphoma, which occurs ultimately in 30% to 50% of these patients.[66,67,96] Mittal and associates[85] reported an initial local control rate of 93%, with an ultimate control rate of 100% after retreatment with surgery or irradiation with an average total dose of 2500 cGy. Other recommended total effective doses for orbital pseudotumors vary from 1600 cGy to 2000 cGy.[46,74]

SKIN

Keloids

Certain persons have a tendency to react to skin trauma with excessive production of fibrous tissue that extends beyond the wound, becomes hyalinized, and does not regress spontaneously. These keloids become unsightly masses, and they frequently cause itching and pain. They may occur in susceptible individuals after infection, burns, or, most commonly, surgical wounds. Scars over the sternal region, shoulder, and back are particularly likely to spread, and large, cherry-like masses in the ear lobes after piercing are common. Although suture tension and stitch infection in the wound may be contributing factors, the recurrence rate after excision is very high even in their absence, and surgical treatment alone is not recommended.[25]

The preferred treatment is excision followed by a procedure tailored to prevent fibroblast proliferation leading to recurrence. Although good results have been reported with local injections of triamcinolone, postoperative radiation therapy is effective and is more comfortable for patients.[35,48,59,82]

Radiation therapy is usually started within 24 hours after excision, using 100 kV to 140 kV with a 1-mm to 7-mm Al half-value layer (HVL). The radiation field is custom shaped with lead, with a 0.5-cm margin around the suture lines. The ear lobes, when treated, are taped away from the face, and a direct anterior or posterior field is used with a small cone. If the lobe is more than 1 cm thick and the wound extends around it, a higher-energy beam is needed. The total dose is 1000 cGy to 1500 cGy given in two or three fractions in 2 weeks. The recurrence rate after local irradiation of 1200 cGy in four fractions of 300 cGy each given at weekly intervals was reported as 2.4% (nine of 375 patients). For this series, 345 (92%) of 375 patients had excellent esthetic results.[13]

Kovalic and Perez[73] followed 75 patients with 113 treated sites for a mean time of 9.75 years. Most of the patients were treated to a dose of 1200 cGy in three fractions over 3 days delivered with superficial x-rays. The overall local control rate was 73%. No advantage to starting radiation therapy within 1 day of surgery was demonstrated. Significant prognostic factors were size greater than 2 cm, previous surgery, and keloids occurring in men (Table 74-2).

Treatment of established keloids by irradiation alone is not as successful, but it may be attempted if surgery is not indicated (*e.g.*, in an elderly patient with a large symptomatic lesion or in presternal and shoulder keloids that commonly recur even after combined treatment). Inalsingh[59] reported good results with 400 cGy given once a month for one to five treatments, using energies between 60 kV and 90 kV. Electron-beam therapy, alone or postoperatively, was reported to be effective by King and Salzman.[69] They used 1-MeV to 3-MeV electrons in 1000-cGy treatments, for one to three fractions. Doornbos and co-workers[34] recommended using 1500 cGy in three treatments if kilovoltage irradiation is used. They reported 90% local control

TABLE 74–2
Prognostic Factors and Their Significance in Keloids

PROGNOSTIC FACTOR	h	% NER*	*P* VALUE
Time between excision and XRT			
≤24 hours	74k, 50p*	72	0.82
>24 hours	26k, 17p	69	
Earlobe keloids	84k	75	0.1038
Non-earlobe keloids	29k	58	
No previous therapy	64k	81	0.0153
Previous therapy	45k	58	
Race:			
White	10p	60	0.313
Black	65p	75	
Sex:			
Male	10p	27	0.0004
Female	65p	77	
Size:			
≤2 cm	48k	85	0.0004
>2 cm	33k	47	
Total dose:			
≤1200 cGy	87k	70	0.3267
>1200 cGy	17k	81	

**NER: no evidence of recurrence;* p: *patients; k: keloids.*
(Kovalic JJ, Perez CA: Int J Radiat Oncol Biol Phys 17:77, 1989)

without reexcision, when treatment is delivered within a year of recurrence.

Plantar Warts

Plantar warts can be extremely painful and disabling. Surgical treatment, including dessication and curettage, leads to incapacity during the long period of healing and may leave painful scarring. A blunt dissection technique has been advocated by Pringle and Helms.[95] Bunney and co-workers[14] recommend a nonsurgical approach using a salicylic acid, lactic acid, and collodin preparation covered by a small piece of plastic and applied daily for 12 weeks. Coskey[28] reported success in 81 of 121 children using salicylic ointment for plantar warts.

Intralesional injection of bleomycin appears effective in the treatment of resistant warts. A cure rate of 77% for extremity warts was reported in a controlled trial with 38 patients and 143 warts. Complete resolution was found in 67% after two injections of bleomycin.[3] Others have reported resolution rates as high as 95% after intralesional bleomycin therapy.[15,101] Static electricity and topical ointments containing salicylic acid are also effective.[57,102]

Radiation treatment for plantar warts can be simple, safe, and effective. Hawley[54] reported the results for 243 patients treated by irradiation with a 87% cure rate after a single treatment of 1000 cGy with 100 kV and a HVL of 4.3-mm Al, using close lead shielding. He does not believe preliminary paring is necessary. The wart usually separates and falls off in 3 to 4 weeks, without sequelae.

Keratoacanthoma

Keratoacanthomas are benign skin tumors that arise from the hair follicles. They tend to spontaneously regress, but on many occasions, additional treatment is needed.[43,79] Caccialanza and Sopelana[19] reported the effectiveness of superficial irradiation in 52 patients treated with 4000 cGy in 400-cGy fractions twice weekly. Complete regression was achieved in all patients with excellent esthetic results.

Hemangiomas

Cutaneous Lesions

Treatment of cavernous hemangiomas of the skin in infants by repeated doses of radium in surface applicators was commonplace many years ago. It was discarded because there is a radiation hazard to the patient and the staff and because the treatment is usually unnecessary. After an initial growth phase, most of these lesions regress spontaneously and disappear by the patient's fifth year.[88] A few, however, may require treatment because of growth and expansion that interfere with vision or eating. Nordberg and Sundberg,[88] who reported treatment of more than 800 patients, gave indications for early treatment: major rapidly growing facial hemangiomas that may cause cosmetic and psychologic difficulty and possibly those lesions in the perineum, where there is danger of maceration and infection.

The classification used at Radiumhemmet is based on the clinical appearance of the hemangioma.[4] The strawberry type (cavernous hemangioma) is the most commonly treated lesion because of responsiveness to radiation, but they also show a strong tendency toward spontaneous regression. The port wine stain (capillary hemangioma) is rather resistant to irradiation.[40] Furst and associates[40] reported the results of irradiation in 20,012 patients with hemangiomas. Most patients (99%) were younger than 2 years of age at the time of treatment. All lesions improved, 72% with excellent cosmetic results and the remainder with some blemish but nonetheless acceptable results.

The technique is dictated by the depth and extent of the lesion. For minor superficial hemangiomas, contact radiation therapy is most suitable, using 50 kV, 0.5-mm Al added filter, and a 20-mm skin-to-source distance, resulting in an HVL of 3 mm in soft tissue. The surface dose is 800 cGy to 900 cGy given in one treatment. A second treatment of 600 cGy to 800 cGy may be given several months later if there is continued growth. Compression during treatment can be used for thicker lesions, or a 1.0-mm Al filter and 40-mm skin-to-source distance can be used, which increases the HVL in tissue to 4 mm to 6 mm. Some thick tumors may require higher energy and longer treatment distances, usually with smaller doses. A tangential beam is sometimes indicated to spare underlying tissue. There has been little experience with electron-beam therapy, but it seems rational that results are comparable.

Central Nervous System

Arteriovenous malformations (AVM) of the brain are clusters of abnormal arteries and veins that shunt blood from the arterial system to the venous system. Surgical excision is considered the treatment of choice for small accessible lesions. Embolization is also used, but not all lesions can be treated with this technique. Wolkov and Bagshaw[114] reported on a small series of patients with AVM of the brain and spinal cord who had good responses to megavoltage treatment with local fields and doses of 4500 cGy to 5500 cGy given in 5 weeks in 200-cGy fractions. Follow-up ranged from 5 to 20 years. There were no complications reported, and all patients were stable.

Single doses of 1500 cGy to 2500 cGy with 6-MV linear accelerator stereotactic techniques have been used to sclerose AVM and prevent hemorrhage. Radiosurgery, though controversial, is also safe and sometimes effective for this problem.[68,105]

For extracerebral cavernous hemangiomas of the middle fossa, a preoperative dose of 3000 cGy has been reported to increase resectability and decrease intraoperative hemorrhage.[106]

Ocular Angiomas

Orbital hemangiomas of childhood occur most frequently in the anterior orbit and eyelid. They are generally harmless and often spontaneously regress. However, a number of these lesions become symptomatic, causing hemorrhage and visual loss. Plowman and Harnett[94] reported a lens-sparing technique for orbital irradiation and successfully managed such difficult cases with this approach. They recommend 1200 cGy in eight fractions of 150 cGy each.

Cavernous Hemangioma of the Liver

Cavernous hemangioma of the liver is a congenital anomaly, asymptomatic in most patients unless the lesion bleeds. This benign vascular tumor has been found at autopsy in 2% to 3% of asymptomatic patients. The incidence of clinically significant lesions is substantially lower. Fever or anemia occurs in 6% of patients. Clinically evident hepatomegaly exists in 50% of these patients, and simultaneous hemorrhage, thrombocytopenia, and hypofibrogenemia have also been described, but rarely.[109]

Trastek and co-workers[110] followed 36 patients for 1 to 15 years (mean, 5.5 years) and reported enlargement in four patients, shrinkage in three, and no change in the others. None had any change in treatments. Most reports in the literature are of patients who underwent surgery, with the expected complications and morbidity.

Radiation therapy has been delivered using different schedules. Techniques and results for patients treated with doses ranging from 1000 to 3000 cGy in 1 to 3 weeks for hemangioma of the liver are summarized in Table 74-3. The recommended doses are 1000 cGy or less for children and 2000 cGy to 3000 cGy in 3 to 4 weeks for adults. If no response is observed in 4 to 6 months, an additional 1000 cGy to 1500 cGy in 1 to 2 weeks may be given.

SOFT TISSUES

Bursitis and Tendonitis

Bursitis and tendonitis most commonly affect the shoulders. These disorders are caused by degenerative and inflammatory changes in the supraspinatus and infraspinatus tendons that lead to calcium deposition, inflammation of the surface of the subdeltoid bursa, and even rupture and discharge of calcific material into the bursa. Calcification may occur without symptoms, or there may be pain, tenderness, and limitation of motion in acute, subacute, or chronic forms. Typical symptoms may also exist without demonstrable calcifications on radiographic examination.

Radiation treatment, particularly for patients with acute disease, was once commonplace but has been supplanted by treatment with antiinflammatory drugs (*e.g.*, salicylates, phenylbutazones, indomethacin) combined with rest or aspiration with injection of corticosteroids and procaine. It is probably true, however, that radiation treatment is equally effective and is sometimes successful if invasive local treatments are not.[84] An opposing view is held by Plenk,[93] who in a small controlled series of 38 patients, could find no treatment-related difference in the course or duration of the disease.

Limited fields encompass the joint only, using either opposed or occasionally a single anterior field. A daily dose of 150 cGy to 200 cGy is given on 3 to 5 successive days for a total of 600 cGy to 1000 cGy. One or two additional treatments may be added after 1 or 2 weeks in chronic cases, in which results are much less satisfactory.

Desmoids and Fibromatoses

Desmoids are low-grade, locally invasive, but nonmetastasizing tumors of connective tissue origin, probably related to other fibromatoses, such as keloids, Peyronie's disease, plantar and palmar fibromatosis, fibromatosis colli, and progressive myositis fibrosa.[104] Growth of these tumors is slow, and pain is a late symptom; tumors are usually large before treatment is sought. The neck and shoulder girdle are common sites of involvement.[56,107] These tumors are deeply infiltrative and nonencapsulated, and they are associated with a high rate (70%) of local failure.[36,61]

Wide surgical excision is the treatment of choice, but if the lesion is extensive and inoperable because of location or infiltration, radiation treatment has provided good re-

TABLE 74–3
Radiation Therapy for Hemangioma of the Liver

INVESTIGATOR	PATIENT AGE (YR) AND SEX	TREATMENT (cGy)	RESPONSE	COMPLICATIONS	RECOMMENDATIONS
Issa[60]	54 (F)	^{60}Co 2500/2 wk TD†	Slow, marked	None	2000 to 3000 cGy in 3 to 4 wk; if no response in 3 to 4 mo, then additional treatment of 1000–1500 cGy in 10 to 15 d
	27 (F)	OrthoV 2000/5 wk TD	Slow, marked	None	
Park and Phillips[91]	55 (M)	250 kV 1500/12 d TD	Gradual, complete	None	2000/10 d (adults); 400–600 cGy (infants); then reevaluate later
	48 (M)	1 MV 1300	Gradual, complete	Fever	
	4 (M)	250 kV 1900/4 wk	Gradual, marked	Fever	
	67 (M)	^{60}Co 1450/11 d	Slow regression	Malaise, no fever	
	51 (F)	1 MV 2000/2 wk	Not evaluated	Died 11 mo + RT	
Okasaki et al[89]	41 (M)	6 MV 940/50/32 d	No regression; died 6 months later	Easy fatigue	<3000 cGy in fractions
	39 (F)	6 MV 1900/50/54 d /100	Transient regression	Mild pancytopenia, nausea	
	*	6 MV 2940/100/41 d /200	Regression		
	32 (F)	6 MV 3050/100/67 d /150	Marked regression	Lymphadenopathy, fever	
	31 (F)	6 MV 3080/150 /200	Regression	None	

* *Repeat.*
† *TD: tumor dose; RT: radiation therapy.*

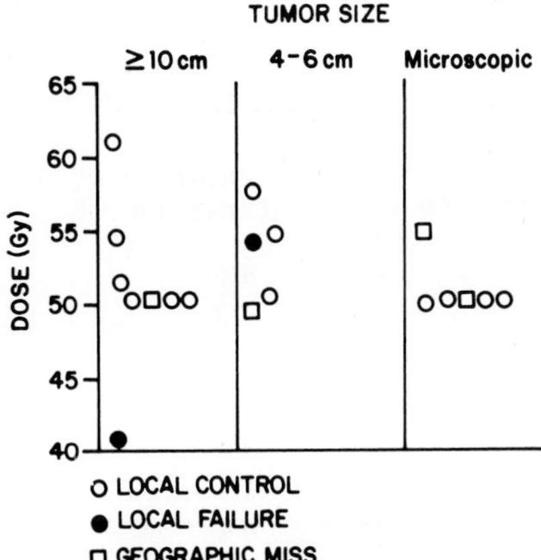

FIGURE 74–2. Scattergram comparing local tumor control with radiation dose and tumor size. (Leibel SA, Wara WM, Hill DR, et al: Int J Radiat Oncol Biol Phys 9:1167, 1983)

sults.[45,47,56,65,75,107] Amputation of an extremity should be considered only if irradiation has failed.

The recommended dose is 5000 cGy to 6000 cGy given in 6 to 7 weeks in 200-cGy daily fractions (Fig. 74-2). Portals should be generous, encompassing the entire aponeurotic compartment or operative fields (Fig. 74-3). Bataini and associates[12] reported no recurrences up to 10 years after irradiation after patients received a total dose of more than 5000 cGy.

Greenberg and colleagues[47] reported long-term control in eight of nine desmoid tumors and two of three neurofibromas treated with doses of 5400 cGy to 6800 cGy after surgical excision.

Leibel and associates[75] described local control in 13 (68%) of 19 patients, 15 of them irradiated (5000–6000 cGy) after surgical recurrences. Eight of the patients had unresectable disease greater than 10 cm in diameter (Table 74-4). In six patients who developed postirradiation recurrences, only one lesion was in the treated field; the other five were marginal. The 5-year relapse free survival rate was 72%. In patients with palpable tumor, regression is slow, with the mass sometimes taking years to disappear completely. Morbidity is minimal, but it depends on tumor location and the proximity of sensitive adjacent normal tissue structures.[100]

Peyronie's Disease

Painful angulation of the erect penis was described by Peyronie in 1743. It is caused by inflammatory lesions of the corpora cavernosa that progress to hard plaques, nodules, or bands that may be localized or extensive. The plaque, or mass, is usually on the dorsum of the penis with curvature or angulation in the direction of the plaque, which may precede the development of pain. The cause is unknown; it is very likely a connective tissue disorder like Dupuytren's contracture of the palm. Although the disease tends to resolve spontaneously over a period of months to years and some authors question the value of radiation therapy, others believe that the treatment is quite effective And hastens regression, with earlier relief of symptoms.[7,21,37,55,81,113] Local corticosteroid injections, systemic corticosteroids, or procarbazine is also effective in some patients.

During radiation treatment, careful lead shielding of the gonads, pubic hair, and glans (if not involved) is required. The penis can be drawn through a hole in a lead sheet, and a single dorsal field may be used. Effective reported doses range from 500 cGy in one fraction, which may be repeated in 1 month, to 300 cGy daily for six or seven fractions. Helvie and Ochsner[55] recommended 300 cGy at 4- to 6-week intervals to a maximum dose of 2400 cGy. Most of their patients improved with doses of 900 cGy to 1200 cGy. Most patients treated by Mira and colleagues[86] received 1000 cGy to 1400 cGy in about 2 weeks with similar results. Ariaturai and associates[7] reported excellent results using 100 kV for a weekly dose of 250 cGy weekly given for four fractions.

BONE

Ameloblastoma

Ameloblastomas usually occur in the jaw, particularly the mandible, and rarely metastasize. Treatment by curettage is often employed, but recurrence is common; adequate initial resection may be preferable.[30,41,100] Many patients, however, have tumors that cannot be completely excised (particularly those in the maxilla) or may be inoperable for other reasons. These lesions have responded well to irradiation, and doses of 5000 cGy to 6000 cGy in 5 to 6 weeks have produced complete regression,

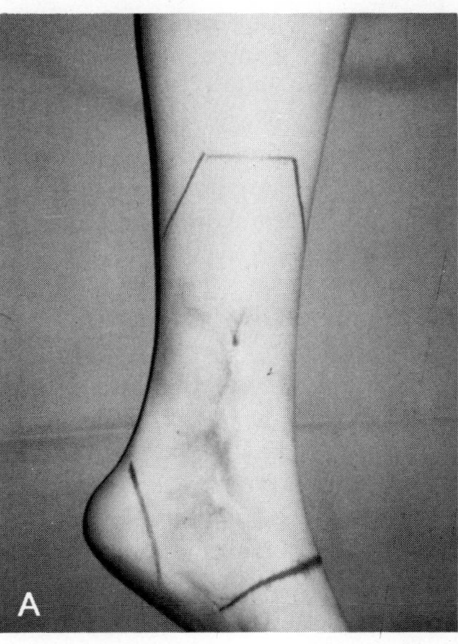

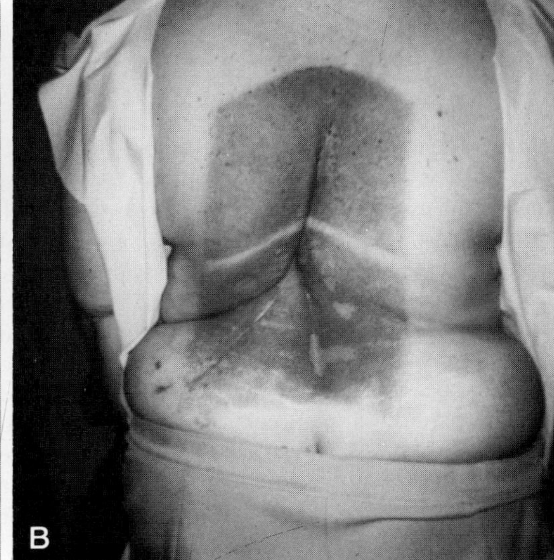

FIGURE 74–3. (**A**) Portal for irradiation for fibromatosis of the leg. (**B**) Photograph of a 35-year-old woman with extensive fibromatosis of the spinal muscles and soft tissues. The patient was treated with a combination of 18-MeV electrons and 4-MV photons for a total dose of 5000 cGy in 6 weeks. The dry desquamation outlines the treatment portal. The patient remains symptom free 5 years after therapy.

TABLE 74–4
Local Control of Desmoid Tumors According to Primary Site and Size of Tumor at Time of Treatment

SITE	TUMOR SIZE ≥10 CM	<10 CM	MICROSCOPIC	LOCAL CONTROL
Shoulder girdle–arm	3/4	1/1	0/1	4/6
Arm		1/2	1/1	2/3
Buttock–pelvis	1/1	1/2	0/1	2/4
Pelvis	1/1			1/1
Hip–thigh	1/1		2/2	3/3
Abdominal wall			1/1	1/1
Mesentery	0/1			0/1
Total	6/8	3/5	4/6	13/19

(Leibel SA, Wara WM, Hill DR, et al: Int J Radiat Oncol Biol Phys 9:1167, 1983)

even of large tumors.[10,20,100] Gardner also recommends the use of irradiation for unfavorable lesions, mainly those located in the posterior maxilla.[42]

Aneurysmal Bone Cysts

Aneurysmal bone cysts are nonneoplastic vascular-cystic lesions that usually appear as expansive, eccentric cavities in the metaphyseal ends of bones, not involving the epiphysis, and protruding into the soft tissues. Treatment is primarily surgical, curettage or resection, if there is no resultant interference with function. Recurrence rates after curettage only have been reported to be as high as 30% to 60%.[23] Radiation treatment is reserved for patients whose lesions are surgically inaccessible or difficult to curette properly because of size and location and continue to grow or repeatedly recur after curettage. Cysts of the spine and pelvis are especially suitable for radiation treatment. Doses of 4000 cGy in 4 weeks with a megavoltage beam, using parallel opposing fields, have produced excellent results; 3500 cGy may be sufficient.[80] Jereb and Smith[62] have reported a large tumor of the innominate bone in a 10-year-old patient that showed excellent response after 2000 cGy in 2 weeks. Ameli[5] recommends a total dose of irradiation not to exceed 2000 cGy followed by a two-stage operation for aneurysmal bone cysts of the spine.

Vertebral Hemangiomas

Vertebral hemangiomas are not uncommon. They are usually diagnosed by the typical radiographic appearance of rarefaction with vertical dense trabeculations of a honeycombed pattern, often extending into the lacunae, pedicles, and transverse or spinous processes. There may be vertebral enlargement; collapse of the body is rare. Most are asymptomatic and require no treatment, but there may be local pain and tenderness. Expansion of the vertebra, extension of the tumor into the extradural space, hemorrhage, or the rare compression fracture may lead to cord compression. Surgical decompression may be required after preliminary arteriography but may be difficult because of hemorrhage. Usually only limited removal of the tumor is possible, and postoperative radiation treatment is recommended.[83,111] There have been a few reports of good results with radiation therapy without surgical decompression.[38,76] A tumor dose of 2000 cGy to 3000 cGy in 2 or 3 weeks is probably sufficient.

Heterotopic Bone Formation

Heterotopic bone formation occurs in 30% of patients undergoing hip arthroplasty.[98] Patients develop ossification in the soft tissues postoperatively, limiting motion. This appears 3 to 6 weeks after surgery, and the process is complete, although not fully calcified, in 8 weeks. The incidence may be as high as 60% among patients who have osteoarthritis, ankylosing spondylitis, or previous myositis ossificans. Treatment is surgical, and recurrence can be prevented by early postoperative radiation treatment.[29] A dose of 2000 cGy is usually given in 2 weeks, using anterior and posterior portals.[78] Radiation treatment should be given early; it is of little value after ectopic bone is visible on radiographic examination. Twenty-eight patients were irradiated postoperatively at UCLA from 1980 to 1986; treatment consisted of 2000 cGy in ten fractions or 1000 cGy in five fractions. There were no differences between the groups in side-effects or recurrence of heterotopic bone formation. There were no failures in patients treated within the fourth postoperative day.[108]

For 46 consecutive hips treated with 1000 cGy, Anthony and associates[6] reported a 4.9% development of heterotopic bone, compared with a rate of 3.2% for another group receiving 2000 cGy. A nonirradiated historic control group showed a 68.5% incidence of heterotopic bone. Lo and associates[77] reported on single-dose 700-cGy treatment within 72 hours of surgery in 23 patients. Their failure rate of 4% appears to be comparable to previous regimens.

GLANDULAR TISSUE

Gynecomastia

Enlargement of the breasts with accompanying tenderness is a common side-effect of estrogen therapy in the treatment of prostatic cancer. It is easily prevented by breast irradiation before administering estrogen; irradiation is not effective if estrogen has been given first. Alafthan and Holsti[1] treated 78 patients in whom the left breast received radiation therapy, the right breast received no treatment, and estrogen therapy was started after 14 days. Gynecomastia occurred in 90% of the control breasts and in only 17% of those that had been irradiated. Only two of 70 patients who received radiation therapy developed severe pain or gynecomastia in a group treated by Cook and Rodriguez-Antunez.[26]

Therapy with 100 to 200 kV, a HVL of 2-mm to 4-mm Al, a skin-to-source distance of 20 cm to 25 cm or therapy with 200 kV, HVL of 0.5-mm to 1.0-mm Cu, a skin-to-source distance of 50 cm, 9 MeV electrons (appositional 6-cm to 8-cm diameter portals) and ^{60}Co or 4-MV photon beams (with tangential portals) can be used; 900 cGy is given as a single dose or 400 cGy to 500 cGy daily for three treatments. It is probably safe to start the hormone treatment within 2 or 3 days after completion of radiation therapy.

In addition to prophylactic treatment, Chou and colleagues[22] reported pain control in ten of 11 patients treated for painful gynecomastia after diethylstilbestrol therapy with 2000 cGy in five fractions or 4000 cGy in 20 fractions. Pain relief was obtained for 2 weeks to 14 months, with an average of 3.6 months. They recommend a dose of 2000 cGy in five treatments of 400 cGy each for these patients.[22]

Ovarian Castration

The controversy over the use of prophylactic or therapeutic castration in premenopausal women with breast cancer is still unresolved, although the tendency is to delay treatment until required.[63,87] Some of the earlier trials are flawed by the use of radiation doses that were quite low, such as 650 cGy in one treatment, with the return of menstrual bleeding in some patients. Because the position of the ovaries varies, the whole pelvis should be treated. Using anterior and posterior fields and ^{60}Co or megavoltage beam, 2000 cGy is delivered to the midplane in five fractions. Today, most patients receive tamoxifen for ovarian suppression, and irradiation is not required.

Parotitis

Acute postoperative parotitis is now a rarity because of better patient care, particularly hydration, antibiotics, and attention to oral hygiene. Typically it occurs 4 to 6 days after surgery in debilitated, seriously dehydrated patients with decreased salivary secretion and dry mouth. Treatment includes correction of dehydration, mouth care, and antibiotic therapy. Stimulation of salivation by lemon or orange juice and gum chewing and probing of Stensen's duct have been recommended but may not be necessary.[49,115]

Radiation treatment combined with these measures is effective and may avoid the necessity for incision and drainage. The response is often rapid and dramatic, with marked improvement in the general condition of the patient within 12 to 14 hours. There is decreased pain, induration, and swelling, and all evidence of disease is gone in 3 to 6 days. In a series of 68 patients reported by Gustafson,[49] there was prompt resolution without abscess in 52 (76%), and only 16 required drainage. A total dose of 750 cGy to 1000 cGy is given in three to five fractions with orthovoltage x-rays, ^{60}Co, or 9-MeV to 12-MeV electrons through a lateral portal encompassing the parotid gland with 2-cm margins.

REFERENCES

1. Alafthan O, Holsti LR: Prevention of gynecomastia by local roentgen irradiation in estrogen-treated prostatic carcinomas. Scand J Urol Nephrol 3:183, 1969
2. Alaniz-Camino F: The use of post-operative beta radiation in the treatment of pterygia. Ophthalmic Surg 13:1022, 1982
3. Amer M, Diab N, Ramadan A, et al: Therapeutic evaluation for intralesional injection of bleomycin sulfate in 143 resistant warts. J Am Acad Dermatol 18:1313, 1988
4. Andren G: The radium treatment of haemangiomata, lymphangiomata and naevi pigmentose. Experiences from Radiumhemmet. Acta Radiol 8:1909, 1927
5. Ameli NO, Abbassioun K, Saleh, et al: Aneurysmal bone cyst of the spine. J Neurosurg 63:685, 1985
6. Anthony P, Keys H, McCollister E, et al: Prevention of heterotopic bone formation with early postoperative irradiation in high risk patients undergoing total hip arthroplasty: Comparison of 10.0 Gy vs 20.0 Gy schedules. Int J Radiat Oncol Biol Phys 3:365, 1987
7. Ariaturai SV, Kimball WR, Wilson ARA, et al: Radiation therapy in the treatment of Peyronie's disease. [Abstract] Int J Radiat Oncol Biol Phys 9(suppl 1):105, 1983
8. Assegadoo ER: Surgery, thio-tepa and corticosteroids in the treatment of pterygium. Am J Opthalmol 74:960, 1972
9. Asad MI, Baum J: Optimal time for postoperative irradiation of pterygia. Am J Ophthalmol 94:1450, 1987
10. Atkinson CH, Harwood AR, Cummings BJ: Ameloblastoma of the jaw: A reappraisal of the role of megavoltage irradiation. Cancer 53:869, 1984
11. Bahrassa C, Datta R: Postoperative beta radiation treatment of pterygium. Int J Radiat Oncol Biol Phys 9:679, 1983
12. Bataini JP, Belber C, Mazapraud A: Desmoid tumors in adults. The role of radiotherapy in their management. Am J Surg 155:754, 1986
13. Borok TL, Bray M, Silclair I, et al: Role of ionization irradiation for 393 keloids. Int J Radiat Oncol Biol Phys 15:865, 1988
14. Bunney MH, Hunter JAA, Ogilvie MM, et al: The treatment of plantar warts in the home. Practitioner 207:107, 1971
15. Bunney MH, Nolan MW, Buxton DK, et al: The treatment of resistant warts with intralesional bleomycin: A controlled clinical trial. Br J Dermatol 111:197, 1984
16. Bureau of Radiological Health: A Review of the Use of Ionizing Radiation for the Treatment of Benign Disease, vol 1, pp 1–2. Rockville, MD, US Department of Health, Education and Welfare, 1977
17. Cameron ME: Pterygium throughout the world. Springfield, IL, Charles C Thomas, Publisher, 1965
18. Campbell OR, Amendola BE, Brady LW: Recurrent pterygia: results of postoperative treatment with strontium applicators in 48 eyes of 42 patients. Radiology 174:565–566, 1990
19. Caccilanza M, Sopelana N: Radiation therapy of keratoacanthomas: results in 55 patients. Int J Radiat Oncol Biol Phys 16:475, 1988
20. Chandhuri P: Ameloblastoma of the upper jaw. J Laryngol Otol 89:457, 1975
21. Chesey J: Peyronie's disease. Br J Urol 47:209, 1975
22. Chou JL, Easley JD, Feldmeier JJ, et al: Effective radiotherapy in palliating mammalgia associated with gynecomastia after DES therapy. Int J Radiat Oncol Biol Phys 15:749, 1988
23. Clough JR, Price CGH: Aneurysmal bone cyst: Pathogenesis and long term results of treatment. Clin Orthop 97:52, 1973
24. Cohen M, Jones DEA, Greene D: Central axis depth dose for use in radiotherapy. Br J Radiol 45(suppl 11): , 1972
25. Converse JM: Reconstructive Plastic Surgery, p 175. Philadelphia, WB Saunders, 1968
26. Cook S, Rodriguez-Antunez A: Pre-estrogen irradiation of the breast to prevent gynecomastia. AJR 117:662, 1963
27. Cooper JS: Postoperative irradiation of pterygia: Ten more years of experience. Radiology 128:753, 1978
28. Coskey RJ: Treatment of plantar warts in children with a salicylic acid-podophyllin-cantharidin product. Pediatr Dermatol 2:71, 1984

29. Coventry, MD, Scanlon PW: The use of radiation to discourage ectopic bone. J Bone Joint Surg [A] 63:201, 1981
30. Crawley WA, Levin S: Treatment of the ameloblastoma: A controversy. Cancer 42:357, 1978
31. Donaldson SS, Bagshaw MS, Kriss JP: Supervoltage orbital radiotherapy for Graves' opthalmopathy. J Clin Endocrinol Metab 37:276, 1973
32. Donaldson SS, Kriss JP, McDougall IR, et al: Orbital irradiation in the treatment of Graves' opthalmopathy: Results in 141 consecutive patients. [Abstract] Int J Radiat Oncol Biol Phys 8:112, 1982
33. Donaldson SS, McDougall IR, Egbert PR, et al: Treatment of orbital pseudomotor (idiopathic orbital inflammation) by radiation therapy. Int J Radiat Oncol Biol Phys 6:79, 1980
34. Doornbos FS, Stoffel JR, Hass AC, et al: The role if kilovoltage in the treatment of keloids. [Abstract] Int J Radiat Oncol Biol Phys 15(suppl 1):230, 1988
35. Doyle, DE, Passey V: Keloid management and it present status. Eye Ear Nose Throat Mon 54:239, 1975
36. Enzinger FM, Shiroki M: Musculoaponeurotic fibromatosis of the shoulder girdle. Cancer 20:1131, 1967
37. Feder BH: Peyronie's disease. J Am Geriatr Soc 19:947, 1971
38. Ferber L, Lampe I: Hemangioma of vertebra associated with compression of the cord: Response to radiation therapy. Arch Neurol Psychiatry 47:19, 1942
39. Fitzpatrick PJ, Macko S: Lymphoreticular tumors of the orbit. Int J Radiat Oncol Biol Phys 10:333, 1984
40. Furst CJ, Lundell M, Holm LE: Radiation therapy of hemangiomas 1909–1959. A cohort based on 50 years of clinical practice at Radiumhemmet Stockholm. Acta Oncol 26:33, 1987
41. Gardner DG, Pecak AJM: Treatment of ameloblastoma. Cancer 46:2514, 1980
42. Gardner DG: Radiotherapy in the treatment of ameloblastoma. Int J Oral Maxillofac Surg 17:201, 1988
43. Ghadially FI: Keratoacanthoma. In Fitzpatrick TB, Eisen AZ, Wolff K, Freedberg IM, Ausren KF (eds): Dermatology in General Medicine, 3rd ed, vol 1, pp 776–772. New York, McGraw-Hill, 1987
44. Godfrey AM, Salaman JR: Radiotherapy in the treatment of acute rejection of human renal allografts. Lancet 1:938, 1976
45. Goodwin PN, Quimby EH, Morgan RH: Physical Foundations of Radiology, 4th ed, p 195. New York, Harper & Row, 1970
46. Gordon PS, Juillard GJF, Selch MT, et al: Orbital lymphomas and pseudolymphomas treated with radiotherapy. Radiology 159:797, 1986
47. Greenberg HM, Goebel R, Weichselbaum RR: Radiation treatment of aggressive fibromatoses. Int J Radiat Oncol Biol Phys 7:305, 1981
48. Griffith BH, Monroe CW, McKinney P: A follow-up study on the treatment of keloids with triamcinolone acetonide. Plast Reconstr Surg 46:145, 1970
49. Gustafson JR: Acute parotitis. Surgery 29:786, 1951
50. Halperin EC, Ballinger RR: The role of irradiation in solid organ transplantations. Int J Radiat Oncol Biol Phys 15:979, 1988
51. Halperin EC, Delmonico PL, Nelson PW, et al: The use of local irradiation following renal transplant. Int J Radiat Oncol Biol Phys 10:981, 1984
52. Hamburger J, Crosnier J: Experience with 45 renal homotransplants in man. Lancet 1:985, 1965
53. Harnett AN, Doughty D, Hirst A, et al: Radiotherapy in benign orbital disease. II. Ophthalmic Graves' disease and orbital histiocytosis X. Br J Ophthalmol 72:289, 1988
54. Hawley SJ: Roentgen therapy in some nonmalignant conditions. Radiology 59:225, 1952
55. Helvie WW, Ochsner SF: Radiation therapy in Peyronie's disease. South Med J 65:1192, 1972
56. Hill DR, Newman H, Phillips TL: Radiation therapy of desmoid tumors. AJR 117:84, 1973
57. Hughes E, Marshall H, Mehlmauer M, et al: Human warts, permanently removed by static electricity. Cutis 31:319, 1983
58. Hume DN, Wolf JS: Modification of renal homograft rejection by irradiation. Transplantation 5:1174, 1967
59. Inalsingh CH: An experience in treating 501 patients with keloids. Johns Hopkins Med J 134:284, 1974
60. Issa P: Cavernous haemangioma of the liver: The role of radiotherapy. Br J Radiol 41:26, 1968
61. Jacobson HM, Parsons JT, Springfield DS, et al: Aggressive fibromatosis: A 15-year experience at a single institution. [Abstract] Am J Clin Oncol 8:18, 1985
62. Jereb B, Smith J: Giant aneurysmal bone cyst of the innominate bone treated with irradiation. Br J Radiol 53:489, 1980
63. Kennedy BJ, Fortuny IE: Therapeutic castration in the treatment of advanced breast cancer. Cancer 17:1197, 1964
64. Khorsand J, Karakousis CP: Desmoid tumors and their management. Am J Surg 149:215, 1985
65. Kiel KD, Suit HD: The use of radiation therapy in the management of aggressive fibromatoses (desmoid tumors): Massachusetts General Hospital experience, 1972–1981. [Abstract] Int J Radiat Oncol Biol Phys 8(suppl 1):126, 1982
66. Kim RY: Orbital pseudotumors: Histopathologic classification and results of radiation therapy. Ala Med 56:43, 1987
67. Kim YH, Fayos JV: Primary orbital lymphoma: A radiotherapeutic experience. Int J Radiat Oncol Biol Phys 1:1099, 1976
68. Kimmig B, Sturm V, Enzenhart R, et al: Stereotactic single high dose radiation therapy of cerebral arterio-venous malformation (AVM) using a linear accelerator. [Abstract] Int J Radiat Oncol Biol Phys 15:226, 1988
69. King GD, Salzman FA: Keloid scars: Analysis of 89 patients. Surg Clin North Am 50:595, 1970
70. Kleis W, Pico G: Thio-tepa therapy to prevent postoperative pterygium occurrence and neovascularization. Am J Ophthalmol 76:371, 1973
71. Knowles DM, Jakobiec FA: Orbital lymphoid neoplasms. Cancer 46:576, 1980
72. Kopicky J, Order SE: Survey and analysis of radiation therapy of benign disease. In A Review of the Use of Ionizing Radiation for the Treatment of Benign Disease, vol II, pp 13–442. Rockville, MD, US Department of Health, Education, and Welfare, Bureau of Radiological Health, 1977
73. Kovalic JJ, Perez CA: Radiation therapy following keloidectomy: A 20-year experience. Int J Radiat Oncol Biol Phys 17:77, 1989
74. Lanciano R, Atlas S, Rubenstein J, et al: The results of radiotherapy for orbital pseudotumor. [Abstract] Int J Radiat Oncol Biol 13(suppl 1):136, 1987
75. Leibel SA, Wara WM, Hill DR, et al: Desmoid tumors: Local control and patterns of relapse following radiation therapy. Int J Radiat Oncol Biol Phys 9:1167, 1983
76. Lindquist I: Vertebral hemangioma with compression of the spinal cord. Acta Radiol 35:400, 1951
77. Lo TCM, Healy WL, Covall DJ, et al: Heterotopic bone formation after hip surgery: Prevention with single dose post-operative hip irradiation. Radiology 168:851, 1988
78. MacLennon I, Keys HM, Evarts CM, et al: Usefulness of postoperative hip irradiation in the prevention of heterotopic bone formation in a high risk group of patients. Int J Radiat Oncol Biol Phys 10:49, 1984
79. Mackie RM: Tumours of the skin. In Rook A, Wilkinson DS, Ebling FJ, Champran RH, Burton JL (eds): Textbook of Dermatology, vol 3, 4th ed, pp 2375–2478. London, Blackwell Scientific, 1986
80. Marks RD, Scruggs HJ, Wallace KM, et al: Megavoltage therapy in patients with aneurysmal bone cysts. Radiology 118:421, 1976
81. Martin CL: Long time study of patients with Peyronie's disease treated with irradiation. AJR 114:492, 1972
82. May H: Plastic Reconstructive Surgery, pp 189–190. Philadelphia, FA Davis, 1971
83. McAllister VL, Kendall BE, Bull JWD: Symptomatic verteberal hemangiomas. Brain 98;71, 1975
84. Milone FP, Copeland MM: Calcific tendonitis of the shoulder joint. AJR 85:901, 1961
85. Mittal BB, Deutsch M, Kennerdell J, Johnson B: Parocular lymphoid tumors. Radiology 159:793, 1986
86. Mira JG, Chahbazian CM, del Regato JA: The value of radio-

therapy for Peyronie's disease: Presentation of 56 new case studies and review of the literature. Int J Radiat Oncol Biol Phys 6:161, 1980
87. Nissen-Meyer R: The role of prophylactic castration in the therapy of human mammary cancer. Eur J Cancer 3:395, 1967
88. Nordberg VB, Sundberg J: Indications and methods for radiotherapy of cavernous hemangiomas. Acta Radiol Ther 1:257, 1963
89. Okazaki N, Yoshino M, Yoshida T, et al: Radiotherapy of hemangioma cavernosum of the liver. Gastroenterology 73:353, 1977
90. Palmer D, Greenberg P, Corne HP, et al: Radiation therapy for Graves' ophthalmopathy: A retrospective analysis. Int J Radiat Oncol Biol Phys 13:1815, 1987
91. Park, WC Phillips R: The role of radiation therapy in the management of hemangiomas of the liver. JAMA 212:1496, 1970
92. Pilepich MV, Sicard GA, Breaux SR, et al: Renal graft irradiation in acute rejection. Transplantation 35:208. 1983
93. Plenk HP: Calcifying tendonitis of the shoulder: A critical study of the value of x-ray therapy. Radiology 59:384, 1952
94. Plowman PN, Harnett AN: Radiotherapy in benign orbital disease. I Complicated ocular angiomas. Br J Ophthalmol 72:281, 1983
95. Pringle WM, Helms DC: Treatment of plantar warts by blunt dissection. Arch Dermatol 108:79, 1973
96. Rao DV, Cosby K, Smith M, et al: Lymphomas and pseudolymphomas of the orbit. [Abstract] Int J Radiat Oncol Biol Phys 8(suppl 1):114, 1982
97. Ravin JG, Sisson JC, Knapp WT: Orbital radiation for the ocular changes of Graves' disease. Am J Ophthalmol 79:285, 1975
98. Ritter MA, Vaughan RB: Ectopic ossification after total hip arthroplasty: Predisposing factors, frequency and effect on results. J Bone Joint Surg [A] 59:345, 1977
99. Sandler H, Rubenstein J, Fowble B, et al: Results of radiotherapy for thyroid ophthalmopathy. [Abstract] Int J Radiat Oncol Biol Phys 15:209, 1988
100. Shaw HJ, Katsikas KD: Ameloblastoma of the maxilla: A clinical study with four cases. J Laryngol Otol 58:873, 1973
101. Shumer SM, O'Keefe EJ: Bleomycin in the treatment of recalcitrant warts. J Am Acad Dermatol 9:91, 1983
102. Steele K, Shirodaria R, O'Hare H, et al: Monochloroacetic acid and 60% salicylic acid as a treatment for simple plantar warts: Effectiveness and mode of action. Br J Dermatol 118:537, 1988
103. Stockdale AD, Casson Am, Col MA: Radiotherapy and conservative surgery in the management of musculo-aponeurotic fibromatosis. Int J Radiat Oncol Biol Phys 15:851, 1988
104. Stout AP, Raffaele L: Tumors of soft tissues. In Atlas of Tumor Pathology, 2nd series, fasc I. Washington, DC, Armed Forces Institute of Pathology, 1967
105. Saunders WM, Winstron KR, Siddon RL, et al: Radiosurgery for arteriovenous malfunction of the brain using a standard linear accelerator: Rationale and technique. Int J Radiat Oncol Biol Phys 15:441, 1988
106. Shibata S, Mori K: Effect of radiation therapy on extracerebral cavernous hemangioma in the middle fossa. J Neurosurg 67:919, 1987
107. Suit HD, Russel WO: Radiation therapy of soft tissue sarcomas. Cancer 36:759, 1975
108. Sylvester JE, Greenberg P, Selch MT: The use of postoperative irradiation for the prevention of heterotopic bone formation after total hip replacement. Int J Radiat Oncol Biol Phys 14:471, 1988
109. Takagi H: Diagnosis and management of cavernous hemangioma of the liver. Semin Surg Oncol 1:12, 1985
110. Trastek VF, et al: Cavernous hemangiomas of the liver: Resect or observe? Am J Surg 145:49, 1983
111. Unni KK, Irvius JC, Beabout JW, et al: Hemangioma, hemangiopericytoma, and hemangioendothelioma (angiosarcoma) of bone. Cancer 27:1403, 1971
112. Van den Brenk HAA: Results of prophylactic postoperative irradiation in 1300 cases of pterygium. AJR 103:723, 1968
113. Williams JL, Thomas CG: The natural history of Peyronie's disease. J Urol 103:75, 1970
114. Wolkov HB, Bagshaw MA: Radiation therapy in the management of vascular malformations in the central nervous system. [Abstract] Int J Radiat Oncol Biol Phys 8(suppl 1):91, 1982
115. Yonkers AJ, Krous HF, Yarrington CT: Surgical parotitis. Laryngoscope 82:1239, 1972

75

○ ○ ○ • • •

Total-Lymphoid Irradiation in the Management of Autoimmune Diseases and Organ Transplantation

Richard T. Hoppe
Samuel Strober

Total-lymphoid irradiation (TLI), which encompasses most of the body's lymphoid tissue, is a curative form of treatment for early-stage Hodgkin's disease. *In vitro* tests of immune function in patients who have been treated with TLI reveal abnormalities not present in untreated patients. Animal models for TLI have facilitated characterization of these immunologic disturbances, and clinical studies of humans have been initiated to exploit TLI for immunomodulation in promoting transplantation tolerance and treating autoimmune diseases.

IMMUNOSUPPRESSIVE EFFECTS OF IRRADIATION IN HUMANS

Total-Lymphoid Irradiation for Hodgkin's Disease

The immunosuppressive effects of TLI in patients treated for Hodgkin's disease were detailed by Fuks and associates[16] in an analysis of 227 patients. They observed a marked depression of the circulating lymphocyte count, persisting for about 2 years after TLI, with subsequent gradual recovery. Quantitation of lymphocyte populations revealed differential long-term effects of TLI on specific lymphocyte subsets. The total number and percent of T cells (T-cell lymphocytopenia) had decreased in most patients, with a compensatory increase in the total number and percent of B cells (B-cell lymphocytosis). After long-term follow-up, there was a reversal of the normal T-cell : B-cell ratio. Furthermore, a differential sensitivity of various T-cell subsets to TLI was observed.[42,49] The T-cell lymphocytopenia is secondary to a decrease in the number of helper T cells, with a normal or almost normal number of suppressor T cells. This produces a reversal of the helper : suppressor T-cell ratio to a value less than 1.0; normal controls or untreated patients have helper : suppressor T-cell ratios greater than 1.0.

Functional lymphocyte assays revealed an impaired ability to respond to mitogens such as phytohemagglutinin (PHA), which persisted for at least 10 years.[16] The ability to respond to allogeneic cells in the mixed lymphocyte reaction was markedly impaired at the completion of TLI, but gradual recovery was later observed. Impaired reactivity of lymphocytes in the autologous mixed lymphocyte reaction persisted for long as 15 years.[13]

TLI also alters cutaneous delayed hypersensitivity reactions. Patients with untreated Hodgkin's disease often have an impaired ability to respond to neoantigens such as 2,5-dinitrochlorobenzene (DNCB).[19] Patients with intact responses to DNCB may lose that response after TLI.[16] Gradual recovery of DNCB reactivity is observed in most of these patients, but almost one third remain anergic.

Despite the degree and severity of the immunosuppression observed *in vitro,* only modest immunologic complications, such as herpes zoster infection, have been reported in these patients.[29] Other opportunistic infections are seen infrequently after TLI.

Local or Regional Irradiation for Cancer

Immunologic abnormalities may be detected after limited irradiation, but the severity of those changes is less profound than after TLI. Regional irradiation has lymphopenic effects.[24,57] Several studies have looked at the effects of regional irradiation on lymphocyte subpopulations.[27,45]

The total lymphocyte counts remained depressed as long

as 10 years after treatment, primarily due to a decrease in the number of T cells, but the B cells showed no significant decrease compared with the controls. Suppressor or cytotoxic T cells recovered to normal levels within 5 to 6 years, but cells with the helper or inducer phenotype were still significantly decreased after 10 years.

IMMUNOSUPPRESSIVE EFFECTS OF TOTAL-LYMPHOID IRRADIATION IN ANIMALS

After identifying the immunologic abnormalities induced by TLI in humans, a variety of animal models were developed to further define these immunosuppressive effects. Slavin and colleagues[55] developed a technique for treating mice with TLI. Shielding was provided for the skull, lungs, long bones of the extremities, a portion of the pelvis, and the tail. Most of the lymphoid tissue, including the mediastinum, thymus, and mesentery, was irradiated. Animals were treated with 250-kV orthovoltage x-rays for 200 cGy per day, 5 days per week, to a total dose of 3400 cGy. Adult BALB/c mice treated in this fashion developed changes in lymphocyte number, T- and B-cell percentages, and functional immunologic impairment similar to that observed in patients treated with TLI for Hodgkin's disease.[56] However, recovery from these abnormalities appeared to be accelerated compared with those in humans studies.

The influence of TLI on the primary antibody response was measured by Zan-Bar and colleagues.[70] TLI was able to modify the primary immune response but was unable to obliterate immunologic memory.

Similar animal models were developed for other species, and comparable degrees of *in vitro* immune abnormality were demonstrated.[54] Similar fractionation programs proved feasible in other rodent species, such as the rat. However, in larger mammals, including dogs and nonhuman primates, hematologic tolerance did not permit the delivery of 3400 cGy TLI in 17 fractions. Alternative dose and fractionation programs were identified that were associated with minimal morbidity and yet induced a similar degree of clinical immunosuppression. These TLI programs consisted of 80 cGy to 100 cGy fractions, two to five fractions per week, for cumulative doses of 800 cGy to 2000 cGy.[36,39]

Enhancement of Allograft Survival

Attempts were made to use TLI as a means of immunosuppression to promote organ transplantation in animals. When BALB/c (H-2d) mice were irradiated and then engrafted with skin from a histoincompatible C57BL/Ka (H-2b) mouse, graft survival increased fivefold compared with unirradiated controls.[55] Subsequent studies in mice examined the ability of TLI to promote bone marrow engraftment as well as skin graft survival.[56] Most BALB/c mice treated with TLI, followed by infusion of bone marrow cells from C57BL/Ka donors, developed chimerism. These chimeric BALB/c mice showed no evidence of graft-*versus*-host disease (GVHD). When BALB/c mice pretreated with TLI received both bone marrow cells and skin grafts from C57BL/Ka donors, chimerism developed, and permanent skin graft survival was demonstrated. These chimeric animals showed specific tolerance for C57BL/Ka skin grafts. Studies in rats revealed similar results and demonstrated permanent survival of heart allografts in TLI-treated animals infused with bone marrow cells from the heart donor, despite major histocompatibility differences.[54]

Experiments were performed to explain the lack of GVHD in the TLI-treated mouse chimeras.[60] These studies showed that the induction of tolerance was mediated by nonspecific suppressor cells that developed after TLI, but the maintenance of tolerance was mediated by specific suppressor cells generated by the donor-host cell interactions.

Laboratory experience using TLI to enhance organ graft survival in animals is now extensive. Important issues being addressed include the evaluation of different dose and fractionation programs, the combined use of TLI and pharmacologic immunosuppression, comparison of pretransplant and posttransplant TLI, and the possible effect of TLI on the enhancement of xenograft survival.[30] Table 75-1 provides examples of some of the transplantation experiments that have been performed.

In addition to organ transplantation, successful tumor allotransplantation in mice and tumor xenograft growth in rats have been demonstrated after TLI and donor bone marrow infusion or cyclophosphamide.[22,23] These studies suggest the possible use of TLI-treated animals as hosts for human tumor xenotransplants, facilitating the *in vivo* study of human tumors.

Autoimmune Diseases

Animal models of autoimmune diseases have been examined for the possible influence of TLI (Table 75-2). Experimental data from two of these systems are reviewed.

NZB/NZW F_1 hybrid mice develop an autoimmune disease characterized by antinuclear antibodies and a fatal immune-complex glomerulonephritis, similar to the nephritis observed in human systemic lupus erythematosus. Kotzin and Strober[31] examined the impact of fractionated TLI (17 fractions of 200 cGy, including the kidneys) on the development of nephritis. After animals with low-grade proteinuria were irradiated, the survival rate 6 months after TLI was 90%, compared with only 25% in the controls. Deaths in the control animals were related to progressive renal disease. In another experiment, animals that had already developed high-grade proteinuria were given TLI or sham irradiation. In the sham group, there were no survivors 6 weeks later, compared with a survival rate of 75% in

TABLE 75–1
Fractionated Total-Lymphoid Irradiation to Enhance Allograft Survival in Animals

ANIMAL	TRANSPLANTED ORGAN
Mouse	Skin[55]
	Bone marrow[56]
Rat	Skin[5]
	Heart[3,46]
	Islet cells[7]
	Pancreas[37]
Dog	Bone marrow[18]
	Kidney[25]
	Heart[61]
Pig	Kidney[15]
	Bone marrow[15]
Baboon	Liver[39]
	Kidney[39]
	Pancreas[12]
Rhesus monkey	Heart[4]
Cynomolgus monkey	Kidney[19]

TABLE 75–2
Fractionated Total-Lymphoid Irradiation in Animal Models of Autoimmune Diseases

ANIMAL	AUTOIMMUNE DISEASE	RESULTS OF IRRADIATION (TO 3400 cGy)
NZB/NZW F_1 mouse[31]	Immune complex glomerulonephritis	TLI in mice with low-grade proteinuria yielded survival of 90% (*vs* 25% in controls); 10% of TLI mice developed high-grade proteinuria (*vs* 75% of controls). TLI in mice with high-grade proteinuria yielded 75% survival (*vs* 0% in controls) and 80% reversal of proteinuria
MRL/1 mouse[65]	T-cell proliferation, arthritis, glomerulonephritis	100% survival 6 months after TLI (*vs* 8% in controls). 0% arthritis after TLI (*vs* 25% in controls). 10%–20% glomerulonephritis after TLI (*vs* 90% in controls).
Lewis rat[50]	Adjuvant arthritis induced by *M. butyricum*	Control animals rapidly developed arthritis during first 100 days. TLI significantly reduced severity of arthritis. TLI plus paw irradiation yielded best outcome.
Sprague-Dawley rat[35]	Collagen arthritis	Animals pretreated with TLI had decreased incidence, delayed onset, and decreased severity of arthritis *vs* control animals, but no effect if TLI administered after the arthritis had already developed.
Inbred LEW rat[34]	Accelerated autologous form of nephrotoxic serum nephritis	TLI-treated rats showed improved histopathology and decreased albuminuria *vs* controls ($P < 0.02$)
	Autologous immune complex nephritis	TLI-treated rats had significant reductions in albuminuria ($P < 0.0001$) and serum creatinine ($P < 0.005$) levels and incidence of lipemia ($P < 0.005$) *vs* controls.
Juvenile strain 3 guinea pig[17]	Chronic experimental allergic encephalomyelitis	TLI delayed time to relapse and decreased the extent of demyelinization compared with controls.

the TLI group. Among the irradiated animals that were still alive, almost 80% had a reversal of the high-grade proteinuria.

An animal model of adjuvant arthritis in rats has been used to test the efficacy of agents used to treat rheumatoid arthritis. Adjuvant arthritis can be induced by a subcutaneous injection of mineral oil combined with *Mycobacterium butyricum* into one of the rat paws. Schurman and associates[50] induced adjuvant arthritis in a group of Lewis rats and treated them with either TLI (17 fractions of 200 cGy), paw irradiation (three doses of 200 cGy), or both TLI and paw irradiation. Rats that were treated with TLI developed significantly less inflammation than the control group. The inflammation and deformity measured in rats treated with paw irradiation alone was slightly reduced compared with the controls. The arthritis activity in animals treated with both TLI and low-dose paw irradiation was the most dramatically altered.

Tolerance to Xenogeneic Proteins

An obstacle to the use of murine monoclonal antibody therapy in humans is the development of human antimouse immunoglobulin antibodies. Preliminary experiments suggest that pretreatment with TLI may alter the pattern of antimouse immunoglobulin antibody production.[33] Lowder and colleagues[33] treated cynomolgus monkeys with TLI (17 fractions of 100 cGy), followed by intravenous infusion of anti-Leu-2a, -3a, and -5 murine monoclonal antibodies. The TLI-treated animals demonstrated a marked delay in the development of antimouse immunoglobulin antibody (<1% of control animals).

HUMAN TRANSPLANTATION

Renal Transplantation

Soon after the first successful transplantation studies in laboratory animals, investigators began to study the utility of TLI in facilitating allograft survival in humans (Table 75-3).

Najarian and associates[40] reported early results in renal transplantation from the University of Minnesota. Their patients were at high risk for rejection because of prior graft rejection and previous splenectomy. They were treated with concurrent mantle and inverted-Y irradiation in 100-cGy to 150-cGy fractions to total doses of 1600 cGy to 4150 cGy (mean, 2739 cGy). The duration of TLI ranged from 24 to 124 days and the delay from the completion of TLI to transplant was 1 to 330 days. After transplant, all patients were maintained on low-dose azathioprine (<1.5 mg/kg/day, titrated according to blood counts) and prednisone (0.4–2.0 mg/kg/day initially, followed a tapered dose). Twenty patients were treated between 1979 and 1981. The best results were achieved with TLI doses of about 2500 cGy administered in 100-cGy fractions and with a minimum delay of less than 2 weeks from completion of TLI to transplant. An initial dose of prednisone of at least 2.0 mg/kg/day was optimal. Tests of immune function indicated a rapid peripheral blood T-cell depletion and loss of *in vitro* responsiveness to mitogens and allogeneic cells.

A recent report reveals 1-year graft survival and patient survival rates of 70%.[63] These compare favorably with the 45% graft survival rate and 70% patient survival rate in historic controls treated with conventional immunosuppression (*e.g.*, azathioprine, prednisone, antilymphocyte globulin). However, in a later group of patients treated with cyclosporine-A plus prednisone, the graft survival rate was 70%, and the patient survival rate was 81%. Although cyclosporine-A was not significantly superior to TLI, the investigators concluded that cyclosporine-A was preferable because of its ease of administration and avoidance of the problem of urgent identification of a suitable kidney for prompt transplantation after TLI.

A collaborative program was developed at Stanford University and the Pacific Medical Center in San Francisco. TLI was used in an attempt to minimize posttransplant immunosuppression.[47] Patients were treated to the mantle and inverted-Y/spleen fields concurrently with 100-cGy fractions, two to three times per week. Treatment was continued to a total dose of 2000 cGy. If leukopenia or thrombocytopenia occurred, TLI was interrupted; when resumed, the mantle was completed

TABLE 75–3
Fractionated Total-Lymphoid Irradiation to Facilitate Renal Transplantation

INVESTIGATION	NO. OF PATIENTS	TLI DOSE (cGy)	PHARMACOLOGIC IMMUNOSUPPRESSION	COMMENTS
University of Minnesota[63]	20	1600–4500 (mean 2739)	Azathioprine (<1.5 mg/kg/d) Prednisone (0.4–2.0 mg/kg/d, tapered)	Eligible patients had rejected a prior graft. All patients had splenectomy. Rejection episodes treated with prednisone pulses.
Stanford University/ Pacific Medical Center[48]	25	2000	Antithymocyte globulin (ATG) (2 mg/kg/d qod × 6) Prednisone (0.2 mg/kg/d, taper to 0.15 mg/kg/d)	"Backburner" irradiation employed while awaiting a suitable kidney. Maintenance prednisone was 7.5–10 mg/d. Rejections treated with prednisone pulse (4 mg/kg) ± ATG ± azathioprine.
University of Leuven[1]	17	2000–3000	Prednisone (15 mg/d, tapered to 10 mg/d)	All patients (except one) had splenectomy. Rejection treated with prednisone pulse and azathioprine.
University of Rome[10]	14	2500–3500	Prednisolone (15 mg/d) Antilymphocyte globulin (12 mg/kg/d × 60 d)	TLI did not include the spleen. After 2 months, azathioprine 3(0.8–1.0 mg/kg/d) was substituted for ATG.
	14	1500–2000	Cyclosporine-A (12 mg/kg/d)	TLI did not include the spleen.
University of Witwatersrand[38]	6	2100–3200		TLI was actually "whole torso," shielding only ribs and lungs.
	12	800–1220	Cyclosporine-A (10–12 mg/kg/d × 8 d, then tapered) Prednisone (30 mg/d, tapered to 10 mg/d by 90 d)	TLI was actually "whole torso." "Backburner" irradiation employed while awaiting a suitable kidney. Rejection episode treated wth azathioprine.

first, then the inverted-Y/spleen field, to a total dose of 2000 cGy each. If a donor kidney was not identified within one week, a "backburner" regimen was used in which the inverted-Y/spleen field was treated with 100-cGy fractions, once per week, until a donor kidney was identified. After TLI, patients received rabbit antithymocyte globulin (usually six injections) and low-dose prednisone.

Twenty-five patients were treated on the Stanford-Pacific Medical Center protocol.[48] Four grafts were rejected, and six patients died with a functioning graft intact. Fifteen patients were alive with functioning grafts at 19 to 37 months, twelve of whom were receiving prednisone maintenance therapy only (average dose, 9.8 mg/day). This study confirmed the possibility of decreasing pharmacologic immunosuppression after TLI. Graft survival rates at 1, 2, and 3 years were 76%, 68%, and 53%, respectively. Patient survival rates at the same intervals were 87%, 77%, and 70%.

The Stanford patients underwent detailed studies of immune function.[48] The total lymphocyte counts and helper T-cell counts were markedly depressed; there was a decrease in the mixed lymphocyte reaction, and responses decreased to PHA, Con-A, and pokeweed mitogen. Subsets of suppressor or cytotoxic lymphocytes, as defined by the Leu-9.3 antigen, were studied. In controls, the Leu-9.3 – subpopulation of cells, which suppress immunoglobulin synthesis, is roughly equivalent in size to the Leu-9.3+ subpopulation (cytolytic cells). In TLI-treated patients, the Leu-9.3-:Leu-9.3+ ratio was approximately ten, largely due to an increase in size of the Leu-9.3 – population.

Among the Stanford patients who were monitored for more than 1.5 years, nine patients were evaluated for the development of specific immune tolerance.[8] In all of these patients, the mixed lymphocyte reaction against a panel of normal stimulator cells returned to normal. Suitably controlled experiments with cryopreserved donor cells revealed a pattern of specific unresponsiveness in seven patients, (*i.e.*, they demonstrated specific unresponsiveness to donor cells in the mixed lymphocyte reaction, but the response to control allogeneic cells was normal).

At the University of Leuven, Belgium, a protocol for patients with end-stage diabetic nephropathy was developed.[68] This program combined TLI and low-dose prednisone. After splenectomy, patients were treated to the mantle and inverted-Y fields in 100-cGy fractions. Initially the dose range was 2000 cGy to 2500 cGy; later patients were treated with 3000 cGy. After transplant, patients received prednisone, approximately 15 mg/day initially, tapered to 10 mg/day. Between 1981 and 1984, 17 patients received transplants.[1] Thirteen patients were alive at the time of last follow-up (six for more than 1 year). Although all 13 had functioning grafts, most had at least one rejection episode during the follow-up period. The 1-year graft survival rate was 80%. *In vitro* assessment of immune response was similar to that reported in other renal transplant studies.[69]

Other TLI protocols have been used in Rome and Johannesburg.[10, 38] Studies of TLI in renal transplantation continue at some of these centers. Important issues that remain to be resolved include the optimal fractionation scheme and total dose of TLI, the optimal form of pharmacologic immunosuppression after transplant, especially various combinations of TLI with cyclosporine-A, and the possible role of posttransplant TLI to prevent or treat rejection.

Bone Marrow Transplantation

Although early animal studies characterized the successful engraftment of bone marrow after TLI, there has been only minimal experience using TLI to enhance bone marrow engraftment in humans.[43,51,53] All of the experience has been in patients with aplastic anemia.

Investigators at the University of Minnesota[43] substituted single-dose TLI (750 cGy) for whole-body irradiation in a program combined with cyclophosphamide (50 mg/kg/day × 4) for previously transfused patients with aplastic anemia. Single-fraction TLI may not provide the same degree of immunosuppression as fractionated TLI and may simply reflect a less toxic form of whole-body irradiation. Nevertheless, the results of this group of patients were promising. Grafting was prompt in 36 of the 40 patients, and subsequent marrow graft rejection occurred in only one patient, despite the fact that 28 of 40 patients had received more than 20 prior transfusions. Chronic GVHD developed in 31% of these patients, and idiopathic interstitial pneumonitis was observed in only 15%. The 2-year survival rate was 72%.

Two small experiences using fractionated TLI have been reported from the Hadassah University Hospital in Jerusalem and the Memorial Hospital in New York.[51,53] Both of these studies are too small to provide evaluable data; however, they suggest that the outcome may be the same as for other programs incorporating total-body irradiation, but with fewer toxic effects.

Miscellaneous Organ Transplantation

There have been anecdotal reports of hepatic, pancreatic, and cardiac transplantation in patients who have been pretreated with TLI.[10,28,38] However, there has not been a large enough experience to define the role of TLI in these settings.

Recent data from Stanford suggest a possible role of post-transplant TLI for treating rejection in cardiac transplant recipients.[26] A protocol was developed for patients who demonstrated biopsy evidence of graft rejection despite treatment with cyclosporine-A, prednisone, azathioprine, and OKT3 antibodies. The treatment program includes TLI to mantle and inverted-Y/spleen fields concurrently, using 80-cGy fractions for one or two fractions per week to a maximum total dose of 800 cGy. The total dose administered is titrated according to the CD4 (helper T cell) count, and treatment is discontinued if the CD4 count falls and remains below 100 cells/mm^3. Promising results have been observed in the first three patients, who have required only 240 cGy to 540 cGy TLI to achieve the desired effect on CD4 counts.

CLINICAL TRIALS OF IRRADIATION FOR AUTOIMMUNE DISEASES

Rheumatoid Arthritis

The first human autoimmune disease to be treated with TLI was rheumatoid arthritis (Table 75-4). Initial trials were conducted at Stanford University and Harvard University.[32,66] The patients selected had severe rheumatoid arthritis with active synovitis and significant disability, and they had been treated unsuccessfully with nonsteroidal antiinflammatory agents, gold, and penicillamine. All patients would have been suitable candidates for cytotoxic therapy with agents like azathioprine or cyclophosphamide. These drugs, although effective in controlling advanced disease, may be accompanied by significant side-effects. Investigational treatment with TLI was therefore deemed appropriate.

In the Stanford trial, the TLI regimen consisted of mantle field treatment with 2000 cGy in ten fractions of 200 cGy in 2 weeks, followed immediately by treatment to the inverted-Y/spleen field with 2000 cGy in 13 fractions of 150 cGy over 3 weeks.[32] The fields treated are shown in Figure 75-1. Patients were evaluated carefully at least twice before initiation of therapy and serially thereafter with specific attention to joint tenderness and joint swelling (an assessment of 78 different joints), duration of morning stiffness, and a global composite score that consisted of 14 subjective and objective variables. Patients also underwent serial immunologic monitoring.

During TLI, many patients felt subjectively worse. There was little measurable change in disease activity for at least 1 month after TLI. Morning stiffness was the first parameter to show improvement, with the joint score and global composite scores improving later. Generally, improvement was reported within 3 months, with an average improvement of 61% in joint tenderness, 49% in joint swelling, 72% in morning stiffness, and 45% in the global composite score. Overall, nine of 11 patients had more than 35% improvement in all four clinical parameters. Further follow-up revealed that improvement persisted throughout the follow-up period without any tendency for disease to regress to baseline levels.[14]

Immunologic evaluation after TLI revealed impaired ability of peripheral blood lymphocytes to respond to mitogens such as PHA and Con-A and also to allogeneic lymphocytes in the mixed lymphocyte reaction.[32] There was a significant inhibition of pokeweed mitogen-induced immunoglobulin synthesis.

TABLE 75–4
Fractionated Total-Lymphoid Irradiation for the Management of Autoimmune Diseases in Humans

AUTOIMMUNE DISEASE	NO. OF PATIENTS	TLI DOSE (cGy)	INVESTIGATION
Rheumatoid arthritis	32	2000	Stanford University[64]
	11	2000	University of Erlangen-Nurenberg[21]
	20	750 *vs* 2000	St. Vincent's, Dublin[20]
	12	3000	Joint Center, Boston[6]
Lupus nephritis	17	2000	Stanford University[58]
Systemic lupus erythematosus	2	2000	Hadassah University, Jerusalem[2]
Multiple sclerosis	20	1980	Univ. Medicine and Dentistry, NJ[9]
Chronic demyelinating polyneuropathy	3	2000	University of Colorado[44]

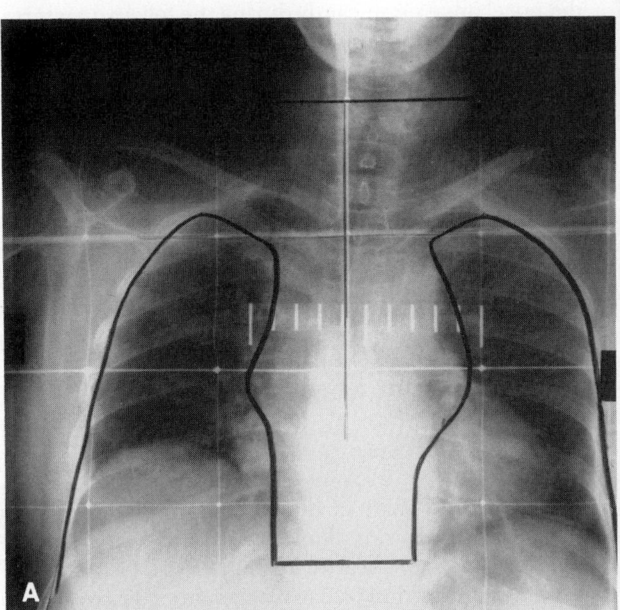

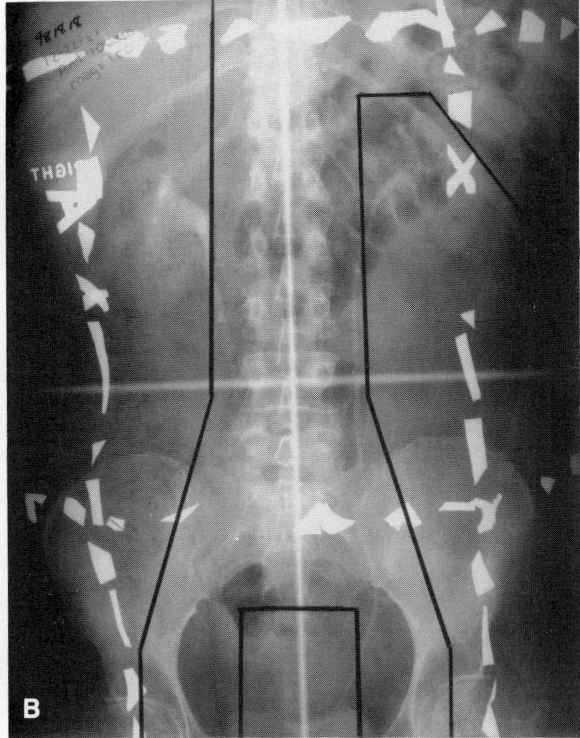

FIGURE 75–1. Setup film for patient being treated with total lymphoid irradiation for autoimmune disease. (**A**) Mantle setup (compare with Fig. 62–4). The blocks are designed to shield a maximum amount of lung. They are drawn tightly around the mediastinum and hila and extend superiorly into the infraclavicular region, even on the anterior port. A low upper border (just above the thyroid notch) is chosen to minimize xerostomia, and a larynx block is placed anteriorly during the actual treatment. Humeral head blocks are not employed when rheumatoid arthritis is treated. (**B**) Inverted-Y setup. The superior border of the inverted-Y area is matched to the inferior border of the mantle. The entire spleen is included in the field and is localized by CT scan or technetium radionuclide scan if necessary. Notice the contrast localization of the kidneys; this should not be employed in lupus nephritis.

Despite clinical improvement after TLI, there was no alteration in serum factors like rheumatoid factor. Analysis of lymphocyte populations revealed a significant decrease in the total number of T cells. A preferential effect on the helper or inducer population led to an excess of the suppressor or cytotoxic cells observed after completion of TLI.

Complications of treatment included mild systemic effects, such as nausea and fatigue, and local effects, including dysphagia, xerostomia, and esophagitis. Herpes zoster infections occurred occasionally. One patient with Felty's syndrome developed an exacerbation of that syndrome during TLI, and another patient with rheumatoid lung disease developed progression of pulmonary symptoms after completing TLI. Patients with a history of Felty's syndrome or rheumatoid lung disease were subsequently excluded from the trial. Occasionally, bacterial infections developed during or after treatment with TLI.

The Harvard treatment program used a higher dose and more protracted course of treatment.[66] Patients received 3000 cGy to the mantle field followed by a 2-week split, then 3000 cGy to the para-aortic-spleen field, another 2-week split, and 3000 cGy to the pelvic nodes. The usual duration of treatment was 13 to 15 weeks. The improvement in these patients observed at 6 months was similar to that reported by the Stanford group.

In a follow-up evaluation of ten of these patients 15 to 40 months after TLI, significant improvement was reported for several parameters of disease activity.[6] However, the investigators reported four deaths among their original 12 patients; two died of infection and two of cardiopulmonary disease. They also found significant morbidity, including xerostomia in eight patients that was serious enough to cause weight loss greater than 10 kg in four patients and the loss of four or more teeth in three patients. There were four episodes of serious bacterial infection, including two deaths.

Differences in xerostomia at Stanford and in Boston may have been secondary to differences in dose (3000 cGy in Boston *versus* 2000 cGy at Stanford) and design of the mantle field (upper border at the mastoid tip or inferior portion of mandible in Boston *versus* the top of the larynx at Stanford). The greater frequency of infections in the Boston patients may have been caused by the higher dose employed and patient selection factors, especially age. The average age of the Boston patients was 60 years, but at Stanford, it was only 51 years.

Another pilot study was carried out at the University of Erlangen-Nurenburg in West Germany.[21] The fractionation program and TLI fields were very similar to those used at Stanford. Eleven patients were treated, and all demonstrated improvement. However, these patients were elderly (average, 66 years), and complications were significant, including four deaths.

In a later Stanford study, patients were randomized to two different dose schedules, with total doses of 2000 cGy or 200 cGy.[62] In the 200-cGy program, patients were treated with 20-cGy fractions to the mantle to a total dose of 200 cGy followed by 20-cGy fractions to the inverted-Y/spleen field to a total dose of 200 cGy. The high-dose program was significantly more beneficial in achieving improvements in joint tenderness, morning stiffness, and the global composite score. The high-dose group also had less joint swelling after TLI than did the low-dose group, but the differences were not statistically significant. Immunologic monitoring showed that patients treated with the 200-cGy TLI program developed none of the immunologic abnormalities previously identified after 2000-cGy TLI.

Another randomized trial was conducted at St. Vincent's Hospital in Dublin.[20] Twenty patients were randomized to one of two dosage schedules: 2000 cGy (200-cGy fractions) or 750 cGy (75-cGy fractions). The TLI technique was similar to that used at Stanford except that the spleen was not irradiated. Patients treated with 750-cGy TLI improved significantly in four of seven measurements of disease activity, and patients treated with 2000-cGy TLI improved in six of seven parameters. Three patients in the low-dose group and four in the high-dose group demonstrated major reductions in disease activity. Sustained peripheral blood lymphopenia, selective decrease in the helper T-cell population, and impaired response to mitogens *in vivo* occurred in both groups. Because the 750-cGy program was accompanied by less acute toxicity than the 2000-cGy TLI program, the investigators concluded that the lower dose was preferable.

More than 30 patients have now been treated with 2000-cGy TLI in various clinical trials at Stanford.[64] The overall rate of significant improvement (≥25% improvement in three of four disease activity parameters) is 75%, and these improvements have persisted during follow-up of up to 4 years. However, 25% of these patients have required immunosuppressive drug therapy to maintain their responses. Four patients (12.5%) died, including one 58-year-old patient of myocardial infarction, a 68-year-old patient of pulmonary embolism, and a 70-year-old woman and a 71-year-old man of complications of rheumatoid lung disease.

A more detailed analysis of the complications in patients treated with TLI at Stanford has been reported and compared to that of a matched group of patients treated with cytotoxic therapy, such as cyclophosphamide, azathioprine, and methotrexate.[52] Hospitalization associated with infection was more common in the TLI group. However, other complications, including gastrointestinal intolerance, oral ulcers, and abnormal liver enzymes, were more common in the drug-treated group. The risk of developing herpes zoster infections and the risk of mortality were the same in both groups.

Lupus Nephritis

A trial testing the efficacy of TLI for severe lupus nephritis has been reported from Stanford (Table 74-4).[59] Patients selected for the study had nephritis that failed to respond to high-dose prednisone or in whom prednisone could not be reduced below 0.5 mg/kg/day. TLI was administered according to the same protocol used in treating rheumatoid arthritis. The pelvic lymph nodes were not irradiated in premenopausal women. Intravenous contrast was not used to visualize the kidneys at the time of setup. The kidneys were localized by ultrasound, renal scanning, or noncontrast CT scanning. During treatment, in addition to monitoring the blood counts, the serum creatinine and BUN levels were determined weekly.

In the most recent report of this series, 17 patients had been treated with a follow-up of 12 to 75 months.[58] The mean serum albumin level before TLI was 2.5 g/dl. This value increased promptly after TLI, reaching a mean of 3.1 g/dl within 3 months ($P<0.001$). Urinary protein decreased from 7.0 g/24 hours to 3.7 g/24 hours during the same period ($P<0.001$). Serum parameters of disease activity improved as well, with an increase in the serum complement ($P<0.001$) and decrease in anti-DNA antibodies ($P<0.005$). The serum creatinine levels did not change significantly during the follow-up interval; however, the mean daily dosage of prednisone was reduced from an average of 37.4 mg to 10.3 mg after 3 years. Steroid therapy had been completely discontinued in seven patients, although four of these seven required reinstitution of prednisone because of arthralgias, fatigue, or recrudesence of renal disease.

Complications in these patients included modest neutropenia (four patients) and thrombocytopenia (one patient). There were three episodes of localized bacterial infection requiring hospitalization and antibiotic therapy and four episodes of localized herpes zoster infections. These complications were not as severe as would be expected with cytotoxic therapy in a similar population of patients.

Multiple Sclerosis

One controlled study of the efficacy of TLI for patients with chronic progressive multiple sclerosis has been carried out at the New Jersey Medical School in Newark (Table 74-4).[9] Forty patients were randomized to receive either TLI or sham irradiation. The TLI treatment consisted of 1980 cGy in 180-cGy fractions to an extended mantle that included the spleen and the para-aortic nodes to the level of L1, followed immediately by 1980 cGy in 180-cGy fractions to an inverted-Y field.[11] The dose to the spinal cord was limited to 1000 cGy by the use of spinal cord blocking.

During a mean follow-up interval of 21 months, the TLI-treated patients suffered significantly less functional decline than the sham irradiated patients ($P<0.01$).[9] TLI was associated with a fall in the percentage of helper T cells, and clinical improvement seemed to be correlated with a decrease in the ratio of helper and suppressor T cells.[67]

Pending Treatment of Autoimmune Disease

The future of TLI for the treatment of autoimmune diseases rests with the continuation of carefully conducted controlled clinical trials.[71] It is still premature to treat these patients outside the context of a clinical trial. The relative impact of TLI compared with other forms of immunosuppression must be assessed and both the efficacy and optimal of TLI for different autoimmune diseases defined more precisely. The actuarial risk of each complication must be measured carefully and compared with other therapies.

REFERENCES

1. Ang KK, Vanrenterghem Y, Waer M, et al: Kidney allograft tolerance in diabetic patients after total lymphoid irradiation (TLI). Radiother Oncol 3:193, 1985
2. Ben-Chetrit E, Gross DJ, Braverman A, et al: Total lymphoid irradiation in refractory systemic lupus erythematosus. Ann Intern Med 105:58, 1986
3. Bentley FR, Sutherland DER, Rynasiewicz JJ, et al: Synergistic effect of posttransplant total lymphoid irradiation and pharmacologic immunosuppression with low-dose anti-lymphocyte globulin or cyslosporine on prolongation of rat heart allograft survival. Transplant Proc 15:671, 1983
4. Bieber CP, Jamieson S, Raney A, et al: Cardiac allograft sur-

vival in rhesus primates treated with combined total lymphoid irradiation and rabbit antithymocyte globulin. Transplantation 28:347, 1979

5. Blum JE, DeSilva SM, Drachman DB, et al: Low-dose-rate total lymphoid irradiation: A new method of rapid immunosuppression. Int J Radiat Oncol Biol Phys 15:547, 1988
6. Brahn E, Helfgott SM, Belli JA, et al: Total lymphoid irradiation therapy in refractory rheumatoid arthritis. Arthritis Rheum 27:481, 1984
7. Britt LD, Scharp DW, Lacy PE, et al: Transplantation of islet cells across major histocompatibility barriers after total lymphoid irradiation and infusion of allogeneic bone marrow cells. Diabetes 31:63, 1982
8. Chow D, Saper V, Strober S: Renal transplant patients treated with total lymphoid irradiation show specific unresponsiveness to donor antigens in the mixed leukocyte reaction (MLR). J Immunol 138:3746, 1987
9. Cook SD, Devereux C, Troiano R, et al: Effect of total lymphoid irradiation in chronic progressive multiple sclerosis. Lancet 1:405, 1986
10. Cortesini R, Molajoni ER, Monari C, et al: Total lymphoid irradiation in clinical transplantation: Experience in 30 high-risk patients. Transplant Proc 17:1291, 1985
11. Devereux CK, Vidaver R, Hafstein MP, et al: Total lymphoid irradiation for multiple sclerosis. Int J Radiat Oncol Biol Phys 14:197, 1988
12. DuToit DF, Heydenrych JJ, Smit B, et al: Prolongation of segmental and pancreaticoduodenal allografts in the primate with total-lymphoid irradiation and cyclosporine. Transplantation 44:346, 1987
13. Engleman EG, Benike CJ, Hoppe RT, et al: Autologous mixed lymphocyte reaction in patients with Hodgkin's disease: Evidence for a T-cell defect. J Clin Invest 66:149, 1980
14. Field EH, Strobber S, Hoppe RT, et al: Sustained improvement of intractable rheumatoid arthritis after total lymphoid irradiation. Arthritis Rheum 26:937, 1983
15. Fradelizi D, Mahouy G, deRiberolles C, et al: Allograft tolerance in pigs after fractionated lymphoid irradiation. II. Kidney graft after conventional total lymphoid irradiation and bone marrow cell grafting. Transplantation 31:365, 1981
16. Fuks Z, Strober S, Bobrove AM, et al: Long term effects of radiation on T and B lymphocytes in peripheral blood of patients with Hodgkin's disease. J Clin Invest 58:803, 1976
17. Gottlieb M.: Personal communication
18. Gottlieb M, Strober S, Hoppe RT, et al: Engraftment of allogeneic bone marrow without graft-*versus*-host disease in mongrel dogs using total lymphoid irradiation. Transplantation 29:487, 1980
19. Haas G, Halperin E, Doseretz D, et al: Prolonging the immunosuppressive effects of lymphoid irradiation by suppression of T cell recovery prior to organ transplantation. Transplant Proc 17:1294, 1985
20. Hanley JG, Hassan J, Moriarty M, et al: Lymphoid irradiation in intractable rheumatoid arthritis. A double-blind, randomized study comparing 750-rad treatment with 2,000-rad treatment. Arthritis Rheum 29:16, 1986
21. Herbst M, Fritz H, Sauer R: Total lymphoid irradiation of intractable rheumatoid arthritis. Br J Radiol 59:1203, 1986
22. Hoogenhout J, Kazem I, Jerusalem CR, et al: Growth pattern of tumor xenografts in wistar rats after treatment with cyclophosphamide, total lymphoid irradiation and/or cyclosporin A. Int J Radiat Oncol Biol Phys 9:871, 1983
23. Hoppe RT, Dorie MJ: Successful murine tumor allotransplantation after total lymphoid irradiation. J Immunol 128:2387, 1982
24. Hoppe RT, Fuks Z, Strober S, et al: Long-term effects of radiation on T and B lymphocytes in the peripheral blood after regional irradiation. Cancer 40:2071, 1977
25. Howard RJ, Sutherland DER, Lum CT, et al: Kidney allograft survival in dogs treated with total lymphoid irradiation. Ann Surg 193:196, 1981
26. Hunt S, Strober S, Hoppe R, et al: Total lymphoid irradiation for therapy of intractable cardiac allograft rejection. J Heart Lung Transplant 10:211, 1991
27. Job G, Pfreundschuh M, Bauer M, et al: The influence of radiation therapy on T-lymphocyte subpopulations defined by monoclonal antibodies. Int J Radiat Oncol Biol Phys 10:2077, 1984
28. Kahn DR, Hong R, Greenberg AJ, et al: Total lymphatic irradiation and donor bone marrow for human heart transplantation. Transplantation Proc 13:215, 1981
29. Kaplan HS: Hodgkin's Disease, pp 366–441. Cambridge, MA, Harvard University Press, 1980
30. Knechtle SJ, Halperin EC, Bollinger RR: Xeongraft survival in two species combinations using total-lymphoid irradiation and cyclosporine. Transplantation 43:173, 1987
31. Kotzin BL, Strober S: Reversal of NZB/NZW disease with total lymphoid irradiation. J Exp Med 150:371, 1979
32. Kotzin BL, Strober S, Engleman EG, et al: Treatment of intractable rheumatoid arthritis with total lymphoid irradiation. N Engl J Med 305:969, 1981
33. Lowder JN, Miller RA, Hoppe R, et al: Suppression of anti-mouse immunoglobulin antibodies in subhuman primates receiving murine monoclonal antibodies against T cell antigens. J Immunol 138:401, 1987
34. Lowry RP, Forbes RDC, Carpenter CB, et al: Immune reactivity and immunosuppressive intervention in experimental nephritis. II. Effect of TLI on the course of two models of nephritis in the inbred rat. J Immunol 132: 1007, 1984
35. McCune WJ, Buckley JA, Belli JA, et al: Immunosuppression by fractionated total lymphoid irradiation in collagen arthritis. Arthritis Rheum 25:532, 1981
36. Modry DL, Strober S, Hoppe RT, et al: Total lymphoid irradiation: experimental models and clinical application in organ transplantation. Heart Transplant 2:122, 1983
37. Mullen Y, Shibukawa RL: Use of total lymphoid irradiation in transplantation of rat fetal pancreas. Diabetes 31(suppl 4):69, 1982
38. Myburgh JA, Smit JA, Meyers AM, et al: Total lymphoid irradiation in renal transplantation. World J Surg 10:369, 1986
39. Myburgh JA, Smit JA, Stark JH, et al: Total lymphoid irradiation in kidney and liver transplantation in the baboon: Prolonged graft survival and alterations in T cell subsets with low cumulative dose regimens. J Immunol 132:1019, 1984
40. Najarian JS, Ferguson RM, Sutherland DER, et al: Fractionated total lymphoid irradiation as preparative immunosuppression in high-risk renal transplantation: Clinical and immunological studies. Ann Surg 196:442, 1982
41. Pennock JL, Reitz BA, Bieber CP, et al: Survival of primates following orthotopic cardiac transplantation treated with total lymphoid irradiation and chemical immune suppression. Transplantation 32:467, 1981
42. Posner MR, Reinherz E, Lane H, et al: Circulating lymphocyte populations in Hodgkin's disease after mantle and paraaortic irradiation. Blood 61:705, 1983
43. Ramsay NK, Kim TH, McGlave P, et al: Total lymphoid irradiation and cyclophosphamide conditioning prior to bone marrow transplantation for patients with severe aplastic anemia. Blood 62:622, 1983
44. Rosenberg NL, Lacy JR, Kennaugh RC, et al: Treatment of refractory chronic demyelinating polyneuropathy with lymphoid irradiation. Muscle Nerve 8:223, 1985
45. Rotstein S, Blomgren H, Petrini B, et al: Long-term effects on the immune system following local radiation therapy for breast cancer. I. Cellular composition of the peripheral blood lymphocyte population. Int J Radiat Oncol Biol Phys I11:921, 1985
46. Sadeghi AM, Downing TP, Bieber CP, et al: Heterotopic cardiac allograft in rats: Prolonged survival with low-dose preoperative and postoperative total lymphoid irradiation combined with low-dose cyclosporin. Heart Transplant II:209, 1983
47. Sampson D, Levin BS, Hoppe RT, et al: Clinical observations of the use of total lymphoid irradiation in human cadaver renal transplantation. Transplant Proc 17:1299, 1985
48. Saper V, Chow D, Engleman Ed, et al: Clinical and immunological studies of cadaveric renal transplant recipients given total-lymphoid irradiation and maintained on low-dose prednisone. Transplantation 45:540, 1988
49. Schoeppel S, Hoppe RT, Engleman E, et al: Lymphocyte subsets in Hodgkin's disease (HD) patients (PTS) treated with

irradiation. Proceedings of the American Association of Cancer Research 27:329, 1986

50. Schurman DJ, Hirshman HP, Strober S: Total lymphoid and local joint irradiation in the treatment of adjuvant arthritis. Arthritis Rheum 24:38, 1981
51. Shank B, Bonfiglio P, Dinsmore R, et al: Immunosuppression for sensitized aplastic anemia patients: Comparison of TLI with TBI. Int J Radiat Oncol Biol Phys 10:174, 1984
52. Sherrer Y, Bloch D, Strober S, Fries J: Comparative toxicity of total lymphoid irradiation and immunosuppressive drug treated patients with intractable rheumatoid arthritis. J Rheumatol 14:46, 1987
53. Slavin S, Naprastek E, Weshler Z, et al: Bone marrow transplantation for severe aplastic anemia in HLA identical siblings using total lymphoid irradiation (TLI) and cyclophosphamide. Transplant Proc 15:668, 1983
54. Slavin S, Reitz B, Bieber CP, et al: Transplantation tolerance in adult rats using total lymphoid irradiation: Permanent survival of skin, heart, and marrow allografts. J Exp Med 147:700, 1978
55. Slavin S, Strober S, Fuks Z, et al: Long-term survival of skin allografts in mice treated with fractionated total lymphoid irradiation. Science 193:1252, 1976
56. Slavin S, Strober S, Fuks Z, et al: Induction of specific tissue transplantation tolerance using fractionated total lymphoid irradiation in adult mice: Long-term survival of allogeneic bone marrow and skin grafts. J Exp Med 146:34, 1977
57. Stjernsward J, Jondal M, Vanky F, et al: Lymphopenia and change in distribution of human B- and T-lymphocytes in peripheral blood induced by irradiation for mammary carcinoma. Lancet 1:1352, 1972
58. Strober S, Farinas MC, Field EH, et al: Treatment of lupus nephritis with total lymphoid irradiation. Observations during a 12–79 month follow-up. Arthritis Rheum 31:850, 1988
59. Strober S, Field E, Kotzin B, et al: Treatment of intractable lupus nephritis with total lymphoid irradiation. Ann Intern Med 102:450, 1985
60. Strober S, King DP, Gottlieb M, et al: Induction of transplantation tolerance after total lymphoid irradiation: Cellular mechanisms. Federation Proceedings 40:1463, 1981
61. Strober S, Modry DL, Hoppe RT, et al: Induction of specific unresponsiveness to heart allograft in mongrel dogs treated with total lymphoid irradiation and antithymocyte globulin. J Immunol 132:1013, 1984
62. Strober S, Tanay A, Field E, et al: Efficacy of total lymphoid irradiation in intractable rheumatoid arthritis. A double-blind, randomized trial. Ann Intern Med 102:441, 1985
63. Sutherland DER, Ferguson RM, Rynasiewicz JJ, et al: Total lymphoid irradiation versus cyclosporin for retransplantation in recipients at high risk to reject renal allografts. Transplant Proc 15:460, 1983
64. Tanay A, Field EH, Hoppe RT, et al: Long-term followup of rheumatoid arthritis patients treated with total lymphoid irradiation. Arthritis Rheum 30:1, 1987
65. Theophilopoulos AN, Balderas R, Shawler DL, et al: Inhibition of T cell proliferation and SLE-like syndrome of MRL/1 mice by whole body or total lymphoid irradiation. J Immunol 125:2137, 1980
66. Trentham DE, Belli JA, Anderson RJ, et al: Clinical and immunological effects of fractionated total lymphoid irradiation refractory rheumatoid arthritis. N Engl J Med 305:976, 1981
67. Troiano R, Cevereux C, Oleske J, et al: T cell subsets and disease progression after total lymphoid irradiation in chronic progressive multiple sclerosis. J Neurol Neurosurg Psychiatry 51:980, 1988
68. Vanrenterghem Y, Waer M, Ang KK, et al: Renal cadaveric transplantation after total lymphoid irradiation in patients with diabetes (TLI). Kidney Int 23(suppl 14):569, 1983
69. Waer M, Vanrenterghem Y, Ang KK, et al: Comparison of the immunosuppressive effect of fractionated total lymphoid irradiation (TLI) vs conventional immunosuppression (CI) in renal cadaveric allotransplantation. J Immunol 132:1041, 1984
70. Zan-Bar I, Slavin S, Strober S: Effect of total lymphoid irradiation (TLI) on the primary and secondary antibody response to sheep red blood cells. Cell Immunol 6:167, 1979
71. Zvaifler NJ: Fractionated total lymphoid irradiation: A promising new treatment for rheumatoid arthritis? Yes, no, maybe. Arthritis Rheum 30:109, 1987

76

Radiation Therapy in Palliative Cancer Management

A. Robert Kagan

The aim of palliative irradiation for incurable cancer is to improve the quality of life that remains; it may prolong life, but it should not be used to prolong death. The decision not to administer irradiation to an informed patient should not be censured; as Wangensteen stated, "The limitation of the method constitutes no reflection upon its user, save insofar as he fails to recognize it."

Many factors influence the decision to give palliative irradiation: survival time, severity and length of side-effects, potential hospitalization for treatment of complications, and possible benefit and cost. Other factors also prevent straightforward decisions. Psycho-oncologic radiation therapy may be demanded by the referring physician, the patient, or the patient's family. Second opinions are frequently sought by the patient with incurable disease. For every expert radiation oncologist, there are other experts who may render a contrary opinion.

CLINICAL ASSESSMENT

In the United States, most patients with metastases are referred for irradiation late in the course of the disease, when systemic therapy is failing. Besides the sites of serious metastases described for poor-risk patients, nonambulation, anemia, hypercalcemia, and four or more sites of metastases are poor prognostic signs that usually diminish the effectiveness of irradiation. The median survival of patients whose metastatic breast cancer is confined to the skeleton is 24 months; for estrogen receptor-negative patients, it is one third less. Median survival for patients with visceral site metastases is approximately 15 months after first relapse in the liver. Patients referred to the radiation oncologist who have three or more sites of metastasis or have failed hormonal therapy and second-line chemotherapy have a median survival of 6 months.[11,12,22,99] Symptomatic patients with cancer of the prostate in whom hormonal therapy has failed have a median survival of 4 to 8 months.[20] Patients with multiple myeloma have a median survival of 40 ± 10 months; if systemic therapy has failed, the median survival decreases to about 10 months.[50]

There are necessary steps in accepting a patient for palliative irradiation:

1. Establish a treatment goal. A patient with a solitary metastasis and a long recurrence interval (<5% of patients) may be treated with curative intent, but a patient with multiple metastases and a short recurrence interval should be treated with a short, palliative course of therapy.
2. Communicate the treatment goal. The treatment goal must be clearly communicated to the patient, family, and other members of the treatment team.
3. Determine that the metastasis is the cause of the symptoms. A patient with flank pain cannot be assumed to have T12 radiculopathy. Flank pain may be caused by liver, pleural, rib, or retroperitoneal metastasis. T12 disease should be evident on an imaging study before beginning treatment. Many of the symptoms of sciatica can arise from cord compression at the T10 to L1 level, from metastases to the lumbar vertebrae, or from metastases to the sacral or innominate bone regions.
4. Avoid radiation-induced sequelae. More than 90% of the patients treated for metastases die directly or indirectly of their cancer. Adding radiation side-effects to symptoms that may or may not be successfully palliated is poor management.
5. Consider the complexity of treatment. Palliative treatment techniques may be complicated. Blocking of overlapping portals over the spinal cord, retreatment of the brain, face, and eye, and prevention of lung irradiation are just a few of the problems. Complex palliative irradiation is best carried out in a department with modern machinery, competent technologic and physics personnel, and a physician properly trained in radiation oncology.
6. Consider the patient's condition. Desperately ill patients rarely improve with palliative irradiation, and providing it may drain the resources of the department without significant benefit to the patient.

DOSIMETRY

Although errors can occur in estimating dose, more frequently an overlap of adjacent fields leads to inadvertent retreatment and erroneous underestimation of the total dose administered, which may be the result of poor record keeping.

Overlap of adjacent fields may occur in the spine if several segments are sequentially irradiated (Fig. 76-1) or in the pelvis if a patient returns for treatment of the femoral head and acetabulum after earlier treatment for metastasis to the lumbosacral spine (Fig. 76-2). Irradiation to the spinal cord should never be overlapped. With the beam divergence on simulator films, the exact bottom and top of the spinal portal can only be estimated; simulator fields centered over the top and bottom of the field are accurate but are rarely obtained. Using a tape to measure from the coccyx to the portal center may help. If adjacent vertebral portals overlap, a 2-cm to 3-cm length of spinal cord must be blocked. A cord shield blocks most, but not all, of the transmission dose. The dose under the cord block is the summation of the transmission dose and the scattered dose. The scattered dose depends on the width of the cord block; more scattered dose exists with a 2-cm-wide block than with a 3-cm-wide block. We recommend a 3-cm shadow width and a length of 2 cm, because variations of positioning and setup occur, especially with patients who are in severe pain and have difficulty lying flat without movement.

Palliative irradiation of orbital metastases after irradiation of the cranium, or vice versa, creates overlap (Fig. 76-3). The use of photons with wedges or electrons (heterogenicity of bone absorption) for orbital irradiation can minimize but not eliminate this overlap. A common error about treating the face stems from a lack of appreciation of photon interaction at depth. For example, in the treatment of a patient with metastatic scalp nodules or with a history of skin cancer treated with 250 kVp, the brain may be unintentionally treated to tolerance levels after irradiation for brain metastasis. Retreatment of skin due to flash irradiation beyond the skin surface, especially after extensive chemotherapy, may produce severe dermatitis and necrosis.

Dosimetry errors can occur as a result of irregularly shaped fields, changing anteroposterior separation, or gaps. These areas, which are machine-specific, increase the dose above the central-axis dose at the periphery of long fields (25–30 cm); these isodose areas do not disappear at some depth. Depending on the length of the field and the depth of irradiation, a 5% to 12% increase in dose can occur. A change of 5 cm or more in the anteroposterior diameter of the treatment field can make a difference of 10% to 15% in the tumor dose that is greatest at the periphery of the field. The dose in the gap depends on the addition of adjacent field penumbras. The smaller the penumbra of the beam, the more critical is the position of the gap in ensuring dose homogeneity in routine treatment. Because they have a wider penumbra, the beams from ^{60}Co teletherapy machines may be less likely to produce cold and hot spots in the

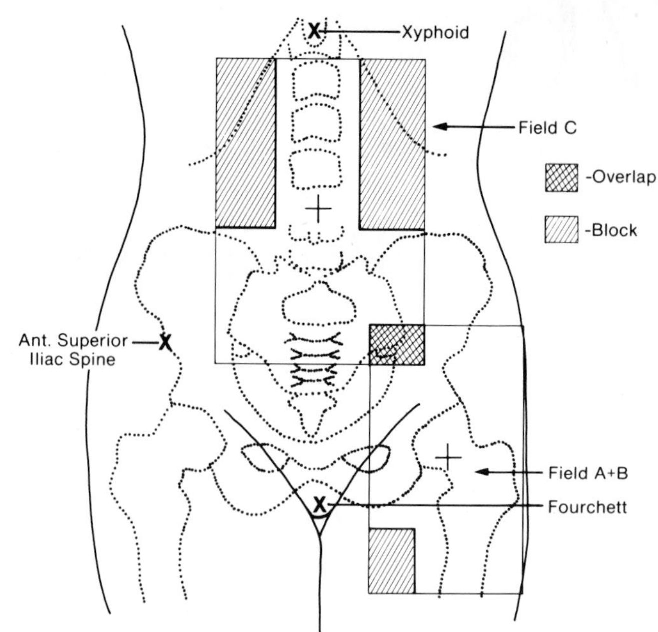

FIGURE 76–2. An unintentional overlap of a lumbosacral portal and an acetabular-femoral portal irradiated months apart, possibly overirradiating a segment of gut.

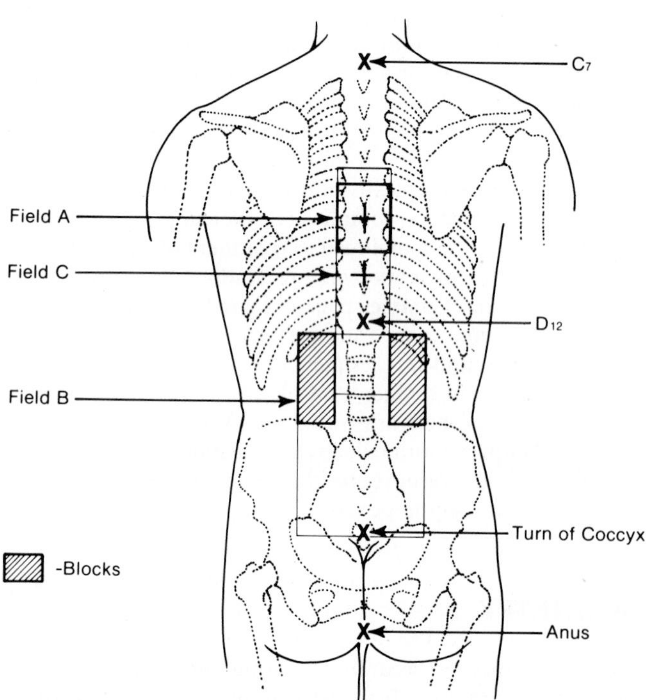

FIGURE 76–1. Multiple portals over the spine showing abutment of fields C and B and retreatment of the same vertebrae using fields A and C, possibly overdosing the spinal cord.

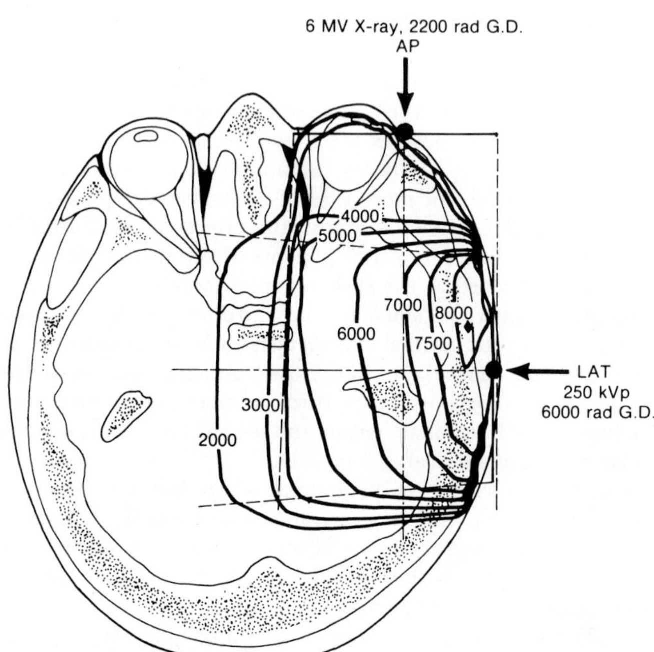

FIGURE 76–3. Irradiation of the skin and eye on two occasions may result in excess doses of over 6000 cGy to the brain.

gap. Gap calculations should be obtained for optimal results (Chap. 9).

PALLIATION OF ADVANCED REGIONAL CARCINOMA

Complete remission of large carcinomas is rare; despite intensive irradiation, the length and overall quality of the patient's life often are not substantially changed.

Large tumors need high radiation doses; however, we do not recommend large doses such as 5000 cGy in 4 weeks or 6000 cGy in 6 weeks for palliation because normal tissue injury may occur at these levels.[13] For a patient with an advanced primary carcinoma, we recommend a homogeneous dose of 2000 cGy in four or five fractions and evaluation of tumor response in 3 to 4 weeks, depending on the expected radiosensitivity of the tumor. If there is no response, poor radioresponsiveness is likely, and no further irradiation is indicated; if a complete or partial response occurs, the oncologist may add more irradiation or await possible regrowth and repeat the 2000 cGy in four or five fractions.

Lung Cancer

Most patients with advanced lung cancer have chronic obstructive pulmonary disease with airway obstruction, and some have forced expiratory volume of less than 1000 ml per second and arterial oxygen pressure (PaO_2) below 60 mm Hg. Small ($\leq$3 cm) endobronchial lesions causing atelectasis, pneumonia, or dyspnea can be successfully palliated for long-term control. However, large ($\geq$12 cm) hilar or combined extrabronchial-endobronchial lesions are poorly controlled. Palliative regimens of 4000 cGy to 4400 cGy at daily doses of 300 cGy to 400 cGy for 4 days weekly, with or without a planned interruption, deliver approximately 1500 to 1700 ret. A spinal cord block is used to ensure that only 1300 ret is delivered to the cord; a portal film should be used to verify accurate cord blocking. Intraluminal radiations are reported to be effective in doses from 1500 cGy in two fractions to 3000 cGy in four fractions.

Esophageal invasion leading to tracheoesophageal fistula after irradiation is a serious problem. Dysphagia can be caused by compression or invasion, which can be successfully palliated if the carcinomatous mass is radioresponsive.

Hemoptysis in a patient with pulmonary carcinoma is common; it often decreases in 72 hours and resolves in 1 week after irradiation. Bleeding may persist in a patient with a bleeding disorder (*e.g.*, alcoholic patient with severe liver disease). Irradiation is indicated for persistent hemoptysis.

Many patients with cancer of the lung have chest pain. Successful palliation depends on the cause. Bone and pleural pain improve if included in the portal, but intercostal nerve or brachial plexus involvement is rarely resolved, although partial improvement may occur. Volumes should be restricted to 100 cm^2 to 150 cm^2.

Esophageal Obstruction

Malignant esophageal obstruction is rarely caused by anything other than esophageal carcinoma, although cancer of the lung may cause esophageal compression.[60] Metastatic carcinomas, such as cancer of the breast, to the mediastinal lymph nodes may cause dysphagia.[32] Radiation therapy can give temporary relief, but the obstructive symptoms usually recur if the patient lives longer than 6 months; 1200 cGy intraluminal radiation, at 1 cm, or external-beam irradiation is equally effective.[25,51] Endoscopic laser therapy is a practical alternative to maintain patency or to allow placement of an intraluminal prosthesis. Esophageal tubes should be considered only in the most debilitated patients.[41,59] The radiation oncologist must realize that blockage of an esophageal tube by food or migration of the tube, which occurs frequently and may happen during irradiation, can cause symptoms simulating growing carcinoma. The use of tubes is not suitable for high esophageal lesions. Gastrostomy for feeding purposes does not prevent the morbidity of aspiration.

Urinary Hemorrhage or Obstruction

Advanced cancer causing urinary hemorrhage or obstruction is most commonly a postoperative recurrence of adenocarcinoma of the rectum, recurrent bladder carcinomas, or recurrent hormone-resistant cancers of the prostate or cervix. Surgery, irradiation, or chemotherapy is not recommended for the terminally ill patient.[101] Stents can be advanced through an obstructed ureter, beginning at the ureterovesical orifice (retrograde) or at the dilated renal pelvis (antegrade), and can remain during the patient's life. A nephrostomy is not desirable, because the external appliances complicate the life of a patient who will soon die of the cancer, often never leaving the hospital. Indwelling urethral catheters and suprapubic catheter drainage by way of cystostomy can decompress the lower urinary tract. An attempt to irradiate to relieve acute obstruction is not recommended. The value of this type of irradiation for further palliation, beyond the relief of obstruction provided by an indwelling tube, has not been established. After the obstruction is mechanically corrected, irradiation should be given only if the area has not been previously irradiated and local symptoms warrant it.

Repeat irradiation should be undertaken with a great deal of caution. In low-irradiated patients, doses of 5000 cGy in 25 fractions or 2000 cGy in five fractions, with reevaluation in 3 to 4 weeks for assessment of response and administration of additional 2000 cGy in five fractions, or 4000 cGy in 15 fractions are methods of temporizing until extensive metastases occur. The use of large (400 cGy) or small (200 cGy) daily fractions depends on the amount of bowel included in the treatment portal (field size). After abdominoperineal resection, 60% of the small bowel may be included in a pelvic portal extending to the S1 vertebra. Large daily fractions should be confined to portals smaller than 15 cm × 15 cm.[92]

Pelvic Pain

Pelvic pain caused by malignant disease, including pain from sciatica, is caused by pelvic bone or lumbosacral neuroplexus involvement.[2] For treatment, a mass must be defined by bone scan, plain radiography, or computed tomography (CT) scan; however, posterior root ganglia and peripheral nerves may be affected by diffuse dural tumor infiltration that cannot be localized by imaging studies. Rarely, pelvic pain can also be caused by carcinomatous spinal meningitis, by spinal cord compression, and by vertebral metastasis, especially in carcinoma of the prostate or breast.

In patients with cancer of the rectum, particularly after abdominoperineal resection, vaginal or CT examination may reveal a presacral mass. Patients with "neuritic" pain after cystectomy (cystectoprostatovesiculectomy) may have a paravaginal mass or a mass in the region of the prostate. In patients with cancer of the cervix who have leg edema, hydronephrosis, and back pain, "sciatic" pain or "obturator" pain is often associated with advanced or recurrent pelvic disease. Symptoms and signs are rarely caused by benign disease or postirradiation fibrosis.[26]

In our experience, pelvic pain can be helped by irradiation if the area causing the pain is well defined. A patient referred for pelvic pain in whom all the appropriate imaging studies yield negative results should be followed, and the physical examination or imaging studies should be repeated if clinically warranted. Treatment through a portal directed to the pelvis is an alternative. Marked pain relief may be achieved with only minor shrinkage of the pelvic mass. Substantial relief of pain from osteolytic defects in the pelvic bones or vertebrae occurs despite absence of recalcification.[27] Total and daily doses depend on the field size and amount of fixed bowel or history of bowel disease, such as diverticulitis, predisposing to radiation injury. For pelvic masses, most of our patients have received 3000 cGy in ten fractions, four times weekly; 4000 cGy in ten fractions delivered in two courses of five fractions given 3 weeks apart or 2000 cGy in four or five fractions weekly may be used for portals up to 144 cm^2. Very large fractions, 700 cGy to 1000 cGy single daily doses, should be avoided, because of increased morbidity. Meoz and associates[64] reported five (17%) of 30 patients receiving three fractions of 1000 cGy each delivered every 2 to 3 weeks. Bowel obstruction or perforation occurred in four patients. An update of this approach was reported by Spanos and coworkers[92] for 46 patients. Four (11%) patients with grade 3 disease and seven (19%) with grade 4 disease had gastrointestinal toxic effects, particularly late small bowel injury. However, recently the Radiation Therapy Oncology Group (RTOG) published a report of 142 patients with advanced pelvic malignancy who received twice-daily high-fractionation palliative irradiation (370 cGy twice daily on two consecutive days, repeated 2 to 3 times every 3 to 6 weeks for total doses of 2960 cGy to 4440 cGy).[91] The major and moderate complication rate was only 1.4% (two of 142 patients).

Opposed portals are used most often; multiple portals should be considered if the anteroposterior diameter is greater than 22 cm and photons of higher energy (10 MV) are unavailable. A three-field technique or double arc, 120-degree rotation can be used for presacral masses with bladder and some bowel sparing. Meticulous care must be given to the perineum, including the vulva or scrotum because severe radiation epidermitis may occur.

PALLIATION OF METASTATIC DISEASE

Supraclavicular Nodal Recurrence or Metastasis

Supraclavicular lymph node recurrences are relatively frequent findings in patients with advanced or recurrent tumors of the breast, lung, occasionally the head and neck, or abdominal or pelvic viscera, such as the colon, uterus, bladder, or prostate. Frequently these lymph nodes are treated electively because it is more difficult to control the disease, even for palliation, as they enlarge. If the supraclavicular region is the first site of recurrent disease or distant metastasis, an incisional biopsy should be carried out to confirm the clinical suspicion. In general an anteroposterior oblique field, with the patient in a supine position, the head turned to the opposite side of the lymphadenectomy, is irradiated; this area extends from the upper neck to the subclavicular region. If possible, the spinal cord should be excluded from the irradiated volume, with lateral angulation of the beam (10–15 degrees). Doses of approximately 4500 cGy to 5000 cGy in 4 weeks to 6000 cGy in 6 weeks should be delivered, calculated at a depth of 3 cm to 4 cm. If the patient has advanced disease and the expectation of survival is short, a dose of 4000 cGy in 3 weeks may be adequate for transient palliation. When doses over 5000 cGy are delivered, the last 1000 cGy should be done with reduced portals (boost).

Brachial plexopathy secondary to irradiation or carcinomatous lymphadenopathy can occur in the supraclavicular area.[1,37] A distinct mass, which sometimes can be appreciated only by CT scan, usually indicates recurrence, but severe skin changes implicate radiation injury as a cause of painful neuropathy.[75] Doses biologically greater than 7000 cGy in 6 weeks, usually resulting from overlap of irradiation portals, suggest radiation injury. Occasionally, vertebral metastasis, epidural compression, or a second primary occurrence of Pancoast tumor may be the cause. Surgical exploration of the supraclavicular region has been recommended for diagnosis; however, cancer extant at exploration may be missed, and severe healing difficulties can occur if the exploration has been through a heavily irradiated site.

Metastasis to Orbital Region

Cancer of the breast can metastasize to the retroorbital tissues, but a retroorbital metastasis is more often part of the metastatic process involving the cranial bones. The signs are usually painful proptosis and diplopia; visual acuity may remain intact or be impaired because of retinal detachment. Enophthalmos has been reported.[78]

In solitary metastasis to the orbital region, other conditions should be eliminated. Hyperthyroidism, meningioma, or pseudotumor of the orbit can also occur in the patient who has a history of breast cancer or lymphoma. Orbital fine-needle aspiration and immunocytologic preparation are recommended if the diagnosis is disputed.

If the projected survival of the patient warrants it (>2 years), the radiation therapist should consider designing treatment portals so that the lens receives only a portion of the dose, although sometimes this cannot be done without diminishing the dose to the tumor.[17,29,31] If the orbital metastasis is solitary or the recurrence-free interval is greater than 3 years, a dose higher than 3000 cGy given over an interval greater than 2 weeks may be indicated. Right-angled wedges, a direct anterior or lateral portal, and even the type of energy used in irradiation have advantages and disadvantages.

The base of the skull must be evaluated carefully for associated lesions. If warranted, irradiation should also be directed to the base of the skull.

Although at least one third of the patients have bilateral involvement, most investigators have treated only the affected eye. Response is marked improvement in vision in one third of these patients, some improvement in another third, and a poor response in the remainder.

Liver Metastasis

Selected patients irradiated for liver metastasis have a median survival of 4 months.[42,49] Our patients have reported pain relief, but we have not been impressed with decrease in liver size. Liebel[57] reported 187 evaluable patients treated with 2000 cGy in seven fractions in a randomized RTOG study to test misonidazole as a radiation sensitizer. The median survival was 4.2 months with a response rate of 80%. CT scan assessment of 164 patients demonstrated a complete response in one patient. Radiation-induced hepatitis was not observed. Although 2800 cGy to 3000 cGy in 200-cGy fractions to the entire liver may be well tolerated, we have observed radiation hepatitis at lower doses after chemotherapy with mechlorethamine, vincristine, procarbazine, prednisone, and 5-fluorouracil. Localized portions of the liver can be treated to higher doses. Oblique portals may be helpful.[79]

The exact role of liver irradiation in the management of liver metastasis remains undefined. Important responses are subjective, but treatment should be based on objective responses.[56,57,71,103]

Intraluminal irradiation of the bile duct for extrahepatic obstruction has been used. Malignant portal lymphadenopathy is usually larger than 2 cm, and the bypass tube is left in place, making evaluation of this method difficult.[6] Jaundice is most often due to diffuse hepatic malignancy rather than focal extrahepatic lymphadenopathy.

Brain Metastasis

Most metastases to the brain are supratentorial and multiple.[7] Differential diagnosis includes abscess, meningoma, demyelinating disease, and infarction and intracerebral hematoma, most commonly in the elderly, detectable by magnetic resonance imaging (MRI).[18,23,86] It is prudent to have a positive imaging study, because paraneoplastic syndromes occur.[35] Estimates of median overall survival of 3 to 5 months have not changed in 10 years.[4] At least half of treated patients die of intracranial metastases.

We have found the following functional scale valuable in predicting prognosis in such patients:

Level I: fully functional; able to work
Level II: fully functional; not able to work
Level III: stays in bed; needs help half the time
Level IV: requires help all the time

Patients with level I function have a median survival of 26.9 weeks; in level IV patients, it is only 4.6 weeks. Corticosteroids are recommended to improve neurologic function, but neither survival nor length of response is affected.

Occasionally, metastasis to the cerebellum with severe ataxia or a large single metastasis in the cerebral hemisphere can best be palliated by removal; the most favorable factor is a disease-free survival greater than 1 year.[21] Most reports of an operative removal of solitary metastatic lesion to the brain cover 20 years.[15,36,62,72] Prognostic factors in this subset are of questionable value because of "superselectivity."[87,90] Nonetheless, irradiation is needed after craniotomy because local recurrence is double when only an operative procedure is performed. The median survival increases from 6 to 12 months in patients who receive postoperative irradiation to the skull with doses equivalent to 4000 cGy in 20 fractions.[63,70,90] Five-year survival has been reported even in patients with solitary cerebral metastasis from cancer of the lung.[84]

Sheline and Brady[88] summarized the dose-time associations, emphasizing the RTOG data; 2000 cGy in 1 week or 3000 cGy in 2 weeks is as effective for palliation as any other dose-time regimen.[16,19,53,55] However, RTOG conducted two randomized studies comparing several fractionation schedules and total doses of irradiation for the palliative treatment of brain metastasis (Fig. 76-4).[9] Improvement in neurologic function, duration of improvement, time to progression, and survival were the same in the various treatment groups. There was significant relief of symptoms such as headache, motor loss, and impaired mentation.[9] We have encountered significant neurologic morbidity, despite use of steroids and analgesics, in patients given large fractions of 750 cGy and 1000 cGy. Data supporting 5000 cGy in 25 fractions for brain metastases are suspect because of patient selection. Multiple daily fractionation and reirradiation are not helpful.[28,47]

Biologic doses greater than 2000 cGy in 1 week may be considered for testicular carcinoma or choriocarcinoma because patients with these diseases may be cured.[58,100] Rustin and associates have questioned the necessity of brain irradiation for choriocarcinoma.[81]

Opposed fields from the supraorbital ridge to the mastoid can easily be applied to a cooperative patient. However, if the lesion is in the inferior portion of the frontal or temporal lobe, the portal must descend from the infraorbital ridge to the external auditory meatus (Fig. 76-5). A lens block or a fixed shield may be considered in this instance. Patients who respond to 2000 cGy in four or five fractions or 3000 cGy in ten to 12 fractions and have a recurrence can be treated again with similar doses.

Bone Metastasis

An ambulatory patient who has localized pain, a positive imaging study compatible with metastasis, fewer than four sites of metastasis without serious sites (metastasis to nervous system, lymphangitic metastasis to lung, and rapidly advancing liver metastasis), and no hypercalcemia is an excellent candidate for

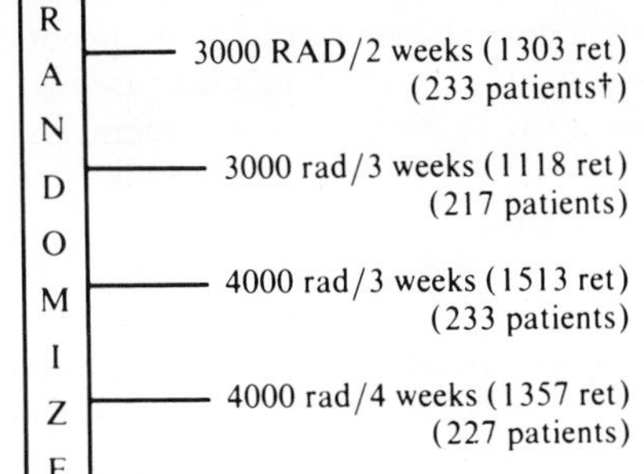

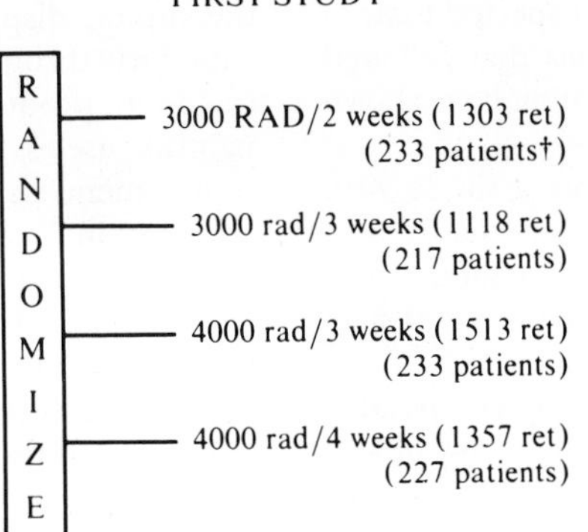

FIGURE 76–4. Radiation Therapy Oncology Group brain metastases protocol. (Borgelt B, Gelber R, Kramer S, et al: Int J Radiat Oncol Biol Phys 6:2, 1980)

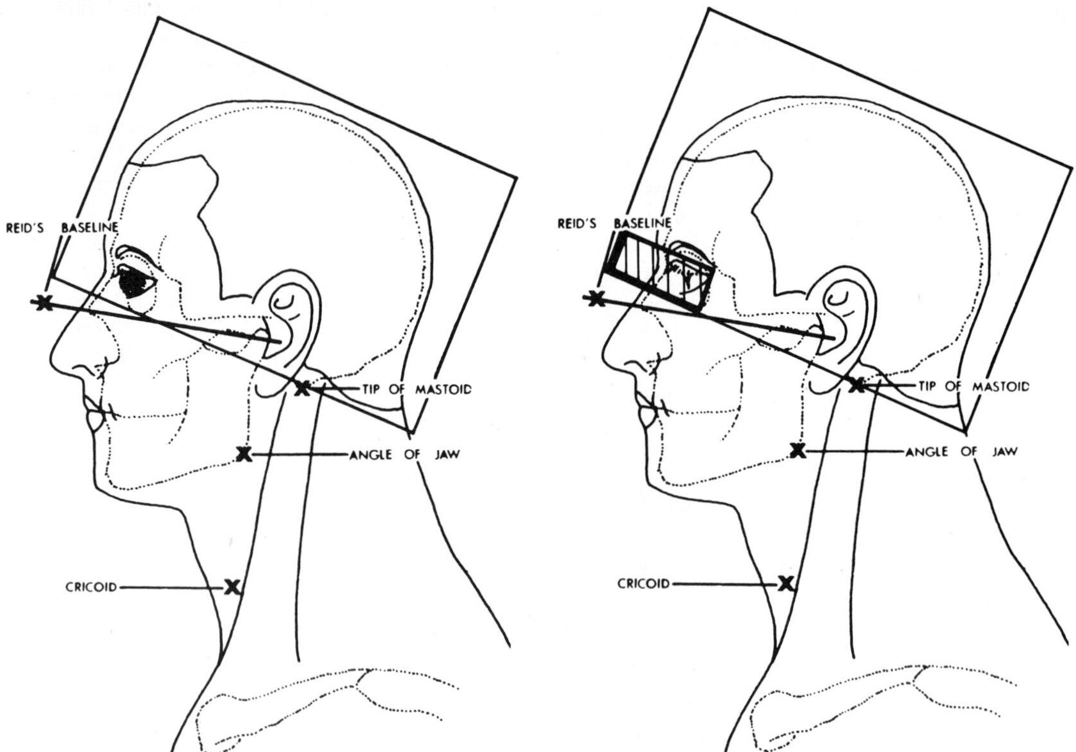

FIGURE 76–5. Metastases in inferior aspects of the temporal and frontal lobes require that the inferior border of the portal be at the line drawn from the inferior orbital ridge to the mastoid tip. A lens or orbital block should be used.

successful long-term palliation. The signs and symptoms of bony metastasis should correlate with an imaging study; if not, follow-up in 1 to 2 weeks, and not irradiation, is recommended. Not all patients in pain and with a history of cancer have metastases; almost one third may have benign disease.[33,48,68,77,96,97] We recommend percutaneous needle biopsy for a first occurrence of metastasis if it is associated with equivocal imaging study findings or is a solitary recurrence suspected after a disease-free interval of more than 2 years.[65] Needle biopsy may be especially helpful in determining cancer regrowth or necrosis in an area that has already been irradiated. Osteoradionecrosis of the femoral head, which may be the result of steroid use, may simulate metastasis.

Half-body irradiation, in a single or fractionated dose, has been reported.[80] Upper hemibody irradiation (skull to L4), lower hemibody irradiation, and mid-hemibody irradiation (diaphragm to obdurator foramen) are being evaluated in the treatment of occult and overt metastasis, and doses above 800 cGy (no lung correction) have been associated with an increase in pneumonitis. The doses for patients with myeloma have been reduced to 300 cGy because of previously unsuspected toxicity to the bone marrow at 600 cGy. Most studies that followed multidrug chemotherapy by hemibody irradiation have shown significant toxic effects.

Although hemibody irradiation takes only a single visit, premedication is mandatory. The side-effects necessitate overnight hospitalization or a recovery room in the radiation therapy department. So far, it appears that the incidence of pain relief is similar to that seen with localized radiations.[83,98]

In the asymptomatic patient, we don't recommend irradiation if there is a positive bone scan, except in the case of suspected metastasis in the weight-bearing bones, such as the femoral neck-trochanteric region and humerus.

If pain increases during irradiation, the physician must be alert to the progress of the irradiated lesion, to the growth of lesions outside the field of irradiation, or to development of a pathologic fracture. If half of the combined measured cortex is missing on lateral and anteroposterior views, the probability of fracture is high.[82] Even without severe cortical destruction, patients with painful lesions larger than 3 cm in a long bone should be given a sling, splints, casts, crutches, brace, or wheelchair to limit weight-bearing activities.[30,73] In our experience, osteolytic lesions of metastatic carcinomas that are negative on bone scan but positive on radiograph are prone to fracture.

After a pathologic fracture occurs, internal fixation is necessary to immobilize the bone, decrease pain, and accelerate healing and ambulation of the patient. Monitoring a lytic lesion after irradiation is difficult. After irradiation, femoral lesions must be followed every 3 months. Pain should be relieved, and the lytic lesions should not grow (Fig. 76-6). Any lesion affecting the superomedial aspect of the acetabulum, however, is especially serious, because this area transmits the patient's weight to the head of the femur. Even if irradiation completely destroys the tumor, displacement of the femoral head medially and superiorly through weakened bone and irradiated tumor tissue can occur, producing a migration of the femur and an unstable, painful, useless hip.[39] Surgical intervention, most often hip replacement, has an immediate palliative effect.

Hoskin[46] reviewed 16 nonrandomized and three randomized studies of localized radiation therapy for bone pain. He concluded that there is no dose effect, that single or multiple fractions produce identical effects, and that generally 70% of patients have relief of bone pain at the irradiated site by 3 months.[74] Of those patients alive at the end of 1 year, half still have relief of pain at the irradiated site. Response rates are lower and of shorter duration in patients with cancer of the lung.[5]

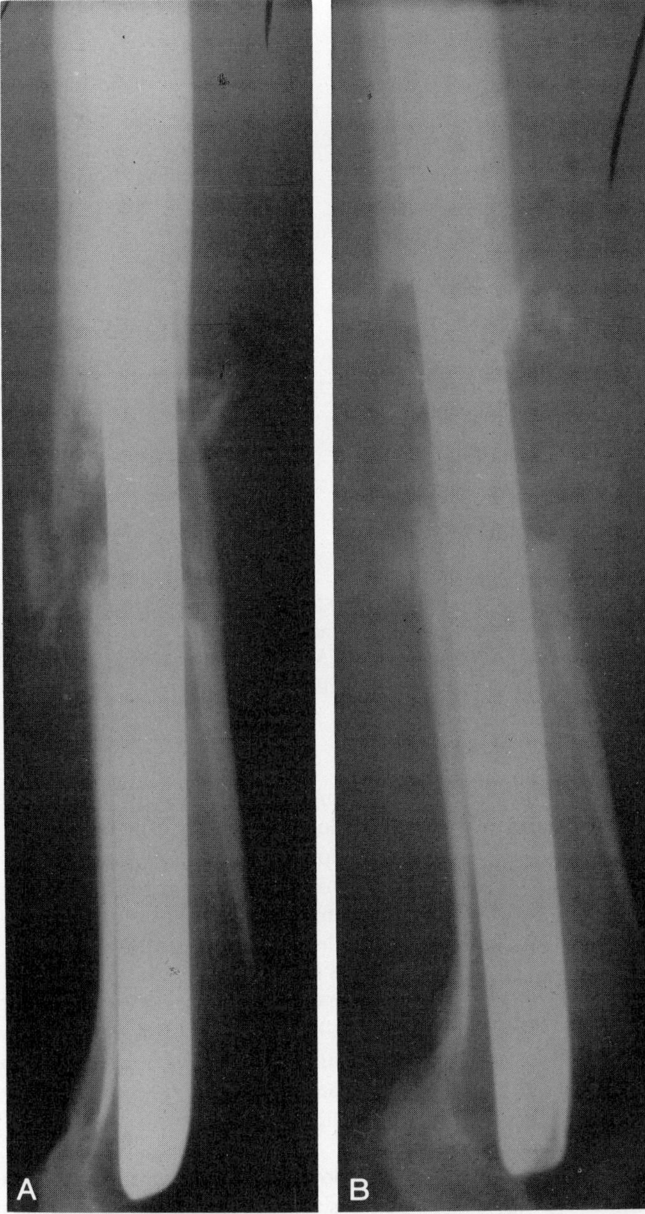

FIGURE 76–6. (**A**) X-ray film shows a metastatic lesion from an undetermined primary tumor in a 40-year-old male smoker treated by intramedullary rod and irradiation. (**B**) X-ray film of the same patient referred 6 months later for irradiation of a hilar mass causing vocal cord paralysis. The progressive lesion indicates a poorly responsive tumor.

Doses of 800 cGy in one fraction, 2000 cGy in five fractions, and 3000 cGy in ten fractions give equal response rates. RTOG carried out a randomized study on 1016 patients with symptomatic osseous metastasis (266 solitary, 750 multiple), who were treated with different doses of irradiation (Fig. 76-7). Fifty-four percent of the patients achieved complete relief, and 83% had partial relief of pain. There was no significant difference in pain relief with the various schedules.[95] Reanalysis of the RTOG study on palliation of symptomatic osseous metastasis demonstrated that the patients receiving 3000 cGy in ten fractions or 4000 cGy in 15 fractions had a higher percentage of complete relief compared with patients receiving lower doses (Fig. 76-8).[8] Patients whose life expectancy is predicted to exceed 1 year should be considered for larger doses at lower daily doses, such as 4000 cGy to 5000 cGy in 20 to 25 fractions. The entire bone

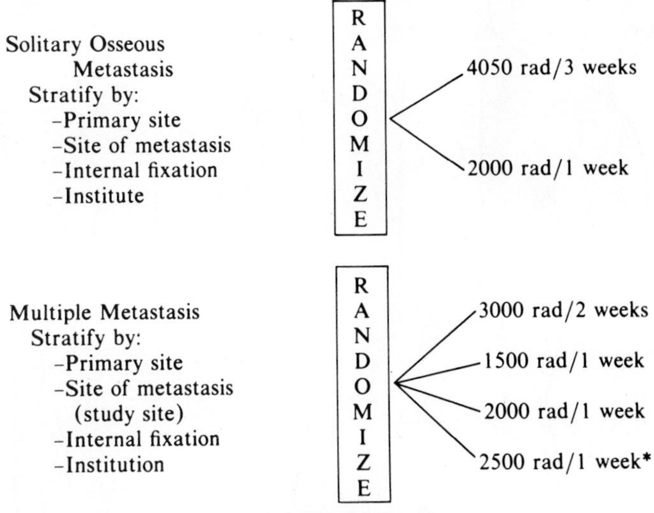

FIGURE 76–7. Radiation Therapy Oncology Group bone metastases protocol. *When spinal cord is in field: 2000 rad = 1 week. (Tong C, Gillick L, Hendrickson FR: Cancer 50:894, 1982)

harboring the metastasis should be treated, even if the defect appears localized (Figs. 76-9 and 76-10).

Patients who have had a prosthetic device inserted with methylmethacrylate ("hyperthermic" bone cement) often have tumor that invades the soft tissues, indicating the need for postoperative irradiation. Even with supervoltage radiation, most metal rods reduce the transmitted dose from a homolateral portal by 5% to 20%.

Metastases (or myeloma) to the pituitary or the sphenoid sinus may be successfully treated by irradiation. Usually the entire calvaria, or at least the base of skull, should be included in the portal.

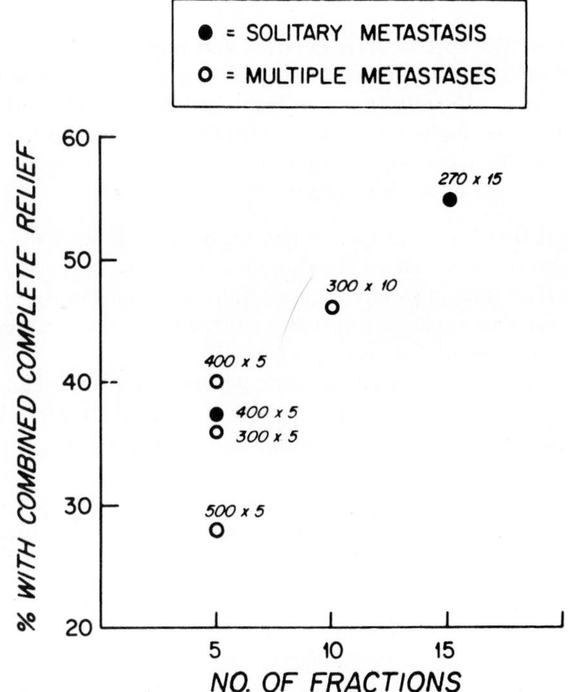

FIGURE 76–8. Radiation Therapy Oncology Group reevaluation of bone metastases protocol results. (Blitzer PH: Cancer 55:1470, 1985)

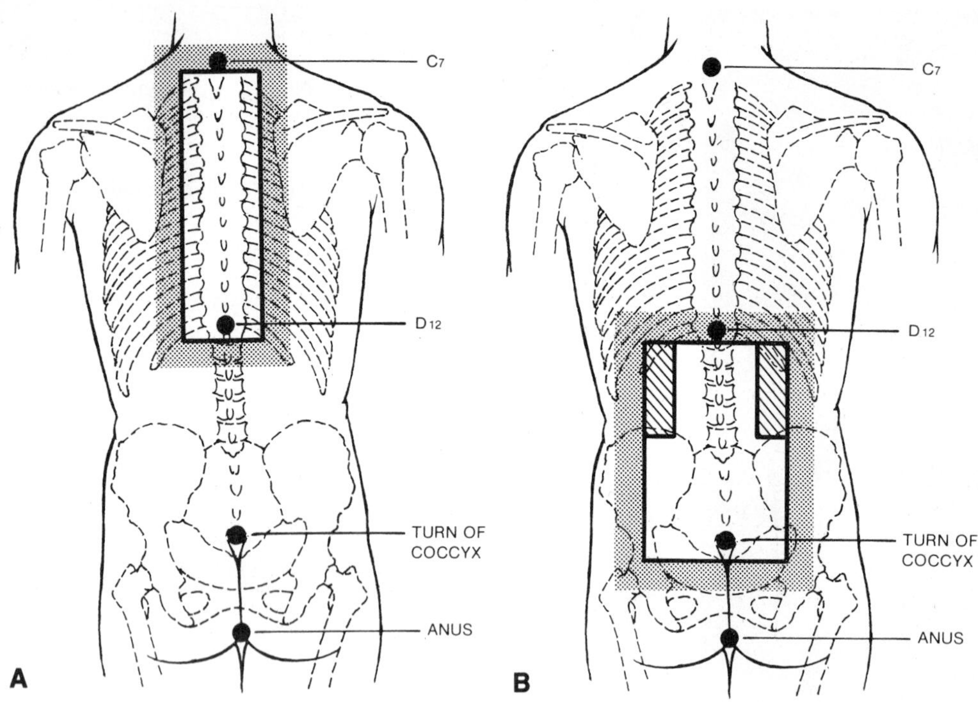

FIGURE 76–9. Examples of portals used to treat bone metastases in (**A**) the thoracic or (**B**) lumbosacral spine.

Harbert[38] suggested radionuclide therapy in patients resistant to other means of management. Although ^{32}P-orthophosphate has been used, he suggests ^{89}Sr ($SrCl_2$) as a better isotope because of less myelosuppression but warns that the dose and dosimetry of ^{89}Sr are more uncertain.[54]

Radioiodine therapy of metastatic differentiated carcinoma is effective; nevertheless, we advocate external irradiation for bone metastasis.

Cord Compression from Metastasis to the Epidural Space

Despite widespread bony deposits and even partial vertebral collapse, cord compression is rare, but when it occurs, it may become catastrophic. Because many patients are referred by a medical oncologist, it is important for the radiation oncologist to have a plan for management that includes neurosurgical consultation for these situations:

1. If there is no history of cancer, because about half of all cord compressions are due to nonmalignant causes
2. If an imaging study suggests bony fragments in the spinal canal or a collapsed vertebra (anterior resection and reconstruction of the vertebrae)
3. If previous lesions in the patient have demonstrated limited radioresponsiveness or the type of lesion is known to have limited radioresponsiveness, such as kidney and colon tumors or melanoma
4. If there is not a vertebral metastasis at the level of the cord block, with the exception of cases of known lymphoma, neuroblastoma, and leukemia

Epidural compression of the spinal cord is most commonly caused by a vertebral metastasis breaking through the posterior bony spinal canal and invading the epidural space. If a posterior laminectomy is done, tumor resection anterior to the cord is minimal.[3] Unless the tumor is posterior, irradiation, not laminectomy, determines ultimate outcome.

Clinically, cord compression can be divided into two types. In the first, sensory radiculopathy precedes weakness by months. In this situation, an epidural mass slowly compresses the cord, and use of steroids gives the radiation oncologist time to deliver a course of irradiation and the cancer time to regress. In the second and unfavorable scenario, sensory and motor dysfunction occur quickly, and the patient presents with paraplegia or, despite the ability to contract muscles, cannot move against gravity. Paraplegia usually means cord infarction and is irreversible. Sometimes in an unclear situation, raising the steroid dose from 16 mg of dexamethasone to 64 mg or higher decreases the neurologic deficit, ruling out the suspected diagnosis of cord infarction.

Knowing that the neurologic deficit has improved with steroid therapy assists the physician to select the patient who is most likely to benefit from irradiation, providing the tumor is radioresponsive.[50]

Although cord compression is generally a preterminal event, with most patients dying within 3 to 6 months, longer-term survival does occur.[40,66] In many patients, there is abundant warning of pending cord compression; the median duration of the first and second signs is in weeks. Patients who have marked vertebral tenderness or sensory radiculopathy should be suspected of having early cord compression and considered for urgent (not emergency) irradiation after MRI or CT scans. MRI can demonstrate the entire spinal cord, but the CT scan must be directed to a smaller vertebral region to be practical. The ease of obtaining and performing these two relatively new imaging studies, compared with myelography, should translate into earlier diagnosis (Fig. 76-11).[85]

In a review of patients treated for malignant cord compression from 1960 to 1980, Findlay[24] concluded that irradiation and steroid therapy were as effective as surgery with or without irradiation. In a recent series managed mostly by radiation and steroid therapy, 30% of presenting patients were ambulatory and 50% of patients were ambulatory until death, emphasizing earlier diagnosis, less use of surgery, and overall better palliation.[102]

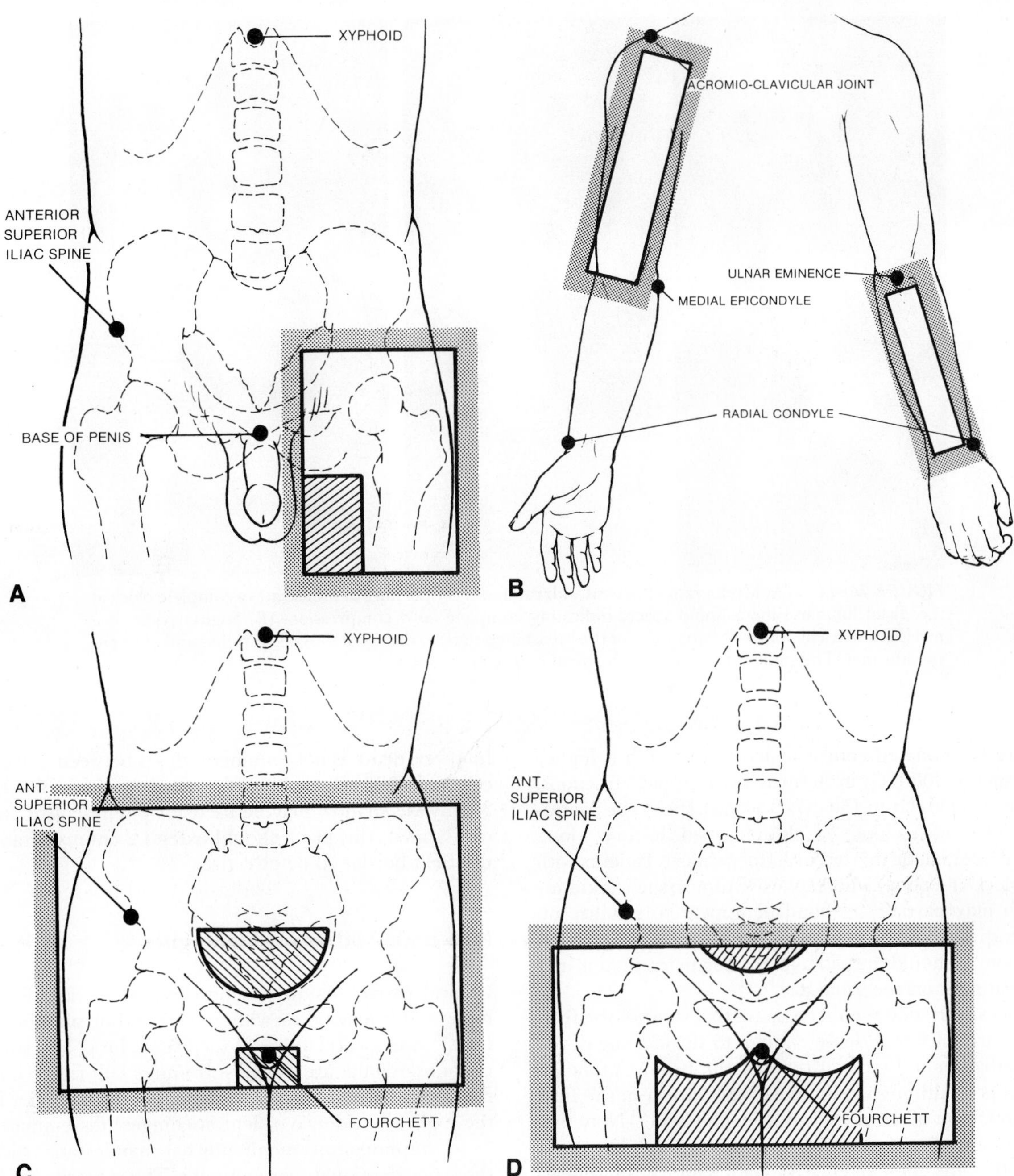

FIGURE 76–10. Typical portals for palliation of bone metastases.

We do not routinely request a myelogram from above and below to outline the epidural deposit; however, there are probably other epidural metastases, especially if the block is complete. Although much notoriety has been given to pedicle erosion, over 80% of metastatic tumors to the epidural space come from the adjacent vertebral body. The major exceptions are lymphomas and neuroblastomas, which gain access to the epidural space from a paraspinal soft tissue mass (replaced lymph node). Doses of 2000 cGy in four to five fractions are effective.[50,76] Patients are maintained on steroids, and dose tapering occurs 2 weeks after the completion of irradiation. The tumor dose is usually taken at 5 cm to 6 cm. However, lateral simulation roentgenograms may show that the lower lumbar vertebra (cauda equina) may be as deep as 8 cm to 10 cm or that the spinal canal in children is closer to the surface. The tumor volume should include the affected vertebra.

Photons are more suitable to irradiate the spinal canal and the vertebrae. The choice of electrons must be made very carefully; for example, in a neck with an anteroposterior diameter of 9 cm after laminectomy, using 20-MeV electrons, the cord will receive 95% and the minimal tumor dose to the vertebrae will be 80%. However, with intact spinous processes, the minimal tumor dose to the vertebrae will be 50%; and if the anteroposterior diameter of the neck is larger than 9 cm, the minimal dose to the vertebrae will be 0%. ^{60}Co or 6 MV will give approximately 85% to the spinal canal and a minimal vertebral dose of 70%. With photons, attention to the lung dose in the thorax is important, especially with a wide posterior portal or two oblique portals. If there is an associated paraspinous mass, the portal size must be enlarged over the common 8-cm-wide portal size; and if the mass extends anteriorly, the tumor depth will be greater than the anterior surface of the vertebral body.

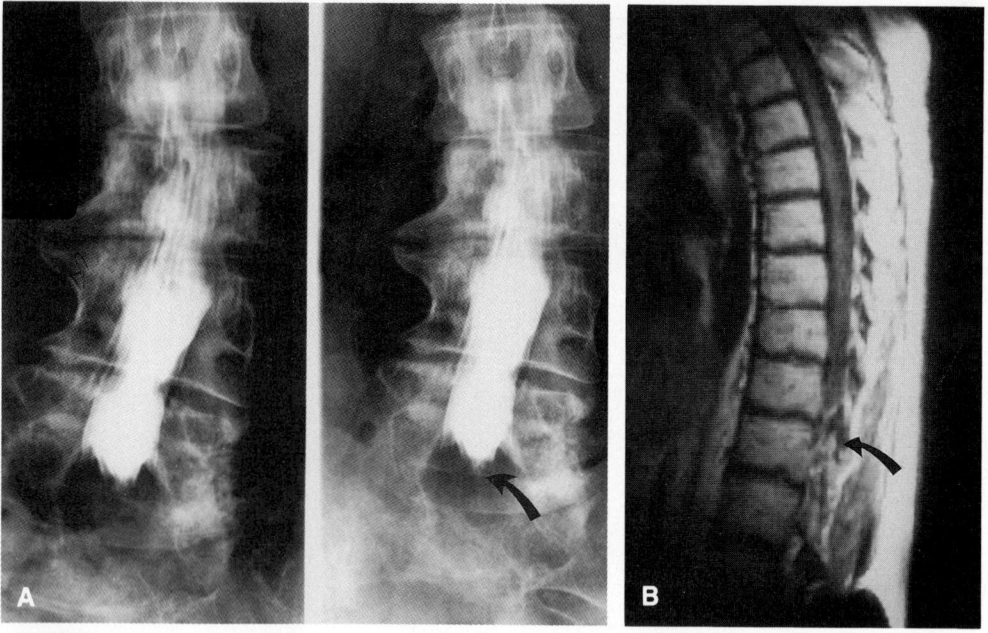

FIGURE 76–11. (**A**) Myelogram of patient with carcinoma of the lung demonstrates a complete block at the distal lumbar subarachnoid space, indicating complete cord compression. (**B**) Sagittal view of a myelogram in a patient with carcinoma of the breast metastatic to the distal thoracic vertebra and adjacent spinal canal. The patient presented with spinal cord compression.

A more fractionated course of irradiation with a higher total dose, such as 4000 cGy in 20 fractions, 5000 in 25 fractions, or 5500 cGy to 6000 cGy in 150-cGy fractions, should be considered in a patient with a long, "stable" metastatic history, a long disease-free interval, or thyroid or kidney cancer. Patients with complete block or a poor radioresponsive tumor, such as kidney lesion, who may partially respond or appear to stabilize on steroid therapy, should be monitored carefully for progression on irradiation, as should the patients who began irradiation and steroids treatment on the same day.[93,94]

Postoperatively, one should be aware that some of the fixation devices are thick and dense enough to shield some of the photon irradiation and most of the electron beam irradiation from the tumor. Although recurrences can appear in the field of irradiation, most of them occur outside the field.[61] Nonetheless, retreatment of a portion of the spinal cord may become a problem at the time of recurrence. If death is imminent, repeating 2000 cGy in four or five fractions can be recommended, because radiation myelitis takes about 5 months to begin. If, however, death is not imminent, doses between 150 cGy to 170 cGy and 3600 cGy to 4000 cGy may be given. A block casting a 3-cm-wide shadow may be used for a segment of cord that is overlapped; this block should extend 2 cm inside and outside the field border to be effective.

Metastatic Malignant Meningitis

Clinical carcinomatous leptomeningeal metastasis is uncommon, and it may occur without cerebral or pulmonary metastasis.[43] Adenocarcinomas of the breast, lung, and stomach and melanosarcomas are the most frequent culprits. Primitive neuroectodermal and anaplastic gliomas of the posterior fossa have the highest incidence of leptomeningeal dissemination.[69]

Lymphomatous meningitis has manifestations identical to those of carcinomatous meningitis. The extensive infiltration of peripheral nerves that occurs in lymphoma is unknown in carcinoma. CT scans may show enlarged lymph nodes or a paraver-

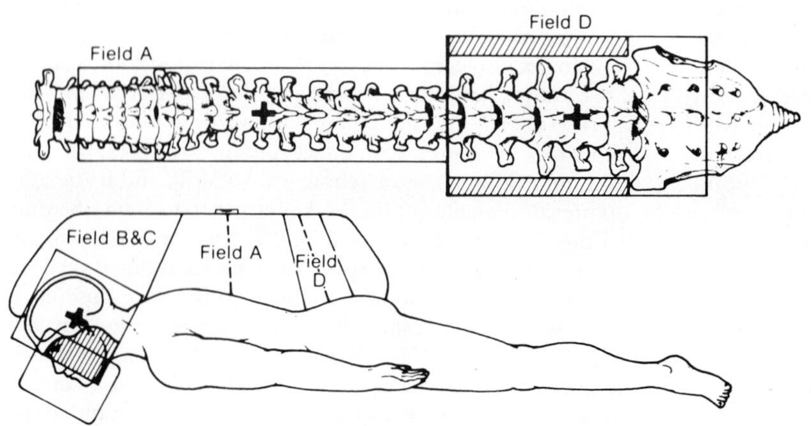

FIGURE 76–12. Diagram of craniospinal irradiation shows how a 30-cm cervicothoracic field is planned. The cranial field is angled with a 0.5-cm gap; the lumbosacral field is abutted at an angle; and the fields are marked on a jig, the top of which is parallel to the table.

tebral mass, which should be irradiated in conjunction with therapy for the lymphomatous meningitis. The results of treatment by craniospinal irradiation alone or combined with intrathecal methotrexate therapy are generally disappointing because of bulky extraneurologic lymphoma or disease resistant to chemotherapy, and the results in no way compare with the better response observed in leukemic meningitis.[44]

We try not to consider a patient for cranial irradiation until the abnormal cytology is cleared by intrathecal chemotherapy; dosages from 2000 cGy in 1 week to 3000 cGy in 3 to 4 weeks can be delivered; lens blocks may be used. Spinal irradiation is reserved for lymphomatous or leukemic meningitis resistant to chemotherapy. The dose approximates 2000 cGy to 3000 cGy; one lateral cranial portal and all the spinal portals are treated daily (Fig. 76-12). Craniospinal reirradiation, once every 8 weeks for 2 years, for leukemic meningitis is being investigated. A single continuous field with the patient's head turned to one side eliminates the need for field junctions.[52]

REFERENCES

1. Ampil FL: Radiotherapy for carcinomatous brachial plexopathy. Cancer 56:2185, 1985
2. Ampil FL: Palliative irradiation of carcinomatous lumbosacral plexus neuropathy. Int J Radiat Oncol Biol Phys 12:1681, 1986
3. Aprin H: Metastatic tumors of the spine. Spine 2:301, 1987
4. Baglan RJ, Marks JE: Comparison of symptomatic and prophylactic irradiation of brain metastases from oat cell carcinoma of the lung. Cancer 47:41, 1981
5. Barak F, Werner A, Walach N, et al: The palliative efficacy of a single high dose of radiation in treatment of symptomatic osseous metastases. Int J Radiat Oncol Biol Phys 13:1233, 1987
6. Bellotti JE, Kagan RA, Wollin M, Olch A, Chan SL: An assessment of the clinical and dosimetric role of intraluminal curietherapy in cancer of the upper gastrointestinal tract and biliary tree. Endocurietherapy/Hyperthermia Oncology 5(2):91–99, 1989
7. Bentson JR, Steckel RJ, Kagan AR: Diagnostic imaging in clinical cancer management: Brain metastases. Invest Radiol 23:335, 1988
8. Blitzer PH: Reanalysis of the RTOG study of the palliation of symptomatic osseous metastasis. Cancer 55:1468, 1985
9. Borgelt B, Gelber R, Kramer S, et al: The palliation of brain metastases: Final results of the first two studies by the Radiation Therapy Oncology Group. Int J Radiat Oncol Biol Phys 6:1, 1980
10. Bruckman JE, Bloomer WD: Management of spinal cord compression. Semin Oncol 5:135, 1978
11. Coleman RE, Rubens RD: The clinical course of bone metastases from breast cancer. Br J Cancer 55:61, 1987
12. Coleman RE, Rubens RD: Bone metastases and breast cancer. Cancer Treat Rev 12:251, 1985
13. Cohen L. Creditor M: Isoeffect tables for tolerance of irradiated normal human tissues. Int J Radiat Oncol Biol Phys 9:233, 1983
14. Cryar AK, Morgan J, Rock JP, et al: Pituitary metastasis: Lung cancer presenting as bitemporal hemianopsia with diabetes insipidus and anterior pituitary deficiency. Henry Ford Hosp Med 35:185, 1987
15. Datz FL: Cerebral edema following iodine-131 therapy for thyroid carcinoma metastatic to the brain. J Nucl Med 27:637, 1986
16. D'Elia F, Bonucci I, Biti GP, et al: Different fractionation schedules in radiation treatment of cerebral metastases. Acta Radiol Oncol 25:181, 1986
17. Dobrowsky W: Treatment of choroid metastases. Br J Radiol 61:140, 1988
18. Drayer BP: Imaging of the aging brain. Radiology 166:797, 1988
19. Egawa S, Tukiyama I, Akine Y, et al: Radiotherapy of brain metastases. Int J Radiat Oncol Biol Phys 12:1621, 1986
20. Eisenberger MA: Chemotherapy for prostate carcinoma. In Consensus Development Conference on the Management of Clinically Localized Prostate Cancer. NCI Monogr 7:151, 1988
21. Fadul C, Misulis KE, Wiley RG: Cerebellar metastases: Diagnostic and management considerations. J Clin Oncol 5: 1107, 1987
22. Falkson G, Gelman RS, Tormey DC, Falkson CI, Wolter JM, Cummings FJ: Treatment of metastatic breast cancer in premenopausal women using CAF with or without oophorectomy: An Eastern Cooperative Oncology Group study. J Clin Oncol 5:881, 1987
23. Ferrante L, Mastronardi L, Acqui M, et al: Neuroradiologic evaluation of a multiple sclerosis case with acute onset. RAYS (Roma) 12:15, 1987
24. Findlay GFG. Adverse effects of the management of malignant spinal cord compression. J Neurol Neurosurg Psychiatry 47:761, 1984
25. Flores AD: New radiotherapy modalities in the management of cancer of the esophagus and cardia, p 124. [Abstract] In Brachytherapy Working Conference, 5th International Selectron Users' Meeting, Hague, Netherlands, September 1, 1988
26. Foley KM: Pain syndromes in patients with cancer. Med Clin North Am 71:169, 1987
27. Fossa SD: Palliative pelvic radiotherapy in patients with hormone-resistant prostatic cancer in prostate cancer. In: Murphy GP (ed): Proceedings of the Second International Symposium on Prostate Cancer, pp 479–485. New York, Alan Liss, 1987
28. Franchin G, Minatel E, Roncadin M, et al: Accelerated split course regimen in the treatment of brain metastases. Radiother Oncol 12:39, 1988
29. Freedman MI, Folk JC: Metastatic tumors to the eye and orbit. Arch Opthalmol 105:1215, 1987
30. Galasko CSB: The role of the orthopaedic surgeon in the treatment of bone pain. Cancer Surv 7:103, 1988
31. Glassburn JR, Klionsky M, Brady LW: Radiation therapy for metastatic disease involving the orbit. Am J Clin Oncol 7:145, 1984
32. Goldberg RI, Rams H, Stone B, et al: Dysphagia as the presenting symptom of recurrent breast carcinoma. Cancer 60:1085, 1987
33. Goodkin R, Carr BI, Perrin RG: Herniated lumbar disc disease in patients with malignancy. J Clin Oncol 5:667, 1987
34. Greenberg HS, Deck MDF, Vikram B, et al: Metastasis to the base of the skull: Clinical findings in 43 patients. Neurology 31:530, 1981
35. Grunwald GB, Klein R, Simmonds MA, et al: Autoimmune basis for visual paraneoplastic syndrome in patients with small-cell lung carcinoma. Lancet I:658, 1985
36. Hankins JR, Miller JE, Salcman M, et al: Surgical management of lung cancer with solitary cerebral metastasis. Ann Thorac Surg 46:24, 1988
37. Hans S, Lindner DW, Webster JD: Brachial plexus neuropathy from metastatic testicular seminoma: Prolonged survival after surgery and radiation therapy. Urology 25:398, 1985
38. Harbert JC: Nuclear Medicine Therapy, pp 207–220. Thieme, New York, 1987
39. Harrington KD: The management of acetabular insufficiency secondary to metastatic malignant disease. J Bone Joint Surg [A] 63:653, 1981
40. Harrison KM, Muss HB, Ball MR, McWhorter M, Case D. Spinal cord compression in breast cancer. Cancer 55:2839, 1985
41. Haynes JW, Miller PR, Steiger Z, et al: Celestin tube use: Radiographic manifestations of associated complications. Radiology 150:41, 1984
42. Heimdal K, Hannisdal E, Fossa SD: Survival after palliative radio-therapy of liver metastases. Acta Oncol 27:63, 1988

43. Henson RA, Urich H: Cancer and the Nervous System: The Neurological Manifestations of Systemic Malignant Disease. Boston, Blackwell, 1982
44. Hitchins RN, Bell DR, Woods RL, Levi JA: A prospective trial of single-agent versus combination chemotherapy in meningeal carcinomatosis. J Clin Oncol 5:1655, 1987
45. Holte H, Saeter G, Dahl IMS, et al: Progressive loss of vision in patients with high-grade non-Hodgkin's lymphoma. Cancer 60:2521, 1987
46. Hoskin PJ: Scientific and clinical aspects of radiotherapy in the relief of bone pain. Cancer Surv 7:69, 1988
47. Hazuka MB, Kinzie JJ: Brain metastases: Results and effects of re-irradiation. Int J Radiat Oncol Biol Phys 15:433, 1988
48. Kagan AR, Stekel RJ, Bassett LW, et al: Radiologic contributions to cancer management: Bone metastasis. AJR 147:305, 1986
49. Kagan AR: Dose-time relationships in the palliation of metastasis to liver, lung, brain and bone by radiations. Front Radiat Ther Oncol 22:165, 1988
50. Kagan AR: Radiation therapy for metastases and myeloma. Spine 2: 343, 1988
51. Kaul TK, Rowland CG, Pagliero KM: Carcinoma of oesophagus: treatment with radical surgery or brachytherapy, p 126. [Abstract] In Branchytherapy Working Conference, 5th International Selectron Users' Meeting, Hague, Netherlands, September 1, 1988
52. Kim TH, Ramsay NK, Steeves RA, Nesbit ME: Intermittent central nervous system irradiation and intrathecal chemotherapy for central nervous system leukemia in children. Int J Radiat Oncol Biol Phys 13: 1451, 1987
53. Kjaer M, Engelholm SA: The clinical course and prognosis of patients with renal adenocarcinoma with solitary metastasis. Int J Radiat Oncol Biol Phys 8:1691, 1982
54. Kloiber R, Molnar CP, Barnes M: Sr-89 therapy for metastatic bone disease: scintigraphic and radiographic follow-up. Radiology 163:719, 1987
55. Kramer S, Hendrickson F, Zelen M, et al: Therapeutic trials in the management of metastatic brain tumors by different time/dose fraction schemes of radiation therapy. NCI Monogr 46:213, 1977
56. Kumar PP, Good RR, Linder J: Complete response of granulosa cell tumor metastatic to liver after hepatic irradiation: A case report. Obstet Gynecol 67:95S, 1986
57. Leibel SA, Pajak TF, Massullo V, Order SE, Komaki RU, Chang CH, Wasserman TH, Phillips TL, Lipshutz J, Durbin LM: A comparison of misonidazole sensitized radiation therapy to radiation therapy alone for the palliation of hepatic metastases: Results of a Radiation Therapy Oncology Group randomized prospective trial. Int J Radiat Oncol Biol Phys 13:1057, 1987
58. Lester ST, Morhis JG, Hornback NB, et al: Brain metastases and testicular tumors: Need for aggressive therapy. J Clin Oncol 2:1397, 1984
59. Lipinski JK, Conway SS, Kottler RE, et al: The radiology of eosophageal tubes for malignant strictures. Clin Radiol 33:453, 1982
60. Little AG, Ferguson MK, DeMeester TR, et al: Esophageal carcinoma with respiratory tract fistula. Cancer 53:1322, 1984
61. Loeffler JS, Glickman AS, Tefft M, Gelch M. Treatment of spinal cord compression: A retrospective analysis. Med Pediatr Oncol 11:347, 1983
62. Magilligan DJ, Duvernoy C, Malik G, et al: Surgical approach to lung cancer with solitary cerebral metastasis: Twenty-five years' experience. Ann Thorac Surg 42:360, 1986
63. Mandell L, Hilaris B, Sullivan M, et al: The Treatment of single brain metastasis from non-oat cell lung carcinoma. Cancer 58:641, 1986
64. Meoz RT, Spanos WJ, Doss L, Johnson R, Wasserman TH: Misonidazole combined with large-fraction pelvic irradiation in the treatment of patients with advanced pelvic malignancies: Preliminary report of an ongoing RTOG phase I-II study. Am J Clin Oncol 6:417, 1983
65. Mink J: Percutaneous bone biopsy in the patient with known or suspected osseous metastases. Radiology 161:191, 1986
66. Murray PK. Functional outcome and survival in spinal cord injury secondary to neoplasia. Cancer 55:197, 1985
67. Noseda A, Louis O, Mockel J, et al: Case report: Diabetes insipidus from metastatic oat cell carcinoma: Recovery after brain irradiation. J Med Sci 289:27, 1985
68. O'Rourke T, George CB, Redmond J, et al: Spinal computed tomography and computed tomographic metrizamide myelography in the early diagnosis of metastatic disease. J Clin Oncol 4:576, 1986
69. Packer RJ, Siegel KR, Sutton LN, Litmann P, Bruce DA, Schut L: Leptomeningeal dissemination of primary central nervous system tumors of childhood. Ann Neurol 18:217, 1985
70. Patchell RA, Cirrincione C, Thaler HT, et al: Single brain metastases: Surgery plus radiation or radiation alone. Neurology 36:447, 1986
71. Patt YZ, Boddie AW, Charnsangavej C, et al: Hepatic arterial infusion with floxuridine and cisplatin: Overriding importance of antitumor effect versus degree of tumor burden as determinants of survival among patients with colorectal cancer. J Clin Oncol 4:1356, 1986
72. Pellettieri L, Sjolander U, Jakobsson KE: Prognostic evaluation before operative extirpation and radiotherapy of solitary brain metastasis. Acta Neurochir (Wien) 86:6, 1987
73. Pongracz N, Zimmerman R, Kotz R: Orthopaedic management of bony metastases of renal cancer. Semin Surg Oncol 4:139, 1988
74. Price P, Hoskin PJ, Easton D, et al: Low dose single fraction radiotherapy in the treatment of metastatic bone pain: A pilot study. Radiother Oncol 12:297, 1988
75. Rapoport S, Blair DN, McCarthy SM, et al: Brachial plexus: correlation of MR imaging with CT and pathologic findings. Radiology 167:161, 1988
76. Rate WR, Solin LH, Turrisi AT. Palliative radiotherapy for metastatic malignant melanoma: brain metastases, bone metastases, and spinal cord compression. Int J Radiat Oncol Biol Phys 15:859, 1988
77. Redmond J, Friedl KE, Cornett P: Clinical usefulness of an algorithm for the early diagnosis of spinal metastatic disease. J Clin Oncol 6:154, 1988
78. Reifler DM: Orbital metastasis with enophthalmos: A review of the literature. Henry Ford Hosp Med J 33:171, 1985
79. Rostock RA, Fishman EK, Zinreich ES, Lee DJ: Computed tomography in radiation therapy treatment planning of hepatic metastases. J Comput Assist Tomogr 9:755, 1985
80. Rubin P, Heilmann H-P: Large field trials. Int J Radiat Oncol Biol Phys 14:S65, 1988
81. Rustin GJS, Newlands ES, Bagshawe KD, et al: Successful management of metastatic and primary germ cell tumors in the brain. Cancer 57:2108, 1986
82. Ryan JR, Rowe DE, Salciccioli GG: Prophylactic internal fixation of the femur for neoplastic lesions. J Bone Joint Surg [A] 58:1071, 1976
83. Salazar OM, Rubin P, Hendrickson FR, et al: Single-dose half-body irradiation for palliation of multiple bone metastases from solid tumors. Cancer 58:29, 1986
84. Sarma DP, Weilbaecher TG: Long-term survival after brain metastasis from lung cancer. Cancer 58:1366, 1986
85. Sarpel S, Sarpel G, Yu E, Hyder S, Kaufman B, Hindo W, Ezdinli. Early diagnosis of spinal-epidural metastasis by magnetic resonance imaging. Cancer 59:1112, 1987
86. Sculier JP, Feld R, Evans WK, et al: Neurologic disorders in patients with small cell lung cancer. Cancer 60:2275, 1987
87. Seitz W, Karcher KH, Binder W: Radiotherapy of metastatic renal cell carcinoma. Semin Surg Oncol 4:100, 1988
88. Sheline GE, Brady LW: Radiation therapy for brain metastases. J Neurooncol 4:219, 1987
89. Sherry MM, Greco FA, Johnson DH, et al: Metastatic breast cancer confined to the skeletal system. Am J Med 81:381, 1986
90. Smalley SR, Schray MF, Laws ER, et al: Adjuvant radiation therapy after surgical resection of solitary brain metastasis: Association with pattern of failure and survival. Int J Radiat Oncol Biol Phys 13:1611, 1987
91. Spanos WJ, Guse C, Perez C, Grigsby P, Doggett RLS, Poulter C: Phase II study of multiple daily fractionation in the pallia-

tion of advanced pelvic malignancies: Preliminary report of RTOG 85–02. Int J Radiat Oncol Biol Phys 17(3):659–661, 1989

92. Spanos WJ, Wasserman T, Meoz R, et al Palliation of advanced pelvic malignant disease with large fraction pelvic radiation and misonidazole: Final report of RTOG phase I/II study. Int J Radiat Oncol Biol Phys 13:1479, 1987
93. Sundaresan N, Scher H, DiGiacinto GV, Yagoda A, Whitmore W, Choi IS: Surgical treatment of spinal cord compression in kidney cancer. J Clin Oncol 4:1851, 1986
94. Tomita T, Galicich, Sundaresan N: Radiation therapy for spinal epidural metastases with complete block. Acta Radiol Oncol 22:135, 1983
95. Tong C, Gillick L, Hendrickson FR: The palliation of symptomatic osseous metastases: Final results of the study by the Radiation Therapy Oncology Group. Cancer 50:893, 1982
96. Tumeh SS, Beadle G, Kaplan WD: Clinical significance of solitary rib lesions in patients with extraskeletal malignancy. J Nucl Med 26:1140, 1985
97. Van Lom KJ, Kellerhouse LE, Pathria MN, et al: Infection versus tumor in the spine; criteria for distinction with CT. Radiology 166:851, 1988
98. Wilkins MF, Keen CW: Hemi-body radiotherapy in the management of metastatic carcinoma. Clin Radiol 38:267, 1987
99. Williams MR, Todd JH, Ellis IO, et al: Oestrogen receptors in primary and advanced breast cancer: An eight-year review of 704 cases. Br J Cancer 55:67, 1987
100. Yordan EL, Schlaerth J, Gaddis O, et al: Radiation therapy in the management of gestational choriocarcinoma metastatic to the central nervous system. Obstet Gynecol 69:627, 1987
101. Zadra JA, Jewett MAS, Keresteci AG, et al: Nonoperative urinary diversion for malignant ureteral obstruction. Cancer 60:1353, 1987
102. Zevallos M, Chan PYM, Munoz L, Wagner J, Kagan AR: Epidural spinal cord compression from metastatic tumor. Int J Radiat Oncol Biol Phys 13:875, 1987
103. Zinser JW, Hortobagyi GN, Buzdar AU, Smith TL, Fraschini G: Clinical course of breast cancer patients with liver metastases. J Clin Oncol 5:773, 1987

77

Supportive Care in Radiation Oncology

Marvin Rotman
Richard J. Torpie

The radiation oncologist, concerned with the disease process and technical intricacies of treatment, usually has not been involved in managing the supportive aspects of caring for the patient. Yet at a very critical time in the course of treatment, the radiation oncologist becomes the one most responsible for overseeing the total care of the cancer patient. The intensive nature of radiation therapy, with daily treatment for some weeks, initiates a special relationship between the physician and patients with curable disease or those requiring palliation.

Supportive care generally involves prevention and correction of tissue dysfunction, augmentation of nutrition, metabolic and electrolyte regulation, rehabilitation, and pain and infection control. This chapter offers an overview of a considerable volume of literature dealing with issues that were once the domain of a rather small group of physicians, nutritionists, and psychologists. The discussion also highlights emotional and psychosocial considerations.

EMOTIONAL CONSIDERATIONS

Premorbid Personality Traits

There are many studies indicating the role of premorbid personality traits and stressful life events, such as the recent loss of a sibling, in the clinical onset of cancer.[46,49,55,59,97] LeShan and Worthington[60] investigated the relationship between stressful life events and cancer and reported in a controlled study that 77% of patients with cancer, but only 14% of controls, endured the loss of a major relationship 6 months to 8 years before the diagnoses of tumors.

The patient's personality before the development of the tumor determines in large measure his or her emotional reaction to it and, ultimately, therapeutic relief. Some personality patterns observed include impaired self-awareness, a predisposition toward hopelessness, and poor emotional expression.[2,55,93] The current thinking on mechanisms of psychogenically induced pathology focuses on the ability of the person to cope with stressful situations; if coping is inadequate, the inherent emotional deficits are compounded.

The concept of chronic stress leading to abnormal hormonal and immunologic function has been employed in several animal and human studies.[6,64,67,84] Riley[84] showed that mice infected with mammary tumor virus and caged under stressful conditions, such as noise and bleeding, have a significantly greater incidence and shorter latency period for breast carcinoma than a control group caged under less stressful conditions. Several studies have concluded that the ratio of a woman's corticoid to androgenic steroids can be used to predict the course of her breast neoplasm.[10,64,67]

Patient Reaction

When patients are first seen in the radiation oncology department, they have invariably undergone the trauma of a battery of investigative procedures, have been subjected to the rigors of hospitalization, and possibly have been told they have cancer. To compound these difficulties, they are confronted by an array of complex and bewildering machinery and a even by a large body of misinformation about the nature and role of irradiation in the treatment of their disease.

Major fears stem from equating the need for irradiation with inoperability and therefore incurability. Their apprehensions are often derived from a physician who has indicated that irradiation is the treatment for them because their tumor "cannot be removed by surgery." They also worry about "being burned" or disfigured, an inability to perform normal bodily functions, and sterility or a loss of sexuality.[86] Women with genitourinary and breast tumors and men with prostate or testicular cancers often suffer from feelings of shame and unattractiveness, adding anxieties about rejection and abandonment to the fears of pain and mutilation.

Many patients do not express their depressive reactions. A preliminary analysis of an extensive pretreatment interview devised by DeLeon and associates[24] of more than 100 patients in metropolitan New York showed this contradiction. Most of these patients did not reveal any degree of hopelessness, anger, or depression in their overt attitudes toward the future. The overwhelming primary emotional reaction was that of denial, accompanied by an internalization of the experience of the diagnosis of cancer. They exhibited surprising passivity and considerable repression; most were docile and expressed little negative reaction when told they would need radiation treatment.

The patient may feel that cancer is a judgment or curse for some unknown sin or past misdeed, in which case the patient actually derives a secondary gain from the illness by satisfying some unconscious need for punishment.[86]

The patient with a diagnosis of recurring cancer often experiences a deeper distress and greater lack of support than at the time of the original diagnosis of potentially curable diseases. Feelings of helplessness, loss of control, and loss of self-image are heightened by the breakdown of spiritual and cultural values and by family and economic crises. It is the palliative patient who deserves our greatest attention, because too often the attitude of others creates feelings of expendability. The most dreaded fears of the cancer patient are of isolation and abandonment, concerns that can be relieved by simple measures of care, comfort, and concern.

Family Reaction

The beliefs and reactions of family members sometimes mirror those of the patients. They often perceive irradiation as a futile procedure in a hopeless situation. One common misconception is that the patient becomes radioactive and contaminated after radiation treatments. The family may react by becoming overly protective or conversely by abandoning the patient. Parental response to a child with cancer reflects myriad stresses and demands that tax relationships inside and outside the family circle. The physician-family relationship in these cases depends on factors such as the age of the child at onset of illness, the degree of physical morbidity caused by the particular cancer, the likely prognosis, and especially the presence of preexisting emotional problems within the affected family.[101]

Sometimes the patient and family may direct and express their resentment and anger toward the physician during or after the initial interview. These reactions are often a displacement of fear of the illness itself. It is important for the physician not to be provoked by these emotional reactions and reject or dismiss the patient. The oncologist should understand that the emotional outburst will soon abate and was never meant to be a personal attack.

Physician-Patient Rapport

The need to improve the quality of the interpersonal relationship between the physician and patient is obvious. The first step is to achieve a rapport with the patient and understand the person's underlying fears. This entails the physician's ability to communicate verbally and nonverbally, to convey a positive affect of care, concern, and warmth, to anticipate the patient's difficulties in following treatment regimens, and to transfer information in a manner that promotes the patient's cooperation.

The basic interview is one of the best methods to evaluate and relieve needs and fears and to deliver information to the patient about cancer and radiation therapy.[13,31,86]

During the physical examination, the radiation oncologist should try to determine the degree of the patient's anxiety. A pilot study at New York Medical College[86] demonstrated marked fluctuations blood pressure of patients while in the treatment room, which was related to the absence or lack of information.[25] Central to all anxieties is the fear of the unknown; it is essential that the patient become more knowledgeable about the disease and its treatment.

The first pretreatment meeting is the most propitious time to develop physician-patient rapport. It is best that the patient, spouse, and other close family members attend this initial discussion. Doing so creates a sense of team approach and permits the airing of questions and emotions that facilities treatment. The oncologist should use simple language and avoid ambiguity and excessive optimism or pessimism. At no point should the patient or family be lied to, an ill-advised approach that only causes anxiety, confusion, and misunderstanding. Usually, the most difficult aspect of disease information to be imparted is that of prognosis. The best overall attitude is to be generally reassuring; hope should never be denied, even in the worst situations.[33]

Alternatives to the interview include an audiovisual presentation introducing people, procedures, and practical aspects of the treatment; a chance to talk with a long-term survivor of the same disease could be vastly reassuring to a cancer patient; group therapy sessions under the supervision of a psychologist may indicate a positive and realistic attitude toward life in these depressed patients.

Every oncologist is faced with patient noncooperation and the resultant incomplete administration of the prescribed treatment regimen. There is increasing evidence that this noncooperation is related to the failure of the physician to communicate the specified treatment effectively to the patient, the subtle or overt antagonism of some physicians, and the lack of opportunity given patients to express feedback.[31]

The quality of patient-physician relationship may influence the outcome of treatment. For example, studies have shown that postoperative recovery is affected by a patient's preoperative levels of fear and anxiety, that human interaction has major effects on cardiac function, and that an improved patient-physician rapport can significantly lower narcotic dosage and hospital occupancy.[57,63]

The relationship with the patient needing palliative treatment depends on accurate assessment of the shared therapeutic goals of the physician and the patient. Palliation must not be provided in an emotional vacuum.

Lippincott[62] stated that there is a need for understanding the patient in these situations and one's own needs, history, and expectations. A firm philosophy allowing honesty with one's self and with the patient, the ability to tell the truth and to listen with enough sensitivity not to burden the patient, and a recognition of the communication and emotional changes taking place are important features in the care of the dying patient, along with the skills to reduce pain and suffering.

Certain oncologists find themselves unable to interact with patients once cure is unobtainable. They may become angry or annoyed with patients who are not responding well to treatment.[69] Doctors usually tend to view the patient's lack of progress or even death as personal failures. Consequently, they may prescribe prolonged or ill-advised treatment plans that preclude life's termination and death as a signified event.

Special Emotional Problems of the Dying Patient

With the dying patient, it is important to create a conceptual time frame for the process of gradual and inevitable death. Kubler-Ross[56] established a time intensity scale for the adjustment stages of dying (Fig. 77-1). The early stages include short-lived shock at disclosure, strong denial, and anger.

It is denial that is most poorly understood. Denial, as it

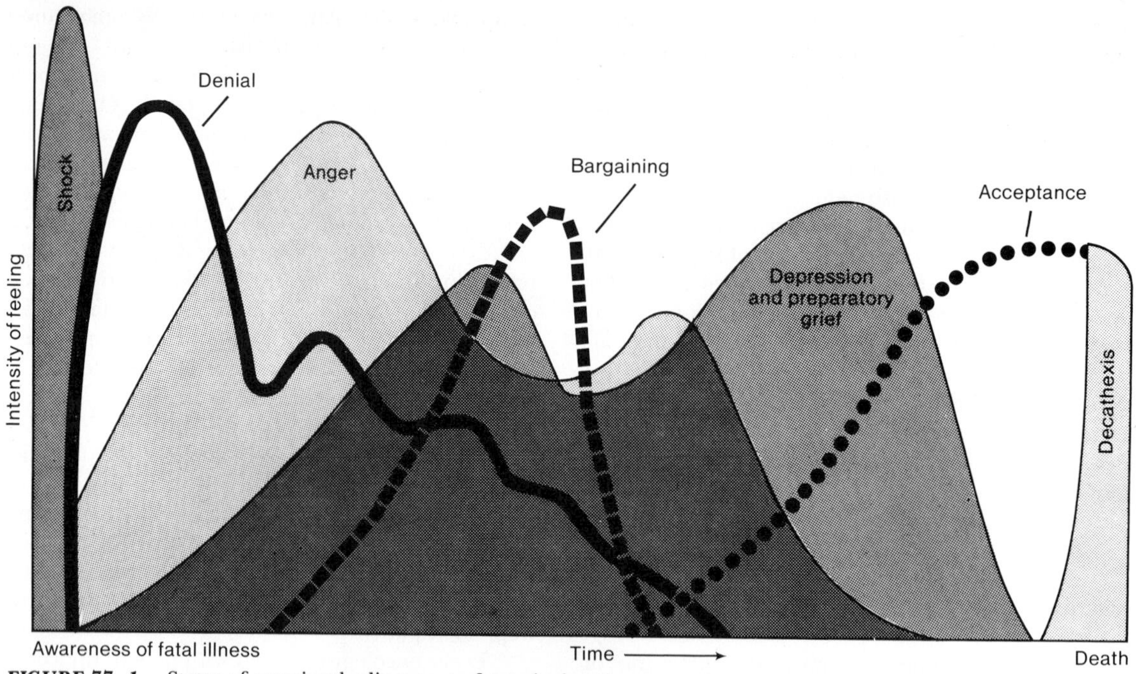

FIGURE 77–1. States of emotional adjustment of terminal patients.

originates from the patient, is a potent psychologic defense that protects the mind from the concept of its own annihilation. Freud[39] observed that the ego cannot envision its own lack of future. Denial may vary from negligible to intense, from distortion and seemingly not hearing, to displacement and untypical behavior. It should be respected by the physician, but the physician should never hide behind the patient's denial.

The fine work of Abrams[1] on the changing patterns of communication of the cancer patient and the work of others show the importance of listening and communicative skills in working with these patients, some of whom are followed over many years and others of whom have only a short time to live.[34,38,44,51,53,69,71,77,83,92,108,109] Some preterminal patients are caught up in a conspiracy of silence based on physician denial or the well-meaning initial intent of families who have decided "not to tell." This deception in the face of advancing symptoms only further isolates the patient and interferes with all the shared meaningful ritualism of death and grieving. According to Stehlin and Beach,[99] "Nothing is more pathetic than the incurable patient who knows the truth about his condition, even though he has not been officially told, and would desperately need to talk to someone about his problems."

Shore[96] observed that feelings of anger and helplessness are often not expressed and that there may be a subtle parrying of what the patient perceives is "allowed" by the therapist, because in effect the patient gives clues as to what he or she can emotionally manage. It is important to allow the expression of this grief so that sorrow can facilitate acceptance. This process is overwhelmingly emotional and cannot be managed by the physician alone, who must have help from other disciplines.

Participation in the bereavement process after the death of the patient may help the surviving family, oncologist, and medical staff to deal with their own grief.[92,95] Simple measures of respect, such as letters and telephone calls, show that the patient was valued. Deutsch[26] has pointed out the emotional penalties exacted by the unconscious: "Every unresolved grief is given expression in some form or the other and must be expressed in full . . . and must be carried to completion." Modern studies verify these penalties for unresolved grief of the physician and staff; they include depression, displacement of anger, increased use of drugs and alcohol, suicide, somatic complaints, emotional burnout, disordered clinical judgment, and retreat from the painful responsibilities of care.[94,95] In addition, Cassel[11] indicated that attempts at palliation of dying patients may be disordered.

Studies that address the psychosocial factors surrounding all aspects of treatment with radiation (curative and palliative) have only recently appeared in the literature.[12,34,30,38,48,74,80,86,106] These have examined the emotional perspectives of the medical staff and have stressed the importance of preparatory information, support for the family, and the need for interventional psychotherapy.

PATHOLOGIC CONSIDERATIONS

Some aspects of patients care are related to prevention and amelioration of the side-effects of irradiation on various organic systems. The amount of discomfort or disability experienced by a patient is related to the type of tissue affected, how vital it is to the organ or host, the ability of the tissue to restore itself, and the type of therapy administered.[35,65,76,87]

Skin

In the early decades of radiation therapy, skin reactions were the major impediment to delivery of tumoricidal doses. For lack of better means of dose measurement, the concept of "skin erythema dose" was established, based on consistent skin changes after irradiation with low-voltage machines.[78]

The skin overlying the intergluteal folds, the perineum, the axillae, and the retromammary sulcus are particularly prone to undesirable reactions because of excessive moisture and warmth. Further, these areas are especially likely to develop bacterial and fungal infections. The skin-sparing effect of supervoltage irradiation may be nullified by treatment over areas covered with bandages or clothes. The combined use of irradiation and systemic chemotherapeutic agents, such as doxorubicin (Adriamycin) and dactinomycin (actinomycin D), increases skin damage. The "recall phenomenon" originally described by D'Angio and associates[22] for skin reactions manifested after dactinomycin and irradiation may eventually apply to several other drugs, an important matter to consider in this decade of multimodal therapy.

The principles for treatment of reactions are similar to those for burns. Erythematous areas are kept dry and well aerated. For dry desquamation and pruritus, topical agents should be avoided, but parenteral agents like Benadryl may be used. However, agents such as baby powder and cornstarch frequently bring considerable relief to patients and should be applied after each treatment. If moist desquamation occurs, fundamental aspects of care are maintenance of hygiene to avoid secondary infection and the promotion of reepithelization. Mild antiseptics, such as 2% gentian violet and diluted solutions of hydrogen peroxide, are beneficial. Vitamins A and D or steroid ointments can relieve the discomfort associated with this side-effect and actually enhance the healing process by their antimoisture and antiinflammatory effects. Fungal infections like moniliasis are controlled with nystatin ointment. Chronic skin changes, such as skin necrosis and ulceration, may require skin grafting. A program of manual massage, physical therapy, and oral or topical triiodothyronine may alleviate the problems associated with subcutaneous fibrosis.[88]

Dental Tissues

Controlled clinical trials have shown that dental prophylaxis can reduce radiation-induced decay and necrosis by one third to one half in patients whose initial dental status is reasonably satisfactory. This is a critical factor in improving radiation tolerance and minimizing postirradiation dental problems in head and neck cancer patients. Patients must be encouraged to clean teeth regularly, using effective plaque and tartar removal techniques. Adding regular fluoride applications gives the teeth some protection against acidic degradation. The method recommended is to use custom-fitted dental plates soaked in a sodium fluoride solution or gel that are held in the mouth for 5 minutes every day; this procedure must be continued indefinitely. The use of supersaturated solutions of calcium phosphate to remineralize the teeth can reinforce the stability of the teeth and prevent plaque formation.

Teeth that are already severely decayed should be extracted before beginning radiation therapy. There is no need to remove healthy teeth because they have considerable tolerance for even high doses of radiation, especially if a program of strict oral hygiene is followed.

Radiation damage to the periodontal membrane may cause tooth decay, despite all prophylactic efforts. Decay can also arise as an indirect result of the changes in salivary viscosity and acidity with irradiation.[21,79] Normal salivary action serves to buffer and dilute acids produced by food fermentation and to cleanse teeth of sucrose-metabolizing bacteria. Without this action, large numbers of cariogenic organisms can adhere to tooth surfaces and form plaques. In the calcified area, an acidic attack on the tooth surface is initiated, and once established, dental caries provide a route of infection that may lead to mandibular or maxillary necrosis.

Postirradiation management of dental decay or necrosis must be conservative. Tooth extraction should be a last resort. If possible, the use of synthetic or porcelain fillings, root canal therapy, antibiotics, zinc peroxide applications, analgesics, and more frequent fluoride applications should be implemented.

Head and Neck Tissues

Supportive care in treatment of head and neck cancer includes the preventive maintenance of good oral hygiene. There is also a need for strict adherence to a diet that ensures adequate nutrition during the course of treatment. A variety of tissue responses to irradiation combine to make normal nutrition difficult, and it is important for patients to compensate for this factor. As a result of dryness of the mouth, mastication becomes progressively more difficult. There is also altered taste sensations, distaste for seasoned foods, and anorexia.

This is exacerbated by an increased susceptibility of the oropharyngeal mucosa to exogenous irritants and infections. The ensuing side-effects often cause considerable discomfort and pain and may prevent the administration of adequate doses of radiation.

In the first weeks of irradiation, a so-called pseudotumor effect may appear in which the mucosa overlying the tumor area becomes highlighted.[95] In the final weeks, a whitish pseudomembrane may develop within the irradiated mucosa overlying a superficially ulcerated base. Occasionally, tumor erosion and necrosis may precipitate hemorrhaging, but this is rare.

Patients should be encouraged to embark on an oral hygiene regimen before the treatment program begins. Mouth rinsing five to six times a day is recommended, especially after meals. A lukewarm solution of a tablespoon each of salt and baking soda in a quart of water should be prepared. Bathing the tissues in a mouthful of the solution for 5 minutes at a time alleviates some of the painful side-effects. Over-the-counter mouthwashes and diluted hydrogen peroxide solutions are less effective.

It is beneficial to encourage patients to consume foods and fluids that do not irritate the mucous membranes and that pass easily through the upper digestive tract; a dietitian may play an important role at this point. A mixture of aspirin and glycerine (aspirin mucilage) or a 2% viscous xylocaine solution can be used to alleviate sore throat or dysphagia. In extreme cases of dysphagia, a gastrostomy or hyperalimentary parenteral feeding may be required to maintain high nutrition and a positive nitrogen balance.

Gastrointestinal Tract

Irradiation of the esophageal and gastric areas leads mainly to nausea, vomiting, dyspepsia, and anorexia after about 2 or 3 weeks of treatment. Esophageal mucositis and edema can lead to dysphagia. Upper abdominal or para-aortic irradiation with doses as low as 3000 cGy to the stomach infrequently produce an alarming hematemesis. The symptom probably is caused by the malignant disease process, radiation treatment, drugs, diet, and psychologic stress. Radiation-induced gastric ulcers can cause obstruction or perforation, but they are rare occurrences with doses of less than 4500 cGy given in 4.5 to 5 weeks.

With small and large bowel irradiation, emesis and anorexia may develop. The most common symptom, however, is diarrhea. The strophic mucositis and reduced absorptive capacity of damaged intestinal villi can lead to malabsorption, steatrorrhea, generalized wasting, and megaloblastic anemia.

Nausea and vomiting are often, but not always, responsive

to drugs. The phenothiazines, such as prochlorperazine (Compazine), are generally useful. Marijuana has been effective for some patients in controlling nausea and vomiting caused by chemotherapy, and it may have a role to play in relieving intractable emesis caused by radiation therapy. It is known that the minimum effective clinical dose of the active marijuana ingredient, tetrahydrocannabinol (THC), is 40 mg to 80 mg, but the average marijuana "toke" contains only 18 mg or less of active THC.[9] The severe cerebral side-effects that result from doses high enough to be effective can be controlled by phenothiazines.

Other symptoms may be controlled by altering diet. Dyspepsia, gastritis, and radiation "ulcer" are amenable to a regimen of a bland diet combined with antacids, sedatives, and antispasmodics.[54] Diet changes can also be effective in controlling diarrhea. A low-residue diet, together with the use of Kaopectate or opiate drugs like codeine and diphenoxylate (Lomotil), is often sufficient remedy. However, it may be necessary to suspend treatment for a few days.

Diarrhea is the most common side-effect of pelvic and abdominal irradiation. Important factors have been found to be decreased fat absorption, characterized by high fecal fat values, and decreased serum glycerol trioleate,[82] lactase enzyme deficiency,[103] and fecal bile salt alterations.[3] Ileal dysfunction may be secondary to irradiation. It can cause choleraic enteropathy, resulting in the passage of unreabsorbed bile acids into the colon, where they induce water and electrolyte secretion. Initial studies have suggested that cholestyramine, a drug that binds bile acids before they pass through to the colon, can be effective in preventing radiation-induced diarrhea when administered in dosages of 4 g three times a day.[6,47]

Other substances being considered for the control of diarrhea are a number of salicylate and other antiprostaglandin compounds, on the presumption that irradiation increases prostaglandin secretion. It is known that certain prostaglandin fractions cause diarrhea in patients,[50] and salicylates are known to block prostaglandin biosynthesis at low concentrations.[107] A pilot study at the Royal Marsden Hospital showed that 12 of 15 women with diarrhea caused by pelvic irradiation failed to respond to conventional therapy but showed clinical improvement after treatment with aspirin.[66] Furthermore, chronic radiation-induced enteritis has been shown to be susceptible to combinations of salicylates and sulphonamides, such as salicylazosulphapyridine.[41]

Urinary Tract

Before any urinary problem is treated, it is essential to do repeated urinalyses, urine cultures, and antibiotics and sensitivity tests if bacteria are present. The symptoms of radiation cystitis (*i.e.*, pain, burning, and urgency) may be relieved by 200 mg of phenazopyridine (Pyridium) given three times a day, which has a topical analgesic effect on the bladder mucosa.[43] Tumor breakdown and blockage may be another cause of bladder spasms, and intermittent irrigations can provide relief. If the symptoms continue and cultures are normal, it may be necessary to resort to a combination of broad-spectrum antibiotics. A urinary antispasmodic, such as mixture of potassium citrate and tincture of hyoscyamus, is often effective.[37]

An occasional late complication in patients receiving pelvic irradiation, systemic cyclophosphamide, or both is hemorrhagic cystitis. Conservative management for this condition is often successful. Acidification of urine, bladder washouts with Mercurochrome (1 in 200 dilution), potassium permanganate solution, or 1% to 2% formaldehyde solution, and blood transfusions are all worth trying.[37] However, the chronic nature of the condition often leads to overenthusiastic surgical procedures, such as urinary diversion with or without cystectomy or ligation of the internal iliac artery.[81] The source of the bleeding is known to be delicate telagiectatic arterioles or capillaries at the base of ulcerated areas of bladder mucosa.[58] Lapides[58] successfully treated hemorrhagic cystitis by cautious electrocoagulation of telangiectatic vessels.

The normal mucosa of the urinary bladder is protected by a layer of mucin composed in part of glycosamine glycan (GAG). Radiation may break the normal protective barrier laid down by the transitional cell mucosa lining, giving rise to a bacterial infection and interstitial cystitis. Hematuria may develop as a result of the cystitis. Exogenous GAG-like compounds, such as pentosanpolysulfate (PPS), have none of the identical activities in adhering to the bladder surface as the endogenous GAG. Forty-five percent of the patients receiving PPS experienced a persistent remission of radiation cystitis, but remission occurred in only 24% of patients receiving a placebo.[73]

In some malignancies, such as leukemias, lymphomas, and multiple myelomas, there may be rapid dissolution of tumor masses as a result of irradiation. In these cases, renal function requires constant protection to prevent shutdown secondary to uric acid deposits.[43] Administration of allopurinol, an antigout drug, in doses of 100 mg administered three times a day, effectively prevents uric acid breakdown by inhibiting the production of xanthine oxidase, an essential enzyme in the process.

NUTRITIONAL SUPPORT

Cachexia

The reasons for the common occurrence of weight loss in malignant disease are not fully understood, but some of the factors involved are anorexia, cancerous involvement of the digestive organs, infection, and tumor growth.

Cachexic patients show signs of anorexia, weight loss, early satiety, and asthenia.[105] Anorexia may be initiated by physiologic changes in taste perception, affecting, for example, the appreciation of sweetness or salinity.[28] A 50% incidence of the loss of pleasurable taste and a 30% incidence of aversion to meat was found by DeWys.[27] Aberrations in the metabolism of zinc may be responsible for these changes.[42] Other factors in anorexia may be psychologic reactions to the disease, complications of the disease, and side-effects of the treatment. An interesting suggestion is that certain metabolites of cancer, such as peptides and nucleotides, directly maintain the state of anorexia by affecting peripheral and central nervous system receptor and responder cells.[104]

An imbalance between caloric intake and expenditure is characteristic of cachexia and is manifested clinically as weight loss. The imbalance may be accentuated by malabsorption, external nutrient loss (vomiting and diarrhea), increased basal metabolic rate, and even tumor-host competition for nutrients. As the condition develops, there is a reduction in caloric intake, and essential nutrients in the metabolic pool are depleted. Aberrations are found in the metabolism of fats, carbohydrates, minerals, vitamins, and hormones; electrolyte and acid-base abnormalities develop, and the patient's immunocompetence is comprised.

Nutritional Therapy

In 86% of anergic patients given nutritional support, immunocompetence was restored.[45] In this group of responding patients, there was an 11% mortality rate, but the mortality rate was 100% among patients in whom immune function was not restored. Further, there was a mortality rate of 50% among patients who became anergic after surgery, radiation therapy, or chemotherapy, compared with only 14% for patients whose immunocompetence was preserved.

The usual result of anorexia, altered metabolism, and changes in eating behavior in cancer patients is protein-calorie malnutrition.[7,45] In severe malnutrition, provision of adequate calories is critical: calories from other sources have eight times the impact of protein on weight gain.[40] For every 100 calories administered, only about 2.5 g of protein should be included. If possible, feeding through the alimentary tract is preferable to the intravenous route.

There are commercially available formulas tailored to specific nutrient and metabolic requirements to cope with different physiologic abnormalities.[8] DeWys and Herbst[29] found that patients preferred milk-based products to synthetic nutritional products; however, 70% of noncaucasians have lactose intolerance problems.[40] It has been shown that the use of feeding supplements during radiation treatment or chemotherapy is an effective method of reversing weight loss and maintaining normal serum protein levels.[20]

Hyperalimentation

Total parenteral nutrition, initially described by Dudrick and co-workers,[32] can ensure proper nutrition and create an anabolic state in patients who are incapable of adequate oral food intake or have significantly deficient alimentary absorption. Intravenous hyperalimentation is an effective adjunct in antineoplastic therapy in both animal and human radiation therapy trials.[17,20,32,98]

In patients with obstructive lesions of the esophagus further compromised with radiation esophagitis, the discontinuation of oral feedings and the institution of parenteral feeding provides a respite from secretory and mechanical functions and facilitates eventual repair. Copeland and colleagues[18] reported that 95% of 39 malnourished patients treated with radiation therapy and intravenous hyperalimentation were able to complete their intended courses of therapy. Intravenous hyperalimentation was used for an average of 37.6 days, and the average weight gain was 7 to 8 pounds. After intravenous hyperalimentation is terminated, most patients are able to maintain their improved weights.[15]

Treatment consists of correction of fluid deficits and electrolyte abnormalities after hospital admission. A high caloric hyperosmolar solution containing 6 g nitrogen, 20% glucose, and essential vitamins and minerals is infused through a catheter placed in the subclavian vein. In the average patient, approximately 2000 ml of this fluid is infused over a 24-hour period and provides about 2000 calories.[15,32] Intravenous lipid solutions, a mixture of triglycerides, mostly long-chain unsaturated fatty acids, allow reduction of dextrose concentrations below 12.5% and permit the use of peripheral veins for intravenous alimentation.

The potential risks of intravenous hyperalimentation, such as subclavian vein thrombosis, thrombophlebitis, and sepsis, can be decreased to within 2% if it is undertaken by a special team of physicians, nurses, and technicians and if the parenteral feeding catheter is not used for other purposes, such as blood withdrawal, transfusion, or central venous pressure monitoring.[16] Uncommon complications include hyperglycemia, azotemia, anemia, electrolyte imbalance, hypervitaminosis, and acidosis. Problems associated with infusion of hypertonic solutions, such as osmotic diuresis, can be prevented by reducing the concentration of protein hydrolysate from 6% to 3.5%. Although intravenous hyperalimentation has been reported to stimulate tumor growth in rats, it has not been similarly confirmed in human clinical studies.[16,18,100]

Elemental Diet

An alternative to intravenous hyperalimentation for patients in relentless carabolic states secondary to severe radiation enteritis is a diet that allows for total absorption in the proximal small intestine.[70] The low-fat content and elemental nature of these diets do not stimulate pancreatic, biliary, and gastrointestinal secretions. The diet contains 7 g nitrogen or 45 g essential amino acids and 1000 calories per 1000 ml solution. Given orally or through feeding tubes, approximately 3000 ml can be given a day for extended periods without the problems of sepsis associated with intravenous hyperalimentation.[72]

PAIN CONTROL

Radiation therapy is the most effective means of achieving sustained palliation of pain from cancer. Pain constitutes the single most frequent symptom for which patients are referred for palliative radiation.

Perception of pain and individual reactions are extremely variable and are influenced by factors as age, sex, and anxiety. Petrie[75] identified augmentors, deducers, and moderates as three types of individuals with distinct responses to the magnitude of pain. Anxiety is considered to be the single most important factor that intensifies the experience of pain.[102] Anxiety in this instance may be related to a fear of the unknown or in response to the continuous reminder that something harmful is occurring within the body.[4,102]

It is important that the oncologist realize that it is the memory or anticipation of pain that is a major reason for the increasingly higher doses of analgesics or narcotics demanded by the patient in pain. If this anticipation is removed, drug requirements can soon be reduced. Oral narcotic combinations, such as the Brompron's mixture along with prochlorperazine or chlorpromazine, used in a standardized program have been shown by Saunders[91] and others to be effective in obtaining a pain-free state without a clouded sensorium.[14,68]

Fractionated radiation therapy is manifestly successful in the management of painful metastatic and primary bone disease. However, Cox[19] and Barkley[5] have pointed with caution to the use of large-dose rapid fractionation in soft tissue because of the incidence of severe complications.

Hemibody radiation in patients with widespread bony disease in selected patients suggests is a safe and often dramatic method of achieving palliation of pain.[66] Rubin and associates[89] reviewed the potential for sequential hemibody irradiation for the relief of pain secondary to metastatic disease. Doses of 600 cGy to 800 cGy administered with assiduous detail, premedication, and necessary hospitalization may provide rapid pain relief, which is considered to be excellent in almost 20% of patients and to be good in another 40%. Patients must be carefully selected because toxic reactions can be severe.

In some situations, radiation therapy is only partially effective, as in actual induration of nervous tissue (*e.g.*, celiac or brachial plexus infiltration). Interruption or blocking of painful nervous impulses can be effected by surgery, anesthetic blocks, or electric stimulation.

INFECTION CONTROL

Altered humoral and cellular responses, decrease and malfunction of granulocytes, and changes in endogenous microflora of the host contribute to increased susceptibility to infection in cancer patients; multimodal treatment of cancer patients renders them vulnerable to opportunistic organisms. Infections can potentially offset the significant gains made in patient survival and are important causes of morbidity and mortality in cancer patients.[52]

Gram-negative bacteria have emerged as the most significant cause of infections in cancer patients and are frequently found in lesions of the lungs, alimentary tract, and skin.[52,111] *Pseudomonas, Bacteroides, Escherichia coli, Klebsiella,* and *Proteus* are common gram-negative organisms causing infection in these patients. Fungal infections are commonly caused by *Candida albicans, Aspergillus* organisms, and cryptococci. The herpesvirus group is responsible for the largest number of viral infections in cancer patients. *Pneumocystis carinii* is a protozoal parasite increasingly responsible for pulmonary infections in leukemic patients.

It is estimated that febrile episodes in virtually all patients with solid tumors and 75% of patients with leukemia or lymphomas are caused by infection. The anergic and sometimes debilitated status of these patients necessitates prompt and radical search for the infective agent or agents. While culture results are awaited, it may judicious to initiative vigorous broad-spectrum antibiotic therapy. A combination of carbenicillin and gentamicin is considered the most effective treatment available before isolation of the infecting pathogen(s).[111] Amphotericin B is most commonly used in the treatment of fungal infections. After diagnosis by biopsy or aspirate examination, *P. carinii* infections are treated with pentamidine isethionate.[110] Continued use of steroids and chemotherapeutic agents may facilitate viral infections.

REFERENCES

1. Abrams RD: The patient with cancer: His changing pattern of communication. N Engl J Med 274:317, 1966
2. Abse DW, Wilkins MN, van duCastle RL, et al: Personality and behavioral characteristics of lung cancer patients. J Psychosom Res 18:101, 1974
3. Anderson H, Bosaeus I, Nystrom C: Bile salt malabsorption in the radiation syndrome. Acta Radiol 17:312, 1978
4. Bard M: The price of survival for cancer victims. Transaction 3:10, 1966
5. Barkley HT: Accelerated treatment. Cancer 55:2112, 1985
6. Berk RN, Seay DG: Cholerheic enteropathy as a cause of diarrhea and death in radiation enteritis and its prevention with cholestyramine. Radiology 104:153, 1972
7. Blachburn GL, Bothe A: Assessment of malnutrition in cancer patients. Cancer Bull 30:88, 1978
8. Bounous G, LeBel E, Shuster J, et al: Dietary protection during radiotherapy. Strahlentherapie 149:476, 1975
9. Boyd JB (ed): The Clinical Cancer Letter. 2:1, 1979
10. Bulbrook RD, Greenwood FC, Hayward JL: Selection of breast cancer patients for adrenalectomy or hypophysection by determination of urinary 17-hydrocorticosteroids and aetiocholanolene. Lancet 1:1154, 1960
11. Cassel EJ: The nature of suffering and the goals of medicine. N Engl J Med 306:639, 1982
12. Cassileth BR, Lusk EJ, Strouse TB, et al: A psychological analysis of cancer patients and their next of kin. Cancer 55:72, 1985
13. Cassileth BR, Volckmar D, Goodman RL: The effect of experience on radiation therapy patients' desire for information. Int J Radiat Oncol Biol Phys 6:493, 1980
14. Catalano R: Medical management of pain caused by cancer. Semin Oncol 2:378, 1975.
15. Copeland EM, MacFadyen BV, Dudrick SJ: Intravenous hyperalimentation in cancer patients. J Surg Res 16:241, 1974
16. Copeland EM, MacFadyen BV, Dudrick SJ: The use of hyperalimentation in patients with potential sepsis. Surg Gynecol Obstet 138:377, 1974
17. Copeland EM, MacFadyen NV, Lanzotti V, et al: Intravenous hyperalimentation as an adjunct to cancer chemotherapy. Am J Surg 129:167, 1975
18. Copeland EM, Souchon EA, MacFadyen BV, et al: Intravenous hyperalimentation as an adjunct to radiation therapy. Cancer 39:609, 1977
19. Cox JD: Large dose fractionation (hypofractionation). Cancer 55: 2105, 1985
20. Crossland SG, Higgins GC: Nutrition supplements in head and neck radiation therapy. [Abstract] JPEN 1:27A, 1977
21. Daly TE: Dental care in the irradiated patient. In Fletcher GH (ed): Textbook of Radiotherapy, 2nd ed, pp 157–165. Philadelphia, Lea & Febiger, 1973
22. D'Angio GJ, Farber S, Maddock CL: Potentiation of x-ray effects by actinomycin D. Radiology 73:175, 1959
23. Davis MS: Variations in patients' compliance with doctors' advice: An empirical analysis of patterns of communications. Am J Pub Health 58:274, 1968
24. DeLeon G: Personal communication, August 1979
25. DeLeon G: Stimulus control of human systolic pressure. Psychol Sci 6:63, 1966
26. Deutsch H: Absence of grief. Psychoanal Q 6:12, 1937
27. DeWys WD: Abnormalities of taste as a remote effect of a neoplasm. Ann NY Acad Sci 230:427, 1974
28. DeWys WD: Anorexia as a general effect on cancer. Cancer 43:2013, 1979
29. DeWys WD, Herbst SH: Oral feeding in the nutritional management of the cancer patient. Cancer Res 37:2429, 1977
30. Diamond NH, Whittington R, Lichtenberg P, et al: Shared control in the practice of radiation oncology. In Torpie RJ, Liegner LM, Chang CH, et al (eds): Radiation Therapy and Thanatology, p 98. Springfield, IL, Charles C Thomas, 1984
31. Dimatteo MR: A social-psychological analysis of physician patient rapport: Toward a science of the art of medicine. J Soc Issues 35:12, 1979
32. Dudrick SJ, Wilmore DW, Vars HM, et al: Long-term parenteral nutrition with growth, development and positive nitrogen balance. Surgery 64:134, 1968
33. Dunphy JE: Annual discourse: On caring for the patient with cancer. N Engl J Med 295:313, 1976
34. Eisler KR: The Psychiatrist and the Dying Patient. New York, International Universities Press, 1955
35. Ellis F: Nominal standard dose and the ret. Br J Radiol 44:101, 1971
36. Fletcher GH (ed): Textbook of Radiotherapy, 3rd ed, pp 92–102. Philadelphia, Lea & Febiger, 1980
37. Fletcher GH (ed): Textbook of Radiotherapy, 2nd ed, pp 620–665. Philadelphia, Lea & Febiger, 1973
38. Forester B, Kornfield DS, Fleiss JL: Psychotherapy during radiotherapy: Effects on emotional and physical distress. Am J Psychiatry 142:22, 1985
39. Freud S: Thoughts for the Time on War and Death, vol XIV. London, Hogarth Press and Institute of Psychoanalysis, 1957
40. Gastineau CF: Nutrition in stress and starvation. Dialog Nutr 1:1, 1976
41. Goldstein F, Khoury J, Thornton JJ: Treatment of chronic

radiation enteritis and colitis with salicylazosulfapyridine and systemic corticosteroid. Am J Gastroenterol 65:201, 1978
42. Good RA, Fernandes G, West A: Nutrition, immunity and cancer: A review. Clin Bull 9:3, 1979
43. Goodman LS, Gilman A: The Pharmacological Basis of Therapeutics, p 768. London, MacMillan & Co, 1970
44. Hackett T, Weisman A: Denial as a factor in patients with heart disease and cancer in care of patients with fatal illness. Ann NY Acad Sci 164:802, 1969
45. Harvey KB, Bothe A, Blackburn GL: Nutritional assessment and patient outcome during oncological therapy. Cancer 43:2065, 1979
46. Headley DB: Premorbid psychological factors of cancer. Biol Psychol Bull 5:1, 1977
47. Hensinkveld RS, Mannis MR, Aristabal SA: Control of radiation-induced diarrhea with cholestyramine. Int J Radiat Oncol Biol Phys 4:687, 1978
48. Holland J: Psychological aspects of oncology: Symposium on psychiatry in internal medicine. Med Clin North Am 61:737, 1977
49. Holmes TH, Masuda M: Life change and illness susceptibility. In Dohrenwend BS, Dohrenwend BP (eds): Stressful Life Events: Their Nature and Effects. New York, John Wiley & Sons, 1974
50. Horton EW, Main IHM, Thompson CJ, et al: Effect of orally administered prostaglandin E_1 on gastric secretion and gastrointestinal motility in man. Gut 9:655, 1968
51. Howell DA: A child dies. J Pediatr Surg 1:2, 1965
52. Inagaki J, Rodriguez V, Bodey GP: Causes of death in cancer patients. Cancer 33:568, 1974
53. Kastenbaum R, Aisenberg R: The Psychology of Death. New York, Springer-Verlag, 1972
54. Katz D, Siegel HI: Erosive gastritis and acute gastrointestinal mucosal lesions. In Glass GBJ (ed): Progress in Gastroenterogy, vol 1, p 67. New York, Grune & Stratton, 1968
55. Kissen D: The significance of personality in lung cancer men. Ann NY Acad Sci 125:820, 1966
56. Kubler-Ross, E: On Death and Dying. New York, MacMillan, 1969
57. Langer EJ, Janis IL, Wolfer JA: Reduction of psychologic stress in surgical patients. J Exp Soc Psychol 11:155, 1975
58. Lapides J: Treatment of delayed intractable hemorrhagic cystitis following radiation or chemotherapy. J Urol 104:707, 1970
59. LeShan L: Psychological states as factors in the development of malignant disease: A critical review. JNCI 22:1, 1959
60. LeShan L, Worthington RE: Personality as a factor in the pathogenesis of cancer: A review of the literature. Br J Med Psycol 29:49, 1956
61. Levy MH: Palliative care. Semin Oncol 12:335, 1985
62. Lippincott RC: The physician's responsibility to the dying patient: Symposium on therapeutic problems. Med Clin North Am 56:677, 1972
63. Lynch JJ, Thomas SA, Mills ME, et al: The effects of human contact on cardiac arrhythmia in coronary care patients. J Nerv Ment Dis 158:88, 1974
64. Marmorston J, Geller PJ, Weiner JM: Pretreatment urinary hormone patterns and survival in patients with breast cancer, prostate cancer or lung cancer. Ann NY Acad Sci 164:483, 1969
65. Mendelsohn ML: The biology of dose-limiting tissues. In Bond VP, Suit HD, Marcial V (eds): Time and Dose Relationships in Radiation Biology as Applied to Radiotherapy, pp 154–173. Upton, NY, Brookhaven National Laboratory Report 50203 (C-57), 1969
66. Mennie AT, Dalley V: Aspirin in radiation induced diarrhea. Lancet 1:1131, 1973
67. Moore FD, Woodrow SI, Aliapoulios MA, et al: Carcinoma of the breast. N Engl J Med 277:411, 1967
68. Mount BM, Ajemian I, Scott JF: Use of the Brompton mixture in treating the chronic pain of malignant disease. Can Med Assoc J 115:122, 1976
69. Natterson J, Kundson AG: Observations concerning fear of death in fatally ill children and their mothers. Psychosom Med 22:456, 1960
70. Nealon TF Jr, Grossi CE, Steier M: Use of elemental diets to correct catabolic states prior to surgery. Ann Surg 180:9, 1974
71. Norton J: Treatment of a dying patient. Psychoanal Study Child 18:541, 1964
72. Page CP, Ryan JA, Haff RC: Continual catheter administration of an elemental diet. Surg Gynecol Obstet 142:184, 1976
73. Parsons CL, Schmidt JD, Pollen JJ: Successful treatment of interstitial cystitis with sodium pentosanpolysulfate. J Urol 130:51, 1983
74. Peck A, Boland J: Emotional reactions to radiation treatment Cancer 40:180, 1977
75. Petrie A: Individuality in Pain and Suffering, p 1. Chicago, University of Chicago Press, 1967
76. Phillips TL, Wharam MD, Margolis LW: Modification of radiation injury to normal tissues by chemotherapeutic agents. Cancer 35:1678, 1975
77. Plank EN: Death on a children's ward. Med Times 92:638, 1964
78. Quimby EH: The skin erythema dose with a combination of two types of radiation. Am J Roentgenol 46:621, 1927
79. Rafla S, Rotman M (eds): Introduction to Radiotherapy, pp 59–60. St. Louis, CV Mosby, 1974
80. Rainey LC: Effects of preparatory patient education for radiation oncology patients. Cancer 56:1056, 1985
81. Ram MD: Complications of radiotherapy for carcinoma of the bladder. Proc R Soc Med 63:93, 1970
82. Reeves RJ, Sanders AP, Isley JK, et al: Fat absorption studies in patients undergoing ^{60}Co teletherapy and/or radium application. AJR 94:848, 1965
83. Richmond JB, Waisman HA: Psychologic aspects on management of children with malignant disease. J Dis Child 89:42, 1955
84. Riley V: Mouse mammary tumors: Alteration of incidence as apparent function of stress. Science 189:465, 1975
85. Rotman M, John MJ, Moon SH, et al: Limitations of adjunctive surgery in carcinoma of the cervix. Int J Radiat Oncol Biol Phys 5:327, 1979
86. Rotman M, Rogow L, DeLeon G. et al: Supportive therapy in radiation oncology. Cancer 39:744, 1977
87. Rubin P, Cooper R, Phillips TL: The dose-limiting organs in radiation oncology. In Set RTL: Radiation Oncology, Radiation Biology and Radiation Pathology Syllabus, pp 2–7. Chicago, American College of Radiology, 1975
88. Rubin P, Casarett GW: Skin and adenexa. In Rubin P, Casarett GW (eds): Clinical Radiation Pathology, 2nd ed, p 62. Philadelphia, WB Saunders, 1978
89. Rubin P, Salazar O, Zagars G, et al: Systemic hemibody irradiation for overt and occult metastases. Cancer 55:2210, 1985
90. Salazar OM, Rubin P, Keller B, et al: Systemic (half-body) radiation therapy: Response and toxicity. Int J Radiat Oncol Biol Phys 4:951, 1978
91. Saunders C: The Management of Terminal Illness. London, Hospital Publications, 1967
92. Saunders CM: The Management of Terminal Disease. In The Management of Malignant Disease Series, vol 1. London, Edward Arnold Publishers, 1978
93. Schmale AH, Iker HP: The effect of hopelessness and the development of cancer. Psychosom Med 28:714, 1966
94. Schoenberg B, Carr A, Kutscher A, et al: Loss and Grief: Psychological Management in Medical Practice. New York, Columbia University Press, 1970
95. Schoenberg B, Carr A, Kutscher A, et al: Psychosocial Aspects of Terminal Care. New York, Columbia University Press, 1972
96. Shore ME: Treating the depressed cancer patient: Sorrow, sadness, and somatic illness. Symposium, Eighth Annual Conference on Psychosomatic Disorders, Jefferson Medical College. New York, Praeger, 1987
97. Snell L, Graham S: Social trauma as related to cancer of the breast. Br J Cancer 25:721, 1971
98. Soucher EA, Copeland EM, Watson P, et al: Intravenous

hyperalimentation as an adjunct to cancer chemotherapy with 5-fluorouracil. J Surg Res 18:451, 1975

99. Stehlin JS, Beach KH: Psychological aspects of cancer therapy: A surgeon's viewpoint. JAMA 197:100, 1966
100. Steiger E, Oram-Smith J, Miller E, et al: Effects of nutrition on tumor growth and tolerance of chemotherapy. J Surg Res 18:455, 1975
101. Steinhauer PD, Mushin DN, Rae-Grant G: Psychological aspects of chronic illness. Pediatr Clin North Am 21:825, 1974
102. Sternbach RA: Pain: A Psychophysiological Analysis, pp 12–22. New York, Academic Press, 1968
103. Stryker JA, Mortel R, Hepner GW: The effect of pelvic radiation in lactase absorption. Int J Radiat Oncol Biol Phys 4:859, 1979
104. Theologides A: Anorexia producing intermediary metabolites. Am J Clin Nutr 29:552, 1976
105. Theologides A: Cancer cachexia. Cancer 43:2004, 1979
106. Torpie RJ, Liegner LM, Chang CH, et al: (eds): Radiation Therapy and Thanatology. Springfield, IL, Charles C Thomas, 1984
107. Vane JR: Inhibition of prostaglandin synthesis as a mechanism of action for aspirin. Nature New Biol 231:232, 1971
108. Weisman AD: On Death and Dying: A Psychiatric Study of Terminality. New York, Behavioral Publications, 1972
109. Weisman AD: The Coping Capacity: On the Nature of Being Mortal. New York, Human Sciences Press, 1984
110. Western KA, Perera DR, Schultz MG: Pentamidine isethionate in the treatment of *Pneumocystis carinii* pneumonia. Ann Int Med 73:675, 1970
111. Yates JW: Problems of neoplastic disease infections. Semin Drug Treat 3:27, 1973

Index

Page numbers followed by *f* indicate figures; those followed by *t* indicate tabular material.

B

C

D

E

F

G

H

N

O

P

Q

R

U

V

W

X

ISBN 0-397-51162-0